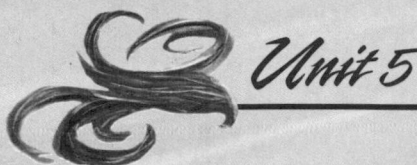
Unit 5

PSYCHOSOCIAL BASIS
FOR NURSING PRACTICE

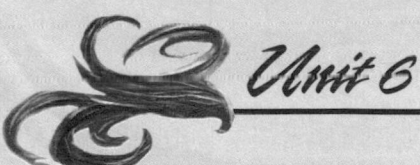
Unit 6

SCIENTIFIC BASIS FOR
NURSING PRACTICE

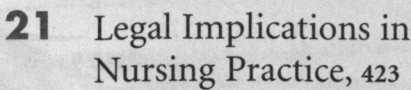
Unit 7

BASIC HUMAN NEEDS

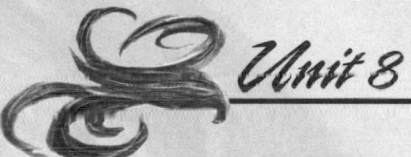
Unit 8

CLIENTS WITH
SPECIAL NEEDS

**New 2002 CDC Hand Hygiene
Guidelines, see page ii**

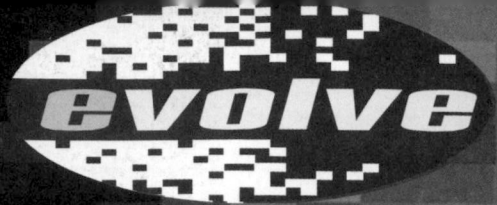

The Latest *Evolution* in Learning.

Evolve provides online access to free learning resources and activities designed specifically for the textbook you are using in your class. The resources will provide you with information that enhances the material covered in the book and much more.

Visit the Web address listed below to start your learning evolution today!

▶▶ *LOGIN: http://evolve.elsevier.com/Potter/fundamentals/*

Evolve Student Learning Resources for Potter, Perry: *Fundamentals of Nursing*, fifth edition offers the following features:

- **Web Links**
  An exciting resource that lets you link to hundreds of websites carefully chosen to supplement the content of this textbook. The Weblinks are regularly updated, with new ones added as they develop.

- **Content Updates**
  New and updated information related to this textbook.

- **Frequently Asked Questions**
  Common questions related to the topics covered in this textbook.

Think outside the book...*evolve.*

FUNDAMENTALS
OF NURSING

OVERVIEW OF CDC HAND HYGIENE GUIDELINES

The Centers for Disease Control and Prevention recently released new recommendations for hand hygiene in health care settings. Hand hygiene is a term that applies to either handwashing, use of an antiseptic hand rub, or surgical hand antisepsis. Evidence suggests that hand antisepsis, the cleansing of hands with an antiseptic hand rub is more effective in reducing nosocomial infections than plain handwashing.

Follow these guidelines in the care of all patients

- Continue to wash hands with either a non-antimicrobial or an antimicrobial soap and water whenever the hands are visibly soiled.
- Use an alcohol-based hand rub to routinely decontaminate the hands in the following clinical situations: (Note: if alcohol-based hand rubs are not available, the alternative is hand washing)
  - Before and after client contact.
  - Before donning sterile gloves when inserting central intravascular catheters.
  - Before performing non-surgical invasive procedures (e.g. urinary catheter insertion, nasotracheal suctioning).
  - After contact with body fluids or excretions, mucous membranes, nonintact skin, and wound dressings.
  - If moving from a contaminated-body site (rectal area or mouth) to a clean-body site (surgical wound, urinary meatus) during client care.
  - After contact with inanimate objects (including medical equipment) in the immediate vicinity of the client).
  - After removing gloves.
- Before eating and after using a restroom, wash hands with a non-antimicrobial or an antimicrobial soap and water.
- Antimicrobial-impregnated wipes (i.e., towelettes) are not a substitute for using an alcohol-based hand rub or antimicrobial soap.
- If exposure to Bacillus anthracis is suspected or proven, wash hands with a non-antimicrobial or an antimicrobial soap and water. The physical action of washing and rinsing hands is recommended because alcohols, chlorhexidine, iodophors, and other antiseptic agents have poor activity against spores.

Method for decontaminating hands

When using an alcohol-based hand rub, apply product to palm of one hand and rub hands together, covering all surfaces of hands and fingers, until hands are dry. Follow the manufacturer's recommendations regarding the volume of product to use.

Follow these guidelines for surgical hand antisepsis

- Surgical hand antisepsis reduces the resident microbial count on the hands to a minimum.
  - The CDC recommends using an antimicrobial soap, and to scrub hands and forearms for the length of time recommended by the manufacturer, usually 2–6 minutes. The Association of Operating Room Nurses recommends 5 to 10 minutes. Refer to agency policy for time required.
  - When using an alcohol-based surgical hand-scrub product with persistent activity, follow the manufacturer's instructions. Before applying the alcohol solution, prewash hands and forearms with a non-antimicrobial soap and dry hands and forearms completely. After application of the alcohol-based product as recommended, allow hands and forearms to dry thoroughly before donning sterile gloves.

General Recommendations for Hand Hygiene

- Use hand lotions or creams to minimize the occurrence of irritant contact dermatitis associated with hand antisepsis or handwashing.
- Do not wear artificial fingernails or extenders when having direct contact with clients at high risk (e.g., those in intensive-care units or operating rooms).
- Keep natural nails tips less than 1/4-inch long.
- Wear gloves when contact with blood or other potentially infectious materials, mucous membranes, and nonintact skin could occur.
- Remove gloves after caring for a client. Do not wear the same pair of gloves for the care of more than one client, and do not wash gloves between uses with different clients.
- Change gloves during client care if moving from a contaminated body site to a clean body site.

(From Centers for Disease Control and Prevention (Morbidity and Mortality Weekly Report [MMWR], October 25, 2002 51 (RR16): 1-44 www.cdc.gov/handhygiene)

FUNDAMENTALS
OF NURSING

Fifth Edition

With over 1100 illustrations

PATRICIA A. POTTER, RN, MSN, PhD (Cand), CMAC

Research Scientist
Barnes-Jewish Hospital
St. Louis, Missouri

ANNE GRIFFIN PERRY, RN, MSN, EdD

Professor and Co-Coordinator, Adult Health Specialty
Saint Louis University School of Nursing
Saint Louis University Health Sciences Center
St. Louis, Missouri

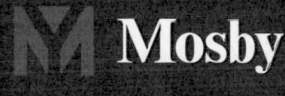

Mosby

An Affiliate of Elsevier Science

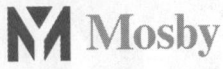
An Affiliate of Elsevier Science

Vice President, Nursing Editorial Director: *Sally Schrefer*
Senior Editor: *Susan Epstein*
Developmental Editor: *Sharon Malchow*
Project Manager: *John Rogers*
Senior Production Editor: *Cheryl A. Abbott*
Designer, Chapter and Cover Art: *Kathi Gosche*
Photography: *Rick Brady*

Fifth EDITION
Copyright ©2001 by Mosby, Inc.

Previous editions copyrighted 1985, 1989, 1993, 1997

NOTICE

Pharmacology is an ever-changing field. Standard safety precautions must be followed, but as new research and clinical experience broaden our knowledge, changes in treatment and drug therapy may become necessary or appropriate. Readers are advised to check the most current product information provided by the manufacturer of each drug to be administered to verify the recommended dose, the method and duration of administration, and contraindications. It is the responsibility of the treating physician, relying on experience and knowledge of the patient, to determine dosages and the best treatment for each individual patient. Neither the publisher nor the editor assumes any liability for any injury and/or damage to persons or property arising from this publication.

Permissions may be sought directly from Elsevier's Health Sciences Rights Department in Philadelphia, USA: phone: (+1)215-238-7869, fax: (+1)215-238-2239, email: healthpermissions@elsevier.com. You may also complete your request on-line via the Elsevier Science homepage (http://www.elsevier.com), by selecting 'Customer Support' and then 'Obtaining Permissions'.

Mosby, Inc.
An Affiliate of Elsevier Science
11830 Westline Industrial Drive
St. Louis, MO 63146

Printed in the United States

International Standard Book Number   0-323-01141-1

03 04 GW/KPT 9 8 7 6 5

Contributors

DENISE E. ANTLE, BSN, MSN, RN, CCRN
CV/Critical Care Clinical Nurse Specialist
Genesis Medical Center
Davenport, Iowa

MYRA A. AUD, MSN(R), PhD(CAND.)
Doctoral Student
Saint Louis University
St. Louis, Missouri

ELIZABETH AYELLO, PhD, MS, BSN, RN,
CS, CWOCN
Clinical Assistant Professor
New York University, Division of Nursing
New York, New York

JULIE K. BAYLOR, MSN, RN
Assistant Professor of Nursing
Bradley University
Peoria, Illinois

JAN BOUNDY, RN, PhD
Professor/Coordinator
Saint Francis Medical Center College of Nursing
Peoria, Illinois

PEGGY BRECKINRIDGE, MSN, FNP
Associate Professor
College of Health Sciences
Roanoke, Virginia

JUDITH C. BROSTRON, RN, BA, JD, LLM
Attorney
Lashly and Baer
St. Louis, Missouri

MAUREEN CARTY, MSN, RN, OCN
Oncology Clinical Nurse Specialist
Genesis Medical Center
Davenport, Iowa

KATHRYN ANN CAUDELL, PhD, RN, AOCN
Clinical Research and Education Manager
Amgen, Inc.
Thousand Oaks, California

MARY F. CLARKE, BSN, MA, RN
Informatics Nurse Specialist
Genesis Medical Center
Davenport, Iowa

JUDITH A. COLLINS, MA, BSN, ARNP, CS
Psychiatric Liaison Clinical Nurse Specialist
Genesis Medical Center
Davenport, Iowa

RUTH DAVIDHIZAR, RN, BSN, MSN, DNS,
CS, FAAN
Dean of Nursing
Bethel College
Mishawaka, Indiana

MARGARET ECKER, BA, MS (MFA), PNP
Clinical Nurse Specialist
UCLA Children's Hospital
Los Angeles, California

MARTHA ELKIN, RN, MSN
Lactation Consultant
Stephens Memorial Hospital
Norway, Maine

SUSAN JANE FETZER, RN, BA, BSN, MSN,
MBA, PhD
Assistant Professor
University of New Hampshire
Durham, New Hampshire

LEAH FREDERICK, MSN, RN, CIC
Infection Control Consultant
Infection Control Consultants
Scottsdale, Arizona

JOYCE NEWMAN GIGER, EdD, RN, CS,
FAAN
Professor, Graduate Studies
School of Nursing, University of Alabama at
   Birmingham
Birmingham, Alabama

CYNTHIA S. GOODWIN, MSN, RN
Instructor, School of Nursing and Health Professions
University of Southern Indiana
Evansville, Indiana

AMY HALL, RN, BSN, MS, PhD(CAND.)
Assistant Professor
Saint Francis Medical Center College of Nursing
Peoria, Illinois

LOIS C. HAMEL, MS, RN, CS, PhD(CAND.)
Adult Nurse Practitioner/Adjunct Assistant Professor
University of New England/University of Vermont
    Medical School
Portland, Maine

JUDITH ANN KILPATRICK, BSN, MSN, RNC
Lecturer
Widener University
Chester, Pennsylvania

CARL A. KIRTON, RN, BSN, MA, ACRN,
ANP-CS
Clinical Assistant Professor of Nursing
New York University
New York, New York

KRISTINE L'ECUYER, RN, BSN, MSN
Adjunct Assistant Professor
Saint Louis University School of Nursing
St. Louis, Missouri

VIRGINIA LESTER, RN, BSN, MSN, CNS
Assistant Professor
Angelo State University
San Angelo, Texas

ANNE R. LEWIS, BSN, MA, RN
Neuroscience Clinical Nurse Specialist
Genesis Medical Center
Davenport, Iowa

RUTH LUDWICK, BSN, MSN, PhD, RN, C
Associate Professor
Kent State University, School of Nursing
Kent, Ohio

KATHLEEN MULRYAN, BSN, MSN
Professor of Nursing
LaGuardia Community College
Long Island City, New York

ELAINE K. NEEL, BSN, MSN
Nursing Instructor
Methodist Medical Center of Illinois, School of Nursing
Peoria, Illinois

SHELLEY-RAE PHELER, MSN, BSN, RN
Maternal Child/Pediatric Clinical Nurse Specialist
Genesis Medical Center
Davenport, Iowa

PATSY L. RUCHALA, RN, BSN, MSN, DNSc
Director Master's Programs in Nursing
Saint Louis University School of Nursing
St. Louis, Missouri

NANCY SEMENZA, RN, BSN, MS, PhD (CAND.)
Nursing Faculty, Adjunct
MacMurray College
Jacksonville, Illinois

BOBBI SHATTO, BSN, MSN
Adjunct Instructor
Saint Louis University School of Nursing
Saint Louis, Missouri

SHARON SOUTER, RN, BSN, MSN
Nursing Program Director
New Mexico State University at Carlsbad
Carlsbad, New Mexico

ELIZABETH SPEAKMAN, RN, MEd
Associate Professor of Nursing/Doctoral Candidate,
    Columbia University
Community College of Philadelphia
Philadelphia, Pennsylvania

PATRICIA A. STOCKERT, BSN, MS,
PhD (CAND.)
Associate Professor
Saint Francis Medical Center College of Nursing
Peoria, Illinois

PAMELA BECKER WEILITZ, RN, MSN(R),
CS, ANP
Adult Nurse Practitioner
Washington University School of Medicine,
    University Care
St. Louis, Missouri

RITA WUNDERLICH, MSN(R), PhD(CAND.),
CCRN
Lecturer
Southern Illinois University—Edwardsville
Edwardsville, Illinois

Reviewers

To the memory of my parents,
William and Grace Potter.
The gifts of their love, wisdom, and work ethic endure and continue to inspire.

Patricia A. Potter

To Pat, whose intellectual curiosity and commitment to excellence continue to set the standard for this textbook. Her belief in our profession and promotion of clinical scholarship help to shape the standards of practice and meet the challenges of contemporary nursing practice.

Anne Griffin Perry

Preface to the Student

This book was designed for you, the busy student. It was designed to welcome you to nursing and to help you learn all of the fundamental nursing concepts and skills in a visually appealing, easy-to-use format. The writing style is clear and engaging, with hundreds of full-color drawings and photographs to illustrate the text. Numerous special features are included to help you learn, understand, and apply the content. Check out some of these special features.

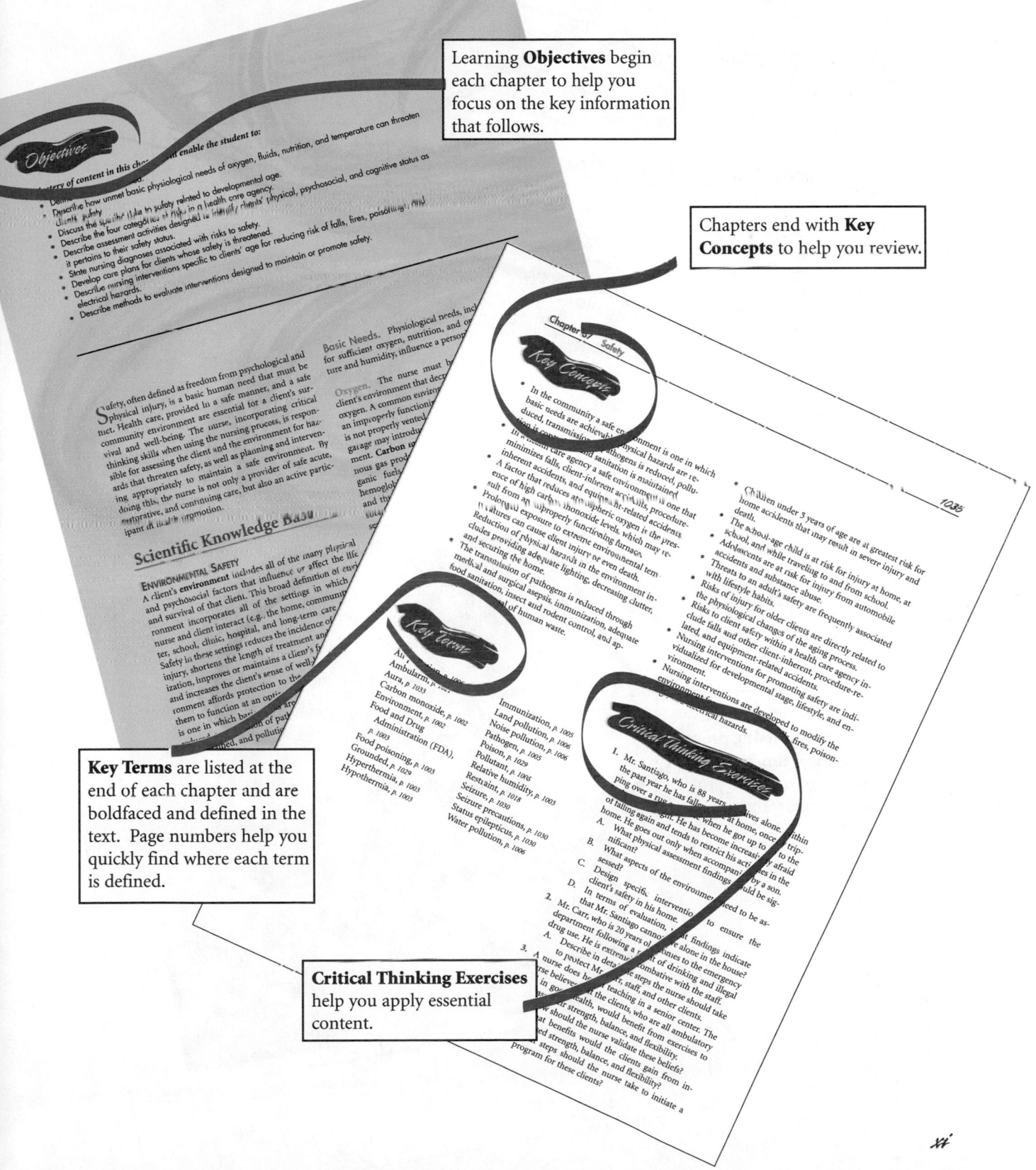

Learning **Objectives** begin each chapter to help you focus on the key information that follows.

Chapters end with **Key Concepts** to help you review.

Key Terms are listed at the end of each chapter and are boldfaced and defined in the text. Page numbers help you quickly find where each term is defined.

Critical Thinking Exercises help you apply essential content.

1011

medications, use of restraints, and use of medical devices). All of this information and experience is referred to by the nurse as he or she conducts a detailed assessment of a specific client. For example, while assessing a specific client's knowledge re-garding typical locations within the home where dangers commonly exist. If a client has a visual impairment, the nurse will apply previous experiences in caring for clients with visual changes to anticipate how to thoroughly assess the client's needs. Critical thinking directs the nurse to anticipate what needs to be assessed and how to make conclusions about available data.

Safety and the Nursing Process

ASSESSMENT

To conduct a thorough client assessment, the nurse considers possible threats to the client's safety, as well as ____ environment ___ client in the any individual risk factors. Wh___ home, a home hazard assessment is necess___ 37-1). The nurse should walk through the home with the client and discuss how the client normally conducts daily activities. Getting a sense of the client's routines helps the nurse recognize hazards that are not as obvious. For example, if a client typically uses certain items in a kitchen that require the client to use a footstool, the nurse can anticipate the need to assess risks for falls. Including the family in the assessment may also help reveal hazards or risks.

When the client is cared for within a health care facility, the nurse must determine if any hazards exist in the immediate care environment. Does the placement of equipment or furniture pose barriers when the client a___ tempts to ambulate? Does positioning of the client's sta___ allow the client to reach items on a bedside table or sta___? In what way are self-care items in a bathroom arranged ___ accessibility? The nurse also collaborates with clinical engineering staff to make sure that equipment has been assessed to ensure proper function and condition.

A nursing history will include data about the client's level of wellness to determine if any underlying conditions exist that pose threats to safety. For example, the nurse will give special attention to assessing the client's gait, muscle strength and coordination, balance, and vision. A review of the client's developmental status must be considered as assessment information is analyzed. The nurse will also re-view if the client is taking any medications or undergoi___ any procedures that pose risks. For example, use of diu___ ics increases the frequency of voiding and may res___ the client having to use toilet facilities more often. F___ ten occur with clients who must get out of bed qu___ cause of urinary urgency. An example of a proce___ may pose risks is use of an electric aquatherm___ Chapter 47).

Client Expectations. Clients generally expect to be safe in their home and in the health care setting. However, there are times when a client's view of what is safe does not agree with that of the nurse. For this reason, any assessment must include the client's understanding of his or her perception of risk factors. This will be important later as the nurse attempts to make changes in the client's environment. Clients usually do not purposefully put themselves in jeopardy. When clients are uninformed or inexperienced, threats to their safety can occur. Clients must always be consulted on ways to reduce hazards in their environment.

NURSING DIAGNOSIS

After completing ___ assessment of the client's ___ fety status, the nurse reviews any clusters ___ data show-ing ___ ___ assessing that safety is threate___ Iden-tification or defining characteristics from the da___ direct the nurse in identifying appropriate nursing diagn___ (Box 37-4). The diagnostic process requires accura___ ___ of defining characteristics, as well as the re-lated factors ___ ___ ___ is for selecting nurs-ing therapies. For example, *risk for inj___ ___ to barri___ paired mobility* and *risk for injury related to barri___* require different nursing interventions. The client with altered mobility may require ambulatory aids and physical therapy. When the related factor is barri-ers in the home, the nurse intervenes to make changes that will create a safer environment. At times, as in the example in Box 37-5, multiple related factors may app___

PLANNING

During planning the nurse critically synthesizes in-formation from multiple sources (Figure 37-6). Critical ___ ___ that the client's plan of care integrates all that the nurse has learned about the client, as well as the key critical thinking elements. For example, the nurse will refl___ ___ knowledge regarding the services other disci-pl___ ____national therapy) can provide in helping

Box 37-4

1010

KNOWLEDGE
- Basic human needs
- Potential risks to the client's safety from physical hazards, lifestyle, risks associated with health care environment, and environmental risks
- Influence of developmental stage on safety needs
- Influence of illness/medications on the client's safety

STANDARDS
- Apply intellectual standards of accuracy, significance, competence, and fairness when assessing for threats to the client's safety
- Apply ANA standards for nursing practice

ASSESSMENT
- Identify actual and potential threats to the client's safety
- Determine impact of the underlying illness on the client's safety
- Identify the presence of risks for the client's developmental stage

EXPERIENCE
- Caring for clients whose mobility or sensory impairments increase threats to safety
- Personal experience in caring for younger siblings or children

ATTITUDES
- Demonstrate perseverance when necessary to identify all threats to the client's safety
- Be responsible for collecting unbiased, accurate data regarding threats to the client's safety
- Display fairness to objectively evaluate risks to the client's safety in the home or community

Figure 37-5 *Synthesis Model for Safety Assessment Phase.*

The 5-step **Nursing Process** provides a consistent, logical framework.

This unique model clearly shows how **nursing process** and **critical thinking** come together to help you provide the best care for your clients.

Sample Nursing Care Plans highlight key assessment data that lead to the nursing diagnosis.

Client **Goals** and **Expected Outcomes** establish direction for nursing care.

Intervention Classification labels help you think in terms of this widely used system.

Rationales for each of the interventions help you to understand *why*.

Procedural Guidelines provide streamlined, step-by-step instructions for performing basic skills.

Client Teaching boxes tell you what and how to teach clients and how to evaluate learning.

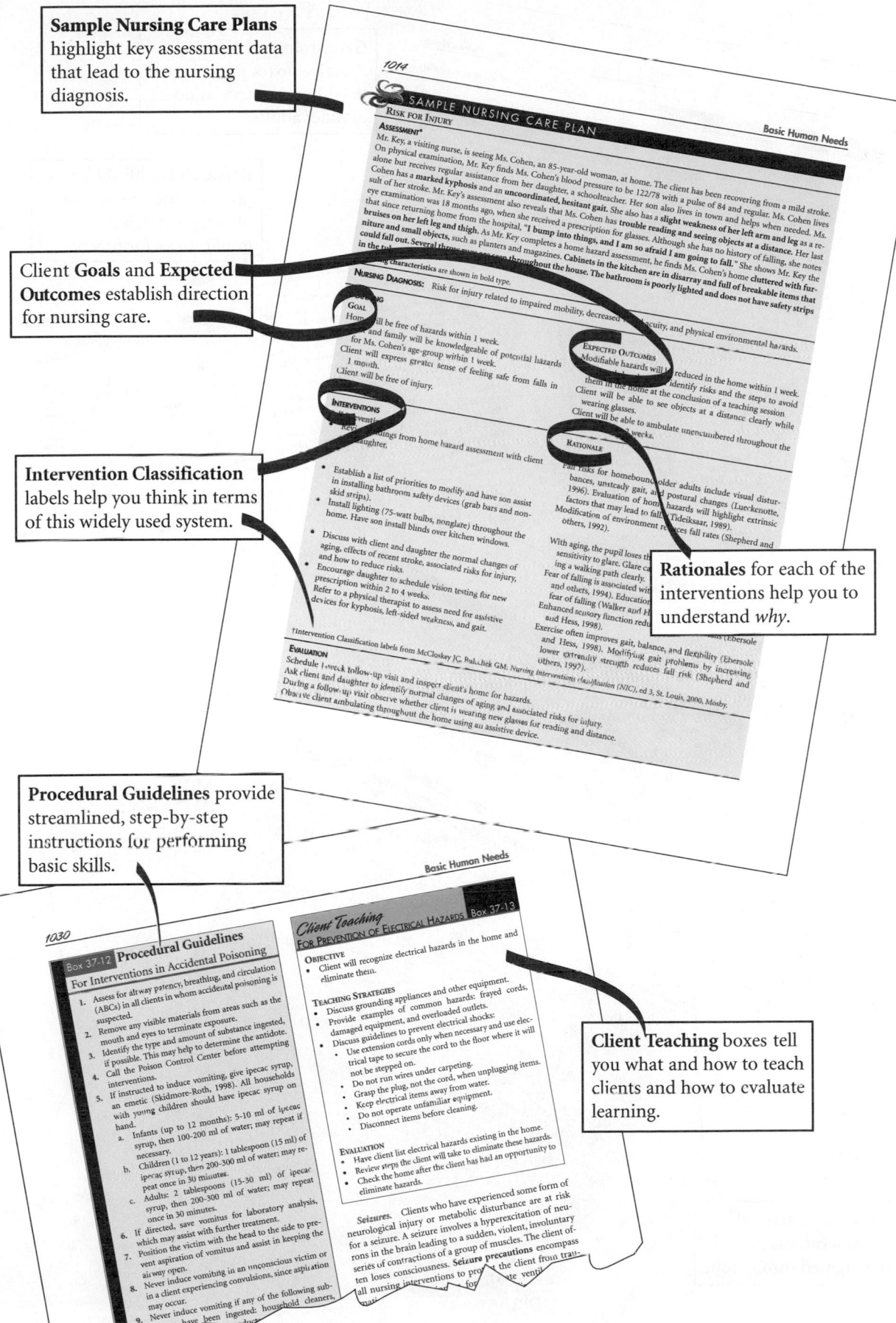

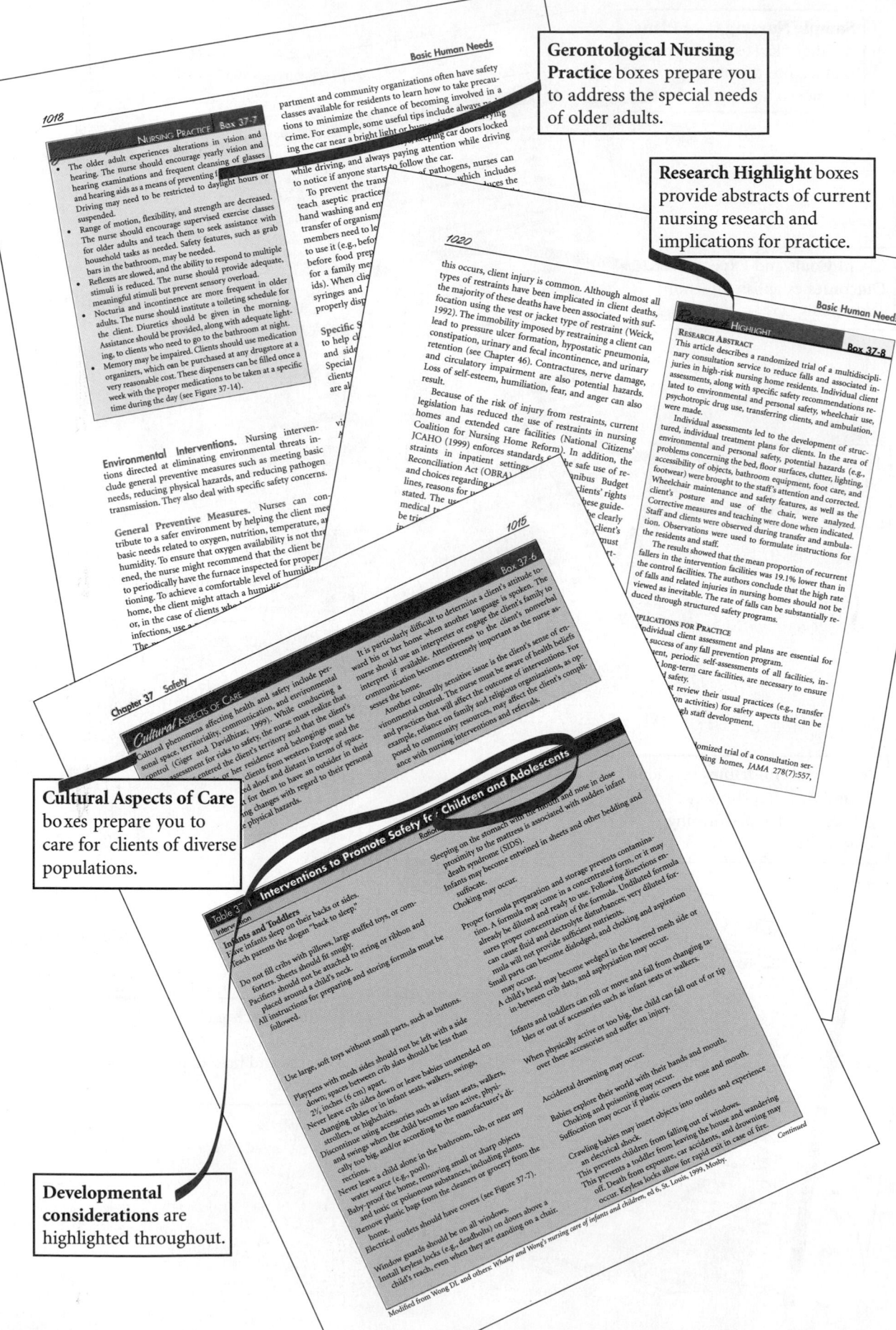

Gerontological Nursing Practice boxes prepare you to address the special needs of older adults.

Research Highlight boxes provide abstracts of current nursing research and implications for practice.

Cultural Aspects of Care boxes prepare you to care for clients of diverse populations.

Developmental considerations are highlighted throughout.

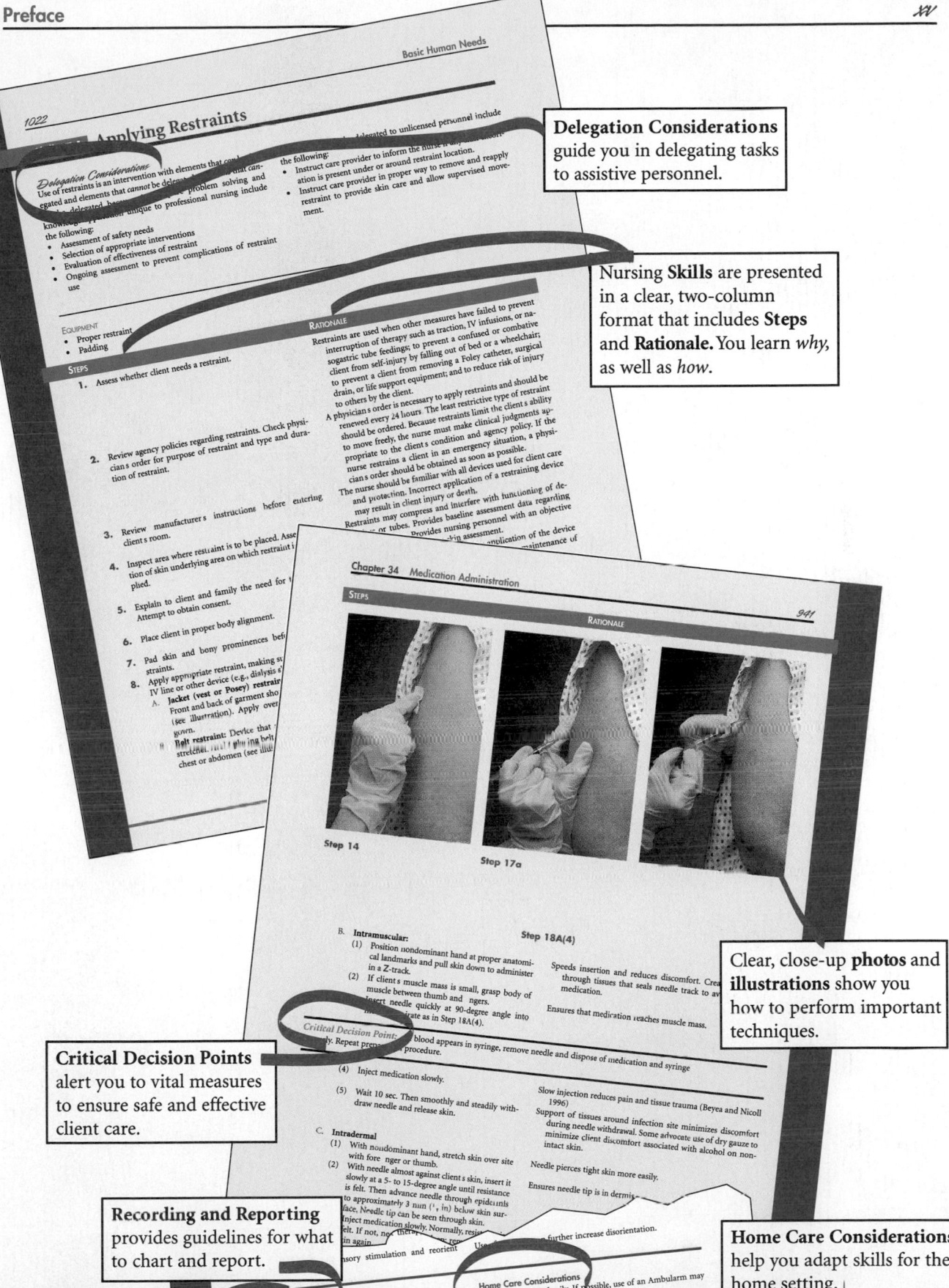

Delegation Considerations guide you in delegating tasks to assistive personnel.

Nursing **Skills** are presented in a clear, two-column format that includes **Steps** and **Rationale.** You learn *why*, as well as *how*.

Clear, close-up **photos** and **illustrations** show you how to perform important techniques.

Critical Decision Points alert you to vital measures to ensure safe and effective client care.

Recording and Reporting provides guidelines for what to chart and report.

Home Care Considerations help you adapt skills for the home setting.

Preface to the Instructor

The future of nursing promises dynamic change and continual challenges. Nurses of tomorrow need a broad knowledge base from which to provide care. The role of the nurse includes assuming the lead in preserving nursing practice and demonstrating its contribution to the health care of our nation. Nurses of tomorrow, therefore, need to become critical thinkers, client advocates, clinical decision makers, and client educators within a broad spectrum of care services.

The fifth edition of *Fundamentals of Nursing* has been revised to prepare today's students for the challenges of tomorrow. This textbook is designed for beginning students in all types of professional nursing programs. The comprehensive coverage provides fundamental nursing concepts, skills, and techniques of nursing practice and a firm foundation for more advanced areas of study.

This revision introduces an innovative, visual approach to teaching critical thinking in nursing practice. We have developed a five-dimensional model that we believe will help students understand not only the elements of critical thinking but also how to apply them in every client-care situation. By clearly demonstrating the synergistic relationship between critical thinking and the nursing process, we provide a logical, comprehensive model for nursing care that students can readily understand and use.

Fundamentals of Nursing provides a contemporary approach to nursing practice, discussing the entire scope of primary, acute, and restorative care. The increased focus on primary care includes health promotion for clients in the home and community-based settings, addressing the commonalties and uniqueness of various settings. The important themes of managed health care, cultural diversity, client education, nursing research, care of the older adult, and critical thinking are integrated throughout to prepare students for practice. We are indebted to the many educators and students who have shared their thoughts, visions, and ideas with us, and we credit each of them as valuable collaborators for this revision.

Features

We have carefully developed this fifth edition with the student in mind. We have designed this text to welcome the new student to nursing, communicate our own love for the profession, and promote learning and understanding. Key features of the text include the following:

CLASSIC FEATURES
- **Comprehensive** coverage and readability of all fundamental nursing content.
- **Full-color** text to enhance visual appeal and instructional value.

- **Nursing process** provides a consistent organizational framework.
- Important nursing **skills** are presented in a clear, two-column format with rationale for all steps; whenever possible, rationale are based on research.
- Covers **health promotion, acute and tertiary care, and restorative care** to address today's practice in various settings.
- **Cultural diversity** is presented in Chapter 7, stressed in clinical examples throughout the text, and highlighted in special boxes.
- **Nursing research** principles and concepts are presented in Chapter 25. **Research Highlight** boxes integrated throughout the text provide abstracts of nursing research and implications for practice.
- **Client education** is presented in Chapter 23 and stressed in boxes that list teaching objectives, strategies, and evaluation for clinical topics throughout the text.
- **Gerontologic nursing** principles are addressed in Chapter 12, as well as in special boxes throughout the text.
- **Diverse clinical settings** are discussed, including clinics, extended care facilities, and the home, as well as acute care settings.
- A series of **Nursing Process** boxes in clinical chapters demonstrate *how* to apply the 5-step process to client care.
- **Sample Nursing Care Plans** provide clinical scenarios that highlight key assessment data and feature NIC classifications, client goals, and expected outcomes.

NEW FEATURES
- **6 new/expanded chapters:**
  - Community-Based Nursing Practice
  - Leadership, Delegation, and Quality Management
  - Theoretical Foundations of Nursing Practice
  - Nursing Healing and Caring
  - Developmental Theories
  - Complementary and Alternative Therapies
- **New and expanded content:**
  - Caring for older parents/family members
  - Contemporary research on women's health, and child and adolescent health
  - Laboratory tests
  - Delegation to assistive personnel
- **Critical thinking** in clinical chapters is presented through a visual **five-dimensional model** that demonstrates the ongoing assimilation of knowledge, critical thinking attitudes, intellectual and professional standards, and experience in relationship to clinical decision making and the nursing process.
- **NIC classifications** are included in Sample Nursing Care Plans.
- **Critical pathways** from progressive agencies across the country address collaborative care in the home, as well as acute care.

- **Procedural Guidelines** boxes provide streamlined, step-by-step instructions for performing very basic skills.
- The chapter on the **profession of nursing** expands coverage of practice opportunities and roles, career options, and paths.
- A **health promotion/wellness** thread is used consistently throughout the text.
- **Skills** highlight **delegation considerations** and include select research-based **interventions, critical decision points, recording and reporting** guidelines, and **home care considerations.**
- **Diversity in caring** includes clients with cultural diversity, as well as socioeconomic and sexual diversity.
- **Free CD-Companion** in each text includes Butterfield's **Fluids and Electrolytes** program, Skills Checklists, and Glossary. **Case Studies** will introduce the five-dimensional critical thinking model and provide interactive practice in applying it to client scenarios.

ANCILLARIES

- **Study Guide** provides an ideal supplement to help students understand and apply the content of the text. Each chapter includes four sections:
  - *Preliminary Reading* includes a chapter assignment from the text.
  - *Comprehensive Understanding* identifies topics and main ideas from the text in outline format. By completing the outline, students learn to extract key information from the chapter. Once completed, these outlines serve as ideal review tools for exams.
  - *Review Questions* are NCLEX style multiple choice questions that require students to provide rationale for their answers.

- *Application of Critical Thinking Synthesis Model* expands the case study from the chapter's Sample Care Plan and asks students to develop a step in the synthesis model based on the nurse and client in the scenario. This helps students learn to apply both content learned and the critical thinking synthesis model.

  Procedure Performance Checklists are included so that students can evaluate skill competency.
- **Instructor's Resource Manual With Test Bank** in NCLEX format
  ISBN: 0-323-01142-X
- **Computerized Test Bank** (cross-platform CD)
  ISBN: 0-323-01143-8
- **Electronic Image Collection** includes all non-borrowed illustrations in the text and can be used with Power Point to create classroom lectures
  ISBN: 0-323-01144-6

• • •

We are pleased to note the growing number of men currently involved in the practice of nursing, and we acknowledge their dedication, skill, and professionalism. We have therefore made every effort to eliminate any gender-specific pronouns. In a very few instances, we have used she to refer to the nurse and he to refer to the client in order to clearly communicate to the reader.

The development of this textbook resulted from the combined efforts of many talented professionals committed to excellence. We appreciate their dedication and enthusiasm. Throughout the text we have attempted to acknowledge the contributions of our professional nurse colleagues who make a difference in the lives of their clients and the communities they serve. We are very proud to be associated with such fine individuals.

Patricia A. Potter
Anne Griffin Perry

Acknowledgments

We wish to give special recognition to the editorial and production teams who have helped to make this textbook a reality. We especially wish to thank:

- Suzi Epstein, Senior Editor, and Shari Malchow, Developmental Editor, for their guidance and support. This text is truly a team effort. Their leadership has ensured a quality textbook with innovative design and informative content. Both Suzi and Shari provide insight, humor, and passion to help us create an excellent text.
- Cheryl Abbott, for her detailed and methodical approach to the very important production process. She is a critical part of the *Fundamentals* team.
- Kathi Gosche, Book Designer, whose innovative design gives the book its exciting and attractive visual appeal.
- Rick Brady, Annapolis, Maryland, for his photographic contributions that bring visual life to each page.
- Anne Arundel Medical Center, Annapolis, Maryland; Natural Healing of Annapolis; Bowie Health Center, Bowie, Maryland; Columbia Lighthouse for the Blind, Washington, D.C.; Larkin Chase Convelescent Center, Bowie, Maryland; South County Senior Center, Anne Arundel County, Maryland; and Goucher College, Dance Depart, Baltimore, Maryland—our thanks for their contributions to the diverse array of photographs that help bring the text to life.
- Jack Reuter, for his computer expertise, which provides clear, detailed illustrations to enhance and complement the text.
- Our contributors and reviewers, whose painstaking critique of content and design ensures a high-quality textbook. Their work often goes unnoticed; however, they have helped to set the standard for a comprehensive and accurate text.
- To the professional managers and nursing staff at Barnes-Jewish Hospital, the faculty and students of Jewish College of Nursing and Allied Health, the nursing faculty of Saint Louis University School of Nursing, and the nursing staff of Saint Louis University Hospital. We hope to capture and reveal the accomplishments they achieve daily through the case studies, clinical examples, and photographic images within the text. Their example of clinical excellence motivates us to develop an instructive textbook.

The creation of a nursing textbook is no small feat. We continue to be very grateful to the faculty and students who use our text. The partnership that we have forged during the last two decades has been a very rewarding one. We hope to continue to meet the standard of excellence you, our readers, expect.

Contents

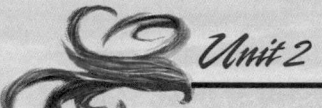
Unit 2

CARING THROUGHOUT THE LIFE SPAN

Unit 3

CRITICAL THINKING IN NURSING PRACTICE

Unit 4

PROFESSIONAL STANDARDS IN NURSING PRACTICE

Unit 5

PSYCHOSOCIAL BASIS FOR NURSING PRACTICE

30   Stress and Adaptation, 643
Bobbi Shatto, BSN, MSN

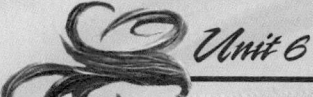

Unit 6

SCIENTIFIC BASIS FOR NURSING PRACTICE

31   Vital Signs, 668
Susan Jane Fetzer, RN, BA, BSN, MSN, MBA, PhD

32   Health Assessment and Physical Examination, 724
Elaine K. Neel, BSN, MSN

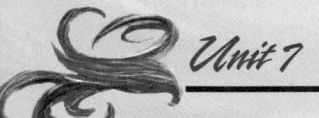

Unit 7

BASIC HUMAN NEEDS

Unit 8

CLIENTS WITH SPECIAL NEEDS

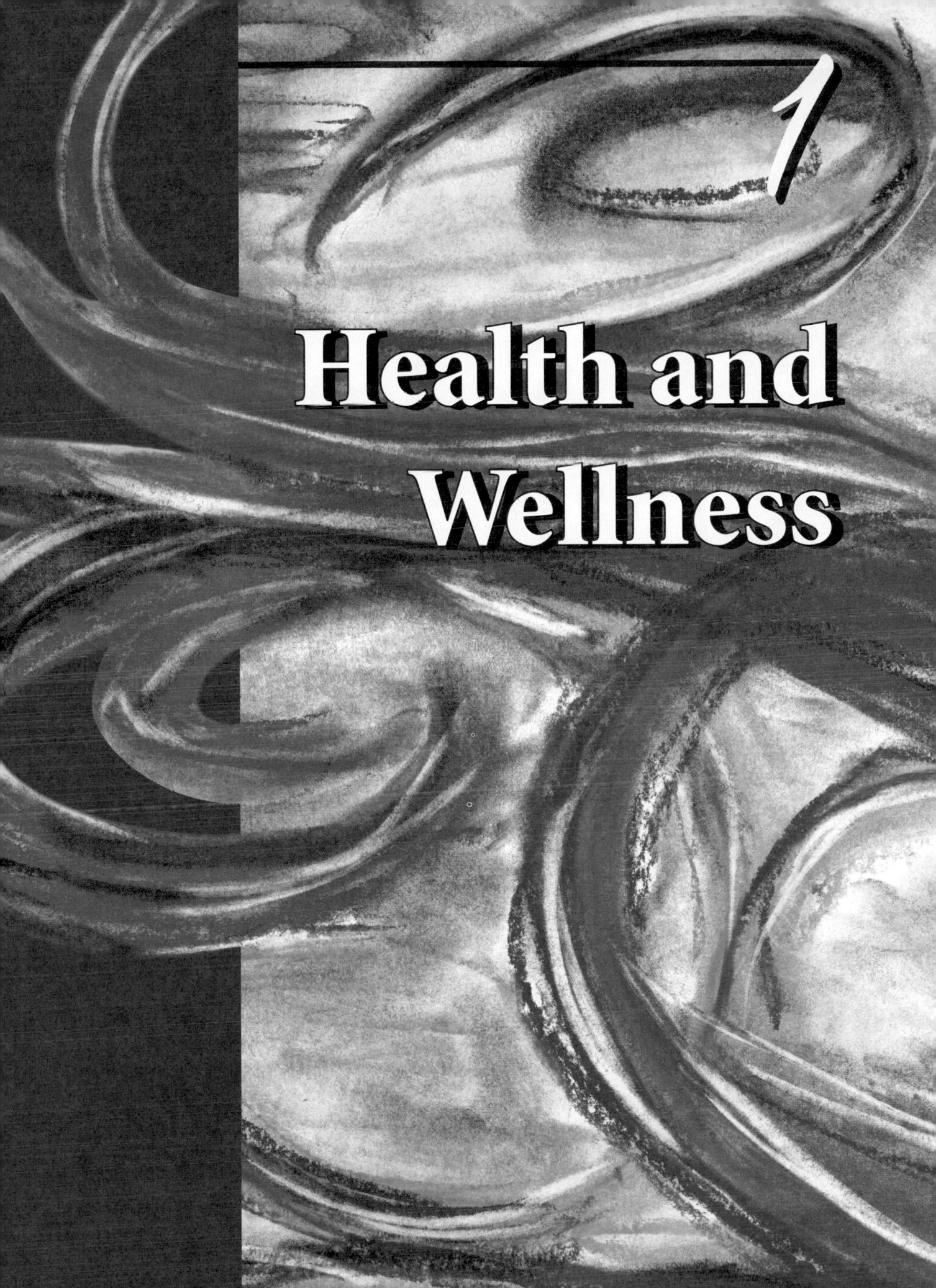

Health and Wellness

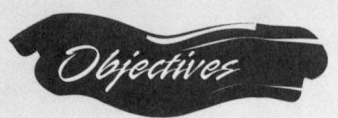

Mastery of content in this chapter will enable the student to:

- Define the key terms listed.
- List the two general *Healthy People 2010* public health goals for Americans.
- Discuss the definition of health and related concepts.
- Discuss the health-illness continuum, health belief, health promotion, basic human needs, and holistic health models to understand the relationship between the client's attitudes toward health and health practices.
- Describe health promotion and illness prevention activities.
- Discuss the three levels of preventive care and four types of risk factors.
- Describe variables influencing health beliefs and practices.
- Describe variables influencing illness behavior.
- Describe the impact of illness on the client and family.
- Discuss the nurse's role in health and illness.

I n the past, most individuals and societies viewed good health, or wellness, as the opposite or absence of disease. This simple attitude ignores states of health between disease and good health. Health is a multidimensional concept and must be viewed from a broader perspective. The concept of health includes a sense of independence, optimism, a sense of psychological well-being, and a state of physical, emotional, social, and spiritual wellness (Plawecki, 1997). A person's state of health directly influences his or her daily choices, independence, individuality, and lifestyle; therefore health is an integral aspect of an individual's identity (Plawecki, 1997). An assessment of the client's state of health is an important aspect of nursing.

Nurses use models of health to understand the relationships between the concepts of health, wellness, and illness. Nurses are in a unique position to assist clients in achieving and maintaining optimal levels of health. Nurses understand the challenges of today's health care system and embrace the opportunity to use wellness activities to promote health and prevent illness. In an era of cost containment and advanced technology, nurses can be a vital link to improved health of individuals and society.

Nurses also identify actual and potential risk factors that predispose a person or a group to illness. Risk factor modification strategies may be used by the nurse in an attempt to promote health or prevent illness.

When illness does occur, different attitudes about illness cause people to react in different ways to illness or that of a family member. Medical sociologists call the reaction to illness, **illness behavior**. Nurses who understand how clients react to illness can minimize the effects of illness and assist clients and their families in maintaining or returning to the highest level of functioning.

Healthy People Documents

In 1979 an influential document, *Healthy People: The Surgeon General's Report on Health Promotion and Disease Prevention* was published. This report introduced national goals for improving the health of Americans by 1990. It outlined priority objectives for preventive services, health protection, and health promotion that address improvements in health status, risk reduction, public and professional awareness of prevention, health services and protective measures, and surveillance and evaluation. The report served as a framework for the 1990s as the United States began to focus more on health promotion and disease prevention instead of illness care. The strategy announced by the Secretary of Health and Human Services requires a cooperative effort by government, voluntary and professional organizations, businesses, and individuals. Widely cited by popular media, in professional journals, and at health conferences, it has inspired health promotion programs throughout the country.

In 1990 *Healthy People 2000: National Health Promotion and Disease Prevention Objectives* was published as a follow-up effort to reduce preventable deaths, disabilities, and diseases for Americans by the year 2000 (U.S. Department of Health and Human Services (USDHHS). The *Healthy People 2000* initiative focused on three broad public health goals for Americans: (1) to increase the span of healthy life, (2) to reduce health disparities, and (3) to achieve access to preventive services. The document has undergone many comprehensive reviews. The Depart-

The authors acknowledge the contribution of Carole Edelman to this chapter in the previous edition of this text.

ment of Health and Human Services continually chronicles progress toward achieving the objectives. Many states have used the *Healthy People 2000* document in setting their own health objectives.

More than 340 organizations with national membership have been involved in the development of the latest document, *Healthy People 2010* (Maiese and Fox, 1998). The two overarching goals for *Healthy People 2010* are (1) to increase quality and years of healthy life and (2) to eliminate health disparities (USDHHS, 1998). The 2010

Healthy People 2010: Focus Areas   Box 1-1

PROMOTING HEALTHY BEHAVIORS
Physical activity and fitness
Nutrition
Tobacco use

PROMOTING HEALTHY AND SAFE COMMUNITIES
Educational and community-based programs
Environmental health
Food safety
Injury/violence prevention
   Injuries that cut across intent
   Unintentional injuries
   Violence and abuse
Occupational safety and health
Oral health

IMPROVING SYSTEMS FOR PERSONAL AND PUBLIC HEALTH
Access to quality health services
   Preventive care
   Primary care
   Emergency services
   Long-term care and rehabilitative services
Family planning
Maternal, infant, and child health
Medical product safety
Public health infrastructure
Health communication

PREVENTING AND REDUCING DISEASES AND DISORDERS
Arthritis, osteoporosis, and chronic back conditions
Cancer
Diabetes
Disability and secondary conditions
Heart disease and stroke
Human immunodeficiency virus (HIV) infection
Immunization and infectious diseases
Mental health and mental disorders
Respiratory diseases
Sexually transmitted diseases
Substance abuse

Modified from U.S. Department of Health and Human Services: *Healthy people 2010 objectives: draft for public comment,* Washington, DC, 1998, Office of Disease Prevention and Health Promotion (http://web.health.gov/healthypeople/2010Draft/object.htm).

---

document has grown in size and includes 26 focus areas (previously called priority areas) with 521 objectives. The document is divided into four areas: (1) promoting healthy behaviors, (2) promoting healthy and safe communities, (3) improving systems for personal and public health, and (4) preventing and reducing diseases and disorders (Box 1-1).

Definition of Health

Defining good health is difficult. The World Health Organization (WHO) defines **health** as a "state of complete physical, mental and social well-being, not merely the absence of disease or infirmity" (WHO, 1947). Many other aspects of health need to be considered. Health is a state of being that people define in relation to their own values, personality, and lifestyle. Each person has a personal concept of health. Individuals' views of health can vary among different age-groups, gender, race, and culture (Pender, 1996). Pender (1996) explains that "all people free of disease are not equally healthy."

To help clients identify and reach health goals, the nurse must discover and use information about their concepts of health to set individual goals. Pender (1996) suggests that for many people, conditions of life rather than pathological states are what define health. Life conditions can have positive or negative effects on health long before an illness is evident (Pender, 1996). Life conditions may include socioeconomic variables such as environment, diet, and lifestyle practices or choices, as well as many other physiological and psychological variables.

Health and illness must be defined in terms of the individual. Health can include conditions previously considered to be illness. For example, a person with epilepsy who has learned to control seizures with medication and who functions at home and at work may no longer consider himself or herself ill. Nurses' attitudes toward health and illness should consider the total person, as well as the environment in which the person lives, to individualize nursing care and enhance meaningfulness of the client's future health status.

Models of Health and Illness

A model is a theoretical way of understanding a concept or idea. Models represent different ways of approaching complex issues. Because health and illness are complex concepts, models are used to understand the relationships between these concepts and the client's attitudes toward health and **health behaviors.**

Health beliefs are a person's ideas, convictions, and attitudes about health and illness. They may be based on factual information or misinformation, common sense or myths, or reality or false expectations. Because health beliefs usually influence health behavior, they can positively or negatively affect a client's level of health. Positive health behaviors are activities related to maintaining, attaining, or regaining good health and preventing illness. Common positive health behaviors include immunizations, proper sleep patterns, adequate exercise, and nutrition. Negative health behaviors include practices actually or potentially harmful to health, such as smoking, drug or alcohol abuse, poor diet, and refusal to take necessary medications.

Nurses have developed the following health models to understand clients' attitudes and values about health and illness so that effective health care can be provided. These nursing models allow nurses to understand and predict clients' health behavior, including how they use health services and adhere to recommended therapy.

HEALTH-ILLNESS CONTINUUM MODEL

According to a **health-illness continuum model,** health is a dynamic state that fluctuates as a person adapts to changes in the internal and external environments to maintain a state of physical, emotional, intellectual, social, developmental, and spiritual wellbeing. **Illness** is a process in which the functioning of a person is diminished or impaired in one or more dimensions when compared with the person's previous condition. Because health and illness are relative qualities, existing in varying degrees, it may be more useful to consider health and illness in terms of a point on a scale or continuum rather than as an absolute state (Figure 1-1).

High-level wellness and severe illness (premature death) are at opposite ends of the continuum. According to Neuman (1990), "health on a continuum is the degree of client wellness that exists at any point in time, ranging from an optimal wellness condition, with available energy at its maximum, to death, which represents total energy depletion." A nurse can determine a client's level of health at any point on the health-illness continuum.

Central to the health-illness continuum model are risk factors, which are important in identifying the level of health. Risk factors include genetic and physiological variables, such as age, lifestyle, and environment. As a person progresses through the developmental stages, certain risk factors are more common than others. An adolescent, for example, is more likely than an adult to experience stressors related to body image and self-concept, and an older adult is more likely than a child to develop cardiac illness.

The way clients view their levels of health depends on their attitudes toward health, values, beliefs, and perceptions of their physical, emotional, intellectual, social, developmental, and spiritual wellbeing. Stubblefield (1995) notes that "nurses are intuitively aware of the positive effects of an optimistic outlook on their clients' response to illness."

The drawback of the health-illness continuum is that it is not always easy to describe a client's level of health in terms of one point between two extremes. For example, is a man with a broken leg who has adapted to limited mobility more or less healthy than a physically healthy man experiencing severe depression after the death of his spouse? The health-illness continuum is most effective when used to compare a client's present level of health with the client's own previous level of health. Subsequently it is useful as the nurse helps the client set goals to attain a future level of health.

HEALTH BELIEF MODEL

Rosenstoch's (1974) and Becker and Maiman's (1975) **health belief model** (Figure 1-2) addresses the relationship between a person's belief and behaviors. It provides a

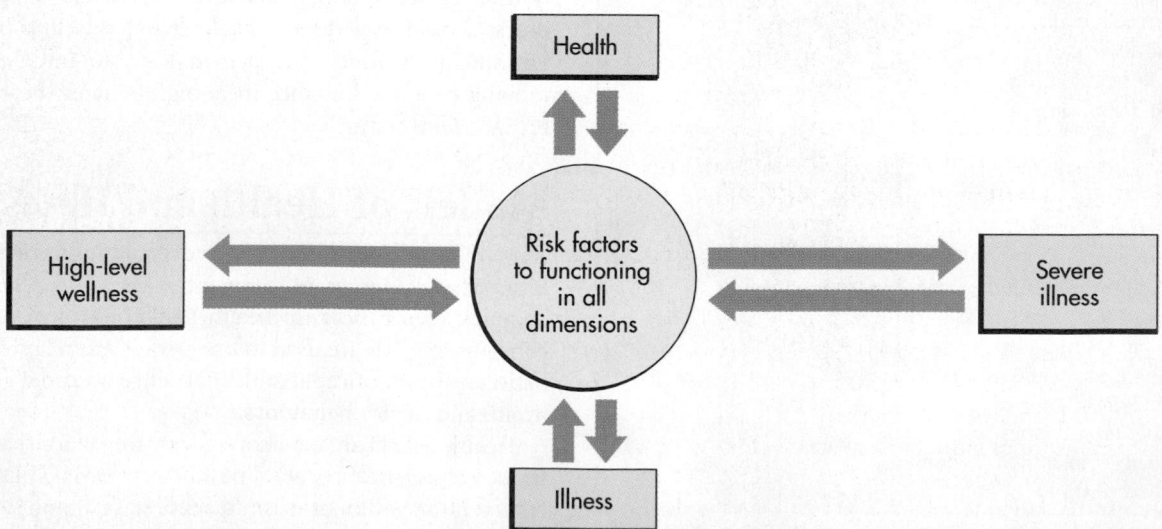

Figure 1-1 The health-illness continuum, ranging from high-level wellness to severe illness, provides a method of identifying a client's level of health. Level of health is a reflection of the client's level of functioning in all dimensions.

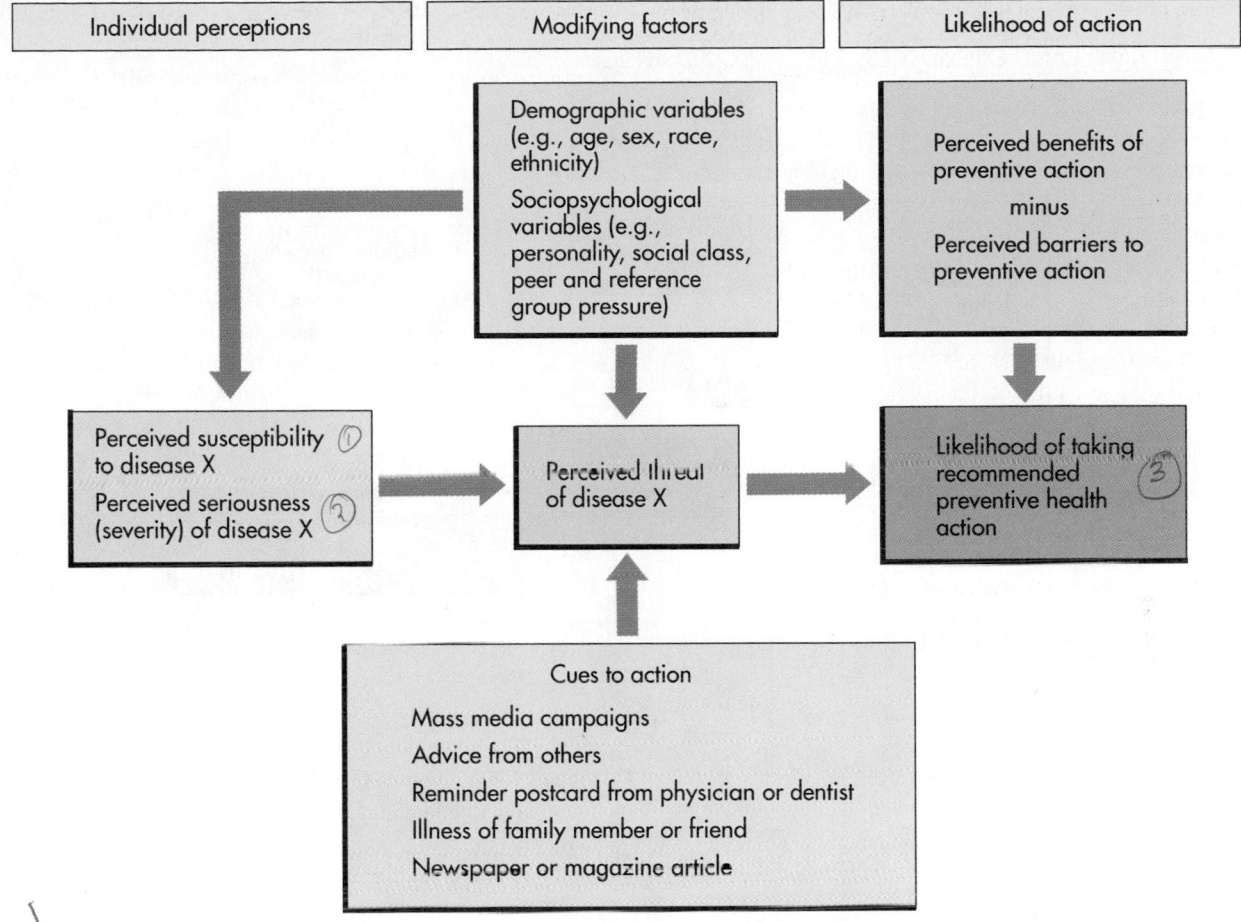

| Individual perceptions | Modifying factors | Likelihood of action |

Figure 1-2 Health belief model.
Data from Becker M, Maiman L: Sociobehavioral determinants of compliance with health and medical care recommendations, *Med Care* 13(1):12, 1975.

way of understanding and predicting how clients will behave in relation to their health and how they will comply with health care therapies.

The first component on this model involves the individual's perception of susceptibility to an illness. For example, a client needs to recognize the familial link for coronary artery disease. After this link is recognized, particularly when one parent and two siblings have died in their fourth decade from myocardial infarction, the client may perceive the personal risk of heart disease.

The second component is the individual's perception of the seriousness of the illness. This perception is influenced and modified by demographic and sociopsychological variables, perceived threats of the illness, and cues to action (e.g., mass media campaigns and advice from family, friends, and medical professionals).

The third component—the likelihood that a person will take preventive action—results from the person's perception of the benefits and barriers of taking action. Preventive action may include lifestyle changes, increased adherence to medical therapies, or a search for medical advice or treatment.

The health belief model helps nurses to understand factors influencing clients' perceptions, beliefs, and behavior in order to plan care that will most effectively assist clients in maintaining or restoring health and preventing illness.

HEALTH PROMOTION MODEL

The health promotion model proposed by Pender (1982, 1993, 1996) was designed to be a "complementary counterpart to models of health protection" (Figure 1-3, p. 6). It defines health as a positive, dynamic state, not merely the absence of disease (Pender, 1993, 1996). Health promotion is directed at increasing a client's level of wellbeing (Pender, 1993, 1996). The health promotion model describes the multidimensional nature of persons as they interact within their environment to pursue health (Pender, 1996). The model focuses on the following three areas: (1) client's cognitive perceptual factors (individual perceptions), (2) modifying factors (demographic and social), and (3) participation in health-promoting behaviors (likelihood of action). The model also organizes cues into a pattern to explain the likelihood of a client's developing

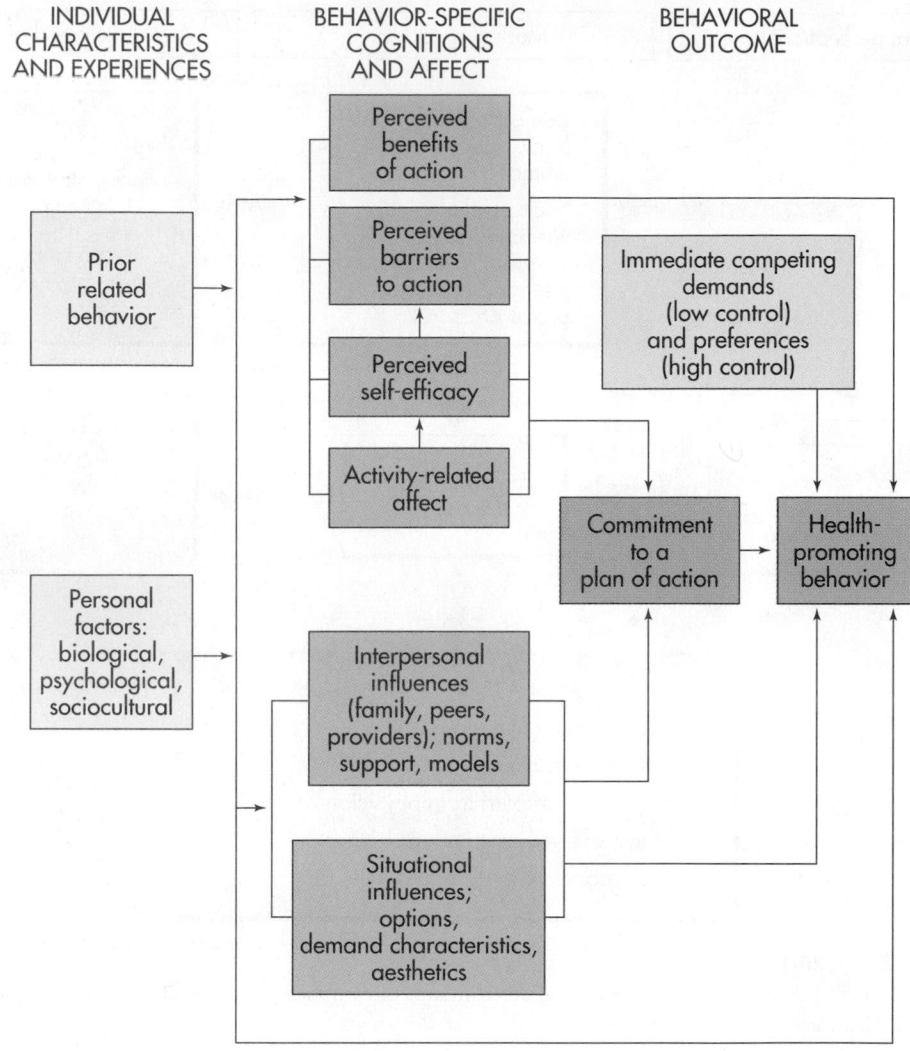

Figure 1-3 Health promotion model.
Redrawn from Pender NJ: *Health promotion and nursing practice*, ed 3, Stamford, Conn, 1996, Appleton & Lange.

health-promoting behaviors (Pender, 1993, 1996). The focus of this model is to explain the reasons why individuals engage in health activities. It is not designed for use with families or communities.

BASIC HUMAN NEEDS MODEL

Basic human needs are elements that are necessary for human survival and health (e.g., food, water, safety, and love). Although each person has other unique needs, the basic human needs are shared by all people, and the extent to which basic needs are met is a major factor in determining a person's level of health.

Maslow's hierarchy of needs is a model that nurses can use to understand the interrelationships of basic human needs (Figure 1-4). According to this model, certain human needs are more basic than others; that is, some needs must be met before other needs (e.g., fulfilling the physiological needs before the needs of love and belonging).

This model can provide a basis for nursing clients of all ages in all health settings. However, when the model is applied, the focus of care is on the client's needs rather than on strict adherence to the hierarchy. In all cases an emergent physiological need takes precedence over a higher-level need. In some situations it is unrealistic to expect a client's basic needs to occur in the fixed hierarchical order. To provide the most effective care, the nurse needs to understand the relationships of different needs and the factors that determine the priorities for the client.

HOLISTIC HEALTH MODELS

Health care has begun to take a more holistic view of health by considering emotional and spiritiual well-being, as well as other dimensions of an individual, as important aspects of physical wellness. The **holistic health model** of nursing attempts to create conditions that promote optimal health. In this model, nurses using the nursing process consider

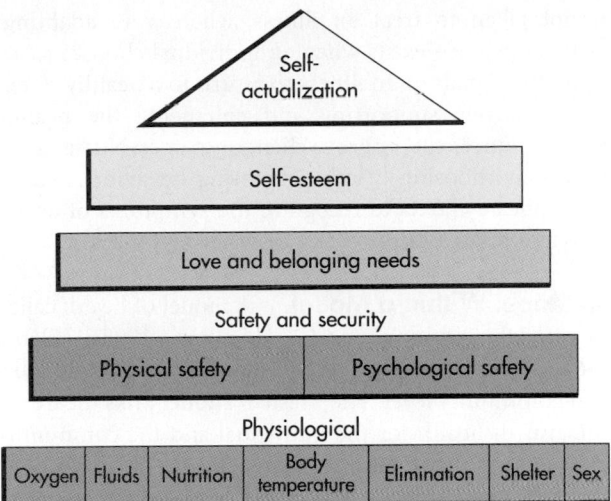

Figure 1-4 Maslow's hierarchy of needs. Redrawn from Maslow AH: *Motivation and personality,* Upper Saddle River, NJ, 1970, Prentice Hall.

clients the ultimate experts regarding their own health and respect clients' subjective experience as relevant in maintaining health or assisting in healing. In the holistic health model, clients are involved in their healing process, thereby assuming some responsibility for health maintenance (Edelman and Mandle, 1998). By being involved in their own health care, clients are able to gain personal control over their health and illness (Schuster, 1997).

Nurses use holistic nursing interventions, such as music therapy, reminiscence, relaxation therapy, therapeutic touch, massage therapy, biofeedback, and guided imagery, because they are effective, economical, noninvasive, nonpharmacological complements to traditional medical care. Holistic interventions can be used to augment standard treatments, to replace interventions that are ineffective or debilitating, and to promote or maintain health (Mornhinweg and Voigner, 1995). These holistic strategies, which can be used in all stages of health and illness, are integral in the expanding role of nursing.

Most holistic therapies are easily learned and can be applied to almost any nursing setting and in all stages of health and illness. For example, reminiscence may be used in the geriatric population to help relieve anxiety for a client dealing with memory loss or for a cancer patient dealing with the difficult side effects of chemotherapy. Music therapy may be used in the operating room to create a soothing environment. Relaxation therapy may be useful in any setting to distract a client during a painful procedure, such as a dressing change. Breathing exercises are commonly taught to help clients deal with the pain associated with labor and delivery.

Recently there has been an increase in the numbers of people using alternative and complementary medical therapies. These therapies are used either alone or in conjunction with conventional medicine (see Chapter 35). These therapies incorporate theories of the holistic health model and recognize the natural healing abilities of the body. In a recent study, Astin (1998) found that people use alternative medicine not because they are dissatisfied with conventional medicine, but because alternative therapies are more congruent with their values, beliefs, and philosophical orientations toward health and life.

Nurses should be aware that their clients may have previous knowledge or experience with alternative and complementary therapies and may therefore be accepting of holistic nursing interventions. Nurses can help all clients recognize the many options available and assist them in making choices to enhance health.

EMERGING MODELS OF HEALTH

Wellness-Illness Model. Jensen and Allen (1993) propose a wellness-illness model that describes the relationship between health, disease, wellness, and illness as distinct parts of a process involving the changing person in the changing world. In this model, health is viewed as an objective process characterized by stability, balance, and integrity of functioning. Disease, also an objective process, is viewed as a dysfunction or alteration in functioning. Disease is measured by laboratory tests and direct observation. In contrast, wellness is the subjective experience of health (Benner and Wrubel, 1989). Illness, then, is the human experience of disease and may be perceived as loss, challenge, threat, punishment, or gain (Lipowski, 1969, 1983).

In this model, wellness-illness is affected by intrapersonal, interpersonal, health-disease–related, and extrapersonal factors. Intrapersonal factors include personality, past experiences, and emotional state. Interpersonal factors include social supports and relationships. Health-disease–related factors include health promotion orientation, functional status, visibility of disease-health, and severity and prognosis of disease. Extrapersonal factors are sociocultural and economic (Jensen and Allen, 1993).

Simplified, wellness-illness is viewed as the human experiences of actual or perceived function-dysfunction states that are influenced by the way the individual perceives or views the experience of health-disease.

The HEALTH-Healing/Disordering Model. McCabe (1995) constructed a model of healing based on current literature on the phenomenon of healing and the lived experiences of nurses who use holistic and complementary therapies in their practice of nursing. The proposed model may have significance for any health care practitioner as a means to understand the health care provider's role in the process of healing. In the model (Figure 1-5, p. 8), health is a dynamic process conceptualized as a functional state. Illness is deviation from a normal state in which disordering processes occur.

According to McCabe (1995):

The HEALTH-Healing/Disordering model is a conceptual map. It is not to be interpreted as a fixed sequence of events, but rather as an energy field wherein health processes are seen as dynamic potentials. Out of these potentials events may arise sequentially or spontaneously. The HEALTH-Healing/Disordering model denotes a concept of health *which incorporates both healing and disordering processes as aspects of health.*

In the model, the middle circle represents a normal state of health wherein minor fluctuations occur on a daily basis and can be perceived as temporary tiredness, constipation, indigestion, or a headache. A normal state of health is challenged (shifting) by any disordering influence that renders an individual susceptible to illness. Symptoms of an illness are known as signaling and act to summon the healing response. The healing response corrects everyday fluctuations in physical and nonphysical health status; its strength is dependent on the total health of the individual. This model views healing as purposeful with a goal to recreate integrated function in an impaired system. The choices made by the individual during the illness phase or disordering phase will affect the individual's adaptation and ability to return to a previous or improved state of health. As health returns, a reordering process occurs. An adapting-compromising pattern exists when care is not taken to treat an illness, whereas an adapting-evolving pattern exists when an individual chooses to act upon the signals of an illness to return to a healthy state.

By actively supporting and enhancing the healing process, nurses can improve client outcomes. Nurses assist clients in choosing health-promoting behaviors. Nurses also educate clients to recognize the symptoms of an illness and how to respond to a disordering process.

A Model Within a Model.   A model of health called "a model within a model" (Collins, 1995) (Figure 1-6) addresses the determinants of health on an individual and community level. The "nested" model links the determinants of health for the individual and the community and suggests that they are interdependent. In this model, the individual consists of five "environments" of health determinants. The health of the individual is affected by a

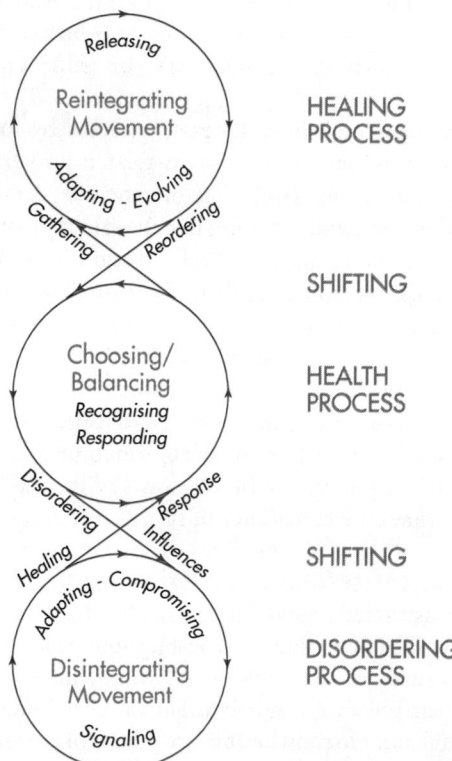

Figure 1-5   The HEALTH-Healing/Disordering model. Redrawn from McCabe P: Exploring the phenomenon of healing: healing as a health capacity, *Aust J Holistic Nurs* 2(1):13, 1995.

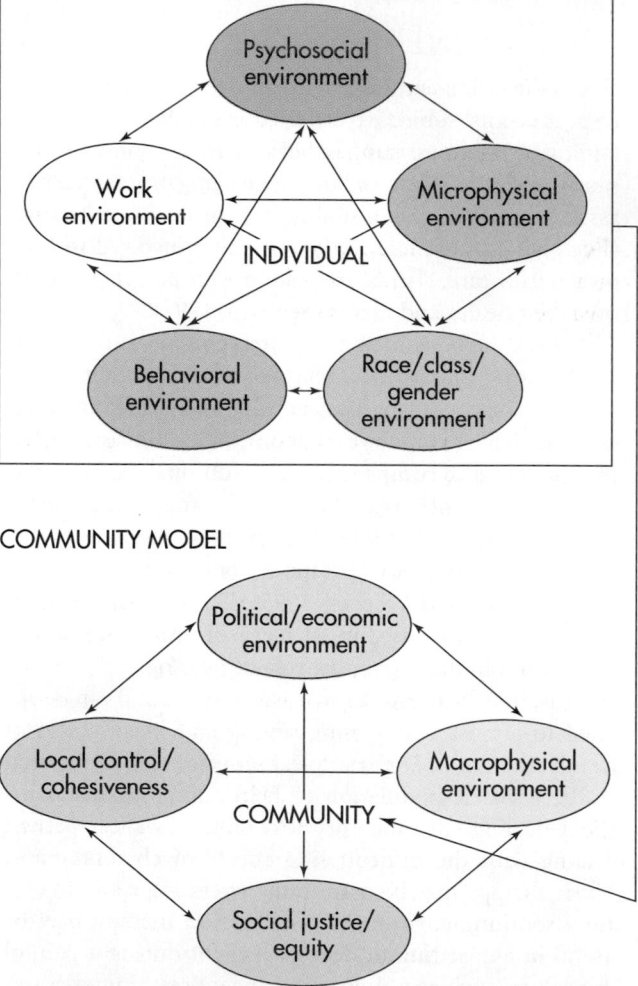

Figure 1-6   A nested model of health. Note that the individual is located within the community model. Redrawn from Collins T: Models of health: pervasive, persuasive and politically charged, *Health Promot Int* 10(4):320, 1995.

combination of these factors, as well as by the individual's biological makeup. The individual is "nested" as the center of a community. The community consists of four categories of social determinants of health. "The determinants of a healthy community are expected to have an impact on the determinants of individual health" (Collins, 1995). A reciprocal relationship ensues with the individual when individual change leads to community change.

The model has implications for both health promotion practice and health public policy. The author believes that the model encourages health promotion program developers (educators) to consider broader aspects of an issue. For example, rather than focusing on an individual behavior such as smoking cessation, an educational program could use a multifaceted approach to the issue by including psychosocial benefits of smoking and political and economic aspects of tobacco production and cigarette advertising (Collins, 1995).

Variables Influencing Health Beliefs and Practices

There are many variables that can influence a client's health beliefs and practices. Internal and external variables can influence how a person thinks and acts. As previously stated, health beliefs usually influence health behavior, or health practices, and likewise can positively or negatively affect a client's level of health. Therefore understanding the effects of these variables allows the nurse to plan and deliver individualized care.

INTERNAL VARIABLES

Internal variables include a person's developmental stage, intellectual background, perception of functioning, and emotional and spiritual factors.

Developmental Stage. A person's thought and behavior patterns change throughout life. The nurse must consider the client's level of growth and development when using his or her health beliefs and practices as a basis for planning care. The concept of illness of a child, adolescent, or adult is dependent on the individual's developmental stage. Fear and anxiety are common among ill children, especially if thoughts about illness, hospitalization or procedures are based on lack of information or lack of clarity of information. Good communication through provision of age-appropriate explanations aimed at increasing a client's understanding and knowledge of illness or procedures provides the foundation for effective treatment (Moss-Morris, and Paterson, 1995). Emotional development may also influence personal beliefs about health-related matters. For example, the nurse uses different techniques for teaching about contraception to an adolescent than would be used for an adult. Knowledge of the stages of growth and development helps the nurse pre-

dict the client's response to the present illness or the threat of future illness. The planning of nursing care is then adapted to these expectations, as well as to the client's abilities to participate in self-care.

Intellectual Background. A person's beliefs about health are shaped in part by the person's knowledge (or misinformation) about body functions and illnesses, educational background, and past experiences. These variables influence how a client thinks about health. In addition, cognitive abilities shape the *way* a person thinks, including the ability to understand factors involved in illness and to apply knowledge of health and illness to personal health practices. Cognitive abilities also relate to a person's developmental stage. A nurse considers intellectual background so that these variables can be incorporated into nursing care (Edelman and Mandle, 1998).

Perception of Functioning. The way people perceive their physical functioning affects health beliefs and practices. When nurses assess a client's level of health, they gather subjective data about the way the client perceives physical functioning, such as level of fatigue, shortness of breath, or pain. They also obtain objective data about actual functioning, such as blood pressure, height measurements, and lung sound assessment. This information allows nurses to more successfully plan and implement individualized care.

Emotional Factors. The client's degree of calm or stress can influence health beliefs and practices. The manner in which a person handles stress throughout each phase of life will influence the way the person reacts to illness. A person who generally is very calm may have little emotional response during illness, whereas an individual unable to cope emotionally with the threat of illness may either overreact to illness and assume it is life threatening or deny the presence of symptoms and not take therapeutic action (see Chapter 30).

Spiritual Factors. Spirituality is reflected in how a person lives his or her life, including the value and beliefs exercised, the relationships established with family and friends, and the ability to find hope and meaning in life. Spirituality serves as an integrating theme in peoples' lives (see Chapter 28). Religious practices are one way that people exercise spirituality. There are some religions that restrict the use of certain forms of medical treatment. Nurses must understand clients' spiritual dimensions to involve them effectively in nursing care. Ross (1995) suggests that hospitalization can precipitate spiritual distress; therefore clients' spiritual needs should be addressed, since the spiritual dimension is important for the attainment of an overall sense of health, well-being, and quality of life.

The concept of a spiritual wellness program has been

introduced in some long-term care facilities (Anderson, 1998). In this program, a spiritual wellness staff uses a holistic approach to care in order to address the needs of older residents, their family members, and the staff. Whereas a traditional medical model focuses on physical health, a social/relational model identifies a person's core identity to provide the care the client needs.

EXTERNAL VARIABLES

External variables influencing a person's health beliefs and practices include family practices, socioeconomic factors, and cultural background.

Family Practices. The way that clients' families use health care services generally affects their health practices. Their perceptions of the seriousness of diseases and their history of preventive care behaviors (or lack of them) can influence how clients will think about health.

Socioeconomic Factors. Social and psychosocial factors can increase the risk for illness and influence the way that a person defines and reacts to illness. Psychosocial variables include the stability of the person's marital or intimate relationship, lifestyle habits, and occupational environment. A person generally seeks approval and support from social networks (neighbors, peers, and co-workers), and this desire for approval and support affects health beliefs and practices. Najman (1993) suggests that the five social categories that constitute the majority of those in poverty are single parents and their children, older adults, the unemployed, members of racial and ethnic minorities, and the disabled. In addition, data point to a consistent pattern of higher mortality rates for the economically most disadvantaged.

Social variables partly determine how the health care system provides medical care. Because the health care system is organized in certain ways, it determines how clients can obtain care, the treatment method, the economic cost to the client, and potential reimbursement to the health care agency or client.

Like social variables, economic variables may affect a client's level of health by increasing the risk for disease and influencing how or at what point the client enters the health care system.

A person's compliance with the treatment that is designed to maintain or improve health is also affected by economic status. A person who has high utility bills, a large family, and a low income tends to give a higher priority to food and shelter than to costly drugs or treatment, or expensive foods for special diets.

Cultural Background. Cultural background influences beliefs, values, and customs. It influences the approach to the health care system, personal health practices, and the nurse-client relationship. Cultural background may also influence an individual's beliefs about causes of illness, as well as remedies or practices to restore health. Cultural differences can affect the dynamics of health care, in that one of the major characteristics of each culture is the way it deals with the problems of pain, suffering, and death (Dimou, 1995). If nurses are not aware of their own and other cultural patterns of behavior and language, they may not be able to recognize and understand a client's behavior and beliefs and may have difficulty interacting with the client. As with family and socioeconomic variables, cultural variables must be incorporated into a client's care plan (see Chapter 7).

Health Promotion, Wellness, and Illness Prevention

Health care has become increasingly focused on health promotion, wellness, and illness prevention. The rapid rise of health care costs has motivated people to seek ways of decreasing the incidence and minimizing the results of illness or disability.

The concepts of health promotion, wellness, and illness prevention are closely related and, in practice, overlap to some extent. All are focused on the future; the difference between them involves motivations and goals. **Health promotion** activities such as routine exercise and good nutrition, help clients maintain or enhance their present levels of health. **Wellness** education teaches people how to care for themselves in a healthy way and includes topics such as physical awareness, stress management, and self-responsibility. Wellness has been described as the ongoing and dynamic process of striving to achieve optimum health (Plawecki, 1997). **Illness prevention** activities such as immunization programs protect clients from actual or potential threats to health.

Nurses emphasize health promotion, wellness-enhancing strategies, and illness prevention activities as important forms of health care because they assist clients in maintaining and improving health. Health promotion activities motivate people to act positively to reach more stable levels of health. Wellness strategies are designed to help persons achieve new understanding and control of their lives. Illness prevention activities motivate people to avoid declines in health or functional levels.

The goal of a total health program is to improve a client's level of well-being in all dimensions, not just physical health. Total health programs are based on the belief that many factors can affect a person's level of health. The following categories are identified as important determinants of health status (Edelman and Mandle, 1998):

Tobacco use
Nutrition
Alcohol use
Habituating drug use
Driving
Exercise

Sexuality and contraceptive or barrier use
Family relationships
Risk factor modification
Coping and adaptation

Health can be influenced by individual practices, such as poor eating habits and little or no exercise. It can also be affected by physical stressors, such as a poor living environment, exposure to air pollutants, and an unsafe environment. Hereditary and psychological stressors, such as emotional, intellectual, social, developmental, and spiritual factors, can also influence one's level of health. Total health programs are directed at individuals changing their lifestyle by developing habits that can improve their level of health.

Other programs are aimed at specific health care problems. For example, support groups exist to help people with human immunodeficiency virus (HIV) infection. Exercise programs encourage participants to exercise regularly to reduce their risk of cardiac disease. Stress reduction programs teach participants to cope with stressors and reduce their risks for multiple illnesses, such as infections, gastrointestinal disease, and cardiac disease.

Some health promotion, wellness education, and illness prevention programs are operated by health care agencies; others are independently operated. Many corporations have developed on-site health promotion activities for employees. Likewise, colleges and community centers offer health promotion and illness prevention programs. Nurses may be actively involved in these programs or may be consultants or give referrals. The goal of these activities is to improve the client's level of health through preventive health services, environmental protection, and health education.

Health promotion is an emerging field with proactive attempts to prevent illness or disease. Health promotion activities can be passive or active. With **passive strategies of health promotion,** individuals gain from the activities of others without acting themselves. The fluoridation of municipal drinking water and the fortification of homogenized milk with vitamin D are examples of passive health promotion strategies. With **active strategies of health promotion,** individuals are motivated to adopt specific health programs. Weight reduction and smoking cessation programs require clients to be actively involved in measures to improve their present and future levels of wellness while decreasing the risk of disease.

Health is acquired and maintained by engaging in activities that promote and maintain wellness (Plawecki, 1997). An individual takes responsibility for health and wellness by making appropriate lifestyle choices. Lifestyle choices are important in that they affect a person's quality of life. Positive lifestyle choices and the avoidance of negative lifestyle choices may also play a role in the prevention of illness. Northam (1996) adds that prevention of illness serves humanitarian, as well as economic, purposes. Prevention of illness can reduce anxiety, stress, pain, and

suffering. At the same time, prevention of illness enables the ongoing attainment of life goals, including work, family and education (Northam, 1996). Prevention of illness has an economic impact in that it decreases health care costs.

An understanding of risk factors, behavior, risk factor modification, and behavior modification are integral components of health promotion, wellness, and illness prevention activities. Nurses in all areas of practice often have opportunities to assist clients in adopting activities to promote health and decrease risks of illness.

LEVELS OF PREVENTIVE CARE

Nursing care oriented to health promotion, wellness, and illness prevention can be understood in terms of health activities on primary, secondary, and tertiary levels (Figure 1-7, p. 12).

Primary Prevention. **Primary prevention** is true prevention; it precedes disease or dysfunction and is applied to clients considered physically and emotionally healthy. Primary prevention aimed at health promotion includes health education programs, immunization, and physical and nutritional fitness activities. It can be provided to an individual or to a general population, or it can focus on individuals at risk for developing specific diseases. Wellness activities (Edelman and Mandle, 1998) are synonymous with the activities identified for primary prevention by Leavell and Clark (1965) in Figure 1-7. Primary prevention includes all health promotion efforts, as well as wellness activities that focus on maintaining or improving the general health of individuals, families, and communities (Edelman and Mandle, 1998).

Secondary Prevention. **Secondary prevention** focuses on individuals who are experiencing health problems or illnesses and who are at risk for developing complications or worsening conditions. Activities are directed at diagnosis and prompt intervention, thereby reducing severity and enabling the client to return to a normal level of health as early as possible (Pender, 1993; Edelman and Mandle, 1998). A large portion of nursing care related to secondary prevention is delivered in homes, hospitals, or skilled nursing facilities. It includes screening techniques and treating early stages of disease to limit disability by averting or delaying the consequences of advanced disease.

Tertiary Prevention. **Tertiary prevention** occurs when a defect or disability is permanent and irreversible. It involves minimizing the effects of long-term disease or disability by interventions directed at preventing complications and deterioration (Edelman and Mandle, 1998). Activities are directed at rehabilitation rather than diagnosis and treatment. Care at this level aims to help clients achieve as high a level of functioning as possible, despite

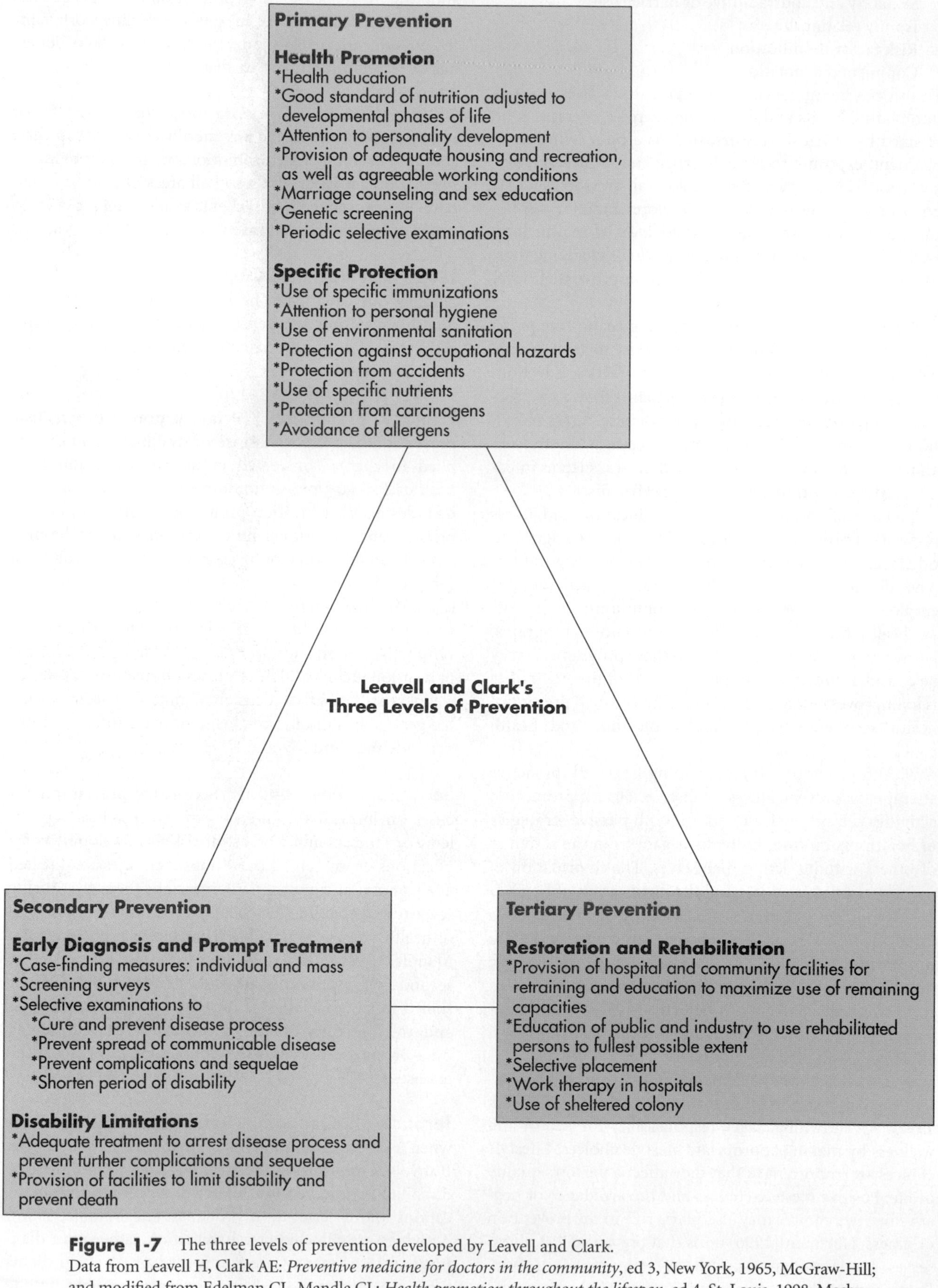

Primary Prevention

Health Promotion
*Health education
*Good standard of nutrition adjusted to
 developmental phases of life
*Attention to personality development
*Provision of adequate housing and recreation,
 as well as agreeable working conditions
*Marriage counseling and sex education
*Genetic screening
*Periodic selective examinations

Specific Protection
*Use of specific immunizations
*Attention to personal hygiene
*Use of environmental sanitation
*Protection against occupational hazards
*Protection from accidents
*Use of specific nutrients
*Protection from carcinogens
*Avoidance of allergens

**Leavell and Clark's
Three Levels of Prevention**

Secondary Prevention

Early Diagnosis and Prompt Treatment
*Case-finding measures: individual and mass
*Screening surveys
*Selective examinations to
  *Cure and prevent disease process
  *Prevent spread of communicable disease
  *Prevent complications and sequelae
  *Shorten period of disability

Disability Limitations
*Adequate treatment to arrest disease process and
 prevent further complications and sequelae
*Provision of facilities to limit disability and
 prevent death

Tertiary Prevention

Restoration and Rehabilitation
*Provision of hospital and community facilities for
 retraining and education to maximize use of remaining
 capacities
*Education of public and industry to use rehabilitated
 persons to fullest possible extent
*Selective placement
*Work therapy in hospitals
*Use of sheltered colony

Figure 1-7   The three levels of prevention developed by Leavell and Clark.
Data from Leavell H, Clark AE: *Preventive medicine for doctors in the community*, ed 3, New York, 1965, McGraw-Hill;
and modified from Edelman CL, Mandle CL: *Health promotion throughout the lifespan*, ed 4, St. Louis, 1998, Mosby.

the limitations caused by illness or impairment. This level of care is called preventive care because it involves preventing further disability or reduced functioning.

Risk Factors

A **risk factor** is any situation, habit, social or environmental condition, physiological or psychological condition, developmental or intellectual condition, or spiritual or other variable that increases the vulnerability of an individual or group to an illness or accident. The presence of risk factors does not mean that a disease will develop, but risk factors increase the chances that the individual will experience a particular disease or dysfunction. Nurses and other health care professionals are concerned with risk factors, sometimes called health hazards, for several reasons. Risk factors play a major role in how a nurse identifies a client's health status. They can also influence health beliefs and practices if a person is aware of their presence. Risk factors can be placed in the following interrelated categories: genetic and physiological factors, age, physical environment, and lifestyle.

GENETIC AND PHYSIOLOGICAL FACTORS

Physiological risk factors involve the physical functioning of the body. Certain physical conditions, such as being pregnant or overweight, place increased stress on physiological systems (e.g., the circulatory system), increasing susceptibility to illness in these areas. Heredity, or genetic predisposition to specific illness, is a major physical risk factor. For example, a person with a family history of diabetes mellitus is at risk for developing the disease later in life. Other documented genetic risk factors include family histories of cancer, heart disease, kidney disease, or mental illness.

AGE

Age increases or decreases susceptibility to certain illnesses (e.g., the risk of heart disease increases with age for both sexes). The risks of birth defects and complications of pregnancy increase in women bearing children after age 35. Many kinds of cancer pose a greater risk for persons over age 45 than for younger persons. Age risk factors are often closely associated with other risk factors such as family history and personal habits. Nurses need to educate their clients about the importance of regularly scheduled checkups for their age-group (Figure 1-8).

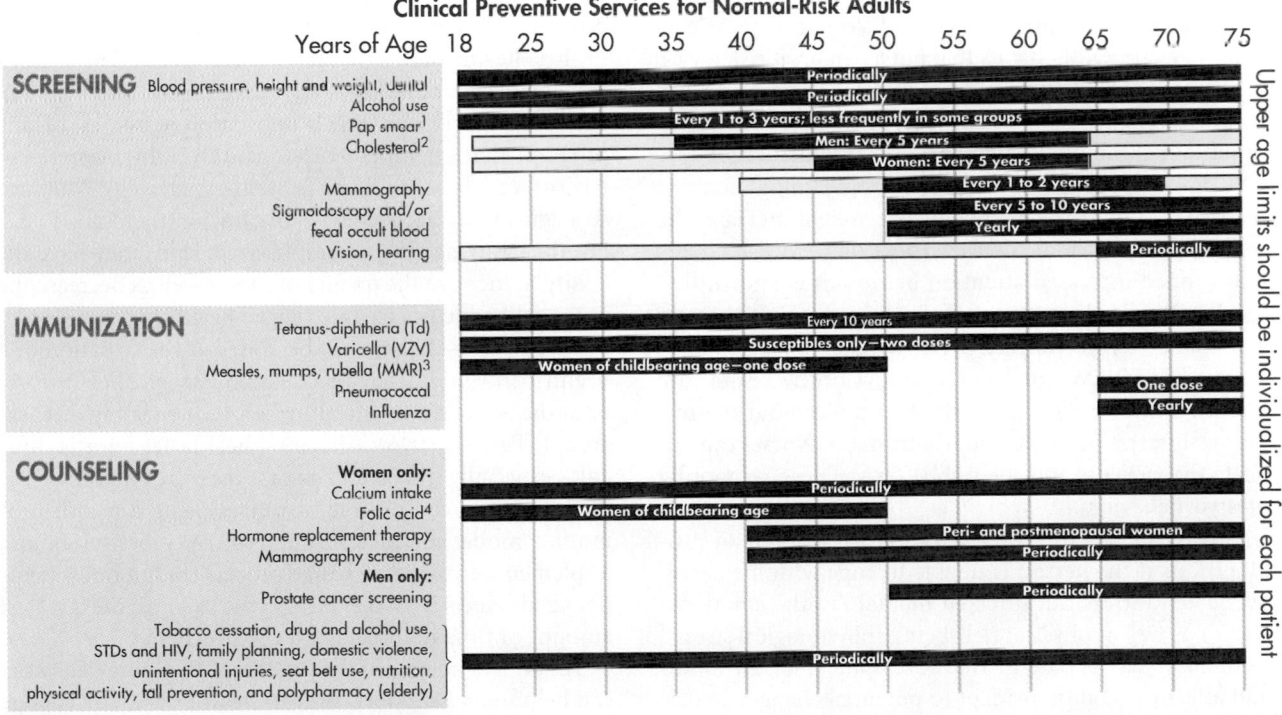

Figure 1-8   Clinical Preventive Services for normal-risk adults.
Redrawn from *Clinician's handbook of preventive services*, ed 2, Germantown, Md, 1998, International Medical Publishers.

ENVIRONMENT

The physical environment in which a person works or lives can increase the likelihood that certain illnesses will occur. For example, some kinds of cancer and other diseases are more likely to develop when industrial workers are exposed to certain chemicals or when people live near toxic waste disposal sites. Screening for these environmentally based risk factors are directed at the short-term effects of the exposure and the potential for long-term effects (Edelman and Mandle, 1998).

Blackburn (1994) reports that researchers have demonstrated how low income acts as a key health hazard by increasing exposure to health hazards such as poor housing, pollution (air, water, noise), lack of safe play areas, and poor social support networks. For example, in the home the environment may include conditions that pose risks to an individual or family, such as unclean, poorly heated or cooled, or overcrowded dwellings. These conditions can increase the likelihood that infections and other diseases will be contracted and spread.

LIFESTYLE

Many activities, habits, and practices involve risk factors. Lifestyle practices and behaviors can also have positive or negative effects on health. Practices with potential negative effects are risk factors; these include overeating or poor nutrition, insufficient rest and sleep, and poor personal hygiene. Other habits that put a person at risk for illness include tobacco use, alcohol or drug abuse, and activities involving a threat of injury, such as skydiving or mountain climbing. Some habits are risk factors for specific diseases. For example, excessive sunbathing increases the risk of skin cancer, and being overweight increases the risk of cardiovascular disease. These lifestyle risk factors have gained increased attention because it is known that many of the leading causes of death in the United States are related to lifestyle patterns or habits. This also represents a huge impact on the economics of the health care system. Therefore it is important to understand the impact of lifestyle behaviors on health status. Nurses can educate their clients and the public on wellness-promoting lifestyle behaviors.

Stress can be a lifestyle risk factor if it is severe or prolonged, or if the person is unable to cope with life events adequately. Stress can threaten mental health (emotional stress), as well as physical well-being (physiological stress). Both may play a part in the development of an illness and affect the ability to adapt to potential changes associated with an illness, as well as the ability to survive a life-threatening illness. Stress may also interfere with health promotion activities and the ability to implement needed lifestyle modifications. Emotional stressors may result from life events such as divorce, pregnancy, death of a spouse or family member, and financial instabilities. Job-related stressors, for example, may overtax a person's cognitive skills and decision-making ability, leading to "men-

tal overload" or "burnout" (see Chapter 30). Stress can also threaten physical well-being and has been associated with illnesses such as heart disease, cancer, and gastrointestinal disorders (Pender, 1996). Life stressors should be reviewed as part of a comprehensive risk factor analysis.

The goal of risk factor identification is to merely assist clients in visualizing those areas in their life that can be modified or even eliminated to promote wellness and prevent illness. More comprehensive health risk appraisals, using a variety of available health risk appraisal forms, can be done in order to estimate a person's specific health threats based on the presence of various risk factors (Edelman and Mandle, 1998). It is important to understand that implementation of a health risk appraisal must be linked with educational programs and other community resources in order to result in necessary lifestyle changes and in risk reduction (Pender, 1996).

Risk Factor Modification and Changing Health Behaviors

Identifying risk factors is the first step in health promotion, wellness education, and illness prevention activities. Health hazards should be discussed with the client following a comprehensive nursing assessment; then the client can decide if he or she wants to maintain or improve his or her health status by taking risk reduction actions (Edelman and Mandle, 1998). Risk factor modification, health promotion or illness prevention activities, or any program that attempts to change unhealthy lifestyle behaviors can be considered a wellness strategy. Wellness strategies that teach clients to care for themselves in a healthier way need to be emphasized, since they have the ability to increase the quality of life, as well as decrease the potential high costs of unmanaged health problems.

Attempts to change may be aimed at the cessation of a health-damaging behavior (tobacco use, alcohol misuse) or at the adoption of a healthy behavior (healthy diet, exercise) (Pender, 1996). Changing health behavior is difficult, especially those behaviors that are ingrained in lifestyle patterns. The role of nurses using a health promotion model for identification of risky behaviors and implementation of the change process cannot be overemphasized, since it is the nurse who spends the greatest amount of time in direct contact with clients.

An understanding of the process of changing behaviors can help nurses support difficult **health behavior change** in their clients. It is believed that change involves movement through a series of stages (Figure 1-9). Prochaska and DiClemente (1992) and Conn (1994) have identified five stages of change from no intention to change (precontemplation) to maintaining a changed behavior (maintenance stage). Nursing implications for each stage are discussed in Table 1-1. As individuals attempt a change in behavior, relapse followed by recycling through the stages occurs frequently. When relapse occurs, the person will return to the contemplation or precontemplation stage before attempting the change again. Relapse can be viewed as a learning process, and what is learned from relapse can be applied to the next attempt to change. It is important to understand what occurs at the various stages of the change process in order to time the implementation of interventions (wellness strategies) adequately and to provide appropriate care at each stage (Pender, 1996).

Most behavior change programs are designed (and have a chance of success) for those people who are ready to take action regarding their health behavior problems. Only a minority of people are actually in this action stage (Prochaska, 1991). Further work needs to be done to design interventions and wellness strategies for people in all stages of health behavior change. Changes will be maintained over time only if they are integrated into an individual's overall lifestyle. Maintenance of healthy lifestyles can prevent hospitalizations and potentially lower the cost of health care. Nurses can assist clients with their adaptation to a changed and healthier lifestyle.

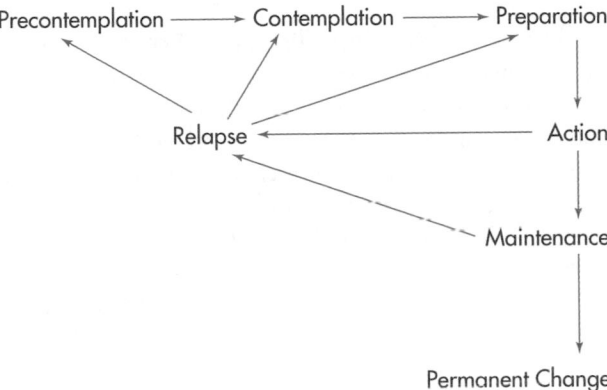

Figure 1-9 Stages of health behavior change.
Redrawn from Conn VS: A stage based approach to helping people change health behaviors, *Clin Nurs Spec* 8[4]:187, 1994; and Prochaska JO and others: In search of how people change: applications and addictive behaviors, *Am Psychol* 47[9]:1102, 1992.

Illness

Illness is a state in which a person's physical, emotional, intellectual, social, developmental, or spiritual functioning is diminished or impaired compared with previous experience. Cancer is a disease process, but one client with leukemia who is responding to treatment may continue to function as usual, whereas another client with breast cancer who is preparing for surgery may be affected in dimensions other than the physical.

Illness, therefore, is not synonymous with disease; although nurses must be familiar with different kinds of diseases and their treatments, they are concerned more with illness, which may include disease but also the effects on functioning and well-being in all dimensions.

Table 1-1 **Stages of Health Behavior Change**		
	Definition	Nursing Implications
Precontemplation	Not intending to make changes within the next 6 months.	Client will not be interested in information about the behavior and may be defensive when confronted with the information.
Contemplation	Considering a change within the next 6 months.	Ambivalence may be present, but clients will more likely accept information as they are developing more belief in the value of change.
Preparation	Make small changes in preparation for a change in the next month.	Client believes advantages outweigh disadvantages of behavior change. May need assistance in planning for the change.
Action	Actively engaged in strategies to change behavior. This stage may last up to 6 months.	Be aware of previous habits that may prevent action on new behaviors. Identify barriers and facilitators of change.
Maintenance Stage	Sustained change over time. This stage begins 6 months after action has started and continues indefinitely.	Changes need to be integrated into the client's lifestyle.

Modified from Prochaska JO, DiClemente CC: Stages of change in the modification of problem behaviors, *Prog Behav Modif* 28:184, 1992; and Conn VS: A staged-based approach to helping people change health behaviors, *Clin Nurs Spec* 8(4):187, 1994.

ACUTE ILLNESS AND CHRONIC ILLNESS

Acute illness and chronic illness are two general classifications of illness used in this chapter. Both acute and chronic illnesses have the potential to be life threatening. An **acute illness** usually has a short duration and is severe. The symptoms appear abruptly, are intense, and often subside after a relatively short period. An acute illness may affect functioning in any dimension. A **chronic illness** persists, usually longer than 6 months, and can also affect functioning in any dimension. The client may fluctuate between maximal functioning and serious health relapses that may be life threatening. A person with a chronic illness is similar to a person with a disability in that both have limitations (of varying degrees) in function resulting from either a pathological process or an injury. Mechanic (1995) notes that "a chronic disabling disease interferes with ongoing life adaptations by making the performance of routine tasks more challenging." In addition, the social surroundings and physical environment in which the individual lives can impact the abilities, motivation, and psychological maintenance of the disabled person.

Chronic illnesses and disabilities remain a leading health problem in North America for older adults and children. Issues of coping and living with a chronic illness can be complex and overwhelming. A major role for nursing is to provide client education aimed at helping clients manage their illness or disability. The goal of managing a chronic illness is to reduce the occurrence of symptoms or to improve the tolerance of symptoms. In a recent study, McWilliam and others (1996) found that older people with chronic illnesses tended to focus not on their chronic illness, but on their own activities and attitudes toward the illness. By focusing on a client's life and health, nurses can assist clients in creating alternatives and solutions to respond positively to challenges in the environment (McWilliam and others, 1996). By enhancing wellness, nurses may help improve the quality of life for clients living with chronic illnesses or disabilities.

ILLNESS BEHAVIOR

People who are ill generally act in a way that medical sociologists call illness behavior. It involves how people monitor their bodies, define and interpret their symptoms, take remedial actions, and use the health care system (Mechanic, 1982). Personal history, social situations, social norms, and the opportunities and constraints of community institutions can all affect illness behavior (Mechanic, 1995). Although there is a large variability in the way people react to an illness, illness behavior displayed in sickness can be used to manage life adversities (Mechanic, 1995). In other words, if people perceive themselves to be ill, illness behaviors can be coping mechanisms. For example, illness behavior can result in clients being released from roles, social expectations, or responsibilities. For a homemaker, for example, the "flu" may be viewed as an added stressor, or it may be a temporary release from child care and household responsibilities.

Illness behavior may become abnormal when it is disproportionate to the present problem and the client persists in the sick role (Clark and Smith, 1997). For example, a normal sick role during the acute phase following a stroke may be the avoidance of physical activity. This behavior would be inappropriate if it persisted during rehabilitation (Clark and Smith, 1997). Beckingham (1995) believes that for many clients a period of "convalescence" is necessary after an illness. It is a gradual and personal process in which clients recover at their own pace and, when healed, are able to relinquish the sick role (Beckingham, 1995).

Variables Influencing Illness Behavior. Just as health behavior is affected by internal and external variables, so is illness behavior. The influences of these variables, as well as the stage of illness behavior the client is in, may affect the likelihood of seeking health care, compliance with therapy, and therefore health outcomes. Based on an understanding of these variables and behaviors, nurses can plan individualized care to assist clients in coping with their illness at various stages of illness. The goal of nursing is to promote optimal functioning in all dimensions throughout an illness.

Internal Variables. Internal variables influencing the way clients behave when they are ill are their perceptions of symptoms and the nature of the illness. If clients believe that the symptoms of their illnesses disrupt their normal routine, they are more likely to seek health care assistance than if they do not perceive the symptoms to be disruptive. If clients believe that the symptoms are serious or perhaps life threatening, they are also more likely to seek assistance. Persons awakened by crushing chest pains in the middle of the night generally view this symptom as potentially serious and life threatening, and they will probably be motivated to seek assistance. However, such a perception can also have the opposite effect. Individuals may fear serious illness, react by denying it, and not seek medical assistance.

The nature of the illness, either acute or chronic, can also affect a client's illness behavior. Clients with acute illnesses are likely to seek health care and comply readily with therapy. On the other hand, a client with a chronic illness, in which the symptoms may not be cured, but only partially relieved, may not be motivated to comply with the therapy plan. Chronically ill clients may become less actively involved in their care, may experience greater frustration, and may comply less readily with care. Because nurses generally spend more time than other health care professionals with chronically ill clients, they are in the unique position of being able to assist these clients in overcoming problems related to illness behavior.

A client's coping skills, as well as his or her locus of control, are other internal variables that affect the way the client behaves when ill (see Chapter 30).

External Variables.   External variables influencing a client's illness behavior include the visibility of symptoms, social group, cultural background, economic variables, accessibility of the health care system, and social support. The visibility of the symptoms of an illness can affect body image and illness behavior. A client with a visible symptom may be more likely to seek assistance than a client without such a visible symptom.

Clients' social groups may assist them in recognizing the threat of illness or support the denial of potential illness. Families, friends, and coworkers all may influence clients' illness behavior. Clients often react positively to social support while practicing positive health behaviors. A person's cultural and ethnic background teaches the person how to be healthy, how to recognize illness, and how to be ill. The effects of disease and its interpretation vary according to cultural circumstances.

Economic variables influence the way a client reacts to illness. Because of economic constraints, a client may delay treatment and in many cases may continue to carry out daily activities. Clients' access to the health care system is closely related to economic factors. The health care system is a socioeconomic system that clients must enter, interact within, and exit. For many clients, entry into the system is complex or confusing, and some clients may seek nonemergency medical care in an emergency department because they do not know how otherwise to obtain health services. The physical proximity of clients to a health care agency often influences how soon they enter the system after deciding to seek care.

Impact of Illness on the Client and Family

Illness is never an isolated life event. The client and family must deal with changes resulting from illness and treatment. Each client responds uniquely to illness, and therefore nursing interventions must be individualized. The client and family commonly experience behavioral and emotional changes, as well as changes in roles, body image and self-concept, and family dynamics.

BEHAVIORAL AND EMOTIONAL CHANGES
People react differently to illness or the threat of illness. Individual behavioral and emotional reactions depend on the nature of the illness, the client's attitude toward it, the reaction of others to it, and the variables of illness behavior.

Short-term, non–life-threatening illnesses evoke few behavioral changes in the functioning of the client or family. A husband and father who has a cold, for example, may lack the energy and patience to spend time in family activities and may be irritable and prefer not to interact with his family. This is a behavioral change, but the change is subtle and does not last long. Some may even consider such a change a normal response to illness.

Severe illness, particularly one that is life threatening, can lead to more extensive emotional and behavioral changes, such as anxiety, shock, denial, anger, and withdrawal. These are common responses to the stress of illness. The nurse can develop interventions to assist the client and the family in coping with and adapting to this stress because the stressor itself cannot usually be changed.

IMPACT ON BODY IMAGE
Body image is the subjective concept of physical appearance (see Chapter 26). Some illnesses result in changes in physical appearance, and clients and families react differently to these changes. These reactions of clients and families to changes in body image depend on the following:

The type of changes (e.g., loss of a limb or an organ)
Their adaptive capacity
The rate at which changes take place
Support services available

When a change in body image occurs, such as results from a leg amputation, the client generally adjusts in the following phases: shock, withdrawal, acknowledgment, acceptance, and rehabilitation. Initially the client may be shocked by the change or impending change and may depersonalize it and talk about it as though it were happening to someone else. As the client and family recognize the reality of the change, they become anxious and may withdraw, refusing to discuss it. Withdrawal is an adaptive coping mechanism that can assist the client in making the adjustment. As the client and family acknowledge the change, they move through a period of grieving. At the end of the acknowledgment phase, they accept the loss. During rehabilitation the client is ready to learn how to adapt to the change in body image through use of a prosthesis or changing lifestyles and goals.

IMPACT ON SELF-CONCEPT
Self-concept is a mental self-image of strengths and weaknesses in all aspects of personality. Self-concept depends in part on body image and roles but also includes other aspects of psychology and spirituality (see Chapters 26 and 28). The impact of illness on the self-concepts of clients and family members may be more complex and less readily observed than role changes.

Self-concept is important in relationships with other family members. A client whose self-concept changes because of illness may no longer meet family expectations, leading to tension or conflict. As a result, family members may change their interactions with the client. In the course of providing care, a nurse is able to observe changes in the client's self-concept (or in the self-concepts of family members) and develop a care plan to help them adjust to the changes resulting from the illness.

IMPACT ON FAMILY ROLES
People have many roles in life, such as wage earner, decision maker, professional, child, sibling, or parent. When an

illness occurs, parents and children try to adapt to major changes resulting from a family member's illness. Role reversal is common (see Chapter 8). If a parent of an adult becomes ill and cannot carry out usual activities, the adult child often assumes many of the parent's responsibilities and in essence becomes a parent to the parent. Such a reversal of the usual situation can lead to stress, conflicting responsibilities for the adult child, or direct conflict over decision making.

Such a change may be subtle and short term or drastic and long term. An individual and family generally adjust more easily to subtle, short-term changes. In most cases they know that the role change is only temporary and will not require prolonged adjustment phases. Long-term changes, however, require an adjustment process similar to the grief process (see Chapter 29). The client and family often require specific counseling and guidance to assist them in coping with the role changes.

IMPACT ON FAMILY DYNAMICS

Because of the effects of illness on the client and family, family dynamics often change. Family dynamics is the process by which the family functions, makes decisions, gives support to individual members, and copes with everyday changes and challenges. If a parent in a family becomes ill, family activities and decision making often come to a halt as the other family members wait for the illness to pass, or they delay action because they are reluctant to assume the ill person's roles or responsibilities. Because of the effects of illness, family dynamics often change. The nurse must view the whole family as a client under stress, planning care to help the family regain the maximal level of functioning and well-being (see Chapter 8).

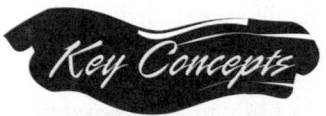

Key Concepts

- Health and wellness are not merely the absence of disease and illness.
- A person's state of health, wellness, or illness depends on individual values, personality, and lifestyle.
- According to the health-illness continuum model, health and illness are in a dynamic, relative relationship.
- The health belief model considers factors influencing health beliefs.
- The health promotion model increases individual well-being and self-actualization.
- Holistic health models of nursing promote optimal health by incorporating active participation of clients in improving their health state.
- Holistic nursing interventions can be used by nurses to augment standard medical therapy.
- Health beliefs and practices are influenced by internal and external variables and should be considered when planning care.
- Health promotion activities help maintain or enhance health.
- Wellness education teaches clients how to care for themselves.

- Illness prevention activities protect against health threats and thus maintain an optimal level of health.
- Nursing incorporates health promotion, wellness, and illness prevention activities rather than simply treating illness.
- The three levels of preventive care are primary, secondary, and tertiary.
- Risk factors threaten health, influence health practices, and are important considerations in illness prevention activities.
- Risk factors involve genetic or physiological variables, age, environment, and lifestyle.
- Improvement in health may involve a change in health behaviors.
- Illness behavior, like health practices, is influenced by many variables and must be considered by the nurse when planning care.
- Illness can have many effects on the client and family, including changes in behavior and emotions, family roles and dynamics, body image, and self-concept.

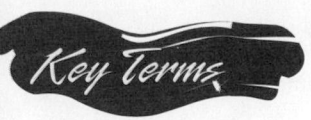

Key Terms

Critical Thinking Exercises

1. How would you describe your current state of health:
   excellent, good, fair, or poor? What definition of
   health did you use to make this judgment? List the
   current health promotion, wellness, and illness prevention activities that you regularly engage in. Are
   there any areas that need to be improved or changed?
   What will influence your ability to adopt any needed
   changes?

2. Assess the lifestyle patterns of someone you know.
   Identify risk factors that increase this person's vulnerability to illness or susceptibility to disease. Are there
   risk factors present that could be modified?

3. With this same individual, how could you approach
   the subject of risk factor modification? What influences exist that will assist the individual in making a
   change? What barriers exist that may prevent maintenance of a change in health behavior? What resources
   are available to you and to this individual that may assist in the change process?

4. Have you witnessed illness behavior of yourself or
   someone you know? Did you (or they) respond differently to an acute versus a chronic illness? Evaluate
   the different responses you remember. Explore how
   the various internal and external variables influenced
   your reactions and behaviors. Was there an impact on
   the individual's self-concept or on family roles and
   dynamics?

References

American Nurses Association: *Clinician's handbook of preventive services: put prevention into practice,* Washington, DC, 1994, The Association.

Anderson D: The spiritual wellness paradigm: a new approach for long-term care organizations, *Health Prog* 79(3):40, 1998.

Astin J: Why patients use alternative medicine: results of a national study, *JAMA* 279(19):1548, 1998.

Becker M, Maiman L: Sociobehavioral determinants of compliance with health and medical care recommendations, *Med Care* 33(1):1021, 1975.

Beckingham C: Relinquishing the sick role: convalescence and rehabilitation, *Aust J Adv Nurs* 12(3):15, 1995.

Benner P, Wrubel J: *The primacy of caring: stress and coping in health and illness,* Reading, Mass, 1989, Addison-Wesley.

Blackburn C: Low income, inequality and health promotion, *Nurs Times* 90(39):42, 1994

Clark M, Smith D: Abnormal illness behaviour in rehabilitation from stroke, *Clin Rehabil* (11):162, 1997.

Collins T: Models of health: pervasive, persuasive and politically charged, *Health Promot Int* 10(4):317, 1995.

Conn VS: A staged-based approach to helping people change health behaviors, *Clin Nurs Spec* 8(4):187, 1994.

Dimou N: Illness and culture: learning differences, *Patient Educ Couns* 26:153, 1995.

Edelman CL, Mandle CL: *Health promotion throughout the life span,* ed 4, St. Louis, 1998, Mosby.

Jensen L, Allen M: Wellness: the dialectic of illness, *Image J Nurs Sch* 25(3):220, 1993.

Leavell H, Clark A: *Preventive medicine for the doctor in his community,* ed 3, New York, 1965, McGraw-Hill.

Lipowski Z: Psychological reports of disease, *Ann Intern Med* 71:1197, 1969.

Lipowski Z: Psychosocial reactions to physical illness, *Can Med Assoc J* 128:1069, 1983.

Maise D, Fox C: Laying the foundation for Healthy People 2010, *Pub Health Rep* 113:92, 1998.

McCabe P: Exploring the phenomenon of healing: healing as a health capacity, *Aust J Holistic Nurs* 2(1):13, 1995.

McWilliam C and others: Creating health with chronic illness, *Adv Nurs Sci* 18(3):1, 1996.

Mechanic D: The epidemiology of illness behavior and its relationship to physical and psychological distress. In Mechanic D: *Symptoms, illness behavior, and help seeking,* New York, 1982, Prodist.

Mechanic D: Sociological dimensions of illness behavior, *Soc Sci Med* 41(9):1207, 1995.

Mornhinweg G, Voigner R: Holistic nursing interventions, *Orthop Nurs* 14(4):20, 1995.

Moss-Morris R, Paterson J: Understanding children's concepts of health and illness: implications for developmental therapists, *Phys Occup Ther Pediatr* 14(3/4):95, 1995.

Najman JM: Health and poverty: past, present and prospects for the future, *Soc Sci Med* 36(2):157, 1993.

Neuman B: Health as a continuum based on the Neuman systems model, *Nurs Sci Q* 3:129, 1990.

Northam S: Access to health promotion, protection, and disease prevention among impoverished individuals, *Pub Health Nurs* 13(5):353, 1996.

Pender NJ: *Health promotion and nursing practice,* Norwalk, Conn, 1982, AppletonCenturyCrofts.

Pender NJ: Health promotion and illness prevention. In Werley HH, Fitzpatrick JJ, editors: *Annual review of nursing research,* New York, 1993, Springer.

Pender NJ: *Health promotion and nursing practice,* ed 3, Stamford, Conn, 1996, Appleton & Lange.

Plawecki H: Holistic health interventions: the same difference, *J Gerontol Nurs* 23(11):44, 1997.

Prochaska JO: Assessing how people change, *Cancer* 67(3, suppl):805, 1991.

Prochaska JO, DiClemente CC: Stages of change in the modification of problem behaviors, *Prog Behav Modif* 28:184, 1992.

Rosenstoch I: Historical origin of the health belief model, *Health Educ Monogr* 2:334, 1974.

Ross L: The spiritual dimension: its importance to patients' health, well-being and quality of life and its implications for nursing practice, *Soc Sci Med* 32(5):457, 1995.

Schuster J: Wholistic care: healing a sick system, *Nurs Manage* 28(6):56, 1997.

Stubblefield C: Optimism: a determinant of health behavior, *Nurs Forum* 39(1):19, 1995.

U.S. Department of Health and Human Services, Public Health Service: *Healthy people 2000: national health promotion and disease prevention objectives,* Washington, DC, 1990, U.S. Government Printing Office.

U.S. Department of Health and Human Services, Public Health Service: *Healthy people 2010 objectives: draft for public comment,* Washington, DC, 1998, Office of Disease Prevention and Health Promotion.

World Health Organization Interim Commission: *Chronicle of WHO,* Geneva, 1947, The Organization.

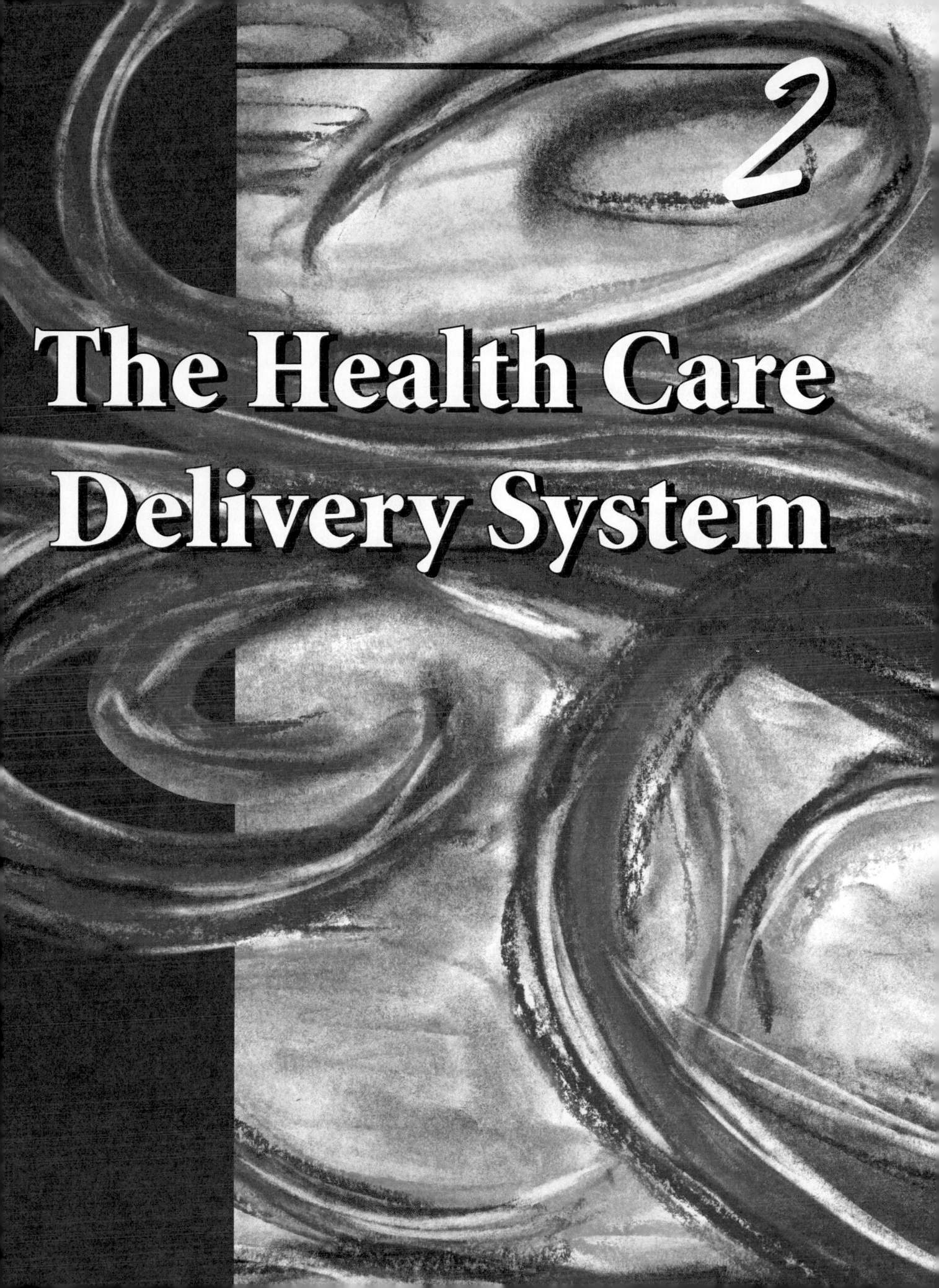

The Health Care Delivery System

2

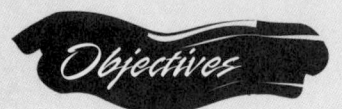
Objectives

Mastery of content in this chapter will enable the student to:

- Define the key terms listed.
- Discuss the effects that managed health care is having on the health care environment.
- Explain the rationale for regulatory and competitive approaches used to control health care costs.
- Discuss and compare the methods for financing health care.
- Describe the six levels of health care.
- Explain the relationship between levels of health care and levels of prevention.
- Discuss the role of nurses in different health care delivery settings.
- Explain why population-based care can ultimately improve quality of health care while lowering costs.
- Discuss the factors a professional nurse must consider when delegating tasks to assistive personnel.
- Describe the quality measures used to evaluate health care delivery performance.
- Explain the role nursing has in promoting client satisfaction.
- Discuss nursing's role within delivery of care.

The U.S. health care system has been experiencing constant change since the mid 1980s. Before that time, the cost of health care was a function of whatever resources were needed by physicians and other health care professionals to diagnose and treat a client's health problems. Hospitals were "cash cows," and insurance companies paid fee-for-service, full charges for any services. A client with health insurance had relatively easy access to almost any physician, including specialists, that he or she desired. Few limits were established for the utilization of resources in health care. However, with the costs of health care spiraling and no end in sight, employers (who pay employees' insurance), **third-party payers** (insurance groups), and the government began to search for new approaches that would reduce health care costs.

The United States has the best medical care system in the world, with the best-educated physicians and nurses and the most sophisticated hospitals (Grace, 1997). Health care is provided in diverse settings, offering every technological advance. The quality of health care has been undisputed. However, problems exist. Access to health care services is an issue, particularly for the underinsured and those who have restrictions imposed by their managed care organizations. Continuity of services does not exist in all organizations. As a client moves from one physician or service to another, little information is passed on about the client's needs or planned treatment. The question being asked is, how can health care in the United States be financed so that health care services are produced efficiently, costs are effectively controlled, and quality is maintained or improved? In response to the cost issue, there have been hospital and health system mergers, closure of costly health care facilities, merging of allied health support services, and changes in the way care is delivered

to clients at the bedside. In the center of this controversy lies nursing.

Nursing is a caring discipline. The values of our profession are rooted in helping individuals to regain, maintain, or improve their health, prevent illness, find comfort, and retain their individuality and dignity. The health care system of the new millennium has become less service oriented and significantly more business oriented in light of cost-saving initiatives. As a result, the practice of nursing is changing. In the face of rapid change, nursing must lead the way and retain its values for client care while meeting the challenges of new roles and new responsibilities in the health care environment. To become leaders in health care, nurses must understand the health care system and the issues that affect how care is provided to clients and their families.

Health Care Regulation and Competition

In the United States, total health expenditures grew from $41.9 billion in 1965 to $425 billion in 1985 (Grace, 1997). This occurred in an environment where there were no incentives to control use of inappropriate diagnostic tests or treatments. Whatever physicians chose to order for a client's care and treatment, insurers paid for. This was the case even if treatments were not medically sound. Rising costs were also due to an aging population, increased numbers of people who were not part of the workforce, and increasing costs of insurance to employers (Garg and others, 1997). As a result, both regulatory and competitive approaches have been used in an attempt to control health care spending.

Examples of regulatory or government interventions are certificates of need, professional standards review organizations, and prospective payment systems. Certificates of need (CONs) aim to control the structure of health care by limiting the development of hospital capacity (Garg and others, 1997). The National Health Planning and Resources Development Act of 1974 required every state to have a CON law to review plans by health care institutions for any building expenses over $150,000 or any change in beds or services. The concept is designed to prevent hospitals in a community from having all of the same services. Its influence on cost control has been minimal, since most review boards have approved all proposals presented to them.

Professional standards review organizations (PSROs) were created to review the quality, quantity, and cost of hospital care provided through **Medicare** (Garg and others, 1997). Medicare-qualified hospitals were required to have utilization review (UR) committees supervised by physicians. The committees reviewed admissions, diagnostic testing, and therapeutic interventions provided by physicians to hospitalized Medicare clients in an effort to identify unnecessary costs of care. If a given physician was overutilizing diagnostic testing unnecessarily, the UR committee might submit a warning or recommendation. There is debate as to whether the program has reduced costs or whether the cost of the program exceeded any savings.

The **prospective payment** system (PPS), established by Congress in 1983, eliminated cost-based reimbursement. Hospitals serving Medicare clients were no longer paid for costs of services. Instead, inpatient hospital services for Medicare clients were bundled into 468 **diagnosis-related groups (DRGs)**.

Each group has a fixed reimbursement amount with adjustments for case severity, rural/urban/regional labor costs, and teaching costs (Box 2-1). Hospitals are reimbursed a set dollar amount for each DRG, regardless of the client's length of stay or use of services in the hospital. The PPS has a major effect in making hospitals realize that cost control is serious. In fact, many hospitals were forced to close because their overhead was higher than the volume of procedures. When clients were hospitalized for lengthy periods, hospitals were forced to absorb the portion of costs not reimbursed. Soon after DRGs were implemented, hospitals began to increase discharge planning activities, and hospital lengths of stay began to shorten. During the first 3 years of the PPS, inflation in hospital expenses was reduced (Garg and others, 1997).

Competitive approaches to contain health care costs have supplemented and in some cases replaced regulatory approaches. Competition in economic terms means rivalry between sellers of comparable goods for customers (Garg and others, 1997). In other words, hospital systems compete with one another so that customers (insurers, employers, and clients) will choose the health care services

---

Clinical Scenario of a DRG Example   Box 2-1

Mr. Truman was admitted to the hospital on November 1 after experiencing chest pain and shortness of breath. He had undergone cardiac surgery almost 10 years before but was beginning to have recurrent chest pain, even at rest. He was scheduled for a cardiac catheterization, but it was delayed until November 3. The physician also referred Mr. Truman for diet counseling for a low-cholesterol diet. The cardiac catheterization proceeded without complications, and surgery was unnecessary. Mr. Truman remained hospitalized overnight to ensure that no problems developed. He was discharged on November 4.

Principal diagnosis: Heart ischemia

Secondary diagnosis: Disturbances of heart, functional, long-term effect of cardiac surgery

DRG assigned: DRG 125: circulatory disorders except acute myocardial infarction with cardiac catheterization without complex diagnosis

Assigned or allowed length of stay: 2.2 days

Actual length of stay: 3.1 days

Payment calculation (based on 2.2 days): Payment per discharge × DRG weight = $3400 × 0.7015 = $2385

Actual hospital costs for Mr. Truman: $2960

Loss for hospital: $575

---

that cost less, assuming that quality is not sacrificed. The market encourages hospitals and other health care institutions to keep their prices down. Two common competitive approaches have been managed care, or **health maintenance, organizations (MCOs, HMOs)** and **preferred provider organizations (PPOs)**.

Under **managed care**, payment is prospective and capitated. The provider or health care system receives a predetermined, fixed amount of payment for each client enrolled in the program. In this case the MCO becomes a financial risk bearer, as well as client care provider (Garg and others, 1997). The organization's focus of care shifts from individual illness care to concern for the health of its covered population. If people stay healthy, the cost of medical care declines. Systems of managed care focus on three values: the capacity to contain or reduce costs, the ability to increase client satisfaction, and the ability to improve the health or functional status of the individual (Pew Health Professions Commission, 1995). A managed care program has the health care needs of its clients funneled through a gatekeeper/case management function. Clients must see their **primary care** provider (e.g., medical internist, family practitioner, pediatrician), who coordinates all care and limits access to costly medical specialists and hospitalization. Nurse practitioners and physician assistants are often integrated into the role of gatekeeper in managing select client populations. The managed care system is having an impact on the numbers of clients hospitalized. Clearly, there is a shift from inpatient to outpatient care. Only the acutely ill or those in need of major surgery are being admitted to hospitals. Once they are admitted, plans begin immediately for their discharge home or to other facilities.

Third-party payers contract selectively with hospitals and physician groups in providing medical care to their covered population. Typically, a payer identifies a subset of hospitals and physicians to be "preferred providers" on the basis of a predetermined rate of reimbursement (Garg and others, 1997). The payer then directs clients to those hospitals and physicians through financial incentives such as lower co-payments and deductibles. It is to the physicians' and hospitals' advantage to control costs and provide quality service so as to retain preferred provider referrals.

NURSING IMPLICATIONS

Health care organizations are influenced daily by both regulatory and competitive approaches to control costs and maintain quality health care services. These pressures alter the amount and the way that organizations are paid for producing health care services, directly affecting employers' demand for nurses and transforming the economic environment in which nurses work (Buerhaus, 1997). Nursing is vulnerable, since it typically makes up a large percentage of a health care institution's labor budget. It is easy for an organization to change the care delivery model and hire fewer nurses, with the idea that costs will be reduced with minimal sacrifice to quality. However, recent nursing research has shown that when the proportion of hours of care delivered on a patient care unit by registered professional nurses (RNs) is reduced, there are adverse client outcomes (Blegen and others, 1998). Nursing units with a lower proportion of hours of care delivered by RNs saw greater negative outcomes (e.g., medication errors, pressure sore rates, and client complaints). Organizations must carefully judge whether client care is jeopardized when RNs are replaced by assistive personnel.

Despite the threats posed to nursing, the profession has the talent, knowledge, and initiative to make a significant difference in health care. In the eyes of a health care employer, the most valuable employees will be those who contribute the most to the organization's ability to survive in a competitive and rapidly changing financial environment (Buerhaus, 1997). For example, nursing has already made valuable contributions in developing ways to provide cost-effective outpatient care, reducing unnecessary hospitalizations. Nurse practitioners (see Chapter 19) are being hired by many MCOs to manage the care of select client populations, partnering with physicians and thus reducing the labor costs within physicians' offices. Finally, nurses are in key positions to critically examine their practice and discover new ways to deliver care that are cost-effective while guaranteeing excellent quality to clients. Nursing research (see Chapter 25) is one avenue that gives nurses the innovations needed to improve client care.

Financing Health Care

With MCOs leading the way, health care financing is more complicated. It is not necessary for each nurse to become a financial expert. However, it is important for nurses to understand the basics of health care financing so that they can recognize how professional employers and clients are affected. Table 2-1 summarizes health plans most common in the health care environment.

PAYMENT MECHANISMS

In addition to the various health care plans clients acquire to cover health care costs, there are payment mechanisms nurses should understand. The type of payment mechanism that an organization chiefly relies on will affect its cost-control approaches.

Capitation.   **Capitation** is a payment mechanism in which a provider (e.g., health care network or managed care organization) receives a fixed amount per client (e.g., enrollee) (Appleby, 1996). The aim of capitation is to build a payment plan for select diagnoses or surgical procedures that includes the best standards of care, including essential diagnostic and treatment procedures at the lowest cost. For example, if heart surgery is to be capitated, the health care plan will develop practice protocols for common medical services (e.g., pharmaceuticals, diagnostic tests, and surgical treatment). The protocols will ensure thoroughness and a measure of consistency in the way physicians, covered by the capitated plan, deliver care. The plan will also decide what tests and procedures will and will not be included in the primary care physician's portion of the capitated rate. Capitation may be global or partial (Grimaldi, 1995). A global payment covers inpatient, physician, and other outpatient services ordinarily covered by conventional insurance. Certain services may not be covered. Partial-capitation payment applies to subsets of services, such as all necessary hospital inpatient acute care services, physician services, and infusion therapy.

Under capitation the role of specialists and hospitals is defined so that each provider receives a "piece of the pie." Therefore it does a hospital no good to bill for additional services in an attempt to increase revenue. Payment is capped. No additional monies are available if the client's care requires more than what is typically included in the capitated rate. The risk of capitation is that clients may receive less care than might be optimal, particularly if standards of care change. However, the aim is to establish payment on strong clinical standards. If physicians involved in a capitated plan do not have input in developing the guidelines for payment, serious problems can arise. Tests or procedures deemed necessary by physicians might not be included in the guidelines if financial advisors are the ones who recommend clinical standards. Subspecialty care is so tightly controlled that clients may be unable to access new and innovative treatment approaches. In that case,

Table 2-1   Health Care Plans

Type	Definition	Characteristics
Managed care organization (MCO)	Provides comprehensive, preventive, and treatment services to a specific group of voluntarily enrolled persons. Structures include a variety of models: *Staff model:* Physicians are salaried employees of the MCO. *Group model:* MCO contracts with single group practice. *Network model:* MCO contracts with multiple group practices and/or integrated organizations. **Independent practice association (IPA):** MCO contracts with physicians who usually are not members of groups and whose practices include fee-for-service and capitated clients.	Focus on health maintenance, primary care. All care provided by a primary care physician. Referral needed for access to specialists and hospitalization.
Medicare MCO	Program same as MCO but designed to cover health care costs of senior citizens.	Premium generally less than supplemental plans.
Preferred provider organization (PPO)	One that limits an enrollee's choice to a list of "preferred" hospitals, physicians, and providers. An enrollee pays more out-of-pocket expenses for using a provider not on the list.	Contractual agreement exists between a set of providers and one or more purchasers (self-insured employers or insurance plans). Comprehensive health services at a discount to companies under contract. Focus on health maintenance.
Exclusive provider organization (EPO)	One that limits an enrollee's choice to providers belonging to one organization. May or may not be able to use outside providers at additional expense.	Limited contractual agreement. Less access to select specialists.
Medicare	Federally funded national health insurance program in the United States for people over age 65. Part A provides basic protection for medical, surgical, and psychiatric care costs based on diagnosis-related groups (DRGs). Part B is a voluntary medical insurance; covers physician and certain outpatient services.	Payment for plan deducted from monthly individual Social Security check. Covers services of nurse practitioners. Does not pay full cost of certain services. Supplemental insurance is encouraged.
Medicaid	Federally funded, state-operated program of medical assistance to people with low incomes. Individual states determine eligibility and benefits.	Finances a large portion of maternal and child care for the poor. Reimburses for nurse midwifery and other advanced practice nurses (varies by state). Reimburses nursing home funding.
Private insurance	Traditional fee-for-service plan. Payment computed after services are provided on basis of number of services used.	Policies typically expensive. Most policies have deductibles that clients must meet before insurance pays.
Long-term care insurance	Supplemental insurance for coverage of long-term care services. Policies provide a set amount of dollars for an unlimited time or for as little as 2 years.	Very expensive. Good policy has a minimum waiting period for eligibility, payment for skilled nursing, intermediate or custodial care, and home care.

clients clearly might not receive necessary services, and quality of care is threatened.

Fee-for-Diagnosis Framework.   Medicare and other prospective payment plans use fee-for-diagnosis billing. A health care organization receives a fixed dollar amount for the treatment of an episode of illness. The amount of a fee is calculated on the basis of the client's principal medical diagnosis, secondary diagnoses, age and gender, and the usual treatment appropriate for the client's health problem. DRGs are an example of a fee-for-diagnosis framework.

Fixed Payment.   Most reimbursement through MCOs occurs through a fixed payment system. The program provides comprehensive preventive and treatment services to a specific group of voluntary enrolled persons under a fixed, prepaid plan. Clients of an MCO, for example, make periodic payments in advance for expected costs of benefits. The MCO's promise to deliver specifically defined services within a fixed, prepaid system offers providers (e.g., hospital or physician group) an incentive to contain costs and unnecessary use of services. Providers receive a fixed payment based on an individual client's medical condition or surgical procedure. The formulas are similar to those seen in Medicare DRG payments. Typically, an acute care payment is based on the anticipated number of days required for treatment of a specific condition or surgical procedure. Home health reimbursement is often based on the number of required visits.

Direct Contracting.   Employers, looking for ways to reduce health care costs, contract directly with providers at a package price for all needed care and services and agree to work cooperatively on improving efficiency and outcomes. Contracting may be established with selected health care systems anywhere in the country. The key is managing high-cost cases like organ transplantation or respiratory failure. Employees have more choices in selecting a contracting physician, since the company usually contracts with a wide variety of physicians and hospitals who have established evidence of excellent clinical care.

Levels of Health Care

The health care industry is moving toward health care practices that emphasize managing health rather than managing illness. The progress is slow because the delivery system has been illness oriented, with services being fragmented and episodic instead of well coordinated over the length of a client's illness or health problem. A wellness perspective places focus on the health of populations rather than just that of individuals (see Chapter 3). With this new perspective, health care systems are moving toward **integrated delivery networks (IDNs).** An IDN is a

set of providers organized to deliver a coordinated continuum of care to an enrolled population in return for capitated payment. This integrated system can reduce duplication of services, coordinate care across settings, and ensure that clients receive care in the most appropriate and cost-effective settings (Curran, 1997).

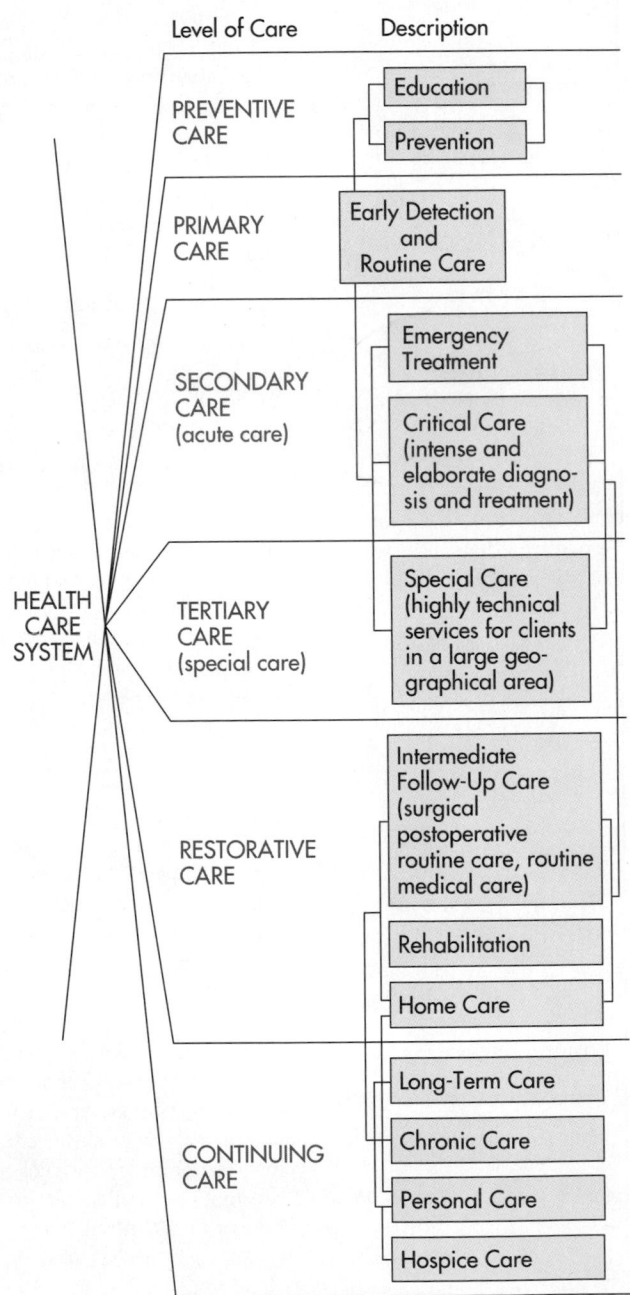

Figure 2-1   Spectrum of health services delivery. Modified from Cambridge Research Institute: *Trends affecting the U.S. health care system*, 262, Health Planning Information Series, Human Resources Administration, Public Health Service, Department of Health, Education, and Welfare, Washington, DC; 1976, revised and updated 1992, U.S. Government Printing Office.

The health care system provides six levels of care (Figure 2-1). Levels of care describe the scope of services and settings where health care is offered to clients in all stages of health and illness. For example, the secondary level of care is the traditional acute care setting where clients who present signs and symptoms of disease are diagnosed and treated. The restorative care level includes those settings and services where clients who are recovering from illness or disability receive rehabilitation and supportive care. Levels of care are not the same as levels of prevention (see Chapter 1). Levels of prevention instead describe the focus of health-related activities: avoiding disease (health promotion and disease prevention [primary prevention]), curing disease (secondary prevention), and diminishing complications (tertiary prevention). At any level of care (e.g., primary or tertiary), nurses and other health care providers might offer a variety of levels of prevention. The nurse working in an acute care hospital setting, for example, might monitor the recovery of a client following open heart surgery, while also providing health promotion information to the family concerning diet and exercise.

It is important to understand how levels of care are organized and delivered. Each level creates different requirements and opportunities for the nurse. In addition, changes unique to each level of care have developed as a result of health care reform. There is greater emphasis being placed on the importance of wellness and primary and preventive care. More resources are being dedicated to these levels of care, particularly health promotion. Nursing has the chance to provide leadership to communities and health care systems that are aligning resources to better serve their populations. Critical to the success of improving health care delivery will be the ability to find strategies that better address client needs at all levels of care.

A broad variety of health care services (Box 2-2) are available to clients and families, depending on the nature and extent of a health problem and the level of care required. The types of services offered also depend on the site in which clients seek health care.

PREVENTIVE AND PRIMARY CARE SERVICES

Primary care has been defined by the Institute of Medicine (1994) as the "provision of integrated, accessible health care services by clinicians who are accountable for addressing a large majority of personal health services, developing a sustained partnership with clients, and practicing in the context of family and community." The emphasis is on personal health services. More and more in settings where primary care and preventive care are delivered, health promotion is a major theme. Health promotion services are a key to quality health care. Successful programs are designed to help clients acquire healthier lifestyles and achieve a decent standard of living (see Chapter 1). Health promotion programs can lower the overall costs of health care by reducing the incidence of

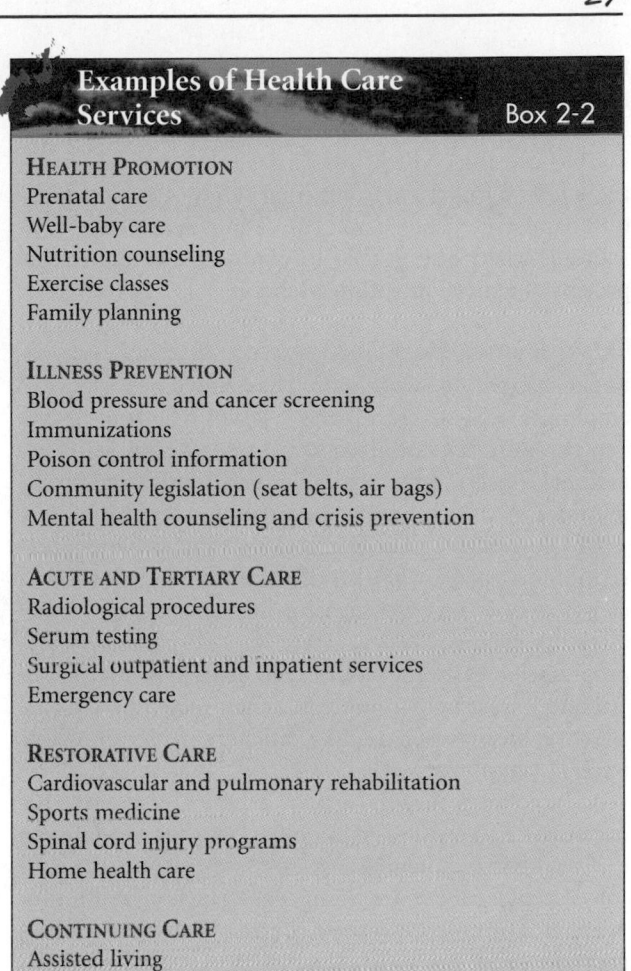

Examples of Health Care Services   Box 2-2

HEALTH PROMOTION
Prenatal care
Well-baby care
Nutrition counseling
Exercise classes
Family planning

ILLNESS PREVENTION
Blood pressure and cancer screening
Immunizations
Poison control information
Community legislation (seat belts, air bags)
Mental health counseling and crisis prevention

ACUTE AND TERTIARY CARE
Radiological procedures
Serum testing
Surgical outpatient and inpatient services
Emergency care

RESTORATIVE CARE
Cardiovascular and pulmonary rehabilitation
Sports medicine
Spinal cord injury programs
Home health care

CONTINUING CARE
Assisted living
Psychiatric day care

disease, minimizing complications, and thus reducing the need to use more expensive health care resources. Preventive care is more disease oriented and focused on reducing and controlling risk factors for disease through activities such as immunization and occupational health programs.

School Health Services. Often we think of school health services as the school nurse sitting in an office and offering first aid and symptom management to children who become ill during class sessions. In actuality, effective school health services are comprehensive programs that integrate health promotion principles throughout a school's curriculum. School health services protect and promote the health of all students and school personnel. School health nurses are specialized in school nursing practice. The American Nurses Association (ANA) (1983) published *Standards of School Nursing Practice*, which addresses issues such as program management, interdisciplinary collaboration, and community health systems. The school nurse develops programs that foster children's growth, positive life skills for successful coping, and acquisition of knowledge and skills for self-care, and that reinforce positive health attitudes (Pender, 1996). Specific nursing interventions in the school setting include health education, parent programming and counseling, communicable disease control, physical assessment, screening, crisis intervention, environmental safety, nutrition planning, and emergency care. The school nurse role is rewarding when one is able to contribute to the overall process of education within a school.

Occupational Health Services. Recently, occupational health in the work setting has gained importance as employers seek to reduce the costs of health insurance benefits for injured or ill workers. Occupational health is a national concern, affecting individuals, families, and communities. A comprehensive occupational health program geared to health promotion and accident or illness prevention can increase worker productivity, decrease absenteeism, reduce use of expensive medical care, and lower disability claims (Pender, 1996). An occupational health program increases the health-enhancing potential of social and physical environments. When such programs are effective, businesses have little difficulty in recruiting and retaining employees.

Occupational health nurses conduct environmental surveillance (hazardous equipment, injuries occurring in the workplace, potential stressors), direct nursing care (physical assessment, screening, emergencies), health education, communicable disease control, counseling, administration, and research (Clemen-Stone, McGuire, and Eigsti, 1998). Recurring issues that nurses face in the work site are drug testing, right-to-know issues, concerns related to acquired immunodeficiency syndrome (AIDS), and exposure to environmental hazards. One of the nurse's roles is to help ensure that workers who have been injured are recovered and able to return to the work site safely. Some businesses try to reintroduce employees back into the workforce as soon as possible following illness or injury, even if they assume a different job temporarily. The nurse can help to optimize the work experience by creating programs that involve workers in health promotion and in creating a safe work environment.

Physicians' Offices. Physicians' offices have traditionally provided primary care for most of the population. Physicians in office practices tend to focus on the diagnosis and treatment of specific illnesses rather than on health promotion. However, this trend is slowly changing. More health care plans are requiring enrollees to have regular physical examinations, or checkups, with their primary care physician. During these visits physicians and nurse practitioners screen for possible health problems, identify clients' health promotion practices, and make recommendations to minimize or control risk factors. The addition of advanced practice nurses to physicians' offices looks beyond diagnosis and treatment to the holistic needs of clients. The advanced practitioner's time spent with a client addresses education, counseling, and community referrals (see Chapter 19).

RNs are often employed in physicians' offices to assume the role of office or practice manager. This includes supervision of secretarial and medical assistant staff and medical record personnel. The office manager is a problem solver who helps with referral questions, managing the flow of clients through the office, and dealing with physician concerns. The nurse can also be an important bridge to the physician in becoming closely familiar with their population of clients, in identifying trends in the types of problems clients present, and in recognizing opportunities to increase health promotion activities.

Clinics. Clinics that assess and treat ambulatory clients on an outpatient basis are often called ambulatory health services. A clinic may be affiliated with a hospital, medical school, group practice, MCO, church, or community organization (Clemen-Stone, McGuire, and Eigsti, 1998). The nature of the clinic affiliation often determines the type of services the clinic provides. For example, hospital clinics offer diagnostic and treatment services. A clinic in a community organization may offer primary care such as immunizations or screening services (e.g., high blood pressure, tuberculosis, and glaucoma testing). There are also clinics that offer comprehensive care to specific client populations (e.g., well-baby, mental health, and allergy clinics). Hospital emergency departments often serve as ambulatory clinics for neighborhoods or towns with no formal outpatient clinic facility or primary care physicians. Emergency departments can also serve as "fast track" clinics to refer clients to primary care providers who accept new clients. This ensures that clients develop relationships with a stable and consistent physician rather than relying on episodical emergency care.

Community health nurses play an important role in planning and providing clinic health care services. A comprehensive assessment of community needs is critical to ensure that clinic programs address the health status, lifestyle patterns, and cultural diversity of its clients. Often a neighborhood clinic becomes a focal point for a community. The successful clinic recognizes the work and lifestyle patterns of its clients and establishes a strong network of relationships with churches, schools, and businesses. Those networks become important for clients' continued care following hospitalization.

Nursing Centers. Nurse-managed clinics, or community nursing centers, have developed over the past 20 years to provide high-quality nursing services with a focus on health promotion and health education, disease prevention, chronic disease management, and support for self-care and caregivers (Riesch, 1992; Barger and Rosenfeld, 1993). Nurses control practice and client care in nursing centers. Typically, nursing centers serve vulnerable populations such as minority and ethnic groups of low-income status, the elderly, and the disabled. Riesch (1992) identified three criteria for nursing centers: direct access by the client to the nurse, a nursing model of care, and holistic reimbursed services. Nurses in advanced practice roles, such as nurse practitioners and clinical nurse specialists, typically manage the nursing center. However, public health nurses are also actively involved. The public health nurse's chief concern is the health of the community. Community health problems related to family dysfunction, illegal drug use, violent crimes, and poverty will have a direct effect on clients using the nursing center.

Many of the centers operate in association with academic centers to combine teaching and research in a nurse-controlled environment (Phillips and Steel, 1994; Zachariah and Lundeen, 1997). The clinics maintain a collaborative and consultative relationship with physicians. This is necessary in most states to guarantee reimbursement for nursing services. The services offered in a nurse-managed clinic are varied (Box 2-3). It is how the services are delivered that makes a nurse-managed clinic unique. The nurse in an advanced practice role combines nursing and medical knowledge within a perspective of client-centered care (Phillips and Steel, 1994). The advanced practice nurse stresses education and self-care. Clients with chronic illness are taught to partner with family members or friends to do the work of managing their illness. The public health nurse works to improve the conditions within the home and the community. A nurse-managed clinic designs services to help people assume more responsibility for their health and to acquire necessary coping skills. Scott and Moneyham (1995) learned that the design of the services and actions of the nurses in a nursing center supported clients' need for respect, which helped to build the necessary confidence needed for self-care. Over the long term, advanced practice nurses are very effective in improving client outcomes by enabling clients to maintain maximal function within their home and community.

Block and Parish Nursing. Two nontraditional settings where preventive and primary care can be found are in block and parish nursing. Both fill in gaps of the formal health care system, usually with older clients or those unable to leave the home (Clemen-Stone, McGuire, and Eigsti, 1998). **Block nursing** happens where the nurse lives, and services are available based on need rather than on the availability of reimbursement (Jamieson, 1990). Nurses who live within a neighborhood, through networks of friends, church groups, Girl Scouts, or Boy Scouts, collaborate to offer services to people in the community. These services might include running errands to the grocery store or pharmacy, transporting clients to a physician's office, providing respite care to family members, and being homemaker aides. Parish nursing is the same as block nursing, except churches and synagogues offer the site and support system for the program's activities.

Volunteer Agencies. **Volunteer agencies** are not-for-profit health care agencies established nationally or within a community to meet a specific need. Examples are the American Lung Association and the Alzheimer Association and, in Canada, the Canadian Lung Association and the Canadian Heart Foundation. Most volunteer agencies do not provide treatment but have programs designed to provide education for the prevention and detection of specific illnesses. In addition, some volunteer agencies provide financial support for training of physicians and nurses, as well as for biomedical research directed at the prevention, detection, or treatment of certain diseases. Many volunteer agencies are staffed in part by professional nurses, while at the same time many health professionals donate time and resources to agencies within their specialty.

Primary Health Care in the Community. Primary care focuses on personal health services. In contrast, **primary health care** is an approach for building interventions that lead to improved health outcomes for an entire population (Shoultz and Hatcher, 1997). The primary health care model (Figure 2-2, p. 30) focuses on collaboration of health professionals, community members, and others working in multiple sectors, emphasizing health promotion, development of health policies, and prevention of diseases for all individuals. A closer look at each sector finds that they are all linked and that events within each sector have an impact, either positive or negative, on each other and on the outcome of the population's health (Hatcher and others, 1994). For example, the health problems that commonly affect members of a lower socioeconomic level can often be traced to poor community services (e.g., water treatment, waste disposal, air quality, and transportation services). A primary health care approach requires a multisectoral approach by addressing many of the determinants of health (Shoultz and Hatcher, 1997).

Nurse-Managed Clinic Services   Box 2-3

Day care
Recreation
Physical and developmental assessment
Health risk appraisal
Wellness counseling
Health education
Youth and family support services
Employment readiness
Psychosocial counseling
Care and prevention of common diseases
Acute and chronic care management
Home care services

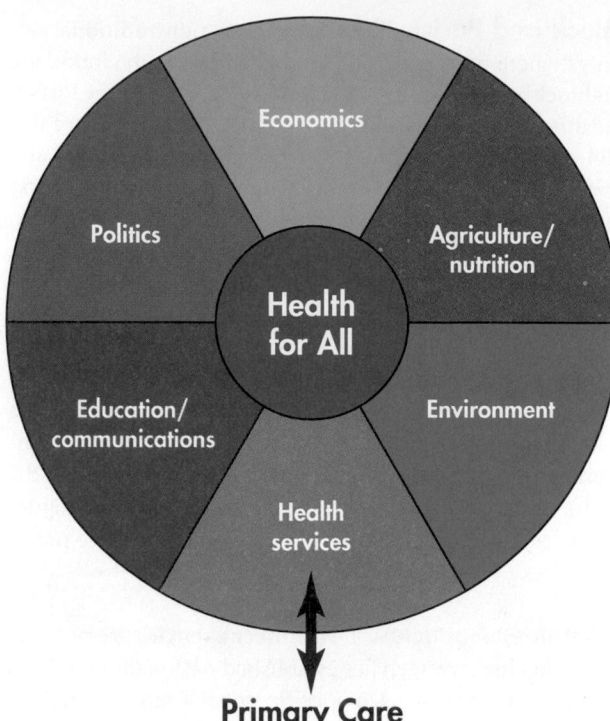

Primary Care

Figure 2-2 Primary health care model: a multisectoral or intersectoral approach.
Copyright 1996 by Hatcher P, Shoultz J, Patrick W.

Primary care is a key component of the primary health care model. However, primary health care looks beyond primary care, with essential elements that include health education, proper nutrition, maternal/child health care, family planning, immunizations, and control of locally endemic diseases. Chapter 3 provides a more comprehensive discussion of primary health care in the community.

Secondary and Tertiary Care

Diagnostic and treatment services are generally the most commonly used services of the health care delivery system. With the arrival of managed care, these services are being delivered in primary care settings. For example, more physicians are performing simple surgeries in office surgical suites. However, once a client develops a more complicated problem and the primary care provider is not able to care for a particular condition, a medical specialist is needed. This often requires hospitalization of the client.

Hospitals. Hospital emergency departments and urgent care centers, critical care units, and inpatient medical-surgical units are the sites where secondary and tertiary levels of care are provided. In these settings nurses work closely with all members of the health care team to plan, coordinate, and deliver care for clients who are seriously ill. Nurses must constantly monitor and evaluate whether care is effective and how it can be improved.

Nurses are also recognizing that in a busy, stress-filled location such as an inpatient nursing unit, client satisfaction is a priority. Clients are more educated than ever before and have higher expectations of services in a competitive environment. Acute care nurses must respond to client needs and expectations so as to form effective care partnerships.

With the arrival of prospective payment and managed care, a hospitalized client with a given medical diagnosis or who undergoes surgery is expected to be cared for and discharged within a projected time period. Emphasis is on efficiency and the use of only those resources that are necessary to adequately care for the client until discharge. Case management (see p. 41) is one approach to coordinating a client's care throughout the hospital stay. The multidisciplinary team approach ensures that the client has a well-designed discharge plan. In some institutions diagnostic and treatment services have been redesigned to be more efficiently delivered on nursing units. Services such as x-ray and laboratory services are often available on nursing units, thus minimizing the need to transfer and transport clients across multiple diagnostic and treatment areas. Another approach is the introduction of multiskilled workers who are able to perform the services (e.g., phlebotomy, x-ray, electrocardiographic [ECG]) once delivered by several different staff members. Customer service is the philosophy of acute care organizations.

Perhaps one of the biggest influences on hospital nursing is client acuity. Hospitalized clients are very ill and in need of comprehensive and specialized tertiary health care. Clients may still be relatively ill when discharged. Therefore nurses rarely see clients who have gained complete symptom relief or who are not requiring some level of intense intervention. The care of hospitalized clients requires the nurse to have the knowledge and skills for using critical thinking and applying the nursing process (see Unit 3). This requires the nurse to have contact with clients on an ongoing basis and to be able to recognize changes in their clinical condition. When working with assistive personnel (see p. 38), it is important for nurses to recognize their priority in client assessment and clinical decision making.

The services provided by hospitals vary considerably. Small rural hospitals may only offer limited emergency and diagnostic services, as well as general inpatient services. In comparison, large urban medical centers offer comprehensive, state-of-the-art diagnostic services, trauma and emergency care, surgical intervention, intensive care units, inpatient services, and rehabilitation facilities. Larger hospitals also offer professional staff from a variety of specialties such as social service, respiratory therapy, physical and occupational therapy, and speech therapy. The focus in hospitals is to provide the highest quality of care possible so that clients can be discharged early, but safely, to the home or a facility that can adequately manage remaining health care needs.

Hospitals are classified as public or private and as for-profit or not-for-profit institutions. Public hospitals are not-for-profit institutions that exist throughout Canada and the United States. A public hospital is financed and operated by a government agency at the local, state, provincial, or national level. Many clients in public hospitals either cannot afford to pay for care or are underinsured. Private hospitals may be for-profit or not-for-profit institutions and are operated by groups such as churches, corporations or businesses, or charitable organizations. Many hospitals have merged to form large hospital system networks. The majority of clients who enter private hospitals have some type of personal health insurance or health care plan, including Medicare or **Medicaid.** The profit status of a hospital influences how revenue can be used for services and taxation purposes.

A nurse who works within a hospital has the opportunity to work in a variety of roles and different departments (see Chapter 19). Staff nurses provide comprehensive nursing and medical therapies, educate clients and families, facilitate family support, and coordinate health care services and discharge planning. As the depth of nursing knowledge increases, many nurses specialize in their practice. This allows them to become expert in the care of select client populations (e.g., oncology or pulmonary). Other opportunities for nurses within a hospital setting may include the role of client educator, nurse manager, clinical nurse specialist, and infection-control coordinator.

Intensive Care.

An intensive care unit (ICU) or critical care unit is a hospital unit in which clients receive close monitoring and intensive medical care. The units are equipped with the most advanced technologies, such as computerized cardiac monitors, mechanical ventilators, and blood perfusion devices. Although many of these devices can be found on regular nursing units, the clients hospitalized within ICUs are being monitored and maintained on multiple devices at the same time. Nursing and medical staff within an ICU are educated on critical care principles and techniques. It is the most expensive delivery site for medical care because of the staffing pattern required to deliver care and the related volume of treatments and procedures the clients must undergo.

Subacute Care.

Subacute care units are designated sites that provide medical specialty care for clients who need a greater intensity of care than is generally provided in a skilled nursing facility but who no longer require acute care (Stahl, 1994). Subacute care units are located in hospitals, skilled nursing facilities, and rehabilitation facilities. Generally, clients who have suffered an acute illness, injury, or worsening of a chronic disease and who require continued hospitalization are candidates for subacute care. Typical clients seen on subacute care units include those being rehabilitated following cerebrovascular accidents, trauma, and respiratory failure. The clients require

a transitional phase of stabilization and often still have intensive medical, social, and familial needs. Clients receive goal-oriented treatment given immediately after or instead of acute care hospitalization to treat one or more specific, active, complex medical conditions or to administer technically complex treatments (Stahl, 1994). Many of the clients who require subacute care are **outliers** (clients with extended lengths of stay, well beyond the allowed inpatient DRG days). Thus a hospital can transfer a client to a subacute care unit and reduce its financial burden, since the stay on the unit meets different reimbursement guidelines. However, recent changes in reimbursement are causing many hospitals to reevaluate this type of in-hospital unit.

Psychiatric Facilities.

Clients who suffer emotional and behavioral problems such as depression, violent behavior, and eating disorders often require special counseling and treatment in psychiatric facilities. Located in hospitals, independent outpatient clinics, or private mental health hospitals, psychiatric facilities offer inpatient and outpatient services, depending on the seriousness of the problem. Clients may enter these facilities voluntarily or involuntarily. Hospitalization involves relatively short stays for stabilizing clients and then transferring them to outpatient treatment centers. A comprehensive multidisciplinary treatment plan involving clients and families is established for clients with psychiatric illness. Medicine, nursing, social work, and activity therapy collaborate to develop a plan of care that will enable clients to return to functional states within the community. At discharge from inpatient facilities, clients are usually referred for follow-up care at clinics or with counselors.

Rural Hospitals.

Access to health care in rural areas has been a serious problem. Most rural hospitals have had a severe shortage of primary care providers. Many have been forced to close because of economic failure. In 1989 the Omnibus Budget Reconciliation Act (OBRA) directed the Department of Health and Human Services to create a new health care entity, the rural primary care hospital (RPCH). An RPCH provides 24-hour emergency care, with no more than six inpatient beds for providing temporary care for 72 hours or less to clients needing stabilization before transfer to a larger hospital. Physicians, nurse practitioners, or physician assistants staff the RPCH (Sharp, 1991). The RPCH can provide inpatient care to acutely ill or injured persons before they are transferred to better-equipped facilities. Basic radiological and laboratory services are also available.

With health care reform, more big-city health care systems are branching out and establishing affiliations or mergers with rural hospitals. The rural hospitals provide a referral base to the larger tertiary care medical centers. Recently, federal laws have granted higher cost-based rates of payment from Medicare and Medicaid to certified rural health clinics (Montague, 1994). This improves the hospitals' financial standing. The number of these clinics has grown significantly in the last few years, improving access to health care for millions of citizens.

Nurses who work in rural hospitals or clinics often function independently in the absence of a physician. Competence in physical assessment, clinical decision making, and emergency care is essential. Nurse practitioners use medical protocols or work under collaborative agreements with staff physicians.

RESTORATIVE CARE

Clients recovering from acute or chronic illnesses or who have disabilities usually require a continuing level of care that is needed until they return to their previous level of function or reach a new level of function limited by their illness or disability. The goal of restorative care is to assist an individual in regaining maximal functional status, enhancing the individual's quality of life while promoting client independence and self-care. With the emphasis on early discharge from hospitals, there are few clients who do not require some level of restorative care. For example, surgical clients will require ongoing wound care, activity and exercise management, and sometimes diet interventions until they have recovered to a point where they can independently resume normal activities of daily living.

The intensity of care has increased in restorative care settings, since clients leave hospitals earlier. It is not uncommon to have clients in the home setting still receiving intravenous (IV) fluids (see Chapter 40), enteral nutrition (see Chapter 43), and oxygen therapy (see Chapter 39). The restorative health care team is an interdisciplinary group of health professionals that includes the client and family or significant others. In restorative settings, nurses recognize early that success is dependent on effective partnering with clients and their families. Clients and families require a clear understanding of goals for physical recovery, the rationale for any physical limitations, and the purpose and potential risks associated with therapies. The more clients and families are involved in restorative care, the more likely it is that they will be motivated to follow treatment plans and clients will be able to achieve optimal functioning.

The restorative care team functions as a unit to assist clients in achieving a level of function that will enable them to return to their community. As a whole, the team engages in clinical decision making involving assessment, diagnosis, planning, implementation, and evaluation (American Congress of Rehabilitation Medicine, 1992). Each health care professional participates and contributes from the specific focus of his or her respective discipline (McCourt, 1993). For example, if a client has a functional problem related to mobility, the physical therapist focuses on the physical adjustments to enhance mobility while the nurse focuses on planning activities to increase activity tolerance during mobility.

Home Health Care.   **Home health care** is that component of a continuum of comprehensive health care whereby health services are provided to individuals and families in their home for the purpose of promoting, maintaining, or restoring health, or of maximizing the level of independence while minimizing the effects of disability and illness (Stanhope, 2000). Services provided by a home health agency include medically related professional and paraprofessional services and equipment for health maintenance, education, illness prevention, diagnosis and treatment of disease, palliation, and rehabilitation. Home health care is unique, with health care providers practicing in the client's environment. For this reason, knowledge of family dynamics, cultural practices, spiritual values, and communication principles is just some of the knowledge that nurses must apply in making critical decisions regarding client and family care. Services are planned, coordinated, and made available by providers organized for the delivery of home care through the use of employed staff, contractual arrangements, or a combination of both. Nursing is the primary service offered under Medicare; however, home health care might also include medical services; physical, occupational, speech, and respiratory therapy; and nutritional therapy. Home health equipment or durable medical equipment (DME) is any medically related product adapted for home use.

For the purpose of this chapter, home health care is discussed under the category of restorative care, since a good percentage of home health services occurs following hospitalization. However, all levels of care can occur within

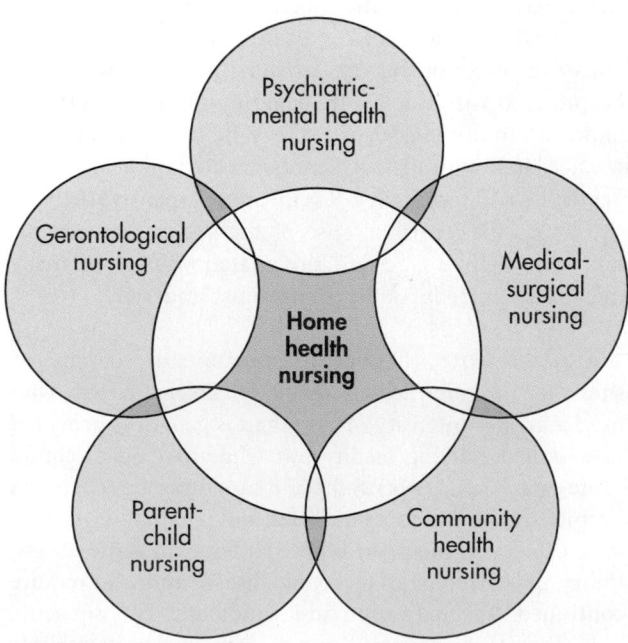

Figure 2-3   Home health nursing synthesizes community health nursing and other nursing specialties.

the home setting. Stanhope (2000) notes that home health care involves a primary preventive focus (community health), as well as secondary and tertiary prevention (care of individuals). Figure 2-3 shows that home health nursing is a synthesis of community health nursing (see Chapter 3) and selected knowledge and skills from other nursing specialties.

Home health care agencies provide skilled and intermittent professional services and home health aide services. These services usually are delivered once or twice a day, up to 7 days a week. Some of the services offered by home health care agencies are summarized in Box 2-4. Approved home care agencies usually receive reimbursement for services from the government (such as Medicare and Medicaid in the United States), private insurance, and private pay. The government has strict regulations for governing reimbursement for home health care services. An agency cannot simply charge for a service and expect to receive full reimbursement. Most professional services are reimbursed at the costs for providing the service by government programs. Commercial payers often negotiate contract rates or provide reimbursement for billed charges. Chapter 3 discusses the role of the home health nurse.

Rehabilitation. Rehabilitation is the restoration of a person to the fullest physical, mental, social, vocational, and economic usefulness possible (Clemen-Stone, McGuire, and Eigsti, 1998). Clients require rehabilitation after a physical or mental illness, injury, or chemical addiction. Rehabilitation was once available primarily for clients with illnesses or injury to the nervous system and/or musculoskeletal system, but the health care delivery system has expanded its scope of such services. Today, specialized rehabilitation services, such as cardiovascular and pulmonary rehabilitation programs, help clients and families adjust to necessary changes in lifestyle and learn to function with the limitations of their disease. **Drug rehabilitation centers** help the client become free from drug dependence and return to the community.

Rehabilitation services include physical, occupational, and speech therapy (Box 2-5). Ideally, rehabilitation be-

---

Home Health Care Services   Box 2-4

WOUND CARE
Sterile dressing changes, debridement and irrigations, packing, and instructing clients and families in wound care techniques

RESPIRATORY CARE
Oxygen therapy, mechanical ventilation, suctioning, and care of tracheotomies

VITAL SIGNS
Monitoring blood pressure and cardiopulmonary status; instructing clients and families in vital sign measurement

ELIMINATION
Ostomy care, appliance application, skin care, and irrigation; insertion of indwelling and intermittent urinary catheters, irrigation, and instructing families in catheter management; home dialysis.

NUTRITION
Administration of tube feedings and enternal feedings; assessment of nutrition and hydration status.
Instructing clients and families in tube feedings

REHABILITATION
Ambulation and gait training, use of assistive devices, range-of-motion exercises, and instructing clients and families on transfer techniques

MEDICATIONS
Monitoring compliance; administering injections; and instructing clients and families on drug information, medication preparation, and steps to take in the event of side effects

INTRAVENOUS THERAPY
Administration of blood products, analgesic and chemotherapeutic agents, and long-term hydration
Instructing clients and families on use of intravenous devices, steps to take in the event of disconnection or accidental fluid infusion, and side effects

LABORATORY STUDIES
Blood glucose monitoring (including client and family instruction) and drawing blood for specific diagnostic purposes

---

Common Rehabilitation Services   Box 2-5

PHYSICAL THERAPY
Therapeutic exercises, gait training, use of ambulatory assist devices, massage, application of heat and cold to joints and muscles, hydrotherapy, and electric stimulation of nerves

OCCUPATIONAL THERAPY
Treatment through purposeful activity of people whose ability to perform activities of daily living is impaired: design, fabrication, and application of orthoses; guidance in selection and use of adaptive equipment; therapeutic exercises to enhance functional performance; prevocational evaluation and training; and consultation for adaptation of the physical environment for the handicapped or wheelchair-bound client

SPEECH THERAPY
Treatments and counseling in the prevention or correction of speech and language disorders: measurement and evaluation of language abilities, auditory processes, and speech production and clinical treatment of clients with speech and language disorders

gins the moment a client enters a health care setting for treatment. For example, some orthopedic programs now have clients undergo physical therapy exercises before major joint repair so as to enhance their recovery postoperatively. Initially, rehabilitation may focus on the prevention of complications related to the illness or injury. As the condition stabilizes, rehabilitation is directed at maximizing the client's functioning and level of independence.

Rehabilitation occurs in many health care settings, including rehabilitation institutions, outpatient settings, and the home. Frequently clients needing long-term rehabilitation (e.g., stroke and spinal injury clients) have severe disabilities affecting their ability to carry out activities of daily living. When rehabilitation services are provided in outpatient settings, clients receive treatment at specified times during the week but remain at home the rest of the time. Specific rehabilitation strategies are applied to the home environment so that maximal levels of function and independence can be achieved.

Extended Care Facilities.

An **extended care facility** provides intermediate medical, nursing, or custodial care for clients recovering from acute or chronic illnesses or disabilities. Extended care facilities include intermediate care and skilled nursing facilities. Some include long-term care and assisted living facilities (see Continuing Care). At one time, extended care facilities cared primarily for older adults. However, as hospitals manage clients toward early discharge, there is a greater need for intermediate care settings for clients of all ages. For example, a young client who has experienced a traumatic accident may be transferred to an extended care facility for rehabilitative or supportive care until discharge to the home becomes a safe option. The growth of extended care facilities will increase as the number of older adults grows.

An intermediate care facility, or **skilled nursing facility**, offers skilled care from a licensed nursing staff. This may include administration of IV fluids, wound care, long-term ventilator management, and physical rehabilitation. Extensive supportive care is provided until clients can move back into the community or into residential care. Extended care facilities provide around-the-clock nursing coverage. Nurses employed in such a setting have expertise similar to that of nurses working in acute care inpatient settings. In addition, the nurse should have a background in gerontological nursing principles.

CONTINUING CARE

Clients across the life span often have long-term health care needs as a result of developing disabilities, progression of chronic disease, or permanent impairment from injuries. These individuals require personal, social, and health care services to maintain a quality of life that offers security and dignity. Continuing, or long-term, care offers services over a prolonged period of time to people who have lost or never acquired functional capacity (Kane and Kane, 1987). The need for continuing health care services

is growing in the United States and Canada. People are living longer, and many of those have no immediate family members to care for them. A decline in the number of children families choose to have, the aging of care providers, and the increasing rates of divorce and remarriage complicate this problem. Continuing care may be provided within institutional settings (nursing facility), communities (adult day care), or the home (home health) (Lueckenotte, 2000).

Nursing Facilities.

The language of continuing, or long-term, care can be confusing. The nursing home has been the dominant setting in which continuing care has been provided (Lueckenotte, 2000). With the Omnibus Budget Reconciliation Act of 1987, the term *nursing facility* became the term for nursing homes and other skilled nursing facilities where long-term care is provided.

The number of people in the United States who lived in nursing homes, or nursing facilities, in 1998 was 1.6 million (Meyer, 1998). A nursing facility provides 24-hour intermediate and custodial care for clients of any age with chronic or debilitating illnesses. The majority of clients in nursing facilities are older adults. Nursing facilities have been under attack for years because of claims regarding inadequate care and abuse. Many of the claims have been justified. However, the nursing facility industry has become one of the most highly regulated industries in the United States. These regulations have raised the standard of services provided. One regulatory area that deserves special mention is that of resident rights. Nursing facilities must recognize their residents as active participants and decision makers in their care and life in institutional settings (Lueckenotte, 2000). This also means that family members are active partners in the planning of residents'

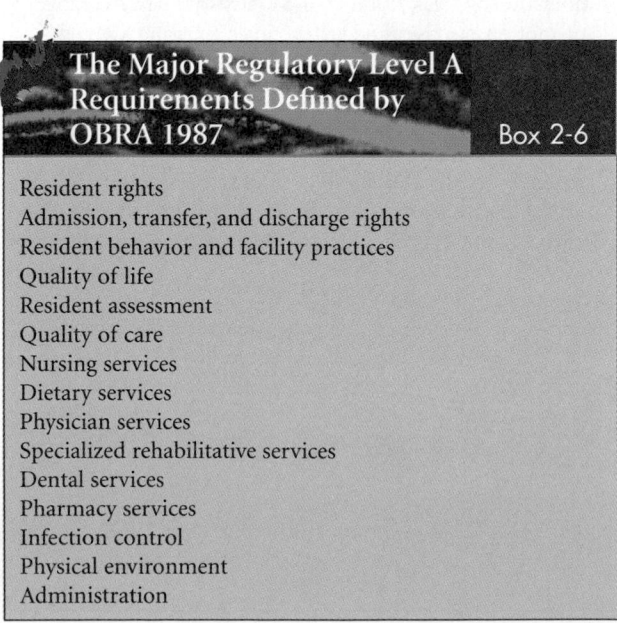

The Major Regulatory Level A Requirements Defined by OBRA 1987   Box 2-6

Resident rights
Admission, transfer, and discharge rights
Resident behavior and facility practices
Quality of life
Resident assessment
Quality of care
Nursing services
Dietary services
Physician services
Specialized rehabilitative services
Dental services
Pharmacy services
Infection control
Physical environment
Administration

From Lueckenotte A: *Gerontologic nursing*, ed 2, St. Louis, 2000, Mosby.

care. Box 2-6 summarizes the types of standards currently established for nursing facilities.

Interdisciplinary functional assessment of residents is the cornerstone of clinical practice within nursing facilities (Lueckenotte, 2000). Government regulations require that each resident be comprehensively assessed, with care planning decisions made within a prescribed time period. A client's functional ability and long-term physical and psychosocial well-being are the focus. The Resident Assessment Instrument (RAI) must be completed on all residents. The RAI consists of the Minimum Data Set (MDS)(Box 2-7), Resident Assessment Protocols (RAPs), and utilization guidelines of each state. The RAI ultimately can provide a national database for nursing facilities so that policy makers can better understand the health care needs of this long-term care population.

Assisted Living.
Assisted living is one of the fastest-growing industries within the United States. With over 30,000 facilities in the United States in 1998 (Meyer, 1998), assisted living offers an attractive long-term care setting with a homier environment and greater resident autonomy. Clients are generally in need of some assistance with activities of daily living but remain relatively independent within a partially protective setting. Usually people keep all personal possessions in their residences. Facilities range from hotel-like buildings with hundreds of units to modest group homes that house a handful of seniors. Services within an assisted living facility might include meals, social and recreational programs, personal laundry and housekeeping, transportation, an emergency call system, and health checks (Kane and Wilson, 1993).

Minimum Data Set and Examples of Resident Assessment Protocols   Box 2-7

MINIMUM DATA SET
Resident's background
Cognitive, communication/hearing, and vision patterns
Physical functioning and structural problems
Mood, behavior, and activity pursuit patterns
Psychosocial well-being
Bowel and bladder continence
Health conditions
Disease diagnoses
Oral/nutritional and dental status
Skin condition
Medication use
Special treatments and procedures

RESIDENT ASSESSMENT PROTOCOLS (EXAMPLES)
Delirium
Falls
Pressure ulcers
Psychotropic drug use

The greatest limitation to assisted living is that most residents pay privately (Meyer, 1998). There are no government fee caps and little regulation. This severely limits the choices in long-term care for those individuals with limited financial resources. Many states are under pressure to provide financial assistance through Medicaid. Assisted living is seen as a cheaper alternative to nursing homes. Twenty-eight states pay some assisted living costs, and more are considering the option (Meyer, 1998).

Respite Care.
The need to care for family members within the home creates great physical and emotional burdens for adult caregivers. The caregiver is usually an adult who not only has the responsibility for providing care to a loved one (e.g., spouse, parent, or sibling), but often must also maintain a full-time job and manage the routines of daily living. **Respite care** is a service that provides short-term relief or time off for persons providing home care to the ill or disabled (e.g., children, psychiatric clients, or frail older adults). Adult day care is one form of respite care. However, respite care can also be provided within the home by health professionals and trained volunteers. The caregiver is able to leave the home for errands or for just some social time while a responsible person stays in the home to care for the loved one.

Adult Day Care Centers.
Adult day care centers provide a variety of health and social services to specific client populations who live alone or with family in the community. The centers' services allow family members to maintain their lifestyles and employment and still provide home care for their relatives (Lueckenotte, 2000). Day care centers may be associated with a hospital or nursing facility or exist as independent centers. Frequently clients do not require hospitalization but need continuous health care services while their families or support persons work. These clients include older adults needing daily physical rehabilitation, individuals with emotional illnesses needing daily counseling, and individuals with chemical dependence problems who are involved in rehabilitation programs. The centers usually operate 5 days per week during typical business hours and usually charge on a per diem basis. Adult day care centers reduce the cost of health care and allow clients to retain more independence by living at home.

Services offered in day care settings include transportation to and from the facility, assistance with personal care, nursing and therapeutic services (e.g., counseling and rehabilitation), meals, and recreational activities (Lueckenotte, 2000). Nurses working in day care centers provide continuity between care delivered in the home and in the center. For instance, nurses can ensure that the client continues to take prescribed medication and administer specific treatments. Knowledge of community needs and resources is essential in providing adequate support of clients who often spend only a few hours a week in the day care setting (Ebersole and Hess, 1998).

Hospice.   A **hospice** is a system of family-centered care designed to allow clients to live and remain at home with comfort, independence, and dignity while alleviating the strains caused by terminal illness. The focus of hospice care is palliative care, not curative treatments (see Chapter 29). Hospice can benefit a client in the terminal phases of any disease, such as cardiomyopathy, multiple sclerosis, AIDS, and cancer.

A client entering a hospice has reached the terminal phase of illness (generally, the final 6 weeks), and the client, family, and physician have agreed that no further treatment could reverse the disease process. An attempt is made to provide care that ensures death with dignity in the client's home. Occasionally a client must be admitted to a hospice unit within a hospital or independent location. The client and family must accept the fact that the hospice will not use emergency measures such as cardiopulmonary resuscitation to prolong life. Instead, the hospice uses a multidisciplinary approach to provide pain control and comfort measures.

Hospice nurses work in institutional and community settings. They are committed to the philosophy and objectives of the facilities for which they work. They provide care and support for the client and the family during the terminal phase and at the time of death, and they continue to offer bereavement counseling and follow-up to the family following the client's death. Many hospice programs provide respite care, which is important in maintaining the health of the primary caregiver and family.

Canadian Health Care System

The Canadian people believe passionately in health insurance coverage as a right of citizenship (Kerr, 1997). The Canadian Medicare health care plan is an integrated system that provides universal coverage to all citizens and a uniform, comprehensive package of benefits, with no consumer billing. Hospital care and physician services are insured through the plan. The citizens have free choice of medical providers. All financial arrangements occur between the providers and the government insurer. The government negotiates directly with providers to establish health care rates. Canada has substantially lower health care costs than the United States (Kerr, 1997). The Canadian health plan provides an extensive range of services while containing costs, principally by controlling the rates of increase in physicians' fee schedules.

Access to specialized medical care (e.g., cardiologists, oncologists) has been limited in Canada, and as a result, half of all Canadian physicians are general practitioners (Terris, 1991). When comparisons were made with the United States, Terris (1991) found that only 10% of physicians practicing in the United States were primary care physicians. Since that time, the number of primary care physicians in the United States has grown. Unlike in the United States, clients in Canada may experience long waiting periods for elective procedures. Access is also a problem, with a sparse population scattered over a vast territory. To ensure the survival of the Canadian system, measures are needed to guarantee that universal availability and access to services are balanced by the provision of reasonably comprehensive services in a publicly funded, nonprofit, affordable system (Kerr, 1997). Canada is facing higher costs from high public use of services. The Canadian system is beginning to focus more on health promotion through a community-based model of care.

Issues in Health Care Delivery

The climate in health care today is influencing health care professionals, as well as consumers. In the midst of an evolving health care system, nurses must be prepared to participate fully and effectively within the new, managed care environment. Berwick (1994) has noted that "only those who provide care can in the end change care." As nurses struggle with issues of how to maintain health care quality while reducing costs, they need to acquire the knowledge, skills, and values that will allow them to practice competently and effectively as professionals.

Consumers of health care want to access appropriate, cost-effective, quality health care. Society generally believes that all people have a right to health care. Access to care refers to the consumer's ability to easily use a broad range of health care providers at a variety of community health care sites (American Organization of Nurse Executives [AONE], 1994). Furthermore, access should not be limited to those individuals who are healthy or who can afford insurance. It is important for clients to be able to acquire needed health services easily, in cost-effective settings. Consumers also want health care institutions to be accountable for quality and to show the benefit gained from using their services.

Nursing plays a major role in the health care delivery system. Nursing services are necessary for virtually every client seeking care at any level. Every nurse practicing today needs to appreciate that health care is a business. The success of any health care business depends on nursing's participation in being accountable for high-quality care and collaborating to help create the systems and strategies to ensure that clients receive cost-effective and efficient care.

COMPETENCY OF HEALTH CARE PROVIDERS

As the health care system changes, so must the competencies of its professionals. A consumer of health care should expect that the standards of nursing care and practice in any health care setting are appropriate, safe, and efficacious. There are two principal mechanisms designed to ensure competent professional nursing practice: standards of formal education programs and continuing education in-service organizations. An established nursing education program must set professional standards for its students and meet educational outcomes based on national accreditation guidelines. Program graduates should be able to assume entry-level positions within health care settings and perform competently within their defined responsibilities. Health care organizations, such as hospitals or home care agencies, ensure quality by establishing policies, procedures, and protocols that meet national accrediting standards. Competency is further promoted with organizations providing appropriate, ongoing in-service education. An additional assurance that high-quality standards are met by professionals is provided through certification of individuals in general and specialty practices.

The Pew Health Professions Commission investigated the trends in health care and the preparation of professionals, and identified six critical competencies needed for health professions by the year 2005 (Shugars, O'Neil, and Bader, 1991):

1. Be able to care for the community's health.
2. Practice primary care and prevention.
3. Promote healthy lifestyles.
4. Involve clients and families in health care decision making.
5. Assess and use technology appropriately.
6. Accommodate expanded accountability.

The Pew Commission's recommendations clearly show a prioritization for health care professionals to become more competent in health promotion efforts.

POPULATION-BASED CARE

The health care delivery model has traditionally been focused on the treatment of disease rather than on the promotion of health. Emphasis on specialization, fragmentation of medical services, and barriers in access to services are all symptoms of a disease-focused health care system. This must change if the health of our citizens is to improve and if the costs of health care are to be controlled.

Approximately 52% of all diseases are a product of unhealthy lifestyles and behavioral choices that result in ill health (Grace, 1997). To improve the health of the population, there is a need to refocus health care in ways that better inform the public and redistribute resources for health promotion and disease prevention efforts. Nursing can make a significant contribution in educating the public about its health. For example, there is a need to help young people learn to acquire healthy lifestyles for long and productive lives. Nurses in schools, nursing centers, and clinics should develop and institute programs promoting health habits, including good nutrition, adequate sleep, and routine exercise. Every school curriculum in the country should contain content on the effects of drug (including tobacco) and alcohol abuse (Grace, 1997). Systematic programs are needed in every community to conduct health screenings so as to detect health problems at their earliest stages. Prenatal care, adolescent health monitoring, and health and fitness assessment for seniors are just some examples. Nursing's involvement must not be simply at an individual client level but at a community level as well (see Chapter 3).

REDESIGNING ACUTE CARE DELIVERY

The changes created by managed care include the overhaul of acute care delivery. Hospitals are the source of high health care costs due to labor, high-cost technology and pharmaceuticals, and high utilization of diagnostic and treatment resources. Major efforts have arisen in restructuring hospital departments and redesigning the delivery of care to clients.

Work Redesign.
Health care organizations, hospitals in particular, are looking for ways to reduce costs, gain efficiency, reduce the duplication of tasks, and reduce the overall size of the workforce. **Work redesign** is a concept that refers to changing the actual structure and ultimately the responsibilities of the jobs people perform (Tonges, 1992). Specifically, health care institutions are looking at how care is delivered to clients. Are there ways to make work more efficient, help care providers become more productive, and improve clients' satisfaction with the level of care delivered?

Most hospitals can point to inefficiencies in services as a source of increasing costs. The work of client care involves a variety of care providers and ancillary staff who often duplicate the work of one another. In work redesign, an analysis is made of the work process being performed (e.g., the admission of clients). Each task or activity (e.g., history taking, delivering supplies, or gathering specimens) associated with the process is reviewed to determine if it is necessary or appropriate. Then the analysis asks who is performing the task and should that person be doing it (Tonges, 1992).

In many work redesign efforts it becomes obvious that indirect, or nonnursing, care activities (e.g., gathering supplies, delivering meals, cleaning client units) take up a good amount of the professional nurse's time. Work redesign on a client care unit involves identifying care activities that can be safely and appropriately assigned to less costly labor, such as assistive personnel. Many hospitals have developed positions such as the patient service representative. This staff member provides no direct client care but assumes a role that combines the elements of the housekeeping, dietary, supply clerk, and unit maintenance aspects of a nurse's aide role (Tonges, 1992). Instead of three different staff members performing the work, one multiskilled worker provides indirect care activities.

The best use of the RN's time requires efficient use of ancillary personnel (licensed practical nurses [LPNs]) and assistive personnel. The best approach is redesigning delivery of care to involve all levels of staff in the redesign process. RNs, for example, identify the types of care processes (e.g., client assessment and education) that influence client outcomes. RNs and LPNs review skills (e.g., IV therapy) that require their knowledge and experience.

Licensure issues, as well as state nurse practice acts, are reviewed and clarified. Then the RNs and LPNs identify the types of tasks they believe can be safely delegated to multiskilled **assistive personnel**. This process helps all staff understand their unique role so as to minimize duplication of effort and ensure better teamwork.

Assistive Personnel.   Professional nurses in hospitals and skilled care facilities are finding themselves in situations where more support is needed to do the daily, repetitive tasks of client care. Many institutions have fewer RNs to care for hospitalized clients who are acutely ill. The RN is expected to coordinate care delivery for groups of clients, perform assessments, make professional judgments and clinical decisions, deliver and change therapies as needed, and provide client counseling and education. At the same time, clients still require basic supportive care activities (e.g., daily hygiene and nutritional support). A professional nurse simply cannot do all of the work necessary to care for a group of clients. An issue that concerns many hospital nurses is that they have more to do and less time to do it in, and they are worried that quality of care and client safety might suffer (Lumsdon, 1995).

More institutions are hiring assistive personnel to provide support to RNs and LPNs in the health care setting. Assistive personnel might include certified nurse assistants, trained technicians, or staff who transfer from non–client care areas (e.g., dietary, housekeeping) to clinical areas. One problem with assistive personnel is the inconsistency in training. Certified nurse assistants receive excellent preparation for basic client care responsibilities, but often their focus is in long-term care. There are many assistive personnel who receive only in-house training and minimal clinical preparation for their roles. Assistive personnel must become competent and demonstrate consistent performance in the nursing care skills delegated by RNs. Then and only then can the RN have a level of trust in assistive personnel so that they can team together and deliver client care safely and effectively.

Delegation.   When delegating responsibilities to a competent individual, the RN still remains accountable for the overall nursing care of the client (Parkman, 1996). The nurse must exercise good judgment in deciding what tasks to delegate and in what situations. Chapter 4 covers the guidelines for safe and appropriate delegation.

QUALITY HEALTH CARE

Quality health care is difficult to define. Research has shown that what clients define as quality health care may not necessarily be the same as what health professionals define as quality (Gerteis and others, 1993). Unless health care providers can define quality, the purchasers of health care will buy services based on price alone. The health care system that can deliver a given service (e.g., delivery of a baby and mother-infant care) for the cheapest price will become the primary provider of that service. Health care providers are trying to define and measure quality in terms of outcomes. An outcome is a measure of what actually does or does not happen as a result of a process of care; it is the end result (desirable or undesirable) of care delivered (Donabedian, 1966; Bernstein and Hilborne, 1993). Examples of outcomes are the readmission rates for surgical clients, the functional health status of clients following discharge (e.g., ability and time frame for returning to work), and the rate of infection following surgery. Health plans throughout the United States are now relying on the Health Plan Employer Data and Information Set (HEDIS) as a quality measure (Greene, 1998). Participating health plans provide vital statistics on more than 70 quality indicators, allowing employers to check on the performance of different health plans. HEDIS is the database of choice for the Health Care Financing Administration (HCFA), which requires the information from Medicare MCOs. One of the most common outcome measures is client satisfaction. The Joint Commission on the Accreditation of Health Care Organizations (JCAHO) (2000) requires health care organizations to determine how well an organization meets client needs and expectations. Organizations are using outcomes such as client satisfaction as a basis to redesign how care is managed and delivered in hopes of improving quality in the long term.

Client Satisfaction.   Almost every major health care organization measures certain aspects of client satisfaction. The Picker/Commonwealth Program for Patient-Centered Care was established to explore clients' needs and concerns, as defined by clients, and to promote models of care that make the experience of illness and hospitalization more humane (Gerteis and others, 1993). After interviewing hundreds of clients and their families, seven broad "dimensions" of care were identified that most affect clients' experiences with health care (Box 2-8). The seven dimensions cover much of what is the scope of nursing practice. A close look shows that most of the dimensions, which can be reflected in client satisfaction, can be applied to almost any health care setting.

The Picker/Commonwealth program has developed a survey that measures client satisfaction along the seven dimensions. The survey looks globally at client perceptions of care in an attempt to understand how all hospital departments influence client satisfaction. The survey is conducted through telephone interviews after the client is discharged from the health care setting. Many other companies have developed similar client satisfaction surveys that are mailed to clients. Staff involved in client care receive the satisfaction scores as feedback regarding their success in meeting client expectations. It is the responsibility of staff to identify the unique issues that influence client satisfaction for their area. Client satisfaction findings become the basis for many quality improvement studies (see Chapter 4).

| The Dimensions of Client-Centered Care | Box 2-8 |

RESPECT FOR CLIENT'S VALUES, PREFERENCES, AND EXPRESSED NEEDS

Clients expect to be treated with dignity and respect.

Clients want to be informed and involved in decisions about their care.

Clients' perception of needs should not be completely different from those identified by a care provider.

COORDINATION AND INTEGRATION OF CARE

Clients' feelings of powerlessness can be reduced by a competent and caring staff.

Clients look for someone to be in charge of care and to communicate clearly with other health team members.

Clients look to have services and procedures well coordinated.

Clients need to know at all times whom to call for help.

INFORMATION, COMMUNICATION, AND EDUCATION

Clients expect to receive accurate and timely information about their clinical status, progress, or prognosis.

Clients and families need to be informed of major changes in therapies or status.

Tests and procedures must be explained clearly in language clients understand.

Clients and family members want to know how to manage care on their own to the extent they desire or are able.

PHYSICAL COMFORT

Physical care that comforts clients is one of the most elemental services caregivers can provide.

Nurses should respond in a timely and effective way to any request for pain medication, explain the extent of pain clients can expect, and offer alternatives for pain management.

Clients expect privacy and to have their cultural values respected.

The health care setting environment should be clean and comfortable.

EMOTIONAL SUPPORT AND RELIEF OF FEAR AND ANXIETY

Clients look to care providers to share their fears and concerns.

Clients need to understand the impact illness will have on their ability to care for themselves and their family.

Clients worry about their ability to pay for their medical care. Are there staff who can help with those worries?

INVOLVEMENT OF FAMILY AND FRIENDS

Care providers must recognize and respect the family and friends on whom clients rely for support.

Clients have the right to determine if family members are to be involved in decisions about their care.

Clients expect those family or friends who will provide physical support and care after discharge to be properly informed.

TRANSITION AND CONTINUITY

Clients want information about medications to take, dietary or treatment plans to follow, and danger signals to look for after hospitalization or treatment.

Clients expect to have their continuing health care needs met after discharge with well-coordinated services.

Clients and family members expect access to any necessary health care resources after discharge.

Data from Gerteis M and others: *Through the patient's eyes,* San Francisco, 1993, Jossey-Bass.

It is important for nurses to recognize the need to identify client expectations. The seven dimensions of care can be a useful guide. By learning early what a client expects in regard to information, comfort, and availability of family and friends, the nurse can better plan client care. When should the nurse ask about a client's expectations? It should become a routine question when the client first enters a health care setting and episodically as care continues. For example, many clients receive analgesics for pain relief on a prn, or as-needed, basis. The nurse may wish to say, "The medication is here when you need it," and then ask, "Would you like me to offer it when it is available or would you prefer to ask for it?" Client expectations are an important measure of the evaluation of nursing care.

Client Perceptions of Nurse Caring.

Caring has historically denoted the task of giving physical care to another person (Williams, 1997). Today it has become clear that caring also has an affective dimension, incorporating a humanistic approach. During a time of change within health care, it is critical for nurses to recognize that caring is central to nursing and necessary for cure to take place

(see Chapter 6). Research has shown that clients place emphasis on the tasks of nursing care, yet they also want nurses to be kind, friendly, considerate, and careful in the way care is administered (Williams, 1997). It is therefore important for nurses to always apply a caring approach in their practice. Whether the nurse is giving a bath, assessing a client's pain, or administering a medication, the nurse's tone of voice, facial expression, and selection of words convey the extent to which the nurse cares about an individual. Many argue that caring is the art of nursing. It is the expression of this art that can make a difference to a client's sense of well-being and satisfaction with nursing care (Box 2-9, p. 40).

THE CONTINUUM OF HEALTH CARE

When an individual presents a health problem, there is the potential of requiring a variety of services to enable the person to regain or maintain his or her health. Management of a client during an episode of illness should occur smoothly across the continuum of care. This means that a client can easily access all services along the continuum from primary to continuing care, without delays, du-

Research HIGHLIGHT   Box 2-9

RESEARCH ABSTRACT

This study explored the relationship between nurse caring and client satisfaction. The Holistic Caring Inventory (HCI) measures clients' perceptions of nurse caring, specifically the humanistic caring component of the nurse-client interaction (Latham, 1990). The inventory contains four dimensions of caring: physical caring (addressing clients' physical well-being), interpretive caring (assists clients in discussing and interpreting the meaning of their feelings), spiritual caring (focuses on spiritual needs of clients), and sensitive caring (sensitivity to individual feelings and needs). The Patient Satisfaction Inventory (PSI) was developed for hospitalized clients (Hinshaw and Atwood, 1982). The 25-item survey has three dimensions of satisfaction with nursing care that include technical and professional activities, trust, and educational activities.

Ninety-four hospitalized medical clients from two rural hospitals were asked to complete both the HCI and the PSI. Findings revealed that the clients' overall satisfaction with nursing care was low. However, the clients in the study indicated that caring was evident, and that they were more satisfied when they perceived their nurses to be caring. Sensitive caring was the best predictor of client satisfaction.

IMPLICATIONS FOR PRACTICE

- Nursing care should not focus simply on completion of the tasks of nursing, but on the interpersonal relationship between nurse and client as well.
- Time and resources should be planned based on clients' subjective, interpersonal, and caring needs.
- Nurses must learn more about the caring behaviors that are supportive of clients, such as showing respect, appreciating clients as individuals, being hopeful for clients, and checking frequently on client needs.

REFERENCE

Williams SA: The relationship of patients' perceptions of holistic nurse caring to satisfaction with nursing care, *J Nurs Care Qual* 11(5):15, 1997.

plication of services, or poorly coordinated treatment plans. An integrated health care system has as its aim the delivery of care across the continuum. However, in most settings the levels of care do not function as an integrated system (Fowler and Stokes, 1996). At best, they operate in a coordinated manner in which clients are smoothly transferred from one level of care (e.g., hospital) to another (e.g., skilled nursing facility). At worst, they exist as independent levels, with each level operating autonomously. Nursing plays a role in developing models for supporting clients through a continuum of care.

Discharge Planning. Managing a client through a particular level of care is commonly achieved through discharge planning. **Discharge planning** is a centralized, co-ordinated, multidisciplinary process that ensures that the client has a plan for continuing care after leaving a health care agency. The process helps in the transition of the client from one environment to another (e.g., from hospital to rehabilitation facility, from rehabilitation facility to home). The transition from hospital to home is one of the more problematic ones for clients (Gerteis and others, 1993). Too often, discharge planning seems to be more focused on anticipating obstacles to discharge from a health care facility to avoid extra costs. But clients worry about how they will care for themselves and their families and manage their illness over the long term. Nurses can help to anticipate and identify clients' continuing needs before the actual time of discharge and coordinate health team members so that an effective and appropriate discharge plan is implemented.

Discharge planning begins the moment a client is admitted to a health care facility. The nurse knows that a surgical client will require continued wound care on discharge home, whereas the client with newly diagnosed diabetes will need to be able to take prescribed medications. There are certain clients who are more in need of discharge planning because of the risks they present (Box 2-10). However, any client who is being discharged from a health care facility with remaining functional alterations and/or who must follow certain restrictions or therapies for recovery needs discharge planning. All caregivers who care for a client with a specific health problem must participate in discharge planning. The process is truly multidisciplinary. For example, the diabetic client visiting an education center requires the collaboration of a nurse educator, dietitian, and physician to ensure that the client returns home with the right information to manage his or her condition. A client who has experienced a stroke will not be discharged from the hospital until plans have been established with physical and occupational therapists to begin a program of rehabilitation.

Effective discharge planning often requires referrals to various health care disciplines. The nurse is often the first to recognize the client's needs. In many agencies a physician's order is needed for a referral, especially when specific therapies are planned (e.g., physical therapy). It is best to have clients participate in referral processes so that they are involved early in any necessary decision making. Some tips on making the referral process successful include the following:

- Make a referral as soon as possible. Always think and anticipate the client's needs.
- Inform the care provider receiving the referral of as much information about the client as possible. This avoids duplication of effort and exclusion of important information.
- Involve the client and family in the referral process: selecting the necessary referral and explaining the service to be provided, the reason for the referral, and what to expect from the service.

Examples of JCAHO Standards for Admission and Discharge   Box 2-10

NURSING AND HEALTH TEAM RESPONSIBILITIES
Before Hospital Admission
Identifies and uses available information sources about the client's needs.
Communicates with other care settings and organizations.
During Admission
The hospital:
  Provides services consistent with its mission, population served, and settings.
  Makes arrangements with other organizations and settings to facilitate the client's admission.
  Clients are referred and transferred to meet their needs based on intensity, risk, and staffing level.
  When appropriate, clinical consultants and contractual arrangements are used for referrals and transfers.
In the Hospital
Services flow continuously from assessment through treatment and reassessment.
The client's care is coordinated between practitioners.
Before Discharge
The need for discharge planning assessment is determined.
  The hospital has a way of identifying those clients for whom discharge planning is critical.
Education prepares the client for discharge.
At Discharge
The client is directly referred to practitioners, settings, and organizations to meet his or her continuing needs.
The use and value of continuing care to meet the client's needs are reassessed.
The hospital provides information or data to help others meet the client's continuing care needs.

Modified from Joint Commission on Accreditation of Healthcare Organizations: *Manual of hospital accreditation: 1998 standards,* Chicago, 2000, The Commission.

- Determine what the referral discipline recommends for the client's care and incorporate this into the treatment plan as soon as possible.
- Referrals must be made to agencies approved by a client's insurer.

Good discharge planning depends on comprehensive client and family education (see Chapter 23). It is critical for clients to know what to do when they get home, how to do it, and what to observe for when problems develop. The JCAHO (2000) requires the following instruction before clients leave health care facilities:

- Safe and effective use of medications and medical equipment
- Instruction on potential food-drug interactions and counseling on nutrition and modified diets
- Rehabilitation techniques to support adaptation to and/or functional independence in the environment
- Access to available community resources as needed

- When and how to obtain further treatment
- The client's and family's responsibilities in the client's ongoing health care needs and the knowledge and skills needed to carry out those responsibilities
- Maintenance of good standards for personal hygiene and grooming

Good discharge planning involves the client from the beginning, uses the strengths of the client in planning, provides resources to meet the client's limitations, and is focused on improving the client's long-term outcomes.

Care Delivery Models.   One approach to improving the continuum of care for a client is in the development of care delivery models that coordinate care at individual levels of care and across multiple levels of care. Today, care delivery requires a multidisciplinary approach. All members of the health care team must be involved. Nurses again play a key role, because of ongoing contact with clients, in managing and coordinating the client's care in an efficient, value-driven, and competent manner.

Care Management and Critical Pathways.   In the past, caregivers from all disciplines, such as nursing, medicine, and social work, managed a client's care within a hospital by contributing their own plans of care. There has always been an objective to coordinate the work of all caregivers so that a single plan was followed with favorable outcomes. This was not always easy to do, depending on the nursing delivery-of-care model or the collaboration of all caregivers. For example, team nursing was so focused on the tasks of nursing care that little effort was given to ensure continuity of discharge planning and participation by all caregivers. Frequently, members of the team were unaware of each discipline's plan.

A successful care delivery approach is care management: structuring accountability for client outcomes at the care delivery level within a unit or area of care (Zander, 1994). With care management, typically one caregiver (e.g., a primary nurse or a nurse coordinator) coordinates care from admission through discharge within a care setting. This may involve coordination of care on a single nursing unit, on multiple units, or during home care. A single, multidisciplinary plan is implemented so that all caregivers work with one plan to achieve the same client outcomes. A popular tool used in care management is a critical pathway. A **critical pathway** is a multidisciplinary treatment plan that sequences clinical interventions over a projected length of stay or a projected time frame for specific case types (Figure 2-4, pp. 42-43), such as normal vaginal delivery, home visits for a client following hip replacement, or an outpatient diagnostic test. A pathway is developed by members of all disciplines that normally care for the particular client type. The interdisciplinary team reviews the best practice patterns in determining the type of interventions and desired outcomes that should make up a critical pathway. One

BARNES

CARE PATH
100 CHEMOTHERAPY

①

SERVICE	PHYSICIAN
PRIMARY NURSE	PRIMARY NURSE

DC DATE	ADM DATE	DATE OF SURGERY	
			A-8

PROBLEM NUMBER	*IF APPLICABLE	PATIENT PROBLEMS / NURSING DIAGNOSES
#1	LACK OF KNOWLEDGE	
#2	ALTERATION IN NUTRITION R/T DECREASED INTAKE, NAUSEA, VOMITING, ANOREXIA, INCREASED CALORIC REQUIREMENT	
#3	POTENTIAL FOR INFECTION R/T MYELOSUPPRESSION, IMMUNOSUPPRESSION	
#4	POTENTIAL ALTERATION IN MUCOUS MEMBRANES R/T STOMATITIS, ESOPHAGITIS, VAGINITIS	
#5	ALTERATION IN URINARY ELIMINATION R/T NEPHROTOXIC EFFECTS OF CHEMOTHERAPY, POTENTIAL FOR HEMORRHAGIC CYSTITIS	
#6	POTENTIAL FOR INJURY R/T THROMBOCYTOPENIA, SEDATION	

PROBLEM NUMBER		PRE-ADMIT	DAY 1	DAY 2
#2 #3 #4 #5 #6 #7 #8	ASSESSMENT / MONITORING	Evaluate IV access Evaluate response to previous treatment **Patient tolerated previous treatment without complications** Patient has adequate IV access (peripheral or VAD)	Nutritional status Nausea, vomiting Weight Bowel function I & O Pain / comfort Skin / mucous membrane integrity Fall prevention Understanding of therapy / knowledge deficits Emotional response / coping mechanisms IV / vascular access site condition / type Results of CBC, SMA6 Vital signs **Pt will have stable vital signs** **Pt will have adequate urinary output without evidence of hematuria**	Nausea, vomiting Effectiveness of antiemetics Bowel function I & O Pain / comfort Skin / mucous membrane integrity Patient response to treatment Emotional response / coping mechanisms IV / vascular access site condition Vital signs **Pt will have stable vital signs** **Pt will have adequate urinary output without evidence of hematuria**
#2 #7	CONSULTS	*Surgery for access placement	*SW - Emotional support, community resources, financial resources *Dietary - If patient has lost 5% of TBW within one month BHH / *BHIV - If portion of tx to be done at home. If nursing required at home. *CNS *Pastoral Care *Psychological Resource Nurse (Gyn / Onc only)	*SW consult completed *Dietary consult completed *CNS consult completed
	PROC. TEST	CBC *SMA 6 *Cr Cl	**CBC / SMA6 results adequate for chemotherapy administration**	*SMA 6 *Mg
#4 #5 #8	TREATMENT		Initiate and monitor IV fluid Administer antiemetic therapy Initiate chemotherapy regimen Initiate oral hygiene	Monitor IV fluid Administer antiemitic Rx Continue chemotherapy regimen Continue oral hygiene Determine accuracy of IV rate - determine if rate needs to be increased with MD approval to facilitate DC

Figure 2-4 Chemotherapy care path.
Courtesy Barnes-Jewish Hospital, St. Louis, Mo.

			DAY 1	DAY 2
	ACTIVITY		Up with assistance	Up with assistance
			Institute fall prevention protocol	Continue fall prevention protocol
	MEDS / IV		Initiate IV access within 2 hours of admission	
			IV site / VAD without redness, swelling, tenderness and with adequate blood return	**IV site / VAD without redness, swelling, tenderness and with adequate blood return**
#2	NUTRITION		Diet as tolerated	Diet as tolerated
			Pt will have 2 or less episodes of nausea / vomiting	**Pt will have 2 or less episodes of nausea / vomiting**
			Pt will have 2 or less episodes of diarrhea	**Pt will have 2 or less episodes of diarrhea**

#1
 	
#7
	PATIENT / FAMILY EDUCATION		**Develop and Initiate Teaching Plan**
			1. Reason for and implication of chemotherapy
			2. Method of administration
			3. Anticipated length of therapy
			4. Names of drugs
			5. Review of each drug
			6. Side effects / management
			  A. Nausea / vomiting
			  B. Anorexia
			  C. Diarrhea
			  D. Constipation
			  E. Alopecia
			  F. Stomatitis
			  G. Skin changes
			  H. Fatigue
			  I. Myelosuppression
			  J. Sexuality implications
			  *K. Renal toxicity
			  *L. Hemorrhagic cystitis
			  *M. Cardiotoxicity
			  *N. Neurotoxicity
			  *O. Ototoxicity
			7. Resources:
			  Cancer Information Center (CIC)
			  American Cancer Society
			  Support groups (refer to CIC)
			*Care of VAD
			Informed consent signed (If chemotherapy is investigational)
			 Give drug information and symptom management sheets to pt
			Pt will have written information outlining chemotherapy drug names, method of administration, common side effects and their management
			Pt will have information regarding support groups, community resources and Cancer Information Center
				Reassess comprehension
				Reinforce teaching
				Teach signs and symptoms to report to MD after discharge
				1. Severe nausea, vomiting, diarrhea, constipation
				2. Temperature greater than 38.5°C
				3. Sore which will not heal
				4. Spontaneous bleeding / bruising
				5. Cough which does not resolve
				6. Frequent, painful urination or blood in urine
				7. Rash of any kind
				8. Sudden weight gain or loss
				9. Pain of unusual intensity or distribution
				
				Medications to **AVOID** without MD order:
				Aspirin
				Antibiotics
				Anticonvulsants
				Anticoagulants
				Barbiturates
				Antihypertensives
				Cough medications
				Darvon
				Hypoglycemics
				Diuretics
				Hormones
				Tranquilizers
				Nasal spray
				Vitamins

	DISCHARGE PLANNING	Evaluate for appropriateness of home infusional therapy	**Pt / family verbalizes understanding of Care Path. Plan of care mutually set with pt / family.**	
#1 #7	PSYCHOSOCIAL / EMOTIONAL NEEDS		Provide opportunity to discuss implications / issues relating to disease / treatment **Patient / family exhibits positive coping skills related to disease / treatment**	Provide opportunity to discuss implications / issues relating to disease / treatment **Patient / family exhibits positive coping skills related to disease / treatment**
	SIGNATURES			

3

100

3100-22 REV. 9/92

Figure 2-4, cont'd

model for a pathway is the **CareMap**. Initially developed at the New England Medical Center in Boston, a CareMap describes the clinical work of each professional discipline and department as it relates to clients' and families' measurable outcomes of care (Zander, 1992). The CareMap is unique in that it incorporates day-to-day expected outcomes, as well as those outcomes anticipated at discharge or at the end of a treatment phase.

For each day, the CareMap outlines clinical assessments, treatments and procedures, dietary interventions, activity and exercise therapies, patient education, and other discharge planning activities necessary to ensure a smooth, uneventful course of recovery. The CareMap tells caregivers what care should be given and when, so that the client is discharged on time and in as healthy a condition as possible. Outcomes incorporated into the CareMap give nurses, physicians, and other care providers important signs for determining if care is appropriate and if the client is responding as desired. In many agencies CareMaps are designed to be documentation tools as well. There will always be clients who do not follow a CareMap's course of recovery. If a client does not proceed as predicted, and if interventions or outcomes do not occur as planned, the team analyzes these variances (see Chapter 18) to decide how to revise the CareMap. When a CareMap is used 24 hours a day by each professional caring for a client, care management toward outcomes is tightly structured (Zander, 1992). In many hospitals a primary nurse (see Chapter 4) coordinates the client's progress through the CareMap. The nurse is responsible for communicating with other caregivers so that the client's progress is uninterrupted.

Case Management.   Case management is a delivery-of-care approach that coordinates and links health care services to clients and their families at single levels of care (e.g., during hospitalization), as well as across levels of care (e.g., from the hospital, to home, to the clinic). Various models have been used in the past to arrange and connect health and social services for clients who have ongoing health problems. Case management is the coordination of client care across care areas, between agencies, and (where possible) extending into wellness (Zander, 1994). In case management, clinicians, either as individuals or as part of a collaborative group, oversee the management of case-type–based care (e.g., clients with specific diagnoses) and are usually held accountable to some standard of cost management and quality. Nurses and other health care professionals work together on an interdisciplinary team focusing on daily evaluation of client progress toward specific outcomes, modifying care based on their evaluation, and preparing clients for timely discharge or transition to other care areas (Lynn and Kelly, 1997). Case management involves managing a client's care across a continuum and is one approach that comes close to providing integration of services. For example, in one model a client with a

chronic disease such as congestive heart failure may be assigned a nurse as a case manager in a medical outpatient clinic. Whenever the client is hospitalized, the same case manager coordinates care so that all providers understand the client's unique needs. When the client is discharged, the case manager will determine if home care or other services are necessary to sustain and support the client's health status. The case manager may visit the client in the home to ensure that health promotion behaviors are being maintained. Institutions have different case management models, based on their services and the needs of clients.

In many institutions case managers are often clinical nurse specialists or primary nurses who have demonstrated an expert level of nursing practice. The case manager becomes accountable for short- and long-range clinical outcomes for an assigned client, as well as overall financial outcomes. The case manager partners with the physician and other care providers to ensure that diagnostic and treatment approaches are appropriate and delivered promptly. Duplication of services and use of unnecessary resources are effectively managed. In addition, the case manager establishes a plan of care with the client, coordinates any consultations, updates the client and family on progress in care, and facilitates discharge to an appropriate health care facility or the home. Case management has been found to make positive contributions to the perceived quality of care delivered by both staff and case managers. Insurance companies are employing case managers for their served population.

Patient-Focused Care.   The concept of patient-focused care was first implemented in 1989 as a cost saving initiative that would maintain quality client care (Clouten and Weber, 1994). It involves bringing all care providers and services to the client, rather than taking the client to the services. Cross-trained caregivers from multidisciplinary backgrounds form self-governed teams, responsible for the "whole" work process that delivers care to clients (Clouten and Weber, 1994). The assumption is that if the tasks that are normally provided by ancillary personnel (e.g., phlebotomy, ECG testing, physical therapy, and respiratory therapy) are moved closer to clients, the number of staff involved and number of steps needed to get the work done will be reduced. Hospitals realize cost savings, and clients perceive better overall care and service. A typical patient-focused care unit has its own admitting, pharmacy, laboratory, and radiology areas. Variations of patient-focused care models exist within different hospitals. However, in some agencies the cost of bringing services to all client care areas has in fact become too costly.

The Future of Health Care

This discussion on the health care delivery system began with the issue of change. Change often creates chaos, but it also creates opportunities to improve the way we do things. The issue in designing and delivering health care is the health and welfare of our population. Health care in the United States has not yet created the perfect continuum of services. However, many health care organizations are striving to find ways to redesign their services, reduce unnecessary costs, improve access to services, and guarantee high-quality client care. Professional nursing finds itself to be an important player in the future of health care delivery.

The ANA (1991) published *Nursing's Agenda for Health Care Reform,* which made recommendations for a restructured health care system, a federally defined standard package of essential health services, a phase-in of essential services for vulnerable client populations, and steps to reduce health care costs. In addition, the *Agenda* recommended provisions for long-term care and insurance reform. The *Agenda* continues to be relevant and timely with the dawn of a new century. The document offers useful strategies designed to provide better-quality health care services to the population, such as the institution of case management. The ANA was futuristic and challenged nurses to become active participants in developing a better health care system. The components of the *Agenda* still apply as nursing strives to participate in the leadership needed to influence the future of health care. The traditional medical model for health care is no longer responsive to the holistic needs of clients. Successful achievement of nursing's agenda will shift the focus of health care from illness and cure to wellness and care (ANA, 1991).

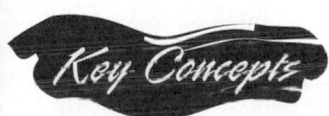

Key Concepts

- Health care regulatory controls include measures that control building of facilities; review quality, quantity, and costs of Medicare services; and eliminate cost-based reimbursement.
- A competitive approach to controlling health care costs includes managed care.
- Managed care programs are designed in principle to contain or reduce costs, improve client satisfaction, and improve the health of individuals.
- With capitated payment, no additional monies are available if a client's care requires more than what is typically included in a capitated rate.
- Levels of care describe the scope of services and settings where health care is offered to clients in all stages of health and illness.
- Nursing centers typically serve vulnerable populations and are unique in providing a nursing model of care with holistic services.
- Primary health care looks beyond personal health services and instead focuses on determinants of health for a population.
- Although hospitalized clients are acutely ill, there is an emphasis on efficient use of resources and timely discharge.

- The intensity of care has increased in restorative care settings because of earlier hospital discharges.
- The standards of care within nursing facilities have increased with the introduction of government regulations.
- Assisted living is one of the fastest growing industries in health care, allowing older adults to remain relatively independent within a partially protective setting.
- Although the Canadian health care system guarantees health care to all citizens, it has problems with access and availability of specialized care services.
- The professional nurse is accountable for remaining competent within the rapidly changing health care environment.
- The nurse can influence client satisfaction by understanding a client's expectations and by giving compassionate care.
- Discharge planning and case management are two approaches designed to ease a client's transition from one level of care to another.
- CareMaps are multidisciplinary plans of care for each day of a client's expected length of stay or episode of treatment.

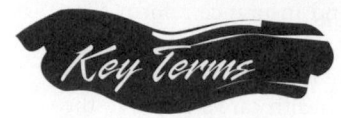

Key Terms

Critical Thinking Exercises

1. Mrs. Jackson is a 52-year-old woman who is employed as a faculty member at a major university. She
was in a car accident 1 week ago, suffering a fractured
left leg and bruised ribs. She hopes to return to work
before the semester is over. Her nursing care needs
have primarily involved pain management, good skin
care around her cast, and exercise therapy. She will
continue to wear a leg cast for about 6 weeks.

    What level of health care will Mrs. Jackson require
before returning to work?

2. Discuss the following scenario with three or four of
your classmates: Patricia is a graduate nurse, assigned
to work on a busy medical nursing division. She has
just attended a staff meeting where her head nurse
talked about the importance of cost control and discharging clients as quickly and efficiently as possible.
Patricia is caring for Mrs. Wilms, a 72-year-old woman
with diabetes and poor vision, who lives alone. Mrs.
Wilms was placed on new medications just that morning. To Patricia's surprise, the physician caring for Mrs.
Wilms announces that Mrs. Wilms must be discharged
that evening. The physician says, "The hospital is pres-
suring me to get clients home as soon as we can."
Patricia considers how to handle this situation, since
she also must care for four other clients.

What problems does this situation create for Mrs.
Wilms? For Patricia? Is the quality of health care for
Mrs. Wilms threatened? How might Patricia respond
to the physician's order without compromising the
quality of care Mrs. Wilms requires? How might the
discharge have been planned better?

References

American Congress of Rehabilitation Medicine: *Guide to interdisciplinary practice in rehabilitation settings,* Skokie, Ill, 1992,
The Congress.

American Nurses Association: *Standards of school nursing practice,* Kansas City, Mo, 1983, The Association.

American Nurses Association: *Nursing's agenda for health care reform,* Kansas City, Mo, 1991, The Association.

American Organization of Nurse Executives: The consumer
health care reform agenda, *Nurs Manage* 25(5):17, 1994.

Appleby C: Managed care's true values, *Hosp Health Netw*
70(8):20, 1996.

Barger S, Rosenfeld P: Models in community health care, *Nurs
and Health Care* 14(8):426, 1993.

Bernstein SJ, Hilborne LH: Clinical indicators: the road to quality care? *Jt Comm J Qual Improv* 19(11):501, 1993.

Berwick DM: Eleven worthy aims for clinical leadership of health
system reform, *JAMA* 272:797, 1994.

Blegen M and others: Nurse staffing and patient outcomes, *Nurs
Res* 47(1):43, 1998.

Buerhaus PI: How changes in payment systems are affecting
nurses. In McCloskey JC, Grace HK, editors: *Current issues in
nursing,* ed 5, St. Louis, 1997, Mosby.

Cambridge Research Institute: *Trends affecting the U.S. health
care system,* 262, Health Planning Information Series, Human Resources Administration, Public Health Service, Department of Health, Education, and Welfare, Washington,
DC; 1976, revised and updated 1992, U.S. Government
Printing Office.

Clemen-Stone S, McGuire SL, Eigsti DG: *Comprehensive community health nursing,* ed 5, St. Louis, 1998, Mosby.

Clouten K, Weber R: Patient focused care . . . playing to win, *Nurs
Manage* 25(2):34, 1994.

Curran C: The future of academic health centers in a cost-driven
market. In McCloskey JC, Grace HK, editors: *Current issues in
nursing,* ed 5, St. Louis, 1997, Mosby.

Donabedian A: Evaluating the quality of medical care, *Milbank
Mem Fund Q* 44:166, 1966.

Ebersole P, Hess P: *Toward healthy aging,* ed 5, St. Louis, 1998,
Mosby.

Fowler FJ, Stokes J: Case management for multiprovider systems,
TCM 2:63, 1996.

Garg ML and others: Controlling health care costs: regulation
versus competition. In McCloskey JC, Grace HK, editors:
Current issues in nursing, ed 5, St. Louis, 1997, Mosby.

Gerteis M and others: *Through the patient's eyes,* San Francisco,
1993, Jossey-Bass.

Gerteis M and others: What patients really want, *HMQ* 11:2,
third quarter, 1993.

Grace HK: From a medical care system for a few to a comprehensive health care system for all. In McCloskey JC, Grace HK, editors: *Current issues in nursing,* ed 5, St. Louis, 1997, Mosby.

Greene J: Blue skies or black eyes? *Hosp Health Netw* 72(8):27, 1998.

Grimaldi P: Variations on the capitation theme, *Nurs Manage* 26(12):12, 1995.

Hatcher PA and others: Impacts: a primary health care game to develop global health consciousness, *J Fam Community Health* 17(2):74, 1994.

Hinshaw AS, Atwood JR: A patient satisfaction instrument: precision by replication, *Nurs Res* 31:170, 1982.

Institute of Medicine: *Defining primary care: an interim report,* Washington, DC, 1994, National Academy Press.

Jamieson MK: Block nursing: practicing autonomous professional nursing in the community, *Nurs Health Care* 11(5):250, 1990.

Joint Commission on Accreditation of Healthcare Organizations: *Manual of hospital accreditation: 2000 standards,* Chicago, 2000, The Commission.

Kane R, Kane R: *Long term care: principles, programs, and policies,* New York, 1987, Springer.

Kane R, Wilson K: *Assisted living in the United States: a new paradigm for residential care for frail older persons?* Washington, DC, 1993, American Association of Retired Persons.

Kerr JCR: The Canadian health care system: overview and issues. In McCloskey JC, Grace HK, editors: *Current issues in nursing,* ed 5, St. Louis, 1997, Mosby.

Latham CL: Humanistic caring: personal influences, coping processes, psychological outcomes and coping effectiveness, *Dissertation Abstracts Int* No. 9030761, 1990.

Lueckenotte A: *Gerontologic nursing,* ed 2, St. Louis, 2000, Mosby.

Lumsdon K: Will nursing ever be the same? *Hosp Health Netw* 69(23):31, 1995.

Lynn MR, Kelley B: Effects of case management on the nursing context: perceived quality of care, work satisfaction, and control over practice, *Image J Nurs Sch* 29(3):237, 1997.

McCourt A: *The specialty practice of rehabilitation nursing: a core curriculum,* ed 3, Skokie, Ill, 1993, The Rehabilitation Nursing Foundation of the Association of Rehabilitation Nurses.

Meyer H: The bottom line on assisted living, *Hosp Health Netw* 72(14):22, 1998.

Montague J: Rural and primary care across the nation, *Hosp Health Netw* 68(8):60, 1994.

Parkman CA: Delegation: are you doing it right? *Am J Nurs* 96(9):43, 1996.

Pender NJ: *Health promotion in nursing practice,* ed 3, St. Louis, 1996, Mosby.

Pew Health Professions Commission: *Health professions education and managed care: challenges and necessary responses,* San Francisco, 1995, UCSF Center for the Health Professions.

Phillips DL, Steel JE: Factors influencing scope of practice in nursing centers, *J Prof Nurs* 10(2):84, 1994.

Riesch SK: Nursing centers: state of the art survey results. In *Nursing centers: meeting the demand for quality health care,* NLN Pub No. 21-2311, New York, 1992, National League for Nursing.

Scott CB, Moneyham L: Perceptions of senior residents about a community-based nursing center, *Image J Nurs Sch* 27(3):181, 1995.

Sharp N: Rural healthcare: new opportunities for nurses, *Nurs Manage* 22(3):22, 1991.

Shoultz J, Hatcher PA: Looking beyond primary care to primary health care: an approach to community-based action, *Nurs Outlook* 45(1):23, 1997.

Shugars D, O'Neil E, Bader J, editors: *Health America: practitioners for 2005,* Durham, NC, 1991, Pew Health Professions Commission.

Stahl D: Subacute care: the future of health care, *Nurs Manage* 25(10):34, 1994.

Stanhope M: Community health nurse in home health and hospice care. In Stanhope M, Lancaster J, editors: *Community health nursing: process and practice for promoting health,* ed 5, St. Louis, 2000, Mosby.

Terris M: Global budgeting and the control of hospital costs, *J Public Health Policy* 12(1):61, 1991.

Tonges MC: Work designs: sociotechnical systems for patient care delivery, *Nurs Manage* 23(1):27, 1992.

Williams SA: The relationship of patients' perceptions of holistic nurse caring to satisfaction with nursing care, *J Nurs Care Qual* 11(5):15, 1997.

Zachariah R, Lundeen SP: Research and practice in an academic community nursing center, *Image J Nurs Sch* 29(3):255, 1997.

Zander K: Quantifying, managing and improving quality, *New Definition* 7(2):1, 1992.

Zander K: Responsive restructuring. IV. Care management and case management, *New Definition* 9(2):1, 1994.

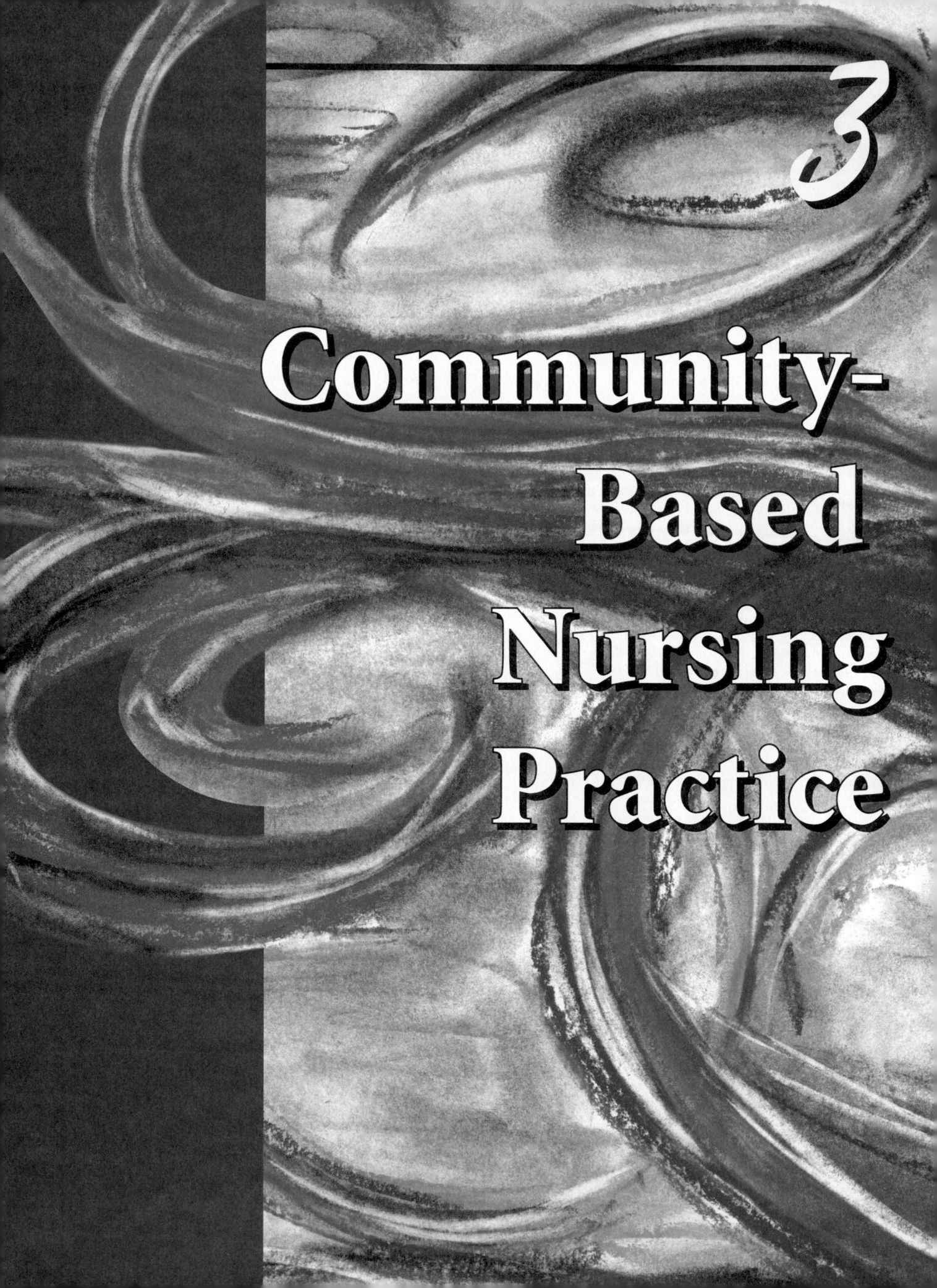

3

Community-Based Nursing Practice

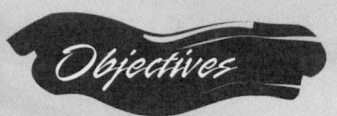

Mastery of content in this chapter will enable the student to:

- Define the key terms listed.
- Explain the relationship between public health and community health nursing.
- Differentiate community health nursing from community-based nursing.
- Discuss the role of the community health nurse.
- Discuss the role of the nurse in community-based practice.
- Explain the characteristics of clients from vulnerable populations that influence a nurse's approach to care.
- Describe the competencies important for success in community-based nursing practice.
- Describe elements of a community assessment.

Historically, nurses have played an active role in the care of people who live in families and communities. Florence Nightingale created district nursing in England, whereby cities were divided into nursing districts and assigned committees of "friendly visitors" to provide health care to the needy (Kalisch and Kalisch, 1977). In 1893 Lillian Wald organized the first visiting nurse service. The nurses in the Henry Street Settlement delivered health care to the poor residents of New York City (Stanhope and Lancaster, 2000). Mary Breckenridge founded the Frontier Nursing Service following World War I in an effort to provide health care for individuals in rural and inaccessible areas in the Appalachian sections of Kentucky (Stanhope and Lancaster, 2000). In each case where a nursing leader or pioneer made a difference, his or her work aimed to improve the living conditions of a population, to make health care more accessible, and to provide illness care within the client's home.

Today, the health care climate is changing, with a gradual transition from acute care delivered in hospital settings to care in the community. There is a greater focus on keeping individuals healthy and well, on providing illness care in the client's home environment, and on containing costs (Ayers, Bruno, and Langford, 1999). With this new focus, nursing is in a particularly advantageous position to play an important role in health care delivery. The focus of keeping individuals healthy and well has always been appropriate to the holistic practice of professional nursing. Nursing's rich history in the development of community health services makes the profession a leader in being able to understand the types of services people require and demand. Community health nursing and community-based nursing are components of health care delivery necessary to improve the health of the general public.

Achieving Healthy Populations and Communities

To gain an understanding of community health and community-based nursing, it is helpful to first understand the perspective of public health practice. The Institute of Medicine (1995) published a report defining **public health** as "what we, as a society, do collectively to assure the conditions in which people can be healthy." Emphasis is on the health of the entire population. Government-funded agencies have historically supported public health programs that improve the safety and adequacy of food supplies, provide a safe water supply and adequate sewage disposal, and improve personal behavior (e.g., reproductive health). Public health policy has largely been responsible for the dramatic gain in life expectancy for Americans during the last century (Stanhope and Lancaster, 2000).

Today, the challenges in public health are many. Social lifestyles, political policy, and economic initiatives have all influenced some of the major public health problems, including the following: an increase in sexually transmitted diseases, environmental pollution, underimmunization of infants and children, and the appearance of new fatal diseases (e.g., acquired immunodeficiency syndrome [AIDS] and Ebola virus infection). More than ever before, a commitment is needed to reform the health care system and bring attention to the health care needs of all communities.

The U.S. Public Health Service emphasizes the essential functions and services of public health that have had the greatest influence on improving the health of the entire population (Figure 3-1, p. 50). The essential services listed in the figure represent the outcomes of the three core functions that exist at all levels of the government: assessment, policy development, and assurance (U.S. Public Health Service, 1993). Assessment includes systematic

PUBLIC HEALTH IN AMERICA

Vision:
Healthy people in healthy communities

Mission:
*Promote physical and mental health and
prevent disease, injury, and disability*

Public health

- Prevents epidemics and the spread of disease
- Protects against environmental hazards
- Prevents injuries
- Promotes and encourages healthy behaviors
- Responds to disasters and assists communities in recovery
- Assures the quality and accessibility of health services

Essential public health services

- Monitors health status to identify community health problems
- Diagnoses and investigates health problems and health hazards in the community
- Informs, educates, and empowers people about health issues
- Mobilizes community partnerships to identify and solve health problems
- Develops policies and plans that support individual and community health efforts
- Enforces laws and regulations that protect health and ensure safety
- Links people to needed personal health services and assures the provision of health care when otherwise unavailable
- Assures a competent public health and personal health care workforce
- Evaluates effectiveness, accessibility, and quality of personal and population-based health services
- Researches for new insights and innovative solutions to health problems

Source: Essential Public Health Services Work Group of the Core
    Public Health Functions Steering Committee

Membership: American Public Health Association
     Association of State and Territorial Health Officials
     National Association of County and City Health Officials
     Institute of Medicine, National Academy of Sciences
     Association of Schools of Public Health
     Public Health Foundation
     National Association of State Alcohol and Drug Abuse Directors
     National Association of State Mental Health Program Directors
     U.S. Public Health Service
      Centers for Disease Control and Prevention
      Health Resources and Services Administration
      Office of the Assistant Secretary for Health
      Substance Abuse and Mental Health Services Administration
      Agency for Health Care Policy and Research
      Indian Health Service
      Food and Drug Administration

Figure 3-1   Public health in America.
From U.S. Public Health Service: *The core functions project,* 1993, Office of Disease Prevention and Health
Promotion.

data collection on the population, monitoring of the population's health status, and making information available on the health of the community (Stanhope and Lancaster, 2000). Examples of assessment include gathering information on **incident rates** for cancer or flu immunization rates for older adults, and reporting the number of annual traffic accidents. Policy development refers to health professionals providing leadership in developing policies that support the population's health. An example is using research-based findings in developing policies such as the use of seat belts or fluoridation of the water. Assurance refers to the role of public health in making sure that essential community-wide health services are available (Stanhope and Lancaster, 2000). Examples of assurance include the provision of prenatal care to the uninsured and establishing educational programs to ensure the competency of public health professionals. Population-based public health programs focus on disease prevention, health protection, and health promotion. This focus provides the foundation for health care services at all levels (see Chapter 2) (Figure 3-2).

The five levels of services in the health services pyramid must be part of a health care system with health as a goal (U.S. Public Health Service, 1995). When the lower services are effective, there is a greater likelihood of the higher tiers contributing efficiently to health improvement of the population. For example, if the water supply to a community is poor, it becomes more difficult to en-

force health promotion efforts and to prevent the occurrence of disease. On the other hand, when a community has the resources for mosquito control and immunizations offered in public schools, primary preventive care services can focus on child developmental problems and child safety. The principles of public health practice aim at achieving a healthy environment for all individuals to live in. These principles can be applied with individuals, families, and the communities in which they live. Nursing plays a role in all levels of the health services pyramid. By using public health principles, the nurse is able to better understand the types of environments in which clients live and the types of interventions necessary to help keep clients healthy.

Community Health Nursing

Frequently the terms *community health nursing* and *public health nursing* are used interchangeably. There are similarities. A public health focus requires understanding the needs of a **population,** or a collection of individuals who have in common one or more personal or environmental characteristics (Stanhope and Lancaster, 2000). Examples of populations might include high-risk infants, older adults, or a cultural group such as Native Americans. A public health professional must understand factors that influence health promotion and health maintenance of groups, the trends and patterns influencing the incidence of disease within populations, environmental factors contributing to health and illness, and the political processes used to affect public policy. A public health nurse requires preparation at the basic entry level to hold a baccalaureate degree in nursing that includes educational preparation and clinical practice in public health nursing. A specialist in public health is prepared at the graduate level with a focus in the public health sciences (*Consensus Conference,* 1985).

Community health nursing is a nursing approach that merges knowledge from the public health sciences with professional nursing theories to safeguard and improve the health of populations in the community (Ayers, Bruno, and Langford, 1999). The focus of such nursing care is somewhat broader than that of public health, with an emphasis on the health of a community. In addition to considering the needs of populations, the community health nurse is prepared to provide direct care services to subpopulations within a community. These subpopulations may be a clinical focus in which the nurse has gained expertise (e.g., a case manager who follows older adults recovering from stroke and sees the need for community rehabilitation services, or a nurse practitioner who gives immunizations to clients with the objective of managing communicable disease within the community). By focusing on subpopulations, the community health nurse cares for the community as a whole and considers the individual or family to be only one member of

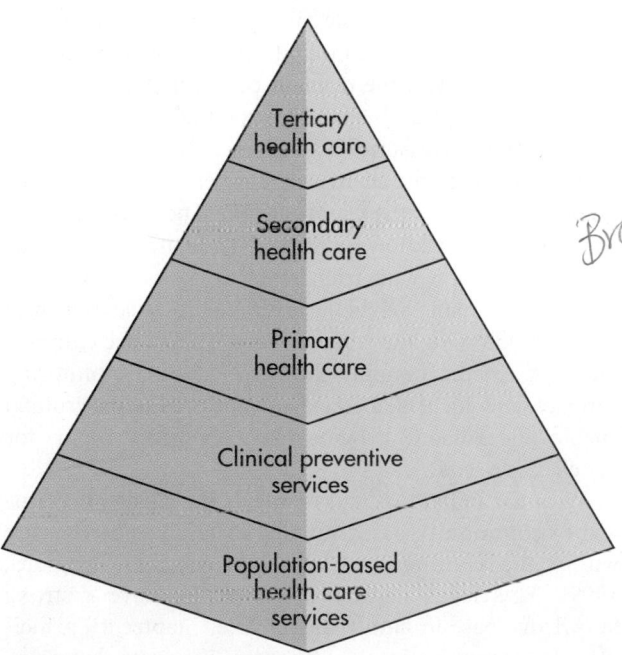

Figure 3-2 Health services pyramid.
From Stanhope M, Lancaster J: *Community health nursing: a process and practice for promoting health,* ed 5, St. Louis, 2000, Mosby.

a group at risk. Competence as a community health nurse requires the ability to use interventions that take into account the broad social and political context in which community problems occur and are resolved (Stanhope and Lancaster, 2000). The educational requirements for entry-level nurses practicing in community health nursing roles are not as clear-cut as those for public health nurses. An advanced degree may not be required by a hiring agency. However, nurses with a graduate degree in nursing who practice in community settings are considered community health nurse specialists, regardless of their public health experience (Stanhope and Lancaster, 2000).

NURSING PRACTICE IN COMMUNITY HEALTH

Population-focused nursing practice requires a unique set of skills and knowledge. In the health care delivery system, nurses who become expert in community health practice may have advanced nursing degrees, yet the baccalaureate-prepared generalist can also become quite competent in formulating and applying population-focused assessments and interventions (Diekemper, SmithBattle, and Drake, 1999). The expert community health nurse comes to understand the needs of a population or community through experience with individual families and working through their social and health care issues. Critical thinking becomes important for the nurse who applies knowledge of public health principles, community health nursing, family theory, and communication in finding the best approaches in partnering with families. Diekemper, SmithBattle, and Drake (1999) interviewed community health nurses to hear their stories and to understand what population-focused practice involves. Often community health nurses see their practice evolve "naturally" as they serve families and communities. This is best supported when the working environment does not restrict the nurse's ability to work closely with members of the community.

A successful community health nursing practice involves building relationships with the community and being responsive to changes within the community (Diekemper, SmithBattle, and Drake, 1999). An example is seeing a need (e.g., the incidence of grandparents assuming child care responsibilities) and establishing an instructional program in cooperation with local schools to assist and support grandparents in caregiving. The community health nurse is socially responsive, becoming an active part of a community, knowing its members, its needs, and its resources, and then working to establish effective health promotion and disease prevention programs. This may require working with highly resistant systems (e.g., welfare system) and trying to encourage them to be more responsive to the needs of a population. Skills of client advocacy, communicating people's concerns, and designing new systems in cooperation with existing systems help to make community nursing practice effective.

Community-Based Nursing

Community-based nursing involves the acute and chronic care of individuals and families that enhances their capacity for self-care and promotes autonomy in decision making (Ayers, Bruno, and Langford, 1999). Although care takes place in community settings such as the home or a clinic, the focus is nursing care of the individual or family. The nurse's competence is based on critical thinking and decision making at the level of the individual client—assessing health status, selecting nursing interventions, and evaluating outcomes of care. Because direct care services are provided where clients live, work, and play, it is important for community-based nursing to remain individual and family oriented and to appreciate the values of a community (Zotti, Brown, and Stotts, 1996).

The philosophical foundation for community-based nursing is the human ecological model, which conceptualizes human systems as open and interactive with the environment (Chalmers and others, 1998). In an ecological model the individual is viewed within the larger systems of family, community, culture, and society. The social interaction units seen in Figure 3-3 depict four circles: the inner circle of the client and the immediate family, the second circle of people and settings that have frequent contact with the client and family, the third circle of the local community and its values and policies, and the outer circle of larger social systems such as government and church (Ayers, Bruno, and Langford, 1999). A nurse in a community-based practice must understand the interaction of all of the units while caring for the client and family in their natural environment. The nurse will typically become involved in the domain of the first three circles when providing health care. For example, a home health nurse working with a newly diagnosed diabetic client will work closely with the client and family to establish a comprehensive plan for the client's health. The nurse may become involved in knowing the habits or lifestyle patterns when the client is with friends and co-workers to anticipate ways to plan the client's exercise schedule and meal routines. Knowing the resources available in the community (e.g., medical supply shops for glucose monitoring supplies and local diabetes association support groups) enables the nurse to provide comprehensive support for the client's needs.

With the individual and family as the clients, the context of community-based nursing is family-centered care within the community (Ayers, Bruno, and Langford, 1999). This focus requires the nurse to have a strong knowledge base in family theory (see Chapter 8), principles of communication (see Chapter 22), group dynamics, and cultural diversity (see Chapter 7). The nurse learns to partner with clients and families so that ultimately the client and family assume responsibility for their health care decisions. The family becomes involved in planning,

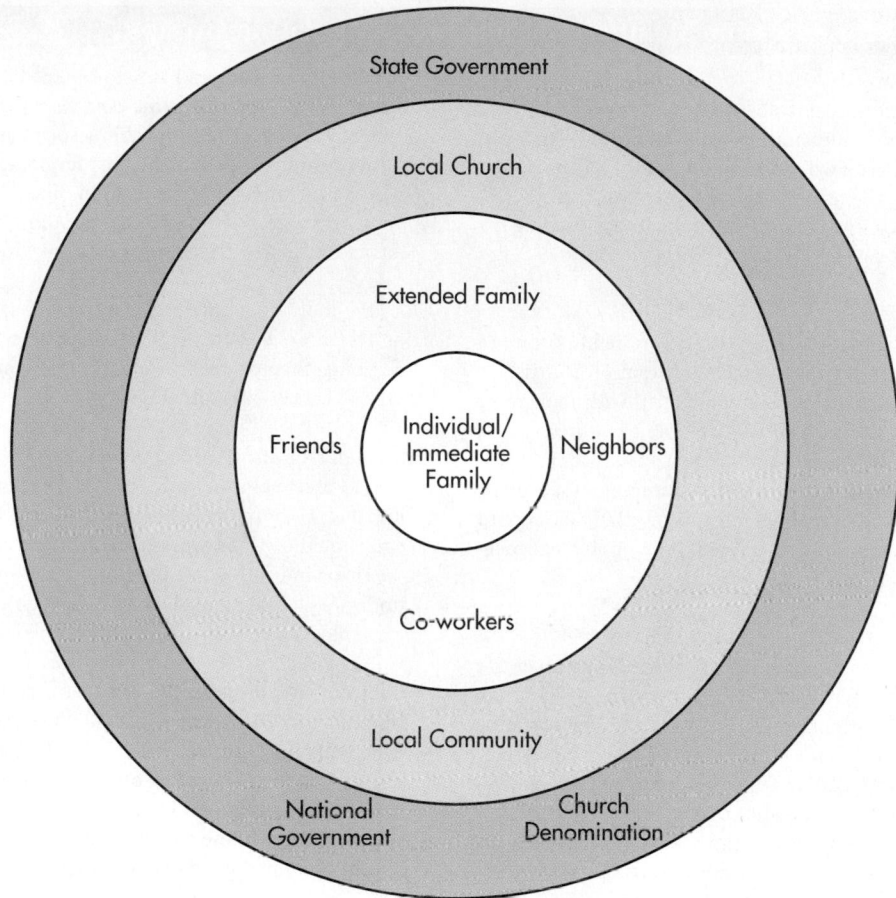

Figure 3-3 These concentric circles represent the social interaction units of the human ecology model.
From Ayers M, Bruno AA, Langford RW: *Community-based nursing care: making the transition,* St. Louis, 1999,
Mosby.

decision making, implementation, and evaluation of health care approaches.

VULNERABLE POPULATIONS

Although the community-based nurse cares for clients from diverse cultures and backgrounds, and with various health conditions, changes in the health care delivery system have made high-risk groups the nurse's principal clients. Home health nurses, for example, are not likely to visit low-risk mothers and babies. Instead, adolescent mothers or mothers with drug addiction are more likely to receive home care services. **Vulnerable populations** of clients are those who are more likely to develop health problems as a result of excess risks, who have limits in access to health care services, or who are dependent on others for care. Individuals living in poverty, older adults, homeless persons, individuals in abusive relationships, substance abusers, severely mentally ill persons, and new immigrants are examples of vulnerable populations. Vulnerable individuals and their families often belong to more than one of these groups. Frequently these clients come from varied cultures, have different beliefs and

values, face language barriers, and have few sources of social support (Chalmers and others, 1998). Their special needs form the backdrop for the challenges nurses face in caring for increasingly complex acute and chronic health conditions.

To become competent in the care of vulnerable populations, it is especially important for nurses in community-based practice to become culturally competent. Chapter 7 addresses factors influencing individual differences within cultural groups and the nurse's role in providing culturally appropriate care. To be culturally competent, the nurse must be more than just sensitive to a client's cultural uniqueness. The nurse must be able to appraise and understand a client and family's cultural beliefs, values, and practices to determine their specific needs and the interventions that will most likely be successful in improving their state of health. The nurse cannot judge or evaluate a client's beliefs and values about health in terms of the nurse's own culture. Communication and caring practices become critical in learning a client's perceptions of his or her problems and then planning health care strategies that will be meaningful, culturally appropriate, and successful.

Guidelines for Assessing Members of Vulnerable Population Groups   Box 3-1

SETTING THE STAGE

Create a comfortable, nonthreatening environment.

Learn as much as you can about the culture of the clients you work with so that you will understand cultural practices and values that may influence their health care practices.

Provide culturally competent assessment by understanding the meaning of language and nonverbal behavior in the client's culture.

Be sensitive to the fact that the individual or family you are assessing may have other priorities that are more important to them. These might include financial or legal problems. You may need to give them some tangible help with their most pressing priority before you will be able to address issues that are more traditionally thought of as health concerns.

Collaborate with others as appropriate; you should not provide financial or legal advice. However, you should make sure to connect your client with someone who can and will help them.

NURSING HISTORY OF AN INDIVIDUAL OR FAMILY

You may have only one opportunity to work with a vulnerable person or family. Try to complete a history that will provide all the essential information you need to help the individual or family on that day. This means that you will have to organize in your mind exactly what you need to ask, and no more, and why the data are necessary.

It will help to use a comprehensive assessment form that has been modified to focus on the special needs of the vulnerable population group with whom you work. However, be flexible. With some clients, it will be both impractical and unethical to cover all questions on a comprehensive form. If you know that you are likely to see the client again, ask the less pressing questions at the next visit.

Be sure to include questions about social support, economic status, resources for health care, developmental issues, current health problems, medication, and how the person or family manages their health status. Your goal is to obtain information that will enable you to provide family-centered care.

Does the individual have any condition that compromises his or her immune status, such as AIDS, or is the individual undergoing therapy that would result in immunodeficiency, such as cancer chemotherapy?

PHYSICAL EXAMINATION OR HOME ASSESSMENT

Again, complete as thorough a physical examination (on an individual) or home assessment as you can. Keep in mind that you should collect only data for which you have a use.

Be alert for indications of physical abuse, substance use (e.g., underweight, being inadequately clothed).

You can assess a family's living environment using good observational skills. Does the family live in an insect- or rat-infested environment? Do they have running water, functioning plumbing, electricity, and a telephone? Is perishable food (e.g., mayonnaise) left sitting out on tables and countertops? Are bed linens reasonably clean? Is paint peeling on the walls and ceilings? Is ventilation adequate? Is the temperature of the home adequate? Is the family exposed to raw sewage or animal waste? Is the home adjacent to a busy highway, possibly exposing the family to high noise levels and automobile exhaust?

From Stanhope M, Lancaster J: *Community health nursing: process and practice for promoting health*, ed 5, St. Louis, 2000, Mosby.

Vulnerable populations typically experience poorer outcomes than those clients with ready access to resources and health care services. Dramatically shorter life spans and higher morbidity rates pose real threats to members of ethnically and racially diverse minority groups (Porter and Villarruel, 1993). Members of vulnerable groups frequently have cumulative risks or combinations of risk factors that make them more sensitive to the adverse effects of individual risk factors that others might overcome (Nichols and others, 1986). It becomes essential for the community-based nurse to assess members of vulnerable populations by taking into account the multiple stressors that affect their clients' lives. It is also important to learn the clients' strengths and resources for coping with stressors. Box 3-1 summarizes guidelines to follow when assessing members of vulnerable population groups.

Poor and Homeless Persons.   People who live in poverty are more likely to live in hazardous environments, work at high-risk jobs, eat less nutritious diets, and have multiple stressors in their life. When the life expectancy of European Americans and African-Americans have been compared, the causes of the differences have been found to be related to low socioeconomic status rather than race (Kochanek and others, 1994). Clients with low income not only lack financial resources, but also are forced to live in poor living environments and face practical problems such as poor or unavailable transportation. Homeless clients have even fewer resources than the poor. They do not have the advantage of shelter and must cope with finding a place to sleep at night and finding food. Exacerbations of chronic health problems are common because the homeless have no place to store medications if they can afford them and cannot obtain nutritious meals. In addition, they lack a healthy balance of rest and activity because of the necessity to walk throughout the day to meet basic needs and because of vagrancy laws that prohibit loitering (Sebastian, 1985). There is a high incidence of mental illness, personality disorder, and substance abuse among the homeless population. The nurse must help homeless people identify the resources they may have (e.g., mobile health care unit, Figure 3-4), their eligibility

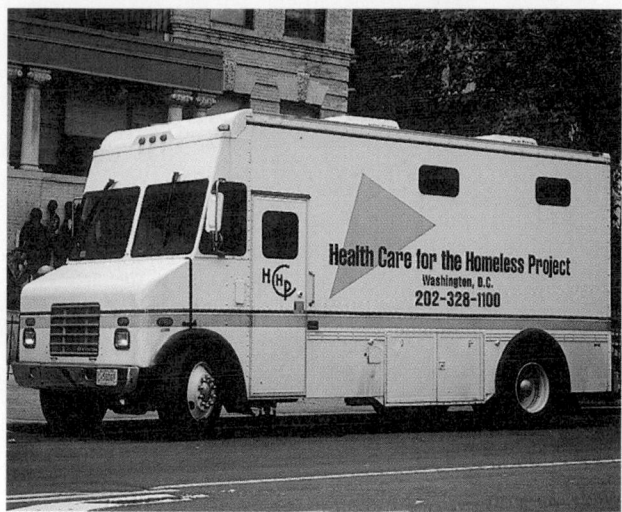

Figure 3-4   The homeless population has unique health care needs.

for assistance, and the interventions that may promote an increased ability to improve their health status (Scholler-Jaquish, 1995) (Table 3-1, p. 56).

Abused Clients.
Physical, emotional, and sexual abuse, as well as neglect, are major public health problems affecting older adults, women, and children (Sebastian, 1996). Risk factors for abusive relationships include mental health problems, substance abuse, socioeconomic stressors, and dysfunctional family relationships. An important principle in dealing with clients at risk or who may have suffered abuse is to provide protection. The nurse must interview clients at a time when their privacy is ensured and the individual suspected of being the abuser is not present. Clients who have been abused fear retribution if they discuss their problems with a health care provider. Most states have abuse hot lines that must be notified when an individual has been identified as being at risk.

Substance Abusers.
Substance abuse is a blanket term used to describe more than the use of illegal drugs. This term also includes the abuse of alcohol and prescribed medications such as antianxiety agents and narcotic analgesics. A client with substance abuse has health and socioeconomic problems. The socioeconomic problems result from the financial strain of the cost of drugs, criminal convictions from illegal activities used to obtain drugs, communicable disease from sharing drug paraphernalia, and family breakdown. For example, health problems for cocaine users can include nasal and sinus disorders and cardiac alterations that can be fatal (Sebastian, 1996). Health care providers who objectively assess substance use in terms of the amount, frequency,

and type of use will gain useful information to assist the substance abuser. Frequently these clients may avoid health care for fear of judgmental attitudes by health care providers and concern over being turned in to criminal authorities.

Severely Mentally Ill Persons.
When a client has a severe mental illness such as schizophrenia or severe personality disorders such as bipolar disorder there are multiple health and socioeconomic problems that must be explored. Many clients with pervasive mental illnesses are homeless or marginally housed. Others lack the ability to maintain employment or to even care for themselves on a daily basis. Clients suffering from pervasive mental illness require medication therapy, counseling, housing, and vocational assistance. The mentally ill are no longer routinely hospitalized in long-term psychiatric institutions. Instead, the goal is to offer community resources within their community; however, comprehensive service networks have not developed in every community (Stanhope and Lancaster, 2000). Many clients are left with fewer and more fragmented services, with little skill in surviving and functioning within the community. There is an increased number of young mentally ill persons who have had only episodic hospital care. Collaboration with multiple community resources is a key to helping the pervasively mentally ill obtain adequate health care.

Older Adults.
With the increase in the older adult population, there is a simultaneous increase in the number of clients suffering from chronic disease and a greater demand for health care services. Health promotion and prevention of disease are infrequently associated with older adults because of the image of aging and its association with poor health and disease (Birchfield, 1996). However, it is important for the nurse to view health promotion from a broad context. This begins with the understanding of what health means to older adults and the steps they can take to maintain their own health (Box 3-2, p. 57). When individuals feel empowered to control their own health, disability from chronic disease can be reduced. There is an opportunity to improve the lifestyle of older adults and their quality of life. Table 3-2 describes the major health problems encountered by older adults and the role of community health nurses.

COMPETENCY IN COMMUNITY-BASED NURSING
A nurse in community-based practice must have a variety of skills and talents to be successful in assisting clients with their health care needs and in developing relationships within the community. The Pew Health Professions Commission, in response to the *Healthy People 2000* initiative (see Chapter 1), recommended competencies for health care professionals that included the practice of prevention and caring for the community's health (Box 3-3, p. 59). Being able to apply the nursing process (see Unit 3)

Table 3-1	**Nursing Interventions for Care of the Homeless**	
Level of Prevention		
Primary Intervention	Secondary Intervention	Tertiary Intervention
Stage 1: Prevent or Reduce Frequency of Homeless Experiences		
Improvement of physical environment (community, home)	Health screening	Control of spread of disease
Provision of adequate housing	Referral programs	Treatment of tuberculosis and acquired immunodeficiency syndrome (AIDS)
Health education	Case management	Drug and alcohol treatment programs
Sex education	Case finding	Treatment of mental illnesses
Drug and alcohol education	Screening for iron, tuberculosis, human immunodeficiency virus (HIV), hemoglobin, substance use	Strengthening of support systems
Good nutrition	Diagnostic services	
Pregnancy and nutrition	Treatment of acute illnesses	
Advocacy	Treatment of potentially life-threatening illnesses (e.g., rehydration of young children)	
Support of legislation that helps the poor		
Increased minimum wage		
Child day care		
Access to health care		
Stage 2: Assist Homeless in Reducing Factors That Keep Them Homeless and in Gaining Skills to Move Into Higher Level of Functioning		
Teaching regarding effective coping behaviors	Screening for chronic illnesses	Treatment for major mental illnesses
Teaching regarding avoidance of potentially violent situations	Leg ulcers	Treatment for major illnesses and injuries
Advocacy	Drug abuse	Detoxification programs
Health education	Trauma	Management of chronic illnesses
Interpersonal skills training	Hypertension	Management of AIDS symptoms
Development of interrelationships with service providers	Cancer	
Recommendations regarding food and handling and exposure to infectious diseases	Immunizations	
Teaching regarding importance of good nutrition	Monitoring of psychiatric status and compliance with medical regimen	
Referrals for legal assistance	Monitoring for status of infectious diseases	
	Provision of on-site care in shelters and service centers	
Stage 3: Increase Amount of Interaction With Service Providers and Acceptance of Resources		
Advocacy	Case management	Protection from violence
Outreach program	Mobile treatment programs	Promotion of wet and dry detoxification
Promotion of legislation regarding homeless mentally ill	Monitoring for changes in health status	Treatment for major illnesses
Promotion of legislation for care to homeless	Provision of access to basic nutritional needs	Help for persons in getting into mental health programs
Location of homeless through outreach programs		Supervised housing
Multiservice programs in service sites		Promotion of increased independence

Modified from Scholler-Jaquish A: Homelessness in America. In Smith CM, Maurer FA, editors: *Community health nursing: theory and practice,* Philadelphia, 1995, WB Saunders.

in a critical thinking approach ensures good, individualized nursing care for specific clients and their families. Additional competencies reviewed here enable the nurse to deliver care within the context of the client's community so that long-term success is more likely.

Case Manager.   Chapter 2 describes briefly the case management model for care delivery. In community-based practice, case management is an important competency. It is the ability to establish an appropriate plan of care based on assessment of clients and families and to co-

| Research HIGHLIGHT | Box 3-2 |

RESEARCH ABSTRACT

A sample of 30 elderly women (10 African-Americans, 10 Chinese-Americans, and 10 European-Americans), all over 60 years of age, were asked to participate in in-depth interviews and complete a series of surveys designed to determine their health promotion practices. Interviews were conducted in the older adults' homes. Themes and core categories were identified by the researchers. The participants defined health as being able to enjoy one's life, doing things one desires to do, feeling good, and living without pain. Health promotion measures identified included the following: exercise ("get moving"), getting a regular checkup, knowing how to care for self, eating right, and keeping busy. Despite similar health promotion measures among subjects, there were differences in how members of each ethnic group defined each category. For example, "get moving" meant walking to African-Americans, walking and doing Tai Chi to Chinese-Americans, and joining an exercise club or walking or dancing to European-Americans. The researchers also found that language and transportation barriers and distrust of the health care system can influence success with health promotion activities.

IMPLICATIONS FOR PRACTICE
- Nurses must learn how members of an ethnic group interpret health-promoting measures.
- Community health nurses need to integrate ethnic differences into their care.
- Programs to improve access to and use of preventive services should be linguistically appropriate and culturally sensitive.

REFERENCE

Zhan L and others: Promoting health: perspectives from ethnic elderly women, *J Community Health Nurs* 15:31, 1998.

ordinate needed resources and services for the client's well-being (Kenyon and others, 1990). Generally, a community-based nurse will assume responsibility for the case management of multiple clients. This usually involves clients who are at greatest risk for needing extensive coordination of health care services (e.g., clients with neurological disease, trauma victims, psychiatric clients, and clients with complex medical conditions). The greatest challenge is coordinating the activities of multiple providers and payers, in different settings, throughout a client's continuum of care (Box 3-4, p. 59). Although the nurse may be employed and located in one setting, the nurse will influence the selection and monitoring of care provided in other settings by formal and informal caregivers (Stanhope and Lancaster, 2000). An effective case manager eventually learns the roadblocks, deficits, and even the opportunities that exist within the community that influence the ability to find solutions for clients'

health care needs. Case management with individual clients and families reveals the big picture of health services and the health status of a community.

Collaborator. A nurse who practices community-based nursing must be competent in working not only with individuals and their families, but also with other related health care disciplines. Collaboration, or working in a combined effort with all those involved in care delivery, is required for a mutually acceptable plan to be obtained that will achieve common goals (Ayers, Bruno, and Langford, 1999). For example, when a client is discharged home with terminal cancer, the home health nurse must be able to collaborate with hospice staff, social workers, and pastoral care to initiate a plan to support the client and family. For collaboration to be effective, there must be mutual trust and respect for each professional's abilities and contributions. Similarly, clients must share trust in the health care providers. Teamwork is central to being able to explore client issues and those of team members, knowing the contributions each professional can offer, clarifying roles, and developing a plan of care that client and health care providers can accept and support.

Educator. Community-based nurses must also demonstrate competency in client education. The nurse will have the opportunity to work with single individuals, as well as groups of clients. A nurse who is competent in establishing relationships with community service organizations by being accessible and knowing the needs of the organization's clients can offer educational support to a wide range of client groups. Perinatal classes, infant care, child safety, and cancer screening are just some of the health education programs in which a nurse in community practice may participate.

With the goal of helping clients assume responsibility for their own health care, the role of educator takes on greater importance in community-based nursing than in episodic care (Ayers, Bruno, and Langford, 1999). Clients and families are expected to gain the skills and knowledge needed to learn how to give care themselves. Chapter 23 covers client education principles. In community-based practice the nurse must assess a client's learning needs and readiness to learn within the context of the individual, the systems the individual interacts with (e.g., family, business, school), and the resources available for support. Teaching skills likewise must be adapted so that the nurse can instruct within the home setting and make the learning process meaningful. The nurse in community-based practice has the opportunity to follow clients over time. Planning for return demonstration of skills, use of follow-up phone calls, and referral to community support and self-help groups give the nurse the opportunity to provide continuity in instruction and to reinforce important instructional topics. Evaluation of client learning occurs over time, requiring the nurse's patience and commitment.

Table 3-2	**Major Health Problems in Elders and Community Health Nursing Roles**
Problem	**Community Health Nursing Roles**
Hypertension	Monitor blood pressure and weight; educate about nutrition and antihypertensive drugs; teach stress management techniques; promote an optimal balance between rest and activity; establish blood pressure screening programs; assess client's current lifestyle and promote lifestyle changes; promote dietary modifications by using techniques such as a diet diary.
Cancer	Obtain health history; promote monthly breast self-examinations and yearly Pap smears and mammograms for older women; promote regular physical examinations; encourage smokers to stop smoking; correct misconceptions about processes of aging; provide emotional support and quality of care during diagnostic and treatment procedures.
Arthritis	Help adult avoid the false hope and expense of arthritis quackery; educate adult about management of activities, correct body mechanics, availability of mechanical appliances, and adequate rest; promote stress management; counsel and assist the family to improve communication, role negotiation, and use of community resources.
Visual impairment (e.g., loss of visual acuity, eyelid disorders, opacity of the lens)	Provide support in a well-lighted, glare-free environment; use printed aids with large, well-spaced letters; assist adult with cleaning eyeglasses; help make arrangements for vision examinations and obtain necessary prostheses; teach adult to be cautious of fraudulent advertisements.
Hearing impairment (e.g., presbycusis)	Speak with clarity at a moderate volume and pace and face audience when performing health teaching; help make arrangements for hearing examination and obtain necessary prostheses; teach adult to be cautious of fraudulent advertisements.
Confusional states	Provide complete assessment; correct underlying causes of disease (if possible); provide for a protective environment; promote activities that reinforce reality; assist with adequate personal hygiene, nutrition, and hydration; provide emotional support to the family; recommend applicable community resources such as adult day care, home health aides, and homemaker services.
Alzheimer's disease	Maintain optimal functioning, protection, and safety; foster human dignity; demonstrate to the primary family caregiver techniques to dress, feed, and toilet adult; provide frequent encouragement and emotional support to caregiver; act as an advocate for client when dealing with respite care and support groups; ensure that clients' rights are protected; provide support to maintain family members' physical and mental health; maintain family stability; recommend financial services if needed.
Dental problems	Perform oral assessment and refer as necessary; emphasize regular brushing and flossing, proper nutrition, and dental examinations; encourage clients with dentures to wear and take care of them; allay fears about dentist; help provide access to financial services (if necessary) and access to dental care facilities.
Drug use and abuse	Obtain drug history; educate adult about safe storage, risks of drug, drug-drug, and drug-food interactions, and general information about drug (e.g., drug name, purpose, side effects, dosage); instruct adult about presorting techniques (using small containers with one dose of drug that are labeled with specific administration times).
Substance abuse	Arrange and monitor detoxification if appropriate; counsel adults about substance abuse; promote stress management to avoid need for drugs or alcohol; encourage adult to use self-help groups such as Alcoholics Anonymous and Al-Anon; educate public about dangers of substance abuse.

From Stanhope M, Lancaster J: *Community health nursing: process and practice for promoting health*, ed 4, St. Louis, 1996, Mosby.

Counselor. The role of counselor assists clients in identifying and clarifying health problems and in choosing appropriate courses of action to solve those problems (Ayers, Bruno, and Langford, 1999). A counselor is responsible to provide information, listen objectively, and be supportive, caring, and trustworthy. Counselors do not make decisions; they help clients reach decisions that best suit them (Stanhope and Lancaster, 2000). The nurse in community-based practice will face many situations where counseling is an important skill. Clients and families often require assistance in first identifying and clarifying health problems. For example, a client who repeatedly vocalizes a problem in being unable to follow a prescribed diet may actually have the problem of being unable to afford nutritious foods or have family members who do not support good eating habits. The nurse may discuss with the client factors that block or aid problem resolution, identify a range of solutions, and then discuss which solutions are most likely to be successful. The nurse encourages the client to make decisions and fosters confidence in the choice that is made.

An important factor in the nurse's ability to be an ef-

Pew Commission Competencies for Health Care Practitioners   Box 3-3

CARE FOR THE COMMUNITY HEALTH
Broad understanding of health determinants (environmental, socioeconomic, behavioral, genetic, medical)
Ability to work with others in the community to integrate services to prevent illness and promote and protect health

EXPAND ACCESS TO EFFECTIVE CARE
Participation in efforts that promote health care access for individuals, families, and communities

PROVIDE CONTEMPORARY CLINICAL CARE
Possession of up-to-date clinical skills that meet the public's health care needs

EMPHASIZE PRIMARY CARE
Ability and willingness to function in new health care settings
Participation in interdisciplinary arrangements designed to meet primary health care needs

TAKE PART IN COORDINATED CARE
Ability to work as effective team member in organized settings
Emphasis on quality, cost-effective, and integrated services

ENSURE COST-EFFECTIVE, APPROPRIATE CARE
Ability to balance cost and quality in decision-making processes

PRACTICE PREVENTION
Emphasis on primary and secondary preventive strategies with all people

INVOLVE CLIENTS AND FAMILIES IN DECISION-MAKING PROCESS
Expectation of active participation in health care decisions by individuals and their families
Active involvement of client and family in evaluation of quality and acceptability of care received

PROMOTE HEALTHY LIFESTYLES
Ability to assist individuals, families, and communities in maintaining healthy behaviors

ASSESS AND USE TECHNOLOGY APPROPRIATELY
Understanding of, and ability to use, increasingly complex technology

IMPROVE THE HEALTH CARE SYSTEM
Understanding of determinants and operations of the health care system from political, economic, social, and legal perspectives
Ability to improve the operations and accountability of the health care system

MANAGE INFORMATION
Ability to manage and use large volumes of scientific, technological, and client information

UNDERSTAND THE ROLE OF THE PHYSICAL ENVIRONMENT
Ability to assess, prevent, and mitigate impact of environmental hazards on the public

PROVIDE COUNSELING ON ETHICAL ISSUES
Participation in discussions of ethical issues in health care that affect the public and the health care system
Provision of counseling to clients about pertinent ethical issues

ACCOMMODATE EXPANDED ACCOUNTABILITY
Responsiveness to increasing levels of public, governmental, and third-party participation in, and scrutiny of, the shape and direction of the health care system

PARTICIPATE IN A RACIALLY AND CULTURALLY DIVERSE SOCIETY
Appreciation of growing diversity of the population
Understanding of health status and care needs from different cultural perspectives

CONTINUE TO LEARN
Anticipation of changes in health care and maintenance of professional competency throughout practice life

Data from Pew Health Professions Commission: *Health America: practitioners for 2005,* Durham, NC, 1991, The Commission.

Factors Affecting Solutions in the Case Management Process   Box 3-4

Medical necessity
Access to primary care physicians
Family members
Durable medical equipment suppliers
Health maintenance organization (HMO) management

Insurance regulations
Other health care providers
Care standards
Care quality
Costs

Data from Hicks LL, Stallmeyer JM, Coleman JR: *The role of the nurse in managed care,* Washington, DC, 1993, American Nurses Publishing.

fective counselor is knowing what a community can offer clients. Frequently clients must go outside their own family to obtain the support that is necessary to improve their health status. Directing clients to appropriate resources requires the nurse to know those resources well; what services do agencies provide, who are the staff who can be accessed quickly, what reimbursement limitations affect access, and is there coordination between agencies within the community?

Client Advocate.   Client advocacy perhaps is even more important today in community-based practice because of the confusion surrounding access to health care services. Clients often need someone to help them walk through the system, identifying where to go for services, how to reach the individuals with the appropriate authority, what services to request, and how to follow through with the information they received. The community-based nurse may be the one who presents the client's point of view so that appropriate resources can be obtained. The nurse will provide the information necessary for clients to make informed decisions in utilizing and choosing services appropriately. Then the nurse supports clients in defending those decisions. There are similar principles used in both counseling and advocacy.

Change Agent.   A community-based nurse also must be competent as a change agent. This involves seeking to implement new and more effective approaches to problems (Ayers, Bruno, and Langford, 1999). The nurse may act as a change agent within a family system or intercede with problems that reside within the client's community. The nurse might identify any number of problems (e.g., quality of community child care services, availability of older adult day care services, or the status of neighborhood violence). The nurse may act to empower individuals and their families to creatively solve problems or become instrumental in creating change within a health care agency. As a change agent, the nurse gathers and analyzes facts and implements programs. This requires the nurse to be very familiar with the community itself. Many communities are resistant to change, preferring to provide services in an established manner as they always have. Before the nurse can analyze necessary facts, it becomes necessary to manage conflict between the health care providers involved in the client's care, clarify their roles, and clearly identify the needs of the clients. If the community has a history of poor problem-solving, the nurse may have to focus on developing problem-solving capabilities (Stanhope and Lancaster, 2000). Box 3-5 describes the factors that increase the likelihood of change being accepted and adopted. Each factor should be considered as having potential in helping the nurse successfully bring about change. For example, if a nurse is trying to improve a client's adherence to routine health care visits, it may be useful to offer an alternative site, such as a nursing clinic,

---

Success Factors in Adopting Change   Box 3-5

The innovation or change must be perceived as more advantageous than other alternatives. The nature of the innovation determines what specific type of relative advantage (e.g., social, economic, community good) is important to those who adopt the change.

The innovation or change must be compatible with existing values, past experiences, and needs of potential adopters. A change agent will determine needs of clients and recommend changes that fulfill those needs.

The innovation or change must be tried on a limited basis. New ideas that can be experimented with are usually adopted more quickly. Clients trying out a new technology can find out how it works in their own situation.

Simple innovations or changes are more readily adopted than those that are complex. An innovation must be easy to understand and use.

An innovation is more quickly adopted when its results are clearly communicated and visible to others.

Data from Rogers EM: *Diffusion of innovations*, ed 4, New York, 1995, Free Press.

---

that is closer and has more convenient hours for the client to visit. Helping a client learn to perform blood glucose monitoring may be facilitated by having the client try out more than one type of monitor model and choose the one easiest to operate.

Community Assessment

When a nurse practices within a community setting, it is important to learn how to assess the community at large. This is the environment where the nurse's clients live and work. Without an adequate understanding of that environment, any effort to promote the client's health and to institute necessary change is unlikely to be successful. The community can be viewed as having three components: structure or locale, the people, and the social systems. A complete assessment involves a careful look at each component to begin to identify needs for health policy, health program development, and service provision (Box 3-6). When assessing the structure or locale, the nurse should travel around the neighborhood or community and observe its design, the location of services, and the locations where residents congregate. An assessment of the population may best be performed by accessing statistics on the community from a local public health department or public library. Information pertaining to necessary social systems, such as schools or health care facilities, may best be acquired by visiting various sites and learning about their services.

Once the nurse has a good understanding of the community, any individual client assessment is then performed against that background. For example, consider the situation of the nurse assessing a client's home for safety. Does the client have secure locks on doors? Are windows secure and intact? Is lighting along walkways and entry ways operational? The nurse will conduct the assessment, knowing, at the same time, the level of community violence and the resources that are available to the client when help is necessary. No individual client assessment should occur in isolation from the environment and conditions of the client's community.

Changing Clients' Health

The nurse in community-based practice will care for clients from diverse backgrounds and in diverse settings. It is relatively easy over time to become familiar with the resources that are available within a particular community practice setting. Likewise, with practice a nurse is able to learn how to identify the unique needs of individual clients. However, the challenge is how to promote and protect a client's health within the context of the community. Can a client with lung disease, for example, have the quality of life necessary when a community has a serious environmental pollution problem? Likewise, the nurse brings together the resources necessary to improve the continuity of care that clients receive. The nurse can be a key figure in reducing the duplication of health care services and locating the best services for a client's needs.

Perhaps the most important theme to consider to be an effective community-based nurse is to understand clients' lives. This begins by being able to establish strong, caring relationships with clients and their families (see Chapter 6). This becomes more difficult as the amount of time that professional nurses have to spend with clients continues to decline. However, the expert nurse becomes able to advise, counsel, and teach effectively after being accepted into the client's family and by understanding what truly makes the client unique. The day-to-day activities of family life are the variables that influence how the nurse must adapt nursing interventions. The time of day a client goes to work, the availability of the spouse and client's parents to provide child care, and the family values that shape views about health are just a few examples of the many factors nurses must consider in community-based practice. Once the nurse acquires a picture of a client's life, interventions designed to promote health and prevent disease can be introduced so that the picture becomes enhanced.

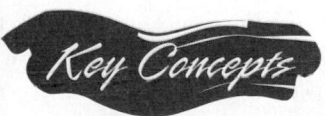

Key Concepts

- The principles of public health practice aim at achieving a healthy environment for all individuals to live in.
- Essential public health functions include assessment, policy development, and assurance.
- When population-based health care services are effective, there is a greater likelihood of the higher tiers of services contributing efficiently to health improvement of the population.
- The community health nurse cares for the community as a whole and considers the individual or family to be only one member of a group at risk.

- A successful community health nursing practice involves building relationships with the community and being responsive to changes within the community.
- The community-based nurse's competence is based on decision making at the level of the individual client.
- Within the ecological model of community-based nursing, the individual is viewed within the larger systems of family, community, culture, and society.
- Vulnerable individuals and their families often belong to more than one vulnerable group.

- The special needs of vulnerable populations form the backdrop for the challenges nurses face in caring for these clients' increasingly complex acute and chronic health conditions.
- When European Americans' and African-Americans' life expectancy have been compared, the causes of differences have been found to be related to low socioeconomic status rather than race.
- Exacerbations of chronic health problems are common among the homeless because they have few resources.
- An important principle in dealing with clients at risk or who may have suffered abuse is protection of the client.
- Clients who are substance abusers may often avoid health care for fear of being turned in to criminal authorities.
- In community-based practice it is important to understand what health means to older adults and the steps they can take to maintain their own health.
- A community-based nurse must be competent as a collaborator, educator, counselor, change agent, and client advocate.
- Factors that increase the likelihood of a change being accepted and adopted include simplicity, visibility to others, "trialability," compatibility with values, and advantage.
- Assessment of a community includes three elements: structure or locale, the people, and the social systems.
- An important theme to consider to be an effective community-based nurse is to understand clients' lives.

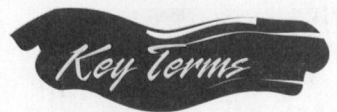

Key Terms

Community-based nursing, *p 52*

Community health nursing, *p 51*

Incident rates, *p 51*

Population, *p 51*

Public health, *p 49*

Vulnerable populations, *p 53*

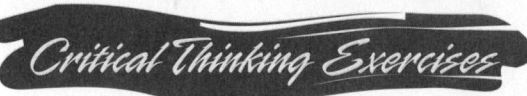

Critical Thinking Exercises

1. As a nurse managing a severely disabled child, you learn that there is an absence of respite services to provide parental support and limited educational resources in your community. What role of the community-based nurse would be important to establish a special education day care service, operated by volunteer educators?

2. Mr. Crowder is a 42-year-old man with emphysema and glaucoma who visits the nursing clinic periodically. Your assessment reveals that he is homeless and that he currently spends nights in a shelter two blocks away. He has been able to acquire medications for his breathing and eyedrops for his glaucoma from clinic funds, but he lost his inhaler 3 days ago. What factors might you consider in attempting to improve Mr. Crowder's adherence to medication administration?

3. Conduct a community assessment of an area that you have visited infrequently. Observe the community locale by driving through the more populated area. Look for the following services: hospital, clinic, drugstore, grocery, schools, park or playground, and police and fire departments.

References

Ayers M, Bruno AA, Langford RW: *Community-based nursing care: making the transition*, St. Louis, 1999, Mosby.

Birchfield PC: Elder health. In Stanhope M, Lancaster J: *Community health nursing: process and practice for promoting health*, ed 4, St. Louis, 1996, Mosby.

Chalmers KI and others: The changing environment of community health practice and education: perceptions of staff nurses, administrators, and educators, *J Nurs Educ* 37:109, 1998.

Consensus Conference on the Essentials of Public Health Nursing Practice and Education, Rockville, Md, 1985, U.S. Department of Health and Human Services, Bureau of Health Professions, Division of Nursing.

Diekemper M, SmithBattle L, Drake MA: Bringing the population into focus: a natural development in community health nursing practice, part I, *Public Health Nurs* 16:3, 1999.

Hicks LL, Stallmeyer JM, Coleman JR: *The role of the nurse in managed care*, Washington, DC, 1993, American Nurses Publishing.

Institute of Medicine, Board on Health Promotion and Disease Prevention, Project on Public Health Performance Monitoring, Washington, DC, 1995.

Kalisch P, Kalisch BJ: *Nursing involvement in the health planning process*, DHEW Pub No. HRA 78-25, Hyattsville, Md, 1977, U.S. Department of Health, Education, and Welfare.

Kenyon V and others: Clinical competencies for community health nursing, *Public Health Nurs* 7:33, 1990.

Kochanek KD and others: Why did black life expectancy decline from 1984 through 1989 in the United States? *Am J Public Health* 84(6):938, 1994.

Nichols J and others: A proposal for tracking health care for the homeless, *J Community Health* 11(3):204, 1986.

Pew Health Professions Commission: *Health America: practitioners for 2005*, Durham, NC, 1991, The Commission.

Porter CP, Villarruel AM: Nursing research with African American and Hispanic people: guidelines for action, *Nurs Outlook* 41(2): 59, 1993.

Rogers EM: *Diffusion of innovations*, ed 4, New York, 1995, Free Press.

Scholler-Jaquish A: Homelessness in America. In Smith CM, Maurer FA, editors: *Community health nursing: theory and practice*, Philadelphia, 1995, WB Saunders.

Sebastian JB: Homelessness: a state of vulnerability, *Fam Community Health* 8(3):11, 1985.

Sebastian JG: Vulnerability and vulnerable populations: an introduction. In Stanhope M, Lancaster J, editors: *Community health nursing: process and practice for promoting health*, ed 4, St. Louis, 1996, Mosby.

Stanhope M, Lancaster J: *Community health nursing: process and practice for promoting health*, ed 4, St. Louis, 1996, Mosby.

Stanhope M, Lancaster J: *Community health nursing: process and practice for promoting health*, ed 5, St. Louis, 2000, Mosby.

U.S. Public Health Service: *The core functions project*, 1993, Office of Disease Prevention and Health Promotion.

U.S. Public Health Service: *A time for partnership: prevention report*, Rockville, Md, December 1994/January 1995, Office of Disease Prevention and Health Promotion.

Zhan L and others: Promoting health: perspectives from ethnic elderly women, *J Community Health Nurs*, 15:31, 1998.

Zotti ME, Brown P, Stotts RC: Community-based nursing versus community health nursing: what does it all mean? *Nurs Outlook* 44(5):211, 1996.

4

Leadership, Delegation, and Quality Management

Sheila O'Brien

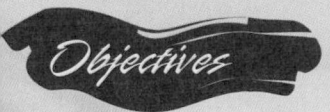

Objectives

Mastery of content in this chapter will enable the student to:

- Define the key terms listed.
- Differentiate between leadership and management.
- Explain the types of change health care organizations are experiencing.
- Discuss the relationship between types of change and types of leadership.
- Describe a leadership style appropriate to use in a specific management situation.
- Differentiate types of nursing care delivery models.
- Discuss ways a nurse manager can support staff involvement in a decentralized decision-making model.
- Discuss clinical care coordination skills in nursing practice.
- Explain a staff nurse's role in team communication.
- Discuss the skills necessary for appropriate delegation of nursing care activities.
- Differentiate total quality management and quality improvement.
- Explain the importance of defining quality before developing a quality improvement program.
- Discuss the elements of the Joint Commission on Accreditation of Healthcare Organizations' (JCAHO's) 10 steps for quality improvement.

The changing health care delivery system is influencing health professionals, clients, and health care organizations (see Chapter 2). With the emphasis on cost control affecting how organizations are organized and delivering client services, there is a need to rethink values and to develop social and organizational approaches that improve the manner in which the activities of the organization are conducted (Kurz, Hernandez, Haddock, 1988; Tebbitt, 1997). There is a need for progressive leaders and appropriate management systems to be in place to use strategic problem-solving approaches that will enable health service organizations to survive. Organizations will require strong, innovative leaders who can foster and implement change without compromising their mission of quality health care service.

Nursing leaders are in a position to take the initiative in creating the vision and culture needed for professional nursing practice to grow and prosper. The nurse executive must be proactive, innovative, and entrepreneurial in seeking opportunities for new programs and services that support excellent client care (Bolster and Petit, 1990; Tebbitt, 1997). Nurse managers play a pivotal role in creating a practice environment that supports staff in their ability to deliver care in the face of ongoing environmental uncertainty. Clinical staff must manage clinical outcomes for clients while also taking a leadership role in meeting organizational goals and objectives. To succeed, nursing leaders are recognizing the importance of staff members' playing a more active role, not only in client care, but in organizational management activities as well. For example, staff nurses are setting standards of care, deciding scheduling and staffing issues, and monitoring quality improvement outcomes. Health care settings are following a trend of fewer managers and more **self-directed work teams.** This makes the development of leadership and management skills of equal importance to developing clinical skills: through theory, application, and practice.

Leadership and Management

In discussing the concepts of **leadership** and **management,** it is important to distinguish the difference between a process an individual uses to achieve a goal or task versus a function within an organization. Leadership is the use of one's skills to direct and influence others to perform to the best of their ability (Dossett, 1992). It is an interpersonal process that involves a relationship between followers and the person who is leading. A leader is not simply someone who has been appointed to an important job or position. Effective leaders must be able to make people want to accomplish something and to therefore get the work done (Dossett, 1992). A leader can be in any type of organizational position; however, the benefits to an organization are greater when leaders assume the more influential positions within an organization.

The word *management* comes from a word meaning "hand." Management involves handling the day-to-day operations of a work group to achieve a desired outcome. The concept is functional by definition. Management functions, summarized in Box 4-1, are diverse, requiring ongoing problem solving and the ability to work with people. Managers are not automatically leaders. However, effective managers often become leaders.

Common Management Functions

Box 4-1

PLANNING

Planning includes determining long- and short-term objectives of an institution or unit and the actions that must be taken to achieve these objectives.

Example: The nursing staff of a medical oncology unit established the following objective: improve clients' satisfaction with pain control. Actions taken to achieve the objective included implementation of an objective measure to assess clients' pain more accurately (see Chapter 42) and implementation of noninvasive pain-control measures.

STAFFING

Staffing includes selecting the personnel to carry out these actions and placing them in positions appropriate to their knowledge and skills.

Example: The manager of the nursing unit selected a staff committee to interview applicants for a new clinical nurse specialist position.

ORGANIZING

Organizing includes mobilizing human and material resources so institutional objectives can be achieved.

Example: The staff development personnel from the hospital were called in to plan with the new nurse specialist and to assist in teaching classes on pain assessment for the medical oncology unit staff.

DIRECTING

Directing includes motivating and leading personnel to carry out the actions needed to achieve the institution's or unit's objectives.

Example: The manager involved staff in selecting members for the nursing practice committee. The manager gave them the objective of communicating the new standards of care for pain management on the unit. The committee met weekly for the first month to review pain management literature for oncology clients and to share the information with all staff on the unit. Posters were displayed in the staff lounge. The nurse manager met with all staff to discuss ways in which new pain management interventions could best be incorporated into their practice.

CONTROLLING

Controlling includes comparing results with predetermined standards of performance and taking corrective action when performance does not meet standards.

Example: The practice committee established two outcome measures: client satisfaction with pain control and staff competency, which is measured on a test of knowledge of noninvasive pain-control techniques. The manager set the expectation that the staff would participate in additional training if competency levels were not met. Satisfaction results from all clients were reviewed weekly by the practice committee. If satisfaction results showed no improvement, the committee investigated causes and redesigned approaches.

DECISION MAKING

Decision making includes identifying a problem, searching for solutions, and selecting the alternative that best achieves the decision maker's objectives.

Example: Three months after staff had been trained and new practice guidelines for pain assessment had been implemented, the manager reviewed client records and found documentation of pain assessment to be consistently reported. The practice committee met with the manager to identify approaches that might improve quality of documentation without adding unnecessary charting requirements.

Data from Gustafson D: The functions of a nurse manager in a health care setting. In Sullivan EJ, Decker PJ, editors: *Effective management in nursing,* ed 3, Redwood City, Calif, 1992, Addison-Wesley.

A distinctive characteristic of leadership is that it fosters change. Change, along with the ability to manage it in a constructive and proactive manner, is central to the concept of leadership. A leader takes an active role in shaping the ideas and goals of an organization (Zaleznik, 1992). Leaders help to develop new approaches for tackling problems and are able to instill a level of excitement in their followers.

Management is more impersonal and passive. A management focus involves keeping individuals on course and directed toward organizational goals, to remain productive. Management requires good negotiation and balancing of the different views of a staff. In comparing management and leadership, one may note that effective management requires problem solving, whereas effective leadership sees the problem before it occurs.

LEADERSHIP IN CHANGE

Leaders in health care organizations must be prepared to deal with constant change. This requires an understanding of the types of change, how they influence an organization, and the strategies that best manage change. There are three types of change occurring in health care organizations: technical change (alteration of means but not goals), transition (alteration of goals but not means), and transformation (alteration of both means and goals) (Kurz, Hernandez, and Haddock, 1988). Change that is technical involves both technological innovation and structural modifications in the design of an organization. For example, many organizations have implemented integrated computer systems, changing the way client documentation is recorded, tests and supplies are ordered, and information is relayed to caregivers. Technological innovations, like the computer system, can dramatically change how work groups function. Implementation must be carefully designed to ensure that the innovation is compatible with the needs of the workers and the organization, that it provides a perceived advantage, and that it offers demonstrable benefits (Rogers, 1983). Another example of technical change is the realignment of services within a hospital, requiring a different administrative structure or hierarchy.

Transitional change involves a shift in the goals of an organization while the means remain the same (Kurz, Hernandez, and Haddock, 1988). The workforce remains intact; however, the nature and scope of work can change significantly, depending on the complexity or number of goals established. An example is when an institution shifts from providing specialty care to providing primary care.

Transformation involves an alteration of both the means and the goals of an organization. A major upheaval occurs with transformation, changing the nature of the work, why it is performed, and who performs it. This has occurred in health care organizations that have experienced mergers of culturally different institutions, a shifting in focus from inpatient to outpatient care, a redesign of acute care delivery processes, and a reduction in managerial oversight.

The type of change that an organization undergoes is important to understand. There are different types of leadership best suited to the nature of an organization and the type of change it experiences.

TYPES OF LEADERSHIP

The health care environment is very complex. There are professionals from diverse backgrounds (e.g., nurses, physicians, pharmacists, and social workers), as well as a wide variety of trained support staff who attempt to collaborate in delivering quality client care. Each group is influenced by its own culture, values, and unique client orientation. At the same time, each group strives to meet the goals of the organization in which it works. With such diversity in the health care workforce, managing and leading health care providers can be very challenging.

The humanistic orientation of health care made it relatively easy for professionals and others to collaborate when health care was primarily service oriented. All efforts were focused on serving clients, maintaining or improving their health with whatever resources were necessary. Now that health care has assumed a business focus, many professionals and support staff sense that a conflict exists between the goal of delivering quality care versus an organization's goal for cost control. The client's welfare may no longer appear to be the priority. Add to this conflict the element of ongoing change, and it is easy to recognize that leadership within health care can be very difficult. The fundamental changes that are occurring in health care require strong leaders. Burns (1978) has defined two types of leadership that are relevant in today's health care environment: transactional and transformational.

Transactional Leadership. **Transactional leadership** is based on exchange theory, involving the exchange of rewards (compensation) for services (getting work done). The transactional form of leadership involves two behavior patterns: contingent reward and management by exception (Kurz, Hernandez, and Haddock, 1988). A leader

using contingent reward identifies tasks to be done to accomplish a goal, explains tasks to subordinates, and indicates the outcomes if tasks are performed and goals are accomplished. Typical rewards include praise, recognition, or a pay increase. Management by exception involves intervention with subordinates only when something goes wrong. It is a punitive approach that is usually not effective by itself. Management by exception is often used with physicians or nurses, especially by the professionals themselves (Kurz, Hernandez, and Haddock, 1988).

The function of transactional leadership is to maintain an organization's operation rather than change it. This does not mean that transactional leadership avoids change. Instead, it is an approach that provides stability to an organization. A transactional leader works within a culture and competently supervises and coordinates the day-to-day management of a work unit, such as a nursing division, where nursing staff are encouraged and recognized in providing their care and in accomplishing client outcomes. The leader tries to maintain the system through control of current procedures or through improvement in them. The leader also responds to workers' needs if they can be met by getting the work done. Transactional leaders recognize and clarify role and task requirements. They also assume that workers maintain motivation to support the manager's plan.

Transactional leadership maintains the status quo; however, it can be used to successfully implement technical and transitional change. Both types of change may indeed create change within a system but not a change of the system itself (Kurz, Hernandez, and Haddock, 1988). The system will remain recognizable after change has occurred. For example, a teaching hospital will add new technologies for specialty practices and research, but it remains a teaching hospital. A transactional leader can adapt to change and achieve organizational goals by clarifying workers' expectations about the outcomes of their effort and by reducing role conflict and confusion (Kurz, Hernandez, and Haddock, 1988). It is common to find transactional leadership at all levels of health care management.

Transformational Leadership. **Transformational leadership** occurs when one or more persons engage with others in such a way that the leader and follower raise one another to higher levels of motivation (Burns, 1978). It is a process that can lead to organizational transformation, whereby workers are motivated to do more than they originally expected. In contrast to the transactional leader, the transformational leader changes a work culture. There are three patterns of transformational leadership behavior: charisma, intellectual stimulation, and individualized consideration (Kurz, Hernandez, and Haddock, 1988).

Charisma is the endowment of a high level of esteem or popularity. The leader is a change agent who can motivate others to commit to a path of long-term change. The charismatic leader is visionary, advocating where an organization needs to be in the future and making it meaningful to subordinates. Being able to take risks and stand for an idea also characterizes the charismatic leader.

Through intellectual stimulation, the transformational leader is able to create in others an awareness of problems and their solutions. Strategic and critical thinking are essential characteristics in this leader who encourages curiosity and innovation among workers. Rather than viewing inquiry and curiosity as insubordination, the transformational leader turns problems into opportunities. This is theorized to develop employees' ability to assess and problem solve creatively as leaders in their own right (McDaniel and Wolf, 1992).

The final pattern of behavior in a transformational leader is individualized consideration. Employees hold the key to success when implementing change or any organizational initiative. The transformational leader is able to develop and empower staff so that the person and the organization benefit in the end.

Transformational leadership can successfully implement transformational change if the processes of transactional leadership are already in place (Kurz, Hernandez, and Haddock, 1988). The process is systematic, consisting of purposeful and organized searches for change. A transformational leader moves resources from areas of lesser productivity to areas of greater productivity. The leader is able to overcome subordinate and even organizational resistance, set the vision for the future, create commitment to the vision, and implement any necessary innovations. Effective management of people is the key to a transformational leader's success. Transformational leadership has been largely unrecognized in health care systems (Kurz, Hernandez, and Haddock, 1988). However, McDaniel and Wolf (1992) studied the leadership qualities of nursing administrators in one health care facility and found a relationship between the transformational qualities of its nurse executives and high staff retention and low staff turnover. The transformational approach matches well with professionals' needs and for work requiring high levels of decision making and autonomy.

LEADERSHIP BEHAVIOR AND STYLES

Regardless of the type of leader one is, the characteristics of a leader are found to be less important than what a leader chooses to do. Research has shown two major dimensions of leadership behavior: initiating structure and consideration (Dossett, 1992). *Initiating structure* refers to behavior in which a leader organizes and defines the work to be accomplished and establishes well-defined work patterns and channels of communication. For example, a nurse manager defines a philosophy of nursing practice for a nursing unit, selects a nursing care delivery model (e.g., primary nursing), determines staffing numbers, works with staff to develop standards of care for their client population, and sets expectations as to how client needs and nursing interventions are clearly communi-

cated among nursing staff members. The manager becomes a leader by setting a clear vision for an environment of nursing practice.

Consideration refers to behavior that conveys mutual trust, respect, warmth, and rapport between manager and staff (Dossett, 1992). In the same example, the nurse manager meets regularly with staff one-on-one and in small groups. The manager welcomes input from staff on ways to improve the operations of the nursing unit. The manager deals with each employee fairly, based on the expectations set for the unit. Staff sense that they are treated as professionals and expected to work together to become an efficient work team.

Nursing students can practice developing consideration in working with other nurses and health care providers in a clinical setting. Using free time to assist others, seeking out the opinion of colleagues, listening to others' ideas and suggestions, and participating openly and noncritically in conferences are ways to establish considerate work behavior.

Styles.   The literature describes a variety of **leadership styles,** or clusters of behaviors that characterize the manner in which a manager uses interpersonal behaviors to influence accomplishment of a work unit's goals (Dossett, 1992). The styles range from total control to extreme permissiveness. Box 4-2 describes each style and the situations in which each can best be used. A manager may use more than one type of style with a group of employees, but typically one style predominates. The situational style is the most flexible, combining four styles in one. This text highlights the situational leadership style.

Situational Leadership.   The situational style of leadership suggests that it is the situation itself, within any work setting, that is a major determinant of the extent to which leadership behaviors or characteristics influence the leader's effectiveness (Stogdill, 1974). There is no single best leadership style. The more managers adapt their leadership styles to work situations and the needs and abilities of staff, the more effective the managers will be. There are four typical styles for situational leadership. The leader may use all four styles at any one time, depending on the size of the work group, the maturity of the staff, and the situations the work group encounters. The four styles are as follows:

1. *Directing:* The leader provides specific instructions and supervises the accomplishment of tasks. There is high direction and low supportive behavior. Leaders give detailed instructions, state specific expectations, enforce rules and policies, and tell employees what to do, how to do it, and when to do it. Directing works best with new employees, employees with repeated performance problems, and crisis work situations.

2. *Coaching:* The leader monitors the accomplishment of tasks while also explaining decisions, asking for

Leadership Styles   Box 4-2

AUTOCRATIC LEADERSHIP

Autocratic leadership is an approach wherein the leader retains all authority and is primarily concerned with task accomplishment. The leader assigns clearly defined tasks and establishes one-way communication with the work group, making decisions alone. The leader stresses prompt, orderly performance and uses power to pressure those who fail to follow expectations. This leadership style can be appropriate in situations where most members of a work group are novices or in situations in which immediate action is required and there is no time for group decisions.

Examples: Crisis situation (e.g., cardiac arrest of a client) or an event that creates major disorder (e.g., a community disaster).

DEMOCRATIC LEADERSHIP

Democratic leadership is a people-centered approach that is primarily concerned with human relations and teamwork. Employees are given more control and participation in decision making. This approach facilitates goal accomplishment while stressing the self-worth of each employee. The democratic style works best with mature employees who work well together as groups. This style may demand more of the leader, but it is often valued for contributing to the growth and development of the staff.

SITUATIONAL LEADERSHIP

Situational leadership is a comprehensive approach that incorporates the leader's style, the maturity of the work group, and the situation at hand. There is no single best leadership style; rather, the style used by the manager depends on the situation and maturity of the subordinates. Four typical styles are used: directing, coaching, supporting, and delegating.

LAISSEZ-FAIRE LEADERSHIP

Laissez-faire leadership is a "free run," or permissive, style of leadership. The leader gives up control completely and chooses to avoid responsibility by delegating all decision making to the work group. The leader fails to establish goals or policies and abstains from leading. The work group receives little or no direction. This style may be somewhat effective with a highly motivated, mature work group.

feedback or suggestions, and recognizing good performance. There is high directive and high supportive behavior. Typically, the leader and staff have jointly developed a work plan.

3. *Supporting:* The leader supports the efforts of others, facilitates their goal accomplishment, and shares responsibility for decision making. There is high supportive and low directive behavior. The leader is willing to try new ideas of staff and uses **consensus decision making** to choose a course of action. The leader values growth and not perfection, collaboration and not competition (Cox, 1995).

4. *Delegating:* The leader gives the responsibility for decision making and problem solving to mature staff

who have demonstrated their competence (Hersey and Blanchard, 1988). There is low supportive and low directive behavior. The leaders recognize that there is more than one right way to do things and gives authority to staff that matches their level of responsibility.

The approach of gradually giving up control and giving increasing decision-making authority to staff is in keeping with modern management theory regarding staff **empowerment.** This means fostering the growth of others and facilitating their development so that they are less and less dependent on the leader. Staff know when they can make decisions confidently on their own (e.g., intervening and resolving client and family complaints, dealing with unclear medical orders from a physician, or resolving conflicts between fellow staff nurses).

The cornerstone of situational leadership is the flexibility of the manager in adapting to the needs of the individual or work group. In a typical work setting the manager may be "directive" in dealing with staff who are in orientation while acting as a "coach" for those on another shift who are more experienced but still need some guidance. The "supporting" style may be apparent as the manager works with a staff practice committee and assists members in solving a problem with another department. A manager who relies on seasoned staff nurses to monitor quality-of-care issues and regularly report results of studies is using the "delegating" style to promote staff development. Obviously, it is important to carefully assess the developmental level or job maturity of staff in matching leadership style. The situational leadership style is growth producing for both manager and staff.

Building a Nursing Team

Nurses are creative professionals who want to enjoy their work and achieve success in delivering the very best care to their clients (Trofino, 1996). They are also self-directed and, if properly led and motivated, can solve even the most complex problems. An empowering work environment is one that brings out the best in a professional, concentrating on effective client care systems (e.g., documentation systems, referral mechanisms, physician-nurse collaboration), supporting risk taking and innovation, focusing on results and rewards, and offering professional opportunities for growth and advancement.

Building an empowered nursing team begins with the nurse executive. The executive's position within an organization is critical in uniting the strategic direction of an organization with the philosophical values and goals of nursing (Box 4-3). The nurse executive speaks the language of multiple disciplines in planning and setting aside resources needed for effective client care delivery (Tebbitt, 1997). Perhaps the most important responsibility of the nurse executive is to establish a vision for nursing that lays the groundwork that enables managers and staff to exer-

Characteristics of a Nurse Executive Box 4-3

A nurse executive:

Is a currently licensed registered nurse qualified by advanced education and management practice

Is responsible for the administration and management of the nursing organization, whether that be a department or division that is centralized or decentralized in structure

Has the authority, responsibility, and accountability for defining the discipline of nursing and for establishing and approving nursing practice standards, policies, and procedures to be developed consistent with current research and nationally recognized professional standards, and adhered to wherever nursing is practiced throughout the organization

Is an active member of the organization's leadership team, responsible for participating in setting the strategic direction for the organization and collaborating with organizational leaders

Participates with leaders from the governing board, management, medical staff, and clinical areas in planning, promoting, and conducting organization performance improvement activities

Modified from American Hospital Association: Role and function of the hospital nurse executive. In *Management advisory,* Chicago, 1990, American Organization of Nurse Executives; and Joint Commission on Accreditation of Healthcare Organizations: *A comprehensive accreditation manual for hospitals,* Chicago, 1997, The Commission.

Developing a Vision for a Nursing Unit Box 4-4

WHAT IS THE NURSING UNIT'S PURPOSE OR MISSION?
Why do we exist?
Who are our customers (internal and external)?
What makes us unique?
What is unique about our clients?

HOW WILL STAFF WORK WITH CLIENTS AND FAMILIES?
Placing client and family needs first
Involving clients and families in all aspects of care
Making communication a priority

WHAT ARE THE STANDARDS OF THE WORK UNIT?
All staff will be competent.
Each staff member is accountable for the care delivered to clients.
Staff will work collaboratively with all members of the health care team.

KEY VALUES
Creating an environment of caring
Being self-motivated and self-managed
Supporting a learning environment

cise excellent nursing practice. A vision is a shared image of a possible and desirable future state for an organization or work unit (Senge, 1990). It is a philosophy of how the work of a unit is managed (Gregory, 1995). A vision is derived from the personal visions each employee has for his or her work team (Box 4-4). In the case of a nursing unit, a shared vision is a pronouncement of a professional nursing staff's values and concerns for how clients should be viewed and cared for. Integral to this vision is the selection of a client care delivery model and management structure that support professional nursing practice.

NURSING CARE DELIVERY MODELS

Since the time of Florence Nightingale there have been a variety of nursing care delivery models, methods by which nursing care is provided for clients. The essence of nursing is in how nurses care for their clients (Duchene, 1992). Ideally, the vision nurses establish for the care of clients should drive the selection of a care delivery model. However, too often the scarcity of nursing resources and business initiatives from the health care organization influence the final decision. Care delivery must be effective in helping nurses achieve desirable outcomes for their clients. Key factors contributing to success are decision-making authority for nurses who provide direct care and effective methods of communicating with colleagues, physicians, and other health care providers (Duchene, 1992).

Total Patient Care. **Total patient care delivery** is the original care delivery model developed during Florence Nightingale's time. A registered nurse (RN) is responsible for all aspects of one or more clients' care. The nurse works directly with the client, family, physician, and health team members. The model typically has a shift-based focus. The same nurse does not necessarily care for the same client over time. Continuity of care from shift to shift or day to day can be a problem if staff do not clearly communicate client needs to one another.

Functional Nursing. **Functional nursing,** first developed in the 1950s during a nursing shortage, involves the division of tasks, with one nurse assuming responsibility for certain tasks (e.g., hygiene and nursing therapies) while another nurse assumes responsibility for others (e.g., medication administration). Nurses tend to become highly competent with the tasks that are repeatedly assigned to them. The major disadvantages of functional nursing are problems with continuity, absence of a holistic view of clients, and the possibility that care becomes mechanical (Duchene, 1992). Functional nursing is task focused, not client focused. Communication is not always clear, since no one nurse is responsible for the overall care of the client.

Team Nursing. **Team nursing** involves the delivery of nursing care by staff of various educational preparations. An RN leads a team made up of other RNs, licensed practical nurses (LPNs), and assistive personnel (e.g., nurse assistants or technicians). The team members provide direct client care to groups of clients, under the direction and coordination of the RN team leader. In this model, assistive personnel are often given client assignments rather than nursing tasks. This poses a risk if assistive personnel are not prepared to perform all care required by a client. Problems can develop with team nursing if the role of the RN versus that of assistive personnel has not been clearly defined.

The team leader coordinates care of the team by communicating with physicians and other health care personnel and resolving problems met by team members. The team leader also is responsible for coordinating each client's nursing plan of care. Limitations to the model include the lack of time the team leader can spend with clients. Depending on the mix of staff, this may mean that clients see an RN infrequently. Risks exist if an RN is unable to make ongoing client assessments and be involved in important clinical decision making. There also may be no attempt to assign the same nurse to the same client each day, potentially causing lack of continuity of care. An advantage of team nursing is the collaborative style that encourages each member of the team to help others.

Primary Nursing. The **primary nursing** model was developed with the aim of placing RNs at the bedside and improving the professional relationships between staff (Manthey, 1980). The model was more popular in the 1970s and early 1980s as hospitals began to employ more RNs. Primary nursing is not a staffing model, prescribing a specific number or percentage of RNs. In other words, it is not necessary to have a staff composed entirely of RNs to practice primary nursing. Instead, primary nursing is a model of care delivery that focuses on the relationship between an RN and his or her clients. In this model, an RN assumes responsibility for a caseload of clients over time. Typically, the RN selects the clients for his or her caseload and cares for the same clients during their hospitalization or stay in a health care setting. The RN assesses the client's needs, develops a plan of care, and ensures that nursing interventions are delivered. In the absence of the primary nurse, associate nurses (e.g., other RNs or LPNs) follow the prescribed nursing plan of care. If there are differences in opinion as to client needs, associates and primary nurses collaborate to modify the plan.

Primary nursing is one care delivery model designed to maintain continuity of care across shifts, days, or visits. It can be applied in any setting, including clinics, an emergency department, and home health. Care consistently managed by a single professional can potentially reduce cost by minimizing delays in therapies, improving collaboration with other professionals, and enhancing the client-nurse relationship.

There have been studies attempting to show the importance of professional nursing care to client outcomes. Generally speaking, studies suggest that a higher RN ratio seems to be associated with better client outcomes (Aiken

and others, 1994; Blegen and others, 1998). In reviewing these studies, it is important to ask what care delivery model is represented. Gardner (1991) was able to compare primary and team nursing, showing that costs were reduced and quality was better with a primary nursing approach.

Case Management. Case management is a care delivery approach that coordinates and links health care services to clients and their families (see Chapter 2). A nursing case management model involves a professional nurse assuming responsibility for client care from admission through and following discharge (Duchene, 1992). What is unique about case management is that clinicians, either as individuals or as part of collaborative groups, oversee the management of case type–based care (e.g., clients with specific diagnoses) and are usually held accountable to some standard of cost management and quality outcome. A case manager coordinates a client's acute care in the hospital and then may follow the client once he or she is discharged home. Case managers may not provide direct care; instead they collaborate and supervise the care delivered by other staff members. The case manager frequently oversees a caseload of clients with complex nursing and medical problems. Depending on the setting, case managers may be nurses, social workers, or physician/RN teams.

Many organizations use CareMaps in a case management delivery system (see Chapter 2). The CareMaps are multidisciplinary treatment plans that are designed for clients of a specific case type. The case manager, along with members of the health care team, uses the CareMap to deliver timely interventions in a coordinated plan of care. CareMaps eliminate the guesswork in client care by having all members of the health care team working from the same plan.

MANAGEMENT STRUCTURE

With a vision for nursing established, it is the manager who directs and supports staff in the realization of that vision. It takes an excellent manager and excellent staff to create an enriching work environment where nursing practice thrives.

The nurse executive supports managers by establishing a management structure that will help to achieve organizational goals and provide appropriate support to care delivery staff (Table 4-1). Tebbitt (1997) notes that leadership is not measured in the power exercised over others, but rather in the power released in others through the nurse executive's ability to influence the structure in which staff works. The leader facilitates change in staff attitudes and behaviors, gains their commitment, and sets examples of professional excellence.

A **decentralized management** structure has an advantage over others in creating an environment where managers and staff become more actively involved in shaping a health care organization's identity and determining its

Table 4-1	**Examples of Management Structures**
Structural Approach	Characteristics
Centralized management	Single administrator leads organization, with directors overseeing departmental responsibilities. Typically, decisions are made by virtue of a person's position in an organization. Decisions are made from top down, with minimal input from staff. Managers tend to have minimal responsibility or accountability for 14-hour operation of nursing unit.
Decentralized management	Structure may appear similar to that of centralized organization. Often there are fewer directors. Decisions are made on basis of knowledge by those staff who are best informed about a problem or issue. Managers often have 24-hour accountability and responsibility for staff, budget, and day-to-day management of work unit.
Matrix	Traditional hospital departments become reorganized into business units. Staff may report to more than one manager.

success. Staff have more say in problem solving, choosing strategies, and evaluating the outcomes of their work. Working in a decentralized structure has the potential for greater collaborative effort, increased competency of staff, and ultimately a greater sense of professional accomplishment.

CREATING AN EMPOWERED WORK ENVIRONMENT

Progressive organizations achieve more when employees at all levels are actively involved. As a result, the role of nurse manager is critical in terms of the management of effective nursing units or groups. The diverse responsibilities assumed by nurse managers are highlighted in Box 4-5. To develop an empowered nursing staff, managers must understand how to get decision making down to the lowest level possible. **Decentralized decision making** requires all staff to become involved. This means that they must be kept well informed and given the opportunity by managers to participate in problem-solving activities. On a nursing unit it is important for RNs, LPNs, assistive personnel, and unit secretaries to have the opportunity to participate in resolving issues that affect their work. Leadership by a manager should not be measured in terms of services or projects completed, but in terms of growth in competence, as well as a sense of autonomy, responsibility, and personal satisfaction felt by staff (Tebbitt, 1997). Key elements to empowering staff and establishing decentralized decision making are responsibility, authority, and accountability (Cox, 1995).

Responsibility refers to the duties and activities for which an individual is employed to perform. A professional nurse's responsibilities in a given role are outlined in a job description describing the nurse's duties in client care and in participating as a member of the nursing unit.

Responsibility reflects ownership; it must be allocated by the individual who oversees the employee, and it must be accepted by the employee. Managers must be sure that staff clearly understand their responsibilities, particularly in the face of change. For example, when hospitals partic-

Responsibilities of the Nurse Manager	Box 4-5

Assist staff in establishing annual goals for the unit and systems needed to accomplish goals.

Monitor professional nursing standards of practice on the unit.

Develop an ongoing staff development plan, including one for new employees.

Recruit new employees (interview and hire).

Conduct routine staff evaluations.

Establish self as a role model for positive customer service (customers include clients, families, and other health care team members).

Submit staffing schedules for the unit.

Conduct regular client rounds and problem solve client or family complaints.

Establish and implement a unit quality improvement plan.

Review and recommend new equipment for the unit.

Conduct regular staff meetings.

Conduct rounds with physicians.

Establish and support staff and interdisciplinary committees.

ipate in work redesign (see Chapter 2), client care delivery models can change significantly. It is the manager's responsibility to clearly define the RN's role within the new care delivery model. If decentralized decision making is in place, professional staff have a voice in identifying the new RN role. Each RN on the work team is responsible for knowing his or her role and how it is to be implemented on the busy nursing unit. For example, a primary nurse is responsible for completing a nursing assessment of all assigned clients and for developing a plan of care that addresses each of the client's nursing diagnoses (see Unit 3). As the plan of care is delivered, the primary nurse is responsible for evaluating whether the plan is successful. This responsibility becomes a work ethic for the nurse in delivering excellent client care.

Authority refers to the right to act in areas where an individual has been given and accepts responsibility (Cox, 1995). For example, a primary nurse managing a caseload of clients may discover that members of the nursing team did not follow through on a discharge teaching plan for an assigned client. The primary nurse has the authority to consult with other nurses and to learn why recommendations on the plan of care were not followed. The primary nurse has the final authority in selecting the best course of action for the client's care.

Accountability refers to an individual being answerable for his or her actions. It involves follow-up and a reflective analysis of one's decisions to evaluate their effectiveness (Cox, 1995). A primary nurse is accountable for his or her clients' outcomes. In the preceding example regarding a discharge teaching plan, the nurse is accountable for what the client learns about continuing self-care at home. The nurse demonstrates accountability in checking on the client and family after discharge and in reviewing with the nursing team whether continuity in teaching occurred.

A successful decentralized nursing unit exercises the three elements of decision making on an ongoing basis. An effective manager sets the same expectations for all staff in how decisions are made. Staff must routinely meet to discuss and negotiate how to maintain an equality and balance in the elements. Staff must feel comfortable in expressing differences in opinion and challenging ways in which the team functions, while at the same time recognizing their own responsibility, authority, and accountability. Ultimately, decentralized decision making becomes a vehicle for realizing the unit's vision of what professional nursing care should be.

Supporting Staff Involvement.

When a decentralized decision-making model exists on a nursing unit, the results can be exciting. The work environment promotes participation, and all staff benefit from the knowledge and skills of the entire work group. If staff learn to value knowledge and the contributions of colleagues, better client care becomes an outcome. The nursing manager nurtures and supports staff involvement through the following approaches:

- *Establishment of nursing practice problem-solving committees or professional* **shared governance** *councils.* Chaired by senior clinical staff, these groups are empowered to establish and maintain care standards for nursing practice on their work unit. The committees review and establish standards of care, develop policy and procedures, resolve client satisfaction issues, or develop new documentation tools (Figure 4-1). Mechanisms are established to ensure that all staff have input on practice issues.
- *Nurse/physician collaborative practice.* A nursing unit's care delivery model influences how nurse and physician collaboration can best be fostered. If the unit

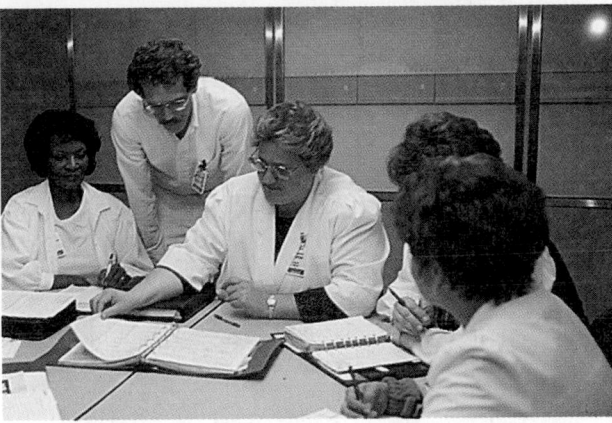

Figure 4-1 Staff collaborating on practice issues.

practices team nursing, it is important for team leaders to regularly participate in physician rounds. If the unit practices primary nursing, the physician should communicate either with each primary nurse or with the associate nurse who is assuming care for the client on that day. In a home health or extended care setting the staff should be able to contact physicians with minimal delay and be able to work together on decisions regarding client care. The manager avoids taking care of problems for staff. Instead, staff learn to keep physicians informed about what is important regarding their clients. Open communication is critical. Physicians are invited to attend practice committees when clinical problems are addressed and to present timely in-service programs on new medical procedures or research findings.

- **Interdisciplinary** *collaboration.* The emphasis on efficiency in health care delivery brings all members of the health care team together. Whenever systems or programs are redesigned, interdisciplinary involvement is crucial because most health care processes involve more than one discipline. At the client care level, nursing staff must recognize the importance of prompt referrals and timely communication with other health professionals. Interdisciplinary collaboration is fostered by including representatives of the various disciplines in practice projects, in-service programs, conferences, and staff meetings.
- *Staff communication.* Perhaps one of the manager's greatest challenges, especially if a work group is large, is communication with staff. It is difficult to ensure that all staff receive the same message: the correct message. In the present health care environment, staff quickly become uneasy and distrusting if they fail to hear about planned changes on their work unit. However, a manager cannot assume total responsibility for all communication. Instead, the manager can use a variety of approaches to ensure that information

is communicated quickly and accurately to all staff. For example, many managers distribute bi-weekly or monthly newsletters of ongoing unit or health care agency activities. Minutes of committee meetings should be posted in an accessible location for all staff to read. When vital issues regarding the operations of the unit or the organization are to be discussed, the manager should conduct staff meetings. When the unit has practice or quality improvement committees, each member should be assigned responsibility to communicate directly to a select number of staff. In that way, all staff are contacted and given the opportunity for input.

- *Staff education.* A professional nursing staff should always grow in knowledge. It is impossible to remain knowledgeable of current medical and nursing practice trends without ongoing education. The nurse manager is responsible for making learning opportunities available so that staff remain competent in their practice. This involves planning in-service programs, sending staff to continuing education classes and professional conferences, and having staff present case studies or practice issues during staff meetings. Staff members are responsible for pursuing educational opportunities when they know that their competencies are lacking.

Leadership Skills for Nursing Students.
As nursing students become involved in clinical assignments with clients, it is important that they prepare themselves for leadership roles. This does not mean that they have to quickly learn how to lead a team of nursing staff. Instead, they first learn to become dependable and competent providers of client care. Just as is the case with the staff nurse, the nursing student has a responsibility for the care given to his or her clients and must assume accountability for that care. Even though the student has limited authority and consults with instructors and staff regarding decisions, the student must not avoid making decisions in client care. The student can learn to become a leader by making good clinical decisions, learning from mistakes and seeking guidance, collaborating closely with professional nurses, and striving to improve his or her performance during each client interaction.

There are certain leadership skills that the nursing student can learn to use, including clinical care coordination, team communication, delegation, and knowledge building.

Clinical Care Coordination.
A student must acquire the skills necessary so that client care can be delivered in a timely and effective manner. In the beginning, this might involve only one client but eventually will involve groups of clients. Clinical care coordination includes clinical decision making, priority setting, use of organizational skills and resources, time management, and evaluation.

When a nurse begins an assignment with a client, the first activity involves a focused but complete assessment of the client's condition that enables the nurse to make an accurate clinical decision as to the client's needs and required nursing therapies. The nurse uses a critical thinking approach, applying previous knowledge and experience to the decision-making process (see Chapter 13). The nursing process is the framework used by the nurse in determining the level of care required, implementing the plan of care, and evaluating its results (see Unit 3). If the nurse fails to make accurate clinical judgments about a client, there can be undesirable outcomes. The client's condition might worsen or remain the same when the potential for improvement has been lost. An important lesson in organizational skills is to be thorough. The nurse must learn to attend to the client, look for any cues (obvious or subtle) that point to a pattern of findings, and direct the assessment to explore the pattern further. Accurate clinical decision making keeps the nurse focused on the proper course of action. A student nurse should never hesitate to ask for assistance when a client's assessment reveals a changing clinical condition.

After forming a picture of the client's total needs, the nurse must then decide on what client needs or problems need to be cared for first. Prioritizing is discussed in Chapter 16. If a client is experiencing serious physiological or psychological problems, the nurse's priority becomes clear. It becomes essential to act immediately to stabilize the client's condition. If the client is in no acute distress, priority setting might be based on the client's basic needs. For example, a client who is immobilized in traction might report being uncomfortable from being in the same position. A service worker arrives in the room to deliver a meal tray. Instead of immediately assisting the client with the meal, the nurse instead repositions the client and offers basic hygiene measures. Making the client comfortable first will likely enable him or her to become more interested in eating.

Priorities must also be made on the basis of client expectations (see Chapter 2). The nurse might have an excellent plan of care established, but if the client is resistant to certain therapies or disagrees with the nurse's approach, little success will be gained. Working closely with the client and showing a caring attitude is important. The nurse shares the priorities defined with the client to establish a level of agreement and cooperation.

Implementing a plan of care requires the nurse to be efficient and well organized. A nurse learns to become efficient by combining various nursing activities—in other words, doing more than one thing at a time. For example, during medication administration or while obtaining a specimen, the nurse combines therapeutic communication skills, teaching interventions, and assessment and evaluation. The nurse always tries to establish and strengthen relationships with clients and uses any client contact as an opportunity to convey important information. Client interaction also provides the nurse the opportunity to convey caring and interest in the client. The nurse always attends to the client's behaviors and responses to therapies to assess if any new problems are developing and to evaluate responses to interventions.

A well-organized nurse approaches any planned procedures by having all of the necessary equipment available and making sure the client is prepared. Being sure the client is comfortable and well informed will increase the likelihood of the procedure going smoothly. Sometimes the nurse requires the assistance of colleagues to perform or complete a procedure. It is always wise to have the work area organized and preliminary steps completed before asking colleagues for assistance.

As the nurse begins to deliver care based on established priorities, events may occur within the health care setting that can interfere with plans. For example, just as a nurse begins to provide morning hygiene for a hospitalized client, an x-ray technician may enter to take a chest film. Once the x-ray film is completed, a phlebotomist may arrive to draw a sample of blood. In such a case the nurse's priorities may seem to conflict with the priorities of other health care personnel. It is important to always keep the client's needs as the center of attention. The client may have experienced symptoms earlier that required a chest film and laboratory work. In such a case it is important to be sure that the diagnostic tests are completed. In another example, a client may be waiting to visit family, and a chest film may be a routine order from 2 days earlier. The client's condition may have since stabilized, and the x-ray technician may be willing to return later to shoot the film. In this situation attending to the client's hygiene and comfort so that family can visit is more of a priority at this time.

Another important aspect of clinical care coordination is appropriate use of resources. Resources in this case include members of the health care team. In any setting, the administration of client care occurs more smoothly when staff work together. Students should never hesitate to have staff assist them, especially when there is an opportunity to make a procedure or activity more comfortable and safer for the client. For example, assistance in turning, positioning, and ambulating clients is frequently necessary when clients experience impaired mobility. Having a staff member assist with handling equipment and supplies during more complicated procedures such as catheter insertion or dressing change can help make procedures more efficient. This is an excellent way for students to learn how to work with assistive personnel. There are also times when the student must recognize personal limitations and use professional resources for assistance. For example, the student may assess a client and find relevant clinical signs and symptoms but be unfamiliar with the underlying physical condition. Consulting with an RN leads to confirmation of findings and assurance that the proper course of action will be taken for the client. Throughout a nurse's

professional career there are always new experiences. A leader knows his or her own limitations and seeks professional colleagues for guidance and support.

Much of the stress experienced by nurses results from the perception that client needs must be met all at once (Gustafson, Duchene, and Baker, 1992). This is, of course, impossible, especially when the nurse is caring for more than one client. One way to manage this stress is through the use of **time management** skills. These skills involve learning how, where, and when to use one's time. Because the nurse has a limited amount of time with clients, it is essential to remain goal oriented and to use time wisely. The nurse learns early the importance of using client goals as a way to identify priorities. However, the nurse must also learn how to establish personal goals and time frames. For example, a nurse may be caring for two clients on a busy surgical nursing unit, one of whom underwent surgery the day before and the other of whom is anticipating discharge the next day. Clearly, the first client's goals center on restoring physiological function impaired as a result of the stress of surgery. The second client's goals center on adequate preparation to assume self-care at home. The nurse, in reviewing the therapies required for both clients, must learn how to organize his or her time so that the activities of care, as well as client goals, can be achieved. The nurse must anticipate when care will be interrupted for medication administration, any diagnostic testing, and planned therapies such as dressing changes and client ambulation. In addition, the nurse must be able to use time throughout the day to keep the charge nurse informed, document ongoing client care information, and consult with colleagues on care issues. Time management requires an ability to anticipate the day's activities, to combine activities when possible, and to not be interrupted by nonessential activities. Box 4-6 summarizes principles of time management.

One of the most important aspects of clinical care coordination is that of evaluation (see Chapter 18). It is a mistake to think that evaluation occurs at the end of an activity. Evaluation is an ongoing process. Once a nurse assesses a client's needs and begins therapies directed at a specific problem area, the nurse should immediately evaluate whether therapies are effective and the client's response. Evaluation compares actual client outcomes with those that are expected. For example, a clinic nurse may assess the condition of a diabetic client's foot ulcer to determine if healing has progressed since the last clinic visit. When expected outcomes are not being met, evaluation reveals the need to continue current therapies for a longer period of time, revise approaches to care, or introduce new therapies.

Keeping a focus on evaluation of the client's progress lessens the chances of becoming distracted by the tasks of care. It is common to assume that staying focused on planned activities will ensure that care is being performed appropriately. However, task orientation does not ensure good client outcomes. The competent nurse learns that at the heart of good organizational skills is constant inquiry into the client's condition and progress toward an improved level of health.

Team Communication. As part of a nursing team, each nurse is responsible for open, professional communication. Regardless of the setting, nurses learn that an enriching, professional environment is one where staff members respect one another's ideas, share information, and keep one another informed. On a busy hospital unit this means keeping colleagues informed about clients with emerging problems, physicians who have been called for consultation, and unique approaches that solved a complex nursing problem. In a clinic setting it may mean sharing unusual diagnostic findings or conveying important information regarding a client's source of family support. One way of fostering good team communication is by setting expectations of one another. An efficient team knows they can count on all members when needs arise. Sharing expectations of what and when to communicate is a step toward establishing a strong work team.

Delegation. Most hospitals today hire assistive personnel (see Chapter 2). As members of the nursing team, assistive personnel provide an additional resource to the RN and LPN for providing client care. An important management behavior for nurses to acquire is the art of delegating client care activities to assistive personnel. **Delegation** refers to the transferring of responsibility for the performance of an activity or task while retaining accountability

for the outcome (American Nurses Association [ANA], 1995).

It is important to recognize that in regard to delegation to assistive personnel, tasks are delegated, not clients. Leah Curtin (1994), a distinguished nursing leader and editor of the journal *Nursing Management,* wrote that unlicensed personnel should not be at the bedside, but at the nurse's side. This means that assistive personnel should not be assigned sole responsibility for the care of clients. Instead, it is the professional nurse in charge of client care who decides what activities assistive personnel may perform independently and what activities must be performed by the RN and assistant in partnership. For example, an RN will always be responsible for the assessment of a client's ongoing status, but if a client is stable, the RN may delegate vital sign monitoring to the assistive personnel. The RN is the one in most settings who makes judgments during client care as to when delegation is appropriate. The LPN directs care in many long-term care facilities. The National Council of State Boards of Nursing has provided some guidelines for delegation of tasks in accordance with RN's legal scopes of practice (Box 4-7). As the leader of the health care team, the RN must know how to give clear instructions, effectively prioritize client needs and therapies, and be able to give staff members timely and meaningful feedback.

The art of effective delegation is a skill nursing students need to observe and practice to improve their own management skills. When a nurse delegates, he or she gives someone else the authority to carry out a care task, but the RN remains accountable for the overall nursing care of the client (Parkman, 1996). A nurse cannot simply assign assistive personnel to tasks without considering the implications. The nurse assesses a client and determines a plan of care before identifying which tasks someone else can perform. When directing assistive personnel, the RN must determine the degree of supervision that may be required. Is it the first time a staff member performed the task? Does the client present a complicating factor whereby the RN's assistance is necessary? Does the staff member have prior experience with a particular type of client in addition to having received training on skill performance? The RN's final responsibility is to evaluate whether a task was performed properly by assistive personnel and whether desired outcomes were realized.

Appropriate delegation begins with knowing what skills can be delegated. This requires the RN to be familiar with the state's nurse practice act, institutional policies and procedures, and the institution's job description for assistive personnel. These standards help to define the necessary level of competency of assistive personnel.

A state's nurse practice act defines the scope of an RN's practice. It defines those activities that only RNs can perform (e.g., client assessment and planning care). Most states identify the delegation and supervision of work as an RN's responsibility (Parkman, 1996). However, each state will address the specifics of delegation differently.

An institution's policies and procedures and job description for assistive personnel provide specific guidelines in regard to what tasks or activities can be delegated. The job description should specify any required education and the types of tasks assistive personnel can perform, either independently or with RN direct supervision. Institutional policy helps in defining the amount of training required of assistive personnel while employed. Procedures specify who is qualified to perform a given nursing procedure, whether supervision is necessary, and the type of reporting required. Job descriptions, policies, and procedures should comply with state laws and regulations (Parkman, 1996). Nurses should have a means to easily access policies or have supervisory staff who can inform them as to assistive personnel's job duties.

Competency of assistive personnel is an important issue because there is no consistent standard for training across institutions. To delegate, the RN must know that assistive personnel are competent to perform a given procedure. This means that the RN should be familiar with the institution's training program. Frequently RNs eventually become directly involved as preceptors in assistive personnel's training. The RN is assigned for a limited time to directly supervise a staff member and observe his or her performance of skills. Participating in the training of assistive personnel and the continual refining of their skills can reduce the fear and mistrust of working with these staff members (Parkman, 1996).

Over time, effective delegation requires that trust develop between the RN and assistive personnel. A purpose of delegation is to improve efficiency. Asking a staff member to obtain an ordered specimen while the nurse attends to a client's pain medication request effectively prevents a delay in the client's gaining pain relief. Efficient delegation requires constant communication—sending clear messages and listening so that all participants understand expectations regarding client care. An RN should provide clear instructions when delegating tasks. These instructions may initially focus on the procedure itself, as well as on the unique needs of a given client. As the RN becomes more familiar with a staff member's competency, trust builds and fewer instructions may be needed, but clarification of clients' specific needs will always be necessary. Delegation can also provide job enrichment. A nurse shows trust in colleagues by delegating tasks to them and showing staff that they are important players in the delivery of care. Assistive personnel respond positively when they are actively included as part of the nursing team.

Another important step in delegation is evaluation of the staff member's performance and the client's outcomes. When assistive personnel do a good job, it is important to provide praise and recognition. If the staff member's performance is not satisfactory, the RN must give constructive and appropriate feedback. The RN should always give specific feedback in regard to any mistakes that were made, explaining how the mistakes could have been avoided. Giving feedback in private is the professional way and preserves the staff member's dignity. Frequently when the performance of assistive personnel does not meet expectations, the cause is due to inadequate training or assignment to too many tasks. The RN may discover the need to review a procedure with staff and offer demonstration or even recommend that additional training be scheduled with the education department. If too many tasks are being delegated, this might be a nursing practice issue. All staff should discuss the appropriateness of delegation on their unit. Some assistive personnel may need help in learning how to prioritize. In some cases RNs may need to learn that they are overdelegating.

The availability of assistive personnel as members of the nursing team can be a positive contribution to a nursing unit. The RN must accept the responsibilities associated with delegation and learn to delegate well. When RNs delegate well, they are able to use the resources of assistive personnel to the client's advantage, as well as their own. Box 4-8 summarizes important requirements for proper delegation.

Knowledge Building. All professional nurses recognize the importance of pursuing knowledge to remain competent. A leader recognizes that there is always something new to learn. Opportunities for learning occur with each client interaction, each encounter with a professional colleague, and each meeting or class session where health care professionals gather to discuss clinical care issues. There is always someone who has had different experi-

Requirements for Delegation   Box 4-8

Determine the complexity of client needs or the nature of the work to be delegated.

Introduce assistive personnel to the client and family and clarify their care responsibilities.

Determine that the work is consistent with the staff member's job description and normal duties.

Clearly communicate expectations and desired results using measurable terms; convey trust and sufficient authority.

Obtain the staff member's voluntary acceptance of the work request.

Keep communication lines open while giving direction, instruction, and supervision.

Compare actual results with expectations; give feedback; praise and reward the staff member's efforts.

Show appreciation for a job well done.

Modified from Wywialowski E: *Managing client care,* St. Louis, 1993, Mosby.

ences and knowledge. In-service programs, work shops, and collegiate courses offer innovative and current information on the rapidly changing world of health care. To become a leader, a nurse actively pursues learning opportunities, both formal and informal, and learns to share knowledge with the professional colleagues he or she encounters.

Quality Management

Within a health care environment where business initiatives and client care activities create constant demands on all levels of staff, it is sometimes difficult to reflect and take the time to consider how improvements can be made in the way work is done. If you would ask a busy staff nurse who just completed caring for six clients, "How can you improve what you just did," you likely might get a skeptical look. It would be easy for the nurse to say that he or she is just too busy to take the time to think about how changes can be made. This is the case unless the nurse works for an organization where **total quality management (TQM)** is a well-integrated philosophy.

Health care organizations cannot ignore the need for improvement. It is a must for customer satisfaction and business survival. TQM has become the philosophy for change within many business organizations. It is a philosophy that influences every single department and thus every single employee of an organization. TQM requires employees to think differently and therefore to act differently from what may be their usual habit (Triolo and others, 1997). An organization that accepts TQM as a work principle acknowledges that perfection is never reached, recognizes that an attempt to improve is not a condemnation of the past, and accepts that change is a continuous process. Table 4-2 summarizes principles and conditions for TQM.

In a well-established TQM program, customer service is a priority. Customers of health care include anyone who uses the products, services, or processes within an organization (National Association for Healthcare Quality, 1994).

Customers are more interested today in the quality of health care because of rising costs and because they are more informed. They want easy access to services, timely and safe delivery of services, coordinated care, and effective services that result in desired outcomes. In a TQM philosophy the term *customer* is not intended to devalue how health care providers perceive their client relationships (Triolo and others, 1997). Instead, it is intended to broaden each staff member's concept of relationships with others in doing work. In addition to clients, customers may include families, physicians, other health care professionals, and even product suppliers. To make improvements in how health care is provided, each employee of a health care organization must be willing to work with others.

Another important principle of TQM is that work is accomplished through processes (such as medication delivery and client education), and that processes make up systems (Triolo and others, 1997). If clients' outcomes are to be improved, there is a need to examine and improve processes. Typically, many individuals are involved in a single process. For example, medication delivery might seem to be simply the concern and responsibility of the

Table 4-2 **Principles and Conditions for Total Quality Management**	
Principles	Conditions in the Work Environment
Continuous quality improvement	Employee involvement
Knowledge of customer expectations, needs	Empowerment
Processes of customer-supplier relationships	An environment that supports risk taking
Belief in people	Teamwork
Statistical analysis	Data collection and analysis skills
Costs of poor quality	Group interaction skills
	Structure and management to enable improvement
	Tools to facilitate the improvement

nurse. But consider that physicians prescribe the medications, the pharmacy must prepare the medications, secretaries communicate orders and changes, transporters often deliver medications to work areas, and the nurse finally administers the medications. With so many individuals involved in most work processes, strong leadership, good collaboration, effective communication, and support of staffs' ideas are essential factors for TQM to be successful. TQM begins with executive leaders and then is integrated through the work of managers and staff. The following section explores the influence a TQM philosophy can have on nursing practice and the involvement of staff nurses.

QUALITY IN NURSING PRACTICE

The Joint Commission on Accreditation of Healthcare Organizations (JCAHO) (1997) defines **quality improvement (QI)** as an approach to the continuous study and improvement of the processes of providing health care services to meet the needs of clients and others. Quality improvement is one of the principles underlying TQM (Triolo and others, 1997). Among the processes that most directly influence clients are those that constitute nursing practice. The quality of nursing practice is a principal responsibility of nursing managers and their staff. Each professional nurse must learn to evaluate his or her success in delivering appropriate and effective client care. Does the nurse perform competently? Is appropriate care delivered? What outcomes does the client experience? These questions drive any QI effort.

The nurse must recognize that good client outcomes are a product of all the individual actions that relate directly or indirectly to the care received by a client (Scoble and Hembrough, 1993). The outcomes of care are a measure of the performance of the entire health care team. Managing quality ultimately becomes a multidisciplinary effort.

With all disciplines contributing to client care, the nurse manager and staff assume the critical role in recognizing trends in nursing practice, identifying when recurrent problems develop, and initiating opportunities to improve the quality of care. For example, after reviewing clients who have undergone hip surgery, the nurse manager asks, "Do clients regain functional mobility without severe pain?" "Is rehabilitation delayed?" and "Are there complications of wound infection?" An effective nurse manager will enforce a work ethic that has nursing staff continually improving on how care is administered. The first step is to define quality of nursing practice.

Quality Defined.

Before the nurse manager and staff can measure trends in nursing practice, they first must know the standards or guidelines that define quality. In other words, to judge if clients with hip surgery have functional mobility impaired by pain, there must be an agreement as to how functional clients should become after

surgery and how pain is assessed. Similarly, to judge if rehabilitation has been delayed, there must be a standard for when clients begin rehabilitation. Quality of care and nursing practice is not something arbitrarily defined. The process is ongoing, involving all members of a nursing department. It therefore occurs at an administration level and at a work unit level. A definition of quality begins with the mission, vision, and philosophy of the nursing department. These statements lay the foundation of values that define how all nurses within an organization are to perform and the services that are to be made available to clients. A well-written set of values for a nursing department then provides direction for professional standards and care guidelines that when administered should guarantee excellent client outcomes. Figure 4-2 provides a framework for quality nursing care.

Professional Standards.

Professional standards are authoritative statements used by the profession in describing the responsibilities for which its practitioners are accountable (Peters, 1995). Standards are an organization's interpretation of the professional's competency. Whenever a work unit such as a nursing staff attempts to define quality, professional performance is a critical element. When the process is done well, the staff will be able to recognize evidence of quality standards in all aspects of their work. The adherence to professional standards is measured through professional outcomes. Examples of professional standards are summarized in Box 4-9.

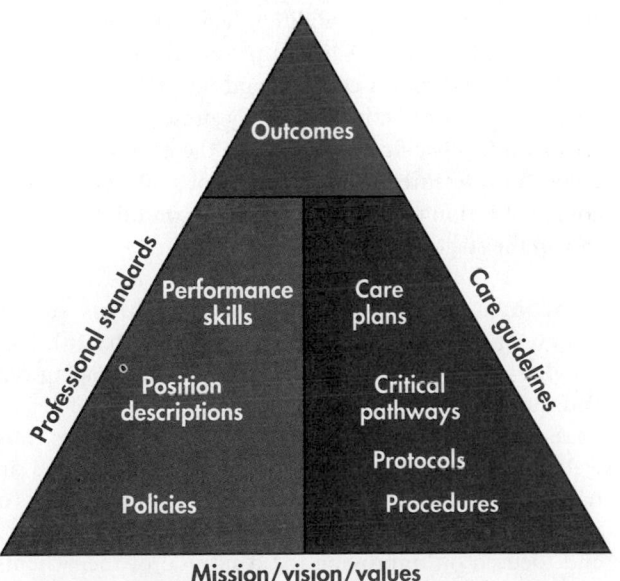

Figure 4-2 Framework for quality.
Data from Peters DA: Outcomes: the mainstay of a framework for quality care, *J Nurs Care Qual* 10(1):61, 1995.

Care Guidelines. Care guidelines are systematically developed statements to assist in determining how diseases, disorders, and other health conditions can be most effectively and appropriately prevented, diagnosed, treated, and clinically managed (ANA, 1991). Guidelines may be developed by single disciplines or be multidisciplinary in focus. There may be care guidelines jointly developed by nurses from similar clinical areas or from a single, unique clinical unit. An example of a nursing clinical protocol is one used for instructing clients newly diagnosed with diabetes. The effectiveness of clinical guidelines is measured through client outcomes.

Care guidelines include procedures, care plans (see Chapter 16), protocols and critical pathways (see Chapter 2). Procedures are step-by-step descriptions of how to perform a psychomotor skill. An example is the nursing skill for changing a sterile dressing. Depending on complexity, skills include cognitive abilities (e.g., assessment steps) and manual dexterity. Clinical protocols outline steps to be taken in treating a certain condition (Peters, 1995). A specific course of action is usually prescribed in specific terms under specific conditions. In the example of treatment for pressure ulcers, a protocol will establish the course of action to take in treating the condition, depending on the stage of the ulcer.

Outcomes. Outcomes are the conditions to be achieved as a result of care delivery (see Chapter 16). They provide the backbone for organizing and managing care and quality (Peters, 1995). An **outcome** tells whether interventions are effective, whether clients progress, how well standards are being met, and whether changes are necessary. When a nursing staff is able to think in terms of outcomes, their actions become much more purposeful and focused on improving the condition of their clients' health. There are two types of outcomes important to differentiate (Peters, 1995):

1. *Professional outcomes:* A measure of the professional caregiver's performance. Professional standards of care, institutional policies, and job descriptions set expectations for how care is to be delivered and the professional nurse's responsibility in care delivery. *Example:* The RN is responsible for the ongoing assessment of clients' status and will communicate changes in a client's condition to appropriate health team members.

2. *Client outcomes:* A measure of the client's status after receiving care. All clients have outcomes reflected in their nursing plan of care. Client outcomes are also defined in other clinical guidelines, such as critical pathways (see Chapter 2) and clinical protocols. *Example:* Following use of reminiscent therapy, a client will be able to discuss concerns regarding the client's terminal illness.

Developing Quality Improvement Teams. It makes sense for health care providers who are most familiar with client care activities to collaborate on QI efforts. For example, if a team of nursing staff identifies an opportunity to improve the timeliness and efficiency of the admission process to their unit, it makes sense to include admitting, transporters, pharmacy, and physicians in the improvement effort. In many health care organizations there are organization-wide and unit-based QI teams or committees. The organization-wide teams are composed of staff from all departments within a hospital. The problems these teams seek to solve usually affect processes that occur on all units within an organization. For example, the redesign of a client documentation system requires participation by all disciplines who enter information in the medical record. These organizational QI teams are given the responsibility to create innovations to make work more efficient and to improve the quality of care provided. In contrast, unit-based QI teams identify clinical priorities for a work unit. Client understanding of discharge instructions and the associated education process is an example of a unit-based QI project for a nursing unit. Unit-based teams are ideally participative, decentralizing decision making and accountability for practice and placing them at the staff level. An effective QI program leads to improved clinical practice, better participation by professional staff members, and increased sophistication of evaluation. It also achieves better client outcomes.

Components of a QI Program. A well-organized QI program focuses on processes or systems that significantly contribute to outcomes. A systematic approach is needed organizationally to ensure that everyone speaks the same language with regard to QI projects. The JCAHO's 10 steps to quality improvement (Box 4-10) are incorporated within many health care organizations' programs. In addition to the JCAHO's model, there are numerous process improvement models to be found across the country (Table 4-3). The models have similar elements, such as process or problem identification, and they are cyclical in nature (Keill and Johnson, 1994). Each requires use of a scientific approach to problem solving, similar to the nursing process, which often requires returning to various steps in the model to evaluate and then reassess work that needs to be done. An organization may use the JCAHO's 10-step program to organize their QI program but use a QI model such as FOCUS-PDCA (see Table 4-3) to structure problem analysis and resolution.

Responsibility for a QI Program. Organizational leadership must create a work culture that supports continuous–quality improvement (QI) beliefs and practice. Most organizations have a director responsible for TQM or system CQI activities. In nursing care areas, home health sections, or clinics, a nurse manager is responsible for supporting a unit-based program. Individual staff are responsible for monitoring practice, making decisions about ways to improve practice, and evaluating results.

Scope of Service. Each nursing care area involved in the care of a select group of clients provides a well-defined set of services. A unit's scope of service includes the types of clients who receive nursing care and the types of processes involved in delivering care. An example might be a general medicine unit in a hospital that cares for middle-age and older adult clients who have diabetes, heart disease, and gastrointestinal disorders. Such a unit would be involved in processes that include intravenous administration, diabetes education, referrals for cardiac diagnostic testing, and endoscopy. An understanding of the scope of service allows staff to focus on quality issues related to typical client groups.

Key Aspects of Service. Unit-based committees review activities or services considered most important in providing quality service to clients. It is a way of prioritizing activities within the unit's scope of service. To identify the greatest opportunity for improving quality, nurses consider those activities that are high-volume, high-risk, and problem areas. Aspects of care are high volume if over 50% of the unit's clients receive that service. A high-risk aspect of care is one that could result in trauma or death for the client, or litigation or loss of professional license. Problem-prone aspects of care are those that have the potential to produce problems for the client, staff, or institution (Patton and Stanley, 1993). In the example of the medicine unit, if a high volume of clients are diabetic and if the unit has seen a problem of readmissions resulting from poor glucose control, an opportunity may exist to improve client education and counseling.

Developing Quality Indicators. A **quality indicator** is a quantitative measure of an important aspect of service that determines whether the service conforms to established standards or requirements. The quality indicator is the focus for a QI project, with the staff monitoring criteria that will show whether indicator standards have been met. There are three types of indicators: structure, process, and outcome.

Structure indicators evaluate the structure or systems for delivering care; an example is adherence in checking if emergency carts are adequately stocked or if forms documenting restraint use are completed correctly. **Process indicators** evaluate the manner in which care is delivered (e.g., the process of pain assessment, recovery of clients

---

JCAHO's 10 Steps for Quality Improvement Box 4-10

1. Establish responsibility and accountability for a QI program.
2. Define the scope of service for a clinical area.
3. Define the key aspects of service for the clinical area.
4. Develop quality indicators to monitor the outcomes and appropriateness of care delivered.
5. Establish thresholds for evaluation of indicators.
6. Collect and analyze data from monitoring activities.
7. Evaluate results of monitoring activities to determine the need for change in practice.
8. Resolve problems through development of action plans.
9. Reevaluate to determine if the plan was successful.
10. Communicate QI results to the organization.

Modified from Joint Commission on Accreditation of Healthcare Organizations: *An introduction to quality improvement in health care*, Chicago, 1991, The Commission.

Table 4-3 **Models for Process Improvement**		
PRIDE	FOCUS-PDCA	FADE
Process—select one to improve	Find process to improve	Focus on a problem
Relevant dimensions of performance measurement	Organize team that knows process	Analyze the problem
Interpret data and evaluate variance	Clarify current knowledge of process	Develop a plan
Design or redesign the process	Understand causes of process variation	Execute the plan
Execute the plan	Select process improvement	
Improve—validate by remeasuring	PDCA: Plan, Do, Check, Act	

Modified from Keill P, Johnson T: Optimizing performance through process improvement, *J Nurs Car Qual* 9(1):1, 1994.

from sedation, and clients' referral to community services). **Outcome indicators** as described earlier, evaluate the end result of care delivered (e.g., incidence of nosocomial infection and adherence to medication therapy). Outcomes are the most important indicators in any QI program, but structural and process indicators cannot be ignored.

Processes of care are obviously closely related to outcomes and the structure in which a process of care occurs, enhances, or hinders the effectiveness of care (Donabedian, 1988). When a unit-based team selects a QI indicator, it is important that the indicator be relevant. It is often appropriate to measure a process, as well as the expected outcome, to know if standards of care are being met. In the example of the medicine unit, staff may choose to measure their success in implementing the process of diabetes instruction early while also measuring the outcome of whether clients learn to administer insulin correctly. When a unit-based team sits together to select quality indicators for a QI project, it helps to ask what processes and related outcomes are in need of improvement and are most likely to make a significant contribution to how nursing care is being practiced. Processes to improve may include the following:

A weak process that is causing problems (e.g., poor pain management for clients with sickle cell anemia)

A stable process that is adequate, but that can benefit from improvement (e.g., waiting time for ambulatory surgery clients)

A process linked to negative outcomes (e.g., care of intravenous access sites with the occurrence of phlebitis)

Establishing Thresholds for Evaluation.   After selecting a quality indicator, staff members must determine ways to quantitatively measure the indicator. The occurrence of an indicator, or the percentage of times the indicator is observed (e.g., the number of clients having surgery who can successfully explain their discharge instructions) is a common measure. A threshold is a standard for determining whether a problem exists. A measurement that falls below the threshold indicates a problem. For example, a staff may set a threshold that states that 95% of older adult clients over age 65 who visit a clinic will receive flu shots. If monitoring of records shows that only 90% of clients scheduled visits to have flu shots, the threshold is not being met. Staff will then thoroughly review the factors interfering with successful client education and adherence. When QI is an ongoing process, staff continuously work to improve outcomes or performance by raising thresholds.

It is important to understand that almost all processes have variation. For example, consider the process of diabetic instruction and the associated outcome of clients administering insulin. Possible variations in the process might include the time when teaching begins, materials used in instruction, and learner motivation. Outcome variations might include accuracy in injection site selection and proficiency in preparing the insulin in a syringe. Setting specific thresholds may not always be achievable. The intent in any QI program is to seek ways to continuously improve. This includes defining the acceptable level of performance and allowing for normal variability.

Data Collection and Analysis.   The process of data collection and analysis can be simple or complex. The importance, however, is in obtaining accurate results that help in making appropriate decisions regarding quality care issues. Many organizations have made QI so important that formal research studies are conducted (see Chapter 25). In this case the process of data collection and analysis is very formal and well designed. Statistical techniques are used to determine if problems that have been identified are significant. Similarly, if a QI project involves introduction of a new practice or procedure, statistics can show whether the improvement made a significant difference in outcomes.

When formal research is not conducted, staff may become involved in simple evaluation studies involving the collection of data on frequencies and percentages for a predetermined number of clients or cases. Evaluation studies offer valuable information on practice trends and whether problems are evident. What is important in data collection is to collect data on the right criteria and to then have adequate data from which to make decisions. QI teams usually have access to resources within their organization who can help determine how much information is needed for QI analysis. In the example of diabetic instruction and insulin administration, staff might monitor criteria that include use of recommended teaching materials, staff's compliance with teaching standards, and each client's score on a return demonstration test. When sufficient data have been collected, the QI team can determine whether problems exist and analyze their possible causes. For example, if diabetic clients perform poorly on their test, staff can analyze whether standards are inconsistently met or if teaching is unnecessarily delayed.

Evaluation of Care.   Monitoring of quality indicators evaluates whether a specifically defined process reaches desired outcomes. If results exceed or meet a threshold, or if performance is within controls set for a process, no problem has been identified and the process is performing well. When thresholds for satisfactory care are not met or when performance is below the control limits set, staff must try to find the cause of problems. For example, if diabetic clients score an average of only 70% on a return demonstration test, staff must determine the reasons. This step requires nurses and colleagues to honestly review practice activities and look for opportunities to reinforce nursing care standards or improve practice.

When a process is not working well, one of the models for QI (e.g., FOCUS-PDCA) may be used. This allows staff to find the aspect of the process to improve, organize an expert team who knows the process, clarify knowledge about the process, understand any sources of variation, and select an improvement or solution. The process may take several team meetings before the group can agree on the actions to take. In the case of diabetic instruction, it would be important to have staff nurses, dietitians, diabetes nurse specialists, and pharmacists involved as part of the QI team. Many of these staff members might have been on the original QI committee. However, once a problem is identified, additional team members may be needed. The team collaborates to discover what are the factors associated with a practice problem. Eventually the team recommends approaches for improving the process with the goal of achieving desired outcomes.

Resolution of Problems.   After evaluating quality problems, staff develop action plans to improve the process and outcomes. It is important to establish actions that will be successful. For example, the action of merely notifying staff that a problem exists is unlikely to change practice or improve outcomes. An action plan should be more direct. In FOCUS-PDCA, staff *P*lan the action or improvement to make, *D*o or implement the change, *C*heck or analyze results of the change, and then *A*ct on the findings. For example, the QI team may discover that clients are not administering insulin correctly because they do not have all of the necessary information. (Staff are not beginning teaching as soon as clients learn that insulin will be a form of therapy. Staff are also found to have trouble acquiring necessary teaching materials for instruction.) In this case the team may recommend having the pharmacy send instructional materials when insulin is sent to the unit and having a clinical pharmacist assist with instruction on insulin therapy. The staff nurses and nurse specialist may develop a practice protocol that outlines specific content to teach until the client learns to administer injections. Collectively, the team may develop an innovative approach that is designed to get appropriate information to clients more quickly and efficiently so that learning can take place.

Evaluation of Improvement.   After implementing an action plan, the staff must reevaluate its success. In the example, staff members may repeat monitoring of the teaching process and the results of client testing to see if improvement has been made. The change may be positive or negative. For example, if client test scores improve, the team has successfully improved outcomes. Similarly, if test scores show no improvement or even worsen, a new plan of action is needed. The QI process is similar to the nursing process (see Unit 3) in that when desired outcomes are not met, the staff reinstitutes the QI process.

Communication of Results.   The results of QI activities must be communicated to staff in all appropriate organizational departments. If findings and results are not communicated, practice changes will likely not occur. Regular discussions of QI activities through staff meetings, newsletters, and memos are examples of communication strategies. Often a QI study reveals information requiring organization-wide change. In this case the organization must be responsible for responding to the problem with the resources needed to make changes. Revision of policies and procedures, modification of standards of care, and implementation of system changes are examples of ways that an organization may respond.

• • •

The incorporation of a QI program within a health care setting benefits the client, the professional staff, and the institution. With a focus on client and professional outcomes, QI activities lead to a selection of interventions that result in improved client care. Professional staff members learn from their own practice, identify opportunities to change practice, and gain greater satisfaction from improved client outcomes. An institution benefits from an improved level of care delivery that reduces excessive or unnecessary use of resources and improves client satisfaction.

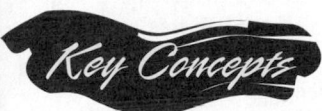
Key Concepts

- Change, along with the ability to manage it, is central to the concept of leadership.
- Management involves keeping individuals on course and directed toward organizational goals.
- An organization that changes its goals, as well as its management structure, undergoes transformational change.
- A function of transactional leadership is to maintain an organization's operation by providing stability in day-to-day management.
- A transformational leader changes a work culture through charisma, intellectual stimulation, and individual consideration.

- In situational leadership a leader may use any one of four different styles depending on the size of a work group, maturity of staff, and the work group's situation.
- An empowered nursing staff has decision-making authority to change how they practice.
- The nurse executive establishes a vision for nursing that lays the groundwork that enables nursing managers and staff to exercise nursing practice.
- Continuity of nursing care can be compromised in total patient care delivery, functional nursing, and team nursing.
- A professional nurse's job description outlines a nurse's professional responsibilities and sets guidelines for professional outcomes.
- Clinical care coordination begins with thorough organizational skills, critical thinking, appropriate use of resources, and the ability to prioritize clients' needs.
- An enriching professional environment is one where staff respect one another's ideas, share information, and keep one another informed.
- Delegation involves transferring responsibility for performing an activity while retaining accountability for the outcome.
- Knowing whether the right task is being delegated requires knowledge of one's state nurse practice act and institutional policies and procedures.
- An important responsibility for the nurse who delegates nursing care is evaluation of the staff member's performance and client outcomes.
- When total quality management is part of an organization's philosophy, every staff member becomes involved in finding ways to improve or change work processes so as to promote customer satisfaction.
- A well-organized quality improvement program focuses on processes or systems that significantly contribute to outcomes.

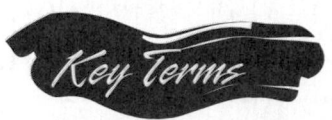

Key Terms

Critical Thinking Exercises

1. It is a busy morning, and Josh has just completed making rounds on his five clients. One of his clients, Mrs. Robinson, is a 60-year old woman who requested that Josh reposition her in bed because of discomfort in her right leg. Mrs. Robinson had surgery on her right leg to repair a fracture and has a dressing that extends along the right thigh. Nancy is a nurse assistant who is working with Josh this morning. Josh approaches Nancy and says, "Would you please go into Mrs. Robinson's room and help turn her." What, if anything, is inapppropriate with Josh's delegation?

2. Linda is the manager of a busy clinic. Her philosophy of leadership has been use of decentralized decision making. In addition to a staff dietitian, pharmacist, and social worker, there are three staff nurses under her supervision: Lisa, Jeff, and Nina. Lisa has worked at the clinic for over 10 years and has assisted Linda in managing the clinic when Linda is absent. Jeff just joined the clinic team about 6 months ago but has shown good progress as a clinician. Nina has been a staff member for 1 year after having worked in an operating room for 5 years. Nina has had difficulty in completing her work on time and has received counseling from Linda. The clinic is starting a new service, diabetic education, and Linda wants the nursing staff to be involved as part of the clinic's multidisciplinary team. Linda has been asked by the clinic director to develop standards of care for client and family instruction. What leadership approaches might Linda use? How might she apply situational leadership principles in involving Lisa, Jeff, and Nina in this project?

3. Assume that you are part of a quality improvement (QI) work team. Your team receives a report from the manager that the rate of infection in clients who have in-dwelling Foley catheters is high. The QI team agrees that a problem exists. Refer to Chapter 44 for the procedure on care and maintenance of an in-dwelling Foley catheter. Knowing that the outcome of infection is undesirable, what criteria might your team monitor in determining possible causes for the incidence of urinary infection in your clients?

References

Aiken LH and others: Lower Medicare mortality among a set of hospitals known for good nursing care, *Med Care* 32:771, 1994.

American Hospital Association: Role and function of the hospital nurse executive. In *Management advisory,* Chicago, 1990, American Organization of Nurse Executives.

American Nurses Association: Task force on nursing practice standards and guidelines: working paper, *J Nurs Qual Assur* 5:1, 1991.

American Nurses Association: Position statement on registered nurse utilization of assistive personnel, *Am Nurse* 25(2):7, 1995.

Blegen MA and others: Nurse staffing and patient outcomes, *Nurs Res,* 47: 43, 1998.

Bolster CJ, Petit B: Quest for health care value will drive nontraditional opportunities for patient care executives, *Aspen's Advisor Nurse Exec* 5(7):4, 1990.

Burns JM: *Leadership,* New York, 1978, Harper & Row.

Curtin L: The heart of patient care, *Nurs Manage,* 25(5):7, 1994.

Cox S: *Managing the workplace 2000,* Seminar conducted at Barnes-Jewish Hospital, St. Louis, fall 1995.

Donabedian A: The quality of care: how can it be assessed? *JAMA* 160:1743, 1988.

Dossett D: Leadership skills. In Sullivan EJ, Decker PJ, editors: *Effective management in nursing,* ed 3, Redwood City, Calif, 1992, Addison-Wesley.

Duchene P: Organizing care. In Sullivan EJ, Decker PJ, editors: *Effective management in nursing,* ed 3, Redwood City, Calif, 1992, Addison-Wesley.

Gardner KA: A summary of findings of a five-year comparison study of primary and team nursing, *Nurs Res* 40:113, 1991.

Gregory CS: Creating a vision for a nursing unit, *Nurs Manage* 26(1):38, 1995.

Gustafson D: The functions of a nurse manager in a health care setting. In Sullivan EJ, Decker PJ, editors: *Effective management in nursing,* ed 3, Redwood City, Calif, 1992, Addison-Wesley.

Gustafson D, Duchene P, Baker L: Stress and time management. In Sullivan EJ, Decker PJ, editors: *Effective management in nursing,* Redwood City, Calif, 1992, Addison-Wesley.

Hersey P, Blanchard K: *Management of organizational behavior: utilizing human resources,* ed 5, Englewood Cliffs, NJ, 1988, Prentice-Hall.

Joint Commission on Accreditation of Healthcare Organizations: *An introduction to quality improvement in health care,* 1991, The Commission.

Keill P, Johnson T: Optimizing performance through process improvement, *J Nurs Care Qual* 9(1):1, 1994.

Kurz R, Hernandez SR, Haddock CC: Organizational change, transformational leadership, and leadership development. In Fottler M, Hernandez S, Joiner C, editors: *Strategic management of human resources in health services organizations,* New York, 1988, John Wiley & Sons.

Manthey M: *The practice of primary nursing,* St. Louis, 1980, CV Mosby.

National Association for Healthcare Quality: *Guide to health care quality management,* Deerfield, Ill, 1994, The Association.

National Council of State Boards of Nursing: *Delegation: concepts and decision-making process,* Chicago, 1995, The Council.

McDaniel C, Wolf GA: Transformational leadership in nursing service, *J Nurs* 22:60, 1992.

Parkman CA: Delegation: are you doing it right? *Am J Nurs* 96(9):43, 1996.

Patton S, Stanley J: Bridging quality assurance and continuous quality improvement, *J Nurs Care Qual* 7(2):15, 1993.

Peters DA: Outcomes: the mainstay of a framework for quality care, *J Nurs Care Qual* 10(1):61, 1995.

Rogers EM: *Diffusion of innovations,* ed 4, New York, 1983, Free Press.

Senge PM: *The fifth discipline,* New York, 1990, Doubleday.

Scoble KB, Hembrough B: Nursing clinical pertinence review: a step toward quality improvement, *J Nurs Care Qual,* 7(2):52, 1993.

Stogdill RM: *Handbook of leadership: a survey of the literature,* New York, 1974, Free Press.

Tebbitt BV: Nurse executives: who are they, what do they do, and what challenges do they face? In McCloskey JC, and Grace HK, editors: *Current issues in nursing,* ed 5, St. Louis, 1997, Mosby.

Triolo PK and others: Total quality management, redesign, reengineering: what's the difference? In McCloskey JC, and Grace HK, editors: *Current issues in nursing,* ed 5, St. Louis, 1997, Mosby.

Trofino J: Vision: a professional model for nursing practice, *Nurs Manage* 27(3):43, 1996.

Wywialowski E: *Managing client care,* St. Louis, 1993, Mosby.

Zaleznik A: Managers and leaders: are they different? *Harv Bus Rev* 70:126, 1992.

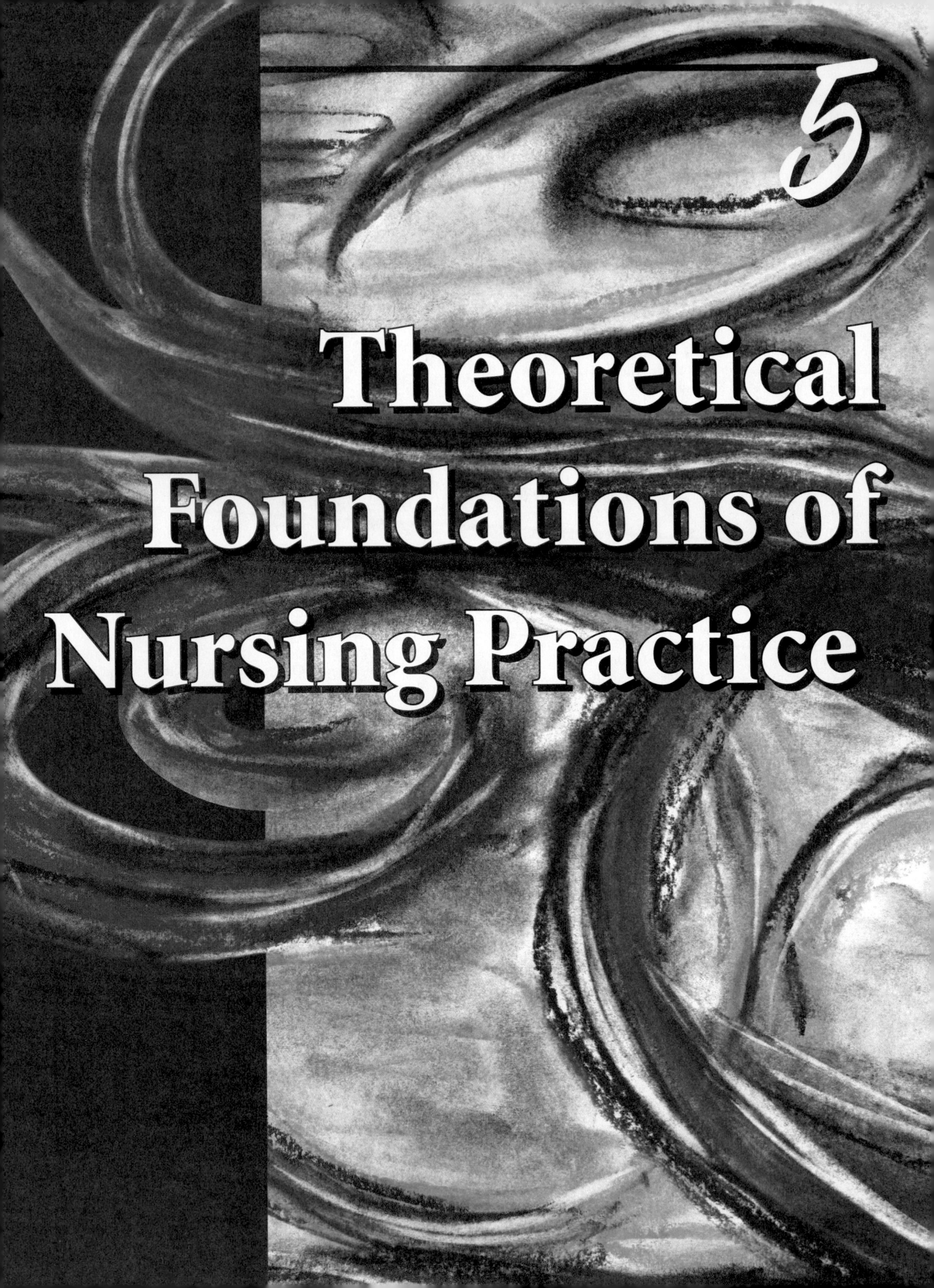

5

Theoretical Foundations of Nursing Practice

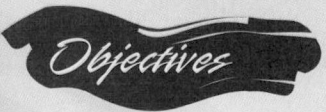

Mastery of content in this chapter will enable the student to:

- Define the key terms listed.
- Define nursing theory.
- Describe types of nursing theories.
- Describe the relationship between theory, the nursing process, and client needs.
- Describe the historical development of nursing theory.
- Discuss selected theories from other disciplines.
- Discuss selected nursing theories.
- Describe the relationship between theory and knowledge development in nursing.

M odern nursing is an art and a science involving the application of knowledge and skills related to basic social sciences, physical sciences, biobehavioral sciences, ethics, contemporary issues, and nursing knowledge. Nursing as a profession is unique because it addresses the many responses of individuals and families to their health problems.

Expertise in nursing is a result of knowledge and clinical experience. The expertise required to interpret clinical situations and make clinical judgments is the essence of nursing care and is the basis for the advancement of nursing practice and the development of nursing science (Benner and Tanner, 1987; Carnevali and Thomas, 1993). Nurses learn from experience. They also learn and grow professionally by becoming familiar with nursing theory and finding ways to apply theory in their practice. Well-developed theories can form the basis for the nurse's approach to client care. The nurse must use critical thinking skills to select the appropriate theoretical base to support clinical judgments about the care needed for clients based on knowledge, experience, attitudes, and standards of care (Alfaro-LeFevre, 1995). Clinical judgment involves conscious reasoning and intuitive responses based on the nursing assessment (Tanner, 1993).

Theory

A **theory** is a set of concepts, definitions, relationships, and assumptions or propositions that project a purposive, systematic view of phenomena by designing specific interrelationships among concepts for the purposes of describing, explaining, predicting, and/or prescribing (Marriner-Tomey and Alligood, 1998; Chinn and Kramer, 1999). A **nursing theory** is a conceptualization of some aspect of nursing communicated for the purpose of describing, explaining, predicting, and/or prescribing nursing care (Barnum, 1994; Meleis, 1997). For example, Orem's (1991) self-care deficit theory can be used to explain the

factors within a clients' living situation that support or interfere with the client's self-care ability. Theory provides nurses with a perspective to view client situations, "a way to organize data," and a method to analyze and interpret information. Theory allows the nurse to plan and implement care purposefully and proactively (Raudonis and Acton, 1997). Application of nursing theory in practice depends on the nurse's knowledge of nursing and interdisciplinary theoretical models and how these models relate to each other (Marriner-Tomey and Alligood, 1998).

Why nursing theory? Why is there a need for theoretical models as a basis for practice? These are questions frequently asked by students and professionals within the discipline of nursing. Meleis (1997) notes that theoretical thinking is integral to all roles of the discipline: the clinician, the educator, the researcher, the administrator, and the consultant.

The development of nursing science, conceptual models, and theory is a scholarly activity. Theory is the goal of all scientific work; theorizing is a central process in all scientific endeavors; and theoretical thinking is essential to all professional undertakings (Meleis, 1997).

Nursing is a learned profession, a science, and an art (Rogers, 1990). Nurses need a theoretical base to exemplify the science and art of the profession when they promote health and wellness for their clients, whether the client is an individual, a family, or a community.

COMPONENTS OF A THEORY

As previously stated, a theory is a set of concepts, definitions, relationships, and assumptions or propositions to explain phenomena (Figure 5-1). They provide a foundation of knowledge for the direction and delivery of nursing care. For example, in Newman's systems model (1972), the goal of nursing is to assist individuals, families, and groups in attaining and maintaining a maximal level of total wellness by purposeful interventions. Neuman's sys-

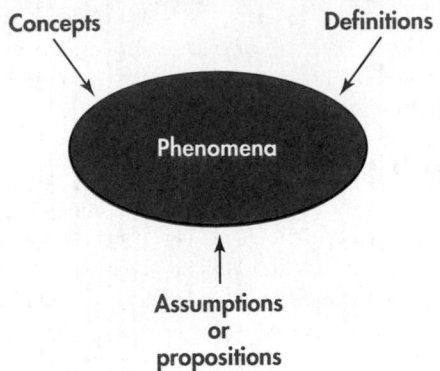

Figure 5-1 Components of a nursing theory.

tems model focuses on nursing care for the client as a whole, in compassing all aspects of the client's life.

CONCEPT

A theory also consists of interrelated concepts. **Concepts** are mental formulations of an object or event that comes from individual perceptual experience (Torres, 1986; Marriner-Tomey and Alligood, 1998). It is an idea, a mental image. Concepts help to describe or label phenomena (Marriner-Tomey and Alligood, 1998). Again using Neuman's systems model (1972) as an example, there are concepts that affect the client system. Some of these concepts are physiological, psychological, sociocultural, environmental, health and wellness, prevention, stressors, and defense mechanisms (Meleis, 1997).

DEFINITION

The **definition**s included within the description of a theory convey the general meaning of the concepts in a manner that fits the theory. These definitions also describe the activity necessary to measure the constructs, relationships, or variables within a theory (Marriner-Tomey and Alligood, 1998; Chinn and Kramer, 1999). For example, Neuman's systems model defines clients as people who are anticipating stress or who are dealing with stress. Nurses focus their care on responses that could be labeled stressful, and these responses are within the domain of nursing (Meleis, 1997).

ASSUMPTIONS

Assumptions are statements that describe concepts or connect two concepts that are factual and are accepted as truths. Assumptions are the "taken for granted" statements that determine the nature of the concepts, definitions, purpose, relationships, and structure of the theory (Meleis; 1997; Chinn and Kramer, 1999). The assumptions in Neuman's systems model are that clients are dynamic; the relationships between the concepts influence a client's protective mechanisms and determine a client's response; clients have a normal range of responses; stressors attack flexible lines of defense followed by the normal lines of de-

fense; and nurses's actions are focused on primary, secondary, and tertiary prevention (Neuman, 1972).

Phenomena. Nursing theories focus on the phenomena of nursing and nursing care. **Phenomena** are aspects of reality that can be consciously sensed or experienced (Meleis, 1997). Within a specific discipline, phenomena reflect the domain or territory of the discipline. In nursing, phenomena reflect the domain of nursing practice. In Neuman's systems model (1972), phenomena include all client responses, environmental factors, and nursing actions.

TYPES OF THEORY

The general purpose of a theory is important because it specifies the context and situation in which the theory applies (Chinn and Kramer, 1999). Theories have different purposes and may be classified by levels of abstraction (grand theories versus middle-range theories) or the goals of the theory (descriptive or prescriptive). Theories may describe, predict, or prescribe activities for the phenomena of interest.

Grand Theories. **Grand theories** are broad in scope and complex (Chinn and Kramer, 1999). These theories require further specification through research before they can be fully tested. A grand theory is not intended to provide guidance for specific nursing interventions, but to provide the structural framework for broad, abstract ideas (Fawcett, 1995). Grand theories contain summative concepts that incorporate smaller-range theories. An example of a grand theory is Parse's theory of human becoming (1989). In this theory the person is unitary, an indivisible being who interrelates with the environment while co-creating health.

Middle-Range Theories. **Middle-range theories** are more limited in scope and less abstract. These theories address specific phenomena or concepts and reflect nursing practice (Meleis, 1997). Middle-range theories may address specific nursing phenomena (e.g., uncertainty, social support, incontinence). For example, Mishel's theory of uncertainty in illness (1988, 1990) focuses on clients' experiences while living with continual uncertainty. The nurse assists the client in appraisal of and adaptation to the uncertainty and the illness response.

Descriptive Theories. **Descriptive theories** are the first level of theory development. They delineate phenomena, speculate on why phenomena occur, and describe the consequences of phenomena. They have the ability to explain, relate, and in some situations predict nursing phenomena (Meleis, 1997). Examples of these theories are those that describe the life processes of a client, such as the developmental theories discussed in Chapter 9. Descriptive nursing theories do not direct specific nursing activities in specific clinical situations, but they have the potential for guiding future nursing research to refine the theory.

Prescriptive Theories.

Prescriptive theories address nursing therapeutics and the consequences of interventions. These types of theories predict the consequence of a specific nursing intervention. In nursing, a prescriptive theory should designate the prescription (i.e., nursing interventions), the conditions under which the prescription should occur, and the consequences (Meleis, 1997). Prescriptive theories are action oriented, which tests the validity and predictability of a nursing intervention. These theories guide nursing research for the development of specific nursing interventions.

THEORETICAL MODELS

A **theoretical model** refers to global ideas about the individuals, groups, situations, or events of interest to a specific discipline. Theories focus more specifically on the events and phenomena of the discipline (Fawcett, 1992). Theory is specific enough to contribute to a sound basis of nursing practice (Chinn and Kramer, 1999). Development of theory or nursing science involves generating knowledge. Although this knowledge can be used with knowledge from other disciplines, it is designed to advance and support nursing practice and health care (Hinshaw, 1989; Chinn and Kramer, 1999).

There are multiple nursing theories, some of which are presented in this and other chapters in the text. These theories can help the student to gain insight into theory development, to understand the influence of theories from other disciplines and nursing on clinical practice and client care, and to use them in developing innovative nursing interventions. Levine (1995) supports the need for a variety of nursing theories, because there is no global theory of nursing that fits every situation. The strength of nursing practice lies in the diversity of its nurses: their experiences, their commitment, and their professionalism (Levine, 1995).

Components of Nursing Theoretical Models.

Within any scientific discipline there are specific components of the domain. A **domain** is the perspective and territory of the discipline. The domain contains the subject, central concepts, values and beliefs, phenomena of interest, and the central problems of the discipline. Components of a discipline's domain are described in a paradigm. A **paradigm** is a term used to denote the linkages of science, philosophy, and theory accepted by a discipline (Marriner-Tomey and Alligood, 1998).

Nursing's Paradigm.

Nursing's paradigm directs the activity of the nursing profession, including knowledge, philosophy, theory, educational experience, practice orientation, research methodology, and literature identified with the profession (Meleis, 1997; Marriner-Tomey and Alligood, 1998). Nursing identified its domain in a paradigm that includes four linkages of interest: the person, health, environment/situation, and nursing.

Person refers to the recipient of care, including individual clients, families, and the community. The person is central to the care being provided. Because the person's needs are multidimensional, it is important that nursing provides care that is individualized to the client's needs.

Health is defined in different ways by the client, the clinical setting, and the health care profession (see Chapter 1). It is the goal of nursing care. The American Nurses Association (ANA)(1995) defines health as "a dynamic state of being in which the developmental and behavioral potential of the individual is realized to the fullest extent possible." Health is dynamic and continuously changing. The nurse is challenged to provide care based on the client's individualized level of health and health care needs at the time of care delivery.

Environment/situation includes all possible conditions affecting the client and the setting in which health care needs occur. For example, a client's level of health and health care needs can be influenced by factors in the home, school, workplace, or community. An adolescent girl with immune-mediated (or type I diabetes) may need to adapt her care regimen to physical activities of school, to the demands of a part-time job, and to the timing of social events, such as her prom. There is continuous interaction between the client and the environment. This interaction can have positive and negative effects on the person's level of health and health care needs.

Nursing is the "diagnoses and treatment of human responses to actual or potential health problems (ANA, 1995)." For example, a nurse does not diagnose the client's heart condition but instead develops nursing diagnoses of fatigue, change in body image, and altered coping. From these nursing diagnoses, the nurse creates an individualized plan of care (see Unit 3). Nurses use critical thinking skills and integrate knowledge, experience, attitudes, and standards into the individualized plan of care for each client.

Historical Perspective

Historically, nursing theories were studied in an isolated academic environment independent of nursing practice. Many nurses argued that theories were not relevant to what occurs in clinical practice. There is, however, a contemporary move toward nursing science–or evidenced–based practice (Donaldson, 1995). For nursing to grow as a profession, knowledge is needed to predict with confidence the types of nursing interventions that will improve client outcomes. Nurses now and in the future need to have models of care from which their practice is based (Parse, 1990; Dean, 1995).

As nursing continues to evolve, nurses theorize about

the nature of nursing practice, the principles on which practice is based, and the proper goals and functions of nursing. Theoretical nursing models are used to identify the domain and goals of nursing practice, provide knowledge to improve practice, and guide research. Nursing theories provide the nurse with goals for assessment, nursing diagnoses, care planning, and interventions; common ground for communication; and professional autonomy and accountability. They also guide future directions for nursing research, practice, education, and administration (Meleis, 1997; Chinn and Kramer, 1999) (Box 5-1).

A historical review demonstrates that nursing has developed a growing body of knowledge (Table 5-1). Nursing concepts and theories have evolved since Florence Nightingale, who, in establishing the discipline of nursing, spoke with firm conviction about the "nature of nursing as a profession that required knowledge distinct from medical knowledge" (Nightingale, 1860; Schuyler, 1992). The overall goal of this knowledge has been to explain the practice of nursing as different and distinct from the practice of medicine, psychology, and social work (Fawcett, 1995; Chinn and Kramer, 1999).

A significant milestone influencing the development of nursing concepts and theory was the establishment of the peer-reviewed journal *Nursing Research* in 1952. This journal reports on the scientific investigations being conducted by nurses and other professionals. The journal has encouraged scientific productivity and provides the framework for inquiry into theory-based nursing (Meleis, 1997).

In the mid-1950s nursing leaders began to formulate theoretical views of nursing and concerns about subjects to include or exclude from nursing curricula. Columbia University Teachers College offered master's and doctoral programs in nursing education and administration (Meleis, 1997). Several prominent nurse theorists graduated from this institution; these include Peplau, Henderson, Hall, Abdellah, King, Wiedenbach, and Rogers.

During the 1960s Yale University School of Nursing defined nursing even further than Nightingale. "Nursing was considered a process rather than an end, an interaction rather than content, and a relationship between two human beings rather than an interaction between unrelated nurse and patient" (Meleis, 1997). In addition, the ANA's 1965 position paper defined nursing and concluded that one of the most significant goals for nursing was theory development. The ANA supported and lobbied for the need for continuing efforts to develop the body of nursing knowledge to ultimately create a nursing science (ANA, 1965; Meleis, 1997). As a result, federal support was provided to nurses pursuing masters and doctoral degrees.

Theory development was emphasized from the mid-1960s to 1970. A series of symposiums, sponsored by Case Western Reserve University, was held to assist in the development of nursing theory. During the mid-1970s the

Goals of Theoretical Nursing Models   Box 5-1

Identify domain and goals of nursing.

Provide knowledge to improve nursing administration, practice, education, and research.

Guide research to establish empirical knowledge base for nursing.

Identify area to be studied.

Identify research techniques and tools that will be used to validate nursing interventions.

Identify nature of contribution that research will make to advancement of knowledge.

Formulate legislation governing nursing practice, research, and education.

Formulate regulations interpreting nurse practice acts so that nurses and others better understand laws.

Develop curriculum plans for nursing education.

Establish criteria for measuring quality of nursing care, education, and research.

Guide development of nursing care delivery system.

Provide systematic structure and rationale for nursing activities.

National League for Nursing (NLN), the accrediting institution for nursing education programs, made theory-based curriculum a requirement for accreditation. Schools of nursing were encouraged to use a conceptual framework in the development and implementation of their curricula (Meleis, 1997).

Relationship of Theory to the Nursing Process and Client Needs

Theory is the generation of nursing knowledge for use in practice. Process is the method for applying the theory or knowledge. The integration of theory and process is the basis for professional nursing (Torres, 1986).

The nursing process, a tool for nursing practice, was introduced first by Orlando (1961) and is a framework for contemporary nursing practice (see Unit 3). The nursing process is the procedure for organizing nursing care in which the first step, assessment, initiates the act of nursing (Barnum, 1994). The goals of the nursing process are noted in the theoretical work by Abdellah, Henderson, Orem, Orlando, Travelbee, and Weidenbach (Meleis, 1997). Together they provide nursing with a perspective on assessment, diagnosis, planning, implementation, and evaluation (Abdellah and others, 1960; Henderson, 1966); create a process of defining and attaining goals (King, 1981), and emphasize clients' perceptions of their health status (Meleis, 1997).

The nursing process offers a systematic approach for nursing practice and enhances research opportunities.

| Table 5-1 | **Chronology of Conceptual Models in Nursing (1952–1989)** | |
Year of First Major Publication	Theorist	Key Emphasis
1952	Hildegard E. Peplau	Interpersonal process is maturing force for personality.
1960	Faye G. Abedllah Irene L. Beland Almeda Martin Rugh V. Matheney	Patient's problems determine nursing care.
1961	Ida Jean Orlando	Interpersonal process alleviates distress.
1964	Ernestine Weidenbach	Helping process meets needs through art of individualizing care.
1966	Lydia E. Hall	Nursing care is person directed toward self-love.
1966	Joyce Travelbee	Meaning in illness determines how people respond.
1967	Myra E. Levine	Holism is maintained by conserving integrity.
1970	Martha E. Rogers	Person-environment are energy fields that evolve negentropically.
1971	Dorothea E. Orem	Self-care maintains wholeness.
1971	Imogene M. King	Transactions provide a frame of reference toward goal setting.
1974	Sr. Callista Roy	Stimuli disrupt an adaptive system.
1976	Josephine G. Paterson Loretta T. Zderad	Nursing is an existential experience of nurturing.
1978	Madeleine M. Leininger	Caring is universal and varies transculturally.
1979	Jean Watson	Caring is moral ideal: mind-body-soul engagement with another.
1979	Margaret A. Newman	Disease is a clue to preexisting life patterns.
1980	Dorothy E. Johnson	Subsystems exist in dynamic stability.
1981	Rosemarie Rizzo Parse	Indivisible beings and environment co-create health.
1989	Patricia Benner and Judith Wrubel	Caring is central to the essence of nursing. It sets up what matters, enabling connection and concern. It creates possibility for mutual helpfulness.

From Chinn PL, Kramer ML: *Theory and nursing: a systematic approach*, ed 5, St. Louis, 1999, Mosby.

The process is adaptable to different clients and different care settings. In addition, the nursing process is compatible with many other systems in the health care delivery system (e.g., computer-generated care plans, patient information systems, patient acuity systems) (Barnum, 1994).

The nursing process is central to the domain of nursing (Meleis, 1997). However, the nursing process is not a theory. It provides the process for the delivery of nursing care, not the knowledge component of the discipline. There are, however, attempts to build a comprehensive theory from the process. First, there is an attempt to use the nursing process in conjunction with other theories that lack a process element. Second, there is an effort to organize nursing diagnoses and interventions as complementary pieces (Barnum, 1994). However, nurse theorists are divided as to whether the nursing process model is compatible with current and emerging theories (Meleis, 1997).

Interdisciplinary Theories

To practice in today's health care systems, nurses need a strong scientific knowledge base from nursing and other disciplines, such as the physical, social, and behavioral sciences. Knowledge from these other disciplines includes relevant theories that explain phenomena. An **interdisciplinary theory** explains a purposive and systematic view of phenomena specific to the discipline of inquiry, such as Freud's psychoanalytic theory in the discipline of psychology.

SYSTEMS THEORY

A system is made up of separate components. The parts rely on one another, are interrelated, share a common purpose, and together form a whole. The system has a specific purpose or goal and uses a process to achieve that goal. The content is the product and information obtained from the system.

Input is the information that enters the system. **Output** is the end product of a system. **Feedback** is the process through which the output is returned to the system. Systems can either be open or closed. An open system interacts with its environment. There is an exchange of information between the system and the environment. Factors that change the environment can also have an impact on the system. A closed system is one that does not interact with the environment. An example of a closed system is a chemical reaction occurring under specific conditions.

One example of a system is the nursing process (Figure 5-2). The purpose of the nursing process is to provide systematic and individualized client care. The process is the five components: assessment, nursing diagnosis, planning, implementation, and evaluation. The content is the information obtained and used from each component. The

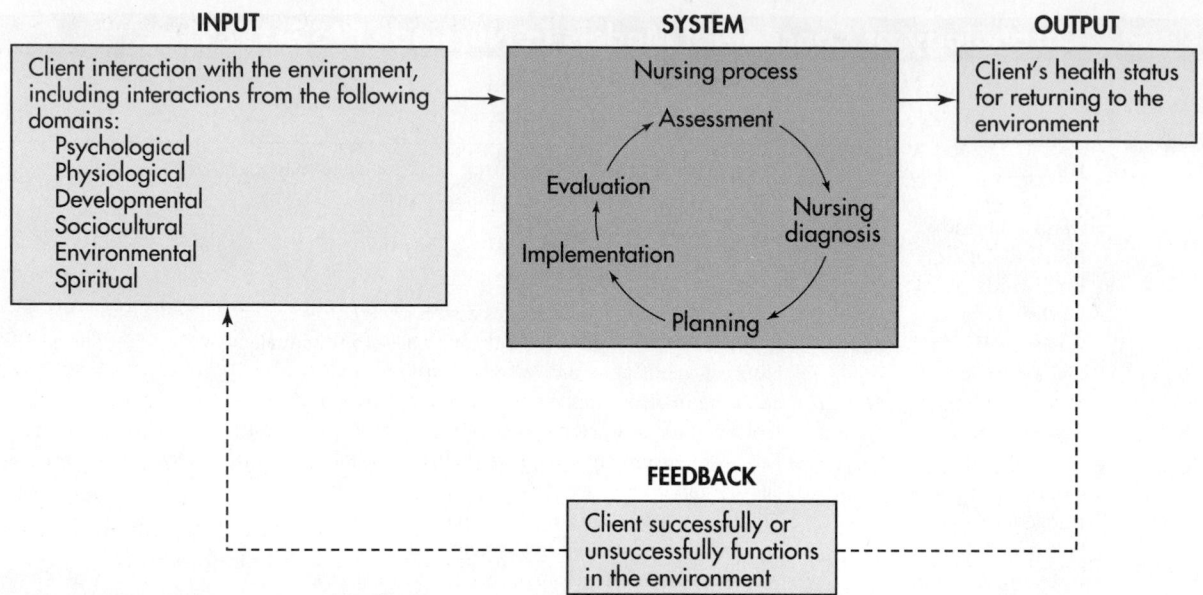

Figure 5-2   Nursing process as a system.

nursing process is an open system because it interacts with its environment, continually changing as the client's nursing needs change. Input to the system comes from the client's assessment data (e.g., how the client interacts with the environment). The output, the client's response to nursing interventions (e.g., the client's status for returning to the environment) is returned as feedback to the system; for example, the client successfully or unsuccessfully functions in the environment.

Nursing theories may have a systems model as the theoretical base. For example, Neuman (1972, 1995) defines a total-person model of wholism and an open-systems approach. As an open system, the person interacts with the environment. The environment is both external and internal, and the person interacts with stressors from the environment that affect the system.

BASIC HUMAN NEEDS

Maslow's hierarchy of needs is an interdisciplinary theory that is useful for designating priorities of care. The hierarchy of human needs arranges the basic needs in five levels of priority (see Chapter 1). The most basic, or first, level includes physiological needs, such as air, water, and food. The second level includes safety and security needs, which involve physical and psychological security. The third level contains love and belonging needs, including friendship, social relationships, and sexual love. The fourth level encompasses esteem and self-esteem needs, which involve self-confidence, usefulness, achievement, and self-worth. The final level is the need for self-actualization, the state of fully achieving potential and having the ability to solve problems and cope realistically with life's situations. Basic physiological and safety needs are usually the first priority. However, the nurse may encounter situations in which

there are no emergent physical or safety needs, but in which high priority must be given to the psychological, sociocultural, developmental, or spiritual needs of the client.

Clients entering the health care system generally have unmet needs. For example, a person brought to an emergency department experiencing acute pneumonia has an unmet need for oxygen, the most basic physiological need. An older woman in a high-crime area may be concerned about physical safety and, while hospitalized, have a need for psychological security because of fear that her home will be burglarized. A widowed homemaker whose children have moved away may feel that she does not belong or is not loved. Nurses in all practice settings strive to help clients and their families meet these needs.

The hierarchy of needs is a useful way for nurses to plan individualized care for a client. One need may take priority over another (such as restoration of an adequate airway before the nurse educates the client in adjusting to an emotional conflict). The nurse uses priorities to organize nursing diagnoses, develop goals and expected outcomes, and select nursing interventions (see Chapter 16).

HEALTH-AND-WELLNESS MODELS

Health-and-wellness models are designed to help health care professionals understand the relationships between these two concepts and the client's attitudes toward health and health practices. Knowledge of these models assist nurses in understanding and predicting the client's health behaviors, including use of health care services and adherence to recommended therapies. Chapter 1 includes a variety of models that explain and predict client behavior related to health promotion activities. An understanding of these models is important when meeting the health promotion and disease prevention needs of the client.

STRESS AND ADAPTATION

Stress and adaptation are universal and dynamic. Everyone experiences stress and attempts to adapt to these stressors. Stressors and stress responses are physiological and behavioral. As a result, the models that explain the stress response are usually biobehavioral and provide the framework for care of clients experiencing stress. Chapter 30 explains the more prominent theories and demonstrates how these models are used in nursing practice.

DEVELOPMENTAL THEORIES

Human growth and development is an orderly predictive process that begins with conception and continues through death. There are a variety of well-tested theoretical models that describe and predict behavior and development at various phases of the life continuum. Chapter 9 details these theories, and Chapters 10 through 12 demonstrate changes in growth and development in various age-groups.

PSYCHOSOCIAL THEORIES

Nursing is an eclectic discipline that strives to meet the holistic needs of client's in their physiological, psychological, sociocultural, developmental, and spiritual domains. There are theoretical models that explain and/or predict client responses in each of these domains. For example, Chapter 7 discusses models for understanding diversity and implementing care to meet the diverse needs of the client. Chapter 8 describes family theory and how to meet the needs of the family when the family is the client or when the family is the caregiver. Chapter 29 discusses several models of grieving and demonstrates how to assist the clients through loss, death, and grief.

Selected Nursing Theories

Definitions and theories of nursing can help the nursing student understand how the roles and actions of nurses fit together in nursing. The following sections describe, in chronological order of theory development, concepts basic to selected nursing theories (Table 5-2).

NIGHTINGALE'S THEORY

Contemporary authors are beginning to explore Florence Nightingale's work as a potential theoretical and conceptual model for nursing (Meleis, 1997; Marriner-Tomey and Alligood, 1998). Meleis (1997) notes that Nightingale's concept of the environment as the focus of nursing care and her suggestion that nurses need not know all about the disease process are early attempts to differentiate between nursing and medicine.

Nightingale did not view nursing as being limited to the administration of medications and treatments but rather as being oriented toward providing fresh air, light, warmth, cleanliness, quiet, and adequate nutrition (Nightingale, 1860; Torres, 1986). Through observation

and data collection, she linked the client's health status with environmental factors and initiated improved hygiene and sanitary conditions during the Crimean War.

Torres (1986) notes that Nightingale provided basic concepts and propositions that could be supported and used for practice in nursing. Nightingale's "descriptive theory" provides nurses with a way to think about nursing with a frame of reference that focuses on clients and the environment (Torres, 1986). Nightingale's letters and writings direct the nurse to act on behalf of the client. Her principles were visionary and encompassed the areas of practice, research, and education. Most important, her concepts and principles shaped and delineated nursing practice (Marriner-Tomey and Alligood, 1998). Nightingale taught and used the nursing process, noting that "vital observation [assessment] . . . is not for the sake of piling up miscellaneous information or curious facts, but for the sake of saving life and increasing health and comfort."

PEPLAU'S THEORY

Hildegard Peplau's theory (1952) focuses on the individual, the nurse, and the interactive process; the result is the nurse-client relationship (Torres, 1986; Yamashita, 1997). According to this theory, the client is an individual with a felt need, and nursing is an interpersonal and therapeutic process. Nursing's goal is to educate the client and family and to help the client reach mature personality development (Chinn and Kramer, 1999). The nurse strives to develop a nurse-client relationship in which the nurse serves as a resource person, counselor, and surrogate.

For example, when the client seeks help, the nurse and client first discuss the nature of the problem and nurse explains the services available. As the nurse-client relationship develops, the nurse and client mutually define the problem and potential solutions. The client gains from this relationship by using available services to meet needs, and the nurse assists the client in reducing anxiety related to the health care problem. Peplau's theory is unique in that the collaborative nurse-client relationship creates a "maturing force" through which interpersonal effectiveness assists in meeting the client's needs (Beeber, Anderson, and Sills, 1990). When the original needs have been resolved, new needs may emerge. The nurse-client interpersonal relationship is characterized by the following overlapping phases: orientation, identification, explanation, and resolution (Chinn and Kramer, 1999).

Peplau's theory and ideas were developed to provide a design for the practice of psychiatric nursing. Nursing research on anxiety, empathy, behavioral tools, and tools to evaluate verbal responses resulted from Peplau's conceptual model (Marriner-Tomey and Alligood, 1998).

HENDERSON'S THEORY

Virginia Henderson defines nursing as assisting the individual, sick or well, in the performance of those activities that will contribute to health, recovery, or a peaceful death

Table 5-2 Summary of Nursing Theories

Theorist	Goal of Nursing	Framework for Practice
Nightingale—1860	To facilitate "the body's reparative processes" by manipulating client's environment (Torres, 1986)	Client's environment is manipulated to include appropriate noise, nutrition, hygiene, light, comfort, socialization, and hope.
Peplau—1952	To develop interaction between nurse and client (Peplau, 1952)	Nursing is a significant, therapeutic, interpersonal process (Peplau, 1952). Nurses participate in structuring health care systems to facilitate natural ongoing tendency of humans to develop interpersonal relationships (Marriner-Tomey and Alligood, 1998).
Henderson—1955	To work independently with other health care workers (Marriner-Tomey and Alligood, 1998), assisting client in gaining independence as quickly as possible (Henderson, 1964); to help client gain lacking strength (Torres, 1986)	Nurses help client to perform Henderson's 14 basic needs (Henderson, 1966).
Abdellah—1960	To provide service to individuals, families, and society; to be kind and caring but also intelligent, competent, and technically well prepared to provide this service (Marriner-Tomey, Alligood, 1998)	This theory involves Abdellah's 21 nursing problems (Abdellah and others, 1960).
Orlando—1961	To respond to client's behavior in terms of immediate needs; to interact with client to meet immediate needs by identifying client's behavior, reaction of nurse, and nursing action to be taken (Torres, 1986, Chinn and Kramer, 1999)	Three elements—client behavior, nurse reaction, and nurse action—compose nursing situation (Orlando, 1961).
Hall—1962	To provide care and comfort to client during disease process (Torres, 1986)	The client is composed of the following overlapping parts: person (core), pathological state and treatment (cure), and body (care). Nurse is caregiver (Marriner-Tomey and Alligood, 1998; Chinn and Kramer, 1999).
Wiedenbach—1964	To assist individuals in overcoming obstacles that interfere with the ability to meet demands or needs brought about by condition, environment, situation, or time (Torres, 1986)	Nursing practice is related to individuals who need help because of behavioral stimulus. Clinical nursing has the following components: philosophy, purpose, practice, and art (Chinn and Kramer, 1999).
Levine—1966	To use conversation activities aimed at optimal use of client's resources	This adaptation model of human as integral whole is based on "four conversation principles of nursing" (Levine, 1973).
Johnson—1968	To reduce stress so that client can move more easily through recovery process	This theory of basic needs focuses on seven categories of behavior. Individual's goal is to achieve behavioral balance and steady state by adjustment and adaptation to certain forces (Johnson, 1980; Torres, 1986).
Rogers—1970	To maintain and promote health, prevent illness, and care for and rehabilitate ill and disabled client through "humanistic science of nursing" (Rogers, 1970)	"Unitary man" evolves along life process. Client continuously changes and coexists with environment.
Orem—1971	To care for and help client attain total self-care	This is self-care deficit theory. Nursing care becomes necessary when client is unable to fulfill biological, psychological, developmental, or social needs (Orem, 1991).
King—1971	To use communication to help client reestablish positive adaptation to environment	Nursing process is defined as dynamic interpersonal process between nurse, client , and health care system.
Travelbee—1971	To assist individual or family in preventing or coping with illness, regaining health, finding meaning in illness, or maintaining maximal degree of health (Marriner-Tomey and Alligood, 1998)	Interpersonal process is viewed as human-to-human relationship formed during illness and "experience of suffering."

Table 5-2	**Summary of Nursing Theories**—cont'd	
Theorist	Goal of Nursing	Framework for Practice
Neuman—1972	To assist individuals, families, and groups in attaining and maintaining maximal level of total wellness by purposeful interventions	Stress reduction is goal of systems model of nursing practice (Torres, 1986). Nursing actions are in primary, secondary, or tertiary level of prevention.
Patterson and Zderad—1976	To respond to human needs and build humanistic nursing science (Patterson and Zderad, 1976; Chinn and Kramer, 1999)	Humanistic nursing requires participants to be aware of their "uniqueness" and "commonality" with others (Chinn and Kramer, 1999).
Leininger—1978	To provide care consistent with nursing's emerging science and knowledge with caring as central focus (Chinn and Kramer 1999)	With this transcultural care theory, caring is the central and unifying domain for nursing knowledge and practice.
Roy—1979	To identify types of demands placed on client, assess adaptation to demands, and help client adapt	This adaptation model is based on the physiological, psychological, sociological, and dependence-independence adaptive modes (Roy, 1980).
Watson—1979	To promote health, restore client to health, and prevent illness (Marriner-Tomey and Alligood, 1998)	This theory involves philosophy and science of caring; caring is interpersonal process comprising interventions that result in meeting human needs (Torres, 1986).
Parse—1981	To focus on human being as living unity and individual's qualitative participation with health experience (Parse 1990; Marriner-Tomey and Alligood, 1998)	The individual continually interacts with environment and participates in maintenance of health (Marriner-Tomey and Alligood, 1998). Health is continual, open process rather than state of well-being or absence of disease (Parse 1990; Marriner-Tomey and Alligood, 1998; Chinn and Kramer, 1999).
Benner and Wrubel—1989	To focus on client's need for caring as a means of coping with stressors of illness (Chinn and Kramer, 1999)	Caring is central to the essence of nursing. Caring creates the possibilities for coping and enables possibilities for connecting with and concern for others (Benner and Wrubel, 1989).

and that the individual would perform unaided if he or she had the necessary strength, will, or knowledge (Harmer and Henderson, 1955; Henderson, 1966). The process of nursing strives to do this as rapidly as possible, and the goal is independence.

Henderson organized the theory into 14 basic needs of the whole person and include phenomena from the following domains of the client: physiological, psychological, sociocultural, spiritual, and developmental. Together the nurse and client work in unison to meet these needs and attain client-centered goals.

ABDELLAH'S THEORY

The nursing theory developed by Faye Abdellah and others (1960) emphasizes delivering nursing care for the whole person to meet the physical, emotional, intellectual, social, and spiritual needs of the client and family. When using this approach, the nurse needs knowledge and skills in interpersonal relations, psychology, growth and development, communication, and sociology, as well as a knowledge of the basic sciences and specific nursing skills. The nurse is a problem solver and decision maker. The nurse formulates an individualized view of the client's needs, which may occur in the following four areas:

1. Comfort, hygiene, and safety
2. Physiological balance
3. Psychological and social factors
4. Sociological and community factors

From these four areas, Abdellah and others (1960) identified 21 specific client needs, which are often referred to as Abdellah's 21 nursing problems.

LEVINE'S THEORY

Formulated in 1966 and published in 1973, Myra Levine's nursing theory views the client as an integrated being who interacts with and adapts to the environment. Health is viewed in terms of conservation of energy. Levine's four conservation principles of nursing are as follows:

1. Conservation of client energy
2. Conservation of structural integrity
3. Conservation of personal integrity
4. Conservation of social integrity

JOHNSON'S THEORY

Dorothy Johnson's theory of nursing (1968) focuses on how the client adapts to illness and how actual or potential stress can affect the ability to adapt. The goal of nursing is to reduce stress so that the client can move more easily through recovery. Johnson describes basic needs in terms of the following categories of behavior:

1. Security-seeking behavior
2. Nurturance-seeking behavior
3. Master of oneself and one's environment according to internalized standards of excellence
4. Taking in nourishment in socially and culturally acceptable ways
5. Ridding the body of waste in socially and culturally acceptable ways
6. Sexual and role-identity behavior
7. Self-protective behavior

According to Johnson, the nurse assesses the client's needs in these categories of behavior, called behavioral subsystems. Under normal conditions the client functions effectively in the environment. When stress disrupts normal adaptation, however, behavior becomes erratic and less purposeful. The nurse identifies this inability to adapt and provides nursing care to resolve problems in meeting the client's needs.

ROGERS' THEORY

In her theory, Martha Rogers (1970) considers the individual (unitary human being) as an energy field coexisting within the universe. The individual is in continuous interaction with the environment and is a unified whole, possessing personal integrity and manifesting characteristics that are more than the sum of the parts (Rogers, 1970; Lutjens, 1995). The unitary human being is a "four dimensional energy field identified by pattern and manifesting characteristics that are specific to the whole and which cannot be predicted from the knowledge of parts" (Marriner-Tomey and Alligood, 1998). The four dimensions used in Rogers' theory—energy fields, openness, pattern and organization, and dimensionality—are used to derive principles related to human development.

Rogers views nursing primarily as a science and is committed to nursing research and theory development. Nursing therefore incorporates knowledge of the basic sciences and physiology, as well as nursing knowledge:

> The science of nursing aims to provide a body of abstract knowledge growing out of scientific research and logical analysis and capable of being translated into nursing practice. Nursing's body of scientific knowledge is a new product specific to nursing.... Nursing is a humanistic science.

OREM'S THEORY

Dorothea Orem (1971) developed a definition of nursing that emphasizes the client's self-care needs. Orem defines self care as a learned, goal-oriented activity directed toward the self in the interest of maintaining life, health, development, and well-being. Orem (1991) describes her philosophy of nursing in this way:

> Nursing has as a special concern man's needs for self-care action and the provision and management of it on a continuous basis in order to sustain life and health, recover from disease or injury, and cope with their effects. Self-care is a requirement of every person–man, woman, and

child. When self-care is not maintained, illness, disease, or death will occur. Nurses sometimes manage and maintain required self-care continually for persons who are totally incapacitated. In other instances, nurses help persons to maintain required self-care by performing some but not all care measures, by supervising others who assist clients, and by instructing and guiding individuals as they gradually move toward self-care.

Thus the goal of Orem's theory is to help the client perform self-care. According to Orem, nursing care is necessary when the client is unable to fulfill biological, psychological, developmental, or social needs. The nurse determines why a client is unable to meet these needs, what must be done to enable the client to meet them, and how much self-care the client is able to perform. The goal of nursing is to increase the client's ability to independently meet these needs (Hartweg, 1995).

KING'S THEORY

Imogene King's goal attainment theory (1971, 1981, 1987) focuses on three dynamic interacting systems: personal, interpersonal, and social (King, 1997). A personal relationship forms between client and nurse. The nurse-client relationship is the vehicle for the delivery of nursing care, which is a dynamic interpersonal process in which the nurse and client are affected by each other's behavior, as well as by the health care system (King, 1971, 1981). The nurse's goal is to use communication to assist the client in reestablishing or maintaining a positive adaptation to the environment.

NEUMAN'S THEORY

Betty Neuman's theory (1972) defines a total-person model for nursing, incorporating a wholistic concept and an open-systems approach (Marriner-Tomey and Alligood, 1998). To Neuman, the person is a dynamic composite of physiological, sociocultural, developmental, psychological, and spiritual components that function as an open system. As an open system, the person interacts with, adjusts to, and is adjusted by the environment, which is viewed as a stressor (Chinn and Kramer, 1999). The internal environment consists of those influences (intrapersonal) within the client. The external environment consists of influences (interpersonal) outside the client. The created environment is the client's attempt to create a safe setting, which may be made up of conscious or unconscious mechanisms (Reed, 1995). Each environment has potential threats from stressors, which disrupt the system. Neuman's model includes intrapersonal, interpersonal, and extrapersonal stressors (Neuman, 1995; Marriner-Tomey and Alligood, 1998).

Neuman believes that nursing is concerned with the whole person. The goal of nursing is to assist individuals, families, and groups in attaining and maintaining a maximal level of total wellness (Neuman and Young, 1972). The nurse assesses, manages, and evaluates client systems. Nursing focuses on the variables affecting the client's response to the stressor (Chinn and Kramer, 1999). Nursing actions are in the primary, secondary, and tertiary levels of prevention. Primary prevention focuses on strengthening a line of defense through the identification of actual or potential risk factors associated with stressors. Secondary prevention strengthens internal defenses and resources by establishing priorities and treatment plans for identified symptoms, and tertiary prevention focuses on readaptation. The principal goal in tertiary prevention is to strengthen resistance to stressors through client education and to assist in preventing a recurrence of the stress response (Marriner-Tomey and Alligood, 1998; Chinn and Kramer, 1999).

ROY'S THEORY

Sister Callista Roy's adaptation theory (Roy and Obloy, 1979; Roy, 1980, 1984, 1989) views the client as an adaptive system. According to Roy's model, the goal of nursing is to help the person adapt to changes in physiological needs, self-concept, role function, and interdependent relations during health and illness (Marriner-Tomey and Alligood, 1998). The need for nursing care arises when the client cannot adapt to internal and external environmental demands. All individuals must adapt to the following demands:

1. Meeting basic physiological needs
2. Developing a positive self-concept
3. Performing social roles
4. Achieving a balance between dependence and independence

The nurse determines what demands are causing problems for a client and assesses how well the client is adapting to them. Nursing care is then directed at helping the client adapt. For example, a postoperative client who has a significant blood loss and now has a low hematocrit value needs nursing interventions designed to assist the client in adapting to the associated fatigue. The nurse may design interventions to allow sufficient rest.

WATSON'S THEORY

Jean Watson's philosophy of transpersonal caring (1979, 1985, 1988) defines the outcome of nursing activity in regard to the humanistic aspects of life (Marriner-Tomey and Alligood, 1998). The action of nursing is directed at understanding the interrelationship between health, illness, and human behavior. Nursing is concerned with promoting and restoring health and preventing illness.

Watson's model is designed around the caring process, assisting clients in attaining or maintaining health or in dying peacefully. This caring process requires that the nurse be knowledgeable about human behavior and human responses to actual or potential health problems, individual needs, how to respond to others, and strengths and limitations of the client and family, as well as those of the nurse. In addition, the nurse comforts and offers compassion and empathy to clients and their families. Caring

represents all of the factors the nurse uses to deliver health care to the client (Watson, 1987).

PARSE'S THEORY

Rosemarie Parse's theory of human becoming (1987, 1989, 1995) states that clients are open, mutual, and in constant interaction with the environment. Health is a process of the individual relating to the environment. Health is a lived experience, which is continually changing. The client redefines health as the interaction evolves with the environment.

The nurse assists the client in interaction with the environment and co-creating health. The person experiences continued growth and development. The nurse assists the client in this growth by sustaining a safe and protective environment. Physiological and psychosocial needs are interrelated and cannot be treated as separate subsystems of the individual. The nursing process is accepted by Parse (1989).

BENNER AND WRUBEL'S THEORY

The primacy of caring is a model proposed by Patricia Benner and Judith Wrubel (1989). In this model, caring is central. Caring creates possibilities for coping, enables possibilities for connecting with and concern for others, and allows for the giving and receiving of help (Chinn and Kramer, 1999).

As defined in this theory, caring means that persons, events, projects, and things matter to people. Caring itself presents a connection. Caring represents a wide range of involvement, (e.g., caring about one's family, caring about one's friendships, and caring about one's clients). Benner and Wrubel see the personal concern as an inherent feature of nursing practice. In caring for one's clients, nurses help clients recover, noticing those interventions that are successful and can guide future care giving. Chapter 6 describes this theory and other theoretical perspectives on caring within the nursing context.

• • •

Application of nursing theory in practice depends on nurses having knowledge of the theories, as well as an understanding of how the theories relate to one another. Theories are the organizing frameworks for the science of nursing and the substantive approaches for nursing care. They provide critical thinking structures to guide clinical reasoning and problem solving.

The Link Between Theory and Knowledge Development in Nursing

Nursing has its own body of knowledge. This knowledge is theoretical and practical (Meleis, 1997). Theoretical knowledge includes and "reflects on the basic values, guiding principles, elements, and phases of a conception of nursing" (Meleis, 1997). The goals of theoretical knowledge stimulate thinking and create a broad understanding of the "science" and practices of the nursing discipline (King and Fawcett, 1997).

Practical knowledge is not organized in the same manner as theoretical knowledge. Practical knowledge is based on nurses' experience. Practical knowledge is the "art" of nursing. It is achieved through personal knowing gained through practice, reflection on experiences, synthesis, and integration of the art, science, and practice of nursing.

An earlier discussion in this chapter described the types of nursing theories and indicated that theories provided direction to nursing research. This relationship between nursing theory and nursing research is one component of the discipline's knowledge development.

Chinn and Kramer (1999) note that one view of the relationship between theory-linked research and theory is a spiral (Figure 5-3). This spiral represents the interaction between theory and research and an underlying assumption that research increases nursing's knowledge base. Research is linked to theory in two ways: generation of theory and testing of theory (Fawcett, 1993; Meleis, 1997; Chinn and Kramer, 1999).

Theory-generating research is designed to discover and describe relationships of phenomena without imposing preconceived notions (e.g., hypotheses) of what the phenomena under study mean (Chinn and Kramer, 1999). In theory-generating research, the investigator makes observations with an open mind in order to view a phenomena in a new way.

Theory-testing research is used to determine how accurately a theory describes nursing phenomena. The investigator has some preconceived notions as to how the phenomena are described and generates research questions or hypotheses to test the assumptions of the theory. No one study can test all components of a theory; the theory is tested through a variety of research activities.

The result of theory-generating or theory-testing research is to increase nursing's knowledge base. As a result, nurses are able to incorporate research-based interventions into the practice of the discipline (King and Fawcett, 1997). As these research activities continue, not only does the knowledge and science of nursing increase, but clients

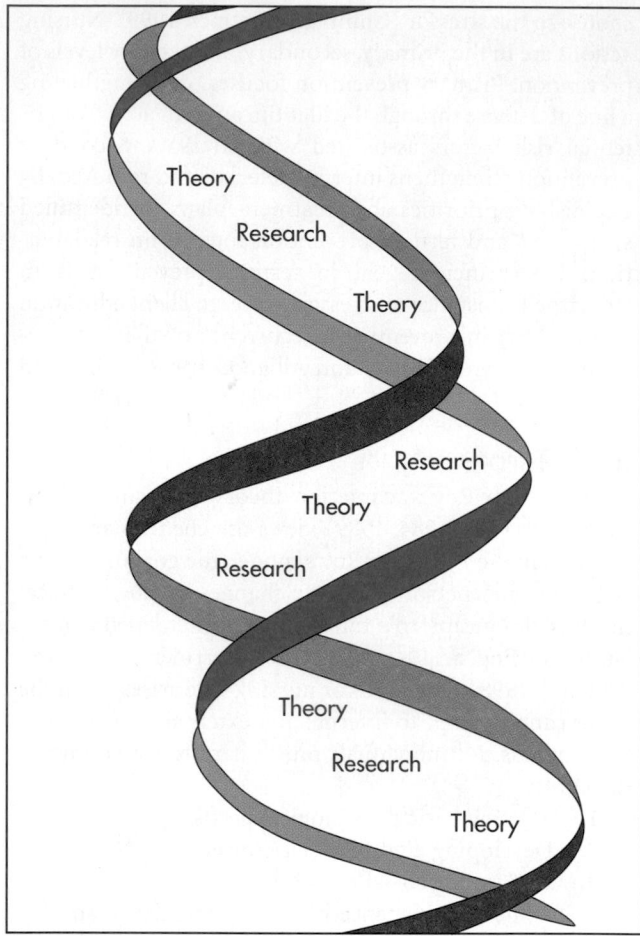

Figure 5-3   Theory-research spiral of knowledge. From Chinn PL, Kramer ML: *Theory and Nursing: a systematic approach*, ed 4, St. Louis, 1995, Mosby.

are the recipients of best evidence–based nursing practice (see Chapter 25).

As an art, nursing relies on knowledge gained from practice and reflection of past experiences. As a science, nursing draws on scientifically tested knowledge that is applied in the practice setting (Kikuchi, Simmons, and Romyn, 1996). But it is the "expert nurse" who transports the art and science of nursing into the scientific realm of creative caring.

Key Concepts

- Conceptual and theoretical nursing models provide knowledge to improve practice, guide research and nursing curricula, and identify the domain and goals of nursing practice.
- Theory is the goal of all scientific work, theorizing is a central process in all scientific endeavors, and theoretical thinking is essential to all professional undertakings.
- A theory is a set of concepts, definitions, relationships, and assumptions that project a systematic view of phenomena by designing specific interrelationships among concepts for the purposes of describing, explaining, predicting, and/or prescribing.
- A nursing theory is a conceptualization of some aspect of nursing communicated for the purpose of describing, explaining, predicting, and/or prescribing nursing care.
- Theories may be classified by levels of abstraction or the goals of the theory.
- Grand theories are broad in scope and complex. These theories provide the structural framework for broad, abstract ideas.
- Middle-range theories are more limited in scope and less abstract. These theories address specific phenomena or concepts and reflect practice.
- A theoretical model refers to global ideas about the individuals, groups, situations, or events of interest to a specific discipline.
- Nursing's paradigm identifies four linkages of interest to the profession: the person, health, environment/situation, and nursing. Nurse theorists agree that these four components are integral to the development of theory.
- Theory is the generation of nursing knowledge used for practice. Process is the method for applying the theory or knowledge. The integration of theory and process is the basis for professional nursing.
- Theories from nursing and other disciplines help the nursing student understand how the roles and actions of nurses fit together in nursing.
- Nursing is an applied discipline with its own body of knowledge that can be theoretical and practical.
- Practical knowledge is achieved through personal knowing, which is achieved through practice, reflection on experiences, synthesis, and integration of the art, science, and practice of nursing.
- Theory-generating research is designed to discover and describe relationships without imposing preconceived notions (e.g., hypotheses) of what the phenomena under study mean.
- Theory-testing research is used to determine how accurately a theory describes nursing phenomena.

Key Terms

Assumptions, *p. 88*
Concepts, *p. 88*
Definition, *p. 88*
Descriptive theory, *p. 88*
Domain, *p. 89*
Environment/situation, *p. 89*
Feedback, *p. 91*
Grand theory, *p. 88*
Health, *p. 89*
Input, *p. 91*
Interdisciplinary theory, *p. 91*

Middle-range theory, *p. 88*
Nursing, *p. 89*
Nursing theory, *p. 87*
Nursing's paradigm, *p. 89*
Output, *p. 91*
Paradigm, *p. 89*
Person, *p. 89*
Phenomena, *p. 88*
Prescriptive theory, *p. 89*
Theoretical model, *p. 89*
Theory, *p. 87*

Critical Thinking Exercises

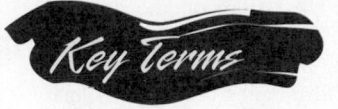

1. Part of your education includes experiences in different types of health care settings. Take a theory and explain how it might apply in different health care settings.
2. What differences would you expect between the application of the theory in a hospital, skilled care facility, and community-based facility? Would you expect any commonalities?
3. Describe how theory-generating research and theory-testing research are similar and how they are different.

References

Abdellah FG and others: *Patient-centered approaches to nursing,* New York, 1960, Macmillan.

Alfaro-LeFevre R: *Critical thinking in nursing: a practical approach,* Philadelphia, 1995, WB Saunders.

American Nurses Association, Committee on Education: *A position paper,* New York, 1965, The Association.

American Nurses Association: *Nursing and social policy statement,* Kansas City, Mo, 1980, The Association.

American Nurses Association: *Nursing's social policy statement,* Washington, DC, 1995, The Association.

Barnum BJS: *Nursing theory: analysis, application, evaluation,* ed 4, Philadelphia, 1994, JB Lippincott.

Beeber L, Anderson CA, Sills GM: Peplau's theory in practice, *Nurs Sci Q* 3(1):6, 1990.

Benner P, Tanner C: How expert nurses use intuition, *Am J Nurs* 87(1):23, 1987.

Benner P, Wrubel J. *The primacy of caring: stress and coping in health and illness,* Menlo Park, Calif, 1989, Addison-Wesley.

Carnevali DL, Thomas MD: *Diagnostic reasoning and treatment decision making in nursing,* Philadelphia, 1993, JB Lippincott.

Chinn PL, Kramer MK: *Theory and nursing: integrated knowledge development,* ed 5, St. Louis, 1999, Mosby.

Dean H: Science and practice: the nature of knowledge. In Omery A, Kasper CE, Page GG, editors: *In search of nursing science*, Thousand Oaks, Calif, 1995, Sage Publications.

Donaldson SK: Nursing science for nursing practice. In Omery A, Kasper CE, Page GG, editors: *In search of nursing science*, Thousand Oaks, Calif, 1995, Sage Publications.

Fawcett J: Contemporary conceptualization of nursing: philosophy or science? In Kikuchi J, Simmons H, editors: *Philosophic inquiry in nursing*, Newbury Park, Calif, 1992, Sage Publications.

Fawcett J: *Analysis and evaluation of conceptual models of nursing*, ed 3, Philadelphia, 1995, FA Davis.

Harmer D, Henderson V: *Textbook of the principles and practice of nursing*, ed 5, Riverside, NJ, 1955, Macmillan.

Hartweg DL: Dorothea Orem: self-care deficit theory. In McQuiston CM, Webb AA, editors: *Foundations of nursing theory*, Thousand Oaks, Calif, 1995, Sage Publications.

Henderson V: The nature of nursing, *Am J Nurs* 64:62, 1964.

Henderson V: *The nature of nursing*, New York, 1966, Macmillan.

Hinshaw AS: Nursing science: the challenge to develop knowledge, *Nurs Sci Q* 2(4):162, 1989.

Johnson DE: Theory in nursing: borrowed and unique, *Nurs Res* 11:206, 1968.

Johnson DE: The behavioral system for nursing. In Riehl JP, Roy C, editors: *Conceptual models for nursing practice*, ed 2, New York, 1980, Appleton-Century-Crofts.

Kikuchi JF, Simmons H, Romyn D: *Truth in nursing inquiry*, Thousand Oaks, Calif, 1996, Sage Publications.

King IM: *Toward a theory for nursing*, New York, 1971, John Wiley & Sons.

King IM: *Toward a theory for nursing: systems, concepts, process*, New York, 1981, John Wiley & Sons.

King IM: King's theory of goal attainment. In Parse RR, editor: *Nursing science: major paradigms, theories, critiques*, Philadelphia, 1987, WB Saunders.

King IM: King's theory of goal attainment in practice, *Nurs Sci Q*, 10(4):180, 1997.

King IM, Fawcett J: *The language of nursing theory and metatheory*, Sigma Theta Tau International, Indianapolis, 1997, Center Nursing Press.

Levine ME: *An introduction to clinical nursing*, ed 2, Philadelphia, 1973, FA Davis.

Levine, ME: The rhetoric of nursing theory, *Image J Nurs Sch* 27:11, 1995.

Lutjens LRJ: Martha Rogers: the science of unitary human beings. In McQuiston CM, Webb AA, editors: *Foundations of nursing theory*, Thousand Oaks, Calif, 1995, Sage.

Marriner-Tomey A, Alligood MR: *Nursing theorists and their work*, ed 4, St Louis, 1998, Mosby.

Meleis, AI: *Theoretical nursing: development and progress*, ed 3, Philadelphia, 1997, JB Lippincott.

Mishel MH: Uncertainty in illness, *Image J Nurs Sch* 20(4):225, 1988.

Mishel MH: Reconceptualization of the uncertainty in illness theory, *Image J Nurs Sch*, 22(4):256, 1990.

Neuman B: *The Neuman systems model*, ed 3, Norwalk, Conn, 1995, Appleton & Lange.

Neuman BM, Young RJ: A model for teaching total person approach to patient problems, *Nurs Res* 21:264, 1972.

Nightingale F: *Notes on nursing: what it is and what it is not*, London, 1860, Harrison & Sons.

Orem DE: *Nursing: concepts of practice*, New York, 1971, McGraw-Hill.

Orem DE: *Nursing: concepts of practice*, ed 4, New York, 1991, McGraw-Hill.

Orlando IJ: *The dynamic nurse-patient relationship: function, process, and principles*, New York, 1961, GP Putnam's & Sons.

Parse RR: *Nursing science: major paradigms, theories, and critiques*, Philadelphia, 1987, WB Saunders.

Parse RR: Man-living-health: a theory of nursing. In Reihl-Sisca J, editor: *Conceptual models for nursing practice*, ed 3, Norwalk, Conn, 1989, Appleton & Lange.

Parse RR: Nursing theory–based practice: a challenge for the 90s, *Nurs Sci Q* 3(2):53, 1990.

Parse RR: *Illumination: the human becoming theory in practice and research*, New York, 1995, National League for Nursing.

Patterson JG, Zderad LT: *Humanistic nursing*, New York, 1976, John Wiley & Sons.

Peplau HE: *Interpersonal relations in nursing*, New York, 1952, GP Putnam's Sons.

Raudonis BM, Acton GJ: Theory-based nursing practice, *J Adv Nurs* 26(2\1):138, 1997.

Reed KS: Betty Neuman: the Neuman systems model. In McQuiston CM, Webb AA, editors: *Foundations of nursing theory*, Thousand Oaks, Calif, 1995, Sage Publications.

Rogers ME: *An introduction to the theoretical basis of nursing*, Philadelphia, 1970, FA Davis.

Rogers ME: Nursing: science of unitary, irreducible, human beings: update 1990. In Barrett EAM, editor: *Visions of Rogers's science-based nursing*, Pub No. 15-2285, New York, 1990, National League for Nursing.

Roy C: The Roy adaptation model. In Riehl JP, Roy C, editors: *Conceptual models for nursing practice*, New York, 1980, Appleton-Century-Crofts.

Roy C: *Introduction to nursing: adaptation model*, ed 2, Englewood Cliffs, NJ, 1984, Prentice Hall.

Roy C: The Roy adaptation model. In Riehl JP, Roy C, editors: *Conceptual models for nursing practice*, ed 3, New York, 1989, Appleton-Century-Crofts.

Roy C, Obloy SM: The practitioner movement: toward a science of nursing, *Am J Nurs* 79:1698, 1979.

Schuyler CB: Florence Nightingale. In Nightingale F: *Notes on nursing: what it is and what it is not*, commemorative ed, Philadelphia, 1992, JB Lippincott.

Tanner CA: Rethinking clinical judgement. In Diekelman NL, Notter ML, editors: *Transforming RN education: dialogue and debate*, ed 2, New York, 1993, NLN Press.

Torres G: *Theoretical foundations of nursing*, Norwalk, Conn, 1986, Appleton-Century-Crofts.

Watson J: *Nursing: the philosophy and science of caring*, Boston, 1979, Little, Brown.

Watson J: *Nursing: human science and human care*, Norwalk, Conn, 1985, Appleton-Century-Crofts.

Watson J: Nursing on the caring edge: metaphorical vignettes, *ANS Adv Nurs Sci* 10(1):10, 1987.

Watson J: *Nursing: human science, human care: a theory of nursing*, Pub No. 15-2236, New York, 1988, National League for Nursing.

Yamashita M: Family caregiving: application of Neuman's and Peplau's theories, *J Psychiat Ment Health Nurs*, 4(6):401, 1997.

6

Nursing Healing and Caring

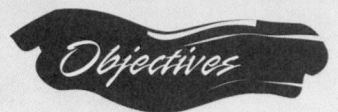

Mastery of content in this chapter will enable the student to:

- Define the key terms listed.
- Discuss the role that caring plays in building a nurse-client relationship.
- Compare and contrast theoretical perspectives on the concept of caring.
- Discuss the potential implications when nurses' and clients' perceptions of caring might differ.
- Discuss how an ethic of care influences the way nurses deal with client care dilemmas.
- Describe how providing presence can be applied when performing a nursing procedure.
- Describe the therapeutic benefit of listening to clients' stories.
- Explain the relationship between knowing a client and clinical decision making.

H ave you ever been ill or experienced a problem requiring health care intervention? Think about that experience for a moment. Then consider the following two scenarios and select the situation that you believe most successfully conveys a sense of caring:

Case STUDY

A nurse enters a client's room, greets the client warmly while touching the client lightly on the shoulder, makes eye contact, sits down for a few minutes and asks about the client's thoughts and concerns, listens to the client's story, looks at the IV hanging in the room, briefly examines the client, and then checks the vital sign summary on the bedside computer screen before departing the room.

A second nurse enters the client's room, looks at the IV hanging in the room, checks the vital sign summary sheet on the bedside computer screen, and acknowledges the client but never sits down or touches the client. Eye contact with the client is from the nurse's lofty vertical position to the client's vulnerable horizontal position. The nurse asks a few brief questions about the client's symptoms and then departs.

There is little doubt that the first scenario presents the nurse in specific acts of caring. The nurse's calm presence, parallel eye contact, attention to the client's concerns, and physical closeness all convey a person-centered, comforting approach. In contrast, the second scenario conveys a sense of indifference and interest only in the tasks of nursing care. During times of illness or when a person seeks the professional guidance of a nurse, caring is essential in helping the individual reach positive outcomes.

Caring has been recognized as being central to nursing practice, but perhaps it has never been more important than today. The pressure and time constraints characteristic of most health care settings can result in nurses and other health professionals becoming cold and indifferent to client needs. Technological advances often take a front seat in health care, with little regard for the interpersonal connections that are critical in therapeutic client relationships. Benner (1989) warns that technological advances can be dangerous and unfeasible without a context of skillful and compassionate care. It is time to value and embrace the caring practices and expert knowledge that are an important part of nursing practice. A nurse who is able to engage clients in a caring and compassionate manner and recognizes the therapeutic gain in caring will make enormous contributions to the health and well-being of those clients.

Theoretical Views on Caring

Caring is a universal phenomenon that influences the ways in which people think, feel, and behave in relation to one another. Caring in nursing has been studied from a variety of philosophical and ethical perspectives since the time of Florence Nightingale. A number of nursing scholars have developed theories on caring because of its importance not only to the practice of nursing, but also to the existence of humankind. This chapter does not detail all of the theoretical positions on caring, but it should help beginning nurses understand that caring is at the heart of a nurse's ability to work with people in a respectful and therapeutic way. Caring actualizes a cherished value in nursing: the individualization of client care.

CARING IS PRIMARY
Patricia Benner (1984, 1989) would quickly argue that her work on expertise in nursing practice and the central role

of caring is not theory in the traditional sense. Theories are typically designed to explain, predict, and describe specific phenomena. For example, a theory on pain control might propose that distracting a person's focus from the painful experience will minimize the person's discomfort. Theories can be very mechanistic, often ignoring the context or situation in which phenomena occur. The theory on pain control likely would ignore the unique cultural and social factors that influence how people respond to pain. In other words, theories often try to treat occurrences of phenomena all in the same way.

Benner, in contrast, does not try to predict or control phenomena. Instead, she attempts to give nurses a rich, holistic understanding of nursing practice and caring through the interpretation of expert nurses' real stories. After hearing and analyzing the stories nurses tell about their clients, Benner is able to describe the essence of excellent nursing practice, which is caring.

Caring as defined by Benner (1989) means that persons, events, projects, and things matter to people. It is a word for being connected. Because caring determines what matters to a person, it describes a wide range of involvements, from parental love to friendship, from caring for one's work to caring for one's pet, to caring for and about one's clients. Caring also reveals what is stressful and the available options for coping. If something does not matter to an individual, it will not likely create stress or the need for coping. Benner (1989) notes: "Caring creates possibility." Personal concern for some person, event, or thing provides motivation and direction for people. Caring is the essential requisite for coping. Benner sees the personal concern of caring as an inherent feature of nursing practice, whereby nurses help clients to recover in the face of illness, to give meaning to that illness, and to maintain or reestablish connection. Caring makes nurses notice which interventions are successful, and this concern then guides future caregiving.

Clients are not all the same. Each brings a different background of experiences, values, and cultural perspectives to a situation, such as a health care encounter. Caring is thus always specific and relational for each nurse-client encounter. Benner's theory of nursing practice focuses on caring to help individuals in their unique situations cope with the stress of illness (Benner, 1989).

It is also important to understand how Benner (1989) describes the relationship between health, illness, and disease. Health is not the absence of illness, nor is illness identical with disease. Health is a state of being that people define in relation to their own values, personality, and lifestyle. Health exists along a continuum (see Chapter 1). Illness is the experience of loss or dysfunction, whereas disease is the manifestation of an abnormality at the cellular, tissue, or organ level. A client may have a disease (e.g., arthritis or diabetes) but not experience the sense of being ill. An individual does not seek health care until there is a disruption, loss, or concern. For example, a client may have had diabetes for a number of years but not sense being ill until the disease begins to cause serious visual impairment, threatening the ability to work. Illness therefore has meaning within the context of the person's life. Any symptoms a person feels are experienced as interruptions or a health worry. Benner (1989) argues that since illness is the human experience of loss or dysfunction, any treatment or intervention given without consideration of its meaning to the individual is likely to be worthless. Expert nurses understand the difference between health, illness, and disease. Through caring relationships, nurses learn to listen to clients' stories about their illness so that an understanding of the meaning of illness can be obtained. With this understanding, therapeutic, client-centered care can be provided. Benner notes that understanding the meaning of the illness for the person is a form of healing.

THE ESSENCE OF NURSING AND HEALTH

From a transcultural perspective, Madeleine Leininger (1978) describes the concept of care as the essence and central, unifying, and dominant domain that distinguishes nursing from other health disciplines. Care is also an essential human need, necessary for the health and survival of all individuals. Care, unlike cure, is oriented to assisting an individual or group in improving a human condition. Acts of caring refer to the direct or indirect nurturant and skillful activities, processes, and decisions that assist people in ways that are empathetic, compassionate, and supportive, and that are dependent on the needs, problems, and values of the individual being assisted. Leininger's studies of numerous cultures around the world have found that care helps protect, develop, nurture, and provide survival to people. Care is vital to recovery from illness and to the maintenance of healthy life practices.

Leininger (1988) stresses the importance for nurses to understand both universal and nonuniversal folk and professional caring behaviors in order to be effective in the care of clients. Even though human caring is a universal phenomenon, the expressions, processes, and patterns of caring vary among cultures. For example, the New Guinea people of Melanesia value surveillance and protection as basic elements of care, whereas Southern rural African-Americans in the United States value concern and support as care. Caring is very personal, and thus its expression will differ for each client. For caring to achieve cure, nurses must learn those culturally specific behaviors that reflect human care processes in different cultures.

TRANSPERSONAL CARING

The managed care system of health care is increasingly removed from nursing's caring values and expertise. As a result, Jean Watson (1979, 1988) describes a new consciousness that is emerging, allowing nursing to raise new questions about what it means to be a nurse, to be ill, and to be caring and healing. Rejecting the disease orientation to health care, nursing instead is beginning to embrace caring as a moral ideal and an end in and of itself. Watson's transpersonal caring theory (1988) places care before cure, with caring becoming the ethical standard by which nursing care is measured. Caring preserves human dignity in a cure-dominated health care system.

Caring encompasses a metaphysical or almost spiritual dimension. Caring-healing is communicated through the consciousness of the nurse to the individual being cared for (Watson, 1988). Caring-healing consciousness takes place during a single caring moment between nurse and client. An interconnectedness forms between the one cared for and the one caring. Transpersonal caring expands the limits of openness and allows access to the higher human spirit, thus expanding human consciousness. Both the nurse and client are influenced through the transaction, for better or for worse.

Watson also argues that the human caring process has an energy field greater than that possessed by each individual. The caring-healing consciousness can promote healing and release a person's own inner power and resources.

SWANSON'S THEORY OF CARING

In the development of her caring theory, Kristen Swanson (1991) conducted interviews with three different groups: women who had miscarried, parents and professionals in a newborn intensive care unit, and socially at-risk mothers who had received long-term, public health interven-

tion. All groups were in a perinatal situation or context and had experienced the phenomenon of caring. Each group was asked questions regarding how caring was experienced or expressed in their situation. Swanson's theory of caring is a composite of the three studies. The theory describes caring as consisting of five categories or processes (Table 6-1). Caring is defined by the theorist as a nurturing way of relating to a valued other, toward whom one feels a personal sense of commitment and responsibility. The theory supports the claim that caring is a central nursing phenomenon but not necessarily unique to nursing practice.

The contributions by Swanson (1991) are valuable in providing direction for how to develop useful and effective caring strategies. Each of the caring processes has subdimensions that can serve as the basis for nursing interventional approaches. For example, if a caring-based nurse counseling program for at-risk mothers were developed, the researcher would develop strategies to help nurses learn how to know and be with clients, based on the subdimensions of caring. Future research is needed to determine if Swanson's caring theory applies to other populations of clients.

SUMMARY OF THEORETICAL VIEWS

In reading and critiquing nursing theorists' views on caring, one finds certain common themes. Caring is highly relational. The nurse and the client enter into a relation-

Table 6-1	**Swanson's Theory of Caring**	
Caring Process	Definitions	Subdimensions
Knowing	Striving to understand an event as it has meaning in the life of the other	Avoiding assumptions Centering on the one cared for Assessing thoroughly Seeking cues Engaging the self or both
Being with	Being emotionally present to the other	Being there Conveying ability Sharing feelings Not burdening
Doing for	Doing for the other as he or she would do for the self if it were at all possible	Comforting Anticipating Performing skillfully Protecting Preserving dignity
Enabling	Facilitating the other's passage through life transitions (e.g., birth, death) and unfamiliar events	Informing/explaining Supporting/allowing Focusing Generating alternatives Validating/giving feedback
Maintaining belief	Sustaining faith in the other's capacity to get through an event or transition and face a future with meaning	Believing in/holding in esteem Maintaining a hope-filled attitude Offering realistic optimism "Going the distance"

From Swanson K: Empirical development of a middle-range theory of caring, *Nurs Res* 40(3):161, 1991.

ship that is much more than one person simply "doing tasks for" another. There is a mutual give and take that develops as nurse and client begin to know and care for one another. Frank (1998) described a personal situation when he was suffering from cancer: "What I wanted when I was ill, was a mutual relationship of *persons* who were also clinician and client." It was important for the author to be seen as one of two fellow human beings, not the dependent client being cared for by the expert technical clinician. Caring may seem highly invisible at times, when a nurse and client enter a relationship of respect, concern, and support. The nurse's empathy and compassion become a natural part of every client encounter. However, the nurse-client relationship can become very visible when caring is absent. A nurse's disinterest or avoidance of a client's request, for example, will quickly convey an uncaring attitude. Benner and Wrubel (1989) relate the story of one expert clinical nurse specialist who learned from a client what caring is all about:

> I felt that I was teaching him a lot, but actually he taught me. One day he said to me (probably after I had delivered some well-meaning technical information about his disease), "You are doing an OK job, but I can tell that every time you walk in that door you are walking out."

Clients can tell quickly when nurses fail to relate to them. In contrast, when caring is practiced, the client senses a commitment on the part of the nurse and is will-ing to enter into a relationship that allows the nurse to gain an understanding of the client and his or her experience of illness. This allows the nurse to become a coach and partner rather than a detached provider of care services.

Another theme that is common in the theories of caring is understanding the context of the person's life and illness. It is difficult to show caring to another individual without gaining an understanding of who they are and their perception of their illness. With experience, the nurse appreciates the value of learning about the client's situation: how was the illness first recognized? How did the client feel? How does the illness affect the client's daily life practices? What values and beliefs influence the client's response? Knowing the context of a client's illness helps the professional nurse to choose and individualize interventions that will actually help the client. This approach will be more successful than simply selecting interventions on the basis of the client's symptoms or disease process.

Clients' Perceptions of Caring

Swanson's theory of caring (1991) provides an excellent beginning to understanding the behaviors and processes that characterize caring. There have been other researchers who have studied caring from clients' perceptions (Table 6-2). The identification of those behaviors that clients per-

Table 6-2   Nurse Caring Behavior (as Perceived by Clients)

Riemen (1986)		Mayer (1986)	Brown (1986)
Perceptions of Female Clients	Perceptions of Male Clients	Perceptions of Cancer Clients and Their Families	Perceptions of Hospitalized Adult Clients
Responding to client's uniqueness	Being physically present so client feels valued	Knowing how to give injections and manage equipment	Providing a reassuring presence
Being perceptive and supportive of client's concerns	Returning voluntarily without being called	Being cheerful	Providing information
Being physically present	Making client feel comfortable, relaxed, and secure	Encouraging clients to call if they have problems	Demonstrating professional knowledge and skill
Having attitudes and displaying behaviors that make client feel valued as a human being	Attending to comfort and needs of client before doing tasks	Putting client first	Assisting with pain
Return to client voluntarily without being asked	Using a kind, soft, pleasant, gentle voice and attitude	Anticipating that first experiences are the hardest	Taking more time than actually needed
Showing concern that is comforting and relaxing			Promoting autonomy
Using a soft, gentle voice			Recognizing individual qualities and needs
Invoking feelings of security			Keeping client under watch
Invoking feelings in client of wanting to reciprocate			

ceive as caring helps to emphasize what clients expect from their caregivers. Clients have always been known to value how effective nurses are in performing tasks, but, clearly, clients also value the affective dimension of nursing care (Williams, 1997). Establishing a reassuring presence, recognizing an individual as unique, and keeping a close, attentive eye on the client are recurrent caring behaviors that researchers have identified. All clients are unique; however, understanding common behaviors that clients associate with caring will help the beginning student learn to express caring in practice.

The study of clients' perceptions is important because health care is now placing great emphasis on client satisfaction (see Chapter 2). What clients experience in their interactions with institutional services and health care professionals, and what they think of that experience, will determine how clients use the health care system and how they will benefit from it (Gerteis, 1993). It is believed that when clients sense that health care providers are interested in them as people, clients will be more willing to follow recommendations and therapeutic plans. Williams (1997) studied the relationship between clients' perceptions of four dimensions of caring and their satisfaction with nursing care (Box 6-1). Clients in the study indicated that they were more satisfied when they perceived nurses to be caring. As institutions look to ways of improving client satisfaction, creating an environment of caring is a necessary and worthwhile goal. Clients' satisfaction with nursing care is the most important factor in their decision to return to a hospital (Risser, 1975; Bader, 1988).

As a nurse begins clinical practice, it is important to consider how clients perceive caring and what are the best approaches to providing care. The behaviors that researchers have associated with caring offer an excellent starting point. But it is also important to understand clients and their unique expectations. Researchers have learned that frequently clients and nurses differ in their perceptions of caring (Mayer, 1987). For that reason, the nurse must focus on building a relationship that allows him or her to learn what is important to the client. A client who is fearful of having an intravenous catheter inserted may benefit more from the novice nurse's acquiring assistance from a staff member who can quickly and skillfully insert the catheter than from the novice nurse's attempt to relieve anxiety through a lengthy description of the procedure. Knowing who clients are will help the nurse to select those caring approaches that are most appropriate to the client's needs.

Ethics of Care

Caring is interpreted by many as being a moral imperative. Through caring for other human beings, ultimately human dignity is protected, enhanced, and preserved. Watson (1988) suggests that caring, as a moral ideal, provides the stance from which one intervenes as a nurse.

Research HIGHLIGHT   Box 6-1

RESEARCH ABSTRACT

Hospitalized clients interact with nurses more than with other health care providers. Clients generally see nursing care as an important factor in satisfaction with their overall care. Ninety-four hospitalized medical clients were studied to assess their perceptions of the extent to which holistic nursing care was received and whether there was a relationship between clients' perceptions of holistic caring and their satisfaction with nursing care. Clients completed the Holistic Caring Inventory (HCI), a 40-item survey designed to measure the holistic, humanistic, caring component of the health care provider–client interaction. The HCI incorporates four dimensions of caring: physical, interpretive, spiritual, and sensitive. The clients also completed a client satisfaction survey that included three dimensions of satisfaction with nurses and their care; technical-professional activities, trust, and educational activities. The study demonstrated a positive correlation between holistic caring and overall client satisfaction. Sensitive caring was the strongest predictor of client satisfaction. In addition, clients indicated that they valued technical skills, competency, and timely physical care.

IMPLICATIONS FOR PRACTICE

* Clients do value the affective aspect of nursing care as much as physical care.
* Nurses should gain an increasing knowledge of what caring behaviors are, through education and clinical practice review.
* Sensitive caring behaviors (e.g., listening, helping clients find meaning in their feelings, showing concern, and helping clients to discuss their feelings) may improve client outcomes.

REFERENCE

Williams SA: The relationship of patients' perceptions of holistic nurse caring to satisfaction with nursing care, *J Nurs Care Qual*, 11(5):15, 1997.

This stance is critical for ensuring that nurses practice ethical standards for good conduct, character, and motives.

Chapter 20 explores the importance of ethics in professional nursing. The term *ethics* refers to the ideals of right and wrong behavior. In any client encounter, a nurse must know what behavior is ethically appropriate. Traditionally, ethical appropriateness is based on standards of practice and the ethical guidelines of beneficence, nonmaleficence, justice, and autonomy. An ethic of care is unique in that the guidelines for making professional decisions are not based solely on intellectual or analytical principles. Instead, an ethic of care places caring at the center of decision making. Should an indigent client be cared for? Is it caring to place a disabled relative in a long-term care facility?

An **ethic of care** is concerned with relationships between people and with a nurse's character and attitude toward others. Caring knowledge is gained through personal and emotional involvement with others and by joining them in their moral struggles (Cooper, 1991). Practitioners who function from an ethic of care are sensitive to unequal relationships that can lead to an abuse of one person's power over another—intentional or otherwise. In health care settings clients and families are often on unequal footing with professionals because of the client's illness, lack of information, regression caused by pain and suffering, and unfamiliar circumstances. An ethic of care places the nurse as the client's advocate, solving ethical dilemmas by attending to relationships and by giving priority to each client's unique personhood.

Caring in Nursing Practice

It is impossible to prescribe ways that will guarantee a nurse's becoming a caring professional. Scholars disagree as to whether caring can be taught or is more fundamentally a way of being in the world. For those who find caring a normal part of their life, caring is a product of their culture, values, experiences, and relationships with others. Persons who do not experience care in their lives often find it difficult to act in caring ways. As nurses deal with health and illness in their practice, they grow in the ability to care. Expert nurses understand the differences and relationships among health, illness, and disease and become able to see clients in their own context, interpret their needs, and offer caring acts that improve clients' health.

PROVIDING PRESENCE

When one reviews the various studies of caring, providing **presence** (being with a client) is a valued behavior. To provide presence is to have a person-to-person encounter that conveys a closeness and sense of security. The ability to provide presence, to be with another person in a way that acknowledges one's shared humanity, is at the core of nursing as a caring practice (Benner, 1989). Presence is more than mere physical presence, although the physical closeness is important. Presence also represents a being "in tune" with each other, an awareness of each individual's uniqueness (Simons, 1987).

When a nurse establishes presence, eye contact, body language, voice tone, listening, and having a positive and encouraging attitude act together to create an openness and understanding. The message conveyed is that the other's experience matters to the one caring (Swanson, 1991). Being able to establish presence with a client also enhances the nurse's ability to learn from the client. As a result, the nurse's ability to provide adequate and appropriate nursing care is strengthened.

It is especially important to establish presence when clients are experiencing stressful events or situations. Awaiting a doctor's report of test results, preparing for an unfamiliar procedure, and planning for a return home after serious illness are just a few examples of events in the course of a person's illness that can create unpredictability and dependency on care providers. The nurse's presence can help to allay anxiety and fear related to stress. Giving reassurance and thorough explanations about a procedure, remaining at the client's side, and coaching the client through the experience all convey a presence that is invaluable to the client's well-being.

COMFORTING

Clients face situations that can be embarrassing, frightening, painful, and exhausting. Whatever the feeling or symptom, clients look to nurses to provide comfort. Comforting provides both an emotional and physical calm.

The use of touch is one comforting approach whereby the nurse reaches out to clients to communicate concern and support. Touch may involve holding a client's hand, giving a back massage, or gently positioning a body part. Because touch can convey many messages, it must be used with discretion.

Comforting also involves the skillful and gentle performance of a nursing procedure. An expert nurse has learned that any procedure is more effective when it is administered carefully and in consideration of any client concern. If a client is anxious about having a procedure, such as the insertion of a nasogastric tube, the nurse affords comfort through a full explanation of how the procedure will be done and what the client will feel. In addition, comfort is associated with the nurse's expressed confidence in being able to perform the procedure safely and successfully. For example, the confidence an expert nurse shows when preparing supplies, positioning the client, and gently manipulating and inserting the nasogastric tube helps the client to relax and feel more at ease. Throughout a procedure the nurse talks quietly with the client to provide reassurance and support.

Chapters 38 and 42 review principles of hygiene and comfort. Both chapters describe measures that can be used to effectively provide comfort for a client. But, it is not simply the "doing for" that is comforting; rather, it is the nurse's comforting approach. For example, a client who is undergoing chemotherapy may suffer fatigue and have ulcerative lesions of the mouth. Anyone can provide mouth care. However, for the mouth care to be comforting, the nurse may choose a time, outside of a routine, that best meets the client's needs. Perhaps the nurse times the mouth care to coincide with 30 minutes after an analgesic has been administered. The nurse provides gentle, cleansing mouth care, dims the room lights, repositions the client, offers some encouraging words, and allows the client to rest peacefully.

LISTENING

Caring involves an interpersonal interaction that is much more than two persons simply talking back and forth. In a caring relationship the nurse establishes trust, opens lines of communication, and listens to what the client has to say

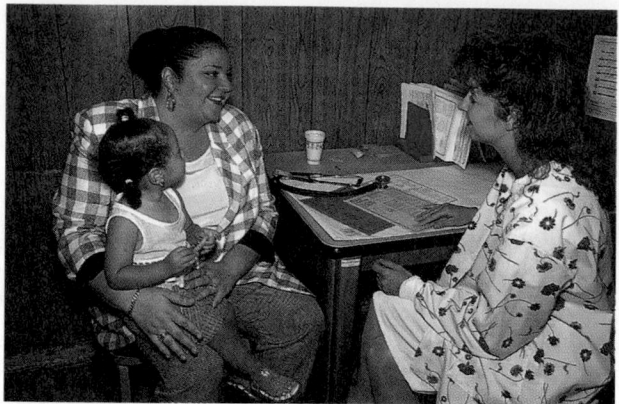

Figure 6-1 Nurse listening to client.

(Figure 6-1). Listening is key, because it can convey the nurse's full attention and interest. Listening to the meaning of what a client says helps create a mutual relationship.

When an individual becomes ill, he or she usually has a story to tell about the meaning of the illness. Any critical or chronic illness affects all of a client's life choices and decisions, sometimes affecting the individual's identity. Being able to tell that story helps the client break the distress of illness. Thus, a story needs a listener. Frank (1998) described his own feelings during his experience with cancer: "I needed a [health care professional's] gift of listening in order to make my suffering a relationship between *us,* instead of an iron cage around *me.*" He needed to be able to express what he needed when he was ill. The personal concerns that are part of a client's illness story determine what is at stake for the client. Caring for a client enables the nurse to be a participant in the client's life. A nurse must be able to give clients their full, focused attention as their stories are told. Listening should not simply be a task, but instead a gift; otherwise, its efficacy is lost (Frank, 1998).

When an ill person chooses to tell his or her story, it involves reaching out to another human being. Telling the story implies a relationship that can only develop if the clinician exchanges his or her stories as well. Frank (1998) argues that professionals do not routinely take seriously their own need to be known as part of a clinical relationship. Yet, unless the professional acknowledges this need, there is no reciprocal relationship, only an interaction (Campo, 1997). There is pressure on the clinician to know as much as possible about the client, but it isolates the clinician from the client. By contrast, knowing and being known each supports the other (Frank, 1998).

As clinicians, nurses will hear and share a variety of stories from clients. Within a clinical relationship there is a hierarchy of needs. The stories of deeply ill persons have priority. Clinicians may tell parts of their own stories but do so in response to the ill person's story (Frank, 1998). To give the gift of listening is to appreciate receiving the gift of a client's story.

Learning to listen to a client is sometimes difficult. It is easy to become distracted by tasks at hand, colleagues shouting instructions, or other clients waiting to have their needs attended to. However, the time one takes to listen (and listen effectively) is worthwhile both in the information gained and in the strengthening of the nurse-client relationship. Listening involves paying attention to the individual's words and tone of voice, and entering his or her frame of reference. By observing the expressions and body language of the client, the nurse can find cues to help assist the client in exploring ways to achieve greater peace, take action, or do whatever a situation requires (Hungelmann and others, 1996). Chapter 22 discusses additional listening techniques.

KNOWING THE CLIENT

One of the five caring processes described by Swanson (1991) is knowing the client. The concept comprises both the nurse's understanding of a specific client and the nurse's subsequent selection of interventions (Radwin, 1995). To know a client means that the nurse avoids assumptions, centers on the client, and engages in a caring relationship with the client that reveals information and cues that facilitate critical thinking and clinical judgments (see Chapter 13). Knowing the client is at the core of the process by which nurses make clinical decisions. By establishing a caring relationship, the mutuality that develops helps the nurse to better know the client as a unique individual and to then choose the most appropriate and efficacious nursing therapies.

The caring relationships that a nurse develops over time, coupled with the nurse's growing knowledge and experience, provide a rich source of meaning when clinical changes in a client occur. Expert nurses develop the ability to detect changes in clients' conditions almost effortlessly. Clinical decision making, perhaps the most important responsibility of the professional nurse, involves various aspects of knowing the client: responses to therapies, routines and habits, coping resources, physical capacities and endurance, and body typology and characteristics (Tanner and others, 1993). Additional factors that the experienced nurse knows about clients are their experiences, behaviors, feelings, and perceptions (Radwin, 1995). When clinical decisions are made accurately in the context of knowing a client well, improved client outcomes will result. Swanson-Kaufman (1986) notes that when care is based on knowing the client, it is perceived by clients as personalized, comforting, supportive, and healing.

The most important thing for a beginning nurse to recognize is that knowing a client is much more than simply gathering data about the client's clinical signs and condition. Of course, this information must be gathered. But success in knowing the client lies in the relationship that is established. To know a client is to enter into a caring, social process that results in a "bonding" whereby the client comes to feel known by the nurse (Lamb and Stempel,

1994). The bonding then sets the stage for the relationship to evolve into "working" and "changing" phases so that the nurse can help the client become involved in his or her care and accept help when needed.

SPIRITUAL CARING

Remen (1988) suggests that healing is not a matter of mechanism, such as treatments or medications, but rather a work of spirit. It is an individual's intrinsic spirit that seems to be a factor in the healing process. Spiritual health is achieved when a person finds a balance between his or her own life values, goals, and belief systems and those of others. Research has shown a link between spirit, mind, and body. An individual's beliefs and expectations can and do have effects on the person's physical well-being (Coe, 1997).

Establishing a caring relationship with a client involves an interconnectedness between the nurse and the client. This is the reason why Watson (1979) describes the caring relationship in a spiritual sense. Spirituality offers a sense of connectedness as well, intrapersonally (connected with oneself), interpersonally (connected with others and the environment), and transpersonally (connected with the unseen, God, or a higher power). When a caring relationship is established, the client and the nurse come to know one another so that both move toward a healing relationship by:

Mobilizing hope for the client and for the nurse

Finding an interpretation or understanding of illness, symptoms, or emotions that is acceptable to the client

Assisting the client in using social, emotional, or spiritual resources

Chapter 28 describes in detail the significance that spirituality plays in an individual's health.

FAMILY CARE

People inhabit their worlds in an involved way. Each individual experiences life through relationships with others. Caring for an individual thus cannot occur in isolation from that person's family. As a nurse, it is important to know the family almost as thoroughly as one knows a client (Figure 6-2). The family is an important resource. Success with nursing interventions often depends on the family's willingness to share information about the client, their acceptance and understanding of therapies, whether the interventions fit with the family's daily practices, and whether the family can support and deliver the therapies recommended.

Mayer (1986) identified 10 nurse caring behaviors that were perceived as most helpful by families of clients with cancer (Box 6-2). Assuring the client's well-being and helping the family to become active participants are critical for family members. Although specific to families of clients with cancer, the behaviors offer useful guidelines for developing a caring relationship with all families. The nurse begins a relationship by learning who makes up the client's family and what their role is in the client's life. Showing the family care and concern for the client creates an openness that then enables a relationship to form with the family. Caring for the family (Chapter 8) takes into consideration the context of the client's illness and the stress it imposes on all members.

The Challenge of Caring

For many nurses, being able to assist individuals during a time of need is the reason for entering the profession. Caring has been part of the nursing discipline since its beginning. The profession of nursing, unlike medicine, can care and assist people without medical diagnoses or new technologies and treatments. Caring is a motivating force for people to become nurses and it becomes the source of

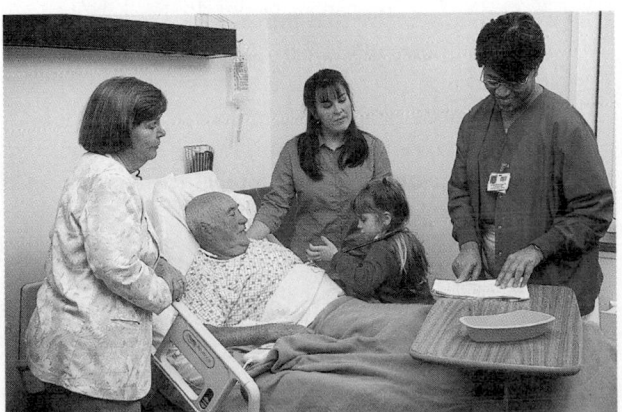

Figure 6-2   Nurse discusses client's health care needs with family.

Nurse Caring Behaviors as Perceived by Families   Box 6-2

Being honest
Giving clear explanations
Keeping family members informed
Trying to make the client comfortable
Showing interest in answering questions
Providing necessary emergency care
Assuring the client that nursing services will be available
Answering family members' questions honestly, openly, and willingly
Allowing clients to do as much for themselves as possible
Teaching the family how to keep the relative physically comfortable

Data from Mayer DK: Cancer patients' and families' perceptions of nurse caring behaviors, *Top Clin Nurs* 8(2):63, 1986.

satisfaction when nurses know they have made a difference in their clients' lives.

It is becoming more of a challenge to care in today's health care system. Being a part of the helping professions is difficult and demanding. Nurses are given less time to spend with clients, making it much harder to know who they are. Leininger (1988) notes that advanced technology threatens human concerns. A reliance on technology and cost-effective health care strategies and efforts to standardize and refine work processes all undermine the nature of caring. Too often clients become just a number, with their real needs either overlooked or ignored.

Paul Morrison (1989) surveyed nurses' perceptions about themselves as professional carers. Although the study involved only a small number of experienced nurses, the results posed some interesting questions for all nurses. The nurses were asked to compare "themselves" with an "ideal self" in regard to eight different objectives: compassionate, safe, selfish, lacking awareness, empathetic, insecure, tolerant, and kind. Any differences between perceptions of "themselves" and the "ideal self" suggested a need for personal change. The study found discrepancies, with nurses perceiving themselves as lacking certain skills within their caring role. Morrison described various reasons that might explain the discrepancies. The nurses might have set unrealistic expectations for themselves, making it difficult to live up to standards. The group also might have lacked appropriate training or knowledge for the caring role. Most important, the system of values prevalent within their "organizational culture" might have differed from the values held by the nurses working in that organization. When organizations fail to reinforce and provide ways for nurses to practice caring, nurses are less likely to meet their personal expectations. When these expectations cannot be met, nurses feel grief and loss in being unable to care for clients adequately.

Human beings cannot be treated like machines or robots if health care is to make a positive difference in their lives. Instead, health care must become more humanizing. As professionals, nurses play an important role in making care an integral part of health care delivery. This begins by nurses making caring a part of the philosophy and environment in the workplace. Incorporating care concepts into standards of nursing care establishes the guidelines for professional conduct. Finally, during the day to day practice with clients and families, nurses must be committed to caring and be willing to establish the relationships necessary for personal, compassionate, and meaningful nursing care to be delivered.

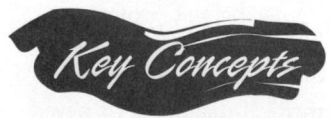

Key Concepts

- A nurse who is able to engage clients in a caring and compassionate manner and recognizes the therapeutic gain in caring will contribute to the health and well-being of those clients.
- According to Benner, caring describes a wide range of involvements and reveals what the available options are for coping.
- Since illness is the human experience of loss or dysfunction, any treatment or intervention given without consideration of its meaning to the individual is likely to be worthless.
- The expressions, processes, and patterns of caring vary among cultures.
- Swanson's theory of caring includes five caring processes: knowing, being with, doing for, enabling, and maintaining belief.
- Caring is highly relational, involving a mutual give and take that develops as nurse and client begin to know and care for one another.
- To care for another individual, one must understand the context of the person's life and illness.

- Client's perceptions of nurse caring include establishing a reassuring presence, recognizing an individual as unique, and keeping a close, attentive eye on the client.
- Clients tend to be more satisfied with nursing care when they perceive that nurses care.
- An ethic of care places caring at the center of decision making.
- When a nurse establishes presence, eye contact, body language, voice tone, listening, and having a positive and encouraging attitude act together to create openness and understanding.
- Comforting involves the use of touch and the skillful and gentle performance of nursing care procedures.
- Listening involves paying attention to an individual's words and tone of voice, and entering into his or her frame of reference.
- Knowing the client is at the core of the process by which nurses make clinical decisions.
- A nurse demonstrates caring by helping family members become active participants in a client's care.

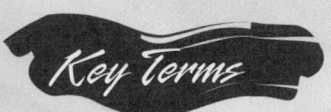
Key Terms

Caring, *p. 102*   Ethic of care, *p. 106*
Comforting, *p. 107*   Presence, *p. 107*

Critical Thinking Exercises

1. Lindsey is a student nurse assigned to care for Mrs. Lowe, a 62-year-old client being treated for lymphoma (cancer of the lymph nodes). The charge nurse informs Lindsey that the nurse who does intravenous procedures will be up shortly to insert a long term, percutaneous intravascular catheter for Mrs. Lowe's chemotherapy. This is the first day Lindsay has cared for Mrs. Lowe, but she has learned that the client has not had an intravenous line previously. In what way can Lindsay provide presence and be comforting for Mrs. Lowe?

2. During your next clinical practicum, select a client to talk with for at least 15 to 20 minutes. Ask the client to tell you about his or her illness. Review the skills of listening in this chapter and in Chapter 22. Immediately after your discussion, reflect on the discussion with the client and answer the following questions:
   A. What do you believe the client was trying to tell you about his or her illness?
   B. Why was it important for the client to share his or her story?
   C. What did you do that made it easy or difficult for the client to talk with you?
   D. Would you rate yourself a good listener? If not, why not? If so, explain.

3. The next time you are assigned to a clinical agency, ask to read their philosophy and standards of care documents. Does the language in the documents represent a caring ethic?

References

Bader MM: Nursing care behaviors that predict patient satisfaction, *J Nurs Qual Assur* 2:11, 1988.

Benner P: *From novice to expert,* Menlo Park, Calif, 1984, Addison-Wesley.

Benner P, Wrubel J: *The primacy of caring: stress and coping in health and illness,* Menlo Park, Calif, 1989, Addison Wesley.

Brown L: The experience of care: patient perspectives, *Top Clin Nurs* 8(2):56, 1986.

Campo R: *The poetry of healing: a doctor's education in empathy, identification, and desire,* New York, 1997, WW Norton.

Coe RM: The magic of science and the science of magic: an essay on the process of healing, *J Health Soc Behav* 38(3):1, 1997.

Cooper M: Principle-oriented ethics and the ethic of care: a creative tension, *ANS Adv Nurs Sci* 14(2):22, 1991.

Frank AW: Just listening: narrative and deep illness, *Fam Syst Health* 16(3):197, 1998.

Gerteis M and others: What patients really want, *Health Manage Q* 15:2, 1993.

Hungelmann J and others: Focus on spiritual well-being: harmonious interconnectedness of mind-body-spirit—use of the JAREL spiritual well-being scale, *Geriatr Nurs* 17(6):262, 1996.

Lamb G, Stempel G: Nursing case management from the client's view: growing as insider-expert, *Nurs Outlook* 42(7):7, 1994.

Leininger M: *Care: the essence of nursing and health,* Detroit, 1988, Wayne State University Press.

Leininger M: *Transcultural nursing: concepts, theories and practices,* New York, 1978, John Wiley & Sons.

Mayer DK: Cancer patients' and families' perceptions of nurse caring behaviors, *Top Clin Nurs* 8(2):63, 1986.

Mayer DK: Oncology nurses' versus cancer patients' perceptions of nurse caring behaviors: a replication study, *Oncol Nurs Forum* 14(3):48, 1987.

Morrison P: Nursing and caring: a personal construct theory study of some nurses' self-perceptions, *J Adv Nurs* 14:421, 1989.

Radwin L: Knowing the patient: a process model for individualized interventions, *Nurs Res* 44:364, 1995.

Remen RN: Spirit: resource for healing, *Noetic Sci Rev,* p 61, autumn 1988.

Riemen DJ: The essential structure of a caring interaction: doing phenomenology. In Munhall PL, Oiler CJ: *Nursing research: a qualitative perspective,* Norwalk, Conn, 1986, Appleton-Century-Crofts.

Risser NL: Development of an instrument to measure patient satisfaction with nurses and nursing care in primary care settings, *Nurs Res* 24:45, 1975.

Simons JE: Science update: patients' and nurses' perception of caring, *Res Rev* 4:2, 1987.

Swanson KM: Empirical development of a middle-range theory of caring, *Nurs Res* 40(3):161, 1991.

Swanson-Kauffman K: Caring in the instance of unexpected early pregnancy loss, *Top Clin Nurs* 8(2):37, 1986.

Tanner C and others: The phenomenology of knowing the patient, *Image J Nurs Sch* 25:273, 1993.

Watson MJ: *Nursing: the philosophy and science of caring,* Boston, 1979, Little, Brown.

Watson MJ: New dimensions of human caring theory, *Nurs Sci Q* 1:175, 1988.

Williams SA: The relationship of patients' perceptions of holistic nurse caring to satisfaction with nursing care, *J Nurs Care Qual* 11(5):15, 1997.

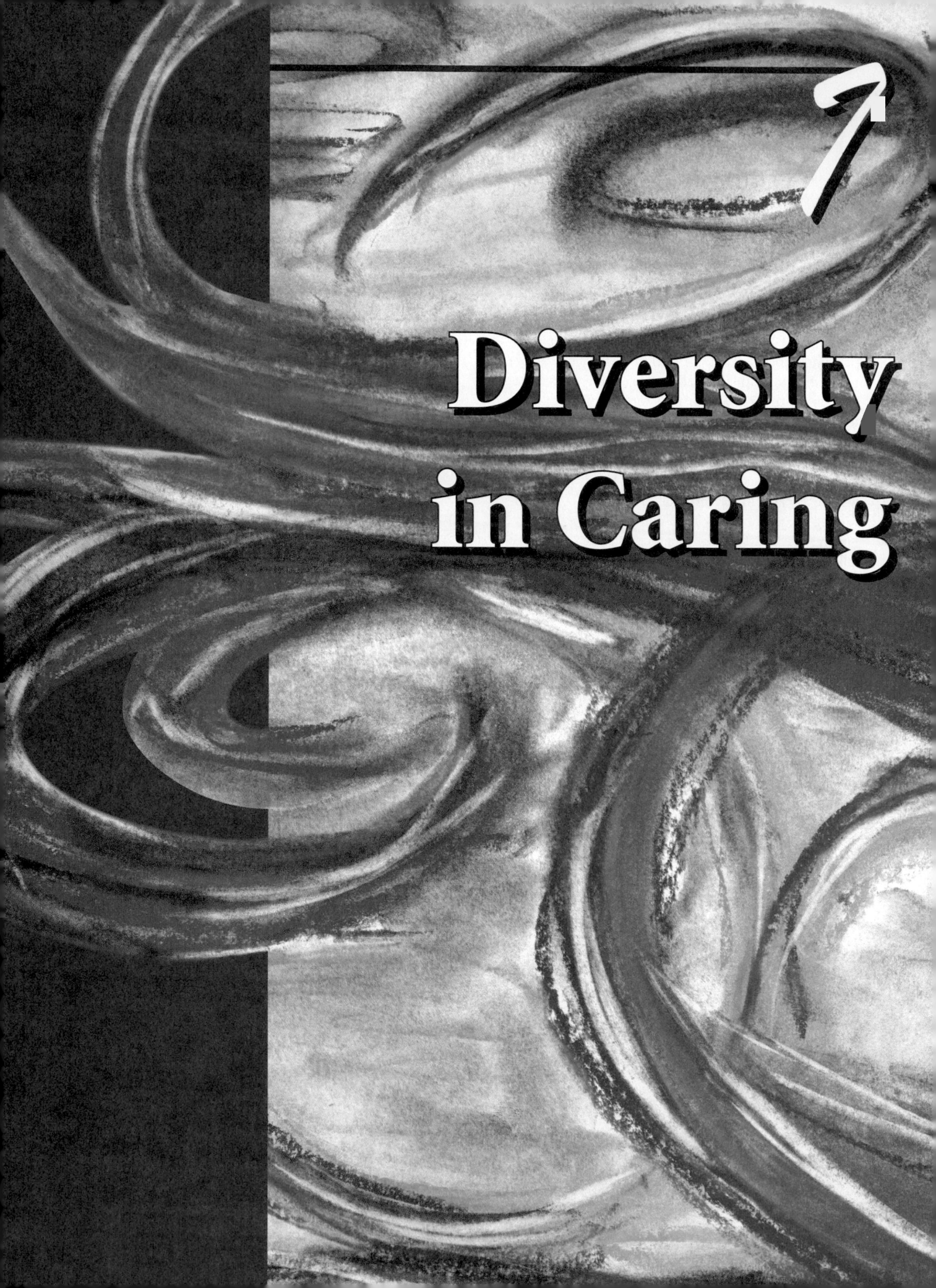

Diversity
in Caring

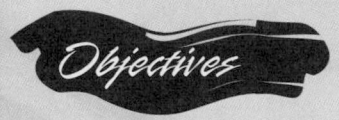

Objectives

Mastery of content in this chapter will enable the student to:

- Define the key terms listed.
- Describe the communication problems encountered when caring for clients and families from multicultural backgrounds.
- Identify how orientation to time and space may affect the nursing care needs of clients and families.
- Describe how cultural behavior is acquired in a social setting.
- Identify types of health care practices, including folk beliefs, that may have significant impact on wellness, illness, and health-seeking behaviors of persons from various cultural groups.
- Describe biological variations present in individuals and families from different racial backgrounds.
- Discuss ways to develop cognitive and psychomotor skills to render culturally competent care.
- Discuss the term *cultural stereotyping* and its relevance to rendering culturally competent care.

The demographic profile of the United States suggests that this country is rapidly becoming a heterogeneous, multicultural, society. This is evidenced by the changes in the 1990 census and the futuristic projections for the next 30 years. In 1998, 70.9% of the population in the United States were white of European descent, 12.9% were African-American, 11.4% were Hispanic, 4.1% were Asian-American, and 0.9% were Native American (U.S. Department of Commerce, Bureau of the Census, 1998). It is projected that by the year 2020 only 53% of the U.S. population will be white of European descent. It is further projected that by the year 2021 the number of Asian-Americans and Hispanics will have tripled, while the number of African-Americans will have doubled (U.S. Department of Commerce, Bureau of the Census, 1993c).

In light of the rapidly changing demographic profile of the United States, it is imperative that nurses develop an understanding about culture and its relevance to competent care. There is no magic recipe for the delivery of culturally competent and appropriate care, because there is as much variation within certain races, cultural groups, or ethnic groups as there is across cultural groups. However, when the informed nurse takes into account the significance of culture, clients are approached with a more informed perspective. Transcultural nursing represents and reflects the need for respect and acknowledgment of the wholeness of all human beings (Figure 7-1). It is essential to remember that regardless of race, ethnicity, culture, or cultural heritage, every human being is culturally unique.

Important Definitions

To understand transcultural nursing, the nurse must develop a basic understanding of key concepts such as cul-

ture, cultural values, cultural behavior, ethnicity, race, biracialism, biculturalism, minority, ethnocentrism, and stereotyping.

Culture is a patterned behavioral response that develops over time through social and religious customs and intellectual and artistic activities. Culture is also a result of acquired mechanisms that may have innate influences but are primarily affected by internal and external environmental stimuli. It is shaped by values, beliefs, norms, and practices that are shared by members of the same cultural group. Culture guides our thinking, doing, and being and becomes patterned expressions of who we are. Patterned expressions of culture are passed down from one generation to the next. The term *culture* implies a dynamic, ever-changing, active or passive process.

Cultural values are unique, individual expressions of a particular culture that have been accepted as appropriate over time. They guide actions and decision making that facilitate self-worth and self-esteem.

Cultural behavior, or how a person acts in certain situations, is socially acquired, not genetically inherited. Patterns of cultural behaviors are learned through a process called enculturation or socialization. This process involves acquiring knowledge and internalizing values. Most people achieve competence in their own culture through enculturation. Children learn to behave culturally by watching adults and making inferences about the rules for behavior (Nolt, 1992).

Ethnicity is frequently, and perhaps incorrectly, used to mean race. The term *ethnicity* includes more than biological identification. Ethnicity in its broadest sense refers to groups whose members share a common social and cultural heritage that is passed on to successive generations. The most important characteristic of ethnicity is that members of an ethnic group feel a sense of identity.

The authors acknowledge the contribution of Dr. Rachel Spector to this chapter in the previous edition of this text.

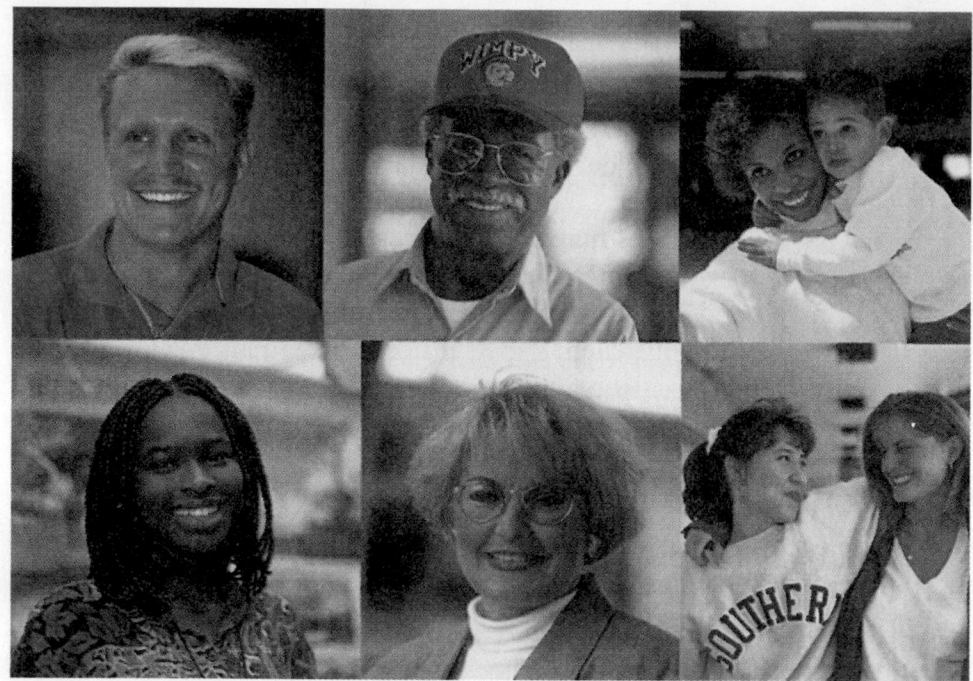

Figure 7-1   Ethnic and cultural diversity makes health care challenging and rewarding.
From Birchenall J: *Mosby's textbook for the home care aide,* St. Louis, 1997, Mosby.

The term *ethnic minority* is often used because it may be less offensive to people of color than other terms. **Ethnic minority** takes into account ethnicity, race, and the relative status of the groups of persons included in the category. Were it not for the use of the word *minority,* perhaps this terminology would be less culturally offensive to some groups of people (i.e., **ethnic people of color**). According to some sources, use of the term **people of color** might be the preferable option, particularly in situations where sensitivity to racial preferences needs to be heightened.

In contrast to the term *ethnicity* is the term **race,** which is related to biology. Members of a particular group share distinguishing physical features such as skin color, bone structure, or blood group. Ethnic and racial groups can and do overlap, because in many cases the biological and cultural similarities reinforce one another (Bullough and Bullough, 1982).

When an individual belongs to two racial groups, the individual is considered **biracial.** For the individual who is biracial, physical attributes such as skin color, the shape of the eyes, or hair may have a profound impact on acceptance by others. One problem associated with biracialism is the inability of the individual to identify with or find acceptance in either one of the biologically related racial and cultural groups (Giger and others, 1994). It is the total exclusion and sense of not belonging to either of the two particular racial groups that creates the dilemma. The term **bicultural** is used to describe a person who has two

cultures, lifestyles, and sets of values. When an individual is bicultural, conflicts may be created when attempts are made to adapt to the value systems inherent to both cultures. To be both biracial and bicultural may create psychological stress for some individuals.

A **minority** can consist of a particular racial, religious, or occupational group that constitutes less than a numerical majority of the population. Using this definition, it is obvious that all kinds of people can belong to various kinds of minorities. Often a group is designated as a minority because of its lack of power, assumed inferior traits, and/or supposedly undesirable characteristics. In any society, cultural groups can be arranged into a hierarchical power structure. Dominant groups are considered powerful, whereas minority groups are considered inferior and as lacking power. The term *minority* is not necessarily synonymous with numbers. For example, in the United States, females compose a larger numerical percentage (51%) than do males (49%) but are considered to be in the minority (U.S. Department of Commerce, Bureau of the Census, 1998).

It is not uncommon for people to look at the world from their own particular cultural viewpoint. In other words, people tend to view the world through **ethnocentrism** in the sense that they believe their way is best. Nurses must remember that their beliefs are not necessarily the best and that other people's ideas are not "ignorant" or "inferior." In addition, nurses must remember that the ideas of lay individuals may be valid for them and, more important, will influence their health care behavior and consequently their health status.

Stereotyping is the assumption that all people in a similar cultural, racial, or ethnic group are alike and share the same values and beliefs. An excellent example of stereotyping is an African-American nurse being assigned to care for an African-American client simply because of ethnicity and race. It is stereotypical when the assumption is that all African-Americans are alike and that therefore the African-American nurse is likely to be more sensitive to the needs of the African-American client. Race and ethnicity do not, in and of themselves, make us "resident experts" on the belief and value systems of other individuals.

Transcultural Nursing

Transcultural nursing is viewed as a culturally competent practice field that is client centered and research focused. Although transcultural nursing is viewed as client centered, it is important for nurses to remember that culture can and does influence how clients are viewed and the care they are given.

Every individual is culturally unique, and nurses are no exception. Therefore, nurses must use caution to avoid projecting their own cultural uniqueness and world views on the client if culturally appropriate care is to be provided. Nurses must carefully identify their own cultural beliefs and values and then separate them from the client's beliefs and values. To deliver culturally sensitive care, the nurse must remember that each individual is unique and a product of past experiences, beliefs, and values that have been learned and passed down from one generation to the next.

According to Stokes (1991), nursing as a profession is not "culturally free" but rather is "culturally determined." Nurses must recognize and understand this fact to avoid becoming grossly ethnocentric (Stokes, 1991). The more nurses know about their clients' cultural beliefs and values, the more culturally sensitive will be the care they provide. Nurses must continually assess and evaluate each client's responses and never assume that all individuals within a specific cultural group will think and behave in a similar manner. Nurses must remember that there is as much diversity within a cultural group as there is across cultural groups. The goal of transcultural nursing is to discover culturally relevant facts about the client that can be used to provide culturally appropriate and competent care. Although transcultural nursing is becoming a highly specialized field, every nurse who is entrusted with the care of clients must make every effort to deliver culturally sensitive care that is free of inherent biases based on gender, race, or religion.

As awareness of transcultural health care has increased, so has the use of the term **cultural competence.** There are many definitions for the term *cultural competence.* For the beginning nursing student, Giger and Davidhizar (1999) provide a clear, understandable definition. They view cultural competence as a dynamic, fluid, continuous process whereby an individual, system, or health care agency finds meaningful and useful care delivery strategies based on knowledge of the cultural heritage, beliefs, attitudes, and behaviors of those to whom they render care. To develop cultural competence, it is essential for the health care professional to use knowledge gained from conceptual and theoretical models of culturally appropriate care. The culturally competent nurse develops meaningful interventions to promote optimal health among individuals regardless of racial or ethnic group, gender or sexual identity, or cultural heritage.

To provide culturally appropriate and competent care, it is important to remember that each individual is culturally unique and as such is a product of past experiences, cultural beliefs, and cultural norms. Cultural expressions become patterned responses and give each individual a unique identity. Although there is as much diversity within cultural and racial groups as there is across and among cultural and racial groups, knowledge of general baseline data relative to the specific cultural or racial group is an excellent starting point for providing culturally appropriate care.

Culturally diverse health care can and should be rendered in all clinical settings. Knowledge of culturally relevant information will assist the nurse in planning and implementing a treatment regimen that meets the unique needs of each client.

Culturally Diverse Nursing Care

Culturally diverse nursing care refers to the variability in nursing approaches needed to provide culturally appropriate and competent care. As we move to the twenty-first century, it will be necessary for nurses to use transcultural knowledge in a skillful and artful manner to render culturally appropriate and competent care to a rapidly changing, heterogeneous client population. Culturally diverse nursing care must take into account six cultural phenomena that vary with application and use, yet are evident in all cultural groups: (1) communication, (2) space, (3) social organization, (4) time, (5) environmental control, and (6) biological variations. It is these elements that make up **Giger and Davidhizar's transcultural assessment model** (Figure 7-2).

In response to the need for a practical assessment tool for evaluating cultural variables and their effects on health and illness behaviors, a transcultural assessment model is offered that greatly minimizes the time needed to conduct a comprehensive assessment in an effort to provide culturally competent care. Before applying this model, the nurse must understand the concepts and assumptions that it is based on.

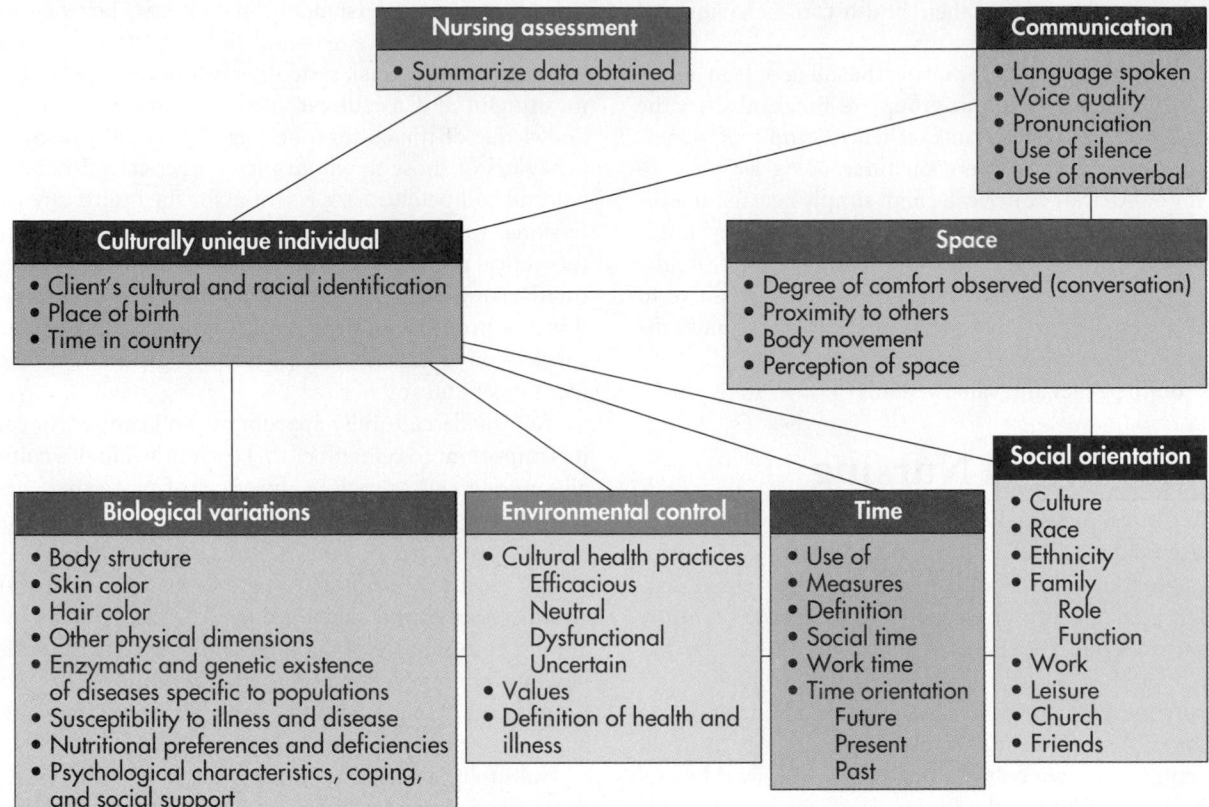

Figure 7-2 Giger and Davidhizar's transcultural assessment model.
From Giger JN, Davidhizar RE: *Transcultural nursing: assessment and intervention,* ed 3, St. Louis, 1999, Mosby.

COMMUNICATION

The word *communication* is derived from the verb *communicate* meaning "to make common, share, participate, or impart." **Communication,** however, goes further than this definition implies and embraces the entire realm of human interaction and behavior. All behavior, whether verbal or nonverbal, in the presence of another individual is communication (Watzlawich, Beavin, and Jackson, 1967; Haber, 1997). Communication provides the means by which people connect. It establishes a sense of commonality with others and permits the sharing of information, signals, or messages in the form of ideas and feelings.

Communication and culture are closely intertwined. Communication is the means by which culture is transmitted and preserved (Delgado, 1983). Culture influences how feelings are expressed and what verbal and nonverbal expressions are appropriate. Cultural patterns of communication are embedded early and are found in childrearing practices (Capirci and others, 1996). The communication practices of persons in individual cultural groups affect the expression of ideas and feelings, decision making, and communication strategies. The communication of an individual reflects, determines, and consequently molds the culture (Kretch, Crutchfield, and Ballachey, 1962; Hedlund, 1992).

In other words, a culture may be limited and molded by its communication practices.

Sensitivity to communication variances is needed to accurately assess and intervene in multicultural situations. The potential for misunderstanding the client is accentuated when the nurse and the client are from different ethnic, racial, and cultural groups. Although the most significant variations occur when two people speak different languages, difficulties can also be encountered when the nurse and client speak variations of English.

Whether the nurse relates to the client in an interview setting, during the process of client care, in a more informal level on the hospital unit, or in the clinic, the guidelines in Box 7-1 will increase the likelihood that the nurse-client relationship will be positive.

SPACE

Personal **space** is the area that surrounds a person's body. It includes the space and the objects within the space. Individuals tend to divide surrounding space into regions of front, back, right, and left. Physical distancing from others varies with the setting and is culturally learned. Generally, in Western culture there are three primary dimensions of space: the intimate zone (0 to 18 inches), the

Guidelines for Communicating With Culturally Diverse Clients   Box 7-1

- *Plan care based on the communicated needs and cultural background.* When care is being planned for persons from other cultures, it must be consistent with the lifestyle and unique needs of the client that have been communicated to the nurse and mutually agreed on (Geissler, 1991; Grossman, 1996). To establish an appropriate plan, it is essential for the nurse to learn about the customs and beliefs of the culture of the clients receiving care. The nurse should encourage the client to communicate cultural interpretations of health, illness, and health care. A client's perception of illness will affect not only communication, but also the care that is planned. Sensitivity to the uniqueness of each client is required if the nurse is to work effectively, particularly with clients from different cultures.

- *Modify communication approaches to meet cultural needs.* A factor that commonly interferes with care delivery to a person from another culture is confusion and fear concerning the treatment process. The fact that a non-English-speaking client is ill and receiving treatment can interfere with the client's normal ability to communicate. The nurse must be attentive to signs of anxiety and respond in a reassuring manner in keeping with the person's cultural orientation.

  Some cultures are primarily oral and do not rely on a written form of communication. In such cases the spoken word holds greater meaning and power. For example, Hmongs are considered an oral cultural group. For these individuals the formation of and acceptance in a social group is primarily dependent on the spoken word (Shadick, 1993). When interacting with individuals from an oral culture, the nurse must remember that if the teaching-learning process is to be effective, instruction must be oral.

- *Understand that respect for the client and communicated needs is central to the therapeutic relationship.* The need to communicate respect for the client is a nursing concept that crosses all cultural boundaries. Regardless of the language spoken or the cultural orientation, communication is increased and interpersonal distance is reduced by the nurse whose approach focuses on individuals and their emotional and physical needs. Communication of respect is central to a focus on emotional needs. Respect for clients is communicated by a kind and attentive approach whereby the nurse clearly listens to what the client says. Active listening techniques are used, such as encouraging clients to share thoughts and feelings by reflecting back what has been heard. The nurse should be attentive to how listening is communicated in the client's culture. For example, for some persons listening may be indicated by eye contact, whereas for others listening may mean having the listener turn a listening "ear." Predictions about what the client is trying to express may be made to encourage elaboration. At the heart of the task of hearing is the art of listening

(Martin, 1995). Listening communicates genuine interest and caring. The feeling of being heard is powerful, reducing distance and drawing people together into positive interpersonal interactions. An attitude of flexibility, respect, and interest can bridge barriers of distance imposed by culture and role.

- *Communicate in a nonthreatening manner.* The interview should be started in an unhurried manner with adherence to acceptable social and cultural amenities. It is usually wise to start with general social topics. During the information-gathering stage, general rather than specific questions should be asked. The interviewer should allow time for the respondent to give what appears to be unrelated information. In some cultures a direct approach appears rude and uncaring. For example, persons of European background and Hispanics often value "small talk" and will not relate optimally to the nurse who talks only about illness-related matters. Many persons, specifically Asians and Hispanics, respond better to a nondirective approach with open-ended questions than to direct questions and answers (Giger and Davidhizar, 1999).

  The appearance of being too busy, of not having time to listen, of not giving sufficient time for an answer, and of not really wanting to hear are equally effective in "cutting off" the client. Clients will be encouraged to talk by a nurse who "wants" to hear.

- *Use validating techniques in communication.* Although validating techniques are always important, they are especially important when the client is from a different culture. The nurse should be alert for feedback indicating that the client does not understand and should use restating and validating techniques, such as "Did I hear and understand you correctly?" When the nurse has difficulty understanding, it may help to find out precisely what the topic is (e.g., "Are you telling me where you're having pain?"). By determining the topic, the number of words can be decreased. If the message is not understood, it may be helpful to have the client try to convey the message in another way (e.g., through pointing or imitation). The nurse should never pretend to understand a message. People usually know when they are understood. By pretending, the nurse conveys to the client that the message is not important (Pore, 1995).

- *Adopt special approaches when the client speaks a different language.* A client who enters the health care system without being able to speak the same language as the caregivers enters a frightening and frustrating world. Without the availability of words, the nurse must relate to the client on an affective level. A tone and facial expression of caring can be pivotal in alleviating the client's fear. Locating an interpreter should be a priority when caring for these clients.

personal zone (18 inches to 3 feet), and the social or public zone (3 to 6 feet). The intimate zone may be used for comforting, protecting, and counseling and is reserved for people who are considered close. The personal zone usually is maintained with friends or in some counseling interactions. Touch can occur in the intimate and personal zones. The social zone is usually used when impersonal business is conducted or with people who are working together. Sensory involvement and communication are often less intense in the social zone. Wide variations of these general dimensions do occur and are often influenced by cultural background.

Although there are variations in spatial requirements from individual to individual, persons in the same cultural group tend to act similarly. For example, in Vietnam, families and extended families live comfortably in fairly small areas. As a result, families of this cultural group may find it necessary to remain close to their loved one and participate in the actual health care. Since individuals are usually not consciously aware of their personal space requirements, they frequently have difficulty understanding a different cultural pattern. It is important for the nurse to be aware of the effects of culture on the client's spatial needs and use sensitivity in responding to the client's need for personal space.

SOCIAL ORGANIZATION

Social organization refers to how a cultural group organizes itself around particular units, such as families, racial or ethnic groups, religious groups, and community or social groups. For members of some cultural groups, such as Chinese-Americans, Mexican-Americans, Vietnamese-Americans, and Puerto Rican-Americans, the family is the single most important unit of organization. In some cases family causes take on more significance than personal, cultural, or even national causes. Persons in some cultural groups tend to extend their families beyond normal bloodlines and thus have a large number of persons who they refer to as family.

Cultural behavior, or how one acts in certain situations, is socially acquired, not genetically inherited, and thus is usually learned in the family. Patterns of cultural behavior are important to the nurse because they provide explanations for behavior related to life events.

In most cultures, next to the family, religion is the second most important social organization. Some people may integrate religion and religious practices within their social activity. For example, Korean Christian churches provide a social anchor for Koreans in the community through youth groups and baby-sitting cooperatives, as well as traditional Christian practices. However, many persons, particularly those with strong religious convictions, tend to think of religion in an entirely different way. For some people, religion is seen in the context of a person's communion with a higher being, and religious experiences fall outside of ordinary experiences (see Chapter 28).

TIME

The concept of the passage of time is very familiar to most people regardless of cultural heritage. Cultural groups construct systems of time that measure social events and agricultural activities. Many cultures, especially Western industrialized cultures, use time to schedule future activities. It must be remembered that a sense of time is not innate but is developed early as a result of experiences linked to the individual's culture. Thus the sense of time results from learning and becomes a part of human nature. The Chinese-American cultural group's time orientation is linked to past events. Cultural groups such as Native Americans or Mexican-Americans may be oriented to present time. In contrast, the dominant American cultural group's time orientation is to the future.

ENVIRONMENTAL CONTROL

Environmental control refers to the ability of an individual from a particular cultural group to plan activities to coordinate with nature. Environmental control also refers to the individual's perception of his or her ability to control factors in the environment. This definition in itself implies that the concept of environment is broader than just the place where an individual resides or where treatment occurs. What a person believes about the causes of illness will affect his or her behavior in preventing and treating illness. These beliefs and practices are important and must be considered when caring for culturally diverse clients.

People and their environment have a reciprocal relationship. There is a continuous exchange between individuals and the environment. When the exchange is goal directed, the interaction is functional and useful. For example, a person's sleep-wake cycle is usually coordinated with sunlight and darkness. It is functional in that a cyclical period of rest occurs. However, if the exchange with the environment is chaotic and lacks goal direction, the interaction is no longer functional. For example, the person who experiences a long international flight may experience multiple time zone changes that alter the sleep-wake cycle. In this case the person experiences periods of irritability, fatigue, and decreased problem-solving abilities.

Perceptions of Health and Illness.   In the broadest sense, health may be viewed as a balance between the individual and the environment. Health practices such as eating nutritiously, subscribing to preventive health services available in the community, and installing hazard- and pollution-control devices are all believed to have a positive effect on the individual, who in turn can positively affect the environment (Spector, 1996).

How one experiences and copes with illness is based on the individual's explanation of sickness. Nurses must incorporate both personal and cultural reactions of the client to illness, disease, and discomfort to give culturally appropriate nursing care. Just as culture influences health-related behavior, it also has a profound effect on expectations and perceptions of sickness. Nurses must keep in mind the fact that perceptions of health and illness are shaped by cultural factors. As a direct result of cultural shaping, individuals vary in health care behaviors, health status, and health-seeking attitudes.

Cultural Health Practices.

Cultural health practices are categorized as efficacious (beneficial), neutral, dysfunctional, or uncertain. According to Western medical standards, efficacious cultural health practices are those practices that are viewed as beneficial to the client's health status, although they can differ vastly from modern scientific practices. Because efficacious health practices can promote effective nursing care, nurses need to actively encourage the use of these practices among and across cultural groups. For example, some Mexican-Americans may subscribe to the theory of "hot" and "cold." For example, headaches may have a causative agent that is believed to have a hot or cold quality not related to temperature. If the causative agent is believed to have a hot quality, then cold herbs may be placed on the person's head to absorb the heat (Giger and Davidizhar, 1999).

Neutral cultural health practices have no effect on the health status of an individual. Although some health care practitioners may consider neutral health practices irrelevant, the nurse must remember that such practices may be extremely important because they may be linked to beliefs that are closely integrated with an individual's behavior (Pillsbury, 1982). For example, Southeast Asian women believe that sitting in a door frame or on a step will complicate labor. Therefore when they are in waiting or examination rooms, these women will avoid sitting near a door (Giger and Davidizhar, 1999).

Dysfunctional cultural health practices are harmful. The nurse must be aware of practices that are dysfunctional and should work to establish educational training programs that will help individuals identify dysfunctional health practices and develop beneficial practices. For example, a Canadian study (Hilsop and others, 1992) noted that women of Canadian Native population did not participate in routine gynecological screening and that their mortality from cervical cancer was higher than in other groups. In this example the nurse needs to teach the client about the benefits of routine screening and assist the client in blending cultural beliefs with contemporary screening practices.

Uncertain health practices are those that have no proven effect. These include such things as swaddling a newborn infant to maintain body temperature and using an abdominal binder for the mother and infant to prevent umbilical hernias. However, these practices are based on tradition and provide comfort to the individuals who practice such activities.

The nurse should always identify the client's health practices and respect them. Unless these practices are harmful, they should be incorporated into the client's individualized plan of care. One of the most prevalent types of cultural health practices is folk medicine.

Folk Medicine.

Folk medicine is one of humankind's earliest uses of the natural environment and is the use of herbs, plants, minerals, and animal substances to prevent and treat illnesses. Folk medicine is practiced in a variety of countries and cultural groups. These remedies have been passed down from generation to generation. Many of the remedies are herbal, and the customs and rituals related to the use of herbs vary among cultural groups.

An individual's worldview largely determines beliefs about disease and the appropriate treatment interventions. For example, a belief in magic may lead to the assumption that a disease is a result of human behavior and that a cure can be achieved by magical techniques. A religious belief may lead to the assumption that disease is a result of supernatural forces and that a cure can be achieved by appealing to those forces.

Classification of Illness.

The folk medicine system classifies illnesses or diseases as natural or unnatural. This division is common among Haitians, persons from Trinidad, Mexicans and Mexican-Canadians, African-Canadians, and some southern white Americans (Snow, 1983). According to this belief system, natural events have to do with the world as God made it and intended it to be. Thus natural laws allow a measure of predictability for daily life. Unnatural events imply the exact opposite, because they upset the harmony of nature. Unnatural events can therefore be viewed as events that interrupt the plan intended by God and, at their very worst, represent the forces of evil and the machinations of the devil.

The classification of an illness affects the type of cure or practitioner sought. All illnesses can be viewed as representing disharmony and conflict in some particular area of life and thus tend to fall into two general categories: natural illnesses/environmental hazards and unnatural illnesses/divine punishment.

Natural illnesses in the folk medicine belief system are those that occur because of dangerous agents, such as cold air or impurities in the air, food, and water. Natural illnesses are based on the fact that everything in nature is connected and that events can be both interpreted and directed by an understanding of these relationships.

Unnatural illnesses are thought to occur because an individual has become so grave a sinner that God withdraws his favor. In fact, illnesses may be attributed to punishment for failure to abide by rules of proper behavior given to man by God (Gregory, 1988). The cause of unnatural illnesses, for those who subscribe to these beliefs, is based on the continual battle between the forces of good and evil as personified in God and the devil.

Comparison of Folk Medicine and Traditional Medicine.

To develop an understanding of folk medicine as a system, the system itself must be examined along with the ecological model, the Western medical system, alternative therapies, and religious systems. Every medical system is based on the philosophy of survival of the human organism. All medical systems have an adaptive nature. As such, the term *medical system* can be defined as the pattern of cultural traditions and social institutions that evolves from deliberate behavior to improve health status regardless of the outcome of a particular behavior (Dunn, 1975).

The ecological model is closely related to the folk medicine system. Ecology focuses on three areas: (1) biological, or the branch of biology that deals with the relationship between organisms and the environment; (2) social, or the relationship between people and institutions, and the interdependence between the two; and (3) cultural, or the relationship between culture and the environment, which also includes culture and societies in the environment. Ecological dimensions of health care can assist the nurse in providing plausible explanations as to why certain individuals contract specific diseases and why other individuals do not.

In contrast to the folk medicine system, which attempts to explain illness in terms of balances between individuals and the physical, social, and spiritual worlds, is the Western medical system of diagnoses and scientific explanations for illness. Western medical practices focus on preventive and curative medicine, whereas folk medicine practices focus on personal rather than scientific behavior. In the folk medicine system, it may make all the sense in the world to burn incense and to avoid certain individuals, cold air, and the "evil eye."

In alternative therapy the mind and the body are seen as a whole. Acupuncture, holistic healing, therapeutic touch, aromatic therapy, meditation, guided imagery, and a variety of other techniques prevail as viable alternative therapies (see Chapter 35). Practitioners of alternative therapies include homeopaths, naturopaths, massage therapists, and reflexologists (Cronsberry, 1996). These therapies continue to gain popularity.

Some religious groups have elaborate rules concerning health care behaviors, including such things as the giving and receiving of health care. Religious experiences are based on cultural beliefs and may include such things as blessings from spiritual leaders, apparitions of dead relatives, and even miracle cures. Healing power based on religion may also be found in animate, as well as inanimate, objects. Religion can and does dictate social, moral, and dietary practices that are designed to assist an individual in maintaining a healthy balance and that play a vital role in illness prevention. An example of a religious system is the Amish. For the Amish, religion and custom are inseparable and blend together as a way of life. Religious considerations determine the hours of work, one's occupation, the means and destination of travel, and one's choice of friends and mates. The Amish believe that the human body was created by God and should not be tampered

with. Some Amish believe that although medication may help, it is God who heals (Randall-David, 1989).

The nurse must keep in mind that regardless of a client's beliefs and practices, there is still safety in harmony and balance, and that there may be danger in anything that is done to the extreme. In other words, it is bad for the body to eat too much, drink too much, or stay out too late (Giger and Davidhizar, 1999).

BIOLOGICAL VARIATIONS

It is a well-known fact that people differ culturally. Less recognized and understood are the **biological variations** that exist among people in various racial groups. It is becoming more evident to nurses that a body of scientific knowledge does exist concerning biological differences. Information about biocultural differences is increasing in the literature, resulting in a field of study known as biocultural ecology. The purpose of biocultural ecology is to study the interactions among culture, human biology, and ecology/environment. Biocultural ecology studies diverse human populations by means of this three-way interaction system and focuses on specific, localized individuals and populations within a given environment. Data relative to all of the variables significant to people within a racial group are essential for complete understanding of the people. Not only are no two persons alike, but no two cultural or racial groups are alike, and all phenomena relative to both individuals and cultural or racial groups must be understood.

Nursing practice in the United States is primarily based on biological baselines of the white race. Because studies on biological baselines in growth and development, nutrition, and other biological phenomena have been conducted using primarily white subjects, standardized norms available to the nurse do not recognize biological variations existing among different racial groups. Therefore values uniracially normed are inappropriate when applied across racial groups. In the United States, white-standardized values for factors related to growth and development, nutrition, and susceptibility to disease are often applied to African-Americans, Asian-Americans, and Native Americans. Therefore significant deviations from the norm that may be labeled "nonnormal" might be more appropriately labeled "nonwhite" (Overfield, 1995). In fact, biological variations among racial groups are so diverse that multiple dimensions are encompassed.

Nurses continue to be challenged to integrate the cultural needs of their clients into the plan of care. Each cultural group has its own unique communication patterns, space and time orientation, social organization, perception of environmental control, and biological variations (Table 7-1). When cultural preferences are included within a plan of care, the client's ability to adhere to the prescribed therapies increases. As a result, there is blending of the client's cultural heritage, health care needs, and individualized therapies of care.

Table 7-1 Cross-Cultural Examples of Cultural Phenomena Affecting Nursing Care

Nations of Origin	Communication	Space	Time Orientation	Social Organization	Environmental Control	Biological Variations
Asian China Hawaii Philippines Korea Japan Southeast Asia (Laos, Cambodia, Vietnam)	National language preference Dialects, written characters Use of silence Nonverbal and contextual cuing	Noncontact people	Present	Family; hierarchical structure, loyalty Devotion to tradition Many religions, including Taoism, Buddhism, Islam, and Christianity Community social organizations	Traditional health and illness beliefs Use of traditional medicines Traditional practitioners: Chinese doctors and herbalists	Liver cancer Stomach cancer Coccidioidomycosis Hypertension Lactose intolerance
African West Coast (as slaves) Many African countries West Indian Islands Dominican Republic Haiti Jamaica	National languages Dialect, pidgin, creole, Spanish, and French	Close personal space	Present over future	Family, many female, single parents Large, extended family networks Strong church affiliation within community Community social organization	Traditional health and illness beliefs Folk medicine tradition Traditional healer: rootworker	Sickle cell anemia Hypertension Cancer of the esophagus Stomach cancer Coccidioidomycosis Lactose intolerance
Europe Germany England Italy Ireland Other European countries	National languages Many learn English immediately	Noncontact people Aloof Distant Southern countries: closer contact and touch	Future over present	Nuclear families Extended families Judeo-Christian religions Community social organizations	Primary reliance on modern health care system Traditional health and illness beliefs Some remaining folk medicine traditions	Breast cancer Heart disease Diabetes mellitus Thalassemia
Native American 500 Native American tribes Aleuts Eskimos	Tribal languages Use of silence and body language	Space very important and has no boundaries	Present	Extremely family oriented Biological and extended families Children taught to respect traditions Community social organizations	Traditional health and illness beliefs Folk medicine tradition Traditional healer: medicine man	Accidents Heart disease Cirrhosis of the liver Diabetes mellitus
Hispanic countries Spain Cuba Mexico Central and South America	Spanish or Portuguese primary language	Tactile relationships Touch Handshakes Embracing Value physical presence	Present	Nuclear family Extended families *Compadrazzo:* godparents Community social organizations	Traditional health and illness beliefs Folk medicine tradition Traditional healers: *curandero, espiritista, partera, señora*	Diabetes mellitus Parasites Coccidioidomycosis Lactose intolerance

Compiled by Rachel Spector, RN, PhD.

Application of Giger and Davidhizar's Transcultural Assessment Model

Giger and Davidhizar's transcultural assessment model (See Figure 7-2), introduced earlier, provides a method for the nurse to identify the client's unique health care needs, which include cultural health practices. The assessment model in Box 7-2 expands the model and provides details that will be helpful when assessing an individual client. The following discussion shows how the variations can be seen in several cultural groups. It should be kept in mind that these discussions are general in nature and that each client must be assessed as an individual.

AFRICAN-AMERICANS

According to the U.S. Census Bureau, in 1998 there were approximately 34,333,000 African-Americans residing in the United States, representing approximately 12.7% of the American population (U.S. Department of Commerce, Bureau of the Census, 1998). Although African-Americans live throughout the United States, the states with the greatest number of African-Americans are New York, California, Texas, Florida, and Georgia.

Some of the health problems noted particularly in African-Americans are thought to be a result of varying genetic pools and hereditary immunity. However, many of these problems have been found to be more closely associated with economic status than with race. Three intervening and reinforcing variables include poverty, discrimination, and social and psychological barriers. These variables are thought to be so profound in their effect on some African-Americans that they tend to keep these individuals from using the health care services that are available. These variables may also explain why morbidity and mortality rates are higher among African-Americans than among the rest of the general population. Although underrepresented in the general population, African-Americans remain overrepresented in the health statistics for life-threatening illness.

The life expectancy for African-Americans continues to lag behind that for whites. The life expectancy for African-Americans is 71.0 years, compared with 76.4 years for whites (U.S. Department of Commerce, Bureau of the Census, 1993c). African-Americans continue to have a higher infant mortality (11.2 per 1000 live births in 1993) than white Americans (9.4 per 1000 live births in 1993) (National Center for Health Statistics, 1993, 1998). In 1997 the rate of deaths for African-American males was 55% higher for heart disease, 26% higher for cancer, 180% higher for stroke, and 100% higher for lung disease than for the rest of the general U.S. population (National Center for Health Statistics, 1998).

Communication. The communication patterns of some African-Americans are unique in dialect and language usage. The dialect that is spoken by some African-Americans is substantially different from Standard English in pronunciation, grammar, and syntax. Some may refer to this dialect as "black English" (Giger and Davidhizar, 1999). Black English, as it spoken today, is a combination of various African languages with the languages of other cultural groups such as the Dutch, the French, and the English. Historically, it is thought that the first African-Americans in this country had a need for a common language. This common language ultimately led to a restructuring of grammar of all language, including English.

The use of Standard English versus black English varies among African-Americans and in some instances may be related to educational level and socioeconomic status, although this is not always the case. The use of black English has served as a unifying factor for African-Americans in maintaining their cultural and ethnic identity. It is not uncommon for some African-Americans to speak Standard English when serving in a professional capacity or when socializing with whites and then revert back to black English when interacting in an all–African-American setting. Some African-Americans who have not mastered Standard English may feel insecure in certain situations where they are required and expected to use Standard English. When confronted with such situations, they may become very quiet.

Space.   The nurse who works with African-Americans may feel somewhat uncomfortable because these cultures generally dictate a much closer personal space (Sue, 1981). Within a home setting, African-Americans may have multiple families residing together. The activities that occur in the space generally involve many members of the family. Therefore when providing care in the home, the nurse must remember that activities of other household members need to be assessed as well.

Social Organization.   Historically, because of legalized segregation, African-Americans were separated or isolated from the mainstream of society. Even today, African-Americans may maintain separate and sometimes unequal lifestyles as compared with other Americans. Evidence of the failure to assimilate on the part of many African-Americans is seen in the existence of predominantly African-American neighborhoods, churches, colleges and universities, and public elementary and high schools.

Characteristics of the Family System.   In 1998, 46.0% of African-Americans families were matrifocal (female headed with no husband present), as compared with 13.0% of white families (U.S. Department of Commerce, Bureau of the Census, 1998). Even when there is a man present in the home, African-American families are oriented around women. This has implications for the nurse because, within the African-American family structure, the wife and/or mother is often charged with the respon-

CULTURALLY UNIQUE INDIVIDUAL

1. Place of birth
2. Cultural definition
   What is . . .
3. Race
   What is . . .
4. Length of time in country (if appropriate)

COMMUNICATION

1. Voice quality
   A. Strong, resonant
   B. Soft
   C. Average
   D. Shrill
2. Pronunciation and enunciation
   A. Clear
   B. Slurred
   C. Dialect (geographical)
3. Use of silence
   A. Infrequent
   B. Often
   C. Length
      (1) Brief
      (2) Moderate
      (3) Long
      (4) Not observed
4. Use of nonverbal
   A. Hand movement
   B. Eye movement
   C. Entire body movement
   D. Kinesics (gestures, expression, or stances)
5. Touch
   A. Startles or withdraws when touched
   B. Accepts touch without difficulty
   C. Touches others without difficulty
6. Ask these and similar questions:
   A. How do you get your point across to others?
   B. Do you like communicating with friends, family, and acquaintances?
   C. When asked a question, do you usually respond (in words or body movement, or both)?
   D. If you have something important to discuss with your family, how would you approach them?

SPACE

1. Degree of comfort
   A. Moves when space invaded
   B. Does not move when space invaded
2. Distance in conversations
   A. 0 to 18 inches
   B. 18 inches to 3 feet
   C. 3 feet or more
3. Definition of space
   A. Describe degree of comfort with closeness when talking with or standing near others
   B. How do objects (e.g., furniture) in the environment affect your sense of space?
4. Ask these and similar questions:
   A. When you talk with family members, how close do you stand?
   B. When you communicate with co-workers and other acquaintances, how close do you stand?
   C. If a stranger touches you, how do you react or feel?
   D. If a loved one touches you, how do you react or feel?
   E. Are you comfortable with the distance between us now?

SOCIAL ORGANIZATION

1. Normal state of health
   A. Poor
   B. Fair
   C. Good
   D. Excellent
2. Marital status
3. Number of children
4. Parents living or deceased?
5. Ask these and similar questions:
   A. How do you define social activities?
   B. What are some activities that you enjoy?
   C. What are your hobbies, or what do you do when you have free time?
   D. Do you believe in a Supreme Being?
   E. How do you worship that Supreme Being?
   F. What is your function (what do you do) in your family unit/system?
   G. What is your role in your family unit/system (father, mother, child, advisor)?
   H. When you were a child, what or who influenced you the most?
   I. What is/was your relationship with your siblings and parents?
   J. What does work mean to you?
   K. Describe your past, present, and future jobs
   L. What are your political views?
   M. How have your political views influenced your attitude toward health and illness?

TIME

1. Orientation to time
   A. Past oriented
   B. Present oriented
   C. Future oriented
2. View of time
   A. Social time
   B. Clock oriented
3. Physiochemical reaction to time
   A. Sleeps at least 8 hours a night
   B. Goes to sleep and wakes on a consistent schedule
   C. Understands the importance of taking medication and other treatments on schedule
4. Ask these and similar questions:
   A. What kind of timepiece do you wear daily?
   B. If you have an appointment at 2 PM, what time is acceptable to arrive?
   C. If a nurse tells you that you will receive a medication in "about a half hour," realistically, how much time will you allow before calling the nurses' station?

From Giger JN, Davidhizar RE: *Transcultural nursing: assessment and intervention*, ed 3, St. Louis, 1999, Mosby.

Continued

Giger and Davidhizar's Transcultural Assessment Model—cont'd   Box 7-2

ENVIRONMENTAL CONTROL

1. Locus of control
   A. Internal locus of control (believes that the power to effect change lies within)
   B. External locus of control (believes that fate, luck, and chance have a great deal to do with how things turn out)
2. Value orientation
   A. Believes in supernatural forces
   B. Relies on magic, witchcraft, and prayer to effect change
   C. Does not believe in supernatural forces
   D. Does not rely on magic, witchcraft, or prayer to effect change
3. Ask these and similar questions
   A. How often do you have visitors at your home?
   B. Is it acceptable to you for visitors to drop in unexpectedly?
   C. Name some ways your parents or other persons treated your illnesses when you were a child.
   D. Have you or someone else in your immediate surroundings ever used a home remedy that made you sick?
   E. What home remedies have you used that worked? Will you use them in the future?
   F. What is your definition of "good health"?
   G. What is your definition of illness or "poor health"?

BIOLOGICAL VARIATIONS

1. Conduct a complete physical assessment noting:
   A. Body structure (small, medium, or large frame)
   B. Skin color
   C. Unusual skin discolorations
   D. Hair color and distribution
   E. Other visible physical characteristics (e.g., keloids, chloasma)
   F. Weight
   G. Height
   H. Check lab for variances in hemoglobin, hematocrit, and sickle cell phenomena if black or Mediterranean
2. Ask these and similar questions:
   A. What diseases or illnesses are common in your family?
   B. Has anyone in your family been told that there is a possible genetic susceptibility for a particular disease?
   C. Describe your family's typical behavior when a family member is ill?
   D. How do you respond when you are angry?
   E. Who (or what) usually helps you to cope during a difficult time?

   F. What foods do you and your family like to eat?
   G. Have you ever had any unusual cravings for:
      (1) White or red clay dirt?
      (2) Laundry starch?
   H. When you were a child, what types of foods did you eat?
   I. What foods are family favorites or are considered traditional?

NURSING ASSESSMENT

1. Note whether the client has become culturally assimilated or observes own cultural practices.
2. Incorporate data into plan of nursing care:
   A. Encourage the client to discuss cultural differences; people from diverse cultures who hold different worldviews can enlighten nurses.
   B. Make efforts to accept and understand methods of communication.
   C. Respect the individual's personal need for space.
   D. Respect the rights of clients to honor and worship the Supreme Being of their choice.
   E. Identify a clerical or spiritual person to contact.
   F. Determine whether spiritual practices have implications for health, life, and well-being (e.g., Jehovah's Witnesses may refuse blood and blood derivatives; an Orthodox Jew may eat only kosher food high in sodium and may not drink milk when meat is served).
   G. Identify hobbies, especially when devising interventions for a short or extended convalescence or for rehabilitation.
   H. Honor time and value orientations and differences in these areas. Allay anxiety and apprehension if adherence to time is necessary.
   I. Provide privacy according to personal need and health status of the client (NOTE: the perception of and reaction to pain may be culturally related).
   J. Note cultural health practices.
      (1) Identify and encourage efficacious practices.
      (2) Identify and discourage dysfunctional practices.
      (3) Identify and determine whether neutral practices will have a long-term ill effect.
   K. Note food preferences.
      (1) Make as many adjustments in diet as health status and long-term benefits will allow and that dietary department can provide.
      (2) Note dietary practices that may have serious implications for the client.

sibility for protecting the health of the family members. The African-American woman is expected to assist each family member in maintaining good health and in determining treatment if a family member is ill.

Some African-American families are composed of large networks and tend to be very supportive during times of crisis and illness. Large-network groups can have both positive and negative effects on wellness, illness, and recovery behaviors. Nonetheless, the nurse should include all of the members in the network in the planning and implementation of health care.

Time.   In African-Americans, just as in individuals from other cultural groups, the perception of time varies according to social and cultural factors. Some African-Americans who have become assimilated into the dominant culture are very time conscious and take pride in punctuality. These individuals are likely to be future oriented and believe that saving and planning are important. (Poussaint and Atkinson, 1970). On the other hand, some African-Americans react primarily to the present situation and are not future oriented. Such individuals are not likely to value time. Thus they do not value the concept of punctuality and may not keep appointments or may arrive much later than the scheduled time. It is the belief of some African-Americans that time is flexible and that events will begin when they arrive. This belief has been translated down through the years to imply an acceptable lateness among some African-Americans of 30 minutes to an hour.

Environmental Control.   African-Americans in the United States are a highly heterogeneous group; thus it is impossible to make a blanket statement about their health care beliefs and practices. Many health care beliefs that are exhibited by African-Americans in the United States are derived from their African ancestry. For example, in West Africa, where a vast majority of African-Americans originated, man was perceived as a being from which the body and soul could not be separated (Smith, 1976). Man was also perceived as a holistic individual with many complex dimensions. Religion was interwoven into health care beliefs and practices. (West Africans continue even today to believe that illness is a natural occurrence resulting from disharmony and conflict in some area of the individual's life.) Since life was centered around the entire family, illness was perceived as a collective event and subsequently a disruption of the entire family system. The traditional West African healers always involved the individual's entire family in the healing process, even when the disorder was thought to be somatic in origin. Thus the traditional West African healer based treatment on the premise of wholeness, the necessity for reincorporation of the client into the family system, and involvement of the entire family system in the care and treatment of the individual (Smith, 1976).

Cultural Health Practices.   Some African-Americans who were reared in the rural South were treated by folk practitioners and may not have encountered a physician until they reached adulthood. Therefore these people are more likely to turn to a neighborhood folk practitioner when they become ill. Folk medicine is still used within the African-American community, perhaps because of humiliation encountered in the mainstream health care system, lack of money, and lack of trust in health care workers. Today, some African-Americans go to physicians primarily to get medications that require a prescription, not because they believe the physician is superior in knowledge or training.

In the African-American culture, illness is often attributed to demons and evil spirits. Some may perceive illness as either a natural or an unnatural occurrence. The illness is classified as natural because of unprotected exposure to a natural element, such as exposure to a cold virus. Unnatural illnesses are those perceived as a punishment from God or the work of the devil (Giger and Davidhizar, 1999). In some families the diagnosis of cancer may be perceived as a punishment from God for past behavior.

Traditional principles regarding the cause and prevention of illness may not be part of the cultural beliefs of some African-American clients. Cultural beliefs about prevention of an illness may focus on avoiding people believed to carry evil spirits. Prayer and a well-balanced diet are considered helpful.

Biological Variations.   Several categories of diseases occur with higher incidence in the African-American population. The illnesses highlighted in this section include human immunodeficiency virus (HIV) infection, hypertension, cardiovascular disease, sickle cell anemia, and alcoholism.

Human Immunodeficiency Virus Infection.   Since the first reported case of acquired immunodeficiency syndrome (AIDS) in 1981, HIV/AIDS has become a major cause of morbidity and mortality among African-Americans. Ward and Duchin (1998) reported that, for the first time, the number of African-Americans with the diagnosis of AIDS was approximately equal to the number of reported cases in whites. In fact, these researchers noted that the death rate from AIDS was 4 times greater for African-American men (178.0 per 100,00) than for white men (138.0 per 100,000). African-American women fared even worse, with a death rate 9 times greater than that for white women, (53,000 per 100,000, compared with 6 per 100,000 for white women) (Ward and Duchin, 1998).

Hypertension.   The incidence of hypertension is significantly higher in African-Americans. The onset of hypertension occurs at an earlier age, and the elevation in blood pressure is more severe and associated with a higher mortality, especially in cardiovascular diseases. The Joint National Committee (1997) concluded that the prevalence of hypertension increases with age at a greater rate for African-Americans than for whites. In addition, the prevalence is greater in African-American men in the young adult and middle years. In later years hypertension is equally distributed among African-American men and women.

Cardiovascular Disease.   Cardiovascular disease remains the leading cause of morbidity and mortality in the United States for all demographic groups. The major causes of death due to cardiovascular disease are myocardial infarction and cerebrovascular accident, which is the third leading cause of all deaths (National Health Statistics, 1998). Liao and Cooper (1995) noted that for the first time since the category of coronary heart disease was recorded in vital statistics, the age-adjusted mortality rate for myocardial infarction in black men exceeded that of whites. Data from the 1997 Heart and Stroke Statistics Update indicated that the age-adjusted death rate from myocardial infarction was highest among African-American men and women (267.9% and 190.3% per 100,000, compared with 165.3% and 99.2% per 100,000 for white men and women). According to Woods (1998), African-American women tend to develop coronary heart disease much earlier than white women. In addition, the death rate for African-American women under age 55 is twice that of white women. Until age 75 the mortality from coronary heart disease is higher in African-American women than in women of other racial backgrounds (Woods, 1998).

Sickle Cell Anemia.   Sickle cell anemia is the most common genetic disorder in the United States. This illness predominantly affects African-Americans. This is a chronic, incurable disorder that includes symptoms of chronic anemia and fatigue, and in acute crises hospitalization is required to manage joint pain, thrombosis, and fever. One problem frequently associated with this disorder is substance abuse. People with sickle cell anemia are at greater risk for substance abuse to gain control of the joint pain.

Alcoholism.   Alcoholism is one of the biggest health problems in the African-American community, contributing to reduced longevity. There are high incidences of acute and chronic alcohol-related diseases among African-Americans, such as alcoholic fatty liver; hepatitis; cirrhosis of the liver; heart disease; cancers of the mouth, larynx, tongue, esophagus, and lung; and unintentional injuries and homicide (Ronan, 1987).

Several causes of alcohol abuse and misuse in African-Americans have been identified in the literature. A primary factor is economics. Many African-American men drink as a result of unemployment, which leads to depression and frustration because of the inability to meet financial commitments. Williams (1986) concluded that unemployment is correlated with a high risk for alcohol problems among African-Americans. Availability is also a factor.

Research suggests that several areas must be addressed to increase the likelihood of successful treatment outcomes. The first step is to get the African-American alcoholic client into a treatment program. Programs that are located within the community and that are accessible to public transportation are more likely to be used, except by the upwardly mobile African-American, who is more likely to seek private services outside the community. The African-American church can, and in some instances does, serve a dual role in this first step because it can provide a facility and, at the same time, act as a referral source.

Implications for Nursing Practice.   Because some African-Americans may believe that good health is equated with one's ability to read the signs of nature or being in "God's good graces," education and spiritual support may be important interventions. The nurse may want to educate the client and family on causation of illness within the context of the client's cultural beliefs. In addition, the client's religious community can play an integral role in health promotion and health care. Some client's may even equate the wearing of specific jewelry with frightening away evil spirits; as a result, the jewelry may become an important intervention in maintaining and restoring health.

HISPANICS

In 1998 there were 28,438,000 Hispanics residing in the United States (U.S. Department of Commerce, Bureau of the Census, 1998). Of the number of Hispanics residing in this country, approximately 63% are Mexican, 10% are Puerto Rican, 3% are Cuban, and 24% are of other Latin American origin. Hispanics are the fastest-growing group of people in the United States today and are expected to become the largest ethnic minority group in the United States within the first decade of the twenty-first century. Between 1980 and 1990 the number of Hispanics residing in the United States grew by 53% (U.S. Department of Commerce, Bureau of the Census, 1993a). This tremendous growth is related to higher birth rates than in the rest of the general population and a substantial influx of immigrants from Mexico, Central America, and South America (U.S. Department of Commerce, Bureau of the Census, 1993b). Projections indicate that the Hispanic population will double its current size by the year 2020 and triple its current size by 2050 (U.S. Department of Commerce, Bureau of the Census, 1993e).

A major issue for some Hispanics is lack of citizenship. Many Mexican-Americans gain entry into the United States by simply walking across the border. The lack of citizenship is a barrier to gaining education, skills, stable jobs, decent living conditions, and government benefits. Preoccupation with possible discovery and deportation for illegal aliens is related to the symptoms of posttraumatic stress disorder (Cervantes, Synder, and Padilla, 1989).

The plight of the illegal alien has expanded since enactment of the Immigration and Reform and Control Act of 1986. In an attempt to control illegal immigration into the United States, employers are now required to verify citizenship status within 24 hours after hiring an employee. Sanctions are being placed against employers who fail to meet this requirement or who hire illegal aliens knowingly. Noncitizens who apply for federal public assistance funds must verify that they are not undocumented aliens.

Communication.

Because many Hispanics rely on Spanish to communicate with other people, it is often very frightening for them to participate in the American health care system. It is also frustrating for the nurses giving them care. The nurse who works with bilingual Hispanics must remember that often, under stress, these clients may revert to their first language, Spanish. Family members may provide invaluable assistance both in reducing stress and in translating the client's needs. The Spanish language is spoken in many dialects; Hispanics may speak 1 of more than 50 dialects.

Some Hispanics are tactile in their relationships. The degree and extent of tactility depends on the country of origin. When being interviewed, some Hispanics may engage in "small talk" before approaching the business of the interview. Verbal expression is more likely to be elaborate and indirect, whereas confrontation and arguments are thought to be rude and disrespectful. Self-disclosure is reserved for those who are known well. Kidding is seen as rude, deprecating, and offensive and is likely to generate a negative response.

Eye contact has special importance to some Hispanics, such as Mexican-Americans, especially when children are involved. *Mal ojo* ("evil eye") is a folk illness that affects infants and children (Dorsey and Jackson, 1976). This condition is believed to occur when an individual who possessed special powers stares at a child without touching the child (Foster, 1978). It is believed that the only way to break the spell is for the individual who has given the "evil eye" to touch the child.

Space.

Some Hispanics value physical presence, including the presence of family members. It is important for some Hispanics to see relatives face to face, to embrace, to touch, and to just be with each other. Hispanics as a group demonstrate a great need for group togetherness. This pattern of togetherness begins with the parent-child relationship and continues into adulthood. It is important for the nurse to have the client's family present whenever possible.

Social Organization.

The foundation of most Hispanic communities is the nuclear family (parents and children). The nuclear family is a priority. For members of some groups, such as Mexican-Americans, Puerto Rican–Americans, and Cuban-Americans, this priority may restrict relocation by sustaining emotional attachment to people, places, and things. In the Hispanic culture, this attachment to family can also cause resistance to changes of all kinds.

For many Hispanics, extended family relationships have special significance, and the family is perhaps the most significant social organization (Murrillo, 1978). The major dominating theme of the traditional Hispanic family is the need for collective achievement of the family as a group. Thus family collective and other family needs supersede the needs of individual members. Also, any dishonor or shame that an individual member experiences is considered a reflection on the entire family. The Hispanic family takes pride in family endeavors and generally does not seek help from outsiders to solve problems or meet needs. Many Hispanic families place a great deal of value on having many relatives live nearby. The local extended family is tightly integrated, has frequent face-to-face encounters, and provides one another with mutual aid.

Within the Hispanic family the father has the dominant role, assuming responsibility for being head of the house and the decision maker. For the male family member there is a strong sense of machismo that is not compatible with the loss of self-esteem or authority. The wife or mother of the family has the primary role of keeping the family cohesive. Although the mother may influence family decisions, she does not have a dominant role in the family.

Roman Catholicism is the prominent religion practiced by many Hispanics. Common religious practices are baptism, confirmation, communion, weddings, and funerals. During times of crisis, some Hispanics may rely on the priest and family for prayers. When a family member is ill, rituals that are practiced include promise making, offering candles, visiting shrines, and offering prayers. Illness and death are considered as "God's will." Grief behaviors tend to be demonstrative (Lawson, 1990).

Time.

Hispanics are usually characterized as having a present time orientation and of being unable or reluctant to incorporate the future into their plans. For example, the Mexican custom of the siesta in some ways represents the belief that rest (or the present) has a priority over work.

It is important for the nurse to remember that personal ethnocentric attitudes toward time may negatively affect the planning of care for clients with a different time orientation. Some Hispanics may be late for an appointment not because of reluctance or lack of respect, but because they are more concerned with a current activity than with planning ahead to be on time. Perceptions and understanding of acute and chronic illness may also be affected.

For example, some Hispanics may first seek out the most accessible and affordable care, which may be with a folk healing practitioner.

Environmental Control.   Some Hispanics are more likely to believe in an external locus of control than are persons in the dominant culture. This belief that the outcome of circumstances is controlled by external forces is conveyed socially. Some Hispanics perceive life as being under the constant influence of the divine will. There is also a fatalistic belief that one is at the mercy of the environment and has little control over what happens. Associated with this view is the belief that personal efforts are unlikely to influence the outcome of a situation; thus some Hispanics do not believe that they are personally responsible for present or future successes or failures. This belief in an external locus of control may precipitate feelings of hopelessness regarding the future and positive change.

Cultural Health Practices.   An external locus of control influences the way in which an individual views health. Some individuals may believe that health is a result of good luck or a reward from God for good behavior. For some Hispanics, health is a state of equilibrium in the universe wherein the forces of "hot," "cold," "wet," and "dry" must be balanced. This concept is thought to have originated with the early Hippocratic theory of health and the four humors. According to the Hippocratic theory, the body humors—blood, phlegm, black bile, and yellow bile—vary in both temperature and moisture. Persons who subscribe to this theory believe that health exists only when these four humors are in balance. Thus health can be maintained by diet and other practices that keep the four humors in balance. Illness, on the other hand, is believed to be misfortune or bad luck, a punishment from God for evil thoughts or actions, or a result of the imbalance of hot and cold or wet and dry.

The concept of balance dominates much of the Hispanic worldview regarding the cause and treatment of illness. Good health infers that one is in proper balance with God, as well as with the family, fellow men, and the church. Illness is often believed to be a result of an imbalance in the social or spiritual aspects of life.

Folk Medicine.   Operating within the *curanderismo* folklore system of beliefs and practices are several levels of healers. The first healer sought out is a member of the family; if the case is or becomes more complicated, healers within the community are sought. The family member healer is generally female and is respected for her knowledge of folk medicine. This individual may be a wife/mother, grandmother, or revered older adult relative. The healing practices are passed down in the family from mother to daughter. If the client does not improve, there is usually an intermediary person who directs the client to the *jerbero* or *curandero*.

The *jerbero* is a folk healer who specializes in using herbs and spices for preventive and curative purposes. This person grows and distributes herbs and spices and explains how to use them effectively (Richardson, 1982).

The more serious physical and mental/emotional illnesses are brought to the *curandero* (male folk healer) or *curandera* (female folk healer). The *curandero* perceives life as being under the consistent influence of the divine will. People are born as sinners, with death being a result of their sins. The central focus of these healers' treatment is relieving clients of their sins. Suffering is seen as a component of illness, and death is seen as failure to be cured of sin (Ruiz, 1985).

Brujos/brujas (witches) may not be sought out until other forms of healing have been tried. The practitioners of witchcraft use several kinds of magic. Black magic is practiced by both male witches (*brujos*) and female witches (*brujas*), and red magic and green magic are thought to empower a witch to solve love problems by assuming an animal form (Wanderer and Rivera, 1986).

Biological Variations.   Several categories of diseases occur with high incidence in Hispanics. The following section highlights the impact of diabetes mellitus, hypertension, heart disease, communicable diseases, obesity, and HIV infection in this cultural group.

Diabetes Mellitus.   In Mexican-Americans not only is the incidence of diabetes 5 times the national average, but complications are also more frequent (Reinert, 1986). Hispanics suffer primarily from type 2 (adult-onset) diabetes, with diabetes ranking as the third-leading cause of death for Hispanic women between the ages of 45 and 74 (Vasquez, 1997).

Hypertension.   Hypertension is also found with increased prevalence among Hispanics (National Center for Health Statistics, 1993). Pernicious anemia, most often seen in older adults, has been shown to occur in those of Latin America origin at a younger age than in white clients (Carmel, Johnson, and Weiner, 1987).

Cardiovascular Disease.   Hispanics in the San Antonio Heart Study were found to be less knowledgeable than non-Hispanic whites about preventing heart attacks and not engaging in risk-reducing behaviors (Hazuda and others, 1983). Derenowski (1990) noted that cardiovascular risk reduction and changes in lifestyle are necessary components of education for some Mexican-Americans. In providing this education, however, the nurse must remember to address cultural differences such as health values, ethnic care practices, family life patterns, and dietary practices. The whole family should be committed to developing and sustaining the lifestyle changes if they are to be successful.

Communicable Diseases.   It is essential for the nurse working with Hispanics to realize that approximately 85% of the health problems common to Hispanics involve communicable diseases (National Center for Health Statistics, 1993, 1998). These include respiratory tract infections, diarrhea, skin disorders, nutritional problems (particularly during the first year of life), macroscopic parasitosis, and amebiasis. In the United States the population group that is most at risk for the incidence and transmittal of tuberculosis includes newly arrived immigrants, including Mexicans (Hood and Jackson, 1989; Phipps, 1997). Since there is a high prevalence of tuberculosis in Mexico, it is thought that Mexican-Americans may have a higher predisposition for tuberculosis than other Americans.

Hepatitis C has also been found to occur at a higher rate among Hispanics. It is estimated that more people could die from the complications of hepatitis C than from AIDS (Cronin, 1997). Some 70% of cases result in liver damage that leads to death. Once hepatitis C is diagnosed, lifestyle changes such as avoiding alcohol can prolong the length and quality of life for persons with this disease.

Obesity.   There is a growing incidence of childhood obesity noted among Hispanics, particularly among Mexican-Americans. Alexander and Blank (1988) suggest that the increasing incidence of obesity in Mexican-American children may be a result of mothers believing that a fat baby is a healthy baby. The mothers in this study had a greater body mass index than did mothers in a control group. These subjects also had "pushier" feeding practices with their children. To prevent the complications of adult obesity stemming from childhood obesity, nurses should identify mothers and their children who are at risk for obesity and encourage a weight reduction program.

Human Immunodeficiency Virus Infection.
Nationwide cases of HIV infection among Hispanics are occurring at triple the rate among non-Hispanics (Caudle, 1993). Because of the unsanitary working and housing conditions of migrant farm workers and limited opportunity to protect themselves, the opportunity for higher risk for HIV infection exists. A study of farm workers in Florida found the rate of HIV infection to be 5%, 10 times higher than in the general population (HIV Surveillance Report, 1997). In a study of 587 subjects interviewed in Harris County, Texas, community health centers, only 58% of Hispanics indicated that they understood that the use of condoms during sexual intercourse decreased the risk of contracting AIDS (Aruffo, Coverdale, and Vallbona, 1991).

Implications for Nursing Practice.   In addition to cultural differences, English may be a second language for Mexican-American clients. For some clients, Spanish is their only language, and it is very frightening to not understand English or to have to rely on others for communication. It is important that the nurse establish methods for communication early in the caregiving situation. These communication interventions must meet the client's and health care provider's needs simultaneously, they must be reliable, and they must be understood by all.

Because some Mexican-American clients may rely on folk and alternative therapies, the nurse should recognize the importance of folk medicine practices mentioned earlier. Mexican-American clients also need to be encouraged to practice their religious beliefs and receive support from members of their religious community. Acknowledging the client's reliance on folk health practices, as well as religious beliefs, will promote a more individualized plan of care.

ASIAN-AMERICANS

In 1998 there were 10,071,000 persons of Asian descent residing in the United States (U.S. Department of Commerce, Bureau of the Census, 1998). Of the number of Asian-Americans residing in this country, 16% are Chinese, 13% are Filipino, 10% are Japanese, 9% are Asian Indian, 7% are Korean, and the remaining 45% are from all other Asian groups (World Almanac, 1997; Information Please Almanac, 1998). Pacific Islanders are not included in these data.

Communication.   There is no single unifying language among Asian-Americans other than English. Since Asian-Americans come from a number of Asian countries, many languages are spoken, including Japanese, Mandarin, Korean, and Hmong. Of the number of Asian-Americans residing in this country, 65.2% speak Asian or a Pacific Islander language at home and 56% do not speak English well (U.S. Department of Commerce, Bureau of the Census, 1993d).

Although most Asian-Americans are from countries that have for hundreds of centuries had both a written and spoken form of language, some are not. For example, Hmongs are primarily an oral cultural group. Some Hmongs have never learned to read Hmong or any other language (Shadick, 1993).

What are frequently viewed as unique Asian-American characteristics in language and behaviors reflect some of the values inherent to this ethnic group. For example, some Asian-Americans view constant verbal communication as unnecessary. These individuals believe that it is more important to communicate through actions and demonstration of attitudes and feelings than through words. A talkative person is considered to be a "show-off" or insincere.

As a cornerstone of Asian-American society, respect is evident in communication (Huynh, 1987). Regardless of their language, the commonalty that most Asian-Americans share is their desire to communicate respect. The word *yes* is used in English to express agreement and does not reflect an attitude of respect or disrespect. In contrast, for some Asian-Americans, *yes* may indicate respect, but not necessarily agreement.

Traditionally, the high value of emotional self-control and the general esteem for correct behavior has limited the use of touch in communication for some Asian-Americans. Physical behavior, including backslapping, is not considered proper for well-bred persons. Touch is generally reserved for loved ones and then is used only in moderation.

In most Asian-American cultures respect is also conveyed through nonverbal communication. From the time they can stand alone, Asian American children are taught to cross the arms over the chest, lower the head, and bend the upper torso slightly forward when greeting an older adult or a guest coming into the house. Forms of this behavior continue throughout life in all situations requiring respect. Deference to others shows a Confucian and Buddhist influence in that how something is done is often more important than what is done.

Respect is also shown by avoiding eye contact when talking with someone to whom one is not equal in education, social standing, age, or sex. For example, bowing the head slightly to avoid eye contact when entering the presence of an older person conveys respect. Using both hands to give something to an adult, especially an older adult, also conveys respect. The head is considered sacred, and care should be taken in touching and patting it. Feet are the lowliest body members and should be kept on the floor.

Open expression of emotions is considered in bad taste except in very private circumstances. Emotions interfere with self-control and can be considered weaknesses. Romantic overtures are reserved for home or private settings, and wildly joyous scenes in public are not considered appropriate. One exception to the usual restraint is the expected behavior of a widow at the grave on the burial of her husband, when she may wail or attempt to throw herself into the grave.

Space. Beliefs about space are deeply rooted in the Asian-American culture. For the traditional Asian-American, intimate-zone activities are confined to private settings. Holding hands in public, especially with members of the opposite sex, is considered in poor taste. Hugging or emotionally touching in public, even by close friends or family members, is embarrassing to the traditional Asian-American onlooker (Hoang and Erickson, 1982).

Social Organization. For most Asian-Americans the family is the basic institution of society and as such provides lifelong protection and guidance to the individual (Figure 7-3). The roles and structure of the family are generally well defined, with extensive terminology designating kinship relationships. In most Asian-American families the father is the head of the household but shares the rights and authority with his spouse.

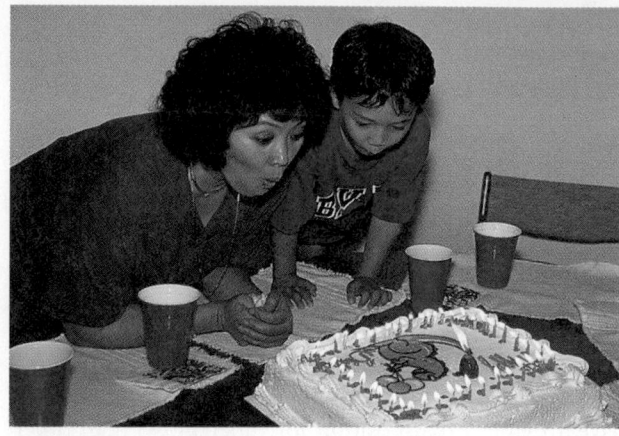

Figure 7-3   Blending of Asian culture and American practices at a child's birthday party.

The immediate family includes parents, unmarried children, sometimes the husband's parents, and sons with their wives and children. The extended family may include other close relatives who live in the same community. For some Asian-American families the eldest son has the responsibility of carrying on the family name, of taking over for the parents when they become older, and of following through with religious and ancestral observances.

Stress of Role Reversal.   Many Asian Americans (e.g., Hmongs, Vietnamese, Laotians) were forced to reverse traditional roles after arriving in the United States. Persons who were traditionally "providers" became the "recipients." For example, Vietnamese-American women, initially on arriving in this country, are more likely to gain employment, since "women's jobs" such as maids, sewing machine operators, and food service workers are more plentiful than male-oriented unskilled jobs. Thus the Asian-American man is often forced to reverse roles with the wife, becoming the recipient instead of the provider. Likewise, Asian-American children often assume the role of translator for non–English-speaking parents. Because Vietnamese-American children have assimilated very rapidly into the U.S. society, they are more likely than their parents to find gainful employment. Among some Asian-American families, role reversals create intergenerational conflicts (Gold, 1992).

Religion.   The religious beliefs of most Asian-Americans have been strongly influenced by several different religions, including Buddhism, Confucianism, and Taoism. The practice of Buddhism was introduced from China and India in the second century AD. Buddhism is considered less an organized orthodoxy than a state of mind using the Four Noble Truths taught by Buddha, which, simply stated, are (1) life is suffering; (2) suffering is caused by desire; (3) suffering can be eliminated by eliminating desire; and (4) to eliminate desire, one must follow the eightfold path of right understanding, purpose, speech, conduct, vocation, effort, thinking, and meditation. The Four Noble of Truths of Buddhism have played a large part in molding the Asian-American characteristics of stoicism, strong self-control, and apparent passivity.

Confucianism is of Chinese origin and is a code of ethics rather than a true religion. Confucianism emphasizes hierarchy of society; worship of ancestors; and respect for age, customs, teacher, and family.

Time.   Most Asian cultures date back thousands of years, and this antiquity is reflected in an orientation to time that places emphasis on the past. Emphasis is placed on ancestors and their wishes, memories, and graves. Most Asian-Americans have been oriented to think of time in terms of cycles, events, or occurrences (Hoang and Erickson, 1982). Some Asian-Americans, even those who are not Buddhist, have some belief in reincarnation. This cultural heritage makes time less of a fixed point (here and gone) and more of a recurring reality. This results in a less stressful and less time-conscious pace than that commonly experienced in the West. Being late or early is not considered a problem. The nurse should be aware that the concept of illness prevention requires both a future and a present time orientation, which is difficult for some traditional Asian-Americans to understand. Illness prevention is a difficult concept if a person lacks a scientific understanding of the relative meaning of health, illness, and the disease processes. The nurse should also be aware that some Asian-Americans may feel that luck and fate play a significant role in suffering and that illness may be considered a result of spiritual failure or punishment. For some Asian-Americans, the act of seeking medical care is influenced by a number of factors, including time orientation.

Environmental Control.   Traditional Asian-Americans tend to combine Chinese medicine with scientific techniques brought in from the West (Tran, 1972, 1980, 1989). The explanation of the causes of illness for some Asian-Americans can be divided into three types: naturalistic (folk medicine), supernaturalistic (animistic beliefs), and metaphysical (the theory of "hot" and "cold"). None of these theories excludes the others, and a client may explain illness by aspects of all three. A fourth explanation of illness (i.e., germs) is offered by some.

Cultural Health Practices.   The naturalistic explanation for illness encourages a search for a natural or obvious cause of the symptoms, such as rotten food, "poisonous water," or an obvious cause-and-effect relationship. To counteract the effects of these natural elements, an informal body of knowledge has been collected about indigenous medicinal herbs, therapeutic diets, and simple med-

ical and hygienic measures. The information is usually transmitted orally and often treated with secrecy, remaining inside the clan or extended family.

The supernaturalistic explanation for disease lays the blame on supernatural powers, such as gods, demons, or spirits. The illness is considered a punishment for a fault, for a violation of religious or ethical codes, or for an act of omission causing displeasure to a deity. In the supernaturalistic theory, disease may be caused by black magic or an evil incantation of an enemy who has bought the services of a sorcerer (Westermeyer and Winthrob, 1979).

Metaphysical explanation is built on the theory that nature and the body operate within a delicate balance between two opposite elements: the yin and the yang (e.g., female and male, dark and light, or hard and soft). In medicine the opposites are expressed as "hot" and "cold," and health is a result of a balance between hot and cold elements. This results in harmonious functioning of the organs, as well as harmony with the environment. An excess or shortage in either direction causes discomfort and illness. All illnesses, foods, medications and herbs are classified along a continuum according to their hot and cold qualities. Hot medications and foods are used for balance in cold diseases, and vice versa.

Biological Variations.   Several categories of diseases occur with high incidence in Asian-Americans. The following section highlights the impact of cancer, diabetes mellitus, and coronary heart disease in this cultural group.

Cancer.   Cancer of the stomach, esophagus, and liver occurs more frequently among Japanese-Americans than among their white counterparts (Tominaga, 1985; Rhoads, Glober, and Stemmerman, 1991; Overfield, 1995). It is believed that eating dried salted fish is a predisposing factor for gastric cancer (Nomura, 1982; Nomura, Stemmerman, and Heilbrun, 1985). In addition, diets high in salt-cured foods and nitrites and low in vitamin C have been commonly associated with a greater incidence of stomach cancer. Also, drinking hot tea may contribute to the development of esophageal cancer.

Diabetes Mellitus.   Pockets of high incidences of diabetes and obesity have been noted among the Japanese in Hawaii (Kawate and others, 1978). These higher incidences may be a result of a combination of diet and lifestyle.

Cardiovascular Disease.   Longitudinal research noting the incidence of coronary heart disease has been conducted on the Japanese in Japan, in Hawaii, and on the U.S. mainland. The mortality from coronary heart disease (as well as breast and colon cancer) has been attributed to variations in diets and lifestyles of Asians, Hawaiians, and mainland Japanese. Coronary artery mortality is lowest in Japan, intermediate in Hawaii, and highest on the U.S.

mainland (Reed and others, 1982; Yano, Reed, and McGee, 1984).

Cerebrovascular disease mortality appears to be opposite that for coronary artery disease. There is a higher incidence in Japan, an intermediate incidence in Hawaii, and the lowest incidence on the U.S. mainland (Syme and others, 1975; Yano, Reed, and Kagan, 1985).

Implications for Nursing Practice.

It is important for the nurse to remember that there are many countries of origin for Asian-Americans. Each of these countries has its own customs, beliefs, and language or dialects. However, there are some universal interventions that can be used for this culturally diverse population.

First, when English is the second language, the nurse and other health care providers must establish a communication method. It is frightening to be sick and not understand the language of the health care providers. During stressful situations it is not uncommon for individuals to revert to their primary language.

Whenever possible, the nurse should try to incorporate Eastern medical practice into the plan of care. For example, the use of relaxation or acupuncture may be very effective for some Asian-American clients. Since these types of alternative therapies are also becoming popular in traditional health care practices, the nurse does have access to practitioners of alternative therapies (see Chapter 35).

NATIVE AMERICANS

According to the census, there were 1,900,000 Native Americans among 10 different tribes living in the United States in 1990. The Cherokee and Navajo tribes have the largest populations. Indian populations are found in Arizona, Oklahoma, New Mexico, Alaska, California, North Carolina, South Dakota, New York, Montana, Washington, and Minnesota (U.S. Department of Commerce, Bureau of the Census, 1995). Providing culturally appropriate nursing care is complicated by the fact that each nation or tribe of Native Americans has its own language and religion, and belief system practices differ significantly among groups, as well as among members of the same tribe (Vogel, 1970).

There is a clear distinction between American Indians and the Alaska Natives. Thus when the term *Native Americans* is used it is intended to imply tribes residing in the continental United States. Today, although many Native Americans remain on reservations and in rural areas, an equal number also reside in cities (U.S. Department of Commerce, Bureau of the Census, 1995).

The basic authority for health care for American Indians and Alaska Natives is provided by the Snyder Act of 1921. The Bureau of Indian Affairs assumed responsibility as a federal branch for providing health care services for the Navajo people until 1954. In 1954 this responsibility was transferred to the Indian Health Service.

Communication.

There is no common language that unites Native Americans. Each tribe has its own distinct language. For example, the language spoken by the Navajo is classified as "Athapaskan" because historically it is thought to have been derived from the languages used by the people of Lake Athapaskan in Northwest Canada. The Navajo language is also similar to the languages spoken by some people living in Alaska, some people on the northern coast of the Pacific Ocean, and the people of the Apache tribe. Many Native Americans maintain the tradition of speaking in their native language, as well as English. Since some Native Americans do not speak English, it may be necessary to find a translator familiar with the specific language. Translating is often difficult, since many Native American languages do not have one single word that is similar to an English word, which makes translating difficult. When a Native American interpreter is used, this person must be knowledgeable about medical terminology, as well as the cultural aspects of the Native American lifestyle.

Instead of using the handshake on meeting another person, some Native Americans extend their hand and lightly touch the hand of the person they are greeting. Other examples of the use of touch in the Navajo culture include the tradition of massaging a newborn baby as a bonding experience between mother and baby. Another tradition is to give a small gift and prepare a small feast for the family when the baby laughs for the first time, because this token of esteem touches the hearts of all of the people around the baby. Another example is the taboo against touching a dead person or animal killed by lightning, which is extended to touching articles associated with the deceased individual or animal involved. This traditional taboo is not extended to animals whose death resulted from natural causes.

Some Native Americans believe that it is disrespectful to engage in eye contact. Although this is a common practice overall, the nurse must recognize that this practice might cause discomfort for the Native American client.

Space.

For some Native Americans there is no such thing as imaginary space. Space is so real a concept that it may not be located in any dimension other than real space. For example, space may not be located in the realm of thought; there is no abstract space. For some Native Americans space such as that found in a room or a house is the same as a small universe (Hall, 1966).

Since some Native Americans place an extremely high value on personal space, and because they also believe that it has imaginary boundaries, some may experience difficulty adjusting to unfamiliar spaces. It is important for the nurse to familiarize the client with the space provided during hospitalization and when personal space is limited during health care administration.

Social Organization. Native Americans are extremely family oriented, but the term *family* has a much broader meaning than just the nuclear family (Figure 7-4). The biological family is the center of social organization and includes all members of the extended family. There are some tribes (e.g., the Navajo) who are traditionally a matriarchal society. This means that when a couple marry, the husband makes his home with his wife's relatives, and his family becomes one of several units that live in a group of adjacent hogans or other dwellings. The family is considered so important in the Navajo culture that to be without relatives is to be really poor. Children learn from infancy that the family and the tribe are of paramount importance.

Historically, Native Americans have been guided by sacred myths and legends that describe the tribe's evolution from inception to the present time. Supernatural beings portrayed in these stories symbolize the culture, in which religion and healing practices are blended with each other. Values and beliefs intrinsic to their culture and religion form the Navajo day-to-day living experiences.

Time. The cultural interpretation of time has a temporal focus that views human life as existing in a three-point range that includes past, present, and future (Kluckhohn and Strodtbeck, 1961). Native Americans are viewed as being primarily present time oriented. However, it should be noted that some Native Americans are also perceived as being both past and present time oriented.

It is important for the nurse to remember that since Native Americans are often perceived as being present oriented, time is viewed as being on a continuum with no beginning and no end (Primeaux, 1977). In some Indian homes there are no clocks, since Indian time is casual, present oriented, and relative to present tasks that need to be accomplished in a present time frame. Since certain tasks are associated with present needs, it may be difficult for the nurse to counsel and advise a Native American client about crucial future events such as taking medications. The present time orientation of a Navajo client may result in eating two meals today, four meals tomorrow, no meals the next day, and three meals the day after. This becomes an important nursing implication if a client is told to take a medication with meals, particularly if the medication is to be taken 3 times a day. Another indication of Native Americans' present time orientation is related to the failure to keep clinical appointments.

Environmental Control. Some Native Americans have an external locus of control. Although they believe that man is not subjugated to the effects of nature, they also believe that it is essential for man to put forth effort to live in harmony with nature and its elements.

Cultural Health Practices. Traditional Native American concepts focus on the need for the individual to be in harmony with the surrounding environment and with the family. Health and religion cannot be separated within the Native American world. The linkage between traditional religion and healing ceremonies found among Native Americans is obvious.

Native American Healers. Native American Healers spend many years learning their skills and serving as apprentices. There are a variety of healers within each tribe, including herbalists, diagnosticians, and medicine men. Medicine men and medicine women have *jists,* or medicine bundles, containing symbolic and sacred items, including corn pollen, feathers, stones, arrowheads, and other instruments used for healing and blessing.

The nurse should keep in mind that a Navajo client needs to feel in harmony with the environment. Therefore the environment must be structured in such a way that this harmony is promoted. If a nurse were to deny or not allow the client the opportunity to achieve harmony with other people, animals, plants, nature, weather, and supernatural forces, the client would not be able to obtain a sense of assuredness in relation to physical, social, psychological, and spiritual health.

Biological Variations. Several categories of diseases occur with high incidence in Native Americans. The following section highlights the impact of diabetes mellitus, sexually transmitted diseases, alcoholism, and suicide in this cultural group.

Diabetes Mellitus. Type 2 diabetes is a major health problem for Native Americans, occurring as early as the teens or early 20s. The earlier onset leads to an earlier onset of complications, as well as excessive mortality in the early and middle adult years. Age-specific death rates for

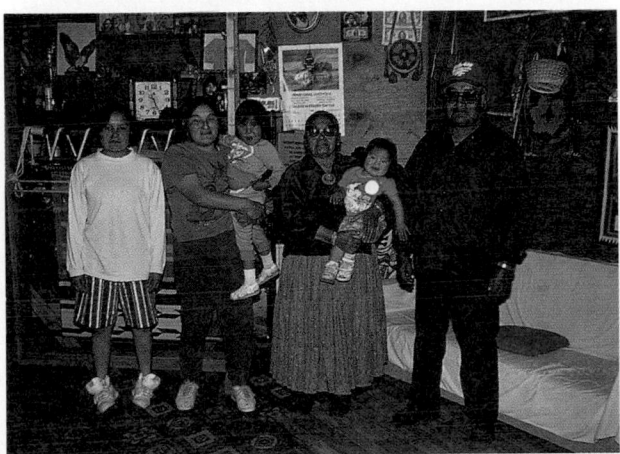

Figure 7-4 American Indian family in front of a display at a local festival.

diabetes appear to be 2.6 times higher for Native Americans between 25 and 54 years of age than for the rest of the general U.S. population (U.S. Department of Health and Human Services, Indian Health Service, 1992). In addition, the complications from diabetes among Native Americans are appearing with distressing frequency.

Sexually Transmitted Diseases.   American Indians and Alaska Natives in a 13-state area had twice the reported gonorrhea and syphilis morbidity of the rest of the general population. In addition, in some states they also had the highest incidence of hepatitis B. The number of persons who are HIV seropositive is reported to be low in these groups. It is important to remember, however, that although there has been a relatively lower number of cumulative AIDS cases among American Indians and Alaska Natives, the incidence of AIDS is steadily increasing among this population (U.S. Department of Health and Human Services, Indian Health Service, 1992).

Alcoholism.   In whites, alcohol is metabolized "fairly efficiently" by the liver enzyme dehydrogenase. In contrast, in Native Americans and Asians, it is metabolized by aldehyde dehydrogenase (ALDH), which works faster, often causing circulatory and unpleasant effects such as facial flushing and palpitations (Kudzma, 1992). Studies have indicated that American Indians experience marked facial flushing and other vasomotor symptoms after ingesting alcohol, as compared with their white and African-American counterparts, who experience less severe reactions.

Approximately 85% to 90% of American Indians have been found to have the high-activity variant of ALDH, which means that the alcohol they consume is rapidly converted to acetaldehyde. However, the next step, conversion of acetaldehyde to acetic acid, is delayed in 35% to 70% of American Indians. It is because of these enzyme differences that a majority of American Indians experience a rapid onset initially and thereafter a slow decrease in blood acetaldehyde levels (Goedde, 1983). Alcoholism exists among Native Americans in very high percentages. The age-adjusted alcoholism death rate for American Indians and Alaska Natives has decreased 61% since its peak in 1973 of 66.1 deaths per 100,000 population. This is largely due to multiple efforts of the Indian Health Service for prevention and treatment.

Suicide.   Suicide is another major contributor to death in Native Americans. Men are at higher risk than women for suicide (U.S. Department of Health Services, Indian Health Services, 1992). The mental health of Native Americans is complicated by the pressures created by traditional cultural demands, attempts at assimilation into the Western culture, and the availability of alcohol. Suicide is associated with alcohol abuse, which in turn is a symptom of a people attempting to assimilate in a rapidly changing society.

Implications for Nursing Practice.   The Native Americans are proud people with a rich heritage in the United States. However, their access to health care may be somewhat limited because of the high unemployment percentages within the tribal setting. As a result, the use of screening and prevention may often be overlooked. The nurse can begin to educate the client with regard to health maintenance practices.

In addition, this culture is rich in traditional folk methods for health and illness. Whenever possible, incorporating these practices into a plan of care can assist the client in combining traditional folk medicine with Western principles of care. Such a practice demonstrates mutual respect for the client's culture and standard medical practice. The family can be of great assistance to the nurse in incorporating some of the folk methods into the plan of care.

• • •

It is essential to understand differences in individuals as they relate to cultural heritage. It is also important to appreciate that each client and family are culturally unique and bring to the care environment this uniqueness. In addition, the nurse who gives care also brings to the client-nurse relationship a personal cultural heritage. It is essential to refrain from imposing personal values and beliefs on the client and to respect the uniqueness and differences each brings to the care environment.

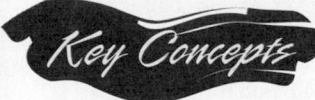

Key Concepts

- Culture is a patterned behavioral response that develops over time as a result of being imprinted on the mind through social and religious structures and intellectual and artistic manifestations.
- Patterns of cultural behaviors are learned through a process called enculturation or socialization.
- The way that culture influences behaviors, attitudes, and values depends on many factors and thus may not be the same for individual members of a cultural group.
- Transcultural nursing is viewed as a culturally competent practice field that is client centered and research focused. Although transcultural nursing is viewed as client centered, it is important for nurses to remember that culture can and does influence how clients are viewed and the care they are given.
- Giger and Davidhizar's transcultural assessment model provides a method for the nurse to identify the client's unique health care needs, which include cultural health practices.
- The nurse should have an understanding of the prevalent characteristics of members of four major groups in North America: African-Americans, Hispanics, Asian-Americans, and Native Americans.
- To provide culturally appropriate and competent care, it is important to remember that each individual is culturally unique and as such is a product of past experiences, cultural beliefs, and cultural norms.
- Culturally diverse nursing care refers to the variability in nursing approaches needed to provide culturally appropriate and competent care.
- Culturally diverse nursing care must take into account six cultural phenomena that vary with application and use, yet are evident in all cultural groups: (1) communication, (2) space, (3) social organization, (4) time, (5) environmental control, and (6) biological variations.
- Cultural health practices are categorized as efficacious (beneficial), neutral, dysfunctional, or uncertain.
- Folk medicine is practiced in a variety of countries and cultural groups. These remedies have been passed down from generation to generation. Many of the remedies are herbal, and the customs and rituals related to the use of herbs vary among cultural groups.

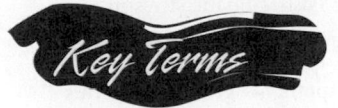

Key Terms

Bicultural, *p. 114*
Biological variations, *p. 120*
Biracial, *p. 114*
Communication, *p. 116*
Cultural behavior, *p. 113*
Cultural competence, *p. 115*
Cultural values, *p. 113*
Culturally diverse nursing care, *p. 115*
Culture, *p. 113*
Environmental control, *p. 118*
Ethnic minority, *p. 114*
Ethnic people of color, *p. 114*

Ethnicity, *p. 113*
Ethnocentrism, *p. 114*
Folk Medicine, *p. 119*
Giger and Davidhizar's transcultural assessment model, *p. 115*
Minority, *p. 114*
People of color, *p. 114*
Race, *p. 114*
Social organization, *p. 118*
Space, *p. 116*
Stereotyping, *p. 115*
Transcultural nursing, *p. 115*

Critical Thinking Exercises

1. What impact does culture have on cultural beliefs, illness, and wellness behaviors?
2. In what ways does communication present barriers to culturally competent care, even when the nurse and the client speak the same language?
3. In what ways do time orientation; spatial needs; and efficacious, neutral, or dysfunctional health care practices affect compliance or adherence to a particular treatment regimen?

References

Alexander M, Blank J: Factors related to obesity in Mexican American preschool children, *Image J Nurs Sch* 20(2):79, 1988.

Aruffo J, Coverdale J, Vallbona C: AIDS knowledge in low-income and minority population, *Public Health Rep* 106(2):115, 1991.

Birchenall J: *Mosby's textbook for the home care aide,* St. Louis, 1997, Mosby.

Bullough VL, Bullough B. *Health care for the other Americans,* East Norwalk, Conn, 1982, Appleton-Century-Crofts.

Capirci, O, and others: Gestures and words during the transition in two-word speech. *J Child Lang* 23:645, 1996.

Carmel R, Johnson C, Weiner J: Pernicious anemia in Latin Americans is not a disease of the elderly, *Ethnology* 147(11): 1995, 1987.

Caudle P: Providing culturally sensitive health care to Hispanic patients, *Nurse Pract* 18(12):40, 1993.

Centers for Disease Control: *HIV surveillance report: estimated incidence of AIDS and deaths of persons with AIDS, adjusted for delays in reporting, by quarter-year of diagnosis/death, United States, January 1985 through December 1997,* vol 9(2), Atlanta, 1997 Genga.

Cervantes R, Synder S, Padilla A: Posttraumatic stress in immigrants from Central America and Mexico, *Hosp Community Psychiatry* 40 (6):615, 1989.

Cronin M, Billboard campaign spotlights growing hepatitis C epidemic, *Seattle Times,* p A1, July 30, 1997.

Cronsberry T: Alternative cancer therapies, *Can Nurs* p. 35, April 1996.

Delgado M: Hispanics and psychotherapeutic groups, *Int J Psychother* 33 (4):507, 1983.

Derenowski J: Coronary heart disease in Hispanics, *Cardiovasc Nurs* 4(4):13, 1990.

Dorsey P, Jackson H: Cultural health traditions: the Latino-Chino perspective. In Branch MF, Paxton PP, editors: *Providing safe nursing care for ethnic people of color,* Norwalk, Conn, 1976, Appleton-Century-Crofts.

Dunn FL: Transcultural Asian medicine and cosmopolitan medicine as adaptive systems. In Leslie E, editor: *Asian medical systems: a comparative study,* Berkeley, 1975, University of California Press.

Foster G: Relationship between Spanish and Spanish American folk medicine. In Martinez RA, editor: *Hispanic culture and health care: fact, fiction, folklore,* St. Louis, 1978, Mosby.

Geissler E: Transcultural nursing and nursing diagnosis, *Nurs Health Care* 12(4):190, 1991.

Giger JN and others: Cultural factors influencing mental health and mental illness. In Taylor C, editor: *Essentials of psychiatric nursing,* St. Louis, 1994, Mosby.

Giger JN, Davidhizar RE: *Transcultural nursing: assessment and intervention,* ed 3, St. Louis, 1999, Mosby.

Goedde H: Population genetic studies on aldehyde dehydrogenase isoenzyme deficiency and alcohol sensitivity, *Am J Hum Genet,* 35:769, 1983.

Gold S: Mental health and illness in Vietnamese refugees, *West J Med* 157 (3):290, 1992.

Gregory D: Nursing practice in native communities. In Baumgart A, Larson J, editors: *Canadian nursing faces the future,* St. Louis, 1988, Mosby.

Grossman D: Cultural dimensions in home health care nursing, *Am J Nurs* 96(7):33, 1996.

Haber J: Therapeutic communication. In Haber J and others, editors: *Comprehensive psychiatric nursing,* ed 5, St. Louis, 1997, Mosby.

Hall ET: *The hidden dimension,* New York, 1966, Doubleday.

Hazuda H and others: Ethnic differences in health knowledge and behaviors related to the prevention and treatment of coronary heart disease, *Am J Epidemiol,* 117:717, 1983.

Hedlund N: Communication. In Beck CK, Rawlins RP, Williams S, editors: *Mental health–psychiatric nursing: a holistic life approach,* ed 3, St. Louis, 1992, Mosby.

Hilsop TG and others: Participation in the British Columbia cervical cytology screening programme by native Indian women, *Can J Public Health* 83(5):344, 1992.

Hoang G, Erickson R: Guidelines for providing medical care for Southeast Asian refugees, *JAMA* 248 (6):710, 1982.

Hood L, Jackson N: Caring for the patient with TB, *Adv Clin Care,* 4(4):14, 1989.

Huynh TD: *Introduction to Vietnamese culture,* San Diego, Calif, 1987, Multifunctional Resource Center, San Diego State University.

Information please almanac, Boston, 1998, Houghton Mifflin.

Joint National Committee: *The report of the Joint National Committee on detection, evaluation, and treatment of high blood pressure,* Washington, DC, 1997, National Institutes of Health, National Heart, Lung, and Blood Institute.

Kawate R and others: Preliminary studies of the prevalence and mortality of diabetes mellitus in Japanese in Japan and on the island of Hawaii, *Adv Metab Dis* 9:201, 1978.

Kluckhohn K, Strodtbeck F: *Variations in value orientations,* New York, 1961, Row, Peterson.

Kretch D, Crutchfield R, Ballachey E: *Individual in society,* New York, 1962, McGraw-Hill.

Kudzma E: Drug responses: all bodies are not created equal, *Am J Nurs* 92:48, 1992.

Lawson I: Culturally sensitive support for grieving, *J Matern Child Nurs* 15(2):76, 1990.

Liao Y, Cooper R: Continued adverse trends in coronary heart disease mortality among blacks, 1980-1991, *Public Health Rep* 110:572, 1995.

Martin B: The difficult art of listening, *Gospel Herald* 88(48):1, 1995.

Murrillo N: The Mexican American family. In Hernandez CA, Huang MJ, Wagner NN, editors: *Chicanos: social and psychological perspectives,* St. Louis, 1978, Mosby.

National Center for Health Statistics: *Health, United States, 1998,* DHHS Pub No. (PHS) 91-1232, Hyattsville, Md, 1998, U.S. Department of Health and Human Services, Public Health Services.

National Center for Health Statistics: *Healthy people 2000 review (1993): healthy United States,* 1992, Hyattsville, Md, 1993, U.S. Department of Health and Human Services, Public Health Service.

Nolt S: *A history of the Amish,* Intercourse, Pa, 1992, Good Books.

Nomura A: Stomach cancer. In Schottenfeld D, Fraumeni J, editors: *Cancer epidemiology and prevention,* Philadelphia, 1982, WB Saunders.

Nomura A, Stemmerman G, Heilbrun L: Gastric cancer among the Japanese in Hawaii: a review, *Hawaii Med J,* 44 (8):301, 1985.

Overfield RT: *Biologic variations in health and illness: race, age and sex differences,* ed 2, Reading, Mass, 1995, Addison-Wesley.

Phipps WJ: The patient with pulmonary problems. In Long, BC, Phipps WJ, Cassmeyer V, editors: *Medical surgical nursing: concepts and clinical practice,* ed 6, St. Louis, 1997, Mosby.

Pillsbury B: Doing the month: confinement and convalescence of Chinese women after childbirth. In Kay M, editor: *Anthro-pology of human birth,* Philadelphia, 1982, FA Davis.

Pore S: I can't understand what my patient is saying, *Adv Nurs Pract,* July 1995, p. 17.

Poussaint A, Atkinson C: Black youth and motivation, *Black Scholar,* 1:43, 1970.

Primeaux M: Caring for the American Indian patient, *Am J Nurs* 77(1):91, 1977.

Randall-David E: *Strategies for working with culturally diverse communities and clients,* Washington, DC, 1989, U.S. Department of Health and Human Services.

Reed D and others: Acculturation and coronary heart disease among Japanese men in Hawaii, *Am J Epidemiol,* 115 (6):894, 1982.

Rhoads GG, Glober GA, Stemmerman GN: A review of some tumors of interest for demographic study in Hawaii, *Hawaii Med J,* 50 (9):326, 1991.

Richardson L: Caring through understanding. II. Folk medicine in the Hispanic population, *Imprint* 29(2):21, 1982.

Reinert B: The healthcare beliefs and values of Mexican Americans, *Home Healthcare Nurse* 4(5):23, 1986.

Ronan L: Alcohol-related health risks among Black Americans, *Alcohol Health Res World* 12:36, 1987.

Ruiz P: Cultural barriers to effective medical care among Hispanic-American patients, *Ann Rev Med* 36:63, 1985.

Shadick K: Development of a transcultural health education program for the Hmong, *Clin Nurse Spec,* 7(2):48, 1993.

Smith JA: The role of the Black clergy as allied health care professionals in working with Black patients. In Luckraft D, editor: *Black awareness: implications for Black care,* New York, 1976, American Journal of Nursing Co.

Smith L: Cultural competence for nurses: canonical correlation of two culture scales, *J Cult Divers* 5(4):120, 1988.

Snow LF: Traditional health beliefs and practice among lower class Black Americans, *West J Med* 139(6):820, 1983.

Spector R: *Cultural diversity in health and illness,* Stamford, Conn, 1996, Appleton & Lange.

Stokes G: A transcultural nurse is about, *Senior Nurse* 11(1):40, 1991.

Sue D: *Counseling the culturally different: theory and practice,* New York, 1981, John Wiley & Sons.

Syme S and others: Epidemiologic studies of coronary heart disease and stroke in Japanese men living in Japan, Hawaii and California: an introduction, *Am J Epidemiol* 102(6):477, 1975.

Tominaga S: Cancer incidence in Japanese in Japan, Hawaii, and Western United States, *Nat Cancer Institute Monogr* 69:83, 1985.

Tran TM: The family and the management of mental health problems in Vietnam. In Lebra WP, editor: *Transcultural research in mental health,* Honolulu, 1972, University of Hawaii Press.

Tran TM: *Indochinese patients,* Falls Church, Va, 1980, Action for Southeast Asians.

Tran TM: Personal communication, October 1989.

U.S. Department of Commerce, Bureau of the Census: *Population profiles of the United States: 1993,* Hyattsville, Md, 1993a, U.S. Government Printing Office.

U.S. Department of Commerce, Bureau of the Census: *Population projections of the United States by age, sex, race, and Hispanic origin: 1992-2050,* Hyattsville, Md, 1993b, U.S. Government Printing Office.

U.S. Department of Commerce, Bureau of the Census: *Race and Hispanic origins in the United States and regions,* Hyattsville, Md, 1993c, U.S. Government Printing Office.

U.S. Department of Commerce, Bureau of the Census: *We the American Blacks,* Hyattsville, Md, 1993d, U.S. Government Printing Office.

U.S. Department of Commerce, Bureau of the Census: *We the American Hispanics,* Hyattsville, Md, 1993e, U.S. Government Printing Office.

U.S. Department of Commerce, Bureau of the Census: *Top 25 American Indian tribes for the United States: 1990 and 1980,* Internet release, August 1995.

U.S. Department of Commerce, Bureau of the Census: *Population profiles of the United States,* Internet update, June 30, 1998, Hyattsville, Md, 1998, U.S. Government Printing Office.

U.S. Department of Health and Human Services, Indian Health Service: Prevalence of HIV and AIDS in American Indians and Alaska Natives, *IHS Prim Care Provider* 17(5):66, 1992.

Vasquez S: Diabetes alert: high-fat, genetics make Hispanics prone to the disease, *Rocky Mountain News,* p 3d, May 20, 1997.

Vogel VJ: *American Indian medicine,* 1970, Norman, Okla, University of Oklahoma Press.

Wanderer J, Rivera G: Black magic beliefs and white magic practice: the common structures of intimacy, tradition and power, *Soc Sci J* 23(4):419, 1986.

Ward J, Duchin J: U.S. epidemiology of HIV and AIDS. In Volberding P, Jacobson M, editors: *AIDS clinical review,* New York, 1998.

Watzlawich P, Beavin J, Jackson D: *Pragmatics of human communication,* New York, 1967, WW Norton.

Westermeyer J: The role of ethnicity in substance abuse. In Stimmel B, editor: *Cultural and sociological aspects of alcoholism and substance abuse,* New York, 1984, Haworth Press.

Westermeyer J, Winthrob R: "Folk" explanations of mental illness in rural Laos, *Am J Psychiatry,* 136(7):901, 1979.

Williams M: Alcohol and ethnic minorities: Native American update, *Alcohol Health Res Works* 11(2):5, 1986.

Woods S: Can aspirin prevent coronary heart disease in women? *Womens Health Prim Care* 1:210, 1998.

World almanac, Mahwah, NJ, 1997, A K-111 Communications Co.

Yano K, Reed DM, Kagan A: Coronary heart disease, hypertension and stroke among Japanese-American men in Hawaii: the Honolulu Heart Program, *Hawaii Med J* 44(80):297, 1985.

Yano K, Reed D, McGee D: Ten year incidence of coronary heart disease in the Honolulu: heart program: relationship to biologic and lifestyle characteristics, *Am J Epidemiol* 119(5):653, 1984.

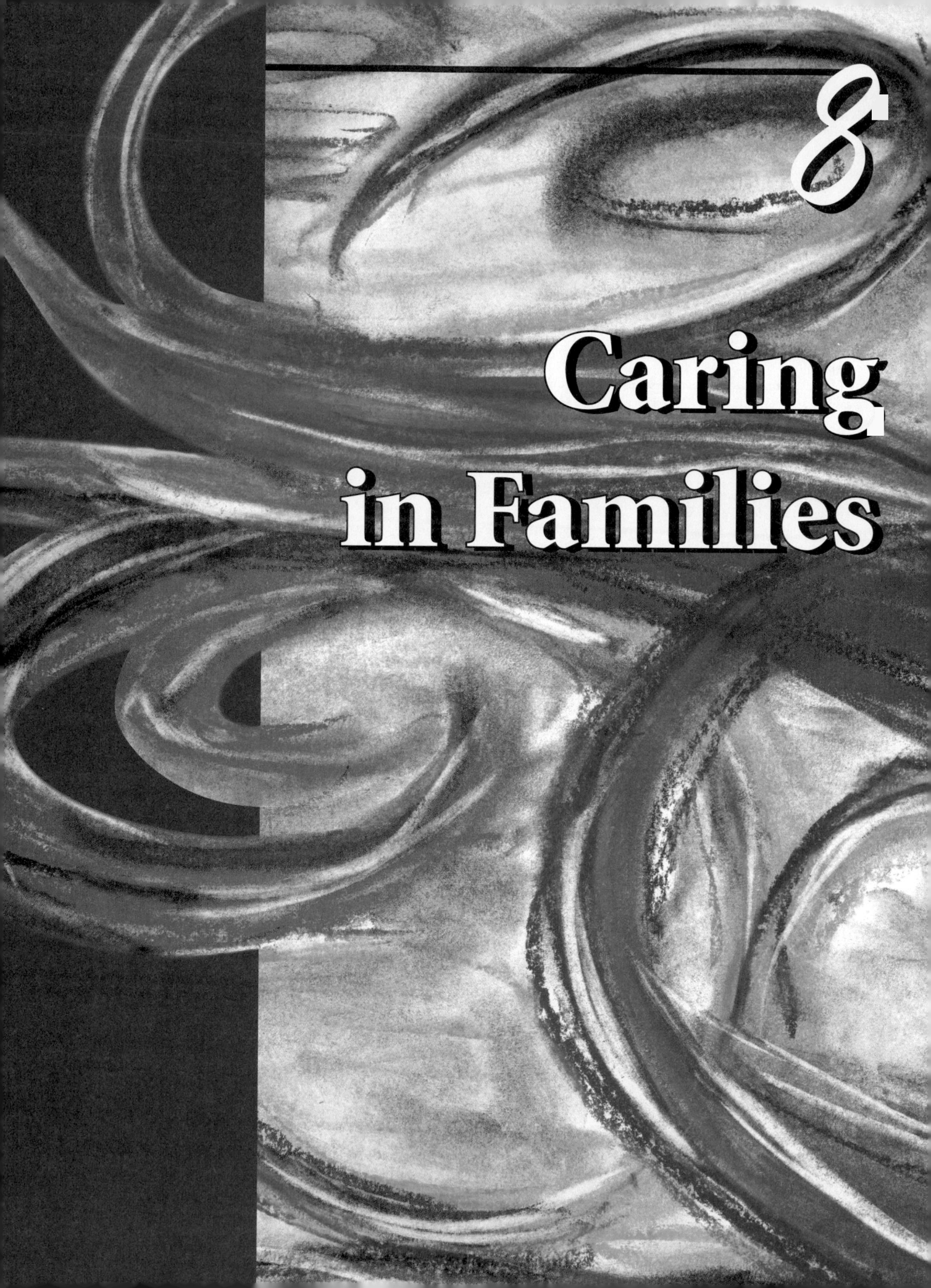

8

Caring
in Families

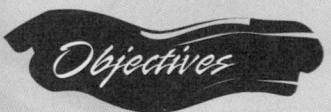

Objectives

Mastery of content in this chapter will enable the student to:

- Define the key terms listed.
- Discuss how the term *family* can be defined to reflect family diversity.
- Examine current trends in the American family.
- Describe theoretical approaches to the study of families.
- Explain how family structure and patterns of functioning affect the health of family members and the family as a whole.
- Discuss the way family members influence one another's health.
- Assess families as caregivers.
- Interpret external and internal factors that promote family health.
- Compare family as context to family as client and explain the way that these perspectives influence nursing practice.
- Use the nursing process to provide for the health care needs of the family.

The Family

Major changes have occurred in the concept and structure of the family, but it is clear that the family remains the central institution in American society. The current general assumption is that although the family is in transition and may look very different from the families of the 1950s, it is here to stay. It is true that contemporary families face many challenges; they are, however, characterized by three important attributes: durability, resiliency, and diversity.

Family durability is the term for the intrafamilial system of support and structure that may extend beyond the walls of the household. The players may change, the parents may remarry, and the children may or may not leave home as adults, but the "family" is considered to transcend long periods and inevitable lifestyle changes.

Family resiliency is the ability to cope with expected and unexpected stressors. The family's ability to adapt to role changes, developmental milestones, and crises shows resilience. The goal of the family is not only to survive "the challenge," but also to thrive and to grow as a result of the newly gained knowledge.

Family diversity is the attention to uniqueness. Some families will be experiencing marriage for the first time and having children in later life, when others are grandparents at the same age. Every person within this familial unit has specific needs, strengths, and important developmental considerations. Nurses are responsible for first understanding the makeup (configuration), structure, function, and coping capacity of the family and then seeing how to build on their relative strengths to overcome their weaknesses.

The authors acknowledge the contribution of Dr. JoEtta Vernon to this chapter in the previous edition of this text.

CONCEPT OF FAMILY

The term *family* evokes a visual image of adults and children living together in a satisfying, harmonious manner. Families are, however, as diverse as the individuals that compose them, and clients have deeply ingrained values about their families that deserve respect. Thus the nurse must think of *family* as defined by each individual. In other words, the nurse can think of the **family** as a set of relationships that the client identifies as family or as a network of individuals who influence each other's lives whether or not there are actual biological or legal ties.

DEFINITION: WHAT IS A FAMILY?

Defining *family* would at first appear to be a simple undertaking. However, different definitions have resulted in heated debates among social scientists and legislators. The choice of a definition is not an insignificant matter. It determines who is included on health insurance policies, who has access to children's school records, who can file joint tax returns, and who has eligibility for sick-leave benefits or public programs. The family can be defined biologically, legally, or as a social network with personally constructed ties and ideologies. To some clients, family may include only persons related by marriage, birth, or adoption. To others, aunts, uncles, close friends, cohabitating persons, and even pets are considered family. The nurse's personal beliefs do not have to coincide with those of the client. To provide individualized care, the nurse understands that families take many forms and have diverse cultural and ethnic orientations. In other words, the nurse can think of the family as a set of relationships that the client identifies as family or as a network of individuals who influence each other's lives (Figure 8-1).

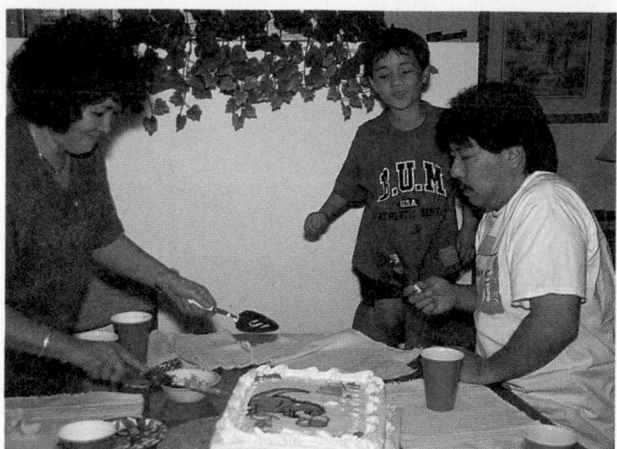

Figure 8-1   Family celebrations and traditions strengthen the role of the family.

FAMILY FORMS

Family forms are patterns of people considered by family members to be included in the family. Although all families have some things in common, each family form has unique problems and strengths. The nurse needs to have an open mind about what constitutes a family so that potential resources and concerns are not overlooked. Several family forms are displayed in Box 8-1.

Current Trends and New Family Forms

Although the institution of the family remains strong, the family itself is changing. The "typical" family (two biological parents and children) is no longer the norm. People are marrying later, women are delaying childbirth, and couples are choosing to have fewer children or none at all. The number of people living alone is expanding rapidly and represents approximately 25% of all households. Divorce rates have tripled since the 1950s, and although the rate appears to have stabilized, it is estimated that 60% of marriages will end in divorce (U.S. Bureau of the Census, 1997). About 90% of young Americans are likely to marry, and between 66% and 75% of those who divorce remarry. The median interval between divorce and remarriage is about 3 years. Men are more likely to remarry than women, younger persons are more likely to remarry than older persons, and divorcees are more likely to remarry than widows or widowers. Remarriage often results in a blended family with a complex set of relationships among stepparents, stepchildren, half brothers and sisters, and extended family members.

Marital roles are also more complex as families increasingly comprise two wage earners. The majority of women work outside the home, and about 63% of mothers are in the workforce (U.S. Bureau of the Census, 1997).

Family Forms   Box 8-1

NUCLEAR FAMILY
The **nuclear family** consists of husband and wife (and perhaps one or more children).

EXTENDED FAMILY
The **extended family** includes relatives (aunts, uncles, grandparents, and cousins) in addition to the nuclear family.

SINGLE-PARENT FAMILY
The **single-parent family** is formed when one parent leaves the nuclear family because of death, divorce, or desertion, or when a single person decides to have or adopt a child.

BLENDED FAMILY
The **blended family** is formed when parents bring unrelated children from prior or foster parenting relationships into a new, joint living situation.

ALTERNATE PATTERNS OF RELATIONSHIPS
These relationships include multiadult households, "skip-generation" families (grandparents caring for grandchildren), communal groups with children, "nonfamilies" (adults living alone), cohabiting partners, and homosexual couples.

Balancing employment and family life creates a variety of challenges in terms of child care and household work. Concerns that maternal employment is detrimental for children are unsubstantiated (Nichols, 1994; Harvey, 1999). However, finding quality substitute child care is a major issue for parents. Managing household tasks can also be a major issue. Research demonstrates that although equal division of labor receives verbal approval, the majority of household tasks remain "women's work." There is some evidence that the fathering role is changing. Fathers are now expected to participate more fully in day-to-day parenting responsibilities. Twenty-two percent of children (ages 0 to 4), as reported by the U.S. Bureau of the Census in 1997, have their fathers as caretakers whether or not the fathers are employed.

The number of single-parent families doubled from the 1970s to the 1990s but now appears to be stabilizing at about 29% of all families with children. Although 83% of single-parent families are headed by mothers, father-only families are on the rise. Forty-one percent of children are living with mothers who have never married; many of these children are a result of an adolescent pregnancy (U.S. Bureau of the Census, 1997). Adolescent pregnancy is an ever-increasing concern. The majority of these adolescents continue to live with their families. A teenage pregnancy tends to have long-term consequences for the mother and often severely stresses family relationships and resources. Teenage fathers also have stressors placed on them when their partner becomes pregnant. As a result, both of these adolescents are often struggling with the normal tasks of development and identity but now are also forced to accept a responsibility that they may not be ready for physically, emotionally, socially, and/or financially.

Although unable to marry by law, many homosexual couples define their relationship in family terms. Approximately half of all gay male couples live together, compared with three fourths of lesbian couples. These couples have become more open about their sexual preferences and more vocal about their legal rights. Some homosexual families include children, either through adoption or artificial insemination, or from prior relationships.

The fastest-growing age-group is 65 years of age and over. For the first time in history the average American has more living parents than children, and children are more likely to have living grandparents and even great-grandparents. This "graying" of America has had an impact on the family life cycle that has perhaps been most significant for the middle generation. These individuals are finding that they must balance the needs of their offspring and the needs of their aging parents. This balance often occurs at the expense of their own well-being and resources, earning them the title of the "sandwiched generation" (Schwartz, 1979). Caring for a frail or chronically ill relative is a primary concern for a growing number of families, and it is not uncommon for people in their 60s and 70s to be the major caregivers of each other predominantly, as well as of their own elderly parents. Box 8-2 provides a list of family nursing gerontological concerns.

Grandparents are also increasingly being called on to raise their grandchildren. This parenting responsibility is due to a number of societal factors: the increase in the divorce rate, dual-income families, and single parenthood. Most often it is a consequence of legal intervention when parents are deemed unfit or renounce their parental obligations.

Families face many challenges, including changing structures and roles in the changing economic status of society. Here we observe the lack of parental supervision, role modeling, and positive interaction with caring adults because more single parents or dual-income families are spending so much time on the job. In addition to family challenges related to divorce, changing structures and roles, and the aging of its older members, there are four further trends that social scientists identify as threats or concerns facing the family: (1) changing economic status (e.g., declining family income, lack of access to health care), (2) homelessness, (3) family violence, and (4) human immunodeficiency virus (HIV).

CHANGING ECONOMIC STATUS
Making ends meet is a daily concern because of the declining economic status of families. Although two-income families have become the norm, real family income has not increased since 1973. Families at the lower end of the income scale have been particularly affected, and single-

---

NURSING PRACTICE   Box 8-2

- The nurse must consider caregiver strain; caregivers are usually either spouses, who may also be an older adult and may have declining physical stamina, or middle-age children, who often have other responsibilities.
- Later-life families have a different social network than younger families because friends and same-generation family members may have died or been ill themselves. The nurse may need to look for social support within the community and church affiliation.
- Greater physical health impairment increases the risk of the older adult's depression.
- As in the other stages of life, members of later-life families need to be working on developmental tasks (see Chapter 12).
- Abuse of older adults in families occurs across all social classes. Spouses are the most frequent abusers. Unexplained bruises and skin trauma should not be ignored but should be reported by nurses to state protective agencies.

---

parent families are especially vulnerable. According to the Children's Defense Fund, 40% of all children in young families were living in poverty in 1990 (Clemen-Stone, McGuire, and Eigsti, 1998). Forty percent of all children lacked employer health coverage in 1990, and only about 25% of all infants were born to mothers who had received early prenatal care.

HOMELESSNESS
During the 1980s a new homeless population became apparent. Whereas formerly, homeless persons were primarily men residing in "skid row," the "new homeless" was increasingly being made up of women and entire families. Being homeless affects all aspects of family life. Finding food and shelter is the focus of daily existence; family relationships, physical health, and emotional stability are severely strained. The National Coalition for the Homeless estimates that only about 43% of homeless children are able to attend school. Obstacles such as residency requirements, transportation, and poor nutrition can be overwhelming, however, and dropout rates are high and performance tends to be poor. Homeless children are at serious risk for developing long-term health, psychological, and socioeconomic problems, thus posing a major challenge for our entire society (Lindsey, 1994).

FAMILY VIOLENCE
The statistics regarding family violence are even more disturbing. Clemen-Stone, McGuire, and Eigsti (1998) state that 2.7 million children were reported as being abused or neglected in 1991, up from 1.1 million in the preceding 11 years, and in the 4 years between 1986 and 1990 the need

for foster care increased by almost 50%. The infliction of emotional and/or physical pain on family members occurs in more than half of all households in the United States. Emotional, physical, and sexual abuse occurs toward spouses, children, and older adults and across all social classes. Research spanning two decades has demonstrated that the cause of family violence is complex and multidimensional. Factors associated with violence include stress, poverty, social isolation, psychopathology, and learned family behavior. Although abuse may end when one leaves a specific family environment, negative long-term physical and emotional consequences are often evident.

HUMAN IMMUNODEFICIENCY VIRUS

The statistics regarding HIV/acquired immunodeficiency syndrome (AIDS) are approaching a leveling in incidence. However, the number of HIV-infected persons is high, and new infections continue to occur. The AIDS-related mortality is down, indicating that people with HIV are living longer and better lives; however, if the "improvements in . . . [client] survival are not matched by reductions in HIV incidence, the population of HIV-infected persons will increase" (Ward and Duchin, 1997-1998). The characteristics of HIV are changing over time, although the rates of incidence have not changed much since about 1992 (Centers for Disease Control and Prevention [CDC], 1998). The rates appear highest in African-Americans and Hispanics, and a fifth of the persons with AIDS are women. The increasing incidences are now seen with intravenous (IV) drug use and heterosexual transmission. Finding that one is HIV positive is devastating, not only for the individual, but for the family and friends as well. As with all serious illnesses, caring for a family member who develops active HIV infection is emotionally and financially devastating. Unfortunately, a diagnosis of HIV often carries the additional burdens of guilt, social stigma, lifestyle conflicts, and isolation that affect all family members.

Theoretical Approaches: An Overview

There are a number of different perspectives that can be applied when working with or studying families. General systems and developmental theories are the two perspectives most fully incorporated in this chapter. Family scholars often look at families from three additional general perspectives: functionalism, social conflict, and symbolic interactionism.

FUNCTIONAL THEORY OR FUNCTIONALISM

Functionalism is considered a "conservative" theory that emphasizes stability and harmony of the family unit. The family is viewed as a universal, necessary, social institution that fulfills the needs of individuals and society.

SOCIAL CONFLICT APPROACH

As opposed to stability and harmony, this theory assumes that conflict and change are expected features of life. The family is assumed to consist of two kinds of power imbalances: those based on gender and those based on age.

SYMBOLIC INTERACTIONISM

This approach is based on the assumption that all interactions have different meanings to different individuals in different situations and that individuals interact only in relation to other people. According to this approach, a family can be understood only by knowing about its past experiences and the meaning that the individual members place on former and current situations.

• • •

The primary theoretical approaches to the family include general systems theory and developmental theory. Both of these perspectives and their concepts provide the foundation for family assessment.

General Systems Theory

FAMILY AS AN OPEN SOCIAL SYSTEM

The family is viewed as an open social system that exists in and interacts with the larger systems (suprasystems) of the community (e.g., political, religious, school, and health care systems). The family system consists of interrelated parts (family members) that form a variety of interaction patterns (subsystems). As with all systems, the family system has both implicit and explicit goals, which vary according to the stage in the family life cycle, family values, and individual concerns of the family members.

STRUCTURE

Families also have a structure and a way of functioning. Structure and function are closely related and continually interact with one another. Structure is based on organization (i.e., the ongoing membership of the family and the pattern of relationships). Relationships can be numerous and complex. For example, a woman's relationships may include wife-husband, mother-son, mother-daughter, employee-boss, and colleague-colleague, each with different demands, roles, and expectations. Patterns of relationships form power and role structures within the family. These structures can be determined by observing family behavior and asking questions that identify who makes the decisions, how they are made (power structure), and who performs which tasks (role structure).

Structure may enhance or detract from the family's ability to respond to stressors. Very rigid or very flexible structures can impair functioning. A rigid structure specifically dictates who is permitted to accomplish a task, and it may also limit the number of persons outside the immediate family who are allowed to assume these tasks. For example, the mother might be considered the only acceptable person to provide emotional support for the children, or the husband might be considered the only one to provide financial support. A change in the health status of the person responsible for a task places a burden on the family because no other person is available or considered acceptable to assume that task.

An extremely open structure can also present problems for the family. Consistent patterns of behavior that lead to automatic action do not exist, and enactment of roles is overly flexible. A common example is an inconsistent parenting role. The parent sometimes is a strict authoritarian figure and at other times treats the child as a "best friend and confidant." This type of conduct can cause family members to become confused about what behavior is appropriate and who can be relied on for support. A general feeling of instability is created. During a crisis or rapid change, family members do not have a defined structure to "fall back on," and family disintegration can be a result.

FUNCTION

Friedman (1992) describes functioning as what the family does. Family functioning focuses on the processes used by the family to achieve its goals. These processes include communication among family members, goal setting, conflict resolution, caregiving, nurturing, and use of internal and external resources. The reproductive, sexual, economic, and educational goals that were once considered universal family goals no longer apply to all families. Although many families pursue these goals at various times during their development, they provide psychological support to their members throughout the life span. When the psychological needs of family members are not met, symptoms of family dysfunction are the usual consequence.

Family goals are more easily achieved when communication is clear and direct. Clear communication enhances problem solving and conflict resolution, and it can facilitate coping with life-threatening stressors (Box 8-3). Another family process, facilitating goal achievement, includes the ability to nurture and promote growth. Families must have available, and must be able to use, internal and external resources. A social network is useful as an external resource. Social relationships within the community act as buffers, particularly during times of stress, and reduce a family's vulnerability.

Developmental Stages Theory

Families, like individuals, change and grow over time. Although families are far from identical to one another, they tend to go through certain stages. Each developmental stage has its own challenges, needs, and resources and includes tasks that need to be completed before the family can successfully move on to the next stage. Societal changes and an aging population have precipitated

Research HIGHLIGHT   **Box 8-3**

RESEARCH ABSTRACT

Researchers explored themes in the bereavement experience of inner-city adolescents. Eight bereaved adolescents (median age 13, five girls, three boys) from poverty-level families attending an inner-city junior high school were observed in a semistructured group setting. Data were gathered using audiotaped recordings of eight group discussions examining the bereavement experiences of these adolescents. Chaos and stress were major themes pervading each discussion session. There was a lack of family and social support and a fear for their future. Avoidance was the major coping strategy used by the adolescents.

IMPLICATIONS FOR PRACTICE

- Inner-city adolescents need to be assessed carefully when they have experienced loss of significant others.
- Provision of mental health services in schools could provide intervention services for current and future problems.

REFERENCE

Van Epps J, Opie ND, Goodwin T: Themes in the bereavement experience of inner city adolescents, *J Child Adolesc Psychiatr Nurs* 10(1):25, 1997.

changes in the stages and transitions in the family life cycle. For example, adult children are not leaving the nest as predictably or as early as in the past, and many are returning home. In addition, more people are living into their 80s and 90s. Sixty-five is now considered the "backside of middle-age," and the length of the midlife stage in the family life cycle has increased, as has the later stage in family life.

McGoldrick and Carter's classic model of family life stages (1985) is based on expansion, contraction, and realignment of family relationships that support the entry, exit, and development of the members. This model provides the nurse with the emotional aspects of transition and the changes and tasks necessary for the family to proceed developmentally (Table 8-1). Thus the nurse can promote behaviors to achieve essential tasks and help families prepare for later transitions. It should be noted that this model does not address diverse family forms, such as blended families, single-parent families, or cohabiting partners.

THE FAMILY AND HEALTH

The health of the family is influenced by its relative position in society. Although American families exist within the same culture, they live in very different ways. The structure, function, and health of any family are a reflection and result of many variables. These variables include social class, economic resources, and racial and ethnic

Table 8-1   Stages of the Family Life Cycle

Family-Life-Cycle Stage	Emotional Process of Transition: Key Principles	Changes in Family Status Required to Proceed Developmentally
Between families: unattached young adult	Accepting parent-offspring separation	Differentiation of self in relation to family of origin Development of intimate peer relationships Establishment of self in work
Joining of families through marriage: newly married couple	Commitment to new system	Formation of marital system Realignment of relationships with extended families and friends to include spouse
Family with young children	Accepting new generation of members into system	Adjusting marital system to make space for children Taking on parental roles Realignment of relationships with extended family to include parenting and grandparenting roles
Family with adolescents	Increasing flexibility of family boundaries to include children's independence	Shifting of parent-child relationships to permit adolescents to move into and out of system Refocus on midlife material and career issues Beginning shift toward concerns for older generation
Launching children and moving on	Accepting multitude of exits from and entries into family system	Renegotiation of marital system as dyad Development of adult-to-adult relationships between grown children and their parents Realignment of relationships to include in-laws and grandchildren Dealing with disabilities and death of parents (grandparents)
Family in later life	Accepting shifting of generational roles	Maintaining own or couple functioning and interests in the face of physiological decline; exploration of new familial and social role options Support for more central role for middle generation Making room in system for wisdom and experience of older adults; supporting older generations without overfunctioning for them Dealing with loss of spouse, siblings, and other peers, and preparation for own death; life review and integration

Modified from McGoldrick M, Carter E: The stages of the family life cycle. In Henslin J, editor: *Marriage and family in a changing society*, New York, 1985, Free Press; and Walsh F: *Normal family processes*, New York, 1982, Guilford Press.

background. For some minority groups and the poor, patterned differences in family living are consequences of inequalities deeply rooted in society. Class and ethnicity can produce differences in the access of families to society's resources and rewards, and this access creates differences in family life, most significantly in different life chances for its members.

Distribution of wealth greatly affects the capacity to maintain health. Low educational preparation, poverty, and decreased amounts of support compound on one another, magnifying each other's impact *of* sickness in the family, and magnifying the amount of sickness *in* the family. Economic stability increases a family's access to adequate health care, creates more opportunity for education, increases sound nutrition, and decreases stress.

The family is the primary social context in which health promotion and disease prevention take place. The family strongly influences health behaviors of its mem-

bers. In turn, the health status of each individual influences how the family unit functions and its ability to achieve goals. When the family satisfactorily functions to meet its goals, its members tend to feel positive about themselves and their family. Conversely, when they do not meet goals, families view themselves as ineffective.

Good health may not be highly valued; in fact, detrimental practices may be accepted. In some cases a family member may provide mixed messages about health. For example, a parent may continue to smoke while telling children that smoking is bad for them. Family environment is crucial because health behavior reinforced in early life has a strong influence on later health practices. In addition, the family environment can be a crucial factor in an individual's adjustment to a crisis. Although relationships can be strained when confronted with illness, research indicates that family members have the potential to be a primary force for coping.

ATTRIBUTES OF HEALTHY FAMILIES

Ruebin Hill's classic work (1958) noted that it is possible to explain the reactions of crisis-proof and crisis-prone families. The crisis-proof, or effective, family is able to integrate the need for stability with the need for growth and change. This family has a flexible structure that allows adaptable performance of tasks and acceptance of help from outside the family system. The structure is flexible enough to allow adaptability but not so flexible that the family lacks cohesiveness and a sense of stability. The effective family has control over the environment and exerts influence on the immediate environment of home, neighborhood, and school. The ineffective, or crisis-prone, family may lack or believe it lacks control over these environments.

Recently health promotion research has started to focus on the stress-moderating effect of **hardiness** as a factor that contributes to long-term health. Family hardiness has been defined as "the internal strengths and durability of the family unit, characterized by a sense of control over the outcome of life events and hardships, a view of change as beneficial and growth-producing, and as an active rather than passive orientation in responding to stressful life events" (Danielson, and Hamel-Bissel, 1993).

Family Nursing

To begin working with families, nurses must have a scientific knowledge base in family theory, as well as an adequate knowledge base in family nursing. Although the past and present health care systems tend to emphasize the individual, nursing's attempt to include families when providing care dates back to Florence Nightingale. A family-focused approach has been most evident when caring for children because of the recognition that the family is central in a child's life. Family nursing is based on the assumption that all people regardless of age are a member of some type of family group. The goal of the family nurse is to help the family and its individual members reach and maintain maximum health. Family nursing is the focus of the future across all practice settings and is emphasized in all health care environments.

Nursing scholars have proposed different approaches for family nursing practice. Friedman (1992) suggests three focuses: (1) the individual with family as context, (2) relationships within the family (relational), and (3) processes within the family (transactional). A very similar approach is a focus on (1) the individual within the context of the family, (2) the family with the individual as context, and (3) the whole family as the unit of care. The perspective that a nurse uses is related to the clinical setting, the clinical problem, and realistic and practical considerations. Dealing with very complex family system problems often requires an interdisciplinary approach. The nurse must always be aware of the limits of nursing practice and make referrals when appropriate.

For the purposes of this chapter, family nursing practice is conceptualized as having three levels of approaches: (1) **family as context**, (2) **family as client**, and (3) the newest model, called **family as system**, which includes both relational and transactional concepts. If only one family member is receptive to nursing care, it is realistic and practical to view the family as context. When all family members are involved in the day-to-day care of one another, nursing intervention with one individual necessitates some change in the activities of the others, suggesting that family as client would be the best approach. Both family as context and family as client are approaches that can be useful in providing effective nursing care. The newest model, family as system, believes that a person should not be thought of as *either* an individual *or* a family member, but as *both*. Newby (1996) states that the family is viewed as an irreducible whole that cannot be understood by only examining the individual members of the family. In using this theoretical framework, nurses would consider the family to be in a constant state of change that is innovative and continuous. In more simple terms, it merely suggests that nurses must learn to view the family as more complex than a combination of individual members.

FAMILY AS CONTEXT

When the nurse views the family as context, the primary focus is on the health and development of an individual member existing within a specific environment (i.e., the client's family). Although the nurse focuses the nursing process on the individual's health status, the nurse also assesses the extent to which the family provides the individual's basic needs. These needs vary, depending on the individual's developmental level and situation. Since families provide more than just material essentials, their ability to help the client meet psychological needs must also be considered. Family members may need direct interventions themselves.

FAMILY AS CLIENT

When the family as client is the approach, family processes and relationships (e.g., parenting or family caregiving) are the primary focuses of nursing care. Family patterns versus individual characteristics are assessed by the nurse. The nursing process concentrates on the extent to which these patterns and processes are consistent with reaching and maintaining family and individual health.

FAMILY AS SYSTEM

It is important to understand that although theoretical and practical distinctions can be made between the family as context and the family as client, they are not necessarily mutually exclusive, and both are often used simultaneously, such as with the perspective of the family as system. The following clinical scenario illustrates the differences:

If the family is viewed as context, the nurse (Susan) focuses on the client (Patrick) as an individual. Susan assesses Patrick's knowledge of high-sodium foods, strategies for reducing the number of high-sodium foods in his diet, realistic opportunities to reduce the number and extent of perceived stressors in Patrick's work and family environment, and Patrick's knowledge and skill in stress management, such as relaxation or biofeedback techniques.

If the family is viewed as client, Susan assesses Patrick's family's current dietary patterns and their desire and resources for changing the patterns as a result of Patrick's hypertension. The nurse determines the demands placed on Patrick and the family. The family's capabilities to support Patrick's efforts at changing eating patterns and use of stress management techniques are also assessed.

Using the family as system, elements of both of the above perspectives are used. The decision and application is very individualized, based on the nursing assessment and clinical judgment. For instance, Susan decides, based on her assessment, that the cultural impact of diet on the family is great. The decision is made by the family for all members to adjust their diet to incorporate Patrick's needs, but Patrick decides that he is the only one who needs to join the gym to work on exercise and stress management. This combination of decisions is based on several factors: (1) Patrick wanting time away alone to "unwind," (2) the family's financial priorities to place their income toward living expenses and college savings, and (3) the family's schedules not allowing easy access to the gym. They will however, all decide to exercise as a family on the weekends, once per day for at least 45 minutes (walking, jogging, bicycling, or roller blading).

Nursing Process for the Family

Nurses interact with families in a variety of community-based and clinical settings. Family nursing process is the same, regardless of the setting or whether the focus is on the family as context or as client. It is also the same process as that used with individual clients. Three beliefs underlie the family approach to the nursing process:

1. That all individuals must be viewed within their family context
2. That families have an impact on individuals
3. That individuals have an impact on families

ASSESSING THE NEEDS OF THE FAMILY

Family assessment is essential to provide adequate family care and support. Box 8-4 shows an example of a family assessment tool. Although the family as a whole differs from individual members, the measure of family health is more than a summation of the health of all members. Areas unique to family assessment are the form, structure, and function of the family; its developmental stage; and its progress toward or accomplishment of developmental tasks (e.g., how many members are in the family, how many are living together, what stage of development [parenting or midlife] applies to the family.)

The nurse begins assessment by determining the client's definition of and attitude toward family and the extent to which the family can be incorporated into nursing care. To determine family form and membership, the nurse can ask whom the client considers family or with whom the client shares strong emotional feelings. If the client is unable to express a concept of family, the nurse can ask with whom the client lives, spends time, and shares confidences and then ask whether the client considers them to be family or like family. To further assess the family structure, the nurse asks questions that determine the power structure and patterning of roles and tasks (e.g., "Who decides where to go on vacation?" "How are tasks divided in your family?" "Who mows the lawn?" "Who usually prepares the meals?").

The nurse assesses family functions such as the ability to provide emotional support for members, the ability to cope with its current health problem or situation, and the appropriateness of its goal setting and progress toward achievement of developmental tasks (Figure 8-2). The nurse also assesses whether the family is able to provide and allocate sufficient economic resources and whether its social network is extensive enough to provide support.

A family's cultural background (see Chapter 7) is an important variable when assessing the family because race and ethnicity can affect structure, function, health beliefs, values, and the way events are perceived (Box 8-5). The United States is increasingly more diverse. A large number of immigrants enter the country daily, adding both to the number and to the variety of the many ethnic groups that make up the population. American health care institutions tend to operate from a white, middle-class perspective, and immigrant populations may have particular difficulty understanding and "fitting into" the system. Cultural assessment educators encourage the use of a "culturagram," which assesses and empowers culturally diverse families

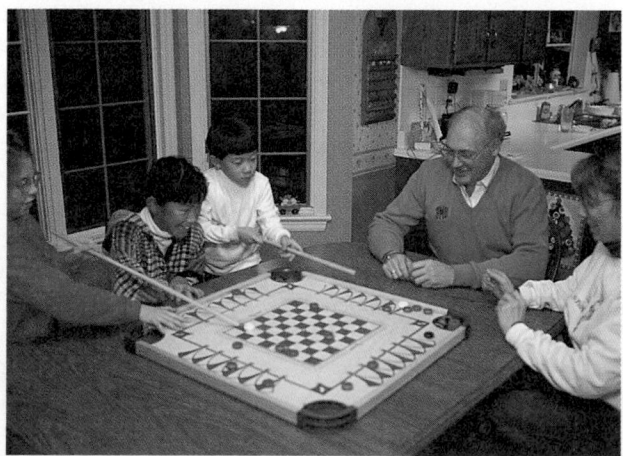

Figure 8-2 Observing family interactions assists in understanding family functioning.

Family Assessment Tool   Box 8-4

The family assessment tool is used when the beginning student interviews family members and observes family interaction. It is a guideline only and is not meant to be all-inclusive. The student must also ensure that individual health histories accompany this assessment.

FAMILY FORM AND STRUCTURE

Names of adults   Ages

_____

Relationship _____
                              (Single, married, divorced, separated, cohabiting)
Names of children   Ages

_____

_____

_____

Others living in home (include age, sex, relationship)

_____

Cultural background (include pertinent health beliefs, child-rearing practices, related health concerns)

_____

Developmental stage _____
Progress toward accomplishment of developmental tasks _____
Concerns related to developmental stage _____
Do family members consider pets a part of the family? What types? How many? Any concerns about their care?

_____

RESOURCES

Significant relatives and friends not occupying immediate residence _____
Strengths and coping skills _____
How does the family obtain health services? _____
Membership in community groups (e.g., church affiliation) _____
Education (formal and informal) _____
Finances (ability to meet current and future needs) _____

FAMILY PATTERNS

Persons working outside the home _____
Type of work _____ Number of hours _____
Satisfaction with work _____
How are the housekeeping tasks accomplished? _____
Are family members satisfied with the way tasks are divided? _____
How are child-rearing responsibilities divided? _____
Who makes the major decisions in the family? _____
Who makes day-to-day decisions? _____
Are family members satisfied with the way decisions are made? _____

FAMILY FUNCTION

Goals
Long term _____
Short term _____
Individual family member's goals _____
Are individual and family goals appropriate, considering their current health problem and status? _____
How are individual family members and the family as a whole coping with their current health problem and status?

_____

COMMUNICATION

Do husband and wife communicate regularly and effectively with each other? _____
Are family members able to communicate openly and honestly with each other? _____
Is conflict openly expressed and discussed? _____
Do family members respect one another's point of view? _____
Do family members offer emotional support to each other? _____

Perception of certain events can vary across cultural groups and have particular impact on families. For example, the death of a grandparent may take on greater significance in families whose culture emphasizes veneration of older family members. Stressors such as rape may have an especially devastating effect on Hispanic women and their families, since great importance is placed on female virginity (Congress, 1994).

Intergenerational support and patterns of living arrangements can be related to cultural background. For example, older Chinese, African-American, Japanese, and Hispanic persons are more likely to live in extended family households than are their white counterparts (Kamo, Zhou, 1994).

Health beliefs differ among various cultures, which may affect the decision of a family and its members about when and where to seek help. For example, Asians rarely consider symptoms as psychological and are not likely to go to mental health clinics (Congress, 1994).

and encourages ethnic-sensitive practice. This tool assesses a variety of factors such as language spoken in the home, impact of crisis events, and values regarding family, education, and work.

Drawing conclusions based on cultural backgrounds requires critical thinking and careful consideration. It is imperative to remember that categorical generalizations can be misleading (e.g., all Asian-Americans are good at math). As many caution, overgeneralizations in terms of racial and ethnic group characteristics do not lead to greater understanding of the culturally diverse family. Culturally different families can vary in meaningful and significant ways; however, neglecting to examine similarities can lead to inaccurate assumptions and stereotyping. Some studies reveal a lack of cultural differences in certain family processes. For example, more similarities than differences exist in parenting behaviors among white, African-American, Hispanic, and Asian-American parents.

FAMILY-FOCUSED CARE

Nursing practice is enhanced by a family-focused approach (St. John and Rolls, 1996). When the nurse has established a relationship with a family, it is important to identify potential and external resources so that effective nursing care approaches can be implemented. The assessment provides this information. Any plan for nursing care must be clearly understood by the family and mutually agreed on by all members. Whatever goals the nurse sets in caring for the family must be concrete and realistic, compatible with the family's developmental stage, and acceptable to family members. The nurse collaborates closely with all appropriate family members when determining what they hope to achieve with regard to the family's health.

Collaboration with family members is essential, whether the family is the client or the context of care. A positive collaborative relationship is based on mutual respect and trust (Figure 8-3). The nurse's ability to care facilitates the building of trust (see Chapter 6). The family must feel "in control" as much as possible. By offering alternative actions and asking family members for their own ideas and suggestions, the nurse can help to reduce the family's feelings of powerlessness. For example, offering options for how to prepare a low-fat diet or how to rearrange the furnishings of a room to accommodate a family member's disability gives the family an opportunity to express their preferences, make choices, and ultimately feel as though they have contributed. Collaboration also extends to other health care professionals: it is impossible to be all things to all families. Collaborating with other disciplines increases the likelihood of a comprehensive approach to the family's health care needs, and it ensures better continuity of care. Using other disciplines is particularly important when discharge planning from a health care facility to home or an extended care facility is necessary.

When the family is viewed as the client, the nurse will aim to support communication between all family members. This ensures that the family remains informed as to the nurse's intent and progress in providing health care. Often the nurse must support conflict resolution between family members so that each member can confront and resolve problems in a healthy way. The nurse also helps family members use the external and internal resources that are necessary. Ultimately, the nurse's aim is to help the family reach a point of optimal function, given the family's resources, capacities, and desire to become healthier.

A family-focused approach when the family is context requires that the nurse help family members better understand the illness of its member(s) and its effects. Whenever a family member becomes ill, there are implications for how the family's routines, rituals, and daily

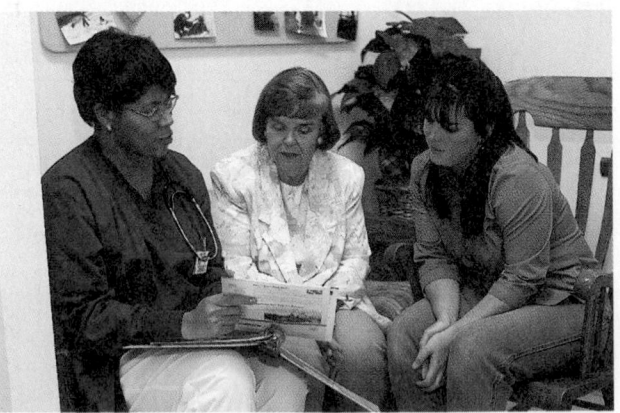

Figure 8-3 Nurse and family members.

practices are affected. For example, when a client returns home after recovering from a stroke, there can be significant changes regarding the work that is performed by various family members, the assistance that the stroke victim may require, and changes in the home environment to ensure the family member's safety. Often the person who has had to assume the majority of household responsibilities becomes ill and essentially changes roles with another family member. Long-term planning focuses on new, adaptive patterns so that the family can reach optimal individual health and family functioning. Collaboration with a family therapist, family social worker, or both can provide additional perspectives on the proper approach to care.

IMPLEMENTING FAMILY-CENTERED CARE

Whether caring for a client with the family as context or directing care to the family as client, nursing interventions aim to increase family members' abilities in certain areas, to remove barriers to health care, and to do things that the family cannot do for itself. The nurse guides the family in problem solving, provides practical services, and conveys a sense of acceptance and caring by listening carefully to family members' concerns and suggestions. One of the roles the nurse will need to adopt is that of educator. As a nurse, providing accurate health information about diagnosis, necessary self-care activities and the projected course of the condition helps the family caregiver to interpret behavior correctly and not to "blame" the client. Caregivers are not born with the knowledge of how to be caregivers, and older adults are not born with the knowledge of how to accept dependency (Box 8-6).

HEALTH PROMOTION

Implementation of family nursing care always includes health promotion. This encourages clients and families to reach their optimal levels of wellness. Identifying attributes that contribute to healthy, resilient families has been a focus of ongoing research for at least three decades. "Strong" families that adapt to expected transitions and unexpected crises and change tend to be characterized by clear communication among members, good problem-solving skills, a commitment to each other and to the family unit, and a sense of cohesiveness and spirituality. Health promotion programs aimed at enhancing these attributes are available for families and children in many communities. The nurse must be aware of family-oriented offerings so that families can be referred as needed. Health promotion behaviors that the nurse needs to encourage are often tied to the developmental stage of the family (e.g., adequate prenatal care for the childbearing family, effective parenting, and adherence to immunization schedules for child-rearing family) (Box 8-7).

Health education is a process by which information is shared by nurse and client in a two-way fashion.

Research HIGHLIGHT   **Box 8-6**

RESEARCH ABSTRACT

A study comparing 76 African-American and 86 Hispanic caregivers of relatives with Alzheimer's disease sought to determine the factors characterizing the process and outcomes of family caregiving. The study documents the personal strain and role strain in each ethnic group. Findings revealed that Hispanics were more vulnerable to each type of strain. This may be explained by the facts that Hispanics cared for more impaired relatives, were younger, and lacked expressive supportive relationships when compared with African-Americans.

IMPLICATIONS FOR PRACTICE
- Nurses must determine what meaning caregiving has for cultural groups and its effect on daily functioning.
- There is a need for the development of more sensitive assessment tools for caregiver strain, appropriate nursing interventions, and family and community supports.

REFERNCE
Cox C, Monk A: Strain among caregivers: comparing the experiences of African-American and Hispanic caregivers of Alzheimer's relatives, *Int J Aging Hum Dev* 43(2):93, 1996.

Family/client needs for information may be recognized through direct questioning, but they are generally far more subtle. The nurse may recognize that the father is fearful of cleaning the newborn's umbilical cord, or that an elderly woman is not using her cane or walker safely. Respectful communication is required. Often the subtle needs for information can be approached by saying, "I notice you are trying to not touch the umbilical cord; I see that a lot." Or "You use the cane the way I did before I was shown a way to keep from falling or tripping over it; do you mind if I show you?" The nurse's assuming a humble position before coming across as an authority on the subject often decreases the client's defenses and makes the client more willing to listen without feeling embarrassed.

One approach for meeting goals and promoting health is the use of family strengths. Families do not look at their own system as one that has inherent, positive components. The nurse can help the family become aware of its own unique strengths, thereby increasing its potential and capabilities. Family strengths include clear communication, adaptability, healthy child-rearing practices, support and nurturing among family members, and the use of crisis for growth. The nurse can help the family focus on these strengths instead of its problems and weaknesses. For example, the nurse can point out that a couple's 10-year marriage must have endured many crises and transitions. Therefore they are likely to have the capabilities to adapt to this latest challenge.

Client Teaching FOR FAMILY CAREGIVERS ABOUT NEWBORN CARE   Box 8-7

OBJECTIVES
- Client/family will be able to explain the purpose of cord care for the newborn.
- Client/family will be able to perform cord care correctly by return demonstration.
- Client/family will know who/when/where/why/how to call if problems develop.

TEACHING STRATEGIES
- Explain the following to the parents/grandparents/mature children:
  1. The umbilical cord does not have nerve endings, and if the baby cries, it is because of the cold alcohol near its skin, and because of being exposed to the cooler air.
  2. The cord needs to be kept dry to promote its "falling off" without risk of infection.
  3. Tub baths will have to wait until the cord falls off.
  4. Diapers will need to be rolled down so that the cord stays dry (and the penis needs to be pointed down for boys).

5. The cord will fall off at around 2 weeks of age.
6. Signs and symptoms of infection include a red ring around the umbilical area, foul smell, moist oozing cord, drainage at the site, and either a high or very low core temperature in the newborn.
- Allow them to watch the nurse perform cord care correctly and ask them to repeat for return demonstration.
- Offer them the opportunity to ask questions and repeat the skill as often as necessary for their comfort.

EVALUATION
- Ask the client and family to explain the reasons and strategies used to care for the cord.
- Review with the family and provide feedback during their demonstrations. Frame it positively and provide gentle encouragement.
- Remind them that the hospital nursing staff is available 24 hours a day, 365 days a year, for questions. They will refer the client/family to their own physician if there are problems or complications that are in need of medical evaluation.

CHALLENGES FOR FAMILY NURSING

Delegation in the management of nursing care activities can become a challenge in family nursing. Often nurses are trying to make an impact on family health by delegating duties to family members or to other members of the health care team. For example, the nurse helps family members learn how to provide certain types of procedures to care for an ill family member. With earlier discharge and more complex family needs at the time of discharge, planning for discharge begins with the initiation of care by the registered nurse.

Discharge planning with a family involves an accurate assessment of what will be needed for care at the time of discharge, along with any shortcomings in the home setting. For example, if a postoperative client will be discharged to home and the elderly husband does not feel comfortable with the dressing changes required, the nurse first finds out if there is anyone else in the family or neighborhood who would or could do this. If not, the nurse arranges for a home health service referral. If the client also needs exercises and strength training, then perhaps a physical therapy referral is required.

In newborn nursing, a home health referral is usually done for at least a follow-up phone call or one home visit. In many areas it is a free service for one visit. The nurse assesses the mother's physical, emotional, and informational needs regarding self and newborn care. The family is also assessed in terms of the situational crisis that a new member to a family creates. Usually this is a developmental crisis/stressor that provides the family with an opportunity for growth. The home health nurse examines roles, relationship strains, communication patterns, and whether all family members' health is optimized. Are such

needs as food, love, clothing, shelter, safety, security, and warmth being met?

Cultural sensitivity (see Chapter 7) in family nursing requires recognizing not only the diverse ethnic, cultural, and religious backgrounds of nurses dealing with the clients, but also the difference and similarities even within the same family. Different-age family members may ascribe to different folk remedies, health care beliefs, and religious influences. As nurses, we will encounter cultures in which we do not hold the same basic values, and it is our job as nurses to support the beliefs of these clients, not convince them to see our views. Geissler (1998) demonstrates how one of the best ways to learn about other cultures is to spend time simply observing their interactions, if possible. But learning can also be through the media, including documentaries, novels, newspaper articles, ethnographies, and research studies. We can visit markets and ethnic restaurants to learn about their foods and see the role that foods play in different cultures' health and illness. In family-centered care, we can choose to learn more by observing religious ceremonies, rituals, the symbolism in the arts and crafts of clients, and celebrations (e.g., marriage, births, graduations, and even clients' unique treatments of loss and death). Using effective and respectful communication techniques enables the nurse to determine the family's strengths and areas for potential problems.

Acute Care

Because family is becoming more of the focus, nursing will need to take more of a role in emphasizing family and client needs within the context of health care delivery in a managed care environment. Nurses need to be ever mindful of the early discharge states, paired with the increasing numbers of people within the household now being employed outside the home. These factors are challenges to the nurse to prepare family members to assist with health care or to locate appropriate community resources. Often when family members assume the role of caregiver, they may lose support from significant others. The nurse must be sure that families are willing to assume care responsibilities.

Family nursing requires a holistic view not only of the client but of the family as well. Nursing care in the acute environment can become very complex, making it a challenge for the client to feel cared for and to keep family members involved. A helpful tool is an independent journal in which clients and family members can communicate their thoughts, ideas, and reactions. The client or family members can use the journal as an open communication tool, updating entries based on their needs and observations of the acute care experience. It may also be helpful for a family member to use the journal as a record of care activities. The journal can be used to record data about when the client was turned, who visited, when the last pain medication was administered, and any special client requests. This information helps clients and families who are trying to "keep up" with what is happening in the acute care environment.

Restorative Care

In restorative care settings the challenge in family nursing is in trying to maintain clients' functional abilities within the context of the family. This includes having home health nurses help clients remain in their homes following acute injuries, surgery, or illness. It may also entail finding ways to better the lives of chronically ill and disabled individuals and their families. One way the nurse can best provide family care is through support of family caregivers. Family caregiving involves the routine provision of services and personal care activities for a family member by spouses, siblings, or parents. Caregiving activities might include personal care (bathing, feeding, grooming), monitoring for complications or side effects of medications, instrumental activities of daily living (shopping or housekeeping), and the ongoing emotional support and decision making that is necessary. Whenever an individual becomes dependent on another family member for care and assistance, there is significant stress affecting both the caregiver and the care recipient. In addition, the caregiver must continue to meet the demands of his or her normal lifestyle (e.g., raising children, working full time, or dealing with personal problems or illness). In many cases older adult children are caring for their parents or older relatives. Without adequate preparation and support from health care providers, caregiving can predispose the family to serious problems, including a decline in the health of the caregiver and that of the care receiver, dysfunctional relationships, and even abusive relationships.

Despite its demands, caregiving can be a positive and rewarding experience (Picot, Youngblut, and Zeller, 1997). Within the last 10 years, more attention has been given to the positive elements in caregiving that sustain family involvement. As a nurse, it is important to have a more holistic view of what caregiving involves. It is more than simply a series of tasks. Caregiving occurs within the context of a family. Whether it is a wife caring for a husband or a daughter caring for a mother, caregiving is an interactional process. The interpersonal dynamics between family members influence the ultimate quality of caregiving. Thus the nurse can play a key role in helping family members develop better communication and problem-solving skills to build the relationships needed for caregiving to be successful. Researchers have identified variables such as caregiver and care recipient expectations of one another influencing caregiving quality. Carruth (1996) has studied the concept of **reciprocity**, acknowledging the importance of the capability of care recipients to share exchanges that contribute to a caregiver's perception of self-worth. When the caregiver knows that the care recipient appreciates his or her efforts and values the assistance provided, a healthier and more satisfying caregiving relationship will exist.

Providing care and support for family caregivers often involves using available family and community resources. Establishing a caregiving schedule enabling all family members to participate, having extended family members share any financial burdens posed by caregiving, and having distant relatives send cards and letters communicating their support can be very useful. Use of community resources might include locating a service required by the family or providing respite care so that the family caregiver has time away from the care recipient. Examples of services that may be beneficial to families include caregiver support groups, housing and transportation services, food and nutrition services, housecleaning, legal and financial services, home health care, hospice, and mental health resources (Hogstel, 1998). Before referring a family to a community resource, it is critical that the nurse understand the family's dynamics and know whether support is desired or welcomed. Often a family caregiver will resist help, feeling obligated to be the sole source of support to the care recipient. The nurse must be sensitive to family relationships and help caregivers understand the normalcy of caregiving demands. Given the appropriate resources, caregivers can acquire the skills and knowledge necessary to effectively care for the loved ones within the context of the home while maintaining rich and rewarding personal relationships.

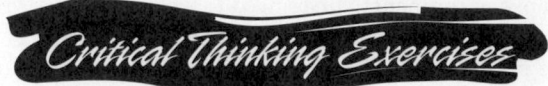

Key Concepts

- The family influences the lives of its members.
- Family members influence one another's health beliefs, practices, and status.
- Because the concept of family is highly individual, the nurse should base care on the client's attitude toward the family rather than on an inflexible definition of family.
- The family's structure, functioning, and relative position in society significantly influence its health and ability to respond to health problems.
- Two theories that help nurses assess families are the systems perspective and the developmental stages perspective.
- The family can be viewed as an important context for the individual family member, the family unit can be viewed as the client, or the family unit can be viewed as a system (simultaneously viewing the family as both client and family in context).
- Measures of family health involve more than a summation of individual members' health.
- The family's health is influenced by its social class, economic stability, and racial and ethnic background.
- Family members as caregivers are often spouses who may be either older adults themselves or adult children trying to work full time, care for aging parents, and launch teenagers successfully.
- Health promotion through health education is an important tool in family nursing practice.
- Cultural sensitivity is paramount to family nursing. Members may subscribe to differing beliefs, traditions, and restrictions even within the same generation.
- Family nursing requires that nurses continually examine the current trends in the American family and its health care implications.
- Family caregiving is an interactional process that occurs within the context of the relationships among its members.

Critical Thinking Exercises

1. Saundra is a home health nurse visiting a family consisting of an older adult mother and her daughter. In trying to gain a better understanding of this family and how it functions, Saundra learns about additional family members and the social and religious groups in which they participate. She also assesses the mother and daughter carefully in an effort to understand their personal values, beliefs, and concerns. To understand the caregiving relationship between mother and daughter, Saundra assesses the history of the relationship and the meaning it has for both family members. What theoretical approach is Saundra using in assessing this family?

2. Mr. Lee is a 70-year-old client who is being discharged from the hospital following a broken hip. The nurse determines the level of the client's mobility and the extent to which it will influence his ability to ambulate within his home. The nurse makes recommendations for rearranging furniture and placing extra chairs along Mr. Lee's usual walking path. After learning how dependent Mrs. Lee normally is on the client's ability to assist with daily activities, the nurse makes recommendations to the family for Mrs. Lee to hire a temporary housekeeper. Has the nurse provided care to the Lee family as context, client, or system?

3. Mr. and Mrs. Baillargeron, both in their early 50s, are the youngest members of large Catholic French Canadian families. They are employed full time and have two teenage children of their own. Both sets of their parents are in their 80s and have chronic health problems. All of their brothers and sisters are geographically farther away. How can you assist Mr. and Mrs. Baillargeron in developing extended resources to aid in caring for their parents and at the same time maintain the responsibilities of their own family unit?

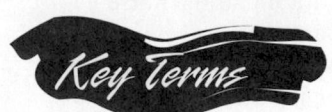

Key Terms

Blended family, *p. 140*
Extended family, *p. 140*
Family, *p. 139*
Family as client, *p. 145*
Family as context, *p. 145*
Family as system, *p. 145*
Hardiness, *p. 145*
Nuclear family, *p. 140*
Reciprocity, *p. 151*
Single-parent family, *p. 140*

References

Carruth AK: Development and testing of the caregiver reciprocity scale, *Nurs Res* 45:92, 1996.

Centers for Disease Control and Prevention, U.S. Public Health Service: *HIV/AIDS surveillance reports* 10(2), 1998.

Clemen-Stone S, McGuire SL, Eigsti DG: *Comprehensive community health nursing*, St. Louis, 1998, Mosby.

Congress EP: The use of culturagrams to assess and empower culturally diverse families, *Fam Soc J Contemp Hum Serv* 23:531, 1994.

Cox C, Monk A: Strain among caregivers: comparing the experiences of African-American and Hispanic caregivers of Alzheimer's relatives, *Int J Aging Hum Dev* 43(2):93, 1996.

Danielson CB, Hamel-Bissel BP: *Families: health and illness*, St. Louis, 1993, Mosby.

Friedman M: *Family nursing: theory and assessment*, ed 3, New York, 1992, Appleton-Century-Crofts.

Geissler EM: *Pocket guide to cultural assessment*, ed 2, St. Louis, 1998, Mosby.

Harvey E: Short-term and long-term effects of early parental employment on children: the National Longitudinal Survey of Youth, *Dev Psychol*, 1999.

Hill R: Generic features of families under stress, *Soc Casework* 39:145, 1958.

Hogstel MO: *Community resources for older adults: a guide for case managers*, St. Louis, 1998, Mosby.

Kamo Y, Zhou M: Living arrangements of elderly Chinese and Japanese in the United States, *J Marriage Fam* 56(3):544, 1994.

Lindsey EW: Homelessness. In McHenry PC, Price SH, editors: *Families and change: coping with stressful events*, London, 1994, Sage Publications.

McGoldrick M, Carter E: The stages of the family life cycle. In Henslin J, editor: *Marriage and family in a changing society*, New York, 1985, Free Press.

Newby NM: Chronic illness and the family life-cycle, *J Adv Nurs* 23(4):786, 1996.

Nichols SY: Work and family stress. In McHenry PC, Price SJ, editors: *Families and change: coping with stressful events*, London, 1994, Sage Publications.

Picot SJF, Youngblut J, Zeller R: Development and testing of a measure of perceived caregiver rewards in adults, *J Nurs Meas* 5:33, 1997.

St. John W, Rolls C: Teaching family nursing: strategies and experiences, *J Adv Nurs* 23(1):91, 1996.

Schwartz AN: Psychological dependency: an emphasis on the later years. In Ragan P, editor: *Aging parents*, Los Angeles, 1979, Andrus Gerontology Center, University of Southern California.

U.S. Bureau of the Census: *Statistical abstract of the United States: full, 1994, and census information polls in 1997*, Washington, DC, 1997, The Bureau; http//:www.census.gov.

Van Epps J, Opie ND, Goodwin T: Themes in the bereavement experience of inner city adolescents, *J Child Adolesc Psychiatr Nurs* 10(1):25, 1997.

Walsh F: *Normal family processes*, New York, 1982, Guilford Press.

Ward JW, Duchin JS: The epidemiology of HIV and AIDS in the United States, *AIDS Clin Rev*, p 1, 1997-1998.

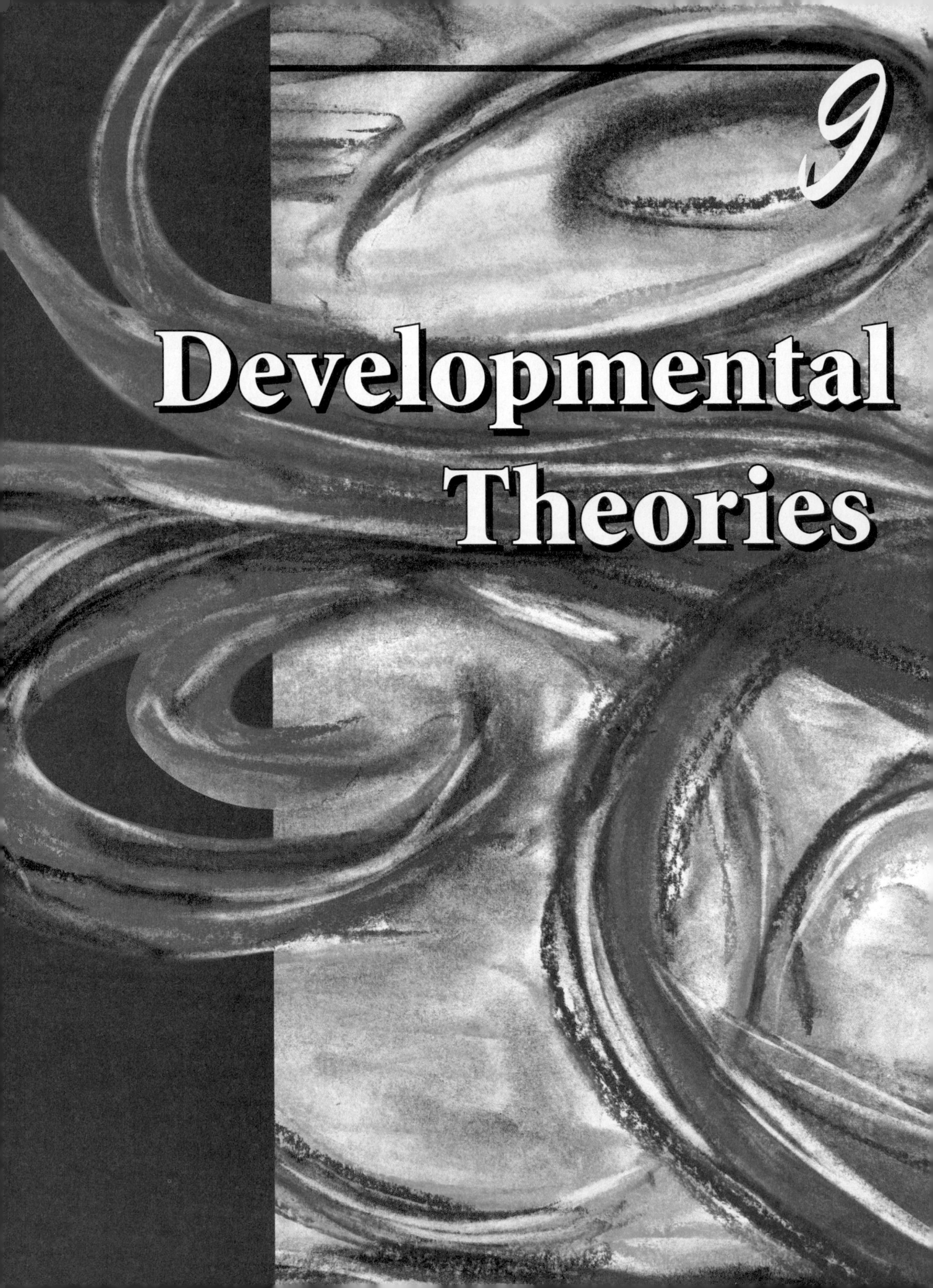

Developmental Theories

9

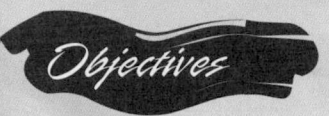
Mastery of content in this chapter will enable the student to:

- Define the key terms listed.
- Describe biophysical developmental theories under the categories of genetic theory, nongenetic cellular theories, and the physiological theories of aging.
- Describe and compare the psychosocial theories proposed by Freud, Erikson, Havighurst, and Gould.
- Identify the characteristics of temperament.
- Describe Piaget's theory of cognitive development.
- Discuss how Kohlberg built upon Piaget's stages of moral development.
- Discuss Gilligan's criticism of Kohlberg's moral developmental stage theory.
- Apply developmental theories when planning interventions in the care of clients.

Role of Theories

A theory is an organized and logical set of statements about a subject. Human developmental theories are models intended to account for how and why people become as they are (Thomas, 1997). Theories provide the framework to clarify and organize existing observations and to try to explain and predict human behavior (Schroeder, 1992). It is important to recognize the complexities of human development and the theories that explain human development.

Developmental theories are important because nurses assess and treat a person's response to an illness. Understanding developmental theory provides the basis for nurses to understand those responses seen in their clients.

Growth Versus Development

It is important for nurses to know the difference between growth and development. Growth refers to the quantitative changes that can be measured and compared to norms, for example, taking the height and weight of a pediatric client and comparing the measurements to the standardized growth charts. Development implies a progressive and continuous process of change leading to a state of organized and specialized functional capacity, for example, a child's progressions from rolling over to crawling to walking are developmental changes. These changes can be measured quantitatively but are more distinctly measured in qualitative changes (Haywood, 1993). Theories explaining human development were developed through study of limited cultural and gender-based populations, and the ability to generalize these theories to other groups may be limited.

Four Areas of Theory Development

To help the reader understand the number of developmental theories, this chapter has been grouped into four main areas of theory development: biophysical, psychosocial, cognitive, and moral development. The areas of learning theory and spiritual development are covered in Chapters 23 and 28, respectively.

Biophysical development attempts to describe the way our physical bodies grow and change. These changes are quantified and can be compared against established norms. Biophysical developmental theory is defined as the process of biological maturation.

Psychosocial developmental theories attempt to describe the development of the human personality and behavior. This development is thought to occur with varying degrees of influence from the internal biological forces and the external societal/cultural forces.

Cognitive development is focused on rational thinking processes that include the changes in how people come to perform intellectual operations. These operations are related to the ways persons learn to understand the world in which they live.

Moral development focuses on the description of moral reasoning. Moral reasoning is how people think about the rules of ethical or moral conduct but does not predict what a person would actually do in a given situation. Moral development is the ability of an individual to distinguish right from wrong and to develop ethical values on which to base his or her actions (Rich and DeVitis, 1985).

Biophysical Developmental Theories

Biophysical development is how our physical bodies grow and change. The changes that occur as a newborn infant grows into adulthood can be quantified and compared against established norms. How does the physical body age? What are the triggers that move the body from the physical characteristics of childhood, through adolescence, to the physical changes of adulthood? Thinking of this process in the terms of developmental theory is a way to organize current findings about why that developmental process occurs.

Biophysical developmental theory is defined as the process of biological maturation. Biophysical development was described by Gesell, who initiated the study and development of a theory based on his observations of children as related to their physical growth. The other theories covered in this section are named by how they define the aging process; they are not linked to any one person but instead are being studied by a number of different scientists.

GESELL'S THEORY OF DEVELOPMENT

Arnold Gesell (1880-1961) was a psychologist who also obtained his medical degree to help him explain the physiological processes he was observing in the behavior of the children he studied. Through extensive observations in the 1940s, he developed behavior norms that still serve as a primary source of information for childhood development today.

Fundamental to Gesell's theory of development is that although each child's pattern of growth (development) is unique, this pattern is directed by the activity of the genes. Environmental factors can support, inflect, and modify the pattern, but they do not generate the progressions of development (Gesell, 1948). Gesell found the pattern of maturation as a fixed developmental sequence in all humans. Sequential development is seen in fetuses, where there is a specified order of development of the various organ systems (Crain, 1992). After birth, children grow according to their genetic blueprint and gain skills in an orderly fashion, but at each individual's own pace. For example, most children will learn first how to crawl before they learn how to walk, but not every child develops those skills at exactly the same time. Gesell was clear to point out that the environment does play a part in the development of the child, but it does not have any part in the sequence of development. Gesell believed that a child could not be pushed to develop faster than that child's own unique timetable. Although Gesell felt genes controlled the person's development, he did not know the process by which the genes programmed development in an individual.

There are many other theories of biophysical development, but each falls into one of three categories: the ge-

Table 9-1	**Biophysical Theories**
Theory Category	Specific Theories
Genetic theories—how DNA molecules transfer information that determines function and life span of cells	Programmed cell death Radiation influence on DNA molecule Error theory of aging
Nongenetic cellular theories—how changes in the molecules and structural elements impair a cell's effectiveness	Wear and tear theory Cross-linking theory Free radical theory
Physiological theories of aging—theories related to the performance of a single organ or impairment of the physiological control mechanisms	Caloric intake and effect on aging Effect of stress on immune system Effect of stress alone on the body

netic theories of aging, nongenetic cellular theories, and the physiological theories of aging (Table 9-1).

GENETIC THEORIES OF AGING

The genetic theories of aging try to define how the DNA molecules transfer information to the formation of proteins, which determines the function and life span of specific cells (Shock, 1977; Schroeder, 1992; Cavanaugh, 1993; Eliopoulos, 1999). Why do members of families who have parents and grandparents who have lived a long life, live longer than members of families whose parents die before the age of 50? This programmed cell death is a function of physiological processes that cause cells to trigger processes in other cells and self-destruct. It is unknown how this self-destruct program is triggered. Currently, considerable research is being done that explores this theory of aging (Eliopoulos, 1999).

One DNA theory looks at how exposure to radiation shortens the life span. Laboratory studies have shown that animals have a shortened life span when exposed to nonlethal does of radiation. It is felt that this can occur in humans, which is supported by the fact that ultraviolet light causes wrinkling of the skin and promotes skin cancer. The error theory of cellular aging looks at how errors in the genetic code can occur by the process of transporting DNA information in the production of the protein and enzyme molecules required by the cell (Shock, 1977; Schroeder, 1992; Cavanaugh, 1993; Eliopoulos, 1999). When these errors occur, the altered protein or enzyme synthesis leads to defective cellular structure and function.

NONGENETIC CELLULAR THEORIES

Nongenetic cellular theories look at the cellular level (as opposed to the DNA) and how changes that take place in the molecules and structural elements of cells impair their effectiveness (Shock, 1977; Schroeder, 1992; Cavanaugh, 1993; Eliopoulos, 1999). The wear-and-tear theory works on the premise that our bodies just "wear out." This theory can explain some specific processes of aging (such as osteoarthritis) that contribute to aging, but it does not explain general aging.

Cross-linking theory finds that certain proteins within human cells interact with molecules to form cross-links that alter the physical and chemical properties of the molecules involved. These molecules then no longer function the same way as they did before and accumulate over time. These processes occur in arteries, muscles, and skin tissues and account for age-related changes in the body. This theory is the premise for the research described in Box 9-1.

The free radical theory proposes that aging is due to unstable molecules that are highly reactive chemicals causing cellular damage and thereby impairing the functioning of the organ. The rate of the formation of these free radicals is accelerated by radiation but inhibited by the presence of antioxidants, lathyrogens, prednisolone, and penicillamine. This theory has spurred research in the inhibitory properties of the antioxidants (especially vitamins A, C, and E) and how these vitamins counteract the effects of free radicals, thereby extending life.

PHYSIOLOGICAL THEORIES OF AGING

Physiological theories of aging look at either the breakdown in the performance of a single organ or in the impairment of the physiological control mechanisms (Shock, 1977; Schroeder, 1992; Cavanaugh, 1993; Eliopoulos, 1999). Under this category, various theories relate to single organs or metabolic processes being tested. One theory looks at how many calories one eats. Reducing calories lowers the risk of premature death and can slow down the normative age-related changes, which is supported by the facts we currently know about the problems caused by obesity, high cholesterol levels, and vitamin deficiencies.

Stress alone or in combination as an effect on the immune system are the bases for two other theories being tested to describe the theory of aging. Some theorists suggest that alterations in the effectiveness of the immune system are responsible for aging. The body may lose its ability to distinguish its own proteins from foreign ones and will attack and destroy its own tissues. The second immunological theory proposes that, as the body ages, it is less able to fight off infection, which is felt to be a factor in the development of chronic diseases such as cancer, diabetes, and cardiovascular disease (see Chapter 30).

• • •

The biophysical theories all attempt to describe the processes of why our bodies age. Gesell went as far as to propose that it is our biological body that determines our behavioral development (Figure 9-1). The psychosocial

---

Research HIGHLIGHT   **Box 9-1**

NATURE VERSUS NURTURE: RESEARCH INTO BRAIN DEVELOPMENT

RESEARCH ABSTRACT

Through the use of magnetic resonance imaging (MRI), positron emission tomography (PET), magnetic resonance spectroscopy (MRS), and functional MRI (fMRI), a number of researchers have been able to map the brain as we have never been able to before. At birth, a baby's brain contains 100 billion neurons. Although the brain contains almost all of the nerve cells it will ever have, the wiring between the nerve cells has not been established. The firing of neurons that occurs through stimulation received through the senses builds the connections between the neurons, creating the physical structure of the brain. The first 3 years of life see the most activity related to the firing between the neurons, and many pathways are established during that time. By the age of 10, those pathways that have not been repeatedly used are lost. Children who do not play much or are rarely touched develop brains 20% to 30% smaller than normal for their age. Contrary to not receiving enough stimulation, other children may be hypersensitive to sensory stimulation, causing the brain to "shut down." These children are at risk for developing autism, and parents must find ways to decrease disorienting noises and lights for this child. Parents also play an important role in setting up the neural circuitry that helps children regulate their responses to stress. If a child is exposed to abuse early in life, the circuitry in the brain is then wired to respond to even the slightest threat with a full stress response (e.g., elevated heart rate and release of stress hormones).

IMPLICATIONS FOR PRACTICE

- Because nursing applies research from not only its own discipline but that of other disciplines, this research is important to encourage and foster normal growth and development. Nurses involved with child-bearing and child-rearing families can teach parents about how the neurons develop pathways. Repeated experiences are what develop the connections in the brain, so the types of experiences a child has programs the brain to respond. Finding the right balance of experiences and stimulation, and at the same time protecting the child from harmful stimulation, is important information to share with parents.
- Adults are also affected by this research. The old "if you don't use it, you lose it" theory applies to the neural pathways. Adults are encouraged to continue to learn new things to maintain the neural pathway connections, which help to maintain memory and cognitive functioning.

REFERENCE
From Nash JM: Fertile minds, *Time*, 149(5):8, 1997.

Table 9-2 Comparison of Major Developmental Theories

Developmental Stage (Approximate Age)	Freud (Psychosexual Development)	Erikson (Psychosocial Development)	Piaget (Logical and Cognitive Development) Piaget (Moral Development)	Kohlberg (Development of Moral Reasoning)
Infancy (Birth to 18 months)	Oral stage	Trust versus mistrust Ability to trust others/sense of own trustworthiness versus withdrawal and estrangement	Sensorimotor period Stage 1—reflexes cause actions Stage 2—repeats pleasing actions Stage 3—makes interesting action last, finds partially hidden object	
Early childhood/toddler (18 months to 3 years)	Anal stage	Autonomy versus shame and doubt Self-control without loss of self-esteem Ability to cooperate/express self versus compulsive compliance; defiance	Stage 4—coordinates more than one action, finds hidden object Stage 5—tries new actions to see what happens Stage 6—holds idea for later action Preoperational period Preconceptual—uses symbols (language, play) to recall past, represent present, and anticipate future	
Preschool (3-5 years)	Phallic stage (Oedipus complex; Electra complex)	Initiative versus guilt Realistic sense of purpose/able to evaluate own behavior versus self-denial/self-restriction	Intuitive—increased use of symbols; ability to see simple relationships Egocentric—can see things from only one point of view *Heteronomous morality—follows rules of those in authority*	Level I—preconventional level Stage 1—punishment and obedience orientation—obeys rules to avoid punishment

Age period	Freud	Erikson	Piaget	Kohlberg
Childhood (6-12 years)	Latent stage	Industry versus inferiority Realization of competence/perseverance versus feeling one will never be any good, withdrawal from school and peers	Concrete operations period Developing logical thinking related to concrete tasks that are immediate and physically present	Level I—preconventional level Stage 2—instrumental relativist orientation—conforms to obtain rewards or favors
Early adolescence (12-14 years)	Genital stage	Identity versus identity diffusion Coherent sense of self/plan to actualize abilities versus feelings of confusion/indecisiveness or antisocial behavior	Formal operations period Stage 1 (preconventional)—ability to think in abstract manner develops, scientific reasoning emerges Concern about satisfying own needs *Autonomous morality—moral judgments based on mutual respect for the rules and mutual regard for person*	Level II—conventional level Stage 3—good boy-nice girl orientation—seeks good relations and approval of family group; orientation to interpersonal relations of mutuality
Middle adolescence (14-16 years)	Genital stage	Identity versus identity diffusion	Formal operations period Stage 2 (conventional)—ability to order ideas—and possibilities	Level II—conventional level Stage 4—society-maintaining orientation—obedience to law and order in society; maintenance of social order—shows respect for authority
Late adolescence (17-21 years)	Genital stage	Identity versus identity diffusion	Formal operations period Stage 3—true formal thought: construction of all possible combinations of relations; deductive hypothesis testing	Level III—postconventional level Stage 5—social contract orientation—concern with individual rights and legal contract; social contract; utilitarian lawmaking perspective Level III—postconventional level Stage 6—universal ethical principle orientation—higher law and conscience orientation; orientation to internal decisions of conscience but without clear rationale or universal principles

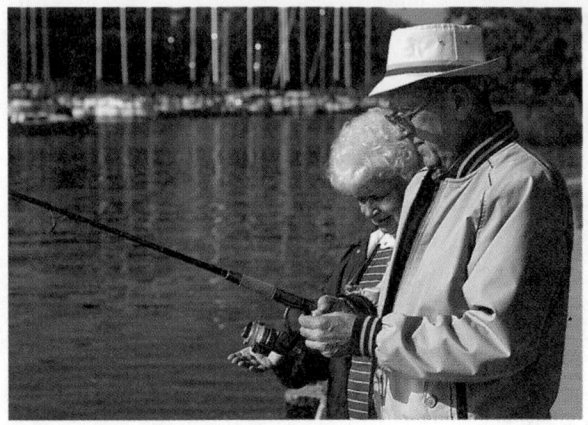

Figure 9-1   A retired couple enjoying fishing together. From Sorrentino S: *Assisting with patient care*, St. Louis, 1999, Mosby.

theories look at the process of development from a very different perspective.

Psychosocial Theory

The **psychosocial theories** attempt to describe human development from the perspective of personality, thinking, and behavior (Table 9-2). Human behavior is extremely complex and therefore difficult to capture within one theory. Many theorists have devoted their entire lifetime to the development of a consistent understanding of how we become successful human beings.

SIGMUND FREUD

The first person to provide a formal, structured theory of personality development was Sigmund Freud (1856-1939). Writing at the turn of the century from observations of his psychoanalytic patients, he built his theory (Ashburn, 1978; Crain, 1992). His theory is grounded in the belief that two internal biologic forces essentially drive psychological change in the child: sexual and aggressive energies. Motivation for behavior is to achieve pleasure and avoid pain created by these forces. These forces come into conflict with the reality of the world, and maturational changes occur.

His **psychoanalytic model of personality development** has five psychosexual developmental stages associated with a sequencing of sensual pleasurable zones. In his theory, the definition of sexual is anything that produces bodily pleasure (Crain, 1992).

Stage 1: Oral (Birth to 12 to 18 Months).   Initially sucking, oral satisfaction is not only vital to life, but extremely pleasurable in its own right. Late in this stage, the infant begins to realize that the mother/parent is some-

thing separate from self. Disruption in the physical or emotional availability of the parent (e.g., mental disability, chronic illness) could have an impact on the infant's development.

Stage 2: Anal (12 to 18 months to 3 Years).   The focus of pleasure changes to the anal zone. Children become increasingly aware of the pleasurable sensations of this body region with interest in the products of their effort. This is the stage when the child is first asked to withhold pleasure to meet parental/societal expectations through the toilet-training process.

Stage 3: Phallic or Oedipal (3 to 6 Years).   It is during this stage that the sexual organ gains prominence. According to Freud, the boy becomes more interested in the penis; the girl becomes aware of the absence of the penis. These are times of exploration and imagination as the child fantasizes about the parent as the first love interest. Freud believed that sexual wishes are temporarily driven underground through the action of the developing superego, or conscience, as the resolution of this stage.

Stage 4: Latency (6 to 12 Years).   This is a stage in which Freud believed that the aggressive and sexual urges, submerged in the unconscious at the end of the oedipal stage, are channeled into productive activities that are socially acceptable. Latency was thought to be a time of minimal sexual interest or activity. Within the educational and social worlds of the child, there is much to learn and accomplish. This is where the child places energy and effort.

Stage 5: Genital (Puberty Through Adulthood).   This is Freud's final stage. He did not formally continue his theory into adulthood. This is a time of turbulence when earlier sexual urges reemerge to be dealt with. Freud believed that the task of moving from the sexual attachment to the parent of childhood to the separation and emotional independence of the adult sexual partner is difficult to achieve.

Components of the Personality.   Through these stages the components of personality develop. Freud believed that the functions of these components govern adult life. These components are the id, the ego, and the superego. The id, basic instinctual impulses driven to achieve pleasure, is the most primitive part of the personality and originates with the infant. The ego represents the reality components mediating conflicts with the world when the person is driven by the id. The ego helps us judge reality accurately, regulate impulses, and make good decisions. The third component, superego, performs inhibiting, restraining, and prohibiting actions. Often referred to as the conscience, the superego is initially derived from the standards of outside social forces (parent, teacher).

The goal of development as seen by Freud was the development of balance between the pleasures of the world and the domination of guilt and shame. The fully developed adult would have a strong sense of conscience that allowed the experience of pleasure within a clear appraisal of reality. Although Freud's theory has been soundly criticized for gender and cultural biases, it is clear that he gave other theorists a basis for observation of emotion and behavior. He started with a nearly clean slate and developed a complex theory of personality development.

ERIK ERIKSON

Freud had a strong influence on his psychoanalytic followers, including Carl Jung, Alfred Adler, and others who continued to develop and define his theory. One of the most notable was Erik Erikson (1902-) who was a student of Anna Freud. (Erikson, 1963, 1997; Maier, 1965) Erikson extended Freud's model by placing psychoanalytic theory within a social/cultural perspective. He believed that development was an evolutionary process based on sequencing biological, psychological, and social events. He added three new stages of the adult's years detailing the completion of the life cycle. He believed that the maturation of bodily functions was linked with expectations of society and culture in which the person live.

Erikson defined **eight stages of life,** the first five coinciding with Freud's stages. He believed that social and cultural expectations compel the individual to establish equilibrium related to a specific developmental task at hand. Each task is framed as opposing tendencies, such as the adolescent's need to develop a sense of personal identity challenged by many confusing choices. These tasks are triggered by life forces.

Each stage builds on the successful resolution of the previous developmental conflict. Readiness for the task is necessary for success. Erikson believed that ideal resolution of developmental conflicts involves achievement of balancing positive features of the conflict experience with the negative. For example, the infant's trust is built through consistent, reliable caregiving; some frustration is experienced when needs occasionally go unmet. The person achieves a general trust with the ability to differentiate that all people are not equally trustworthy. Research built upon this concept is presented in Box 9-2. In adult life, the person must have some skepticism to avoid being cheated by unsavory people. This is the function of Erickson's concept of balance.

Eight Stages of Life
Acquiring Trust While Overcoming the Sense of Mistrust (Birth to 1 Year).
Starting with oral satisfaction, the infant learns to trust the caregiver as well as self. Trust is achieved when the infant will let the caregiver out of sight without undo distress. The caregiver is representative of the greater world. The infant has learned not only to trust others but also self. Key to this stage is the caregiver's confidence that he or she is doing things in a way

| *Research* HIGHLIGHT | Box 9-2 |

EFFECT OF MOTHER'S POSTPARTUM DEPRESSION ON LONG-TERM SEQUELAE OF CHILD'S DEVELOPMENT

RESEARCH ABSTRACT

An analysis of nine studies looked at the potential long-term sequelae for children whose mothers had experienced postpartum depression. It has been well known that there are short-term effects of postpartum depression on the maternal-infant interaction, but the long-term effects have not been documented. The results showed a small but significant effect was found on a child's cognitive and emotional development when the mother experienced postpartum depression.

IMPLICATIONS FOR PRACTICE
- Early recognition and treatment of a woman's postpartum depression has long-term effects on not only the mother but her child as well.
- Clinicians must start identifying those women at risk for developing depression after delivery.
- Interventions that target the risk factors associated with postpartum depression could be started prenatally and must be continued through the postpartum period.
- By decreasing the incidence of postpartum depression, the adverse effects on child development can be prevented.

REFERENCE

Beck CT: The effects of postpartum depression on child development: a meta-analysis, *Arch Psychiatr Nurs* 12(1):12, 1998.

that is good for the infant. The parent's struggle with building the sense of competence can be assisted by the nurse's use of anticipatory guidance and other educative interventions. The parent may need to have guidance to understand the importance of a safe environment when meeting the child's need to explore through creeping and crawling before walking.

Acquiring Autonomy While Combating a Sense of Shame and Doubt (1 to 3 Years). The growing child now realizes, in part through bowel and bladder control experiences, that there is a choice of holding on or letting go. There is also opportunity to learn that parents and society have expectations about these choices. Choices include activities related to relationships, personal desires, and manipulative objects such as toys. We observe the child's changing abilities to share toys and withhold wishes to have his own way. The manner in which the regulation of autonomy occurs with empathetic guidance and support from caregivers has an impact on the achievement of successful control without loss of self-esteem. The nurse can model empathetic guidance that indicates support for and understanding of the challenges of the

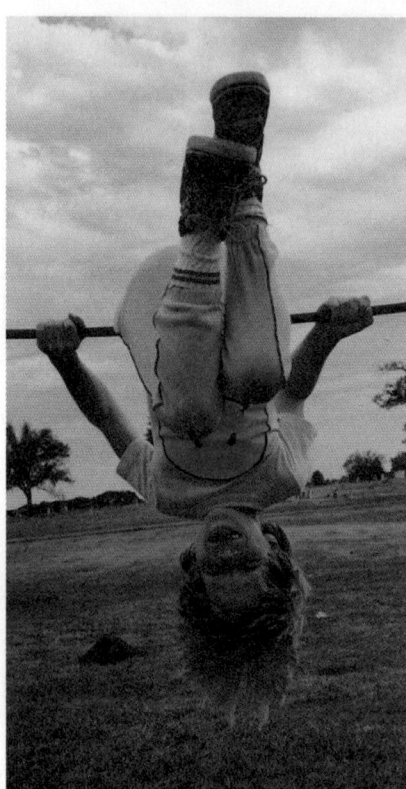

Figure 9-2 Play is therapeutic at any age and provides a means for release of tension and stress in the environment. From Wong DL: *Nursing care of infants and children,* ed 6, St. Louis, 1999, Mosby.

stage rather than harsh or violence-prone discipline for the toddler.

Acquiring Initiative and Overcoming a Sense of Guilt (3 to 6 Years).   Children can now begin to make plans, set goals, and mark achievement with efforts based on wants or urges. This is a time of expanding physical and intellectual abilities (Figure 9-2). The child may make plans in the sandbox that may extend into another child's space. When conflict occurs, autonomy may be thwarted, leading to frustration and guilt. Social prohibitions in the form of the superego occur, causing the failure of the plan. A crisis may occur when the plans fail. Guilt may occur if the caregiver's responses to the crisis are too punitive. Teaching cooperative behaviors to the child can help the family avoid the risks of parental violence or childhood behavior disorders associated with risk for altered development. (Box 9-3) (North American Nursing Diagnosis Association [NANDA], 1999)

Acquiring a Sense of Industry While Fending Off a Sense of Inferiority (6 to 11 Years).   Children are eager to apply themselves to learning socially productive skills and tools. They learn to work and play with their peers. Lack of achievement occurs in part because children

---

⟨ **NURSING DIAGNOSES** Box 9-3
GROWTH AND DEVELOPMENT

GROWTH, ALTERED, RISK FOR
Prenatal Risk Factors
   Altered nutrition
   Substance use/abuse
Individual Risk Factors
   Caregiver and/or individual maladaptive feeding behaviors
   Chronic illness
   Substance abuse
Environmental Risk Factors
   Deprivation
   Poverty
   Violence
Caregiver Risk Factors
   Abuse
   Mental illness
   Mental retardation
   Severe learning disability

DEVELOPMENT, ALTERED, RISK FOR
Prenatal Risk Factors
   Substance abuse
   Lack of, late, or poor prenatal care
   Poverty
Individual Risk Factors
   Congenital or genetic disorders
   Brain damage (hemorrhage in postnatal period, shaken baby, abuse, accident)
   Chronic illness
   Failure to thrive
   Inadequate nutrition
   Behavior disorders
   Substance abuse
Environmental Risk Factors
   Poverty
   Violence
Caregiver Risk Factors
   Abuse
   Mental illness
   Mental retardation
   Severe learning disability

lack adult capacities; this may create a sense of inadequacy and inferiority for children as they judge their performance. Imagine a learning disabled child struggling to learn to read. Because of a biological difference and the delayed achievement, this child may have difficulty avoiding a sense of inferiority. Erikson believed that the adult's attitudes toward work can be traced to successful achievement of this task (Erikson, 1963).

Acquiring a Sense of Identity While Overcoming Role Confusion (Puberty).   Dramatic physiological changes associated with sexual and aggressive drives mark this stage. There are also new social demands, opportunities, and conflicts that relate to the emergent identity and separation from family. This is the milieu in which identity development begins. Alternatives are tried with the goal of achieving some perspective or direction to answer "Who am I?" Acquiring a sense of identity is essential for making adult decisions such as choice of vocation or marriage partner. Each adolescent moves in his or her unique way into society as an interdependent member (Figure 9-3). The nurse can provide education and anticipatory guidance for the parent about the changes and challenges to the adolescent.

Achieving a Sense of Intimacy While Avoiding Isolation (Young Adult).

Young adults, having developed as sense of identity, deepen their capacity to love others and care for them through work (Table 9-3). This is the time to become fully participative in the community, enjoying adult freedom and responsibility. If young persons have not achieved a sense of personal identity, they may experience feelings of isolation from others and the inability to form attachments. Their willingness to share and mutually regulate their lives with another marks the completion of this task. The hospitalized young adult may have privacy needs related to the achievement of intimacy for which the nurse can make accommodations.

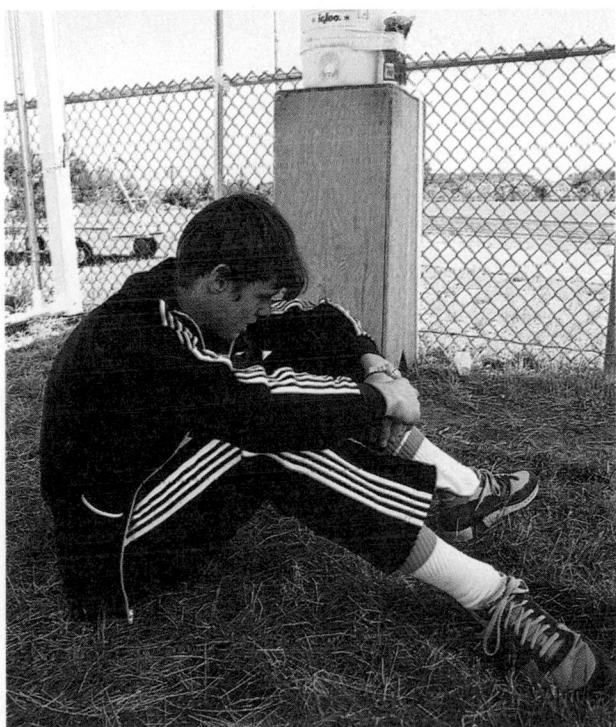

Figure 9-3 Adolescents use being alone as a method of coping with stress. Health professionals need to assess whether this method also indicates an attempt to cope with depression. From Wong DL and others: *Nursing care of infants and children,* ed 6, St. Louis, 1999, Mosby.

Achieving a Sense of Generativity While Avoiding Self-Absorption and Stagnation (Middle Age).

Following the successful development of an intimate relationship, the adult can focus on raising the next generation, building the basis of trust for a child. The ability to sacrifice one's own needs to care for others is possible with or without the production of offspring. The emphasis on independent achievement so prevalent in our culture can create the situation in which adults become too absorbed in their own success, causing neglect of the caring for others.

Acquiring a Sense of Integrity While Avoiding Despair (Old Age).

As the aging process creates physical and social losses, the adult may also suffer loss of status and function, such as through retirement or illness. These external struggles are also met with internal struggles, such as the search for meaning in life. Meeting these challenges creates the potential for growth and wisdom. Many elders review their lives with a sense of satisfaction even with the inevitable mistakes. Others see themselves as failures with marked contempt and disgust.

Nurses are in positions of influence within their communities and can contribute to the valuing of persons at all ages and stages. Erikson stated, "healthy children will not fear life, if their parents have integrity enough not to fear death" (Erikson, 1963). Erikson did significant research during his academic career with varied cultural traditions and gender groups. He believed his theory to be widely applicable.

ROBERT HAVIGHURST

Influenced by Erikson's work and his observation of the **developmental tasks** critical to healthy development, Robert Havighurst (1900-) defined a series of essential tasks that arise from predictable internal and external pressures (Table 9-3) (Ashburn, 1978). These pressures include increasing physical maturity, cultural pressure of society, and the individual's personal goals and aspirations.

Looking at the developmental tasks defined by Havighurst, it is clear that more than one source of pressure might be present. Increasing physical maturity would be associated with the development of skills such as walking, talking, or eating. Cultural pressure creates the conditions necessary to learn social behaviors and ethical norms. Although the adolescent girl may be physically able to accomplish the task of having a child, the preparation and timing for the onset of parenthood can also be considered from a perspective of cultural pressure from both the youth and adult cultures. The desire to have a child might also grow out of the individual's personal goal or aspiration to be a parent.

Havighurst believed that there are critical periods when the individual is most receptive to the learning necessary to achieve success in performing these tasks. Effective learning and achievement of tasks during one period leads

Table 9-3 **Adult Developmental Theorists**			
Adult Stages (Approximate Ages)	Erickson	Gould	Havighurst

Early-early adult (16-22 years)	Intimacy versus isolation
	Ability to form intimate relationships
		Theme: "I have to get away from my parents."
		Gradually establishing control of self as an adult
			Early adulthood stage
			    Selecting a mate
			    Learning to live with a marriage partner
			    Starting a family
			    Rearing children
			    Getting started in an occupation
			    Taking on civic responsibilities
			    Finding a congenial social group

Middle-early adult (22-28 years)			
Late-early adult (28-34 years)		Theme: "Is what I am the only way for me to be?" Demonstrating independent competence while overcoming failures	
Middle adult (34-45 years)	Adulthood Generativity versus stagnation productivity and creativity	Theme: "Have I done the right thing?" Learning to live with ambivalence without need to prove self Beginning sense of time to effect wanted results	Middle age Assisting teenage children to become responsible adults Achieving adult social and civic responsibility Reaching and maintaining satisfactory performance in one's occupation
Middle adult (continued) (40-50 years)		Theme: "The die is cast." Believing that possibilities are limited Seeing time as having an end point Decreased negativism	Developing adult leisure-time activities Relating to one's spouse as a person Accepting and adjusting to the physiologic changes of middle age Adjusting to aging of parents
Middle adult (continued) (50-60 years)		Middle adult (continued) Increased feelings of self-satisfaction Realize mortality and concern for health	
Late adult/old age (60-85 years)	Integrity versus despair, disgust		Later maturity Adjusting to decreasing physical strength and health Adjusting to retirement and reduced income Adjusting to death of a spouse Establishing an affiliation with one's age-group Adopting and adapting social roles in a flexible way Establishing satisfactory physical living arrangements

to happiness and success with later tasks. Failure leads to unhappiness, disapproval by society, and difficulty with later tasks. An example might be the struggle that adolescents might experience in preparing for a work career after having failed to develop fundamental skills in reading and calculating.

As an educator, Havighurst believed that schools have considerable responsibility in helping a child attain success necessary to lead to achievement of later adult development. His theory is a structure of both nonrecurrent tasks specific to a stage of development, such as learning to walk, and recurrent tasks that reemerge in new ways, such as learning to get along with age-mates. Havighurst's theory is limited in its cultural application according to critics who believe that it describes developmental milestones from the perspective of middle-class norms within the American culture. It would be difficult to fit all cultural or ethnic mores within this theoretical framework.

ROGER GOULD

Psychiatrist Roger Gould reviewed the work of other theorists and also found that a lack of understanding of the adult years contributed to the maturing and changing of personality (Table 9-3) (Gould, 1972). He conducted extensive research at UCLA that supported stage theory in adult development with a set of **development themes.** Gould found that over the adult years, persons dismantle the protective thinking developed during childhood. Shedding these beliefs marked a shift from childhood into adult consciousness over a period of years.

These themes start in the 20s with "I have to get away from my parents." This is challenged in minor ways before the end of high school but culminates as young persons begin to live away from home. The move away from the influence of the parent is gradual as they establish themselves as adults.

The second theme, from the early 30s, "Is what I am the only way for me to be?" occurs when young adults experience the consequences of the decisions to start an independent life, taking on a personal identity separate from the parent. Everything does not work out magically as might have been expected. There are failures to be overcome. Acceptance for who they are is essential as is acceptance of their own growing children as unique and separate.

The third theme, in the mid to late 30s, "Have I done the right thing? Is there time to change?" recognizes the complexities of adult decisions. The impact of a growing family and aging parents influences this theme. There is a beginning sense of time left to effect wanted results.

The fourth theme, identified in the 40s, "The die is cast," is indicative of resignation and the belief that possibilities are limited. Personality is set. Changes in career are believed to be less likely to be successful. Parents are blamed for the lack of choices. Regret is faced for mistakes made with children.

During the 50s a decrease in negativism occurs. Gould finds a realization of mortality with a concern for the state of health. There is less responsibility for the welfare of the children and more attachment to the spouse, as might be expected.

Gould believes his research describes a sequential process taking place between the internal life (personality) of the adult and the outer world (culture, lifestyle). He points out that these are generalizations but believes the sequencing if not the age specifics to be true for most people (Gould, 1972). Gould's theoretical work can focus the nurse's appreciation of the life issues of the adult client.

STELLA CHESS AND ALEXANDER THOMAS

Psychiatrists Stella Chess and Alexander Thomas conducted a 20-year longitudinal study of children from a wide range of populations, including normal children of middle-class parents born in the United States and Puerto Rican–American working-class parents as well as mentally challenged children. The breadth of the data allowed them to look at the behavior of persons from childhood to early adulthood as they interacted with their environment. Their work defined temperament from an operational perspective.

Temperament is a behavioral style demonstrated when one approaches people or situations. It is evident at birth and is predictive of the adult's personality (Chess and Thomas, 1986). There is evidence that one's environment can heighten, diminish, or modify in other ways the characteristics of temperament.

The nine characteristics identified by Chess and Thomas include the following:

1. *Activity level:* the intensity or frequency of motor activity. The parent might be distressed by the persistent difficulty in diapering the overactive infant or remark about how nonreactive the child is.

2. *Rhythmicity:* regularity in repetitive biological function. Some individuals have a very strong sense of daily rhythm and have difficulty when schedules change.

3. *Adaptability:* the ease or difficulty with which initial responses to new situations can be modified. Parents might comment on the difficulty the child has in moving from the crib to the junior bed at nighttime. Some children adjust rapidly after initial distress and others do not.

4. *Approach withdrawal:* the behavior when a new experience is introduced. When observing a child, the nurse might observe an initial period of curiosity or persistent withdrawal and fear.

5. *Intensity of response:* the degree or amount of energy invested in reacting to a situation. The parent might describe the lengthy bedtime battles that take place in the home compared to others who have a brief protest from their child.

6. *Threshold of responsiveness:* level of external stimulation needed to get a reaction. The parent might describe the sensitivity to environmental sensation that keeps the infant from resting, sleeping, or just being comfortable.

7. *Quality of mood:* general state of cheerfulness or unhappiness. Parents will describe whether it is enjoyable to be with their child.

8. *Distractibility:* ease of altering ongoing behavior by external stimuli. The nurse might observe that it is very difficult to get the child to concentrate on a task when there is anyone else present in the room.

9. *Persistence and attention span:* the length of time an activity is pursued and the ability to tolerate frustration in that activity despite obstacles. One child might give up a task immediately after the first challenge is faced, whereas another would continue the battle until it is completed.

Taken together, the assessment of a child's characteristics leads to the formation of a personality structure. The three personality types are the easy child, the difficult child, and the slow-to-warm child. These personalities were found by Thomas and Chess (1977) to be associated with varied incidence and risk for development of behavioral problems. The easy child was identified in 40% of the research subjects with 18% having behavioral problems. The difficult child was seen in 10% of the subjects with 70% of the problems. The slow-to-warm child was identified 15% of the time and accounted for 40% of the problems. One of the factors in the development of problems for these children was the ability of the parent(s) and the environment to be flexible and to understand the needs of the child given the personality structure.

Chess and Thomas make it very clear in their discussion of the research that temperament is not a theory in and of itself. They believe that an appreciation of temperament must be incorporated into any theory to make that theory complete. As nurses observe infants and children, it is clear that infants come into the world with a unique approach to what they will experience. It is the world's challenge to respond in a manner that is useful to each individual.

Cognitive Developmental Theory

JEAN PIAGET'S THEORY OF COGNITIVE DEVELOPMENT

Jean Piaget (1896-1980), a Swiss biologist and philosopher, was most interested in the child's development of intellectual organization, how we think. He created a theory of **cognitive development**, which includes four periods and recognizes that children move through these specific periods at different rates but in the same sequence or order (Maier, 1965; Crain, 1992). His theory was built on years of observing children as they explored, manipulated, and tried to make sense out of the world in which they lived. In Piaget's theory external or internal forces did not shape thinking, although he acknowledged their presence in the process.

Piaget's theory includes four general periods of development with a number of stages within each (see Table 9-2).

Period I: Sensorimotor Intelligence (Birth to 2 Years).   During a time of unparalleled changes, the infant develops the schema or action pattern for dealing with the environment. These schemas may include hitting, looking, grasping, or kicking. Schema become self-initiated activities, for example, the infant learning that sucking achieves a pleasing result generalizes the action to suck fingers, blanket, or clothing. Successful achievement leads to greater exploration.

There are circular reactions when the infant experiences something and repeats it until successful. The child goes on to create these reactions through his or her own effort and keep it going. Last, the child can perform two actions to achieve a purpose. For example, the child wishes to grab a toy but is blocked by the parent's hand; the child then pushes the parent's hand away and gets the toy. Later the child tries more than one action in a situation, such as exploring several ways to keep the water from flowing out of the bathtub.

Finally, observations find the child seeming to think before acting. Thinking is inferred in a situation where a child, being unsuccessful in achieving expected results from an action, pauses before trying something new. Moving from random acts to thoughtful choices within one developmental period demonstrates the enormous achievements during this period.

Period II: Preoperational Thought (2 to 7 Years).

Period II is a time when children learn to think with the use of symbols and images. This requires that the child must reorganize thinking all over again. Play is the initial method of nonlanguage use of symbols. Imitation and make-believe play are ways to represent experience. Nursing interventions during this period will recognize the use of play as the way the child understands the events taking place. Parents can be assisted in the use of play materials such as thermometers, blood pressure equipment, and play needles that will allow the child to communicate feelings about health care procedures they experience.

Later, language develops and broadens possibilities for thinking about the past or the future. Children can now communicate about events with others. As the language fits into a logical form, it mirrors the thinking process at the time.

Children are frequently egocentric in this period in that they are unable to distinguish their perspective from that of another person. This is a time of parallel play. Parallel play can be observed as children engage in activities side-by-side without a common goal. One child might interfere with another's play to fulfill his or her own need. This action may create conflict as the child works to understand others. While assisting children in resolving conflict before violence occurs, the nurse can observe the children learning to handle differences in their own ways. The experiential learning compliments the natural changes in thinking as children live with the responses of others to their actions.

Period III: Concrete Operations (7 to 11 Years).

Children achieve the ability to think systematically during Period II but only when they can refer to concrete objects or activities. For example, these concrete experiences are things that can be seen, felt, tasted. They can now describe a process without actually performing it. At this time they are able to coordinate two concrete perspectives in social as well as scientific thinking. In other words, they can appreciate the difference between their perspective and that of a friend. Children can begin to cooperate and share with new information about the act they perform. The parent will be able to adjust their approaches to guide the child into helpful activities within the home, such as bargaining about chores in exchange for wishes for privileges (TV time, play with friends)

Period IV: Formal Operations (11 Years to Adulthood).
The individual's thinking moves to abstract and theoretical subjects in the formal operations period. Thinking can venture into such subjects as achieving world peace, finding justice, and seeking meaning in life. Adolescents can organize their thoughts in their minds. They have the capacity to reason with respect to possibilities. New cognitive powers allow the adolescent to do more far-reaching problem solving including their futures and that of others. This thinking matures with experience in the adult years.

Piaget believed that the sequencing of these stages occurs for all children but that the rate of achievement may vary. He also theorized that this would be true in all cultures. He acknowledged that biological maturation plays a role in this developmental theory but believed that rates of development depend upon the intellectual stimulation and challenge in the environment of the child.

Moral Developmental Theory

Moral developmental theories try to explain "how individuals acquire moral values and how such values help guide the way those persons treat other people" (Thomas, 1997). Although various psychosocial and cognitive theorists have addressed moral development within their respective theories, Piaget and Kohlberg are the two who have done the most to propose a theory of moral development (see Table 9-2).

JEAN PIAGET'S MORAL DEVELOPMENTAL THEORY
Piaget studied boys, 5 to 13 years of age, from middle-class backgrounds. He noted that the child's environment and the stage of cognitive development influence the child's moral development. Piaget notes a natural shift in moral development that occurs around the same time as the cognitive transition from preoperational to operational thought (Kurtines and Gewirtz, 1984). In his theory of moral development, Piaget terms his two stages the heteronomous morality and autonomous morality. In the stage of heteronomous morality children follow the rules set up by those in authority, such as their parents, teachers, clergy, or police. When a person reaches the stage of autonomous morality, moral judgments are based on mutual respect for the rules and also mutual regard for the person. The person at this stage starts to consider information related to the subjective intent in making moral judgments that involve others.

Piaget first saw the child following the rules without understanding the rules. Children see these rules as fixed and handed down by adults or by God, so they cannot change them. Young children base their moral decisions on the extent of the consequences to the action, not necessarily on the action itself. For example, a young child will not eat a cookie before supper not because the mother said not to, but because the child is afraid of the punishment that would result if he or she did.

Around 10 or 11 years of age, children's cognitive ability matures and the rules children follow are understood within the context of community life, the interaction with those around them. Children understand that the rules can be changed if everyone agrees to change the rules. Moral maturity is the internalization of the principles, the desire to weigh all the relationships and circumstances before making a decision. Rules are the tools that humans use to get along (Duska and Whelan, 1975; Crain, 1992).

LAWRENCE KOHLBERG'S MORAL DEVELOPMENTAL THEORY
Kohlberg expanded on Piaget's moral developmental theory during his graduate work in psychology at the University of Chicago. Kohlberg initially interviewed boys at ages 10, 13, and 16. Kohlberg felt that Piaget did not go far enough in the development of his stages. From a series of moral dilemmas, he identified six stages of moral development under three levels (Kohlberg, 1981). Kohlberg found a link between moral development and Piaget's cognitive development; a child's moral development did not advance if the child's cognitive development did not also mature. In this way, Kohlberg's **theory of moral development** follows Piaget's cognitive developmental theories (see Table 9-2).

Level I: Preconventional Level.
At Level I the person reflects on moral reasoning based on personal gain. This closely correlates with Piaget's first stage, in that the person's moral reason for acting, the "why," relates to the consequences the person believes will occur. These consequences can come in the form of punishment or reward. It is at this level that children may view illness as a punishment for fighting with their siblings or not obeying their parents. The nurse must be aware of this thinking and reinforce teaching that the child cannot become ill because of wrongdoing.

Stage 1: Punishment and Obedience Orientation.
In this first stage, the child's response to a moral dilemma is in terms of absolute obedience to authority and the law. A child in this stage reasons: "I must follow the rules otherwise I will be punished." The child's avoidance of punishment or the unquestioning deference to authority are characteristic motivations. A child will be home on time for supper because the parents said the child needed to be.

Stage 2: Instrumental Relativist Orientation.
This second stage is where a child recognizes there is more than one right view; a teacher may have one view that is different than the child's parent. The decision to do something morally right is based on satisfying one's own needs, and

occasionally the needs of others. Punishment is perceived not as proof of the child being wrong (as in Stage 1), but something that one wants to avoid. Children at this stage will follow their parent's rule about being home in time for supper because they do not want to be confined to their room for the rest of the evening if they do not get home on time.

Level II: Conventional Level.
At Level II, the person sees moral reasoning based on his or her own personal internalization of societal and others' expectations. A person wants to fulfill the expectations of the family, group, or nation and also develop a loyalty to and actively maintain, support, and justify the order. Moral decision making at this level moves from "What's in it for me?" to "How will it affect my relationships with others?" Nurses may observe this when family members make end-of-life decisions for their loved ones; individual members may struggle with this moral dilemma. Grief support will involve an understanding of the level of moral decision making of each family member.

Stage 3: Good Boy–Nice Girl Orientation.
Stage 3 correlates with Piaget's second stage of moral development. The individual wants to win approval and maintain the expectations of one's immediate group. "Being good" means to have good motives, show concern for others, and keep mutual relationships through trust, loyalty, respect, and gratitude. One earns approval by "being nice." A person in this stage may stay after school and do odd jobs to win the teacher's approval.

Stage 4: Society-Maintaining Orientation.
Individuals expand their focus from a relationship with others to societal concerns at Stage 4. Moral decisions take into account this societal perspective. Right behavior is doing one's duty, showing respect for authority, and maintaining the social order. Adolescents may choose not to attend a party where they know beer will be served, not because they are afraid of getting caught, but because they know that it is not right.

Level III: Postconventional Level.
The person finds a balance between basic human rights and obligations and societal rules and regulations in this level. Individuals move away from moral decisions based on authority or conformity to groups to define their own moral values and principles. Individuals at this stage start to look at what an ideal society would be like.

Stage 5: Social Contract Orientation.
Having reached Stage 5, an individual may follow the societal law but recognizes the possibility of changing the law to improve society. The individual also recognizes that different social groups may have different values but believes that all rational people would agree on basic rights, such as liberty and life.

Individuals at this stage make more of an independent effort to think out what society ought to value, not related to what the society as a group would value, as would occur in Stage 4. The United States Constitution is based on this morality. An individual at this stage recognizes laws as social contracts that the citizens have agreed to uphold but believes that there must be a mechanism to change unfair laws by democratic means (Crain, 1992).

Stage 6: Universal Ethical Principle Orientation.
Stage 6 defines "right" by the decision of conscience in accord with self-chosen ethical principles. These principles are abstract, like the Golden Rule, and appeal to logical comprehensiveness, universality, and consistency (Kohlberg, 1981). For example, the principles of justice would require the individual to treat everyone in an impartial manner, respecting the basic dignity of all people, and would guide the individual to base decisions on an equal respect for all (Figure 9-4). Stage 5 emphasizes the basic rights and the democratic process, whereas Stage 6 defines the principles by which agreements will be most just.

Nurses need consciousness of their moral reasoning level. Recognizing their own moral developmental level

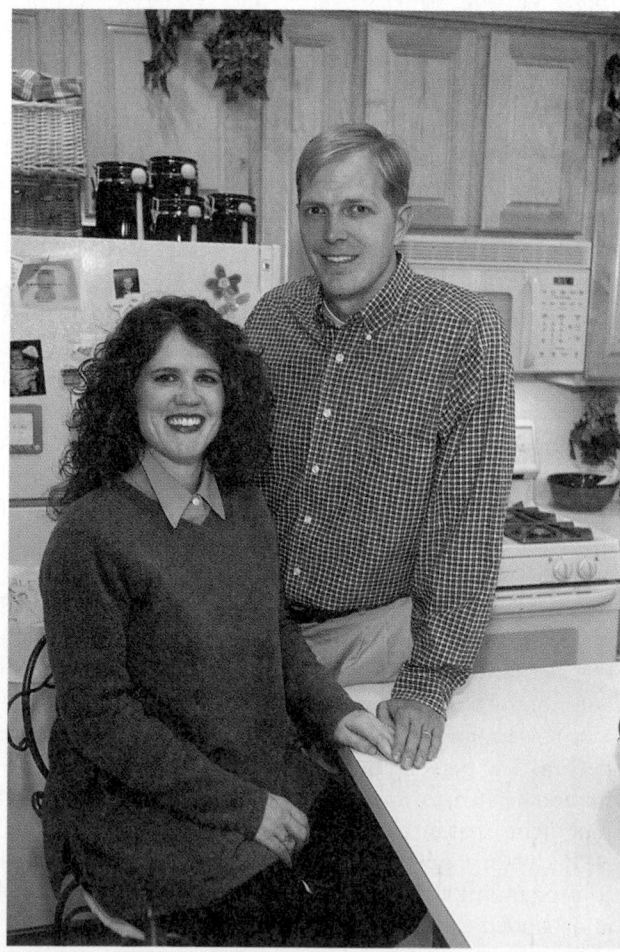

Figure 9-4 Adults must take responsibility for themselves.

will be essential in helping clients clarify their own decisions without the nurse's beliefs and values dominating the client's decision-making process. Nurses may also find that the level of moral decision making influences decisions made by the health care team. This can be exemplified in the following scenario. The nurse is caring for a homeless person and believes that all clients deserve the same level of care. The case manager, being responsible for resource allocation, complains about the client's length of stay and the amount of resources being expended on this one client. The nurse and the case manager are in conflict because of their different levels of moral decision making within their practices.

Further research on the part of Kohlberg made him question Stage 6 as he found that very few subjects consistently reasoned at this stage. He concluded that his research method of using moral dilemmas did not draw out difference between Stages 5 and 6. He termed Stage 6 a "theoretical stage" and no longer scored individuals as achieving this stage in his research.

Kohlberg's Critics.

Kohlberg constructed a systemized way of looking at moral development. He has been recognized as a leader in moral developmental theory. He does have his critics. Many of the differences arise from the choice of research subjects. Most of Kohlberg's subjects were males of the Western philosophical traditions.

Research attempting to support Kohlberg's theory with individuals raised in the Eastern philosophies has found that those study participants never rose above Stages 3 or 4 of Kohlberg's model. Does that mean that they have not reached higher levels of moral development, as most of the adults raised in the Western traditions? Or is it that Kohlberg's research design did not allow a way to measure those raised within a different culture?

Kohlberg has also been criticized for age and gender bias. Kohlberg himself in later studies identified that Stage 5 may not be reached until adulthood (Kohlberg, 1973). Gender bias was raised as a criticism by Carol Gilligan (1982), an associate and coauthor with Kohlberg. Her research looked at moral development and concentrated on the differences that may be related to gender.

Gilligan's Argument.

Gilligan, a psychologist and researcher, started questioning the differences she observed in the way men and women approach and answer moral dilemmas. All developmental theories are subject to this gender bias, according to Gilligan, and it has only been recently that our society has researched and recognized the differences between men and women, in the way they think and how they have been raised to make decisions.

Gilligan proposes that Kohlberg's theory is biased in favor of men. She believes there may be parallel ways that men and women develop, with one not being superior to the other. Basic to Gilligan's argument is the developmental difference in relationships and issues of dependency between women and men (Gilligan, 1982; Crain, 1992; Schroeder, 1992). Separation and individuation are critically tied to male development, as separation from the mother is essential for the boy in his development of masculinity. Girls do not need to separate from their mothers to achieve feminine identity; it is through this attachment to their mother that their identity is formed. Most developmental theories use achievement of increasing separation as a developmental norm. When women are measured against this norm as it relates to their need to maintain relationships, they are seen as failures or less evolved developmentally.

Male moral development may focus on logic, justice, and social organization, whereas female moral development focuses on interpersonal relationships. Interestingly, studies using Gilligan's critique as the research design have been inconclusive. As a result, Gilligan's position remains controversial (Cavanaugh, 1993).

Conclusion

Developmental theories have been described that assist nurses to use critical-thinking skills when asking how and why people respond as they do. From the diverse set of theories included in this chapter, it is clear how complex human behavior is. No one theory successfully describes human growth and development in all of its complexity. Theorists themselves demonstrate their own values and beliefs in their focus and the subjects chosen for their work. They work within a cultural and historical perspective. As nurses apply the theories, it is important to keep this in mind.

Growth and development is not a linear process, as most theories tend to be, but multidimensional. The theories included are meant to be the basis for a meaningful observation of an individual's pattern of growth and development. All theories require validation through research to become fact. They are important guidelines for understanding important human processes that can allow nurses to begin to predict human responses.

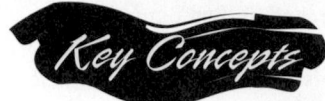

Key Concepts

- Nurses care for human beings at various developmental stages. Developmental theory provides a basis for nurses to assess and understand the responses seen in their clients.
- Humans continue to develop throughout their lives. Development does not end at adolescence; persons grow and develop throughout their life span.
- Theory is a way to account for how and why people grow up as they do. Theories provide a framework and a way to clarify and organize existing observations to explain and try to predict human behavior.
- Growth refers to the quantitative changes that can be measured and compared to norms.
- Development implies a progressive and continuous process of change leading to a state of organized and specialized functional capacity. These changes can be measured quantitatively but are more distinctly measured in qualitative changes.
- Biophysical development explores theories of why individuals age from a biological standpoint.
- Cognitive development focuses on the rational-thinking processes that include the changes in how children and adolescents perform intellectual operations.
- Developmental tasks are age-related achievements, the success of which leads to happiness whereas failure may lead to unhappiness, disapproval, and difficulty in achieving later tasks.
- Developmental crisis is when a person is having great difficulty in meeting tasks of the current developmental period.
- Socialization is the outside influence a person receives from family, peers, and society.
- Psychosocial theories attempt to describe the development of the human personality with varying degrees of influence from the internal biological forces and the external societal/cultural forces.
- Temperament is a behavioral pattern that is inherent in the individual and persists throughout a lifetime.
- Moral development attempts to define how moral reasoning matures for an individual.

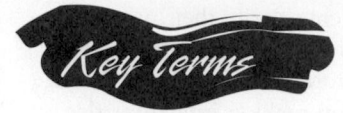

Key Terms

Biophysical development, *p. 155*

Cognitive development, *p. 155*

Erikson's eight stages of life, *p. 161*

Freud's psychoanalytic model of personality development, *p. 160*

Genetic theories of aging, *p. 156*

Gould's development themes, *p. 156*

Havighurst's developmental tasks, *p. 163*

Kohlberg's theory of moral development, *p. 167*

Moral development, *p. 155*

Nongenetic cellular theories, *p. 156*

Physiological theories of aging, *p. 156*

Piaget's theory of cognitive development, *p. 166*

Piaget's theory of moral development, *p. 167*

Psychosocial developmental theories, *p. 155*

Psychosocial theories, *p. 160*

Critical Thinking Exercises

1. A 7-year-old boy has been diagnosed with immune-mediated diabetes. A nurse must begin the educational process for him and his family. What developmental tasks must the nurse determine are already accomplished by the client and his family to design an effective educational program and meet the needs of a family now faced with a chronic illness in one of its members? Based on his cognitive development, how would the nurse approach teaching him about his diabetes?

2. A 76-year-old female has just been diagnosed with breast cancer. She also has severe cardiovascular disease that limits her choices of treatment. Her oncologist has recommended a series of chemotherapy that her cardiologist believes would be fatal. Her family is urging her to do all that is recommended. The client, who is in good spirits despite her diagnosis, chooses palliative care. Based on her developmental stage, how can you help the family adjust to her choice?

3. A 45-year-old executive from a local corporation enters the emergency department with intense chest pain. Upon evaluation, it is determined that he has severe cardiovascular disease and requires open heart surgery. His children, ages 13 and 17, and wife accompany him to the hospital. They live a very expensive lifestyle, and he is the sole wage earner for the family. The oldest son is planning to enroll in an eastern Ivy League school in the fall. After the client settles in his room, he asks for computer access to complete some work before surgery. How will the nurse assist this client in changing his lifestyle while understanding his developmental tasks?

References

Ashburn SS: Selected theories of development. In *The process of human development: a holistic approach,* Boston, 1978, Little, Brown.

Beck CT: The effects of postpartum depression on child development: a meta-analysis, 1998, *Arch Psychiatr Nurs* 12(1): 12, 1998.

Cavanaugh JC: *Adult development and aging,* ed 2, Pacific Grove, Calif, 1993, Brooks/Cole.

Chess S, Thomas, A: *Temperament in clinical practice,* New York, 1986, Guilford Press.

Crain W: *Theories of development: concepts and applications,* ed 3, Englewood Cliffs, NJ, 1992, Prentice Hall.

Duska R, Whelan M: *Moral development: a guide to Piaget and Kohlberg,* New York, 1975, Paulist Press.

Eliopoulos C: *Manual of gerontologic nursing,* St. Louis, 1999, Mosby.

Erikson E: *Childhood and society,* New York, 1963, Norton.

Erikson E: *The lifecycle completed,* New York, 1997, Norton.

Gesell A: *Studies in child development,* New York, 1948, Harper.

Gilligan C: *In a different voice: psychological theory and women's development,* Cambridge, Mass, 1982, Harvard University Press.

Gould RL: The phases of adult life: a study in developmental psychology, *Am J Psychiatry* 129:5, November 1972.

Haywood K: *Life span motor development,* Champaign, Ill, 1993, Human Kinetics Publishers.

Kohlberg L. Continuities in childhood and adult moral development revisited. In Baltes PB, Schaie KW, editors: *Life-span developmental psychology,* New York, 1973, Academic Press.

Kohlberg L. *The philosophy of moral development: moral stages and the idea of justice,* San Francisco, 1981, Harper & Row, Publishers.

Kurtines WM, Gewirtz JL: *Morality, moral behavior, and moral development,* New York, 1984, John Wiley & Sons.

Maier HW: *Three theories of child development,* New York, 1965, Harper & Row.

North American Nursing Diagnosis Association: *Nursing diagnoses: definitions & classification, 1999–2000,* Philadelphia, 1999, The Association.

Nash JM: Fertile minds, *Time,* 149(5):8, 1997.

Rich JM, DeVitis JL: *Theories of moral development,* Springfield, Ill, 1985, Charles C. Thomas Publisher.

Schroeder BA: *Human growth and development,* St. Paul, Minn, 1992, West Publishing Co.

Shock N: Biological theories of aging. In Birren JE, Schaie LW, editors: *Handbook of the psychology of aging,* New York, 1977, Van Nostrand Reinhold Co.

Sorrentino S: *Assisting with patient care,* St. Louis, 1999, Mosby.

Thomas A, Chess S: *Temperament and development,* New York, 1977, Brunner/Mazel.

Thomas RM: *Moral development theories: secular and religious: a comparative study,* Westport, Conn, 1997, Greenwood Press.

Wong DL: *Nursing care of infants and children,* ed 6, St. Louis, 1999, Mosby.

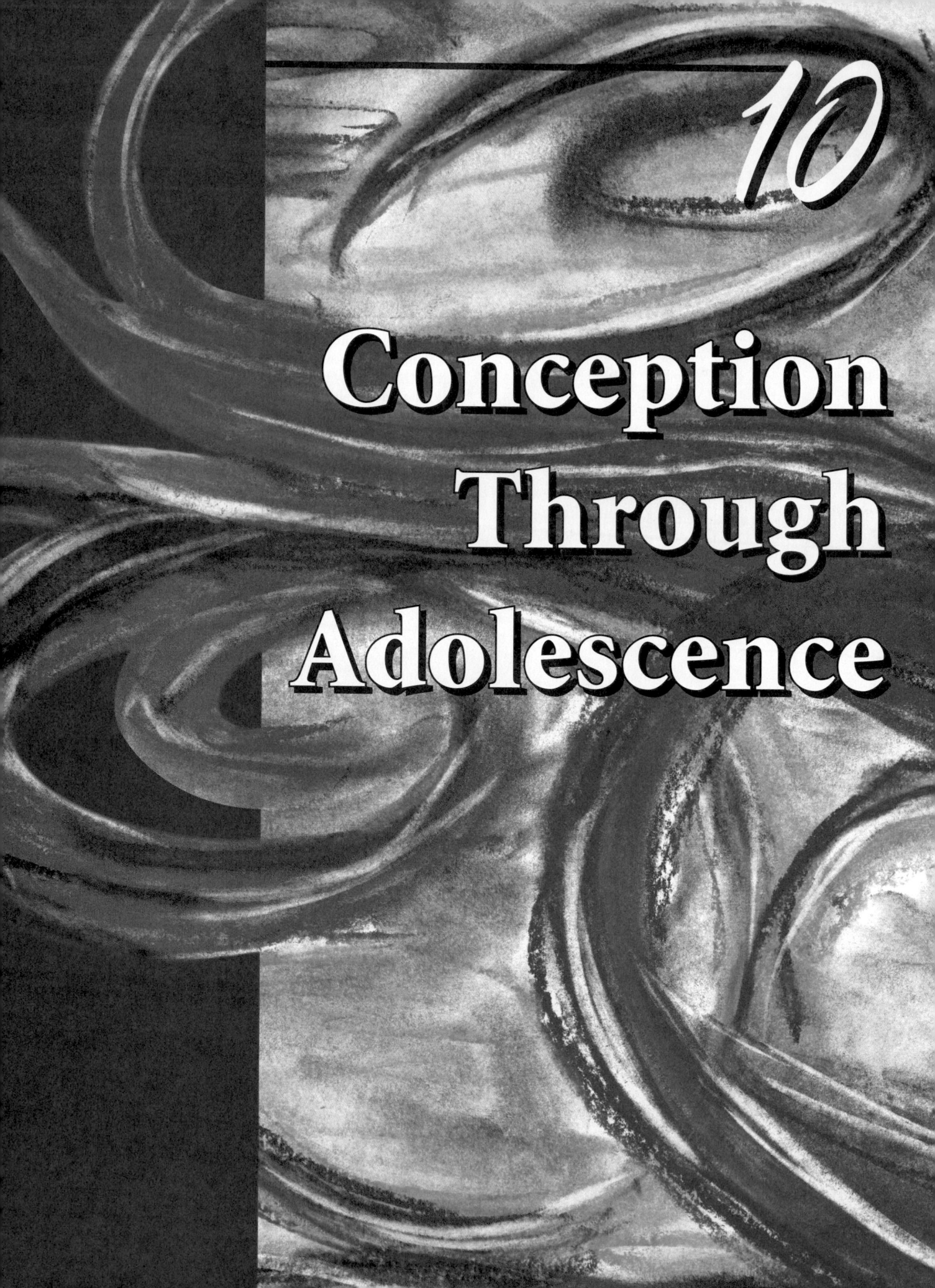

10

Conception Through Adolescence

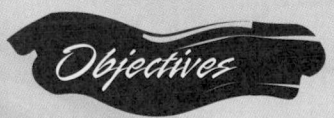

Objectives

Mastery of content in this chapter will enable the student to:

- Define the key terms listed.
- Identify basic principles of growth and development.
- Discuss factors influencing growth and development.
- Discuss physiological and psychosocial health concerns during the transition of the child from intrauterine to extrauterine life.
- Describe characteristics of physical growth of the unborn child and from birth to adolescence.
- Describe cognitive and psychosocial development from birth to adolescence.
- Describe the interactions that occur between parent and child.
- Describe variables influencing how children learn about and perceive their health status.
- Explain the role of play in the development of the child.
- Identify factors that contribute to self-esteem in youth.
- Describe the influence of the school environment on the development of the child.
- Plan culturally appropriate health promotion activities for children of all backgrounds.
- Discuss ways in which the nurse can help parents meet their children's developmental needs.

Understanding children and their growth and development is essential to promoting health and establishing healthful patterns. The nurse must have a clear understanding of the normal ranges of expected growth and development in all stages. Age groups identified in the developmental stages are arbitrarily assigned and should be used as a guideline for the majority of children.

Nursing practice based on principles of growth and development is organized and directed at helping children and their families adapt to changing internal and external conditions. This chapter discusses principles and concepts of growth and development and their application to health promotion from conception through adolescence. A good understanding of growth and development is essential for individualizing the care of all children.

Growth and Development

Human growth and development are orderly, predictable processes beginning with conception and continuing until death (see Chapter 9). All persons progress through definite phases of growth and development, but the pace and behavior of this progression are highly individual. Children learn to walk before they can run, but one child may walk at 10 months, and another may not walk until 15 months of age.

The ability to progress through each developmental phase influences the holistic health of the individual. The success or failure experienced within a phase may affect the

The authors acknowledge the contributions of Dr. Janice Rumfelt and Joyce Hamlin to this chapter in the previous edition of this text.

ability to complete subsequent phases. If an individual experiences repeated developmental failures, inadequacies result. However, if the individual experiences repeated successes, competencies that maintain and promote health result. A child not learning to walk by 18 or 20 months, for example, demonstrates delayed gross motor ability that slows exploration and manipulation of the environment. A child walking by 10 months is able to explore and find stimulation in the environment, thereby enhancing learning.

DEFINITIONS

Growth and development are synchronous processes that are interdependent in the healthy individual. Growth, development, maturation, and differentiation depend on a sequence of endocrine, genetic, constitutional, environmental, and nutritional influences (Seidel and others, 1995). A person experiences growth or quantitative change and developmental or qualitative change.

Physical Growth. **Physical growth** is the quantitative, or measurable, aspect of an individual's increase in physical measurements. Measurable growth indicators include changes in height, weight, teeth, skeletal structures, and sexual characteristics. For example, children generally double their birth weight by 5 months of age and their birth height by 36 months.

Development. **Development** occurs gradually over time. The individual advances from a lower to a higher level of complexity. An individual's capacities are expanded through growth, learning, and maturation. Increased capacity for functioning results from a mastery of several smaller skills. For instance, an observable change for preschoolers is participating in telephone conversations with their parents. Before developing this capacity, they must develop a small vocabulary, learn to put words together in phrases and sentences, and develop a cognitive understanding of **object permanence** (that a person or object out of sight still exists).

Maturation.

Maturation is the process of aging. The individual begins to adapt and show competence in new situations. Maturation can be described as a more qualitative type of change. It involves an individual's biological ability, physiological condition, and desire to learn more mature behavior. To mature, the individual may have to relinquish previous behavior and learning, integrate new patterns into existing behavior, or both. Maturation influences the sequence and timing of the changes associated with growth and development. For example, the infant relinquishes crawling for walking because walking permits more extensive investigation of the environment and more learning. However, the infant cannot walk until the biological ability and structures to perform the action (i.e., increased muscle cells and tone) have developed.

Differentiation.

Differentiation is the process by which cells and structures become modified and develop more refined characteristics. It is a simple-to-complex development of activities and functions. Embryonal cells begin as vague and undifferentiated and develop into complex, highly diversified cells, tissues, and organs.

CRITICAL PERIODS OF DEVELOPMENT

Stages of growth and development involve the concept of critical periods of development. A **critical period** is a specific span of time during which the environment has its greatest impact on the individual. During these critical periods some form of sensory stimulation is necessary for developmental progression. Without stimulation, task completion is difficult or unattainable. For example, the toddler who has not been encouraged to learn to walk during a set time may have difficulty learning to walk at another time. Therefore developmental progression depends on the timing and degree of stimulation, as well as on the readiness to be stimulated by the environment. A stimulus provided too early may not be useful. For example, an 18-month-old child cannot learn to write, regardless of the intensity of the stimuli.

Stages of Growth and Development

Human growth and development are continuous and intricate, complex processes that are often divided into stages organized by age groups, such as from conception to adolescence. Although this chronological division is arbitrary, it is based on the timing and sequence of developmental tasks that the child must accomplish to progress to another stage (Box 10-1).

MAJOR FACTORS INFLUENCING GROWTH AND DEVELOPMENT

The human being is a complex, open system influenced by natural forces from within and from the environment (Table 10-1). Interaction between these forces affects development.

Selecting a Developmental Framework for Nursing

Providing developmentally appropriate nursing care is easier when planning is based on a theoretical framework (see Chapter 9). An organized, systematic approach ensures that the child's needs are assessed and met by the plan of care. If nursing care is delivered only as a series of isolated actions, some of the child's developmental needs may be overlooked. A developmental approach encourages organized care directed at the child's current level of functioning to motivate self-direction and health promotion. For example, nurses might encourage toddlers to feed themselves to advance their developing independence and thus promote their sense of autonomy. Or understanding an adolescent's need to be independent should prompt the nurse to establish a contract about the care plan and its implementation.

Conception

From the moment of conception, human development proceeds at a predictive and rapid rate. Intrauterine health problems are caused by both genetic and environmental factors. During the prenatal period, the embryo grows from a single cell to a complex, physiological being. All major organ systems develop in utero, with some functioning before birth (Figure 10-1). The psychosocial being also begins to emerge during gestation.

INTRAUTERINE LIFE

Intrauterine life that reaches full term lasts 10 lunar or 9 calendar months, 40 weeks, or 280 days. The length of pregnancy is computed using **Nagele's rule,** which counts back 3 months from the last menstrual period (LMP) and adds 7 days. Only one sperm penetrates the ovum. Fertilization of the ovum takes place in the outer one third of the fallopian tube and occurs within 24 hours of the ovum's release. Once fertilization takes place, the material from both cell nuclei unites. The organism then has its full genetic complement in one pair of sex chromosomes and 22 pairs of autosomal chromosomes. The ovum and the sperm each contribute one chromosome to each pair. It is through this mechanism that genetically programmed diseases (such as Down syndrome) and genetically deter-

Developmental Age Periods
Box 10-1

PRENATAL PERIOD: CONCEPTION TO BIRTH

Germinal: Conception to approximately 2 weeks

Embryonic: 2 to 8 weeks

Fetal: 8 to 40 weeks (birth)

A rapid growth rate and total dependency make this one of the most crucial periods in the developmental process. The relationship between maternal health and certain manifestations in the newborn emphasizes the importance of adequate prenatal care to the health and well-being of the infant.

INFANCY PERIOD: BIRTH TO 12 OR 18 MONTHS

Neonatal: Birth to 28 days

Infancy: 1 to approximately 12 months

The infancy period is one of rapid motor, cognitive, and social development. Through mutuality with the caregiver (parent), the infant establishes a basic trust in the world and the foundation for future interpersonal relationships. The critical first month of life, although part of the infancy period, is often differentiated from the remainder because of the major physical adjustments to extrauterine existence and the psychologic adjustment of the parent.

EARLY CHILDHOOD: 1 TO 6 YEARS

Toddler: 1 to 3 years

Preschool: 3 to 6 years

This period, which extends from the time the children attain upright locomotion until they enter school, is characterized by intense activity and discovery. It is a time of marked physical and personality development. Motor de-velopment advances steadily. Children at this age acquire language and wider social relationships, learn role standards, gain self-control and mastery, develop increasing awareness of dependence and independence, and begin to develop a self-concept.

MIDDLE CHILDHOOD: 6 TO 11 OR 12 YEARS

Frequently referred to as the school age, this period of development is one in which the child is directed away from the family group and is centered around the wider world of peer relationships. There is steady advancement in physical, mental, and social development with emphasis on developing skill competencies. Social cooperation and early moral development take on more importance with relevance for later life stages. This is a critical period in the development of a self-concept.

LATER CHILDHOOD: 11 TO 19 YEARS

Prepubertal: 10 to 13 years

Adolescence: 13 to approximately 18 years

The period of rapid maturation and change known as adolescence is considered to be a transitional period that begins at the onset of puberty and extends to the point of entry into the adult world—usually high school graduation. Biologic and personality maturation are accompanied by physical and emotional turmoil, and there is redefining of the self-concept. In the late adolescent period the child begins to internalize all previously learned values and to focus on an individual, rather than a group identity.

From Wong DL: *Whaley and Wong's nursing care of infants and children,* ed 6, St. Louis, 1999, Mosby.

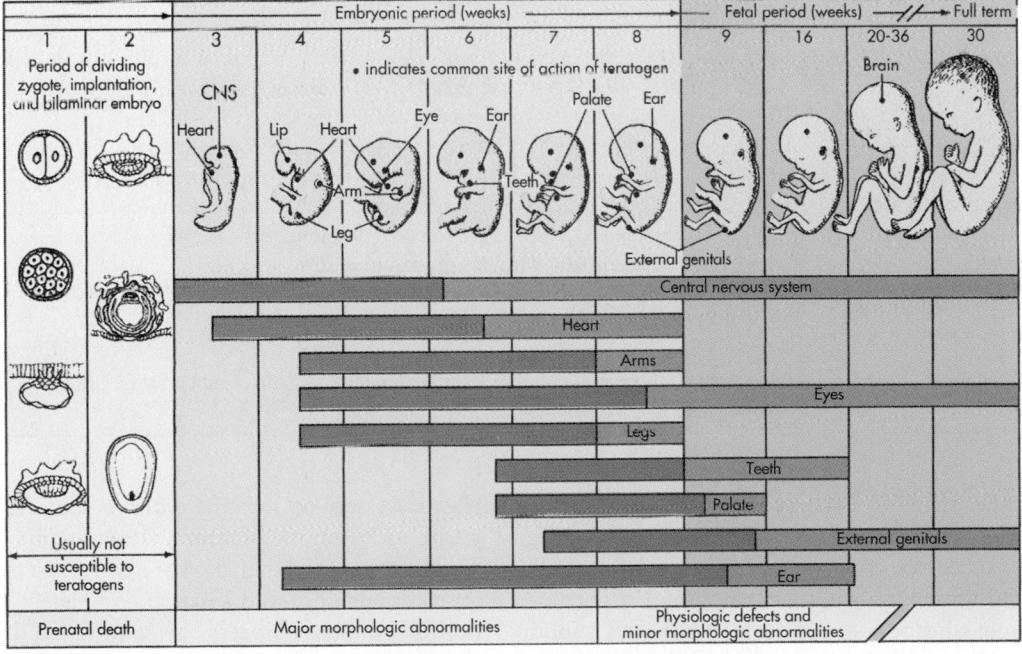

Figure 10-1 Periods of organ differentiation.
From Moore KL, Pernaud TV: *The developing human: clinically oriented embryology,* ed 5, Philadelphia, 1993, WB Saunders.

Table 10-1	**Major Factors Influencing Growth and Development**
Factors	Relevant Influences
Forces of Nature	
Heredity	Genetic endowment determines sex, race, hair and eye color, physical growth, stature, and to some extent psychological uniqueness.
Temperament	Temperament is characteristic psychological mood with which the child is born and includes behavioral styles of easy, slow-to-warm, and difficult. It influences interactions between the individual and environment.
External Forces	
Family	Family purpose is to protect and nurture its members.
	Family functions include means for survival, security, assistance with emotional and social development, assistance with maintenance of relationships, instruction about society and world, and assistance in learning roles and behaviors.
	Family influences through its values, beliefs, customs, and specific patterns of interaction and communication.
	Ordinal position and sex influence individual's interaction and communication in family.
Peer group	Peer group provides new and different learning environment.
	Peer group provides different patterns and structures of interaction and communication, necessitating different style of behavior.
	Functions of peer group include allowing individual to learn about success and failure; to validate and challenge thoughts, feelings, and concepts; to receive acceptance, support, and rejection as unique person apart from family; and to achieve group purposes by meeting demands, pressures, and expectations.
Life experiences	Life experiences and learning processes allow individual to develop by applying what has been learned to what needs to be learned.
	Learning process involves series of steps: recognition of need to know task; mastery of skills to perform task; mastery of task; expertise in performing task, which expands capabilities; integration into whole functioning; and use of accumulated skills and experiences to develop repertoire of effective behavior.
Health environment	Level of health affects individual's responsiveness to environment and responsiveness of others to the individual.
Prenatal health	Preconception (e.g., genetic and chromosomal factors, maternal age, health) and postconception (e.g., nutrition, weight gain, use of tobacco and alcohol, medical problems, use of prenatal services) factors affect fetal growth and development.
Nutrition	Growth is regulated by dietary factors. Adequacy of nutrients influences whether and how physiological needs, as well as subsequent growth and development needs, are met.
Rest, sleep, and exercise	Balance between rest or sleep and exercise is essential to rejuvenating body. Disturbances diminish growth, whereas equilibrium reinforces physiological and psychological health.
State of health	Illness or injury potentially hampers growth and development. Nature and duration of health problem influences its impact. Prolonged injury or illness may cause inability to cope and respond to demands and tasks of developmental stages.
Living environment	Factors affecting growth and development include season, climate, home life, and socioeconomic status.

mined characteristics (such as eye color) are transmitted from parent to child.

The fertilized ovum, or **zygote,** passes through the fallopian tube to the uterus within 3 to 4 days. During this time the zygote continues to divide. Within 3 days a solid ball of cells, the **morula,** has formed. The morula continues to develop and forms a central cavity, or **blastocyst.** Even at this early stage of development, cells begin to differentiate in structure and function. Cells at one end of the

blastocyst develop into the **embryo,** and those at the opposite end form the **placenta.** Between days 6 and 10, enzymes are secreted that allow the blastocyst to burrow into the endometrium and become completely covered. This portion of the process is known as **implantation.** Chorionic villi, fingerlike projections, develop to obtain oxygen and nutrition from the maternal blood supply and dispose of carbon dioxide and waste products.

Before implantation the embryo is relatively protected

from the external environment, but with implantation it becomes more vulnerable to the larger maternal environment via exchange of materials through the placenta. The placenta produces essential hormones that help maintain the pregnancy. Because the placenta is extremely porous, noxious materials such as viruses and drugs can also pass from mother to child. The effect of noxious agents on the unborn child depends on the developmental stage in which exposure takes place, with the embryonic stage being the most crucial. The embryonic stage lasts from day 15 until approximately 8 weeks after conception. This is a crucial stage in the development of organ systems and the main external features. The period of gestation is frequently divided into three periods called trimesters.

First Trimester

Physical Changes. During the first trimester, the first 3 calendar months, the uterus continues to be a pelvic organ. After implantation, fetal cells continue to differentiate and develop into essential organ systems. These processes of cellular change (differentiation) and staged organ change (development) occur at different rates and times, and each organ is extremely vulnerable to environmental insult. Interference with growth can cause the congenital absence of an organ system or extensive structural or functional alterations. Because several organ systems develop at the same time, disruption of one system often occurs with disruption of others. Figure 10-1 shows the approximate times of critical differentiation for some of the major organ systems and their overlapping of development. Toward the end of the first trimester, it is possible to elicit fetal heart tones (FHTs) by fetoscope or ultrasound.

Health Promotion. Agents capable of producing adverse effects in the fetus are called **teratogens.** Some teratogens produce defects only if the fetus is exposed to the agent when the vulnerable organ is developing. The nurse educates the mother about avoiding exposure to teratogenic agents. One such teratogen is the rubella or German measles virus, which can cause spontaneous abortion, stillbirth, or birth defects of the eyes, ears, and heart, primarily when exposure is in the first trimester.

Many drugs are teratogenic during rapid organ growth (**organogenesis**) in the first trimester. Past and present use of home remedies, herbs, and prescription, over-the-counter, and illegal drugs must be carefully assessed. Barbiturates, anticoagulants, antimicrobials, alcohol, cancer chemotherapeutics, and hydantoin anticonvulsants are only a few of the chemical agents associated with fetal abnormalities, and many other agents are still under investigation. Benefits of any drug needed to maintain the mother's health must be weighed against potential harm to the fetus. Abuse of drugs such as cocaine and LSD may result in preterm labor and chromosomal breakage, respectively. Smoking has been shown to reduce birth weight and increase the incidence of fetal and neonatal death (Lowdermilk, Perry, and Bobak, 1999). Infants exposed prenatally to alcohol can develop fetal alcohol syndrome (FAS), fetal alcohol effect (FAE), or an alcohol-related birth defect (ARBD) (Coles 1993). Although the effect on the fetus of maternal caffeine use is controversial, the safest policy is to avoid it. With this knowledge, the nurse can explore lifestyle changes that can help a pregnant woman protect the health of her **fetus.**

The diet of a woman both before and during pregnancy has a significant effect on the development of the infant in utero. It has been repeatedly demonstrated that mothers who eat well have fewer complications of pregnancy and childbirth and bear healthier babies than those with inferior nutritional intake (Grodner, Anderson, and DeYoung, 1996). An adequate folic acid intake is encouraged for any woman contemplating pregnancy (Box 10-2). Folic acid intake is believed to be responsible for decreasing the incidence of neural tube defects. The consequences of maternal malnutrition on fetal development make the attention to improvements in the nutritional state of pregnant women critical.

Second Trimester

Physical Changes. During the second trimester, the end of month 3 through month 6, the uterus becomes an abdominal organ. Measurement of the height of the uterus, above the symphysis pubis, is one indicator of fetal growth. The height of the uterus can also indicate approximate gestational age and high-risk situations. The **fundus, or top of the uterus,** typically measures 1 cm for each week of gestation up to 36 weeks. A 16-week gestation should measure 16 cm above the top of the symphysis pubis. Between 16 and 20 weeks, the mother begins to feel fetal movement. This feeling of life is referred to as **quickening.**

Some organ systems continue basic development while the functional capabilities of others are refined. By the end of the sixth month, most organ systems are complete and can function. The fetus is therefore considered viable, or capable of life outside the uterus, if given intensive environmental support. The fetus weighs about 0.7 kg (1½ pounds) and is approximately 30 cm (12 inches) long. Fingers and toes are differentiated, rudimentary kidneys function, and the sex of the fetus can be determined. The fetus is covered with **vernix caseosa,** a cheeselike substance coating the skin. **Lanugo,** or fine hair, covers most of the body. These substances protect the thin, fragile skin and decrease in amount as the pregnancy nears its completion; thus infants born before 38 weeks' gestation have more of these protective coverings than full-term infants.

Health Promotion. In the second trimester the fetal heartbeat becomes audible to stethoscope auscultation, and the mother becomes aware of fetal movement. Both events are highly significant to the parents because they provide tangible evidence of the pregnancy and reassure them that the fetus is alive. Therefore the nurse should focus on these events during prenatal care.

Client Teaching ABOUT FOLIC ACID FOR WOMEN CONTEMPLATIING PREGNANCY   Box 10-2

OBJECTIVE
Client will consume 0.4 mg of folic acid (vitamin B₉) every day.

TEACHING STRATEGIES
* Educate females of childbearing age about the benefits of folic acid to a developing fetus.
* Discuss the need for women to have an adequate daily intake of folic acid because the moment of conception is not always known. Folic acid is a water-soluble vitamin and is readily excreted in the urine.
* Encourage consumption of 0.4 mg of folic acid daily. This amount may be consumed in food sources; however, ado-

lescents are usually deficient. Deficiency is not related to socioeconomic status.
* Discuss foods rich in folic acid, such as green leafy vegetables, liver, kidney, and asparagus. More limited amounts may be found in milk, poultry, and eggs.
* Assist clients to develop menus with folic acid–rich foods.
* Encourage clients to take a daily multivitamin to supplement dietary intake.

EVALUATION
Review client's 3-day diet intake diary.

Changes in maternal behavior during this period include planning for the birth, concern for personal safety, and preoccupation with health and appearance. The nurse can help the woman adapt to these changes and plan for the impending birth. This is often a good time for education about gestational events and appropriate maternal rest, nutrition, dental care, physical activity, posture, employment, and infant feeding options.

Due to dramatic changes occurring in the renal system, it is possible for a mother to have an asymptomatic urinary tract infection. Urinary tract infections greatly increase the risk of preterm labor. Proper voiding habits should be discussed with the mother during this time.

The mother should be educated to recognize potential complications and preterm labor as well as the appropriate actions to take with each. With advances in modern technology, it is possible for 500-g babies of 24 to 26 weeks' gestation to survive; however, there may be significant risk of morbidity. **Prematurity** is identified as any infant between 20 and 37 weeks' gestation. Causes for prematurity are poorly understood and may be the result of maternal, fetal, or placental problems. Maternal risk factors include physiological stresses such as renal and cardiovascular disease, diabetes mellitus, or uterine and cervical abnormalities. Research has also demonstrated an increased risk among mothers living in poverty, smokers, and mothers receiving poor antenatal care (Lowdermilk, Perry, and Bobak, 1999). Multiple pregnancies and fetal infections are two of the potential fetal factors for prematurity. Placental factors include abruptio placentae and placenta previa. **Tocolysis,** the use of therapeutic interventions to stop labor, is implemented when labor occurs before 37 weeks and continued until the fetus is closer to its due date. Interventions can include intravenous (IV) fluids, medications, and bed rest.

THIRD TRIMESTER
Physical Changes.   During the last 3 months of intrauterine life the fetus grows to approximately 50 cm (19 to 20 inches) in length. Subcutaneous fat is stored, and weight increases to between 3.2 and 3.4 kg (7 to 7 1/2

pounds). The skin thickens, lanugo begins to disappear, and the fetal body becomes rounder and fuller.

A tremendous spurt in brain growth begins during this trimester and lasts well into the first few years of life. The central nervous system has established its total number of neurons and connections between neurons, and myelination of nerve fibers progresses at a rapid rate.

At the end of the third trimester the normal fetus is physically able to make the transition from intrauterine to extrauterine life. The cardiac system can change its circulation to end bypassing of the lungs. The lungs are capable of maintaining the inflated state for gas exchange. The primitive temperature maintenance systems, reflexes, and sensory organs are ready for use.

Health Promotion.   Exposure to noxious agents and the absence of essential nutrients can cause damage to the central nervous system and result in alteration of high-level cognitive functions. The nurse can increase the mother's awareness of these dangers through counseling and help her evaluate the quality of her nutritional intake. Thoughts of delivering a healthy infant are foremost in the mother's mind as she focuses on preparing her mind and body for the delivery. Parents often seek information regarding the childbirth process and breast-feeding.

Discussion of childbirth preparation methods and birth environment should begin during this trimester. Advanced preparation for the nurse in childbirth education is available and can be especially helpful for group teaching situations. Depending on the mother's location, many different types of childbirth education groups are available. Some groups are for first-time parents and may be focused on the adolescent or the older (35 years or more) mother. Other classes may focus on the repeat mother who needs a refresher course, the cesarean section mother, or the mother who wants to attempt a vaginal birth after a cesarean section (**VBAC**). Because some areas may have limited access to childbirth classes, parents should be encouraged to investigate local classes early.

Birth-setting choices should also be discussed at this time. Hospitals have been the more traditional setting for childbirth for the past 60 years. Many hospitals have taken a family-centered approach to childbirth. The woman is placed in a private room that has a more homelike atmosphere. It is not unusual to find wooden furniture, a couch, rocking chair, or television in these rooms. Depending on the facility, the mother may spend her entire hospitalization in the same room or may be moved into another room after delivery. The majority of births in this country take place in the hospital because it is homelike and emergency backup is available in case of difficulties.

In some areas of the country, freestanding birthing centers are available for those who do not prefer the hospital setting. Women delivering in this setting are required to attend childbirth and parenting classes, and the pregnancy must be considered low risk. Physicians and midwives with hospital privileges may attend births in this facility. Mothers must understand that there is always a possibility of transfer to a hospital if the conditions warrant.

A small percentage of mothers choose to deliver at home. Home birth has been popular in Sweden and the Netherlands but has a limited following in this country. Control over the birth process seems to be the most attractive factor for mothers who do not believe they will have choices in a hospital setting. Another advantage is that the entire family or other persons close to the family can be part of the event. The main reason home birth has met with opposition in this country is due to the concern that the mother and baby may be exposed to unnecessary risks. Emergency situations in the home are much more difficult to handle. Certain precautions should be take if home delivery is going to be pursued. The two most important considerations are (1) the mother must be low-risk and (2) the care provider must be well trained with adequate supplies available. Providing support and reassurance about the pregnancy's progression and the decisions that need to be made are appropriate nursing actions at this stage.

Cognitive Changes.   Relationships between prenatal events and cognitive development are difficult to establish. However, periods of diminished oxygen (anoxia) during fetal life are known to cause deficits in later cognitive functioning, and inadequate prenatal nutrition has been associated with lower brain weight. The large volume of research on developmental outcomes in low-birth-weight (LBW) and very low-birth-weight (VLBW) infants indicates these infants have an increased risk for learning disorders, school failures, **temperament** problems, neurological and motor impairment, and developmental delays. Many additional factors affect the infants' temperament. Such factors include prenatal exposure to drugs, maternal analgesia during labor, and length of gestation (Medoff-Cooper 1995). Research demonstrates a positive relationship between a supportive home environment and cognitive development in LBW infants (Feingold, 1994). The implication of this research is that families of LBW infants

must be assessed for need of nursing interventions that may facilitate a supportive home environment for optimal cognitive outcomes.

Psychosocial Changes.   Little information is available about the relationship between prenatal factors and the child's psychosocial development. Some authorities believe that nutritional deficiencies of the fetus can significantly influence later psychosocial development. This is especially true if maternal malnutrition occurs during the period of rapid brain growth because a permanent reduction in brain cells may occur (Wong, 1999).

Transition From Intrauterine to Extrauterine Life

The transition from intrauterine to extrauterine life requires rapid changes in the newborn. The nurse assesses the newborn's ability to make these changes and plans for appropriate nursing interventions. Gestational age and development, exposure to depressant drugs before or during labor, and the newborn's own behavioral style influence adjustment to the external environment. Therefore initial assessment encompasses a variety of physical and psychosocial elements. The nurse also provides opportunities for the parents and child to develop close emotional bonds.

PHYSICAL CHANGES

An immediate assessment of the newborn's condition is performed to determine the physiological functioning of the major organ systems. The most extreme physiological change occurs when the newborn leaves the in utero circulation and develops independent respiratory functioning. Nursing care is directed at maintaining an open airway, stabilizing and maintaining body temperature, and protecting the newborn from infection.

The most widely used assessment tool is the **Apgar score.** Heart rate, respiratory effort, muscle tone, reflex irritability, and color are rated to determine overall status. The Apgar assessment is generally conducted at 1 and 5 minutes after birth and may be repeated until the newborn's condition stabilizes. Table 10-2 outlines the scoring criteria of physiological functioning. A total score of 0 to 3 signifies severe distress, a score of 4 to 6 represents moderate difficulty, and a score of 7 to 10 indicates little difficulty in adjusting to extrauterine life. The nurse can use the Apgar score to determine areas requiring further assessment and careful observation. In addition, the nurse monitors the newborn's body temperature and other vital signs until they stabilize.

PSYCHOSOCIAL CHANGES

After immediate physical evaluation and application of identification bracelets, the nurse promotes the parents

Table 10-2 Apgar Scoring			
Sign	Score 0	Score 1	Score 2
Heart rate	Absent	Slow (below 100)	Over 100
Respiratory effort	Absent	Slow, irregular, hypoventilation	Good, crying lustily
Muscle tone	Flaccid	Some flexion of extremities	Active motion, well flexed
Reflex irritability	No response	Crying, some motion	Vigorous cry
Color	Blue, pale	Pink body, blue hands and feet	Completely pink

Modified from Wong DL: *Whaley and Wong's nursing care of infants and children,* ed 6, St. Louis, 1999, Mosby.

and newborn's need for close physical contact. Early parent-child interaction encourages parent-child attachment. Physical factors (e.g., fatigue, hunger, and health) and emotional factors (e.g., happiness and needs for affection and touch) are assessed.

Merely placing the family together does not promote closeness. The parents and newborn must be capable and desirous of exploring and responding to each other. Most healthy newborns are awake and alert for the first half-hour after birth. This is an opportune time for parent-child interaction to begin. Close body contact, often including breast-feeding, is a satisfying way for most families to start. If immediate contact is not possible, the nurse incorporates it into the care plan as early as possible, which may mean bringing the newborn to an ill parent or bringing the parents to an ill or premature child.

Bonding occurs when parents and newborn elicit reciprocal and complementary behavior. Parental bonding behaviors include attentiveness and physical contact. Newborn bonding behavior involves maintenance of contact with the parent. Preterm, ill newborns and ill mothers have more difficulty forming this bond if separation is prolonged. The bonding process is further complicated if parents are unable to care for the usual infant needs. The nurse should give the parents support throughout the early attachment process, particularly if the newborn or mother is ill or if the newborn is separated from the parents.

HEALTH RISKS

Airway patency is best ensured by removing nasopharyngeal and oropharyngeal secretions with suction or a bulb syringe. Because hypothermia increases oxygen needs, the newborn's body temperature must be stabilized and maintained. The newborn may be placed directly on the mother's abdomen and covered in warm blankets; be dried and wrapped in warm blankets, being sure to keep the head well covered; or placed unclothed in an infant warmer with a temperature probe in place. For newborns unable to sustain adequate body temperature, isolettes and incubators, which supply radiant heat, are preferred.

Prevention of infection is a major concern in the care of the newborn, whose immune system is immature. Good hand-washing technique is the most important factor in protecting the newborn and nurse from infection.

Cover gowns do not need to be worn while providing care for the healthy newborn once the blood and amniotic fluid have been removed from the infant's skin. Other precautions include wearing gloves when touching mucous membranes or nonintact skin such as in a new wound (i.e., fresh circumcision) and when drawing blood (e.g., heel stick) (Garner, 1996).

The most commonly used prophylactic treatment against ophthalmic conjunctivitis is erythromycin (0.5%) because it prevents *Neisseria gonorrhoeae* and other infections, which can be transmitted during passage through an infected vaginal canal. Application should occur during the newborn's initial assessment.

The stump of the moist umbilical cord is an excellent medium for bacterial growth. The cord should be cleansed by application of 70% alcohol at each diaper change. Until the cord dries and falls off, the diaper should be folded below the umbilicus to prevent accumulation of moisture.

Newborn

The **neonatal period** is the first month of life. During this stage the newborn's physical functioning is mostly reflexive, and stabilization of major organ systems is the body's primary task. Behavior greatly influences interaction between the newborn and the environment and caregivers. For example, the average 2-week old smiles spontaneously and is able to regard the mother's face. The impact of these reflexive behaviors is generally a surge of maternal feelings of love that prompt the mother to cuddle the baby.

Nurses can apply their knowledge of this stage of growth and development to promote newborn and parental health. If the nurse understands, for example, that the newborn's cry is generally a reflexive response to an unmet need (such as hunger), parents can be assisted in identifying ways to meet those needs, such as counseling the parents to feed their baby on demand rather than on a rigid schedule.

PHYSICAL CHANGES

A comprehensive nursing assessment is performed as soon as the newborn's physiological functioning is stable, generally within a few hours after birth. At this time the nurse measures height, weight, head circumference, temperature, pulse, and respirations and observes general appearance, body functions, sensory capabilities, reflexes and responsiveness.

The average newborn weighs 3400 g (7 pounds, 8 ounces), is 50 cm (20 inches) in length, and has a head circumference of 35 cm (14 inches). Up to 10% of birth weight is lost in the first few days of life, primarily through fluid losses by respiration, urination, defecation, and low fluid intake. Birth weight is usually regained by the second week of life, and a gradual pattern of increase in weight, height, and head circumference is evident. During the first month, these increases average 4 to 8 ounces in weight per week, 0.6 to 2.5 cm (1/4 to 1 inch) in length, and 2 cm in head circumference.

The newborn's heart rate ranges from 120 to 160 beats per minute. The average blood pressure is 74/46 mm Hg. The newborn's respiratory movements are primarily abdominal and vary in rate and rhythm, with an average rate of 30 to 50 breaths per minute. The axillary temperature ranges from 36° to 37.5° C (97.7° to 99.5° F) and generally stabilizes within 24 hours after birth.

Normal physical characteristics include the continued presence of lanugo on the skin of the back; cyanosis of the hands and feet for the first 24 hours; and a soft, protuberant abdomen. Skin color varies according to racial and genetic heritage and gradually changes during infancy. **Molding,** or overlapping of the soft skull bones, allows the fetal head to adjust to various diameters of the maternal pelvis and is a common occurrence with vaginal births. The bones readjust within a few days, producing a rounded appearance. The sutures and **fontanels** are usually palpable at birth. The diamond shape of the anterior fontanel and the triangular shape of the posterior fontanel between the unfused bones of the skull are shown in Figure 10-2.

Neurological function is assessed by observing the newborn's level of activity, alertness, irritability, responsiveness to stimuli, and the presence and strength of reflexes. Normal reflexes include blinking in response to bright lights and startling in response to sudden, loud noises. Table 10-3 describes other commonly evaluated reflexes. An absence of any of the reflexes indicates prematurity, possible trauma, or central nervous system complications. Because the newborn depends largely on reflexes for response to environment, assessment of these characteristic responses is vital.

Normal behavioral characteristics of the newborn include periods of sucking, crying, sleeping, and activity. Movements are generally sporadic, but they are symmetrical and involve all four extremities. The relatively flexed fetal position of intrauterine life continues as the newborn attempts to maintain an enclosed, secure feeling. Newborns normally watch the caregiver's face, reflexively smile, and respond to sensory stimuli, particularly the primary caregiver's face, voice, and touch.

The first hour of the unmedicated newborn's life is spent in a primarily quiet alert state with wide-open eyes

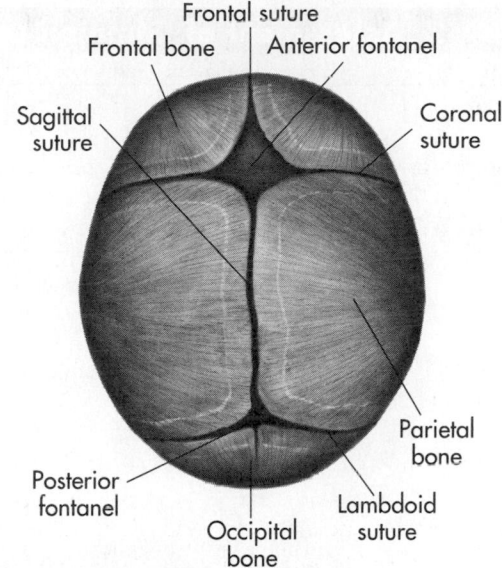

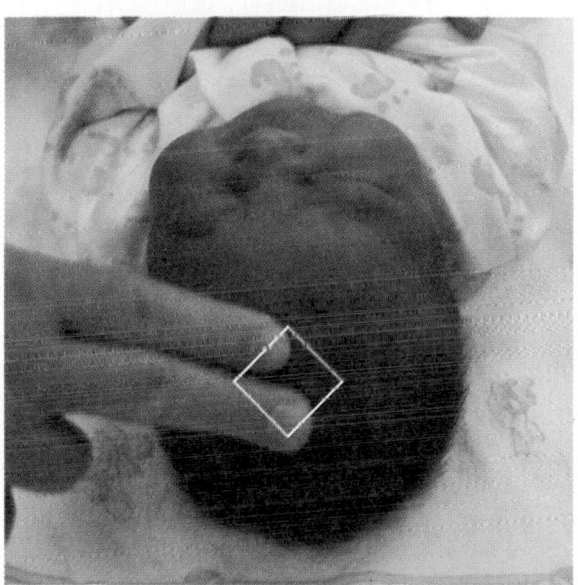

Figure 10-2   Fontanels and suture lines.
From Wong DL: *Whaley and Wong's nursing care of infants and children,* ed 6, St. Louis, 1999, Mosby.

and vigorous sucking activity. Then infants sleep almost continuously for the next 2 to 3 days to recover from the exhausting birth process. Thereafter sleep periods vary from 20 minutes to 6 hours with little day-night differentiation (Figure 10-3). Infant behavior is characterized by five distinct states that are highly influenced by environmental stimuli. It is important for parents to understand these states (summarized in Table 10-4) and their implications for parental interaction. In accordance with the recommendations of the American Academy of Pediatrics (AAP) (1997b), infants who are put down for sleep should be positioned on their side or back to decrease the risk of sudden infant death syndrome (SIDS). Co-sleeping or bed

Table 10-3   Assessment of Common Localized Reflexes in the Newborn

Reflexes	Expected Behavioral Responses
Localized	
EYES	
Blinking or corneal reflex	Infant blinks at sudden appearance of bright light or at approach of object toward cornea. Reflex persists throughout life.
Doll's eye	As head is moved slowly to right or left, eyes lag behind and do not immediately adjust to new position of head. Reflex disappears as fixation develops. Persistent occurrence indicates neurological damage.
NOSE	
Sneeze	Nasal passages respond spontaneously to irritation or obstruction. Reflex persists throughout life.
Glabellar	Tapping briskly on glabella (bridge of nose) causes eyes to close tightly.
MOUTH AND THROAT	
Sucking	Infant begins strong sucking movements of circumoral area in response to stimulation. Reflex persists throughout infancy, even without stimulation, such as during sleep.
Gag	Stimulation of posterior pharynx by food, suction, or passage of tube causes infant to gag. Reflex persists throughout life.
Rooting	Touching or stroking cheek along side of mouth causes infant to turn head toward that side and begin to suck. Reflex should disappear at about age 34 mo but may persist up to 12 mo.
Extrusion	When tongue is touched or depressed, infant responds by forcing it outward. Reflex disappears by 4 mo.
Cough	Irritation of mucous membranes of larynx or tracheobronchial tree causes coughing. Reflex persists throughout life and is usually present first day after birth.
Swallowing	Appropriate swallowing of liquid introduced into mouth. Can also be elicited by directing a puff of air at infant's face.
EXTREMITIES	
Grasp	Touching palms of hands or soles of feet near base of digits causes flexion of hands and toes. Palmar grasp lessens after 3 mo and is replaced by voluntary movement. Plantar grasp lessens by 8 mo.
Babinski	Stroking outer sole of foot upward from heel and across ball of foot causes toes to hyperextend and hallux to dorsiflex. Reflex disappears after age 1 yr (see the illustration below)
MASS	
Moro	Sudden jarring or change in equilibrium causes sudden extension and abduction of extremities and fanning of fingers, with index finger and thumb forming **C** shape, followed by flexion and adduction of extremities. Legs may weakly flex. Infant may cry. Reflex disappears after 3-4 mo and is usually strongest during first 2 mo.
Startle	Sudden, loud noise causes abduction of arms with flexion of elbows. Hands remain clenched. Reflex disappears by 4 mo.
Dance or step	If infant is held so that sole of foot touches hard surface, there is reciprocal flexion and extension of leg, stimulating walking. Reflex disappears after 3-4 wk and is replaced by deliberate movement.
Crawl	When placed on abdomen, infant makes crawling movements with arms and leg. Reflex disappears at about 6 wk.
Placing	When infant is held upright under arms and dorsal side of foot is briskly placed against hard object, such as table, leg lifts as if foot is stepping on table. Age of disappearance varies.

Modified from Wong DL: *Whaley and Wong's nursing care of infants and children*, ed 6, St. Louis, 1999, Mosby.
Illustration redrawn from Wong DL: *Whaley and Wong's nursing care of infants and children*, ed 6, St. Louis, 1999, Mosby.

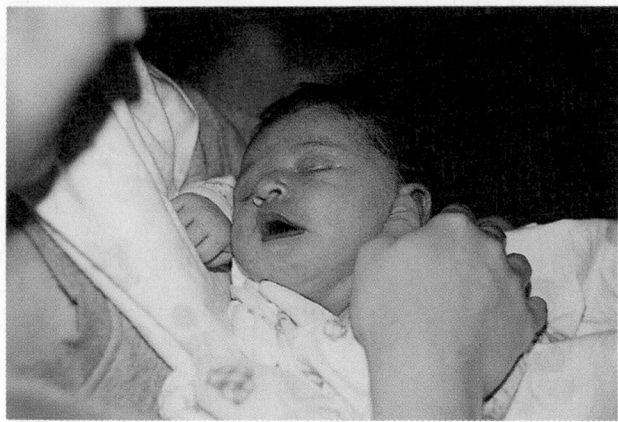

Figure 10-3   Newborn sleep periods have little day-night differentiation.

Research HIGHLIGHT   Box 10-3

RESEARCH ABSTRACT

Sudden infant death syndrome is the sudden, unexpected, and unexplained death of a seemingly healthy infant. It is the primary cause of infant death outside the neonatal period. Although studied extensively, the etiology appears unclear. This study explored the evolution of the various recommendations for infant positioning. In 1992, the AAP suggested an association between the prone position and SIDS. In 1996, the AAP stressed the need for infants to be placed in a supine or side-lying position to decrease the risk of SIDS. The supine position is preferred and offers the lowest risk of SIDS in healthy newborns.

IMPLICATIONS FOR PRACTICE

*   Nurses provide education to parents and caregivers on a daily basis. Current AAP recommendations should be provided to the parents and caregivers.
*   Recognize that many parents may be reluctant to use the supine position for fear of aspiration.
*   Share information that is consistent with the safety of the supine position and the rarity of aspiration.

REFERENCE

From Lockridge T: Now I lay me down to sleep: SIDS and infant sleep positions, *Neonatal Network* 16(6):25, 1997.

sharing has also been reported to be possibly associated with an increased risk for SIDS (Mitchell, 1996). Safeguards include proper positioning; removing stuffed animals, soft bedding, and pillows; and avoiding overheating of the infant (Box 10-3). Smoking should be avoided during pregnancy and around the infant (AAP, 1997a).

COGNITIVE CHANGES

Early cognitive development begins with innate behavior, reflexes, and sensory functions. Newborns initiate reflex activities, learn behaviors, and learn their desires. For example, newborns learn to turn to the nipple and learn that crying results in parent response of feeding, diapering, and cuddling.

Sensory functions contribute to cognitive development in the newborn. At birth, children can focus on objects about 8 to 10 inches from their faces and can perceive forms. A preference for the human face is apparent. Auditory and vestibular systems function from birth. These sensory capabilities allow newborns to elicit stimuli rather than simply receive them. Parents should be taught the importance of providing sensory stimulation, such as talking to their babies and holding them to see their faces. This allows infants to seek or take in stimuli, thereby enhancing learning and promoting cognitive development.

It is debatable whether infant crying is the precursor of refined language. However, crying elicits a response, and caregivers discriminate cry patterns. Crying therefore has significance to newborns and parents. For newborns, crying is a means of communication to provide cues to parents. Some babies cry because their diapers are wet or they are hungry or want to be held. Others cry just to make noise or because they need a change in position or activity. Their crying may frustrate the parents if they cannot see an apparent cause. With the nurse's help, parents can learn to recognize infants' cry patterns and take appropriate action when necessary.

PSYCHOSOCIAL CHANGES

During the first month of life, parents and newborns normally develop a strong bond that grows into a deep attachment. Interactions during routine care enhance or detract from the attachment process. Feeding, hygiene, and comfort measures consume much of infants' waking time. These interactive experiences provide a foundation for the formation of deep attachments. Newborns are active participants in this process.

If parents or children experience health complications after birth, attachment and bonding may be compromised. Infants' behavioral cues may be weak or absent, and caregiving may be less mutually satisfying. Tired, ill parents have difficulty interpreting and responding to their infants. Children who have congenital anomalies are often too weak to be responsive to parental cues and require special supportive nursing care. For example, infants born with heart defects may tire easily during feedings. They may rest frequently after several bursts of sucking and fall asleep after taking 1 to 1½ ounces. Infants may awaken after 1½ hours, crying because they are hungry again. Mothers, not understanding that the crying is a physiologically dictated sequence of events, may think that the infants are being fussy or that they are inadequate. Both infants and mothers derive decreasing pleasure from feeding experiences. In this case, however, bonding is not enhanced and may even be reduced unless nursing intervention breaks the sequence of events.

Table 10-4 **States of Sleep and Activity**		
State/Behavior	Duration	Implications for Parenting
Regular Sleep		
Closed eyes	4-5 hours/day	Infant not aroused by external stimuli.
Regular breathing	10-20 minute	Usual house noises can continue.
Occasional body jerks	sleep cycles	Leave infant alone even for brief cries.
Irregular Sleep		
Closed eyes	12-15 hours/day	External stimuli may arouse infant.
Irregular breathing	20-45 minute	Periodic groaning or crying is usual; not an indication of
Slight muscle twitching of body	sleep cycles	discomfort.
Drowsiness		
Eyes may be open	Variable	Most stimuli arouse infant.
Irregular breathing		Pick infant up during this time rather than leave in crib.
Active body movement		
Alert Inactivity		
Responds to environment by active body movement and staring at close-range objects	2-3 hours/day	Satisfy infant's needs such as hunger. Place infant in area of activity. Place toys/objects within infant's view.
Waking and Crying		
May begin with whimpering and slight body movements	1-4 hours/day	Remove intense internal/external stimuli. Repeat activities that were effective during alert inactivity.
Progresses to strong, angry cry and uncoordinated thrashing of extremities		Rock and swaddle to decrease crying.

HEALTH RISKS

Hyperbilirubinemia refers to an excessive amount of accumulated bilirubin in the blood and is characterized by a yellow coloring of the skin, or jaundice. The accumulation occurs when the infant's body is unable to balance the destruction of red blood cells (RBCs) and the use or excretion of by-products. The balance can be upset by prematurity, breast-feeding, excess production of bilirubin, certain disease states, or a disturbance in the liver. Because bilirubin is highly toxic to neurons, an infant with levels greater than 18 mg/100 ml is at risk for brain damage. Phototherapy is used to help break down the bilirubin for easier excretion. Special care must be given to properly shielding the infant's eyes to protect exposure to the light. Because excretion of the extra bilirubin can cause watery stools, adequate fluid balance in the infant must be maintained.

HEALTH CONCERNS

Screening. The nurse coordinates screening tests and other laboratory tests as indicated by the newborn's state of health. Blood tests can be used to determine **inborn errors of metabolism** (IEM). This term applies to genetic disorders caused by the absence or deficiency of a substance, usually an enzyme, essential to cellular metabolism that results in abnormal protein, carbohydrate, or fat me-

tabolism. Although IEMs are rare, they account for a significant proportion of health problems in children. Neonatal screening can detect phenylketonuria (PKU), hypothyroidism, and galactosemia and thus allow appropriate treatment that can prevent permanent mental retardation and other health problems. This testing is mandatory in most of the United States.

Circumcision. Circumcision is a common and controversial procedure in this country. The controversy surrounds the risks and benefits, especially with respect to pain control. Risks have been identified as hemorrhage, infection, adhesions, and meatal stenosis. Benefits include prevention of penile cancer and urinary tract infections, and preservation of male body image to be consistent with peers (Wong, 1999). Parents should give informed consent prior to the procedure. Because of the newborn's unstable physiological state during the first day, circumcision is not recommended to take place during this time. Care of the site depends on the type of method used for the procedure. If a Gomco clamp is used, petroleum jelly may be applied to a gauze dressing and then to the site to prevent adherence to the diaper. This type of dressing is not necessary when a plastibell is used. The newborn should be checked frequently for evidence of swelling or oozing and the ability to void.

Infant

Infancy, the period from 1 month to 1 year of age, is characterized by rapid physical growth and change. This is the only period marked by such dramatic physical changes and marked development. Psychosocial development advances, aided by the progression from reflexive to more purposeful behavior. Interaction between infants and the environment is greater and more meaningful. Infants who giggle and roll over in response to tickling are interacting more with their social environments and are displaying a greater response than when they merely smile in response to a hug. During this first year of life the nurse can easily observe the adaptive potential of infants because qualitative and quantitative changes in growth and development occur so rapidly.

PHYSICAL CHANGES

Steady and proportional growth of the infant is more important than absolute growth values. Charts of normal age- and gender-related growth measurements enable the nurse to compare growth with norms for a child's age. Using growth charts, the nurse can also evaluate an individual infant's growth patterns by recording measurements of weight, length, and head circumference at selected intervals. Measurements recorded over time are the best way to monitor growth and identify problems. An infant with a growth problem may be generally below the expected norms at all intervals or may experience an acute, brief interference with growth. An infant with a feeding problem may be below the expected norm for weight.

Size increases rapidly during the first year of life; birth weight doubles in approximately 5 months and triples by 12 months. An average weight gain is 1½ pounds the first 5 months and ¾ pound for months 7 to 12. Height increases an average of 1 inch during each of the first 6 months and ½ inch the next 6 months. This 50% increase in birth height occurs primarily in the trunk, with the chest diameter approximating that of the head by the first birthday (Wong, 1999). The fontanels become smaller; the posterior fontanel closes at about 2 months; the anterior at about 12 to 18 months.

Physiological functioning stabilizes, and by the end of the first year, the heart rate is 80 to 150 beats per minute, the blood pressure averages 90/50 mm Hg, and the respiratory rate is 30 to 35 breaths per minute. Patterns of body function also stabilize, as evidenced by predictable sleep, elimination, and feeding routines. Motor development proceeds steadily in a cephalocaudal direction. Table 10-5 identifies milestones in gross motor and fine motor development.

COGNITIVE CHANGES

The infant learns by experiencing and manipulating the environment. Developing motor skills and increasing mobility expand an infant's environment and, with developing visual and auditory skills, enhance cognitive development. For these reasons Piaget (1952) named his first stage of cognitive development, which extends until around the third birthday, the sensorimotor period. The characteristics of each of the three subphases of this period that occur during the first year of life are described in Chapter 9.

Before the acquisition of language the extraordinary development of the mind occurs through the child's developing senses and motor abilities. For example, a 1-month old can follow the path of a moving object. Improved visual acuity and eye-hand coordination allow grasping and exploration of objects. In addition, rudimentary color vision begins by 2 months and improves throughout the first year, making the environment more interesting to see and explore. The infant's hearing also

Table 10-5 **Milestones in Infant Motor Development**				
Month 3	Month 6	Month 9	Month 12	Month 15
Gross Motor				
Lifts head 90 degrees when prone	Rolls completely over	Attains sitting position independently	Walks holding onto walls and furniture (cruising)	Walks alone
Sits with support	Good head control in sitting position	Creeps on all four extremities	Stands alone	
	Crawls on abdomen with arms	Pulls self to standing position	Takes 1 to 2 steps	
Fine Motor				
Grasps and briefly holds objects and takes them to mouth	Uses palm grasp with fingers encircling object	Crude thumb-finger pincer grasp	Places tiny object, such as raisin, into container	Scribbles with crayon
	Transfers cube from hand to hand	Bangs hand-held cubes together	Makes marks with crayon	Builds tower of two cubes

Modified from Frankenburg WK and others: The Denver II: a major revision and restandardization of the Denver Developmental Screening Test, *Pediatrics* 89(1):91, 1992.

progresses, allowing localization and discrimination of sounds.

Infants need opportunities to develop and use their senses. Nurses must evaluate the appropriateness and adequacy of these opportunities. For example, ill or hospitalized infants may lack the energy to interact with their environments, thereby slowing their cognitive development. On the other hand, continuous stimulation can overwhelm and confuse infants. Infants need to be stimulated according to their temperament, energy, and age. Visual, sensory, and tactile stimulation are as necessary for healthy development as food. The nurse uses stimulation strategies that maximize the development of infants while conserving their energy and orientation. An example of this is the nurse talking to and encouraging an infant to suck on a pacifier while administering the infant's tube feeding.

Language.   Speech is an important aspect of cognition that develops during the first year. Infants proceed from crying, cooing, and laughing to imitating sounds, comprehending the meaning of simple commands, and repeating words with knowledge of their meaning. By 1 year, infants not only recognize their own names but also have two- or three-word vocabularies including *Da-Da, Ma-Ma,* and *no.* The nurse can promote language development by encouraging mothers to name objects on which their infants' attention is focused.

PSYCHOSOCIAL CHANGES

Separation.   During their first year, infants begin to differentiate themselves from others as separate beings capable of acting on their own. Initially, infants are unaware of the boundaries of self, but through repeated experiences with the environment, they learn where the self ends and the external world begins. As infants determine their physical boundaries, they begin to respond to others (Figure 10-4). Two- and 3-month-old infants begin to smile responsively rather than reflexively. Similarly, they can recognize differences in people when their sensory and cognitive capabilities improve. By 8 months, most infants can differentiate a stranger from a familiar person and respond differently to the two. Close attachment to the primary caregivers, most often parents, is usually established by this age. Infants seek out these persons for support and comfort during times of stress. The ability to distinguish self from others allows infants to interact and socialize more within their environments. By 9 months, for example, infants play simple social games such as patty-cake and peekaboo. More complex interactive games such as hide-and-seek involving objects are possible by age 1.

Trust Versus Mistrust.   Erikson (1963) describes the psychosocial developmental crisis for the infant as trust versus mistrust. He explains that the quality of parent-

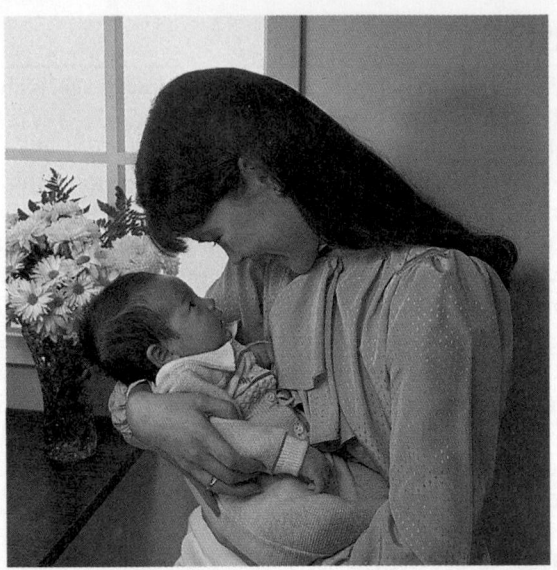

Figure 10-4   Smiling at and talking to an infant encourages the infant to respond, which increases interaction with parent or caregiver.

infant interactions determines development of trust or mistrust. Parents who meet needs for warmth and comfort, love and security, and food when infants express these needs promote a sense of trust, whereas those who meet the needs of infants at their own convenience or not at all allow a sense of mistrust to develop (see Chapter 9).

The nurse assesses the availability and appropriateness of experiences contributing to psychosocial development. Hospitalized infants may have difficulty establishing physical boundaries because of repeated bodily intrusions and painful sensations. Limiting these negative experiences and providing pleasurable sensations are interventions that support early psychosocial development. Extended separations from parents complicate the attachment process and increase the number of caregivers with whom the infant must interact. Ideally, the parents should provide the majority of care during hospitalization. When parents are not present, an attempt should be made to limit the number of caregivers who have contact with the infant and to follow the parents' directions for care. These interventions will foster the infant's continuing development of trust.

Play.   Play is a meaningful set of activities through which individuals interact with their environment and relate to others. Play provides opportunities for the infant to develop many motor skills. Much of infant play is exploratory as they use their senses to observe and examine their own bodies and objects of interest in their surroundings. Activities such as the infant's placement of his toes in his mouth provide him with pleasure, information about his own body, and help form his early self-concept. Play becomes manipulative as the child learns control of the hands. Adults can facilitate infant learning by planning activities that promote the development of milestones and providing toys that are safe for the infant to explore with the mouth and manipulate with the hands, such as rattles, wooden blocks, plastic stacking rings, squeezable stuffed animals, and busy boxes. Infants most frequently engage in solitary (one-sided) play but do enjoy watching others, particularly the antics of their siblings. Infants need to be played with and stimulated through interactions with others. They delight in activities such as peekaboo and patty-cake.

HEALTH RISKS

Injury Prevention.   Injury is a major cause of death in children 6 to 12 months old. An understanding of the major developmental accomplishments during this time period will allow for injury prevention planning. Table 10-6 lists the main types of injuries occurring in this age group and possible prevention strategies based on major developmental accomplishments.

Automobile injuries are the leading cause of death in children older than 1 year. Many of these deaths occur when the child is not properly restrained. All infants must be restrained in a U.S. federally approved car seat restraint. Infant restraints may also convert into a toddler type of restraint (Figure 10-5). The infant should always be placed in a restraint that is rear facing in the backseat of the vehicle. Placing an infant in a rear-facing restraint in the front seat of a vehicle is extremely dangerous in any vehicle with a passenger-side air bag (Figure 10-6).

Child Maltreatment.   Child maltreatment includes intentional physical abuse or neglect, emotional abuse or neglect, and sexual abuse (Wong, 1999). More children suffer from neglect than any other type of maltreatment. Many suffer from more than one type of maltreatment. The Child Protective Services agencies reported that of the 1 million children suffering from maltreatment, half suffered from some type of neglect, one quarter from physical abuse, and 13% from sexual abuse. More than half, 56%, were under the age of 4 years. Of the 996 deaths reported to Child Protective Services, most were under the age of 3 (U.S. Department of Health and Human Services [USDHHS], 1997). All 50 states have a mandatory reporting law for all health professionals to report suspected abuse. No one profile fits a victim of maltreatment. Although signs and symptoms vary, Box 10-4 includes possible findings of child maltreatment. A combination of signs and symptoms or a pattern of injury should arouse suspicion. It is important for the health care provider to be aware of certain disease processes and cultural practices. Lack of awareness of normal variants such as mongolian spots or cultural practices such as coining will cause the health care provider to arouse undue suspicion of abuse. Box 10-5 identifies conditions that can be mistaken for sexual abuse.

HEALTH CONCERNS

Health Perception.   The foundation for children's perceptions of their health status is laid early in life. Internal body sensations and experiences with the outside world affect self-perceptions. The nature of this influence and the value of nursing interventions to alter later perceptions are unknown. It is known, however, that parents tend to label children who are ill in early life as more vulnerable than their siblings and that this labeling may affect the children's perceptions of their own health. In addition,

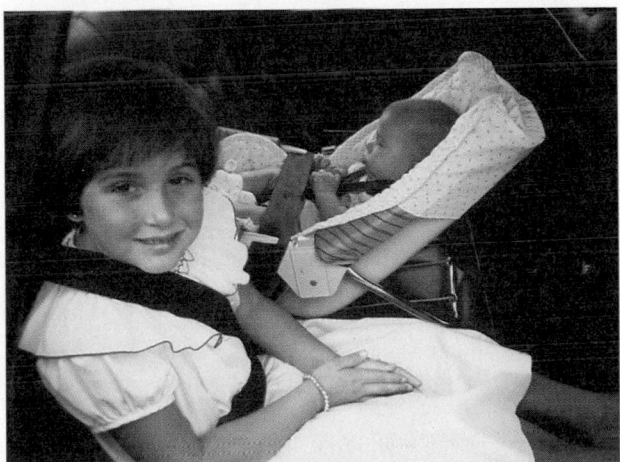

Figure 10-5   Federally approved infant car restraint. Note placement in middle of backseat and use of car lap/shoulder belt for older child.

From Wong DL: *Whaley and Wong's nursing care of infants and children,* ed 6, St. Louis, 1997, Mosby.

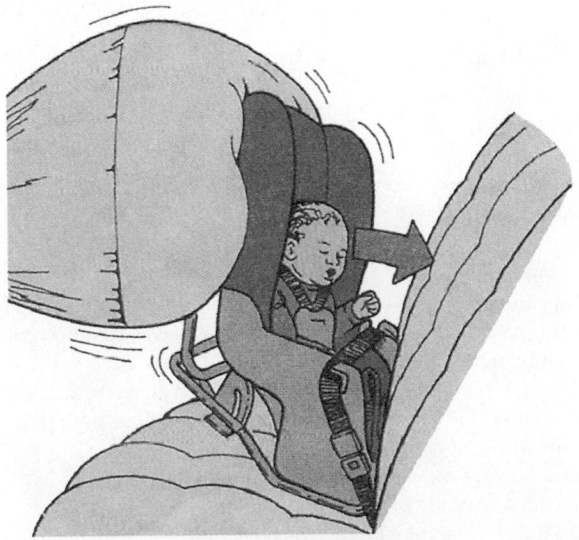

Figure 10-6   An air bag could strike a child safety seat, seriously injuring the infant.

Redrawn from Health alert, *AAP News* 10(4):22, 1994.

Table 10-6 **Injury Prevention During Infancy**

Age: Birth-4 Months
MAJOR DEVELOPMENTAL ACCOMPLISHMENTS

Involuntary reflexes, such as the crawling reflex, may propel infant forward or backward, and the startle reflex may cause the body to jerk

May roll over

Increasing eye-hand coordination and voluntary grasp reflex

INJURY PREVENTION

Aspiration

Not as great a danger to this age-group, but should begin practicing safeguarding early (see under Age: 4-7 Months)

Never shake baby powder directly on infant; place powder in hand and then on infant's skin; store container closed and out of infant's reach

Hold infant for feeding; do not prop bottle

Know emergency procedures for choking*

Use pacifier with one-piece construction and loop handle

Suffocation/drowning

Keep all plastic bags stored out of infant's reach; discard large plastic garment bags after tying in a knot

Do not cover mattress with plastic

Use a firm mattress and loose blankets; no pillows

Make sure crib design follows federal regulations and mattress fits snugly—crib slats <2⅜ in (6 cm) apart

Position crib away from other furniture and away from radiators

Do not tie pacifier on a string around infant's neck

Remove bibs at bedtime

Never leave infant alone in bath

Do not leave infant under 12 months alone on adult or youth mattress

Falls

Always raise crib rails

Never leave infant on a raised, unguarded surface

When in doubt as to where to place child, use the floor

Restrain child in infant seat and never leave child unattended while the seat is resting on a raised surface

Avoid using a high chair until child can sit well with support

Poisoning

Not as great a danger to this age-group, but should begin practicing safeguards early (see under Age: 4-7 Months)

Burns

Install smoke detectors in home

Use caution when warming formula in microwave oven; always check temperature of liquid before feeding

Check bathwater

Do not pour hot liquids when infant is close by, such as sitting on lap

Beware of cigarette ashes that may fall on infant

Do not leave infant in the sun for more than a few minutes; keep exposed areas covered

Wash flame-retardant clothes according to label directions

Use cool-mist vaporizers

Do not leave child in parked car

Check surface heat of car restraint before placing child in seat

Motor vehicles

Transport infant in federally approved, rear-facing car seat,* preferably in backseat

Do not place infant on the seat or in lap

Do not place child in a carriage or stroller behind a parked car

Do not place infant or child in front passenger seat with an air bag

Bodily damage

Avoid sharp, jagged objects

Keep diaper pins closed and away from infant

Age: 4-7 Months
MAJOR DEVELOPMENTAL ACCOMPLISHMENTS

Rolls over

Sits momentarily

Grasps and manipulates small objects

Resecures a dropped object

Has well-developed eye-hand coordination

Can focus on and locate very small objects

Mouthing is very prominent

Can push up on hands and knees

Crawls backward

INJURY PREVENTION

Aspiration

Keep buttons, beads, syringe caps, and other small objects out of infant's reach

Keep floor free of any small objects

Do not feed infant hard candy, nuts, food with pits or seeds, or whole or circular pieces of hot dog

Exercise caution when giving teething biscuits, because large chunks may be broken off and aspirated

Do not feed infant while child is lying down

Inspect toys for removable parts

Keep baby powder, if used, out of reach

Avoid storing large quantities of cleaning fluid, paints, pesticides, and other toxic substances

Discard used containers of poisonous substances

Do not store toxic substances in food containers

Discard used button-sized batteries; store new batteries in safe area

Know telephone number of local poison control center (usually listed in front of telephone directory)

From Wong DL: *Whaley and Wong's nursing care of infants and children*, ed 6, St. Louis, 1999, Mosby.
*Home care instructions for care of the choking infant and for use of child safety seats are available in Wong DL: *Wong and Whaley's clinical manual of pediatric nursing*, ed 5, St. Louis, 2000, Mosby.
†Information available from U.S. Consumer Product Safety Commission; (800) 638-CPSC.

Table 10-6   Injury Prevention During Infancy—cont'd

Suffocation

Keep all latex balloons out of reach

Remove all crib toys that are strung across crib or playpen when child begins to push up on hands or knees or is 5 months old

Falls

Restrain in a high chair

Keep crib rails raised to full height

Poisoning

Make sure that paint for furniture or toys does not contain lead

Place toxic substances on a high shelf or in locked cabinet

Hang plants or place on high surface rather than on floor

Burns

Keep faucets out of reach

Place hot objects (cigarettes, candles, incense) on high surface

Limit exposure to sun; apply sunscreen

Motor vehicles

See under Age: Birth-4 Months

Bodily damage

Give toys that are smooth and rounded, preferably made of wood or plastic

Avoid long, pointed objects as toys

Avoid toys that are excessively loud

Keep sharp objects out of infant's reach

Age: 8-12 Months

MAJOR DEVELOPMENTAL ACCOMPLISHMENTS

Crawls/creeps

Stands, holding onto furniture

Stands alone

Cruises around furniture

Walks

Climbs

Pulls on objects

Throws objects

Is able to pick up small objects; has pincer grasp

Explores by putting objects in mouth

Dislikes being restrained

Explores away from parent

Increasing understanding of simple commands and phrases

INJURY PREVENTION

Aspiration

Keep lint and small objects off floor, furniture, and out of reach of children

Take care in feeding solid table food to ensure that very small pieces are given

Do not use beanbag toys or allow child to play with dried beans

See also under Age: 4-7 Months

Suffocation/drowning

Keep doors of ovens, dishwashers, refrigerators, coolers, and front-loading clothes washers and dryers closed at all times

If storing an unused appliance, such as a refrigerator, remove the door

Supervise contact with inflated balloons; immediately discard popped balloons and keep uninflated balloons out of reach

Fence swimming pools

Always supervise when near any source of water, such as cleaning buckets, drainage areas, toilets

Keep bathroom doors, closed

Eliminate unnecessary pools of water

Keep one hand on child at all times when in tub

Falls

Fence stairways at top and bottom if child has access to either end†

Dress infant in safe shoes and clothing (soles that do not "catch" on floor, tied shoelaces, pant legs that do not touch floor)

Avoid walkers, especially near stairs

Ensure that furniture is sturdy enough for child to pull self to standing position and cruise

Poisoning

Administer medications as a drug, not as a candy

Do not administer medications unless so prescribed by a practitioner

Replace medications and poisons immediately after use; replace caps properly if a child-protector cap is used

Have syrup of ipecac in home; use only if advised

Burns

Place guards in front of or around any heating appliance, fireplace, or furnace

Keep electrical wires hidden or out of reach

Place plastic guards over electrical outlets; place furniture in front of outlets

Keep hanging tablecloths out of reach (child may pull down hot liquids or heavy or sharp objects)

because infants and children depend on others for their health care, their experiences with caregivers influence their health attitudes and behavior. The nurse has a responsibility to educate parents and other caregivers about health promotion behavior that will positively affect perception of health and self.

Nutrition.   The quality and quantity of nutrition influence the infant's growth and development. The nurse helps parents select and provide a nutritionally adequate diet for their infant. The nurse must understand that nutrition is influenced by many variables (e.g., family culture, food preferences, slow eating, or food allergies) and

PHYSICAL NEGLECT

Suggestive Physical Findings

Failure to thrive

Signs of malnutrition, such as thin extremities, abdominal distention, lack of subcutaneous fat

Poor personal hygiene, especially of teeth

Unclean and/or inappropriate dress

Evidence of poor health care, such as nonimmunized status, untreated infections, frequent colds

Frequent injuries from lack of supervision

Suggestive Behaviors

Dull and inactive; excessively passive or sleepy

Self-stimulatory behaviors, such as finger-sucking or rocking

Begging or stealing food ⎫
Absenteeism from school ⎬ in older child
Drug or alcohol addiction ⎪
Vandalism or shoplifting ⎭

EMOTIONAL ABUSE AND NEGLECT

Suggestive Physical Findings

Failure to thrive

Feeding disorders, such as rumination

Enuresis

Sleep disorders

Suggestive Behaviors

Self-stimulatory behaviors such as biting, rocking, sucking

During infancy, lack of social smile and stranger anxiety

Withdrawal

Unusual fearfulness

Antisocial behavior, such as destructiveness, stealing, cruelty

Extremes of behavior, such as overcompliant and passive or aggressive and demanding

Lags in emotional and intellectual development, especially language

Suicide attempts

PHYSICAL ABUSE

Suggestive Physical Findings

Bruises and welts

On face, lips, mouth, back, buttocks, thighs, or areas of torso

Regular patterns descriptive of object used, such as belt buckle, hand, wire hanger, chain, wooden spoon, squeeze or pinch marks

May be present in various stages of healing

Burns

On soles of feet, palms of hands, back, or buttocks

Patterns descriptive of object used, such as round cigar or cigarette burns, "glovelike" sharply demarcated areas from immersion in scalding water, rope burns on wrists or ankles from being bound, burns in the shape of an iron, radiator, or electric stove burner

Absence of "splash" marks and presence of symmetric burns

Stun gun injury—lesions circular, fairly uniform (up to 0.5 cm), and paired approximately 5 cm apart (Frechette and Rimsza, 1992)

Fractures and dislocations

Skull, nose, or facial structures

Injury may denote type of abuse, such as spiral fracture or dislocation from twisting of an extremity or whiplash from shaking the child

Multiple new or old fractures in various stages of healing

Lacerations and abrasions

On backs of arms, legs, torso, face, or external genitalia

Unusual symptoms, such as abdominal swelling, pain, and vomiting from punching

Descriptive marks such as from human bites or pulling out of hair

Chemical

Unexplained repeated poisoning, especially drug overdose

Unexplained sudden illness, such as hypoglycemia from insulin administration

Suggestive Behaviors

Wariness of physical contact with adults

Apparent fear of parents or of going home

Lying very still while surveying environment

Inappropriate reaction to injury, such as failure to cry from pain

Lack of reaction to frightening events

Apprehensiveness when hearing other children cry

Indiscriminate friendliness and displays of affection

Superficial relationships

Acting-out behavior, such as aggression, to seek attention

Withdrawal behavior

SEXUAL ABUSE

Suggestive Physical Findings

Bruises, bleeding, lacerations or irritation of external genitalia, anus, mouth, or throat

Torn, stained, or bloody underclothing

Pain on urination or pain, swelling, and itching of genital area

Penile discharge

Sexually transmitted disease, nonspecific vaginitis, or venereal warts

Difficulty in walking or sitting

Unusual odor in the genital area

Recurrent urinary tract infections

Presence of sperm

Pregnancy in young adolescent

Suggestive Behaviors

Sudden emergence of sexually related problems, including excessive or public masturbation, age-inappropriate sexual play, promiscuity, or overtly seductive behavior

Withdrawn behavior, excessive daydreaming

Preoccupation with fantasies, especially in play

Poor relationships with peers

Sudden changes, such as anxiety, loss or gain of weight, clinging behavior

In incestuous relationships, excessive anger at mother for not protecting daughter

Regressive behavior, such as bed-wetting or thumb-sucking

Sudden onset of phobias or fears, particularly fears of the dark, men, strangers, or particular settings or situations (e.g., undue fear of leaving the house or staying at the daycare center or the baby-sitter's house)

Running away from home

Substance abuse, particularly of alcohol or mood-elevating drugs

Profound and rapid personality changes, especially extreme depression, hostility, and aggression (often accompanied by social withdrawal)

Rapidly declining school performance

Suicidal attempts or ideation

From Wong DL: *Whaley and Wong's nursing care of infants and children,* ed 6, St. Louis, 1999, Mosby.

Conditions That Can Be Mistaken for Sexual Abuse   Box 10-5

Accidental straddle injuries
Accidental impaling injuries
Nonspecific vulvovaginitis and proctitis
Group A β-streptococcal vaginitis and proctitis
Diaper dermatitis
Foreign bodies
Lower extremity girdle paralysis as in myelomeningocele
Defects that cause chronic constipation, Hirschsprung disease, anteriorly displaced anus
Chronic gastrointestinal disease, Crohn disease
Labial adhesions
Anal fissures

Modified from Brouder AE, Montelone JA: *Child maltreatment: a clinical guideline and reference,* St. Louis, 1994, GW Medical.

that no diet is effective for all children or for one age group.

Feeding Alternatives.   Supplying essential nutrients to the infant is the nurse's and parents' goal. The nurse should support the parents' choice of feeding methods and facilitate a successful feeding process. Breast-feeding is recommended for infants because breast milk contains the essential nutrients of protein, fats, carbohydrates, and immunoreactive proteins that bolster the ability to resist infection and it is considered the most complete nutritional source until 6 months of age. Breast-feeding has been associated with a decreased frequency of gastroenteritis, otitis media, and food allergies.

However, if breast-feeding is not possible or not desired by the parent, an acceptable alternative is iron-fortified commercially prepared formula. Commercially prepared formulas are popular because they are convenient, contain standard ingredients, and are fortified with vitamins and minerals. Infants receiving powered or concentrated formulas may be at risk for lead poisoning from tap water or other illnesses from untested well water. Bottled water is a relatively safe alternative for those at risk for contaminated water supplies (Wong, 1999). All types of cow's milk—skim, 2%, or whole—or imitation milks are not recommended in the first year because of the infant's decreased ability to digest the contained fat. Cow's milk also contains more sodium and protein and less iron (Grodner, Anderson, and DeYoung, 1996). The renal solute load in cow's milk is too heavy for the immature infant kidneys to handle. Because cow's milk is low in iron and high in calcium and phosphorus, absorption of iron may be decreased, causing anemia.

The average 1-month-old infant takes approximately 18 to 21 ounces of breast milk or formula per day. This amount increases slightly during the first 6 months and decreases when solid foods are introduced. The amount of formula per feeding and the number of feedings vary among infants. The addition of solid foods is not recommended before the age of 6 months because the gastrointestinal tract is not sufficiently mature to handle these complex nutrients and infants are exposed to food antigens that may produce food protein allergies. Developmentally, infants are not ready for food prior to 6 months. The extrusion (protrusion) reflex causes food to be pushed out of the mouth. The introduction of cereals, fruits, vegetables, and meats during the second 6 months of life provides iron and additional sources of vitamins. These become especially important when children are taken off breast milk or formula and begun on whole cow's milk after the first birthday. Well-cooked table foods are also tolerated by 1 year. The amount and frequency of feedings vary among infants, so the nurse should discuss differing feeding patterns with parents.

Honey has been used to sweeten water and coat pacifiers. The use of honey should be discouraged in infants less than 1 year because of the potential for infant botulism poisoning (AAP, 1997).

Supplementation.   The need for dietary vitamin and mineral supplements depends on the infant's diet. Full-term infants are born with some iron stores. The breast-fed infant absorbs adequate iron from breast milk during the first 4 to 6 months of life. After 6 months, iron-fortified cereal is generally considered an adequate supplemental source. Because iron in formula is less readily absorbed than that in breast milk, formula-fed infants should receive iron-fortified formula throughout the first year.

Adequate concentrations of fluoride to protect against dental caries are not available in human milk, and therefore fluoridated water or supplemental fluoride is generally recommended. The presence of fluoride in formula depends on the type of formula and the source of water used in preparing the concentrated forms. Fluoride supplementation may be necessary.

Overfeeding.   The association between overfeeding, infant obesity, and later adult obesity is still controversial. However, early feeding experiences can influence later eating habits. The nurse should therefore emphasize balanced nutrition and good dietary habits through feeding experiences mutually satisfying for the parents and infant. Eating habits are frequently affected by the sociocultural background of the family. Certain cultures regard "a fat baby as a healthy baby." Because some cultures consider a fat baby to be a sign of good mothering, any suggestion to limit intake or slow weight gain may be seen as a threat. It is important for the nurse to develop an understanding of the cultural influences to develop effective nursing interventions (Box 10-6).

Cultural ASPECTS OF CARE   Box 10-6

Cultural practices and beliefs have a significant influence on the choice of infant feeding methods. Although cultural norms exist, application of the norms may not be appropriate for all individuals. Immigrants to the United States from poorer countries may choose to bottle-feed their infants because it is believed to be better and more modern. Others may choose bottle-feeding because of a desire to adapt to American culture.

Many cultures choose not to give the infants colostrum. Filipinos, Mexican-Americans, Vietnamese, Hmong, Koreans, Nigerians and Indians are a few of the 50 known cultures that delay breast-feeding until the milk has "come in." Other cultures may begin breast-feeding immediately after delivery and offer the breast each time the infant cries.

Cultural attitudes regarding breast-feeding, modesty, and dietary beliefs are important considerations for the nurse. The balance between energy forces may be the basis for food selections. "Hot" foods in some cultures are considered to be the best. "Hot" does not refer to the temperature of the foods. Chicken and broccoli are considered "hot." "Cold" foods include fresh fruits and vegetables. Families may bring desired foods into the health care setting.

Dentition.   The average age for the first tooth to erupt is 7 months, but there is considerable variation among infants because of their genetic endowment. An occasional infant is born with a tooth whereas others remain toothless at 1 year. The order of tooth eruption is fairly predictable with the lower central incisors being first to appear, closely followed by the upper central incisors. Most 1-year-olds have six teeth.

Teething may result in considerable discomfort for some infants and little or none for others. The inflammation of the gums as the tooth prepares to emerge may result in a low-grade fever and irritability. Some have increased drooling, biting, or finger sucking. The use of a frozen teething ring or ice cube wrapped in a washcloth is soothing. Over-the-counter teething medications to rub on the inflamed gums and appropriate doses of acetaminophen are helpful when the infant is irritable and has difficulty eating or sleeping.

Most dentists recommend that parents cleanse their infant's teeth after each feeding. This can be accomplished very simply and quickly with a wet washcloth and the parent's finger. Dietary considerations should also be addressed with the parents. Prolonged breast- or bottle-feeding, especially bottle propping when the infant is likely to fall asleep and leave milk in the mouth to surround the teeth, should be discouraged due to the development of dental caries (American Academy of Pediatric Dentistry, 1996).

Immunizations.   The widespread use of immunizations has resulted in the dramatic decline of infectious diseases over the past 50 years and is therefore a most important factor in health promotion during childhood. Although most immunizations can be given to persons of any age, it is recommended that the administration of the primary series begin soon after birth and be completed during early childhood. Table 10-7 provides the 1998 recommended childhood schedule for routine active vaccination of infants and children (Centers for Disease Control and Prevention [CDC], 1998b).

Complacency and fear regarding the side effects of vaccines, especially diphtheria and tetanus toxoids and pertussis vaccine (DTP), have resulted in large numbers of children not receiving appropriate immunizations during recent years. Vaccines are among the safest and most reliable drugs used. Minor side effects may occur; however, serious reactions are rare. Parents should receive instructions regarding the potential side effects of immunizations. High fever and extreme irritability should be reported to their health care provider. As with all medications, some contraindications exist. In general, no vaccines should be given during a severe febrile illness. This precaution avoids adding possible side effects to an ill child. The side effects could be misinterpreted as additional symptoms from the illness, or illness symptoms could be misinterpreted as vaccination side effects.

Sleep.   Sleep patterns vary among infants, with many having their days and nights mixed up until 3 to 4 months of age. By this time, most infants are nocturnal and sleep between 9 and 11 hours. Total daily sleep averages 15 hours. Most infants take one or two naps a day by the end of the first year. Sleep disturbances with a physiological basis are rare, with the possible exception of colic. More common sleep disturbances are described in Table 10-8.

Toddler

Toddlerhood ranges from the time when children begin to walk independently until they walk and run with ease, which is from 12 to 36 months. The toddler is characterized by increasing independence bolstered by greater physical mobility and cognitive abilities. Toddlers are increasingly aware of their abilities to control and are pleased with successful efforts with this new skill. This success leads them to repeated attempts to control their environments. Unsuccessful attempts at control may result in negative behavior and temper tantrums. These behaviors are most common when parents thwart the initial independent action. Parents cite these as the most problematic behaviors during the toddler years and at times express frustration with trying to set consistent and firm limits while simultaneously encouraging independence.

PHYSICAL CHANGES

The rapid development of motor skills allows the child to participate in self-care activities such as feeding, dressing,

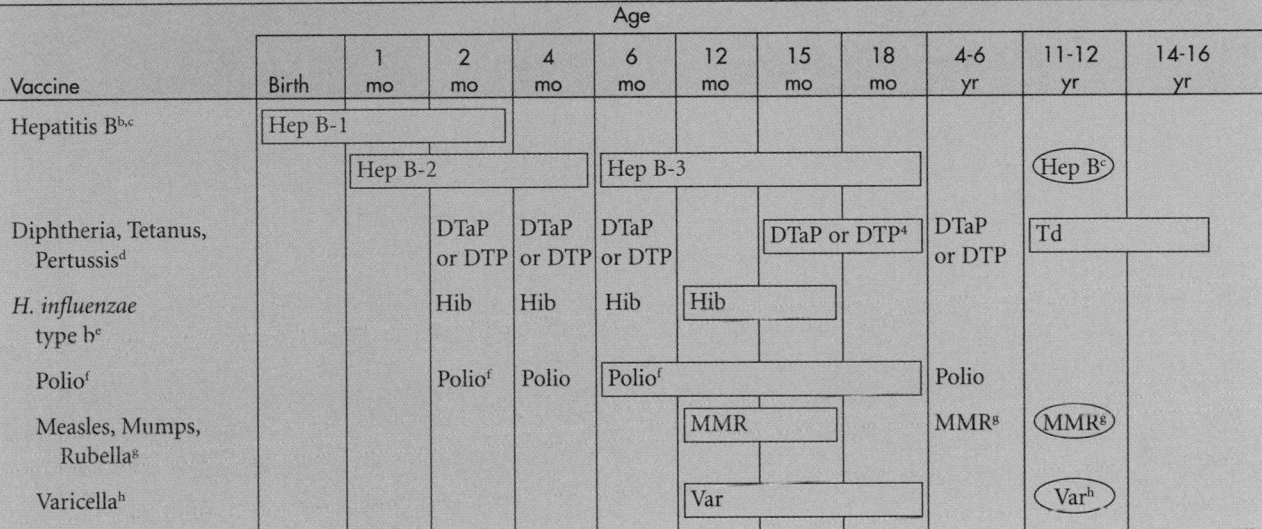

Table 10-7   Recommended Childhood Immunization Schedule

United States, January–December 1998

Vaccines[a] are listed under the routinely recommended ages. [Bars] indicate range of acceptable ages for immunization. Catch-up immunization should be done during any visit when feasible. (Ovals) indicate vaccines to be assessed and given if necessary during the early adolescent visit.

Vaccine	Birth	1 mo	2 mo	4 mo	6 mo	12 mo	15 mo	18 mo	4-6 yr	11-12 yr	14-16 yr
Hepatitis B[b,c]	Hep B-1									(Hep B[c])	
		Hep B-2			Hep B-3						
Diphtheria, Tetanus, Pertussis[d]		DTaP or DTP	DTaP or DTP	DTaP or DTP		DTaP or DTP[4]			DTaP or DTP	Td	
H. influenzae type b[e]		Hib	Hib	Hib	Hib						
Polio[f]		Polio[f]	Polio	Polio[f]					Polio		
Measles, Mumps, Rubella[g]						MMR			MMR[g]	(MMR[g])	
Varicella[h]						Var				(Var[h])	

Modified from Wong DL: *Whaley and Wong's nursing care of infants and children*, ed 6, St. Louis, 1999, Mosby.

Approved by the Advisory Committee on Immunization Practices (ACIP), the American Academy of Pediatrics (AAP), and the American Academy of Family Physicians (AAFP).

[a]This schedule indicates the recommended age for routine administration of currently licensed childhood vaccines. Some combination vaccines are available and may be used whenever administration of all components of the vaccine is indicated. Providers should consult the manufacturers' package inserts for detailed recommendations.

[b]Infants born to HBsAg-negative mothers should receive 2.5 μg of Merck vaccine (Recombivax HB) or 10 μg of SmithKline Beecham (SB) vaccine (Engerix-B). The 2nd dose should be administered at least 1 month after the 1st dose. The 3rd dose should be given at least 2 months after the second, but not before 6 months of age.

Infants born to HBsAg-positive mothers should receive 0.5 ml of hepatitis B immune globulin (HBIG) within 12 hours of birth, and either 5 μg of Merck vaccine (Recombivax HB) or 10 μg of SB vaccine (Engerix-B) at a separate site. The 2nd dose is recommended at 1–2 months of age and the 3rd dose at 6 months of age.

Infants born to mothers whose HBsAg status is unknown should receive either 5 μg of Merck vaccine (Recombivax HB) or 10 μg of SB vaccine (Engerix-B) within 12 hours of birth. The 2nd dose of vaccine is recommended at 1 month of age and the 3rd dose at 6 months of age. Blood should be drawn at the time of delivery to determine the mother's HBsAg status; if it is positive, the infant should receive HBIG as soon as possible (no later than 1 week of age). The dosage and timing of subsequent vaccine doses should be based upon the mother's HBsAg status.

[c]Children and adolescents who have not been vaccinated against hepatitis B in infancy may begin the series during any visit. Those who have not previously received 3 doses of hepatitis B vaccine should initiate or complete the series during the 11- to 12-year-old visit, and unvaccinated older adolescents should be vaccinated whenever possible. The 2nd dose should be administered at least 1 month after the 1st dose, and the 3rd dose should be administered at least 4 months after the 1st dose and at least 2 months after the 2nd dose.

[d]DTaP (diphtheria and tetanus toxoids and acellular pertussis vaccine) is the preferred vaccine for all doses in the vaccination series, including completion of the series in children who have received 1 or more doses of whole-cell DTP vaccine. Whole-cell DTP is an acceptable alternative to DTaP. The 4th dose (DTP or DTaP) may be administered as early as 12 months of age, provided 6 months have elapsed since the 3rd dose, and if the child is unlikely to return at 15–18 months. Td (tetanus and diphtheria toxoids) is recommended at 11–12 years of age if at least 5 years have elapsed since the last dose of DTP, DTaP or DT. Subsequent routine Td boosters are recommended every 10 years.

[e]Three H. influenzae type b (Hib) conjugate vaccines are licensed for infant use. If PRP-OMP (PedvaxHIB [Merck]) is administered at 2 and 4 months of age, a dose at 6 months is not required.

[f]Two poliovirus vaccines are currently licensed in the US: inactivated poliovirus vaccine (IPV) and oral poliovirus vaccine (OPV). The following schedules are all acceptable to the ACIP, the AAP, and the AAFP. Parents and providers may choose among these options:

1. 2 doses of IPV followed by 2 doses of OPV
2. 4 doses of IPV
3. 4 doses of OPV

The ACIP recommends 2 doses of IPV at 2 and 4 months of age followed by 2 doses of OPV at 12–18 months and 4–6 years of age. IPV is the only poliovirus vaccine recommended for immunocompromised persons and their household contacts.

[g]The 2nd dose of MMR is recommended routinely at 4–6 years of age but may be administered during any visit, provided at least 1 month has elapsed since receipt of the 1st dose and that both doses are administered beginning at or after 12 months of age. Those who have not *previously* received the second dose should complete the schedule no later than the 11- to 12-year visit.

[h]Susceptible children may receive varicella vaccine (Var) at any visit after the first birthday, and those who lack a reliable history of chickenpox should be immunized during the 11- to 12-year-old visit. Susceptible children 13 years of age or older should receive 2 doses, at least 1 month apart.

Table 10-8 Selected Sleep Disturbances During Infancy and Early Childhood

Disorder/Description	Management
Nighttime Feeding* Child has a prolonged need for middle-of-night bottle- or breast-feeding Child goes to sleep at the breast or with a bottle Awakenings are frequent (may be hourly) Child returns to sleep after feeding; other comfort measures (e.g., rocking or holding) are usually ineffective	Increase daytime feeding intervals to 4 hours or more (may need to be done gradually) Offer last feeding as late as possible at night; may need to gradually reduce amount of formula or length of breast-feeding Offer no bottles in bed Put to bed *awake* When child is crying, check at progressively longer intervals each night; reassure child but do not hold, rock, take to parent's bed, or give bottle or pacifier
Developmental Night Crying Child age 6-12 months with undisturbed nighttime sleep now awakes abruptly; may be accompanied by nightmares	Reassure parents that this phase is temporary Enter room immediately to check on child but keep reassurances *brief* Avoid feeding, rocking, taking to parent's bed, or any other routine that may initiate trained night crying
Trained Night Crying* (Inappropriate Sleep Associations) Child typically falls asleep in place other than own bed (e.g., rocking chair or parent's bed) and is brought to own bed while asleep; on awakening, cries until usual routine is instituted (e.g., rocking)	Put child in own bed when *awake* If possible, arrange sleeping area separate from other family members When child is crying, check at progressively longer intervals each night; reassure child but do not resume usual routine
Refusal to Go to Sleep* Child resists bedtime and comes out of room repeatedly Nighttime sleep may be continuous, but frequent awakenings and refusal to return to sleep may occur and become a problem if parent allows child to deviate from usual sleep pattern	Evaluate if hour of sleep is too early (child may resist sleep if not tired) Assist parents in establishing consistent before-bedtime routine and enforcing consistent limits regarding child's bedtime behavior If child persists in leaving bedroom, close door for progressively longer periods Use reward system with child to provide motivation
Nighttime Fears Child resists going to bed or wakes during the night because of fears Child seeks parent's physical presence and falls asleep easily with parent nearby, unless fear is overwhelming	Evaluate if hour of sleep is too early (child may fantasize when nothing to do but think in dark room) Calmly reassure the frightened child; keeping a night-light on may be helpful Use reward system with child to provide motivation to deal with fears Avoid patterns that can lead to additional problems (e.g., sleeping with child or taking child to parent's room) If child's fear is overwhelming, consider desensitization (e.g., progressively spending longer periods of time alone; consult professional help for protracted fears) Distinguish between nightmares and sleep terrors (confused partial arousals).

Modified from Ferber R: Behavioral "insomnia" in the child, *Psychiatr Clin North Am* 10(4):641, 1987.
*Guidelines for parents in dealing with these sleep problems are in Wong DL: *Wong and Whaley's clinical manual of pediatric nursing,* ed 5, St. Louis, 2000, Mosby.

and toileting. In the beginning the toddler walks in an upright position with a broad-stanced gait, protuberant abdomen, and arms out to the sides for balance. Soon the child begins to navigate stairs, using a rail or the wall to maintain balance while progressing upward, placing both feet on the same step before continuing. Success provides courage to attempt the upright mode for descending the stairs in the same manner. Locomotion skills soon include running, jumping, standing on one foot for several seconds, and kicking a ball. Most toddlers can ride tricycles, climb ladders, and run well by their third birthday. Fine motor capabilities move from scribbling spontaneously to drawing circles and crosses accurately. By 3 years the child draws simple stick people and can usually stack a tower of small blocks. Increased locomotion skills, the ability to undress, and development of sphincter control allow toilet training if the toddler has developed the necessary cognitive abilities. Parents often consult nurses for an assessment of readiness for toilet training. The nurse needs to remind parents to look for cues that the child is ready or interested in toileting and that patience, consistency, and a nonjudgmental attitude, in addition to the child's readiness, are essential to successful toilet training.

The cardiopulmonary system becomes stable in the toddler years. The heart and respiratory rates slow to an average of 110 beats and 25 breaths per minute, respectively, and the blood pressure varies slightly from infancy. The average blood pressure for a toddler is 90/50 mm Hg.

The anterior fontanel closes between 12 and 18 months of age, ending the period of most rapid growth of the skull and brain. Routine measurement of head circumference should be done until 3 years of age.

The rate of increase in weight and length slows. By 2½ years the child weighs 4 times the birth weight. Height during toddlerhood increases by approximately 3 inches a year, mainly as a result of increases in leg length. The average height of 2-year-olds is 34 inches. Slowed growth rates are accompanied by decreased caloric need and smaller food intake (**physiological anorexia**), which leads some parents to worry about the adequacy of dietary intake. Parents need encouragement to offer the child appropriate servings of food from the food pyramid and to avoid force feeding or allowing the child to fill up on foods that are high in fat and sugar. The nurse can reassure parents that the child's nutrition is adequate by demonstrating the child's satisfactory status on a growth grid.

COGNITIVE CHANGES

Toddlers' completion of the development of object permanence, their ability to remember events, and their beginning ability to put thoughts into words at about 2 years of age signal their transition from Piaget's sensorimotor stage of cognitive development to the **preoperational thought** stage (Piaget, 1952). Toddlers recognize that they are separate beings from their mothers, but they are un-

able to assume the view of another. They use symbols to represent objects, places, and persons. This function is demonstrated when children imitate the behavior of another that they viewed earlier (e.g., pretend to shave like daddy), pretend one object is another (use a finger as a gun), and use language to stand for absent objects (e.g., request bottle).

Language. The 18-month-old child uses approximately 10 words. The 24-month-old child has a vocabulary of up to 300 words and is generally able to speak in short sentences. "Who's that?" and "What's that?" typify questions asked during this period. Verbal expressions such as "me do it" and "that's mine" demonstrate the 2-year-old child's use of pronouns and desire for independence and control. Despite the expanded vocabulary of an older toddler, most parents comment that their child's favorite word is *no* until well into the third year.

Because children's moral development is closely associated with their cognitive abilities, the moral development of toddlers is only beginning and is also egocentric. Toddlers do not understand concepts of right and wrong. However, they do grasp the fact that some behaviors bring pleasant results (positive reinforcement) and others elicit unpleasant results (negative reinforcement). Therefore until toddlers achieve a higher level of cognitive function, they behave simply to avoid the unpleasant and seek out the pleasant (Wong, 1999).

PSYCHOSOCIAL CHANGES

According to Erikson (1963), a sense of autonomy emerges during toddlerhood. Children strive for independence by using their developing muscles to do everything for themselves and become the master of their bodily functions. Their strong wills are frequently exhibited in negative behavior when caregivers attempt to direct their actions. Temper tantrums may result when toddlers are frustrated by parental restrictions. Parents need to provide toddlers with graded independence, allowing them to do things that do not result in harm to themselves or others. This prevents them from doubting their ability to do things that they are capable of learning or feeling a sense of shame for those things that they have done. Firm consistent limits, patience, and support allow toddlers to develop socially acceptable behavior, which is the goal of parental guidance. Young toddlers who want to learn to hold their own cups may benefit from two-handled cups with spouts and plastic bibs with pockets to collect the milk that spills during the learning process.

Socially, toddlers remain strongly attached to their parents and fear separation from them. In their presence they feel safe, and their curiosity is evident in their exploration of the environment. Mothers of toddlers are rarely allowed any bathroom privacy because closing of the door results in incessant crying until the door is opened.

The child continues to engage in solitary play during

toddlerhood but also begins to participate in parallel play, which is playing beside rather than with another child. Toddlers who are just learning what belongs to them are often possessive of their toys. They learn the joy of sharing when they offer parents toys to hold and the parents express pleasure.

Health Risks

The newly developed locomotion abilities and insatiable curiosity of toddlers make them a danger to their own well-being. Toddlers need close supervision at all times and particularly when in environments that have not been childproofed. Poisonings occur frequently because children near 2 years of age are interested in placing any object or substance in their mouths to learn about it. Fortunately, ingestions do not always result in death, but they do have many negative consequences such as chemical pneumonia. The wise parent removes or locks up all possible poisons, including plants, cleaning materials, and medications. These parental actions create a safer environment for exploratory behavior. Toddlers' lack of awareness regarding the danger of water and their newly developed walking skills combine to make drowning a major cause of accidental death in this age group. Limit setting is extremely important for toddlers' safety. Automobile safety requires toddlers to remain in car seats, even though they say (often loudly) that they would prefer to move freely about the car. Children often learn to release the car restraints, and parents must be firm in their resolve not to drive unless the children are securely restrained. Toddlers completely depend on their parents for physical safety. Table 10-9 identifies developmental abilities acquired during this age period and injury prevention strategies.

Health Concerns
Health Perceptions.
Toddlers' perceptions of their own health are limited by their cognitive capabilities. Children increasingly recognize internal body sensations but have difficulty pinpointing their location. Therefore children often associate generalized responses with illness. Children who deviate radically from their usual patterns of eating, sleeping, or playing require assessment to determine whether these alterations result from illness. During this stage, children begin to internalize the labels that parents or health care professionals give to the somatic states. That is, if the parents label particular sensations, such as abdominal discomfort, an "illness," children begin to label related sensations similarly. At the same time, children observe and mimic parents' health care practices. Health beliefs and practices are therefore being significantly shaped, even in these early years.

Nutrition.
Most toddlers change from breast milk or formula to cow's milk, consuming three to four 8 ounce servings per day. Nutritional requirements are increasingly met by solid foods from the food pyramid. Because the consumption of more than a quart of milk per day usually decreases the child's appetite for these essential solid foods and results in inadequate iron intake, the nurse should advise parents to limit milk intake to 2 to 3 cups per day. Children are usually not offered low fat or skim milk until age 2 because they need the fat for satisfactory physical and intellectual growth. The healthy toddler requires a balanced daily intake of bread and grains, vegetables, fruit, dairy products, and proteins. Because parents frequently overestimate the size of a normal serving for their child, the nurse can reduce their anxiety about inadequate intake by pointing out the normal serving size.

Children who are ill, are undergoing surgery, or have diseases involving ingestion, absorption, or use of nutrients require special dietary considerations. Alterations in the type of foods and caloric requirements may be necessary. Children on strict vegetarian diets also require careful planning to ensure adequate, balanced protein intake. Regardless of children's health status, several basic principles of nutrition apply. Mealtime has psychosocial and physical significance. If the parents struggle to control toddlers' dietary intake, problem behavior and conflicts may result. Toddlers often develop "food jags," or the desire to eat one food repeatedly. Rather than becoming disturbed by this behavior, parents should be encouraged by the nurse to offer a variety of nutritious foods at meals and to provide only nutritious snacks between meals. Serving finger foods to toddlers allows them to eat by themselves and to satisfy their need for independence and control. Small, reasonable servings allow toddlers to eat all of their meals.

Preschooler

The **preschool period** refers to those years between 3 and 5. Children refine the mastery of their bodies and eagerly await the beginning of formal education. Many people consider these the most intriguing years of parenting because children are less negative, can more accurately share their thoughts, and can more effectively interact and communicate. Physical development continues to slow, whereas cognitive and psychosocial development are rapid.

Physical Changes

Several aspects of physical development continue to stabilize in the preschool years. Heart and respiratory rates range from 60 to 100 beats and 23 to 25 breaths per minute, respectively. Blood pressure rises slightly to an average of 92/56 mm Hg. Children gain about 5 pounds per year; the average weight at 3 years is 32 pounds, at 4 years is 37 pounds, and at 5 years is about 41 pounds. Preschoolers grow 2½ to 3 inches per year, double their birth length around 4 years, and stand an average of 43 inches tall by their fifth birthday. The elongation of the

Table 10-9 Injury Prevention During Early Childhood

Developmental Abilities Related to Risk of Injury	Injury Prevention
	Motor vehicles
Walks, runs, and climbs	Use federally approved car restraint; if restraint is not available, use lap belt
Able to open doors and gates	Supervise child while playing outside
Can ride tricycle	Do not allow child to play on curb or behind a parked car
Can throw ball and other objects	Do not permit child to play in pile of leaves, snow, or large cardboard container in trafficked area
	Supervise tricycle riding
	Lock fences and doors if not directly supervising children
	Teach child to obey pedestrian safety rules
	Obey traffic regulations; walk only at crosswalks and when traffic signal indicates it is safe to cross
	Stand back a step from curb until it is time to cross
	Look left, right, and left again and check for turning cars before crossing street
	Use sidewalks; when there is no sidewalk, walk on left, facing traffic
	Wear light colors at night, and attach fluorescent material to clothing
	Drowning
Able to explore if left unsupervised	Supervise closely when near any source of water, including buckets
Has great curiosity	Keep bathroom doors and lid on toilet closed
Helpless in water, unaware of its danger; depth of water has no significance	Have fence around swimming pool and lock gate
	Teach swimming and water safety (not a substitute for protection)
	Burns
Able to reach heights by climbing, stretching, standing on toes, and using objects as a ladder	Turn pot handles toward back of stove
	Place electric appliances, such as coffee maker, frying pan, and popcorn popper, toward back of counter
Pulls objects	Place guardrails in front of radiators, fireplaces, or other heating elements
Explores any holes or opening	Store matches and cigarette lighters in locked or inaccessible area; discard carefully
Can open drawers and closets	Place burning candles, incense, hot foods, ashes, embers, and cigarettes out of reach
Unaware of potential sources of heat or fire	Do not let tablecloth hang within child's reach
Plays with mechanical objects	Do not let electric cord from iron or other appliance hang within child's reach
	Cover electrical outlets with protective devices
	Keep electrical wires hidden or out of reach
	Do not allow child to play with electrical appliance, wires, or lighters
	Stress danger of open flames; teach what "hot" means
	Always check bathwater temperature; adjust hot-water heater temperature to 48.9°C (120°F) or lower; do not allow children to play with faucets
	Apply a sunscreen with SPF 15 or higher when child is exposed to sunlight
	Poisoning
Explores by putting objects in mouth	Place all potentially toxic agents (including plants) in a locked cabinet or out of reach
Can open drawers, closets, and most containers	Replace medications and poisons immediately; replace child-resistant caps properly
	Refer to medications as drugs, not as candy
Climbs	Do not store large surplus of toxic agents
Cannot read warning labels	Promptly discard empty poison containers; never reuse to store a food item or other poison
Does not know safe dose or amount	Teach child not to play in trash containers
	Never remove labels from containers of toxic substances
	Have syrup of ipecac in home; use only if advised
	Know number and location of nearest poison control center (usually listed in front of telephone directory)
	Falls
Able to open doors and some windows	Keep screen in window, nail securely, and use guardrail
	Place gates at top and bottom of stairs
Goes up and down stairs	Keep doors locked or use child-resistant doorknob covers at entry to stairs, high porch, or other elevated area, such as laundry chute
Depth perception unrefined	Remove unsecured or scatter rugs
	Apply nonskid mat in bathtub or shower
	Keep crib rails fully raised and mattress at lowest level

Continued

Table 10-9 Injury Prevention During Early Childhood—cont'd

Developmental Abilities Related to Risk of Injury	Injury Prevention
	Place carpeting under crib and in bathroom
	Keep large toys and bumper pads out of crib or playpen (child can use these as "stairs" to climb out), then move to youth bed when child is able to crawl out of crib
	Avoid using walkers, especially near stairs
	Dress in safe clothing (soles that do not "catch" on floor, tied shoelaces, pant legs that do not hang on floor)
	Keep child restrained in vehicles; never leave unattended in shopping cart or stroller
	Supervise at playgrounds; select play areas with soft ground cover and safe equipment
	Choking and suffocation
Puts things in mouth	Avoid large, round chunks of meat, such as whole hot dogs (slice lengthwise into short pieces)
May swallow hard or nonedible pieces of food	Avoid fruit with pits, fish with bones, dried beans, hard candy, chewing gum, nuts, popcorn, grapes, marshmallows
	Choose large, sturdy toys without sharp edges or small removable parts
	Discard old refrigerators, ovens, and so on; if storing old appliance, remove doors
	Keep automatic garage door transmitter in inaccessible place
	Select safe toy boxes or chests without heavy, hinged lids
	Keep venetian blind strings out of child's reach.
	Remove drawstrings from clothing
	Bodily damage
Still clumsy in many skills	Avoid giving sharp or pointed objects—such as knives, scissors, or toothpicks— especially when walking or running
Easily distracted from tasks	Do not allow lollipops or similar objects in mouth when walking or running
Unaware of potential danger from strangers or other people	Teach safety precautions (e.g., to carry fork or scissors with pointed end away from face)
	Store all dangerous tools, garden equipment, and firearms in locked cabinet
	Be alert to danger of animals, including household pets
	Use safety glass and decals on large glassed areas, such as sliding glass doors
	Teach personal safety
	Teach name, address, and phone number and to ask for help from appropriate people (cashier, security guard, policeman) if lost; have identification on child (sewn in clothes, inside shoe)
	Avoid personalized clothing in public places
	Teach child to never go with a stranger
	Teach child to tell parents if anyone makes child feel uncomfortable in any way
	Always listen to child's concerns regarding others' behavior
	Teach child to say "no" when confronted with uncomfortable situations

From Wong DL: *Whaley and Wong's nursing care of infants and children*, ed 6, St. Louis, 1999, Mosby.

legs results in more slender appearing children. Little difference exists between the sexes, although boys are slightly larger with more muscle and less fatty tissue.

Large and fine muscle coordination improves. Preschoolers run well, walk up and down steps with ease, and learn to hop. By 5 years they can usually skip on alternate feet, jump rope, and begin to skate and swim. Improving fine motor skills allows intricate manipulations. They learn to copy crosses and squares. Triangles and diamonds are usually mastered between age 5 and 6. Scribbling and drawing help to develop fine muscle skills and eye-hand coordination needed for the printing of letters and numbers.

Children need opportunities to learn and practice new physical skills. Nursing care of healthy and ill children includes an assessment of the availability of these opportu-

nities. Although children with acute illnesses benefit from rest and exclusion from usual daily activities, children who have chronic conditions or who have been hospitalized for long periods need ongoing exposure to developmental opportunities. The parents and nurse weave these opportunities into the children's daily experiences, depending on their abilities, needs, and energy level.

COGNITIVE CHANGES

Preschoolers continue to master the preoperational stage of cognition. The first phase of this period, known as preconceptual thought (2 to 4 years), is characterized by perceptual-bound thinking, in which children judge persons, objects, and events by their outward appearance or what seems to be (Piaget, 1952). For example, children may determine that an 8-ounce glass full of fluid contains more than a 10-ounce glass that also contains 8 ounces of fluid because they center their thoughts on the fullness of the glass. Even if they watch the 8 ounces of fluid from the full glass being poured into the 10-ounce glass and the 8-ounce glass refilled, they will still assert that the full 8-ounce glass contains more because they cannot attend to the transfer. Thinking is hindered by their limited attention and attending skills. **Artificialism,** the misconception that everything in the world has been created by humanity, may result in children asking questions such as who built the mountains. Another misconception of preschool thinking, **animism,** the attribution of life to inanimate objects, often results in statements such as "Trees cry when their branches are broken." A third misconception is a type of reasoning called immanent justice, the notion that the world is equipped with a built-in code of law and order. It may result in children's beliefs that matches burned them because they were not supposed to handle them.

Around the age of 4 years, the intuitive phase of preoperational thought develops, and children's ability to think more complexly is demonstrated by their ability to classify objects according to size or color and by questions such as "Why do they call it the thirty-first day of the month instead of the thirty last?" Egocentricity persists, but during these 3 years, it begins to be replaced with social interaction, as is illustrated by the 5-year-old child who offers a bandage to a child with a cut finger. Children become aware of cause-and-effect relationships, as illustrated by the statement "The sun sets because people want to go to bed." Early causal thinking is also evident in preschoolers' transductive thoughts (reasoning occurs from one particular to another). If two events are related in time or space, children link them in a causal fashion. The hospitalized child, for example, may reason, "I cried last night, and that's why the nurse gave me the shot." As children near age 5, they begin to use or can be taught to use rules to understand causation. They then begin to reason from the general to the particular. This forms the basis for more formal logical thought. The child can now reason, "I get a shot twice a day, and that's why I got one last night."

Preschoolers' knowledge of the world remains closely linked to concrete (perceived by the senses) experiences. Even their rich fantasy life is grounded in the perception of reality. The mixing of the two aspects can lead to many childhood fears and may be misinterpreted by adults as lying when children are actually presenting reality from their perspective.

The greatest fear of this age group appears to be that of bodily harm, and it can be seen in children's fear of the dark, animals, thunderstorms, and medical personnel. This fear often interferes with their willingness to allow nursing interventions such as measurement of vital signs. Preschoolers may cooperate if they are allowed to help the nurse measure the blood pressure of a parent or if they are allowed to manipulate the nurse's equipment.

The preschooler's moral development expands to include a beginning understanding of behaviors considered socially right or wrong. The child continues to be motivated, however, by the wish to avoid punishment or the desire to obtain a reward. The primary difference between this stage of moral development and that of a toddler is that a preschooler is better able to identify behaviors that elicit rewards or punishment and begins to label these behaviors as right or wrong.

Language. Preschoolers' vocabularies continue to increase rapidly, and by the age of 5 children have more than 2000 words that they can use to define familiar objects, identify colors, and express their desires and frustrations. Language is more social, and questions expand to "Why?" and "How come?" in the quest for information. Phonetically similar words such as *die* and *dye* or *wood* and *would* may cause confusion in preschool children. The nurse avoids such words when preparing children for procedures and assesses comprehension of explanations.

PSYCHOSOCIAL CHANGES

The world of preschoolers expands beyond the family into the neighborhood where children meet other children and adults. Their curiosity and developing initiative lead to the active exploration of the environment, the development of new skills, and the making of new friends. Preschoolers have a surplus of energy that permits them to plan and attempt many activities that may be beyond their capabilities, such as pouring milk from a gallon container into their cereal bowls. Guilt arises within children when they overstep the limits of their abilities and feel they have not behaved correctly. Children who in anger have wished their sibling were dead experience guilt if that sibling becomes ill. Children need to be taught that "wishing" for something to happen does not make it occur. Erikson (1963) recommends that parents help their children strike a healthy balance between initiative and guilt by allowing them to do things on their own while setting firm limits and providing guidance.

During times of stress or illness, preschoolers may revert to bed-wetting or thumb sucking and want the parents to feed, dress, and hold them. Box 10-7 lists potential sources of stress in the preschooler. These dependent behaviors are often confusing and embarrassing to parents, who can benefit from the nurse's reassurance that they are the child's normal coping behaviors. The nurse should provide experiences that these children can master. Such successes help children return to their prior level of independent functioning. As language skills develop, children should be encouraged to talk about their feelings. Play is also an excellent way for preschoolers to vent frustration or anger and is a socially acceptable way to deal with stress.

Play. The play of preschool children becomes more social after the third birthday as it shifts from parallel to associative play. All participants engage in similar if not identical activity; however, there is no division of labor, and no rigid organization or rules. Most 3-year-old children are able to play with one other child in a cooperative manner in which they make something or play designated roles such as mother and baby. By age 4, children play in groups of two or three, and by 5 years the group has a temporary leader for each activity.

In many play activities, preschoolers display awareness of social context. Sex-role identification is strengthening, and children most often assume roles of persons of their own sex. Children frequently mimic or repeat social experiences. This tendency is especially significant for the nurse working with hospitalized children. Through play, children may express questions, fears, anger, and misunderstanding about their illnesses and care. The nurse should be alert to such clues and ensure that children can play within energy limits. Play can provide a healthy outlet for frustration when children have been subjected to painful or restrictive experiences against their will.

Pretend play involving imaginary situations depends on children's ability to retain images of things they have seen or heard. This sociodramatic play involving other children occupies about a third of 5-year-old children's playtime. Pretending allows children to learn to understand other's points of view, develop skills in solving social problems, and become more creative. Some children have imaginary playmates. These playmates serve many purposes—friends when they are lonely, they can accomplish what the child is still attempting and can experience what the child wants to forget or remember. Imaginary playmates are a sign of health and allow the child to distinguish between real and fantasy. Children who watch a great deal of television engage less frequently in imaginative play, possibly because they develop the habit of passively absorbing images rather than generating their own (Wong, 1999)

HEALTH RISKS

As fine and gross motor skills develop and the child becomes more coordinated with better balance, falls become much less of a problem. Guidelines for injury prevention in the toddler also apply to the preschooler. The nurse

---

Sources of Stress in Preschoolers   Box 10-7

THREE-YEAR-OLD

Infantile behavior—Reverts to babyish ways; can't completely let go of babyhood

Stubbornness—Although is developing an interest in social relationships and a concept of "we," may lapse into uncooperative behavior

Possessiveness—Guards belongings and may be bossy about them

Jealousy—Particularly when it comes to parents' love

Separation anxiety

Stranger anxiety

Confusion—Cannot always discriminate between fantasy and reality

White lies—May result from wishful thinking, fantasy, and desire to please or impress

Imaginary playmate—Often blamed for misdeeds

Fears—May be precipitated by imagination, may also fear dogs or other animals

Speech—May stutter or stumble over words

Activity level—Seems to be in perpetual motion; may exhaust himself or herself

Eating—May forget to eat or lose interest in food

Nap or bedtime—May fear bad dreams, the dark, or missing out on some fun while asleep

Destructiveness—May damage or destroy objects

Questions—Continually asks "why," and is upset if trusted adults do not respond or do not know the answer

FOUR-YEAR-OLD

Insecurity—May develop nervous habits such as nail biting, facial tics, thumb sucking, genital manipulation, eye blinking, or nose picking; may insist on bringing a familiar item from house to preschool

Exaggerations—May attempt to boost self-image with boasts

Companionship—Enjoys interacting with friends, although there may be many quarrels

Silliness—Tends to engage in silly play; likes words and is fascinated by rhyming syllables or foul language; is disciplined for lack of control

Property rights—Protects belongings; may become bossy

Sex—Interested in the human body; may engage in exhibitionism

Activity level—Enjoys running, jumping, and slamming doors; may be punished for disruptive behavior

Fears—Picks up fears from adults; may fear dark room, snakes and lizards, or anything perceived as "creepy"

Attention—Likes to talk and is frustrated if ignored or put off; whines to get own way

FIVE-YEAR-OLD

Approval—Parents' love and acceptance are vital; seeks praise

School—May have difficulty adjusting to kindergarten

Separation anxiety—Particularly fears loss of mother

Infantile behavior—May occasionally lapse into babyish behavior as a result of realizing that babyhood has ended

Worrying—May develop irrational fears, take information out of context, or fret over a misinterpreted, overheard conversation

Masturbation—Is concerned about being "bad"

Belongings—Protects possessions

Showing off—Performs in order to gain praise

Procrastination—May dillydally now and then

Name-calling—Insults others to boost self-image but is upset when she or he is the victim of mockery

Modified from Kuczen B: *Childhood stress: don't let your child be a victim,* New York, 1982, Delacorte Press.

should alert parents of children in this age group to the risks of poisoning and pedestrian–motor vehicle accidents.

HEALTH CONCERNS

Little research has explored preschoolers' perceptions of their own health. Parental beliefs about health, children's bodily sensations, and their ability to perform usual daily activities help children develop attitudes about their health. Preschoolers are usually quite independent in washing, dressing, and feeding. Alterations in this independence can influence their feelings about their own health.

Nutrition. Nutrition requirements for the preschooler vary little from the toddler. The average daily intake is 1800 calories. Parents may still worry about the amount of food their child is consuming. The quality of the food is more important than quantity in most situations. Preschoolers consume about half of the average adult portions. Finicky eating habits are characteristic of the 4-year-old, however the 5-year-old is more interested in trying new foods.

Sleep. Preschoolers average 12 hours of sleep a night and take infrequent naps. Sleep disturbances are not uncommon during these years. Disturbances may range from trouble getting to sleep to nightmares to prolonging bedtime with extensive rituals. Frequently, the child has had an overabundance of activity and stimulation. Helping them to slow down prior to bedtime usually results in less resistance.

School-Age Children and Adolescents

School-age children and adolescents lead demanding, challenging lives. The developmental changes between ages 6 and 18 are diverse and span all areas of growth and development. Physical, psychosocial, cognitive, and moral skills are developed, expanded, refined, and synchronized so that the individual may become an accepted and productive member of society. The environment in which the individual develops skills also expands and diversifies. Instead of the principal limits of family and close friends, the environment may include the school, community, and church. Because of expectations for development, increasing skill and knowledge base, and environmental expansion, the individual experiences new difficulties and dilemmas. With age-specific assessment, the nurse must review the appropriate developmental expectations for each age group. For example, before assessing risk-taking behaviors, the nurse recognizes that adolescents normally strive to achieve a sense of identity while developing a moral code compatible with society.

The nurse needs to direct school-age children and adolescents toward normal developmental behaviors, assisting them in maximizing their abilities and using them to cope. By helping children and adolescents achieve a necessary developmental balance, the nurse promotes health. Table 10-10 provides an overview of developmental behavior typical of school-age children and adolescents. The nurse must also increasingly involve the child or adolescent in charting a developmental course. Because preadolescents have increased cognitive and social skills, they are better able to plan developmental activities. Not only can they describe their feelings about the changes, but they can also think through these changes. Problem solving becomes more purposeful and sophisticated and results in the achievement of the outcomes that they desire. This paced, active participation may initiate a style of involvement in lifelong self-care.

School-age children and adolescents must cope with changes involving all areas of development. For example, 6-year-old children are confronted with new authority figures, teachers, as well as new rules and restrictions. They need to cooperatively work and play with a large group of children of various cultural backgrounds. School-age children must meet the challenge of developing cognitive skills that enhance their reasoning and allow them to learn to read, write, and manipulate numbers. Because of the stress of these changes, a child may develop physical and psychosocial health problems (e.g., increased susceptibility to upper respiratory infections, school maladjustment, inadequate peer relationships, or learning disorders). The nurse designs health promotion interventions that are based on the child's developmental stage.

School-Age Child

During these "middle years" of childhood, the foundation for adult roles in work, recreation, and social interaction is laid. In industrialized countries this **school-age** period begins when the child starts elementary school around the age of 6 years. **Puberty,** around 12 years of age, signals the end of middle childhood. Great developmental strides are made during these years when children develop competencies in physical, cognitive, and psychosocial skills. During these years children become "better" at things; for example, they can run faster and farther as proficiency and endurance develop.

The school or educational experience expands the child's world and is a transition from a life of relatively free play to a life of structured play, learning, and work. The school and home influence growth and development, requiring adjustment by the parents and child. The child must learn to cope with rules and expectations presented by the school and peers. Parents must learn to allow their child to make decisions, accept responsibility, and learn from life's experiences.

Table 10-10 Developmental Behaviors of School-Age Children and Adolescents

School-Age Children	Adolescents

Relationships With Parents

Children gradually learn that parents are less than perfect; they can be disillusioned with them and wish that friends' parents were their own. Sometimes they believe that they must be adopted. They rely on parents for unconditional love, security, guidance, and nurturing.

Adolescents desire for increasing independence and autonomy and continuing need for some dependence and limit setting by parents place strain on their relationship. Effective communication and democratic parenting are best tools for meeting this challenge.

Relationships With Siblings

School-agers seem to be at odds with one another at home; yet they are each others' best defenders away from home. Younger children often idolize older siblings, and this frequently leads to competition. Older children may envy attention that younger siblings require and be quite bossy and somewhat abusive.

Younger siblings rarely understand their adolescent siblings' need for privacy to think, dream, and talk with peers. Adolescents often enjoy interacting with and guiding younger brothers and sisters when timing is convenient for them and they can remain in control.

Relationships With Peers

During primary grades (6-7 years), children of both sexes play together, depending on who is available and interested. Around age 8, social groupings of same-sex peers form. These "gangs" allow children to declare their independence from parental rules and establish their own secret codes or languages and rules of membership and behavior. This period is often referred to as *secret society* of childhood. Preadolescent (10-12 years) friendships are characterized by having best friend of same sex. These relationships may be transient, but they are intense and allow discussion of all areas of life. Some interest in heterosexual relationships develops but they usually are not reciprocal.

Peer group is factor of critical influence to adolescents, who have increasing need for recognition and acceptance. Companionship offered by peer groups provides secure environment for individuals to try out new ideas and share similar feelings and attitudes. Adolescents often form cliques with peers from same socioeconomic group with similar interests. Cliques, which are highly exclusive, help their members, who have strong emotional bonds, develop their identities. The crowd, which is more impersonal than the clique, offers opportunities for heterosexual interaction and social activities. The crowd also maintains rigid membership requirements; clique membership is usually prerequisite for crowd membership.

Self-Concept

Children's feelings of competence regarding mastery of tasks are key elements in forming self-esteem. Children need to receive positive feedback from teachers and parents regarding their efforts. It is important for children to develop skills in at least one area such as reading, music, or swimming. Pets that require children's care and attention reward them with unconditional love and promote feelings of self-worth.

Formal and informal peer groups are primary force in shaping self-concept of group members. Popularity and recognition within peer group enhance self-esteem and reinforce self-concept. Total immersion in peer group may make it appear that adolescents have no original thoughts and are incapable of making decisions. Adolescents who withdraw from peers into isolation struggle with developing identity.

Fears

There is decline in fears related to body safety such as storms, dogs, darkness, noises, scrapes, and scratches. Fears of supernatural such as ghosts and witches persist and decline slowly. New fears related to school and family occur. They fear ridicule from teachers and friends and disapproval and rejection of parents. They also become frightened about death and items that they hear on news such as war and destruction of environment.

Fears in this age group center around peer group acceptance, body changes, loss of self-control, and emerging sexual urges. Adolescents constantly examine their bodies for changes and signs of imperfection. Any defect, real or imagined, is cause of endless worry. Adolescents' developing awareness of economic and political problems may result in fear of going to war with its resulting death and destruction.

Table 10-10 Developmental Behaviors of School-Age Children and Adolescents—cont'd

School-Age Children	Adolescents
Coping Patterns To deal with stress, school-agers use problem solving and defense mechanisms including regression, denial, aggression, and suppression. Several categories of coping behaviors of hospitalized school-agers include inactivity (total silence, lack of activity, and apathy), orientation or precoping (looking and listening, walking around and exploring, and asking questions), cooperation (compliance with care), resistance (attempt to get away from the situation by turning away or making physical or verbal attacks), and controlling (assuming responsibility for self-care and suggesting how things could be done).	Repertoire of coping behaviors has expanded with experiences adolescents have gained from life and from developing cognitive maturity. By age 15, most use full range of defense mechanisms, including rationalization and intellectualization. Adolescents' problem-solving abilities have matured, and they can reason through philosophical discussions and complex situations that require abstract thinking and proposition of hypotheses. Some adolescents use avoidance coping strategies in which the problem is denied or repressed and an attempt is made to reduce tension by engaging in chemical abuse or avoiding people.
Morals Children learn rules from parents, but their understanding of rules or reasons for them is limited until about 10 years. Before that, they are concerned with own needs first and may cheat to win. After 10, justice is based on "eye for an eye," and punishment should correct situation (e.g., if children break something, they should pay to have it fixed).	According to Kohlberg (1964), as youths approach adolescence they reach conventional level, where internalization of expectations of their family and society begins. Initially there is considerable conformity to rules to win praise or approval from others and to avoid social disapproval or rejection; later, they seek to avoid criticism from persons of authority in institutions.
Diversional Activity School-agers play cooperatively in group activities such as jumping rope, hopscotch, soccer, and baseball. Play becomes competitive, and children often have difficulty learning to lose. Teasing, insults, dares, superstitions, and increased sensitivity are characteristics of this age.	Many teenagers develop special interests in certain sports and concentrate on developing maximal skills therein. Recreational activities are often determined by what is popular with peers and what can provide independence from parents (e.g., computers, cars).
Nutrition Children have definite likes and dislikes. Few nutritional deficiencies occur in this age group. Children have voracious appetites after school and need quality snacks such as fruit and sandwiches to avoid empty calorie foods such as chips and candy.	Total nutritional needs become greater during adolescence. Girls' caloric needs decrease, and their need for protein increases slightly. Iron needed by adolescents is almost twice that of adult men, and growth spurt increases calcium demand.

PHYSICAL CHANGES

The rate of growth during these early school years is slower than any time since birth but continues steadily. A particular child may not follow the pattern precisely. The school-age child appears slimmer than the preschooler, as a result of changes in fat distribution and thickness (Edelman and Mandle, 1994). Growth accelerates at different times for different children. The average increase in height is 2 inches per year, and weight, which is more variable, increases by 4 to 7 pounds per year. An average 6-year-old is 45 inches tall and weighs 46 pounds; the average 12-year-old is 59 inches tall and weighs 88 pounds. Many children double their weight during these middle childhood years (Wong, 1999).

School provides children with the opportunity to compare themselves with large numbers of children of the same age. The physical examination usually required for the first grade is an excellent opportunity for the nurse to discuss with the child and parents the influences of genetic endowment, nutrition, and exercise on height and weight. Annual measurement of height and weight may reveal alterations in growth that are symptoms of the onset of a variety of childhood diseases.

Boys are slightly taller and heavier than girls during these early school years. Approximately 2 years before puberty, children experience a rapid acceleration in skeletal growth. Girls, who reach puberty first, begin to surpass boys in height and weight, which causes embarrassment to both sexes. These changes may begin as early as 9 years in girls but do not usually occur in boys before 12 years of age.

Cardiovascular functioning is refined and stabilized during the school-age years. The heart rate averages 70 to 90 beats per minute, the blood pressure normalizes to approximately 110/70 mm Hg, and the respiratory rate stabilizes to 19 to 21 breaths per minute. Lung growth is minimal and respirations become slower, deeper, and more regular. However, by the end of this period the heart is 6 times the size it was at birth and has generally reached its adult size.

School-age children become more graceful during the school years because their large muscle coordination improves and their strength doubles. Most children practice the basic gross motor skills of running, jumping, balancing, throwing, and catching during play, resulting in refinement of neuromuscular function and skills. Individual differences in the rate of mastering skills and ultimate skill achievement become apparent. Individual differences in motor skills are established by participation in activities and games requiring coordinated muscle movements and innate ability.

Fine motor skills lag behind gross motor skills but progress at approximately the same rate. As control is gained over fingers and wrists, children become proficient in a wide range of activities.

Most 6-year-old children can hold a pencil adeptly and print letters and words, but by age 12 the child can make detailed drawings and write sentences in script. Painting, drawing, playing computer games, and modeling allows children to practice and improve newly refined skills.

Nurses should encourage children and have parents encourage them to pursue these activities. Table 10-11 describes specific gross motor and fine motor skills and their use in self-care activities.

The improved fine motor capabilities of youngsters in middle childhood allow them to become very independent in bathing, dressing, and taking care of other personal needs. They develop strong personal preferences in the way these needs are met. Illness and hospitalization threaten children's control in these areas. Therefore it is important to allow them to participate in care and maintain as much independence as possible. Children whose care demands restriction of fluids cannot be allowed to decide the amount of fluids they will drink in 24 hours, but they can help decide the type of fluids and keep an accurate record of intake.

Assessment of neurological development is often based on fine motor coordination. This assessment may include penmanship, stacking ability, and performance of sequential, rapid, alternating movements such as touching the finger to the nose and then to the examiner's finger (smooth movement without tremors is the normal response). Fine motor coordination is critical to success in the typical American school, where children must be able

Table 10-11   Motor Development in the School-Age Child

6-7 Years	8-10 Years	11-12 Years
Fine Motor Skills		
Uses knife to butter bread and learns to cut tender meat	Uses knife and fork simultaneously	Learns to peel apples and potatoes
Cuts, folds, and pastes paper	Learns to thread needle and tie knot	Sews simple garments on machine
Prints with pencil	Uses hammer, saw, and screwdriver	Builds simple objects like birdhouse
Draws man with 12-16 details	Becomes proficient at writing cursive	Enjoys using decorative script
Copies triangle at 6 years and diamond by 7 years	Uses symbols in drawing (e.g., bird, star)	Begins to use creative and artistic talents
Colors within lines of picture	Builds simple models of cars and planes and does simple handcrafts	Builds complex models of cars and planes and does complex handcrafts
Needs assistance to clean teeth thoroughly	Learns to play jacks and marbles	Learns to play musical instrument
	Can learn to floss teeth effectively and be independent in tooth care	Becomes proficient in caring for teeth with braces and other appliances
Gross Motor Skills		
Remains in constant motion	Can catch, throw (70 feet), and hit baseball	Can do standing broad jump of 5 feet
Moves more cautiously at 7 years than at 6 years	Engages in alternate rhythmic hopping in 2-2, 2-3, or 3-3 pattern	Can do standing high jump of 3 feet
Hops and jumps into small squares	Engages in complex styles of skipping rope accompanied by verbal jingles	Plays games involving simultaneous use of two or more complex motor skills such as roller skating, ice hockey, or dance skating
Learns to roller skate, skip rope, ride bicycle, and swim		
Self-Care		
Takes bath without supervision	Learns to clean bathroom after bath	Dusts, vacuums, and straightens own room
Often returns to finger feeding	Enjoys fixing own snacks and sack lunch	Learns to cook simply prepared foods
Learns to brush and comb hair in acceptable fashion without help	Learns to part hair and insert hair ribbons and barrettes	Washes, dries, and fixes own hair in braids, curls, and ponytails
Puts on most clothes but may need assistance with shirttails, sashes, and final adjustments	Dresses self completely and can help younger siblings with clothes	Learns to sort, wash, dry, and press own clothing
	Can make own bed	Learns to care for fingernails and toenails

to hold pencils and crayons and use scissors and rulers. The opportunity to practice these skills through schoolwork and play is essential to the acquisition of coordinated, complex behaviors.

Other physical changes take place during the school-age years. Steady skeletal growth in the trunk and extremities occurs, and small- and long-bone ossification is present but not complete by age 12. Facial bones grow and remodel, as indicated by the presence of frontal and sphenoid sinuses by age 8 or 9 (Seidel and others, 1995). Dental growth is prominent during the school-age years. The first permanent or secondary teeth erupt at approximately 6 years of age. Development of the permanent teeth has been occurring for some time prior to eruption. The root is absorbed leaving the crown, which causes the tooth to become loose and fall out. This makes room for the new permanent teeth. Eruption usually begins with the 6-year molar and follows the same order as with the primary teeth. By 12 years, all primary teeth have been shed, and the majority of permanent teeth have erupted. Fig. 10-7 illustrates the pattern and timing of dental shedding and eruption. Infrequent or inadequate dental care remains a persistent problem for many American children.

As skeletal growth progresses, body appearance and posture change. Earlier posture, which was characterized by a stoop-shouldered, slightly lordotic stance and prominent abdomen, changes to a more erect posture. It is essential that children, especially girls after the age of 12 years, be evaluated for scoliosis, the lateral curvature of the spine.

Eye shape alters because of skeletal growth. This improves visual acuity, and normal adult 20/20 vision is achievable. Screening for vision and hearing problems is easier, and results are more reliable because school-age children can more fully understand and cooperate with the test directions. The school nurse typically assesses the dental, visual, and auditory status of school-age children and refers those with possible deviations to a health care provider, such as their family practitioner or pediatrician.

COGNITIVE CHANGES

Cognitive changes provide the school-age child with the ability to think in a logical manner about the here and now but not about abstraction. The thoughts of school-age children are no longer dominated by their perceptions, and thus their ability to understand the world greatly expands. Around 7 years of age, children enter Piaget's third stage of cognitive development, known as **concrete operations,** in which they are able to use symbols to carry out operations (mental activities) in thought rather than in action. They begin to use logical thought processes with concrete materials (objects, people, and events they can touch and see).

Children in the concrete operational stage are considerably less egocentric than younger children and develop the ability to **decenter,** which enables them to concentrate on more than one aspect of a situation. Decentering has developed when children can look at two lines of dots unequal in length and recognize that they have the same number of dots even though the spaces in between dots differ (. . . . and . . . .). They also develop **reversibility,** the ability to trace their line of thinking back to its origin. An example would be the recognition that not only does 3 + 2 = 5 but that 5 − 3 = 2 and 5 − 2 = 3.

Decentering and reversibility allow the child to use conservation, the ability to recognize that the amount or quantity of a substance remains the same even when its shape or appearance changes. For instance, two balls of clay of equal size remain the same amount of clay even when one is flattened and the other remains in ball shape.

Seriation, the ability to place objects in order according to their increasing or decreasing size, develops by age 7 or 8. This is easily measured by asking the child to arrange a group of pencils according to their length. The younger child usually aligns the tops of the pencils, whereas the child of 7 or 8 uses a methodical approach to line them up from the longest to the shortest.

The mental process of **classification** becomes more complex during the school years. The young child can separate objects into groups according to shape or color, but the school-age child understands that the same element can exist in two classes at the same time. For example, the school-age child could be shown a group of 16 wooden

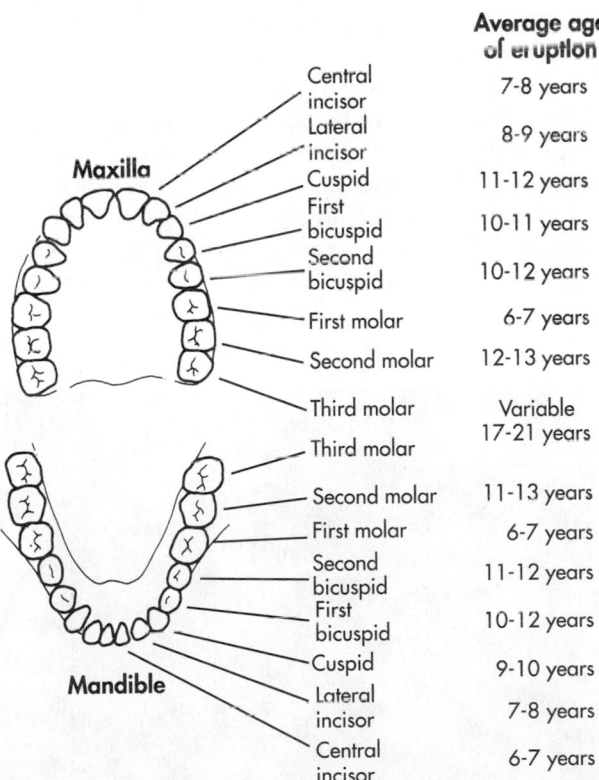

	Average age of eruption
Central incisor	7-8 years
Lateral incisor	8-9 years
Cuspid	11-12 years
First bicuspid	10-11 years
Second bicuspid	10-12 years
First molar	6-7 years
Second molar	12-13 years
Third molar	Variable 17-21 years
Third molar	
Second molar	11-13 years
First molar	6-7 years
Second bicuspid	11-12 years
First bicuspid	10-12 years
Cuspid	9-10 years
Lateral incisor	7-8 years
Central incisor	6-7 years

Maxilla

Mandible

Figure 10-7 Sequence of eruption of secondary teeth. From Wong DL: *Whaley and Wong's nursing care of infants and children,* ed 6, St. Louis, 1999, Mosby.

green beads and 4 wooden red beads and asked if there were more green beads or more wooden beads. The school-age child would recognize there were three classes of beads (red, green, and wooden) and would answer there were more wooden beads, whereas the preschool child would recognize only two classes of beads and answer green.

Middle childhood youngsters can use their newly developed cognitive skills to solve problems. Some individuals are better than others at problem solving because of native intelligence, education, and experience, but all children can improve these skills. Middle school-age children who are good problem solvers demonstrate the following characteristics: a positive attitude that the problem can be solved with persistence, a concern for accuracy, the ability to divide the problem into parts for study, and the ability to avoid guessing while searching for facts. Techniques that adults can use to help children improve their problem solving strategies include helping them define the problem and its nature, plan their solution carefully, and evaluate their plan and the solution (Dacey and Travers, 1991). Nurses can use these strategies to help school-age children understand their illness and assume responsibility for their general health.

Language Development.
Language growth is so rapid during middle childhood that it is no longer possible to match age with language achievements. The average 6-year-old child has a vocabulary of about 3000 words that quickly expands with exposure to peers and adults and reading ability. Children improve their use of language and expand their structural knowledge. They become more aware of the rules of syntax, the rules for linking words into phrases and sentences. They can also identify generalizations and exceptions to rules. They accept language as a means for representing the world in a subjective manner and realize that words have arbitrary, rather than absolute, meanings. They can use different words for the same object or concept, and they understand that a single word may have many meanings. Many school-age children use "bad language" to gain peer status and to shock adults. It often begins with bathroom language and progresses to sexual or genital words. Children begin to think about language, which enables them to appreciate jokes and riddles. By the end of this period their use of language is similar to adults.

PSYCHOSOCIAL CHANGES

Erikson (1963) identifies the developmental task for school-age children as industry versus inferiority. During this time, children strive to acquire competence and skills necessary for them to function as adults. School-age children who are positively recognized for success feel a sense of worth. Those faced with failure can feel a sense of mediocrity or unworthiness, which may result in withdrawal from school and peers.

Moral Development.
The need for a moral code and social rules becomes more evident as school-age children's cognitive abilities and social experiences increase. For example, 12-year-old children are able to consider what society would be like without rules because of their ability to reason logically and their experiences with group play. They view rules as necessary principles of life, not just dictates from authorities. In the early school years, children strictly interpret and adhere to rules. As they develop, they make more flexible judgments and evaluate rules for applicability to a given situation. School-age children consider motivations and the actual behavior when making judgments about the way that their behaviors affect themselves and others. The ability to be flexible when applying rules and to take the perspective of others is essential in developing moral judgments. These abilities are present at times in earlier years but are more consistently displayed in later school years.

Peer Relationships.
Group and personal achievements become important to the school-age child. Success is important in physical and cognitive activities. Play involves peers and the pursuit of group goals. Although solitary activities are not eliminated, they are overshadowed by group play. Learning to contribute, collaborate, and work cooperatively toward a common goal becomes a measure of success (Figure 10-8).

The school-age child prefers same-sex peers to opposite-sex peers. Strong gender identity is evidenced by the close network of same-sex companions that a child maintains. In general, girls and boys view the opposite sex negatively. Peer influence becomes quite diverse during this stage of development. Conformity is evidenced in mannerisms, clothing styles, and speech patterns, which are reinforced and influenced by contact with peers. During this time period, clubs and peer groups become prominent.

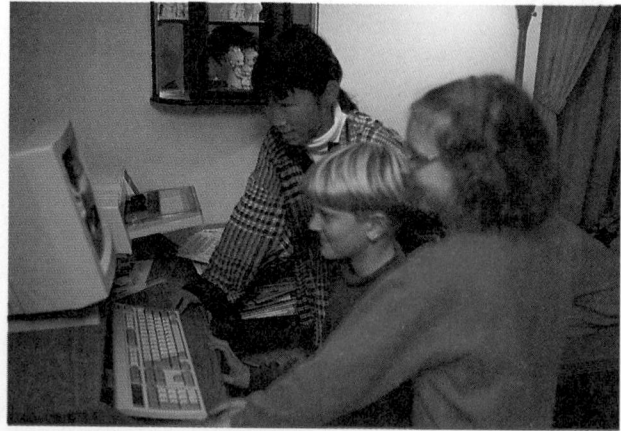

Figure 10-8   School-age children gain a sense of achievement when playing with peers.

Group identity increases as the school-age child approaches adolescence.

Sexual Identity.
Freud described middle childhood as the latency period because he felt that children of this period had little interest in their sexuality. Today many researchers believe that school-agers have a great deal of curiosity about their sexuality. Some may experiment, but this play is usually transitory. Emotional consequences are a result of how the behavior is dealt with by the parents or how the child believes the action would be interpreted from the parents' point of view. Children's curiosity about adult magazines or meanings of sexually explicit words is also an example of their sexual interest.

While the child goes through the adjustments in this stage, the nurse assists in promoting health. This is done by helping the parents and child to identify potential stressors and by designing interventions to minimize stress and the child's stress response. Interventions must include parent, child, and teacher for maximal success. Box 10-8 provides an overview of stressors commonly encountered by school age children and appropriate nursing interventions.

HEALTH RISKS
Accidents and injuries are a major health problem affecting school-age children. Motor vehicle accidents and accidents related to recreational activities or equipment are the leading causes of death or injury. These unintentional injuries account for nearly half of all childhood deaths (Table 10-12).

Although falls account for a major portion of pediatric hospital admissions, they account for less than 5% of pediatric deaths resulting from injury. More children die from automobile accidents than from all major preventable childhood diseases. The rates of injury and death have begun to decrease with the institution of automobile child restraint laws.

School-age children are also significantly affected by cancer, birth defects, homicide, and heart disease (Wong, 1999). In this age group, these problems have a relatively low mortality rate but a high morbidity rate compared to accidents. Cancers are the second leading cause of death in children 1 to 14 years of age. Leukemia is the most frequent type, with brain tumors and lymphoma second and third, respectively.

Infections account for the majority of all childhood illnesses; respiratory infections are the most prevalent. The common cold remains the chief illness of childhood. Certain groups of children are more prone to disease and disability, often as a result of barriers to health care. Mental retardation, learning disorders, sensory impairments, and malnutrition are far more prevalent among children living in poverty (USDHHS, 1992).

Poverty and prevalence of illness are highly correlated. Access to care is often very limited; health promotion and preventative health care are minimal. Infant mortality, dental problems, poor nutrition, and lack of immunizations continue to be major health concerns for uninsured or impoverished families. Involvement with social reform, environmental change, and the method of delivery of health care is necessary if the nurse wants to positively influence the health of children. Children's developing cognitive and psychomotor skills make it possible for them to become more involved in health promotion and the management of chronic illness.

HEALTH CONCERNS
Perceptions.
During the school-age years, identity and self-concept become stronger and more individualized. Perception of wellness is based on readily observable facts such as presence or absence of illness and adequacy of eating or sleeping. Functional ability is the standard by which personal health and the health of others are judged.

Antwerp and Spaniolo (1991) have developed a questionnaire that can be used as a tool to assess and promote healthy lifestyles among school-agers (Figure 10-9). This tool increases children's and parents' awareness of activities that promote health and prevent injury. It also provides data that allow the nurse or health educator to assess the health education needs of children.

Health Education.
The school-age period is a crucial period for the acquisition of behaviors and health practices for a healthy adult life. Since cognition is advancing during the period, effective health education must be developmentally appropriate. Promotion of good health practices is a nursing responsibility. Programs directed at health education are frequently organized and conducted in the school. Pender (1996) identifies the critical functions of school-based health promotion programs (Box 10-9).

During these programs, the nurse focuses on the development of behaviors that positively affect children's health status. School-age children should receive age-appropriate human immunodeficiency virus (HIV) education that begins in the fourth grade (McGinnis and DeGraw, 1991). Other topic areas for elementary health education curricula that are consistent with *Healthy People 2000* include tobacco and alcohol use prevention (USDHHS, 1992).

Nurses also instruct parents regarding health promotion appropriate for the school-age child. Parents need to recognize the importance of annual health maintenance visits for immunizations, screenings, and dental care. When their school-age child reaches 10 years of age, parents need to begin discussions in preparation for upcoming pubertal changes. Topics should include introductory information regarding menstruation, sexual intercourse, and reproduction. Nurses should provide age-appropriate written materials to aid parents in their efforts. The settings where health promotion activities can occur are varied. These include the classroom, school nurse's office,

Potential Sources of Stress in Middle Childhood*

Box 10-8

SOURCES OF STRESS FOR THE SIX-YEAR-OLD

Expectations—Parents, teachers, and other adults begin to demand more

School—First grade introduces the child to the more formal academic setting; it may be the child's first experience away from home all day

Activity level—May find it difficult to sit still for long periods of time; may have frequent accidents, such as spilling milk

Competition—The child wants to be "first" or best

Shyness—May initially be shy in a new situation but usually recovers quickly

Aggression—May become hostile or aggressive; temper tantrums peak

Sensitivity—Begins to read body language or facial expressions and becomes upset when disapproval is sensed

Teasing—Engages in teasing, but becomes upset when on the receiving end

Decisions—Has difficulty coping with increasing independence

Jealousy—Sibling rivalry is common

Fears—Usually center around newly found independence and might include fear of getting lost or fear of making an embarrassing social blunder

SOURCES OF STRESS FOR THE SEVEN-YEAR-OLD

Moodiness—Is often moody, unhappy, or pensive

Approval—Continues to need praise and approval from peer group and parents

Modesty—Demands privacy when in the bathroom or dressing

Organization—Is comfortable with rules, regulations, routines, and order; becomes upset when they are disrupted

Interruptions—Hates to be disturbed when intensely involved in an activity

Idols—Has a desire to be more like an admired idol

Friendship—Becomes more selective about playmates

SOURCES OF STRESS FOR THE EIGHT-YEAR-OLD

Self-criticism—Is very critical of personal ability and performance

Parental authority—Is beginning to resent parental authority

Loneliness—Likes frequent interaction with friends; may hate to miss school

Praise—Continues to seek approval but can identify when praise is not genuine

Independence—Many begin to stay alone for brief periods of time while parents run errands; with resulting feelings of uneasiness

SOURCES OF STRESS FOR THE NINE-YEAR-OLD

Rebelliousness—Occasionally tests independence by rebelling

Opposite sex—Engages in sex-segregated play, expresses an aversion to the opposite sex

Fair play—Has a keen sense of what is fair and is vehement in demanding personal rights when a situation is perceived as unfair

Interruptions—Continues to dislike interruptions but will usually resume an activity after an interruption

Propriety—Has a sense of propriety and will often be upset if siblings or parents offend the child's notion of decorum or dignity

SOURCES OF STRESS FOR THE TEN- TO TWELVE-YEAR-OLD

Sexual maturation—Girls, in particular, may become self-conscious regarding obvious signs of development

Social issues—A new level of awareness can generate concern regarding pressing societal problems

Size—Both boys and girls may be upset by the fact that the girls are taller; the extremely small or extremely large child may be concerned about his or her size

Shyness—If the child already has a problem in this area, it is likely to become more pronounced at this stage

Opposite sex—May become interested, yet shy, around members of the opposite sex

Confusion—Too much freedom can cause the child to flounder

Health—It is not uncommon for a child to become a hypochondriac during this period of development

Money—Child is anxious to earn and handle money, but often uses poor judgment

Competition—Continues to be highly competitive and looks to peer group for prestige

Burnout—Child may become vigorously involved in so many activities that he or she finally becomes exhausted

Self-concept—May engage in teasing, scapegoating, or vicious attacks to temporarily boost his or her self-image; guilt often ensues; may be self-conscious about attempting a new skill

Parents—Often becomes highly critical or intolerant of parents

Idols—Continues hero worshipping

Fair play—Continues to have a highly developed sense of fair play

Drugs and sex—May be tempted to experiment with drugs or sex because "everyone" is doing it

Peer pressure—Becomes a powerful motivating force

Self-criticism—Child may be highly critical of personal performance

From Kuczen B: *Childhood stress: don't let your child be a victim,* New York, 1982, Delacorte Press.
*Violence is a universal stress at all ages.

Table 10-12 Injury Prevention During School-Age Years

Developmental Abilities Related to Risk of Injury	Injury Prevention
	Motor vehicles
Is increasingly involved in activities away from home	Educate child regarding proper use of seat belts while a passenger in a vehicle
	Maintain discipline while a passenger in a vehicle (e.g., keep arms inside, do not lean against doors or interfere with driver)
Is excited by speed and motion	Remind parents and children that no one should ride in the bed of a pickup truck
	Emphasize safe pedestrian behavior
Is easily distracted by environment	Insist on wearing safety apparel (e.g., helmet) where applicable, such as when riding a bicycle, motorcycle, moped, or all-terrain vehicle
Can be reasoned with	
	Drowning
Is apt to overdo	Teach child to swim
May work hard to perfect a skill	Teach basic rules of water safety
	Select safe and supervised places to swim
Has cautious, but not fearful, gross motor actions	Check sufficient water depth for diving
	Swim with a companion
Likes swimming	Use an approved flotation device in water or boat
	Advocate for legislation requiring fencing around pools
	Learn CPR
	Burns
Has increasing independence	Make sure smoke detectors are in homes
	Set hot water temperatures to (120°-130°F) to avoid scald burns
Is adventuresome	Instruct child in behavior in areas involving contact with potential burn hazards (e.g., gasoline, matches, bonfires or barbecues, lighter fluid, firecrackers, cigarette lighters, cooking utensils, chemistry sets); avoid climbing or flying kites around high-tension wires
Enjoys trying new things	Instruct child in proper behavior in the event of fire (e.g., fire drills at home and school)
	Teach child safe cooking (use low heat, avoid any frying, be careful of steam burns, scalds, or exploding foods, especially from microwaving)
	Poisoning
Adheres to group rules	Educate child regarding hazards of taking nonprescription drugs and chemicals, including aspirin and alcohol
May be easily influenced by peers	Teach child to say "no" if offered illegal or dangerous drugs or alcohol
Has strong allegiance to friends	Keep potentially dangerous products in properly labeled receptacles—preferably locked and out of reach
	Bodily damage
Has increased physical skills	Help provide facilities for supervised activities
Needs strenuous physical activity	Encourage playing in safe places
	Keep firearms safely locked up except during adult supervision
Is interested in acquiring new skills and perfecting attained skills	Teach proper care of, use of, and respect for devices with potential danger (power tools, firecrackers)
Is daring and adventurous, especially with peers	Teach children not to tease or surprise dogs, invade their territory, take dogs' toys, or interfere with dogs' feeding
Frequently plays in hazardous places	Stress eye, ear, or mouth protection when using potentially hazardous objects or devices or when engaged in potentially hazardous sports (e.g., baseball)
Confidence often exceeds physical capacity	Teach safety regarding use of corrective devices (glasses); if child wears contact lenses, monitor duration of wear to prevent corneal damage
Desires group loyalty and has strong need for friends' approval	Stress careful selection, use, and maintenance of sports and recreation equipment such as skateboards and in-line skates
	Emphasize proper conditioning, safe practices, and use of safety equipment for sports or recreational activities
Attempts hazardous feats	Caution against engaging in hazardous sports, such as those involving trampolines
Accompanies friends to potentially hazardous facilities	Use safety glass and decals on large glassed areas, such as sliding glass doors
	Use window guards to prevent falls.
	Teach name, address, and phone number and to ask for help from appropriate people (cashier, security guard, policeman) if lost; have identification on child (sewn in clothes, inside shoe)
Delights in physical activity	Teach stranger safety:
Is likely to overdo	Avoid personalized clothing in public places
Growth in height exceeds muscular growth and coordination	Caution child to never go with a stranger
	Have child tell parents if anyone makes child feel uncomfortable in any way
	Always listen to child's concerns regarding others' behavior
	Teach child to say "no" when confronted with uncomfortable situations

From Wong DL: *Whaley and Wong's nursing care of infants and children,* ed 6, St. Louis, 1999, Mosby.

Date _____

Child's first name _____

Child's age _____   Grade _____

Lifestyle Questionnaire for School-Age Children*

Activities that promote health	Yes	No	Sometimes
1. I sleep at least 8 hours every night.			
2. I brush my teeth twice a day.			
3. I visit the dentist every year.			
4. I watch less than 2 hours of TV every day.			
5. I exercise (running, biking, swimming, active sports) one hour every day.			
6. I eat fruits.			
7. I eat vegetables.			
8. I limit my intake of salty snacks and high-sugar snacks.			
9. I have a physical examination every 2 or 3 years.			
10. I stay away from cigarettes.			
11. I stay away from alcohol.			
Injury prevention	**Yes**	**No**	**Sometimes**
12. I wear a seat belt in an automobile.			
13. I look both ways when crossing streets.			
14. I follow bike safety rules.			
15. I stay away from lighters or matches.			
16. I never ride ATVs (all-terrain vehicles).*			
17. I wear a helmet when I go on bike trips.			
18. I swim with a buddy.			
19. I wear a life jacket when I ride in a boat.			
20. I take medicine only with my parent's permission.			
21. I stay away from real guns.			
22. I tell my parents where I am going.			
23. I say "no" to drugs.			
24. Our home has a smoke detector that works.			
25. Our home has a fire extinguisher.			
26. If there is a fire, I know a safe way out of my house.			
Feelings	**Yes**	**No**	**Sometimes**
27. I think it is okay to cry.			
28. I enjoy my family.			
29. It is easy for me to fall asleep at night.			
30. My appetite is good.			
31. I like myself just the way I am.			

*The American Academy of Pediatrics recommends that children do not ride on these vehicles.

Figure 10-9   Lifestyle questionnaire for school-age children.
From Antwerp CV, Spaniolo AM: Checking out children's lifestyles, *MCN Am J Matern Child Nurs* 16(3):144, 1991.

school-based clinic, community-based clinic, or in the community itself.

Examples of topics that encourage positive behaviors by children are dental health and treatment for a cold. A comprehensive list of health promotion topics is presented in Table 10-13.

Safety. Since accidents are the leading cause of death and injury in the school-age period, safety is a priority health teaching consideration. Nurses can contribute to the general health of children by educating them about safety measures to prevent accidents. At this age, children should be encouraged to take responsibility for their own safety.

Nutrition. Nurses can contribute to meeting national policy goals by promoting healthy lifestyle habits, including nutrition. School-age children should participate in educational programs that enable them to plan, select, and prepare healthy meals and snacks. These foods should be consistent with the U.S. Department of Agriculture food guide pyramid nutritional guidelines limiting intake of total and saturated fats and increasing the intake of complex carbohydrates, fruits, and vegetables. Box 10-10 outlines several learning activities appropriate for this age group. Additionally, nurses need to promote an increase in the number of children involved in daily physical activity.

Although actual growth may slow down during the school-age period, the body is preparing for a pubertal growth spurt (Grodner, Anderson, and DeYoung, 1996). A buildup of weight may occur at this time. Additional weight should not be a concern if moderate eating habits are in place with the child. Obesity may become a problem because children often rush into the home after school or play and eat the most easily obtainable and appealing foods. Unfortunately, these foods are often nutritionally poor and calorie laden. Providing nutritious snacks is often the best way for a parent to ensure good nutritional intake. Parents should provide ready access to fresh fruit, raw vegetables, cheese, popcorn, and high-protein snacks such as skim-milk pudding and hot chocolate. Children can learn a great deal about the food pyramid and a balanced diet by helping to prepare their own lunches and snacks. Nurses should encourage parents to provide children with a variety of foods in adequate amounts to support growth and energy for play. Activity levels vary from day to day, and children's appetites and consumption of food vary accordingly. When children are overweight, they should be encouraged to increase their expenditure of calories through exercise and vigorous play. Children who become overweight have lower self-esteem, have difficulty keeping up with other children in physical activities, and are often rejected by their peers. Nurses can help families and children prevent obesity through proper nutrition and exercise.

Today's families may often eat in fast-food restaurants

Critical Functions of School-Based Health Promotion Program | Box 10-9

Promote acquisition of knowledge and skills for competent self-care and informed decision making about health.
Reinforce positive health attitudes.
Structure environment and social influences to support health promoting behaviors.
Facilitate growth and self-actualization.
Sensitize students to aspects of the environment and Western culture that are detrimental to health and well-being.
Foster positive life skills that enhance successful coping.

Modified from Pender N: *Health promotion in nursing practice*, ed 3, Norwalk, Conn, 1996, Appleton & Lange.

Table 10-13 **Health Promotion in the School-Age Period**

School-Age Health Concerns	Health Promotion Interventions
Nutrition	Provide nutrition education that promotes healthy lifestyle: food guide pyramid; limiting fat intake to 30% of calories, saturated fat to 10% of calories.
Oral hygiene	Provide examples of low cariogenic snacks.
	Review mechanics of dental hygiene: brushing, flossing.
	Stress importance of biannual dental checkups.
Infections	Provide immunization information and follow-up.
	Teach infection prevention practices (hand washing, care of minor skin injuries).
	Teach concepts of viral and bacterial illness.
Tobacco, alcohol, and drug use	Provide tobacco use prevention programs.
	Provide information regarding the hazards of drug use.
Human sexuality	Provide information about sexual maturation and reproduction in age-appropriate manner.
	Encourage parents to view their child's sexual curiosity as part of the developmental process.
	Discuss with parents the learning needs of their child regarding sexuality.
	Provide age-appropriate HIV education.

School-Based Interventions to Promote Nutrition Education

Box 10-10

Have young children collect pictures of healthy foods and make a poster for display in the school cafeteria.

Make healthy foods (fruits, vegetables, whole grains, low-fat snacks) available in school vending machines and at school sporting events.

Discourage the use of high-fat foods (candy bars) as part of school fund-raising projects.

Avoid the use of food as rewards for behavior; use verbal praise and token gifts to reinforce healthy eating and physical activity.

Have teachers and school personnel model healthy eating habits.

Ask children to select foods from a fast-food restaurant menu and to identify those foods high in fat, cholesterol, and sodium.

Ask each child to keep a diary of foods eaten in 1 day; using the Food Guide Pyramid, evaluate these foods.

Incorporate nutrition education into other classes (such as using a computer to analyze the nutritional content of foods).

Have students keep a diary to identify cues for their eating behavior (e.g., hunger, stress, other people, social situations).

Teach students how to read and discuss the nutrition labels on foods.

Ask students to examine television commercials, magazine advertisements, and billboards to identify social influences on eating and physical activities.

Use role-playing to help students learn to cope with social and peer pressures to eat specific foods.

Have students identify environmental barriers to healthy eating.

Have students prepare nutritious foods, plan menus, and develop a recipe book of healthy foods.

Involve parents in nutrition education through homework assignments or by inviting parents to attend student-led nutrition fairs.

Modified from Center for Communicable Diseases: Guidelines for school programs to promote lifelong healthy eating, *J Sch Health* 67:9, 1996.

where the food is high in fat, calories, and salt. Nurses need to encourage healthy food choices in these situations. Selections should include meats that are not breaded and are broiled, shakes that are made with low-fat yogurt or skim milk, and fruits and vegetables that are fresh or prepared in a low-calorie manner.

Preadolescent

Professionals in behavioral science often refer to the transitional period between childhood and adolescence as **preadolescence.** Others have referred to this period as late childhood, early adolescence, and pubescence. Physically it refers to the beginning of the second skeletal growth spurt, when physical changes such as the development of pubic hair and female breasts begins. These physical changes that announce the approach of puberty begin about 2 years earlier in girls than boys. In addition, children become much more social, and their behavioral patterns become much less predictable. This preparatory period often includes experimentation with makeup by girls and an interest in music and performers that are popular among older adolescents. Both sexes usually develop "best friends" with whom they share intimate feelings. New interest in the opposite sex develops. Youths of both sexes often develop a friendship with adults other than their parents (ego ideal), which allows them to acquire information about grown-ups.

Adolescent

Adolescence is the period of development during which the individual makes the transition from childhood to adulthood, usually between 13 and 20 years. The term *adolescent* usually refers to psychological maturation of the individual, whereas *puberty* refers to the point at which reproduction becomes possible. The hormonal changes of puberty result in changes in the appearance of the young person, and mental development results in the ability to hypothesize and deal with abstractions. Adjustments and adaptations are needed to cope with these simultaneous changes and the attempt to establish a mature sense of identity. In the past, many have referred to adolescence as a stormy and stressful period filled with inner turmoil, but today it is recognized that most teenagers successfully meet the challenges of this period. Adaptations required push the adolescent to develop coping mechanisms and styles of behavior that will be used or adapted throughout life. These challenges may cause the adolescent to be moody and difficult. Within adolescence, three subphases exist: early adolescence (11 to 14 years), middle adolescence (15 to 17 years), and late adolescence (18 to 20 years). Opportunities, challenges, changes, skills, pressures, and physical, cognitive, and psychosocial development vary widely between the subphases (Table 10-14).

The nurse's understanding of development provides a unique perspective for helping teenagers and parents anticipate and cope with the stresses of adolescence. Nursing activities, particularly education, can promote healthy development. These activities occur in a variety of settings and can be directed at the adolescent, parents, or both. For example, the nurse can conduct seminars in a high school to provide practical suggestions for solving problems of concern to a large group of students, such as treating acne or making responsible decisions about drugs or alcohol use. Similarly, a group education program for parents about how to cope with teenagers would promote parental understanding of adolescent development. These programs can be held in the school, clinic, private office, or

Table 10-14 Growth and Development During Adolescence

Early Adolescence (11-14 years)	Middle Adolescence (14-17 years)	Late Adolescence (17-20 years)
Growth		
Rapidly accelerating growth	Growth decelerating in girls	Physically mature
Reaches peak velocity	Stature reaches 95% of adult height	Structure and reproductive growth almost complete
Secondary sex characteristics appear	Secondary sex characteristics well-advanced	
Cognition		
Explores newfound ability for limited abstract thought	Developing capacity for abstract thinking	Established abstract thought
Clumsy groping for new values and energies	Enjoys intellectual powers, often in idealistic terms	Can perceive and act on long-range operations
Comparison of "normality" with peers of same sex	Concern with philosophic, political, and social problems	Able to view problems comprehensively
		Intellectual and functional identity established
Identity		
Preoccupied with rapid body changes	Modifies body image	Body image and gender role definition nearly secured
Trying out of various roles	Very self-centered; increased narcissism	Mature sexual identity
Measurement of attractiveness by acceptance or rejection of peers	Tendency toward inner experience and self-discovery	Phase of consolidation of identity
Conformity to group norms	Has a rich fantasy life	Stability of self-esteem
	Idealistic	Comfortable with physical growth
	Able to perceive future implications of current behavior and decisions; variable application	Social roles defined and articulated
Relationships With Parents		
Defining independence-dependence boundaries	Major conflicts over independence and control	Emotional and physical separation from parents completed
Strong desire to remain dependent on parents while trying to detach	Low point in parent-child relationship	Independence from family with less conflict
No major conflicts over parental control	Greatest push for emancipation; disengagement	Emancipation nearly secured
	Final and irreversible emotional detachment from parents; mourning	
Relationships With Peers		
Seeks peer affiliations to counter instability generated by rapid change	Strong need for identity to affirm self-image	Peer group recedes in importance in favor of individual friendship
Upsurge of close, idealized friendships with members of the same sex	Behavioral standards set by peer group	Testing of male-female relationships against possibility of permanent alliance
Struggle for mastery takes place within peer group	Acceptance by peers extremely important—fear of rejection	Relationships characterized by giving and sharing
	Exploration of ability to attract the opposite sex	
Sexuality		
Self-exploration and evaluation	Multiple plural relationships	Forms stable relationships and attachment to another
Limited dating, usually group	Decisive turn toward heterosexuality (if is homosexual, knows by this time)	Growing capacity for mutuality and reciprocity
Limited intimacy	Exploration of "self-appeal"	Dating as a male-female pair
	Feeling of "being in love"	Intimacy involves commitment rather than exploration and romanticism
	Tentative establishment of relationships	
Psychologic Health		
Wide mood swings	Tendency toward inner experiences; more introspective	More constancy of emotion
Intense daydreaming	Tendency to withdraw when upset or feelings are hurt	Anger more apt to be concealed
Anger outwardly expressed with moodiness, temper outbursts, and verbal insults and name-calling	Vascillation of emotions in time and range	
	Feelings of inadequacy common; difficulty in asking for help	

From Wong DL: *Whaley and Wong's nursing care of infants and children,* ed 6, St. Louis, 1999, Mosby.

community center. To learn more about specific topics or problems, the nurse must identify teenagers' needs and desires. Involvement produces more active, interested learners.

PHYSICAL CHANGES

Physical changes occur rapidly in adolescence. Sexual maturation occurs with the development of primary and secondary sexual characteristics. Primary characteristics are physical and hormonal changes necessary for reproduction, and secondary characteristics externally differentiate males from females. Four main focuses of the physical changes are:

1. Increased growth rate of skeleton, muscle, and viscera
2. Sex-specific changes, such as changes in shoulder and hip width
3. Alteration in distribution of muscle and fat
4. Development of the reproductive system and secondary sex characteristics

Wide variation exists in the timing of physical changes associated with puberty between sexes and within the same sex. Girls tend to begin their physical changes earlier than boys. Variations are more pronounced in boys. Cultural variations exist in rapidity of growth. For example, African-American youths obtain a greater proportion of their adult stature earlier. The sequence of pubertal growth changes is the same in most individuals (Table 10-15).

Visible and invisible changes take place during puberty. All of these changes are created by hormonal changes within the body when the hypothalamus begins to produce gonadotropin-releasing hormones, which signal the pituitary to secrete gonadotropic hormones. Gonado-

tropic hormones stimulate ovarian cells to produce **estrogen** and testicular cells to produce **testosterone.** These hormones contribute to the development of secondary sex characteristics such as hair growth and voice changes and play an essential role in reproduction. The changing concentrations of these hormones are also linked to acne and body odor. Understanding these hormonal changes enables the nurse to reassure adolescents and educate them about body care needs.

Boys who mature early have been shown by some research to be more poised, relaxed, good-natured, skilled in athletic activities, and more likely to be school leaders than boys who mature late. In contrast, girls who mature early have been found to be less sociable and more shy and introverted, perhaps from feeling so conspicuous (Edelman and Mandle, 1994).

The ranges of normal are stressed. As with increases in height and weight, the pattern of sexual changes is more significant than their time of onset. Large deviations from normal frames require investigation. Being like peers is extremely important for adolescents (Figure 10-10). Any deviation in the timing of the physical changes can be extremely difficult for them to accept. The nurse should therefore provide emotional support for adolescents undergoing assessment of early or delayed puberty. Even adolescents whose physical changes are occurring at the normal times may seek confirmation of and reassurance about their normalcy.

Height and weight increases usually occur during the prepubertal growth spurt. The growth spurt for girls generally begins between 8 and 14 years of age. Height increases 2 to 8 inches, and weight increases by 15 to 55 pounds. The male growth spurt usually takes place be-

Table 10-15 **Average Sequences of Physiological Changes in Adolescence**		
Characteristics	Girls*	Boys*
Beginning of skeletal growth spurt	8-14½ (peak: 12)	10½-16 (peak: 14)
Beginning of breast development	8-13	
Enlargement of testes and scrotal sac		10-13½
Appearance of straight, pigmented pubic hair, which gradually becomes curly	8-14	10-15
Early voice changes (cracks)		11-14½
Enlargement of penis and prostate gland		11-14½
Menarche	10-18 (average: 12¼)	
Spermatogenesis (ejaculation of sperm)		11-17 (average: 13½)
Ovulation and completion of breast development	14-18 (average: 15½)	
Appearance of downy facial hair		12-17
Appearance of axillary (underarm) hair and increased output of oil and sweat-producing glands, which may lead to acne	10-16	12-17
Widening and deepening of female pelvis, with deposition of subcutaneous fat that gives rounded appearance to body	10-18	
Increase in shoulder width		11-21
Deepening of voice in males, with appearance of coarse and pigmented facial hair and appearance of chest hair		16-21

*Age range is in years.

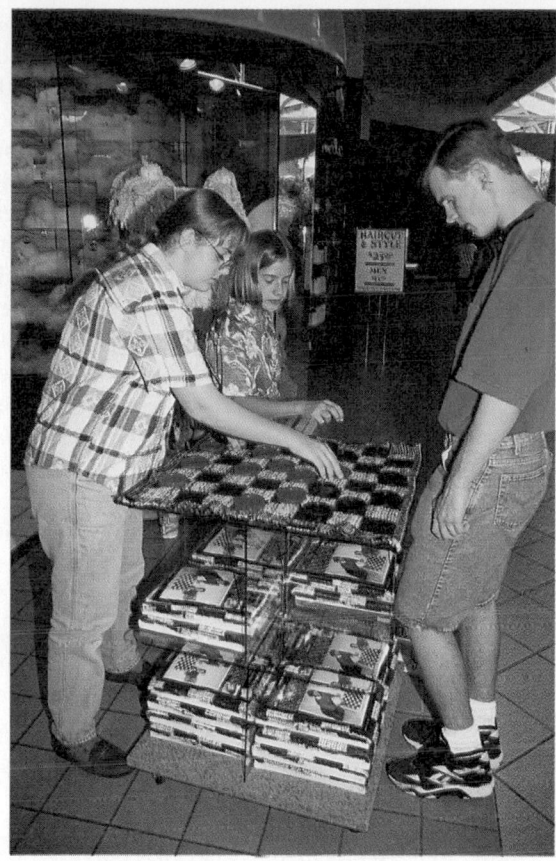

Figure 10-10   Interacting with peers helps to increase in self-esteem during puberty.

tween 10 and 16 years of age. Height increases approximately 4 to 12 inches, and weight increases by 15 to 65 pounds. The final 20% to 25% of adult height and 50% of adult weight is gained during this time period (Wong 1999).

Girls attain 90% to 95% of their adult height by **menarche** (the onset of menstruation) and reach their full height by 16 to 17 years of age, whereas boys continue to grow taller until 18 to 20 years of age. Fat is redistributed into adult proportions as height and weight increase, and gradually the adolescent torso takes on an adult appearance.

Although there are individual and sex differences, growth follows a similar pattern for both sexes. Growth in the length of the extremities occurs earliest, making the hands and feet appear very large and the legs very long; the individual often appears awkward and clumsy. At the same time the lower jaw and nose become longer and the forehead higher and wider as the baby face of childhood disappears. Next the thighs widen; then the shoulders broaden, and growth of the trunk proceeds. Widening of the female hips and broadening of the male shoulders continue throughout adolescence.

Personal growth curves help the nurse assess physical development. The individual's sustained progression along the curve, however, is more important than a comparison to the norm. The nurse charts growth measurements during routine health assessments to evaluate changes.

Adolescents are sensitive about physical changes that make them different from peers. For this reason they are generally interested in the normal pattern of growth and their personal growth curves. Consequently, the nurse should share this information to reassure adolescents that their own patterns are normal.

COGNITIVE CHANGES

Changes that occur within the mind and the widening social environment of the adolescent result in formal operations, which is the highest level of intellectual development, according to Piaget. Without an appropriate educational environment, young persons who possess sufficient neurological development to reach this stage may not attain it, and those who are guided toward rational thinking may reach this stage early.

The adolescent develops the ability to solve problems through logical operations. The teenager can think abstractly and deal effectively with hypothetical problems. When confronted with a problem, the teenager can consider an infinite variety of causes and solutions. For the first time the young person can move beyond the physical or concrete properties of a situation and use reasoning powers to understand the abstract. School-age individuals think about what is, whereas adolescents can imagine what might be. These newly developed abilities allow the individual to have more insight and skill in playing games such as video games, computer games, and board games that require abstract thinking and deductive reasoning about many possible strategies. A teenager can even solve problems requiring simultaneous manipulation of several abstract concepts. Development of this ability is important in the pursuit of an identity. For example, newly acquired cognitive skills allow the teenager to define appropriate, effective, and comfortable sex-role behaviors and to consider their impact on peers, family, and society. The ability to think logically about these behaviors and their outcomes encourages the adolescent to develop personal thoughts and means of expressing sexual identity. In addition, a higher level of cognitive functioning makes the adolescent receptive to more detailed and diverse information about sexuality and sexual behaviors. For example, sex education can include an explanation of physiological sexual changes and birth control measures.

By midadolescence there is an introspective quality emerging with regard to cognition. At this time adolescents believe an "imaginary audience" (Elkind, 1984) provides them with an evaluative means and a sense of being unique. This concept may account for some typical adolescent behaviors, including self-consciousness and the desire for privacy.

Elkind (1984) also describes another characteristic of cognitive function, the personal fable. This is a story created by the adolescent that is not true. This concept may account for many undesirable risk-taking behaviors, since the adolescent believes he or she is immune from negative consequences.

The complex development of thought during this period leads adolescents to question society and its values. Although adolescents have the capability to think as well as an adult, they do not have experiences on which to build. It is common for teenagers to consider their parents too narrow minded or too materialistic. Cognitive abilities and performance vary greatly among adolescents. In fact, an adolescent may perform at different levels in different situations based on past experiences, formal education, and motivation in the use of logic and effective deductive reasoning.

Language Skills.
Language development is fairly complete by adolescence, although vocabulary continues to expand. The primary focus becomes communication skills that can be used effectively in various situations. Adolescents need to communicate thoughts, feelings, and facts to peers, parents, teachers, and other persons of authority. The skills used in these diverse communication situations are varied. Adolescents must select the person with whom to communicate, decide on the exact message, and choose the way to transmit the message. For example, the way teenagers tell parents about failing grades is not the same as the way that they tell friends. Adolescents develop different skills and styles of communication and learn how and when to use them most effectively. These diverse communication skills are used and refined throughout life. Good communication skills are critical for adolescents to overcome peer pressure to participate in nonhealthy behaviors.

PSYCHOSOCIAL CHANGES
The search for personal identity is the major task of adolescent psychosocial development. Teenagers must establish close peer relationships or remain socially isolated. Erikson (1963) sees identity (or role) confusion as the prime danger of this stage and suggests that the cliquishness and intolerance of differences seen in adolescent behavior are defenses against identity confusion (Erikson, 1968). Adolescents work at becoming emotionally independent from their parents, while retaining family ties. In addition, they need to develop their own ethical systems based on personal values. Choices about vocation, future education, and lifestyle must be made. The various components of total identity evolve from these tasks and compose adult personal identity that is unique to the individual. Behaviors indicating negative resolution of the developmental task for this age are indecisiveness and the inability to make an occupational choice.

Sexual Identity.
Achievement of sexual identity is enhanced by the physical changes of puberty. In Freud's view, these physiological changes of puberty reactivate the libido, the energy source that fuels the sex drive. This is evidenced by the teenager's interest in heterosexual relationships with partners outside of the family and the practice of masturbation. The physical evidence of maturity encourages the development of masculine and feminine behaviors. If these physical changes involve deviations, the person has more difficulty developing a comfortable sexual identity. Adolescents depend on these physical clues because they want assurance of maleness or femaleness and because they do not wish to be different from peers (Figure 10-11). Without these physical characteristics, achieving sexual identity is difficult. Other influences are cultural attitudes and expectations of sex-role behavior and available role models. The masculine and feminine behaviors that teenagers see affect the way that they express sexuality.

Group Identity.
Adolescents seek a group identity because they need esteem and acceptance. Similarity in dress or speech is common in teenage groups. Popularity is a major concern. Trends in the desire for popularity have not changed much in recent years. Peer groups provide the adolescent with a sense of belonging, approval, and the opportunity to learn acceptable behavior. Popularity with opposite-sex and same-sex peers is important. The strong need for group identity seems to conflict at times with the search for personal identity. It is as though adolescents require close bonds with peers so that they can later redefine themselves against this group identity.

Family Identity.
The movement toward stronger peer relationships is contrasted with adolescents' movements away from parents. Although financial independence for

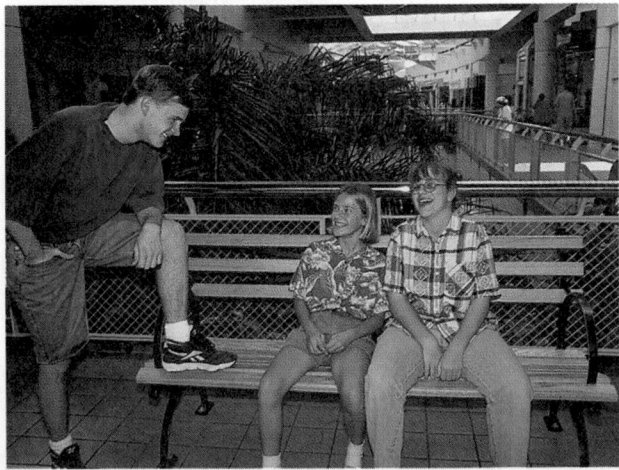

Figure 10-11 Adolescents acquire sexual identity during social interactions.

adolescents is not the norm in American society, many adolescents work part time, using their income to bolster independence. When adolescents cannot have a part-time job because of studies, school-related activities, and other factors, parents can provide allowances for clothing and incidentals, which encourage adolescents to develop decision-making and budgeting skills.

Some adolescents and families have more difficulty during these years than others. Adolescents need to make choices, act independently, and experience the consequences of actions. This testing, however, is best done against a firm, supportive, family foundation. The family needs to allow independence while providing a haven in which adolescents can contemplate actions. Families unable to provide this support complicate movement toward identity formation. Support to the family and adolescent may be essential to their success.

Nurses can assist families to consider ways that are appropriate for them to foster the independence of their adolescent while maintaining family structure. Many of these discussions often involve curfews, jobs, and participation in family chores. Emancipation from the immediate family is most successful when accomplished gradually, resulting in separation from the family and family ties that last a lifetime.

Vocational Identity.

The selection of an occupation or a vocational direction in life provides a goal for adolescents. Because of society's changing needs, adolescents must be future oriented when making these choices. However, adolescents do not know which jobs will be available or which jobs will be rewarding 10 or 20 years in the future, so selecting a career is a complicated task. The nurse should provide emotional support during this process and should help adolescent clients select courses of action that promote self-satisfaction, identity, and continued opportunity for growth.

Moral Identity.

The development of moral judgment depends heavily on cognitive and communication skills and peer interaction. Although moral development begins in early childhood, it is consolidated in adolescence because of the presence of certain skills. Adolescents learn to understand that rules are cooperative agreements that can be modified to fit the situation, rather than absolutes. Regarding rules, adolescents learn to use their own judgment rather than use the rules to avoid punishment as in earlier years. Kohlberg (1964) explains moral development in terms of stages (see Chapter 9). At the highest level, morality is derived from individual principles of conscience. Adolescents judge themselves by internalized ideals, which often leads to conflict between personal and group values. Group values become less significant in later adolescence.

Not all adolescents attain the same level of moral development. There is, however, a general forward movement through the stages of moral development, and the sequence of the stages is similar for all individuals even when their time of achievement varies. Kohlberg's moral development (1964) has a focus on justice based on reciprocity and equal respect. Females have been found to be more likely to give caring responses to moral problems. Males have been found to give more justice-oriented responses.

Psychosocial Moratorium.

According to Erikson (1968), adolescence provides a time-out period when society allows the physically mature teenager to delay the assumption of adult responsibilities. This is time for youth to try a variety of ideological and vocational roles before making a commitment. This **psychosocial moratorium** ends in the selection of values and a consolidation of identity.

Health Identity.

Another component of personal identity is perception of health. This component is of specific interest to health care providers. Healthy adolescents evaluate their own health according to feelings of well-being, ability to function normally, and absence of symptoms (Wong, 1999).

Research indicates that adolescents participate in health-related self-care practices (McCaleb and Edgil, 1994). Interventions to improve health perception might, therefore, concentrate on the adolescent period. The rapid changes during this period make health promotion programs especially crucial. Adolescents try new roles, begin to stabilize their identity, and acquire values and behaviors from which their adult lifestyle will evolve.

HEALTH RISKS

Accidents.

Accidents remain the leading cause of death in adolescence. Motor vehicle accidents, which are the most common cause of death, resulted in almost half of the fatalities among 16- to 19-year-olds (Edelman and Mandel, 1994). Such accidents are often associated with alcohol intoxication or drug abuse. Bicycling fatalities were 4 to 7 times more likely to occur in males than females. Other frequent causes of accidental death in teenagers are drowning and firearms. Feelings of being indestructible lead to risk-taking behavior. The 1997 Youth Risk Behavior Surveillance System addressed several behaviors related to areas of injury in high school students. Results indicated that 19.3% never or rarely use a seat belt; 36.2% of those riding a motorcycle and 88.4% of those riding a bicycle never or rarely used a helmet; 36.6% had ridden with someone who had been drinking alcohol; 8.5% had carried a weapon to school during the month before the survey; 14.8% had been in a fight during the year before; 4% had missed at least 1 day of school in the previous month due to feeling unsafe at or on the way to school; and 20.5% had seriously considered suicide in the previous year (CDC, 1998c).

Homicide. Homicide is the second leading cause of death in the 15- to 24-year-old age group. Males and African-Americans have shown the greatest increases. Individuals 12 years of age and older are most likely to be killed by an acquaintance or gang member and most frequently with a firearm. Firearm homicides are 6 times greater in metropolitan than nonmetropolitan areas and are the leading cause of death in 15- to 19-year-old African-American males (Fingerhut, Ingram, and Feldman, 1992).

Suicide. Suicide is the third leading cause of death in adolescents between 15 and 24 years of age (Hawton, 1990). Depression and social isolation commonly precede a suicide attempt, but suicide probably results from a combination of several factors. Nurses should be alert to the following warning signs, which often occur for at least a month before suicide is attempted:

 Decrease in school performance

 Withdrawal

 Loss of initiative

 Loneliness, sadness, and crying

 Appetite and sleep disturbances

 Verbalization of suicidal thought

Other associated suicide risk factors are listed in Box 10-11. The nurse must be able to identify the factors associated with adolescent suicide risk and precipitating events.

 Immediate referrals to mental health professionals need to be made when assessment suggests that adolescents may be considering suicide. Guidance can help them focus on the positive aspects of life and strengthen coping abilities.

Substance Abuse. Substance abuse is in fact a concern to those who work with adolescents. Adolescents may believe that mood-altering substances create a sense of well-being or improve level of performance. All adolescents are at risk for experimental or recreational substance use, but those who have unconventional values or come from unstable homes are more at risk for chronic use and physical dependency. Some adolescents believe that substance use makes them more mature. In 1994, it was estimated that teenage drug use had declined 54% since 1979, and of those using drugs, the majority used marijuana (U.S. Substance Abuse and Mental Health Services Administration [SAMHSA], 1995). Abuse of acetaminophen, aspirin, and ibuprofen were almost 4 times more likely to send an adolescent to the emergency department than marijuana, cocaine, or LSD (SAMHSA, 1994).

 Tobacco use continues to be a problem among adolescents. The 1997 Youth Risk Behavior Surveillance System reported that 70% of students in the survey had tried cigarettes, 36.4% had smoked on 1 or more days in the last month, and 16.7% reported frequent cigarette use.

Factors Associated With Suicide Risk   Box 10-11

PAST HISTORY

Previous suicide attempt

Family member friend has made a suicide attempt

History of child abuse or neglect

Past psychiatric hospitalization

Death of a parent when child was young

INDIVIDUAL FACTORS

Hopelessness

Marked, persistent depression

Alcohol or drug abuse

Impulsive

Difficulty tolerating frustration

Feelings of self-hatred or excessive guilt, feelings of humiliation

Thinking disorder (wishes to join a deceased person, hears voices telling to kill self)

Physical/body image problems (delayed puberty, chronic illness, disability, attention deficit hyperactivity disorder, learning disorders)

Gender identity concerns; gay or lesbian in an unsupportive environment

Sees self as totally helpless—a victim of fate

A need to do things perfectly

FAMILY FACTORS

Difficult home situation—long, bitter parent-child conflict

Hostile parents

Overt rejection by one or both parents

Divorce or separation of parents

Recent or impending move

Family breakup or parental loss

Exposure to unrealistically high parental expectations

Parental indifference with very low expectations

SOCIAL/ENVIRONMENTAL FACTORS

Firearms in the home

Incarceration

Lack of effective social support system

Isolation

Exposure to suicide of another

Few social, vocational, educational opportunities

From Wong DL: *Whaley and Wong's nursing care of infants and children,* ed 6, St. Louis, 1999, Mosby.

Students were also asked about the use of smokeless tobacco. Use of chewing tobacco and snuff was reported by 9.3% (CDC, 1998c). An attempt to decrease availability to those under 18 years of age resulted in a law that requires proof of age to purchase cigarettes. However, 66.7% of those currently using cigarettes reported not being asked for identification (CDC, 1998c).

Eating Disorders. The number of eating disorders is on the rise in adolescent girls, and knowledge of growth progression may be a way to discourage radical weight-reduction activities. If an adolescent deviates radically from the usual pattern, further assessment is necessary to identify the cause. Areas to include in the assessment are past and present diet history, food records, eating habits, attitudes, health beliefs, and socioeconomic and psychosocial factors (Freidman and others, 1998). Weight extremes resulting from excessive or inadequate caloric intake are common during the adolescent years. Allowing the adolescent to see when and how the weight curve changed can be a first step in identifying the problem and implementing dietary changes.

Although anorexia nervosa and bulimia are classified as separate disorders, there is significant overlap between the two eating disorders (Friedman and others, 1998). Anorexia nervosa is considered a clinical syndrome with both physical and psychosocial components. The majority of clients are adolescents and young women. Attending a highly competitive high school and being from a professional, upper middle-class family increases the risk for this disorder. Persons with anorexia nervosa have an intense fear of gaining weight and refuse to maintain body weight at the minimal normal weight for their age and height.

Bulimia nervosa is most identified with binge eating and behaviors to prevent weight gain. Behaviors include self-induced vomiting, misuse of laxatives and other medications, and excessive exercise (Friedman and others, 1998). Because adolescents rarely volunteer information about behaviors to prevent weight gain, it is important to take a thorough dietary history. Bulimia is considered a biopsychosocial illness. Both anorexic and bulimic clients have a strong awareness of society's emphasis on being thin.

Sexual Experimentation.

Sexual experimentation is common among adolescents. Peer pressure, physiological and emotional changes, and societal expectations contribute to early heterosexual and homosexual relations. According to the Centers for Disease Control and Prevention (1999), 54% of adolescents between grades 9 and 12 have admitted to having sexual intercourse at least once. The degree of sexual activity among teenagers may not change significantly, but the degree of informed, consenting participation can. Data from the Centers for Disease Control and Prevention (1991) indicate that 22% of teenagers report having sexual relations with at least four partners. Two prominent consequences of adolescent sexual activity are sexually transmitted disease and pregnancy.

Sexually Transmitted Disease.

Sexually transmitted disease (STD) annually afflicts around 10 million persons under the age of 25 years. This high degree of incidence makes it imperative that sexually active adolescents be screened for STDs, even when they have no symptoms. The annual physical examination of a sexually active adolescent should include a thorough sexual history and a careful examination of the genitalia so that condylomata acuminata (genital warts), herpes, *Phthirius pubis* (crab lice), primary syphilitic chancres, and other STDs are not missed. Recommended tests for women include Papanicolaou (Pap) smears, cervical cultures for gonorrhea and *Chlamydia* species, and syphilis tests; for men, urethral cultures for gonorrhea and *Chlamydia* species and syphilis tests are recommended. If men have participated in homosexual activities, rectal and pharyngeal cultures also need to be taken to check for gonorrhea. The health care provider can be proactive by using the interview process to identify risk factors in the adolescent. Once identified, the risk factors should lead to a strong message of prevention (CDC, 1998a).

Human immunodeficiency virus, which causes acquired immunodeficiency syndrome (AIDS), is transmitted through unprotected sexual intercourse, the use of shared needles, and through infected blood products. Therefore the risk-taking behaviors of adolescent sexual activity and drug use make adolescents vulnerable to the threat of AIDS. Approximately 30,000 HIV-infected adolescents live in the United States today; AIDS is the sixth leading cause of death among individuals between 15 and 24 years of age (CDC, 1994). Adolescents who have placed themselves at risk for AIDS should be tested for HIV.

Pregnancy.

Adolescent pregnancy is a common occurrence in the United States; 1 of every 10 female 15- to 19-year olds get pregnant, and many choose to keep their babies. Pregnancy rates are higher among older adolescents than they are among younger adolescents (Guttmacher Institute, 1994). Adolescent pregnancy occurs across socioeconomic class, in public and private schools, among all ethnic and religious backgrounds, and in all parts of the country. Two factors believed to account for adolescent childbearing levels and trends are the adult childbearing levels and trends and poverty as reflected in race (Males, 1996). Poverty also correlates with higher birthrates among childbearing adults. Multiple studies have identified a diverse set of risk factors for teenage pregnancy; however, there is limited agreement among the studies.

HEALTH CONCERNS

Perceptions.

One area of concern is the formation of healthy habits of daily living. Emphasis on exercise, sleep, nutrition, and stress-reduction habits is increasing. The nurse must recognize the importance of these habits and identify ways to adapt them to each adolescent. To do this the nurse must assess the individual's positive and negative habits and attitudes about health. Extensive and long-term follow-up is required if individualized interventions are to succeed. The nurse needs to be aware of the prevalence of health problems and make assessments accordingly.

Health Education. Community and school-based health programs for adolescents are focused on health promotion and illness prevention. Nurses are involved in community health through screening and teaching programs. Through their efforts in the school and community, nurses can make a contribution in meeting the *Healthy People 2000* objectives (US DHHS, 1992). Appropriate topics for adolescents are listed in Table 10-16.

The services provided to adolescents must be easily accessed and confidential. Nelson (1995) finds that for adolescents to reveal intimate information about their risk-taking behaviors, they must first feel comfortable and respected as individuals. Large numbers of school-based clinics have been developed and implemented to respond to adolescents' needs.

Nurses can play an important role in preventing injuries and accidental deaths. Injury prevention activities and support of organizations that promote responsible behavior, including Mothers Against Drunk Driving (MADD) and Drug Abuse Resistance Education (DARE), and encouraging students to participate in Students Against Drunk Driving (SADD) are types of important activities. Stimulating adolescents to discuss alternatives to driving when under the influence of drugs or alcohol prepares them to consider alternatives when such an occasion arises. The nurse must identify those adolescents at risk for abuse, provide education to prevent accidents related to substance abuse, and provide counseling to those in rehabilitation.

The nurse must provide sex education and counseling. Nurses play a key role in counseling teenagers on ways to avoid pregnancies. After pregnancy has occurred, the nurse can assist them in obtaining medical care and developing skills that will enhance their infants' development.

Extensive educational efforts to prevent the spread of AIDS and other STDs in this age group are a nursing responsibility. Education may occur in the school or community and be formal, informal, one-on-one, or in a group setting. Speakers and organizations can be used to help in the educational process.

Rural Adolescents. Fifty percent of adolescents live in the rural South, 27% live in the rural Midwest, and the remaining adolescents are fairly evenly distributed among the two remaining regions of the United States. Areas of concern for these adolescents include limited access to health care, limited health care insurance, limited privacy, lack of transportation to health care, poverty, and farming accidents.

Nurses can play an important role in improving the health of the adolescent. Decreasing barriers to care, health promotion education, development of coping strategies, and assessment of health beliefs are important areas for the nurse to address.

Minority Adolescents. An examination of 1990 census figures indicates that demographic changes are taking place in the nation. According to the Children's Defense Fund (1991), minority groups make up approximately 30% of the U.S. population. By the next century, it is expected that minorities as a group will become the majority. Minority adolescents have been identified as experiencing a greater percentage of health problems and barriers to health care.

Issues of concern for these adolescents living in a high-

Table 10-16 **Health Promotion During the Adolescent Period**	
Adolescent Health Concerns	Health Promotion Intervention
Unintentional injuries	Advise adolescent to take driver's education course and to wear seat belts. Inform the adolescent of risk associated with drinking and driving; use of drugs. Promote helmet use by adolescent bicyclists and motorcyclists. Ensure adolescent receives proper orientation to the use of all sports equipment. Encourage adolescent to swim with a "buddy."
Firearm use and violence	Teach conflict resolution skills.
Tobacco, alcohol, and drug use	Screen for tobacco (including smokeless), alcohol, and drug use and inform of the risks of use.
Suicide	Offer suicide prevention information. Teach methods to deal with a suicidal peer. Promote suicide alternatives.
Sexually transmitted diseases	Provide adolescent with information regarding disease, mode of transmission, and related symptoms. Encourage abstinence from sexual activity; or if sexually active, the use of condoms. Provide accurate information about the consequences of sexual activity.

risk environment include learning or emotional difficulties, death related to violence, unintentional injuries, increased rate for adolescent pregnancy, STDs, and AIDS.

Poverty is a major factor negatively affecting the lives of minority adolescents. Limited access to health services is common. Nurses can make a significant contribution to improving access to appropriate health care for adolescents.

Nurses must be able to identify effective coping strategies that enable minority adolescents to overcome stresses inherent in their environment (Ryan-Wenger and Copeland, 1994). Health promotion initiatives must be based on topics of concern for these adolescents.

Nurses working in the community must adopt culturally sensitive interventions to meet the needs of minority adolescents and their families (Spector, 1991). They must be able to communicate in another language by speaking it or using an interpreter. Teaching materials need to be written in the appropriate language. Information regarding health beliefs and healing practices must be assessed. With knowledge about various cultures and the means to care for minority adolescents, the nurse acts as an advocate to ensure accessibility of appropriate services.

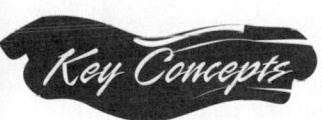

Key Concepts

- Growth and development are orderly, directional, predictable, interdependent, and complex processes that continue throughout life.
- A developmental perspective helps the nurse understand commonalities and variations in each stage and the impact they have on the client's health.
- During critical periods of development, a multitude of factors can foster or hinder optimal physical, cognitive, and psychosocial development.
- Growth and development are influenced by the inner forces of heredity and temperament and the outer forces of family, peers, life experiences, and environmental elements.
- Because the embryo and fetus grow and develop throughout the intrauterine period, genetic factors and environmental factors (teratogens) may result in impairments in any body system in utero.
- Physiological, cognitive, and psychosocial development continue from conception through adolescence, and the nurse must be familiar with normal parameters to determine potential problems and promote normal development.
- Physical growth during the school years is slow and steady until the skeletal growth spurt just before puberty.
- The major psychosocial developmental task of the school-age child is the development of a sense of industry, which is gained through personal achievements and results in positive self-esteem.

- Cognitively, the young school-age child develops conservation, the mental operation that allows thought processes to become more logical.
- The prepubertal growth spurt usually occurs 2 years earlier in girls than in boys; during this time, development of secondary sexual changes begins.
- Preadolescents move forward to the last stage of cognitive development, formal operations, in which they begin to think in an abstract manner, reflect on thought processes, and plan for the future.
- Adolescence begins with puberty, when primary sexual characteristics begin to develop and secondary sexual characteristics complete development.
- The adolescent is able to solve complex mental problems, use deductive reasoning, and hypothesize about the future.
- The adolescent's rapid change in physical appearance heightens self-consciousness and concerns regarding body image.
- Accidents are the major cause of death in all age groups.
- Motor vehicle accidents are the major cause of accidental death in adolescence.
- Sexually transmitted diseases are the most common communicable diseases among adolescents.
- Adolescents begin the long process of emancipation from their parents and need parental support to accomplish this in a timely manner.

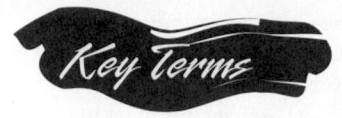

Key Terms

Adolescence, *p. 212*
Animism, *p. 199*
Apgar score, *p. 179*
Artificialism, *p. 199*
Blastocyst, *p. 176*
Bonding, *p. 180*
Classification, *p. 205*
Concrete operations, *p. 205*
Critical period, *p. 174*
Decenter, *p. 205*
Development, *p. 173*
Differentiation, *p. 174*
Embryo, *p. 176*
Estrogen, *p. 214*
Fetus, *p. 177*
Fontanel, *p. 181*
Fundus, *p. 177*
Hyperbilirubinemia, *p. 184*
Implantation, *p. 176*
Inborn errors of metabolism, *p. 184*
Infancy, *p. 185*
Lanugo, *p. 177*
Maturation, *p. 174*
Menarche, *p. 215*
Molding, *p. 181*
Morula, *p. 176*
Nagele's rule, *p. 174*
Neonatal period, *p. 180*

Object permanence, *p. 174*
Organogenesis, *p. 177*
Physical growth, *p. 173*
Physiological anorexia, *p. 195*
Placenta, *p. 176*
Preadolescence, *p. 212*
Prematurity, *p. 178*
Preoperational thought, *p. 195*
Preschool period, *p. 196*
Psychosocial moratorium, *p. 217*
Puberty, *p. 201*
Quickening, *p. 177*
Reversibility, *p. 205*
School-age, *p. 201*
Seriation, *p. 205*
Sexually transmitted disease (STD), *p. 219*
Temperament, *p. 179*
Teratogens, *p. 177*
Testosterone, *p. 214*
Tocolysis, *p. 178*
Toddlerhood, *p. 192*
VBAC, *p. 178*
Vernix caseosa, *p. 177*
Zygote, *p. 176*

Critical Thinking Exercises

1. Mrs. Kim is attending a health clinic for newly pregnant mothers. A major area for discussion of health promotion is focused on teratogens. How should the nurse explain what a teratogen is and what types of exposure should be avoided? What types of lifestyle changes should be discussed?
2. Two-year-old Jamal has been admitted to the hospital because of pneumonia. His parents wish to participate in his care when they are present but will not be able to be with him continuously. The mother plans to spend the late evening and night at the hospital but will continue to work during the day. The father will visit on his way to work in the morning. Identify nursing measures that will minimize separation anxiety for Jamal.
3. Six-year-old Jackie has been admitted to the hospital for osteomyelitis of her right foot and is receiving in-

travenous antibiotic therapy. What strategies can the nurse use in her daily care to reduce her fears? How can the nurse establish a trusting relationship with Jackie?
4. Twelve-year-old Elizabeth is brought to the pediatric clinic for a physical examination. She is concerned about her lack of physical development compared to her peers. Discuss ways to educate Elizabeth about puberty and the variations that occur.
5. Fifteen-year-old Daniel is in skeletal traction with a fractured femur. Discuss ways to meet Daniel's needs for diversional activity.

References

American Academy of Pediatrics, Committee on Infectious Diseases: *1997 Red Book report of the Committee on Infectious Disease*, ed 24, Elk Grove Village, Ill, 1997a, The Academy.

American Academy of Pediatrics, Task Force on Infant Positioning and SIDS: Does bed sharing affect the risk of SIDS? *Pediatrics* 100(2):272, 1997b.

American Academy of Pediatric Dentistry: Reference Manual 1996-1997, *Pediatr Dent* 18(6):24,1996.

Antwerp CV, Spaniolo AM: Checking out children's lifestyles, *MCN Am J Matern Child Nurs* 16(3):144, 1991.

Brouder AE, Montelone JA: *Child maltreatment: a clinical guideline and reference,* St. Louis, 1994, GW Medical.

Center for Communicable Diseases: Guidelines for school programs to promote lifelong eating habits, *J Sch Health* 67:9, 1996.

Centers for Disease Control and Prevention: *Survey: teen health and sex habits*, Atlanta, 1991, The Centers.

Centers for Disease Control and Prevention: *HIV/AIDS surveillance report*, Atlanta, 1994, The Centers.

Centers for Disease Control and Prevention: 1998 guidelines for the treatment of sexually transmitted disease, *MMWR Morbid Mortal Wkly Rep,* 47(RR-1):1, 1998a.

Centers for Disease Control and Prevention: Measles, mumps and rubella—vaccine use and strategies for the elimination of measles, mumps, rubella, and congenital rubella and control of mumps: recommendations of the Advisory Committee on Immunization Practices (ACIP) *MMWR Morbid Mortal Wkly Rep,* 47(RR-8):1, 1998b.

Centers for Disease Control and Prevention: Youth risk behavior surveillance—United States, *MMWR Morbid Mortal Wkly Rep,* 47(55-3):1 1998c.

Centers for Disease Control and Prevention: Trends in HIV related sexual risk behaviors among high school students—selected U.S. cities, *MMWR Morbid Mortal Wkly Rep,* 48(21):400, 1999.

Children's Defense Fund: *The state of America's children,* Washington, DC, 1991.

Coles C: Impact of prenatal alcohol exposure on the newborn and the child, *Clin Obstet Gynecol* 36(2):255, 1993.

Dacey J, Travers J: *Human development across the lifespan,* Dubuque, Iowa, 1991, Brown.

Edelman C, Mandle C, editors: *Health promotion throughout the life span,* ed 3, St. Louis, 1994, Mosby.

Elkind D: *All grown up and no place to go,* Reading, Mass, 1984, Addison-Wesley.

Erikson EH: *Childhood and society,* ed 2, New York, 1963, Norton.

Erikson EH: *Identity: youth and crises,* New York, 1968, Norton.

Feingold C: Correlates of cognitive development in low-birth-weight infants from low-income families, *J Pediatr Nurs* 9(2):91, 1994.

Ferber R: Behavioral "insomnia" in the child, *Psychiatr Clin North Am* 10(4):641, 1987.

Fingerhut L, Ingram D, Feldman J: Firearm homicide among black teenage males in metropolitan countries, *JAMA* 267(22):3054, 1992.

Frankenburg WK and others: The Denver II: a major revision and restandardization of the Denver Developmental Screening Test, *Pediatrics* 89(1):91, 1992.

Friedman S and others: *Comprehensive adolescent health care,* ed 2, St. Louis, 1998, Mosby.

Garner J: Guidelines for isolation precautions in hospitals, *Infect Control Hosp Epidemiol* 17(1):54, 1996.

Grodner M, Anderson S, DeYoung S: *Foundations and clinical applications of nutrition: a nursing approach,* St. Louis, 1996, Mosby.

Guttmacher Institute: *Sex and America's teenagers,* New York, 1994, Alan Guttmacher Institute.

Hawton K: *Suicide and attempted suicide among children and adolescents,* 1990, Sage.

Kohlberg L: Development of moral character and moral ideology. In Hoffman ML, Hoffman LNW, editors: *Review of child development research,* vol 1, New York, 1964, Russel Sage Foundation.

Kuczen B: *Childhood stress: don't let your child be a victim,* New York, 1982, Delacorte Press.

Lockridge T: Now I lay me down to sleep: SIDS and infant sleep positions, *Neonatal Network* 16(6):25, 1997.

Lowdermilk D, Perry S, Bobak I: *Maternity nursing,* ed 5, St. Louis, 1999, Mosby.

Males M: *The scapegoat generation: America's war on adolescents,* Monroe, Me, 1996, Common Courage Press.

McCaleb A, Edgil A: Self-concept and self-care practices of healthy adolescents, *J Pediatr Nurs* 9(4):233, 1994.

McGinnis J, DeGraw C: Healthy Schools 2000: creating partnerships for the decade, *J Sch Health* 61:292, 1991.

Medoff-Cooper B: Infant temperament: implications for parenting from birth through 1 year, *J Pediatr Nurs* 10(3):141, 1995.

Mitchell E: Co-sleeping and sudden infant death syndrome, *Lancet* 348:1466, 1996.

Moore KL, Pernaud TV: *The developing human: clinically oriented embryology,* ed 5, Philadelphia, 1993, WB Saunders.

Nelson J: HIV in adolescents, *MCN Am J Matern Child Nurs* 20:34, 1995.

Pender N: *Health promotion in nursing practice,* ed 3, Norwalk, Conn, 1996, Appleton & Lange.

Piaget J: *The origins of intelligence in children,* New York, 1952, International Universities Press.

Ryan-Wenger NM, Copeland SG: Coping strategies used by black school-aged children from low-income families, *J Pediatr Nurs* 9(1):33, 1994.

SAMHA: Annual emergency room data, U.S. Department of Health and Human Services Pub No. SMA 94-2080, Rockville, Md, 1994.

Seidel H and others: *Mosby's guide to physical examination,* ed 3, St. Louis, 1995, Mosby.

Spector R: *Cultural diversity in health and illness,* Norwalk, Conn, 1991, Appleton & Lange.

U.S. Department of Health and Human Services: *Healthy People 2000: national health promotion and disease prevention objectives,* Boston, 1992, Jones & Bartlett.

U.S. Department of Health and Human Services: Child maltreatment 1995: reports from the states to the National Child Abuse and Neglect Data System, Washington, DC, 1997.

U.S. Substance Abuse and Mental Health Services Administration: Preliminary estimates from the 1994 national household survey on drug abuse, Rockville, Md, 1995.

Wong DL: *Whaley and Wong's nursing care of infants and children,* ed 6, St. Louis, 1999, Mosby.

Wong DL: *Wong and Whaley's clinical manual of pediatric nursing,* ed 5, St. Louis, 2000, Mosby.

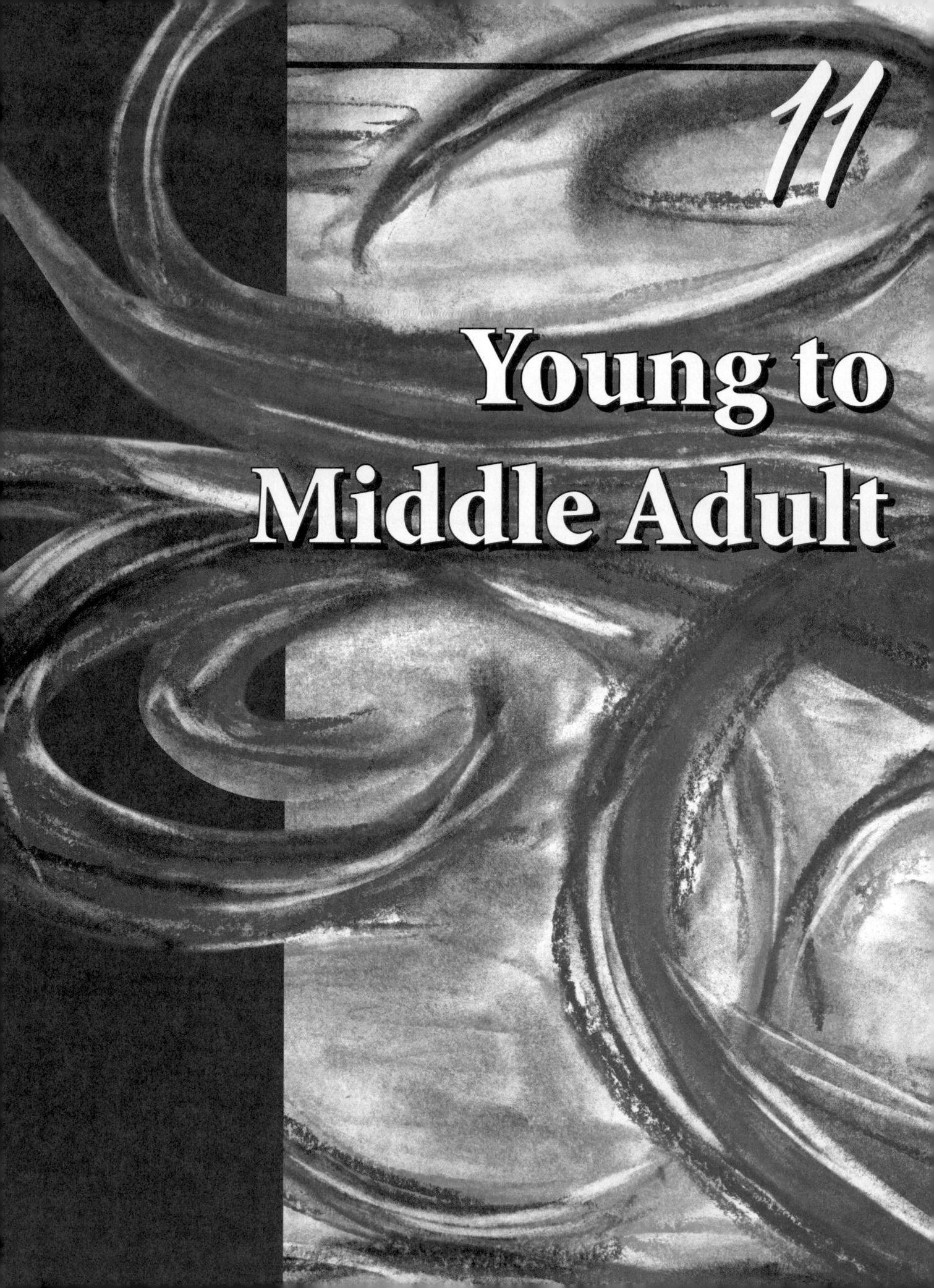

11

Young to Middle Adult

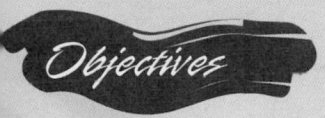
Objectives

Mastery of content in this chapter will enable the student to:

- Define the key terms listed.
- Discuss developmental theories of young and middle adults.
- List and discuss major life events of young and middle adults and the childbearing family.
- Describe developmental tasks of the young adult, the childbearing family, and the middle adult.
- Discuss the significance of family in the life of the adult.
- Describe normal physiological changes in young and middle adulthood and in pregnancy.
- Discuss cognitive and psychosocial changes occurring during the adult years.
- Describe health concerns of the young adult, the childbearing family, and the middle adult.
- Apply the nursing process to administer care to young and middle adults.

Young and middle adulthood is a period of challenges, rewards, and crises. Challenges may include the demands of work and raising families, although adults can also be rewarded by successes in their career endeavors and in their personal lives. Also, adults face such crises as caring for their aging parents, the possibility of job loss in a changing economic environment, and dealing with their own developmental needs as well as those of their family members.

Adult development involves orderly changes in characteristics and attitudes. Developmental changes are based on earlier characteristics that help shape subsequent behavior and characteristics. Each person's development, however, is a unique process (Haber and others, 1997). The changes experienced by young adults include the natural processes of maturation and socialization. Young adults pass through alternating periods of stability and change. During periods of stability, they make certain choices and build structures around them. In periods of change, they reevaluate these choices and consider new alternatives (Erikson, 1968, 1982).

Young adulthood is the period between the late teens and the mid- to late 30s (Edelman and Mandle, 1998). Young adults comprise approximately 26% of the population. During young adulthood, individuals increasingly separate from their families of origin, establish career goals, and decide whether to marry and begin families or remain single. Young adults are active and must adapt to new experiences.

Middle age occurs between the mid- to late 30s and the mid-60s. The transition into middle age occurs when young persons become aware that changes in reproductive and physical abilities signify the beginning of another stage in life. This is a time of continuing transitions when individuals may reassess their goals in life and add new goals. In 1990, almost 84 million persons in the United States were between the ages of 35 and 64, or approximately 34% of the U.S. population were middle-age adults (U.S. Department of Commerce, 1992).

People are said to have reached **maturity** when they have reached a balance of growth in physiological, psychosocial, and cognitive areas. Mature individuals feel comfortable with the abilities, knowledge, and responses that they have developed over the years. They look at the world with a broad view, based on a blend of insight, emotion, and imagination. They take on problems that can be solved but recognize and learn to live with unsolvable problems.

Mature people are open to suggestions and can accept constructive criticism without a major loss of self-esteem. They weigh other persons' input and recommendations when making decisions but are not overly influenced or intimidated by others. Above all, mature people develop by learning from their own and others' experiences.

Other characteristics of maturity are related to interpersonal communication and behavior. Mature persons acknowledge accomplishments and shortcomings. Mature adults confront tasks openly, use decision-making techniques to solve problems, and are accountable and responsible for their actions.

Classic work by such developmental theorists as Levinson and others (1978), Diekelmann (1976), Erikson (1963, 1982), and Havighurst (1972) has attempted to describe the phases of young and middle adulthood and related developmental tasks (see Chapter 9 for an in-depth discussion of developmental theories). It has been proposed that intellectual and moral development differ between men and women. According to Gilligan (1993), women struggle with the issues of care and responsibility, and in turn their relationships progress toward a maturity of interdependence. As women progress toward adulthood the moral dilemma changes from how to exercise their rights without interfering in the rights of others to "how to lead a moral life," which includes obligations to themselves and their families and people in general (Gilligan, 1993).

As women entered professional arenas, they hoped to develop the caring and nurturing roles in their male colleagues (Gordon, 1991). Women have long recognized that, without caring, the perceived quality of life is changed. As a result women maintained caring in the home and educational and work environments. However, women became frustrated in their development because the responsibility of caring was not shared, and frequently nurturing became a gender-specific responsibility.

In many cultures familial authority has historically been associated with the male. Men have traditionally assumed the overwhelming majority of positions of power. Boys learn how to be men by absorbing messages about manliness from parents, siblings, peers, teachers, television, and action movies. These messages encourage boys to be competitive, focus on external success, rely on their intellect, withstand physical pain, and repress their vulnerable emotions. Traditional masculine roles include providing and protecting. Recently, however, men have been characterized as moving into greater disequilibrium. Faced with a societal structure that differs greatly from the norms of 20 years ago, many men are challenged with determining what it means to be a man and how to feel good about it in today's society (Sheehy, 1995). As a provider, for example, a man is traditionally viewed as the primary supporter of the family. More women, however, have been successful in entering the workforce and pursuing careers, and in some age groups, men's incomes have declined, as much as 24% among young adult men. In fact, in the 1980s the driving force in the U.S. economy was earnings by women (Sheehy, 1995).

Developmental theories provide nurses with a basis for understanding the life events and developmental tasks of the young and middle adult. Each young or middle adult, however, brings unique characteristics and needs to his or her developmental stage. Clients may present challenges to nurses who themselves may be young or middle adults coping with the demands of their respective developmental period. Nurses must be careful to recognize the needs of their clients even if they are not experiencing the same challenges and events.

Young Adult

PHYSICAL CHANGES
The young adult has completed physical growth by the age of 20. An exception to this is the pregnant or lactating woman. The physical, cognitive, and psychosocial changes and the health concerns of the pregnant woman and the childbearing family are extensive.

Young adults are usually quite active, experience severe illnesses less commonly than older age groups, tend to ignore physical symptoms, and often postpone seeking health care. Physical characteristics of young adults begin to change as middle age approaches. Unless clients have illnesses, assessment findings are generally within normal limits.

Nonetheless, clients in this developmental stage may benefit from a personal lifestyle assessment (see Chapter 1). A personal lifestyle assessment can help nurses and clients identify habits that increase the risk for cardiac, malignant, pulmonary, renal, or other chronic diseases. A personal lifestyle assessment of the young adult includes assessment of general life satisfaction; hobbies and interests; habits such as diet, sleeping, exercise, sexual habits, and use of caffeine, alcohol, and illicit drugs; home conditions, including housing, economic condition, type of health insurance, and pets; and occupational environment, including type of work, exposure to hazardous substances, and physical or mental strain. Military records, including dates and geographical area of assignments, may also be useful in assessing the young adult for risk factors.

COGNITIVE CHANGES
Rational thinking habits increase steadily through the young and middle adult years. Formal and informal educational experiences, general life experiences, and occupational opportunities dramatically increase the individual's conceptual, problem-solving, and motor skills.

Identifying preferred occupational areas is a major task of young adults. When people know their skills, talents, and personality characteristics, educational preparation, and occupational choices are easier and more satisfying. Many young adults, however, either lack the resources or the support systems to facilitate further education or the development of skills necessary for many positions in the workplace. As a result, some young adults may have limited occupational choices.

An understanding of how adults learn assists the nurse in developing teaching plans (see Chapter 23). Adults enter the teaching-learning situation with a background of unique life experiences, including illness. Therefore the nurse always views adults as individuals. Their compliance with regimens such as medications, treatments, or lifestyle changes such as smoking cessation, involves decision-making processes. When determining the amount of information that the individual needs to make decisions about the prescribed course of therapy, the nurse should consider those factors that may affect the individual's compliance with the regimen, including educational level, socioeconomic factors, and motivation and desire to learn.

Because young adults are continually evolving and adjusting to changes in the home, workplace, and personal lives, their decision-making processes should be flexible. The more secure young adults are in their roles, the more flexible and open they are to change. Insecure persons tend to be more rigid in making decisions.

PSYCHOSOCIAL CHANGES

The emotional health of the young adult is related to the individual's ability to address and resolve personal and social tasks. The young adult is usually caught between wanting to prolong the irresponsibility of adolescence and wanting to assume adult commitments. Certain patterns or trends, however, are relatively predictable. Between the ages of 23 and 28, the person refines self-perception and ability for intimacy. From 29 to 34 the person directs enormous energy toward achievement and mastery of the surrounding world. The years from 35 to 43 are a time of vigorous examination of life goals and relationships. Alterations are made in personal, social, and occupational lives. Often the stresses of this reexamination result in a "midlife crisis" in which marital partner, lifestyle, and occupation may change.

During the young adult years, people generally give more attention to occupational and social pursuits. During this period individuals attempt to improve their socioeconomic status. Upward mobility is sought through career choices. Recent trends toward corporate downsizing, however, are leading to fewer high-level positions. Subsequently, many young adults are facing the added stress of greater competition in the workplace for fewer positions. For many young adults, a dual-income family is also needed to achieve and maintain middle-class status. Career and personal counseling can help individuals identify career choices and set realistic goals.

Ethnic and gender factors have a sociological and psychological influence in an adult's life, and these factors can pose a distinct challenge for nursing care. Each person holds culture-bound definitions of health and illness. Nurses and other health professionals bring with them distinct practices for the prevention and treatment of illness. Knowing too little about a client's self-perception or beliefs regarding health and illness may create conflict between the nurse and the client. Changes in the traditional role expectations of both men and women in young and middle adulthood have also led to greater challenges for nursing care. Women often continue to work during the child-rearing years, and many women struggle with the enormity of balancing three careers: wife, mother, and employee. This is a potential source of stress for the adult working woman. Men are more aware of parental and household responsibilities and find themselves having more responsibilities at home while achieving their own career goals (Haber and others, 1997). An understanding of ethnicity, race, and gender differences enables the nurse to provide individualized care (see Chapter 7).

Support from the nurse, access to information, and appropriate referrals provide opportunities for achievement of a client's potential. Because health is not merely the absence of disease but involves wellness in all human dimensions, the holistic, humanistic nurse acknowledges the importance of the young adult's psychosocial needs and needs in other dimensions.

The young adult must make decisions concerning career, marriage, and parenthood. Although each person makes these decisions based on individual factors, the nurse should understand the general principles involved in these aspects of psychosocial development while assessing the young adult's psychosocial status.

Lifestyle.   Lifestyle habits such as smoking, stress, lack of exercise, and poor personal hygiene increase the risk of future illness. Family history of cardiovascular, renal, endocrine, or neoplastic disease increases the risk of illness as well. The nurse's role in health promotion is to identify factors that increase the young adult's risk for health problems and to provide client education and support to reduce unhealthy lifestyle behaviors.

Those lifestyle habits that activate the stress response (see Chapter 30) increase the risk of illness. Smoking is a well-documented risk factor for pulmonary, cardiac, and vascular diseases in smokers and the individuals who receive secondhand smoke. Inhaled cigarette pollutants increase the risk of lung cancer, emphysema, and chronic bronchitis. The nicotine in tobacco is a vasoconstrictor that acts on the coronary arteries, increasing the risk of angina, myocardial infarction, and coronary artery disease. Nicotine also causes peripheral vasoconstriction and may lead to vascular problems.

Prolonged stress increases wear and tear on the body's adaptive capacities. Stress-related diseases such as ulcers, emotional disorders, and infections can occur (see Chapter 30).

Career.   Young men and women hope to have careers that will enable them to realize the occupational dreams of their childhood. They may formulate short- and long-term goals in traditional or nontraditional careers. A successful vocational adjustment is important in the lives of most men and women. Successful employment not only ensures economic security but also leads to friendships, social activities, support, and respect from co-workers.

Two-career marriages are increasing. The two-career marriage has benefits and liabilities. In addition to increasing the family's financial base, the person who works outside the home is able to expand friendships, activities, and interests. However, stress may occur in a two-career family. These stressors can result from a transfer to a new city; increased expenditures of physical, mental, or emotional energy; child care demands; or household needs.

Male and female stereotypes of the past are decreasing. Men are becoming more involved in child-rearing and homemaking duties. Women are becoming active in house and automobile maintenance. To avoid stress in a two-career family, neither partner can assume all responsibilities. For some families a solution may be to limit recreational expenses and instead hire someone to do routine housework. Others may set up an equal division of household, shopping, and cooking duties.

Sexuality.

The development of secondary sexual characteristics occurs during the adolescent years (see Chapter 10). Physical development is accompanied by the ability to perform sexual acts. The young adult usually has emotional maturity to complement the physical ability and is therefore able to develop mature sexual relationships. Young adults who have failed to achieve the developmental task of personal integration may, however, develop relationships that are superficial and stereotyped (Haber and others, 1997).

Masters and Johnson (1970) have contributed important information about the physiological characteristics of the adult sexual response. Detailed discussion of the sexual response occurs in Chapter 27.

The psychodynamic aspect of sexual activity is as important as the type or frequency of sexual intercourse to young adults. Psychological beliefs and expectations give feelings of pleasure and satisfaction to adults. To maintain total wellness, adults should be encouraged to explore various aspects of their sexuality and be aware that their sexual needs and concerns evolve. As the rate of early initiation of sexual intercourse continues to increase, young adults are at risk for sexually transmitted diseases. Consequently they need education regarding the mode of transmission, prevention, and symptom recognition and management.

Childbearing Cycle.

Conception, pregnancy, birth, and the puerperium are major phases of the childbearing cycle. The changes during these phases are complex. Women experience significant changes in physiological condition, emotion, and body image during the second trimester of pregnancy and during the early puerperium (Fishbein and Burggraf, 1998).

Education such as Lamaze classes can prepare pregnant women, their partners, and other support persons to participate in the birthing process (Figure 11-1). Social support has also been reported to have a positive impact on pregnant women and their families. Schaffer and Lia-Hoagberg (1997) reported that social support positively affected both the adequacy of prenatal care and prenatal health behaviors. Another study revealed a positive association between social support and the reduction of low birth weight in African Americans (Norbeck, DeJoseph, and Smith, 1996). A current trend in some health care agencies is to provide a lay **doula** or support person to be present during labor to assist women who have no other source of support.

Lactation, or the process of breast-feeding, offers many advantages to both the new mother and baby. For the inexperienced mother, breast-feeding may also be a source of anxiety and frustration. Women who have had no contact with other mothers who breast-feed and who have had little or no contact with newborns require assistance to breast-feed successfully. The nurse must be alert for signs that the mother needs information and assistance. Direct observation of the breast-feeding mother-infant dyad (pair) alerts the nurse to such problems as proper positioning of either the mother and infant or ineffective sucking by the infant.

The personal and social changes occurring in the lives of a couple after the birth of a baby cannot be underestimated (Figure 11-2). The nursing assessment of the couple's response to the birthing experience and parent-child bonding are discussed in a later section of this chapter.

Types of Families.

During young adulthood most individuals experience singlehood and the opportunity to be on their own. Those who eventually marry experience several changes as they take on new responsibilities. Many married couples choose to become parents. Middle adults who remain single experience unique challenges and opportunities as well.

Singlehood.

Social pressure to get married is not as great as it once was, and many young adults do not expect to be married until their late 20s or early 30s, or not at all (Sheehy, 1995). For young adults who remain single, parents and siblings become the nucleus for a family, although the single young adult maintains independence from parental controls. Close friends and associates of the single young adult may also be viewed as the individual's "family."

One cause for the increased single population is the expanding career opportunities for women. Women enter the job market with greater career potential and have greater opportunities for financial independence. More single individuals are choosing to live together outside of

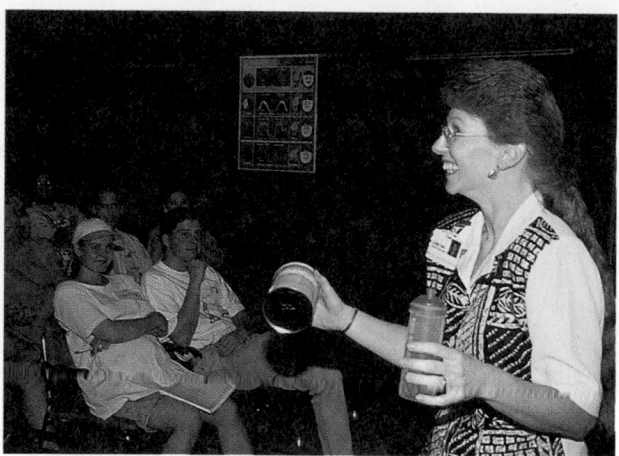

Figure 11-1   Nurse providing Lamaze class for expectent young adults.

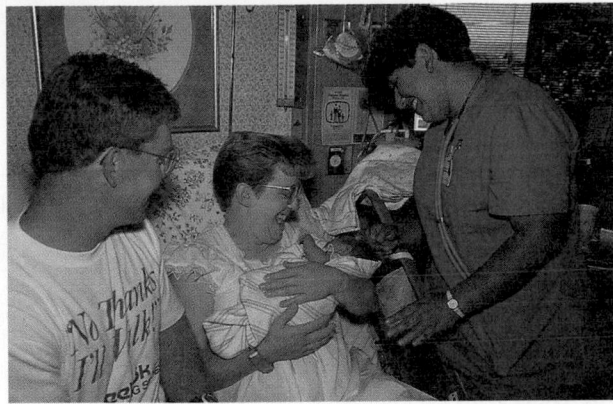

Figure 11-2 Parent-child nurturing is important in adapting to a newborn.

Modified from Stanhope M, Lancaster J: *Community health nursing: process and practice for promoting health*, ed 4, St. Louis, 1996, Mosby.

Ten Hallmarks of Emotional Health	Box 11-1

A sense of meaning and direction in life
Successful negotiation through transitions
Absence of feelings of being cheated or disappointed by life
Attainment of several long-term goals
Satisfaction with personal growth and development
When married, feelings of mutual love for partner; when single, satisfaction with social interactions
Satisfaction with friendships
Generally cheerful attitude
No sensitivity to criticism
No unrealistic fears

marriage as well as become parents either biologically or through adoption. Similarly, many married couples choose to separate or divorce if they find their marital situation unsatisfactory.

Marriage. Every couple's relationship is unique. Although no rules guarantee a successful marriage, some guidelines are useful for building a happy marriage. Before marriage the couple ideally should complete five tasks. First, the partners should make certain that their emotions are based on love rather than physical or sexual attraction. Second, both partners should explore their motivation for wanting to marry. Third, they should focus on developing clear communication. Fourth, they should understand that any annoying behavior patterns and habits are unlikely to change after marriage. Last, they should determine their compatibility in important beliefs and values.

When establishing a household and family, the married couple must begin to work as a team. They have the following tasks:

Establishing an intimate relationship
Deciding on and working toward mutual goals
Establishing guidelines for power and decision-making issues
Setting standards for extrafamily interactions
Finding companionship with other people for a social life
Choosing morals, values, and ideologies acceptable to both

These major tasks of adults require considerable maturity and self-esteem. When accomplished, however, they provide the foundation for a stable relationship. Growth in marriage extends over many years. Success in solving the challenging problems that occur in any marriage offers marital partners insight into each other.

A marital relationship involves different developmental stages. The establishment stage begins at the wedding and continues as the couple attempts to function as a dyad. The couple learns patterns of sexual expression and ways to live intimately with each other. They must learn styles of conflict resolution, decision making, and role patterns. In addition, each partner may experience a sense of loss of individuality and self in the transition from *me* to *we*.

The family orientation stage is directed at childbearing and child-rearing activities. Parenting roles must be defined and practiced. Nurturing and socialization needs of the children can put pressure on the couple's intimate relationship. In addition, parents' images of the "perfect parent" conflict with reality.

Parenthood. The availability of contraception makes it easier for today's couples to decide when and if to start a family. One factor influencing this decision is the reason for wanting a child. Social pressures may encourage a couple to have a child or may influence them to limit the number of children they have. Economic considerations frequently enter into the decision-making process because having and bringing up children are expensive. General health status and age are also considerations in decisions about parenthood because couples are getting married later and are postponing pregnancies.

Hallmarks of Emotional Health. Most young adults have the physical and emotional resources and support systems to meet the many challenges, tasks, and responsibilities they face. During psychosocial assessment of young adults, the nurse can assess for 10 hallmarks of emotional health (Box 11-1) that indicate successful maturation in this developmental stage.

HEALTH RISKS
Risk Factors. Risk factors for the young adult's health originate in the community, lifestyle, and family history.

Family History. A family history of a disease may put a young adult at risk for developing it in the middle or older adult years. For example, a young man whose father and paternal grandfather had myocardial infarctions (heart attacks) in their 50s has a risk for a future myocardial infarction. The presence of certain chronic illnesses in the family increases the family member's risk of developing a disease. This family risk is distinct from hereditary disease.

Personal Hygiene Habits. As in all age groups, personal hygiene habits in the young adult can be risk factors. Sharing eating utensils with a person who has a contagious illness increases the risk of illness. Poor dental hygiene increases the risk of periodontal disease. Gingivitis (inflammation of the gums) and periodontitis (loss of tooth support) can be avoided through oral hygiene (see Chapter 38).

Violent Death and Injury. Violence is the greatest cause of mortality and morbidity in the young adult population. Death and injury can occur from physical assaults, motor vehicle or other accidents, and suicide attempts. In 1996 the death rate (per 100,000 population) for 25- to 34-year-olds in the United States due to homicide was 13.4; the death rate due to motor vehicle accidents was 19.1; and the death rate due to suicide in this age group was 14.5 (U.S. Department of Health and Human Services [USDHHS], 1998).

While recent media attention has focused on the increase in violent crime among youth, adults still commit the majority of crimes. Eighty-four percent of all arrests for murder and 77% of all arrests for weapons violations in 1993 involved adults (Children's Defense Fund, 1995). Factors that may predispose to violence, with subsequent injury or death, include poverty, family breakdown, child abuse and neglect, repeated exposure to violence, and ready access to guns. It is important that the nurse perform a thorough psychosocial assessment, including such factors as behavior patterns, history of physical abuse and substance abuse, education, work history, and social support systems, to detect personal and environmental risk factors for violence.

Substance Abuse. Substance abuse directly or indirectly contributes to mortality and morbidity in young adults. Intoxicated young adults may be severely injured in motor vehicle accidents that may result in death or permanent disability to other young adults as well.

Dependence on stimulant or depressant drugs can result in death. Overdose of a stimulant drug ("upper") can stress the cardiovascular and nervous systems to the extent that death occurs. The use of depressants ("downers") can lead to an accidental or intentional overdose and death.

Caffeine is a naturally occurring legal stimulant that is readily available in carbonated beverages, chocolate-containing foods, coffee and tea, and over-the-counter medications, such as cold tablets, allergy and analgesic preparations, and appetite suppressants. It is the most widely ingested stimulant in North America. Caffeine can stimulate catecholamine release, which, in turn, stimulates the central nervous system; increases gastric acid secretion, heart rate, and basal metabolic rate; alters blood pressure; increases diuresis; and relaxes smooth muscle (Mitchell, 1997). Consumption of large amounts of caffeine can result in restlessness, anxiety, irritability, agitation, muscle tremor, sensory disturbances, heart palpitations, nausea, or vomiting and diarrhea in some individuals.

Substance abuse is not always diagnosable, particularly in its early stages. Nonjudgmental questions about use of legal drugs (prescribed drugs, tobacco, and alcohol), use of soft drugs (marijuana), and use of more problematic drugs (cocaine or heroin) should be a routine part of any physical assessment. Important information may be obtained by making specific inquiries about past medical problems, changes in food intake or sleep patterns, or problems of emotional lability. Reports of arrests because of driving while intoxicated, wife or child abuse, or disorderly conduct should alert the health care provider to probe the possibility of drug abuse more carefully.

Unplanned Pregnancies. Unplanned pregnancies, although more common among adolescents, account for 55% of pregnancies in young and middle adult women (Alan Guttmacher Institute, 1994). Unplanned pregnancies can have long-term physical and emotional effects in the young adult years. Unplanned pregnancies are a continual source of stress. Often young adults have educational and career goals that take precedence over family development. Interference with these goals can affect future relationships and affects later parent-child relationships.

Determination of situational factors that may affect the progress and outcome of an unplanned pregnancy is important. Exploration of problems such as financial, career, and living accommodations; family support systems; potential parenting disorders; depression; and coping mechanisms is important in assessing the woman with an unplanned pregnancy.

Sexually Transmitted Diseases. Sexually transmitted diseases (STDs) are a major health problem in the 1990s. STDs include syphilis, chlamydia, gonorrhea, genital herpes, and AIDS. Sexually transmitted diseases have immediate effects such as discharge, discomfort, and infection. They may also lead to chronic disorders, which can result from genital herpes; infertility, which can result from gonorrhea; or even death, which results from acquired immunodeficiency syndrome (AIDS). These diseases may occur in sexually active persons, and it is estimated that there are 4 million new infections of chlamydia each year, 3 million new infections of gonorrhea, and

100,000 new infections of syphilis (Ament and Whalen, 1996).

Environmental or Occupational Factors.   A common environmental or occupational risk factor is exposure to airborne particles, which may cause lung diseases and cancer. Such lung diseases include silicosis from inhalation of talcum and silicon dust and emphysema from inhalation of smoke. Cancers resulting from occupational exposures may involve the lung, liver, brain, blood, or skin (Table 11-1). Questions regarding occupational exposure to hazardous materials should be a routine part of the nurse's assessment.

HEALTH CONCERNS

Health Promotion.   Young adults are generally active and have a minimum of major health problems. However, their lifestyles may put them at risk for illnesses or disabilities during their middle or older adult years. Young adults may also be genetically susceptible to certain chronic diseases such as diabetes mellitus and familial hypercholesterolemia (McCance and Huether, 1998). Crohn's disease, a chronic inflammatory disease of the small intestine, most commonly occurs between 15 and 35 years of age. Many young adults have misconceptions regarding transmission and treatment of STDs. Partners are encouraged to know one another's previous sexual history and sexual practices. The nurse should be alert for STDs when clients come to clinics with complaints of urological or gynecological problems (see Chapter 32). Young adults should be assessed for their knowledge of genital self-examinations.

Infertility.   **Infertility** is a man's, woman's, or couple's involuntary inability to conceive. To most health professionals, it is the inability to conceive after a year or more of regular sexual intercourse. An estimated 15% to 20% of otherwise healthy adults are infertile, and many infertile clients are young adults. However, about half of the couples evaluated and treated in infertility clinics become pregnant. In about 10% to 20% of couples the cause of infertility is unknown and they remain infertile. In the remaining 30% the cause of the infertility is diagnosed but the couples remain infertile because of endometriosis, blocked fallopian tubes, or decreased sperm motility. For some infertile couples the nurse may be the first resource identified. Nursing assessment of the infertile couple should include comprehensive histories of both the male and female partners to determine factors that may have affected fertility as well as pertinent physical findings (Lowdermilk, Perry, and Bobak, 1997).

Exercise.   Exercise patterns can affect health status. Exercise that produces a sustained increase in the pulse rate for 15 to 20 minutes 3 times a week improves cardiopulmonary function by decreasing blood pressure and heart rate. In addition, exercise decreases fatigability, insomnia, tension, and irritability. The nurse should conduct a thorough musculoskeletal assessment, including joint mobility and muscle tone, and psychosocial assessment for improved tolerance to stress to determine the effects of exercise.

Routine Health Screening.   Poor adherence to routine screening examinations can put the client at risk for severe illnesses because of failed early detection. Clients should be encouraged to perform monthly breast self-examination (BSE) or genital self-examination (see Chapter 32). The nurse's role is extremely important in educating female clients about BSE and the current breast screening recommendations since breast cancer is the most common major cancer among women in the United States with a steadily increasing incidence (Lowdermilk, Perry, and Bobak, 1997). Routine assessment of the skin for recent changes in color or presence of lesions and changes in their appearance should be encouraged. Prolonged exposure to ultraviolet rays of the sun by the adolescent and young adult can increase the risk for development of skin cancer later in life.

Psychosocial Health.   The psychosocial health concerns of the young adult are often related to stress, such as job or family stress. As noted in Chapter 30, stress can be valuable because it motivates a client to change. However, if the stress is prolonged and the client is unable to adapt to the stressor, health problems can develop.

Occupational Chemical	Cancer
	Occupational Hazards
Table 11-1	**Associated With Cancers**
Asbestos	Mesothelioma (pleural and peritoneal)
	Lung cancer
Vinyl chloride (plastics)	Liver cancer (hemangiosarcoma)
	Brain cancer
	Lung cancer
Benzene	Leukemia, predominantly acute myelogenous
Bischloromethane ether	Oat cell carcinoma of the lungs
Chromium	Cancer of nasal or paranasal sinus, lung, larynx
	Lung cancer
Arsenic	Cancer of lung, larynx, skin
Coal tar pitch, coke oven emissions	
Iron oxide	Cancer of lung, larynx
Nickel	Lung cancer
Petroleum distillates	Cancer of lung, larynx

From Stanhope M, Lancaster J: *Community health nursing: process and practice for promoting health,* ed 4, St. Louis, 1996, Mosby.

Job Stress.   Job stress can occur every day or from time to time. Most young adults are able to handle day-to-day crises (Figure 11-3). Situational job stress may occur when a new boss enters the workplace, a deadline is approaching, or the worker is given new or greater numbers of responsibilities. A recent trend in today's business world and risk factor for job stress is corporate downsizing, leading to increased responsibilities for employees with fewer positions within the corporate structure. Job stress also occurs when a person becomes dissatisfied with a job or responsibilities. Because individuals perceive jobs differently, the types of job stressors vary from client to client. The nurse's assessment of the young adult should include a description of the usual work performed and present work if different. Job assessment also includes conditions and hours, duration of employment, changes in sleep or eating habits, and evidence of increased irritability or nervousness.

Family Stress.   Family stressors can occur at any time in family life (see Chapter 8). Family life has peaks, when everyone in the family works together, and valleys, when everyone appears to pull apart. Situational stressors occur during events such as births, deaths, illnesses, marriages, and job losses. Because of the multiplicity of changing relationships and structures in the emerging young adult family, stress is frequently high. Stress may be related to a number of variables, including the work trajectories of both husband and wife, and may lead to dysfunction in the young adult family. This may be reflected in the fact that the highest divorce rate occurs during the first 3 to 5 years of marriage for young adults under the age of 30. When a client seeks health care and presents stress-related symptoms, the nurse should assess for the occurrence of a life change event.

Each family has certain predictable roles or jobs for members. These roles enable the family to function and be an effective part of society. One necessary role is the family leader. In most families one parent is the leader, or both parents act as coleaders. In single-parent families the parent or occasionally a member of the extended family is the family leader. When this changes as a result of illness, a situational crisis may occur. The nurse should assess environmental and familial factors, including support systems and coping mechanisms commonly used by family members.

Pregnant Woman and Childbearing Family.   A developmental task for most young adult couples is the decision to begin a family. Although the physiological changes of pregnancy and childbirth occur only in the woman, cognitive and psychosocial changes and health concerns affect the entire childbearing family, including the baby's father, siblings, and grandparents.

Health Practices.   Women who are anticipating pregnancy benefit from good health practices before concep-

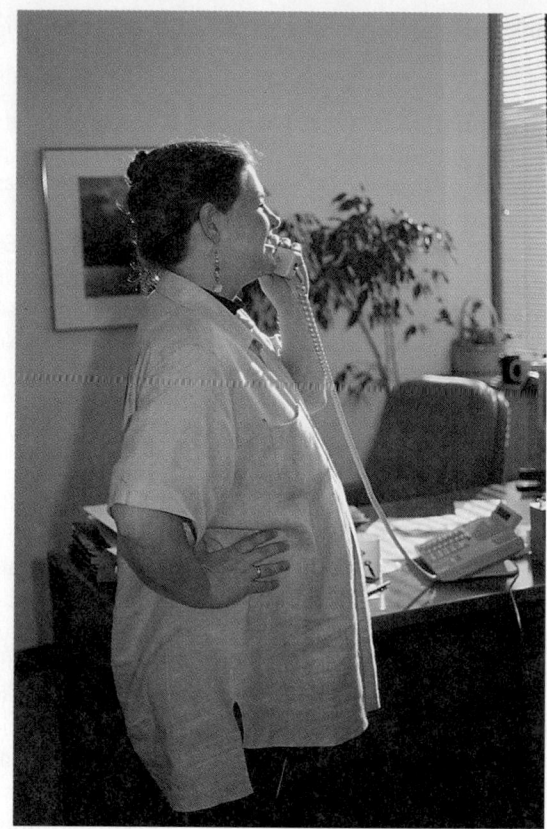

Figure 11-3   The ability to handle day-to-day challenges at work minimizes stress.

tion; these include a balanced diet, exercise, dental checkups, avoidance of alcohol, and cessation of smoking. Women trying to become pregnant should not try weight-reduction diets. The physiological changes and needs of the pregnant woman vary with each trimester (Table 11-2).

Prenatal Care.   **Prenatal care** is the routine examination of the pregnant woman by an obstetrician, nurse practitioner, or certified nurse-midwife. Prenatal care includes assessment of the pregnant woman's weight; blood pressure; urine for glucose, acetone, and protein; and measurement of the fundus. Information should be provided from the beginning regarding sexually transmitted diseases, other vaginal infections, and urinary infections that could adversely affect the fetus. In addition, the pregnant woman may be counseled about exercise patterns, diet, and child care. Regular health care can address health concerns such as preeclampsia, eclampsia, gestational diabetes, excessive weight gain, and the high-risk infant.

First Trimester.   All women experience some physiological changes in the first trimester, but some changes affect only certain women. These changes include **morning sickness,** increased urination, lack of energy, and changes in nutritional intake. The nurse must be familiar with

Table 11-2 Major Physiological Changes During Pregnancy

Signs and Symptoms	Causes
First Trimester	
Amenorrhea	Fertilization of egg by sperm
Morning sickness	Increased serum hormone levels
Breast changes	Increased estrogen levels
Enlargement	
Tenderness	
Darkened and enlarged nipples	
Urinary frequency	Pressure of uterus on bladder
Fatigue	Increases in hormone levels
	Increased nutritional demands
	Decreased nutritional intake resulting from morning sickness
Second Trimester	
Integumentary changes	Increased levels of melanocyte-stimulating hormone
Pigmented nipple and breast	
Hyperpigmentation of abdominal line (linea nigra)	
Mottling of cheeks or forehead (chloasma or "mask of pregnancy")	
Local or generalized pruritus	
Hypertrophy of gums causing gingival swelling and bleeding	Proliferation of interdental papillary blood vessels, resulting in local inflammation and hyperplasia
Increasing size of uterine fundus	Growth of fetus
Sensation of movement or gaslike movements (quickening)	Fetal movement
Braxton Hicks contractions	Expanding uterus and preparation of uterus for labor
Third Trimester	
Increased colostrum	Hormonal influence; preparation of breasts for lactation
Increased urinary frequency	Pressure on bladder from enlarged fetus

Data from Lowdermilk D, Perry S, Bobak I: *Maternity and women's health care*, ed 6, St. Louis, 1997, Mosby; and Dickason E, Silverman B, Kaplan J: *Maternal-infant nursing care*, St. Louis, 1998, Mosby.

these physiological changes, their causes, and helpful interventions.

During this period signs of pregnancy are usually not observable by others. If a woman frequently has morning sickness, however, her family, friends, and co-workers may suspect that she is pregnant. The newly pregnant woman needs routine prenatal care.

Second Trimester. During the second trimester, growth of the uterus and fetus results in some of the physical signs of pregnancy. Morning sickness has usually disappeared, and the woman's energy level is restored if her nutritional intake has caught up with her metabolic demands. The urinary frequency ceases, and she is able to sleep through the night.

If this is the woman's first pregnancy, she may be able to see and feel the enlarged uterus. However, it is common for her abdomen to stay relatively flat. In subsequent pregnancies she may "show" as early as the beginning of the second trimester.

Third Trimester. During the third trimester increases in **Braxton Hicks contractions** (irregular, short contractions), fatigue, and urinary frequency occur. Close to the onset of labor, the woman may experience a burst of energy during which she cleans house and prepares for the baby by shopping for baby supplies. This period is called **nesting.** Many experts in obstetrics and seasoned veterans of pregnancy believe that nesting indicates a rapidly approaching time of delivery.

Puerperium. The **puerperium** is a period of approximately 6 weeks after delivery. During this time the woman's body reverts to its prepregnant physical status. The nurse should assess the woman's knowledge of and ability to care for both herself and for her newborn baby. Assessment of parenting skills and maternal-infant interactions is particularly important.

Cognitive Changes. Cognitive changes during pregnancy, primarily involving sensory perception and needs for education, affect both parents and may occur gradually or quickly.

Sensory Perception. The pregnant woman generally experiences changes in sensory perception. Temporary changes occur in visual and hearing acuity, taste, and smell. Many pregnant women frequently stroke the abdomen, possibly because of a change in the sensation of touch or other sensory need. The woman may be using the sensation of touch to initiate bonding with her child.

Needs for Education. The entire childbearing family needs education about pregnancy, labor, delivery, breastfeeding, and integration of the newborn into the family structure. Traditionally, childbirth classes help parents plan for the birth of the child and focus on the normal physiological changes of pregnancy, the processes of labor and delivery, methods of pain control, symptoms of impending labor, and care of the newborn (Box 11-2). Many health care centers also have sibling and grandparent preparation classes. Not all pregnant women, however, attend childbirth classes for a variety of reasons. Childbirth education classes may not be accessible to women of all socioeconomic classes, and women may choose not to attend because of cultural beliefs about childbirth or lack of knowledge about the importance of childbirth education.

Psychosocial Changes. Like the physiological changes of pregnancy, psychosocial changes may occur at various times during the 9 months of pregnancy and in the puerperium. The major categories of psychosocial changes involve body image, role, sexuality, coping mechanisms, and stresses during the puerperium. Table 11-3 summarizes these psychosocial changes and implications for nursing intervention.

Health Concerns. The pregnant woman and her partner have many health questions. For example, they may wonder whether the pregnancy and baby will be normal. The majority of the health needs related to pregnancy can be met with proper prenatal care (Figure 11-4).

Acute Care. The young adult years are generally a time of good physical and emotional health. Potential health hazards may be related to lifestyle. Acute care for young adults is frequently related to accidents, substance abuse, exposure to environmental and occupational hazards, stress-related illnesses, respiratory infections, gastroenteritis, influenza, urinary tract infections, and minor surgery. An acute minor illness can cause a disruption in life activities of the young adult and increase stress in an already hectic lifestyle. Dependency and limitations posed by treatment regimens can also increase frustration for the young adult. To give young adults a sense of maintaining control of their health care choices, it is important to keep

Research HIGHLIGHT   Box 11-2

RESEARCH ABSTRACT

Pregnancy and the birth of a child can be a stressful time for both parents. Eighty-three couples were studied to determine whether the use of father-focused perinatal classes with an emphasis on teaching coping skills to relieve psychological stress and on increasing social network support would positively influence spousal relations during pregnancy. Forty couples were in the traditional childbirth classes, and 43 couples were in the experimental classes. Results showed that men in the father-focused classes had a greater decrease in psychological symptoms than men in the traditional classes. Fathers in the father-focused classes also showed significantly greater improvement in spousal relationships than those in the traditional classes. Both groups increased from pretest to posttest in the use of social support as a means of coping, but this increase was greater for men in the father-focused group.

IMPLICATIONS FOR PRACTICE

- Nurses must realize that fathers are an integral part of the childbearing process and may also experience stress and anxiety related to the pregnancy either along with or independent from their partners.
- A family-centered philosophy of nursing care should result in perinatal education that includes consideration for fathers along with the traditional attention to expectant women.
- Nurses can serve as a resource for couples to assist them in the identification and use of coping strategies and the reduction of stress.

REFERENCE

Deimer G: Expectant fathers: influence of perinatal education on stress, coping, and spousal relations, *Res Nurs Health* 20(4):281, 1997.

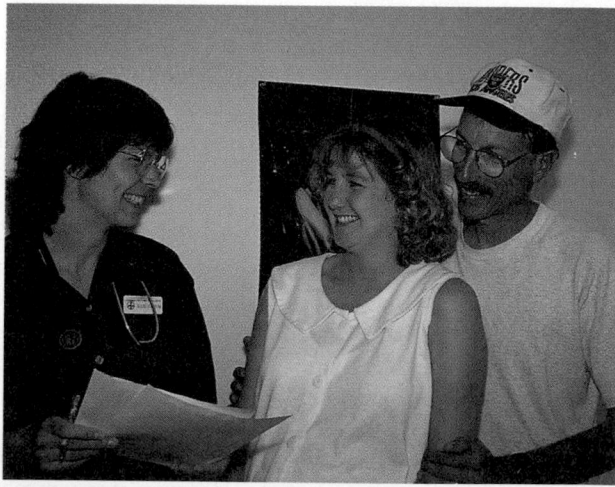

Figure 11-4 Ongoing prenatal care reduces complications of pregnancy.

Table 11-3 Major Psychosocial Changes During Pregnancy

Category	Implications for Nursing
Body image	Morning sickness and fatigue may contribute to poor body image
	Client may feel big, awkward, and unattractive during third trimester when fetus is growing more rapidly
	Increase in breast size may make the woman feel more feminine and sexually appealing
	May take extra time with hygiene and grooming, trying new hairstyles and makeup
	Begins to "show" during the second trimester and starts to plan maternity wardrobe
	General feeling of well-being when woman can feel the baby move and hear the heartbeat
Role changes	Both partners think about and can have feelings of uncertainty about impending role changes
	May have feelings of ambivalence about becoming parents and concern about ability to be parents
Sexuality	Need reassurance that sexual activity will not harm fetus
	Desire for sexual activity may be influenced by body image
	May desire cuddling and holding rather than sexual intercourse
Coping mechanisms	Need reassurance that childbirth and child rearing are natural and positive experiences, but can also be stressful
	Often unable to cope with particular stressors such as finding new housing, preparing the nursery, or participating in childbirth classes
Stresses during puerperium	May return home from hospital fatigued and unfamiliar with infant care
	May experience physical discomfort or feelings of anxiety or depression
	May be necessary for woman to return to work soon after delivery with subsequent feelings of guilt, anxiety, or, possibly, sense of freedom or relief

them informed about their health status and involve them in health care decisions.

Restorative and Continuing Care.   Chronic conditions are not common in young adulthood, but they can occur. Chronic illnesses such as hypertension, coronary artery disease, and diabetes may have their onset in young adulthood without being known to the young adult until later in life. Causes of chronic illness and disability in the young adult can include accidents, multiple sclerosis, rheumatoid arthritis, AIDS, and cancer. Chronic illness and disability can affect the accomplishment of important developmental tasks in young adulthood. The threat to the young adult's independence that is caused by chronic illness or disability can result in the need to change personal, family, and career goals. Nursing interventions for the young adult faced with chronic illness or disability should include potential developmental problems related to sense of identity, the establishment of independence, reorganization of intimate relationships and family structure, and launching of a chosen career (Lewis, Heitkemper, and Dirkson, 2000).

Middle Adult

In middle adulthood, the individual makes lasting contributions through involvement with others. Generally the middle adult years begin around the early to mid-30s and last through the late 60s (Edelman and Mandle, 1998), corresponding to Levinson's developmental phases of

"settling down" and the "payoff years." During this period, personal and career achievements have often already been experienced. Many middle adults find particular joy in assisting their children and other young people to become productive and responsible adults. They may also begin to help aging parents. Using leisure time in satisfying and creative ways is a challenge that, if met satisfactorily, enables middle adults to prepare for retirement.

While most middle adults have achieved socioeconomic stability, recent trends in corporate downsizing have left many middle adults either jobless or forced to accept lower paying jobs. Economists at the Agency for Health Care Policy and Research have revealed that in 1996, 75% of U.S. workers were offered health insurance by their employers, an increase from 72% in 1987. However, the number of workers who turned down employer-offered health insurance coverage has more than doubled over the past decade, from 2.6 million in 1987 to 6 million in 1996. During that same time period, health insurance premiums rose by 90%, and fewer employers have shared the cost of health insurance plans that include coverage for dependents (Cooper and Schone, 1997). As a result, a greater proportion of the population is currently unable to afford adequate health insurance coverage (Scanlon, Chernew, and Lave, 1997).

Men and women must adjust to inevitable biological changes. As in adolescence, middle adults use considerable energy to adapt self-concept and body image to physiological realities and changes in physical appearance. High self-esteem, a favorable body image, and a positive attitude toward physiological changes are fostered when adults engage in physical exercise, balanced diets, adequate sleep, and good hygiene practices that promote vigorous, healthy bodies.

PHYSICAL CHANGES

Major physiological changes occur between 40 and 65 years of age. Table 11-4 summarizes these normal devel-

opmental changes that the nurse considers when conducting a physical examination.

The most visible changes are graying of the hair, wrinkling of the skin, and thickening of the waist. Balding commonly begins during the middle years, but it may also occur in young male adults. Decreases in hearing and visual acuity are often noted during this period. According to national health care statistics, approximately 23% of all

Table 11-4 Physical Assessment Findings in the Middle Adult

Body System	Findings
Integument	Intact condition
	Appropriate distribution of pigmentation
	Slow, progressive decrease in skin turgor
	Graying and loss of hair (Baldness patterns in males are established by age 55; hair loss after this time might have other causes.)
Head and neck	Symmetry of scalp, skull, and face
	Normal accessory organs of vision
Eyes	Visual acuity by Snellen chart that is less than 20/50
	Pupillary reaction to light and accommodation
	Normal visual fields and extraocular movements
	Normal retinal structures
Ears	Normal auditory structures and acuity
Nose, sinuses, and throat	Patent nares and intact sinuses, mouth, and pharynx
	Location of trachea at midline
	Nonpalpable lateral thyroid lobes
Thorax and lungs	Increased anteroposterior diameter
	Respiratory rate 16-20 breaths per minute and regular
	Ratio of respiratory rate to heart rate: 1:4
	Normal tactile fremitus, resonance, and breath sounds
Heart and vascular system	Normal heart sounds
	Systole: S_1 less than S_2 at base
	Diastole: S_1 greater than S_2 at apex
	Point of maximal impulse: at fifth intercostal space in midclavicular line and 2 cm or less in diameter
	Vital signs
	Temperature: 36.7°-37.6° C (97°-99.6° F)
	Pulse: 60-100 (conditioned athlete ≈ 50)
	Blood pressure: 95-140/60-90 mm Hg
	Respirations: 12-20 breaths per minute
	All pulses palpable
Breasts	Decreased size resulting from decreased muscle mass
	Normal nipples
Abdomen	No tenderness or organomegaly
	Decreased strength of abdominal muscles
Female reproductive system	Change in menstrual cycle and in duration and quality of menstrual flow
	"Hot flashes"
	Change in cervical mucosa
Male reproductive system	Normal penis and scrotum
	Prostatic enlargement in some individuals
Musculoskeletal system	Decreased muscle mass
	Decreased range of joint motion
Neurological system	Appropriate effect, appearance, and behavior
	Lucidity and appropriate level of cognitive ability
	Intact cranial nerves
	Adequate motor responses
	Responsive sensory system

visits to office-based physicians by adults aged 44 to 64 are for a primary diagnosis of glaucoma (USDHHS, 1995). Often these physiological changes have an impact on self-concept and body image. The most significant physiological changes during middle age are menopause in women and the climacteric in men.

Menopause.   Menstruation and ovulation occur in a cyclical rhythm in the woman from adolescence into middle adulthood. **Menopause** is the disruption of this cycle, primarily because of the inability of the neurohormonal system to maintain its periodic stimulation of the endocrine system. The ovaries no longer produce estrogen and progesterone, and the blood levels of these hormones drop markedly. Menopause typically occurs between 45 and 60 years of age (see Chapter 27). Approximately 10% of women have no symptoms of menopause other than cessation of menstruation, 70% to 80% are aware of other changes but have no problems, and approximately 10% experience changes severe enough to interfere with activities of daily living (Lowdermilk, Perry, and Bobak, 1997).

Climacteric.   The **climacteric** occurs in men in their late 40s or early 50s (see Chapter 27). It is caused by decreased levels of androgens. Throughout this period and thereafter, a man is still capable of producing fertile sperm and fathering a child. However, penile erection is less firm, ejaculation is less frequent, and the refractory period is longer.

COGNITIVE CHANGES

Changes in the cognitive function of middle adults are rare except with illness or trauma. The middle adult can learn new skills and information. Some middle adults enter educational or vocational programs to prepare themselves for entering the job market or changing jobs.

PSYCHOSOCIAL CHANGES

The psychosocial changes in the middle adult may involve expected events, such as children moving away from home, or unexpected events, such as a marital separation or the death of a close friend. These changes may result in stress that can affect the middle adult's overall level of health. Nurses should assess the major life changes occurring in the middle adult and the impact that the changes have on that person's state of health. Nursing assessment should also include individual psychosocial factors such as coping mechanisms and sources of social support.

In the middle adult years, as children depart from the household, the family enters the postparental family stage. Time and financial demands on the parents decrease, and the couple faces the task of redefining their own relationship. As grandchildren arrive, grandparenting styles must be chosen. It is during this period that many middle-age adults begin to take on a healthier lifestyle. Although not advisable to wait until this stage in life to think about

health promotion, "better late than never" does apply. Assessment of health promotion needs for the middle adult include adequate rest, leisure activities, regular exercise, good nutrition, reduction or cessation in the use of tobacco or alcohol, and regular screening examinations. Assessment of the middle adult's social environment is also important, including relationship concerns; communication and relationships with children, grandchildren, and aging parents; and caregiver concerns with their own aging or disabled parents.

According to Erikson's developmental theory, the primary developmental task of the middle years is to achieve generativity (Erikson, 1968, 1982). Generativity is the willingness to care for and guide others. Middle adults can achieve generativity with their own children or the children of close friends or through guidance in social interactions with the next generation. If middle adults fail to achieve generativity, stagnation occurs. This is shown by excessive concern with themselves or destructive behavior toward their children and the community. For example, the National Committee to Prevent Child Abuse indicated that in 1993 there were 3 million reported cases of abuse or neglect; and although recent media coverage has reinforced the increase in youth violence, federal statistics indicate that greater than 80% of the increase in violent crime since the early 1980s is attributable to adults (Children's Defense Fund, 1995).

Career Transition.   Career changes may occur by choice or as a result of changes in the workplace or society. In recent decades, middle adults more often change occupations for a variety of reasons, including limited upward mobility, decreasing availability of jobs, and seeking an occupation that is more challenging to the individual. In some cases technological advances or other changes force middle adults to seek new jobs. Such changes, particularly when unanticipated, may result in stress that can affect health, family relationships, self-concept, and other dimensions.

Sexuality.   After the departure of their last child from the home, many couples recultivate their relationships and find increased marital and sexual satisfaction during middle age. The onset of menopause and the climacteric can affect the sexual health of the middle adult. A woman may desire increased sexual activity because pregnancy is no longer possible.

During middle age a man may notice changes in the strength of his erection and a decrease in his ability to experience repeated orgasm. Other factors influencing sexuality during this period include work stress, diminished health of one or both partners, and the use of prescription medications, for example, antihypertensive agents, with side effects that may influence sexual desire or functioning. Both partners may experience stresses related to sexual changes or a conflict between their sexual needs and self-perceptions and social attitudes or expectations (see Chapter 27).

Family Types.
Psychosocial factors involving the family may include the stresses of singlehood, marital changes, transition of the family as children leave home, and the care of aging parents.

Singlehood.
In 1990, 10% of adults between the ages of 35 and 59 years of age in the United States had never been married (U.S. Department of Commerce, 1992). Many of those are college-educated people who have embraced the philosophy of choice and freedom, have delayed marriage, and have delayed parenthood. Some middle-age adults who have chosen to remain single, however, have also opted to become parents either biologically or through adoption. Many single middle-age adults may have no relatives but share a family-type relationship with close friends or work associates. Consequently, some single middle-age adults may feel isolated during traditional "family" holidays such as Thanksgiving or Christmas. In times of illness, middle-age adults who have chosen to remain single and childless may have to rely on other relatives or friends, increasing caregiving demands of those family members who may also have other caregiving responsibilities. Nursing assessment of single middle-age adults should include a thorough assessment of psychosocial factors, including the individual's definition of family and available support systems.

Marital Changes.
Marital changes that may occur during middle age include death of a spouse, separation, divorce, and the choice of remarrying or remaining single. A widowed, separated, or divorced client goes through a period of grief and loss in which it is necessary to adapt to the change in marital status. Normal grieving progresses through a series of phases, and resolution of grief may take a year or more. The nurse should assess effective coping of the middle-age adult to the grief and loss associated with certain life changes.

If a single middle-age adult decides to marry, the stressors of marriage are similar to those for the young adult. In addition, the couple may have to cope with the social expectations and pressures related to marriage.

Family Transitions.
The departure of the last child from the home may be a stressor. Many parents welcome freedom from child-rearing responsibilities, whereas others feel lonely or without direction because of this change. Eventually parents must reassess their marriage and are able to resolve conflicts and plan for the future. Occasionally this readjustment phase may lead to marital conflicts, separation, and divorce.

Care of Aging Parents.
Increasing life spans in the United States and Canada have led to increased numbers of older adults in the population. Therefore greater numbers of middle-age adults must address the personal and social issues confronting their aging parents. Many middle adults find themselves in the **"sandwich generation"** caught between the responsibilities of caring for dependent children and those of caring for aging and ailing parents. The needs of the caregivers is an area that continues to grow.

Housing, employment, health, and economic realities have changed the traditional social expectations between generations in families. The middle adult and the older adult parent may have conflicting priorities related to their relationship while the older adult strives to remain independent. Negotiations and compromises help in defining and resolving problems. Nurses deal with middle and older adults in the community, long-term care facilities, and hospitals. The nurse can help identify the health needs of both groups and can assist the multigenerational family in determining the health and community resources available to them as they make decisions and plans. The nurse should also assess family relationships to determine family members' perceptions of responsibility and loyalty in relation to caring for older adult members. Assessment of environmental resources (e.g., number of rooms in the house, stairwells) in relation to the complexity of health care demands for the older adult is also important.

HEALTH CONCERNS
Health Promotion.
Physiological concerns for the middle adult include stress, level of wellness, and the formation of positive health habits.

Stress and Stress Reduction.
Because middle adults are experiencing physiological changes and face certain health realities, their perceptions of health and health behaviors are often important factors in maintaining health. Today's complex world makes individuals more prone to stress-related illnesses such as heart attacks, hypertension, migraine headaches, ulcers, colitis, autoimmune disease, backache, arthritis, and cancer. In 1996, the death rate (per 100,000 population) attributable to heart attacks was 8.4 for 35- to 44-year-olds; 36.9 for 45- to 54-year-olds; and 111.4 for 55- to 64-year-olds. For the same year and age groups, the death rates attributable to hypertensive heart disease were 2.0, 6.5, and 14.2, respectively (U.S. DHHS, 1998).

When adults seek health care, the nurse's focus on the goal of wellness can guide clients to evaluate health behaviors, lifestyle, and environment. Attention to risk factors that can be altered to improve the client's health, such as stress, obesity, use of tobacco, excessive alcohol consumption, poor nutrition, and unsafe sexual practices, can increase the quality of life and add years to it.

Throughout life, people are exposed to many stressors (see Chapter 30). After these stressors are identified, the client and nurse can work together to intervene and modify the stress response. Specific interventions for stress reduction can fall into three categories. First, the frequency of stress-producing situations is minimized. Together the nurse and client identify approaches to prevent stressful situations, such as habituation, change avoidance, time blocking, time management, and environmental modification. The second category is psychophysiological preparation to increase stress resistance, such as increasing self-esteem, improving assertiveness, redirecting goal alternatives, and reorienting cognitive appraisal. Last, the physiological response to stress is avoided. The nurse uses relaxation techniques (see Chapter 30), imagery, and biofeedback to recondition the client's response to stress. Chapter 29 explains these general interventions in greater detail.

Levels of Wellness.   The nurse must be able to assess the health status of the middle adult client. Such assessment offers direction for planning nursing care and is useful in evaluating the effectiveness of nursing interventions. Table 11-4, which shows the physical changes of the middle adult, can be used with other standard assessment techniques as a guide for physical assessment (see Chapter 32).

Forming Positive Health Habits.   A habit is a person's usual practice or manner of behavior. This behavior pattern is reinforced by frequent repetition until it becomes the individual's customary way of behaving. Some habits support health, such as exercise and brushing and flossing the teeth each day. Other habits involve risk factors to health, such as smoking or eating foods with little or no nutritional value.

During assessment the nurse frequently obtains data indicating positive and negative health behaviors by the client. Examples of positive health behaviors include regular exercise; adherence to good dietary habits; avoidance of excess consumption of alcohol; participation in routine screening and diagnostic tests (laboratory work for serum cholesterol, mammography) for disease prevention and

health promotion; and lifestyle changes to reduce stress. In the planning, implementation, and evaluation phases, the nurse helps the client maintain habits that protect health and offers healthier alternatives to poor habits.

Health teaching and health counseling are often directed at improving health habits (Box 11-3). The more fully the nurse understands the dynamics of behavior and habits, the more likely interventions will help the client to achieve or reinforce health-promoting behaviors.

To help clients form positive health habits the nurse becomes a teacher and facilitator. By providing information about how the body functions and how habits are formed and changed, the nurse raises clients' levels of knowledge regarding the potential impact of behavior on health. A nurse cannot change clients' habits. Clients have control of and are responsible for their own behaviors. The nurse can explain psychological principles of changing habits and offer information about health risks. The nurse can also offer positive reinforcement (such as praise and rewards) for health-directed behaviors and decisions. Such reinforcement increases the likelihood that the behavior will be repeated. Ultimately, however, the client decides which behaviors will become habits of daily living.

The nurse may assist young and middle adults in considering factors such as prevention of STDs, substance abuse, and accident prevention, in relation to decreasing health risks. For example, clients should be provided with factual information on sexually transmitted disease causes, symptoms, and transmission. The nurse should discuss methods of protection during sexual activity with the client in an open and nonjudgmental manner and reinforce the importance of practicing "safe sex" (see Chapter 27). The nurse can provide counseling and support for clients seeking treatment for substance abuse. The nurse can assist clients to recognize and alter unsafe habits and potential health hazards (see Chapter 37). The nurse should also encourage clients to express their feelings to promote problem solving and recognition of risk factors by clients themselves.

Client Teaching ABOUT POSITIVE HEALTH HABITS   Box 11-3

OBJECTIVE
- Client will increase exercise patterns to include three mile walks per week to assist weight loss and improve cardiopulmonary functions.

TEACHING STRATEGIES
- Review with client the daily work schedule and identify potential times for exercise.
- Inform client about the effect of exercise on weight control and improved cardiac function.
- Demonstrate how to calculate target heart rate and assess pulse correctly.

- Provide warm-up and cool-down exercises and demonstrate how to do them.
- Instruct client about support shoes for walking exercises.

EVALUATION
- Have client keep log of exercise periods.
- Have client demonstrate pulse measurement.
- Have client demonstrate warm-up and cool-down exercises.
- Inspect client's feet for blisters or sores.

Barriers to change do exist (Box 11-4). Unless these barriers are minimized or eliminated, it is futile to encourage the client to take actions that are going to be blocked.

Psychosocial Concerns.   Two common psychosocial health concerns of the middle adult are anxiety and depression.

Anxiety.   Anxiety is a critical maturational phenomenon related to change, conflict, and perceived control of the environment (Haber and others, 1997). Adults often experience anxiety in response to the physiological and psychosocial changes of middle age. Such anxiety can motivate the adult to rethink life goals and can stimulate productivity. For some adults, however, this anxiety precipitates psychosomatic illness and preoccupation with death. In this case the middle adult views life as being half or more over and thinks in terms of the time left to live.

Clearly, a life-threatening illness, marital transition, or job stressor increases the anxiety of the client and family. The nurse may need to use crisis intervention or stress management techniques to help the client adapt to the changes of the middle adult years (see Chapter 30).

Depression.   Depression is a mood disorder that manifests itself in many ways. Although the most frequent age of onset is between ages 25 and 44, it is common among adults in the middle years and may have many causes (Haber and others, 1997). The risk factors for depression include being female; disappointments or losses at work, school, or in family relationships; departure of the last child from the home, and family history. In fact, the incidence of depression in women is twice that of men (Haber and others, 1997). Persons experiencing mild depression describe themselves as feeling sad, blue, downcast, down in the dumps, and tearful. Other symptoms include alterations in sleep patterns such as difficulty in sleeping (insomnia) or sleeping too much (hypersomnia), irritability, feelings of social disinterest, and decreased alertness. Physical changes such as weight loss or weight gain, headaches, or feelings of fatigue regardless of the

amount of rest may also be depressive symptoms. Depression that occurs during the middle years is commonly characterized by moderate-to-high anxiety and physical complaints. Mood changes and depression are common phenomena during menopause. Depression may be worsened by the abuse of alcohol or other substances. Nursing assessment of the depressed middle adult includes focused data collection regarding individual and family history of depression, mood changes, cognitive changes, behavioral and social changes, and physical changes. Assessment data should be collected from both the client and the client's family, since family data may be particularly important, depending on the level of depression being experienced by the middle adult.

Community Health Programs.   Community health programs for young and middle adults are designed to prevent illness, promote health, and detect disease in the early stages. Nurses can make valuable contributions to the community's health by taking an active part in the planning of screening and teaching programs.

Family planning, birthing, and parenting skills are program topics in which adults might be interested. Health screening for diabetes, hypertension, eye disease, and cancer is a good opportunity for the nurse to perform assessment and provide health teaching and health counseling.

Health education programs can promote changes in behavior and lifestyle. The nurse as health teacher offers information that enables the client to make decisions about health practices within the context of health pro-

---

Barriers to Change   Box 11-4
EXTERNAL BARRIERS
Lack of facilities
Lack of materials
Lack of social supports
INTERNAL BARRIERS
Lack of knowledge
Lack of motivation
Insufficient skills to effect change in health habits
Undefined short- and long-term goals

Cultural ASPECTS OF CARE   Box 11-5
Lack of understanding of differences between ethnic cultural beliefs and practices may promote misunderstanding and frustration for nurses providing health care to clients from other cultures. According to Spector (1996), Hispanic subgroups comprise the second largest group in the United States. Hispanic-American adults' primary health care problems are the barriers faced when they seek health care. These problems include language, poverty, and time orientation. The Hispanic tendency to place little value on the exact time of day makes appointment keeping very frustrating for the client and the nurse.
Poverty may predispose middle-age adults from many ethnic groups to such conditions as tuberculosis, malnutrition, depression, and dental problems. In particular, inadequate economic resources is a burden for many middle-age adult women. African-American, Hispanic, and Native American women have high rates of poverty, especially if they are single heads of households. Because of lack of health insurance and the high cost of health care, many middle-age women postpone obtaining adequate health care and delay important health screening such as mammography and Papanicolaou (Pap) smears. Cultural competency is crucial in providing health care, particularly for at-risk populations.

motion for young to middle adults. The nurse must be sure that educational programs are culturally appropriate (see Box 11-5). Changes to more positive health practices during young and middle adulthood may lead to fewer or less complicated health problems as an older adult. During health counseling the nurse and client design a plan of action that addresses the client's health and well-being. Through objective problem solving, the nurse helps the client grow and change.

Regardless of the age of its members and its structure, the family faces certain health tasks. The nurse as health teacher and counselor understands the autonomy of the family and supports it while promoting family health.

Nursing roles include community-centered care, hospital-based acute care, and restorative care. Participation in community health programs for the adult or family often requires many nursing roles and skills.

Acute Care.

Acute illnesses and conditions experienced in middle adulthood are similar to those of young adulthood. Injuries and acute illnesses in middle adulthood, however, may take a longer recovery period because of the slowing of recuperative processes. As well, acute illnesses and injuries experienced in middle adulthood are more likely to become chronic conditions. For those middle adults who are in the "sandwich generation," stress levels may also increase as the middle adult tries to balance responsibilities related to employment, family life, care of children, and care of aging parents while recovering from an injury or acute illness.

Restorative and Continuing Care.

Chronic illnesses such as diabetes mellitus, hypertension, rheumatoid arthritis, chronic obstructive pulmonary disease, or multiple sclerosis may affect the roles and responsibilities assumed by the middle adult. Strained family relationships, modifications in family activities, increased health care tasks, increased financial stress, the need for housing adaptation, social isolation, medical concerns, and grieving may all result from chronic illness. The degree of disability and the client's perception of both the illness and the disability determine the extent to which lifestyle changes will occur. A few examples of the problems experienced by clients who develop debilitating chronic illness during adulthood include role reversal, changes in sexual behavior, and alterations in self-image. Along with the current health status of the chronically ill middle adult, the nurse must assess the knowledge base of both the client and family. This assessment should include the medical course of the illness and the prognosis for the client, the coping mechanisms of the client and family, adherence to treatment and rehabilitation regimens, and the need for community and social services, along with appropriate referrals.

Key Concepts

- Adult development involves orderly and sequential changes in characteristics and attitudes that adults experience over time.
- Many changes experienced by the young adult are related to the natural process of maturation and socialization.
- Maturity is reached when the young adult attains a balance of growth in the physiological, psychosocial, and cognitive areas.
- Young adults are in a stable period of physical development, except for changes related to pregnancy.
- Cognitive development continues throughout the young and middle adult years.
- Emotional health of young adults is correlated with the ability to address and resolve personal and social problems.
- Young adults must choose a career and decide whether to remain single or marry and begin a family.
- Pregnant women need to understand physiological changes occurring in each trimester.

- Cognitive and psychosocial changes and health concerns during pregnancy and the puerperium affect the parents, the siblings, and often the extended family.
- Prenatal care reduces maternal and fetal mortality and morbidity.
- Midlife transition begins when a person becomes aware that physiological and psychosocial changes signify passage to another stage in life.
- Two significant physiological changes of the middle years are menopause in women and the climacteric in men.
- Cognitive changes are rare in middle age except in cases of illness or physical trauma.
- Psychosocial changes for middle adults may be related to career transition, sexuality, marital changes, family transition, and care of aging parents.
- Health concerns of middle adults commonly involve stress-related illnesses, health assessment, and adoption of positive health habits.

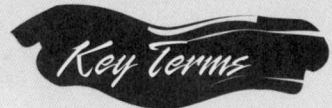

Key Terms

Braxton Hicks contrac-
tions, *p. 233*

Climacteric, *p. 237*

Doula, *p. 228*

Infertility, *p. 231*

Lactation, *p. 228*

Maturity, *p. 225*

Menopause, *p. 237*

Morning sickness, *p. 232*

Nesting, *p. 233*

Prenatal care, *p. 232*

Puerperium, *p. 233*

Sandwich generation, *p. 238*

Critical Thinking Exercises

1. Joan K. is a 24-year-old woman who smokes two packs of cigarettes per day. She began smoking when she was 14 years old. Joan complains to the nurse at the clinic, "I just can't seem to kick the habit no matter how hard I try." What information does the nurse need to know to assist Joan in quitting smoking?

2. James D., age 48, married, and the father of 13- and 16-year-old sons has recently had to assume the responsibility of caring for his 78-year-old mother after she suffered a stroke. Describe the nurse's role in assisting James in caring for his mother.

References

Alan Guttmacher Institute: *Sex and America's teenagers,* New York, 1994, Alan Guttmacher Institute.

Ament L, Whalen E: Sexually transmitted diseases in pregnancy: diagnosis, impact, and intervention, *J Obstet Gynecol Neonatal Nurs* 25(8):657, 1996.

Cooper P, Schone B: More offers, fewer takers for employment-based health insurance: 1987 and 1996, *Health Aff* 16(6):142, 1997.

Dickason E, Silverman B, Kaplan J: *Maternal-infant nursing care,* St. Louis, 1998, Mosby.

Diekelmann J: The young adult: the choice is health or illness, *Am J Nurs* 76:1276, 1976.

Diemer G: Expectant fathers: influence of perinatal education on stress, coping, and spousal relations, *Res Nurs Health* 20(4): 281, 1997.

Edelman C, Mandle C: *Health promotion throughout the lifespan,* ed 4, St. Louis, 1998, Mosby.

Erikson E: *Childhood and society,* ed 2, New York, 1963, WW Norton.

Erikson E: *Identity: youth and crisis,* New York, 1968, WW Norton.

Erikson E: *The life cycle completed: a review,* New York, 1982, WW Norton.

Fishbein E, Burggraf E: Early postpartum discharge: how are mothers managing, *J Obstet Gynecol Neonatal Nurs* 27(2): 142, 1998.

Gilligan C: *In a different voice,* Cambridge, Mass, 1993, Harvard University Press.

Gordon S: *Prisoners of men's dreams: striking out for a new feminine future,* Boston, 1991, Little, Brown.

Haber J and others: *Comprehensive psychiatric nursing,* St. Louis, 1997, Mosby.

Havighurst R: Successful aging. In Williams RH, Tibbits C, Donahue W, editors: *Process of aging,* vol 1, New York, 1972, Atherton.

Levinson D and others: *The seasons of a man's life,* New York, 1978, Knopf.

Lewis S, Heitkemper M, Dirksen S: *Medical-surgical nursing,* ed 4, St. Louis, 2000, Mosby.

Lowdermilk D, Perry S, Bobak, I: *Maternity and women's health care,* ed 6, St. Louis, 1997, Mosby.

Masters W, Johnson V: *Human sexual response,* Boston, 1970, Little, Brown.

McCance K, Huether S: *Pathophysiology: the biologic basis for disease in adults and children,* ed 3, St. Louis, 1998, Mosby.

Mitchell M: *Nutrition across the life span,* Philadelphia, 1997, WB Saunders.

Norbeck J, DeJoseph J, Smith R: A randomized trial of an empirically-derived social support intervention to prevent low birthweight among African American women, *Soc Sci Med* 43(6):947, 1996.

Scanlon D, Chernew M, Lave J: Consumer health plan choice: current knowledge and future directions, *Annu Rev Public Health* 18:507–528, 1997.

Schaffer M, Lia-Hoagberg B: Effects of social support on prenatal care and health behaviors of low-income women, *J Obstet Gynecol Neonatal Nurs* 26(4):433, 1997.

Sheehy G: *New passages: mapping your life across time,* New York, 1995, Random House.

Spector, R: *Cultural diversity in health and illness,* ed 4, East Norwalk, Conn, 1996, Appleton & Lange.

Stanhope M, Lancaster J: *Community health nursing: process and practice for promoting health,* ed 4, St. Louis, 1996, Mosby.

U.S. Department of Commerce: *1990 Census of population: general population characteristics, United States,* Washington, DC, 1992, Bureau of the Census.

U.S. Department of Health and Human Services, Public Health Service: *Advance data: office visits for glaucoma: United States, 1991–92,* 262, Hyattsville, Md, 1995, Centers for Disease Control and Prevention, National Center for Health Statistics.

U.S. Department of Health and Human Services, Public Health Service: *National vital statistics report: deaths: final data for 1996,* 47(9), Hyattsville, Md, 1998, Centers for Disease Control and Prevention, National Center for Health Statistics.

12

Older Adult

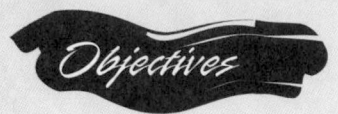

Mastery of content in this chapter will enable the student to:

- Define the key terms listed.
- Describe common myths and stereotypes about older adults.
- Discuss the significance of nurses' attitudes toward older adults.
- Describe the types of community-based and institutional health care services available to older adults.
- Describe some of the biological and psychosocial theories of aging.
- Identify common developmental tasks of older adults.
- Discuss common physiological changes of aging.
- Discuss the cognitive changes seen in some older adults.
- Differentiate among delirium, dementia, and depression.
- Discuss issues related to psychosocial changes of aging.
- Identify nursing interventions related to the physiological, cognitive, and psychosocial changes of aging.
- Identify the health concerns of older adults.

Older adulthood traditionally begins after retirement, usually between 65 and 75 years of age. The number of people in this age group is increasing at a dramatic rate. Demographers project a continuing increase in the older-adult population well into the next century (Figure 12-1). While the size of the group as a whole is increasing, the rate of increase is greatest for persons 85 years of age and older (Ebersole and Hess, 1998). Because the amount of time spent by health professionals in all settings with older adults is increasing, health care professionals must focus on ways to identify and meet this group's special needs. Older adults and health professionals must work together to address concerns related to acute and chronic health problems, changes in the health care system, and economic, social, and ethical issues.

The cultural, ethnic, and racial diversity of the older-adult population in the United States is also growing. Minority groups accounted for 15% of persons over age 65 in 1996 (American Association of Retired Persons [AARP], 1997). Population estimates for 2030 suggest that members of minority groups will make up 25% of the older-adult population. The percentage of older African-Americans is expected to increase from 7.9% to 11%. The number of older adults of Hispanic origin will also increase.

Nursing care of older adults poses special challenges because of great variation in their physiological, cognitive, and psychosocial health status. Older adults also vary widely in their levels of functional ability. The majority are active, involved, productive members of their communities. A smaller number have lost the ability to care for themselves, are confused or withdrawn, and are unable to make decisions concerning their needs. Most older adults live in noninstitutional settings, with 67% living in family settings with spouse, children, relatives, or nonrelatives

and 32% living alone. Only 4% of all older adults reside in institutions such as nursing homes (AARP, 1997). Many older adults (90%) report having at least one chronic health condition (Eliopoulos, 1998). The most common chronic conditions are arthritis, dental problems, hypertension, heart disease, visual problems, osteoporosis, hearing problems, depression, vascular disease, and functional dependency (Rubenstein and Nahas, 1998).

Nursing assessment of an older adult is a complex and challenging process. It must take into account five key points to ensure an age-specific approach: (1) the interrelation between physical and psychosocial aspects of aging, (2) the effects of disease and disability on functional status, (3) the decreased efficiency of homeostatic mechanisms, (4) the lack of standards for health and illness norms, and (5) altered presentation and response to specific disease (Lueckenotte, 1996a).

The physical and psychosocial aspects of aging are closely related. For the older person, a reduced ability to respond to stress, the experience of multiple losses, and the physical changes associated with normal aging may combine to place the person at high risk for illness and functional deterioration. Although the interaction of these physical and psychosocial factors can be serious, the nurse should not assume that all older adults have signs, symptoms, or behaviors representing disease and decline. The older adult's strengths and abilities must also be identified during the assessment.

Aging does not inevitably lead to disease and disability. Most older people remain functionally independent despite the increasing prevalence of chronic disease. How-

The authors acknowledge the contribution of Annette Giesler Leukenotte to this chapter in the previous edition of this text.

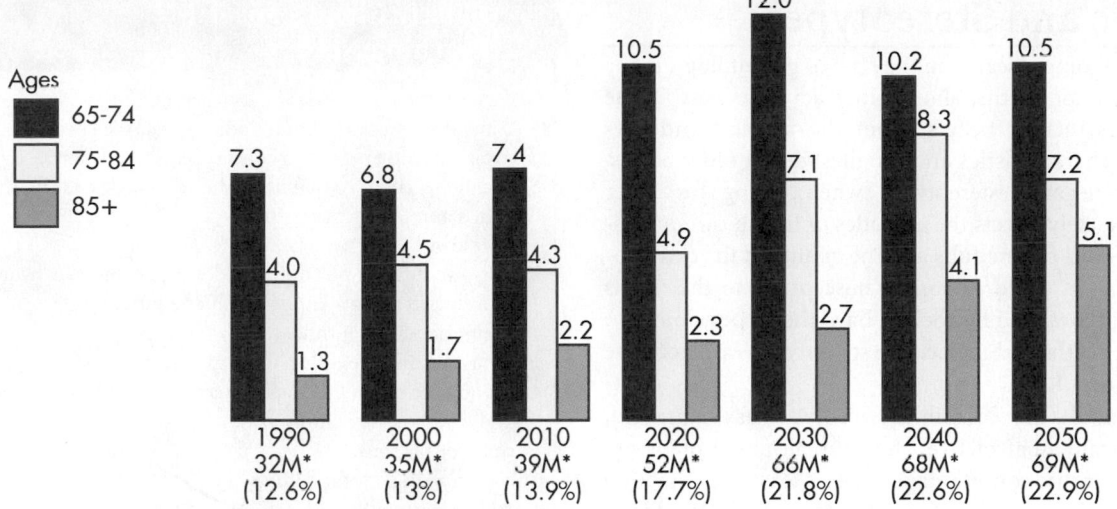

*Total number (in millions rounded off) of U.S. population over 65; below, percent of total population.

Figure 12-1   The coming surge in the numbers of elderly.
From American Association of Homes and Services for the Aging: States reach out to CCRC resident groups, *Provider News* 10(4):7, 1995.

ever, chronic disease does increase the older adult's vulnerability to functional decline (Guralnik, 1994). Therefore nursing assessment of physical and psychosocial function is important because it can provide valuable clues to the effect of a disease or illness on functional status.

Declining physiological function and increased prevalence of disease, especially in the oldest old, is due in part to a reduction in the ability to respond to stress through homeostatic mechanisms. The deficits in adaptability are most evident in neuroendocrine interaction, as well as in the separate responses of these two systems (Ebersole and Hess, 1998). The nurse should therefore assess older adults for the presence of stressors and their physical and emotional manifestations.

The established norms for diagnostic testing, pathological conditions, and growth and development in older people are constantly changing as more scientific studies are conducted. There is an ongoing debate about what constitutes normal in any of these areas (Abrams, Beers, and Berkow, 1995). However, most experts agree that older adults should be viewed and treated individually to compensate for the lack of definitive standards. The nurse can then compare the older person's own past patterns of health and function with present health status to determine the overall plan of care.

The classic signs and symptoms of diseases may be absent, blunted, or atypical in older adults (Lueckenotte, 1996a). This may be due to age-related changes in organ systems and homeostatic mechanisms, progressive loss of physiologic and functional reserves, or coexisting acute or chronic conditions (Emmett, 1998). As a result, the older adult with a urinary tract infection may present with con-

fusion, loss of appetite, weakness, dizziness, or fatigue instead of fever, dysuria, frequency, or urgency (Abrams, Beers, and Berkow, 1995). The older adult with pneumonia may have tachycardia, tachypnea, and confusion without the more common symptoms of fever and productive cough. Instead of substernal chest pain and diaphoresis, the older adult with a myocardial infarction may experience no pain, epigastric discomfort, referred pain, restlessness, hypotension, or confusion.

Terminology

As the number of older adults increases, the specialty of gerontological nursing is gaining importance. Several terms are used, at times interchangeably, to describe this specialty. Knowledge of the most frequently used terms and their definitions clarifies the differences and improves communication.

Geriatrics is the branch of medicine dealing with the physiological and psychological aspects of aging and with diagnosis and treatment of diseases affecting older adults. **Gerontology** is the study of all aspects of the aging process and its consequences. **Gerontological nursing** is concerned with assessment of the health and functional status of older adults; diagnosis, planning, and implementing health care and services to meet the identified needs; and evaluating the effectiveness of such care. This is the term most often used by nurses specializing in this field. **Gerontic nursing,** a seldom-used term, considers the nursing care of older adults to be the art and practice of nurturing, caring, and comforting rather than merely the treatment of disease (Lueckenotte, 1996b).

Myths and Stereotypes

Despite ongoing research in the field of gerontology, many false beliefs, or myths, about older adults persist. These stereotypes include beliefs about the physical and psychosocial characteristics and the lifestyles of older adults. Applying negative stereotypes when caring for older adults adversely affects the attitudes of health care professionals toward older adults and the quality of the care provided. Nurses, while personally susceptible to the myths and stereotypes held by society, have the responsibility to dispel the myths and replace the stereotypes with accurate information.

Older adults are sometimes stereotyped as ill, disabled, and physically unattractive. However, although many experience chronic conditions or have at least one disability that limits their performance of activities of daily living (ADLs), only 28% of older adults describe their health as poor or fair (AARP, 1997). Other common misconceptions hold that older adults are not interested in sex and that any interest in sexual activities is abnormal and should be discouraged. Yet older adults report continued enjoyment of sexual relationships.

Some people believe that older adults are forgetful, confused, rigid, bored, and unfriendly and that they are unable to understand and learn new information. Yet centenarians, the oldest of the old, are described as having an optimistic outlook on life, good memories, broad social contacts and interests, and tolerance for others (Ebersole and Hess, 1998). And although the process of learning may be affected by age-related changes in vision or hearing or by reduced energy and endurance, older adults are lifelong learners. The nurse should use teaching techniques that compensate for sensory changes, provide additional time for remembering and responding, and present concrete rather than abstract material to facilitate learning by older adults. Other effective teaching techniques draw on the older adult's past experiences and correspond to the identified interests of the older adult rather than to the content areas believed important by the health care professional. Box 12-1 presents additional teaching strategies that the nurse can use to address the special learning needs of older adults.

Stereotypes about lifestyles include mistaken notions about living arrangements and finances. Most older adults live in noninstitutional settings, either with family members or alone. Only 4% live in institutions such as nursing homes (AARP, 1997). Misconceptions about the financial status of older adults range from beliefs that many are affluent to beliefs that many are poor. According to the American Association of Retired Persons (1997), 10.8% of persons over age 65 have incomes below the poverty level with another 7.6% classified as near poor. However, the median net worth (assets minus liabilities) of older households was above the average for all households in the United States in 1995.

Elderly Client's Special Learning Needs   Box 12-1

Make sure the client is ready to learn before trying to teach. Watch for clues that would indicate that the client is preoccupied or too anxious to comprehend the material.

Sit facing the client so that he or she can watch your lip movements and facial expressions.

Speak slowly.

Keep your tone of voice low; elderly persons can hear low sounds better than high-frequency sounds.

Present one idea at a time.

Emphasize concrete rather than abstract material.

Give the client enough time in which to respond because elderly persons' reaction times are longer than those of younger persons.

Focus on a single topic to help the client concentrate.

Keep environmental distractions to a minimum.

Defer teaching if the client becomes distracted or tired or cannot concentrate for other reasons.

Invite another member of the household to join the discussion.

Use audio, visual, and tactile cues to enhance learning and help the client remember information.

Ask for feedback to ensure that the information has been understood.

Use past experience; connect new learning to that already learned.

Compensate for physical discomfort and sensory decrements.

Support a positive self-image in the learner.

Use creative teaching strategies.

Respond to identified interests of learners.

Emphasize and integrate emotional and personal values in the acquisition of skills and ideas.

Modified from Fielo S. Rizzolo M: Handle with caring: meeting elderly clients' special learning needs, *Nurs Health Care* 9(4):193, 1988.

In a society that values attractiveness, energy, and youth these myths and stereotypes lead to the undervaluing of older adults. Some people believe that older adults become worthless after they leave the workforce. Others consider the knowledge and experience of older adults to be too old-fashioned to have any current value. These notions underlie the concept of **ageism,** which is discrimination against people because of increasing age, just as people who are racists and sexists discriminate because of skin color and gender. Ageism, unopposed, has the potential to undermine the self-confidence of older adults, limit their access to care, and distort caregivers' understanding of the uniqueness of each older adult (Cutillo-Schmitter, 1996).

Today there are laws banning discrimination on the grounds of age. The economic and political power of older adults also acts against ageism. Older adults are a significant proportion of the consumer economy. As voters and activists in various issues, they influence the formation of public policy. Their participation adds a unique perspective on social, economic, and technological issues because they have experienced almost 100 years of developments. In the past 100 years, we have gone from riding in horse-drawn carriages to observing space shuttle flights. Gaslights and steam power have given way to electricity and nuclear power. Typewriters and carbon paper have been replaced by computers and copier machines. Older adults have lived through the Great Depression. Older adults have also experienced two world wars and wars in Korea, Vietnam, and the Persian Gulf. Older adults have seen changes in health care as the era of the family doctor gave way to the age of specialization. After witnessing the government initiatives that established the Social Security system, Medicare, and Medicaid, older adults are currently living with the changes imposed by health care reform. Having lived through all of these events and changes, older adults have stories and examples of coping with change to share.

Nurses' Attitudes Toward Older Adults

It is important for nurses to assess their attitudes toward older adults, their own aging, and the aging of their family, friends, and clients because these attitudes influence nursing care. Positive attitudes are based in part on a realistic portrayal of the characteristics and health care needs of older adults. In the past, negative attitudes about aging and older adults have contributed to the persistence of stereotypes of older adults as dependent and less attractive than younger clients. Nursing care, under the influence of these attitudes, has often ignored the opportunity to respect older adults and actively involve them in care decisions and activities. At times institutional settings such as hospitals and nursing homes have treated older adults as objects to be acted upon rather than independent, dignified adults. Involving older adults in decision making and in the definition of desired outcomes leads to greater client satisfaction with the quality of care. Individualized care, where the older adult takes priority over tasks, requires knowing the older adult, developing a relationship, encouraging the older adult to make choices about care, and facilitating the older adult's participation in care activities (Happ and others, 1996). Older adults expect their nurse-caregivers to be attentive, caring, and knowledgeable (Santo-Novak, 1997). Whether in acute care, institutional long-term care, or home care, listening to the concerns and priorities of the older adult leads to more realistic care planning and evaluation.

The attitude of the nurse toward older adults comes in part from personal experiences with older adults, education, employment experiences, and attitudes of co-workers and employing institutions. The nurse's own age, either as a factor contributing to the amount of experience or as a factor reflecting the nurse's own aging, also contributes to the nurse's attitude toward older adults. Given

Cultural ASPECTS OF CARE   Box 12-2

The racial and ethnic diversity of the older-adult population in the United States challenges nurses to be sensitive to the cultural aspects of care. Culture influences the values of a group and provides a framework for the beliefs, attitudes, and behaviors of individual members of a group. However, each individual embodies the values of a culture in unique ways. Each individual must be viewed as an individual, not a stereotypical member of a group.

Nurses working with individuals from ethnic groups other than their own must be sensitive to different beliefs about health, communication with health care providers, disease causation, disease treatment, response to symptoms, and family roles during illness. Culture also influences beliefs about aging; the roles, activities, and behaviors appropriate for older adults; and the response of younger adults and children to older adults.

The nurse must consider the older adult's culture while planning and delivering nursing care. The nurse's cultural sensitivity begins with consideration of her own culture's values. Then, as the nurse learns about other cultures, the nurse recognizes how the older adult's perspectives on health and illness are related to culture. Culture influences the role of the nurse and the role of the client. Culture influences the responses of the client to the nurse's questions about symptoms. Culture influences the acceptability of nursing interventions to the client. When the expectations of the nurse and the client about the style and content of health care differ, assessments may not represent the true situation of the client, interventions may be misdirected, and the health of the client may suffer.

the increasing number of older adults in health care settings, cultivation of positive attitudes toward older adults and knowledge about aging and the health care needs of older adults are priorities for nurses (Box 12-2).

Theories of Aging

Theorists have tried to describe the complex biopsychosocial process of aging. Although several theories have been developed, there is no single universally accepted theory that predicts and explains the complexities of the aging process. The nurse must be aware of the scientific attempts to explain the aging process and the concepts included in the theories. Although the theories are in various stages of development and have limitations, nurses can use them to increase understanding of the phenomena affecting the health and well-being of older adults.

BIOLOGICAL THEORIES

There are two types of biological theories of aging: **stochastic theories** and **nonstochastic theories** (Abrams, Beers, and Berkow, 1995). Stochastic theories consider that aging is caused by random damage that accumulates over time. Nonstochastic theories hold that the occurrence of aging changes are predetermined by mechanisms within the body.

Stochastic Theories.
The stochastic theories of biological aging propose that the physiological changes of the aging process are due to the accumulation of various types of cellular damage (Ebersole and Hess, 1998). In the free radical theory, damage from exposure to free radicals alters cell membrane structure and function. The principal source of free radicals, highly reactive molecules, is oxygen metabolism (Abrams, Beers, and Berkow, 1995). Current research is examining the role that antioxidant compounds such as vitamin E play in protecting cells from the damaging effects of free radicals. In the somatic mutation theory, the damage involves mutation of chromosomes after exposure to radiation or chemicals. In the wear-and-tear theory, damage from internal and external sources leads to the progressive failure of the body to repair itself.

Nonstochastic Theories.
Nonstochastic theories of aging assume that there is a physiological mechanism that controls the process of aging. The programmed aging theory proposes the existence of a biological clock that controls cell behavior and length of life span (Maddox, 1996). Aging follows an orderly path. In the pacemaker theory neurohormones regulate development and aging throughout the life span. Normally these regulators maintain the homeostatic balance of the body. Theorists suggest that changes in the neurohormonal controls account for such common features of aging as reproductive system changes, loss of muscle strength, reduced ability to respond to stress, and reduced ability to maintain homeostasis (Ebersole and Hess, 1998). The immunologic theory considers changes in the immune system responsible for some of the effects of aging.

PSYCHOSOCIAL THEORIES
Psychosocial theories of aging attempt to explain changes in behavior, roles, and relationships that occur as individuals age. As with biological theories of aging, there is no single theory that is universally accepted. The theories also reflect the values held by the theorist and society at the time the theory was first articulated. There are three classic psychosocial theories of aging: disengagement theory, activity theory, and continuity theory (Ebersole and Hess, 1998).

Disengagement Theory.
The disengagement theory of Cummings and Henry (1961) states that aging people withdraw from customary roles and engage in more introspective, self-focused activities. Older adults and their society mutually draw back from each other. After a period of transition during which roles in the workplace and the community change, the older adult is centered in self rather that in others or in the community. Aging is suc-

cessful to the degree that the older adult and society withdraw from each other. Although criticized by some for oversimplifying the aging process and by older adults for promoting withdrawal from society, the theory represented beliefs about aging that were held at that time. The theory is still valuable for the discussion it stimulates (Maddox, 1996).

Activity Theory.
Unlike the disengagement theory, the activity theory asserts that the continuation of activities performed during middle age is necessary for successful aging (Lemon, Bengston, and Peterson, 1972). When specific activities may not be continued because of circumstances unique to an individual, replacement of those activities chosen by the older adult is important. Socially active older people are more likely to adjust well to aging. Studies since then have shown that older adults with greater social involvement have higher morale and life satisfaction and more positive adjustment and mental health than those with less social involvement.

Critics, however, note that aging is too complex to be characterized in such a simple manner. They argue that this theory assumes that older adults have the same needs as middle-age persons. In addition, this theory does not address the impact of biological changes or the presence of multiple losses on the ability of older people to continue to replace activities. The general consensus of the critics is that many other variables affect responses to aging, which this theory does not adequately explain.

Continuity Theory.
The continuity or developmental theory (Neugarten, 1964) states that personality remains the same and behavior becomes more predictable as people age. Personality and behavior patterns developed during a lifetime determine the degree of engagement and activity in older adulthood. According to this theory, personality is a critical factor in determining the relationship between role activity and life satisfaction. This psychosocial theory is viewed by some as a promising one because it addresses the complexities of the aging process and people's adaptive ability. Critics argue that it too is simplistic and does not consider the many factors that affect one's response to the aging process.

Developmental Tasks for Older Adults

Theories of aging are closely linked to the concept of developmental tasks appropriate for distinct stages of life. Although no two individuals age in the same way, either biologically or psychosocially, frameworks outlining tasks appropriate developmentally for older adults have been developed. Seven developmental tasks for older adults are listed in Box 12-3.

Developmental Tasks of the
Older Adult   Box 12-3

Adjusting to decreasing health and physical strength
Adjusting to retirement and reduced or fixed income
Adjusting to death of a spouse
Accepting self as aging person
Maintaining satisfactory living arrangements
Redefining relationships with adult children
Finding ways to maintain quality of life

Older adults face the necessity of adjustment to the physical changes that accompany aging. The extent and timing of these changes vary from individual to individual, but as body systems age, changes in appearance and functioning occur. These changes are not associated with a disease but are normal changes. The presence of disease may alter the timing of the changes or their impact on daily life. Structural and functional changes associated with aging are described in the section on physiological development.

Some older adults find it difficult to accept themselves as aging. This is seen in benign behaviors as some older adults, both men and women, understate their ages when asked, adopt younger styles of clothing, or attempt to conceal physical evidence of aging with cosmetics. But other older adults deny their own aging in ways that are potentially problematic. For example, some older adults may deny functional declines and refuse to ask for assistance with tasks that place their safety at great risk. Others avoid activities designed to benefit older adults, such as senior citizen centers and senior health promotion activities, and thus do not receive these benefits. Acceptance of personal aging does not mean retirement into inactivity, but it does require a realistic review of strengths and limitations.

Older adults retired from employment outside the home are challenged to cope with the loss of that work role. Older adults who worked at home and the spouses of those who worked outside the home also face role changes as they age. Because retirement is usually anticipated, persons can plan ahead to make financial plans and to consider replacement activities. Many older adults welcome retirement as a time to pursue new interests and hobbies, to participate in volunteer activities, to continue their education, or to start a new business career. Retirement plans for some older adults include changes of residence such as moving to a different city or state or moving to a different type of housing within the same area.

Reasons other than retirement may also lead to changes of residence. For example, physical impairments may require relocation to a smaller, single-level home. Severe health problems may require the older adult to live with relatives or friends. A change in living arrangements for the older adult may require an extended period of adjust-

ment during which assistance and support from health care professionals, friends, and family members are needed.

The majority of older adults are faced with the deaths of spouses. In 1995 almost half (47%) of all older women were widows (AARP, 1997). Some older adults must cope with the death of adult children and grandchildren. All experience the deaths of friends. These deaths represent both losses and reminders of personal mortality. Coming to terms with these deaths is often difficult. By assisting older adults through the grieving process, the nurse can help them resolve the issues posed by these deaths.

The redefining of relationships with children that occurred as those children grew up and left home continues as older adults experience the challenges of aging. A variety of issues may arise, including, but not limited to, role reversal, control of decision making, dependence, conflict, guilt, and loss. How these issues surface in situations and how they are resolved depends in part on the past relationship between the older adult and the adult children. All the involved parties bring past experiences and powerful emotions to the table. When adult children assist the older adults of their family, they must find ways to balance the demands of their own children and their careers. Adult children also debate how much assistance to provide and how much decision-making authority to assume. As adult children and aging parents negotiate the parameters of the changed roles, nurses may act as counselors to both the parents and the children. Nurses can assist adult children by listening and by helping them distinguish between changes and behaviors related to illness, normal aging changes, and their parents' lifelong preferences and patterns of behavior.

In the face of the changes that come with aging, older adults must find ways to maintain their quality of life. What defines quality of life varies from person to person (Figure 12-2). Nurses must listen to what the older adult considers to be most important rather than making assumptions about that individual's priorities. Together the nurse and the older adult may set objectives that lead to the maintenance of quality of life. Whether it is defined as maintenance of social relationships, continuing to live alone, or continuing activities such as driving or gardening, older adults look to the nurse for assistance.

These developmental tasks are common to most older adults. Many of these tasks are associated with losses experienced in varying degrees by older adults. The more common losses are of health, significant others, a sense of being useful, socialization, income, and independent living. The way that older adults adjust to the changes of aging depends on the individual. For some, adaptation and adjustment are relatively easy. For others, coping with aging changes may require the assistance of family, friends, and health care professionals. The nurse must be sensitive to the effect of such losses on older adults and their families and be prepared to offer support.

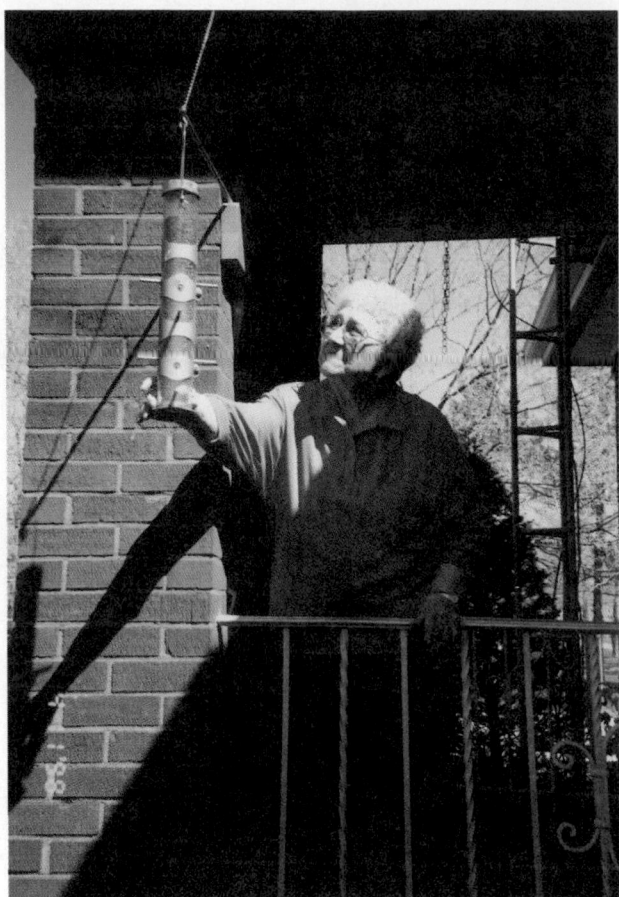

Figure 12-2   Older adults achieve a quality of life through participation in a variety of activities.

Community-Based and Institutional Health Care Services

General health care services are described in Chapter 2. However, five types of community-based and institutional health care services are used by older adults.

RETIREMENT COMMUNITIES

Retirement communities offer alternatives to living in a single-family dwelling or apartment. The communities have apartment-style units with design features that support the independence of older adults and supportive services. Residents may choose among services such as meals, housekeeping, transportation, emergency response systems, and planned social activities. Physical fitness activities and other health-promoting activities may also be provided.

HOME CARE

Home health care and homemaker services prevent or delay institutionalization for older adults who need assistance with daily living. Care is provided by professional nurses and therapists or nonprofessional staff, such as homemaker aides.

ADULT DAY CARE

Adult day care offers health and rehabilitative services for the older adult and respite from caregiving activities to family caregivers. Clients of day care centers are usually not seriously ill, although they may have chronic conditions, disabilities, or cognitive impairments that limit independence.

RESPITE CARE

Respite care is temporary relief for the primary caregiver of a dependent older adult. Service is provided in the home or in an institution. Respite care enables the caregiver to be away from home for a few hours or, when residential institutions are utilized, away from home for several days or weeks.

LONG-TERM CARE

Declining health, decreased physical strength, cognitive impairment, increased dependence, and fewer caregiver resources may make it necessary for an older adult to move to a long-term care facility. Licensed long-term care facilities include assisted living facilities (also called residential care facilities or board-and-care homes) and several types of nursing homes.

Assisted living facilities provide relatively independent older adults with supervision, assistance, and limited health care services in a homelike setting. The amount of assistance provided is less than that available in a nursing home, and residents are usually given some options in the type of service or the amount of assistance received. Residents may maintain their own activities and social engagements or attend the activities scheduled by the facility. Assisted living facilities are an alternative to nursing home placement for some frail older adults when living alone at home is no longer feasible.

Nursing homes provide personal care assistance, professional nursing services, supervision of prescribed medical care, rehabilitation services, and psychosocial services. The probability of entering a nursing home for at least a brief stay increases with age. Nursing home residents may be classified into two groups according to length of stay: short-term and long-term residents.

The subacute care industry and managed care are market forces that have changed the face of the traditional nursing home population by increasing the number of short-term residents. Short-term residents are usually admitted to the nursing home directly from the hospital and seek skilled nursing care and rehabilitation services. Their goals include discharge from the nursing home to their own home, a family caregiver's home, or an assisted living facility. Long-term residents reside in nursing homes for longer than 6 months. Long-term residents include older adults who are very frail, whose medical conditions are unstable or complex, and who lack the financial resources or caregivers necessary for intensive 24-hour-per-day home care. They are often older and may have greater cognitive deficits and functional impairments than the nursing home residents who return home after a brief stay.

The decision to move to a nursing home as a long-term resident is not easily made. Family caregivers may consider nursing home placement when in-home care becomes increasingly difficult for family caregivers (Chenier, 1997). The decision to enter a nursing home should come only after the older adult and the family have considered the full range of long-term care choices. Although that decision is never final and once admitted to a nursing home a resident may be discharged to home or to another facility, many older adults view the nursing home as their final residence. During the decision-making period, the actual move to the nursing home, and the time after admission, the nurse's role is to support the older adult and the family and to provide information about the selection of a good nursing home.

Table 12-1	Techniques for Assessing Older Adults With Sensory Problems
Sensory Alteration	**Assessment Technique**
Visual disturbance	Position self in full view of client
	Provide diffuse, bright light; avoid glare
	Make sure client's glasses are worn and in good working order
	Face client when speaking; do not cover mouth
Hearing deficit	Speak directly to client in clear, low tones at a moderate rate; do not cover mouth
	Articulate consonants with special care
	Restate if client does not understand question initially
	Speak toward "good" ear
	Reduce background noises
	Make sure client's hearing aid is worn and is working properly

Assessing the Needs of Older Adults

Gerontological nursing offers creative approaches for maximizing the potential of older adults. With comprehensive assessment information regarding the older adults's strengths, resources, and limitations, the nurse and the older adult identify needs and problems and select interventions that maintain the older adult's physical abilities and create an environment for psychosocial and spiritual well-being. A thorough assessment requires the nurse to actively engage the older adult and provide the older adult enough time to share important information about his or her health. The nurse assesses for changes in physiological development, cognition, and psychosocial behavior.

Obtaining a comprehensive assessment of an older adult may take more time than the assessment of a younger adult because of the longer life and medical history and the potential complexity of that history. By planning to spend extra time with the assessment, the nurse and the older adult are less likely to feel rushed. During the assessment process, the nurse may find it necessary to allow rest periods or to conduct the assessment in several sessions because of the reduced energy and limited endurance experienced by some frail older adults.

Sensory changes may also affect data gathering. The nurse's choices of communication techniques will be influenced by any visual or hearing impairments experienced by the older adult. If older adults are unable to un-

derstand the nurse's visual or auditory cues, assessment data may be inaccurate or misleading. For example, if older adults have difficulty hearing the nurse's questions, inappropriate responses may lead the nurse to believe that they are confused. Table 12-1 suggests techniques to be used during the assessment of older adults with sensory problems.

Memory deficits will affect the accuracy and completeness of the data collected. Information contributed by a family member or other caregiver may be necessary to supplement the older adult's recollection of past medical events and information such as allergies and immunizations. Tact must be used when involving another person in the assessment interview with the older adult. The additional person supplements the answers of the older adult with the consent of the older adult, but the older adult remains the focus of the interview.

PHYSIOLOGICAL CHANGES
Perception of well-being can define quality of life. Understanding the older adult's perceptions about health status is essential for accurate assessment and development of clinically relevant interventions. Older adults' concepts of health generally depend on personal perceptions of functional ability. Therefore older adults engaged in activities of daily living usually consider themselves healthy, whereas those whose activities are limited by physical, emotional, or social impairments may perceive themselves as ill.

There are normal physiological changes anticipated in

Table 12-2 Normal Physiological Changes of Aging

System	Normal Findings
Integument	
Skin color	Spotty pigmentation in areas exposed to the sun; pallor even in absence of anemia
Moisture	Dry, scaly condition
Temperature	Cooler extremities; decreased perspiration
Texture	Decreased elasticity; wrinkles; folding, sagging condition
Fat distribution	Decreased amount on extremities; increased amount on abdomen
Hair	Thinning and graying on scalp; often, decreased amount of axillary and pubic hair and hair on extremities; decreased facial hair in men; possible chin and upper lip hair in women
Nails	Decreased growth rate
Head and neck	
Head	Sharp and angular nasal and facial bones; loss of eyebrow hair in women; bushier eyebrows in men
Eyes	Decreased visual acuity; decreased accommodation; reduced adaptation to darkness; sensitivity to glare
Ears	Decreased pitch discrimination; diminished light reflex; diminished hearing acuity
Nose and sinuses	Increased nasal hair; decreased sense of smell
Mouth and pharynx	Use of bridges or dentures; decreased sense of taste; atrophy of papillae of lateral edges of tongue
Neck	Nodular thyroid gland; slight tracheal deviation resulting from muscle atrophy
Thorax and lungs	Increased anteroposterior diameter; increased chest rigidity; increased respiratory rate with decreased lung expansion; increased airway resistance
Heart and vascular system	Significant increase in systolic pressure with slight increase in diastolic pressure; usually insignificant changes in heart rate at rest; common diastolic murmurs; easily palpated peripheral pulses; weaker pedal pulses and colder lower extremities, especially at night
Breasts	Diminished breast tissue; pendulous, flabby condition
Gastrointestinal system	Decreased salivary secretions, which may make swallowing more difficult; decreased peristalsis; decreased production of digestive enzymes, including hydrochloric acid, pepsin, and pancreatic enzymes; constipation; reduced motility
Reproductive system	
Female	Decreased estrogen; decreased uterine size; decreased secretions; atrophy of epithelial lining of vagina
Male	Decreased levels of testosterone; decreased sperm count; decreased testicular size
Urinary system	Decreased renal filtration and renal efficiency; subsequent loss of protein from kidney; nocturia; decreased bladder capacity; increased incontinence
Female	Urgency and stress incontinence resulting from decrease in perineal muscle tone
Male	Urinary frequency and retention resulting from prostatic enlargement
Musculoskeletal system	Decreased muscle mass and strength; bone demineralization (more pronounced in women); shortening of trunk as result of intervertebral space narrowing; decreased joint mobility; decreased range of joint motion; enhanced bony prominences
Neurological system	Decreased rate of voluntary or automatic reflexes; decreased ability to respond to multiple stimuli; insomnia; shorter sleeping periods

Data from Ebersole P, Hess P: *Toward healthy aging: human needs and nursing response,* ed 5, St. Louis, 1998, Mosby.

older adults (Table 12-2). These physiological changes are not pathological processes but may render older adults vulnerable to some common clinical conditions. Some older adults experience all of these changes, and others experience only a few. The body changes continuously with age, but the effects on particular older adults depend on health, lifestyle, stressors, and environmental conditions. The nurse should know about these normal changes to provide appropriate care for older adults and to assist them in adapting to the changes.

General Survey.   The general survey begins during the initial nurse-client encounter and includes a quick, but

careful, head-to-toe scan of the older adult that could be written as a concise description. An initial inspection of an older adult might reveal eye contact and facial expression appropriate to the situation, facial wrinkles, gray hair, loss of body mass in the extremities, and an increase of body mass on the trunk.

Integumentary System.   The skin loses resilience and moisture in older adulthood. The epithelial layer thins, and elastic collagen fibers shrink and become rigid. Wrinkles of the face and neck reflect lifelong patterns of muscle activity and facial expressions, the pull of gravity on tissue, and diminished elasticity.

Spots and lesions may also be present on the skin. Smooth, brown, irregularly shaped spots (age spots, or senile lentigo) initially appear on the backs of the hands and on forearms. Small, round, red or brown cherry angiomas may be found on the trunk. Seborrheic lesions or keratoses may appear as irregular, round or oval, brown, watery lesions. Years of sun-exposure contribute to the aging of the skin and may lead to premalignant and malignant lesions. Examination of skin lesions must rule out three malignancies related to solar exposure: melanoma, basal cell carcinoma, and squamous cell carcinoma (Abrams, Beers, and Berkow, 1995).

Pressure ulcers are a particular risk for frail older adults who have many of the factors that lead to their development (see Chapter 47). Multiple factors play a role in pressure ulcer formation, including reduced mobility, inactivity, diminished sensory perception, excessive moisture on skin surfaces or in skin folds, friction and shearing factors, loss of subcutaneous fat over bony prominences, poor nutrition, and arteriolar pressure (Maklebust, 1997).

Head and Neck.   The facial features of the older adult become more pronounced from loss of subcutaneous fat and skin elasticity. Facial features may appear asymmetrical because of missing teeth or improperly fitting dentures. In addition, common vocal changes include a rise in pitch and a loss of power and range.

The older adult's visual acuity declines. This may be the result of retinal damage, reduced pupil size, development of opacities in the lens, or loss of lens elasticity. **Presbyopia,** a progressive decline in the ability of the eyes to accommodate for close, detailed work, is common. There is a reduced ability to see in darkness and to adapt to abrupt changes from dark areas to light areas (and the reverse). Older adults also have increased sensitivity to the effects of glare. Changes in color vision and discoloration of the lens make it difficult to distinguish between blues and greens and among pastel shades.

Auditory changes are often subtle. The earliest losses of hearing acuity may be ignored until compensatory attempts such as turning up the volume on televisions and radios are commented on by friends and family members. A common age-related change in auditory acuity is called **presbycusis.** Presbycusis affects the ability to hear high-pitched sounds and sibilant consonants such as *s, sh,* and *ch.* Before assuming presbycusis, inspect the external auditory canal for the presence of cerumen. Impacted cerumen is an easily treated cause of diminished hearing acuity.

Taste buds atrophy and lose sensitivity. The older adult is less able to discern among salty, sweet, sour, and bitter tastes. The sense of smell is also decreased, further reducing taste. Salivary secretion is reduced.

Thorax and Lungs.   Because of changes in the musculoskeletal system, the configuration of the thorax sometimes changes. After age 55 respiratory muscle strength begins to decrease (Abrams, Beers, and Berkow, 1995). The anteroposterior diameter of the thorax increases. Vertebral changes due to osteoporosis lead to dorsal kyphosis, the curvature of the thoracic spine sometimes called "dowager's hump" because of the increased incidence in older women. Calcification of the costal cartilage can cause decreased mobility of the ribs. The chest wall gradually becomes stiffer. Lung expansion decreases. If kyphosis or chronic obstructive lung disease is present, breath sounds are distant.

Heart and Vascular System.   Decreased contractile strength of the myocardium results in a decreased cardiac output. The decrease is significant when the older adult is stressed by anxiety, excitement, illness, or strenuous activity. The body tries to compensate for decreased cardiac output by increasing the heart rate during exercise. However, after exercise, it takes longer for the older adult's rate to return to baseline.

Systolic and/or diastolic blood pressures may be abnormally elevated. More than 50% of older adults have systolic or diastolic hypertension. Although common, hypertension is not a normal aging change and predisposes an older adult to heart failure, stroke, renal failure, coronary heart disease, and peripheral vascular disease (Abrams, Beers, and Berkow, 1995).

Peripheral pulses are frequently weaker, although still palpable, in the lower extremities than in the upper extremities. Older adults may complain that their lower extremities are cold, particularly at night.

Breasts.   Decreased muscle mass, tone, and elasticity result in smaller breasts in older women. In addition, the breasts sag. Atrophy of glandular tissue, coupled with more fat deposits, results in a slightly smaller, less dense, and less nodular breast. Gynecomastia, enlarged breasts in men, may be due to medication side effects, hormonal changes, or obesity. Both older men and women are at risk of breast cancer development.

Gastrointestinal System and Abdomen.   Aging leads to an increase in the amount of fatty tissue in the trunk. As a result, the abdomen increases in size. Because muscle tone and elasticity decrease, it also becomes more protuberant. Gastrointestinal function changes include a slowing of peristalsis and alterations in secretions. The older adult may experience these changes as the development of intolerance to certain foods and discomfort due to delayed gastric emptying. Alterations in the lower gastrointestinal tract may lead to constipation, flatulence, or diarrhea.

Reproductive System.   Changes in the structure and function of the reproductive system occur as the result of hormonal alterations. Female menopause is related to a reduced responsiveness of the ovaries to pituitary hormones and a resultant decrease in estrogen and progesterone levels. In men, there is no definite cessation of fertility associated with aging. Spermatogenesis begins to decline during the fourth decade but continues into the ninth. The changes in reproductive structure and function, however, do not affect libido. Less frequent sexual activity can result from illness, death of a sexual partner, decreased socialization, or loss of sexual interest.

Urinary System.
Hypertrophy of the prostate gland may develop in older men. This hypertrophy enlarges the gland, and pressure is displaced to the neck of the bladder. As a result, urinary retention, frequency, incontinence, and urinary tract infections occur. In addition, prostatic hypertrophy can result in difficulty initiating voiding and maintaining a urinary stream. Cancer of the prostate is the second most common cause of cancer death in men. Although over 50% of men over age 70 have evidence of prostate cancer on biopsy of prostate tissue, most of these cancers are asymptomatic and less than 3% of the men with this evidence will die of prostatic cancer (Abrams, Beers, and Berkow, 1995).

Older women, particularly those who have had children, can experience stress incontinence, in which an involuntary release of urine occurs when they cough, sneeze, or lift an object. This is a result of a weakening of the perineal and bladder muscles. Other types of urinary incontinence are urge, overflow, functional, and mixed incontinence. The risk factors for urinary incontinence include age, menopause, diabetes, hysterectomy, stroke, and obesity. Although for women over age 60 the estimates of prevalence of any urine loss is 40% and of daily incontinence 7% to 17%, urinary incontinence is an abnormal condition in older women (Luft and Vriheas-Nichols, 1998).

Musculoskeletal System.
With aging, muscle fibers are reduced in size. Muscle strength diminishes in proportion to the decline in muscle mass. Bone mass also declines. Older adults who exercise regularly do not lose as much bone and muscle mass or muscle tone as those who are inactive. Postmenopausal women have a greater rate of bone demineralization than older men although osteoporosis is also a problem for older men (Kessenich and Rosen, 1996). Women who maintain calcium intake throughout life and into menopause have less bone demineralization than those who do not. Older men with poor nutrition and decreased mobility are also at risk for bone demineralization.

Neurological System.
The number of neurons in the nervous system begins to decrease in the middle of the second decade, which can lead to functional changes. The changes can affect the special senses described earlier. In addition, the older adult may experience a decreased sense of balance or uncoordinated motor responses.

Age-Related Sleep Changes	Box 12-4

Total sleep time decreases until age 80, then increases slightly.
Time in bed increases after age 65.
Onset to sleep is lengthened (>30 minutes in about 32% of women and 15% of men).
Awakenings are frequent, increasing after age 50 (>30 minutes of wakefulness after sleep onset in over 50% of older subjects).
Naps are more common, although only about 10% report daily napping.
Sleep is subjectively and objectively lighter (more stage I, less stage IV, more disruptions).
Frequency of abnormal breathing events is increased.
Frequency of leg movements during sleep is increased.

From Ebersole P, Hess P: *Toward healthy aging: human needs and nursing response,* ed 5, St. Louis, 1998, Mosby.

Alterations in the quality and the quantity of sleep are frequently reported by older adults (see Chapter 41). Reports include difficulty falling asleep, difficulty staying asleep, difficulty falling asleep again after waking during the night, waking too early in the morning, and excessive daytime napping. Age-related sleep changes are summarized in Box 12-4.

COGNITIVE CHANGES
A common misconception about aging is that cognitive impairments are widespread among older adults. Because of this misconception, older adults fear that they are, or soon will be, cognitively impaired and younger adults assume that older adults are confused and no longer able to handle their affairs. Disorientation, loss of language skills, loss of the ability to calculate, and poor judgment are not normal aging changes (Eliopoulos, 1998). Structural and physiological changes within the brain, such as reduction in the number of cells, deposition of lipofuscin and amyloid in cells, and change in neurotransmitter levels, are seen in older adults with cognitive impairment and without cognitive impairment.

Three common conditions affecting cognition are **delirium, dementia,** and **depression.** Distinguishing between these three conditions is challenging, but essential (Foreman and others, 1996). Table 12-3 compares the clinical features of delirium, dementia, and depression. To select appropriate nursing interventions, the nurse should be able to distinguish among these three conditions. Appropriate nursing interventions are specific to the cause of the cognitive impairment. The use of techniques such as reality orientation, validation therapy, and reminiscence also depends on the nature of the cognitive impairment.

Delirium.
Delirium, or acute confusional state, is a potentially reversible cognitive impairment that is often due to a physiological cause. Delirium may also be due to environmental factors such as sensory deprivation or unfa-

Table 12-3 A Comparison of the Clinical Features of Delirium, Dementia, and Depression

Clinical Feature	Delirium	Dementia	Depression
Onset	Acute/subacute, depends on cause, often at twilight or in darkness	Chronic, generally insidious, depends on cause	Coincides with major life changes, often abrupt
Course	Short, diurnal fluctuations in symptoms, worse at night, in darkness, and on awakening	Long, no diurnal effects, symptoms progressive yet relatively stable over time	Diurnal effects, typically worse in the morning, situational fluctuations, but less than with delirium
Progression	Abrupt	Slow but uneven	Variable, rapid or slow but even
Duration	Hours to less than 1 month, seldom longer	Months to years	At least 6 weeks, can be several months to years
Awareness	Reduced	Clear	Clear
Alertness	Fluctuates, lethargic or hypervigilant	Generally normal	Normal
Attention	Impaired, fluctuates	Generally normal	Minimal impairment, but is easily distracted
Orientation	Generally impaired, severity varies	Generally normal	Selective disorientation
Memory	Recent and immediate impaired	Recent and remote impaired	Selective or "patchy" impairment, "islands" of intact memory
Thinking	Disorganized, distorted, fragmented, incoherent speech, either slow or accelerated	Difficulty with abstraction, thoughts impoverished, judgment impaired, words difficult to find	Intact but with themes of hopelessness, helplessness, or self-deprecation
Perception	Distorted, illusions, delusions, and hallucinations, difficulty distinguishing between reality and misperceptions	Misperceptions usually absent	Intact, delusions and hallucinations absent except in severe cases
Psychomotor behavior	Variable, hypokinetic, hyperkinetic, and mixed	Normal, may have apraxia	Variable, psychomotor retardation or agitation
Sleep/wake cycle	Disturbed, cycle reversed	Fragmented	Disturbed, usually early morning awakening
Associated features	Variable affective changes, symptoms of autonomic hyperarousal, exaggeration of personality type, associated with acute physical illness	Affect tends to be superficial, inappropriate and labile, attempts to conceal deficits in intellect, personality changes, aphasia, agnosia may be present, lacks insight	Affect depressed, dysphoric mood, exaggerated and detailed complaints, preoccupied with personal thoughts, insight present, verbal elaboration
Assessment	Distracted from task, numerous errors	Failings highlighted by family, frequent "near miss" answers, struggles with test, great effort to find an appropriate reply, frequent requests for feedback on performance	Failings highlighted by individual, frequently answers "don't know," little effort, frequently gives up, indifferent toward test, does not care or attempt to find answer

Data from Foreman: A comparison of the clinical features of delirium, dementia, and depression, *Geriatr Nurs* 17(5):229, 1996.

miliar surroundings or psychosocial factors such as emotional distress or pain. Although delirium may occur in any setting, an older adult in the acute care setting is especially at risk because of predisposing factors (psychological, environmental, psychosocial) in combination with the medical condition that led to the hospital admission.

The physiological causes of delirium can be metabolic, structural, or infectious (Abrams, Beers, and Berkow, 1995). The metabolic causes include conditions such as electrolyte imbalances, chronic endocrine abnormalities, anoxia or transient ischemia, hypoglycemia, postictal and postconcussion states, and drug effects. Structural causes include space-occupying lesions such as primary or metastatic brain tumors, subdural hematomas, and brain hemorrhages and cerebrovascular conditions such as vascular occlusion, cerebral infarction, subarachnoid hemorrhage, and cerebral hemorrhage. Delirium in older adults is sometimes seen with infection, including pneumonia and urinary tract infections.

Delirium is characterized by fluctuations in cognition, mood, attention, arousal, and self-awareness (Abrams, Beers, and Berkow, 1995). Other features include illusions, hallucinations, occasional incoherent speech, disturbed sleep-wake cycle, and disorientation. The onset of delirium is typically sudden, and there are rapid fluctuations in symptoms and severity. The presence of delirium requires prompt assessment and intervention. The cognitive impairment secondary to delirium is usually reversed once the cause of delirium is identified and treatment started unless there has been permanent damage to the brain. Being potentially reversible is one of the characteristics differentiating delirium from dementia.

Dementia.   Dementia is a generalized impairment of intellectual functioning that interferes with social and occupational functioning. Cognitive function deterioration leads to a decline in the ability to perform basic and instrumental activities of daily living. Unlike delirium, dementia is characterized by a gradual, progressive, irreversible cerebral dysfunction. Because of the close resemblance between delirium and dementia, the presence of delirium must be ruled out whenever dementia is suspected.

The most common form of dementia is **Alzheimer's disease,** named after Dr. Alois Alzheimer, who published the first description. Alzheimer's disease, also called senile dementia of the Alzheimer type (SDAT) or dementia of the Alzheimer type (DAT), is characterized by brain atrophy and the development of senile plaques and neurofibrillary tangles in the cerebral hemispheres. The cause of the disease is not known, and although several theories are being studied, none are definitive.

Symptoms that may indicate Alzheimer's disease include difficulty learning and retaining new information and difficulty handling complex tasks that require completion of a series of steps (Agency for Health Care Policy and Research [AHCPR], 1996). When reasoning ability is affected, the ability to develop a suitable response to a problem is impaired. Changes in the ability to be oriented in space may make driving a car hazardous or finding the way home from familiar locations difficult. Language skill may be affected, leading to difficulty finding the correct words in conversation or in writing. Behavioral symptoms vary widely. Some individuals with Alzheimer's disease appear more passive and less responsive whereas others exhibit behaviors that are exaggerated forms of earlier behavior styles. Early recognition of Alzheimer's disease is important because medications are available that offer some hope for slowing the progression of the disease.

The progression of Alzheimer's disease has been divided into three stages (Filley, 1995). However, the progression of the disease in each individual with Alzheimer's disease is unique to that person and may not closely follow the stages as outlined. In the early stage the primary symptom is memory loss. In addition to short-term memory loss, the older adult may have difficulty concentrating, loss of interest in usual activities, and disorientation to time. Clinical signs of depression may be present. The earliest symptoms of Alzheimer's disease may be very subtle and may be dismissed by the older adult's family as insignificant. The older adult may attempt to conceal the effects of memory loss, to compensate for them, or to deny them.

Because the older adult in the middle stage of Alzheimer's disease is less able to remember the cues that lead to understanding the environment, confusion increases. Communication skills, both verbal and written, are lost. The older adult is disoriented to place and time and may be unable to follow simple instructions. Safety becomes a concern, and the older adult needs almost constant supervision. Wandering behaviors, inside and outside the home, are common. Nocturnal wandering may occur as sleep patterns change. Behavior related to dressing, bathing, grooming, eating, and toileting may change. Episodes of incontinence may occur. Supervision and assistance with these activities of daily living is necessary.

In the final stage of Alzheimer's disease long-term memory, as well as short-term memory, is affected. Personal identity seems to be lost. Family members may not be recognized. More and more help is needed with all activities of daily living until the older adult is completely dependent on a caregiver. Mobility decreases until bed rest is required. In spite of a good diet including supplements and assistance with eating, the older adult loses weight. Immobility, incontinence, and weight loss lead to skin breakdown. Resistance to infection decreases.

Another common form of dementia is **vascular dementia,** which is also called multiinfarct dementia. Vascular dementia results from interruptions in blood flow to the brain as in cerebrovascular disease or anoxia secondary to cardiac arrest (Robinson, 1998). The onset of vascular dementia is usually sudden, although the diagnosis may not be made until the cumulative effect of a series of small vascular events becomes clinically apparent.

Although older adults with this form of dementia may display symptoms similar to dementia of the Alzheimer's type, vascular dementia is distinguished by periods of remission, preservation of personality, insight, and lability of emotion.

Other forms of dementia include the dementias that occur in some individuals with Parkinson's disease, acquired immunodeficiency syndrome (AIDS), and Huntington's chorea (Robinson, 1998). Dementia may also follow head injury, as with dementia pugilistica, in which the injuries are sustained in the sport of boxing.

Nursing management of older adults with any form of dementia is complex. Interventions must consider the needs of the older adult with dementia and the needs of the family. Those needs change as the progressive nature of dementia leads to increased cognitive deterioration. In addition to the physical needs of the older adult, safety needs and psychosocial needs must be considered. The older adult's family needs information and support. Understanding of the stages of dementia and of strategies to address situations common to the stages will decrease the stress of the family caregivers. Meeting the needs of the older adult related to dementia is made more complex by preexisting acute and chronic physical conditions, sensory impairments, depression, and environmental stressors. Environmental stressors include unfamiliar environments, such as hospitals, and conditions within any environment, such as glare, excessive noise, hurried activities, and unfamiliar persons. Environmental stressors are poorly understood by the older adult with dementia. These misunderstandings lead to increased confusion and agitation. Misunderstanding the environment and feeling threatened, the older adult may respond with aggressive gestures or acts, increased voice volume, restlessness, and hostility. Acute agitation may also be due to side effects of medications, infection, pain, urinary retention, or fecal impaction (Lehninger, Ravindran, and Stewart, 1998). To meet the needs of the older adult with dementia, nursing care objectives are individualized and promote the use of remaining functional abilities.

Depression.   Delirium and depression, both reversible disorders, are often mistaken for irreversible dementia in the older adult because cerebral dysfunction and cognitive impairment occur with these conditions, as well as with dementia. Consequently, older adults with such disorders may not be appropriately assessed and treated, and a reversible disorder may become irreversible.

Late-life depression may be experienced by 20% of older adults (Butler and Lewis, 1995). Depression reduces happiness and well-being, contributes to physical and social limitations, complicates the treatment of concomitant medical conditions, and increases the risk of suicide. From 20% to 25% of older adults with dementia of the Alzheimer's type also experience depression (Butler and Lewis, 1995; Tueth, 1995). When dementia and depression

occur together, the distress of the older adult and the family is increased.

Cognitive Impairment Related to Alcohol Abuse.
It is estimated that up to 15% of community-dwelling older adults are heavy drinkers (Gambert, 1997). Studies of alcohol abuse in older adults report two patterns: a lifelong pattern of heavy drinking that continues and a late-onset pattern when heavy drinking begins late in life. Frequently cited causes of excessive alcohol use are depression, loneliness, and lack of social support.

In addition to its physiological effects, alcohol abuse can affect cognitive functioning. Normal physiological changes that occur with aging increase the susceptibility of older adults to the effects of alcohol (Gambert, 1997). A greater proportion of alcohol is delivered to the brain because of changes in the distribution of body fluids and the proportion of body fat to muscle. The ratio of alcohol to brain cell increases and even moderate alcohol intake can lead to cognitive impairment. Other effects of alcohol ingestion that may compound cognitive impairment include hypothermia, hypoglycemia, and electrolyte imbalance. When the abuse of alcohol has been long-term, there may be cerebral, cerebellar, sensory, and peripheral nervous system damage.

Abuse of alcohol may be underidentified in older adults. The clues to create suspicion of alcohol abuse are subtle, and the assessment may be complicated by coexisting dementia or depression. Suspicion of alcohol abuse increases when there is a history of repeated falls and accidents, a change in behavior or personality, social isolation, recurring episodes of memory loss and confusion, a history of skipping meals or medications, and difficulty managing household tasks and finances (Zimberg, 1996). When abuse of alcohol is suspected, treatment includes age-specific approaches that acknowledge the stresses experienced by the older adult and encourage involvement in activities that match the older adult's interests and boost feelings of self-worth. The identification and treatment of coexisting depression is also important.

PSYCHOSOCIAL CHANGES
The psychosocial changes that occur with aging involve changes in roles and relationships. Roles and relationships within the family change as parents become grandparents, adult children become caregivers for aging parents, or spouses become widows or widowers. Group membership roles and relationships change as the older adult retires from work, moves from a familiar neighborhood, or stops attending social activities because of declining health status.

The nurse assesses the nature of the psychosocial changes facing an older adult and the adaptation of the older adult to those changes. In the assessment the nurse asks how the older adult feels about self, self in relation to others, and self as aging. Areas to be addressed during the assessment include the family, intimate relationships, past and present occupation, finances, housing, social networks, activities, and spirituality. Specific topics related to these areas include retirement, housing and environment, social isolation, sexuality, and death.

Retirement.
Retirement is often mistakenly associated with passivity and seclusion. In actuality, it is a stage of life characterized by transitions and role changes. The psychosocial stresses of retirement may be related to role changes with spouse or within the family and to loss of role. There may also be problems related to social isolation and finances.

The age of retirement varies. The use of age 65 as a determinant of old age or retirement age has its origins in German social reforms in the nineteenth century. Adopted as the age indicating eligibility for Social Security benefits, age 65 has taken on meanings that were not originally intended. Retirement, which may be mandatory or voluntary, occurs at a variety of ages. But whether it occurs at age 55, age 65, or age 75, retirement is one of the major turning points in life.

Preretirement planning is an important advisable task for middle-age individuals. People who plan in advance for retirement generally have a smoother transition into retirement. Preretirement planning is more than financial planning, although financial planning is important. Planning begins with consideration of the "style" of retirement desired and includes an inventory of interests, current skills, and general health. Meaningful retirement planning is critical because retirement can last for 30 or more years.

Retirement has an impact on more individuals than the retired person. Spouses, adult children, and grandchildren are all affected. When the spouse is still working, the retired person faces time alone. For example, the working spouse may have new ideas about the amount of participation in housework expected of the retired person. Friction may develop when the plans of the retired person conflict with the work responsibilities of the working spouse. The working spouse may also have expectations of the retired person that need clarification. For couples the adjustment to retirement is affected by the quality of their communication with each other, their process of decision making about issues such as money or activities, their adherence to either traditional or shared role orientations, and their level of affection and intimacy (Ebersole and Hess, 1998). Adult children may expect the retired person to become an automatic baby-sitter for the grandchildren.

Loss of the work role has a major impact on some retired persons. When so much of life has revolved around work and the personal relationships at work, the loss of the work role may be devastating. Personal identity may be rooted in the work role, and with retirement a new identity must be constructed. The structure imposed on daily life by a work schedule is also lost with retirement. Also lost are the social exchanges and interpersonal support that occur in the workplace. In the adjustment to retirement the older adult is challenged to develop a personally meaningful schedule and a supportive social network.

The most powerful factors that influence the retired person's satisfaction with life are health status, the option to continue working, and sufficient income (Ebersole and Hess, 1998). Positive preretirement expectations also contribute to satisfaction in retirement. The nurse can help the older adult and family prepare for retirement by discussing with them several key areas, including relations with spouse and children, meaningful activities to replace the work role, adjusting or rebuilding social networks, issues related to income and health promotion and maintenance, and long-range planning, including wills and advance directives.

Social Isolation.
Many older adults experience social isolation, and the degree of isolation experienced may increase with age. There are two forms of isolation. Isolation may be a choice, the result of a desire not to interact with others. Isolation may also be a response to conditions that inhibit the ability or the opportunity to interact with others (Ebersole and Hess, 1998). Although some older adults may choose to be isolated or to continue a lifelong pattern of reduced interaction with others, other older adults do not choose isolation but are vulnerable to its imposition.

The vulnerability of older adults to isolation is increased in the absence of supportive others such as may occur with loss of the work role or relocation to unfamiliar surroundings. Impaired hearing, diminished vision, and reduced mobility also contribute to reduced interaction with others and isolation. Reduced mobility includes limitations in mobility such as impaired ambulation, inability to use assistive devices independently, or inability to negotiate barriers to access, and the loss of the ability to drive. Because the loss of the ability to drive may limit older adults' ability to live independently, this restriction of mobility potentially affects more than socialization.

Some older adults withdraw from social interaction because of feelings of rejection (Ebersole and Hess, 1998). Societal attitudes about what is attractive and attitudes about aging as unattractive result in feelings of rejection for some older adults. These older adults see themselves as unattractive and rejected because of changes in their personal appearance due to normal aging changes or because of body image changes following illness or surgery. Society, including health care professionals, also considers some behaviors and situations to be unacceptable. Older adults who are confused or incontinent, who are unable to communicate, who are institutionalized, or who are poor or homeless are examples of older adults who may be isolated by society. The societal trend toward the geographic dispersion of families leads to decreased opportunities for interaction among family members. Some older adults consider this to be rejection by their families.

Patterns of Isolation — Box 12-5

Type 1: Lifelong extrovert isolated by condition or situation
- Ameliorate the situation to the greatest extent possible.
- Seek to bring in contact with individuals and groups through Internet, distance learning.
- Assist to identify like individuals who may enjoy frequent telephone contact.
- Establish pen-pal network.

Type 2: Retiree whose contacts were mostly through work and who is now bereft of socialization opportunities
- Seek ready-made groups with some shared interests, often similar to work skills and expertise.
- Interest person in volunteer activities that will use particular skills.
- Provide opportunities to express particular skills in arenas where others will appreciate abilities.

Type 3: Active extrovert who withdraws later in life because of events causing shame, e.g., divorce, alcoholism, poverty
- Assist with grief resolution, suggest counseling, seek support, self-help group.
- Help find resources addressing specific alienating condition.

Type 4: Lifelong isolate
- Assist in finding resources to augment areas of interest, hobbies.
- Initiate dyadic interactions if individual is willing.

From Ebersole P, Hess P: *Toward healthy aging: human needs and nursing response*, ed 5, St. Louis, 1998, Mosby.

The nurse can assist lonely older adults in rebuilding social networks and reversing the patterns of isolation (Ebersole and Hess, 1998). Box 12-5 displays four patterns of isolation and suggested interventions. Many communities have outreach programs designed to make contact with isolated older adults. Outreach programs may meet nutritional needs, such as Meals on Wheels; socialization needs, such as daily telephone calls by volunteers; or need for activities, such as outings. Social service agencies in most communities welcome older adults as volunteers and provide the opportunity to serve as well as being served. Other organizations within communities such as churches, colleges, unions, and libraries offer a variety of programs for older adults that increase the opportunity to meet people with similar activities, interests, and needs.

Sexuality.   Sexuality is increasingly recognized as important in the care of older adults. All older adults, whether healthy or frail, need to express sexual feelings. Sexuality involves love, warmth, sharing, and touching, not just the act of intercourse. Sexuality is linked with identity and validates the belief that people can give to others and have the gift appreciated.

Maintaining sexual health requires integration of somatic, emotional, intellectual, and social aspects of the sexual being. To help the older adult achieve or maintain sexual health, the nurse needs to understand the physical changes in sexual response (see Chapter 27). The nurse should provide privacy for any discussion of sexuality and should maintain a nonjudgmental attitude. Open-ended questions inviting the older adult to explain sexual activities or concerns may elicit more information than a list of closed-ended questions about specific activities or symptoms. Older adults may appreciate information about the typical age-related changes in sexuality. Information about the prevention of sexually transmitted diseases should be included when appropriate.

The older adult's libido does not decrease, although frequency of sexual activity may decline. An older woman who does not understand physical changes affecting sexual activity may be concerned that her sex life is nearly over with the onset of menopause. The older man may feel the same when he discovers a change in the firmness of his erection, a decreased need for ejaculation with each orgasm, or a longer recovery period between episodes of intercourse.

In addition to physical changes affecting sexual functioning, many older adults are prescribed medications that depress sexual activity, such as antihypertensives, antidepressants, sedatives, or hypnotics. Some drugs increase libido in older adults. For example, phenothiazines increase sexual desire in women, and levodopa has a similar effect in men.

While considering the older adult's need for sexual expression, the nurse must not ignore the equally important need to touch and be touched. Touch is an overt expression with many meanings and is an important part of sexuality. Touch can complement traditional sexual methods or serve as an alternative sexual expression when physical intercourse is not desired or possible and thus can serve as an important method of achieving intimacy (Wallace, 1996). The nursing student needs to recognize that knowledge of older adults' sexual and intimacy needs will increase with professional growth. As information about the older adult is obtained, the nurse will be able to incorporate this information into the nursing care plan.

Alternative sexual practices, as well as the sexuality of older adults, are often difficult for some people to support or understand (Wallace, 1996). Older gay men and lesbians make up approximately 10% of the population over age 65 (Ebersole and Hess, 1998). Little information is available regarding older adult homosexuals and their health care needs. Older lesbian women and older heterosexual women have similar health care needs (Wojciechowski, 1998). Nurses need to be aware of their own beliefs and the impact those beliefs may have on their ability to assist older homosexuals with meeting their sexual needs.

The nurse assists older adults in achieving sexual health. However, a counselor for one or both partners may be needed to describe methods for sexual satisfaction. In addition, the nurse may help other health care professionals understand the sexual behavior of older adults. Not all nurses feel comfortable counseling older adults about sexual health. The nurse need not feel obligated to do so. However, the nurse should recognize the need for assistance. If the nurse is uncomfortable with discussing sexuality, another health care professional (e.g., a social worker or psychologist) should be consulted.

Housing and Environment.

The extent of the older adult's ability to live independently strongly determines housing choices. Changes in social roles, family responsibilities, and health status influence older adults' living arrangements. Some choose to live with family members. Others prefer their own homes or apartments near their families. Leisure or retirement communities provide older people with living and social opportunities in a one-generation setting. Federally subsidized housing, where available, offers apartments with communal, social, and, in some cases, food service arrangements.

When assisting older adults with housing needs, the nurse should assess their activity level, financial status, access to public transportation and community activities, environmental hazards, and support systems. Housing choices should also look to the future needs of the older adults in so far as these can be anticipated. A housing unit with only one floor and without exterior steps may be a prudent choice for the older adult with severe arthritis who has already had some lower extremity joint replacement surgeries and anticipates the need for future surgeries.

Housing and environment are important because they can have a major impact on the health of older adults. The environment can support or hinder physical and social functioning, enhance or drain energy, and complement or tax existing physical changes such as vision and hearing. For example, red, orange, and yellow are easiest for older adults to see. Older adults have difficulty distinguishing between green and blue and among pastel shades. To help older adults in health care settings find their rooms, pictures or other decorations near their doors have been used as landmarks. Door frames and baseboards in a color that contrasts with the color of the wall improve perception of the boundaries of halls and rooms. Glare from highly polished floors, metallic fixtures, and windows is poorly tolerated.

Furniture should be comfortable and designed for the musculoskeletal changes of older adults. Older adults should examine furniture carefully for size, comfort, and function before purchasing it. Furniture should be easy to get into and out of and should provide back support. Dining room chairs should be tested for comfort during meals and for height in relation to the table. Older adults may prefer transferring out of a wheelchair to another chair for meals because some styles of wheelchairs do not let older adults sit close enough to the table to eat comfortably. Raising the table to clear the wheelchair arms may bring the table closer to the older adult but may make it too high for comfortable use. To make getting out of bed easier and safer, the height of the bed should allow the older adult's feet to be flat on the floor when the older adult is sitting on the side of the bed.

The nurse assesses environmental needs of older adults to increase independence and functional ability. Safety is also a major concern. Assessment of safety includes assessment of the risks within the environment and the older adult's ability to recognize and respond to the risks. Risks include factors leading to injury within the home, such as water heaters set at excessively hot temperatures or throw rugs that could cause a fall, and factors outside of the home, such as deteriorating sidewalks and steps or a high incidence of street crime.

Death.

Part of the life history of an older adult is the experience of the death of family members and friends (Chapter 29). This includes the experience of the loss of the older generations of their families and sometimes, sadly, the loss of a child. By age 75, 63% of women have experienced the death of a husband and 20% of men, the death of a wife (Ebersole and Hess, 1998). As the older adult ages, friends are gradually lost to death as those friends grow older. In spite of these experiences, it would be wrong to assume that the older adult is comfortable with the idea of death.

A common misconception is that the death of an older adult is a blessing and the culmination of a full life. Even as death approaches, many older adults still have unfinished business and are not prepared to die. Families and friends may not be ready to let go of the older adult. The nurse may be the person to whom the older adult and their family or friends turn to cope with death and loss. With knowledge and skills the nurse can help make the dying process a time of fulfillment and growth while enlisting the support, understanding, and assistance of family and friends of the dying older adult.

Health Risks

The three most common causes of death in older adults are heart disease, cancer, and stroke. Other frequently reported causes of death are lung disease, accidents/falls, diabetes, kidney disease, and liver disease. All of these causes of death have preventive measures that could potentially reduce the frequency of these conditions and delay disability and/or death (Rubenstein and Nahas, 1998). Table 12-4 provides examples of preventive measures for each of these causes of death in older adults. Nurses have opportunities to participate in activities such as health screenings and fairs that can identify older adults at risk and advise them about preventive measures. Nurses in acute care and long-term care settings also have opportunities to assess the health status of older adults, to intervene in acute situations, and to plan with older adults strategies to reduce risk and manage chronic conditions. Each contact with an older adult, regardless of setting, offers opportunities to teach and counsel.

Table 12-4 Major Causes of Death in Elderly People and Preventability

Rank	Cause	%*	Primary†	Secondary†	Examples
1	Cardiovascular	47	++	+	Control risk factors: smoking, hypertension, hypercholesterolemia. Exercise regularly. Take aspirin, estrogens.
2	Cancer	20	++	++	Control risk factors: tobacco, radiation, sunlight. Screen for cancer of breast, colon, skin, prostate, uterus, mouth.
3	Stroke	11	++	+	Control risk factors: hypertension, tobacco. Take aspirin, anticoagulants in atrial fibrillation. Secondary prevention: screen for carotid artery plaques, emboli.
4	Lung disease	6	++	±	Avoid risk factors: tobacco, allergens. Immunization: influenza, pneumococcal infection.
5	Accidents/falls	2	+	+	Reduce risk factors: weakness, imbalance, polypharmacy, environmental hazards. Careful exercise.
6	Diabetes	2	0	±	Screening may allow earlier intervention.
7	Kidney disease	1	+	±	Control hypertension and diabetes. Treat infections.
8	Liver disease	1	++	0	Avoid toxic substances (e.g., alcohol). Immunization.

From Rubenstein L, Nahas R: Primary and secondary prevention strategies in the older adult, *Geriatr Nurs* 19(1):11, 1998.

*Percentage of all deaths occurring in people age 65 years and older.

†Effectiveness of primary and secondary preventive measures: ++, Very effective; +, effective; ±, equivocal; 0, not effective.

Addressing the Health Concerns of Older Adults

Nursing interventions for older adults are directed toward improving or maintaining the older adult's health needs and concerns. Although various interventions cross all three levels of care, health promotion, acute care, and restorative care, there are approaches unique to each level. When planning interventions it is important to incorporate the older adult's routines or rituals when possible because the older adult feels more secure when routines are continued. The interventions generally are aimed at promoting independence and supporting self-care abilities.

HEALTH PROMOTION AND MAINTENANCE: PHYSIOLOGICAL CONCERNS

Older adults value good health (Box 12-6). A state of wellness provides energy, vitality, and a zest for life (Clark, 1998). The factors that lead to wellness in advanced age have not been fully identified, but four important factors seem to be genetics, good luck, good health habits, and preventive measures (Rubenstein and Nahas, 1998). The nurse is unable to do anything about an older adult's genetic heritage or luck, but the nurse is in a unique position to establish health maintenance programs that promote older adults' wellness and to recommend preventive measures. Senior citizens' centers, churches, schools, shopping malls, libraries, and hospital lobbies can be used as settings to conduct screening tests and present information on health topics. Using creative approaches, the nurse can include health promotion activities for older adults in all health care settings.

Approximately 90% of adults over 65 have at least one chronic health condition, and chronic conditions are more than 4 times more common among older adults than in other age groups (Eliopoulos, 1998). The effect of chronic conditions on the lives of older adults varies widely, but, in general, chronic conditions diminish the well-being and threaten the independence of older adults. Nursing interventions are often directed at the management of these conditions, but interventions can also be preventive, either primary or secondary (Rubenstein and Nahas, 1998). The goal of primary preventive measures is the prevention of the onset of a disease. Examples of primary preventive measures include avoiding smoking to prevent heart disease and lung cancer and receiving immunization to prevent influenza, pneumococcal pneumonia, and tetanus. Secondary preventive measures attempt to identify an established disease in a presymptomatic stage for the purpose of early cure or prevention of progression. Examples of secondary preventive measures include screening for early detection of cancer and screening for depression. Table 12-5 lists 10 conditions and additional examples of preventive measures.

Most older adults are interested in their health and are capable of taking charge of their lives. They want to remain independent and to prevent disability. Initial screenings establish baseline data that can be used to determine wellness, identify health needs, and design health maintenance programs. Following initial screening sessions, nurses can share with older adults information on nutrition, exercise, medications, and safety precautions. Information on specific conditions such as hypertension or arthritis or on self-care procedures such as foot and skin care may also be provided. By providing information about health promotion and self-care, nurses can significantly improve the health and well-being of older adults.

The use of self-help strategies is especially appropriate for older adults with limited financial and social resources. Many older adults monitor their own or their spouses' blood pressures, attend health fairs, plan special diets, and care for spouses with chronic disease. The self-help net-

---

Research HIGHLIGHT   **Box 12-6**

RESEARCH ABSTRACT

Nurses and older adults are concerned with self-care and health promotion. This study examines what active older adults say they do to keep healthy and what wellness activities they relate to staying fit, remaining independent, and enhancing well-being. A sample of 28 older adults between ages 57 and 83 completed a questionnaire with open-ended questions about nutrition, rest, sleep, fitness, activity, stress management, social support, environmental safety, quality of life, zest for living, and staying independent and energetic.

The respondents associated being healthy and staying independent with remaining active. Good nutrition was described as important. Most respondents described sleeping 6 to 8 hours a night with additional rest during the day as needed and believed that adequate rest was positively linked to feeling well and remaining active. All of the respondents felt that they handled stress well using techniques that ranged from refusal to pursue stressful issues, diversional activities, positive thinking, prayer, or discussion with others. The respondents looked after their own safety by being careful and using common sense. All of the respondents kept in touch with family and friends and reported positive feelings about these contacts. Keeping active was described as important for feeling energetic and independent. Enhanced quality of life and zest for living were associated with staying active, eating healthily, exercising, balancing activity and rest, staying in touch with family, managing stress, choosing activities they like, reading the Bible, and "feeding the life of the mind."

IMPLICATIONS FOR PRACTICE

- Older adults believe that activity is important for staying fit and remaining independent.
- Older adults believe that their own positive actions contribute to enhanced quality of life.
- Although some older adults identify family problems as stressors, regular interaction with family members is generally associated with positive feelings and viewed as a source of support.
- The self-care behaviors that the active older adults in this study found helpful may be suggested to other active older adults and to less active older adults as measures to improve health and well-being.

REFERENCE

Clark C: Wellness self-care by healthy older adults, *Image J Nurs Sch* 30:351, 1998.

---

work of older adults is extensive. For example, while shopping, older adults may exchange information about the best physician for cataract surgery, a hospital that provides the best care, and nursing homes to avoid.

Heart Disease.   Heart disease is the leading cause of death in older adults. Common cardiovascular disorders

are hypertension and coronary artery disease. Hypertension is diagnosed when repeated blood pressure measurements of 90 mm Hg or greater diastolic and 140 mm Hg or greater systolic are present. In coronary artery disease partial or complete blockage of one or more coronary arteries leads to myocardial ischemia and myocardial infarction. The risk factors for both hypertension and coronary artery disease include smoking, obesity, lack of exercise, and stress. Additional risk factors for coronary artery disease include hypertension, hyperlipidemia, and diabetes mellitus.

Nursing interventions for hypertension and coronary artery disease address weight reduction, exercise, dietary changes limiting salt and fat, stress management, and smoking cessation. Client teaching includes information about medications, blood pressure monitoring, nutrition, stress reduction techniques, and the symptoms indicating the need for emergency care.

Cancer.   Malignant neoplasms are the second most common cause of death among older adults. Nurses participate in programs to educate older adults about early detection, treatment, and risk factors. Examples include smoking cessation, teaching breast self-examination (see Chapter 32), and encouraging all older adults to have annual screening for fecal occult blood. It is also important to educate older adults about the signs of cancer and encourage prompt reporting of nonhealing skin lesions, unexpected bleeding, change in bowel habits, and unexplained weight loss (Rubenstein and Nahas, 1998). Detection is complicated when symptoms are mistakenly identified as part of the normal aging process.

Stroke (Cerebrovascular Accident).   Cerebrovascular accidents, the third leading cause of death in the United States, occur as brain ischemia or brain hemorrhage (Abrams, Beers, and Berkow, 1995). In brain ischemia there is an inadequate supply of blood to areas of the brain due to blockage of blood vessels or general circulatory failure. Brain hemorrhage, either subarachnoid hemorrhage or intracerebral hemorrhage, is less common than brain ischemia. Risk factors for cerebrovascular accidents include hypertension, hyperlipidemia, diabetes mellitus, history of transient ischemic attacks, and family history of cardiovascular disease. Treatment usually includes hospitalization for days or months, depending on the degree of brain damage. Cerebrovascular accidents may impair the functional abilities of older adults and limit their ability to live independently. The scope of nursing interventions ranges from teaching older adults about risk reduction strategies to care of the older adult after a cerebrovascular accident and during recovery and rehabilitation.

Smoking Cessation.   Cigarette smoking has been recognized as a risk factor in the four most common causes

Table 12-5   Major Chronic Conditions in Old Persons: Preventability

Rank	Cause	%*	Primary†	Secondary†	Examples
1	Arthritis	45-55	+	±	Avoid joint stress. Early treatment of rheumatoid arthritis.
2	Dental problems	40-60	+	+	Oral hygiene. Dental prophylaxis. Screening and early intervention.
3	Hypertension	35-45	++	±	Avoid salt and stress. Exercise. Regular screening.
4	Heart disease	30-40	++	+	Control risk factors: smoking, hypertension, hypercholesterolemia. Regular exercise. Take aspirin, estrogens.
5	Visual problems	30-40	±	+	Avoid excessive ultraviolet light. Screening and refraction.
6	Osteoporosis	25-60	++	±	High calcium intake. Estrogen replacement. Exercise.
7	Hearing problems	20-35	+	+	Avoid excess noise. Screening and amplification.
8	Depression	10-20	±	+	Screening and treatment.
9	Vascular disease	10-20	+	±	Control risk factors: smoking, hypertension, hypercholesterolemia. Regular exercise. Take aspirin, estrogens.
10	Functional dependency	10-15	±	+	Exercise and other activity. Screening, assessment, and specific treatment and therapies.

From Rubenstein L, Nahas R: Primary and secondary prevention strategies in the older adult, *Geriatr Nurs* 19(1):11, 1998.

*Percentage of persons age 65 years and older with the condition (prevalence)

†Effectiveness of primary and secondary preventive measures: ++, very effective; +, effective; ±, equivocal

---

of death for older adults: heart disease, cancer, stroke, and lung disease. Smoking cessation is a health promotion strategy for older adults just as it is for younger adults. Older smokers can still benefit from smoking cessation (Boyd, 1996). In addition to reducing risk, smoking cessation may stabilize existing conditions such as chronic obstructive pulmonary disease (COPD). Smoking cessation may even contribute to the extension of life or of independent functioning.

There are four sequential approaches that nurses may use to encourage smoking cessation (Boyd, 1996). First, the nurse asks the older adult about smoking, including the type of tobacco product used, the frequency of smoking, and the number of years smoking. Then, the nurse provides information about the ill effects of smoking and the benefits of quitting. Finally, the nurse recommends quitting. If smoking cessation is rejected, the nurse should suggest a reduction in smoking. Assistance in developing a plan for quitting is offered, and various strategies such as the use of gum containing nicotine or nicotine patches and asking family members to reduce smoking are discussed. Lastly, the nurse, on subsequent visits with the older adult, offers encouragement and assistance in modifying the plan as necessary. Although some mistakenly believe that older adults do not want to quit smoking or are unable to quit, some older adults do choose to quit smoking and do succeed.

Nutrition.   How older adults meet their needs for good nutrition is influenced by lifelong eating habits and situational factors. Lifelong eating habits based in tradition, ethnicity, and religion influence choices of what foods are eaten and how those foods are prepared (Ebersole and Hess, 1998). Situational factors affecting nutrition include access to food stores, adequate finances, the physical and cognitive capability for food preparation, and a place to store food and prepare meals.

The nutritional needs of older adults are affected by their levels of activity and by clinical conditions. Level of activity has implications for the total amount of calories with more sedentary older adults usually needing fewer calories than more active older adults. However, caloric requirements are not determined solely by activity. Additional calories may be required in clinical situations such as recovery from surgery, whereas calories may be restricted when the older adult is diabetic or overweight. Beyond caloric requirements, therapeutic diets may restrict fat, sodium, or simple sugars or may increase fiber or foods high in calcium, iron, vitamin A, or vitamin C.

Good nutrition for older adults includes appropriate caloric intake and limited intake of fat, salt, refined sugars, and alcohol (Fishman, 1996). Although the nutritional guidelines displayed in the food guide pyramid (see Chapter 43) are the basic recommendations for older adult nutrition, some older adults do not follow these guidelines. Protein intake may be lower than recommended if older adults have trouble chewing meat or have reduced finances. Fat intake may be higher than recommended because of the substitution of fast-food restaurant meals for meals prepared at home or because of methods of cooking featuring fried foods and sauces using butter and cream. Extra salt and sugar may be used while cooking or at the table to compensate for a diminished sense of taste. Vitamin intake may be reduced if shopping for fresh fruits and vegetables is difficult.

Older adults with dementia have special nutritional needs. As their memory and their functional skills decline with the progression of dementia, they lose the ability to remember when to eat, how to prepare food, and, eventually, how to feed themselves. At the same time their caloric needs may increase because of the energy expended in pacing and wandering activities. Nurses and other caregivers of older adults with dementia should routinely monitor weight and food intake, serve food that is easy to eat, provide assistance with eating, and offer food supplements as needed to maintain weight (Yen, 1997). Mealtime interventions for older adults with dementia also provide opportunities for socialization and practice with functional skills.

Dental Problems.

Dental problems are common in older adults and include problems with natural teeth and dentures. Dental caries, gingivitis, broken or missing teeth, and ill-fitting or missing dentures may affect nutritional adequacy, cause pain, and lead to infection. The nurse can help prevent dental and gum disease through education about routine dental care (see Chapter 38). The nurse can also help older adults find dental services that offer reduced rates and that are accessible to those with impaired mobility.

Exercise.

Older adults should be encouraged to maintain physical exercise and activity. The primary benefits of exercise include maintaining and strengthening functional ability and promoting a sense of enhanced well-being. An exercise such as walking builds endurance, increases muscle tone, improves joint flexibility, strengthens bones, reduces stress, and contributes to weight loss (Butler, 1998). Other benefits of a program of exercise include improvement of cardiovascular function, improved plasma lipoprotein profiles, increased metabolic rate, increased gastrointestinal transit time, and improved sleep quality (Butler and others, 1998b). Frail older adults who exercise may experience improved mobility, gait, and balance plus less difficulty getting up from a chair or climbing stairs. Exercise may also have a positive effect on anxiety and depression (Gunnarsson and Judge, 1997).

Before beginning a formal exercise program, an older adult should have a physical examination, which may include a stress cardiogram or stress test. This provides information about cardiovascular function during sustained exercise. Older adults with unstable cardiac disease should not participate in exercise training (Butler and others, 1998a). Exercise programs for sedentary older adults who have not been exercising should begin conservatively and progress slowly (Gunnarsson and Judge, 1997). Walking is a preferred exercise of many older adults. Other exercises can be incorporated into the older adult's activities of daily living. For example, arm circles and leg circles can be performed while watching television.

The nurse should plan an exercise program that meets physical needs while allowing for physical impairments and encourage the older adult to persevere with the exercise program. Safety considerations include wearing shoes and clothing appropriate to the exercise, drinking water before and after exercising, avoiding outdoor exercise when the weather is very warm or very cold, and exercis-

ing with a partner. Nurses should instruct the older adult to stop exercising and seek help if chest pain or tightness, shortness of breath, dizziness or light-headedness, or palpitations are experienced during exercise (Gunnarsson and Judge, 1997).

Arthritis.

Arthritis is a common condition in older adults, especially in women. The degree to which the mobility of older adults is impaired depends on the extent of the disease and joints affected. The impact of arthritis on the lives of older adults is a combination of the changes in joint range of motion and stability and the amount of pain experienced. Arthritis has no cure, but recently developed pharmacological agents can decrease pain and swelling and therefore increase joint motion. Nursing interventions are aimed at promoting comfort, functional ability, and safety. Education about self-care techniques, joint protection, and exercises for flexibility and strength is also important.

Falls.

Falls are a safety concern of many older adults. Falls may lead to fear of additional falls, withdrawal from usual activities, and loss of independence. Hospitalization and placement in a nursing home for rehabilitation or long-term placement may be required. Approximately 30% of older adults who live independently in their own homes will fall at least once a year (Tibbitts, 1996). A fracture will be sustained in 5% of those falls, and in 1% of the falls a hip fracture will occur. Falls are more frequent and more serious for older adults over age 85.

The risk factors leading to falls are a combination of health-related issues and environmental hazards (Tideiksaar, 1996). Health-related issues include impaired vision; cardiovascular conditions such as postural hypotension or syncope; conditions affecting mobility such as arthritis, muscle weakness, and foot problems; conditions affecting balance; alterations in bladder function such as frequency or incontinence; cognitive impairment, and adverse medication reactions. Environmental hazards include, but are not limited to, poor lighting, slippery or wet floors, stairs or sidewalks in poor repair, shoes in poor repair or with slippery soles, and household items that could be tripped over, such as throw rugs, foot stools, and electric extension cords.

Nursing interventions are directed toward the management of health-related conditions and the reduction of environmental hazards. Older adults taking medications with adverse effects such as postural hypotension, dizziness, or sedation can be instructed to be aware of these potential effects and to take precautions such as changing position slowly or holding onto sturdy furniture if unsteady. Simple interventions in the home such as rearranging furniture to provide a clear pathway to the bathroom and providing a night-light in the bathroom can reduce falls related to nighttime trips to the toilet. Picking up throw rugs and other items on the floor reduces slipping and tripping. Nurses can also instruct older adults in the safe use of assistive devices such as canes, walkers, and wheelchairs.

Sensory Impairments.
The older adult usually has changes in vision, hearing, taste, and smell that are a result of normal aging. Chapter 48 describes in detail the nursing interventions used to maintain and improve sensory function.

Reports of age-related changes in pain perception are controversial, and both health care professionals and lay persons believe that pain is a natural part of aging and disease (Ferrell and Rivera, 1996). This misperception results in underreporting of pain and prevents appropriate use of pain relief measures in older adults. The causes of pain in older adults include acute and chronic conditions (e.g., trauma, infection, and neuropathies). Many factors influence the management of pain, including cultural influences on the meaning and expression of pain for older adults, fears related to the use of analgesic medications, and the problem of pain assessment with cognitively impaired older adults. Nurses caring for older adults are challenged to advocate for appropriate and effective pain management (see Chapter 42).

Medication Use.
Adults over 65 are the greatest users of medications with approximately 66% of older adults using prescription and nonprescription drugs (Abrams, Beers, and Berkow, 1995). Older adults use 30% of all prescription medications (Hayes, 1998). Most older adults use at least one drug daily; many use several drugs daily. The most commonly used medications are cardiovascular drugs, antihypertensives, analgesics, antiarthritic agents, sedatives, tranquilizers, laxatives, and antacids (Eliopoulos, 1998). **Polypharmacy,** the concurrent use of many medications, increases the risk for adverse reactions. While polypharmacy may reflect inappropriate prescribing, it may be necessary in situations where an older adult has multiple acute and chronic conditions. However, periodic and thorough review of all medications being used is important to restrict the number of medications used to the fewest necessary. The nurse's role with an older adult undergoing drug therapy is to ensure the greatest therapeutic benefit with the least amount of harm.

Older adults are at risk for adverse reactions because of age-related changes in the absorption, distribution, metabolism, and excretion of drugs (Table 12-6). Medications may also interact with one another, adding or negating the effect of another drug. Medications may also cause confusion; affect balance and mobility; cause dizziness, nausea, and vomiting; or lead to constipation, urinary frequency, or incontinence. Because of these effects some older adults are unwilling to take medications. Other older adults, perhaps as many as 50%, take their medications incorrectly because they do not understand the instructions about their medications (Hayes, 1998).

When drugs are used in the management of confusion, special care is necessary. The sedatives and tranquilizers sometimes prescribed for acutely confused older adults may themselves cause or exacerbate confusion. Drugs used to manage confused behaviors should be carefully administered, taking into account age-related changes in body systems that can affect the pharmacokinetic activity. When confusion has a physiological cause, that cause, rather than the confused behavior, should be specifically treated. When confusion varies by time of day or is related to environmental factors, the nurse can use creative, nonpharmacological measures such as making the environment more meaningful, providing adequate light, encouraging use of assistive devices (glasses, hearing aids), or even making telephone calls to friends or family members to let older adults hear reassuring voices.

Managing medications is a very important component of maintaining and promoting good health in old age. The nurse works collaboratively with the older adult to ensure safe and appropriate use of all medications, both prescribed and over-the-counter medications (Box 12-7). The older adult should be taught the names of all drugs being taken, when and how to take them, and the desirable and undesirable effects of the drugs. The nurse also teaches how to avoid adverse effects and/or interactions of drugs and how to establish and follow an appropriate self-administration pattern. Strategies for reducing the risk for an adverse medication reaction in the older adult include reviewing the medications with the older adult at each visit, examining for potential interactions with food or other drugs, simplifying and individualizing the drug regimen, taking every opportunity to inform the older adult and family about all aspects of medication use, and encouraging the older adult to question the physician, advanced practice nurse, and/or pharmacist about all prescribed drugs and all over-the-counter drugs.

For some older adults on large numbers of medications, safely managing medications can be a complex activity that can easily become overwhelming. Nurses can provide valuable assistance to their older adult clients as they carry out this important self-care activity.

HEALTH PROMOTION AND MAINTENANCE: PSYCHOSOCIAL HEALTH CONCERNS
Interventions supporting the psychosocial health of older adults resemble those for other age groups. However, some interventions are more crucial for older adults experiencing social isolation, cognitive impairment, or stresses related to retirement, relocation, or approaching death. These interventions include therapeutic communication, touch, reality orientation, validation therapy, reminiscence, and interventions to improve body image.

Therapeutic Communication.
With therapeutic communication the nurse perceives and respects the older adult's uniqueness. The nurse who communicates effectively will be accepted as one who shares a genuine concern for the older adult's welfare. The nurse cannot simply enter an older adult's environment and immediately es-

Table 12-6 Age-Related Changes Affecting Drug Therapy in the Elderly

Change	Effect	Nursing Measures
Drier mucous membrane of oral cavity	Tablets and capsules may stick to roof or sides of mouth and not be swallowed, or dissolve in and irritate mouth.	Offer fluids before drug administration to moisten mouth and ample fluids during administration. Inspect client's mouth or advise client to inspect mouth for any tablet or capsule that may not have been swallowed (dentures and reduced oral sensations may cause client to be unaware of presence of medication). Unless contraindicated, break large tablets to facilitate swallowing.
Decreased circulation to lower bowel and vagina; lower body temperatures	Suppositories require more time to melt and can be expelled undissolved.	Explore possibility of using alternative route. Allow more time for suppository to melt. Check client or advise to check that the suppository has melted before getting out of bed to resume activities.
Decreased tissue elasticity; reduced muscle mass and activity	Poor seal of tissues after injection and oozing or poor absorption may result.	Use Z-track injection technique for injections to facilitate sealing. Cleanse any medication that has oozed onto skin.
Decreased pain sensation	Infection or other problem at injection site may not be detected.	Check injection sites regularly.
Decreased cardiac efficiency	Greater risk exists for circulatory overload during intravenous administration of medications.	Monitor intravenous drip closely. Observe for signs of circulatory overload, such as rise in blood pressure, rapid respirations, coughing, or shortness of breath.
Less gastric acid	Slower absorption of drugs that require low gastric pH may result.	Ensure that gastric acid is not further reduced by other drugs such as antacids.
Increase in adipose tissue compared, with lean body mass; decreased cardiac output	Drugs stored in adipose tissue (lipid-soluble drugs) have increased tissue concentrations and decreased plasma concentrations and accumulate and remain in body longer. Plasma levels of drugs can increase while less is deposited in reservoirs (particularly true of water-soluble drugs).	Ensure that dosages are adjusted for age. Become familiar with adverse effects of drugs being administered and observe for these effects.
Reduced serum albumin levels	The administration of protein-bound drugs together can result in drugs competing for the same protein molecules. Some drugs may not effectively bind and may be less effective.	Advise physician of other protein-bound drugs client is taking when new protein-bound drug is prescribed. Highly protein-bound drugs include acetazolamide, amitriptyline, cefazolin, chlordiazepoxide, chlorpromazine, cloxacillin, digitoxin, furosemide, hydralazine, nortriptyline, phenylbutazone, phenytoin, propranolol, rifampin, salicylates, spironolactone, sulfisoxazole, and warfarin. Ensure that serum albumin level is evaluated along with blood level of drug. (If serum albumin level is low, client is at greater risk for toxicity despite normal or low blood levels of drug.)
Reduced number of functioning nephrons; decreased glomerular filtration rate; reduced blood flow	Biologic half-life is extended, and drugs take longer to be filtered from body; risk of adverse reactions is increased.	Ensure that age-adjusted dosages are prescribed for drugs excreted through renal system.

From Eliopoulos C: *Manual of gerontologic nursing*, ed 2, St. Louis, 1998, Mosby.

Client Teaching ABOUT DISCHARGE INSTRUCTIONS FOR SAFE MEDICATION USE   Box 12-7

OBJECTIVES

- The client will be knowledgeable about the prescribed medications.
- The client will have a reduced risk of adverse medication reactions.

TEACHING STRATEGIES

- Match the teaching strategies to the individual characteristics and needs of the client.
- Adapt the strategies to physical, sensory, and cognitive deficits.
- Address pain, anxiety, and other comfort issues before teaching.
- Provide a well-lit, quiet, comfortable environment.
- Ask the client about including a family member or friend.
- Utilize a slow, clear, concise style for the verbal delivery of material.
- Use large-print, specifically written materials to reinforce the verbal information.
  - Written materials should be at a fourth- to fifth-grade reading level.

- Written materials should be on white or cream, low-gloss paper with black print and a font size that is at least 14 point and easy to read.
- Use a format for the written materials that includes the following:
  - General information about the medication (purpose)
  - How to take the medication (dose, schedule, method)
  - Outcomes (anticipated effects, side effects, emergency information)

EVALUATION

- Ask the client to repeat the name of the medication and the reason for its use.
- Ask the client to describe when, how much, and how the client will take the medication.
- Ask the client what are the expected effects of the medication.
- Ask the client to describe when it would be necessary to call the doctor or nurse.

Modified from Hayes K: Randomized trial of geragogy-based medication instruction in the emergency department, *Nurs Res* 47:211, 1998.

---

tablish a therapeutic relationship, but must first be knowledgeable and skilled in communication techniques.

Touch.   Throughout life touch tells us about our environment and the people around us. Gentle touch conveys affection and friendliness. A firm handclasp may convey security. Older adults may be deprived of touching when separated from family or friends. An older adult who is isolated, dependent, or ill; who fears death; or who lacks self-esteem has a greater need for touch.

The nurse should recognize that older adults may be suffering from touch deprivation. Older adults may demonstrate this need for touch by reaching for the nurse's hand. Unfortunately older men are sometimes wrongly accused of sexual advances when they reach out to touch others. When nurses use touch, it should not be in a condescending way such as patting an older adult on the head. Touch should convey respect and sensitivity. The nurse should not be surprised if the older adult reciprocates because of an unmet need for intimacy.

Touch is a therapeutic tool that nurses can use to help comfort the older adult. It can provide sensory stimulation, induce relaxation, provide physical and emotional comfort, orient the person to reality, convey warmth, and communicate interest. It is a powerful physical expression of a relationship.

Reality Orientation.   **Reality orientation** is a communication technique used to make an older adult more aware of time, place, and person. The purposes of reality orientation include restoring a sense of reality, improving the level of awareness, promoting socialization, elevating independent functioning, and minimizing confusion, disorientation, and physical regression.

Although the nurse can use reality orientation techniques in any health care setting, they may be especially useful in the acute care setting. The older adult experiencing a change in environment, surgery, illness, or emotional stress is at risk for becoming disoriented. Environmental changes, such as the bright lights, unfamiliar noises, and lack of windows in specialized units of a hospital, often lead to disorientation and confusion. Absence of familiar caregivers is also disorienting. When anesthesia, sedatives, tranquilizers, analgesics, and physical restraints are used, disorientation is increased. The nurse should anticipate and monitor for disorientation and confusion as possible consequences of hospitalization, relocation, surgery, loss, or illness and should incorporate interventions based on reality orientation into the care plan.

Once used as a therapy with disoriented individuals and groups of cognitively impaired individuals, the principles of reality orientation offer useful guidelines for communicating with acutely confused individuals. The key elements of reality orientation include frequent reminders of person, time, and place; the use of environmental aids such as clocks, calendars, and personal belongings; and stability of environment, routine, and staff (Eliopoulos, 1998). Communication is always respectful, patient, and calm. The nurse answers questions from the older adult simply and honestly with sensitivity and a caring attitude.

Validation Therapy.

Validation therapy is an alternative approach to communication with a confused older adult. Where reality orientation insists that the confused older adult agree with our statements of time, place, and person, validation therapy accepts the description of time and place as stated by the confused older adult. In validation therapy, statements and behaviors of the confused older adult are not confronted. They are believed to represent an inner need or feeling. By listening with sensitivity and validating what is expressed, the nurse conveys respect, reassurance, and understanding. Validation does not involve reinforcing the confused older adult's misperceptions, but reflects a sensitivity to hidden meanings in statements and behaviors. Validating or respecting confused older adults' feelings in the time and place that is real to them is more important than insisting on the literally correct time and place (Day, 1997).

Reminiscence.

Reminiscence is recalling the past. Many older adults find enjoyment in sharing past experiences. As a therapy, reminiscence uses the recollection of the past to bring meaning and understanding to the present and to resolve current conflicts (Eliopoulos, 1999). Looking back to positive resolutions to problems reminds the older adult of coping strategies used successfully in the past. Reminiscing is also a way to express personal identity. Reflection on past achievements supports self-esteem. For some older adults the process of looking back on past events uncovers new meanings for those events.

During the assessment process, the nurse may use reminiscence to assess self-esteem, cognitive function, emotional stability, unresolved conflicts, coping ability, and expectations for the future (Eliopoulos, 1999). Reminiscence also occurs during direct care activities. Taking time to ask questions about past experiences and listening attentively conveys to an older adult the nurse's attitudes of respect and concern (Puentes, 1998).

Although reminiscence is often used in a one-on-one situation of nurse and older adult, reminiscence can also be a group therapy for cognitively impaired or depressed older adults. The nurse organizes the group and selects strategies. The group's size, structure, process, goals, and activities are adapted to meet its members' needs.

Body-Image Interventions.

The way that older adults present themselves has a significant impact on body image and feelings of isolation. Some physical characteristics of older adulthood are socially desirable, such as distinguished-looking gray hair. Other features are also impressive, such as a lined face that displays character or wrinkled hands that convey a lifetime of hard work. Too often, however, society sees older people as incapacitated, deaf, obese, or shrunken in stature. Consequences of illness and aging that threaten the older adult's body image include invasive diagnostic procedures, pain, surgery, loss of sensation in a body part, skin changes, loss of scalp hair, and incontinence. Body image is also affected by the use of devices such as dentures, hearing aids, artificial limbs, indwelling catheters, ostomy devices, and enteral feeding tubes.

The importance to the older adult of presenting a socially acceptable image must be considered. When older adults have acute or chronic illnesses, the related physical dependence makes it difficult for them to maintain body image. The nurse by assisting with grooming and hygiene has a direct influence on the older adult's appearance. It takes little effort to assist the older adult with combing hair, cleaning dentures, shaving, or changing clothing. The older adult does not choose to have an objectionable appearance. The nurse should also be sensitive to odors in the environment. Odors created by urine and some illnesses are often present. By controlling odors, the nurse may prevent visitors from shortening their stay or not coming at all.

Older Adults and the Acute Care Setting

Older adults in the acute care setting need special attention to help them adjust to the acute care environment and to meet their basic needs for comfort, safety, nutrition/hydration, and skin integrity. Older adults in the acute care setting are at increased risk for adverse events such as delirium, dehydration, malnutrition, nosocomial infections, urinary incontinence, and falls.

The risk for delirium is increased when hospitalized older adults experience immobilization, infection, dehydration, pain, and hypoxia. Multiple medications and multiple medical diagnoses are also risk factors for delirium (Simon, Jewell, and Brokel, 1997). Nonmedical causes of delirium include placement in unfamiliar surroundings, separation from supportive family members, and stress. Impaired vision or hearing contributes to confusion and interferes with attempts to reorient the older adult. When the prevention of delirium fails, interventions begin with treatment of the cause. Supportive interventions include encouraging family visits, providing memory cues (clocks, calendars, name tags), and compensating for sensory deficits. Reality orientation techniques may be useful.

Older adults are at greater risk for dehydration and malnutrition during hospitalization (Sullivan, Sun, and Walls, 1999). Standard procedures such as limiting food and fluids in preparation for tests may place older adults at increased risk for dehydration and malnutrition. The risk for dehydration and malnutrition is also increased when older adults are unable to reach beverages or to feed themselves while in bed or connected to medical equipment. Interventions include getting the client out of bed, providing beverages and snacks frequently, and including favorite foods and beverages in the diet plan.

The increased risk for nosocomial infections in older adults is related to age-related reductions in immune system response. The use of indwelling urinary catheters accounts for 80% of nosocomial urinary tract infections (Lee and Burnett, 1998). Other nosocomial infections include surgical site infection, pneumonia, and bloodstream infections (Russell, 1999). Prevention begins with hand washing and measures to minimize the risk of infection from procedures (Chapter 33). Prevention also includes measures to increase the older adult's resistance to infection.

Older adults in acute care settings are also at risk for becoming incontinent of urine (**transient incontinence**). Causes of transient urinary incontinence include delirium, untreated urinary tract infection, excessive urine production, medications, restricted mobility, and constipation or impaction (Bradway, Hernly, and the NICHE Faculty, 1998). Interventions for transient urinary incontinence are geared to correcting contributing factors. The interventions may include an individualized plan to provide voiding opportunities and modification of the environment to improve access to the toilet. Indwelling urinary catheters should be avoided if possible. Measures to prevent skin breakdown should be used.

The increased risk for skin breakdown is related to changes in aging skin and to situations that arise in the acute care setting such as immobility, incontinence, and malnutrition. The key points in the prevention of skin breakdown are avoiding pressure, reducing shear forces and friction, providing skin care and moisture management, and providing nutritional support (Maklebust, 1997).

Older adults in the acute care setting are at risk for falling and sustaining injuries. Many of the falls occur as the older adult gets out of bed without assistance. Sedating medications may increase unsteadiness. Medications causing orthostatic hypotension may also increase the risk for falls because of the blood pressure drop when the older adult gets out of a bed or chair. The increase in urine output from diuretics increases the risk for falling by increasing the number of attempts to get out of bed to void. Attempts to get out of bed when physically restrained may lead to injury when the older adult becomes entangled in the restraint. Equipment such as wires from monitors, intravenous tubing, urinary catheters, and other medical devices become obstacles to safe ambulation. Impaired vision may prevent the older adult from seeing tripping hazards such as trash cans. Confused older adults who may try to get out of bed although weak, unsteady, or drowsy may benefit from reality orientation or the presence of family members and friends. Interventions to reduce the risk for falling include assistance with ambulation, strengthening exercises, medication monitoring, assistance with toileting, and removal of tripping hazards.

Older Adults and Restorative Care

Restorative care refers to two types of ongoing care. The first type of restorative care continues the convalescence from acute illness or surgery that began in the acute care setting. The second type of restorative care addresses chronic conditions that affect day-to-day functioning. Both types of restorative care take place in private homes and in long-term care settings.

Interventions during convalescence from acute illness or surgery are directed toward regaining or improving the prior level of independence in activities of daily living (ADLs). Interventions that began in the acute care setting should be continued and later modified as convalescence progresses. To achieve this continuation, the acute care setting's discharge information should include information on the ongoing interventions (e.g., exercise routines, wound care routines, medication schedules, vital sign monitoring, and blood glucose monitoring). Interventions should also address the restoration of interpersonal relationships and activities at either their previous level or at the level desired by the older adult.

When restorative care addresses chronic conditions, the goals of care include stabilizing the chronic condition, promoting health, and promoting independence in activities of daily living. Interventions to stabilize the chronic condition may focus on regulation or prevention. An example of a regulatory intervention is the monitoring of blood glucose levels in diabetes. An example of prevention is a smoking cessation program for the older adult with chronic obstructive pulmonary disease.

Health promotion for older adults, as addressed in this chapter, applies to all older adults. Health promotion interventions should occur in all health care settings. For example, nurse-directed programs in long-term care have improved ambulation, reversed urinary incontinence, and reduced confusion.

Interventions to promote independence in ADLs address physical ability, cognitive ability, and safety. The physical ability to perform ADLs requires strength, flexibility, and balance. Accommodation must be made for impairments of vision, hearing, and touch. The cognitive ability to perform ADLs requires the ability to recognize, judge, and remember. Cognitive impairments, such as Alzheimer's disease, may interfere with safe performance of ADLs, although the older adult is still physically capable of the activities. Interventions to promote independence in ADLs adapt these requirements to the needs and lifestyle of the older adult. Safety is always considered because it is not enough to be able to perform any of the ADLs. The older adult should be able to perform the ADLs with only an amount of risk that is acceptable to the older adult.

Restorative care measures focus on activities to prevent, improve, reduce, or eliminate problems. Priorities of care are established, client goals and expected outcomes are determined, and appropriate interventions are selected. This is done with the older adult's participation so that the interventions are understood and conflicts in approaches or priorities can be avoided. Consideration by the nurse of the older adults' lifetime experiences, as well as the values and sociocultural patterns developed, serves as the basis for planning individual care. When the older adult's cognitive status prevents participation in health care deci-

sions, families must be included. Families and friends are rich sources of data because they knew the older adult before the impairment. Frequently, they can provide explanations for the older adult's behaviors and suggest methods of management. Thoughtful assessment and planning leads to goals of care that consider the influence of normal aging changes, facilitate an optimal level of comfort and coping, and promote independence in self-care activities.

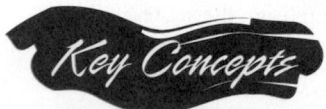

Key Concepts

- The number of older adults, especially older adults over age 85, is increasing.
- Because nurses' attitudes toward older adults influence the quality of care, those attitudes should be based on accurate information about older adults, rather than myths and stereotypes.
- The biological and psychosocial theories of aging offer possible explanations for the changes seen in aging.
- Older adults adapt to physical changes in all organ systems as they age.
- Older adults and their adult children redefine their mutual relationships.
- Changes in social roles, family responsibility, and health status influence the choice of living arrangements appropriate for the older adult.
- Health care services for older adults are available in community-based and institutional settings.
- The physical changes that accompany aging are considered to be normal, not pathological, although they may predispose the older adult to disease.
- Cognitive impairment is not normal in older adults and requires assessment and intervention.
- Cognitive impairment includes acute, potentially reversible disorders and chronic, irreversible, progressive disorders.
- Areas affected by psychosocial changes of aging include retirement, social isolation, change in housing, death, and sexuality.
- Nursing interventions for psychosocial concerns include therapeutic communication, touch, reality orientation, validation therapy, reminiscence, and interventions to improve body image.
- The leading causes of death in the older population are cardiovascular disease, cancer, stroke, lung disease, accidents/falls, diabetes, kidney disease, and liver disease.

- Nurses are able to establish health programs that promote older adults' wellness and to recommend preventive measures.
- Health promotion recommendations for older adults include good nutrition, regular exercise, smoking cessation, measures to reduce the risk for falls, and measures to reduce adverse medication reactions.
- Acute care settings place older adults at risk for delirium, dehydration, malnutrition, nosocomial infections, urinary incontinence, and falls.
- Restorative nursing interventions, whether accomplished in the older adult's home or in long-term care institutions, stabilize chronic conditions, promote health, and promote independence in activities of daily living.

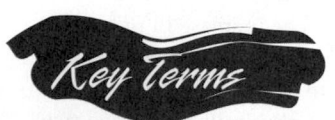

Key Terms

Ageism, *p. 246*
Alzheimer's disease, *p. 256*
Delirium, *p. 254*
Dementia, *p. 254*
Depression, *p. 254*
Geriatrics, *p. 245*
Gerontic nursing, *p. 245*
Gerontological nursing, *p. 245*
Gerontology, *p. 245*
Nonstochastic theories, *p. 247*

Polypharmacy, *p. 265*
Presbycusis, *p. 253*
Presbyopia, *p. 253*
Reality orientation, *p. 267*
Reminiscence, *p. 268*
Stochastic theories, *p. 247*
Transient incontinence, *p. 269*
Validation therapy, *p. 268*
Vascular dementia, *p. 256*

Critical Thinking Exercises

1. Mr. Brown, age 73, has come to the clinic for a routine check of his blood pressure and cholesterol level. The policy of the clinic is to review all medications at every clinic visit. What concerns related to safe medication use will you discuss with Mr. Brown?

2. Mrs. Shephard's daughter has come with her to the clinic. She is concerned about her mother's memory. She tells you that although her mother's memory is usually excellent with only occasional forgetting of names or the location of keys, this has suddenly changed. Two days ago Mrs. Shephard phoned her daughter 6 times in 2 hours asking where her husband (the late Mr. Shephard) was and when told of his death 4 years ago denied this fact. When her daughter arrived at her house to check on her, she found that Mrs. Shephard had emptied the contents of all the closets onto the floor and accused her daughter of theft. Mrs. Shephard has spent the last two nights at her daughter's house for safety. Suspecting delirium, what biophysiological areas and conditions should you consider as potentially reversible causes?

3. On her visit to the clinic you note that Mrs. Johnson, a frail 86-year-old, has lost 15 pounds since her visit 1 month ago. Mrs. Johnson lives alone now since the death of her husband 2 months ago. Her children live out of town. What areas will you include in your assessment?

References

Abrams W, Beers M, Berkow R: *The Merck manual of geriatrics,* ed 2, Whitehouse Station, NJ, 1995, Merck.

Agency for Health Care Policy and Research: *Early identification of Alzheimer's disease and related dementias,* Quick reference guide for clinicians, no. 18, 1996.

American Association of Retired Persons: *A profile of older Americans,* Washington, DC, 1997, The Association.

Boyd N: Smoking cessation: a four-step plan to help older patients quit, *Geriatrics* 51(11):53, 1996.

Bradway C, Hernly S, the NICHE faculty: Urinary incontinence in older adults admitted to acute care, *Geriatr Nurs* 19:98, 1998.

Butler R: Tell your patients to take a walk, *Geriatrics* 53(5):15, 1998.

Butler R, Lewis M: Late-life depression: when and how to intervene, *Geriatrics* 50(8):44, 1995.

Butler R and others: Physical fitness: how to help older patients live stronger and longer, *Geriatrics* 53(9):26, 1998a.

Butler R and others: Physical fitness: benefits of exercise for the older patient, *Geriatrics* 53(10):46, 1998b.

Chenier M: Review and analysis of caregiver burden and nursing home placement, *Geriatr Nurs* 18(3):121, 1997.

Clark C: Wellness self-care by healthy older adults, *Image J Nurs Sch* 30:351, 1998.

Cummings E, Henry W: *Growing old: the process of disengagement,* New York, 1961, Basic Books.

Cutillo-Schmitter T: Aging: broaden our view for improved nursing care, *J Gerontol Nurs* 22(7):31, 1996.

Day C: Validation therapy: a review of the literature, *J Gerontol Nurs* 23(4):29, 1997.

Ebersole P, Hess P: *Toward healthy aging: human needs and nursing response,* ed 5, St. Louis, 1998, Mosby.

Eliopoulos C: *Manual of gerontologic nursing,* ed 2, St. Louis, 1998, Mosby.

Emmett K: Nonspecific and atypical presentation of disease in the older patient, *Geriatrics* 53(2):50, 1998.

Ferrell B, Rivera L: Pain. In Lueckenotte A, editor: *Gerontologic nursing,* St. Louis, 1996, Mosby.

Fielo S, Rizzolo M: Handle with caring: meeting elderly client's special learning needs, *Nurs Health Care* 9(4):193, 1988.

Filley C: Alzheimer's disease: it's irreversible but not untreatable, *Geriatrics* 50(7):18, 1995.

Fishman P: *Healthy people 2000:* what progress toward better nutrition? *Geriatrics* 51(4):38, 1996.

Foreman M: A comparison of the clinical features of delirium, dementia, and depression, *Geriatr Nurs* 17(5):229, 1996.

Foreman M and others: Assessing cognitive function, *Geriatr Nurs* 17(5):228, 1996.

Gambert S: Alcohol abuse: medical effects of heavy drinking in late life, *Geriatrics* 52(6):30, 1997.

Gunnarsson O, Judge J: Exercise at midlife: how and why to prescribe it for sedentary patients, *Geriatrics* 52(5):71, 1997.

Guralnik J: Understanding the relationship between disease and disability, *J Am Geriatr Soc* 42:1128, 1994.

Happ M and others: Individualized care for frail elders: theory and practice, *J Gerontol Nurs* 22(3):7, 1996.

Hayes K: Randomized trial of geragogy-based medication instruction in the emergency department, *Nurs Res* 47:211, 1998.

Kessenich C, Rosen C: Osteoporosis: implications for elderly men, *Geriatr Nurs* 17(4):171, 1996.

Lee V, Burnett E: A case report: special needs of hospitalized elders, *Geriatr Nurs* 19:185, 1998.

Lehninger F, Ravindran V, Stewart J: Management strategies for problem behaviors in the patient with dementia, *Geriatrics* 53(4):55, 1998.

Lemon B, Bengston V, Peterson J: An exploration of the activity theory of aging: activity types and life satisfaction among inmovers to a retirement community, *J Gerontol* 27:516, 1972.

Lueckenotte A: Gerontologic assessment. In Lueckenotte A, editor: *Gerontologic nursing,* St. Louis, 1996a, Mosby.

Lueckenotte A: Overview of gerontologic assessment. In Lueckenotte A, editor: *Gerontologic nursing,* St. Louis, 1996b, Mosby.

Luft J, Vriheas-Nichols A: Identifying the risk factors for developing incontinence: can we modify individual risk? *Geriatr Nurs,* 19(2):66, 1998.

Maddox M: Theories of aging, In Lueckenotte A, editor: *Gerontologic Nursing,* St. Louis, 1996, Mosby.

Maklebust J: Pressure ulcers: decreasing the risk for older adults, *Geriatr Nurs* 18(6):250, 1997.

Neugarten B: *Personality in middle and late life,* New York, 1964, Atherton.

Puentes W: Incorporating simple reminiscence techniques into acute care nursing practice, *J Gerontol Nurs* 24(2):15, 1998.

Robinson B: Diagnosis of irreversible dementia: how extensive the evaluation? *Geriatrics* 53(1):49, 1998.

Rubenstein I, Nahas R: Primary and secondary prevention strategies in the older adult, *Geriatr Nurs* 19(1):11, 1998.

Russell B: Nosocomial infections, *Am J Nurs* 99(6):24J, 1999.

Santo-Novak D: Older adults' descriptions of their role expectations of nursing, *J Gerontol Nurs* 23(1):32, 1997.

Simon L, Jewell N, Brokel J: Management of acute delirium in hospitalized elderly: a process improvement project, *Geriatr Nurs* 18:150, 1997.

Sullivan D, Sun S, Walls R: Protein-energy undernutrition among elderly hospitalized patients, *JAMA* 281:2013, 1999.

Tibbitts G: Patients who fall: how to predict and prevent injuries, *Geriatrics* 51(9):24, 1996.

Tideiksaar R: Preventing falls: how to identify risk factors, reduce complications *Geriatrics* 61(2):43, 1996.

Tueth M: How to manage depression and psychosis in Alzheimer's disease, *Geriatrics* 50(1):43, 1995.

Wallace M: Touch and intimacy. In Lueckenotte A, editor: *Gerontologic nursing*, St. Louis, 1996, Mosby.

Wojciechowski C: Issues in caring for older lesbians, *J Gerontol Nurs* 24(7):28, 1998.

Yen P: Weight loss resulting from Alzheimer's disease, *Geriatr Nurs* 18(3):132, 1997.

Zimberg S: Treating alcoholism: an age-specific intervention that works for older patients, *Geriatrics* 51(10):45, 1996.

13

Critical Thinking and Nursing Judgment

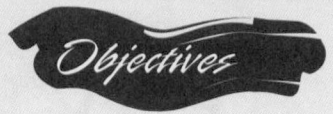

Mastery of content in this chapter will enable the student to:

- Define the key terms listed.
- Discuss the nurse's responsibility in making clinical decisions.
- Describe the components of a critical thinking model for clinical decision making.
- Discuss critical thinking skills used in nursing practice.
- Explain the relationship between clinical experience and critical thinking.
- Discuss the effect attitudes for critical thinking have on clinical decision making.
- Explain how professional standards influence a nurse's clinical decisions.
- Discuss the relationship between ethical nursing practice and critical thinking.
- Discuss how reflection can improve knowledge of nursing.
- Discuss the relationship of the nursing process to critical thinking.

Nurses in clinical practice face an endless variety of situations involving clients, family members, health care staff, and peers. Each situation poses new experiences with new problems involving clients' care, different approaches to resolving problems, and different perspectives on the best way to proceed. Within clinical situations, it is important for the nurse to think critically so that the client ultimately receives the very best nursing care. Critical thinking is not a simple step-by-step, linear process that can be learned overnight. It is a process that can be acquired only through hard work, commitment, and an active curiosity toward learning. Ideally, critical thinking becomes a habit of mind, a part of each nurse's character (Facione and Facione, 1996).

Clinical Decisions in Nursing Practice

Nurses have the important responsibility of making accurate and appropriate clinical decisions. Decision making is one skill that separates professional nurses from technical or ancillary personnel (Hughes and Young, 1992). When given the responsibility to assist persons in maintaining, regaining, or improving their health, a nurse must be able to think critically to problem solve and find the best solution for a client's needs. Most clients have problems for which there are no clear textbook solutions. Their clinical symptoms, the information clients share about themselves, and the situation in which the nurse meets them do not automatically present the nurse with a clear picture of the client's needs and what actions should be taken to meet those needs. Instead the nurse must learn to question, to wonder, and then to be self-directed in exploring

different perspectives and interpretations and finding one that can best help the client (Whiteside, 1997).

The nurse learns to adjust what she or he knows or needs to know to make appropriate clinical decisions. Nurses must learn how to make sense of what can be learned about a client, by reflecting on previous knowledge and experience, listening to other caregivers' views, identifying the nature of the client's problems, and selecting the best solutions for improving the client's health. Over time, the nurse gains the expertise to test and refine nursing approaches, to learn from successes and failures, and to apply new knowledge (e.g., nursing research findings). The ability to think critically through the application of knowledge and experience, problem solving, and decision making is central to professional nursing practice.

Clients present to the nurse various experiences, behaviors, social perspectives, values, and signs and symptoms of health alterations. To add to the complexity of clinical decision making, these variables can change while caring for a given client. In the presence of such variation, it is the nurse who observes the client closely, examines ideas and **inferences** about client problems, considers scientific principles relating to the problems, recognizes the problems, and develops an approach to care. The nurse thinks creatively, seeks new knowledge as necessary, acts quickly when events change, and makes sound decisions that promote the client's well-being. Even more importantly, every clinical experience becomes a lesson that informs the nurse about the next practice experience (Paul and Heaslip, 1995). No nursing action or interaction with a client is trivial or ordinary (Fox, 1980). Although the responsibility of making clinical decisions may seem frightening to a new student, it is what makes nursing a rewarding and challenging profession.

Critical Thinking Defined

Thinking and learning are interrelated, lifelong processes (Chaffee, 1994). As a person selects a career path, it is important for that individual to become more aware and skilled in thinking. Over time, the knowledge and practical experiences gained help individuals to broaden their ability to make thoughtful observations and judgments.

Critical thinking is the active, organized, cognitive process used to carefully examine one's thinking and the thinking of others (Chaffee, 1994). It involves use of the mind in forming conclusions, making decisions, drawing inferences, and reflecting (Gordon, 1995). It means taking nothing for granted. A critical thinker identifies and challenges assumptions, considers what is important in a situation, imagines and explores alternatives, applies reason and logic, and thus makes informed decisions. For a new student nurse, critical thinking begins when the student seriously questions, and in a continuing way tries to answer, again and again: "What do I really know about this nursing care situation and how do I know it?" (Paul and Heaslip, 1995). For example, "What do I really know about caring for an older adult, and how do I know it?"; "What do I really know about Mr. Yount's pain, and how do I know it?" Critical thinking presupposes a certain basic level of intellectual humility (e.g., acknowledging one's own ignorance) and a commitment to think clearly, precisely, and accurately and to act on the basis of genuine knowledge. When the nurse directs critical thinking toward understanding and assisting clients in finding solutions to their health problems, the process becomes purposeful and goal oriented.

The American Philosophical Association (APA) has recognized critical thinking to be purposeful and self-regulatory judgment that results in interpretation, analysis, evaluation, and inference (Facione, 1990). Through critical thinking, a person addresses problems, considers choices, and chooses an appropriate course of action. It is clear that critical thinking requires not only cognitive skills but a person's habit to ask questions, to remain well informed, to be honest in facing personal biases, and always to be willing to reconsider and think clearly about issues (Facione, 1990). The APA identified core critical thinking skills that when applied to nursing are useful in showing the complex nature of clinical decision making (Table 13-1). Being able to apply all of these skills takes experience and the thoughtful consideration of the knowledge gained in the clinical care of clients. Facione and Facione (1996) describe elements that increase the tendency to think critically in an ideal critical thinker (Box 13-1).

The nurse who is a good critical thinker faces problems without forming a quick, single solution and instead is focused on the options for what to believe and do (Kataoka-Yahiro and Saylor, 1994). This requires discipline to avoid premature decision making. Learning to think critically helps a nurse to care for clients as their advocate and to make better-informed choices about their care. Critical thinking is more than just solving problems, instead it is

Table 13-1	**Critical Thinking Skills Proposed by the American Philosophical Association**	
Skill	Description	Nursing Practice Applications
Interpretation	Categorization Decoding sentences Clarifying meaning	Be systematic in data collection. Look for patterns to categorize data (e.g., nursing diagnoses [see Chapter 15]). Clarify any data you are uncertain about.
Analysis	Examining ideas Identifying arguments Analyzing arguments	Be open minded as you look at information about a client. Do not make careless assumptions. Do the data reveal what you believe is true, or are there other options?
Evaluation	Assessing claims Assessing arguments	Look at all situations from an objective view. Use criteria (e.g., expected outcomes) to determine results of any actions or interactions. Reflect on your own behavior.
Inference	Examining evidence Speculating or conjecturing alternatives Making conclusions	Look at the meaning and significance of findings. Are there relationships between findings? Do the data about the client help you in seeing that a problem may exist?
Explanation	Stating results Justifying procedures Presenting arguments	Support your findings and conclusions. Use knowledge to select strategies you use in the care of clients.
Self-regulation	Self-examination Self-correction	Reflect on your experiences. Identify in what way you can improve your own performance. What will make you feel that you have been successful?

Data from Facione P: *Critical thinking: a statement of expert consensus for purposes of educational assessment and instruction. The Delphi report: research findings and recommendations prepared for the American Philosophical Association,* ERIC Doc No. ED 315-423, Washington, DC, 1990, ERIC.

> ## Dispositions Toward Critical Thinking
> Box 13-1
>
> *Being inquisitive:* eagerness to acquire knowledge
> *Being systematic:* valuing organization, focus, and diligence in any inquiry
> *Being analytical:* use of reason and evidence to resolve problems
> *Truth seeking:* honesty and objectivity with findings, even if they do not support one's own beliefs or preconceptions
> *Being open minded:* tolerance of divergent views
> *Critical thinking self-confidence:* trust in one's own reasoning powers
> *Cognitive maturity:* prudence in making, suspending, or revising judgment; recognition that some problems have more than one option

> ## Tips on Facilitating Critical Thinking
> Box 13-2
>
> - When possible, work alongside another nurse colleague and discuss with one another what was done for a client, how the client responded, and whether the nursing care was effective.
> - During a clinical conference focus on common health concerns that clients assigned to your clinical group have experienced (e.g., pain management, coping with crisis, impaired mobility). Discuss the significant features or characteristics of these health concerns.
> - Maintain a journal of your experiences with clients. Be sure to include these elements: identification, description, significance, and implications (Baker, 1996). Telling a story or drawing a picture are two ways to identify the situation or experience you wish to reflect on. Describe in detail what you felt, thought, and did. Analyze the significance of the experience by considering feelings, thoughts, and possible meanings. Describe the implications of the experience in terms of your own clinical practice or self-perceptions as a learner. Refer to the journal often when you care for clients in similar situations.
> - Talk with peers who have observed your clinical work. Ask if their observations are the same as yours.
> - Keep all written care plans or clinical papers. Use them frequently as a resource.
> - Take time to reflect, both after having cared for a client and before caring for new clients with similar conditions.
> - Discuss your experiences with colleagues with whom you are comfortable and whose decisions you trust.
> - Participate in videotaping of actual or simulated client encounters. Have an instructor guide discussion on approaches that were effective.

an attempt to continually improve. The nurse learns to focus on problem prevention and maximizing a client's potential (Alfaro-LeFevre, 1995). A critical thinker learns from each clinical experience and pursues each new opportunity with an openness and renewed purpose to excel in practice.

REFLECTION

One important aspect of critical thinking is **reflection** (Box 13-2). This is a process of thinking back or recalling an event to discover the meaning and purpose of that event (Miller and Babcock, 1996). As a nurse, reflection involves thinking back on a client situation or experience to explore the information and other factors that influenced the handling of the situation (Saylor, 1990). Reflection requires adequate knowledge and is necessary for self-evaluation, to review one's successes and mistakes. O'Neill and Dluhy (1997) caution that new clinicians should not question every judgment they make. An emphasis on reflection can deter thinking in a clinical situation because of the second-guessing it can create.

The process of reflection helps the nurse to seek and understand the relationships between concepts learned in the classroom and real-life clinical incidents. Reflection helps the nurse judge personal performance and make judgments about standards of practice. It is a process that helps make sense out of an experience and facilitates the incorporation of the experience into one's view of self as a professional (Baker, 1996).

Engaging in reflection is very individualized (Miller and Babcock, 1996). Not everyone reflects in the same way. Some individuals make mental pictures of the information they contemplate, some prefer quiet thought, whereas others may prefer to reflect on new knowledge by discussing it with others. Learning to be reflective takes practice. A nurse who chooses to reflect on a clinical experience must be open to new information and be able to look at the client's perspective as well as his or her own.

Learning from experience with clients can create an "aha" feeling, because reflection reveals behavior significant to the nurse's professional development. The worth of reflection is evident in the actions that result from it (Dewey, 1933). Through reflection, the nurse recognizes that the actions taken were either successful or unsuccessful. The next time a similar experience arises, the nurse uses approaches that were successful or revises an approach to ensure a successful outcome.

One common approach to reflection is journaling. A clinical journal is an objective and subjective chronicle that reflects a student's attitudes, feelings, and cognitive learning throughout a clinical experience (Callister, 1993). The student keeps a written record, similar to a diary, of clinical experiences and/or interactions with colleagues. Writing journal entries assists a student nurse in developing observation skills and describing clinical practice (Heinrich, 1992). It also helps a student to define more clearly the meaning of any critical incidents (Patton and others, 1997). The journal can become a rich resource for the student to revisit important experiences and gain insight into the thoughts and actions that make up clinical practice.

LANGUAGE

Another important aspect of critical thinking is the use of language. Thinking and language are closely related processes. The ability to use language is closely associated with the ability to think meaningfully (Miller and Babcock, 1996). To become a critical thinker, a nurse must be able to use language precisely and clearly. When language is sloppy (vague, inaccurate), it reflects similar thinking.

As nurses care for clients it becomes important not only to communicate clearly with clients and families but then to be able to clearly communicate findings to other health professionals. When a nurse uses incorrect terminology, jargon, or vague descriptions, communication is ineffective. This may become obvious if the client is unable to cooperate with nursing therapies or if members of the nursing team do not follow through on the nurse's recommendations. Critical thinking requires a framing of one's thoughts so that the focus and resultant message are clear. It helps to reflect on one's language and to consider whether what one communicates expresses an idea, position, or judgment precisely and clearly.

INTUITION

Expertise in nursing involves the ability to think critically about the knowledge required for a client's care and the knowledge the nurse brings to a nursing care situation. A knowledgeable nurse who enters into a client encounter immediately and intuitively recognizes the importance of the nursing care situation (Paul and Heaslip, 1995). Each clinical experience is a lesson for the next one. The expert nurse practices intuitively on the basis of a deep knowledge base that is applied in daily practice.

Intuition is the "immediate apprehension that something is so without benefit of conscious reasoning" (Guralnik, 1972). It is a common experience that all persons have after interacting with their environments. A nurse gains intuitive knowledge by learning to describe accurately in precise nursing language the common client responses in nursing care situations (Paul and Heaslip, 1995). For example, an experienced neurosurgical nurse may enter the room of a head injury client and know immediately if the client's behavior change suggests an increase in intracranial pressure. This is known intuitively, without benefit of a blood pressure measure or intracranial monitoring data. Similarly, a home health nurse may know by looking at a client's expression and a quick check of the surroundings that the client is likely depressed. This is known intuitively, without benefit of a detailed assessment of the client's mood or recent behaviors. At a moment's notice these nurses have knowledge available to them without having to exercise conscious reasoning.

What is important to remember is that quality nursing practice does not depend solely on intuition. Just as it is critical to know what knowledge we have, it is even more critical to know what we do not know. If nurses do not recognize how much they do not know in relation to what they do know, then they are courting malpractice and endangering the health and well-being of their clients (Paul and Heaslip, 1995).

Each clinical situation must be carefully thought through. Even if a nurse believes intuitively that a client is experiencing an expected change, it is important to confirm that finding through appropriate clinical observations and measurements. The neurosurgical nurse will assess the client's level of consciousness, measure the blood pressure and intracranial pressure readings, and note what medications have been given in the last hour. Thoughtful analysis of what the nurse knows, plus a review of the most current clinical data, allows the nurse to make an accurate and sound clinical decision. Prejudices, biases, and failure to acknowledge one's limitations do not result in thoughtful, professional practice.

Levels of Critical Thinking in Nursing

As a nurse gains new knowledge and matures into a competent professional, the ability to critically think expands. Kataoka-Yahiro and Saylor (1994) identify three levels of critical thinking in nursing: basic, complex, and commitment.

At the basic level of critical thinking a learner trusts that experts have the right answers for every problem. Thinking is concrete and based on a set of rules or principles. For example, a nurse uses an institution's procedure manual to confirm how to insert a foley catheter. The student nurse follows the procedure step-by-step without adjusting the procedure to meet a client's unique needs (e.g., positioning to accommodate the client's pain). For basic critical thinkers, answers to complex problems are either right or wrong, and one right answer usually exists for each problem. This is an early step in the development of reasoning ability (Kataoka-Yahiro and Saylor, 1994), revealing that the individual has had limited experience in critical thinking. Despite the tendency to be governed by others, a person learns to accept the diverse opinions and values of experts (e.g., instructors, staff nurse role models). Inexperience, weak competencies, and inflexible attitudes can restrict a person's ability to move to the next level of critical thinking.

In the complex level of critical thinking a person begins to detach from authorities and analyze and examine alternatives more independently. Kataoka-Yahiro and Saylor (1994) note that the nurse's best answer to a problem at this level is "It depends." The person's thinking abilities and initiative begin to change. A nurse realizes that alternative, perhaps conflicting, solutions do exist. Consider the case of Mr. Rosen, a 36-year-old man who underwent hip surgery. The client is having pain but refusing his ordered analgesic. His physician is concerned the client will not progress as planned, delaying rehabilitation. In discussing the importance of rehabilitation with Mr. Rosen, the nurse realizes the client's conviction to avoid taking pain medication. The nurse learns that the client practices meditation at home and decides to discuss this as an option with the client for pain control.

In complex critical thinking each solution has benefits and risks that the nurse weighs before making a final decision. There are options. Thinking can become more creative and innovative. There is a willingness to consider deviations from standard protocols or policies when complex situations develop. Nurses learn a variety of different approaches for the same therapy.

The third level of critical thinking is commitment. The individual anticipates the need to make choices without assistance from others and then assumes accountability for them. At this level the nurse does more than just consider the complex alternatives a problem poses. At the commitment level, the nurse chooses an action or belief based on the alternatives available and stands by it. Sometimes an action may be no action, or the nurse may choose to delay an action until a later time but does so as a result of experience and knowledge. Because the nurse assumes accountability for the decision, attention is given to the results of the decision and a determination of whether it was appropriate. Committed critical thinkers act in support of the client and support of the professional beliefs that underlie the discipline of nursing.

Critical Thinking Competencies

Critical thinking competencies are the cognitive processes a nurse uses to make judgments. There are three types of competencies: general critical thinking, specific critical thinking in clinical situations, and specific critical thinking in nursing (Kataoka-Yahiro and Saylor, 1994). General critical thinking processes include the **scientific method, problem solving,** and **decision making.** General critical

thinking competencies are not unique to nursing but are used in other disciplines and in nonclinical situations. Specific critical thinking competencies in clinical situations include **diagnostic reasoning,** clinical inferences, and clinical decision making. These competencies are used by physicians, social workers, nurses, and other health care professionals in deciding about the clinical care and support of clients. The specific critical thinking competency in nursing is the **nursing process.** The format for the nursing process is unique to nursing and offers one approach to critical thinking in clinical decision making.

SCIENTIFIC METHOD

The scientific method is one approach to reasoning that is used in nursing, medicine, and a variety of other disciplines. It is a process that moves from observable facts of experience to reasonable explanations of those facts (Bandman and Bandman, 1995). It is an approach to verify that a set of facts agree with reality. Components of the scientific method are summarized in Table 13-2. Some nurse researchers use the scientific method when testing research questions in nursing practice situations. For example, a nurse researcher might observe that terminally ill clients in a hospice program often have difficulty communicating their feelings to family members. After interviewing family members, the nurse learns more about what causes this problem and considers the possibility that family members might have poor communication skills. The nurse asks the question, "Can family members who receive instruction on communication principles provide support to loved ones with a terminal illness?" The nurse might design a study that involves formal instruction in communication skills and uses a support group to help family members practice and apply the skills. Once the course is completed, the nurse may ask clients to interpret their feelings about communication with loved ones. The nurse hopes that results from the study will give other nurses working in hospice settings useful approaches for improving family communication. The scientific method is one formal way to approach a problem, plan a solution, test the solution, and come to a conclusion.

Table 13-2 **Steps of the Scientific Method**	
Step	Example in Practice
Identify the problem to be investigated.	Family members have difficulty communicating with a dying loved one.
Collect data about the problem.	Review previous studies about grieving families. Review literature on methods for improving communication. Talk with dying clients about feelings they think are important to communicate.
Formulate a hypothesis to explain the problem.	Family members who receive instruction on ways to communicate with dying loved ones will be perceived as more supportive by the dying family member.
Test the hypothesis through experimentation.	Include family members in a group session on communication approaches. Have the family members use the new approaches when communicating with their dying loved ones.
Evaluate the hypothesis.	Interview the clients to determine if they perceive family members to be more supportive.

PROBLEM SOLVING

Problem solving involves obtaining information and using information to reach acceptable solutions when there is a gap between what is occurring and what should be occurring. When a person starts to water the lawn and finds that the water is not flowing from the nozzle, a quick problem-solving approach involves looking for kinks in the hose. An example of problem solving in a clinical situation might involve a nurse entering a client's room and finding the client lying in a twisted manner. The nurse knows that the client underwent back surgery and is supposed to remain in as straight an anatomical alignment as possible to avoid stress on the surgical area. The nurse suspects the client is having pain but instead learns quickly through questioning that he is uncomfortably cold. The nurse repositions the client and provides an additional blanket for warmth. Returning to the client's room 30 minutes later, the nurse finds the client asleep. The nurse obtained information that clarified the client's source of discomfort and tested a solution that was successful. Effective problem solving also involves the nurse evaluating a solution over time to be sure that it is still effective. It may become necessary to try different options if a problem recurs. Having solved a problem in one situation allows the nurse to apply that knowledge to future client situations.

DECISION MAKING

In decision making, a person is faced with a problem or situation where a choice must be made as to a course of action. Decision making is an end point of critical thinking that leads to problem resolution. For example, decision making occurs when a person decides on the choice of a physician. To make a decision, an individual must recognize and define the problem or situation (need for a physician to provide medical care), assess all options (consider recommended physicians or choose one whose office is close to home), weigh each option against a set of criteria (experience, friendliness, reputation), test possible options (talk directly with the physicians), consider the consequences of the decision (examine pros and cons of selecting one physician over another), and then make a final decision. Although the set of criteria seem to follow a sequence of steps, decision making involves moving back and forth in considering all criteria. Using such a process leads to a conclusion that is informed and supported by evidence and by reasons (Bandman and Bandman, 1995). Another example involves a nurse deciding on a choice of dressings for a client with a surgical wound. Several criteria are usually considered when selecting a dressing: location and size of the wound, presence and type of drainage, and whether an infection is present. The nurse considers all available options of the dressing materials, which ones will be most effective given the client's wound status, and the extent to which the client will be mobile and applying stress to the dressing. The nurse may actually try different dressings over the course of a day before making the final

choice. The nurse's ability to decide on the type of dressing is based on knowledge, experience, and an assessment of this particular client's unique needs. Use of all of this information increases the likelihood of a sound decision.

DIAGNOSTIC REASONING AND INFERENCES

As soon as a nurse receives information about a client in a particular clinical situation, diagnostic reasoning begins. It is a process of determining a client's health status (O'Neill and Dluhy, 1997). For example, a client may present symptoms that can be indicative of dementia and depression. The nurse must retrieve knowledge regarding symptoms and then reason in a direct and precise way to determine the nature of the client's problem. Diagnostic reasoning enables the nurse to assign meaning to the behaviors, physical signs, and reported client symptoms. The process involves a series of clinical judgments made during and after data collection, resulting in an informal judgment or formal diagnosis (Carnevali and Thomas, 1993). Formulating a nursing diagnosis (see Chapter 15) is an example of diagnostic reasoning. Another example of diagnostic reasoning involves the nurse who makes ongoing clinical assessments on the basis of a client's known medical problem. Nurses do not make medical diagnoses, but they do monitor clients closely and compare their signs and symptoms with those that are common to a diagnosis. This process assists in making clinical inferences or judgments about a client's progress. When certain symptoms present themselves, the nurse considers all variables influencing the client in addition to the medical diagnosis and then infers if the client is doing better or worse.

Consider this clinical example. Mrs. Spellman had a myocardial infarction (heart attack) just 10 months ago. She must periodically be monitored for possible chest pain, shortness of breath, and/or irregularity of vital signs (signs and symptoms of recurrent cardiac problems). If Mrs. Spellman has a regular heart rate, denies discomfort, and is breathing normally without difficulty, the nurse makes a diagnostic decision that the client's cardiac status is currently stable. The nurse must critically analyze changing clinical situations so that a client's status can immediately be determined. This allows the nurse to initiate appropriate therapies, for example, activity restriction, so that the client's condition does not worsen. In addition, any diagnostic conclusions made by the nurse will help the physician pinpoint the nature of a problem more quickly and select proper medical therapies.

CLINICAL DECISION MAKING

When a nurse approaches a clinical problem, such as a client who has an injury to the skin or who is anxious about having surgery, a decision must be made on choosing the best approach for reaching a mutually desired goal. This may mean minimizing the severity of the problem, or it might mean resolving the problem completely. The clinical-decision-making process requires thoughtful reasoning so that the best options for the client are chosen on the basis of the client's condition and the priority of the problem. Nurses make clinical decisions all of the time in an attempt to improve a client's health or to maintain ongoing wellness.

When making clinical decisions, the nurse first asks why a decision is necessary. For example, Mrs. Little is an 87-year-old client who lives alone. Her daughter, Marie, lives just a few minutes away and is Mrs. Little's primary caregiver. During a recent clinic visit the nurse, Ruth, observes a bruised area of the skin over Mrs. Little's right hip. Mrs. Little describes it as a scrape that she received when she slipped on the edge of her bathtub. Knowing the client's age and the physiological changes that occur with aging, Ruth knows a decision is needed about whether Mrs. Little is living in a safe environment. Ruth must also make decisions about what actions are needed to promote healing and prevent further injury. Before a decision can be made Ruth must take into account the client's home environment and whether repeated injuries have been part of the client's history.

Strader (1992) notes that criteria for decision making must be established so that the appropriate choices can be made. Criteria should include the following:

What needs to be achieved? (healing of the skin, a safe home environment)

What needs to be preserved? (mobility, nutrition, and comfort, and safety)

What needs to be avoided? (further tissue injury or infection and further falls)

After considering each of the criteria, the nurse sets priorities as they relate to the client's situation (see Chapter 16). Because different clients bring different variables to a situation, an activity may be more of a priority in one situation and less of a priority in another. For example, if a client is physically dependent, unable to eat, and incontinent of urine, the nurse recognizes skin integrity as a greater priority than if the client were immobile but continent of urine and able to eat a normal diet. The nurse must not assume that a certain condition is an automatic priority. For example, a client who has surgery is anticipated to experience a certain level of pain, which often becomes a priority of nursing care. However, if the client is experiencing severe anxiety that heightens pain perception, it may become necessary to focus on ways to relive the anxiety before pain relief measures can be effective.

After determining the order of priority of the client's problems, the nurse chooses the nursing interventions most likely to relieve each problem. A wide range of choices may be available from nurse-administered interventions to client self-care strategies. The nurse collaborates with the client and then selects, tests, and evaluates each approach. The nurse tries to anticipate what might go wrong and considers alternative approaches to minimize or prevent problems. For example, Ruth will talk with Mrs. Little's daughter about having someone check the condition of Mrs. Little's bathroom to see if there are any obstacles creating a risk for falls. A complete home safety assessment would be most helpful. Based on the findings, Ruth makes recommendations to Marie on ways to minimize any hazards or obstacles so that further injury is less likely.

Nurses make decisions about individual clients, and they also make decisions about groups of clients. A nurse who works on a busy hospital unit is likely to care for several clients. The nurse uses criteria such as the clinical condition of the client, risks involved in treatment delays, and the clients' expectations of care to determine which clients have the greatest priorities for care. For example, a client who is having a sudden drop in blood pressure along with a change in consciousness requires the nurse's attention immediately as opposed to the client who needs to be assisted for a walk down the hallway. The nurse visits the client who has had no visitors and has recently been given a diagnosis of cancer before checking on the recovering surgical client whose family has just arrived. For nurses to be able to manage the wide variety of problems associated with groups of clients (Box 13-3), skillful, prioritized decision making is critical.

NURSING PROCESS AS A COMPETENCY

Nurses apply the nursing process as a competency when delivering client care. The nursing process consists of five steps: assessment, diagnosis, planning, implementation, and evaluation. Specifically, the process is a systematic approach that is used by nurses to gather client data, critically examine and analyze the data, identify the client's response to a health problem, design expected outcomes, take appropriate action, and then evaluate whether the action is effective. The process incorporates general and specific critical thinking competencies in a manner that focuses on a particular client's unique needs. The format for the nursing process is unique to the discipline of nursing and provides a common language and process for nurses to "think through" clients' clinical problems (Kataoka-Yahiro and Saylor, 1994). The nursing process is a systematic and comprehensive approach for nursing care.

Clinical Decision Making for Groups of Clients   Box 13-3

Identify the problems of each client.

Compare clients and determine which problems are most urgent on the basis of basic needs, the client's changing or unstable status, and problem complexity.

Anticipate the time it will take to attend to priority problems.

Decide how to combine activities to resolve more than one problem at a time.

Consider how to involve the client as a decision maker and participant in care.

Thinking and Learning

Learning is a lifelong process. Our intellectual and emotional growth involve acquiring new knowledge and refining the ability to think, problem solve, and make judgments. To learn one must be flexible and always open to new information. The science of nursing is growing rapidly, and there will always be new information for nurses to apply in practice. Learning and thinking are inseparable. Over time, as nurses have new experiences and apply the knowledge gained, they become better able to form assumptions, present ideas, and make valid conclusions.

A professional nurse must learn to think and to anticipate. This involves looking ahead and asking, What is a client's status, how might it change, and how can nursing knowledge be applied to improve the client's condition? A nurse cannot allow thinking to become routine or standardized. Instead, a nurse learns to look beyond the obvious, recognizing that each client is unique. This does not mean that the nurse knows nothing about a client until having met him or her. A nurse's experience with other clients aids in recognizing patterns of behavior, seeing commonalities in signs and symptoms, and anticipating reactions to therapies. Thinking about those experiences enables the nurse to better anticipate client needs and recognize problems when they develop.

Nursing practice is always changing. As new knowledge becomes available, professional nurses must challenge traditional ways of doing things and discover those interventions that are most effective, have scientific relevance, and result in better client outcomes. The nurse's ability to think critically demonstrates a commitment to learning and enhances the ability to positively influence nursing practice.

Critical Thinking Model

Models serve to explain concepts. Because critical thinking and clinical decision making are complex, a model can help to explain all of the factors involved in making decisions and judgments about clients. Kataoka-Yahiro and Saylor (1994) have developed a model of critical thinking for nursing judgment (Figure 13-1). The model defines the outcome of critical thinking as nursing judgment that is relevant to nursing problems in a variety of settings. According to the model, when a nurse enters into any clinical experience there are five components of critical thinking that lead the nurse to make the clinical judgments that are necessary for safe, effective, nursing care (Box 13-4).

SPECIFIC KNOWLEDGE BASE

The first component of critical thinking is the nurse's specific knowledge base. This varies according to the nurse's educational experience, including basic nursing education, continuing education courses, and additional college de-

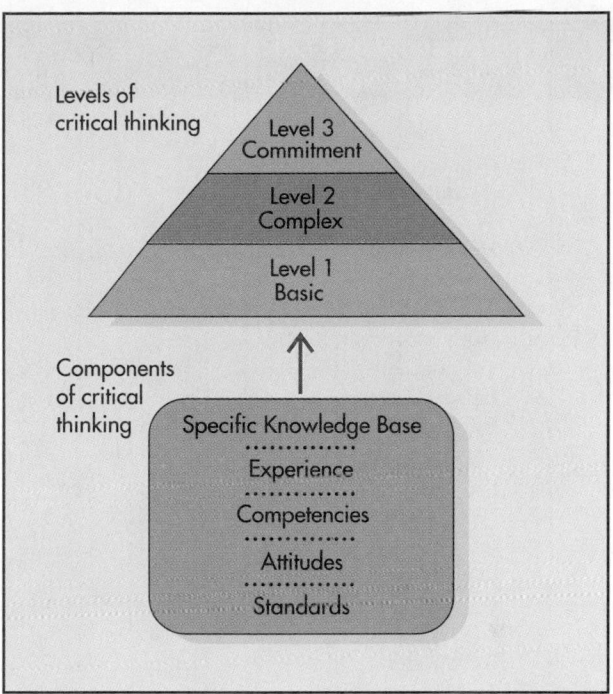

Figure 13-1   Critical thinking model for nursing judgment. Redrawn from Kataoka-Yahiro M, Saylor C: A critical thinking model for nursing judgment, *J Nurs Educ* 33(8):351, 1994. Modified from Glaser, 1941; Miller and Malcolm, 1990; Paul, 1993; and Perry, 1970.

grees that the nurse may pursue. A nurse's knowledge base includes information and theory from the basic sciences, humanities, and nursing. Nurses utilize their knowledge base in a unique way from other health care disciplines regarding how they think about client problems. The broad knowledge base gives the nurse a more holistic view of clients and their health care needs. The depth and extent of knowledge influence the nurse's ability to think critically about nursing problems (Figure 13-2).

Consider this clinical example: Robert Perez previously earned a degree in education and taught high school for 1 year. He is just starting his third year of study in his nursing program. He has successfully completed his required courses in the sciences, health ethics, introduction to nursing concepts, and communication principles. His first clinical course is in health promotion with a clinical assignment on a general medicine clinic. Although still a novice to nursing, his preparation and knowledge base will help him in knowing how to interview clients and begin to make clinical decisions about clients' health promotion practices.

EXPERIENCE

The second component of the critical thinking model is experience in nursing. Unless a nurse has the opportunity to practice and make decisions about client care, critical

Components of Critical Thinking in Nursing   Box 13-4

I. Specific knowledge base in nursing
II. Experience in nursing
III. Critical thinking competencies
    A. General critical thinking competencies
    B. Specific critical thinking competencies in clinical situations
    C. Specific critical thinking competency in nursing
IV. Attitudes for critical thinking
    A. Confidence   G. Perseverance
    B. Independence   H. Creativity
    C. Fairness   I. Curiosity
    D. Responsibility   J. Integrity
    E. Risk taking   K. Humility
    F. Discipline
V. Standards for critical thinking
    A. Intellectual standards
        1. Clear   9. Deep
        2. Precise   10. Broad
        3. Specific   11. Complete
        4. Accurate 12. Significant
        5. Relevant   13. Adequate
        6. Plausible   (for purpose)
        7. Consistent 14. Fair
        8. Logical
    B. Professional standards
        1. Ethical criteria for nursing judgment
        2. Criteria for evaluation
        3. Professional responsibility

Modified from Kataoka-Yahiro M, Saylor C: A critical thinking model for nursing judgment, *J Nurs Educ* 33(8):351, 1994.
Data from Paul R: The art of redesigning instruction. In Willsen J, Blinker AJA, editors: *Critical thinking: how to prepare students for a rapidly changing world*, Santa Rosa, Calif, 1993, Foundation for Critical Thinking.

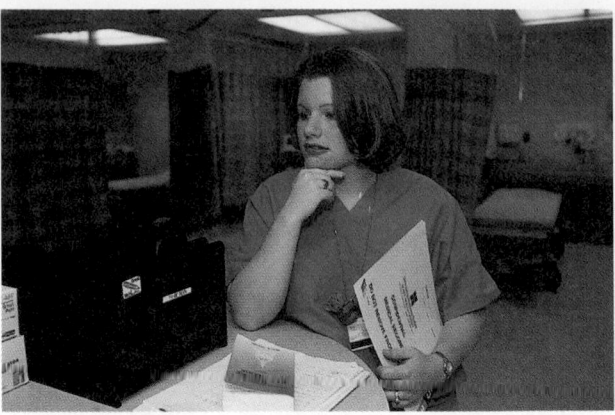

Figure 13-2 The nurse utilizes a broad knowledge base to think critically about nursing problems.

thinking in clinical decision making will not develop. A nurse learns from observing, sensing, talking with the client, and then reflecting actively on the experience. Clinical experience is the laboratory for testing nursing knowledge. The nurse will learn that "textbook" approaches lay important groundwork for practice, but adaptations or revisions in approaches must be made to accommodate the setting, the unique qualities of the client, and the experience the nurse has gained from using the approaches for previous clients. Benner (1984) notes that the expert nurse understands the context of a clinical situation, recognizes cues suggesting patterns, and interprets them as relevant or irrelevant. This level of competency comes only from experience. Perhaps the best lesson to be learned by a new nursing student is to value all client experiences, which become stepping-stones for building new knowledge and stimulating innovative thinking.

During the previous summer, Robert worked as a nurse assistant in a nursing home. This experience provided him with valuable time spent in interacting with older adult clients and in giving basic nursing care. As Robert thinks about his clinical experience at the clinic, he recognizes he still has a lot to learn. However, each client has provided him valuable learning experiences. Specifically, he has been able to acquire good interviewing skills and understand the importance of the family in an individual's health, and he has learned the role nurses play as advocates for clients. His time in the physical assessment laboratory and the time he worked in the nursing home have helped him begin to be a watchful observer. Robert also knows that his previous experience as a teacher will help him apply educational principles in his nursing role.*

CRITICAL THINKING COMPETENCIES

The model for critical thinking includes the competencies discussed on p. 278. When the nurse is involved in the clinical care of clients, the specific critical thinking competency utilized is the nursing process.

ATTITUDES FOR CRITICAL THINKING

The fourth component of the critical thinking model is attitudes. Paul (1993) has identified 11 attitudes that are central features of a critical thinker (see Box 13-4). These attitudes are the values that an individual must practice or show to be a successful critical thinker. Attitudes of inquiry involve an ability to recognize that problems exist and to accept the general need for evidence in support of what is asserted to be true (Watson and Glaser, 1980). Critical thinking attitudes offer guidelines for how to approach a problem or decision-making situation. An important part of critical thinking is interpreting, evaluating, and making judgments about the adequacy of various arguments and available data. Knowing when more information is needed, knowing when information is misleading, and recognizing one's own knowledge limits are examples of how critical thinking attitudes play a key role in eventual decision making. Table 13-3 summarizes how critical thinking attitudes can be applied in nursing practice.

Confidence. To be confident is to feel certain in one's ability to accomplish a task or goal. Confidence grows with experience and a maturity in recognizing one's strengths and limitations. Confidence is not arrogance or the feeling of superiority. Instead confident critical thinkers remain aware of the balance between what they know and what they do not know. Critical thinkers have a realistic view of the knowledge and experience they bring to situations, a condition that promotes confidence. Clients recognize nurses who are confident in their decisions by the manner in which they speak and in the way they perform their responsibilities. Confidence builds trust between the nurse and client and is often instrumental in achieving client outcomes.

Thinking Independently. As persons mature and gain new knowledge, they learn to consider a wide range of ideas and concepts before forming an opinion or making a judgment. This does not mean they discount other people's ideas. All sides of a given situation should be considered. However, a critical thinker does not accept another person's ideas without question. To think independently, one challenges the ways others think and looks for rational and logical answers to problems. Independent thinking and reasoning is essential to the improvement and expansion of nursing practice.

Fairness. A critical thinker deals with situations in a just manner. This means that bias or prejudice does not enter into a decision. For example, regardless of how a nurse feels about obesity, he or she should not allow personal attitudes to influence the way care is delivered to a client who is overweight. Fairness helps one to look at a situation objectively, analyzing all viewpoints, to understand the situation completely before arriving at a decision.

Responsibility and Accountability. When caring for clients, a nurse has a responsibility to perform nursing care activities correctly based upon standards of practice, the minimum level of performance accepted to ensure high-quality care. Part of a professional nurse's responsibility is remaining competent in performing nursing ther-

Table 13-3 Critical Thinking Attitudes and Applications in Nursing Practice

Critical Thinking Attitude	Application in Practice
Confidence	Learn how to introduce yourself to a client. Speak with conviction when you begin a treatment or procedure. Do not lead a client to think that you are uncertain of being able to perform care safely. Always be prepared before performing a nursing activity.
Thinking independently	Read the nursing literature, especially when there are different views on the same subject. Talk with colleagues and share ideas about nursing interventions.
Fairness	Listen to both sides in any discussion. If a client or family member complains about a colleague, listen to the story and then speak with the colleague as well. Weigh all facts.
Responsibility and authority	Ask for help if you are uncertain about an aspect of client care. Report any problems immediately. Follow standards of practice in your care.
Risk taking	If your knowledge causes you to question a physician's order, do so. Offer alternative approaches to nursing care when colleagues are having little success with clients.
Discipline	Be thorough in whatever you do. Use known criteria for activities such as assessment and evaluation. Take time to be thorough.
Perseverance	Be wary of an easy answer. If colleagues give you information about a client, and some fact seems to be missing, go clarify information or talk to the client directly. If problems of the same type continue to occur on a nursing division, bring colleagues together, look for a pattern, and find a solution.
Creativity	Look for different approaches if interventions are not working. A client may need a different positioning technique or a different instructional approach that will suit his or her unique needs.
Curiosity	Always ask "why." A clinical sign or symptom can indicate a variety of problems. Explore and learn more about the client so as to make the right clinical judgments.
Integrity	Recognize when your opinions may conflict with those of a client; review your position, and decide how best to proceed to reach mutually beneficial outcomes.
Humility	Recognize when you need more information to make a decision. When you are newly assigned to a clinical division and you are unfamiliar with the clients, ask to be oriented to the area. Ask RNs regularly assigned to the area for assistance. Read the professional journals regularly to keep updated on new approaches to care.

apies and in making clinical decisions about clients. A nurse who intervenes for a client must be answerable or accountable for the results of any nursing actions. An accountable nurse is reliable and willing to recognize when nursing care is ineffective. Nurses demonstrate their responsibility and accountability in making decisions in response to a client's rights, needs, and interests. Ultimately, the nurse assumes accountability for whatever decisions and resultant actions are made on the client's behalf.

Risk Taking.   When a person takes a risk in an action or decision, it often is perceived that a loss may be at stake. Driving 30 miles an hour over the speed limit is a risk that might result in injury to the driver and an unlucky pedestrian. But risk taking does not have to cause injury. Risk taking can be desirable, particularly when the result is a positive outcome. A critical thinker is willing to take risks in trying different approaches to solving problems. The willingness to take risks often comes from experience with similar problems. In nursing, risk taking frequently results in client care innovations. Nurses in the past have taken risks in trying different approaches to skin and wound care, pulmonary hygiene, and pain management, to name a few. When taking a risk, the nurse considers all options, analyzes any potential danger to a client, and then acts in a well-reasoned, logical, and thoughtful manner.

Discipline.   To be a good critical thinker one must use discipline. A disciplined thinker misses few details and follows an orderly approach when making decisions or taking action. For example, Chapter 42 describes how an in-depth assessment of a client's pain ensures the selection of the most appropriate nursing interventions. Disciplined thinking does not lessen a person's creativity, rather it ensures that any decision is made systematically with a comprehensive approach.

Perseverance.   A critical thinker is determined to find effective solutions to client care problems. This is especially important when problems remain unresolved or when they reoccur. The nurse learns as much as possible about a problem, tries various approaches to care, and continues to seek additional resources until a successful approach is found. A critical thinker who perseveres is not satisfied with minimal effort. Achieving the highest level of quality in care is important.

Creativity.   Creativity involves original thinking. This means finding solutions outside of standard, acceptable procedure. Miller and Babcock (1996) describe creativity as a great motivator that enables one to generate options and alternative approaches and to see the future. Often clients pose problems that require unique approaches. A client's clinical problems, social support systems, and living environment are just a few examples of factors that can make the simplest nursing procedure more compli-

cated if the nurse does not consider a creative approach for the client's situation.

Curiosity.   Probably the favorite question of a critical thinker is, "Why?" In any clinical situation, a nurse learns a great deal of information about a client. As the nurse analyzes client information, data patterns emerge that are not always clear. Having a sense of curiosity motivates the nurse to inquire further and to investigate a clinical situation so that all the information needed to make a decision is obtained.

Integrity.   Critical thinkers question and test personal knowledge and beliefs as rigorously as they test the knowledge and beliefs of others. Personal integrity builds trust from peers and subordinates. A person of integrity is honest and willing to admit to any mistakes or inconsistencies in his or her own ideas and beliefs. Critical thinkers strive to adhere to high standards of practice even in the face of adversity.

Humility.   It is important to admit one's own limitations in knowledge and skills. Critical thinkers admit what they do not know and try to acquire the knowledge needed to make a proper decision. A client's safety and welfare may be at risk if a nurse is unable to admit to his or her inability to deal with a practice problem. The nurse must rethink a situation, pursue additional knowledge, and then use the information to form an opinion, draw a conclusion, and take action.

STANDARDS FOR CRITICAL THINKING

The fifth component of critical thinking includes intellectual and professional standards. These standards are the criteria for determining the soundness, justness, and appropriateness of critical decisions and judgments.

Intellectual Standards.   Paul (1993) identified 14 intellectual standards (see Box 13-4) that are universal for critical thinking. When a nurse considers a client problem, it is important to apply standards such as preciseness, accuracy, and consistency to ensure that clinical decisions are sound or valid.

For example, during a clinic visit Mrs. Lamar is examined by Robert, who finds an ulcer on the client's left foot. A quick check of the client's medical record reveals a description of the ulcer from a clinic visit 2 weeks earlier. The client is receiving a topical medication for the ulcer. To be consistent in his assessment, Robert uses the same assessment criteria applied during the last examination. He methodically inspects the affected area of the skin, asks if the client is experiencing discomfort, measures the size of the ulcer, and notes the appearance of any drainage. The wound location and appearance are described in Mrs. Lamar's medical record using specific anatomical terms. Robert examines Mrs. Lamar further to ensure that his findings are accurate and to determine if any other ulcers are present. He adds an assessment of the client's ability to ambulate, knowing that the ulcer could impair function. By applying appropriate intellectual standards, Robert is able to determine that the ulcer is healing and has improved since the last visit.

The use of intellectual standards involves a rigorous approach to clinical practice and demonstrates that critical thinking cannot be done haphazardly.

Professional Standards.   Professional standards for critical thinking refer to ethical criteria for nursing judgments (see Chapter 20), criteria to be used for evaluation, and criteria for professional responsibility. Application of professional standards requires that nurses use critical thinking for the good of individuals or groups (Kataoka-Yahiro and Saylor, 1994). Standards also ensure that the highest level of quality is promoted.

The conscientiousness and caring that nurses display are often a reflection of their ethical standards. Client care requires more than just the application of scientific knowledge. Being able to focus on a client's values and beliefs helps a nurse to make clinical decisions that are just, faithful to the client's choices, and beneficial to the client's well-being. Critical thinkers maintain a sense of self-awareness through conscious awareness of their beliefs, values, feelings, and the multiple perspectives that clients, family members, staff, and peers present in clinical situations (Ludwick and Sedlak, 1998).

Critical thinking also requires the use of criteria for evaluation when clinical judgments are made. These criteria may be based on standards of nursing care, recognized in the professional literature or developed by clinical agencies or professional organizations. The evaluation criteria set the minimum requirements necessary to ensure quality of care. For example, CareMaps (see Chapter 2) used in managing the care of clients with designated medical diagnoses include recommended interventions and outcomes that are used for evaluating the client's clinical progress. The outcomes provide evaluation criteria with which clinical staff can make sound and consistent judgments. Evaluation criteria also include norms established through research in nursing practice to be used when determining the clinical status of a client. Box 13-5 summarizes types of evaluation criteria nurses commonly use in their daily practice.

The standards of professional responsibility that a nurse strives to achieve are those standards cited in nurse practice acts, national regulatory and treatment guidelines, institutional practice guidelines, and professional organizations' standards of practice. The American Nurses Association Standards of Care (see Chapter 19) and the Agency for Health Care Policy and Research (AHCPR) treatment guidelines for pressure ulcers (see Chapter 47) are examples. These standards "raise the bar" for the responsibilities and accountabilities that a nurse must assume in guaranteeing quality health care to the public.

Critical Thinking Synthesis

Critical thinking is a reasoning process by which individuals reflect on and analyze their own thoughts, actions, and decisions and those of others (Ludwick and Sedlak, 1998). As was described earlier, critical thinking is nonlinear. In other words, it is not simply a prescribed series of ordered steps that one follows to make a decision. A critical thinker applies one critical thinking skill almost simultaneously while thinking about the outcomes of other critical thinking skills and addressing the problem at hand (Facione and Facione, 1996). For example, while assessing a client's current pain, a nurse must analyze his or her interpretation of the source of pain, analyze the relevance of the pain to the client's overall clinical situation, and evaluate the consequences of treatment choices. Critical thinking is ongoing with information being analyzed from many sources.

The nursing process is the traditional critical thinking competency that allows nurses to make clinical judgments and take actions based on reason. A process is a series of steps or components leading to achievement of a goal. The nursing process includes five steps, but what is important to understand is that the nursing process is circular. A nurse will assess a client's condition, determine an appropriate diagnosis, plan care based on the nursing diagnosis, implement the plan, and evaluate the results of care. This suggests the nursing process is linear, but it is often necessary to then reassess the client for changes in the original problem or the occurrence of new problems. In addition, a nurse may implement a plan of care but, because of the client's response, revise the plan by changing the type of intervention. The nursing process is continuous until the client's health is improved, restored, or maintained (Figure 13-3, p. 286).

If one places the nursing process within the context of the critical thinking model, one is able to see two processes occurring together (Figure 13-4, p. 287). As the nurse engages in the nursing process for the care of a specific client, the nurse is also synthesizing critical thinking knowledge, experience, standards, and attitudes simultaneously. The nurse who is assessing a client's pain does not focus only

---

Examples of Evaluation Criteria   Box 13-5

Character of pain: Onset, duration, location, severity, type or description of pain, precipitating factors, relieving factors, other related symptoms
Medication effectiveness: Change in physical signs or symptoms, development of side effects, extent of desired action
Client instruction: Client's ability to recount information learned, client's ability to perform learned skill correctly, client's success in adapting knowledge or skill in the home

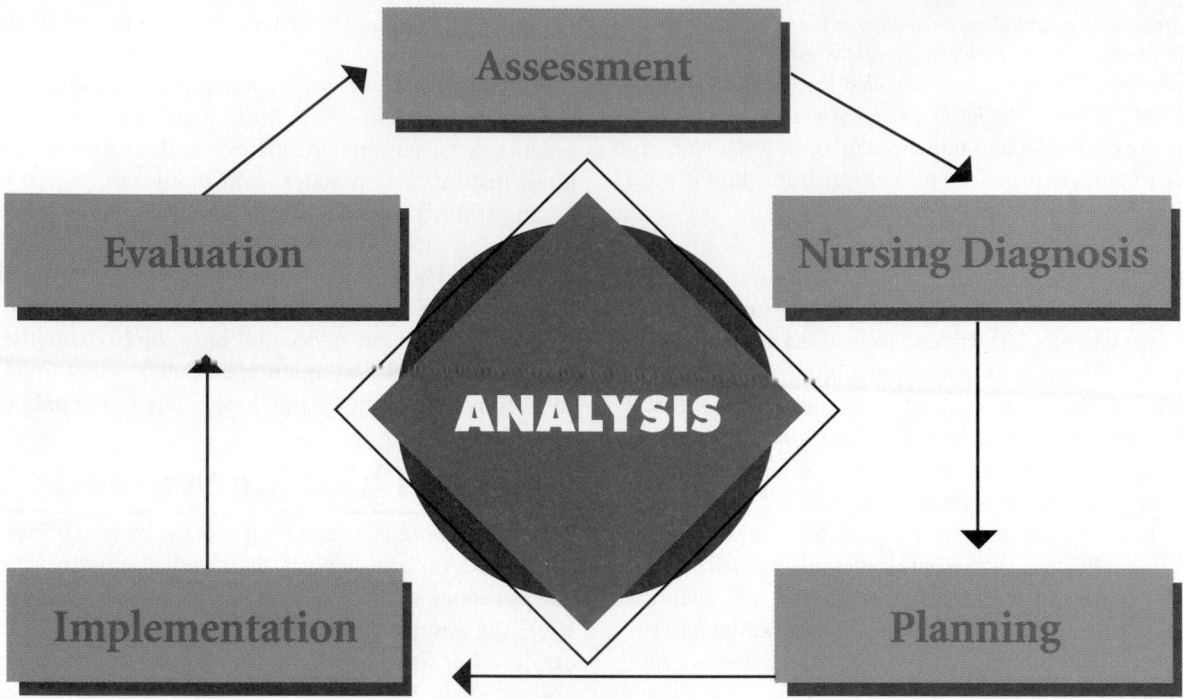

Figure 13-3   Five-step nursing process model.

on what the client reports about the pain and what the nurse is able to observe and measure. The nurse is also reflecting on prior experience with clients who have had similar pain so as to compare and contrast this new client's response. The nurse is referring to the information scientific texts have to offer about how the pain might be relieved. The nurse also displays the proper intellectual standards in being sure the pain assessment is accurate and objective. Finally, the nurse exercises the attitudes necessary for the client to be cared for fairly and responsibly. The clinical chapters within this textbook unite the nursing process and critical thinking model into one approach for the comprehensive care of clients.

Nursing Process Overview

The three characteristics of a process are purpose, organization, and creativity (Bevis, 1978). Purpose is the goal or aim of the process. The nursing process is used to diagnose and treat human responses to health and illness (American Nurses Association, 1980). Organization is the series of steps or components needed to achieve the goal. The five steps of the process are dynamic but inclusive of the clinical-decision-making activities and clinical skills nurses use to help clients meet agreed on outcomes for better health. Creativity is characteristic of the nursing process because the process is continually changing in response to a client's needs. For example, after a nurse has

evaluated the results of nursing care and finds that the client has not improved, the nurse can reassess a client's condition to update data, redefine problems, and select new interventions. The nursing process is a blueprint for care. Critical thinking is the cognitive process the nurse uses when developing and implementing the nursing process.

The nursing process provides a creative, organized structure and framework for the delivery of nursing care, yet it is flexible enough to be used in all settings. When nurses use the nursing process, they are able to identify a client's health care needs, determine priorities, establish goals and expected outcomes of care, establish and communicate a client-centered plan of care, provide appropriate nursing interventions, and evaluate the effectiveness of nursing care. At any time in the care of a client, a nurse may move back and forth from one step of the process to another should new data emerge. For example, while sitting with a client to discuss a plan of care, the nurse may recognize a new symptom the client is experiencing and assess its status before continuing. The nurse must always be thinking and recognizing what step of the process is being used. Bandman and Bandman (1995) describe the whole nursing process as a series of means-ends relationships. The means are the nurse's accurate assessment, diagnosis, and treatment of the client and the ends are the client's increased level of function and well-being.

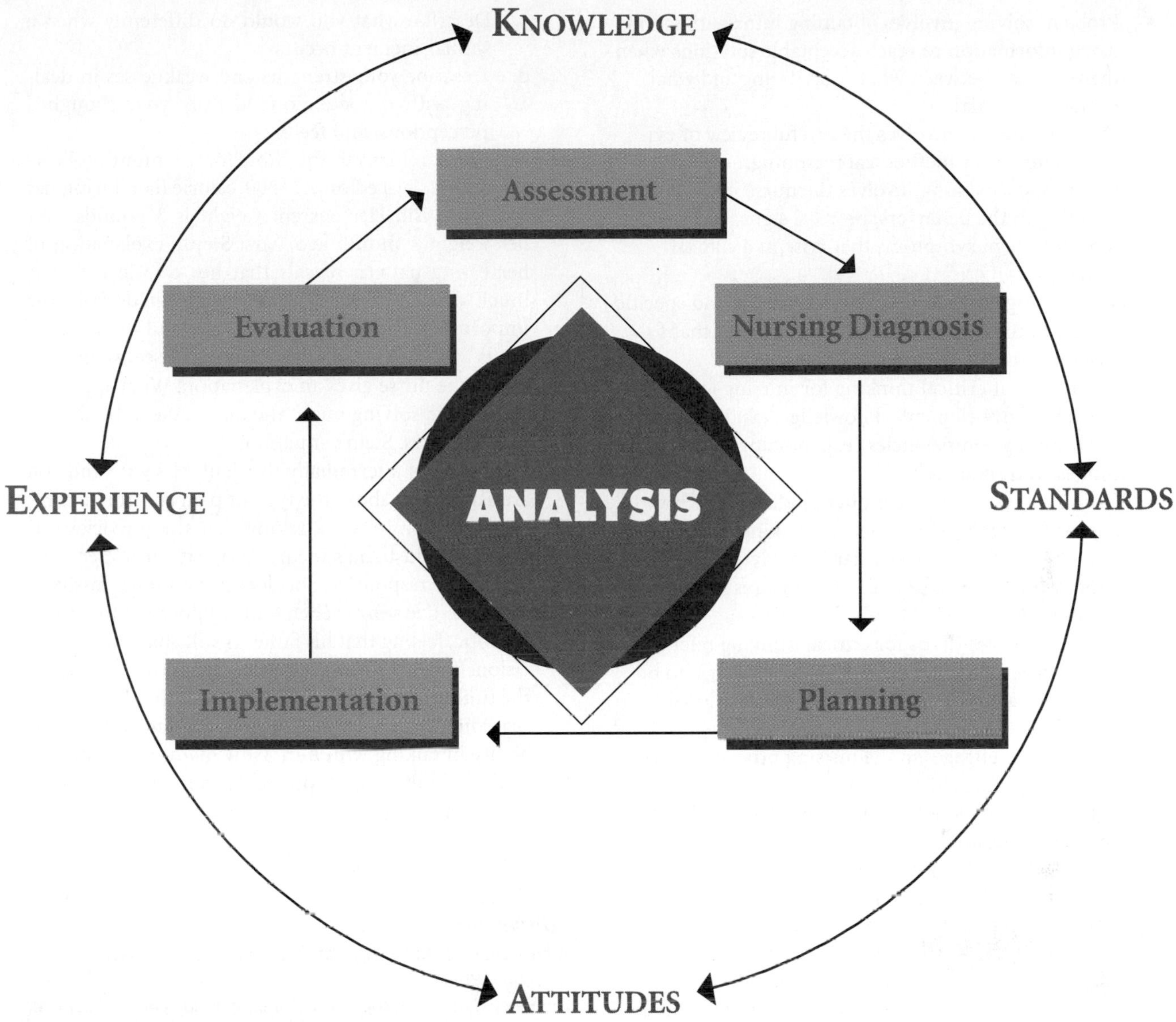

KNOWLEDGE

Assessment

Evaluation

Nursing Diagnosis

EXPERIENCE

ANALYSIS

STANDARDS

Implementation

Planning

ATTITUDES

Figure 13-4   Synthesis of critical thinking with the nursing process competency.

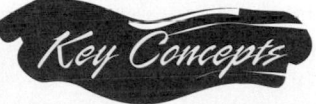

Key Concepts

- Decision making is one skill that separates professional nurses from technical or ancillary personnel.
- Critical thinking is purposeful and goal oriented, involving the identification and challenging of assumptions, consideration of what is important in a situation, the exploration of alternatives, and application of reason and logic in making informed decisions.
- The nurse who is a good critical thinker faces problems without forming a quick, single solution and instead is focused on the options for what to believe and do.

- Reflection is a form of self-evaluation that helps the nurse judge personal performance and make judgments about standards of practice.
- The use of language in critical thinking requires a framing of one's thoughts so that the focus and resultant message are clear.
- Each clinical experience is a lesson for the next one, with a nurse building an intuitive knowledge base that can be applied in daily practice.
- The three levels of critical thinking in nursing are basic, complex, and commitment.

- Problem solving involves obtaining information and using information to reach acceptable solutions when there is a gap between what is occurring and what should be occurring.
- Decision making involves the careful review of evidence and use of methodical reasoning.
- Diagnostic reasoning involves the nurse in assigning meaning to the behaviors, physical signs, and reported client symptoms that arise in a clinical situation.
- The nursing process incorporates general and specific critical thinking competencies in a manner that focuses on a particular client's unique needs.
- The model of critical thinking for nursing judgment consists of five elements: knowledge, experience, critical thinking competencies (e.g., nursing process), attitudes, and standards.
- Critical thinking attitudes offer guidelines for how to approach a problem or decision-making situation.
- The use of intellectual standards involves a rigorous approach to clinical practice that ensures a high quality of nursing care.
- Professional standards for critical thinking refer to ethical criteria for nursing judgments, criteria to be used for evaluation, and criteria for professional responsibility.
- As the nurse engages in the nursing process for the care of a specific client, the nurse is also synthesizing critical thinking knowledge, experience, standards, and attitudes simultaneously.

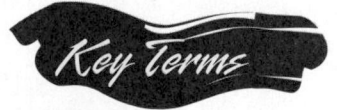

Key Terms

Critical thinking, *p. 275*
Decision making, *p. 278*
Diagnostic reasoning, *p. 278*
Inferences, *p. 274*
Intuition, *p. 277*

Problem solving, *p. 278*
Reflection, *p. 276*
Nursing process, *p. 278*
Scientific method, *p. 278*

Critical Thinking Exercises

1. Select a day and write a journal entry describing any one of the following experiences *that stimulated your thinking:* an interaction you had with a client, an interaction you had with your spouse or one of your children, or an interaction you had with someone you were trying to help. For the entry, discuss each of the following:
   a. Describe, as thoroughly as you can, what you did.
   b. Describe your decision-making process.
   c. Describe what you would do differently when a similar incident occurs.
   d. Describe your strengths and weaknesses in dealing with the situation. Identify your thoughts, perceptions, and feelings.
2. Mrs. Stein returns to the clinic for a 1-month follow-up. She was placed on an 1800-calorie diet during her previous visit. Her current weight is 3 pounds over her weight 1 month ago. Mrs. Stein's explanation of her eating pattern reveals that her calorie intake is much too high. The nurse begins to again describe the importance of the 1800-calorie diet and the types of foods Mrs. Stein should eat. The client seems inattentive as the nurse gives an explanation. What approach to problem solving might the nurse take to better understand Mrs. Stein's situation?
3. Mr. Spicer is a terminally ill client. His wife and son are asking you about the type of pain control he is receiving. Mrs. Spicer is asking that the physician increase her husband's medication, even if it means he will not be responsive. She does not want her husband to suffer. The son is vehemently opposed to too much narcotic, feeling that his father is still able to make decisions for himself. Mr. Spicer remains alert much of the time and is able to talk with you about his feelings regarding death. He seems to appreciate your availability in talking with him. How might you apply the critical thinking attitudes of fairness, responsibility, and creativity in this case study?

References

Alfaro-LeFevre, R: *Critical thinking in nursing: a practical application,* Philadelphia, 1995, WB Saunders.

American Nurses Association: *Nursing social policy statement,* Kansas City, Mo, 1980, The Association.

Baker CR: Reflective learning: a teaching strategy for critical thinking, *J Nurs Educ* 35(1):19, 1996.

Bandman EL, Bandman B: *Critical thinking in nursing,* ed 2, Norwalk, Conn, 1995, Appleton & Lange.

Benner P: *From novice to expert,* Menlo Park, Calif, 1984, Addison Wesley.

Bevis EM: Curriculum building in nursing: a process, St. Louis, 1978, Mosby.

Callister, LC: The use of student journals in nursing education: making meaning out of clinical experience, *J Nurs Educ* 32(4):185, 1993.

Carnevali DL, Thomas MD: *Diagnostic reasoning and treatment decision making in nursing,* Philadelphia, 1993, JB Lippincott.

Chaffee J: *Thinking critically,* ed 3, Boston, 1994, Houghton Mifflin.

Dewey J: *How we think.* In Regnery H; editor: *Essays in experimental logic,* Chicago, 1933, University of Chicago.

Facione N, Facione P: Externalizing the critical thinking in knowledge development and clinical judgment, *Nurs Outlook* 44:129, 1996.

Facione P: *Critical thinking: a statement of expert consensus for purposes of educational assessment and instruction. The Delphi report: research findings and recommendations prepared for the American Philosophical Association*, ERIC Doc No. ED 315-423, Washington, DC, 1990, ERIC.

Fox RC: The evolution of medical uncertainty, *Milbank Memorial Fund Quarterly/Health and Society* 58(1):1, 1980.

Glaser E: *An experiment in the development of critical thinking*, New York, 1941, Bureau of Publications, Teachers College, Columbia University.

Gordon M: *Nursing diagnosis: process and application,* ed 3, St. Louis, 1995, Mosby.

Guralnik DB, editor: *Webster's New World Dictionary,* college ed 2, Toronto, 1972, Nelson, Foster & Scott.

Heinrich KT: The intimate dialogue: journal writing by students, *Nurse Educator* 17(6):17, 1992.

Hughes KK, Young WB: Decision making: stability of clinical decisions, *Nurse Educator* 17(3):12, 1992.

Kataoka-Yahiro M, Saylor C: A critical thinking model for nursing judgment, *J Nurs Educ* 33(8):351, 1994.

Ludwick R, Sedlak CA: Ethical issues and critical thinking: students' stories, *Nurs Connect* 11(3), 1998.

Miller M, Malcolm N: Critical thinking in the nursing curriculum, *Nurs Health Care* 11:67, 1990.

Miller MA, Babcock DE: *Critical thinking applied to nursing,* St. Louis, 1996, Mosby.

O'Neill ES, Dluhy NM: A longitudinal framework for fostering critical thinking and diagnostic reasoning, *J Adv Nurs* 26:825, 1997.

Patton JG and others: Enhancing the clinical practicum experience through journal writing, *JONE* 36(5):238, 1997.

Paul RW: The art of redesigning instruction. In Willsen J, Blinker AJA, editors: *Critical thinking: how to prepare students for a rapidly changing world,* Santa Rosa, Calif, 1993, Foundation for Critical Thinking.

Paul RW, Heaslip P: Critical thinking and intuitive nursing practice, *J Adv Nurs* 22:40, 1995.

Perry W: *Forms of intellectual and ethical development in the college years: a scheme,* New York, 1979, Holt, Rinehart, & Winston.

Saylor CR: Reflection and professional education: art, science, and competency, *Nurse Educator* 15(2):8, 1990.

Strader M: Critical thinking. In Sullivan EJ, Decker PJ, editors: *Effective management in nursing,* ed 3, Redwood City, Calif, 1992, Addison Wesley Nursing.

Watson G, Glaser E: *Watson-Glaser critical thinking appraisal manual,* New York, 1980, MacMillan.

Whiteside C: A model for teaching critical thinking in the clinical setting, *Dimens Crit Care Nurs* 16(3):152, 1997.

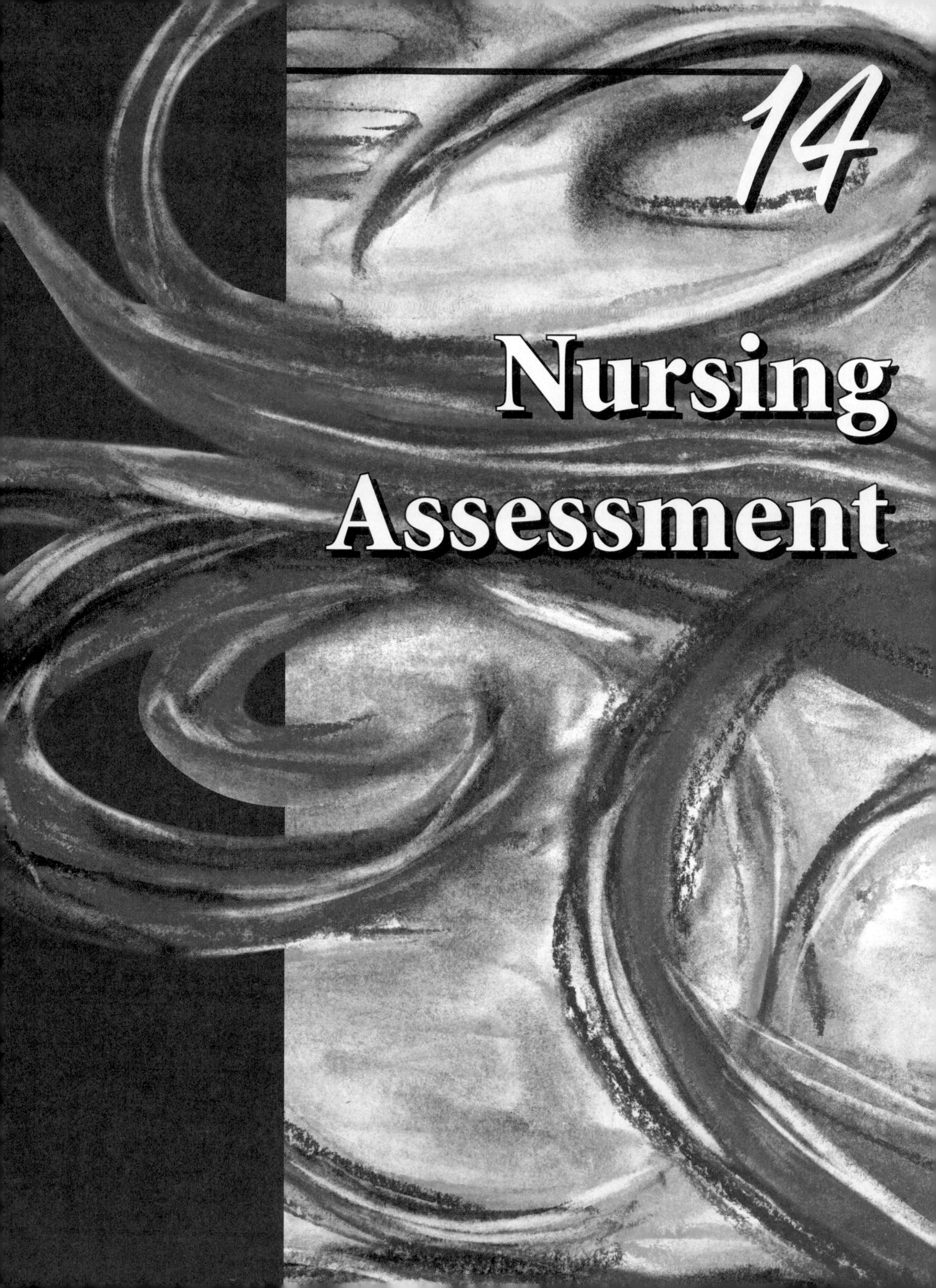

14

Nursing
Assessment

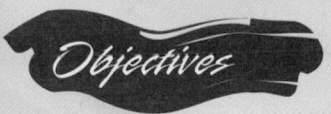
Mastery of content in this chapter will enable the student to:

- Define the key terms listed.
- Discuss the purpose of nursing assessment.
- Explain the relationship between data collection, data analysis, and critical thinking.
- Explain the difference between a comprehensive and a problem-oriented assessment.
- Explain why client expectations are important to include in assessment.
- Describe how assessment is a flexible approach to problem solving.
- Differentiate between objective and subjective data.
- State the sources of data for a nursing assessment.
- Describe the four interviewing techniques.
- State the purpose of a nursing history.
- State the purpose of a physical examination.
- Conduct and record a nursing assessment.

Nursing is unique because of its broad focus on understanding and managing a person's health. A competent nurse must have an adequate knowledge of physiology, pathophysiology, psychopathology, social and behavioral sciences, and medical treatment to safely perform and provide therapies. For example, when a physician orders a medication such as insulin, the nurse must know the drug's effect, the symptoms the client might have if side effects develop, and the actions to take when problems occur. In this same example the nurse must also have knowledge of therapeutic communication, dimensions of daily living that affect a person's health situation, and principles of adult learning to instruct and support the client in daily self-administration of insulin injections. The nurse has two focuses in clinical practice: as a primary provider of nursing care and as a collaborator with other disciplines (Carpenito, 1997).

Nursing Process Overview

The nursing process enables the nurse to organize and deliver nursing care. To successfully apply the nursing process, the nurse integrates elements of critical thinking to make judgments and take actions based on reason. The nursing process is used to identify, diagnose, and treat human responses to health and illness (American Nurses Association [ANA], 1995). The nursing process includes five steps: assessment, nursing diagnosis, planning, implementation, and evaluation (see Chapter 13). It is a dynamic, continuous process as the client's needs change. The use of the nursing process promotes individualized nursing care and assists the nurse in responding to client needs in a timely and reasonable manner to improve or maintain the client's level of health.

The nursing process involves scientific reasoning (Table 14-1). The nurse makes inferences about the meaning of a client's response to a health problem or generalizes about the client's functional state of health. A pattern will begin to form, for example, if the client is having acute back pain and his or her mobility is limited. The nurse continues to gather more information until an accurate classification of the client's problem is determined, such as the following nursing diagnosis: impaired physical mobility related to acute back pain. The clear definition of the client's problem provides the basis for nursing interventions and evaluation of outcomes. The nurse's interventions are designed to relieve the pain so as to improve the client's mobility.

The nursing process is simply one variation of scientific reasoning that allows nurses to organize, systematize, and conceptualize nursing practice (Bandman and Bandman, 1995). It is a general approach to client systems of individuals, families, groups, or communities. It is an approach that allows nurses to differentiate their practice from that of physicians and other health care professionals. When nurses think critically, the client becomes an active participant and the ultimate outcome is a comprehensive, individualized approach to care.

A Critical Thinking Approach to Assessment

Our present health care system requires the nurse to solve problems accurately, thoroughly, and quickly. The nurse

Table 14-1	Comparison of Steps in Problem Solving, the Scientific Method, and the Nursing Process		
Problem Solving	Copi and Cohen's Seven-Step Scientific Method*	Nursing Process	
Encountering problem	The problem	Assessing	
	Preliminary hypothesis		
Collecting data	Collecting additional facts		
Identifying exact nature of problem	Formulating hypotheses	Forming a nursing diagnosis	
Determining plan of action	Deducing further consequences	Planning (outcome identification)	
Carrying out plan	Testing consequences	Implementing	
Evaluating plan in new situation	Application	Evaluating	
Plan of action			

*Copi IM, Cohen C: *Introduction to logic,* ed 9, New York, 1994, Macmillan.

must be able to review information from a variety of sources and to make critical judgments. During a nursing **assessment,** the nurse systematically collects, verifies, analyzes, and communicates data about a client. This phase of the nursing process includes two steps: collection and verification of data from a primary source (the client) and secondary sources (family, health professionals) and the analysis of that data as a basis for nursing diagnoses (Bandman and Bandman, 1995). The purpose of the assessment is to establish a database about the client's perceived needs, health problems and responses to these problems, related experiences, health practices, goals, values, lifestyle, and expectations from the health care system. The information contained in the **database** is the basis for developing nursing diagnoses and planning individualized nursing care, which is evaluated and refined as needed throughout the time the nurse cares for the client.

The nurse must apply principles of critical thinking when conducting a client assessment (see Chapter 13). As the nurse initiates the assessment component for a specific client, the nurse is also synthesizing critical thinking knowledge, experience, standards, and attitudes simultaneously (Figure 14-1). The nurse brings knowledge from the physical, biological, and social sciences to the assessment. This knowledge enables the nurse to ask relevant questions and collect relevant physical assessment data related to the client's expectation of care or underlying health care needs. Communication skills and knowledgeable assessment skills enable the nurse to collect complete, accurate, and relevant data. Prior clinical experience contributes to the skills of assessment. Validation of abnormal assessment findings and observation of assessments by skilled professionals enable the nurse to gain competency in the assessment process. The nurse applies standards of practice, accepted standards of normal for physical assessment data, and the intellectual standards of accuracy, significance, completeness, and fairness when assessing clients. The nurse brings attitudes such as fairness, perse-

verance, integrity, and confidence to the nurse-client relationship so that a complete assessment database is obtained.

The assessment must be relevant to a particular health problem. The nurse uses critical thinking to collect and analyze data to determine what is relevant for the assessment database. The nurse's clinical problem solving is sometimes stepwise; sometimes branching, when data from new problems are recognized; and at other times cyclical, when the nurse must reassess and validate information. For example, in an urgent care setting, when a client enters the facility because of a possible ankle fracture, the nurse would gather information regarding the injury, intensity, type, and location of pain, initial first aid measures, medication allergies, and perhaps when the client last ate. In some settings, the nurse collects data on a standardized form, which is designed to collect targeted relevant data in a timely, efficient manner (Gordon, 1994). In a community-based setting the assessment focuses on the client's illness, circle of family and friends, and resources within the community (Bryans and McIntosh, 1996).

It is important for a nurse to learn to critically think about what to assess. The independent judgment of when a question or measurement is appropriate is influenced by the nurse's clinical knowledge and experience (Gordon, 1994). When a nurse first encounters a client, there is a chance for a quick overview. This overview is usually based on the nurse's specialty of practice or the treatment situation. For example, an emergency department nurse uses the A-B-C (airway-breathing-circulation) approach, and a psychiatric nurse may focus on the client's reality, anxiety level, and potential for violence (Carnevali and Thomas, 1993). It is possible that other important cues may be missed with such an intense focused assessment. However, the nurse interprets cues from the client to know how in-depth an assessment should be. Assessment is dynamic; it should allow the nurse to freely explore relevant problems as they appear.

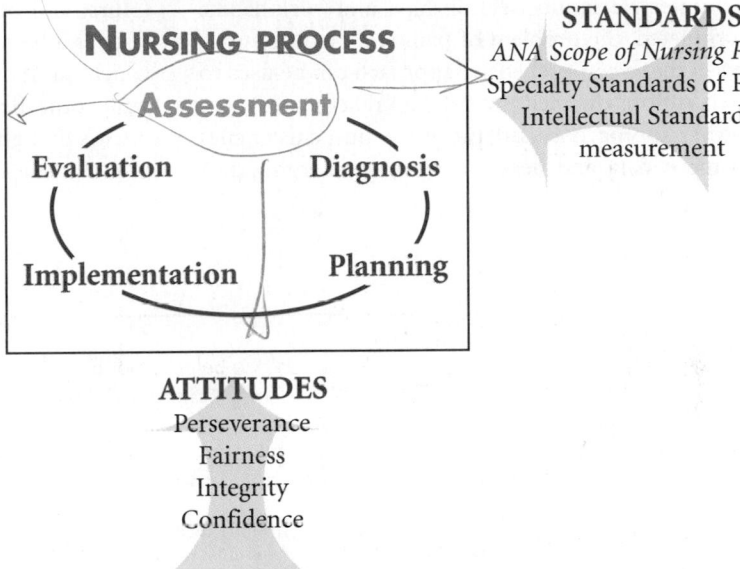

KNOWLEDGE
Underlying disease process
Normal growth and development
Normal psychology
Normal assessment findings
Health promotion
Assessment skills
Communication skills

EXPERIENCE
Previous client care experience
Validation of assessment findings
Observation of assessment techniques

STANDARDS
ANA Scope of Nursing Practice
Specialty Standards of Practice
Intellectual Standards of
measurement

NURSING PROCESS
Assessment
Evaluation   Diagnosis
Implementation   Planning

ATTITUDES
Perseverance
Fairness
Integrity
Confidence

Figure 14-1   Critical thinking and the assessment process.

The initial overview of the client's situation allows the nurse to use key assessment data to respond to priorities, such as the onset of pain. It is important for the nurse to recognize that the client's situation can change at any time during assessment and that data collection must be accurate, relevant, and appropriate for the client's situation.

Carnevali and Thomas (1993) suggest two approaches to collecting comprehensive data. One is a structured comprehensive database format, such as Gordon's 11 functional health patterns (Box 14-1), and the other is a problem-oriented approach focusing on the client's presenting situation.

The comprehensive approach moves from general to specific. For example, a nurse may use a history form organized by Gordon's functional patterns. Data are collected in all 11 categories and then reviewed to see if patterns of problems are revealed. For each of the 11 patterns the nurse assesses clients by organizing patterns of behavior and physiological responses that pertain to a functional health category. The nurse then compares assessment data with the client's baseline (e.g., usual blood pressure, weight, and nutritional intake); established norms based on age, gender, height, and weight; and cultural, social, or other norms, such as religious practices,

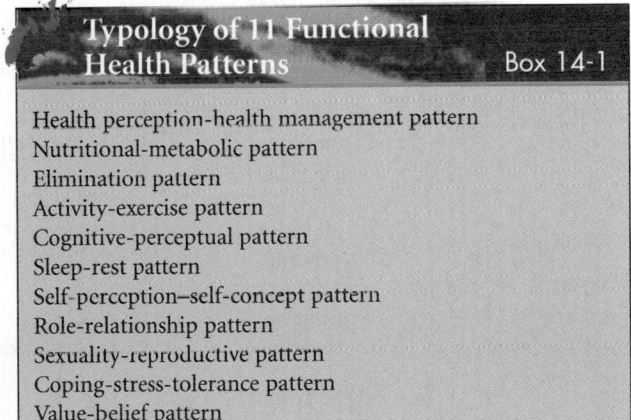

Typology of 11 Functional Health Patterns   Box 14-1

Health perception–health management pattern
Nutritional-metabolic pattern
Elimination pattern
Activity-exercise pattern
Cognitive-perceptual pattern
Sleep-rest pattern
Self-perception–self-concept pattern
Role-relationship pattern
Sexuality-reproductive pattern
Coping-stress-tolerance pattern
Value-belief pattern

From Gordon M: *Nursing diagnosis: process and application,* ed 3, St. Louis, 1994, Mosby.

ethnic dietary guidelines, and health care practices (Gordon, 1987). The assessment of each of the 11 patterns represents the interaction of the client and the environment, which Gordon calls biopsychosocial integration. No one health pattern can be understood without knowledge of the other patterns (Gordon, 1991). Description and evaluation of health patterns assist the nurse in identifying functional patterns (client strengths) and dysfunctional patterns (nursing diagnoses), which assist in developing the nursing care plan (Gordon, 1987, 1991).

The second method for assessment is the problem-focused approach to assessment. The assessment begins with problematic areas such as pain and spreads out to relevant areas of the client's life. A comprehensive pain assessment begins with a review of the nature of the pain itself and then broadens to categories such as the influence of pain on lifestyle, family relationships, and work habits. Once completed, the problem of pain will be thoroughly analyzed so that a comprehensive approach can be used to plan interventions directed toward pain relief.

Whatever approach is used, the nurse must cluster cues of assessment data and begin to identify emerging pat-

terns and potential problems. To do this well, a nurse critically anticipates. In other words, the nurse always tries to stay a step ahead of the assessment. Once a question has been asked of a client or an observation has been made, the information often branches to an additional series of questions or observations (Figure 14-2). The risk the nurse takes in not anticipating assessment questions is to fail to recognize problems or to dismiss relevant problems (Hurst and others, 1991). Knowing how to frame questions is a basic skill, refined over time. The nurse decides which questions are relevant to the situation while at the same time being sure the assessment is complete. The nurse's thoughts about the client proceed from something given, a cue or data, to a conclusion. The extent of a

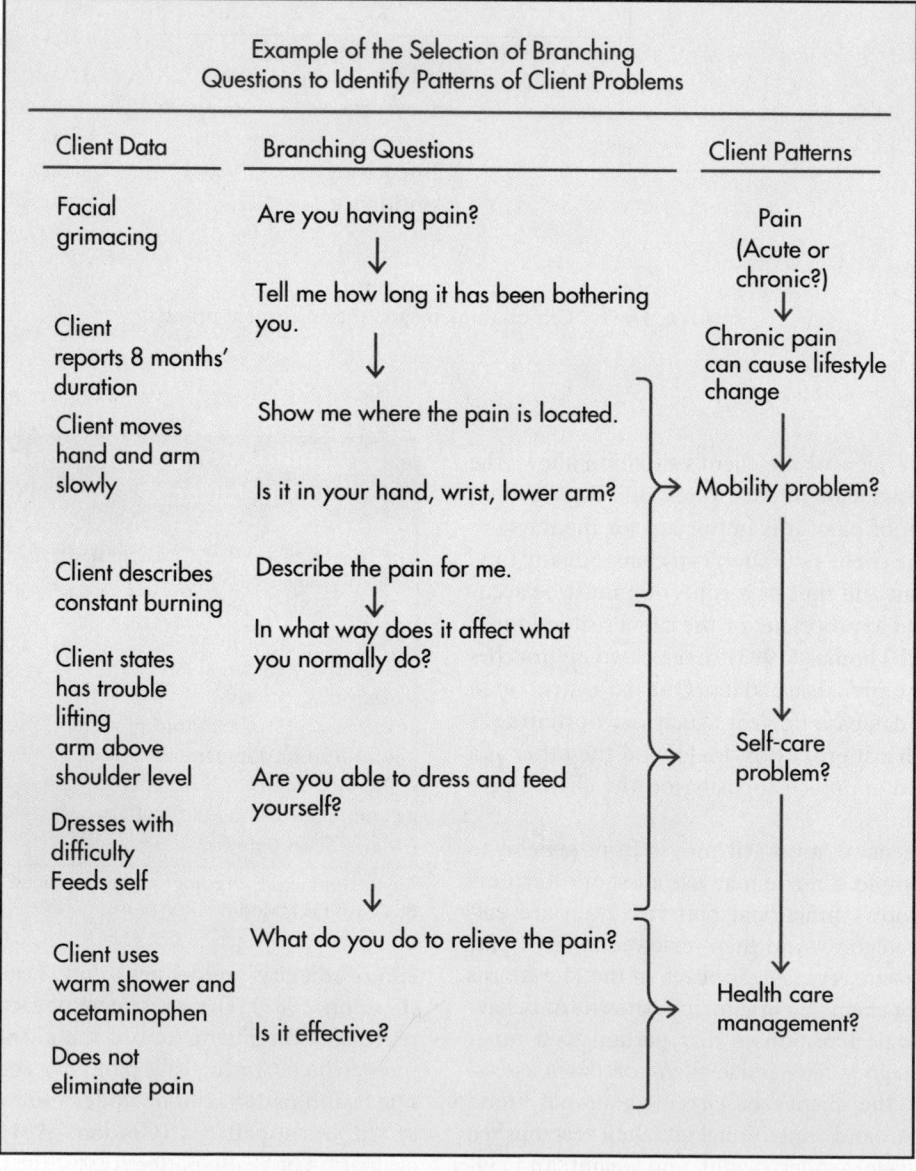

Figure 14-2 Example of branching logic for selecting assessment questions.

nurse's ability to grasp the meaning of all the data being collected and analyzed is related to the nurse's knowledge and experience.

Assessment is used in the nurse's collaborative role. The nurse makes clinical observations of a client, reports the client's situation relative to a medical problem, and then follows delegated medical activities prescribed by the physician. In the independent role of a health care provider, the nurse assesses a client's health care needs and institutes nursing interventions to maintain or improve the client's health. Accurate assessment is crucial to ensure needs are properly identified and the right course of action is implemented by the nurse.

ORGANIZATION OF DATA GATHERING

Accurate assessment makes it possible to develop appropriate nursing diagnoses (see Chapter 15) and to devise appropriate goals, expected outcomes, and strategies for a client. Before the assessment is initiated, the nurse must organize the assessment process and determine which data must be collected. The faculty of Ohio State University developed one methodology for teaching nursing students problem-solving techniques (Ryan-Wenger, 1990). The approach emphasizes how assessment requires a level of detail to ensure accuracy (Table 14-2). Steps in the assessment phase are outlined to provide clearer direction for how nurses make client care decisions.

It is important for the nurse's assessment to first consider the nurse-client interaction. Why has the client sought health care? What is the purpose of any nurse-client interaction? Who will be involved? What knowledge does the nurse have about the situation that brings the nurse and client together? These factors influence the nurse's success in developing a relationship with the client that leads to a directed, purposeful, and comprehensive assessment.

As a nurse conducts an assessment, there are considerable interactions (verbal and nonverbal) between the nurse and client. In addition, the client presents physiological responses such as posturing, breathing patterns, and body movement that relay information to the nurse. The nurse must use all senses to accurately assess client behavior.

Our senses collect experiences that we classify and judge (Bandman and Bandman, 1995). For example, when a nurse observes a client having difficulty breathing, sense impressions are formed that the client is in trouble. These sense impressions are sources of knowledge and often reliable clues that lead the nurse to more deliberate assessment. The skills of physical examination (see Chapter 32) enable the nurse to explore physical findings accurately and in detail, such as measurement of respiratory rate, rhythm, and depth. When making judgments the nurse connects sense experiences to nursing knowledge to ensure accurate reasoning.

As a client and nurse interact, the nurse asks relevant questions to gather more data. This requires practice for the beginning nurse to become proficient. If the nurse prematurely stops asking questions, the database can be incomplete and the resultant conclusions, made in the form of nursing diagnoses, can be inaccurate. Any **inferences** about the client or about the nurse's own behavior toward the client are separated from actual data.

DATA COLLECTION

The nurse collects data that are descriptive, concise, and complete. Assessment does not include inferences or interpretative statements that are unsupported with data. Descriptive data originate in the client's perception of a symptom, the perceptions and observations of the family, the nurse's observations, or reports from other members of the health care team. It is important to encourage clients to tell their story about their illness or health care problem. For example, a client may describe pain as a "sharp, throbbing pain in the abdomen." The nurse's observation may be, "The client lies on the right side holding the abdomen. Facial grimacing present." The nurse conducts a focused examination and records only observations and avoids interpreting behavior (e.g., "The client tolerates pain poorly"). Concise data briefly describe the information obtained. The information is summarized in a short format using correct medical terms (e.g., "Client describes a constant, sharp, throbbing pain in the upper right quadrant of the abdomen. Pain began 18 hours before hospitalization, 2 hours after a high-fat meal. Pain was not relieved by antacids"). Complete data collection results from obtaining all information relevant to the actual or potential health problem. To confirm that complete data have been collected, the nurse might ask, "Do I have the information to answer the questions, When, where, and what are the duration and influencing factors?" For example, a nurse in an outpatient clinic uses these questions to write the assessment of a client seeking treatment for recurrent headaches.

The collection of inaccurate, incomplete, or inappropriate data may lead to incorrect identification of the client's health care needs and subsequent inaccurate, incomplete, or inappropriate nursing diagnoses. Inaccurate data result if the nurse fails to collect information relevant to a specific area or if the nurse is disorganized or unskilled in assessment techniques. Data are incomplete if the nurse neglects to obtain all information about a specific area, jumps to conclusions about a potential problem, or makes assumptions without validation. Inappropriate data are unrelated to the area being assessed.

Types of Data

During assessment, the nurse obtains two types of data, subjective and objective. **Subjective data** are clients' perceptions about their health problems. Only clients can provide this kind of information. For example, the pres-

Table 14-2 **A Methodology for Nursing Assessment**

Element	Nursing Activity
Nurse-client interaction	Identify purpose of the nurse-client interaction (e.g., to provide hygiene care, administer a tube feeding, interact with an anxious client).
	Identify the system of study along with important subsystems (e.g., the client, nurse-client, group of clients, community).
	Recognize relationships between client and the environment that influence client's behavior and/or nurse-client interaction.
	Know the purpose of each nursing experience and type of client to prepare for the interaction. For example, practice hygiene skills before giving hygiene care.
Recording nurse and client behavior	Nurse and client are affected by each other's behavior and characteristics. Observe own verbal and nonverbal behavior to assess effect on client.
	Use all senses to accurately observe and record client's verbal/nonverbal behavior.
	Use tools and instruments (stethoscope, thermometer, height/weight chart) to accurately measure behavior and physiological signs.
Questions and inferences	Ask relevant questions to gather more data. *Do not be satisfied with simple answers.* For example:
	Nurse: Are you feeling nauseated?
	Client: Yes.
	Nurse: Tell me when it began; are you having other symptoms?
	Be aware of inferences about your own behavior: "My nervousness is showing;" "The client and I are not communicating well." *Keep inferences separate from data.* Use appropriate follow-up questions to clarify.
	The client responds to questions asked, and other data are collected to support or refute inferences.
Identifying patterns	Based on knowledge and data, identify patterns of nurse and client behavior. A pattern is similar to a nursing diagnosis and is defined as a particular behavior occurring over time (e.g., client walks 4 miles a day—has a pattern of regular exercise), or a pattern may be a cluster of behavior (e.g., client has shortness of breath, increased heart rate, rapid respirations following routine exercise—indicating poor activity tolerance).
	Identify positive and negative patterns. A positive pattern might be a client's spiritual strengths; a negative pattern might be poor eating habits. It is important to recognize and maintain positive health patterns as well as to decrease effects of negative health patterns.
	Identify interaction patterns based on observation of nurse-client interaction. For example, nurse asks questions and client responds in one-word phrases with no eye contact.
Apply theories and concepts	Concepts and theories help to support, refute, or give meaning to observed patterns. For example, while administering medication a student identifies a pattern of grief over a client's loss of a spouse and supports the finding by documentation that expression of guilt, crying, and poor eating habits are signs of dysfunctional grieving.
	Previously identified patterns are assessed for their potential or real effect on a client. Patterns with a negative effect on health (e.g., poor compliance in taking medication) are noted. Patterns that positively affect health (e.g., getting regular sufficient sleep) are reviewed.
	Also consider patterns of nurse behavior or client-nurse interaction that have positive or negative effects.
Validation	Document interpretation of patterns of data with reliable sources (e.g., literature, other nurses, family, health care professionals).

From Ryan-Wenger NM: A nursing process methodology, *Nurs Outlook* 38(4):190, 1990.

ence of pain or the meaning of an illness are subjective findings. Only clients can provide information about a symptom's frequency, duration, location, and intensity. Subjective data may include feelings of anxiety, physical discomfort, or mental stress. Although only clients can provide subjective data relevant to these feelings, the nurse must be aware that these problems can result in physiological changes, which are identified through objective data collection.

Objective data are observations or measurements made by the data collector (Figure 14-3). Assessment of a client's wound and identification of the size of a localized body rash are examples of observed objective data. The measurement of objective data is based on an accepted **standard,** such as the Fahrenheit or Celsius measure on a thermometer or centimeters on a measuring tape. Body temperature and blood pressure are examples of measured objective data.

Sources of Data

Subjective data are obtained from the client, family, significant others, health care team members, and health records. Objective data are obtained though physical ex-

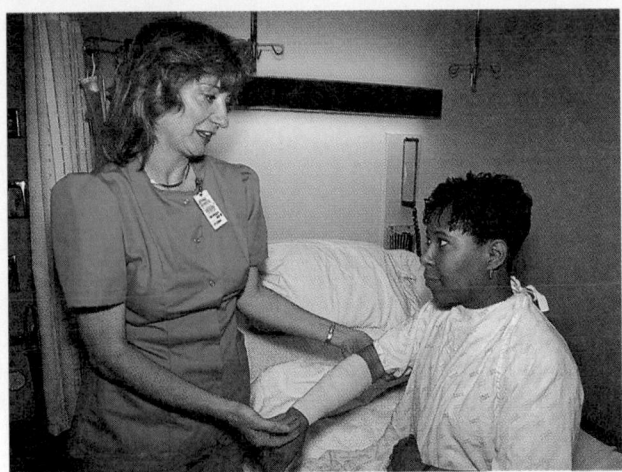

Figure 14-3   Nurse palpates temperature of skin to assess quality of circulation.

amination, results of diagnostic and laboratory tests, and pertinent nursing and medical literature. The nurse's own past experiences with similar types of clients is an additional source of data. Each source provides information about the client's level of wellness, anticipated prognosis, risk factors, health practices and goals, and patterns of health and illness, as well as information relevant to the client's health care needs.

CLIENT

In most situations the client is the best source of information. The client who is oriented and answers questions appropriately can provide the most accurate information about health care needs, lifestyle patterns, present and past illnesses, perception of symptoms, and changes in activities of daily living. It is important, however, to consider the setting where the nurse interacts with a client. A client experiencing acute symptoms in an emergency department will not be able to offer the same depth of information as one who comes to a primary care clinic for a routine checkup.

FAMILY AND SIGNIFICANT OTHERS

Families and significant others can be interviewed as primary sources of information about infants or children and critically ill, mentally handicapped, disoriented, or unconscious clients. In cases of severe illness or emergency situations, families may be the only available sources of data about a client's health-illness patterns, current medications, allergies, onset of illness, and other information needed by nurses and physicians.

The family and significant others are also important secondary sources of information. It is important to include them in assessment of the client when appropriate. Often spouses or close friends will sit in during an assessment and provide their view of the client's health problems or needs. Not only can they supply information

about the client's current health status, but also they often are able to indicate when changes in the client's status occurred and how the client's functioning was affected. Finally, family and friends can make pertinent observations about the client's needs that can affect the way care is delivered.

HEALTH CARE TEAM MEMBERS

The health care team consists of physicians, nurses, allied health professionals, and nonprofessional employees working in a health care setting (see Chapter 19). Because assessment is an ongoing process, the nurse must communicate with other health care team members, including physical therapists, social workers, community health workers, and spiritual advisers, whenever possible. Health care team members can provide information about the way the client interacts within the health care environment; the client's reaction to information about diagnostic tests; and, in acute and restorative care settings, how the client responds to visitors. Every member of the health care team is a potential source of information, and the team can identify and communicate data and verify information from other sources.

MEDICAL RECORDS

The present and past medical records of the client can verify information about past health patterns and treatments or can provide new information. By reviewing medical records, the nurse can identify patterns of illness, previous responses to treatment, and past methods of coping.

OTHER RECORDS

Other records such as educational, military, and employment records may contain pertinent health care information (e.g., immunizations, prior illnesses). If the client received services at a community health center or day care clinic, the nurse should obtain data from these records but must first obtain written permission from the client or guardian to see them. Any information obtained is confidential and is treated as part of the client's legal medical record (see Chapter 21).

LITERATURE REVIEW

Reviewing nursing, medical, and pharmacological literature about an illness helps the nurse complete the database. The review increases the nurse's knowledge about the symptoms, treatment, and prognosis of specific illnesses, and established standards of therapeutic practice. The knowledgeable nurse is able to obtain pertinent, accurate, and complete information for the assessment database.

NURSE'S EXPERIENCE

Benner (1984) notes that a nurse's expertise develops after testing and refining propositions, questions, and principle-based expectations. For example, after a nurse has cared for a client with abdominal pain there are lessons learned. The nurse will recognize more quickly the behavior the client showed while in acute pain. The nurse will have noted the extent to which positioning techniques helped the client to relax and have less discomfort. The principle of administering a pain medication regularly rather than when the client requests it, to achieve better pain control, will have been tested. Critical thinking is strengthened by practical experience and the opportunity to make decisions. A nurse's ability to make an assessment will improve from using past experience, applying relevant knowledge, and focusing on data collection that avoids wasteful consideration of unnecessary information.

Methods of Data Collection

The nurse uses the interview, the nursing health history, the physical examination, and results of laboratory and diagnostic tests to establish the database. Each method allows the nurse to collect complete information about the client's past and present level of wellness.

INTERVIEW

The first step in establishing the database is to interview the client. The **interview** is a pattern of communication initiated for a specific purpose and focused on a specific content area. In nursing, the major purposes of the interview are to obtain a nursing health history, identify health needs and risk factors, and determine specific changes in level of wellness and pattern of living. Perhaps most important, the interview should help clients relate their own interpretation and understanding of their condition. This means the nurse and client must be partners during the interview rather than the nurse controlling the interview. Unless an interview allows a client to express needs, the interaction may be unsuccessful.

An interview may be focused, as in the case of a client admitted to the emergency department; or it can be comprehensive, as is the case of a new client requiring a complete physical examination. The interviewer obtains information about the client's health, lifestyle, support systems, patterns of illness, patterns of adaptation, strengths and limitations, and resources. As the nurse listens and considers the information shared, the client may be directed to give more detail or discuss a topic that seems to reveal a possible problem. Since the client's report will include subjective information, the nurse uses data from the interview to later validate with objective data. For example, if the client reports difficulty in walking, the nurse will later assess the client's gait and muscle strength.

When conducting the interview, the nurse uses specific communication skills to focus attention on the client's level of wellness. The nurse also helps the client understand the changes that are occurring or will occur once health care begins. This chapter describes communication skills and the interview, whereas Chapter 22 discusses the total communication process and details the various communication techniques necessary for nursing practice.

The nursing interview achieves several objectives (Box 14-2). First, the **nurse-client relationship** is initiated. A nurse-client relationship is the association between the nurse and the client that has a mutual concern, the client's well-being. This relationship builds a professional interpersonal closeness that develops and aids in the investigation and discussion of the client's responses to health and illness. This relationship encourages the sharing of information, ideas, and emotions and enables the nurse to express a level of caring for the client (see Chapter 6).

During the interview the nurse obtains information about a client's physical, developmental, emotional, intellectual, social, and spiritual dimensions. Physical and developmental information reflects normal functioning and the pathological changes in a person's pattern of living induced by illness, trauma, or developmental crisis. Emotional information includes the behavioral responses to changes in health and pattern of living. Relevant emotional information includes mood, perceptions, body image, self-concept, and attitudes about sexuality. Intellectual information includes intellectual performance, problem-solving ability, educational level, communication patterns, and attention span. Social information involves environmental, cultural, ethnic, or social patterns that can affect the present or future level of wellness. The nurse also collects information about values, beliefs, and religious practices, which are part of the spiritual dimension.

The interview also provides the nurse with the opportunity to observe the client. The nurse observes interactions between the client and family and between the client and the health care environment; the nurse also observes the use of eye contact, nonverbal communication, and other body language. While observing this behavior, appearance, and interaction with the environment, the nurse determines whether the data obtained by observation are consistent with those obtained by verbal communication. For example, if the client states no concern about an upcoming diagnostic test but appears anxious and irritable,

Objectives of the Nursing Interview   Box 14-2

Establish a therapeutic relationship with the client.

Establish the nurse's sense of caring for the client as an individual.

Introduce the client to the facility in a manner that is not threatening.

Gain insight about the client's concerns.

Determine the client's expectations of health care providers and the health care delivery system.

Obtain cues about parts of the data collection phase that require in-depth investigation (branching).

the data conflict. Observations during an interview lead the nurse to gather additional objective information to form accurate conclusions.

The interview is a mechanism by which the client can obtain information as well. If a positive nurse-client relationship has been established, the client will feel comfortable asking the nurse questions about the health care environment, treatments, diagnostic testing, and available resources. The client needs this information to participate in decision making regarding goals and the plan of care. It is important for the nurse to ask the client about his or her expectations of health care providers. In addition, the interview is a first step toward establishing a therapeutic relationship between the nurse and client so that health interventions such as education or counseling can occur. To interview a client successfully and achieve the purpose and objectives of the interview, the nurse needs skills in initiating the nurse-client relationship, using the various types of interview techniques, and moving from one phase of the interview to the next.

Types of Interview Techniques.   The client's personality and health care needs, the health care setting, and the nurse's skill and experience affect the interview process. An emergency situation may require a type of interview technique in which the nurse asks focused questions pertaining to the client's physical status. This approach moves quickly in an effort to problem solve and identify what factors or conditions are causing alterations in the client's health. A client entering an extended care facility with a chronic illness requires an interview approach that includes more elaboration and description of data. In this case the nurse is able to collect a full picture of the client's health, living habits, familial and social resources, and the client's expectations for health care.

The interview in an emergent setting usually centers on the present illness or trauma, precipitating factors, medications, and allergies. In contrast, an interview with a client undergoing extensive rehabilitation may focus on past and present illnesses, coping strategies, family and community resources, daily living activities, and present limitations and goals for rehabilitation. The nurse uses many interview techniques to elicit the necessary information from the client or another source.

In a setting where the nurse is able to obtain a complete nursing history, it is helpful to begin by trying to find out, in the client's own words, what the health problem is and what is likely causing it. Remember, clients are the best resource in most cases in being able to relate their health history. The nurse begins by asking the client a question to elicit the client's story. For example, the nurse may begin by asking, "So, can you tell me what brings you to the clinic today?" or "Tell me about the problems you are having."

The nurse uses **open-ended questions** to obtain a response of more than one or two words. This technique leads to a discussion in which clients actively describe their health status. This method strengthens the nurse-client relationship because it shows that the nurse wants to invest time in hearing the client's thoughts. The nurse will encourage and let the client tell the story all the way through. The nurse's intent is reinforced through the use of good eye contact and listening skills. In addition the nurse may use **back channeling,** which includes active listening techniques such as "all right" or "uh-huh," which indicate the nurse has heard what the client says.

As the client tells his or her story, the nurse encourages a full description without trying to control the direction the story takes. This may require the nurse to probe with further open-ended statements such as, "Is there anything else you can tell me?" or "What else is bothering or affecting you?" It can also be very helpful to end the client's story by asking the client what might be causing his or her problem. This is described as the client's "explanatory model" (Lipkin and others, 1995). A physician is interested in a causal explanation so as to zone in on possible symptoms and their physical causes. In contrast, a nurse is interested in a causal explanation to understand the client's perceptions and the meaning the problem has for the client. The client's sense of the cause of the problem will help to direct the nurse's subsequent focused assessment.

Once a client has told his or her story, the nurse will apply a **problem-seeking interview** technique. This approach will take the information provided in the client's story to more fully describe and identify the client's specific problems. For example, a client may report experiencing indigestion over the course of several days and acknowledge having some diarrhea and loss of appetite. The client's explanation for the cause relates to a recent travel schedule that might have changed the client's eating habits. The nurse will focus on the symptoms the client identifies, as well as the general indigestion problem, by asking **closed-ended questions** that limit the client's answers to one or two words such as "yes" or "no." For example, the nurse might ask, "How often does the diarrhea occur?" or "Do you have pain or cramping?" or "Are you having nausea?"

The closed-ended questions require concise answers and are used to clarify previous information or provide additional information (Ivey, 1988). The questions do not encourage the client to volunteer more information than is directly requested. This type of questioning helps the nurse to acquire specific information about health problems such as symptoms, precipitating factors, or relief measures. As closed-ended questions reveal more information, the nurse may need to have the client elaborate more historical information. For example, after hearing the client relate an explanation for the cause of the problem, the nurse will ask the client to describe a normal day's food intake and how the client's travel schedule changed his or her eating pattern.

A good interviewer leaves with a complete story that

contains enough details for understanding the client's perceptions of his or her problem, as well as the information needed to guide the selection of nursing interventions. Quality nursing care begins with having a full and rich description of the client's health care problems and needs.

Phases of the Interview.

The interview involves orientation, working, and termination phases. Before interviewing the client, the nurse prepares by considering the purpose of the interview and collects data from all available sources and creates an environment conducive to an interview. If it is likely the interview will lead the nurse to perform any skills (e.g., obtaining a blood glucose level), a review of those skills is useful for a beginning nurse. An interview with a hospitalized client should be scheduled for a time when interruptions by other health care professionals or family will be minimal and the client will not be receiving visitors. An environment in which the client is comfortable and relaxed is also conducive to a good interview. A client interviewed at home may prefer that the interview take place in a bedroom away from other family members or in the living room with a spouse present. Remember to let the client decide when to involve family. Finally, the nurse selects a place private enough to allow the client to be comfortable when providing personal information.

Orientation Phase.

Before beginning, the nurse reviews the purpose for the interview, the types of data to be obtained, and the methods most appropriate for conducting the interview. The interview helps establish the nurse-client relationship, which influences the ability of the nurse to establish trust with the client. While conducting the interview, the nurse remains aware that the client is forming an impression about nursing.

Establishing the Nurse-Client Relationship.

Perhaps the most difficult client interview for a nurse to conduct is the first. It is an important time for the nurse to establish a relationship that fosters trust and confidence with a client. For some clients, being interviewed by a nurse is a new experience. An important goal for the initial interview is to lay the groundwork for the nurse to understand the client's needs and to begin a relationship that allows the client to become an active partner in decisions about care.

After the orientation phase of an interview, a client should begin to feel more comfortable speaking with the nurse. This is important, because the working phase requires the nurse to gather information of a more personal and focused nature. The nurse consciously communicates a sense of trust and confidentiality to clients. Illnesses that cause people to seek help are often accompanied by anxiety, helplessness, disruption of family relationships, and changes in self-image. Frequently clients are asked to provide very personal information about themselves and their families. Generally people share such information only with close friends, and there is a certain amount of trust that this information will not be shared with others. The nurse assures clients that interviews are confidential before asking them to share personal information.

Finally, the nurse-client relationship is enhanced by the professionalism and competence conveyed by the nurse. The nurse's attitude, professional manner, and appearance encourage a supportive therapeutic relationship with the client. Their free communication allows for ongoing identification of health care needs and objectives. The nurse is involved with the client and family and becomes an advocate for the client. The nurse acts for the client and encourages others to put the client's needs high on their list of priorities.

The nurse opens the interview by explaining the purposes of the interview (Figure 14-4). The nurse also discusses the types of questions that will be asked and the client's role in the process. Then the nurse spends a few minutes becoming acquainted with the client (Box 14-3). The case study in Box 14-3 will be used in subsequent chapters to demonstrate the steps of the nursing process.

In the case study, Mr. Coffey introduced his role to Mr. Brown. He reviewed the interview process and its objectives, confidentiality, and length. The nurse and client agreed mutually on an interview time. Before beginning the interview, Mr. Coffey asked his client if he had any questions. Mr. Coffey's answer about the oxygen allowed Mr. Brown to clarify his concern so that he would not be distracted during the interview. Mr. Coffey asked an open-ended question about Mr. Brown's family to encourage him to talk.

Working Phase.

As the interview progresses, the nurse asks questions to form a database from which the nursing care plan will be developed. The four techniques of interviewing are implemented as needed. In addition, the nurse

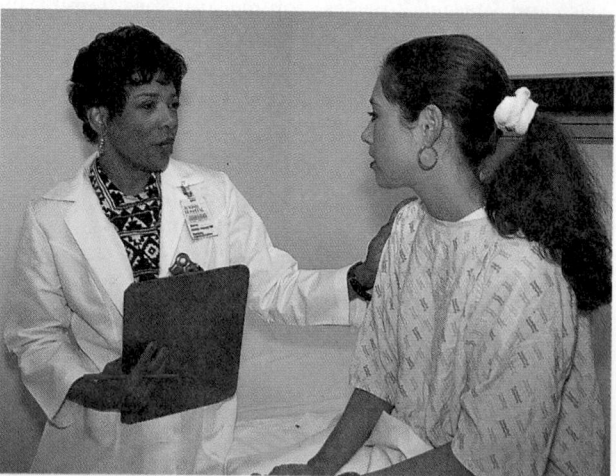

Figure 14-4 Nurse explains the purpose of the interview.

Case S T U D Y   BOX 14-3

Mr. Coffey is preparing an admission history on Mr. Brown, a 21-year-old man hospitalized for the first time.

Mr. Coffey: Good afternoon, Mr. Brown. I'm Joe Coffey, and I'm the nurse who will be managing your care during your hospital stay and through discharge to your home.

Mr. Brown: Hi, Joe. Please call me Bill. What do you mean by managing my care?

Mr. Coffey: That means I'm responsible for coordinating your nursing care with the rest of the nurses while you're hospitalized. I will work with them to plan for your discharge back to your home. Although other nurses will sometimes take care of you when I'm off, I'm the nurse who plans your care. Once you're discharged, I'll call you at home to see how you are doing and if you have any questions.

Mr. Brown: I guess that's a lot like being a coach. You may not play the game, but you're responsible for winning or losing.

Mr. Coffey: I suppose that's one way of looking at it. To better plan your care I will be asking some questions about your health. We call this a health interview. Any information you give me is confidential. The total interview should take about 20 to 30 minutes. Is it okay if I begin the interview in a few minutes?

Mr. Brown: How about giving me a half hour? My wife is about to leave. She needs to go pick up the kids at day care. That way we can have some time together. I'll be ready after that.

Mr. Coffey: That's fine. Since you're in a private room, I will do the health interview here. (Mr. Brown nods.)

Thirty minutes later, Mr. Coffey returns to the room.

Mr. Coffey: Okay. Before I get started, do you have any questions for me?

Mr. Brown: Yes. Why is there an outlet for oxygen on the wall above my bed? Does that mean that I'm really sick—did they put me in a special room?

Mr. Coffey: No, that's not it. Every bed in this hospital has an oxygen outlet located on the wall above the head of the bed. The reason is that this hospital has a central oxygen delivery system, and when a patient needs oxygen, we're able to supply it quickly, easily, and safely.

Mr. Brown: Okay. I wasn't actually worried. I was basically just curious. That was the only piece of equipment I couldn't explain.

Mr. Coffey: (pause) Bill, you mentioned that you and your wife have children in day care. Tell me a bit about your family.

Strategies for Effective Communication   Box 14-4

Silence is helpful for making observations and provides the client with time to organize thoughts and present complete information to the interviewer.

Attentive listening demonstrates interest in the client's needs, concerns, and problems. Listening can be facilitated by maintaining eye contact, remaining relaxed, and using appropriate touch techniques.

Conveying acceptance demonstrates the interviewer's willingness to listen to the client's beliefs, values, and practices without being judgmental.

Related questions are planned. When asking these questions, the nurse uses words and word patterns in the client's normal sociocultural context.

Paraphrasing provides an opportunity for the interviewer to validate information from the client without changing the meaning of the statement. Paraphrasing is the interviewer's formulation of what the client has said in more specific words.

Clarifying facilitates correct communication of information. It is achieved by asking the client to restate the information or by providing an example.

Focusing eliminates vagueness in communication, limits the area of discussion, and helps the interviewer direct attention to the pertinent aspects of a client's message.

Stating observations provides the client with feedback about how the interviewer observes behavior, action, facial expression, or activities.

Offering information allows the interviewer to clarify treatments, initiate health teaching, and identify and correct misconceptions.

Summarizing condenses the data into an organized review. It validates data because the client has the opportunity to confirm that they are correct. Summarizing indicates the end to a particular part of the interview.

---

uses 10 communication strategies (Box 14-4) to facilitate communication and ensure that nurse and client clearly understand each other (see Chapter 22).

Termination Phase.   As in the other phases of the interview, termination requires skill on the part of the interviewer. Ideally the client should be given a clue that the interview is coming to an end. For example, the nurse may say, "There are just two more questions," or "We'll be finished in 5 to 6 minutes." With this method the client can maintain attention without being distracted by wondering how much longer the interview will last. Also, the client may ask any final questions before the interview ends.

The nurse should be as organized during this phase as during the opening. The interview is terminated in a friendly manner, with the nurse indicating specifically when there will be additional contact. For example, an appropriate way to end an interview would be, "Thank you for your help. The information you have shared will be helpful in planning your care. Another nurse will be caring for you this evening, but I'll be back on duty tomorrow morning. Do you have any other questions? Is there anything I can do for you now?"

The nurse's interviewing skills and techniques are essential to developing a good database. The skillful inter-

BARNES HOSPITAL
ST. LOUIS, MISSOURI

Brown, William
4823 Independence Dr.
Yorktown, MO

Person to Contact: Hannah (wife)   Emergency Phone: 555-4821

Why you came to the hospital? "To find out why I've had diarrhea for 3 weeks"

Allergies (food, drugs, latex, environment)? Penicillin

Items brought in from home?
- ☐ Medications   ☐ Dentures
- ☐ Contacts   ☑ Glasses
- ☐ Hearing Aid

Did you bring:
- ☐ Money   ☐ Jewelry   ☐ Credit Cards   ☐ Checkbook/Checks   ☐ Other _____
- *(These need to be locked up with security or sent home. Hospital will not be responsible for valuables left in room)* All sent home c̄ Hannah Brown

	MEDICINE NAMES	Dose & How Often Taken	Reason You Take Medicine	Time of Last Dose
Prescribed by a Doctor	immodium	2 tabs	diarrhea	2° ago
Non-Prescription	acetaminophen		headaches	2 wks ago

Do you have any problems with your medicines?
No - "but it isn't working"

Do you smoke? ☑ Yes ☐ No   Do you use "street" drugs? ☐ Yes ☑ No   How much caffeine do you drink or eat?
Do you chew tobacco? ☐ Yes ☑ No   How much alcohol do you drink? _____   4 cups coffee

Medical History:
- ☐ Heart Disease
- ☐ Lung Disease
- ☐ Liver Disease
- ☐ Immune Disorders
- ☐ Other _____
- ☐ Epilepsy
- ☐ Stroke
- ☐ Diabetes
- ☐ TB
- ☐ Cancer
- ☐ Hepatitis
- ☐ High Blood Pressure
- ☐ Rheumatic Disease
- ☐ Sexually Transmitted Disease: _____
- ☐ Chicken Pox/Shingles
- ☐ Fainting/Dizzy Spells
- ☐ Stomach Problems
- ☐ Bladder Problems
- ☐ Menstrual Disease
- ☐ Circulation Problems
- ☐ Swelling
- ☐ Bleeding

HISTORY COMMENTS:

Could you be pregnant?   ☐ Yes   ☐ No   N/A   When was you last Period? _____

What surgeries or procedures have you had? (Date)

Family Health History: ☐ Hypertension   ☐ Diabetes   ☐ Heart Disease   ☐ Stroke   ☐ Cancer   ☐ Other _____

Which of the following have you had in the past 12 months?
- ☐ Self Breast Exam
- ☐ Mammogram (over 40)
- ☐ Prostate Check
- ☑ Testicular Check
- ☑ Glaucoma Check
- ☐ Pelvic Exam
- ☑ Rectal Check (over 40)
- ☐ Hearing Check
- ☑ Dental Exam
- ☑ Vision Check

Are your immunizations current?   ☑ Yes   ☐ No   ☐ Unknown
(Call ID Specialist)

Figure 14-5   Nursing health history for Mr. Brown.
Courtesy Barnes-Jewish Hospital, St. Louis, Mo.

Are you on a special diet? *"no - but diarrhea occurs after all meals"*	How is your appetite? *poor last week*
Any foods you can't eat and why? *"everything causes diarrhea"*	Any difficulty eating or swallow- *no*
Nutritional supplements/or diet substitutions (e.g., vitamins, artificial sweeteners salt, substitutes)	Weight loss/gain (amount) in the last 12 months? *15 lb. weight loss in last 3 weeks*

How often do you have a BM? *diarrhea*
Do you have any difficulty having a bowel movement?
☐ use laxatives   ☐ hemorrhoids
☐ use stool softeners   ☐ black/tarry

Do you have any difficulty urinating? *no*
☐ burning   ☐ blood   ☐ leaking   ☐ frequency

Do you tire easily?   ☑ Yes   ☐ No
Do you get regular exercise?   ☐ Yes ☐ No
What kind? _____   How often? _____

Have you fallen recently?   ☐ Yes   ☑ No
Usually walk $\frac{1}{1}$ mile/day - hasn't done this for $\frac{1}{1}$ mo.

What activities do you need help with?
☐ Feeding/eating   ☐ Meal preparation
☐ Dressing   ☐ Transportation
☐ Grooming/bathing   ☐ Housework
☐ Taking medications   ☐ Handling finances
☐ Toileting   ☐ Grocery shopping
☐ Moving/positioning

☐ Walking on level surfaces
☐ Walking on stairs
☐ Paying for Medicines

(RN consider appropriate consults)

Aides used at home:
☑ Eye glasses   ☐ Contact lenses
☐ Hearing aid   ☐ Cane
☐ Walker   ☐ Wheelchair
☐ Prosthesis: _____
DENTURES: ☐ Upper   ☐ Lower
PARTIALS: ☐ Upper   ☐ Lower

Is it difficult for you to carry out prescribed health care regimens (Diet, Activity, Medications)?   ☐ Yes   ☐ No
If YES, explain: *During last week, increased fatigue, increased abdominal pain*

How much sleep do you normally get? *8 hrs.*

What helps you fall asleep? *nothing*

Who do you live with?   ☐ Alone   ☐ Spouse only   ☑ Family   ☐ Friends   ☐ Nursing Home

Who helps you at home?   ☑ Spouse   ☐ Family   ☐ Friends   ☐ Home Health   ☐ Visiting Nurse

Do you have concerns about your family while you are in the hospital?
no

What major changes have you had in your life in the past 12 months?
none

Do you feel you deal successfully with stress?   ☑ Yes   ☐ No
"Afraid that I have cancer"

Would you like additional resources?   ☑ Yes   ☐ No

Do you have concerns that your illness/hospitalization will affect:
☐ appearance   ☐ job   ☐ male/female roles   ☐ how you feel about yourself

Is religion important in your life?   ☐ Yes   ☐ No
yes - Methodist

Will this illness/hospitalization interfere with any religious beliefs/practices?   ☐ Yes   ☑ No

What do you expect from us while in the hospital?
"To stop my diarrhea + pain" and "to tell me I don't have cancer"

Do you have a Living Will?   ☑ Yes   ☐ No
Do you have a copy with you?   ☑ Yes   ☐ No

Do you have a Power of Attorney?   ☑ Yes   ☐ No

Patient/Significant Other Signature: Relationship: *William Brown*	Date *7/3*	Staff Signature: Title: *Gary Jones, RN*	Date *7/3*

☐ REVIEWED BY REGISTERED NURSE   SIGNATURE: *Gary Jones, RN*   DATE: *7/3*

TO BE COMPLETED BY STAFF ONLY

Patient provided:
Patient instructed:
☑ Admit kit   ☑ ID band   ☑ Sensitivity/Allergy band on patient   ☑ Allergy sticker on chart
☑ Valuables policy   ☑ Waiver signed   ☑ Smoking   ☑ Visitation
☑ Nursing call/Emergency   ☑ TV/phone   ☐ Fall precautions/band on wrist
☑ Patient's Rights/responsibilities   ☑ Received copy of Personal Directions for My Healthcare

Time patient arrived on Division: *0850*   SIGNATURE: *Gary Jones*

Figure 14-5—cont'd

viewer is able to adapt interview strategies based on the client's responses. Pertinent health data are obtained when the nurse is prepared for the interview and is able to carry out each interview phase with minimal interruption.

NURSING HEALTH HISTORY

The **nursing health history** is data collected about the client's level of wellness (present and past), family history, changes in life patterns, sociocultural history, spiritual health, and mental and emotional reactions to illness. The nursing history is obtained during an interview, and it is a major component in conducting an assessment. The objective is to identify patterns of health and illness, risk factors for physical and behavioral health problems, deviations from normal, and available resources for adaptation. Although many health history forms are structured, the nurse learns to use the questions as starting points (Figure 14-5). A good assessor learns to refine and broaden questions as needed so that the client's unique needs are correctly assessed.

Patterns of a client's health and illness are identified by collecting data about the physical and developmental, intellectual, emotional, social, and spiritual dimensions (Figure 14-6). Incorporating data from all dimensions enables the nurse to develop a complete plan of care. Although many formats for the nursing health history have been given in the literature, all contain similar basic components.

Biographical Information. Biographical information is factual demographic data about the client. The client's age, address, occupation and working status, mar-

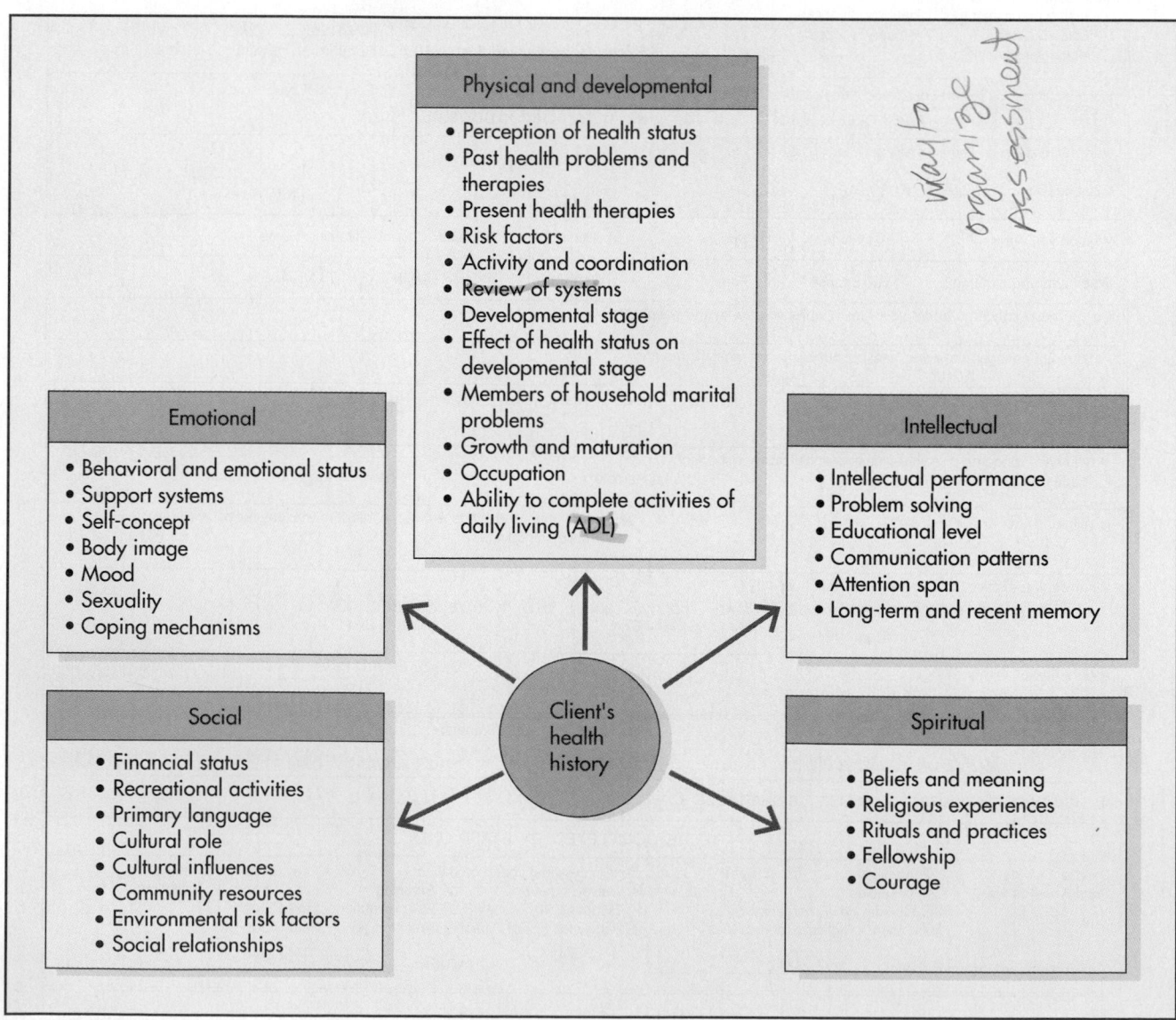

Figure 14-6 Dimensions for gathering data for a health history.

ital status, and types of insurance coverage should be included.

Reason for Seeking Health Care. The nurse asks why the client sought health care, because the information contained on the initial admission form may differ greatly from the client's subjective reason for seeking health care. The client's statement is not diagnostic, instead it is the client's perception of reasons for seeking health care. Clarification of the client's perception identifies potential areas for education, counseling, or community resources required throughout all phases of diagnosis and recovery. When recorded, the statement is enclosed in quotation marks to indicate the client's words.

Client Expectations. The assessment of client expectations is not the same as the reason for seeking medical care, although they are often related. It is becoming more important for nurses to acknowledge what is important to the client who is seeking health care. Failure to identify a client's expectations of health care providers and a health care institution can result in poor client satisfaction. Client satisfaction is becoming a standard measure of quality for all hospitals throughout the country (see Chapter 2).

Clients typically have expectations in the following areas:

Information needed to care for their health problems independently
Caring and compassion expressed by care providers
Timeliness of caregivers' response to client requests
Relief of pain and symptoms
Involvement in decision making
Cleanliness of the care environment

The initial interview can establish the client's expectations when entering the health care setting. Later, as the client has had interactions with health care providers, it is valuable to assess if the client's expectations have been met.

Present Illness. If an illness is present, nurses gather essential and relevant data about the onset of symptoms. The nurse determines when the symptoms began, whether they began suddenly or gradually, and whether they are always present or come and go. The nurse also asks about the duration of symptoms. In the section of the history on present illness, the nurse records specific information such as location, intensity, and quality of a symptom. For example, when the client indicates the symptom of pain, the nurse asks the client to point to or outline the area of the body affected, asks the client to rate the intensity on a scale of 1 to 10, and has the client describe what the pain feels like (see Chapter 42). The nurse needs to know whether any action precipitates the symptoms, makes them worse, or provides relief.

It is also appropriate to learn clients' expectations of the health care providers. The nurse determines whether clients expect to be "cured," "free of pain," or "able to care for themselves." This information assists in establishing the goals of nursing care, as well as in determining whether clients' expectations of themselves and the health care providers are realistic. In addition, such expectations provide the nurse with information on client perceptions about patterns of illness or changes in lifestyle.

Past Health History. The information collected about past history provides data on the client's health care experiences. The nurse assesses whether the client has ever been hospitalized or has undergone surgery. Also essential in planning nursing care are descriptions of allergies, including allergic reactions to food, latex, drugs, or pollutants. If an allergy is present, the specific reaction and treatment are noted on the assessment form.

The nurse also identifies habits and lifestyle patterns. Use of alcohol, tobacco, caffeine, over-the-counter drugs, or routinely taken medications can place the client at risk for diseases involving the liver, lungs, heart, nervous system, or thought processes. Noting the type of habit, as well as the frequency and duration of use, provides essential data.

Assessing patterns of sleep (see Chapter 41), exercise (see Chapter 36), and nutrition (see Chapter 43) is important when planning nursing care. The plan of care within a health care setting should match a client's lifestyle patterns as much as possible. Frequently, variations in sleep, activity, and nutritional patterns can be accommodated.

Family History. The purpose of the family history is to obtain data about immediate and blood relatives. The objectives are to determine whether the client is at risk for illnesses of a genetic or familial nature and to identify areas of health promotion and illness prevention (see Chapter 1). The family history also provides information about family structure, interaction, and function that may be useful in planning care (see Chapter 16). For example, a cohesive, supportive family can be a resource in helping a client adjust to an illness or disability and should be incorporated into the plan of care. On the other hand, if the client's family is not supportive, it may be better to not involve them in care, particularly if the family history reveals that the client is experiencing stress related to familial relationships.

Environmental History. The environmental history provides data about clients' home environments and any support systems that they or family members may need to use. Information pertaining to the home environment may include function of utilities, layout of rooms in the house, and the presence of any barriers or risks to client safety. In addition, the environmental history identifies exposure to pollutants that can affect health, existence of high crime that prevents clients from walking around their neighborhoods, and available resources that can assist clients in returning to the community.

Psychosocial History. A complete psychosocial history will reveal the client's support system, which may include spouse, children, other family members, and close friends. The psychosocial history includes information about ways that the client and family typically cope with stress (see Chapter 30). The same behavior, such as taking a walk, reading, or talking with a friend, can be used as a nursing intervention if the client experiences stress while receiving health care. The nurse also learns if the client has experienced any recent losses that create a sense of grief (see Chapter 29).

Spiritual Health. Life experiences and events are shaped by one's spirituality. The spiritual dimension represents the totality of one's being and is difficult to assess quickly (see Chapter 28). A nurse reviews with clients their beliefs about life, their source for guidance in acting on beliefs, and the relationship they have with family in exercising their faith. Rituals and religious practices as a way to express spirituality are also assessed.

Review of Systems. The **review of systems (ROS)** is a systematic method for collecting data on all body systems. The systems that are assessed depend on the client's condition and urgency in initiating care. During the ROS, the nurse asks the client about the normal functioning of each system and any noted changes. Such changes are usually subjective data because they are described as perceived by the client.

As the nurse proceeds through the nursing health history, assessment data are recorded in a clear, concise manner using appropriate terminology. A clear, concise record is necessary for use by other health care professionals (see Chapter 24).

Gordon's **functional health patterns** (1994) serve as one way to focus or organize an approach for collecting the nursing assessment (see Box 14-1). Information from the nursing health history provides a systematic description of the 11 functional health patterns and the client's perception, evaluation, and explanation of any particular problems. The 11 patterns establish the nursing database because the historical and current information about all health patterns is collected and the information is used as baseline criteria against which any future changes are evaluated (Gordon, 1991, 1994). Assessments of functional health patterns and biomedical systems are easily integrated and aid in completing the client's physical and behavioral assessment database.

PHYSICAL EXAMINATION

The physical examination and collection of diagnostic and laboratory data involve the gathering of objective, observable information undistorted by client perceptions (see Chapter 32). The **physical examination** is the taking of vital signs and other measurements and the examination of all body parts using the techniques of inspection, palpa-

tion, percussion, auscultation, and olfaction. The examiner looks for abnormalities that may yield information about past, present, and future health problems. The physical examination is conducted after the nursing health history so that historical data can be verified. In addition, new data (e.g., appearance of the client's skin and muscle strength) are obtained during the examination.

Throughout the examination, data are measured against a standard, which is an established rule or basis of comparison in measuring or judging capacity, quantity, content, and value of objects in the same category. The term **norm** is frequently used interchangeably with the term *standard* in the literature. Selected standards are reliable and relevant for the category being compared. For example, established standards for ideal height and weight are used to determine whether an individual is taller or shorter than the standard or is overweight or underweight. There are standards for blood pressure ranges for clients of select age groups. The nurse conducts the physical examination to verify information and collect further data, which are compared with the standards to determine whether the findings are normal or abnormal.

Before conducting the physical examination, the nurse prepares the client, environment, and necessary equipment. The nurse informs the client about the process of the physical examination, specifically its purposes, the nurse's role, the client's role, and the approximate duration.

Order of Examination. The physical examination is carried out in a systematic manner similar to the ROS in the health history. This component of assessment usually begins with data on the client's height, weight, and vital signs (see Chapter 31). Next the examiner writes a general statement about client perceptions and the client's level of health. This statement, called the general survey, includes information about mental status, body development, nutritional status, sex and race, chronological versus apparent age, behavior, appearance, and speech (Chaper 32). Last is a head-to-toe examination of the body systems. The examiner describes and records objective data obtained, using clear, concise, and appropriate language.

Physical Examination Techniques. The nurse uses **inspection, palpation, percussion, auscultation, and olfaction** to thoroughly examine a client. Each technique requires that certain principles be followed to ensure accurate data collection. Throughout an examination the nurse works closely with a client to minimize any anxiety or discomfort. Chapter 32 describes each of the examination techniques in detail.

DIAGNOSTIC AND LABORATORY DATA

The final source of assessment data is the results of diagnostic and laboratory tests. The tests are ordered by physicians or advanced practice nurses. It is important for the nurse to review the results to verify alterations identified in the nursing health history and physical examination. They include baseline information about the response to illness and information about the effects of later treatment measures. Laboratory data can help to identify actual or potential health care problems not previously noted by the client or examiner.

Laboratory data are compared with the established norms for a particular test, age group, and sex. The nurse identifies variations from normal and interprets findings according to the disease process and treatments. In addition, laboratory data can be used to evaluate the success or failure of nursing and medical interventions.

Laboratory tests are selected according to the client's symptoms or disease. However, common tests may be used for a large number of clients. Specific laboratory tests and the nursing responsibilities associated with them are detailed in Units 7 and 8.

Formulating Nursing Judgments

To be useful, assessment data must refer to the intended purpose of nursing and relate to the client's health problems (Bandman and Bandman, 1995). These interrelated concepts are the basis for nursing judgments. The nurse critically chooses the type of information to collect about a client, interprets the information to determine abnormalities, conducts further observations to clarify information, and then names the client's problem(s) in the form of nursing diagnoses (see Chapter 15).

DATA INTERPRETATION

The nurse may collect extensive information about a client. Through a process of inferential reasoning and judgment the nurse decides what information has meaning in relation to the client's health status (Gordon, 1994). Inferential reasoning involves the process of attaching new meaning to known clinical data. For example, consider the following situation: When entering the client's room at 6 AM the nurse notices the client's bed linen is pulled down to the end of the bed and twisted in a lump, with the blanket on the floor. (Inference: the bed linen is in disarray.) Closer inspection finds the client sitting up in the chair next to the bed, holding his incision firmly, breathing slowly, and stating, "I didn't get much sleep last night." (Inference: the client received inadequate sleep.)

In this example of inference in practice, one nurse will infer inadequate sleep and then assess further the nature of the problem. In this case, assessment of the client's comfort level may reveal important additional cues. Another nurse may not make the second inference, and simply tidy up the bed and leave the room. Interpretation of data summarizes the data and provides a focus for attention (Gordon, 1994).

Problem assessment means collecting, estimating, and judging the value and significance of data (Lauri, 1982). This means the nurse is always thinking and analyzing data about a client to make accurate and meaningful interpretations of the client's problems. Assessment enables the nurse to understand problems further, to judge the extent of the problem, and to trace relationships between problems (Vitale and others, 1978). This is the heart of critical thinking and clinical problem solving. To prevent errors, the nurse validates and verifies any inferences or assumptions. Validation is obtained by comparing data with another source. For example, while summarizing an interview the nurse asks the client about accuracy of the most pertinent information. Findings gained in a physical examination can be validated with another nurse or with the medical record summary.

DATA CLUSTERING

After collecting and validating subjective and objective data and interpreting the data, the nurse organizes the information into meaningful clusters. This is dependent on recognizing significant cues. There are times when assessment data point clearly to a certain nursing diagnosis. For example, a client who has recently been diagnosed with diabetes, has had no opportunity to talk with a physician, and is asking questions about insulin obviously has a problem related to inadequate knowledge. As the nurse clusters cues, such as the client asking questions and reporting no previous experience with insulin use, a pattern of meaning forms. Clustering of data helps to focus on identification of the correct problem. In the case of the diabetic client, data interpretation is relatively simple and routine; the nurse recognizes similarity to past situations.

During data clustering certain cues alert the nurse's thinking processes more than others (Gordon, 1994). These cues help to generate nursing diagnoses. The nurse becomes experienced in recognizing features of health problems, such as pain, anxiety, or immobility. Over time the nurse stores knowledge from previous experiences so that more complicated clustering becomes recognizable. This explains the difference in the skill of a beginning nurse and a more expert nurse.

During data clustering, the nurse organizes data and focuses attention on client functions needing support and assistance for recovery. The next step is to form nursing diagnoses from the clusters of data to develop specific nursing interventions for the client's care. Box 14-5 demonstrates focused data clustering using the system-oriented assessment and functional health pattern assessment completed on Mr. Brown.

Data Documentation

Data documentation is the last part of a complete assessment. Thoroughness and accuracy are necessary when recording data. If an item is not recorded, it is lost and unavailable to the database.

Focused Data Clustering for Mr. Brown
Box 14-5

SYSTEM-ORIENTED FORMAT

Integumentary System

Intact, flushed skin that is hot and dry to touch

Dry oral mucosa, coated tongue, and cracked lips

Gastrointestinal System

Distended, firm abdomen that is tender to palpation in lower quadrants

Hyperactive bowel sounds in all quadrants

History of diarrhea and cramping for 3 weeks

Poor nutritional intake over last week

Medical Record

Laboratory tests indicating elevated white blood cell (WBC) count and hematocrit level: hypernatremia

Abdominal x-ray examination showing gas-filled loops of bowel

Admitting diagnosis of gastroenteritis

FUNCTIONAL HEALTH PATTERN FORMAT

Activity and Exercise Pattern

Statement of increased fatigue when walking

Demonstration of ability to perform activities of daily living (ADLs)

Fatigued, dyspneic, and diaphoretic appearance when performing ADLs

Increased pulse from 90 to 126 beats per minute during ADLs

Sleep and Rest Pattern

Report of difficulty in falling and remaining asleep

Denial of use of sleeping aids

Coping-Stress-Tolerance Pattern

Anxiety about illness

Pain

Medical Record

Previous history of decreased activity tolerance and poor sleeping 2 weeks before hospital admission for congestive heart failure

Chest x-ray film showing pulmonary congestion

Thoroughness in data documentation is essential for two reasons. First, all data pertinent to a client's status are included. Even information that does not seem to indicate an abnormality should be recorded. It may become pertinent later, serving as a baseline for a change in status. A general rule of thumb is that if it is assessed it should be recorded. Second, observation and recording of client status is a legal and professional responsibility. The nurse practice acts in all states and the ANA Policy Statement (1995) and Standards of Clinical Practice (1991) mandate accurate data collection and recording as independent functions essential to the role of the professional nurse (see Chapter 19).

Being factual is easy after it becomes a habit. The basic rule is to record all observations. When recording data, a nurse should pay attention to facts and should make an effort to be as descriptive as possible. Anything heard, seen, felt, or smelled should be reported exactly. Conclusions about such data become nursing diagnoses. Because assessment includes the collection and documentation of subjective and objective data, the nurse should make certain that the database is complete and factual before data clustering. Premature clustering can lead to inaccurate nursing diagnoses. In situations in which the client has just been admitted or when the client's status is changing rapidly, it is better to continually collect and document the new data and delay clustering.

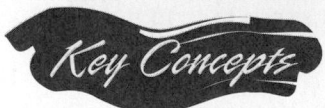

Key Concepts

- Good assessment requires the nurse to apply knowledge and experience in making the necessary observations and measurements to gather data about clients.
- Written data statements should be descriptive, concise, and complete and should not include inferences or interpretative statements.
- Collection of inaccurate, incomplete, or inappropriate data may result in incorrect identification of the client's health care needs.

- The nature and amount of data in assessment are always changing, requiring a nurse to anticipate and ask questions to be sure assessment is accurate and complete.
- Gordon's 11 functional health patterns are a framework for a comprehensive assessment that moves inquiry from the general to the specific so that patterns of problems can be identified.
- Subjective data are the client's perceptions.

- Good assessment requires communicating with all health care team members.
- Families can be an important source of information about the client's health status.
- The interview enables a nurse to establish a nurse-client relationship through caring, which fosters the sharing of ideas for a thorough assessment.
- The problem-solving interview technique explores in-depth data about specific problems.
- An interview includes an orientation, working, and termination phase.
- An interview with a client seeking health care should include assessment of the client's expectations.
- To form a nursing judgment, the nurse critically assesses a client, interprets the information gathered, conducts further assessment for clarification, and names the client's problems.
- The nursing health history involves data about level of wellness, past medical history, family history, environmental history, psychosocial and cultural history, and a review of the body systems.
- Laboratory and diagnostic tests add to the database and verify data gathered through the nursing health history and physical examination.

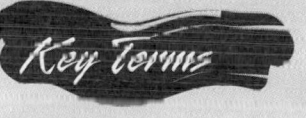

Key Terms

Assessment, *p. 292*	Nursing health history,
Auscultation, *p. 306*	*p. 304*
Back channeling, *p. 299*	Objective data, *p. 296*
Closed-ended questions,	Olfaction, *p. 306*
p. 299	Open-ended questions, *p. 299*
Database, *p. 292*	Palpation, *p. 306*
Functional health patterns,	Percussion, *p. 306*
p. 306	Physical examination, *p. 306*
Inference, *p. 295*	Problem-seeking inter-
Inspection, *p. 306*	view, *p. 299*
Interview, *p. 298*	Review of systems (ROS),
Norm, *p. 306*	*p. 306*
Nurse-client relationship,	Standard, *p. 296*
p. 298	Subjective data, *p. 295*

Critical Thinking Exercises

1. Mrs. Kinsey is a 61-year-old woman who is being seen at home following hospitalization for her arthritis. She greets you at the door, and you enter the home. The two of you sit down at the kitchen table. You notice many unwashed dishes in the sink, and the counter is covered with stacks of mail. On the kitchen table are six bottles of medication. What inferences might you make from your observations? How might you assess the client to gather more objective information about her health status?

2. Miss Fong has been assigned to your care for the first time. The nurse from the previous shift tells you she had surgery on her left lower leg and has a very large bandage. During the night she required an analgesic to help her sleep. She is able to drink liquids without nausea. You know that one of your responsibilities is to do an assessment of the client's condition. What are three priorities you would focus assessment on?

3. Mr. Rossi comes to the clinic with the following history: for the last 3 days he has had ringing in his ears and dizziness. Within the last 24 hours he has experienced nausea and headache as well. Identify three different open-ended questions that will prompt Mr. Rossi to discuss his condition.

References

American Nurses Association: *Nursing's social policy statement*, Washington, DC, 1995, The Association.

American Nurses Association: *Standards of clinical nursing practice*, Washington, DC, 1991, The Association.

Bandman EL, Bandman B: *Critical thinking in nursing*, ed 2, Norwalk, Conn, 1995, Appleton & Lange.

Benner P: *From novice to expert: excellence and power in clinical practice*, Menlo Park, Calif, 1984, Addison-Wesley.

Bryano A, McIntosh J: Decision making in community nursing; an analysis of the stages of decision making as they relate to community nursing, *J Adv Nurs* 24(1): 24, 1996.

Carnevali DL, Thomas MD: *Diagnostic reasoning and treatment decision making in nursing*, Philadelphia, 1993, JB Lippincott.

Carpenito LJ: *Nursing diagnosis*, ed 7, Philadelphia, 1997, JB Lippincott.

Cohen BJ and others: Educators' responses to changes in the health care system, *J NY State Nurses Assoc* 28(2):4, 1997.

Gordon M: *Nursing diagnosis: process and application*, ed 2, St. Louis, 1987, Mosby.

Gordon M: *Manual of nursing diagnoses: 1991–1992*, St. Louis, 1991, Mosby.

Gordon M: *Nursing diagnosis: process and application*, ed 3, St. Louis, 1994, Mosby.

Hurst K and others: The recognition and non-recognition of problem-solving stages in nursing practice, *J Adv Nurs* 16:1444, 1991.

Ivey AE: *Intentional interviewing and counseling: facilitating client development*, ed 2, Pacific Grove, Calif, 1988, Brooks/Cole.

Lauri S: Development of the nursing process through action research, *J Adv Nurs* 7:301, 1982.

Lipkin M and others: *The medical interview: clinical care, education, and research*, New York, 1995, Springer-Verlag.

Ryan-Wenger NM: A nursing process methodology, *Nurs Outlook* 38(4):190, 1990.

Vitale B and others: *A problem-solving approach to nursing care plans*, St. Louis, 1978, Mosby.

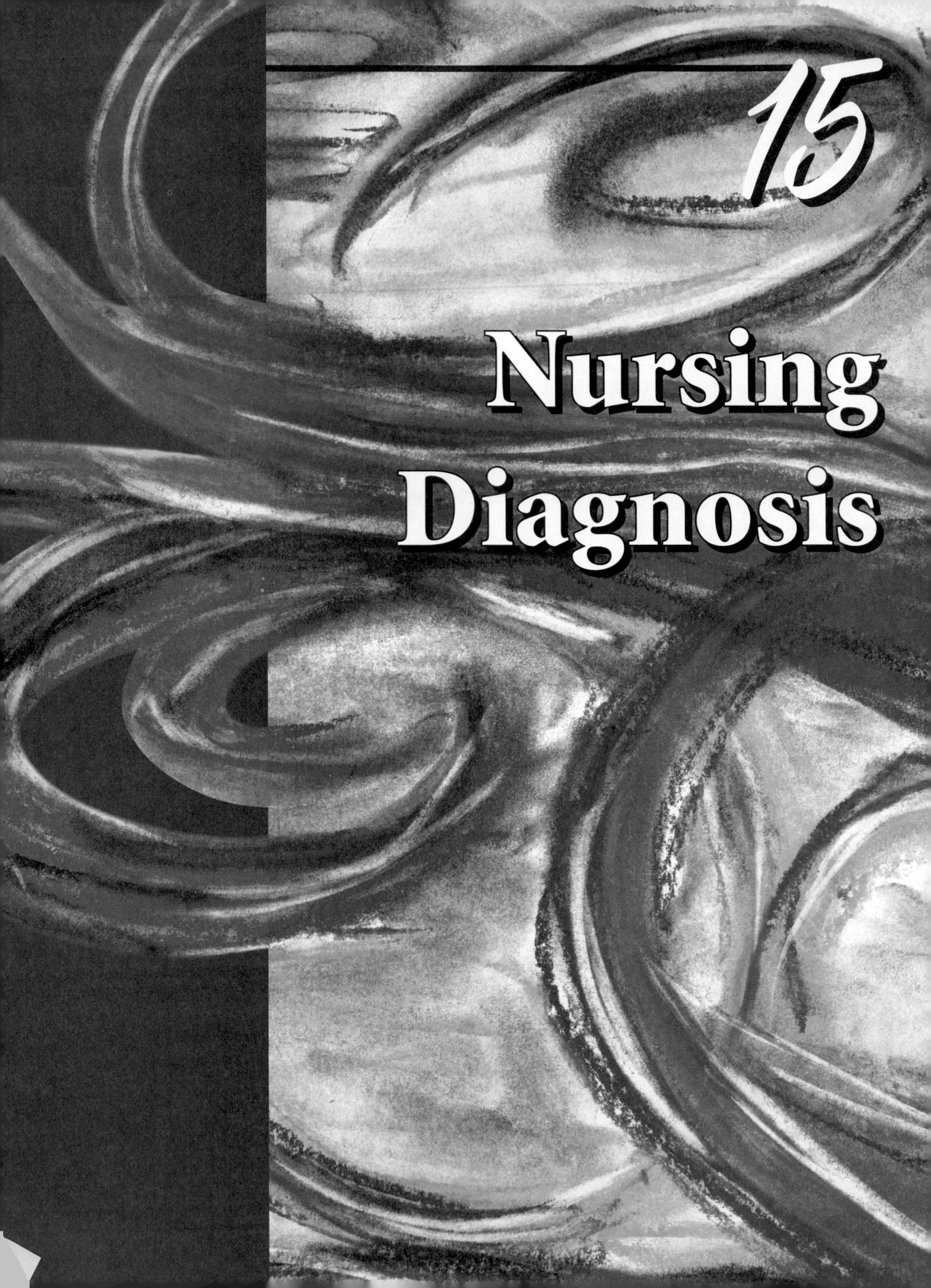

15

Nursing Diagnosis

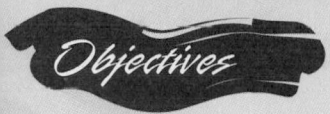

Mastery of content in this chapter will enable the student to:

- Define the key terms listed.
- Describe the way defining characteristics and the etiological process individualize a nursing diagnosis.
- List and discuss the steps of the nursing diagnostic process.
- Demonstrate the nursing diagnostic process.
- Differentiate between a nursing diagnosis and a medical diagnosis.
- Explain what makes a nursing diagnosis correct.
- Discuss the advantages of nursing diagnoses for the client and the nursing profession.
- Discuss the limitations of nursing diagnoses.
- Formulate nursing diagnoses from a nursing assessment.

After completing the nursing assessment, the nurse proceeds to the process of forming appropriate nursing diagnoses. A nursing diagnosis is a clinical judgment about individual, family, or community responses to actual or potential health problems or life processes. A **nursing diagnosis** is a statement that describes the client's actual or potential response to a health problem that the nurse is licensed and competent to treat. *Impaired skin integrity related to decreased mobility* and *risk for infection related to poor nutritional intake* are examples of nursing diagnoses. Nursing diagnoses provide the basis for selection of nursing interventions to achieve outcomes for which the nurse is accountable (Rantz and LeMone, 1997). Outcomes and interventions are selected in relationship to particular nursing diagnoses (McCloskey and Bulechek, 2000).

Having gathered a comprehensive assessment of the client's health status, the nurse now moves to apply critical thinking to formulating judgments about the client's health. The nurse uses her knowledge and experience and applies standards and critical thinking attitudes to interpret the assessment data in a meaningful and relevant way to make judgments about the client's responses to health problems. These judgments are essentially nursing diagnoses. The reasons for formulating a nursing diagnosis after analyzing assessment data are to identify health problems involving the client and family and to provide direction for nursing care. The statement of a nursing diagnosis is the result of a diagnostic process during which the nurse uses critical thinking and takes into account the physical, developmental, intellectual, emotional, social, and spiritual data obtained during assessment.

A nursing diagnosis is a statement that describes the client's actual or potential response to a health problem. The client's actual and potential responses are obtained from the assessment database, a review of pertinent literature, the client's past medical records, and consultation with other professionals, all of which are collected during assessment. Last, the client's actual or potential responses require interventions from the domain of nursing practice (Carpenito, 1997).

Evolution of Nursing Diagnosis

Nursing has attempted to define itself professionally and functionally since the writings of Nightingale, who stated that the purpose of nursing care was to put patients in the best condition for nature to act upon them (Nightingale, 1860). Initially, nursing school curricula were organized around disease entities or medical models as frameworks for describing the role of the nurse in providing nursing care. However, in the mid-1950s and early 1960s, nursing leaders and educators started to revise curricula around **client-centered problems** (Carpenito, 1995, 1997). Nursing diagnosis was first introduced in the nursing literature in 1950 (McFarland and McFarlane, 1989). Fry (1953) proposed that nursing could be more creative by the formulation of nursing diagnoses and an individualized nursing care plan. This placed more emphasis on the nurse's independent practice compared with the dependent practice driven by physicians' orders. Initially, nursing diagnoses were not supported by professional nursing, and in 1955 the *Model Nurse Practice Act* of the American Nurses Association (ANA) excluded diagnosis or prescriptive therapies (ANA, 1955). As a result, nurses were hesitant to use nursing diagnostic labels in their practice.

However, Henderson, Abdellah, and other theorists encouraged defining nursing in terms of client problems. These early theorists, by defining nursing action in terms of client-centered problems, were partly responsible for

North American Nursing Diagnosis Association (NANDA) Accepted Nursing Diagnoses

Box 15-1

Activity intolerance
Activity intolerance, risk for
Adaptive capacity, decreased: intracranial
Adjustment, impaired
Airway clearance, ineffective
Anxiety
Anxiety, death
Aspiration, risk for
Body image disturbance
Body temperature, altered, risk for
Bowel incontinence
Breastfeeding, effective
Breastfeeding, ineffective
Breastfeeding, interrupted
Breathing pattern, ineffective
Cardiac output, decreased
Caregiver role strain
Caregiver role strain, risk for
Communication, impaired verbal
Community coping, ineffective
Community coping, potential for enhanced
Confusion, acute
Confusion, chronic
Constipation
Constipation, colonic
Constipation, perceived
Constipation, risk for
Coping, defensive
Coping, family: potential for growth
Coping, ineffective family: compromised
Coping, ineffective family: disabling
Coping, ineffective individual
Decisional conflict (specify)
Denial, ineffective
Dentition, altered
Development, altered, risk for
Diarrhea
Disuse syndrome risk for
Diversional activity deficit
Dysreflexia
Dysreflexia, autonomic, risk for
Energy field disturbance
Environmental interpretation syndrome, impaired
Failure to thrive, adult
Family processes, altered
Family processes, altered: alcoholism
Fatigue
Fear
Fluid volume deficit
Fluid volume deficit, risk for
Fluid volume excess
Fluid volume imbalance, risk for
Gas exchange, impaired
Grieving, anticipatory
Grieving, dysfunctional
Growth, altered, risk for
Growth and development altered

Health maintenance, altered
Health-seeking behaviors (specify)
Home maintenance management, impaired
Hopelessness
Hyperthermia
Hypothermia
Incontinence, stress
Incontinence, total
Incontinence, urge
Incontinence, urinary, functional
Incontinence, urinary, reflex
Incontinence, urinary urge, risk for
Infant behavior, disorganized
Infant behavior, disorganized: risk for
Infant behavior, organized: potential for enhanced
Infant feeding pattern, ineffective
Infection, risk for
Injury, perioperative positioning: risk for
Injury, risk for
Knowledge deficit (specify)
Latex allergy response
Latex allergy response, risk for
Loneliness, risk for
Management of therapeutic regimen, community: ineffective
Management of therapeutic regimen, families: ineffective
Management of therapeutic regimen, individual: effective
Management of therapeutic regimen, individual: ineffective
Memory, impaired
Mobility, impaired bed
Mobility, impaired physical
Mobility, impaired wheelchair
Nausea
Noncompliance (specify)
Nutrition, altered: less than body requirements
Nutrition, altered: more than body requirements
Nutrition, altered: risk for more than body requirements
Oral mucous membrane, altered
Pain
Pain, chronic
Parent/infant/child attachment, altered: risk for
Parental role conflict
Parenting, altered
Parenting, altered, risk for
Peripheral neurovascular dysfunction, risk for
Personal identity disturbance
Poisoning, risk for
Posttrauma syndrome
Posttrauma syndrome, risk for
Powerlessness
Protection, altered
Rape-trauma syndrome
Rape-trauma syndrome: compound reaction
Rape-trauma syndrome: silent reaction
Relocation stress syndrome
Role performance, altered
Self-care deficit, bathing/hygiene
Self-care deficit, dressing/grooming

North American Nursing Diagnosis Association: *Definitions and classifications, 1999–2000*, Philadelphia, 1999, The Association.

North American Nursing Diagnosis Association (NANDA) Accepted Nursing Diagnoses—cont'd

Box 15-1

Self-care deficit, feeding
Self-care deficit, toileting
Self-esteem, chronic low
Self-esteem, situational low
Self-esteem disturbance
Self-mutilation, risk for
Sensory/perceptual alterations (specify) (visual, auditory, kinesthetic, gustatory, tactile, olfactory)
Sexual dysfunction
Sexuality patterns, altered
Skin integrity, impaired
Skin integrity, impaired, risk for
Sleep deprivation
Sleep pattern disturbance
Social interaction, impaired
Social isolation
Sorrow, chronic
Spiritual distress (distress of the human spirit)
Spiritual distress, risk for
Spiritual well-being, potential for enhanced

Suffocation, risk for
Surgical recovery, delayed
Swallowing, impaired
Thermoregulation, ineffective
Thought processes, altered
Tissue integrity, impaired
Tissue perfusion, altered (specify type) (renal, cerebral, cardiopulmonary, gastrointestinal, peripheral)
Transfer ability, impaired
Trauma, risk for
Unilateral neglect
Urinary elimination, altered
Urinary retention
Ventilation, inability to sustain spontaneous
Ventilatory weaning response, dysfunctional
Violence, risk for: directed at others
Violence, risk for: self-directed
Walking, impaired
Wheelchair transfer ability, impaired

the interest and eventual use of nursing diagnosis in contemporary nursing education, practice, administration, and research (see Chapter 5).

In 1973, the first national conference for the classification of nursing diagnosis was held to identify nursing functions and establish a classification system. Over the years, participants of these conferences have developed the nursing diagnostic categories (Box 15-1). In 1982 a professional association, the **North American Nursing Diagnosis Association (NANDA),** was established. The purpose of NANDA was "to develop, refine, and promote a taxonomy of nursing diagnostic terminology of general use for professional nurses" (Kim, McFarland, and McLean, 1984). In other words, NANDA's work provides a common language for the health problems nurses deal with. Just as the medical diagnosis diabetes mellitus informs physicians about the nature and treatment of a specific disease, the nursing diagnosis *impaired skin integrity* informs nurses about the nature of and care activities required for this specific health problem. The ANA has officially sanctioned NANDA as the organization to govern the development of a classification system of nursing diagnoses (Carpenito, 1993).

Nursing diagnosis was first incorporated into the ANA's *Standards of Nursing Practice* in 1971 (ANA, 1973), and it remains in the current standards (ANA, 1991). In 1980 and 1995, the ANA supported nursing diagnosis in *Nursing: A Social Policy Statement,* which defined nursing as "the diagnosis and treatment of human responses to actual or potential health problems" (ANA, 1980, 1995). In 1987 the definition of nursing diagnosis was strengthened

in the refined definition of nursing in ANA's paper *Scope of Nursing Practice,* which defines nursing as the diagnosis and treatment of human responses to health and illness (ANA, 1987).

As nursing curricula continue to incorporate nursing diagnosis into the educational preparation of nurses, the research in this field will continue to grow. As a result, new diagnostic labels are continually developed, researched, and added to the NANDA listing, which is by no means complete. The continued evolution of nursing diagnosis draws from the collective wealth of nursing knowledge. Through the ongoing collaboration of nursing educators, administrators, researchers, and practitioners, the further development of nursing diagnoses has the potential to enrich the nursing profession.

Definition

Nursing literature contains many definitions for nursing diagnosis (Table 15-1). These definitions evolved as the profession's acceptance of nursing diagnosis strengthened. Common components of these definitions include nursing, client, and health problems. In addition, each definition implies that the nurse uses critical thinking skills to analyze the client's assessment data to form nursing diagnoses.

The definition of a nursing diagnosis presented in this text is designed to assist the student in using diagnoses as a framework for delivering nursing care. The formulation of nursing diagnoses, like all components of the nursing process, enables the student to critically plan individualized nursing care.

dn't need to learn

Table 15-1 **Definitions of Nursing Diagnosis**

Author	Definition
Abdellah (1957)	"The determination of the nature and extent of nursing problems presented by the individual patients or families receiving nursing care."
Durand, Prince (1966)	"A statement of a conclusion resulting from a recognition of a pattern derived from a nursing investigation of the patient."
Gebbie, Lavin (1975)	"The judgment or conclusion that occurs as a result of nursing assessment."
Bircher (1975)	"An independent nursing function. . . . An evaluation of a client's personal responses to his or her human experience throughout the life cycle, be they developmental or accidental crises, illness, hardship, or other stresses."
Aspinall (1976)	"A process of clinical inference from observed changes in patient's physical or psychological condition; if it is arrived at accurately and intelligently, it will lead to identification of the possible causes of symptomatology."
Gordon (1976)	"Actual or potential health problems which nurses, by virtue of their education and experience, are capable and licensed to treat."
Roy (1982)	"Nursing diagnosis is a concise phrase or term summarizing a cluster of empirical indicators representing patterns of unitary man."
Shoemaker (1984)	"A nursing diagnosis is a clinical judgment about an individual, family, or community that is derived through a deliberate, systematic process of data collection and analysis. It provides the basis for prescriptions for definitive therapy for which the nurse is accountable. It is expressed concisely and includes the etiology of the condition when known."
Carpenito (1997)	"A nursing diagnosis is a statement that describes the human response (health state or actual/potential altered interaction pattern) of an individual or group which the nurse can legally identify and for which the nurse can order the definitive interventions to maintain the health state or to reduce, eliminate, or prevent alteration."
NANDA (1990) Kim (1997)	"A nursing diagnosis is a clinical judgment about individual, family, or community responses to actual and potential health problems and life processes. Nursing diagnoses provide the basis for selection of nursing interventions to achieve outcomes for which the nurse is accountable."

Critical Thinking and the Nursing Diagnostic Process

Critical thinking is a complex process (see Chapter 13). Its use in formulating a nursing diagnosis is essential (Figure 15-1). As nursing care expands into a variety of health care settings, more aspects of critical thinking are required in diagnostic reasoning and judgment (Gordon, 1994).

DIAGNOSTIC PROCESS

The **diagnostic process** includes decision-making steps the nurse uses to develop a diagnostic statement (Carnevali and Thomas, 1993; Liukkonen, 1992). This process includes gathering the assessment database, analyzing and interpreting data, identifying client needs, and formulating nursing diagnoses. The diagnostic process is dynamic and requires the nurse to reflect on existing assessment data and health care needs of the client (Da Cruz and Acuri, 1998). Clinical situations demand that diagnostic reasoning be used to identify and validate pertinent assessment data to support a nursing diagnosis. Data validation and clustering follow assessment and lead to analysis and interpretation of data (Figure 15-2).

Nursing diagnosis is the step of the nursing process that enables the nurse to individualize care for the client. During the diagnostic phase, the nurse uses scientific knowledge and experience to analyze and interpret data collected about the client. The nurse then identifies the client's health care problems and writes nursing diagnoses, which form the basis for a plan of care. The use of standard formal nursing diagnostic statements endorsed by NANDA serves several purposes (see Box 15-1). Each diagnosis has a precise definition that gives all members of the health care team a clear understanding of the client's needs. Also, because the nursing diagnosis deals with the client's response to the illness or condition rather than the medical diagnosis, it distinguishes the nurse's role from the physician's role and helps the nurse to focus on the role of nursing.

ANALYSIS AND INTERPRETATION OF DATA

In the assessment phase, data are initially collected from a variety of sources and validated. The nurse then applies reasoning and begins to look for patterns in the assessment data. Patterns form as data is sorted into clusters or categories (see Figure 15-2). The database is continually revised to include changes in the client's physical and

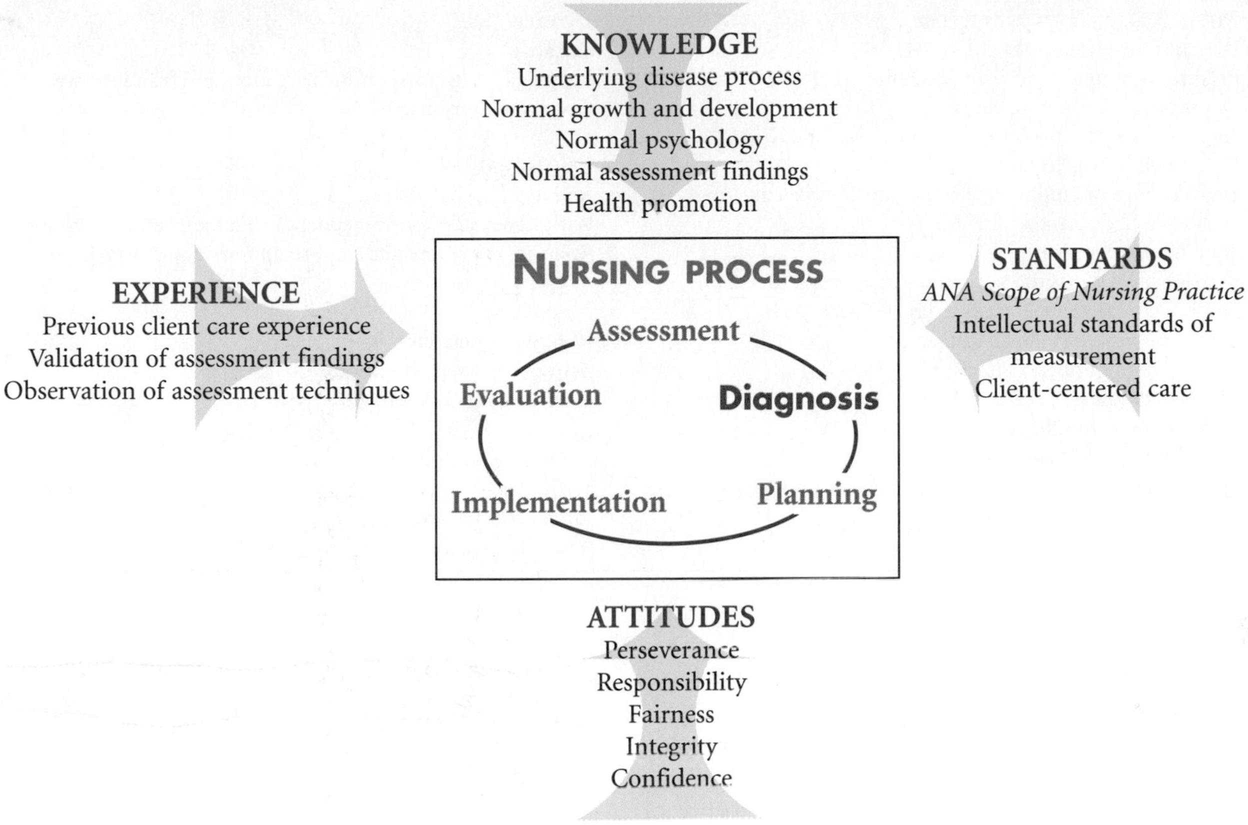

KNOWLEDGE
Underlying disease process
Normal growth and development
Normal psychology
Normal assessment findings
Health promotion
EXPERIENCE
Previous client care experience
Validation of assessment findings
Observation of assessment techniques
NURSING PROCESS
Assessment
Evaluation
Diagnosis
Implementation
Planning
STANDARDS
ANA Scope of Nursing Practice
Intellectual standards of measurement
Client-centered care
ATTITUDES
Perseverance
Responsibility
Fairness
Integrity
Confidence

Figure 15-1 Critical thinking and the nursing diagnostic process.

emotional status and the results of laboratory and diagnostic tests.

Data analysis involves recognizing patterns or trends, comparing them with normal healthful standards, and coming to a reasoned conclusion about the client's response to a health problem. When looking for a pattern or trend, the nurse examines the data in the database. A cluster is a set of signs or symptoms that are grouped together in a logical order. This is the pattern that emerges. Alone these signs or symptoms tell the nurse little, and no diagnostic conclusion can be made. However, when these signs are placed or clustered together as a group, the nurse sees a relationship between and among these assessment findings. For example, Box 15-2 includes a summary of relevant data from Mr. Brown's assessment. Singularly these symptoms could be related to multiple nursing diagnoses, but analyzing these together the nurse begins to think about functional health patterns and the potential effect that Mr. Brown's illness may have on his independence. When the nurse recognizes a pattern and identifies a relationship among patterns, client-centered needs begin to emerge.

Clusters and patterns the nurse recognizes contain defining characteristics. **Defining characteristics** are the clinical criteria or assessment findings that support (vali-

Data validation
Data clustering
Interpretation of data
Identification of client needs
Formulation of nursing diagnoses

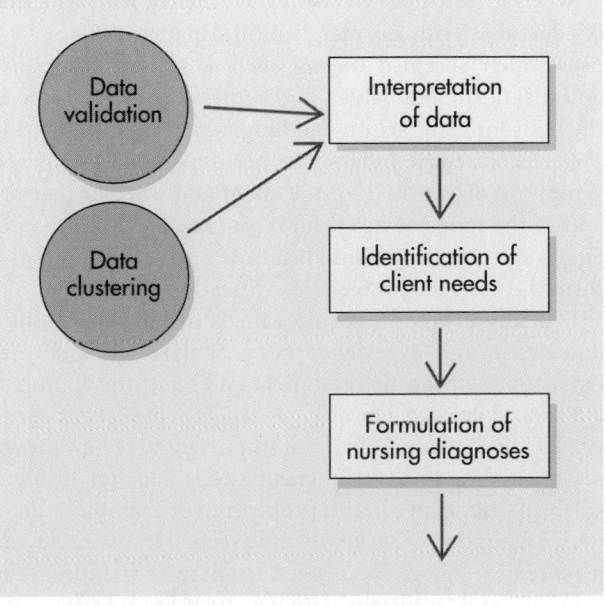

Figure 15-2 Nursing diagnostic process.

| Summary of Relevant Data From Mr. Brown's Complete Assessment | Box 15-2 |

PHYSICAL AND DEVELOPMENTAL
Diarrhea for 3 weeks
Productive cough upon rising each morning
Occasional rales in lung bases
15-pound weight loss 3 weeks before hospitalization
Hemoglobin 12 g/100 ml
Slight change of emphysema shown on chest roentgenogram
Distended abdomen
Squamous cell cancer
Biopsy obtained during outpatient colonscopy June 24
Smoked for 20 years, 2 packs a day (40 pack-years)
Family history of stomach cancer
Family history of heart attack
Married 40 years
Self-employed for 20 years
One adult son, 35 years old
Two sisters, 50 and 48, with no major health problems

INTELLECTUAL
Talkative
Frequently asks nurses if he has cancer and "can it be treated?"
Good attention span

EMOTIONAL
Anxious
Withdrawn after biopsy report of squamous cell cancer
Awaiting colon resection and temporary colostomy

SOCIAL
Walks with neighbor
Active in his neighborhood
Married with children

SPIRITUAL
Methodist
Attends church weekly
Reads Bible daily

date) the presence of a diagnostic category. Clinical criteria are objective or subjective signs and symptoms, clusters of signs and symptoms, or risk factors. Multiple defining characteristics resulting from assessment data support the nursing diagnosis (Carpenito, 1995, 1997). Absence of these characteristics suggests that the proposed diagnosis should be rejected. Defining characteristics that either support or eliminate a particular diagnosis must be examined. This requires a nurse to know nursing diagnoses and the defining characteristics and related factors (Kim, McFarland, and McLean, 1997). Accuracy is achieved when all characteristics are evaluated, nonrelevant ones are eliminated, and relevant ones are confirmed (Collier and others, 1996).

The identified pattern is then compared with data that is consistent with normal, healthful patterns. The nurse uses widely accepted norms, such as normal laboratory and diagnostic test values, and professional knowledge as the basis for comparison and judgment. When comparing patterns, the nurse judges whether the grouped signs and symptoms are normal for the client and whether they are within the range of healthful responses. Defining characteristics that are not within healthy norms are isolated and form the basis for problem identification (Box 15-3).

Nursing diagnoses requires the nurse to draw from a knowledge and experience base, analyze and interpret data, apply diagnostic reasoning, and select the appropriate descriptor (diagnostic label) for the client need (Collier and others, 1996). It is important to review the assessment data to identify client needs and not to focus solely on the client's health problems. For example, a client with a diagnosis of *social isolation related to relocation into a retirement village* has a need to increase friends, social supports, and familiarity with new surroundings. Working with the client to resolve this nursing diagnosis may ulti-

| Example of Data Analysis: Mr. William Brown | Box 15-3 |

RECOGNIZE PATTERN (CLUSTER OF DEFINING CHARACTERISTICS)
Diarrhea for 3 weeks
Ribbon-shaped or watery stools
Distended abdomen
Cramping before and during each bowel movement

COMPARE WITH NORMAL STANDARDS
Soft, formed stool daily
Abdomen soft, nondistended
Defecation nonpainful

MAKE A REASONED CONCLUSION
Bowel elimination problem

mately result in improving the client's independence and level of wellness and can help the client avoid future health problems. When client needs/problems are identified, it is important for the nurse to remember that the formulation of nursing diagnoses are not solely the result of illness or physiological alterations.

IDENTIFICATION OF CLIENT NEEDS

Before formulating the nursing diagnosis, the nurse identifies the client's general health care problems. For example, after receiving clusters of data, such as dyspnea, increased respiratory rate, and cough, the nurse may recognize that the client has a general respiratory problem. However, before a nurse can effectively give care, the problem must be more specifically defined. When identifying these problems, the nurse considers all assessment data and focuses on pertinent and abnormal data (Gordon, 1994). It may help the inexperienced nurse to think of this identification phase as the general health care problem and the formulation of the nursing diagnosis as the specific health care problem. The nurse moves from general to specific.

To identify the client's needs, the nurse first determines what the client's health problems are and whether they are actual or potential problems. An **actual health problem** is one that is perceived or experienced by the client, such as a disruption in sleep related to a noisy environment. An **at risk health problem** is identified when the nurse makes a clinical judgment that an individual, family, or community is more vulnerable to development of a problem than others in the same or similar situation (Carpenito, 1997). The diagnoses alert the nurse to the need for preventive interventions (Gordon, 1994). For example, during the postoperative course, a smoker is at *risk for ineffective airway clearance related to incisional pain.*

FORMULATION OF THE NURSING DIAGNOSIS

Once patterns and clusters of data are sorted and client needs are identified, the nurse is ready to formulate nursing diagnoses.

NANDA has identified five types of nursing diagnoses. An actual nursing diagnosis is a judgment that is clinically validated by the presence of major defining characteristics. The presence of such a diagnosis indicates that sufficient assessment data are available to establish the nursing diagnosis (Collier and others, 1996).

A risk nursing diagnosis describes human responses to health conditions/life processes that may develop in a vulnerable individual, family, or community (NANDA, 1999). For example, a client with a spinal cord injury that limits mobility is at *risk for impaired skin integrity.* The key assessment for this type of diagnosis is the presence of data that support the client's vulnerability. Such data include physiological, psychosocial, familial, lifestyle, and environmental factors that increase the client's vulnerability to, or likelihood of developing, the condition.

A possible nursing diagnosis describes a suspected problem for which current and available data are insufficient to validate the problem (Collier and others, 1996). This type of diagnosis, such as *fluid volume deficit,* has relevance in that the nurse is directed to gather further data and relevant cues to confirm or eliminate the diagnosis. For example, a client has a history of nausea, vomiting, and diarrhea for 3 days. Further data about the client's overall level of health, age, skin turgor, intake and output, and analysis of laboratory data are needed before the nursing diagnosis can be validated. However, because of the symptoms listed earlier, *fluid volume deficit* is a possible nursing diagnosis.

Syndrome diagnosis is a diagnostic label given to a distinct cluster of nursing diagnoses that frequently go together and present a clinical picture (NANDA, 1999; Collier and others, 1996). This type of diagnosis is a useful and efficient way to describe a complex problem without documenting each component of the problem as a distinct nursing diagnosis. To date NANDA (1999) has approved only three syndrome diagnoses. When writing these diagnoses, only the diagnostic label is used (Box 15-4).

A wellness nursing diagnosis is a clinical judgment about an individual, group, or community in transition from a specific level of wellness to a higher level of wellness (NANDA, 1999). This type of diagnosis is used when the client wishes to or has achieved an optimal level of health, for example, *family coping: potential for growth related to unexpected birth of twins.* The nurse and the family unit work together to adapt to the stressors associated with twins and identify the family's strengths and resources, as well as their needs. In doing so, the nurse incorporates the client's strength into a plan of care, with the outcome directed at an enhanced level of coping.

Nursing Diagnosis Statement

The nursing diagnosis statement (that is, how the actual diagnosis is stated) flows from the diagnostic process. Throughout this text, nursing diagnoses are stated in a two-part diagnostic statement, using a format accepted by NANDA (McLean, 1987; NANDA, 1990): the diagnostic label followed by a statement of related factors (Table 15-2). The diagnostic label is a category approved by NANDA (see Box 15-1). The related factor is a condition that causes or is associated with a client's actual or potential response to the health problem. The related factor can be altered or resolved by nursing interventions, thus resulting in a resolution of the diagnosis. This two-part format is accepted by most nursing leaders (Gordon, 1994; Carpenito, 1997). The related factor individualizes a client's nursing diagnosis, providing direction for the selection of appropriate interventions. Table 15-3 compares three nursing diagnoses with different causes and the related nursing interventions.

NURSING DIAGNOSES Box 15-4

CLIENTS WITH RISK FOR DISUSE SYNDROME

Activity intolerance, risk for
Body image disturbance
Constipation
Infection, risk for
Injury, risk for
Mobility, impaired physical
Powerlessness
Thought processes, altered
Tissue integrity, impaired

Table 15-2	NANDA Nursing Diagnosis Format	
Diagnostic Statement	Related Factors
Constipation	Inadequate dietary fiber
	Effects of medications
	Inadequate fluid intake
	Decreased activity
Fatigue	Discomfort
	Excessive role demands
	Increased energy requirement
Skin integrity, impaired	Fluid retention
	Excessive secretions
	Immobilization
	Altered circulation

The "related to" phrase identifies the etiology, or cause, of the problem. This is not a cause-and-effect statement, but rather it indicates that the etiology can contribute to or be associated with the problem (Figure 15-3). Including the phrase requires the nurse to use critical thinking skills to individualize subsequent interventions.

The **etiology,** or cause, of the nursing diagnosis must be within the domain of nursing practice and a condition that responds to nursing interventions. In some settings, the nurse mistakenly records medical diagnoses as the etiology of the nursing diagnosis. This is incorrect. Nursing interventions cannot change the medical diagnosis. However, nursing interventions can be directed at etiological factors and the diagnostic label. For example, the nursing diagnosis *pain related to breast cancer* is incorrect. Nursing actions cannot affect the medical diagnosis of breast cancer.

Rewording the diagnosis to read *pain related to impaired skin integrity secondary to mastectomy incision* results in nursing interventions directed at improving comfort through pain control and incision care.

As the client's health status changes, nursing diagnoses are modified. If a health problem has been resolved, the nursing diagnosis no longer exists. When the client's physiological and emotional status changes, the health problem may remain relevant, but the etiology may change. Therefore the nurse must modify the nursing diagnoses by changing the etiology. If a new problem arises, the nurse develops new nursing diagnoses reflecting changes in the client's needs and status.

The modification of nursing diagnoses is ongoing. As the level of nursing care and level of wellness change, these changes are reflected in the statement of nursing diagnoses. Outdated nursing diagnoses do not accurately reflect the client's current needs.

SUPPORT OF THE DIAGNOSTIC STATEMENT

Nursing assessment data must support the diagnostic label, and the related factors must support the etiology. To collect complete, relevant, and correct assessment data it may help to identify assessment activities that produce specific kinds of data. For example, asking the client about the quality and perception of pain results in subjective data. However, palpating an area, which may elicit a painful grimace, provides objective information. Likewise, asking a client to describe the perception of an irregular heartbeat elicits subjective information, and using auscultation to obtain a pulse produces an objective measurement of heart rate and rhythm. Box 15-2 contains a summary of the relevant assessment data for Mr. Brown that may lead to the identification of an actual or potential

Table 15-3	Comparison of Interventions for Nursing Diagnoses With Different Etiologies	
Nursing Diagnoses	Interventions
Client A	
Ineffective airway clearance related to obesity	Place client in high Fowler's position.
	Have client cough and deep breathe every 2 hours while awake.
	Start weight-reduction diet (1200 calories) to decrease obesity.
Feeding self-care deficit related to inability to bend arms secondary to bilateral arm casts	Encourage family to visit during meals.
	Be certain staff or family members are available to feed client.
	Provide high-calorie milkshakes with straw at 3 and 8 PM.
Anxiety related to social isolation secondary to protective isolation	Plan staffing patterns to include visits to client's room 4 times a day.
	Provide diversional activities.
Client B	
Ineffective airway clearance related to poor coughing technique	Teach client deep breathing and coughing.
	Splint client's abdominal incision during coughing.
Feeding self-care deficit related to inability to grasp feeding utensils	Provide large-handled eating utensils.
	Offer finger foods cut in large pieces for between-meal snacks: 10-2-8.
Social isolation related to effects of neighborhood	Provide client with phone numbers and location of local senior citizens' center.
	Draw client a map of neighborhood stores, restaurants, and libraries.

health care problem. Table 15-4 demonstrates data clustering, identification of client need, and formulation of nursing diagnoses from Mr. Brown's assessment data.

Table 15-5 uses the two nursing diagnoses, *ineffective airway clearance* and *self-esteem disturbance,* to demonstrate how defining characteristics and probable related factors assist in the development of the total diagnostic label.

Sources of Diagnostic Error

The diagnostic process is not error free. In the diagnostic process the nurse relies on four areas. First, there must be an assessment database. Second, the nurse analyzes and interprets these data. Third, the data are clustered into meaningful groups. Last, the nurse identifies client problems that result in the identification of the diagnostic label. Each of these four areas is a potential source of diagnostic error, which can alter the health outcomes of the client (Box 15-5).

ERRORS IN DATA COLLECTION

This type of error occurs during the assessment process (see Chapter 14). The nurse must be knowledgeable and skilled in physical examination (see Chapter 32). If data are incomplete, omitted, or inaccurate, nursing diagnoses may be missed. If data collection is disorganized, the diagnostic process is scattered.

The following practices are essential during assessment to avoid data collection errors. First, prior to assessment,

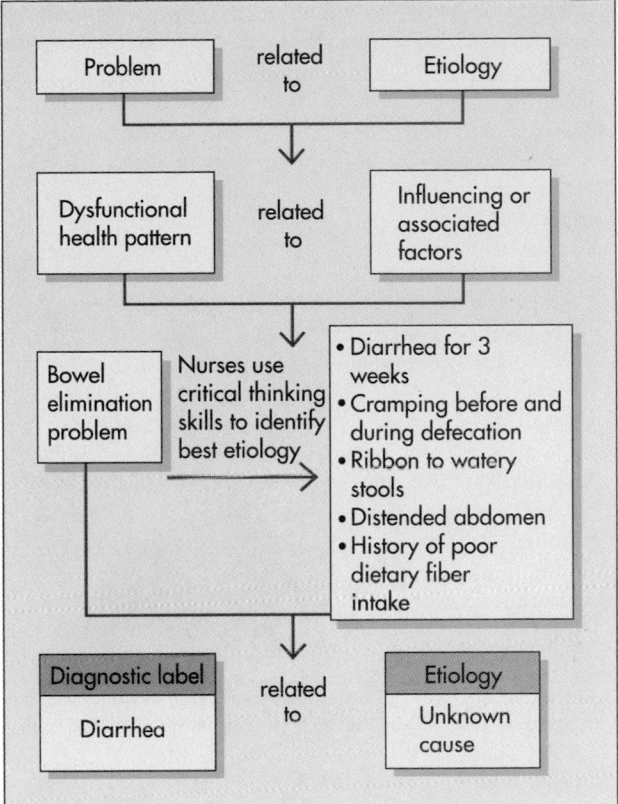

Figure 15-3 Relationship between diagnostic statement and format.
Redrawn from Hickey P: *Nursing process handbook,* St. Louis, 1990, Mosby.

Table 15-4 Foundation of Nursing for Mr. Brown

Clustering Data	Identification of Client Need	Nursing Diagnosis Formulation
Diarrhea for 3 weeks Distended abdomen Family history of stomach cancer	Alteration of elimination patterns	Diarrhea related to irritation
Weight loss: 15 pounds	Excessive weight loss	Altered nutrition: less than body requirements related to inability to absorb nutrients because of chronic diarrhea for 3 weeks
Anemia, hemoglobin level of 10 g/100 ml 40 pack-year history of smoking Slight change of emphysema shown on chest x-ray film Crackles auscultated in lung fields Productive cough on rising each morning	Risk for postoperative respiratory complications	Ineffective airway clearance after surgery related to incisional pain
Temporary colostomy Abdominal incision Client resistance to viewing of abdomen	Change in body image	Self-esteem disturbance related to change in body image
Client verbalization of fear of stomach cancer Client withdrawal after biopsy report Anxiety	Changes in interpersonal interactions	Ineffective individual coping related to fear about unknown prognosis

Table 15-5   Defining Characteristics and Etiologies to Support Nursing Diagnoses

Assessment Activities	Defining Characteristics	Nursing Diagnoses	Etiologies ("Related to")
Auscultate lungs.	Abnormal breath sounds	Ineffective airway clearance	Decreased energy or fatigue
Observe respiration.	Changes in rate or depth of respiration		Tracheobronchial infection, obstruction, or secretion
Observe cough.	Cough		Pain
Inspect skin color.	Cyanosis		
Ask client about shortness of breath and observe for it.	Dyspnea		
Ask client about smoking.	Smoking history		
Observe client's grooming.	Verbal or nonverbal response to actual or perceived change in structure or function	Self-esteem disturbance	Biophysical factors (e.g., amputation or loss of function of extremity)
Observe client's willingness to participate in rehabilitation.	Missing or impaired body part, not looking at or touching body or body part		Cognitive or perceptual factors (e.g., expressions of worthlessness and sorrow)
Review history of trauma injury.	Trauma to body. Refusal to acknowledge change		Psychosocial factors (e.g., withdrawal behavior or excessive crying)

Defining characteristics and relevant etiologies are from Kim MJ, McFarland GK, McLean AM: *Pocket guide to nursing diagnoses,* ed 7, St. Louis, 1997, Mosby and are derived from the NANDA classification.

Sources of Diagnostic Error   Box 15-5

COLLECTING
Lack of knowledge or skill
Inaccurate data
Missing data
Disorganization

INTERPRETING
Inaccurate interpretation of cues
Failure to consider conflicting cues
Using an insufficient number of cues
Using unreliable or invalid data
Failure to consider cultural influences or developmental stage

CLUSTERING
Insufficient cluster of cues
Premature or early closure
Incorrect clustering

LABELING
Wrong diagnostic label selected
Condition is a collaborative problem
Failure to validate nursing diagnosis with client
Failure to seek guidance

the nurse critically reviews his or her level of comfort and competence with interview and physical assessment skills. The beginner should approach assessment in steps. For example, the first experience may be completing an interview of a family member or collecting physical assessment data on one body system. The learner then moves on to more complex assessments.

Second, the nurse must determine the accuracy of data collected. For example, the nurse who auscultates abnormal lung sounds for the first time may be unsure of what is being heard through the stethoscope. Inaccurate assessment data means that data from clients are misinterpreted, inappropriate interventions may be selected, and the quality of care is jeopardized (Lunney, 1998). To minimize the risk of inaccuracy, the nurse must have a more experienced colleague validate findings or explain why they are incorrect.

Third, when developing assessment skills, the nurse needs to check completeness of assessment data. Reviewing client assessments in clinical or classroom settings provides the nurse with a constructive learning opportunity to determine when assessments are complete or when further revisions are needed.

Last, errors in data collection are reduced when an organized approach is used for the assessment. Prior to assessment the nurse should have the appropriate forms and examination equipment. The nurse can achieve an organized assessment if the environment is private, quiet, and comfortable for the client.

ERRORS IN INTERPRETATION AND ANALYSIS OF DATA

Following assessment the nurse reviews the database. During this review the nurse determines if data are accurate and complete. The nurse reviews the data to validate that subjective data are supported by measurable objective physical findings when necessary. When data are not appropriately validated, there may be an inaccurate match between the clinical cues and the diagnosis (Lunney, 1998). The nurse may also review supportive literature to ensure an adequate knowledge base to form a correct nursing diagnosis. Last, the nurse begins to identify and organize relevant assessment patterns to support the presence of client problems.

ERRORS IN DATA CLUSTERING

Errors in data clustering occur when data are clustered prematurely, incorrectly, or not at all (Gordon, 1982, 1994). Premature closure of clustering occurs when the nurse makes the nursing diagnosis before all data have been grouped. Incorrect clustering occurs when the nurse tries to make the nursing diagnosis fit the signs and symptoms obtained. The nursing diagnosis should be derived from the data, not the reverse. An incorrect nursing diagnosis affects quality of care.

ERRORS IN THE DIAGNOSTIC STATEMENT

The last type of error that can occur is the manner in which the nursing diagnosis is stated. There are some common guidelines to reduce errors in the diagnostic statement itself. The statement should be worded in appropriate, concise, and precise language, which involves using correct terminology reflecting the client's response to the illness or condition. A diagnostic statement such as "unhappy and worried about health" can lead to errors. The language needs to be more precise and appropriate, such as *ineffective individual coping related to fear of medical diagnosis.* Also, the problem and etiology portions must be within the scope of nursing to diagnose and treat.

Avoiding and Correcting Errors. Concise wording ensures that the nursing need can be easily communicated to other nurses and health care professionals. Box 15-6 lists suggestions for writing nursing diagnoses.

Nursing diagnoses are easy to write if the nurse remembers that the problem portion of the statement is concerned with the client's response to the illness or condition and that the etiology portion must be within the scope of nursing to diagnose and treat. The following suggestions should help the nurse to avoid the most common errors in formulating nursing diagnoses accurately:

1. Identify the client's response, not the medical diagnosis (Carpenito, 1995, 1997). Because the medical diagnosis requires medical interventions, it is legally inadvisable to include it in the nursing diagnosis. The diagnosis, pain related to myocardial infarction, should be changed to *pain related to physical exertion.*

Avoiding Diagnostic Errors   Box 15-6

Identify client's response to illness.
State a NANDA diagnostic statement.
Identify an etiology treatable by nursing.
Identify a client need associated with a treatment or test.
Identify client's response to equipment.
Identify client's, not nurse's, problem.
Identify client's problem, not interventions.
Identify client's problem, not goals.
Avoid prejudicial statements.
State the etiology legally.
Identify a problem and an etiology.
Identify only one client problem in a diagnostic statement.

---

2. Identify a NANDA diagnostic statement rather than the symptom. Nursing diagnoses are derived from a cluster of defining characteristics; one symptom is insufficient for problem identification. For example, cough related to excessive mucus production should be written as *ineffective breathing pattern related to increased airway secretions.*

3. Identify a treatable etiology rather than a clinical sign or chronic problem. Nursing interventions are directed toward correcting the etiology of the problem. A diagnostic test or a chronic dysfunction is not an etiology or nursing intervention. Altered respiratory function related to abnormal arterial blood gas levels can be correctly stated as *altered peripheral tissue perfusion related to inadequate oxygen intake.*

4. Identify the problem caused by the treatment or diagnostic study rather than the treatment or study itself. Clients experience many responses to diagnostic tests and medical treatment. These responses are the area of nursing concern. The diagnosis, cardiac catheterization related to angina, should be restated to read *anxiety related to lack of knowledge about cardiac catheterization.*

5. Identify the client response to the equipment rather than the equipment itself. Clients are often unfamiliar with medical technology. The diagnosis, anxiety related to cardiac monitor, can be changed to *knowledge deficit regarding the need for cardiac monitoring.*

6. Identify the client's problems rather than the nurse's problems. Nursing diagnoses are always client centered and form the basis for goal-directed care. Potential complications related to poor vascular access indicates a nursing problem in initiating and maintaining intravenous therapy. The diagnosis *potential for infection related to presence of invasive lines* properly centers attention on client needs.

7. Identify the client problem rather than the nursing intervention. Nursing interventions are planned to alleviate client problems. Failure to state a diagnostic label results in an inability to evaluate problem reso-

lution. The statement, offer bedpan frequently because of altered elimination patterns, should be changed to identify the problem and etiology. *Diarrhea related to food intolerance* corrects the misstatement and allows proper implementation of the nursing process.

8. Identify the client problem rather than the goal. Goals are established in terms of client problems. If the problem is not identified, evaluation of problem resolution is difficult. Client needs high-protein diet related to potential alteration in nutrition should be changed to *potential altered nutrition: less than body requirements related to inadequate nutritional intake* to allow for planning to correct the etiology.

9. Make professional rather than prejudicial judgments. Nursing diagnoses are based on subjective and objective client data and should not include the nurse's personal beliefs and values. The nurse's judgment can be removed from potential impairment of skin integrity related to poor hygiene habits by changing the etiology to lack of knowledge about perineal care.

10. Avoid legally inadvisable statements (Carpenito, 1995, 1997). Statements that imply blame, negligence, or malpractice can result in litigation. The diagnosis, recurrent angina related to insufficient medication, implies inadequate prescription by the physician. Correct problem identification might read *pain related to improper use of medications*.

11. Identify the problem and etiology. Be careful to avoid a circular statement. Such statements are vague and give no direction to nursing care. Alteration in comfort related to pain can be changed to identify the client problem and the cause: *ineffective breathing pattern related to incisional pain*.

12. Identify only one client problem in the diagnostic statement. Every problem has different specific expected outcomes. Confusion during the planning step occurs when multiple problems are included in a nursing diagnosis. It is, however, permissible to include multiple etiologies contributing to one client problem. Pain and anxiety related to difficulty in ambulating should be restated as two nursing diagnoses, such as *impaired mobility related to pain in right knee* and *anxiety related to difficulty in ambulating*.

In addition, there are three incorrect ways to state the diagnostic label: statement of nursing diagnoses as medical diagnoses, use of medical terminology to describe the cause, and statement of the nursing diagnosis as an intervention (Table 15-6). These are errors because they shift the focus of the statement from nursing to medicine or shift the focus from the cause to the intervention. As expertise with the diagnostic process is gained, the likelihood of errors is reduced, and the nurse is able to develop nursing diagnoses based on the actual or potential nursing needs of the client. Errors in the diagnostic process result in the development of an incomplete or inappropriate nursing care plan.

NURSING DIAGNOSIS AND MEDICAL DIAGNOSIS

Nursing diagnosis focuses on and defines the nursing needs of the client (Gordon, 1994). It reflects the client's level of health or response to a disease or pathological process, an emotional state, a sociocultural phenomenon, or a developmental stage. A **medical diagnosis** predominately identifies a specific disease state. The medical focus is on the diagnosis and treatment of the disease.

Medical and nursing diagnoses are developed using assessment databases. In both professions the diagnostic label directs the direction of care. However, the nursing database is global and includes an in-depth assessment of the physiological, psychological, sociocultural, developmental, and spiritual dimensions of the client. Medicine's database includes the physiological systems and the personal and social systems. The personal and social systems may be limited to a family medical history and the economic and insurance history of the client (Gordon, 1994).

The goals and objectives of a nursing diagnosis differ

Table 15-6   Examples of Errors in Formulating the Nursing Diagnostic Statement

Correct Statement	Stated as Medical Diagnosis	Stated in Medical Terminology	Stated as Nursing Intervention
Diarrhea related to unknown cause	Diarrhea	Alteration in bowel elimination related to lesion in descending colon	Offer bedpan frequently because of diarrhea.
Altered nutrition: less than body requirements related to chronic diarrhea for 3 weeks	Potential malnutrition	Alteration in nutrition: less than body requirements owing to malnutrition	Provide high-protein diet due to high risk for altered nutrition.
Self-esteem disturbance related to change in body image	Avoidance reaction to colostomy	Disturbance in self-concept owing to colostomy	Encourage client to interact with others.

from those of a medical diagnosis. The goal of a nursing diagnosis is to direct a plan of care to assist clients and their families to adapt to their illness and to resolve health care problems. The goals of a medical diagnosis are to identify and to design a treatment plan for curing the disease or the pathological process.

The objective of a nursing diagnosis is development of an individualized plan of care so that the client and family are able to cope with changes and to meet the challenges resulting from health problems. The objective of the medical diagnosis is to prescribe treatment. For example, a 20-year-old college student is admitted with right lower quadrant abdominal pain. The physician makes a medical diagnosis of appendicitis, and the client undergoes an emergency appendectomy to remove the infected appendix. After the appendectomy the nurse develops several nursing diagnoses, one of which is impaired physical mobility related to pain secondary to an abdominal incision. The nursing care will be directed at gradually increasing the client's mobility to preoperative levels.

Nursing Diagnoses: Application to Care Planning

The use of nursing diagnoses is a mechanism for identifying the domain of nursing. The formulated nursing diagnoses provide direction for the planning process and the selection of nursing interventions to achieve the desired outcomes. The care plan (see Chapter 16) is a mechanism for demonstrating accountability (Carpenito, 1997). In addition, the nursing diagnoses and subsequent care plan assist in communicating to other professionals the client-centered problems through the nursing care plan, consultations, discharge planning, and client care conferences (Figure 15-4).

ADVANTAGES OF NURSING DIAGNOSES

Nursing diagnoses are advantageous for both nurses and clients. They facilitate communication among nurses about a client's level of wellness and assist in discharge planning. The health care delivery system today requires greater numbers of health care professionals. As more people become responsible for the care of a client, it is essential that these professionals are able to clearly communicate about the client's problems. Nursing diagnoses facilitate communication in several ways. The initial list of nursing diagnoses is an easily obtainable reference to the client's current health care needs. Nursing diagnoses also help prioritize the client's needs. As the nurse communicates with other professionals, the use of nursing diagnoses encourages organized communication relevant to the client's goals and priorities.

Nursing diagnoses are also used for charting in the progress notes, writing referrals, and providing effective transition of care from one unit to another, from one

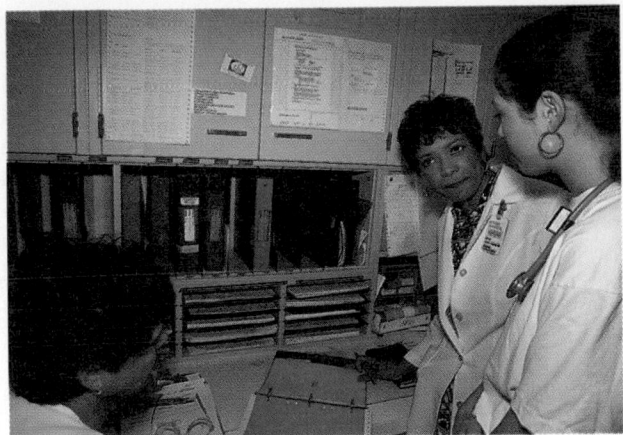

Figure 15-4 Nurses discuss client's health care needs.

clinic to another, or from the hospital to the community. Discharge planning is the set of decisions and activities designed to give continuity and coordination to nursing care. Discharge planning is necessary when a client is discharged from one hospital to another or from the hospital to a community-based agency. In discharge planning, nursing diagnoses are the mechanism for communicating and delineating care the client still requires (Gordon, 1994; Carpenito, 1997).

Nursing diagnoses can also serve as a focus for quality improvement (Gordon, 1994). Quality improvement is the monitoring and evaluation of process and outcomes to identify opportunities for improvement (see Chapter 18). The nursing diagnosis is a method of identifying the focus of nursing activity. When focusing on the nursing diagnosis, the reviewer can determine whether nursing care was correct and delivered according to standards of practice.

The benefits of nursing diagnoses for the profession are also important for the client and family. Better communication among health care professionals helps eliminate potential problems in giving care and maintains a focus on meeting the client's health care goals. Similarly, the ultimate reason for improvement and peer review is to ensure that high-quality care is given to clients and families. Furthermore, the client benefits from the individualization of nursing care resulting from appropriate goal setting, correct selection of priorities, selection of appropriate interventions, and establishment of outcome criteria.

LIMITATIONS OF NURSING DIAGNOSES

Nursing diagnoses have limitations, and the beginning practitioner should be aware of their existence. Because of the continuous evolution of the terms and use of nursing diagnoses, the language can occasionally be verbose and contain jargon. This may limit the use of nursing diagnoses to only nursing professionals and result in confusion among other members of the health care team (Seahill, 1991; Carpenito, 1997).

Imprecise language of the diagnosis may incorrectly "label" a client. One such diagnostic label is noncompliance. The term is value laden and incomplete (Stantis and Ryan, 1982). In addition, the evolution of a standardized terminology in the form of a taxonomy has resulted in confusion about the language of the diagnostic label (Lunney, 1986; Porter, 1986). The 1986 National Conference for the Classification of Nursing Diagnosis first proposed a taxonomic structure for an organizational framework of current and future diagnostic labels (McLean, 1987). To date, the revised taxonomic structure serves as a classification system for nursing diagnosis (Carpenito, 1997).

The evolving taxonomy can limit nursing practice. Nursing diagnoses, developed by the Task Force of the National Group for the Classification of Nursing Diagnoses, are only the beginning of a total classification system. Through formulation and use of other nursing diagnoses, the taxonomy will grow and expand the focus of professional nursing.

Key Concepts

- The diagnostic process includes critical analysis and interpretation of data, identification of client problems, and formulation of nursing diagnoses.
- The interpretation of data requires the nurse to validate and cluster data.
- Nursing diagnoses state the actual or potential problems of the client's health status.
- Nursing diagnoses are written for the physical, developmental, intellectual, emotional, social, and spiritual dimensions of the client.
- Nursing diagnoses are necessary to develop a plan of care that will help the client and family adapt to changes resulting from an illness or change in lifestyle.
- The "related to" factor of the diagnostic statement assists the nurse in individualizing a client's nursing diagnoses and provides direction for the selection of appropriate interventions.
- Nursing diagnostic errors can occur by errors in data collection, interpretation and analysis of data, clustering of data, or in the diagnostic statement.
- Nursing diagnoses improve communication between nurses and other health professionals.
- Nursing diagnoses can serve as a focus for quality assurance and improvement and peer review.

Key Terms

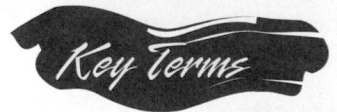

Actual health problem, *p. 317*

At risk health problem, *p. 317*

Client-centered problems, *p. 311*

Critical thinking, *p. 314*

Defining characteristics, *p. 315*

Diagnostic process, *p. 314*

Etiology, *p. 318*

Medical diagnosis, *p. 322*

North American Nursing Diagnosis Association (NANDA), *p. 313*

Nursing diagnosis, *p. 311*

Critical Thinking Exercises

1. Your client's nursing Kardex contains a care plan for bathing/hygiene and toileting self-care deficit related to decreased mobility of right arm. What data do you need from the assessment database to determine whether the nursing diagnosis is relevant?
2. Using a client's assessment cluster data from the history and physical examination components, identify which trends are fully supported by data and which trends need more data. (Using multicolored highlighters can assist with this exercise.)
3. How do you organize assessment data to derive nursing diagnoses that reflect client response to illness, hospitalization, and lifestyle changes?

References

American Nurses Association: *Model nurse practice act,* Washington, DC, 1955, The Association.

American Nurses Association: *Standards of nursing practice,* Washington, DC, 1973, The Association.

American Nurses Association: *Nursing: a social policy statement,* Washington, DC, 1980, The Association.

American Nurses Association: *Scope of nursing practice,* Washington, DC, 1987, The Association.

American Nurses Association: *Standards of clinical nursing practice,* Washington, DC, 1991, The Association.

American Nurses Association: *Nursing: a social policy statement,* Washington, DC, 1995, The Association.

Carnevali DL, Thomas MO: *Diagnostic reasoning and treatment decision making in nursing,* Philadelphia, 1993, JB Lippincott.

Carpenito LJ: *Nursing diagnoses: application to clinical practice,* ed 5, Philadelphia, 1993, JB Lippincott.

Carpenito LJ: *Nursing diagnoses: application to clinical practice,* ed 6, Philadelphia, 1995, JB Lippincott.

Carpenito LJ: *Nursing diagnoses: application to clinical practice,* ed 7, Philadelphia, 1997, JB Lippincott.

Collier IC and others: *Writing nursing diagnoses: a critical thinking approach,* St. Louis, 1996, Mosby.

Da Cruz DALM, Acuri EAM: The influence of nursing diagnosis on information processing on undergraduate students, *Nurs Diagn* 9(3):93, 1998.

Fry VS: The creative approach to nursing, *Am J Nurs* 53:301, 1953.

Gordon M: *Nursing diagnoses: process and practice,* New York, 1982, McGraw-Hill.

Gordon M: *Nursing diagnosis: process and application,* ed 3, St. Louis, 1994, Mosby.

Hickey P: *Nursing process handbook,* St. Louis, 1990, Mosby.

Kim MJ, McFarland GK, McLean AM, editors: *Classification of nursing diagnoses: proceedings of the fifth conference (NANDA),* St. Louis, 1984, Mosby.

Kim MJ, McFarland GK, McLean AM: *Pocket guide to nursing diagnoses,* ed. 7, St. Louis, 1997, Mosby.

Liukkonen A: The nurse's decision-making process and the implementation of psychogeriatric nursing in a mental hospital, *J Adv Nurs* 17(3):356, 1992.

Lunney M: Nursing diagnoses: refining the system, *Am J Nurs* 82:456, 1986.

Lunney M: Accuracy of nurses' diagnoses: foundation of NANDA, NIC, and NOC, *Nurs Diagn* 9(2):83, 1998.

McCloskey JC, Bulechek GM: *Nursing interventions classification,* ed 3, St. Louis, 2000, Mosby.

McFarland GK, McFarlane EA: *Nursing diagnosis and intervention: planning for patient care,* St. Louis, 1989, Mosby.

McLean AM, editor: *Classification of nursing diagnoses: proceedings from the seventh conference (NANDA),* St. Louis, 1987, Mosby.

Nightingale F: *Notes on nursing: what it is and is not,* London, 1860, Harrison & Sons.

North American Nursing Diagnosis Association: *Proceedings of the ninth national conference,* Orlando, Fla, March 17–21, 1990.

North American Nursing Diagnosis Association: *Definitions and classifications, 1999-2000,* Philadelphia, 1999, The Association.

Porter EJ: Critical analysis of NANDA nursing diagnoses taxonomy, part I, *Image J Nurs Sch* 18:137, 1986.

Rantz MJ, LeMone P. *Classification of nursing diagnoses: proceedings of the twelfth conference, North American Nursing Diagnosis Association,* Glendale, Calif, 1997, CINAHL Information Systems.

Seahill L: Nursing diagnosis vs. goal-oriented treatment planning in child psychiatry, *Image J Nurs Sch* 23:95, 1991.

Stantis MA, Ryan J: Noncompliance, an unacceptable diagnosis, *Am J Nurs* 82:941, 1982.

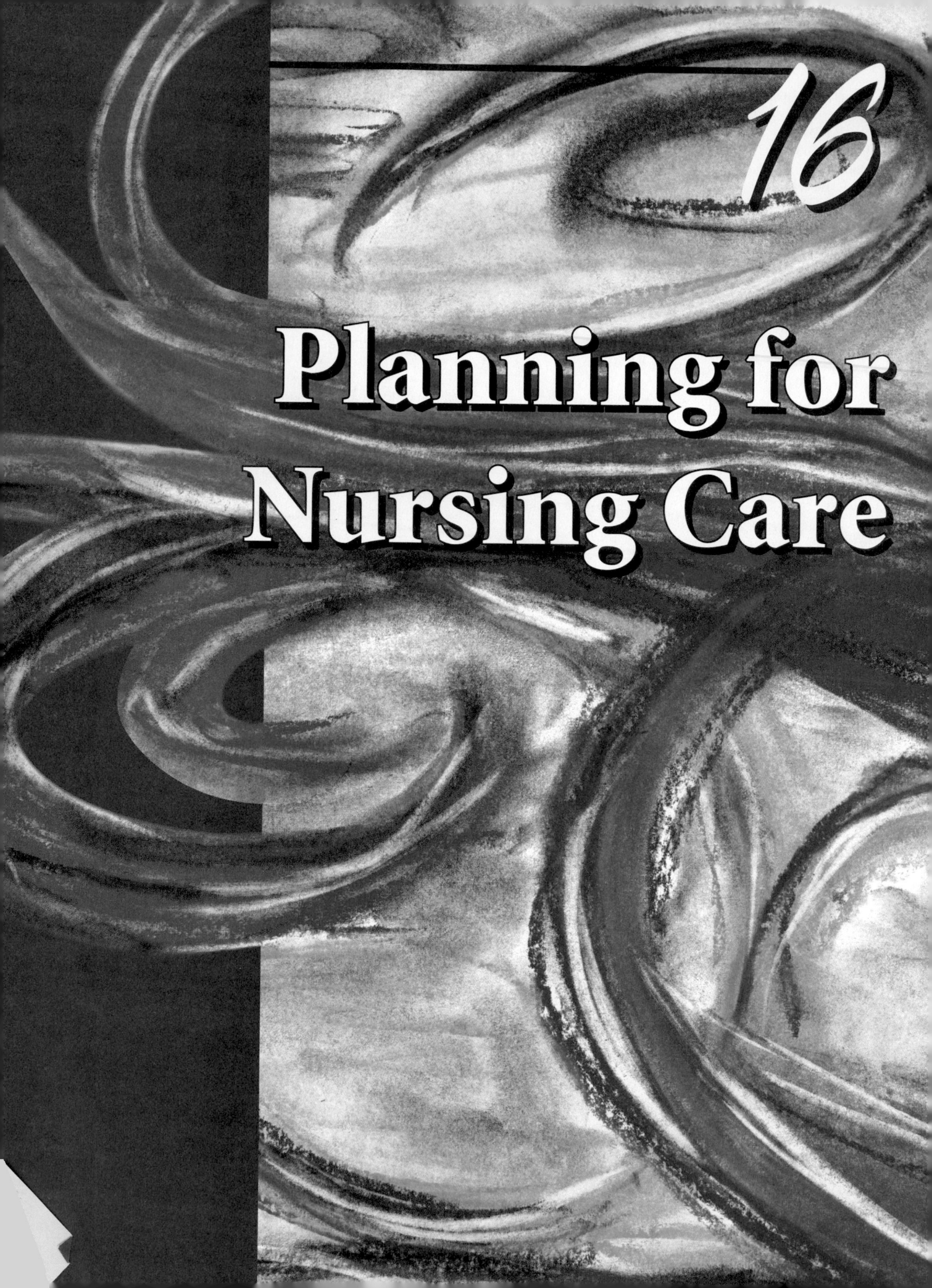

16

Planning for Nursing Care

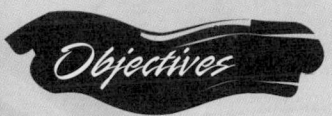

Mastery of content in this chapter will enable the student to:

- Define the key terms listed.
- Discuss the process of priority setting.
- Describe goal setting.
- Discuss the difference between a goal and an expected outcome.
- List the seven guidelines for writing an outcome statement.
- Discuss the process of selecting nursing interventions.
- Define the three types of nursing interventions.
- Discuss the differences between nurse-initiated, physician-initiated, and collaborative interventions.
- List the purposes of critical pathways.
- Describe the differences between care plans used in hospital and community health settings.
- Describe the similarities and differences between nursing care plans and critical pathways.
- Develop a care plan from a nursing assessment.
- List the six steps involved in consultation.
- Discuss the consultation process.

Nursing assessment and the formulation of nursing diagnoses are essential to the planning step of the nursing process. **Planning** is a category of nursing behaviors in which client-centered goals and expected outcomes are established and nursing interventions are selected to achieve the goals and outcomes of care. During planning, priorities are set. In addition to collaborating with the client and family, the nurse consults with other members of the health care team, reviews pertinent literature, modifies care, and records relevant information about the client's health care needs and clinical management.

Establishing Priorities

After formulating specific nursing diagnoses, the nurse uses critical thinking skills to establish priorities for the client's diagnoses by ranking them in order of importance. Priorities are established to help the nurse anticipate and sequence nursing interventions when a client has multiple problems or alterations (Carpenito, 1997).

Establishing priorities is not merely a matter of numbering the nursing diagnoses on the basis of severity or physiological importance. Obviously, basic physiological needs must be addressed first; however, some clients may have sociocultural or psychological needs that have greater priority than nonemergent physiological needs. Rather, priority selection is the method the nurse and client use to mutually rank the diagnoses in order of importance based on the client's desires, needs, and safety.

Maslow's hierarchy of needs (1970) can be one useful method for designating priorities. The hierarchy of human needs arranges the basic needs in five levels of priority (see Chapter 5). The most basic, or first, level includes

physiological needs such as air, water, and food. The second level includes safety and security needs, which involve physical and psychological security. The third level contains love and belonging needs, including friendship, social relationships, and sexual love. The fourth level encompasses esteem and self-esteem needs, which involve self-confidence, usefulness, achievement, and self-worth. The final level is the need for self-actualization, the state of fully achieving potential and having the ability to solve problems and cope realistically with life's situations. Basic physiological and safety needs are usually first priority. However, the nurse may encounter situations in which there are no emergent physical or safety needs, but in which high priority must be given to the psychological, sociocultural, developmental, or spiritual needs of the client.

Clients entering the health care system generally have unmet needs. For example, a person brought to an emergency department experiencing acute pneumonia has an unmet need for oxygen, the most basic physiological need. An older woman living in a high-crime area may be concerned about physical safety and, while hospitalized, may have a need for psychological security from fear that her home will be burglarized. A widowed homemaker whose children have moved away may feel that she does not belong or is not loved. Nurses in all practice settings encounter clients with unmet needs. Nursing care includes helping clients, and often the family, meet these needs.

Priorities are classified as high, intermediate, or low. Priorities depend on the urgency of the problem, the nature of the treatment indicated, and the interactions among the nursing diagnoses. Nursing diagnoses that, if untreated, could result in harm to the client or others have the highest priorities (Gordon, 1994). For example, risk for violence, impaired gas exchange, and decreased cardiac output are high-priority nursing diagnoses. High priorities can occur in both the psychological and physiological dimensions, and the nurse should avoid classifying only physiological nursing diagnoses as high priority.

Intermediate-priority nursing diagnoses involve the nonemergent, non–life-threatening needs of the client. Low-priority nursing diagnoses are client needs that may not be directly related to a specific illness or prognosis.

Whenever possible, the client should be involved in priority setting. In some situations the client and nurse assign different priority rankings to nursing diagnoses. If both place different values on health care needs and treatments, these differences can be resolved through open communication. However, when the client's physiological and emotional needs are at stake, the nurse needs to assume primary responsibility for setting priorities.

When the nurse uses clinical judgment and diagnostic reasoning to assign priorities to nursing diagnoses, the needs of the client, the resources of the health care system, and the limitations of time are considered (Gordon et al, 1994; Kataoka-Yahiro and Saylor, 1994) Table 16-1 displays priority settings and rationales. These priorities involve client needs and resources and limitations of the health care system.

Critical Thinking in Establishing Goals and Expected Outcomes

Before delivering any form of nursing care, the nurse must decide what the end point of nursing care should be for the client. In other words, appropriate goals and expected outcomes of care must be developed. Establishing goals and expected outcomes requires that the nurse critically evaluate the preestablished priority diagnoses, the urgency of the problems, and the resources of the client and the health care delivery system (Bandman and Bandman, 1995). Goals and expected outcomes are specific statements used to indicate anticipated client behavior or responses from nursing care. After assessing, diagnosing, and establishing priorities about the client's health care needs, the nurse formulates goals and expected outcomes with the client for each nursing diagnosis (Gordon, 1994). Figure 16-1 illustrates the relationships among nursing diagnoses, goals, expected outcomes, and nursing interventions.

The purposes for writing goals and expected outcomes are twofold: first, to provide direction for individualized nursing interventions, and second, to set standards of determining the effectiveness of the interventions.

Each goal and expected outcome statement must have a time frame for evaluation. The time element depends on the nature of the problem, etiology, overall condition of the client, and treatment setting.

GOALS OF CARE

Individualized nursing diagnoses and priority setting helps determine the goals of care. Bulechek and McCloskey (1992), define **goals** as guideposts to the selection of nursing interventions and criteria in the evaluation of nursing interventions. Mutual goal setting is an activity that includes the client and family to prioritize the goals of care, then develop a plan of action to achieve those goals (McCloskey and Bulechek, 1994).

To create a plan of care the nurse uses critical thinking skills to develop goals and expected outcomes that are relevant to the client needs as evidenced by the assessment

Table 16-1 **Priority Setting**	
Nursing Diagnoses	Rationale
High Priority	
Diarrhea related to unknown cause	Prompt resolution of diarrhea and cause prevents further decline in physiological and emotional status.
Ineffective individual coping related to anxiety of unknown diagnosis	Prompt intervention for ineffective coping will help client prepare for a diagnostic test, treatment, or diagnosis.
Ineffective airway clearance after surgery related to abdominal incisional pain	Because of the risk of postoperative pulmonary complications, nurse will institute aggressive pulmonary hygiene (Chapter 39) and client education.
Intermediate Priority	
Altered nutrition: less than body requirements related to chronic diarrhea for 3 weeks	This nursing diagnosis does not affect client's immediate physiological or emotional status. Possible surgery will also assist in resolving diagnosis.
Low Priority	
Risk for infection related to history of smoking for 20 years	This nursing diagnosis reflects client's long-term needs.

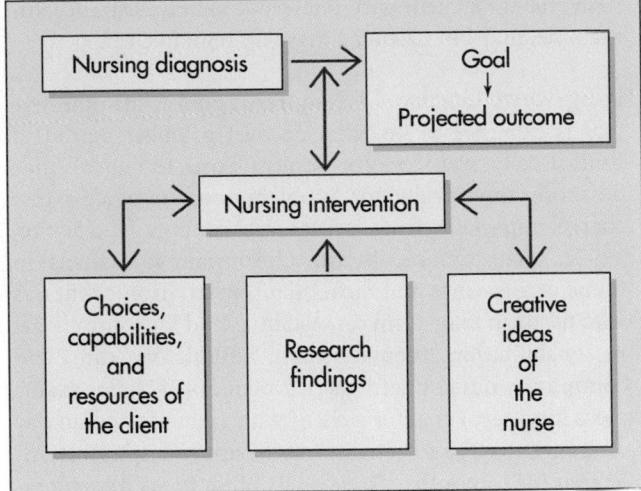

Figure 16-1 From diagnosis to outcome.
Redrawn from Gordon M: *Nursing diagnosis: process and application,* ed 3, St. Louis, 1994, Mosby.

database and the nursing diagnoses. As the goals and expected outcomes are developed, the nurse is also simultaneously synthesizing critical thinking knowledge, experience, standards, and attitudes that pertain to the client's present health care needs (Figure 16-2).

The nurse's knowledge from scientific, sociobehavioral, and nursing disciplines enable the planning of goals. For example, a client who has pneumonia may have a nursing diagnosis of *impaired gas exchange.* The nurse's knowledge of the pathophysiology of pneumonia and the normal anatomy and physiology of the lung tissue, coupled with the knowledge of respiratory care principles, allows her to establish the goal "client will achieve clear lung sounds to auscultation by 8/10." Similarly the nurse's knowledge base suggests that indications of improved gas exchange will be effected in outcomes such as return of oxygen saturation to normal range, absence of pulmonary secretions. Finally, experience with other clients with pulmonary alterations allows the nurse to select interventions that were successful previously.

Role of the Client in Goal Setting. A **client-centered goal** is a specific, measurable objective designed to

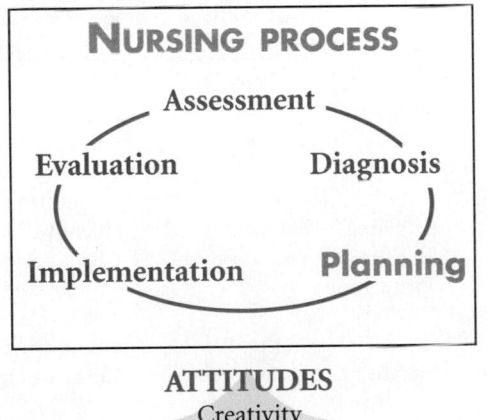

Figure 16-2 Critical thinking and the process of planning care.

reflect the client's highest possible level of wellness and independence in function. Client-centered goals require active involvement by the client. Goals should be realistic and based on client needs and resources.

For clients to participate in goal setting, they should be alert and have some degree of independence in completing activities of daily living, problem solving, and decision making. This is important as the nurse and client partner together throughout the client's care. If the clients' cognitive and physical impairments are so severe that they cannot actively participate in goal setting, the nursing team acts in their behalf to develop client-centered goals. When developing goals, the nurse acts as an advocate for the client to develop nursing interventions to promote the client's return to health or to prevent further deterioration in the client's level of wellness or cognitive and physical functioning (Carpenito, 1995, 1997). As the nurse gains experience, the knowledge acquired forms a basis for clinical decision making and goal setting (Miller and Babcock, 1996).

Goals should not only meet the immediate needs of the client but should also strive toward prevention and rehabilitation. Two types of goals, short-term goals and long-term goals, are developed for the client depending upon the nature of the client's need or problems and the nature of the nursing services provided.

Short-Term Goals.   A **short-term goal** is an objective that is expected to be achieved in a short time, usually less than a week (Carpenito, 1997). With the present health care system and shorter hospital stays, short-term goals are the direction for the immediate care plan. A short-term goal for a client with ineffective airway clearance, for example, may be "Client's lungs will remain clear."

Long-Term Goals.   A **long-term goal** is an objective that is expected to be achieved over a longer period of time, usually over weeks or months. Long-term goals may be more appropriate for problem resolution after discharge, especially from acute care settings (Carpenito, 1997). Long-term goals are appropriate for clients in home care settings and those adapting to chronic illnesses who reside in long-term care facilities and for some clients in rehabilitation, mental health, ambulatory care, and community nursing settings (Carpenito, 1997). For example, a long-term goal for a client with an ineffective airway clearance may be to remain free of upper respiratory infection for 6 months. These goals often focus on prevention, rehabilitation, discharge, and health education. Failure to set long-term goals may prevent the client from receiving continuity of care.

Goal setting establishes the framework for the nursing care plan. Mr. Brown was introduced in Chapter 14. It is now 1 day after Mr. Brown had surgery for a bowel resection. His operative course had some complications. His blood loss was greater than anticipated, and his hemoglobin level is now 8.5 g. His fatigue has worsened, and his tolerance of routine postoperative leg exercises and ambulation is poor. Table 16-2 shows the progression from nursing diagnoses to goals and expected outcomes for Mr. Brown. Through goals, the nurse is able to provide continuity of care and promote optimal use of time and resources. Ultimately the goal leads to the development of expected outcomes.

Table 16-2   Examples of Goal Setting With Expected Outcomes for Mr. Brown

Nursing Diagnoses	Goals	Expected Outcomes
Ineffective individual coping related to fear of negative prognosis	Client will openly discuss diagnosis.	Client will ask pertinent questions about diagnosis by 7/5. Client will express fears by 7/5. Client will identify at least two strategies for dealing with fears by 7/6.
Ineffective airway clearance related to incisional pain	Client's lungs will remain clear throughout postoperative period.	Client will turn, cough, and deep breathe every hour. Client achieves incentive spirometer goal of 90% every 2 hours. Client pain level remains ≤ 4 on a scale of 0-10.
Knowledge deficit regarding postoperative care at home related to inexperience	Client will state four postoperative risks before discharge.	Client drinks 2 to 3 L of fluid every day by 7/5. Client will name three signs of wound infection by 7/5. Client will demonstrate aseptic wound care by 7/5. Client will state home activity restrictions by 7/5.
Altered peripheral tissue perfusion related to postoperative venous status and risk for thrombophlebitis	Client will maintain adequate tissue perfusion by discharge.	Client performs active range of motion exercises every 2 hours while restricted to bed. Client's toes remain warm, dry with capillary refill of ≤ 2 seconds. Client increases ambulation by 50 feet every day.

EXPECTED OUTCOMES

An **expected outcome** is the specific, step-by-step objective that leads to attainment of the goal and the resolution of the etiology for the nursing diagnosis. An outcome is a measurable change of the client's status in response to nursing care (Gordon and others, 1994; Carpenito, 1997). Client outcomes have been referred to as the ultimate definition of effectiveness and efficiency, and there is an increased emphasis on identifying and measuring the results of nursing interventions and practice (Deaton, 1998). Outcomes are the desired responses of a client's condition in the physiological, social, emotional, developmental, or spiritual dimensions. This change in condition is documented through observable or measurable client responses. The expected outcomes determine when a specific, client-centered goal has been met and later assist in evaluating the response to nursing care and resolution of the nursing diagnosis (see Table 16-2).

Expected outcomes have several functions. Projected before nursing actions are selected, expected outcomes provide a direction for nursing activities (Gordon, 1994). Outcomes include observable client behavior and measurable criteria for each goal. They provide a projected time span for goal attainment and an opportunity to state any additional resources that may be required to achieve the goal, including additional equipment, personnel, or knowledge. Finally, the nurse uses expected outcomes as criteria to evaluate the effectiveness of nursing activities.

When writing expected outcomes, the nurse should ensure that the outcome statement is written in measurable behavioral terms. This allows the nurse to note specifically the behavior expected for resolution of the client's problem. The expected outcome statements should be written sequentially, with time frames. This provides the nurse with an order for the interventions, as well as a time reference for resolution of the problem.

Several expected outcomes are usually developed for each goal and nursing diagnosis. The rationale for the multiple expected outcomes is that few client problems can be resolved by one nursing action. In addition, the listing of the step-by-step expected outcomes gives the nurse practical guidance in planning interventions.

In the current health care environment, much attention is given to measuring outcomes of nursing interventions. The Iowa Intervention Project has published a classification of nursing outcomes and has linked the outcome states to nursing diagnoses (Johnson, Mass, and Moorhead, 2000). These nursing outcomes are dependent on delivery-of-care setting. For example, outcomes in a critical care setting are not necessarily appropriate for a community-based setting or a rehabilitation facility. Outcomes are also dependent on the acute or chronic disease state of the client (Chase, 1998). It is important to reflect on the goals and expected outcomes of care to ensure that they are specific to the care delivery setting, the client, the discipline delivering the care, and the underlying medical diagnosis.

Developing a plan of care must also incorporate the role of other health care disciplines, the family, and community resources. The nurses also uses information gained from previous experiences to determine what has worked or not worked in similar situations. This clinical testing of interventions helps the nurse to be more therapeutic for each new client. As goals and expected outcomes are developed, the nurse must be aware and committed to accepted standards of practice from nursing and other disciplines in designing safe and relevant client-centered care. In the planning of care the nurse displays attitudes such as creativity, perseverance, and humility to develop a plan of care that is individualized to the client/family needs and has measurable outcomes of care.

GUIDELINES FOR WRITING GOALS AND EXPECTED OUTCOMES

There are seven guidelines for writing goals and expected outcomes. These seven guidelines involve client-centered, singular, observable, measurable, time-limited, mutual, and realistic factors.

Client-Centered Factors.   Because nursing care is directed by nursing diagnoses, the goals and expected outcomes focus on the client and underlying diagnosis (Chase, 1998). These statements reflect expected client behavior and responses as a result of nursing interventions.

A common error in writing goals and expected outcomes is to write the statement as an intervention. A correct outcome statement is "client will ambulate in the hall 3 times a day." A common error is to write "nursing assistant will ambulate client in the hall 3 times a day."

Singular Factors.   Each goal and expected outcome statement should address only one behavioral response. This singularity provides a more precise method to evaluate client response to the nursing action. An incorrect outcome statement may read "client's lungs will be clear to auscultation, and respiratory rate will be 20 per minute by 8/22," and the lungs are clear but the respiratory rate is 28 per minute after nursing actions. It is difficult to determine whether the expected outcome has been achieved. By splitting the statement into two parts, "lungs will be clear to auscultation by 8/22" and "respiratory rate will be 20 per minute by 8/22," the nurse can determine specifically the outcome that has been achieved. In addition, singularity assists the nurse in modification of the care plan.

Observable Factors.   Nursing is under pressure to objectively demonstrate the effectiveness of nursing interventions on the client's level of health (Head, Mass, and Johnson, 1997). One way to address this challenge is to design expected outcomes that are observable. Through observation the nurse notes if change has taken place. Observable changes can occur in physiological findings, the client's level of knowledge, and behavior. The results can be obtained by directly asking the client about the

Table 16-3   Nursing Interventions Classification (NIC) Taxonomy

Domain 1	Domain 2	Domain 3
Level 1 Domains		
1. **Physiological: Basic** Care that supports physical functioning	2. **Physiological: Complex** Care that supports homeostatic regulation	3. **Behavioral** Care that supports psychosocial functioning and facilitates life-style changes
Level 2 Classes		
A *Activity and Exercise Management:* Interventions to organize or assist with physical activity and energy conservation and expenditure	G *Electrolyte and Acid-Base Management:* Interventions to regulate electrolyte/acid base balance and prevent complications	O *Behavior Therapy:* Interventions to reinforce or promote desirable behaviors or alter undesirable behaviors
B *Elimination Management:* Interventions to establish and maintain regular bowel and urinary elimination patterns and manage complications due to altered patterns	H *Drug Management:* Interventions to facilitate desired effects of pharmacological agents	P *Cognitive Therapy:* Interventions to reinforce or promote desirable cognitive functioning or alter undesirable cognitive functioning
C *Immobility Management:* Interventions to manage restricted body movement and the sequelae	I *Neurologic Management:* Interventions to optimize neurologic functions	Q *Communication Enhancement:* Interventions to facilitate delivering and receiving verbal and nonverbal messages
D *Nutrition Support:* Interventions to modify or maintain nutritional status	J *Perioperative Care:* Interventions to provide care before, during, and immediately after surgery	R *Coping Assistance:* Interventions to assist another to build on own strengths, to adapt to a change in function, or to achieve a higher level of function
E *Physical Comfort Promotion:* Interventions to promote comfort using physical techniques	K *Respiratory Management:* Interventions to promote airway patency and gas exchange	S *Patient Education:* Interventions to facilitate learning
F *Self-Care Facilitation:* Interventions to provide or assist with routine activities of daily living	L *Skin/Wound Management:* Interventions to maintain or restore tissue integrity	T *Psychological Comfort Promotion:* Interventions to promote comfort using psychological techniques
	M *Thermoregulation:* Interventions to maintain body temperature within a normal range	
	N *Tissue Perfusion Management:* Interventions to optimize circulation of blood and fluids to the tissue	

From McCloskey JC, Bulechek GM: *Nursing interventions classification (NIC)*, ed 3, St. Louis, 2000, Mosby.

condition or can be observed using assessment skills. Examples of outcomes involving assessment skills are "lungs will be clear on auscultation by 8/22" and "purulent wound drainage will cease by 9/12."

Measurable Factors.   Goals and expected outcomes are written to give the nurse a standard against which to measure the client's response to nursing care. Examples are "body temperature will remain 98.6," and "apical pulse will remain between 60 and 100 beats per minute." A goal or an outcome that is stated in measurable terms allows the nurse to objectively quantify changes in the client's status.

Common mistakes are made when the nurse uses vague qualifiers such as *normal, stable, acceptable,* or *sufficient* in the expected outcome statement. Vague qualifiers

have different meanings to different people. Using such terms results in guesswork in determining the client's response to care. Terms specifically describing quality, quantity, frequency, and weight allow the nurse to evaluate whether the expected outcome was achieved.

Time-Limited Factors.   The time frame for each goal and expected outcome indicates when the expected response should occur. Time frames assist the nurse and client in determining that progress is being made at a reasonable rate. When the date of evaluation arrives, the nurse assesses the client to determine whether that particular expected outcome has been reached. If the outcome is unmet, but it is still appropriate for the client's care, another future evaluation date is set.

Table 16-3 Nursing Interventions Classification (NIC) Taxonomy—cont'd

Domain 4	Domain 5	Domain 6	Domain 7
4. Safety Care that supports protection against harm	**5. Family** Care that supports the family unit	**6. Health System** Care that supports effective use of the health care delivery system	**7. Community** Care that supports the health of the community
U Crisis Management: Interventions to provide immediate short-term help in both psychological and physiological crises *V Risk Management:* Interventions to initiate risk-reduction activities and continue monitoring risks over time	*W Childbearing Care:* Interventions to assist in understanding and coping with the psychological and physiological changes during the childbearing period *Z Childrearing Care:* Interventions to assist in rearing children *X Lifespan Care:* Interventions to facilitate family unit functioning and promote the health and welfare of family members throughout the lifespan	*Y Health System Mediation:* Interventions to facilitate the interface between patient/family and the health care system *a Health System Management:* Interventions to provide and enhance support services for the delivery of care *b Information Management:* Interventions to facilitate communication among health care providers	*c Community Health Promotion:* Interventions that promote the health of the whole community *d Community Risk Management:* Interventions that assist in detecting or preventing health risks to the whole community

Mutual Factors. Mutual setting of goals and expected outcomes ensures that the client and nurse agree on the direction and time limits of care. Mutual goal setting can increase the client's motivation and cooperation. During this mutual setting of goals and outcomes, the nurse does not impose personal values on the client. However, the nurse must also be aware of standards of practice, client safety, and basic human needs. Using experience and acquired knowledge, the nurse may need to direct some of the goals and expected outcomes to keep the client physically and emotionally stable and safe.

Realistic Factors. Short-term, realistic goals and expected outcomes can quickly provide the client and nurse

with a sense of accomplishment. In turn, this sense of accomplishment can increase the client's motivation and cooperation. When establishing realistic goals, the nurse, through assessment, must know the resources of the health care facility, family, and client; the client's physiological, emotional, cognitive, and sociocultural potential; and the economic cost and resources available to reach expected outcomes in a timely manner. Establishing goals and expected outcomes without a thorough assessment of client, environment, or resources can be frustrating to the client and nurse because the plan then contains unrealistic goals.

. . .

Critical Thinking in Designing Nursing Interventions

Nursing interventions, strategies, or actions are selected after goals and expected outcomes are established (see Figure 16-1). Nursing interventions are those actions designed to assist the client in moving from the present level of health to that which is described in the goal and measured with the expected outcomes (Gordon, 1994). Implementation of these interventions occurs during the implementation phase of the nursing process (see Chapter 17).

Choosing suitable nursing interventions is a decision-making process (Bulechek and McCloskey, 1994; Alfaro-LeFevre, 1995). The nurse uses critical thinking by applying attitudes and standards and synthesizing information from the client's assessment data, knowledge, and experience to select interventions that will successfully meet established goals and expected outcomes for each diagnostic statement (Carnevali and Thomas, 1993). In addition, to initiate the intervention the nurse must be competent in three areas: (1) know the scientific rationale for the intervention, (2) possess the necessary psychomotor and interpersonal skills, and (3) be able to function within a particular setting to use the available health care resources effectively (Bulechek and McCloskey, 1992).

The Iowa Intervention Project has linked nursing interventions to nursing diagnostic labels (Table 16-3). Linking interventions to nursing diagnoses is one method for selecting interventions. The nurse must also determine that the interventions are individualized to the client's needs.

TYPES OF INTERVENTIONS

There are three categories of nursing interventions: nurse-initiated, physician-initiated, and collaborative interventions. Category selection is based on client needs. One client may require all three categories, whereas another client may need only nurse- and physician-initiated interventions.

Nurse-Initiated Interventions.   **Nurse-initiated interventions** are the independent response of the nurse to the client's health care needs and nursing diagnoses. This type of intervention is an autonomous action based on scientific rationale that is executed to benefit the client in a predicted way related to the nursing diagnosis and client-centered goals (Bulechek and McCloskey, 1994). Nurse-initiated interventions involve aspects of professional nursing practice encompassed by licensure and law. These interventions require no supervision or direction from others. For example, interventions for increasing a client's knowledge about adequate nutrition or activities of daily living related to hygiene are independent nursing actions.

In delineating the scope of nursing practice, the

Essential Features of Contemporary Nursing Practice   Box 16-1

Attention to the full range of human experiences and responses to health and illness without restriction to a problem-focused orientation

Integration of objective data with knowledge gained from an understanding of the patient or group's subjective experience

Application of scientific knowledge to the processes of diagnosis and treatment

Provision of a caring relationship that facilitates health and healing

From American Nurses Association: *Nursing's social policy statement,* Washington, DC, 1995, The Association.

American Nurses Association (ANA) (1995) listed examples of essential features of contemporary nursing practice (Box 16-1). This list, with the continuing work of North American Nursing Diagnosis Association (NANDA), the Nursing Interventions Classification (NIC) project at the University of Iowa, and nurse researchers, clarifies and elaborates the realm of independent nursing practice.

Nurse-initiated interventions do not require a physician's order or an order from another professional. Physicians frequently include in their written orders the specifics of independent nursing interventions. However, according to the nurse practice acts in a majority of states, nursing actions pertaining to activities of daily living, health education, health promotion, and counseling are in the domain of nursing practice. These acts delineate the legal scope of the practice of nursing within the geographical boundaries of the jurisdiction (see Chapter 21).

Physician-Initiated Interventions.   **Physician-initiated interventions** are based on the physician's response to a medical diagnosis. The nurse intervenes by carrying out physicians' written orders (Bulechek and McCloskey, 1994). Administering a medication, implementing an invasive procedure, changing a dressing, and preparing a client for diagnostic tests are examples of such interventions. It is not always within the legal practice of nursing for the nurse to prescribe and order these treatments, but it is within the practice of nursing for the nurse to complete such orders and to individualize approaches to their administration. For example, a physician may order a dressing change twice a day, an intravenous (IV) medication every 6 hours, and a bone scan for a client. The nurse incorporates each of these orders into the client's plan of care so that they are safely and efficiently completed.

Each physician-initiated intervention requires specific

nursing responsibilities and technical nursing knowledge. For example, when administering medications, the nurse is responsible for knowing the classification of the drug, its physiological action, normal dosage, side effects, and nursing interventions related to its action or side effects (see Chapter 34).

With an invasive procedure or dressing change, the nurse is responsible for knowing when the procedure is necessary, the clinical skills necessary to complete it, and its expected outcome and possible side effects. The nurse is also responsible for adequate preparation of the client and proper communication of the results.

When a specific diagnostic or laboratory test is ordered by a physician, the nurse is responsible for scheduling the test, preparing the client, and knowing the normal findings and nursing implications associated with it.

Collaborative Interventions. **Collaborative interventions** are therapies that require the knowledge, skill, and expertise of multiple health care professionals. For example, Mr. Joseph is a 68-year-old man who is a hemiplegic from a recent cerebrovascular accident (stroke) and also has a long-term history of dementia. His cognitive functions are limited, he is at risk for problems related to impaired sensation and mobility, and he is unable to independently complete activities of daily living. In order for Mr. Joseph to maintain his present level of health, he requires multiple interventions, including nursing interventions to prevent pressure ulcers, physical therapy interventions to prevent musculoskeletal changes from immobility, and occupational therapy interventions for eating and hygiene needs. The care for this client requires the coordination of collaborative interventions from multiple health care professionals, all directed toward the long-term goal of maintaining Mr. Joseph's present level of health.

• • •

Nurse-initiated, physician-initiated, and collaborative interventions require critical thinking and decision making. When encountering physician-initiated or collaborative interventions, the nurse does not automatically implement the therapy but must determine whether it is appropriate for the client. Every nurse encounters an inappropriate or incorrect order at some time. The nurse with a strong knowledge base recognizes the error and seeks to correct it. The ability to recognize incorrect therapies is particularly important when administering medications or implementing procedures. An error can occur in writing the order or transcribing it to the **Kardex** or medication administration record (MAR). Clarifying an order is competent nursing practice, and it protects the client and members of the health care delivery system. The nurse carrying out an incorrect or inappropriate intervention is as much in error as the person who wrote or transcribed the original order and is liable for any complica-

tions resulting from the error. Chapter 21 explains legal issues affecting nursing practice.

SELECTION OF INTERVENTIONS

When selecting interventions for a client, the nurse, using clinical decision-making skills, deliberates about six factors. These factors are elaborated in Box 16-2: (1) characteristics of the nursing diagnosis, (2) expected outcomes, (3) research base (nursing knowledge) for the interventions, (4) feasibility of the intervention, (5) acceptability to the client, and (6) competencies of the nurse (Bulechek and McCloskey, 1987, 1994; McCloskey and Bulechek, 1998). To achieve this the nurse also reviews standardized

---

Choosing Nursing Intervention Box 16-2

CHARACTERISTICS OF THE NURSING DIAGNOSIS
Interventions must be directed toward altering the etiological factors or signs and symptoms associated with the diagnostic label.
Interventions may be directed toward altering or eliminating risk factors, which are associated with "risk for" nursing diagnoses.

EXPECTED OUTCOMES
Outcomes are stated in measurable terms and used to evaluate the effectiveness of the interventions.

RESEARCH BASE
Review clinical nursing research related to diagnostic label and client problem.
Review articles that describe the utilization of research findings in similar clinical situations and settings.

FEASIBILITY
Interaction of nursing interventions with treatments being provided by other health professionals.
Cost: Is intervention both clinically effective and cost efficient?
Time: Are time and personnel resources well managed?

ACCEPTABILITY TO THE CLIENT
Treatment plan must be congruent with client's goals and health care values.
Mutually decided nursing goals.
Client must have required self-care abilities or have a person who can assist with health care.

COMPETENCIES OF THE NURSE
Knowledgeable of scientific rationale for the intervention.
Possession of necessary psychosocial and psychomotor skills to complete interventions.
Ability to function within setting and effectively and efficiently use health care resources.

Modified from Bulechek GM, McCloskey JC: Nursing interventions: what they are and how to choose them, *Holistic Nurs Pract* 1(3):36, 1987.

care plans, critical pathways, policy or procedure manuals, textbooks, and nursing and related health care literature; and collaborates with other health care professionals. During deliberation, the nurse reviews previous experiences, client needs, and priorities to select nursing interventions that have the best potential for achieving the expected outcomes. As the nurse gains experience, this deliberation process becomes more efficient and experience based (Benner, 1984).

Research of standardized care plans, critical pathways, policy and procedure manuals, textbooks, and nursing and related literature addresses usual problems and nursing actions for given conditions. Although they are written in general terms, the nurse may use these resources to acquire new knowledge. This knowledge assists in the individualization of the intervention.

Collaboration completes the selection of interventions. Through collaboration the nurse is able to tap the best resources to individualize the nursing actions. During collaboration the nurse includes the client and/or family to select suitable interventions. The collaboration process is discussed in a later section of this chapter.

The Nursing Interventions Classification (NIC) project, developed at the University of Iowa, is a system to classify 336 direct care treatments that nurses perform (McCloskey and Bulechek, 2000). The purpose of the NIC is to provide standardization of language for nursing treatments, which will facilitate communication and documentation of care (Carter and others, 1995). Standardized nursing language generates data that accurately represent nursing practice (Keenan and Aquilino, 1998). NIC is evolving and is practice oriented; it is designed to enable nurses in all practice settings to have a standard classification system for documenting nursing care. The classification is designed to be comprehensive, including independent and collaborative interventions that cover all specialty areas (Carter and others, 1995).

Classifications are subdivided into six domains, which make up the taxonomy of nursing interventions (see Table 16-3). The taxonomy has five advantages. First, the domains and classes help clinicians locate and select interventions appropriate to their clients. Second, it helps in the design and revision of curricula for beginning and advanced nurses. Third, the structure of the taxonomy permits numerical coding, which can facilitate computer use and ease in analysis of data (Iowa Intervention Project [IIP], 1993). This feature assists in furthering nursing knowledge through nursing research. Fourth, the taxonomy can easily be expanded to include more interventions. Last, the taxonomy provides a mechanism to effectively determine the cost of nursing care (IIP, 1993; Carter and others, 1995).

Initially the nurse will usually have more interventions than are necessary to meet a client's desired outcome. Some are discarded as inappropriate, others are adapted to the client's needs and abilities. As a result, the list of possible interventions is narrowed down to those suitable to the client (Redman, 1997). These interventions are then written on the nursing care plan.

Planning Nursing Care

There are multiple methods to communicate a client's nursing care. One is the nursing care plan, which includes the nursing diagnoses, goals, expected outcomes, and specific nursing activities and strategies. In many settings nursing care plans are being integrated into multidisciplinary plans of care. The nursing component of a multidisciplinary plan is easily recognizable.

A second method is critical pathways. **Critical pathways** are multidisciplinary treatment plans that prescribe interventions and the time frame for achieving expected outcomes for select clients over a projected length of stay (London, 1993).

PURPOSE OF CARE PLANS

The **nursing care plan** is a written guideline for client care. Written care plans document the client's health care needs. In addition, the written care plan communicates to other nurses and health care professionals the client's pertinent assessment data, a list of problems, and therapies. A written care plan is designed to decrease the risk of incomplete, incorrect, or inaccurate care.

The care plan is organized so that any nurse can quickly identify the nursing actions to be delivered. In hospitals and outpatient and community-based settings, the client often receives care from more than one nurse, physician, or allied health professional. The written nursing care plan makes possible the coordination of nursing care, subspecialty consultations, and scheduling of diagnostic tests.

The care plan can also identify and coordinate resources used to deliver nursing care. The listing of specific equipment and supplies necessary for nursing actions is an economically efficient mechanism for selecting equipment. If all equipment and supplies are included in the care plan, the nurse's time is used more effectively in providing care.

The nursing care plan enhances the continuity of nursing care by listing specific nursing actions necessary to achieve the goals of care. These nursing activities can be carried out daily. A correctly formulated nursing care plan facilitates the continuity of care from one nurse to another. As a result, all nurses have the opportunity to deliver high-quality, consistent care.

Written nursing care plans organize information exchanged by nurses in change-of-shift reports. Nurses focus these reports on nursing care and treatments delineated in care plans. At the end of shifts, nurses discuss care plans with the next caregivers. Thus all nurses are able to discuss current and pertinent information about the client's care plan.

The written care plan also includes the long-term needs of the client. Incorporating the goals of the care plan into discharge planning is particularly important for a client who will be undergoing long-term rehabilitation in the community. A complete care plan enhances the continuity of nursing care between nurses in the hospital and community.

When developing an individualized care plan, the nurse involves the family and client. The family is a resource that can be used to help the client meet health goals. In addition, meeting some of the family's needs can improve the client's level of wellness.

The last item documented on the nursing care plan is the expected outcome criteria used in evaluation of care. Proper listing of the criteria provides the nurse with objective statements that help determine whether the goals of care have been achieved.

The complete care plan is the blueprint for nursing action. It provides direction for implementation of the plan and a framework for evaluation of the client's response to nursing actions.

CARE PLANS IN VARIOUS SETTINGS

The format of the nursing care plan varies from one health care setting to another. For example, in a hospital setting a care plan may consist of columns for assessment, goals, interventions, and expected outcomes. In a community health setting the care plan may be narrative, but includes client needs, goals, plan, and expected outcomes. Although the format of the care plan varies from setting to setting, its overall purpose is to provide a written guideline for care so that the health care needs of the client and subsequent therapies are communicated among the health care team.

The nursing care plan developed for the client returning home is usually based solely on long-term health needs. In addition, the client, family, and significant others are more involved and assume more responsibility for care because the client is receiving nursing care in the home.

Same-day surgeries and earlier discharges from hospitals require the nurse to plan discharge needs on the care plan the moment the client enters a health care agency. Incomplete assessments and the absence of measurable outcome criteria may extend client stays in short-term, 1-day surgical centers. As a result, there can be confusion among the health care team as to when the client could safely be discharged from the setting.

Institutional Care Plans.
Institutional (staff) care plans are concise documents that become part of the client's medical record. Many hospitals use the Kardex nursing care plan. Kardex is a trade name for a card-filing system that allows quick reference to the particular needs of the client for certain aspects of nursing care. Information about medica-

tions, activity levels, level of self-care, diet, treatments, and procedures is usually included on the outside of the card. The nursing care plan is commonly placed on the inside (Figure 16-3). Each institution has its own format for the Kardex, but the basic information contained on it is universal. The care plan section of the Kardex also has institutional variations. One institution might use a three-column nursing care plan, which includes the problem, goal, and nursing action. Another institution may incorporate a four-column nursing care plan, which includes the nursing diagnosis, goal, nursing action, and evaluation.

Computerized Care Plans.
The use of computers and the need to efficiently organize the nurse's time have resulted in standardized care plans, which are forms created for a specific nursing diagnosis or clinical area (e.g., coronary care, abdominal surgery, postpartum, and same-day surgery units). For example, the nurse selects a nursing diagnosis and then individualizes a standard care plan by making selections from menus. Each care plan lists generalized nursing diagnoses, goals, outcome criteria, and interventions for specific clients (Figure 16-4).

After completing a nursing assessment, the nurse determines whether a standardized form should be used for that particular client. Even if the care plan is generally appropriate for a client, the nurse must add or delete information on the standardized form to individualize it for the client's needs. Failure to do so can result in incomplete and inaccurate care.

Computerized/standardized nursing care plans are a method to streamline and augment care planning, and provide documentation for third-party reimbursement (Hirtzel-Trexler, 1994). They are designed to incorporate current practice guidelines to achieve the desired client outcomes for a specific group of clients. In addition these plans encourage the nurse to incorporate individual client care needs into the plan of care (Hirtzel-Trexler, 1994).

Student Care Plans.
Nursing students learn to write and use a nursing care plan as part of their education. The student care plan is essential for learning the problem-solving technique, the nursing process, skills of written communication, and organizational skills needed for nursing care. Most important, by using the nursing care plan students can apply the knowledge gained from nursing and medical literature and the classroom to a practice situation.

The student care plan is more elaborate than a care plan in a hospital or community health care agency because its purpose is to teach the process of planning care. To learn the care planning process, the student must progress in a step-by-step manner, beginning with assessment and ending with evaluation. Student care plans vary from one educational program to another and between beginning and more advanced students. Some educational

Medical Diagnosis and other pertinent medical information:

10/25 LBP c̄ RLE Sciatica
10/26 Laminectomy L4-L5 c̄ Bone Graft

1083   13160   23-4
Smith, Phil

Condition	Satis	PMH:
Allergies (Drugs, food, other)	PCN, ASA, Codeine	DM

| Adm. Date | 10/23 | Age | 64 | Religion | Cath. | Mode of Travel | |
| Service | Ortho | Doctor | Ford | Resident | Kowalski | Inter | |

FREQUENTLY ORDERED ITEMS		Date	Specimens/Daily Lab	Date	Treatments
Temp.					
Pulse & Resp.	＞ q4°	10/25	Adm. Blood work	10/24	BR and Logroll q2°
BP		10/25	UA c̄ Micro		
		10/25	BS		
I & O	q 8°				
Weights					
Spot Checks					
Chest P.T.					
Incentive Spirometer					
P.T					

ACTIVITIES		NUTRITION	Date	Diagnostic Procedures
Ad lib		Diet Regular		
Ambulate	x 2		10/25	Myelogram
Chair				CT Scan
BRP				
Bedrest		Feedings	10/25	CXR
Self Bath			10/25	ECG
Tub		Assist c meals		
Shower		FLUID BALANCE		
Bed	✓	Force		
Assist.		D E N		
		Restrict		
		D E N		

Family:

NURSING CARE PLAN

Date	Nursing Diagnosis	Expected Outcomes	Nursing Plan/Orders
10/26	Pain related to incisional Swelling	1. Client use of PCA decreases by 10/28. 2. Client respiratory expansion ↑ by 10/27.	1. Encourage client to Log Roll when Turning. 2. Instruct client in relaxation exercizes.
10/27	Impaired physical mobility related to pain	1. Client increases ambulation from BID to QID or greater by 10/28. 2. Client assumes ADL by 10/29.	1. Ambulate in Hall c̄ client 20 min. after administration of analgesic. 2. Encourage family to walk client. 1. Allow client extra time to do self-care for hygiene needs.

Discharge Planning:	Destination:	Transportation:	Probable Date:	Referral Agencies:	Appointment:
				Supplies:	

Patient Name

Figure 16-3   Nursing care plan on a nursing Kardex.

institutions model the student care plan on the care plan used in the affiliated health care agency. The only modification may be that the instructor requires the beginning student to include the scientific rationale for the nursing interventions selected (Table 16-4). A **scientific rationale** is the reason that, based on supporting literature, a specific nursing action was chosen.

Care Plans for Community-Based Settings.   Planning care for clients in community-based settings, for example, clinics, community centers, or client's homes, in-

volves using the same principles of nursing practice. However, in these settings the nurse must complete a more comprehensive community, home, and family assessment. In this setting, the client/family unit is in equal partnership with health care professionals (Bond, Phillips, and Rollins, 1994). Ultimately the client/family must be able to independently provide the majority of health care. The nurse designs a plan to (1) educate the client/family about the necessary care techniques, (2) teach the client/family how to integrate care within family activities, and (3) allow the client/family to assume a greater percentage of

NURSING STANDARD CARE PLAN

Nursing Diagnosis: INEFFECTIVE BREATHING PATTERN

Related to: _____
(respiratory muscle fatigue, anxiety, pain, impaired respiratory
mechanics such as chest tubes, incisions, anatomy)

Date Initiated/ Initials	Expected Outcomes	Date to be Met/Initials	Date Met/ Initials
_____	Patient will verbalize understanding of _____ .	_____	_____
_____	Patient will demonstrate ability to perform _____ .	_____	_____
_____	Patient will pace and schedule activities.	_____	_____
_____	Patient will use relaxation techniques for breathing control.	_____	_____
_____	Patient will maintain respiratory rate of _____ with PaC02 of _____ .	_____	_____
_____	Other: _____		

Relevant baseline data: _____
_____

Referrals: (date contacted)

☐ Nurse Specialist: _____ ☐ Home Care: _____ ☐ Social Work: _____
☐ Other: _____ ☐ Other: _____

Date Initiated/ Initials	Nursing Interventions	Date Inactivated/ Initials
	1. Assess respiratory function for rapid, shallow, irregular, or slow breathing, dyspnea, use of accessory muscles, breath sounds, restlessness, confusion, and cyanosis every _____ .	
	2. Monitor patient's mental status/LOC every _____ .	
_____ _____ _____	3. Maintain adequate airway by: ☐ a. cough/splinting every _____ ☐ b. suction every _____ ☐ c. incentive spirometry every _____	_____ _____
	4. Pace and schedule activity to avoid dyspnea resulting from fatigue. Schedule is _____	
	5. Provide physical and emotional support during episodes of respiratory distress by: _____	
_____ _____ _____ _____ _____	6. Provide teaching specific to patient or support person's needs. Initiate individual plan: ☐ a. pursed lip breathing ☐ b. coughing/splinting techniques (specify) _____ _____ ☐ c. relaxation techniques (specify) _____ _____ ☐ d. diaphragmatic breathing _____ _____ ☐ e. other: _____ _____	_____ _____ _____ _____ _____
_____ _____ _____ _____	7. Other interventionsl specific to patient: a. _____ b. _____ c. _____ d. _____	_____ _____ _____ _____
	Signature/Initials: _____	

☐ **PLAN OF CARE MUTUALLY SET WITH PATIENT AND/OR FAMILY**

Figure 16-4 Standardized nursing care plan.
Courtesy Barnes-Jewish Hospital, St. Louis, Mo.

BARNES

CARE PATH®
501
LUNG TRANSPLANT EVALUATION

SERVICE		PHYSICIAN	
PRIMARY NURSE		PRIMARY NURSE	
DC DATE	ADM DATE	DATE OF SURGERY	

A-8

Problem Number	PATIENT PROBLEMS / NURSING DIAGNOSES
#1	LACK OF KNOWLEDGE R/T LUNG TRANSPLANT EVALUATION EXPERIENCE
#2	DECREASE IN EXERCISE CAPACITY R/T IMPAIRED OXYGENATION/VENTILATION/DECONDITIONING
#3	POTENTIAL FOR ALTERATION IN COPING R/T SITUATIONAL CRISIS/TRANSITION
#4	POTENTIAL FOR ALTERATION IN FAMILY PROCESSES R/T SITUATIONAL CRISIS/TRANSITION
#5	POTENTIAL FOR ALTERATION IN NUTRITION R/T INAPPROPRIATE INTAKE/DYSPNEA
#6	IMPAIRED GAS EXCHANGE R/T ALVEOLAR-CAPILLARY MEMBRANE CHANGE/ALTERED BLOOD FLOW *IF APPROPRIATE

#	1 - 12	1 - 12	1 - 2, 6 - 8, 12	2, 10, 12	1
	ASSESSMENT / MONITORING	**CONSULTS**	**PROCEDURES / TEST**	**TREATMENT**	**ACTIVITY**
PRE ADMIT		Transplant office to preschedule following as needed for pt.: 2-D Echo, Quant. V-Q, Resting RVG, PFTs, MRI, Cardiac Cath, Chest CT, Transesophageal echocardiogram			
DAY 1	Braden scale Respiratory status Fall prevention Assess/individualize pt. problem list	Notify consults as per orders. Check with transplant P.A. for additional tests which may be needed. SMA 6 and 12, CBC, CMV, HSV, EBV, Vz titers, HbsAq, HbsAb, HIV, Hep. A, Hep. C titers, T & S, PT, PTT, HLA (A, B, C, DR) Typing, incl. cytotoxic screen, u/a - routine & micro, CXR-AP & lat	Apply skin tests 07 08 Nursing, Pulm. Rehab., 08 & H.O. 10 11 12 Psychologist 13 14 CDL 15 16 PFTs 17 Chaplain 18 19 Cardialogy Consult 20	Appropriate bed surface for Braden scale O$_2$ • at rest _____ • Activity _____ CPT x1 x2 x3 x4 by Nursing, Physical Therapy, family Aerosols x1 x2 x3 x4 (Self)	Continue activity as done at home
	SIGNATURE	**INIT.**	**SIGNATURE**	**INIT.**	**SIGNATURE**	**INIT.**

3100-45 (REV. 10/93)

Copyright 1993, Barnes Hospital - All Rights Re-

501

Figure 16-5 Critical pathway.
Courtesy Barnes-Jewish Hospital, St. Louis, Mo.

					2

BARNES

CARE PATH®
501
LUNG TRANSPLANT EVALUATION

CNS	DIETARY	RT	
HOME HEALTH	OT	OTHER	
PT	SW	OTHER	A-8

Problem Number	PATIENT PROBLEMS / NURSING DIAGNOSES
#7	POTENTIAL FOR INEFFECTIVE AIRWAY CLEARANCE R/T EXCESSIVE SECRETIONS/FATIGUE
#8	INEFFECTIVE BREATHING PATTERN R/T INCREASED WORK OF BREATHING
#9	POTENTIAL FOR INFECTION R/T ALTERED NUTRITION/CHRONIC DISEASE
#10	POTENTIAL FOR INJURY R/T PHYSICAL DECONDITIONING
#11	SPIRITUAL DISTRESS R/T CHALLENGED BELIEF AND VALUE SYSTEM
#12	POTENTIAL FOR ALTERED SKIN INTEGRITY R/T POOR NUTRITION/DECREASED MOBILITY

1	1, 5, 9, 12	1 - 12	1 - 12	1, 2, 4, 11	INITIALS (SEE KEY AT BOTTOM)		
MEDS / IVS	NUTRITION	PATIENT / FAMILY EDUCATION	DISCHARGE PLANNING	PSYCHOSOCIAL/ EMOTIONAL/ SPIRITUAL NEEDS			
		Give LTE manual, 6200 pt. letter.					
Pt. to do self meds.; Initiate IV access within 2 hrs. of admission	Continue home diet	Lung transplant evaluation Review tests for day 1 & 2 Personalize instruction to pts. individual learning needs. **Pt./family able to verbalize purpose and any special preparation for follow-up care for tests.**	Plan of care has been mutually set with pt./ family. Educational and DC planning needs will be assessed. **Pt./family verbalizes understanding of care path.**	Allow pt./ family to verbalize concerns and questions and relate problems back to appropriate discipline.			

SIGNATURE	INIT.	SIGNATURE	INIT.	SIGNATURE	INIT.

Figure 16-5, cont'd   Critical pathway.

care in graduated increments (Bond, Phillips, and Rollins, 1994; Lund, 1994). Last, the plan is designed to include nurses' and the client's/family's evaluation of expected outcomes.

Critical Pathways.

Critical pathways allow staff from all disciplines, such as medicine, nursing, pharmacy, and social work, to develop integrated care plans for a projected length of stay or number of visits for clients with a specific case type. For example, the pathway in Figure 16-5 is for a lung transplant evaluation, which recommends on a day-by-day basis the client's activities, consults, procedures, and discharge planning activities, and educational topics expected for client's progression through the transplantation process. The nurse and other health team members use the pathway to monitor a client's progress and as a documentation tool. Due to the arrival of managed care (Chapter 2), documentation tools that integrate the standards of care for multiple disciplines are necessary. Critical pathways meet this need, and charting by exception is frequently the method of choice (Chapter 24).

Initially, critical pathways were developed to manage clients in acute care settings. However, these pathways are now integrated into community-based settings (e.g., home care, restorative care settings, same day surgery) (Leininger and Laux, 1998). When using critical pathways to plan care, many other forms (e.g., the nursing care plan, flow sheets, nurses' notes) are eliminated because all the pertinent components are included on the pathway format.

Writing the Nursing Care Plan

The nursing diagnosis with the highest priority is the beginning point for the nursing care plan and is followed by other nursing diagnoses in order of assigned priority. In this example we will show how to write a care plan in a five-column format. In the assessment column (column 1), the nurse includes all data relevant to the corresponding nursing diagnosis. The nurse includes the previously developed goals in the next column (column 2). At this point, the nurse begins to translate the short- and long-term goals into action plans that anticipate the needs of the client, coordinate nursing care, and select appropriate nursing measures.

The nurse writes the action plan in the implementation column (column 3) of the care plan. Each nursing action is written to include information necessary to implement nursing care. It may help the beginning nurse to ask whether the stated interventions answer the following questions:

What is the intervention?

When should each intervention be implemented?

How should the intervention be performed?

Who should be involved in each aspect of intervention? In addition, the nurse should understand the scientific rationale (column 4) for a specific intervention. Nonspecific nursing interventions result in incomplete or inaccurate nursing care, lack of continuity among caregivers, and poor use of resources.

Common omissions in writing nursing interventions include action, frequency, quantity, method, or person to perform them. These errors can occur if the nurse is unfamiliar with the planning process. Table 16-5 illustrates these types of errors by showing incorrect and correct statements of nursing interventions.

Column 5 of the nursing care plan contains the projected outcome criteria previously identified. Listing the criteria on the care plan gives a written estimation of when

Table 16-4 Scientific Rationale for the Student Care Plan

NURSING DIAGNOSIS: Risk for impaired skin integrity related to immobility resulting from coma
DEFINITION: Risk for impaired skin integrity is the state in which an individual's skin is at risk of being adversely altered.

Assessment	Goals	Implementation	Rationale	Expected Outcomes
Fever: higher than 102° F for 72 hours Diaphoresis Incontinence of urine	Skin remains intact Muscle mass is retained over bony prominences	Turn client every 2 hours in following sequence: 8 AM—supine 10 AM—left side Noon—prone Repeat, beginning with supine position. Administer antipyretics as ordered.	Critical time for skin tissue breakdown is between 1 and 2 hours of constant pressure.	No skin breakdown is noted. Skin color, temperature, and capillary return are normal. Client is afebrile within 24 hours.
Decreased skin turgor No skin breakdown noted		Keep client's skin dry at all times.	Moisture increases maceration of skin and promotes bacterial growth.	Skin remains dry and intact. Skin turgor is improved within 24 hours.

Data from Kim MJ, McFarland GK, McLane AM: *Pocket guide to nursing diagnoses,* ed 7, St. Louis, 1997, Mosby.

Table 16-5 **Frequent Errors in Writing Nursing Interventions**		
Type of Error	Incorrectly Stated Nursing Intervention	Correctly Stated Nursing Intervention
Failure to precisely or completely indicate nursing actions	Nurse assistant will turn client every 2 hours.	Nurse assistant will turn client every 2 hours, using the following schedule: 8 AM—supine 10 AM—left side Repeat at 4 PM Noon—prone and 2 AM 2 PM—right side
Failure to indicate frequency	Nurse assistant will observe client cough and deep breathe.	Nurse assistant will observe client cough and deep breathe at 10 AM—2 PM—6 PM—10 PM.
Failure to indicate quantity	Primary nurse will provide hydrogen peroxide (H_2O_2) mouthwash to client every 2 hours while awake: 8-10-12-2-4-6-8-10.	Primary nurse will provide 50 ml of H_2O_2 mouthwash to client every 2 hours while awake: 8-10-12-2-4-6-8-10.
Failure to indicate method	Primary nurse will change client's dressing once a shift: 6 AM—2 PM—10 PM.	Primary nurse will replace client's dressing, with Neosporin ointment to wound and two dry 4×4 dressings secured with hypoallergenic tape, once a shift: 2 PM—10 PM—6 AM.
Failure to indicate person to perform the action	Irrigate nasogastric (NG) tube every 2 hours (even) round the clock with 30 ml of normal saline (NS).	Primary nurse will irrigate NG tube every 2 hours (even) around the clock with 30 ml NS.

the goal of care is to be achieved. The nurse can enter when outcomes are met, thus indicating when a particular nursing diagnosis is no longer relevant to the client's plan of care.

Writing Critical Pathways

The writing of a critical pathway is a lengthy process, involving all members of a multidisciplinary health care team. Often it takes many weeks of research and review for a team to agree on the components of a critical pathway. Once developed, critical pathways become a case management tool that delineates desired interventions and client outcomes within specific time frames (Windle, 1994). To write and use a critical pathway the nurse must understand each component of the nursing process (Zander and McGill, 1994). Critical pathways are multidisciplinary, outcome-based care plans.

Critical pathways delineate specific care but also provide a mechanism for timely revision of the plan of care (Zander, 1988). This method of care delivery reframes the work of nursing and other disciplines so that it is clear to the health care team and to the client and family (Zander and McGill, 1994; Zander, 1998). When writing a critical pathway; the team must be familiar with other pathways developed in the agency and the literature as it is related to a specific disease or surgical procedure. The pathway developed for a medical condition or procedure delineates related nursing diagnoses and the interventions to be administered by all health team members. Expected outcomes are developed during the planning phase, and a specific time interval for achieving the outcome is included. In addition, the critical pathway is written so that all members of the health care team can document delivery of care or changes in a client's status (Chapter 24).

Consulting Other Health Care Professionals

Planning nursing care involves consultation with other members of the health care team (Figure 16-6). **Consultation** may occur at any step in the nursing process, but it is needed most often in the planning and intervention steps, when the nurse is more likely to identify a problem requiring additional knowledge, skills, or resources (Lund, 1994). Consultation is a process in which the expertise of a specialist is sought to identify ways to handle problems in client management or the planning and implementation of programs. Consultation is based on the problem-solving approach, and the consultant is the stimulus for change.

In clinical nursing, consultation is used to solve problems in the delivery of nursing care or the use of resources. Nurse consultants are most frequently approached for advice about difficult clinical problems. Nurses are consulted for their clinical expertise, client education skills, or staff education skills.

Nurses also consult with other members of the health care team, such as physical therapists, nutritionists, and

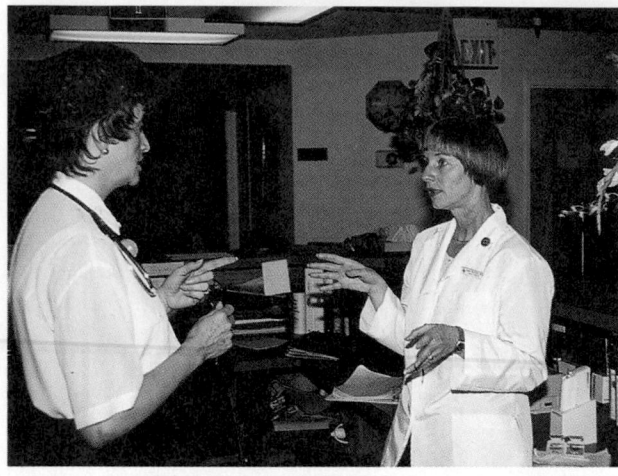

Figure 16-6　Consultation and planning care.

social workers. Again, the consultant focuses on problems in nursing.

When to Consult

The need for consultation in nursing occurs when the nurse has identified a problem that cannot be solved using personal knowledge, skills, and resources. Consultation increases the nurse's knowledge about the problem and helps in learning skills and obtaining the resources needed to solve the problem. After the consultation, the nurse may be able to resolve similar problems in the future. For example, a nurse encountering a client with a recent colostomy might request a consultation from an enterostomal therapist to determine the materials needed to clean the colostomy site and the specific techniques to use during the procedure.

Consultation is also used when the exact problem remains unclear. A consultant objectively entering a situation can more clearly assess and identify the exact nature of the problem, whether it is client, personnel, or equipment oriented. An unbiased consultant can often objectively identify the problem and outline a method for resolving it.

How to Consult

The first step in the consultation process is identification of the general problem area, which will give the consultant a starting point for identifying the problem. Second, the consultation should be directed to the appropriate professional, who may be another nurse or another member of the health care team.

Third, the nurse provides the consultant with pertinent assessment information and resources about the problem area. Pertinent information includes a brief assessment of the problem, interventions used to resolve the problem, and the outcome of those interventions. Other resources can include the client's complete nursing assessment and medical record, nurses and other members of the health team, and the client's family.

Fourth, the nurse should not provide biased information to the consultant. Consultants are in the clinical setting to identify and resolve a nursing problem, and biasing them can hinder problem resolution. Bias can be avoided by not overloading consultants with subjective and emotional conclusions about the client and problem.

Fifth, the nurse requesting consultation should be available to discuss the findings and recommendations. When a consultation is requested, the nurse provides a private, comfortable atmosphere in which the consultant and client can meet. However, this does not mean that the nurse leaves the environment. A common mistake is turning the whole problem over to the consultant. The consultant is not there to take over the problem but is there to assist the nurse in resolving it. The nurse requesting assistance should request the consultation for a day when both are scheduled to work and a time when distractions are minimal.

Finally, the nurse incorporates the consultant's recommendations into the plan of care. The changes in care must be communicated in writing on the nursing care plan or Kardex and verbally to all nursing and other health care providers. The success of the advice depends on the implementation of the problem-solving techniques suggested. The nurse should also provide feedback to the consultant regarding the outcome of the recommendations.

Consultants are a valuable adjunct to nursing care. In clinical nursing practice, competent and experienced nurses encounter problems beyond their knowledge or experience. Professional and competent nurses recognize their limitations, seek appropriate consultation, and learn from the findings and recommendations.

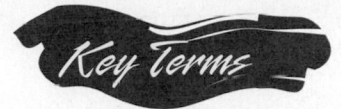

Key Concepts

- During the planning component, client goals are determined and prioritized, expected outcomes of nursing care are developed, and a nursing care plan is written.
- Nursing care is planned and organized around specific nursing diagnoses, resulting in individualized care plans.
- Goals include prevention, rehabilitation, and addressing the crisis or urgent needs of the client.
- Goal setting establishes a framework for the care plan.
- Using expected outcomes, the nurse measures the effectiveness of the care plan.
- The care plan is a written guideline for care so that care can be given effectively, efficiently, and is understood by all members of the health care team.
- Critical pathways are multidisciplinary treatment plans that predict the interventions and outcomes to be met for selected clients over a projected length of stay.
- Care plans and critical pathways increase communication among nurses and facilitate the continuity of care from one nurse to another and from one health care setting to another.
- The planning of individualized care requires involvement of the client and family.
- The care plan is a method for teaching students to transfer knowledge gained from nursing and medical literature and the classroom into practical experience.
- Correctly written nursing interventions include actions, frequency, quantity, method, and the person to perform them.
- Nurse-initiated or independent nursing interventions can solve the client's problems without consultation or collaboration with physicians or other health care professionals.
- Physician-initiated or dependent nursing interventions are completed with a physician's order, but require nursing judgment or decision making.
- Planning nursing care often involves consultation with other members of the health care team.

Key Terms

Client-centered goal, *p. 329*
Collaboration, *p. 336*
Collaborative interventions, *p. 335*
Consultation, *p. 343*
Critical pathway, *p. 336*
Expected outcome, *p. 331*
Goals, *p. 328*
Kardex, *p. 335*

Long-term goal, *p. 330*
Nurse-initiated interventions, *p. 334*
Nursing care plan, *p. 336*
Physician-initiated interventions, *p. 334*
Planning, *p. 327*
Scientific rationale, *p. 338*
Short-term goal, *p. 330*

Critical Thinking Exercises

1. How do you link goals and expected outcomes of nursing care from nursing diagnoses?
2. What criteria do you use to determine expected outcomes for a given set of client-centered goals?
3. What criteria do you use to select interventions?
   A. What client cultural information is needed?
   B. What health care resource information is needed?
   C. What assessments do you make regarding your competency to perform a specific skill?

References

Alfaro-LeFevre R: *Critical thinking in nursing: a practical approach*, Philadelphia, 1995, WB Saunders.

American Nurses Association: *Nursing's social policy statement*, Kansas City, Mo, 1995, The Association.

Bandman EL, Bandman B: *Critical thinking in nursing*, ed 2, Norwalk, Conn, 1995, Appleton & Lange.

Benner P: *From novice to expert: excellence and power in clinical nursing practice*, Menlo Park, Calif, 1984, Addison-Wesley.

Bond N, Phillips P, Rollins JA: Family-centered care at home for families with children who are technology dependent, *Pediatr Nurs* 20:123, 1994.

Bulechek GM, McCloskey JC: Nursing interventions: what they are and how to choose them, *Holistic Nurs Pract* 1(3):36, 1987.

Bulechek GM, McCloskey JC: *Nursing interventions: treatments for nursing diagnoses*, ed 2, Philadelphia, 1992, WB Saunders.

Bulechek GM, McCloskey JC: Nursing interventions classification: defining nursing care. In McCloskey JC, Grace H, editors: *Current issues in nursing*, ed 4, St. Louis, 1994, Mosby.

Carnevali DL, Thomas MD: *Diagnostic reasoning and treatment decision making in nursing*. Philadelphia, 1995, JB Lippincott.

Carpenito LJ: *Nursing diagnoses: application to clinical practice*, ed 6, Philadelphia, 1995, JB Lippincott.

Carpenito LJ: *Nursing diagnoses: application to clinical practice*, ed 7, Philadelphia, 1997, JB Lippincott.

Carter J and others: Using the nursing interventions classification to implement Agency for Health Care Policy and Research guidelines, *J Nurs Care Qual* 9(2):166, 1995.

Chase S: Teaching baccalaureate nursing students to project outcomes to nursing interventions, *Nurs Diagn* 9(2):62, 1998.

Deaton C: Outcomes measurement, *J Cardiovasc Nurs* 12(4):49051, 1998.

Gordon M: *Nursing diagnosis: process and application,* ed 3, St. Louis, 1994, Mosby.

Gordon M et al: Clinical judgment: an integrated model, *Adv Nurs Sci* 16:55, 1994.

Head B, Mass M, Johnson M: Research and development: outcomes for home and community nursing in integrated delivery systems, *Caring* 16(1):50, 1997.

Hirtzel-Trexler BJ: Commentary on practice guidelines: a standard whose time has come, *AONE's Leadership Perspectives* 2(2):22, 1994.

Iowa Intervention Project: the NIC taxonomy structure, *Image J Nurs Sch* 25:1816, 1993.

Johnson M, Mass M, Moorhead S: *Nursing outcomes classification,* ed. 2, St. Louis, Mo, 2000, Mosby.

Kataoka-Yahiro M, Saylor C: A critical thinking model for nursing judgment, *J Nurs Educ* 33(8):351, 1994.

Keenan G, Aquilino ML: Standardized nomenclatures: keys to continuity of care, nursing accountability and nursing effectiveness, *Outcomes Management for Nursing Practice* 2(2):81, 1998.

Kim MJ, McFarland GK, McLane AM: *Pocket guide to nursing diagnosies,* ed 7, St. Louis, 1997, Mosby.

Leininger SM, Laux LH: The continuum of health care: highlights of orthopaedic and general medical pathways, *Home Health Care Management and Practice* 10(4):1, 1998.

London J: On the right path: collaborative case management makes nurses partners in the care-planning process, *Health Progr* 164(5):36, 1993.

Lund SM: Family-centered nurse coordinator-early childhood intervention: development and implementation of the CNS role, *Clinical Nurse Specialist* 8:109, 1994.

Maslow AH: *Motivation and personality,* ed 2, New York, 1970, Harper & Row.

McCloskey JC, Bulechek GM: Standardizing the language for nursing treatments: an overview of the issues, *Nurs Outlook* 42:56, 1994.

McCloskey JC, Bulechek GM: *Nursing interventions classification (NIC),* ed 3, St. Louis, 2000, Mosby.

McCloskey JC, Bulechek GM: Nursing interventions core to specialty practice, *Nurs Outlook* 46(2):67, 1998.

Miller MA, Babcock DE: *Critical thinking applied to nursing,* St. Louis, 1996, Mosby.

Redman BK: *The practice of patient education,* ed 8, St. Louis, 1997, Mosby.

Windle PE: Critical pathways: an integrated documentation tool, *Nurs Manage* 25(9):80, 1994.

Zander K: Nursing case management: resolving the DRG paradox, *Nurs Clin North Am* 23:503, 1988.

Zander K: Historical development of outcomes-based care delivery, *Crit Care Nurs Clin North Am* 10(1):1, 1998.

Zander K, McGill R: Critical and anticipated recovery paths: only the beginning, *Nurs Manage* 25(8):34, 1994.

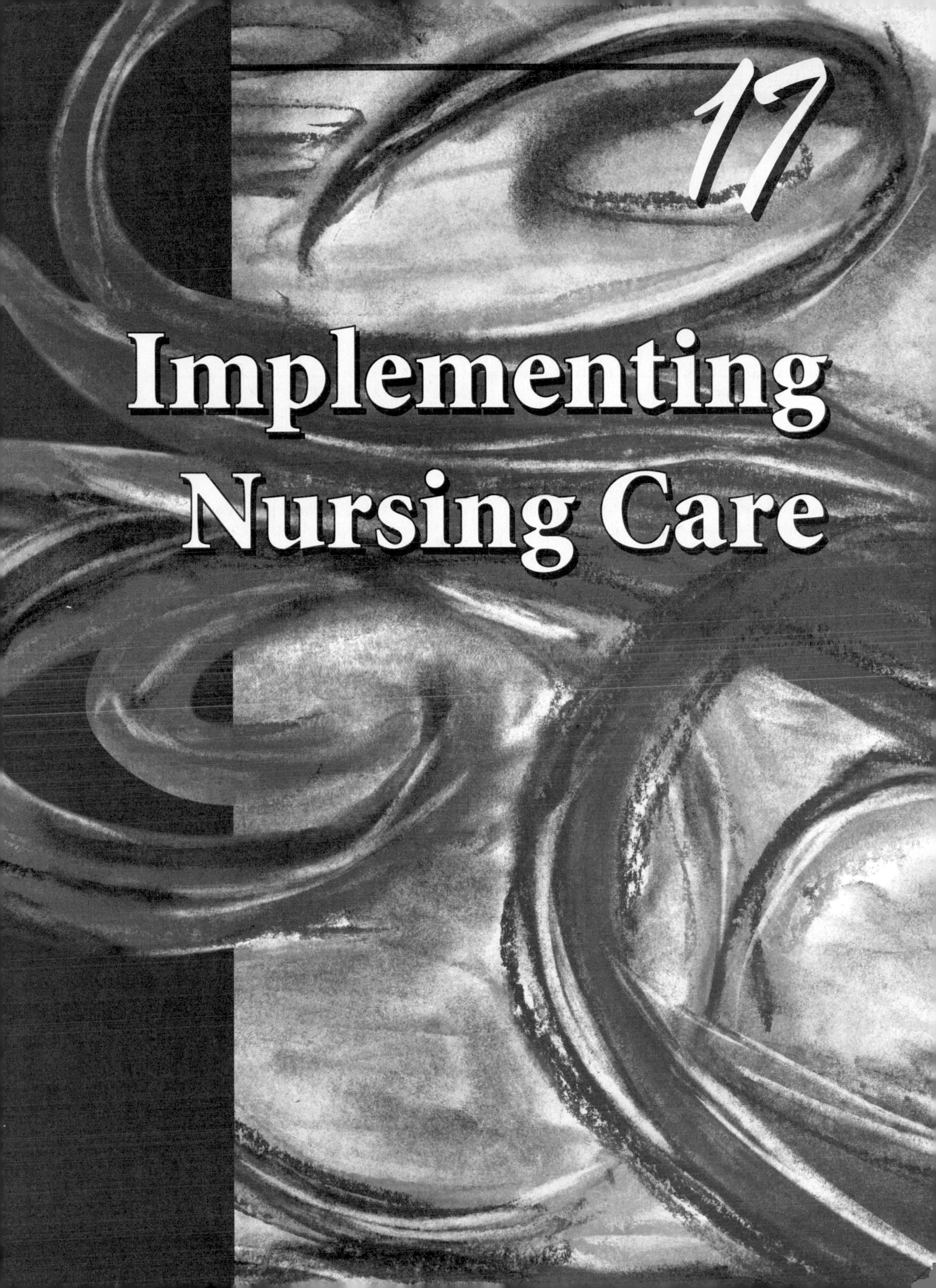

17

Implementing Nursing Care

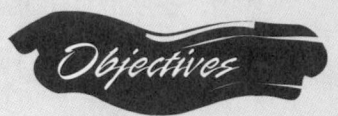

Mastery of content in this chapter will enable the student to:

- Define the key terms listed.
- Explain the relationship of implementation to the diagnostic process.
- Discuss the differences between protocols and standing orders.
- Describe the link between critical thinking and selecting nursing interventions.
- Describe the role of the Nursing Interventions Classification (NIC) project in advancing nursing knowledge.
- Describe the five different implementation methods.
- Select appropriate implementation methods for an assigned client.

I mplementation, a component of the nursing process, begins after the care plan has been developed. With the care plan based on clear and relevant nursing diagnoses, the nurse then selects and initiates interventions that are most likely to support or improve the client's health status. In theory, implementation of the nursing care plan follows the planning component of the nursing process. However, in many health care settings implementation may begin directly after assessment. For example, immediate implementation is necessary when the nurse identifies urgent needs of the client in situations such as cardiac arrest or sudden death of a loved one.

Implementation describes a category of nursing behaviors in which the actions necessary for achieving the goals and expected outcomes of nursing care are initiated and completed. Implementation includes nursing interventions for performing, assisting, or directing the performance of activities of daily living; counseling and teaching the client or family; providing direct care to achieve client-centered goals; delegating, supervising, and evaluating the work of staff members; and recording and exchanging information relevant to the client's continued health care.

A **nursing intervention** is any action taken by the nurse to help the client move from a present health state to the health state described in the expected outcomes (Gordon, 1994). The client may require intervention in the form of medication; treatment for the current condition; client-family education; treatment to prevent future health problems; or social, emotional, or physical support. Interventions that promote culturally sensitive care increase the potential for the attainment of the goals and expected outcomes of nursing care (Doswell and Erlem, 1998).

Implementation is a continuous process and interacts with the other components of the nursing process. As the nurse carries out interventions, the client's condition can change or the client may respond to the interventions as expected. For implementation to be effective, the nurse must also be knowledgeable about the types of nursing interventions, the implementation process, and specific implementation methods.

Types of Nursing Interventions

Implementation puts the care plan into action. After the plan has been developed according to client needs and priorities, the nurse performs specific nursing interventions, which include nurse-initiated, physician-initiated, and collaborative treatments (McCloskey and Bulechek, 2000) (see Chapter 16). At times, nursing interventions are based on protocols or standing orders. A clear understanding of the types of interventions is necessary for safe nursing practice.

INDEPENDENT NURSING INTERVENTIONS

Chapter 16 discusses independent nursing interventions. These interventions are the independent response of the nurse to the client's health care needs and nursing diagnoses. These are autonomous actions based on scientific rationale that is executed to benefit the client in a predicted way in relation to the nursing diagnoses and client-centered goals (Bulechek and McCloskey, 1990). These independent interventions involve aspects of professional nursing practice encompassed by licensure and law.

PROTOCOLS AND STANDING ORDERS

A **protocol** is a written plan specifying the procedures to be followed during care of a client with a select clinical condition or situation, such as care of a postoperative client. Nurses providing primary care for clients in an outpatient setting follow treatment and diagnostic protocol. In such a setting, nurses assess the client and identify abnormalities. The protocol delineates the conditions that nurses are permitted to treat, such as controlled hypertension, and the types of treatment they are permitted to administer, such as well-baby immunizations.

A protocol can also be strictly within the framework of nursing, such as a protocol for admission and discharge, pain management, or initiating cardiopulmonary resuscitation (CPR). Protocols are also used in interdisciplinary settings for diagnostic testing and physical, occupational, and speech therapies.

A **standing order** is a document containing orders for the conduct of routine therapies, monitoring guidelines, and/or diagnostic procedures for specific clients with identified clinical problems. The orders direct the conduct of client care in various clinical settings. Standing orders are approved and signed by the physician in charge of care before their implementation. They are commonly found in critical care settings, where client's needs can change rapidly and require immediate attention. Such a standing order might specify a certain drug, such as lidocaine or propranolol, for an irregular heart rhythm. After assessing the client and identifying the irregular rhythm, the critical care nurse gives the specified medication without first notifying the physician. Standing orders are also common in the community health setting, in which the nurse encounters situations that do not permit immediate contact with a physician. Thus standing orders and protocols give the nurse legal protection to intervene appropriately in the client's best interest.

· · ·

Before implementing any therapy, including those in protocols and standing orders, the nurse must use sound judgment in determining whether the intervention is correct and appropriate. Second, the nurse implementing any intervention has the responsibility to obtain correct theoretical knowledge and develop the clinical competency necessary to perform the intervention. Nursing responsibility is equally great for all types of interventions.

Critical Thinking in Implementing Nursing Interventions

Nurses using the nursing process make two major types of decisions. During the diagnostic process, the nurse forms conclusions, makes decisions, and draws inferences about the client's assessment data and health care needs (Miller and Babcock, 1996). The nurse then uses a methodological, systematic, research-based approach to plan and select appropriate nursing interventions (Gordon, 1994).

The student must carefully select the interventions best suited to achieve expected outcomes and know how nurse-initiated, physician-initiated, and collaborative in-

terventions differ (see Chapter 16). Several factors make decision making more difficult when choosing among nurse-initiated (independent) nursing interventions (Snyder, Egan, and Nojima, 1996). One factor is the absence of objective data concerning the probable effects or results of the interventions (Stewart and Archbold, 1993). To date, the research-based literature documenting the effectiveness and consequences of independent nursing interventions is scant. A second factor is that nurse-initiated interventions are often not mutually exclusive. Frequently they must be administered with therapies in other disciplines. For example, the nurse may need to include relaxation, massage, and guided imagery techniques with prescribed analgesics for pain management (see Chapter 42). The third factor is a lack of common intervention language that can deter collaboration, development of research-based practice, and reimbursement for nursing services (Snyder, Egan, and Nojima, 1996). The Nursing Interventions Classification (NIC) project at the University of Iowa is a major effort to define interventions performed by nurses for clients with select nursing diagnoses. These classifications will help to advance the knowledge base of nursing (McCloskey and Bulechek, 2000). The ongoing development of the NIC will help to differentiate nursing practice from the practice of other health care professionals (Box 17-1). The interventions are arranged in a taxonomy that organizes the interventions into seven domains of care. The taxonomy can assist the nurse in planning the nursing interventions to achieve the goals of care (see Chapter 16).

The critical thinking model discussed in Chapter 13 explains what is involved in making decisions for implementing nursing care (Figure 17-1). The nurse implements the care plan using the knowledge bases that were necessary for care planning (see Chapter 16) and to complete the planned interventions most effectively. In addition, the nurse applies prior clinical experiences in using specific interventions. Thus to each clinical situation the nurse brings an experiential base of what has worked and what did not work in certain situations. Before implementing a plan of care, the nurse is aware of both professional and the agency's standards of practice. It is important to know what the guideline are for frequency of procedures and to whom the procedures may be delegated. Attitudes of independent thinking and responsibility and authority will enable the nurse to reflect on the care delivered. Creativity and self-discipline will guide the nurse in reviewing, modifying, and implementing activities. This model is effective in teaching the student clinical decision making. However, the beginning student or practitioner still needs supervision from an instructor or experienced nurse to guide the decision-making process.

When making decisions about implementing care, the nurse may want to consider the following components determining nursing interventions (Snyder, 1985):

• The set of all possible nursing actions (e.g., pain-

Purposes of the Nursing Interventions Classification Project
Box 17-1

1. Standardization of the nomenclature (e.g., labeling, describing) of nursing treatments. Needed to standardize the language nurses use to describe specific behaviors when delivering nursing care.
2. Expansion of nursing knowledge about links between diagnoses, treatments, and outcomes. These links will be determined through the study of actual client care using a database that the classification will generate.
3. Development of nursing and health care information systems. Information systems will standardize a system for describing the treatments that nurses perform.
4. Teaching decision making to nursing students. Defining and classifying nursing interventions will help in teaching beginning nurses how to determine a client's need for care and respond appropriately. In addition, a classification of nursing interventions will make it easier to identify nursing interventions requiring higher knowledge and skill levels.
5. Determination of the cost of services provided by nurses.
6. Planning for resources needed in all types of nursing practice settings.
7. Language to communicate the unique functions of nursing.
8. Articulate with the classification systems of other health care providers.

From McCloskey JC, Bulechek GM: *Nursing interventions classification (NIC)*, ed 3, St. Louis, 2000, Mosby.

control measures, including analgesia, relaxation, and positioning).

- A listing of all possible consequences associated with each possible nursing action, such as relief of pain, no relief of pain, and adverse reaction to analgesia.
- The determination of the probability that each of the consequences will occur. For example, the client's pain decreased with previous analgesia and positioning; therefore adverse reactions are unlikely.
- A judgment based on the value of that consequence to the client. For example, the client's pain will most likely be decreased with analgesia and positioning.

Implementation Process

The nurse must adequately and thoroughly prepare before implementing the care plan. This preparation ensures efficient, safe, and effective nursing care. The implementation component of the nursing process has five steps: reassessing the client, reviewing and revising the existing nursing care plan, organizing resources and care delivery, anticipating and preventing complications, and implementing nursing interventions.

Case STUDY
BOX 17-2

A nursing care plan has been developed for Mrs. Coyle (Table 17-1). The nursing diagnosis of *altered urinary elimination related to perineal swelling after vaginal delivery* provided the focus for the plan. Before inserting the straight catheter, the nurse reassesses Mrs. Coyle to determine if she has voided spontaneously. Spontaneous voiding of 150 ml of urine would indicate that the straight catheterization procedure was no longer appropriate. However, if Mrs. Coyle had not voided or had voided a small amount (less than 150 ml) of urine, the straight catheter would still be appropriate.

REASSESSING THE CLIENT

Assessment is a continuous process that occurs each time a nurse interacts with a client. When new data are gathered and a new client need is identified, the nurse modifies the care plan. During the initial phase of implementation, the nurse reassesses the client. This is a partial assessment and may focus on one dimension of the client, such as level of comfort, or on one system, such as the cardiovascular system. The reassessment provides a way to determine whether the proposed nursing action is still appropriate for the client's level of wellness. When new data are obtained and a new client need is identified, the nurse must modify the nursing care plan (Box 17-2).

The reassessment phase of the implementation component thus provides a mechanism for the nurse to determine whether the proposed nursing action is appropriate. Although the nursing care plan was developed according to the nursing diagnoses identified during assessment, changes in the client's status can necessitate modification of planned nursing care.

REVIEWING AND REVISING THE EXISTING NURSING CARE PLAN

Before beginning care, the nurse reviews the care plan and compares it with assessment data to validate the stated nursing diagnoses and determine whether the nursing interventions are the most appropriate for the clinical situation. If the client's status has changed and the nursing diagnosis and related nursing interventions are no longer appropriate, the nursing care plan needs to be modified (see Chapter 16).

Modification of the existing written care plan includes several steps. First, data in the assessment column are revised to reflect the client's current status. New data entered in the care plan should be dated to inform other members

KNOWLEDGE
Expected effects of interventions
Role of other health care disciplines
Health care resources
(e.g., fiscal, equipment, personnel)
Anticipated client responses to care
Interpersonal skills
Counseling theory
Teaching/learning principles
Delegation and supervision principles

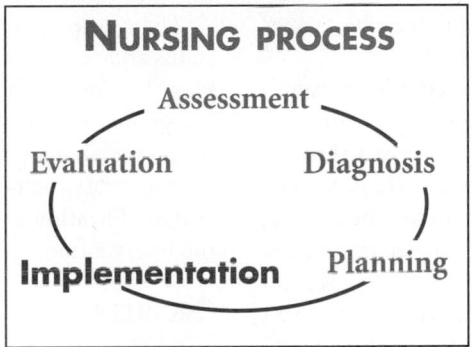

EXPERIENCE
Previous client care experience
Knowledge of
successful interventions

NURSING PROCESS

Assessment

Evaluation   Diagnosis

Implementation   Planning

STANDARDS
Standards of practice (e.g., ANA,
subspecialty) and
evidence-based practice guidelines (e.g., AHCPR)
Agency's policies/procedures
for guidelines of nursing
practice and delegation

ATTITUDES
Independent thinking
Responsibility
Authority
Creativity
Discipline

Figure 17-1   Critical thinking and the process of implementing care.

Table 17-1 **Sample Nursing Care Plan**

NURSING DIAGNOSIS: Altered urinary elimination related to perineal swelling after vaginal delivery.
DEFINITION: Altered urinary elimination is the state in which an individual experiences a disturbance in urinary elimination.*

Assessment	Goals	Implementation	Evaluation
Client has not voided in 8 hours. Fluid intake for last 8 hours is 2400 ml. Client states that she "feels the urge to void" and experiences bladder discomfort. Bladder is palpable to 2 cm below umbilicus.	Achieve emptying of bladder (8/17).	Insert straight catheter, using sterile technique, if client has not voided in 8 hours and bladder is palpable.	1000 ml of clear yellow urine is returned via straight catheter (8/16). Bladder is not palpable (8/16). Client no longer has urge to void (8/17). Client no longer complains of bladder discomfort (8/17).

*Data from Kim MJ, McFarland GK, McLane AM: *Pocket guide to nursing diagnoses,* ed 7, St. Louis, 1997, Mosby.

of the health care team of the time that the change occurred.

Second, nursing diagnoses are revised. Nursing diagnoses that are no longer relevant are deleted, and new nursing diagnoses are added and dated. Because the client's status and health care needs have changed, the priorities, goals, and expected outcomes also must be revised. The revisions are also dated on the care plan.

Third, specific implementation methods are revised to correspond to the new nursing diagnoses and client goals. This revision reflects the client's present status. In addition, revised implementation can include the client's specific needs for health care resources.

Finally, the nurse determines what methods of evaluation will be used. For example, a preoperative care plan was developed for Mr. Brown. As he progressed through the postoperative period, his nursing needs changed. The nurse made modifications in the care plan for one nursing diagnosis: *ineffective breathing pattern after surgery related to abdominal incisional pain* (Table 17-2). On the second postoperative day the nurse assessed the client and noted decreased chest wall movements, crackles that were auscultated in the right lower lobes, and an elevated temperature (39°C [102.2°F]). Mr. Brown had a standing order

for a chest x-ray examination, which was taken immediately and revealed the collapse of alveoli in the right lower lobe. The nursing diagnosis was revised to read, *ineffective airway clearance related to abdominal incisional pain*. The nursing diagnostic label was revised because of the presence of right lower lobe crackles and decreased chest wall movement. The goal of maintaining a patent airway was still appropriate. Specific new nursing interventions were developed to assist in achieving a patent airway. Finally, the nurse determined the method of evaluation for the new clinical problem.

The astute nurse is sensitive to changes in the client's status and readily incorporates these changes into the care plan. The health status of the client changes continuously. Therefore the care plan needs to be flexible to incorporate necessary changes. An out-of-date or incorrect care plan compromises the quality of nursing care, whereas review and modification enable the nurse to provide timely nursing interventions to best meet the client's needs.

ORGANIZING RESOURCES AND CARE DELIVERY

A facility's resources include equipment and skilled personnel. Organization of equipment and personnel makes efficient, skilled client care possible (see Chapter 4). After

---

Table 17-2   Modified Nursing Care Plan for Mr. Brown

NURSING DIAGNOSIS: Ineffective airway clearance related to abdominal incisional pain.
DEFINITION: Ineffective airway clearance is the state in which an individual is unable to clear secretions or obstructions from the respiratory tract to maintain airway patency.*

Assessment	Goals	Implementation	Evaluation
Smoked two packs/day for 20 years; chest x-ray film showing slight change of emphysema; crackles auscultated in lung field; scheduled for abdominal surgery	Maintain a patent airway (11/8).	Demonstrate turn, cough, and deep breathing exercise to client.† Have client perform exercises every 2 hours while awake.	Productive cough produced. Airway clear to auscultation.
Modified 24 Hours After Surgery			
Decreased chest wall movements; crackles in base that do not clear with coughing	Promote airway clearance (11/8).	Administer chest physiotherapy to all lobes of the lung: 8-12-4-8-12-4.† Have Mr. Brown cough and deep breathe every 2 hours around the clock.† Suction nasotracheal area every 2 hours if client is unable to cough productively.† Teach client to splint incision with pillow before and during coughing.	Lung fields are clear on auscultation. Client becomes afebrile. Chest x-ray film demonstrates atelectasis resolving. Client does not report increased pain during coughing.

*Data from Kim MJ, McFarland GK, McLane AM: *Pocket guide to nursing diagnoses*, ed 7, St. Louis, 1997, Mosby.
†Intervention categories supported by NIC. From McCloskey JC, Bulechek GM: *Nursing interventions classification (NIC)*, ed 3, St. Louis, 2000, Mosby.

a plan of care is determined, the nurse prepares the necessary supplies and decides on the time and provider of care. Preparation for care delivery also involves preparing the environment and client for nursing intervention.

Equipment.
Most nursing procedures, from bed making to client teaching, require some equipment or supplies. The nurse analyzes each planned intervention for needed items and their availability. Equipment should be in working order to ensure safe use.

All necessary supplies should be gathered and put in a convenient location, usually where they will be used, before implementation. Extra supplies should be available in case of mishaps. By having extra sterile gloves, for example, the nurse anticipates the possibility of a break in sterile technique. However, extra supplies should not be opened unless they are needed; this controls health care costs. The nurse also arranges the supplies in the order in which they will be used. Following the procedure the nurse appropriately returns any unopened supplies.

Personnel.
As the nurse prepares to intervene, he or she must consider the competencies of personnel available and the model of care delivery being used. Determining staff members' competencies involve knowing what they have been trained to perform. Agency policies also help to clarify what interventions can be performed by various levels of staff. Nursing care delivery systems vary among facilities and must be considered when allocating resources. The system by which nursing is organized determines the way in which personnel are designated for client care delivery. The most common types of nursing delivery systems are functional, team, total client care, primary nursing, and case management (see Chapter 2).

Three categories of functions are inherent to professional nursing practice: direct client care, delegation, and coordination. These functions assume varying levels of importance, depending on the nursing system.

A functional nursing system divides client care into a series of tasks, each of which is delegated to the lowest level of personnel having the requisite skill and competency to complete the task. For example, the task of bed making is a task that can be performed by assistive personnel, licensed practical nurses (LPNs), and registered nurses (RNs). Medications can be administered only by LPNs and RNs. Blood products can be administered only by RNs. Each staff member performs the task he or she is competent to perform for clients on the unit. Assistive personnel are assigned to clients requiring the most basic skills. The client may be ultimately cared for by a number of people who concentrate on their own tasks (see Chapter 4).

A team nursing system is a method of care delivery in which a small group of personnel, supervised by a professional nurse, delivers care to a number of clients. The team leader is responsible for the client and the care plan, delegates client care to team members, and coordinates the team's efforts. Cooperation and collaboration are hallmarks of good team nursing (Figure 17-2).

With total client care, an RN is responsible for the total care of a number of clients throughout a shift. Client care is totally individualized; the nurse assigned to the client is responsible for direct client care, coordination with other departments for services, and contribution to the care plan. Direct client care is emphasized. When assigning clients, the unit manager should assign nurses to the same clients to ensure continuity of care. There is no delegation under this system; the nurse on each shift independently gives care and is responsible for the care plan during that time (see Chapter 4).

A primary nursing system assigns a primary nurse who is responsible for all aspects of a specific client's nursing care from admission to discharge. When the primary nurse is off duty, an associate nurse assumes care of the client. If a problem arises, the associate nurse confers directly or indirectly with the primary nurse, who retains full authority and responsibility for the client's nursing care plan (see Chapter 4).

Case management is an organized system for delivering health care to an individual client or a group of clients through an episode of illness. This system includes assessment and development of a plan of care, coordination of all services, referral, and follow-up. These functions are usually assigned to one individual, commonly an RN (see Chapter 4).

Regardless of the type of nursing care delivery system in a particular agency, continuity of individualized care is a primary consideration when assigning and organizing personnel.

Environment.
Environmental factors influence the delivery and reception of care. The surroundings in which

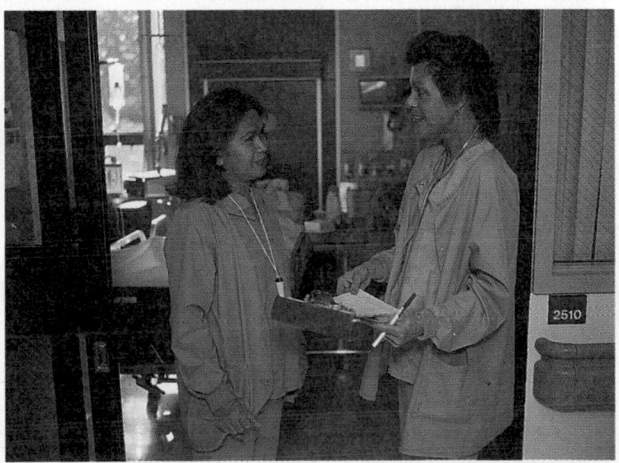

Figure 17-2 Collaboration with other health care providers results in effective interventions.

nursing activities occur should be safe and conducive to the implementation of the therapy. Client safety is always the first concern. If the client has sensory deficits, physical disability, or an alteration in level of consciousness, the environment must be arranged to prevent injury. Having special rooms, rearranging furniture and equipment, having rooms free of clutter, and providing for additional personnel are examples of creating safe surroundings.

The client benefits most from nursing interventions when surroundings are compatible with activities. Privacy promotes relaxation when body parts are exposed. Reducing distractions enhances a client's learning opportunities. Provision of adequate space and lighting provides for efficiency when procedures are performed.

Client.

Before beginning to perform interventions, the nurse should make the client as physically and psychologically comfortable as possible. Symptoms such as nausea, dizziness, or pain, for example, frequently interfere with a client's full concentration and cooperation. Administering comfort measures before initiating interventions enables the client to participate more fully. In the case of analgesic administration, for example, if client alertness is needed, the dose of pain medication should be sufficient to relieve discomfort but not impair mental faculties.

Even if symptoms are not a factor, the client should be made physically comfortable during interventions. Controlling environmental factors, positioning, and taking care of other physical needs should precede initiation of interventions. The nurse should also consider the client's level of endurance and plan only the amount of activity that the client can comfortably tolerate.

Awareness of the client's psychosocial needs helps the nurse to create a favorable emotional climate. Some clients feel reassured by having a significant other present to lend encouragement and moral support. Other strategies include planning sufficient time or multiple opportunities for the client to work through and ventilate feelings and anxieties. Adequate preparation allows the client to obtain maximal benefit from each intervention.

Anticipating and Preventing Complications.

Risks to the client arise from both illness and treatment. The nurse must identify these risks, evaluate the relative benefit of the treatment versus the risk, and initiate risk prevention measures.

Many client conditions place the client at risk for additional complications. For example, the client with preexisting left-sided paralysis following a stroke 2 years earlier is at risk for developing a pressure ulcer following orthopedic surgery, which requires traction and bed rest. The nurse's knowledge of pathophysiology helps in the early identification of complications that can occur. Scientific rationales for how certain interventions can prevent or minimize complications help the nurse to evaluate the

usefulness of preventive measures. If the client's postoperative pain is not controlled, the risk for pressure ulcer development increases because the client may be unwilling or unable to change position frequently, because of pain. The nurse knows that changing a client's position removes pressure from the skin and underlying tissues.

Some nursing procedures also pose risks for the client. The nurse needs to be aware of potential complications and institute precautionary measures. For instance, the client receiving feedings through a nasogastric tube is at risk for aspiration. The nurse should elevate the head of the bed and have pharyngeal suction equipment at the bedside before initiating the feedings.

Identifying Areas of Assistance.

Some nursing situations require the nurse to acquire assistance by seeking additional personnel, knowledge, and/or nursing skills. Before implementing care, the nurse reviews the plan to determine the need for assistance and the type required.

Situations requiring additional personnel vary. Assistance may be needed in performing a procedure, comforting a client, or preparing the client for a procedure. For example, a nurse assigned to care for an overweight, immobilized client may need additional personnel to help turn, transfer, and position the client. The nurse needs to determine the number of additional personnel and when they are needed. The nurse then explains the type of assistance needed, when it is needed, and how the client has responded in the past when more than one caregiver is needed to perform the intervention.

Some nursing situations require additional knowledge and skills, as well as additional personnel. A nurse needs additional knowledge when administering a new medication or implementing a new procedure. Such information can be obtained from a hospital's formulary or procedure book. If the nurse still is uncertain about the new medication or procedure, other members of the health care team can be consulted.

Because of the continual growth of health care professions and related technology, a nurse may lack the skills to perform a new procedure. When this occurs, information about the procedure is obtained from the literature and the agency's procedure book. Next, all equipment necessary for the procedure is collected. Finally, another nurse who has completed the procedure correctly and safely provides assistance and guidance. The assistance can come from another staff nurse, a supervisor, an educator, or a nurse specialist. Requesting assistance occurs frequently in all types of nursing practice and is a learning process that continues throughout educational experiences and into professional development.

IMPLEMENTING NURSING INTERVENTIONS

A variety of interventions can be selected by the nurse in administering care. Each has implications for appropriate use with clients. The nurse selects from the following nursing intervention methods to achieve the goals of nursing care:

>   Performing, assisting, or directing the performance of activities of daily living
>   Counseling and teaching the client and family
>   Providing direct care to achieve client-centered goals
>   Delegating, supervising, and evaluating the work of other staff members
>   Recording and exchanging information relevant to the client's continued care

Nursing practice includes cognitive, interpersonal, and psychomotor (technical) skills. Each type of skill is needed to implement interventions. The nurse is responsible for knowing when one of these methods is preferred over another and for having the necessary theoretical knowledge and psychomotor skills to implement each. A later section introduces the general theoretical information for each method and refers to subsequent chapters that detail the necessary theoretical and psychomotor skills.

Cognitive Skills.   Cognitive skills involve the application of nursing knowledge. This ensures that no nursing intervention is automatic. The nurse must continually think and anticipate so that client care is well designed, individualized, and appropriate. For example, the nurse must know the rationale for each therapeutic intervention, understand normal and abnormal physiological and psychological responses, be able to identify client learning and discharge needs, and recognize the client's health promotion and illness prevention needs.

Interpersonal Skills.   Interpersonal skills are essential to effective nursing action. The nurse must communicate clearly with the client, family, and other members of the health care team. Caring and trust are conveyed when nurses communicate openly and honestly. Client teaching and counseling must be done to the level of the client's understanding and expectations. The nurse must also be sensitive to the client's emotional response to the illness and treatment. Proper use of interpersonal skills enables the nurse to be perceptive to the client's verbal and nonverbal communication (see Chapter 22).

Psychomotor Skills.   Psychomotor skills are those skills used when providing direct care to clients, such as changing a dressing, giving an injection, or suctioning a tracheostomy. With time and practice the nurse learns to perform skills smoothly, confidently, and efficiently. This ensures safe performance and conveys that the nurse is competent. The nurse has a professional responsibility to acquire necessary psychomotor skills. In the case of a new skill, nurses assess their level of competency and obtain the necessary resources to ensure that the client receives the treatment safely.

Implementation Methods

The nurse carries out the nursing care plan by using several implementation methods. For example, a client with the nursing diagnosis of *impaired physical mobility related to bilateral arm casts* may require assistance in performing activities of daily living. A client with the diagnosis of *ineffective individual coping related to fear of the medical diagnosis* may require counseling as a method of nursing intervention. A client with the diagnosis of *knowledge deficit* needs client health education focused on the area of need. The totally immobilized or disoriented client requires direct care nursing interventions. Another method of implementation involves the supervision and evaluation of other members of the health care team.

For each nursing diagnosis the nurse identifies appropriate interventions, each of which requires specific theoretical knowledge and clinical skills.

ASSISTING WITH ACTIVITIES OF DAILY LIVING

Activities of daily living (ADLs) are activities usually performed in the course of a normal day; they include ambulating, eating, dressing, bathing, brushing the teeth, and grooming. Conditions resulting in the need for assistance with ADLs can be acute, chronic, temporary, permanent, or rehabilitative. An acute disease is characterized by symptoms that are usually severe and are present for a relatively short time, usually less than 6 months. An episode of acute disease results in recovery to a state of health and activity comparable to the state before the disease, passage into a chronic phase of the disease, or death. An example is the postoperative client who is unable to independently complete all ADLs. While progressing through the postoperative period, the client gradually depends less on nurses for completing ADLs.

A chronic disease persists longer. Although the symptoms are usually less severe than those of the acute phase of the same disease, chronic disease may result in complete or partial disability. A client with partial paralysis after a cerebrovascular accident may have a chronic impairment requiring long-term assistance with ADLs.

The client's need for assistance with ADLs may be temporary, permanent, or rehabilitative. In the case of temporary assistance with ADLs, the client needs assistance during a specific period. A client with impaired mobility because of bilateral arm casts has a temporary need for assistance. After the casts are removed, the client will gradually assume responsibility for ADLs. However, a client with a total self-care deficit related to an irreversible injury high in the cervical spinal cord has a permanent need for assistance. It is unrealistic for the nurse to plan a rehabilitation program with the goal that this client will be able to independently complete all ADLs. However, through restorative care, the client will learn new ways to perform ADLs, thus becoming more independent .

Through assessment, the nurse collects data that verify the need for assistance with ADLs. Client's whose assessment data reveal fatigue, limitations in mobility, confusion, and pain, for example, may need assistance with ADLs. This assistance can range from partial assistance to complete care. In clients with chronic conditions, assistance with ADLs can change from day to day.

When clients need assistance with ADLs, the nurse must also assess client preferences. For example, a client whose activities are limited because of mobility restrictions, pain, or fatigue may prefer to have assistance with partial hygiene but maintain independence in feeding and grooming activities. Another client may wish to have assistance with ADLs spaced throughout the day and maintain independence in all ADLs. Involving the client in planning the timing and types of interventions aimed at meeting individualized ADLs can be a significant boost to the client's self-esteem and willingness to become more independent in some aspects of care.

COUNSELING

Counseling is an implementation method that helps the client use a problem-solving process to recognize and manage stress and to facilitate interpersonal relationships among the client, family, and health care team. Nurses provide counseling to help the client accept actual or impending changes resulting from stress. Counseling involves emotional, intellectual, spiritual, and psychological support. A client and family who need nursing counseling have normal adjustment difficulties and are upset or frustrated, but they are not necessarily psychologically disabled. For example, more families are now taking care of their older adult relatives who have physical disabilities following surgery, stroke, or chronic illnesses. These families need assistance in adjusting to the demands placed on the caregiver. Likewise, the recipient of care also needs assistance in adjusting to the disability. Clients with psychiatric diagnoses require therapy by nurses specializing in psychiatric nursing or by social workers, psychiatrists, or psychologists.

Many counseling techniques are used to foster cognitive, behavioral, developmental, experiential, and emotional growth in clients (Box 17-3). Counseling encourages individuals to examine available alternatives and decide which choices are useful and appropriate. When clients are able to examine alternatives, they can develop a sense of control and are able to better manage stress. To assist clients in need of counseling techniques, the nurse must be able to identify the need for counseling and possess communication skills to develop a therapeutic relationship (Sundeen and others, 1998).

Clients or families needing counseling include persons who must adjust lifestyle patterns, as in smoking cessation, weight reduction, or increasing activity. Clients coping with chronic or disabling diseases require counseling to help them adapt to changes in lifestyle or body image as

---

Counseling Strategies and Selected Examples Used by Nurses   Box 17-3

BEHAVIOR MODIFICATION
Client changes from smoking to meditating to cope with stress.
Client uses exercise as a health promotion activity.

BEREAVEMENT COUNSELING
Nurse assists client in productive reminiscing of loved one.
Nurse supports client in removing loved one's belongings from home.

BIOFEEDBACK
Regulation of stress
Control of eating urges

RELAXATION EXERCISES
Progressive muscle relaxation exercises
Meditation

CRISIS INTERVENTION
Therapy designed to assist in coping with crisis
Anticipatory guidance to recognize and avoid modifiable crises

GUIDED IMAGERY
Pain control
Anxiety control

PLAY THERAPY
Assist children in coping with loss and grief.
Assist children in coping with chronic illness.
Assist children in becoming competent in self-care activities.

---

the disease progresses. During life-threatening illnesses, clients and families need counseling to cope with the possibility of death.

TEACHING

Counseling is closely aligned with teaching. Both involve using communication skills to effect a change in the client. However, with counseling, the change results in the development of new attitudes and feelings, whereas in teaching, the focus of change is intellectual growth or the acquisition of new knowledge or psychomotor skills (Redman, 1997).

Teaching is an implementation method used to present correct principles, procedures, and techniques of health care to clients and to inform clients about their health status (see Chapter 23). As a nursing responsibility, teaching is implemented in all health care settings, such as in acute care, home care, and community-based settings (Figure 17-3). The nurse is responsible for assessing the learning needs of clients and is accountable for the quality of education delivered.

The teaching-learning process is an interaction between the teacher and the learner in which specific learning objectives are presented (Redman, 1997). This process provides the organizational structure and framework for client education. The teaching-learning process is much like the basic nursing process.

During assessment the nurse determines the client's learning needs and readiness to learn. The nurse then interprets the data to formulate nursing diagnoses reflecting the identified needs. During planning the nurse and client establish goals for learning. Implementation is the initiation of the teaching strategies designed to achieve the learning goal. Finally, evaluation measures the learning that has occurred. The purpose of the teaching-learning process is to develop and implement a teaching plan individualized for the client's needs, level of knowledge, and learning resources. The goal is to give clients the knowledge and skills necessary to assume health-related behaviors.

Providing Direct Nursing Care

To achieve the therapeutic goals for the client, the nurse initiates interventions to compensate for adverse reactions, uses preventive measures in providing care, applies correct techniques in administering care and preparing the client for special procedures, and initiates lifesaving measures in emergency situations. The following sections briefly discuss the nursing interventions in these areas. The specific knowledge and skills needed to carry out these nursing procedures are detailed in subsequent chapters.

Compensation for Adverse Reactions

An **adverse reaction** is a harmful or unintended effect of a medication, diagnostic test, or therapeutic intervention. Adverse reactions can follow any nursing interventions. Nursing actions that compensate for adverse reactions reduce or counteract the reaction. To intervene, the nurse must have knowledge of the potential undesired effects.

For example, when applying a moist heat compress, the nurses assesses the area requiring the compress. Following application of the compress, the nurse reassesses the area for any adverse reaction, such as excessive reddening of the skin from the heat or skin maceration from the moisture of the compress. When completing a physician-directed intervention, such as medication administration, the nurse understands the known and potential side effects of the drug. After administration of the medication, the nurse assesses the client for any adverse effects. The nurse should be aware of drugs that can counteract the side effects. For example, a client may have an unknown hypersensitivity to penicillin and may develop hives after three doses. The nurse records the reaction and stops further administration of the drug. The nurse also consults the physician's standing orders and administers diphenhydramine (Benadryl), an antihistamine and antipruritic medication, to reduce the allergic response and to relieve the itching.

When caring for a client who is undergoing or has undergone a particular diagnostic test, the nurse must understand the test and any potential adverse effects. For example, a client has not had a bowel movement in 24 hours after a barium enema. Because bowel impaction is a potential side effect of a barium enema, the nurse increases fluid intake and instructs the client to let the nursing personnel know when a bowel movement occurs.

Therapeutic interventions may also have potential adverse effects. Although adverse effects are not common, they do occur (Box 17-4). The nurse learns potential adverse effects. Ultimately, the nurse wants to prevent any adverse effects. However, it is imperative that the nurse recognize the signs and symptoms of an adverse reaction and intervene in a timely manner.

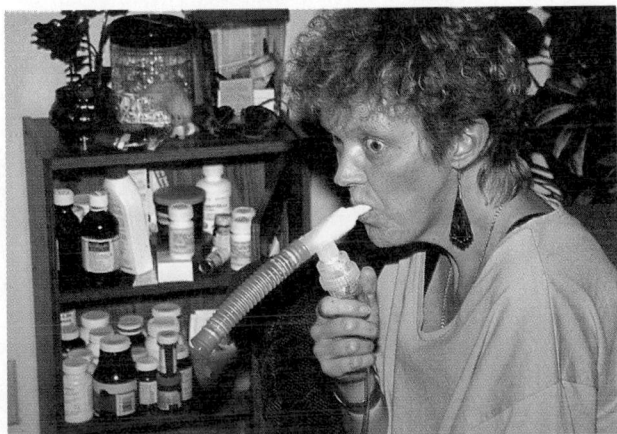

Figure 17-3 Teaching client in home setting to use an aerosol medication delivery device.

Case STUDY   BOX 17-4

Ms. Rice, RN, assesses a stage I pressure ulcer on Mr. Blaskowitz's sacrum. She develops interventions designed to prevent further skin breakdown and promote wound healing. She obtains an order for an alternating air mattress and film dressing (Tegaderm). Ms. Rice also changes Mr. Blaskowitz's turning schedule from every 2 hours to every hour while awake and every 2 hours while asleep (2200 to 0700 hours). After the second day of treatment, Ms. Rice reassesses Mr. Blaskowitz's skin and notes stage I pressure ulcers on both heels; the sacral ulcer has also progressed to a stage III ulcer. To counteract the continued skin breakdown, the nurse discontinues the air mattress and obtains an order for the Clinitron bed, Tegaderm for the heel ulcers, and a hydrogel dressing for the sacral ulcer (see Chapter 47).

PREVENTIVE MEASURES

Preventive nursing actions promote health and prevent illness to avoid the need for acute or rehabilitative health care. Prevention includes assessment and promotion of the client's health potential, application of prescribed measures (e.g., immunizations), health teaching, and identification of risk factors for illness and/or trauma.

Consider, for example, the case of Mrs. Schmidt, who is providing in-home care to an older parent, maintaining a career, and caring for two school-age children as a single parent. Mrs. Schmidt and the nurse agree that the client is experiencing a great deal of stress. The nurse can implement preventive measures to assist the client in controlling some of the stress. The nurse initiates stress-reducing interventions, such as relaxation therapy, for Mrs. Schmidt (see Chapter 30). In addition, the nurse assists Mrs. Schmidt in identifying community agencies and resources, such as respite care (see Chapter 3). The nurse teaches Mrs. Schmidt how to provide hygiene, nutrition, and medications. Together, the nurse and Mrs. Schmidt identify signs and symptoms that indicate whether her parent's health status is changing and what actions should be taken.

Preventive nursing interventions aimed at promoting health and preventing illness are needed in all types of care settings and with all age-groups. As changes in the health care system continue, there is and will be greater emphasis on health promotion and illness prevention (see Chapter 1).

CORRECT TECHNIQUES IN ADMINISTERING CARE AND PREPARING A CLIENT FOR PROCEDURES

The administration of direct nursing care requires the nurse to be experienced in the methods followed in performing specific procedures such as administering medications, changing clients' dressings, or inserting Foley catheters. These methods include protecting the nurse and client from injury, using proper infection-control practices, using an organized approach, and positioning clients correctly. When techniques are integrated within a procedure, the ultimate outcome is safe and effective.

To carry out a procedure, the nurse must be knowledgeable about the procedure itself, the frequency, the steps, and the expected outcomes. In a hospital the nurse completes many procedures each day. Some of these procedures might be new, so before conducting a new procedure the nurse assesses personal competencies and determines the need for assistance, new knowledge, or new skills.

LIFESAVING MEASURES

A **lifesaving measure** is implemented when a client's physiological or psychological state is threatened. The purpose of the lifesaving measure is to restore physiological or psychological equilibrium. Such measures include administering emergency medications, instituting cardiopulmonary resuscitation (Figure 17-4), restraining a

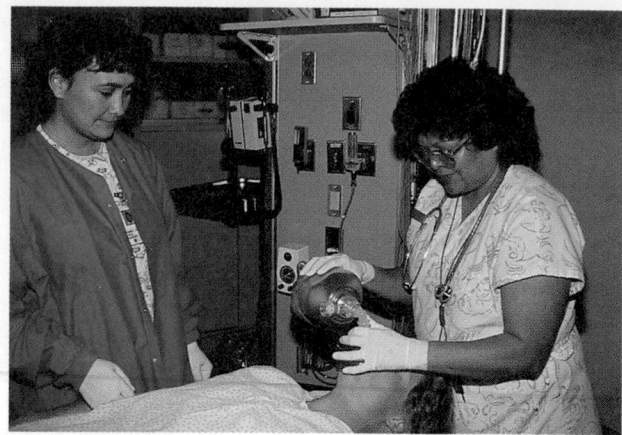

Figure 17-4   Initiating artificial respiration.

confused or violent client, and obtaining immediate counseling from a crisis center for a severely anxious client.

The initiation of lifesaving measures is an essential component of nursing practice. As with any procedure, the nurse must be knowledgeable about the lifesaving procedure itself, steps, and expected outcomes. If an inexperienced nurse faces a situation requiring emergency measures, the proper nursing action may be to get an experienced professional.

ACHIEVING GOALS OF CARE

The client's health care goals can be achieved by providing an environment conducive to meeting such goals; adjusting care in accordance with the client's expressed or implied needs; stimulating and motivating clients, thereby enabling them to achieve self-care and independence; and encouraging clients to accept care or adhere to the treatment regimen. For each nursing intervention, the nurse and client work together to meet the mutually developed goals. The nurse assumes a more active or more passive role depending on the intervention.

Nurses can help create a health care environment conducive to achieving clients' goals. Ideally, the nurse creates an environment that provides clients with adequate privacy for meeting basic needs and allows them to feel safe and free to interact with the health care team. An early step in establishing an appropriate environment is to orient clients and families to the health care agency. If it is a hospital, clients need to be oriented to their rooms, the health care team, and other clients. Clients in clinics should be oriented to clinic policies and procedures, the location of restrooms and cafeterias, and the health care team. When clients receive care in the home, the nurse should take time to acquaint clients and their families with the purposes and expectations of the home visits.

Whether clients are in the hospital, outpatient clinic, or a community setting, the nurse takes measures to provide privacy. Obviously, clients need privacy to carry out activities of hygiene, grooming, and elimination. In addition, they need privacy to talk with family, friends, or members of the health care team. In an environment of privacy, clients may feel free to share concerns, ask questions about their diagnosis and treatment, and resolve personal problems.

Nursing care and other therapeutic measures are designed to meet the client's needs. As a further aid in the attainment of health care goals, the nursing care plan should be flexible so that the client is not placed in a fixed routine. Obviously, the degree of flexibility depends on the nature of the need, the severity of the client's disability or illness, and the client's dependence on nursing care. However, even the smallest degree of flexibility, giving the client an opportunity to have some choice about the type or timing of nursing care, is valuable.

Clients with severe and chronic diseases should be encouraged to increase their levels of self-care and independence. To avoid discouraging clients, it is best to attempt to achieve this nursing goal gradually. The care plan is implemented so that clients successfully achieve one level of independence before attempting the next (Box 17-5).

In the case study presented in Box 17-5, each day includes achievable tasks for Mr. Porter. Placing the tasks in sequential order has been done for the following reasons: (1) each task was developed with the knowledge that Mr. Porter could indeed successfully complete the activity, (2) a sequence of successes will motivate Mr. Porter to continue with the plan, and (3) the sequence was designed to gradually increase Mr. Porter's activity tolerance.

Clients with chronic diseases may need to adhere to many treatment modalities. **Client adherence** means that clients and families invest time in carrying out the required home treatments. For example, a client with chronic obstructive pulmonary disease (COPD) may need to spend several hours a day performing respiratory therapies designed to keep the airway open and maintain an acceptable level of wellness.

Some treatment plans include the need for the client and family to adjust to functional changes as a result of medications. For example, a client with high blood pressure being treated with atenolol (Tenormin) occasionally feels increasingly fatigued during the early stages of treatment. Another client with cancer who is undergoing chemotherapy may have changes in energy level and body image as a result of the medication.

Finally, adherence to treatment plans can require an increased financial investment by the client and family. For example, for a client who has cardiac disease, a two-story house may no longer be suitable because the client is unable to climb stairs without feeling short of breath. Thus the client and family may need to invest in a new house or have their present home modified.

Investments of time, money, and personal resources for a long period can be discouraging. The discouraged client may neglect the treatment regimen. After the client begins to reduce adherence to treatment, levels of wellness may decline.

Nurses are able to intervene and assist the client in adhering to the treatment plan. Adequate discharge planning and education of the client and family help promote a smooth transition from one health care setting to another or to the home. They also help increase the client's level of knowledge about the treatment plan. Counseling helps the client and family adapt to change resulting from the disease process or treatment. Continuity of care also provides a supportive professional who is familiar with the client's pattern of living, pattern of wellness, and treatment. In addition, reinforcing successes with the treatment plan encourages the client to adhere to the regimen.

DELEGATING, SUPERVISING, AND EVALUATING THE WORK OF OTHER STAFF MEMBERS

Depending on the system of health care delivery, the nurse who develops the care plan frequently does not perform all of the nursing interventions. Some activities may be delegated to other members of the health care team and coordinated by the nurse. Noninvasive interventions such as skin care, range-of-motion exercises, ambulation, grooming, and hygiene measures can be assigned to a nursing assistant. An LPN can perform these measures in addition to certain invasive tasks (e.g., catheterization, dressing care, and suctioning). When a nurse delegates aspects of a client's care to another staff member, the nurse assigning tasks is responsible for ensuring that each task is appropriately assigned and is completed according to the standard of care, and that the direct care interventions are

---

𝒞ase STUDY   BOX 17-5

Mr. Porter is a 50-year-old executive, husband, and father of three teenagers. He is recovering from a severe myocardial infarction (heart attack) and cardiac arrest. For the past 3 days, all of Mr. Porter's hygiene and grooming needs have been met by the nursing staff. Mr. Porter has expressed doubts about ever getting his energy back and being able to care for himself. Mr. Martin, a student nurse, assesses Mr. Porter and develops a nursing care plan. One of the goals is complete self-care by Mr. Porter within 1 week. With the help of his instructor, Mr. Martin implements the following plan, which is designed to achieve the overall goal of independence in various phases:

Day 1 Wash face, shave, and comb hair
Day 2 Feed himself meals, wash face, shave, and
    comb hair
Day 4 Perform grooming activities and feed himself
Day 6 Shower

delegated to those personnel competent to provide the specific type of care (McCloskey and others, 1996).

COMMUNICATING NURSING INTERVENTIONS

Nursing interventions are written and/or communicated orally. Written nursing interventions are incorporated into the nursing care plan and client's medical record. The care plan usually reflects proposed nursing interventions. After the interventions are completed, the client's response to the treatment is recorded on the appropriate record (see Chapter 24). This information usually includes a brief description of the nursing assessment, the specific procedure, and the client's response.

Documenting a brief description of pertinent assessment findings and the client's response in the client's medical record validates the need for a specific nursing intervention. Writing the time and the details of the intervention documents that the procedure was completed.

Nursing interventions are also communicated orally from one nurse to another or to other health care professionals. Unless communication is timely and accurate, caregivers can be uninformed, interventions may be needlessly duplicated, procedures may be delayed, or tasks may be left undone (Gerteis and others, 1993). Clients can quickly tell when members of the health care team communicate inconsistent messages, indicating that no one is in charge. Nurses commonly communicate orally when conferring with colleagues, changing shifts, transferring a client to another unit, or discharging a client to another health care agency. Whether the nursing intervention is written or communicated orally, the language should be clear, concise, and to the point.

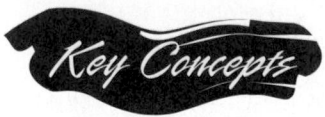

Key Concepts

- Implementation requires the nurse to reassess the client, review and modify the existing care plan, identify areas in which assistance is needed, implement nursing interventions, and communicate nursing interventions.
- The care plan is modified as a client's level of wellness and health care needs change.
- The implementation of nursing care may require additional knowledge, nursing skills, and personnel.
- Counseling helps the client use problem solving to recognize and manage stress and facilitates interpersonal relationships among the client, family, and health care team.
- Teaching is used to present correct principles, procedures, and techniques of health care to clients; inform clients about their health status; and refer clients and families to appropriate resources.
- Nursing actions to achieve therapeutic goals include compensation for adverse reactions, preventive measures, correct techniques for administering care and preparing the client for procedures, and lifesaving measures.
- Nursing actions that achieve the attainment of health care goals include providing a conducive environment, adjusting care to fit the client's needs, and stimulating and motivating the client.

- Delegating care to other personnel involves ensuring that the individuals are skilled in the tasks and that they complete them according to the standard of care.
- To complete any nursing procedure, the nurse must be knowledgeable about the procedure, its frequency, the steps, and the expected outcomes.
- After implementation, the nurse writes in the client's record a brief description of the nursing assessment, specific procedures, and the client's response to nursing care.

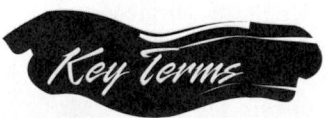

Key Terms

Activities of daily living (ADLs), *p. 355*
Adverse reaction, *p. 357*
Client adherence, *p. 359*
Counseling, *p. 356*
Implementation, *p. 348*
Lifesaving measure, *p. 358*

Nursing intervention, *p. 348*
Preventive nursing actions, *p. 358*
Protocol, *p. 348*
Standing order, *p. 349*
Teaching, *p. 356*

Critical Thinking Exercises

1. Mrs. Allen has a long-term history of osteoarthritis. At present, she plans to move into an older adult assisted living retirement complex. She voices sadness at leaving her home and neighbors; however, most of all she worries about maintaining her independence. Although she knows she can get assistance with daily activities, she wants to be able to learn how to accomplish her personal care and conserve energy. What types of nursing interventions are appropriate for direct care activities for Mrs. Allen or a care provider? What activities do you think Mrs. Allen may need assistance with? What are important areas of teaching for Mrs Allen? How will you design interventions to counsel Mrs. Allen?

2. You are assigned to ambulate Mr. Clay, who had abdominal surgery 24 hours ago. Mr. Clay weighs 270 pounds and is 6 feet tall. He has a patient-controlled analgesia (PCA) system for pain control. His intravenous (IV) fluids are running at 100 ml/hr, and he has two IV antibiotics scheduled to run every 6 hours. What questions do you need to answer before you attempt to ambulate this client?

3. Your client needs a complicated wound irrigation and dressing change. What measures will you take to reduce the risk of an adverse reaction to this intervention?

References

Bulechek GM, McCloskey JC: Nursing interventions taxonomy development. In McCloskey JC, Grace HK, editors: *Current issues in nursing,* ed 3, St. Louis, 1990, Mosby.

Doswell WM, Erlem JA: Multicultural issues and ethical concerns in the delivery of nursing care interventions, *Nurs Clin North Am* 33(2):353, 1998.

Gerteis M and others, editors: *Through the patient's eyes,* San Francisco, 1993, Jossey-Bass Health Series.

Gordon M: *Nursing diagnosis: process and application,* ed 3, St. Louis, 1994, Mosby.

Kim MJ, McFarland GK, McLane AM: *Pocket guide to nursing diagnoses,* ed 7, St. Louis, 1997, Mosby.

McCloskey JC, Bulechek GM: *Nursing interventions classification (NIC),* ed 3, St. Louis, 2000, Mosby.

McCloskey JC and others: Nurses' use and delegation of indirect care interventions, *Nurs Econ* 14(1):22, 1996.

Miller MA, Babcock DE: *Critical thinking applied to nursing,* St. Louis, 1996, Mosby.

Redman BK: *The practice of patient education,* ed 8, St. Louis, 1997, Mosby.

Snyder M: *Independent nursing interventions,* New York, 1985, John Wiley & Sons.

Snyder M, Egan EC, Nojima Y: Defining nursing interventions, *Image J Nurs Sch* 28(2):137, 1996.

Stewart BJ, Archbold PG: Nursing intervention studies required outcomes measures that are sensitive to change, part II, *Nurs Res Health* 17:77, 1993.

Sundeen SJ and others: *Nurse-client interaction: implementing the nursing process,* ed 6, St. Louis, 1998, Mosby.

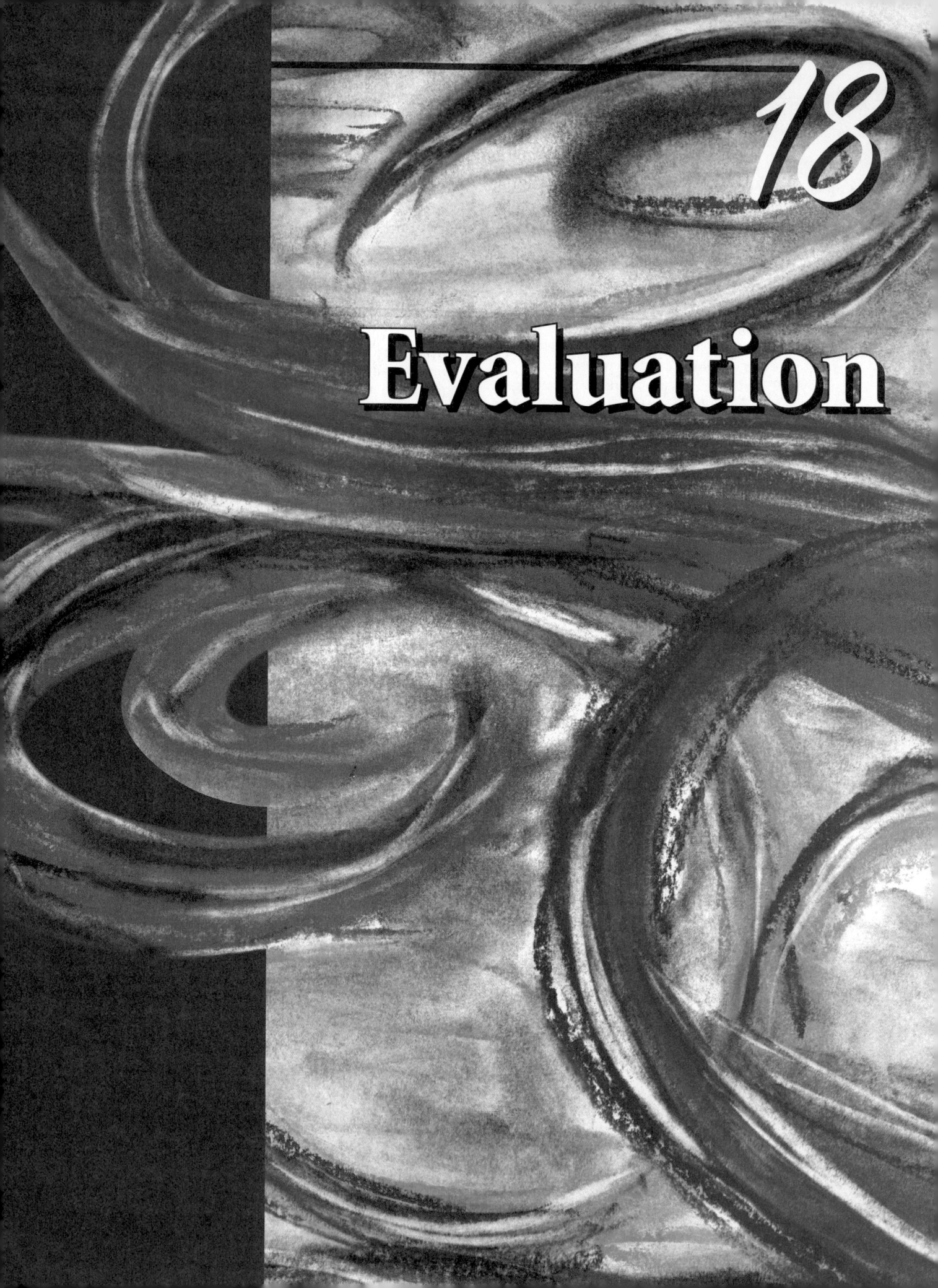

18

Evaluation

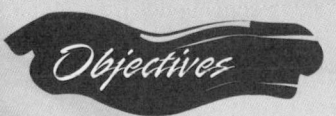

Mastery of content in this chapter will enable the student to:

- Define the key terms listed.
- Explain the relationship between expected outcomes and goals of care.
- Explain how evaluation involves critical thinking.
- Give examples of evaluation measures used to determine a client's progress toward outcomes.
- Evaluate nursing actions selected for a client.
- Describe how evaluation can lead to revision or modification of a plan of care.
- Explain the interaction between evaluation and quality improvement (QI).

Nurses must be critical thinkers. The nursing process is a series of nursing actions based on and supported by clinical judgments. The previous chapters describe how the nurse uses critical thinking skills to gather client data, form nursing diagnoses, develop a plan of care, and implement the care plan. Evaluation, the final step of the nursing process, is crucial to determine whether, after application of the nursing process, the client's condition or well-being improves.

Whenever a nurse delivers care and provides therapy, certain questions must be asked: Was the therapy effective in improving the client's well-being? Did the client benefit? It is important to evaluate each client according to the level of wellness or recovery the health care team and client have established in the goals of care. The emphasis is on client outcomes. The nurse evaluates whether the client's behaviors or responses reflect a reversal or improvement in a nursing diagnosis or in maintenance of a healthy state. The **evaluation** step of the nursing process measures the client's response to nursing actions and the client's progress toward achieving goals. Data are collected on an ongoing basis to measure changes in functioning, in daily living, and in availability or use of external resources (Carnevali and Thomas, 1993). Evaluation is one of the most critical phases of the nursing process because it supports the basis of the usefulness and effectiveness of nursing practice, which is client driven and client centered (Lin, 1996). During evaluation the nurse decides if the previous steps of the nursing process were effective by examining the client's responses and comparing them with the behaviors stated in the expected outcomes.

Another aspect of evaluation involves measurement of the quality of nursing care provided in a health care setting (see Chapter 4). Nurses evaluate each client's progress and recovery, but this is not enough. A health care organization must be accountable and responsible for evaluating and improving the quality of nursing and other client care services being provided to all clients. The quality of health care is a focus of the Joint Commission on Accreditation of Healthcare Organizations (JCAHO) and **professional standards review organizations (PSROs).** The JCAHO (1999) defines quality of care as the "degree to which health services for individuals and populations increase the likelihood of desired health outcomes and are consistent with current professional knowledge." Each health care professional must be competent, but to achieve high-quality care, an organization must have the right systems and processes to provide care that is appropriate and efficacious. There are always opportunities to improve because client care is complex, involving numerous variables. The larger the organization, the greater the variables influencing how care is delivered. Nursing plays a key role in helping an organization find ways to improve the quality of client care. The emphasis is on client outcomes, professional practice, and the systems in which professionals practice.

Critical Thinking Skills and Evaluation

Evaluation of care requires the nurse to reflect on client responses to nursing interventions and to determine their effectiveness in promoting the client's well-being. It is evaluation that makes a nurse a critical thinker (Figure 18-1). Preparation for evaluation requires that the nurse be knowledgeable in characteristics of improved care in all client domains, expected and unexpected outcomes of interventions from nursing and other disciplines, characteristics of improved family and group dynamics, and community resources. Previous client care experiences add to the nurse's knowledge base. Professional and regulatory standards of care, as well as agency standards, are applied when evaluating care. The nurse applies attitudes of critical thinking to objectively evaluate the existing care plan and to make appropriate modifications.

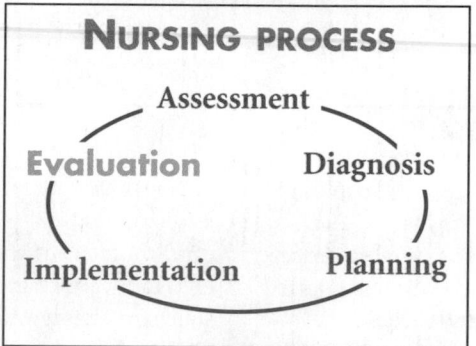

KNOWLEDGE
Characteristics of improved physiological,
psychological, spiritual, and sociocultural status
Expected outcomes of pharmacological, medical,
nutritional, and other therapies
Unexpected outcomes of pharmacological,
medical, nutritional, and other therapies
Characteristics of improved family and group
dynamics
Community resources

EXPERIENCE
Previous client care experience

NURSING PROCESS
Assessment
Evaluation   Diagnosis
Implementation   Planning

STANDARDS
Expected outcomes of care
Specialty standards of practice

ATTITUDES
Creativity
Responsibility
Perseverance
Humility

Figure 18-1   Critical thinking and evaluation.

While caring for clients, the nurse compares subjective and objective data gathered from the client, other nurses or caregivers, and the family to determine the degree of success in meeting expected outcomes established during planning. If outcomes are met, the overall goals for the client are also met. The nurse compares client behaviors and responses assessed before the delivery of nursing interventions with the behaviors and responses that occur following nursing care. The nurse applies knowledge about the client's condition, considers previous experience with similar clients, and reviews data from the assessed baseline to critically analyze whether the client's condition is changing. Critical thinking directs the nurse to analyze the findings from evaluation. Is the client's condition improved? Can the client improve, or are there physical factors preventing recovery? Does the client's motivation or willingness to pursue healthier behavior influence his or her response to therapies?

Evaluation is the step in the nursing process whereby the nurse continually redirects nursing care to best meet client needs. For example, when evaluating a client for a change in vital signs, the nurse applies knowledge of disease processes and physiological responses to interpret whether a change has indeed occurred and whether the change is desirable. A client in acute pain may present an increased heart rate and increased muscular tension. The nurse knows that this is a sympathetic nervous system response to painful stimuli. After administering a pain medication and repositioning the client, the nurse will return to evaluate whether vital signs have returned to either a more acceptable level or to the client's pre-pain baseline. Positive evaluations occur when established outcomes are achieved, leading the nurse to conclude that the dosage of medication and nursing intervention effectively met the client's goal of improved comfort. Negative evaluations or undesired results indicate that the intervention was not effective in minimizing or resolving the actual problem or in avoiding a potential problem. New data about the client's condition indicate the client's ability to meet the established outcome. As a result, the nurse must change the care plan and try different therapies or a different approach in administering existing therapies.

This sequence of critically evaluating and revising therapies continues until problems are appropriately resolved.

The nurse must realize that evaluation is dynamic and ever changing, depending on the client's nursing diagnoses and condition; as problems change, so, too, may expected outcomes. A client whose health status continuously changes requires more frequent evaluation. In addition, priority diagnoses are often evaluated first. For example, a nurse evaluates a client's acute pain before evaluating the status of a knowledge deficit.

GOALS

As hospital stays become shorter, many clients are discharged before all goals are met and all nursing diagnoses are resolved. When preparing a client for discharge, the nurse evaluates the status of each nursing diagnosis and writes an evaluative statement identifying the client's progress toward goal achievement and problem resolution. Appropriate revisions to the care plan are made for home or follow-up care (e.g., an extended care facility). The nurse must clearly distinguish between goals that have been met and goals that require continued intervention. A home health nurse will probably revise interventions to adapt them to the client's home.

A goal specifies the expected behavior or response that indicates resolution of a nursing diagnosis or maintenance of a healthy state. It is a summary statement of what is to be accomplished when all expected outcomes have been met. The nurse evaluates goals after comparing evaluative findings with all expected outcomes. When a goal has been accomplished, the nurse knows that interventions have been successful toward improving the client's well being.

EXPECTED OUTCOMES

It is imperative for nurses to measure the outcome of care. The Nursing Outcomes Classification (NOC) project is designed to provide the language for the evaluation step of the nursing process. The purposes of NOC are: (1) to identify, label, validate, and classify nursing-sensitive client outcomes and indicators; (2) to field test and validate the classification; and (3) to define and test measurement procedures for the outcomes and indicators (Johnson and Mass, 1997). This project is complementary to the work of the North American Nursing Diagnosis Association (NANDA) and the Nursing Interventions Classification (NIC) project.

Client-expected outcomes help define the effectiveness, efficiency, and measurement of the results of nursing interventions and practice (Deaton, 1998). These outcomes are also dependent on the acute or chronic disease state of the client, the delivery care setting, the discipline delivering the care, and the underlying medical diagnosis (Chase, 1998).

Expected outcomes are the expected results of a goal-oriented process (see Chapter 16). They are statements of progressive, step-by-step responses or behaviors that the client needs to accomplish to achieve the goals of care provided. When outcomes are achieved, the related factors for a nursing diagnosis no longer exist. For example, for a nursing diagnosis of *impaired skin integrity related to pressure of physical immobilization,* the client must achieve the goal of attaining intact skin in the area of injury. This will be accomplished by meeting the outcomes of "the skin lesion will be clean without drainage in 3 days" and showing evidence of healing through "reduction in size (by 1 cm) and inflammation in 1 week." If the outcomes are met, the nurse has successfully eliminated pressure over the skin and used therapies that have healed the skin lesion. Expected outcomes have short time frames (depending on the health care setting) and include as few as one or two intervention sessions.

After a specified interval or when all interventions in the plan of care have been completed, the nurse evaluates the client's ability to demonstrate the behavior or response stated in the outcomes. Evaluation of each expected outcome and its place in the sequence of care is essential. Failure to evaluate each expected outcome results in an inability to determine the place in which the sequence faltered. In other words, the nurse is not able to revise and redirect the plan of care at the most appropriate time. Achievement of expected outcomes has the potential to demonstrate specifically how planned nursing interventions can improve the client's level of health (Kelly and others, 1994; Beecroft, 1995).

If the client achieves the expected outcomes, the nurse either continues the care plan or discontinues interventions because the goal of care is met. If evaluation determines that the expected outcomes were not met or only partially met, the nurse begins reassessment and revision of the care plan. For greatest accuracy, outcome data should be captured as close to the source as possible, including direct data capture for clients and their families (Zielstorff, 1995).

Evaluation of Goal Achievement

The purpose of nursing care is to assist the client in resolving actual health problems, preventing the occurrence of potential problems, and maintaining a healthy state. Evaluation of the goals of care determines whether this purpose was accomplished. The nurse matches the client's behavior (e.g., self-administration of insulin or anxiety-free behavior) or physiological response (e.g., decrease in size of pressure ulcer or fall in body temperature) with the behavior or response specified in the goal. For example, during an initial assessment, a client may report acute abdominal pain, rate the pain as 8 on a scale of 0 to 10 (see Chapter 42), and grimace or hold the abdomen during attempts to move in bed. This baseline is used by the nurse to identify the nursing diagnosis of *pain* and establish the goal of "client will perceive a reduction in pain within 48 hours." The nurse's evaluation determines whether the outcomes that reflect goal accomplishment were met. Did the interventions of positioning, proper and timely administration of analgesics, and use of relaxation successfully reduce the client's pain? Outcomes may include "client will rate pain as 3 on a scale of 0 to 10 in 24 hours" and "client will position self without nonverbal signs of discomfort." After providing appropriate comfort measures, the nurse reassesses the client by measuring the subjective report of pain, observing facial expressions, and noting whether the client initiates turning and repositioning. The new data or client responses are compared with outcome criteria to determine whether predicted changes have occurred (Table 18-1). To objectively evaluate the degree of success in achieving a goal, the nurse should use the following steps:

1. Examine the goal statement to identify the exact desired client behavior or response.
2. Assess the client for the presence of that behavior or response.
3. Compare the established outcome criteria with the behavior or response.
4. Judge the degree of agreement between outcome criteria and the behavior or response.
5. If there is no agreement (or only partial agreement) between the outcome criteria and the behavior or response, what is/are the barriers? Why did they not agree?

There are different degrees of goal attainment. If the client's response matches or exceeds the outcome criteria, the goal is met. If the client's behavior begins to show changes but does not yet meet criteria set, the goal is partially met. If there is no progress, the goal is not met (Table 18-2). A clearly defined goal with specific outcomes is easily measured (see Chapter 16).

EVALUATIVE MEASURES AND SOURCES

Evaluative measures are simply the assessment skills and techniques used to collect data for evaluation (e.g., auscultation of lung sounds, observation of a client's skill performance, discussion of the client's feelings, and inspection of the skin) (Figure 18-2). In fact, they are the same as assessment measures but are performed at the point of care when decisions are made about the client's status and progress. The intent of assessment is to identify what if any problems exist. The intent of evaluation is to determine if the known problems have improved, worsened, or otherwise changed.

The data collected during evaluation are critically analyzed and compared with expected outcomes to determine whether changes in the client's health status occurred (see Table 18-1). After caring for a client over a long period, the nurse is able to make subtle comparisons of responses and behaviors. Previous experience coupled with a scientific knowledge base is key to critical thinking. The accuracy of any evaluation improves when the nurse is familiar with the client's behavior and physiological status. Evaluation is also more exact after the nurse has seen more than one client with a similar type of problem.

The primary source of data for evaluation is the client. However, the nurse also uses the family and other caregivers. Documentation and reporting are of critical importance in the evaluation process. Written nursing progress notes, assessment flow sheets, and information shared among nurses during change-of-shift reports (see

Table 18-1	Evaluation Measures to Determine the Success of Goals and Expected Outcomes		
Goals	**Evaluative Measures**	**Expected Outcomes**	
Client's pressure ulcer will heal within 7 days.	Inspect color, condition, and location of pressure ulcer.	Erythema will be reduced in 2 days.	
	Measure diameter of ulcer daily.	Diameter of ulcer will decrease in 5 days.	
	Note odor and color of drainage from ulcer.	Ulcer will have no drainage in 2 days.	
		Skin overlying ulcer will be closed in 7 days.	
Client will tolerate ambulation to end of hall by 11/20.	Palpate client's radial pulse before exercise.	Pulse will remain below 110 beats per minute during exercise.	
	Palpate client's radial pulse 10 minutes after exercise.	Pulse rate will return to resting baseline within 10 minutes after exercise.	
	Assess respiratory rate during exercise.	Respiratory rate will remain within two breaths of client's baseline rate.	
	Observe client for dyspnea or breathlessness during exercise.	Client will deny feeling of breathlessness.	
Client will have improved grief resolution by 1/15.	Ask client about frequency of periods of crying, sadness.	Client reports decreased frequency of crying, sadness in 2 months.	
	Review client's sleeping log.	Client has periods of 6-7 hours of sleep without interruption within 10 days.	
	Review client's dietary intake.	Client has no weight loss in 1 month.	

Table 18-2 **Examples of Objective Evaluation of Goal Achievement**			
Goals	Outcome Criteria	Client Response	Evaluation Findings
Client will self-administer insulin by 12/18.	Client prepares insulin dosage in syringe by 12/17. Client demonstrates self-injection by 12/18.	Client prepared accurate dosage in syringe on 12/17. Client administered morning insulin dosage; self-injection was correctly performed on 12/18.	Client has progressed and achieved desired behavior.
Client's lungs will be free of secretions by 11/30.	Coughing will be nonproductive by 11/29. Lungs will be clear to auscultation by 11/30. Respirations will be 20 per minute by 11/30.	Client coughed frequently and productively on 11/29. Lungs were clear to auscultation on 11/30. Respirations were 18 per minute on 11/29.	Client will require continued therapy. Condition is improving.
Client will be able to perform self-care measures without discomfort in 2 days.	Client will rate pain as 3 on a scale of 10 within 2 days. Client will initiate bathing within 2 days.	Client rates severe right-sided abdominal pain as 5 on a scale of 10 while attempting bathing on day 2.	Client's condition still indicates a problem. Continued therapy with possibly new care measures is required.

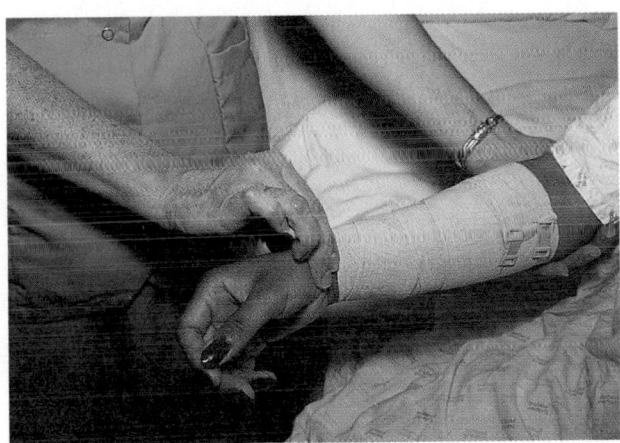

Figure 18-2   Nurse evaluates circulation following application of elastic wrap bandage.

Chapter 24) should communicate a client's progress toward meeting expected outcomes and goals for the nursing plan of care. If a client is cared for using a critical pathway or CareMap (see Chapter 24), the nurse and team members clearly know what outcomes are to be met for a given day (Figure 18-3). The CareMap as a documentation tool includes expected outcomes that the care team predicts will be met during the client's projected length of stay. The nurse and other team members refer to the outcomes on the CareMap on an ongoing basis. If there is variance (unexpected outcomes or outcomes occurring at a different time than expected), the nurse reports these responses and revises the plan of care as needed. By having

outcomes clearly documented on either a CareMap or other documentation form, the nurse and other health care providers clearly know what to evaluate. All members of the health care team should have a sense of the client's progress. Each nurse summarizes data on an ongoing basis to ensure that the client is progressing to a better level of health.

Care Plan Revision and Critical Thinking

As goals are evaluated, adjustments to the care plan are made as indicated. If a goal was successfully met, that portion of the care plan is discontinued. Unmet and partially met goals require the nurse to continue intervention. After a nurse reassesses a client, nursing diagnoses may be modified or added with appropriate goals and expected outcomes, and interventions are established (Table 18-3). The nurse also redefines priorities. This is an important step in critical thinking—knowing how the client is progressing and how problems either resolve or worsen. The nurse's careful monitoring and early detection of problems are a client's first line of defense (Benner, 1984, Benner and others, 1996). Benner describes the importance of nurses learning how to anticipate the client's future course. Clinical judgments are based on the nurse's observations of what is occurring with a specific client and not merely what may happen to clients in general. Frequently changes are very subtle. Evaluation must be client specific, based on a close familiarity with each client's behavior, physical

SERVICE ORTHO_____ PHYSICIAN_____ CARE PATH 804
PRIMARY NURSE_____ ADM DATE _____
DC DATE _____

	PATIENT PROBLEMS/NURSING DIAGNOSIS
#1	Pain
#2	Impaired physical mobility
#3	Lack of knowledge
#4	High risk for injury

PROBLEM NUMBER		ED ADM DATE	MED CLEARANCE	DAY DOS	DAY POD 1
	ASSESSMENT MONITORING	Total Nursing Admission/Assessment Assess for hip or leg deformity Assess skin condition q shift NV status check	Assess NV status q 4o	Dressing D/I HMV patent to SS NV assessment q 1o x4 then q 2o to hip/LE Assess bowel sounds Assess lung sounds Assess abdominal distention Skin assessment q shift	Dressing D/I HMV patent to SS NV assessment q 2o Assess bowel sounds Assess lung sounds Assess abdominal distention Skin assessment q shift
	CONSULTS	Pre-Screening		Consults… P.T. O.T. S.W.	Initiate… P.T. O.T.
	PROCEDURE/ TEST	Admit labs CBC, 6, PT/PTT SMA 12, T & S UA with micro EKG CXR Hip x-ray Overhead frame Trapeze Advance 2000 bed	Medical clearance tests	X-ray post op m PAR/OU CBC, 6 post op in PAR	CBC, 6 Hgh/Hct > than transfuse
	TREATMENT	Traction (skeletal or Buck's 5lb) Foley cath Ice to hip prn I/O I.S. every 2o WA TCDB every 2o	Bucks tx I.S. every 2o Foley cath care	HMV I/O I.S. every 1o TCDB every 2o Foley cath care Check hip dressing	DC Foley cath I/O I.S. every 1o TCDB every 2o Check hip dressing
	ACTIVITY	Bedrest Turn 45° every 2°	Bedrest Turn 45° every 2°	Bedrest Turn every 2°	Chair BID MD to determine weight bearing status Stand with walker and P.T. Assist with ADL's
	MEDS/IVS	Heplock 20 gauge of > Prn analgesic LOC AAOC	PRN analgesics Flush HL every 8o IVF's stated after MN day before surgery	IVF's PCA Ancef x6 doses #1/#2	IVF to KVO PCA Ancef #3/4/5
	NUTRITION	Req. NPO after MN	Req. NPO after MN	Clear/full liquids	Advance to regular
	PATIENT/ FAMILY EDUCATION	Nursing Pre-op teaching Use of I.S. Traction Post-op routine Potential need for 730cu	Nursing Continue — pre-op post-op teaching	Reinforce pre-op Post-op teaching i.e., activity, I/O, I.S., PCA, diet	P.T./Nursing Wt bearing status Transfers OOB to chair
	DISCHARGE PLANNING	Nursing Assess condition at home Determine need for: Social Services P.T. O.T. Home Health **Pt./Family verbalizes understanding of Care Path. Plan of care has been mutually set with pt/family**	**High risk screening** Social Worker		Initiate P.T.
	PSYCHO-SOCIAL/ EMOTIONAL	Provide emotional support		Provide emotional support	Give positive feedback on activity
	VARIANCE				
	SIGNATURES				

Figure 18-3 Portion of total hip care path. Note outcomes in bold and expected DC (discharge) outcomes. Courtesy Barnes-Jewish Hospital, St. Louis, Mo.

DAY POD 2	DAY POD 3	DAY POD 4	DAY POD 5	DC OUTCOMES
Dressing D/I DC HMV per HO dressing over old HMV site NV assessment q shift	Incision line clean, dry, well approximated 4 x 4 over old HMV site D/I Minimal HMV site drainage Afebrile	Incision line clean, dry, well approximated No drainage from old HMV site	Staples/sutures removed per H.O. if not on Prednisone (If on Prednisone — remove 14 days in office/clinic) Check walker/crutches to go home with patient for safety	No signs or symptoms infection No evidence of dislocation
		Potential evaluation Home Health		
		Hip x-ray taken CBC		Wound clean and dry Hgh/Hct stable
I.S. every 2o WA	I.S. every 2o WA	I.S. every 4o WA		Lungs clear or WNL
Check hip dressing				
Chair BID P.T. BID Assist with ADL's	Chair		Chair TID R.T.–bid Transfers OOB indep. Amb. indep. with walker and steady gait Indep. with ADL's	Ind. ambulate with steady gait/walker Uses O.T. equipment correctly to perform self care activity
IVF's chd to HL DC PCA DC Ancef after #6 Initiate p.o. pain medications	DC H.L. if Hct > 28 p.o. pain medications	p.o. pain medications	p.o. pain meds	Pain controlled with p.o. analgesics
Regular	Regular	Regular	Regular	
P.T./Nursing	P.T./Nursing OT–instructions	P.T./Nursing	P.T./Nursing	Able to verbalize and demonstrate correct precautions/weight bearing status. Able to verbalize understanding of home care exercises.
ADL Equipment form OT– reacher, etc.	Follow-up with P.T. concerning DC plans ADL training with O.T. Initial eval. of DC by S.W.		DC pt with discharge instructions, prescriptions, home equipment	DC to appropriate level of care with MD/clinic follow-up
Verbal praise for accomplishment	Accepting D/C plan and motivated to learn	DC plan accepted	DC plan accepted with positive attitude	Demonstrated appropriate coping and emotional response

Figure 18-3, cont'd

Table 18-3 **Modification of Nursing Care Plan for Mr. Brown**			
Reassessment	Nursing Diagnosis	Goals and Expected Outcomes	Interventions
40-pack year history of smoking	Ineffective airway clearance related to poor control of incisional pain	Client's pain will be reduced. *Expected outcomes:* Client will use PCA* more frequently within 24 hours.	Instruct client on proper use of PCA* and rationale for regular use of medication.
Right middle lobe infiltrate present on chest x-ray film			
Rales present in right middle lobe		Client will splint incision before each cough and deep breathing exercise.	Demonstrate correct splinting procedure. Allow for return demonstration by client.
Achieves only 60% to 70% of incentive spirometry goal because of incisional pain		Client's level of pain decreases to 3-4 on a scale of 0-10 within 36 hours.	
Reluctant to turn, cough, and deep breathe because of incisional pain		Client's lungs will become clear. *Expected outcomes:*	
Does not splint abdominal incision		Client's lungs will become clear to auscultation within 36 hours.	Assist client with splinting procedure.
Oral temperature of 39.8° C (103.6° F)		Client will achieve 90% of incentive spirometry goal.	Instruct and assist client with incentive spirometry.
Infrequent, irregular use of PCA*		Client's oral temperature will return to normal within 36 hours.	
Rates incisional pain as 7 on a scale of 0-10		Client will turn, cough, and deep breathe.	Turn, cough, and deep breathe client every hour.

*PCA, Patient-controlled analgesia.

status, and reaction to caregivers. Critical thinking skills promote accurate evaluation, which leads to the appropriate revision of ineffective care plans and discontinuation of therapy that has been successful (see Figure 18-1).

DISCONTINUING A CARE PLAN

After determining that expected outcomes and goals have been achieved, the nurse confirms this evaluation with the client. If the nurse and client agree that the expected outcomes have been met, the nurse discontinues that care plan. For example, a client has the nursing diagnosis of *knowledge deficit regarding self-administration of insulin related to inexperience.* To achieve the ultimate goal of accurate client administration of insulin, the nurse establishes outcomes, including "client will describe the purpose of insulin by 9/20," "client will correctly prepare insulin in syringe by 9/20," and "client will administer insulin injection independently by 9/22." The nurse evaluates the information with the client and learns whether the client understands explanations and is comfortable in applying the information. In addition, the nurse will observe the client's preparation of the medication and actual self-injection. Once outcomes are met successfully, it is unnecessary to teach additional information about insulin administration. The care plan can be documented as discontinued.

This ensures that other nurses will not unnecessarily continue the care plan. Continuity of care assumes that care provided is relevant to client needs. Significant time is wasted when achieved goals are not communicated.

MODIFYING A CARE PLAN

When goals are not met, the nurse identifies the variables or factors that interfered with goal achievement. Usually a change in the client's condition, needs, or abilities makes alteration of the care plan necessary. For example, when teaching self-administration of insulin, the nurse discovers that the client has a literacy problem or a visual impairment that prevents the reading of insulin dosages on the syringe. As a result, original outcomes cannot be met. Thus the nurse uses new interventions and revises outcomes to meet the goal of care.

Lack of goal achievement may also result from an error in nursing judgment or failure to follow each step of the nursing process. Clients frequently have very complex problems. The nurse should always remember the possibility of overlooking or misjudging something. When there is failure to achieve a goal, no matter what the reason, the entire nursing process sequence is repeated to discover changes that need to be made to promote, maintain, or restore the client's health.

Reassessment.

A complete reassessment of all client factors relating to the nursing diagnosis and etiology is necessary when modifying a plan. Reassessment requires critical thinking when the nurse compares new data about the client's condition with previously assessed information. Often a nurse applies intuitive knowledge from experiences with other clients to direct the reassessment process. Encounters over time with clients and families who have similar health problems give nurses a strong background of knowledge to use for anticipating client needs and planning care. For example, consider Mr. Landis, who has the nursing diagnosis of *pain related to trauma of a surgical incision.* Two days following surgery, the client continues to have a poor appetite despite the fact that there are no obvious surgical complications. If the client continues to have pain, the nurse may automatically associate loss of appetite with discomfort. However, the experienced nurse may recall a previous client who became almost depressed following surgery. After exploring the problem further, the nurse learns that Mr. Landis's family has not been visiting, the client is fearful of losing his job, and in addition to experiencing loss of appetite, the client is not sleeping well. Although the client continues to have pain, a new priority diagnosis may be *anticipatory grieving related to losses associated with illness.* Focusing on this diagnosis may improve the client's appetite. As in the original assessment, data are collected from all available sources. Depending on the nurse's findings, it often becomes necessary to assess variables that were not covered on the initial assessment.

Reassessment ensures that the database is accurate and current. It may also reveal the missing link (i.e., a critical piece of new information that was overlooked and thus interfered with goal achievement). All new data are sorted, validated, and clustered to analyze and interpret differences from the original database. The nurse documents reassessment data to alert other nursing staff to the client's status.

Nursing Diagnoses.

After reassessment, the nurse determines what nursing diagnoses are accurate for the situation. The nurse asks whether the correct diagnosis was selected and whether it and the etiological factor are current. The problem list should then be revised to reflect the client's changed status. A new diagnosis may be made. If a previous diagnosis no longer accurately reflects the problem, it should be discontinued and a modified statement should be entered. For example, if the nurse finds that a client with diabetes has a serious visual impairment, it may be unlikely that the client will be able to self-administer insulin. The nurse's assessment may reveal that a family member is available as a resource. To develop a plan designed to educate an alternate caregiver about the administration of insulin, the nurse then establishes a new diagnosis: *altered health maintenance related to visual impairment.*

A nurse's care is based on an accurate list of nursing diagnoses. Accuracy is more important than the number of diagnoses selected. As the client's condition changes, the diagnoses do, too.

Goals and Expected Outcomes.

When care plans are revised, the nurse reviews goals and expected outcomes for needed changes. Even the goals for unchanged nursing diagnoses should be examined for appropriateness. Determining that each goal and expected outcome is realistic for the problem, etiology, and time frame is particularly important. Unrealistic expected outcomes and time frames make goal achievement difficult.

The nurse clearly documents goals and expected outcomes for new or revised nursing diagnoses so that all team members are aware of the revised care plan. When the goal is still appropriate but has not yet been met, the nurse may change the evaluation date to allow more time. All goals and expected outcomes should be client centered, with realistic expectations for client achievement.

Interventions.

The evaluation of interventions examines two factors: the appropriateness of the interventions selected and the correct application of the implementation process. The appropriateness of an intervention may be based on the standard of care for a client's health problem. A **standard of care** is the minimum level of care accepted to ensure high quality of care to clients. Standards of care define the types of therapies typically administered to clients with defined problems or needs. If the client who is postoperative for abdominal surgery has a specific nursing diagnosis, such as *ineffective airway clearance,* the standard of care established by a nursing department for this problem may include pain-control measures with coughing or deep breathing exercises to help the client breathe more easily with a clear airway. The nurse reviews the standard of care to determine whether the right interventions have been chosen or whether additional ones are required.

Appropriateness of care may be achieved by increasing or decreasing the frequency of interventions. The nurse uses judgment based on previous experience, as well as the client's actual response to therapy. For example, if a client continues to have congested lung sounds, the nurse increases the frequency of coughing exercises to remove secretions.

During evaluation the nurse may determine that some planned interventions are designed for an inappropriate level of nursing care. If the level of care needs to be changed, a different action verb, such as *assist* in place of *provide,* may be substituted. Sometimes the level of care is appropriate but the interventions are unsuitable because of a change in the expected outcome. In this case the interventions should be discontinued and new ones planned.

During implementation the nurse evaluates the client's

response during and immediately after intervention. Evaluation must be integrated with ongoing nursing care activity. If the response is favorable, implementation continues. Reevaluation occurs when the intervention proves to be unsuccessful. The nurse then examines the other components of implementation, such as client and environment preparation, anticipated complications, or use of personal or technical skills during care delivery.

Changes in implementation should be guided by the nature of the client's unfavorable response. Consulting with other nurses may yield suggestions for improving the approach to care delivery. Senior nurses are often excellent resources because of their experience. Simply changing the care plan is not enough. The nurse must implement the new plan and reevaluate the client's response to the nursing actions.

Occasionally during evaluation the nurse may discover unmet client needs. This should be anticipated. The nursing process is designed to be a systematic, problem-solving approach to individualized client care, but there is a wide array of variables for each client with a health care problem. Clients with the same health care problem are not treated the same way. As a result, the nurse sometimes makes errors in judgment. The systematic use of evaluation provides a way for nurses to catch these errors in judgment. The nurse consistently incorporates evaluation into practice to minimize errors and ensure that the most appropriate interventions are used.

• • •

Evaluation is the final step of the nursing process, a systematic method for organizing and delivering nursing care. The exclusion of evaluation from the nursing process prevents the nurse from evaluating nursing practice and determining whether the outcomes of client care are beneficial. The regular application of evaluation ensures that a client's care plan is current and appropriate.

Quality Improvement

The evaluation of health care is a process used to determine the quality of care and service provided to clients. Each professional nurse is expected to evaluate his or her success in delivering effective nursing care. However, good client outcomes are a product of all individual actions and interactions that relate directly or indirectly to the care received by a client (Scoble and Hembrough, 1993). The outcomes of care are a measure of the performance of the entire health care team. For example, following surgery for a total hip repair, does the client regain functional mobility without severe pain and without complications such as wound infection? To achieve such results requires collaboration by nurses, physical therapists, physicians, dietitians, and perhaps even infection-control specialists. More and more, emphasis is being placed on monitoring and evaluating the systems and processes that influence client care. This process is receiving more attention than ever before because of the increasing costs of health care.

Today's consumers are more informed and thus more interested in the quality of health care because of rising costs. Accrediting and regulatory agencies are attempting to set a uniform set of standards so that quality comparisons can be made across health care institutions (Health Care Advisory Board, 1994). There are wide variations in the quality of health care within and among institutions. High costs of care do not necessarily ensure high quality, and therefore there is significant room for improvement within all health care organizations. The focus of quality improvement at one point was only on hospitals. Now even health care plans (see Chapter 2) are being asked to demonstrate quality, since their coverage often restricts employers and consumers from choosing their provider of health care.

As health care institutions look for ways to differentiate themselves from other organizations, quality of care is the answer (see Chapter 4). Nursing has participated in the monitoring of quality for many years, and for this reason, nurses are leading the efforts within organizations to better understand how to measure quality of care. The JCAHO (1999) defines **quality improvement (QI)** as an approach to the continuous study and improvement of the processes of providing health care services to meet the needs of clients and others. Staff within an organization work together in teams to identify what opportunities exist for improving care and what actions are necessary to achieve success. The purpose of QI is not to identify problems retrospectively, but to identify opportunities prospectively to improve the quality of care or service (Patton and Stanley, 1993). There are several dimensions of performance that a health care institution should include to have a comprehensive QI program (Box 18-1). Assessment of whether an organization is doing the right thing or doing the right thing well should be the focus of QI activities.

EVALUATION OF CARE

Monitoring of quality indicators evaluates whether specifically defined processes are reaching desired outcomes. If results are exceeding or meeting a threshold, or if performance is within the controls set for a process, no problem has been identified and the process is performing well. When thresholds for satisfactory care have not been met or when performance is below the control limits set, staff must attempt to determine the cause of problems. For example, if clients who receive diabetic instruction are able to score only an average of 70% on a return demonstration test, staff must determine the reasons for this. This step requires nurses and colleagues to honestly review practice activities and look for opportunities to reinforce nursing care standards or improve practice.

Dimensions of Performance   Box 18-1

DOING THE RIGHT THING

Efficacy of a procedure or treatment (e.g., pain management, skin care) in relation to a client's condition. Does the procedure or treatment produce the desired result?

Appropriateness of a test, procedure, or service to meet the client's needs. Is the level of care given the level of care considered necessary (e.g., use of pulse oximetry instead of arterial blood gases)?

DOING THE RIGHT THING WELL

Availability of a needed test, procedure, treatment, or service to the client who needs it (e.g., appointment scheduling in clinics, access to emergency care)

Timeliness with which a needed test, procedure, treatment, or service is provided to the client (e.g., response time for stat x-ray, delays in operating room cases)

Effectiveness with which tests, procedures, treatments, and services are provided (e.g., success with established standard of care on a CareMap in meeting client outcomes)

Continuity of the services provided to the client with respect to other services, practitioners, and providers over time (e.g., prompt and appropriate referrals to home health; use of a teaching plan preadmission, during a hospital stay, and postadmission)

Safety of the client (and others) to whom the services are provided (e.g., use of physical restraints, use of standard precautions)

Efficiency with which services are provided, showing the relationship between outcomes and the resources used to deliver care (e.g., readmission rate to hospital, comparing client's functional status with the cost of providing care)

Respect and caring with which services are provided (e.g., client satisfaction ratings, informing clients about advance directives)

EVALUATION OF IMPROVEMENT

After implementing an action plan to improve quality of care, staff must reevaluate the success of the plan. In the example of Mr. Brown (see Table 18-3), staff will repeat monitoring of the teaching process and the results of client testing to see if improvement has been made. The change may be positive or negative. For example, if the client's test scores improve, the team has successfully improved outcomes. Similarly, if test scores show no improvement or even worsen, a new plan of action will be needed. The QI process is similar to the nursing process. When desired outcomes (QI criteria) are not met, staff will reinstate the QI process.

Providing health care in a timely, competent, and cost-effective manner is a complex and challenging process. Evaluation is a means for addressing this challenge. This chapter on the evaluation process has discussed multiple methods to determine the effectiveness of care and to make necessary modifications to continuously provide client-centered care for clients.

Evaluation of care is a professional responsibility, and it is a crucial component of nursing care. Evaluation can focus on a single client's plan of care, or it can focus on the delivery of care provided by an agency or a specific nursing division within an agency. Through the continuous evaluation of care, nurses are in a position to improve client care.

• • •

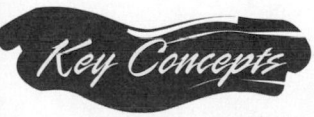

Key Concepts

- Evaluation determines a client's response to nursing actions and the extent to which goals of care have been met.
- Evaluation involves critical thinking because the nurse determines the optimal way to deliver nursing care.
- The nurse compares the client's response to nursing actions with expected outcomes established during planning.
- Expected outcomes are stated in behavioral terms to describe the desired effect of nursing actions.

- Evaluation measures are assessment skills used to collect data for evaluation.
- The nursing care plan is modified based on data obtained during evaluation.
- As a result of evaluation, client priorities may change.
- Evaluation enables the nurse to determine why the care plan was successful or unsuccessful.
- For nurses to be accountable for their practice, they must know the outcomes of care.

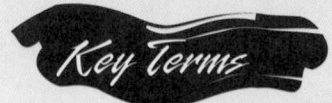
Key Terms

Critical Thinking Exercises

1. Mr. Vicar has been visiting the clinic for more than a month. He visits weekly for follow-up care for a chronic venous stasis ulcer of the left leg. The nurse's note at the time of his first visit contained the following information: "Ulcer with irregular margins, 4 cm wide by 5 cm long, approximately 0.5 cm deep, draining foul-smelling purulent yellowish drainage. Only subcutaneous tissue visible. Skin around ulcer, brownish rust in color. Zinc oxide and calamine gauze applied to ulcer; elastic wrap bandage applied to gauze. Client instructed to return in 2 weeks." As the nurse who is caring for the client on the follow-up visit, what expected outcomes would you anticipate for the goal of "wound will demonstrate healing within 4 weeks"? What evaluative measures would you use to determine if the wound was healing?

2. Ms. Acad is a 55-year-old woman who experienced a heart attack and is now recovering on a medical cardiology unit. Her primary nurse has identified the need to teach Ms. Acad about activity restriction, diet, stress management, and medications. Ms. Acad will likely be in the hospital for 3 more days. Explain why evaluation is important in this case. How will the nurse's evaluation of Ms. Acad's learning influence the plan of care at discharge?

3. As a nurse on a neurological unit, you care for a number of clients with parkinsonism, a disorder that causes an unsteady gait, muscle weakness, and muscular rigidity. Over the last month five clients with parkinsonism have fallen. Develop a quality indicator and monitoring criteria to measure this practice problem.

References

Beecroft PC: Making the connections to patient outcomes: why outside observers make no mention of the hidden knowledge work of nurses, *Clin Nurse Spec* 9(6):285, 1995.

Benner P: *From novice to expert: excellence and power in clinical nursing practice,* Menlo Park, Calif, 1984, Addison-Wesley.

Benner P, Stannard D, Hooper PL: A "thinking-in-action" approach to teaching clinical judgement: a classroom innovation for acute care advanced practice nurses, *Adv Pract Nurs Q* 1(4):70, 1996.

Carnevali DL, Thomas MD: *Diagnostic reasoning and treatment decision making in nursing,* Philadelphia, 1993, JB Lippincott.

Chase S: Teaching baccalaureate nursing students to project outcomes to nursing interventions, *Nurs Diagn* 9(2):62, 1998.

Deaton C: Outcomes measurement, *J Cardiovasc Nurs* 12(4):49, 1998.

Health Care Advisory Board: *Next generation of outcomes tracking: implications for health plans and systems,* vol 2, *Quality measures,* Washington, DC, 1994, The Board.

Johnson M, Mass ML, Moorhead S: *Nursing outcomes classification,* ed 3, St. Louis, 2000, Mosby.

Joint Commission on Accreditation of Healthcare Organizations: *1999 Accreditation manual for hospitals,* vol 1, *Standards,* Chicago, 1999, The Commission.

Kelly KC and others: The medical outcomes study: a nursing perspective, *J Prof Nurs* 10(4):209, 1994.

Lin C: Patient satisfaction with nursing care as an outcome variable: dilemmas for nursing evaluation researchers, *J Prof Nurs* 1294:207, 1996.

Patton S, Stanley J: Bridging quality assurance and continuous quality improvement, *J Nurs Care Qual* 7(2):15, 1993.

Scoble KB, Hembrough B: Nursing clinical pertinence review: a step toward quality improvement, *J Nurs Care Qual* 7(2):52, 1993.

Zielstorff RD: Capturing and using clinical outcome data: implications for information systems design, *J Am Med Inform Assoc* 2(3):191, 1995.

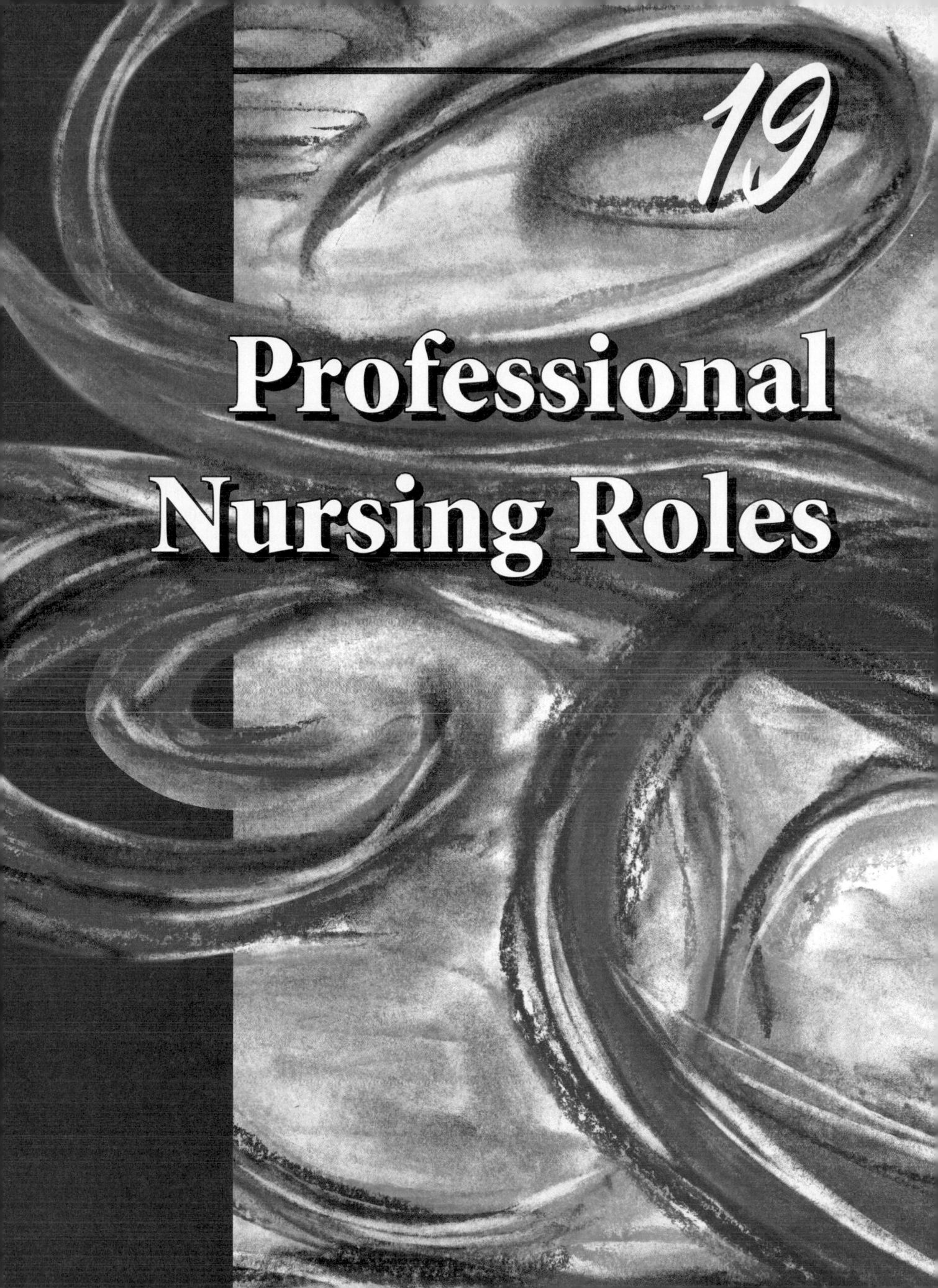

19

Professional Nursing Roles

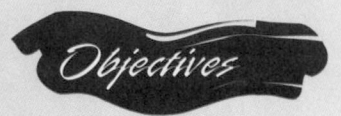

Mastery of content in this chapter will enable the student to:

- Define the key terms listed.
- Discuss the historical development of professional nursing roles.
- Describe educational programs available for professional registered nurse education.
- List and describe practice settings for nurses.
- Describe the roles and career opportunities for nurses.
- List the five characteristics of a profession and discuss how nursing demonstrates these characteristics.
- Discuss the influence of social and economic changes on nursing practices.

N ursing is an art and a science involving many activities, concepts, and skills related to basic social sciences, physical sciences, ethics, contemporary issues, and other areas. Nursing is a unique profession because it addresses the responses of individuals and families to health promotion, health maintenance, and health problems. Nurses assume many simultaneous roles: direct care provider, clinical decision maker, client and family advocate researcher, and educator. This role has evolved from the day of Florence Nightingale (1860), when nurses provided care, performed housekeeping duties, washed the linen, prepared and served meals, and maintained and stocked supplies.

A professional registered nurse provides a specified service according to standards of practice and follows a code of ethics. The foundation for professional practice arises from theories of nursing, relevance to basic social values, educational preparation, motivation, autonomy, a sense of commitment, a sense of community, and a code of ethics (Bernhard and Walsh, 1995).

Nursing has developed many philosophies and definitions of nursing. The following definition, written by Virginia Henderson (1966) and adopted by the **International Council of Nurses (ICN)** in 1973, is a concise, mutually agreed on statement:

> The unique function of the nurse is to assist the individual, sick or well, in the performance of those activities contributing to health, its recovery, or to a peaceful death that the client would perform unaided if he had the necessary strength, will, or knowledge. And to do this in such a way as to help the client gain independence as rapidly as possible.

The profession of nursing is complex and multifaceted, with nurses practicing in many settings. Individuals can become a registered nurse through a variety of educational programs. Multiple career opportunities are available as nurses advance their education and increase clinical competencies.

Expertise in nursing is a result of knowledge and clinical experience. The expertise required to interpret clinical situations and make complex decisions is the essence of nursing care and is the basis for the advancement of nursing practice and the development of nursing science (Benner, 1984; Carnevali and Thomas, 1998). Critical thinking skills are essential to nursing (see Chapter 13). When providing nursing care, the nurse makes clinical judgments about the care needed for clients based on fact, experience, and standards of care (Alfaro-LeFevre, 1995). Knowledge, expertise, and lifelong learning are gained through the continual process of critical thinking.

The profession of nursing has evolved as society, health care needs, and policies change. Nursing responds and adapts to changes, meeting new challenges as they arise. The evolution of nursing has brought the profession to one of the most challenging and exciting times in history. There are limitless opportunities to improve the health and quality of the lives of clients and communities as the nursing profession and nursing practice are continually developed.

Historical Perspective

The historical roots of nursing enable both students and practicing professionals to prepare for the health care needs of the twenty-first century. Nursing is a melding of knowledge from the physical sciences, humanities, social sciences, and clinical competencies needed to meet the individual needs of clients and their families. Knowledge of the profession's history increases the nurse's awareness and promotes an understanding of the social and intellectual origins of the discipline (Keeling and Ramos, 1995) (Box 19-1). Although the general goals of nursing have remained relatively the same over the centuries, advancing science has influenced the practice of nursing and society's changing needs.

Milestones in Nursing History

Box 19-1

300 AD Entry of women into nursing.

1100-1200 AD Formation of Hospital Brothers of St. Anthony's.
Formation of the Brothers of Misericordia, Italy.
Formation of the Alexian Brothers.

1633 Sisters of Charity founded.

1809 Mother Elizabeth Seton introduced the Sisters of Charity into America, later known as the Daughters of Charity.

1836 Deaconess Institute of Kaiserwerth, Germany, founded.

1846 Nightingale received the *Yearbook of the Institution of Deaconess at Kaiserwerth.*

1860 Establishment of the Nightingale Training School for Nurses at St. Thomas' Hospital in London, England.

1860 Florence Nightingale published *Notes on Nursing: What It Is and What It Is Not.*

1860-1865 Dorthea Lynde Dix served as superintendent of the Union Army female nurses; Mary Ann Ball (Mother Bickerdyke) organized ambulance services, searched for wounded, and supervised nurses; Harriett Tubman tended to soldiers and led over 300 slaves to freedom through the Underground Railroad Movement.

1874 First training school in Canada founded: St. Catherine's, Ontario.

1882 United States ratified the American Red Cross, founded by Clara Barton.

1884 Mary Agnes Snively assumed directorship of Toronto General Hospital.

1890 Establishment of the Nurses' Associated Alumni of the United States and Canada.

1893 First community health service for the poor: Henry Street Settlement.

1894 Isabel Hamptom Robb was the first superintendent of the Johns Hopkins Training School in Baltimore, Maryland.

1896 Nurses' Associated Alumnae of the United States and Canada (NAAUSC) founded.

1897 Initial discussion of nursing code of ethics.

1899 Canadian affiliation removed from NAAUSC.

1901 First university affiliated nursing program. Army Nurse Corps established.

1902 Sigma Theta Tau was formed by six student nurses from Indiana University.

1907 First professor of nursing, Mary Adelaide Nutting.

1908 Navy Nurse Corps established; Canadian National Association of Trained Nurses (later changed to the Canadian Nurses Association, 1924) founded.

1911 NAAUSC became the American Nurses Association (ANA).

1920 Graduate nurse midwifery programs were established.

1923 Goldmark Report: Rockefeller Foundation–funded survey identified need for increased financial support to university-based schools of nursing.

1926 ANA Code of Ethics proposed.

1948 Brown Report: Dr. Esther Lucille Brown concluded that all nursing education programs should be affiliated with universities and have their own budgets. She recommended a broad academic education within a university and 2 years of nursing education focused on technical skills.

1949 Association of Operating Room Nurses formed.

1952 Dr. Mildred Montag established the associate degree nursing program.
Nursing Research, a journal reporting on the scientific investigations of nursing, was established.

1953 National League for Nursing (NLN), in collaboration with universities, developed graduate nursing education.

1960 Yale University School of Nursing defined nursing as a profession, interaction, and relationship between two human beings.

1965 Jerome Lysaught directed the National Commission on Nursing and Nursing Education Report. Recommended that nursing roles and responsibilities be clarified in relation to other health care professionals and that increased financial support and career opportunities were needed to attract and retain nurses; ANA position paper defined nursing.

1969 American Association of Critical Care Nurses (AACN) formed.

1975 Oncology Nursing Society formed.
NLN required theory-based curriculum for accreditation.

1985 ANA published *Code for Nurses With Interpretive Statements.*

1996 The Pew Report.

1996 Institute of Medicine (IOM) Report.

From its earliest history, nursing was a form of community service to protect and preserve the family. Nursing began as a desire to keep people healthy and to provide comfort and assurance to the sick. Historically, men and women have held the role of nurse. In the prehistoric period, women were responsible for gathering the herbs, roots, and plants that were used to heal the sick. Religious leaders performed ceremonies and rituals to drive out sickness and evil spirits.

EARLY CIVILIZATION

Sixteenth-century BC Egypt was a society that valued health and preventive medicine. The Egyptians believed that these values appeased their gods and the spirits of the dead (Ellis and Hartley, 1997). Ancient Egyptians developed plans for hygiene and food preparation to reduce disease transmission (Cherry and Jacob, 1999). Egyptian women served as care providers to the sick and elderly and during childbirth for the aristocracy (Ellis and Hartley, 1997).

Early Hebrews (1400 to 1200 BC) developed dietary laws that protected the public by prescribing what foods could and could not be eaten together and providing guidelines for the safe eating of the meat of slaughtered animals. Hebrew priests and widows or maidens tended to the sick in their homes. People with a suspected communicable disease were quarantined until well (Cherry and Jacob, 1999).

Greek philosophers (1500 to 1000 BC) believed that illness and health were controlled by the gods and goddesses of Greek mythology (Cherry and Jacob, 1999). Hippocrates (460-362 BC), the father of medicine, believed that disease and illness was due to natural rather than supernatural causes (Kalisch and Kalisch, 1995).

Ancient Chinese (551 to 479 BC) used massage, hydrotherapy, and exercise as preventive health measures (Giger and Davidhizar, 1999). They also used many herbs, minerals, and acupuncture to heal the sick (Cherry and Jacob, 1999).

By the time of the Roman Empire (27 BC to 476 AD), trained physicians staffed hospitals and adopted medical practices from conquered countries. Both men and woman cared for the sick (Cherry and Jacob, 1999).

CHRISTIANITY

The entry of women into nursing can be traced to approximately 300 AD (Donahue, 1996). Christians taught that men and women are equal before God and appealed to women "to carry on His work in behalf of all who were in distress" (Shryock, 1959). The founding of the Benedictine order in the sixth century increased the number of men entering nursing. Although the Benedictines were scholars, librarians, teachers, and agriculturists, nursing the sick eventually became the chief function and duty of their community life (Donahue, 1996).

MIDDLE AGES

During the Middle Ages (1100 to 1200 AD) charitable institutions were started to care for the aged, sick, and poor (Deloughery, 1998). Nurses delivered custodial care and depended on physicians or priests for direction. Nurse midwifery, one of the oldest nursing roles, flourished during the Middle Ages. Medicine, nursing, and society recognized and accepted their role in assisting women in childbearing.

Secular groups were also formed to meet specific health care needs. The Hospital Brothers of St. Anthony cared for victims of the disease called St. Anthony's fire, the Brothers of Misericordia in Italy provided transportation services for the ill, and the Alexian Brothers (a group still active today) cared for victims of bubonic plague.

FIFTEENTH TO NINETEENTH CENTURY

The Crusades expanded health care by establishing hospitals and nursing orders for men. The Alexian Brothers and other secular groups were formed in response to the bubonic plague and the need to care for the victims. After the Crusades, large cities began to develop and grow with the decline of feudalism. The extensive population growth in cities led to certain health problems (Box 19-2) and an increased need for health care.

The lack of hygiene and sanitation, and the increasing

Problems Associated With Illnesses During the Growth of Cities   Box 19-2

Overcrowding
Poor ventilation
Poor heating and cooling
Poor sanitation, garbage collection, and plumbing
Poor water supply
Inadequate methods of preserving foods
Ignorance of elementary hygiene practices

---

poverty in urban centers resulted in serious health problems in the fifteenth to seventeenth centuries. Societal factors, such as laws punishing the poor and the Window Tax, which led to decreased ventilation because landlords bricked in windows to avoid paying the tax, created conditions and health needs to which nursing responded.

Christianity greatly influenced the development of nursing. One of the earliest records of Christian nursing was the formation of the Order of the Deaconesses, a group of public health or visiting nurses. Deaconess appointments by the bishops were highly valued and given only to women of high social standing (Deloughery, 1998). The need for nurses and increasing nursing responsibilities was due to the economic growth of the eighteenth century, the smallpox epidemics, and the Revolutionary War.

The Sisters of Charity, founded in 1633 by St. Vincent de Paul, cared for people in hospitals, asylums, and poorhouses. The sisters became widely known as visiting nurses because they cared for sick people in their homes. The first supervisor of the Sisters of Charity was Louise de Gras, a widow of high social standing who entered the order and was later known as Sr. Louise de Marillac. She established perhaps the first educational program to be associated with a nursing order and recruited intelligent, refined, and compassionate women (Donahue, 1996). The program included experiences in the care of the sick in the hospital, as well as home visits. In 1809 the Sisters of Charity was introduced in America by Mother Elizabeth Seton; later their name was changed to the Daughters of Charity (Donahue, 1996).

In the eighteenth century the further growth of cities brought an increase in the number of hospitals and an expanded role for nurses. Smallpox epidemics in the French colonies and during the Revolutionary War in the English colonies increased the need for nursing services. Because there was little formal nursing education, nursing skills and knowledge were generally passed on by experienced nurses.

During the nineteenth century, Protestant churches revived the Deaconess order. The Deaconess Institute at Kaiserswerth, Germany, was established in 1836 by Pastor

Theodore Fliedner (Donahue, 1996). The regeneration of this nursing order was stimulated by the recognition of the need for the services of nurses.

FLORENCE NIGHTINGALE

The founder of modern nursing, Florence Nightingale, established the first nursing philosophy based on health maintenance and restoration in *Notes on Nursing: What It Is and What It Is Not* (Nightingale, 1860). Her views on nursing were derived from a spiritual philosophy, developed in her adolescence and adulthood (Macrae, 1995), and reflected the changing needs of society. She saw the role of nursing as having "charge of somebody's health" based on the knowledge of "how to put the body in such a state to be free of disease or to recover from disease" (Nightingale, 1860). During the same year, she developed the first organized program for training nurses, the Nightingale Training School for Nurses at St. Thomas' Hospital in London.

Nightingale was the first practicing nurse epidemiologist (Cohen, 1984). Her religious roots were seen in the statistical analyses that connected poor sanitation with cholera and dysentery. She viewed nursing as a search for truth in finding answers to health care questions or discovering and using God's laws of healing in nursing practice (Macrae, 1995).

In 1853 Nightingale went to Paris to study with the Sisters of Charity and was later appointed superintendent of the English General Hospitals in Turkey. During this period she brought about major reforms in hygiene, sanitation, and nursing practice and reduced the mortality rate at the Barracks Hospital in Scutari, Turkey, from 42.7% to 2.2% in 6 months (Woodham-Smith, 1983; Donahue, 1996).

THE CIVIL WAR

The Civil War (1860 to 1865) stimulated the growth of nursing in the United States. Clara Barton, founder of the American Red Cross, tended soldiers on the battlefields, cleansing their wounds, meeting their basic needs, and comforting them in death. The U.S. Congress ratified the American Red Cross in 1882 after 10 years of lobbying by Barton. Dorothea Lynde Dix, Mary Ann Ball (Mother Bickerdyke), and Harriet Tubman also influenced nursing during the Civil War (Donahue, 1996). As superintendent of the female nurses of the Union Army, Dix organized hospitals, appointed nurses, and oversaw and regulated supplies to the troops. Mother Bickerdyke organized ambulance services, supervised nurses, and walked abandoned battlefields at night, looking for wounded soldiers. Harriet Tubman was active in the Underground Railroad movement and assisted in leading over 300 slaves to freedom (Donahue, 1996).

After the Civil War, nursing schools in the United States and Canada began to pattern their curricula after the Nightingale School. The first training school in Canada, St. Catherine's in Ontario, was founded in 1874 (Donahue, 1996). In 1884 Mary Agnes Snively took over the directorship of the Toronto General Hospital, and in 1908 she helped form the Canadian National Association of Trained Nurses, which became the **Canadian Nurses Association (CNA)** in 1924.

The first African-American professional nurse was Mary Mahoney. She was concerned with relationships between cultures and races, and as a noted nursing leader, she brought forth an awareness of cultural diversity and respect for the individual, regardless of background, race, color, or religion.

Isabel Hampton Robb, a graduate of St. Catherine's in Ontario, was the first superintendent of the Johns Hopkins Training School in Baltimore, Maryland, in 1894. As one of her many contributions to nursing, she helped found the Nurses' Associated Alumnae of the United States and Canada in 1896; this organization became the **American Nurses Association (ANA)** in 1911. She authored many nursing textbooks, including *Nursing: Its Principles and Practice for Hospital and Private Use* (1894), *Nursing Ethics* (1900), and *Educational Standards for Nurses* (1907), and was one of the original founders of the *American Journal of Nursing* (Donahue, 1996).

Nursing in hospitals expanded in the late nineteenth century. However, nursing in the community did not increase significantly until 1893, when Lillian Wald and Mary Brewster opened the Henry Street Settlement, which focused on the health needs of poor people who lived in tenements in New York City (Donahue, 1996). Nurses working in this settlement were some of the first to demonstrate autonomy in practice because they frequently encountered situations that required quick and innovative problem solving and critical thinking without the supervision or direction of a physician. The poor people also needed nursing therapies aimed at maintaining wellness through proper nutrition, hygiene, and shelter. Wald described her activities with the Henry Street Settlement in the textbooks *The House on Henry Street* (1915) and *Windows on Henry Street* (1934).

TWENTIETH CENTURY

In the early twentieth century a movement toward a scientific, research-based defined body of nursing knowledge and practice was seen. Nurses began to assume expanded and advanced practice roles. Mary Adelaide Nutting, a member of the first graduating class at Johns Hopkins Hospital and successor to Isabel Hampton Robb as superintendent of the Johns Hopkins Training School, was instrumental in the affiliation of nursing education with universities. She became the first professor of nursing at Columbia University Teachers College in 1907 (Donahue, 1996).

In 1923 the Rockefeller Foundation funded a survey of nursing education, the Goldmark Report. The report concluded that nursing education needed increased financial support and suggested that the money be given to university schools of nursing. As a result, the Rockefeller Foundation funded the expansion of several nursing programs, including those at Yale and Vanderbilt universities and the University of Toronto.

As nursing education developed, nursing practice also expanded. In 1901 the Army Nurse Corps was established, followed in 1908 by the Navy Nurse Corps. By the 1920s nursing specialization was developing. Graduate nurse-midwifery programs were initiated, and beginning in the 1950s specialty nursing organizations, such as the Association of Operating Room Nurses (1949), American Association of Critical-Care Nurses (1969), and Oncology Nursing Society (1975), were formed.

NATIONAL COMMISSION ON NURSING AND NURSING EDUCATION

In 1965 the National Commission on Nursing and Nursing Education explored issues that included the supply of and demand for nurses, clarification of nursing roles and functions, education of nurses, and career opportunities available to nurses. Their report, often called the Lysaught report after Jerome P. Lysaught, the director of the study, called for clarification of nursing roles and responsibilities in relation to those of other health care professionals. It also advocated greater financial support for nurses and more career opportunities to attract nurses and retain them in the profession (Lysaught, 1970).

As nursing practice and education evolved to meet the needs of society, nursing's code of ethics, initially discussed in 1897, was revised to meet the scientific advancement. The first written ANA Code of Ethics was proposed in 1926 to "create a sensitiveness to ethical situations and to formulate general principles which result in the formation of conscious and critical judgment resulting in action in specific situations" (ANA, 1926). Again, as technology and the needs of society changed, the code underwent multiple revisions, the most recent being the *Code for Nurses With Interpretive Statements* (ANA, 1985) (see Chapter 20).

Today, the profession is faced with multiple challenges. Nurses and nurse educators are revising nursing practice and curricula to meet the ever-changing needs of society. Advances in technology, the rising acuity of clients, and early discharge from health care institutions require nurses to have a strong and current knowledge base from which to practice. Nursing practice is moving toward multiple care settings that are based in institutions, the community, and home care agencies. The challenge now is to prepare professional nurses to deliver complex, multifaceted care in the client's home.

NURSING THEORIES

Nurses theorize about the nature of nursing practice, the principles on which practice is based, and the proper goals and functions of nursing in society. Conceptual and theoretical nursing models are used to provide knowledge to improve practice, guide research and curricula, and identify the domain and goals of nursing practice (see Chapter 5). **Nursing theories** guide future directions for nursing research, practice, education, and administration (Meleis, 1997; Marriner-Tomey and Alligood, 1998; Chinn and Kramer, 1999).

Nursing as a Profession

PROFESSIONALISM

Nursing is not simply a collection of specific skills, and the nurse is not simply a person trained to perform specific tasks. Nursing is a profession. No one factor absolutely differentiates a job from a profession, but the difference is important in terms of how nurses practice. When we say a person acts "professionally," for example, we imply that the person is conscientious in actions, knowledgeable in the subject, and responsible to self and others. Professions possess the following primary characteristics:

A profession requires an extended education of its members, as well as a basic liberal foundation.

A profession has a theoretical body of knowledge leading to defined skills, abilities, and norms.

A profession provides a specific service.

Members of a profession have autonomy in decision making and practice.

The profession as a whole has a code of ethics for practice.

Nursing clearly shares, to some extent, each of these characteristics. However, nursing as a profession still faces controversial issues as nurses strive for greater professionalism.

EDUCATION

As a profession, nursing requires that its members possess a significant amount of education. The issue of standardization of nursing education and entry into practice is a major controversy today. The ANA's 1965 position paper on nursing education emphasizes the role of education in the profession (Box 19-3). In 1984 the ANA described two levels of practice: the associate nurse and the professional nurse, which required a baccalaureate degree in nursing. The **National League for Nursing (NLN)** also supported a proposal that required associate and diploma graduates to take the same licensing examination. Most nurses agree that nursing education is important to practice and that it must respond to changes in health care created by scientific and technological advances.

THEORY

The practice of professional nursing and nursing knowledge has been developed through nursing theories. Theoretical models serve as frameworks for nursing curricula and clinical practice. Nursing theories also lead to

Nursing is a helping profession and, as such, provides services which contribute to the health and well-being of people.

Nursing is of vital consequence to the individual receiving services; it fills needs which cannot be met by the person, by the family, or by other persons in the community.

The demand for services of nurses will continue to increase.

The professional practitioner is responsible for the nature and quality of all nursing care that clients receive.

The services of professional practitioners of nursing will continue to be supplemented and complemented by the services of nurse practitioners who will be licensed.

Education for those in the health professions must increase in depth and breadth as scientific knowledge expands.

In addition to those licensed as nurses, the health care of the public, in the amount and to the extent needed and demanded, requires the services of large numbers of health occupation workers to function as assistants to nurses. These workers are presently designated: nurses' aides, orderlies, assistants, attendants, etc.

The professional association must concern itself with the nature of nursing practice, the means for improving nursing practice, the education necessary for practice, and the standards for membership in the professional association.

From American Nurses Association: *A position paper: educational preparation for nurse practitioners and assistants to nurses,* Kansas City, Mo, 1965, The Association.

further research that increases the scientific basis of nursing practice (see Chapter 5).

SERVICE

Nursing has always been a service profession, although in the past the service was usually viewed as a charitable one. Today, nursing is a vital and indispensable component of the health care delivery system. Nurses today and in the future need a more consumer-focused and service-based practice. Clients are more aware and educated through written and visual media, as well as the Internet. The nurse needs to work with the client and family, individualizing care, considering cultural and religious differences, and providing support for the entire family and extended family. Respect for the client's time is shown by providing services on time, scheduling tests to meet the consumer's needs, and reducing waiting times in outpatient and emergency settings.

AUTONOMY

Autonomy is an essential element to professional nursing. Autonomy means that a person is reasonably independent and self-governing in decision making and practice. In the past, physicians, hospital administrators, and others in the health care delivery system have found nursing autonomy difficult to understand and support. Nurses attain in-

creased autonomy through higher levels of education. Through clinical competence and diverse practice settings, nurses are increasingly taking on independent roles in nurse-run clinics, collaborative practice, and advanced nurse practice settings.

With increased autonomy come greater responsibility and accountability. Accountability means that the nurse is responsible, professionally and legally, for the type and quality of nursing care provided. The nurse is accountable for keeping abreast of technical skills and knowledge needed to perform nursing care. The nursing profession itself regulates accountability through nursing audits and standards of practice.

CODE OF ETHICS

Nursing has a **code of ethics** that defines the principles by which nurses' function. In addition, nurses incorporate their own values and ethics into practice. The ANA has a number of publications that address ethics and human rights in nursing. The *Code for Nurses With Interpretive Statements* provides a guide for carrying out nursing responsibilities that provide quality nursing care and provides for the ethical obligations of the profession (ANA, 1985). Other areas include ethical guidelines for conducting nursing research (ANA, 1995); ethical dilemmas and how the nurse would handle the situation (ANA 1993); and guidelines for reporting incompetent, unethical, or illegal practices (ANA, 1994). Together, these guidelines provide the nurse with a framework for conducting practice. Chapter 20 gives several examples of specific statements of nursing's code of ethics.

Educational Preparation

PROFESSIONAL REGISTERED NURSE EDUCATION

There are various educational routes for becoming a professional **registered nurse (RN)**. Initially, hospital schools of nursing were developed to educate nurses to work within those institutions. As nursing increasingly defined its own body of knowledge, formalized educational processes developed to ensure a consistent level of education in institutions. Such consistency was also necessary for RN licensure.

Currently in the United States an individual can become an RN by completion of an associate degree, diploma, or baccalaureate degree program. In Canada there are currently only diploma and baccalaureate degree programs.

Associate Degree Education.   The associate degree program in the United States is a 2-year program that is usually offered by a university or junior college. This program focuses on the basic sciences and theoretical and clinical courses related to the practice of nursing. Graduates of this type of program take the state board examination for RN licensure.

Diploma Education. The diploma program in the United States is a 2- or 3-year hospital-based program. Diploma programs focus on the basic sciences and on theoretical and clinical courses related to nursing practice, usually with a substantial clinical component. Some diploma programs are affiliated with colleges or universities, which grant college credit for nonnursing courses. Graduates of a diploma program receive a diploma from the hospital and are eligible to take the state board examination for RN licensure. In the United States, diploma programs are declining in numbers. In Canada, diploma programs are offered in community colleges or hospitals and are 2-year programs (or 3 years in some hospital-based programs) that are comparable to associate degree programs in the United States.

Baccalaureate Education. The baccalaureate degree program usually encompasses 4 years of study in a college or university. The program focuses on the basic sciences and on theoretical and clinical courses, as well as courses in the social sciences, arts, and humanities to support nursing theory. In Canada the degree of Bachelor of Science in Nursing (BScN) or Bachelor in Nursing (BN) is equivalent to the degree of Bachelor of Science in Nursing (BSN) in the United States. The American Association of Colleges of Nursing (AACN) published the *Essentials of Baccalaureate Education for Professional Nursing: A Final Report* (1998). This document delineated essential knowledge, practice and values, attitudes, personal qualities, and professional behavior for the baccalaureate-prepared nurse. The goal of this document was to provide standards by which "faculty can measure the content of the curriculum and the performance of the graduate" (American Association of Colleges of Nursing, 1998).

RN completion programs are available at many colleges and universities. These programs are designed to assist the practicing RN in obtaining a baccalaureate degree in nursing. The Internet, computerized learning programs, shared faculty via teleconferencing, and weekend and evening options provide the practicing RN many options for degree completion. Some innovative universities have programs at the baccalaureate level in an accelerated 12-month program when the candidate already has a baccalaureate degree in a basic science.

ACCREDITATION

To be accredited, nursing programs must meet certain criteria established by the National League for Nursing Accrediting Commission (NLNAC). This voluntary accreditation is available for basic nursing education programs and master's degree programs in nursing. The NLNAC is responsible for the accreditation of all levels of nursing education. The purposes of the accreditation of education programs in nursing are to (NLNAC, 1999):

Uphold agreed upon standards for educational quality and public accountability.

Assure the public of accurate information regarding nursing in education programs at any level.

Foster continuous development and improvement in the quality of educational programs in nursing.

Evaluate nursing programs in relation both to their stated purpose and the agreed upon standards and criteria for accreditation.

Involve institutional administrators and the faculty, staff, and students of nursing programs in the process of continuous self-examination.

Bring together practitioners, administrators, faculty, staff, and students in improving nursing quality and the preparation of students for their responsibilities to society. Provide for external peer-review.

LICENSURE

In the United States, RN candidates must pass the National Council Licensure Examination for Registered Nurses (NCLEX-RN), which is administered by the individual State Boards of Nursing. Regardless of educational preparation, the examination for RN licensure is exactly the same in every state in the United States. This provides a standardized minimum knowledge base for the client population nurses serve.

In Canada the CNA Testing Service (CNATS) administers the test to qualified candidates in each province. Whether nurses can practice in a state or province other than their own depends on the agreement between the states or provinces involved.

RN licensure for practice in the United States requires that the student complete a prescribed course of study from program approved by the State Board of Nursing in the state in which the student is seeking licensure. The process for licensure application is unique to each state. In some states a minimum number of continuing education courses is required to maintain licensure. In Canada a Provincial Board of Nursing must approve the program in the province in which the student is seeking licensure.

CERTIFICATION

Beyond the NCLEX-RN, the nurse may choose to work toward certification in a specific area of nursing practice. Minimum practice requirements are set, based on the certification the nurse is seeking. National nursing organizations, such as the ANA, have many types of certification that the nurse can work toward. After passing the initial examination, the nurse maintains certification by ongoing continuing education and clinical or administrative practice.

As expressed by the ANA (1969), the purpose of a graduate education in nursing is to prepare advanced practice nurses who are capable of improving nursing care through the advancement of nursing theory and sciences.

MASTER'S DEGREE PREPARATION

A person completing a graduate program can receive the degree of Master of Arts (MA) in nursing, Master in Nursing (MN), or Master of Science in Nursing (MSN).

This provides the advanced clinician with strong skills in nursing science and theory with emphasis in the basic sciences and research-based clinical practice. A master's degree in nursing can be valuable for nurses seeking roles of nurse educator, clinical nurse specialist, nurse administrator, or nurse practitioner. These roles are described later in this chapter.

DOCTORAL PREPARATION

The first nursing doctorate program opened in 1953 at the University of Pittsburgh. Professional doctoral programs in nursing (DSN or DNSc) emphasize the application of research findings to clinical nursing. Other programs emphasize more basic research and theory and award the degree of Doctor of Philosophy (PhD) in nursing. The need for nurses with doctorate degrees is rising. Expanding clinical roles, new areas of nursing such as nursing informatics, and rapidly advancing technology are just a few reasons for increasing the number of doctorally prepared nurses. It is important to continue to do research in areas such as nursing theory, basic science, and clinical practice to expand nursing knowledge. Doctorally prepared nurses are needed to educate the beginning nurse and those seeking advanced academic and clinical preparation.

CONTINUING AND IN-SERVICE EDUCATION

Because nursing is a dynamic profession, continuing education programs help nurses remain current in nursing skills, knowledge, and theory. **Continuing education** involves formal, organized, and educational programs offered by State Nurses Associations (Figure 19-1) and educational and health care institutions. As expressed by the ANA (1994), the goals of continuing education in nursing are to improve and maintain nursing practice, promote and exercise leadership in effecting change in health care delivery systems, and fulfill professional learning needs. Other goals include helping nurses become specialized in a particular area of practice and teaching nurses' new skills and techniques.

In general, continuing education programs are short term and are designed for all nurses. The ANA or the State Board of Nursing is the accrediting agency for these programs. The ANA awards continuing education units on completion of specific courses. Some states require nurses to take continuing education courses for license renewal. An **in-service education** program is instruction or training provided by a health care agency or institution. An in-service program is held in the institution and is designed to increase the knowledge, skills, and competencies of nurses and other health care professionals employed by the institution. For example, a hospital might offer an in-service program to inform nurses about primary nursing before it is implemented at the hospital.

All nurses have access to continuing education and in-service programs organized and conducted by a university, private hospital, private continuing education service, or the employing institution or agency. Such programs assist the practicing nurse in acquiring new knowledge and skills necessary for today's highly technical and fast-changing health care delivery system.

Education continues to be important after the nurse begins practice, whether the practice setting focuses on the adult or child, the chronically or acutely ill, or the home or hospital. Nursing encompasses an ever-widening range of roles. Multiple career paths and goals are open to new and experienced practitioners.

LICENSED PRACTICAL NURSE EDUCATION

A licensed practical or vocational nurse is trained in basic nursing techniques and direct client care. The **licensed practical nurse (LPN)** or **licensed vocational nurse (LVN)** practices under the supervision of a registered nurse in a hospital or community health practice setting. An LPN, or in Canada a registered nurse's assistant (RNA), generally receives 1 year of education and training in a hospital, community college, or other agency. The LPN or LVN is licensed by a board after completing the educational program and passing the licensure examination.

• • •

Nurses practice in a variety of settings, in many roles within those settings, and with other caregivers in the allied health professions. Administrators in hospitals and other health care agencies and institutions guide the practice of nursing only in part. State and provincial Nurse Practice Acts establish specific legal regulations for practice, and professional organizations establish standards of practice as criteria for nursing care.

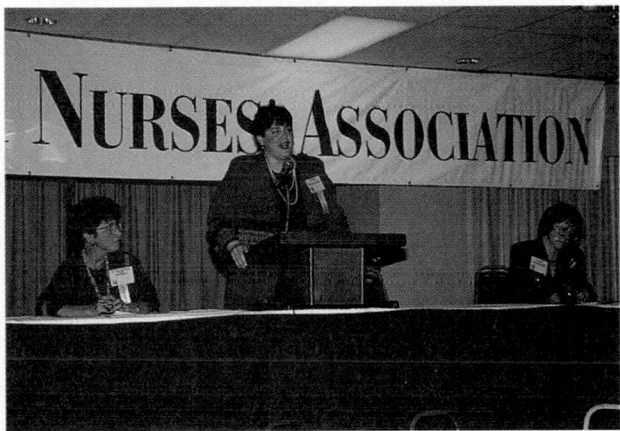

Figure 19-1   Participating at State Nurses Association meetings provides continuing education and networking opportunities.

Nursing Practice

AMERICAN NURSES ASSOCIATION DEFINITION OF NURSING PRACTICE

In 1955 the ANA published the following official definition of nursing practice:

> The practice of professional nursing means the performance for compensation of any act in the observation, care, and counsel of the ill, injured, or infirm or in the maintenance of health or prevention of illness of others, or in the supervision and teaching of other personnel, or the administration of medications and treatments as prescribed by licensed physician or dentist, requiring substantial specialized judgment and skill and based on knowledge and application of the principles of biological, physical, and social sciences. The foregoing shall not be deemed to include acts of diagnosis or prescription of therapeutic or corrective measures.

This early definition by the ANA is significant in its attempt to define nursing practice in a fairly specific manner. Nonetheless, it tends to stress nursing's dependent role, an emphasis no longer accepted. In 1965 the ANA Committee on Education issued a position paper that presents a fuller definition of nursing as a helping profession that, as such, provides services that contribute to the health of people, and emphasizes nursing as an independent profession:

> Nursing is a vital consequence to the individual receiving services; it fills needs that cannot be met by the person, family, or other persons in the community.

Three essential components of professional nursing are care, cure, and coordination. The care aspect is more than "to take care of"; it is also "caring for" and "caring about." Caring is dealing with human beings under stress, frequently over long periods of time. The caring component of nursing provides comfort and support in times of anxiety, loneliness, and helplessness. It involves listening, evaluating, and intervening appropriately (see Chapter 6).

The promotion of health and healing is the cure aspect of professional nursing. To cure is to assist clients in understanding their health problems and helping them cope. The cure aspect involves the administration of medications and treatments, and the use of clinical nursing judgment in determining, on the basis of client outcomes, whether the plan of care needs to be maintained or changed. It is knowing when and how to use existing and potential resources to help patients move toward recovery and adjustment by mobilizing their own resources.

Professional nursing practice shares responsibility for the health and welfare of all people in the community and participates in programs designed to prevent illness and maintain health. It also coordinates and synchronizes medical and other professional and technical services that affect patient care. A professional nurse supervises, teaches, and directs all those involved in nursing care.

In 1979 the Committee of Chairpersons of the ANA determined that the Congress for Nursing Practice should define the nature and scope of nursing practice. The Congress for Nursing Practice is the part of the ANA concerned with legal aspects of nursing practice, public recognition of the significance of nursing practice to health care, and implications for nursing practice of trends in health care. In 1980 the Congress for Nursing Practice defined nursing as the diagnosis and treatment of human responses to actual or potential health problems (ANA, 1980). This definition involves the following characteristics of nursing: phenomena, theory application, nursing action, and evaluation of the effects of action. Phenomena are the human responses to actual or potential health problems. The nurse identifies the client's responses by assessing health status and obtaining data. The nurse applies nursing theory to understand these responses. The nurse takes actions to resolve actual or potential health care problems. The nurse then evaluates the effects of the actions on the client's responses. These four characteristics are related to the nursing process, which is described in Unit 3.

CANADIAN NURSES ASSOCIATION DEFINITION OF NURSING PRACTICE

The CNA's *A Definition of Nursing Practice* and *Standards for Nursing Practice* (1986) defined nursing as a

> . . . dynamic, caring, helping relationship in which the nurse assists the client to achieve and maintain optimal health. The nurse fulfills this purpose by applying knowledge and skills from nursing and related fields using the nursing process, the substance of which is determined by a conceptual model(s) for nursing.

Founded in 1908, the CNA provides leadership to practicing nurses in the Canadian provinces through its actions and activities to allow Canadian nurses to meet the health care demands of the Canadian society.

STANDARDS OF NURSING PRACTICE

As an independent profession, nursing has increasingly set its own standards for practice. Standards of nursing practice serve as objective guidelines for nurses to provide care and as a means to evaluate care. Standards of nursing practice are developed and established based on strong scientific research and the work of nurse clinical experts. They provide a method to assure clients that they are receiving high-quality care, that the nurses know exactly what is necessary to provide nursing care, and that measures are in place to determine whether the care meets the standards. The ANA has published *Standards of Professional Performance* (Table 19-1), and the CNA has published *Standards for Nursing Practice* (Box 19-4).

STANDARDS OF CARE

Competent levels of nursing care are described by the *Standards of Clinical Practice* (Table 19-2). The levels of care are demonstrated through the nursing process: as-

Table 19-1   ANA Standards of Professional Performance

Standard	Definition	Measurement Criteria
I: Quality of care	The nurse systematically evaluates the quality and effectiveness of nursing practice.	Participates in quality-of-care activities. Practice changes are a result of quality-of-care activities. Quality-of-care activities are used to initiate changes throughout the health care delivery system.
II: Performance appraisal	The nurse evaluates one's own nursing practice in relation to professional practice standards and relevant statutes and regulations.	Engages in performance appraisal on a regular basis. Seeks constructive feedback regarding one's own practice. Takes action to achieve goals identified during performance appraisal. Participates in peer review as appropriate. Practice reflects knowledge of current professional practice standards, laws, and regulations.
III: Education	The nurse acquires and maintains current knowledge and competency in nursing practice.	Participates in ongoing educational activities related to clinical knowledge and professional issues. Seeks experiences to maintain clinical skills. Seeks knowledge and skills appropriate to the practice setting.
IV: Collegiality	The nurse interacts with, and contributes to the professional development of, peers and other health care providers as colleagues.	Shares knowledge and skills with colleagues. Provides peers with constructive feedback regarding their practice. Interacts with colleagues to enhance one's own professional nursing practice. Contributes to an environment that is conducive to clinical education of nursing students as appropriate. Contributes to a supportive and healthy work environment.
V: Ethics	The nurse's decisions and actions on behalf of patients are determined in an ethical manner.	Practice is guided by the *Code for Nurses.* Maintains patient confidentiality. Acts as a patient advocate. Delivers care in a nonjudgmental and nondiscriminatory manner that is sensitive to patient diversity. Delivers care in a manner that preserves patient autonomy, dignity, and rights. Seeks available resources in formulating ethical decisions.
VI: Collaboration	The nurse collaborates with the patient, family, and other health care providers in providing patient care.	Communicates with the patient, significant others, and health care providers regarding patient care and nursing's role in the provision of care. The nurse collaborates with the patient, family, and other health care providers in the formulation of overall goals and the plan of care and in the decisions related to care and delivery of services. Consults with health care providers for patient care as needed. Makes referrals, including provisions for continuity of care, as needed.

VII: Research	The nurse uses research findings in practice.	Utilizes best available evidence, preferable research data, to develop the plan of care and interventions.
		Participates in research activities as appropriate to the nurse's education and position. Such activities may include:
		    Identifying clinical problems suitable for nursing research
		    Participating in data collection
		    Participating in a unit, organization, or community research committee
		    Sharing research activities with others
		    Conducting research
		    Critiquing research for application to practice
		Using research findings in the development of policies, procedures, and practice guidelines for patient care.

VIII: Resource utilization	The nurse considers factors related to safety, effectiveness, and cost in planning and delivering patient care.	Evaluates factors related to safety, effectiveness, availability, and cost when practice options would result in the same expected patient outcome. Assists the patient and family in identifying and securing appropriate and available services to address health-related needs. Assigns or delegates tasks as defined by the state nurse practice acts and according to the knowledge and skills of the designated caregiver. Assigns or delegates tasks based on the needs and condition of the patient, the potential for harm, the stability of the patient's condition, the complexity of the task, and the predictability of the outcome. Assists the patient and family in becoming informed consumers about the cost, risks, and benefits of treatment and care.

Modified from American Nurses Association: *Standards of clinical practice,* ed 2, Washington, DC, 1998, The Association.

sessment, diagnosis, outcome identification, planning, implementation, and evaluation. The nursing process is the foundation of clinical decision making and includes all significant actions taken by nurses in providing care to clients. Within these standards are the nursing responsibilities for diversity: safety, education, health promotion, treatment, self-care, and planning for the continuity of care (ANA 1998). Standards of care are important if a legal dispute arises over whether a nurse practiced appropriately in a particular case (see Chapter 21).

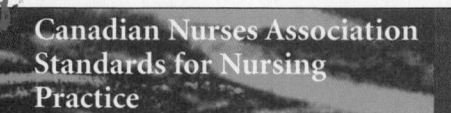

Canadian Nurses Association Standards for Nursing Practice   Box 19-4

Nursing practice requires that a conceptual model(s) for nursing be the basis of practice.
Nursing practice requires the effective use of the nursing process.
Nursing practice requires that the helping relationship be the nature of the client-nurse interaction.
Nursing practice requires nurses to fulfill professional responsibilities.

Modified from Canadian Nurses Association: *A definition of nursing practice. Standards for nursing practice,* Ottawa, 1986, The Association.

Nurse Practice Acts

In all states in the United States and all provinces in Canada, Nurse Practice Acts regulate the licensure and practice of nursing. Each state or province defines for itself the scope of nursing practice, but most have similar practice acts. The definition of nursing practice published by the ANA in 1955 (see p. 384) is in some ways representative of the scope of nursing practice as defined in most states and provinces. In the last decade, however, many states have revised their Nurse Practice Acts to reflect nursings' growing autonomy and the expanded roles of nurses in practice. The 1955 ANA prohibition against diagnosis and treatment, for example, has been removed from nurse practice acts in many states or rephrased to differentiate between nursing diagnosis and treatment, and medical diagnosis and treatment.

Practice Settings

Nursing practice settings are expanding as a result of changes in the health care delivery system. Nurses need an educational basis to prepare them to address the ever-changing health care needs of their clients, develop research skills to monitor client outcomes, and increase their psychomotor skills and cognitive knowledge as technology increases (AACN 1993). There is a greater emphasis on community-based practice, and the knowledge base for this practice developed from traditional and nontraditional methods. Table 19-3 gives statistics on the numbers of nurses in practice settings.

Hospitals, Skilled Nursing, and Restorative Settings

Hospital nursing is the largest group of practicing nurses. Hospitals may be acute, long-term, or rehabilitation care facilities. Nurses employed in the acute care setting care for clients with severe, multisystem illness and complex medical, psychological, and social problems. These clients are usually more dependent and more seriously ill than clients in the past, compounded by shorter hospitalizations. As a result, nursing practice in acute care settings has become more specialized and complex. Organ transplantation, advanced technological equipment used to support clients in the critical care setting, and opportunistic infections contribute to a higher percentage of critically ill clients in hospitals.

The clinical area of practice determines the skills and knowledge needed to practice in this setting. Advances in technology have required the nurse to be not only knowledgeable about nursing practice, but also computer literate, able to manage multiple pieces of complex equipment and remain customer focused.

Current reimbursement practices of private and federal or state insurance groups have resulted in shorter hospital stays (see Chapter 2). Clients are being discharged from hospitals sooner and often require continued nursing care at home. The hospital-based professional nurse needs to be knowledgeable about community-based resources and able to anticipate the client's home health care needs. Through early discharge planning and collaborating with case managers, physicians, social workers, and home health care agencies, the client's needs are evaluated and care is planned.

Nursing services in the hospital operate 24 hours a day, 7 days a week. Differing staffing patterns are used to meet the need for nursing care, including 8-hour shifts, 12-hour shifts, or 10-hour shifts that overlap during the early morning, late afternoon, and night. Many hospitals have alternative staffing patterns to help attract staff, such as 12-hour weekends only, or 4-hour or 6-hour shifts to assist during peak care times. The roles and responsibilities of nurses employed in hospitals vary because hospitals differ widely in size and organizational structure. Hospital floors may be specialized by case type, such as neurology or orthopedics, or may be simply medicine and general surgery. University-affiliated hospitals often have many areas of specialization. All hospitals accredited by the Joint Commission on Accreditation of Hospitals and Organizations (JCAHO) require an RN as the chief nurse executive who is responsible for the nursing care and standards for the organization.

Increases in health care costs, reduction in insurance reimbursement, increasing numbers of health maintenance organizations (HMOs), and a larger population of capitated clients have challenged hospitals and other health care institutions to develop creative ways of meeting the budget. Many organizations have changed the skill mix of direct care providers. More assistive personnel are being employed to help reduce staff costs and help provide direct care while reducing ancillary care providers, such as phlebotomy or transport.

An increasing older adult population and more complex supportive care measures have given rise to an in-

Table 19-2   ANA Standards of Care

Standard	Measurement Criteria
Assessment The nurse collects patient health data.	Data collection involves the patient, significant others, and health care providers when appropriate. The priority of data collection is determined by the patient's immediate condition or needs. Pertinent data are collected using appropriate assessment techniques. Relevant data are documented in a retrievable form. The data collection process is systematic and ongoing.
Nursing Diagnosis The nurse analyzes the assessment data in determining diagnoses.	Diagnoses are derived from the assessment data. Diagnoses are validated with the patient, significant others, and health care providers, when possible. Diagnoses are documented in a manner that facilitates the determination of expected outcomes and plan of care.
The nurse identifies expected outcomes individualized to the patient.	Outcomes are derived from the diagnoses. Outcomes are mutually formulated with the patient and health care providers, when possible. Outcomes are culturally appropriate and realistic in relation to the patient's present and potential capabilities. Outcomes are attainable in relation to resources available to the patient. Outcomes include a time estimate for attainment. Outcomes provide direction for continuity of care. Outcomes are documented as measurable goals.
Planning The nurse develops a plan of care that prescribes interventions to attain expected outcomes.	The plan is individualized to the patient and patient's condition or needs. The plan is developed with the patient, significant others, and health care providers, when appropriate. The plan reflects current nursing practice. The plan provides for continuity of care. Priorities for care are established. The plan is documented.
Implementation The nurse implements the interventions identified in the plan of care.	Interventions are consistent with the established plan of care. Interventions are implemented in a safe and appropriate manner. Interventions are documented.
Evaluation The nurse evaluates the patient's progress toward attainment of outcomes.	Evaluation is systematic, ongoing, and criterion-based. The patient, significant others, and health care providers are involved in the evaluation process, when appropriate. Ongoing assessment data are used to revise diagnoses, outcomes, and the plan of care as needed. Revisions in diagnoses, outcomes, and the plan of care are documented. The effectiveness of interventions is evaluated in relation to outcomes. The patient's responses to interventions are documented.

From American Nurses Association: *Standards of clinical nursing practice,* ed 2, Washington, DC, 1998, The Association.

creased need for skilled nursing facilities. Older adults may not have a spouse to help with home care, and often children work or have families of their own. Skilled nursing facilities provide for care needs that cannot be met in the home and that require nursing support and care planning. Skilled nursing facilities are an intermediate step between the hospital and home.

The increasing numbers of older adults, clients with chronic illnesses, and clients with functional impairments have resulted in the growth of long-term care facilities. Long-term care is provided in institutions such as chronic disease hospitals, psychiatric hospitals, and nursing homes. Nursing homes are the most common agencies providing in-house, long-term care.

Table 19-3 **Demographics for Today's Registered Nurses**		
	United States*	Canada†
Licensed nurses	2.2 million	260 thousand
Employed nurses	1.8 million	220 thousand
Gender:		
Female	95.7%	95.8%
Male	4.3%	4.2%
Race:		
White/Caucasian	90%	—
African-American	4%	—
Asian/Pacific Islanders	3.4%	—
Hispanics	1.4%	—
American Indian/Alaska Natives	0.4%	—
Age:		
<30 years	4.0%	—
30-49 years	>60%	—
Education:		
Diploma program	10%	77.6%
Associate degree	59%	—
Bachelor's degree	31%	20.8%
Master's degree	7.5%	1.5%
Doctorate	0.5%	0.1%
Hospitals	66%	62.4%
Nursing homes/extended care	7%	11.8%
Community/public health	10%	7.1%
Home care	—	4.4%
Ambulatory care	8%	—
Other (physician office, nursing education)	10%	14.3%

*Data from American Nurses Association: Nursing facts: today's registered nurse—number and demographics. From *Sixth national sample of registered nurses,* March 1992, U.S. Department of Health and Human Services, Public Health Service, Division of Nursing, Health Resources and Services Administration.

†Data from Canadian Nurses Association, Policy Regulation and Research Division: *1998 RN data statistics,* Ottawa, Canada, 1999, The Association.

Restorative care facilities generally employ many types of health care professionals. The goal of these institutions is to teach disabled clients to achieve a maximal level of function and to teach families to help them reach that level (see Chapter 2).

COMMUNITY-BASED PRACTICE SETTINGS

The number of nurses employed in community-based practice settings is increasing substantially. The rising cost of institutional care creates the need for community-based nursing services aimed at health promotion, disease prevention, and restorative care (see Chapter 3).

Nursing in community-based settings is focused on health promotion and maintenance, education and management, and coordination and continuity of restorative care within the client's community. Community-based nurses assess the health needs of individuals, families, and communities, and help clients cope with threats to health and problems of illness. Whereas institutional health care focuses on the individual and family, community-based nursing is also directed toward the health of the commu-

nity and the interaction of individuals within that community. A community can be a particular location, such as an urban or rural area, or a group of people related by occupation, school, or another common interest or characteristic. Thus community-based nurses are employed in a variety of practice settings, including community and occupational health centers, schools, home health care agencies, health clinics, and private practices.

Community Health Centers. Community health centers offer comprehensive programs for health maintenance and promotion, education and management, and coordination of care within the community. Community health centers provide ambulatory care (care sought by clients able to come to the centers), as well as care within the home.

Nurses employed in these centers often work more independently than nurses in institutional settings did. Community health centers also employ other health professionals, but nurses generally provide most of the care and may in fact own and operate the facility (Figure 19-2).

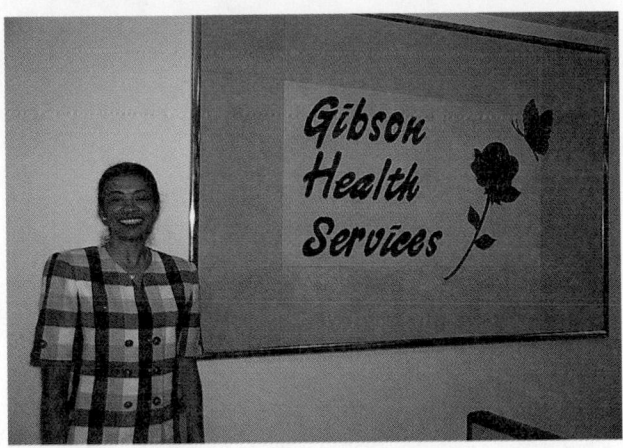

Figure 19-2   Nursing provides opportunities to create local health care centers.

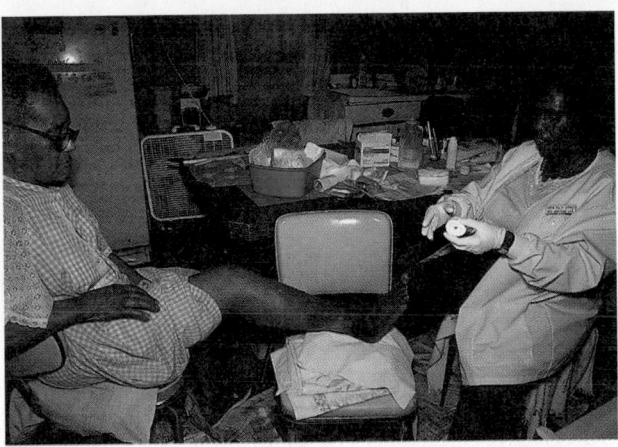

Figure 19-3   Nurse teaching a client about care in the home setting.

In some settings physicians are called in only when specific needs arise. Examples of community health centers are Planned Parenthood clinics and family care and mental health centers.

Schools.   Community-based health services are common in schools and on college campuses. Nursing services include health education in disease prevention, health promotion, and sex education. In addition, nurses working in schools may provide care for students with non-emergent acute illnesses, such as upper respiratory tract infections, influenza, infections with other opportunistic pathogens, and minor cuts and abrasions. School nurses also make referrals for students and their families when additional, more specialized health care is needed.

Occupational Health Settings.   Many large companies provide health services to employees in occupational health centers located on the premises. Nursing care in these settings involves five areas. The nurse may develop programs aimed at increasing health and safety in the workplace by reducing the number of occupational accidents, the risk of occupational disease, or the transmission of a contagious disease among the workers. The nurse may provide programs for health promotion, disease prevention, and health education. As corporations realize that health promotion and disease prevention provide a better workforce, the nurse may take a more active role in risk factor identification for heart disease, provide education for breast self-examination, and assist employees with health promotion and maintenance plans. They may also assist in supervised exercise programs for employees with known health problems; the nurse also treats nonemergent acute illness and provides first aid. In emergency situations such as heart attacks or trauma, the nurse gives emergency care and arranges transportation to a hospital. The nurse also refers employees to additional health resources when necessary.

Home Health Care Agencies.   A client often needs specific nursing care that can be given efficiently in the home. Nurses in these agencies provide home-based nursing care to clients discharged from that particular institution. Other agencies providing home health care include The Visiting Nurse Association, public health nursing agencies, hospices, and private home care agencies.

The nurse who functions in the home must also be skilled at teaching. Rising health care costs have limited the duration and frequency of visits. As a result, the home health care nurse often teaches the client or family to competently perform nursing activities and self-care. Caring for the client in the home environment requires the nurse to be flexible, resourceful, creative, and self-confident, as well as clinically competent (see Chapter 3) (Figure 19-3).

Other Settings.   There are many settings in which nurses practice and where their roles and responsibilities vary widely. A nurse may be employed in a physician's office, a managed care organization, or a health care consultation service. A nurse may practice in solo or joint practice with other nurses and other health care professionals who provide care independently to well or stable client groups. Nurses are also employed in educational and research positions.

Regardless of the practice setting, nurses are challenged to deliver quality care. Nursing research linking quality client outcome studies with cost-effectiveness reveals that nurses are meeting the challenge. Nurses are an active voice at all levels of government, speaking out about health care issues and providing information to the public.

Roles and Functions of the Nurse

FUNCTIONS

Contemporary nursing requires that the nurse possess knowledge and skills in a variety of areas. In the past, the principal role of nurses was to provide care and comfort as they carried out specific nursing functions. However, changes in nursing have expanded the role to include increased emphasis on health promotion and illness prevention, as well as concern for the client as a whole. The contemporary nurse functions in the interrelated roles of caregiver, clinical and ethical decision maker, protector and client advocate, case manager, rehabilitator, comforter, communicator, and teacher.

Caregiver.   As **caregiver,** the nurse helps the client regain health through the healing process. Healing is more than just curing a specific disease, although treatment skills that promote physical healing are important to caregivers. The nurse addresses the holistic health care needs of the client, including measures to restore emotional, spiritual, and social well-being. The caregiver helps the client and families set goals and meet those goals with a minimal cost of time and energy.

Clinical Decision Maker.   As **clinical decision maker,** the nurse uses critical thinking skills throughout the nursing process to provide effective care. Before undertaking any nursing action, whether it is assessing the client's condition, giving care, or evaluating the results of care, the nurse plans the action by deciding the best approach for each client (see Unit 3). The nurse makes these decisions alone or in collaboration with the client and family (Figure 19-4). In each of these situations, the nurse collaborates and consults with other health care professionals (Keeling and Ramos, 1995).

Protector and Client Advocate.   As protector, the nurse helps maintain a safe environment for the client and takes steps to prevent injury and protect the client from possible adverse effects of diagnostic or treatment measures. Confirming that a client does not have an allergy to a medication and providing immunization against disease in a community-based practice are examples of the nurse's protective role (see Chapter 37).

In the role of **client advocate,** the nurse protects the client's human and legal rights and provides assistance in asserting those rights if the need arises. The nurse advocates for the client, keeping in mind the client's religion and culture. For example, the nurse may provide additional information for a client who is trying to decide whether or not to accept a treatment, or the nurse may assist with communication within the family. The nurse may also defend clients' rights in a general way by speaking out

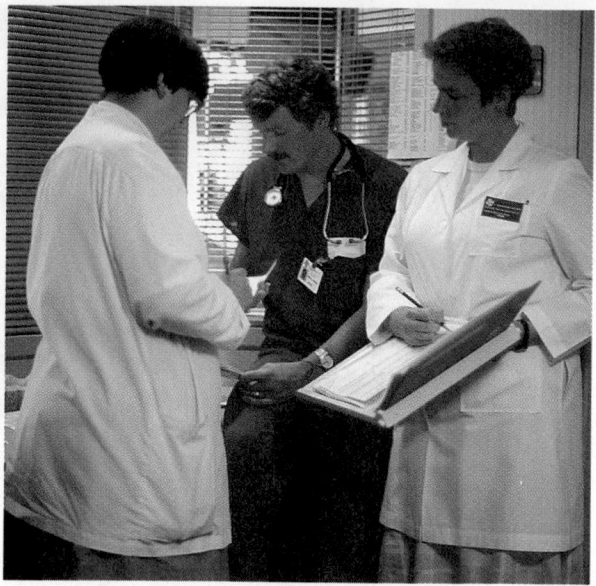

Figure 19-4   Decision making is at the core of nursing practice.

against policies or actions that might endanger their well-being or conflict with their rights.

Case Manager.   As **case manager,** the nurse coordinates the activities of other members of the health care team, such as nutritionists and physical therapists, when managing a group of clients' care. A hospital or an insurance provider may employ the case manager. The role of that person is to review the care being provided to the client and assist with delays, such as in testing or making arrangements for discharge. The hospital-based case manager may be part of the quality improvement department. In addition to identifying client's who need additional help with posthospitalization plans, they also assist in coding for insurance and quality monitoring. Many insurance providers have case managers that review the client's chart and, based on protocols and criteria, either approve or deny hospital days. The insurance case manager is also available to assist the in-hospital case manager with complex clients.

Rehabilitator.   Rehabilitation is the process by which individuals return to maximal levels of functioning after illness, accidents, or other disabling events. Frequently clients experience physical or emotional impairments that change their lives, and the nurse helps them adapt as fully as possible. Rehabilitative and restorative care activity range from teaching clients to walk with crutches to helping clients cope with lifestyle changes often associated with chronic illness.

Comforter.   The role of comforter, caring for the client as a person, is a traditional and historical one in nursing and has continued to be important as nurses have assumed new roles. Because nursing care must be directed to the whole person, rather than simply the body, comfort and emotional support often help give the client strength to recover. While carrying out nursing activities, nurses can provide comfort by demonstrating care for the client as an individual with unique feelings and needs. As comforter, nurses should help the client reach therapeutic goals rather than encourage emotional or physical dependence (see Chapter 42).

Communicator.   The role of communicator is central to all other nursing roles. Nursing involves communication with clients and families, other nurses and health care professionals, resource persons, and the community. Without clear communication, it is impossible to give care effectively, make decisions with clients and families, protect clients from threats to well-being, coordinate and manage client care, assist the client in rehabilitation, offer comfort, or teach. The quality of communication is a critical factor in meeting the needs of individuals, families, and communities (see Chapter 22).

Teacher/Educator.   As teacher, the nurse explains to clients concepts and facts about health, demonstrates procedures such as self-care activities, determines that the client fully understands, reinforces learning or client behavior, and evaluates the client's progress in learning. Some client teaching can be unplanned and informal, such as when a nurse responds to a question about a health issue in casual conversation. Other teaching activities may be planned and more formal, such as when the nurse teaches a client with diabetes to self-administer insulin injections. The nurse uses teaching methods that match the client's capabilities and needs and incorporates other resources, such as the family, in teaching plans (see Chapter 23).

CAREER ROLES

The preceding roles and functions apply to all nurses in most practice settings. Career roles, on the other hand, are specific employment positions or paths. Because of increasing educational opportunities for nurses, the growth of nursing as a profession, and a greater concern for job enrichment, the nursing profession offers expanded roles and different kinds of career opportunities. Examples of career roles include nurse educators, advanced practice nurses, nurse managers and administrators, nurse researchers, nurse risk managers, quality improvement nurses, medical-legal consultants, and product consultants.

Clinician.   Most nurses enter the profession with the goal of providing direct care. The nurse providing direct client care accounts for the majority of the practicing nurses. Until recently, this has been in the acute care hospital setting. As health care returns to the home care set-

ting, there will be increasing opportunities for nurses to provide direct care in the clients' home. The clinical nurse provides direct care to the client, using the nursing process and critical thinking skills. The focus is restorative and curative. The clinical nurse provides education to the client and family to promote health maintenance and self-care. In collaboration with other health care team members, the clinician focuses on returning the client to his or her home and usual state of health.

Nurses may choose to practice in a medical-surgical setting or concentrate on a specific area of practice, such as critical care or emergency care. Most specialty care areas require some experience as a medical-surgical nurse and additional continuing or in-service education. Many intensive care unit (ICU) and emergency department nurses are required to have training in advanced cardiac life support and certification in critical care, emergency nursing, or trauma nursing. Hospital-based nurses may also choose to practice in specialty areas such as transplantation, rehabilitation, or oncology. Larger medical centers offer more opportunity to concentrate practice in a single area.

Nurse Educator.   A **nurse educator** works primarily in schools of nursing, staff development departments of health care agencies, and client education departments. Nursing educators generally have a background in clinical nursing, which provides them with practical skills and theoretical knowledge. A faculty member in a school of nursing prepares students to function as a nurse. Nursing faculty members are responsible for teaching current nursing practice theory and necessary skills in laboratories and clinical settings. Nurse educators in nursing schools are usually required to have graduate degrees in nursing and additional education in the educational process. Many hold doctorate or advanced degrees in nursing, education, or administration, such as a master's degree in business administration (MBA). Generally, they have a specific clinical, administrative, or research specialty and advanced clinical experience.

Nurse educators in staff development departments of health care institutions provide educational programs for nurses within their institution. These programs include orientation of new personnel, critical care nursing courses, assisting with clinical skill competency, safety training, and instruction about new equipment or procedures. These nursing educators often participate in the development of nursing policies and procedures.

The primary focus of the nurse educator in an agency's department of client education is to teach ill or disabled clients and their families how to provide care in the home. These nurse educators may be specialized and certified, such as a certified diabetic educator (CDE) or an ostomy care nurse, and see only a discrete population of clients. In most health care agencies, however, the budget does not permit a separate client education department. Therefore the responsibility falls to the staff nurse to plan and provide client and family education.

Advanced Practice Nurse.

The **advanced practice nurse (APN)** is generally the most independent functioning nurse. An APN has a master's degree in nursing, advanced education in pharmacology and physical assessment, and certification and expertise in a specialized area of practice (ANA, 1996). The APN may work in primary, acute, or restorative care, or in a community health care agency. The APN functions as a clinician, educator, case manager, consultant, and researcher within his or her area of practice, to plan or improve the quality of nursing care for the client and family. The term *advanced practice nurse* is an umbrella term for an advanced clinical nurse that includes nurse practitioners, clinical nurse specialists, certified registered nurse anesthetists, and nurse-midwives.

Clinical Nurse Specialist.

The **clinical nurse specialist (CNS)** is an APN with nursing expertise in a specialized area of practice and may work in any practice setting. Traditionally, the CNS has practiced most often in the hospital setting. The CNS may specialize in a specific disease, such as diabetes mellitus, cancer, or cardiac problems, or in a specific field, such as pediatrics or gerontology. The CNS functions as an expert clinician, educator, case manager, consultant, and researcher to plan or improve the quality of care provided to the client and family (Figure 19-5).

Nurse Practitioner.

The **nurse practitioner** provides health care to clients, usually in an outpatient, ambulatory care, or community-based setting. Nurse practitioners provide care for clients with complex problems and provide a more holistic approach, attending to symptoms of nonpathological conditions, comfort, and comprehensiveness of care. A significant percentage of primary care encounters extend beyond the boundaries of medicine and demand the expertise of the nurse. The nurse practitioner is able to establish a collaborative provider-client relationship. A nurse practitioner may work with a specific group of clients or with clients of all ages and health care needs. The major nurse practitioner categories are adult, family, pediatric, obstetrics-gynecology, and geriatric nurse practitioner. A nurse practitioner has the knowledge and skills necessary to detect and manage self-limiting acute and chronic stable conditions. The nurse practitioner's educational preparation includes a master's degree in nursing and additional education in the practitioner program.

An adult nurse practitioner (ANP) provides primary, ambulatory care to adults with a nonemergent acute or chronic illness and in some settings tertiary care. ANPs work collaboratively with one or more primary care physicians.

A family nurse practitioner (FNP) provides primary

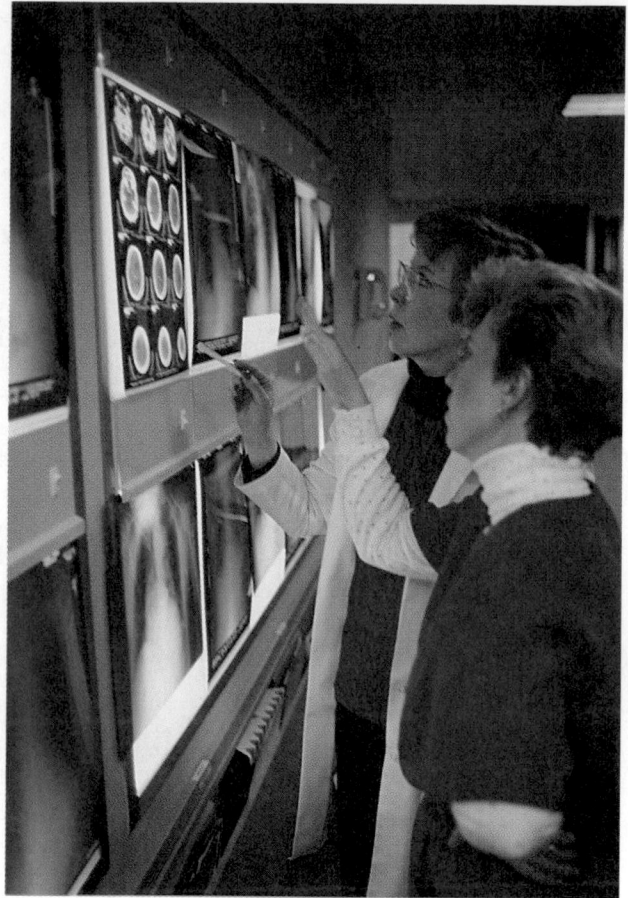

Figure 19-5 Nurse specialist consults on a difficult client case.

ambulatory care for families, usually in collaboration with a family care physician. The FNP meets the family's general health care needs, manages some illnesses by providing direct care, and guides or counsels the family as needed.

A pediatric nurse practitioner (PNP) provides health care to infants and children. PNPs practice in hospital, ambulatory care, and emergency care and physicians' offices.

A women's health nurse practitioner (WHNP) provides primary ambulatory care to women seeking obstetrical or gynecological health care.

The **acute care nurse practitioner** is a new role. It was developed in 1995 to meet the increasing need for an APN to function in the absence of a physician or house staff physician. The first certification examination by the American Nurses Credentialing Center (ANCC) was held in 1996. The acute care nurse practitioner is a generalist, usually based in internal medicine, focusing on the care of the hospitalized patient. The difference between the CNS and the acute care NP can be difficult to distinguish. Usually the CNS has a specialized body of knowledge, such as cardiovascular or oncology, and the ACNP has a broader clinical focus.

The **geriatric nurse practitioner (GNP)** is an ANP with specialization in care of the older adult. GNP's are trained in the special needs of the aging adult, with emphasis on health promotion, health maintenance, and functional status. The GNP works with the client and family to promote independence and self-care. The client population is usually age 65 and older.

Certified Nurse-Midwife. A **certified nurse-midwife (CNM)** is an RN who is also educated in midwifery and is certified by the American College of Nurse-Midwives. The practice of nurse-midwifery involves providing independent care for women during normal pregnancy, labor, and delivery, as well as care for the newborn. It may include some gynecological services such as routine Papanicolaou (Pap) smears, family planning, and treatment for minor vaginal infections. A CNM practices with a health care agency that provides medical consultation, collaborative management, and referral.

Certified Registered Nurse Anesthetist. A **certified registered nurse anesthetist (CRNA)** is an RN who has received advanced training in an accredited program in anesthesiology. Nurse anesthetists provide surgical anesthesia under the guidance and supervision of an anesthesiologist, who is a physician with advanced knowledge of surgical anesthesia.

Nursing Administrator. A **nurse administrator** manages client care and the delivery of specific nursing services within a health care agency. Nursing administration begins with positions such as the charge nurse or assistant nurse manager. Experience and additional education may lead to a middle-management position, such as nurse manager of a specific patient care area(s) or house supervisor, or to an upper-management position, such as assistant or associate director or director of nursing services.

Nurse manager's positions usually require at least a baccalaureate degree in nursing, and director and nurse executive positions generally require a master's degree. Chief nurse executive and vice president positions in large health care organizations often require preparation at the doctorate level. Nurses may have advanced degrees such as a master's degree in business administration (MBA), hospital administration (MHA), or public health (MPH).

In today's health care organizations, directors may have responsibility for more than nursing personnel. Responsibilities may include a particular service or product line, such as medicine or cardiology, and include supportive functions and personnel such as medicine clinics, cardiac diagnostics, or outpatient services such as cardiac catheterization. In addition, the director may be responsible for ancillary personnel such as cardiology technicians, respiratory therapists, social workers, and dietitians.

Vice presidents of nursing or chief nurse executives often have responsibilities for all clinical functions within the hospital. This may include all ancillary personnel who provide and support patient care services. The nursing administrator needs to be skilled in business and management, as well as understand all aspects of nursing and client care. Functions of administrators include budgeting, staffing, strategic planning of programs and services, employee evaluation, and employee development (Douglas, 1996).

Nurse Researcher. The **nurse researcher** investigates problems to improve nursing care and to further define and expand the scope of nursing practice (see Chapter 25). The nurse researcher may be employed in an academic setting, hospital, or independent professional or community service agency. The minimum educational requirement is a doctoral degree, with at least a master's degree in nursing.

Military Nursing. There are many opportunities to provide nursing care in the armed forces. All branches of the United States military, except the marines, have a nursing corps. Entry into the military as an RN requires a BSN degree. Individuals who already possess a BSN degree can enlist, or individuals who have been accepted to an accredited baccalaureate nursing program can join the service and complete their education while in the military. Military nursing can be a lifelong career, with opportunities to practice in a variety of practice settings, such as primary care, hospital care, long-term care, and facilities overseas. After discharge, many nurses continue in the reserves, serving 1 weekend per month and 2 full-time weeks per year. Salaries are competitive with civilian positions and are based on achieving rank requirements.

HEALTH CARE TEAM

In most practice settings the nurse works with other health care professionals to provide total care for clients. The health care team comprises four general types of professionals, including nurses, physicians, allied health professionals such as therapists and technicians, and other specialists such as social workers and chaplains. The involvement of many different persons in the client's health care, however, may cause a fragmenting of care. Because nurses have the greatest opportunity to interact with all of the other professionals in the health care team, they often have the role of coordinating and integrating services within a managed care system.

Physician. A **physician** is a professional who has earned the degree of Doctor of Medicine (MD) or Doctor of Osteopathy (DO). The physician has completed a required curriculum, has had a specific period of postgraduate training, and has passed a licensing examination. A physician is licensed for the medical diagnosis and treatment of clients (Figure 19-6).

The current trend in health care is the development of primary care physicians. Schools of medicine have now developed primary care programs to train physicians in managing a client's care over the life span. In addition, there are many physicians who specialize in a single area of medicine, such as a cardiologist who specializes in heart diseases or an oncologist who specializes in cancer. Physicians may choose to become a general surgeon or specialize in a specific area of surgery, such as orthopedics or vascular surgery.

Nurses work with physicians in many capacities. One nurse may work in a setting in which most nursing care depends on the physician's orders, or an intensive care nurse may follow written standing orders that permit more independent nursing actions. A clinical nurse specialist or nurse practitioner may function collaboratively with a physician, or a nurse and physician may work together to teach a newly diagnosed diabetic client and the family about the disease and home care.

Physician Assistant.
A **physician assistant (PA)** is trained in certain aspects of the practice of medicine to provide support to physicians, including conducting physical examinations, performing diagnostic procedures, assisting in the operating room or emergency department, and completing treatments such as cast application and suturing. PAs practice in hospitals, clinics, or private physicians' offices. Their practice is skill based to assist the physician. They are required to practice under the direction and supervision of the physician. PAs practice in the

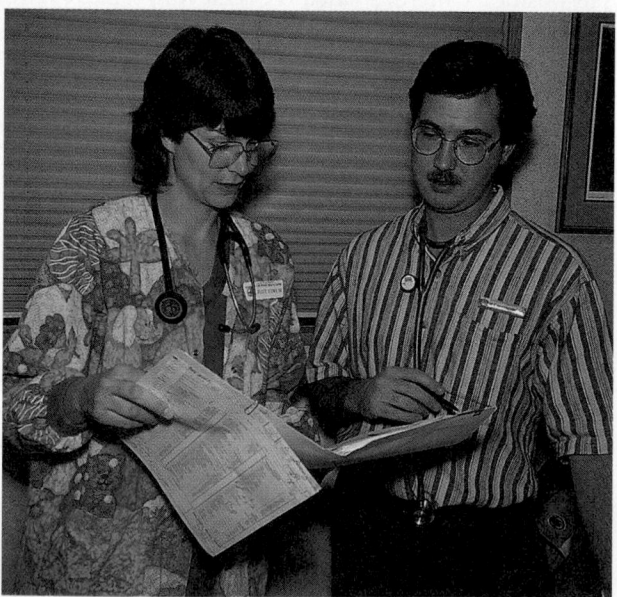

Figure 19-6   The nurse collaborates with the physician regarding a question about patient care.

United States but not in Canada. In some states PAs may prescribe medications.

Allied and Other Health Care Professionals
Therapist.   There are a number of personnel who carry the title of therapist, including physical therapists, respiratory therapists, occupational therapists, and massage therapists.

A **physical therapist (PT)** is licensed to assist in the examination, testing, and treatment of physically disabled or handicapped people through the use of special exercises, the application of heat and cold, the use of sonar waves, and other techniques. A PT usually receives training in a 6-year college program leading to a master's degree in physical therapy. A PT practices in hospitals, clinics, rehabilitation centers, and community-based agencies.

An **occupational therapist (OT)** is licensed or certified to develop and use adaptive devices that help chronically ill or handicapped clients carry out activities of daily living. OTs usually receive education and training in 4-year college programs and, like PTs, work in a variety of settings.

A **respiratory therapist (RT)** is licensed to deliver treatment designed to improve clients' ventilatory function or oxygenation. Educational and training programs vary. They range from 6-month training programs to educational programs in 4-year colleges. An RT is usually employed in an institutional health care setting.

A massage therapist is a certified therapist educated in the use of massage therapy for the relief of muscular ailments. New to many hospitals, it is an alternative therapy that is being used to assist in the treatment of musculoskeletal injury. Often, the massage therapist works closely with the physical therapist to provide care.

Nurses work with therapists in a collaborative capacity (Figure 19-7). Care initiated by therapists is frequently continued and evaluated by nurses. Nurses and therapists together consider the client's progress and develop goals and discharge plans that include the client and family. In addition, nurses refer clients to therapists for further care. For example, a nurse caring for a person with severe pulmonary disease may refer the client to a physical therapist to learn exercises for strengthening the upper arm muscles, to an OT to learn energy-saving techniques for activities of daily living, and to an RT for techniques to promote airway clearance.

Pharmacist.
A **pharmacist** is a licensed professional who formulates and dispenses medications. The pharmacist's education ranges from a baccalaureate degree to a doctorate in pharmacology. A pharmacist practices in an institutional or outpatient setting. The pharmacist may practice only within a pharmacy or may be involved in client care conferences or in the development of medication administration systems (see Chapter 34). Some clinical pharmacists in acute care settings have responsibility for managing clients on total parental nutrition (TPN).

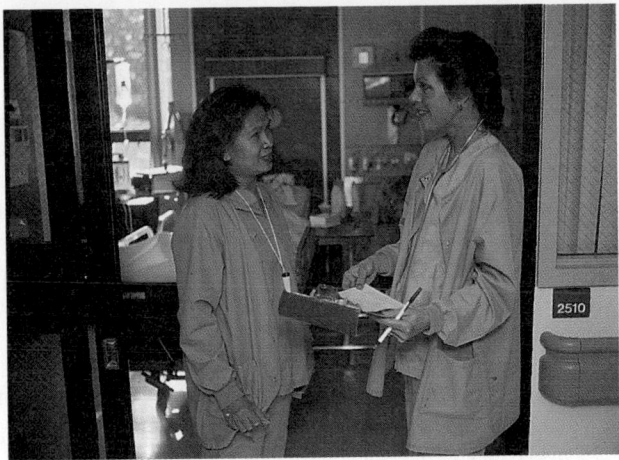

Figure 19-7 Collaboration with other health care providers results in effective interventions.

They monitor the client's laboratory values and write orders for the TPN.

The pharmacist is a valuable resource for nurses. For example, the nurse can request information about new drugs from the pharmacist. The nurse must always know the action, desired effect, correct dosage, and side effects of all drugs administered. If this information is unavailable in standard reference books such as textbooks or hospital formularies, the nurse should consult the pharmacist. Pharmacists also provide information about which drugs are compatible and which can be mixed or administered together. In addition, pharmacists can tell the nurse which over-the-counter drugs may interact adversely with pre-scribed drugs so that this information can be incorporated into the discharge teaching plan.

Social Worker.   A **social worker** is trained to counsel clients and families. Counseling services may include pro-viding emotional support for clients and families during severe or terminal illnesses, arranging placement in ex-tended care facilities, and locating financial resources. The social worker generally has a baccalaureate or master's de-gree in social work and is employed in every type of agency in the health care system. A nurse frequently refers clients to a social worker, and they work together to iden-tify resources for meeting clients' present and future health care needs.

Pastoral Care.   **Pastoral care** offers spiritual support and guidance to clients and families and may be provided by an agency or institution or by a religious affiliation within the community. Spiritual advisors are ministers, priests, nuns, rabbis, or lay members of religious congre-gations. A client may request to see a chaplain or spiritual advisor, or the nurse may initiate a referral.

Assistive Personnel/Nursing Assistant.   **Assistive personnel (AP)** or a nursing assistant (NA) provides assis-tance to the RN with tasks and functions that require min-imal critical thinking. These staff members work under the direction and supervision of the RN. The RN uses crit-ical thinking skills to determine which tasks are appropri-ately delegated to the AP or NA, ensuring safe and appro-priate client care. In some hospitals and skilled nursing facilities, APs may have responsibilities for phlebotomy and procedures such as Foley catheterization, intravenous (IV) dressing changes, and discontinuing IV lines. The RN uses critical thinking skills to determine which tasks are appropriately delegated to the AP or NA based on assess-ment of the client, thereby ensuring safe and appropriate care.

Clerical/Secretarial Staff.   The clerical/secretarial staff provide support to the health care team and to the client and family. They are often the first staff personnel the client and family meet. They are invaluable in assisting with the organization of tests, procedures, and support services. The clerical/secretarial staff have expertise in ob-taining resources and arranging for services both in the hospital and for discharge.

Professional Nursing Organizations

A **professional organization** is created to deal with issues of concern to those practicing in the profession. In North America the major professional nursing organizations are the American Nurses Association (ANA), Canadian Nurses Association (CNA), and National League for Nursing (NLN). The CNA and ANA were formed in the late nineteenth century to improve standards of health and the availability of health care, to foster high standards for nursing, and to promote the professional development and general and economic welfare of nurses. The ANA and CNA are part of the International Council of Nursing (ICN). The objectives of the ICN parallel those of the CNA and ANA: promoting national associations of nurses, improving standards of nursing practice, seeking a higher status for nurses, and providing an international power base for nurses.

The NLN is concerned with the improvement of nurs-ing education, nursing service, and health care delivery in the United States. In Canada the Canadian Association of University Schools of Nursing and the Canadian Asso-ciation of Practical and Nursing Assistants perform simi-lar functions.

Nursing students also take part in organizations such as the National Student Nurses Association (NSNA) in the United States and the Canadian Student Nurses Asso-ciation (CSNA) in Canada. These organizations consider issues of importance to nursing students and often cooperate in activities and programs with the professional organizations.

Some professional organizations focus on specific areas such as critical care, nursing administration or research, or nurse-midwifery. These organizations seek to improve the standards of practice, expand nursing roles, and foster the welfare of nurses within the specialty areas. In addition, professional organizations present education programs and publish journals. Some representative specialty organizations are discussed in the following paragraphs.

The Association of Operating Room Nurses (AORN) in the United States and the National Conference of Operating Room Nurses in Canada are concerned with continuing education for operating room nurses, higher standards for operating room care, and increased research activities.

The Association of Women's Health, Obstetrical, and Neonatal Nurses (AWHONN) includes Canadian and American nurses and promotes standards of practice in obstetrical and gynecological nursing, encourages professional growth for its members, and is an accrediting body for advanced programs in obstetrical and gynecological nursing.

The National Association of Pediatric Nurse Associates/ Practitioners (NAPNAP) is a national organization for nurses prepared by training or experience to give primary care to children. NAPNAP works in conjunction with the American Academy of Pediatrics.

The American Association of Critical-Care Nurses (AACN) is a national organization of nurses working in critical care areas. It is concerned with nursing education, practice, and research as they involve critical care nursing.

Societal Influences on Nursing

There are many external forces that affect nursing. These include the demographic changes, the aging population, cultural diversity, heightened consumer awareness, economic influences, the changing health care delivery system, and political agendas.

DEMOGRAPHIC CHANGES

Demographic changes affect the population as a whole. Changes that have influenced health care in recent decades include the population shift from rural areas to urban centers; the increasing life span; the higher incidence of chronic, long-term illness; and the increased incidence of diseases such as alcoholism and lung cancer. Nursing as a profession responds to such changes by exploring new methods for providing care, by changing educational emphases, and by establishing practice standards in new areas. To better meet the changing health care needs of clients, the nurse also responds to demographic changes in the population served by the practice setting.

CULTURAL DIVERSITY

As the people of the world move about, nurses are confronted with many cultures different from their own. The nurse must now have an awareness of how different cultures view health and illness (see Chapter 7). Nurses are challenged to be culturally aware and competent. Care that is not culturally competent may be more costly and may be ineffective (Sullivan 1999). *Healthy People 2010* is one example of meeting the health of multiple cultures by defining goals and objectives for health (U.S. Department of Health and Human Services [USDHHS] 1998).

CONSUMER'S MOVEMENT

The consumer's movement is a heightened awareness of the value and costs of products and services. It has influenced health care by calling for new kinds of health care agencies, such as health maintenance organizations, new forms of health insurance, and concern about the rising costs of health care (see Chapter 2). Consumers are also more knowledgeable about health and illness and are becoming more vocal in their desire for high-quality care. Because nurses generally interact with clients more than other health care professionals do, they must often answer questions about the quality and costs of health care. Health care consumers are also more aware of their rights as clients. The nurse supports these rights in the role of client advocate.

HEALTH PROMOTION AND WELLNESS

There is also a greater emphasis in society on health promotion, health maintenance, and illness prevention. Exercise, nutrition, and healthy lifestyles are subjects that interest many people. Nursing has responded to this greater concern for health promotion by providing programs in the community such as health fairs and wellness programs; educational programs for specific diseases; and client and family teaching activities in hospitals, clinics, primary care facilities, and other health care settings. Health promotion activities are an important part of the role of a nurse (see Chapter 1).

WOMEN'S MOVEMENT

The women's movement has brought about many changes in society as women have increasingly sought economic, political, occupational, and educational equality. Nursing is responding in two ways. Because most nurses are women, they are increasingly asserting their equal rights as human beings, employees, and health care professionals. The women's movement has encouraged nurses to seek greater autonomy and responsibility in providing care. The women's movement has caused female clients to seek more responsibility for and control for their bodies, health, and lives in general. As women become more aware of their own unique needs and qualities, they seek health care that can help them meet those needs and reach their full potential.

HUMAN RIGHTS MOVEMENT

The human rights movement is changing the way society views the rights of all of its members, including minorities, clients with terminal illness, pregnant women, and older adults. Many groups have special health care needs, and nursing has responded by respecting all clients as individuals with a right to good care and with basic human rights. Nurses advocate the rights of all clients, but they have also recognized the special needs of some groups and thus have created bills of rights for dying, hospitalized, and pregnant clients, as well as other groups, to ensure that quality care is provided without sacrificing these rights.

Trends in Nursing

This chapter has emphasized that nursing is not a static, unchanging profession but is continuously growing and evolving as society changes, as health care emphases and methods change, as lifestyles change—and as nurses themselves change. To speak of nursing at all is to speak of nursing as it is at a given time, and in this sense, this chapter is about trends in nursing.

The current philosophies and definitions of nursing demonstrate the holistic trend in nursing—to address the whole person in all dimensions, in health and illness, and in interaction with the family and community. Nursing continues to draw on the social sciences and other fields as the focus of nursing care expands.

One trend in nursing education is the growing number of students receiving basic nursing education in community colleges and universities. Professional nursing organizations continue to stress the importance of advanced education for nurses seeking new and expanded roles.

Nursing practice trends include a growing variety of employment settings in which nurses have greater independence, autonomy, and respect as members of the health care team. Nursing roles continue to expand and develop, broadening the focus of nursing care and providing a more holistic and all-encompassing domain. Nursing is now not only drawing from traditional nursing and medicine, spiritual, and emotional realms, but also expanding into alternative therapies such as healing touch, massage therapy, and natural herbs and vitamins.

Trends in nursing as a profession include the growing emphasis on the aspects of nursing that characterize it as a profession, including education, theory, service, autonomy, and ethical codes. The activities of nursing's professional organizations reflect all of the trends in nursing education and practice. Finally, all of the influences of society on nursing also reflect trends in contemporary nursing.

Two other trends need to be discussed: the increasing political influence of nursing and nursing's influence on health care policy and practice.

POLITICAL INFLUENCE OF PROFESSIONAL NURSING

Historically, nurses' involvement in politics has been limited. Individual nurses such as Florence Nightingale, Lillian Wald, Margaret Sanger, and Lavinia Dock have influenced decision making in areas such as sanitation, nutrition, and birth control. Nurses as a large and potentially powerful group have not accomplished as much as have many of the group's individuals. The women's movement, however, has inspired nurses to address health care issues. In addition, as more college-educated people enter the profession, they bring to nursing the activism and involvement of the university campus.

In 1974 the ANA formed the Nurses Coalition in Politics (N-CAP), which was the first political action committee (PAC) for nurses. This organization, which was later renamed ANA-PAC, is a major PAC that is sought for support for candidates seeking federal offices.

The ability to influence or persuade an individual holding a government office to exert the power of that office to affect a desired outcome is known as political power or influence. Traditionally, nurses have been uncomfortable with politics because of its male domination. Nurses are becoming more aware of historical precedents established by nurses in the political arena and thus are becoming more politically astute. Advanced education in the political arena is helping to position nurses to successfully compete in politics and political issues. Nurses' involvement in politics is receiving greater emphasis in nursing curricula, professional organizations, and health care settings. Professional nursing organizations have employed lobbyists to urge state legislatures and the U.S. Congress to improve the quality of health care.

The ANA works for the improvement of health standards and the availability of health care services for all people, fosters high standards of nursing, stimulates and promotes the professional development of nurses, and advances their economic and general welfare. The purposes are unrestricted by considerations of nationality, race, creed, lifestyle, color, sex, or age. The ANA employs RNs as lobbyists at the federal level, and state nursing organizations also hire lobbyists and legislative specialists to work on state nursing issues and assist with federal efforts. Finally, lobbyists working on behalf of nursing are employed in Washington, D.C., by professional organizations such as the American Federation of Teachers, NLN, American College of Nurse-Midwives, American Public Health Association, and AACN. These groups aim to remove financial barriers to health care, increase the quality of nursing care available, increase economic rewards to nurses, and expand professional nursing roles.

In addition, individual nurses can influence policy decisions at all governmental levels, and organized nursing's unified efforts, such as with Nursing's Agenda for Health Care Reform (ANA 1991), will be critical to exert nurses' influence early in the political process (Hall-Long, 1995). Specific strategies include integration of public policy into nursing curricula, early socialization and participation in professional organizations, diverse settings for clinical practice, and running for public office (Hall-Long, 1995). If nurses become serious students of social needs, activists in influencing policy to meet those needs, and generous contributors of time and money to nursing and their organizations and to candidates working for universal good health care, then the future is bright indeed.

NURSING'S INFLUENCE ON HEALTH CARE POLICY AND PRACTICE

Nurses are becoming more involved in health care reform. Nursing's Agenda for Health Care Reform supports the creation of a health care system that ensures access, quality, and services at affordable costs. The plan for reform focuses on primary health care services and the promotion, restoration, and maintenance of health (ANA, 1991).

Healthy People 2010 (USDHHS, 1998) is a document for public health policy for the new millennium (see Chapter 1). It outlines goals for vulnerable populations, such as low-income groups, minorities, and persons with disabilities (Lancaster, 1999).

Political activism and commitment are a part of professionalism, however, and politics are an important aspect of the delivery of health care. Therefore nurses should view politics as a reality that includes the arts of influence, compromise, and social interaction. Nurses have been involved in a different sort of politics in schools of nursing and in health care settings when seeking additional resources, more self-direction, and accountability with authority. The skills gained in such experiences can be transferred to the politics of health care policy making.

As long as nurses maintain involvement in health care policy and practice, misinformed outsiders cannot attempt to impose their will on nursing and nursing practice. Nonnursing groups, often led by other health care providers, have made attempts to impose institutional licensure, mandatory continuing education, curtailment of advanced nursing practice, and other constraints on the nursing profession. Nursing should have its own voice in decisions made in these and numerous other areas affecting the practice and quality of nursing care. Although nurses have often successfully prevented infringement on the profession's self-governance, the future of nursing requires that nurses individually and collectively seek a greater influence on health care policies affecting nursing practice.

Key Concepts

- Nursing has responded to the health care needs of society, which were influenced by economic, social, and cultural variables of a specific era.
- The Canadian Nurses Association and the American Nurses Association were established in the late nineteenth century.
- Nursing education became affiliated with universities early in the twentieth century.
- Expansion of nursing into the military occurred in the early twentieth century, and the development of specialty nursing organizations began in the 1950s and has continued to the present.
- The Lysaught report (1970) emphasized the need for clarification of nursing roles and responsibilities, greater financial support for nurses, and more career opportunities.
- Nursing definitions reflect changes in the practice of nursing and help bring about changes by identifying the domain of nursing practice and guiding research, practice, and education.
- Educational preparation of the registered nurse can be through one of three programs in the United States or two programs in Canada.

- Nursing standards provide the guidelines for implementing and evaluating nursing care.
- The multiple roles and functions of the nurse include caregiver, decision maker, protector, client advocate, case manager, rehabilitator, comforter, communicator, and teacher.
- Specific employment positions include nurse educator, advanced practice nurse, nurse practitioner, certified nurse-midwife, nurse anesthetist, administrator, and researcher.
- The health care team is multidisciplinary and may include a nurse, physician, physician assistant, physical therapist, occupational therapist, respiratory therapist, massage therapist, pharmacist, social worker, and spiritual advisor.
- Nursing is a profession encompassing educational preparation for the nurse, nursing theory, a provided service, autonomy, and a code of ethics.
- Professional nursing organizations deal with issues of concern to specialist groups within the nursing profession.
- Changes in society, such as increased technology, new demographic patterns, consumerism, health promo-

tion, and the women's and human rights movements, have led to changes in nursing.

- Nurses are becoming more politically sophisticated and, as a result, are able to increase nursing's influence on health care policy and practice.

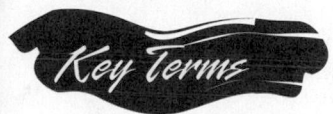
Key Terms

Acute care nurse practitioner (ACNP), *p. 392*

Advanced practice nurse (APN), *p. 392*

American Nurses Association (ANA), *p. 379*

Assistive personnel (AP), *p. 395*

Canadian Nurses Association (CNA), *p. 379*

Caregiver, *p. 390*

Case manager, *p. 390*

Certified nurse-midwife (CNM), *p. 393*

Certified registered nurse anesthetist (CRNA), *p. 393*

Client advocate, *p. 390*

Clinical decision maker, *p. 376*

Clinical nurse specialist (CNS), *p. 392*

Code of ethics, *p. 381*

Continuing education, *p. 383*

Geriatric nurse practitioner (GNP), *p. 393*

In-service education, *p. 383*

International Council of Nurses (ICN), *p. 376*

Licensed practical nurse (LPN), *p. 383*

Licensed vocational nurse (LVN), *p. 383*

National League for Nursing (NLN), *p. 380*

Nurse administrator, *p. 393*

Nurse educator, *p. 391*

Nurse practitioner, *p. 392*

Nurse researcher, *p. 393*

Nursing theory, *p. 380*

Occupational therapist (OT), *p. 394*

Pastoral care, *p. 395*

Pharmacist, *p. 394*

Physical therapist (PT), *p. 394*

Physician, *p. 393*

Physician assistant (PA), *p. 394*

Professional organization, *p. 395*

Registered nurse (RN), *p. 381*

Respiratory therapist (RT), *p. 394*

Social worker, *p. 395*

Critical Thinking Exercises

1. You are assigned to teach a Hispanic male client about his hypertension and medication regimen. What must the nurse consider in developing a plan of care?

2. You are part of a selection team to hire an advanced practice nurse for the cardiovascular rehabilitation unit. Based on your knowledge of advanced practice nurses, what role would you recommend and why?

3. Part of your education includes experiences in different types of health care settings. How would your role in the primary care setting be different from your role the acute care setting?

References

Alfaro-LeFevre R: *Critical thinking in nursing: a practical approach,* Philadelphia, 1995, WB Saunders.

American Association of Colleges of Nursing: *Nursing education's agenda for the twenty-first century,* Washington, DC, 1993, The Association.

American Association of Colleges of Nursing: *Essentials of baccalaureate education for professional nursing: a final report,* Washington, DC, 1998, The Association.

American Nurses Association: *A code of ethics, Am J Nurs* 26:621, 1926.

American Nurses Association: ANA news, *Am J Nurs* 55:1474, 1955.

American Nurses Association: *A position paper: educational preparation for nurse practitioners and assistants to nurses,* Kansas City, Mo, 1965, The Association.

American Nurses Association: *Statement on graduate education in nursing,* New York, 1969, The Association.

American Nurses Association: *Nursing and social policy statement,* Kansas City, Mo, 1980, The Association.

American Nurses Association: *Code for nurses with interpretive statements,* ANA Pub No. G-56, Kansas City, Mo, 1985, The Association.

American Nurses Association: *Nursing's agenda for health care reform,* Washington, DC, 1991.

American Nurses Association: Nursing facts: today's registered nurse—number and demographics. From *Sixth national sample of registered nurses,* March 1992, U.S. Department of Health and Human Services, Public Health Service, Division of Nursing, Health Resources and Services Administration.

American Nurses Association: *Ethical dilemmas in contemporary nursing practice,* Washington, DC, 1993, American Nurses Publishing.

American Nurses Association: *Standards for nursing professional development: continuing education and staff development,* ANA Pub No. COE-17, Washington, DC, 1994, American Nurses Publishing.

American Nurses Association: *Nursing and social policy statement,* Washington, DC, 1995, American Nurses Publishing.

American Nurses Association: *Scope and standards of advanced practice registered nursing,* Pub No. ADV-1, Washington, DC, 1996, American Nurses Publishing.

American Nurses Association: *Standards of clinical nursing practice,* ed 2, Washington, DC, 1998, The Association.

Benner P: *From novice to expert: excellence and power in clinical nursing practice,* Menlo Park, Calif, 1984, Addison-Wesley.

Bernhard LA, Walsh M: *Leadership: the key to the professionalization of nursing,* ed 3, St. Louis, 1995, Mosby.

Canadian Nurses Association: *A definition of nursing practice. Standards for nursing practice,* Ottawa, 1986, The Association.

Canadian Nurses Association, Policy Regulation and Research Division: *1998 RN data statistics,* Ottawa, Canada, 1999, The Association.

Carnevali DL, Thomas MD: *Diagnostic reasoning and treatment decision making in nursing,* Philadelphia, 1998, JB Lippincott.

Cherry B, Jacob SR: *Contemporary nursing: issues, trends, and management,* St. Louis, 1999, Mosby.

Chinn PL, Kramer MK: *Theory and nursing: integrated knowledge development,* ed 5, St. Louis, 1999, Mosby.

Cohen IB: Florence Nightingale, *Sci Am* 250(128):137, 1984.

Deloughery C: *Issues and trends in nursing,* ed 3, St. Louis, 1998, Mosby.

Donahue MP: *Nursing: the finest art: an illustrated history,* ed 2, St. Louis, 1996, Mosby.

Douglas LM: *The effective nurse: leader and manager,* ed 5, St. Louis, 1996, Mosby.

Ellis JR, Hartley CL: *Nursing in today's world: challenges, issues and trends,* Philadelphia, 1997, JB Lippincott.

Giger JN, Davidhizar RE: *Transcultural nursing: assessment and intervention,* ed 3, St. Louis, 1999, Mosby.

Hall-Long BA: Nursing's past, present and future political experiences, *Nurs Health Care* 16:24, 1995.

Henderson V: *The nature of nursing,* New York, 1966, Macmillan.

Kalisch P, Kalisch B: *The advance of American nursing,* ed 3, Philadelphia, 1995, JB Lippincott.

Keeling AW, Ramos MC: The role of nursing history in preparing nursing for the future, *Nurs Health Care* 16:30, 1995.

Lancaster J: *Nursing issues in leading and managing change,* St. Louis, 1999, Mosby.

Lysaught JP: *An abstract for action,* New York, 1970, McGraw-Hill.

Macrae J: Nightingale's spiritual philosophy and its significance for modern nursing, *Image J Nurs Sch* 27:8, 1995.

Marriner-Tomey A, Alligood MR: *Nursing theorists and their work,* ed 4, St. Louis, 1998, Mosby.

Meleis AI: *Theoretical nursing: development and progress,* ed 3, Philadelphia, 1997, JB Lippincott.

National League for Nursing Accrediting Commission: *Accreditation standards and criteria,* New York, 1999, The Commission.

Nightingale F: *Notes on nursing: what it is and what it is not,* London, 1860, Harrison & Sons.

Shryock RH: *The history of nursing: an interpretation of the social and medical factors involved,* Philadelphia, 1959, WB Saunders.

Sullivan EJ: *Creating nursing's future: issues, opportunities, and challenges,* St. Louis, 1999, Mosby.

U.S. Department of Health and Human Services: *Healthy people 2010:* objectives: draft for public comment, Washington DC, 1998, Office of Disease and Health Promotion, The Department.

Woodham-Smith C: *Florence Nightingale,* New York, 1983, McGraw-Hill.

20

Ethics
and
Values

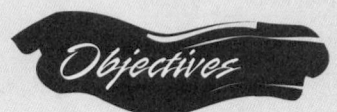

Objectives

Mastery of content in this chapter will enable the student to:

- Define the key terms listed.
- Discuss how values can influence client care.
- Describe the process and techniques of values clarification.
- Use a values clarification strategy to examine personal values.
- Describe basic philosophies of ethics.
- Describe the nursing perspective in ethics.
- Apply a method of ethical analysis to a clinical situation.
- Identify the major functions of institutional ethics committees.
- Discuss informed consent and advance directives.
- Identify contemporary ethical issues and nursing implications.

The term **ethics** refers to the study of philosophical ideals of right and wrong behavior. In professional practice such as nursing, a **code of ethics** provides guidelines for safe and compassionate care. Nurses and other health care professionals agree to national codes of ethics that define practice and offer to the public a definition of professional practice standards. This chapter reviews this aspect of ethics. Built on the foundation of basic medical and nursing ethics, the field of **bioethics** has developed during the past two decades. Along with the development of extraordinary technical advances in the treatment and management of disease has come concerns and conflict about ethical implementation of the new technologies. The study of bioethics guides the often complicated negotiations that characterize contemporary decisions about health care. Some new medical interventions challenge society's established definitions of autonomy and quality of life. This chapter also reviews the development of bioethics and reviews the vital role that the nursing profession plays.

Discussion and resolution of ethical issues requires critical thinking skills. Unlike the resolution of clinical problems, however, the resolution of ethical issues involves the negotiation of closely held personal values and philosophies, not facts or measurable clinical data. Resolution of ethical issues often incorporates not only the nurse's personal values, but also the interpretation of the client's personal values, based on the unique perspective of nurses. Its process works best in a climate where skills of values clarification and negotiation are protected and nurtured.

Ethics

Ethics is the study of good conduct, character, and motives. It is concerned with determining what is good or valuable for all people. Acts that are ethical often reflect a commitment to standards beyond personal preferences—standards on which individuals, professions, and societies agree.

BASIC TERMS

To discuss ethics, it is helpful to establish a basic vocabulary. Although the terms may have a certain meaning in a larger context, they provide specific meanings within the context of ethics that further the understanding and discussion about ethical matters. These basic terms include autonomy, beneficence, nonmaleficence, justice, and fidelity (Table 20-1).

Autonomy. **Autonomy** refers to a person's independence. As a standard in ethics, autonomy represents an agreement to respect another's right to determine a course of action. Respect for another's autonomy is fundamental to the practice of health care. It serves to justify the inclusion of clients in all aspects of decision making regarding their health care. The agreement to respect autonomy involves the recognition that clients are "in charge of their own destiny in matters of health and illness" (O'Neil, 1995). For example, the purpose of the preoperative consent that clients must read and sign before surgery is the assurance in writing that the health care team respects the client's independence by obtaining permission to proceed.

The authors acknowledge the contribution of Dr. Valerie J. Yancy to this chapter in the previous edition of this book.

Table 20-1   **Principles of Health Care Ethics**

Definitions	Nursing Implications
Autonomy Independence, self-determination, self-reliance	Display respect for all persons; support client's right to informed consent; autonomy is truly exercised when members of the health care team agree to the importance of autonomy.
Justice Fairness or equity	Ensure fair allocation of resources such as nursing care to all clients; determine the order in which clients should be treated (e.g., clients at greatest risk are treated first).
Fidelity Faithfulness; striving to keep promises	Keep promises made to clients, families, and other professionals; avoid abandonment of clients, even when client goals differ from health care provider goals.
Beneficence Actively seeking benefits; promotion of good	Promote actions that benefit clients; seek benefits that provide the least harm; consider client's best interest above self-interest.
Nonmaleficence Actively seeking to do no harm	Avoid deliberate harm, risk of harm, and harm that occurs during performance of nursing actions; seek to do the least harm if benefits must result in some harm.

The consent process implies that a client may refuse treatment, and in most cases the health care team must agree to follow the client's wishes. Health care professionals agree to abide by a standard of respect for the client's autonomy (Box 20-1).

Beneficence.   **Beneficence** refers to taking positive actions to help others. The practice of beneficence encourages the urge to do good for others. Commitment to beneficence helps to guide difficult decisions wherein the benefits of a treatment may be challenged by risks to the client's well-being or dignity. A child's immunization may cause discomfort during administration, but the benefits of protection from disease, both for the individual and for society, outweigh the temporary discomforts. The agreement to act with beneficence also requires that the best interests of the client remain more important than self-interest. For example, a nurse will not simply follow medical orders but will act thoughtfully to understand client needs and then work actively to help meet those needs.

Nonmaleficence.   Maleficence refers to harm or hurt; thus **nonmaleficence** is the avoidance of harm or hurt. In health care ethics it is important to remember that ethical practice involves not only the will to do good, but also the equal commitment to do no harm. The health care professional tries to balance the risks and benefits of a plan of care while striving to do the least harm possible. This principle is often helpful in guiding discussions about new or controversial technologies. For example, a new bone marrow transplant procedure may promise a chance at cure. The procedure, however, may require long periods of pain

and suffering. These discomforts should be considered in light of the suffering that the disease itself might cause, and in light of the suffering that other treatments might

---

Cultural ASPECTS OF CARE   Box 20-1

In his essay "Autonomy Under Duress," Leonard Harris (1992) challenges the notion that respect for autonomy guarantees respect for all persons. He is concerned that the definition of autonomy is influenced by the culture of the people using the term. His concerns led him to conclude that there can be limits to the value of respect for autonomy. His argument is based on his experience as an African-American. "If race-targeted advertising such as cigarette and alcohol advertising elicits less social consternation than we might hope, one reason may be that the target is not invested by physicians and society in general with ties of affection, compassion, . . . and value among those empowered to create change." Society may claim respect for autonomy, and health care providers specifically commit to this respect in their professional practices. Nonetheless, Harris argues, certain groups of poor or historically underserved peoples may not enjoy equal respect for autonomy. The respect they enjoy is lessened as a result of racial prejudice. Respect for autonomy applied in this way promotes harm. Harris does not argue to abandon the concept of autonomy. He does warn, however, that an honest appraisal of its use is critical. Harris recommends a thorough self-examination to ensure that when the term *autonomy* is applied, it is applied with respect, compassion, and value, as though no differences existed between classes or races of people.

cause. The commitment to provide least harmful interventions illustrates the term *nonmaleficence.* The standard of nonmaleficence promotes a continuing effort to consider the potential for harm even when it may be necessary to promote health.

Justice.
Justice refers to fairness. Health care providers agree to strive for justice in health care. The term often is used during discussions about resources. What constitutes a fair distribution of resources may not always be clear. In these cases national discussion about just distribution of resources often helps to clarify methods for achieving fairness. For example, in the United States the number of candidates awaiting liver transplants is approximately three times larger than the number of available organs for transplantation. Decisions about who should receive available organs are always difficult. Criteria set by a national multidisciplinary committee strive for justice by ranking recipients according to need. These criteria are preferable to resorting to selling organs for profit, which would favor recipients with the most money, and preferable to distributing them by lottery, which would result in random distribution without regard to justice.

Fidelity.
Fidelity refers to the agreement to keep promises. A commitment to fidelity explains the reluctance to abandon clients, even when disagreement arises about decisions that a client may make. The standard of fidelity also includes an obligation to follow through with care offered to clients. For example, if a nurse assesses a client for pain and then offers a plan to manage the pain, the standard of fidelity encourages the nurse to monitor the client's response to the plan. Professional behavior by the nurse includes revision of the plan as necessary to try to keep the promise to reduce pain.

PROFESSIONAL NURSING
Code of Ethics.
A code of ethics is a set of ethical principles that are accepted by all members of a profession. A profession's ethical code is a collective statement about the group's expectations and standards of behavior. Codes serve as guidelines to assist nurses and other professional groups when conflict or disagreement arises about correct practice or behavior. The nursing code of ethics, as in other professions, sets forth ideals of conduct. The American Nurses Association (ANA), the International Council of Nurses (ICN), and the Canadian Nurses Association (CNA) have established widely accepted codes that professional nurses attempt to follow. These codes differ somewhat in specific emphasis, but they reflect the same basic principles, including responsibility, accountability, advocacy, confidentiality, and veracity (Boxes 20-2 to 20-4). Nurses agree to responsibility for specific actions and accountability for the consequences. To practice responsibly, professional nurses also agree to maintain competence in their practice and to use competence in the application of judgment.

> ### American Nurses Association
> ### Code of Ethics   Box 20-2
>
> The nurse provides services with respect for human dignity and the uniqueness of the client unrestricted by considerations of social or economic status, personal attributes, or the nature of health problems.
>
> The nurse safeguards the client's right to privacy by judiciously protecting information of a confidential nature.
>
> The nurse acts to safeguard the client and the public when health care and safety are affected by the incompetent, unethical, or illegal practice of any person.
>
> The nurse assumes responsibility and accountability for individual nursing judgments and actions.
>
> The nurse maintains competence in nursing.
>
> The nurse exercises informed judgment and uses individual competence and qualifications as criteria in seeking consultation, accepting responsibilities, and delegating nursing activities to others.
>
> The nurse participates in activities that contribute to the ongoing development of the profession's body of knowledge.
>
> The nurse participates in the profession's efforts to implement and improve standards of nursing.
>
> The nurse participates in the profession's efforts to establish and maintain conditions of employment conducive to high-quality nursing care.
>
> The nurse participates in the profession's effort to protect the public from misinformation and misrepresentation and to maintain the integrity of nursing.
>
> The nurse collaborates with members of the health professions and other citizens in promoting community and national efforts to meet the health needs of the public.

From American Nurses Association: *Code for nurses with interpretive statements,* Kansas City, Mo, 1985, The Association.

Accountability.
Accountability refers to the ability to answer for one's own actions. A nurse is accountable to self most of all. In addition, the nurse balances accountability to the client, the profession, the employer, and society. For example, a nurse may know that a client who will be discharged soon remains confused about how to administer insulin. The action that a nurse takes in response to this situation will be guided by the sense of accountability. The client, the institution, and society rely on the good judgment of the nurse and trust that the nurse will take action in response to this situation. The nurse may request more hospitalization to provide further teaching or arrange home care to continue teaching at home. The goal is the prevention of injury to the client. The nurse's sense of accountability guides actions that achieve this goal (see Box 20-5).

To remain accountable to society, nursing professionals agree to evaluate practices and actions and to take action to preserve nursing excellence. The Joint Commission on Accreditation of Healthcare Organizations (JCAHO), a national accreditation association, recommends standards for the delivery of nursing care. These standards provide a basic structure against which nursing care is objectively measured. Accountability is best ensured and measured when

---

International Council of Nurses Code for Nurses*

Box 20-3

The fundamental responsibility of the nurse is fourfold: to promote health, to prevent illness, to restore health, and to alleviate suffering.

The need for nursing is universal. Inherent in nursing is respect for life, dignity, and rights of man. It is unrestricted by considerations of nationality, race, creed, color, age, sex, politics, or social status.

Nurses render health services to the individual, the family, and the community and coordinate their services with those of related groups.

NURSES AND PEOPLE

The nurse's primary responsibility is to those people who require nursing care.

The nurse, in providing care, promotes an environment in which the values, customs, and spiritual beliefs of the individual are respected.

The nurse holds in confidence personal information and uses judgment in sharing this information.

NURSES AND PRACTICE

The nurse carries personal responsibility for nursing practice and for maintaining competence by continual learning. The nurse maintains the highest standards of nursing care possible within the reality of a specific situation.

The nurse uses judgment in relation to individual competence when accepting and delegating responsibilities.

The nurse when acting in a professional capacity should at all times maintain standards of personal conduct which reflect credit upon the profession.

NURSES AND SOCIETY

The nurse shares with other citizens the responsibility for initiating and supporting action to meet the health and social needs of the public.

NURSES AND CO-WORKERS

The nurse sustains a cooperative relationship with co-workers in nursing and other fields. The nurse takes appropriate action to safeguard the individual when his care is endangered by a co-worker or any other person.

NURSES AND THE PROFESSION

The nurse plays the major role in determining and implementing desirable standards of nursing practice and nursing education.

The nurse is active in developing a core of professional knowledge.

The nurse, acting through the professional organization, participates in establishing and maintaining equitable social and economic working conditions in nursing.

From International Council of Nurses: *ICN code for nurses: ethical concepts applied to nursing,* Geneva, 1973, Imprimeries Populaires.
*New Code will be published May, 2000.

---

quality of care has been defined. National organizations such as the JCAHO and ANA provide these definitions and offer standards of practice to achieve quality, as well as a structure for evaluation of continuing practice (JCAHO, 1999). The following activities serve to support standards of the JCAHO and ANA in the nursing professions:

Evaluation of new professional practices and reassessment of existing ones

Maintenance of standards of health care

Facilitation of personal reflection, ethical thought, and personal growth

Provision of a basis for ethical decision making

Responsibility. The term **responsibility** refers to the characteristics of reliability and dependability. The term implies an ability to distinguish between right and wrong. In professional nursing, responsibility includes a duty to perform actions well and thoughtfully. When administering a medication, for example, a nurse is responsible for assessing the client's need for the drug, for giving it safely and correctly, and for evaluating the response to it. By agreeing to act responsibly, the nurse gains trust from clients, colleagues, and society.

Confidentiality. The concept of **confidentiality** in health care enjoys widespread acceptance in the United

States. Health care providers go to great lengths to ensure that client privacy is respected. Medical records may not be copied or forwarded without a client's consent. Health care information, including laboratory results, diagnosis, and prognosis, is not shared with others without specific client consent. This practice even includes preventing other family members or friends of the client from acquiring health care information. Conflicting obligations may arise when a client wants to keep information from insurance companies to preserve coverage or from employers to preserve a job. The commitment to confidentiality is particularly challenged as medical records become computerized. Preservation of confidentiality is often in competition with the need to facilitate access to information. In the case of computer access, health care institutions work to protect confidentiality by using special access codes that limit what certain employees can find on a computer system.

Veracity. A part of the ANA code of conduct addresses the issue of veracity, another aspect of reliability. **Veracity** in general means accuracy or conformity to truth. As a part of the nursing code of ethics, veracity guides nurses to practice truthfulness. Although in most circumstances veracity is an obvious asset, the practice of truthfulness may be challenged during the delivery of health care. A nurse

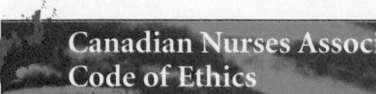

may have to balance competing interests in certain cases. For example, a spouse may make an urgent plea that a client not be given news of a poor prognosis. In this case principles generally in effect that may take precedence over the spouse's wishes include respect for the client's autonomy and the principle of veracity. In some instances it may be tempting to tell a child that a medicine tastes good when it does not, or that a procedure will not hurt when it

probably will, to achieve a level of compliance. Professional codes of ethics guide the nurse to tell the truth, however, and it is a rare circumstance where other principles would support another behavior.

Values

Nursing is essentially a work of intimacy. The tasks of nursing require the nurse to be in very close contact with clients, both physically and emotionally. This kind of contact is usually not acceptable in conventional public relationships. As a result of this intimacy, the work of nursing involves the negotiation of values, whether those values be of the client, the physician, the employer, or other groups. To negotiate values, it is important to have clarity about one's own values: what they are, where they came from, and how they stand in relationship to other's values and to society's values.

A **value** is a personal belief about the worth of a given idea, attitude, custom, or object that sets standards that influence behavior (Maslow, 1959; Rokeach, 1973). The values that an individual holds reflect cultural and social influences, relationships, and personal needs. Values vary among people and develop and change over time. Understanding one's own value system and assessing the value systems of others helps to facilitate decision making while ensuring respect for client autonomy.

VALUE FORMATION

People acquire values in many ways. An understanding of values begins in earliest childhood and is influenced by the way a child is raised. Children develop through different stages of cognitive and emotional growth. The classic works of Piaget (1932), Kohlberg (1981), and Gilligan (1982) provide descriptions of this intricate process (Table 20-2). Basically, as children become more complex cognitively, they become more capable of complex emotional behavior as well. Since a fundamental part of value formation involves the ability to identify strong feelings and to act on them, the acquiring of values depends in large part on experiences within the family.

The character of parenting influences what children come to value as adults. In some cultures children may be prized and indulged until they reach school age and then must face more rigorous discipline as they enter school and the world outside the family. In other cultures children may be raised according to strict gender expecta-

- Discussing life values with clients helps them make meaningful choices in ethical situations. Many older adults have special needs—hearing deficits, cognitive or memory impairments, multiple chronic illnesses, and isolation—that may affect the communication process. The nurse should be prepared to devote the time necessary to communicate with older adults. Listening to older adult clients tell their life stories may give the nurse important moral information about client values.

- Older adult clients may not as readily accept offered medical interventions. Although refusals of treatment may be contrary to the professional's value system, care should be taken to develop a relationship of trust and support with the client to determine his or her values.

- Because of decreasing physical capabilities and cultural bias, older adults are often thought of as mentally incompetent for many decisions. The nurse should support a client's autonomy by directing choices and questions to the client, not a younger relative or caretaker.

- Many older persons have not been as influenced by ideas of client autonomy as younger generations. The nurse should understand that some older adults are uncomfortable questioning or disagreeing with medical authorities. They may view assertiveness as a violation of trust.

- Older persons living in nursing homes should have assistance in preparing advance directives. In collaboration with the client, family, and medical team the nurse can encourage discussions to determine how nursing home residents want their medical care to proceed if they become unable to speak for themselves.

tions. For example, girls assume household duties early in their lives and boys acquire more physical or labor-related skills. In still other cultures children are raised quite separately from adult activities, in communal settings with less exposure to adult socialization or patterning opportunities. These variations in child rearing result in variations in values and variations in adult behavior. The fundamental urge to love and nurture children takes on many different expressions and produces many different kinds of value systems with which we must contend, as individuals and as professionals.

Once children begin to experience life outside the family, they experience a broad range of influences on value

formation. Religious institutions are often charged with the primary responsibility for teaching and enforcing values. Schools, governments, and other social institutions also play a role. The nature of the role depends to a large degree on the nature of the institution. Religions with a strict code of behavior might teach the value of obedience, whereas religions with a focus on helping the poor might focus on the value of charity. A young person who begins to learn about other religions might experience conflict over these differences. Institutional lessons may undergo change from one generation to another. A basic task of the young adult is the identification of values within the context of the community. Over time, an individual acquires values by choosing some that are strongly held in the community and perhaps discarding or transforming others.

Finally, individual experience influences what we come to value. A person who suffers much loss early in life, of a parent or sibling, may grow to value certain things very differently than someone whose life has been free of suffering. A person whose employment has been menial may form certain values that reflect experience of a lack of dignity in the workplace. An appreciation of the source of these differences may promote respectful and effective communication. Within health care, nurses and other providers agree to respect the wide variety of value systems that clients may hold and to try to understand how these differences affect client health and wellness.

VALUES CLARIFICATION

To better articulate one's point of view, it will be helpful to clarify one's own values. One's values constitute an important part of the way one sees the world, and they influence how a person interprets confusing or conflicting information. As individuals mature and experience new situations, their values change. It would be unusual if any one value remained the primary motivating factor throughout a person's life. Value changes may involve a reordering of values or the replacement of old values with new ones. As a result of changing values, a person may modify attitudes and behavior. The willingness to change shows a healthy attitude toward life and the ability to adapt to new experiences.

To adopt new values, a person must first be aware of existing values and how those values affect behavior. To achieve awareness of personal values, it may be helpful to practice the process of **values clarification.** This is a process of self-discovery that helps a person gain insight into values. It is not a set of rules designed to interfere with

Table 20-2 **Modes of Value Transmission**	
Descriptions	Implications
Modeling	
Persons act in a way to show others the preferred way to behave.	Children initially wish to be like their parents; thus parents can model values they perceive as significant.
People acquire values from a variety of role models.	Modeling may not lead to socially acceptable behavior (e.g., viewing another's aggressive behavior).
	Unless parents point out the most desirable values, children can follow any role model.
Moralizing	
Parents and teachers hold standards for right and wrong and rigidly force children to conform to their sets of values.	This approach can be very authoritarian.
	Moralizing parents may be unwilling to consider alternative values for children.
	With this approach, one way is often the only way.
	Young persons reared by moralizing adults often have difficulty with making independent choices.
Laissez-Faire	
At times, people acquire values by behaving informally without restrictions or limitations.	Parents want children to be free to explore a variety of life experiences.
	Children are encouraged to be inquisitive and learn from experiences.
No one value system is right for everyone, and children form values without parents' rigid guidelines.	Parents may refrain from discipline.
	A limitation is that no one assumes responsibility for children's behavior.
	Conflict and confusion may arise if children have no direction.
Responsible Choice	
Balance of freedom and restriction allows children to select values that lead to personal satisfaction and parental support. Children's choices are more limited, as compared with the laissez-faire approach.	Values are not strictly imposed by parents.
	As children choose values, parents, other family members, and teachers allow them to explore, within boundaries, new behaviors and their consequences.
	Children who can freely discuss their behavior and its effects will learn to understand their own values.
Reward and Punishment	
Offering rewards for certain valued behaviors serves to control behavior. When children fail to assume certain behaviors, parents administer punishment.	Parents may choose to use either form of value transmission more frequently.
	Using rewards can be a positive approach to strengthen preferred values.
	Punishment may teach that violence is acceptable.

conscientious decision making, and it does not suggest that a specific set of values should be accepted by all persons. If persons hold a particular value, they have personally chosen, interpreted, justified, and preferred that value over others. Louis Raths (1979) pioneered values clarification as an approach to individual appraisal of values. A person clarifying values learns to make choices when alternatives are presented and determines whether choices are carefully made. The result of values clarification is greater self-awareness and personal insight (Box 20-6).

Cultural values are those adopted as a result of the social setting in which a person lives. Cultural values vary according to the community and the needs of the community. **Ethnocentrism** refers to the belief that one's own culture is superior. As Kirkpatrick and Deloughery (1995) explain, the nurse who holds this belief "may assess and plan intervention for the client, as well as evaluate the effectiveness of what was done, based on personal perceptions and values, without taking into account the perceptions and beliefs of the client." The exercise in Box 20-7 illustrates the wide variety of cultural values that affect perception of health care issues.

The nursing profession has identified professional values that it prizes and nurtures in all members. The

<table>
<tr><td colspan="2">

Three Steps of Values Clarification   Box 20-6

CHOOSING ONE'S BELIEFS AND BEHAVIORS
Choosing from alternatives
Choosing freely
Considering all consequences

PRIZING ONE'S BELIEFS AND BEHAVIORS
Prizing and cherishing the choice
Publicly affirming the choice

ACTING ON ONE'S BELIEFS
Making the choice part of one's behavior
Acting with a pattern of consistency and repetition

</td></tr>
</table>

Modified from Raths LS, Harmin M, Simon SB: *Values and teaching,* ed 2, Columbus, Ohio, 1979, Merrill Publishing.

American Association of Colleges of Nursing (AACN) conducted a national survey of nurses and published the results (Table 20-3). The consensus among nursing leaders across the United States was to recommend seven values essential for the professional nurse: altruism, equality, esthetics, freedom, human dignity, justice, and truth. The description of these values includes samples of personal qualities and behaviors that demonstrate the values.

By understanding one's own point of view, the nurse will become better prepared to understand a client's values, as well as the values of other members of the health care team. The ultimate test of a value system lies in its ability to guide individuals through dissent or confusion. The technologies of contemporary medicine often cause ethical dilemmas wherein competing points of view leave members of the health care team or the team and the client in conflict. Values clarification plays a significant role in the resolution of these dilemmas. In addition, nurses strengthen their ability to advocate for a client when nurses are able to identify personal values and then accurately identify the values of the client.

Once the nurse has mastered the skill of clarifying personal values, it will be possible to turn to the client and apply similar practices that improve the nurse's ability to construct and implement health care interventions. Values clarification can promote a consciousness raising through which clients gain an awareness of personal priorities, identify ambiguities in values, and resolve major conflicts between values and behavior. The nurse may help the client clarify the meaning and significance of values and emotions. The goal of values clarification with a client is effective nurse-client communication. As the client becomes more willing to express problems and feelings, the nurse can better establish an individualized plan of care. The nurse who learns about the client's values and needs can devise a successful plan of care to promote well-being.

A useful method for values clarification with a client is

Cultural Values Exercise   Box 20-7

If persons from a variety of cultures were given this questionnaire, some would strongly agree with the beliefs listed on the left and others would strongly agree with the opposite viewpoint listed on the right. Circle 1 if you strongly agree or 2 if you moderately agree with the statement on the left. Circle 3 if you moderately agree or 4 if you strongly agree with the statement on the right.

1.	Preparing for the future is an important activity and reflects maturity.	1 2 3 4	Life has a predestined course. The individual should follow that course.
2.	Vague answers are dishonest and confusing.	1 2 3 4	Vague answers are sometimes preferred because they avoid embarrassment and confrontation.
3.	Punctuality and efficiency are characteristics of a person who is both intelligent and concerned.	1 2 3 4	Punctuality is not as important as maintaining a relaxed atmosphere, enjoying the moment, and being with family and friends.
4.	When in severe pain, it is important to remain strong and not to complain too much.	1 2 3 4	When in severe pain, it is better to talk about the discomfort and express frustration.
5.	It is self-centered and unwise to accept a gift from someone you do not know well.	1 2 3 4	It is an insult to refuse a gift when it is offered.
6.	Addressing someone by their first name shows friendliness.	1 2 3 4	Addressing someone by their first name is disrespectful.
7.	Direct questions are usually the best way to gain information.	1 2 3 4	Direct questioning is rude and could cause embarrassment.
8.	Direct eye contact shows interest.	1 2 3 4	Direct eye contact is intrusive.
9.	Ultimately, the independence of the individual must come before the needs of the family.	1 2 3 4	The needs of the individual are always less important than the needs of the family.

Modified from Renwick GW, Rhinesmith SH: *An exercise in cultural analysis for managers,* Chicago, 1995, Intercultural Press.

Table 20-3   Essential Nursing Values and Behaviors*

Essential Values	Attitudes and Personal Qualities	Professional Behaviors
Altruism Concern for the welfare of others	Caring Commitment Compassion Generosity Perseverance	Gives full attention to the client when giving care Assists other personnel in providing care when they are unable to do so Expresses concern about social trends and issues that have implications for health care
Equality Having the same rights, privileges, or status	Acceptance Assertiveness Fairness Self-esteem Tolerance	Provides nursing care based on the individual's needs irrespective of personal characteristics Interacts with other providers in a nondiscriminatory manner Expresses ideas about the improvement of access to nursing and health care
Esthetics Qualities of objects, events, and persons that provide satisfaction	Appreciation Creativity Imagination Sensitivity	Adapts the environment so that it is pleasing to the client Creates a pleasant work environment for self and others Presents self in a manner that promotes a positive image of nursing
Freedom Capacity to exercise choice	Confidence Hope Independence Openness Self-direction Self-discipline	Honors individual's right to refuse treatment Supports the rights of other providers to suggest alternatives to the plan of care Encourages open discussion of controversial issues in the profession
Human Dignity Inherent worth and uniqueness of an individual	Consideration Empathy Humaneness Kindness Respectfulness Trust	Safeguards the individual's right to privacy Addresses individuals as they prefer to be addressed Maintains confidentiality of clients and staff Treats others with respect regardless of background
Justice Upholding moral and legal principles	Courage Integrity Morality Objectivity	Acts as a health care advocate Allocates resources fairly Reports incompetent, unethical, and illegal practice objectively and factually
Truth Faithfulness to fact or reality	Accountability Authenticity Honesty Inquisitiveness Rationality Reflectiveness	Documents nursing care accurately and honestly Obtains sufficient data to make sound judgments before reporting infractions of organizational policies Participates in professional efforts to protect the public from misinformation about nursing

From American Association of Colleges of Nursing: *Essentials of college and university education for professional nursing,* Washington, DC, 1986, The Association, reprinted from American Nurses Association: *Code for nurses,* Kansas City, Mo, 1976, The Association.
*The values are listed in alphabetical rather than priority order.

structured communication. Simple strategies that promote the process of sharing feelings can be quite effective. For example, responding to a client by repeating the client's sentence as a question ("You wish you could be at home?") will encourage the client to elaborate. Avoiding questions that can be answered with a yes or no encourage the client to answer in greater detail. Rather than asking, "Do you want to live at home with your daughter?" the nurse might say, "Tell me how you feel about living at home with your daughter."

The character of a nurse's response to a client can motivate the client to examine personal thoughts and actions. When the nurse makes a clarifying response, it should be brief, and nonjudgmental. For example, when talking with a client who exercises rarely, about home arrangements the nurse might say, "I see, so what does your daughter think of the situation?" An effective clarifying response encourages the client to think about personal values after the exchange is over without imposing one's own values onto the client's. In this way, the nurse respects the client's self-direction and avoids inappropriately introducing personal values into the conversation. Although values clarification can occur in any setting, it is often most successful when the nurse has contact with the client over several occasions.

In summary, values clarification plays an important role in communication between people. Especially when the topic concerns issues of personal health, private habits, and quality of life, participants in a discussion will benefit from a clarity of values. The nurse who appreciates values will accurately identify differences between personal opinion and the values that others embrace. Through values clarification, the nurse better serves the needs of clients, especially when values differ. The respect demonstrated for the client's differences and the skill used in helping the client clarify values promote a nurse's ability to teach and to heal.

Bioethics

Just as health care and society itself have changed radically in the past two decades, so, too, has the practice of ethical consideration of health care issues. Perhaps the most striking change in the philosophy of health care delivery is the change in the relationship between health care provider and health care recipient. Half a century ago, health care was delivered in a way that seems like a father taking care of children, by today's standards. A sick person would seek a physician's care and advice and then usually follow the advice without question. The assumption in that culture was that the physician knew everything about sickness and the client knew very little. Issues of client consent and concepts of shared knowledge did not begin until relatively recently.

In an infamous research project conducted in this century, a population of African-American men with syphilis were observed, untreated, for many years so that more could be learned about the progress of syphilis, even though treatment modalities were available, and even though the transmission of syphilis was well understood. Studies such as this one eventually came under close scrutiny as the concept of consent gained recognition in society (Twenty years after, 1992). In many ways, the notion of autonomy was developed to explain and define a society's growing desire to protect clients from scientific endeavors. The notion of client autonomy reflects a change in society's definition of power and knowledge.

PHILOSOPHICAL CONSTRUCTIONS

Philosophical discussion about health care issues has progressed over time, just as developments in health care and society itself have progressed. The methods for discussion and the philosophical constructs that shape the discussions have also changed. Ethics began as a standard reference point for the determination of right action. It has now grown into a field of study that is filled with differences of opinion, competing systems of values, and deeply meaningful efforts to understand human interaction with new technologies. The following discussion introduces the reader to a variety of contemporary ethical systems. The list is neither exclusive nor comprehensive.

Deontology.   A traditional ethical theory, **deontology** proposes a system of ethics that is perhaps most familiar to practitioners in health care. Its foundations are often associated with the work of the eighteenth-century philosopher Immanuel Kant (1724–1804). Deontology defines actions as right or wrong based on their "right-making characteristics such as fidelity to promises, truthfulness, and justice" (Beauchamp and Childress, 1989). It locates the essence of right or wrong within these principles. Deontology specifically does not look to consequences of actions to determine rightness or wrongness. Instead, it critically examines a situation for the existence of essential rightness or wrongness. Ethical terms such as justice, autonomy, and beneficence serve to define right or wrong. Deontology proposes that we determine the presence or absence of each of these principles in an individual situation as a guide for determination of right action. If an act is just, respects autonomy, and provides good, then the act will be ethical. This process depends on a mutual understanding and acceptance of these principles.

Difficulty arises when a person must choose between conflicting principles, which is often the case in health care ethical dilemmas. For example, how to apply the principle of respect for autonomy can be confusing when dealing with the health care of children. The health care team may recommend a certain course of treatment, but the parent may disagree or even refuse the recommendation. Whose autonomy should receive the respect? The parent's? Who should speak for the child's best interest? Society often struggles to understand who should be ultimately responsible for the well-being of children. A commitment to respect autonomy does not guarantee that controversy can be avoided.

Utilitarianism.

A utilitarian system of ethics proposes that the value of something is determined by its usefulness. This philosophy may also be known as **consequentialism,** since its main emphasis is on the outcome or consequence of action. A third term associated with this philosophy is **teleology,** from the Greek word *telos,* meaning "end," or the study of ends or final causes. Its philosophical foundations were first proposed by John Stuart Mill (1806–1873), a British philosopher and social commentator. The greatest good for the greatest number of people is the guiding principle for determining right action in this system. As with deontology, this theory relies on the application of a certain principle, namely, measures of "good" and "greatest" (Beauchamp and Childress, 1989). The difference between utilitarianism and deontology is in the focus on consequences or outcomes. Utilitarianism measures the effect that an act will have; deontology looks to the presence of principle regardless of outcome.

Individuals or groups of individuals may have conflicting definitions of "greatest good." For example, research suggests that education regarding safe sex practices may reduce the spread of human immunodeficiency virus (HIV). But some argue that education about sex should be provided in the family and that sex education in public schools diminishes the role and the value of family. For some, the greater good is defined as educating the greatest number of people in the most effective way possible. For others, the greater good is the preservation of family values and the protection of individual choices regarding sex education of children. The concepts of utilitarianism provide guidance, but they do not inevitably provide answers with universal agreement.

Feminist Ethics.

A newer philosophy focuses on feminism and bioethics. Feminist ethicists consider their work a critique of conventional ethics, as well as a critique of social values. Their work focuses on continuing inequalities between people (Holmes and Purdy, 1992; Wolf, 1996). They look to the nature of relationships between people for guidance in the definition and processing of ethical dilemmas. Writers with this perspective concentrate on more practical solutions than on ethical theory.

Changes in the consideration of women have changed society in many ways. New approaches to old problems, and identification of new problems to solve, have arisen. These changes reflect new perspectives on women's relationship to family, to work, to science, and to society (Sherwin, 1992). For example, until the early 1980s conventional teaching held that moral development, in general, reached its highest stages more often in men than in women. According to this theory, moral development occurred in measurable, predictable stages. The most com-

plex stage incorporated a sense of justice, with young girls not reaching this sense as often as young boys (Kohlberg, 1981). Research from the early 1980s disputed these findings. Carol Gilligan (1982) proposed that Kohlberg's tools to measure moral development were **gender biased.** Gilligan went on to build a new theory of moral development based on her findings. Her theories attempted to accommodate gender differences. Specifically, she concluded that young girls tend to pay attention to community and to individual circumstances, and that young boys tend to process dilemmas through ideals or principles determined abstractly.

Feminist ethics philosophy builds on the idea that principles may distract participants from dealing with larger issues of community. Feminist ethicists value the role of relationships and the stories about relationships. They emphasize the importance of stories and the role of community over an attention to universal principles. In fact, they argue that it is impossible for anyone to be unbiased or not influenced by relationships to people. They even propose that the natural human urge to be influenced by relationships is a positive value (Wolf, 1996).

This system of ethics also addresses issues of gender inequality, proposing that an inequality of attention to women can be remedied by routinely asking, in the midst of any ethical dilemma, how bioethical decisions will affect women (Sherwin, 1992). For example, in a discussion regarding the ethics of fetal surgery (surgical intervention before birth of the child), feminist ethics would propose that questions about the effects of the intervention on the mother are at least as important as questions about the effects on the fetus. Furthermore, feminist ethics philosophy might even value the mother's autonomy above the autonomy of the fetus. In another example, in response to an argument in the literature of ethics that health care services to the very old should be allocated in deference to younger people, the feminist critique works to define and protect the point of view of women. In our society there are more older women than older men, and they tend to be poorer and more alone than older men. Bell (1992) concludes, "If age becomes a standard for limiting the provision of health care, the limits that will be set will affect women more drastically than they affect men." Feminist bioethicists' insistence on gender-based investigations in all ethical discussion would ensure that social facts such as these are addressed.

Ethics of Care.

This ethical theory explores the notion of care as a central activity of human behavior and one that deserves special attention in health care. Those who write about **ethics of care** are often interested in a clear distinction between an ethical theory based on principles, which is considered a male-biased theory, from an ethical theory based on care, which is more female biased, especially as it promotes nurturing of clients and caregivers. Ethics of care and feminist ethics are closely related. Since nursing is primarily a profession of women, the ethics-of-care philosophy has often found supporters from within the profession of nursing.

Supporters of ethics of care conceptualize the activity of care. Nel Noddings (1984) uses the designation "the one-caring" to identify the individual moral agent who provides care or cares for the client and "the cared-for" to refer to the client or patient. In adopting this language, Noddings hopes to emphasize the role of feelings but not at the expense of conventional principles such as autonomy and beneficence. Edmund Pellegrino (1985), a physician, has written on the moral obligation of physicians and nurses to incorporate complex notions of care into a definition of professional behavior. He describes many aspects of care, including the ability and obligation to appreciate, understand, and even share the pain or condition of a client.

Several contemporary nurse authors have proposed a specific philosophy regarding nursing ethics of care that conceptualizes the work of nursing as it is distinct from physician practice. The writers pay special attention to the nursing point of view and nursing practice (Fry, 1989; Leininger, 1988; Watson, 1994). As Leininger (1988) has written, care has been the "central and unifying domain for the body of knowledge and practices in nursing." The ethics-of-care philosophy in nursing suggests that ethical dilemmas will be solved by attention to relationships and by attention to clients' stories. By paying attention in this way, the nurse can promote fundamental acts of caring. This attention to relationships distinguishes ethics of care from ethics based on universal principles. The ethics-of-care philosophy does not rely on universal principles whose content is derived from purely intellectual, analytical processes (Watson, 1994).

The word *care* derives from an old English term, *caru,* meaning "sorrow" or "troubled state of mind." Contemporary use generally implies feeling concern or interest in one who has sorrow, or perhaps even sharing that concern to the point of becoming sorrowful oneself as a show of support. A variation from that meaning suggests taking care of in the sense of providing for or protecting against trouble.

If the term *care* is used too loosely, however, it has a tendency to become sentimental and ineffective. Critics of ethics of care warn that sentimentalizing nursing serves to belittle it—that the nursing point of view may be seen as less strong or less important than the facts associated with medical findings (Boyer and Nelson, 1990). Nonetheless, restating common ethical dilemmas in the language of care provides new and refreshing access to discussion and, hopefully, solution. Is it caring to place a disabled relative in an extended care facility? Should the indigent be cared for? If so, how? Is a shortened hospital stay an expression of caring? How, and for whom? The ethics-of-care philosophy tries to locate ethical discourse at the level where these activities of relationship are located, rather than in an intellectual discussion.

The goal of the ethics-of-care philosophy in nursing is at least twofold: to encourage a broad sense of relationship in ethical discourse and to distinguish nursing as a practice from others to promote understanding of its value to society.

CONSENSUS IN BIOETHICS

The process of addressing ethical issues, especially ethical dilemmas, often becomes a process of negotiation of differences. Each of the above philosophical points of view represents a potential justification for a particular stand on an issue. None of them guarantees a solution. A growing body of writing addresses the potential for group process to facilitate the solution of dilemmas. The understanding of group process, how to promote it, how to protect individuals, how to incorporate principles and social values into the process—all of these things become part of the study of consensus building. Those who study consensus turn to academic fields for help in understanding, including sociology and psychology, as well as philosophy, medicine, and nursing.

Bioethics consensus promises to diminish ethnocentricity by encouraging respect for unusual points of view while still striving to come to agreement between all participants (Moreno, 1995). Bioethics consensus proposes a methodology for processing moral conflict with equal regard for different points of view. It is a technique with a philosophical agenda to promote respect and agreement, rather than a philosophy or moral system itself. Critics of consensus are concerned that group process that is motivated to find agreement will decrease efforts to identify social, religious, or personal values (Callahan, 1993). Like feminist ethicists, critics of bioethics consensus worry that the attention given to resolution will promote avoidance of larger issues of community health in favor of individual cases of conflict.

NURSING POINT OF VIEW

The health care team is truly multidisciplinary, regardless of where the client may be on the wellness-illness continuum. The days of a single practitioner who guides care from the cradle to the grave are gone. Furthermore, economic changes in the delivery of health care in the United States have resulted in large changes in the management of health care systems (see Chapter 2). Professional nurses have come to play vital roles in the fiscal management of health care units and in the clinical management of clients' care in both outpatient and inpatient settings. A client will inevitably interact with a nurse on any journey through the health care system. Although precise understanding of the differences between nurses and other health care professionals may be elusive, most would agree that the differences are real and important.

When ethical dilemmas arise, the nurse's point of view plays a vital and essential role. The nurse will often acquire information about a client that is not available to any of the other disciplines involved. Nurses usually interact with clients over longer time intervals than do other disciplines. In addition, since nurses may be involved in very intimate physical acts such as bathing, feeding, and special procedures, clients and families are revealing information not generally solicited by physicians or social workers. Details about family life at home, information about coping styles or personal preferences, and details about fears and insecurities may come out during nursing interventions (Shannon, 1997).

On the other hand, it is important for nurses to remember that care of any one client has become multidisciplinary and fragmented. The nursing point of view is part of a larger picture that is best built by all members of the health care team, including the client and family. Managers and administrators from many different professional backgrounds may also contribute to ethical discourse with their knowledge of systems, allocation of resources, financial possibilities, or constraints (Figure 20-1).

Wherever the ethical issue arises, the nursing point of view is valuable and often essential. It is both an obligation and a privilege for the professional nurse to accumulate information on the issues, examine personal values, and share knowledge with clients and colleagues in an effort to address the difficult issues that constitute ethical dilemmas in health care.

How to Process an Ethical Dilemma

Ethical problems can cause distress and confusion for both clients and caregivers. Controversy is the very nature of ethical problems, and few people like conflict. To overcome controversy and determine a course of action, ethical issues are processed carefully and deliberately. Participants refrain from making decisions solely on an

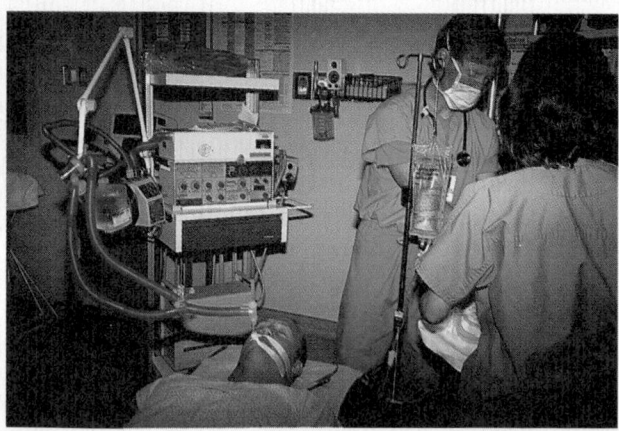

Figure 20-1   Nurses collaborate with other professionals in making ethical decisions.

emotional level, but preserve the free expression of feelings. As discussed previously, however, an ethical outcome is not obtained by considering only what people want and feel. A pattern or guide for thinking through ethical conflicts or dilemmas is very helpful.

Wherever an ethical dilemma is resolved—in a committee setting, at the bedside, or in a family conference—the nurse applies a careful, critical processing of the dilemma. Resolving an ethical dilemma is similar to the nursing process. It requires deliberate, systematic thinking (Miller and Babcock, 1996). Processing an ethical dilemma differs from the nursing process insofar as it requires negotiation of differences, incorporation of conflicting ideas, and an effort to respect differences of opinion. The process of negotiating ethical dilemmas may in part be the process of understanding ambiguities.

Each step in the processing of an ethical dilemma resembles steps in critical thinking. The nurse begins with gathering information and moves through assessment, planning, intervention, and evaluation. The first step guides the nurse in determining whether the problem is an ethical one. Not all problems are ethical in nature. The nurse learns to distinguish ethical problems from questions of procedure, legality, or medical diagnosis. To distinguish an ethical problem from other problems, Curtin and Flaherty (1982) recommend that the nurse decide whether the problem has one or more of the following characteristics:

- It cannot be resolved solely through a review of scientific data. To make this determination, it will be necessary to gather detailed information about the situation. This information may come from medical records, health care literature, consultation with colleagues, or with the client and the client's family. What at first appears to be a dilemma may resolve on the nurse's learning, for example, that a review of a diagnostic procedure reveals a different prognosis.
- It is perplexing. One cannot easily think logically or make a decision about the problem. Or, the nurse may disagree with a decision that others are making, and the difference of opinion is perplexing.
- The answer to the problem will have a profound relevance for several areas of human concern.

A part of gathering information includes an examination of one's own values as they relate to the issues. The distinction between personal opinion and the facts of the case, or the opinions of others, is essential for resolution to proceed. To clarify the true ethical issues in any situation, a nurse needs to be aware of personal responses. People come to different conclusions about the same situation with no malice intended toward other people. Remembering this will help the nurse arbitrate conversations.

After reviewing relevant information and personal values, a clear statement of the ethical problem becomes the groundwork to begin negotiation. Discussions are more likely to remain focused and constructive when all parties agree on the statement of the dilemma. These discussions are next facilitated by listing possible courses of action as they occur to the group. Possibilities may occur at any time during deliberations. After alternatives are considered, persons in an ethical conflict come to a point of resolution or agreement, and action is taken. Decisions are made that can be evaluated in an ongoing manner (Box 20-8).

Documentation of the ethical process can take a variety of forms. Whenever the process involves a family conference or results in a change in the management plan, the process should be documented in the medical record. Some institutions may use a formal consultation format whenever a request for discussion comes to the ethics committee. If the ethical dilemma does not directly affect client care, however, documentation may occur by means of minutes from a meeting or in a memorandum to affected parties. In the following case study, the nursing concerns and the family conferences would be recorded in the medical record and in nursing flow sheets.

On your unit, a young 35-year-old woman has been hospitalized in the final stages of a struggle with brain cancer. She is a single mother with two young children at home. Although she has been treated by conventional, as well as some experimental treatments, the tumor continues to grow, and the medical team has agreed that further treatment

---

How to Process an Ethical Dilemma   Box 20-8

Step 1. Is this an ethical dilemma? If a review of scientific data does not resolve the question, the question is perplexing, and the answer will have profound relevance for several areas of human concern, then an ethical dilemma may exist.

Step 2. Gather all of the information relevant to the case. To be sure it is a true dilemma, it will be important to review all pertinent information. Occasionally an overlooked fact may provide quick resolution. At this point, client, family, institutional, and social perspectives are important sources of relevant information.

Step 3. Examine and determine your own values on the issues. Values clarification provides a foundation for clarity and for confidence during discussions that will be necessary for resolution of a dilemma.

Step 4. Verbalize the problem. A clear, simple statement of the dilemma may not always be easy, but it is essential for the next step to take place.

Step 5. Consider possible courses of action. To respect all sides of an issue, it is helpful to list potential actions, especially when the list will reflect opinions that conflict.

Step 6. Negotiate the outcome. Sometimes courses of action that seem unlikely at the beginning of the process take on new possibility as they are put to rational and respectful consideration. Negotiation requires a confidence in one's own point of view and a deep respect for the opinions of others.

Step 7. Evaluate the action.

---

would be futile. You have cared for this client during past admissions, and during an especially open discussion, she expressed wishes to explore "do not resuscitate" (DNR) orders. During the current admission, her primary physician is out of town. The attending physician does not know the client personally, but he has spent time with her. He has reviewed the clinical data and agrees that the client is entering the terminal stage of her disease. In his opinion, however, the client is not ready to discuss end-of-life issues. In fact, he states that on offering the option to discuss DNR, the client declined. You have asked him to convene a family conference to discuss DNR orders, but he refuses to do so, since in his opinion the client is not ready to participate.

Step 1. Is this an ethical dilemma? What may at first appear to be a question of ethics may be resolved by clarifying one's knowledge base about clinical facts. A review of policy and procedure, or of standards of care, may explain legal obligations that determine a course of action, regardless of personal opinion. If the question remains perplexing, and the answer will have profound relevance for several areas of human concern, then an ethical dilemma may exist.

The single mother's situation meets the criteria for an ethical dilemma. Further review of scientific data will probably not contribute to a resolution of the dilemma, but it is important to review the data carefully to make this determination. The disagreement does not revolve around whether the client is in a terminally ill state, so further clinical information will not change the basic question: Should the client have an opportunity to discuss DNR orders at this time? The question is perplexing. Basically, two professional team members disagree on an assessment of a client's readiness to confront the very difficult issues related to dying. The answer to the question "Is this client ready to discuss end of life?" has important human implications. If she is not ready, then raising the issues may cause anguish and fear in the client and her family. If she is ready and the team avoids discussion, she may suffer unnecessarily in silence. If she is very close to death, then the lack of a DNR order will necessitate the application of cardiopulmonary resuscitation (CPR) in a futile situation. As a nurse, you know that CPR can cause pain. If applied in a situation where further life is unlikely, then CPR could prolong suffering and reduce dignity.

Step 2. Gather as much information as possible that is relevant to the case. Since resolution to dilemmas may arise from unlikely sources, it is helpful to incorporate as much knowledge as possible at every step of the process. At this point, the information could include looking at laboratory and test results, the clinical state of the client in question, and perhaps current literature about the diagnosis or condition of the client. It may include careful investigation into the psychosocial concerns of the client, as well as those of the client's significant others. A client's religious, cultural, and family orientation are part of the nurse's assessment.

You obtain all of the clinical information that is pertinent to the question. It may be helpful in this case to determine if the client retains most cognitive functions, even though her brain tumor is aggressive. You review the chart and discuss this aspect with the physician, and you agree that the client is fully competent, but definitely afraid, and overwhelmed by the prognosis. Since the dilemma exists because two professionals do not agree on a client's state of mind, it may be helpful to reassess the client, or even to request that an independent person assess the client's readiness to discuss end-of-life issues. Sometimes family members or significant others in the client's life will hold important clues to a client's psychological state of mind.

Step 3. Examine and determine your own values on the issues. This step is important for all participants in the discussion. It is at this stage that the nurse, and others, will practice values clarification and try to differentiate between their own values and the values of the client and other team members. Part of the goal is the accurate formation of one's own opinion. An equally essential part of the goal is the establishment of respect for others' opinions.

At this point, you stop to reflect on your own values. You realize that your own religious practices would not prohibit you from deciding to forego further treatment if you were in the client's condition. You also realize that you do not yet have family members who rely on you, such as children or elderly parents. This client's religious practices are perhaps more strictly constructed than your own. Her religion discourages actions that diminish life in any way, and you realize that she may have come to see a DNR order as giving up, or as "acting like God." In addition, you understand that the attending physician has not had time to know this client like her own physician has or like you have. You continue to believe that the client would be capable of a discussion, in spite of her statements to the physician. In fact, you believe that she would benefit from a discussion, since perhaps the combination of an unfamiliar caretaker and declining physical health have silenced her even though her fears and concerns persist.

Step 4. Verbalize the problem. Once all of the relevant information has been gathered, then accurate definition of the problem may proceed. It is helpful to try to state the problem in a few sentences. By agreeing to a statement of the problem, the group can proceed with discussion in a focused way.

Here, the problem seems to be this: Should this client discuss DNR at this time? What are the benefits and what constitute risks of a DNR order at this time? An important question also seems to be on the table regarding the client's current state of mind: Is she afraid to speak? Is she feeling cut off from her normal network (a primary physician)? Are these feelings contributing to confusion about DNR decisions?

Step 5. Consider possible courses of action. What options are available within the context of the situation and the client's value.

Once you have asked the basic question, other questions and possible courses of action arise. Should you initiate a discussion with the client independently of the physician? Would you be outside your professional domain if you facilitated a DNR order? What if your assessment were incorrect? Would you contribute not to the dignity but to the distress of the client? The answers to these questions may be elusive, since

they depend on an understanding of client feelings and values that are not necessarily obvious. Even if legally the nurse cannot actually write a DNR order, this fact does not relieve the nurse of troubling questions, since the ability to influence a physician's or client's decision regarding DNR remains.

Step 6. Negotiate the outcome. This step represents the most important and delicate part of the process. These negotiations may happen informally at the bedside or in the charting room. Or a formal ethics meeting may be necessary. Wherever negotiations occur, the nurse has an obligation to speak for the nursing point of view. The nurse's point of view, by definition, represents a unique contribution to the discussion.

If an ethics committee meeting is convened, then the discussion will usually be multidisciplinary by definition. A facilitator or chairperson will ensure that all points of view are examined and that all pertinent issues are identified. A decision or recommendation is the usual outcome of discussion. In the best of circumstances, participants discover a course of action that meets criteria for acceptance by all. Occasionally, however, participants may leave the discussion disappointed or even opposed to the decision. But in a successful discussion, all members will have agreed on an action or decision that can be implemented.

The discussion focuses on the disagreement between your assessment and the physician's regarding the client's readiness to discuss end-of-life issues. The principles involved during the discussion include beneficence and nonmaleficence: Which plan would provide the most good for this client, a DNR order or no order? A separate question addresses the client's point of view: Would a discussion with the client promote well-being or promote anguish? The principle of autonomy reveals that a troublesome question remains: Does the client want something different from what she is expressing?

With several members of the health care team present, the discussion proceeds. You present your point of view. You continue to sense that the client is ready to discuss DNR orders, but that she may be reluctant to trust the circumstances of this admission. But you also respect the attending physician and his analysis and continue to have concerns that the client may have experienced a change of mind between the last admission and this one. In the end, the team proposes the following: a formal meeting with the client, where you, the attending physician, and a supportive family member, are all present. You support this proposal since you sense that it will maximize the support of the client's existing network. In addition, you recognize that in a trusting environment, the client is most likely to express her fears, insecurities, and wishes most accurately. Team members agree to keep the discussion open ended, and exploratory. You suggest that rather than asking if the client wants a DNR order, perhaps the team could wait for her to bring up the issue. In this way, the team could be assured of her consent and willingness to participate in the discussion.

Step 7. Evaluate the action.

At the meeting the client in fact opens up. She expresses relief at the chance to explore her options and feelings. Pain management issues are clarified. She wants to discuss a DNR order but requests a visit from her priest before making a final decision.

Institutional Ethics Committees

Most health care institutions use an ethics committee to process ethical dilemmas. These committees are generally multidisciplinary and include representatives who are nurses, as well as representatives from other disciplines. Some institutions, especially hospitals, may maintain a council specifically for nurses. These councils serve to educate nurses and others about the ethical process. They may also assume responsibility for policies that guide nursing practice in the care of clients near the end of life. An ethics committee can be especially helpful for the nurse who feels powerless or confused in the presence of an ethical dilemma. Access to an ethics committee or council provides an important resource for the nurse who identifies an ethical conflict or dilemma (Box 20-9).

Processing ethical issues in institutional settings is a community activity, involving input from clients, families, professionals, and administrators. To help facilitate ethical discourse and provide the educational and policy resources necessary to create a climate sensitive to ethical challenges, health care institutions turn to ethics committees. Ethics committees typically serve several purposes, including education, policy recommendation, and case consultation or review. The case review function of ethics committees is accessible to any involved person, including nurses, physicians, clients, and families of clients.

The functions of institutional ethics committees undergo revision and expansion as health care systems change (Smith, 1994). The shift of health care delivery from hospital to community settings has prompted the development of committees in new settings that address the range of social and ethical issues that arise outside of acute care facilities. For example, home care agencies, long-term care facilities, or even ambulatory care settings may set up ethics committees to review difficult situations when they arise and to educate employees and clients about current ethical issues. The JCAHO regularly issues

standards that promote the support of ethical discourse in all delivery settings. Ethics committees serve as a source of policy development to support and protect ethical practice within institutions (Heitman, 1993).

Institutional ethics committees constitute an important part of the fabric that is professional nursing. Ethical issues may be addressed in many other settings, however. Ethical situations can be handled by means of sensitive intervention by the professionals involved. Nurses can provide the insight and skills to solve ethical problems within the context of family conferences, staff meetings, and other settings. Many problems begin when people feel misled or are not aware of their options and do not know when to speak up about their concerns. Formal help from an ethics committee may be sought after other avenues of communication have been pursued. Ethics committees do not replace important relationships; however, they complement relationships and offer a valuable resource for strengthening them.

Issues in Bioethics

Ethical conflict arises in a wide variety of circumstances (Table 20-4). Certain issues common to many health care settings deserve special mention. The concept of informed consent has been developed over the past three decades (see Chapter 21). Its application is often under scrutiny. A corollary to informed consent may be found in the concept of **advance directives,** documents that intend to indicate a client's wishes in the event that the client becomes incapacitated. Both informed consent and advanced directives require that the client and health care providers grapple with definitions of quality of life, another complex issue that often arises within the context of issues in bioethics. Finally, it has become difficult to discuss any of these issues without addressing the perplexing problem of allocation of scarce resources.

INFORMED CONSENT

The goal of informed consent has been to protect the client's ability to participate as fully as possible in decisions regarding personal health. The primary means of meeting this goal has been to share knowledge about clinical findings and management plans as they are implemented. In certain well-defined situations the client must provide written evidence of consent, as in a surgical consent or as in a consent to participate in an experimental regimen.

The practice of informed consent has wide acceptance and respect. Health care providers now go to great lengths to share information that promotes informed consent. Institutional policies and civil law protect the client's right to informed consent. Its practice represents a clear effort to respect the autonomy of clients and in this way also represents a fundamental shift from the paternalism that was more common earlier in this century.

Primary Functions of Ethics Committees   Box 20-9

To offer education in ethics to diverse populations: clients, families, professionals, institutional staff, and community members

To assist institutions in the development and review of policies related to ethical responsibilities

To ensure that policies are implemented and understood by ever-changing groups of practitioners

To serve as resource persons or consultants for specific client situations with ethical dimensions

Table 20-4 **Contemporary Issues in Bioethics**	
Topic	Potential Nursing Implications
Reproductive rights	How do you feel about minors and their ability to seek and receive health care for sexually related issues? If you were a nurse in a clinic setting, how would you approach assessment of an adolescent's sexual activity?
Genetic engineering	Genetic testing may alert a client to a preexisting condition, such as Lou Gehrig's disease. Since no cure currently exists for this disease, how would you counsel a client to approach the test? Does fidelity to the client and respect for autonomy require that you "tell all," or does the principle of nonmaleficence suggest that the information is troublesome and should not be obtained?
Advances in management of infertility	New technologies in fertility often produce multiple-embryo pregnancies. How do you feel about selective abortion in these cases, wherein some embryos may be sacrificed early in the pregnancy to secure the health of the mother and the remaining fetuses? You may be called on to care for very premature infants who are the product of new techniques in fertility management. These infants may be very fragile and require prolonged hospitalization with multiple surgeries and other invasive procedures. How would you define futile care in such a situation?
Physician-assisted suicide	Some states have made it easier for physicians and nurses to participate in the suicide of certain clients. If you were asked to administer drugs or otherwise assist, how would you feel about it? How would you resolve a respect for autonomy with your personal views?

A commitment to the concept of informed consent does involve controversy, however. The concept depends on competence on the part of the provider to communicate well and on the competence of the client to understand. It is not always easy to secure these competencies. Studies on communication skills demonstrate that health care providers are more likely to share information with clients who have similar cultural backgrounds to the provider. Providers may be more likely to give directives or advice than to truly share knowledge with clients who they perceive to be less educated or less intelligent (Todd, 1982).

ADVANCE DIRECTIVES

In 1990 the **Patient Self-Determination Act (PSDA)** became law and was implemented in all health care institutions in the United States. Under the PSDA, clients must be provided with information about their rights to formulate written directions regarding care that they wish to receive in the event that they become incapacitated. Advance directives may include a living will, a document that lists the medical treatment a person chooses to omit or refuse if the person becomes unable to make decisions and is terminally ill. Advance directives may also include the naming of a relative or trusted friend to make medical decisions in the event of the client's incapacitation. This friend or relative is said to have durable power of attorney for health care. A routine part of any admission to a hospital now usually includes inquiry about the client's advance directives, and if they exist, they are included as part of the medical record.

The intent of the advance directive concept is valuable and important. To nurture and protect the voice of clients at what may be their most vulnerable moment is a laudable goal (Figure 20-2). However, the implementation of this concept has been imperfect at best. Although the law has definitely raised public awareness of the issue, many people remain uncomfortable addressing the very difficult issue of dying and avoid dealing with an advance directive. Many people who are admitted to hospitals do so without the advantage of an advance directive. Even when an advance directive is in place, however, its implementation can be controversial or insecure. A long-range study, published in 1995, examined the experiences of dying for several thousand clients (Box 20-10). The study found that most people's wishes were ignored, even when the wishes were reenforced by a written document, a personal meeting, and the assignment of a registered nurse to coordinate regular communication between the client and the health care team. The study made the following conclusion: "Enhancing opportunities for more client-physician communication, although advocated as the major method for improving client outcomes, may be inadequate to change established practices" (SUPPORT, 1995). Even when nurses and others took special measures to communicate client preferences, the process of dying seemed to have a life of its own, unaffected by client preferences. Individuals, institutions, and our society at large continue to grapple with this very challenging effort to ensure client participation throughout the dying process.

Advance directives cannot address the very difficult situation in which conflict or uncertainty exists concerning a child. When a child faces difficult medical management decisions or is determined to be dying, society promotes the role of parent in decision making. But what about parents who are divorcing or a parent who has been abusive, or when parents even in a solid marriage disagree? The determination of the right action and the incorporation of the beliefs and feelings of those who love and care for the

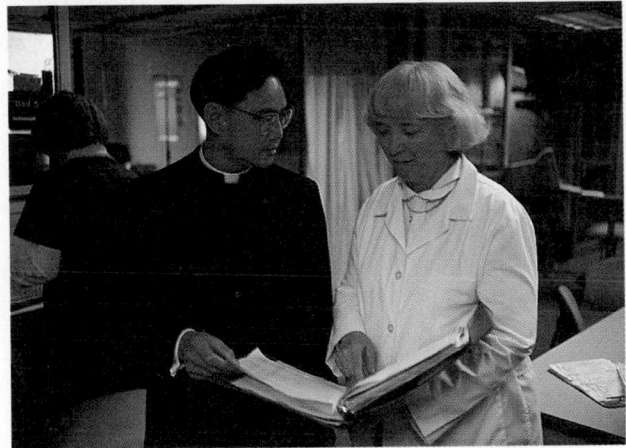

Figure 20-2 Advance directives convey a client's choices about the level of care to be given in times of critical illness.

child into that determination can be deeply challenging tasks, even in light of a commitment to shared knowledge (Nelson and Nelson, 1995).

QUALITY OF LIFE

It is difficult to imagine a concept whose definition is more personal or more elusive than quality of life. For each individual, quality of life is something that is intensely personal and particular. Yet society uses quality-of-life measures to help determine the benefits of medical intervention, and as a result, discussions about quality of life abound. Some social scientists have proposed formulas or other objective measuring devices that can be applied to individual situations (Jacoby, 1992; Fallowfield, 1990). These formulas might take into account the age of the client, the client's ability to live independently, and the client's ability to contribute to society in a gainful way. Such a formula might help a committee determine the relative merits of giving an organ to one recipient over another, for example. Or, a quality-of-life measure could help a client and family decide on the merits of a certain risky intervention, such as an organ transplant or experimental drug management. The question of quality of life is paramount to discussions about futile care, physician-assisted suicide, and DNR discussions.

The definition of quality has been especially challenged by the population of disabled persons in the past few decades. The national movement to pay respect to the abilities of the "disabled" has raised the visibility of quality-of-life issues and forced a reconsideration of the definition of quality. Many school districts, for example, have stopped sequestering physically or mentally challenged children and choose instead to "mainstream" them, or place them in conventional classrooms. Public places have been made accessible to people who must use wheelchairs (Figure 20-3). Economic security has been en-

| Research HIGHLIGHT | Box 20-10 |

RESEARCH ABSTRACT
Providers at five teaching hospitals in the United States studied the process of dying and the effectiveness of communication between clients and providers during the process of dying. In phase I of the study, the investigators followed over 4000 clients in terminal stages of their illnesses. They found striking shortcomings in the quality of communications between clients and providers. Less than half of the physicians knew when their clients preferred avoiding CPR. For half the clients, families reported that the client suffered moderate to severe pain at least half the time.

In phase II, the study team constructed interventions to improve these outcomes and then measured again. The interventions included assigning a special nurse to each family to facilitate and clarify client preferences. The nurse could organize family conferences, make entries into the medical record, and provide other appropriate interventions. Still, at the end of phase II, outcomes were essentially unchanged from those of phase I.

The researchers conclusions were thoughtful and troubling. "Perhaps," they surmised, "physicians and patients in this study acknowledged problems with the care of the seriously ill patients as a group. However, when involved with their own situation or engaged in the care of their individual patients, they felt they were doing the best they could, were satisfied they were doing well, and did not wish to directly confront problems or face choices." In the end, the researchers urged the reexamination of individual and collective commitments to the goal of management of dying wherein pain and unnecessary prolongation of life are reduced and communication between providers and families is enhanced.

IMPLICATIONS FOR PRACTICE
- Nurses can play a key role in bringing health care providers, clients, and families together in end-of-life care.
- When disagreements arise over end-of-life care, the nurse must seek ways to gain consensus.

REFERENCE
SUPPORT Principal Investigators: A controlled trial to improve care for seriously ill hospitalized patients, *JAMA* 274(20):1591, 1995.

hanced by laws that protect people who may be physically or otherwise challenged from discrimination. These changes have greatly increased the integration of disabled persons into general society, and many people have had to reconsider basic definitions of quality. These social changes are not without controversy, but they remind society at large, and health care workers specifically, that definitions of quality are not necessarily written in stone. Society as a whole benefits from these lessons.

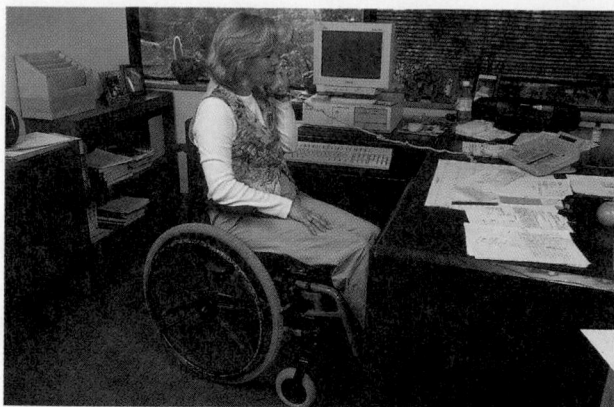

Figure 20-3 Measures can be made to provide accessibility in the work environment.

ALLOCATION OF SCARCE RESOURCES

The concept of scarce resources once was used primarily to assist with discussion of organ transplantation. The term *scarce resource* usually referred to the difficult but common situation wherein far more recipients existed than organs available for transplantation. However, the term has grown to have greater implication as society in the United States is faced with the unequal availability of all health care resources. More than 14% of people living in the United States have no health insurance, and many of those people are women and children. Furthermore, the national costs of health care grow astronomically: in 1991, the United States spent 13.2% of its gross national product on health care; by 1993 that percentage had risen above 18% (Nelson and Nelson, 1996). The growth of managed care reflects a national and economic effort to

control these spiraling costs, but the successes are few, and they generally raise controversy as providers and clients alike struggle with a sense of chaos and lost control.

Although this issue is often larger than a nurse's individual relationship with a client, the application of ethical process or discussion is still applicable. The discussion about allocation of scarce resources easily accommodates the language of ethical principles: respect for autonomy requires that a client not only be able to make an informed choice, but that the treatment chosen be available. Issues of justice apply when certain treatments are available only to certain populations. Processing these thoughts in a way that suggests a clear plan of action, however, is challenging. The individual nurse is still left to ponder personal thoughts. Should resources be focused on research for treatment of devastating disease or on prevention? Which activity is more valuable, research or delivery of care? If public funds are made available for a very expensive intervention, will other populations suffer a diminished level of basic care?

• • •

The courage and intelligence to act, both as an advocate for clients and as a professional member of the health care team, comes only after a committed effort to learn and to understand ethical principles. The professional nurse has a unique point of view regarding clients, the health care system that supports clients, and the institutions that make up the health care system. The nurse has both a duty and the privilege to articulate that point of view. Learning the language of ethical discourse is a part of the skill necessary to exercise this duty and privilege. In addition, review and consideration of various ethical principles assists nurses in forming of personal points of view, a necessary ingredient in the negotiation of difficult ethical situations.

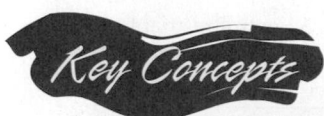

- Ethics refers to the study of philosophical ideals of right and wrong behavior.
- Bioethics refers specifically to ethical issues that affect health and the delivery of health care.
- A code of ethics provides a foundation for professional nursing.
- Professional nursing promotes accountability, responsibility, and advocacy.
- Professional nurses maintain competence in practice and assume responsibility for nursing judgments.
- The primary functions of advocacy are to inform and to support.

- Professional nurses have a commitment to clients, the profession, and society to provide high-quality health care.
- Basic standards of ethics in health care include autonomy, beneficence, nonmaleficence, justice, and fidelity.
- Personal ethics grow from personal values.
- A child acquires values from parents, other family members, school, church, and other social institutions.
- Values clarification helps a nurse to explore personal values and feelings and to decide how to act on personal beliefs.

- Values clarification promotes effective reasoning and decision making.
- Ethical problems arise from differences in values, changing professional roles, technological advances, and social issues that influence quality of life.
- A standard process for thinking through ethical dilemmas helps providers resolve conflict or uncertainty about right actions.
- Critical thinking is an important part of processing ethical dilemmas.
- Feelings and beliefs may also play an important role in the resolution of ethical problems.
- Ethical dilemmas may occur in any segment of the health care delivery system.
- The nurse's point of view provides a unique and valuable voice in the resolution of ethical dilemmas.

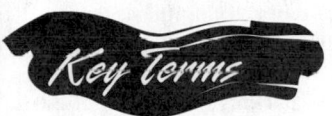

Key Terms

Accountability, *p. 404*

Advance directives, *p. 417*

Autonomy, *p. 402*

Beneficence, *p. 403*

Bioethics, *p. 402*

Code of ethics, *p. 402*

Confidentiality, *p. 405*

Consequentialism, *p. 412*

Cultural values, *p. 408*

Deontology, *p. 411*

Ethics, *p. 402*

Ethics of care, *p. 412*

Ethnocentrism, *p. 408*

Fidelity, *p. 404*

Gender biased, *p. 412*

Justice, *p. 404*

Nonmaleficence, *p. 403*

Patient Self-Determination Act (PSDA), *p. 418*

Responsibility, *p. 405*

Teleology, *p. 412*

Value, *p. 406*

Values clarification, *p. 407*

Veracity, *p. 405*

Critical Thinking Exercises

1. Complete the "cultural values" exercise (Box 20-7) with your classmates or with members of another class of professionals. Compare the answers and discuss the differences.

2. You are caring for a 17-year-old client who has been admitted for treatment of sickle cell crisis. She needs fluid management and comfort management. Even though she is receiving narcotics around the clock, she continues to complain of pain. She also complains about her roommate, the food, and the intravenous line. She comes from a community far from the hospital, and her mother cannot visit every day. She has an older brother who has been convicted of possession of illegal drugs. Discuss your approach to this client. Rank her needs. What is your priority action, based on what you know so far? Examine and describe your opinions about pain, pain management, and addiction.

3. You are a clinic nurse in an small community clinic. A 45-year-old male client has been coming to the clinic for several years for treatment and support of his acquired immunodeficiency syndrome (AIDS). During recent months he has lost his long-term companion to AIDS. In addition, both his parents died many years ago. His clinical condition has deteriorated. His vision is failing, his nutritional status is difficult to maintain, and he has been hospitalized 3 times in the past 3 months for pneumonia. He asks for your help in planning his suicide. Discuss your response to his request. Begin by an examination of your personal feelings about suicide. Include a discussion about your understanding of AIDS: Where does it come from? Who gets the disease? Why? What are your feelings and opinions about people with AIDS? Construct your response, keeping in mind the ethical principles of fidelity, autonomy, beneficence, and nonmaleficence. Since all of these principles collide in this example, it will be important to identify each and recognize personal responses to the role that each plays in this narrative. Just as important is the role that one imagines they play for the client, especially as they differ from one's own. For the sake of this discussion, it is illegal in your state for nurses to prescribe medicines? What are your possible courses of action?

References

American Association of Colleges of Nursing: *Essentials of college and university education for professional nursing,* Washington, DC, 1986, The Association.

American Nurses Association: *Code for nurses with interpretive statements,* Kansas City, Mo, 1985, The Association.

Beauchamp T, Childress J: *Principles of biomedical ethics,* ed 3, New York, 1989, Oxford University Press.

Bell NK: If age becomes a standard for rationing health care. In Holmes HB, Purdy LM, editors: *Feminist perspectives in medical ethics,* Bloomington, 1992, Indiana University Press.

Boyer JR, Nelson JL: A comment on Fry's "The Role of Caring in a Theory of Nursing Ethics," *Hypatia* 5(3), 153, 1990.

Callahan D: Why America accepted bioethics, *Hastings Cent Rep* 23(6 suppl), 58, 1993.

Canadian Nurses Association: *Code of ethics for nursing,* Ottawa, November, 1997, The Association.

Curtin L, Flaherty MJ: *Nursing ethics: theories and pragmatics,* Bowie, Md, 1982, Brady.

Deloughery G: *Issues and trends in nursing,* ed 3, St. Louis, 1998, Mosby.

Fallowfield L: *The quality of life: the missing measurement in health care,* London, 1990, Souvenir Press.

Fry ST: The role of caring in a theory of nursing ethics, *Hypatia* 4(2), 89, 1989.

Gilligan C: *In a different voice,* Cambridge, Mass, 1982, Harvard University Press.

Harris L: Anatomy under duress. In Flack HE, Pellegrino ED, editors: *African-American perspectives on biomedical ethics,* Washington, DC, 1992, Georgetown University Press.

Heitman E: A proactive role for the ethics committee or ethics consultant: meeting the JCAHO standards on patient rights, *Trends Healthcare Law Ethics* 8(4):11, 1993.

Holmes HB, Purdy LM, editors: *Feminist perspectives in medical ethics,* Bloomington, 1992, Indiana University Press.

International Council of Nurses: *Ethical concepts applied to nursing,* Geneva, 1973, Imprimeres Populaires.

Jacoby A: Epilepsy and the quality of everyday life, *Soc Sci Med* 34(6):657, 1992.

Joint Commission on Accreditation of Healthcare Organizations: *1999 accreditation manual for hospitals,* vol 1, Standards, Chicago, 1998, The Commission.

Kirkpatrick SM, Deloughery GL: Cultural influences on nursing. In Deloughery GL, editor: *Issues and trends in nursing,* ed 2, St. Louis, 1995, Mosby.

Kohlberg L: *Essays on moral development,* vols 1-3, San Francisco, 1981, Harper & Row.

Leininger M: *Caring: an essential human need,* Detroit, 1988, Wayne State University Press.

Maslow A: *New knowledge in human values,* New York, 1959, Harper & Row.

Miller MA, Babcock, DE: *Critical thinking applied to nursing,* St. Louis, 1996, Mosby.

Moreno J: *Deciding together: bioethics and moral consensus,* New York, 1995, Oxford University Press.

Nelson HL, Nelson JL: *The patient in the family: an ethics of medicine and families,* New York, 1995, Routledge.

Nelson HL, Nelson JL: Justice in the allocation of health care resources. In Wolf S, editor: *Feminism and bioethics,* New York, 1996, Oxford University Press.

Noddings N: *Caring: a feminist approach to ethics and moral education,* Berkeley, 1984, University of California Press.

O'Neil J: Ethical decision making and the role of nursing. In Deloughery GL, editor: *Issues and trends in nursing,* ed 2, St. Louis, 1995, Mosby.

Pellegrino ED: The caring ethic: the relation of physician to patient. In Bishop AH, Scudder JR editors: *Caring, curing, coping: nurse, physician, and patient relations,* Birmingham, 1985, University of Alabama Press.

Piaget J: *The moral development of the child,* New York, 1932, Free Press.

Raths LE, Harmin M, Simon SB: *Values and teaching,* ed 2, Columbus, Ohio, 1979, Merrill Publishing.

Renwick GW, Rhinesmith SH: *An exercise in cultural analysis for managers,* Chicago, 1995, Intercultural Press.

Rokeach M: *The nature of human values,* New York, 1973, Free Press.

Shannon SE: The roots of interdisciplinary conflict around ethical issues, *Crit Care Nurs Clin North Am* 9(1):13, 1997.

Sherwin S: *No longer patient: feminist ethics and health care,* Philadelphia, 1992, Temple University Press.

Smith M: The future of healthcare ethics committees, *Trends Healthcare Law Ethics* 9(2):7, 1994.

SUPPORT Principal Investigators: A controlled trial to improve care for seriously ill hospitalized patients, *JAMA* 274(20): 1591, 1995.

Todd AD: *Intimate adversaries,* Philadelphia, 1982, University of Pennsylvania Press.

Twenty years after: the legacy of the Tuskegee syphillis study, *Hastings Cent Rept* 22, November–December 1992.

Watson J, editor: *Applying art and science of human caring,* New York, 1994, National League of Nursing Press.

Wolf SM, editor: *Feminism and bioethics,* New York, 1996, Oxford University Press.

Legal Implications in Nursing Practice

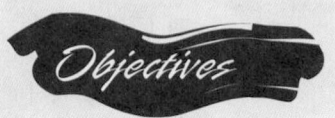

Mastery of content in this chapter will enable the student to:

- Define the key terms listed.
- Explain legal concepts that apply to nurses.
- Describe the legal responsibilities and obligations of nurses.
- List sources for standards of care for nurses.
- Define legal aspects of nurse-client, nurse-physician, nurse-nurse, and nurse-employer relationships.
- Give examples of legal issues that arise in nursing practice.

Safe nursing practice includes an understanding of the legal boundaries within which nurses must function. As with all aspects of nursing today, an understanding of the implications of the law supports critical thinking on the nurse's part. Nurses must understand the law to protect themselves from liability and to protect their clients' rights. Nurses need not fear the law but rather should view the information that follows as the foundation for understanding what is expected by our society from professional nursing care providers. The laws in our society are fluid and constantly changing to meet the needs of the persons the laws are intended to protect. As technology has expanded the role of the nurse, the ethical dilemmas associated with client care have increased and often become legal issues as well. The public is better informed than in the past about their rights to health care. Although federal laws apply to all of the states, nurses must also be aware that laws vary widely across the country. It is important for nurses to know the laws in their state that affect their practice. Nurses' familiarity with the laws enhances their ability to be client advocates.

Licensure

All registered nurses are licensed by the State Board of Nursing of the state in which they practice. The requirements for licensure vary among states, but most states have minimum education requirements and require a licensure examination. All states use the National Council Licensure Examinations (NCLEX) for registered nurse and licensed practical nurse examinations. Licensure permits persons to offer special skills to the public, but it also provides legal guidelines for protection of the public.

A license can be suspended or revoked by the State Board of Nursing if a nurse's conduct violates provisions in the licensing statute. For example, nurses who perform illegal acts such as selling or taking controlled substances jeopardize their license status. Because a license is viewed as a property right, due process must be followed before a license can be suspended or revoked. Due process means that nurses must be notified of the charges brought against them and that the nurses have an opportunity to defend against the charges in a hearing. Hearings for suspension or revocation of a license do not occur in court but are usually conducted by a hearing panel of professionals. Some states provide administrative and judicial review of such cases after nurses have exhausted all other forms of appeal.

Legal Limits of Nursing

Professional nurses must understand the legal limits influencing their daily practice. This, coupled with good judgment and sound decision making, ensures safe and appropriate nursing care.

SOURCES OF LAW

The legal guidelines that nurses must follow are derived from statutory law, regulatory law, and common law. **Statutory law** is created by elected legislative bodies such as state legislatures and the U.S. Congress. An example of state statutes are the Nurse Practice Acts found in all 50 states. These **Nurse Practice Acts** describe and define the legal boundaries of nursing practice within each state. An example of a federal statute enacted by the U.S. Congress is the Americans With Disabilities Act (1995). This statute protects the rights of handicapped individuals in the workplace, in educational institutions, and throughout our society. **Regulatory law,** or **administrative law,** is created by administrative bodies such as State Boards of Nursing when they pass rules and regulations. An example of regulatory law is the duty to report incompetent or unethical nursing conduct to the State Board of Nursing. **Common law** is created by judicial decisions made in courts when individual legal cases are decided. An example of common law is informed consent and the client's right to refuse treatment.

The authors acknowledge the contribution of Penny S. Brooke to this chapter in the previous edition of this text.

Statutory law is either civil or criminal. **Criminal laws** prevent harm to society and provide punishment for crimes (Black, 1990). There are two classifications of **crimes.** A **felony** is a crime of a serious nature that has a penalty of imprisonment for greater than 1 year or even death. A **misdemeanor** is a less serious crime that has a penalty of a fine or imprisonment for less than 1 year. An example of criminal conduct for nurses would be misuse of a controlled substance.

Civil laws protect the rights of individual persons within our society and encourage fair and equitable treatment among people (Black, 1990). Generally, violations of civil laws cause harm to an individual or property. The damages for civil laws involve the payment of money, unlike criminal laws, which are punished by imprisonment.

TORTS

A **tort** is a civil wrong made against a person or property. Torts may be classified as unintentional or intentional. An example of an unintentional tort is negligence or malpractice. **Malpractice** is negligence committed by a professional such as a nurse or physician. Intentional torts are willful acts that violate another's rights. Examples are assault, battery, invasion of privacy, and deformation of character.

Intentional Torts

Assault. **Assault** is any intentional threat to bring about harmful or offensive contact. No actual contact is necessary. The law protects clients who are afraid of harmful contact. It is an assault for a nurse to threaten to give a client an injection or to threaten to restrain a client for an x-ray procedure when the client has refused consent. The key issue is the client's consent. In a lawsuit wherein assault is alleged, the client's consent would bar the claim of assault against a nurse.

Battery. **Battery** is any intentional touching without consent. The contact can be harmful to the client and cause an injury, or it can be merely offensive to the client's personal dignity. A battery always includes an assault, which is why the terms *assault* and *battery* are commonly combined. In the example of a nurse threatening to give a client an injection without the client's consent, if the nurse actually gives the injection, it is considered battery. Battery can also result if the health care provider performs a procedure that exceeds the client's consent. For example, if the client gives consent for an appendectomy and the physician performs a tonsillectomy, battery has occurred. Once again, the key issue is the client's consent.

In some situations consent is implied. For example, if a client gets into a wheelchair or transfers to a stretcher after being advised that it is time to be taken for an x-ray procedure, the client has given implied consent to the procedure. If the client learns that an x-ray film of the head instead of the foot is to be taken and the client refuses to have the x-ray film taken, the consent has been revoked or withdrawn.

Invasion of Privacy. The tort of invasion of privacy protects the client's right to be free from unwanted intrusion into his or her private affairs. The four types of invasion of privacy torts are intrusion on seclusion, appropriation of name or likeness, publication of private or embarrassing facts, and publicity placing one in a false light (Prosser and Keeton, 1988).

Clients are entitled to confidential health care. For example, in a classic case, reporters published photographs of a female client in her hospital room without her consent. A claim for invasion of privacy was upheld. This case is an example of intrusion on seclusion or publication of private, embarrassing facts (*Barber v Time Magazine*, 1942).

Another form of invasion of privacy is the release of a client's medical information to an unauthorized person, such as a member of the press or the client's employer. The information that is contained in a client's medical record is a confidential communication. It should be shared with health care providers for the purpose of medical treatment only.

Hospitals should not make copies of the client's medical record available to anyone without the client's written authorization to release the information and a written request from the party requesting the information (Infante, 1996). The nurse should not disclose the client's confidential medical information without the client's consent. For example, a nurse should respect a wish not to inform the client's family of a terminal illness. Similarly, a nurse should not assume that a client's spouse or family members know all of the client's history, particularly with respect to private issues such as mental illness, medications, pregnancy, abortion, birth control, or sexually transmitted diseases.

An individual's right to privacy may conflict with the public's right to know. In one case a married couple was filmed by a television crew while attending a hospital program in which they participated. The couple had previously told no one but their immediate family that they were involved in the in vitro fertilization program and had been assured that there would be no publicity or public exposure. After the newscast they were subjected to phone calls and embarrassing questions. The couple filed a lawsuit. The court held that the husband and wife stated a claim for invasion of privacy and that even though the in vitro fertilization program may have been of public interest, the identity of the plaintiffs was a private matter (*YG v Jewish Hospital*, 1990).

Many states, through their respective public health departments, require that certain infectious or communicable diseases be reported. Sometimes the client is a public figure whose physical condition is considered newsworthy (Prosser and Keeton, 1988). There are also cases in which information is given out about a scientific discovery or a major medical breakthrough, as with the first heart transplant case or the first artificial heart recipient. If an event falls into any of these categories, information should be channeled through the public relations department of the institution to ensure that invasion of privacy does not occur. The nurse should not independently attempt to decide the legality of disclosing information.

Defamation of Character.   **Defamation of character** is the publication of false statements that result in damage to a person's reputation. The statements must be published with malice in the case of a public official or public figure. **Malice** means that the person publishing the information knows it is false and publishes it anyway or that it is published with reckless disregard as to the truth or falsity of the statement. If the statement is presented orally, it is called **slander.** If the statement is made in writing, it is called **libel.** For example, if a nurse tells people erroneously that a client has venereal disease and the disclosure affects the client's business, the nurse could be held liable for slander.

Unintentional Torts

Negligence.   **Negligence** is conduct that falls below the standard of care. The standard of care is established by law for the protection of others against an unreasonably great risk of harm (Black, 1990). For example, if a driver of a car acts unreasonably in failing to stop at a stop sign, it is negligence. In general, courts define negligence in car accident cases and other negligence cases as the failure to use that degree of care that an ordinarily careful and prudent person would use under the same or similar circumstances (Missouri Approved Instructions, §11.02).

Malpractice.   Malpractice is one type of negligence; it is referred to as professional negligence. Nursing malpractice results when nursing care falls below the standard of care. Nurses can be found liable for malpractice if the following criteria are established: (1) the nurse (defendant) owed a duty to the client (plaintiff); (2) the nurse did not carry out that duty; (3) the client was injured; and (4) the nurse's failure to carry out the duty caused the injury. Even though nurses do not intend to injure clients, if nurses give care that does not meet the appropriate standards, they may be held liable for negligence. Negligence may involve failing to check a client's arm band and then administering medication to the wrong client. Negligence may also involve administering a medication to a client even though it has been documented that the client has an allergy to that medication. In general, courts define nursing negligence as the failure to use that degree of skill or learning ordinarily used under the same or similar circumstances by members of the nursing profession (Missouri Approved Instructions, §11.06) (Box 21-1).

The best way for nurses to avoid being liable for negli-

> ### Common Negligent Acts   Box 21-1
>
> Medication errors that result in injury to clients
> Intravenous therapy errors resulting in infiltrations or phlebitis
> Burns to clients caused by equipment, bathing, or spills of hot liquids and foods
> Falls resulting in injury to clients
> Failure to use aseptic technique where required
> Errors in sponge, instrument, or needle counts in surgical cases
> Failure to give a report, or giving an incomplete report, to an oncoming shift
> Failure to adequately monitor a client's condition
> Failure to notify a physician of a significant change in a client's status

---

gence is to follow standards of care (see p. 429); give competent health care; communicate with other health care providers; document assessments, interventions, and evaluations fully; and develop empathetic rapport with the client. Poor client relations are leading causes of lawsuits (Rutherford, 1994; Ladebauche, 1995). A client who believes that the nurse performed duties correctly and was concerned with his or her welfare is unlikely to initiate a lawsuit. In addition, if a nurse is brought into a lawsuit, careful, complete, and thorough documentation is one of the best defenses. Nurses should also know the current nursing literature in their areas of practice. They should know and follow the policies and procedures of the institution in which they work. Nurses should be sensitive to common sources of client injury, such as falls and medication errors. Finally, nurses must communicate with the client, explain the tests and treatment to be performed, document that specific explanations were provided to the client, and listen to the client's concerns about the treatment. Any significant changes in the client's condition must be reported to the physician and documented in the chart.

STUDENT NURSES

Student nurses are liable if their actions cause harm to clients. If a client is harmed as a direct result of a nursing student's actions or lack of action, the liability for the incorrect action is generally shared by the student, instructor, hospital or health care facility, and university or educational institution. Student nurses should never be assigned to perform tasks for which they are unprepared, and they should be carefully supervised by instructors as they learn new skills. Although student nurses may not be considered employees of the hospital, the institution has a responsibility to monitor the acts of student nurses. Student nurses are expected to perform as professional nurses would in providing safe client care. Faculty members are usually responsible for instructing and observing students, but in some situations staff nurses serving as preceptors may share these responsibilities. Every nursing school should provide clear definitions of preceptor and faculty responsibility.

When students are employed as nursing assistants or nurses' aides when not attending classes, they should not perform tasks that do not appear in a job description for a nurses' aide or assistant. For example, even if a student has learned to administer intramuscular medications in class, this task may not be performed by a nurse's aide. If a staff nurse overseeing the nursing assistant or aide knowingly assigns work without regard for the person's ability to safely conduct the task defined in the job description, the staff nurse will also be liable. If students employed as nurse's aides are requested to perform tasks that they are not prepared to safely complete, this information should be brought to the supervisor's attention so that the needed help can be obtained.

Legal Liability in Nursing

Minimizing Liability Through Effective Documentation and Client Relationships

Nurses can reduce their chances of being named in lawsuits by following standards of care, giving competent health care, and developing an empathetic rapport with clients. In addition, careful, complete, and objective documentation serves as evidence of the standard of nursing care provided (see Chapter 24). Timely and truthful documentation is important to provide the communication necessary among the health care team members. Documentation is used in many ways that benefit the client and demonstrate that the nurse is an effective care provider. Good documentation also keeps other health care providers up to date on the most recent treatments received by the client so that ongoing care can be safely provided. Nurses must be certain that documentation is legible and signed.

A number of courts have stated that when a health care provider negligently alters or loses medical records relevant to a malpractice claim, the health care provider must demonstrate why these events occurred. An institution has a duty to maintain nursing records. These duties are established by statutes and accreditation regulations. Nursing notes contain substantial evidence needed to understand the care received by a client. If records are lost or incomplete, the court will presume that the care that cannot be reviewed was negligent and therefore the cause of the client's injuries. The hospital can, however, provide evidence that it was not negligent and that the injury was not a result of care (Reagan Report, 1994).

Contracts

A **contract** is a written or oral agreement between two people in which goods or services are exchanged (Black,

1990). For a contract to be legally binding, there must be consent, consideration, and competent parties. The law provides a remedy for a breach of the contract.

Employment Contracts. Many nurses are hired without a formal written contract. An oral contract is as legally binding as a written one but may be more difficult to prove. A breach of contract occurs if either party fails to carry out the agreed-on obligations. Even though nurses' employment agreements generally are not in the form of a written contract, some states acknowledge that the employee handbooks and manuals that describe the nurse's responsibilities may be interpreted as the written form of the agreement between the hiring institution and the nurse. Without a written contract, it becomes difficult to prove the terms of the agreement between the employer and the employee nurse, but the court will look to any evidence of what was reasonably agreed on between the nurse and the employer. Nurses should become aware of the state law related to firing "for cause" or "no cause" in the state in which they work. It is important for nurses to understand the employment laws in the state in which they work.

By accepting a job, a nurse enters into an agreement with an employer. The nurse agrees to perform professional duties competently and to adhere to the policies and procedures of the institution. During an employment interview, a prospective employee may want to document what was agreed on. The document should be dated and signed and kept in a safe place. In return, the employer agrees to pay for the nursing services and also to furnish the facilities and equipment in proper working order to enable the nurse to provide efficient and competent care. If nurses sign a contract without reading the agreement, they will be held to the terms of the agreement. Not reading a legally binding contract before signing is no excuse. Institutional policies, procedures, and employee handbooks may be interpreted as the written terms of a nurse's employment contract.

Nurses also enter into contractual arrangements with clients. Nurses agree to give competent care, and the clients agree to pay for the services. When clients sign admission forms on entering a health care institution or agree to nursing care in any health care setting, they initiate the contract. Many private duty nurses have specific written contracts with their clients. It is from such contracts that the client and the nurse identify the specific expectations of both parties.

Insurance. Insurance is a contract wherein for an agreed-on amount of money one party undertakes to compensate the other for loss on a specified subject by specified perils (Black, 1990). For example, a car insurance premium insures a specific car against collision and liability that may result if an accident occurs. The reason that insurance companies can stay in business and make a profit is because they take in more money in insurance premiums than they pay out in claims.

Health Insurance. Health insurance is a contract that provides for payment of physician bills, hospital bills, diagnostic tests, laboratory work, and sometimes medications and dental work. Historically, health insurance was either "service benefit" or "indemnity coverage." Service benefit plans paid the hospital directly and provided full coverage for services such as hospitalization. Indemnity coverage paid the amount specified in the policy to the enrollee, and the enrollee was responsible if the hospital's charges exceeded the insurance payment. Managed care is a system of controlling health care costs while maintaining quality in an attempt to keep the premiums for health insurance coverage affordable (see Chapter 2).

Right to Continue Group Health Coverage. Since most insured individuals and their families obtain health insurance coverage from their employers, Congress passed legislation to allow a terminated employee the ability to maintain group health insurance coverage for a specified period of time as long as the premium is paid. The Consolidated Omnibus Budget Reconciliation Act of 1985 (COBRA) applies to private employers and state and local entities that employ 20 or more employees and sponsor a group health plan. The employee qualifies for COBRA if he or she loses his or her insurance benefits by terminating or being terminated from his or her employment (other than for gross misconduct) or through a reduction in hours. The spouse and the dependents of the employee also qualify if the covered employee loses coverage by termination, death, divorce, legal separation, eligibility for Medicare, or cessation of dependent child status under the plan.

The qualified beneficiary can purchase continuous coverage for 18 months for a termination or reduction in hours, or 36 months for most other events. The beneficiary has to pay the premium on the group health policy, and the employer cannot charge the beneficiary more than 102% of the total cost of the plan for other beneficiaries similarly situated. The right to coverage terminates before the 18 or 36 months if the employer ceases to provide insurance or if the beneficiary fails to make the premium payments, becomes covered under another group health plan that does not exclude or limit coverage for a preexisting condition, or becomes eligible for Medicare. COBRA means that an employee and his or her family will not lose health insurance coverage between jobs and will not have to purchase individual health insurance policies that are much more expensive than employer-sponsored group health coverage. Nurses should take advantage of this privilege, as well as making clients aware of the availability of COBRA.

Portability of Health Insurance. One of the ways that insurance companies keep costs down is by not in-suring certain preexisting conditions that clients have when they obtain the group health insurance coverage. For example, if a client has heart disease, an insurer may agree to provide health insurance for the client for all medical problems except heart disease. The Health Insurance Portability and Accountability Act of 1996 (HIPAA) limits the extent to which health plans may impose preexisting condition limitations and prohibits discrimination in health plans against individual participants and beneficiaries based on health status. HIPAA requires insurers of plans marketed to 2 to 50 employees to guarantee coverage and renewability to small employers who seek coverage. It also requires insurers to make coverage available to certain individuals who had previously had group coverage. Under HIPAA the insurer can only limit coverage for a preexisting condition for 12 months in most cases. The period of any such preexisting condition exclusion is reduced by the aggregate of the periods of creditable coverage unless the employee goes for more than 63 days without any coverage. This means that if an employee has group health insurance coverage with his job for at least 12 months and then changes jobs, the second employer cannot impose a preexisting condition exclusion on the individual. Similarly, if the employee is terminated from his first job and then elects COBRA for 18 months in between jobs, when he starts his second job no preexisting coverage exclusions can be imposed on him. The advantages of HIPAA are that employees can change jobs without losing coverage as a result of a preexisting coverage exclusion as long as they have had 12 months of continuous group health insurance coverage.

Malpractice Insurance. Malpractice or professional liability insurance is a contract between the nurse and the insurance company. Malpractice insurance provides for a defense when a nurse is sued for professional negligence or medical malpractice. As part of the insurance contract, the insurance company pays for any judgment or settlement of the case and also pays for the attorney's fees generated in the representation of the nurse. Nurses employed by health care institutions generally are covered by that institution's insurance and do not need to purchase any supplemental insurance unless the nurse plans to practice nursing outside of the employing institution. The employing institution's insurance, however, only covers nurses while they are working within the scope of their employment. Because nurses are professionals and it is often difficult to separate their private lives from their professional skills, they should consider purchasing individual professional liability insurance, even if the employing institution has coverage. A nurse who is called on by neighbors and friends to provide nursing care on a volunteer basis would not be covered by the hospital's policy if the neighbor or friend filed suit.

Nurses should consult their lawyers on what types of policies to purchase and what rights or duties, if any, exist under the policy. If the employing institution and the nurse are sued in a professional liability case, even though the nurse has insurance with the hospital, the nurse should notify his or her private insurance carrier of the lawsuit. If both the hospital policy and the private policy are considered primary and the hospital loses as a result of the nurse's acts, theoretically the hospital could sue the nurse's private insurer to recover its losses. Most private insurance policies for nurses, however, are considered excess policies and only begin covering the nurse after all of the primary (hospital) insurance coverage has been exhausted. Since the hospital insurance coverage is generally much greater than the private insurance coverage, hospitals very rarely sue nurses' private insurers.

Mothers and Babies. The Newborns and Mothers Health Protection Act of 1996 was passed as a result of what was referred to as "drive-through deliveries," which were attempts to cut utilization of services and limit coverage for hospital stays for mothers and newborns. The statute provides that group health plans, insurance companies, and health maintenance organizations offering health coverage for hospital stays in connection with the birth of children are required to provide such coverage for a minimum time period of not less than 48 hours for a mother and newborn after a normal vaginal delivery and not less than 96 hours after a cesarean section. The minimum time periods do not apply in a case where the decision to discharge the mother or the newborn child is made by the attending physician in consultation with the mother.

Mental Health. Health plans are free to eliminate coverage for certain specialties such as maternity care without violating the Newborn and Mothers Health Protection Act of 1996. They can also impose limits on the amount of coverage that they will pay for certain illnesses. But if mental health benefits are provided, a recent federal statute regulates restrictions on mental health benefits. The Mental Health Parity Act of 1996 forbids health plans from placing lifetime or annual limits on mental health coverage that is less generous than those placed on medical or surgical benefits.

GOOD SAMARITAN LAWS

Nurses may act as Good Samaritans by providing emergency assistance at an accident scene. Good Samaritan laws have been enacted in almost every state to encourage health care professionals to assist in emergency situations (Good Samaritan Law, 1998). These laws limit liability and offer legal immunity for nurses who help at the scene of an accident. They also provide that a nurse can assist a minor in an emergency at the scene of an accident or competitive sports event before obtaining the parent's consent. If a nurse stops at the scene of an automobile accident and gives appropriate emergency care, such as applying pressure to stop hemorrhage, the nurse is acting within accepted standards, even though proper equipment was not available. If the client subsequently develops complications

as a result of the nurse's actions, the nurse is immune from liability as long as he or she acted without gross negligence. Nurses should check their own state's Good Samaritan statute, since some states (e.g., Minnesota and Vermont) require nurses to stop and help in an emergency.

Standards of Care

Standards of care are the legal guidelines for nursing practice. Nursing standards of care are defined in the Nurse Practice Acts and by the State Board of Nursing of each state, by the federal and state laws regulating hospitals and other health care institutions, by the professional and specialty nursing organizations, and by the written policies and procedures of employing institutions (Nursing Practice Act, 1998). In a malpractice lawsuit, nursing standards of care are used to measure nursing conduct and to determine whether the nurse acted as any reasonably prudent nurse would act under the same or similar circumstances. A breach of the nursing standard of care is one element that must be proved in the tort of nursing negligence or malpractice.

The law defines the standards of care that nurses must follow. All state legislatures have passed Nurse Practice Acts that define the scope of nursing practice. Since assistance personnel have been employed, some State Boards of Nursing have defined the registered nurse's responsibilities specifically and developed position statements and guidelines to help licensed nurses delegate safely (Sheehan, 1998). Nurse Practice Acts establish educational requirements for nurses, distinguish between nursing and medical practice, and generally define the scope of nursing practice. The rules and regulations enacted by the State Board of Nursing define the practice of nursing more specifically. For example, a state board may develop a rule regarding intravenous therapy. All nurses are responsible for knowing the provisions of the Nurse Practice Act for the state in which they work, as well as the rules and regulations enacted by the State Board of Nursing and other regulatory administrative bodies.

Professional organizations are another source for defining standards of care. The American Nurses Association (ANA) has developed standards for nursing practice, policy statements, and similar resolutions. The standards delineate the scope, function, and role of the nurse and establish clinical practice standards. For example, the standards for community health nursing practice include data collection, diagnosis, planning, treatment, and evaluation. Nursing specialty organizations also have standards of practice defined for certification of nurses who work in specialty areas such as the operating room (OR) or critical care. These standards also serve as guidelines to determine whether nurses perform their duties appropriately.

The Joint Commission on Accreditation of Healthcare Organizations (JCAHO, 1999) requires that accredited hospitals have written nursing policies and procedures.

Anatomy of a Lawsuit   Box 21-2

Petition—elements of the claim: The plaintiff outlines what the defendant nurse did wrong and how as a result of that alleged negligence the plaintiff was injured.

Answer: The nurse admits or denies each allegation in the petition. Anything that is not admitted must be proved.

Discovery

Interrogatories: Written questions requiring answers under oath. Usual questions concern witnesses, insurance, experts, and which health care providers the plaintiff has seen before and after the incident.

Medical records: The defendant obtains all of the plaintiff's relevant medical records for treatment before and after the incident.

Witnesses' depositions: Questions are posed to the witness under oath to obtain all relevant, nonprivileged information about the case.

Parties' depositions: The plaintiff and defendants (doctor, nurse, hospital personnel) are almost always deposed.

Other witnesses: Factual witnesses, both neutral and biased, are deposed to obtain information and their version of the case. This may include family members on the plaintiff's side and other medical personnel (e.g., nurses) on the defendant's side.

Treating physicians' depositions: Before subsequent treating, physicians' depositions may be taken to establish issues such as those concerning preexisting conditions, causation, the nature and extent of injuries, and permanency.

Experts: The plaintiff selects experts to establish the essential legal elements of the case against the defendant. The defendant selects experts to establish the appropriateness of the nursing care.

Trial: Usually occurs at least 2 to 3 years, and sometimes as long as 6 to 8 years, after the filing of the petition. (Only about 5% of cases are tried. Most are dismissed or settled. Settlement means that money has been paid for the case to be dismissed, usually without any admission of liability.)

PROOF OF NEGLIGENCE

The nurse owed a duty to the client.

The nurse did not carry out the duty or breached the duty (failure to use that degree of skill and learning ordinarily used under the same or similar circumstances by members of their profession).

The client was injured:

  Medical bills, lost wages

  Pain and suffering

  Perinatal damages

  Wrongful death damages

The client's injury was caused by the nurse's failure to carry out that duty ("but for" the breach of duty the client would not have been injured).

The written policies and procedures of the employing institution detail how nurses are to perform their duties. These internal standards of care are usually quite specific and are generally found in ring binders on most nursing units. For example, a policy/procedure outlining the steps that should be taken when changing a dressing or administering medication provides specific information about how nurses are to perform these tasks. Some hospitals are also now using procedural textbooks to outline the institution's general policies and procedures. Nurses must know the policies and procedures of their employing institution because the same standard of care should be used by all nurses in the health care institution (Autonberry, 1995). Institutional policies and procedures must conform to state and federal laws and cannot conflict with legal guidelines that define acceptable standards of care.

In a lawsuit for malpractice or nursing negligence, a nursing expert is called to testify to the jury about the standards of nursing care as applied to the facts of the case (Box 21-2). The standards of care are used by the jury to determine whether the nurse acted appropriately. Nurse experts must base their opinions on existing standards of practice established by Nurse Practice Acts, professional organizations, institutional policies and procedures, federal and state hospital licensing laws, standards of the JCAHO, job descriptions, and current nursing literature (Ladebauche, 1995).

Usually, general duty nurses are responsible for meeting the same standards as other general duty nurses in similar settings. However, specialized nurses such as nurse anesthetists, intensive care nurses, certified nurse-midwives, or OR nurses are held to standards of care and skill exercised by those in the same specialty as defined by applicable standards. All nurses should know the standards of care that they are expected to meet within their specific specialty and work setting. Ignorance of the law or of standards of care is not a defense against malpractice. However, at the time of trial, the standard of care is what the nurse experts testify that standard to be and ultimately what the jury believes (Carroll, 1996).

One of the first and most important cases to discuss a nurse's liability was *Darling v Charleston Community Memorial Hospital.* This 1966 Illinois Supreme Court case has been adopted in almost every state. It involved an 18-year-old man with a fractured leg. The emergency department physician applied a cast with insufficient padding. The man's toes became swollen and discolored, and he developed decreased sensation. He complained to the nursing staff many times. Although the nurses recognized the symptoms as signs of impaired circulation, they failed to tell their supervisor that the physician did not respond to their calls or the client's needs. Gangrene developed, and the man's leg had to be amputated. Although the physician was held liable for incorrectly applying the cast, the nursing staff was also held liable for failing to adhere to the standards of care for monitoring and reporting the client's symptoms. Even though the nurses attempted to contact the physician, this case holds that when the physician fails to respond, the nurse must go over the physician's head to make sure that the client is appropriately treated.

The best way for nurses to keep up with the current legal issues affecting nursing practice is to read the nursing literature in their practice area. Current nursing literature deals with the changing obligations and standards of care for nurses, explains pertinent state and federal laws, and keeps the nurse up to date on any new rules or regulations and case law.

CONFIDENTIALITY

Nursing standards for what constitutes confidential information are based on professional ethics (see Chapter 20). The ideals of privacy and sensitivity to the needs and rights of clients who may not choose to have nurses intrude on their lives, but who depend on nurses for their care, guide the nurse's judgment. The nurse's sense of fairness and professionalism demand that confidential information not be shared with others. A client's medical record is confidential. There are several state and federal statutes that protect the confidentiality of medical information. Unless the client consents, nurses should not disclose confidential client information.

CONSENT

A signed consent form is required for all routine treatment, hazardous procedures such as surgery, some treatment programs such as chemotherapy, and research involving clients (JCAHO, 1999). A client signs general consent forms when admitted to the hospital or other health care facility (Figure 21-1). Separate special consent or treatment forms must be signed by the client or a representative before specialized procedures or treatments are performed.

State statutes provide the designation of individuals who are legally able to give consent to medical treatment (Consent to Surgical or Medical Treatment, 1998). Nurses should know the law in their own states and be familiar with the policies and procedures of their employing institution regarding consent (Box 21-3).

If a client is deaf, illiterate, or speaks a foreign language, an interpreter should be available to explain the terms of consent. A client under the effects of a sedative is not able to clearly understand the implications of an invasive procedure. Every effort should be made to assist the client in making an informed choice.

Nurses must be sensitive to the cultural issues of consent. The nurse must understand the way in which clients and their families communicate and make important decisions. It is essential for nurses to understand the various cultures with which they interact. The cultural beliefs and values of the client may be very different from those of the nurse. It is important for nurses not to impose their own cultural values on the client. Insensitivity toward and stereotyping of different ethnic groups are of equal concern. A conscious awareness of the different values and be-

---

Statutory Guidelines for Legal Consent for Medical Treatment
Box 21-3

Those who may consent to medical treatment are governed by state law but generally include the following:
I. Adults
   A. Any competent individual 18 years of age or older for himself or herself
   B. Any parent for his or her unemancipated minor
   C. Any guardian for his or her ward
   D. Any adult for the treatment of his or her minor brother or sister (if an emergency and parents are not present)
   E. Any grandparent for a minor grandchild (if an emergency and parents are not present)
II. Minors
   A. For his or her child and any child in his or her legal custody
   B. For himself or herself in the following situations:
       1. Lawfully married or a parent (emancipated)
       2. Pregnancy (excluding abortions)
       3. Venereal disease
       4. Drug or substance abuse
   C. Unemancipated minors may not consent to abortions without one of the following:
       1. Consent of one parent
       2. Self-consent being granted by court order
       3. Consent specifically given by a court

---

liefs held by various cultures is essential for sensitive nursing care.

Informed Consent.   **Informed consent** is a person's agreement to allow something to happen, such as surgery, based on a full disclosure of risks, benefits, alternatives, and consequences of refusal (Black, 1990). Informed consent not only requires that a person be given all relevant information required to reach a decision regarding treatment, but also requires that the person be capable of understanding the relevant information and does in fact give consent. One who performs a procedure on a client without informed consent may be found civilly liable for committing battery.

The following factors must be verified for a consent to be valid (Prosser and Keeton, 1988):
1. The person giving the consent must be mentally and physically competent and be legally an adult (usually over 18 years of age or emancipated).
2. The consent must be given voluntarily; no forceful measures may be used to obtain it.
3. The person giving the consent must thoroughly understand the procedure, its risks and benefits, and alternative procedures.
4. The person giving consent has a right to have all questions answered satisfactorily and confirm his or her understanding of the treatment to be given.

TERMS AND CONDITIONS OF ADMISSION

NECESSARY MEDICAL TREATMENT
Recognizing the need for hospital care for the child whose name appears herein, consent is hereby given for hospital services rendered under the general and specific instructions of the attending physician and treatment to be necessary for the safety, welfare, and health of the child.

PROFESSIONAL CARE
The patient is under the professional care of an attending physician who arranges for services for the care and treatment of the patient. The attending physician is usually selected by the patient's parent or guardian but may when not designated or under emergency circumstances be otherwise selected.

RELEASE OF INFORMATION
The Hospital is authorized to furnish information from the patient's medical record to any insurer, compensation carrier, or welfare agency who may be providing financial assistance for hospital care.

PHOTOGRAPHS
Photographs of the patient may be taken under the supervision of The Hospital by members of the staff or other persons for teaching, medical research purposes, or for publicity as deemed proper by The Hospital, and the taking of pictures, unless specifically denied in writing, shall not be deemed an invasion of privacy.

PERSONAL VALUABLES
The Hospital shall not be liable for loss or damage to any personal property of the patient brought into The Hospital.

PAYMENT FOR HOSPITAL CARE
I/We do hereby assume financial responsibility for and agree to make payment in full to The Hospital for all charges for services or medical supplies furnished the patient. Payment is to be made within 30 days as bills are presented, with settlement in full or arrangements for same to be made in the Financial Counseling Department before departure of the patient.

I/We do certify that the financial information given is true, accurate, and complete to the best of my/our knowledge and further authorize The Hospital to investigate any and all financial information given on this admission under their normal investigative procedures.

I/We do hereby assign and authorize payment directly to The Hospital and physician(s) of all hospitalization or insurance benefits and physician-fee benefits and guarantee to pay any balance with the understanding that the account is not settled or closed until after the insurance benefits are received by The Hospital and if there is a remaining balance I/we agree to pay the same. I/We are aware of the above contents.

I/We hereby certify that I/we have read all parts of this Admission Form and agree and accept all terms and conditions hereon and state that all representations made by me/us are true.

I am aware of the above contents.

A photocopy of the agreement shall be considered as valid and as effective as the original.

SIGNED	ADDRESS	PHONE
RELATIONSHIP TO PATIENT	DATE	
WITNESS	DATE	
SECOND WITNESS (TELEPHONE CONSENTS)	DATE	

Figure 21-1   Sample consent form for admission to the hospital.

Informed consent is part of the physician-client relationship. Because nurses do not perform surgery or direct medical procedures, in most situations, obtaining clients' informed consent does not fall within the nursing duty. Even though the nurse assumes the responsibility for witnessing the client's signature on the consent form, the nurse does not legally assume the duty of obtaining informed consent (Figure 21-2). The nurse's signature witnessing the consent means that the client voluntarily gave consent, that the client's signature is authentic, and that the client appears to be competent to give consent

(Sullivan, 1998). When nurses provide consent forms for clients to sign, the clients should be asked if they understand the procedures for which consent is being given. If clients deny understanding or the nurse suspects they do not understand, the nurse must notify the physician or nursing supervisor and must make certain that clients are informed before signing. Some consent forms also have a line for the physician to sign after explaining the risks and alternatives to a client. Such a form is helpful in a court case when a client alleges that consent was not informed. A client refusing surgery or other medical treatment must

INFORMED CONSENT FOR AMNIOCENTESIS

I. I hereby request and authorize Doctor _____ to perform a diagnostic amniocentesis (pass a needle through the abdominal wall and withdraw some of the amniotic fluid). I further request that an attempt be made to perform the following test(s) on my unborn child:

  A. Chromosome analysis _____ (Initial)

  B. Alpha-fetoprotein _____ (Initial)

  C. Acetylcholinesterase _____ (Initial)
      (If indicated)

  D. _____ _____ (Initial)

II. I consent to the performance of an ultrasound examination for the purpose of dating the pregnancy, locating the placenta and selecting a site for placement of the needle.

III. I understand that:

  A. the procedure of amniocentesis involves a small risk to both mother and fetus and that these risks include; discomfort at the site where the needle was inserted, cramping, bloody spotting, leakage of amniotic fluid, intrauterine infection and miscarriage.

  B. there is a possibility that growing the fetal cells may not be successful and that repeat amniocentesis would then be required.

  C. although the likelihood of an error is considered to be extremely small, a complete and correct diagnosis of the condition of the fetus based on the test(s) performed cannot be guaranteed.

  D. the results provided of normal chromosomes or normal biochemical status of the fetus does not eliminate the possibility that the child may have birth defects and/or mental retardation because of other disorders.

  E. in the case of twins, the results may apply to only one of the pair.

  F. in some Rh negative mothers Rh sensitization has occurred following amniocentesis.

IV. I have had my questions answered and understand and accept the risks and limitations of this test.

Signed: _____ (Patient)

         _____ (Spouse)

         _____ (Witness)

         Date: _____

Figure 21-2 Sample consent form for a special procedure.

be informed about any harmful consequences of refusal. If the client persists in refusing the treatment, this rejection should be written, signed, and witnessed.

If a client participates in an experimental treatment program or submits to use of experimental drugs or treatments, an even more detailed and stringently regulated informed consent form is used. The Food and Drug Administration (FDA) and an organization's institutional review board (IRB) review the information in the consent form for research involving human subjects. The client may withdraw from the experiment at any time (see Chapter 25).

Parents are usually the legal guardians of pediatric clients, and therefore they are the persons who must sign consent forms for treatment. If the parents are divorced, the parent with legal custody must give consent. Occasionally a parent or guardian refuses treatment for a child. In those cases the court may intervene on the child's behalf.

In some instances obtaining informed consent is difficult. If, for example, the client is unconscious, consent must be obtained from a person legally authorized to give consent on the client's behalf. Other surrogate decision makers may have legally been delegated this authority through special process of attorney documents or through court guardianship procedures. If a person has been declared legally incompetent in a judicial proceeding, consent must be obtained from the person's legal guardian (Coker and Johns, 1994). In emergency situations, if it is impossible to obtain consent from the client or an authorized person, the procedure required to benefit the client or save a life may be undertaken without liability for failure to obtain consent. In such cases the law assumes that the client would wish to be treated.

Psychiatric clients must also give consent. They retain the right to refuse treatment until a court has legally determined that they are incompetent to decide for themselves.

Legal Relationships in Nursing Practice

PHYSICIANS' ORDERS

The physician is responsible for directing medical treatment. Nurses are obligated to follow physician's orders unless they believe the orders are in error or would harm clients. Therefore all orders must be assessed, and if one is found to be erroneous or harmful, further clarification from the physician is necessary. If the physician confirms the order and the nurse still believes it is inappropriate, the supervising nurse should be informed. A nurse should not proceed to perform a physician's order if it is foreseeable that harm will come to the client. The nursing supervisor should be informed and given a written memorandum detailing the events in chronological order, the reasons for refusing to carry out the order should also be written to protect the nurse from disciplinary action. The supervising nurse should help resolve the questionable order. A medical consultant may be called in to help clarify the appropriateness or inappropriateness of the order. A nurse carrying out an inaccurate or inappropriate order may be legally responsible for any harm suffered by the client.

In a malpractice lawsuit against a physician and a hospital, one of the most frequently litigated issues is whether the nurse kept the physician informed of the client's condition. To inform a physician properly, nurses must perform a competent nursing assessment of the client to determine the signs and symptoms that are significant in relation to the attending physician's tasks of diagnosis and treatment. Nurses must be certain to document that the physician was notified and document his or her response, the nurse's follow-up, and the client's response.

VERBAL ORDERS

The physician should write all orders, and the nurse must make sure that they are transcribed correctly. Verbal orders are not recommended because they increase the possibilities for error. If a verbal order is necessary (e.g., during an emergency), it should be written and signed by the physician as soon as possible, usually within 24 hours. The nurse should be familiar with the institution's policy and procedures regarding verbal orders.

"DO NOT RESUSCITATE" ORDERS

A difficult area regarding physician orders involves an order of "no code" or "do not resuscitate" (DNR) for a terminally ill client. Many physicians are reluctant to write such orders because they fear legal repercussions for "abandoning" a client. A "no code" order should be written, not given verbally. The physician should regularly review DNR orders in case the client's condition warrants a change. Partial code or "slow code" verbal instructions have been suggested as a way for a physician to avoid writing a "no code" order. However, "slow codes" may be defined differently by various institutions and may be interpreted as not performing resuscitative procedures as a competent person would. If resuscitative procedures are performed more slowly than recommended by the American Heart Association, they may be interpreted as being below the standard of care and therefore become the basis for a lawsuit.

Cardiopulmonary resuscitation (CPR) is an emergency treatment that is provided without client consent. It is a procedure that is performed on an appropriate client unless a DNR order is written in the client's chart. Since 1988, when New York first adopted legislation regarding DNR orders, over 20 states have drafted similar statutes (New York DNR Statute, 1988). The statutes assume that all clients will be resuscitated unless there is a DNR order in the chart in writing. Adult clients may consent to a DNR order orally or in writing after being given the appropriate information by the physician. An oral consent requires two witnesses, one of whom must be a physician affiliated with the hospital. A written consent requires two adult witnesses. If the client lacks the capacity to give consent, a surrogate may give consent for the client if two physicians say that within reasonable medical certainty the client has a terminal condition, the client is terminally unconscious, resuscitation would be medically futile, or resuscitation would impose extraordinary burden on the client in light of the client's medical condition and the expected outcome of resuscitation. If no surrogate is available to give consent, the DNR order can still be written but only if the physician is reasonably medically certain that the resuscitation would be futile. The statutes provide that the attending physician must review the DNR orders every 3 days for hospitalized clients or every 60 days for clients in residential health facilities.

SHORT STAFFING

During nursing shortages or staff downsizing periods, the issue of inadequate staffing may arise. The JCAHO (1999) requires institutions to have guidelines for determining the number (staffing ratios) of nurses required to give care to a specific number of clients. Legal problems may arise if there are not enough nurses to provide competent care. If nurses are assigned to care for more clients than is reasonable, they should bring this information to the attention of the nursing supervisor. If nurses are required to accept assignments, they should make written protest to nursing administrators. Although these protests may not relieve nurses of responsibility if a client suffers an injury because of inattention, it would show that they were attempting to act reasonably. Whenever a written protest is made, nurses should keep a copy of this document in their own personal file. Most administrators recognize that knowledge of a potential problem shifts some of the responsibility to the institution. Nurses should not walk out when staffing is inadequate, because charges of abandonment could be made. A nurse who refuses to accept an assignment may be considered insubordinate, and clients will not benefit from having even less staff available. It is important to know the institution's policies and procedures on how to handle such reports before the situation arises.

FLOATING

Nurses are sometimes required to "float" from the area in which they normally practice to other nursing units. In one case a nurse in obstetrics was assigned to an emergency department. A client entered the emergency department and complained of chest pain. The client was given an increased dosage of lidocaine by the obstetrical nurse and died after suffering irreversible brain damage and cardiac arrest. The nurse lost the malpractice lawsuit. Nurses who float should inform the supervisor of any lack of experience in caring for the type of clients on the nursing unit. They should also request and be given orientation to the unit. A supervisor can be held liable if a staff nurse is given an assignment he or she cannot safely handle. In the case of *Winkelman v Beloit Memorial Hospital* (1992), the court remarked that if an employer wishes to rotate nurses to areas outside of their usual area of expertise, the employer should provide the training and education to prepare nurses to work in an area outside of their normal assignment. Before accepting employment, nurses should find out the institution's policies regarding floating and have an understanding as to what is expected. For example, nurses should not be floated to areas where they have not been adequately cross-trained.

Legal Issues in Nursing Practice

Legal issues in nursing practice reflect changing trends in the lifestyles of people in our society. The following topics are examples of recent developments in the law.

SURROGATE PREGNANCY CONTRACTS AND ADOPTION

Several states have statutes that prevent enforcement of surrogate parenting agreements. In such agreements couples agree to pay pregnancy and birth expenses to a woman who is artificially impregnated and gives birth to the couple's baby. In states where there is no challenge to surrogacy itself and no governing statute, if a dispute arises between the parties, the courts need to become involved to determine the rights and responsibilities of the parties, as well as the enforceability of any contractual agreements between the parties. Other states have "baby selling" statutes that prohibit the exchange of money for adoption and thus make most surrogacy contracts unenforceable. In the case of *In the Matter of Baby M* (1988), a New Jersey Court held that a surrogacy contract that involved the payment of money was illegal. In a 1993 California case, *Johnson v Calvert*, the court held that the payments were to compensate the surrogate for services and labor and not for giving up parental rights. Legal and public policy considerations determine whether surrogacy statutes are enforceable. All states have statutes regulating adoption and prohibit a mother from giving final consent to the adoption of her child before birth or before the passage of a waiting period after birth. Therefore after the child is delivered by the surrogate, the child is adopted by the intended parents.

ABORTION ISSUES

In 1973 in the case of *Roe v Wade*, the U.S. Supreme Court ruled that there is a fundamental right to privacy, which includes a woman's decision to have an abortion. The court ruled that during the first trimester a woman could end her pregnancy without state regulation because the risk of natural mortality from abortion is less than with normal childbirth. During the second trimester the state has an interest in protecting maternal health, and the state may enforce regulations regarding the person performing the abortion and the abortion facility. By the third trimester, when the fetus becomes viable, the state's interest is to protect the fetus, so the state can therefore prohibit abortion except when necessary to save the mother.

In 1989 in the case of *Webster v Reproductive Health Services*, the court substantially narrowed the *Roe v Wade* case. States may require viability tests before conducting abortions if the fetus is thought to be over 28 weeks' gestational age. States may also require a minor's parental consent or a judicial decision that the minor is mature and can self-consent.

In the case of *Planned Parenthood of Southeastern Pennsylvania v Casey* (1992), informed consent was upheld in that the physician must present the woman with a description of the nature of the abortion procedure, the health risk related to abortion and childbirth, the probable gestational age of the fetus, and the availability of state-published material about medical assistance, adoption agencies, and child support from the father. The court also upheld a mandatory 24-hour waiting period between when the materials are provided to the client and when the abortion is performed. An emancipated minor must get informed consent of one parent or a judicial determination that the minor is mature and can give her own informed consent.

To make a case of ADA discrimination, the plaintiff must prove:

That he or she has a disability:

Has a physical or mental impairment that substantially limits one or more major life activities

Has a record of such impairment *or*

Is regarded as having such impairment

That he or she is otherwise qualified (can perform the essential functions of the job with or without reasonable accommodations)

IMPLICATIONS FOR PRACTICE

Health care workers with disabilities (i.e., HIV infection) are protected in the workplace.

Health care workers may not discriminate against HIV-positive clients.

AMERICANS WITH DISABILITIES ACT

The Americans With Disabilities Act (ADA) (1995) is a very broad reaching civil rights statute. It protects the rights of disabled people and is the most extensive law on how employers must treat health care workers and clients infected with the human immunodeficiency virus (HIV). The Supreme Court ruled in 1998 in *Bragdon v Abbott* that even asymptomatic HIV constitutes a disability within the meaning of the ADA. This means that the HIV-positive individual who does not have acquired immunodeficiency syndrome (AIDS), which is a cluster of symptoms, is still protected by the ADA (Box 21-4).

HUMAN IMMUNODEFICIENCY VIRUS

HIV is found in clients in virtually every segment of nursing practice, from clients with AIDS on medical-surgical units, to mothers and infants in perinatal units, to pediatric clients with hemophilia. Nurses must use standard precautions when caring for all clients (see Chapter 33). Nurses have the responsibility to safeguard themselves and others from exposure to infectious material. Therefore items or areas contaminated with body fluids must be appropriately handled, discarded, and/or decontaminated.

Co-workers who refuse to work with HIV-infected people can leave companies open to indirect charges of discrimination if the employer does not monitor the work environment. Issues of disclosure, privacy, and confidentiality are an important concern when working with HIV-infected clients or peers. Several cases have held that the health care provider may be obligated to disclose the fact that he or she is infected with HIV. The ADA regulations protect the privacy of infected people by giving individuals the opportunity to decide whether to disclose their disability.

Health care workers are not required to be tested for HIV as a condition of employment. If a health care worker is contaminated by a client whose HIV status is unknown, the health care worker cannot check the client's blood for HIV without the client's consent. The statute provides that the client must be provided "consultation" before being tested for HIV and during the reporting of the test result.

DEATH AND DYING

Many legal issues surround the event of death, including a basic definition of the actual point at which a person is considered dead. There are essentially two standards for the determination of death. The cardiopulmonary standard requires irreversible cessation of circulatory and respiratory functions. The whole-brain standard requires irreversible cessation of all functions of the entire brain, including the brain stem. The reason for the development of different definitions is to facilitate recovery of organs for transplantation. Even though the client may be legally "brain dead," the client's organs may be healthy for donation to other clients. The Uniform Determination of Death Act (1980) has been adopted in most states and provides that either the cardiopulmonary definition or the whole-brain definition may be used to determine death. Nurses must be aware of legal definitions of death because they must document all events that occur when the client is in their care. Nurses may also be assigned the responsibility of discussing the possibility of organ donation with a dying client's family.

Consent for an autopsy must have been given previously by the decedent before death or may be given by a close family member at the time of death. In many states there is an order of priority for the giving of consent for autopsies, such as (1) decedent, in writing; (2) durable power of attorney; (3) surviving spouse; and (4) surviving child, parent, brother, or sister in the order named (Autopsy Consent, 1998). Death is to be reported and investigated by the coroner when there are reasonable grounds to believe that the person died as a result of violence, homicide, suicide, accident, or death occurring in any unusual or suspicious manner. The coroner should be also be contacted if a client's death is unforeseen and sudden and the client has not been seen by a physician in over 36 hours.

In other situations involving death, nurses have specific legal duties. For example, nurses have the legal obligation to treat the deceased person's remains with dignity (see Chapter 29). Wrongful handling of a deceased person's remains could cause emotional harm to the survivors. In one case, for example, survivors sued when a mislabeling of bodies led to an Orthodox Jew's body being prepared for a Roman Catholic funeral and a Roman Catholic's body being prepared for Jewish burial.

RIGHT TO REFUSE TREATMENT

The doctrine of informed consent ensures the client the right to refuse medical treatment. The right of a competent client to refuse medical treatment was upheld in the *Bouvia v Superior Court* case in 1986. That case allowed the discontinuation of the client's tube feedings at her request. The courts have also upheld the right of a competent client to refuse medical treatment for religious reasons. Christian Scientists refuse medical treatment based on religious beliefs, and Jehovah's Witnesses accept medical treatment but refuse blood transfusions for religious beliefs. In the absence of a truly compelling reason otherwise, the right to make those choices are protected. The U.S. Supreme Court stated in the *Cruzan v Director Missouri Department of Health* case in 1990 that "we assume that the U.S. Constitution would grant a constitutionally protected competent person the right to refuse lifesaving hydration and nutrition." In cases involving the client's right to refuse or withdraw medical treatment, the courts balance the client's interest with the state's interest in protecting life, preserving medical ethics, preventing suicide, and protecting innocent third parties. Children are generally considered innocent third parties. While the courts will not force adults to undergo treatment that is refused for religious reasons, they will grant an order allowing hospitals and doctors to treat children of Christian Scientists or Jehovah's Witnesses who have denied consent for treatment of their minor children.

Where clients are incompetent and are unable to make health care decisions, the courts balance the state's interest with what the client would have wanted. The courts attempt to substitute their judgment as to what the client would have chosen if the client were competent. The Supreme Court held in the Cruzan case that states had the right to require "clear and convincing evidence" of an incompetent client's prior wishes when making determinations to discontinue life-sustaining treatment. In that case nutrition and hydration were recognized as life-sustaining medical treatment that could be withdrawn.

Every state now requires "clear and convincing evidence" of the client's choice but states differ as to what standard satisfies the amount of evidence required. If there is no evidence of the client's prior choice, most states allow treatment to be stopped based on other factors, including the best interest of the client balanced with the state's interest.

PHYSICIAN-ASSISTED SUICIDE

In 1994 the State of Oregon passed the Oregon Death With Dignity Act, which was the first statute that permitted physician-assisted suicide. The statute provided that a competent individual with a terminal disease, defined as an "incurable and irreversible disease that has been medically confirmed and will, within reasonable medical judgment, produce death within 6 months," could make an oral and written request for medication to end his or her life in a humane and dignified manner. The written request had to be signed and witnessed by two individuals. The attending physician had to refer the individual to a

consulting physician and refer the individual for counseling, if appropriate. The attending physician also had to have the individual notify his or her next of kin and provide information regarding the medication so that an informed decision could be made. There was a 15-day waiting period between the initial oral request and the writing of the prescription and no less than a 48-hour waiting period between the written request and the writing of the prescription. The individual had a right to rescind the request at any time and had to be able to self-administer the medication. The courts in Oregon prevented enforcement of the statute.

In *Compassion in Dying v Washington* (1996) and *Quill v Vacco* (1996), challenges to state statutes that made assisting in suicide a criminal act in Washington and New York respectively were filed with the courts. The lower courts both held that the criminal statutes were unconstitutional. The cases were heard by the Supreme Court, and on June 26, 1997, the Supreme Court held in *Washington v Glucksberg* that there is no fundamental constitutional right to assisted suicide. In making its ruling, the Supreme Court did not preclude the states from passing legislation legalizing assisted suicide. The Supreme Court also relied on the fact that there are no legal barriers to obtaining pain medication and that dying patients in Washington and New York could "obtain palliative care, even when doing so would hasten their deaths."

Nurses must be aware of the issues surrounding physician-assisted suicide. Other states have proposed similar legislation. The ANA's position statement on assisted suicide (1994) defines assisted suicide as making a means of suicide (e.g., pills or a weapon) available to a client with knowledge of the client's intention to commit suicide (Price and Murphy, 1995). The ANA believes that nurses should not participate in assisted suicide.

ADVANCE DIRECTIVES

Many clients have living wills, special medical directives, or medical powers of attorney identifying health care surrogates. The *Patient's Self-Determination Act* (1992) requires health care institutions to provide written information to clients concerning the clients' rights under state law to make decisions, including the right to refuse treatment and formulate advance directives. Under the act, it must be documented in the client's record whether the client has signed an advance directive. The hospital is also required to ensure that state law is followed and provide education for the staff and the public concerning living wills and durable powers of attorney. The nurse should be familiar with the institution's policies complying with the act.

Living Wills. **Living wills** are documents instructing physicians to withhold or withdraw life-sustaining procedures when death is imminent. These procedures are considered as prolonging the dying process rather than promoting life. Each state providing for living wills has its own requirements for executing them. Generally, two witnesses, neither of whom can be a relative or physician, are needed when the client signs the document. If health care workers follow the directions of the living will, they are immune from liability.

Medical special directives also must be legally prepared with the appropriate witnessing of the client's signature. They give directions to health care providers on the client's desires in specific critical situations. Health care surrogate statutes are sometimes also referred to as durable powers of attorney. Clients execute these documents to appoint someone to make health care decisions if and when they are no longer able to make decisions on their own behalf.

ORGAN DONATIONS

An individual who is at least 18 years of age may make an anatomical gift (defined as a "donation of all or part of a human body to take effect upon or after death.") The gift must be made in writing and signed by the donor. If the donor cannot sign, the document must be signed by another individual and two witnesses. In many states adults may sign the back of their driver's license, indicating consent to organ donation. Pursuant to the Uniform Anatomical Gift Act of 1987, which has been adopted in nearly 20 states, unless the gift is revoked by the donor before death, no further consent is required after the donor's death.

In most states Required Request laws mandate that at the time of admission to a hospital, a qualified health care provider must ask each patient over 18 whether they are an organ or tissue donor. If the answer is affirmative, a copy of the document should be obtained. If the answer is negative and the attending physician consents, the option to make or refuse an anatomical gift should be discussed. Documentation should be placed in the client's medical record. Required Request laws came about because of the shortage of suitable organs for transplantation. Required Request laws are also part of the Uniform Anatomical Gift Act (1987), which addresses many issues involving organ donation, including the rights and duties at death. The physician who certifies death shall not be involved in the removal or transplantation of organs (see Chapter 29).

The National Organ Transplant Act of 1984 prohibits the purchase or sale of organs. The act also provides civil and criminal immunity to the hospital and physician who acts in accordance with the act. The act also protects the donor's estate from liability for injury or damage that may result from the use of the gift. Organ transplantation is extremely expensive. Clients in end-stage renal disease are eligible for Medicare coverage for a kidney transplant, but other transplants have to be paid for by private insurance. The United Network for Organ Sharing has a contract with the federal government and sets policies and guidelines for the procurement of organs. Most clients who require organ transplantation have to be placed on a waiting list for an organ in their geographical area. Recently, the geographical system has changed to give priority to clients who demonstrate the greatest need. Nurses must be familiar with their employing institution's policies and procedures regarding organ donation.

Legal Issues in Nursing Specialties

Within every specialty of nursing there are legal issues that affect nursing practice. Some of the more common legal issues follow.

COMMUNITY HEALTH NURSING

Nurses work in various sites outside of institutionalized nursing settings. Included in community settings are occupational or industrial work sites where nurses provide preventive and ongoing primary care to workers. Nurses also work in public or community health, where preventive services such as immunizations and well-child care are provided in schools, homes, and clinics. Nurses are professionals who are accountable for the autonomous judgments they make while working in a community setting. The community health nurse must work collaboratively with other health care team members to verify that the care provided and information shared is timely and accurate.

It is important that nurses, especially those employed in community health settings, understand the public health laws. State legislatures enact statutes under the Health Code, which describes the reporting laws for communicable diseases, school immunizations, and laws intended to promote health and reduce health risks in communities. The Centers for Disease Control and Prevention (CDC) (*http://www.CDC.gov*) and the Occupational Health and Safety Act (OHSA) (*http://www.osha.gov*) also provide guidelines on a national level for safe and healthy communities and work environments. The purposes of public health laws are protection of the public's health, advocating for the rights of people, regulating health care and health care financing, and ensuring professional accountability for the care provided. Community health nurses have the legal responsibility to enforce the laws enacted to protect the public's health. These laws may include reporting suspected abuse and neglect, reporting communicable diseases, ensuring that required immunizations have been received by clients in the community, and reporting of other health-related issues enacted to protect the public's health.

EMERGENCY DEPARTMENT

As a result of clients being transferred from private hospitals to public hospitals without appropriate screening and stabilization (referred to as "patient dumping"), Congress enacted the Emergency Medical Treatment and Active Labor Act (1986). This act provides that when a client comes to the emergency department or the hospital, an appropriate medical screening must be done within the hospital's capacity. If an emergency condition exists, the client may not be discharged or transferred until the condition is stabilized. The client can be discharged or transferred before he is stable, however, if the client requests in writing to be transferred or discharged after being informed of the benefits and risks, or if a physician certifies that the benefits of transfer outweigh the risks. The transfer must always be appropriate, which means (1) that the receiving facility agrees to the transfer, has space for the client, and has qualified personnel to receive the client; (2) the medical records must be forwarded to the receiving hospital; and (3) the client must be transported by qualified personnel and transportation equipment.

Nursing of Children

Every state with child abuse legislation requires that suspected child abuse or neglect must be reported. Health care professionals such as nurses are mandated to report suspected cases. To encourage reports of suspected cases, states provide legal immunity for the reporter if the report is made in good faith. Health care professionals who do not report suspected child abuse or neglect may be held liable for civil or criminal legal action.

As in all areas of nursing practice, negligence involving pediatric clients is possible, and the nurse is responsible for preventing a child in his or her care from accidentally coming to harm. Cribs, which sometimes have a restraining device over the top, are designed to keep infants and toddlers from climbing out of bed and injuring themselves. All poisonous substances and sharp objects should be kept out of the reach of small children. When possible, small children should be kept under constant watch to minimize opportunities for accidental harm.

Medical-Surgical Nursing and Geriatrics

Many hospitals and long-term care facilities are considered to be "restraint free." Adults who are disoriented or confused, however, may require some form of restraining device to prevent accidental self-injury. Standards of care, laws, and regulations concerning the use of restraints and supervision required apply to nursing practice with medical-surgical and other clients. In the general hospital and long-term care settings, the most frequent indications for restraints are as follows: (1) risk of injury to self (falls) or others, (2) interference with treatment, and (3) disruptive or disturbing behavior (Ortiz-Pruitt, 1995). The FDA has set forth guidelines for the use of restraints (U.S. Department of Health and Human Services, 1992). Side rails and bed alarms are available on most hospital beds for use with adult clients. The nurse must know when and how to use restraints correctly. A physician's order including the purpose for the restraint is required to physically restrain a client. Orders for a restraint are limited to 24 hours. After a client is restrained, the nurse is required to make frequent client assessments and to periodically release restraints (see Chapter 37). A client who falls out of bed and becomes injured or who suffers injury from improper restraint application may bring a lawsuit against the nurses and the institution.

The *Resident's Rights* section of the *Medicaid Statute* (1988) regulates the use of physical or chemical restraints in nursing facilities. The statute provides that restraints may be imposed (1) only to ensure the physical safety of the resident or other residents and (2) only on the written order of a physician that specifies the duration and circumstances under which the restraints are to be used (except in emergency circumstances until such an order could reasonably be obtained).

Critical Care Nursing

Critical care nurses require special training and ongoing in-service education with regard to advanced client monitoring and management of critical illness. The staffing ratio in an intensive care setting should be one nurse for each client, depending on the severity of the clients' conditions. The JCAHO recommends these ratios because of the intensity of care required by such clients (JCAHO, 1999). These clients usually require careful observation and assessment of their conditions, as well as treatments, procedures, and medications. If a nurse is assigned to three or four intensive care clients, is unable to give appropriate care, and a client suffers harm, the nurse is liable for accepting the client assignment.

Potential legal problems for critical care nurses are associated with the use of electronic monitoring devices. No monitor is totally reliable, and the nurse must not completely depend on it. Therefore the nurse's continual assessment of a client is necessary to help document the accuracy of electronic monitoring. There may also be electrical hazards to the nurse and the client. The equipment should be checked routinely by biomedical engineers to ensure that it is in proper working order and to make sure that a client will not receive an electrical shock.

Operating Room Nursing

Sponge, needle, and instrument counts are routine standards in the operating room to prevent lawsuits. Even though the physician inserts sponges and instruments into the surgical wound, the physician relies on the nurse's counts at the end of the procedure. Generally, when the chart records a correct sponge count and the client suffers an injury because of a retained sponge, the hospital is liable because the nurse charted a correct count when it was not correct.

Every piece of equipment must be carefully used to prevent injury to the client. Laser equipment has created the potential for burns and other tissue injuries (Merriman, 1995). There can also be liability for nurses because of incorrect positioning or insufficient padding placed when positioning the client.

PSYCHIATRIC NURSING

A client can be admitted to a psychiatric unit involuntarily or on a voluntary basis. A petition for involuntary detention must be filed with the court within 96 hours of the client's initial detention. A hearing must be conducted within 2 days of the filing of the involuntary petition. If the judge determines that the client is a danger to self or others, the judge will grant the involuntary detention, and the client can be detained for 21 more days for psychiatric treatment.

Potentially suicidal clients are admitted to psychiatric units. If the client's history and medical records indicate suicidal tendencies, the client must be kept under supervision. Lawsuits result from clients' attempts at suicide within the hospital. The allegations in the lawsuits are that the health care provider failed to provide adequate supervision and failed to safeguard the facilities. Documentation of precautions against suicide is essential.

HOME HEALTH CARE NURSING

With the increased focus on managed care, hospital stays are much shorter, and as a result many clients may be discharged from the acute care setting at an earlier time in their disease process and still require nursing care (Fiesta, 1995). Nursing care may range from assistance with daily living activities to ventilator care. The nurse has greater responsibility and autonomy in the home.

Home health care, however, differs from the acute care setting because in the hospital setting, hospital personnel and physicians are available to assess client changes. In the home the nurse must know when to call in the supervisor or the physician. Nurses must know the policies and procedures of the employing institution, particularly with respect to the chain of command, equipment failure, and informed consent (Sullivan, 1994). The chain of command generally refers to the hierarchy of supervisors and physicians to report to if problems arise. Most of all, nurses must be sure to document their assessments and interventions so that any claim of inadequate or improper care can be defended.

THE NURSE AS AN ADVOCATE

Nurses serve as client advocates by protecting the rights of clients to be informed and to participate in decisions regarding the care they will receive. The nurse may also become an advocate when a health risk is identified for which there is no legal guidance. The nurse may become actively involved as a lobbyist through the legislative and administrative processes. Nurses serve as client advocates when they become involved to improve health care. A lobbyist is a person who informs decision makers and educates them regarding the needs of clients and the safe practice of nursing. Nurses must serve as experts in educating lawmakers and policy makers on the needs of clients and the community.

THE NURSE AS RISK MANAGER

Risk management is a system of ensuring appropriate nursing care. All nurses should be risk managers. The steps involved in risk management include identifying possible risks, analyzing them, acting to reduce the risks, and evaluating the steps taken. One tool used in risk management is the **incident report** (Figure 21-3).

For nurses in practice, the underlying rationale for quality improvement and risk management programs is the highest possible quality of care. Some insurance companies, medical and nursing organizations, and the JCAHO require the use of quality improvement and risk management procedures (JCAHO, 1999).

Risk management also requires good documentation. The nurse's documentation can be the nurse's memory of what actually was done for a client and can serve as proof that the nurse acted reasonably and safely. Documentation should be thorough, accurate, and performed in a timely manner (see Chapter 24). To protect the nurse and the client, the nurse should document the care given and the details associated with it (Eggland, 1995). Charting "physician notified" may be insufficient if at the time the nurse is being questioned about the lawsuit, he or she does not recall which physician and what specific facts were told to the physician. When a lawsuit is filed, very often the nurse's notes are the first thing reviewed by an attorney. The nurse's assessments and the reporting of significant changes in the assessments are very important factors in defending a lawsuit. Therefore the nurse should identify the physician contacted, the information communicated to the physician, and the physician's response.

PROFESSIONAL INVOLVEMENT

Nurses must be involved in their professional organizations and on committees that define the standards of care for nursing practice. If current laws, rules and regulations, or policies under which nurses must practice do not re-

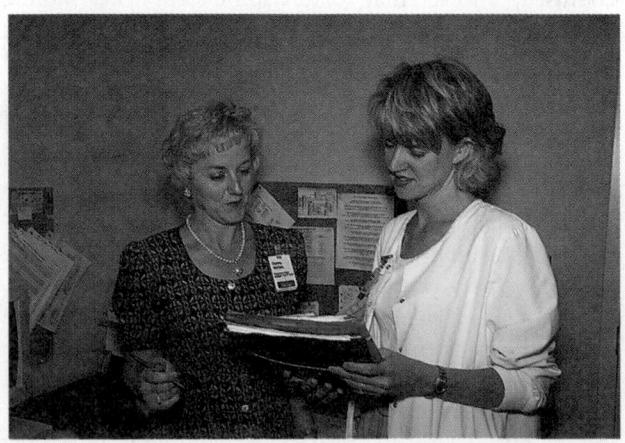

Figure 21-3   Nurses discussing an incident report.

flect reality, nurses must become involved in lobbying to see that the scope of nursing practice is accurately defined. Nurses must be willing to represent nursing and the client's perspective on community boards as well. The viewpoint of nurses becomes more powerful and nurses become more effective as a profession when they are organized and cohesive.

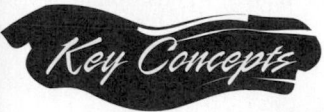

Key Concepts

- With increased emphasis on client rights, nurses in practice today must understand their legal obligations and responsibilities to clients.
- Registered nurses and licensed practical nurses are licensed by the state in which they practice; licensing is based on educational requirements, the passing of an examination, and other criteria.
- The civil law system is concerned with the protection of a person's private rights, and the criminal law system deals with the rights of individuals and society as defined by legislative statutes.
- Nurses should act and speak carefully to avoid frightening, coercing, or physically intimidating clients (assault).
- Informed consent allows physical procedures to be carried out in a lawful manner, without fear of battery.
- A nurse can be found liable for malpractice if the following criteria are established: the nurse (defendant) owed a duty to the client (plaintiff), the nurse did not carry out that duty, the client was injured, and the nurse's failure to carry out the duty caused the client's injury.
- All clients are entitled to confidential health care and freedom from unauthorized release of information.
- Student nurses are expected to perform as professional nurses, should be assigned only to tasks for which they are prepared, and should be carefully supervised.
- Under the law, practicing nurses must follow standards of care, which originate in Nurse Practice Acts, the guidelines of professional organizations, and the written policies and procedures of employing institutions.
- Nurses are responsible for confirming that informed consent has been given for any surgery or other medical procedure before the procedure is performed.
- Nurses are responsible for performing all procedures correctly and exercising professional judgment as they carry out physicians' orders.
- Nurses are obligated to follow physicians' orders unless they believe the orders are in error or could be detrimental to clients.

- Staffing standards determine the ratio of nurses to clients, and if the nurse is required to care for more clients than is reasonable, a formal protest should be made to the nursing administration.
- Legal issues involving death include documenting all events surrounding the death, treating a deceased person with dignity, and obtaining consent for an autopsy from the decedent (before death) or a close family member (after death).
- A competent adult can legally give consent to donate specific organs, and nurses may serve as witnesses to this decision.
- All nurses should know the laws that apply to their area of practice.
- Depending on state laws, nurses are required to report possible criminal activities such as child abuse, as well as certain communicable diseases.
- Nurses are client advocates and ensure quality of care through risk management and lobbying for safe nursing practice standards.
- Nurses must file incident reports in all situations when someone could or did get hurt.

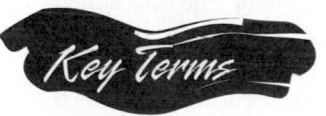

Key Terms

Administrative law, *p. 424*	Libel, *p. 426*
Assault, *p. 425*	Living wills, *p. 437*
Battery, *p. 425*	Malice, *p. 426*
Civil laws, *p. 425*	Malpractice, *p. 425*
Common law, *p. 424*	Misdemeanor, *p. 425*
Contract, *p. 427*	Negligence, *p. 426*
Crimes, *p. 425*	Nurse Practice Acts, *p. 424*
Criminal laws, *p. 425*	Regulatory law, *p. 424*
Defamation of character, *p. 426*	Risk management, *p. 440*
	Slander, *p. 426*
Felony, *p. 425*	Standards of care, *p. 429*
Incident report, *p. 440*	Statutory law, *p. 424*
Informed consent, *p. 431*	Tort, *p. 425*

Critical Thinking Exercises

1. Nurse Smith and Nurse Jones are getting on an elevator to go down to the cafeteria. There are several visitors present in elevator, as well as hospital personnel. Nurse Smith and Nurse Jones are talking about a patient who is in the intensive care unit who has just tested positive for HIV. They identify the patient as the man in Room 14B. One of the visitors on the elevator who overhear this information is a woman who is engaged to the client in Room 14B.
   A. Have Nurse Smith and Nurse Jones breached a client's right to confidential health care?
   B. Will the client in Room 14B have any legal cause of action against the nurses?
   C. Even though the client's fiancée may have a right to know the HIV status of her future husband, is there any duty on the part of the nurses to disclose confidential information to the fiancée?

2. While transporting a client down the hall on a stretcher, Nurse Black stops to chat with an orderly. The side rails on the stretcher are down, and while Nurse Black has her back to the stretcher, the client rolls over, falls off the stretcher, and fractures his hip. In a lawsuit by the client against Nurse Black, what must the client establish to prove negligence against the nurse?

3. During the client's labor and delivery of her first child, she developed a fever of 38.9° C (102° F). When the client was fully dilated, Nurse White called the physician and informed him that the client was fully dilated. At that time, the physician said that he would be at the hospital within 30 minutes. After the doctor hung up the phone, he fell asleep again and did not arrive at the hospital for 1½ hours. The baby suffered brain damage as a result of a bacterial infection. In the client's lawsuit against the physician and the nurse:
   A. Did the nurse have any obligation to call the physician back when he did not arrive at the hospital within 30 minutes?
   B. If the nurse was unable to contact the physician, should she have notified her supervisor or called the head of obstetrics?
   C. The physician testified at the trial that the nurse did not advise him of the fever and that if he had known about it, he would have ordered antibiotics and gotten to the hospital sooner. Should the nurse have advised the physician of the fever when she called him about the dilation?
   D. If the fever developed after she hung up the phone, should she have called the physician back to notify him of the fever?
   E. The client's nurse expert testified that the nurse was negligent because she did not tell the physician that the patient had an elevated temperature.

What sources for the standard of care did the nurse expert use to establish nursing negligence?

4. Sally Green, a 16-year-old girl, is the mother of a newborn baby. While driving in her car, without having her newborn baby in an appropriate baby carrier, Sally Green has a car accident. Her newborn baby suffers a head injury. Physicians tell Sally Green that her baby has suffered severe brain damage and that she cannot be maintained without life support. They request her consent to have the baby's organs donated for transplant.
   A. Since Sally Green is a minor, is she able to give consent?
   B. Does the hospital have any duty to report Sally Green to the Division of Family Services for failure to have her child in a protective seat?
   C. If Baby Green should suffer a cardiac arrest, can the nurses and doctors perform CPR on the baby without consent?

References

American Nurses Association: *Position statement on assisted suicide,* Unpublished manuscript, 1994.

Autonberry D: Risk management and non-employed nurses, *Nurs Manage* 26(9):70, 1995.

Black HC: *Black's law dictionary,* ed 6, St. Paul, Minn, 1990, West Publishing.

Carroll M: Nursing malpractice and corporate negligence, *J Nurs Law* 3(3):53, 1996.

Coker L, Johns A: Guardianship for elders: process and issues, *J Gerontol Nurs* 20(12):25, 1994.

Eggland E: Charting tips: avoiding incomplete charting, *Nurs 95,* p 73, October 1995.

Fiesta J: Home care liability, part I, *Nurs Manage* 26(11):24, 1995.

Infante M: Legally speaking: the legal risks of managed care, *RN* 59(3):57, 1996.

Joint Commission on Accreditation of Healthcare Organizations: *Accreditation manual for hospitals,* Chicago, 1999.

Ladebauche P: Limiting liability to avoid malpractice litigation, *MCN Am J Matern Child Nurs* 20:243, 1995.

Merriman J: How have changes in health care affected perioperative nurses' liability? *AORN J* 61(1):258, 1995.

Missouri Approved Instructions: *Definition: negligence of adult,* § 11.02.

Missouri Approved Instructions: *Definition: negligence of health care providers,* § 11.06.

Ortiz-Pruitt J: Physical restraint of critically ill patients: a human issue, *Crit Care Nurs Clin North Am* 7(2):363, 1995.

Price D, Murphy P: Assisted suicide: new ANA policy reflects difficulty of issue, *J Nurs Law* 2(2):53, 1995.

Prosser W, Keeton W: *Prosser and Keeton on the law of torts,* ed 5, St. Paul, Minn, 1988, West Publishing.

Reagan Report on Nursing Law, 35 RRNS, December 7, 1994.

Rutherford M: Legally speaking: small patients, big legal risks, *RN* 57:51, September 1994.

Sheehan J: Directing UAPs—safely: unlicensed assistive personnel, *RN* 61(6):53, 1998.

Sullivan G: Legally speaking: home care: more autonomy, more legal risks, *RN* 57:63, May 1994.

Sullivan G: Getting informed consent: role of nurses in obtaining informed consent from patients, *RN* 61(4):59, 1998.

U.S. Department of Health and Human Services, Food and Drug Administration: *Safety alert*, Rockville, Md, 1992, The Department.

Statutes

Americans With Disabilities Act (ADA), 42 USC §§121.010-12213 (1995).

Autopsy Consent, Mo Rev Stat §194.115 (1998).

Consent to Surgical or Medical Treatment, Mo Rev Stat §431.061 (1998).

Consolidated Omnibus Budget Reconciliation Act (COBRA), 29 USC §1161 et seq (1985).

Emergency Medical Treatment and Active Labor Act (EMTALA), 42 USC §1395 (dd) (1986).

Good Samaritan Law, Mo Rev Stat §537.037 (1998).

Health Insurance Portability and Accountability Act of 1996 (HIPAA), Public Law No. 104 (1996).

Mental Health Parity Act of 1996, 29 USC §1885 (1996).

National Organ Transplant Act, Public Law 98–507 (1984).

New York DNR Statute, NY Public Health Laws §2962 (1988).

Newborns and Mothers Health Protection Act of 1996, 29 USC §1185(a) (1996).

Nursing Practice Act, Mo Rev Stat §§335.011–335.096 (1998).

Oregon Death With Dignity Act, Ore Rev Stat §§127.800–127.897 (1994).

Patient Self-Determination Act, 42 CFR 417 (1992).

Resident's Rights, Medicaid Statute, 42 USCA §1396R (1988).

Uniform Determination of Death Act (1980).

Uniform Anatomical Gift Act (1987).

Cases

Barber v Time Magazine, 159 SW2d 291 (1942).

Bouvia v Superior Court, 225 Cal Rptr 297 (1986).

Bragdon v Abbott, 524 U.S. 624 (1998).

Compassion in Dying v Washington, 79 F3d 790 (9th Cir 1996).

Cruzan v Director Missouri Department of Health, 497 U.S. 261 (1990).

Darling v Charleston Community Memorial Hospital, 33 Ill 2d 326 (Ill 1966).

Johnson v Calvert, 851 P 2d 776 (Cal 1993).

In the Matter of Baby M, 537 A 2d 1227 (NJ 1988).

Planned Parenthood of Southeastern Pennsylvania v Casey, 505 U.S. 883 (1992).

Quill v Vacco, 80 F3d 716 (2nd Cir 1996).

Roe v Wade, 410 U.S. 113 (1973).

Washington v Glucksberg, 521 U.S. 702 (1997).

Webster v Reproductive Health Services, 492 U.S. 490 (1989).

Winkelman v Beloit Memorial Hospital, 484 NW2d 211 (W 1992).

YG v Jewish Hospital, 795 SW2d 488 (Mo App 1990).

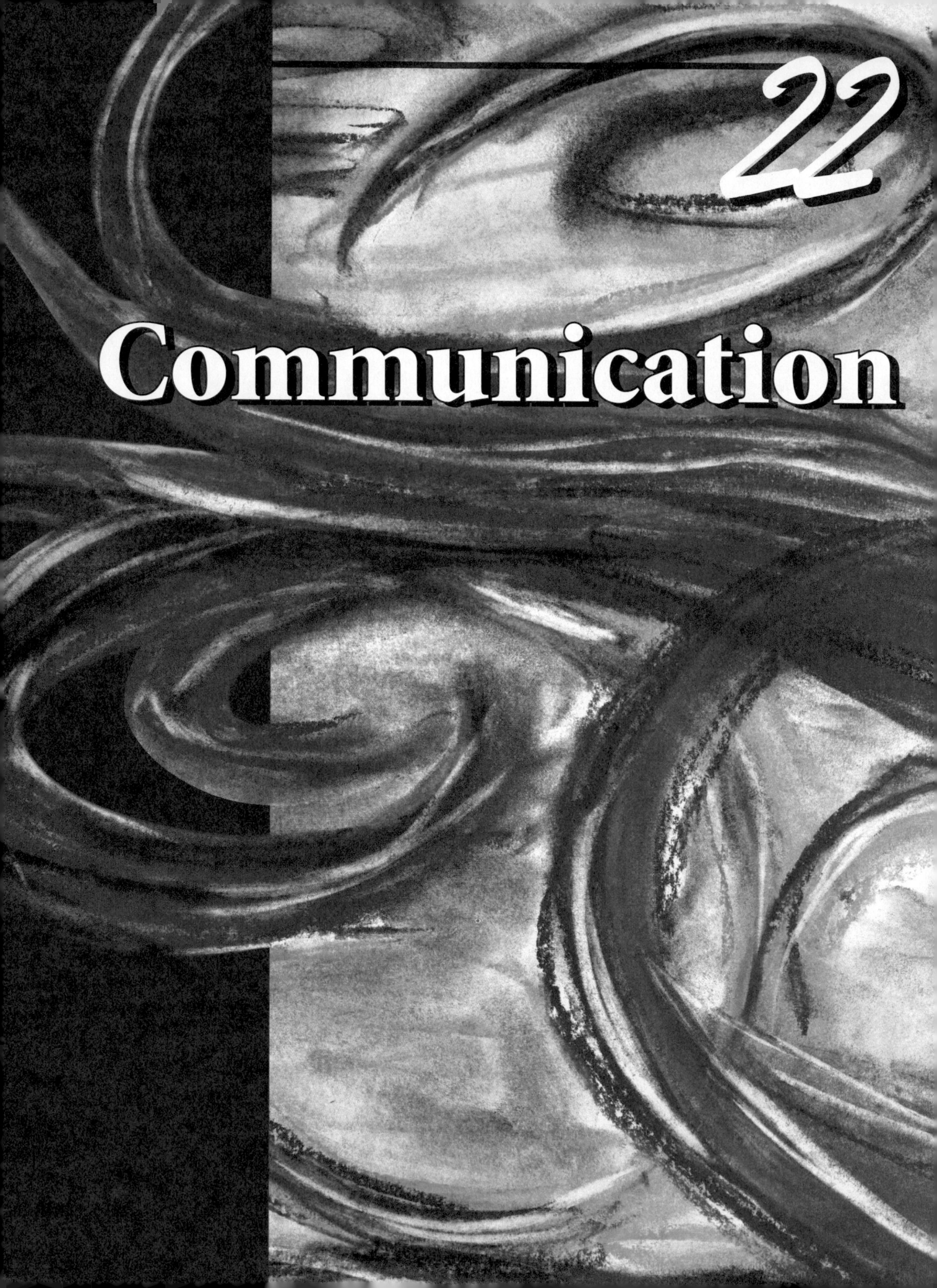

Communication

22

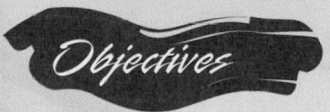

Mastery of content in this chapter will enable the student to:

- Define the key terms listed.
- Describe aspects of critical thinking that are important to the communication process.
- Describe the five levels of communication and their uses in nursing.
- Describe the basic elements of the communication process.
- Identify significant features and therapeutic outcomes of nurse-client helping relationships.
- List nursing focus areas within the four phases of a nurse-client helping relationship.
- Identify significant features and desired outcomes of nurse–health team member relationships.
- Describe qualities, behaviors, and communication techniques that affect professional communication.
- Discuss effective communication techniques for clients at various developmental levels.
- Identify client health states that contribute to impaired communication.
- Discuss nursing care measures for clients with special communication needs.

Communication and Nursing Practice

Communication is a process in which people affect one another through the exchange of information, ideas, and feelings. Interpersonal communication is basic to human interaction and essential for nursing practice. Communication is part of the art of nursing—the intentional creative use of oneself, based on skill and expertise, to transmit emotion and meaning to another. It is a process that requires interpretation, sensitivity, imagination, and active participation (Jenner, 1997). It is an exchange of energy, an act of sharing that is used to establish and maintain relationships with others.

Nurses interact with many persons in the course of their profession. Competency in communication helps the nurse maintain effective relationships within the entire sphere of professional practice and helps meet legal, ethical, and clinical standards of care. Failure to communicate causes serious difficulty, increases liability, and threatens professional credibility.

The qualities, behaviors, and therapeutic communication techniques described in this chapter characterize professionalism in helping relationships. Although the term *client* is often used, the same principles can be applied when communicating with any person, in any nursing situation.

COMMUNICATION AND INTERPERSONAL RELATIONSHIPS

At the core of nursing are caring relationships formed between the nurse and those affected by the nurse's practice

The authors acknowledge the contributions of Martina Jones and Jeffrey C. McManemy to this chapter in the previous edition of this text.

(Chapter 6). Communication is the means to establish these helping-healing relationships. The caring nurse communicates with others in a manner that expresses awareness and respect for persons as individuals, with knowledge and consideration for their specific needs. This involves an unconditional acceptance of persons as they are, together with a vision of what they are capable of becoming (Sundeen and others, 1998). Nurses with expertise in communication can express caring by becoming sensitive to self and others, promoting and accepting the expression of positive and negative feelings, and developing helping-trust relationships. Caring is also demonstrated by instilling faith and hope, promoting interpersonal teaching and learning, providing a supportive environment, assisting with gratification of human needs, and allowing for the expression of spiritual forces and phenomena (Watson, 1985).

The nurse's ability to relate to others is a very important aspect of interpersonal communication. This includes the nurse's ability to take initiative in establishing and maintaining communication, to be authentic (one's self), and to respond appropriately to the other person. Good interpersonal communication also requires the nurse to develop a sense of mutuality, a belief that the nurse-client relationship is a partnership and that both are equal participants. Nurses must honor the fact that people can be very complex and ambiguous. There is often more communicated than first meets the eye, and client responses are not always what the nurse might expect. It is very helpful for the nurse to purposefully focus on positive intentions for the other person and to use the technique of re-imagining a possible future (Hartrick, 1997) so that a vision of hope and better health can be shared.

A new perspective of human relationships suggests a multidimensional energy field that permeates and connects everything to each other, providing a matrix for physical, emotional, mental, and spiritual being. It is highly organized and basically synergistic, which means that the action of separate entities together have a greater total effect than the sum of their individual parts (Brennan, 1987). Considering these principles, it is not surprising that nurses often perceive the strong sense of connection to others that occurs within a helping relationship. Nurses know that attitudes and emotions are easily transmitted and are often aware that the relationship between helper and client becomes a vehicle for healing (Hover-Kramer, Mentgen, and Scandrett-Hibdon, 1996). Most nurses embrace the profession's view of the holistic nature of people and have experienced synergy in human interaction when client and nurse together accomplish much more than either can alone.

Accepting that humans are energy-based beings means that nurses of the twenty-first century must look at communication in new ways. All communication contains stimuli with the potential to influence others (Curtis, Floyd, and Winsor, 1997). Like any powerful therapeutic agent, the nurse's communication can result in both harm and good. Every nuance of posture, every small expression and gesture, every word chosen, every attitude held—all have the potential to hurt or heal, affecting others through the transmission of human energy. Knowing that intention and behavior directly influence human energy fields, and therefore health, gives nurses tremendous ethical responsibility to do no harm to those entrusted to their care. Communication must be respected for its potential power and not carelessly misused to hurt, manipulate, or coerce others. Good communication empowers others and enables people to know themselves and make their own choices, an essential aspect of the healing process. Nurses have wonderful opportunities to bring about good things for themselves, their clients, and their colleagues through this kind of therapeutic communication.

DEVELOPING COMMUNICATION SKILLS

Moving from novice to expert in communication, as in any aspect of nursing, requires both an understanding of the communication process and reflection about one's communication experiences within the nursing role. Nurses who have developed good critical thinking skills make the best communicators. They are able to draw upon theoretical knowledge about communication and integrate this knowledge with what has been learned through personal experience. They can interpret messages received from others, analyze their content, make inferences about their meaning, evaluate their effect, explain rationale for communication techniques used, and self-examine personal communication skills (Creasia and Parker, 1996).

Other qualities of good critical thinking are also important to the communication process. Being inquisitive and desiring to know more about a person or to understand a situation motivates the nurse to communicate. Being systematic is important, because good communicators tend to seek and provide information in an organized,

focused, and diligent way. Being analytical helps the nurse examine communication for congruency between verbal and nonverbal behavior, identify recurrent themes, and examine the impact of the communication on the participants. Being a truth seeker is important in trying to understand or clarify the true meaning of what is being communicated. Being open minded helps the nurse enter into a situation without preconceived ideas about the nature of the communication. Being self-confident is important because the nurse who conveys confidence and comfort while communicating can more readily establish interpersonal helping-trust relationships and convey competence in the professional role. Being mature is important since, in a helping relationship, the other person's needs take priority over one's own.

It is challenging to understand human communication within interpersonal relationships. Each person's perceptions are influenced by many factors, including the individual's own cultural conditioning, educational background, and personal experience (Knapp and Vangelisti, 1996). Critical thinking can help the nurse overcome **perceptual biases,** human tendencies that interfere with accurately perceiving and interpreting messages from others. People often assume that others would think, feel, act, react, and behave as they would in similar circumstances. They tend to distort or ignore information that goes against their expectations, preconceptions, or stereotypes (Beebe, Beebe, and Redmond, 1999). By thinking critically about personal communication habits, the nurse can learn to control these tendencies and become more effective in interpersonal relationships.

As communication skills develop, the nurse's competence in the nursing process will also grow. Communication skills must be integrated throughout the nursing process as nurses collaborate with clients and health team members to achieve goals (Box 22-1). Nurses use communication skills to gather, analyze, and transmit information and to accomplish the work of each phase. Assessment, diagnosis, planning, implementation, and evaluation all depend on effective communication among nurse, client, family, and others on the health care team. Although the nursing process is a reliable framework for client care, it will not work well unless the nurse masters the art of effective interpersonal communication and forms helping relationships with others.

The nature of the communication process requires that nurses constantly make decisions about what, when, where, why, and how to convey messages to others. The nurse's decision making is always contextual—the unique features of any situation influence the nature of the decisions made. For example, the explanation of the importance of following a prescribed diet to a client with a newly diagnosed medical condition will differ from the explanation to a client who has repeatedly chosen not to follow diet restrictions. Effective communication techniques can be easily learned, but their application is more difficult. Deciding which techniques best fit each unique nursing

Communication Throughout the Nursing Process Box 22-1	**Challenging Communication Situations** Box 22-2

ASSESSMENT
Verbal interviewing and history taking
Visual and intuitive observation of nonverbal behavior
Visual, tactile, and auditory data gathering during physical examination
Written medical records, diagnostic tests, and literature review

NURSING DIAGNOSIS
Intrapersonal analysis of assessment findings
Validation of health care needs and priorities via verbal discussion with client
Handwritten or computer-mediated documentation of nursing diagnosis

PLANNING
Interpersonal or small-group health team planning sessions
Interpersonal collaboration with client and family to determine implementation methods
Written documentation of expected outcomes
Written or verbal referral to health team members

IMPLEMENTATION
Delegation and verbal discussion with health care team
Verbal, visual, auditory, and tactile health teaching activities
Provision of support via therapeutic communication techniques
Contact with other health resources
Written documentation of client's progress in medical record

EVALUATION
Acquisition of verbal and nonverbal feedback
Comparison of actual and expected outcomes
Identification of factors affecting outcomes
Modification and update of care plan
Verbal and/or written explanation of revisions of care plan to client

Silent, withdrawn persons who do not express any feelings or needs
Sad, depressed persons who have slow mental and motor responses
Angry, hostile persons who do not listen to explanations
Sullen, uncooperative persons who resent being asked to do something
Talkative, lonely persons who want someone with them all the time
Demanding persons who want someone to wait on them or meet their requests
Ranting and raving persons who blame nursing staff unfairly
Sensory impaired persons who cannot hear or see well
Verbally impaired persons who cannot articulate words
Gossiping, catty persons who violate confidentiality and cause friction
Bitter, complaining persons who are negative about everything
Mentally handicapped persons who are frightened and distrustful
Confused, disoriented persons who are bewildered and uncooperative
Foreign-born persons who speak very little English
Anxious, nervous persons who cannot cope with what is happening
Grieving, crying persons who have had a major loss
Screaming, kicking toddlers who want their mother
Unresponsive, comatose persons who cannot communicate at all
Flirtatious, sexually inappropriate persons
Loud, obscene persons causing a disturbance or violating a rule

situation is challenging. Throughout this chapter, brief clinical examples guide students in the use of effective communication techniques. Situations that challenge the nurse's decision-making skills and call for careful use of therapeutic techniques often involve the types of persons described in Box 22-2. Since the best way to acquire skill is through guided practice, it is useful for students to discuss and role play these scenarios prior to experiencing them in the clinical setting. Consider that clients, family, nurse colleagues, assistive personnel, physicians, or other health team members might be involved and decide which communication techniques might be most effective.

Levels of Communication

Nurses use different levels of communication in their professional role. The nurse's communication skills need to include techniques that reflect competence in each level.

INTRAPERSONAL COMMUNICATION

Intrapersonal communication is a powerful form of communication that occurs within an individual. This level of communication is also called self-talk, self-verbalization, self-instruction, inner thought, and inner dialogue (Balzer-Riley, 1996). People's thoughts strongly influence perceptions, feelings, behavior, and self-concept. Intrapersonal communication creates a set of conditions through which life is experienced. Nurses should be aware of the nature and content of their thinking and try to replace negative, self-defeating thoughts with positive assertions. Positive self-talk can be used as a tool to improve the nurse's or client's health and self-esteem. In forms such as guided imagery, it can be used to enhance coping and reduce stress. Self-instruction can provide a mental rehearsal for difficult tasks or situations so individuals can deal with them more effectively. Nurses and clients can use intrapersonal communication to develop self-awareness and a positive self-concept that will enhance appropriate self-expression.

INTERPERSONAL COMMUNICATION

Interpersonal communication is one-to-one interaction between the nurse and another person that often occurs face to face. It is the level most frequently used in nursing situations and lies at the heart of nursing practice. It takes place within a social context and includes all the symbols and cues used to give and receive meaning. Since meaning resides in persons and not in words, messages received may be different from messages intended. Nurses work with people who have different opinions, experiences, values, and belief systems, so meaning must be validated or mutually negotiated between participants. Meaningful interpersonal communication results in exchange of ideas, problem solving, expression of feelings, decision making, goal accomplishment, team building, and personal growth.

TRANSPERSONAL COMMUNICATION

Transpersonal communication is interaction that occurs within a person's spiritual domain. Many persons use prayer, meditation, guided reflection, religious rituals, or other means to communicate with their "higher power." Nurses who value the importance of human spirituality often use this form of communication with clients and for themselves. Sellers and Haag (1998) found that nurses enhance the spirituality of clients and their families through prayer; active listening and therapeutic communication; conveying acceptance, respect, and a nonjudgmental attitude; instilling hope; and using presence and touch. Brown-Saltzman (1997) reviewed nursing literature and also found that meditative prayer and prayers of silence are effective approaches the nurse can use in caring for self and others.

SMALL-GROUP COMMUNICATION

Small-group communication is interaction that occurs when a small number of persons meet together. This type of communication is usually goal directed and requires an understanding of group dynamics. When nurses work on task forces or committees, lead client support groups, form research teams, or participate in client care conferences, a small-group communication process is used. Small groups are more effective when they are a workable size, have an appropriate meeting place, suitable seating arrangements, and cohesiveness and commitment among group members (Hybels and Weaver, 1998).

PUBLIC COMMUNICATION

Public communication is interaction with an audience. Nurses have opportunities to speak with groups of consumers about health-related topics, present scholarly work to colleagues at conferences, or lead classroom discussions with peers or students. Public communication requires special adaptations in eye contact, gestures, voice inflection, and use of media materials to communicate messages effectively. Effective public communication increases audience knowledge about health-related topics, health issues, and other issues important to the nursing profession.

Basic Elements of the Communication Process

Communication is an ongoing, dynamic, and multidimensional process. Its basic elements are shown in Figure 22-1 and described below. This simple linear model under represents a very complex process but helps the nurse identify its essential components. Nursing situations have many unique aspects that influence the nature of communication and interpersonal relationships. In nonprofessional roles, people rarely analyze the meaning of every gesture or word. In the professional role, the nurse must use critical thinking to focus on each aspect of communication so interactions can be purposeful and effective.

REFERENT

The **referent** motivates one person to communicate with another. In a health care setting, sights, sounds, odors, time schedules, messages, objects, emotions, sensations, perceptions, ideas, and other cues initiate communication. The nurse who knows what stimulus initiated communication can develop and organize messages more efficiently and better perceive meaning in another's message. A client request for help prompted by difficulty breathing brings a different nursing response than a request prompted by boredom.

SENDER AND RECEIVER

The **sender** is the person who encodes and delivers the message, and the **receiver** is the person who receives and

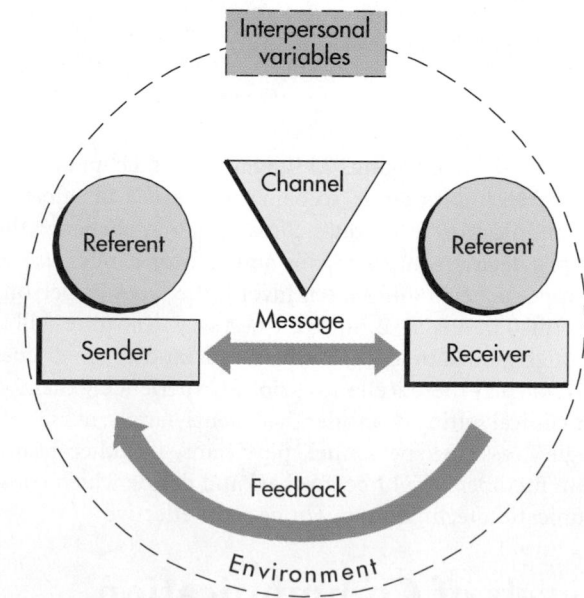

Figure 22-1 Communication as active process between sender and receiver.

decodes the message. The sender puts ideas or feelings into a form that can be transmitted and is responsible for the accuracy of its content and emotional tone. The sender's message acts as a referent for the receiver, who is responsible for attending to, translating, and responding to the sender's message. Sender and receiver roles are fluid and change back and forth as two persons interact; sending and receiving may even occur simultaneously. The more the sender and receiver have in common and the closer the relationship, the more likely they will accurately perceive one another's meaning and respond accordingly.

MESSAGES

The **message** is the content of the communication. It may contain verbal, nonverbal, and symbolic language. Messages are interpreted by those who receive them through personal perceptions that may or may not distort the meaning intended by the sender. Two nurses can provide the same information yet convey very different messages according to their personal communication styles, or one nurse can send the same message to two persons and be understood differently by each. Nurses can send effective messages by expressing themselves clearly, directly, and in a manner familiar to the receiver. Watching the listener for nonverbal cues that suggest confusion or misunderstanding helps the nurse know whether the message needs to be clarified. Communication can be difficult when participants have different levels of education and experience. "Your incision is well approximated without purulent drainage" means the same as "Your wound edges are together, and there are no signs of infection," but a client more easily understands the latter. The nurse must be sure clients can read before sending messages in writing.

CHANNELS

Channels are means of conveying and receiving messages through visual, auditory, and tactile senses. Facial expressions send visual messages, spoken words travel through auditory channels, and touch uses tactile channels. The more channels the sender uses to convey a message, the more clearly it is usually understood. For example, when teaching about insulin self-injection, the nurse talks about and demonstrates the technique, gives the client printed information, and encourages hands-on practice with the vial and syringe. Nurses use verbal, nonverbal, and mediated (technological) communication channels. They send and receive information in person, by informal or formal writing, over the telephone or pager, by audiotape and videotape, through fax and electronic mail, and through computer interactive and information sites.

FEEDBACK

Feedback is the message returned by the receiver. It indicates whether the meaning of the sender's message was understood. Senders need to seek verbal and nonverbal feedback to ensure that good communication has oc-

curred. To be effective, the sender and receiver must be sensitive and open to each other's messages, clarify the messages, and modify behavior accordingly. In a social relationship, both persons assume equal responsibility for seeking openness and clarification, but the nurse assumes primary responsibility in the nurse-client relationship.

INTERPERSONAL VARIABLES

Interpersonal variables are factors within both the sender and receiver that influence communication. **Perception** is one such variable that provides a uniquely personal view of reality formed by one's expectations and experiences. Each person senses, interprets, and understands events differently. A nurse might say, "You have been very quiet since your family left. Is there something on your mind?" One client might perceive the nurse's question as caring and concerned; another might perceive the nurse as invading privacy and be less willing to talk. Other interpersonal variables include educational and developmental levels, sociocultural backgrounds, values and beliefs, emotions, gender, physical health status, and roles and relationships. Variables associated with illness, such as pain, anxiety, and medication effects, can also affect nurse-client communication.

ENVIRONMENT

The **environment** is the setting for sender-receiver interaction. For effective communication, the environment should meet participant needs for physical and emotional comfort and safety. Noise, temperature extremes, distractions, and lack of privacy or space may create confusion, tension, and discomfort. Environmental distractions are common in health care settings and can interfere with messages sent between people, so nurses must try to control the environment as much as possible to create favorable conditions for effective communication.

Forms of Communication

Messages are conveyed verbally and nonverbally, concretely and symbolically. As people communicate, they express themselves through words, movements, voice inflection, facial expressions, and use of space. These elements can work in harmony to enhance a message or conflict with one another to contradict and confuse it.

VERBAL COMMUNICATION

Verbal communication uses spoken or written words. Verbal language is a code that conveys specific meaning as words are combined. The most important aspects of verbal communication are discussed below.

Vocabulary. Communication is unsuccessful if senders and receivers cannot translate each other's words and phrases. When a nurse cares for a client who speaks another language, an interpreter may be necessary. Even those who speak the same language use subcultural variations of certain words: *dinner* may mean a noon meal to one person and the last meal of the day to another. Medical jargon (technical terminology used by health care providers) may sound like a foreign language to clients unfamiliar with the health care setting and should be used only with other health team members. Children have a more limited vocabulary than adults. They may use special words to describe bodily functions or a favorite blanket or toy. Teenagers often use words in unique ways that are unfamiliar to adults.

Denotative and Connotative Meaning.

A single word can have several meanings. The denotative meaning is shared by individuals who use a common language: *baseball* has the same meaning for everyone who speaks English, but *code* denotes cardiac arrest primarily to health care providers. The connotative meaning is the shade or interpretation of a word's meaning influenced by the thoughts, feelings, or ideas people have about the word. Families who are told a loved one is in serious condition may believe that death is near, but to nurses *serious* may simply describe the nature of the illness. Nurses should carefully select words that cannot be easily misinterpreted, especially when explaining a client's medical condition or therapy. Even a much-used phrase such as "I'm going to take your vital signs" can be unfamiliar to an adult or frightening to a child.

Pacing.

Conversation is more successful at an appropriate speed or pace. Nurses should speak slowly enough to enunciate clearly. Talking rapidly, using awkward pauses, or speaking slowly and deliberately can convey an unintended message. Long pauses and rapid shifts to another subject may give the impression that the nurse is hiding the truth. Pacing is improved by thinking before speaking and by developing awareness of the cadence of one's speech.

Intonation.

Tone of voice dramatically affects a message's meaning. Depending on intonation, even a simple question or statement can express enthusiasm, anger, concern, or indifference. The nurse must be aware of voice tone to avoid sending unintended messages. For example, clients may interpret a nurse's patronizing tone of voice as condescending, and further communication may be inhibited. A client's voice tone often provides information about his or her emotional state or energy level.

Clarity and Brevity.

Effective communication is simple, brief, and direct. Fewer words result in less confusion. Clarity is achieved by speaking slowly, enunciating clearly, and using examples to make explanations easier to understand. Repeating important parts of a message also clarifies communication. Phrases such as "you know" or "OK?" at the end of every sentence detract from clarity. Brevity is achieved by using short sentences and words that express an idea simply and directly. "Where is your pain?" is much better than "I would like you to describe for me the location of your discomfort."

Timing and Relevance.

Timing is critical in communication. Even though a message is clear, poor timing can prevent it from being effective. For example, the nurse should not begin routine teaching when a client is in severe pain or emotional distress. Often the best time for interaction is when a client expresses an interest in communicating. If messages are relevant or important to the situation at hand, they are more effective. When a client is facing emergency surgery, discussing the risks of smoking is less relevant than explaining perioperative procedures.

NONVERBAL COMMUNICATION

Nonverbal communication is message transmission through body language, without using words. It includes facial expressions, vocal cues, eye contact, gestures, posture, touch, odor, physical appearance, dress, silence, and the use of space, time, and objects. Nonverbal communication often reveals true feelings because it is hard to control: a colleague who says nothing is wrong but has tears in her eyes is probably in distress. Nonverbal cues add depth to verbal messages and help the nurse judge their reliability. Becoming an astute observer of nonverbal behavior takes practice, concentration, and sensitivity to others. Nurses should avoid sending "mixed messages" through nonverbal communication. Saying "this won't hurt a bit" while wearing a sarcastic grin will not relieve anxiety or establish trust!

Personal Appearance.

Personal appearance includes physical characteristics, facial expression, manner of dress and grooming, and adornments. These factors help communicate physical well-being, personality, social status, occupation, religion, culture, and self-concept. First impressions are largely based on appearance. Nurses learn to develop a general impression of client health and emotional status through appearance, and clients develop a general impression of the nurse's professionalism and caring in the same way.

Posture and Gait.

Posture and gait are forms of self-expression. The way people sit, stand, and move reflect attitudes, emotions, self-concept, and health status. For example, an erect posture and a quick, purposeful gait communicate a sense of well-being and confidence. Leaning forward conveys attention. A slumped posture and slow shuffling gait may indicate depression, illness, or fatigue.

Facial Expression.

The face is the most expressive part of the body. Facial expressions convey emotions such as surprise, fear, anger, disgust, happiness, and sadness.

Some persons have an expressionless face, or flat affect, which reveals little about what they are thinking or feeling. An inappropriate affect is a facial expression that does not match the content of a verbal message, for example, smiling when describing a sad situation. People can be unaware of the messages their expressions convey. For example, a nurse may frown in concentration while doing a procedure and the client may interpret this as anger or disapproval. Clients often closely observe nurses. Consider the impact a nurse's facial expression might have on a person who asks, "Am I going to die?" The slightest change in the eyes, lips, or facial muscles can reveal the nurse's feelings. Although it is hard to control all facial expression, the nurse should try to avoid showing shock, disgust, dismay, or other distressing reactions in the client's presence.

Eye Contact.
People signal readiness to communicate through eye contact. Maintaining eye contact during conversation shows respect and willingness to listen. Eye contact also allows people to closely observe one another. Lack of eye contact may indicate anxiety, defensiveness, discomfort, or lack of confidence in communicating. However, persons from Asian cultures may consider eye contact intrusive, threatening, or harmful and minimize or avoid its use. Eye movements communicate feelings and emotions. Looking down on a person establishes authority, whereas interacting at the same eye level indicates equality in the relationship. Rising to the same eye level of an angry person helps establish one's autonomy.

Gestures.
Gestures emphasize, punctuate, and clarify the spoken word. Gestures alone carry specific meanings, or they may create messages with other communication cues. A finger pointed toward a person may communicate several meanings, but when accompanied by a frown and stern voice, the gesture becomes an accusation or threat. Pointing to an area of pain may be more accurate than describing the pain's location.

Sounds.
Sounds such as sighs, moans, groans, or sobs also communicate feelings and thoughts. Combined with other nonverbal communication, sounds help send clear messages. Sounds can be interpreted in several ways: moaning can convey pleasure or suffering, and crying can communicate happiness, sadness, or anger. The nurse must validate such nonverbal messages with the client to interpret them accurately.

Territoriality and Personal Space.
Territoriality is the need to gain, maintain, and defend one's right to space. Territory is important because it provides people with a sense of identity, security, and control. Territory can be separated and made visible to others, such as a fence around a yard or a bed in a hospital room. Personal space is invisible, individual, and travels with the person. During interpersonal interaction, people maintain varying distances between each other depending on their culture, the nature of their relationship, and the situation. When personal space becomes threatened, people respond defensively and communicate less effectively. Situations dictate whether the interpersonal distance between nurse and client is appropriate. Examples of nursing actions within zones of personal space are listed in Box 22-3, along with zones of touch. Nurses frequently move into clients' territory and personal space due to the nature of caregiving. The nurse must convey confidence, gentleness, and respect for privacy, especially when actions require intimate contacts or involve a client's vulnerable zone.

SYMBOLIC COMMUNICATION
Good communication requires awareness of **symbolic communication,** the verbal and nonverbal symbolism used by others to convey meaning. Art and music are

---

Zones of Personal Space and Touch   Box 22-3

ZONES OF PERSONAL SPACE
Intimate zone (0 to 18 inches)
Holding a crying infant
Performing physical assessment
Bathing, grooming, dressing, feeding, and toileting a client
Changing a client's dressing

Personal zone (18 inches to 4 feet)
Sitting at a client's bedside
Taking the client's nursing history
Teaching an individual client
Exchanging information at change of shift

Social zone (4 to 12 feet)
Making rounds with a physician
Sitting at the head of a conference table
Teaching a class for clients with diabetes
Conducting a family support group

Public zone (12 feet and greater)
Speaking at a community forum
Testifying at a legislative hearing
Lecturing to a class of students

ZONES OF TOUCH
Social zone (permission not needed)
Hands, arms, shoulders, back

Consent zone (permission needed)
Mouth, wrists, feet

Vulnerable zone (special care needed)
Face, neck, front of body

Intimate zone (great sensitivity needed)
Genitalia

forms of symbolic communication that may be used by the nurse to enhance understanding and promote healing. Dreams, drawings, metaphorical language, a child's play, and even the symptoms of illness are all symbolic forms of self-expression that have rich messages for health care providers (Seigel, 1989).

METACOMMUNICATION

Metacommunication is important to effective interpersonal interaction. It is "communication about communication" so that the deeper "message within a message" can be uncovered and understood (Wood, 1999). Metacommunication can help people better understand what they have communicated. For example, the nurse observes a young client holding his body rigidly erect and his voice is sharp as he says, "Going to surgery is no big deal." The nurse replies, "You say having surgery doesn't bother you, but you look and sound tense. I'd like to help." This is metacommunication, and it may result in further exploration of the client's feelings and concerns.

Professional Nursing Relationships

Professional relationships are created through the nurse's application of knowledge, understanding of human behavior and communication, and commitment to ethical behavior. Having a philosophy based on caring and respect for others will help the nurse be more successful in establishing relationships of this nature.

NURSE-CLIENT HELPING RELATIONSHIPS

Helping relationships are the foundation of clinical nursing practice—the essential element of care with every client, in every situation (Edelman and Mandle, 1998). In such relationships, the nurse assumes the role of professional helper and comes to know the client as an individual who has unique health needs, human responses, and patterns of living. The relationship is therapeutic, promoting a psychological climate that facilitates positive change and growth. As Fortinash and Holoday-Worret (2000) noted, the nurse's therapeutic use of communication is the mechanism by which clients can achieve successful outcomes to the problems currently preventing them from achieving optimum health. There is an explicit time frame, a goal-directed approach, and a high expectation of confidentiality. The nurse establishes, directs, and takes responsibility for the interaction, and the client's needs take priority over the nurse's needs. The relationship is also characterized by the nurse's nonjudgmental acceptance of the client. Acceptance conveys a willingness to hear a message or to acknowledge feelings. It does not mean the nurse must always agree with the other person or approve of the client's decisions or actions.

A helping relationship between nurse and client does not just happen—it is created with care and skill and is built on the client's trust in the nurse. Nursing theorist Imogene King (1971) calls the nurse-client relationship "learning experiences whereby two people interact to face an immediate health problem, to share, if possible, in resolving it, and to discover ways to adapt to the situation." Clients are helped to clarify needs and goals, problem solve, cope with situational or maturational crises, clarify and strengthen values, reduce stress and anxiety, and gain insight and self-understanding (Edelman and Mandle, 1998).

The nurse-client relationship is characterized by a natural progression of four goal-directed phases that often begin before the nurse meets the client and continue until the caregiving relationship ends (Box 22-4). Even a brief interaction uses an abbreviated version of the same preinteraction, orientation, working, and termination phases. For example, the student nurse may gather client information to prepare in advance for caregiving, meet the client and establish trust, accomplish health-related goals through use of the nursing process, and say goodbye at the end of the day.

Socializing is often an important initial component of interpersonal communication. It helps people get to know one another and relax. It is easy, superficial, and not deeply personal, whereas therapeutic interactions are often more intense, difficult, and uncomfortable. A nurse often uses social conversation to help the client feel comfortable and lay a foundation for a closer relationship: "Hi, Mr. Simpson, I hear it's your birthday today. How old are you?" A friendly, informal, and warm communication style helps establish trust, but nurses must get beyond social conversation to talk about issues or concerns affecting the client's health. During social conversation, clients may ask personal questions about the nurse's family, place of residence, and so forth. Students often wonder whether it is appropriate to reveal such information. The skillful nurse uses judgment about what to share and provides minimal information or deflects such questions with gentle humor and refocuses conversation back to the client.

Creating a therapeutic environment depends on the nurse's ability to communicate, to provide comfort, and to help clients meet their needs. Bottorff, Gogag, and Engelberg-Lotzkar (1995) found that comforting strategies used by nurses included gentle humor, physical comfort measures, emotionally supportive statements, and comforting and connecting touch. The nurses provided information, supported clients' active decision making, and offered opportunities for clients to engage in social exchange.

Nurses often encourage clients to share personal stories, which is called narrative interaction. Through narrative interactions, nurses may begin to understand the context of others' lives and learn what is meaningful for them from their perspective (Canales, 1997). For example, a nurse asked a client to tell about a time in his life when he

Phases of the Helping Relationship   Box 22-4

PREINTERACTION PHASE

Before meeting the client the nurse:

Reviews available data, including the medical and nursing history

Talks to other caregivers who may have information about the client

Anticipates health concerns or issues that may arise

Identifies a location and setting that will foster comfortable, private interaction

Plans enough time for the initial interaction

ORIENTATION PHASE

When the nurse and client meet and get to know one another, the nurse:

Sets the tone for the relationship by adopting a warm, empathetic, caring manner

Recognizes that the initial relationship may be superficial, uncertain, and tentative

Expects the client to test the nurse's competence and commitment

Closely observes the client and expects to be closely observed by the client

Begins to make inferences and form judgments about client messages and behaviors

Assesses the client's health status

Prioritizes the client's problems and identifies the client's goals

Clarifies the client's and nurse's roles

Forms contracts with the client that specify who will do what

Lets the client know when to expect the relationship to be terminated

WORKING PHASE

When the nurse and client work together to solve problems and accomplish goals, the nurse:

Encourages and helps the client to express feelings about his or her health

Encourages and helps the client with self-exploration

Provides information needed to understand and change behavior

Encourages and helps the client to set goals

Takes actions to meet the goals set with the client

Uses therapeutic communication skills to facilitate successful interactions

Uses appropriate self-disclosure and confrontation

TERMINATION PHASE

During the ending of the relationship, the nurse:

Reminds the client that termination is near

Evaluates goal achievement with the client

Reminisces about the relationship with the client

Separates from the client by relinquishing responsibility for his or her care

Achieves a smooth transition for the client to other caregivers as needed

---

had to make a hard decision. He related the following story:

> When I was a young man, I worked on the family farm. An uncle died and left me some money. All of a sudden I could afford to go to college, but Dad didn't want me to go because he needed me there. I had to decide whether to stay or go, and it was real hard, because at first I just wanted to get away. I talked to our preacher, and he said it was up to me, to pray about it and do what my heart told me to. So I stayed. Oh, I've thought from time to time what I might have made of myself, but I never regretted it. I had a good life in farming.

From this brief story, the nurse understood that it was important to the client to put his family's needs above his personal desires and that seeking spiritual guidance was an important component of his decision making.

Nurses also provide information and use strategies that help clients understand and change behavior. Lewis and Zahlis (1997) found that nurses use "coaching behavior" with clients in several dimensions. For example, coaching behavior in the dimension of exploring solutions might include working with a client to help generate a list of ideas that might alleviate or resolve the client's problem. The nurse uses contracts with clients to establish mutually agreed-upon health goals and expectations for behavioral change. The nurse uses immediacy, which means helping clients to focus on their present choices and actions, rather than what has happened in the past.

The nurse and client work as a team. The nurse offers others the opportunity to make choices, even as simple as choosing a bath time or which prn medication to take. The nurse also acts as an advocate to keep the client informed of health care alternatives and give support in decision making.

A good way to encourage autonomy is to collaborate with others. For example, the nurse can ask clients and family members for input and suggestions about goals, interventions, and evaluation of the plan of care. This type of mutuality (give-and-take, creative mutual exchanges) has been shown to balance power and respect and to promote productive provider-client communication (Henson, 1997). It gives the other person a greater sense of purpose and direction, encourages personal responsibility for health, helps establish priorities for care, gives the opportunity for self-expression, and strengthens the client's problem-solving ability. Research has shown that successful collaboration requires an active and committed involvement by both client and nurse and a joint effort toward problem solving. Such a relationship will enhance the client's well-being and the nurse's feeling of success (Box 22-5) (Paavilainen and Astedt-Kurki, 1997).

Research HIGHLIGHT   Box 22-5

RESEARCH ABSTRACT

This qualitative research study describes the client-nurse relationship as experienced by public health nurses in community settings. The purposes were to examine ways the client and public health nurse cooperate with one another and to identify what facilitates efficient collaboration. Nurses told personal stories through written essays and focused interviews, and the content of their narrative was analyzed. Results were that successful collaboration requires an active and committed involvement by both client and nurse, and a joint effort to help the client cope with his or her situation. Results also suggested that what happens in a client-nurse relationship is extremely important to both parties in the dyad.

IMPLICATIONS FOR PRACTICE

- For successful collaboration, there must be a shared understanding of the ultimate goal of nursing (health promotion, health maintenance, health restoration, or peaceful death).
- Open and sincere interactions build confidence and can create a sense of confidentiality and trustworthiness that facilitate client cooperation.
- The client's well-being and the public health nurse's feeling of success will depend to a great extent on the kind of relationship they can construct.

REFERENCE

Paavilainen E, Astedt-Kurki P: The client-nurse relationship as experienced by public health nurses: toward better collaboration, *Public Health Nurs* 14(3): 137, 1997.

NURSE-FAMILY RELATIONSHIPS

Many nursing situations, especially those in community and home health settings, require the nurse to form helping relationships with entire families. The same principles that guide one-to-one helping relationships also apply when the client is a family unit, although communication within families requires additional understanding of the complexities of family dynamics, needs, and relationships. Collaboration among nurse, client, and family caregivers is especially important. Robinson (1996) found that nurse-family health care relationships are pivotal to making positive change and that healing was facilitated when the nurse related to the family as an attentive listener, compassionate stranger, nonjudgmental collaborator, and mirror of family strengths. Conversely, Fowler (1997) found that inadequate communication can lead to misunderstandings, client and provider dissatisfaction, and even termination of home care provider-client relationships.

NURSE–HEALTH TEAM RELATIONSHIPS

Nurses are members of a larger health care community and often function in roles that require interaction with multiple health team members. Many elements of the nurse-client helping relationship are also applied in these collegial relationships, which are focused on accomplishing the work and goals of the clinical setting. Communication in such relationships may be geared toward team building, facilitating group process, collaboration, consultation, delegation, supervision, leadership, and management (Chapter 4). A variety of communication skills are needed, including presentational speaking, persuasion, group problem solving, providing performance reviews, and writing business reports.

Both social and therapeutic interactions are needed between the nurse and health team members to build morale and strengthen relationships within the work setting. Everyone has interpersonal needs for acceptance, inclusion, identity, privacy, power and control, and affection (Stewart and Logan, 1998). Nurses need friendship, support, guidance, and encouragement from one another to cope with the many stressors imposed by the nursing role and must extend the same caring communication used with clients to build positive relationships with colleagues and co-workers.

NURSE-COMMUNITY RELATIONSHIPS

Many nurses form relationships with community groups by participating in local organizations, volunteering for community service, or becoming politically active. Nurses in a community-based practice must be able to establish relationships with their community to be effective change agents (Chapter 3).

Communication within the community occurs through channels such as neighborhood newsletters, public bulletin boards, newspapers, radio, television, and electronic information sites. Nurses can use these forms of communication to share information and discuss issues important to community health.

Elements of Professional Communication

Professional appearance, demeanor, and behavior are important in establishing the nurse's trustworthiness and competence. They communicate that the nurse has assumed the professional helping role, is clinically skilled, and is focused on the client. Nothing harms nursing's professional image like an individual nurse's inappropriate appearance or behavior.

A professional is expected to be clean, neat, well-groomed, conservatively dressed, and scent- and odor-free. Professional behavior should reflect warmth, friendliness, confidence, and competence. Professionals speak in a clear well-modulated voice, use good grammar, listen to others, help and support teammates, and communicate effectively. Being on time, organized, well prepared, and equipped for the responsibilities of the nursing role also communicate one's professionalism.

COURTESY

Common courtesy is part of professional communication. To practice courtesy, the nurse says hello and goodbye, knocks on doors before entering, uses self-introduction and states his or her purpose, addresses people by name, says please and thank you to team members, and apologizes for inadvertently making an error or causing someone distress. Being discourteous causes the nurse to be perceived as rude or insensitive. It sets up barriers between nurse and client and causes friction among team members.

USE OF NAMES

Self-introduction is especially important. The nurse's failure to give a name, indicate status (e.g., registered nurse or licensed practical nurse) or acknowledge the client can create uncertainty about the interaction and convey an impersonal lack of commitment or caring. Making eye contact and smiling at others gives them recognition. Addressing others by name conveys respect for human dignity and uniqueness. Since using last names is respectful in most cultures, nurses usually use the client's last name in the initial interaction, then use the first name if it is requested by the client. The nurse should ask others how they would like to be addressed and let them know personal preference. Using first names is appropriate for infants, young children, confused or unconscious clients, and close team members. Avoid terms of endearment such as "honey," "dear," "Grandma," or "sweetheart." Avoid referring to clients by diagnosis, room number, or other attribute, which is demeaning and sends the message that the nurse does not care enough to know the person as an individual.

PRIVACY AND CONFIDENTIALITY

Maintaining confidentiality is an important aspect of professional behavior. It is essential that the nurse safeguard the client's right to privacy by carefully protecting information of a sensitive, private nature (Chapter 21). Sharing personal information or gossiping about others violates nursing ethical codes and practice standards. It sends the message that the nurse cannot be trusted and damages interpersonal relationships. Team members directly involved in the client's care should be given only relevant information about the client's status. Respect for clients is demonstrated when the nurse treats others with dignity and maintains their physical and emotional privacy.

TRUSTWORTHINESS

Trust is relying on someone without doubt or question. Being trustworthy means helping others without hesitation when help is needed. To foster trust, the nurse communicates warmth and demonstrates consistency, reliability, honesty, and competence. Sometimes it is not easy for a client to ask for help. Trusting another person involves risk and vulnerability, but it also fosters open, therapeutic communication and enhances the expression of feelings, thoughts, and needs. Without trust, a nurse-client relationship rarely progresses beyond social interaction and superficial care. Avoid dishonesty at all costs. Knowingly withholding key information, lying, or distorting the truth violates both legal and ethical standards of practice.

AUTONOMY AND RESPONSIBILITY

Autonomy is the ability to be self-directive in accomplishing goals and advocating for others. Nurses who are autonomous take responsibility for their own thoughts, feelings, and behavior. They take initiative in problem solving and communicate in a manner that reflects what they really need and want (Burden, 1997). Nurses support client autonomy by respecting and upholding the person's right to his or her own values and decisions.

ASSERTIVENESS

Assertiveness is standing up for one's rights without violating those of others (Stanhope and Lancaster, 1996). Nurses who are skilled in assertive communication techniques are more likely to advocate for clients and peers who are vulnerable, afraid, or experiencing a threat to their human rights (Mallik, 1997). Nurses can also teach assertiveness skills to others as a means for promoting personal health. Assertive people express feelings and emotions confidently, spontaneously, and honestly. They make decisions and control their lives more effectively than nonassertive individuals. They can better deal with criticism and manipulation by others and learn to say no, set limits, and resist intentionally imposed guilt.

Assertive responses are characterized by feelings of security, competence, power, optimism, and professionalism. They are good tools for dealing with criticism, change, negative conditions in personal or professional life, and conflict or stress in relationships. Assertive responses often contain "I" messages, such as "I want," "I need," "I think," or "I feel." Simple assertive messages are usually stated in three parts referencing the nurse, the other individual's behavior, and its impact: "I need you to tell me right away if Mrs. Harrison's blood pressure drops, so we can treat it quickly." The nurse can state a more complex assertive message by also including the action that prompted the need for the message, a subjective interpretation of the action, the effects of the action, a request of the other person, and one's intentions if the request is not met (Berko, Rosenfeld, and Samovar, 1997). For example, a nurse might say to a colleague, "When you talked to the nurse manager without letting me know there was a problem, I assumed you weren't comfortable coming to me about it. I was surprised and hurt, and expect that you'll come to me first in the future. If you don't, it will damage our friendship."

Communication Within the Nursing Process

In the following section the focus of the nursing process is on providing care for clients who need special assistance with communication. However, the nursing intervention section contains examples of therapeutic communication techniques that are appropriate strategies for use in any interpersonal nursing situation.

ASSESSMENT

Assessment of a client's ability to communicate includes gathering data about the many contextual factors that influence communication. The word *context* refers to all the parts of something that help determine its meaning. Situations have several aspects that influence the nature of communication, interpersonal relationships, and client needs (Beebe, Beebe, and Redmond, 1999). These include the participants' internal factors and characteristics, the nature of their relationship, the situation prompting communication, the environment, and the sociocultural elements present. Box 22-6 lists the major factors influencing communication within these contexts. Assessing these situational aspects helps the nurse make sound decisions during the communication process. The case study on p. 457 illustrates how the nurse might consider these influencing factors in a client situation.

As the example illustrates, working with physiologically unstable clients and families in an emotionally charged emergency care setting requires sensitive, highly focused, prioritized communication. Had Amy known Mr. and Mrs. Hudson in a long-term home care relationship, an entirely different type of communication might have taken place.

Physical and Emotional Factors.   In client assessment, it is especially important to focus on the psychophysiological factors that influence communication. There are many altered health states and human responses that limit communication. Persons with hearing or visual impairments have fewer channels through which to receive messages (Chapter 48). Facial trauma, laryngeal cancer, or endotracheal intubation may prevent movement of air past vocal cords or mobility of the tongue, resulting in inability to articulate words. An extremely breathless person must use oxygen to breathe rather than speak. Persons with aphasia after a stroke or in late-stage Alzheimer's disease often cannot understand or form words. Certain mental illnesses such as psychoses or depression may cause clients to demonstrate flight of ideas, constant verbalization of the same words or phrases, a loose association of ideas, or slowed speech patterns. Persons with high anxiety may be unable to perceive environmental stimuli or hear explanations. Finally, unresponsive or heavily sedated persons cannot send or respond to verbal messages.

Review of the client's medical record helps provide relevant information about the client's ability to communicate. The medical history and physical examination may document physical barriers to speech, neurological deficits, and pathophysiology affecting hearing or vision. Reviewing the client's medication record is also important. For example, opiates, antidepressants, neuroleptics, hypnotics, or sedatives may cause a client to slur words or

---

Contextual Factors Influencing Communication   Box 22-6

PSYCHOPHYSIOLOGICAL CONTEXT
The internal factors influencing communication:
Physiological status (e.g., pain, hunger, weakness, dyspnea)
Emotional status (e.g., anxiety, anger, hopelessness, euphoria)
Growth and development status (e.g., age, developmental tasks)
Unmet needs (e.g., safety/security, love/belonging)
Attitudes, values, and beliefs (e.g., meaning of illness experience)
Perceptions and personality (e.g., optimist/pessimist, introvert/extrovert)
Self-concept and self-esteem (e.g., positive or negative)

RELATIONAL CONTEXT
The nature of the relationship between the participants:
Social, helping, or working relationship
Level of trust between participants
Level of self-disclosure between participants
Shared history of participants
Balance of power and control

SITUATIONAL CONTEXT
The reason for the communication:
Information exchange
Goal achievement
Problem resolution
Expression of feelings

ENVIRONMENTAL CONTEXT
The physical surroundings in which communication takes place:
Privacy level
Noise level
Comfort and safety level
Distraction level

CULTURAL CONTEXT
The sociocultural elements that affect the interaction:
Educational level of participants
Language and self-expression patterns
Customs and expectations

use incomplete sentences. The nursing progress notes may reveal other factors that contribute to communication difficulties, such as the absence of family members who could provide more information about a confused client.

Communicating directly with clients provides information about their ability to attend to, interpret, and respond to stimuli. If clients have difficulty communicating, it is important to assess how they are affected by the problem. Persons with the nursing diagnosis of impaired verbal communication have described feelings of discomfort, fear, and frustration (Fowler, 1997). The client who cannot communicate effectively will often have difficulty expressing needs and responding appropriately to the environment. A client who is unable to speak can be at risk for injury unless an alternate communication method can be found. If there are barriers that make it difficult to communicate directly with the client, family or friends become important sources of data about the client's communication patterns and abilities.

Developmental Factors.   Aspects of a client's growth and development also influence nurse-client interaction. For example, an infant's self-expression is limited to crying, body movement, and facial expression, whereas older children can express their needs more directly. The nurse adapts communication techniques to the special needs of infants and children. Communication with children and their parents requires special considerations. The nurse can include the parents, child, or both as sources of information about the child's health, depending on the child's age. A young child can be given toys or other distractions so the parent can give full attention to the nurse. Children are especially responsive to nonverbal messages, and sudden movements, loud noises, or threatening gestures can be frightening. Children often prefer to make the first move in interpersonal contacts and do not like adults to stare or look down at them. A child who has received little environmental stimulation may be behind in language development, thus making communication more challenging.

Age alone does not determine an adult's capacity for communication. However, as persons age, their ability to communicate may be affected by many different factors. Mandel and Schulman (1997) state that 2 of every 10 older adults have disorders that limit self-expression and comprehension, often compounded by factors such as depression or dementia. Normal changes of aging include decreases in hearing, vision, strength, and endurance. Older adults may need more time to recall information during history taking and more time to learn new material during client teaching because of changes in short-term memory. They may repeat themselves or share the same stories over and over without realizing it.

Sociocultural Factors.   Culture is a blueprint for thinking, feeling, behaving, and communicating. Nurses need to be aware of the typical patterns of interaction that

C̶a̶s̶e̶ STUDY   BOX 22-7

Mr. Hudson is brought into the emergency department with severe chest pain and difficulty breathing. Amy, his nurse, knows she has to stay in a professional helping role and build trust quickly with this stranger. She does so by staying calm, using his name, introducing herself, and conveying that she will stay with him and help him through this crisis. Because he is physiologically unstable, Amy avoids social conversation, focuses questions on his immediate symptoms, and uses brief, simple instructions and explanations. His need for oxygen makes conversing stressful, so she encourages him to rest quietly as medications take effect. Because he has never been in a hospital and is surrounded by unfamiliar sights, sounds, and sensations, she helps interpret what is going on in his environment using everyday language. Mrs. Hudson is extremely anxious, so Amy uses calming touch and patiently repeats her explanations. As soon as she can, Amy takes Mrs. Hudson to a quiet, private area with a telephone and helps her plan whom she needs to call. She listens attentively and empathetically as Mrs. Hudson expresses her fear and provides her with tissues and a hug when she starts to cry. Because Mrs. Hudson is asking God why this had to happen and pleading with Him to spare her husband's life, Amy offers to call the hospital chaplain to stay with her, and Mrs. Hudson gratefully accepts.

characterize various cultures. For example, European Americans are more open and willing to discuss private family matters, whereas Latin-, African-, and Asian-Americans may be reluctant to reveal personal or family information to strangers. Latin- and Asian-Americans value a quiet demeanor and self-restraint; to be open or argumentative is thought to reflect negatively on family honor. Native Americans also value silence and are comfortable with it.

Foreign-born persons may not speak or understand English. Those who speak English as a second language often experience difficulty with self-expression or language comprehension. To practice cultural sensitivity in communication, the nurse understands that persons of different cultures use different degrees of eye contact, personal space, gestures, loudness of voice, pace of speech, touch, silence, and meaning of language. The nurse makes a conscious effort not to interpret messages through his or her cultural perspective but to consider the communication within the context of the other individual's background. The nurse avoids stereotyping, patronizing, or making fun of other cultures.

Gender.   Gender is another factor that influences how we think, act, feel, and communicate. Male and female communication patterns tend to differ, which can sometimes create barriers to effective communication (Wood, 1996; Beebe, Beebe, and Redmond, 1999).

Males tend to use communication to achieve goals, establish individual status and authority, and compete for attention and power. They typically prefer to talk about topics that do not expose personal feelings. Men tend to speak directly when giving criticism or orders. They use more banter, teasing, and playful put-downs. Men usually want others to know of their accomplishments.

Females tend to use communication to build connections with others, include others, and cooperate with, respond to, show interest in, and support others. Women enjoy discussing feelings and personal issues and find closeness in dialogue. They tend to downplay their achievements. Women speak indirectly, couching criticism and commands in praise or vagueness to avoid causing offense or hurt feelings. A male nurse might say to his colleague, "Help me turn Jeremy." A female nurse might say, "Jeremy needs to be turned," expecting her colleague to understand the implied request for help. Research has shown there are differences in the way male and female nurses use silence, touch, and humor in their practice (Perry, 1996).

To practice gender sensitivity in communication, the nurse recognizes the differences in male and female patterns and does not misinterpret messages sent by someone of the opposite gender. The nurse avoids conversation with sexual overtones, gender-denigrating jokes, and male-female stereotyping.

NURSING DIAGNOSIS

Most individuals experience difficulty with some aspect of communication. Persons who are free of illness or disability may lack skills in attending, listening, responding, and self-expression. Most often, the nurse's care is directed toward those individuals who experience more serious impairments in communication.

The primary nursing diagnostic label used to describe the client who has limited or no ability to communicate verbally is *impaired verbal communication*. This is the state in which an individual experiences a decreased or absent ability to use or understand language in human interaction (Kim, McFarland, and McLane, 1997). A client will have defining characteristics such as the inability to articulate words, stuttering, or slurring, which the nurse clusters together to form the diagnosis. This diagnosis is useful for a wide variety of clients with special problems and needs related to communication, such as impaired perception, reception, and articulation. Although a client's primary problem may be impaired verbal communication, the associated difficulty in self-expression or altered communication patterns may also contribute to other nursing diagnoses. For example, such persons may experience anxiety, social isolation, ineffective individual or family coping, powerlessness, or impaired social interaction.

The related (contributing) factors for impaired verbal communication focus on the causes of the communication disorder. These can be physiological, mechanical, anatomical, psychological, cultural, or developmental in nature. For example, a deaf older adult with untreated cataracts who also has expressive aphasia secondary to a stroke has the following nursing diagnosis: *impaired verbal communication related to limited vision, absent hearing, and the inability to articulate words.* Nursing interventions would then be planned to compensate for the client's visual and hearing deficits and inability to speak. Accuracy in the identification of related factors is necessary so that the nurse selects interventions that can effectively resolve the diagnostic problem.

PLANNING

Once the nurse has identified the nature of the client's communication dysfunction, several factors must be considered as the care plan is designed. Motivation is a factor in improving communication, and clients often require encouragement to try different approaches that involve significant change. It is especially important to involve the client and family in decisions about the plan of care to determine whether suggested methods are acceptable. The nurse needs to make sure basic comfort and safety needs are met before introducing new communication methods and techniques. Adequate time must be allowed for practice, and participants need to be patient with themselves and one another if effective communication is to be achieved. When the focus is on practicing communication, the nurse should arrange for a quiet, private place that is free of distractions such as television or visitors. Communication aids may be needed, such as a writing board for a client with a tracheostomy or a special call system for a client who is paralyzed.

The nurse may need to collaborate with other health team members who have expertise in communication strategies. Speech therapists can help clients with aphasia, interpreters may be needed for clients who speak a foreign language, and psychiatric nurse specialists might help angry or highly anxious clients to communicate more effectively.

Expected outcomes for the client with impaired communication are important to identify. In general, effective nursing interventions will result in the client experiencing a sense of trust in the nurse and health team. The client will be able to attend to appropriate stimuli, transmit clear and understandable messages, and demonstrate congruent verbal and nonverbal messages. He or she will send and receive feedback during the communication process. The client will demonstrate decreased frustration, or increased satisfaction, with the communication process.

At times nurses care for well clients whose difficulty in sending, receiving, and interpreting messages interferes with healthy interpersonal relationships. In this case, impaired communication may be a contributing factor to other nursing diagnoses such as *impaired social interaction* or *ineffective individual coping*. Nurses can plan interventions to help such clients improve their communication skills. For example, the nurse can model effective communication techniques and provide feedback regarding the client's communication. Role play can help clients rehearse situations in which they have difficulty communicating. Expected outcomes for a client in this situation might include demonstrating the ability to appropriately express needs, feelings, and concerns; demonstrating improved interpersonal interaction skills; communicating thoughts and feelings more clearly; developing problem-solving skills; engaging in appropriate social conversation with peers and staff; and increasing feelings of autonomy and assertiveness.

IMPLEMENTATION

In carrying out any plan of care, nurses need to use communication techniques that are appropriate for the client's individual needs. Before learning how to adapt communication methods to help clients with serious communication impairments, it is necessary to learn the communication techniques that serve as the foundation for professional communication.

The most basic nursing interventions used in communication are **therapeutic communication techniques.** Therapeutic communication techniques are specific responses that encourage the expression of feelings and ideas and convey the nurse's acceptance and respect. Learning these techniques helps the student develop awareness of the variety of nursing responses available for use in different situations. Although some of the techniques may seem artificial at first, skill and comfort will increase with practice. Tremendous satisfaction will result as therapeutic relationships and outcomes are achieved.

Therapeutic Communication Techniques

Active Listening.   **Active listening** means listening attentively with one's whole being—mind, body, and spirit. It includes listening for conversational themes, acknowledging and responding, giving appropriate feedback, and paying attention to the other person's total communication, including the content, the intent, and the feelings expressed (Berko, Rosenfeld, and Samovar, 1997). Active listening allows the nurse to better understand the entire message being communicated and is an excellent way to build trust. In many nursing situations, the other person simply needs someone to listen.

To listen attentively, the nurse faces the client at a distance of about 3 feet, removes any physical barriers, maintains eye contact, assumes a relaxed posture and sits quietly, leans forward slightly, and nods in acknowledgment when clients talk about important points or look for feedback. Fidgeting, breaking eye contact, daydreaming during conversation, or only pretending to listen convey the message that what the other person has to say is not important. It inhibits conversation and undermines trust.

Being available means offering oneself and expressing a willingness to listen, talk, or be physically present with another person when the person needs it. By expressing availability, even though the other person may not make his or her needs known, the nurse shows a caring attitude. Going out of one's way to avoid another person communicates unwillingness to face discomfort or resolve conflict. Clients often sense when they are being avoided, and negative behavior may increase as a result.

Availability and active listening are often described as nursing **presence,** an intersubjective encounter between a nurse and a client in which the nurse encounters the client as a unique human being in a unique situation and chooses to "spend" himself or herself on the client's behalf (Doona, Haggerty, and Chase 1997). Presence is the nursing quality of "being there" for the client, not only physically present but also listening attentively from a perspective of humanistic caring: "I'll stay with you awhile. If you want to talk, I'll be glad to listen."

Sharing Observations.   Nurses make observations by commenting on how the other person looks, sounds, or acts. Stating observations often helps the client communicate without the need for extensive questioning, focusing, or clarification. This technique can help start a conversation with quiet or withdrawn persons. The nurse does not state observations that might embarrass or anger the client, such as telling someone "You look a mess!" Even if such an observation is made with humor, the client can become resentful.

Sharing observations differs from making assumptions, which means drawing unwarranted conclusions about the other person without validating them. Making assumptions puts the client in the position of having to contradict the nurse. Examples might include the nurse interpreting fatigue as depression or assuming that untouched food indicates lack of interest in meeting nutritional goals. Making observations is a gentler and safer technique: "You look tired . . . ," "You seem different today . . . ," or "I see you haven't eaten anything."

Sharing Empathy.   **Empathy** is the ability to understand and accept another person's reality, to accurately perceive feelings, and to communicate this understanding to the other. Balzer-Riley (1996) states "When clients or colleagues are hurting, confused, troubled, anxious, alienated, terrified, doubtful of self-worth, or uncertain as to identity, then understanding is called for." To express empathy, the nurse reflects understanding of the importance of what has been communicated by the other person on a feeling level. Such empathic understanding requires the nurse to be both sensitive and imaginative, especially if the nurse has not had similar experiences. Although nurses are rarely empathetic in every situation, it is an important goal to work for, a key to unlocking concern and communicating support for others. Statements reflecting empathy are highly effective because they tell the person that the nurse heard feeling content, as well as factual content, of the communication. Empathy statements are neutral and nonjudgmental. They can be used to establish trust in difficult situations. For example, the nurse might say to an angry client who has lost mobility after a stroke: "It must be very frustrating to know what you want and not be able to do it."

Sharing Hope.   Nurses recognize that hope is essential for healing and learn to communicate a "sense of possibility" to others. Appropriate encouragement and positive feedback are important in fostering hope and self-confidence and for helping people achieve their potential and reach their goals. The nurse can give hope by commenting on the positive aspects of the other person's behavior, performance, or response. Sharing a vision of the future and reminding others of their resources and strengths can also strengthen hope. Clients can be reassured that there are many kinds of hope and that meaning and personal growth can come from illness experiences. For example, the nurse might say to a client discouraged about a poor prognosis: "I believe you will find a way to face your situation, because I have seen your courage and creativity in the past."

Sharing Humor.   Humor is an important but underused resource in nursing interactions. Beck (1997) found that humor does several things. It helps nurses deal effectively with difficult situations and clients and creates a sense of cohesiveness between nurses and their clients and also among nurses themselves. It helps decrease client anxiety, depression, and embarrassment. Humor can be planned and routine or unexpected and spontaneous, and it creates lasting effects beyond the immediate moment for both nurses and clients. According to Wooten (1993), humor can help promote well-being by changing perspective, releasing tension, and giving a feeling of superiority or mastery. Laughter can be good "medicine" when nurses use humor to help clients adjust to stress imposed by illness. Laughter helps to relieve stress-related tension and pain by decreasing serum cortisol levels, increasing immune system activity, and stimulating endorphin release from the hypothalamus. Humor can increase the nurse's effectiveness in providing emotional support to clients and can humanize the illness experience. Laughter provides both a psychological and physical release for both nurse and client. Humor can help others to interact more

openly and comfortably and can make nurse's own humanity more apparent.

Wooten advises that nurses should establish professional competency and caring before using humor, take care of the client's comfort and security needs first, and test receptivity to humor with small, safe doses. Avoid sexual, religious, or ethnic humor. Use gentle humor, or hoping humor, by telling jokes, sharing humorous incidents or situations, using props (such as giving an angry client a squirt gun), and using puns. Nurses should realize that humor can backfire: not everyone will appreciate a light approach due to mood, stress, or physical discomfort. Nurses need to avoid using humor to mask their own fears and discomforts or their inability to communicate with others.

A kind of dark, negative humor is sometimes used after difficult or traumatic situations as a way to survive intact and defuse unbearable tension and stress. This coping humor has a high potential for being misinterpreted as callous or uncaring by persons not involved in the situation. For example, student nurses are sometimes offended and wonder how staff can laugh and joke after unsuccessful resuscitation efforts. When nurses use coping humor within earshot of clients or their loved ones, great emotional distress can result.

Sharing Feelings.   Emotions are subjective feelings that result from one's thought and perceptions. Feelings are not right, wrong, good, or bad, although they may be pleasant or unpleasant. If feelings are not expressed, stress and illness can worsen. Nurses can help clients express emotions by making observations, acknowledging feelings, encouraging communication, giving permission to express "negative" feelings, and modeling healthy emotional self-expression. At times, clients may direct anger or frustration prompted by their illness toward the nurse, who should not take such expressions personally. Acknowledging clients' feelings communicates that the nurse listened to and understood the emotional aspects of their illness situation.

When nurses care for clients they must be aware of their own emotions, because feelings are difficult to hide. Students may wonder whether it is helpful for the nurse to share feelings with clients. Sharing emotion makes nurses seem more human and can bring people closer. It is appropriate to share feelings of caring, or even cry with others, as long as the nurse is in control of how those feelings are expressed and does so in a way that does not burden the client or break confidentiality. Clients are perceptive and can sense a nurse's emotions. It is usually inappropriate to discuss negative personal emotions such as anger or sadness with clients. A social support system of colleagues is helpful, and employee assistance programs, peer group meetings, and the use of interdisciplinary teams such as social work and pastoral care provide other means for nurses to safely express feelings away from clients.

Using Touch.   In today's fast-paced technical environments, nurses are required more than ever to bring the sense of caring and human connection to their clients. Touch is one of the nurse's most potent forms of communication. Nurses are privileged to experience more of this intimate form of personal contact than almost any other professional. Many messages, such as affection, emotional support, encouragement, tenderness, and personal attention, are conveyed through touch. Comfort touch, such as holding a hand, is especially important for vulnerable clients who are experiencing severe illness with its accompanying physical and emotional losses. Research has found that nurses use touch not connected with procedures to get a client's attention, arouse them from sleep, begin a nursing intervention, add emphasis to explanations, make requests, bring comfort, emphasize or point things out, tease, thank, and reprimand (Routasalo, 1996) (Figure 22-2).

Seed (1995) found that students may initially find giving intimate care to be stressful, especially when caring for clients of the opposite gender, and that students learn to cope with intimate contact by changing their perception of the situation. Since much of what nurses do involves touching, nurses must learn to be sensitive to other's reactions to touch and use it wisely. Touch should be as gentle or as firm as needed and delivered in a comforting, nonthreatening manner. There are times when touch should be withheld; for example, highly suspicious or angry persons may respond negatively or even violently to the nurse's touch.

Using Silence.   It takes time and experience to become comfortable with silence. Most people have a natural tendency to fill empty spaces with words, but sometimes what those spaces really need is time for the nurse and client to observe one another, sort out feelings, think how to say

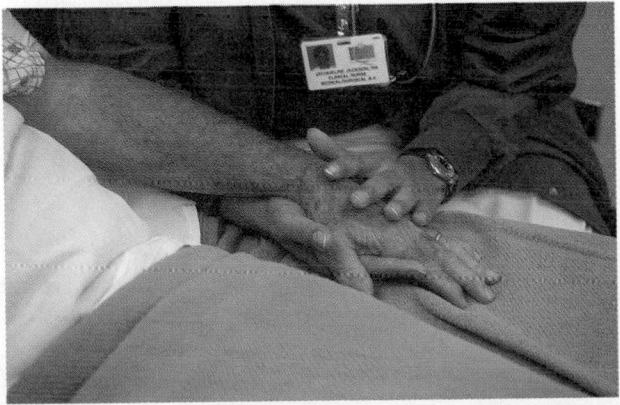

Figure 22-2   The nurse uses touch to communicate.

things, and consider what has been communicated. Upon losing her voice, one nurse found her nurse-client relationships actually improved (Kacperek, 1997). She noted that the skilled use of nonverbal communication through silence, facial expression, touch, and close physical proximity facilitated active listening and helped to develop empathy, intuition, and presence between herself and her clients.

Silence is particularly useful when people are confronted with decisions that require much thought. For example, silence may help a client gain confidence needed to share the decision to refuse medical treatment. Silence also allows the nurse to pay particular attention to nonverbal messages such as worried expressions or loss of eye contact. Remaining silent demonstrates the nurse's patience and willingness to wait for a response when the other person is unable to reply quickly. Silence may be especially therapeutic during times of profound sadness or grief.

Asking Relevant Questions.   Asking questions allows nurses to seek information needed for decision making. Nurses should ask only one question at a time and fully explore one topic before moving to another area. During client assessment, questions follow a logical sequence and usually proceed from general to more specific. Open-ended questions allow the client to take the conversational lead and introduce pertinent information about a topic: "What happens when you and your husband argue?" Focused questions are used when more specific information is needed in an area: "What do you argue about most often?" The nurse should allow clients to fully respond to an open-ended question before asking more focused questions. Closed-ended questions elicit a yes, no, or one-word response: "How many arguments did you have last week?" They are generally less useful during therapeutic exchanges, although they may be needed during assessment.

Asking too many questions can be dehumanizing, because seeking factual information does not allow the nurse or client to establish a more meaningful relationship or deal with important emotional issues. It may be a way for the nurse to ignore uncomfortable areas in favor of more comfortable, neutral topics. A useful exercise is to try conversing without asking the other person a single question. By giving general leads ("tell me about it . . ."), making observations, paraphrasing, focusing, providing information, and so forth, nurses can discover much of importance that would have remained hidden if questions alone were used during the communication process.

Providing Information.   Providing relevant information tells other persons what they need or want to know so they can make decisions, experience less anxiety, and feel safe and secure. It is also an integral aspect of health teaching. It is usually not helpful to hide information from clients, particularly when they seek it. If a physician withholds information, the nurse needs to clarify the reason. Clients have a right to know about their health status and what is happening in their environment. Information of a distressing nature needs to be communicated with sensitivity, at a pace appropriate to what the client can absorb, and in general terms at first: "John, your heart sounds have changed from earlier today, and so has your blood pressure. I'll let your doctor know." The nurse provides information that enables others to understand what is happening and what to expect: "Mrs. Evans, John is getting an echocardiogram right now. This test uses painless sound waves to create a moving picture of his heart structures and valves and should tell us what is causing his murmur."

Paraphrasing. Paraphrasing is restating another's message more briefly using one's own words. Through paraphrasing, the nurse sends feedback that lets others know whether their messages were understood. Practice is required to paraphrase accurately. If the meaning of a message is changed or distorted through paraphrasing, communication may become ineffective. For example, a client may say, "I've been overweight all my life and never had any problems. I can't understand why I need to be on a diet." Paraphrasing this statement by saying, "You don't care if you're overweight or not," is incorrect. It would be more accurate to say, "You're not convinced you need a diet because you've stayed healthy."

Clarifying. To check whether understanding is accurate, the nurse can restate an unclear or ambiguous message to clarify the sender's meaning. Instead of restating the message, the nurse can also ask the other person to rephrase it, explain further, or give an example of what the person means. Without clarification, the nurse may make invalid assumptions and miss valuable information. Despite efforts at paraphrasing, the nurse may not understand the client's message and should let the client know if this is the case: "I'm not sure I understand what you mean by 'sicker than usual.' What is different now?"

Focusing. Focusing is used to center on key elements or concepts of a message. If conversation is vague or rambling or clients begin to repeat themselves, focusing is a useful technique. The nurse does not use focusing if it interrupts clients while discussing an important issue. Rather, the nurse uses focusing to guide the direction of conversation to important areas: "We've talked a lot about your medications, but let's look more closely at the trouble you're having in taking them on time."

Summarizing. Summarizing is a concise review of key aspects of an interaction. Summarizing brings a sense of satisfaction and closure to an individual conversation and is especially helpful during the termination phase of a nurse-client relationship. By reviewing a conversation, participants focus on key issues and can add additional relevant information as needed. Beginning a new interaction by summarizing a previous one helps the client recall topics discussed and shows the client that the nurse has analyzed communication. Summarizing also clarifies expectations, as in this example of a nurse manager who has been working with a dissatisfied employee: "You've told me a lot of things about why you don't like this job and how unhappy you've been. We've also come up with some possible ways to make things better, and you've agreed to try some and let me know if any of them help."

Self-Disclosing. To use self-disclosure, the nurse reveals personal experiences, thoughts, ideas, values, or feelings in context of the relationship with the intent of helping the other person. This is not therapy for the nurse; rather, it shows clients that their experiences can be understood and are not unique. Such personal statements are intentionally revealed to the other person for the purposes of modeling and educating, fostering a therapeutic alliance, validating reality, and encouraging autonomy (Sundeen and others, 1998). Self-disclosures should be relevant and appropriate and made to benefit the client rather than the nurse. They are used sparingly so the client is the focus of the interaction: "That happened to me once, too. It was devastating, and I had to face some things about myself that I didn't like. I went for counseling, and it really helped. . . . What are your thoughts about seeing a counselor?"

Confronting. To confront someone in a therapeutic way, the nurse helps the other person become more aware of inconsistencies in his or her feelings, attitudes, beliefs, and behaviors (Stuart and Sundeen, 1998). This technique improves client self-awareness and helps the client recognize growth and deal with important issues. Confrontation should be used only after trust has been established, and it should be done gently, with sensitivity: "You say you've already decided what to do, yet you're still talking a lot about your options."

Nontherapeutic Communication Techniques. Certain communication techniques can hinder or damage professional relationships. These specific techniques are referred to as non-therapeutic or blocking and will often cause recipients to activate defenses to avoid being hurt or negatively affected. Nontherapeutic techniques tend to discourage further expression of feelings and ideas and may engender negative responses or behaviors in others.

Asking Personal Questions. "Why don't you and John get married?" Asking personal questions that are not relevant to the situation, simply to satisfy the nurse's curiosity, is not appropriate professional communication. Such questions are nosy, invasive, and unnecessary. If clients wish to share private information, they will. If the nurse needs to know more about the client's interpersonal roles and relationships, a question such as "How would you describe your relationship with John?" can be asked.

Giving Personal Opinions.   "If I were you, I'd put your mother in a nursing home." When the nurse gives a personal opinion, it takes decision making away from the client. It inhibits spontaneity, stalls problem solving, and creates doubt. Personal opinions differ from professional advice. At times, clients need suggestions and help to make choices. Suggestions are presented to clients as options because the final decision rests with the client. Remember, the problem and its solution belong to the other person and not the nurse. A much better response would be, "Let's talk about what options are available for your mother's care."

Changing the Subject.   "Let's not talk about your problems with the insurance company. It's time for your walk." Changing the subject when another person is trying to communicate something important is rude and shows a lack of empathy. It tends to block further communication, and the sender may then withhold important messages or fail to openly express feelings. Thoughts and spontaneity are interrupted, ideas become tangled, and information provided may be inadequate. In some instances, changing the subject can serve as a face-saving maneuver or may be necessary due to circumstances. If this happens, reassure the client you will return to his concerns: "After your walk, let's talk some more about what's going on with your insurance company."

Automatic Responses.   "Older adults are always confused." "Administration doesn't care about the staff." Stereotypes are generalized beliefs held about people. Making stereotyped remarks about others reflects poor nursing judgment and can threaten nurse-client or team relationships. A cliché is a stereotyped comment such as "you can't win them all" that tends to belittle the other person's feelings and minimize the importance of his or her message. These automatic phrases communicate that the nurse is not taking concerns seriously or responding thoughtfully. Another kind of automatic response is parroting, repeating what the other person has said, word for word. Parroting is easily overused and is not as effective as paraphrasing. A simple "oh?" can give the nurse time to think if the other person says something that takes one by surprise.

A nurse who is task-oriented automatically makes the task or technical procedure the entire focus of interaction with clients, missing opportunities to communicate with them as individuals and meet their needs. Task-oriented nurses are often perceived as cold, uncaring, and unapproachable. When students first perform technical skills, it is difficult to integrate therapeutic communication due to the need to focus on the procedure. In time, the nurse can learn to integrate communication with high-visibility tasks and accomplish several goals simultaneously.

False Reassurance.   "Don't worry, everything will be all right." When a client is seriously ill or distressed, the nurse may be tempted to offer hope to the client with statements such as "You'll be fine" or "There's nothing to worry about." When a client is reaching for understanding, false reassurance from the nurse may discourage open communication. Offering reassurance not supported by facts or based in reality can do more harm than good. Although it might be intended kindly and have the secondary effect of helping the nurse avoid the other person's distress, it tends to block conversation and discourage further expression of feelings. A more facilitative nursing response would be "It must be difficult not to know what the surgeon will find. What can I do to help?"

Sympathy.   "I'm so sorry about your amputation, it must be terrible to lose a leg." **Sympathy** is concern, sorrow, or pity felt for the client generated by the nurse's personal identification with the client's needs. Sympathy is a subjective look at another person's world that prevents a clear perspective of the issues confronting that person. While sympathy is a compassionate response to another's situation, it is not as therapeutic as empathy. The nurse's own emotional issues can prevent effective problem solving and impair good judgment. Stuart and Sundeen (1998) explain that sympathy can cause problems in a helping relationship, because helpers who share the client's needs may be unable to help the client select realistic solutions for problems. A more empathetic approach would be "Losing your leg has been a major change. How has it affected your life?"

Asking for Explanations.   "Why are you so anxious?" A nurse may be tempted to ask the other person to explain why the person believes, feels, or has acted in a certain way. Clients frequently interpret "why" questions as accusations or think the nurse knows the reason and is simply testing them. Regardless of client perception of the nurse's motivation, "why" questions can cause resentment, insecurity, and mistrust. If additional information is needed, it is best to phrase a question to avoid using the word why. "You seem upset. What's on your mind?" is more likely to help the anxious client to communicate.

Approval or Disapproval.   "You shouldn't even think about assisted suicide, it's not right." Nurses must not impose their own attitudes, values, beliefs, and moral standards on others while in the professional helping role. Other people have the right to be themselves and make their own decisions. Judgmental responses by the nurse often contain terms such as *should, ought, good, bad, right,* or *wrong.* Agreeing or disagreeing sends the subtle message that nurses have the right to make value judgments about client decisions. Approving implies that the behavior being praised is the only acceptable one. Often the client shares a decision with the nurse, not in an effort to seek approval but to provide a means to discuss feelings. On the other hand, disapproving implies that the client must meet the nurse's expectations or standards. Instead, the nurse should help clients explore their own beliefs and decisions. The nursing response "I'm surprised you are considering assisted suicide. Tell me more about it . . ." gives the client a chance to express ideas or feelings without fear of being judged.

Defensive Responses. "No one here would intentionally lie to you." Becoming defensive in the face of criticism implies the other person has no right to an opinion. The sender's concerns may be ignored when the nurse focuses on the need for self-defense, defense of the health care team, or defense of others. When clients express criticism, nurses should listen to what they have to say. Listening does not imply agreement. To discover reasons for the client's anger or dissatisfaction, the nurse must listen uncritically. By avoiding defensiveness the nurse can defuse anger and uncover deeper concerns: "You believe people have been dishonest with you. It must be hard to trust anyone."

Passive or Aggressive Responses. "Things are bad, and there's nothing I can do about it." "Things are bad, and it's all your fault." Passive responses serve to avoid conflict or sidestep issues. They reflect feelings of sadness, depression, anxiety, powerlessness, and hopelessness. Aggressive responses provoke confrontation at the other person's expense. They reflect feelings of anger, frustration, resentment, and stress. Nurses who lack assertive skills may also use triangulation, complaining to a third party rather than confronting the problem or expressing concerns directly to the source. This lowers team morale and draws others into the conflict situation. Assertive communication is a far more professional approach for the nurse to take.

Arguing. "How can you say you didn't sleep a wink, when I heard you snoring all night long?" Challenging or arguing against perceptions denies that they are real and valid to the other person. They imply that the other person is lying, misinformed, or uneducated. The skillful nurse can give information or present reality in a way that avoids argument: "You feel like you didn't get any rest at all last night, even though I thought you slept well since I heard you snoring."

Adapting Communication Techniques for the Client with Special Needs.
Interacting with those who have conditions that impair communication requires special thought and sensitivity. Such clients benefit greatly when the nurse adapts communication techniques to their unique circumstances or developmental level. For example, the nurse caring for a client with impaired verbal communication related to cultural differences may provide a table of simple words in the client's language. The nurse and client use the table to help communicate about basic needs such as food, water, toileting, pain relief, sleep, and so forth.

The nurse's actions are directed at meeting the goals and expected outcomes identified in the plan of care, addressing both the communication impairment and its contributing factors. Box 22-8 lists many methods available to encourage, enhance, restore, or substitute for verbal communication. The nurse must be sure that the client is physically able to use the chosen method and that it does not cause frustration by being too complicated or difficult.

Box 22-9 provides general guidelines for communicating with persons at preadult developmental levels. Students may consult pediatric nursing textbooks for more detailed information about communication and establishing nurse-client relationships with children and their parents.

In helping older adults with impaired communication, the primary goal is to establish a reliable communication system that is easily understood by all health care team members, since nursing care of the older adult is ideally delivered through an interdisciplinary model. Effective communication involves adapting to any special needs resulting from sensory, motor, or cognitive impairments that may be present. Nurses can also encourage older adults to share life stories and reminisce about the past, which has a therapeutic effect and increases their sense of well-being. The nurse should avoid sudden shifts from subject to subject. It is helpful to include the client's family and friends and to become familiar with the client's favorite topics for conversation.

EVALUATION
The nurse and client determine whether the plan of care has been successful by evaluating the client communication outcomes established during planning. The nurse evaluates nursing interventions to determine what strategies or interventions were effective and what client changes resulted because of the interventions. For example, if using a pen and paper proves frustrating for a nonverbal client whose handwriting is shaky, the care plan can be revised to include use of a picture board instead. If expected outcomes are not met or progress is not satisfactory, the nurse needs to determine what factors influenced the outcomes, then modify the plan of care.

Nurses can evaluate the effectiveness of their own communication by making process recordings, written records of their verbal and nonverbal interactions with clients. Process recording analysis reveals how the nurse can improve personal communication techniques to make them more effective. Box 22-10 contains a sample communication analysis of such a record. Analysis of a process recording enables the nurse to evaluate the following:

- Determine whether he or she encouraged openness and allowed the client to "tell his story," expressing both thoughts and feelings.
- Identify any missed verbal or nonverbal cues or conversational themes.

CLIENTS WHO CANNOT SPEAK CLEARLY (APHASIA, DYSARTHRIA, MUTENESS)

Listen attentively, be patient, and do not interrupt.

Ask simple questions that require "yes" or "no" answers.

Allow time for understanding and response.

Use visual cues (e.g., words, pictures, and objects) when possible.

Allow only one person to speak at a time.

Do not shout or speak too loudly.

Encourage the client to converse.

Let client know if you have not understood him.

Collaborate with speech therapist as needed.

Use communication aids:

   Pad and felt-tipped pen or magic slate

   Communication board with commonly used words, letters, or pictures denoting basic needs

   Call bells or alarms

   Sign language

   Use of eye blinks or movement of fingers for simple responses ("yes" or "no")

CLIENTS WHO ARE COGNITIVELY IMPAIRED

Reduce environmental distractions while conversing.

Get client's attention prior to speaking.

Use simple sentences and avoid long explanations.

Avoid shifting from subject to subject.

Ask one question at a time.

Allow time for client to respond.

Be an attentive listener.

Include family and friends in conversations, especially in subjects known to client.

CLIENTS WHO ARE UNRESPONSIVE

Call client by name during interactions.

Communicate both verbally and by touch.

Speak to client as though he or she could hear.

Explain all procedures and sensations.

Provide orientation to person, place, and time.

Avoid talking about client to others in his or her presence.

Avoid saying things client should not hear.

CLIENTS WHO DO NOT SPEAK ENGLISH

Speak to client in normal tone of voice (shouting may be interpreted as anger).

Establish method for client to signal desire to communicate (call light or bell).

Provide an interpreter (translator) as needed.

Avoid using family members, especially children, as interpreters.

Develop communication board, pictures, or cards.

Translate words from native language into English list for client to make basic requests.

Have dictionary (English/Spanish and so forth) available if client can read.

COMMUNICATING WITH INFANTS

Use firm touch and gentle physical contact such as cuddling, patting, or rocking.

Hold infant so he or she can see the parents.

Talk softly to the infant.

COMMUNICATING WITH TODDLERS AND PRESCHOOLERS

Interact with parents before communicating with child.

Assume a position that is at the child's eye level.

Allow children to touch and examine objects that will come in contact with them.

Offer a choice only if one exists.

Focus communication on the child, not on the experience of others.

Don't use analogies—small children are very literal, direct, and concrete.

Use simple words and short sentences.

Keep unfamiliar equipment out of view until it is needed.

Keep facial expression congruent with activity (don't smile while doing something painful).

Communicate through transition objects such as dolls, puppets, or stuffed animals before questioning a young child directly.

COMMUNICATING WITH CHILDREN

Allow time for the child to feel comfortable.

Avoid sudden or rapid advances, broad smiles, staring, or other threatening gestures.

Talk to the parent if the child is initially shy.

Give older children the opportunity to talk without the parents present.

Speak in a quiet, unhurried, and confident voice.

Use correct scientific/medical terminology.

Give correct reason for why something is done or how equipment works.

State directions and suggestions specifically and positively.

Be honest and let the child know what to expect and how to participate.

Allow the child to express concerns and fears; allow time for questions.

Use a variety of communication techniques such as drawing or play.

COMMUNICATING WITH ADOLESCENTS

Give undivided attention.

Listen, listen, listen.

Be courteous, calm, and open minded.

Try not to overreact. If you do, take a break.

Avoid judging or criticizing.

Avoid the "third degree" of continuous questioning.

Choose important issues when taking a stand.

Make expectations clear.

Respect their privacy and views.

Praise good points and tolerate differences.

Encourage expression of ideas and feelings.

Modified from Wong D and others: *Whaley and Wong's nursing care of infants and children,* ed 6, St. Louis, 1999, Mosby.

Sample Communication Analysis

Box 22-10

Nurse: "Good morning, Mr. Simpson."
(Smiles, approaches bed holding clipboard)
Acknowledging by name, social greeting to begin conversation

Client: "What's good about it?"
(Arms crossed over chest, frowning, direct stare)
Nonverbal signs of anger

Nurse: "You sound unhappy."
(Pulls up chair and sits at bedside)
Sharing observation, nonverbal communication of availability

Client: "You'd be unhappy, too, if nobody would answer your questions."
(Angry voice tone, challenging expression)
Further expression of feelings facilitated by nurse making accurate observation

Nurse: "Are you saying that you need some information you haven't been able to get?"
Clarifying what has been implied

Client: "Oh, I've tried to get it, alright. But nothing does any good."
Feeling powerless

Nurse: "I'd like to hear more about it."
(Leans forward slightly, lays clipboard in lap)
Offering self, removing barriers to active listening

Client: "You're probably just like all the rest of the incompetents in this hospital. Why should I talk to you?"
Testing and challenging nurse

Nurse: "This hospital has a fine staff, Mr. Simpson. I'm sure no one would intentionally keep information from you."
Feeling threatened and being defensive, a nontherapeutic technique

Client: "All right then: Why wouldn't that girl tell me what my blood sugar was?"

Nurse: "I'm not sure. If I were you, I'd forget about it and get a fresh start."
Giving advice and using cliché, which was nontherapeutic; would have been better to acknowledge that client had a right to know the information

Nurse: "I'm going to test your glucose in a minute, and I'll tell you the results." (does test) "Your blood sugar was 350."
Providing information, demonstrating trustworthiness

Client: "That's up pretty high, isn't it?"
(Worried facial expression)
Feeling very concerned about test results

Nurse: (Nods) . . . long pause . . .
Nonverbal affirmation, use of silence to allow client time to absorb information and gather thoughts

Client: "I'll never be normal again."
(Tears in eyes and voice)
Expressing feelings, which is therapeutic

Nurse: "This illness has changed a lot of things for you, hasn't it?"

Empathy statement, acknowledging implied feelings

Client: "I'm sorry, I shouldn't cry. I'm acting like a baby."
Embarrassed about showing his emotions

Nurse: "I don't think you're acting like a baby. I think being able to express your feelings is important and healthy."
(Hands him tissue box)
Sharing perception, giving professional opinion, meeting comfort needs

Client: "I'm so afraid complications will set in since my blood sugar is high."
(Stares out window)
Feels free to express deeper concerns, but they are hard to face

Nurse: "What kinds of things are you worried about?"
Open-ended question to seek information

Client: "I could lose a leg, like my mother did. Or go blind. Or have to live hooked up to a kidney machine for the rest of my life. I could go crazy!"

Nurse: "Go crazy? I'm not sure what you mean."
(Puzzled and faintly alarmed facial expression)
Concerned about meaning, trying to clarify

Client: "Go crazy from worrying, I guess."
(Both laugh)
Use of humor defuses tension

Nurse: "You've been thinking about all kinds of things that could go wrong, and it adds to your worry not to be told what your blood sugar is."
Summarizing to let client "hear" what he has communicated

Client: "I always think the worst."
(Shakes head in exasperation)
Expressing insight into his "inner dialogue"

Nurse: "I'll pass along to the tech that it's OK to tell you your glucose levels. And later this afternoon, I'd like us to talk more about some things you can do to help avoid these complications and set some goals for controlling your glucose."
(Stands up, keeps looking at client)
Providing information, encouraging collaboration and goal setting
Giving nonverbal cue that conversation is nearing end

Client: "OK, if you can stand an old pessimist like me."
(Smiles, appears relaxed)
Trust established, willing to work with nurse; anxiety lessened

Nurse: "Old pessimists are my biggest challenge! Seriously, I'm glad you let me know what was going on, and I'd like to help."
Humor, positive reinforcement for client's willingness to communicate

- Examine whether nursing responses blocked or facilitated the client's efforts to communicate.
- Determine whether nursing responses were positive and supportive or superficial and judgmental.
- Examine the type and number of questions that were asked.
- Determine the type and number of therapeutic communication techniques used.
- Discover any missed opportunities to use humor, silence, or touch.

Evaluation of the communication process will help nurses gain confidence and competence in interpersonal skills. Becoming an effective communicator greatly increases the nurse's professional satisfaction and success. There is no skill more basic, no tool more powerful.

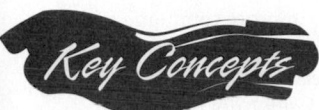

Key Concepts

- Communication is a powerful therapeutic tool and an essential nursing skill used to influence others and achieve positive health outcomes.
- Communication involves the entire human being, including body, mind, emotions, and spirit.
- Critical thinking facilitates communication through creative inquiry, focused self-awareness and awareness of others, purposeful analysis, and control of perceptual biases.
- Nurses consider many contexts and factors influencing communication when making decisions about what, when, where, how, why, and with whom to communicate.
- Communication is most effective when the receiver and sender accurately perceive the meaning of one another's messages.
- Message transmission is influenced by the sender's and receiver's physical and developmental status, perceptions, values, emotions, knowledge, sociocultural background, roles, and environment.
- Effective verbal communication requires appropriate intonation, clear and concise phrasing, proper pacing of statements, and proper timing and relevance of a message.
- Effective nonverbal communication complements and strengthens the message conveyed by verbal communication so that the receiver is less likely to misinterpret the message.
- Nurses use intrapersonal, interpersonal, transpersonal, small-group, and public interaction to achieve positive change and health goals.

- Helping relationships are strengthened when the nurse demonstrates caring by establishing trust, empathy, autonomy, confidentiality, and professional competence.
- Effective communication techniques are facilitative and tend to encourage the other person to openly express ideas, feelings, or concerns.
- Ineffective communication techniques are inhibiting and tend to block the other person's willingness to openly express ideas, feelings, or concerns.
- The nurse must blend social and informational interactions with therapeutic communication techniques so that others can explore feelings and manage health issues.
- Methods that facilitate communication with children include sitting at eye level; interacting with parents; using simple, direct language; and incorporating play activities.
- Older-adult clients with sensory, motor, or cognitive impairments require the adaptation of communication techniques to compensate for their loss of function and special needs.
- Clients with impaired verbal communication require special consideration and alterations in communication techniques to facilitate the sending, receiving, and interpreting of messages.
- Desired outcomes for clients with impaired verbal communication include increased satisfaction with interpersonal interactions, the ability to send and receive clear messages, and attending to and accurately interpreting verbal and nonverbal cues.

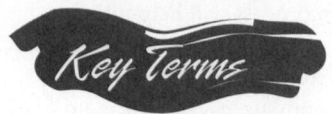

Key Terms

Active listening, *p. 459*

Assertiveness, *p. 455*

Autonomy, *p. 455*

Channels, *p. 449*

Communication, *p. 445*

Empathy, *p. 459*

Environment, *p. 449*

Feedback, *p. 449*

Interpersonal communication, *p. 448*

Interpersonal variables, *p. 449*

Intrapersonal communication, *p. 447*

Message, *p. 449*

Metacommunication, *p. 452*

Nonverbal communication, *p. 450*

Perception, *p. 449*

Perceptual biases, *p. 446*

Presence, *p. 459*

Public communication, *p. 448*

Receiver, *p. 448*

Referent, *p. 448*

Sender, *p. 448*

Small-group communication, *p. 448*

Symbolic communication, *p. 451*

Sympathy, *p. 463*

Therapeutic communication techniques, *p. 459*

Transpersonal communication, *p. 448*

Verbal communication, *p. 449*

Critical Thinking Exercises

1. Mrs. Maria Ramirez, an American of Puerto Rican descent, is faced with the difficult decision of whether or not to continue chemotherapy in the face of a rapidly spreading malignancy. What communication techniques could the nurse use to help her at this point, and what traps must the nurse avoid in such a situation?

2. Jan, a nurse colleague, is having difficulty standing up to a physician who has an abrupt, intimidating communication style. She often ends up with a lot of unspoken anger, developing tension headaches and easily becoming tearful. What could the nurse do to help?

3. Mr. Hess, a client with Parkinson's disease living at an extended care facility, has a stiff, expressionless face. He sits slumped in a recliner chair all day and seems lost in his own world, rarely looking at or interacting with anyone. When he does talk, he mumbles in a soft voice and his words are difficult to understand. What kinds of things could the nurse do to establish a helping-healing relationship with Mr. Hess?

4. Jennifer Hughes, a new graduate, is very discouraged. In school, she had felt a great deal of anxiety about her own performance, and even now she finds it difficult to be positive about herself or her job. What knowledge about communication could she use to help improve her situation?

References

Balzer-Riley J: *Communications in nursing,* ed 3, St. Louis, 1996, Mosby.

Beck C: Humor in nursing practice: a phenomenological study, *Int J Nurs Stud* 34(5):346, 1997.

Beebe S, Beebe S, Redmond M: *Interpersonal communication: relating to others,* ed 2, Boston, 1999, Allyn & Bacon.

Berko M, Rosenfeld L, Samovar L: *Connecting: a culture-sensitive approach to interpersonal communication competency,* ed 2, Philadelphia, 1997, Harcourt Brace.

Bottorff J, Gogag M, Engelberg-Lotzkar M: Comforting: exploring the work of cancer nurses, *J Adv Nurs* 22(6):1077, 1995.

Brennan B: *Hands of light: a guide to healing through the human energy field,* New York, 1987, Bantam.

Brown-Saltzman K: Replenishing the spirit by meditative prayer and guided imagery, *Semin Oncol Nurs* 13(4), 1997.

Burden N: Using self-responsibility to improve communications: one nurse's perspective, *J Perianesth Nurs* 12(1):25, 1997.

Canales M: Narrative interaction: creating a space for therapeutic communication, *Issues Ment Health Nurs* 18(5), 1997.

Creasia J, Parker P: *Conceptual foundations of professional nursing practice,* St. Louis, 1996, Mosby.

Curtis D, Floyd J, Winsor J: *Business and professional communication,* ed 2, Dubuque, Iowa, 1997, Kendall/Hunt.

Doona M, Haggerty L, Chase S: Nursing presence: an existential exploration of the concept, *Sch Inq Nurs Pract* 11(1):3, 1997.

Edelman C, Mandle C: *Health promotion throughout the lifespan,* ed 4, St. Louis, 1998, Mosby.

Fortinash K, Holoday-Worret P: *Psychiatric mental health nursing,* ed 2, St. Louis, 2000, Mosby.

Fowler S: Impaired verbal communication during short-term oral intubation, *Nurs Diagn* 8(3):93, 1997.

Hartrick G: Relational capacity: the foundation for interpersonal nursing practice, *J Adv Nurs* 26(3):523, 1997.

Henson R: Analysis of the concept of mutuality, *Image J Nurs Sch* 29(1):77, 1997.

Hover-Kramer D, Mentgen J, Scandrett-Hibdon S: *Healing touch: a resource for health care professionals,* Boston, 1996, Delmar.

Hybels S, Weaver R: *Communicating effectively,* ed 5, Boston, 1998, McGraw-Hill.

Jenner C: The art of nursing: a concept analysis, *Nurs Forum* 32(4):5, 1997.

Kacperek L: Non-verbal communication: the importance of listening, *Br J Nurs* 6(5), 1997.

Kim M, McFarland G, McLane A: *Pocket guide to nursing diagnoses,* ed 7, St. Louis, 1997, Mosby.

King I: *Toward a theory for nursing,* New York, 1971, John Wiley & Sons.

Knapp M, Vangelisti A: *Interpersonal communication and human relationships,* ed 3, Boston, 1996, Allyn & Bacon.

Lewis F, Zahlis E: The nurse as coach: a conceptual framework for clinical practice, *Oncol Nurs Forum* 24(10):1695, 1997.

Mallik M: Advocacy in nursing: perceptions of practicing nurses, *J Clin Nurs* 6(4):303, 1997.

Mandel E, Schulman M: Overcoming communication disorders in the elderly, *Patient Care* 31(2):55, 1997.

Paavilainen E, Astedt-Kurki P: The client-nurse relationship as experienced by public health nurses: toward better collaboration, *Public Health Nurs* 14(3):137, 1997.

Perry B: Influence of nurse gender on the use of silence, touch, and humor, *Int J Palliative Nurs* 2(1):7, 1996.

Robinson C: Health care relationships revisited, *J Fam Nurs* 2(2):152, 1996.

Routasalo P: Non-necessary touch in the nursing care of elderly people, *J Adv Nurs* 23(5):904, 1996.

Seed A: Crossing the boundaries: experiences of neophyte nurses, *J Adv Nurs* 21(6):1136, 1995.

Seigel B: *Peace, love and healing,* New York, 1989, Harper & Row.

Sellers S, Haag B: Spiritual nursing interventions, *J Holist Nurs* 16(3):338, 1998.

Stanhope M, Lancaster J: *Community health nursing: process and practice for promoting health,* ed 4, St. Louis, 1996, Mosby.

Stewart J, Logan C: *Together: communicating interpersonally,* ed 5, Boston, 1998, McGraw-Hill.

Stuart G, Sundeen S: *Principles and practice of psychiatric nursing,* ed 6, St. Louis, 1998, Mosby.

Sundeen S and others: *Nurse-client interaction: implementing the nursing process,* ed 6, St. Louis, 1998, Mosby.

Watson J: *Nursing: human science and health care,* Norwalk, Conn, 1985, Appleton-Century-Crofts.

Wong D: *Whaley and Wong's nursing care of infants and children,* ed 6, St. Louis, 1999, Mosby.

Wood J: *Gendered relationships,* Mountain View, Calif, 1996, Mayfield.

Wood J: *Interpersonal communication,* ed 2, Cincinnati, 1999, Wadsworth.

Wooten P: *Jest for the health of it!* making humor work, *J Nurs Jocularity* 3:(4)40, 1993.

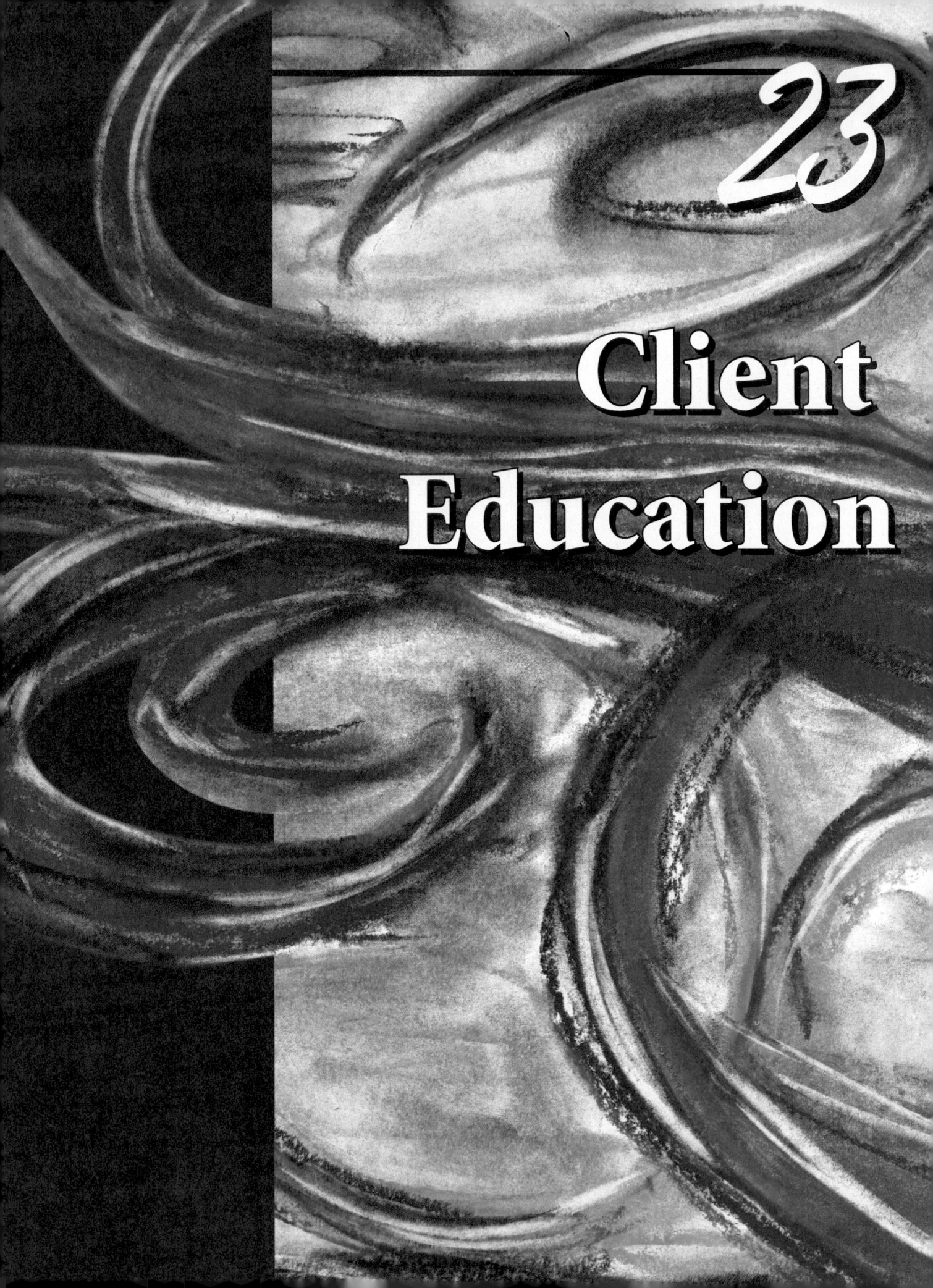

23

Client
Education

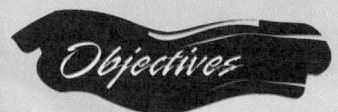

Objectives

Mastery of content in this chapter will enable the student to:

- Define the key terms listed.
- Identify appropriate topics for a client's health education needs.
- Describe the similarities and differences between teaching and learning.
- Identify the role of the nurse in client education.
- Identify the purposes of client education.
- Describe how to incorporate communication principles into client education.
- Describe the domains of learning.
- Identify basic learning principles.
- Differentiate factors that determine the readiness to learn from those that determine the ability to learn.
- Compare and contrast the nursing and teaching processes.
- Write learning objectives for a teaching plan.
- Describe characteristics of a good learning environment.
- Describe ways to incorporate teaching with routine nursing care.
- Identify methods for evaluating learning.
- Discuss guidelines for effective documentation of client education.

Client education has become one of the most important roles for nurses working in any health care setting. Teaching prenatal care to healthy mothers in a physician's office, instructing parents visiting a clinic about immunization of children, and teaching people who have had heart attacks about newly prescribed medications are all examples of client education. Clients and family members have the right to health education so that they are able to make intelligent, informed decisions about their health and lifestyle. Educating clients has become even more important for several reasons. For example, many clients now receive treatments in their homes or in an outpatient setting. In addition, hospitalized clients are being discharged earlier. All of these situations require the nurse to provide adequate education to ensure the achievement of client outcomes. Furthermore, effective health education is essential to care for increasing numbers of clients in the community and to minimize the effects of preventable diseases.

Shorter hospital stays, increased demands on nurses' time, and the need to give acutely ill clients concise, meaningful information as soon as possible emphasize the importance of quality client education (Babcock and Miller, 1994). As nurses try to find the best way to educate clients, the general public has become more assertive in seeking knowledge and understanding of their health and the resources available within the health care system. Providing clients with needed information about health care is necessary to ensure continuity of care from the hospital to the

home (Chachkes and Christ, 1996). A well-designed, comprehensive teaching plan that fits a client's learning needs can reduce health care costs, improve the quality of care, and help clients gain optimal wellness and increased independence.

The significance of client education is enhanced because of the client's right to know and to be informed about the diagnosis, prognosis, treatments, and risks. Educational materials provided should be readily understandable. It is negligent to assume that clients will learn on their own. Accurate, timely teaching is needed for clients to make decisions about their health and improve their overall health status. More attention is being paid in courts of law as to whether clients are adequately informed about ways to manage their health. Competent professional nursing practice includes client education. The nurse can provide effective education only by identifying clients' learning needs and by using the most appropriate teaching strategies.

Standards for Client Education

Client education has long been a standard for professional nursing practice. According to Virginia Henderson (1966), part of a nurse's role is to "improve the patient's level of understanding and therefore promote health." Various accrediting agencies set guidelines for providing client education in health care institutions. These guidelines ensure that the client and family receive information necessary to maintain the client's optimal level of health (Barnes, 1993). Health care institutions in the United States are ac-

The authors acknowledge the contribution of Mary Kay Knight Macheca to this chapter in the previous edition of this text.

Client Education Standards   Box 23-1

STANDARD 1

The client's learning needs, abilities, preferences, and readiness to learn are assessed.

The assessment considers cultural and religious practices, emotional barriers, desire and motivation to learn, physical and cognitive limitations, language barriers, and the financial implications of care choices.

When called for by the age of the client and the length of stay, the hospital assesses and provides for clients' academic education needs.

Clients are educated about the safe and effective use of medication, according to law and their needs.

Clients are educated about the safe and effective use of medical equipment.

Clients are educated about potential drug-food interactions and provided counseling on nutrition and modified diets.

Clients are educated about rehabilitation techniques to help them adapt or function more independently in their environment.

Clients are informed about access to additional resources in the community.

Clients are informed about when and how to obtain any further treatment the client may need.

The hospital makes clear to clients and families what their responsibilities are regarding the patient's ongoing health care needs and gives them the knowledge and skills they need to carry out their responsibilities.

With due regard for privacy, the hospital teaches and helps clients maintain good standards for personal hygiene and grooming, including bathing, brushing teeth, caring for hair and nails, and using the toilet.

STANDARD 2

Client education is interactive.

STANDARD 3

When the hospital gives discharge instructions to the client or family, it also provides these instructions to the organization or individual responsible for the client's continuing care.

STANDARD 4

The hospital plans, supports, and coordinates activities and resources for client and family education.

The hospital identifies and provides the educational resources required to achieve its educational objectives.

The client and family educational process is collaborative and interdisciplinary, as appropriate to the plan of care.

Modified from Joint Commission on Accreditation of Healthcare Organizations: *Accreditation manual of hospitals,* Chicago, 2000, The Commission.

credited by the Joint Commission on Accreditation of Healthcare Organizations (JCAHO). According to the JCAHO (2000), the goal of client and family education is to promote healthy behaviors and encourage the client's involvement both in the delivery of health care and in health care decisions, to improve outcomes. In 1994 client education became a separate chapter in the JCAHO standards manual, placing greater emphasis on the importance of client education and its interdisciplinary focus (Miller and Capps, 1997). Box 23-1 lists JCAHO's standards for client education. The successful accomplishment of these standards enhances client recovery and depends on participation of all health care professionals. Educational efforts must take into consideration the client's psychosocial, spiritual, and cultural values, as well as his or her desire to actively participate in the educational process (JCAHO, 2000). Evidence of successful client education must be documented in the client's medical record. Standards such as these help to direct nurses in client education.

Purposes of Client Education

The goal of educating others about their health is to assist individuals, families, or communities in achieving optimal levels of health (Edelman and Mandle, 1998). *Nursing's Agenda for Health Care Reform* by the American Nurses Association (ANA) (1991) recommends a restructuring of the health care system—focusing on wellness and care rather than illness and cure. The emphasis is on maintaining health. Clients now know more about health and want to be involved in health maintenance. Nurses need to provide education about health and health care in places that are convenient and familiar to clients (ANA, 1991). Comprehensive client education includes three important purposes, each involving a separate phase of health care (Box 23-2).

MAINTENANCE AND PROMOTION OF HEALTH AND ILLNESS PREVENTION

The public has recently become more health conscious. Participation in fitness clubs, diet programs, regular exercise activities, and health screening programs are examples of ways that people pay attention to their health.

The nurse is a visible, competent resource for clients intent on improving physical and psychological well-being. In the school, home, clinic, or workplace, the nurse provides information and skills that allow clients to assume healthier behaviors (see Box 23-2). For example, in childbearing classes, nurses teach expectant parents about physical and psychological changes in the woman and about fetal development. After learning about normal childbearing, the mother is more likely to eat healthy foods, engage in physical exercise, and avoid substances that might harm the fetus. Promoting healthy behavior through education increases self-esteem by allowing

Topics for Health Education   Box 23-2

HEALTH MAINTENANCE AND PROMOTION AND ILLNESS
PREVENTION
First aid
Avoidance of risk factors (e.g., smoking, alcohol)
Stress management
Growth and development
Hygiene
Immunizations
Prenatal care and normal childbearing
Nutrition
Exercise
Safety (in home and health care setting)
Screening (e.g., blood pressure, vision, cholesterol level)

RESTORATION OF HEALTH
Client's disease or condition
   Anatomy and physiology of body system affected
   Cause of disease
   Origin of symptoms
   Expected effects on other body systems
   Prognosis
   Limitations on function
   Rationale for treatment
   Medications
   Tests and therapies

Nursing measures
   Surgical intervention
Expected duration of care
Hospital or clinic environment
Hospital or clinic staff
Long-term care
Methods for client participation in care
Limitations posed by disease or surgery

COPING WITH IMPAIRED FUNCTIONS
Home care
   Medications
   Intravenous therapy
   Diet
   Activity
   Self-help devices
Rehabilitation of remaining function
   Physical therapy
   Occupational therapy
   Speech therapy
Prevention of complications
   Knowledge of risk factors
   Implications of noncompliance with therapy
   Environmental alterations

---

clients to assume more responsibility for their health.
Greater knowledge can result in better health maintenance
habits. When clients become more health conscious, they
are more likely to seek early diagnosis of health problems
(Redman, 1997).

RESTORATION OF HEALTH

Injured or ill clients need information and skills that will
help them regain or maintain their levels of health (see
Box 23-2). Clients recovering from illness or injury and
adapting to the resultant changes often seek information
about their conditions. However, clients who find it difficult to adapt to illness may become passive and uninterested in learning. The nurse learns to identify clients' willingness to learn and help motivate interest in learning.

   The family can be a vital part of a client's return to
health and may need to know as much as the client. If the
nurse excludes the family from a teaching plan, conflicts
may arise. For example, if the family does not understand
a client's need to regain independent function, their efforts may cause the client to become unnecessarily dependent and slow the client's recovery. The nurse should not
assume that the family should be involved and must first
assess the client-family relationship.

COPING WITH IMPAIRED FUNCTIONING

Not all clients fully recover from illness or injury. Many
must learn to cope with permanent health alterations.

New knowledge and skills are often necessary for clients to
continue activities of daily living (see Box 23-2). For example, a client whose ability to speak is lost after surgery
of the larynx must learn new ways of communicating. The
client with severe heart disease learns to modify risk factors that might cause further heart damage.

   In the case of serious disability, the client's family needs
to understand and accept these changes. The family's ability to provide support can result from education, which
begins as soon as the client's needs are identified and the
family displays a willingness to help. The nurse teaches
family members to assist the client with health care management (e.g., giving medications through gastric tubes
and doing passive range-of-motion exercises). Families of
clients with alterations such as alcoholism, mental retardation, or drug dependence also learn to adapt to the
emotional effects of these chronic conditions.

   A nurse learns to recognize the information to teach to
clients at different levels of wellness by assessing clients'
needs and abilities. Learning occurs when information is
practical and useful to the learner (Redman, 1997).
Comparing the desired level of health with the actual state
enables the nurse to plan effective teaching programs.

Teaching and Learning

It is impossible to separate teaching from learning.
Teaching is an interactive process that promotes learning.

It consists of a conscious, deliberate set of actions that help individuals gain new knowledge, change attitudes, adopt new behaviors, or perform new skills (Babcock and Miller, 1994; Redman, 1997). A teacher provides information that prompts the learner to engage in activities that lead to a desired change.

Learning is the purposeful acquisition of new knowledge, attitudes, behaviors, and skills (Babcock and Miller, 1994). Complex patterns are required if the client is to learn new skills or change existing attitudes (Redman, 1997). A new mother exhibits learning when she demonstrates to the nurse how to bathe her newborn. Learning is also demonstrated when a client preparing for abdominal surgery demonstrates deep breathing and coughing while splinting the abdomen with a pillow. Generally, teaching and learning begin when a person identifies a need for knowing or acquiring an ability to do something. Teaching is most effective when it responds to the learner's needs. The teacher assesses these needs by asking questions and determining the learner's interests. Interpersonal communication is essential for successful teaching to occur (see Chapter 22).

ROLE OF THE NURSE IN TEACHING AND LEARNING

Nurses have an ethical responsibility to teach their clients. In *A Patient's Bill of Rights,* the American Hospital Association (1992) indicates that clients have the right to make informed decisions about their care. The information required to make informed decisions must be presented clearly and be relevant and current. The nurse should anticipate clients' needs for information based on their physical condition or treatment plan. The nurse's responsibility is to teach the information that clients and their families need. The nurse often clarifies information provided by physicians and other health care providers and may become the primary source of information needed for adjusting to health problems.

Clients and their families often ask nurses for health information. For example, a client may request information about a new medication, or family members may question the reason for their mother's pain. The leader of a support group for teenage mothers may ask the nurse to explain the importance of healthy food choices for children. Identification of the need for teaching is easy when clients request information. Often, however, a client's need for teaching may be less obvious.

To be an effective educator, the nurse must do more than just pass on facts. The nurse must carefully determine what clients need to know and find the time when they are ready to learn. When nurses value client education and are able to implement it, clients are better prepared to assume health care responsibilities. The relationship between client education and favorable client outcomes is an important nursing research issue (Rankin and Stallings, 1996; Redman, 1997) (Box 23-3).

Research HIGHLIGHT   **Box 23-3**

RESEARCH ABSTRACT

The purpose of health education programs is to stimulate a change in behavior. However, studies about the effectiveness of different types of educational programs are varied. This study evaluated the effectiveness of a structured client-centered educational program. It was hypothesized that clients who received structured information would have better knowledge of risk factors associated with hypertension than those who received unstructured information while hospitalized. A sample of 40 clients with an average age of 67 (range 47 to 90) participated in the study. The sample was split into two equal groups. One group, the control group, received information routinely provided during the hospital stay. The other group, the experimental group, received information through a structured educational program. Both groups' knowledge of hypertension was measured within 24 hours of admission and then at 8 weeks and 1 year after discharge. Both groups had a poor understanding of hypertension on admission. At 8 weeks after discharge, knowledge of the control group did not improve, but the experimental group did demonstrate a significant improvement in knowledge that persisted 1 year after discharge.

IMPLICATIONS FOR PRACTICE

- Improvement in knowledge is enhanced by providing structured information.
- Structured educational programs improve client outcomes.
- Nurses should develop more structured client-centered educational programs.
- Nurses need to improve informal teaching interventions.

REFERENCE

Zernike W, Henderson A: Evaluating the effectiveness of two teaching strategies for patients diagnosed with hypertension, *J Clin Nurs* 7(1):37, 1998.

TEACHING AS COMMUNICATION

The teaching process closely parallels the communication process (see Chapter 22). Effective teaching depends in part on effective interpersonal communication. A teacher applies each element of the communication process while imparting information to learners. Thus the teacher and learner become involved together in a teaching process that increases the learner's knowledge and skills.

The steps of the teaching process can be compared with those of the communication process (Table 23-1). In teaching, the referent is the need to provide the client with information. The client may request information, or the nurse may perceive a need for information because of a client's health restrictions or the recent diagnosis of an illness. The nurse then identifies specific learning objectives. A **learning objective** describes what the learner will be able to do after successful instruction.

The nurse is the sender who wants to convey a message

Table 23-1 **Comparison of Terms Used in Teaching and Communication**	
Communication	Teaching
Referent Idea that initiates reason for communication	Perceived need to provide person with information; establishment of relevant learning objectives by teacher
Sender Person who conveys message to another	Teacher who performs activities aimed at helping other person to learn
Intrapersonal Variables (Sender) Knowledge, values, emotions, and sociocultural influences that affect sender's thoughts	Teacher's philosophy of education (based on learning theory); knowledge of teaching content; teaching approach; experiences in teaching; teacher's emotions and values
Message Information expressed or transmitted by sender	Content or information taught
Channels Methods used to transmit message (e.g., visual, auditory, touch)	Methods used to present content (e.g., visual and auditory materials, touch, taste, smell)
Receiver Person to whom message is transmitted	Learner
Intrapersonal Variables (Receiver) Knowledge, values, emotions, and sociocultural influences that affect receiver's thoughts	Willingness and ability to learn (e.g., physical and emotional health, education, experience, developmental level)
Feedback Information revealing that true meaning of message was received	Determination of whether learning objectives were achieved

to the client. The nurse promotes learning by communicating in a language recognizable to the learner. Many intrapersonal variables influence the nurse's style and approach. The nurse's attitudes, values, emotions, and knowledge influence the way the nurse delivers information. Past experiences with teaching are also helpful as the nurse chooses the best way to present the necessary content.

The message or content to be taught is delivered clearly and precisely. The nurse organizes information to be taught in a logical sequence so that the client will more easily understand skills or ideas. Each lesson progresses from the simple to the more complex skills or ideas (Babcock and Miller, 1994).

The nurse may use a variety of ways to present teaching content. All of the senses are channels for presenting information. The auditory channel is the simplest, as in a lecture or discussion. The learning process becomes more stimulating and effective, however, when several sensory channels are used together. For example, a client with newly diagnosed heart disease will learn how to measure a pulse best by actually feeling the pulsation of the radial artery.

The receiver in the teaching-learning process is the learner. A number of intrapersonal variables affect motivation and ability to learn. Clients are ready to learn when they express a desire to do so and are more likely to receive the message when they understand the content. Attitudes, anxiety, and values influence the ability to understand a message. The ability to learn depends on factors such as emotional and physical health, education, the stage of development, and previous knowledge.

An effective teacher provides a mechanism for evaluating the success of a teaching plan and providing feedback. Examples of ways to evaluate teaching sessions include having a client demonstrate a newly learned skill or asking the client to describe how the correct dosage schedule for a new medication will be incorporated into a daily routine. Feedback must show the success of the learner in achieving objectives; that is, the learner verbalizes information or provides a return demonstration of skills learned.

Domains of Learning

Learning occurs in three domains: cognitive (understanding), affective (attitudes), and psychomotor (motor skills)

(Bloom, 1956). Any topic to be learned may involve one or all domains or any combination of the three. The nurse often works with clients who need to learn in each domain. For example, clients diagnosed with diabetes must learn how diabetes affects the body and how to control blood glucose levels for healthier lifestyles (cognitive domain). In addition, clients must learn to accept the chronic nature of diabetes (affective domain). Finally, many clients living with diabetes must learn to test their blood glucose levels at home (psychomotor domain). The characteristics of learning within each domain affect the teaching and evaluation methods used. Understanding each learning domain prepares the nurse to select proper teaching techniques. However, the nurse needs to also be able to apply the basic principles of learning to any teaching method.

COGNITIVE LEARNING

Cognitive learning includes all intellectual behaviors and requires thinking (Babcock and Miller, 1994). Bloom (1956) classified cognitive behaviors in an ordered hierarchy. The simplest behavior is acquiring knowledge, whereas the most complex is evaluation.

Knowledge. Using knowledge is acquiring new facts or information and being able to recall them. For example, the client learns about a prescribed medication and is able to describe its purpose and potential side effects.

Comprehension. Comprehension is the ability to understand the meaning of learned material. For example, the client is able to explain specifically how a new medication will improve a physical condition.

Application. Application involves using abstract, newly learned ideas in a concrete situation. For example, the client develops a medication schedule according to normal mealtimes to ensure optimal desired effects of the medication.

Analysis. Analysis involves relating ideas in an organized way. It allows a person to distinguish important from unimportant information. For example, the client is able to distinguish which side effects are more likely to be experienced from a medication and to compare them with the effects experienced by another person.

Synthesis. Synthesis is the ability to recognize parts of information as a whole. For example, the client experiences side effects from a medication and is able to take preventive steps.

Evaluation. Evaluation is a judgment of the worth of a body of information for a given purpose. For example, the client is able to recognize the need for more information about a medication (e.g., insulin) to plan a safe exercise program.

AFFECTIVE LEARNING

Affective learning deals with expression of feelings and acceptance of attitudes, opinions, or values. Values clarification (see Chapter 20) is an example of affective learning. The simplest behavior in the hierarchy is receiving, and the most complex is characterizing (Krathwohl and others 1964).

Receiving. Receiving is being willing to attend to another person's words. For example, a woman shows a willingness to listen to a nurse explain the surgical procedure for removal of a breast by being attentive and maintaining eye contact while the nurse is talking.

Responding. Responding involves active participation through listening and reacting verbally and nonverbally. The person feels satisfied from the response. For example, the client asks the nurse about what the incision will look like after the surgery.

Valuing. Valuing means attaching worth to an object or behavior. This is shown through the learner's behavior. The person is motivated to act out the behavior. For example, the client who expresses concern about the appearance of a surgical incision before having a breast removed refuses to look at the incision and wears a gown with a high neck after the surgery.

Organizing. Organizing is developing a value system by identifying and organizing values and resolving conflicts. For example, the client learns to accept changes created by surgery and is willing to participate in social activities.

Characterizing. Characterizing involves acting and responding with a consistent value system. The person behaves consistently when values are tested or challenged. For example, the client assumes a normal lifestyle after having breast surgery and is able to discuss positive self-feelings with others.

PSYCHOMOTOR LEARNING

Psychomotor learning involves acquiring skills that require the integration of mental and muscular activity, such as the ability to walk or to use an eating utensil. The simplest behavior in the hierarchy is perception, whereas the most complex is origination (Redman, 1997; Rankin and Stallings, 1996).

Perception. Perception is being aware of objects or qualities through the use of sense organs. A person associates a sensory cue with the task to perform. For example, a new mother recognizes that different pitches of her newborn's cry indicate that the baby either needs to be fed or is tired.

Set. A set is a readiness to take a particular action. There are three sets: mental, physical, and emotional. For example, a person who has recently been injured in a motor vehicle accident uses judgment to determine the best way to arise from a wheelchair (mental readiness). Before getting out of the wheelchair, the person aligns and postures properly (physical readiness). The client makes a commitment (emotional set) to regularly perform strengthening exercises to facilitate recovery from the sustained injuries.

Guided Response.   A guided response is the performance of an act under the guidance of an instructor. This involves imitation of a demonstrated act. For example, a client prepares an insulin injection after watching a nurse's demonstration. The nurse provides immediate reinforcement after the client correctly performs the self-injection.

Mechanism.   A mechanism is a higher level of behavior whereby a person has gained confidence and skill in performing behavior. Usually the skill is more complex or involves several more steps than a guided response. For example, a client is able to fill the insulin syringe for different insulin doses.

Complex Overt Response.   A complex overt response involves performing a motor skill involving a complex movement pattern. The person performs the skill smoothly and accurately without hesitation. For example, a client who is recently paralyzed as a result of a spinal tumor is able to perform self-catheterization and does not acquire a urinary tract infection.

Adaptation.   Adaptation occurs when a person is able to change a motor response when unexpected problems arise. For example, a new mother who is breast-feeding and who is returning to work learns how to collect breast milk, store it, and coordinate pumping times with her baby's feeding demands and her work schedule.

Origination.   Origination is a highly complex motor act that involves creating new movement patterns. A person acts on the basis of existing psychomotor skills and abilities. For example, a client who has motor deficits from a cerebrovascular accident must learn to eat, dress, and walk while on a rehabilitation unit.

Basic Learning Principles

To teach effectively and efficiently, the nurse must first understand how people learn. Learning depends on the motivation to learn, the ability to learn, and the learning environment. Motivation addresses a person's desire to learn (Redman, 1997). The client's willingness to become involved in learning influences a nurse's teaching approach. Previous knowledge, attitudes, and sociocultural factors influence motivation.

The ability to learn depends on physical and cognitive attributes, developmental level, physical wellness, and intellectual thought processes. If a learning ability is impaired, such as with a client in pain, the nurse should postpone teaching activities or modify teaching strategies to better meet the needs of the learner.

The environment also affects the ability to learn. One of the nurse's major tasks is to manipulate environmental conditions to facilitate learning. For example, when the environment is noisy, the nurse modifies conditions, such as shutting the door or turning off the television, to enhance learning. This can be particularly challenging for a nurse in a busy health care setting.

MOTIVATION TO LEARN

Attentional Set.   An attentional set is the mental state that allows the learner to focus on and comprehend the material. People often use mental pictures to visualize ideas. While a nurse explains how to give support to a dying client, the family members might envision grasping the fragile hand of their dying family member. Before learning anything, clients must give attention to, or concentrate on, the information to be learned.

Physical discomfort, anxiety, and environmental distractions can influence the ability to attend. Any physical condition that impairs the ability to concentrate (e.g., pain, fatigue, anxiety, or hunger) interferes with learning. Therefore the nurse determines the client's level of comfort and energy before beginning a teaching plan and ensures that the client is comfortable enough for discussion. Nonverbal cues can also reveal that a client is not ready to learn.

Anxiety may increase or decrease the ability of a person to pay attention. Anxiety is uneasiness or uncertainty resulting from anticipating a threat or danger. When faced with change or the need to act differently, a person feels anxious. Learning requires a change in behavior and thus produces anxiety. A mild level of anxiety may motivate learning. However, a high level of anxiety prevents learning from occurring. It incapacitates a person, creating an inability to attend to anything other than to relieve the anxiety.

Environmental distractions interfere with the ability to attend to a teacher and to learning activities. Unplanned interruptions or an uncomfortable environment is not conducive to learning.

Motivation.   Motivation is a force that acts on or within a person (e.g., an idea, emotion, or a physical need) that causes the person to behave in a particular way (Redman, 1997). If a person does not want to learn, it is unlikely that learning will occur. Motivation may result from a social, task, or physical motive.

Social task mastery and physical motives stimulate a person to learn. Social motives are a need for connection, social approval, or self-esteem. People normally seek out others with whom they can compare opinions, abilities, and emotions. For example, new parents often seek validation of ideas and parenting techniques from others whom they have identified as role models in their social environment or health care workers with whom they have established a rapport.

Task mastery motives are based on needs such as achievement and competence. For example, a high school senior who has diabetes begins to test blood glucose levels and make decisions about insulin dosages in preparation for leaving home and establishing independence. The ability to successfully manage diabetes provides the motivation to master the task or skill. After a person succeeds at a task, the person is usually motivated to achieve more.

Often client motives are physical. A client with a physical change in function may be motivated to learn. Knowledge that is necessary for survival, problem recognition, and critical decision-making skills creates a stronger stimulus for learning than knowledge that merely promotes health (Babcock and Miller, 1994; Rankin and Stallings, 1996). Teaching strategies reflect the relative importance of each kind of physical motive.

Not all persons are interested in maintaining health. A client with lung disease may continue to smoke. An obese client may worsen a heart condition by refusing to follow a low-fat diet. No therapy will have an effect unless a person is motivated by the belief that health is important. The trend in health care is to treat clients in their homes after they recover from the acute phase of illness. Such treatment is successful only if clients follow the recommendations of the caregivers. **Compliance** is a client's adherence to the prescribed course of therapy. The nurse must assess the client's motivation to learn and what the client needs to know in order to adhere to the prescribed therapy. The nurse must also determine interventions that will stimulate learning and positive behavior changes.

Use of Theory to Enhance Motivation and Learning.
Health education often involves changing attitudes and values that are not altered by simple teaching of facts. Therefore nurses use various interventions, based on theory, when developing client education plans. The client's ideas, beliefs, and motivation must be assessed in order for learning to occur. For example, when a client is a busy executive with high blood pressure, the nurse can use the client's desire to succeed and the concern that illness will impair the ability to work as motivating factors.

Because of the complexity of the client education process, several theories and models have been used to guide the conceptual development of client education (Redman, 1997). Using a theory that matches the client's needs in practice helps the nurse provide effective client education. Social learning theory provides one of the most useful approaches to client education because it explains the characteristics of the learner and guides the educator in developing effective teaching interventions that result in enhanced learning and improved motivation (Rankin and Stallings, 1996; Bandura, 1997).

According to social learning theory, people continuously attempt to control events that affect their lives. This allows people to attain desired outcomes and avoid undesired outcomes, resulting in improved motivation. **Self-efficacy,** a concept included in social learning theory, refers to a person's perceived ability to successfully complete a task. When people believe that they can execute a particular behavior, they are more likely to actually perform the behavior consistently and correctly. Personal efficacy beliefs influence how much effort is expended in controlling a situation, how long people will try to overcome obstacles in the face of adversity, how people cope with demands, and the outcomes people attain (Bandura, 1997).

Self-efficacy beliefs arise from four sources: enactive mastery experiences, vicarious experiences, verbal persuasion, and physiological and affective states (Bandura, 1997). Enactive mastery experiences refer to the client's perceived ability to successfully complete a desired behavior. For example, the confidence of an older adult client learning to prepare low-fat meals is enhanced as the client successfully prepares meals that are low in fat and taste good. Actually performing a behavior provides the greatest source of efficacy beliefs.

Vicarious experiences are gained through modeling someone else's behavior. For example, the older adult client learning how to prepare low-fat meals models techniques learned from the nurse during the cooking class. This is especially important for those who are learning new skills or behaviors.

Verbal persuasion occurs when significant others express faith in one's capabilities. Providing verbal encouragement often improves a client's self-efficacy. For example, the nurse provides positive reinforcement as the client describes low-fat ingredients used when preparing meals.

Finally, physiological and affective states also affect self-efficacy. If a client perceives physiological and/or emotional improvement as a result of a desired behavior, perceived levels of self-efficacy will improve. For example, the client who believes that a diet low in fat will lead to a healthier life will be more likely to change behaviors than one who does not believe in the benefits of a low-fat diet.

Understanding the four sources of self-efficacy allows nurses to develop interventions that will improve clients' abilities to adopt healthy behaviors. For example, a nurse wishing to teach a child recently diagnosed with asthma to correctly use an inhaler expresses personal beliefs in the child's ability to use the inhaler (verbal persuasion). Then the nurse demonstrates how to use the inhaler (vicarious experience). Once the demonstration is complete, the child uses the inhaler (enactive mastery experience). As the child's wheezing and anxiety decrease after the correct use of the inhaler, the child experiences positive feedback, further enhancing the child's confidence to use the inhaler (physiological and affective states). Interventions such as these enhance perceived self-efficacy, which in turn improves the achievement of desired outcomes. As a result of the positive outcomes associated with self-efficacy, other health behavior theorists have included self-efficacy in their theories. For example, self-efficacy is incorporated into the health promotion model (Pender, 1996) and the health belief model (Rosenstock, Strecher, and Becker, 1988). Health behavior theories that do not include self-efficacy as a concept often have difficulty predicting the adoption of healthy behaviors (Bandura, 1997).

Psychosocial Adaptation to Illness. A temporary or permanent loss of health is difficult for clients to accept. The process of grieving gives clients time to adapt psychologically to the emotional and physical implications of illness. The stages of grieving (see Chapter 29) encompass a series of responses that clients experience during illness. People experience these stages at different rates and sequences, depending on their self-concept before illness, the severity of the illness, and the changes in lifestyle

that the illness creates. Effective, supportive care guides the client through the grieving process.

Readiness to learn is significantly related to the stage of grieving (Table 23-2). When they are unwilling or unable to accept the reality of illness, clients cannot learn. However, properly timed teaching can facilitate adjustment to illness or disability.

The nurse identifies the client's stage of grieving on the basis of typically displayed behaviors. When the client enters the stage of acceptance, the stage compatible with learning, the nurse introduces a teaching plan. Continuous assessment of the client's behaviors determines the stages of grieving. Teaching continues as long as the client remains in a stage conducive to learning.

Active Participation. Learning is facilitated when the client is actively involved in the educational session

Table 23-2   Relationship Between Psychosocial Adaptation to Illness and Learning

Stage	Client's Behavior	Learning Implications	Rationale
Denial or disbelief	Client avoids discussion of illness ("There's nothing wrong with me"), withdraws from others, and disregards physical restrictions. Client suppresses and distorts information that has not been presented clearly.	Provide support, empathy, and careful explanations of all procedures while they are being done. Let client know you are available for discussion. Explain situation to family or significant other if appropriate. Teach in present tense (e.g., explain current therapy).	Client is not prepared to deal with problem. Any attempt to convince or tell client about illness will result in further anger or withdrawal. Provide only information client pursues or absolutely requires.
Anger	Client blames and complains and often directs anger toward nurse or others.	Do not argue with client but listen to concerns. Teach in present tense. Reassure family/significant other of client's normalcy.	Client needs opportunity to express feelings and anger; client is still not prepared to face future.
Bargaining	Client offers to live better life in exchange for promise of better health ("If God lets me live, I promise to manage my disease better").	Continue to introduce only reality. Teaching only in present tense.	Client is still unwilling to accept limitations.
Resolution	Client begins to express emotions openly, realizes that illness has created changes, and begins to ask questions.	Encourage expression of feelings. Begin to share information needed for future, and set aside formal times for discussion.	Client begins to perceive need for assistance and is ready to accept responsibility for learning.
Acceptance	Client recognizes reality of condition, actively pursues information, and strives for independence.	Focus teaching on future skills and knowledge required. Continue to teach about present occurrences. Involve family/significant other in teaching information for discharge.	Client is more easily motivated to learn. Acceptance of illness reflects willingness to deal with its implications.

(Edelman and Mandle, 1998). A client's involvement in learning implies an eagerness to acquire knowledge or skills. It also improves the opportunity for the client to make decisions during teaching sessions. For example, to manage the disease, a client with a diagnosis of diabetes learns to change insulin dosages as a result of blood glucose levels taken at home. The nurse assists the client in choosing a blood glucose meter and creating a daily schedule that incorporates personal lifestyle patterns, as well as requirements for diabetes management (Figure 23-1).

ABILITY TO LEARN

Developmental Capability.
Cognitive development influences the client's ability to learn. A nurse can be a competent teacher, but if the client's intellectual abilities are not considered, teaching will be unsuccessful. Sometimes a nurse has shared teaching booklets and brochures and then discovered that the client cannot read. Learning, like developmental growth, is an evolving process. The nurse must know the client's level of knowledge and intellectual skills before beginning a teaching plan. For example, reading a thermometer or measuring liquid or solid food portions requires the ability to perform mathematical calculations. Reading a medication label or instructions in a teaching booklet requires reading and comprehension skills. Learning to regulate insulin dosages requires problem-solving skills. Following directions when performing self-care in accordance with limitations requires comprehension and application skills.

A requisite level of maturation and cognitive development must exist before an individual is capable of learning new information. It is wrong to assume that a client has a certain level of knowledge; instead, the nurse assesses the client's level of knowledge. Learning occurs more readily when new information complements existing knowledge.

Learning in Children.
The capability for learning and the type of learning behaviors that can be acquired depend on the child's maturation. Without proper biological, motor, language, and personal-social development, many types of learning cannot take place. However, learning can occur in children of all ages. Intellectual growth moves from the concrete to the abstract as the child matures. Therefore information presented to children must be understandable, and the expected outcomes must be realistic, based on the child's developmental stage (Table 23-3). Teaching aids that are developmentally appropriate should also be used (Figure 23-2). Learning occurs when behavior changes as a result of experience or growth (Wong, 1997).

Adult Learning.
Teaching adults differs from teaching children: Because adults become independent and self-directed as they mature, they are often able to identify their own learning needs. These learning needs arise out of problems or tasks that result from real-life situations. Although adults may tend to be self-directed learners, they may become dependent in new learning situations (Cravener, 1996). The amount of information that can be provided and learned and the amount of time that can be spent with the adult client varies depending on the client's personal situation and readiness to learn. An adult's readiness to learn is often associated with his or her developmental stage and what other events are occurring in his or her life (Merriam, 1996). Needs or issues that are perceived as extremely important to the adult must be resolved before learning can occur.

Adults have a wide variety of personal and life experiences to draw on. Therefore adult learning is enhanced when they are encouraged to use these experiences to solve problems (McKenna, 1995; Cravener, 1996; Merriam,

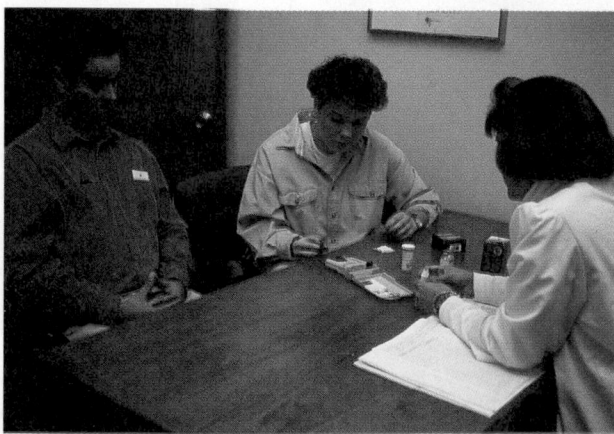

Figure 23-1 The nurse involves the client in choosing and learning to use a blood glucose meter.
Courtesy Steve Frazier, Barnes-Jewish Hospital, St. Louis, Mo.

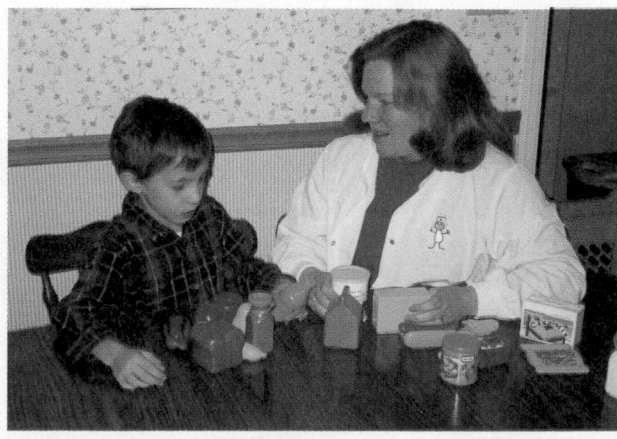

Figure 23-2 The nurse uses developmentally appropriate food models to teach healthy eating behaviors to the school-age child.

Table 23-3 Developmental Capacities for Learning

Learning Capacity	Teaching Methods
Infant	
Infant relies on parents for basic needs.	Keep routines (e.g., feeding, bathing) consistent.
Infant learns to trust adults when they convey love and compassion.	Hold infant firmly while smiling and speaking softly to convey sense of trust.
Infant explores environment through senses.	Have infant touch different textures (e.g., soft fabric, hard plastic).
Toddler	
Toddler learns to understand words and express feelings verbally.	Use play to teach procedure or activity (e.g., handling examination equipment, applying bandage to doll).
Toddler learns by associating words with objects.	Offer picture books that describe story of children in hospital or clinic.
Toddler likes to explore environment through play.	Use simple words such as *cut* instead of *laceration* to promote understanding.
Preschooler	
Vocabulary grows.	Use role playing, imitation, and play to make it fun for preschoolers to learn.
Preschooler uses language without comprehending meaning of words, especially concepts (e.g., right or left, time).	Encourage questions and offer explanations. Use simple explanations and demonstrations.
During play, child expresses feelings more through actions than words.	Encourage children to learn together through pictures and short stories of how to perform hygiene.
Preschooler asks questions and imitates adults.	
School Age Child	
Child interacts with adults and peers outside family.	Teach psychomotor skills needed to maintain health. (Complicated skills, such as learning to use a syringe, may take considerable practice.)
Child begins to acquire ability to relate series of events and actions to mental representations that can be expressed verbally and symbolically.	Offer opportunities to discuss health problems and answer questions.
Child is able to make judgments.	
Child matures physically.	
Play becomes more formal and imaginative.	
Child is inquisitive and asks many questions about health.	
Adolescent	
Adolescent struggles between childlike feelings of dependence and independence of adults.	Help adolescent learn about feelings and need for self-expression.
Teenager wants to be in control but, during illness, fears loss of self-concept or body image.	Allow adolescents to make decisions about health and health promotion (e.g., safety, sex education, substance abuse).
Adolescent is able to solve abstract problems.	Use problem solving to help adolescents make choices.
Teenager learns best when immediate benefit is gained.	
Young or Middle Adult	
Adult complies with health teaching because client fears the results.	Encourage participation by setting mutual goals.
Learning occurs when adult values information being taught.	Encourage independent learning.
	Offer information so that adult can understand effects of health problem.
Older Adult	
Often, there is decline in visual and auditory acuity, which impairs perception of stimuli.	Teach when client is alert and rested.
Sensory alterations, mobility limitations, and physical coordination problems affect capacity to learn.	Involve adult in discussion or activity.
Sleep-wake cycles are more fragmented.	Focus on wellness and the person's strength.
Older adult takes pride in being independent.	Use approaches that enhance sensorially impaired client's reception of stimuli (see Chapter 48).
There is no decline in intelligence with age.	Keep teaching sessions short.

1996). Furthermore, educational topics and goals need to be developed in collaboration with the adult client. Adult clients are ultimately responsible for changing their own behavior. Assessing what the adult client currently knows, teaching what the client wants to know, and setting mutual goals will improve the outcomes of client education (Fox, 1998).

Physical Capability.   The ability to learn often depends on the client's level of physical development and overall physical health. To learn psychomotor skills, a client must possess the necessary level of strength, coordination, and sensory acuity. For example, it is useless to teach a client to transfer from a bed to a wheelchair if the client has insufficient upper body strength. An older client with poor eyesight or the inability to grasp objects tightly cannot learn to apply an elastic bandage. Therefore the nurse should not overestimate the client's physical development or status. The following physical attributes are required to learn psychomotor skills:

Size (height and weight match the task to perform or the equipment to use [e.g., crutch walking])

Strength (ability of the client to follow a strenuous exercise program)

Coordination (dexterity needed for complicated motor skills, such as using utensils or changing a bandage)

Sensory acuity (visual, auditory, tactile, gustatory, and olfactory; sensory resources needed to receive and respond to messages taught)

Any condition (e.g., pain) that depletes a person's energy will also impair the ability to learn. A client who spends a morning undergoing rigorous diagnostic studies is unlikely to be capable of the effort needed for any learning discussion. When an illness becomes aggravated by complications, such as a high fever or respiratory difficulty, teaching should be postponed. After working with a client, the nurse assesses the client's energy level by noting the client's willingness to communicate, the amount of activity initiated, and the client's responsiveness toward questions. The nurse may halt teaching temporarily if the client needs rest. The nurse achieves greater teaching success when the client is an active participant in learning.

LEARNING ENVIRONMENT

Factors in the physical environment where teaching takes place make learning either a pleasant or a difficult experience. The nurse chooses a setting that helps the client focus on the learning task. The number of persons being taught, the need for privacy, the room temperature, the room lighting, noise, the room ventilation, and the room furniture are important factors when choosing the setting.

The ideal environment for learning is a room that is well lit and has good ventilation, appropriate furniture, and a comfortable temperature (Figure 23-3). A darkened room interferes with the client's ability to watch the

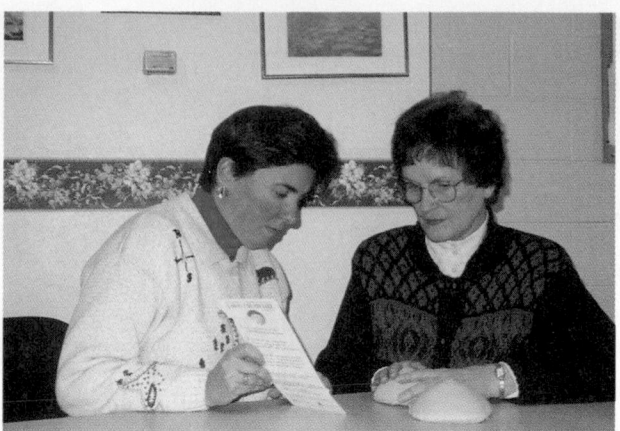

Figure 23-3 Choosing comfortable, pleasant environments enhances the learning experience. The nurse is explaining the breast self-examination procedure to the client.

nurse's actions, especially when demonstrating a skill or using visual aids such as posters or pamphlets. A room that is cold, hot, or stuffy will make the client too uncomfortable to attend to the nurse's activities. Comfortable furniture helps eliminate distractions, such as the need to change position or shift body weight.

It is also important to choose a quiet setting. A quiet setting offers privacy; infrequent interruptions are best. The nurse can provide privacy even in a busy hospital by closing cubicle curtains or taking the client to a quiet spot. In the home a bedroom might separate the client from household activities. If the client desires it, family members or significant others may share in discussions. However, a client may be reluctant to discuss the nature of the illness when others, even close family members, are in the room.

Teaching a group of clients requires a room that allows everyone to be seated comfortably and within hearing distance of the teacher. The size of the room should not overwhelm the group, tempting participants to sit outside the group along the room's perimeter. Arranging the group to allow participants to observe one another further enhances learning. More effective communication occurs as learners observe others' verbal and nonverbal interactions.

Integrating the Nursing and Teaching Processes

A relationship exists between the nursing and teaching processes. With the nursing process, a thorough assessment reveals the client's health care needs. The nursing diagnoses identified are individualized to the client's unique needs. A care plan is individualized, prescribing nursing therapies designed to improve or maintain the client's level of health. Evaluation determines the level of success in meeting goals of care.

While diagnosing a client's health care problems, the nurse may also identify the need for education. When education becomes a part of the care plan, the teaching process begins. Like the nursing process, the teaching process requires assessment, in this case, analyzing the client's needs, motivation, and ability to learn (Table 23-4). A diagnostic statement specifies the information or skills that the client requires. The nurse sets specific learning objectives and implements the teaching plan using teaching and learning principles to ensure that the client acquires knowledge and skills. Finally, the teaching process requires an evaluation of learning based on learning objectives.

The nursing and teaching processes are not the same. The nursing process requires assessment of all sources of data to determine a client's total health care needs. The teaching process focuses on the client's learning needs and willingness and capability to learn. Table 23-4 compares the teaching and nursing processes.

ASSESSMENT

Success in teaching a client requires the nurse to assess all factors influencing relevant content, the client's ability to learn, and the resources available for instruction. Learning needs, identified by both the client and the nurse, determine the choice of teaching content. An effective assessment is the basis on which instruction can be individualized to each client (Redman, 1997).

Expectations of Learning.   Clients have the ability to identify learning needs based on the implications of living with their illness. To meet these learning needs, the nurse assesses what clients view as important information to know. The nurse identifies what information clients perceive as necessary in many ways. For example, the nurse asks clients to identify perceived learning needs and their importance and listens to questions raised by the client or family about health issues. When a client feels a need to know something, the nurse recognizes that the client will likely be receptive to information presented.

Nurses also use assessment tools to determine the perceived learning needs of clients. For example, the "Everything You Ever Wanted to Know About Heart Disease" questionnaire asks clients to respond to how important it is to know about educational topics related to coronary artery disease, including anatomy and physiology of the heart, exercise, smoking, and dietary restrictions (Czar and Engler, 1997). After having clients respond to the questions on the tool, the nurse identifies the perceived learning needs of the clients and the perceived importance of each need. This assessment tool provides an efficient way for nurses to determine appropriate information to share with their clients.

Learning Needs.   In addition to the perceived learning needs of the client, the nurse also determines the information that is critical for the client to learn. Learning needs change depending on the client's current health sta-

Table 23-4 **Comparison of the Nursing and Teaching Processes**		
Basic Steps	**Nursing Process**	**Teaching Process**
Assessment	Collect data about client's physical, psychological, social, cultural, developmental, and spiritual needs from client, family, diagnostic tests, medical record, nursing history, and literature.	Gather data about client's learning needs, motivation, ability to learn, and teaching resources from client, family, learning environment, medical record, nursing history, and literature.
Nursing diagnosis	Identify appropriate nursing diagnoses based on assessment findings.	Identify client's learning needs on basis of three domains of learning.
Planning	Develop individualized care plan. Set diagnosis priorities based on client's immediate needs. Collaborate with client on care plan.	Establish learning objectives, stated in behavioral terms. Identify priorities regarding learning needs. Collaborate with client on teaching plan. Identify type of teaching method to use.
Implementation	Perform nursing care therapies. Include client as active participant in care. Involve family/significant other in care as appropriate.	Implement teaching methods. Actively involve client in learning activities. Include family/significant other participation as appropriate.
Evaluation	Identify success in meeting desired outcomes and goals of nursing care. Alter interventions as indicated when goals are not met.	Determine outcomes of teaching-learning process. Measure client's ability to achieve learning objectives. Reinforce information as needed.

tus. Because a client's health status is dynamic, assessment is an ongoing activity. The nurse assesses the following:

Client's level of understanding of current health status, implications of illness, types of therapy, and prognosis. This information helps to determine a client's perception of the threat of illness and its effect on lifestyle.

Information or skills needed by the client to perform self-care and to understand the implications of a health problem. Health care team members anticipate learning needs related to specific health problems. For example, the nurse anticipates a client's need to learn the physical restrictions imposed by major surgery before the procedure, or the nurse teaches a boy who has just entered high school to perform testicular self-examination.

Client's experiences that influence the need to learn. For example, a woman who is pregnant for the third time is more likely to be familiar with the implications of pregnancy than a woman who is pregnant for the first time.

Information that family members or significant others require to support the client's needs. The amount of information needed depends on the extent of the family's role in helping the client.

Motivation to Learn.
The nurse asks questions that define the client's motivation. These questions help to determine whether the client is prepared and willing to learn. Although a client may have a variety of learning needs, a lack of motivation seriously threatens the success of the teaching plan. The nurse assesses the following motivational factors:

Client's behavior (e.g., attention span, tendency to ask questions, memory, and ability to concentrate during the teaching session).

Client's health beliefs and perception of the severity and susceptibility of a health problem, and the benefits and barriers to treatment.

Client's perceived ability to complete a required health behavior.

Client's desire to learn.

Client's attitudes about health care providers (e.g., role of client and nurse in making decisions). Mutually set goals are more likely to be achieved by the client.

Client's knowledge of information to be learned. The client must play an active role in seeking health-based information.

Pain, fatigue, anxiety, or other physical symptoms that can interfere with the ability to maintain attention and participate. In acute care settings a client's physical condition can easily detract from learning.

Client's sociocultural background. A client's beliefs and values about health and various therapies may be influenced by sociocultural norms or tradition (see Chapter 7).

Client's learning style preference. When various options are available for learning (e.g., brochures, videotape, and discussion), a client may perceive one approach as being more interesting. For example, TenHave and others (1997) found that people receiving cardiovascular nutrition education who had less than an eighth-grade reading level preferred audiotapes over printed instructions.

Ability to Learn.
The nurse determines the client's physical and cognitive levels. Health care providers often underestimate the client's cognitive deficits. Many factors can impair the ability to learn, including body temperature, electrolyte levels, oxygenation status, and blood glucose level. In any health care setting, several of these factors may influence a client at one time. The nurse assesses the following factors related to the ability to learn:

Physical strength, movement, and coordination. The nurse determines the extent to which the client can perform skills.

Sensory deficits (see Chapter 48) that may affect the client's ability to understand or follow instruction.

Client's reading level. This can be difficult to assess because a functionally illiterate client is often able to conceal it by using excuses such as not having the time or not being able to see. To assess the client's reading level and level of understanding, the nurse asks a client to read instructions from a teaching brochure and then explain its meaning.

Client's developmental level. This influences the approaches chosen by the nurse during teaching (see Table 23-3).

Client's cognitive function, including memory, knowledge, association, and judgment.

Teaching Environment.
The environment for a teaching session must be conducive to learning. The nurse assesses the following factors when seeking a place to teach clients:

Distractions or persistent noise. A quiet area should be set aside for teaching.

Comfort of the room, including ventilation, temperature, lighting, and furniture.

Room facilities and available equipment.

Resources for Learning.
A client may require the support of family members or significant others. In this case the nurse assesses the readiness and ability of family and friends to learn the information necessary for the care of the client. The nurse needs to understand the home environment. Assessment of resources also includes a review of any teaching tools available. The nurse assesses the following resources for learning:

Family members' perceptions and understanding of the client's illness and its implications. Family members' perceptions should match those of the client; otherwise, conflicts may arise in the teaching plan.

Client's willingness to have family members and significant others involved in the teaching plan and to provide health care. Information about the client's health care is confidential unless the client chooses to share it. Sometimes it is difficult for the client to accept the help of family members, especially when bodily functions are involved.

Family's or significant other's willingness to participate in care. If the client chooses to share information regarding his or her health status with family members, the family members must be assessed for their abilities and willingness to participate in care of the client. Not all family members may be responsible, willing, or able to assist in care.

Resources within the home. These include persons willing to assist the client with procedures, such as bathing or taking medications; financial or material resources, such as obtaining health care equipment; and architectural resources, such as arrangement of rooms or stairways.

Teaching tools, including brochures, audiovisual materials, or posters. Printed material should present current information that is written clearly and logically and that matches the client's reading level. Currently, printed educational materials often surpass clients' reading levels (Bauman, 1997; Mumford, 1997).

NURSING DIAGNOSIS

After assessing information related to the client's ability and need to learn, the nurse interprets data and clusters defining characteristics to form diagnoses that reflect the client's specific learning needs (Box 23-4). This ensures that teaching will be goal directed and individualized. If a client has several learning needs, nursing diagnoses allow for priority setting (Box 23-5).

Several nursing diagnoses apply to learning needs. Each diagnostic statement describes the specific type of learning need and its cause. Classifying diagnoses by the three learning domains helps the nurse to focus specifically on subject matter and teaching methods.

Some health care problems can be managed or eliminated through education. In these situations, the related factor of the diagnostic statement is *knowledge deficit*. For example, an older adult client may have difficulty managing a medication regimen because of the number of medications that must be taken at different times of the day. In this case educating the client about the medications may improve the client's ability to schedule and take the medications as directed.

Some nursing diagnoses also indicate that teaching may be inappropriate. The nurse may identify conditions that cause barriers to effective learning (e.g., nursing diagnosis of *pain* or *activity intolerance*). In these cases the nurse delays teaching until the nursing diagnosis is resolved or the health problem is controlled.

PLANNING

After determining the nursing diagnoses that identify a client's learning needs, the nurse develops a teaching plan, determines goals and expected outcomes, and in-

SAMPLE NURSING DIAGNOSTIC PROCESS   Box 23-4

LEARNING NEEDS

Assessment Activities	Defining Characteristics	Nursing Diagnosis
Have client describe what has been explained about planned surgery.	States cannot remember what physician said at office visit Provides inaccurate description of purpose and implications of surgery	Knowledge deficit (cognitive) regarding impending surgery related to lack of exposure and recall and misinterpretation of information
Observe verbal and nonverbal response to discussion.	Asks many questions about surgical process and what to expect Exhibits anxiety (talks fast, does not maintain eye contact)	
Review medical record for past history of surgery.	Has not had any surgery in the past	
Have client describe how to walk with crutches.	States has not received information about use of crutches Asks questions about how to use crutches	Knowledge deficit (psychomotor) regarding use of crutches related to lack of exposure
Have client demonstrate three-point crutch walking on level surfaces and up stairs.	Uses crutches inappropriately Cannot go up or down stairs on crutches	

volves the client in selecting learning experiences (see care plan). Expected outcomes (or learning objectives) guide the choice of teaching strategies and approaches with a client. Client participation ensures a more relevant, meaningful plan.

Developing Learning Objectives. The first step in forming a teaching plan is developing learning objectives. A learning objective identifies the expected outcome of a planned learning experience and helps establish priorities for learning. Despite all planning, a particular instructional session often leads to unanticipated learning. It may be difficult to anticipate all objectives for a teaching session. However, objectives cause a teacher to plan teaching sessions so that time is maximized and the best resources are available for learning. Objectives are either short term or long term. Short-term objectives relate to the client's immediate learning needs, such as knowing the nature of gallbladder disease to understand an upcoming test. Long-term objectives relate to acquisition of the knowledge and skills that are needed to permanently adapt to a health problem (e.g., learning to plan a diet within restrictions caused by ulcerative colitis). Like a goal of care, a long-term objective is usually all-encompassing. Short-term objectives can be compared with outcomes of care.

The objectives established by the nurse and client guide the teaching plan. Poorly determined objectives can create confusion throughout the teaching-learning process. Thus a learning objective includes the same criteria as outcomes in a nursing care plan (see Chapter 16), including the following:

Singular behaviors
Observable or measurable content
Timing or conditions under which the objective is measured
Goals mutually set between the nurse and client

Each objective is a statement of a singular behavior that identifies the learner's ability to do something after a learning experience. A behavioral objective contains an active verb, describing what the learner will do after the objective is met, such as *will empty* colostomy bag, *will administer* an injection, or *will verbalize* drug dosages. The verb should have few interpretations (e.g., verbalize, demonstrate, identify, describe, label, classify, or select) and be stated in terms of how the client is to demonstrate learning, rather than what or how the teacher is to teach (Redman, 1997). Singular behaviors are easier to evaluate at the end of instruction.

Behavioral objectives are measurable and observable and indicate how learning will be evidenced (e.g., "will perform *three-point crutch gait*" or "will prepare *foods without using salt*"). The objective describes precise behaviors and content. An example of a vague or nonspecific objective might be "will be familiar with chronic renal failure." This example does not explain what the learner is to do, and it raises questions about how the behavior can be measured. If content is missing, the objective cannot guide teaching and learning. The precise behaviors and content set the standard for feedback that reflects learning and forms the basis for evaluation of the teaching plan.

An objective is more precise when it describes the conditions or timing under which the behavior occurs. Conditions or time frames should be realistic and designed for the learner's needs (e.g., "will identify the side effects of aspirin by discharge"). It also helps to consider conditions under which the client or family will typically perform the learning behavior (e.g., "will walk from bedroom to bathroom using crutches"). The criteria for acceptable performance set a standard by which achievement of objectives is measured. A teacher sets criteria on the basis of a desired level of accuracy, success, or satisfaction. For example, a client undergoing therapy for a fractured leg will walk on crutches *to the end of the hall within 3 days*. Criteria are more acceptable when they are mutually established by the teacher and learner. However, the nurse serves as a resource in setting the minimum criteria for success. Criteria on which the client and nurse agree help define the expected behaviors and the quality of performance. The client also uses these criteria for self-evaluation, which is a powerful motivator of behavior.

After formulating objectives, the nurse and client work to establish a teaching plan. During planning, the nurse integrates basic teaching principles and develops a well-timed, organized teaching plan.

Integrating Basic Teaching Principles. Teaching priorities should reflect the priorities of the nursing diagnoses. When developing a teaching plan, the nurse considers the principles that improve its effectiveness. The realm of teaching deals with teachers' behavior, the reason teachers behave the way they do, and effects of their behavior on learners. There is no single correct way to teach, since each learning situation determines the best way to teach. The principles of teaching are, in effect, techniques that incorporate the principles of learning.

Setting Priorities. Priorities for teaching are based on the client's immediate needs, nursing diagnoses, and the

SAMPLE NURSING CARE PLAN

CLIENT EDUCATION

ASSESSMENT*

As Nancy is preparing Mr. Holland for his colon resection, which is scheduled in 1 week, she begins to assess his knowledge of the surgery, why he is having it, and what he can expect postoperatively. Mr. Holland's medical record reflects that he spoke with his physician and scheduled the surgery 2 weeks ago. Mr. Holland reports that he has had Crohn disease for 15 years. Although he has a good understanding of his illness and states why he must have the surgery, **he cannot remember all that the physician told him about his surgery.** He is **extremely anxious, gets teary eyed, and verbalizes many questions** about what will happen to him after the surgery. He is **unable to verbalize** how to cough and deep breathe or the importance of activity postoperatively.

*Defining characteristics are shown in bold type.

NURSING DIAGNOSIS:
Knowledge deficit (cognitive) regarding implications of surgery and postoperative care related to lack of recall and exposure to information.

PLANNING

GOALS

Client will describe preoperative care by 12/10.

Client will participate in preoperative and postoperative surgical care procedures during hospitalization.

EXPECTED OUTCOMES

Client will verbalize preoperative care planned for the day before surgery by 12/10, including expected laboratory tests, visit by surgeon and anesthesiologist, time of surgery, and how his significant others will be notified of his progress through surgery.

Client will demonstrate deep breathing and range-of-motion exercises by 12/10.

Client will verbalize what to expect during the postoperative period, including pain management, purpose of nasogastric (NG) tube, progression of diet, and related rationale by 12/10.

INTERVENTIONS†

Learning Readiness Enhancement

- Determine readiness to learn and learning needs.
- Describe anticipated preoperative routine, including what laboratory tests will be drawn, who will speak with him before surgery, when the surgery is scheduled to occur, how his family will be notified during surgery, anticipated bowel preparation, and the need to be NPO after midnight.

Learning Facilitation

- Give client brochure on preoperative care during educational session.

- Explain, demonstrate, and have client perform return demonstration of coughing and deep breathing, and range-of-motion exercises.
- Describe anticipated postoperative care with rationale, including pain management, use of nasogastric (NG) tube, and progression of diet. Allow client to see and touch NG tube and patient-controlled analgesia pump.

- Make follow-up phone call 48 hours before surgery to answer questions and reinforce information.

RATIONALE

Client must demonstrate readiness to learn, and information presented must be perceived as important, for the adult to learn effectively (Fox, 1998).

Explaining to clients what to expect before surgery can reduce anxiety, enhance coping, and improve outcomes (Redman, 1997).

Early timing and reinforcement of preoperative teaching may improve knowledge of surgery routines, facilitate return to preoperative activity levels, and enhance client satisfaction (Lookinland and Pool, 1998).

Improving self-efficacy by using role modeling and having the client perform behaviors enhances healthy behaviors (Bandura, 1997).

Providing structured education about postoperative procedures and allowing clients to see and touch equipment before surgery enhances learning and decreases anxiety. Understanding the importance of care helps enhance compliance with postoperative routine (Redman, 1997).

Repetition and learning information over time will enhance the client's understanding of information (Redman, 1997).

†Intervention Classification labels from McCloskey JC, Bulechek GM: *Nursing interventions classification (NIC)*, ed 3, St. Louis, 2000, Mosby.

EVALUATION

Have client describe what to expect before and after surgery.

Observe client as he demonstrates coughing and deep breathing, and range-of-motion exercises.

Assess level of pain and progression of activity level and diet postoperatively.

Observe client's verbal and nonverbal behavior before and after surgery.

learning objectives established for the client. Priorities also depend on what the client perceives to be most important, the client's anxiety level, and the amount of time available to teach. A client's learning needs must be set in order of priority to conserve the time and energy of the client and nurse. For example, a client recently diagnosed with coronary artery disease has a knowledge deficit related to the new illness and its implications. The client will benefit most by first learning about the correct way to take nitroglycerin and how long to wait before calling for help when chest pain occurs. Once these needs related to basic survival are met, then other topics, such as exercise and nutritional changes, can be discussed.

Timing.   When is the right time to teach? Before a client enters a hospital? When a client first enters a clinic? At discharge? At home? Each may be appropriate because clients continue to have learning needs and opportunities as long as they stay in the health care system. The nurse should plan teaching activities for a time when the client is most attentive, receptive, and alert. The client's activities should be organized to provide time for rest and teaching-learning interactions.

Timing can be difficult because emphasis is placed on a client's early discharge from a hospital. For example, it may take several days after surgery for a client to become free of discomfort so that attention can be given to learning. By the time the client feels ready to learn, discharge may already be scheduled. Therefore nurses need to anticipate educational needs of clients before they occur. For example, the nurse educates a pregnant woman about care of the newborn 1 month before the expected delivery date, or a client scheduled to have a hip replacement receives information about what to expect during and after the surgery the week before admission. Anticipating a client's educational needs can improve the client's outcomes. Lookinland and Pool (1998) discovered that women scheduled for open abdominal surgery who received structured education before admission to the hospital were discharged sooner, experienced better functional status, and were more satisfied with their care when compared with women who received unstructured information after admission.

The duration of teaching sessions also influences learning ability. Prolonged sessions cause concentration and attentiveness to decrease. Frequent sessions lasting 20 minutes are more easily tolerated and retain the client's interest in the material. However, factors such as shorter hospital stays and lack of insurance reimbursement for outpatient education sessions may necessitate longer teaching sessions. The nurse assesses a client's loss of concentration by observing for nonverbal cues, such as poor eye contact or slumped posture. After loss of concentration is noted, the session should be stopped. However, teaching sessions should not be too brief. The client needs time to comprehend the information and to give feedback.

Teaching sessions should be held frequently enough to document the client's learning. The frequency of sessions depends on the learner's abilities and the complexity of the material. For example, a child newly diagnosed with diabetes will require more visits to an outpatient center than the elderly client who has had diabetes for 15 years and who lives in a nursing home. Intervals between teaching sessions should not be so long that the client might forget information. For a client discharged from a hospital, home health nurses must reinforce learning.

Organizing Teaching Material.   A good teacher gives careful consideration to the order of information presented. An outline of content helps organize information into a logical sequence. Material should progress from simple to complex ideas because a person must learn the simple facts and concepts before learning how to make associations or complex interpretations of ideas. For example, to teach a woman how to feed her husband who has a gastric tube, the nurse first teaches the wife how to measure the tube feeding and how to manipulate the equipment. Once this is accomplished, the process of administering the feeding occurs.

The nurse begins any instruction with essential content. Clients are more likely to remember information that is taught in the beginning of a teaching session. For example, after surgical removal and postsurgical treatment of a malignant breast tumor, the chance for cancer recurrence makes learning the signs of metastasized breast cancer crucial. The nurse starts with essential information and then completes a teaching session with informative but less critical content. Key points should be summarized. Repetition also reinforces learning. A concise summary of key topics helps the learner remember the most important information (Murphy and Davis, 1997).

Maintaining Learning Attention and Participation. Active participation is key to learning. Persons learn better when more than one of the body's senses are stimulated. Audiovisual aids and role playing are good teaching strategies. By actively experiencing a learning event, the person will be more likely to retain the knowledge gained.

A teacher's actions can also increase learner attention and interest. When conducting a discussion with a learner, the teacher should stay active by changing the tone and intensity of his or her voice, making eye contact, and using gestures that accentuate key points of discussion. An effective teacher often uses as much energy as the learner, talking and moving among a group rather than remaining stationary behind a lectern or table. A learner remains interested in a teacher who is actively enthusiastic about the subject under discussion.

Building on Existing Knowledge.   A client learns best on the basis of preexisting cognitive abilities and knowledge. Thus a teacher is more effective by presenting information that builds on a learner's existing knowledge. A client quickly loses interest if a nurse begins with familiar information. For example, a client who has lived with multiple sclerosis for several years must begin a new medication that is given subcutaneously. Before teaching the client how to prepare the medication and give the injection, the nurse asks the client about previous experience with injections. On assessment, the nurse learns that the client's father had diabetes and that the client administered the insulin injections. The nurse individualizes the teaching plan for this client by building on the client's previous knowledge and experience with insulin injections.

Selection of Teaching Methods. During planning the nurse chooses appropriate teaching methods and encourages the client to offer suggestions. A teaching method is the way that the teacher delivers information and is based on the client's learning needs (Box 23-6). For example, a client with a psychomotor deficit learns best through demonstrations and supervised practice. The client masters skills by manipulating equipment and practicing manual skills. Discussions, question-and-answer sessions, and formal lectures are effective methods for promoting cognitive learning. Clients with intellectual deficits are given the opportunity to explore new ideas, recognize new relationships, and apply knowledge to their

unique needs. A highly effective method for stimulating affective learning is group discussion. More than one method may be used for instruction.

Availability of Teaching Resources. The nurse is the primary member of the health care team responsible for ensuring that all client educational needs are met. However, sometimes client needs are highly complex. In these cases the nurse identifies appropriate health education resources within the health care system or the community during the planning stage. Resources for client education include diabetes education clinics, cardiac rehabilitation programs, prenatal classes, and support groups. When clients receive education and support from these types of resources, the nurse is responsible for obtaining a referral if necessary, encouraging clients to attend these resources, and reinforcing information taught. Resources that specialize in a particular health need are integral to successful client education.

Writing Teaching Plans. In all health care settings, nurses develop written teaching plans for use by colleagues. When one nurse, such as a primary nurse, is responsible for developing the initial teaching plan, all information about the client is incorporated appropriately. The teaching plan includes topics for instruction, re-

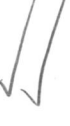

Appropriate Teaching Methods Based on Client's Learning Needs   Box 23-6

COGNITIVE

Discussion (one-on-one or group)
  May involve nurse and one client or nurse with several clients
  Promotes active participation and focuses on topics of interest to client
  Allows peer support
  Enhances application and analysis of new information
Lecture
  Is more formal method of instruction because it is controlled by teacher
  Helps learner acquire new knowledge and gain comprehension
Question-and-answer session
  Designed specifically to address client's concerns
  Assists client in applying knowledge
Role play, discovery
  Allows client to actively apply knowledge in controlled situation
  Promotes synthesis of information and problem solving
Independent project (computer-assisted instruction), field experience
  Allows client to assume responsibility for completing learning activities at own pace
  Promotes analysis, synthesis, and evaluation of new information and skills

AFFECTIVE

Role play
  Allows expression of values, feelings, and attitudes
Discussion (group)
  Allows client to acquire support from others in group
  Permits client to learn from others' experiences
  Promotes responding, valuing, and organization
Discussion (one-on-one)
  Allows discussion of personal, sensitive topics of interest or concern

PSYCHOMOTOR

Demonstration
  Provides presentation of procedures or skills by nurse
  Permits client to incorporate modeling of nurse's behavior
  Allows nurse to control questioning during demonstration
Practice
  Gives client opportunity to perform skills using equipment in a controlled setting
  Provides repetition
Return demonstration
  Permits client to perform skill as nurse observes
  Provides excellent source of feedback and reinforcement
Independent projects, games
  Require teaching method that promotes adaptation and origination of psychomotor learning
  Permit learner to use new skills

sources (e.g., equipment, teaching booklets, referrals to special educational programs), recommendations for involving family, and objectives of the teaching plan. A plan may be lengthy or in outline form.

The setting influences the complexity of any teaching plan. In an acute care setting, plans are concise and focused on the primary learning needs of the client because there is limited time for teaching. A home health care teaching plan or outpatient clinic plan may be more comprehensive in scope because nurses often have more time to instruct clients and clients are often less anxious in outpatient settings.

A plan should provide continuity of instruction, particularly when several nurses are involved in caring for the client. The more specific the plan, the easier it is for nurses to follow through. To enhance communication among nurses and to avoid duplication, the nurse should know the point at which the last teaching session ended.

IMPLEMENTATION

The successful implementation of a teaching plan is dependent on the nurse's ability to critically analyze assessment data when identifying learning needs and developing the teaching plan. The nurse carefully evaluates the learning objectives and determines which teaching and learning principles will most effectively and efficiently assist the client in meeting expected goals and outcomes. Implementation involves believing that each interaction with a client is an opportunity to teach. The nurse maximizes opportunities for effective learning and uses a diversified approach to create an active learning environment.

Teaching Approaches.   A nurse's approach in teaching is different from teaching methods. Some situations require a teacher to be directive. Others may require a nondirective approach. An effective teacher concentrates on the task and uses teaching approaches according to the learner's needs. A learner's needs and motives can change over time. Thus the teacher must always be aware of the need to modify teaching approaches.

Telling.   The telling approach is useful when limited information must be taught (e.g., preparing a client for an emergent diagnostic procedure). If a client is highly anxious but it is vital for information to be given, telling can be effective. When using telling, the nurse outlines the task to be done by the client and gives explicit instructions. There is no opportunity for feedback with this method.

Selling.   The selling approach uses two-way communication. The nurse paces instruction based on the client's response. Specific feedback is given to the client who shows success in learning. For example, the client learns a step-by-step procedure for changing a dressing. The nurse

uses information from the client to adapt the teaching approach.

Participating.   The participating approach involves the nurse and client setting objectives and participating in the learning process together. The client helps decide content, and the nurse guides and counsels the client with pertinent information. In this method, there is opportunity for discussion, feedback, mutual goal setting, and revision of the teaching plan. For example, a parent caring for a child with leukemia and receiving chemotherapy must learn how to care for the child at home and how to recognize problems that need to be reported immediately. The parent and the nurse collaborate on developing an appropriate teaching plan that will facilitate the parent's learning and the child's discharge from the hospital. After each teaching session is completed, the parent and nurse review the objectives together, determine if the objectives were met, and plan what will be covered in the next session.

Entrusting.   The entrusting approach provides the client the opportunity to manage self-care. Responsibilities are accepted, and tasks are performed correctly and consistently by the client. The nurse observes the client's progress and remains available to assist without introducing more new information. For example, a client has been managing diabetes well for 10 years. Because of the development of a complication of diabetes, the client must now walk instead of jog during exercise. The client understands how to adjust insulin when exercising to prevent hypoglycemia. The nurse instructs the client about the newly prescribed exercise therapy and allows the client to adjust insulin dosages independently.

Reinforcing.   The principle of reinforcement applies to the process of learning; however, the teacher must often be the source of reinforcement. **Reinforcement** is using a stimulus that increases the probability for a response. A learner who receives reinforcement before or after a desired learning behavior is likely to repeat the behavior. Feedback is a common form of reinforcement.

Reinforcers are positive or negative. Positive reinforcement, such as a smile or spoken approval, produces desired responses. Although negative reinforcement, such as frowning, complaining, or criticizing, can decrease an undesired response, people usually respond better to positive reinforcement (Babcock and Miller, 1994). The effects of negative reinforcement are less predictable and often undesirable.

Three types of reinforcers are social, material, and activity. When a nurse works with a client, most reinforcers are social ones (e.g., smiles, compliments, words of encouragement, or physical contact), which are used to acknowledge a learned behavior. Examples of material reinforcers are food, toys, and music. These work best with young children. Activity reinforcers rely on the principle that a person is motivated to engage in an activity if he or she is promised that after its completion the opportunity to engage in more desirable activity will be available. For example, a client will more likely go to a mental health counseling session if he or she is given the chance to go outside for a walk with the nurse afterward.

Choosing an appropriate reinforcer involves giving careful thought and attention to individual preferences. Observing behavior often helps reveal the best reinforcer to use. Reinforcers should never be used as threats and are not always effective with every client. A young child responds more to social reinforcers than do older children or adults. An adult with whom the nurse has a good relationship is more effectively reinforced than an adult with whom the nurse has a poor relationship.

Incorporating Teaching With Nursing Care.

Many nurses find that they can teach more effectively while delivering nursing care. For example, while hanging blood, the nurse explains why the blood is needed and the symptoms indicated with transfusion reactions that should be reported immediately. Another example is the nurse who explains a drug's side effects while administering the medication. An informal, unstructured style relies on the positive therapeutic relationship between nurse and client, which fosters a spontaneity in the teaching-learning process. This does not suggest that teaching should occur without a formal plan. When the nurse follows a teaching plan informally, the client feels less pressure to perform and learning becomes more of a shared activity. Teaching during routine care is efficient and cost-effective (Figure 23-4).

Instructional Methods.

Instructional methods that are used depend on the client's learning needs, the time available for teaching, the setting, the resources available, and the nurse's own comfort level with teaching. Skilled teachers are flexible in altering teaching methods accord-

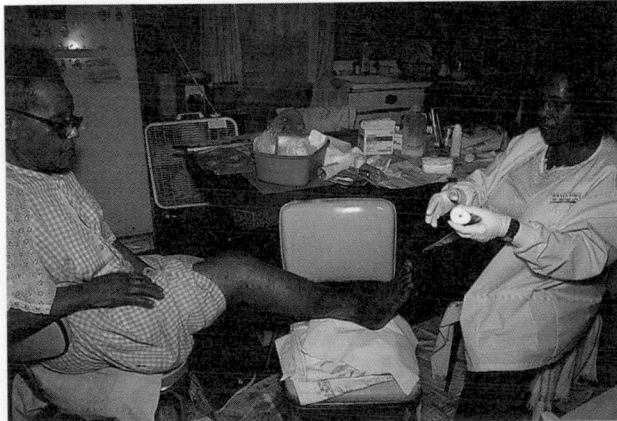

Figure 23-4 The nurse incorporates teaching about wound care during a home visit.

ing to the learner's responses. An experienced teacher uses a variety of techniques and teaching aids. A nurse cannot expect to be an expert educator when first entering nursing practice. Learning to become an effective educator takes time and practice.

When first starting to teach clients, it helps to remember that clients perceive the nurse as an expert. However, this does not mean that the nurse must have all of the answers. It simply means that clients expect that the nurse will keep them appropriately informed. The nurse can provide an effective teaching plan, keeping it simple and focused on clients' needs. A variety of teaching methods can be used, and a variety of teaching aids are usually available.

One-on-One Discussion.   Perhaps the most common method of instruction used by a nurse is one-on-one discussion. When teaching a client at the bedside, in a physician's office, or in the home, the nurse directly shares information. Various teaching aids can be used during the discussion, depending on the client's learning needs. Information is usually given in an informal manner, allowing the client to ask questions or share concerns. The nurse uses unstructured and informal discussion when helping the client understand the implications of illness and ways to cope with health stressors.

Group Instruction.   A nurse uses group instruction with clients or families for one of the following reasons (Redman, 1997).

Groups are an economical way to teach a number of clients at one time.

The experience of being part of a group may be the most likely way for clients to meet learning objectives.

Group instruction often involves both lecture and discussion. Lectures are highly structured and are efficient in helping groups of clients learn standard content about a subject. For example, a nurse might teach groups of clients about the warning signs of breast cancer, the health risks of smoking, or the normal development of a fetus. A lecture does not ensure that learners are actively thinking about the material presented; thus discussion and practice sessions are essential (Redman, 1997).

After hearing information from a lecture, learners need the opportunity to share ideas and seek clarification. Group discussions allow clients and families to learn from each other as they review common experiences. A productive group discussion helps participants solve problems and arrive at solutions toward improving each member's health. To be an effective group leader, the nurse must be able to guide participation. Acknowledging a look of interest, asking questions, and summarizing key issues foster group involvement. However, not all clients benefit from group discussions, and sometimes the physical or emotional level of wellness may prohibit participation.

Preparatory Instruction.   Clients frequently face unfamiliar tests or procedures that create significant anxiety. Providing information about procedures helps clients form realistic images of what to anticipate. This is a common expectation of clients in acute care settings because information helps to give them a sense of control. When the experience matches expectations, the client is more likely to attend to the nurse's future explanations. A nurse gains respect when preparatory explanations prove useful. The nurse uses the following guidelines for giving preparatory explanations:

Physical sensations during the procedure are described but not evaluated. For example, when drawing a blood specimen, the nurse explains that the client will feel a sticking sensation as the needle punctures the skin.

The cause of the sensation is described, preventing misinterpretation of the experience. For example, the nurse explains that a needle stick burns because the alcohol used to cleanse the skin enters the puncture site.

Clients are prepared only for aspects of the experience that have commonly been noticed by other clients. For example, the nurse explains that it is normal for a tight tourniquet to cause a person's hand to tingle and feel numb.

The client finds comfort in knowing what to expect. When the nurse's descriptions accurately portray the actual experience, the client is able to cope more effectively with stress from procedures and therapies (Redman, 1997). The known is less threatening than the unknown.

Demonstrations.   Demonstrations are useful methods for teaching psychomotor skills such as conflict resolution skills, preparation of a syringe, bathing an infant, crutch walking, or measuring a pulse. The client is able to observe a skill before practicing it. Demonstrations are most effective when learners first observe the teacher and then practice the skill in mock or real situations (**return demonstrations**). Nurses commonly use demonstrations for teaching motor skills; however, motor skills are not learned separately from attitudes and factual knowledge (Redman, 1997). A demonstration should be combined with discussion to clarify concepts and feelings. An effective demonstration requires advanced planning:

1. Be sure the learner can easily see the demonstration. Position the learner to provide a clear view of the skill being performed.
2. Review the rationale and steps of the procedure.
3. Assemble and organize equipment. Be sure that all equipment works.
4. Perform each step in sequence while analyzing the knowledge and skills involved.
5. Determine when explanations are to be given, considering the client's learning needs.
6. Judge proper speed and timing of the demonstration, based on the client's cognitive abilities and anxiety level.

The nurse demonstrates a skill in the same order in which the client will perform it. The demonstration involves the following:

Performing each step slowly and accurately

Encouraging the client to ask questions so that each step is understood

Explaining the rationale for each step

Allowing the client to observe each step

Avoiding a hurried approach

Allowing the client to handle equipment and practice the skill under supervision

The client demonstrates the procedure to ensure that learning has occurred. The independent demonstration should occur under the same conditions that will be experienced at home or in the place where the skill is to be performed. For example, if a client is learning to walk with crutches, the nurse simulates the home environment. If short, narrow steps lead to the client's bedroom, the client should learn to climb similar stairs in the hospital.

Analogies.   Learning occurs when a teacher translates complex language or ideas into words or concepts that the client understands. In addition, the client benefits by integrating new information into daily routines. **Analogies** supplement verbal instruction with familiar images that make complex information more real and understandable (Redman, 1997). For example, when explaining arterial blood pressure an analogy would be the flow of water through a hose. To use analogies, the nurse uses the following general principles:

Be familiar with the concept.

Know the client's background, experience, and culture.

Keep the analogy simple and clear.

Role Playing.   A nurse uses role play for teaching ideas and attitudes. During role play, people are asked to play themselves or someone else. The technique involves rehearsing a desired behavior. For example, a nurse teaches a parent to respond to a child's behavior by pretending to be a child who is having a temper tantrum. This scenario allows the parent to practice responding in this situation. Afterward, the nurse evaluates the parent's response and determines whether an alternative approach would have been more appropriate. As a result of role play, clients are taught the skills required and feel more confident in being able to perform them independently.

Discovery.   Discovery is a useful technique for teaching clients problem solving, application, and independent thinking. During individual or group discussion, a nurse poses a pertinent problem or situation for clients to solve. For example, clients with heart disease are asked to plan a meal that is low in cholesterol and fat. The clients in the group decide which foods would be appropriate. The nurse asks the group members to present their diet, providing an opportunity to identify mistakes and reinforce correct information.

Speaking the Client's Language.   It is important to use words a client can understand. Medical jargon can be confusing. Clients understand fewer medical words than health care professionals predict. The problem of **functional illiteracy,** the inability to read above a fifth-grade level, is also real. The National Adult Literacy Survey (NAdLitS), conducted in 1992, assessed the extent of literacy skills in Americans over the age of 16. Participants in this survey completed simulations of daily life experiences. Once the participants completed the survey, they were classified according to their literacy level, with level 1 representing the lowest level of literacy and level 5 being the highest level of literacy. Results from the NAdLitS placed 21% to 23% (about 40 to 44 million) of Americans over the age of 16 in level 1. These people demonstrated only rudimentary reading and writing skills. About 8 million people were unable to perform even the simplest literacy tasks. Approximately 25% to 28% (about 50 million) of adults in America were placed in level 2. These adults had a limited ability to perform tasks that required integration or synthesis of information. Although illiteracy existed among all races, African-American, American Indian/Alaska Native, Hispanic, and Asian/Pacific Islander adults were more likely to be classified into the lowest two literacy levels when compared with Caucasian (white) adults (National Center for Education Statistics, 1996).

To compound the problem, the readability of printed health education material has been researched extensively and has been shown to range from elementary school level to college level (Owen and others, 1993). For example, Mumford (1997) evaluated the readability of 24 nurse-designed client education materials. The readability formulas used in this study indicated that the reading levels of these materials ranged between the ninth and fifteenth grades and required an average of an eleventh-grade education to be understood. Thus it appears that written health information available to a client often exceeds a client's reading ability, despite recommendations for information that is easier to comprehend.

Implications of illiteracy include an impaired ability to analyze instructions or synthesize information and incorporate it into a behavior task. Also, many illiterate adults have not acquired the problem-solving skills of drawing conclusions and inferences from experience, and they will not ask questions to obtain or clarify information that has been presented. Nursing interventions that can be used when caring for clients who are illiterate are summarized in Box 23-7.

The nurse must also have knowledge of the client's cultural background and beliefs, as well as the client's ability to understand instructions developed outside of his or her native language. Cultural diversity is increasing and poses a great challenge to the nurse who is providing culturally sensitive care. When educating clients of different ethnic groups, the nurse must (Ranking and Stallings, 1996; Edelman and Mandle, 1998):

Become aware of the distinctive aspects of each culture.

Collaborate with other nurses and educators to assist in dealing with cultural diversity.

Enlist the help of people in the cultural group to share values and beliefs.

Use input and experiences of ethnic nurses in providing care to members of their own community.

Nurses also must assess for intergenerational conflict of values (Babcock and Miller, 1994). This occurs when immigrant parents uphold their traditional values and their children, who are exposed to American values in social encounters, develop beliefs similar to those of their American peers. This conflict in values must be considered when pro-

---

| *Client Teaching* FOR THE ILLITERATE CLIENT | Box 23-7 |

OBJECTIVES
- Client will understand information presented.
- Client will perform desired behaviors accurately.

TEACHING STRATEGIES
- Use simple terminology to enhance the client's understanding.
- Avoid medical jargon if possible or, if necessary, explain medical terms using basic one- or two-syllable words.
- Keep teaching sessions short and to the point.
- Include the most important information at the beginning of the session.
- Relate information to personal experiences or real-life situations.
- Use simple analogies when appropriate.
- Frequently ask the client for feedback to determine whether the client comprehends information.

- Ask for return demonstrations (provides opportunity to clarify instructions and time to review procedures).
- Provide teaching materials that reflect the reading level of the client, with attention given to short words and sentences, large type, and simple format (generally, information written on a fifth-grade reading level is recommended for adult learners).
- Reinforce the most important information at the end of the session.

EVALUATION
- Ask the client to verbalize understanding of information taught.
- Observe and evaluate the client's ability to perform desired behaviors.

Data from Murphy PW, Davis TC: When low literacy blocks compliance, *RN* 60(10):58, 1997.

viding information to families or groups that are composed of members from different generations.

To enhance client education in culturally diverse populations, nurses must know when and how to provide education so that cultural values are respected. Teaching regarding interventions or desired behaviors may need to be modified to mediate cultural differences (Box 23-8). Effective educational strategies may require the nurse to use different patterns of communication.

Using Teaching Tools.   Many teaching tools are available for nurses to use when instructing a client. Selection for the right tool depends on the instructional method chosen, the client's learning needs, and the client's ability to learn (Table 23-5). For example, a printed pamphlet may not be the best tool to use for a client with poor reading comprehension, and an audiotape may be the best choice for a client with visual impairment.

Special Needs of Children and Older Adults.   A nurse's choice of instructional methods and application of teaching-learning principles are based on a client's age and developmental level. Children, adults, and older adults learn differently. The nurse adapts teaching strategies to each learner.

Children pass through several developmental stages (see Unit 2). In each developmental stage, children acquire new cognitive and psychomotor abilities that respond to different types of learning (Figure 23-5). For example, a nurse teaches school-age children about health as they acquire the ability to see things through the point of view of others. Dental hygiene, nutrition, safety measures, and sex education are examples of topics that may be presented to school children of varying ages. Parental input is incorporated in planning health education for children.

Older adults experience numerous physical and psychological changes as they age (see Chapter 12). These changes not only increase the educational needs of older adults, but they can also create barriers to learning unless adjustments are made in nursing interventions.

Sensory changes such as visual and hearing deficits require teaching methods that enhance older adult clients' functioning. For example, the nurse sits to face clients with hearing problems and speaks in a low tone of voice during discussions. Clients with visual problems can benefit from the use of printed materials containing large print. Older adults learn and remember effectively if the learning is paced properly and the material is relevant to

---

𝒞𝓊𝓁𝓉𝓊𝓇𝒶𝓁 ASPECTS OF CARE   Box 23-8

Asians and Pacific Islanders are the second largest ethnic group in the United States. They share many traditional values, including the value of the extended family, maintenance of harmony and avoidance of conflict, and respect for authority figures. Asian folk medicine and philosophies are strongly influenced by the Chinese; Asians use a variety of herbs to promote healing (Edelman and Mandle, 1998).

Wallace, Awan, and Talbot (1996) developed a culturally sensitive, interdisciplinary program for Asian women who had diabetes. After developing an understanding of the Asian culture, 20 Asian women with diabetes were interviewed, through an interpreter, to gain further insight into their health beliefs and culture. Feedback from these interviews was used to develop a 10-week diabetes management program. After completing the program, the participants demonstrated improved knowledge about diabetes, exercised more, and had instituted healthy diet changes. They were also able to express their feelings about their illness. There was a notable increase in their self-confidence. The women realized that they could help themselves.

In this culture men are usually the respected authority figures. Therefore they often do the shopping, complicating the women's abilities to change dietary habits. It is hoped that as a result of the improved knowledge and self-confidence, these women will be able to improve their diet and other diabetes management skills.

The program also benefited the health care team. The health care providers developed a better understanding of the culture and beliefs of the Asian population. Therefore they enhanced their communication skills and were able to provide more effective care. Continued efforts to understand and meet the needs of culturally diverse populations will enhance the ability of nurses to provide effective client education.

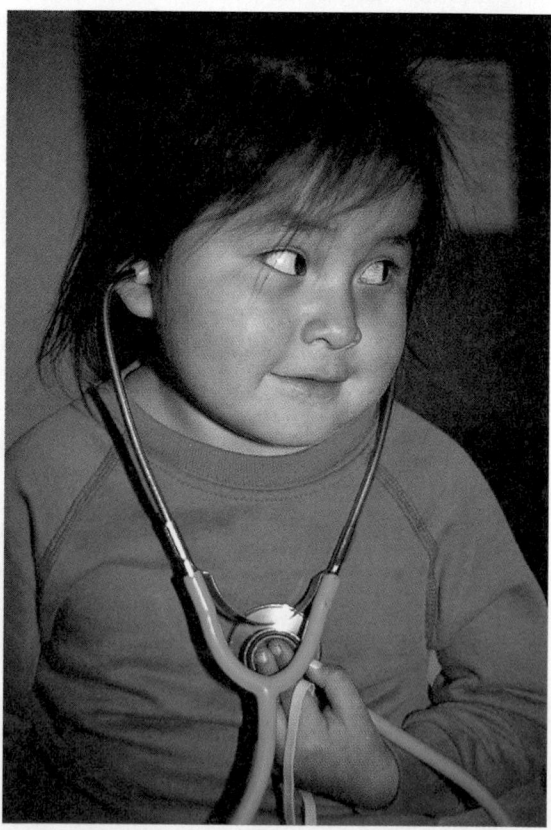

Figure 23-5   The preschool child learns not to be afraid of medical equipment by being allowed to handle the stethoscope and imitating its use.

Table 23-5 Teaching Tools for Instruction

Description	Learning Implications
Printed Material Written teaching tools available as pamphlets, booklets, brochures	Material must be easily readable for learner. Information must be accurate and current. Method is ideal for understanding complex concepts and relationships.
Programmed Instruction Written sequential presentation of learning steps requiring that learners answer questions and that teachers tell them whether they are right or wrong	Instruction is primarily verbal, but teacher may use pictures or diagrams. Method requires active learning, giving immediate feedback, correcting wrong answers, and reinforcing right answers. Learner works at own pace.
Computer Instruction Use of programmed instruction format in which computers store response patterns for learners and select further lessons on basis of these patterns (programs can be individualized)	Method requires reading comprehension, psychomotor skills, and familiarity with computer.
Nonprint Materials DIAGRAMS Illustrations that show interrelationships by means of lines and symbols	Method demonstrates key ideas, summarizes, and clarifies key concept.
GRAPHS (BAR, CIRCLE, OR LINE) Visual presentations of numerical data	Graphs help learner to grasp information quickly about single concept.
CHARTS Highly condensed visual summary of ideas and facts that may highlight series of ideas, steps, or events	Charts demonstrate relationship of several ideas or concepts. Method helps learners know what to do.
PICTURES Photographs or drawings used to teach concepts in which the third dimension of shape and space is not important	Photographs are more desirable than diagrams because they more accurately portray the details of the real item. Drawings are pertinent for removing the superfluous detail present in real objects.
PHYSICAL OBJECTS Use of actual equipment, objects, or models to teach concepts or skills	Models are useful when real objects are too small, large, or complicated or are unavailable. Learners can manipulate objects that are to be used later in skill.
OTHER AUDIOVISUAL MATERIALS Slides, audiotapes, television, and videotapes used with printed material or discussion	Materials are useful for clients with reading comprehension problems and visual deficits.

the learner's needs and abilities (Rankin and Stallings, 1996; Tiivel, 1997). Although older adults have slower cognitive function and reduced short-term memory, nurses can facilitate learning in several ways to support behaviors that maximize the individual's capacity for self-care (Box 23-9). When teaching older clients, information must be based on the client's previous level of understanding, and reachable, short-term goals should be established. Family members who may be assuming partial care for the client must also be included. However, the nurse must be sensitive to the client's desire for assistance, since offering unwanted support may result in negative outcomes and may be perceived as nagging and interference. Furthermore, not all relationships between older adults and other family members are therapeutic. Because of the high incidence of abuse and neglect of older adults, the nurse needs to assess family dynamics before including family members in educational sessions (Burke and Walsh, 1997).

EVALUATION

Client education is not complete until the nurse evaluates outcomes of the teaching-learning process (see care plan, p. 487). The nurse determines whether clients

Nurses can facilitate learning by using the following interventions when providing client education to older adults:

- Present information slowly.
- Speak in a low tone of voice (lower tones are easier to hear than higher tones).
- Allow ample time for understanding of the material.
- Emphasize concrete material that applies to current situations.
- Reduce environmental distractions.
- Provide information in frequent, small amounts.
- Reinforce important information.
- Relate new material to previous life experiences.
- Build on existing knowledge.
- Establish mutually set goals.
- Allow clients to progress at their own pace (older adults are more cautious, so it may take longer to adopt a behavior change).
- Use group experiences if appropriate to enhance problem solving.
- If written material is used, assess the client's ability to read and use information that is printed in a large font size and in a color that contrasts highly with the background (e.g., black 14 point font print on buff-colored paper).

Data from: Edelman CL, Mandle, CL: *Health promotion throughout the lifespan*, ed 4, St. Louis, 1998, Mosby; Lusis S: The challenges of nursing elderly surgical patients, *AORN J* 64(6):954, 1996; Rankin SH, Stallings, KD: *Patient education: issues, principles, practices*, ed 3, Philadelphia, 1996, JB Lippincott; Tiivel J: Increasing the effectiveness of your teaching program for the elderly: assessing the client's readiness to learn, *Perspectives* 21(3):7, 1997.

have learned the material. Evaluation reinforces learners' correct behavior, helps learners realize how they should change incorrect behavior, and helps the teacher determine adequacy of teaching (Cronbach, 1977; Redman, 1997). The evaluation process of client education includes the following (Babcock and Miller, 1994; Rankin and Stallings, 1996; Redman, 1997):

Noting barriers that impeded successful learning

Measuring the extent to which the learning objectives have been met by the client

Identifying any learning objectives that needed clarification

Indicating teaching interventions that were ineffective, including teaching methods

Noting areas that required clarification, correction of misconceptions, or reinforcement

The nurse evaluates success by observing the client's performance of each expected behavior (see care plan, p. 487). Success depends on the client's ability to meet the established performance criteria.

Direct observation of client behaviors is useful when determining how a person will act in the future. In direct observation the nurse has the client demonstrate the behaviors described in the learning objectives. If the evalua-

tion process indicates a knowledge or skill deficit, the nurse repeats or modifies the teaching plan. Watching a client demonstrate a skill helps the nurse to know whether the correct technique is being used. However, a client may choose to behave differently later. Therefore observation works best in real-life situations (Babcock and Miller, 1994).

Oral and written questioning are other useful evaluation methods. A client's success in cognitive learning can be measured verbally by the client answering questions about a specific topic that was taught. Questions measure behaviors that are not easily observed. The nurse should carefully phrase questions to ensure that the learner understands them and that objectives are truly measured.

Another form of evaluation includes self-reports (oral and written) and self-monitoring (written). This involves the client or family member providing information independently. An example might include a client's written log of the foods eaten during a specific week, matched against a newly prescribed diet. The nurse relies on the client's honesty and memory in self-reporting.

Because of the increasing importance of client satisfaction (see Chapter 2), nurses should evaluate whether clients have the information they want. Have their expectations been met? A client may want specific information that he or she knows will be necessary to continue a normal lifestyle at home. Nurses must include client expectations as a part of their evaluation. For example, during teaching sessions the nurse periodically asks clients if they understand what is being taught. At the end of the teaching session, the nurse asks clients to identify information that was not provided that should have been covered. Clients may also be given the opportunity to evaluate a teaching session (or the nurse doing the teaching) in writing. Questionnaires used in these situations ask clients to express their satisfaction with the education they received. At times, written evaluations may be more truthful than evaluations obtained in a face-to-face situation.

Evaluation may reveal new learning needs or the existence of new factors that may interfere with the client's ability to learn. Alternative teaching methods often help clarify information or skills that the client was unable to comprehend or perform originally. When a client has difficulty in an acute care setting, the nurse may make a referral to resources, such as home health care or an outpatient clinic, for further education and evaluation. Like the nursing process, the teaching-learning process is continuous and ever changing.

Documentation of Client Teaching. Because client teaching often occurs informally between nurse and client (e.g., during medication administration or physical examination), it is difficult to document it consistently. Nurses often fail to take the time to write down material that is taught. However, because a nurse is legally responsible for providing accurate, timely client information that promotes continuity of care, it is essential to document the outcomes of teaching. Many institutions have special forms that allow easy documentation. For instance, teaching flow sheets are excellent records that document the plan, implementation, and evaluation of learning. Smalley (1997) suggests documenting the following regarding client education:

- *Assessment of learning needs.* Documenting assessment data provides important information needed when developing the teaching plan.
- *Specific content.* Specifically describing subject matter enables other nurses to follow up and reinforce teaching (e.g., "Explained side effects of Inderal" or "Demonstrated umbilical cord care"). Note the date, time, and specific person or persons taught. Avoid generalizations (e.g., "medications taught") that leave staff uninformed about what content has been taught.

- *Method of teaching.* Knowing the methods used in instruction (e.g., demonstrations or discussion) helps staff follow up more efficiently or offer alternative teaching methods if learning does not occur. When resources such as pamphlets or audiovisual materials are used, the nurse documents this in the client's record.
- *Reinforced information.* Documenting information that has been reinforced helps determine learning needs that have not been met or learning needs that were not identified in the initial assessment.
- *Evaluation of learning.* Documenting evidence of learning (e.g., a return demonstration or the ability to verbalize the purpose and side effects of a medication) informs staff about the client's progress and determines information that still must be taught.

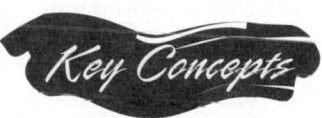

Key Concepts

- In the health care system today, there is greater emphasis on providing quality health education.
- The nurse must ensure that clients, families, and communities receive information needed to maintain optimal health.
- Health education is aimed at the promotion, restoration, and maintenance of health.
- Teaching is most effective when it is responsive to the learner's needs.
- Teaching is a form of interpersonal communication, with the teacher and student actively involved in a process that increases the student's knowledge and skills.
- The ability to learn depends on a person's physical and cognitive attributes.
- The ability to attend to the learning process depends on physical comfort and anxiety levels and the presence of environmental distraction.
- A person's health beliefs influence the willingness to gain knowledge and skills necessary to maintain health.
- Teaching must be timed to coincide with the client's readiness to learn.
- Clients of different age-groups require different teaching strategies as a result of developmental capabilities.
- The client should be an active participant in a teaching plan, agreeing to the plan, helping choose instructional methods, and recommending times for instruction.
- Learning objectives describe what a person is to learn in behavioral terms.

- A combination of teaching methods improves the learner's attentiveness and involvement.
- A teacher is more effective when presenting information that builds on a learner's existing knowledge.
- A teacher who uses reinforces, such as praise or encouragement, for a behavior is increasing the probability of the behavior recurring.
- The older adult learns most effectively when information is slowly paced and presented in small amounts.
- A nurse evaluates a client's learning by observing performance of expected learning behaviors under desired conditions.
- Effective documentation describes the entire process of client education, promotes continuity of care, and demonstrates that educational standards have been met.

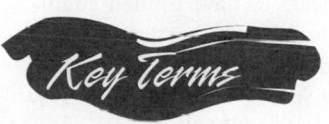

Key Terms

Affective learning, *p. 476*

Analogies, *p. 492*

Cognitive learning, *p. 476*

Compliance, *p. 478*

Functional illiteracy, *p. 493*

Learning, *p. 474*

Learning objective, *p. 474*

Motivation, *p. 477*

Psychomotor learning, *p. 476*

Reinforcement, *p. 490*

Return demonstrations, *p. 492*

Self-efficacy, *p. 478*

Teaching, *p. 473*

Critical Thinking Exercises

1. Susan, a manager of a preschool, has noticed that many of the children in the preschool are missing days because of illness. Susan states, "These kids always seem to be sick. They seem to get the same thing over and over again." The teachers at the preschool have asked Susan to contact you to educate the 3- and 4-year-olds about the need to use tissues and proper hand washing in hopes of keeping the children healthier. What teaching methods would you employ while teaching these children?

2. Kay, who is a 50-year-old nurse, has recently had a myocardial infarction (heart attack). Her medical history reflects that she has a family history of heart disease and has had hypertension and high serum cholesterol levels for 15 years. She reports eating a diet high in fat and says that she does not exercise regularly. Kay experienced chest pain for 2 days that worsened with activity before she sought medical attention. She states, "The reason why I can't change my diet is because my husband won't eat low-fat food, and I had a heart attack because I have been worried about my husband's health." List your teaching priorities for this client.

3. Anne, who is 20 years old, has just delivered a healthy baby boy. According to her CareMap, now that she is on the mother-baby unit, you are to review her teaching plan with her and individualize it to meet her needs. You ask Anne to review the teaching plan with you. You ask her to read the medical center's baby care pamphlet and discuss its content with you. You discover that although the pamphlet is written at a fifth-grade level, Anne is unable to comprehend the information in the brochure. When you ask her how well she can read and write English, she responds, "I can read and write well." Describe how you would individualize Anne's teaching plan to effectively teach her how to care for her baby.

4. George, who is 70 years old, has had a cerebrovascular accident (CVA). Before his CVA, he was very active socially, went to work 2 days a week, and golfed 3 to 4 days a week. He is about to start the rehabilitation process. Although he appears to have limited cognitive deficits, he will need to use a walker at home. He states, "Walkers are for old people." Describe how you will approach George and what factors you will consider as you teach him how to use his walker.

References

American Hospital Association: *A patient's bill of rights,* Chicago, 1992, The Association.

American Nurses Association: *Nursing's agenda for health care reform,* Kansas City, Mo, 1991, The Association.

Babcock DE, Miller MA: *Client education: theory and practice,* St. Louis, 1994, Mosby.

Bandura A: *Self-efficacy: the exercise of control,* New York, 1997, WH Freeman.

Barnes LP: Patient education standards, *MCN Am J Matern Child Nurs* 18(1):45, 1993.

Bauman A: The comprehensibility of asthma education materials, *Patient Educ Counsel* 32:S51, 1997.

Bloom BS, editor: Taxonomy of educational objectives, *Cognitive domain,* vol 1, New York, 1956, Longman.

Burke MM, Walsh MB: *Gerontologic nursing: wholistic care of the older adult,* ed 2, St. Louis, 1997, Mosby.

Chachkes E, Christ G: Cross cultural issues in patient education, *Patient Educ Counsel* 27:13, 1996.

Cravener PA: Principles of adult health education, *Gastroenterol Nurs* 19(4):140, 1996.

Cronbach LJ: *Educational psychology,* ed 3, New York, 1977, Harcourt Brace Jovanovich.

Czar ML, Engler MM: Perceived learning needs of patients with coronary artery disease using a questionnaire assessment tool, *Heart Lung* 26(2):109, 1997.

Edelman CL, Mandle CL: *Health promotion throughout the lifespan,* ed 4, St. Louis, 1998, Mosby.

Fox VJ: Postoperative education that works, *AORN J* 67(5):1010, 1998.

Henderson V: *The nature of nursing: a definition and its implications for practice, research, and education,* New York, 1966, Macmillan.

Joint Commission on Accreditation of Healthcare Organizations: *Accreditation manual of hospitals,* Chicago, 2000, The Commission.

Krathwohl DR and others: *Taxonomy of educational objectives: the classification of educational goals, Handbook II, Affective domain,* New York, 1964, David McKay.

Lookinland S, Pool M: Study on effect of methods of preoperative education in women, *AORN J* 67(1):203, 1998.

Lusis S: The challenges of nursing elderly surgical patients, *AORN J* 64(6):954, 1996.

McCloskey JC, Bulechek GM: *Nursing interventions classification (NIC),* ed 3, St. Louis, 2000, Mosby.

McKenna G: Learning theories made easy: humanism, *Nurs Stand* 9(31):29, 1995.

Merriam SB: Updating our knowledge of adult learning, *J Contin Educ Health Prof* 16:136, 1996.

Miller B, Capps E: Meeting JCAHO patient-education standards, *Nurs Manage* 28(5):55, 1997.

Mumford M: A descriptive study of the readability of patient information leaflets designed by nurses, *J Adv Nurs* 26(5):985, 1997.

Murphy PW, Davis TC: When low literacy blocks compliance, *RN* 60(10):58, 1997.

National Center for Education Statistics: *1992 National adult literacy survey,* 1996; http://nces.ed.gov/nadlits/.

Owen and others: Reading, readability, and patient education, *Cardiovasc Nurs* 29(2):9, 1993.

Pender NJ: *Health promotion in nursing practice,* ed 3, Stamford, Conn, 1996, Appleton & Lange.

Rankin SH, Stallings KD: *Patient education: issues, principles, practices,* ed 3, Philadelphia, 1996, JB Lippincott.

Redman BK: *The practice of patient education,* ed 8, St. Louis, 1997, Mosby.

Rosenstock IM, Strecher VJ, Becker MH: Social learning theory and the health belief model, *Health Educ Q* 15:175–183, 1988.

Smalley R: Taking charge: patient education: we have a better system now, *RN* 60(6):19, 24, 1997.

TenHave TR and others: Literacy assessment in a cardiovascular nutrition education setting, *Patient Educ Counsel* 31(2):139, 1997.

Tiivel J: Increasing the effectiveness of your teaching program for the elderly: assessing the client's readiness to learn, *Perspectives* 21(3):7, 1997.

Wallace P, Awan A, Talbot J: Health advice for Asian women with diabetes, *Prof Nurse* 11(12):794, 1996.

Wong DL: *Whaley and Wong's essentials of pediatric nursing,* ed 5, St. Louis, 1997, Mosby.

Zernike W, Henderson A: Evaluating the effectiveness of two teaching strategies for patients diagnosed with hypertension, *J Clin Nurs* 7(1):37, 1998.

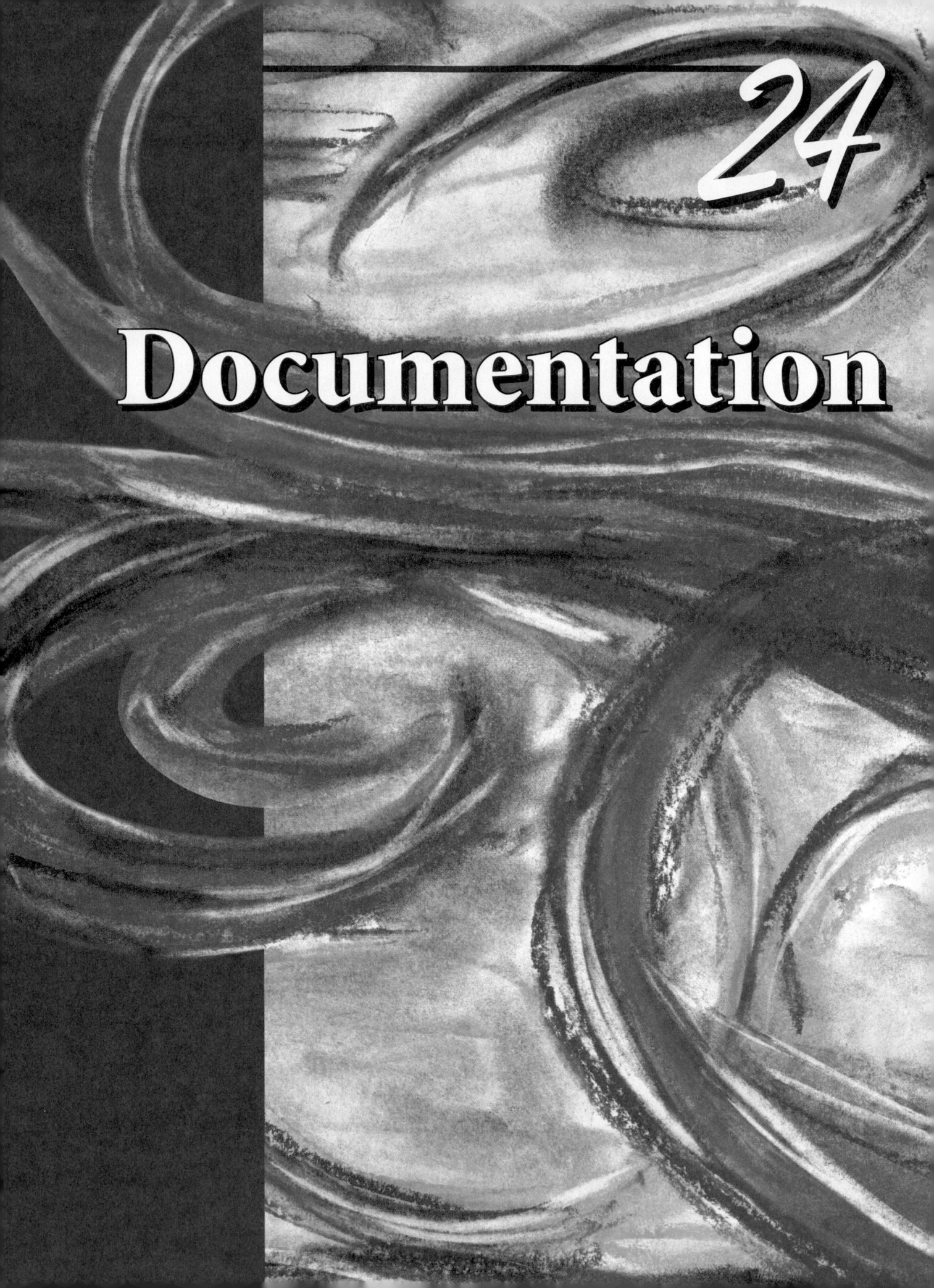

Documentation

24

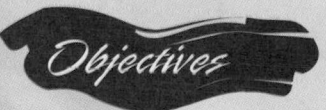

Mastery of content in this chapter will enable the student to:

- Define the key terms listed.
- Discuss the relationship between documentation and health care financial reimbursement.
- Identify purposes of a health care record.
- Describe guidelines for effective documentation and reporting.
- Discuss legal guidelines for recording.
- Describe the different methods used in record keeping.
- Discuss the advantages of standardized documentation forms.
- Identify elements to include when documenting a client's discharge plan.
- Describe the role of critical pathways in multidisciplinary documentation.
- Identify the important aspects of long-term care documentation.
- Discuss issues related to computerization in documentation.
- Describe the purpose and content of a change-of-shift report.
- Explain how to verify telephone orders.

D ocumentation is a vital aspect of nursing practice. Although the destination of changes in health care is not clear, the direction toward lower costs and more efficient care delivery is unmistakable. Nursing documentation must be both comprehensive and flexible enough to retrieve critical data, to maintain quality and continuity of care, to track client outcomes, and to reflect current standards (Eggland, 1995).

Accreditation agencies such as the Joint Commission on Accreditation of Healthcare Organizations (JCAHO) specify guidelines for documentation. Under the prospective payment system, hospitals are reimbursed a set dollar amount by Medicare for each **diagnosis-related group (DRG)** (Box 24-1). Everything that is done for a client must be documented in the medical record for the health care institution to recover its costs.

As members of the health care team, nurses need to communicate information about clients accurately and in a timely, effective manner. The quality of client care depends on caregivers' ability to communicate with one another. All health care providers require the same information about clients so that they can plan an organized, comprehensive care plan. Unless the client's care plan is communicated to all members of the health care team, care becomes fragmented, repetition of tasks occurs, and therapies may be delayed or even omitted. The result of inadequate communication may affect client outcomes, resulting in delayed recovery.

The health care environment creates many challenges for accurately documenting and reporting the care deliv-

ered to clients. The quality of care, the standards of regulatory agencies, the reimbursement structure in the health care system, and the legal guidelines for nursing practice make documentation and reporting an extremely important responsibility of a nurse.

Multidisciplinary Communication Within the Health Care Team

Client care requires effective communication among members of the health care team. **Reports** include both oral and written exchanges of information between caregivers (Figure 24-1). At the end of a work shift in hospitals and other agencies giving round-the-clock care, nurses give a verbal report to nurses on the next shift. A physician may call a nursing unit to receive a verbal report on a client's condition and progress. The laboratory submits a written report providing the results of diagnostic tests.

A client's **record** or chart is permanent legal documentation of information relevant to a client's health care management. With each hospital or health care agency visit, information about the client's health care is recorded, providing an ongoing account of the client's health care status and needs.

Information is also communicated through discussions among team members. Discussions allow a review of information so that problems are identified and solutions are recommended. For example, discharge planning conferences often involve members of all disciplines (e.g., nursing, social work, dietary, medicine, and physical ther-

The authors acknowledge the contribution of Dr. Rick Daniels to this chapter in the previous edition of this text.

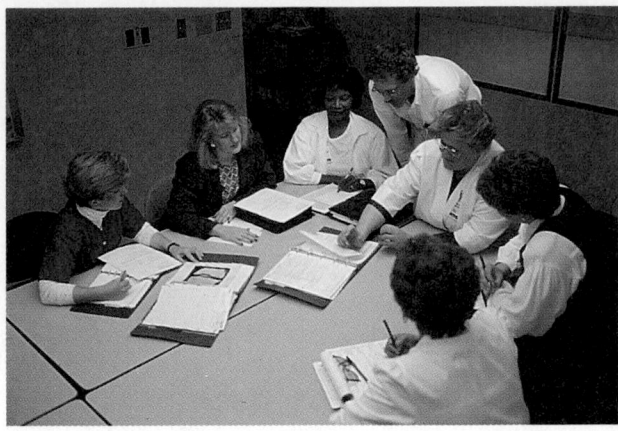

Figure 24-1   Staff communicate information about their
clients during a change-of-shift report.

apy), who meet to discuss the client's progress toward established discharge goals. **Consultations** are another form
of discussion whereby one professional caregiver gives formal advice about the care of a client to another caregiver.
An acute care nurse may make a referral to or consult with
a dietitian in the management of diet therapy for a client
with a diagnosis of diabetes. Referrals, consultations, and
conferences must be documented in a client's permanent
record so that all caregivers can benefit from the information and plan care accordingly.

Documentation

Documentation is defined as anything written or printed
that is relied on as a record of proof for authorized persons. Effective documentation reflects the quality of care
and provides evidence of each health care team member's
accountability in giving care.

Several types of records are used to communicate information about clients. All records contain basically the
following information:

   Client identification and demographic data
   Informed consent for treatment and procedures
   Admission nursing history
   Nursing diagnoses or problems
   Nursing or multidisciplinary care plan
   Record of nursing care treatment and evaluation
   Medical history
   Medical diagnosis
   Therapeutic orders
   Medical and health discipline's progress notes
   Reports of physical examinations
   Reports of diagnostic studies
   Summary of operative procedures
   Discharge plan and summary

PURPOSES OF RECORDS

A record is a valuable source of data that is used by all
members of the health care team. Its purposes include
communication, financial billing, education, assessment,
research, auditing, and legal documentation.

Communication.   The record is a means by which
health care team members communicate contributions to
the client's care, including individual therapies, content of
important discussions, client education, and use of referrals for discharge planning. Staff also communicate the
client's response to therapies. The plan of care should be
clear to anyone reading the chart. When a staff member is
caring for a client, the record should communicate the
measures needed to maintain continuity and consistency
of care.

Financial Billing.   The client care record is a document that shows the extent to which health care agencies
should be reimbursed for services. Diagnosis-related
groups have become the basis for establishing reimbursement for client care. Detailed recording helps in establishing codable diagnoses that are used to determine a DRG.
The nurse's contribution to documentation can help clarify the type of treatment a client receives. When client
charges exceed the length of stay allowed for a particular
DRG, appropriate documentation is essential to justify the
additional time.

Education.   Students of nursing and other health-
related disciplines use the medical record as an educational resource. A client's record contains a variety of information, including diagnoses, signs and symptoms of
disease, successful and unsuccessful therapies, diagnostic
findings, and client behaviors. An effective way to learn the
nature of an illness and the individual client's response to
it is to read the client care record. No two clients have
identical records, and patterns of information can be identified in records of clients who have similar health problems. With this information students learn the patterns to
look for in various health problems and become better
able to anticipate the type of care required for a client.

Assessment.   A nursing history and initial assessment is completed when a client is admitted to a nursing care unit. This usually contains biographical data (e.g., age, marital status), method of admission, reason for admission, a brief medical-surgical history (e.g., previous surgeries or illnesses), allergies, current medication (prescribed and over-the-counter), the client's perceptions about illness or hospitalization, and a review of health risk factors. A physical assessment of all body systems is either incorporated into the nursing history or included on a separate form.

The record provides data that nurses use to identify and support nursing diagnoses and plan proper interventions for care. Information from the record adds to the nurse's observations and assessment. It is unnecessary for the nurse to collect information that is already available. If there is reason to believe that the information is inaccurate, information should be verified.

The medical progress notes detail the physician's findings at the time of assessment. Before caring for any client, the nurse refers to the medical record for new, relevant assessment findings. The nurse is able to enter a client's room, anticipate the status of the client, and then conduct an individualized assessment of the client.

Assessment data entered accurately by each health care team member reveals the client's health status. For example, after inspection of a wound the nurse may conclude that healing is delayed. The record will give much additional information, including the client's appetite, descriptions of the wound's previous appearance, and laboratory results indicating the presence or absence of infection. Such information can help explain the reasons for and implications of changes in client condition.

Research.   Statistical data relating to the frequency of clinical disorders, complications, use of specific medical and nursing therapies, recovery from illness and deaths can be gathered from client records. Records are a valuable resource for describing characteristics of the client populations in a health care agency.

A nurse may use client's records during a research study to collect information on certain factors. For example, if a nurse uses a new method of pain control for a group of clients, the records provide data on the success of therapy. Recording entries that describe the type and dose of analgesic medications used and clients' subjective reports of pain relief could be used to evaluate pain-control measures. Nurses may also research records of previously discharged clients to identify nursing care problems. For example, a study to determine the incidence of infection in clients with specific types of intravenous catheters might be performed by means of a chart review.

Auditing.   A regular review of information in client records gives a basis for evaluation of the quality and appropriateness of care provided in an institution. The JCAHO requires hospitals to establish quality improvement programs for conducting objective, ongoing reviews of client care. The JCAHO has established standards for the type of information to be found in the client's record, such as indications that a plan of care is developed with the client as a participant and that discharge planning and client education have occurred. The JCAHO asks institutions to establish standards for quality care. Nurses monitor or review records throughout the year to determine the degree to which quality improvement standards are met (see Chapter 4). Deficiencies identified during monitoring are shared with all members of the nursing staff so that corrections in policy or practice can be made. Quality improvement programs keep nurses informed of standards of nursing practice to maintain excellence in nursing care.

Medical records are also audited to review charges for the client's care. Private insurance carriers and auditors from the federal government review records to determine the reimbursement that a client or a health care agency receives. Accurate documentation of supplies and equipment that have been used ensures that costs are recovered and that clients receive the care they require.

Legal Documentation.   Accurate documentation is one of the best defenses for legal claims associated with nursing care. The record serves as a description of exactly what happened to a client. Nursing care may have been excellent; however, "care not documented is care not done" in a court of law. Nurses need to indicate all instructions and referrals in the medical record (Mandell, 1994).

Four common communication problems in malpractice caused by inadequate documentation are (1) not charting the correct time when events occurred, (2) failing to record verbal orders or failing to have them signed, (3) charting actions in advance to save time, and (4) documenting incorrect data (Martin, 1994). Table 24-1 provides guidelines for legally sound documentation.

The law protects information about clients that is gathered by examination, observation, conversation, or treatment. Nurses may not discuss a client's status with other clients or staff uninvolved in the client's care. Nurses are legally and ethically obligated to keep information about clients' illnesses and treatments confidential. Only staff directly involved in care have legitimate access to the records. Clients frequently request copies of their medical records, and they have the right to read those records. Each institution has policies for controlling the manner in which records are shared. In most situations clients are required to give written permission for release of medical information. Nurses are responsible for protecting records from all unauthorized readers.

When nurses and other health care professionals have a legitimate reason to use records for data gathering, research, or continuing education, appropriate authorization must be obtained according to agency policy. Student nurses and faculty may be required to present identifica-

Table 24-1   Legal Guidelines for Recording

Guidelines	Rationale	Correct Action
Do not erase, apply correction fluid, or scratch out errors made while recording.	Charting becomes illegible: it may appear as if you were attempting to hide information or deface record.	Draw single line through error, write word *error* above it; then record note correctly.
Do not write retaliatory or critical comments about client or care by other health care professionals.	Statements can be used as evidence for nonprofessional behavior or poor quality of care.	Enter only objective descriptions of client's behavior; client comments should be quoted.
Correct all errors promptly.	Errors in recording can lead to errors in treatment.	Avoid rushing to complete charting; be sure information is accurate.
Record all facts.	Record must be accurate and reliable.	Be certain entry is factual; do not speculate or guess.
Do not leave blank spaces in nurse's notes.	Another person can add incorrect information in space.	Chart consecutively, line by line; if space is left, draw line horizontally through it and sign your name at end.
Record all entries legibly and in ink.	Illegible entries can be misinterpreted, causing errors and lawsuits; ink cannot be erased; records are photocopied and stored on microfilm.	Never erase entries or use correction fluid, and never use pencil.
If order is questioned, record that clarification was sought.	If you perform order known to be incorrect, you are just as liable for prosecution as the physician is.	Do not record "physician made error." Instead, chart that "Dr. Smith was called to clarify order for analgesic."
Chart only for yourself.	You are accountable for information you enter into chart.	Never chart for someone else (exception: if caregiver has left unit for day and calls with information).
Avoid using generalized, empty phrases such as "status unchanged" or "had good day."	Specific information about client's condition or case can be accidently deleted if information is too generalized.	Use complete, concise descriptions of care.
Begin each entry with time, and end with your signature and title.	This guideline ensures that correct sequence of events is recorded; signature documents who is accountable for care delivered.	Do not wait until end of shift to record important changes that occurred several hours earlier; be sure to sign each entry.

tion indicating access to the record is authorized. The nurse should know the location of the record at all times. The record is stored by the health care agency after treatment ends.

GUIDELINES FOR QUALITY DOCUMENTATION AND REPORTING

Quality documentation and reporting are necessary to enhance efficient, individualized client care. Quality documentation and reporting have five important characteristics: they are factual, accurate, complete, current, and organized.

Factual.   A record contains descriptive, objective information about what a nurse sees, hears, feels, and smells. An objective description is the result of direct observation and measurement. The use of inferences without supporting factual data is not acceptable because it can be misunderstood. The use of words such as *appears, seems,* or *ap-*

parently are not acceptable because they suggest that the nurse did not know the facts. For example, the description "the client seems anxious" does not accurately communicate facts and does not inform another caregiver of the details regarding the behaviors exhibited by the client that led to the use of the word *anxious.* The phrase *seems anxious* is a conclusion without supported facts. Documentation needs to clearly explain the nurse's observations of the client's behaviors. When recording subjective data, document the client's exact words within quotation marks whenever possible (Eggland, 1995). For example, "Client states, 'I feel very nervous, and out of control.'" Any objective findings that are related to the client's anxiety, such as an increased blood pressure and pulse rate, can also be added.

Accurate.   The use of exact measurements ensures that a record is accurate. The nurse makes descriptions such as "Intake, 360 ml of water" rather than "Client drank an adequate amount of fluid." Measurements are later used as a means to determine whether a client's condition has changed. Charting that an abdominal wound is "5 cm in length without redness, drainage, or edema" is more accurate than "large wound is healing well." Use of an institution's accepted abbreviations, symbols, and system of measures (e.g., metric) ensures that all staff members will use the same language in their reports and records. Use abbreviations carefully to avoid misinterpretation. For example, od (every day) can be interpreted to mean O.D. (right eye). To avoid any chance of error, abbreviations are spelled in their entirety when terminology is confusing.

Correct spelling is important and demonstrates a level of competency and attention to detail. Many terms can easily be confused or misinterpreted (e.g., *dysphagia* or *dysphasia* and *dram* or *gram*). Some spelling errors can also cause serious treatment errors; for example, medications such as digitoxin and digoxin or morphine and Numorphan are similar and must be transcribed carefully to ensure that the client receives the correct medication.

JCAHO standards (1995) require that "all entries in medical records are dated and a method is established to identify the authors of entries." Records need to reflect accountability during the time frame of the entry. This is best accomplished when nurses chart their own observations and actions. Each entry in a client's record is identified with the caregiver's full name or initials and status, such as "Julie Smith, RN." Each time initials are used, the full name and status must previously appear on the same page so the individual entering initials can be readily identified. A nursing student enters full name and educational institution, such as "David Jones, SN (student nurse), OHSU (Oregon Health Sciences University)." The signature holds that nurse accountable for information recorded. If information was inadvertently omitted from the record, it is acceptable for nurses to ask colleagues to chart information after they leave work. The entry needs to clearly show what was done and by whom (e.g., "At 11 AM Sam Turner, RN, called and reported that at 8 AM Demerol 100 mg IM was administered to client for abdominal pain" [Kopf, 1993]).

Complete.   The information within a recorded entry or a report needs to be complete, containing concise, appropriate and thorough information about a client's care. Concise data are easy to understand. Clear, succinct recording and reporting gives essential information, avoiding unnecessary words and irrelevant detail.

Criteria for thorough communication exist for certain health problems or nursing activities (Table 24-2). The nurse makes written entries in the client's medical record, describing nursing care that is administered and the client's response. An example of a thorough nurses' note follows:

1915 Client verbalizes sharp, throbbing pain localized along radial side of right ankle, beginning approximately 15 minutes ago after twisting his foot on the stairs. Pain increased with movement, slightly

Table 24-2 Examples of Criteria for Reporting and Recording

Topic	Criteria to Report or Record
Assessment	
Subjective data	Description of episode in quotation marks
	Location, severity, onset, precipitating factors, frequency and duration, aggravating and relieving factors
Client behavior (e.g., anxiety, confusion, hostility)	Onset, behaviors exhibited, precipitating factors
Objective data (e.g., rash, tenderness, breath sounds)	Onset, location, description or quality of findings, aggravating or relieving factors
Nursing Interventions and Evaluation	
Treatments (e.g., enema, bath, dressing change)	Time administered, equipment used (if appropriate), client's response (objective and subjective changes) compared to previous treatment; for example, "client denied pain during dressing change" or "client reported severe abdominal cramping during enema"
Medication administration	Time administered, preliminary assessment (e.g., pain level, vital signs), client response or effect of medication; for example, "client reports pain level 2 (scale 0-10) 30 minutes after Tylenol was given" or "pruritis and hives developed over lower abdomen 1 hour after penicillin was given"
Client teaching	Information presented, method of instruction (e.g., discussion, demonstration, videotape, booklet), client response, including questions and evidence of understanding such as return demonstration or change in behavior
Discharge planning	Client goals or expected outcomes, progress toward goals, need for referrals

relieved with elevation. Pedal pulses equal bilaterally. Right ankle circumference 1 cm larger than left. Ice applied. Percocet 2 tabs given for pain. Physician notified. Lee Turno, RN.

Current.   Timely entries are essential in the client's ongoing care (JCAHO, 1999b). To increase accuracy and decrease unnecessary duplication, many health care agencies use bedside records, which facilitate immediate documentation of information as it is collected from a client. Activities or findings to communicate at the time of occurrence include the following:

Vital signs

Administration of medications and treatments

Preparation for diagnostic tests or surgery

Change in status

Admission, transfer, discharge, or death of a client

Treatment for a sudden change in status

This information is often included in flow sheets kept at the bedside. Nurses often also keep a work sheet when caring for several clients, making notes as the care occurs to ensure that entries recorded later in the record are accurate. Most health care agencies use military time, a 24-hour system that avoids misinterpretation of AM and PM times (Figure 24-2). Instead of two 12-hour cycles in standard time, the military clock is one 24-hour time cycle. For example, 1:00 PM is 1300 military time; 10:22 AM is 1022 military time.

Organized.   The nurse communicates information in a logical order. For example, an organized note describes the client's pain, nurse's assessment and interventions, and the client's response. To write notes in an organized fashion the nurse needs to think about the situation and sometimes make notes of what is to be included before beginning to write in the permanent legal record.

STANDARDS

Documentation needs to follow JCAHO standards to maintain institutional accreditation and to lessen liability. Current standards require that all clients who are admitted to a health care institution have an assessment of physical, psychosocial, environmental, self-care, client education, and discharge planning needs (JCAHO, 1999b). In addition, the JCAHO stresses the importance of evaluating client outcomes, including the client's response to treatments, teaching, or preventive care.

The nursing service department of each health care agency selects the method that is used to document client care. The method reflects the philosophy of the nursing department and incorporates the standards of care. For example, if a nursing department's standards of practice use nursing diagnosis or a framework such as Gordon's functional health patterns (Gordon, 1998), the documentation system uses nursing diagnoses and health patterns in care plans and other forms.

Because the nursing process shapes a nurse's approach and direction of care, good documentation reflects the nursing process. Assessment data are recorded to offer to all health care team members a database from which to draw conclusions about the client's problems. Information describing the client's problems or diagnoses then directs caregivers to choose an appropriate care plan with nursing therapies. Evaluation of care communicates the client's status, degree of progress, and success in meeting expected outcomes of care.

The JCAHO requires documentation within the context of the nursing process, as well as evidence of client and family teaching and discharge planning. If more than one discipline regularly cares for a client, the JCAHO also expects a multidisciplinary care plan.

NARRATIVE DOCUMENTATION

Narrative documentation is the traditional method for recording nursing care. It is simply the use of a storylike format to document information specific to client conditions and nursing care. Narrative charting, however, has many disadvantages, including the tendency to have repetitious information, to be time consuming, and to require the reader to sort through much information to locate desired data.

Problem-Oriented Medical Records.   The **problem-oriented medical record (POMR)** is a method of documentation that places emphasis on the client's problems. Data are organized by problem or diagnosis. Ideally each member of the health care team contributes to a single list of identified client problems. This assists in coordinating a common plan of care. The POMR has the following major

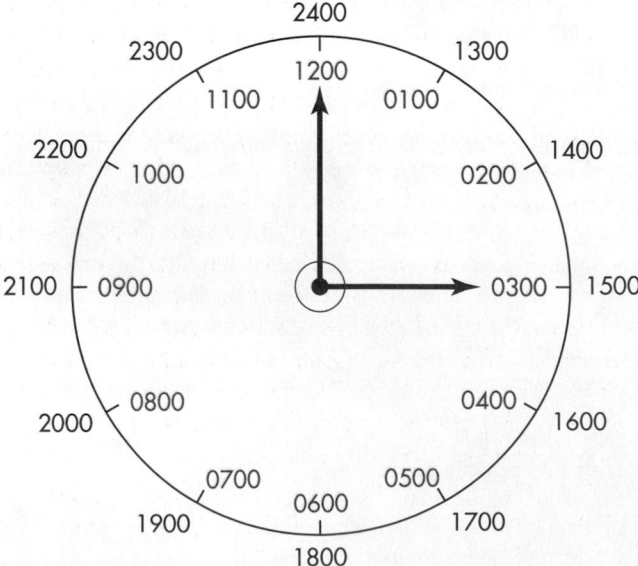

Figure 24-2   Military time clock.

sections: database, problem list, care plan, and progress notes.

Database.   The database section contains all available assessment information pertaining to the client (e.g., history and physical examination, the nurse's admission history and ongoing assessment, the dietitian's assessment, laboratory reports, and radiological test results). The database is the foundation for identifying client problems and planning care. As new data become available, the database is revised. It accompanies clients through successive hospitalizations or clinic visits.

Problem List.   After data are analyzed, problems are identified and a single list is made. The problems include the client's physiological, psychological, social, cultural, spiritual, developmental, and environmental needs. The problems are listed in chronological order and filed in the front of the client's record to serve as an organizing guide for the client's care. New problems are added as they are identified. When a problem has been resolved, the date is recorded and it is highlighted or a line is drawn through the problem and its number.

Nursing Care Plan.   A care plan is developed for each problem by the disciplines involved in the client's care (see Chapter 16). Nurses document the plan of care in a variety of formats. Generally these plans of care include nursing diagnoses, expected outcomes, and interventions.

Progress Notes.   Health care team members monitor and record the progress of a client's problems (Box 24-2). The information can be expressed in various formats of structured notes. One method is **SOAPIE:** S—subjective data (verbalizations of the client), O—objective data (that which is measured and observed), A—assessment (diagnosis based on the data), P—plan (what the caregiver plans to do), I—intervention, and E—evaluation. **SOAP** is also a format used.

   In the **PIE** format the assessment information is documented on special flow sheets. The narrative note includes P—problem, I—intervention, and E—evaluation. The PIE notes are numbered or labeled according to the client's problems. Resolved problems are dropped from daily documentation after the nurse's review. Continuing problems are documented daily.

   Focus charting or **DAR** notes include D—data (both subjective and objective), A—action or nursing intervention, and R—response of the client (i.e., evaluation of effectiveness). One distinction of focus charting is its movement away from charting only problems, which has a negative connotation. Instead the notes are structured according to client concerns: a sign or symptom, a condition, a nursing diagnosis, a behavior, a significant event, or a change in a client's condition. Documentation is written in accordance with the nursing process, nurses are en-

couraged to broaden their thinking to include any client concerns, not just problem areas, and critical thinking is encouraged. Focus charting is easily understood by caregivers and adaptable to most health care settings. Focus charting helps promote effective documentation (Lampe, 1994).

Source Records.   In a **source record** the client's chart is organized so that each discipline (e.g., nursing, medicine, social work, or respiratory therapy) has a separate section in which to record data. One advantage of a source record is that caregivers can easily locate the proper section of the record in which to make entries. Table 24-3 lists the components of a source record.

   A disadvantage of the source record is that information is not organized by client problems, so that details about a

---

Examples of Progress Notes Written in Different Formats   Box 24-2

SOAP

1/19/95 Knowledge deficit related to inexperience regarding surgery
4:30 PM
 S—"I'm worried about what it will be like after surgery."
 O—"Client asking frequent questions about surgery. Has had no previous experience with surgery. Wife present, acts as a support person.
 A—Knowledge deficit regarding surgery related to inexperience. Client also expressing anxiety.
 P—Explain routine preoperative preparation. Demonstrate and explain rationale for TCDB exercises. Provide explanation and teaching booklet on postoperative nursing care. S. Lazarus, RN

PIE

 P—Knowledge deficit regarding surgery related to inexperience.
 I—Explained to client normal preoperative preparations for surgery. Demonstrated TCDB exercises. Provided booklet to client on postoperative nursing care.
 E—Client demonstrates TCDB exercises correctly. Needs review of postoperative nursing care. S. Lazarus, RN

FOCUS CHARTING

 D—BP in left arm 90/60, client's skin diaphoretic, client responds to name.
 A—Placed client in Trendelenburg's position, increased IV fluid rate to 100 ml/hr per protocol, called Dr. Arkin.
 R—Client remains responsive, BP in left arm 94/68, 3 min after increasing fluids. S. Wilson, RN

 D—Twisting in bed, grimacing with movement, states has sharp lower back pain.
 A—Administered morphine sulfate 10 mg IM.
 R—Verbalized relief within 15 minutes, lying quietly. T. Newson, RN

Table 24-3 Organization of Traditional Source Record

Sections	Contents
Admission sheet	Specific demographic data about client: legal name, identification number, sex, age, birth date, marital status, occupation and employer, health insurance, nearest relative to notify in an emergency, religious preference, name of attending physician, date and time of admission
Physician's order sheet	Record of physician's orders for treatment and medications, with date, time, and physician's signature
Nurse's admission assessment	Summary of nursing history and physical examination
Graphic sheet and flow sheet	Record of repeated observations and measurements such as vital signs, daily weights, and intake and output
Medical history and examination	Results of initial examination performed by physician, including findings, family history, confirmed diagnoses, and medical plan of care
Nurses' notes	Narrative record of nursing process: assessment, nursing diagnosis, planning, implementation, and evaluation of care
Medication records	Accurate documentation of all medications administered to client: date, time, dose, route, and nurse's signature
Physician's progress notes	Ongoing record of client's progress and response to medical therapy and review of disease process
Health care discipline's records	Entries made into record by all health-related disciplines: radiology, social work, and laboratories
Discharge summary	Summary of client's condition, progress, prognosis, rehabilitation, and teaching needs at time of dismissal from hospital or health care agency

specific problem may be distributed throughout the record. For example, the nurse describes the character of abdominal pain and use of relaxation therapy and analgesic medication in the nurses' notes. The physician's notes describe the progress of the client's bowel obstruction and the plan for surgery in a separate section of the record. The results of x-ray examinations that show the location of the bowel obstruction are in the test results section of the record. The method by which source records are organized does not show how information from the disciplines is related or how care is coordinated to meet all of the client's needs.

The notes section is where nurses enter a narrative description of nursing care and the client's response (Box 24-3). It is also a section for documenting care that is provided by the physician in the nurse's presence. The nurse may record key diagnostic test results from other sections of the record in the nurses' notes if they are of major importance in the care of the client.

CHARTING BY EXCEPTION

Charting by exception is an innovative approach that is used to streamline documentation. Charting by exception reduces repetition and time spent in charting. It is a shorthand method for documenting normal findings and routine care based on clearly defined standards of practice and predetermined criteria for nursing assessments and interventions. Clearly defined standards of practice that specify nurses' responsibilities to clients provide the framework for routine care of all clients. With standards integrated into documentation forms, such as predefined

Sample Narrative Note   Box 24-3

8/6 1100   Client states, "I'm having a hard time catching my breath." Respirations, labored at 28/min; P, 96; BP, 112/70. Client using intercostal muscles during inhalation. Breath sounds auscultated, crackles over both lower lobes. Chest excursion equal bilaterally. Elevated head of bed to Fowler's position. Obtained arterial blood gas analysis at 1045 order. Results are pH, 7.34, PCO_2, 44 mm Hg; PO_2, 80 mm Hg. Dr. Stein called. Applied O_2 at 4 L/min per mask as ordered. Remained at bedside to calm client. P. Haske, RN

normal assessment findings or predetermined interventions, a nurse need only document significant findings or exceptions to the predefined norms. In other words, the nurse writes a progress note only when the standardized statement on the form is not met. Assessments are standardized on forms so that all caregivers evaluate and document findings consistently (Figure 24-3).

Because the standard assessments are located in the chart, client data are already present on the permanent record, so nurses do not have to keep temporary notes for later transcription and caregivers have easy access to current data. The assumption with charting by exception is that all standards are met unless otherwise documented. When nurses see entries in the chart, they know that something out of the ordinary has been observed or has

BARNES-JEWISH HOSPITAL

Nursing Shift Assessment C-6

Requested by: CAROL

789651458 X

Collins, Phil

S.S.

Dr.

Unit: Bed:

Search Interval   From: 05-Dec-1999 at 07:00
                  To: 06-Dec-1999 at 14:51

Patient Assessment

		Monday 12/06 07:00
N/S	**NEUROSENSORY STANDARD** Alert and awake. If asleep awakens to name. Verbal appropriate, clear, and understandable. Swallows without coughing. Oriented to time, place, person and situation. Behavior is appropriate to situation. Moves all extremities well, ambulates with steady gait.	Within Normal Limits
RESP	**RESPIRATORY STANDARD** Respirations are even and unlabored. Nailbeds and mucous membranes are pink. Patent airway. Lung sounds clear to auscultation. No cough noted	Within Normal Limits
CARD	**CARDIOVASCULAR STANDARD** Regular palpable pulses. Skin pallor within patient's norm. Skin warm and dry. No edema.	Within Normal Limits
SKIN	**SKIN INTEGRITY STANDARD** Skin and mucous membranes intact without notable lesions or impaired integrity. Mucous membranes moist and pink. Braden Score greater than 17.	* Exception as noted below
	Braden Risk Assessment	Mobility: Slightly Limited (3) Sensory: Slightly Limited (3) Moisture: Occasionally Moist (3) Activity: Walks Occasionally (3) Nutrition: Adequate (3) Friction/Shear: Potential Problem (2) Total Score 17
	Casts, Splints, Braces Type:Fiberglass Cast Site:Right Lower Leg	Maintains correct anatomical position No pressure areas noted Distal extremity pink warm to touch Palpable distal pulse Capillary Refill <3 seconds Sensation normal Able to move distal phalanges.
	VASCULAR ACCESS STANDARD IV SITE: Site free of redness, swelling, pain, bleeding, drainage, IV patent, dressing occlusive and intact.	
NUTR	**NUTRITION STANDARD** Tolerating prescribed diet without nausea and vomiting. Eating at least 75% of each meal without difficulty. Feeds self.	Within normal limits
	Diet Type	Regular
GI	**GASTROINTESTINAL STANDARD** Abdomen soft. Bowel sounds active all 4 quadrants. No pain with palpation. Having bowel movements within patient's normal pattern, consistency, and color.	Within Normal Limits
CU	**GENITOURINARY STANDARD** Continent of urine. Urine clear and yellow to amber color.	Within Normal Limits
PSYCH	**PSYCHOSOCIAL STANDARD** Accepts situation and facial expressions are appropriate. Family support available and patient receives visitors. Able to communicate without assistance.	Within Normal Limits
EDU	Health Status Teaching	
	Tests/Procedures/Therapies	
	Medication Teaching	
	Nutrition Teaching	
	Medical Equipment Teaching	
HMGT	Equipment	
	Charted By	cl

Signatures:
cl   C. Logan, rn

Printed: 06-Dec-1999 at 14:51

Figure 24-3 Nursing care record.
Courtesy Barnes-Jewish Hospital, St. Louis, Mo.

BARNES

**CARE PATH® 405
MULTIPLE SCLEROSIS
EXACERBATION**

SERVICE NEUROLOGY	PHYSICIAN
PRIMARY NURSE	PRIMARY NURSE

DC DATE	ADM DATE	DATE OF SURGERY	A-8

Problem Number	PATIENT PROBLEMS / NURSING DIAGNOSES
#1	SELF CARE DEFICIT R/T MUSCLE WEAKNESS, PAIN, COORDINATION OR PARALYSIS
#2	IMPAIRED PHYSICAL MOBILITY R/T MUSCLE WEAKNESS
#3	ALTERATION IN ELIMINATION R/T NEUROMUSCULAR IMPAIRMENT
#4	LACK OF KNOWLEDGE R/T UNFAMILIARITY WITH TREATMENT AND DISEASE PROCESS

* IF APPROPRIATE

DATE #	1, 2 ASSESSMENT / MONITORING	1, 2 CONSULTS	3 PROCEDURES / TEST	1, 2, 3 TREATMENT	1 ACTIVITY
DAY 1	Assess for fall prevention Assess for skin breakdown Assess neuro status and information processing Assess urinary elimination Assess bowel function VS q shift with NC Notify House Officer for Temp ≥ 37.9 Malaise, change in bladder habits, weakness Monitor VS q 30 min. during 1st dose of Solumedrol infusion. House Officer to remain with pt. for 1st 15 min. of infusion.	Physical Therapy evaluation *Occupational Therapy *Social Work *Pastoral Care *Speech-communication and swallow	EKG prior to 1st dose of Solumedrol and after 1st dose completed *MRI *LP Straight cath for PVR *Straight cath q 6 hrs. Guaiac all stools Notify House Officer if + on guaiac Monitor blood glucose 2 hrs. after Solumedrol Notify House Officer if ≥ 250 I & O	Urinalysis	Up with assist Out of bed in chair at least TID for ½ hr. periods
DAY 2	Assess for fall prevention Assess for skin breakdown Assess neuro status and information processing Assess urinary elimination Assess bowel function Notify House Officer if no BM after 48 hrs. VS routine with NC Notify House Officer for Temp ≥ 37.9 Malaise, change in bladder habits, weakness **Skin remains intact** **Pt. maintains bowel function** **Pt. remains free of injury**	Evaluation completed Frequency of tx and pain established Social Work-Consult Occupational Therapy to address functional performance *Foot care nurse if indicated	Speech-Functional communication established Bedside swallow evaluation completed within 24 hrs. **Stool remains guaiac negative**		

SIGNATURE	INIT.	SIGNATURE	INIT.	SIGNATURE	INIT.

405

Figure 24-4   Critical path for multiple sclerosis exacerbation.
Courtesy Barnes-Jewish Hospital, St. Louis, Mo.

					2

BARNES
CARE PATH® 405 MULTIPLE SCLEROSIS EXACERBATION

CNS	DIETARY	RT
HOME HEALTH	OT	OTHER
PT	SW	OTHER

A-8

Problem Number	PATIENT PROBLEMS / NURSING DIAGNOSES

1, 2, 3	2	4	1, 2, 3, 4	1, 2, 4	INITIALS (SEE KEY AT BOTTOM)		
MEDS / IVS	NUTRITION	PATIENT / FAMILY EDUCATION	DISCHARGE PLANNING	PSYCHOSOCIAL/ EMOTIONAL/ SPIRITUAL NEEDS			
IV-Hep lock flush q shift with NS Solumedrol 250mg/100cc NS q 6 hrs.-given over ½-1 hr. times 12-30 doses Zantac 150 mg PO BID Oscal 500 mg with Vit. D - 1 tab BID Docusate Sodium 100 mg q hs Mylanta 30cc PO pc and hs Dalmane 15-30 mg or Restoril 15-30 mg q hs	*Low sodium Advance diet as tolerated Maintain hydration	Orient to unit Provide information on Solumedrol therapy **Pt. verbalizes understanding of Solumedrol Protocol and IV Therapy**	**Pt./family understands goal of therapy. Pt./family verbalizes understanding of disease process. Pt./family understands safety needs. Pt./family verbalizes understanding of care path. Plan of care has been mutually set with pt./family.**	*Social Work for crises intervention *Pastoral Care- emotional and spiritual			
Evaluate time schedule for Solumedrol to minimize sleep interruption	**Pt. caloric needs met body weight maintained. Pt. adequate fluid intake of 3,000/day.**		Social Work- consult with nursing, MD, and therapists to assess pt. needs. Social Work assessment completed.	Pastoral Care- Pt./family support needs assessed. **Social Work- high risk screening form completed.**			

SIGNATURE	INIT.	SIGNATURE	INIT.	SIGNATURE	INIT.

Figure 24-4, cont'd Critical path for multiple sclerosis exacerbation.

occurred. For that reason when changes in a client's condition have developed, it is easy to track them.

Charting by exception can pose legal risks if nurses are not disciplined in documenting exceptions. This is particularly important when clients' conditions change. Thorough and precise descriptions of what happens to clients and the actions taken are essential.

CASE MANAGEMENT AND CRITICAL PATHWAYS

The **case management** model of delivering care (see Chapter 2) incorporates a multidisciplinary approach to documenting client care. In many organizations the standardized plan of care is summarized into critical pathways for a specific disease or condition. The **critical pathways** are multidisciplinary care plans that include key interventions and expected outcomes within an established time frame. The nurse and other team members such as physicians, dietitians, social workers, physical therapists, and respiratory therapists use the same critical pathway to monitor the client's progress during each shift or in the case of home care, every visit. Critical pathways reduce duplication and the amount of charting (Woodyard and Sheetz, 1993). In general the critical pathway identifies the expected outcomes for each day of care (Figure 24-4). Unexpected occurrences, unmet goals, and interventions not specified within the clinical pathway time frame are called **variances** (Eggland, 1995). A negative variance occurs when the activities on the clinical pathway are not completed as predicted or the client does not meet the expected outcomes. An example of a negative variance is when a postoperative client develops pulmonary complications requiring oxygen therapy and monitoring with pulse oximetry. A positive variance occurs when a client progresses more rapidly than expected (e.g., use of a Foley catheter may be discontinued a day early). A variance

analysis is necessary to review the data for trends and for developing and implementing an action plan to respond to the identified client problems (Box 24-4). In addition, variances may result from changes in the client's health or may occur as a result of other health complications not associated with the primary reason for which the client requires care (Hospital Case Management, 1993). The nurse's responsibility is to address the variance and to justify the actions taken to manage the critical pathway deviation (Iyer and Camp, 1999). Over time, the reoccurrence of similar variances may lead the health care team to revise a critical pathway.

COMMON RECORD-KEEPING FORMS

A variety of forms are available that are specially designed for the type of information nurses routinely document. The categories within a form are usually derived from institutional standards of practice or guidelines established by accrediting agencies.

Nursing History.   A nursing history form is completed when a client is admitted to a nursing care unit. The history form guides the nurse through a complete assessment to identify relevant nursing diagnoses or problems (see Chapter 14). Data on history forms provide baseline data that can be compared with changes in the client's condition. Each institution designs a nursing history form differently, based on the standards of practice and philosophy of nursing care.

Graphic Sheets and Flow Sheets.   **Flow sheets** are forms that allow nurses to assess the client and document vital signs and routine repetitive care, such as bath, ambulation, meals, weights, and safety and restraint checks, quickly and effectively using a coding system (Figure 24-5). If something on the flow sheet is unusual or changes significantly a focus note is needed. For example, if a client's blood pressure becomes dangerously high, the nurse completes a focus assessment and records this as well as action taken in the progress notes. Flow sheets provides a quick, easy reference for the health care team members in assessing a client's status. Critical care and acute care units commonly use flow sheets for all types of physiological data (Box 24-5).

Nursing Kardex.   In some settings information that is needed for the daily care of clients is readily accessible in the nursing Kardex (see Chapter 16). The **Kardex** is a form or card that is kept in a portable "flip-over" file or notebook at the nurses' station. Most Kardex forms have two parts, an activity and treatment section and a nursing care plan section, that organize information for quick reference as nurses give change-of-shift reports or make walking rounds. An updated Kardex eliminates the need for repeated referral to the chart for routine information throughout the day. In many institutions Kardex entries

---

Example of Variance Documentation   Box 24-4

A 56-year-old client is on a surgical unit 1 day after cholecystectomy. He is beginning to have an elevated temperature, his breath sounds are decreased bilaterally in the bases of both lobes of the lungs, and he is slightly confused. Ordinarily, 1 day after surgery the client should be afebrile with lungs clear. The following is an example of the variance documentation for this client.

9/23/xx 1000   Breath sounds diminished bilaterally at the bases. T, 100.4; P, 92; R, 24/min; oxygen sat, 84. Daughter states he is "confused" and did not recognize her when she arrived a few minutes ago. Oxygen started at 2 L per standing orders. Will monitor pulse oximetry and vital signs every 15 minutes. Physician notified of change in status. Daughter at bedside.

are done in pencil because of the need for frequent revisions as the client's needs change. In settings in which the Kardex is a permanent part of the client's record, entries are made in ink.

Information commonly found in the Kardex includes the following:

Basic demographic data (e.g., age and religion)

Primary medical diagnosis

Current physician's treatment orders to be carried out by the nurse (e.g., dressing changes, ambulation, glucose monitoring)

Nursing orders (e.g., education sessions, symptom relief measures, counseling)

Scheduled tests and procedures

Safety precautions to be used in the client's care

Factors related to activities of daily living

Acuity Recording Systems.

Staffing patterns can be determined by measuring and documenting the acuity levels of the clients on a particular nursing unit. The client-to-staff ratios established for a unit depend on a composite gathering of data for the 24-hour interventions that are necessary for each client receiving care. **Acuity recording** requires that staff assign a numerical rating scale to interventions, thereby obtaining a numeric level of acuity for each client. For example, an acuity system might rate bathing clients from 1 to 5 (1 is totally dependent, 5 is independent). A client returning from surgery requiring frequent monitoring and extensive care may be listed with an acuity level of 1. On the same continuum another client awaiting discharge after a successful recovery from surgery has an acuity level of 5. Accurate acuity ratings are necessary to justify over time the numbers and qualifications of staff needed to safely care for clients.

Standardized Care Plans.

Many institutions have attempted to make documentation easier for nurses with **standardized care plans.** The plans, based on the institution's standards of nursing practice, are preprinted, established guidelines that are used to care for clients who have similar health problems. After a nursing assessment is completed, the staff nurse identifies the standard care plans that are appropriate for the client. The care plans are placed in the client's medical record. Modifications can be made in ink to the standardized plans to individualize the

therapies. Most standardized care plans also allow the nurse to write in specific goals or desired outcomes of care and the dates by which these outcomes should be achieved.

One advantage of standardized care plans is establishment of clinically sound standards of care for similar groups of clients. These standards can be useful when quality improvement audits are conducted. Another advantage is education. Nurses learn to recognize the accepted requirements of care for clients. The standardized care plans can also improve continuity of care among professional nurses.

The use of standardized care plans is controversial. The major disadvantage is the risk that the standardized plans inhibit nurses' identification of unique, individualized therapies for clients. When standardized care plans are used in a health care facility, the nurse remains responsible for an individualized approach to care. Standardized care plans cannot replace the nurse's professional judgment and decision making. In addition, care plans need to be updated on a regular basis to ensure that content is current and appropriate. There is the trend among many hospitals to computerize care plans. With such a system, daily computer-generated care plans are printed and incorporate several nursing diagnoses or problems in a single care plan. Such a system facilitates the process of revision and individualization of plans.

Discharge Summary Forms.

Much emphasis is placed on preparing a client for an efficient, timely discharge from a health care institution. A prospective payment system based on DRGs encourages health care institutions to be more efficient and to discharge the client as soon as possible. However, it is important to ensure that a client's discharge results in desirable outcomes. The earlier a client is discharged, the more likely it is that a hospital will be fully reimbursed. Multidisciplinary involvement in discharge planning helps to ensure that a client leaves the hospital in a timely manner with the necessary resources.

Ideally discharge planning begins at admission. Nurses revise the plan of care as the client's condition changes. There needs to be evidence of the involvement of the client and family members in the discharge planning process so that the client and family have the necessary information and resources to return home. The *JCAHO* (1999a) has established standards for client education necessary for effective discharge planning:

Instruction in potential food-drug interactions, nutrition intervention, and modified diets

Rehabilitation techniques to support adaptation to and/or functional independence in the environment

Access to available community resources

When and how to obtain further treatment or follow-up care

The client's and family's responsibilities in the client's care

Oregon Health Sciences University
Hospitals and Clinics

ACUTE CARE
24 HOUR FLOW SHEET
4 YEARS TO ADULT

ACCOUNT NO.
MED. REC. NO.
NAME
BIRTHDATE

DATE ______________ WEIGHT ________________ YESTERDAY'S WEIGHT ______________

ISOLATION ______________________________________

TIME																									
F C																									F C
103.1 39.5																									103.1 39.5
102.2 39.0																									102.2 39.0
101.3 38.5																									101.3 38.5
100.4 38.0																									100.4 38.0
99.5 37.5																									99.5 37.5
98.6 37.0																									98.6 37.0
97.7 36.5																									97.7 36.5
96.8 36.0																									96.8 36.0
95.9 35.6																									95.9 35.6
95.0 35.0																									95.0 35.0
PULSE RADIAL																									PAIN LEVEL
PULSE APICAL																									
RESP.																									0-NONE
B/P																									10-SEVERE
PAIN																									
SA O_2 O_2																									

	DAYS / INITIALS: RN: CNA:		EVENINGS / INITIALS: RN: CNA:		NIGHTS / INITIALS: RN: CNA:
HYGIENE	☐ BED BATH ☐ SHOWER ☐ ORAL CARE ☐ CATHETER CARE COMMENTS:______	HYGIENE	☐ BED BATH ☐ SHOWER ☐ ORAL CARE ☐ CATHETER CARE COMMENTS:______	HYGIENE	☐ BED BATH ☐ SHOWER ☐ ORAL CARE ☐ CATHETER CARE COMMENTS:______
ACTIVITY	☐ BED REST CHAIR:______ AMBULATE:______SLEEP:_____HRS COMMENTS:______	ACTIVITY	☐ BED REST CHAIR:______ AMBULATE:______SLEEP:_____HRS COMMENTS:______	ACTIVITY	☐ BED REST CHAIR:______ AMBULATE:______SLEEP:_____HRS COMMENTS:______
SAFETY	☐ SAFETY POLICY ☐ RESTRAINTS TYPE:______ ☐ SITTER COMMENTS:______	SAFETY	☐ SAFETY POLICY ☐ RESTRAINTS TYPE:______ ☐ SITTER COMMENTS:______	SAFETY	☐ SAFETY POLICY ☐ RESTRAINTS TYPE:______ ☐ SITTER COMMENTS:______

	BREAKFAST	LUNCH	DINNER
DIET			
% TAKEN			
% SNACKS			
ASSIST (S - SELF, P-PARTIAL, F - FEED)			

RESOURCES/EQUIPMENT USED TO PROVIDE PATIENT CARE:
SCD ☐ K PAD ☐ TRAPEZE ☐ __________ ☐
NUMBER OF IV PUMPS SINGLE ________ DOUBLE ________
NUMBER OF SUCTION UNIITS ________
SPECIAL BED ________
OTHER ________

8.1-4A (1) (10/94) 0748-1054

8.1-4A (1)

Figure 24-5 Twenty-four hour client care record.
Courtesy Oregon Health Sciences University Hospitals and Clinics, Portland, Ore.

DATE:					
START DATE/ TIME	STANDARDS AND INTERVENTIONS	✔ — ASSESSMENT STANDARD OR PROTOCOL MET. INTERVENTION CARRIED OUT	✳ — VARIANCE FROM STANDARDS OR ORDERED INTERVENTIONS. SEE NARRATIVE ENTRY.	→ — VARIANCES REMAIN. NO CHANGES FROM LAST NARRATIVE ENTRY.	

RN INITIALS

ASSESSMENT STANDARDS

PROTOCOLS / INTERVENTIONS

TEACHING

ASSESSMENT STANDARDS: ADULTS AND PEDIATRIC PATIENTS ABOVE 4 YEARS.   All normal assessments include patient without subjective

NORMAL NEUROLOGICAL ASSESSMENT:
- alert and oriented X3 (person, place, time)
- behavior appropriate to situation
- PERL
- full range of motion with symmetry of strength
- no paresthesia
- verbalization clear and coherent
- swallows without coughing or choking on liquids or solids
- gait steady if patient ambulatory
- clear vision (corrective lenses allowable)

PEDIATRIC:
- alert and oriented appropriately for developmental age
- verbalization/vocalization appropriate for developmental age
- tracks and recognizes objects appropriately for developmental age (if unable to assess clear vision)

NORMAL RESPIRATORY ASSESSMENT:
- rate appropriate for age while at rest
- respirations quiet, regular and unlabored
- equal and clear breath sounds over both lung fields
- nail beds and mucous membranes pink
- sputum and nasal drainage clear if present

NORMAL CARDIOVASCULAR ASSESSMENT:
- regular apical or radial pulse
- capillary refill less than 3 seconds
- no edema
- peripheral pulse palpable and of equal quality
- pink nail beds and mucous membranes

NORMAL GASTROINTESTINAL ASSESSMENT:
- abdomen soft and non-distended
- no pain with palpation
- bowel tones present
- tolerates prescribed diet without problem
- bowel movements appropriate in color, volume, and consistency for intake
- if NG present, drainage clear to light green in color, heme negative
- continent

NORMAL GENITOURINARY ASSESSMENT:
- able to empty bladder q shift without urgency, frequency, pain, or post-void feeling of fullness or distention
- urine clear yellow to amber without foul odor.
- absence of vaginal or penile drainage
- continent
- if catheter present, patent and draining freely.

PEDIATRIC: urine output 1-3 cc/kg/hour

NORMAL NEUROVASCULAR (CMS) ASSESSMENT:
- pink nail beds
- warm
- full range of motion
- capillary refill less than 3 seconds
- palpable peripheral pulses
- no edema
- no paresthesia

NORMAL MUSCULOSKELETAL ASSESSMENT:
- absence of joint tenderness, swelling, redness, or increased temperature
- full range of motion all joints
- no muscle weakness

NORMAL INTEGUMENTARY ASSESSMENT:
- skin color consistent with race
- skin warm, dry, and intact
- mucous membranes moist and without lesions
- no rashes, petechiae, or purpura
- no signs of infestation

Figure 24-5, cont'd Twenty-four hour client care record.

Medication instructions, including when to take each medication and why, the dose, the route, precautions and possible adverse reactions, and when and how to get prescriptions refilled

In addition to the JCAHO standards, a common standard in nursing practice is to educate clients about the nature of their disease process, its likely progress, and the signs and symptoms of complications to look out for (Eggland, 1995).

When a client is discharged from inpatient care, a discharge summary is prepared by the various members of the health care team and given to the client or family, or home health care, rehabilitation, or long-term care agency (JCAHO, 1999). Discharge summary forms (Figure 24-6) make the summary concise and instructive. A summary form emphasizes previous learning by the client and family and care that should be continued in any restorative care setting. When given directly to clients the form may be attached to pamphlets or teaching brochures.

HOME HEALTH CARE DOCUMENTATION

The home health care business continues to grow with shorter hospitalizations and larger numbers of older adults requiring home health care services. Medicare has specific guidelines for establishing eligibility for home health care reimbursement. In the fulfillment of these Medicare guidelines, documentation by home health care nurses has become a concern: 50% of the nursing time is spent in documentation (Braunstein, 1993).

Documentation in the home health care system has different implications than in other areas of nursing. One primary difference is that the majority of care is witnessed by the client and family rather than the nurse. Nurses must have astute assessment skills to gather the needed information about changes in the client's health care status. In addition, documentation systems need to provide the entire health care team with the necessary information to be able to work together effectively (Box 24-6). The docu-

---

Home Health Care Forms for Documentation   Box 24-6

The usual forms used to document home care include:
Client assessment
Referral source information/intake form
Discipline-specific care plans
Physician's plan of treatment
Medication sheet
Clinical progress notes
Miscellaneous (conference notes, verbal order forms, telephone calls)
Discharge summary
Reports to third-party payers

Modified from Iyer PW, Camp NH: *Nursing documentation: a nursing process approach*, St. Louis, 1999, Mosby.

---

mentation is both the quality control and the justification for reimbursement from Medicare, Medicaid, or private insurance companies. Nurses need to document all their services for payment (e.g., direct skilled care, client instructions, skilled observation, and evaluation visits) (JCAHO, 1999a).

Some parts of the record are needed in the home with the client; other information is needed in an office setting. Thus duplication of documentation is necessary, or agency policies are needed regarding what forms nurses need to leave at their office versus what forms need to be taken into the homes. Computerized client records are evolving as one means of addressing these different needs. With the use of modems and laptop computers it is becoming possible for the records to be available in multiple locations, which allows greater access to the multidisciplinary needs that are often present in home health care.

LONG-TERM HEALTH CARE DOCUMENTATION

An increasing number of older adults require care in long-term health care facilities. Since many individuals will live in this setting for the rest of their lives, they are referred to as **residents** rather than clients. Nursing personnel face challenges much different from those in the acute care setting, which require a significantly different basis for nursing documentation (Iyer and Camp, 1999).

In long-term care, governmental agencies are instrumental in determining the standards and policies for documentation. For example, the Omnibus Budget Reconciliation Act of 1987 included extremely significant Medicare and Medicaid legislation for long-term care documentation, including assessments, individualized care plans, and qualifications for health care providers (e.g., registered nurses, licensed practical nurses, nurse's aides). In addition, the department of health in each state governs the frequency of written nursing records of the residents in long-term care facilities. Since residents are often stable, daily documentation is done using flow sheets. Assessments done several times a day in the acute care setting may be required only weekly or monthly in the long-term care setting.

Long-term care agencies are also developing skilled care units with clients requiring increased levels of care in response to the demands for shorter hospital stays. Long-term care documentation supports a multidisciplinary approach in the assessment and planning process. Communication among such health care providers as nurses, social workers, recreational therapists, and dietitians is essential in the regulated documentation process. The fiscal support for long-term care residents hinges on the justification of nursing care as demonstrated in documentation of the services rendered.

COMPUTERIZED DOCUMENTATION

Nurses have been using computerized systems for supplies, equipment, stock medications, and diagnostic test-

Barnes Hospital

PATIENT DISCHARGE SUMMARY

C-16

Date 10/17/--   Time _____ 1030

MEANS: ☐ Ambulatory ☒ Wheelchair ☐ Stretcher

METHODS: ☒ M.D. order ☐ AMA with release ☐ AMA with release   Addressograph Plate

Afebrile 24 hours? ☒ Yes ☐ No   TPR 36⁸-72-16 _____   B/P 124/72 _____

☐ Physician notified of irregularities

DISCHARGED TO: ☐ Home   ☐ Nursing Home   ☒ Home with Home Health Care   ☐ Other

   If discharged to Nursing Home or other facility/service:

   Name _____   Address/Phone _____

☐ Release of information form signed   ☐ Chart copied   ☐ Transfer form completed   ☐ Transportation Arranged

DISCHARGE CONSIDERATIONS:

☐ Valuables from cashier   ☐ PTA meds returned   ☐ Scripts given
☒ NA   ☒ NA   ☒ NA

DISCHARGE INSTRUCTIONS

FOR PROBLEMS OR FOLLOW-UP:

   Physician Dr. Stan Jones _____   Phone 362-5000   Appt. 10/24/91 _____

   Other: _____

   _____

Activity: __To remain in bed with Ⓛ foot elevated on two pillows. May be up only__ to go to the bathroom.

Diet: __To follow 1800 calorie ADA diet as instructed by the dietitian. For questions__ about diet, call the dietitian (Sue Marlin) 362-3184.

Medications: __To take usual dosage of 30 units NPH insulin and 8 units of regular__ insulin every morning before breakfast.

Wound Care: __Change dressings to Ⓛ foot daily using moistened fine mesh gauze__ with dry 4x4 gauze and wrap dressings with 4 kling gauze.

Teaching Materials Given: __Copy of "Controlling Your Diabetes" and "Diabetic Menu__ Planning."

Special Instructions: __Call doctor for increased pain, redness, swelling or drainage from__ Ⓛ foot wound. Barnes Home Health nurses will be visiting daily to change dressing to Ⓛ foot.

My discharge instructions have been explained and a copy has been given to me.

Patient/Significant Other *John Owens* _____   Relation HUSBAND _____

Nurse B. Rand, RN _____

Figure 24-6 Discharge summary form.
Courtesy Barnes-Jewish Hospital, St. Louis, Mo.

ing for some time. In some settings nurses are also using computerized documentation. Software programs allow nurses to quickly enter specific assessment data, and the information is automatically transferred to different reports. Computers also help generate nursing care plans and document all facets of client care.

Computer systems have not been limited to facilities with major expenditure budgets. Rural health care organizations have shown that, despite fiscal constraints, commercially available software is affordable. A 53-bed hospital in Jefferson, Iowa, was able to implement a sophisticated, computerized, client-centered documentation system. A community acquired immunodeficiency syndrome (AIDS) clinic in Santa Clara, California, implemented computerized documentation in its telephone triage system (Henry and others, 1994). The high volume of client contacts made computerized documentation a valuable tool for the triage nurses.

Computerized documentation systems are drastically changing. Typical user interfaces (e.g., keyboard and monitor) require typing skills and can result in data entry errors. **Graphic user interfaces** (e.g., touch pads, mouse, and icons) are not well suited for nursing. Pen-based or **automated speech-recognition** (ASR) or voice-recognition technology may eventually become extremely effective for nursing documentation (Box 24-7). A notebook-sized computer is available, allowing nurses to document with ease and flexibility not possible in the current systems (Trofino, 1993).

The development of a complete **computer-based patient care record** (CPCR) is envisioned as a trend for client records. The CPCR will be a comprehensive system that uses many components of data collection. The idea for this system of record keeping stemmed from the Computer-Based Patient Record Institute, which was formed in 1992. This group comprised vendors, health care providers, and professional organizations. The new CPCR provides a much broader scope than the current charting systems (Box 24-8). The CPCR permits the nurse to have an instrumental role in development of this form of documentation (Simpson, 1991a, 1991b).

There are legal risks associated with computerized documentation. Any given person could theoretically access a computer station within a hospital and gain information on almost any client. Confidentiality of access to computerized records is a major issue. Security requires the use of a password to enter and sign off computer files. A good system requires periodic changes in personal passwords to prevent unauthorized persons from tampering with records. In addition, most staff have access only to clients in their work area. Select staff may be given authority to access all client records.

Nurses need to know how to correct charting errors on a computer. As with any documentation method, data that has been part of the record is not deleted. Incorrect entries must be corrected, indicating who made the correction and when.

The transition to computerized documentation presents both opportunities and challenges to nurses and nurse managers (Figure 24-7). The successful implementation of a computerized documentation system requires preparation, involvement, and commitment of the entire nursing staff.

Benefits of Automated Speech-Recognition (ASR) Technology   Box 24-7

The following are benefits of ASR:

Comprehensive nursing documentation with minimal nursing effort

Decreased charting errors and omissions

Consistent documentation patterns

Increased interdisciplinary communication

Considerable time savings for the nurse

Clear, concise, legible documentation

Increased compliance with Joint Commission on Accreditation of Healthcare Organization standards (written into the software)

Objectives of Computer-Based Patient Care Recording (CPCR)   Box 24-8

Improved uniformity, accuracy, and retrievability of data about client care

Confidentiality of health care information ensured in the system

Access for authorized health care providers from any department

Ability to retrieve information selectively and choose various formats for examining it

Assistance with clinical application, including analysis tools, risk assessment, and clinical reminders

Support for data collection in a manner that adequately supports health care providers' direct entry and stores information according to a defined vocabulary

Easy access to client data, fast retrieval, and versatile data display that facilitates improved health care delivery

Availability of a lifelong record of health-related events incorporating records from various settings and time periods

Modified from National Coordination Office for Computing, Information, and Communications: *High Performance Computing and Communications FY 1997 Implementation plan,* Washington, DC, 1996, U.S. Government Printing Office; http://www.ccic.gov/pubs/imp97/136.html.

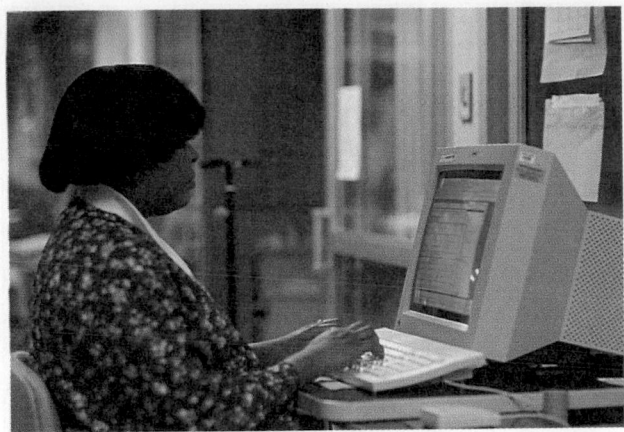

Figure 24-7 Computerized documentation systems can improve uniformity, accuracy, and retrievability of data.

Reporting

Nurses communicate information about clients so that all team members can make appropriate decisions about their care. Four types of reports made by nurses are change-of-shift reports, telephone reports, transfer reports, and incident reports.

CHANGE-OF-SHIFT REPORTS

At the end of each shift nurses report information about their assigned clients to the nurses working on the next shift. The purpose of the report is to provide continuity of care among nurses who are caring for a client. For example, if one nurse finds a certain pain-relief measure effective for a client, it is important that the information be relayed to the next nurse caring for the client so that pain-control interventions can be continued.

A **change-of-shift report** may be given orally in person, by audiotape recording, or during "walking-planning" rounds at each client's bedside. Oral reports are given in conference rooms, with staff members from both shifts participating. An advantage of oral reports is that it allows staff members to ask questions or clarify explanations. When nurses make rounds, the client and family members also have the opportunity to participate in any decisions. The nurses can see the client together to perform needed assessments, evaluate progress, and discuss the interventions best suited to the client's needs. An audiotape report is given by the nurse who has completed care for the client and is left for the nurse on the next shift to review. Taped reports can improve efficiency by allowing staff to report when time is available.

Because of the many responsibilities nurses have to assume, it is important that a change-of-shift report be conducted quickly and efficiently (Table 24-4). A good report describes clients' health status and lets staff on the next shift know exactly what kind of care the clients will require. A change-of-shift report should not simply be a reading of the client's Kardex. The Kardex is readily available to read by all staff. Instead, significant facts about clients are reviewed (e.g., the condition of wounds or episodes of chest pain) to provide a baseline for comparison during the next shift. Data about clients need to be objective, current, and concise.

An organized report follows a logical sequence. To prepare for the report, the nurse gathers information from work sheets, the client's Kardex (if used), and the client's care plan. A systematic approach such as using the nursing process can provide staff with critical information that is needed to continue care. The following is an example of a change-of-shift report:

Background information: Cy Tolan in bed 4, a 32-year-old client of Dr. Lang, is scheduled for a colon resection this morning. He has had ulcerative colitis for 2 years. He was admitted last night with slight abdominal discomfort. This is his first experience with surgery. He knows he may require a colostomy.

Assessment: Mr. Tolan expressed difficulty falling asleep last night. He had several questions about surgery. Early in the night he called for assistance several times.

Nursing diagnosis: His chief nursing care problems are anxiety related to inexperience with surgery and risk for body image disturbance.

Teaching plan: He asks appropriate questions about surgery. Staff on evenings explained postoperative routines. I reinforced information with him early in the night. He stated that he felt less anxious.

Treatments: A cleansing enema was administered until clear at 9 PM; no blood was noted in the return. He complained of some abdominal cramping immediately afterward, but that subsided. He received a Dalmane 15 mg PO at 11:30 PM, and I gave him a back rub. He was awake at 6:30 AM and stated he slept OK.

Family information: His wife remained with him last evening until the end of visiting hours. She has returned and is in the room this morning.

Discharge plan: Mr. Tolan is a very active person at home. He plays tennis and basketball and swims. Mrs. Tolan is concerned about how he might react to a colostomy. I suggest making a referral to the enterostomal therapist early, if the colostomy is performed.

Priority needs: Right now, Mr. Tolan is relaxing in his room. The operative permit has been signed. All preoperative procedures have been completed except for his preop medications, due on call to the operating room.

When giving a report, the nurse discusses clients or family members in a professional manner. It is often necessary to describe the interactions among clients, nurses, and fam-

Table 24-4 **Comparison of Do's and Dont's of Change-of-Shift Report**	
Do's	**Dont's**
Provide only essential background information about client (i.e., name, sex, age, physician's diagnosis, and medical history).	Don't review all routine care procedures or tasks (e.g., bathing, scheduled changes).
Identify client's nursing diagnosis or health care problems and their related causes.	Don't review all biographical information already available on Kardex.
Describe objective measurements or observations about client's condition and response to health problem: emphasize recent changes.	Don't use critical comments about client's behavior, such as "Mrs. Wills is so demanding."
Share significant information about family members as it relates to client's problems.	Don't make assumptions about relationships between family members.
Continuously review ongoing discharge plan (e.g., need for resources, client's level of preparation to go home).	Don't engage in idle gossip.
Relay to staff significant changes in the way therapies are given (e.g., different position for pain relief, new medication).	Don't describe basic steps of a procedure.
Describe instructions given in teaching plan and client's response.	Don't explain detailed content unless staff members ask for clarification.
Evaluate results of nursing or medical care measures (e.g., effect of back rub or analgesic administration).	Don't simply describe results as "good" or "poor." Be specific.
Be clear about priorities to which oncoming staff must attend.	Don't force oncoming staff to guess what to do first.

ily members in behavioral terms. The nurse needs to avoid using judgmental language such as *uncooperative, difficult,* or *bad* when describing such behaviors.

It is important to include assistive personnel in the change-of-shift report. Assistive personnel are part of the team and can contribute more when they also know a client's condition and the nursing team's priorities in care. The registered professional nurse (RN) can use the report to emphasize to assistive personnel the tasks to be done.

TELEPHONE REPORTS

Nurses inform physicians of changes in a client's condition and communicate information to nurses on other units about client transfer. The laboratory staff or a radiologist may report results of diagnostic tests. Persons involved with a telephone report need to provide clear, accurate, and concise information. In many cases information in a telephone report is documented when significant events or changes in a client's condition have occurred. To document a phone call, the nurse includes when the call was made, who made it (if other than the writer of the information), who was called, to whom information was given, what information was given, and what information was received, for example, "At 10:22 AM called Dr. M's office; S. Thomas, RN, will inform Dr. M that Mr. Rush's STAT potassium level drawn at 8:00 AM was 3.2. C. Towns, RN."

TELEPHONE ORDERS

Telephone orders (TOs) involve a physician stating a prescribed therapy over the phone to a registered nurse. Clarifying messages is important when a nurse accepts physician's orders over the telephone. The order needs to be verified by repeating it clearly and precisely. Then the nurse writes the order on the physician's order sheet in the client's permanent record and signs it. An example follows: "1/16/95: 7:20 PM Darvocet-N PO 1 tab now and q4h prn. T.O. Dr. Reiss/Carol Towns, RN" The physician later verifies the telephone order legally by signing it within a set time period (e.g., 24 hours). Telephone orders are frequently given at night or during an emergency and need to be used only when absolutely necessary. Certain guidelines can be used to prevent errors in receiving telephone orders (Box 24-9).

TRANSFER REPORTS

Clients may transfer from one unit to another to receive different levels of care. For example, clients transfer from an intensive care unit or the recovery room to general nursing units when the client no longer requires such intense monitoring. To promote continuity of care, **transfer reports** may be given by phone or in person. When giving a transfer report, nurses include the following information:

1. Client's name, age, primary physician, and medical diagnosis

If the physician sounds hurried over the phone, use clarification questions to avoid misunderstandings.

Clearly determine the client's name, room number, and diagnosis.

Repeat any prescribed orders back to the physician.

Write a telephone order to include date and time given; name of client, nurse, and physician; and the complete order.

Follow agency policies; some institutions require telephone (and verbal) orders to be reviewed and signed by two nurses.

Have the physician cosign the order within the time frame required by the institution (usually 24 hours).

2. Summary of progress up to the time of transfer
3. Current health status (physical and psychosocial)
4. Current plan of care
5. Any critical assessments or interventions to be completed shortly after transfer (helps receiving nurse to establish priorities of care)
6. Any special considerations, such as isolation status or resuscitation status
7. Need for any special equipment

After completion of the transfer report, the receiving nurse needs an opportunity to ask questions about the client's status. In some cases written documentation must include a record of information reported.

INCIDENT REPORTS

An incident is any event that is not consistent with the routine operation of a health care unit or routine care of a client. Examples of incidents include client falls, needle-stick injuries, a visitor having symptoms of illness, medication administration errors, accidental omission of ordered therapies, and circumstances that led to injury or a risk for client injury. Analysis of incident reports helps with the identification of trends in systems and unit operations that provide justification for changes in policies and procedures or for in-service seminars. **Incident reports** are an important part of a unit's quality improvement program (see Chapter 21).

When an incident occurs, the nurse involved in the incident or the nurse who witnesses an injury completes an incident report. The report is completed even though an injury does not occur or is not apparent. Most institutions have incident report forms, which are sent to the risk management office for review and follow-up action. For example, the employee health department might review all incidents involving employee needle-stick injuries, and the legal department may review incidents for which the potential for a lawsuit against the hospital exists.

When a client or visitor is involved in an incident, the nurse observing the incident deals with the situation and then completes a report describing details of the incident. In many cases a physician is notified and determines actions to be taken to determine if any injury has been suffered. If a client is affected, the physician documents the examination and findings in the client's medical record. The nurse documents only an objective description of what was actually observed and follow-up care that occurred and does not specify in the medical record that an incident report was prepared. Examples of an accurate and an inaccurate note follow:

Accurate note: 2200 Heard a thump. Client found on floor, complained of aching pain in left hip, pain rated 8 (scale 0-10). Noted external rotation and shortening of left leg. Lifted into bed using Hoyer lift. VS: BP, 142/88; P, 90; R, 22. Side rails up, call light within reach, instructed to remain in bed. Dr. Smith notified, portable x-ray ordered.

Incomplete note: Client fell out of bed, complained of pain in left hip. Noted external rotation and shortening of left leg. Dr. Smith notified.

One of the more common types of incidents is a medication error (see Chapter 34). An incident report for a medication error needs to include the following: (1) an accurate, concise description of the medication error, (2) all pertinent related information (e.g., actions taken, staff involved), and (3) record of any adverse reactions the client has had (Parisi, 1994).

Nurses become involved in client-related incidents at some point in their careers. The following list provides guidelines for correctly completing an incident report:

The nurse who witnessed the incident or who found the client at the time of the incident files the report.

Describe specifically what happened in concise, objective terms.

Describe objectively the client's condition when the incident was discovered.

Report any measures taken by oneself, other nurses, or physicians at the time of the incident.

Do not interpret or attempt to explain the cause of the incident or blame anyone.

Submit the report as soon as possible to the appropriate administrator.

Keep a written account of the incident report for personal files.

Do not photocopy the report since the copy could be subpoenaed in court.

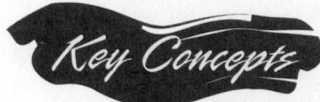

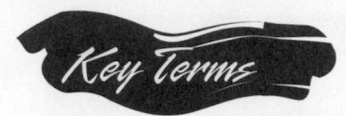

- The medical record is a legal document and requires information describing the care that is delivered to a client.
- All information pertaining to a client's health care management that is gathered by examination, observation, conversation, or treatment is confidential.
- Multidisciplinary communication is essential within the health care team.
- Accurate record keeping requires an objective interpretation of data with precise measurements, correct spelling, and proper use of abbreviations.
- A nurse's signature on an entry in a record designates accountability for the contents of that entry.
- Any change in a client's condition warrants immediate documentation to keep a record accurate.
- The medical record is a client's bill or financial record that serves as the basis for reimbursement.
- Problem-oriented medical records are organized by the client's health care problems.
- The intent of SOAP, SOAPIE, PIE, or DAR charting is to organize entries in the progress notes by the nursing process.
- Critical pathways provide members of the health care team a way to document their contributions to the client's total plan of care.
- Medicare guidelines for establishing a client's home health care cost reimbursement is the basis for documentation by home health care nurses.
- Long-term care documentation is multidisciplinary and closely linked with fiscal requirements of outside agencies.
- Computerized information systems provide information about clients in an organized and easily accessible fashion.
- The major purpose of the change-of-shift report is to maintain continuity of care.
- Rounds allow nurses to perform needed assessments, evaluate clients' progress, and determine the best interventions for a client's needs.
- When information pertinent to care is communicated by telephone, the information needs to be verified.
- Incident reports objectively describe any event that is not consistent with the routine care of a client.

Accreditation, *p. 501*
Acuity recording, *p. 513*
Automated speech-recognition, *p. 518*
Case management, *p. 512*
Change-of-shift report, *p. 519*
Charting by exception, *p. 508*
Computer-based patient care record, *p. 518*
Consultations, *p. 502*
Critical pathways, *p. 512*
DAR, *p. 507*
Diagnosis-related group (DRG), *p. 501*
Documentation, *p. 502*
Flow sheets, *p. 512*

Focus charting, *p. 507*
Graphic user interface, *p. 518*
Incident reports, *p. 521*
Kardex, *p. 512*
PIE, *p. 507*
Problem-oriented medical record (POMR), *p. 506*
Record, *p. 501*
Reports, *p. 501*
Residents, *p. 516*
SOAP, *p. 507*
SOAPIE, *p. 507*
Source record, *p. 507*
Standardized care plans, *p. 513*
Transfer reports, *p. 520*
Variances, *p. 512*

Critical Thinking Exercises

1. Joseph Page is an 80-year-old man admitted with a diagnosis of possible pneumonia. He complains of general malaise and a frequent productive cough, worse at night. Vital signs are as follows: blood pressure, 150/90 mm Hg; pulse rate, 92 beats per minute; respirations, 22 breaths per minute; and temperature, 38.5° C (101.2° F). During your initial assessment he coughs violently for 40 to 45 seconds without expectorating. His lungs have wheezes and rhonchi in both bases and are otherwise clear. He states, "It hurts in my chest when I cough." Differentiate between objective and subjective data in this case example.

2. The nurse positions Mr. Page in a semi-Fowler's position, encourages increased fluid intake, and gives Tylenol 650 mg PO as ordered for fever. One hour later the client is resting in bed. Vital signs are as follows: blood pressure, 130/86 mm Hg; pulse rate, 86 beats per minute; respirations, 22 breaths per minute; and temperature, 37.7° C (99.8° F). He states he has been unable to sleep. His fluid intake has been 200 ml of water. Use the given information to write a nurse's progress note using each of the following formats: SOAPIE, PIE, and DAR.

3. At the end of your shift 6 hours later you have identified *fluid volume deficit* as a nursing diagnosis for Mr. Page. Since his admission he has had fluid intake of about 600 ml, and his urine output was 300 ml of dark concentrated urine. His temperature is back up to 38.4° C (101° F), his mucous membranes are dry, and he states he feels very weak. Using the nursing care records (see Figure 24-3), record significant data. List what should be included in the change-of-shift report.

4. Several days later, following treatment with intravenous antibiotics, Mr. Page is feeling much better and preparations are being made for discharge. He is to take Keflex 500 mg every 6 hours for the next 10 days, continue to drink extra fluids, and get extra rest. He lives alone. Although he is generally cooperative, he does not like drinking water or taking pills. He is to make an appointment with his physician for 1 week from today and should call the physician if he develops symptoms of recurrence. Write a discharge summary that is concise and instructive.

References

Anonymous: Keep focus on the big picture when tackling variance analysis, *Hospital Case Management* 1(18):1, 1993.

Braunstein ML: The electronic patient records solution, *Caring* 12(7):30, 1993.

Eggland ET: Charting smarter: using new mechanisms to organize your paperwork, *Nursing 95* 25(9)34, 1995.

Gordon M: *Manual of nursing diagnosis: 1998–1999*, St. Louis, 1998, Mosby.

Henry SB and others: A computer-based approach to quality improvement for telephone triage in a community AIDS clinic, *Nurs Adm Q* 18(2):65, 1994.

Iyer PW, Camp NH: *Nursing documentation: a nursing process approach*, St. Louis, 1999, Mosby.

Joint Commission on Accreditation of Healthcare Organizations: *Standards for the accreditation of home care*, Chicago, 1999a, The Joint Commission.

Joint Commission on Accreditation of Healthcare Organizations: *Standards for the accreditation of hospitals*, Chicago, 1999b, The Joint Commission.

Kopf R: Are your medical records a legal asset or liability? Legal documentation guidelines, *J Nurs Law* 1(1):5, 1993.

Lampe S: *Focus charting: documentation for patient-centered care*, Minneapolis, 1994, Creative Nursing Management.

Mandell M: Not documented: not done, *Nursing 94* 24(8):62, 1994.

Martin F: Documentation tips: to help you stay out of court, *Nursing 94* 24(6):63, 1994.

Parisi S: What to do after a med error, *Nursing 94* 24(6):59, 1994.

Simpson R: Computer-based patient records: the Institute of Medicine's vision, part I, *Nurse Manage* 22(10):24, 1991a.

Simpson R: Computer-based patient records: the Institute of Medicine's vision, part II, *Nurse Manage* 22(11):26, 1991b.

Trofino J: Voice-activated nursing documentation: on the cutting edge, *Nurs Manage* 24(7):40, 1993.

Woodyard LW, Sheetz, J: Critical pathway patient outcomes: the missing standard, *J Nurs Care Qual* 8(1):51, 1993.

25

Research
as a Basis
for Practice

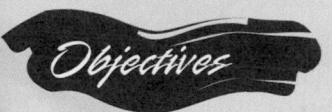

Mastery of content in this chapter will enable the student to:

- Define the key terms listed.
- Compare the various ways to acquire knowledge.
- List the characteristics of scientific investigation.
- Compare methods for developing new nursing knowledge.
- Define nursing research.
- Compare the research process with the nursing process.
- List the National Institute of Nursing Research's priorities for nursing research.
- Explain how the rights of human research subjects are protected.
- Explain the rights of others who assist in human research studies.
- Discuss methods of locating research reports in nursing and related areas.
- Explain how to organize information from a research report.
- Discuss the process of research utilization.

Nursing knowledge, scientific knowledge, and research findings have rapidly expanded over the last few years. Nurses must share a "commitment to the advancement of nursing science and the ethical conduct of nursing science" (American Nurses Association [ANA], 1997). The commitment to the development of this science through a process of systematically generated knowledge to guide nursing practice has been the catalyst for growth of nursing research, along with increased resources to support these research endeavors (Hinshaw, Feetham, and Shaver, 1999).

The scientific knowledge base for professional practice is developed through scholarly inquiry of research literature and the actual conduct of research. The multidisciplinary nature of the nursing profession challenges nurses to be knowledgeable concerning current research in the discipline of nursing, but also to be knowledgeable about the status of research in the behavioral and physical sciences and other health care disciplines.

Nursing research involves a systematic search for and validation of knowledge about issues important to the nursing profession. It is a systematic examination of phenomena important to nursing as a discipline, as well as to nurses, their clients, and their families. Nursing research is important to validate nursing as a profession, to document the effectiveness of nursing interventions, to provide a scientific knowledge base for practice, and to demonstrate accountability of the profession (Polit and Hungler, 1999).

The International Council of Nurses (1986) supports the need for nursing research as a means for improving the health and welfare of people. Nursing research is a way to identify new knowledge, improve professional education and practice, and use resources effectively. In 1983 the National Center for Nursing Research (NCNR) and the International Council of Nurses (ICN) established broad priorities for nursing research. These priorities were to promote the in-depth knowledge base for nursing practice, to recognize nursing research as an integral aspect of nursing practice and education, to facilitate cross-cultural research, to ensure adequate preparation of nurse researchers, and to encourage all national nurse associations to establish ethical research standards (NCNR/ICN, 1990).

Research-based practice is essential if the nursing profession is to meet the needs of society for safe, effective, and efficient care (ANA, 1997). However, nurses need the skills to effectively access and appraise existing research and scientific knowledge. In addition, nurses need the skills to create change in the practice settings to implement research-based interventions (Munhall, Alexander, and le May, 1998).

Historical Perspective

Nursing leaders and organizations have made considerable efforts to increase nurses' awareness of the importance of nursing research as a foundation for practice (Box 25-1). It is agreed that Florence Nightingale's detailed observation about the effects of nursing actions, such as the impact of nutrition and hygiene, during the Crimean War was the initial nursing research study (Polit and Hungler, 1999). In 1923 the Committee for the Study of Nursing Education studied the preparation of educators, administrators, and public health nurses and the clinical experiences of nursing students and published the results in the

Historical Milestones in the Evolution of Nursing Research
Box 25-1

BEFORE 1950

1854 Florence Nightingale is at military hospital in Scutari during the Crimean War.

1858 Nightingale's *Notes on Matters Affecting the Health, Efficiency and Hospital Administration of the British Army* and *Notes on Hospitals* are published in London by Harrison and Sons.

1858 Nightingale is made a fellow of the Royal Statistical Society.

1923 Goldmark report is sponsored by the Committee for the Study of Nursing Education.

1924 Teachers College, Columbia University, offers first doctoral program for nurses, granting an EdD.

1934 New York University offers first PhD in nursing.

1936 Sigma Theta Tau awards first grant for research in the United States.

AFTER 1950

1952 *Nursing Research*, the official research journal of the American Nurses Association (ANA), is published.

1953 Institute of Research and Service in Nursing Education at Teachers College in Columbia University.

1955 The American Nurses Foundation is formed.

1956 Committee on Research and Studies is formed by the ANA.

1957 Western Interstate Commission on Higher Education (WICHE), Southern Regional Educational Board (SREB).

1963 Surgeon General's Consultant Group on Nursing (*Toward Quality in Nursing*).

1964 *International Journal of Nursing Studies* is published.

1966 *International Nursing Index* is published.

1970 Lysaught report: *An Abstract for Action.*

1976 ANA Commission on Nursing Research publishes *Preparation of Nurses, for Participation in Research.*

1981 ANA Commission on Nursing Research publishes *Research Priorities for the 1980s* and *Guidelines for the Investigative Function of Nurses.*

1985 ANA Cabinet on Nursing Research publishes *Directions for Nursing Research: Toward the Twenty-first Century.*

1986 Establishment of the National Center for Nursing Research at the National Institutes of Health.

1989 Clinical Practice Guidelines is published by the Agency for Health Care Policy and Research.

1992 *Healthy People 2000.*

1993 National Center for Nursing Research is renamed the National Institute of Nursing Research.

1999 *Healthy People 2010.*

Goldmark report. The Goldmark report identified gaps in the educational background in nursing education; as a result, the method for educating nurses changed, and more university-based nursing curricula resulted. During the 1940s research activities focused on educational issues. In the 1950s, however, there was an increase in the number of nurses with advanced degrees, and the journal *Nursing Research* was initiated. The University of Pittsburgh offered the first doctoral program in nursing in 1954. There were increases in the availability of private and government monies, and the American Nurses Foundation was established (Polit and Hungler, 1999).

In the 1960s several professional nursing organizations initiated development of nursing research priorities. The Lysaught report recommended increases in research toward nursing practice and nursing education. Terms such as *conceptual framework, conceptual model, nursing process,* and *theoretical base of nursing practice* began to appear in the nursing literature.

During the 1970s nursing studies tended to focus on the roles and characteristics of nurses rather than on problems in delivering professional care to clients. During this time more nurses were receiving doctoral preparation and initiating their own research, and more nursing research journals were published (Box 25-2).

In 1981 the ANA published specific recommendations for studying research at the different nursing education levels. This document has since been updated and refined (ANA, 1997). A study of nursing by the Institute of Medicine (1983) recommended that the federal government increase funds for scientific research in nursing and that steps be taken to establish a national organization to place nursing research "in the mainstream of scientific investigation." Acting on this recommendation in 1985, the

Journals Focusing on Nursing Research (Non-Specialty-Based Journals)
Box 25-2

Decade	Journal Title
1950	*Nursing Research*
1960	*Image—The Journal of Nursing Scholarship*
	International Journal of Nursing Studies
1970	*Advances in Nursing Science*
	Research in Nursing and Health
	Western Journal of Nursing Research
1980	*Applied Nursing Research*
	Journal of Nursing Measurement
	Nursing Scan in Research
	Nursing Science Quarterly
	Scholarly Inquiry for Nursing Practice
1990	*Clinical Nursing Practice*
	Qualitative Health Research
	Measurement of Nursing Outcomes

U.S. Congress overrode two presidential vetoes to establish the NCNR under the National Institutes of Health (NIH).

In 1993 the NCNR was promoted to the National Institute of Nursing Research (NINR), giving it equal status and accountability with the other institutes of the NIH. The NINR (1997) supports:

> ... clinical and basic research to establish a scientific basis for the care of individuals across the life span—from management of patients during illness and recovery to the reduction of risks for disease and disability and the promotion of healthy life styles. According to its mandate the Institute seeks to understand and ease the symptoms of acute and chronic illness, to prevent or delay the onset of disease or disability or slow its progression, and to improve the clinical settings in which care is provided. . . . research extends to problems encountered by patients, families, and care givers. It also emphasizes the special needs of at-risk and underserved populations.

Nurse researchers convene to develop research priorities for the NINR. The current research priorities of the NINR are listed in Box 25-3.

A continual trend for nursing research is outcomes research. Outcomes research in nursing is research designed to assess and document the effectiveness of health care services (Polit and Hungler, 1999). For example, studying the effects of an outpatient education program on the ability of older adult clients to follow a nutrition and exercise program is an outcome study. The emphasis for outcomes research originates from quality assessment and quality assurance functions that originated out of professional standard review organizations (PSROs). This type of research represents a response of the health care industry to the increased demand from policy makers, insurers, and the public to justify care practices and systems in terms of improved client outcomes and costs (Polit and Hungler, 1991; Hinshaw, Feetham, and Shaver, 1999).

National Institute of Nursing Research Priorities for 2000 — Box 25-3

CHRONIC DISEASES OR CONDITIONS
Enhancing adherence to diabetes self-management behaviors
Symptom management of children with asthma

BEHAVIORAL CHANGES AND INTERVENTIONS
Biobehavioral research for effective sleep in health and illness
Acute care of children with posttraumatic brain injury

RESPONDING TO COMPELLING PUBLIC HEALTH CONCERNS
Enhancing end-of-life care
Collaborations with clinical trials networks

Data from National Institute of Nursing Research: *National Institute of Nursing Research, 2000, NINR areas of research opportunity,* Bethesda, Md, 1997, National Institutes of Health; http://www.nih.gov/ninr/NINR/ 2000AoRO.html.

Nursing research also has the support of professional and specialty organizations. In 1991 the ANA revised the *Standards of Clinical Nursing Practice.* Within this document are the *Standards of Professional Performance* (see Chapter 19). Standard 7 recommends that the professional nurse use research findings in practice (ANA, 1991). Thus the ANA recommends that nurses incorporate research findings into clinical practice to restore health, prevent illness, and minimize the effects of acute and chronic disease and disability. Nursing specialty organizations, (e.g., American Association of Critical Care Nurses, Oncology Nursing Society, National Perinatal Nurses Association), all have priorities for nursing research and encourage members to conduct research relevant to the specialty practice.

One cannot overlook the fact that a major contribution to clinical nursing research is the increase in the number of master's and doctorally prepared nurses. In 1965, three universities awarded doctoral degrees in nursing. In 1997, 66 universities awarded doctoral degrees in nursing. As of 1998, doctorally prepared nurses increased to approximately 18,000 as compared with 500 in 1965 (Hinshaw, Feetham, and Shaver, 1999).

Scientific Research in Nursing

Knowledge acquisition is essential in contributing to scientific research in nursing. The expansion of technology, changes in the health care delivery system, and changes in reimbursement all require that nurses must use a **scientific approach** to identify and solve clinical nursing problems and issues.

KNOWLEDGE ACQUISITION

One hallmark of a mature discipline is the development of multiple research methods designed to develop a knowledge base unique to the discipline (Barrett, 1998). Although acquired in many ways, knowledge is information, and discovery is the creative process of obtaining new knowledge. A person continuously takes in information, and, through the processes of critical thinking, evaluates numerous pieces of information to understand experiences.

Tradition.   One way of acquiring knowledge is by tradition. One generation passes knowledge to the next. For example, children often learn about traditional holidays such as Christmas and Passover through traditional or customary family practices. In nursing, certain traditional methods of practice, such as the change-of-shift report, and other daily hospital work practices are passed from one practitioner to the next. Tradition is an efficient way of learning, although it can also limit the ability to seek new ways of doing things. If tradition becomes so ingrained that a person does not question the custom, other, more appropriate or efficient ways may be overlooked.

Information Seeking.   Knowledge is also acquired by seeking information from experts in a particular field. Experts are often asked to solve problems or answer questions. For example, at income tax time an accountant's help is sought to fill out tax forms. Similarly, nursing students often seek the advice of instructors and practicing nurses when assessing and caring for clients. Authority, like tradition, is not infallible, although it is commonly treated as absolute truth.

Another method of seeking information is by investigating knowledge from other disciplines. For example, by using Selye's model of general adaptation, the nurse is able to use knowledge and apply it to clinical situations in which the client is experiencing stress. As a result, nursing interventions are designed to assist the client in reducing the stress response (see Chapter 30).

Experience.   A person also learns through experience. Without this process a person would have to relearn a procedure every time it was performed. Practice leads to the development of routines that help build skills. For example, a student nurse taking a blood pressure measurement for the first time may feel awkward and unsure of hearing the sounds, but with practice the student's technique and confidence improve. Although experience is an important way of learning, it has limitations. A person may continue to do something simply because it was learned that way and may overlook improved or other ways of doing the same thing. If experience causes a person to learn something incorrectly, the person uses knowledge inappropriately.

Problem Solving.   Learning by problem solving is yet another way of gaining knowledge. Trying various ways of resolving client's health care needs, developing new staffing patterns, or evaluating health care products will eventually result in problem solving. This method of learning is practical, but it is unsystematic and often a haphazard way of learning. In nursing, because clients' health status depends on nursing actions, the problem-solving method may lead toward specific research questions.

Critical Thinking.   The nurse can use the skills of critical thinking to analyze information acquired through traditional learning, information seeking, experiential learning, investigating ideas from other disciplines, and problem solving to determine a course of nursing action (see Chapter 13). In addition, the nurse can use the skills of critical thinking to identify and investigate a clinical, professional, or educational issue.

SCIENTIFIC METHOD

The scientific researcher also seeks to explain or understand reality, but the scientist's process of acquiring knowledge is systematic and logical (Polit and Hungler, 1999). This process, or **scientific method,** is the foundation of research. Scientific research is the most reliable and objective of all methods of gaining knowledge.

The scientific method is an advanced, objective means of acquiring and testing knowledge. By use of this method, the researcher attempts to understand, explain, predict, or control a nursing phenomenon (Polit and Hungler, 1999). The method is characterized by systematic, orderly procedures that, although not without fault, seek to limit the possibility for error and minimize the likelihood that any bias or opinion by the researcher might influence the results of research and thus the knowledge gained. Polit and Hungler (1999) describe the characteristics of scientific investigation as follows:

The problem area or what needs to be studied is identified.

The steps of planning and conducting an investigation are undertaken in a systematic, orderly fashion.

Researchers attempt to control external factors that are not under direct investigation but that can influence a relationship between phenomena they are studying. For example, if a nurse were studying the relationship between diet and heart disease, other characteristics such as stress or smoking history would have to be controlled for contributing factors to this disease.

Evidence that is part of experience (**empirical data**) is gathered directly or indirectly through use of observations and assessments and is the basis for discovering new knowledge.

The goal is to understand phenomena in such a way that the knowledge gained can be applied generally, not just to isolated cases or circumstances.

Scientists strive to conduct investigations that contribute to testing or developing theories, thereby advancing the knowledge that can be applied toward increasing understanding of people, places, or life events.

Nursing and the Scientific Approach

In nursing, the scientific method is a systematic approach to generate questions for quantitative and qualitative research to identify and test knowledge (Table 25-1). The scientific method is a system for acquiring knowledge or predicting nursing phenomena (Polit and Hungler, 1999).

Compared with other ways of acquiring knowledge, the scientific method is more orderly and objective in its approach. In the past, much of the information used in nursing practice was borrowed from other disciplines such as biology, physiology, psychology, and sociology. Often this information was applied to nursing without testing or comparing ways of caring for clients. For example, nurses use several methods to help clients sleep. Interventions such as giving a client a back rub, making sure that the bed is clean and comfortable, preparing the environment by dimming the lights, and talking to a worried or anxious

Table 25-1 Types of Research and Related Research Questions

Purpose	Types of Questions: Quantitative Research	Types of Questions: Qualitative Research
Identification		What are the phenomena?
Description	How frequent are the phenomena?	What are the dimensions of the phenomena?
	What are the characteristics of the phenomena?	What is important about the phenomena?
Exploration	What factors are related to the phenomena?	What is occurring with the phenomena?
	What are the forerunners (or antecedents) of the phenomena?	What is the process by which the phenomena are experienced?
Explanation	What are the measurable associations among the phenomena?	How do the phenomena work?
		Why do the phenomena exist?
	What causes the phenomena?	What is the meaning of the phenomena?
	Does the theory explain the phenomena?	How did the phenomena occur?
Predictive	What will happen if an intervention is used?	
	If phenomenon X occurs, will Y follow?	
	How can we make the phenomena happen?	
	Can the phenomena be controlled?	

Modified from Polit DF, Hungler BP: *Nursing research: principles and methods*, ed 6, Philadelphia, 1999, JB Lippincott.

client are frequently used nursing measures and, in general, are logical, commonsense approaches. However, when these measures are considered in greater depth, questions may arise about their applications for different clients in different situations.

Research provides a way for nursing questions and problems to be studied in greater depth within the context of nursing. Frequently nurses rely on personal experience or the statements of nursing experts. If an intervention works for most clients, the nurse may be satisfied with this success without questioning whether there might be a better way. If the intervention is not successful, the nurse might use an approach practiced by a colleague or try a different sequence of accepted measures. Even if an intervention discovered with this approach is effective for one or more clients, it may not be appropriate for other clients in other settings. Approaches must be tested to determine the measures that work best with specific clients.

DEFINITIONS OF SCIENTIFIC AND NURSING RESEARCH

The scientific method is a systematic method of questioning and challenging the validity of scientific assumptions (Polit and Hungler, 1999). Within the scientific method is the scientific approach, which is a logical, orderly, and objective means of generating research questions and testable hypotheses.

Several factors may affect when a researcher uses systematic, controlled methods for studying events or problems. These studies are well organized and follow a specific procedure. In addition, other researchers should be able to reproduce the study or examine the evidence and achieve the same **phenomena** (results). To guide the design of a research study, scientists create a hypothetical proposition (**hypothesis**) about what they expect to see before conducting the study. For example, a researcher may hypothesize that the client's use of relaxation exercises reduces postoperative pain. Scientists generally study the way that

characteristics or events are different or the way that one event is causally associated with another.

When reading research studies, nurses should avoid interpreting results in terms of cause and effect because there is a difference between cause-and-effect and other kinds of relationships. For example, as people get older, they tend to lose their hair, and their skin becomes wrinkled. These factors are related to each other as part of the aging process, but neither causes the other. Researchers often study such relationships without being able to determine why or how these changes take place.

Biomedical research is concerned primarily with discovering the causes and treatments of disease. In contrast, nursing research focuses on the full range of human responses and is directed toward helping well people improve their health status and stay healthy, as well as assisting clients who are sick or disabled by an illness in maintaining or improving their health. For example, the effect of preoperative teaching on postoperative recovery is an area that has been studied extensively. Some studies have examined the effect of preoperative teaching on positive postoperative outcomes (Meeker, 1994; Planchock and Wiggins, 1994). Timmons and Bower (1993) examined the effect of preoperative teaching on clients' understanding of patient-controlled analgesia and their management of postoperative pain. The group receiving preoperative education managed their pain significantly better. Teaching clients what they can expect on the day of surgery and in the immediate postoperative period is now a widely accepted and implemented nursing measure.

Research Methods

Nurses are interested in acquiring knowledge about a wide range of human needs and responses to health problems. Nursing research uses many methods to study clinical problems (Box 25-4). There are two broad approaches to research: quantitative and qualitative methods.

HISTORICAL RESEARCH
Systematic studies designed to establish facts and relationships concerning past events (Polit and Hungler, 1999)

EXPLORATORY RESEARCH
Initial study designed to develop or refine the dimensions of phenomena or to develop or refine a hypothesis about the relationships among phenomena (Polit and Hungler, 1999)

EVALUATION RESEARCH
Study that tests how well a program, practice, or policy is working

DESCRIPTIVE RESEARCH
Study in which the objective is to accurately portray characteristics of persons, situations, or groups and the frequency with which certain events or characteristics occur

EXPERIMENTAL RESEARCH
Study in which the investigator controls the independent variable and randomly assigns subjects to different conditions

QUASI-EXPERIMENTAL RESEARCH
Study in which subjects cannot be randomly assigned to treatment conditions, although the researcher controls the independent variables

CORRELATIONAL RESEARCH
Study that explores the interrelationships among variables of interest without any active intervention by the researcher

QUANTITATIVE RESEARCH

Quantitative research efforts use traditional methods of research, such as experimental, survey, or correlational analysis (Knapp, 1998). **Quantitative nursing research** is the investigation of nursing phenomena that lend themselves to precise measurement and quantification. For example, pain severity, rate of wound healing, and body temperature changes can be quantitatively measured. Quantitative research is rigorous, systematic, objective examination of specific concepts and their relationships to test theory by focusing on numerical data, statistical analysis, and controls to eliminate bias (Knapp, 1998; Polit and Hungler, 1999). The following sections describe some of the quantitative approaches used to answer research questions.

Experimental Research. The hallmark of scientific research is the experiment. In a true **experimental study,** the conditions under which a measure is investigated are tightly controlled. Experimental approaches to studying a problem require that the information about human subjects be collected and quantified in a prescribed manner.

The study usually includes a control or comparison group, which does not receive the nursing measure being investigated. The results for this group are compared with those of a study or experimental group—the group that receives some form of treatment or intervention. The **subjects**—persons selected for the comparison and experimental groups—are chosen at random from among those eligible for the study. Random selection of subjects gives all eligible subjects the same chance to be in the control or experimental (treatment) group and eliminates sampling bias. Designing an experiment to study physical causes of disease is less difficult than designing an experiment that also includes psychological or social aspects of health. For example, to study the relationship between postoperative anxiety and preoperative teaching, the researcher can control one psychological factor by using only subjects having surgery for the first time. However, the researcher cannot control other experiences that the clients may have had, such as hearing a friend's "horror" stories about surgery or reading about surgical experiences in the newspapers. These psychological factors, which cannot be controlled, may influence the subject's level of anxiety.

Quasi-Experimental Research. **Quasi-experimental research** design is one in which the conditions are controlled; however, the subjects are usually not randomly assigned to control group or treatment conditions. Quasi-experimental research is a practical and in some situations less expensive method of answering a research question. When this type of design is used, both the investigator and the reader of the research need to be aware of any weakness resulting from a lack of randomization or control group.

Surveys. Surveys are another type of quantitative research. **Surveys** are designed to obtain information from populations regarding prevalence, distribution, and interrelation of variables within the study population (Polit and Hungler, 1999). They may be conducted for the general purposes of obtaining information about practices, opinions, attitudes, and other characteristics of people (Knapp, 1999). The most basic function of a survey is description. Surveys can amass a large amount of data to describe the population being studied, as well as the topic of study. It is important in survey research that the population sampled is large to keep sampling error at a minimum. The survey items (e.g., questionnaires, interviews) must be constructed carefully and pretested to determine correctness in style, ease of use, and appropriateness for the research question.

Evaluation Research. **Evaluation research** is a form of quantitative research that involves finding out how well a program, practice, procedure, or policy is working (Polit and Hungler, 1999). Ultimately, the purpose of evaluation research is to determine the success of a program. This type of research can determine specifically why a program was successful. When programs are unsuccessful, evaluation research can assist in identifying problems with the program, why it was not successful, or even barriers to implementation of programs.

Quantitative Analysis.   Secondary analysis and meta-analysis are two methods of quantitative analysis that can be used to answer research questions. Secondary data analysis involves the use of data previously gathered in a study and used to test new hypotheses or explore new relationships. This type of analysis provides a method of examining relationships among variables that were previously not analyzed. In addition, secondary analysis can focus on a subgroup of a study population.

Meta-analysis is the application of statistical procedures to findings from similar research reports. The findings from multiple studies on the same topic can be combined into a larger data set. Meta-analysis may be useful in combining several studies with small populations. However, when conducting this type of analysis, the investigator must follow a precise and systematic method of analysis.

· · ·

Nursing studies use many quantitative methods for investigating clinical problems; some may be similar to the experimental approach. Other research methods may be similar to those used in the social sciences, such as anthropology and sociology. The amount of knowledge known about the problem and the type of problem being investigated are factors that determine the methods used. Nursing is a practice discipline that deals with unique physical, emotional, and social problems that people experience in regaining, maintaining, and promoting health.

QUALITATIVE RESEARCH

Qualitative research is used to describe information obtained in a nonnumerical form (e.g., data obtained from transcripts from an unstructured interview). **Qualitative nursing research** is the investigation of phenomena that are not easily quantified or categorized in which inductive reasoning is used to develop generalizations or theories from specific observations or interviews (Morse and Field, 1995; Polit and Hungler, 1999). Qualitative research involves the discovery and understanding of important characteristics and the ways that they might be related. For example, a qualitative research study might involve a survey measuring clients' perceptions of mechanical ventilation (Ketchum and Perry, 1999). When qualitative methods are used, the investigator can use one of several design strategies, some of which are presented here, to study the area of interest.

Ethnography.   **Ethnography** involves the description and interpretation of cultural behavior (Polit and Hungler, 1999). This type of research is closely associated with the field of anthropology, which focuses on the culture of the study population. The goal of this research is to understand the culture of the study population as the culture is practiced in the study environment. For example, Margaret Mead's work in Samoa was undertaken as an ethnographical study in which she collected and analyzed data while living within the community of the Samoans.

Phenomenology.   **Phenomenology** is a research method with roots in philosophy (Polit and Hungler, 1999). The focus of this type of qualitative research is what people experience in regard to daily practices or experiences and how they interpret those experiences. For example, an investigator may want to study the impact of surrogate decision making regarding end-of-life decisions (Jeffers, 1998). The goal of this type of research is to describe fully the lived experience of the surrogate decision maker, the perceptions of the surrogate role, the decision-making process, and the meaning of the decisions. The source of data is from the subject, and the data are usually the result of in-depth conversations. The units of analysis are the conversations, which are coded and analyzed.

Grounded Theory.   **Grounded theory** is a method of collecting and analyzing qualitative data with the aim of developing theories and theoretical propositions that are grounded in real-world observations (Polit and Hungler, 1999). For example, in studying weaning from mechanical ventilation, Wunderlich and Perry (1999) interviewed clients who were successfully weaned from mechanical ventilation. As a result of these interview data, the investigators noted that social support was the most important factor that assisted clients in being weaned from mechanical ventilation. This information, along with findings from another study, begins to define some theoretical concepts for preparing clients to be weaned from mechanical ventilation (Ketchum and Perry, 1999).

Nursing Research and the Nursing Process

The **research process** consists of phases or steps that can be compared and contrasted with those of the nursing process. Both are problem-solving processes used by nurses in practice (Table 25-2), but they are very different. The nursing process is used to determine health needs and plan nursing care for clients. It is used as a basis for gaining and using information about clients to help them restore, maintain, or promote health. Depending on the nursing diagnosis, knowledge from a number of disciplines may be used in the nursing process to help clients solve particular health problems.

In contrast, the research process is used to gain knowledge that can be used in other, similar situations. Nurses may want to gain knowledge about the reason why a par-

Table 25-2	Comparison of the Nursing Process and the Research Process	
Nursing Process	**Research Process**
Assessment	Identification of phenomena
Diagnosis	Research problem
	Hypotheses
Planning	Study design
Goals	Review of literature
Patient outcomes	Theoretical or conceptual framework
Implementation	Data collection
Evaluation	Analysis of results
	Recommendations and implications for further research

Modified from Talbot LA: *Principles and practice of nursing research*, St. Louis, 1995, Mosby.

ticular event happens or the best way to provide care for clients with a certain health problem. The research process is used to gain knowledge that can be applied to a whole group or class of clients.

During the assessment phase of the nursing process, the nurse caring for a client with sleeping difficulties determines factors that might interfere with the ability to sleep. These may include the client's concern about health status, pain, a noisy environment, or a messy or uncomfortable bed. After assessing these aspects, the nurse formulates a nursing diagnosis, plans interventions, implements these interventions, and evaluates the subjective and objective evidence that indicates whether the client is able to sleep.

In contrast, a researcher studying sleeping difficulties seeks new information that can be applied to more than one client. For example, a nurse notices that many clients seem to have a difficult time sleeping the night before a particular diagnostic procedure. Based on work with these clients, the nurse determines that most of them have concerns about the results of the test. In this situation the nurse might design a research study in which some of the clients receive the usual nursing care and others receive care based on relieving anxiety. After collecting information about the effects of the usual care for the one group and the new approach for the other, the nurse researcher compares the results to determine whether clients who received the new care had less difficulty sleeping than those who received the normal care. If the clients receiving the new care slept better, the nurse has acquired new knowledge about how generally to help clients.

CONDUCTING NURSING RESEARCH

In 1997 the ANA published a position statement on the educational preparation for participation in nursing research. In this document, the ANA (1997) noted that all nurses share a "commitment to the advancement of nursing science and the ethical conduct of nursing science."

Nurses conduct research in a variety of settings. Student nurses and practitioners may be asked to participate in studies that investigate client outcomes and the effectiveness of nursing care. These types of research projects are commonly called quality assurance or improvement studies (see Chapter 4). Data are collected to determine the influence nurses have on achievement of client care objectives in a particular clinical setting. Because the results of such research are usually applicable only in one institution, this is not scientific research as discussed earlier. However, such research is important to the institution because the nursing department can use it to demonstrate the contributions made by nurses to client care.

Clinical nursing research should be undertaken by nurses educated to conduct scientific investigations (Figure 25-1). An experienced researcher is usually more qualified than a beginning researcher to undertake a complex, long-term project. Nurses new to research may, however, make important contributions by assisting with data collection, conducting replicated studies (studies previously performed elsewhere), or conducting less complex studies.

Research Preparation.   The preparation of nurse scientists, who have primary responsibility for the conduction of research, is begun at the master's level and is concentrated at the doctoral and postdoctoral levels. However, the ANA's position paper (1997), which describes the participation of nurses in research according to their academic preparation, does include research activities for nurses with various levels of academic preparation.

Associate Degree in Nursing.   Nurses with an associate degree are prepared to participate in research activities (1) through identification of clinical problems in nursing practice; (2) by assisting with organized data collection; and (3) in conjunction with nurses holding more advanced credentials, appropriately using research findings in clinical practice.

Baccalaureate Degree in Nursing.   Nurses with a baccalaureate degree are prepared to read research critically and use existing standards to determine the readiness of the findings for clinical practice. In addition, nurses with this preparation participate in research activities (1) through identification of clinical problems in nursing practice; (2) by assisting experienced investigators in gaining access to clinical sites; (3) by influencing the selection of appropriate methods of data collection; and (4) by collecting data and implementing nursing research findings.

Master's Degree in Nursing.   Nurses with a master's degree are prepared to be active members of a research

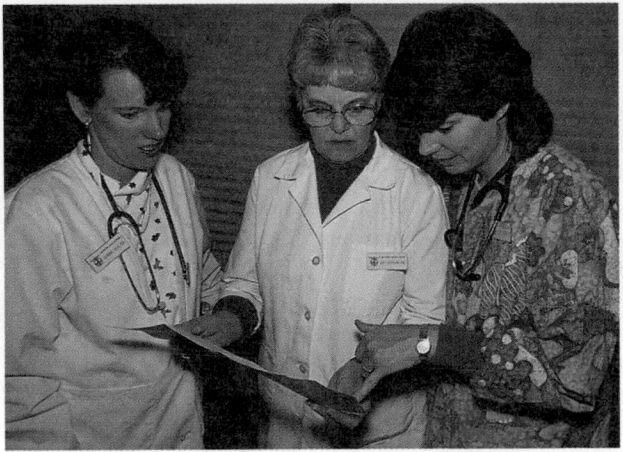

Figure 25-1   Nurses collaborating on research.

team. This level of preparation allows nurses to assume the role of clinical expert and be able to create a climate in which research-based change can be implemented into practice. Master's prepared nurses assume leadership roles in creating an environment for nursing research and integrating the findings into clinical practice.

Doctoral Education.   Nurses are prepared to contribute to nursing knowledge through the conduction of research aimed at advancing the scientific basis of nursing practice. Doctorally prepared nurses are prepared to design studies independently, as well as collaborate with other clinicians and researchers in conducting studies. Doctorally prepared nurses are responsible for acquiring funding for research from public and private sources.

Ethical Issues in Research

The conduction of research must meet ethical standards in which the rights of human subjects are protected. In addition, other research participants (e.g., health care professionals, teachers, students) also have rights as research participants.

RIGHTS OF HUMAN SUBJECTS

To refine existing knowledge and develop new knowledge, clinical research is sometimes directed at trying new procedures whose outcome is doubtful or unknown (ANA, 1985a). This kind of research may conflict with the purpose of nursing practice, which is to meet specific clients' needs. In such cases the researcher is responsible for structuring the investigation to avoid or minimize harm to the subjects. Although it is not always possible to anticipate all potential undesirable effects, researchers are obligated to inform everyone involved about the known potential risks. Other basic human rights must also be observed. These principles are set forth by both the Canadian Nurses Association (CNA) (1983, 1991) and the ANA (1985).

Informed Consent.   **Informed consent** means that research subjects (1) are given full and complete information about the purpose of the study, procedures, data collection, potential harm and benefits, and alternative methods of treatment; (2) are capable of fully understanding the research and the implications of participation; (3) have the power of free choice to voluntarily consent or decline participation in the research; and (4) understand how confidentiality or anonymity are maintained. **Confidentiality** guarantees that any information provided by the subject will not be reported in any manner that identifies the subject and will not be made accessible to people outside the research team (Polit and Hungler, 1999). **Anonymity** occurs when even the researcher cannot link the subject to the data (Polit and Hungler, 1999). The subject is assured of free choice in giving consent, including the right to withdraw from the study at any time (Polit and Hungler, 1999). Procedures for obtaining informed consent must be outlined in the study protocol.

Within the consent document, the investigator must outline in lay language the purpose of the study, the role of the subjects, types of data that are to be obtained, how the data are obtained, the duration of the study, subject selection, procedures, risks to the subject (including financial risks), potential benefits (including the possibility of no benefit), alternatives to participation, and contact information concerning the principal investigator and local institutional review board. This consenting process is done to provide subjects with complete information regarding the study's risks, benefits, and costs.

In addition, the researcher planning to conduct a study must possess the knowledge and skills necessary to undertake the research. Generally, a nurse planning to conduct a study involving psychiatric clients should be familiar with psychiatric nursing principles and theory. Current ANA (1997) and CNA (1983, 1991) guidelines state that qualified nurse researchers have the right to engage in research and have the right of access to resources needed to conduct studies.

Institutional Review Board.   Federal regulations (Code of Federal Regulations, 1993) require that institutions receiving any federal funding or conducting drug or medical device research regulated by the Food and Drug Administration establish institutional review boards (IRBs). Such groups review all studies conducted in the institution to ensure that ethical principles (see Chapter 20) are observed. A major responsibility of an IRB is to determine the risk status of all research projects (Box 25-5).

RIGHTS OF OTHER RESEARCH PARTICIPANTS

Student nurses and practicing nurses may be asked to participate in research as data collectors or may be involved in the care of clients participating in a study. All participants, including health care professionals caring for clients, have the right to be fully informed about the study, its procedures (including the consenting process and risk factors), and any physical or emotional injury that clients could experience as a result of participation. Often the physical risks are more obvious than the emotional risks. Depending on the problem being studied, clients may be asked to give highly personal, intrusive information. Because this type of research can lead to anxiety or stress for some clients, the researcher should prepare all participants, including nurses delivering care, for this possibility and assist them in coping with the effects. Participants also have the right to see review forms from the IRB that certify approval of the study. Any student, nurse, or other participant has the right to refuse to carry out any research procedures if he or she is concerned about their ethical aspects.

Nursing Research in Nursing Practice

RESEARCH REPORT VERSUS CLINICAL ARTICLE

When reading nursing literature, the nurse must be able to distinguish a research report or article from other types of writing. This may not be as simple as it seems. Even if the title has the word *research* in it, the article does not necessarily report the results of a research study. The nurse can determine whether an article reports a research study only by examining its contents. Sometimes, however, an article's title can give a clue to its contents. Phrases such as "a study of" or "comparison of" suggest a research report.

The abstract and the introductory paragraphs of an article can also indicate whether the article is based on research.

An **abstract** is a short summary of the purpose of a study, the subjects included in the research, the way the study was conducted, and the results obtained in the investigation (Box 25-6). An abstract is often quite brief and does not contain all of the essential information in the article. The first few paragraphs of the article should provide further clues about whether it describes a research study. Phrases such as "the purpose of this study was" and "his research was carried out to determine" are indications that the article is a research report. If the article describes only the author's experience with a particular aspect of nursing care, it probably is not a research article. In addition to the abstract, a typical research report has the following parts:

Introduction section: An introductory section presenting the purpose, a summary of literature used to formulate the study, and the hypotheses tested.

Methods section: Description of the methods used to conduct the study, including the sample (what or who was studied), and to collect data, including the device or instrument used to measure empirical information.

Results section: Description of the results obtained in the study, including statistical tests used to analyze data.

Discussion section: Presentation of the author's interpretation of the results, including conclusions and implications that can be drawn from the study.

Reference list: Articles used to support the study.

If the report is written by one of the researchers in the study, it is a **primary source.** Any other article about the study is considered a **secondary source** (e.g., an article in which the author was not directly involved in conducting the study but collected the information from a primary or another secondary source). Most nursing textbooks are secondary sources of information. Authors of these texts incorporate knowledge and information gathered from nursing and related literature, including research written by original investigators.

The fact that a report is a primary source does not guarantee its accuracy, which depends on the ability of researchers to be scientific, impersonal, and impartial in conducting studies. However, a primary source does report firsthand knowledge, whereas a secondary source may include another person's interpretation of the original work.

Locating Research Studies.   Nurses often need to find research articles on subjects that interest them (Figure 25-2). In the health care field a number of resources are useful when searching the literature for research articles.

To locate primary research sources related to a particular subject, the first source is the journals where original research reports are usually published. The most efficient way to locate research articles is to consult a computerized

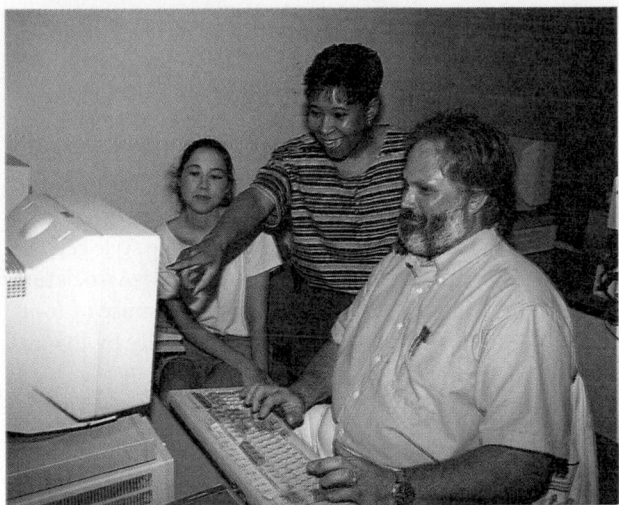

Research HIGHLIGHT   Box 25-6

RESEARCH ABSTRACT

Engaging older adults in a discussion regarding life-sustaining interventions (cardiopulmonary resuscitation [CPR], tube feeding, and mechanical ventilation) is recommended but remains an uncommon practice among health care providers. This study was conducted to determine the short-term impact of a discussion by a physician with homebound older adult clients, ages 60 to 93 years, concerning areas of urgent, life-sustaining interventions. Data were collected using the Zung Depression Scale, Life Satisfaction Index A and B, Locus of Desired Controls, and an interview with the physician. Clients' knowledge of specific urgent care modalities were assessed during the discussion with the physician. Most clients voiced no specific fears of the future. However, some clients lacked a clear understanding of the concepts and terminology regarding CPR, intubation, and tube feeding.

IMPLICATIONS FOR PRACTICE

- Discussing life-sustaining interventions with older adults is not widely used; therefore teaching is an effective nursing strategy, using terminology that the client understands.
- Involving older adult clients in the decision-making process regarding life-sustaining choices may increase their internal locus of control. Nurses should be supportive and encouraging.
- Many older adults have not discussed life-sustaining interventions with significant others.
- Open communication patterns involve a conscious effort by the health care team to clearly present the client's regimen of care and decision-making process.

REFERENCE

Kellogg F and others: Life-sustaining interventions in frail elderly persons, *Arch Intern Med* 152:2317, 1994.

Figure 25-2   Nursing students using the computer to find research articles.

database or an index of journal articles. The *Cumulative Index to Nursing and Allied Health Literature (CINAHL)*, published bimonthly, contains listings from over 300 nursing and allied health journals written in English, as well as publications of the ANA and National League for Nursing. The *International Nursing Index*, published 4 times a year, contains listings from more than 200 nursing journals from around the world. *Index Medicus*, an international index published monthly, includes listings from approximately 2900 biomedical journals, including about 60 nursing journals. The *Hospital Literature Index*, published quarterly, contains listings from journals dealing with planning and providing health care programs and services. These indexes are generally found in reference sections of medical and nursing libraries. In addition, individual subscribers can purchase CD-ROM formats for these databases.

The indexes just mentioned can save time in locating articles. Each index uses a list of key words that form subject headings and subheadings; article listings are grouped or organized under these headings. For example, a person might find subject headings such as *pain* or *primary nursing*, whereas subheadings might include *physiology* or *history*, respectively. An author listing is also available, making it possible to find articles published during a certain period by a specific author. Many nursing and medical libraries provide computerized searches for articles. A list of articles and abstracts is transmitted over telephone lines within hours of being requested. Nurses who have access to computers and modems may access bibliographical services available through the Internet or a database vendor.

Major nursing journals publish research studies or research reports. Some journals, such as *Nursing Research*, are devoted solely to research; other nursing journals, such as the *American Journal of Critical Care*, also publish original reports of research studies. Specialty practice journals publish research articles devoted to the particular specialty.

Secondary literature sources such as books can be helpful in finding primary research sources. Nursing students seeking research articles should use reference lists or bibliographies at the end of textbook chapters. To document the scientific basis for their writing, authors frequently cite primary sources as references, and these references are a valuable resource for nursing students who want more information.

Other secondary resources helpful in finding primary nursing research articles are research reviews such as the *Annual Review of Nursing Research* and the *Review of Research in Nursing Education*. Each volume is devoted to a certain topic. A review can help determine the status of research on a topic and can direct the reader toward other primary research sources. Research reviews are relatively new in nursing.

Organizing Information From a Research Report.

Articles listed in a bibliography or reference section are called **citations.** A citation provides the author's name and information about where ideas or quoted material was originally published. Writers are ethically obligated to give credit to others whose thoughts are used, even if the original author's exact words are not quoted.

There are many ways to list a citation. The style recommended by the American Psychological Association (1994) is widely used. This format avoids the use of footnotes. All citations are arranged alphabetically by the author's name at the end of the report.

The date of publication gives the approximate time the study was conducted. Sometimes researchers define the exact time period in the article because a considerable time (as long as 2 years) may pass between the time a study was completed and the time the article is published. Noting when a study was conducted allows the reader to track the development of knowledge in a particular area.

In nursing, many kinds of clinical problems are studied. The subject of the study provides information about the topics being investigated by nurse researchers. Studies undertaken in a particular problem area can then be collected and evaluated. There are often many ways to investigate a particular research problem. Knowing the way in which researchers studied a question helps students evaluate the thoroughness of the investigation.

A major purpose of scientific research is to increase knowledge about general classes of people or events. Knowledge about the subjects in a research study gives the nurse information about clients to whom the conclusions may be applied. When similar results are obtained with different groups of clients, nurses can be more confident when using the new methods with other clients.

The clinical setting can influence the results of a study. For example, findings from research studies on acute care needs are not necessarily applicable in a long-term care setting. This information is particularly relevant for research involving psychological aspects of nursing care. Different regions of the country have unique traditions and customs. Nursing interventions appropriate for people with certain attitudes and beliefs may not be relevant in regions or settings where attitudes and beliefs differ substantially.

The results summarize the findings about the area of study. When the findings and conclusions are replicated in a number of research studies, the conclusions are more generalizable than in the case of an isolated research project. The effects of preoperative teaching on the postoperative recovery of clients, for example, is a problem area in which collective evidence provides a reasonable scientific foundation for nursing practice.

IDENTIFYING CLINICAL NURSING PROBLEMS

Diers (1979) defined a **clinical nursing problem** as "a difference between two states of affairs, a discrepancy between the way things are and the way they ought to be, or between what one knows and what one needs to know to eliminate the problem." The following questions are raised by this definition:

Given the nursing interventions recommended for clients with a particular health care problem, how might the suggested care be improved so that the results or outcomes of care are better?

Given the knowledge about how to provide nursing care, what additional information would be needed to plan new interventions for clients with a particular health care problem?

Unanswered questions and the desire to improve nursing practice can provide the stimulus for conducting a research study.

Experience can make it possible to identify a researchable clinical nursing problem, but a nurse does not need to have years of clinical practice to identify a nursing problem. Sometimes a person who is relatively new in a situation can more easily see how things could be improved than those who have more experience and who take present conditions for granted. The nurse also considers whether the problem frequently occurs in a particular client group, whether it can be consistently and accurately measured, and whether a possible nursing solution might change the way care is delivered.

Sometimes nursing students or practicing nurses think that their ideas about nursing problems for study are not worthwhile unless they are certain that the proposed clinical study would make a radical change in client care. However, research efforts also may have to refine ideas about a clinical problem before the investigator can test alternative nursing interventions. In fact, some nurse researchers think that more investigative work needs to be conducted to describe the client response before research is designed to test an alternative intervention. In addition, the researcher may have to devise correct ways for measuring results before the study can proceed. All of these factors may discourage a nurse from undertaking a nursing research project. On the other hand, such projects can be viewed as stimulating challenges because much information has yet to be scientifically tested for its relevance to nursing practice.

RESEARCH UTILIZATION

Nurses should read journals that contain research reports, as well as textbooks and other sources, in nursing and related fields. Within those resources, findings from research studies may be suitable for use in nursing practice. For example, this text uses Research Highlight boxes to illustrate how research can progress from the phase of clinical problem investigation to application in day-to-day client care situations. To use findings in clinical practice, the nurse must be aware of the problems already studied and be able to identify relevant research studies.

Not all research related to clinical nursing problems

can or should be applied in practice. The nurse must judge the scientific worth of a study before considering its use in practice. This chapter can provide only a foundation for judging the worth of a research study. Other aspects that should be considered follow (Stetler, 1985, 1994; Stetler and DiMaggio, 1991):

The amount of supportive evidence provided by other scientific studies that have obtained similar results

Determination of whether the subjects and environment in the study are similar to the clients for whom the nurse provides care in the particular practice setting

The theoretical basis for present nursing care and the effectiveness of current theory in solving clinical nursing problems

The feasibility of applying findings, including ethical and legal limitations; institutional policy; changes in the organization of nursing services that might be required; and potential costs in time, money, and equipment

The nurse must take specific steps to make judgments that involve validating the scientific soundness of a study, comparatively evaluating whether any use can be made of the findings, and deciding the type of application that would be appropriate (Box 25-7).

The identification of a clinical problem, such as an increase in pressure ulcer development in a specific group of clients, initiates **research utilization** (Haller, Reynolds, and Horsley, 1979). In this example the research studies about the clinical problem, pressure ulcers, is thoroughly reviewed. The results of these studies are used and evaluated in the clinical practice setting.

When implementing research utilization in practice, it must be remembered that the problem area chosen must have an established research base, be relevant to practice, and be reliably evaluated by nurses in clinical settings. When selecting the problem area, the nurse first determines whether a solid research base exists for changing practice, the scientific merit of the studies that constitute the research base, and the potential risk to the client in implementing the practice change. The final phases include developing a clinical protocol that can be used to implement the change and clinically evaluating the outcomes of the new nursing care to determine its effectiveness.

Nurses often participate in quality assurance or quality improvement studies that evaluate the processes and outcomes (results) of nursing care (see Chapter 18). These studies measure how well nursing interventions are being implemented with specific clients by examining expected outcomes related to the nursing process protocols and procedures of a specific setting. By examining the quality of care provided for clients in their own setting and changing care as needed, nurses can use research to improve the quality of care.

Nurses should not change from accepted to unproven ways of providing client care without careful deliberation and consultation with colleagues. Experimenting with

---

Steps in the Research Utilization Process   Box 25-7

1. Identify and gather research studies appropriate to the clinical problem.
2. Critique the research studies.
3. Determine the merit of each study in terms of applicability to clinical practice.
4. Develop a specific practice innovation based on research findings of studies critiqued.
5. Apply the practice innovation to a defined clinical population.
6. Determine outcomes of the innovation.
7. Evaluate outcomes of the innovation for widespread use.
8. Communicate the innovation and outcomes to nursing staff.
9. Incorporate the innovation into the daily patient care routine.

From Feldman HR: Strategies for teaching nursing research: teaching baccalaureate nursing students, *West J Nurs Res* 18:479, 1996.

Barriers to Research Utilization   Box 25-8

THE RESEARCH ITSELF
Poorly designed and/or implemented research
Research not replicated
Relevant literature not compiled in one place
Poorly supported results
Poorly implemented or written statistical analysis

PRACTICING NURSES
Isolation from knowledgeable colleagues
Nurses too new on the job to implement new ideas
Lack of authority to implement changes

ORGANIZATIONAL SETTINGS
No support of nursing research findings
Changes in the health care environment
Acuity rate
Degree of nursing shortage
Financial constraints to implement change

THE NURSING PROFESSION
Limited research-based journals
Limited federal funding for nursing research
Poor communication between practitioners and researchers
Shortage of appropriate role models

Data from Polit DF, Hungler BP: *Nursing research: principles and methods,* ed 6, Philadelphia, 1999, JB Lippincott; Walsh M: Barriers to research utilization and evidence based practice in A & E nursing, *Emerg Nurse* 5(2):24, 1997; and Carroll DL and others: Barriers and facilitators to the utilization of nursing research, *Clin Nurse Spec* 11(5):207, 1997.

new nursing measures is inappropriate, especially if an increased risk to clients' health is possible.

Barriers to Research Utilization.
Nursing has long been urged to base care on research findings rather than tradition and ritual. The rapid growth of doctorally prepared nurse researchers has enabled the scientific base for nursing practice to grow. There are, however, barriers to utilization of research in clinical settings. Polit and Hungler (1999) and Funk, Tournquist, and Champagne (1995), among others, have tried to identify some of these barriers. Barriers such as those listed in Box 25-8 limit the potential of identifying clinical outcomes of nursing care. However, recognizing and acknowledging the existence of these barriers enable nurses to implement change in practice in a more timely manner.

• • •

Nursing research improves the practice of nursing and raises the standards for the profession. Involvement in nursing research takes place in many ways: designing studies, being part of a research team, collecting data, using research findings to change clinical practice, improving patient outcomes, and maintaining the cost of health care (Titler and others, 1994). Promoting research and research utilization in practice increases the scientific knowledge base for nursing practice. The recipients of these improvements to practice are the consumers of nursing care.

Key Concepts

- People acquire knowledge through tradition, from authorities in a field, through experience, through problem solving and critical thinking, and through application of the scientific method.
- A scientific investigation is an orderly, planned, and controlled way of studying reality that can be applied to general situations and contributes to the testing of theories about people, places, or life events.
- Nursing research is conducted to study the physical or psychosocial responses of people of all ages in health and illness.
- An experimental research study controls factors that could influence the results, includes comparison and experimental treatment groups of subjects, and uses random means for selecting study subjects.
- A qualitative research study organizes information in narrative format so that phenomena can be described and patterns of relationships can be discovered.
- Participation of human subjects in research studies requires the researcher to obtain informed consent of study subjects, maintain the confidentiality of subjects, and protect subjects from undue risk or injury.
- When summarizing data reported in a research study, the nurse should note when, how, where, and by whom the investigation was conducted and who and what were studied.
- A researchable clinical nursing problem is one that is not satisfactorily resolved by present nursing interventions, occurs frequently in a particular group, can be consistently and accurately measured, and has a possible solution within the realm of nursing practice.

- To determine whether research findings can be used as a basis for nursing practice, the nurse should consider the scientific worth of the study, the substantiating evidence provided in other studies, the similarity of the research setting to the nurse's own clinical practice setting, the status of current nursing theory, and factors affecting the feasibility of application.

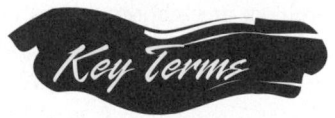

Key Terms

Abstract, *p. 534*
Anonymity, *p. 533*
Biomedical research, *p. 529*
Citations, *p. 536*
Clinical nursing problem, *p. 536*
Confidentiality, *p. 533*
Empirical data, *p. 528*
Ethnography, *p. 531*
Evaluation research, *p. 530*
Experimental study, *p. 530*
Grounded theory, *p. 531*
Hypothesis, *p. 529*
Informed consent, *p. 533*
Nursing research, *p. 525*
Phenomena, *p. 529*

Phenomenology, *p. 531*
Primary source, *p. 534*
Qualitative nursing research, *p. 531*
Quantitative nursing research, *p. 530*
Quasi-experimental research, *p. 530*
Research process, *p. 531*
Research utilization, *p. 537*
Scientific approach, *p. 527*
Scientific method, *p. 528*
Secondary source, *p. 534*
Subjects, *p. 530*
Surveys, *p. 530*

Critical Thinking Exercises

1. The nurse is concerned about learning to properly clean a pressure ulcer. Explain the benefits to the client if the nurse learns how to clean the sore by the scientific method versus trial and error.
2. If you wished to determine the best method for cleaning a pressure ulcer, what type of research method would you use for study?
3. The nurses working on an orthopedic unit decide to study the factors that commonly result in client falls on their unit. Explain why this quality improvement study is not scientific research. How could it be made into a scientific research study?

References

American Nurses Association: *Human rights guidelines for nurses in clinical and other research*, Washington, DC, 1985, The Association.

American Nurses Association: *Standards of clinical practice*, Washington, DC, 1991, The Association.

American Nurses Association: *Position statement: educational preparation for participation in nursing research*, Washington, DC, 1997, The Association.

American Psychological Association: *Publication manual of the American Psychological Association*, ed 4, Washington, DC, 1994, The Association.

Barrett EAM: Unique nursing research methods: the diversity chant of pioneers, *Nurs Sci Q* 11(3):94, 1998.

Canadian Nurses Association: *Ethical guidelines for nursing research involving human subjects*, Ottawa, 1983, The Association.

Canadian Nurses Association: *Code of ethics for nurses*, Ottawa, 1991, The Association.

Carroll DL and others: Barriers and facilitators to the utilization of nursing research, *Clin Nurse Spec* 11(5):207, 1997.

Code of Federal Regulations: *Protection of human subjects*, 45CFR46 (1983, revised as of March 1993), Washington, DC, 1993, U.S. Department of Health and Human Services.

Diers D: *Research in nursing practice*, Philadelphia, 1979, JB Lippincott.

Feldman HR: Strategies for teaching nursing research: teaching baccalaureate nursing students, *West J Nurs Res* 18:479, 1996.

Funk SG, Tournquist EM, Champagne MT: Barriers and facilitators of research utilization: an integrative review, *Nurs Clin North Am* 30(3):395, 1995.

Haller KB, Reynolds MA, Horsley JA: Developing research-based innovation protocols: process, criteria, and issues, *Res Nurs Health* 2:45, 1979.

Hinshaw AS, Feetham SL, Shaver JL: *Handbook of clinical nursing research*, Thousand Oaks, Calif, 1999, Sage Publications.

Institute of Medicine, Division of Health Care Services: *Nursing and nursing education: public policies and private actions*, Washington DC, 1983, National Academy.

International Council of Nurses: *Nursing research: ICN position statement*, Geneva, 1986, The Council.

Jeffers BR: Research for practice: the surrogate's experience during treatment decision making, *Medsurg Nurs*, 7(6):357, 1998.

Kellogg F and others: Life-sustaining interventions in frail elderly persons, *Arch Intern Med* 152:2317, 1994.

Ketchum K, Perry AC: *Patients' perceptions in weaning from mechanical ventilation*, Manuscript submitted for publication, 1999.

Knapp TR: *Quantitative nursing research*, Thousand Oaks, Calif, 1998, Sage Publications.

Meeker BJ: Preoperative education: evaluating postoperative patient outcomes, *Patient Educ Counsel* 23(1):41, 1994.

Morse JM, Field PA: *Qualitative research methods for health professional*, ed 2, Thousand Oaks, Calif, 1995, Sage Publications.

Munhall M, Alexander C, le May A: Appraising the evidence for practice: what do nurses need? *J Clin Effect* 3(2):54, 1998.

National Center for Nursing Research/International Council of Nurses: *Nursing research worldwide: report of the Task Force on International Nursing Research*, Geneva, Switzerland, 1990, The Association.

National Institute of Nursing Research: *National Institute of Nursing Research mission statement*, Bethesda, Md, 1997, National Institutes of Health; http://www.nih.gov/ninr/NINR2000A.RO.html.

Planchock NY, Wiggins MV: Preoperative assessment and teaching: physiological and psychological preparation, *Semin Periop Nurs* 3(2):161, 1994.

Polit DF, Hungler BP: *Nursing research: principles and methods*, ed 6, Philadelphia, 1999, JB Lippincott.

Stetler C: Research utilization: defining the concept, *Image J Nurs Sch* 17:40, 1985.

Stetler CB: Refinement of the Stetler/Marram model for application of research findings to practice, *Nurs Outlook* 42(1):15, 1994.

Stetler CB, DiMaggio G: Research utilization among clinical nurse specialists, *Clin Nurs Spec* 5(3):151, 1991.

Talbot LA: *Principles and practice of nursing research*, St. Louis, 1995, Mosby.

Timmons ME, Bower FL: The effect of structured preoperative teaching on patients' use of patient-controlled analgesia (PCA) and their management of pain, *Orthop Nurs* 12(1):23, 1993.

Titler MG and others: Infusing research into practice to promote quality care, *Nurs Res* 43(50):307, 1994.

Walsh M: Barriers to research utilization and evidence based practice in A & E nursing, *Emerg Nurse* 5(2):24, 1997.

Wunderlich R, Perry AG: Manuscript submitted for publication, 1999.

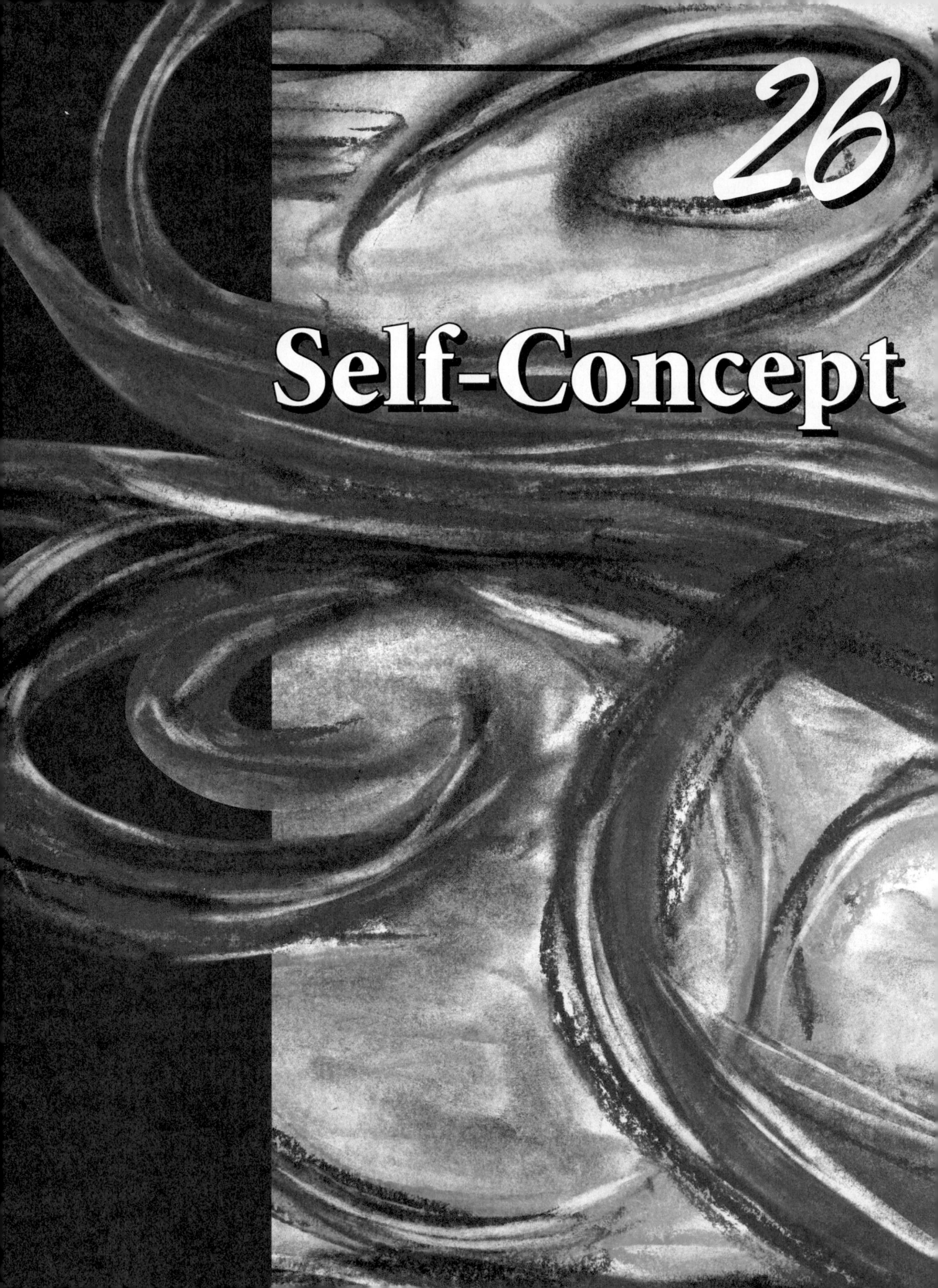

26

Self-Concept

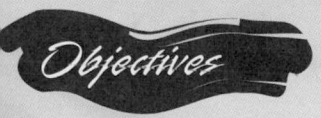

Objectives

Mastery of content in this chapter will enable the student to:

- Define the key terms listed.
- Distinguish the four components of self-concept: identity, body image, self-esteem, and roles.
- Describe stressors that can affect self-concept.
- Relate factors that can lead to role conflict, role ambiguity, and role strain.
- Identify the components of identity confusion.
- Define the components of a healthy self-concept as related to psychosocial and cognitive stages.
- Identify and discuss ways in which the nurse's self-concept and nursing activities can affect the client's self-concept.
- Describe behaviors indicating identity confusion, disturbed body image, low self-esteem, and role conflict.
- Identify important aspects of culture that affect nursing care in support of clients' self-concept.
- Distinguish factors that promote a healthy self-concept.

Scientific Knowledge Base

Our relationship with our self is our most intimate relationship, one of the most important aspects of our life experience, yet it is one of the most difficult to define. What we think and feel about ourselves affects the way in which we care for ourselves physically and emotionally and the way in which we are able to care for others. Individuals who have poor self-concepts often do not feel worthy of care, which influences whether they seek physical and emotional assistance as the need arises.

Self-concept is an individual's knowledge about the self (e.g., "I am good at math") (Sundeen and others, 1998). It is a subjective sense of the self and a complex mixture of unconscious and conscious thoughts, feelings, attitudes, and perceptions. Self-concept provides us with a frame of reference that affects our management of situations and our relationships with others. Self-concept begins to form at a young age. Adolescence is a critical time when many things continually affect the self-concept (Figure 26-1). Discrepancies between certain aspects of personality and self-concept may become sources of stress or conflict.

A person's self-concept and perception of his or her health are closely related to each other. A client's belief in personal good health can enhance his or her self-concept. Statements such as "I'm strong as an ox" or "I've never been sick a day in my life" indicate that a person's thoughts about personal health are positive. Such thoughts can influence self-concept. Illness, hospitalization, and surgery can also affect self-concept. Chronic illness may affect the ability to provide financial support, thereby affecting an individual's self-worth and roles within the family. Negative perceptions regarding health status may be reflected in such statements as "It's not worth it anymore" or "I'll never get any better."

The authors acknowledge the contribution of Dr. Judith A. Chaney to this chapter in the previous edition of this text.

Nursing Knowledge Base

In providing high-quality nursing care to clients, the nurse draws on nursing knowledge—knowledge built over time from the humanities, science and nursing research, and nursing practice. The nurse's broad knowledge base allows for a holistic view of clients, thus allowing problem solving that can best meet each client's needs.

OVERVIEW OF SELF-CONCEPT

Self-concept is developed through a very complex process that involves many variables. The four components of self-concept frequently considered by nurses are identity, body image, self-esteem, and role performance. Self-concept is the psychic representation of an individual, the central core of "I" around which all perceptions and experiences are organized. Self-concept is a dynamic combination formulated over years and based on the following:

Reactions of others to one's body

Ongoing perceptions of the reactions of others to the self

Relationships with self and others

Spiritual identity

Personality structure

Perceptions of stimuli that have an impact on the self

Prior and new experiences

Present feelings about the physical, emotional, and social self

Expectations about the self

A positive self-concept gives a sense of continuity, wholeness, and consistency to a person. A healthy self-concept has a high degree of stability and generates positive or negative feelings toward the self.

Identity forms one of the four integrating principles of self-concept. People are aware of whether they are being

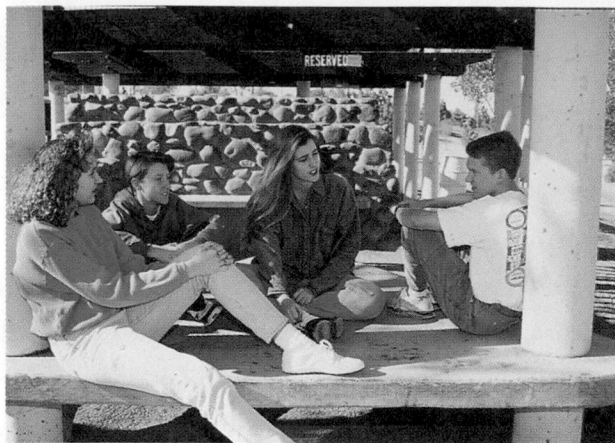

Figure 26-1   Adolescents in group activities can foster self-esteem.

who they really are versus behaving in a particular way because it is expected of them. Being "oneself" is the crux of identity. Identity is often gained from self-observations and from what individuals are told about themselves (Sundeen and others, 1998).

Body image is an individual's mental picture of his or her physical appearance. These mental images are not necessarily consistent with the actual body structure or appearance. Culture and society influence the norms of body image. Body image may change within a few hours, days, weeks, or months, depending on the impact of external stimuli on the body and actual changes in appearance, structure, or function. The way others view a person's body is also influential. For example, a controlling, violent husband might tell his wife that she is ugly and that no one else would want her. Over the years of marriage, she believes this image of herself and incorporates it into her self-concept.

Self-esteem is influenced by both self-evaluation and the responses of others. Self-esteem involves an individual's evaluation of his or her own worth. A person who values himself or herself, despite weaknesses and limitations, and who feels valued by others usually has high self-esteem. A person who feels worthless and who receives little respect from others usually has low self-esteem.

Individuals have self-perceptions based on gender, age, perceived health status, background, family roles, occupational and social roles, and use of leisure time. Basic feelings about the self tend to be constant, even though there is some fluctuation, with good and bad days. An individual's self-perception does not necessarily match the perceptions of others.

A person's ability to contribute in a meaningful way to society often affects his or her self-concept and self-esteem. Individuals who are sick and unable to be involved in society may feel a sense of worthlessness. The nurse's

acceptance of a client as an individual with worth and dignity can be vital in maintaining and improving the client's self-esteem.

COMPONENTS OF SELF-CONCEPT

One way to consider self-concept is to look at the various components that make up self-concept. Four significant components of self-concept that nursing considers are identity, body image, self-esteem, and role performance.

Identity.   **Identity** involves the internal sense of individuality, wholeness, and consistency of a person over time and in various circumstances. The concept of identity thus includes constancy and continuity. Identity implies being distinct and separate from others—being a whole and unique self.

Identity develops over time. A child learns culturally accepted values, behaviors, and roles through **identification.** The child first identifies with parenting figures and later with teachers, peers, and heroes. To form an identity, the child must be able to bring together learned behaviors and expectations into a coherent, consistent, and unique whole (Erikson, 1963).

The achievement of identity is necessary for intimate relationships because one's identity is expressed in relationships with others. Sexuality is a part of one's identity. Sexual identity is a person's image of the self as a man or a woman and the meaning of this image. This image and its meaning depend on culturally determined values that are learned through socialization (see Chapter 27). One's occupation or primary work role also contributes to one's identity.

Body Image.   Body image is made up of a person's perceptions of the body, both internally and externally. It includes feelings and attitudes toward the body. Body image is influenced by personal views of physical characteristics and abilities and by perceptions of others' views.

Body image is affected by cognitive growth and physical development. Normal developmental changes such as physical growth and aging have a more apparent effect on body image than on other aspects of self-concept. A school-age child's body image is different from an infant's. Hormonal changes during adolescence and menopause influence body image. Aging changes (e.g., wrinkles; graying hair; decrease in visual acuity, hearing, and mobility) may also affect body image.

Cultural and societal attitudes and values also influence body image (Box 26-1). In American society, youth, beauty, and wholeness are emphasized—a fact apparent in television programs, movies, and advertisements. Western cultures (particularly in the United States) have been socialized to fear and dread the normal aging process, whereas in Eastern cultures aging is viewed very positively: the older adult is respected.

Body image depends only partly on the reality of the

Recent issues in the study of the self attempt to explain cultural differences between individuals by looking at the differences cultures have in viewing independence versus collectivism. In this case independence refers to an individualism, wherein one is not dependent on or subject to the control or opinion of others. Collectivism, by contrast, refers to persons considered as members of a group or whole with similarity among members.

Often the concepts of individualism and collectivism are viewed in Eastern versus Western cultural terms. In cultures emphasizing collectivism (e.g., Japan and China) the collective self is more complex and intricate in structure and the individualistic self is more simplistic, whereas in cultures where individualism is emphasized (United States, Canada, and Australia) the individual, private self is the most complex. These cultures have different values in regard to the group. People socialize according to their culture. Culture influences what people tend to value in their lives. How people think about themselves, what motivates them, and how they behave are all related to the culture within which people are socialized.

The preceding concept applies to dress and body adornment. In Western cultures people value individual expression through clothing and hairstyles. In Eastern cultures there is a more restrictive code of clothing and hairstyles that is acceptable (although this is changing as society becomes more international). The effect of individualism versus collectivism can be seen in newspapers, movies, and other media from both cultures.

body. When physical changes occur, individuals may or may not incorporate these changes into their body image. Often, for example, people who have experienced significant weight loss do not perceive themselves as thin. Older adults often report that they do not feel different. Then when they look in the mirror, they are surprised by wrinkled skin or gray hair.

Self-Esteem. **Self-esteem** is an individual's sense of self-worth and is based on both internal and external factors. According to Erikson (1963), young children begin to develop a sense of usefulness or industry by learning to act on their own initiative. A child's self-esteem is related to the child's evaluation of his or her effectiveness at school or work, within the family, and in social settings. The evaluation of others also is likely to have a profound influence on the child's self esteem.

Understanding self-esteem can be enhanced by considering the relationship between a person's self-concept and the ideal self. The **ideal self** consists of the aspirations, goals, values, and standards of behavior that a person considers ideal and strives to attain. The ideal self originates in the preschool years and develops throughout life; it is influenced by societal norms and the expectations and demands of parents and significant others. In general, a person whose self-concept comes close to matching the ideal self has high self-esteem, whereas a person whose self-concept varies widely from the ideal self has low self-esteem.

A person's family and society in general set the standards by which individuals evaluate themselves. A child who excels in school and who is liked by peers is likely to have high self-esteem, whereas a child who has difficulty in school and is not liked by peers is likely to develop a low self-esteem.

Self-evaluation is an ongoing mental process. A positive sense of self-worth, or self-esteem, is a basic human need, according to Maslow's hierarchy. An individual's self-esteem affects how he or she functions in the world. A person's self-esteem affects his or her self-concept.

Role Performance. Roles that individuals assume or follow in given situations involve expectations or standards of behavior that have developed in their society or culture. An individual develops role behavior based on patterns established through socialization. Socialization begins just after birth, when an infant responds to adults and adults respond to the infant's behaviors. The patterns are stable and change only minimally during adulthood. A child learns behaviors that are approved by society through the following processes:

Reinforcement-extinction: Certain behaviors become common or are avoided, depending on whether they are approved and reinforced or discouraged and punished.

Inhibition: A child learns to refrain from behaviors, even when tempted to engage in them.

Substitution: A child replaces one behavior with another, which provides the same personal gratification.

Imitation: A child acquires knowledge, skills, or behaviors from members of the social or cultural group.

Identification: A child internalizes the beliefs, behavior, and values of role models into a personal, unique expression of self.

During **socialization,** a child generally develops the skills necessary for functioning in many different roles. Unsuccessful socialization is an inability to function acceptably according to society's values.

Ideal societal role behaviors are often hard to live out in real life where individuals have multiple roles and individual needs. Successful adults learn to distinguish between ideal role expectations and realistic possibilities. To function effectively in roles, people must know the expected behavior and values, must desire to conform to them, and must be able to meet the role requirements. Most individuals have more than one role. Common roles include mother or father, wife or husband, daughter or son, employee or employer, sister or brother, and friend. Each role involves meeting certain expectations. Fulfillment of these expectations leads to rewards. Difficulty or failure in meeting role expectations often contributes to decreased self-esteem.

Role performance is the way in which an individual perceives his or her competency in carrying out significant roles. An individual's perception of competency may or may not match the evaluation of others who relate to the person.

STRESSORS AFFECTING SELF-CONCEPT

Stressors challenge a person's adaptive capacities. Selye (1956) states that stress is the normal wear and tear of life, not the specific result of any one action or typical response to any one thing. The normal process of maturation and development itself is a stressor. Changes that occur in physical, spiritual, emotional, sexual, familial, and socio-cultural health are stressful. A self-concept stressor is any real or perceived change that threatens identity, body image, self-esteem, or role behavior (Figure 26-2)

Different individuals react to the same situation with varying degrees of stress. Perception of a stressor is an important factor that influences the response to it. People learn patterns of behavior as a way of coping with or adapting to stressors. These patterns are often used when a person encounters a new stressor. Some of these patterns of responding to stressors are more adaptive than others. Being able to adapt to stressors is likely to lead to a positive sense of self, whereas failure to adapt often leads to a negative sense of self. An individual's ability to adapt is related to numerous factors, including the number of stressors, duration of the stressor, and health status (see Chapter 30).

Any change in health can be a stressor that affects self-concept. A physical change in the body can lead to an altered body image affecting identity and self-esteem. Chronic illnesses often alter role performance, which may alter one's identity and self-esteem. The case study in Box 26-2 illustrates the interrelationship of the four components of self-concept.

A crisis occurs when a person cannot overcome obstacles with usual methods of problem solving and adapting. Any crisis requires change and thus threatens self-concept. Some crises, such as the case study in Box 26-2, directly affect all four components of self-concept. During self-concept crises, as with other kinds of crises, supportive re-

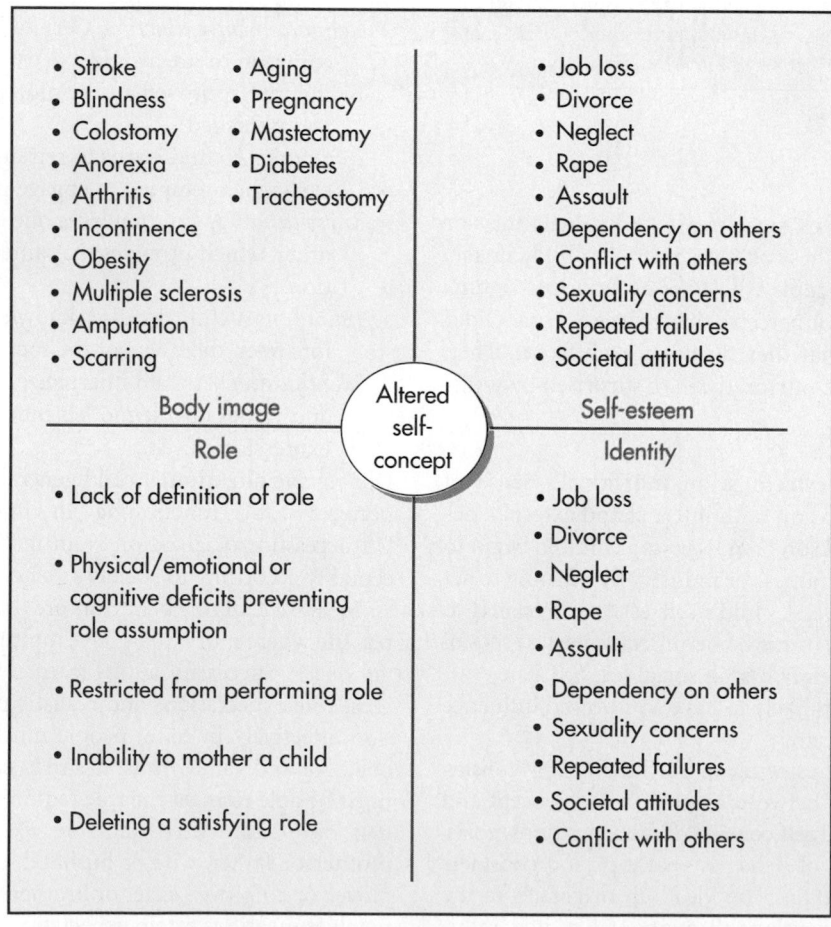

Figure 26-2   Common stressors that can influence self-concept.

sources can be valuable in helping a person learn new ways of coping with and responding to the event or situation to maintain a positive self-concept.

Identity Stressors.

The identity is defined as the "organizing principle of the personality system that accounts for the unity, continuity, uniqueness, and consistency of the personality" (Sundeen and others, 1998). One's identity is affected by stressors throughout life. Adolescence is a time of great change, causing insecurity and anxiety. Adolescents are trying to adjust to the physical, emotional, and mental changes of increasing maturity. Stressors may arise in any of these areas or as a result of conflicts among them.

An adult generally has a more stable identity and thus a more firmly developed self-concept. Cultural and social stressors rather than personal stressors may have more impact on an adult's identity. For example, an adult may have to decide between career and marriage, cooperation and competition, or dependence and independence in a relationship (Sundeen and others, 1998).

Developmental markers such as the initiation of menses, puberty, menopause, retirement, and decreasing physical abilities may affect identity. Identity, like body image, is closely related to appearance and abilities (Figure 26-3). Retirement may mean the loss of an important means of achievement and continued success. People at retirement may begin to question their identities and accomplishments. Loss of a significant other can lead the

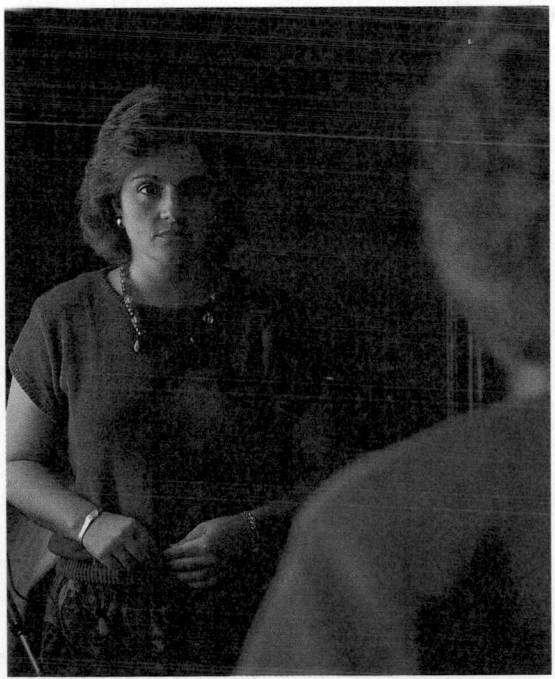

Figure 26-3   An individual's appearance influences self-concept.

> ## Case STUDY   BOX 26-2
>
> Paul, a 48-year-old man, suffers a stroke. The stroke is unexpected and sudden. He was not even aware that he had hypertension, since he had not been getting yearly checkups. Paul awakens in the hospital bed to find that he cannot move even his hand. He cannot care for himself. He cannot even turn himself for days. Finally, he is able to pull himself out of bed and into a chair with the nurse's help. He wonders what lies in store for him. Paul's body image has dramatically changed from that of a man of strength and endurance to that of a helpless individual. Paul worries about his family and what will happen. His daughter, the oldest child, is away at college, and his son is still in high school. Paul and his wife, Meredith, are terrified. Although Meredith works, they have not saved enough money to be able to educate their children without Paul's wages. Paul's role as chief financial provider for the family may be drastically changed if his condition does not change.
>
> Paul's self-esteem wanes as his recovery and rehabilitation move slowly. His self-concept changes from that of a strong laborer, one who did his own plumbing and car repairs, to a man who has to tell his son what to do because he does not have the strength to do these tasks. Although he is now at home in the rehabilitation process, Paul is not able to perform tasks for the family and must wait until his wife and son get home to help him with things that require strength. Paul's adaptation capabilities are stretched to the maximum, although his physician tells him that he is very fortunate to be alive. His life is now changed—for how long he does not know. Paul's identity is not clear to him any more, he has no clear role within the family, his body image has been drastically altered, and his self-esteem is spiraling lower and lower.
>
> Paul continues in outpatient physical therapy. It takes much time and hard work even on simple tasks, but he begins to gain some strength. Paul continues to make gains. He is able to return to work. He has some diminished mental quickness and some muscle weakening, but he is able to perform his job. His self-esteem recovers, and his body image is enhanced. Although he still feels somewhat altered, his capabilities closely resemble his capabilities before the stroke.

surviving individual to reexplore aspects of his or her identity.

Identity confusion results when people do not maintain a clear, consistent, and continuous consciousness of personal identity. It may occur at any stage of life if a person is unable to adapt to identity stressors. Under extreme stress an individual may experience depersonalization, a state in which internal and external realities or the differences between the self and others cannot be determined.

Body Image Stressors.

Changes in the appearance, structure, or function of a body part will require a change in body image. Changes in the appearance of the body, such as an amputation or facial disfigurement, are obvious stressors affecting body image. Mastectomy, colostomy, and ileostomy are surgical procedures that alter the appearance and function of the body, although the changes are not apparent when people are clothed. Even though they are not apparent to others, these bodily changes have a significant effect on the individual. Chronic illnesses such as heart and renal disease involve a change in function, in which the body no longer functions at an optimal level. Even "normal" body changes resulting from the normal developmental process of aging can affect body image. In addition, the effects of pregnancy, significant weight gain or loss, chemotherapy, or radiation therapy change body image.

An individual's perception of body changes may be affected by how the changes came about. For example, paralysis caused by war injuries may be considered acceptable by society. A veteran may be treated as a hero and praised for bravery. Governmental resources will be available for rehabilitation. However, people who have automobile accidents while drunk and suffer paralysis may receive a very different response from society.

The significance of a loss of function or a change in appearance is affected by the individual's perception of the alteration. Body image consists of ideal and real elements. For example, if a woman's body image incorporates breasts as the ideal, the loss of a breast by mastectomy may be a very significant alteration. The greater the importance of the body or a specific body part, the greater the threat felt by a change in body image.

Many people associate success with a specific body part or function. For example, athletes may consider their bodies and physical activities to be the focus of personal success. If they can never again participate in physical activities because of an accident, their adaptation and rehabilitation may be affected. They must revise long-accepted assumptions about themselves and alter their lifestyles. To regain a positive self-concept and self-esteem, and to maintain good health, they must adapt to their body image stressors.

Positive social changes with regard to illness and altered body image have occurred. The media now frequently present positive stories about persons with serious disabilities or who have had major body-altering surgery. These stories provide positive role models for individuals undergoing unusual stressors, as well as for their families, friends, and society as a whole.

Self-Esteem Stressors.

Positive or high self-esteem involves an individual seeing himself or herself as being a good person, worthy of respect and love. A person with low self-esteem tends to feel unloved and often experiences depression and anxiety. Self-esteem fluctuates somewhat with surrounding conditions, although a basic core of positive or negative self-esteem remains fairly constant even with changing circumstances. Most people experience "bad days," when they feel less worthy and competent, but these feelings pass relatively quickly for someone with a positive self-esteem.

Self-esteem stressors vary with developmental stages. Inability to meet parental expectations, harsh criticism, inconsistent punishment, sibling rivalry, and repeated defeats may reduce the level of self-worth of children at various stages of development. Stressors affecting the self-esteem of an adult include failure in work and failures in relationships.

Illness, surgery, or accidents that change life patterns may also influence feelings of self-worth. Chronic illnesses such as diabetes, arthritis, and cardiac dysfunction require changes in accepted and long-assumed behavioral patterns. The more the chronic illness interferes with the ability to engage in activities contributing to feelings of worth or success, the more it affects self-esteem.

Role Stressors.

Roles involve expected behavior patterns associated with one individual's function in various social groups (Sundeen and others, 1998). Throughout life, people undergo numerous role changes. Normal changes associated with growth and maturation result in developmental transitions. Situational transitions occur when parents, spouses, or close friends die or people move, marry, divorce, or change jobs. A health-illness transition is a movement from a state of health or well-being to one of illness or vice versa. Any of these transitions may lead to role conflict, role ambiguity, role strain, or role overload. It is important to recognize that a shift along the continuum from illness to wellness is as stressful as a shift from wellness to illness.

Role conflict results when a person is required to simultaneously assume two or more roles that are inconsistent, contradictory, or mutually exclusive. For example, when a middle-age woman with teenage children assumes responsibility for the care of her older parents, conflicts may arise in relation to being both a parent to her children and the child of her parents. Negotiating a balance of time and energy between her children and parents may create role conflicts. The importance of each conflicting role influences the degree of conflict experienced.

Role ambiguity involves unclear role expectations.

When there are unclear expectations, people are unsure about what to do, how to do it, or both. Such a situation is often stressful and confusing. Role ambiguity is common in the adolescent years. Adolescents are pressured by parents, peers, and the media to assume adultlike roles, yet remain in the role of a dependent child. Role ambiguity is also common in employment situations. In complex, rapidly changing, or highly specialized organizations, employees often become unsure about what is expected of them.

Role strain blends role conflict and role ambiguity. Role strain may be expressed as a feeling of frustration when a person feels inadequate or feels unsuited to a role. Role strain is often associated with gender role stereotypes (Sundeen and others, 1998). Women in positions typically held by men may be perceived by others as less competent, less objective, or less knowledgeable than their male counterparts. Thus they may feel that they must work harder and be better to compete. Men in typically female roles also encounter gender bias, which frequently questions their masculinity.

Role overload involves having more roles or responsibilities within a role than is manageable. Often during periods of illness or change, those involved—either the one who is ill or significant others—find themselves in role overload.

The **sick role** involves the expectations of others and society regarding how one should behave when sick. Role conflict may occur when general societal expectations (take care of yourself and you'll get better) and the expectations of co-workers (need to get work done) collide. The conflict of taking care of oneself while getting everything done can be a major challenge.

The sick role may also involve role ambiguity. People are expected to be dependent and simultaneously participate actively so that they can get well and leave the sick role quickly. However, chronically ill people cannot do this. The sick role is supposed to be temporary, yet the chronically ill must comply with therapy that may be necessary for the remainder of life.

• • •

Self-concept can be altered by stressors affecting identity, body image, self-esteem, or roles. These stressors can also affect health. If people are unable to adapt to such stressors, their health may be at risk. If the resulting identity confusion, disturbed body image, low self-esteem, role conflict, role strain, or role ambiguity is not relieved, illness may result.

DEVELOPMENT OF SELF-CONCEPT

Development of self-concept is a lifelong process. Each stage of development has specific tasks. Successful negotiation of these tasks tends to promote a positive self-concept (Box 26-3). Influential theorists who have considered various components of human development include

---

Self-Concept: Developmental Tasks   Box 26-3

0 TO 1 YEAR
Begins to trust
Distinguishes self from environment

1 TO 3 YEARS
Has control of some language
Begins to be autonomous in thoughts and actions
Likes body
Likes self

3 TO 6 YEARS
Takes initiative
Identifies with a gender
Increases self-awareness
Increases language skills

6 TO 12 YEARS
Is industrious
Interacts with peers
Increases self-esteem with new skill mastery
Aware of strengths and limits

12 TO 20 YEARS
Accepts changed body
Explores goals for future
Feels positive about self
Interacts with those whom he or she finds sexually attractive

MID-20S TO MID-40S
Has intimate relationships with family and significant others
Has stable, positive feelings about self

MID-40S TO MID-60S
Can accept changes in appearance and endurance
Reassesses life goals
Shows contentment with aging

LATE 60S ON
Feels positive about one's life and its meaning
Interested in providing a legacy for the next generation

Erikson, Piaget, Kohlberg, and Gilligan. The following is a brief discussion of the stages of development. For additional information, consult the chapter indicated with each section.

Infant.   What an infant needs initially is a primary caretaker and a relationship with that caretaker. This nurturing role can be fulfilled by a mother, father, or someone responsible for the caretaking of the infant. When the infant has pleasant, nurturing interactions with the caretakers, these are remembered and internalized into the infant's psyche. If the interactions are unsatisfying, painful, or frustrating, this can result in difficulties in establishing a positive self-concept. When an infant's needs are met with reasonable consistency, the infant develops a sense of trust in his or her world (see Chapter 10). During this phase of development the infant begins to differentiate between self and others.

Toddler. Toddlers (1 to 3 years of age) are more mobile and able to interact with others. Their major psychosocial task is the development of autonomy (see Chapter 10). Toddlers move from total dependence to a greater sense of independence and separateness of themselves from others. They also tend to view others and themselves in terms of "all good" or "all bad." They gain skills in feeding themselves and performing basic hygiene tasks. Toddlers learn to coordinate movements and imitate others. They learn control of their bodies through locomotion, toilet training, speech, and socialization skills.

Preschooler. Body boundaries, sense of self, and gender of preschoolers become more definite to them because of a developing sexual curiosity and awareness of differences from others of the same and opposite gender. Learning about the body—where it begins and ends, what it looks like, and what it can do—is basic to self-concept and body image formation. Growing self-awareness includes discovery of feelings; for example, preschoolers learn names for their feelings. They begin to learn how they affect others and how others respond to them. They also learn the rudiments of control over feelings and behavior. The concept of body is reflected in the way children talk, move, draw pictures, and play. Children begin to test roles and imitate people as they identify with the same-sex parent or a family member (see Chapter 10).

Appraisal by a family member becomes self-appraisal. The family is critical to the child's budding self-concept, and negative input at this time creates a decreased self-esteem, which the person as an adult will have to work very hard to overcome.

School-Age Child. Until children attend school, self-concept and body image are based primarily on parental attitudes (see Chapter 10). At school others contribute to the child's self-concept and body image. This can have a counterbalancing effect for children whose families have been extremely critical, or it can be negative if the child experiences a negative educational environment.

As the child enters the school years, growth is steady, and more motor, social, and intellectual skills are acquired. The child's body changes, and his or her sexual identity strengthens. The child's attention span increases, and reading allows expansion of the child's self-concept, through imagination, into other roles, behaviors, and places. The child begins to reason in a more systematic way and is able to apply previous learning to current situations (Piaget, 1963). Through games children interact with peers, develop additional motor and intellectual skills, and thereby

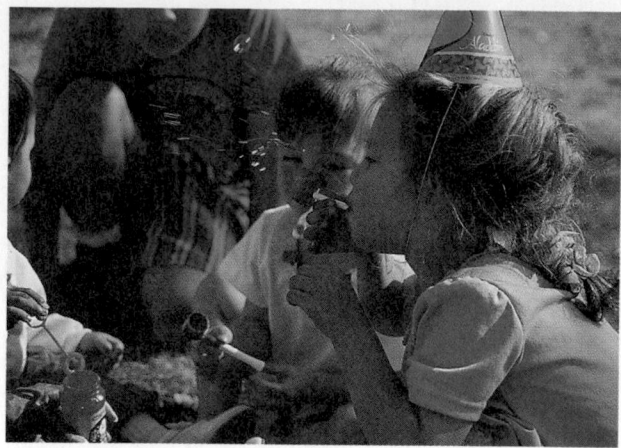

Figure 26-4 A child learns to define self partly through interactions with peers.

expand their self-concept and body image (Figure 26-4). Children express feelings through games, literature, drawing, and music. The nurse can use these to gain clues to children's self-concepts. With increased problem-solving abilities, a greater self-awareness of personal strengths and limitations develops. Self-concept and body image can change at this time because the child is changing physically, emotionally, mentally, and socially.

Adolescent. Adolescence brings physical, emotional, and social upheaval. Throughout sexual maturation, new feelings, roles, and values must be integrated into the self. Rapid growth, noticed by the adolescent and others, is an important factor in body image acceptance and revision (see Chapter 10).

Adolescents are forced to alter their mental pictures of themselves. Physical changes in size and appearance cause changes in self-perception and use of the body. Adolescents spend a great deal of time in front of the mirror for hygiene, grooming, and dressing as they seek to improve their appearance as much as possible. Great distress is felt about perceived body imperfections.

Development of self-concept and body image is closely related to identity formation (Erikson, 1963). According to Gilligan (1982), differences in male and female development during adolescence and young adulthood include boys being more focused on development of individual identity and girls more likely developing identities within the context of relationships. The ways in which adolescent males and females consider moral situations also demonstrate differences. Kohlberg (1969), whose research involved following boys over time to observe moral development, found them to have highly developed moral reasoning concerning equality, reciprocity, justice, and rights. According to Gilligan's research (1982), boys tend to use equality, reciprocity, justice, and rights as the basis for decision making, whereas girls tend to consider caring, relationships between people, and responses that result in good will rather than hurt as their guide for decision making. Being aware of these common gender differences when interacting with clients can assist the nurse in understanding an individual's perceptions of what is important and valued.

Young Adult.

Although physical growth has stopped, cognitive, social, and behavioral changes continue for the rest of life. Young adulthood (early 20s to mid-40s) is a period of choice; it is a period of settling into responsibility, gaining stability in the establishment of employment, and beginning intimate relationships. Self-concept and body image become relatively stable at this time.

Self-concept and body image are social creations, and approval and acceptance are given for normal appearance and proper behavior according to societal standards. Self-concept constantly evolves and can be identified in values, attitudes, and feelings about the self (see Chapter 11).

Middle Adult.

Physical changes such as additional fat deposits, baldness, gray hair, wrinkles, and varicosities confront the middle adult. People realize that they look older, and they may feel older as well. Work may be stressful if middle-age people feel that they have less stamina, endurance, and vigor to cope with the task at hand. This reduced energy level is often a result of lower basal metabolism and reduced muscle tone.

Often middle adulthood is a time of self-reflection and reevaluation. Individuals are likely to reexamine their lives, considering whether they are satisfied with what they have accomplished and how they want to live the rest of their lives (Sheehy, 1995). This time of reflection may be difficult as an individual considers what is right and what is wrong in his or her life. Even though this self-reflection may be difficult at times, it can foster growth and a more integrated self-concept.

Illness or death of loved ones can create concerns about personal health. The person may feel inferior to youth as the previous self-image of a strong and healthy body with boundless energy is replaced with a self-image reflecting the changes of aging. Difficulties in accepting the loss of youth are also caused by fear of the effects of menopause, folklore about sexuality, and social and advertising pressures describing the virtues of youth.

The middle adult years are often the time for a reassessment of life experiences and a redefinition of the self in life roles and values (see Chapter 11). This is called the midlife crisis and might include a reevaluation of career or marriage choices. Successful resolution involves the integration of new qualities into the self-concept. Most people gradually adjust to their slowly changing bodies and accept the changes as part of maturing. Emotionally mature people realize that they cannot return to youth and acknowledge that their own pasts and experiences are valid

and valuable. Middle-age people who are content with their age and have no desire to relive the youthful years exhibit a healthy self-concept.

Older Adult.

Physical changes in older adults can be seen as gradual reductions of structure and function (see Chapter 12). Loss of muscle strength and tone occurs. Osteoporosis, which is a loss of bone density and mass, may increase the risk of fractures and create a "dowager's" hump.

Loss of sensory acuity is a factor that influences older adults in interacting with the environment. The normal process of aging causes decreased visual acuity. Hearing loss can cause negative personality changes, such as suspiciousness, irritability, impatience, or withdrawal, as older people realize that they are less aware of what is happening around them. Many older adults view a hearing aid as another threat to body image. To many older adults, eyeglasses are more socially acceptable because they are worn by all age-groups, but a hearing aid is perceived as direct evidence of age.

Loss of skin tone with accompanying wrinkles may affect self-esteem and cause older persons to feel unattractive in a society that values youth and beauty. Western culture does not discriminate in terms of age and appearance toward men as severely as it does toward women.

Self-concept during older adulthood is influenced by experiences throughout life. It is a time when many people reflect on their lives, reviewing successes and disappointments and thereby creating a unified sense of meaning about themselves and the world (Box 26-4). Helping the younger generation in a positive way often helps an older adult to develop a feeling of leaving a legacy. Self-concept is also influenced by people's present perceived health status.

NURSING PRACTICE   Box 26-4

Reminiscence has been found to support a positive self-concept in older adults. Suggestions for reminiscence include the following:

- Spend time reviewing old photographs and have the older adult tell his or her stories that relate to the pictures.
- Plan sessions where the older adult and a friend can talk about past shared experiences.
- Encourage the person to write about a positive past event.*
- Ask a person to tell you about a memorable event and tape record his or her story (asking permission before you begin), then play the tape back for the person, either at that time or at another time.*
- Encourage the person to write letters to old friends.*

*From Nugent E: Try to Remember . . . reminiscence as a nursing intervention, J Psychosoc Nurs 33(11):7, 1995.

FAMILY EFFECT ON SELF-CONCEPT DEVELOPMENT

The family plays a key role in creating and maintaining its members' self-concepts. Children develop from parents and siblings a basic sense of who they are and how they are expected to live. Negative self-concepts may be cultivated in children, even by well-meaning parents. Parents who are harsh, inconsistent, or have low self-esteem themselves may behave in ways that foster negative self-concepts in their children. To reverse a client's negative self-concept, the nurse may first need to assess the family's style of relating (see Chapter 8). Self-concept change demands hard work and consistency, supported by the entire nursing staff and physicians as well.

THE NURSE'S EFFECT ON THE CLIENT'S SELF-CONCEPT

A nurse's acceptance of a client with an altered self-concept helps promote positive change. When a client's physical appearance has changed, it is likely that both the client and the family will look to nurses and observe their responses and reactions to the changed appearance. Nurses can have a significant impact on clients in this respect. Nursing plans formulated to help a client with an altered self-concept can be enhanced or defeated by the nurse's unconscious values and feelings. It is critical for nurses to assess and clarify the following about themselves:

　　Their own feelings about lifestyle, health, and illness

　　How they react to stress

　　Their awareness of how their nonverbal communication may affect clients and families

　　Their personal values and expectations and how these affect clients

　　Their ability to convey a nonjudgmental attitude in regard to clients

Nurses need to assess themselves honestly before they can begin to understand how they affect their clients with both words and actions. Nurses should pay attention to "triggers," which are heightened feelings that occur in response to a given situation, such as a clients' disability. Nurses should not deny that they have feelings, ideas, values, and expectations or deny that they make judgments. Self-awareness is critical in initially understanding and accepting others. All people make decisions about themselves, the environment, and other people on the basis of personal frames of reference. As professionals, nurses must be prepared to work with people who have different frames of reference from that of the nurse. Nurses who are secure in their own identities more readily accept and thus reinforce clients' identities. However, nurses who are unsure of their own identities may be unable to accept clients and may react as if clients should be something or someone else, thus creating a nonaccepting environment for the client.

Nurses can also have a significant impact on body image. For example, a nurse can influence the body image of a woman who has had a mastectomy in a positive way by showing acceptance of the mastectomy scar. On the other hand, a shocked or disgusted facial expression can contribute to the woman's developing a negative body image. Clients closely watch the reactions of others to their wounds and scars. It is very important for the nurse to monitor responses toward the client. Statements such as "This wound is healing nicely" or "This scar looks good" can be very affirming for the body image of the client.

Inadvertently frowning or grimacing when performing procedures can have profound effects on the client. A nurse who avoids a client should recognize that something is wrong. The nurse's nonverbal behaviors help to convey the level of caring that exists for a client (Figure 26-5). For example, the self-concept of incontinent clients can be threatened by the perception that the caretakers find the situation unpleasant. Nurses should anticipate these reactions, acknowledge them, and focus on the client instead of the unpleasant task or situation. Otherwise, clients may perceive nurses' behaviors as rejection. If nurses can put themselves in the client's position, they can envision measures to ease embarrassment, frustration, anger, and denial.

Critical Thinking Synthesis

Successful critical thinking requires synthesis of knowledge, experience, information gathered from clients, critical thinking attitudes, and intellectual and professional standards. Successful clinical judgment requires the nurse to anticipate the information necessary, analyze the data, and make decisions regarding client care. Critical thinking is always changing. During assessment the nurse must consider all critical thinking elements that contribute to making appropriate nursing diagnoses.

In the case of self-concept, the nurse must integrate knowledge from nursing and other disciplines, including self-concept theory, communication principles, and a con-

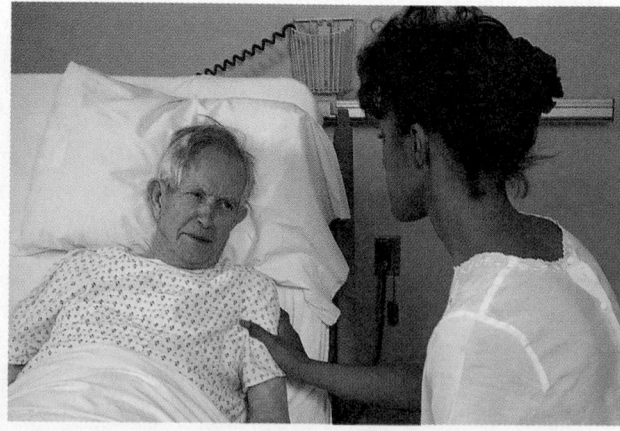

Figure 26-5　Nurses can use touch and eye contact to increase a client's self-esteem.

sideration of cultural and developmental factors. Previous experience in caring for clients with self-concept alterations assists the nurse in adapting care for each new client. Critical thinking attitudes such as integrity ensure that the client receives professional and respectful care. Ethical standards of supporting clients' autonomy and intellectual standards such as relevance ensure that the nurse respects the clients' uniqueness. Self-concept profoundly influences a person's response to illness. A critical thinking approach to care is essential (Figure 26-6).

Self-Concept and the Nursing Process

ASSESSMENT

In assessing self-concept, the nurse should focus on each component of self-concept (identity, body image, self-esteem, and role performance); behaviors suggestive of an altered self-concept (Box 26-5); actual and potential self-concept stressors (see Figure 26-2); and coping patterns. Gathering comprehensive assessment data requires the nurse to critically synthesize information from multiple sources (see Figure 26-6). Much of the data regarding self-concept is most effectively gathered through observation of the client's nonverbal behavior and by paying attention to the content of the client's conversation rather than through direct questioning. The nurse should take note of the manner in which clients talk about the people in their lives, since this can provide clues to both stressful and supportive relationships and to key roles. Using knowledge of developmental stages (see Box 26-2) to determine what areas are likely to be important to the client, the nurse should inquire about these aspects of the per

son's life. For example, the nurse might ask a 65-year-old client about his or her life and what has been important to him or her. This is the stage in life wherein individuals are examining their lives and considering the impact they have had in the world. The individual's conversation will likely provide data relating to role performance, identity, self-esteem, stressors, and coping patterns. At times, specific questions may be useful (Table 26-1).

Coping Behaviors. The nursing assessment should also include consideration of previous coping behaviors; the nature, number, and intensity of the stressors; and the client's internal and external resources. Knowledge of how a client has dealt with stressors in the past can provide insight into the client's style of coping. Not all issues are addressed in the same way by clients, but often one uses a familiar coping pattern for newly encountered stressors. As the nurse identifies previous coping patterns, it is useful to determine whether these patterns have contributed to healthy functioning or created more problems. For example, the use of drugs or alcohol during times of stress often creates additional stressors.

Exploring resources and strengths, such as helpful significant others or prior use of community resources, can be important in formulating a realistic and effective plan. Also pertinent in assessment is determining how the client views the situation. What is viewed as a crisis by one client may be seen as less significant by another client. For example, one client might express great fear and distress over needing to have a colonoscopy and biopsy, whereas another client may see the need for the diagnostic testing as a manageable outgrowth of growing older and take the attitude that if there is something to be concerned about, the client will know about it soon enough.

Significant Others. Valuable data may also evolve out of conversations with family and significant others. Significant others may have insights into the person's way of dealing with stressors and what is supportive to the person. The way in which the person talks about the client and the significant others' nonverbal behaviors may provide information about what kind of support is available for the client.

Client Expectations. Also important in assessing self-concept is the person's expectations. Asking the client how he or she believes interventions will make a difference in his or her problem can provide useful information regarding the client's expectations and an opportunity to discuss the client's goals. For example, a nurse working with a client who is experiencing anxiety related to an upcoming diagnostic study might ask the client about his or her expectations of the relaxation exercise that they have been practicing together. The client's response will provide the nurse with valuable information about the client's beliefs and attitudes regarding the efficacy of the interventions.

Behaviors Suggestive of Altered Self-Concept	**Box 26-5**

Avoidance of eye contact
Overly apologetic
Hesitant speech
Overly critical
Excessive anger
Frequent or inappropriate crying
Puts self down
Excessively dependent
Hesitant to express views or opinions
Lack of interest in what is happening
Passive attitude
Difficulty in making choices
Slumped posture
Unkempt appearance

KNOWLEDGE

- Components of self-concept
- Self-concept stressors
- Therapeutic communication principles
- Nonverbal indicators of distress
- Cultural factors influencing self-concept
- Growth and development concepts
- Pharmacological effects of medications

STANDARDS

- Support the client's autonomy to make choices and express values that support positive self-concept
- Apply intellectual standards of relevance and plausibility for care to be acceptable to the client
- Safeguard the client's right to privacy by judiciously protecting information of a confidential nature

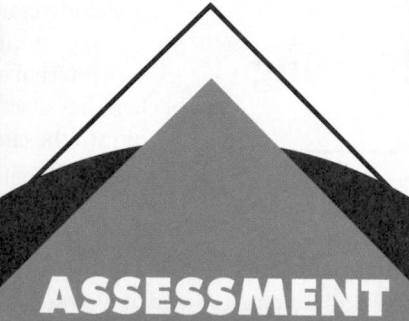

ASSESSMENT

- Observe for behaviors that suggest an alteration in the client's self-concept
- Assess the client's cultural background
- Assess the client's coping skills and resources
- Determine the client's feelings and perceptions about changes in body image, self-esteem, or role
- Assess the quality of the client's relationships

EXPERIENCE

- Caring for a client who had an alteration in body image, self-esteem, role, or identity
- Personal experience of threat to self-concept

ATTITUDES

- Display curiosity in considering why a client might behave or respond in a particular manner
- Display integrity when your beliefs and values differ from the client's; admit to any inconsistencies in your values or your client's
- Take risks if necessary in developing a trusting relationship with the client

Figure 26-6   *Synthesis Model for Self-Concept Assessment Phase.*

Table 26-1 Nursing Assessment of Client's Self-Concept

Assessment Questions*	Responses Reflecting Difficulties With Self-Concept
Identity "How would you describe yourself?"	Derogatory answers (e.g., "I don't know; there's not much that is very exciting about me" or "I'm not good at much of anything") should raise the concern of the nurse.
Body Image "What aspects of your appearance do you like?" "Are there any aspects of your appearance that you would like to change? If yes, describe the changes you would make."	Most people can identify something about their appearance that they like (e.g., "People have always told me I have nice eyes"). If a person cannot identify any appreciated characteristic, this is suggestive of a negative body image and self-esteem. Most people have one or two areas that they would like to change (e.g., "My nose is too big" or "My hips are too big"), but a long list of problem areas should lead the nurse to consider difficulties with self-concept.
Self-Esteem "Tell me about the things you do well."	Statements about not having any strengths or being able to do anything well should raise the concern of the nurse.
Role Performance "What are your primary roles (e.g., partner, parent, friend, sister, professional role)? How do you see yourself carrying out each of these roles?"	The nurse should listen for the number of primary roles identified. A large number of primary roles will put the client at risk for role conflicts and role overload. As with questions above, if the client indicates that he or she does not feel that these roles are adequately covered, the person may be experiencing alterations in self-concept. Although in Western cultures most people carry out many roles and often feel as though some of them are not adequately addressed, listen for the person's perception about his or her overall role competency.

*(In addition to the verbal content of the client's answer, the nurse should note the client's nonverbal behaviors. Hesitant speech, poor eye contact, and hunched posture suggest alterations in self-concept.)

NURSING DIAGNOSIS

Assessment data need careful consideration by the nurse to identify a client's actual or potential problem areas. The nurse will rely on knowledge and experience, apply appropriate standards and attitudes, and look for clusters of defining characteristics that indicate a nursing diagnosis (Box 26-6).

Making nursing diagnoses in the realm of self-concept is complex. Often, isolated data could be defining characteristics for more than one nursing diagnosis (Box 26-7). For example, a client might express feelings of regret and inadequacy. These are defining characteristics for both *anxiety* and *situational low self-esteem*. To make the most appropriate nursing diagnosis in this situation, the nurse must be open to seeing the possibilities of both nursing diagnoses. In fact, the awareness that the client is demonstrating defining characteristics of more than one nursing diagnosis can guide the nurse in gathering specific data to validate and to differentiate the underlying problem. To further assess the possibility of *anxiety* as the nursing diagnosis, the nurse might consider whether the person has any of the following defining characteristics: Is the person experiencing increased muscle tension, shakiness, a sense of being "rattled," or restlessness? These symptoms would suggest *anxiety* as the more appropriate diagnosis. On the other hand, if the person expresses a predominantly negative self-appraisal, including inability to handle situations or events and difficulty making decisions, these characteristics would suggest that the more appropriate nursing diagnosis might be *situational low self-esteem*. To further aid the nurse in differentiating between the two demonstrated diagnoses, information regarding recent events in the person's life and how the person has viewed himself or herself in the past would provide insight into the most appropriate nursing diagnosis. In this example the two nursing diagnoses are closely related. Often in practice the nurse will have to differentiate between several diagnoses. The client may demonstrate several defining characteristics from different diagnoses, but as additional data are gathered, usually, the most appropriate or predominant nursing diagnosis becomes evident.

It is also important that the nurse have sufficient data to correctly identify the factors that have contributed to the nursing diagnosis. These factors will be reflected in the "related to" component of the nursing diagnostic statement. If a thorough database is not gathered before formulating the nursing diagnosis, diagnostic errors are likely. For example, a nurse is caring for a 62-year-old

SAMPLE NURSING DIAGNOSTIC PROCESS   Box 26-6
DISTURBED SELF-CONCEPT

Assessment Activities	Defining Characteristics	Nursing Diagnosis
Observe client's behavior during conversation.	Client demonstrates restlessness, glancing about, facial tension, increased perspiration, and focus on self.	Anxiety related to accidental injury, pain, uncertainty of outcome of upcoming surgery
Ask client, "How are you doing?" or "How do you feel about tomorrow's procedure?"	Client replies, "I'm feeling really scared. You know there is a possibility they may amputate my leg tomorrow. I just don't know how I will manage if it comes to that. I just couldn't sleep last night. There was the pain, and I just kept thinking about all that is happening."	

NURSING DIAGNOSES   Box 26-7
ALTERATIONS IN SELF-CONCEPT

Adjustment, impaired
Anxiety
Body image disturbance
Caregiver role strain
Coping, ineffective individual
Denial, ineffective
Fear
Hopelessness
Loneliness, risk for
Parental role conflict
Parenting altered
Personal identity disturbance
Powerlessness
Rape-trauma syndrome
Role performance, altered
Self-esteem, chronic low
Self-esteem, situational low
Self-esteem disturbance
Self-mutilation, risk for
Spiritual distress (distress of the human spirit)
Violence, risk for: self-directed

woman who was admitted because of chronic back pain. The client demonstrated signs of anxiety (inattentiveness, frequent startling, self-report of poor sleep, diminished appetite, and increased muscle tension). The nurse knew that the client had undergone diagnostic testing to rule out cancer as the cause of the pain. The nurse made the following nursing diagnosis: *anxiety related to the possibility of cancer.* The nurse later learned that the woman was anxious because her grandson had been in a serious motor vehicle accident and was in intensive care. This example illustrates the danger in making a diagnosis without sufficient data. Even though the *anxiety* component of the

nursing diagnosis was correct, the "related to" portion was incorrect. Failure to be accurate and precise regarding the etiology of the anxiety would result in inappropriate nursing interventions. One way to develop an accurate nursing diagnosis is to discuss the problem with the client and with the family. Before involving the family, the nurse needs to consider the client's desires for their involvement and cultural norms regarding who most frequently makes decisions in the family.

To validate critical thinking regarding a nursing diagnosis, the nurse can share observations with the client and allow the client to verify the nurse's perception. This approach often results in the client providing additional data, which further clarifies the situation. In the example above, if the nurse said to the client, "I notice you haven't eaten much of your breakfast or lunch today and that you jumped when I came up behind you. Are you feeling uneasy today?" This could allow the client to verify whether she is in fact anxious and to tell the nurse about her concerns.

PLANNING

During planning the nurse again synthesizes knowledge, experience, critical thinking attitudes, and standards (Figure 26-7). Critical thinking ensures that the client's plan of care integrates all that the nurse knows about the individual, as well as key critical thinking elements. Professional standards are especially important to consider when the nurse develops a plan of care. These standards often establish ethical or scientifically proven guidelines for selecting effective nursing interventions.

The nurse develops an individualized plan of care for each nursing diagnosis (see care plan). The nurse and client set realistic expectations for care. Goals are to be individualized and realistic with measurable outcomes. In establishing goals, the nurse should consult with the client about whether the goals are realistic. Consultation with significant others, mental health workers, and community

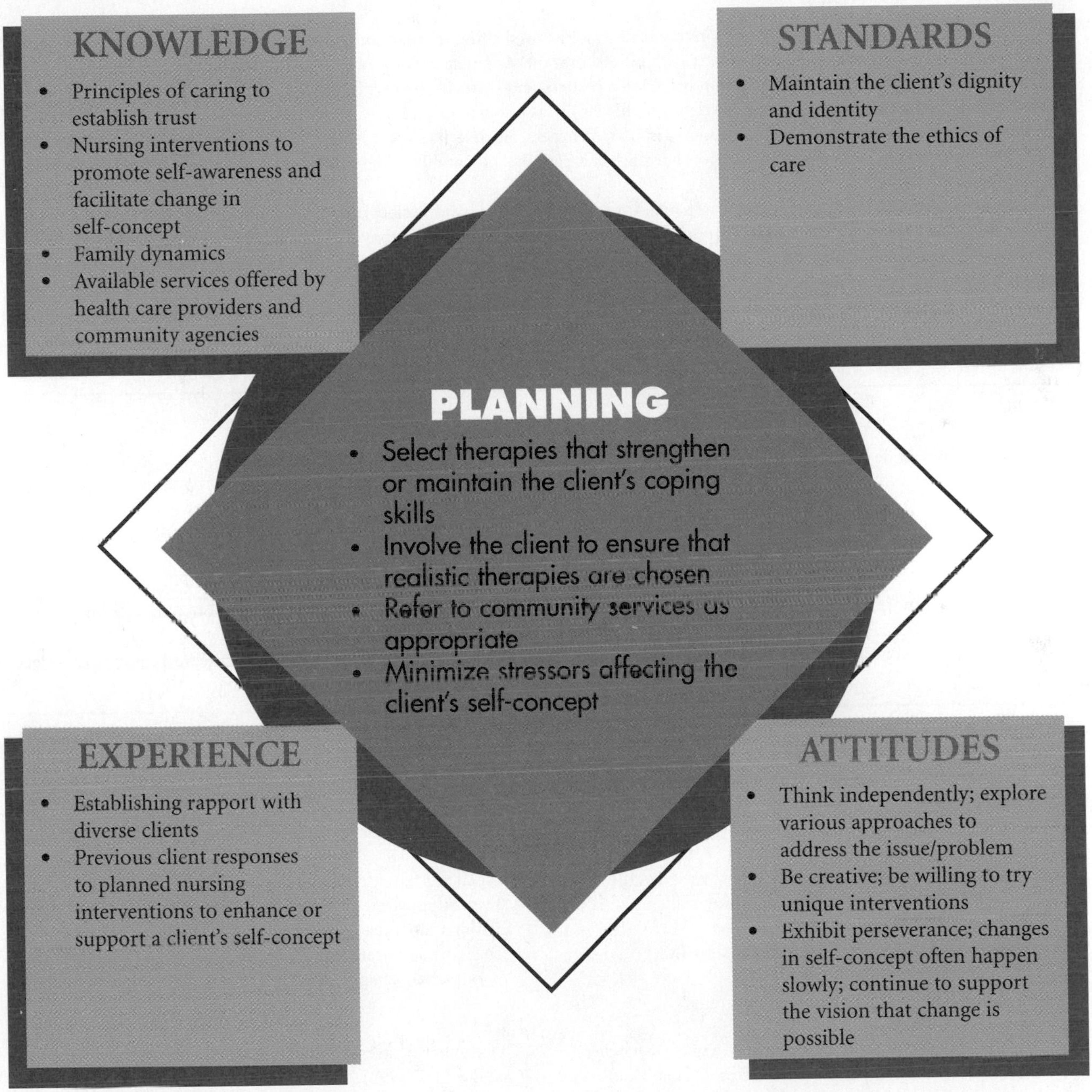

KNOWLEDGE

- Principles of caring to establish trust
- Nursing interventions to promote self-awareness and facilitate change in self-concept
- Family dynamics
- Available services offered by health care providers and community agencies

STANDARDS

- Maintain the client's dignity and identity
- Demonstrate the ethics of care

PLANNING

- Select therapies that strengthen or maintain the client's coping skills
- Involve the client to ensure that realistic therapies are chosen
- Refer to community services as appropriate
- Minimize stressors affecting the client's self-concept

EXPERIENCE

- Establishing rapport with diverse clients
- Previous client responses to planned nursing interventions to enhance or support a client's self-concept

ATTITUDES

- Think independently; explore various approaches to address the issue/problem
- Be creative; be willing to try unique interventions
- Exhibit perseverance; changes in self-concept often happen slowly; continue to support the vision that change is possible

Figure 26-7   *Synthesis Model for Self-Concept Planning Phase.*

SAMPLE NURSING CARE PLAN

ALTERATIONS IN SELF-CONCEPT

ASSESSMENT*

Mr. Johnson is a 45-year-old man who was involved in an automobile accident in which he sustained a crushing blow to his femur. On admission, an open reduction and internal fixation of the femur was done. Since then, he has developed an infection, and the most current x-ray film shows misalignment of the bone fragments. The chart reveals that Mr. Johnson has been in essentially good health up until the time of the accident.

When Jan, the student nurse, first goes in to meet Mr. Johnson, she finds that although he makes eye contact and answers questions, his **answers are brief** and to the point without elaboration. As Jan spends more time with Mr. Johnson, his eye contact increases, but his answers to questions remain brief. He is **restless** and **shifts frequently in the bed**. Mr. Johnson tells Jan that before the accident, he had a nearly ideal life. He describes his family as a source of pleasure and satisfaction. He tells her briefly about a recent trip the family took and the adventures of his two teenagers. He describes his work as OK. He states, "I have been at the plant for 25 years. I know my job. Sometimes it gets boring, but it pays the bills, and I will be able to retire with good benefits if I can just work a few more years."

In gathering the nursing history, Jan learns that Mr. Johnson has had **trouble sleeping** since admission. He says that in addition to the pain, there is just **so much to think about.** Specifically, he says; "You know, **they may not be able to save my leg.**" In reviewing flow sheets since admission, Jan notes that Mr. Johnson's **appetite has been recorded as poor and he usually eats only one fourth to one half of his meals.**

*Defining characteristics are shown in bold type.

NURSING DIAGNOSIS: Anxiety related to accidental injury, pain, and uncertainty of outcome of upcoming surgery and treatment.

PLANNING

GOAL

Client's anxiety will be diminished within 1 week.

EXPECTED OUTCOMES

Client will state that his anxiety/worry is less within 3 days.

Client will discuss his concerns openly with a staff person within 3 days.

Client will perform progressive relaxation exercises within 3 days.

Client's restlessness will decrease within 1 week.

Client will regain normal sleep pattern in 1 week.

Client will report having slept for 4 consecutive hours during the night within 1 week.

Client's weight will remain stable for next month.

Client will report an increased appetite and eat at least three-fourths of his meals within 1 week.

INTERVENTIONS†

Coping Enhancement

- Help client to define his level of anxiety (use terminology the client is comfortable with, e.g., *worry, nervous*).
- Empathize with client that worry is a normal response to what has happened.
- Explore coping skills the client has used in the past. Encourage and support adaptive coping skills used in the past.
- Encourage client to express concerns verbally.

RATIONALE

Anxiety is highly individualized, and different clients manifest anxiety in varying degrees.

Anxiety is a normal response to an actual or perceived danger.

Most clients have developed effective coping skills during their lives. Supporting these coping skills in currently stressful situations can aid adaptation.

Verbalizing a concern can allow the client to be more objective about what is happening.

Calming Techniques

- Decrease the number of new stressors (e.g., answer client's call bell promptly, explain procedures, decrease unnecessary noise).

The number of stressors affects the stress experience (Sundeen and others, 1998).

Pain Management

- Treat pain before it becomes moderate to severe.
- Teach client the importance of seeking pain relief before the pain reaches a rating of 5.

Pain is a stressor that can increase anxiety.

Increasing the client's ability to control his experiences and environment will help to decrease anxiety (Lin and Ward, 1996).

†Intervention Classification labels from McCloskey JC, Bulechek GM: *Nursing interventions classification (NIC)*, ed 3, St. Louis, 2000, Mosby.

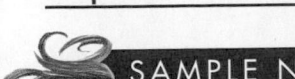

SAMPLE NURSING CARE PLAN — cont'd

ALTERATIONS IN SELF-CONCEPT

INTERVENTIONS†	RATIONALE
Pain Management • Teach client progressive relaxation techniques.	Relaxation is psychophysiologically in opposition to anxiety. Relaxation is energy conserving and nurturing (Sundeen and others, 1998).
Progressive Muscle Relaxation	

†Intervention Classification labels from McCloskey JC, Bulechek GM: *Nursing interventions classification (NIC)*, ed 3, St. Louis, 2000, Mosby.

EVALUATION

Explore with client what his current level of anxiety is.

Ask client how he slept the night before.

Inquire regarding client's appetite and monitor the amount of food eaten from meal trays.

Weigh client daily.

Explore with client his concerns and note areas he discusses.

Observe nonverbal clues regarding eye contact and degree of restlessness during discussion.

---

resources (Box 26-8) can result in a more comprehensive and workable plan. Once a goal has been formulated, the nurse should consider how the clues that alerted him or her to the problem would change if the problem were diminished. These changes should be reflected in the outcome criteria. As an example, a client is diagnosed with *situational low self-esteem related to a recent job loss*. The defining characteristics that she demonstrates are verbalizations of not being able to do anything right lately and expression of shame about losing her job. The nurse formulates the goal that the client's self-esteem will improve within 1 week. Appropriate expected outcomes might include: that the client will discuss a minimum of three areas of her life where she is functioning well and voice the recognition that losing her job is not reflective of her worth as a person.

The care plan presents the goals, expected outcomes, and interventions for a client with an alteration in self-concept. Interventions focus on helping the client adapt to the stressors that led to the self-concept disturbance and on supporting and reinforcing the development of coping methods. Often a client perceives a situation as overwhelming and may feel hopeless about returning to the level of previous functioning. The client may need time to adapt to physical changes. The nurse should look for strengths in both the individual and the family and provide resources and education to turn limitations into strengths. Client teaching creates understanding of why certain events have happened (e.g., nature of a chronic disease, change in relationships, effect of a loss), and often, once this is understood, the sense of hopelessness and helplessness can be lessened.

Often alterations in self-concept are not simple problems to address. The nurse should consider referral to mental health professionals and community resources that may be able to support the client in working with complex problems (see Box 26-8).

Resources in the Community for Supporting Self-Concept   Box 26-8

Adult Children of Alcoholics (ACOA)

Alcoholics Anonymous (AA)

Battered-women's shelters

Big Brothers/Big Sisters (an organization in which adults spend time with children and teenagers who lack positive adult supports)

Boy Scouts and Girl Scouts

Grief support groups

League of Older Americans (LOA)

National Alliance for the Mentally Ill (NAMI)

Overeaters Anonymous (support group for eating disorders)

Reach for Recovery (support group for women who have had mastectomies)

IMPLEMENTATION

Once the goals and outcome criteria have been developed, the nurse considers nursing interventions that would help move the client toward the goals. To develop effective nursing interventions, the nurse should consider the nursing diagnosis and broad interventions that address the diagnosis. These broad, standard interventions should be tailored to the individual client. The nurse develops additional nursing interventions based on the "related to" component of the nursing diagnosis. Developing interventions that affect the etiological or "related to" factors will often decrease the problem reflected in the nursing diagnosis. In the case of Mr. Johnson (see care plan), the "related to" component of the nursing diagnosis focuses the nurse on the areas to explore in talking with the client.

Promoting a Healthy Self-Concept.   Nursing interventions are designed to promote a client's healthy self-concept. Strategies help clients regain or restore the elements that contribute to a strong and secure sense of self. The approaches that nurses choose to use will vary according to the level of care clients require.

Health Promotion.

The nurse may have the opportunity to work with clients to help them develop healthy lifestyle measures that contribute to a healthy self-concept. Measures that support adaptation to stress, such as sound nutrition, regular exercise within the client's capabilities (Box 26-9), measures that facilitate adequate sleep and rest, and stress-reducing practices, may contribute to a healthy self-concept. Nurses are in a unique position to identify lifestyle practices that put a person's self-concept at risk or are suggestive of altered self-concepts. For example, a young teacher visits a clinic, with complaints of being unable to sleep and having difficulty with anxiety attacks. In gathering the nursing history, the nurse may learn of lifestyle practices such as too little rest, a large number of life changes occurring simultaneously, or excessive use of alcohol, which are either suggestive of self-

concept disturbances or put the person at risk for self-concept disturbances. The nurse in this situation talks with the client to determine how she views the various lifestyle elements, to facilitate the client's seeing the behaviors as potentially problematic and to make appropriate referrals or provide needed health teaching (Box 26-10).

Acute Care.

In the acute care setting the nurse is likely to encounter clients who are experiencing threats to their self-concept because of the nature of the treatment and diagnostic procedures. Threats to a person's self-concept can result in anxiety and/or fear. Numerous stressors, including unknown diagnoses, the need to make changes in lifestyle, and change in functioning, may be present and need to be dealt with. In the acute care setting there is often more than one stressor, thus increasing the overall stress level for the client and his or her family.

Nurses in the acute care setting also encounter clients who are faced with the need to adapt to an altered body image as a result of surgery or other physical change. Often a visit by someone who has experienced similar changes and adapted to them (e.g., someone who has had a laryngectomy) may be helpful. The timing of such a visit is important. The nurse needs to be sensitive to the client's level of acceptance of the change. Forcing confrontation with the change before the client is ready could delay the person's acceptance. Signs that a person may be receptive to such a visit would include the client's asking questions related to how to manage a particular aspect of what has happened or looking at the changed area. As the client expresses readiness to integrate the body change into his or her self-concept, the nurse can either let the client know about groups (e.g., the Lost Cord for a person who has had a laryngectomy) that are available or ask the client if he or she would like the nurse to make the contact. Another way in which the nurse can facilitate adjustment to a change in physical appearance is through his or her own response to the wound or change. As the nurse responds with acceptance, this models acceptance for both the client and the family. Assisting and encouraging a client to dress in an attractive manner can also contribute to the client's self-concept.

Restorative Care.

It is often in a long-term nurse-client relationship in a home health or restorative care environment that a nurse has the opportunity to work with a client to reach the goal of attaining a more positive self-concept. Interventions designed to help a client reach the goal of adapting to changes in self-concept or attaining a positive self-concept are based on the premise that the client first develops insight and self-awareness concerning problems and stressors and then acts to solve the problems and cope with the stressors. This approach, outlined by Stuart and Sundeen (1998), involves the following levels of intervention: expanded self-awareness, self-exploration, self-evaluation, planning of realistic goals, and commitment to action (Table 26-2).

Research HIGHLIGHT   Box 26-9

RESEARCH ABSTRACT

The authors explored the effects of 10 weeks of aerobic exercise (a minimum of 30 minutes per session, 4 days a week at $\geq 60\%$ of age-predicted maximum heart rate) on depressive/anxiety symptoms and self-esteem in breast cancer survivors. The research design was one of experimental crossover, meaning that those in the control group for the first 10 weeks did not exercise but were given the same exercise prescription as the experimental group for a subsequent 10 weeks. Findings included the following: Breast cancer survivors who successfully participated in aerobic exercise improved their depression and anxiety profiles. However, self-esteem was not improved. Those who received a physician's recommendation to exercise were significantly more likely to be compliant with the exercise regimen. Those who began exercise closer to the time of surgery improved significantly more than those who had surgery more than 2 years previously.

IMPLICATIONS FOR PRACTICE

- Exercise can improve depression and decrease anxiety.
- The recommendation of a health care provider to engage in exercise improves exercise compliance.
- Beginning an exercise program as soon as possible within the recovery process is most likely to benefit the client in terms of decreased depression and anxiety. Recommendations can be tailored to the client's physical condition, and suggestions can be made to increase exercise as rehabilitation progresses.

REFERENCE

Segar M and others: The effect of aerobic exercise on self-esteem and depressive and anxiety symptoms among breast cancer survivors, *Oncol Nurs Forum* 25(1):107, 1998.

Client Teaching FOR ANXIETY REDUCTION

Box 26-10

OBJECTIVES

- Client will identify physical sensations associated with anxiety.
- Client will describe the location, size, and shape of physical sensations associated with uncomfortable emotional feelings.
- Client will, while maintaining awareness of the size and shape of physical sensations associated with uncomfortable emotional feelings, verbalize whether the size and shape remain constant or change in some way.
- Client's voice will become soft and slower in pacing as the experience unfolds.
- Client will voice feeling more relaxed.
- Client will explain how he or she could use the technique by himself or herself when experiencing anxiety.

TEACHING STRATEGIES

- Explain to the client that often our habitual way of coping with emotional discomfort/anxiety is to ignore it or try to get away from it in some way (e.g., eating, use of substances). Suggest other ways of working with anxiety; paying attention to physical sensations and allowing them to move and change. This way of being with physical manifestations of anxiety can allow one to experience anxiety in a more accepting way. This acceptance can allow one to notice that all experience is constantly changing and that in fact what one sees as unbearable has periods of time when it is intense but also periods when the sensations are less intense.
- To guide the client in using this technique, have the client find a comfortable position. This could be lying in bed with arms at the sides and legs uncrossed or sitting with good body alignment.
- Ask the client to take in several deep breaths and let them go, relaxing onto the chair or bed.
- Ask the client to make contact with the physical sensation experienced in touching the chair or bed.

- Ask the client to describe the location, size, and shape of the sensation. Ask him or her to stay with the physical sensation and every 5 or 10 seconds voice whether the sensation is the same, saying "same" or, if changing, "changing." If the client is quiet for 30 to 60 seconds, you can say, "and now" to remind the client to stay with his or her sensations. If the client notes the sensation changing, ask if it is getting larger or smaller. If larger have the client note, "expanding"; if smaller, note "contracting"; if no change, note "same."
- Continue in this way for 20 to 60 minutes. At the end of this time, ask the person to take in a deep breath, let it go, and then gently open his or her eyes.
- At the completion of this experience, if a person has been able to focus on his or her sensations, he or she is likely to experience a sense of relaxation and a sense of peacefulness.
- Review the steps of the process as outlined above. Young (1997) offers a guided experience using this technique.

EVALUATION

- Ask the client to describe his or her physical sensations at the beginning of the experience.
- Ask the client to describe the location, size, and shape of a physical sensation.
- Ask the client to voice the ongoing characteristic of the physical sensation as either changing or remaining the same. If changing, describe whether it is expanding or contracting.
- Note whether the client's voice quality and speed of speaking change as the experience unfolds.
- Ask the client how he or she is feeling and note his or her response.
- Ask the client if he or she could use this technique when anxiety arises.
- If you have continuing contact with the client, inquire if he or she has used the technique since practicing it with you, and how it went.

Increasing the client's self-awareness is achieved through establishing a trusting relationship that allows the client to openly explore feelings. Open exploration can make the situation less threatening for the client and encourages behaviors that expand self-awareness.

Encouraging the client's self-exploration is achieved by accepting the client's feelings and thoughts, by helping the client to clarify interactions with others, and by being empathetic. The nurse encourages self-expression and stresses the client's self-responsibility.

Assisting the client in self-evaluation involves helping the client to define problems clearly and to identify positive and negative coping mechanisms. The nurse works closely with the client to help to analyze adaptive and maladaptive responses, contrast different alternatives, and discuss outcomes.

Assisting the client in establishing realistic goals involves helping the client to identify alternative solutions and develop realistic goals based on them. This facilitates real change and encourages further goal-setting behaviors. The nurse designs opportunities that result in success, reinforces the client's skills and strengths, and assists the client in getting needed assistance.

Assisting the client in becoming committed to decisions and actions to achieve goals involves teaching the client to move away from ineffective coping mechanisms and develop successful coping strategies. Supporting attempts that are health promoting is essential, because with each success another attempt can be made. Supporting adaptive, flexible coping is critical to intervening in self-concept alterations.

Clients who are experiencing threats to or alterations in self-concept often benefit from collaboration with mental health and community resources to promote increased

Table 26-2 **Levels of Nursing Interventions for Self-Concept Disturbance**		
Principle	Rationale	Nursing Actions
Goal: Expand Client's Self-Awareness		
Work with resources client possesses.	Some resources, such as self-control and self-perception, are needed as foundations for later nursing care.	Confirm identity. Provide support measures to reduce anxiety. Approach client in an undemanding way. Accept and attempt to clarify any verbal or nonverbal communication. Prevent client isolation. Help establish simple routine. Help set limits on inappropriate behavior. Orient client to reality. Reinforce appropriate behavior. Gradually increase activities and tasks that provide positive experiences. Assist in personal hygiene and grooming. Encourage client to care for self.
Maximize client's participation in therapeutic relationship.	Mutuality is necessary for client to assume ultimate responsibility for behavior and coping responses.	Gradually increase client's participation in decisions that affect care. Convey that client is a responsible individual.
Goal: Encourage Client's Self-Exploration		
Show interest in and accept client's feelings and thoughts.	When nurse shows interest in and accepts client's feelings and thoughts, the nurse helps client to do so also.	Attend to and encourage client's expression of emotions, beliefs, behavior, and thoughts—verbally, nonverbally, symbolically, or directly. Use therapeutic communication skills and empathetic responses. Note use of logical and illogical thinking and reported and observed emotional responses.
Help client clarify self-concept and relationships to others through self-disclosure.	Self-disclosure and understanding self-perceptions are prerequisites to bringing about future change; this may in itself reduce anxiety.	Elicit client's perceptions of strengths and weaknesses. Help describe ideal self. Identify self-criticisms. Help describe how client perceives relationships to other people and events.
Be aware and have control of your own feelings.	Self-awareness allows nurse to model authentic behavior.	Be open to your own feelings. Accept your positive and negative feelings. Practice therapeutic use of self: share your feelings with client, describe how another might have felt, and mirror your perception of client's feelings.
Respond empathetically, not sympathetically, emphasizing that power to change lies with client.	Sympathy can reinforce client's self-pity; rather, nurse should communicate that client's life situation is subject to one's own control.	Use empathetic responses and monitor yourself for feelings of sympathy or pity. Reaffirm that client is not helpless or powerless when dealing with problems. Convey verbally and behaviorally that client is responsible for behavior, including choice of maladaptive or adaptive coping responses. Discuss with client scope of choices, areas of strength, and coping resources available.
Goal: Assist Client in Self-Evaluation		
Help client to clearly define problem.	Only after problem is accurately defined can alternative choices be proposed.	Identify relevant stressors with client and ask for appraisal of them. Clarify that client's beliefs influence feelings and behaviors. Mutually identify faulty beliefs, misperceptions, distortions, delusions, and unrealistic goals. Mutually identify areas of strength.

Modified from Stuart GW, Sundeen SJ: *Principles and practice of psychiatric nursing,* ed 6, St. Louis, 1998, Mosby.

Principle	Rationale	Nursing Actions
Explore client's adaptive and maladaptive coping responses to problem.	Examination of client's choices made during coping will help define successful and unsuccessful responses.	Place concepts of success and failure in proper perspective. Explore use of coping resources. Describe how coping responses are chosen and have positive and negative consequences. Contrast adaptive and maladaptive responses. Mutually identify disadvantages of client's maladaptive coping responses.

Goal: Assist Client in Forming Realistic Goals

Principle	Rationale	Nursing Actions
Help client identify alternative solutions.	Only when all possible alternatives have been evaluated can change be effected.	Mutually identify advantages or "payoffs" of client's maladaptive coping responses. Help client understand that one can only change oneself, not others. If client holds inconsistent perceptions, show that the following can change: beliefs or ideals to bring them closer to reality, and environment to make it consistent with beliefs. If self-concept is not consistent with behavior, client can change the following: behavior to conform to self-concept, beliefs underlying self-concept to include behavior, and self-ideal.
Help client conceptualize realistic goals.	Goal setting that includes clear definition of expected change is necessary.	Mutually review use of coping resources. Encourage client to form personal (not nurse's) goals. Mutually discuss emotional and practical consequences of each goal. Help client define concrete change to be made. Encourage client to enter new experiences for growth potential. Use role modeling and role playing when appropriate.

Goal: Assist Client in Becoming Committed to Decision and in Achieving Goals

Principle	Rationale	Nursing Actions
Help client take necessary action to change maladaptive coping responses and maintain adaptive ones.	Ultimate objective in promoting client's insight is to replace maladaptive coping responses with more adaptive ones.	Provide opportunity for success. Reinforce strengths, skills, and healthy aspects of client's personality. Assist client in gaining assistance (e.g., vocational, financial, social services). Use family and groups to enhance client's self-esteem. Allow client sufficient time to change. Provide support and positive reinforcement to maintain progress.

Goal: Assist Client in Acknowledging Goals Achieved and Evaluating Those Not Achieved

Principle	Rationale	Nursing Actions
Help client to purposefully review achievements and explore reasons for any problems or setbacks.	Reinforcement of gains made in strengthening self-concept will motivate continued change.	Mutually review progress made. Affirm achievements with client and family or significant others. Evaluate what contributed most to success. Help client discuss feelings regarding goals not achieved.

Goal: Assist Client to Re-Form Plan for Achieving Goals

Principle	Rationale	Nursing Actions
Support client in reviewing goals.	Insight gained from attempts to change will support further progress.	Review with client the need for further self-evaluation. Encourage client to continue those experiences that were successful.
Identify alternatives not tried previously	Different approaches may be necessary to achieve desired outcomes.	Explore how new coping resources can be applied to continued change. Redefine changes in adaptive behaviors to be made. Continue to reinforce strengths and successes.

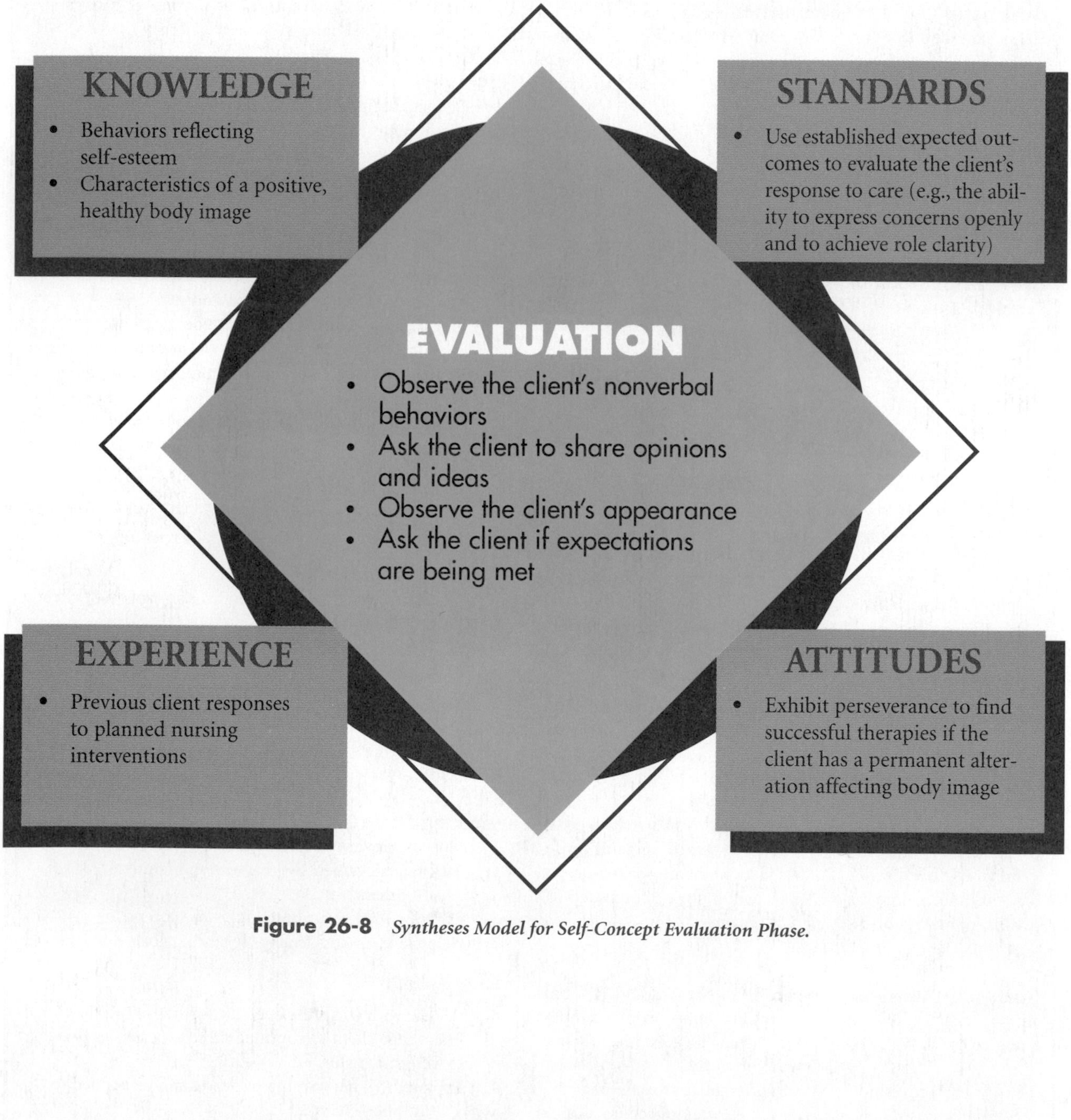

KNOWLEDGE

- Behaviors reflecting self-esteem
- Characteristics of a positive, healthy body image

STANDARDS

- Use established expected outcomes to evaluate the client's response to care (e.g., the ability to express concerns openly and to achieve role clarity)

EVALUATION

- Observe the client's nonverbal behaviors
- Ask the client to share opinions and ideas
- Observe the client's appearance
- Ask the client if expectations are being met

EXPERIENCE

- Previous client responses to planned nursing interventions

ATTITUDES

- Exhibit perseverance to find successful therapies if the client has a permanent alteration affecting body image

Figure 26-8 *Syntheses Model for Self-Concept Evaluation Phase.*

awareness. Knowledge of available community resources, such as counseling and 12-step groups, allows the nurse to make appropriate referrals.

Establishing a therapeutic environment and a therapeutic relationship (see Chapter 22), and increasing self-awareness are critical to successfully intervening with clients who have alterations in self-concept, whether care is focused on health promotion, dealing with an acute process, or addressing restorative care. To support the development of a positive self-concept in a client, the nurse must convey genuine caring for the client (see Chapter 6). Then, and only then, can the nurse establish a partnership with the client to address underlying problems.

EVALUATION

Client Care.   Evaluating success in meeting each client goal and the established expected outcomes requires critical thinking (Figure 26-8). Frequent evaluation of client progress is recommended so that changes can be instituted if necessary. The nurse applies knowledge of behaviors and characteristics of a healthy self-concept when reviewing the actual behaviors clients display. This determines whether outcomes have been met.

Expected outcomes for a client with a self-concept disturbance may include nonverbal behaviors indicating a positive self-concept, statements of self-acceptance, and acceptance of change in appearance or function. Key indicators of a client's self-concept can be his or her nonverbal behaviors. For example a client who has had difficulty making eye contact may demonstrate a more positive self-concept by making more frequent eye contact during conversation. Social interaction, adequate self-care, acceptance of the use of prosthetic devices, and statements indicating understanding of teaching all indicate progress. A positive attitude toward rehabilitation and increased movement toward independence facilitate a return to preexisting roles at work or at home. Patterns of interacting can also reflect changes in self-concept. For example, a client who has been hesitant to express his or her views may more readily offer opinions and ideas as self-esteem increases.

The goals of care may be unrealistic or inappropriate as the client's condition changes. The nurse may need to revise the plan, reflecting on successful experiences with other clients.

Client adaptation to major changes may take a year or longer, but the fact that this period is long does not signify maladaptation. The nurse should look for signs that the client has reduced some stressors and that some behaviors have become more adaptive. Changes in self-concept take time. Self-concept is formed over years. It should not be discouraging that changes in self-concept also require time. Although change may be slow, care of the client with a self-concept disturbance can be rewarding.

Client Expectations.   If the nurse has developed a good rapport with the client, the client may well be able to share how things are going from his or her perspective. The nurse may be able to facilitate this sharing by initiating a review of what has happened over time. This offers the nurse the opportunity to share perceptions and encourages the client to consider and voice how he or she has experienced any changes.

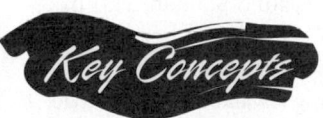

- Self-concept is an integrated set of conscious and unconscious feelings, attitudes, and perceptions about the self.
- Self-concept is influenced by health, family experiences, social and occupational roles, and intellectual and leisure activities.
- The components of self-concept are identity, body image, self-esteem, and role performance.
- Each developmental stage involves factors that are important to the development of a healthy, positive self-concept.
- Identity is particularly vulnerable during adolescence.
- Body image is the mental picture of one's body and is not necessarily consistent with a person's actual body structure or appearance.

- Body image also includes attitudes, emotions, and personality reactions of the person toward the body.
- Body image is influenced by growth and development, cultural and societal values and attitudes, and individual perceptions of the body.
- Body image stressors include changes in physical appearance, structure, or functioning caused by normal developmental changes or illness.
- Self-esteem depends on a person's perception of the ideal self as it compares with the real self.
- Self-esteem stressors include developmental and relationship changes, illness (particularly chronic illness involving changes in what were normal activities), surgery, accidents, and the responses of other individuals to changes resulting from these events.

- Roles are learned through socialization, from one's family, and from one's culture.
- Role stressors, including role conflict, role ambiguity, and role strain, may originate in unclear or conflicting role expectations and may be aggravated by the effects of illness.
- The nurse's self-concept and nursing actions can have an effect on a client's self-concept.
- Planning and implementing nursing interventions for self-concept disturbance involve expanding the client's self-awareness, encouraging self-exploration, aiding in self-evaluation, helping formulate goals in regard to adaptation, and assisting the client in achieving those goals.

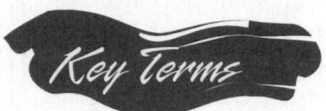

Key Terms

Body image, *p. 542*
Ideal self, *p. 543*
Identification, *p. 542*
Identity, *p. 542*
Identity confusion, *p. 546*
Role ambiguity, *p. 546*
Role conflict, *p. 546*

Role overload, *p. 547*
Role performance, *p. 544*
Role strain, *p. 547*
Self-concept, *p. 541*
Self-esteem, *p. 543*
Sick role, *p. 547*
Socialization, *p. 543*

Critical Thinking Exercises

1. You are assigned to care for a 23-year-old Asian-American client who was in a motor vehicle accident and sustained multiple fractures to his face and a fractured femur (which was fixated through surgery on the eve of admission 4 days ago). He has grown up in the United States; he and his mother came to the United States when he was a young child. He works as a janitor for a local university. He lives with his girlfriend and their 7-month-old daughter. You have been with him for most of the morning and found that he is in moderate pain, which has been treated with morphine. The morphine has decreased his pain rating from a 6 to a 3 but has left him somewhat drowsy. During the morning he has shared with you some of his concerns about when he will be able to return to work. You are in the room when the surgeon tells him about his upcoming surgery. A temporary tracheotomy is planned because of the extensive work needed in the nasal and throat area. After the surgeon leaves, the client tells you that he does not want the tracheotomy. He indicates that he is unclear about what it actually entails, even though the surgeon explained it in fairly simple terms. He says to you, "I just want to get back to my normal self." How would you address his comment regarding "get back to normal" and his lack of understanding regarding the tracheotomy?

2. A 51-year-old man has been transferred to the rehabilitation unit following 2 weeks of hospitalization resulting from an industrial accident in which his pelvis was crushed by a hydraulic press. His pelvis was stabilized with an external fixator. Initially he was paralyzed from T12 down. During the 2 weeks since the accident, feeling and movement have begun to return in his lower extremities. With the return of function there have also been spasms that occur with movement and increase in severity if movement is continued. With the gradual return of functioning, the physicians have been hesitant to give the client a prognosis and have told him that waiting and seeing is what will reveal his returning functioning. The client seems satisfied with this explanation at this point. His main focus is on directing his personal care to minimize risk of infection and to ensure that whoever is caring for him understands the importance of waiting for a muscle spasm to subside before continuing with care. The student is assigned to care for the client for a 4-week rotation. The student will be there once a week for 4 hours. How might the student establish trust and assess the client's concerns about the future?

3. As a part of your community health experience, you are assigned to visit an 85-year-old woman who has gone to her daughter's home after being hospitalized for a fractured hip. The hip was internally fixated, and the client was discharged using a walker. When you go to the home, you find the 65-year-old daughter near tears. She says, "I just don't know if I can do this. She doesn't like anything I cook. She calls me two or three times during the night to help her to the bathroom. And now my husband had been diagnosed with lung cancer." What additional assessment data would you want to gather?

References

Erikson E: *Childhood and society,* ed 2, New York, 1963, WW Norton.

Gilligan C: *In a different voice,* Cambridge, Mass, 1982, Harvard University Press.

Kohlberg L: The cognitive-developmental approach to socialization. In Goshin D, editor: *Handbook of socialization,* Chicago, 1969, Rand McNally.

Lin C, Ward S: Perceived self-efficacy and outcomes expectancies in coping with chronic low back pain, *Res Nurs Health* 19(4):299, 1996.

McCloskey JC, Bulechek GM: *Nursing interventions classification (NIC),* ed 3, St. Louis, 2000, Mosby.

Nugent E: Try to remember . . . reminiscence as a nursing intervention, *J Psychosoc Nurs* 33(11):7, 1995.

Piaget J: *The child's conception of the world,* New York, 1963, Littlefield, Adams.

Segar M and others: The effect of aerobic exercise on self-esteem and depressive and anxiety symptoms among breast cancer survivors, *Oncol Nurs Forum* 25(1):107, 1998.

Seyle H: *The stress of life,* New York, 1956, McGraw-Hill.

Sheehy G: *New passages: mapping your life across time,* New York, 1995, Random House.

Stuart GW, Sundeen SJ: *Principles and practice of psychiatric nursing,* ed 6, St. Louis, 1998, Mosby.

Sundeen S and others: *Nurse-client interaction: implementing the nursing process,* ed 6, St. Louis, 1998, Mosby.

Young S (speaker): *Break through difficult emotions* (cassette recording), Boulder, Colo, 1997, Sounds True.

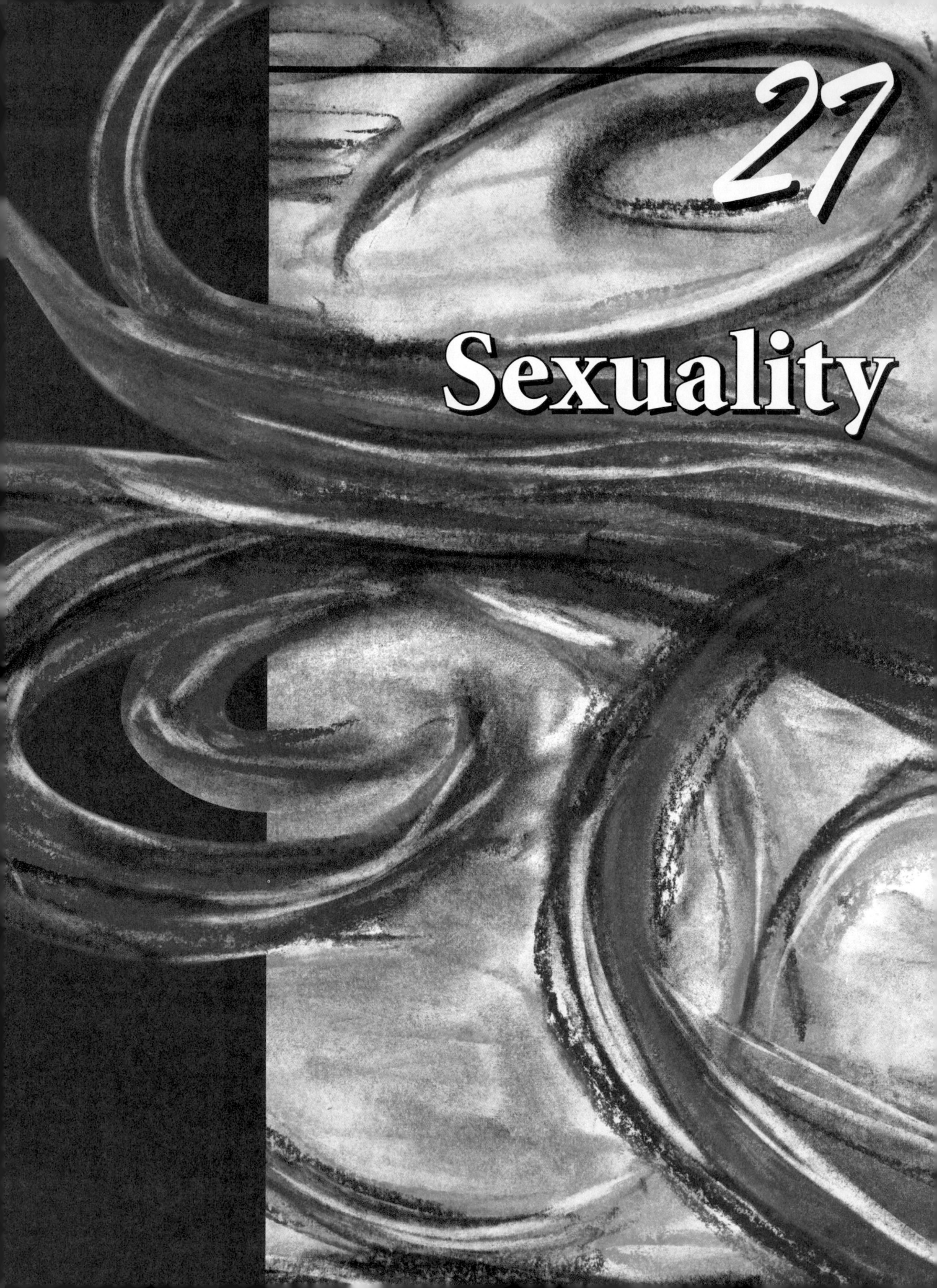

27

Sexuality

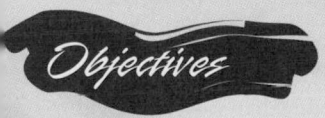
Objectives

Mastery of content in this chapter will enable the student to:

- Define the key terms listed.
- Identify personal attitudes, beliefs, and biases related to sexuality.
- Discuss the nurse's role in maintaining or enhancing a client's sexual health.
- Describe key concepts of sexual development during infancy, childhood, adolescence, and adulthood.
- Describe the sexual response cycle.
- Identify potential causes of sexual dysfunction.
- Assess a client's sexuality.
- Define appropriate nursing diagnoses for clients with alterations in sexuality.
- Identify client risk factors in the area of sexual health.
- Identify and describe nursing interventions to promote sexual health.
- Evaluate a client's sexual health.
- Identify potential referral resources for clients' sexual concerns outside the nurse's level of expertise.
- Use critical thinking skills in assisting clients in meeting their sexual needs.

Sex is a topic that was long considered taboo for proper adult conversation. Gradually, over the last 30 to 50 years, knowledge about sex and the ability to discuss sexual issues have come to be recognized as important for an individual's overall well-being and health. Even though openness to sexual topics and discussion has increased over the years, many adults lack knowledge regarding **sexuality** and are reluctant to raise questions related to sexuality. Common concerns may include postpartum resumption of sexual **intercourse,** normalcy of development, and anxiety over the effects of medications on sexual function. Often a client is hesitant to bring up sexual concerns, yet when the nurse addresses sexuality in a relaxed, matter-of-fact manner, the client may feel it is safe to bring up his or her areas of concern. For the nurse to address sexuality in a relaxed, matter-of-fact manner, the nurse needs to have an adequate knowledge base regarding sexual functioning and sexual issues; well-developed communication skills; knowledge of areas to assess in regard to sexuality; personal comfort in discussing sexuality; and a caring, sensitive attitude. It is also critical that the nurse recognize that sexual issues are value laden. Religious teachings, culturally prescribed **gender roles,** beliefs about **sexual orientation,** and social and environmental climates all influence both the client's and the health care provider's value systems.

Sexuality is more than genital physical activity. Sexuality encompasses our whole being. It includes our sense of femaleness and maleness. Sexuality includes biological, sociological, psychological, spiritual, and cultural dimensions of each person's being. In addition, sexuality is influenced by values, attitudes, behaviors, relationships with others, and the need to establish emotional closeness with others (MacLaren, 1995). **Sexual health** has been defined as an emotional and physical state of well-being that permits enjoyment and the ability to respond to sexual feelings (Boston Women's Health Collective, 1998). Key aspects of sexual health include an acceptance of one's body image, sexual identity, and self-concept (MacLaren, 1995).

Scientific Knowledge Base

For the nurse to plan effectively to assist a client in meeting his or her sexual needs, the nurse must have a sound scientific knowledge base regarding sexuality. A basic understanding of sexual development, sexual orientation, the **sexual response cycle, contraception,** abortion, and **sexually transmitted diseases (STDs)** is necessary.

SEXUAL DEVELOPMENT

As a person grows and develops, so does his or her sexuality. Each stage of development brings changes in sexual functioning and the role of sexuality in relationships.

Infancy. At birth, the infant is identified as female or male. Psychologically the infant is developing trust (Erikson, 1963). Trust in the self involves exploration of the body, including pleasant and unpleasant sensations. Exploration includes the discovery of self-soothing sensations, such as touching the genital area. Parents' and other significant caregivers' responses to these exploratory behaviors can set the tone for the infant's sexual development. Caregivers should be encouraged to accept the infant's exploratory behavior as a normal part of development.

The authors acknowledge the contribution of Judith Roos to this chapter in the previous edition of this text.

Toddler/Preschool Period.   The child from ages 1 to 5 or 6 continues to solidify the sense of **gender identity** and to differentiate socially defined, gender-appropriate behaviors. This learning process occurs in the course of everyday adult-child interactions, from the toys given to the child, clothing worn, games played, and responses encouraged. Children also observe adult behavior, begin to imitate actions of the same-sex parent, and maintain or modify behavior based on parental feedback.

Body exploration continues at this age, and the child may extend exploration to others. Children may role play games of doctor or mommy and daddy exploring each other's bodies in various stages of undress. Nurses can teach parents that this is a normal aspect of sexual development. Rather than responding with shock or punishment, caregivers can respond by simply redirecting play.

School-Age Years.   Children from 6 to 10 years of age expand their horizons from home to include school and the community. Learning and reinforcement of gender-appropriate behavior come from parents and teachers but more significantly from the child's peer group. North American society today defines a broad range of behavior acceptable for girls and boys (e.g., both sexes participate in cooking and sports).

During this time of development, children are likely to continue self-stimulating behavior. Teaching children the difference between behaviors that are culturally acceptable in public and those that need to be private may be appropriate in regard to masturbation.

Older children are likely to have a desire and need for privacy. This should be honored. By the age of 10, many girls and some boys are already beginning some of the changes of puberty. As children enter puberty, their bodies change and they experience increased modesty. School-age children generally have questions regarding the physical and emotional aspects of sex (Finan, 1997a). They need accurate information from home and school about body and emotional changes during this period and what to expect as they move into puberty. Knowledge about normal emotional and physical changes associated with puberty may decrease the anxieties as these changes begin to happen. An uninformed child may be frightened by menstruation or nocturnal emission and view them as evidence of a dreadful disease.

At this age, children may assert their independence by testing the limits of appropriate behavior. Limit testing may be manifested by the use of "dirty words" or by telling jokes with sexual connotations while watching adult reactions. Limit testing is an important part of developing a sense of independence from the family. Parents need to be taught that setting limits on unacceptable behaviors helps children learn societal expectations. Setting limits can be a difficult task. Supporting parents in this role of limit setting can be helpful for both the parent and the child.

Puberty/Adolescence.   The onset of puberty in girls is usually signaled by the development of the breasts. This process, which in part is controlled by heredity, may begin as early as age 8 and may not be complete until the late teenage years. The age of menarche varies widely but usually occurs around age 12. Although the menstrual cycle is initially irregular and ovulation may not occur at first, fertility should always be assumed unless proved otherwise.

Ejaculation in boys does not occur until the sex organs begin to mature, around the age of 12 or 14. Ejaculation may first occur during sleep (nocturnal emission). This may be interpreted as an episode of bed-wetting and even in knowledgeable boys can be very embarrassing. Boys need to understand that although they may not produce sperm with their first ejaculations, they will soon be fertile.

The emotional changes during puberty and adolescence are as dramatic as the physical ones. The adolescent functions within a powerful peer group, with the almost constant anxiety of "Am I normal?" and "Will I be accepted? (Figure 27-1)." Same-sex peers or friends remain influential in defining appropriate behavior, but the task of establishing a romantic relationship begins. Adolescence is a self-centered, egocentric stage. This introspection is necessary to establish a sense of self within the context of family, community, and emotional relationships. Assurance of normalcy in physical and emotional development should be given honestly and often.

The adolescent is faced with many decisions and needs accurate information on topics such as body changes, sexual activity, emotional responses within intimate sexual relationships, STDs, and pregnancy. In the United States 70% of adolescents have had sexual intercourse by the age of 18 (Kenney and others, 1998). A substantial number of these teenagers do not protect themselves from pregnancy or STDs. The dynamics of sexual risk taking are not fully understood, but numerous studies have found correla-

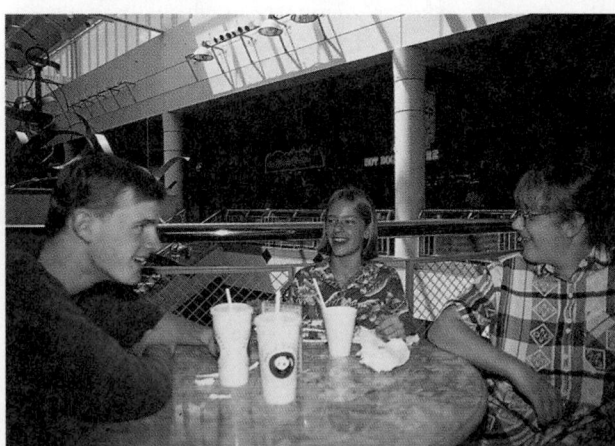

Figure 27-1   Adolescents function within a powerful network of peers as they explore their sexual identity.

tions between drug/alcohol use, sexual abuse, and unsafe sex (Keller, Reinholtz, and Angelini, 1996; Kenney and others, 1998). Adolescents tend to have a sense of being invulnerable, believing that unwanted pregnancy, STDs, and other negative outcomes of sexual behavior are not likely to happen to them (Keller and others, 1996).

Factual information regarding sexuality and sexual activity is important, but equally or perhaps more important is guidance in establishing a personal value or belief system to use as a framework for decision making. In healthy family networks much of this guidance will have been conveyed in the course of child rearing. Parents need to understand the importance of providing information, sharing their values, and promoting sound decision-making skills. Parents and significant others need to be counseled that even with the best guidance and information, adolescents will make their own decisions and must be held accountable for those decisions.

Adolescence is often a developmental phase during which an individual explores his or her primary sexual orientation. Many adolescents will have at least one **homosexual** experience with an individual or in a group. Adolescents may fear that this experience defines their total sexuality as homosexual. This is not true. Many individuals continue with a strictly **heterosexual** orientation after such experiences. However, some teenagers may recognize their preference as distinctly homosexual. This can be frightening and confusing for an adolescent. Support for the adolescent's sexual identity can be important during this time. Support can come from a variety of sources, such as school counselors, clergy, family, or health professionals.

Adulthood.

The adult has gained physical maturation but is continuing to explore and define emotional maturation in relationships. Intimacy and sexuality are issues for all adults whether they are in a sexual relationship, choose to abstain from sex, remain single by choice, are homosexual, or are widowed—whatever circumstances arise. People can be sexually healthy in numerous ways. Sexual activity is often defined as a basic need, but sexual desire can be channeled healthily into other forms of intimacy throughout a lifetime.

As sexually active adults develop intimate relationships, they need to learn techniques of stimulation that are satisfying to both themselves and their sexual partners. Some adults may need permission or affirmation that alternative ways of sexual expression other than penile-vaginal intercourse are normal. Other individuals may require significant education or therapy to achieve mutually satisfying sexual relationships.

Later in the adult years, individuals may be adjusting to the social and emotional changes associated with children moving away from home. This can be a time of renewed intimacy between partners, or it may be a time when formerly intimate partners realize that they no longer care for each other or have common interests. In either case, children leaving home usually herald a time of change in intimate relating.

Changing physical appearance related to aging may lead to concern about sexual attractiveness. In addition to concerns about changes in physical appearance, actual physical changes can affect sexual functioning. Decreasing levels of estrogen in the **perimenopausal** woman may lead to diminished vaginal lubrication and decreased vaginal elasticity. Both of these changes may lead to **dyspareunia.** Decreasing levels of estrogen can also result in a decreased desire for sexual activity. As men age, they are likely to experience an increase in the postejaculatory refractory period, delayed ejaculation, and other changes. Anticipatory guidance regarding these normal changes related to aging can ease concerns regarding functioning. Suggestions such as using vaginal lubrication and creating time for caressing and tenderness can help to ease adjustment to normal changes related to aging. Aging adults may also need to adjust to the impact of chronic illness, medications, aches, pains, and other health concerns on sexuality.

Older Adulthood.

The capacity for sexuality is lifelong. Theoretically, people can engage in sex as far into old age as they choose. The best indicator for continued sexual satisfaction with aging is a regularly active sex life during adulthood and into later life (Masters, Johnson, and Kolodny, 1982). Older adults often face health concerns and societal attitudes that make it difficult for them to continue sexual activity. Although declining physical abilities may make sex as they knew it difficult, learning alternative ways of sexual expression can allow for satisfying sexual activity.

Numerous factors, including lack of a sexual partner or declining health, can affect the sexual activity of the older adult. Yet research has consistently shown that many older adults remain sexually active and value this expression (Johnson, 1996). Nurses working with older adults need to be aware of the sexuality of their clients, assess interest and functioning, and plan accordingly.

SEXUAL RESPONSE CYCLE

Kaplan (1979) identified three phases of the sexual response cycle: desire, arousal, and orgasm. These phases are a result of **vasocongestion** and **myotonia,** the basic physiological responses of sexual arousal. In women, this reaction leads to vaginal lubrication, tumescence of the clitoris and the labia minora and majora, and engorgement of the outer third of the vagina (orgasmic platform). In men, vasocongestion leads to erection of the penis. Myotonia, or neuromuscular tension, gradually increases throughout the body during the excitement and plateau phases. Myotonia peaks during orgasm, resulting in involuntary contractions of the woman's vagina and the man's vas deferens and urethra. Women and men may experience contractions of the arm and leg muscles, facial muscles, and gluteal muscles. After orgasm, vasocongestion and myotonia return to prearousal levels. The phases described are not absolute. Male and female response patterns are similar.

SEXUAL ORIENTATION

Sexual orientation describes the predominant gender preference of a person's sexual attraction over time. Sexual orientation can be toward someone of the opposite sex, the same sex, or both sexes. Human sexual attraction is on a continuum between heterosexual and homosexual orientations. Based on Kinsey's studies (1948, 1953), most people cluster toward the heterosexual end of the continuum; a smaller percentage are at the homosexual (**gay** or **lesbian**) end. Sell and others (1995) reported on a nationally representative sample that found that 21% of males and 18% of females in the United States reported either homosexual behavior or homosexual attraction after age 15. Examination of homosexual behavior separately found that 6.2% of males and 3.6% of females in the United States reported having had sexual contact with someone of the same sex in the previous 5 years.

CONTRACEPTION

There are numerous contraceptive options available to sexually active couples today. The various methods provide varying levels of protection against unwanted pregnancies. Some methods do not require a prescription, whereas other methods do require intervention by a health care provider.

Nonprescription Contraceptive Methods. Nonprescription methods for contraception include abstinence, various barrier methods, and timing of intercourse in regard to the menstrual cycle. Abstinence from sexual intercourse is 100% effective. But abstinence is often a difficult method for both men and women to use consistently. Any act of unprotected intercourse can result in pregnancy.

Barrier methods include over-the-counter spermicidal products (i.e., creams, jellies, foams, and sponges) that are put into the vagina before intercourse to create a spermicide barrier between the uterus and ejaculated sperm. A **condom** is a thin rubber sheath that fits over the penis to prevent entrance of sperm into the vagina. Vaginal spermicides and condoms are most effective when instructions are carefully followed; their combined use has been found to be more effective in preventing pregnancy than the use of either one alone (Braden, 1998).

Effectiveness varies with each contraceptive method and the consistency of use. The percentage of women experiencing an accidental pregnancy using these nonprescription methods ranges from 3% to 12% with consistent and correct use (Braden, 1998). The words *consistent* and *correct* need to be carefully noted. Contraceptive methods are dependent on repeated use around the act of inter-

course. There are likely to be times when no method is used, which greatly increases the chance of pregnancy.

Nonprescription methods of contraception that are based on the physiological changes of the menstrual cycle include the rhythm, basal body temperature, cervical mucus, and fertility awareness methods. These methods require that the female client understand the reproductive cycle of her body and be aware of the subtle signs and signals her body gives during the cycle. These methods also require abstinence from sexual intercourse during designated fertile periods. The failure rate for these methods during the first year of use is 20% (Braden, 1998).

Additional nonprescription methods that clients use include withdrawal and douching. Withdrawal consists of withdrawing the penis from the vagina before ejaculation. There can be some passage of sperm from the penis before ejaculation. Also, sperm that are deposited outside of the vagina can still enter the vagina, uterus, and fallopian tubes. Douching, when used in an attempt to prevent pregnancy, involves douching following intercourse. The intention is to wash sperm from the vagina, but sperm are likely to enter the uterus and fallopian tubes quickly following ejaculation. Neither withdrawal nor douching offers significant protection against an unwanted pregnancy.

Methods Requiring a Health Care Provider's Intervention. Contraceptive methods that require the intervention of a health care provider include hormonal contraception, intrauterine devices (IUDs), the **diaphragm,** the cervical cap, and **sterilization.** Hormonal contraception is available in several forms: oral contraceptive pills, intramuscular injection, subdermal implant, and IUDs. Hormonal contraception alters the hormonal environment to prevent ovulation and thicken cervical mucus.

An IUD is a plastic device inserted by a health care provider into the uterus through the cervical opening. IUDs vary in shape and may contain copper or may be impregnated with progesterone. The presence of the IUD results in the lining of the uterus being less favorable for the implantation of a fertilized ovum.

The diaphragm is a round, rubber dome that has a flexible spring around the edge. It must be used with a contraceptive cream or jelly and is inserted in the vagina so that it provides a contraceptive barrier over the cervical opening.

The cervical cap functions like the diaphragm; however, it covers only the cervix. It may be left in place longer and may be perceived as more comfortable than the diaphragm.

Effectiveness rates are reported as follows: oral contraceptives, 97% to 99.9%; IUDs, 98% to 99.9%; diaphragm, 88% to 94%; and cervical cap, 64% to 91% (Braden, 1998). The variation in rates for the diaphragm and cervical cap relates in part to the need for correct and consistent use during each act of intercourse for the method to be effective. Using a contraceptive method that requires specific action at the time of sexual excitement and activity can decrease the consistency of use.

Sterilization is the most effective contraception method other than abstinence. It should be considered permanent. Female sterilization, or **tubal ligation,** involves cutting, tying, or otherwise ligating the fallopian tubes. In male sterilization, or **vasectomy,** the vas deferens, which carries the sperm away from the testicles, is cut and tied. Both a tubal ligation and a vasectomy are considered minor surgical procedures, although a vasectomy is a less involved procedure and can be performed with the client under local anesthesia in a physician's office.

ABORTION

Abortions have been performed since ancient times. The safety and availability of abortions in the United States have improved since the 1973 Supreme Court decision, *Roe v. Wade.* Abortions are safer and less costly when performed in the early weeks of pregnancy. This is possible with improved pregnancy testing and more accurate early diagnosis. The availability of abortions, however, remains tenuous and uncertain. Public opinion relating to the right to life, results of elections or appointments to political offices or positions, advocacy by "pro-life" and "pro-choice" groups, and the increasing use of violence against women and workers in abortion clinics are all forces that could reshape federal and state laws.

Over 50% of women who have abortions are between the ages of 19 and 24 (Centers for Disease Control and Prevention [CDC] 1998a). Approximately 88% of abortions are performed within the first 12 weeks of pregnancy (CDC, 1998a).

SEXUALLY TRANSMITTED DISEASES

The United States has the highest rate of STDs in the industrialized world (Institute of Medicine, 1997). The highest prevalence is among teenagers and young adults (Youngkin, 1995). Acquired immunodeficiency syndrome (AIDS) continues to receive wide public attention; however, other STDs also need to be considered. Although human immunodeficiency virus (HIV) infection is an STD, it affects a much smaller group and is a different epidemic from that of all other STDs. Therefore for the purposes of this section, it is categorized and discussed separately.

Prevalent STDs include syphilis, gonorrhea, chlamydia, trichomoniasis, and infection with the human papillomavirus (HPV) and herpes simplex virus (HSV) type II (genital warts and genital herpes, respectively). The populations most at risk are teenagers, women and their infants, and ethnic minorities who are poor and lack access to medical care (American Family Physician, 1999).

As the name implies, STDs are transmitted from infected individuals to partners during intimate sexual con-

tact. The site of transmission is usually genital, but it may also be oral-genital or anal-genital. Those persons most likely to be infected share one key characteristic: unprotected sex with multiple partners. Diseases that are caused by bacteria and that can usually be cured with antibiotics include gonorrhea, chlamydia, syphilis, and pelvic inflammatory disease. All clients need to understand that antibiotics need to be taken for the full course of treatment. An emerging concern, however, is that some of these bacterial infections (e.g., gonorrhea and syphilis) are now developing antibiotic-resistant strains. Two diseases—genital herpes and genital warts—are caused by viruses and cannot be cured.

A major problem in dealing with STDs is finding and treating the people who have them. Some people may not even know that they are infected, because symptoms are absent or go unnoticed. Because sexual behavior may include the whole body rather than just the genitalia, many parts of the body are potential sites for an STD. The ears, mouth, throat, tongue, nose, and eyelids can be used for sexual pleasure. The perineum, anus, and rectum are also frequently included in sexual activity. Furthermore, any contact with another person's body fluids around the head or an open lesion on the skin, anus, or genitalia can transmit an STD.

Sometimes people do not seek treatment because they are embarrassed to discuss sexual symptoms or concerns. They may also hesitate to talk about their sexual behavior if they believe that it is not "normal." Oral-genital sex, anal-genital sex, or any sexual behavior that embarrasses the client may hinder the detection of an STD.

The most valuable tool the nurse can develop for providing care in areas of sexuality involves communication skills and a nonjudgmental attitude. By questioning and talking with the client in a caring manner that evokes trust, the nurse can pick up valuable clues about an STD that the client may have missed. The nurse can also begin to assess the client's attitudes toward sexuality and adjust the intervention to make it acceptable to the client's sexual value system.

Human Immunodeficiency Virus Infection.   HIV infection or AIDS is also spread through sexual contact. Although HIV is present in the majority of body fluids, it is really a blood-borne pathogen. For transmission to occur, therefore, some exchange of body fluid, particularly blood, must occur. Primary routes of transmission include contaminated intravenous (IV) needles; anal intercourse, vaginal intercourse, and oral-genital sex; and transfusion of blood and blood products.

Those primarily vulnerable to HIV infection, therefore, are gay men; IV drug users, their partners, and their children; and clients with hemophilia and others who have received contaminated blood. As with other STDs, heterosexual persons who have unprotected sex with multiple partners or who have a partner who has multiple other partners are also at risk.

Odds of transmission of HIV increase with frequent unprotected sex with an infected partner. Transmission of HIV is believed to eventually result in AIDS (CDC, 1998b) individuals who are infected with HIV may have no symptoms or manifest varying degrees of AIDS symptoms. AIDS may take as long as 17 years to present, with the median interval from infection to manifestation being 10 years (CDC, 1998b). Much remains to be learned about this virus, the disease, and those who have no symptoms or do not display the full range of symptoms. There is no cure for the disease, which is usually fatal. Treatments and vaccines are being investigated.

Nursing Knowledge Base

As the nurse plans to assist the client in addressing his or her sexual needs, the nurse also uses critical thinking skills and basic nursing knowledge. The nurse may draw from the following areas of nursing knowledge: sociocultural dimensions of sexuality; the impact of pregnancy and menstruation on sexuality; factors that influence discussion of sexual issues; factors that influence decisions regarding contraception, abortion, STD prevention, and abortion; **infertility;** sexual abuse; and **sexual dysfunction**

SOCIOCULTURAL DIMENSIONS OF SEXUALITY

Sexuality is influenced by cultural rules and norms that determine what is acceptable behavior within the culture. Global cultural diversity creates considerable variability in sexual norms and represents a wide spectrum of beliefs and values (Box 27-1). Common areas of diversity include the meaning of dating and behavior allowed during dating, what is considered arousing, the types of sexual activity commonly practiced, sanctions and prohibitions concerning sexual behavior, who one marries, and who is allowed to marry.

A definitive and comprehensive survey of sexual practices and beliefs in America conducted by University of Chicago researchers confirmed that people are influenced by their social networks and tend to act out social scripts (Michael and others, 1994). Sexual behavior is very similar to any other social behavior (i.e., people behave the way they are rewarded for behaving). They tend to "play by the rules" when choosing someone to have sex with and when choosing someone to marry.

Society plays a powerful role in shaping sexual values and attitudes and in supporting specific expression of sexuality in its members. Each cultural and social group has its own set of rules and norms that guide the behavior of its members. These rules become an integral part of an individual's thinking and underlie sexual behavior, including, for example, how people find partners, who they choose as partners, how they relate to one another, how often they have sex, and what they do when they have sex.

Cultural ASPECTS OF CARE   Box 27-1

Refugees who come to the United States are required to have a physical examination within a year of arriving. Either in relation to this regulation or because of a refugee's more urgent health needs, nurses are likely to encounter individuals of various ethnic origins within various health care settings. Before entry into the United States, refugees often live in camps located near their homeland. Life within these camps is often hard, and refugees may face family disintegration, overcrowding, inadequate nutrition, and poor sanitation. Rape and other types of physical violence are common. Refugees often suffer from emotional distress, including fear, anger, confusion, and grief.

In addition to emotional distress, when refugees seek health services, there are numerous cultural barriers that affect interactions. Languages often differ, and the refugee may speak either no English or minimal English. In some cultures it is inappropriate for individuals to ask questions of health care providers. In addition to these barriers, refugees may be afraid to reveal health problems because of fear that the health problem may affect their remaining in this country. Within various cultures there are also norms that differ from the predominant American customs. For example, in some countries it is appropriate to tell the family, rather than the individual, the diagnosis. In some African countries female circumcision is the norm.

Trained medical interpreters, preferably of the same gender, facilitate communication. Because of the sensitive nature of many health problems, particularly those relating to sexuality (e.g., STDs, pregnancy), use of a medical interpreter for translation is preferable to use of a child or spouse of the individual. Family members are less desirable as translators because they may express their own views and beliefs rather than those of the client. When an interpreter is not available, the nurse will need to speak slowly, say things in different ways, use gestures, and ask the person to repeat to discern understanding (Kang and others, 1998).

Impact of Pregnancy and Menstruation on Sexuality. Many cultures have taboos against sexual intercourse or even male-female contact during menstruation and pregnancy. For example, in the Hindu culture a woman must stay away from worship, cooking, and other members of the family during menstruation. Scientific inquiry has found no physiological contraindication to intercourse during menstruation or during most pregnancies. Female sexual interest tends to fluctuate during pregnancy, with increased interest during the second trimester and often decreased interest during the first and third trimesters. Emotional overtones (e.g., dealing with blood during menstruation or fear of injury to the fetus or mother during pregnancy) may need to be resolved to promote mutual sexual satisfaction.

Discussing Sexual Issues. Sexuality is a significant part of each person's being. Yet sexual assessment and interventions are not always included in health care. The area of sexuality can be emotionally charged for nurses, as well as for clients. Discomfort with talking about sexual issues, lack of information, differences in values between the client and the nurse, and guilt may prevent the nurse from discussing issues regarding sexuality with clients. The most valuable tool that the nurse can develop for providing care in areas of sexuality involves communication skills. Nurses who have difficulty discussing topics related to sexuality should explore their discomfort and develop a plan for addressing their discomfort. If the nurse is uncomfortable with topics related to sexuality, the client is unlikely to share sexual concerns with the nurse.

DECISIONAL ISSUES

There are numerous decisions individuals make regarding their sexuality. Some of those decisions that the nurse is likely to encounter and perhaps influence include decisions regarding contraception and abortion.

Contraception.

The decisions that women and men make regarding contraception can have far-reaching effects on their lives. Pregnancy, whether planned or unplanned, significantly affects the life of the mother and often the father and larger support network. Effects are physical, interpersonal, social, financial, and societal. The choice to use contraception is multifaceted and is not completely understood. Henshaw (1998) estimated the number of unintended pregnancies in the United States at 49%. Of these, 54% ended in abortion. Effective contraception involves factors relating to the sexually active couple, the method of contraception, the couple's understanding of the contraceptive method, the consistency of use, and the compliance with the requirements of the chosen method. Personal characteristics that have been identified as positively influencing contraceptive use include motivation to avoid unintended pregnancy, ability to plan, comfort with sexuality, and previous contraceptive use (Beckman and Harvey, 1996)

Abortion.

Abortion continues to be a hotly debated issue. Women and their partners who are faced with an unwanted pregnancy often consider abortion. The nurse can provide an environment in which the issue of abortion can be openly discussed, allowing exploration of various options with an unwanted pregnancy. Reasons for choosing an abortion vary and may include terminating an unwanted pregnancy or aborting a fetus known to have birth defects. When abortion is chosen as a way of dealing with an unwanted pregnancy, the woman, and often her partner, may experience a sense of loss, grief, and/or guilt. Guilt may surface immediately or may be more covert and manifest as sexual dysfunction or altered perceptions.

Health care providers must sort out personal values related to abortion. The health care provider is entitled to personal views and should not be forced to participate in counseling or procedures contrary to beliefs and values. Nurses should choose specialties or places of employment where their personal values are not compromised and the care of a client in need of health care is not jeopardized.

STD Prevention.

"Safe sex" is a term used to describe responsible sexual behavior aimed at preventing the spread of STDs, including AIDS. Responsible sexual behavior includes knowing one's sexual partner, being able to openly discuss sexual and drug-use history with the partner, not allowing one's decision to be influenced by drugs or alcohol, and using protective devices.

ALTERATIONS IN SEXUAL HEALTH

Infertility.

A group with special health care needs is made up of individuals who want to conceive but cannot. Infertility is defined as the inability to conceive after 1 year of unprotected intercourse. A couple who want to conceive and cannot may experience a sense of failure and may feel that their bodies are somehow defective. A desire to become pregnant can grow until it permeates most waking moments. A woman or her partner may become preoccupied with creating just the right circumstances for conception. With advances in reproductive technology, infertile couples face many choices that involve religious and ethical values and financial constraints.

Choices for the infertile couple include pursuit of adoption, medical assistance with fertilization, or adapting to the probability of remaining childless. Organizations such as RESOLVE or international adoption groups can provide couples with support.

Sexual Abuse.

Sexual abuse is a wide spread health problem in our society. Abuse crosses all socioeconomic and ethnic groups. It is estimated that from one fourth to one half of all females experience some type of sexual abuse before reaching the age of 18 (Guidry, 1995; Bohn and Holz, 1996). Most often this abuse is at the hands of a former intimate partner or family member. Sexual abuse is also an issue for males. Studies indicate that one in six males experiences at least one sexually abusive incident before reaching adulthood (Guidry, 1995). Sexual abuse has far-ranging effects on physical and psychological functioning (Dickinson and others, 1999).

Evidence of sexual abuse in children may be uncovered during history taking or physical examination. Symptoms that should raise suspicion of the possibility of sexual abuse include a child showing an early, exaggerated awareness of sex or exhibiting seductive behavior toward adults; swelling or bruising of the external genitalia, anus, breasts, or buttocks; lacerations of or a foreign substance in the vagina or anus; and an STD in a child under 15 years of age.

Sexual abuse may begin, continue, or even intensify during pregnancy. The abuser may not fit any classic description. Cues that raise a question of possible sexual abuse include extreme jealousy and refusal to leave a woman's side. The overall appearance may be of a very concerned and caring husband or boyfriend when the underlying dynamic is very different from this picture.

When abuse is recognized, support needs to be mobilized for the victim and the family. All family members may require therapy in situations of incest to promote healthy interactions and relationships. Rape victims may need to work through the crisis before feeling comfortable with intimate expressions of affection. The partner may need support in understanding this process and ways to assist the victim. Children who have been sexually molested need to understand that they are not at fault for the incident. The parents must understand that their response is critical to how the child reacts and adapts. The nurse may come in contact with clients confronting these stressors. Nurses are in an ideal position to assess occurrences of sexual violence and to educate individuals regarding community services. Nurses should be aware of resources for referral and support in the community.

Personal and Emotional Conflicts.   Ideally, sex is a natural, spontaneous act that passes easily through a number of recognizable physiological stages and culminates in one or more orgasms. In reality, this sequence of events is more the exception than the rule. Nurses encounter clients who have problems with one or more of the stages of sexual activity, including the feeling of wanting sex, the physiological processes and emotions of having sex, and the feelings experienced after sex. For example, some women who are taking antidepressants have noted that their ability to reach orgasm is negatively affected.

Sexual Dysfunction.   Sexual dysfunction is common. A recent analysis of a large sample of U.S. men and women ages 18 to 59 found that 43% of women and 31% of men reported sexual dysfunction (Laumann and others, 1999). Sexual dysfunction is more prevalent in men and women with poor emotional and physical health. Sometimes the exact cause cannot be determined. Common chronic illnesses that can contribute to sexual dysfunction include diabetes mellitus, kidney disease, alcoholism, neurological disorders, hormone deficiencies, multiple sclerosis, and vascular insufficiency (Sipski and Alexander, 1997) (Tables 27-1 and 27-2). Medication side effects can also contribute to sexual dysfunction (Box 27-2).

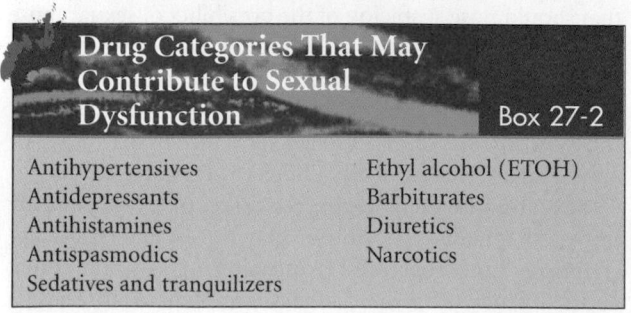

Drug Categories That May Contribute to Sexual Dysfunction	Box 27-2

Antihypertensives	Ethyl alcohol (ETOH)
Antidepressants	Barbiturates
Antihistamines	Diuretics
Antispasmodics	Narcotics
Sedatives and tranquilizers	

Critical Thinking Synthesis

Successful critical thinking requires synthesis of knowledge, experience, information gathered from clients, critical thinking attitudes, and intellectual and professional standards. Clinical judgment requires the nurse to anticipate the information necessary, analyze the data, and make appropriate decisions regarding client care. Critical thinking is always changing. Figure 27-2 demonstrates that the nurse must consider numerous critical thinking elements, as well as client assessment data, that contribute to appropriate nursing diagnoses.

In the case of sexuality the nurse integrates knowledge from nursing and other disciplines. The nurse must have a good understanding, for example, of the human sexual response, safe sex practices, and the risks and behaviors associated with sexual problems to anticipate how to assess a client and then how to interpret findings. Previous experience in caring for clients whose sexuality becomes threatened helps the nurse approach the next client in a more reflective and helpful way. Clients will have different customs and values from those of the nurse. Professional standards call for the nurse to respect each client as an individual. Critical thinking attitudes such as integrity require the nurse to recognize when his or her opinions and values are in conflict with those of the client and to consider how to proceed in a way that is mutually beneficial for the client and the nurse.

Sexuality and the Nursing Process

A person's sexuality has physical, psychological, social, and cultural elements. The nurse must assess all relevant elements to determine a client's sexual well-being. Many nurses find that they are uncomfortable talking about sexuality with clients. To increase comfort in discussing sexuality, the nurse should build a sound knowledge base and be willing to explore personal issues regarding sexuality. The nursing role in addressing sexual concerns can range from ongoing assessment to providing information to counseling to referral. Recognition that the nurse is not expected to have answers to all of the sexual issues and concerns identified can free the nurse to gather an appropriate sexual history database.

ASSESSMENT
Factors Affecting Sexuality.   In gathering a sexual history, the nurse should consider physical, functional, relationship, lifestyle, and self-esteem factors that may influence sexual functioning. Sexual desire varies among individuals; some people want and enjoy sex every day, whereas others want sex only once a month, and still others have no sexual desire and are quite comfortable

Table 27-1 Common Female Sexual Dysfunctions

Description	Possible Causes	Interventions
Preorgasmic (primary) orgasmic dysfunction: impaired ability of woman to have orgasm	Religious prohibitions Restrictive learning environment Fear of losing control Poor communication with partner Inadequate clitoral stimulation Excessive drug or alcohol use Past negative sexual experiences	Provide information on sexual prohibitions and restrictions. Teach sensate focus exercises.* Suggest genital play. Teach Kegel exercises.† Suggest directed masturbation. Encourage nondemand intercourse. Initiate referral to sex therapist. Initiate referral to preorgasmic support group.
Secondary orgasmic dysfunction: impaired ability of woman to have orgasm currently but with history of ability to have orgasm	Low sexual interest Attitude toward partner Causes listed for primary orgasmic dysfunction	Discuss attitude toward partner. Provide information on sexual prohibitions. Teach sensate focus exercises.* Suggest nondemand intercourse. Suggest genital play. Teach Kegel exercises.† Suggest directed masturbation. Encourage partner communication. Initiate referral to sex therapist.
Vaginismus: involuntary constriction of outer third of vagina, making vaginal penetration impossible	Religious prohibitions Sexual prohibitions Experience of sexual assault Painful intercourse Painful pelvic examinations Alcohol abuse Traumatic early experiences with sex Fear of pregnancy, venereal disease, or cancer	Legitimize existence of spasm. Suggest use of vaginal dilators in graduated sizes. Teach Kegel exercises.† Encourage improvement of partner communication. Initiate referral to sensitive, experienced health care provider.
Diminished lubrication	Neurological disease, including but not limited to multiple sclerosis (MS) or cerebrovascular accident (CVA) Aging changes‡	
Dyspareunia: painful intercourse	Negative attitude toward partner Strong religious prohibitions Sexual prohibitions Genital sensitivity Physical problems (e.g., tears, infections, trauma, spasms, lack of lubrication) Roughness during intercourse Lack of arousal Neurological disease, including but not limited to MS or CVA‡ Aging changes‡	Initiate referral to sensitive, experienced health care provider. Treat physical problems. Provide sufficient lubrication. Discuss sexual attitudes. Discuss comfortable positions.
Lack of desire: loss of interest in being sexual	Strong negative emotions Illness Fatigue Drug or alcohol use Avoidance response because of feeling sexually pressured Unresolved anger or fear Depression History of sexual abuse or incest Pain associated with intercourse Neurological disease, including but not limited to MS CVA‡ or Fatigue related to neurological disease, anemia, or cancer treatment‡ Diabetes	Discuss attitude toward partner. Provide information on sexual prohibitions and restrictions. Teach sensate focus exercises.* Teach Kegel exercises.† Encourage genital play. Encourage resolution of conflicts between partners. Initiate referral to mental health professional or sex therapist.

*Series of pleasurable touching exercises that are focused on sensual (not sexual) activities with partner.
†Exercises for pubococcygeus muscle to increase sensation and maintain muscle tone of pelvic floor.
‡Information regarding medical conditions and sexual dysfunction from Sipski M, Alexander C: *Sexual function in people with disability and chronic illness,* Gathersburg, Md, 1997, Aspen.

Table 27-2   Common Male Sexual Dysfunctions

Description	Possible Causes	Interventions
Primary erectile dysfunction: inability of man to penetrate during sexual contact and to sustain an erection to point of penetration (Man may masturbate to ejaculation.)	Extreme religious prohibitions Traumatic initial failure Performance anxiety and fears	Relieve pressure of goal-oriented sexual performance. Discuss sexual prohibitions and restrictions. Provide accurate information. Teach sensate focus exercises.* Restrict intercourse. Encourage female superior position with lubrication. Encourage alternatives to intercourse (e.g., manual stimulation, oral-genital sex). Initiate referral to sex therapist.
Secondary erectile dysfunction: inability of man to maintain or perhaps even experience erection but with a history of penetration at least one time (Man has experienced erectile failure during at least 25% of sexual opportunities.)	Interference with central nervous system caused by drugs, alcohol, stress, fatigue, or surgical procedures Performance anxiety Poor communication with partner Depression Neurological disease, including but not limited to multiple sclerosis (MS) or cerebrovascular accident (CVA)‡ Diabetes‡	Relieve pressure of goal-oriented sexual performance. Discuss sexual prohibitions and restrictions. Provide accurate information. Teach sensate focus exercises.* Teach Kegel exercises to female partner.† Initiate referral to urologist.
Premature ejaculation: consistent premature ejaculation	Fast ejaculation patterning during adolescence Failure to attend to internal cues of approaching ejaculation Lack of sensual self-awareness Performance anxiety Neurological disease, including but not limited to MS or CVA‡	Provide accurate information. Encourage communication with partner. Teach sensate focus exercises.* Teach Kegel exercises to female partner.† Explain stop-start technique. Encourage different positions. Teach retraining of ejaculatory response. Relieve pressure of performance anxiety. Suggest changing tempo of thrusting during intercourse. Initiate referral to sex therapist.
Delayed ejaculation: inability to ejaculate during penetration	Religious restrictions Fear of impregnating Lack of physical interest Active dislike for partner Past traumatic sexual event Infidelity Punishment for masturbation as child Excessive drug or alcohol use	Relieve pressure of goal-oriented sexual performance. Discuss sexual prohibitions and restrictions. Provide accurate information. Teach sensate focus exercises.* Teach Kegel exercises to female partner.† Encourage communication with partner. Initiate referral to mental health professional or sex therapist.

*Series of pleasurable touching exercises that are focused on sensual (not sexual) activities with partner.
†Exercises for pubococcygeus muscle to increase sensation and maintain muscle tone of pelvic floor.
‡Information regarding medical conditions and sexual dysfunction from Sipski M, Alexander C: *Sexual function in people with disability and chronic illness*, Gathersburg, Md, 1997, Aspen.

with that fact. Sexual desire becomes an issue if the person wants to feel sexual desire more often, if the person believes it is necessary to measure up to some cultural norm, or if there is a discrepancy between the sexual desires of the partners in a relationship.

The nurse assesses for factors that typically can influence sexual desire. A person may experience a decrease in sexual desire for physical reasons, such as pain or discomfort during sexual activity. Even imagining that sex could

hurt can lessen sexual desire. Minor illness and fatigue can also decrease sexual desire. Medications (see Box 27-2) can affect sexual desire. Lifestyle factors, such as the use or abuse of alcohol, lack of sleep, or lack of time, can also be influencing factors. Working parents, for example, may feel so overburdened that they perceive sexual advances from a partner as an additional demand on them. When the nurse identifies factors that can potentially affect sexual desire, he or she will confirm them with the client and

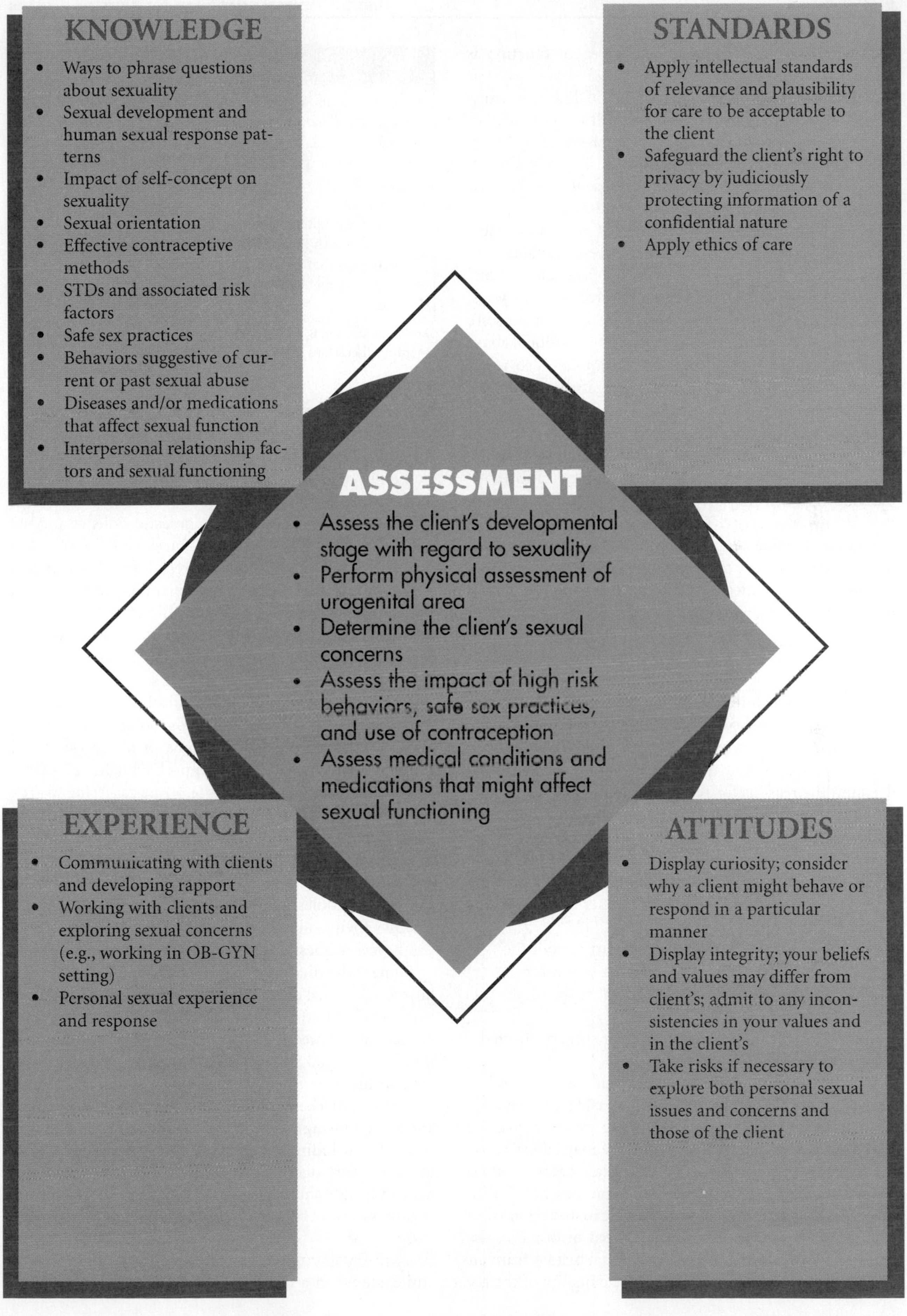

KNOWLEDGE

- Ways to phrase questions about sexuality
- Sexual development and human sexual response patterns
- Impact of self-concept on sexuality
- Sexual orientation
- Effective contraceptive methods
- STDs and associated risk factors
- Safe sex practices
- Behaviors suggestive of current or past sexual abuse
- Diseases and/or medications that affect sexual function
- Interpersonal relationship factors and sexual functioning

STANDARDS

- Apply intellectual standards of relevance and plausibility for care to be acceptable to the client
- Safeguard the client's right to privacy by judiciously protecting information of a confidential nature
- Apply ethics of care

ASSESSMENT

- Assess the client's developmental stage with regard to sexuality
- Perform physical assessment of urogenital area
- Determine the client's sexual concerns
- Assess the impact of high risk behaviors, safe sex practices, and use of contraception
- Assess medical conditions and medications that might affect sexual functioning

EXPERIENCE

- Communicating with clients and developing rapport
- Working with clients and exploring sexual concerns (e.g., working in OB-GYN setting)
- Personal sexual experience and response

ATTITUDES

- Display curiosity; consider why a client might behave or respond in a particular manner
- Display integrity; your beliefs and values may differ from client's; admit to any inconsistencies in your values and in the client's
- Take risks if necessary to explore both personal sexual issues and concerns and those of the client

Figure 27-2 *Synthesis Model for Sexuality Assessment Phase.*

then determine the extent to which sexual function is impaired.

Self-concept issues (see Chapter 26), including identity, body image, role performance, and self-esteem, affect a client's sexuality. Poor body image, particularly when magnified by feelings of rejection or by body-altering surgery, may result in diminished or absent sexual desire. A person's self-esteem can lead to conflicts involving sexuality. If a healthy sense of a sexual self and comfortable sexual behaviors have not been developed, sexuality may cause negative feelings or lead to the suppression of sexual feelings. Sexual self-esteem can be lowered in many ways. Low sexual self-esteem will negatively affect a person's self-concept. Rape, incest, and physical or emotional abuse leave deep scars. Low sexual self-esteem can also result from lack of adequate sex education, negative role models, and attempts to live up to unrealistic personal or cultural expectations.

Issues in a relationship can also affect sexual desire. After the initial glow of a new relationship has faded, couples may find that they are faced with major differences in their values or lifestyles. The degree to which they still feel close to each other and interact on an intimate level depends on their ability to negotiate and compromise. Thus communication between sexual partners plays a crucial role in sexual satisfaction within a relationship.

Sexual Health History.

When taking a nursing history, the nurse should consider including a few questions related to sexual functioning to determine whether the client has any sexual concerns. These questions can be incorporated in the review of systems and addressed in a routine, matter-of-fact manner. The nurse needs to understand the reasons for the question and be able to provide them to the client on request. An opening statement such as, "Sex is an important part of life and can be affected by our health status and vice versa. To better understand your health, it is useful to know . . ." is a possible introduction to these questions. Other questions for adults might include the following:

> How do you feel about the sexual part of your life?
>
> Have you noticed any changes in the way you feel about yourself (as a man, woman, husband, or wife)?
>
> How has your illness, medication, or surgery affected your sex life?
>
> It is not unusual for people with your condition to be experiencing some sexual changes. Have you noticed any changes, or do you have any concerns?

When caring for older adults, the nurse may adjust his or her assessment approach. The American Association of Retired Persons surveyed older adults on how health care providers could better assess their sexuality (Johnson, 1997) and received the suggestions listed in Box 27-3. In addition, when the nurse gathers a sexual history from an older adult, areas to explore include the quality of the re-

---

Geriatric   NURSING PRACTICE   Box 27-3

- Use clear and easy-to-understand words.
- Create an environment that allows for discussion of sexual concerns. The concern can be hard for the client to bring up, so give permission for discussion by bringing up the topic of sexuality. Ask direct questions related to sexuality.
- If you cannot answer questions, offer to find out the answer, refer the client to another source, or provide written materials that address the concern.
- Acknowledge that sexual interest and desire is healthy in old age.

Data from Johnson B: Older adults' suggestions for health care providers regarding discussions of sex, *Geriatr Nurs* 18(2):65, 1997.

---

lationship between partners, the death or loss of a partner, sexual satisfaction and history during middle adulthood, the general health status of both partners, use of prescription and nonprescription medications, and current satisfaction with sexual activity (Finan, 1997b).

In light of the prevalence of domestic violence and sexual abuse, questions relating to abusive relationships can be important. Questions that address domestic violence or abuse should be addressed to the client in private. A question such as "Are you in a relationship in which someone is hurting you?" may open the door for a client to reveal present or previous abuse. An additional question such as "Has anyone ever forced you to have sex you did not wish to participate in?" may more specifically open the door for the client to discuss concerns. Recognizing both subjective and objective signs and symptoms of abuse can aid in recognition of this too common problem (Box 27-4).

It is also significant to explore, while gathering the sexual history for sexually active clients, the client's use of contraception and safe sex practices. Adolescents may respond to a comment that allows them to know that having questions related to sexuality is normal. A lead-in could be, "Many adolescents have questions about STDs or whether their bodies are developing at the right rate. Do you have any questions about sex or other things?"

Some individuals are too embarrassed or do not know how to ask sexual questions directly. The nurse may detect clues that a person has questions if the person expresses concern about how his or her partner may respond now or if the person makes a sexual comment or joke. Observing for and listening to concerns about sexuality takes practice. With experience the nurse develops skill in clarifying and paraphrasing to help individuals express sexual concerns. By including sexuality in the nursing history, the nurse acknowledges that sexuality is an important component of health and creates an opportunity for the person to discuss sexual concerns.

Sexual Dysfunction.

The nurse needs to be able to anticipate when a client is at risk for sexual dysfunction

---

Signs and Symptoms That May Indicate Current Sexual Abuse or a History of Sexual Abuse

Box 27-4

Bruises	Premenstrual syndrome
Lacerations	Sleep pattern disturbances
Abrasions	Nightmares
Burns	Repetitive dreams
Frequent visits to health care providers	Insomnia
Vague symptoms	Depression
Headaches	Anxiety
Gastrointestinal problems	Fear
Eating disorders	Decreased self-esteem
Abdominal pain	Difficulty developing trust
Vaginal pain	Difficulties with intimate relationships
Dysmenorrhea	Substance abuse

Modified from Bohn D, Holz K: Sequelae of abuse: health effects of childhood sexual abuse, domestic battering, and rape, *J Nurse Midwifery* 41(6):442, 1996.

Client Teaching FOR KEGEL EXERCISES

Box 27-5

OBJECTIVE
- Client will demonstrate ability to tighten pubococcygeus muscle and will verbalize methods to assess correct procedures and increasing strength.

TEACHING STRATEGIES
- Explain method to identify proper muscle contraction by sitting on toilet with knees far apart and tighten muscles to stop the flow of urine.
- After muscle is identified, instruct client to contract muscle for a count of 3, hold and release for a count of 3, and repeat this 10 times. Client should do this about 5 times a day.

- Explain that within first week of exercises, client should assess if proper muscle contraction is occurring by placing two fingers in vagina to identify if tightening can be felt or asking partner to identify during sexual intercourse when muscle is tightened.

EVALUATION
- Ask client if she has identified pubococcygeus muscle via finger insertion or partner response.
- During vaginal bimanual examination, ask client to do exercises and assess muscle tone.

(see Tables 27-2 and 27-3). The nurse applies a knowledge base of those conditions that may cause sexual dysfunction while assessing a client's risks. Awareness of the possible effects of physical problems, altered self-concept, medications, and the factors addressed thus far on sexual functioning assist the nurse in conducting a thorough assessment. A client may also bring up the topic of sexual dysfunction, or issues may become evident as the client answers other nursing history questions.

Physical Assessment.   The physical examination is important in evaluating the cause of sexual concerns or problems and may be the best opportunity to teach an individual about sexuality. In examining a woman's breasts and the external and internal genitalia, the nurse has the opportunity to assess the woman's reaction, answer questions, and provide information about the examination of anatomical and physiological structures. A woman can learn to perform a breast self-examination during physical

assessment (see Chapter 32). In addition, the nurse may choose to teach Kegel exercises (Box 27-5). These exercises strengthen the pubococcygeus muscle. Toning of this muscle often decreases as a result of stretching during childbirth and loss of general elasticity during aging. Maintaining good tone helps prevent bladder or rectal prolapse into the vagina (cystocele or rectocele), reduces problems with later urinary incontinence, and can enhance sexual enjoyment through and beyond menopause. During physical assessment of the genitalia, men can be taught to perform testicular self-examination (see Chapter 32). Knowledge of normal scrotal anatomical structures aids men in detecting signs of testicular cancer. The nurse can instruct both men and women on signs and symptoms of STDs during the examination when clients' histories suggest risks for STD.

Client Expectations.   As in the case of any client assessment, it is important to understand the client's expec-

SAMPLE NURSING DIAGNOSTIC PROCESS   Box 27-6
ALTERED SEXUALITY PATTERNS

Assessment Activities	Defining Characteristics	Nursing Diagnosis
Observe readiness to discuss sex through verbalization (e.g., "When can I return to life as normal?" or "There goes my love life") or behavior (e.g., exhibitionism).	Client verbalizes concern that sexual activity may cause another myocardial infarction or death.	Altered sexuality patterns related to fear of recurrent myocardial infarction or death during intercourse.
Ask client and spouse about previous level and method of sexual expression (e.g., frequency, initiator).		
Observe for affectionate behavior (e.g., touching, hand holding, kissing).	Client's spouse exhibits reluctance to touch client.	
In privacy, ask spouse about perceptions of recovery and return to full functioning.	Spouse verbalizes concern that client will need continuous care, attention, and protection.	
Observe for anxiety (e.g., hand wringing).	Client maintains eye contact, shifts position frequently.	

tations regarding his or her care. Questions such as "What would you like to have happen in regard to [expressed concern]?" and "What initial steps might you take?" can help the person identify desired outcomes. It is important for the nurse to set aside personal views and not assume what a client's expectations might be.

NURSING DIAGNOSIS

After completing an assessment and applying critical thought to the diagnostic process (Box 27-6), the nurse selects diagnoses applicable to the client's needs. Possible nursing diagnoses related to sexual functioning are listed in Box 27-7. Clues that may signal at-risk or an actual nursing diagnosis related to sexuality include history of surgery of reproductive organs, changes in appearance, past or current physical or sexual abuse, chronic illness, and developmental milestones such as puberty or menopause. When making nursing diagnoses related to sexual dysfunction, the nurse must have assessed anatom-

NURSING DIAGNOSES   Box 27-7
ALTERATIONS IN SEXUALITY

Body image disturbance
Decisional conflict
Knowledge deficit (contraception/STDs)
Adjustment, impaired
Rape-trauma syndrome
Rape-trauma syndrome, compound reaction
Rape-trauma syndrome, silent reaction
Self-esteem disturbance
Sexual dysfunction
Sexuality pattern, altered

ical, physiological, sociocultural, ethical, and situational issues thoroughly.

As with making any nursing diagnosis, the process in regard to sexuality is often one of clarification with the client to establish that the nursing diagnosis defining characteristics in fact exist and that the client perceives a problem or difficulty with regard to sexuality. Determining the etiological or contributing factors is important, to focus effective planning and to select appropriate nursing interventions. For example, the nursing interventions appropriate for the nursing diagnosis of *self-esteem disturbance* would be different for different etiological factors. *Self-esteem disturbance related to long-standing herpes infection* would lead to counseling and education on how to maintain safe sexual practices. In contrast, *self-esteem disturbance related to sexual abuse* would require counseling and referral to community resources (e.g., Crisis Services, sexual abuse support group).

PLANNING

During planning the nurse again synthesizes information from multiple resources (Figure 27-3). Critical thinking ensures that the client's plan of care integrates all that the nurse knows about the individual, as well as critical thinking elements as they pertain to sexuality. Professional standards are especially important to consider when the nurse develops a plan of care. Maintaining a client's dignity and identity is a significant consideration. For example, conveying respect for a client's gender preferences by including a lesbian or gay partner in the plan to the degree that the client wishes can assist the client in maintaining his or her identity and dignity.

The nurse develops an individualized plan of care for each nursing diagnosis (see care plan) The nurse and

KNOWLEDGE

- PLISSIT model
- Community resources for sex education information
- Community resources for contraception and STD treatment and counseling

STANDARDS

- Maintain the client's dignity and identity
- Promote an environment in which the client's values, customs, and spiritual beliefs are respected
- Report STDs as required by law
- Report cases of suspected abuse as required by law

PLANNING

- Create an atmosphere in which the client can explore sexual concerns
- Refer to appropriate resources for exploration of sexual concerns
- Explore the client's understanding, beliefs, and attitudes regarding sexuality and sexual functioning

EXPERIENCE

- Establishing rapport with diverse clients
- Care of clients with HIV infection
- Care of clients with various sexual orientations

ATTITUDES

- Think independently; explore various approaches to address the issue/problem
- Be creative and try unique interventions
- Demonstrate perseverance— changes in self-concept often happen slowly; continue to support the vision that change is possible
- Take risks by asking about the client's concerns even when the topic is sensitive

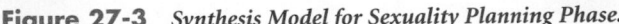

Figure 27-3 *Synthesis Model for Sexuality Planning Phase.*

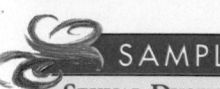

SAMPLE NURSING CARE PLAN

SEXUAL DYSFUNCTION

ASSESSMENT*

Mr. Clements is a 46-year-old black client who was last seen in the office 2 months ago, when he was found to have mild hypertension and was given a prescription for propranolol (Inderal). His blood pressure today is 122/82.

Jack Constant is a 25-year-old nursing student who goes in to talk with Mr. Clements after reading his records, which includes the recent diagnosis of mild hypertension, the order for propranolol, and the current blood pressure reading of 122/82. The record also indicates that Mr. Clements is married and living with his wife.

In talking with Mr. Clements, Jack tells him of the improvement in his blood pressure since his last visit. He inquires if Mr. Clements is taking his medication regularly. Mr. Clements reports that he has been taking his medication regularly. He relates that it scared him when his blood pressure was up because both of his parents had died of strokes. Jack then inquires if he has noted any side effects from the medicine. Mr. Clements says not really, except he is maybe a little more tired than he use to be. Jack then asks the question he formulated, "Some people find that certain blood pressure medications affect their sexual performance. Have you noticed any changes in sexual functioning since you began your medication?" Mr. Clements replies that he finds he just **is not very interested in sex any more** and that this **is becoming somewhat of a problem between him and his wife.** Her interest does not seem to have waned at all, he tells Jack.

Jack asks Mr. Clements when he first began noticing his decreased interest in sex. In thinking back, Mr. Clements says that it started about 2 months ago, sometime around the first of the year. Jack reminds him that this is about the same time he started taking propranolol. Jack then asks Mr. Clements about his sexual relationship with his wife before beginning the propranolol. He learns that the couple use to have intercourse 1 to 3 times per week. Now Mr. Clements reports sometimes having **trouble having an erection.** Jack inquires if anything else has changed in his life since the first of the year, and Mr. Clements denies any changes. Mr. Clements says, "Do you think there may be a relationship between my blood pressure medicine and my lack of interest?" Jack shares that some people have had that experience and suggests that Jack talk it over with the physician when he comes in.

*Defining characteristics are shown in bold type.

NURSING DIAGNOSIS: Sexual dysfunction related to side effects of antihypertensive medication.

PLANNING

GOAL	EXPECTED OUTCOMES
Client will express satisfaction with sexual relationship with wife within 1 month.	Client will report a renewed interest in sex within 1 month Client will report resolution of problem with impotence.

INTERVENTIONS†	RATIONALE
Sexual Counseling	
• Establish trust and respect with client. Offer privacy during conversations.	Conveys sense of caring, increasing likelihood of client's ability to express concerns fully.
• Discuss possible effects of antihypertensive on sexual functioning and encourage client to discuss sexual concerns with physician.	Helps client to understand possible cause for sexual difficulties. Gives client important option to review with physican.
• Encourage client to discuss concerns with his wife. Role play so client can practice ways to approach concerns.	Many of the sexual problems in relationships involve poor communication (Finan, 1997b).
Anxiety Reduction	
• Assure client that there are other blood pressure medications available that can maintain blood pressure control and that do not negatively affect sexual function.	Gives client sense of control knowing that there are options and that blood pressure can continue to be safely managed.

†Intervention Classification labels from McCloskey JC, Bulechek GM: *Nursing interventions classification (NIC),* ed 3, St. Louis, 2000, Mosby.

EVALUATION

Have client discuss satisfaction with sexual function during return office visit.
Ask client to describe perception of conversations with physician and wife.

client together set realistic goals for care. Expected oucomes need to be individualized and realistic.

A useful framework for guiding planning is the PLISSIT model developed by Annon (1976). In this model there are progressively more involved levels of intervention. The *P* stands for permission giving. During assessment the nurse's questions can bring up the topic of sexuality and can give the individual permission to talk about sexual concerns. *LI* stands for limited information, which involves providing basic information regarding sexuality and sexual functioning. An example would be discussing nocturnal emissions with a prepubescent boy to minimize fear that might develop if the boy did not know this was a normal part of development. *SS* stands for specific suggestions whereby the nurse provides specific suggestions regarding a sexual concern or issue. For example, a postmenopausal woman might be concerned about her lack of vaginal lubrication. The nurse might suggest use of a water-based lubricant during sexual intercourse, or the concern expressed might be one that the nurse is not equipped to address. In this case the nurse should refer to another health care provider. The *IT* stands for intensive therapy. At this level of intervention, the nurse's role would be to refer the client to a qualified practitioner, such as a social worker or sex counselor, for individualized therapy.

Planning in the area of sexuality may include referrals to community resources (Box 27-8). Sexual conflicts in marriage or trauma related to sexual abuse or incest may require intensive treatment with a mental health professional or certified sex therapist. For the woman who is currently in an abusive relationship, most communities have battered women's shelters that can provide counseling and serve as a safe haven for the woman while further plans are made.

Community Resources Relating to Sexuality
Box 27-8

Planned parenthood
Sex therapists
Clinical psychologists
Social workers
Health department (often for both family planning and STDs)
Groups that provide education/services for those with particular conditions include:
    American Diabetes Association
    American Heart Association
    Muscular Dystrophy Association
    Muscular Sclerosis Society
Sexual abuse support groups
Women's shelters (for those who have been physically and/or sexually abused)
Hot lines for help (will have lists of community support resources)

IMPLEMENTATION

The nurse's role includes the promotion of sexual health as a component of overall wellness. The nurse can promote sexual health by identifying clients at increased risk (Box 27-9), by providing appropriate information, by helping individuals gain insight into their problems, and by exploring methods to deal with them effectively.

Research HIGHLIGHT
Box 27-9

RESEARCH ABSTRACT

A study was done to compare the rates of sexually transmitted diseases (STDs) in young women who were sexually abused, in those who began sexual activity before age 16, and in those who engaged in high-risk behaviors (inconsistent use of condoms and birth control, alcohol and drug use, multiple sex partners, and having sex on the first date) with young women who did not have similar factors in their experience. Data were gathered through questionaires completed by 1994 young women between the ages of 18 and 22. The young women were recruited from 44 different urban and rural sites, which included health clinics, private health care providers, vocational schools, community colleges, and universities. The study findings showed that young women who were sexually abused, who began sexual activity before age 16, or who engaged in high-risk behaviors were 4 times more likely to have had an STD than young women who had not had these experiences. High-risk behaviors appeared to be more of a risk factor for STDs than sexual abuse or sexual activity before age 16. One third of the young women in the study reported having had sex on a first date or reported another high-risk behavior.

IMPLICATIONS FOR PRACTICE

- Nurses can educate young women about the increased risk of STDs for those who are sexually active at a younger age, for those who have experienced sexual abuse, and for those who engage in high-risk behaviors. Initiating health education in middle and high schools and in the community could help to heighten awareness of risk factors.
- Nurses can act as advocates for sexual abuse awareness and prevention programs in high schools and colleges, organizing opportunities to discuss the issues of sexual abuse and date rape. These sessions would include opportunities for participants to role play ways to handle sexual coercion.
- In gathering a nursing history, areas that need to be addressed include whether the client is or has been sexually active; when sexual activity began; and whether there is a history of sexual abuse and/or risk-taking behaviors.
- Identifying young women at risk could allow the nurse to explore current sexual behaviors and signs and symptoms that would suggest STDs.

REFERENCE

Kenney, Reinholtz, and Angelini: Sexual abuse, sex before age 16, and high-risk behaviors of young females with sexually transmitted diseases, *J Obstet Gynecol Neonatal Nurs* 27(1):54, 1998.

Health Promotion.   Helping clients gain a healthy sexuality involves consideration of factors that influence sexual satisfaction. The nurse needs to educate clients about sexual health, including measures for contraception and prevention of STDs. Regular breast self-examinations and Pap smear are important sexual health measures for women that should be encouraged, as are testicular self-examinations for men.

Exploring an individual's values, discussing levels of satisfaction, and providing sex education require good communication skills. The environment and timing should be structured to provide privacy, comfort, and uninterrupted time. For example, when discussing methods of contraception with a woman, the nurse should provide comfortable chairs in a private area rather than discussing this in the examination room when the client is only partially clothed.

Topics of education vary, depending on the defining characteristics and related factors in the nursing diagnosis (see Box 27-7). Client education may provide guidelines for normal development; for example, the nurse might talk to a toddler's mother regarding a new baby, to a school-age child regarding appearance of pubic hair, or to a 60-year-old man regarding delayed ejaculation. Details of physiological changes should be provided as a part of general health care. Providing client education gives permission for clients to raise questions or concerns regarding personal functioning.

Discussions of healthy sex should include contraception when talking with both men and women of childbearing age. The discussion should include desire for children, usual sexual practices, and acceptable methods of contraception. Factors that need to be considered when discussing contraception include frequency of sexual activity, comfort with genital touching, comfort with sharing contraceptive responsibility with the partner, and comfort with interruption of sexual acts. Formulating questions related to sexuality can be uncomfortable for the nurse. The way in which questions are asked will depend on numerous factors, including the rapport between the client and the nurse, the comfort of both the client and the nurse when discussing sexually related topics, and the client's reason for the health care contact. The nurse might ask, "Are you using contraception with your partner now?" and then follow up, based on the client's answer. If the method of contraception is one that requires participation at the time of intercourse, such as condoms, foam, or a diaphragm, the nurse might ask, "What is it like for you to stop lovemaking to use contraception?" or "Some people find it difficult to use a method consistently that requires remembering or effort each time to actually use the method—has that been a problem for you?" or "How frequently do you have intercourse without protection?" The questions will need to flow from each situation. For clients who do not have a regular contraceptive method, who do not have a reliable contraceptive method, or who

are not satisfied with their current method, the various methods of contraception should be reviewed to provide necessary information for an informed choice. The best method is the one that the person will use consistently.

Individuals having more than one sex partner or whose partner has other sexual experiences need to learn more about safe-sex practices. Information should be provided regarding STD symptoms and transmission, use of condoms, and risky sexual activities (e.g., trauma from penile-anal sex). An area to consider in discussing sexual relating is the emotional risks within a relationship. Role play can be a useful educational tool in helping a person learn to say no or negotiate with a partner to use a condom.

Also significant in maintaining sexual health is regular health examinations. Often STDs, particularly chlamydia and gonorrhea in women and chlamydia in men, are asymptomatic and are only diagnosed during a physical examination with appropriate laboratory work. The annual health examination also provides an easy opportunity to discuss contraception and safe sex practices.

Acute Care.   Nursing interventions that address alterations in sexuality generally are aimed at raising awareness, assisting clarification of issues or concerns, and/or providing information. Nurses who have pursued specialized education in sexual functioning and counseling may provide more intensive sex therapy. Nurses should recognize when an individual's needs exceed their expertise and provide appropriate referral.

The initial intervention often includes exploring present sexual practices with the individual. The individual should be encouraged to investigate and acknowledge social and ethical values and consider the role of sexuality in his or her self-concept. When there is significant discrepancy between values and past or present practices, the person may need referral for more intensive counseling.

Major developmental crises (e.g., puberty, **climacteric,** or menopause) should prompt education about effects on sexuality. Situational crises such as a life change with pregnancy, illness, extreme financial stress, placement of a spouse in a nursing home, or loss and grief affect sexuality. Effects may last for days, months, or years and can generate performance anxieties that lead to continued sexual dysfunction. If an individual is prepared for possible changes in sexual functioning, performance anxieties may be minimized.

Illness and surgery are situational stressors that often affect a person's sexuality. During periods of illness, individuals may experience major physical changes, the effects of drugs or treatments, the emotional stress of a prognosis, concern about future functioning, and separation from significant others. Situational stressors could include survival of a heart attack (myocardial infarction); cancer diagnosis and treatment; or chronic disease such as diabetes, multiple sclerosis, or Parkinson's disease. The nurse should not assume that sexual functioning is not a concern because of an individual's age or severity of prognosis. When concerns are assessed and identified, they can be addressed in the context of the individual's value system.

In response to identified concerns, the nurse may initiate discussion in pertinent areas. It may be appropriate to discuss sexual practices such as oral-genital sex or mutual masturbation as methods of expressing intimate affection when penile-vaginal intercourse is contraindicated. A partner experiencing joint pain may appreciate a discussion of various positions for intercourse. Use of fantasy or a sense of playfulness may add new romance or stimulation to a long-term relationship. A couple may need confirmation or assurance that the thoughts and acting out of nonharmful fantasy is normal and healthy.

Restorative Care.

In the home environment it is important to assist individuals in creating an environment that is comfortable for sexual activity. This may involve making recommendations for ways to arrange the bedroom to accommodate any limitations the individual may have. For example, wheelchair-bound individuals may prefer being able to move the chair close to the side of the bed at an angle that allows for more ease in touching and caressing. Suggestions regarding how to accommodate barriers such as Foley catheters or drainage tubes can contribute to sexual activity.

In the long-term care setting, facilities should make proper arrangements for privacy during residents' sexual experiences (Lueckenotte, 1996). The ideal situation is to set up a pleasant room that can be used for a variety of activities but may also be reserved for private visits with a spouse or partner. If this is not feasible, making arrangements for the roommate of a client to have another place to be can allow a couple time alone.

EVALUATION

Client Care.

The nurse will review client responses to interventions to determine if goals and outcome criteria have been met (Figure 27-4). Critical thinking ensures that the nurse applies what is known about sexuality and the client's unique situation.

Having follow-up discussions with the client or spouse will determine whether goals and outcomes have been achieved. Sexuality is felt more than observed, and sexual expression requires an intimacy that is not amenable to observation. Clients can be asked to relate risk factors, verbalize concerns, and share experiences and their level of satisfaction. The nurse can also observe behavioral cues, such as eye contact, posture, and extraneous hand movements, that indicate comfort or suggest continued anxiety or concern as topics are addressed. As outcomes are evaluated, the individual, spouse, and nurse may need to modify expectations or establish more appropriate time frames in which to achieve the target goals. All involved may need to be reminded of the individual nature of sexual expression and the multiple factors that affect perceptions and responses. Sexual wellness is not an absolute. An individual must define what is acceptable and satisfying. The partner's level of sexual satisfaction must also be considered. Sexual performance is seldom the exclusive focus of sexual satisfaction. Open communication and positive self-esteem are essential factors in effectively resolving concerns.

Client Expectations.

In evaluating the outcomes of interventions related to sexuality, the nurse must consult with the client. Resolution of sexual concerns must meet the client's perceptions of improvement. Sexuality is not an absolute. An individual must define what is acceptable and satisfying. In considering the status of sexual health, the client's partner's perceptions of sexual satisfaction are also significant.

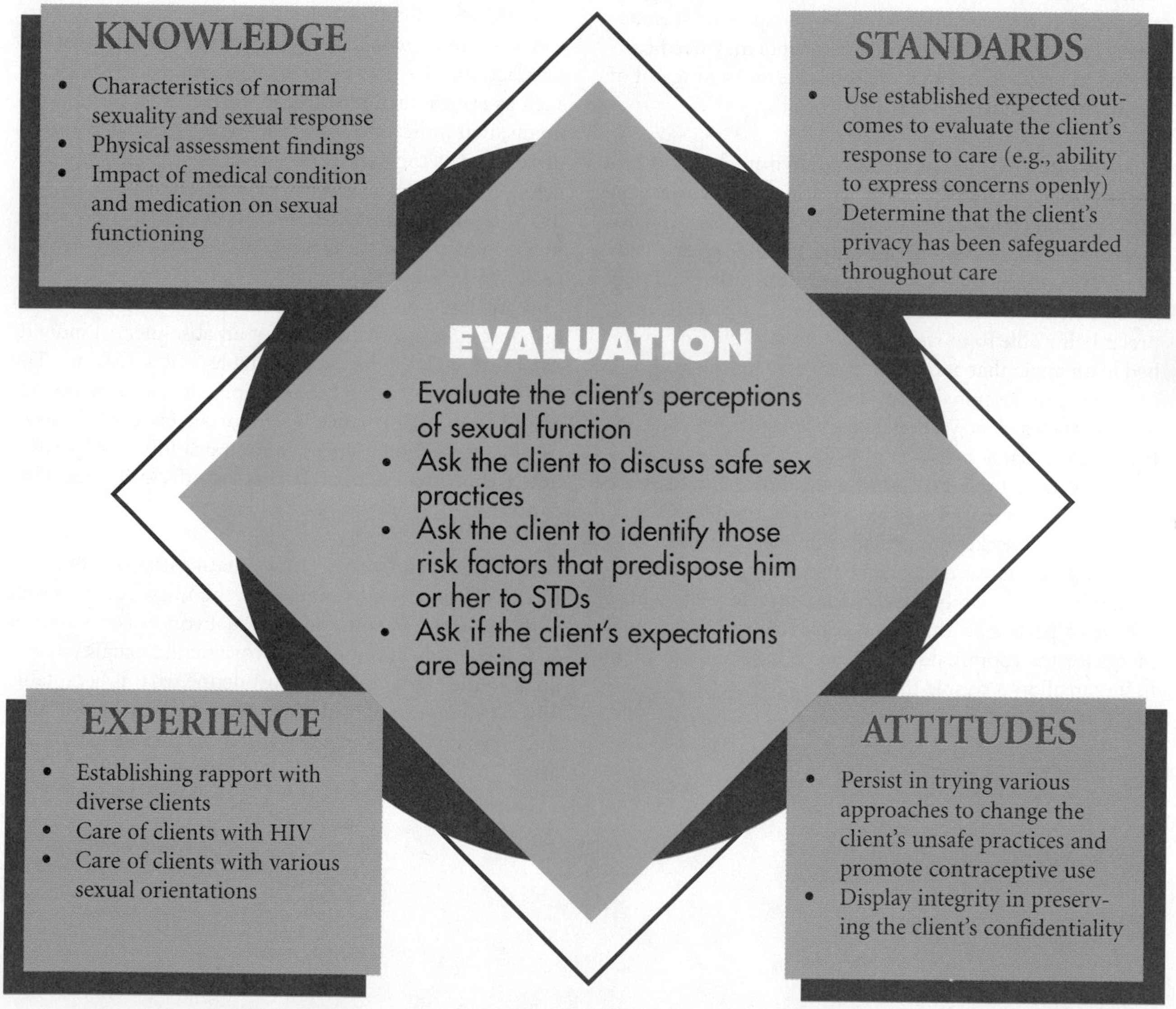

KNOWLEDGE

- Characteristics of normal sexuality and sexual response
- Physical assessment findings
- Impact of medical condition and medication on sexual functioning

STANDARDS

- Use established expected outcomes to evaluate the client's response to care (e.g., ability to express concerns openly)
- Determine that the client's privacy has been safeguarded throughout care

EVALUATION

- Evaluate the client's perceptions of sexual function
- Ask the client to discuss safe sex practices
- Ask the client to identify those risk factors that predispose him or her to STDs
- Ask if the client's expectations are being met

EXPERIENCE

- Establishing rapport with diverse clients
- Care of clients with HIV
- Care of clients with various sexual orientations

ATTITUDES

- Persist in trying various approaches to change the client's unsafe practices and promote contraceptive use
- Display integrity in preserving the client's confidentiality

Figure 27-4   *Synthesis Model for Sexuality Evaluation Phase.*

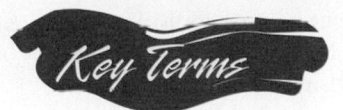

Key Concepts

- Sexuality is related to all dimensions of health; therefore sexual concerns or problems should be addressed as a part of nursing care.
- Sexuality is a part of each individual's identity and includes biological sex, gender identity, gender role, and sexual partner preference.
- Attitudes toward sexuality vary widely and are influenced by religious beliefs, society's values, the media, the family, and other factors.
- Nurses' attitudes toward sexuality also vary and may differ from those of clients; nurses should be sensitive to clients' sexual preferences and needs.
- The three-phase sexual response cycle is one way of understanding the physiological changes of sexual response during desire, arousal, and orgasm.
- Sexual development is a process beginning in infancy and involves some level of sexual behavior or growth in all developmental stages.
- The physiological sexual response changes with aging, but aging does not lead to diminished sexuality.
- Sexual health involves physical and psychosocial aspects and contributes to an individual's sense of self-worth and positive interpersonal relationships.
- Sexual dysfunctions can result from an easily identified etiology or varied and complex etiologies.
- Interventions for sexual dysfunctions depend on the condition and the client; interventions may include giving information, teaching specific exercises, improving communication between partners, and referral to a knowledgeable professional.
- Choice and use of effective contraceptive methods are affected by sexual biases, comfort with touching genitalia, desire for future fertility, financial status, ability to plan sexual contact, and ability to communicate with the sex partner regarding sensitive issues.
- A brief review of sexuality should be included in every nursing assessment of a client's level of wellness.
- Most nursing interventions to enhance a client's sexual health involve providing information and education.
- Evaluation is formulated based on discussion with the individual and possibly his or her partner regarding satisfaction with sexual functioning and through observations of nonverbal behaviors that suggest anxiety.

Key Terms

Climacteric, *p. 584*
Condom, *p. 570*
Contraception, *p. 567*
Diaphragm, *p. 570*
Dyspareunia, *p. 569*
Gay, *p. 570*
Gender identity, *p. 568*
Gender roles, *p. 567*
Heterosexual, *p. 569*
Homosexual, *p. 569*
Infertility, *p. 572*
Intercourse, *p. 567*
Lesbian, *p. 570*
Myotonia, *p. 569*

Perimenopausal, *p. 569*
Sexual dysfunction, *p. 572*
Sexual health, *p. 567*
Sexual orientation, *p. 567*
Sexual response cycle, *p. 567*
Sexuality, *p. 567*
Sexually transmitted diseases (STDs), *p. 567*
Sterilization, *p. 570*
Tubal ligation, *p. 571*
Vaginismus, *p. 575*
Vasectomy, *p. 571*
Vasocongestion, *p. 569*

Critical Thinking Exercises

1. Your current clinical experience is in a family practice office. You are conducting the initial interview with a 48-year-old man who started taking antihypertensives 2 weeks ago. You take his blood pressure and find it to be 136/74. You ask him how he has been doing since his last visit. He looks down at the floor and says, "Oh, OK I guess. Seems like I'm just getting old now." What kind of follow-up would be indicated based on this information?

2. You are assigned to care for a 15-year-old girl who was admitted after a motor vehicle accident. Yesterday she had an internal fixation of a fractured ankle. In gathering her nursing history, you explore sexuality and learn that she has just recently become sexually active with her boyfriend of 3 months. When you ask about safe sex and the use of birth control, she tells you that she knows she does not have to worry about STDs with him because he is just not one of those kinds of boys. In regard to birth control, she says that her boyfriend has reassured her that because he is pulling out before ejaculation, there is no risk of her becoming pregnant. How would you proceed, given this assessment data?

3. You are working on a rehabilitation unit and caring for a 67-year-old man who had a stroke 3 weeks ago. He shares a room with another man who is recovering from a stroke. He has been progressing in his self-care skills and is now able to get around with a cane, feed himself, and do most of his bath. His wife is in fairly good health, and the plan is for him to return home within the next 1 to 2 weeks. As you work with him one morning, he says to you, "You know, one of the

things that is hardest about being here is not being able to sleep in the same bed as Greta. I miss her so much. Even though she visits everyday, it is just not the same." How would you explore his comment, and what planning would you consider?

References

American Family Physician: Briefs, *Am Fam Physician* 59(8):2367, 1999.

Annon JS: The PLISSIT model: a proposed conceptual scheme for the behavioral treatment of sexual problems, *J Sex Educ Ther* (2):1, 1976.

Beckman LF, Harvey SM: Factors affecting the consistent use of barrier methods of contraception, *Obstet Gynecol* 88(10):65S, 1996.

Bohn D, Holz K: Sequelae of abuse: health effects of childhood sexual abuse, domestic battering, and rape, *J Nurse Midwifery* 41(6):442, 1996.

Boston Women's Health Collective: *Our bodies, ourselves for the new century: a book by and for women,* New York, 1998, The Collective.

Braden PS: Contraceptive choice and patient compliance, *J Nurse Midwifery* 43(6):471, 1998.

Centers for Disease Control and Prevention: Abortion surveillance: preliminary analysis—United States, 1996, *MMWR Morb Mortal Wkly Rep* 47(47), 1998a.

Centers for Disease Control and Prevention: 1998 guidelines for treatment of sexually transmitted diseases, 1998, *MMWR Morb Mortal Wkly Rep* 47(RR-1), 1998b.

Dickinson LM and others: Health-related quality of life and symptom profiles of female survivors of sexual abuse, *Arch Fam Med* 8(1):35, 1999.

Erikson EH: *Childhood and society,* ed 2, New York, 1963, WW Norton.

Finan SF: Promoting healthy sexuality: guidelines for the school-age child and adolescent, *Nurse Pract* 22(11):62, 1997a.

Finan SF: Promoting healthy sexuality: guidelines for the early through older adulthood, *Nurse Pract* 22(12):54, 1997b.

Guidry HM: Childhood sexual abuse: role of the family physician, *Am Fam Physician* 51(2):407, 1995.

Henshaw SK: Unintended pregnancy in the United States, *Fam Plann Perspect* 30(1):24, 1998.

Institute of Medicine: *The hidden epidemic: confronting sexually transmitted diseases,* Washington, DC, 1997, National Academy Press.

Johnson B: Older adults and sexuality: a multidimensional perspective, *J Gerontol Nurs* 22(2):6, 1996.

Johnson B: Older adults' suggestions for health care providers regarding discussions of sex, *Geriatr Nurs* 18(2):65, 1997.

Kang D, Kahler LR, Tesar CM: Cultural aspects of caring for refugees, *Am Fam Physician* 57(10):1254, 1998.

Kaplan J: *Disorders of sexual desire,* New York, 1979, Simon & Schuster.

Keller M and others: Adolescents' views of sexual decision-making, *Image J Nurs Sch* 28(2):125, 1996.

Kenney JW, Reinholtz CO, Angelini PO: Sexual abuse, sex before age 16, and high-risk behaviors of young females with sexually transmitted diseases, *J Obstet Gynecol Neonatal Nurs* 27(1):54, 1998.

Kinsey AC and others: *Sexual behavior in the human male,* Philadelphia, 1948, WB Saunders.

Kinsey AC and others: *Sexual behavior in the human female,* Philadelphia, 1953, WB Saunders.

Laumann EO and others: Sexual dysfunction in the United States: prevalence and predictors, *JAMA* 281(6):537, 1999.

Lueckenotte L: *Gerontologic nursing,* St. Louis, 1996, Mosby.

MacLaren A: Primary care for women: comprehensive sexual health assessment, *J Nurse Midwifery* 40(2):104, 1995.

Masters W, Johnson V, Kolodny R: *Human sexuality,* Boston, 1982, Little, Brown.

McCloskey JC, Bulechek GM: *Nursing interventions classification (NIC),* ed 3, St. Louis, 2000, Mosby.

Michael RT and others: *Sex in America: a definitive survey,* New York, 1994, Little, Brown.

Sell RL and others: The prevalence of homosexual behavior and attraction in the United States, the United Kingdom and France: results of national population-based samples, *Arch Sex Behav* 24(6):235, 1995.

Sipski M, Alexander C: *Sexual function in people with disability and chronic illness,* Gathersburg, Md, 1997, Aspen.

Youngkin E: Sexually transmitted diseases: current and emerging concerns, *J Obstet Gynecol Neonatal Nurs* 24(8):743, 1995.

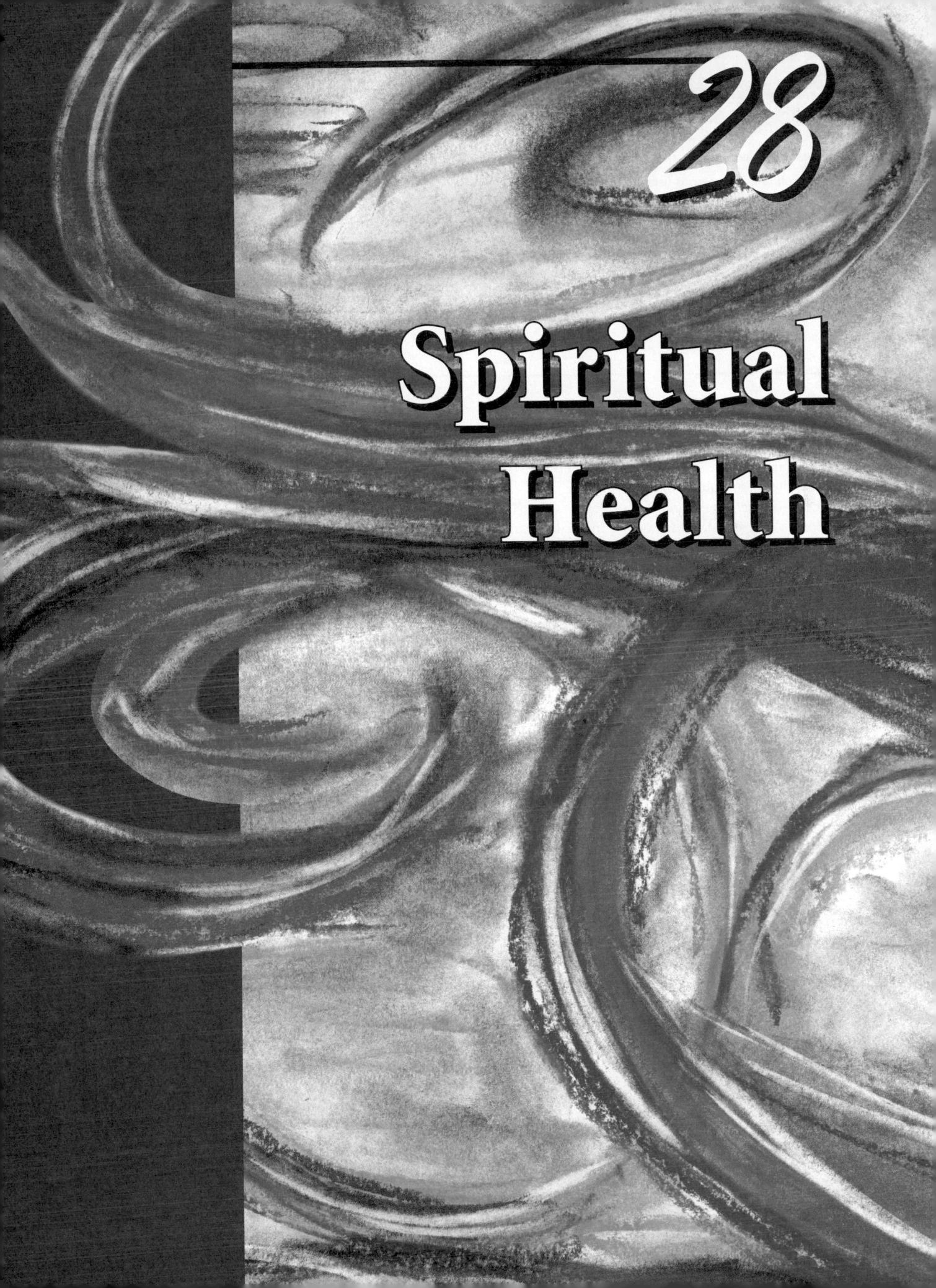

28

Spiritual Health

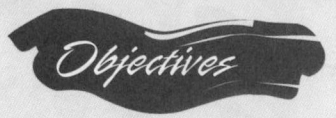

Mastery of content in this chapter will enable the student to:

- Define the key terms listed.
- Discuss the relationship of spirituality to an individual's total being.
- Explain why spiritual care is such a basic part of holistic nursing practice.
- Describe the relationship between faith, hope, and spiritual well-being.
- Compare and contrast the concepts of religion and spirituality.
- Perform an assessment of a client's spiritual well-being.
- Discuss nursing interventions designed to promote spiritual health.
- Evaluate attainment of spiritual health.

The word **spirituality** derives from the Latin word *spiritus,* which refers to breath or wind. The spirit gives life to, or animates, a person. It signifies whatever is at the center of all aspects of a person's life (Dombeck, 1995). A person's health depends on a balance of physical, psychological, sociological, cultural, developmental, and spiritual factors. Spirituality is often identified as the important factor that helps to achieve the balance needed to maintain health and well-being and to cope with illness. The **holistic** view of health is the focus and heart of nursing practice. Holism encourages nurses to constantly look for factors and relationships that affect health and illness.

Too often in nursing, clinicians tend not to emphasize the spiritual dimension of human nature (Calabria and Macrae, 1994), perhaps because it is not scientific enough or it is difficult to measure or quantify. Perhaps it is because there are individuals who do not believe in God or an ultimate being. Frequently spirituality becomes equated with religion and the privacy of an individual's religious orientation. But spirituality is a much broader and more unifying concept than religion. Recently, nurse researchers as well as pastoral care professionals, physicians, social workers, and others have proposed that spirituality has special importance as the integrating theme that unifies all aspects of an individual's health. Florence Nightingale described spirituality as the sense of a presence higher than human, the divine intelligence that creates, sustains, and organizes the universe, and an awareness of our inner connection with this higher reality (Calabria and Macrae, 1994). It is a force intrinsic to human nature and is one of the deepest and most potent resources for healing.

The human spirit is a powerful force that defines our existence, offers a source of hope, and helps to achieve inner harmony (O'Neill and Kenny, 1998). Expert nursing care involves helping clients utilize their spiritual resources as they identify and explore what is meaningful in their lives and as they find ways to cope with the impact of illness and the ongoing stressors of life. Appropriate spiritual care requires the nurse to demonstrate caring that then sets up the possibility of giving help and receiving help and thus establishing meaningful relationships with clients (Benner and Wrubel, 1989).

Scientific Knowledge Base

Recently health care research has begun to show the association between spirituality and health. There may be beneficial health outcomes when an individual is able to engage his or her beliefs in a higher power and sense a source of strength or support. Turner and Clancy (1986) studied clients with chronic low back pain and found that increased use of praying and hoping was related to decreased pain intensity. Prayer is frequently used as a method of coping and is effective in minimizing physical stressors. Remen (1988) suggests that healing is not a matter of mechanism but rather it is a work of spirit. Research has shown, for example, that meditation is successful in treating chronic pain, insomnia, anxiety, and depression (Culligan, 1996).

The relationship between spirituality and healing is not completely understood. However, it is the individual's intrinsic spirit that seems to be the factor in healing. When clients are given a placebo (sugar pill) instead of a prescribed medication, often they improve, not because of the sugar pill but because of their faith in the doctor who prescribed it. The placebo phenomenon shows that healing can take place because of believing.

Research is showing a link between spirit, mind, and body. An individual's beliefs and expectations can and do have effects on the person's physical well-being (Coe, 1997). Many of these effects may be tied to hormonal and neurological function. Prayer, relaxation training, and

The authors acknowledge the contribution of Veronica Peterson to this chapter in the previous edition of this text.

guided imagery, for example, have been shown to enhance immune function and delay disease progression (Kiecolt-Glaser and others, 1985; Bullock and da Cunha, 1992). A person's inner beliefs and convictions can become powerful resources for healing. A nurse will be more successful in helping clients achieve desirable health outcomes after learning to support clients and families spiritually as well as mentally and physically.

Nursing Knowledge Base

CONCEPTS IN SPIRITUAL HEALTH

To provide meaningful and supportive spiritual care, it is important for a nurse to understand the concepts that are at the foundation of spiritual health. The concepts of faith, hope, spiritual well-being, and religion give direction in understanding the views each individual has of life and its value.

Spirituality. Spirituality is a concept that is unique to each individual. Individual's definitions of their own spirituality are influenced by their culture, development, life experiences, beliefs, and ideas about life. An individual's spirituality enables the person to love, have faith and hope, seek meaning in life, and to nurture relationships with others. Spirituality offers a sense of connectedness intrapersonally (connected within oneself), interpersonally (connected with others and the environment), and transpersonally (connected with the unseen, God, or a higher power). Elements of spirituality that are frequently found in the literature include spiritual well-being, spiritual needs, and spiritual awareness. Hungelmann and others (1996) describe **spiritual well-being** as a sense of harmonious interconnectedness between self, others/nature, and an ultimate other that exists throughout and beyond time and space. There are two important characteristics of spirituality about which most authors agree: (1) it is a unifying theme in people's lives, and (2) it is a state of being.

There are individuals who either do not believe in the existence of God (**atheist**) or who believe that any ultimate reality is unkown or unknowable (**agnostic**). However, this does not mean that spirituality is not an important concept for the atheist or agnostic. Atheists search for meaning in life through their work and their relationships with other individuals (Burnard, 1988). Because atheists feel they are alone, they sense a strong responsibility for themselves. They also tend to believe in a joint responsibility for others. In acting for themselves, they feel they should also act for all of mankind (Burnard, 1988). In the case of agnostics, it is important for them to discover or find meaning in what they do or how they live. Burnard (1988) explains that since agnostics find no ultimate meaning for the way things are, they believe that we as people bring meaning to what we do.

Traditionally, nursing's holistic model of health has included the dimensions of physical, psychological, cultural, developmental, social, and spiritual health. One way of viewing the spiritual dimension is an integrated one (Figure 28-1). Each dimension relates to the other, while containing unique features or characteristics. An optional view that better demonstrates the significance of spirituality as an integrating theme in our lives is the unifying approach developed by Farran and others (1989) (Figure 28-2). In the model, spirituality represents the totality of one's being and serves as the overriding perspective that unifies the various aspects of the individual. Clark and

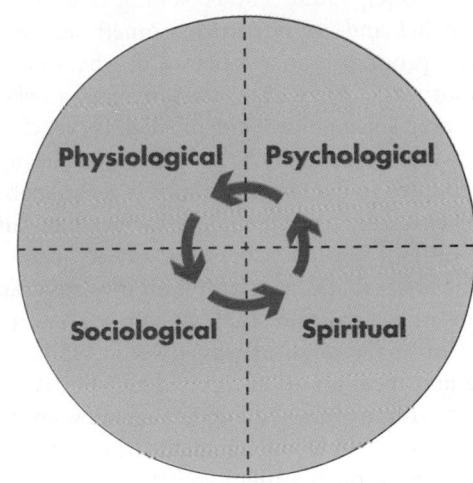

Figure 28-1 The spiritual dimension: an integrated approach.
Redrawn from Farran CJ and others: Development of a model for spiritual assessment and intervention, *J Religion Health* 28(3):185, 1989.

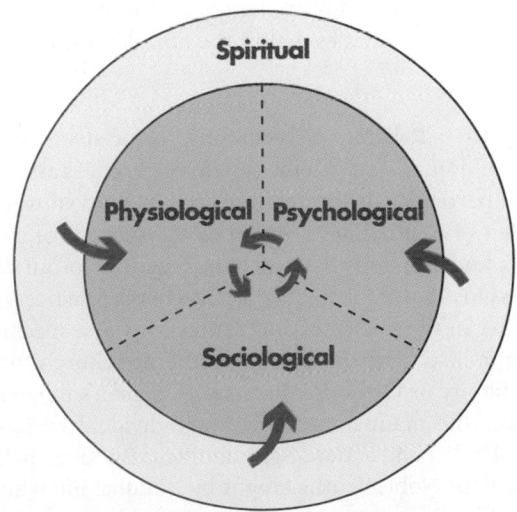

Figure 28-2 The spiritual dimension: the unifying approach.
Redrawn from Farran CJ and others: Development of a model for spiritual assessment and intervention, *J Religion Health* 28(3):185, 1989.

others (1991) stress how the spiritual dimension spreads throughout all other dimensions whether or not a person acknowledges or develops it.

Faith.

The concept of faith has two uses described in the literature. In the first, faith is defined as a cultural or institutional religion, such as Judaism, Buddhism, Islam, or Christianity. Faith as a religion is described in the next section. The second use deals with **faith** as a relationship with a divinity, higher power, authority, or spirit that incorporates a reasoning faith (belief) and a trusting faith (action) (Benner, 1985). The reasoning faith is an individual's belief and confidence in something for which there is no proof. It is an acceptance of what our reasoning cannot reach. Sometimes that involves a belief in a higher power, spirit guide, God, or Allah (Fryback, 1993). However, faith also might be in the manner in which a person chooses to live life. Faith in this sense enables action. For example, a person might believe that having a positive outlook on life is the best way to achieve life's goals. The belief that comes with faith involves **transcendence,** or an awareness of that which one cannot see or know in ordinary physical ways (Reed, 1987). It gives purpose and meaning to an individual's life. A trusting faith deals with the inner resources that allow an individual to act. For example, cancer clients who have faith in a positive outlook on life might pursue more knowledge about their disease and continue to pursue daily activities rather than resign themselves to the disease's symptoms. Hall (1998) studied clients diagnosed with human immunodeficiency virus (HIV) and found that after suffering, spirituality frames individuals' lives. Individuals become open to discover their unique spiritual meaning after a crisis that threatens health. Their faith becomes strengthened, and they are better able to go on with life and engage in activities that fit the new definition of their selves.

Religion.

Religion is commonly associated with the "state of doing," or a specific system of practices associated with a particular denomination, sect, or form of worship. Emblen (1992) defines religion as a system of organized beliefs and worship that a person practices to outwardly express his or her spirituality. Many clients practice a faith or belief in the doctrines and expressions of a specific religion or sect, such as the Lutheran church within Christianity or Orthodox Judaism. A person's religion influences the manner in which an individual exercises a faith of belief and action. For example, a Buddhist believes in the Four Noble Truths taught by Buddha: life is suffering, suffering is caused by desire, suffering can be eliminated by eliminating desire, and to eliminate desire, one must follow an eightfold path (Giger and Davidhizar, 1995). The path includes right understanding, purpose, speech, conduct, vocation, effort, thinking, and meditation. The Buddhist turns inward, holding faith in the im-

portance of self-control, versus the faith of Christians, who look to the teachings of God to provide enlightenment and direction in life.

Religion serves different purposes in people's lives. For some, religion is a set of rules and rituals used to worship a supreme being. For others, religion is a way of life providing nourishment and a connectedness to all of life. In this latter context, religion is more directly associated with spiritual well-being.

When providing spiritual care to clients it is important to understand the differences between religion and spirituality. Religious care is seen as helping clients maintain their faithfulness to their belief systems and worship practices. Spiritual care is seen as helping people maintain personal relationships and a relationship to a higher being or life force, to identify meaning and purpose in life, and to hopefully look beyond the present (Alridge, 1993).

Hope.

Spirituality is frequently identified as a key element in hope. When a person has the attitude of something to live for and look forward to, hope is present. Miller and Powers (1988) describe **hope** as a multidimensional concept consisting of anticipation of a continued good, an improvement, or the lessening of something unpleasant. Hope is energizing, giving individuals a motivation to achieve and the resources to use toward that achievement. Nowotny (1989) notes that hope can be found in all aspects of life as a force that helps individuals cope with any life stressors (Box 28-1). Hope is an invaluable personal resource whenever someone is faced with a loss (Chapter 29) or a challenge that seems difficult to achieve. Hope has purpose and direction and gives reason for being (Post-White and others, 1996).

In studies with cancer clients, having hope has been found to help individuals find meaning in their illness

---

The Concept of Hope   Box 28-1

Hope is future oriented. An individual imagines what is not yet seen.

Hope usually includes active involvement by the individual. Involvement might include goal setting, caring, planning, or praying.

Hope comes from within a person (though its locus or center might be outside the person, as in God or "medicine") and is related to trust.

That which is hoped for is seen by the person as truly possible. Hope is more than a desire or wish.

Hope relates to or involves other people or a higher being. This can involve thoughts, feelings, and actions that involve others.

The outcome of hope is important to the individual. The expectation is often a future outcome that has meaning to the individual.

Modified from Nowotny ML: Assessment of hope in patients with cancer: development of an instrument, *Oncol Nurs Forum* 16(1):57, 1989.

(O'Connor and others, 1990; Fryback, 1993). When clients with cancer face uncomfortable symptoms, increasing disability, or the fear of death, hope enables them to face the discomforts of their disease and continue to value living as fully as possible. There is a difference between ultimate hope (e.g., hope for an afterlife) and intermediate hope (e.g., hope to accomplish some task or achievement in life). However, in either form, hope often offers new meaning to life, especially when a person conquers a disease or disability.

Spiritual Health. Spiritual health is achieved when people find a balance between their life values, goals, and belief systems and their relationship within themselves and with others. Throughout life an individual may grow more spiritual, becoming increasingly aware of the meaning, purpose, and values of life. For example, some people with acquired immunodeficiency syndrome (AIDS) have experienced beneficial, even life-transforming, outcomes as a result of meeting their spiritual needs (O'Neill and Kenny, 1998). Growth, mastery, and empowerment are positive outcomes that can occur when spiritual resources have been utilized. In times of stress, illness, recovery, or loss, a person may turn to previous ways of responding or adjusting to a situation. Often these coping styles lie within the person's spiritual beliefs.

Spirituality begins as children learn about themselves and their relationships with others. Many adults experience spiritual growth by entering into lifelong relationships. An ability to care meaningfully for others and the self is evidence of a healthy spirituality. Older adults often turn to important relationships and the giving of themselves to others as spiritual tasks.

Establishing a connection with a supreme being, beings, or an important meaning or value is one way a person develops spiritually. Followers of Confucianism develop a spirituality through their commitment to a code of ethics that emphasizes a hierarchy of society, worship of ancestors, and respect for age and custom (Giger and Davidhizar, 1995). In the Judeo-Christian context children often begin with a concept of a supreme being as presented to them by their home or religious community. Adolescents often reconsider their childlike concept of a spiritual power, and in the search for an identity, they may either question practices and values or find the spiritual power as the motivation to seek a clearer meaning to life.

As people mature they often turn inward to enduring values and to a concept of a supreme being or a higher meaning that has been sustaining and meaningful. A healthy spirituality in older people is one that gives peace and acceptance of the self and that is often based on a lifelong relationship with a supreme being. Illness and loss can threaten and challenge the spiritual developmental process. It thus becomes important for the nurse to understand the nature and status of a client's belief system and spiritual health.

SPIRITUAL PROBLEMS

When illness, loss, grief, or a major life change affects a person, spiritual resources either help a person move to recovery or spiritual needs and concerns develop. **Spiritual distress** is the disruption of an individual's "life principle," which fills the person's entire being and transcends or exceeds one's biological and psychosocial nature (Kim and others, 1997). A catastrophic illness, for example, can upset a person's spiritual well-being sufficiently to cause doubt and loss of faith. Spiritual distress may cause the person to feel alone or even abandoned by resources that at one time were very nurturing. Individuals may question their spiritual values, raising questions about their whole way of life, purpose for living, and source of meaning. Spiritual distress also occurs when there is conflict between a person's beliefs and prescribed health regimens or the inability to practice usual rituals.

Acute Illness. Sudden, unexpected illness that poses both an immediate and a long-term threat to a client's life, health, and/or well-being can create significant spiritual distress. For example, both the 50-year-old man who has a heart attack and the 20-year-old who is a victim of a motor vehicle accident face crises that may threaten their spiritual health. The illness or injury creates an unanticipated scramble to integrate and cope with new realities (e.g., disability). People look for ways to remain faithful to their beliefs and value systems. They may pray, attend religious services more often, or spend time reflecting on the positive aspects of their lives. Often conflicts can develop around a person's beliefs and the meaning of life. Anger is not uncommon, and clients may express it against God, their families, themselves, or the nurse. The strength of a client's spirituality influences how he or she copes with sudden illness and how quickly he or she can move to recovery. Yim and Vande Creek (1996) have developed a spiritual healing critical pathway for coronary artery bypass clients. Their research has shown that knowledge of a person's spiritual well-being can be used to maximize a client's recovery. Hope and the ability to speak about life values help the individual gain meaning from illness and influence the ability to recover from heart surgery. The pathway identifies where clients are in their spiritual recovery and recommends appropriate interventions that help clients find purpose and worth to move forward and recover.

Chronic Illness. Persons with chronic illness often suffer debilitating symptoms that change the ability to continue their lifestyles. A symptom is more than just a signal for a persistent health problem or a road map for diagnosing a disease. A symptom can give a person permission to take needed rest, be an ominous sign of impending disruption, or even raise feelings about the person's self-worth and strength (Benner and Wrubel, 1989). Symptoms are experienced as meaningful to the individual, and that meaning is shaped by the person's history and the current context of the illness.

With chronic illness independence can be threatened, causing fear, anxiety, and an overall dispiritedness. Dependence on others for routine self-care measures can create a feeling of powerlessness. A person may feel a loss of a sense of purpose in life that affects the inner strength needed to deal with alterations in functioning. A person's spirituality can be a significant factor in how he or she adapts to the changes resulting from chronic illness. Successful adaptation can strengthen a person spiritually. A reevaluation of life may occur. Those who are able to engage and use their spiritual resources will have a much better chance to reestablish a self-identity and live to their potential.

Terminal Illness.   Terminal illness commonly causes fears of physical pain, isolation, the unknown, dying, and

the threat to integrity (Turner and others, 1995). However, when people experience periods of disease remission, they may become asymptomatic for long periods of time and put off the idea of illness and any terminal outcome. Terminal illness creates an uncertainty about what death means and thus can make clients susceptible to spiritual distress. There are also clients who have a spiritual sense of peace that enables them to face death without fear (Box 28-2).

Individuals experiencing a terminal illness will often find themselves reviewing their life and questioning its meaning. Common questions asked might include "Why is this happening to me?" or "What have I done?" Family and friends can be affected just as much as the client. Terminal illness causes members of the family to ask important questions about its meaning and how it will affect their relationship with the client (see Chapter 29).

Fryback (1993) conducted a study to learn how people with a terminal illness describe health. Clients in the study identified the following three domains of health: mental-emotional, spiritual, and physical (Figure 28-3). The spiritual domain was seen as being essential for health and included having a relationship with a higher power, recognizing mortality, and striving for self-actualization. Although many of the participants in the study either attended church or stated a desire to do so, others found that spirituality was not dependent on a religion or church. They associated health with belief in a higher power that

Research HIGHLIGHT   Box 28-2

RESEARCH ABSTRACT
A study was conducted involving 10 men and women in advanced-stage HIV disease who self-identified as having spiritual or religious experiences that had helped them cope with HIV disease. The researcher conducted unstructured interviews to understand how spiritual meaning is structured in advanced stages of the disease. Subjects' spirituality was expressed by referring to God or a higher power as it pertained to their personal faith. People with HIV learn to live and experience life in a context created by the disease itself and in a culture that judges and labels them. Their struggle creates a sense of victimization manifested in feelings of helplessness, depression, and hopelessness. However, positive personal meanings emerge, not only from this rejection but also from the knowledge that they have a terminal illness that will perhaps limit their time to live. Three major themes developed from the study: purpose in life emerges from stigmatization; opportunities for meaning arise from a disease without a cure; and after suffering, spirituality frames the subject's life. These individuals discovered a unique spiritual meaning after a crisis that threatened their health. Living with HIV required clearing one's life of the stressful existence, problematic relationships, and memberships that did not work. Spirituality helped them find peace in themselves and their death.

IMPLICATIONS FOR PRACTICE
• Professional caregivers need to recognize that fear associated with HIV can inform and promote spiritual growth in clients. Questions such as "For what purpose is this happening to me now?" and "What does God want me to do with this?" help clients find meaning in suffering. Caregivers must support clients in being able to express these concerns.

REFERENCE
Hall BA: Patterns of spirituality in persons with advanced HIV disease, *Res Nurs Health* 21:143, 1998.

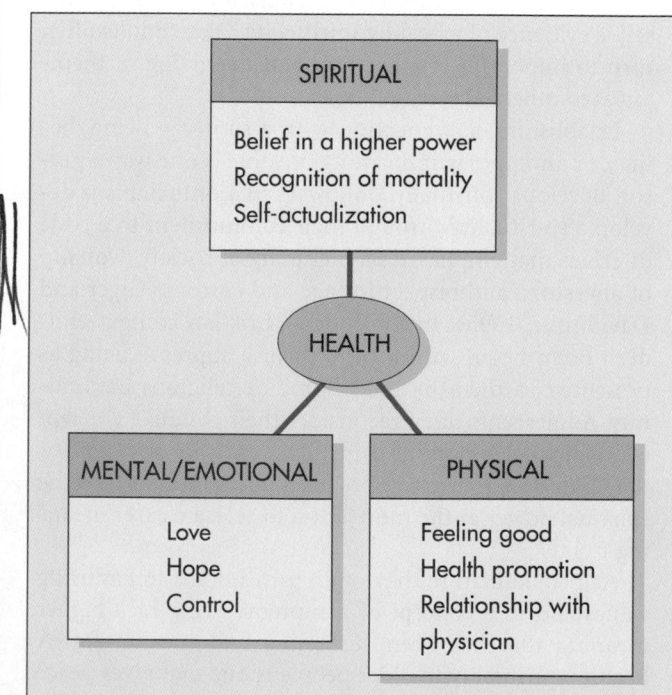

Figure 28-3 Domains of health based on perceptions of terminally ill clients.
Modified from Fryback PB: Health for people with a terminal diagnosis, *Nurs Sci Q* 6(3):147, 1993.

gave them faith and the ability to love (Fryback, 1993). The study revealed that when terminally ill clients have a perception of being unhealthy, it is not due to the disease but to being unable to live their lives fully and do the things they desire.

Near-Death Experience. Nurses may encounter clients who have had a near-death experience (NDE). An NDE has been identified as a psychological phenomenon of people who either have been close to clinical death or may have recovered after being declared dead. It is not associated with a mental disorder (Basford, 1990). Persons who experience an NDE after cardiopulmonary arrest, for example, often tell the same story of feeling themselves rising above their bodies and watching caregivers initiate lifesaving measures. Most individuals describe passing through a tunnel to a bright light, encountering people who had preceded them in death, and feeling an inner tranquillity and peace. Instead of moving toward the light, they learn it is not time for them to die and they return to life.

Clients who have had an NDE are often reluctant to discuss it, thinking family or caregivers will not understand. Isolation and depression can occur. However, individuals experiencing an NDE who can discuss it with family or caregivers find openness to the power of the experience as it is reported. They consistently report positive aftereffects, including a positive attitude and spiritual development (Turner and others, 1995). After a client has survived cardiopulmonary arrest it is important for the nurse to remain open and give the client a chance to explore what happened.

Religious Problems

Clients' religious problems can affect their spirituality. Customary religious practices, if interrupted or changed, may affect the structure or support that religion contributes to the person's sense of well-being.

Change in Denominational Membership or Religious Conversion. Marrying a person with a different religious background or moving to a new community that does not have a branch of a particular religious group, will create, at least initially, loss for an individual. Of course, it can also open up new options. If a loss is felt, the individual experiences separation from a previously valued religious community (Turner and others, 1995). Not only is there a threat of losing the routine rituals one depends on to express one's faith, but there is separation from friends and acquaintances. The extent of the loss is influenced by the choice the individual had in the change, how flexible the person's religious expression is, and what communities of faith are available to the individual.

Loss or Questioning of Faith. Faith is a way of relating to self, community, and a higher power. A person often finds a way to express his or her faith through religious practices. Faith develops over time, along with a person's spiritual growth. Persons who are at an early stage of development of their faith or who find their faith challenged by an event such as acute or chronic illness, terminal disease, or loss of a loved one may become vulnerable to loss of or doubt about their faith (Turner and others, 1995). This can also occur when one is shunned by one's religious community (e.g., a Jehovah's Witness who elects to have surgery requiring a blood transfusion or a traditionally religious person being diagnosed with HIV) or when one seriously questions the position one's religious denomination takes on a public issue (e.g., abortion or euthanasia). A loss or questioning of faith can cause serious guilt and a sense of loneliness even when it can lead to a more mature faith and stronger convictions.

Critical Thinking Synthesis

Dr. Patricia Benner (1984) describes the helping role as an important domain for nursing practice. Clients look to nurses for a different kind of help than that sought from other professionals. Expert nurses acquire the unique ability to know the personal issues affecting clients' willingness to receive and seek help. Expert nurses embrace a holistic philosophy and caring that enables them to offer a level of comfort and support that is often intuitive.

Clinical intuition is a process whereby the nurse knows something about a client that cannot be verbalized, is verbalized with difficulty, or for which a source of knowledge is not known (Young, 1987). Intuition is an aspect of critical thinking. Rew (1989) describes a relationship between spirituality and intuition. Nurses' intuitive experiences happen when they feel especially close to a client or a client's family. Intuition comes from a sense of relatedness to the client. It is a sense of empathy from within. The ability of a nurse to use intuition is vital to expert care.

In a beginning nurse, intuition has not yet evolved to the point where the student can analyze and sense cues that reflect clients' spiritual needs. However, the student can begin to apply critical thinking skills that will prepare the nurse to deliver spiritual care. Critical thinking in this case begins with the knowledge, experience, and critical thinking attitudes and standards that can be applied during client assessment (Figure 28-4). All of these elements work together to enable the nurse to think critically about client situations and needs. Previous experiences in which the nurse has cared for clients who have expressed their spiritual convictions and beliefs and then used them in coping with illness can be very useful. Often this type of experience helps the nurse learn how to relate to the client in a meaningful way. A spiritual assessment is most successful when the nurse applies knowledge that pertains to therapeutic communication, principles of loss and grief, and knowledge of caring practices. This information helps to guide the nurse's approach and selection of assessment

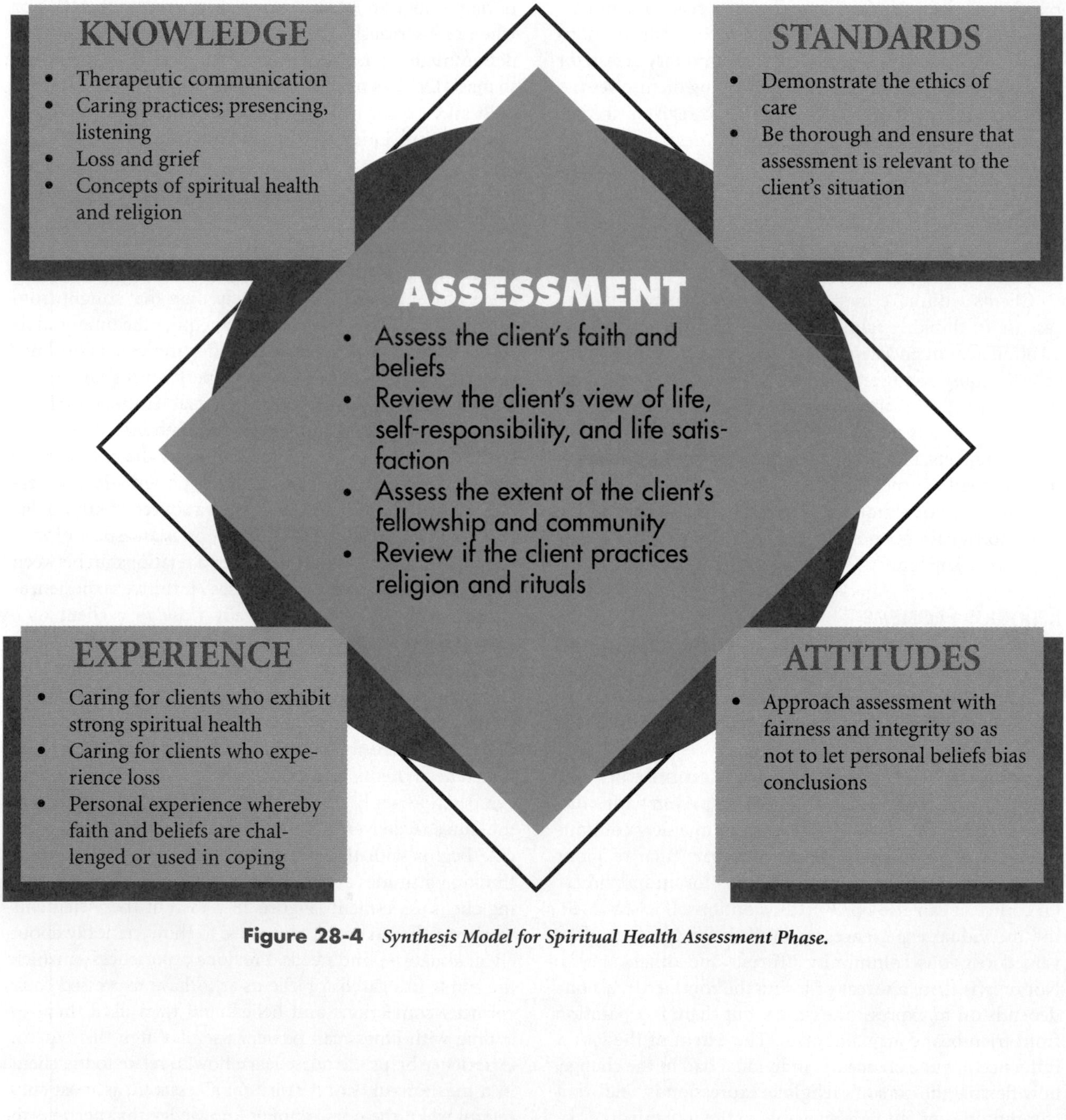

KNOWLEDGE

- Therapeutic communication
- Caring practices; presencing, listening
- Loss and grief
- Concepts of spiritual health and religion

STANDARDS

- Demonstrate the ethics of care
- Be thorough and ensure that assessment is relevant to the client's situation

ASSESSMENT

- Assess the client's faith and beliefs
- Review the client's view of life, self-responsibility, and life satisfaction
- Assess the extent of the client's fellowship and community
- Review if the client practices religion and rituals

EXPERIENCE

- Caring for clients who exhibit strong spiritual health
- Caring for clients who experience loss
- Personal experience whereby faith and beliefs are challenged or used in coping

ATTITUDES

- Approach assessment with fairness and integrity so as not to let personal beliefs bias conclusions

Figure 28-4   *Synthesis Model for Spiritual Health Assessment Phase.*

questions. For example, if the nurse knows that a client has just lost a spouse, knowledge of how clients respond to grief and the use of good listening techniques can be applied in attempting to learn about the client's spiritual resources. The nurse's knowledge base coupled with what he or she knows about spirituality allows the nurse to build a relationship that establishes trust and a respect for the client's views. To provide spiritual care, the nurse must act by applying attitudes of fairness and integrity so that personal beliefs do not bias the nurse's diagnostic conclusions. Finally, an ethic of caring (see Chapter 6) provides the nurse with a framework for decision making. A client's spiritual beliefs may place the client on an unequal footing with professionals because of the influence those beliefs have on the client's choice of therapy. An ethic of care places the nurse as the client's advocate, solving ethical dilemmas by attending to relationships and honoring the client's personal choices.

Nursing Process

At the core of nursing is the commitment to caring. Care for others is an individualized, interactive process by which individuals help each other grow and become actualized (Clark and others, 1991). An element of quality health care is to exhibit caring for the client so that a relationship of trust forms. Trust is strengthened when the caregiver acknowledges and supports the client's spiritual well-being.

Application of the nursing process from the perspective of a client's spiritual needs is not simple. It goes beyond assessing a client's religious practices and rituals. Understanding a client's spirituality and then appropriately identifying the level of support and resources needed requires a new, broader perspective. Heliker (1992) describes the importance of shared community and compassion. *Compassion* comes from the Latin words *pati* and *cum,* meaning "to suffer with." *Community* is derived from the Latin word meaning "fellowship." To be compassionate is to "enter into places of pain, to share in brokenness with other human beings" (Heliker, 1992). To practice compassion as a nurse requires awareness of the very human tie between clients and a healing community.

The nurse must remove from the assessment and care plan any personal biases or misconceptions. Typically one of the questions usually asked on a client's admission form is the client's "religion." Such a question leaves little doubt that the accepted position is that of a "believer" (Burnard, 1988). It is important for nurses to sort out value judgments about other people's belief systems. Working through values clarification exercises can be helpful (see Chapter 20). If the nurse is a believer, does he or she judge harshly the unbeliever? If the nurse is an agnostic or atheist, does he or she dismiss the believer? As nurses, it becomes important to accept and acknowledge others' beliefs and not spend work time trying to convert others to our personal beliefs.

The nurse must be willing to share and discover another person's meaning and purpose in life, sickness, and health. A nurse learns to look beyond a personal view when establishing a client relationship. This means identifying the common values that make us human and respecting the commitments and values that make humans unique. Love, trust, hope, forgiveness, meaning, and community are spiritual needs we all have (Carson, 1989). Learning to share these needs helps the nurse find a way to give clients spiritual care and support.

Another important aspect of spiritual care is recognizing that a client does not have to have a spiritual problem. Clients bring certain spiritual resources that the nurse can engage as resources to help them assume healthier lives, recover from illness, or face impending death. Supporting and recognizing the positive side of a client's spiritually will go a long way toward delivering effective, individualized nursing care.

ASSESSMENT

A nurse's ability to gain a reliable picture of a client's spiritual dimension may be limited by the setting in which the nurse practices. This is especially true if nurses have limited contact with clients, where it is difficult to build therapeutic relationships with them. But once a trusting relationship with a client is established, the nurse and client reach a point of learning together, and spiritual caring can occur. The nurse learns to consciously integrate an attitude of spiritual care into the nursing process. The assessment should focus on aspects of spirituality most likely to be influenced by life experiences, events, and questions in the case of illness and hospitalization. Even conducting an assessment can be therapeutic because it conveys a level of caring and support. The nurse who understands the overall approach to spiritual assessment can enter into thoughtful discussions with the client and gain a greater awareness of the personal resources an individual brings to a situation. These resources ought to be incorporated into an effective plan of care.

A Spiritual Well-Being Screening Tool. The JAREL spiritual well-being scale (Figure 28-5) was developed to provide nurses and other health care professionals with a simple tool for assessing a client's spiritual well-being (Hungelmann and others, 1996). The tool was developed for clients from Christian, non-Christian, and atheist belief systems. Items on the tool comprise three key dimensions: faith/belief, life/self-responsibility, and life-satisfaction/self-actualization. The tool is simple to use, requiring clients to rate their level of agreement with each item on a five-point scale (strongly agree to strongly disagree). For clients with visual or literacy problems, the nurse can read the items and record the client's response. If the client's score on any item, group of items, or particular dimension is low, it may indicate an area to explore further (Hungelmann and others, 1996).

DIRECTIONS: PLEASE CIRCLE THE CHOICE THAT **BEST** DESCRIBES HOW MUCH YOU AGREE WITH EACH STATEMENT. CIRCLE ONLY **ONE** ANSWER FOR EACH STATEMENT. THERE IS NO RIGHT OR WRONG ANSWER.

		Strongly Agree	Moderately Agree	Agree	Disagree	Moderately Disagree	Strongly Disagree
1.	Prayer is an important part of my life.	SA	MA	A	D	MD	SD
2.	I believe I have spiritual well-being.	SA	MA	A	D	MD	SD
3.	As I grow older, I find myself more tolerant of others' beliefs.	SA	MA	A	D	MD	SD
4.	I find meaning and purpose in my life.	SA	MA	A	D	MD	SD
5.	I feel there is a close relationship between my spiritual beliefs and what I do.	SA	MA	A	D	MD	SD
6.	I believe in an afterlife.	SA	MA	A	D	MD	SD
7.	When I am sick I have less spiritual well-being.	SA	MA	A	D	MD	SD
8.	I believe in a supreme power.	SA	MA	A	D	MD	SD
9.	I am able to receive and give love to others.	SA	MA	A	D	MD	SD
10.	I am satisfied with my life.	SA	MA	A	D	MD	SD
11.	I set goals for myself.	SA	MA	A	D	MD	SD
12.	God has little meaning in my life.	SA	MA	A	D	MD	SD
13.	I am satisfied with the way I am using my abilities.	SA	MA	A	D	MD	SD
14.	Prayer does not help me in making decisions.	SA	MA	A	D	MD	SD
15.	I am able to appreciate differences in others.	SA	MA	A	D	MD	SD
16.	I am pretty well put together.	SA	MA	A	D	MD	SD
17.	I prefer that others make decisions for me.	SA	MA	A	D	MD	SD
18.	I find it hard to forgive others.	SA	MA	A	D	MD	SD
19.	I accept my life situations.	SA	MA	A	D	MD	SD
20.	Belief in a supreme being has no part in my life.	SA	MA	A	D	MD	SD
21.	I cannot accept change in my life.	SA	MA	A	D	MD	SD

Figure 28-5   JAREL spiritual well-being scale.
Copyright 1987 by J Hungelmann, E Kenkel-Rossi, L Klassen, R Stollenwerk, Marquette University College of Nursing, Milwaukee, Wisc.

The tool helps the nurse to explore with a client any perceptions or concerns he or she might have. For example, if a client disagrees about accepting life situations, the nurse will need to spend time understanding how an illness is being accepted and managed by the client. Whether a nurse uses a tool like the JAREL scale or directs an assessment with questions that are based on principles of spirituality, it is important to not impose personal value systems on the client. This is particularly true when the client's values and beliefs are similar to those of the nurse, as it can then become very easy to make false assumptions.

Faith/Belief. Each individual has some source of authority and guidance in his or her life. It is that inner voice or outer authority that leads persons to choose and act on their beliefs. The authority can be a supreme being, a code of conduct, a specific religious leader, family or friends, oneself, or a combination of sources. Faith in an authority provides a sense of confidence that guides a person in exercising beliefs and experiencing growth. Knowing a client's source of strength and faith can direct interaction with him or her. The nurse can assess a person's faith in an authority by asking, "To what or whom do you look as a source of strength or faith in life?" or "What is your personal source of strength or hope?"

The nurse must determine if the client has a religious source of guidance that conflicts with medical treatment plans. This can seriously affect the options nurses and other health care providers can offer clients. For example, if a client looks to the Jehovah's Witnesses as a source of authority, blood products cannot be accepted as a form of treatment. Christian Scientists often refuse any medical intervention because they believe that their faith will heal them.

It is also important to understand a client's philosophy of life. Asking the client, "Tell me what is most important in your life" or "Tell me what gives your life meaning," may help to assess what is the basis of the client's belief system regarding meaning and purpose in life. This information reveals the client's spiritual focus and may help to reflect the impact illness, loss, or disability has on the person's life. Depending on a client's religious practices, views about health and the response to illness may influence how nurses provide support (Table 28-1).

| Table 28-1   **Religious Beliefs About Health** | | |
Religious/Cultural Group	Health Care Beliefs	Response to Illness
Hinduism	Accepts modern medical science.	Illness is caused by past sins. Prolonging life is discouraged.
Sikhism	Accepts modern medical science.	Females to be examined by females. Removing the undergarment will cause great distress.
Buddhism	Accepts modern medical science.	May refuse treatment on Holy Days. Nonhuman spirits invading the body cause illness. May want a Buddhist priest. May permit withdrawal of life support. Does not practice euthanasia.
Islam	Must be able to practice the Five Pillars of Islam (see p. 600). May have a fatalistic view of health.	Uses faith healing. Family members are a comfort. Group prayer is strengthening. May permit withdrawal of life support. Does not practice euthanasia.
Judaism	Believes in the sanctity of life. God and medicine must have a balance. Observance of the Sabbath is important. May refuse treatments on the Sabbath.	Visiting the sick is an obligation. They are obligated to seek care. Euthanasia is forbidden. Life supports are discouraged.
Christianity	Accepts modern medical science.	Uses prayer, faith healing. Appreciates visits from clergy. Some will use laying on of hands. Holy communion is commonly used.
Navajos	Concepts of health have a fundamental place in their concept of humans and their place in the universe.	Blessingway is a practice that attempts to remove ill health by means of stories, songs, rituals, prayers, symbols, and sand paintings (Sobralske, 1985).
Appalachians	External locus of control. Life and health are controlled by nature. Accept folk healers. Good Christian members of community are called as servants to minister to disabled (Giger and Davidhizar, 1995).	Dislike hospitals. Tend to be noncompliant in following medical regimens but expect to be helped directly when seeking episodic treatment.

Life and Self-Responsibility.   Hungelmann and others (1996) found that spiritual well-being includes life and self-responsibility. Individuals who can accept change in life, make decisions regarding their life, and are able to forgive others in times of difficulty had a higher level of spiritual well-being. During times of illness clients often are unable to accept limitations or know what to do to regain a functional and meaningful life. Often they display anger toward those whom they feel were associated with their problems. Their sense of helplessness may reflect a diminished spiritual well-being. However, if clients are able to adapt to changes readily and seek solutions for how to deal with any limitations, spiritual well-being may be providing an important coping resource. The nurse assesses to what extent a client understands any limitations or threats posed by an illness and the manner in which the client has chosen to adjust to them. In addition, questions to ask might include "Tell me how you feel about the changes caused by this illness" and "How do these changes affect what you now need to do?"

Life Satisfaction.   Spiritual well-being seems to be tied to a person's satisfaction with life and what he or she has accomplished (Hungelmann and others, 1996). When individuals are satisfied with life and the manner in which they are using their abilities, more energy is available to deal with new difficulties and to resolve problems. A sense of satisfaction with life and oneself gives an individual resources to live for the moment, face difficulties directly, and remain motivated to deal with adversities. Satisfaction with someone or something has been found by Haase and others (1992) to be associated with acceptance. Acceptance is the process of resolving issues within oneself or dealing with life experiences and is closely tied to hope and spirituality. A nurse can assess a client's life satisfaction by asking, "How happy are you with your life?" or

"Tell me to what extent you feel satisfied with what you have accomplished in life."

Fellowship and Community.   Fellowship is one kind of relationship an individual can have with other persons (Farran and others, 1989), including immediate family, close friends, associates at work or school, fellow members of a church, and neighbors. More specifically, this includes the extent of the community of shared faith between clients and their support networks. The nurse can ask, "With whom do you find the greatest source of support in times of difficulty?" When a client knows that others of similar faith care, they can become a source for hope.

The nurse's holistic assessment explores the extent and nature or quality of a person's support networks and their relationship with the client. It is unwise to assume that a given network offers the kind of support a client desires. For example, calling the client's clergy to request a visit might be inappropriate if the client finds little support or fellowship from the individual. Does the client have one significant fellowship or several? What is the level of support received from the community? How does the community express feelings of concern? Do they visit, say prayers, or support the client's immediate family? The nurse needs to learn whether openness exists between the client and those persons with whom a fellowship has formed.

Ritual and Practice.   One of the easiest areas to assess about a client's spirituality is the use of rituals and practice. Rituals include participation in a religious group or private worship, prayer, sacraments such as baptism or communion, fasting, singing, icons, meditating, scripture reading, and making offerings or sacrifices. Different religions have established various rituals for certain life events (Table 28-2). The nurse assesses whether a client's usual rituals or practices have been interrupted as a result of illness or hospitalization. A ritual can provide the client with structure and support during difficult times. Often clients may request the ability to practice rituals during hospitalization. For example, Muslims practice the Five Pillars of Islam with the second pillar requiring a person to pray 5 times a day, facing east (toward Mecca, the holy city of Islam).

Table 28-2 **Religious Practices Related to Birth and Death**		
Religion	Birth Rituals	Death Rituals
Hinduism	No special rituals.	The dying may want to lie on the floor. A priest will tie a thread around the neck or wrist *(do not remove)*. A priest will pour water in the client's mouth. Family will wash the body before cremation.
Sikhism	Allow mother and child to remain together.	The deceased will need the five Ks: *Kesh,* uncut hair; *Kangra,* wooden comb; *Kara,* wrist band; *Kirpan,* sword; *Kach,* shorts.
Buddhism	No special rituals. Baptism later in childhood.	A priest should be called. Last rites and chanting at bedside. Burial or cremation is acceptable.
Shinto	No special rituals.	All jewelry should be removed, and the body is washed and dressed in a white kimono and straw shoes.
Islam	A prayer is said into the infant's ear.	The dying must confess their sins. The body is washed and wrapped in white cloth. The head is turned toward right shoulder. The body faces east, toward Mecca. A prayer called *Kalima* is said.
Judaism	Circumcision on day 8 for Orthodox and Conservative Jews.	Body is washed by burial society, and someone needs to remain with the body for Orthodox and Conservative Jews.
Christianity	Rituals vary. Many will baptize.	Rituals vary greatly among groups. Many give last rites or communion. Prefers burial to cremation.
Church of Jesus Christ of Latter-Day Saints (Mormonism)	Baptism by immersion.	Many give last rites or communion. Prefers burial to cremation.
Navajos	After a child's delivery the umbilical cord is taken from the newborn, dried, and buried near a place that symbolizes what parents want for child's future.	Navajo medicine men and women conduct formal ceremonies.

Vocation. Individuals express their spirituality on a daily basis in life routines, work, play, and relationships (Farran and others, 1989). Spirituality can be used in their vocation in life and be part of their identity. The nurse determines if illness or hospitalization has altered the person's ability to express his or her spirituality. Expression of spirituality may include showing an appreciation for life in the variety of things people do, living in the moment and not worrying about tomorrow, appreciating nature, expressing love towards others, and being productive. The nurse assesses whether the client loses the ability to express a sense of relatedness to something greater than the self (Fryback, 1993). Questions might include "Has your illness affected the way you live your life spiritually?" or "Has your illness affected your ability to express what's important in life for you?" If illness or loss prevents one from exercising his or her spirituality, the nurse must understand the implications psychologically, socially, and spiritually and find ways to offer guidance and support.

Client Expectations. It is important to include in any client assessment a review of the client's expectations for his or her health care. This part of the assessment gives the nurse and the client the chance to share what is most important to the client in terms of what caregivers are expected to provide and what the client hopes to gain. The nurse should not try to anticipate a client's expectations. What a client needs from the perspective of the nurse may have nothing to do with what the client actually expects or wants. Assessing client expectations requires the nurse to ask questions such as "What do you hope we will be able to do for you?" or "Your expectations are important to us; how can we make your care most satisfactory?" During times of loss or crisis, the client might simply desire a trust-ing and open relationship with the nurse. It might also be important that the client perceive caregivers to be accepting of his or her religious rituals. Asking the client what expectations are held of caregivers and then following through in meeting those expectations can be very beneficial in establishing a strong nurse-client relationship.

NURSING DIAGNOSIS

When reviewing a spiritual assessment to identify appropriate nursing diagnoses, the nurse will have learned a great deal about who the client is and the extent that spirituality plays in the client's day-to-day coping. Exploring the client's spirituality may reveal responses to health problems that require nursing intervention, or it may reveal existence of a strong set of resources that enable the client to cope effectively. As a nurse identifies the nursing diagnoses for a client, it is important to recognize the significance that spirituality has for all types of health problems. Pain, fear, anxiety, and self-care deficit are just some examples of common nursing diagnoses that will require the nurse to incorporate spiritual care principles.

There are two nursing diagnoses accepted by the North American Nursing Diagnosis Association that pertain specifically to spirituality. *Potential for enhanced spiritual well-being* is based on defining characteristics that show a pattern of well-being and the interconnectedness that comes from inner faith and hope (Kim and others, 1997). When the nurse's assessment reveals that the client has inner strength through hope and faith, believes in a higher power or unifying force, has a defined purpose and meaning in life, spiritual well-being is a likely diagnosis (Box 28-3).

The presence of this state shows the client has potential resources to draw on when faced with other nursing diag-

---

SAMPLE NURSING DIAGNOSTIC PROCESS — Box 28-3

HEALTH NEEDS RELATED TO SPIRITUALITY

Assessment Activities	Defining Characteristics	Nursing Diagnosis
Ask client to describe his or her source of faith.	Client expresses an inner strength and source of guidance.	Potential for enhanced spiritual well-being
Have client describe level of satisfaction with life.	Life has purpose and meaning.	
Determine who provides the greatest source of strength and support to the client during times of difficulty.	Person has a relatedness and connectedness with self, others, and a higher power or God.	
Ask the client to describe the meaning the stress of an illness poses for his or her life.	Client is passive, verbalizes little on own.	Hopelessness
Observe client's nonverbal cues while listening and being attentive.	Decreased affect and lack of initiative. Turns away from speaker, closes eyes.	
Ask client to describe how he or she feels about the future and the choices available to help client cope with illness.	Shares a despondency about life.	

noses such as chronic pain, fatigue, sensory/perceptual alterations, or body image disturbance. Since the client may not know how to engage the resources to cope with the health problems, the nurse offers support in exploring options.

The nursing diagnosis of *spiritual distress* creates a different clinical picture. Defining characteristics from a nurse's assessment may find patterns that reflect a person's dispiritedness (e.g., expressing concern with the meaning of life and belief systems, anger toward God, verbalizing conflicts about personal beliefs, or asking for spiritual assistance). Critical thinking requires a review of concrete data (e.g., religious rituals and sources of fellowship) and an assessment of previous client experiences, the nurse's own spirituality, and the appraisal of the client's spiritual well-being. Defining characteristics must be validated and clarified with the client before a diagnosis and plan of care are made. With spiritual care, the importance of the nurse's own spiritual well-being and perceptions cannot be overemphasized. The nurse avoids imposing his or her personal beliefs on the client. Each diagnosis must have an accurate related factor so that resulting interventions can be purposeful and goal directed (Box 28-4).

PLANNING

During the planning step of the nursing process, the nurse develops a plan of care for each of the client's nursing diagnoses. Critical thinking is again important because the nurse must reflect on previous experience and apply knowledge and critical thinking attitudes and standards in selecting the most appropriate nursing interventions (Figure 28-6). Prior experience in selecting interventions that support clients' spiritual well-being is invaluable when the nurse considers the best options for clients with similar types of situations or problems. During planning the nurse integrates the knowledge gathered from assessment and knowledge relating to resources and therapies available for spiritual care to develop an individualized

NURSING DIAGNOSES   Box 28-4

CLIENTS IN NEED OF SPIRITUAL SUPPORT

Anxiety
Coping, family: potential for growth
Coping, ineffective family: compromised
Coping, ineffective individual
Family processes, altered
Fear
Grieving, dysfunctional
Hopelessness
Powerlessness
Self-esteem disturbance
Spiritual well-being, potential for enhanced
Spiritual distress

plan of care (see care plan). In other words, the nurse matches the client's needs with those interventions that are supported and recommended in the clinical and research literature. Confidence becomes an important critical thinking attitude as the nurse attempts to build a caring relationship with the client. Confidence works to build trust, enabling nurse and client to enter into a healing relationship together. Attempting to meet or support clients' spiritual needs is not simple, and often the new nurse will require humility in recognizing that additional resources may be needed. The nurse's skills in helping clients interpret and understand the meaning of illness and loss, for example, may be limited. Because spiritual care is so personal, standards of autonomy and self-determination are critical in supporting the client's decisions about the plan of care.

As is the case in developing any plan of care, a spiritual care plan must include realistic and individualized goals along with relevant outcomes. It is important for both nurse and client to collaborate closely in setting goals and choosing related interventions. Setting realistic goals will require the nurse to know the client well. In cases where spiritual care requires helping clients adjust to loss or stressful life situations, goals may be long-term oriented (see care plan). However, short-term outcomes can be established so that the client progressively reaches a more spiritually healthy situation.

Caring must clearly be communicated between the nurse and client. Caring and communication are also integrated themes for whatever nursing interventions are chosen. The personal nature of spirituality requires the client to be able to speak openly with the nurse and to recognize the nurse's interest in his or her needs.

Significant others, such as spouses, siblings, parents, and friends, need to be involved, as appropriate, to lend support. This means that the nurse learns from the assessment what individuals or groups have formed a relationship with the client. These individuals may become involved in all levels of the nurse's plan. The client's support network may assist in giving physical care, providing emotional comfort, and sharing spiritual support.

In a hospital setting, one of the best resources to utilize in planning a client's spiritual care is the hospital's pastoral care department. A health care chaplain has special expertise in dealing with the spiritual problems confronted by clients. These professionals should be part of the health care team, lending insight about how and when to best support clients and families.

If the client participates in a formal religion, members of the clergy or members of the church, temple, mosque, or synagogue may need to be involved in the plan of care. Depending on the client's health status and needs, part of the plan will involve a continuation of appropriate religious rituals. The nurse must make sure that any icons or religious materials such as scriptures or a prayer book are made available.

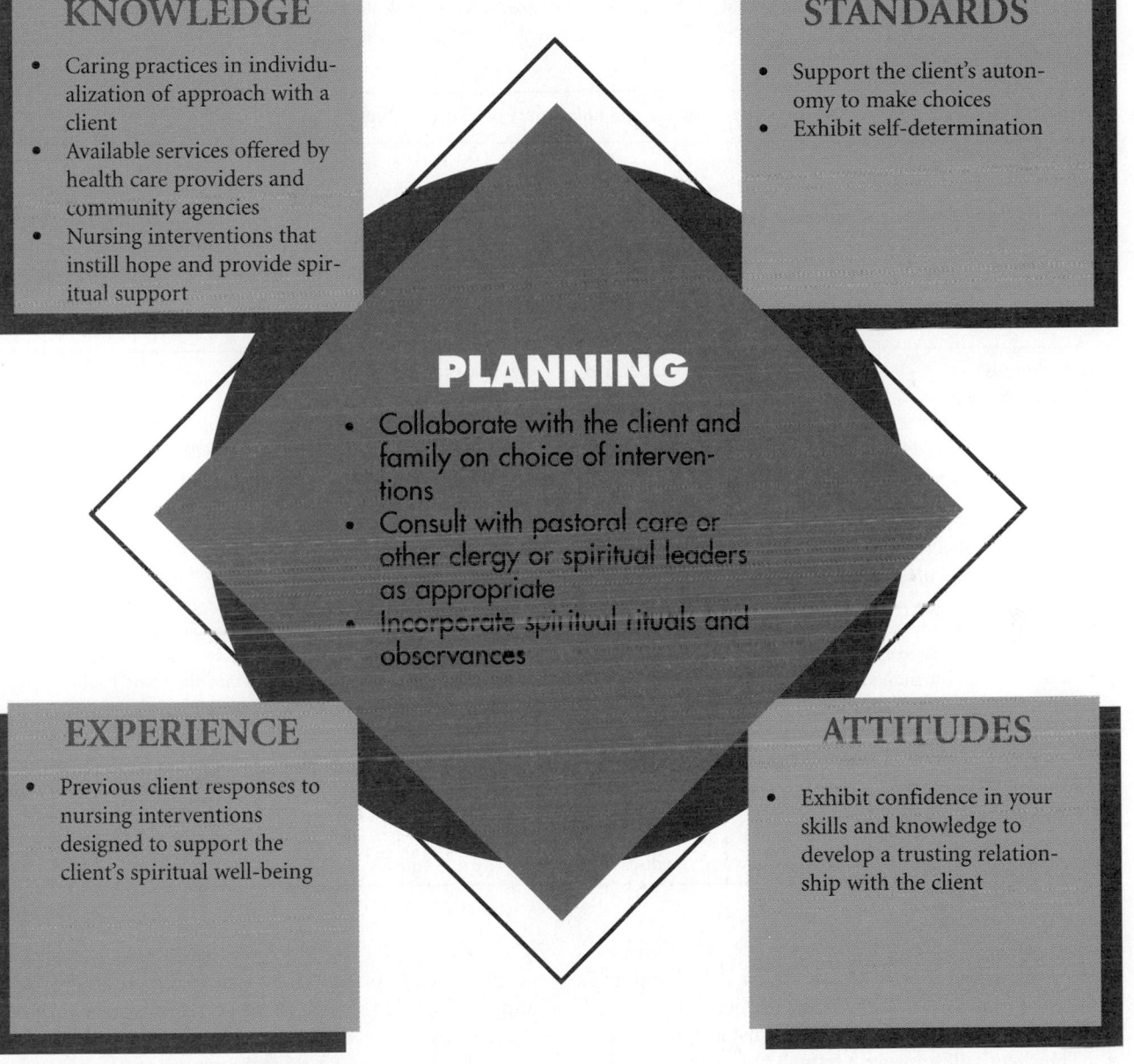

Figure 28-6   *Synthesis Model for Spiritual Health Planning Phase.*

SAMPLE NURSING CARE PLAN

SPIRITUAL WELL-BEING

ASSESSMENT*

James is a 24-year-old who has recently been diagnosed with AIDS. The clinic nurse, Leah, has been talking with James during his last three visits. During that time James expresses a fear of dying. She now talks with James in a private conference area and learns of his **anger with God:** "How can God do this to me? It just can't be happening." Leah attempts to learn more about James's faith and sources of spiritual support. James begins to **cry** and admits that he **feels very alone, "I just don't know what to believe in anymore;** this has happened so suddenly. It is as though God and everyone else has abandoned me. I am so afraid. Life isn't making sense." In further discussion, Leah learns that James has been **unable to sleep,** has little desire for food, and is having **difficulty finding ways to talk with his friends.**

*Defining characteristics are shown in bold type.

NURSING DIAGNOSIS: Spiritual distress related to fear and uncertainty of terminal illness

PLANNING

GOAL

Client will express a sense of purpose.

Client gains a sense of hope.

EXPECTED OUTCOMES

Client will discuss how the experience of having AIDS may have a positive influence in life within 1 month.

Client expresses a sense of confidence in treatments available for AIDS in 2 weeks.

Client begins to talk of the future within 1 month.

INTERVENTIONS†

Hope Instillation

- Plan instructional session to discuss typical course of AIDS, emphasizing the typical pattern of remissions with drug therapy. Review therapies available for treatment.

Spiritual Support

- Encourage client's expression of loneliness through establishing a caring presence.

- Listen to client's feelings and concerns
- Use spiritual resources. Plan discussion session with client that includes an individual(s) with whom client shares a similar faith. Have client discuss his or her ability to cope with AIDS and the meaning it has spiritually.

RATIONALE

Knowledge about disease will help client think as a person living with AIDS rather than dying with AIDS (Hall, 1998). Reality of disease course will help instill hope.

Presencing reflects being in tune with the client and displays caring. It is an effective technique that makes a topic of discussion more approachable (Benner, 1989).

People question and become open to discover their unique spiritual meaning after a crisis that threatens health (Hall, 1998). Provides client a resource from client's community of faith to share concerns.

†Intervention Classification labels from McCloskey JC, Bulechek GM: *Nursing interventions classification (NIC),* ed 3, St. Louis, 2000, Mosby.

EVALUATION

Ask client to discuss what meaning client has gained from experiencing AIDS.

Have client discuss how client plans to adjust to the disease in the future (e.g., continuing work, social activities)

In establishing a plan of care, there are several goals universal to spiritual caregiving for the nurse to consider:

- The client will sense a feeling of trust in caregivers.
- The client will improve personal harmony and connections with members of his or her support system.
- The client's personal quest for meaning and self-awareness will be enhanced.

IMPLEMENTATION

If a client experiences spiritual distress or has a health problem that requires the client to utilize spiritual resources, a compassionate and understanding relation-

ship between nurse and client is necessary. Both the client and nurse must feel free to let go and discover together the meaning illness or loss poses for the client and the impact it has on the meaning and purpose of life. Achieving this level of understanding with a client enables the nurse to deliver care in a sensitive, creative, and appropriate manner.

Health Promotion.   Spiritual care should be a central theme in promoting an individual's overall well-being. Spirituality is one personal resource that affects the balance between health and illness. In settings where health promotion activities occur, clients are often in need of information, counseling, and guidance to make the necessary choices to remain healthy.

Establishing Presence.   Clients have reported that the presence of nurses and their caregiving activities contributes to a sense of well-being and provides hope for recovery (Clark and others, 1991). Behaviors that establish the nurse's presence include giving attention, answering questions, listening, and having a positive and encouraging (but realistic) attitude. The ability to establish presence is part of the art of nursing (Chapter 6). It is not simply being in the same room with a client performing procedures or sharing technical information with a client. Benner (1984) clarifies that presencing involves "being with" a client versus "doing for" a client. Presencing involves offering a closeness with the client, physically, psychologically, and spiritually.

Nurses will work with clients who seek preventive health care because of their predisposing risks for health problems. In addition, clients will have early signs of problems that can be effectively managed without acute exacerbations of disease. When health promotion is the focus of care, the nurse's presence becomes important in instilling confidence in clients' abilities to take the steps necessary to remain healthy. A nurse can convey a caring presence by listening to clients' concerns over possible outcomes should their health become impaired, willingly involving family in discussions about the client's health, displaying self-confidence when health instruction is provided, and supporting the client's faith in the choices he or she makes. The client who seeks health care may be fearful of experiencing an illness that would threaten loss of control and looks for someone to offer competent direction. The nurse's encouraging words of support and the nurse's calm and decisive approach establish a presence that builds trust and well-being.

Trust is fundamental to any relationship. The attitude a nurse conveys when first interacting with a client sets the tone for all conversations (see Chapter 22). Listening to the meaning of what a client says is most important. It involves paying attention to the person's words, tone of voice, and listening carefully to their story. By observing expressions and body language of the client, the nurse learns to find cues to help assist the client in exploring ways to achieve inner peace, take action, or do whatever a situation demands (Hungelmann and others, 1996). Emblen and Halstead (1993) found in their research that nurses listening to clients was the option clients preferred when spiritual care was provided.

Supporting a Healing Relationship.   A nurse learns to look beyond isolated client problems and recognize the broader picture of a client's needs. For example, the nurse does not just look at a client's back pain as a problem to solve with quick remedies, but rather how the pain influences the client's ability to function and achieve goals established in life. A holistic view enables the nurse to establish a helping role. Within a helping role, nurses learn to establish healing relationships (Benner, 1984). Three steps are evident when a healing relationship develops between nurse and client:

1. Mobilizing hope for the nurse as well as for the client
2. Finding an interpretation or understanding of the illness, pain, anxiety, or other stressful emotion that is acceptable to the client
3. Assisting the client to use social, emotional, and spiritual resources (Benner, 1984)

Central to a healing relationship is mobilizing the client's hope. Hope motivates people with strategies to face challenges in life. The nurse can help a client find things to hope for. A newly diagnosed diabetic might hope to learn how to manage the disease so as to continue a productive and satisfying way of life. An adult daughter who has decided to become caregiver to her older-adult parent might hope to be able to protect the parent from injury or worsening disability.

Hope has both short- and long-term implications. From a long-term perspective, hope gives individuals motivation to carry on with life's responsibilities. In the short-term view, hope offers an incentive for constructive coping with obstacles and for finding ways to realize the object of hope (Dufault and Martocchio, 1985). Hope helps a client work toward recovery. To help clients achieve hope, the nurse and client work together to find an explanation of the situation that is acceptable to both. Then the nurse helps the client realistically exercise hope. This might include supporting a client's positive attitude toward life or a desire to be informed and to make decisions.

To further support a healing relationship the nurse must remain aware of the client's spiritual resources and needs. It is always important for a client to be able to express and exercise his or her beliefs and to find spiritual comfort. When life stressors or illness create confusion or uncertainty for the client, the nurse must recognize the possible effect this can have on a client's well-being. How can spiritual resources be used and strengthened? The nurse may begin by encouraging a client to discuss the effect illness has had on personal beliefs and faith. This gives the nurse the chance to clarify any misconceptions or inaccuracies in information. Having a clear sense of what illness may hold for an individual helps the person to apply all resources toward recovery.

Acute Care.   Within acute care settings, clients experience multiple stressors that threaten to overwhelm their coping resources. Support and enhancement of a client's spiritual well-being can be a challenge when the focus of health care seems to be one of treatment and cure rather than care. The nurse works closely with the client and his or her support network in finding ways to make the client's spiritual resources become part of the therapeutic plan of care.

Support Systems.   Use of support systems is of course important in any health care setting. Clark and others (1991) found that support systems provided clients with the greatest sense of well-being during hospitalization. Support systems serve as a human link connecting the client, the nurse, and the client's lifestyle before an illness. Part of the client's caregiving environment is the regular presence of family and friends viewed by the client as supportive. The nurse plans care with the client and the client's support network to promote the interpersonal bonding that is needed for recovery. The support system is a source of faith and hope, and it can be an important resource in conducting the religious rituals on which some clients rely.

When it is known that clients depend on family and friends for support, the nurse encourages them to visit the client regularly. The nurse's encouragement to family to be themselves during visits can facilitate the family's ability to provide the spiritual comfort that they are capable of sharing. Often illness and the treatment environment produce unknowns that intimidate family members and friends. The nurse helps the family feel welcome and uses their support and presence to promote the client's healing. Including family members in prayer, for example, is a thoughtful gesture if it is appropriate to the client's religion and if family members are comfortable participating. Encouraging the family to bring meaningful religious symbols to the client's bedside can offer significant spiritual support.

Another important resource to clients are spiritual advisors and members of the clergy. Many hospitals have pastoral care departments that assist in notifying community clergy of their congregants' admission. If not, the nurse should ask if clients desire to have their clergy notified of their hospitalization. All clergy should be made welcome on nursing units. When requested by clients or families, the nurse should keep clergy informed of any physical, psychosocial, or spiritual concerns affecting the client. The nurse shows respect for clients' spiritual values and needs by willingly cooperating with others giving spiritual care and by facilitating the administration of sacraments, rites, and rituals.

Providing privacy for the client and clergy is a thoughtful and sensitive gesture. The nurse determines the proper routine in a client's religion by asking the clergy, family, or client. Often a client within the hospital may want to discuss spiritual concerns in the evening or late at night, when support services such as clergy and social services are unavailable. The nurse can help to meet the client's needs by careful, skilled, and active listening.

If a client does not have a personal clergy available and desires one, the hospital's pastoral care department is an excellent resource. These highly trained professionals are often able to spend extended time with clients and families to determine their spiritual needs. Pastoral care professionals are expert at giving attention to both how an illness is influencing a person's beliefs and how the beliefs of the person can influence the actual illness and recovery experience.

Diet Therapies.   Food and nutrition are important aspects of client care. Food is also an important component of some religious observances (Table 28-3). As with many aspects of a particular culture or religion, food and the rituals surrounding the preparation and serving of food can be important to a person's spirituality. The nurse can consult with the dietitian to integrate the client's dietary preferences into daily care. In the event that a hospital or other health care agency cannot prepare food in the preferred way, the family may be asked to bring meals fitting into any dietary restrictions posed by the client's condition.

Table 28-3 **Religious Dietary Regulations Affecting Health Care**	
Religion	Dietary Practices
Hinduism	Some sects are vegetarians. The belief is not to kill *any* living creature.
Buddhism	Some are vegetarians, and many will not use alcohol or tobacco and may hesitate to use drugs. Many will fast on Holy Days.
Islam	Eating pork and consuming alcohol are prohibited. Fasting is done during the month of Ramadan.
Judaism	Some observe the kosher dietary restrictions of avoiding pork and shellfish and not preparing and eating milk and meat at the same time.
Christianity	Some Baptists, Evangelicals, and Pentecostals discourage the use of alcohol, caffeine, and tobacco. Some Roman Catholics may fast during Lent, Ash Wednesday, Good Friday, and 1 hour before receiving Communion.
Jehovah's Witnesses	Members may avoid food prepared with or containing blood.
Mormonism	Members abstain from alcohol, caffeine, and tobacco.
Baha'i	Members abstain from alcohol, caffeine, and tobacco.
Russian Orthodox Church	Followers must observe fast days as well as a "no meat" rule on Wednesdays and Fridays. During Lent all animal products, including dairy products and butter, are forbidden.
Native Americans	Food practices are influenced by individual tribal beliefs.

Supporting Rituals.   Nurses can become active in their clients' spiritual care by supporting clients' participation in spiritual rituals and activities. This is especially important for older adults (Box 28-5). Personal care of the client should be planned to allow time for religious readings, spiritual visitations, or attendance at religious services. Some churches and synagogues offer audiotapes of their services for those members who cannot attend in person. Family members can plan a prayer session or an organized reading of scriptures on a regular basis. Arrangements may need to be made with pastoral care staff for the client and family to receive the sacraments. Clergy will routinely offer to make home visits for persons unable to attend religious services. Taped meditations, classical or religious music, and televised religious services provide other effective options. The nurse should be respectful of icons, medals, prayer rugs, or crosses that clients bring to a health setting to be sure they are not accidentally lost, damaged, or misplaced.

Restorative and Continuing Care.

For clients who are recovering from a long-term illness or disability or who suffer chronic or terminal disease, spiritual care becomes especially important. Many of the nursing interventions applicable in health promotion and acute care apply to this level of health care as well.

Prayer.   The act of prayer gives an individual the opportunity to renew personal faith and belief in a higher being in a specific, focused way that may be highly ritualized and formal or quite spontaneous and informal.

Prayer has been shown to be an effective coping resource for physical as well as psychological symptoms. Clients may pray in private or pursue opportunities for group prayer with family, friends, or clergy. The nurse can be supportive of prayer by giving the client privacy if desired, learning if the client wishes to have the nurse participate, and by suggesting prayer when it is known to be a coping resource for the client. If prayer is not suitable for a client, an alternative may be to read from a book selected by the client or from poetry or inspirational texts.

Meditation.   Meditation can be a highly effective means for creating a relaxation response that reduces daily stress. Chapter 42 reviews guided imagery, an approach nurses can use to help clients learn meditation. Individuals who regularly—twice a day, for 10 to 20 minutes—sit quietly in a comfortable position with their eyes closed and repeat a sound, phrase, or sacred word in rhythm with their breathing, gently disregarding intrusive thoughts as they do so, experience decreased metabolism and heart rate, easier breathing, and slower brain waves (Culligan, 1996). Meditation exercises can give individuals relief from chronic pain, insomnia, anxiety, and depression and can help in coping with the side effects of therapies for cancer and AIDS. When clients use meditation in conjunction with their spiritual beliefs, often they report an increased spirituality that is described as experiencing the presence of a power, force, or energy, or what was perceived as God (Box 28-6).

Supporting Grief Work.   Clients who experience terminal illness or who have suffered permanent loss in body function because of a disabling disease or an injury will require the nurse's support in grieving over and coping with their loss. Chapter 29 provides a variety of nursing interventions to use in support of clients' grief work. Supporting a client during times of grief can be strengthened by the nurse's ability to enter into a spiritual relationship with the client, whereby nurse and client come to know one another as individuals. Establishing a pattern of connectedness with a client and with one's self is a process of self-reflecting that allows one to intimately know the self and others (Walton, 1996). The process of gaining intimate insight into the individual self is nurtured in relationships with clients. Interpersonal relationships have the potential to be therapeutic when interactions become meaningful, thus aiding coping and problem solving. Consistent caring, listening, and focusing on the client must occur for intimacy and trust to form. Nurses can prepare themselves for interactions by quieting and centering themselves to focus energy and set the stage for listening. When a connectedness forms between nurse and client, the client's concerns can be better addressed and there is an improved chance that meaningful and relevant interventions will be selected in supporting the client's ability to cope with illness and disability.

NURSING PRACTICE   Box 28-5

- Religious activities and attitudes are very common among older adults. A large proportion of older adults claim that religion helps them to cope both when asked directly about religion as a source of strength in difficult times and when asked indirectly about how they coped with stressful life events (Koenig, 1987).
- The very old are more likely to be interested in the nonorganizational aspects of religion than in active participation (Courtney and others, 1992).
- Consideration and a belief in the afterlife increases as adults grow older. Visits from clergy, social workers, lawyers, and even financial advisors can be made available so clients feel prepared. Leaving a legacy to loved ones prepares the older adult to leave the world with a sense of meaning (Ebersole and Hess, 1998). Legacies may include oral histories, works of art, publications, photographs, or some other object of significance.

Client Teaching FOR MEDITATION TECHNIQUES   Box 28-6

OBJECTIVE
The client will be able to achieve a state of relaxation and a transcendent state of being.

TEACHING STRATEGIES
- Instruct client to select a quiet room in the home where interruptions can be eliminated.
- Peaceful music or the quiet whirring of a fan may be useful in lessening distraction from the meditation exercise.
- Each meditation should involve about 20 minutes.
- Have client practice 2 or more times daily.
- To begin the exercise have the client assume a comfortable position with extremities unencumbered and supported.

- Coach the client in slow, rhythmic, deep breathing.
- Have the client focus on a sound, a thought, or an image.
- Chanting psalms, a poem, or a prayer repeatedly may assist in focusing.
- After meditation have the client think about what became the focus of meditation, what the client learned or felt about himself or herself.

EVALUATION
- Have the client describe the meaning meditation has provided.

EVALUATION

The evaluation of a client's spiritual care requires the nurse to apply critical thinking in determining if efforts at restoring or maintaining the client's spiritual health were successful (Figure 28-7). The nurse will consider knowledge of spirituality and coping theory (see Chapter 30) in evaluating whether the client has been able to adjust to those factors that threaten spiritual well-being. Outcomes established during the planning phase will serve as the standards to evaluate the client's progress. In addition, an ethic of caring ensures that the nurse evaluates any ethical concerns that may arise in the course of the client's spiritual care and support. Critical thinking attitudes are applied to ensure sound nursing judgments. The nurse's evaluation includes a review of the client's response to care and whether the client's expectations were achieved.

Client Care.   Attainment of spiritual health is a lifelong goal. Clients will experience the need to clarify values (see Chapter 20), reshape philosophies, strengthen relationships, and live those experiences that help to shape one's purpose in life. The nurse conducts a plan of therapy for the client's spiritual health while always evaluating whether planned outcomes and goals were achieved. The nurse compares the client's level of spiritual health with the behaviors and perceptions noted in the nursing assessment. For example, if the nurse's assessment finds the client losing hope, the follow-up evaluation will involve a discussion with the client to determine if the client has regained an attitude of something to live for. Family and friends with whom the client seeks to have fellowship can be a useful source of evaluative information. Successful outcomes should reveal the client developing an increased or restored sense of connectedness with family; maintaining, renewing, or reforming a sense of purpose in life and, for some, a confidence and trust in a supreme being or power.

For clients with a serious or terminal illness, evaluation focuses on the goal of helping the client retain faith and hope or expressing openly the uncertainties life poses. The nurse evaluates how the client is accepting his or her illness and whether hope has enabled the client to recognize individual mortality and focus on living for each day. Fryback (1993) found that the terminally ill, regardless of whether they followed a formal religion, held a belief in a higher power, which gave them a sense that God was with them and they were not alone. The nurse must not assume all clients have such faith. However, the nurse's support aims to help clients accept their destiny and to be at peace.

Client Expectations.   The nurse evaluates whether client expectations of the nurse and health care team were met. In regard to spiritual care, this involves evaluating if the client's spiritual practices were respected and if the nurse-client relationship was one of caring and support. Both the client and family should be able to relate if opportunities were offered for religious rituals. With respect to the nurse-client relationship, does the client express trust and confidence in the nurse? Is the client able to discuss those things important to him or her? Is the client comfortable in expressing spiritual needs and hopes to the nurse? Taking time to ask the client to reflect on the quality of the nurse-client relationship is time well spent. Asking the client, "Have I helped you to become comfortable in saying what you feel is important to you spiritually?" or "Do you feel your expectations of me in supporting your spiritual needs, were met?" will determine whether an effective healing relationship was developed.

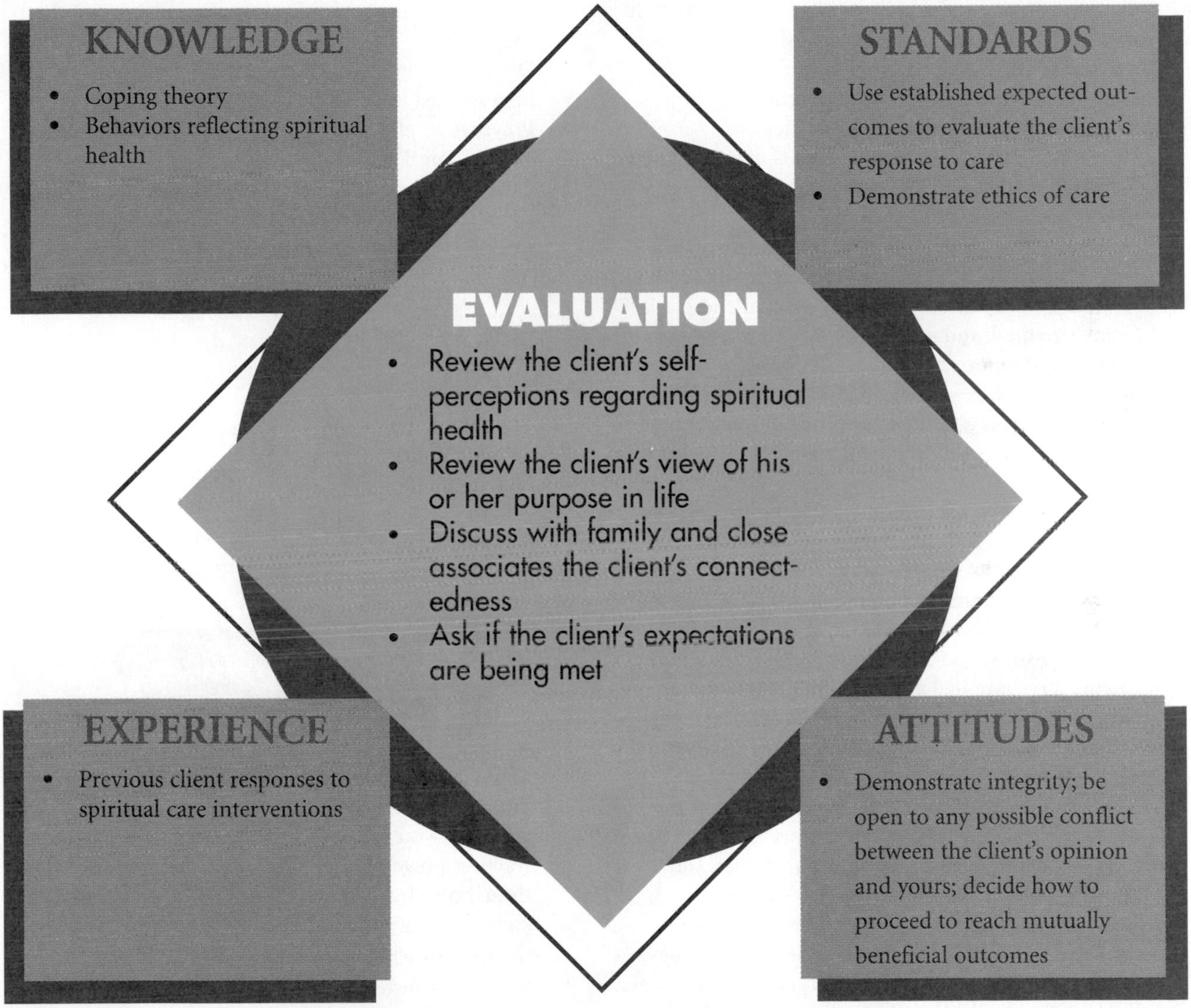

KNOWLEDGE

- Coping theory
- Behaviors reflecting spiritual health

STANDARDS

- Use established expected outcomes to evaluate the client's response to care
- Demonstrate ethics of care

EVALUATION

- Review the client's self-perceptions regarding spiritual health
- Review the client's view of his or her purpose in life
- Discuss with family and close associates the client's connectedness
- Ask if the client's expectations are being met

EXPERIENCE

- Previous client responses to spiritual care interventions

ATTITUDES

- Demonstrate integrity; be open to any possible conflict between the client's opinion and yours; decide how to proceed to reach mutually beneficial outcomes

Figure 28-7 *Synthesis Model for Spiritual Health Evaluation Phase.*

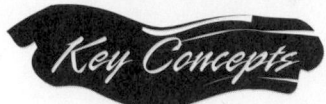

Key Concepts

- Spirituality is the sense of a presence or meaning higher than human that is intrinsic to human nature and a deep resource for healing.
- Spiritual forms of expression can and do have effects on an individual's physical well-being.
- The concept of spirituality as a unifying theme in our lives demonstrates the importance of the spiritual dimension influencing a person's physical, psychological, social, and developmental health.
- Faith in a higher power or in one's choice of how to live life can enable a person to take action.
- Religious care involves helping clients maintain their faithfulness to their belief systems and worship practices.
- Common religious rituals include private worship, prayer, singing, use of a rosary, and scripture reading.
- Hope is a multidimensional concept that energizes, is future oriented, and gives individuals a motivation to achieve and to face difficulties.
- Spiritual health is a balance between a person's life values and goals and their relationship within themselves and others that can be threatened by illness or loss.
- The strength of a client's spirituality influences how he or she copes with sudden illness and how quickly he or she can move to recovery.
- Terminal illness creates an uncertainty about what death means and thus can make clients susceptible to spiritual distress.
- Clients who have had a near-death experience are often reluctant to discuss it and think caregivers will not understand, but being given a chance to explore what happened can be spiritually uplifting.
- A spiritual assessment is most successful when the nurse applies knowledge that pertains to therapeutic communication, principles of loss and grief, and knowledge of caring practices.
- The personal nature of spirituality requires open communication and the establishment of trust between nurse and client.
- If a client's religious beliefs conflict with medical treatment, options to nurses and other health care providers can be limited.
- Anger is a typical response to the limitations posed by illness; however, if clients can seek solutions for how to deal with any limitations, spiritual well-being may be an important coping resource.
- An important part of spiritual assessment is learning who are the client's friends or family who share a community of faith.
- Confidence is a critical thinking attitude that works to build trust, enabling the nurse and client to enter into a healing relationship together.

- In a hospital setting, one of the best resources to utilize in planning a client's spiritual care is the hospital's pastoral care department.
- Central to a healing relationship is mobilizing the client's hope.
- Part of a client's caregiving environment can be the regular presence of family, friends, and spiritual advisors.
- Depending on a client's religion, certain foods may be restricted in the diet.
- Prayer is an effective coping resource for physical and psychological symptoms.
- Establishing a connectedness with a client enables the client to express concerns and progress through grief work.

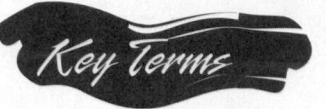

Key Terms

Agnostic, *p. 591*

Atheist, *p. 591*

Faith, *p. 592*

Holistic, *p. 590*

Hope, *p. 592*

Spiritual distress, *p. 593*

Spiritual well-being, *p. 591*

Spirituality, *p. 590*

Transcendence, *p. 592*

Critical Thinking Exercises

1. A client with degenerative joint disease tells you he is afraid he will soon be unable to walk. His affect is blunted, and he often looks away in the distance. His wife tells you that the pain her husband has during walking prevents him from going to church. At one time both husband and wife were very active in church activities. What might you want to learn about the client during your spiritual assessment?
2. Mrs. Stills has been hospitalized with cancer of the ovaries. Her disease has progressed, but she expresses a satisfaction with her life and a faith that God will guide and protect her. She asks you about meditation exercises. In the acute care environment, how might you arrange a teaching session on meditation?
3. Critical thinking is an ongoing process. When you learn that you are assigned to Julio Gonsaga, you note that the Kardex information includes his religion, Catholic, and his place of birth, Cuba. A colleague tells you he can speak some English. The client is 80 years old and reportedly has a bit of a hearing deficit. What knowledge might you wish to reflect on critically before beginning a spiritual assessment of this client?

References

Aldridge D: Is there evidence for spiritual healing? *Adv J Mind-Body Health* 9(4):4, 1993.

Basford TK: *Near death experience: an annotated bibliography,* New York, 1990, Garland.

Benner DG: *Baker encyclopedia of psychology,* Grand Rapids, Mich, 1985, Baker Book House.

Benner P: *From novice to expert,* Menlo Park, Calif, 1984, Addison-Wesley.

Benner P, Wrubel J: *The primacy of caring,* Menlo Park, Calif, 1989, Addison-Wesley.

Bullock BL, da Cunha M: Immune deficiency. In Bullock BL, Rosendahl PP, editors: *Pathophysiology: adaptations and alterations in function,* Philadelphia, 1992, JB Lippincott.

Burnard P: The spiritual needs of atheists and agnostics, *Professional Nurse* 4(3):130, 1988.

Calabria M, Macrae J, editors: *Suggestions for thought by Florence Nightingale: selections and commentaries,* Philadelphia, 1994, University of Pennsylvania Press.

Carson V: *Spiritual dimensions of nursing practice,* Philadelphia, 1989, WB Saunders.

Clark CC and others: Spirituality: integral to quality care, *Holist Nurs Pract* 5(3):67, 1991.

Coe RM: The magic of science and the science of magic: an essay on the process of healing, *J Health Soc Behav* 38(3):1, 1997.

Courtney BC and others: Religiosity and adaptation in the oldest-old. In Poon LW, editor: *The Georgia centenarian study,* Amityville, NY, 1992, Baywood.

Culligan K: Spirituality and healing in medicine, *America,* p 17, August 31, 1996.

Dombeck MB: Dream-telling: a means of spiritual awareness, *Holist Nurs Pract* 9(2):37, 1995.

Dufault K, Martocchio BC: Hope: its spheres and dimensions, *Nurs Clin North Am* 20:379, 1985.

Ebersole P, Hess P: *Toward healthy aging,* ed 5, St. Louis, 1998, Mosby.

Emblen JD: Religion and spirituality defined according to current use in nursing literature, *J Prof Nurs* 8(1):41, 1992.

Emblen JD, Halstead L: Spiritual needs and interventions: comparing the views of patients, nurses, and chaplains, *Clin Nurs Spec* 7(4):175, 1993.

Farran CJ and others: Development of a model for spiritual assessment and intervention, *J Religion Health* 28(3):185, 1989.

Fryback PB: Health for people with a terminal diagnosis, *Nurs Sci Q* 6(3):147, 1993.

Giger JN, Davidhizar RE: *Transcultural nursing: assessment and intervention,* ed 2, St. Louis, 1995, Mosby.

Haase JE and others: Simultaneous concept analysis of spiritual perspective, hope, acceptance, and self-transcendence, *Image J Nurs Sch* 24(2):141, 1992.

Hall BA: Patterns of spirituality in persons with advanced HIV disease, *Res Nurs Health* 21:143, 1998.

Heliker D: Reevaluation of a nursing diagnosis: spiritual distress, *Nurs Forum* 27(4):15, 1992.

Hungelmann J and others: Focus on spiritual well-being: harmonious interconnectedness of mind-body-spirit—use of the JAREL spiritual well-being scale, *Geriatr Nurs* 17(6):262, 1996.

Kiecolt-Glaser JK and others: Psychosocial enhancement of immunocompetence in a geriatric population, *Health Psychol* 4:25, 1985.

Kim MJ and others: *Pocket guide to nursing diagnoses,* ed 7, St. Louis, 1997, Mosby.

Koenig H: *Religion and well-being in later life* (abstract). Proceedings of the Third Congress of the International Psychogeriatric Association, Chicago, 1987.

McCloskey JC, Bulechek GM: *Nursing interventions classification (NIC),* ed 3, St. Louis, 2000, Mosby.

Miller JF, Powers MJ: Development of an instrument to measure hope, *Nurs Res* 37(1):6, 1988.

Nowotny ML: Assessment of hope in patients with cancer: development of an instrument, *Oncol Nurs Forum* 16(1):57, 1989.

O'Connor AP and others: Understanding the cancer patient's search for meaning, *Cancer Nurs* 13:167, 1990.

O'Neill DP, Kenny EK: Spirituality and chronic illness, *Image J Nurs Sch* 30(3):275, 1998.

Post-White J and others: Hope, spirituality, sense of coherence, and quality of life in patients with cancer, *Oncology Nurs Forum* 23(10):1571, 1996.

Reed PG: Spirituality and well-being in terminally ill hospitalized adults, *Res Nurs Health* 10:335, 1987.

Remen RN: Spirit: resource for healing, *Noetic Sci Rev,* p 61, autumn 1988.

Rew L: Intuition: Nursing knowledge and the spiritual dimension of persons, *Holist Nurs Pract* 3(3):56, 1989.

Sobralske M: Perceptions of health: Navajo Indians, *Top Clin Nurs* 7(3):32, 1985.

Turner JA, Clancy S: Strategies for coping with chronic low back pain: relationship to pain and disability, *Pain* 24:355, 1986.

Turner RP and others: Religious or spiritual problem: a culturally sensitive diagnostic category in the DSM-IV, *J Nerv Ment Dis* 183(7):435, 1995.

Walton J: Spiritual relationships, *J Holist Nurs* 14(3):237, 1996.

Yim RJR, Vande Creek L: Unbinding grief and life's losses for thriving recovery after open heart surgery, *Caregiver Journal* 12(2):8, 1996.

Young CE: Intuition and the nursing process, *Holist Nurs Pract* 1(3):52, 1987.

29

Responding to Loss, Death, and Grieving

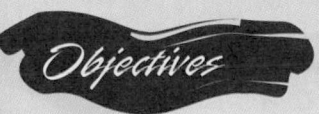

Objectives

Mastery of content in this chapter will enable the student to:

- Define the key terms listed.
- Identify the nurse's role in each phase of the nursing process when helping clients and families (or communities) experiencing loss, grief, or death.
- Describe and compare theorist's phases relating to grief.
- List various factors influencing a client's reaction to loss and the ability to cope.
- Describe characteristics of a person experiencing grief.
- Compare and contrast grief after loss, anticipatory grief, and accommodated grief.
- Develop a plan of care for a client, family, health care worker, and/or a unique group of people experiencing grief.
- Identify nursing diagnoses that can be applied during the grieving process that are within legal, ethical, and cultural guidelines for a client or a family.
- Identify and contrast global losses with personal loss.
- Implement interventions for grieving clients to provide sensitive caring that supports the client and family in their grief work.
- Describe how a nurse meets a dying client's need for comfort and caring.
- Explain ways for the nurse to assist a family in caring for the dying client.
- Discuss important factors in caring for the body after death.
- Discuss the role of the nurse's own loss experience as it influences care of the grieving.

General Concepts of the Grieving Process

LOSS

Loss includes issues beyond the actual death experience; physical death is not the only event that produces a loss. Loss can include the loss of an "ideal child" when the anticipated features, such as gender or hair coloring, are not seen at birth. An example could be that a sixth girl is born to a family that wanted a boy. Loss might involve a middle-age adult who has worked loyally for 20 years but is let go because of downsizing of the company. Loss can be described as the absence of something desired or previously thought to be available. The decreasing ability to move and do activities in the aging client is an example of loss of independence and the return to a less-desired dependent role. When one dreams and makes plans for oneself or another, the potential is present for failure to achieve these goals. One example might be the great sense of loss experienced by a couple who have tried for years to become pregnant and are finally told that they can never have their own children (Thomas and Striegel, 1994-1995). This type of loss changes all of the anticipated future dreams for that individual or couple.

Loss comes in many forms based on the values and priorities learned within one's sphere of influence, including one's family, friends, society, and cultural environment. One classification of categories of loss includes the following: loss of an external object, a known environment, a significant other, an aspect of self, and life (Box 29-1). Loss and death are universal and unique to all individuals, yet each client's death or loss is interpreted differently by the involved persons. The challenge in nursing is to identify the needs of each participant (Attig, 1996).

GRIEF

Grief is the emotional and behavioral responses to loss. Successful mastery of the grieving process after the loss occurs when one adapts through mourning and moves forward in one's own life experiences with a minimum of disruptions (Engel, 1964). Grief is manifested in a variety of ways that are individual and based on personal experiences, cultural expectations, and religious beliefs (Farber and others 1999) (see Chapters 7 and 28). This process leads to a gradual acceptance and adaptation of one's expectations to go on in a world without that which was lost. Grief can be healthy and out of sequence for some individuals. Often grief is repetitive and cyclic. One level of grieving does not have to be sequentially mastered before moving on to recovery. Some individuals work at several levels of recovery at the same time. Grief comes and goes with their life experiences. Some events remind them of their loss and the feelings return even many years later after the initial loss and grief resolution. Events that bring grief back to the surface may include smells, places, foods,

The authors acknowledge the contribution of Sally M. Featherstone to this chapter in the previous edition of this text.

Categories of Losses and Examples	Box 29-1
Category	**Examples**
External objects	Jewelry
	Home
	Car
	Pet
Known environment	City/country
	Moving
	Work changes
	Hospitalization
Significant other	Death
	Divorce
	Separation
	Broken relationship
Aspect of self	Body part/function
	Control
	Memory
	Dignity
	Self-worth
	Hope
	Freedom
Life	Physical death
	Brain death
	Ability to reason

Behavioral Signs of Dysfunctional Grief — Box 29-2

Overactivity without a sense of loss
Alteration in relationships with friends and family
Hostilities against specific persons
Agitated depression with tension, insomnia, feelings of worthlessness, extreme guilt, and even suicidal tendencies
Diminished participation in religious and ritual activities related to the client's culture
Inability to discuss the loss without crying (particularly more than a year after the loss)
False sense of well-being

dates, holidays, clothing, television presentations, or other people (Rando, 1984).

Dysfunctional grief occurs when there is prolonged emotional instability, a withdrawal from usual tasks or activities that previously gave pleasure, and the lack of progression from one level to successful coping with the loss (Box 29-2). One example of dysfunctional grief would include the significant other who is seeking additional "support" for many years after a loss. The significant other is said to have the "secondary gains" of receiving attention when a loved one has passed on and no healthy relationships have developed to help the significant other to cope successfully (Stocker, 1994).

Disenfranchised grief occurs when societal norms do not define the loss as a loss within its traditional definition. The client is not acknowledged for the loss and does not gain support from others (Lendhardt, 1997a). Disenfranchised loss in children might be exhibited as changes in behavior at school, including changes in grades, interests, or relationships. Strategies for counselors to deal with these children have been published by Lendhardt (1997b). Other nontraditional losses that could lead to disenfranchised grief could include the death of a same-sex lover, the loss of innocence, broken relationships, the death of one who is greatly admired, or the loss of a child by abortion. In this case society has defined the "grieving rules" to include who, what, when, how, and under what circumstances it is acceptable to grieve (Horn, 1993). Therefore the survivor's grief must be hidden to avoid negative social pressures. When complications occur in the grieving process, a delay of resolution of grief will result (Rando, 1992-1993).

Anticipatory grief describes the process of grieving before a client has died or a loss has occurred. In this situation future hopes and goals are recognized as impractical, such as when individuals are told that they have only a month to live but they had planned to return to school the next year. Another example might include the cancer client who is slowly wasting away with cancer and the family has accepted the "death" before the "actual physical departure" of the client. Therefore the family will be missing out on any gains that might be obtained while the client is still alive.

Life is a series of expected or unexpected gains and losses. A loss occurs when the child begins to walk and gains a level of independence from the parental caregiver. Walking becomes a loss of the child's dependence on the parent. In another example, anticipatory grief could apply to the parent who realizes that the child who is brain dead will never walk (Spector, 1996).

The more expectations are placed on a child by the parent, the greater is the sense of anticipatory loss felt when goals are not met (Rosenfeld, 1991; Stinson and others, 1992). Feelings and resentments must be grieved to move forward to a healthier lifestyle (Thomas and Striegel, 1994-1995). Acknowledging these feelings becomes the first step toward the healing process. Therefore the goals for the situation must be modified to be realistic or to deal with new expectations based on the actual loss. In the case of a disabled child, the nurse must help develop new goals for the child who will never run, play, or marry, to help the parents find satisfaction in realistic expectations for the child (Rando, 1986). The parent must grieve through the loss for future hopes and deal honestly with the capabilities of the child that exist in the present circumstance (Rando, 1986).

PERSONAL LOSS

Personal loss is any significant loss of someone or something that can no longer be seen, felt, heard, known, or experienced and that requires individual adaptation through the grieving process. Personal losses can include tangible and intangible components, such as perceived beauty, roles, pleasure, and satisfaction with life in general. It is an individual interpretation of the value of the person or object that makes it personal or unique (Cressy, 1997). In contrast, global loss is loss experienced by many; it requires less personal involvement and minimal grieving to adapt to such a change (e.g., in the political arena when a well-liked individual is removed from office because of some hidden problems). The loss is really not personal unless the livelihood of the client is based on that politician's employment. Thus generally the loss is broader with a global loss and may have very little effect on the day-to-day events of the client (Cairns, 1997).

Actual Loss

Actual loss is any loss of a person or object that can no longer be felt, heard, known, or experienced by the individual. The tangible loss is usually understood by all who are aware of its value to the grieving client. Examples could include the loss of an arm, hair, youth, child, spouse, relationship, object, known environment, body functions, and role changes. Lost objects that have been valued by a client include any possession that is worn out, misplaced, stolen, or ruined by disaster. A child may grieve over a familiar toy or blanket. A widow may grieve over the loss of the smell of her deceased husband's pipe on his clothing.

Valuing is unique to each person, but the concept of loss is common or understood by others. The moving of an individual into an assisted living facility represents the loss of familiarity and independence. A maturational loss might include the expected changes that occur with aging, in which impaired mobility and memory make independence a safety issue for older adults as their physical health declines (Sheehan, 1996; Shapiro, 1999), although if one compared two different 99-year-old persons, their needs and activity might be at either extreme.

Perceived Loss

Perceived loss is any loss that is less tangible and uniquely defined by the grieving client, such as the loss of confidence or prestige. By individual interpretation, no actual loss may need to take place. Examples could be the parents' expectation of a tall blond girl and the actual situation that a fat-faced red-headed boy is born. Despite the fact that the red hair is not a death sentence and the child is healthy, it is the expectation of the blond-haired child, idealized during the pregnancy, that is the perceived loss (Stinson and others, 1992). Therefore the loss is in the eye of the beholder. Other examples of perceived loss can include a minor scar or gaining 2 pounds, which may be major disasters to someone who values personal good looks. Individual interpretation makes a difference in how the loss is really uniquely valued and the response that one will have during the grieving process.

Maturational Loss

Maturational Loss includes any change in the developmental process that is normally expected during a lifetime. One example would be the feeling of loss as the child goes to school for the first time. Another would be the loss of dependence felt when the child stops breast-feeding, or the empty nest syndrome felt by the parents whose last child has finally left home. These events are expected, but the feelings of loss persist as grieving occurs to adapt to the change.

Situational Loss

Situational Loss includes any sudden, unexpected, and definable event that is not predictable. Often this type of loss includes multiple situational losses rather than a single loss. A hurricane or massive flooding that has removed houses, possessions, livelihood, the things of the past, and the hopes for tomorrow is one type of situational loss. An automobile accident may leave the driver paralyzed, but the grief of causing the death of another person may be a greater loss than the driver's own injury. People who have survived plane crashes or other catastrophes have stated that therapy was needed to enable them to cope with the severity of the losses, in addition to the reasons for their survival. Survivors feel very guilty that they did not die, and many have trouble with successes after a major disaster. Other survivors often seek tasks or goals that must be completed before their death.

Coping Mechanisms in Grief and Loss

To assist the nurse in comprehending the total picture of a client's loss, various coping mechanisms must be considered (Raphael, 1986). Concepts such as hope, mourning, and closure help to describe some of the assessments performed by health care workers to adequately plan for goals and actions that are individualized. Many aspects of the client's or family's life must be discussed to get adequate knowledge of the client's database. The database helps the nurse to decide the success or failure of the coping mechanisms used by the client to allow further intervention as needed.

Hope is characterized by a confident, yet uncertain, expectation of achieving a goal (Dufault and Martocchio, 1985; Bierman and others, 1998). It is not a single act but a complex series of thoughts, feelings, and actions. Hope can enhance coping skills and even influence survival (Doka, 1993). As a way of assessing their hopefulness, the nurse listens to what the clients say their expectations are for life, the present, and the future. Often in terminal illness the client's hope is focused on milestones, significant events, or for the relief of pain (Weissman and others, 1999). Spiritual distress by a client or a family is often based on their definition of hope or the lack of hope (Stepnick and Perry, 1992). During a loss some clients see hope as encouragement to work toward successful recovery. Other clients may view hope negatively by not seeing any outcomes except futility.

Mourning is the process that follows a loss and includes working through the grief. The processes of grief and mourning are intense, internal, painful, and lengthy. Often the terms *grief, mourning,* and *bereavement* are used interchangeably.

Grief work is a concept in which the individual responds, feels, and behaves in reaction to a loss. The uniqueness of grief work varies from person to person. There can be different types of losses within the same individual, as values influence each loss. Theories about grief and steps used in the process of resolution of grief are covered later in the chapter.

Closure is the point at which the loss has been resolved and the grieving individual can move on with life without focusing on the loss. Closure is not a single point of no return but a series of fluid points in time and may last for years until one day the loss is resolved. As time progresses, less time is spent in the mourning process as the individual returns to a preloss state. An expected period of the return of grief includes sadness on the anniversary date of the loss. For example, if the death of a family member occurred on December 1, often a person will feel concerned or anxious around that time. The individual may not understand the feeling until he or she realizes that this is the anniversary of the date of the loss. Anticipation of the anniversary date allows the survivor to recall pleasant memories that are less painful than when the loss first occurred.

Persons who are grieving try a variety of strategies to cope. The tasks of grief work have been described by the acronym TEAR (Worden, 1982; Harper, 1983).

T   *To* accept the reality of the loss
E   *Experiencing* the pain of loss
A   *Adjustment* to an environment that no longer includes the lost person, object, or aspect of self
R   *Reinvesting* emotional energy into new relationships

The successful completion of these tasks leads to the passage from grief into closure (Maglio, 1991).

Scientific Knowledge Base

The nurse who understands the various effects of different loss situations will recognize and address these issues as a practitioner with the upmost skill to achieve greater success in actually helping clients cope with loss. When dealing with the needs of these clients, scientific knowledge should be integrated from other disciplines to support nursing judgment and the plan of action for the grieving client or family.

Nursing practice, including the care of clients experiencing loss, is based on nursing theory (see Chapter 5). Nursing theory includes the application of knowledge from other disciplines such as psychology, sociology, and education. Nonnursing theories guide the practice of nursing when dealing with the evolving individual in his or her relationship to the environment. These principles help guide the nurse in drawing conclusions and selecting interventions that ultimately may contribute to a new nursing knowledge base. Nursing is in its infancy of development. Proven theories from other disciplines have helped to guide and validate new nursing theories without starting over from scratch (Kübler-Ross, 1969). By borrowing theories, concepts, precepts, conclusions, and research from other disciplines, the nurse researcher uses already-validated concepts to guide the development of new nursing theory (see Chapter 25).

THEORIES OF THE GRIEVING PROCESS

There is no right way or wrong way to grieve a loss. Behaviors and feelings associated with the **grieving process** occur in individuals as a unique pattern of coping mechanisms or the lack of such (McLean, 1999). Losses such as physical changes or deaths are viewed differently based on many factors, which are clarified in the assessment phase of the nursing process. The increasing focus on grief occurs naturally as one comes closer to one's own death. Grief is experienced by all who come in contact with the grieving client, whether these persons are friends, family, staff, social support, or caregivers, including physicians and nurses. The length of a relationship is not always the key to the severity of grieving. Someone can develop a close relationship in a very short time. The dying client may depend extensively on the nurse to support the client when the client feels that the family does not need any other problems and cannot cope with other concerns. Identification of sources of support becomes a major task for the nurse in this situation (Figure 29-1).

Therefore the concepts and theories of grief are only tools that can be used to anticipate potential needs of clients and families and to plan interventions to help them understand their grief while trying to deal with it. Several theorists, including Engel, Kübler-Ross, and Rando, describe stages, phases, steps, or tasks of the grieving process (Table 29-1). The components are not meant to be sequential and separate, but rather an overlapping and interwoven presentation of the common characteristics of

Table 29-1	Comparison of Three Theories of the Grieving Process		
Engel (1964)	**Kübler-Ross (1969)**	**Rando (1991)**
Shock and disbelief	Denial	Avoidance
	Anger	
	Bargaining	
Developing awareness	Depression	Confrontation
Reorganization and restitution	Acceptance	Accommodation

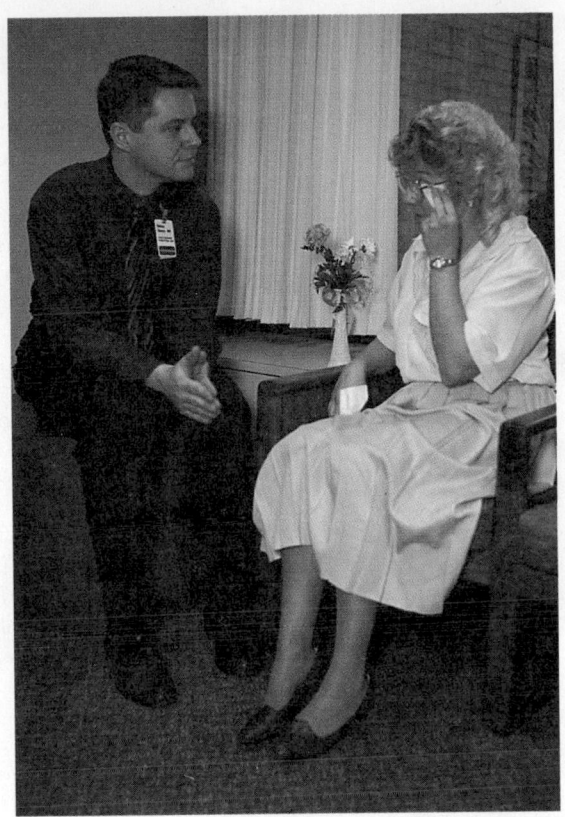

Figure 29-1   Nurses assist family members in finding resources to help with the grieving process.

grieving. The nurse must identify the experience for that client and not just classify the stages or phases experienced by the client or family.

Observation and anticipation of the phases of the grieving process guide the nurse's judgment to help the client work successfully through the grieving process. Behaviors can be best understood in relationship to these phases and should not be taken personally in any way. For example, Kübler-Ross's second stage is that of anger. The nurse should understand that the family is yelling at the nurse because they are upset. The human response is to yell back, but the nurse must try to set aside this urge, because nurses cannot remain therapeutic while yelling back at the family. Although emotions can run high at times, apologizing when one is out of line will help to maintain the therapeutic direction and show a human side. To avoid a knee-jerk reflex type of response, the nurse must stop and recognize these behaviors as those of coping mechanisms. The frustration of the dying client may bring up unresolved past issues that will never be resolved by the death of the client. The nurse must think critically to understand and to intervene appropriately by redirecting the anger to a healthy outlet. Awareness of these phases, then, guides the nurse in anticipating predictable behaviors and

preplanning interventions that might be needed to support effective coping skills and minimize dysfunctional behaviors. By giving support and sharing observations of the client and the family, the nurse can maximize successful coping strategies.

Engel's Theory.   Engel (1964) proposed that the grieving process has three phases that can be applied to grieving and dying persons. In the first phase the individual denies the reality of the loss and may withdraw, sit motionlessly, or wander aimlessly. It may seem to the observer that the person has not realized what the loss means. Physical reactions to death or grief may include the following: fainting, diaphoresis, nausea, diarrhea, rapid heart rate, restlessness, insomnia, and fatigue—all related to the fight-or-flight response, which is produced by increased epinephrine when one is under stress.

In the *second phase* the individual begins to feel the loss acutely and may experience desperation. Suddenly anger, guilt, frustration, depression, and emptiness occur. Crying is typical as the individual becomes preoccupied with the loss.

In the *third phase* the reality of the loss is acknowledged. Anger and depression are no longer needed. The loss is clear to the individual, who begins to reorganize life. By experiencing these phases, a person moves from a lower to a higher level of emotional and intellectual functioning. New self-awareness is developed. Therefore these experiences and growth through the grieving process become the basis from which to draw on for dealing with future losses.

Kubler-Ross's Stages of Dying.   The framework provided by Kübler-Ross (1969) focuses on behavior and includes five stages. In the denial stage individuals act as though nothing has happened and may refuse to believe that a loss has occurred. Statements such as "No, that can't be so," and "It can't be happening to me!" are common.

In the anger stage the individual resists the loss and may "act out" to everyone and everything in the environment. In the bargaining stage there is a postponement of the reality of the loss. The individual attempts to make deals in a subtle or overt manner to prevent the loss. The client frequently seeks opinions of others during this stage. A hospitalized client may show model behavior because of a belief that the staff will find a cure if he or she is a "good client."

The depression stage occurs when the loss is realized and the full impact of its significance is apparent. A person may feel overwhelming loneliness and withdrawal. The depression stage provides an opportunity to work through the loss and to begin problem solving.

The fifth stage begins with acceptance. Physiological reactions cease, and social interactions resume. Kübler-Ross defines acceptance as coming to terms with the situation rather than submitting to resignation or hopelessness.

Rando's Phases of Grieving.

Although the grieving process has a generally predictable course and distinctive symptoms, no two persons progress through it in the same way or over the same time. Some people move forward, regress, and then progress again during the grieving process until resolution of grief occurs. Therefore moving from one descriptor or category to another and back again is very common. Rando (1992-1993) refined the grieving responses into three categories: avoidance, confrontation, and accommodation. In avoidance, shock, denial, and disbelief of the loss occur. In **confrontation** the grieving client is in a highly charged emotional state, in which the client repeatedly faces his or her loss. The grief is most intense and felt most acutely during this second phase. **Accommodation** includes a gradual decline of acute grief and the beginning of an emotional and social reentry into the everyday world. At this point the client learns to live with the loss. To expect clients to progress in some specified manner over a specified time would be incorrect, inappropriate, and possibly harmful (Toth, 1997; Weissman and others, 1999).

• • •

Nursing implications based on Kübler-Ross's stages of dying and Rando's phases of grief are compared later in the chapter under nursing interventions.

According to Harper (1983), certain tasks are identified for facilitating a healthy recovery from a loss. The tasks do not have to be sequential and progressive in nature. They are often overlapping and fluid in nature. Thus the guidance of the family through the tasks can be individually applied to meet each situation. The acronym TEAR, described earlier, is used to describe the tasks that clients work through when coping with grief.

PSYCHOSOCIAL PERSPECTIVES OF LOSS AND GRIEF

Loss and death are universal for all living things. The nurse applies past experiences of losses to understand the feelings that come with a loss (Cairns, 1997). A human's sociological development offers a unique interpretation of life's experience. Death is an overwhelming experience that affects everyone involved in the loss situation or in the death of the individual. According to psychologists, the valuing of individuals is a unique, learned response of a specific culture and society (Binstock and Spector, 1997). Age, gender, status, race, religious beliefs, intellect, achievement, self-expression, and cultural opportunity (Box 29-3) are the basis for an individual to define and qualify the definition of life or death (Cressy, 1997). The nurse is a product of that environment and reflects many of the biases or perspectives gained during sociological development. Concepts, perspectives, and definitions of events of "loss" are described within a cultural bias of a specific society (Witoszek, 1998). Thus the norms for psychosocial patterns of loss and grief are reflected in the caregiver, as well as in the client with the loss.

Cultural ASPECTS OF CARE   Box 29-3

Interpretations of a loss vary greatly with cultural and ethnic backgrounds, in addition to socioeconomic, religious, and racial perspectives. An accurate assessment by the nurse includes therapeutically communicating a willingness to individualize the planned care to meet specific needs of the client and support system. Examples of questions that guide the assessment process are included in Table 29-2. The nurse must further assess the success of the grieving process, as well as the dysfunctional behaviors that indicate additional nursing management (see Box 29-2).

Rituals that are practiced before or at the time of death are further governed by religious practices and traditions within a family unit. For example, the practicing Catholic client would expect the priest to come to administer the "last rites" before death or as soon as possible after death. Jewish people have rituals about the time and date of the burial in relationship to the time of death and the day of the week. Other Jewish practices are very specific descriptors ranging from the type of wood used in the coffin to wooden nails used instead of metal nails. Issues about autopsy, limb disposal, and preservation of the body vary according to the ethnocultural background.

The support system or family is expected to behave a certain way to show value and respect for the client who died. Generally, in the Western hemisphere the grieving process is one that is personal and private, with little show of emotion. In Eastern nations the respect for the dead is shown by loud wailing and physical demonstration of grief for a specified time after the death. A further consideration includes the color of clothing worn both during and after the time of death. This is dictated by ethnocultural perspectives. Some individuals wear dark clothing, whereas others wear bright colors. The time-frame expectations for following these rituals are understood but may evolve with time. In the past, the widow would wear black for a year and then have a coming-out-of-mourning event to show her availability again. Today, this practice has become less formalized and shortened to a few months, without the physical dressing in dark or black clothing. The tradition of a "wake" includes the gathering of friends and family after the funeral to share collectively in grief while bringing food to the family experiencing the loss.

Even within the same ethnocultural background, individuals respond to loss and death to differing degrees. Therefore the challenge for the nurse dealing with these issues is to explore realistically and practically the desires of the client and the support system to clearly identify concepts and approaches for effective guidance through the loss experience.

An individual's expression of grief evolves as the person matures and as personal experiences shape the **coping mechanisms** that the individual uses to handle these stressors (Box 29-4). As psychologists frequently explain, the coping mechanisms that were effective in the past are repeated as a first response to the pain of the loss. When older coping strategies are unsuccessful, new coping

Factors influencing grief in older adults:
- Physical changes accompanying aging
- Loss of employment
- Loss of social respect
- Loss of relationships
- Loss of self-care capabilities
- Fear of loss of control
- Sense of fulfillment and contributions made
- Personality traits
- Feelings of self-worth
- Functional ability retained

mechanisms are attempted (see Chapter 30). Thus by repetition that is based on the successes and failures of different coping mechanisms, the client learns what is needed for his or her own coping when exposed to these losses. Sometimes the number or depths of losses become overwhelming, and familiar coping styles are not successful. Professional assistance is required to help the client and family understand and deal realistically with losses. Dysfunctional or disenfranchised grief develops when society has different expectations than the person experiencing the loss (Rando, 1992-1993). Thus the concepts surrounding the definition of death are, again, based on societal expectations and religious beliefs (Stepnick and Perry, 1992).

With more research and advancements in lifesaving technology, standards of care must be clarified regarding the subtleties of the definitions and characteristics of "life" and "death." These beginning or ending qualities of life must guide legal and ethical choices in health care and be the basis for modifying one's therapeutic approach as lifesaving advances are developed. Concepts are evolving; an abortion can be interpreted differently when technology validates a beating heart by the end of the first month (Catalano, 1995). Some might interpret abortion as murder from the day that the pregnancy is recognized. Others believe that a potential for viability, which occurs much later in the pregnancy, becomes the point at which the abortion does constitute a murder. Society does not take into consideration the individual's unique interpretation of life, and thus society, as a whole, forces the entire population group to follow the leaders who are the loudest in defining the process. The majority may or may not be the defining group. Therefore standards and ethical guidelines are established to guide the nurse in behaving in a professional manner during the loss. The establishment of ethical review boards (see Chapter 20) are mandatory to avoid individual choices that may be less than desirable by another's standards (Murphy, 1999). These boards give rulings of the preferred treatment or approach to manage the care, but in essence it is often the lesser of two evils that is involved. Usually someone will always be unhappy about

the management decision; therefore the client's management may or may not be that which is preferred by the nurse.

In coping with the stress of a loss, physical and mental stressors create a need for the body to adapt. The stimulation of stress responses implies that there is an imbalance in the body and that a threat to one's being has occurred. According to chemists and microbiologists, physical symptoms of stress are related to the fight-or-flight response, with the secretion of adrenaline and noradrenaline. Thus as stress continues, more physiological breakdowns occur, which impairs the overall immune response. When these stressors are not controlled or removed, they cause physical and mental illnesses. The prolonged imbalance and adaptation process experienced by the individual in reaction to the stressors will add additional stress, causing physical and mental changes (Stocker, 1994). To understand the effects of loss, it is important to also understand the stress response and its influence on health (see Chapter 30).

Nursing Knowledge Base

Nursing has traditionally focused on the acute care setting of the hospital, where losses are more physical in nature. As the nurse enters the home setting and the community, the definitions of losses are different. There are new challenges for complex applications of the nursing process wherein every client's situation is different. Solutions for these challenges will become future professional standards as they are validated through research (see Chapter 25).

The nurse must gather information from a multitude of sources to be able to comprehend the needs of the client or family or staff who is dealing with a loss. Dracup and Brown (1998) suggest approaches to asking difficult questions during a loss. Death experiences and individual interpretation are influenced by many factors and may vary according to different circumstances within a person's lifetime. Individualizing the plan of care is based on many other factors in addition to the actual loss experienced by the client or family. Past personal experiences with death or loss, differences between the client and the family in their stages of grief, communication skills and understanding through this process, specific psychological needs, and advancing technology are just a few factors for the nurse to effectively assess to plan for successful outcomes. Trends in terminal or end-of-life care and current legal guidelines direct the acceptable standards of practice that will further affect the plan of action (Murphy, 1999).

DEATH AS A UNIQUE EXPERIENCE
Death affects everyone who knows the dying client. Nurses become a part of that circle of acquaintances through a shared relationship during caregiving. The nurse shares in the loss by empathetic support of the client with newly diagnosed breast cancer or of the client who has given birth

to a child who is less than "perfect." The nurse must learn many values, beliefs, cultural backgrounds, and attitudes about life, death, or loss to be able to deal with the dying client and the client or family experiencing a loss. A personal understanding of these issues will minimize bias in situations where the values, beliefs, and practices vary from those of the client and family (see Chapter 7).

Despite age, gender, status, race, religious beliefs, intellect, achievement, self-expression, and cultural opportunity, the nurse must learn to find value in all clients. By recognizing any bias or preferences that might influence the choices made by the nurse, nursing becomes therapeutic rather than personal in preference (see Chapter 7). By using this understanding, alternatives and options can be openly explored to identify the client's actual needs versus the desired needs of the staff. Based on the client-focused and mutually decided goals, the nurse will accept and follow individualized interventions that are preferred by the dying client. The family's needs are considered, but it must be understood that the client is the primary person responsible for the choices made.

Often the family is at a different "stage" of grieving than the client. Conflicting desires may lead to confusion and delay in the grieving process for the client. By understanding the process of grief for both the family and the client, the nurse can be successful in helping both achieve appropriate grief work (Box 29-5).

COMMUNICATION

Communication is the basis for gathering accurate information regarding the perceptions and feelings of individual clients. Without a complete understanding of the facts, beliefs, and attitudes of the client, the nurse cannot identify the client's needs in an accurate manner. Presumptions and poor communication lead to an ineffective and nontherapeutic relationship in which the opportunity to assist in the grieving process is lost. Therapeutic communication identifies and directs the client's discussion to narrow it down to the needs valued by the client (see Chapter 22). In contrast, nontherapeutic conversations give the nurse only what the client thinks the nurse wants to hear. Inappropriate communication focuses on what the nurse wants and will rob the client of time to work through the loss. Communication includes many other areas in addition to the words that are used. Facial expressions, posture, inflections, lack of eye contact, and spacing are some of the nonverbal influences that result in incomplete information gathering. Inappropriate communication by the nurse and/or the client will result in a distraction from the real issues of grief work; precautions should be taken by the nurse to avoid blocks in communication that will delay or miss the key issues of the loss.

VALUES

Valuing of individuals and self-analysis will guide the nurse into an honest assessment of personal values that

---

Research HIGHLIGHT   **Box 29-5**

RESEARCH ABSTRACT

One of the most profound losses experienced by humans is the death of a spouse. The purposes of this report were to describe the grief experiences of older adults over the first 2 years after the death of their spouse and to compare these experiences with those of younger bereaved spouses. Emotional responses to the loss were similar. Two differences were noted: younger widows experienced a deep despair that was not described by older spouses, and younger spouses experienced feelings of disorganization accompanied by feelings of diminished capacity and fear of emotional breakdown that older spouses did not describe. Perhaps older spouses felt it was acceptable to acknowledge shock and sadness, but despair or fear of breakdown may have had different, more threatening meanings for them. Recommendations for how nurses can meet the needs of bereaved older adults were made.

IMPLICATIONS FOR PRACTICE

- Older bereaved spouses present a unique challenge to nurses, owing to the catastrophic nature of the loss and the complexities of the concerns facing older people in general.
- Acknowledgment of persistent, painful emotions months and years after the loss legitimizes these feelings and may enhance self-acceptance if the feelings are recognized as normal.
- An awareness that older people may be more reluctant to discuss their feelings suggests that nurses must encourage clients to do so by giving permission and making themselves available to the bereaved.

REFERENCE

Anderson KL, Dimond MF: The experience of bereavement in older adults, *J Adv Nurs* 22:308, 1995.

---

might interfere with judgment as a nurse. By opening up to other values, the genuine, sensitive, and honest approach desired toward the client will be easily obtained through directed communications. An inner strength in the nurse allows the nurse to develop the art of being with the grieving and dying. Lack of understanding about oneself will bring in personal bias and values that may be in conflict with those of the client. Perceptions and anticipation must also be based on the client's perspectives of the situation and not on what the nurse guesses to be the problem when no facts are used to support the false conclusion (see Chapter 20). The nurse must be willing to risk involvement with the dying client to be able to share personally with the client and family during this time of loss. Without involvement the nurse is perceived as "cold" and "unfeeling" or "unwilling" to get involved. Often the client views certain topics as taboo and then avoids initiating certain topics to make the nurse feel comfortable in the loss. Personal issues should be initiated by the nurse to help work through the grief process.

ETHICAL ISSUES

Increasing technology in the field of health care is changing the expectations and quality of life and death that can be chosen by clients. Clients' lives can be extended, but often the quality of life becomes sacrificed. Informing clients of legal rights and choices becomes a critical area in nursing documentation to validate the exact choices discussed and the options preferred by the client. Some of the moral and ethical issues faced by today's nurse includes the following: When does "life" or "death" occur? What is death? Who is valued or not valued in society? When does self-determination begin and end? Who can choose the time of one's own death? These are a few of the issues that ethical review boards for health care facilities are wrestling with on an increasingly frequent basis. Many are deciding the choices, not by what is right or wrong, but by which choice is the "lesser of two evils," or "for the greater good of many" (see Chapter 20).

Critical Thinking Synthesis

Successful critical thinking requires a synthesis of knowledge, experiences with loss and grief, and information gathered from clients. Attitudes and intellectual and professional standards should be considered during this process. Clinical judgments require the nurse to anticipate the information necessary, analyze the data, and make decisions regarding client care. Critical thinking is crucial in the application of the nursing process. The application of new data in determining client outcomes is evaluated continually as the nurse focuses on existing problems. During assessment (Figure 29-2) the nurse must consider all elements that build toward making appropriate nursing diagnoses. To understand the process of grief and its impact on the client and family, the nurse must integrate knowledge from nursing and other disciplines, previous experiences, and information gathered from the client and family. In addition, the use of critical thinking attitudes such as perseverance is needed to develop a plan of care to provide successful grief work. Professional standards are based on research outcomes of various agencies. A few agencies that help develop new guidelines for grief work include the following: the Agency for Health Care Policy and Research (AHCPR), the World Health Organization (WHO) and the National Institute for Environmental Health of the National Institutes of Health (NIH), as well as other private research agencies.

Figure 29-2 illustrates the critical thinking model as it applies during the assessment phase by showing the relationship of various components in loss or grief (Paul, Wilsen, and Binker, 1993). The assessment process begins with increasing awareness of components that guide the outcome of grief work. Components illustrated in the assessment phase include knowledge, past experiences, standards, and attitudes, which are assimilated during the nurse's assessment activities. Without the supporting categories the central focus of the nursing assessment becomes incomplete and may lead the nurse to an inadequate conclusion concerning the client's needs. The nurse's past experiences, such as personal loss of a family member or caring for a client in a full-leg cast (with loss of independence), help in understanding a client who is experiencing a similar loss. Knowledge of the stages of grief, intellectual standards, and critical thinking attitudes will increase awareness for the nurse, enabling the nurse to better empathize with the family and client. Through identification of the various stages or concepts of grief and loss according to theorists, the nurse is able to direct the assessment process. Clustering of data will then point to the client's individualized problems. Therefore the nurse can anticipate needs and prepare clients and family members as assessment data are gathered by relating experience and knowledge from a previous situation to the current one.

The Nursing Process and Grief

ASSESSMENT

During assessment the nurse should not assume how or if the client or family experiences grief. The nurse should avoid assuming that a particular behavior indicates grief; rather, the nurse should allow persons to share what is happening in their own way. Perceptions of loss may vary greatly even within the same societal norms. The critical thinking model for assessment illustrates the impact of past experiences, previously learned skills, and coping patterns of the individual that can be brought into the current situation for use as a database for the application of the nursing process during a client's loss.

Assessment of the client and family begins by exploring the meaning of the loss to the individuals involved. Examples of topics to be explored include personal characteristics, the nature of family relationships, support systems, the nature of the loss, cultural and spiritual beliefs, life goals, hope, the phase of grief, the family, risks, and nursing role perceptions (Table 29-2). Many variables affect grief. Consideration of the variables gives the nurse a broad database from which to individualize the plan of care. Examples are meant to be only a beginning guide for database collection.

The nurse interviews the client and family, using honest, open communication by emphasizing listening skills and observing responses and behaviors from a neutral perspective. Impressions are summarized and validated with the client and family so that nursing diagnoses can be made. Other health care workers contribute to the database from which problems are identified and the plan of care is directed. The nurse assesses how the client *is* reacting rather than how the client *should be* reacting. The sequencing of stages or behaviors of grief may occur in order, they may be skipped, or they may reoccur, as explained in the section on theories of grief. Therefore the identification of expected phases should be used only to

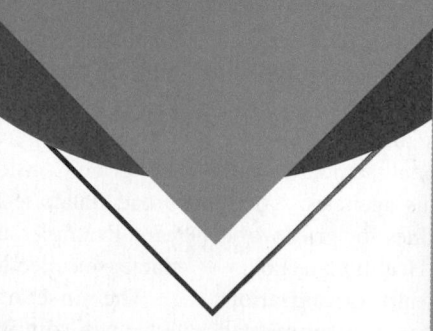

KNOWLEDGE

- Grief process
- Pathophysiology of related illness threatening a loss
- Therapeutic communications principles
- Cultural perspectives on the meaning of loss/death
- Family dynamics in offering social support
- Concepts of caring

STANDARDS

- Apply the principles outlined in the dying person's Bill of Rights
- Demonstrate the ethical principles of health care
- Apply intellectual standards of significance; know what is important to the client

ASSESSMENT

- Assess meaning of loss for this client
- Observe behaviors and other symptoms indicative of grief response
- Note quality and extent of client's family support

EXPERIENCE

- Caring for a client who experienced a physical or emotional loss
- Caring for a client who died
- Personal experience with loss or death of a significant other

ATTITUDES

- Take risks if necessary to develop a close relationship with the client to understand loss

Figure 29-2   *Synthesis Model for Loss, Death, and Grieving Assessment Phase.*

Table 29-2 Assessment Factors for Grieving Client

Factors	Areas/Suggested Questions to Explore
Personal characteristics	Age, sex role, education, socioeconomic status *Examples:* What is a child's response to the loss? What is an older adult's life satisfaction? What spiritual beliefs do you relate to death? Does the age of the dying make a difference? How do you expect your life to change with the loss of your leg? Arm? Breast? Child? How does the gender of the client affect the response to death as described by society? What resources do clients have to cope with a loss (e.g., medical insurance, costs for schooling)?
Nature of relationships	Functions of family, community, society *Examples:* How long have you known the dying client? What role did the dying client play in your family? What is your relationship? Will it change? What contributions have been made by the client? How do you interpret the potential loss? By the client? By the significant other? How will family relationships change as a result of the loss?
Social support system	Availability of health care workers, timing, family needs *Examples:* Who is present? Absent? Supportive? Nonsupportive? Are they always actually available or do they just say, "Call me if you need me"? Are they helpful, or do they avoid the issues offered for discussion by the client? Do they use a listening ear approach rather than a judgmental approach? Is the client's self-esteem built up and supported?
Nature of loss	Death issues: personal, family, or community; private or group; actual versus perceived; functional versus dysfunctional or disenfranchised; recognized or not by society *Examples:* What is your belief about death? How do you define death? Define the loss in your own terms. What factors will help you grieve? What factors will interfere with grieving? What support does the grieving significant other have? Are these persons available when needed? What past experiences have you had? Outcomes? What has helped you cope in the past? What has not? Can you identify coping behaviors?
Cultural and spiritual beliefs	Values, practices, customs, attitudes, clergy, spiritualist *Examples:* How is this person valued based on spiritual and cultural expectations? How does the loss of a limb change this valuing? How does the client or significant other perceive physical death? Meaning of life? How should the body (or part) be treated when removed? What traditions are required to show value of all life? Can religious practices interfere with medical treatment? Who has the right to say "yes" or "no"? Legally? Ethically? Can the court interfere?
Loss of personal life goals	Actual or perceived individual losses affecting future decisions and options *Examples:* What is your goal in life for. . . . ? How was this changed with this diagnosis? Surgery? How have things changed since the accident (e.g., an automobile accident causing permanent quadriplegia)? How will your role change your personal goals? What planning has occurred for your own life? How does your perception of the problem differ from the client's view?

Continued

Table 29-2 **Assessment Factors for Grieving Client**—cont'd	
Factors	Areas/Suggested Questions to Explore

Hope	Goals, worth, adaptations to future changes
	Examples:
	  What do you expect now that. . . . ?
	  How do you feel about yourself?
	  Tell me what you will do now that. . . . ?
	  What do you expect to help you through this. . . . ?

Phases of grief	Relate to a theorist: Kübler-Ross, Engel, Rando
	Examples:
	  Use assessment to classify behavioral theory
	  Contrast the stage of the client to the stage of the significant other
	  Validate feelings expressed in emotions:
	    You seem angry, tell me more about. . . .
	    You seem sad; tell me. . . .
	    What are your feelings about. . . . ?

Family's grief for dying client	Relationships, involvement with dying process
	Examples:
	  Observation of client and family's level of grieving, patterns, rank of leadership, and power
	    person
	  What has helped you deal with problems in the past? What has not helped?
	  What do you perceive as your strength? Weakness?

Risk factors in survivors	High risk, such as sudden death, violent death, length of processes, or loss of a child
	Examples:
	  Prior and subsequent variables: ambivalence, dependence, marked emotions, unresolved
	    issues, mental health problems, mourners' perception of the lack of social support
	  Describe your feelings. Your grieving processes.
	  Who has helped you the most?
	  What are your feelings?
	  Could you really have prevented this?
	  Are you feeling guilty because . . . ?
	  What did you use for early interventions with this problem, and were they helpful?

Nursing role in grief	Stage of nurse's grief, role perceived by nurse, role perceived by client and family, neutral support, therapeutic communication
	Examples:
	  What stage of grief am I in? Am I blaming myself?
	  What could I have done differently?
	  I am really sorry that . . . (acknowledging the loss).
	  How do you see me helping you?
	  Do I need to consult others for better support?

guide the nurse and not to judge the outcomes of the grieving process. Simply classifying a stage of grief will not correct the problem. The application of the theorists' phases will aid in the accurate assessment of the situation. Therefore the nurse can anticipate characteristics or responses during a phase of grieving and be able to plan ahead or educate a client about future expectations.

Psychological and physiological assessment skills are used to gather a complete database about a client and/or family in a loss situation. Inductive and deductive reasoning is needed to analyze the data cues obtained through

assessment (see Chapters 13 and 14). Refining the ability to make judgments through critical thinking involves intellectual and emotional growth that evolve by acquiring new knowledge. Commitment and accountability to oneself and the profession will direct new experiences. Both interviewing and physical assessment skills guide the nurse in the roles of advocate, caregiver, and teacher. Clear guidelines for professional behaviors are reflected by nursing standards for specific situations and state law. These standards of care describe the highest quality desired, but autonomy of the nurse allows for adaptation of these standards to individual needs. Critical thinking skills become the key to addressing the problems to be resolved by the nursing process. The nursing diagnosis, interventions, and evaluation are all guided by ongoing assessments of the situation (see Unit 3).

Client Expectations.   The client expects an accurate assessment of the situation that is based on sound nursing judgment and the application of critical thinking skills. The client expects the nurse to listen with open ears and be able to integrate clues and interpret facts given when the client is under the nurse's care. The assessments are client focused and specific for clear identification of needs. The client further expects the staff to understand and support the significant others involved in the loss. Therefore the client's death does not end the nursing process; the nurse's assessments change focus to the significant others as the nurse's new client.

In the assessment phase the client's expectations of the nurse may vary greatly. In most cases the client and the family desire a compassionate nurse who assists in the recognition of the emotions and feelings associated with the loss and in the application of resources to minimize the problems that can occur with the loss. Furthermore, the nurse is expected to retain dignity and uniqueness in the care of the dying client. To meet these expectations, an accurate assessment must be continually validated by the family and the client. Open, honest, and therapeutic communication must be emphasized at all times through humble and creative approaches (Paul, Willsen, and

Binker, 1993). Establishing rapport and continuing in the support of the client and family is expected. Perseverance and risk of self-involvement during assessments must be considered by the nurse, who must forego his or her own values while helping the client and family (Paul, Willsen, and Binker, 1993). Clients expect a comfortable death or loss that they have been able to participate in by verbalizing desires within options given by state/federal guidelines. Fairness and equality of care despite specific individual characteristics should be expected despite all of the following characteristics: race, creed, nationality, and religion (Paul, Willsen, and Binker, 1993).

NURSING DIAGNOSIS

Based on the nurse's conclusions during the assessment phase, the nurse identifies a nursing diagnosis that accurately reflects needs exhibited by the client or family experiencing the loss (Paul, Willsen, and Binker, 1993; Kim, McFarland, and McLane, 1997). Critical thinking skills are the tools used to apply concepts of assessment, clustering of cues, and drawing a conclusion of the actual or perceived needs of the client. The nurse will cluster defining characteristics and identify the nursing diagnosis applicable to the client's situation (Box 29-6). Goals and outcomes are based on the nursing diagnosis. Without accurate identification of diagnoses based on the client's database, the actual client needs may not be met by the nurse. In turn, planned interventions will be inadequate to meet the needs of the client or family if the nursing diag-

---

SAMPLE NURSING DIAGNOSTIC PROCESS   Box 29-6

GRIEVING

Assessment Activities	Defining Characteristics	Nursing Diagnoses
Observe client's nonverbal behavior when discussing loss.	Client becomes silent and looks away when topic of loss is raised.	Dysfunctional grieving related to loss of health and terminal illness.
Ask client and family to discuss their understanding of loss situation.	Client and family believe that illness is minor and client will fully recover.	
Observe client's behavior related to treatment.	Client attempts activities prohibited by physical condition and refuses to follow prescribed treatment.	
Assess daily activity level.	Client reports difficulty in sleeping, decreased appetite, and difficulty in concentrating.	
Assess ability to perform roles.	Client withdraws from usual decision-making role in family.	
Ask client to discuss future goals and plans.	Client sighs and says, "I have no future."	Hopelessness related to failing physical condition.
Observe client's nonverbal behavior.	Client becomes passive with little affect and turns away from speaker.	
Offer client choices and observe responses.	Client shrugs and says, "What does it matter?"	
Assess activity level.	Client refuses to eat. Client sleeps all the time, keeping blinds pulled and lights out. Client refuses to participate in care.	

nosis is not applicable in this loss. Whether an actual loss or a perceived loss has occurred, the client's behaviors and statements will direct the identification of the need that leads to the nursing diagnosis (Box 29-7).

Accurate validation of each diagnosis will result in an individualized plan of care that is more likely to meet the actual needs of the client or family experiencing a loss (see care plan). The care plan emphasizes the unique characteristics of grief and the reaction to the loss as defined by the particular client. Examples of nursing diagnoses for the client, family, and community (or group) are given in Box 29-7. Each nursing diagnosis is uniquely applied to only the specific circumstance at a client's specific stage of illness or loss. In addition, the goals of care derived from the nursing diagnoses will further guide the evaluation process. Listing specific outcome criteria will guide the interventions and the validation of the goals that were accomplished in helping the client to adapt to a loss.

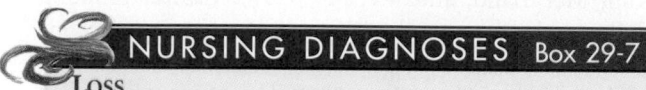

NURSING DIAGNOSES Box 29-7
Loss

Individual
Anxiety
Coping, defensive
Denial, ineffective
Grieving, dysfunctional
Hopelessness
Personal identity disturbance
Powerlessness
Self-esteem disturbance
Spiritual distress (distress of the human spirit)
Thought processes, altered

Family
Caregiver role strain
Coping, ineffective family: compromised
Coping, ineffective family: disabling
Decisional conflict
Home maintenance management, impaired
Hopelessness
Management of therapeutic regimen, families: ineffective
Role performance, altered
Self-care deficit, bathing/hygiene
Self-care deficit, dressing/grooming
Self-care deficit, feeding
Self-care deficit, toileting
Self-esteem, situational low

Community or a Specific Group of People
Community coping, ineffective
Denial, ineffective
Fear
Knowledge deficit
Management of therapeutic regimen, community: ineffective
Posttrauma syndrome
Violence, risk for: self-directed or directed at others

Behavioral symptoms of dysfunctional grief are given in Box 29-2. Exaggerated or prolonged grief responses should be identified. It is also important for the nurse to identify the appropriate related factors for the diagnosis. For example, *dysfunctional grieving related to the loss of a spouse* will require different interventions than *dysfunctional grieving related to the loss of a job and declining health* (Kim, McFarland, and McLane, 1997). The primary nursing diagnosis is based on the defining characteristics identified to support the need of the problem.

One example would be when the nurse identifies the nursing diagnosis as *sleep pattern disturbance related to the fears of "bad dreams" and the loss of a spouse* and defining characteristics include symptoms of fatigue, verbal reports of dreams and not sleeping, and a change in appetite. If the nurse presumed that not sleeping after the death of a spouse was a normal behavior, the nurse would not identify sleeping as a need to be addressed. Therefore the nurse's valuing and knowledge (or lack thereof) about grieving would lead to a conclusion that was not unique to the client. If the factors were not identified in relationship to the loss, then other conclusions would be inaccurately made. For example, the nurse may presume that the lack of sleep was due to other factors such as a change in job, move, financial stressors, change in routine, or other lifestyle modifications, and not related to the loss. The nurse's presumption would be caused by inadequate data collection or a preconceived conclusion that was unrelated to the actual need of the client. Therefore with an inadequate database the nurse might inappropriately refer the client to financial aid or a life management class, rather than dealing with the real issue of the loss. If the nurse had jumped to other conclusions before assessing the actual facts for the client, the nurse would have missed the concept that the spouse's death was causing the fears and the dreams. Therefore the planned interventions would focus not on the real needs of the client, but on the preconceived and inaccurate guess of the nurse.

When identifying nursing diagnoses for the dying client, other problems are identified separately according to specific standards of care for the dying client. Other nursing diagnoses can include areas such as *body image disturbance, impaired physical mobility related to pain,* or *altered role performance.* More physical nursing diagnoses are formed when the client is closer to death and might include the following: *altered urinary elimination and/or bowel incontinence, pain, sensory/perceptual alterations,* and *ineffective breathing pattern.* Successful recovery is not always an expected outcome. The comfort of the dying and the acceptance of the dying process by the family are realistic expectations for the nurse to deal with in the dying situation. With terminal illness, physical assessment of the dying process is ongoing to continue to adapt or validate the actual needs with the changing condition of the client.

PLANNING

Grieving is a natural response to loss, and it has a therapeutic value. It enables people to work through their losses by recollecting their thoughts and feelings as pleasant memories, and it enables people to resume life after adaptation with new insights and direction (Paul, Willsen, and Binker, 1993). The application of critical thinking through exploration, valuing, and organization of data helps to prioritize and emphasize clues given in assessment. Figure 29-3 illustrates the interrelatedness of critical thinking factors during the planning phase of the nursing process. Areas summarized include the knowledge base, attitudes, past experiences, and standards used in the planning of activities.

The nurse's knowledge base includes identification of potential resources that will aid the grieving process, including available organizations, staff, agencies, spiritual or cultural experts, and other factors that would help the client in loss. The standards section of the critical thinking model pulls from guidelines learned to assist in maximizing the outcomes of the client's physical or mental management. Standards are focused on the following: basic care, comfort, privacy, safety, moral and ethical prioritizations of management, and an obligation to the client first, as well as individual choice. Professional standards guide the quality and direction of care for the individual. Attitudes by a client, family, and staff should include a realistic expectation of hope and/or a comfortable death. Open and honest communication is therapeutic to identification and satisfaction of needs. Misconceptions and ignorance of outcomes are avoided by clear understanding on the part of all involved. Past loss experiences of clients, families, and nurses must be analyzed to give insights to responses to the current loss. Sharing of fears by the client should be encouraged by the nurse. Therefore the critical thinking model of planning should guide the mutual decision-making process through therapeutic communication to adapt expectations and apply skills to maintain dignity and self-esteem for a specific client in a specific loss situation.

The potential for ongoing problem identification is vast, and without continuous validation with the client or family experiencing the loss, the nurse would waste time and resources and not meet the current needs of the client (see Chapter 13). Therefore nursing care plans are developed based on realistic goals that are mutually set by the client, family, staff, and other health care workers. The nursing care plan gives direction and depth to interventions suggested to meet the goals of the plan.

General nursing goals for clients with a loss include accommodating grief, accepting the reality of the loss, regaining a sense of self-esteem, and renewing regular activities or relationships that were typical for the client. Physiological, developmental, cultural, psychological, and spiritual needs are the basis for these goals. The nurse

must be tolerant and accept a willingness to spend more time with a dying client, to listen to expressions of grief, and to individualize care to improve quality of life. Without this involvement by the nurse, the client's needs will go unmet.

Pain control, dignity and self-worth preservation, and love and affection are three crucial needs of the dying client. Goals suggested based on these needs could include maintaining comfort; encouraging independence, choice, and hope; establishing or maintaining spiritual comfort; and avoiding isolation (Box 29-8). The nurse's role includes participation to reduce anxiety, ensure feelings of security and worth, and to control the environment for the client. Encouragement and availability can be given to the significant others, which will further ensure that the client has confidence in the caregiver. Anticipation of and assistance with choices by the nurse are expected to relieve the client's and family's concerns and minimize surprises. The client will expect a unique approach to dealing with his or her needs to allow a greater satisfaction in outcomes. Without a clear understanding of the client and family's desires, the nurse will miss the valued issues and leave the client's family or client feeling that the staff was ineffective.

Interdisciplinary teams are helpful to assist in identifying and meeting the needs of those who experience losses. Dietitians, clergy, physicians, social workers, psychologists, and other specialty health care workers can assist in meeting a client's needs. A coordinated group approach to management of a client's needs reassures that little is left to chance or forgotten by a busy nurse. In addition, the loss experienced by the nurse (and others) can be shared with others and support the healing for all who worked with the dying client. However, the client remains the key team member and will direct and decide preferred treatment until he or she is no longer able to participate. Based on the client's wishes, the team can remain as an advocate to follow the client's wishes, even when the client can no longer speak for himself or herself. Emotional stressors increase in all participants of the team. The successful achievement of the desired goals for the dying client is shared according to individual expertise. Conflicts and differences can be openly discussed and solutions found in a healthy manner with the client as the primary focus. By working together, the sharing of experiences, feelings, al-

---

Goals for the Dying Client   Box 29-8

Gaining and maintaining comfort
Maintaining independence in daily activities
Maintaining hope
Achieving spiritual comfort
Gaining relief from loneliness and isolation

SAMPLE NURSING CARE PLAN

GRIEF AND LOSS

ASSESSMENT*

The nurse admits Mr. Miller, a 40-year-old man, from the emergency department to the intensive care unit with a massive my-ocardial infarction after he collapsed at a tennis match. He has had no previous cardiac episodes but does have a family history of severe cardiovascular disease. The **terminal prognosis has been explained by the physician.** As the nurse continues to give updates on his condition to the wife, **the wife asks, "Will he be OK? I am sure that he will be better; his brother recovered from a heart attack!"** She does **not exhibit any understanding** of the seriousness of his condition and the futility of recovery from this exten-sive damage to the heart. The wife calls her husband's office and **reassures them that he will be back in a few weeks. She also con-tinues to make calls to plan a business dinner party later in the week.** The staff have explained organ donation and have tried to encourage her to make a decision about such, but **she keeps saying, "He will be fine, that's not important right now!"**

*Defining characteristics are shown in bold type.

NURSING DIAGNOSIS: Dysfunctional grieving related to husband's sudden illness and absence of expected anticipatory grief.

PLANNING

GOALS

Client's wife will accept impending death of client within 48 hours.

Client's wife will demonstrate effective grieving characteristics.

EXPECTED OUTCOMES

Wife will verbalize within the next 6 hours that death is actu-ally impending.

Wife will not deny reality of loss while waiting.

Wife will make a decision about organ donation within the next 12 hours.

Wife will state several immediate lifestyle changes that will oc-cur as a result of client's hospitalization and death.

Wife will demonstrate feelings of sadness and exhibit anticipa-tory loss within the next 24 hours.

Wife will demonstrate characteristics of grieving as related to theory, such as Kübler-Ross's stages of grief: denial, anger, bargaining, and acceptance.

INTERVENTIONS†

Presence

- Display interest in wife's situation and accept her behaviors of denial.

- Establish trust and a positive regard by creating an atmos-phere of sharing. Offer privacy and security.

Grief Work Facilitation

- Offer encouragement to explore and verbalize feelings of grief.

- Identify personal coping strategies used in the past; evalu-ate effectiveness and offer as needed.

- Include resources of community support: significant other, family, clergy, or other health care workers.

RATIONALE

Recognizing denial (*based on* Kübler-Ross's theory) gives the staff direction for planning unique interventions based on theory (Cressy, 1997).

Loss is directed by psychosocial, spiritual, and cultural expec-tations (Hepburn, 1994).

Privacy offers a place of security to exhibit personal needs and to work through feelings (McLean, 1999). Anxiety about los-ing self-esteem will hinder an honest expression of feelings (McLean, 1999). Rapport is based on mutual trust (Rando, 1986).

Encouragement refocuses on current needs and minimizes dysfunctional adaptation behaviors by facilitating resolution of grief by increasing problem-solving skills (Braza, 1993).

Previously successful coping strategies are the first to be used when one is under stress (Cressy, 1997). Discouraging mal-adaptive behaviors will minimize dysfunctional grieving (Lendhardt, 1997b).

Professionals can use their expertise and skills to direct the grieving process (Catalono, 1995). Trust and relationships already formed will speed the therapeutic communication process (Stocker, 1994).

†Intervention Classification labels from McCloskey JC, Bulechek GM: *Nursing interventions classification (NIC),* ed 3, St. Louis, 2000, Mosby.

SAMPLE NURSING CARE PLAN—cont'd

GRIEF AND LOSS

INTERVENTIONS†—cont'd	RATIONALE
Family • Answer wife's support questions in a nonthreatening and unbiased manner. • Encourage wife to become involved and talk with spouse even if she gets no response; give wife permission to grieve.	Exploration of potential reality allows better-informed choices (Cairns, 1997). Involvement gives the family something tangible to minimize feelings of hopelessness or helplessness (Rando, 1984). Hearing is considered the last sense to leave before death, and saying "good-bye" helps to move to closure of the grieving process (Engel, 1964).

†Intervention classification labels from McCloskey JC, Bulechek GM: *Nursing interventions classification (NIC)*, ed 3, St. Louis, 2000, Mosby.

EVALUATION

Plan a conversation for wife to discuss her feelings about what has happened to her husband.
Within several hours explore with wife her interest in organ donation.
Give wife the opportunity during a conversation to openly grieve.
Ask if wife is ready to explore funeral arrangements with clergy and staff.

---

ternatives, and solutions becomes the basis for dealing with future loss situations. Planning for referral then becomes the key to minimizing an overloaded, emotional situation for the nurse.

IMPLEMENTATION

Nursing management includes different levels of health care, including health promotion, health care in the acute care setting, and health care during the restorative and rehabilitation phases. To deliver the client's plan of care appropriately, the nurse must consider all levels of health. Maslow's hierarchy of needs can guide the prioritization of needs. Health promotion issues can be addressed by increasing family members awareness that unspoken needs are not silly or bad. Stressors that are commonly felt and the depression seen in grieving can be understood when others share the same feelings. Health promotion also includes giving clients and families skills to adapt to loss, including stress management activities, education about definitions of wellness, coping strategies, and available community resources. Both public and private organizations can help various age-groups to adapt to loss, including the White Rose Group for families whose infant has died at birth, Building Bridges for parents and children who have experienced the loss of a family member, Reach for Recovery for clients with mastectomies, Parents Without Partners for the widowed and/or divorced, and hospice for a client anticipating death. A major role of the nurse is to clearly review community resources to direct the options available to individual clients.

In the acute care setting, interventions are focused on the direct care of the client who has either experienced a loss or is facing death, whereas the restorative phase of care focuses on longer-term goals. Rehabilitation in the restorative phase is the maximization of remaining strengths of the client. Success of implementation should focus on the client's feeling better about the loss and adapting behaviors to be able to return to the community (family) after a role change.

A sensitivity to the client is important if the nurse is to function effectively. Nurses need to be sensitive to the culture, ethnicity, lifestyle, and social class of the client and family. Nurses must also be sensitive to the limits and nature of their role as perceived by the client and family. Teaching the family various skills will meet the family's need to be useful and involved in the loss experience (Box 29-9). Interventions and skills should be used appropriately for each client problem (Tables 29-3 and 29-4). When the nurse limits his or her availability and is not willing to invest in a relationship with a client, the nurse fails to become aware of his or her own needs (Doka, 1993). If the nurse is unwilling or unable to give assistance, then the role of the nurse becomes dysfunctional and this will hinder the healing process, since individual needs are not identified and interventions are not planned specifically for the dying client. If the nurse tries to continue in a relationship in which he or she does not feel comfortable, the feelings of failure by the nurse will affect other grief responses. In addition, the client will feel the strain and ask less of the nurse who seems to be having difficulty, even when a need is there.

Therapeutic Communication.   Nursing care of the grieving client and family begins with establishing the significance of the loss. This is difficult if the client is unwilling or unable to express feelings or is experiencing shock or denial. The nurse observes the response to loss and then attempts to identify the client's strengths in dealing with it. The nurse uses open-ended questions and reflective statements to give his or her observations validity (see Chapter 22). Open-ended questions will allow the client to speak

KNOWLEDGE

- Spirituality as a resource for dealing with loss
- Role other health professions play in helping clients deal with loss
- Services provided by community agencies
- Principles of providing comfort

STANDARDS

- Provide privacy for the client and family
- Apply ethical principles of autonomy in supporting the client's choice regarding treatment
- Individualize therapies for the client's self-esteem
- Apply appropriate professional standards for end-of-life care

PLANNING

- Select communication strategies that assist the client/family in accepting and adapting to loss
- Select interventions designed to maintain the client's dignity and self-esteem
- Provide skills/knowledge for the family to manage and understand care for the dying client

EXPERIENCE

- Previous client responses to planned nursing interventions for pain management or loss of a significant other

ATTITUDES

- Be responsible for delivering high-quality supportive care
- Demonstrate an openess to participate in experiencing the loss

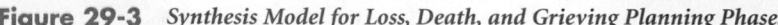

Figure 29-3   *Synthesis Model for Loss, Death, and Grieving Planning Phase.*

Client Teaching FOR THE DYING CLIENT'S FAMILY

Box 29-9

OBJECTIVE
- Family will be able to demonstrate basic client care measures.

TEACHING STRATEGIES
- Describe and demonstrate feeding techniques and selection of foods to facilitate ease of chewing and swallowing.
- Demonstrate bathing, mouth care, and other hygiene measures, and allow family to perform return demonstration.
- Show a video on simple transfer techniques to prevent injury to themselves and the client; help family to practice.
- Instruct family on need to enforce rest periods.

- Teach family to recognize signs and symptoms to expect as the client's condition worsens and information on whom to call in an emergency.
- Discuss ways to support the dying person and listen to needs and fears.
- Solicit questions from family and provide information as needed.

EVALUATION
- Family will perform client care independently.
- Observe family and client interacting using effective communication skills.

Table 29-3 Promoting Comfort in the Terminally Ill Client

Characteristics or Causes	Nursing Implications
Pain	
Pain can be acute or chronic.	Administer narcotic analgesics on regular schedule (see Chapter 42).
Pain from progressive cancer is usually chronic and constant.	Use relaxation, guided imagery, distraction, and peripheral nerve stimulators to provide relief.
	Use combinations of analgesics or other therapies as client's needs change.
	Administer narcotics as ordered. (Oral route for narcotics is preferred, but rectal suppositories, injections, continuous intravenous infusions, and intrathecal infusions are available.)
Any source of physical irritation may worsen pain.	Minimize irritants through skin care, including daily baths, lubrication of skin, frequent repositioning, and dry, clean bed linens.
As client approaches death, mouth remains open, tongue becomes dry and edematous, and lips become dry and cracked.	Provide frequent oral care every 2 to 4 hours. Use soft toothbrushes or foam swabs for frequent mouth care. Apply light film of petroleum jelly to lips and tongue (see Chapter 38).
Blinking reflexes diminish near death, causing drying of cornea.	Remove crusts from eyelid margins and provide eye care. Reduce corneal drying with artificial tears.
Nausea and Vomiting	
Nausea and vomiting result from disease process (e.g., gastric cancer), complications (e.g., bowel obstruction), or medications.	Confer with physician about changing medications when possible. Administer antiemetic before meals. Ask physician about providing relief from obstruction with bowel decompression with insertion of nasogastric tube. Provide mouth care and promptly clean up emesis.
Fatigue	
Metabolic demands of cancerous tumor cause weakness and fatigue.	Set mutual goals with client after identifying valued or desired tasks, and conserve client's energy for only those tasks. Provide frequent rest periods in quiet environment. Time and pace nursing activities to conserve client's energy.
Constipation	
Narcotic medications and immobility slow peristalsis.	Provide preventive care, including increasing fluid intake (e.g., bran, whole grain products, and fresh vegetables in diet) and encouraging exercise.
Lack of bulk in diet or reduced fluid intake may occur with appetite changes.	

Continued

Table 29-3   **Promoting Comfort in the Terminally Ill Client**—cont'd

Characteristics or Causes	Nursing Implications
Diarrhea Diarrhea results from disease process (e.g., colon cancer) and complications of treatment or medications.	Assess for fecal impaction. Confer with physician to change medication if possible. Provide low-residue diet.
Urinary Incontinence Urinary incontinence results from progressive disease (e.g., involvement of spinal cord or reduced level of consciousness).	Protect skin from irritation or breakdown using absorbent pads and clean linen. Prepare for possible use of indwelling urinary or condom catheter.
Inadequate Nutrition Nausea and vomiting can decrease appetite. Depression from grieving may cause anorexia.	Suggest that smaller portions and bland foods may be more palatable. Allow home-cooked meals, which may be preferred by client and gives family chance to participate.
Dehydration As disease progresses, client is less willing or able to maintain oral fluid intake. Certain forms of cancer cause obstruction to portions of gastrointestinal tract.	Provide relief of thirst by using ice chips, sips of fluids, or moist cloth to lips. Provide frequent mouth care.
Ineffective Breathing Patterns Causes include disease progression involving lung tissue capacity, pneumonia, and pulmonary edema. Clients may also be severely anemic, causing reduced oxygen capacity.	Position client upright to improve breathing capacity. Administer supplemental oxygen as ordered. Administer bronchodilator as ordered. Administer narcotics as ordered to suppress cough and ease breathing and apprehension. Suction accumulated secretions from mouth and throat.

about concerns rather than about what the nurse presumes to be the problem. Assumptions and lack of clarification of issues will lead to poor outcomes. Acknowledging grief and showing support, such as a touch on the shoulder, will show genuine concern for the individual and build self-esteem. Trust is begun by showing a desire for involvement with the grieving client. A willingness for involvement will lead to an opportunity to provide a listening ear when the client wants to talk. A lack of commitment and a hurried posture become blocks to communication. The client quickly learns who does and who does not want to listen to shared feelings.

By analyzing the client's response to grief according to theorists, such as Kübler-Ross or Rando, the nurse can make assumptions about the client's phase of grieving (see Table 29-4). If the client starts yelling at everyone, including the nurse who just walked in the door, the nurse can surmise that the client may be in the anger phase and that the anger is not really directed toward the nurse but at the situation. Therefore rather than yelling back at the client,

the nurse can direct communication to acknowledgment of those feelings. For example, the nurse could state the following: "You are obviously upset. I would like you to know that I am available to talk when you are ready." Other suggestions might include the following: "Tell me about your feelings right now," or "I will just sit for a while and wait for you to talk when you are ready." The nurse should not get angry in return and should not generalize about "how everyone feels that way at some time." Therefore the pace and tone of the conversation are directed by the client and not by the needs of the nurse or the family.

Blocks to communication may include denial of the client's grief, false reassurances, avoidance of issues, and focusing on caregivers' needs instead of the client's needs. Examples of blocks by the nurse might include the following: "Go ahead and yell at me, everyone else has today"; "Since you are upset, let us talk about other things today"; "I will come back later when you have become yourself again"; "How dare you yell at me—don't you know how

Table 29-4   Nursing Implications of Rando's Phases of Grief and Kübler-Ross's Stages of Dying

Behaviors	Nursing Implications
Avoidance	
DENIAL	
Denial is immediate response to news of loss or impending loss.	Support emotional needs without reinforcing denial.
Physiological responses may include muscular weakness, tremors, deep sighs, flushed or cold and clammy skin, diaphoresis, anorexia, and discomfort.	Offer to remain with clients without discussing reasons for behavior or need to cope unless they bring it up.
Individuals avoid accepting reality of situation by not making decisions; they may attempt activities that they are no longer able to do, fail to comply with treatment, search for evidence that loss has not or will not occur, and appear artificially happy.	Offer basic care, such as food, drink, oxygenation, comfort, and safety.
Mood swings are common.	
Individuals isolate themselves from sources of accurate information or reject offers of comfort and support.	
ANGER	
Individuals may express anger and retaliate against family, staff, physicians, or Supreme Being.	Provide anticipatory guidance about feelings and their intensity experienced as part of grief; focus especially on anger.
Bereaved may express anger toward deceased.	Do not take anger personally.
Individuals become demanding and accusing.	Meet needs that cause angry response.
Anger may precipitate guilt and lead to anxiety and lowered self-esteem.	Encourage client and family to express their feelings.
Individuals may feel resentful and jealous of others who still have lost object or loved one.	
Individuals may be reluctant to share feelings and thoughts.	
BARGAINING	
Individuals are willing to do anything to avoid loss or change prognosis or fate.	Provide information needed for decision making.
Individuals make bargains with Supreme Being.	
Individuals accept new forms of therapy.	
Confrontation	
DEPRESSION	
Reality and permanence of loss become recognized.	Provide support and empathy. Support crying by offering touch that communicates caring.
Confusion, lack of motivation, disinterest, indecision, and crying are common.	Listen attentively.
Withdrawal from relationships and activities occurs.	Assess risk of harm to self and refer to mental health professional if needed.
Individuals may become quiet and noncommunicative.	
Feelings of loneliness surface.	
Reminiscence about past and lost object begins.	
Individuals may lose interest in appearance.	
Individuals may become suicidal or cope by beginning unhealthy behaviors such as excessive drug use.	
Accommodation	
ACCEPTANCE	
Individuals accept terms of loss and death and begin plans for it.	Offer opportunities to share feelings verbally, in writing or art, or by tape recordings.
Individuals can share feelings about loss.	Allow and encourage review as often as clients want to talk.
Reminiscence about past occurs.	Show acceptance of lability of feelings.
Periods of depression and well-being occur.	Assist in discussing future plans.
Good times begin to outweigh bad times.	
Life begins to stabilize.	

much I am trying to help you?"; or "I am not going to talk to you until you apologize for your behavior."

No topic that a dying client wishes to discuss should be avoided. Listening and helping the client express feelings and thoughts will allow the client to work through all concerns. Compassion and a caring attitude will lead to the final revelation of deeper concerns that the client is less likely to explore except within a "safe" environment. Crying should not be ignored, and the nurse should offer physical support of the need to cry and grieve without abandoning the client. Saying, "I will be back when you stop crying!" gives the client the feeling that it is not acceptable to cry. Therefore there must be something wrong with the client. In some circumstances the tears of the nurse are just as comforting as words. It is therapeutic to show concern and value of the client, especially when the caregiver has worked very closely or for a long time with the client and the family. Showing tears and attending the funerals of long-term care clients will also aid the closure of the grieving for the nurse.

Goals must be explored, and realistic expectations should be given without destroying hope for recovery. Expressing negative outcomes without sharing the potential for positive ones will direct the client to give up (Doka, 1993). Expectations of families and clients will often differ, and the nurse must be available to meet the needs of both, if possible. When anger or denial has interfered with an understanding of expectation outcomes, the nurse should use reassurance and repeatedly validate the significance of outcomes for various therapies to minimize confusion and to meet the actual needs of the client or family experiencing a loss.

End-of-Life Care.
During terminal care, some factors may turn the nurse away from the required care of the client, such as odors, confusion, disfigurement, combativeness, and incontinence. Often clients feel abandoned and lonely, since they are off in a private room with the curtains and doors closed. The nurse must make a special effort to stimulate all senses in a positive manner to maintain a sense of timing, sense of worth, and sense of compassion and to avoid feelings of abandonment in the client. The nurse can schedule visits throughout the day, open curtains and let the light change from the bright of day to the dark of night, and verbally reassure and talk to the client. In addition, the nurse should encourage family members to talk and visit with the client even when the client is unresponsive. Televisions, radios, visitors, calendars, information boards, and staff can maintain orientation and some normalcy in life during the dying process. Often the client is aware of the surroundings well past the point of the ability to respond. Thus the thought is to instill hope and not to express the attitude of hopelessness. The fears related to dying are often related more to loneliness and isolation than to the actual fear of death itself. It is often during the night hours that the client feels most

isolated from the family. Thus the nurse can arrange for the family to stay over with the client so that the client will feel more reassurance.

Giving spiritual comfort means as much to most clients as meeting their physical needs (see Chapter 27). Without a purpose or understanding of the dying process, the client's value and worth as a living human being may be in question. Individual beliefs, customs, and practices held by a client will better guide the nurse in dealing with spiritual needs. The client explores the meaning to life, the purpose of dying, feelings and attitudes, and spiritual answers to life's questions as a step in comprehending the loss experience. The nurse should not dictate or use the bias of his or her own beliefs to tell the client and/or family what to do or how they should act under the circumstances. A neutral-valued approach by the nurse will allow unbiased care.

The client expects the nurse to use whatever knowledge or skill is available to assist in the actual care of the client. Applying communication skills, expressing empathy, praying with the client, reading inspirational literature, and playing music should all be included in the care plan if desired by the client. The nurse will be guided by the family or client regarding the amount of involvement in this area of care. If the nurse's own agenda differs from that of the client, a conflict and therapeutic block may develop that will hinder further sharing of personal feelings. An openness to new and unusual practices will allow rituals and traditions to be a part of the actual care while providing comfort to the family and client.

When supporting the grieving client's family, the nurse must acknowledge their grief, understand the value of the client to the family, and assist them through the dying process. Giving information, sharing concerns, and expressing empathy will show the family that the nurse has been involved in helping the client to die peacefully. Assessment of the family structure will guide the nurse in identifying strengths and those who need additional support.

Involving the family in the care of the dying client may help the family feel a sense of participation and decrease their sense of helplessness during the dying process. In the home the family is closely involved in the client's care, but in the hospital the family must be encouraged to participate in the care (Box 29-10). The family can ease heavy demands of care and should also be encouraged to assist in smaller tasks that they are able to do.

Hospice Care.
Hospice care has existed since the early fifth century (Hospice Care, 1997). The guidelines vary between various facilities, but generally clients accepted into hospice have less than 6 months to live and are considered terminal. The nurse's role in working with hospice agencies emphasizes meeting the primary wishes of the dying client and being open to individual desires of each client (Hospice Care, 1997). Also, the nurse maintains comfort and dignity through choice. Whether the client

Suggestions for Involving the Family in the Care of a Dying Client   Box 29-10

Assist in planning a visitation schedule for family members to prevent the client and family from becoming fatigued.

Allow young children to visit a dying parent when the client is able to communicate.

Be willing to listen to family complaints about the client's care and feelings about the client.

Help family members learn to interact with the dying person (e.g., using attentive listening, avoiding false assurances, conducting conversations about normal family activities or problems).

Allow family members to help with simple care measures such as feeding, bathing, and straightening bed linen. Recognize that family members are often more successful than nursing staff in persuading the client to eat.

When the family becomes fatigued with care activities, relieve them from their duties so that they can acquire needed rest and support. Refer them to resources for meals and lodging.

Support the mutual act of grieving by the client and family. Provide privacy when preferred. Do not discourage open expression of grief by the family and client.

Provide information daily with regard to the client's condition. Prepare the family for sudden changes in the client's appearance and behavior.

Communicate news of impending death when the family is together, if possible. Remember that members can provide support for one another. Convey the news in a private area and be willing to stay with the family.

As death nears, help the family stay in communication with the dying person through short visits, caring silence, touch, and telling the client of their love.

After death, assist the family with decision making, such as selection of a mortician, transportation of family members, and collection of the client's belongings.

Pitorak's Components of Hospice Care   Box 29-11

Coordinated home care with available inpatient beds under hospital administration

Control of symptoms (physical, sociological, psychological, and spiritual)

Physician-directed services

Provision of an interdisciplinary care team of physicians, nurses, spiritual advisers, social workers, and counselors

Medical and nursing services available at all times

Client and family as the unit of care

A bereavement follow-up after a client's death

Use of trained volunteers as a part of the team

Acceptance into the program on the basis of health care needs rather than the ability to pay

Data from Pitorak EF: Establishing a Medicare-certified in-patient unit, *Nurs Clin North Am* 20:311, 1985.

ultimately dies at home or in the hospital, the client's wishes are followed with the understanding that whatever choice is made, is made "for the good of all that is involved." When options are complicated by family needs, hospice will try to work with the client's wishes.

Another role of the nurse is to encourage realistic goals and suggest alternatives for the benefit of all (Box 29-11). If the family cannot meet the client's basic needs, a home health aide or nurse may be available by referral to assist. Respite care is available in many hospice programs to allow for the family to have some time away from the daily care of the dying client. Respite care can include the placement of a client in a temporary facility without the family having to feel guilty about not caring for the client, the use of a temporary replacement caregiver to allow the family time to meet personal care, and emotional support of those who have previously experienced loss. A hospice program emphasizes **palliative treatment** to control symptoms rather than curative treatment, which treats the

disease. The goals are mutually set, and all participants fully understand the options and desires of the client. Efforts by the team are made to meet the client's desires and to encourage the family to stay within those guidelines. Often a visit or visits will be made by the staff of the hospice team to the family even after the death of the client to help the family move through the grieving process successfully. Both home care and hospital care are available based on the current needs of the client. Many clients prefer to die at home in a familiar setting. Others cannot be cared for at home despite the willingness of family and friends to care for the client. The health and welfare issues are viewed from a broader perspective than just the client's desires. The concern for family needs is also taken into consideration.

Other sources of management of the dying client will be very specific for each individual. Some clients may desire greater focus on spirituality needs and request a clergy or a service of their church. Other clients seek nutritional answers, miracles, and other sources of hope despite a financial drain. Nontraditional therapies are encouraged if they give the client hope and do no harm. Explaining realistic options without destroying hope is the key role that the nurse plays in the care of the dying client. The client's and the nurse's attitudes will make the difference between the perceived success or failure of a dying experience.

Care After Death.   Federal and state legislation requires hospitals to formulate policies and procedures based on current laws to validate death, to identify potential donors, and to care for the body after death. For transplantation of organs, the nurse must remember that the need for ventilatory and circulatory support is required until the vital organs can be harvested. The family must clearly understand that the equipment is not keeping the client alive but is keeping the physical body ready for

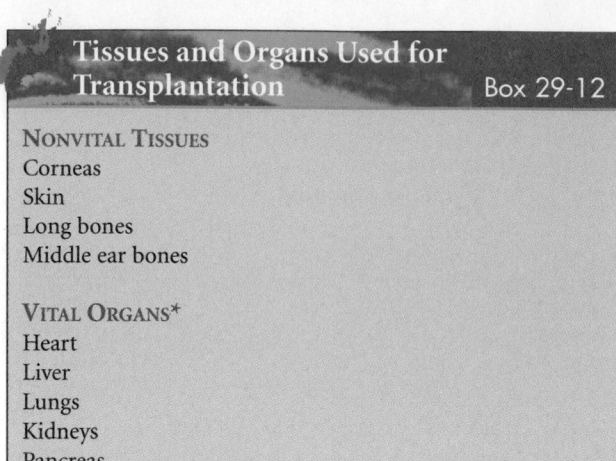

Tissues and Organs Used for Transplantation   Box 29-12

NONVITAL TISSUES
Corneas
Skin
Long bones
Middle ear bones

VITAL ORGANS*
Heart
Liver
Lungs
Kidneys
Pancreas

*These organs are recovered after a client is pronounced clinically dead or brain dead; circulatory and ventilatory support is maintained to perfuse the organs before removal.

transplantation. Brain death must be repeatedly emphasized by all who are participating in the care of the client. Clarification of what defines death should be provided to the family, since these support systems must remain in place even after the person is pronounced "dead." On the other hand, nonvital tissues will not require cardiopulmonary support. Specific guidelines are given by various organ donor banks concerning viable times, conditions, and preservatives, and the representative should be contacted as soon as possible to allow the family to donate effectively if that is the desire of the client or the family (Box 29-12). Organ donation must be agreed on by all of the family if no specific requests were made by the client before the death.

The nurse is responsible for coordination of all aspects of care surrounding the death of the client. The family becomes the new "client" when the actual death has occurred, and the shift of concern moves from the dead client to the living family. Box 29-13 summarizes the physicians and nurse's responsibilities for care after death. The nurse must refocus on the needs of the family after

Care After Death   Box 29-13

1. Physicians must certify the death—time pronounced, therapy used, actions taken.
2. Physicians may request an autopsy, especially for unusual circumstances.
3. Trained staff member provides an option for donation of organs or tissue—personal, religious, and cultural needs should be included during this process (see Chapter 28).
4. Nurses provide dignity and sensitivity to the client and the family.
   a. Check orders for any specimens or special orders needed by the physician.
   b. Make arrangements for staff, minister, or others to stay with the family while preparing the body for viewing; ask for special requests for viewing (e.g., shaving, a special gown, Bible in hand, rosary at the bedside).
   c. Shaving of male clients must be done before removal of the beard. The family may want the client left in the current unshaven state if it was his custom to wear a beard.
   d. Remove all equipment, tubes, supplies, and dirty linens according to protocol (unless organ donation is to take place; in that case leave support systems in place).
   e. Cleanse the body thoroughly, apply clean sheets, and remove all trash from the room.
   f. Position according to protocol—the eyes should be closed by gently holding them down a few minutes; dentures should be in the mouth to maintain facial alignment; packing should not be visible during viewing. Hairpieces may be in place, but no make up is required.

   g. Cover with a clean sheet up to the chin with arms outside covers if possible.
   h. Lower the lighting and spray a deodorizer if possible to remove unpleasant odors.
   i. Give the family the option to view or not to view and go with them.
   j. Clarify that either option is acceptable.
   k. Encourage the family to say goodbye through both touch and talk.
   l. Do not rush this process. Once the family is more comfortable, *ask* if they would like to be left alone. Remind them that they can call you if needed.
   m. Clarify personal belongings that are to stay with the body or who has taken personal items; documentation will require both a descriptor of the objects and the name of who received it, with the time and date.
   n. Discard nothing if items are found after the family is gone—call the family and tell them what was found and ask who might pick it up—describing the articles will be helpful in the decision-making process for the client's family.
   o. Apply name tags according to protocol—such as at the wrist, right big toe, or outside a shroud.
   p. Complete documentation in the nursing notes (see Box 29-14).
   q. Remain sensitive to other hospitalized clients or visitors when transporting the body, such as covering the body with a clean sheet and watching to avoid visitors when moving the body to another part of the hospital or to the exit for the funeral home.
   r. Follow all protocol and policies to meet all legal requirements in caring for the body.

the death and implement actions to meet their current needs.

The nurse must follow policies and procedures that are individually established by each facility. Therefore to be effective in his or her role, the nurse must be familiar and comfortable with these policies before the death. Understanding the physiological changes after death will assist in the timing of care for a dying client (Table 29-5). In larger hospitals several experts are assigned to a team for greater expertise in dealing with dying clients and their families. A multidisciplinary team might include specially trained nurses, physicians, social workers, and chaplains or ministers. However, in a smaller community the nurse might be totally responsible for caring for the body and meeting all the needs of the family of the dying client. In this case the nurse might be assisted by either a floor nurse or a supervisor, who must gain the expertise needed to meet state guidelines. This person must know the details about who does what, when it is done, where it is done, how things are referred, and which forms need to be filled out and sent to whom (e.g., to a social worker, therapist, etc.).

Ministers or priests may be called to assist the family even before the actual death if no bereavement team is available. Some families prefer to grieve alone, whereas other families may desire the support of others. Thus the assessment phase should have identified the needs of the family, as well as those of the client, to develop realistic expectations of the nurse. If expectations are unknown, then simple questions and suggestions for assistance can be offered by anyone who is assisting the family. Priests, ministers, and laymen are available from churches or other organizations. Knowledge of local resources will guide decision making at this time.

After the client's death, there are several guidelines to be considered for effective management that are reviewed in Table 29-4. These actions should guide the nurse to minimize the stress of the situation and to help the grieving family successfully move forward. One aspect in the care of the body is to recognize the actual physiological changes in death and to intervene as necessary (see Table 29-5).

Another area that is difficult for the nurse and the family concerns autopsy. According to Dracup and Brown (1998), getting permission through delicate questioning is difficult at best. Often the doctor will ask for permission for an autopsy, but it is the nurse's job to answer questions and support the family's choices. It is very difficult, according to Dracup and Brown (1998), to approach a grieving family with such a request. Their suggestion is to show the value that an autopsy can have by improving knowledge in the field of medicine. To help the living, the autopsy can lead to new therapies or new understanding of diseases. The more reasons the nurse can think of to support organ donation or autopsy, the more the family will be helped to realize the good that can be accomplished by either donation or research autopsy.

Client expectations, as well as family expectations, will vary in degree and content. A close rapport between staff and the nurse will aid in achieving the greatest success for all. The nurse's role includes staying current with policies and procedures concerning emergency care, the restriction or avoidance of cardiopulmonary resuscitation (CPR) and other medical or nursing techniques, local legal guidelines to support institutional policy, standards of care for the dying, ethical review board options and guidelines, titles, and phone numbers of persons to be called. If the nurse has any disagreement with the care and plan for a specific client, the nurse can discuss these issues with appropriate leadership and/or request not to work under certain circumstances. If the nurse accepts the job of caring for an assigned client, then legally the care is given as written despite the feelings or beliefs of the nurse caregiver. Clarification of the nurse's role and the client's expectations must be very concrete to avoid any problems in client relations during the crisis of a loss.

EVALUATION
Client Care. Although completion of grief work may require months or years, most clients are under the nurse's care for only a short time. The nurse may become frustrated when, just as the client or family begins to

Table 29-5 **Physiological Changes After Death**	
Change	Related Interventions
Stiffening of body (rigor mortis), developing 2 to 4 hours after death (involves contraction of skeletal and smooth muscle from lack of adenosine triphosphate)	Before rigor mortis develops, position body in normal anatomical alignment, close eyelids and mouth, and insert dentures in mouth.
Reduction in body temperature with loss of skin elasticity (algor mortis)	Remove tape and dressings gently to avoid tissue breakdown. Avoid pulling on skin or body parts.
Purple discoloration of skin (livor mortis) in dependent areas from breakdown of red blood cells	Elevate head to prevent facial discoloration.
Softening and liquifying of body tissues by bacterial fermentation	Store body in cool place in hospital morgue or other designated area.

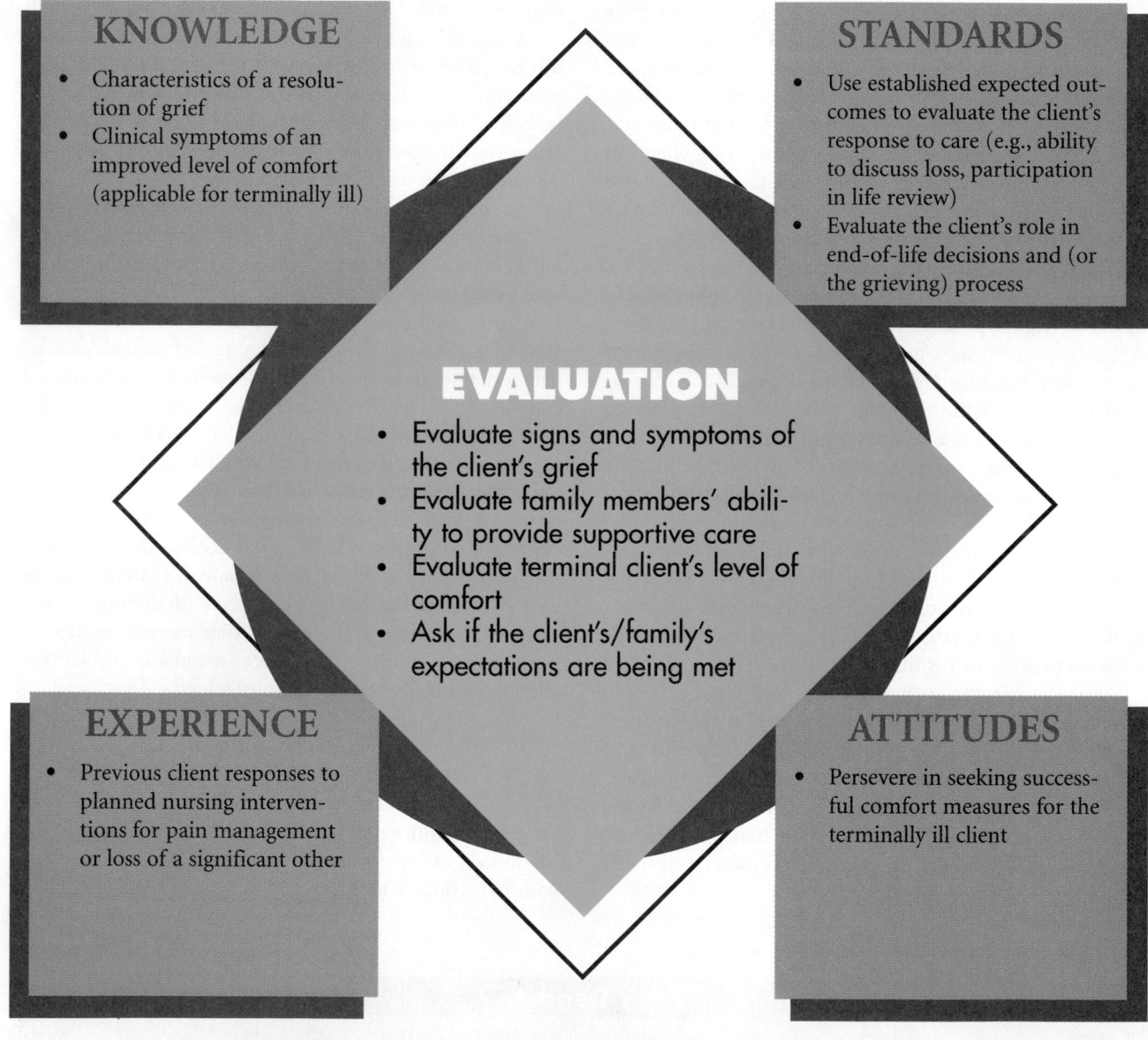

KNOWLEDGE
- Characteristics of a resolution of grief
- Clinical symptoms of an improved level of comfort (applicable for terminally ill)

STANDARDS
- Use established expected outcomes to evaluate the client's response to care (e.g., ability to discuss loss, participation in life review)
- Evaluate the client's role in end-of-life decisions and (or the grieving) process

EVALUATION
- Evaluate signs and symptoms of the client's grief
- Evaluate family members' ability to provide supportive care
- Evaluate terminal client's level of comfort
- Ask if the client's/family's expectations are being met

EXPERIENCE
- Previous client responses to planned nursing interventions for pain management or loss of a significant other

ATTITUDES
- Persevere in seeking successful comfort measures for the terminally ill client

Figure 29-4   *Synthesis Model for Loss, Death, and Grieving Evaluation Phase.*

express grief, the client leaves the health care institution. Grieving is an individual process, and resolution of loss does not follow a set schedule. It is important for the client and family to share experiences and discuss options. The goals and outcomes established with the client and the family become the basis for evaluation. For example, if the goal is to have the client communicate love and caring for the family, the nurse evaluates the verbal and nonverbal communication process for cues related to love. The nurse continues to evaluate the progress and effectiveness of the interventions and the interactions between the family and the client (Paul, Willsen, and Binker, 1993). The critical thinking model emphasizes an integration of all aspects of care to effectively evaluate whether the goals have been met successfully (Figure 29-4).

Client Expectations.
The client expects individualization of care, including comfort, dignity, and cooperation, to maximize the client's quality of life. The success of the evaluation depends partially on the bond formed with the client. Unless the client can fully trust the nurse, the sharing of personal desires is not likely to occur. Other expectations would be the validations that comfort was maintained by decreasing levels of pain on a scale of 0 to 10, by control of symptoms that were not desired, by maintaining of body functions, by completion of unfinished tasks, and by the level of emotional stability observed.

The following are examples of questions that will validate the achievement of the nursing interventions:

Am I meeting your expectations while providing your care?

Would you like me to assist you in a different manner?

Do you have a specific request that I can use in your care at this time?

Is there another problem that we are overlooking or that you feel is of a higher priority?

Are we dealing with your problems in a timely manner?

Through communication and assessment the nurse will continue to evaluate if the outcome criteria were accomplished to support the goals that were chosen from the initial database. Often the evaluation of the client's needs is easy, but the process is more complex as it relates to the family. Once rapport is established, the staff must be ever vigilant to avoid problems that question that rapport.

The Grieving Nurse.
Evaluation should also include the nurse's response to the entire situation. The bond formed between the client and the nurse places the nurse in a similar relationship with the client as that of the family; therefore the nurse must go through the grieving process also. Recognizing the need to grieve will assist the nurse in moving through this process. Often nurses seek out other nurses or health care workers to discuss their own grief (Figure 29-5). Nurses experience additional stressors or losses, including a failure to adapt, when they do not have time or do not allow themselves to grieve.

At this point the nurse develops a bereavement overload. Frustrations, anger, guilt, sadness, helplessness, anxiety, depression, and feelings of being overwhelmed may occur. The nurse's self-care is critical to survival and recovery from loss, not only for his or her own sake, but also for the sake of future clients. Acknowledging the loss begins the process, and mourning the loss may need to take place before the nurse moves on to the next dying client. Individual bereavement work and group support from the staff will provide experiences that can guide future relationships. A personal support system should be in place continually if one is working in areas where a high number of deaths occur. Getting away, sharing opportunities, a nonjudgmental listening ear, open relationships, and stress management will all help nurses to move effectively through their own mourning of lost clients. Without renewal of energy and mutual support opportunities, nurses will not develop closure for each case. Unrelieved grief and stress can lead to diminished well-being and the inability to care for other clients.

Burnout is a popular term used when the stresses exceed the rewards of the job and the individual nurse lacks the support of peers. The nurse, who is always giving, eventually realizes that he or she must also be receiving to be effective. Having a job with increasingly high demands, nurses must be able to modify and acquire new roles that incorporate new trends in health care delivery and ethical decision making about allocation of resources. An understanding of the impact of work on the nurse will allow problem-solving techniques to guide choices without causing dysfunctional responses to loss.

Being informed and up-to-date, practicing within the legal parameters of the nurse's responsibilities, and using current trends in health care, the nurse will be an expert in many fields, including the expertise of caring for the dying client (Catalano, 1995).

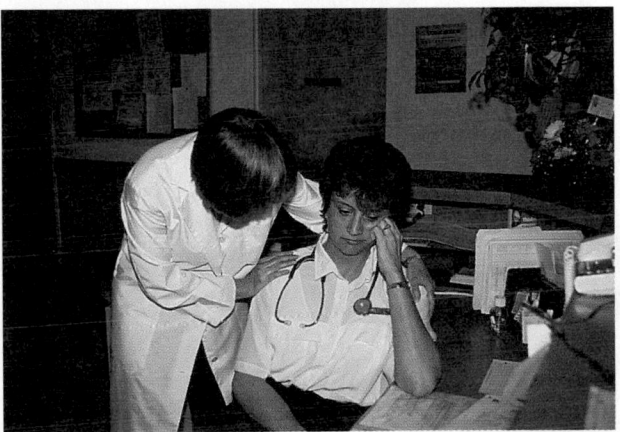

Figure 29-5 Nurses benefit from support of colleagues during their time of loss.

Family Expectations.   The nurse is expected to evaluate the situation in clear and precise terms as stated by the choice of an applicable nursing diagnosis based on an accurate database that is evolving and realistic. These goals are to be met by accomplishing specific, measurable outcome criteria. Sympathy, privacy, and understanding by staff will express to the family that the staff were in tune with their needs during the family's loss. Individual expectations must be clearly discussed with the family, especially when there is a conflict of interest between the client's desires and the family's wishes. Details of expectations should be verbalized and not presumed on anyone's part. By remembering the good things experienced and gained from the care of a client, the family will be helped to move forward in the grieving process.

Documentation

Documentation (see Chapter 24) is the final validation of the success of the application of the nursing process for

---

Documentation of Nursing Notes   Box 29-14

Time of death and actions taken to prevent the death if applicable

Who pronounced the death of the client

Any special preparation and type of donation, including time, staff, and company

Who was called and who came to the hospital—donor organization, morgue, funeral home, chaplin, and individual family members making any decisions

Personal articles left on the body and taped to skin or tubes left in

Personal items given to the family—specific names and descriptors of items

Time of discharge and destination of the body

Location of name tags on the body

Special requests by the family

Any other personal statements that might be needed to clarify the situation

---

the client with a loss or who is in the grieving process. Without clear, precise, and accurate notes in the nursing notes of the chart, communication breakdown will impede progression through the grieving process. Furthermore, the specific descriptions of all events will allow for greater continuity of care between shifts. There are legal guidelines that are supported by each facility's policies and procedures and that must be followed and accurately documented to avoid any breaks in the law. Remember the golden rule of nursing, "If it is not written, it is not done." Box 29-14 lists content to be documented, including the following: who, what, when, how, and why care has been given. Documentation will validate the success of meeting the goals identified for the client or provide a justification for the failure to meet a goal. In addition to these guidelines, the nurse must make sure that the institution's policies are covered in the documentation to minimize legal difficulties at a later date (Youngberg, 1996).

Some medical forms must be signed by a doctor or coroner, but most of the forms must be recorded by the registered nurse. Gathering of this information may have been delegated, but the actual charting of data on the nurse's notes must be done by the registered or licensed vocational nurse. Witnessing of the signing of forms should be done by a licensed professional.

In cases of legal matters the family will expect a clear, concise description of what occurred in the care at the time of death. Opinions are limited, and facts are stated in a nonjudgmental fashion. Both state and federal guidelines will direct what type of information is charted and when it is to be charted. Reading of such a chart by family varies according to state laws, but if it is allowed, the family should be knowledgable of the documentation process. The physician has the final say as to who reads certain parts of the chart. Copies of parts of the chart can be given to family with a written request and the approval of the physician and the hospital. In cases of legal issues surrounding the death or loss, court orders are required for others to view the chart. The nurse must understand and uphold the legal guidelines of documentation at *all* times (see Chapter 24).

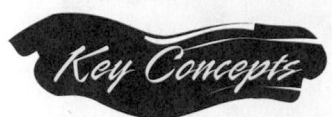

- Loss is a universal response when an important aspect of an individual is no longer present.
- The grieving process involves a set of emotional, cognitive, and behavioral responses to an actual or perceived loss.

- Grieving integrates and accommodates loss to achieve more effective functioning.
- Individuals experience different aspects of the grieving process at different times.
- Individuals can experience either an effective or an ineffective response to a loss.

- Society can dictate the types of acceptable losses and the appropriate responses to such losses.
- The phases of the grieving process vary among theorists but progress from distress and shock to resolution and accommodation by unique rates and sequences.
- Different types of losses may lead to a grief response similar to that occurring following a death.
- The nurse's support of a client's hope can help relieve grieving associated with a loss.
- During assessment the nurse considers physical and behavioral characteristics that suggest the client is grieving.
- Risk factors (e.g., physical health) indicate the possibility that a person who is grieving will suffer physical and psychological illness during bereavement.
- Nursing diagnoses focus on the type of grief experienced by the client, family, or community, as well as the health-related problems common to grieving clients.
- Therapeutic communication helps the nurse assist the grieving and dying client in coping with the loss.
- Nursing interventions to promote return-to-life activities assist the client in accommodating grief and accepting the loss.
- Nursing care of the terminally ill focuses on promoting comfort and improving quality of life.
- As death approaches, the client reviews and analyzes values and beliefs pertinent to the meaning of life and death.
- The nurse assesses whether family members are willing to be involved in a dying client's care before using them as resources.
- Care after death includes caring for the body with dignity and sensitivity.
- The evaluation of nursing care for the grieving and dying client is based on identifiable behavioral changes through the grieving process.
- The nurse's own loss history influences responses to client losses.
- Nurses who work with critically or terminally ill clients experience loss and grief.
- Nurses need to be aware of and mourn their own losses on an ongoing basis to avoid bereavement overload.
- Nurses must remember that a loss is defined by the person and not by the interpretation given by another person or society.
- Nurses need to allow others to help them and to retreat without guilt or shame when bereavement overload occurs.

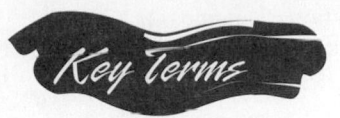

Key Terms

Accommodation, *p. 618*	Grieving processes, *p. 616*
Actual loss, *p. 615*	Grief work, *p. 616*
Anticipatory grief, *p. 614*	Hope, *p. 615*
Burnout, *p. 639*	Loss, *p. 613*
Confrontation, *p. 618*	Maturational loss, *p. 615*
Coping mechanisms, *p. 618*	Mourning, *p. 616*
Disenfranchised grief, *p. 614*	Palliative treatment, *p. 635*
Dysfunctional grief, *p. 614*	Perceived loss, *p. 615*
Grief, *p. 613*	Personal loss, *p. 614*
	Situational loss, *p. 615*

Critical Thinking Exercises

1. A hispanic 28-year-old woman has no living children, and she has just lost her third premature infant. Complications of the pregnancy resulted in a hysterectomy to save her life. She remains very stoic in her responses to the entire loss experience. She states that she has a strong, religious belief system that examines death as a part of the greater scheme of mankind, in which "all things work together for the good..." Identify the types of loss and the stage of loss she has experienced. How can the nurse offer hope and closure? What resources are available in your area to assist the grieving process?

2. While in the grocery store, a former neighbor is seen wandering around lost with a very sad face. The woman explains that her husband of 50 years was recently placed in an institution for late stages of Alzheimer's disease and that he does not recognize her at all anymore. Financially, it has cost her everything to put him into the facility, and now she is living with family. How can you begin to rank the priorities of losses that she is experiencing to identify the most urgent need? What coping strategies or interventions might be suggested to assist her? Should you assess the risk for self-harm?

3. A nursing student has experienced a series of actual and perceived personal losses. On the first day of clinical, her client suddenly dies. She starts crying hysterically in the client's room. The instructor pulls the student aside to talk privately with her. In addition, the student failed her exam the day before the clinical experience because she was unable to focus on her studies. What signs/symptoms would indicate the stage of grieving and the success (or lack thereof) of her present coping strategies? What types of questions might be asked to help her do some critical thinking and problem solving for self-management? What do the

American Nurses Association *Standards of Clinical Nursing Practice* say about the roles of the educator and the student?

References

Anderson KL, Dimond MF: The experience of bereavement in older adults, *J Adv Nurs* 22:308, 1995.

Attig T: *How we grieve: relearning the world,* New York, 1996, Oxford University Press.

Bierman E and others: Assessing access as a first step towards improving the quality of care for very old adults, *J Ambul Care Manage* 21(3):17, 1998.

Binstock W, Spector W: Five priority areas for research on long-term care, *Health Serv Res* 32(5):715, 1997.

Braza K: Families and the grief process, *ARCH Factsheet* 21, March 1993.

Cairns J: *Matters of life and death: perspectives on public health, molecular biology, cancer, and the prospects for the human race,* Princeton, NJ, 1997, Princeton University Press.

Catalano JT: *Ethical and legal aspects of nursing,* ed 2, Springhouse, 1995, Springhouse.

Cressy D: *Birth, marriage, and death: ritual, religion, and the life-cycle in Tudor and Stuart England,* New York, 1997, Oxford University Press.

Doka KJ: *Living with life-threatening illness: a guide for patients, their families, and caregivers,* New York, 1993, Lexington.

Dracup K, Brown CW: Asking difficult questions, *Am J Crit Care* 7(6):399, 1998.

Dufault K, Martocchio BC: Hope: its spheres and dimensions, *Nurs Clin North Am* 20:379, 1985.

Engel GL: Grief and grieving, *Am J Nurs* 64:93, 1964.

Farber SJ and others: Issues in end-of-life care: family practice faculty perceptions, *J Fam Pract* 48(7):525, 1999.

Harper JM: Plateaus of acceptance: pits of pain. In Corr CA, Stillion JM, Ribar MC, editors: *Creativity in death education and counseling,* Hartford, Conn, 1983, Forum for Death Education and Counseling.

Hepburn A: What do we really know about grief counseling? Exploring the contemporary challenges of multiculturalism, post-modernism, and imaginal psychology, *Forum Newslett* 20(6):7, 1994.

Horn M: Grief re-examined, *U.S. New and World Report,* p 81, June 14, 1993.

Hospice Care, *Mayo Clin Health Lett* 15(7):4, 1997.

Kim MJ, McFarland GK, McLane AM: *Pocket guide to nursing diagnoses,* ed 7, St. Louis, 1997, Mosby.

Kübler-Ross E: *On death and dying,* New York, 1969, Macmillan.

Lendhardt AMC: Disenfranchised grief/hidden sorrow: implications for the school counselor, *School Counsel* 44(4):264, 1997a.

Lendhardt AMC: Grieving disenfranchised losses: background and strategies for counselors, *J Hum Educ Dev* 35(4):208, 1997b.

Maglio CJ: *Grief counseling and grief therapy: a cognitive-behavioral perspective,* April 1991.

McLean S: The definition of death: contemporary controversies, *BMJ* 319(7207):42A, 1999.

Murphy WJ: Ethical perspectives in neuroscience nursing practice, *Nurs Clin North Am* 34(3):621, 1999.

Paul R, Willsen J, Binker AJA: *Critical thinking: what every person needs to survive in a rapidly changing world,* ed 3, Santa Rosa, Calif, 1993, Foundation for Critical Thinking.

Pitorak EF: Establishing a Medicare-certified in-patient unit, *Nurs Clin North Am* 20:311, 1985.

Rando TA: *Grief, dying and death,* Champaign, Ill, 1984, Research.

Rando TA: *Loss and anticipatory grief,* Lexington, Mass, 1986, Lexington.

Rando TA: The increasing prevalence of complicated mourning: the onslaught is just beginning, *Omega J Death Dying* 26(1):43, 1992-1993.

Rando TA: *How to go on living when someone you love dies,* New York, 1991, Bantam.

Raphael B: *The anatomy of bereavement,* New York, 1986, Newmarket.

Rosenfeld J: Bereavement and grieving after spontaneous abortion, *Am Fam Physician* 43(5):1679, 1991.

Shapiro RS: In re Edna MF: case law confusion in surrogate decision making, *Theory Med Bioethics* 20(1):45, 1999.

Sheehan G: *Going the distance: one man's journey to the end of his life,* New York, 1996, Villard Books.

Spector W: Functional disability scales. In Spiker B, editor: *Quality of life and pharmacoeconomics in clinical trials,* ed 2, Philadelphia, 1996, Lippincott-Raven.

Stepnick A, Perry T: Preventing spiritual distress in the dying client, *J Psychosoc Nurs* 30(1):17, 1992.

Stinson KM and others: Parents' grief following pregnancy loss: a comparison of mothers and fathers, *Fam Relations* 41(2):218, 1992.

Stocker S: Beyond grief, *Prevention* 46(8):88, 1994.

Thomas V, Striegel P: Stress and grief of a perinatal loss: integrating qualitative and quantitative methods, *Omega J Death Dying* 30(4):299, 1994-1995.

Toth PL: A short-term grief and loss therapy group: group members' experiences, *J Pers Interpers Loss* 2(1):83, 1997.

Weissman DE and others: Pain assessment and management in the long-term care setting, *Theory Med Bioethics* 20(1):31, 1999.

Witoszek N: *Talking to the dead: a study of Irish funerary traditions,* Atlanta, 1998, Rodopi.

Worden JW: *Grief counseling and grief therapy,* New York, 1982, Springer.

Youngberg B: *Nursing and malpractice risks: understanding the law,* ed 3, South Easton, Mass, 1996, Western Schools Press.

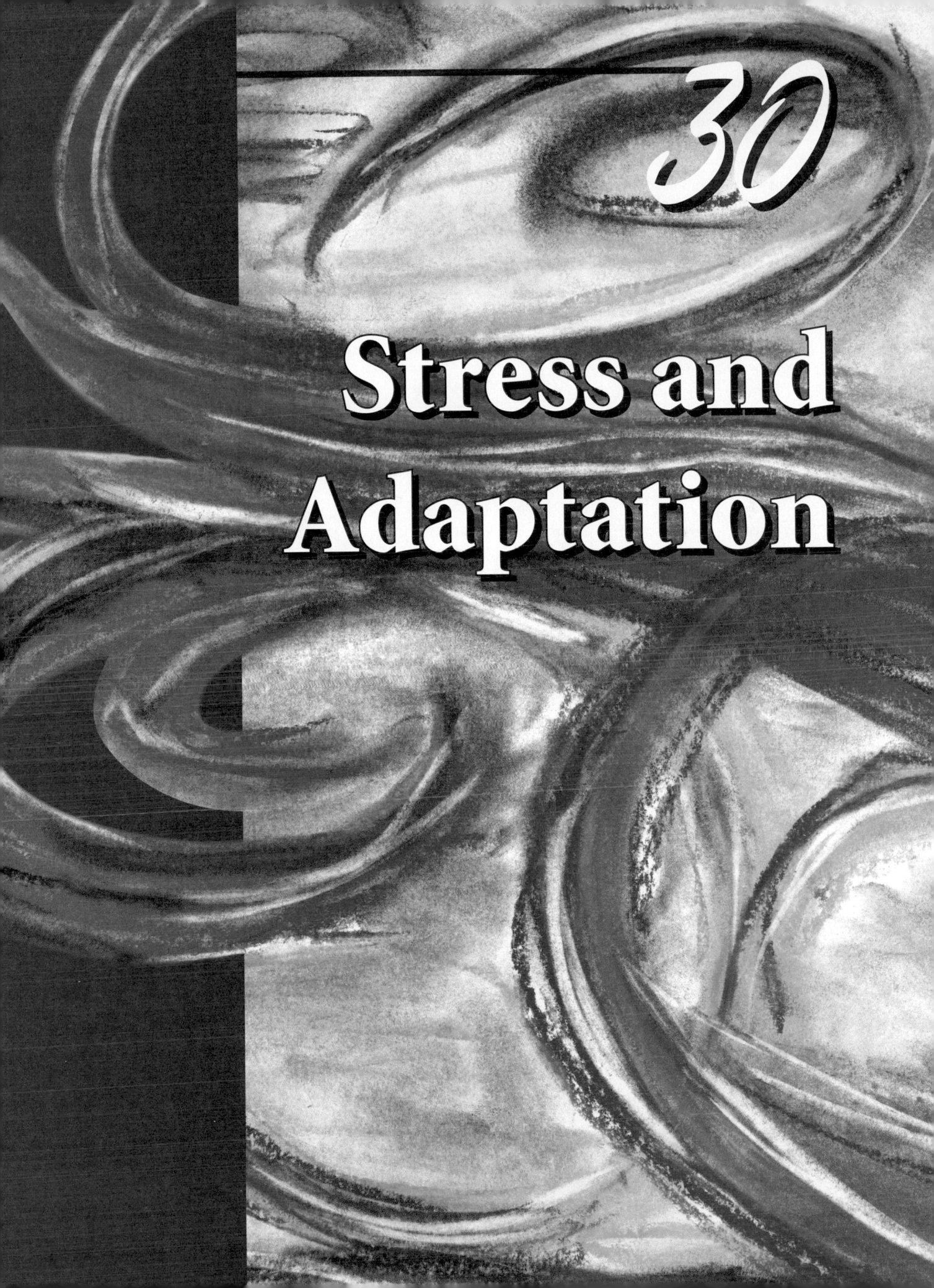

30

Stress and Adaptation

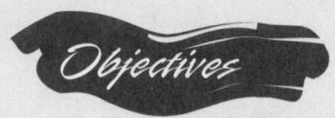
Mastery of content in this chapter will enable the student to:

- Define the key terms listed.
- Discuss the limitations of homeostatic control.
- Compare four models of stress as they relate to nursing practice.
- Describe how adaptation occurs in each of the five dimensions.
- Describe two forms of local physiological adaptation.
- Describe the three phases of the general adaptation syndrome.
- List and discuss behaviors that are responses to stress.
- List and discuss the most common ego-defense mechanisms that are responses to stress.
- Discuss the effects of prolonged stress on each of the five dimensions of a person's functioning.
- Describe stress management techniques that nurses can help clients use and use themselves.
- Discuss techniques of crisis intervention.

Every person experiences forms of **stress** throughout life. Stress can provide the stimulus for change and growth. Some stress is positive and even necessary. However, too much stress can result in poor judgment, physical illness, and inability to cope. A number of studies have proposed a relationship between stressful life events and a wide variety of physical and psychiatric disorders (Mandle and others, 1995; de Anda D and others, 1997; Finlay J and Zigmond M, 1997). Stress affects all dimensions of a person's life.

Claude Bernard, in 1867, was one of the first physiologists to recognize the consequences of stress. He proposed that changes in the internal and external environments disrupted the functioning of an organism and that it was essential for an organism to adapt to a stressor to survive. In 1920 Walter Cannon studied physiological responses to emotional arousal and emphasized the adaptive functions of the "fight-or-flight" reaction. Cannon also noted that these responses were the result of the influence of the emotional state on the body and that the subsequent responses were adaptive and physiological (Robinson, 1990).

Hans Selye (1946) developed a biochemical model of stress known as the **general adaptation syndrome (GAS),** which described physiological events during a stress response. Selye also introduced the concept of **stressors,** which are internal or external stimuli that cause stress (Selye, 1976). Selye's classic research into stress and stressors has been important for health care professionals. Current research in many disciplines is focused on a variety of stress and stress-related concepts.

Scientific Knowledge Base

STRESS AND STRESSORS

Everyone experiences stress from time to time, and normally a person is able to adapt to long-term stress or cope with short-term stress until it passes. Stress can place heavy demands on a person, and if the person is unable to adapt, illness can result. Stress is any situation in which a nonspecific demand requires an individual to respond or take action (Selye, 1976). It involves physiological and psychological responses. Stress can lead to negative or counterproductive feelings or threaten emotional well-being. It can threaten the way a person normally perceives reality, solves problems, and thinks in general and a person's relationships and sense of belonging. Stress can also threaten a person's general outlook on life and health status.

An individual's perception or experience of a major change may initiate the stress response. The stimuli preceding or precipitating the change are called *stressors.* Stressors represent an unmet need and may be physiological, psychological, social, environmental, developmental, spiritual, or cultural. Stressors can be classified as internal or external. **Internal stressors** originate inside a person (e.g., a fever, a condition such as pregnancy or menopause, an emotion such as guilt). **External stressors** originate outside a person (e.g., a marked change in environmental temperature, a change in family or social role, peer pressure).

PHYSIOLOGICAL ADAPTATION

Physiological adaptation to stress is the body's ability to maintain a state of relative balance. This adaptive ability is

---

The authors acknowledge the contribution of Mary E. Walker to this chapter in the previous edition of this text.

a dynamic form of equilibrium in the body's internal environment. The internal environment constantly changes, and the body's adaptive mechanisms continually function to adjust to these changes and thus to maintain equilibrium, or **homeostasis.**

Homeostasis is maintained by physiological mechanisms that control body functions and monitor body organs. For the most part these mechanisms are controlled by the nervous and endocrine systems and do not involve conscious behavior. The body makes adjustments in heart rate, respiratory rate, blood pressure, temperature, fluid and electrolyte balances, hormone secretions, and level of consciousness—all directed at maintaining **adaptation.**

Mechanisms of Physiological Adaptation.

When a person becomes aware of an unmet physiological need, such as food or warmth, deliberate actions can meet the need. For the most part, however, adaptation involves adjustments that the body makes automatically to maintain equilibrium. These homeostatic mechanisms are self-regulatory; in other words, they are automatic. In a person with an illness or injury, however, the mechanisms may not be able to maintain and sustain homeostasis.

Physiological mechanisms of adaptation function through negative feedback, a process by which the controlling mechanism senses an abnormal state, such as lowered body temperature, and makes an adaptive response, such as initiating shivering to generate body heat. Three of the major mechanisms used in adapting to a stressor are controlled by the **medulla oblongata**, the **reticular formation**, and the **pituitary gland.**

Medulla Oblongata.

The medulla oblongata controls vital functions necessary to survival. These include heart rate, blood pressure, and respiration. Impulses traveling to and from the medulla oblongata can increase or decrease these vital functions. For example, regulation of the heartbeat is the result of sympathetic or parasympathetic nervous system impulses traveling from the medulla oblongata to the heart. The heart rate increases in response to pulses from sympathetic fibers and decreases with impulses from parasympathetic fibers.

Reticular Formation.

The reticular formation is a small cluster of neurons in the brain stem and spinal cord. It also controls vital functions and continuously monitors the physiological status of the body through connections with sensory and motor tracts. For example, certain cells within the reticular formation can cause a sleeping person to regain consciousness or increase the level of consciousness when a need arises.

Pituitary Gland.

The pituitary gland, a small gland attached to the hypothalamus, supplies hormones that control vital functions. The pituitary gland produces hormones necessary for adaptation to stress. In addition, the pituitary gland regulates the secretion of thyroid, gonadal, and parathyroid hormones. Hormone secretion, like other homeostatic mechanisms, is normally regulated by a feedback mechanism that continuously monitors hormone levels in the blood. When hormone levels drop, the pituitary gland receives a message to increase hormone secretion. When hormone levels rise, the pituitary gland decreases hormone production.

Limitations of Physiological Mechanisms of Adaptation.

Physiological mechanisms of adaptation work together through complex relationships in the nervous and endocrine systems and other body systems to maintain a relative constancy within the body. In a healthy person these mechanisms affect physiological balance and the body's day-to-day needs are met. However, physiological mechanisms of adaptation can provide only short-term control over the body's equilibrium. They cannot adapt to long-term changes in hormone secretion or vital functions. Thus illness, injury, or prolonged stress can decrease the adaptive capacity. Decreased functioning can result in continued but inadequate homeostatic control or breakdown of the feedback mechanism that allows control. Either form of decreased function can result in further illness or death.

In severe stress situations, for example, the pituitary gland supplies the body with the necessary hormones. However, these hormones may be insufficient in quantity to provide the physiological energy necessary for coping. In such a case the person's condition deteriorates and functioning declines.

MODELS OF STRESS

The origins and effects of stress can be examined in terms of medical and behavioral theoretical models. Stress models are used to identify the stressors for a particular individual and predict that person's responses to them. Each model emphasizes a different aspect of stress. The nurse may use stress models to help a client cope with unhealthy, nonproductive responses to stressors. These models can help the nurse respond in a caring, individualized way.

Response-Based Model of Stress.

The response-based model is concerned with specifying the particular response or pattern of responses that may indicate a stressor. Selye's model of stress (1976) is a model that defines stress as a nonspecific response of the body to any demand made on it. Stress is demonstrated by a specific physiological reaction, the GAS. The GAS is a physiological response of the whole body to stress. It involves the autonomic nervous system and the endocrine system. Thus the response of a person to stress is purely physiological and is never modified to allow cognitive influences (Farrington, 1995).

The response-based model does not consider individual differences in response patterns. For instance, a mountaineer may have no stress response to climbing a mountain. In fact, he may enjoy the difficulties presented to him. For others this same situation could lead to a severe stress response (Farrington, 1995). This lack of flexibility may produce some difficulties for nurses because individual differences must be identified in the assessment phase. However, it may be most useful when determining physiological responses.

Adaptation Model.

The adaptation model is based on the understanding that people experience anxiety and increased stress when they are unprepared to cope with stressful situations. Using this model can assist nurses in planning appropriate interventions.

The adaptation model proposes that four factors determine whether a situation is stressful (Mechanic, 1962). The ability to cope with stress, the first factor, usually depends on the person's experience with similar stressors, support systems, and overall perception of the stressor.

The second factor deals with the practices and norms of the person's peer group. If the peer group considers it normal to talk about a particular stressor, the client may respond by complaining about it or discussing it. This response may help adaptation to the stress, or the client may respond in this way simply to conform to peer group behavior.

The third factor is the impact of the social environment in assisting an individual to adapt to a stressor. For example, a homeless woman with schizophrenia may seek assistance from a clinic nurse practitioner about an acute pelvic infection. The nurse may then assess and make a referral to a local community hospital for intravenous (IV) antibiotic therapy. The nurse and the hospital in this example are resources for the client to reduce the severity of a stressor.

The last factor involves the resources that can be used to deal with the stressor. In the example just given, the client needs transportation to the hospital and Medicaid coverage or financial arrangements that will provide for her care. Both of these factors will influence how she can access the resource to help her cope with the physiological stressor.

Stimulus-Based Model.

The stimulus-based model focuses on disturbing or disruptive events within the environment. The classic research of Holmes and Rahe (1976) that identified stress as a stimulus has resulted in the development of the social readjustment scale, which measures the effects of major life events on illness. The stimulus-based model focuses on the following assumptions (McNett, 1989):

    Life change events are normal, and they require the
        same type and duration of adjustment.
    People are passive recipients of stress, and their per-
        ceptions of the event are irrelevant.
    All people have a common threshold of stimulus, and
        illness results at any point after the threshold.

The scale identifies events that are stressful for most people. This can be very useful when initially assessing a client's level of stress. However, as with the response-based model, the stimulus-based model does not allow for individual differences in perception and response to stressors. Nurses may experience difficulty when attempting to use this model in stress management because of the lack of flexibility for individual adaptation.

Transaction-Based Model.

The transaction-based model views the person and environment in a dynamic, reciprocal, interactive relationship (Lazarus and Folkman, 1984). This model, developed by Lazarus and Folkman, views the stressor as an individual perceptual response rooted in psychological and cognitive processes. The individual's perceptual response allows the individual to be influenced by person-related factors such as beliefs, perception of control, and uncertainty. Stress originates from the relationship between the person and the environment. This model focuses on stress-related processes such as cognitive appraisal and coping (Peirce, 1995).

FACTORS INFLUENCING RESPONSE TO STRESSORS

The response to any stressor depends on physiological functioning, personality, and behavioral characteristics, as well as the nature of the stressor (Box 30-1). Each factor influences the response to a stressor. A person may perceive the intensity or magnitude of a stressor as minimal, moderate, or severe. The greater the magnitude of the stressor, the greater the stress response. Likewise, the scope of a stressor can be described as limited, medium, or extensive. The greater the scope of a stressor, the greater the response of the client to it (Lazarus and Folkman, 1984).

ADAPTATION TO STRESSORS

Adaptation is the process by which the physiological or psychosocial dimensions change in response to stress.

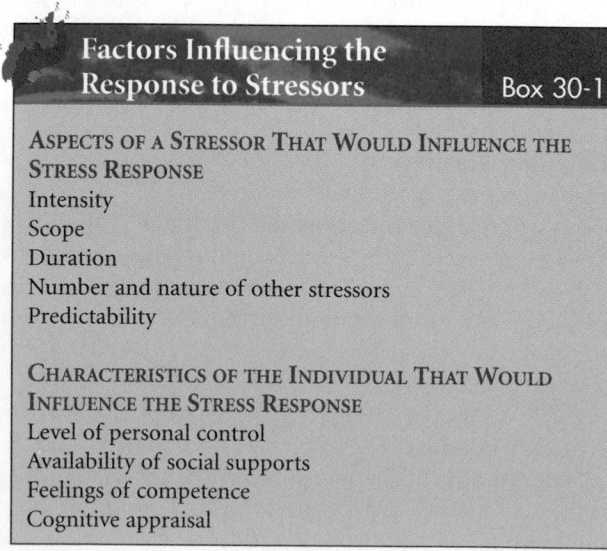

Factors Influencing the Response to Stressors   Box 30-1

ASPECTS OF A STRESSOR THAT WOULD INFLUENCE THE
STRESS RESPONSE
Intensity
Scope
Duration
Number and nature of other stressors
Predictability

CHARACTERISTICS OF THE INDIVIDUAL THAT WOULD
INFLUENCE THE STRESS RESPONSE
Level of personal control
Availability of social supports
Feelings of competence
Cognitive appraisal

Health promotion often focuses on a person's, family's, or community's adaptation to stress. There are many forms of adaptation. Physiological adaptations make possible a physiological homeostasis. A similar process of adaptation, however, may occur in the psychosocial and other dimensions.

Adaptation is an attempt to maintain optimal functioning. Adaptation involves reflexes, automatic body mechanisms for protection, coping mechanisms, and ideally can lead to adjustment or mastery of a situation (Selye, 1976). A stressor that stimulates adaptation may be short term, such as a fever, or long term, such as paralysis of a limb. To function optimally, a person must be able to respond to such stressors and adapt to the required demands or changes. Adaptation requires an active response from the whole person.

Like an individual, a family or group may need to adapt to a stressor. Family adaptation is the process by which a family maintains a balance so that it can fulfill its purposes and tasks, deal with stress, and promote the growth of individual members. For a family to adapt successfully, good communication skills, mutual respect for all family members, adequate resources for adaptation, and previous experience with stressors must exist (Haber and others, 1997).

Dimensions of Adaptation.
Stress can affect the physical, developmental, emotional, intellectual, social, and spiritual dimensions. Adaptive resources exist in each of these dimensions. Therefore, when assessing a client's adaptation to a stress a nurse must consider the total person. Table 30-1 highlights adaptive resources found in each dimension and gives examples of positive and negative outcomes of stressors.

RESPONSE TO STRESS
The total person is involved in responding and adapting to stresses. Most research into stress responses, however, focuses on psychological or emotional and physiological responses, although these dimensions overlap and interact with the other dimensions.

When stress occurs, a person uses physiological and psychological energy to respond and adapt. The amount of energy required and the effectiveness of the attempt to adapt depend on the intensity, scope, and duration of the stressor and the number of other stressors. The stress re-

Table 30-1   Dimensions of Adaptation

Dimension	Adaptive Resources	Example of Stressor	Example of Unsuccessful Outcome	Example of Successful Outcome
Physical	Local adaptation syndrome General adaptation syndrome	Fever	Death	Infection resolved
Developmental	Successful coping in past development task/stages Successful adaptation to past stressors	Retirement	Depression	Role functions altered to other meaningful activities
Emotional	Psychological defense mechanisms Individual personality strengths	Rape	Irrational fear of men	Integration of traumatic memory Serves as advocate for others at rape crisis center
Intellectual	Formal education Ability to problem solve Communication skills Realistic perception of stressor Conscious mobilization of past positive coping strategies	Diagnosis of cancer	Denies presence of cancer and foregoes any treatment	Uses an active problem-solving approach to make decisions about care
Social	Social network that provides support Others who may direct person to needed resources	Alcoholism in a family member	Person with alcoholism withdrawing from family and other social contacts	Active participation of all family members in Alcoholics Anonymous support groups
Spiritual	Prayer groups; support from priest, rabbi, or minister	Ill family member feeling abandoned by God	Withdraws from attending church, won't talk with church members or minister	Begins to seek out friends in the church, volunteers for church-related activities

sponse is adaptive and protective, and the characteristics of this response are the result of integrated neuroendocrine responses (Box 30-2).

Physiological Response.

The classic research by Selye (1946, 1976) has identified the two physiological responses to stress: the **local adaptation syndrome (LAS)** and the general adaptation syndrome (GAS). The LAS is a response of a body tissue, organ, or part to the stress of trauma, illness, or other physiological change. The GAS is a defense response of the whole body to stress.

LAS.   The body produces many localized responses to stress. These include blood clotting, wound healing, accommodation of the eye to light, and response to pressure. All forms of the LAS share the following characteristics:

The response is localized; it does not involve entire body systems.

The response is adaptive, meaning that a stressor is necessary to stimulate it.

The response is short term. It does not persist indefinitely.

The response is restorative, meaning that the LAS assists in restoring homeostasis to the body region or part.

Two localized responses, the reflex pain response and the inflammatory response, are described here as examples of the LAS. Nurses encounter these responses in many health care settings.

Characteristics of the Stress Response   Box 30-2

- Stress response is natural, protective, and adaptive.
- There are normal responses to stressors; stressors encountered in everyday circumstances increase catecholamine excretion, which causes an increase in heart rate and blood pressure.
- Physical and emotional stressors trigger similar responses (specificity versus nonspecificity). Magnitude and patterns may differ.
- There are limits in ability to compensate.
- Magnitude and duration of stressors may be so great that homeostatic mechanisms for adjustment fail, leading to death.
- Repeated exposure to stimuli results in adaptive changes; that is, tissue levels of the enzyme tyrosine hydrolase increase, which increases capacity for the body to produce norepinephrine and epinephrine.
- There are individual differences in response to same stressors.

Modified from Lindsay AM, Carrieri VK, Page GG: Stress response. In Lindsay AM, Carrieri VK, editors: *Pathological phenomenon in nursing: human response to illness,* ed 2, Philadelphia, 1993, WB Saunders.

Reflex Pain Response.   The reflex pain response is a localized response of the central nervous system to pain (see Chapter 42). It is an adaptive response and protects tissue from further damage. The response involves a sensory receptor, a sensory nerve to the spinal cord, a connector neuron within the spinal cord, a motor nerve from the spinal cord, and an effector muscle. An example would be the unconscious, reflex removal of the hand from a hot surface. Another example would be a muscle cramp.

Inflammatory Response.   The inflammatory response is stimulated by trauma or infection. This response localizes the inflammation, thus preventing its spread, and promotes healing. The inflammatory response may produce localized pain, swelling, heat, redness, and changes in functioning. It occurs in three phases. The first phase involves changes in cells and the circulatory system. Initially, narrowing of blood vessels occurs at the injury to control bleeding. Then histamine is released at the injury, increasing blood flow to the area and increasing the number of white blood cells to combat infection. Almost simultaneously, kinins are released to increase capillary permeability to permit the flow of proteins, fluid, and leukocytes to the injury. At this point the localized blood flow decreases, keeping leukocytes in the area to fight infection.

The second phase is characterized by release of exudate from the wound. Exudate is a combination of fluid, cells, and other substances produced in the area of injury. The type and amount of exudate vary from injury to injury and from person to person. Exudate is usually released at the injury, which may be a cut, laceration, or surgical incision.

The last phase is repair of tissue by regeneration or scar formation. Regeneration replaces damaged cells with identical or similar cells. Scar formation replaces original tissue that is not functional. The inflammatory response alerts the nurse that the body is adapting to a local injury. During adaptation the inflammatory response protects the body from infection and promotes healing.

GAS.   The GAS is a physiological response of the whole body to stress. It involves several body systems, primarily the autonomic nervous system and the endocrine system. Some textbooks refer to the GAS as the neuroendocrine response. The GAS consists of the alarm reaction, the resistance stage, and the exhaustion stage (Figure 30-1).

Alarm Reaction.   The alarm reaction involves the mobilization of the defense mechanisms of the body and mind to cope with the stressor. Hormone levels rise to increase blood volume and thereby prepare the person to act. Other hormones are released to increase blood glucose levels to make energy available for adaptation. Increased levels of other hormones—epinephrine and norepinephrine—result in an increased heart rate, increased blood flow to muscles, increased oxygen intake, and greater mental alertness.

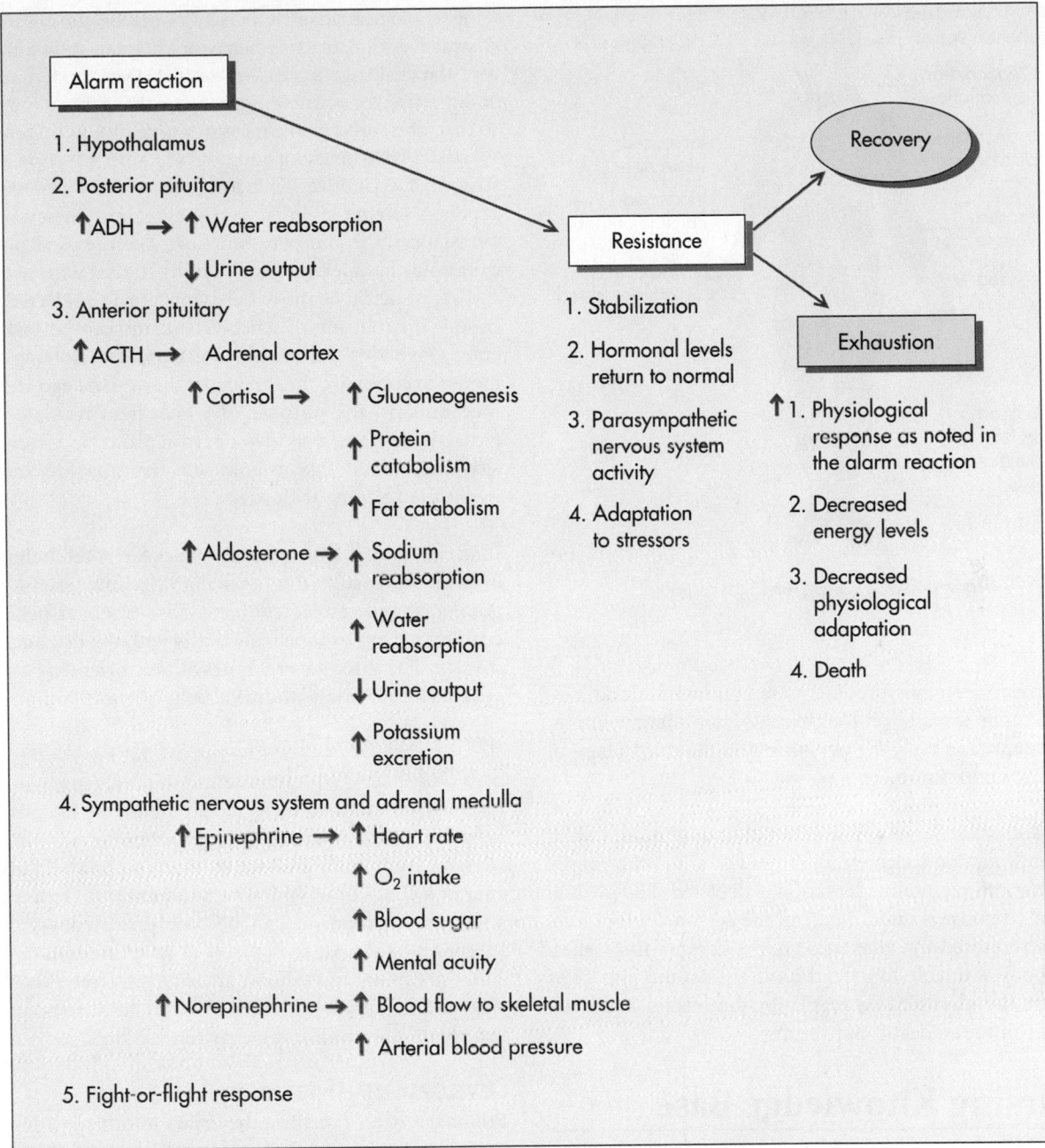

Figure 30-1   General adaptation syndrome (GAS).

This extensive hormonal activity prepares the person for the **fight-or-flight response.** Cardiac output, oxygen intake, and respiratory rate are increased; the pupils of the eyes are dilated to produce a greater visual field; and the heart rate is increased for more energy. Other changes occur to prepare the person to act (Figure 30-2). With this increased mental energy and alertness, the person is prepared to fight or flee the stressor.

During the alarm reaction, the person is faced with a specific stressor. The person's physiological response is extensive, involving major systems of the body, and it may last from a minute to many hours. If the stressor is extreme or remains for a long time, there may be a threat to life. If the stressor is still present after the initial alarm reaction, the person progresses to the second phase of the GAS, resistance.

Resistance Stage.   In the resistance stage the body stabilizes, and hormone levels, heart rate, blood pressure, and cardiac output return to normal. The person is attempting to adapt to the stressor. If the stress can be resolved, the body repairs damage that may have occurred. However, if

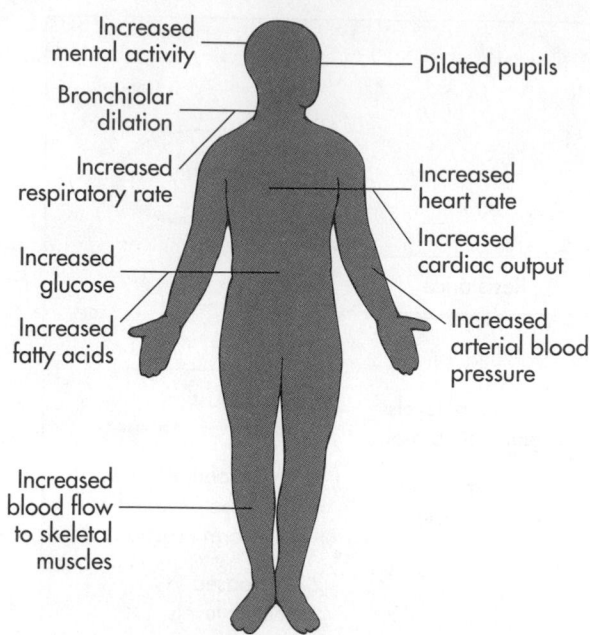

Figure 30-2 Fight-or-flight response.

the stressor remains present, as in continued blood loss, debilitating disease, or long-term severe mental illness, and adaptation fails, the person enters the third phase of the GAS, exhaustion.

Exhaustion Stage.   The exhaustion stage occurs when the body can no longer resist stress and when the energy necessary to maintain adaptation is depleted. The physiological response is intensified, but the person's energy level is compromised and adaptation to the stressor diminishes. The body is unable to defend itself against the impact of the stressor, physiological regulation diminishes, and if the stress continues, death may result.

Nursing Knowledge Base

Nurses are constantly challenged by a variety of stress responses when providing care to clients. Therefore, nurses must possess a thorough understanding of the stress response. Nursing interventions are frequently required when treating symptoms that have arisen from stress. Interventions must consider the client's lifestyle decisions, developmental factors, family dynamics, and psychological issues. By encompassing the studies of many disciplines, the holistic needs of the client can be ascertained.

PSYCHOLOGICAL RESPONSE
Psychological adaptive behaviors influence how a person copes with stress. These behaviors are directed at stress management and are acquired through learning and experience as a person identifies acceptable and successful behaviors.

Psychological adaptive behaviors can be constructive or destructive. Constructive behaviors help an individual accept the challenge to resolve conflict. Even anxiety can be constructive; for example, it can signal that a threat is present so that a person can take measures to reduce its severity.

Destructive behaviors do not help a person cope with a stressor. Destructive behaviors affect reality orientation, problem-solving abilities, personality, and, in severe circumstances, the ability to function. The use of alcohol or drugs may hamper a person's ability to deal with stress.

Psychological adaptive behaviors are also referred to as coping mechanisms. Such mechanisms can be task oriented, involving the use of direct problem-solving techniques to cope with the threats, or they can be **ego-defense mechanisms,** the purpose of which is to regulate emotional distress and thus give a person protection from anxiety and stress. Ego-defense mechanisms are indirect methods of coping with stress.

Task-Oriented Behaviors.   **Task-oriented behaviors** involve using cognitive abilities to reduce stress, solve problems, and resolve conflicts. Task-oriented behaviors enable a person to cope realistically with the demands of a stressor. The three general types of task-oriented behavior are attack behavior, withdrawal behavior, and compromise (Box 30-3).

Ego-Defense Mechanisms.   Ego-defense mechanisms, first described by Sigmund Freud, are unconscious behaviors that offer psychological protection from a stressful event. They are used by everyone and help protect against feelings of worthlessness and anxiety. Occasionally a defense mechanism can become distorted and is no longer able to assist the person in adapting to a stressor. There are many ego-defense mechanisms (see Box 30-3). They are frequently activated by short-term stressors and usually do not result in psychiatric disorders.

DEVELOPMENTAL FACTORS
Prolonged stress can affect the ability to complete developmental tasks. In any developmental stage, a person normally encounters tasks and engages in behaviors characteristic of the stage. In extreme forms, repeated stress can lead to maturational crisis. If parents or the environment prevent a young child from developing a sense of autonomy, the child may experience stress, which is indicated by excessive dependence on others or passive inactive behavior.

INTELLECTUAL FACTORS
Studies have shown that repeated stress can have consequences for brain function, especially in short-term memory (McEwen, 1998). A person's ability to acquire new knowledge or skills may also be impaired. This is especially important information for the nurse who is attempting client teaching. The client may not be able to learn new skills or about a disease process until prolonged

TASK-ORIENTED BEHAVIORS

- Attack behavior is acting to remove or overcome a stressor or to satisfy a need.
- Withdrawal behavior is removing the self physically or emotionally from the stressor.
- Compromise behavior is changing the usual method of operating, substituting goals, or omitting the satisfaction of needs to meet other needs or to avoid stress.

EXAMPLES OF EGO-DEFENSE MECHANISMS

- Compensation is making up for a deficiency in one aspect of self-image by strongly emphasizing a feature considered an asset.
- Conversion is unconsciously repressing an anxiety-producing emotional conflict and transforming it into nonorganic symptoms.
- Denial is avoiding emotional conflicts by refusing to consciously acknowledge anything that might cause intolerable emotional pain.
- Displacement is transferring emotions, ideas, or wishes from a stressful situation to a less anxiety-producing substitute.
- Identification is patterning behavior after that of another person and assuming that person's qualities, characteristics, and actions.
- Regression is coping with a stressor through actions and behaviors associated with an earlier developmental period.

stressors have been resolved or alternate forms of coping have been addressed.

EMOTIONAL BEHAVIORAL ISSUES

Individual personality involves a complex relationship among many factors. The emotional reaction to prolonged stress is determined by examining the client's current lifestyle and stressors, prior experience with stressors, past successful coping mechanisms, role functions, self-concept and **hardiness,** which is a combination of three personality characteristics thought to mediate against stress. These three characteristics are sense of control over life events, commitment to meaningful activities, and anticipation of challenge as an opportunity for growth (Wiebe and Williams, 1992; Tartasky, 1993).

FAMILY FACTORS

The word *family* means different things to different people (see Chapter 8). Each individual has a deeply ingrained value of their perception of a family. The nuclear family of the 1950s has been joined by single-parent families, blended families and alternate patterns of relationship families. The family form itself can be a cause of stress. Single parents face the burden of caring for children on

their own while working and running a home. Adolescent pregnancies are on the increase, and homosexual couples who have children may face the added stress of discrimination. It is important to note that the nurse should always respect the client's ideals of a family. Economic concerns, lack of health care insurance, homelessness, violence, and illness are all factors that can increase the stress within a family. Poor communication habits and maladaptive behaviors among its members can create crisis within a family structure and limit adaptation (Clemen-Stone, McGuire, and Eigsti, 1998).

LIFESTYLE ISSUES

Lifestyle decisions can be important factors that influence stress. An individual may know that smoking can lead to cardiovascular disease or cancer. However, he may choose to continue to smoke because it helps him cope with an unhappy job situation. His child may then ask him to stop smoking. If he is unable or unwilling to quit, he may feel like a failure, therefore precipitating more stress. If he is successful with smoking cessation, then he may feel positive about himself and replace smoking with a daily exercise regime. His child may also feel affirmed because a parent listened to his or her concerns.

Obesity and homosexuality are examples of two other lifestyle issues that can cause a great deal of stress to individuals and their families. When providing care to an obese or homosexual client, the nurse should set aside personal judgments and examine how best to help the client cope effectively.

SOCIOCULTURAL ISSUES

Each social and cultural group has its own views pertaining to stress. Education, poverty, support systems, and accepted coping mechanisms all influence these beliefs (see Chapter 7). Social instability can also play a role in stress and adaptation. McEwen (1998) reported that job instability following the fall of communism and the subsequent increase in cardiovascular disease is a primary reason for the increased death rate in Eastern Europe.

SPIRITUAL CONSIDERATIONS

Spirituality begins early in life and is influenced by culture, beliefs, and life experiences. Just as the concept of family is unique to each person, spirituality is also highly individualized. It is important to note that religion and spirituality are not the same thing. Religion is a system of organized beliefs and worship. Spirituality demonstrates a unique capacity for love, joy, caring, compassion, and for finding meaning in life's difficult experiences (Balzer-Riley, 1996).

During times of stress, some clients will rely on their faith, whereas others may abandon their practices out of disillusionment and anger. Although this is many times a difficult subject for caregivers to approach, it is an essential part of the client's well-being (see Chapter 28).

KNOWLEDGE

- Basic stress response
- Factors influencing stress
- Physiological, emotional, and behavioral risks associated with a stressor
- Basic defense mechanisms
- Cultural influences

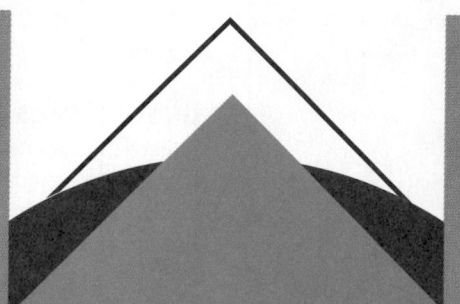

STANDARDS

- Apply intellectual standards of completeness, relevance, precision, and accuracy when assessing the client's stress response

ASSESSMENT

- Identify actual or potential stressors
- Obtain data regarding the client's previous experience with stress
- Determine the impact of illness on the client's lifestyle

EXPERIENCE

- Caring for clients whose illness, lifestyle, family interactions, and personal/professional demands resulted in stress
- Personal experience in dealing with stressful situations

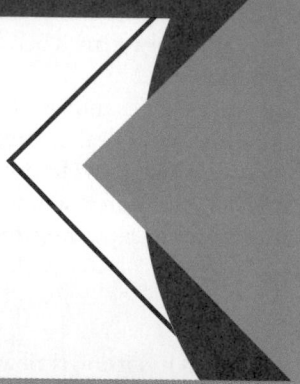
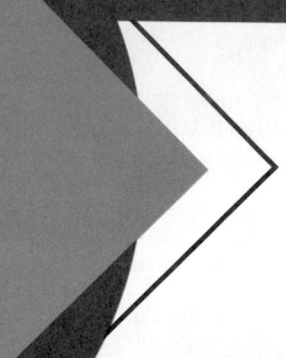
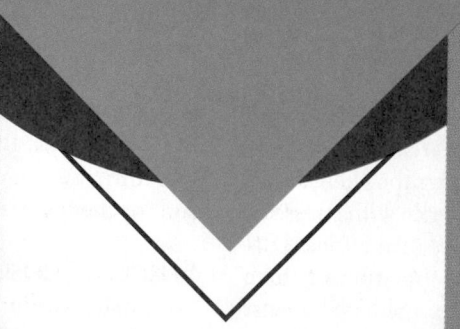

ATTITUDES

- Demonstrate perseverance to identify the client's stressors and response to stressors
- Approach assessment with fairness and integrity to collect data in an unbiased manner and convey that client information remains confidential

Figure 30-3   *Synthesis Model for Stress and Adaptation Assessment Phase.*

Critical Thinking Synthesis

Successful critical thinking requires a synthesis of knowledge, experience, information gathered from clients, critical thinking attitudes, and intellectual and professional standards. Clinical judgments require the nurse to anticipate the information necessary, analyze the data, and make decisions regarding client care. Critical thinking is always changing. During assessment (Figure 30-3) the nurse must consider all elements that build toward making an appropriate nursing diagnosis.

In the case of stress and adaptation, the nurse must integrate knowledge from nursing and other disciplines, previous experiences, and information gathered from clients to understand stress and its impact on the client and family. In addition, the use of critical thinking attitudes such as perseverance is needed to form a plan of care to provide appropriate stress management. To fully understand how stress has affected the client, the nurse must gather complete and accurate data. Cultural and developmental needs must be assessed, and the nurse must use a broad knowledge base to ensure that what the client feels is most important has been addressed.

Physiological Indicators of Stress	Box 30-4

Elevated blood pressure
Increased muscle tension in neck, shoulders, back
Elevated pulse and increased respiration
Sweaty palms
Cold hands and feet
Slumped posture
Fatigue
Tension headache
Upset stomach
Higher-pitched voice
Nausea, vomiting, and diarrhea
Change in appetite
Change in weight
Change in urinary frequency
Abnormal laboratory findings: elevated adrenocorticotropic hormone, cortisol, and catecholamine levels and hyperglycemia
Restlessness: difficulty falling asleep or frequent awakening
Dilated pupils

Nursing Process

ASSESSMENT

Each client has unique perceptions and responses to stress. A person's perception of a stressor is based on beliefs and norms, life experiences and patterns, environmental factors, family structure and function, developmental stage, past experiences with stress, and coping mechanisms.

Because nurses spend a great deal of time with clients and their families or friends, they are in an optimal position to critically analyze coping responses. Stress-response behaviors, both verbal and nonverbal, should be assessed. Nurses also provide care for clients in various settings, and thus they are often able to assess reactions to stress. The nurse assesses for indicators of stress and coping in all dimensions of adaptation and synthesizes that information (see Figure 30-3). Knowledge, experience, and attitudes are especially important when the nurse utilizes critical thinking during the assessment phase of a client's individual plan of care.

Physiological Indicators. Physiological indicators of stress are objective, more readily identified, and can be commonly observed or measured (Box 30-4). However, they are not always observed in all clients experiencing stress, and they vary among individuals. Vital signs are usually elevated, and the client may appear restless and unable to concentrate. These indicators can appear at any stage of stress.

The duration and intensity of the symptoms are directly related to the perceived duration and intensity of the stressor. Physiological indicators arise from a variety of systems. Therefore the assessment of stress involves collecting data from all systems. The link between psychological stress and disease is frequently called the mind-body interaction. Research has shown that stress can affect illness and disease patterns.

During any stage, there may be physical complaints such as nausea, vomiting, diarrhea, or headache. Physical appearance can be changed, posture may be slumped, hygiene and grooming may be poor, and style of dress may differ. Prolonged stress has been linked with cardiovascular and gastrointestinal diseases. Some cancers and immunological disorders, migraine headaches, infertility, **burnout,** and irritability are associated with prolonged, unresolved stressors. In addition, stress is also known to exacerbate neurologic conditions such as Parkinson's disease and Tourette's syndrome (Mandle and others, 1995; Finlay and Zigmond, 1997; McEwen, 1998).

Mild stress situations are stressors that everyone encounters regularly, such as oversleeping, traffic jams, a flat tire, or criticism from a superior. Mild stress situations do not usually produce chronic physiological damage, but moderate and severe stress can create a risk of medical illness or a worsening of a chronic illness. Such situations usually last a few minutes to a few hours. By themselves, these stressors are not significant risks for symptom development. However, multiple mild stressors over a short time can increase risk of illness (Holmes and Rahe, 1976).

Moderate stress situations last longer, from several hours to days. For example, an unresolved disagreement with a co-worker, a sick child, or the prolonged absence of a family member are moderate stress situations.

Severe stress situations are chronic situations that may last several weeks to several years, such as continual marital disagreements, prolonged financial difficulties, and long-term physical illness. The more frequent and longer the stress situation, the higher the health risk (Wiebe and Williams, 1992). The development of stress-related disease can be examined in terms of the health-illness continuum (Figure 30-4). As a person's stress increases, stress behaviors increase gradually, which decreases energy and adaptive responses.

Identifying the mind-body interaction is crucial for predicting the risk of stress-related illness. A nurse also critically assesses the client's perception of stressors, for what may seem a mild stress situation to the nurse may be extremely disturbing to the client.

Psychological Indicators.
Exposure to a stressor results in physiological and psychological adaptive responses. As stated earlier, psychological adaptive behaviors assist the person's ability to cope with stressors. The nurse should assess the client for destructive behaviors that do not help the person cope with a stressor. Conversion, denial, and displacement are examples of destructive ego-defense mechanisms. An example of denial is a high school student who is addicted to cocaine who says he could quit taking drugs whenever he chooses.

To some, the abuse of alcohol or drugs may seem to be an adaptive behavior. In reality, it increases rather than decreases the stress (Box 30-5).

Developmental Indicators.
Infants or young children generally encounter stressors at home. When nurtured in responsive, empathetic environments, they are able to develop healthy self-esteem and ultimately learn healthy adaptive coping responses (Haber and others, 1997). However, the absence of parental figures or their failure to provide the security needed to develop a sense of trust can be stressors. In later life there may be chronic distrust, resulting in withdrawal and disturbed interpersonal relationships.

School-age children normally develop a sense of adequacy. They begin to realize that accumulation of knowledge and mastery of skills can help them accomplish goals, and self-esteem develops through friendships and sharing with peers. At this stage stress is indicated by the inability or unwillingness to develop friendships.

Adolescents normally develop a strong sense of identity but at the same time need to be accepted by peers. Adolescents with strong social support systems report an increased ability to adjust to stressors, but adolescents without social support systems frequently report increased psychosocial problems (DuBois and others, 1992). There are many stressors in this age group, including conflicts involving sexual drive and expected standards of behavior. Prolonged conflict may present as indecision and confusion, rebellion, depression, or anxiety.

Young adults are in transition from youthful experiences to adult responsibilities. They must prepare for careers, living alone and, perhaps, starting families. Conflicts between work and family responsibilities may be a source of stress.

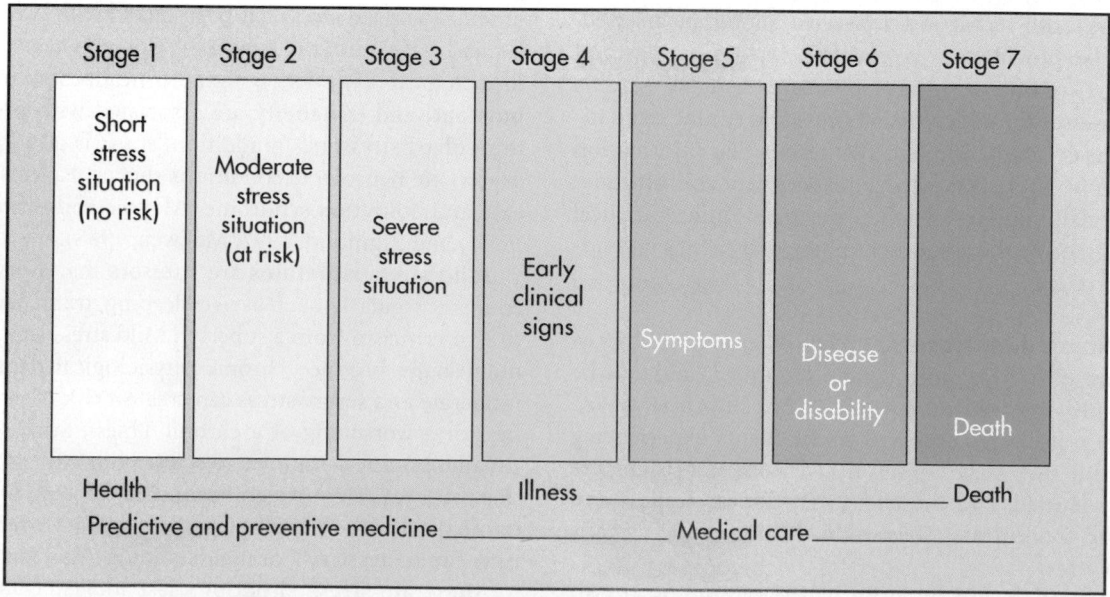

Figure 30-4 Stages of illness development in stress-related diseases.

Alcohol	(beer, wine, "hard" liquor)
Amphetamine	(crank)
Caffeine	(coffee, tea, colas)
Cannabis	(marijuana)
Cocaine	(crack)
Hallucinogens	(LSD, peyote)
Inhalants	(glue, gasoline)
Nicotine	(cigarettes)
Opioids	(morphine, heroin)
Sedatives, hypnotics, anxio-lytics	(diazepam, barbiturates)
Anabolic steroids	
Phencyclidine (PCP)	(angel dust)

Middle-age adults are usually involved in family building, creating stable careers, and perhaps caring for older parents. They are generally able to control desires and in some cases substitute the needs of spouses, children, or parents for their needs. Stress can result, however, if they feel that too many responsibilities have been placed on them. A recent trend is looking at the impact of stressors on the family caregiver's role. Middle adults have been called the sandwich generation because they are frequently responsible for chronically ill parents while raising their own families. Because of the stressors involved, caregivers have reported increases in fatigue, minor illnesses (e.g., colds and influenza), depression, and dissatisfaction with family interaction (Musolf, 1991).

Older adults are commonly faced with adapting to changes in family and perhaps to the deaths of spouses or longtime friends. Older adults must also adjust to changes in physical appearance and physiological functioning (Box 30-6). Major life changes such as retirement also are stressful. Some older adults must cope with relocation to some form of institutionalized living. Moving to a nursing home may be particularly stressful for an older person and can aggravate existing health and emotional problems (Dellasaga and Nolan, 1997).

Emotional Behavioral Indicators.
Emotions are sometimes assessed directly or indirectly by observing a client's behavior. Stress affects emotional well-being in many ways (Box 30-7). Because stress affects each person differently, the nurse should attempt to establish a rapport with the client before assessing the client's emotional status. The client may or may not be aware of his or her behavioral responses. Nonverbal cues such as anger and inappropriate crying are extremely important. Questions that deal with self-worth, current lifestyle, and prior experience with stressors are critical.

Intellectual Indicators.
Prolonged stress can manifest itself in the intellectual dimension and have observable

- Aging is often associated with declines in functional abilities due to the normal aging process. Although this may be true, evidence suggests that coping and adaptation functions are surprisingly well preserved throughout the entire life span (Foster, 1997).
- Health problems are common among the elderly and can be a cause of stress.
- Since many older adults are on a fixed income, the cost of medical care can be a huge stressor. The nurse may need to involve other disciplines such as social services to help the client pay for medications or treatments.
- Loneliness and isolation can be a major stressor for the elderly. Studies have suggested that older people's perceptions of stress are less likely to lead to depression if high social resources are present (Lee and Ellenbacker, 1998).
- Older adults effectively utilize religious coping in response to medical illness and disasters (Foster, 1997).
- Before scheduling a physician's appointment or a needed test, explore the transportation needs of the older client. Dependency is a large stressor for the elderly, and necessary steps should be taken to avoid this issue.

Anxiety
Depression
Burnout
Increased use of chemical substances
Change in eating habits, sleep, and activity pattern
Mental exhaustion
Feelings of inadequacy
Loss of self-esteem
Increased irritability
Loss of motivation
Emotional outbursts and crying
Decreased productivity and quality of job performance
Tendency to make mistakes (i.e., poor judgment)
Forgetfulness and blocking
Diminished attention to detail
Preoccupation (i.e., daydreaming or "spacing out")
Inability to concentrate on tasks
Increased absenteeism and illness
Lethargy
Loss of interest
Proneness to accidents

indicators. A person's ability to acquire new knowledge or skills is impaired. A person's cognitive appraisal of a situation may also be inaccurate. Stress can impede communication between the client and others. A shortened attention span, inability to think clearly, and the tendency to focus narrowly may render the client unable to solve problems and resolve conflicts. Therefore increased dependence on others occurs.

Family Indicators. It is very important for the nurse to understand that nursing interventions for one client can affect the entire family. That is why assessment of the entire family and its members' roles is essential. Culture, structure, and concept of the family are also important when assessing how a family copes with stress. Major life events should be explored. Job instability, death or illness of a family member, and relocation are examples of huge family stressors. The nurse should also assess what the client feels effective emotional support is and if that support is provided by the family structure.

Lifestyle Indicators. At the turn of the century, infectious diseases were the leading causes of death, but since then antibiotics, improved living conditions, increased knowledge of nutrition, and better sanitation methods have lowered the death rate. Now the leading causes of death are diseases involving lifestyle stressors.

There are a variety of lifestyle choices that can create physical and/or psychological stress within a client. Smoking, obesity, drug abuse, and chronic sleep deprivation are examples. Regular exercise, adequate rest, and a nutritious diet are positive lifestyle choices that can reduce stress. The nurse should assess the client for both positive and negative issues in relation to stress. Lifestyle choices such as sex with multiple partners propose a very large stressor in the form of human immunodeficiency virus (HIV) transmission. Smoking and drug or alcohol consumption during pregnancy can cause stress to the fetus and should be thoroughly assessed.

Sociocultural Indicators. Assessing stressors and coping resources in the social dimension involves exploring with the client the amount, type, and quality of social interactions present. Stressors on the family may create dysfunction that affects the client or the family as a whole (Duhamel and Campagna, 1997).

The nurse must also be aware of cultural differences in stress responses or coping mechanisms. For example, an African-American client may prefer obtaining social support from family members rather than professional assistance (Murata, 1994) (Box 30-8).

Spiritual Indicators. People use spiritual resources to adapt to stress in many ways, but stress can also manifest itself in the spiritual dimension. Severe stress may result in anger at the Supreme Being, or the person may view the

---

Cultural ASPECTS OF CARE   Box 30-8

The sharp contrast between Chinese and American cultures can cause a great deal of stress among Chinese-Americans, especially when dealing with health care issues. Western medicine is very technical and has a strong biological base. Chinese culture, including its medicine, is strongly linked to religious and social beliefs. Therefore newly immigrated and first-generation Chinese-Americans often have a high level of stress when seeking Western medicine. Typically they will treat minor or chronic illness with Chinese medical services (herbal remedies, acupuncture, massage therapy, and skin scraping) and seek Western medical services only for acute or serious problems (Giger and Davidhizar, 1995). For this reason, many Chinese-Americans are acutely ill when they first seek medical attention.

It is important for the nurse to respect the differences in culture to reduce the stress of the Chinese client. Language difficulties and cultural differences can lead to frustration, powerlessness, and depression. However, the nurse may not be aware of these feelings because the Chinese client may feel it would inconvenience the health care worker to ask questions. Touching someone's hand and excessive eye contact are considered rude in the Chinese culture, and the nurse can inadvertently add to the stress level of the client (Giger and Davidhizar, 1995). Observing nonverbal behaviors and encouraging clients to verbalize (or obtaining a translator as needed) are very important nursing interventions. The family unit is also an important part of the perceived stress and adaptation of the Chinese. The nurse should include the entire family when developing the plan of care. This will increase the quality of care and better meet the health needs of this population (Lee and Ellenbacker, 1998).

---

stressor as punishment. Stressors such as acute illness or the death of a loved one may threaten a person's meaning of life and can lead to depression. When providing care to a spiritually affected client, a nurse should not judge the appropriateness of religious feelings or practices but should examine how beliefs and values have changed (Box 30-9).

Client Expectations. It is important for the nurse to remember that every person perceives and reacts differently to stress. Culture, life experiences, and family belief systems all play a part in this perception. Research by Raeside (1997) has shown that in the neonatal intensive care unit (NICU), mothers of low-birth-weight babies reported very different environmental stressors than what NICU nurses perceived would be the greatest maternal stressor. The nurses felt that the monitors attached to the baby would create the most stress, whereas the mothers cited the heat of the NICU as most distressing. Complete and accurate assessment of the client and support systems is essential in tailoring care to the individual's needs. The nurse should always ask the client what is expected re-

| Research HIGHLIGHT | Box 30-9 |

RESEARCH ABSTRACT

This study looked at African-American and Anglo-American caregivers of relatives diagnosed with probable Alzheimer's disease. Identifying caregivers who are at risk for emotional problems is an important part of helping the families deal with this debilitating disease. The researcher found that the African-American caregivers reported less occurrence of client disruptive behavior and appraised disruptive behavior as less stressful than did the Anglo-American group. Religious orientation may reduce the perceived stressfulness of behavior problems by providing an interpretation of the situation as part of God's plan, which leads ultimately to a desirable outcome. Life experiences and cultural background may also contribute to the findings. Interventions that develop self-control, self-direction, self-regulation techniques, and problem-solving training were recommended for both groups.

IMPLICATIONS FOR PRACTICE

- Recognize that Anglo-American caregivers of clients with Alzheimer's disease are less likely to utilize religious means as a way of coping with stress than are their African-American counterparts.
- Imagery, meditation, positive reinforcement, and biofeedback are interventions the nurse should discuss with caregivers of relatives with Alzheimer's disease.

REFERENCE

Gonzales E: Resourcefulness, appraisals and coping efforts of family caregivers, *Issues Ment Health Nurs* 18(3):209, 1997.

garding the reduction of stress. This should include achievable goals utilizing reasonable interventions. The very best smoking cessation program does little good if the client does not recognize smoking as a problem. The nurse's own value system should be acknowledged and then set aside so the personal needs of the client can be met.

NURSING DIAGNOSIS

A review of assessment data leads the nurse to cluster data that may indicate a potential or actual stressor and the client's response. Clustering of data, along with the application of the nurse's knowledge and experience with clients in stress, leads to a nursing diagnosis (Box 30-10). For example, changes in appetite and sleeping patterns and increased frequency of headaches are defining characteristics for *ineffective individual coping*, which is a frequent nursing diagnosis for clients experiencing stress.

Identification of a nursing diagnostic label requires the presence of appropriate defining characteristics. The diagnostic label must be supported by the defining characteristics in the database. The nursing diagnosis should identify the probable etiology for the problem. Incorrect identification of the cause of a nursing diagnosis can result in an inappropriate care plan and selected interventions. For example, *ineffective individual coping related to inadequate support system* results in interventions designed to increase the client's support resources (e.g., friends, family, support groups). If the nurse incorrectly identified unmet expectations as the related factor, then the plan of care

SAMPLE NURSING DIAGNOSTIC PROCESS   Box 30-10

CAREGIVER ROLE STRAIN

Assessment Activities	Defining Characteristics	Nursing Diagnosis
Ask client what a typical day is like caring for his wife at home.	Client describes 9 months of maintaining constant care and vigilance over activities of spouse.	Caregiver role strain related to adjustment to recent diagnosis of wife's Alzheimer's dementia.
Determine to what extent the caregiving role interferes with other roles or social functions such as a job.	Client is awakened frequently during the night to find wife wandering in the house. Client reports he regrets not being able to perform duties of church deacon since taking over care of wife. Client states he has no outside activities.	
Explore the caregiver's perception and acceptance of social support and knowledge of community resources.	Client states that he hasn't asked anyone to assist him, but several close friends live nearby. Client has no knowledge of community resources.	
Observe client's behavior and mannerisms during assessment.	Caregiver appears fatigued, sighs occasionally.	

is not directed toward the resolution of the nursing diagnosis (Box 30-11). Stress can result in multiple diagnostic statements. Examples selected here do not represent the entire list. Chapters 26 and 28 include nursing diagnoses associated with unmet self-concept and spiritual needs. This process of nursing diagnosis corresponds with the diagnostic monitoring function domain of nursing practice.

PLANNING

During planning, the nurse again synthesizes information from multiple resources (Figure 30-5). Critical thinking ensures that the clients' plan of care integrates all that the nurse knows about the individual and essential critical thinking elements. Professional standards are especially important to consider when the nurse develops a plan of care. These standards often establish scientifically proven guidelines for selecting effective nursing interventions.

The nurse develops an individualized plan of care for each nursing diagnosis. The nurse and client set realistic expectations for care. Goals are to be individualized and realistic with measurable outcomes. Whenever appropriate, a friend or family member should be involved in planning. Sensitivity to specific cultural stressors and expressions of adaptation also will promote a sense of being cared about when the plan is made.

It is important that the nurse focus on coping strategies that are both realistic and appropriate to the client's needs. For example, a nurse should not be planning client teaching strategies if basic needs such as thirst and rest have not been considered (Box 30-12).

As discussed earlier, stress has been studied by a variety of disciplines. The nurse should determine which of these disciplines to collaborate with on the client's plan of care. Multidisciplinary client care conferences can be instrumental in addressing the holistic needs of the client.

Stress management techniques are designed to match the client's actual and potential stressors. The general

goals for clients who require stress management include the following:

    Reduction in frequency of stress-inducing situations

    Decreased physiological response to stress

    Improved behavioral and emotional responses to stress

    Increased knowledge about the cause of stress

The nurse is responsible for implementing thoughtful interventions that are carried out in several nursing domains (see care plan, on p. 660).

IMPLEMENTATION

Stress management may be seen as a health promotion activity or an intervention that modifies a response to illness. The focus depends on the purpose of the nursing interventions based on the client's needs.

Health Promotion.   Lifestyle decisions can have a dramatic impact on the stress experienced in everyday life. Regular exercise, good nutrition combined with a low-fat diet, adequate rest, effective time management, interactions with positive support systems, and humor are exam-

---

NURSING DIAGNOSES Box 30-11

STRESS

Activity intolerance
Anxiety
Caregiver role strain
Coping, ineffective family: compromised or disabling
Coping, ineffective individual
Fatigue
Fear
Growth and development, altered
Hopelessness
Injury, risk for
Self-esteem disturbance
Sleep pattern disturbance
Spiritual distress

Research HIGHLIGHT   Box 30-12

RESEARCH ABSTRACT

It has been well documented that clients in the intensive care unit (ICU) experience a great deal of stress. A questionnaire regarding clients' perception of environmental stressors was given to 71 ICU clients (2 days after discharge) and 71 ICU nurses. All of the clients had been ventilated at some point during their hospitalization. The results showed that there seemed to be a wide variation in perception of nurses and clients regarding the stress faced by clients in the intensive care unit. The clients' most stressful items included being thirsty, having tubes in your mouth/nose, and not being able to sleep. The nurses ranked being in pain, not being able to communicate, and not being in control of yourself among the most stressful items they felt ICU clients experience. This study was performed in the United Kingdom and replicated a previous study that was performed in the United States. The previous study produced similar results, showing a wide discrepancy between ICU nurses and their clients' perception of environmental stress in the ICU.

IMPLICATIONS FOR PRACTICE

- Basic needs of the client should be assessed frequently.
- Different cultures showed similar tendencies toward the perceptions of environmental stressors.
- There is a need for education of ICU staff with regard to the degree and nature of stressors experienced by clients.

REFERENCE

Cornock M: Stress and the intensive care patient: perceptions of patients and nurses, *J Adv Nurs* 27(3):518, 1998.

KNOWLEDGE

- Role of community resources in assisting client/family adaptation
- Role of health care professionals in stress management
- Impact of diet, exercise, and other health promotion indicators on stress management
- Impact of medication on the client

STANDARDS

- Individualize interventions to meet the client's needs
- Apply ANA code of ethics by safeguarding the client's right to privacy and autonomy in the selection of interventions

PLANNING

- Select nursing interventions to promote adaptation to stress
- Consult with mental health professionals
- Involve the client and family
- Identify community resources accessible to the client

EXPERIENCE

- Previous client responses to planned nursing interventions for improving client's adaptation to stress

ATTITUDES

- Base interventions on client needs and available resources
- Display integrity when creating interventions for the client's lifestyle
- Act independently to seek out resources that could benefit the client

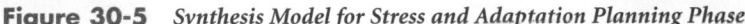

Figure 30-5   *Synthesis Model for Stress and Adaptation Planning Phase.*

SAMPLE NURSING CARE PLAN

CAREGIVER ROLE STRAIN

When Janet Rich first goes to Carl's house, she finds the home to be in slight disarray. The lawn is overgrown, there are dirty dishes in the sink, and an empty can of soup is sitting on the kitchen counter. Carl is standing in the living room folding clothes from a laundry basket, and Evelyn, Carl's wife, is sitting in a chair watching TV. Evelyn was recently diagnosed with Alzheimer's dementia. Carl appears very **tired** and **depressed**. He continues to fold clothes during the visit stating, "There's so much to do that I don't even know where to begin." Carl states that he has **lost 20 pounds in the past 6 months** and that his **appetite has been poor.** Until recently, Evelyn has cooked all of their meals. Carl describes being awakened 3 to 4 times per night to find Evelyn wandering in the house. He states that he has **no outside activities** and his **children live in other states.** He does have **several close friends who live nearby** but **denies any knowledge of community resources.**

*Defining characteristics are shown in bold type.

NURSING DIAGNOSIS: Caregiver role strain related to recent diagnosis of wife's Alzheimer's dementia

---

PLANNING

GOALS

Client will appear rested in 1 week.

Client will maintain a stable weight during next week.
Client will state that he has resumed one outside activity within 1 month.

EXPECTED OUTCOMES

Client will report waking up less frequently during the night within 1 week.
Client will verbalize approaches used to involve others in wife's caregiving activities.
Client will reestablish normal eating pattern within 1 week.
Client will report a balanced routine that incorporates time for own rest or relaxation with 1 week.

INTERVENTIONS*

Caregiver Support

- Assist client in establishing a consistent care routine.
- Discuss ways to simplify care routine such as hiring a neighbor's high school son to mow the lawn, buying frozen meals, having groceries delivered, having a cleaning service twice a month.
- Identify sources of respite care by encouraging client to identify available friends who can assist with caregiving.

- Explore community resources such as home health care, adult day care, and Meals on Wheels with client.
- Teach client stress management techniques.
- Set up monthly health checks for client that include vital sign and weight checks.†

RATIONALE

Routines can help tasks be simplified and more time efficient.
Creates free time for client and may help decrease feelings of being overwhelmed.

Successful caregiving cannot normally occur with only one caregiver. Caregiver may be hesitant to ask for help because of past family conflict (Gulanick and others, 1998).
Feelings of burden have been found to be lower among caregivers with social supports (Solomon and Draine, 1995).
Stress, especially long-term stress, can facilitate physical illness.

†Intervention Classification labels from McCloskey JC, Bulechek GM: *Nursing interventions classification (NIC)*, ed 3, St. Louis, 2000, Mosby.

EVALUATION

Observe for signs of fatigue.
Review new care routines. Ask client what other modifications may need to be made.
Ask client about how community and additional family support is helping to relieve stress.
Ask client to compare past and present energy levels.
Weigh client regularly.
Ask client about recent food intake.

---

ples of habits that can positively affect physical and mental health. Nurses are in an excellent position to educate clients and families about the importance of health promotion and the impact it can have on stress reduction. Helping clients and families to understand their particular stress response and its probable causes is a significant step in stress reduction.

Attempting to eliminate all stressors is unrealistic. However, the nurse can reduce some stressors and thereby provide the client with a greater sense of control. There are several methods that assist in stress reduction.

Time Management.   Persons who use time efficiently generally experience less stress because they feel more in control of their lives. A nurse acting in the teaching-coaching domain may assist clients to prioritize tasks if they are feeling overwhelmed or immobilized.

Controlling the demands of others is essential for effective time management. Few people are able to meet all requests made by others. It is important to learn to recognize which requests can be realistically met, which need to be negotiated, and which ones could be assertively declined. Blocking out a period of time to address specific goals also reduces a sense of urgency and increases feelings of control.

Regular Exercise.
A regular exercise program improves muscle tone and posture, controls weight, reduces tension, and promotes relaxation. In addition, exercise reduces the risk of cardiovascular disease and improves cardiopulmonary functioning. A client who has a history of chronic illness, who is at risk for developing an illness, or who is over the age of 35 should begin a physical exercise program only after discussing it with a physician. In general, for a fitness program to have positive physical effects, a person should exercise at least 3 times a week for 30 to 40 minutes.

Everyone should use warm-up exercises before vigorous exercise such as jogging, aerobic dancing, or tennis. Warm-up exercises stimulate blood flow to the muscles and increase flexibility. They reduce the risk of damage to the musculoskeletal system during exercise. Similarly, after vigorous exercise a person should do cool-down exercises rather than stop abruptly. For example, after jogging or aerobic dancing a person should walk around at a moderate pace, gradually slowing and stopping. Cool-down exercises allow the cardiovascular, pulmonary, musculoskeletal, and metabolic systems to gradually return to their resting states.

Exercise programs are effective in decreasing the severity of stress-related conditions such as hypertension, obesity, tension headaches, fatigue, mental exhaustion, irritability, and depression. Exercise promotes release of endogenous opioids that create a feeling of well-being (McCubbin, 1993).

Nutrition and Diet.
Nutrition and exercise are closely related. Food provides the fuel for activity and increased exercise, which improves circulation and the delivery of nutrients to body tissues.

Everyone is encouraged to maintain weight according to standard ranges for sex, age, and body build. In addition to avoiding overeating or undereating, a person should be aware of the nutritional quality of foods. Too much fat, caffeine, salt, or sugar can upset the body's metabolic functioning; deficiencies in vitamins, minerals, and nutrients can also cause metabolic problems. Poor dietary habits can worsen a stress response and make a person irritable, hyperactive, and anxious. This impairs the ability to meet personal, family, and role responsibilities. Nursing

measures for helping a client meet nutritional needs are detailed in Chapter 43.

Rest.
An established, habitual pattern of sufficient rest and sleep is also important for managing stress. A person experiencing stress should be encouraged to allow time for rest and sleep. Sleep not only refreshes the body but also helps a person become mentally relaxed. A client may need specific help in learning to relax to fall asleep.

Support Systems.
The saying "No man is an island" is of particular importance for stress management. A support system of family, friends, and colleagues who will listen and offer advice and emotional support is beneficial to a person experiencing stress.

Uchino and Garvey's research (1997) suggests that simply having potential access to support is sufficient to foster adaptation to stress. Nurses can use therapeutic communication to teach clients socialization skills if clients do not know how to interact appropriately. All of these methods help clients build stronger support systems. If stress is the result of social isolation, nursing strategies are aimed at helping clients develop new social networks.

Acute Care
Crisis Intervention.
Crisis intervention is a therapeutic technique for helping a client resolve a particular, immediate stress problem. Crisis intervention does not involve an in-depth analysis of a situation but addresses the immediate, urgent need for stress reduction. The goal is to restore the person to the precrisis level of functioning as quickly as possible.

Crises occur when people encounter problems or stress situations with which they are unable to cope in usual ways. A crisis does not necessarily denote occurrence of a traumatic event. However, even if this happens, it can be an opportunity for personal growth if the crisis is successfully mastered (Haber and others, 1997).

Clients and nurses are at risk for two types of crises: situational and developmental. A **situational crisis** arises suddenly in response to an external event or conflict involving a specific circumstance. Symptoms associated with situational crises are transient, and the episode is brief. Situational crises include giving birth, major role changes, acute physical illness, physical assault or rape, family changes such as remarriage or the death of a family member, and unexpected unemployment.

A **developmental crisis** occurs when a person is unable to complete the developmental tasks of a psychosocial stage and is therefore unable to continue developing. A developmental crisis can occur at any point in life if circumstances prevent a person from meeting the challenge of a particular stage.

After determining that a client is experiencing a crisis, the nurse plans and implements specific measures to help resolve it. Aguilera (1998) has developed an approach to intervention that can be used for both types of crises (Figure 30-6).

This approach enables the nurse to understand how a stressful event has led to a state of crisis. Resolution of the crisis depends on the person's realistic perception of the stressful event and use of adequate coping mechanisms. If the crisis has arisen because perception of the event is dis-torted, the nurse helps the client perceive the stressful event realistically. If the crisis has arisen because of a lack of situational support or coping mechanisms, the nurse initiates measures to incorporate regular diet and exercise into the client's lifestyle and suggests appropriate support groups. The nurse then evaluates the extent to which the client is able to resolve the crisis with these means.

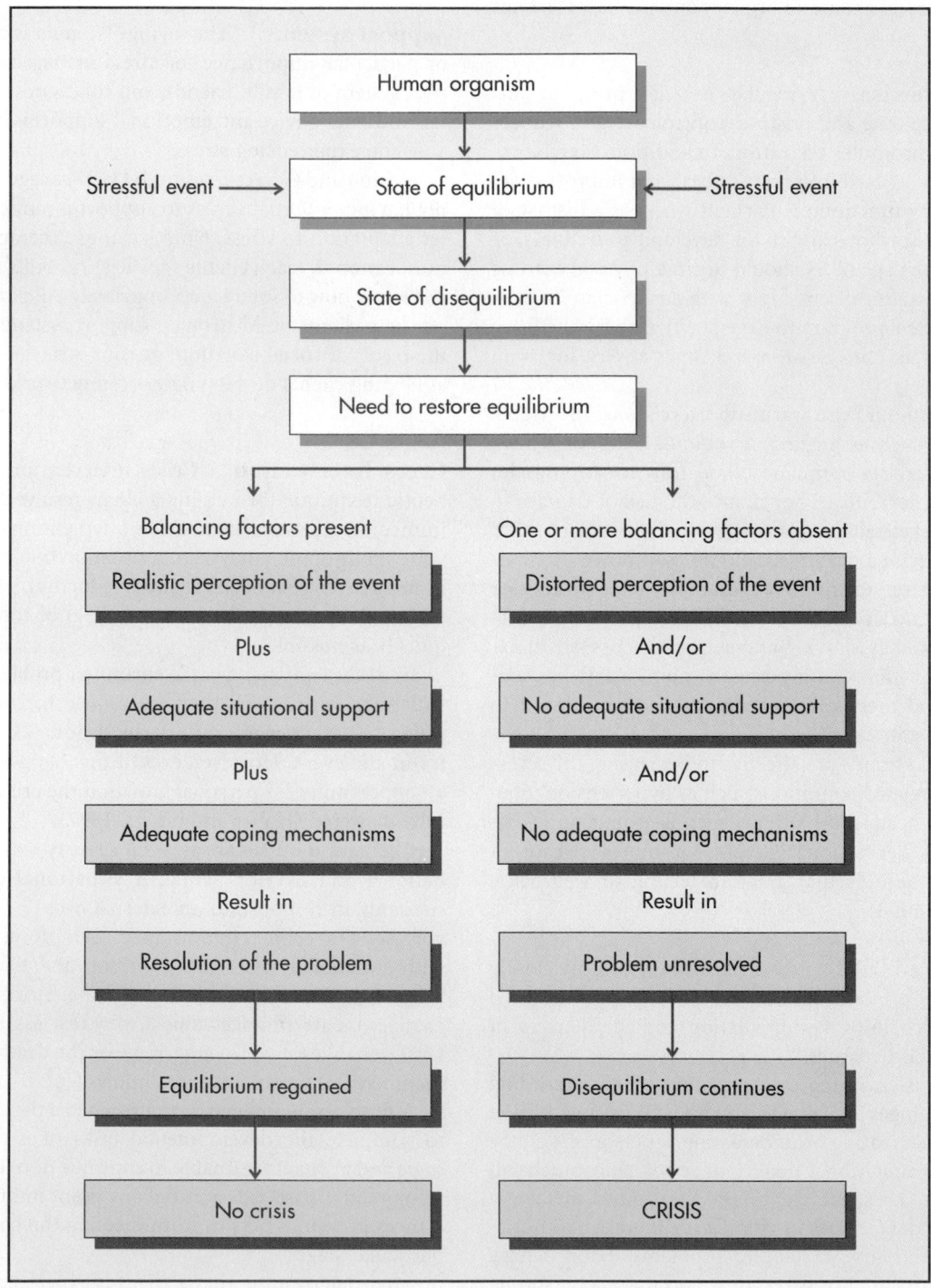

Figure 30-6   Crisis intervention model.
Redrawn from Aguilera DC: *Crisis intervention: theory and methodology,* ed 8, St. Louis, 1998, Mosby.

Restorative Care.   The nurse can assist the client in making lifestyle choices that are healthy and stress reducing. Smoking cessation, humor, spirituality, and stress management techniques are examples of these choices. Although this material is presented with respect to restorative care, the techniques can be utilized in all health care settings.

Humor.   Humor as therapy has been popularized in the lay literature by Norman Cousins (1979). The ability to perceive fun and laugh alleviates stress. The physiological hypothesis is that laughter releases endorphins into the circulation and feelings of stress are relieved. Laughter has been shown to increase the amount of activated T lymphocytes, which stimulates the immune system (Wooten, 1996). Nurses can initiate therapeutic activities by encouraging clients to relate past humorous anecdotes or developing a "humor" scrapbook (Figure 30-7). The nurse will critically examine the client's receptivity to humor first, though, to ensure it is never demeaning or ill timed (Weishaus, 1996).

Enhancing Self-Esteem.   Improvement in a client's self-esteem can assist in positive stress reduction strategies. When clients identify their positive characteristics, it helps them see resources that can be drawn upon to cope with the stressor.

Cognitive restructuring is another intervention that can modify stress responses. This is a technique in which the nurse and client analyze the client's appraisals of a stressor. If these are unrealistic or focused only on negative outcomes, the client is assisted in restructuring the thinking to more realistic, positive patterns. This may be accomplished by encouraging the client to do something for himself or herself (e.g., getting a haircut or taking 30 minutes each day to read a book). This can serve to modulate the emotional reaction and response (Peddicord, 1991; Badger, 1992).

Relaxation Techniques.   Progressive relaxation with and without muscle tension and imagery techniques reduces the physiological and emotional components of stress. Relaxation techniques are learned behaviors and require training and practice sessions. After the client becomes skilled at these techniques, tension is reduced and physiological parameters are changed (Box 30-13).

Examples of these techniques are guided imagery and visualization, progressive muscle relaxation, meditation, and biofeedback. In a critical review of the literature on stress management in the workplace, Murphy (1996) finds that meditation seems to provide the most consistent results for stress reduction, whereas biofeedback is the least effective technique (Box 30-14). It is important to note that relaxation techniques such as biofeedback and hypnosis should be implemented only by those caregivers who are experienced and trained to provide these services.

Spirituality.   Spiritual activities can also have a positive effect in decreasing stress. Practices such as prayer, meditation, or reading religious material may be meaningful resources for a client. According to Foster (1997), older adults effectively use religious coping in response to medical illness and disasters.

Stress Management in the Workplace.   Various studies have reported that 30% to 46% of workers interviewed indicated their job was very stressful or endangered their health. Joseph Dear, former assistant secretary of labor for occupational safety and health, identified work as an emerging occupational hazard. He singled out stress as the working woman's number one problem. Occupational Safety and Health Administration (OSHA) leaders have voiced concern that stress on the job can lead to violence, and Social Security Administration disability

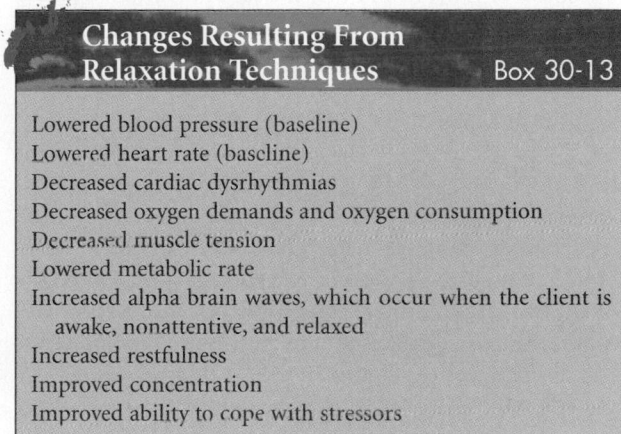

Figure 30-7   Sharing a joke or laughing with clients can assist in reducing stress and supporting a therapeutic relationship.

Changes Resulting From Relaxation Techniques	Box 30-13

Lowered blood pressure (baseline)
Lowered heart rate (baseline)
Decreased cardiac dysrhythmias
Decreased oxygen demands and oxygen consumption
Decreased muscle tension
Lowered metabolic rate
Increased alpha brain waves, which occur when the client is
    awake, nonattentive, and relaxed
Increased restfulness
Improved concentration
Improved ability to cope with stressors

Client Teaching ON MEDITATION FOR A CLIENT WITH ANXIETY   Box 30-14

OBJECTIVES

- Client will report less muscle tension and a heightened sense of relaxation.
- Client will exhibit a decreased pulse rate.

TEACHING STRATEGIES

- Discuss with client the importance of incorporating meditation into daily routine.
- Reinforce that optimal benefits require meditating for 15 to 30 minutes at least once each day.
- Provide a quiet environment. Instruct the client to silence the ringer on the telephone.
- Have the client secure a position that is truly comfortable and where minimal muscular work is needed.
- Reassure client that there is no wrong way to meditate.
- Arrange to have a clock in view so that moving to check time is unnecessary.

- Tell client to pick a word that can be repeated during meditation. Single-syllable words such as *one* are very effective.
- Instruct client to relax all muscle groups beginning with the head and working progressively down to the feet.
- Teach client to breathe in slowly through the nostrils and exhale slowly through the mouth.
- Tell the client that the single-syllable word should be silently repeated while inhaling and exhaling.
- Have the client focus thoughts on this rhythmic chanting and breathing for 10 minutes.
- Instruct client to allow images and thoughts to flow freely.

EVALUATION

- Have client take and report pulse or note difference from prerelaxation rate.
- Ask client to rate self-tension on the scale and report the difference between pre-relaxation and postrelaxation.

Balzer-Riley J: *Communications in nursing,* ed 3, St. Louis, 1996, Mosby.

---

data have shown an increase in stress-related claims (Lusk, 1997).

Most nurses experience stress in their work environments. Stressors can consist of workload, institutional policies, conflict with co-workers, dealing with death and dying, conflict with physicians, and inadequate preparation to deal with emotional needs of clients and families (Farrington, 1995).

Reaction to a job-related stressor depends on the nurse's personality, health status, previous experiences with stress, and coping mechanisms. **Job stress** frequently results in a condition called burnout, which is characterized by a depletion of energy that leaves a continuing sense of helplessness and negativism (Farrington, 1995). The job or profession no longer has positive rewards, and the client may experience anger or apathy.

Nurses are at risk for job stress burnout and benefit from using the same stress management techniques that they teach clients. Nurses should identify specific stressors at work and strive to eliminate them. It is also helpful to gain social support from other nurses to maintain a caring attitude toward clients (Badger, 1995).

EVALUATION

Client Care.   Because clients' perceptions of stress differ, so do their perceptions of stress reduction. Therefore evaluation of nursing interventions directed at stress management must consider whether the client's perception of the stress has declined, whether the client is able to control factors that contribute to the stress, and whether the client is able to independently develop stress reduction strategies (Figure 30-8).

To evaluate interventions directed at stress management, the nurse must objectively measure reduced frequency of stressful situations, decreased physiological response to stress, and improved behavioral and emotional responses to stress. Reports from both the client and family, as well as observations by the nurse, are all important factors.

It is important for the nurse to refer the client to appropriate resources for continuation of care. Lifestyle changes and developing new patterns of coping with stress can be difficult for the client and may take some time. It is also very easy for the client to fall back into old stress-producing habits if adequate, continued support is not given.

Client Expectations.   Clients experiencing stress often have a loss of self-esteem and control. The nurse can help reduce these feelings by maintaining an open line of communication with the client and family members and involving them in all areas of the client's care. This open communication should create an environment in which the client feels comfortable providing important information about which interventions are successful and which are not working. It is critical that the nurse does not create an environment where the client conforms to the "good patient" role. This is a syndrome where the client does not disagree or complain for fear of being perceived as a complainer (Cornock, 1998).

The evaluation process should be ongoing to ensure that the client has an appropriate plan of care. Collaboration among the client, nurse, and all disciplines involved is essential to meeting the expectations of the client.

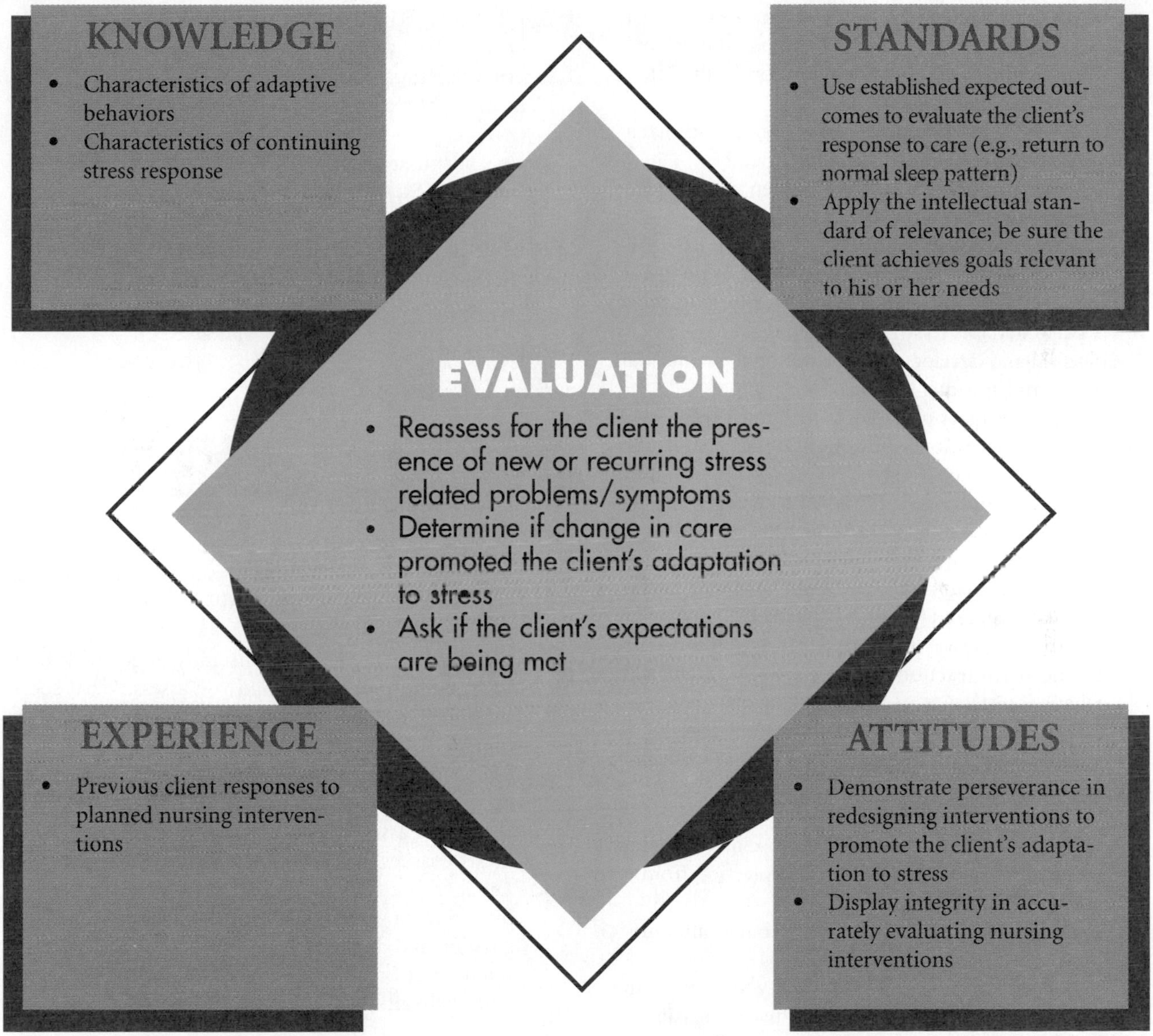

KNOWLEDGE

- Characteristics of adaptive behaviors
- Characteristics of continuing stress response

STANDARDS

- Use established expected outcomes to evaluate the client's response to care (e.g., return to normal sleep pattern)
- Apply the intellectual standard of relevance; be sure the client achieves goals relevant to his or her needs

EVALUATION

- Reassess for the client the presence of new or recurring stress related problems/symptoms
- Determine if change in care promoted the client's adaptation to stress
- Ask if the client's expectations are being met

EXPERIENCE

- Previous client responses to planned nursing interventions

ATTITUDES

- Demonstrate perseverance in redesigning interventions to promote the client's adaptation to stress
- Display integrity in accurately evaluating nursing interventions

Figure 30-8   *Synthesis Model for Stress and Adaptation Evaluation Phase.*

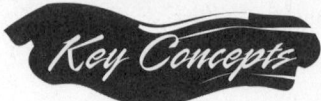

Key Concepts

- Physiological adaptive mechanisms are controlled by the medulla oblongata, reticular formation, and pituitary gland.
- Prolonged stress decreases the adaptive capacity of the body.
- Stress is physiological or psychological tension that can affect a person in any or all human dimensions.
- An individual may encounter stressors in the internal or external environment.
- Stressors necessitate change or adaptation so that a state of equilibrium can be maintained.
- A person's response to stress is influenced by the intensity, duration, and scope of the stressor, by the number of stressors present at one time, predictability, level of personal control, feelings of competence, cognitive appraisal, and availability of social supports.
- A person adapts to stress by using resources in the physical and developmental, emotional, intellectual, social, and spiritual dimensions.
- The two forms of physiological response to stress are the local adaptation syndrome and the general adaptation syndrome.
- The local adaptation syndrome involves several specific responses to stress, including the reflex pain response and the inflammatory response.
- The general adaptation syndrome involves a multisystem physiological response to stress.
- The three stages of the general adaptation syndrome are the alarm reaction, the resistance stage, and the exhaustion stage.
- Psychological responses to stress include task-oriented behaviors and ego-defense mechanisms.
- Task-oriented behaviors include attack behavior, withdrawal, and compromise.
- Ego-defense mechanisms are unconscious behaviors that offer a person psychological protection from stressful feelings or events.
- Stress has an impact on the onset, course, and outcome of illness.
- Prolonged stress decreases the ability to adapt to the stress and affects the person in all five dimensions.
- People generally learn to use short- and long-term strategies to cope with stress.
- Stress management techniques include health-enhancing habits, crisis intervention, and methods of reducing job stress.

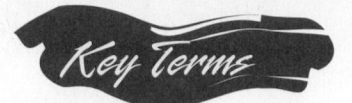

Key Terms

Adaptation, *p. 645*
Burnout, *p. 653*
Crises, *p. 661*
Crisis intervention, *p. 661*
Developmental crisis, *p. 661*
Ego-defense mechanisms, *p. 650*
External stressors, *p. 644*
Fight-or-flight response, *p. 649*
General adaptation syndrome (GAS), *p. 644*
Hardiness, *p. 651*
Homeostasis, *p. 645*
Internal stressors, *p. 644*
Job stress, *p. 664*

Local adaptation syndrome (LAS), *p. 648*
Medulla oblongata, *p. 645*
Mild stress situations, *p. 653*
Moderate stress situations, *p. 653*
Physiological adaptation, *p. 644*
Pituitary gland, *p. 645*
Reticular formation, *p. 645*
Severe stress situations, *p. 654*
Situational crisis, *p. 661*
Stress, *p. 644*
Stressors, *p. 644*
Task-oriented behaviors, *p. 650*

Critical Thinking Exercises

1. You are a nurse working at a community health fair. A man stops by your health assessment booth and tells you he has been apathetic and lethargic since he lost his job 2 months ago. He has begun drinking every evening, and his wife is constantly angry with him. What additional areas would you assess? What social supports would be available in your community for him?

2. John Morgan, who has no family history of heart disease, had a myocardial infarction 3 days ago. What risk-factor assessments do you make? What are some lifestyle issues that will need to be assessed?

3. Lu Chen is a Chinese immigrant who is hospitalized following an automobile accident for a possible concussion and broken finger. What cultural barriers might increase her stress? What can you, as the nurse, do to help alleviate some of that stress?

References

Aguilera DC: *Crisis intervention: theory and methodology,* ed 8, St. Louis, 1998, Mosby.

Badger J: Fourteen tips for managing stress on the job, *Am J Nurs* 95(9):31, 1995.

Badger T: Coping, lifestyle changes, health, perception, and marital adjustment in middle aged women and men with cardiovascular disease and their spouses, *Health Care Women Int* 13:43, 1992.

Balzer-Riley J: *Communications in nursing,* ed 3, St. Louis, 1996, Mosby.

Clemen-Stone S, McGuire SL, Eigsti DG: *Comprehensive community health nursing,* ed 5, St. Louis, 1998, Mosby.

Cornock M: Stress and the intensive care patient: perceptions of patients and nurses, *J Adv Nurs* 27(3):518, 1998.

Cousins N: *Anatomy of an illness,* New York, 1979, Bantam.

de Anda D and others: A study of stress, stressors, and coping strategies among middle school adolescents, *Soc Work Education* 19(2)87, 1997.

Dellasaga C, Nolan M: Admission to care: facilitating role transition amongst family careers, *J Clin Nurs* 6(6)443, 1997.

DuBois D and others: A prospective study of life stress, social support and adaptation in early adolescence, *Child Dev* 63:542, 1992.

Duhamel F, Campagna L: Family care is an increasingly important component of nursing practice, *Can J Cardiovasc Nurs* 8(4)16, 1997.

Farrington A: Stress and nursing, *Br J Nurs* 4(10)574, 1995.

Finlay J, Zigmond M: The effects of stress on central dopaminergic neurons: possible clinical applications, *Neurochem Res* 22(11)1387, 1997.

Foster J: Successful coping, adaptation and resilience in the elderly: an interpretation of epidemiological data, *Psychiatr Q* 68(3)189, 1997.

Giger J, Davidhizar R: *Transcultural nursing,* ed 2, St. Louis, 1995, Mosby.

Gonzales E: Resourcefulness, appraisals, and coping efforts of family caregivers, *Issues Ment Health Nurs* 18(3)209, 1997.

Gulanick M and others: *Nursing care plans: nursing diagnosis and intervention,* ed 4, St. Louis, 1998, Mosby.

Haber J and others: *Comprehensive psychiatric nursing,* ed 4, St. Louis, 1997, Mosby.

Holmes T, Rahe R: The social readjustment scale, *J Psychosom Res* 12:213, 1976.

Lazarus R, Folkman S: *Stress appraisal and coping,* New York, 1984, Springer.

Lee A, Ellenbacker C: The perceived life stressors among elderly Chinese immigrants: are they different from those of other elderly Americans? *Clin Excell Nurse Pract* 2(2)96, 1998.

Linsday AM, Carrieri VK, Page GG: Stress response. In Lindsay AM, Carrieri VK, editors: *Pathological phenomenon in nursing: human response to illness,* ed 2, Philadelphia, 1993, WB Saunders.

Lusk S: Health effects of stress management in the worksite, *AAOHN J* 45(3)149, 1997.

Mandle and others: The efficacy of relaxation response interventions with adult patients: a review of the literature, *J Cardiovasc Nurs* 10(3)4, 1996.

McCubbin J: Stress and endogenous opioids: behavioral and circulatory interactions, *Biol Psychol* 35:91, 1993.

McEwen B: Stress, adaptation and disease, *Ann N Y Acad Sci* 840(5)33, 1998.

McNett SC: Lazarus' theory of stress and coping. In Riegel B, Ehrenreich D, editors: *Psychological aspects of critical care nursing,* Rockville, Md, 1989, Aspen.

Mechanic D: *Students under stress,* Glencoe, Ill, 1962, Free Press.

Murata J: Family stress, social support, violence, and son's behavior, *West J Nurs Res* 16(2):154, 1994.

Murphy L: Stress management in work settings: a critical review of the health effects, *Am J Health Promot* 11(2)112, 1996.

Musolf JM: Easing the impact of the family caregiver's role, *Rehabil Nurs* 16(2):82, 1991.

Peddicord K: Strategies for promoting stress reduction and relaxation, *Nurs Clin North Am* 26(4):867, 1991.

Peirce A: The complex nature of stress, coping and adaptation, *Nurs Lead Forum* 1(3)84, 1995.

Raeside L: Perceptions of environmental stressors in the neonatal unit, *Br J Nurs* 6(16)914, 1997.

Robinson L: Stress and anxiety, *Nurs Clin North Am* 25(4):935, 1990.

Selye H: The general adaptation syndrome and the diseases of adaptation, *Clin Endocrinol* 6:117, 1946.

Selye H: *The stress of life,* ed 2, New York, 1976, McGraw-Hill.

Soloman P, Draine J: Subjective burden among family members of mentally ill adults: relation to stress, coping, and adaptation, *Am J Orthopsychiatry* 65(3):419, 1995.

Tartasky D: Hardiness: conceptual and methodological issues, *Image J Nurs Sch* 25(3):225, 1993.

Uchino BN, Garvey TS: The availability of social support reduces cardiovascular reactivity to acute psychological stress, *J Behav Med* 20(1)15, 1997.

Weishaus G: A lighter side of home care, *Home Health Nurse* 14(11)903, 1996.

Wiebe D, Williams P: Hardiness and health: a social psychophysiological perspective on stress and adaptation, *Br J Soc Clin Psychol* 11(3):238, 1992.

Wooten P: Humor: an antidote for stress, *Holist Nurs Pract* 10(12)49, 1996.

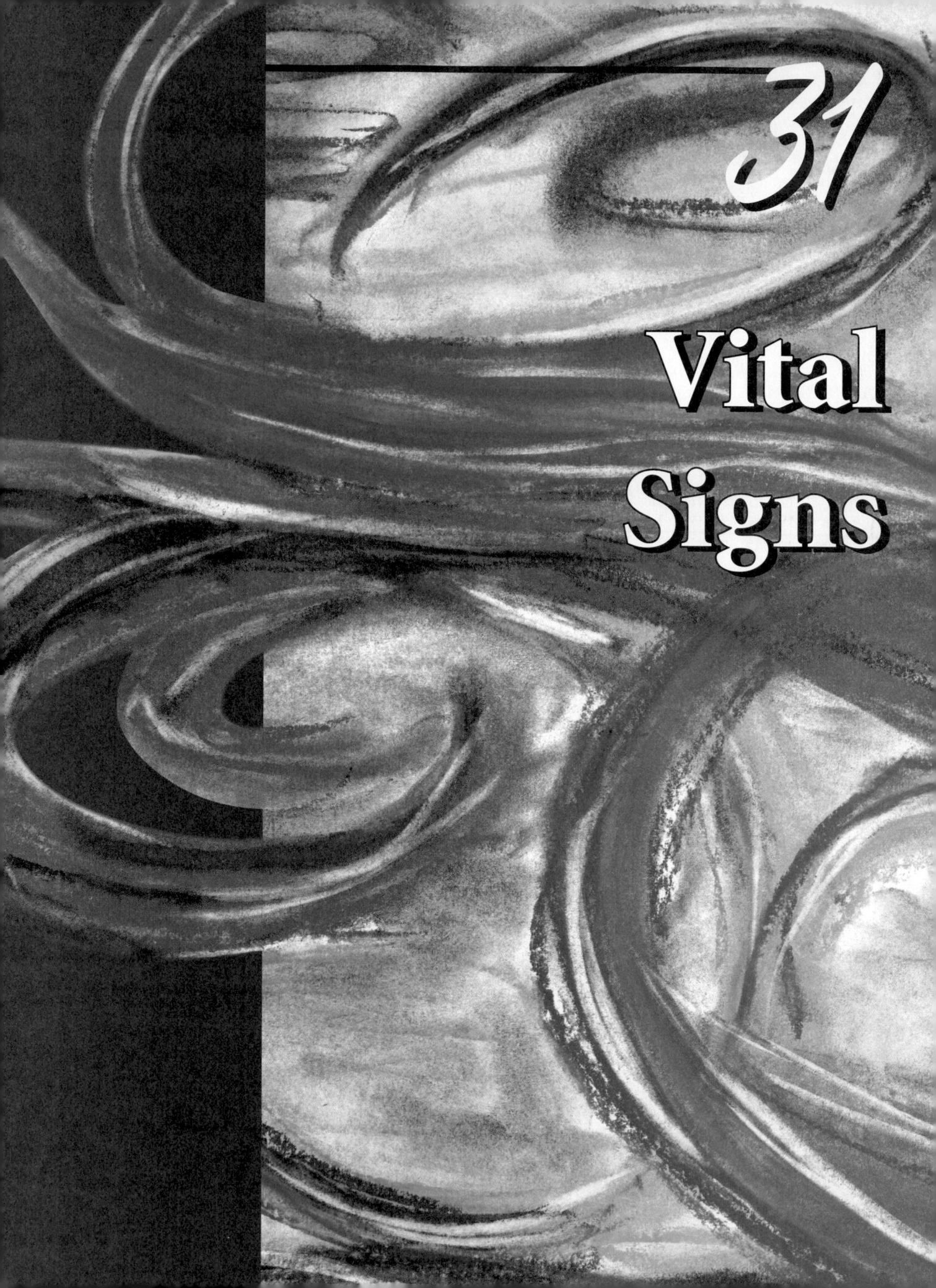

31

Vital Signs

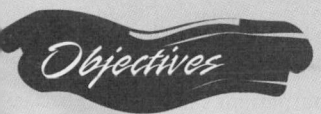

Mastery of content in this chapter will enable the student to:

- Define the key terms listed.
- Explain the principles and mechanisms of thermoregulation.
- Describe nursing measures that promote heat loss and heat conservation.
- Discuss physiological changes associated with fever.
- Accurately assess tympanic, oral, rectal, and axillary temperatures.
- Accurately assess pulse, respirations, oxygen saturation, and blood pressure.
- Explain the physiology of normal regulation of blood pressure, pulse, oxygen saturation, and respirations.
- Describe factors that cause variations in body temperature, pulse, oxygen saturation, respirations, and blood pressure.
- Identify ranges of acceptable vital sign values for an infant, a child, and an adult.
- Explain variations in technique used to assess an infant's, a child's, and an adult's vital signs.
- Describe the benefits and precautions involving self-measurement of blood pressure.
- Identify when vital signs should be taken.
- Accurately record and report vital sign measurements.
- Appropriately delegate vital sign measurement to assistive personnel.

The most frequent measurements obtained by health practitioners are those of temperature, pulse, blood pressure, respiratory rate, and oxygen saturation. As indicators of health status, these measures indicate the effectiveness of circulatory, respiratory, neural, and endocrine body functions. Because of their importance they are referred to as **vital signs.** Many factors, such as the temperature of the environment, the client's physical exertion, and the effects of illness, cause vital signs to change, sometimes outside an acceptable range. Measurement of vital signs provides data to determine a client's usual state of health (baseline data) and response to physical and psychological stress and medical and nursing therapy. A change in vital signs can indicate a change in physiological function. An alteration in vital signs may signal the need for medical or nursing intervention.

Vital signs are a quick and efficient way of monitoring a client's condition or identifying problems and evaluating the client's response to intervention. The basic techniques of inspection, palpation, and auscultation are used to determine vital signs. These skills are simple but should not be taken for granted. Vital signs and other physiological measurements are the basis for clinical problem solving. Assessment of vital signs allows the nurse to identify nursing diagnoses, to implement planned interventions, and to evaluate success when vital signs have returned to acceptable values. When the nurse learns the physiological variables influencing vital signs and recognizes the relationship of vital sign changes to other physical assessment findings, precise determinations of the client's health problems can be made. Vital sign assessment is an essential ingredient when nurses and physicians collaborate to determine the client's health status. Careful measurement techniques ensure accurate findings.

Guidelines for Taking Vital Signs

Vital signs are a part of the database that a nurse collects during assessment. Box 31-1 provides a reference for acceptable values in the adult client. The nurse assesses vital signs whenever a client enters a health care agency. Vital signs are included in a complete physical assessment (see Chapter 32) or obtained individually to assess a client's condition. Establishing a database of vital signs during a routine physical examination serves as a baseline for future assessments. The client's needs and condition determine when, where, how, and by whom vital signs are measured. The nurse must be able to measure vital signs correctly or delegate the measurement of vital signs appropriately to assistive personnel. When vital signs are obtained, the nurse must understand and interpret the values, communicate findings appropriately, and begin interventions as needed. The following guidelines assist the nurse in incorporating vital sign measurement into nursing practice:

- The nurse caring for the client is responsible for vital sign measurement. Measurement of selected vital signs may be delegated to assistive personnel. However, the nurse must analyze the vital signs to interpret their significance and make decisions about interventions.

- Equipment should be functional and appropriate for the size and the age of the client. Equipment used to measure vital signs (e.g., a thermometer) must work properly to ensure accurate findings.
- Equipment should be selected based on the client's condition and characteristics (e.g., an adult-size blood pressure cuff should not be used for a child).
- The nurse knows the client's usual range of vital signs. A client's usual values may differ from the acceptable range for that age or physical state. The client's usual values serve as a baseline for comparison with later findings. Thus a nurse can detect a change in condition over time.
- The nurse knows the client's medical history, therapies, and prescribed medications. Some illnesses or treatments cause predictable vital sign changes. Some medications affect one or more of the vital signs.
- The nurse controls or minimizes environmental factors that may affect vital signs. Assessing the client's temperature in a warm, humid room may yield a value that is not a true indicator of the client's condition.
- The nurse uses an organized, systematic approach when taking vital signs. Each procedure requires a step-by-step approach to ensure accuracy. Organization facilitates efficiency (e.g., respirations can be assessed while taking an oral temperature).
- The manner of approach to the client can alter the vital signs. The nurse approaches the client in a calm, caring manner while demonstrating proficiency in handling the supplies needed for vital sign measurement.
- Based on the client's condition, the nurse collaborates with the physician to decide the frequency of vital sign assessment. In the hospital the physician orders a minimum frequency of vital sign measurements for each client. Following surgery or treatment intervention, vital signs are measured frequently to detect complications. In a clinic or outpatient setting, vital signs are taken before the practitioner examines the client and after any invasive procedures.
- The nurse uses vital sign measurements to determine indications for medication administration. The physician may order certain cardiac drugs to be given only within a range of pulse or blood pressure values. Antipyretics are often administered when temperature is elevated outside of the acceptable range for the client. The nurse does not administer these drugs if the vital sign assessment indicates the measurements are within the specified acceptable range.
- The nurse analyzes the results of vital sign measurement. The nurse is often in the best position to assess all clinical findings about a client. Vital signs are not interpreted in isolation. The nurse must also know other physical signs or symptoms and be aware of the client's ongoing health status.
- The nurse verifies and communicates significant changes in vital signs. Vital signs are documented and communicated to the nurse assuming care of the client. Baseline measurements allow a nurse to identify changes in vital signs. When vital signs appear abnormal, it may help to have another nurse or a physician repeat the measurement. The nurse informs the physician or nurse in charge of abnormal vital signs.
- The nurse develops a teaching plan to instruct the client or caregiver in vital sign assessment.

Regardless of the environment, the nurse is responsible for judging whether more frequent assessments are needed (Box 31-2). Taking vital signs as a basis for determining changes and trends is useful in making therapeutic decisions. As a client's physical condition worsens, it may be

---

Vital Signs: Acceptable Ranges for Adults   Box 31-1

TEMPERATURE RANGE: 36° TO 38° C (96.8° TO 100.4° F)

Average oral/tympanic:	C = 37°	F = 98.6° (Range ± 1° F)
Average rectal:	C = 37.5°	F = 99.5°
Average axilla:	C = 36.5°	F = 97.7°

PULSE
60-100 beats per minute

RESPIRATIONS
12-20 breaths per minute

BLOOD PRESSURE
Average: 120/80 mm Hg
Pulse Pressure: 30-50 mm Hg

When to Take Vital Signs   Box 31-2

When the client is admitted to a health care facility

In a hospital or care facility on a routine schedule according to the physician's order or the institution's standards of practice

Before and after a surgical procedure

Before and after an invasive diagnostic procedure

Before, during, and after the administration of medications that affect cardiovascular, respiratory, and temperature-control function

When the client's general physical condition changes (as with loss of consciousness or increased intensity of pain)

Before and after nursing interventions influencing a vital sign (e.g., before a client previously on bed rest ambulates or before a client performs range-of-motion exercises)

When the client reports nonspecific symptoms of physical distress (e.g., feeling "funny" or "different")

necessary to monitor vital signs as often as every 5 to 15 minutes.

Body Temperature

PHYSIOLOGY

Temperature is the "hotness" or "coldness" of a substance. The body temperature is the difference between the amount of heat produced by body processes and the amount of heat lost to the external environment.

$$\text{Heat produced} - \text{Heat lost} = \text{Body temperature}$$

Despite extremes in environmental conditions and physical activity, temperature-control mechanisms of human beings keep the body's **core temperature** (temperature of the deep tissues) relatively constant (Figure 31-1). However, surface temperature fluctuates depending on blood flow to the skin and the amount of heat lost to the external environment. Because of these surface temperature fluctuations, the acceptable temperature of human beings ranges from 36° to 38° C (96.8° to 100.4° F). The body's tissues and cells function best within the relatively narrow temperature range.

The site of temperature measurement (oral, rectal, axillary, tympanic membrane, esophageal, pulmonary artery, or even urinary bladder) is one factor that determines the client's temperature within this narrow range. For healthy young adults the average oral temperature is 37° C (98.6° F). In clinical practice, nurses learn the temperature range of individual clients. No single temperature is normal for all people.

The measurement of body temperature is aimed at obtaining a representative average temperature of core body tissues. The pulmonary artery offers the most representative readings because of the blood mix from all regions of the body. Measurement of the pulmonary artery temperature is the standard against which all other sites are judged for accuracy. Sites reflecting core temperatures are more reliable indicators of body temperature than sites reflecting surface temperatures (Box 31-3). The temperature value obtained may differ depending on the measurement site.

Regulation.   The balance between heat lost and heat produced, or **thermoregulation,** is precisely regulated by physiological and behavioral mechanisms. For the body temperature to stay constant and within an acceptable range, the relationship between heat production and heat loss must be maintained. This relationship is regulated by neurological and cardiovascular mechanisms. The nurse applies knowledge of temperature-control mechanisms to promote temperature regulation.

Neural and Vascular Control.   The **hypothalamus,** located between the cerebral hemispheres, controls body temperature the same way a thermostat works in the home. A comfortable temperature is the "set point" at which a heating system operates. In the home a fall in environmental temperature activates the furnace, whereas a rise in temperature shuts the system down. The hypothalamus senses minor changes in body temperature. The anterior hypothalamus controls heat loss, and the posterior hypothalamus controls heat production.

When nerve cells in the anterior hypothalamus become heated beyond the set point, impulses are sent out to reduce body temperature. Mechanisms of heat loss include sweating, vasodilation (widening) of blood vessels, and inhibition of heat production. Blood is redistributed to sur-

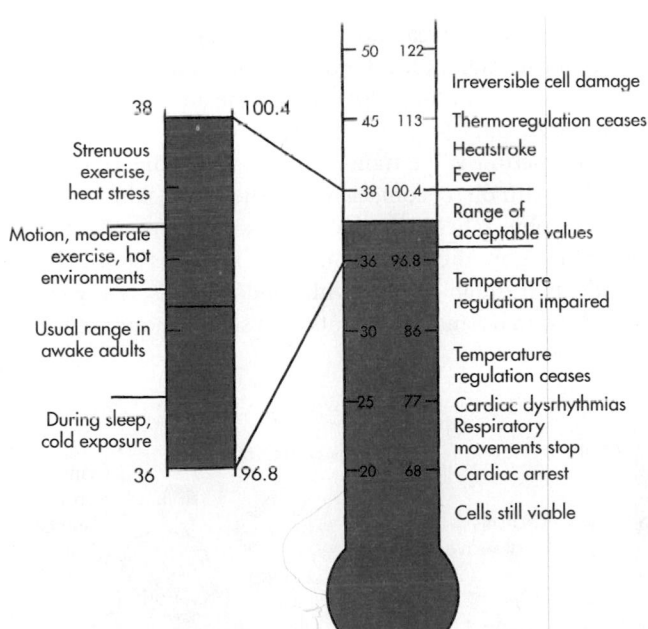

Figure 31-1   Ranges of normal temperature values and physiological consequences of abnormal body temperature. Modified from Thibodeau GA, Patton KT: *Anatomy and physiology,* ed 3, St. Louis, 1996, Mosby.

Core and Surface Temperature Measurement Sites	Box 31-3

Core	Surface
Rectum	Skin
Tympanic membrane	Axillae
Esophagus	Oral
Pulmonary artery	
Urinary bladder	

face vessels to promote heat loss. If the posterior hypothalamus senses the body's temperature is lower than the set point, heat conservation mechanisms are instituted. Vasoconstriction (narrowing) of blood vessels reduces blood flow to the skin and extremities. Compensatory heat production is stimulated through voluntary muscle contraction and muscle shivering. When vasoconstriction is ineffective in preventing additional heat loss, shivering begins. Disease or trauma to the hypothalamus or to the spinal cord, which carries hypothalamic messages, can cause serious alterations in temperature control.

Heat Production.   Heat is produced in the body by metabolism, which is the chemical reaction in all body cells. Food is the primary fuel source for metabolism. Thermoregulation depends on the normal function of heat production processes. Cellular chemical reactions require energy in the form of adenosine triphosphate (ATP). The amount of energy used for metabolism is the metabolic rate. Heat is produced as a by-product of metabolism. Activities requiring additional chemical reactions increase the metabolic rate. As metabolism increases, additional heat is produced. When metabolism decreases, less heat is produced. Heat production occurs during rest, voluntary movements, involuntary shivering, and nonshivering thermogenesis.

- Basal metabolism accounts for the heat produced by the body at absolute rest. The average **basal metabolic rate (BMR)** depends on the body surface area. Thyroid hormones also affect the BMR. By promoting the breakdown of body glucose and fat, thyroid hormones increase the rate of chemical reactions in almost all cells of the body. When large amounts of thyroid hormones are secreted, the BMR can increase 100% above normal. Absence of thyroid hormones can cut the BMR in half, causing a decrease in heat production. Stimulation of the sympathetic nervous system by norepinephrine and epinephrine also increases the metabolic rate of body tissues. These chemical mediators cause blood glucose levels to fall, which stimulates cells to manufacture glucose. The male sex hormone testosterone increases BMR. Men have a higher BMR than women.
- Voluntary movements such as muscular activity during exercise require additional energy. The metabolic rate can increase up to 2000 times normal during exercise. Heat production can increase up to 50 times normal.
- **Shivering** is an involuntary body response to temperature differences in the body. The skeletal muscle movement during shivering requires significant energy. In vulnerable clients shivering can seriously deplete energy sources, resulting in further physiological deterioration. Shivering can increase heat production 4 to 5 times greater than normal. The heat that is produced assists in equalizing the body temperature, and the shivering ceases.

- **Nonshivering thermogenesis** occurs primarily in neonates. Because neonates cannot shiver, a limited amount of vascular brown tissue, present at birth, is metabolized for heat production.

Heat Loss.   Heat loss and heat production occur simultaneously. The skin's structure and exposure to the environment result in constant, normal heat loss through radiation, conduction, convection, and evaporation (Figure 31-2).

Radiation is the transfer of heat from the surface of one object to the surface of another without direct contact between the two (Holtzclaw, 1998). Radiation occurs because heat transfers through electromagnetic waves. Heat radiates from the skin to any surrounding cooler object. Radiation increases as the temperature difference between the objects increases.

Blood flows from the core internal organs carrying heat to skin and surface blood vessels. The amount of heat carried to the surface depends on the extent of vasoconstriction and vasodilation regulated by the hypothalamus. Peripheral vasodilation increases blood flow to the skin to increase radiant heat loss. Peripheral vasoconstriction minimizes radiant heat loss. Up to 85% of the human body's surface area radiates heat to the environment. However, if the environment is warmer than the skin, the body absorbs heat through radiation.

The nurse increases heat loss through radiation by removing clothing or blankets. The client's position enhances radiation heat loss (e.g., standing exposes a greater radiating surface area and lying in a fetal position minimizes heat radiation). Covering the body with dark, closely woven clothing also reduces the amount heat lost from radiation.

Conduction is the transfer of heat from one object to another with direct contact. When the warm skin touches a cooler object, heat is lost. When the temperatures of the two objects are the same, conductive heat loss stops. Heat conducts through contact with solids, liquids, and gases. Conduction normally accounts for a small amount of heat

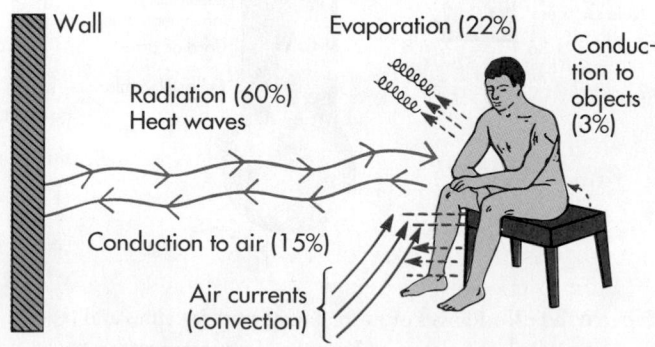

Figure 31-2   Mechanisms of heat loss from the body. Modified from Guyton AC: *Textbook of medical physiology*, ed 9, Philadelphia, 1995, WB Saunders.

loss. The nurse increases conductive heat loss when applying an ice pack or bathing a client with cool water. Applying several layers of clothing reduces conductive loss. The body gains heat by conduction when contact is made with materials warmer than skin temperature.

Convection is the transfer of heat away by air movement. Heat is first conducted to air molecules directly in contact with the skin. Air currents carry away the warmed air. As the air current velocity increases, convective heat loss increases. An electric fan promotes heat loss through convection. Convective heat loss increases when moistened skin comes into contact with slightly moving air.

Evaporation is the transfer of heat energy when a liquid is changed to a gas. During evaporation, approximately 0.6 of a **calorie** of heat is lost for each gram of water that evaporates (Guyton, 1995). The body continuously loses heat by evaporation. About 600 to 900 ml a day evaporates from the skin and lungs, resulting in water and heat loss. This normal loss is considered insensible water loss and does not play a major role in temperature regulation.

By regulating perspiration or sweating, the body promotes additional evaporative heat loss. Millions of sweat glands located in the dermis of the skin secrete sweat through tiny ducts on the skin's surface. When body temperature rises, the anterior hypothalamus signals the sweat glands to release sweat. Sweat evaporates from the skin surface, resulting in heat loss. During exercise and emotional or mental stress, sweating is one way to lose excessive heat produced by the increased metabolic rate. Excessive evaporation can cause skin scaling and itching, as well as drying of the nares and pharynx.

Diaphoresis is visible perspiration primarily occurring on the forehead and upper thorax, though it can also be seen elsewhere on the body. Sweat glands lie deep below the dermis of the skin. The glands secrete sweat, a watery solution containing sodium and chloride, which passes through tiny ducts on the skin's surface. The glands are controlled by the sympathetic nervous system. When the body's temperature rises, sweat glands release sweat, which evaporates from the skin to promote heat loss. A lowered body temperature inhibits sweat gland secretion. Diaphoresis is less efficient when air movement is minimal or when the humidity of the air is high. People who have a congenital absence of sweat glands or a serious skin disease that impairs diaphoresis are unable to tolerate warm temperatures because they cannot cool themselves adequately.

Skin in Temperature Regulation.

The skin's roles in temperature regulation include insulation of the body, vasoconstriction (which affects the amount of blood flow and heat loss to the skin), and temperature sensation. The skin, subcutaneous tissue, and fat keep heat inside the body. When blood flow between skin layers is reduced, the skin alone is an excellent insulator. Persons with more body fat have more natural insulation than do slim and muscular people.

The way that the skin controls body temperature is similar to the way that an automobile radiator controls engine temperature. The engine of an automobile generates a great deal of heat. Water is pumped through the engine's system to collect the heat and carry it to the radiator, where a fan transfers the heat from the water to the outside air. The radiator and fan keep the engine's temperature within safe limits to prevent damage from overheating. In the human body the internal organs produce heat, and during exercise or increased sympathetic stimulation, the amount of heat produced is greater than the usual core temperature. Blood flows from the internal organs, carrying heat to the body surface. The skin is well supplied with blood vessels, especially the areas of the hands, feet, and ears. Blood flow through these vascular areas of the skin may vary from minimal flow to as much as 30% of the blood ejected from the heart (Guyton, 1995). Heat transfers from the blood, through vessel walls, to the skin's surface and is lost to the environment through the heat-loss mechanisms. The body's core temperature remains within safe limits.

The degree of vasoconstriction determines the amount of blood flow and heat loss to the skin. If the core temperature is too high, the hypothalamus inhibits vasoconstriction. As a result, blood vessels dilate, and more blood reaches the skin's surface. On a hot, humid day the blood vessels in the hands are dilated and easily visible. In contrast, if the core temperature becomes too low, the hypothalamus initiates vasoconstriction and blood flow to the skin lessens. Thus body heat is conserved.

The skin is well supplied with heat and cold receptors. Because cold receptors are more plentiful, however, the skin functions primarily to detect cold surface temperatures. When the skin becomes chilled, its sensors send information to the hypothalamus, which initiates shivering to increase body heat production, inhibition of sweating, and vasoconstriction.

Behavioral Control.

Humans voluntarily act to maintain comfortable body temperature when exposed to temperature extremes. The ability of a person to control body temperature depends on (1) the degree of temperature extreme, (2) the person's ability to sense feeling comfortable or uncomfortable, (3) thought processes or emotions, and (4) the person's mobility or ability to remove or add clothes. Body temperature control is difficult if any of these abilities are absent or lost. Infants can sense uncomfortable warm conditions but need assistance in changing their environment. Older adults may need help in detecting cold environments and minimizing heat loss. Illness, a decreased level of consciousness, or impaired thought processes result in an inability to recognize the need to change behavior for temperature control. When temperatures become extremely hot or cold, health-promoting behaviors, such as removing or adding clothing, have a limited effect on controlling temperature. The nurse assesses for variables that place clients at high risk for ineffective thermoregulation.

FACTORS AFFECTING BODY TEMPERATURE

Many factors affect body temperature. Changes in body temperature within an acceptable range occur when the relationship between heat production and heat loss is altered by physiological or behavioral variables. The nurse must be aware of these factors when assessing temperature variations and evaluating deviations from normal.

Age.
At birth the newborn leaves a warm, relatively constant environment and enters one in which temperatures fluctuate widely. Temperature control mechanisms are immature. An infant's temperature may respond drastically to changes in the environment. Extra care is needed to protect the newborn from environmental temperatures. Clothing must be adequate, and exposure to temperature extremes must be avoided. A newborn loses up to 30% of body heat through the head and therefore needs to wear a cap to prevent heat loss. When protected from environmental extremes, the newborn's body temperature is maintained within 35.5° to 37.5° C (95.9° to 99.5° F). Heat production steadily declines as the infant grows into childhood. Individual differences of 0.25° to 0.55°C (0.5° to 1° F) are normal (Wong and others, 1998).

Temperature regulation is unstable until children reach puberty. The normal temperature range gradually drops as individuals approach older adulthood. The older adult has a narrower range of body temperatures than the younger adult. Oral temperatures of 35° C (95° F) are not unusual for older adults in cold weather. However, the average body temperature of older adults is approximately 36° C (96.8° F). Older adults are particularly sensitive to temperature extremes because of deterioration in control mechanisms, particularly poor vasomotor control (control of vasoconstriction and vasodilation), reduced amounts of subcutaneous tissue, reduced sweat gland activity, and reduced metabolism.

Exercise.
Muscle activity requires an increased blood supply and an increased carbohydrate and fat breakdown. This increased metabolism causes an increase in heat production. Any form of exercise can increase heat production and thus body temperature. Prolonged strenuous exercise, such as long distance running, can temporarily raise body temperatures up to 41° C (105.8° F).

Hormone Level.
Women generally experience greater fluctuations in body temperature than men. Hormonal variations during the menstrual cycle cause body temperature fluctuations. Progesterone levels rise and fall cyclically during the menstrual cycle. When progesterone levels are low, the body temperature is a few tenths of a degree below the baseline level. The lower temperature persists until ovulation occurs. During ovulation, greater amounts of progesterone enter the circulatory system and raise the body temperature to previous baseline levels or higher. These temperature variations can be used to predict a woman's most fertile time to achieve pregnancy.

Body temperature changes also occur in women during menopause (cessation of menstruation). Women who have stopped menstruating may experience periods of intense body heat and sweating lasting from 30 seconds to 5 minutes. There may be intermittent increases in skin temperature of up to 4° C (7.2 °F) during these periods, referred to as hot flashes. This is due to the instability of the vasomotor controls for vasodilation and vasoconstriction (Brashers, 1998).

Circadian Rhythm.
Body temperature normally changes 0.5° to 1° C (0.9° to 1.8° F) during a 24-hour period. However, temperature is one of the most stable rhythms in humans. The temperature is usually lowest between 1:00 and 4:00 AM (Figure 31-3). During the day, body temperature rises steadily, until about 6:00 PM, and then declines to early morning levels. Ninety-five percent of clients will have their maximum temperature value at 6:00 PM (Beaudry, VandenBosch, and Anderson, 1996). Interestingly, temperature patterns are not automatically reversed in people who work at night and sleep during the day. It takes 1 to 3 weeks for the cycle to reverse. In general, the circadian temperature rhythm does not change with age.

Stress.
Physical and emotional stress increase body temperature through hormonal and neural stimulation. These physiological changes increase metabolism, which increases heat production. The client who is anxious about entering a hospital or a physician's office may register a higher normal temperature (see Chapter 30).

Environment.
Environment influences body temperature. If temperature is assessed in a very warm room, a client may be unable to regulate body temperature by heat loss mechanisms, and the body temperature will be elevated. If the client has just been outside in the cold without warm clothing, body temperature may be low because of extensive radiant and conductive heat loss. Infants and older adults are most likely to be affected by environmental temperatures because their temperature-regulating mechanisms are less efficient.

Temperature Alterations.
Changes in body temperature outside the usual range affect the hypothalamic set point. These changes can be related to excess heat production, excessive heat loss, minimal heat production, minimal heat loss, or any combination of these alterations. The nature of the change affects the type of clinical problems a client experiences.

Hyperpyrexia, or fever, occurs because heat loss mechanisms are unable to keep pace with excess heat produc-

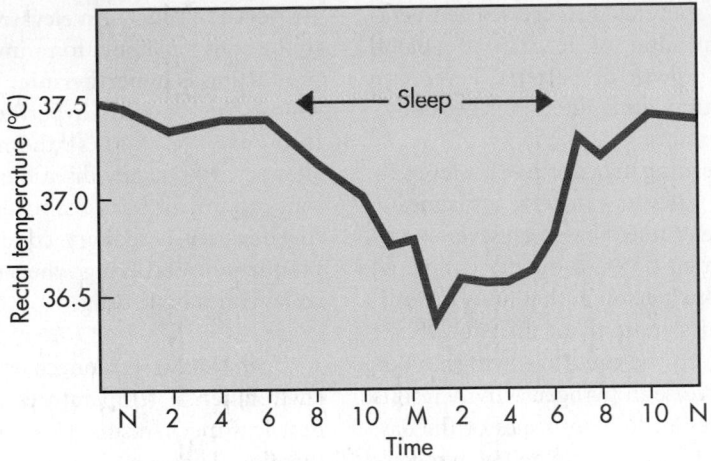

Figure 31-3   Temperature cycle for 24 hours.

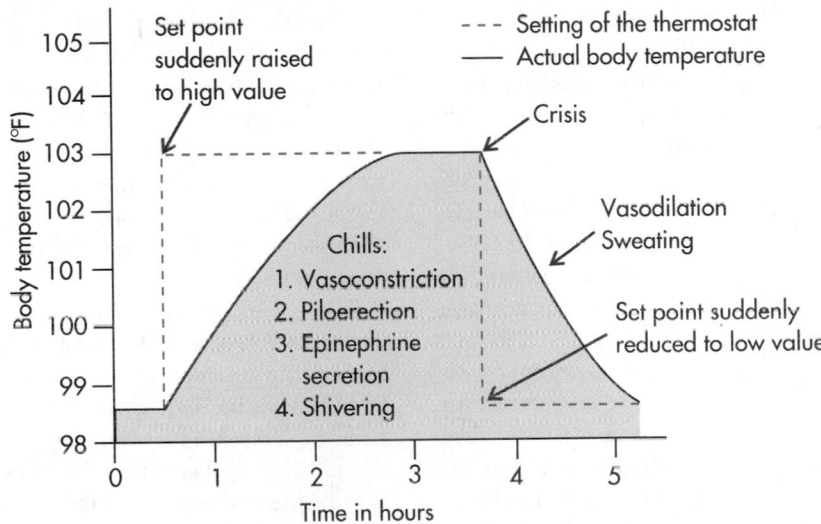

Figure 31-4   Effect of changing the set point of the hypothalamic temperature control during a fever.
Modified from Guyton AC: *Textbook of medical physiology,* ed 9, Philadelphia, 1995, WB Saunders.

tion, resulting in an abnormal rise in body temperature. The level at which a fever threatens health is often a source of disagreement among health care providers. A fever is usually not harmful if it stays below 39° C (102.2° F).

A true fever results from an alteration in the hypothalamic set point. **Pyrogens** such as bacteria and viruses cause a rise in body temperature. When they enter the body, pyrogens act as antigens, triggering the immune system. More white cells are produced to help promote the body's defense against infection. In addition, hormonelike substances are released to further defend against infection. These substances also trigger the hypothalamus to raise the set point. To meet the new higher set point, the body produces and conserves heat. Several hours may pass before the body temperature reaches the new set point.

During this period the person experiences chills, shivers, and feels cold, even though the body temperature is rising (Figure 31-4). The chill phase resolves when the new set point, a higher temperature, is achieved. During the next phase, the plateau, the chills subside and the person feels warm and dry. If the new set point has been "overshot," or the pyrogens are removed (e.g., destruction of bacteria by antibiotics), the third phase of a **febrile** episode occurs. The hypothalamus set point drops, initiating heat loss responses. The skin becomes warm and flushed because of vasodilation. Diaphoresis assists in evaporative heat loss. When the fever "breaks," the client becomes **afebrile.**

Fever is an important defense mechanism. Mild temperature elevations up to 39° C (102.2° F) enhance the body's immune system. During a febrile episode, white blood cell production is stimulated. Increased temperature reduces the concentration of iron in the blood plasma, suppressing the growth of bacteria. Fever also fights viral infections by stimulating interferon, the body's natural virus-fighting substance.

A single temperature reading may not reveal a fever. By analyzing the fever pattern, fevers can serve a diagnostic purpose. A fever can be determined based on several temperature readings at different times of the day compared with the usual range for that person at that time, in addition to physical signs and symptoms of infection. Fever patterns differ depending on the causative pyrogen (Box 31-4). The increase or decrease in pyrogen activity results in fever spikes and declines at different times of the day. The duration and degree of fever depend on the pyrogen's strength and the ability of the individual to respond. The term **fever of unknown origin (FUO)** refers to a fever whose etiology (cause) cannot be determined.

During a fever, cellular metabolism increases and oxygen consumption rises. The body's metabolism increases 13% for every degree Celsius of temperature elevation (Holtzclaw, 1998). Heart and respiratory rates increase to meet the metabolic needs of the body for nutrients. The increased metabolism uses energy that produces additional heat. If the client has a cardiac or respiratory problem, the stress of a fever can be great. A prolonged fever can weaken a client by exhausting energy stores. Increased metabolism requires additional oxygen. If the demand for additional oxygen cannot be met, cellular hypoxia (inadequate oxygen) occurs. Myocardial hypoxia produces angina (chest pain). Cerebral hypoxia produces confusion. Interventions during a fever may include oxygen therapy. The regulatory mechanism used to compensate for fever places a client at risk for fluid volume deficit. Water loss through increased respiration and diaphoresis can be excessive. Dehydration can be a serious problem for older adults and children with low body weight. Maintaining optimum fluid volume status is an important nursing action (see Chapter 40).

Hyperthermia.   An elevated body temperature related to the body's inability to promote heat loss or reduce heat production is **hyperthermia.** Whereas fever is an upward shift in the set point, hyperthermia results from an overload of the body's thermoregulatory mechanisms (Rowsey, 1997). Any disease or trauma to the hypothalamus can impair heat loss mechanisms. **Malignant hyperthermia** is a hereditary condition of uncontrolled heat production, occurring when susceptible persons receive certain anesthetic drugs.

Heatstroke.   Prolonged exposure to the sun or high environmental temperatures can overwhelm the body's heat-loss mechanisms. Heat also depresses hypothalamic function. These conditions cause **heatstroke,** a dangerous heat emergency with a high mortality rate. Clients at risk include those who are very young or very old and those who have cardiovascular disease, hypothyroidism, diabetes, or alcoholism. Also at risk are those who take medications that decrease the body's ability to lose heat (e.g., phenothiazines, anticholinergics, diuretics, amphetamines, and beta-adrenergic receptor antagonists) and those who exercise or work strenuously (e.g., athletes, construction workers, and farmers). Signs and symptoms of heatstroke include giddiness, confusion, delirium, excess thirst, nausea, muscle cramps, visual disturbances, and even incontinence. The most important sign of heatstroke is hot, dry skin.

Victims of heatstroke do not sweat because of severe electrolyte loss and hypothalamic malfunction. Heatstroke with a temperature greater than 40.5° C (105° F) produces tissue damage to the cells of all body organs. Vital signs reveal a body temperature sometimes as high as 45° C (113° F), tachycardia, and hypotension. The brain may be the first organ affected because of its sensitivity to electrolyte imbalances. As the condition progresses, a client becomes unconscious with fixed, unreactive pupils. Permanent neurological damage occurs unless cooling measures are rapidly started.

Heat Exhaustion.   **Heat exhaustion** occurs when profuse diaphoresis results in excess water and electrolyte loss. Caused by environmental heat exposure, the signs and symptoms of fluid volume deficit are common during heat exhaustion. First aid includes transporting the client to a cooler environment and restoring fluid and electrolyte balance.

Hypothermia.   Heat loss during prolonged exposure to cold overwhelms the body's ability to produce heat, causing hypothermia. **Hypothermia** is classified by core temperature measurements (Table 31-1). It can be unintentional, such as falling through the ice of a frozen lake. Hypothermia may be intentionally induced during surgical procedures to reduce metabolic demand and the body's need for oxygen.

Patterns of Fever	Box 31-4
Sustained	A constant body temperature continuously above 38° C (100.4° F) that demonstrates little fluctuation.
Intermittent	Fever spikes interspersed with usual temperature levels. Temperature returns to acceptable value at least once in 24 hours.
Remittent	Fever spikes and falls without a return to normal temperature levels.
Relapsing	Periods of febrile episodes interspersed with acceptable temperature values. Febrile episodes and periods of normothermia may be longer than 24 hours.

Table 31-1	Classification of Hypothermia	
	C	F
Mild	33.1°-36°	91.5°-96.8°
Moderate	30.1°-33°	86.1°-91.4°
Severe	27°-30°	80.6°-86.0°
Profound	<27°	<80.6°

Accidental hypothermia usually develops gradually and may go unnoticed for several hours. When skin temperature drops to 35° C (95° F), the client suffers uncontrolled shivering, loss of memory, depression, and poor judgment. As the body temperature falls below 34.4° C (94° F), heart, respiratory rates, and blood pressure fall. The skin becomes cyanotic. If hypothermia progresses, a client experiences cardiac dysrhythmias, loss of consciousness, and unresponsiveness to painful stimuli. In cases of severe hypothermia a person may demonstrate clinical signs similar to death (e.g., lack of response to stimuli and extremely slow respirations and pulse). The assessment of core temperature is critical when hypothermia is suspected. A special low reading thermometer may be required because standard devices do not register below 35° C (95° F).

Frostbite occurs when the body is exposed to subnormal temperatures. Ice crystals forming inside the cell can result in permanent circulatory and tissue damage. Areas particularly susceptible to frostbite are the earlobes, tip of the nose, and fingers and toes. The injured area is white, waxy, and firm to the touch. The client loses sensation in the affected area. Intervention includes gradual warming measures, analgesia, and protection of the injured tissue.

NURSING PROCESS AND THERMOREGULATION

Knowledge of the physiology of body temperature regulation helps the nurse to assess the client's response to temperature alterations and to intervene safely. Independent measures can be implemented to increase or minimize heat loss, to promote heat conservation, and to increase comfort. These measures add to the effects of medically ordered therapies during illness. Many measures can also be taught to family members, parents of children, or other caregivers.

ASSESSMENT

Sites. There are several sites for measuring core and surface body temperature. The core temperatures of the pulmonary artery, esophagus, and urinary bladder are used in intensive care settings. These measurements require the use of continuous invasive devices placed in body cavities or organs. These devices obtain accurate readings quickly and continually display readings on an electronic monitor.

The sites used most commonly for temperature measurement are also invasive but can be used intermittently. These include the tympanic membrane, mouth, rectum, and axillary sites. Noninvasive chemically prepared thermometer patches can also be applied to the skin. Oral, rectal, axillary, and skin temperature sites rely on effective blood circulation at the measurement site. The heat of the blood is conducted to the thermometer probe. Tympanic temperature relies on the radiation of body heat to an infrared sensor. Because the tympanic membrane shares the same arterial blood supply as the hypothalamus, tympanic temperature is considered a core temperature.

To ensure accurate temperature readings, each site must be measured correctly (Skill 31-1). The temperature obtained varies, depending on the site used, but should be between 36° C (96.8° F) and 38° C (100.4° F). Research findings from numerous studies are contradictory; however, it is generally accepted that rectal temperatures are usually 0.5° C (0.9° F) higher than oral temperatures, and axillary temperatures are usually 0.5° C (0.9° F) lower than oral temperatures (Holtzclaw, 1998). Each of the common temperature measurement sites has advantages and disadvantages (Box 31-5, p. 684). The nurse chooses the safest and most accurate site for the client. The same site should be used when repeated measurements are necessary.

Thermometers. The three types of thermometers used for determining body temperature are glass, electronic, and disposable. The nurse is responsible for being knowledgeable and skilled in the use of the selected measurement device. Each device measures temperature using the **Celsius** or **Fahrenheit** scale. Electronic thermometers allow the nurse to convert scales by activating a switch. When it is necessary to convert temperature readings, the following formulas can be used:

1. To convert Fahrenheit to Celsius, subtract 32 from the Fahrenheit reading and multiply the result by 5/9

$$C = (F - 32°) \times 5/9$$
$$\text{Example: } 40° C = (104° F - 32° F) \times 5/9$$

2. To convert Celsius to Fahrenheit, multiply the centigrade reading by 9/5 and add 32 to the product.

$$F = (9/5 \times C) + 32°$$
$$\text{Example: } 104° F = (9/5 \times 40° C) + 32°$$

Glass Thermometer. The glass thermometer is the most familiar, having been in use since the fifteenth century. It is a glass tube sealed at one end with a mercury-filled bulb at the other. Exposure of the bulb to heat causes the mercury to expand and rise in the enclosed tube. The length of the thermometer is marked with Fahrenheit or Celsius calibrations. The farthest point reached by the mercury in the tube is the temperature reading. The mer-

Text continued on p. 685.

Skill 31-1 Measuring Body Temperature

Delegation Considerations

The skill of temperature measurement can be delegated to assistive personnel.

- Inform caregiver of appropriate route and device to measure temperature.
- Inform and observe caregiver performing proper positioning of clients for rectal temperature measurement.
- Inform caregiver of factors that can falsely raise or lower temperature.

- Inform caregiver of the frequency of temperature measurement.
- Determine that caregiver is aware of the usual values for client.
- Inform caregiver of the need to report any abnormalities that should be reconfirmed by the nurse.

EQUIPMENT

- Appropriate thermometer
- Soft tissue
- Lubricant (for rectal measurements only)

- Pen, pencil, vital sign flow sheet or record form
- Disposable gloves, plastic thermometer sleeve or disposable probe cover

STEPS	RATIONALE
1. Assess for signs and symptoms of temperature alterations and for factors that influence body temperature.	Physical signs and symptoms may indicate abnormal temperature. Nurse can accurately assess nature of variations.
2. Determine any previous activity that would interfere with accuracy of temperature measurement. When taking oral temperature, wait 20 to 30 min before measuring temperature if client has smoked or ingested hot or cold liquids or foods.	Smoking or oral intake of food or fluids can cause false temperature readings in oral cavity.
3. Determine appropriate temperature site and device for client.	Chosen based on advantages and disadvantages of each site (see Box 31-5). Glass thermometer is used for client who is on isolation precautions.
4. Explain way temperature will be taken and importance of maintaining proper position until reading is complete.	Clients are often curious about such measurements and should be cautioned against prematurely removing thermometer to read results.
5. Wash hands.	Reduces transmission of microorganisms.
6. Assist client in assuming comfortable position that provides easy access to temperature site.	Ensures comfort and accuracy of temperature reading.
7. Obtain temperature reading.	
A. **Oral temperature measurement with glass thermometer:**	
(1) Apply disposable gloves.	Maintains standard precautions when exposed to items soiled with body fluids (e.g., saliva).
(2) Hold end (if color-coded, tip will be blue) of glass thermometer with fingertips.	Reduces contamination of thermometer bulb.
(3) Read mercury level while gently rotating thermometer at eye level. If mercury is above desired level, grasp tip of thermometer securely, stand away from solid objects, and sharply flick wrist downward. Continue shaking until reading is below 35.5° C (95.9° F).	Mercury should be below 35.5° C (95.9° F). Thermometer reading must be below client's actual temperature before use. Brisk shaking lowers mercury level in glass tube.
(4) Insert thermometer into plastic sleeve cover (optional).	Protects from contact with saliva.
(5) Ask client to open mouth and gently place thermometer under tongue in posterior sublingual pocket lateral to center of lower jaw (see illustration).	Heat from superficial blood vessels in sublingual pocket produces temperature reading.
(6) Ask client to hold thermometer with lips closed. Caution client against biting down on thermometer.	Maintains proper position of thermometer during recording. Breakage of thermometer may injure mucosa and cause mercury poisoning.
(7) Leave thermometer in place for 3 min or according to agency policy.	Studies vary as to proper length of time for recording. Holtzclaw (1998) recommends 3 minutes.

STEPS	RATIONALE
(8) Carefully remove thermometer, remove and discard plastic sleeve cover in appropriate receptacle if used. Gently rotate until scale appears.	Prevents cross contamination. Ensures accurate reading.
(9) Cleanse any additional secretions on thermometer by wiping with clean soft tissue. Wipe in rotating fashion from fingers toward bulb. Dispose of tissue in appropriate receptacle. Store thermometer in appropriate protective storage container.	Avoids contact of microorganisms with nurse's hands. Wipe from area of least contamination to area of most contamination. Glass thermometers should not be shared between clients unless terminal disinfection is performed between each measurement. Protective storage container prevents breakage and reduces risks of mercury spill.
(10) Remove and dispose of gloves in appropriate receptacle. Wash hands.	Reduces transmission of microorganisms.
B. Oral temperature measurement with electronic thermometer:	
(1) Apply disposable gloves (optional).	Use of oral probe cover, which can be removed without physical contact, minimizes need to wear gloves.
(2) Remove thermometer pack from charging unit. Attach oral probe (blue tip) to thermometer unit. Grasp top of probe stem, being careful not to apply pressure on the ejection button.	Charging provides battery power. Ejection button releases plastic probe cover from tip.
(3) Slide disposable plastic probe cover over thermometer probe until cover locks in place (see illustration).	Soft plastic cover will not break in client's mouth and prevents transmission of microorganisms between clients.
(4) Ask client to open mouth; then gently place thermometer probe under tongue in posterior sublingual pocket lateral to center of lower jaw.	Heat from superficial blood vessels in sublingual pocket produces temperature reading. With electronic thermometer, temperatures in right and left posterior sublingual pocket are significantly higher than in area under front of tongue.
(5) Ask client to hold thermometer probe with lips closed.	Maintains proper position of thermometer during recording.
(6) Leave thermometer probe in place until audible signal occurs and client's temperature appears on digital display; remove thermometer probe from under client's tongue.	Probe must stay in place until signal occurs to ensure accurate reading.
(7) Push ejection button on thermometer stem to discard plastic probe cover into appropriate receptacle.	Reduces transmission of microorganisms.
(8) Return probe to storage position of thermometer unit.	Protects probe from damage. Returning probe automatically causes digital reading to disappear.
(9) If gloves worn, remove and dispose in appropriate receptacle. Wash hands.	Reduces transmission of microorganisms.
(10) Return thermometer to charger.	Maintains battery charge.

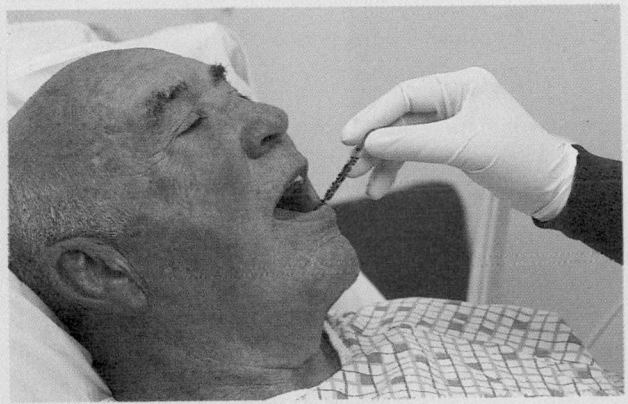

Step 7A(5)

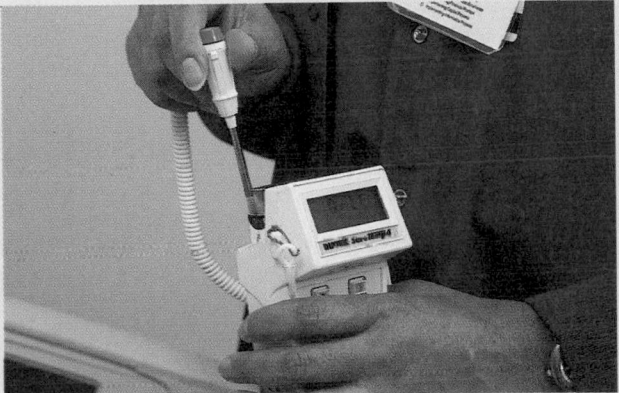

Step 7B(3)

STEPS	RATIONALE
C. **Rectal temperature measurement with glass thermometer:**	
(1) Draw curtain around bed and/or close room door. Assist client to Sims' position with upper leg flexed. Move aside bed linen to expose only anal area. Keep client's upper body and lower extremities covered with sheet or blanket.	Maintains client's privacy, minimizes embarrassment, and promotes comfort. Exposes anal area for correct thermometer placement.
(2) Apply disposable gloves.	Maintains standard precautions when exposed to items soiled with body fluids (e.g., feces).
(3) Hold end (if color-coded, tip will be red) of glass thermometer with fingertips.	Reduces contamination of thermometer bulb.
(4) Read mercury level while gently rotating thermometer at eye level. If mercury is above desired level, grasp tip of thermometer securely, stand away from solid objects, and sharply flick wrist downward. Continue shaking until reading is below 35.5° C (95.9° F).	Mercury should be below 35.5°C (95.9°F). Thermometer reading must be below client's actual temperature before use. Brisk shaking lowers mercury level in glass tube.
(5) Insert thermometer into plastic sleeve cover.	Protects from contact with feces.
(6) Squeeze liberal portion of lubricant on tissue. Dip thermometer's blunt end into lubricant, covering 2.5 to 3.5 cm (1 to 1½ in) for adult.	Lubrication minimizes trauma to rectal mucosa during insertion. Tissue avoids contamination of remaining lubricant in container.
(7) With nondominant hand, separate client's buttocks to expose anus. Ask client to breathe slowly and relax.	Fully exposes anus for thermometer insertion. Relaxes anal sphincter for easier thermometer insertion.
(8) Gently insert thermometer into anus in direction of umbilicus 3.5 cm (1½ in) for adult. Do not force thermometer.	Ensures adequate exposure against blood vessels in rectal wall.
(9) If resistance is felt during insertion, withdraw thermometer immediately. Never force thermometer.	Prevents trauma to mucosa. Glass thermometers can break.

Critical Decision Point: If thermometer cannot be adequately inserted into rectum, remove thermometer and consider alternative method for obtaining temperature.

STEPS	RATIONALE
(10) Hold thermometer in place for 2 min or according to agency policy.	Prevents injury to client. Studies vary as to proper length of time for recording. Holtzclaw (1998) recommends 2 min.
(11) Carefully remove thermometer, remove and discard plastic sleeve cover in appropriate receptacle, and wipe off any remaining secretions with clean tissue. Wipe in rotating fashion from fingers toward bulb. Dispose of tissue in appropriate receptacle.	Prevents cross contamination. Wipe from area of least contamination to area of most contamination.
(12) Read thermometer at eye level. Gently rotate until scale appears.	Ensures accurate reading.
(13) Wipe client's anal area with soft tissue to remove lubricant or feces and discard tissue. Assist client in assuming a comfortable position.	Provides for comfort and hygiene.
(14) Store thermometer in appropriate protective storage container.	Glass thermometers should not be shared between clients unless terminal disinfection is performed between each measurement. Protective storage container prevents breakage and reduces risks of mercury spill.
(15) Remove and dispose of gloves in appropriate receptacle. Wash hands.	Reduces transmission of microorganisms.

STEPS	RATIONALE

D. **Rectal temperature measurement with electronic thermometer:**

(1) Follow steps 7C(1) and 7C(2).

(2) Remove thermometer pack from charging unit. Attach rectal probe (red tip) to thermometer unit. Grasp top of probe stem, being careful not to apply pressure on the ejection button.

Charging provides battery power. Ejection button releases plastic probe cover from tip.

(3) Slide disposable plastic probe cover over thermometer probe until cover locks in place.

Probe cover prevents transmission of microorganisms between clients.

(4) Continue as for C(6), (7), (8), and (9).

(5) Leave thermometer probe in place (see illustration) until audible signal occurs and client's temperature appears on digital display; remove thermometer probe from anus.

Probe must stay in place until signal occurs to ensure accurate reading.

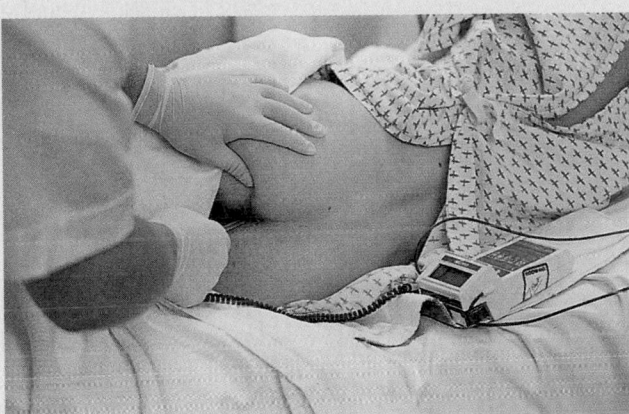

Step 7D(5)

(6) Push ejection button on thermometer stem to discard plastic probe cover into appropriate receptacle.

Reduces transmission of microorganisms.

(7) Return probe to storage position of thermometer unit.

Protects probe from damage. Returning probe automatically causes digital reading to disappear.

(8) Wipe client's anal area with soft tissue to remove lubricant or feces and discard tissue. Assist client in assuming a comfortable position.

Provides for comfort and hygiene.

(9) Remove and dispose of gloves in appropriate receptacle. Wash hands.

Reduces transmission of microorganisms.

(10) Return thermometer to charger.

Maintains battery charge.

E. **Axillary temperature measurement with glass thermometer:**

(1) Wash hands.

Reduces transmission of microorganisms.

(2) Draw curtain around bed and/or close door.

Provides privacy and minimizes embarrassment.

(3) Assist client to supine or sitting position.

Provides easy access to axilla.

(4) Move clothing or gown away from shoulder and arm.

Exposes axilla for correct thermometer placement.

(5) Prepare glass thermometer following Steps 7A(2) and (3).

Mercury must be below client's temperature level before insertion.

STEPS	RATIONALE
(6) Insert thermometer into center of axilla, lower arm over thermometer, and place arm across client's chest (see illustrations).	Maintains proper position of thermometer against blood vessels in axilla.
(7) Hold thermometer in place for 3 min or according to agency policy.	Studies vary as to proper length of time for recording. They concluded that changes after 3 min had little clinical significance.
(8) Remove thermometer, remove plastic sleeve, and wipe off remaining secretions with tissue. Wipe in rotating fashion from fingers toward bulb. Dispose of sleeve and tissue in appropriate receptacle.	Avoids nurse's contact with microorganisms. Wipe from area of least contamination to area of most contamination.
(9) Read thermometer at eye level.	Ensures accurate reading.
(10) Inform client of reading.	Promotes participation in care and understanding of health status.
(11) Store thermometer in appropriate protective storage container.	Glass thermometers should not be shared between clients unless terminal disinfection is performed between each measurement. Storage container prevents breakage and reduces risk of mercury spill.
(12) Assist client in replacing clothing or gown.	Restores sense of well-being.
(13) Wash hands.	Reduces transmission of microorganisms.

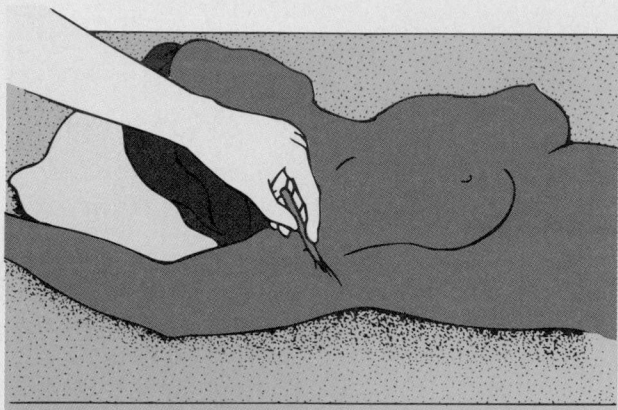 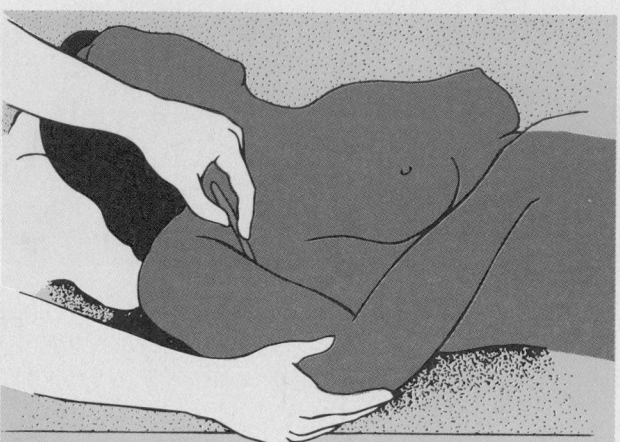

Step 7E(6)

F. **Axillary temperature measurement with electronic thermometer:**

(1) Wash hands.	
(2) Draw curtain around bed and/or close door.	
(3) Position client lying supine or sitting.	Provides easy access to axilla.
(4) Move clothing or gown away from shoulder and arm.	Expose axilla for correct thermometer probe placement.
(5) Remove thermometer pack from charging unit. Be sure oral probe (blue tip) is attached to thermometer unit. Grasp top of probe stem, being careful not to apply pressure on the ejection button.	Charging provides battery power. Ejection button releases plastic cover from probe.
(6) Slide disposable plastic probe cover over thermometer probe until cover locks in place.	Soft plastic cover prevents transmission of microorganisms between clients.
(7) Raise client's arm away from torso, inspect for skin lesion and excessive perspiration. Insert probe into center of axilla, lower arm over probe, and place arm across client's chest.	Maintains proper position of probe against blood vessels in axilla.

STEPS	RATIONALE
(8) Leave probe in place until audible signal occurs and temperature appears on digital display.	Probe must stay in place until signal occurs to ensure accurate reading.
(9) Remove probe from axilla.	
(10) Push ejection button on thermometer stem to discard plastic probe cover into appropriate receptacle.	Reduces transmission of microorganisms.
(11) Return probe to storage position of thermometer unit.	Protects probe from damage. Returning probe automatically causes digital reading to disappear.
(12) Assist client in assuming a comfortable position.	Restores comfort and promotes privacy.
(13) Wash hands.	Reduces transmission of microorganisms.
(14) Return thermometer unit to charger.	Maintains battery charge.

G. **Tympanic membrane temperature with electronic thermometer:**

STEPS	RATIONALE
(1) Assist client in assuming comfortable position with head turned toward side, away from nurse. Right-handed persons should obtain temperature from client's right ear. Left-handed people should obtain temperature from client's left ear. The less acute the angle of approach, the better the probe seal.	Ensures comfort and exposes auditory canal for accurate temperature measurement.
(2) Remove thermometer handheld unit from charging base, being careful not to apply pressure on the ejection button.	Base provides battery power. Removal of handheld unit from base prepares it to measure temperature. Ejection button releases plastic probe cover from tip.
(3) Slide clean disposable speculum cover over otoscope-like lens tip until it locks into place, being careful not to touch lens cover.	Lens cover must be unimpeded by dust, fingerprints, or earwax to ensure clear optical pathway.
(4) Insert speculum into ear canal following manufacturer's instructions for tympanic probe positioning:	Correct positioning of the probe with respect to ear canal ensures accurate readings.
a. Pull ear pinna backward, up, and out for an adult.	The ear tug straightens the external auditory canal, allowing maximum exposure of the tympanic membrane.
b. Move thermometer in a figure-eight pattern.	Some manufacturers recommend movement of the speculum tip in a figure eight pattern that allows the sensor to detect maximum tympanic membrane heat radiation. Gentle pressure seals ear canal from ambient temperature, which can alter readings as much as 2.77° C (5°F). (Braun, Preston, and Smith, 1998).
c. Fit probe snug into canal and do not move.	
d. Point toward nose.	
(5) As soon as probe is in place depress scan button on handheld unit. Leave thermometer probe in place until audible signal occurs and client's temperature appears on digital display.	Depression of scan button causes infrared energy to be detected. Otoscope tip must stay in place until signal occurs to ensure accurate reading.
(6) Carefully remove speculum from auditory meatus.	
(7) Push ejection button on handheld unit to discard plastic probe cover into appropriate receptacle.	Reduces transmission of microorganisms. Automatically causes digital reading to disappear.
(8) If a second reading in necessary, replace probe lens cover and wait 2 to 3 min before inserting the probe tip.	Lens cover must be free of cerumen to maintain optical path. Time allows ear canal to regain usual temperature (Severine and McKenzie, 1997).
(9) Return handheld unit to charging base.	Protects sensory tip from damage.
(10) Assist client in assuming a comfortable position.	Restores comfort and sense of well-being.
(11) Wash hands.	Reduces transmission of microorganisms.
8. Discuss findings with client as needed.	Promotes participation in care and understanding of health status.
9. If temperature is assessed for the first time, establish temperature as baseline if it is within normal range.	Used to compare future temperature measurements.
10. Compare temperature reading with client's previous baseline and acceptable temperature range for client's age group.	Normal body temperature fluctuates within narrow range; comparison reveals presence of abnormality. Improper placement or movement of thermometer can cause inaccuracies. Second measurement confirms initial findings of abnormal body temperature.

Recording and Reporting
- Record temperature in nurses' notes or vital sign flow sheet. Measurement of temperature after administration of specific therapies should be documented in narrative form in nurses' notes.
- Report abnormal findings to nurse in charge or physician.

Home Care Considerations
- Assess temperature and ventilation of client's environment to determine existence of any environmental condition that may influence outcome of client's temperature.
- Assess safe storage of mercury-in-glass thermometers to protect from breakage and mercury spills.

Advantages and Disadvantages of Select Temperature Measurement Sites   Box 31-5

TYMPANIC MEMBRANE SENSOR

Advantages

Easily accessible site

Minimal client repositioning required

Provides accurate core reading

Very rapid measurement (2 to 5 seconds)

Can be obtained without disturbing or waking client

Eardrum close to hypothalamus; sensitive to core

Temperature changes

Unaffected by oral intake of food, fluids, smoking

Can be used for tachypneic clients

Disadvantages

Requires removal of hearing aids before measurement

Should not be used with clients who have had surgery of the ear or tympanic membrane

Requires disposable probe cover

Expensive

Does not accurately measure core temperature changes during and after exercise (Yeo and Scarbough, 1996)

Possible distortion of temperature readings for clients with otitis media

May have lower readings with cerumen impaction (Hasel and Erickson, 1995)

Questions about measurement accuracy in newborns (Bliss-Holtz, 1995)

More variability of measurement than with other core temperature devices (Leick-Rude and Bloom, 1998)

Cannot obtain continuous measurement

RECTUM

Advantages

Argued to be more reliable when oral temperature cannot be obtained

Disadvantages

May lag behind core temperature during rapid temperature changes

Should not be used for children with diarrhea or clients who have had rectal surgery, a rectal disorder, or decreased platelets (Haddock, Merrow, and Swanson 1996)

Should not be used for routine vital signs in newborns (Cusson, Madonia, and Taekman, 1997)

Requires positioning and may be source of client embarrassment and anxiety

Risk of body fluid exposure

Requires lubrication

ORAL

Advantages

Accessible—requires no position change

Comfortable for client

Provides accurate surface temperature reading

Reflects rapid change in core temperature

Disadvantages

Affected by ingestion of fluids or foods, smoke, and oxygen delivery (Holtzclaw, 1998)

Should not be used with clients who have had oral surgery, trauma, history of epilepsy, or shaking chills

Should not be used with infants, small children, or confused, unconscious, or uncooperative clients

Risk of body fluid exposure

AXILLA

Advantages

Safe and noninvasive

Can be used with newborns and uncooperative clients

Disadvantages

Long measurement time

Requires continuous positioning by nurse

Lags behind core temperature during rapid temperature changes

Requires exposure of thorax

Not recommended to detect fever in infants and young children (Haddock, Merrow, and Swanson, 1996)

SKIN

Advantages

Inexpensive

Provides continuous reading

Safe and noninvasive

Does not require disturbing client

Can be used for neonates

Easy to read

Disadvantages

Lags behind other sites during temperature changes, especially during hyperthermia

Adhesion can be impaired by diaphoresis or sweat

Can be affected by environmental temperature

Unreliable during chill phase of fever (Holtzclaw, 1998)

cury will not fluctuate or fall unless the thermometer is shaken vigorously.

The nurse reads a mercury thermometer by using the fingertips to hold it horizontally, with the bulb pointed to the left (Figure 31-5). By rotating the thermometer slowly, the column of silver mercury appears. The calibrated line at the end of the mercury column is the temperature reading. The bulb should not be touched. Touching it might affect the temperature reading or bring the fingers into contact with the client's body secretions. Disposable plastic sleeves may be available to cover the body of the thermometer. Observe standard precautions, including gloves, when using a glass thermometer because of potential contact with body fluids. To reduce the risk of cross contamination a glass thermometer is stored at the client's bedside and sent home when the client is discharged.

Three types of glass thermometers are the oral (slim tip), the stubby, and the rectal (pear-shaped tip) (Figure 31-6). The oral thermometer tip is slender, allowing for greater exposure of the bulb against the blood vessels in the mouth. An oral thermometer usually has a blue tip. The stubby thermometer is shorter and thicker than the oral type. It can be used to measure temperature at any site. The rectal thermometer has a blunt or tapered end designed to prevent trauma to the rectal tissues during insertion. It is usually recognized by a red tip.

The time delay for recordings and breakability are disadvantages of glass thermometers. Mercury is a hazardous material if not properly contained. Accidental breakage of a glass thermometer is a health hazard to the client, nurse, and health care workers. Mercury is highly permeable through skin and mucous membranes; inhaled vapors diffuse rapidly into the blood and are transported to body tissues including the brain. The contents of two mercury glass thermometers in a closed room exceed the permissible exposure limit established by the Occupational Safety and Health Administration (OSHA) (Material Safety Data Sheet, 1989). Steps to take in the event of a mercury spill are presented in Box 31-6.

Advantages of glass thermometers are the low price, wide availability, and reliability. The accuracy of glass thermometers depends on the length of time they have been stored without being used. Generally these thermometers should not be stored more than 6 months (Severine and McKenzie, 1997).

Electronic Thermometer.   The electronic thermometer consists of a rechargeable battery-powered display unit, a thin wire cord, and a temperature-processing probe covered by a disposable plastic sheath (Figure 31-7). One form of electronic thermometer uses a pencil-like probe. Separate nonbreakable probes are available for oral and rectal use. The oral probe can also be used for axillary temperature measurement. Within 20 to 50 seconds of insertion, a reading appears on the display unit. A sound signals when the peak temperature reading has been measured.

Another form of electronic thermometer is used exclusively for tympanic temperature (Figure 31-8). An otoscope-like speculum with an infrared sensor tip detects

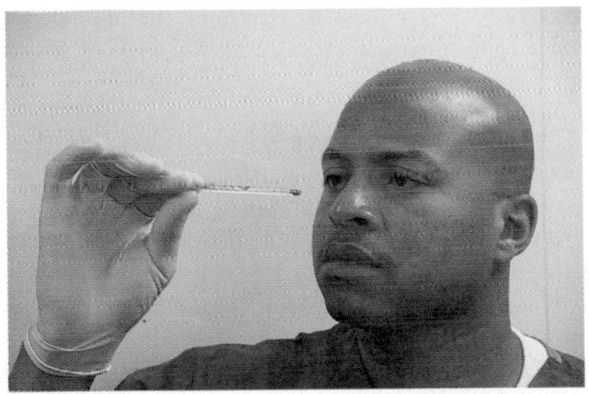

Figure 31-5   Reading a glass thermometer.

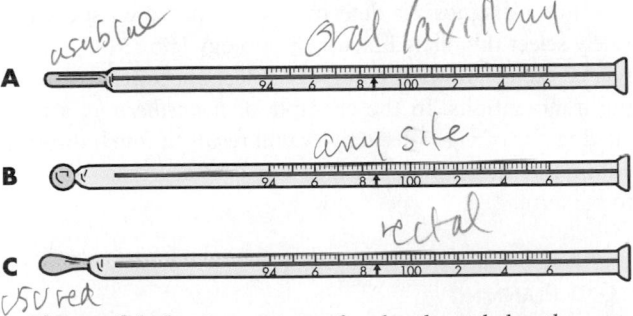

Figure 31-6   Comparison of oral and rectal glass thermometers. **A,** Elongated bulb is for oral or axillary use. **B,** Stubby bulb may be used for any site. **C,** Red bulb indicates rectal use.

Steps to Take in the Event of a Mercury Spill   Box 31-6

1. Do NOT touch spilled mercury droplets. If skin contact has occurred, immediately flush area with water for 15 minutes.
2. If possible, remove client from immediate contaminated environment.
3. Change any clothing or linen that has been contaminated with mercury. Wash hands thoroughly after changing. Wash clothing before reuse.
4. Notify the environmental services department or obtain a mercury spill kit if available.
5. Follow procedures for mercury removal as directed by Material Safety Data Sheet (MSDS). Spills are removed using special absorbent materials, filtered vacuum equipment, and protective clothing.
6. Promote exhaust ventilation to reduce concentration of mercury vapors.
7. Complete occurrence report as directed by institution procedure.

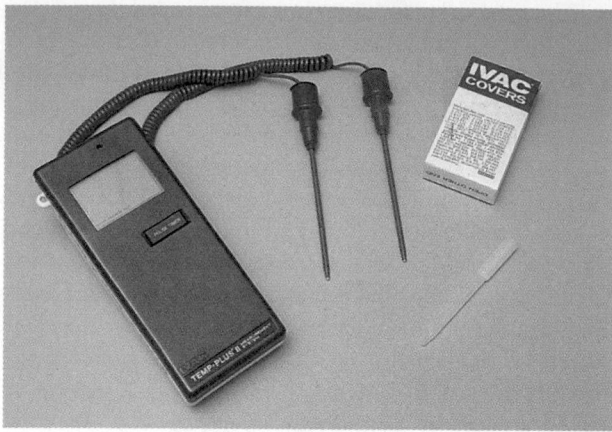

Figure 31-7   Electronic thermometer. Blue probe is for oral or axillary use. Red probe is for rectal use.

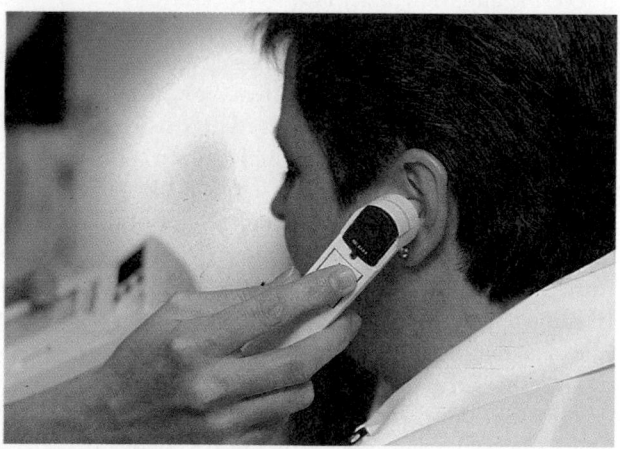

Figure 31-8   Tympanic thermometer with probe cover inserted into auditory canal.

heat radiated from the tympanic membrane. Within 2 to 5 seconds of placement in the auditory canal, a reading appears on the display unit. A sound signals when the peak temperature reading has been measured.

An electronic thermometer using an oral probe is not necessarily more accurate than a glass thermometer. For example, variables that alter oral temperature measurements affect all types of oral thermometers. The greatest advantages of electronic thermometers are that they can be inserted immediately, their readings appear within seconds, and they are easy to read. The plastic sheath is unbreakable and ideal for children. Their expense is a major disadvantage. Electronic thermometer devices measuring axillary temperatures have been reported as less accurate than glass devices.

Disposable Thermometers.   Disposable, single-use thermometers are thin strips of plastic with a temperature

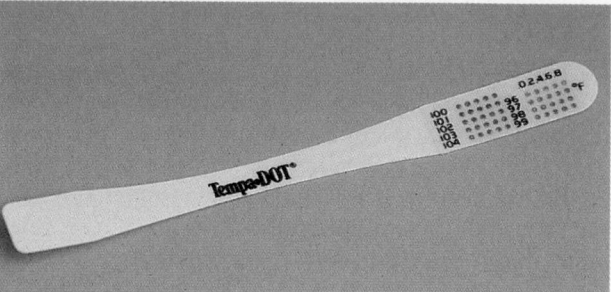

Figure 31-9   Disposable, single-use thermometer strip.

sensor at one end. The sensor consists of a matrix of dot-like indentations that contain chemicals that melt and change color at different temperatures. They are used for oral or axillary temperatures, particularly with children (Figure 31-9). They are inserted the same way as an oral or axillary thermometer and used only once. The thermometer is removed after 3 minutes and read after waiting about 10 seconds for the color change to stabilize.

Another form of disposable thermometer is a temperature-sensitive patch or tape. Applied to the forehead or abdomen, the patch changes color at different temperatures.

Both forms of disposable thermometers are useful to screen clients, especially infants, for altered temperature and are not appropriate for monitoring temperature therapies (Box 31-7). Glass or electronic thermometers are preferred for their accuracy.

NURSING DIAGNOSIS

Assessment of temperature alterations outside an acceptable range leads to a nursing diagnosis. The nurse identifies assessment findings and clusters defining characteristics to form a nursing diagnosis (Box 31-8). For example, an increase in body temperature, flushed skin, skin warm to touch, and tachycardia indicate the diagnosis *hyperthermia*. The nursing diagnosis identifies the client's risk for altered body temperature or an actual temperature alteration. If the client possesses risk factors for temperature alterations, the nurse minimizes or eliminates them.

Once a diagnosis is determined, the nurse must accurately select the related factor or etiology (Box 31-9). The related factor allows the nurse to select appropriate nursing interventions. In the example of *hyperthermia*, a related factor of vigorous activity will result in much different interventions than a related factor of decreased ability to perspire.

PLANNING

During planning the nurse again synthesizes information from multiple resources (see Chapter 16). Critical thinking ensures that the clients' plan of care integrates all that the nurse knows about the individual as well as key

Research HIGHLIGHT   Box 31-7

RESEARCH ABSTRACT

Twenty-four stable postoperative cardiac clients participated in a study to determine the best peripheral method of measuring core body temperature. Ten measures of temperature were compared with temperatures from a pulmonary artery (PA) catheter. Temperatures compared included two tympanic infrared thermometers, electronic thermometers for oral, axillary, and rectal measurements, mercury-in-glass thermometers for oral, axillary and rectal measurements, and chemical indicator thermometer strips for oral and axillary temperatures. Results indicated no significant difference between PA and aural temperatures. The oral chemical indicator thermometer temperatures had lower correlations with PA temperatures than did oral electronic or mercury. Axillary temperatures were significantly lower than PA temperatures. Rectal temperature measurements were significantly higher than PA temperatures but had an excellent correlation with PA temperatures.

IMPLICATIONS FOR PRACTICE

- Oral chemical thermometers should be used for screening and not diagnostic and treatment decisions.
- A single temperature device should be used consistently to track changes in a client's temperature.

REFERENCE

Henker R, Coyne C: Comparison of peripheral temperature measurements with core temperature, *AACN Clin Issues* 6(1):21, 1995.

NURSING DIAGNOSES   Box 31-8

CLIENTS WITH BODY TEMPERATURE ALTERATIONS

Body temperature, altered, risk for
Hyperthermia
Hypothermia
Thermoregulation, ineffective

critical thinking elements. Professional standards are especially important to consider when the nurse develops a plan of care. These standards often establish scientifically proven guidelines for selecting effective nursing interventions.

The nurse develops an individualized plan of care for each nursing diagnosis. The nurse and client set realistic expectations for care. Goals are to be individualized and realistic with measurable outcomes (see care plan).

The plan of care depends on the nurse's assessment of the client's perception and acceptance of the body temperature alteration. Care also depends on the extent to which the client's internal compensatory mechanisms and behaviors have adjusted to the temperature alteration. The client must actively participate in choosing therapies for the care plan. Priorities of care must be set with regard to the extent the temperature alteration affects a client. Safety is a top priority.

Often, other medical problems complicate the care plan. For instance, alterations in body temperature affect the body's requirements for fluids. Clients with heart problems may have difficulty tolerating required fluid replacement therapy.

Clients at high risk for alterations in body temperature require an individualized care plan directed at maintaining normothermia and reducing risk factors. Expected outcomes are established to gauge progress toward returning the body temperature to an acceptable range. For example, the outcome that the client can explain appropriate actions to take during a heat wave is important to establish. The nurse teaches the client and family the importance of thermoregulation and actions to take during excessive environmental heat. Education is particularly important for parents, who need to know how to take action at home when an infant or child develops a temperature alteration.

The severity of a temperature alteration and its effects, together with the client's general health status, will influence the nurse's priorities in the care of a client.

SAMPLE NURSING DIAGNOSTIC PROCESS   Box 31-9

INEFFECTIVE THERMOREGULATION

Assessment Activities	Defining Characteristics Assessment	Nursing Diagnosis
Obtain vital signs, including temperature, pulse, respirations, SpO$_2$.	Increased body temperature above usual range	Ineffective thermoregulation related to aging and inability to adapt to environmental temperature
	Tachycardia	
	Tachypnea	
	Hypoxemia	
Palpate skin.	Warm, dry skin	
Observe client's appearance and behavior while talking and resting.	Restlessness	
	Confusion	
	Flushed appearance	
Review medical history.	Found in unventilated apartment during heat wave; 85 years old with history of dementia	

SAMPLE NURSING CARE PLAN
ELEVATED BODY TEMPERATURE

ASSESSMENT*

Mr. Coburn is a 45-year-old school teacher who arrives at the outpatient clinic with the complaint of malaise. His skin is **warm and dry to touch.** His face is **flushed,** and he appears to have **labored breathing.** He admits to smoking one pack of cigarettes per day and recently began expectorating yellow-green sputum. Vital signs obtained are: blood pressure right arm 116/62, left arm 114/64; right radial **pulse 128,** regular and bounding; **respiratory rate 26;** SpO$_2$ 98% on room air; tympanic **temperature 39.2° C (102.6° F).**
***Defining characteristics** are shown in bold type.

NURSING DIAGNOSIS: Hyperthermia related to infectious process

PLANNING

GOALS

Client will regain normal range of body temperature within next 24 hours.

Client will attain sense of comfort and rest within next 48 hours.

Fluid and electrolyte balance will be maintained during next 3 days.

EXPECTED OUTCOMES

Body temperature will decline at least 1° C (1.8° F) within next 8 hours.

Client will verbalize increased satisfaction with rest and sleep pattern.

Client will report increase in energy level within next 3 days.

Intake will equal output within next 24 hours.

No evidence of postural hypotension during ambulation.

INTERVENTIONS†
Fever Treatment

- Instruct client to reduce external coverings and keep clothing and bed linen dry.

- Instruct client to monitor temperature at home and administer acetaminophen every 4 hours as ordered for temperature over 39° C (102.2° F).

- Instruct client to limit physical activity and increase frequency of rest periods over next 2 days.

- Instruct client to increase oral fluids of choice.

†Intervention Classification labels from McCloskey JC, Bulechek GM: *Nursing interventions classification (NIC),* ed 3, St. Louis, 2000, Mosby.

RATIONALE

Promotes heat loss through conduction and convection.

Antipyretics reduce set point.

Activity and stress increase metabolic rate, contributing to heat production.

Fluids lost through insensible water loss require replacement.

EVALUATION

Ask client to identify temperature and describe energy level.

Ask client about sleep patterns.

Obtain lying, sitting, and standing blood pressures.

Ask client about any dizziness with posture changes.

Ask client to track and report I&O.

IMPLEMENTATION
Health Promotion. Health promotion for client at risk for altered body temperature is directed toward promoting balance between heat production and heat loss. Client activity, temperature of the environment, and clothing are all considered. The nurse teaches clients to avoid strenuous exercise in hot, humid weather; to drink fluids such as water or clear fruity juices before, during, and after exercise; to wear light, loose-fitting, light-colored clothes; to avoid exercising in areas with poor ventilation; to wear a protective covering over the head when outdoors; and to expose themselves to hot climates gradually.

Prevention is the key for clients at risk for hypothermia. Prevention involves educating clients, family members, and friends. Clients most at risk include the very young and the very old and persons debilitated by trauma, stroke, diabetes, drug or alcohol intoxication, sepsis, and Raynaud's disease. Mentally ill or handicapped clients may fall victim to hypothermia because they are unaware of the dangers of cold conditions. Persons without adequate home heating, shelter, diet, or clothing are also at risk. Fatigue, skin color (African-Americans are more susceptible), malnutrition, and hypoxemia also contribute to the risk of frostbite.

Acute Care
Hyperthermia.   The procedures used to intervene and treat an elevated temperature depend on the fever's cause, its adverse effects, and its strength, intensity, and duration. The physician may try to determine the cause of the fever by isolating the causative pyrogen. The nurse obtains necessary culture specimens for laboratory analysis such as urine, blood, sputum, and wound sites (see Chapter 33). Collecting these specimens requires strict aseptic tech-

nique to avoid introducing any outside organisms that might affect the culture results. The physician will order antibiotic medications to be given after the cultures have been obtained. Administering antibiotics destroys pyrogenic bacteria and eliminates the body's stimulus for fever. The nurse administers antibiotics promptly and educates the client regarding the importance of taking and continuing the antibiotic as directed until the course of treatment is complete.

Most fevers in children are of a viral origin, last only briefly, and have limited effects. However, children still have immature temperature control mechanisms and temperatures can rise rapidly. Dehydration and febrile seizures occur during rising temperatures of children between 6 months and 3 years of age. Febrile seizures are unusual in children more than 5 years of age. The extent of the temperature, often exceeding 38.8° C (101.8° F), seems to be a more important factor than the rapidity of the temperature increase (Wong and others, 1998). Children are at particular risk for fluid volume deficit because they can quickly lose large amounts of fluids in proportion to their body weight. The nurse maintains accurate intake and output records and encourages fluids.

The temperature of older adults is normally at the lower end of the temperature range. However, they are very sensitive to slight changes in temperature. The nurse must be aware that a temperature within the normal range may actually be considered a fever in an older adult.

Overall physical condition influences a client's ability to tolerate the increased heart rate, increased respiratory rate, decreased fluid volume, and increased metabolic oxygen demands of fever. Older adults, debilitated clients, and clients with severe burns, neoplastic disease, or a compromised immune system are at high risk for fever-induced complications. Temperatures higher than 39° C (102.2° F) serve little physiological purpose. As core temperature approaches 40° C (104° F), intervention is essential to avoid irreversible damage to cells.

A fever may be a hypersensitivity response to a drug. Drug fevers can be accompanied by other allergy symptoms such as rash or pruritus (itching). Treatment involves withdrawing the medication.

Fever therapy reduces heat production, increases heat loss, and prevents complications. **Antipyretics,** drugs that reduce fever, include corticosteroids and nonsteroidal compounds. Corticosteroids are not used to treat a fever; however, the nurse must be aware of their effect on suppressing the immune system and increasing the client's risk for developing a fever. Clients taking steroids can develop infections without the classic signs appearing. Nonsteroidal drugs such as acetaminophen, salicylates, indomethacin, and ketorolac reduce fever by increasing heat loss. These drugs are commonly prescribed for temperature control.

Nonpharmacological therapy for fever uses methods that increase heat loss by evaporation, conduction, convection, or radiation. Traditionally nurses have used tepid sponge baths, bathing with alcohol water solutions, applying ice packs to axillae and groin areas, and cooling fans. These therapies should be avoided as they lead to shivering. There is no demonstrated advantage of these methods over antipyretic medications, and they may increase client discomfort (Wong and others, 1998). Blankets cooled by circulating water delivered by motorized units increase conductive heat loss. The nurse must follow manufacturer's instructions for applying these hypothermia blankets because of the risk for skin breakdown and "freeze burns." Placing a bath blanket between the client and the hypothermia blanket and wrapping distal extremities (fingers, toes, genitalia) is recommended.

Nursing measures to enhance body cooling must avoid the stimulation of shivering. Shivering is counterproductive because of the heat produced by muscle activity. Vigorous shivering can increase energy expenditure up to 400% (Holtzclaw, 1998). Shivering intensity ranges from palpable but not visible to violent extremity contractions. Wrapping the client's extremities has been recommended to reduce the incidence and intensity of shivering (Holtzclaw, 1998). A dependent nursing intervention for shivering may involve giving medications (e.g., meperidine, butorphanol) that can reduce shivering (Holtzclaw, 1998). Independent nursing measures enhance comfort, reduce metabolic demands, and provide nutrients to meet increased energy needs (Box 31-10).

Heatstroke.   First aid treatment for heatstroke includes moving the client to a cooler environment, reducing clothing covering the body, placing cool wet towels over the skin, and using oscillating fans to increase convective heat loss. Emergency medical treatment may include intravenous (IV) fluids and hypothermia blankets.

Hypothermia.   The priority treatment for hypothermia is to prevent a further decrease in body temperature. The nurse removes wet clothes, provides dry ones, and wraps the client in blankets. In emergencies away from a health care setting, the client lies under blankets next to a warm person. A conscious client benefits from drinking hot liquids such as soup. Placing the client near a fire or in a warm room or placing heating pads next to areas of the body (head and neck) that lose heat the quickest help. When the client reaches an emergency department, treatment depends on the severity of the condition. Warmed intravenous fluids, heating blankets, and warm fluids may be used. Clients are monitored closely for cardiac irregularities and electrolyte imbalances.

Restorative Care.   The nurse educates the client regarding the importance of taking and continuing any antibiotics as directed until the course of treatment for the fever is completed. Children and older adults are at risk for fluid volume deficit because they can quickly lose large amounts of fluids in proportion to their body weight.

Identifying preferred fluids and encouraging oral fluid intake is an important nursing intervention.

☙ EVALUATION

All nursing interventions are evaluated by comparing the client's actual response to the expected outcomes of the care plan. This reveals whether goals of care have been met or if a revision to the plan is needed. After any

---

Nursing Measures for Clients With a Fever   Box 31-10

ASSESSMENT
- Obtain core temperature during each phase of febrile episode.
- Assess for contributing factors such as dehydration, infection, or environmental temperature.
- Identify physiological response to temperature.
  - Obtain all vital signs.
  - Observe skin color.
  - Assess skin temperature.
  - Observe for shivering and diaphoresis.
  - Assess client comfort and well being.
- Determine phase of fever: chill, plateau, fever break.

INTERVENTION (UNLESS CONTRAINDICATED)
- Obtain blood cultures when ordered. Blood specimens are obtained to coincide with temperature spikes when the antigen-producing organism is most prevalent.
- Initiate therapies to minimize heat production.
  - Reduce the frequency of activities that increase oxygen demand such as excessive turning and ambulation.
- Allow rest periods.
  - Limit physical activity.
- Initiate therapies to maximize heat loss.
  - Reduce external covering on client's body to promote heat loss through radiation and conduction. Do not induce shivering.
  - Keep clothing and bed linen dry to increase heat loss through conduction and convection.
- Initiate therapies to meet requirements for increased metabolic rate.
  - Provide supplemental oxygen therapy as ordered to improve oxygen delivery to body cells.
  - Provide measures to stimulate appetite and offer well-balanced meals.
  - Provide fluids (at least 3 L per day for client with normal cardiac and renal function) to replace fluids lost through insensible water loss and sweating.
- Initiate therapies to promote client comfort.
  - Encourage oral hygiene because oral mucous membranes dry easily from dehydration.
  - Control temperature of the environment without inducing shivering.
- Identify onset and duration of febrile episode phases.
- Examine previous temperature measurements for trends.
- Initiate health teaching as indicated.

---

intervention the nurse measures the client's temperature to evaluate for change. In addition, the nurse uses other evaluative measures such as palpation of the skin and assessment of pulse and respirations. If therapies are effective, body temperature will return to an acceptable range, other vital signs will stabilize, and the client will report a sense of comfort.

Pulse

The pulse is the palpable bounding of blood flow noted at various points on the body. It is an indicator of circulatory status. Circulation is the means by which cells receive nutrients and remove waste products of metabolism. For cells to function normally, there must be a continuous blood flow and an appropriate volume and distribution of blood to cells that need nutrients.

PHYSIOLOGY AND REGULATION

Blood flows through the body in a continuous circuit. Electrical impulses originating from the sinoatrial (SA) node travel through heart muscle to stimulate cardiac contraction. Approximately 60 to 70 ml (**stroke volume**) of blood enters the aorta with each ventricular contraction. With each stroke volume ejection, the walls of the aorta distend, creating a pulse wave that travels rapidly toward the distal ends of the arteries. The pulse wave moves 15 times faster through the aorta and 100 times faster through the small arteries than the ejected volume of blood (Guyton, 1995). When a pulse wave reaches a peripheral artery, it can be felt by palpating the artery lightly against underlying bone or muscle. The pulse is the palpable bounding of the blood flow in the peripheral artery. The number of pulsing sensations occurring in 1 minute is the pulse rate.

The volume of blood pumped by the heart during 1 minute is the **cardiac output,** the product of heart rate and the ventricle's stroke volume. In an adult the heart normally pumps 5000 ml of blood per minute. A change in heart rate or stroke volume does not always change the heart's output or the amount of blood in the arteries. For example, if a person's heart rate is 70 beats per minute and the stroke volume is 70 ml, the cardiac output is 4900 ml per minute. What happens if the heart rate drops to 60 beats per minute and the stroke volume rises to 85 ml (Box 31-11)?

Cardiac Output Determination   Box 31-11

Pulse rate × Stroke volume = Cardiac output

70 beats per minute × 70 ml/beat = 4.9 L/min

60 beats per minute × 85 ml/beat = 5.1 L/min

Mechanical, neural, and chemical factors regulate the strength of heart contractions and its stroke volume. But when mechanical, neural, or chemical factors are unable to alter stroke volume, a change in heart rate will result in a change in blood pressure. As heart rate increases, there is less time for the heart to fill. As heart rate increases without a change in stroke volume, blood pressure will decrease. As the heart rate slows, filling time is increased and blood pressure increases. The inability of blood pressure to respond to increases or decreases in heart rate may indicate a health deviation and is reported to the physician.

The cause of an abnormally slow, rapid, or irregular pulse may alter cardiac output. The nurse assesses the heart's ability to meet the demands of the body's tissue for nutrients by palpating a peripheral pulse or by using a stethoscope to listen to heart sounds (apical rate).

ASSESSMENT OF PULSE

Any artery can be assessed for pulse rate, but the radial and carotid arteries are easily palpated peripheral pulse sites. When a client's condition suddenly worsens, the carotid site is the best for quickly finding a pulse. The heart will continue delivering blood through the carotid artery to the brain as long as possible. When cardiac output declines significantly, peripheral pulses weaken and are difficult to palpate.

The radial and apical locations are the most common sites for pulse rate assessment (Figure 31-10). The radial pulse is used by persons learning to monitor their own heart rates (e.g., athletes, persons taking heart medications, and clients starting a prescribed exercise regimen). If the **radial pulse** at the wrist is abnormal or intermittent

resulting from dysrhythmias, or if it is inaccessible because of a dressing, cast, or other encumbrance, the apical pulse is assessed. When a client takes medication that affects the heart rate, the apical pulse may provide a more accurate assessment of heart function. The brachial or apical pulse is the best site for assessing an infant's or young child's pulse because other peripheral pulses are deep and difficult to palpate accurately.

Assessment of other peripheral pulse sites such as the brachial or femoral artery is unnecessary when routinely obtaining vital signs. Other peripheral pulses are assessed when a complete physical is conducted, when surgery or treatment has impaired blood flow to a body part, or when there are clinical indications of impaired peripheral blood flow (see Chapter 32). Table 31-2, p. 695 summarizes pulse sites and criteria for measurement. Skill 31-2 outlines pulse rate assessment.

Use of a Stethoscope.   When assessing the apical rate, the nurse uses a stethoscope (Figure 31-11). The five major parts of the stethoscope are the earpieces, binaurals, tubing, bell chestpiece, and diaphragm chestpiece.

The plastic or rubber earpieces should fit snugly and comfortably in the nurse's ears. The binaurals should be angled and strong enough so the earpieces stay firmly in the ears without causing discomfort. To ensure the best reception of sound, the earpieces follow the contour of the ear canal pointing toward the face when the stethoscope is in place.

Text continued on p. 696.

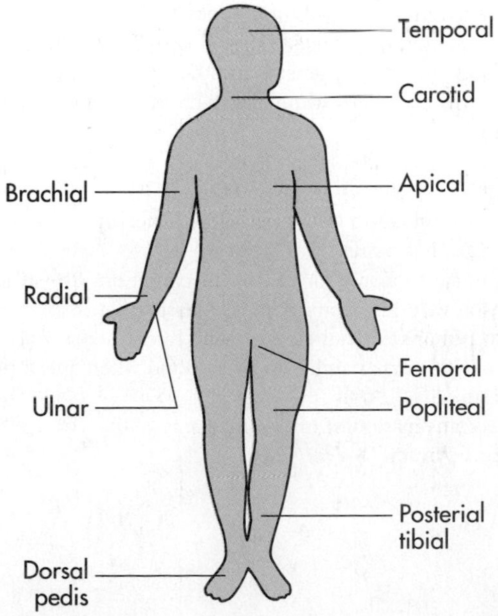

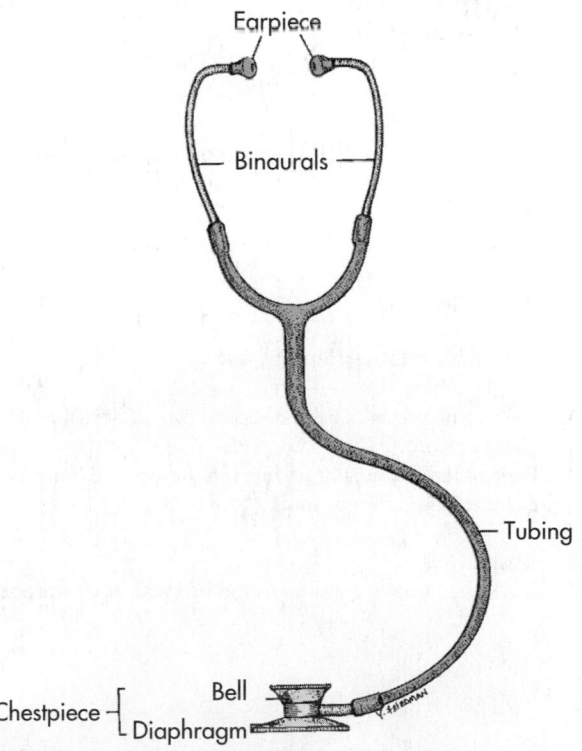

Figure 31-10   Location of pulse points in the body.

Figure 31-11   Parts of a stethoscope.

Skill 31-2 | Assessing the Radial and Apical Pulses

Delegation Considerations

The skill of pulse measurement can be delegated to assistive personnel.

- Inform caregiver of appropriate client position when obtaining apical pulse measurement.
- Inform caregiver of appropriate duration of radial and apical pulse count.

- Inform caregiver of client history or risk for irregular pulse.
- Inform caregiver of frequency of pulse measurement.
- Determine that caregiver is aware of the usual values for the client.
- Inform caregiver of the need to report any abnormalities that should be reconfirmed by the nurse.

EQUIPMENT
- Stethoscope (apical pulse only)
- Wristwatch with second hand or digital display

- Pen, pencil, vital sign flow sheet, or record form
- Alcohol swab

STEPS	RATIONALE
1. Determine need to assess radial or apical pulse: a. Note risk factors for alterations in apical pulse.	Certain conditions place clients at risk for pulse alterations. Heart rhythm can be affected by heart disease, cardiac dysrhythmias, onset of sudden chest pain or acute pain from any site, invasive cardiovascular diagnostic tests, surgery, sudden infusion of large volume of IV fluid, internal or external hemorrhage, and administration of medications that alter heart function.
b. Assess for signs and symptoms of altered stroke volume and cardiac output such as dyspnea, fatigue, chest pain, orthopnea, syncope, palpitations (person's unpleasant awareness of heartbeat), jugular venous distention, edema of dependent body parts, cyanosis or pallor of skin.	Physical signs and symptoms may indicate alteration in cardiac function.
2. Assess for factors that normally influence apical pulse rate and rhythm:	Allows nurse to accurately assess presence and significance of pulse alterations.
a. Age	Acceptable range of pulse rate changes with age (see Table 31-3).
b. Exercise	Physical activity requires an increase in cardiac output that is met by an increased heart rate and stroke volume.
c. Position changes	Heart rate increases temporarily when changing from lying to sitting or standing position.
d. Medications	Antidysrhythmics, sympathomimetics, and cardiotonics affect rate and rhythm of pulse; large doses of narcotic analgesics can slow heart rate; general anesthetics slow heart rate; central nervous system stimulants such as caffeine can increase heart rate.
e. Temperature	Fever or exposure to warm environments increases heart rate; heart rate declines with hypothermia.
f. Emotional stress, anxiety, fear	Results in stimulation of the sympathetic nervous system, which increases heart rate.
3. Determine previous baseline apical rate (if available) from client's record.	Allows nurse to assess for change in condition. Provides comparison with future apical pulse measurements.
4. Explain that pulse or heart rate is to be assessed. Encourage client to relax and not speak.	Activity and anxiety can elevate heart rate. Client's voice interferes with nurse's ability to hear sound when apical pulse is measured.
5. Wash hands.	Reduces transmission of microorganisms.
6. If necessary, draw curtain around bed and/or close door.	Maintains privacy.

STEPS	RATIONALE
7. Obtain pulse measurement.	
A. Radial pulse	
(1) Assist client to assume a supine or sitting position.	Provides easy access to pulse sites.
(2) If supine, place client's forearm straight alongside or across lower chest or upper abdomen with wrist extended straight (see illustration). If sitting, bend client's elbow 90 degrees and support lower arm on chair or on nurse's arm. Slightly flex the wrist with palm down.	Relaxed position of lower arm and extension of wrist permits full exposure of artery to palpation.
(3) Place tips of first two fingers of hand over groove along radial or thumb side of client's inner wrist (see illustration).	Fingertips are most sensitive parts of hand to palpate arterial pulsation. Nurse's thumb has pulsation that may interfere with accuracy.
(4) Lightly compress against radius, obliterate pulse initially, and then relax pressure so pulse becomes easily palpable.	Pulse is more accurately assessed with moderate pressure. Too much pressure occludes pulse and impairs blood flow.
(5) Determine strength of pulse. Note whether thrust of vessel against fingertips is bounding, strong, weak, or thready.	Strength reflects volume of blood ejected against arterial wall with each heart contraction.
(6) After pulse can be felt regularly, look at watch's second hand and begin to count rate: when sweep hand hits number on dial, start counting with zero, then one, two, and so on.	Rate is determined accurately only after nurse is assured pulse can be palpated. Timing begins with zero. Count of one is first beat palpated after timing begins.
(7) If pulse is regular, count rate for 30 sec and multiply total by 2.	A 30-sec count is accurate for rapid, slow, or regular pulse rates.
(8) If pulse is irregular, count rate for 60 sec. Assess frequency and pattern of irregularity.	Inefficient contraction of heart fails to transmit pulse wave, interfering with cardiac output, resulting in irregular pulse. Longer time ensures accurate count.

Critical Decision Point: If pulse is irregular, assess for pulse deficit that may indicate alteration in cardiac output. Count apical pulse while colleague counts radial pulse. Begin apical pulse count out loud to simultaneously assess pulses. If pulse count differs by more than 2, a pulse deficit exists.

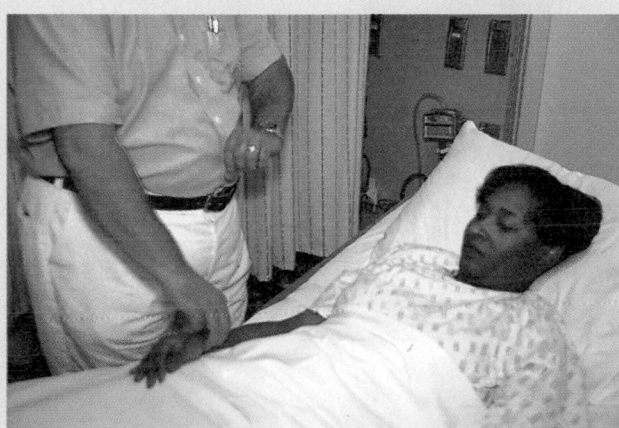

Step 7A(2)

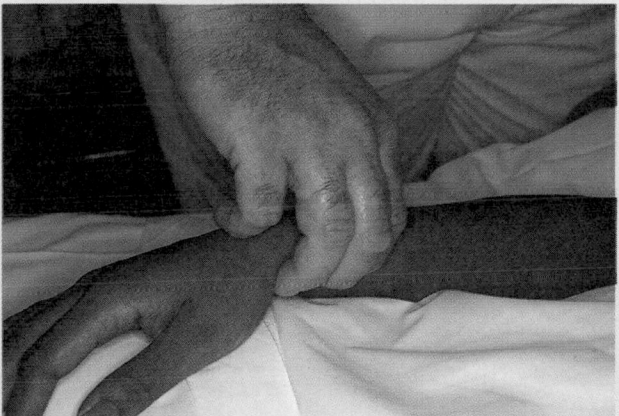

Step 7A(3)

STEPS	RATIONALE
B. Apical pulse	
(1) Assist client to supine or sitting position. Move aside bed linen and gown to expose sternum and left side of chest.	Exposes portion of chest wall for selection of auscultatory site.
(2) Locate anatomical landmarks to identify the point of maximal impulse (PMI), also called the apical impulse. Heart is located behind and to left of sternum with base at top and apex at bottom. Find angle of Louis just below suprasternal notch between sternal body and manubrium; can be felt as a bony prominence. Slip fingers down each side of angle to find second intercostal space (ICS). Carefully move fingers down left side of sternum to fifth ICS and laterally to the left midclavicular line (MCL). A light tap felt within an area 1 to 2 cm ($\frac{1}{2}$ to 1 in) of the PMI is reflected from the apex of the heart.	Use of anatomical landmarks allows correct placement of stethoscope over apex of heart, enhancing ability to hear heart sounds clearly. If unable to palpate the PMI, reposition client on left side. In the presence of serious heart disease, the PMI may be located to the left of the MCL or at the sixth ICS.
(3) Place diaphragm of stethoscope in palm of hand for 5 to 10 sec.	Warming of metal or plastic diaphragm prevents client from being startled and promotes comfort.
(4) Place diaphragm of stethoscope over PMI at the fifth ICS, at left MCL, and auscultate for normal S_1 and S_2 heart sounds (heard as "lub-dub") (see illustration).	Allow stethoscope tubing to extend straight without kinks that would distort sound transmission. Normal sounds S_1 and S_2 are high pitched and best heard with the diaphragm.
(5) When S_1 and S_2 are heard with regularity, use watch's second hand and begin to count rate: when sweep hand hits number on dial, start counting with zero, then one, two, and so on.	Apical rate is determined accurately only after nurse is able to auscultate sounds clearly. Timing begins with zero. Count of one is first sound auscultated after timing begins.
(6) If apical rate is regular, count for 30 sec and multiply by 2.	Regular apical rate can be assessed within 30 sec.
(7) If heart rate is irregular or client is receiving cardiovascular medication, count for 1 min (60 sec).	Irregular rate is more accurately assessed when measured over longer interval.
(8) Note regularity of any dysrhythmia (S_1 and S_2 occuring early or later after previous sequence of sounds; for example, every third or every fourth beat is skipped).	Regular occurrence of dysrhythmia within 1 min may indicate inefficient contraction of heart and alteration in cardiac output.

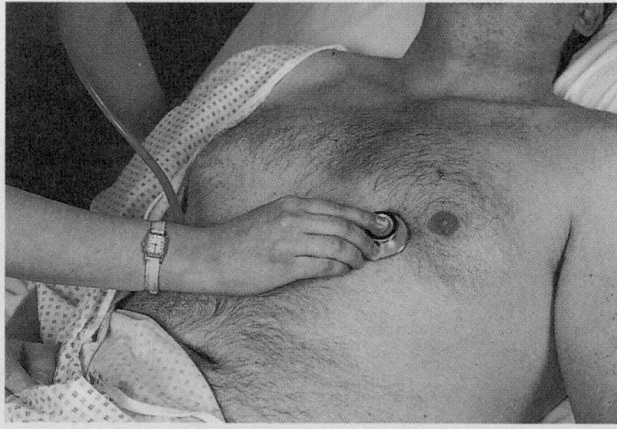

Step 7B(4)

STEPS	RATIONALE
(9) Replace client's gown and bed linen; assist client in returning to comfortable position.	Restores comfort and promotes sense of well-being.
(10) Clean earpieces and diaphragm of stethoscope with alcohol swab as needed (optional).	Controls transmission of microorganisms when nurses share stethoscope.
8. Discuss findings with client as needed.	Promotes participation in care and understanding of health status.
9. Wash hands.	Reduces transmission of microorganisms.
10. Compare readings with previous baseline and/or acceptable range of heart rate for client's age (see Table 31-3).	Evaluates for change in condition and alterations.
11. Compare peripheral pulse rate with apical rate and note discrepancy.	Differences between measurements indicate pulse deficit and may warn of cardiovascular compromise. Abnormalities may require therapy.
12. Compare radial pulse equality and note discrepancy.	Differences between radial arteries indicate compromised peripheral vascular system.
13. Correlate pulse rate with data obtained from blood pressure and related signs and symptoms (palpitations, dizziness).	Pulse rate and blood pressure are interrelated.

Recording and Reporting

- Record pulse rate with assessment site in nurses' notes or vital signs flow sheet. Measurement of pulse rate after administration of specific therapies should be documented in narrative form in nurses' notes.
- Report abnormal findings to nurse in charge or physician.

Home Care Considerations

- Assess home environment to determine room that will afford quiet environment for auscultating apical rate.

Table 31-2 **Pulse Sites**		
Site	Location	Assessment Criteria
Temporal	Over temporal bone of head, above and lateral to eye	Easily accessible site used to assess pulse in children
Carotid	Along medial edge of sternocleidomastoid muscle in neck	Easily accessible site used during physiological shock or cardiac arrest when other sites are not palpable
Apical	Fourth to fifth intercostal space at left midclavicular line	Site used to auscultate for apical pulse
Brachial	Groove between biceps and triceps muscles at antecubital fossa	Site used to assess status of circulation to lower arm Site used to auscultate blood pressure
Radial	Radial or thumb side of forearm at wrist	Common site used to assess character of pulse peripherally and assess status of circulation to hand
Ulnar	Ulnar side of forearm at wrist	Site used to assess status of circulation to hand. Site also used to perform Allen's test
Femoral	Below inguinal ligament, midway between symphysis pubis and anterior superior iliac spine	Site used to assess character of pulse during physiological shock or cardiac arrest when other pulses are not palpable; used to assess status of circulation to leg
Popliteal	Behind knee in popliteal fossa	Site used to assess status of circulation to lower leg
Posterior tibial	Inner side of ankle, below medial malleolus	Site used to assess status of circulation to foot
Dorsalis pedis	Along top of foot, between extension tendons of great and first toe	Site used to assess status of circulation to foot

The polyvinyl tubing should be flexible and 30 to 40 cm (12 to 16 inches) in length. Longer tubing decreases the transmission of sound waves. The tubing should be thick walled and moderately rigid to eliminate transmission of environmental noise and to prevent the tubing from kinking, which distorts sound wave transmission. Stethoscopes can have single or dual tubes. Dual tubes promote sound clarity by minimizing the number of turns the sound wave makes before reaching the earpiece.

The bell and diaphragm compose the stethoscope chestpiece. The diaphragm is the circular, flat portion of the chestpiece covered with a thin plastic disk. It transmits high-pitched sounds created by the high-velocity movement of air and blood. Bowel, lung, and heart sounds are auscultated using the diaphragm. The nurse positions the diaphragm to make a tight seal against the client's skin (Figure 31-12). Enough pressure is exerted to leave a temporary red ring on the client's skin when the diaphragm is removed.

The bell is the bowl-shaped chestpiece usually surrounded by a rubber ring. The ring avoids chilling the client with cold metal when placed on the skin. The bell transmits low-pitched sounds created by the low-velocity movement of blood. Heart and vascular sounds are auscultated using the bell. The nurse applies the bell lightly, resting the chestpiece on the skin (Figure 31-13). Compressing the bell against the skin reduces low-pitched sound amplification and creates a "diaphragm of skin." The bell and diaphragm are rotated into position on the chestpiece, depending on which part the nurse chooses to use. The diaphragm or bell must be in proper position during use for the nurse to hear sounds through the stethoscope. To test, lightly tap to determine which side is functioning. Newer stethoscope models have one chestpiece that combines features of the bell and diaphragm. When the nurse uses light pressure, the chestpiece is a bell, whereas exerting more pressure converts the bell into a diaphragm.

The stethoscope is a delicate instrument and requires proper care for optimal function. The earpieces should be removed regularly and cleaned of cerumen (earwax). The bell and diaphragm are cleaned of dust, lint, and body oils. The tubing should be kept away from the nurse's body oils. Avoid draping the stethoscope around the neck next to the skin. Cleaning the tubing with alcohol can dry and crack the material and is not recommended. Mild soap and water are preferred.

CHARACTER OF THE PULSE

Assessment of the radial pulse includes measurement of the rate, rhythm, strength, and equality. When auscultating an apical pulse, the nurse assesses rate and rhythm only.

Rate. Before measuring a pulse, the nurse reviews the client's baseline rate for comparison (Table 31-3). Some practitioners prefer to make baseline measurements of the pulse rate as the client assumes a sitting, standing, and lying position. Postural changes cause changes in pulse rate because of alterations in blood volume and sympathetic activity. The heart rate temporarily increases when a person changes from a lying to a sitting or standing position.

When assessing the pulse, the nurse must consider the variety of factors influencing the pulse rate (Table 31-4). A combination of these factors may cause significant changes. If the nurse detects an abnormal rate while palpating a peripheral pulse, the next step is to assess the apical rate. The apical rate requires auscultation of heart sounds, which provides a more accurate assessment of cardiac contraction.

The nurse assesses the apical rate by listening for heart sounds (see Chapter 32). The nurse tries to identify the first and second heart sounds (S_1 and S_2). At normal slow rates, S_1 is low pitched and dull, sounding like a "lub." S_2 is higher pitched and shorter, creating the sound "dub." Each

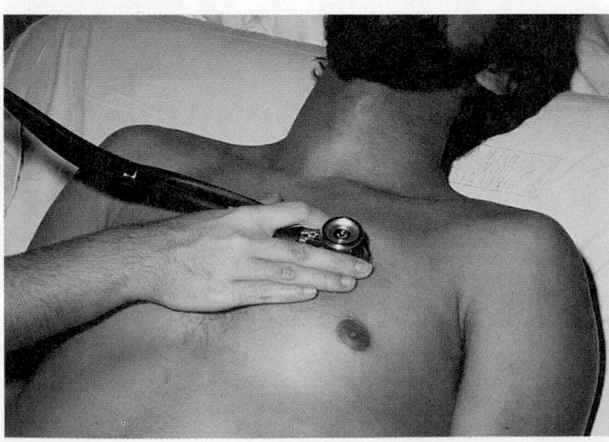

Figure 31-12 Positioning the diaphragm of the stethoscope firmly and securely when auscultating high-pitched heart sounds.

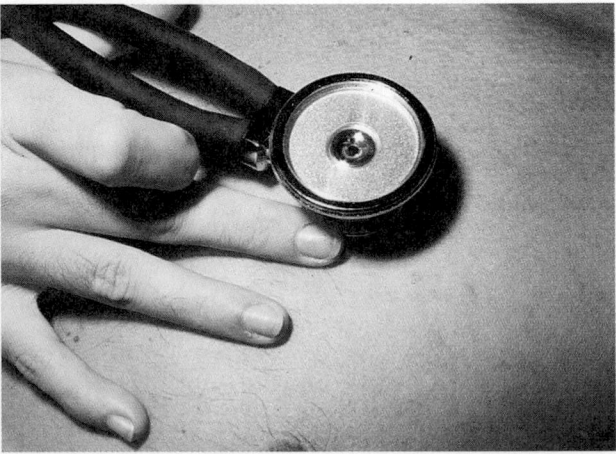

Figure 31-13 Positioning the bell of the stethoscope lightly on the skin to hear low-pitched heart sounds.

set of "lub-dub" is counted as one heartbeat. Using the diaphragm or bell of the stethoscope, the nurse counts the number of lub-dubs occurring in 1 minute.

Peripheral and apical pulse rate assessment may reveal variations in heart rate. Two common abnormalities in pulse rate are tachycardia and bradycardia. **Tachycardia** is an abnormally elevated heart rate, above 100 beats per minute in adults. **Bradycardia** is a slow rate, below 60 beats per minute in adults.

Rhythm. Normally a regular interval occurs between each pulse or heartbeat. An interval interrupted by an early or late beat or a missed beat indicates an abnormal rhythm or **dysrhythmia.** A dysrhythmia threatens the heart's ability to provide adequate cardiac output, particularly if it occurs repetitively. The nurse identifies a dysrhythmia by palpating an interruption in successive pulse waves or auscultating an interruption between heart sounds. If a dysrhythmia is present, the regularity of its occurrence should be assessed. Dysrhythmias may be described as regularly irregular or irregularly irregular.

To document dysrhythmia, a physician may order an electrocardiogram, Holter monitor, or telemetry. An electrocardiogram records the electrical activity of the heart

for a 12-second interval. This test requires placement of electrodes across the client's chest followed by recording of the heart rhythm. The Holter monitor records 24 hours of electrical activity in a small tape recorder that the client wears. Access to the information recorded is not available until after the 24 hours have passed and the data are printed for review. Cardiac telemetry provides continuous monitoring of the heart's electrical activity transmitted to a stationary monitor. Telemetry permits observation of heart rhythm during all of the client's daily activities and thus allows for immediate treatment if the rhythm becomes erratic or unstable.

Children often have a sinus dysrhythmia, which is an irregular heartbeat that speeds up with inspiration and slows down with expiration. This is a normal finding and can be verified by having the child hold his or her breath; the heart rate should then become regular.

An inefficient contraction of the heart that fails to transmit a pulse wave to the peripheral pulse site creates a **pulse deficit.** To assess a pulse deficit the nurse and a colleague assess radial and apical rates simultaneously and then compare rates. The difference between the apical and radial pulse rates is the pulse deficit. For example, an apical rate of 92 with a radial rate of 78 leaves a pulse deficit of 14 beats. Pulse deficits are frequently associated with dysrhythmias.

Strength. The strength or amplitude of a pulse reflects the volume of blood ejected against the arterial wall with each heart contraction and the condition of the arterial vascular system leading to the pulse site. Normally the pulse strength remains the same with each heartbeat. Pulse strength may be graded or described as strong, weak, thready, or bounding. It is included during assessment of the vascular system (see Chapter 32).

Equality. Pulses on both sides of the peripheral vascular system should be assessed. The nurse assesses both radial pulses to compare the characteristics of each. A pulse in one extremity may be unequal in strength or absent in

Table 31-3	Acceptable Ranges of Heart Rate
Age	Heart Rate (Beats per Minute)
Infants	120-160/min
Toddlers	90-140/min
Preschoolers	80-110/min
School-agers	75-100/min
Adolescent	60-90/min
Adult	60-100/min

Data from Hazinski MF: Children are different. In Hazinski MF: *Nursing care of the critically ill child,* ed 2, St. Louis, 1991, Mosby; and Kinney MR and others: *AACN's clinical reference for critical care nursing,* ed 4, St. Louis, 1998, Mosby.

Table 31-4	Factors Influencing Pulse Rates	
Factor	Increase Pulse Rate	Decrease Pulse Rate
Exercise	Short-term exercise.	A conditioned athlete who participates in long-term exercise will have a lower heart rate at rest.
Temperature	Fever and heat.	Hypothermia.
Emotions	Acute pain and anxiety increase sympathetic stimulation, affecting heart rate.	Unrelieved severe pain increases parasympathetic stimulation, affecting heart rate; relaxation.
Drugs	Positive chronotropic drugs such as epinephrine.	Negative chronotropic drugs such as digitalis.
Hemorrhage	Loss of blood increases sympathetic stimulation.	
Postural changes	Standing or sitting.	Lying down.
Pulmonary conditions	Diseases causing poor oxygenation.	

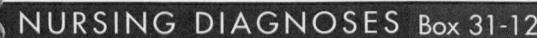

many disease states (e.g., thrombus [clot] formation, aberrant blood vessels, cervical rib syndrome, or aortic dissection). All symmetrical pulses can be assessed simultaneously except for the carotid pulse. The carotid pulse should *never* be measured simultaneously because excessive pressure may occlude blood supply to the brain.

NURSING PROCESS AND PULSE DETERMINATION

Pulse assessment determines the general state of cardiovascular health and the response to other system imbalances. Tachycardia, bradycardia, and dysrhythmias are defining characteristics of many nursing diagnoses and are considered along with other assessment data (Box 31-12). The nursing care plan includes interventions based on the nursing diagnosis identified and the related factor. For example, the defining characteristics of an abnormal heart rate, exertional dyspnea, and a client's verbal report of fatigue lead to a diagnosis of *activity intolerance*. The nurse evaluates client outcomes by assessing the pulse rate, rhythm, strength, and equality following each intervention.

Respiration

Human survival depends on the ability of oxygen (O_2) to reach body cells and for carbon dioxide (CO_2) to be removed from the cells. Respiration is the mechanism the body uses to exchange gases between the atmosphere and the blood and the blood and the cells. Respiration involves **ventilation** (the movement of gases in and out of the lungs), **diffusion** (the movement of oxygen and carbon dioxide between the alveoli and the red blood cells), and **perfusion** (the distribution of red blood cells to and from the pulmonary capillaries). These processes can be assessed independently. The rate, depth, and rhythm of ventilatory movements indicate the quality and efficiency of ventilation. Diagnostic tests that measure O_2 and CO_2 levels in arterial blood offer useful information about both diffusion and perfusion. However, analyzing respiratory efficiency requires integrating assessment data from all three processes. The processes are interdependent. Ventilatory adequacy can affect diffusion and perfusion, which in turn will affect ventilation. Respiration can be affected by various factors (Box 31-13).

PHYSIOLOGICAL CONTROL

Breathing is generally a passive process. Normally a person thinks little about it. The respiratory center in the brain stem regulates the involuntary control of respirations. Adults normally breathe in a smooth, uninterrupted pattern, 12 to 20 times a minute.

Ventilation is regulated by levels of CO_2, O_2, and hydrogen ion concentration (pH) in the arterial blood. The most important factor in the control of ventilation is the level of CO_2 (carbia) in the arterial blood. An elevation in the CO_2 level causes the respiratory control system in the brain to increase the rate and depth of breathing. The increased ventilatory effort removes excess CO_2 by increasing exhalation. However, clients with chronic lung disease have ongoing hypercarbia. For these clients chemoreceptors in the carotid artery and aorta are sensitive to **hypoxemia,** or low levels of arterial O_2. If arterial oxygen levels fall, these receptors signal the brain to increase the rate and depth of ventilation. Hypoxemia helps to control ventilation in clients with chronic lung disease. Because low levels of arterial O_2 provide the stimulus that allows the client to breathe, administration of high oxygen levels can be fatal for clients with chronic lung disease.

MECHANICS OF BREATHING

Although breathing is normally passive, muscular work is involved in moving the lungs and chest wall. Inspiration is an active process. During inspiration the respiratory center sends impulses along the phrenic nerve, causing the diaphragm to contract. Abdominal organs move downward and forward, increasing the length of the chest cavity to move air into the lungs. The diaphragm moves approximately 1 cm (4/10 inch), and the ribs retract upward from the body's midline approximately 1.2 to 2.5 cm ($\frac{1}{2}$ to 1 inch). During a normal, relaxed breath, a person inhales 500 ml of air. This amount is referred to as the **tidal volume.** During expiration the diaphragm relaxes and the abdominal organs return to their original positions. The lung and chest wall return to a relaxed position (Figure 31-14). Expiration is a passive process. The normal rate and depth of ventilation, **eupnea,** is interrupted by sighing. The sigh, a prolonged deeper breath, is a protective physiological mechanism for expanding small airways and alveoli not ventilated during a normal breath.

The accurate assessment of respirations depends on the nurse's recognition of normal thoracic and abdominal movements. During quiet breathing the chest wall gently rises and falls. Contraction of the intercostal muscles between the ribs or contraction of the muscles in the neck and shoulders, the accessory muscles of breathing, is not visible. During normal quiet breathing, diaphragmatic movement causes the abdominal cavity to rise and fall slowly.

ASSESSMENT OF RESPIRATIONS

Respirations are the easiest of all vital signs to assess, but they are often the most haphazardly measured. A nurse

Factors Influencing Character of Respirations   Box 31-13

EXERCISE

Exercise increases rate and depth to meet the body's need for additional oxygen and to rid the body of CO_2.

ACUTE PAIN

Pain alters rate and rhythm of respirations; breathing becomes shallow.

Client may inhibit or splint chest wall movement when pain is in area of chest or abdomen.

ANXIETY

Anxiety increases rate and depth as a result of sympathetic stimulation.

SMOKING

Chronic smoking changes the lung's airways, resulting in increased rate of respirations at rest when not smoking.

BODY POSITION

A straight, erect posture promotes full chest expansion.

A stooped or slumped position impairs ventilatory movement.

Lying flat prevents full chest expansion.

MEDICATIONS

Narcotic analgesics, general anesthetics, and sedative hypnotics depress rate and depth.

Amphetamines and cocaine may increase rate and depth.

Bronchodilators slow rate by causing airway dilation.

NEUROLOGICAL INJURY

Injury to the brain stem impairs the respiratory center and inhibits respiratory rate and rhythm.

HEMOGLOBIN FUNCTION

Decreased hemoglobin levels (anemia) reduce oxygen-carrying capacity of the blood, which increases respiratory rate.

Increased altitude lowers the amount of saturated hemoglobin, which increases respiratory rate and depth.

Abnormal blood cell function (e.g., sickle cell disease) reduces ability of hemoglobin to carry oxygen, which increases respiratory rate and depth.

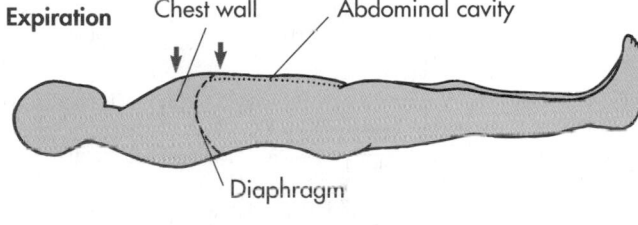

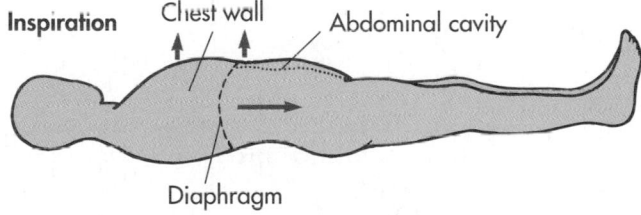

Figure 31-14   Illustration of diaphragmatic and chest wall movement during inspiration and expiration.

Table 31-5	Acceptable Range of Respiratory Rates for Age	
	Age	Rate
	Newborn	30-60
	Infant (6 months)	30-50
	Toddler (2 years)	25-32
	Child	20-30
	Adolescent	16-19
	Adult	12-20

must not estimate respirations. Accurate measurement requires observation and palpation of chest wall movement.

A sudden change in the character of respirations may be important. Because respiration is tied to the function of numerous body systems, the nurse must consider all variables when changes occur. For example, a drop in respirations occurring in a client after head trauma may signify injury to the brain stem. Abdominal trauma may injure the phrenic nerve, which is responsible for diaphragmatic contraction. The nurse must understand the extent of the injury and the implications for the respiratory system.

A skillful nurse does not let a client know that respirations are being assessed. A client aware of the nurse's intentions may consciously alter the rate and depth of breathing. Assessment can best be done immediately after measuring pulse rate, with the nurse's hand still on the client's wrist as it rests over the chest or abdomen. When assessing a client's respirations, the nurse should keep in mind the client's usual ventilatory rate and pattern, the influence any disease or illness has on respiratory function, the relationship between respiratory and cardiovascular function, and the influence of therapies on respirations. The objective measurements of an assessment of respiratory status include the rate and depth of breathing and the rhythm of ventilatory movements (Skill 31-3).

Respiratory Rate.   The nurse observes a full inspiration and expiration when counting ventilation or respiration rate. The respiratory rate varies with age (Table 31-5). The usual range of respiratory rate declines throughout life.

A respiratory monitoring device that aids the nurse's assessment is the apnea monitor. This device uses leads at-

Skill 31-3   Assessing Respirations

Delegation Considerations

The skill of respiration measurement can be delegated to assistive personnel.

- Inform caregiver of appropriate client position when obtaining respirations.
- Inform caregiver of appropriate duration of respiratory rate count.
- Inform caregiver of client history or risk for increased or decreased respiratory rate or irregular respirations.

- Inform caregiver of frequency of respirations measurement.
- Determine that caregiver is aware of the usual values for the client.
- Inform caregiver of the need to report any abnormalities that should be reconfirmed by the nurse.

EQUIPMENT

- Wristwatch with second hand or digital display
- Pen, pencil, vital sign flow sheet or record form

STEPS	RATIONALE
1. Determine need to assess client's respirations: a. Note risk factors for respiratory alterations.	Certain conditions place client at risk for alterations in ventilation detected by changes in respiratory rate, depth, and rhythm. Fever, pain, anxiety, diseases of chest wall or muscles, constrictive chest or abdominal dressings, gastric distention, chronic pulmonary disease (emphysema, bronchitis, asthma), traumatic injury to chest wall with or without collapse of underlying lung tissue, presence of a chest tube, respiratory infection (pneumonia, acute bronchitis), pulmonary edema and emboli, head injury with damage to brain stem, and anemia can result in respiratory alteration.
b. Assess for signs and symptoms of respiratory alterations such as bluish or cyanotic appearance of nail beds, lips, mucous membranes, and skin; restlessness, irritability, confusion, reduced level of consciousness; pain during inspiration; labored or difficult breathing; adventitious breath sounds (see Chapter 32), inability to breathe spontaneously; thick, frothy, blood-tinged, or copious sputum produced on coughing.	Physical signs and symptoms may indicate alterations in respiratory status related to ventilation.

2. Assess pertinent laboratory values:
 A. **Arterial blood gases (ABGs):** Normal ABGs (values may vary slightly within institutions):
    pH 7.35-7.45
    $PaCO_2$ 35-45
    PaO_2 80-100
    SaO_2 94%-98%
	Arterial blood gases measure arterial blood pH, partial pressure of O_2 and CO_2, and arterial O_2 saturation, which reflects client's oxygenation status.

B. **Pulse oximetry (SpO_2):** Acceptable SpO_2 90%-100%; 85%-89% may be acceptable for certain chronic disease conditions; less than 85% is abnormal (see Skill 31-4).	SpO_2 less than 85% is often accompanied by changes in respiratory rate, depth, and rhythm.

C. **Complete blood count (CBC):** Normal CBC for adults (values may vary within institutions):
    (1) Hemoglobin: 14 to 18 g/100 ml, males; 12 to 16 g/100 ml, females.
    (2) Hematocrit: 40% to 54%, males; 38% to 47%, females.
    (3) Red blood cell count: 4.6 to 6.2 million/μl, males; 4.2 to 5.4 million/μl, females.
	Complete blood count measures red blood cell count, volume of red blood cells, and concentration of hemoglobin, which reflects client's capacity to carry O_2.

3. Determine previous baseline respiratory rate (if available) from client's record.	Allows nurse to assess for change in condition. Provides comparison with future respiratory measurements.

STEPS	RATIONALE
4. Be sure client is in comfortable position, preferably sitting or lying with the head of the bed elevated 45 to 60 degrees.	Sitting erect promotes full ventilatory movement.

Critical Decision Point: Clients with difficulty breathing (dyspnea) such as those with congestive heart failure or abdominal ascites or in late stages of pregnancy should be assessed in the position of greatest comfort. Repositioning may increase the work of breathing, which will increase respiratory rate.

STEPS	RATIONALE
5. Draw curtain around bed and/or close door. Wash hands.	Maintains privacy. Prevents transmission of microorganisms.
6. Be sure client's chest is visible. If necessary, move bed linen or gown.	Ensures clear view of chest wall and abdominal movements.
7. Place client's arm in relaxed position across the abdomen or lower chest, or place nurse's hand directly over client's upper abdomen (see illustration).	A similar position used during pulse assessment allows respiratory rate assessment to be inconspicuous. Client's or nurse's hand rises and falls during respiratory cycle.
8. Observe complete respiratory cycle (one inspiration and one expiration).	Rate is accurately determined only after nurse has viewed respiratory cycle.
9. After cycle is observed, look at watch's second hand and begin to count rate: when sweep hand hits number on dial, begin time frame, counting one with first full respiratory cycle.	Timing begins with count of one. Respirations occur more slowly than pulse; thus timing does not begin with zero.
10. If rhythm is regular, count number of respirations in 30 sec and multiply by 2. If rhythm is irregular, less than 12, or greater than 20, count for 1 full min.	Respiratory rate is equivalent to number of respirations per minute. Suspected irregularities require assessment for at least 1 min.

Critical Decision Point: Respiratory rate less than 12 or greater than 20 requires further assessment (see Chapter 32) and may require immediate intervention.

STEPS	RATIONALE
11. Note depth of respirations, subjectively assessed by observing degree of chest wall movement while counting rate. Nurse can also objectively assess depth by palpating chest wall excursion or auscultating the posterior thorax after rate has been counted (see Chapter 32). Depth is described as shallow, normal, or deep.	Character of ventilatory movement may reveal specific disease state restricting volume of air from moving into and out of the lungs.
12. Note rhythm of ventilatory cycle. Normal breathing is regular and uninterrupted. Sighing should not be confused with abnormal rhythm.	Character of ventilations can reveal specific types of alterations.

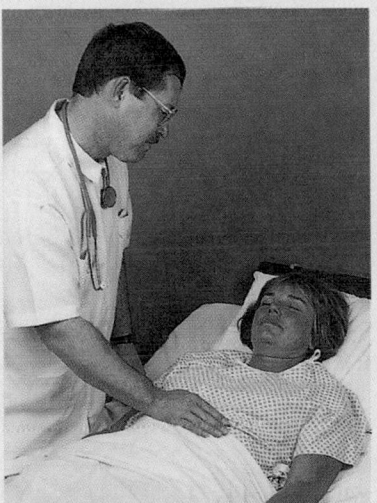

Step 7

STEPS	RATIONALE

Critical Decision Point: Occasional periods of apnea, the cessation of respiration for several seconds, are a symptom of underlying disease in the adult and must be reported to the physician or nurse in charge. An irregular respiratory rate and short apneic pells are usual in a newborn.

STEPS	RATIONALE
13. Replace bed linen and client's gown.	Restores comfort and promotes sense of well-being.
14. Wash hands.	Reduces transmission of microorganisms.
15. Discuss findings with client as needed.	Promotes participation in care and understanding of health status.
16. If respirations are assessed for the first time, establish rate, rhythm, and depth as baseline if within normal range.	Used to compare future respiratory assessment.
17. Compare respirations with client's previous baseline and normal rate, rhythm, and depth.	Allows nurse to assess for changes in client's condition and for presence of respiratory alterations.

Recording and Reporting
- Record respiratory rate and character in nurses' notes or vital sign flow sheet. Indicate type and amount of oxygen therapy if used by client during assessment. Measurement of respiratory rate after administration of specific therapies should be documented in narrative form in nurses' notes.

- Report abnormal findings to nurse in charge or physician.

Home Care Considerations
- Assess for environmental factors in the home that may influence client's respiratory rate such as secondhand smoke, poor ventilation, or gas fumes.

---

tached to the client's chest wall that sense movement. The absence of chest wall movement is interpreted by the monitor as apnea and triggers an alarm. Apnea monitoring is used frequently with infants in the hospital and at home to observe for prolonged apneic events. Noninvasive monitoring provides information that helps the nurse assess the rate, depth, and rhythm of respiration more knowledgeably.

Ventilatory Depth.   The depth of respirations is assessed by observing the degree of excursion or movement in the chest wall. The nurse subjectively describes ventilatory movements as deep, normal, or shallow. A deep respiration involves a full expansion of the lungs with full exhalation. Respirations are shallow when only a small quantity of air passes through the lungs and ventilatory movement is difficult to see. More objective techniques are used if the nurse observes that chest excursion is unusually shallow (see Chapter 32). Table 31-6 summarizes types of respiratory alterations.

Ventilatory Rhythm.   Breathing pattern can be determined by observing the chest or the abdomen. Diaphragmatic breathing results from the contraction and relaxation of the diaphragm and is best observed by watching abdominal movements. Healthy men and children usually demonstrate diaphragmatic breathing. Women tend to use thoracic muscles to breathe; movements are observed in the upper chest. Labored respirations usually involve the accessory muscles of respiration

visible in the neck. When something such as a foreign body interferes with the movement of air in and out of the lungs, the intercostal spaces retract during inspiration. A longer expiration phase is evident when the outward flow of air is obstructed (e.g., asthma).

With normal breathing a regular interval occurs after each respiratory cycle. Infants tend to breathe less regularly. The young child may breathe slowly for a few seconds and then suddenly breathe more rapidly. While assessing respirations, the nurse estimates the time interval after each respiratory cycle. Respiration is regular or irregular in rhythm.

ASSESSMENT OF DIFFUSION AND PERFUSION

The respiratory processes of diffusion and perfusion can be evaluated by measuring the oxygen saturation of the blood. Blood flow through the pulmonary capillaries provides red blood cells for oxygen attachment. After oxygen diffuses from the alveoli into the pulmonary blood, most of the oxygen attaches to hemoglobin molecules in red blood cells. Red blood cells carry the oxygenated hemoglobin molecules through the left side of the heart and out to the peripheral capillaries, where the oxygen detaches, depending on the needs of the tissues.

The percent of hemoglobin that is bound with oxygen in the arteries is the percent of saturation of hemoglobin (or SaO_2). It is usually between 95% and 100%. SaO_2 is affected by factors that interfere with ventilation, perfusion, or diffusion (see Chapter 39). The saturation of venous blood (SvO_2) is lower because the tissues have removed

Table 31-6 Alterations in Breathing Pattern

Alteration	Description
Bradypnea	Rate of breathing is regular but abnormally slow (less than 12 breaths per minute).
Tachypnea	Rate of breathing is regular but abnormally rapid (greater than 20 breaths per minute).
Hyperpnea	Respirations are labored, increased in depth, and increased in rate (greater than 20 breaths per minute). Occurs normally during exercise.
Apnea	Respirations cease for several seconds. Persistent cessation results in respiratory arrest.
Hyperventilation	Rate and depth of respirations increase. Hypocarbia may occur.
Hypoventilation	Respiratory rate is abnormally low, and depth of ventilation may be depressed. Hypercarbia may occur.
Cheyne-Stokes respiration	Respiratory rate and depth are irregular, characterized by alternating periods of apnea and hyperventilation. Respiratory cycle begins with slow, shallow breaths that gradually increase to abnormal rate and depth. The pattern reverses, breathing slows and becomes shallow, climaxing in apnea before respiration resumes.
Kussmaul's respiration	Respirations are abnormally deep, regular, and increased in rate.
Biot's respiration	Respirations are abnormally shallow for two to three breaths followed by irregular period of apnea.

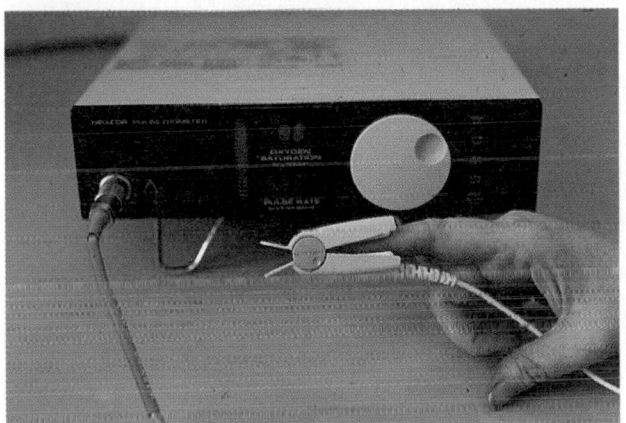

Figure 31-15 Pulse oximeter with spring-tension digit probe.

some of the oxygen from the hemoglobin molecules. A normal value for SvO_2 is 70%. SvO_2 is affected by factors that interfere with or increase the tissue's need for oxygen.

Measurement of Arterial Oxygen Saturation.
The recent development of a reliable device, a pulse oximeter, allows for the indirect measurement of oxygen saturation in the client's vital sign database (Skill 31-4). The pulse oximeter is a probe with a light-emitting diode (LED) and photodetector connected by cable to an oximeter (Figure 31-15). The LED emits light wavelengths that are absorbed by the oxygenated and deoxygenated hemoglobin molecules. The light reflected from the hemoglobin molecules is processed by the oximeter, which calculates pulse saturation (SpO_2). SpO_2 is a reliable estimate of SaO_2 when the SaO_2 is over 70%. Values obtained with pulse oximetry are less accurate at saturations less than 70% (Goodfellow, 1997).

The measurement of SpO_2 is affected by factors that affect light transmission or peripheral arterial pulsations. Selecting the appropriate probe is important to reduce measurement error (Box 31-14) Motion artifact is the most common cause of inaccurate readings (Carroll, 1997). An awareness of these factors allows the nurse's accurate interpretation of abnormal SpO_2 measurements (Box 31-15, p. 706).

Skill 31-4 Measuring Oxygen Saturation (Pulse Oximetry)

Delegation Considerations

The skill of oxygen saturation measurement can be delegated to assistive personnel.

- Inform caregiver to notify nurse immediately of any reading lower than SpO_2 of 90%.
- Inform caregiver of appropriate sensor site, probe, and client position for measurement of oxygen saturation.

- Inform caregiver of frequency of oxygen saturation measurements.
- Determine that caregiver is aware of factors that can falsely lower SpO_2 (Box 30-15).

EQUIPMENT

- Oximeter
- Oximeter probe appropriate for client and recommended by manufacturer

- Acetone or nail polish remover
- Pen, pencil, vital sign flow sheet, or record form

STEPS	RATIONALE
1. Determine need to measure client's oxygen saturation: a. Note risk factors for alteration of oxygen saturation.	Certain conditions place clients at risk for decreased oxygen saturation: acute or chronic compromised respiratory function, recovery from general anesthesia or conscious sedation, or traumatic injury to chest wall with or without collapse of underlying lung tissue, ventilator dependence, changes in supplemental oxygen therapy.
b. Assess for signs and symptoms of alterations in oxygen saturation such as altered respiratory rate, depth, or rhythm; adventitious breath sounds (see Chapter 32); cyanotic appearance of nail beds, lips, mucous membranes, and skin; restlessness, irritability, confusion; reduced level of consciousness; labored or difficulty breathing.	Physical signs and symptoms may indicate abnormal oxygen saturation.
2. Assess for factors that normally influence measurement of SpO_2 such as oxygen therapy, hemoglobin level, and temperature.	Allows nurse to accurately assess oxygen saturation variations. Peripheral vasoconstriction related to hypothermia can interfere with SpO_2 determination.
3. Review client's medical record for physician's order or consult agency policy or procedure manual for standard of care.	Medical order may be required to assess oxygen saturation.
4. Determine previous baseline SpO_2 (if available) from client's record.	Baseline information provides basis for comparison and assists in assessment of current status and evaluation of interventions.
5. Explain purpose of procedure to client and how oxygen saturation will be measured. Instruct client to breathe normally.	Promotes client cooperation and increases compliance. Prevents large fluctuations in minute ventilation and possible error in SpO_2 readings.
6. Assess site most appropriate for sensor probe placement (e.g., digit, earlobe) (see Box 30-14). Site must have adequate local circulation and be free of moisture.	Peripheral vasoconstriction can interfere with SpO_2 determination. Dark nail polish and acrylic nails impede sensor detection of emitted light and produce falsely elevated SpO_2 (Tittle and Flynn, 1997).
7. Wash hands.	Reduces transmission of microorganisms.
8. Position client comfortably. If finger is chosen as monitoring site, support lower arm.	Ensures probe positioning and decreases motion artifact that interferes with SpO_2 determination.
9. Instruct client to breathe normally.	Prevents large fluctuations in respiratory rate and depth and possible changes in SpO_2.
10. If finger is to be used, remove any fingernail polish with acetone from digit to be assessed.	Ensures accurate readings. Opaque coatings decrease light transmission; nail polish containing blue pigment can absorb light emissions and falsely alter saturation.
11. Attach sensor probe to monitoring site. Instruct client that clip-on probe feels like a clothespin on the finger but will not hurt.	Pressure of sensor probe's spring tension on a peripheral digit or earlobe may be unexpected.

STEPS	RATIONALE

Critical Decision Point: Do not attach probe to finger, ear, or bridge of nose if area is edematous or skin integrity is compromised. Do not attach probe to fingers that are hypothermic. Select ear or bridge of nose if adult client has history of peripheral vascular disease. Earlobe and bridge of nose sensors are not used for infants and toddlers because of skin fragility. Disposable adhesive probes contain latex and should not be used if client has latex allergy.

12. Turn on oximeter by activating power. Observe pulse waveform/intensity display and audible beep. Correlate oximeter pulse rate with client's radial pulse. Differences require reevaluation of oximeter probe placement and may require reassessment of pulse rates.

13. Leave probe in place until oximeter readout reaches constant value and pulse display reaches full strength during each cardiac cycle. Read SpO_2 on digital display. Inform client that oximeter will alarm if the probe falls off or if client moves the probe. Read SpO_2 on digital display.

14. If continuous SpO_2 monitoring is planned, verify SpO_2 alarm limits and alarm volume, which are preset by the manufacturer at a low of 85% and a high of 100%. Limits for SpO_2 and pulse rate should be determined as indicated by client's condition. Verify that alarms are on. Assess skin integrity under sensor probe and relocate sensor probe at least every 4 hr.

15. Discuss findings with client as needed.

16. If intermittent or spot-checking SpO_2 measurements are planned, remove probe and turn oximeter power off. Store probe in appropriate location.

17. Assist client in returning to comfortable position.

18. Wash hands.

19. Compare SpO_2 readings with client baseline and acceptable values.

20. Correlate SpO_2 with SaO_2 obtained from arterial blood gas measurements (see Chapter 40) if available.

21. Correlate SpO_2 reading with data obtained from respiratory rate, depth, and rhythm assessment (see Skill 30-3).

(Rationale column)

Pulse waveform/intensity display enables detection of valid pulse or presence of interfering signal. Pitch of audible beep is proportional to SpO_2 value. Double-checking pulse rate ensures oximeter accuracy. Oximeter pulse rate, client's radial pulse, and apical pulse rate should be the same.

Reading may take 10 to 30 seconds, depending on site selected.

Alarms must be set at appropriate limits and volumes to avoid frightening clients and visitors. Spring tension of sensor probe or sensitivity to disposable sensor probe adhesive can cause skin irritation and lead to disruption of skin integrity.

Promotes participation in care and understanding of health status.

Batteries can be depleted if oximeter is left on. Sensor probes are expensive and vulnerable to damage.

Restores comfort and promotes sense of well-being.

Reduces transmission of microorganisms.

Comparison reveals presence of abnormality.

Documents reliability of noninvasive assessment.

Measurements assessing ventilation, perfusion, and diffusion are interrelated.

Recording and Reporting

- Record SpO_2 value on nurses' notes or vital sign flow sheet indicating type and amount of oxygen therapy used by client during assessment. Also record any signs and symptoms of oxygen desaturation in narrative form in nurses' notes. Measurement of SpO_2 after administration of specific therapies should be documented in narrative form in nurses' notes.

- Report abnormal findings to nurse in charge or physician. Assessment of oxygen saturation after administration of specific therapies should be documented in narrative form in nurses' notes.

- Record in nurses' notes client's use of continuous or intermittent pulse oximetry. Documents use of equipment for third-party payors.

Home Care Considerations

- Pulse oximetry is used in home care to noninvasively monitor oxygen therapy or changes in oxygen therapy.

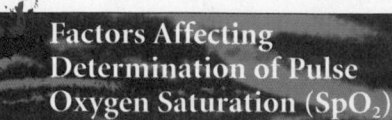

Factors Affecting Determination of Pulse Oxygen Saturation (SpO₂)   Box 31-15

INTERFERENCE WITH LIGHT TRANSMISSION

Outside light sources can interfere with the oximeter's ability to process reflected light.

Carbon monoxide (caused by smoke inhalation or poisoning) artificially elevates SpO₂ by absorbing light similar to oxygen.

Client motion can interfere with the oximeter's ability to process reflected light.

Jaundice may interfere with the oximeter's ability to process reflected light.

Intravascular dyes (methylene blue) absorb light similar to deoxyhemoglobin and artificially lower saturation.

REDUCTION OF ARTERIAL PULSATIONS

Peripheral vascular disease (Raynaud's, atherosclerosis) can reduce pulse volume.

Hypothermia at assessment site decreases peripheral blood flow.

Pharmacological vasoconstrictors (epinephrine, phenylephrine, dopamine) will decrease peripheral pulse volume.

Low cardiac output and hypotension decrease blood flow to peripheral arteries.

Peripheral edema can obscure arterial pulsation.

NURSING DIAGNOSES   Box 31-16

USING RESPIRATORY ASSESSMENT DATA AS DEFINING CHARACTERISTICS

Activity intolerance
Airway clearance, ineffective
Anxiety
Breathing pattern, ineffective
Gas exchange, impaired
Pain
Tissue perfusion, altered
Ventilatory weaning response, dysfunctional

NURSING PROCESS AND RESPIRATORY VITAL SIGNS

Vital sign measurement of respiratory rate, pattern, and depth, along with SpO₂, allows the nurse to assess ventilation, diffusion, and perfusion. The nurse may also conduct other assessments to measure respiratory status (see Chapter 32). Each measurement can provide clues in determining the nature of a client's problem. Respiratory assessment data are defining characteristics of many nursing diagnoses and are considered with other assessment data. The nursing care plan includes interventions based on the nursing diagnosis identified and the related factor (Box 31-16). For example, the defining characteristics of tachypnea, changes in depth of respirations, use of accessory muscles, cyanosis, and a decline in SpO₂ lead to a di-

agnosis of *impaired gas exchange.* The nurse evaluates client outcomes by assessing the respiratory rate, ventilatory depth, rhythm, and SpO₂ following each intervention.

Blood Pressure

Blood pressure is the lateral force on the walls of an artery by the pulsing blood under pressure from the heart. Systemic or arterial blood pressure, the blood pressure in the system of arteries in the body, is a good indicator of cardiovascular health. Blood flows throughout the circulatory system because of pressure changes. It moves from an area of high pressure to an area of low pressure. The heart's contraction forces blood under high pressure into the aorta. The peak of maximum pressure when ejection occurs is the **systolic** blood pressure. When the ventricles relax, the blood remaining in the arteries exerts a minimum or **diastolic** pressure. Diastolic pressure is the minimal pressure exerted against the arterial walls at all times.

The standard unit for measuring blood pressure is millimeters of mercury (mm Hg). The measurement indicates the height to which the blood pressure can raise a column of mercury. Blood pressure is recorded with the systolic reading before the diastolic (e.g., 120/80). The difference between systolic and diastolic pressure is the **pulse pressure.** For a blood pressure of 120/80, the pulse pressure is 40.

PHYSIOLOGY OF ARTERIAL BLOOD PRESSURE

Blood pressure reflects the interrelationships of cardiac output, peripheral vascular resistance, blood volume, blood viscosity, and artery elasticity. A nurse's knowledge of these hemodynamic variables helps in the assessment of blood pressure alterations.

Cardiac Output.   A person's cardiac output (CO) is the volume of blood pumped by the heart (stroke volume [SV]) during 1 minute (heart rate [HR]):

$$CO = HR \times SV$$

The blood pressure (BP) depends on the cardiac output and peripheral vascular resistance (R):

$$BP = CO \times R$$

When volume increases in an enclosed space, such as a blood vessel, the pressure in that space rises. Thus, as cardiac output increases, more blood is pumped against arterial walls, causing the blood pressure to rise. Cardiac output can increase as a result of an increase in heart rate, greater heart muscle contractility, or an increase in blood volume. Changes in heart rate can occur faster than changes in muscle contractility or blood volume. An increase in heart rate may decrease diastolic filling time and end-diastolic volume. As a result there is a decrease in blood pressure.

Peripheral Resistance. Blood circulates through a network of arteries, arterioles, capillaries, venules, and veins. Arteries and arterioles are surrounded by smooth muscle that contracts or relaxes to change the size of the lumen. The size of arteries and arterioles changes to adjust blood flow to the needs of local tissues. For example, when more blood is needed by a major organ, the peripheral arteries constrict, decreasing their supply of blood. More blood becomes available to the major organ because of the resistance change in the periphery. Normally, arteries and arterioles remain partially constricted to maintain a constant flow of blood. Peripheral vascular resistance is the resistance to blood flow determined by the tone of vascular musculature and diameter of blood vessels. The smaller the lumen of a vessel, the greater peripheral vascular resistance to blood flow. As resistance rises, arterial blood pressure rises. As vessels dilate and resistance falls, blood pressure drops.

Blood Volume. The volume of blood circulating within the vascular system affects blood pressure. Most adults have a circulating blood volume of 5000 ml. Normally the blood volume remains constant. However, if volume increases, more pressure is exerted against arterial walls. For example, the rapid, uncontrolled infusion of intravenous fluids elevates blood pressure. When circulating blood volume falls, as in the case of hemorrhage or dehydration, blood pressure falls.

Viscosity. The thickness or viscosity of blood affects the ease with which blood flows through small vessels. The **hematocrit,** or percentage of red blood cells in the blood, determines blood viscosity. When the hematocrit rises and blood flow slows, arterial blood pressure increases. The heart must contract more forcefully to move the viscous blood through the circulatory system.

Elasticity. Normally the walls of an artery are elastic and easily distensible. As pressure within the arteries increases, the diameter of vessel walls increases to accommodate the pressure change. Arterial distensibility prevents wide fluctuations in blood pressure. However, in certain diseases, such as arteriosclerosis, the vessel walls lose their elasticity and are replaced by fibrous tissue that cannot stretch well. With reduced elasticity there is greater resistance to blood flow. As a result, when the left ventricle ejects its stroke volume, the vessels no longer yield to pressure. Instead, a given volume of blood is forced through the rigid arterial walls, and the systemic pressure rises. Systolic pressure is more significantly elevated than diastolic pressure as a result of reduced arterial elasticity.

Each hemodynamic factor significantly affects the others. For example, as arterial elasticity declines, peripheral vascular resistance increases. The complex control of the cardiovascular system normally prevents any single factor from permanently changing the blood pressure. For example, if the blood volume falls, the body compensates with

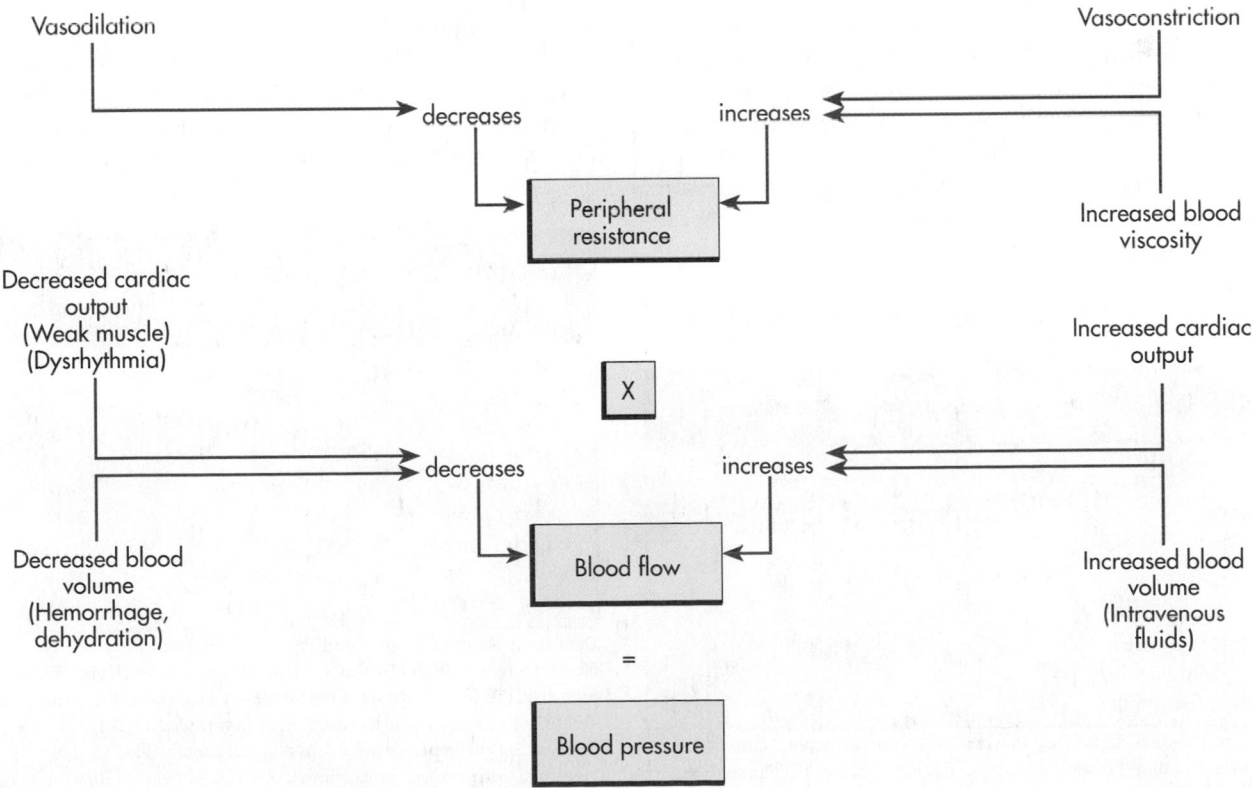

Figure 31-16 Hemodynamic factors that affect blood pressure.

an increased vascular resistance. Figure 31-16 illustrates how hemodynamic variables can affect blood pressure.

FACTORS INFLUENCING BLOOD PRESSURE

Blood pressure is not constant but is continually influenced by many factors during the day. One blood pressure measurement cannot adequately reflect a client's blood pressure. Even under the best conditions, blood pressure changes from heartbeat to heartbeat. Blood pressure trends, not individual measurements, guide nursing interventions. Understanding these factors ensures a more accurate interpretation of blood pressure readings.

Age.   Normal blood pressure levels vary throughout life (Table 31-7). They increase during childhood. The level of a child's or adolescent's blood pressure is assessed with respect to body size and age (Wong and others, 1998). An infant's blood pressure ranges from 65-115/42-80. The normal blood pressure for a 7-year-old is 87-117/48-64. Larger children (heavier and/or taller) have higher blood pressures than smaller children of the same age. During adolescence, blood pressure continues to vary according to body size.

An adult's blood pressure tends to increase with advancing age. The optimal blood pressure for a healthy, middle-age adult is 120/80 with acceptable values of <130/< 85 as the accepted norm (Joint National Committee, 1997) (Table 31-8). Older adults have a rise in systolic pressure related to a decreased vessel elasticity.

Stress.   Anxiety, fear, pain, and emotional stress result in sympathetic stimulation, which increases heart rate, cardiac output, and peripheral vascular resistance. The effects of sympathetic stimulation increase blood pressure.

Race.   The rate of hypertension (high blood pressure) is higher in African-Americans than in European-Americans. African-Americans tend to develop more severe hypertension at an earlier age and have twice the risk for complications such as stroke and heart attack

(Brashers, 1998). Genetic and environmental factors are believed to be contributing factors. Hypertension-related deaths are also higher among African-Americans.

Medications.   Some medications can directly or indirectly affect blood pressure. During blood pressure assessment, the nurse asks whether the client is receiving antihypertensive or other cardiac medications, which lower blood pressure (Table 31-9). Another class of medications affecting blood pressure is narcotic analgesics, which can lower blood pressure.

Diurnal Variation.   Blood pressure levels vary over the course of a day. Blood pressure is typically lowest in the early morning, gradually rises during the morning and afternoon, and peaks in late afternoon or evening. No two persons have the same pattern or degree of variation. Students may find it interesting to have their blood pressure checked by a friend at intervals during 24 hours.

Gender.   There is no clinically significant difference in blood pressure levels between boys and girls. After puberty, males tend to have higher blood pressure readings. After menopause, women tend to have higher levels of blood pressure than men of similar age.

HYPERTENSION

The most common alteration in blood pressure is **hypertension.** It is a major factor underlying deaths from strokes and is a contributing factor to myocardial infarctions (heart attacks). Hypertension is an often asymptomatic disorder characterized by persistently elevated blood pressure. The diagnosis of hypertension in adults is made when an average of two or more diastolic readings on at least two subsequent visits is 90 mm Hg or higher or

Table 31-7	Average Optimal Blood Pressure for Age	
Age	Blood Pressure (mm Hg)	
Newborn (3000 g [6.6 lb])	40 (mean)	
1 month	85/54	
1 year	95/65	
6 years	105/65	
10-13 years	110/65	
14-17 years	120/75	
Middle adult	120/80	
Older adult	140/90	

From National High Blood Pressure Education Program; National Heart, Lung, and Blood Institute; National Institutes of Health: The sixth report of the Joint National Committee on Detection, Evaluation, and Treatment of High Blood Pressure, *Arch Intern Med* 157:2413, 2, 1997.

Table 31-8	Classification of Blood Pressure for Adults Ages 18 and Older*		
Category	Systolic (mm Hg)		Diastolic (mm Hg)
Optimal†	<120		<80
Normal	<130		<85
High normal	130-139		85-89
Hypertension‡			
Stage 1 (mild)	140-159	or	90-99
Stage 2 (moderate)	160-179	or	100-109
Stage 3 (severe)	≥180	or	≥110

Data from National High Blood Pressure Education Program; National Heart, Lung, and Blood Institute; National Institutes of Health: The sixth report of the Joint National Committee on Detection, Evaluation, and Treatment of High Blood Pressure, *Arch Intern Med* 157:2413, 2, 1997.
*Not taking antihypertensive drugs and not acutely ill.
†Optimal with respect to cardiovascular risk is below 120/80 mm Hg. Unusually low readings should be evaluated.
‡Based on average of two or more readings.

Table 31-9 Antihypertension Medications

Medication Type	Names	Action
Diuretics	Furosemide (Lasix), spironolactone (Aldactone), metolazone, polythiazide, benzthiazide	Lower blood pressure by reducing reabsorption of sodium and water by the kidneys, thus lowering circulating fluid volume
Beta-adrenergic blockers	Atenolol (Tenormin), nadolol (Corgard), timolol maleate (Blocadren), propranolol (Inderal)	Combine with beta-adrenergic receptors in the heart, arteries, and arterioles to block response to sympathetic nerve impulses; reduce heart rate and thus cardiac output
Vasodilators	Hydralazine hydrochloride (Apresoline), minoxidil (Loniten)	Act on arteriolar smooth muscle to cause relaxation and reduce peripheral vascular resistance
Calcium channel blockers	Verapamil hydrochloride (Calan), nifedipine (Procardia)	Reduce peripheral vascular resistance by systemic vasodilation
Angiotensin converting enzyme (ACE) inhibitors	Captopril (Capoten), enalapril (Vasotec), lisinopril (Prinivil)	Lower blood pressure by blocking the conversion of angiotensin I to angiotensin II, preventing vasoconstriction; reduce aldosterone production and fluid retention, lowering circulating fluid volume

when the average of multiple systolic blood pressures on two or more subsequent visits is consistently higher than 135 mm Hg. Categories of hypertension have been developed and determine medical intervention (see Table 31-8). One elevated blood pressure measurement does not qualify as a diagnosis of hypertension. However, if the nurse assesses a high reading during the first blood pressure measurement (e.g., 150/90 mm Hg), the client is encouraged to return for another checkup within 2 months.

Hypertension is associated with the thickening and loss of elasticity in the arterial walls. Peripheral vascular resistance increases within thick and inelastic vessels. The heart must continually pump against greater resistance. As a result, blood flow to vital organs such as the heart, brain, and kidney decreases.

Persons with a family history of hypertension are at significant risk. Obesity, cigarette smoking, heavy alcohol consumption, high sodium (salt) intake, sedentary lifestyle, and continued exposure to stress are also linked to hypertension. The incidence of hypertension is greater in diabetic clients, older adults, and African-Americans. When clients are diagnosed with hypertension, the nurse helps to educate them about blood pressure values, long-term follow-up care and therapy, the usual lack of symptoms (the fact that it may not be "felt"), therapy's ability to control but not cure hypertension, and a consistently followed treatment plan that can ensure a relatively normal lifestyle (Joint National Committee, 1997).

HYPOTENSION

Hypotension is generally considered present when the systolic blood pressure falls to 90 mm Hg or below. Although some adults have a low blood pressure normally, for the majority of people, low blood pressure is an abnormal finding associated with illness.

Hypotension occurs because of the dilation of the arteries in the vascular bed, the loss of a substantial amount of blood volume (e.g., hemorrhage), or the failure of the heart muscle to pump adequately (e.g., myocardial infarction). Hypotension associated with pallor, skin mottling, clamminess, confusion, increased heart rate, or decreased urine output is life threatening and should be reported to a physician immediately.

Orthostatic hypotension, also referred to as **postural hypotension,** occurs when a normotensive person develops symptoms and low blood pressure when rising to an upright position. When a healthy individual changes from a lying, to sitting, to standing position, the peripheral blood vessels in the legs constrict. Constriction of the lower extremity vessels when standing prevents the pooling of blood in the legs due to gravity. When clients have a decreased blood volume, their blood vessels are already constricted. When a volume-depleted client stands, there is a significant drop in blood pressure with an increase in heart rate to compensate for the drop in cardiac output. Clients who are dehydrated, anemic, or have experienced prolonged bed rest or recent blood loss are at risk for orthostatic hypotension (Roper, 1996). Some medications can cause orthostatic hypotension if misused, especially in older adult or young clients. Blood pressure should always be measured before administering such medications.

Orthostatic vital sign measurements include obtaining blood pressure and pulse with the client supine, sitting, and standing. When recording orthostatic blood pressure measurements, the nurse records the client's position in addition to the blood pressure measurement. For example: 140/80 supine, 132/72 sitting, 108/60 standing. The readings are obtained 1 to 3 minutes after the client changes position. In most cases, orthostatic hypotension is detected within a minute of standing (Roper, 1996). If or-

Skill 31-5 Measuring Blood Pressure

Delegation Considerations

The skill of blood pressure measurement can be delegated to assistive personnel.

- Inform caregiver of appropriate client position when obtaining blood pressure measurement.
- Inform caregiver if client has alterations affecting the appropriate limb for blood pressure measurement.
- Inform caregiver of appropriate size blood pressure cuff for designated extremity.

- Inform caregiver if client is at risk for orthostatic hypotension.
- Inform caregiver of frequency of blood pressure measurement.
- Determine that caregiver is aware of the usual values for the client.
- Inform caregiver of the need to report any abnormalities that should be reconfirmed by the nurse.

EQUIPMENT

- Mercury or aneroid sphygmomanometer
- Cloth or disposable vinyl pressure cuff of appropriate size for client's extremity
- Stethoscope
- Alcohol swab
- Pen, pencil, vital sign flow sheet or record form

STEPS	RATIONALE
1. Determine need to assess client's BP: a. Note risk factors for alteration in BP.	Certain conditions place clients at risk for BP alteration: history of cardiovascular disease, renal disease, diabetes, circulatory shock (hypovolemic, septic, cardiogenic, or neurogenic), acute or chronic pain, rapid intravenous infusion of fluids or blood products, increased intracranial pressure, postoperative conditions, toxemia of pregnancy.

b. Observe for signs and symptoms of BP alterations:
    (1) High BP (hypertension) is often asymptomatic until pressure is very high. Assess for headache (usually occipital), flushing of face, nosebleed, and fatigue in older adults.
    (2) Low BP (hypotension) is associated with dizziness; mental confusion; restlessness; pale, dusky, or cyanotic skin and mucous membranes; cool, mottled skin over extremities.
	Physical signs and symptoms may indicate alterations in BP.

2. Determine best site for BP assessment. Avoid applying cuff to extremity when intravenous fluids are infusing; an arteriovenous shunt or fistula is present; breast or axillary surgery has been performed on that side; extremity has been traumatized, diseased, or requires a cast or bulky bandage. The lower extremities may be used when the brachial arteries are inaccessible.	Inappropriate site selection may result in poor amplification of sounds, causing inaccurate readings. Application of pressure from inflated bladder temporarily impairs blood flow and can further compromise circulation in extremity that already has impaired blood flow.
3. Select appropriate cuff size.	Improper cuff size results in inaccurate readings (see Table 31-10). If cuff is too small, it tends to come loose as inflated or results in false high readings. If the cuff is too large, false low readings may be recorded.
4. Determine previous baseline BP (if available) from client's record.	Allows nurse to assess for change in condition. Provides comparison with future BP measurements.
5. Encourage client to avoid exercise and smoking for 30 minutes before assessment of BP.	Exercise and smoking can cause false elevations in BP.
6. Have client assume sitting or lying position. Be sure room is warm, quiet, and relaxing.	Maintains client's comfort during measurement. The client's perceptions that the physical or interpersonal environment is stressful affect the BP measurement (Thomas and DeKeyser, 1996).
7. Explain to client that BP is to be assessed and have client rest at least 5 min before measurement. Ask client not to speak when BP is being measured.	Reduces anxiety that can falsely elevate readings. Blood pressure readings taken at different times can be objectively compared when assessed with client at rest. Talking to a client when the BP is being assessed increases readings 10% to 40% (Thomas and DeKeyser, 1996).

STEPS	RATIONALE

8. Wash hands. With client sitting or lying, position client's forearm or thigh, supported if needed. For arm turn palm up; for thigh position with knee slightly flexed.

Reduces transmission of microorganisms. If extremity is unsupported, client may perform isometric exercise that can increase diastolic blood pressure.

9. Expose extremity (arm or leg) fully by removing constricting clothing

Ensures proper cuff application.

10. Palpate brachial artery (arm) or popliteal artery (leg) (see illustration). Position cuff 2.5 cm (1 in) above site of pulsation (antecubital or popliteal space).

Inflating bladder directly over artery ensures proper pressure is applied during inflation.

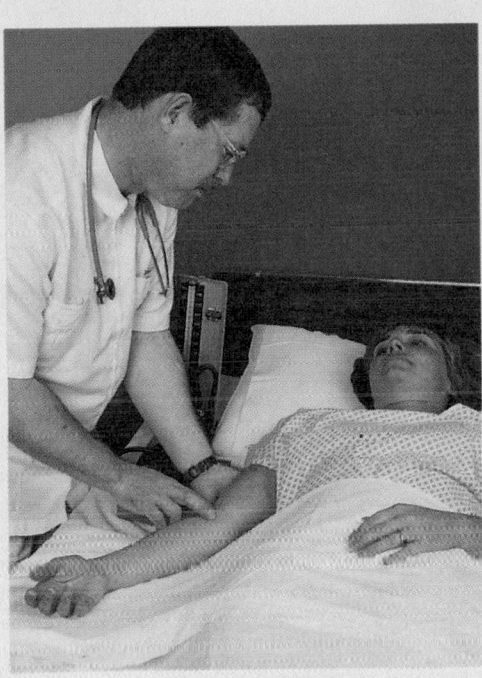

Step 10

11. Apply bladder of cuff above artery by centering arrows marked on cuff over artery. If there are not center arrows on cuff, estimate the center of the bladder and place this center over artery. With cuff fully deflated, wrap cuff evenly and snugly around extremity (see illustrations, p. 712).

Loose-fitting cuff causes false high readings.

12. Position manometer vertically at eye level. Observer should be no farther than 1 m (approximately 1 yd) away

Accurate readings are obtained by looking at the meniscus of the mercury at eye level. The meniscus is the point where the crescent-shaped top of the mercury column aligns with the manometer scale. Looking up or down at the mercury results in distorted readings.

13. If you do not know the client's baseline BP, estimate systolic pressure by palpating the artery distal to the cuff with fingertips of one hand while inflating cuff rapidly to pressure 30 mm Hg above point at which pulse disappears. Slowly deflate cuff and note point when pulse reappears. Deflate cuff fully and wait 30 sec.

Estimating prevents false low readings, which may result in the presence of an auscultatory gap. Maximal inflation point for accurate reading can be determined by palpation. If unable to palpate artery because of weakened pulse, an ultrasonic stethoscope can be used (see Chapter 32). Deflating cuff prevents venous congestion and false high readings.

14. Place stethoscope earpieces in ears and be sure sounds are clear, not muffled.

Each earpiece should follow angle of ear canal to facilitate hearing.

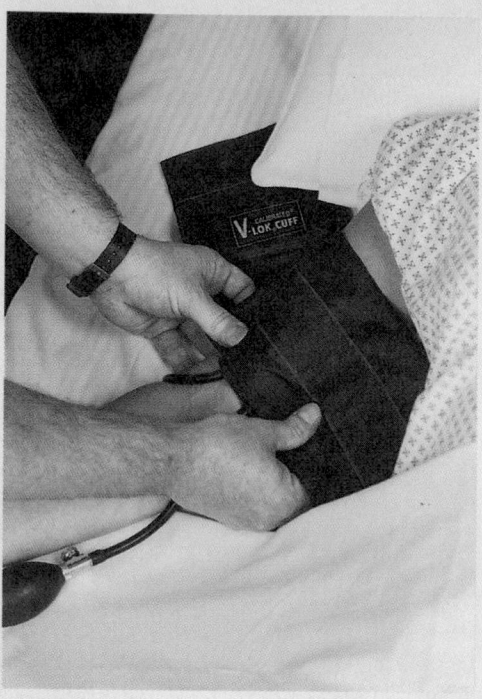 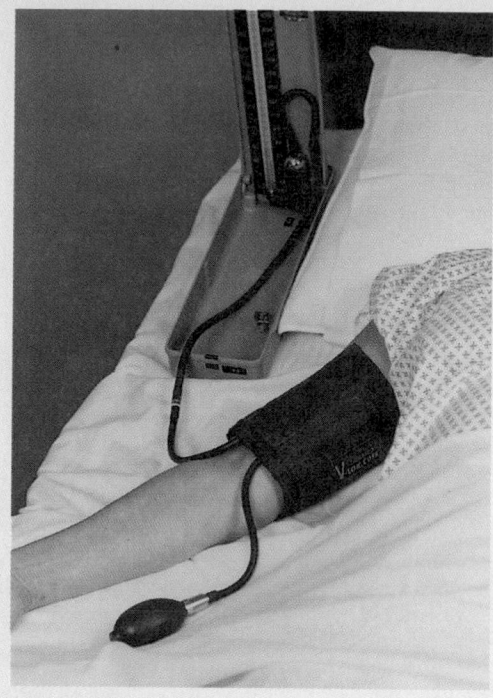

Step 11

15. Relocate brachial or popliteal artery and place bell or diaphragm chestpiece of stethoscope over it. Do not allow chestpiece to touch cuff or clothing (see illustration).

16. Close valve of pressure bulb clockwise until tight. Rapidly inflate cuff to 30 mm Hg above palpated systolic pressure.

17. Slowly release pressure bulb valve and allow mercury or needle of aneroid manometer gauge to fall at rate of 2 to 3 mm Hg/sec.

18. Note point on manometer when first clear sound is heard. The sound will slowly increase in intensity.

19. Continue to deflate cuff, noting point at which muffled or dampened sound appears.

20. Continue to deflate cuff gradually, noting point at which sound disappears in adults. Listen for 10 to 20 mm Hg after the last sound, and then allow remaining air to escape quickly.

21. Remove cuff from extremity unless measurement must be repeated. If this is the first assessment of client, repeat procedure on other extremity.

22. Assist client in returning to comfortable position and cover upper arm if previously clothed.

23. Discuss findings with client as needed.

24. Wash hands.

25. Compare reading with previous baseline and/or acceptable value of blood pressure for client's age.

26. Compare blood pressure in both arms or both legs.

Proper stethoscope placement ensures optimal sound reception. Stethoscope improperly positioned causes muffled sounds that often result in false low systolic and false high diastolic readings.

Tightening of valve prevents air leak during inflation. Inflation ensures accurate measurement of systolic pressure.

Too rapid or slow a decline in mercury level or aneroid pressure can cause inaccurate readings.

First Korotkoff sound indicates systolic pressure.

Fourth Korotkoff sound involves distinct muffling of sounds and is recommended as indication of diastolic pressure in children.

Beginning of the fifth Korotkoff sound is recommended by American Heart Association as indication of diastolic pressure in adults.

Continuous cuff inflation causes arterial occlusion, resulting in numbness and tingling of client's arm.

Comparison of BP in both extremities detects circulation problems. (Normal difference of 5 to 10 mm Hg exists between extremities.)

Restores comfort and promotes sense of well-being.

Promotes participation in care and understanding of health status.

Reduces transmission of microorganisms.

Evaluates for change in condition and alterations.

If using upper extremities, the arm with the higher pressure should be used for subsequent assessments unless contraindicated.

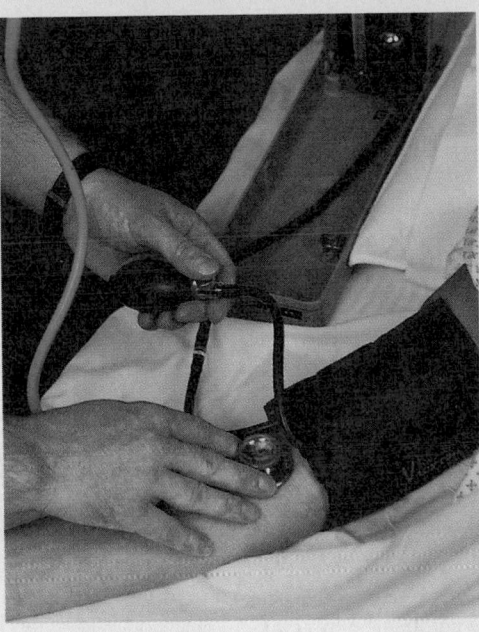

Step 15

27. Correlate blood pressure with data obtained from pulse assessment and related cardiovascular signs and symptoms.	Blood pressure and heart rate are interrelated.

Recording and Reporting
- Inform client of value and need for periodic reassessment.
- Record blood pressure in nurses' notes or vital sign flow sheet. Measurement of blood pressure after administration of specific therapies should be documented in narrative form in nurses' notes.
- Report abnormal findings to nurse in charge or physician.

Home Care Considerations
- Assess home noise level to determine room that will provide quietest environment for assessing BP.
- Consider electronic blood pressure cuff for home if client has hearing difficulties and if client has sufficient financial resources.

thostatic hypotension is assessed, the client is assisted to a lying position and the physician or nurse in charge is notified. While obtaining orthostatic measurements, the nurse observes for other symptoms of hypotension such as fainting, weakness, or light-headedness. Because the skill of orthostatic measurements requires critical thinking and ongoing nursing judgment, this procedure is not delegated to unlicensed assistive personnel.

ASSESSMENT OF BLOOD PRESSURE
Arterial blood pressure may be measured either directly (invasively) or indirectly (noninvasively). The direct method requires the insertion of a thin catheter into an artery. Tubing connects the catheter with electronic monitoring equipment. The monitor displays a constant arterial pressure waveform and reading. Because of the risk of sudden blood loss from an artery, invasive blood pressure monitoring is used only in intensive care settings. The more common noninvasive method requires use of the sphygmomanometer and stethoscope. The nurse measures blood pressure indirectly by auscultation or palpation. Auscultation is the most widely used technique (Skill 31-5).

Blood Pressure Equipment. Before assessing blood pressure the nurse must be comfortable using a sphygmomanometer and stethoscope. A **sphygmomanometer**

comprises a pressure manometer, an occlusive cloth or vinyl cuff that encloses an inflatable rubber bladder, and a pressure bulb with a release valve that inflates the bladder. The two types of manometers are the aneroid and the mercury (Figure 31-17). Both types can be wall mounted or portable.

The aneroid manometer has a glass-enclosed circular gauge containing a needle that registers millimeter calibrations. Before using the aneroid model, the nurse must be sure that the needle points to zero and that the manometer is correctly calibrated. Aneroid sphygmomanometers require biomedical calibration at routine intervals to verify their accuracy. Aneroid manometers have the advantages of being lightweight, portable, and compact. Because metal parts in the aneroid model are subject to temperature expansion or contraction, the aneroid instrument is less reliable than the mercury type.

Mercury manometers are more accurate than aneroid manometers. Repeated calibrations are not necessary. The mercury manometer is an upright tube containing mercury. Pressure created by the inflation of the bladder moves the column of mercury upward against the force of gravity. Millimeter calibrations mark the height of the mercury column. The mercury column must be at zero when the cuff is deflated. To ensure accurate readings, the mercury column should fall freely as pressure is released. Accurate readings are obtained by looking at the meniscus of the mercury at eye level. This is the point where the crescent-shaped top of the mercury column aligns with the manometer scale. Looking up or down at the mercury results in distorted readings. The disadvantages of the mercury manometer are the potential for breakage and the release of mercury. Mercury is a health hazard if not properly contained. Steps to take in the event of a mercury spill are presented in Box 31-6.

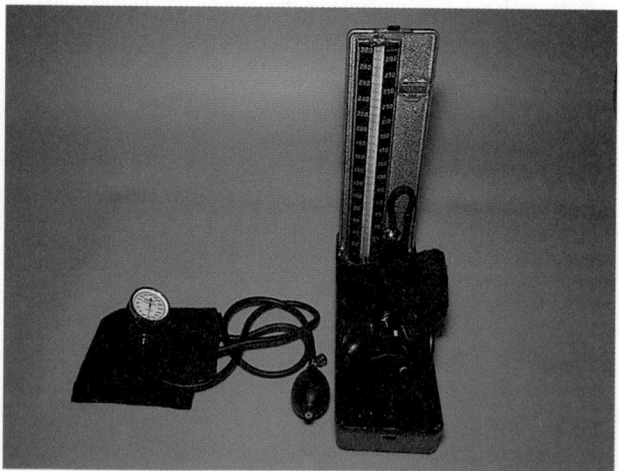

Figure 31-17 Portable sphygmomanometers. *Right*, mercury manometer; *left*, aneroid manometer.

Cloth or disposable vinyl compression cuffs contain the inflatable bladder and come in several sizes. The size selected is proportional to the circumference of the limb being assessed (Figure 31-18). Ideally, the width of the cuff should be 40% of the circumference (or 20% wider than the diameter) of the midpoint of the limb on which the cuff is to be used (National Institutes of Health, 1996). The bladder, enclosed by the cuff, should encircle at least two thirds of the arm of an adult and the entire arm of a child (Joint National Committee, 1997). In children the lower edge of the cuff should be above the antecubital fossa, allowing room for placement of the stethoscope bell or diaphragm. Blood pressure measurements will not be accurate unless the correct size blood pressure cuff is applied appropriately.

Before using a sphygmomanometer the nurse should inspect the parts of the release valve and the pressure bulb. The valve should be clean and freely moveable in either direction. If it sticks or becomes too tightly closed, the deflation of the pressure cuff will be hard to regulate. The pressure bulb is made of tough rubber and should be free of leaks.

Auscultation.   The best environment for blood pressure measurement by auscultation is a quiet room at a comfortable temperature. Although the client may lie or stand, sitting is the preferred position. In most cases blood pressure readings obtained with the client in the supine, sitting, and standing positions are similar. The nurse obtains orthostatic measurements by documenting the patient's blood pressure and pulse rate in all three positions.

The client's position during routine blood pressure determination should be the same during each measurement to permit a meaningful comparison of values. Before assessment the nurse should attempt to control factors responsible for artificially high readings, such as pain, anxiety, or exertion. The client's perceptions that the physical or interpersonal environment is more or less stressful will affect the blood pressure measurement. Blood pressure measurements taken at the client's place of employment or in a physician's office are higher than those taken at the client's home.

During the initial assessment the nurse should obtain and record the blood pressure in both arms. Normally there is a difference of 5 to 10 mm Hg between the arms. In subsequent assessments the blood pressure should be measured in the arm with the higher pressure. Pressure differences greater than 10 mm Hg indicate vascular problems in the arm with the lower pressure.

The nurse asks the client to state his usual blood pressure. If the client does not know, the nurse informs him after measuring and recording the blood pressure. This is a good opportunity to educate a client about optimal values of blood pressure, the risk factors for developing hypertension, and dangers of hypertension.

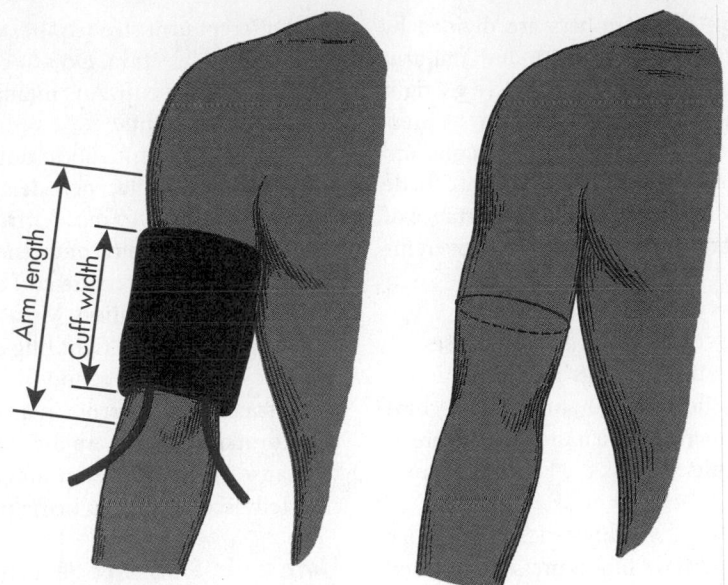

Figure 31-18   Guidelines for proper blood pressure cuff size. Cuff width = 20% more than upper arm diameter, or 40% of circumference and two thirds of arm length.

Indirect measurement of arterial blood pressure works on a basic principle of pressure. Blood flows freely through an artery until an inflated cuff applies pressure to tissues and causes the artery to collapse. After the cuff pressure is released, the point at which blood flow returns and sound appears through auscultation is the systolic pressure.

In 1905, Korotkoff, a Russian surgeon, first described the sounds heard over an artery distal to the blood pressure cuff. The first Korotkoff sound is a clear rhythmical tapping corresponding to the pulse rate that gradually increases in intensity. *Onset of the sound corresponds to the systolic pressure.* With the second Korotkoff sound a murmur or swishing sound occurs as the cuff continues to deflate. As the artery distends, there is a turbulence in blood flow. The third Korotkoff sound is a crisper and more intense tapping. The fourth Korotkoff sounds become muffled and low pitched as the cuff is further deflated. Cuff pressure falls below the pressure within the vessel walls; *this sound is the diastolic pressure in infants and children.* The fifth Korotkoff sound is an absence of sound. *In adolescents and adults, the fifth sound corresponds with the diastolic pressure* (Figure 31-19). In some clients the sounds are clear and distinct. In other clients only the beginning and ending sounds are clear.

The American Heart Association (Joint National Committee, 1997) recommends recording two numbers for a blood pressure measurement: the point on the manometer when the first sound is heard for systolic and the point on the manometer when the fifth sound is heard for diastolic. Some institutions recommend recording the point when the fourth sound is heard as well, especially for

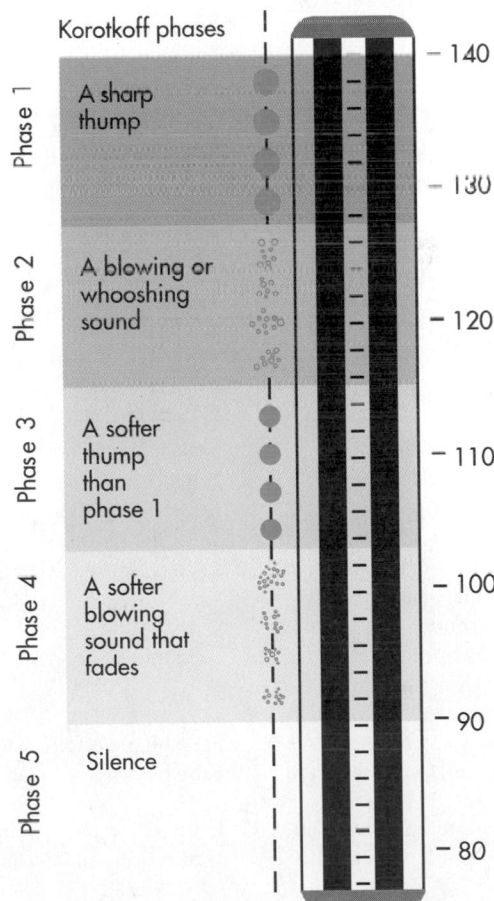

Korotkoff phases

Phase 1   A sharp thump   — 140

— 130

Phase 2   A blowing or whooshing sound   — 120

Phase 3   A softer thump than phase 1   — 110

Phase 4   A softer blowing sound that fades   — 100

— 90

Phase 5   Silence

— 80

Figure 31-19   The sounds auscultated during blood pressure measurement can be differentiated into five Korotkoff phases. In this example blood pressure is 140/90.

clients with hypertension. The numbers are divided by slashed lines (e.g., 120/80 or 120/100/80), and the arm used to measure the blood pressure is noted (e.g., right arm [RA] 130/70), and the client's position when the pressure is assessed (e.g., sitting). Many medical decisions and nursing interventions about a client's health care are made on the basis of blood pressure findings. The importance of obtaining an accurate blood pressure cannot be overemphasized.

Potential Errors in Auscultation.   Several causes exist for error in blood pressure readings if auscultation is not performed correctly. Table 31-10 summarizes common mistakes in measurement. When a nurse is unsure of a reading, a colleague should reassess the blood pressure.

Assessment in Children.   All children 3 years of age through adolescence should have blood pressure checked at least yearly. Blood pressure in children changes with growth and development. The nurse can help parents to understand the importance of this routine screening to detect children who may be at risk for hypertension. The measurement of blood pressure in infants and children is difficult for several reasons.

- Different arm size requires careful and appropriate cuff size selection. Do not choose a cuff based on the name of the cuff. An "infant" cuff may be too small for some infants.
- Readings are difficult to obtain in restless or anxious infants and children. A delay of at least 15 minutes to allow children to recover from recent activities and apprehension is recommended. Preparing the child for the blood pressure cuff's unusual sensation can increase cooperation. Most children will understand the analogy of a "tight hug on your arm."
- Placing stethoscope too firmly on the antecubital fossa can cause errors in auscultation.
- Korotkoff sounds are difficult to hear in children because of low frequency and amplitude. A pediatric stethoscope bell can be helpful.

Ultrasonic Stethoscope.   If a nurse is unable to auscultate sounds because of a weakened arterial pulse, an ultrasonic stethoscope can be used (see Chapter 32). This stethoscope allows the nurse to hear low-frequency systolic sounds and is commonly used when measuring the blood pressure of infants, children, and low blood pressure in adults.

Palpation.   The indirect palpation technique is useful for clients whose arterial pulsations are too weak to create Korotkoff sounds. Severe blood loss and decreased heart contractility are examples of conditions that result in blood pressures too low to auscultate accurately. Only the systolic blood pressure can be assessed by palpation (Box 31-17). The diastolic pressure is difficult to determine by palpation. A subtle change in sensation, usually in the form of a thin, snapping vibration, marks the diastolic level. When the palpation technique is used, the systolic value and the manner in which it was measured are recorded (e.g., RA 90/-, palpated, supine).

The palpation technique is used with auscultation in some instances. In some hypertensive clients, the sounds usually heard over the brachial artery when the cuff pressure is high disappear as pressure is reduced and then reappear at a lower level. This temporary disappearance of

Table 31-10	Common Mistakes in Blood Pressure Assessment
Error	Effect
Bladder or cuff too wide	False low reading
Bladder or cuff too narrow	False high reading
Cuff wrapped too loosely or unevenly	False high reading
Deflating cuff too slowly	False high diastolic reading
Deflating cuff too quickly	False low systolic and false high diastolic reading
Arm below heart level	False high reading
Arm above heart level	False low reading
Arm not supported	False high reading
Stethoscope that fits poorly or impairment of the examiner's hearing, causing sounds to be muffled	False low systolic and false high diastolic reading
Stethoscope applied too firmly against antecubital fossa	False low diastolic reading
Inflating too slowly	False high diastolic reading
Repeating assessments too quickly	False high systolic reading
Inaccurate inflation level	Inaccurate interpretation of systolic and diastolic readings
Multiple examiners using different Korotkoff sounds for diastolic readings	False high systolic and low diastolic reading

Palpating the Systolic Blood Pressure   Box 31-17

1. Apply blood pressure cuff to the upper arm in the same manner as the auscultation method.
2. Continually palpate the radial artery.
3. Inflate blood pressure cuff 30 mm Hg above the point at which the radial pulse can no longer be palpated.
4. Release valve and allow mercury to fall 2 mm Hg/sec.
5. As soon as the radial pulse is palpable, note the manometer reading, the systolic blood pressure.

sound is the **auscultatory gap.** It typically occurs between the first and second Korotkoff sounds. The gap in sound may cover a range of 40 mm Hg and thus may cause an underestimation of systolic pressure or overestimation of diastolic pressure. The examiner must be certain to inflate the cuff high enough to hear the true systolic pressure before the auscultatory gap. Palpation of the radial artery helps to determine how high to inflate the cuff. The examiner inflates the cuff 30 mm Hg above the pressure at which the radial pulse was palpated. The range of pressures in which the auscultatory gap occurs is recorded (e.g., BP RA 180/94 with an auscultatory gap from 180 to 160, sitting).

Assessment of Lower Extremities.

Dressings, casts, intravenous catheters, arteriovenous fistulas or shunts, and axillary lymph node dissection can make the upper extremities inaccessible. Blood pressure must then be measured in the lower extremities. Comparing upper extremity blood pressure with that in the legs is also necessary for clients with certain peripheral vascular abnormalities. The popliteal artery, palpable behind the knee in the popliteal space, is the site for auscultation. The cuff must be wide and long enough to allow for the larger girth of the thigh. Placing the client in a prone position is best. If such a position is impossible, the client should be asked to flex the knee slightly for easier access to the artery. The cuff is positioned 2.5 cm (1 inch) above the popliteal artery with the bladder over the posterior aspect of the midthigh (Figure 31-20). The procedure is identical to brachial artery auscultation. Systolic pressure in the legs is usually higher by 10 to 40 mm Hg than in the brachial artery, but the diastolic pressure is the same.

Automatic Blood Pressure Devices.

Many electronic devices can determine blood pressure automatically (Figure 31-21). These devices are applied when frequent blood pressure assessment is required such as in the critically ill or potentially unstable client, during or after invasive procedures, or when therapies require frequent monitoring (e.g., intravenous heart and blood pressure medications). However, some client conditions are not appropriate for automatic blood pressure devices (Box 31-18).

Whereas the auscultatory technique relies on the detection of Korotkoff sounds, some electronic devices rely on the principle of oscillometry. The system includes either a microphone or a pressure sensor built into the inflatable cuff. The microphone or acoustic system hears Korotkoff sounds and registers diastolic and systolic readings. The pressure sensor or ultrasonic system responds to the pressure waves generated by the movement of blood through the artery. The sensor determines the initial burst of oscillations and translates the information into a systolic pressure reading. The diastolic pressure is measured when the oscillations are lowest, just before they stop (Bridges and Middleton, 1997).

A baseline blood pressure should be obtained using the auscultatory method before applying automatic devices. A comparison assists in evaluation of a client's status and allows proper programming of the device. Once the blood pressure cuff is applied, the nurse can program the device to obtain and record blood pressure readings at preset intervals. Alarm limits can be programmed to alert the nurse

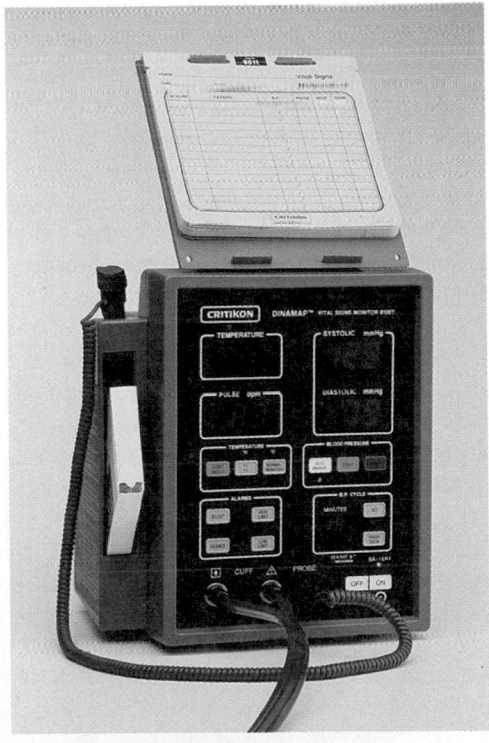

Figure 31-21 Automatic blood pressure monitor. Dinamap Vital Signs Monitor is a trademark of Critikon, Inc. Photo courtesy Critikon, Inc., Tampa, Fla.

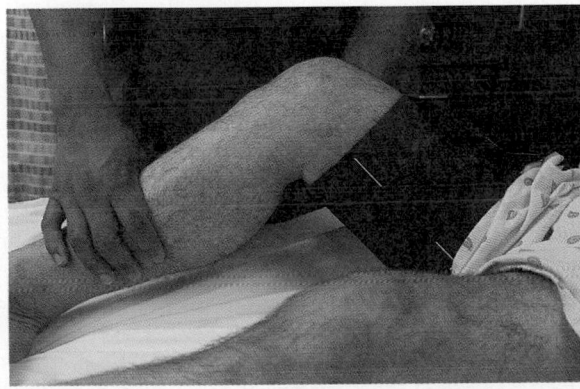

Figure 31-20 Lower extremity blood pressure cuff positioned above popliteal artery at midthigh with knee flexed.

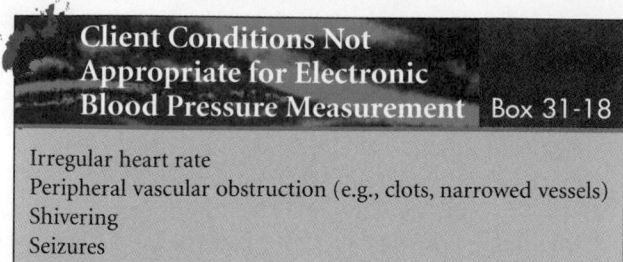

Client Conditions Not Appropriate for Electronic Blood Pressure Measurement   Box 31-18

Irregular heart rate
Peripheral vascular obstruction (e.g., clots, narrowed vessels)
Shivering
Seizures
Excessive tremors
Inability to cooperate
Blood pressure less than 90 mm Hg systolic

if the blood pressure measurement is outside desired parameters.

The advantages of automatic devices are the ease of use and efficiency when repeated or when frequent measurements are indicated. The ability to use a stethoscope is not required. However, automatic devices are more sensitive to outside interference and are susceptible to error. The microphone or pressure sensor must be positioned directly over the artery for proper function. Client movements or vibration or outside noise can interfere with the microphone or sensor signal. Most automatic blood pressure devices are unable to process sounds or vibrations of low blood pressure. The range of device sophistication also can make blood pressure measurement comparisons difficult. The use of automatic blood pressure devices permits assessment of blood pressure during interpersonal interactions. However, the nurse should avoid speaking to the client for at least a minute before initiating a blood pressure recording. Talking to a client when the blood pressure is being assessed can increase readings 10% to 40%.

Self-Measurement of Blood Pressure.

More people measure their own blood pressures because of improved technology in home monitoring devices and a greater interest in health promotion. Two of the more common devices used by the general public include portable home sphygmomanometers and stationary automatic blood pressure machines.

The portable home devices include the mercury and aneroid sphygmomanometers and electronic digital readout devices that do not require use of a stethoscope. The electronic devices inflate and deflate cuffs with the push of a button. The electronic devices may be easier to manipulate but can easily become inaccurate and require recalibration more than once a year. Because of their sensitivity, improper cuff placement or movement of the arm can cause electronic devices to give incorrect readings.

Stationary automatic blood pressure devices can be found in public places such as grocery stores, fitness clubs, banks, airports, or work sites. Users simply rest their arms within the machine's inflatable cuff, which contains a

pressure sensor. The cuff fits over clothing. A visual display tells users their blood pressure within 60 to 90 seconds. The reliability of the stationary machines is limited. Blood pressure values may vary by 5 to 10 mm Hg or more (for both systolic and diastolic values) compared with pressures taken with a manual sphygmomanometer.

Self-measurement of blood pressure has several benefits. Elevated blood pressure may be detected in persons previously unaware of a problem. Persons with high normal blood pressure can provide information about the pattern of blood pressure values. Clients with hypertension can benefit from participating actively in their treatment through self-monitoring, which may help compliance with treatment. The disadvantages of self-measurement include improper use of the device. A client may be needlessly alarmed with one elevated reading. Clients with hypertension may become overly conscious of their blood pressures and make inappropriate self-adjustment of medications.

Consumers can learn to use self-measurement devices if they have the information needed to perform the procedure correctly and if they know when to seek medical attention. The nurse can advise clients of possible inaccuracies in the blood pressure devices, help clients understand the meaning and implications of readings, and teach them proper measurement techniques.

NURSING PROCESS AND BLOOD PRESSURE DETERMINATION

The assessment of blood pressure along with pulse assessment is used to evaluate the general state of cardiovascular health and responses to other system imbalances. Hypotension, hypertension, orthostatic hypotension, and narrow or wide pulse pressures are defining characteristics of certain nursing diagnoses and are considered along with other assessment data (Box 31-19). The nursing care plan includes interventions based on the nursing diagnosis identified and the related factor. For example, the defining characteristics of hypotension, dizziness, pulse deficit, and dysrhythmia lead to a diagnosis of *decreased cardiac output*. The nurse evaluates client outcomes by assessing the blood pressure following each intervention.

Health Promotion and Vital Signs

The emphasis on health promotion and health maintenance, as well as early discharge from hospital settings, has resulted in an increase in the need for clients and their families to monitor vital signs in the home. Teaching considerations affect all vital sign measurements and should be incorporated within the client's plan of care (Box 31-20).

When considering how to teach clients and their families about vital sign measurements and their importance and significance, the client's age is an important factor. With the increased older adult population there is an increased need for caregivers to be aware of changes that are unique to older adults. Box 31-21 identifies some of these variations unique to the older adult.

Recording Vital Signs

Special graphic flowsheets exist for recording vital signs (Figure 31-22). The nurse identifies the institution's procedure for documenting on the graphic or vital sign flow-sheet. In addition to the actual vital sign values, the nurse records in the nurses' notes any accompanying or precipitating symptoms such as chest pain and dizziness with abnormal blood pressure, shortness of breath with abnormal respirations, cyanosis with hypoxemia, or flushing and diaphoresis with elevated temperature. The nurse documents any interventions initiated as a result of vital sign measurement such as administration of oxygen therapy or an antihypertensive medication.

Clients being managed on critical paths or CareMaps may have vital sign values listed as outcomes (see Chapter 18). If a vital sign value is above or below the anticipated outcomes, a variance note is written to explain the nature of the variance and the nurse's course of action. For example, a CareMap for a client who has undergone a thoracotomy may have an outcome during the postoperative period of "afebrile." If the client has a fever, the nurse's variance note may address possible sources of fever (e.g., retained pulmonary secretions) and nursing interventions (e.g., increased suctioning, postural drainage, or hydration).

Client Teaching FOR **HEALTH PROMOTION**   Box 31-20

TEMPERATURE
- Identify client's ability to initiate preventive health measures and recognize alteration in body temperature. Educate clients and family members about measures to prevent body temperature alterations.
- Teach clients risk factors for hypothermia and frostbite: fatigue; malnutrition; hypoxemia; cold, wet clothing; alcohol intoxication.
- Teach clients risk factors for heat stroke: strenuous exercise in hot, humid weather; tight-fitting clothing in hot environments; exercising in poorly ventilated areas; sudden exposures to hot climates; poor fluid intake before, during, and after exercise.
- Teach clients the importance of taking and continuing antibiotics as directed until course of treatment is completed.

PULSE RATE
- Clients taking certain prescribed cardiac medications should learn to assess their own pulse rates to detect side effects of medications. Clients undergoing cardiac rehabilitation should learn to assess their own pulse rates to determine their response to exercise.

BLOOD PRESSURE
- Teach client risk factors for hypertension. Persons with family history of hypertension are at significant risk. Obesity, cigarette smoking, heavy alcohol consumption, high blood cholesterol and triglyceride levels, and continued exposure to stress are factors linked to hypertension (Joint National Committee, 1997).
- Clients with hypertension should learn about their BP values, long-term follow-up care and therapy, the usual lack of symptoms, therapy's ability to control but not cure, and benefits of a consistently followed treatment plan.
- Instruct clients on the importance of appropriate size blood pressure cuff for home use.
- Instruct primary caregiver to take BP at same time each day and after client has had a brief rest. Take BP sitting or lying down, use same position and arm each time pressure is taken.
- Instruct primary caregiver that if it is difficult to hear the pressure, it may be that the cuff is too loose, not big enough, or too narrow; the stethoscope is not over arterial pulse; cuff was deflated too quickly or too slowly; or cuff was not pumped high enough for systolic readings.

RESPIRATIONS
- Clients who demonstrate decreased ventilation may benefit from being taught deep breathing and coughing exercises (see Chapter 49).
- Instruct family member to contact home care nurse of physician if unusual fluctuations in respiratory rate occur.
- Teach client signs and symptoms of hypoxemia: headache, somnolence, confusion, dusky color, shortness of breath, dyspnea.
- Teach client effect of high-risk behaviors such as cigarette smoking on oxygen saturation.

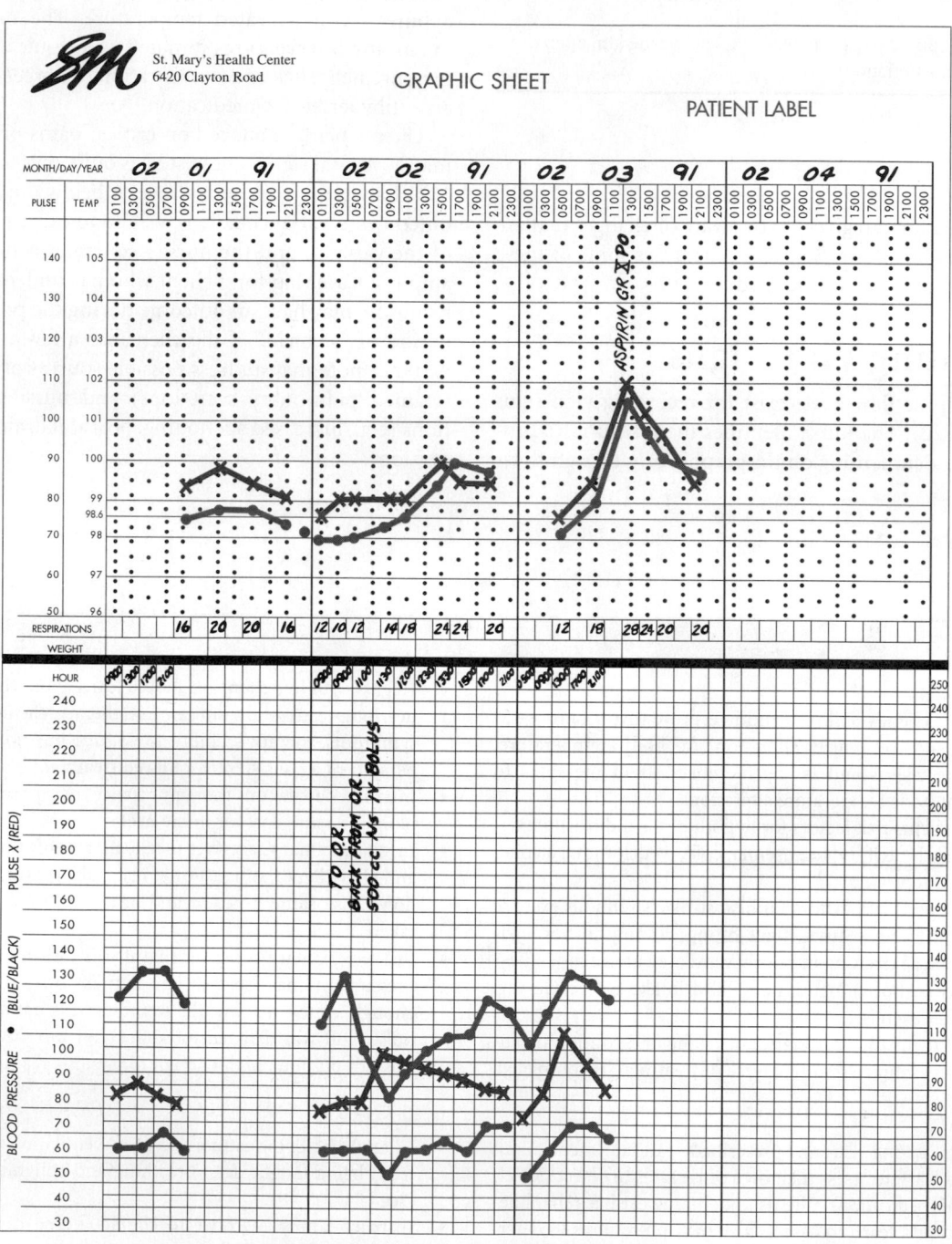

Figure 31-22   Vital signs graphic flow sheet.
Courtesy of St. Mary's Health Center, St. Louis, Mo.

NURSING PRACTICE

Box 31-21

TEMPERATURE

- The temperature of older adults is at the lower end of the normal temperature range, 36° C (96.8° F).
- Temperatures considered within normal range may reflect a fever in an older adult.
- Older adults are very sensitive to slight changes in temperature (Lueckenotte, 1996).
- Environmental temperature plays a greater role in older adults because their thermoregulatory systems are not as efficient (Lueckenotte, 1996).
- A decrease in sweat gland reactivity in the older adult results in a higher threshold for sweating at high temperature, which can lead to hyperthermia and heatstroke (Burke and Walsh, 1997).
- With aging, a loss of subcutaneous fat reduces the insulating capacity of the skin; older men are at especially high risk for hypothermia (Burke and Walsh, 1997).

PULSE RATE

- It is often difficult to palpate the pulse of an older adult or obese client. A Doppler device will provide a more accurate reading.
- The older adult has a decreased heart rate at rest (Lueckenotte, 1996).
- Once elevated, the pulse rate of an older adult takes longer to return to normal resting rate.
- When assessing elderly women with sagging breasts, the breast tissue is gently lifted and the stethoscope placed at the fifth ICS or the lower edge of the breast.
- Heart sounds may be muffled or difficult to hear in older adults because of an increase in air space in the lungs.

BLOOD PRESSURE

- Older adults, especially those who are frail, have lost upper arm mass, requiring special attention to selection of BP cuff size.
- An older adult's BP may elevate with age.
- Older adults have an increase in systolic pressure related to decreased vessel elasticity. The diastolic pressure remains the same, resulting in a wider pulse pressure (Lueckenotte, 1996).
- Older adults are instructed to change position slowly and wait after each change to avoid postural hypotension and prevent injuries.

RESPIRATIONS

- Aging causes ossification of costal cartilage and downward slant of ribs, resulting in a more rigid rib cage, which reduces chest wall expansion. Kyphosis and scoliosis that can occur in older adults may also restrict chest expansion and decrease tidal volume (Lueckenotte, 1996).
- Older adults may depend more on accessory abdominal muscles during respiration than on weakened thoracic muscles (Burke and Walsh, 1997).
- Decreased efficiency of respiratory muscles results in breathlessness at low exercise levels (Lueckenotte, 1996).
- Responses to hypercapnia and hypoxia are reduced 50% in older adults as compared with the young, limiting the ability of older adults to respond to hypoxia with respiratory changes.
- Identifying an acceptable pulse oximeter probe site may be difficult on older adults because of the likelihood of peripheral vascular disease, decreased cardiac output, cold-induced vasoconstriction, and anemia.

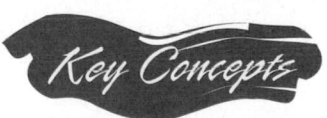

Key Concepts

- Vital signs include the physiological measurement of temperature, pulse, blood pressure, respirations, and oxygen saturation.
- Vital signs are measured as part of a complete physical examination or in a review of a client's condition.
- The nurse assesses vital sign changes with other physical assessment findings, using clinical judgment to determine measurement frequency.
- Knowledge of the factors influencing vital signs assists the nurse in determining and evaluating abnormal values.
- Vital signs provide a basis for evaluating response to nursing interventions.
- Vital signs are best measured when the client is inactive and the environment is controlled for comfort.

- The nurse assists the client in maintaining body temperature by initiating interventions that promote heat loss, production, or conservation.
- A fever is one of the body's normal defense mechanisms.
- The tympanic route is the most accessible and acceptable site for core temperature measurement.
- Rectal temperature measurements should not be performed on newborn infants or adults with rectal alterations.
- To assess cardiac function, pulse rate and rhythm are most easily measured using the radial or apical pulse.
- Respiratory assessment includes measurement to determine the effectiveness of ventilation, perfusion, and diffusion.

- Assessment of respirations involves observing ventilatory movements throughout the respiratory cycle.
- Oxygen saturation is influenced by variables affecting ventilation, perfusion, and diffusion.
- Several hemodynamic variables contribute to blood pressure determination.
- Hypertension is diagnosed only after an average of readings made during two or more subsequent visits reveals an elevated blood pressure.
- Errors in blood pressure measurement can be made by selecting and applying the cuff improperly.
- Changes in one vital sign can influence characteristics of the other vital signs.

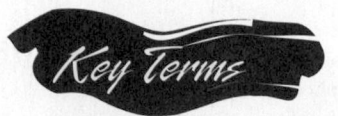

Key Terms

Afebrile, *p. 675*	Hypertension, *p. 708*
Antipyretics, *p. 689*	Hyperthermia, *p. 676*
Auscultatory gap, *p. 717*	Hypotension, *p. 709*
Basal metabolic rate (BMR), *p. 672*	Hypothalamus, *p. 671*
	Hypothermia, *p. 676*
Blood pressure, *p. 706*	Hypoxemia, *p. 698*
Bradycardia, *p. 697*	Malignant hyperthermia, *p. 676*
Calorie, *p. 673*	
Cardiac output, *p. 690*	Nonshivering thermogenesis, *p. 672*
Celsius, *p. 677*	
Conduction, *p. 672*	Orthostatic hypotension, *p. 709*
Convection, *p. 673*	
Core temperature, *p. 671*	Perfusion, *p. 698*
Diaphoresis, *p. 673*	Postural hypotension, *p. 709*
Diastolic, *p. 706*	Pulse deficit, *p. 697*
Diffusion, *p. 698*	Pulse pressure, *p. 706*
Dysrhythmia, *p. 697*	Pyrogens, *p. 675*
Eupnea, *p. 698*	Radial pulse, *p. 691*
Evaporation, *p. 673*	Radiation, *p. 672*
Fahrenheit, *p. 677*	Shivering, *p. 672*
Febrile, *p. 675*	Sphygmomanometer, *p. 713*
Fever, *p. 674*	Stroke volume, *p. 690*
Fever of unknown origin (FUO), *p. 676*	Systolic, *p. 706*
	Tachycardia, *p. 697*
Frostbite, *p. 677*	Thermoregulation, *p. 671*
Heat exhaustion, *p. 676*	Tidal volume, *p. 698*
Heatstroke, *p. 676*	Ventilation, *p. 698*
Hematocrit, *p. 707*	Vital signs, *p. 669*
Hyperpyrexia, *p. 674*	

Critical Thinking Exercises

1. A 47-year-old African-American man is coming to the health clinic for a physical examination by the nurse practitioner for a routine employment physical.

The nursing assistant obtains the following routine vital signs: tympanic temperature, 36.9° C (98.4° F); right radial pulse rate of 96 and irregular; BP, sitting, right arm 162/82, left arm 150/70; SpO$_2$, 95% on room air; respiratory rate 22.

   a. As the admitting nurse, what questions would you ask this client to evaluate his risk for hypertension?

   b. Based on these vital signs, what actions should you take?

2. A teenage mother brings her 3-year-old child to the walk-in health center. She notes that he has been fussy, has not had much of an appetite, and is not his active self. The boy is crying and struggling to get out of his mother's lap during your interview. You note that he is small for his age, but otherwise well developed.

   a. Describe the sequence you would use for obtaining vital signs.

   b. When selecting the appropriate equipment for obtaining the vital signs, what, if any, special considerations are needed?

   c. The unlicensed caregiver reports she has obtained a temperature of 37.7° C (99.8° F). What additional information do you request from the caregiver?

3. A 52-year-old woman is admitted to the medical unit for chronic dyspnea and discomfort in her left chest with deep breathing and coughing. She has been smoking for 35 years and has a 20-year history of emphysema. Over the past 4 months she has lost 10 pounds and currently weighs 110 pounds.

   a. When delegating the vital signs to the unlicensed assistant what information and directions should you provide?

   b. The blood pressure and heart rate are within acceptable ranges. The temperature is 37.5° C (99.5° F) tympanic, the respiratory rate 32 and shallow, the SpO$_2$ 89%. Based on these results, list your actions in priority.

4. An 82-year-old resident in your subacute extended care facility is being treated for pneumonia with antibiotics. She has been on bed rest for the past 2 days. She has a history of hypertension, treated with diuretics, but is otherwise healthy. She has been afebrile for the past 24 hours and is eager to walk to the activity room. She has activity orders "up ad lib."

   a. Should you delegate the ambulation assistance to an unlicensed caregiver?

   b. What places this client at risk for fainting?

   c. Explain to this patient the reason you are obtaining orthostatic measurements.

References

Beaudry M, VandenBosch T, Anderson J: Research utilization: once-a-day temperatures for afebrile patients, *Clin Nurse Spec* 10(1):21, 1996.

Bliss-Holtz J: Methods of newborn infant temperature monitoring: a research review, *Issues Compr Pediatr Nurs* 18:287, 1995.

Brashers VL: *Clinical applications of pathophysiology,* St. Louis, 1998, Mosby.

Braun SK, Preston P, Smith RN: Getting a better read on thermometry, *RN* 61(3):57, 1998.

Bridges EJ, Middleton R: Direct arterial vs oscillometric monitoring of blood pressure: stop comparing and pick one (a decision-making algorithm), *Crit Care Nurse* 17(3):58, 1997.

Burke MM, Walsh MB: *Gerontologic nursing,* St. Louis, 1997, Mosby.

Carroll P: Using pulse oximetry in the home, *Home Health Nurse* 15(2):89, 1997.

Cusson RA, Madonia JA, Taekman JB: The effect of environment on body site temperatures in full-term neonates, *Nurs Res* 46(4):202, 1997.

Goodfellow LM: The oxyhemoglobin in dissociation curve in respiratory management, *Crit Care Nurs Q* 20(2):22, 1997

Guyton AC: *Textbook of medical physiology,* ed 9, Philadelphia, 1995, WB Saunders.

Haddock BJ, Merrow DL, Swanson MS: The falling grace of axillary temperatures, *Pediatr Nurs* 22(2):121, 1996.

Hanna D: Equipment guidelines for pulse oximetry use in pediatrics, *J Pediatr Nurs* 10(2):124, 1995.

Hasel KL, Erickson RS: Effect of cerumen on infrared ear temperature measurement, *J Gerontol Nurs* 21(2):6, 1995

Hazinski MF: *Nursing care of the critically ill child,* ed 2, St. Louis, 1991, Mosby.

Henker R, Coyne C: Comparison of peripheral temperature measurements with core temperature, *AACN Clin Issues* 6(1):21, 1995.

Holtzclaw B: Thermal balance. In Kinney and others, editors: *AACN's clinical reference for critical care nursing,* ed 4, St. Louis, 1998, Mosby.

Joint National Committee on Detection, Evaluation and Treatment of High Blood Pressure: The sixth report of the Joint National Committee on Detection, Evaluation and Treatment of High Blood Pressure, *Arch Intern Med* 157:2413, 1997.

Kinney MR and others: AACN's clinical reference for critical care nursing, ed 4, St. Louis, 1998, Mosby.

Leick-Rude M, Bloom LF: A comparison of temperature taking methods in neonates, *Neonatal Netw* 17(5):21, 1998.

Lueckenotte AG: *Gerontologic nursing,* St. Louis, 1996, Mosby.

Material Safety Data Sheet: *Mercury,* Houston, 1989, Curtin Matheson Scientific.

National High Blood Pressure Education Program; National Heart, Lung, and Blood Institute; National Institutes of Health: The sixth report of the Joint National Committee on Detection, Evaluation, and Treatment of High Blood Pressure, *Arch Intern Med* 157:2413, 1997.

National Institutes of Health: *National Heart, Lung and Blood Institute update on the task force report (1987) on high blood pressure in children and adolescents,* Bethesda, Md, 1996, NIH.

Roper M: Assessing orthostatic vital signs, *Am J Nurs* 96(8):43, 1996.

Rowsey PJ: Pathophysiology of fever. I. The role of the cytokines, *Dimens Crit Care Nurs* 16(4):202, 1997.

Severine JE, McKenzie NE: Advances in temperature monitoring: a far cry from "shake and take," *Nursing 97* 27(5): Supplement, 1997.

Thibodeau GA, Patton KT: *Anatomy and physiology,* ed 3, St. Louis, 1996, Mosby.

Thomas SA, DeKeyser R: Blood pressure, *Annu Rev Nurs Res* 14:3, 1996.

Tittle M, Flynn MB: Correlation of pulse oximetry and co-oximetry, *Dimens Crit Care Nurs* 16(2):88, 1997.

Wong DL and others: *Whaley and Wong's nursing care of infants and children,* ed 6, St. Louis, 1998, Mosby.

Yeo S, Scarbough M: Exercise-induced hyperthermia may prevent accurate core temperature measurement by tympanic membrane thermometer, *J Nurs Meas* 4(2):143, 1996.

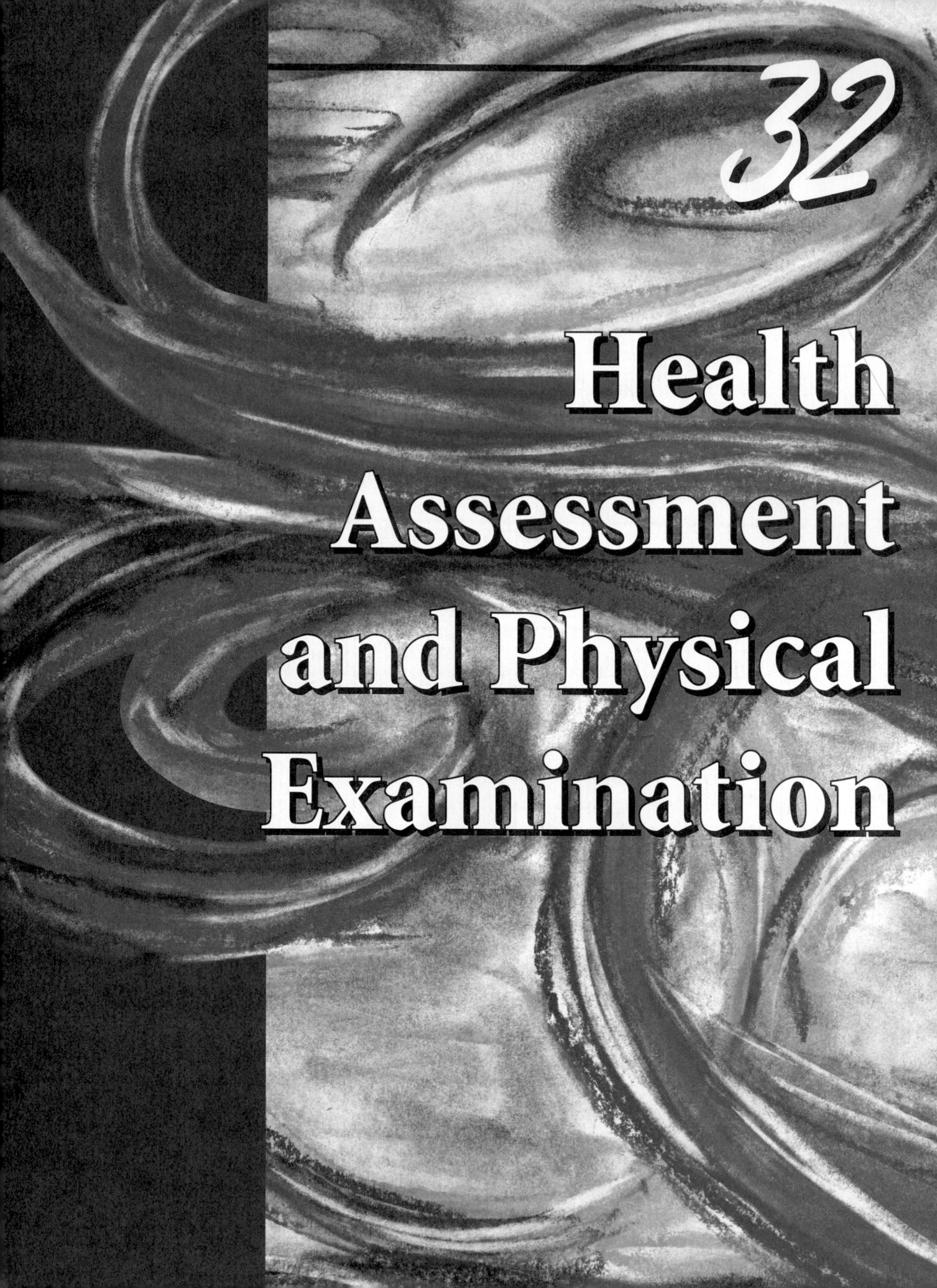

32

Health Assessment and Physical Examination

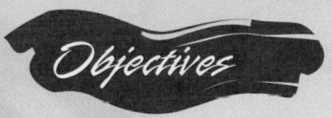

Mastery of content in this chapter will enable the student to:

- Define the key terms listed.
- Discuss the purposes of physical assessment.
- Describe the techniques used with each physical assessment skill.
- Discuss the importance of understanding cultural diversity as it influences the approach to health assessment.
- List techniques used to prepare a client physically and psychologically before and during an examination.
- Describe interview techniques used to enhance communication during history taking.
- Make environmental preparations before an examination.
- Identify information to collect from the nursing history before an examination.
- Discuss normal physical findings in a young and middle-age adult compared with an older adult.
- Discuss ways to incorporate health teaching into the examination.
- Use physical assessment skills during routine nursing care.
- Describe physical measurements made in the assessment of each body system.
- Identify self-screening examinations commonly performed by clients.
- Identify preventive screenings and the appropriate age(s) for each screening to occur.
- Document findings on a physical examination form.
- Communicate abnormal findings to appropriate personnel.

Nurses are most often the first persons to detect changes in clients' conditions, regardless of the setting. For this reason, the ability to think critically and interpret the meaning of client behaviors and presenting physiological changes is very important. The skills of physical assessment and examination provide nurses with powerful tools to detect subtle, as well as obvious, changes in a client's health. Physical assessment enables the nurse to assess patterns reflecting health problems and to evaluate the client's progress following therapy.

The nurse works in a variety of settings, seeking information about clients' health status. The nurse conducts health assessments at health fairs, at screening clinics, in physicians' offices, in acute care agencies, and in the client's home. Health screenings involve measurement of specific physical functions or diagnostic tests to detect persons with high probabilities of having a disease or condition. For example, blood pressure screenings detect the risk for high blood pressure. A tuberculin skin test identifies persons exposed to tuberculosis. Information from health screenings determines the need for more comprehensive examinations.

A complete health assessment involves a more detailed review of a client's condition. The nurse collects a nursing history (see Chapter 14) and performs a behavioral and physical examination. The health history involves a lengthy interview with a client to gather subjective data about the client's level of wellness (present and past), family history, changes in life patterns, sociocultural history, spiritual health, and mental and emotional reactions to illness. The interview is an opportunity for the nurse to establish a relationship with the client that promotes sharing of information. A physical examination is a head-to-toe review of each body system that offers objective information about the client and allows the nurse to make clinical judgments. The client's condition and response affect the extent of the examination. The accuracy of a physical assessment influences the choice of therapies a client receives and the determination of the response to those therapies. Continuity in health care improves when the nurse makes ongoing, objective, and comprehensive assessment.

Purposes of Physical Examination

An examination should be designed for the client's needs. If a client is acutely ill, the nurse recognizes the presenting symptoms and may choose to assess only the involved body systems. A more comprehensive examination is conducted when the client feels more at ease, and the nurse then learns about the client's total health status. A complete physical examination is performed for routine screening to promote wellness behaviors and preventive health care measures; to determine the client's eligibility for health insurance, military service, or a new job; or for the client's admission to a hospital or long-term care facility. The nurse uses physical assessment for the following reasons:

To gather baseline data about the client's health

To supplement, confirm, or refute data obtained in the nursing history

To confirm and identify nursing diagnoses

To make clinical judgments about a client's changing health status and management

To evaluate the physiological outcomes of care

GATHERING A HEALTH HISTORY

The main objective of interacting with clients is to find out what is central to their concerns and to help find solutions. It is important for the nurse to pay attention to clients' worries and to direct an interview and examination so that a clear picture is created of their condition. This means that collection of a health history and a physical examination require patience and a dedication to thoroughness and detail. There are some basic principles that can help in conducting a successful health history (see Chapter 14) and in laying the groundwork for a well-organized physical examination. The interview allows the nurse to form a partnership with the client so that the interview is oriented to the client, not to a disease. Knowing one's own idiosyncrasies (e.g., wanting to be liked, fear of harming the client, or catching a disease) can prevent resultant feelings from harming the relationship with the client.

DEVELOPING NURSING DIAGNOSES AND A CARE PLAN

The nursing health history allows the nurse to gather a complete and detailed database about the client's health status. After collecting a history, the nurse conducts a physical assessment to refute, confirm, or supplement the existing database. The nurse critically thinks about the information provided by the client, applies knowledge from previous clinical care, and methodically conducts an examination to create a clear picture of the client's status. For example, a client may complain of back pain. The nurse asks several questions to clarify the nature of the pain. During the examination the nurse carefully looks for the source of the pain (e.g., discomfort when changing position or a bruise across the client's back) to rule out a variety of potential ailments.

One assessment finding cannot conclusively reveal the nature of an abnormality. A complete assessment is needed to form a definitive diagnosis. The nurse learns to group significant findings into patterns of data that reveal actual or "risk for" nursing diagnoses. In addition, each abnormal finding directs the nurse to gather additional information. Information gathered during an initial physical assessment provides a baseline of the client's functional abilities. The baseline is not necessarily the normal range of physical findings but rather the pattern of findings identified when the client was first assessed. This baseline serves as a comparison for future assessment findings. During a subsequent assessment the nurse can determine whether the client's condition has changed.

The accuracy of the database allows the nurse to develop individualized nursing diagnoses (Table 32-1). Physical assessment findings help determine the etiology of diagnoses so that the nurse can select the correct type of interventions for the care plan. Physical assessment is ongoing, and thus the care plan changes with the client's condition. The nurse monitors the client's progress and responses to therapies to review existing diagnoses and identify new problems.

MANAGING CLIENT PROBLEMS

When caring for clients, the nurse makes many observations and performs a variety of therapies. Yet the nurse's success in giving care depends on the ability to recognize change in status and to modify therapies so that clients gain the most desirable outcome. Physical assessment skills allow the nurse to judge the status of the client's health and direct the management of care. For example, the nurse inspects the skin during a routine bath and finds it excessively dry. The nurse does not use soap and applies body lotion to the skin. The nurse revises the written care plan so that other nurses know the type of skin care to provide. Instruction is also given to the client about skin

Table 32-1 **Development of Individualized Nursing Diagnoses**			
Assessment Method	Findings	Patterns	Nursing Diagnosis
Inspection of skin	Skin along sacral area is intact. There is 3-cm area of redness around coccyx; skin blanches on palpation. No skin lesions are observed.	There is pressure area around coccyx.	Risk for impaired skin integrity.
Palpation of skin	Skin is moist from diaphoresis. There is tenderness to palpation around sacral area. There is good skin turgor.	Skin moisture promotes maceration.	
Historical data	Client suffered fractured left leg. Client is immobilized as a result of left leg traction.	Continued pressure is exerted over sacrum.	

care. Performing the mechanics of physical assessment is relatively simple. The more difficult challenge lies in using findings to make decisions.

EVALUATING NURSING CARE

Nurses become accountable for their nursing care by evaluating the results of nursing interventions. Physical assessment skills enhance the evaluation of nursing measures through monitoring physiological and behavioral outcomes of care. The same physical assessment skills used to assess a condition (e.g., palpation of the client's pulse) can be used as an evaluation measure after care is administered (e.g., an evaluation of a client's tolerance to an exercise plan).

Nurses make accurate, detailed, objective measurements through physical assessment. The measurements determine whether the expected outcomes of care are met.

Cultural Sensitivity

As is the case with any other aspect of nursing, a physical examination must be performed with the nurse respecting the cultural differences of clients. How individuals behave as a result of their cultural heritage influences their willingness to assume responsibility for their health and their tendency to seek professional health care. This is important for the nurse to remember before attempting to conduct a physical examination. A client's health beliefs, use of alternative therapies, nutritional habits, relationships with family, and comfort with the nurse's physical closeness during an examination and history taking must be considered.

It is extremely important for nurses to remain culturally aware and to avoid stereotyping clients on the basis of gender or race. There is a sharp difference between distinguishing cultural characteristics and distinguishing physical characteristics. It is important for nurses to learn common disorders of those ethnic populations within the nurse's community. For example, Navajo Indians often have ear anomalies, Polynesians often suffer clubfoot, and many blacks experience sickle cell disease. Similarly, it is important to know variations in physical characteristics, such as in the skin and musculoskeletal system, that are related to cultural variables. Recognition of cultural diversity helps the nurse to respect a client's uniqueness and to provide care of a higher quality.

Integration of Physical Assessment With Nursing Care

Whether a complete or partial physical assessment is performed, an examination should be integrated into routine care. For example, the nurse can assess the condition of the skin and other body parts during a bed bath. When a client undergoes oral hygiene, the nurse can carefully assess oral cavity structures. As a client ambulates down the hall, the nurse assesses the client's range of motion and gait. This practice makes more efficient use of time. The nurse also learns that physical assessment should become an automatic behavior when the nurse and client interact. Physical assessment skills enable the nurse to gather more comprehensive and relevant assessment findings.

Skills of Physical Assessment

Chapter 14 briefly describes the skills of inspection, palpation, percussion, and auscultation. This chapter provides a more detailed description of those skills and their application in the physical examination.

INSPECTION

Inspection is the process of observation. The nurse inspects body parts to detect normal characteristics or significant physical signs. An experienced nurse learns to make several observations, almost simultaneously, while becoming very perceptive of early warnings of abnormalities. The secret to inspection is to always pay attention to the client, watching all movements and looking very carefully at any body part or area being inspected.

It helps to know normal physical characteristics before trying to distinguish abnormal findings. It is especially important to know normal characteristics of clients of different ages. Dry, wrinkled, inelastic skin is normal in an older adult but not in a young adult. Experience is needed to recognize normal variations among clients, as well as ranges of normal in an individual. Inspection is a simple technique, but it is often underused. For example, when hurrying to complete a bath, a nurse may fail to inspect all skin surfaces and overlook a rash under the client's arm. The quality of an inspection depends on the nurse's willingness to spend time doing a thorough job. To use inspection effectively, the nurse observes the following principles:

Make sure good lighting is available.

Position and expose body parts so that all surfaces can be viewed.

Inspect each area for size, shape, color, symmetry, position, and abnormalities.

If possible, compare each area inspected with the same area on the opposite side of the body.

Use additional light (e.g., a penlight) to inspect body cavities.

Do not hurry inspection. Pay attention to detail.

After inspection of a body part is completed, findings may indicate further examination. Palpation is often used with or after visual inspection.

PALPATION

Further assessment of body parts is made through the sense of touch. Through palpation the hands can make delicate and sensitive measurements of specific physical signs, including resistance, resilience, roughness, texture, and mobility (Table 32-2). The nurse uses different parts of the hand when touching the skin to detect characteristics such as texture and temperature.

The client should be relaxed and positioned comfortably because muscle tension during palpation impairs its effectiveness. Asking the client to take slow, deep breaths enhances muscle relaxation. Placing the arms along the side of the body will decrease abdominal rigidity. Tender areas are palpated last. The nurse asks the client to point out the more sensitive areas and notes any nonverbal signs of discomfort.

Clients appreciate warm hands, short fingernails, and a gentle approach. Palpation may be either light or deep and is controlled by the amount of pressure applied with the fingers or hand. Light palpation always precedes deep palpation. The nurse applies tactile pressure slowly, gently, and deliberately. Light palpation of structures such as the abdomen determines areas of tenderness (Figure 32-1, *A*). The nurse's hand is placed on the part to be examined and depressed about 1 cm (½ inch). Tender areas are examined further for potentially serious abnormalities. The sensation of touch is best preserved with light, intermittent pressure. Heavy, prolonged pressure causes a loss of sensitivity in the nurse's hand.

After light palpation, deeper palpation is used to examine the condition of organs, such as those in the abdomen (Figure 32-1, *B*). The nurse depresses the area being examined approximately 2 to 4 cm (1 to 2 inches) (Seidel and others, 1999). Caution is the rule. A nursing student should not attempt deep palpation without clinical supervision to avoid injuring a client. Deep palpation may be applied with one hand or both hands (bimanually). When the nurse uses bimanual palpation, one hand (sensing hand) is relaxed and placed lightly over the client's skin. The other hand (active hand) applies pressure to the sensing hand. The lower hand does not exert pressure directly and thus retains the sensitivity needed to detect organ characteristics.

The most sensitive parts of the hand, the palmar surface of the fingers and finger pads, are used to assess position, texture, size, consistency, form of a mass, and pulsation (Figure 32-2, *A*). Temperature is best measured using the dorsum or back of the hand (Figure 32-2, *B*) and fingers, where the skin is thinnest. The palm or ulnar surface of the hand (Figure 32-2, *C*) is more sensitive to vibration. The nurse measures position, consistency, and turgor by lightly grasping the body part with the fingertips (Figure 32-2, *D*).

The nurse must not palpate without considering the client's condition. For example, if the client has a fractured rib, extra care is used to locate the painful area. A vital

Table 32-2	Examples of Characteristics Measured by Palpatation
Area Examined	**Criteria Measured**
Skin	Temperature
	Moisture
	Texture
	Turgor and elasticity
	Tenderness
	Thickness
Organs (e.g., liver and intestine)	Size
	Shape
	Tenderness
	Absence of masses
Glands (e.g., thyroid and lymph)	Swelling
	Symmetry and mobility
Blood vessels (e.g., carotid or femoral artery)	Pulse amplitude
	Elasticity
	Rate
	Rhythm
Thorax	Excursion
	Tenderness
	Fremitus

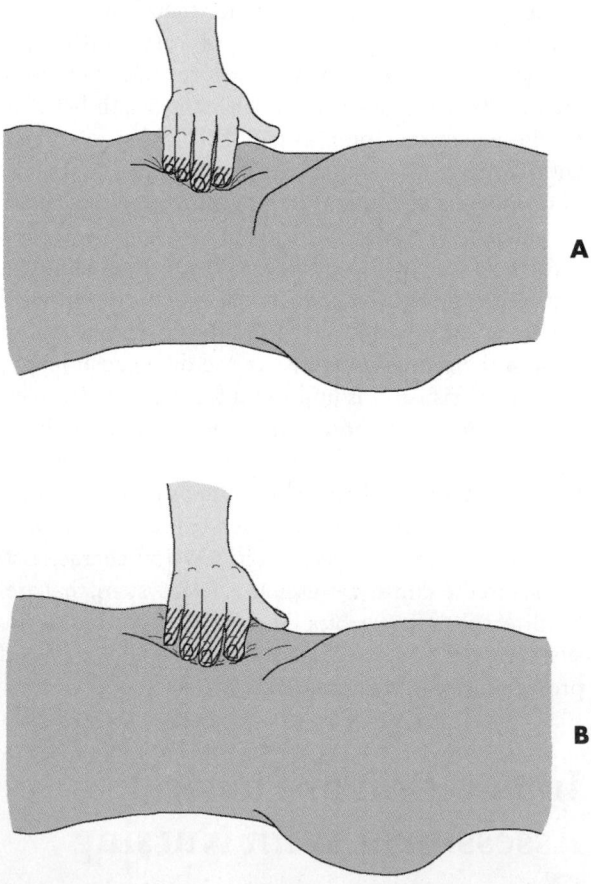

Figure 32-1 **A,** During light palpation, gentle pressure against underlying skin and tissues can detect areas of irregularity and tenderness. **B,** During deep palpation, the nurse depresses tissue to assess the condition of underlying organs.

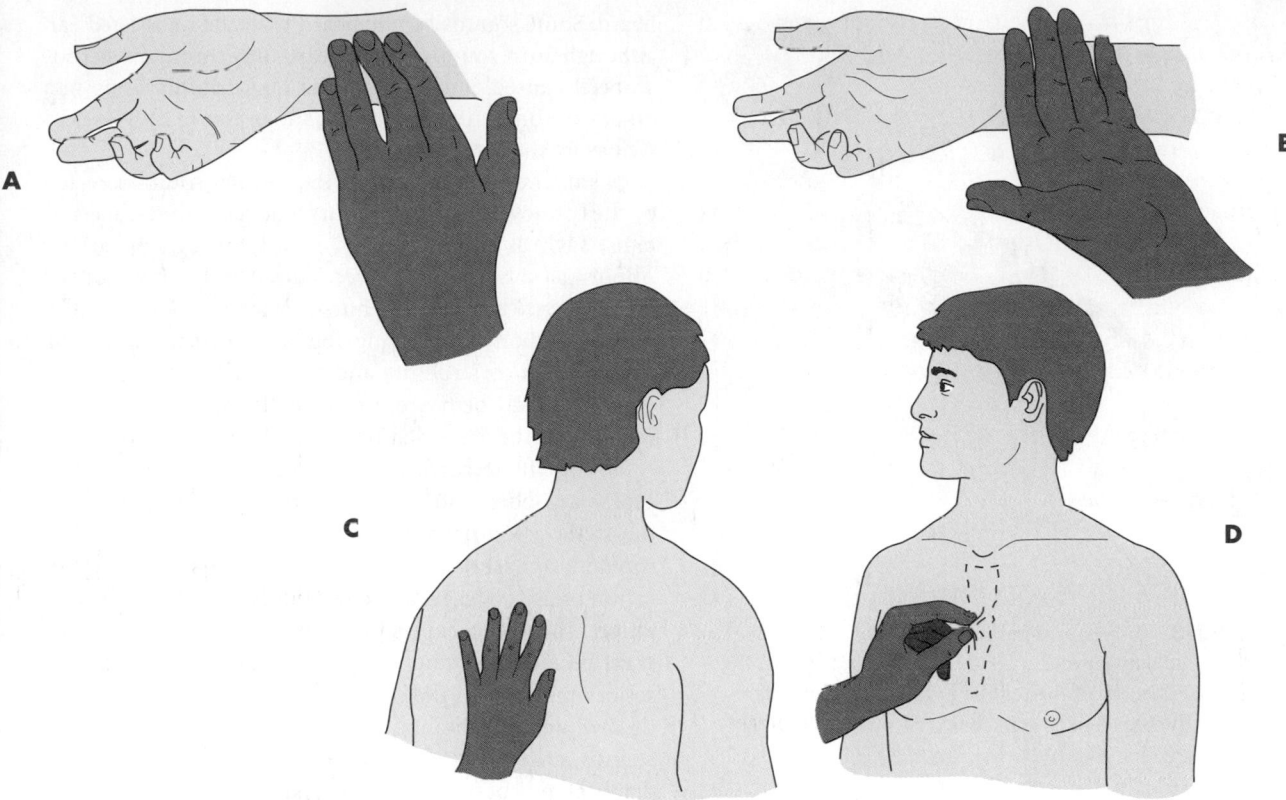

Figure 32-2 **A,** The radial pulse is detected with the pads of the fingertips, the most sensitive part of the hand. **B,** The dorsum of the hand allows the nurse to detect temperature variations in skin. **C,** The nurse uses the bony part of the palm at the base of the fingers to detect vibration. **D,** The nurse grasps the skin with the fingertips to assess turgor.

artery is not palpated with pressure that obstructs blood flow. The nurse also considers the body area being palpated, as well as the reason for using palpation, and must be able to discriminate and interpret the significance of what is sensed.

PERCUSSION

Percussion involves tapping the body with the fingertips to evaluate the size, borders, and consistency of body organs and to discover fluid in body cavities. It requires considerable skill. It is perhaps the least-used assessment skill; however, it can help to confirm other assessment findings. Through percussion the location, size, and density of an underlying structure are determined. Percussion helps verify abnormalities reported from x-ray studies or assessed through palpation and auscultation. For example, if the nurse hears abnormal breath sounds when auscultating the lungs, percussion may rule out the presence of consolidated fluid or air in the pleural space.

Percussion involves striking one object against another, thus producing vibration and subsequent sound waves. When the examiner strikes the body's surface with a finger, vibration is transmitted through the body tissues. Sound waves are heard as percussion tones arising from

vibrations 4 to 6 cm deep in body tissue (Seidel and others, 1999). The character of the sound depends on the density of the underlying tissue. For example, the normal lung transmits sounds with high intensity and low pitch, whereas the more solid liver transmits a high-pitched sound of soft intensity. By knowing the way that densities influence sound, the nurse can locate organs or masses, map their boundaries, and determine their size. An abnormal sound suggests a mass or substance such as air or fluid within an organ or body cavity.

The two methods of percussion are direct and indirect. The direct method involves striking the body surface directly with one or two fingers. The indirect technique is performed by placing the middle finger of the nondominant hand (called the pleximeter) firmly against the body surface, keeping the palm and remaining fingers off the skin. The tip of the middle finger of the dominant hand (called the plexor) strikes the base of the distal joint of the pleximeter (Figure 32-3). The examiner uses a quick, sharp stroke with the plexor finger, keeping the forearm stationary. The wrist remains relaxed to deliver the proper blow. If the blow is not sharp, if the pleximeter is held loosely, or if the palm rests on the body surface, the sound is dampened or softened, preventing transmission of

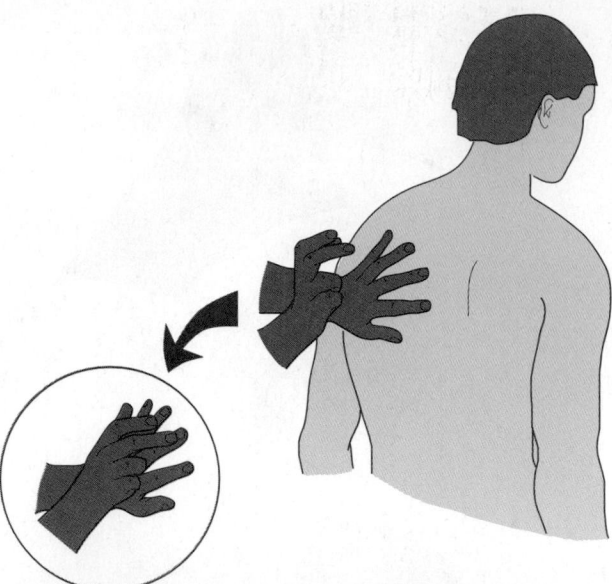

Figure 32-3   To perform indirect percussion, the nurse places the middle finger of the nondominant hand against the body's surface. The tip of the middle finger of the dominant hand strikes the top of the middle finger of the nondominant hand.

sound to underlying structures. The same force must be applied to each area so that an accurate comparison of sounds can be made. A light, quick blow usually produces the clearest sound. Use of direct versus indirect percussion or firm versus light percussion can lead to different interpretations of results.

Percussion produces five types of sounds: tympany, resonance, hyperresonance, dullness, and flatness. Each sound is created by certain types of underlying tissues and is judged by its intensity of pitch, duration, and quality (Table 32-3).

AUSCULTATION

Auscultation is listening to sounds produced by the body. This skill should be carried out last, except during the abdominal examination, after the other techniques have provided information that will assist in interpreting what is

heard. Some sounds can be heard with the unassisted ear, although most sounds can be heard only through a stethoscope. To auscultate correctly, the nurse should listen in a quiet environment, listening for the presence of sound, as well as its characteristics.

A student must first learn the normal sounds created by the cardiovascular, respiratory, and gastrointestinal systems, such as the passage of blood through an artery. Abnormal sounds can be recognized only after normal variations are learned. The nurse becomes more successful in auscultation by knowing the types of sounds arising from each body structure and the location in which they can most easily be heard. Likewise, the nurse becomes familiar with the areas that normally do not emit sounds.

To auscultate correctly, the nurse needs good hearing acuity, a good stethoscope, and knowledge of how to use the stethoscope properly. Nurses with hearing disorders should purchase stethoscopes with greater sound amplification or ask colleagues to check findings through auscultation. The stethoscope should always be placed on naked skin, because clothing obscures sound. Chapter 31 describes the parts of the stethoscope and the general use of the bell and diaphragm. The bell is best for low-pitched sounds, such as vascular and certain heart sounds, and the diaphragm is best for high-pitched sounds, such as bowel and lung sounds.

A nurse must become familiar with the stethoscope before attempting to use it on a client. It helps to practice using it with a friend. A number of extraneous sounds created by movement of the tubing or chestpiece interfere with auscultation of body organ sounds. By deliberately producing these sounds, the nurse learns to recognize and disregard them during the actual examination (Box 32-1). Through auscultation the nurse notes the following characteristics of sounds:

Frequency, or the number of oscillations generated per second by a vibrating object. The higher the frequency, the higher the pitch of a sound, and vice versa.

Loudness, or the amplitude of a sound wave. Auscultated sounds are described as loud or soft.

Quality, or sounds of similar frequency and loudness from different sources. Terms such as *blowing* or *gurgling* describe the quality of sound.

Table 32-3   Sounds Produced by Percussion

Sound	Intensity	Pitch	Duration	Quality	Common Location
Tympany	Loud	High	Moderate	Drumlike	Enclosed, air-containing space; gastric air bubble; puffed-out cheek
Resonance	Moderate to loud	Low	Long	Hollow	Normal lung
Hyperresonance	Very loud	Very low	Longer than resonance	Booming	Emphysematous lung
Dullness	Soft to moderate	High	Moderate	Thudlike	Liver
Flatness	Soft	High	Short	Flat	Muscle

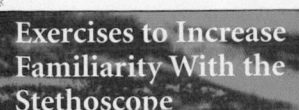

Exercises to Increase Familiarity With the Stethoscope | Box 32-1

Ensure that the earpiece follows the contour of the ear canal. Learn what fit is best for you by comparing amplification of sounds with the earpieces in both directions.

Place the earpieces in your ears with the tips of the earpieces turned toward the face. *Lightly* blow into the diaphragm. Again place the earpieces in your ears, this time with the ends turned toward the back of the head. *Lightly* blow into the diaphragm. After you have learned the right fit for the loudest amplification, wear the stethoscope the same way each time.

Put on the stethoscope and *lightly* blow into the diaphragm. If the sound is barely audible, *lightly* blow into the bell. Sound is carried through only one part of the chestpiece at a time. If the sound is greatly amplified through the diaphragm, the diaphragm is in position for use. If the sound is barely audible through the diaphragm, the bell is in position for use. Rotation of the diaphragm and bell places the chestpiece in the desired position. Leave the diaphragm in position for the next exercise.

Place the diaphragm over the anterior part of your chest. Ask a friend to speak in a normal conversational tone. Environmental noise seriously detracts from hearing the noise created by body organs. When a stethoscope is used, the client and the examiner should remain quiet.

Put the stethoscope on and gently tap the tubing. It is often difficult to avoid stretching or moving the stethoscope's tubing. The examiner should be in a position so that the tubing hangs free. Moving or touching the tubing creates extraneous sounds.

Care of the stethoscope: Earpieces should be removed regularly and cleaned of cerumen (ear wax). The bell and diaphragm are cleaned of dust, lint, and body oils. The tubing should be kept away from nurse's body oils. Avoid draping the stethoscope around the neck next to the skin. Cleansing the tubing with alcohol can dry and crack the material and is not recommended. Mild soap and water are preferred.

Duration, or the length of time that sound vibrations last. The duration of sound is short, medium, or long. Layers of soft tissue dampen the duration of sounds from deep internal organs.

Auscultation requires concentration and practice. Closing your eyes may help to focus on a particular sound. Taking time to listen to a sound is important. The nurse must also consider the part of the body auscultated and the causes of the sounds. For example, the first heart sound is caused by closure of the mitral valve. The nurse learns where sounds can best be heard. The first heart sound is best auscultated at the fifth intercostal space along the midclavicular line. The nurse also learns the characteristics of normal sounds. The first heart sound has the quality of a loud *lub*, whereas the second sound is a *dub*. After the cause and character of

normal auscultated sounds are understood, it becomes easier to recognize abnormal sounds and their origins.

OLFACTION

While assessing a client, the nurse should be familiar with the nature and source of body odors (Table 32-4). Olfaction helps the nurse detect abnormalities that cannot be recognized by any other means. For example, a client with a cast is expected to experience discomfort after an injury. However, the nurse who notes a strong odor will suspect that the discomfort may also be related to wound infection. The discomfort alone does not reveal the presence of infection. Findings from olfaction and other assessment skills allow the nurse to detect serious abnormalities.

Preparation for Examination

Proper preparation of the environment, equipment, and client ensures a smooth physical examination with few interruptions. A disorganized approach when preparing for a physical examination can cause errors and incomplete findings.

INFECTION CONTROL

During an examination the nurse may find clients with open skin lesions or weeping wounds. Examination techniques cause the nurse to contact body fluids and discharge. Standard precautions should be used throughout the examination (see Chapter 33) as appropriate. At times, it becomes necessary to wear gloves during palpation and percussion to reduce contact with microorganisms. If a client has excessive drainage from a wound, the examiner may need to wear a gown.

ENVIRONMENT

A physical examination requires privacy. A well-equipped examination room is preferable. However, in hospitals the examination usually occurs in the client's room, where it may be necessary to use room curtains or dividers around the bed. In the home the nurse may perform an examination in the client's bedroom.

Any examination room should be well equipped for all necessary procedures. Adequate lighting is needed for proper illumination of body parts. Primary lighting can be either daylight or artificial, as long as the light is direct enough to reveal skin characteristics without distortion from shadows. Ideally, an examination room is soundproofed so that clients feel comfortable discussing their conditions. The nurse eliminates sources of noise such as televisions or radios, takes steps to prevent interruptions from others, and makes sure the room is warm enough for the client's comfort.

Sometimes it is difficult to examine clients who are in beds or on stretchers. Special examination tables make clients easily accessible and help them assume special positions. The tables are high and narrow. The nurse must

Table 32-4 **Assessment of Characteristic Odors**		
Odor	Site or Source	Potential Causes
Alcohol	Oral cavity	Ingestion of alcohol, diabetes
Ammonia	Urine	Urinary tract infection
Body odor	Skin, particularly in areas where body parts rub together (e.g., under arms, and breasts)	Poor hygiene, excess perspiration (hyperhidrosis), foul-smelling perspiration (bromidrosis)
	Wound site	Wound abscess
	Vomitus	Undigested food
Feces	Rectal area	Bowel obstruction
		Fecal incontinence
Foul-smelling stools in infant	Stool	Malabsorption syndrome
Halitosis	Oral cavity	Poor dental and oral hygiene, gum disease
Sweet, fruity ketones	Oral cavity	Diabetic acidosis
Stale urine	Skin	Uremic acidosis
Sweet, heavy, thick odor	Draining wound	*Pseudomonas* (bacterial) infection
Musty odor	Casted body part	Infection inside cast
Fetid, sweet odor	Tracheostomy or mucus secretions	Infection of bronchial tree (*Pseudomonas* bacteria)

carefully assist clients so that they do not fall while getting on and off them. A confused, combative, or uncooperative client should not be left unsupervised on an examination table.

Examination tables are often hard and uncomfortable. When the client lies supine, the head of the table can be raised about 30 degrees. The client may also be given a small pillow. When examining a client in bed, the nurse can raise the bed to reach body parts more easily.

EQUIPMENT

Hand washing is done before equipment preparation and before the examination. Hand washing reduces the transmission of microorganisms. The equipment needed for an examination should be clean, readily available, and arranged in order for easy use (Figure 32-4). It should be kept warm as appropriate. The diaphragm of the stethoscope may be briskly rubbed between the hands before it is applied to the skin. Warm water should be run over the vaginal speculum. All equipment must be checked to ensure that it functions properly. The ophthalmoscope and otoscope require good batteries and lightbulbs. Equipment typically used is listed in Box 32-2.

PHYSICAL PREPARATION OF THE CLIENT

The client's physical comfort is vital for a successful examination. Before starting, the nurse asks if the client needs to use the toilet. An empty bladder and bowel facilitate examination of the abdomen, genitalia, and rectum and provide the opportunity to collect urine or fecal specimens. The nurse explains the proper method for collecting specimens and ensures that each specimen is properly labeled. When obtaining specimens, infection-control practices are necessary (see Chapter 33).

Physical preparation involves being sure the client is

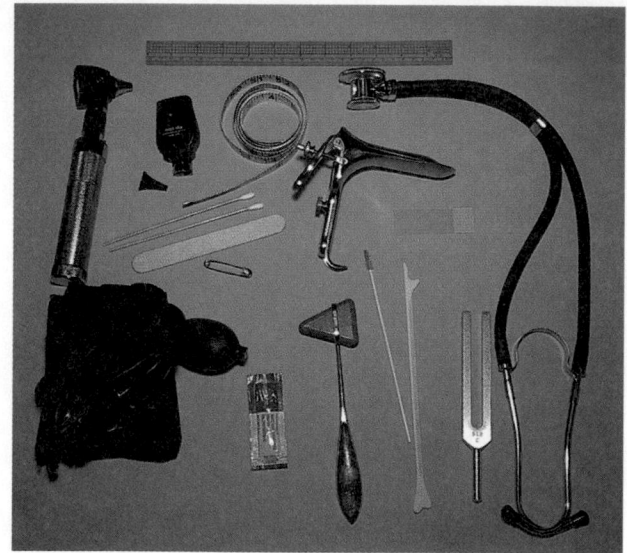

Figure 32-4   Equipment used during a physical examination.

dressed and draped properly. A client in the hospital will likely be wearing only a simple gown. In an outpatient setting the client is instructed to undress and apply a light cover gown. If the examination is limited to certain body systems, it may be unnecessary for the client to undress completely. The client should have privacy during undressing and plenty of time to finish. Walking into the room as the client undresses causes embarrassment. Drapes and gowns are made of linen or disposable paper. After clients have undressed and donned the gown, they should sit or lie down on the examination table with the drape over the lap or lower trunk. The examiner makes

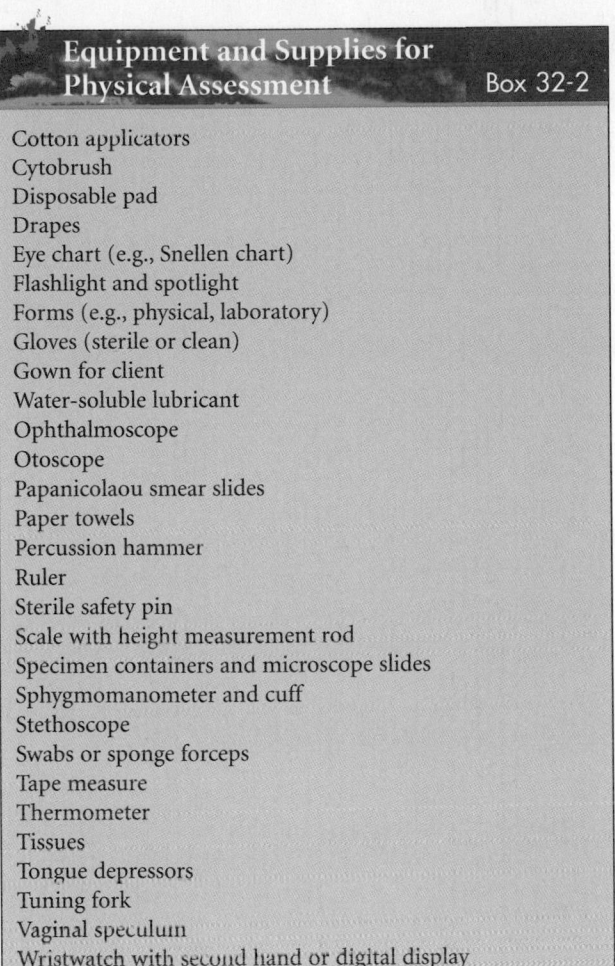

sure that the client stays warm by eliminating drafts, controlling room temperature, and providing warm blankets. A seriously ill client or older adult is more susceptible to chills. The nurse should ask if the client is comfortable. The client may become more relaxed if offered a pillow, sip of water, or tissue.

Positioning. During the examination the nurse asks clients to assume proper positions so that body parts are accessible and clients stay comfortable. Table 32-5 lists the preferred positions for each part of the examination and contains figures illustrating these positions. Clients' abilities to assume positions will depend on their physical strength, mobility, ease of breathing, age, and degree of wellness. Many of the positions, such as the lithotomy and knee-chest positions, are embarrassing and uncomfortable. Therefore clients should be kept in these positions no longer than necessary. The examiner explains the positions and assists clients in attaining them. The drapes are adjusted to be sure that the area to be examined is accessible and that no body part is unnecessarily exposed. More than one position can be assumed for the same part of an examination (e.g., supine and sitting for assessment of the anterior thorax), so the nurse first chooses the position that provides greater accessibility and accuracy in assessing body parts (sitting for assessment of the anterior thorax). However, if clients are too weak or are physically unable to assume a position, the nurse may choose an alternative position. The nurse uses extra care to position older adults so that they may avoid looking into the source of light, which can cause discomfort from glare.

PSYCHOLOGICAL PREPARATION OF THE CLIENT

Clients are easily embarrassed when forced to answer sensitive questions about bodily functions or when body parts are exposed and examined. The possibility that the examiner will find something abnormal also creates anxiety, so reduction of this anxiety may be the nurse's highest priority before the examination. The nurse should convey an open, receptive, and professional approach. A stiff, formal demeanor may inhibit the client's ability to communicate, but a style that is too casual may fail to instill confidence (Seidel and others, 1999). A thorough explanation lets clients know what to expect and what to do so that they can cooperate. The nurse first explains the examination in general terms. Then, as the nurse examines each body system, a more detailed explanation is given.

The nurse uses simple terms when describing the steps of the examination. Complicated terminology confuses clients and adds to their fears. The nurse's manner should be professional, but the voice tone and facial expressions should be relaxed to put clients at ease. The nurse encourages clients to ask questions and mention any discomfort they feel during the assessment. When the client and nurse are of opposite gender, it may be necessary to have a third person of the client's gender in the room, especially when examination of the sexual organs is required. The presence of a third person assures the client that the examiner will behave ethically, and the third person acts as a witness to the examiner's proper conduct.

During the examination the nurse watches the client's emotional responses. The nurse observes whether the client's facial expression conveys fear or concern and whether body movements reveal anxiety, such as frequently pulling the drape around the body or tensing up as the examiner touches the body. The nurse must remain calm and clearly explain each step of the assessment. It may be necessary to stop the examination and ask whether the client feels anxious, afraid, or uncomfortable. The client should not be forced to continue. Postponing the examination until a later time may be advantageous because the findings may be more accurate when the client can cooperate and relax. If the fears result from misconceptions, the nurse clarifies the purpose of the examination and how it is to be performed.

ASSESSMENT OF AGE-GROUPS

The nurse uses different interview styles and approaches to physical examination for clients of different age-groups.

Table 32-5 Positions for Examination

Position	Areas Assessed	Rationale	Limitations
Sitting	Head and neck, back, posterior thorax and lungs, anterior thorax and lungs, breasts, axillae, heart, vital signs, and upper extremities	Sitting upright provides full expansion of lungs and provides better visualization of symmetry of upper body parts.	Physically weakened client may be unable to sit. Examiner should use supine position with head of bed elevated instead.
Supine	Head and neck, anterior thorax and lungs, breasts, axillae, heart, abdomen, extremities, pulses	This is most normally relaxed position. It provides easy access to pulse sites.	If client becomes short of breath easily, examiner may need to raise head of bed.
Dorsal recumbent	Head and neck, anterior thorax and lungs, breasts, axillae, heart, abdomen	Position is used for abdominal assessment because it promotes relaxation of abdominal muscles.	Clients with painful disorders are more comfortable with knees flexed.
Lithotomy*	Female genitalia and genital tract	This position provides maximal exposure of genitalia and facilitates insertion of vaginal speculum.	Lithotomy position is embarrassing and uncomfortable, so examiner minimizes time that client spends in it. Client is kept well draped.
Sims'	Rectum and vagina	Flexion of hip and knee improves exposure of rectal area.	Joint deformities may hinder client's ability to bend hip and knee.
Prone	Musculoskeletal system	This position is used only to assess extension of hip joint.	This position is poorly tolerated in clients with respiratory difficulties.
Lateral recumbent	Heart	This position aids in detecting murmurs.	This position is poorly tolerated in clients with respiratory difficulties.
Knee-chest*	Rectum	This position provides maximal exposure of rectal area.	This position is embarrassing and uncomfortable.

*Clients with arthritis or other joint deformities may be unable to assume this position.

When assessing children, the nurse must be sensitive and anticipate the child's reaction to the examination as a strange and unfamiliar experience. Routine pediatric examinations have a focus on health promotion and illness prevention, particularly for the care of well children who receive competent parenting and have no serious health problems (Wong and others, 1999). The focus of the examination is on growth and development, sensory screening, dental examination, and behavioral assessment. Children who are chronically ill or disabled, foster children, and foreign-born adopted children may require additional examination visits. When examining children, the following tips assist in data collection:

> When obtaining histories on infants and children, gather all or part of the information from parents or guardians.
>
> Perform the examination in a nonthreatening area and provide time for play to become acquainted.
>
> Because parents may think they are being tested by the examiner, offer support during the examination and do not pass judgment.
>
> Call children by their first name, and address the parents as "Mr. and Mrs." rather than by their first names.
>
> Use open-ended questions to allow parents to share more information and describe more of the children's problems.
>
> Interview older children to allow observation of parent-child interactions. Also, older children can often provide details about their health history and severity of symptoms.
>
> Treat adolescents as adults and individuals because they tend to respond best when treated as such.
>
> Remember that adolescents have the right to confidentiality. After talking with parents about historical information, speak alone with adolescents.

A comprehensive health assessment and examination of older adults should include physical data, as well as a review of growth and development, family relationships, group involvement, and religious and occupational pursuits (Ebersole and Hess, 1998). An important part of health assessment involves analysis of the basic activities of daily living (dressing, bathing, toileting, feeding, and continence) that are fundamental to independent living. In addition, the more complex instrumental activities of daily living (using a telephone, preparing meals, managing money) are also assessed. Any examination of an older adult should also include an evaluation of mental status.

Throughout an examination the nurse must recognize that with advancing age the body does not respond vigorously to injury or disease. Therefore older persons do not always exhibit the expected signs and symptoms (Lueckenotte, 1998). Characteristically, older adults present more blunted or atypical signs and symptoms.

Principles to follow during examination of an older adult include the following:

> Do not stereotype aging clients. Most are able to adapt to change and to learn about their health. Similarly, they are reliable historians.
>
> Recognize that sensory or physical limitations can affect how quickly you are able to interview older adults and conduct examinations. Plan for more than one examination session. Sometimes it helps to give clients an initial health questionnaire before they come to a clinic or office (Ebersole and Hess, 1998).
>
> Perform the examination with adequate space; this is especially important for clients with mobility aids such as a cane or walker.
>
> During the examination use patience, allow for pauses, and observe for details. Recognize normalities of later life that would be abnormal in a younger client.
>
> Older clients may find giving certain types of health information stressful. Illness is seen as a threat to independence and a step toward institutionalization.
>
> Perform the examination near bathroom facilities. The client may experience an urgent need to void.
>
> Be alert to signs of increasing fatigue, such as sighing, grimacing, irritability, leaning against objects for support, and drooping of the head and shoulders.

Organization of the Examination

Regardless of the age of a client, a basic physical examination follows a similar approach. A physical examination is composed of individual assessments for each body system. The extent of an examination depends on its purpose and the client's condition. A client who comes to a clinic with symptoms of a severe chest cold will not routinely require a neurological assessment. A client entering the emergency department with an acute illness requires assessment of the body systems most at risk for being abnormal. When a client is admitted to the hospital, a complete examination is usually performed. A client who is receiving a routine health promotion examination may undergo specific preventive screenings, depending on the client's age or health risk (Table 32-6). Clients with specific symptoms or needs often require only portions of an examination. The nurse's judgment is needed to ensure that an examination is relevant and includes the correct observations.

The performance of a complete health assessment follows the format of the nursing history (see Chapter 14). The nurse uses information from the history to focus attention on specific parts of the examination. For example, if the history reveals symptoms of abdominal discomfort, the nurse examines the abdomen carefully. If the client reports difficulties in performing basic activities of daily living, the nurse carefully examines musculoskeletal and neurological function. Findings from the history generally reveal a pattern of related signs and symptoms. The phys-

Table 32-6	**Recommended Preventive Screenings**	
Disease/Condition	Age-Group	Screening Measures
Breast cancer*	Ages 20 to 39	Monthly breast self-examination (BSE)
		Clinical breast examination by health care professional every 3 years
	Ages 40 and up	Monthly BSE
		Annual clinical breast examination by health care professional
		Annual mammogram
Colon/rectal cancer*	Ages 50 and up	Men and women should have one of the following: fecal occult blood test (FDBT) and flexible sigmoidoscopy (if normal, repeat FDBT annually and flexible sigmoidoscopy every 5 years) or double contrast barium enema (if normal, repeat every 5 to 10 years). A digital rectal examination should be done at the same time as above. Earlier screening is needed if risk factors exist.
Ear disorders	All ages	Periodic hearing checks as needed
	Over age 65	Regular hearing checks
Eye disorders	Age 40 and under	Complete eye examination every 3 to 5 years (more if positive history)
	Ages 40 to 64	Complete eye examination every 2 years
	Age 65 and up	Complete eye examination every year
Heart/vascular disorders	Any age on advice of primary care provider	Regular measurement of total blood cholesterol levels and triglycerides; blood pressure screenings
Oral cavity/pharyngeal disorders/cancer	All ages (children, adults, older adults)	Regular dental examinations every 6 months
Ovarian cancer*	Age 18 and up or on becoming sexually active	Annual pelvic examinations by health care professional
Prostate cancer*	Ages 50 and up	Men who have at least a 10-year life expectancy should have a digital rectal examination and prostate specific antigen (PSA) blood test annually. Men at high risk require earlier screening.
Skin cancer*	All ages	Regular skin self-examination
Testicular cancer*	Age 15 and up	Monthly testicular self-examination (TSE)
Uterine cancer* Cervix	Age 18 and up or on becoming sexually active	Annual pelvic examination by health care professional plus an annual Pap test
Endometrium		Annual pelvic examination by health care professional
		Endometrial biopsy at menopause

*Data from American Cancer Society: *1999 cancer facts and figures,* New York, 1999, The Society.

ical examination supplements information from the history to confirm or refute the data.

The examination should be systematic and well organized so that important assessments are not omitted. A head-to-toe approach includes all body systems and helps the nurse anticipate each step. In an adult the nurse begins by assessing the head and neck area, progressing methodically down the body to incorporate all body systems. The following tips help the nurse keep an examination well organized:

Compare both sides of the body for symmetry. A degree of asymmetry is normal (e.g., the biceps muscles in the dominant arm may be more developed than the same muscles in the nondominant arm).

If a client is seriously ill, first assess the systems of the body more at risk for being abnormal. For example, a client with chest pain should undergo a cardiovascular assessment first.

If a client becomes fatigued, offer rest periods between assessments.

Perform painful procedures near the end of the examination.

Record results of the examination in specific anatomical and scientific terms so that any professional can interpret the findings (Figure 32-5).

Use common and accepted medical abbreviations to keep notes brief and concise.

Record quick notes during the examination to avoid keeping the client waiting. Complete any observations at the end of the examination.

A physical assessment form allows recording of information in the same sequence it is gathered.

General Survey

Assessment begins when the nurse first meets the client. The nurse determines the reason the client is seeking health care. Initial data from the general survey begins with a review of the client's primary health problems. The nurse makes mental notes of the client's behavior and ap-

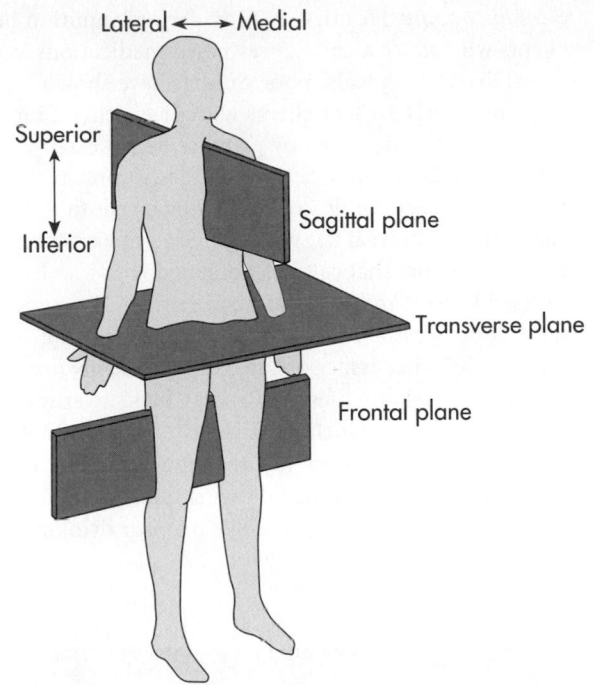

Figure 32-5   The nurse describes assessment findings in terms of the anatomical position within body planes.

pearance. The examination begins with a general survey that includes observation of general appearance and behavior, vital signs, and height and weight measurements. The survey provides information about characteristics of an illness, a client's hygiene and body image, emotional state, recent changes in weight, and developmental status. If abnormalities or problems are found, the affected body system is closely assessed later.

GENERAL APPEARANCE AND BEHAVIOR

Assessment of appearance and behavior begins while the nurse prepares the client for the examination. The review of general appearance and behavior includes the following:

- *Gender and race:* A person's gender affects the type of examination performed and the manner in which assessments are made. Different physical features are related to gender and race. Certain illnesses are more likely to affect a specific gender or race; for example, the incidence of skin cancer is 20 times higher in whites than in blacks, the incidence of pancreatic cancer is higher in African-Americans than in white Americans, and cancer of the bladder is more common in men (American Cancer Society [ACS], 1999).
- *Age:* Age influences normal physical characteristics. The ability to participate in some parts of the examination is also influenced by age.
- *Signs of distress:* There may be obvious signs or symptoms indicating pain, difficulty in breathing, or anxiety. These signs establish priorities regarding what to examine first.

- *Body type:* The nurse observes if a client appears trim and muscular, obese, or excessively thin. Body type can reflect the level of health, age, and lifestyle.
- *Posture:* Normal standing posture is an upright stance with parallel alignment of the hips and shoulders. Normal sitting posture involves some degree of rounding of the shoulders. Observe whether the client has a slumped, erect, or bent posture. Posture may reflect mood or presence of pain. Many older adults assume a stooped, forward-bent posture, with the hips and knees somewhat flexed and the arms bent at the elbows, raising the level of the arms.
- *Gait:* Observe the client walk into the room or at the bedside (if the client is ambulatory). Note whether movements are coordinated or uncoordinated. A person normally walks with the arms swinging freely at the sides, with the head and face leading the body.
- *Body movements:* Observe whether movements are purposeful and note if there are any tremors involving the extremities. Determine if any body parts are immobile.
- *Hygiene and grooming:* The client's level of cleanliness is noted by observing the appearance of the hair, skin, and fingernails. Observe if the client's clothes are clean. Grooming may depend on the activities being performed just before the examination, as well as the client's occupation. Also note the amount and type of cosmetics used.
- *Dress:* Culture, lifestyle, socioeconomic level, and personal preference affect the type of clothes worn. Note if the type of clothing worn is appropriate for the temperature and weather conditions. Depressed or mentally ill persons may be unable to choose proper clothing. An older adult tends to wear extra clothing because of the sensitivity to cold.
- *Body odor:* An unpleasant body odor may result from physical exercise, poor hygiene, or certain disease states. Poor oral hygiene may cause bad breath.
- *Affect and mood:* Affect is a person's feelings as they appear to others. A person's mood or emotional state is expressed verbally and nonverbally. Note if verbal expressions match nonverbal behavior and observe if the client's mood is appropriate for the situation. For example, the mood is inappropriate if the client seems unusually happy after recently being diagnosed with cancer. Observe facial expressions as questions are asked.
- *Speech:* Normal speech is understandable and moderately paced and shows an association with the person's thoughts. Note if the client talks rapidly or slowly. An abnormal pace may be caused by emotions or neurological impairment. Also note if the client speaks in a normal tone with clear inflection of words.
- *Client abuse:* Abuse of children, women, and older adults is a growing and serious health problem. It

may be suspected in clients who have suffered obvious physical injury or neglect (e.g., evidence of malnutrition or presence of bruising on the extremities or trunk). Assess for the client's fear of the spouse or partner, caregiver, parent, or adult child. Note if the partner or caregiver has a history of violence, alcoholism, or drug abuse. Is the person unemployed, ill, or frustrated in caring for the client? Most states mandate a report to a social service center if abuse or neglect is suspected. When abuse is suspected, interview the client in private. It is difficult to detect abuse, since victims often will not complain or report that they are in an abusive situation (Berlinger, 1998). Clients are much more likely to reveal any problems to a nurse when the suspected abuser is absent from the room (Lynch, 1997). Clinical indicators for abuse are summarized in Box 32-3.

- *Substance abuse.* Health care providers' recognition of clients who abuse alcohol, prescribed medications, or illegal drugs is typically poor. Studies have shown that only about 10% of clients who meet criteria for drug abuse are identified by primary health care providers (Caulker-Burnett, 1994). The problem affects all socioeconomic groups. A single visit to a clinic may not reveal the problem. Several visits often reveal behaviors that can be confirmed with a well-focused history and physical examination. The nurse must approach the client in a caring and nonjudgmental way, since issues of substance abuse involve both emotional and lifestyle issues. Clients to suspect for substance abuse include those listed in Box 32-4. When abuse is suspected, it is recommended that the nurse or examiner ask the following questions: Have you ever felt the need to *cut down* on your drinking

---

Clinical Indicators of Abuse   Box 32-3

Physical Findings	Behavioral Findings
CHILD SEXUAL ABUSE	
Vaginal or penile discharge	Problem in sleeping or eating
Blood on underclothing	Fear of certain people or places
Pain or itching in genital area	Play activities recreate the abuse situation
Genital injuries	Regressed behavior
Difficulty sitting or walking	Sexual acting out
Pain while urinating	Knowledge of explicit sexual matters
Foreign bodies in rectum, urethra, or vagina	Preoccupation with other's or own genitals
Venereal disease	
DOMESTIC ABUSE	
Injuries and trauma are inconsistent with reported cause	Attempted suicide
Multiple injuries involving head, face, neck, breasts, abdomen, and genitalia (black eyes, orbital fractures, broken nose, fractured skull, lip lacerations, broken teeth, strangulation marks)	Eating or sleeping disorders
	Anxiety
	Panic attacks
X-rays show old and new fractures in different stages of healing	Pattern of substance abuse (follows physical abuse)
Burns	Low self-esteem
Human bites	Depression
	Sense of helplessness
	Guilt
	Increased forgetfulness
OLDER ADULT ABUSE	
Injuries and trauma are inconsistent with reported cause (cigarette burn, scratch, bruise, or bite)	Dependent on caregiver
	Physically and/or cognitively impaired
Hematomas	Combative
Bruises at various stages of resolution	Wandering
Bruises, chafing, excoriation on wrist or legs (restraints)	Verbally belligerent
Burns	Minimal social support
Fractures inconsistent with cause described	
Dried blood	
Prolonged interval between injury and medical treatment	

Data from Berlinger JS: Why don't you just leave him? *Nursing 98* 28(4):34, 1998; Lynch SH: Elder abuse: what to look for, how to intervene, *Am J Nurs* 97(1):27, 1997; Pace H, Hoag-Apel CM: Stemming the tide of domestic violence, *Point of View Magazine* 33(3):12, 1996; and Shea CA and others: Breaking through the barriers to domestic violence intervention, *Am J Nurs* 97(6):26, 1997.

or drug use? Have people *Annoyed* you by criticizing your drinking or drug use? Have you ever felt bad or *Guilty* about your drinking or drug use? Have you ever used or had a drink first thing in the morning as an *Eye-opener* to steady your nerves or feel normal? If two or more of the CAGE questions are positive, the nurse should strongly suspect abuse and consider how to motivate the client to seek treatment (Stuart and Laraia, 1998).

VITAL SIGNS

Assessment of vital signs (see Chapter 31) should be the first part of the physical examination. Positioning or moving the client during the examination can interfere with obtaining accurate values. However, it is also appropriate for the nurse to measure specific vital signs during assessment of individual body systems. For example, the pulse can be assessed during examination of the peripheral pulses, and the heart and respirations can be assessed during examination of the thorax. Body temperature is always measured during the general survey.

HEIGHT, WEIGHT, AND CIRCUMFERENCE

A person's general level of health can be reflected in the ratio of height to weight. Weight is a routine measure during health screenings and visits to physicians' offices or clinics. Both measures are routine when clients are admitted to a health care setting. A nurse measures infants' and children's height and weight to assess growth and development. In older adults, height and weight coupled with a nutritional assessment are important in determining the cause of and treatment for chronic disease and in assessing the older adult who has difficulty with feeding and other functional activities (Box 32-5). The nurse should look for overall trends in height and weight changes.

A client's weight will normally vary daily because of fluid loss or retention. Progressive weight gain is expected during pregnancy. A downward trend in a frail older adult may indicate serious reduction in nutritional reserves. The assessment screens for abnormal weight changes. The nursing history can help to focus on possible causes for a change in weight (Table 32-7). Before measurement the nurse asks clients their current height and weight. Standardized tables can help reveal the normal expected weight for a client at a given height (see Table 32-8). A weight gain of 5 pounds (2.3 kg) in a day may indicate fluid retention problems. If the client has lost more than 5% of body weight in a month or 10% in 6 months, the loss is significant.

Clients should be weighed at the same time of day, on the same scale, and in the same clothes to allow an objective comparison of subsequent weights. Although measuring body weight may seem routine, care should be taken to be certain of accuracy, since medical and nursing decisions (e.g., drug dosage determinations, lifting, and positioning) may be based on weight changes. Clients capable of bearing their own weight use a standing scale. The nurse calibrates a standard platform scale by moving the large and small weights to zero. The balance beam should be made level and steady by adjusting the calibrating knob. Electronic scales

Table 32-7   Nursing History for Weight Assessment

Assessment Category	Rationale
Ask about total weight lost or gained; compare with usual weight; note time period for loss (e.g., gradual, sudden, desired, or undesired).	Determines severity of problem and may reveal if related to disease process, change in eating pattern, or pregnancy.
If weight loss desired, ask about eating pattern, diet plan followed, usual daily calorie intake, and appetite.	Helps to determine appropriateness of diet plan followed.
If weight loss undesired, ask about anorexia, vomiting, diarrhea, thirst, frequent urination, and change in lifestyle or activity.	Focuses on problems that may cause weight loss (e.g., gastrointestinal problems).
Assess if client has noted changes in social aspects of eating: more meals in restaurants, rushing to eat meals, stress at work, or skipping meals.	Lifestyle changes can contribute to weight changes.
Assess if client takes chemotherapy, diuretics, insulin, psychotropics, steroids, nonprescription diet pills, or laxatives.	Weight gain or loss can be side effect of these medications.

Table 32-8   Height and Weight Table: Weights for Persons 25 to 59 Years According to Build*

Men					Women				
Height		Small frame	Medium frame	Large frame	Height†		Small frame	Medium frame	Large frame
Feet	Inches				Feet	Inches			
5	2	128-134	131-141	138-150	4	10	102-111	109-121	118-131
5	3	130-136	133-143	140-153	4	11	103-113	111-123	120-134
5	4	132-138	135-145	142-156	5	0	104-115	113-126	122-137
5	5	134-140	137-148	144-160	5	1	106-118	115-129	125-140
5	6	136-142	139-151	146-164	5	2	108-121	118-132	128-143
5	7	138-145	142-154	149-168	5	3	111-124	121-135	131-147
5	8	140-148	145-157	152-172	5	4	114-127	124-138	134-151
5	9	142-151	148-160	155-176	5	5	117-130	127-141	137-155
5	10	144-154	151-163	158-180	5	6	120-133	130-144	140-159
5	11	146-157	154-166	161-184	5	7	123-136	133-147	143-163
6	0	149-160	157-170	164-188	5	8	126-139	136-150	146-167
6	1	152-164	160-174	168-192	5	9	129-142	139-153	149-170
6	2	155-168	164-178	172-197	5	10	132-145	142-156	152-173
6	3	158-172	167-182	176-202	5	11	135-148	145-159	155-176
6	4	162-176	171-187	181-207	6	0	138-151	148-162	158-179

Courtesy Metropolitan Life Insurance Company, Statistical Bulletin, 2000.
*Indoor clothing weighing 5 pounds for men and 3 pounds for women.
†Shoes with 1-inch heels.

are automatically calibrated each time they are used. The client stands on the scale platform and remains still (Figure 32-6). Electronic scales automatically display the weight within seconds (Figure 32-7). Stretcher and chair scales are available for clients unable to bear weight. After being transferred to the scale, the client is lifted above the bed by a hydraulic device and the weight is measured on a balance beam or digital display. Caution must be used when transferring clients to and from the scales.

Infants can be weighed in baskets or on platform scales. The nurse removes clothing and weighs infants in dry, disposable diapers to ensure accurate readings. The weight can later be adjusted for the weight of the diaper. The room should be warm to prevent chills. A light cloth or

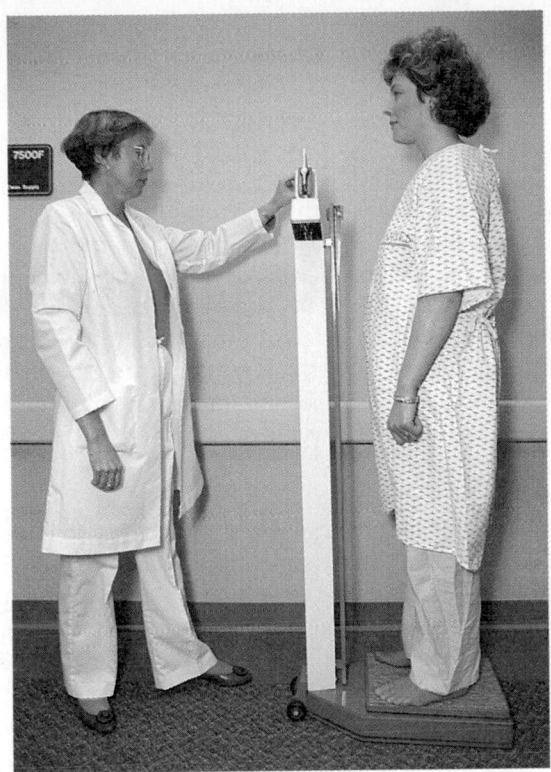

Figure 32-6 The client stands on the scale as the nurse adjusts the balance.

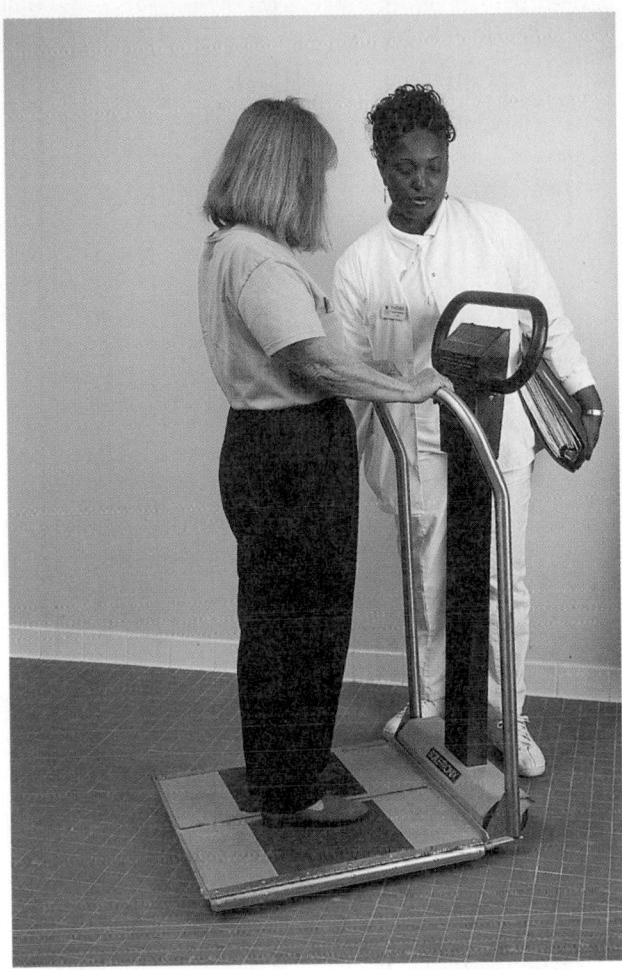

Figure 32-7 Client stands on electronic scale.

paper placed on the scale's surface prevents cross infection from urine or feces. The nurse places infants in baskets or on platforms and holds a hand lightly above them to prevent accidental falls. Weight is measured in ounces and grams.

Different techniques exist for measuring the height of weight-bearing and non–weight-bearing clients. Clients able to stand remove their shoes. A paper towel can be placed on the scale platform or floor so that the client's feet remain clean. A measuring stick or tape is attached vertically to the weight scales or wall. The nurse asks clients to stand erect, exercising good posture. On a standing scale a metal rod, which is attached to the back of the scale, swings out and over the crown of the head (Figure 32-8). A measuring stick or flat book can also be placed on the head when a scale is unavailable. With the rod or stick placed level horizontally at a 90-degree angle to the measuring stick, the nurse measures height in inches or centimeters.

A non–weight-bearing client (such as an infant) is positioned supine on a firm surface. There are portable devices available that provide a reliable means to measure height. The nurse places the infant on the device, having the parent hold the infant's head against the headboard. With the infant's legs straight at the knees, the footboard is placed against the bottom of the infant's feet (Figure

32-9). The infant's length is recorded to the nearest 0.5 cm or ¼ inch.

A more detailed assessment of infants and children requires measurement of the circumferences of the head and chest. The nurse uses a paper measuring tape to record the infant's measurements at each health visit until 2 years of age and then measures the child's head circumference until 6 years of age (Seidel and others, 1999).

Accurate measurements require placement of the measuring tape at the correct anatomical location. The nurse wraps the tape snugly around the child's head at the occipital protuberance and supraorbital prominence. This is the location of the largest circumference. The nurse records the measurement to the nearest 0.5 cm or ⅛ inch. Growth charts indicate the appropriate circumference for the child's age.

A chest circumference can be compared with the head circumference to rule out problems in head or chest size. The nurse firmly wraps the measuring tape around the infant's chest at the nipple line without causing a skin in-

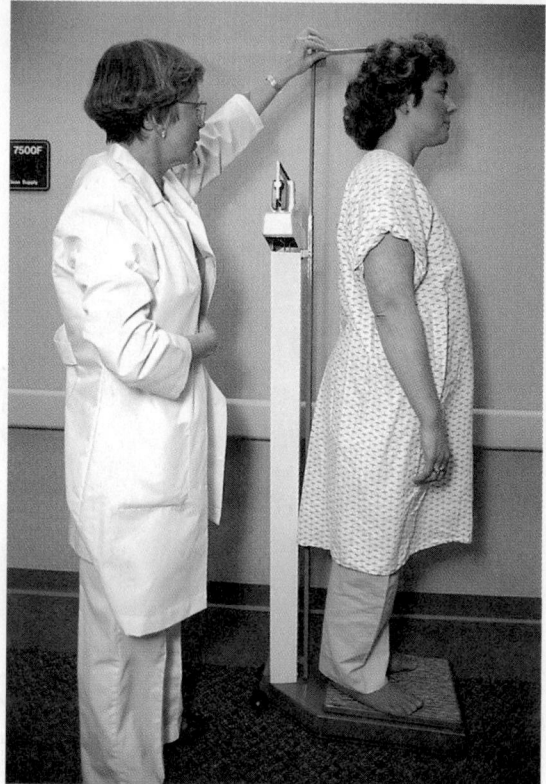

Figure 32-8   The client stands erect to permit accurate measurement of height.

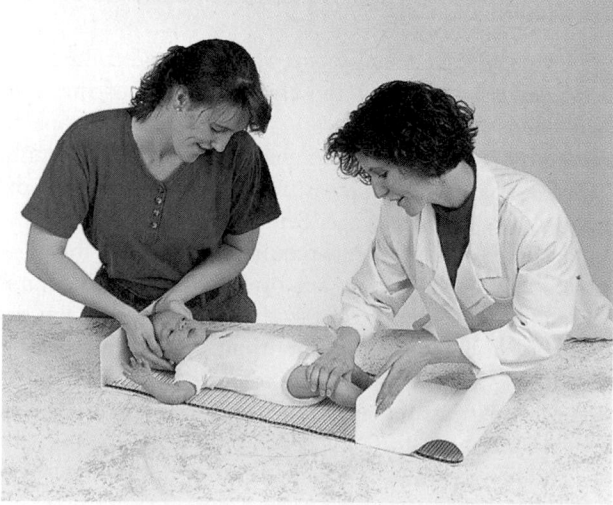

Figure 32-9   Measurement of infant length.
From Seidel HM and others: *Mosby's guide to physical examination*, ed. 4, St. Louis, 1999, Mosby.

dentation. Measurement is taken midway between inspiration and expiration and read to the nearest 0.5 cm or $\frac{1}{5}$ inch.

Skin, Hair, and Nails

The skin provides the body's external protection, regulates body temperature, and acts as a sensory organ for pain, temperature, and touch. Assessment of the **integument** includes the skin, hair, scalp, and nails. The nurse may initially inspect all skin surfaces or may assess the skin gradually while other body systems are examined. The physical assessment skills of inspection, palpation, and olfaction are used to assess the integument's function and integrity.

SKIN

Assessment of the skin can reveal a variety of conditions, including changes in oxygenation, circulation, nutrition, local tissue damage, and hydration. In a hospital setting the majority of clients are older adults, debilitated clients, or young but seriously ill clients. As a result, there are significant risks for skin lesions resulting from trauma to the skin during administration of care, from exposure to pressure during immobilization, or from reaction to various medications used in treatment. Clients most at risk are neurologically impaired clients; chronically ill clients; orthopedic clients; and clients with diminished mental status, poor tissue oxygenation, low cardiac output, or inadequate nutrition. In nursing homes and extended care facilities, clients may be at risk for many of the same problems, depending on their level of mobility and the presence of chronic illness. Nurses must routinely assess the skin to look for primary or initial lesions that may develop. Without proper care, primary lesions can quickly deteriorate to become secondary lesions that require more extensive nursing care. The development of a pressure ulcer, for example, can lengthen a hospital stay unless it is prevented or discovered early and treated properly (see Chapter 47).

The incidence of **melanoma,** an aggressive form of skin cancer, has increased about 4% every year since 1973 (ACS, 1999). In addition, the incidence of highly curable basal cell and squamous cell cancers is also increasing. Cutaneous malignancies are the most common neoplasms seen in clients. The nurse must incorporate performing a thorough skin assessment on all clients with educating them about self-examination (Box 32-6).

The condition of the client's skin reveals the need for nursing intervention. The nurse uses assessment findings to determine the type of hygiene measures required to maintain integrity of the integument (see Chapter 38). Adequate nutrition and hydration become goals of therapy if the nurse identifies alterations in the integument's status (see Chapter 43).

Adequate illumination of the skin is required for accurate observations. The recommended choice is natural or halogen lighting. For detecting skin changes in the dark-skinned client, sunlight is the best choice (Talbot and Curtis, 1996). Room temperature may also affect skin assessment. A room that is too warm may cause superficial vasodilation, resulting in an increased redness of the skin. A cool environment may cause the sensitive client to develop cyanosis around the lips and nail beds (Talbot and Curtis, 1996).

Disposable gloves are required for palpation if open, moist, or draining lesions are present. Although the nurse observes each part of the body during an examination, it helps to make a brief but careful overall visual sweep of the entire body (Seidel and others, 1999). This gives the nurse a good idea of the distribution and extent of any lesions, as well as the overall symmetry of skin color. Because the nurse inspects all skin surfaces, the client must assume several positions. The nursing history for skin assessment is outlined in Table 32-9. If abnormalities are seen during an examination, the nurse palpates the involved areas. Skin odors are usually noted in the folds of the skin, such as the axillae or under the female client's breasts. Figure 32-10 illustrates a normal cross section of the skin.

Color.   Skin color varies from body part to body part and from person to person. Despite individual variations, skin color is usually uniform over the body. Table 32-10 lists common variations. Normal skin pigmentation

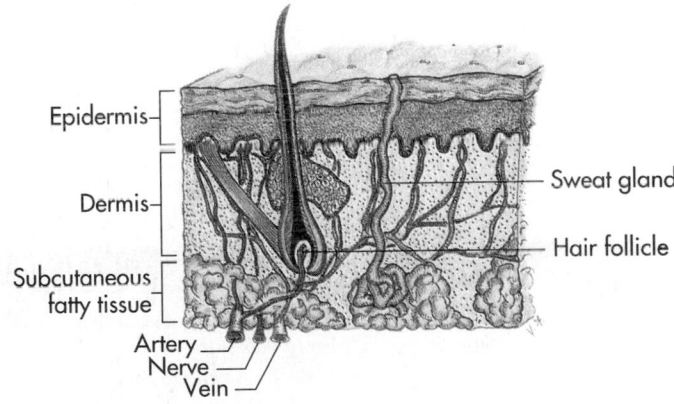

Epidermis
Dermis
Subcutaneous fatty tissue
Artery
Nerve
Vein
Sweat gland
Hair follicle

Figure 32-10   A cross section of the skin reveals three layers: epidermis, dermis, and subcutaneous fatty tissues.

ranges in tone from ivory or light pink to ruddy pink in light skin and from light to deep brown or olive in dark skin. **Basal cell carcinomas** are most commonly seen in sun-exposed areas and frequently occur in a background of sun-damaged skin. In older adults, **pigmentation** increases unevenly, causing discolored skin. While inspecting the skin, the nurse must be aware that color may be masked by cosmetics or tanning agents.

The assessment of color first involves areas of the skin not exposed to the sun, such as the palms of the hands. The nurse notes if the skin is unusually pale or dark. Areas

Table 32-9 Nursing History for Skin Assessment

Assessment Category	Rationale
Ask client about history of changes in the skin: dryness, pruritus, sores, rashes, lumps, color, texture, odor, lesion that does not heal.	Client is best source to recognize change. Skin cancer may first be noticed as a localized change in skin color.
Consider if the client has the following history: age over 50; male; fair, freckled, ruddy complexion; light-colored hair or eyes; tendency to burn easily.	Characteristics are risk factors for skin cancer.
Determine whether client works or spends excessive time outside. If so, ask whether a sunscreen is worn and the level of protection.	Exposed areas such as face and arms will be more pigmented than rest of body. Use of sunscreen is recommended by the American Cancer Society (ACS, 1999).
Determine whether client has noted lesions or changes in skin.	Most skin changes do not develop suddenly. Change in character of lesion might indicate cancer. Bruising indicates trauma or bleeding disorder.
Question client about frequency of bathing and type of soap used.	Excessive bathing and use of harsh soaps can cause dry skin.
Ask if client has had recent trauma to skin.	Injury can cause bruising and changes in skin texture.
Determine whether client has history of allergies.	Skin rashes commonly occur from allergies.
Ask if client uses topical medications or home remedies on skin.	Incorrect use of topical agents may cause inflammation or irritation.
Ask if client goes to tanning parlors, uses sun lamps, or takes tanning pills.	Overexposure of skin to these irritants can cause skin cancer.
Ask if client has family history of serious skin disorders such as skin cancer or psoriasis.	Family history may reveal information about client's condition.
Determine if client works with creosote, coal tar, and/or petroleum products.	Exposure to these agents creates risk for skin cancer.

Table 32-10 Skin Color Variations

Color	Condition	Causes	Assessment Locations
Bluish (cyanosis)	Increased amount of deoxygenated hemoglobin (associated with hypoxia)	Heart or lung disease, cold environment	Nail beds, lips, mouth, skin (severe cases)
Pallor (decrease in color)	Reduced amount of oxyhemoglobin	Anemia	Face, conjunctivae, nail beds, palms of hands
	Reduced visibility of oxyhemoglobin resulting from decreased blood flow	Shock	Skin, nail beds, conjunctivae, lips
Loss of pigmentation	Vitiligo	Congenital or autoimmune condition causing lack of pigment	Patchy areas on skin over face, hands, arms
Yellow-orange (jaundice)	Increased deposit of bilirubin in tissues	Liver disease, destruction of red blood cells	Sclera, mucous membranes, skin
Red (erythema)	Increased visibility of oxyhemoglobin caused by dilation or increased blood flow	Fever, direct trauma, blushing, alcohol intake	Face, area of trauma, sacrum, shoulders, other common sites for pressure ulcers
Tan-brown	Increased amount of melanin	Suntan, pregnancy	Areas exposed to sun: face, arms, areolae, nipples

exposed to the sun, such as the face and arms, will be darker. It is more difficult to note changes such as pallor or cyanosis in clients with dark skin. Usually color hues are best seen in the palms, soles of the feet, lips, tongue, and nail beds. Areas of increased color (hyperpigmentation) and decreased color (hypopigmentation) are common. Skin creases and folds are darker than the rest of the body in the dark-skinned client. The nurse inspects sites where abnormalities are more easily identified. For example, pallor is more easily seen in the face, buccal (mouth) mucosa, conjunctiva, and nail beds. **Cyanosis** (bluish discoloration) is best observed in the lips, nail beds, palpebral conjunctivae, and palms. In recognizing pallor in the dark-skinned client, the nurse would observe that normal brown skin appears to be yellow-brown and normal black skin appears to be ashen gray. The lips, nail beds, and mucous membranes should also be assessed for generalized pallor; if pallor is present, the mucous membranes will be ashen gray. Assessment of cyanosis in the dark-skinned client requires that the nurse observe areas where pigmentation occurs the least (conjunctiva, sclera, buccal mucosa, tongue, lips, nail beds, and palms and soles). In addition, the nurse should verify findings with clinical manifestations (Talbot and Curtis, 1996). The best site to inspect for **jaundice** (yellow-orange discoloration) is the client's sclera. Normal reactive hyperemia, or redness, is most often seen in regions exposed to pressure such as the sacrum, heels, and greater trochanter.

The nurse inspects for any patches or areas of skin color variation. Localized skin changes, such as pallor or **erythema** (red discoloration), may indicate circulatory changes. For example, an area of erythema may be due to localized vasodilation resulting from a sunburn or fever. In the dark-skinned client, erythema is not easily observed, so the nurse must palpate the area for heat and warmth to note the presence of skin inflammation (Talbot and Curtis, 1996). An area of an extremity that appears unusually pale may result from arterial occlusion or edema. It is important to ask if the client has noticed any changes in skin coloring. The client usually knows whether a change has occurred.

A pattern of findings that is becoming more common is that associated with clients who are chemically dependent and are intravenous (IV) drug abusers. Usually clients are in denial about their disease, and it may be difficult to recognize signs and symptoms after just one physical examination (Caulker-Burnett, 1994). A client who takes repeated IV injections may have edematous, reddened, and warm areas along the arms and legs. This pattern suggests recent injections. Evidence of old injection sites appears as hyperpigmented and shiny or scarred areas. Box 32-7 summarizes additional physical findings associated with substance abuse.

Moisture.   The hydration of skin and mucous membranes helps to reveal body fluid imbalances, changes in

---

Physical Findings of the Skin Indicative of Substance Abuse   Box 32-7

Body System	Commonly Associated Drug
Diaphoresis	Sedative hypnotic (including alcohol)
Spider angiomas	Alcohol, stimulants
Burns (especially fingers)	Alcohol
Needle marks	Opioids
Contusion, abrasions, cuts, scars	Alcohol, other sedative hypnotics
"Homemade" tattoos	Cocaine, IV opioids, (prevents detection of injection sites)
Increased vascularity of face	Alcohol
Red, dry skin	Phencyclidine (PCP)

Modified from Caulker-Burnett I: Primary care screening for substance abuse, *Nurse Pract* 19(6):42, 1994; and Friedman L and others: *Source book of substance abuse and addiction*, Baltimore, 1996, Williams & Wilkins.

---

the skin's environment, and regulation of body temperature. Moisture refers to wetness and oiliness. The skin is normally smooth and dry. Skin folds such as the axillae are normally moist. Minimal perspiration or oiliness should be present (Seidel and others, 1999). Increased perspiration may be associated with activity, warm environments, obesity, anxiety, or excitement. The nurse uses ungloved fingertips to palpate skin surfaces and observe for dullness, dryness, crusting, and flaking. Flaking is the appearance of flakes resembling dandruff when the skin surface is lightly rubbed. Scaling involves fishlike scales that are easily rubbed off of the skin's surface. Both flaking and scaling are believed to indicate abnormally dry skin (Hardy, 1996). Excessively dry skin is common in older adults and persons who use excessive amounts of soap during bathing. Other factors causing dry skin include lack of humidity, exposure to sun, smoking, stress, excessive perspiration, and dehydration (Hardy, 1996). Excessive dryness can worsen existing skin conditions such as **eczema** and **dermatitis.**

Temperature.   The temperature of the skin depends on the amount of blood circulating through the dermis. Increased or decreased skin temperature indicates an increase or decrease in blood flow. Localized erythema or redness of the skin often may be accompanied by an increase in skin temperature. A reduction in skin temperature reflects a decrease in blood flow. It is important to remember that if an examination room is cold, the client's skin temperature and color may be affected.

Temperature is more accurately assessed by palpating the skin with the dorsum or back of the hand. The nurse compares symmetrical body parts. Normally the skin temperature is warm. Skin temperature may be the same throughout the body or may vary in one area. Assessment of skin temperature is always done for clients at risk of having impaired circulation, such as after a cast application or vascular surgery. In addition, a nurse can identify a stage I pressure ulcer early when noting warmth and erythema on an area of the skin (see Chapter 47).

Texture. The character of the skin's surface and the feel of deeper portions are its texture. The nurse determines whether the client's skin is smooth or rough, thin or thick, tight or supple, and **indurated** (hardened) or soft by stroking it and palpating it lightly with the fingertips. The texture of the skin is normally smooth, soft, even, and flexible in children and adults. However, the texture is usually not uniform throughout. The palms of the hand and soles of the feet tend to be thicker. In older adults the skin becomes wrinkled and leathery because of a decrease in collagen, subcutaneous fat, and sweat glands.

Localized changes may result from trauma, surgical wounds, or lesions. When irregularities in texture such as scars or hardening are found, the nurse asks if the client has had a recent injury to the skin. Deeper palpation may reveal irregularities such as tenderness or localized areas of induration commonly caused by repeated intramuscular or subcutaneous injections. If the client has diabetes or receives vitamin B_{12} or iron injections, indurated areas may be seen.

Turgor. **Turgor** is the skin's elasticity, which can be diminished by edema or dehydration. Normally the skin loses its elasticity with age. To assess the skin turgor, a fold of skin on the back of the forearm or sternal area is grasped with the fingertips and released (Figure 32-11). Normally the skin lifts easily and snaps back immediately

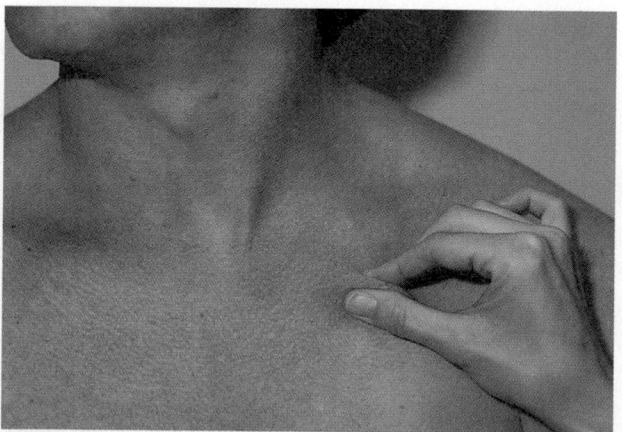

Figure 32-11 Assessment for skin turgor.
From Seidel HM and others: *Mosby's guide to physical examination,* ed, 4 St. Louis, 1999, Mosby.

to its resting position. The back of the hand is not the best place to test for turgor, since the skin is normally loose and thin (Seidel and others, 1999). The skin stays pinched when turgor is poor. The nurse notes the ease with which the skin moves and the speed at which it returns to place. Failure of the skin to reassume its normal contour or shape indicates dehydration. The client with poor skin turgor does not have a resilience to the normal wear and tear on the skin. The skin tends to stay pinched or tented when turgor is poor. A decrease in turgor predisposes the client to skin breakdown.

Vascularity. The circulation of the skin affects the appearance of superficial blood vessels. With aging, capillaries become fragile. Localized pressure areas, found after a client has lain or sat in one position, appear reddened, pink, or pale (see Chapter 47). **Petechiae** are tiny, pinpoint-sized, red or purple spots on the skin caused by small hemorrhages in the skin layers. Petechiae may indicate serious blood-clotting disorders, drug reactions, or liver disease.

Edema. Areas of the skin become swollen or edematous from a buildup of fluid in the tissues. Direct trauma and impairment of venous return are two common causes of **edema.** Edematous areas should be inspected for location, color, and shape. For the client with dependent edema caused by poor venous return, typical sites of edema are the feet, ankles, and sacrum. The formation of edema separates the skin's surface from the pigmented and vascular layers, masking skin color. Edematous skin looks stretched and shiny. The nurse palpates areas of edema to determine mobility, consistency, and tenderness. When pressure from the examiner's fingers leaves an indentation in the edematous area, it is called pitting edema. To check the degree of pitting edema, the nurse presses the edematous area firmly with the thumb for 5 seconds and releases. The depth of pitting, recorded in millimeters determines the degree of edema (Seidel and others, 1999). For example, 1+ edema equals a 2-mm depth.

Lesions. During palpation the nurse may locate skin lesions, which are any pathological skin change (Seidel and others, 1999). The skin is normally free of lesions, except common freckles or age-related changes such as skin tags, **senile keratosis** (thickening of skin), **cherry angiomas** (ruby red papules), and atrophic warts. Lesions may be primary (occurring as initial spontaneous manifestations of a pathological process), such as the wheal of an insect bite, or secondary (resulting from later formation or trauma to a primary lesion), such as a pressure ulcer.

When a lesion is detected, it is inspected for color, location, texture, size, shape, type, grouping (clustered or linear), and distribution (localized or generalized). Any exudate is observed for color, odor, amount, and consistency. The size is best measured by using a small, clear, flexible ruler marked in centimeters. Comparing a lesion with a household measure, such as a coin or eraser, is not reliable (Seidel and others, 1999). Lesions should be measured in centimeters in all dimensions (height, width, depth) when possible.

Palpation determines the lesion's mobility, contour (flat, raised, or depressed), and consistency (soft or indurated). Certain types of lesions present a characteristic pattern. For example, a tumor is usually an elevated, solid lesion larger than 2 cm. Primary lesions, such as macules and nodules, arise from some stimulus to the skin (Box

32-8). Secondary lesions, such as ulcers, occur as alterations in primary lesions. After it is identified, a lesion is closely inspected with good illumination. The lesion is palpated gently, covering its entire area. If the lesion is moist or draining fluid, gloves are worn during palpation.

It helps to ask clients if they have noticed any lesions, their causes, and any recent changes in their character. Further questioning as to how a lesion bothers a client and what has been done to care for it may reveal how a client feels about the disorder. Many clients react with fear and anxiety to rashes or other lesions. Cancerous lesions fre-

Types of Primary Skin Lesions   Box 32-8

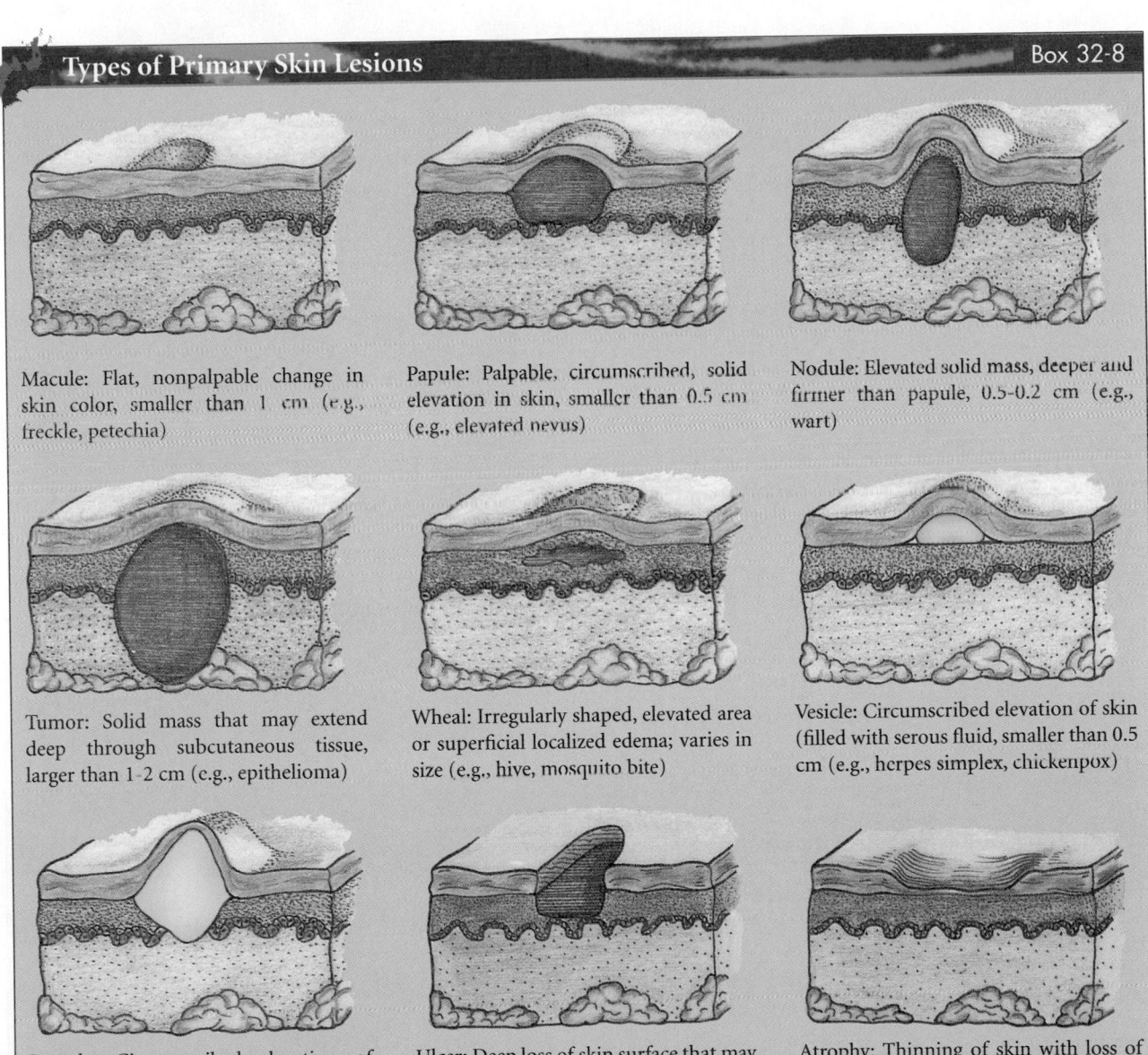

Macule: Flat, nonpalpable change in skin color, smaller than 1 cm (e.g., freckle, petechia)

Papule: Palpable, circumscribed, solid elevation in skin, smaller than 0.5 cm (e.g., elevated nevus)

Nodule: Elevated solid mass, deeper and firmer than papule, 0.5-0.2 cm (e.g., wart)

Tumor: Solid mass that may extend deep through subcutaneous tissue, larger than 1-2 cm (e.g., epithelioma)

Wheal: Irregularly shaped, elevated area or superficial localized edema; varies in size (e.g., hive, mosquito bite)

Vesicle: Circumscribed elevation of skin (filled with serous fluid, smaller than 0.5 cm (e.g., herpes simplex, chickenpox)

Pustule: Circumscribed elevation of skin similar to vesicle but filled with pus; varies in size (e.g., acne, staphylococcal infection)

Ulcer: Deep loss of skin surface that may extend to dermis and frequently bleeds and scars; varies in size (e.g., venous stasis ulcer)

Atrophy: Thinning of skin with loss of normal skin furrow, with skin appearing shiny and translucent; varies in size (e.g., arterial insufficiency)

Skin Malignancies in the Older Adult

Box 32-9

BASAL CELL CARCINOMA

0.5- to 1.0-cm crusted lesion that may be flat or raised and may have a rolled, somewhat scaly border.

Frequently there are underlying, widely dilated blood vessels that can be seen clinically within the lesion.

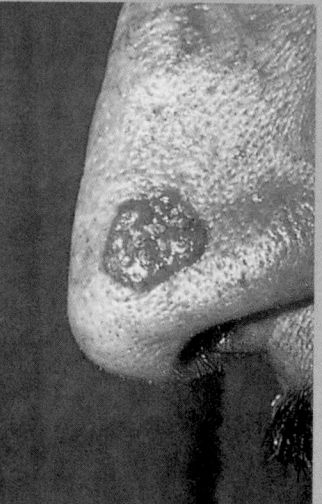

SQUAMOUS CELL CARCINOMA

Occurs more often on mucosal surfaces and nonexposed areas of skin, compared with basal cell.

0.5- to 1.5-cm scaly lesion, may be ulcerated or crusted. Appears frequently and grows more rapidly than basal cell.

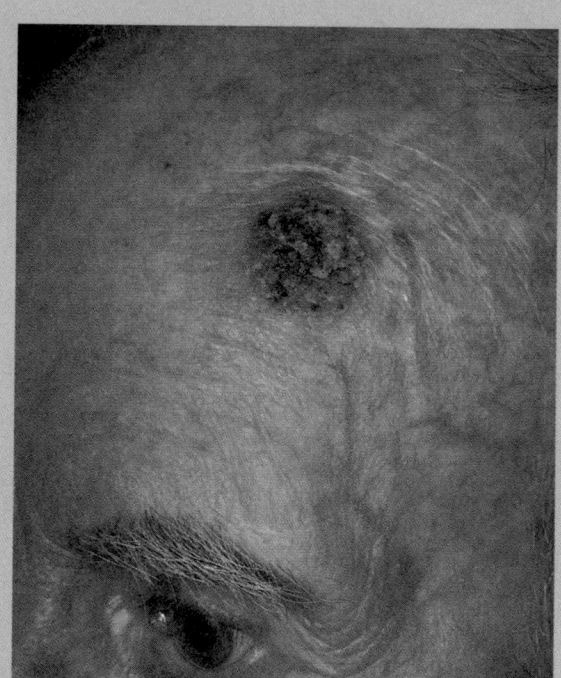

MELANOMA

0.5- to 1.0-cm brown, flat lesion that may arise on sun-exposed or nonexposed skin. Variegated pigmentation, irregular borders, and indistinct margins.

Ulceration, recent growth, or recent change in long-standing mole are ominous signs.

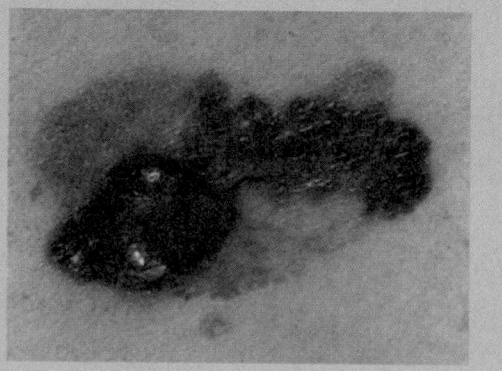

Illustrations from Belcher AE: *Cancer nursing,* St. Louis, 1992, Mosby; Habif TP: *Clinical dermatology: a color guide to diagnosis and therapy,* ed 3, St. Louis, 1996, Mosby; and Zitelli B, Davis H: *Atlas of pediatric physical diagnosis,* ed 2, St. Louis, 1991, Mosby.

quently undergo changes in color and size (Box 32-9). Abnormal lesions are reported to the physician because further examination may be required.

HAIR AND SCALP

The following types of hair cover the body: terminal hair (long, coarse, thick hair easily visible on the scalp, axillae, pubic areas, and in the beard in men) and vellus hair (small, soft, tiny hairs covering the whole body except for the palms and soles). Good lighting allows the nurse to inspect the condition and distribution of hair and the integrity of the scalp. Assessment of the hair occurs during all portions of the examination.

Inspection. Clients are sensitive about personal appearance. During inspection the nurse explains the need to separate parts of the hair to detect problems. If lesions or lice are probable, the nurse wears disposable gloves to avoid infection. Table 32-11 describes the nursing history for assessment of the hair and scalp.

The nurse begins inspection by noting the color, distribution, quantity, thickness, texture, and lubrication of body hair. Scalp hair may be coarse or fine; may be curly or straight; and should be shiny, smooth, and pliant. While separating sections of scalp hair, the nurse observes characteristics of color and coarseness. Color varies from very light blond to black to gray and may show alterations from rinses or dyes. In older adults the hair becomes dull gray, white, or yellow. It also thins over the scalp, axillae, and pubic areas. Older men lose facial hair, whereas older women may develop hair on the chin and upper lip.

Much of the information gathered about characteristics of hair growth comes from the client. The nurse needs to be aware of the normal distribution of hair growth in a man and a woman. At puberty a change in the amount and distribution of hair growth occurs. A client with hormone disorders may experience an unusual distribution and growth. A woman with **hirsutism** has hair growth on the upper lip, chin, and cheeks, with vellus hair becoming coarser over the body. A change in hair growth can negatively affect body image and emotional well-being.

Changes may occur in the thickness, texture, and lubrication of scalp hair. Disturbances such as a febrile illness or scalp disease can result in hair loss. Conditions such as thyroid disease can alter the condition of the hair, making it fine and brittle. Hair loss (**alopecia**), or thinning of the hair, is usually related to genetic tendencies and endocrine disorders such as diabetes, thyroiditis, and even menopause. Poor nutrition can cause stringy, dull, dry, and thin hair. The hair is lubricated from the oil of sebaceous glands. Excessively oily hair is associated with androgen hormone stimulation. Dry, brittle hair occurs with aging and with excessive use of shampoo or other chemical agents. The amount of hair covering the extremities may be reduced as a result of aging and arterial insufficiency and is most commonly seen over the lower extremities. In women, loss of hair should not be confused with shaven legs.

When inspecting the scalp, the nurse asks if the client has noticed anything unusual. The scalp is normally smooth and inelastic, with even coloration. By carefully separating strands of hair, the nurse can thoroughly examine the scalp for lesions, which can easily go unnoticed in thick hair. The nurse notes the characteristics of any scalp lesion. If lumps or bruises are found, the nurse asks if the client has experienced recent trauma to the head. Moles on the scalp are common. The nurse should warn the client that combing or brushing can cause a mole to bleed. Scaliness or dryness of the scalp is frequently caused by dandruff or psoriasis.

Careful inspection of hair follicles on the scalp and pubic areas may reveal lice or other parasites. The three types of lice are *Pediculus humanus capitis* (head lice), *Pediculus humanus corporis* (body lice), and *Pediculus pubis* (crab lice). Head and crab lice attach their eggs to hair. The tiny eggs look like oval particles of dandruff. The lice themselves are difficult to see. Head and body lice are very small with grayish white bodies. Crab lice have red legs. The nurse looks for bites or pustular eruptions in the hair follicles and in areas where skin surfaces meet, such as behind the ears and in the groin. The discovery of lice requires immediate treatment (Box 32-10).

Table 32-11	**Nursing History for Hair and Scalp Assessment**
Assessment Category	**Rationale**
Ask client if wig or hairpiece is being worn and request that it be removed.	Wigs or hairpieces interfere with inspection of hair and scalp. (Client may request to omit this part of examination.)
Determine if client has noted change in growth or loss of hair.	Change may occur slowly over time.
Identify type of shampoo, other hair care products, and curling irons used for grooming.	Excessive use of chemical agents and burning of hair causes drying and brittleness.
Determine if client has recently had chemotherapy (if hair loss noted) or taken a vasodilator (minoxidil) if hair growth noted.	Chemotherapeutic agents kill cells that rapidly multiply, such as tumor cells and normal hair cells. Minoxidil causes excessive hair growth
Has client noted changes in diet or appetite?	Nutrition can influence condition of hair.

Client Teaching DURING HAIR AND SCALP ASSESSMENT

Box 32-10

OBJECTIVE

- Client will perform proper hygiene practices for care of the hair and scalp.

TEACHING STRATEGIES

- Instruct client about basic hygiene practices for care of the hair and scalp (see Chapter 38).
- Instruct clients who have head lice to shampoo thoroughly with pediculicide (shampoo available at drug stores) using cold water, to comb thoroughly with a fine-tooth comb (following product directions); and to discard the comb.
- After combing, remove any detectable nits or nit cases with tweezers or between the fingernails. A dilute solution of vinegar and water may help loosen nits.
- Instruct clients and parents about ways to reduce transmission of lice:
  - Do not share personal care items with others.
  - Vacuum all rugs, car seats, pillows, stuffed animals, mattresses, and upholstered furniture thoroughly. Discard the vacuum bag.

- Seal nonwashable items in plastic bags for 14 days if unable to dry-clean or vacuum.
- Use thorough hand washing.
- Launder all clothing, linen, and bedding in hot soap and water and dry in a hot dryer for at least 20 minutes. Dry-clean nonwashable items.
- Instruct client that his or her partner must be notified if lice were sexually transmitted.
- Avoid physical contact with infested individuals and their belongings, especially clothing and bedding.
- Soak combs, brushes, and hair accessories in lice-killing products for 1 hour or in boiling water for 10 minutes.

EVALUATION

- Have client describe methods used to care for the hair and scalp.
- Have client explain steps taken to reduce lice transmission in the home.

Data from Benenson AS, editor: *Control of communicable diseases manual,* Washington, DC, 1995, American Public Health Association.

Table 32-12	**Nursing History for Nail Assessment**
Assessment Category	**Rationale**
Ask if client has experienced recent trauma or changes in nails (splitting, breaking, discoloration, thickening).	Trauma may change shape and growth of nail. Systemic conditions cause changes in color, growth, and shape. Alterations may occur slowly over time.
Has the client had other symptoms of pain, swelling, presence of systemic disease with fever, or psychological or physical stress?	Can help to indicate if change in nails is due to local or systemic problem.
Question client's nail care practices.	Chemical agents can cause drying of nails. Improper care may damage nails and cuticles.
Determine if client has risks for nail or foot problems (e.g., diabetes, older adulthood, obesity).	Vascular changes associated with diabetes reduce blood flow to peripheral tissues; foot lesions and thickened nails are common. Older adult may have trouble performing foot and nail care because of poor vision, uncoordination, or inability to bend over. Obese clients have difficulty bending over.

NAILS

The condition of the nails can reflect an individual's general state of health, state of nutrition, occupation, and level of self-care. Even a person's psychological state may be revealed by evidence of nail biting. Before assessing the nails, the nurse gathers a brief history (Table 32-12). The most visible portion of the nails is the nail plate, the transparent layer of epithelial cells covering the nail bed (Figure 32-12). The vascularity of the nail bed creates the nail's underlying color. The semilunar, whitish area at the base of the nail bed is called the lunula, from which the nail plate develops.

Inspection and Palpation. The nurse inspects the nail bed for color, cleanliness, and length; the thickness and shape of the nail plate, the texture of the nail; the angle between the nail and the nail bed; and the condition of the lateral and proximal nail folds around the nail. The nurse also palpates the nail base. By inspecting the nails, the nurse can obtain a quick sense about the client's hygiene practices. The nails are normally transparent, smooth, well rounded, and convex, with a nail bed angle of about 160 degrees. The surrounding cuticles are smooth, intact, and without inflammation. If the nails are ragged, dirty, and poorly kept, there is a good indication that either the client practices infrequent nail care or is physically unable to perform care. However, the nurse must consider the client's profession, since some individuals may have dirty nails as part of their employment (e.g., mechanics, coal miners, and farmers) despite excellent nail care. Jagged, bitten, or broken nail edges or cuticles can

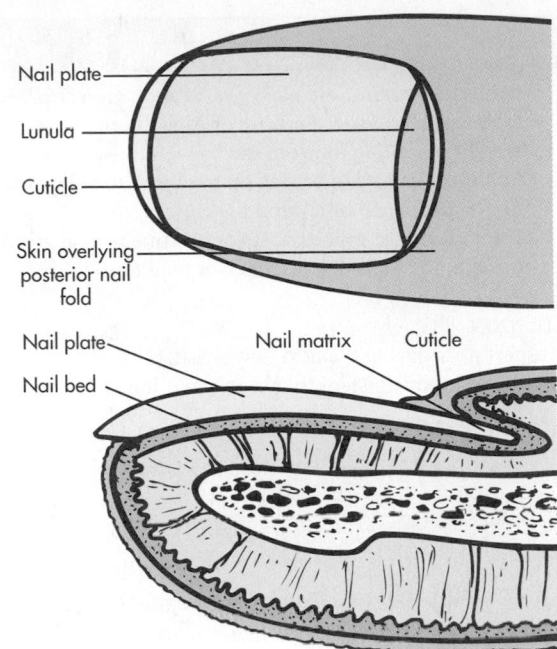

Figure 32-12 Components of the nail unit.
From Thompson JM and others: *Mosby's manual of clinical nursing*, ed 2, St. Louis, 1989, Mosby.

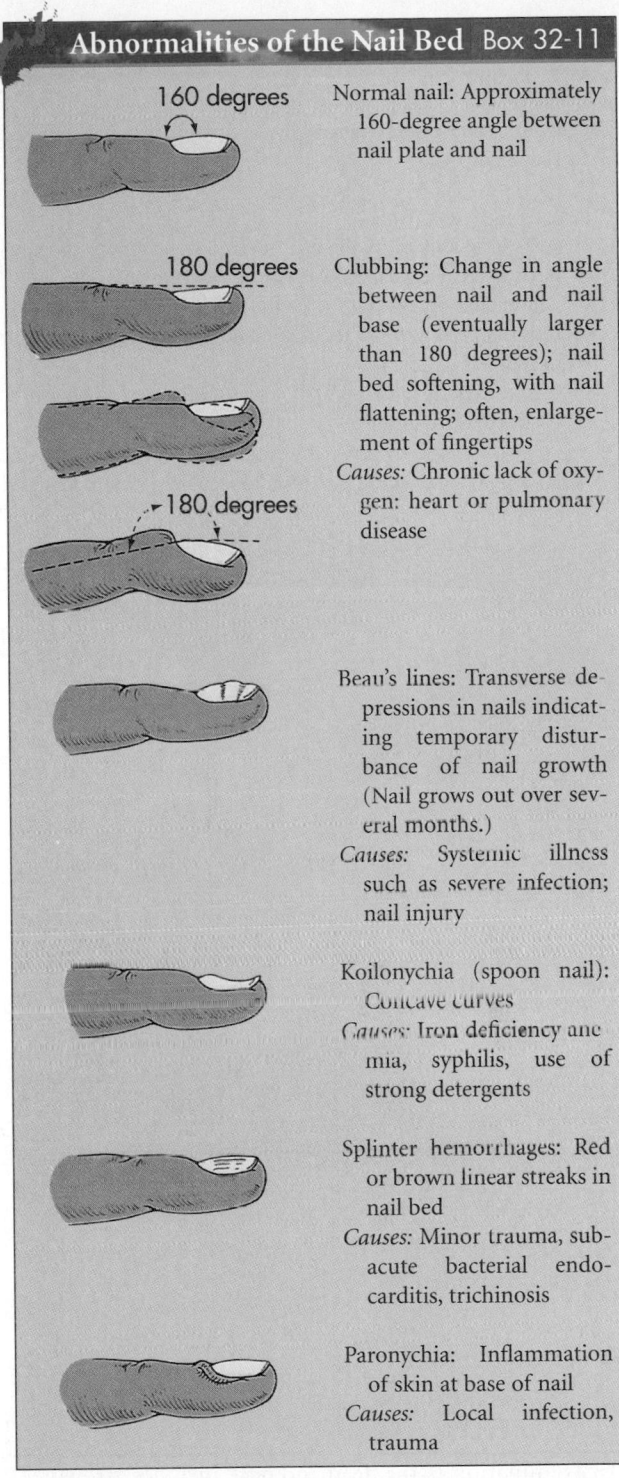

Abnormalities of the Nail Bed Box 32-11

160 degrees — Normal nail: Approximately 160-degree angle between nail plate and nail

180 degrees — Clubbing: Change in angle between nail and nail base (eventually larger than 180 degrees); nail bed softening, with nail flattening; often, enlargement of fingertips
Causes: Chronic lack of oxygen: heart or pulmonary disease

180 degrees

Beau's lines: Transverse depressions in nails indicating temporary disturbance of nail growth (Nail grows out over several months.)
Causes: Systemic illness such as severe infection; nail injury

Koilonychia (spoon nail): Concave curves
Causes: Iron deficiency anemia, syphilis, use of strong detergents

Splinter hemorrhages: Red or brown linear streaks in nail bed
Causes: Minor trauma, subacute bacterial endocarditis, trichinosis

Paronychia: Inflammation of skin at base of nail
Causes: Local infection, trauma

predispose a client to localized infection. Abnormalities such as erythema or swelling should be reported.

In whites the nail beds are pink with translucent white tips. In clients with dark skin, brown or black pigmentation is normally present in longitudinal streaks (Figure 32-13). Splinter hemorrhages can be caused by trauma, cirrhosis, diabetes mellitus, and hypertension. Vitamin, protein, and electrolyte changes can also cause lines or bands in the nail beds.

Nails normally grow at a constant rate, but direct injury or generalized disease can impair growth. With aging, the nails of the fingers and toes become harder and thicker. Longitudinal striations develop, and the rate of nail growth slows. Nails become more brittle, dull, and opaque and may turn yellow in older adults because of insufficient calcium. Also with age, the cuticle becomes less thick and wide. Inspection of the angle between the nail and nail bed normally reveals an angle of 160 degrees (Box 32-11). A larger angle and softening of the nail bed can indicate chronic oxygenation problems. The nurse palpates the nail base to determine firmness and the condition of circulation. The nail base is normally firm.

To palpate, the nurse gently grasps the client's finger and observes the color of the nail bed. Next, gentle, firm, quick pressure is applied with the thumb to the nail bed and released. As the pressure is applied, the nail bed appears white or blanched; however, the pink color should return immediately on release of pressure. Failure of the pinkness to return promptly indicates circulatory insuffi-

ciency. An ongoing bluish or purplish cast to the nail bed occurs with cyanosis. A white cast or pallor results from anemia.

Calluses and corns are commonly found on the toes or fingers. A callus is flat and painless. It results from a thickening of the epidermis. Corns are caused by friction and pressure from shoes and can usually be seen over a bony prominence. During the examination the nurse instructs clients about proper nail care (Box 32-12).

OBJECTIVE
- Client will be able to properly care for fingernails, feet, and toenails.

TEACHING STRATEGIES
- Instruct client to avoid use of over-the-counter preparations to treat corns, calluses, or ingrown toenails.
- Tell clients to cut nails straight across and even with the tops of the fingers or toes. If client has diabetes, tell client to file, not cut, nails.
- Instruct client to shape nails with a file or emery board.
- If client is diabetic:
  - Wash feet daily in warm water. Inspect feet each day in a place with good lighting, looking for dry places and cracks in the skin. Soften dry feet by applying a cream or lotion such as Nivea, Eucerin, or Alpha Keri.
- Do not put lotion between the toes.
- Caution client against using sharp objects to poke or dig under the toenail or around the cuticle.
- Have client see a podiatrist for treatment of ingrown toenails and nails that are thick or tend to split.

EVALUATION
- Inspect nails during the next home visit.
- Have client explain steps to take to avoid injury.

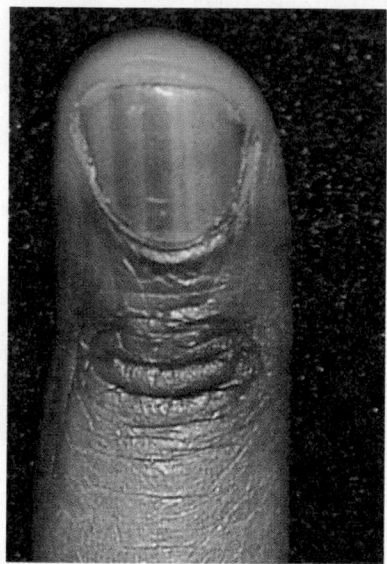

Figure 32-13   Pigmented bands in nail of client with dark skin.
From Seidel HM and others: *Mosby's guide to physical examination,* ed 4, St. Louis, 1999, Mosby.

Head and Neck

An examination of the head and neck includes assessment of the head, eyes, ears, nose, mouth, pharynx, and neck (lymph nodes, carotid arteries, thyroid gland, and trachea). The carotid arteries can also be assessed during assessment of peripheral arteries. Assessment of the head and neck uses inspection, palpation, and auscultation, with inspection and palpation often used simultaneously.

HEAD

Inspection and Palpation.   The nursing history will screen for intracranial injury and local or congenital de-

formities (Table 32-13). The nurse begins by inspecting the client's head position and facial features. The head is normally held upright and still. Holding the head tilted to one side may be an indication of unilateral hearing or visual loss.

The nurse also notes the client's facial features, looking at the eyelids, eyebrows, nasolabial folds, and mouth for shape and symmetry. It is normal for slight asymmetry to exist. If there is facial asymmetry, the nurse notes if all features on one side of the face are affected or if only a portion of the face is involved. Various neurological disorders (e.g., facial nerve paralysis) affect different nerves that innervate muscles of the face.

Examination continues with the nurse noting the size, shape, and contour of the skull. The skull is generally round with prominences in the frontal area anteriorly and the occipital area posteriorly. Local skull deformities are typically caused by trauma. In infants, large heads may result from congenital anomalies or the buildup of cerebrospinal fluid in the ventricles (**hydrocephalus**). Adults may have enlarged jaws and facial bones resulting from **acromegaly,** a disorder caused by excessive secretion of growth hormone. The nurse palpates the skull for nodules or masses. Gentle rotation of the fingertips down the midline of the scalp and then along the sides of the head reveals abnormalities. The nurse then palpates the temporomandibular joint (TMJ) space bilaterally. The nurse places the fingertips just anterior to the tragus of each ear. The fingertips should slip into the joint space as the client's mouth opens, to gently palpate the joint spaces. Normally the movements should be smooth, although it is not unusual to hear or feel a clicking or snapping in the TMJ (Seidel and others, 1999).

EYES

Examination of the eyes includes assessment of visual acuity, visual fields, extraocular movements, and external and internal eye structures. Figure 32-14 shows a cross section

Table 32-13	Nursing History for Head Assessment
Assessment Category	Rationale
Determine if client experienced recent trauma to the head. If so, assess state of consciousness after injury (immediately on return and 5 minutes later), duration of unconsciousness, and predisposing factors (e.g., seizure, poor vision, blackout).	Trauma is major cause for lumps, bumps, cuts, bruises, or deformities of scalp or skull. Loss of consciousness following head injury indicates possible brain injury.
Ask if client has history of headache; note onset, duration, character, pattern, and associated symptoms.	Character of headache can help to reveal causative factors such as sinus infection, migraine, or neurological disorders.
Determine length of time client has experienced neurological symptoms.	Duration of signs or symptoms may reveal severity of problem.
Review client's occupational history for use of safety helmets.	Nature of client's occupation can create a risk for head injury.
Ask if client participates in contact sports, cycling, roller blading, or skateboarding.	Activities require use of safety helmets.

of the eye. The assessment detects visual alterations and determines the level of assistance that clients require when ambulating or performing self-care activities. Clients with visual problems may also need special aids for reading educational materials or instructions (e.g., medication labels). Table 32-14 reviews the nursing history for an eye examination. Box 32-13 describes common types of visual problems.

Visual Acuity.   The assessment of visual acuity, the ability to see small details, tests central vision. The easiest

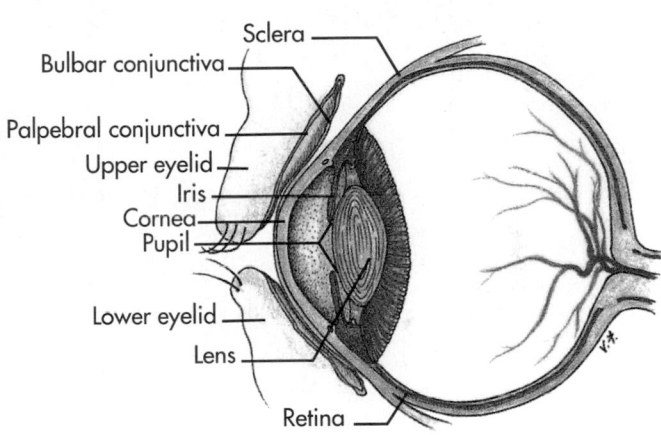

Figure 32-14   Cross section of the eye.

Table 32-14	Nursing History for Eye Assessment	
Assessment Category	Rationale
Determine if client has history of eye disease, eye trauma, diabetes, hypertension, or eye surgery.	Some diseases or trauma can cause risk for partial or complete visual loss. Surgery may have been performed for a visual disorder.
Determine problems that prompted client to seek health care. Ask client about eye pain, photophobia (sensitivity to light), burning, itching, excess tearing or crusting, diplopia (double vision), blurred vision, awareness of a "film" over field of vision, floaters (small, black spots that seem to float across field of vision), flashing lights, or halos around lights.	Common symptoms of eye disease indicate need for physician referral.
Determine whether there is family history of eye disorders or diseases.	Certain eye problems such as glaucoma or retinitis pigmentosa are inherited.
Assess client's occupational history and recreational hobbies; are safety glasses worn?	Performance of close, intricate work can cause eye fatigue. Working with computers may cause eye strain. Certain occupational tasks (e.g., working with chemicals) and recreational activity (e.g., fencing or motorcycle riding) place persons at risk for eye injury unless precautions are taken.
Ask client if glasses or contacts are worn; how often?	Glasses or contacts should be worn during certain portions of examination for accurate assessment.
Determine when client last visited ophthalmologist or optometrist.	Date of last eye examination reveals level of preventive care taken by client.
Assess medications client is taking, including eye drops or ointment.	Determines need to assess client's knowledge of medications. Certain medications can cause visual symptoms.

Common Eye and Visual Problems
Box 32-13

HYPEROPIA

Hyperopia is farsightedness, a refractive error in which rays of light enter the eye and focus behind the retina. Persons are able to clearly see distant objects but not close objects.

MYOPIA

Myopia is nearsightedness, a refractive error in which rays of light enter the eye and focus in front of the retina. Persons are able to clearly see close objects but not distant objects.

PRESBYOPIA

Presbyopia is impaired near vision in middle-age and older adults, caused by loss of elasticity of the lens and associated with the aging process.

ASTIGMATISM

Astigmatism is a condition in which parallel light rays do not focus on a single point on the retina. An uneven curvature of the cornea or lens causes light to be focused on different points.

RETINOPATHY

Retinopathy is a noninflammatory eye disorder resulting from changes in retinal blood vessels. It is a leading cause of blindness.

STRABISMUS

Strabismus is a congenital problem in which the eyes appear crossed. The muscles controlling movement of the eyes are not coordinated.

CATARACTS

A cataract is an increased opacity of the lens, which blocks light rays from entering the eye. Cataracts may develop slowly and progressively after age 35 or suddenly after trauma. Cataracts are one of the most common eye disorders. By age 70, most older adults have some evidence of visual impairment from cataracts.

GLAUCOMA

Glaucoma is intraocular structural damage resulting from elevated intraocular pressure. It is caused by obstruction of the outflow of aqueous humor. Without treatment the disorder can cause blindness.

MACULAR DEGENERATION

Macular degeneration is blurred central vision often occurring suddenly, caused by a progressive degeneration of the center of the retina. It is the most common visual impairment of individuals over age 50 and the most common cause of blindness in older adults. There is no cure.

---

way to assess near vision is to ask clients to read printed material under adequate lighting. If clients wear glasses, they should wear them during the examination. The nurse should know the language clients speak and whether they are able to read. Asking clients to read aloud can help determine literacy. If the client has difficulty reading, move to the next step.

Assessment of distant vision requires use of a Snellen chart (paper chart or projection screen). The chart should be well lighted. Vision is tested without corrective lenses first. The nurse has the client sit or stand 20 feet (6.1 m) away from the chart and try to read all of the letters beginning at any line with both eyes open and then with each eye separately (with the opposite eye covered by an index card or eye cover (Figure 32-15). The client should avoid applying pressure to the eye. The nurse notes the smallest line in which the client can read all of the letters correctly and records the visual acuity for that line. The test is repeated with the client wearing corrective lenses. The nurse does the test rapidly enough that the client does not memorize the chart (Seidel and others, 1999).

If a client is unable to read, the nurse uses an *E* chart or one with pictures of familiar objects. Instead of reading letters, clients tell the nurse which direction each *E* is pointing or the name of the object. The visual acuity score is recorded for each eye and for both eyes.

The Snellen chart has standardized numbers at the end of each line of the chart. The numerator is the number 20,

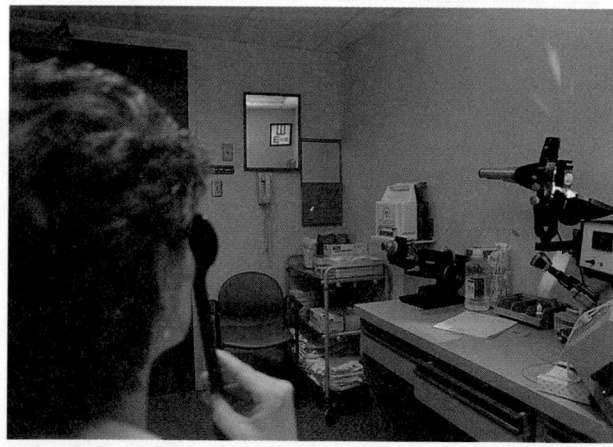

Figure 32-15   Assessment of visual acuity using a projection screen with an *E* chart.

or the distance the client stands from the chart. The denominator is the distance from which the normal eye can read the chart. Normal vision is 20/20. The larger the denominator, the poorer the client's visual acuity. For example, a value of 20/40 means that the client, standing 20 feet away, can read a line that a person with normal vision can read from 40 feet away. The nurse records visual acuity as

$\bar{sc}$ (without correction) or $\bar{cc}$ (with correction), depending on whether or not the client wears glasses or contact lenses.

If clients cannot read even the largest letters or figures of a Snellen chart, the nurse tests their ability to count upraised fingers or distinguish light. The nurse holds a hand 30 cm (1 foot) from the face and instructs clients to count the upraised fingers. To check light perception, the nurse shines a penlight into the eye and then turns the light off. If clients note when the light is turned on or off, light perception is intact.

Near vision can be assessed by asking the client to read a handheld card containing a vision screening chart. The client is instructed to hold the card a comfortable distance (5 to 6 cm, or about 14 inches) from the eyes. The client reads the smallest line possible.

Extraocular Movements.

Six small muscles guide the movement of each eye. Both eyes move parallel to each other in each of the six directions of gaze (Figure 32-16). The client sits or stands 60 cm (2 feet) away, facing the nurse. The nurse holds a finger at a comfortable distance (15 to 30 cm, or 6 to 12 inches) from the client's eyes. The client keeps the head in a fixed position facing the nurse and follows the movement of the finger with the eyes only. The client looks to the right, to the left, and diagonally up and down to the left and right. The nurse's finger moves smoothly and slowly within the normal field of vision.

As the client gazes in each direction, the nurse observes for parallel eye movement, the position of the upper eyelid in relation to the iris, and the presence of abnormal movements. As the eyes move through each direction of gaze, the upper eyelid covers the iris only slightly. By periodically stopping movement of the finger, the nurse can assess **nystagmus,** an involuntary, rhythmical oscillation of the eyes. The nurse can also often initiate nystagmus in clients with normal eye movements by having them gaze to the far left or right. Disturbances in eye movement reflect local injury to eye muscles and supporting structures or a disorder of the cranial nerves innervating the muscles.

The nurse can also check the alignment of the eyes by assessing the corneal light reflex. A weakness or imbalance of the extraocular muscles can cause misalignment. The nurse shines a penlight onto the bridge of the client's nose from 60 to 90 cm (2 to 3 feet) away in a darkened room. The client looks straight ahead. Normally light reflects on the cornea in the same spot on both eyes. If an abnormality is present, the light shines on a different spot on each eye.

Visual Fields.

As a person looks straight ahead, all objects in the periphery can normally be seen. To assess visual fields, the nurse has the client stand or sit 60 cm (2 feet) away, facing the nurse at eye level. The client gently closes or covers one eye (e.g., the left) and looks at the nurse's eye directly opposite. The nurse closes the opposite eye (in this case the right) so that the field of vision is superimposed on that of the client. The nurse moves a finger equidistant from the nurse and client outside the field of vision, then slowly brings it back into the visual field. The client is asked to tell when the nurse's finger is seen. If the nurse sees the finger before the client does, a portion of the client's visual field is reduced. To test temporal field vision, the object should be slightly behind the client. (NOTE: The nurse can see the finger.) The procedure is repeated for each field of vision for the other eye. Clients with visual field problems may be at risk for injury because they cannot see all of the objects in front of them. Older adults commonly have loss of peripheral vision caused by changes in the lens.

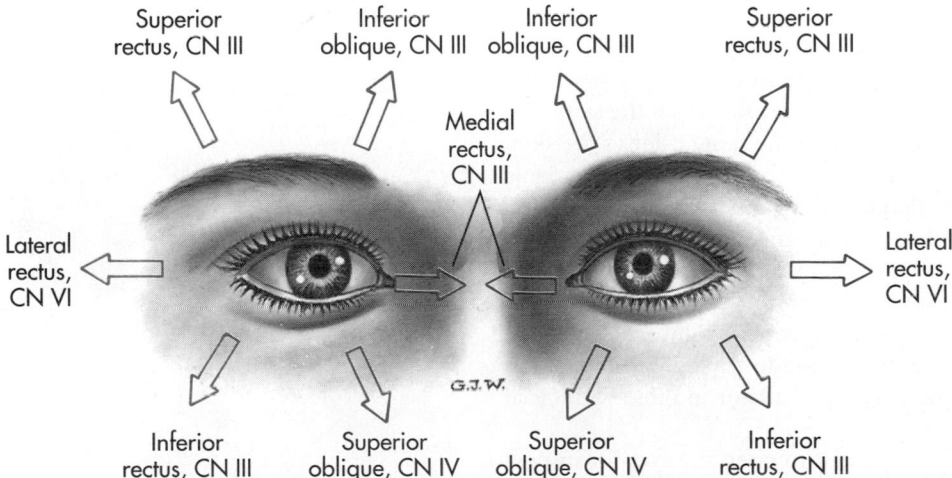

Figure 32-16   Six directions of gaze. The nurse directs the client to follow finger movement through each gaze.
From Seidel HM and others: *Mosby's guide to physical examination,* ed 4, St. Louis, 1999, Mosby.

External Eye Structures. To inspect external eye structures, the nurse stands directly in front of the client at eye level and asks the client to look at the nurse's face.

Position and Alignment. The nurse assesses the position of the eyes in relation to one another. The eyes are normally parallel to each other. Bulging (**exophthalmos**) is usually caused by hyperthyroidism when both eyes are involved. Crossing of eyes (strabismus) results from neuromuscular injury or inherited abnormalities. Tumors or inflammation of the orbit can cause abnormal eye protrusion.

Eyebrows. The eyebrows are normally symmetrical. The eyebrows are inspected for size, extension, texture of hair, alignment, and movement. A loss or absence of hair may indicate a hormonal disturbance or is a result of waxing or plucking. Aging causes loss of the lateral third of the eyebrows. The brows should raise and lower symmetrically. Paralysis of the facial nerve exists if a client cannot move the eyebrows.

Eyelids. The nurse inspects the eyelids for position, color, condition of the surface, condition and direction of the eyelashes, and the client's ability to open, close, and blink. When the eyes are open in a normal position, the lids do not cover the pupil and the sclera cannot be seen above the iris. The lids are also close to the eyeball. An abnormal drooping of the lid over the pupil is called **ptosis** (pronounced "toe-sis") and is caused by edema or impairment of the third cranial nerve. Defects in the position of the lid margins may also be observed. An older adult frequently has lid margins that turn out (**ectropion**) or in (**entropion**). An entropion may lead to the lid's lashes irritating the conjunctiva and cornea, increasing the risk of infection. The eyelashes are normally distributed evenly and curved outward away from the eye. An erythematous or yellow lump (hordeolum or sty) on the follicle of an eyelash indicates an acute suppurative inflammation.

To inspect the surface of the upper lids, the nurse asks clients to close their eyes and raises both eyebrows gently with the thumb and index finger to stretch the skin. The lids are normally smooth and the same color as the skin. Redness indicates inflammation or infection. Lid edema may be due to allergies or to heart or kidney failure. Edema of the eyelids prevents them from closing. Lesions are inspected for typical characteristics and discomfort or drainage. Gloves should be worn if drainage is present.

The lids normally close symmetrically. Failure of the lids to close exposes the cornea to drying. This condition is common in unconscious clients or in those with facial nerve paralysis.

The nurse asks the client to open the eyes for inspection of the lower lids. The same characteristics noted for the upper lids are assessed. Normally a person blinks involuntarily and bilaterally up to 20 times a minute. The blink reflex helps lubricate the cornea. The nurse reports absent or infrequent, rapid, or monocular (one-eyed) blinking.

Lacrimal Apparatus. The anterior surface of the eye, made up of the sensitive cornea and conjunctivae, is moistened or lubricated by tears secreted from the lacrimal gland (Figure 32-17). The gland is located in the upper outer wall of the anterior part of the orbit. Tears flow from the gland across the eye's surface to the lacrimal duct, which is located in the nasal corner or inner canthus of the eye. The lacrimal gland can be the site of tumors or infections. The area of the gland is inspected for edema and redness, and it is palpated gently to detect tenderness. Normally the gland cannot be felt.

The nasolacrimal duct may become obstructed, blocking the flow of tears. If the client complains of excess tearing, the nurse looks for evidence of edema in the inner canthus. Mild palpation of the duct at the lower eyelid just inside the lower orbital rim, not on the side of the nose, may cause a regurgitation of tears.

Conjunctivae and Sclerae. The bulbar conjunctiva covers the exposed surface of the eyeball up to the outer edge of the cornea, and the palpebral conjunctiva is the delicate membrane lining the eyelids. Normally the conjunctiva is transparent, enabling the examiner to view the tiny underlying blood vessels that give it a light pink color. The sclera is seen under the bulbar conjunctiva and normally is the color of white porcelain in whites and light yellow in African-Americans. Sclerae may become pigmented and appear either yellow or green if liver disease is present.

Care must be taken when inspecting the conjunctivae. For adequate exposure of the bulbar conjunctiva, the eyelids must be retracted without placing pressure directly on the eyeball. Both lids are gently retracted, with the thumb and index finger pressed against the lower and upper bony orbits. The client is asked to look up, down, and from side

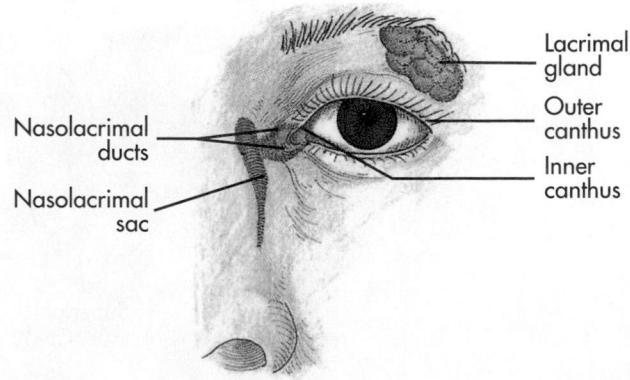

Figure 32-17   The lacrimal apparatus secretes and drains tears, which moisten and lubricate eye structures.

to side. Many clients begin to blink, making the examination difficult. The nurse inspects for color, texture, and the presence of edema or lesions. Normally the conjunctivae are free of erythema. The presence of redness may indicate an allergic or infectious **conjunctivitis.** Bright red blood in a localized area surrounded by normal-appearing conjunctiva usually indicates subconjunctival hemorrhage.

To inspect the palpebral conjunctiva, the nurse must evert the lower eyelids (Figure 32-18). The lower lid is gently depressed with the thumb or index finger. Often the client can depress the eyelid to facilitate examination. A pale conjunctiva results from anemia, whereas a fiery red appearance is a result of inflammation (conjunctivitis). Conjunctivitis is a highly contagious infection. The crusty drainage that collects on eyelid margins can easily spread from one eye to the other. The nurse should wear gloves during the examination. Thorough hand washing is necessary before and after the examination.

Corneas. The cornea is the transparent, colorless portion of the eye covering the pupil and iris. From a side view, the cornea looks like the crystal of a wristwatch. As the client looks straight ahead, the nurse inspects the cornea for clarity and texture while shining a penlight obliquely across the cornea's entire surface. The cornea is normally shiny, transparent, and smooth. However, in an older adult the cornea loses its luster. Any irregularity in the surface may indicate an abrasion or tear that warrants immediate examination by a physician. Both conditions are very painful. The color and details of the underlying iris should be easy to see. In an older adult the iris becomes faded. A thin white ring along the margin of the iris, called an **arcus senilis,** is common with aging but is abnormal in anyone under age 40. To test for the corneal blink reflex, see the cranial nerve test section of this chapter.

Pupils and Irises. The nurse observes the pupils for size, shape, equality, accommodation, and reaction to light. The pupils are normally black, round, regular, and equal in size (3 to 7 mm in diameter) (Figure 32-19). The iris should be clearly visible.

Cloudy pupils indicate cataracts. Dilated pupils can result from glaucoma, trauma, neurological disorders, eye medications (e.g., atropine), or withdrawal from opioids. Constricted pupils may be caused by inflammation of the iris or use of drugs (e.g., pilocarpine, morphine, or cocaine). Pinpoint pupils are a common sign of opioid intoxication (Friedman and others, 1996). When a beam of light is shined through the pupil and onto the retina, the third cranial nerve is stimulated and innervates the muscles of the iris to constrict. Any abnormality along the nerve pathways from the retina to the iris alters the ability of the pupils to react to light. Changes in intracranial pressure, lesions along the nerve pathways, locally applied ophthalmic medications, and direct trauma to the eye may alter pupillary reaction.

Pupillary reflexes (to light and accommodation) should be tested in a dimly lit room. As the client looks straight ahead, the nurse brings a penlight from the side of the client's face, directing the light onto the pupil (Figure 32-20). If the client looks at the light, there will be a false reaction to accommodation. A directly illuminated pupil constricts, and the opposite pupil constricts consensually. The nurse observes the quickness and equality of the reflex. The examination is repeated for the opposite eye.

To test for accommodation, the client is asked to gaze at a distant object (the far wall) and then at a test object (finger or pencil) held by the nurse approximately 10 cm (4 inches) from the bridge of the client's nose. The pupils normally converge and accommodate by constricting when looking at close objects. The pupillary responses are equal. Testing for accommodation is only important if the client has a defect in the pupillary response to light (Seidel and others 1999). If assessment of pupillary reaction is normal in all tests, the nurse records the abbreviation **PERRLA** (pupils equal, round, reactive to light, and accommodation).

Internal Eye Structures. The internal eye cannot be observed without an instrument to illuminate its structures. The **ophthalmoscope** is used to inspect the fundus, which includes the retina, choroid, optic nerve disc, macula, fovea centralis, and retinal vessels. Clients in greatest need of an examination are those with diabetes, hyperten-

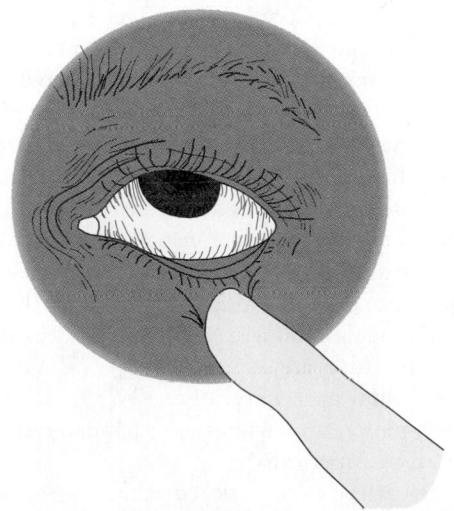

Figure 32-18 Technique for retracting the lower eyelid.

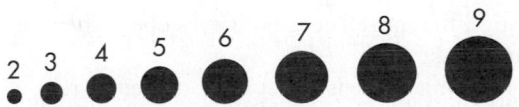

Figure 32-19 Chart depicting pupillary size in millimeters.

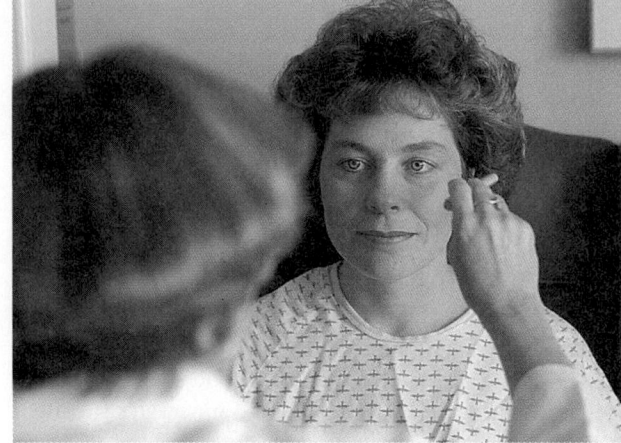

A

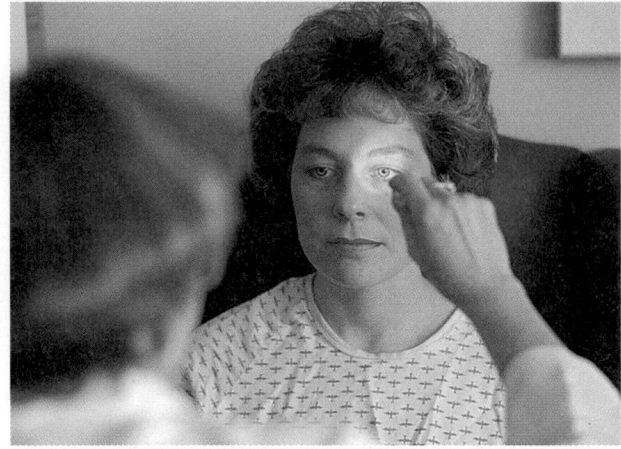

B

Figure 32-20 **A,** To check pupillary reflexes, the nurse first holds the penlight to the side of the client's face. **B,** Illumination of the pupil causes pupillary constriction.

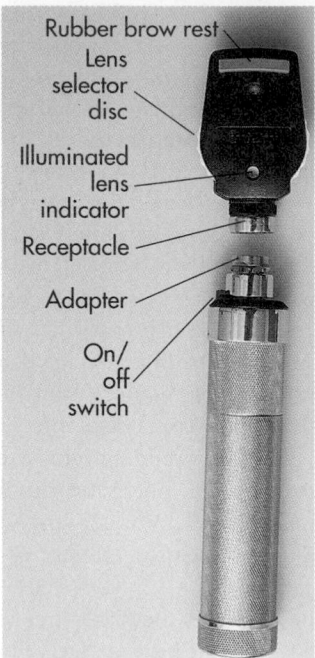

Figure 32-21 Ophthalmoscope.
From Seidel HM and others: *Mosby's guide to physical examination,* ed 4, St. Louis, 1999, Mosby.

sion, and intracranial disorders. The nurse should feel competent in using an ophthalmoscope before attempting this examination.

The ophthalmoscope has a battery tube light source, two dials or disks, and a keyhole viewer (Figure 32-21). The dial at the top of the battery tube changes the light image. Five lenses are available, but the large white light is used for general examination. The dial at the top of the viewer rotates clockwise for selection of the lens, which adjusts the focus for the examiner.

The nurse should practice holding the ophthalmoscope in each hand, using the index finger to rotate the lens dial. The nurse turns the white light on, rotates the lens dial to *0,* and looks through the keyhole, focusing on near objects, such as the palm of the hand. Reading the newspaper with the ophthalmoscope is useful practice. During an examination the nurse keeps both eyes open when looking through the keyhole.

The examination is done in a darkened room. The nurse and client stand or sit in comfortable positions facing each other with their eyes at the same height. The client removes eyeglasses, but contact lenses may be left in place. The ophthalmoscope's light is switched on, and the lens is rotated to 0. The index finger is kept on the lens dial to refocus the ophthalmoscope.

The examiner's right hand and eye are used to examine the client's right eye, and the left hand and eye are used to examine the client's left eye. The ophthalmoscope is held comfortably against the nurse's face. As the client gazes straight ahead with both eyes open, the examiner, at a distance of approximately 25 cm (10 inches) from the client and 25 degrees lateral to the client's central line of vision, shines the light on the pupil (Figure 32-22). A bright orange glow in the pupil, called the red reflex, can then normally be seen. The light from the ophthalmoscope causes the pupil to constrict. The light is slowly moved toward the pupil while the nurse keeps it focused on the red reflex. The nurse must relax and keep both eyes open. As the light approaches the pupil, the nurse begins to see structures of the fundus. Rotating the lens dial brings the internal structures into focus. The examiner inspects the size, color, and clarity of the disc; checks the integrity of the vessels; looks for the presence of retinal lesions; and assesses the appearance of the macula and fovea (Figure 32-23). Normally the following structures are observed:

A clear, yellow optic nerve disc
Reddish pink retina (whites) or darkened retina (African-Americans)
Light red arteries and dark red veins
A 3:2 vein-to-artery ratio in size proportion
The avascular macula

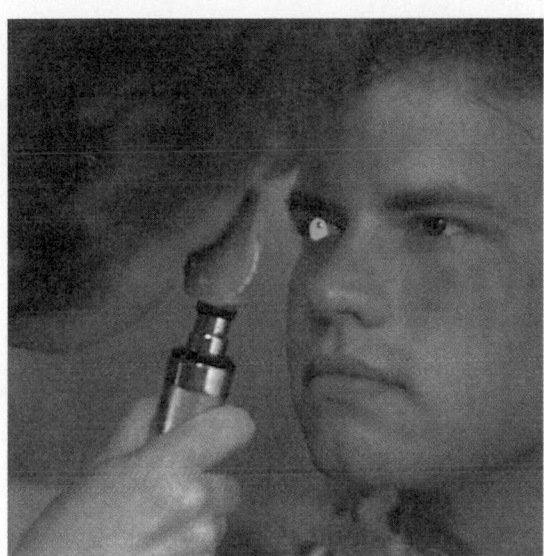

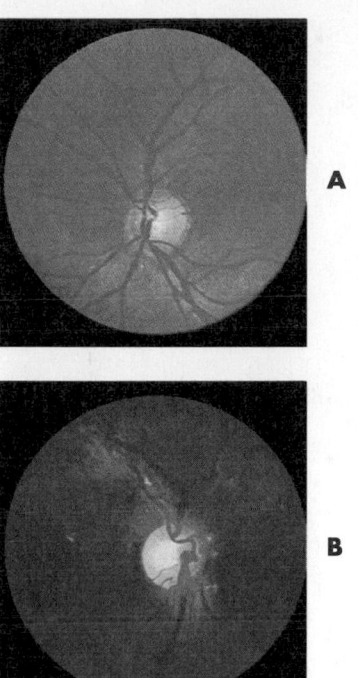

Figure 32-22   To visualize internal eye structures, the nurse moves in toward the pupil with the ophthalmoscope's light focused on the red reflex.

Figure 32-23   Fundus of, **A,** white patient and, **B,** black patient.
Courtesy MEDCOM, Cypress, Calif.

Client Teaching DURING EYE ASSESSMENT   Box 32-14

OBJECTIVES
- Client will follow recommendations for regular eye examinations.
- Client will be able to recognize warning signs and symptoms of eye disease.
- Client will take appropriate safety precautions for visual deficits.

TEACHING STRATEGIES
- Tell client that persons under age 40 should have a complete eye examination every 3 to 5 years (or more often if family histories reveal risks such as diabetes or hypertension).
- Tell client that persons over age 40 for conditions that may develop without awareness (e.g., glaucoma) should have eye examinations every 2 years to screen.
- Tell client that persons over age 65 should have yearly eye examinations.

- Describe the typical symptoms of eye disease (see Box 32-13).
- Instruct older adult to take the following precautions because of normal visual changes: avoid or use caution while driving at night, increase lighting in the home to reduce risk of falls, and paint the first and last steps of a staircase and the edge of each step in between a bright color to aid depth perception.

EVALUATION
- Ask client or family member to report on client's most recent visit to an ophthalmologist.
- Have client describe when to have an eye examination.
- Ask client to describe common symptoms of eye disease.
- Observe the home environment of a client with visual deficits.

If any abnormalities are observed, the client should be examined by an ophthalmologist (Box 32-14). The client's fundus should not be illuminated for extended periods. The bright light of the ophthalmoscope is very irritating and can cause discomfort and tearing. During the examination, the nurse assesses the client for discomfort.

EARS

The ears are easy to examine because of their accessibility. The three parts of the ear are the external, middle, and inner ear (Figure 32-24). The nurse inspects and palpates external ear structures, inspects middle ear structures with an otoscope, and tests the inner ear by measuring hearing

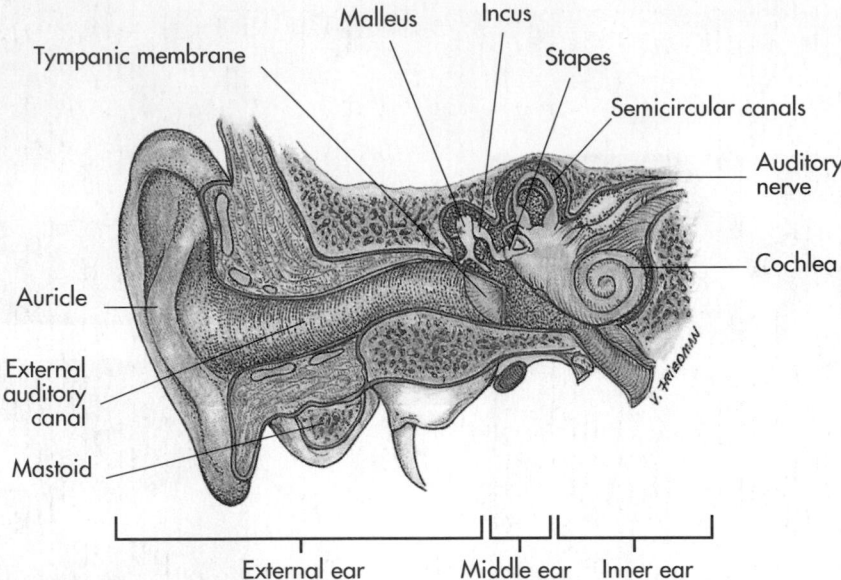

Figure 32-24   Structures of the external, middle, and inner ear.

acuity. External ear structures consist of the auricle, outer ear canal, and tympanic membrane (eardrum). The ear canal is normally curved and approximately (2.5 cm) (1 inch) long in an adult. It is lined with skin containing fine hairs, nerve endings, and glands secreting cerumen. The middle ear is an air-filled cavity containing the three bony ossicles (malleus, incus, and stapes). The eustachian tube connects the middle ear to the nasopharynx. Pressure between the outer atmosphere and the middle ear is stabilized through the eustachian tube.

The inner ear contains the cochlea, vestibule, and semicircular canals. The nurse assesses the ears to determine the integrity of ear structures and the condition of hearing. Nursing history data (Table 32-15) aid in identifying risks for hearing disorders.

Understanding the mechanisms for sound transmission helps the nurse identify the nature of hearing disorders. Sound travels through the ear by air and bone conduction; the following explains the steps of hearing:

1. Sound waves in the air enter the external ear, passing through the outer ear canal.
2. The sound waves reach the tympanic membrane, causing it to vibrate.
3. Vibrations are transmitted through the middle ear by the bony ossicular chain to the oval window at the opening of the inner ear.
4. The cochlea receives the sound vibration.
5. Nerve impulses from the cochlea travel to the auditory (eighth cranial) nerve and to the cerebral cortex.

Disorders of the ear result from several types of problems, including mechanical dysfunction (blockage by ear wax or foreign body), trauma (foreign bodies or noise exposure), neurological disorders (auditory nerve damage), acute illnesses (viral infection), and toxic effects of medications.

Auricles.   With the client sitting comfortably, the nurse inspects the auricle's size, shape, symmetry, landmarks, position, and color (Figure 32-25). The auricles are normally level with each other. The upper point of attachment is in a straight line with the lateral canthus, or corner of the eye. The position of the auricle should also be almost vertical. Ears that are low set or at an unusual angle are a sign of chromosome abnormality (e.g., Down syndrome). The color should be the same as that of the face, without moles, cysts, deformities, or nodules. Redness is a sign of inflammation or fever. Extreme pallor can indicate frostbite.

The nurse palpates the auricles for texture, tenderness, and skin lesions. The auricle is normally smooth, without lesions. If the client complains of pain, the nurse gently pulls the auricle and presses on the tragus and palpates behind the ear over the mastoid process. If palpating the external ear increases the pain, an external ear infection is likely. If palpation of the auricle and tragus does not influence the pain, the client may have a middle ear infection. Tenderness in the mastoid area can indicate mastoiditis.

The nurse inspects the opening of the ear canal for size and discharge. Discharge may be accompanied by an odor. The meatus should not be swollen or occluded. A yellow, waxy substance called **cerumen** is common. Yellow or green, foul-smelling discharge may indicate infection or a foreign body.

Table 32-15 Nursing History for Ear Assessment

Assessment Category	Rationale
Ask if client has experienced ear pain, itching, discharge, vertigo, tinnitus (ringing in ears), or change in hearing.	These signs and symptoms indicate infection or hearing loss.

Assess risks for hearing problem.
  Infants/children: Hypoxia at birth, meningitis, birth weight less than 1500 g, family history of hearing loss, congenital anomalies of skull or face, nonbacterial intrauterine infections (rubella, herpes), maternal drug use, excessively high bilirubin, head trauma
  Adults: Exposure to industrial or recreational noise, genetic disease (Meniere's disease), neurodegenerative disorder
	Risk factors predispose client to permanent hearing loss. It may be difficult to assess infant's hearing status with examination only.

Determine client's exposure to loud noises at work and availability of protective devices.	Prolonged noise exposure can cause temporary or permanent hearing loss.
Note behaviors indicative of hearing loss, such as failure to respond when spoken to, requests to repeat comments, leaning forward to hear, and child's inattentiveness or use of monotonous voice tone.	Persons with hearing loss cope with sensory deficit through a variety of behavioral cues.
Assess if client takes large doses of aspirin or other ototoxic drugs (e.g., aminoglycosides, furosemide, streptomycin, cisplatin, ethacrynic acid).	Medications have side effects of hearing loss.
Determine whether client uses hearing aid.	Determination allows nurse to assess ability to care for device and allows nurse to adjust voice tone to communicate.
If client had recent hearing problem, note onset, contributing factors, affected ear, and effect on activities for daily living.	Nature and severity of hearing problem are determined.
Determine whether client has repeated history of cerumen buildup in ear.	Cerumen impaction is common cause for conduction deafness.

Ear Canals and Eardrums.   The deeper structures of the external and middle ear can be observed only with an **otoscope,** which is an ophthalmoscope with a special ear speculum attached to the battery tube. Speculums come in different sizes to conform to the different sizes of ear canals. For best visualization the largest speculum that fits comfortably into the ear canal should be used.

Before inserting the speculum, the examiner checks for foreign bodies in the opening of the auditory canal. Clients must not move their heads during the examination to avoid damage to the canal and tympanic membrane. Infants and young children often need to be restrained. Infants should lie supine with their heads turned to one side and their arms held securely at their sides. Young children can sit on their parents' laps with their legs held between the parents' knees.

The nurse turns on the otoscope by rotating the dial at the top of the battery tube. To insert the speculum properly, the nurse asks the client to tip the head slightly toward the opposite shoulder. The nurse holds the handle of the otoscope in the space between the thumb and index finger, supported on the middle finger. This leaves the ulnar side of the hand to rest against the client's head, stabilizing the otoscope as it is inserted into the canal (Seidel and others, 1999). Two grips on the otoscope may be used. In one grip, the nurse holds the battery tube along the client's face with the fingers against the face or neck. In the other grip, the inverted otoscope is lightly braced against

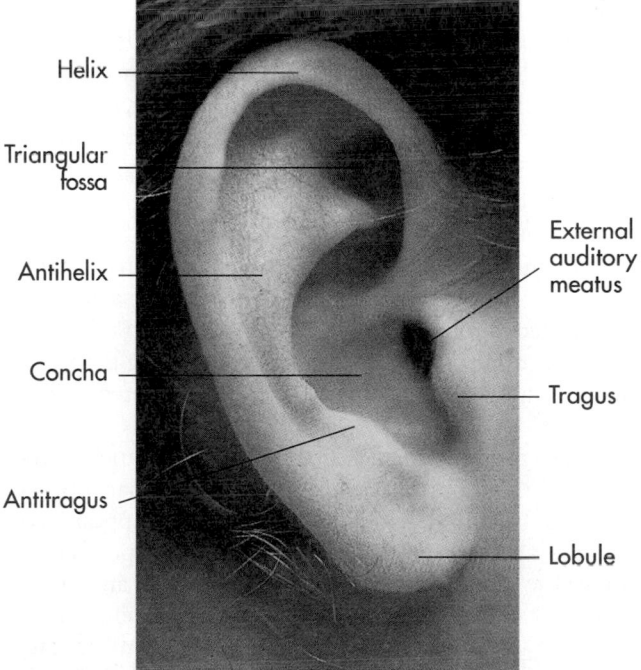

Figure 32-25   Anatomical structures of the auricle.
From Seidel HM and others: *Mosby's guide to physical examination,* ed 4, St. Louis, 1999, Mosby.

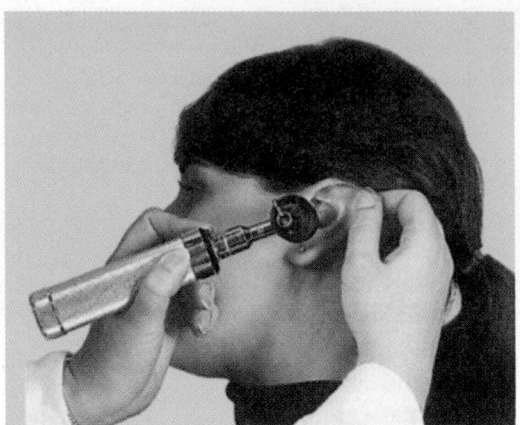

Figure 32-26 Otoscopic examination.
From Seidel HM and others: *Mosby's guide to physical examination*, ed 4, St. Louis, 1999, Mosby.

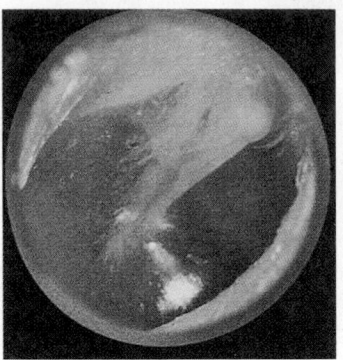

Figure 32-27 Normal right tympanic membrane.
Courtesy Dr. Richard A. Buckingham, Abraham Lincoln School of Medicine, University of Illinois, Chicago.

the side of the client's head or cheek. This grip, used with children, prevents accidental movement of the otoscope deeper into the ear canal. The nurse inserts the scope while pulling the auricle upward and backward in the adult and older child (Figure 32-26). Pulling the auricle gently up, back, and slightly out in the adult or older child straightens the ear canal. In infants the nurse pulls the auricle back and down.

The nurse inserts the speculum slightly down and forward 1 to 1.5 cm (½ inch) into the ear canal. Care is taken not to abrade the sensitive lining of the ear canal, since this can be painful. The skin has little subcutaneous fat between it and the underlying bone. The canal normally has little cerumen and is uniformly pink with tiny hairs in the outer third of the canal. The nurse observes for color, discharge, scaling, lesions, foreign bodies, and cerumen. Normally cerumen is dry (light brown to gray and flaky) or moist (dark yellow or brown) and sticky. Dry cerumen occurs in Asians and Native Americans about 85% of the time (Seidel and others, 1999). A reddened canal with discharge is a sign of inflammation or infection. In other adults, accumulated cerumen is a common problem. Buildup of cerumen can create a mild hearing loss. During the examination the examiner asks about methods that the client uses to clean the ear canal (Box 32-15).

The light from the otoscope allows visualization of the tympanic membrane. The nurse must be familiar with the common anatomical landmarks and their appearances (Figure 32-27). This takes practice. The otoscope is slowly moved so that the entire tympanic membrane and its periphery can be seen. Because the tympanic membrane is angled away from the ear canal, the light from the otoscope appears as a cone rather than a circle. A ring of fibrous cartilage surrounds the oval membrane. The umbo is near the center of the membrane, and the attachment of the malleus is behind it. A knoblike structure at the top of

the tympanic membrane is created by the underlying short process of the malleus. The nurse should check carefully to make sure that there are no tears or breaks in the membrane. The normal tympanic membrane is translucent, shiny, and pearly gray. It is free from tears or breaks. A pink or red bulging membrane indicates inflammation. A white color reveals pus behind it. The membrane is taut, except for the small triangular pars flaccida near the top. If the tympanic membrane is blocked by cerumen, irrigation with warm water will safely remove the wax.

Hearing Acuity.   Often the nurse can tell whether the client has a hearing loss from a response to conversation. The three types of hearing loss are conduction, sensorineural, and mixed. A conduction loss interrupts sound waves as they travel from the outer ear to the cochlea of the inner ear because the sound waves are not transmitted through the outer and middle ear structures. Examples of causes of a conduction loss are swelling of the auditory canal or tears in the tympanic membrane. A sensorineural loss involves the inner ear, auditory nerve, or hearing center of the brain. Sound is conducted through the outer and middle ear structures, but the continued transmission of sound becomes interrupted at some point beyond the bony ossicles. A mixed loss involves a combination of conduction and sensorineural loss.

Clients working or living around loud noises are at risk for hearing loss. Older adults experience an inability to hear high-frequency sounds and consonants (e.g., *S, Z, T,* and *G*). Deterioration of the cochlea and a thickening of the tympanic membrane cause older adults to gradually lose hearing acuity. They are especially at risk for hearing loss due to **ototoxicity** (injury to auditory nerve) resulting from high maintenance doses of antibiotics (e.g., the aminoglycosides).

To begin a hearing assessment, the nurse has the client

Client Teaching DURING EAR ASSESSMENT   Box 32-15

OBJECTIVES
- Client will use proper technique for cleansing the ears.
- Client will follow preventive guidelines for screening of hearing loss.
- Client with hearing loss will communicate effectively.

TEACHING STRATEGIES
- Instruct client about the proper way to clean the outer ear (see Chapter 38), avoiding use of cotton-tipped applicators and sharp objects such as hairpins, which may cause impaction of cerumen deep in the ear canal.
- Tell client to avoid inserting pointed objects into the ear canal.

- Encourage clients over age 65 to have regular hearing checks. Explain that a reduction in hearing is a normal part of aging (see Chapter 48).
- Instruct family members of clients with hearing losses to avoid shouting, speaking instead in low tones, and to be sure the client can see the speaker's face.

EVALUATION
- Ask client to explain the proper technique for cleansing the ears.
- In a follow-up visit, question client about frequency of hearing checks.
- Observe client with hearing loss interacting with family members.

---

remove any hearing aid that is worn. The nurse notes the client's response to questions. Normally the client should respond without excessive requests to have the nurse repeat questions. If hearing loss is suspected, the nurse checks the client's response to the whispered voice. One ear is tested at a time while the client occludes the other ear with a finger. The nurse asks the client to gently move the finger up and down during the test. While standing 30 to 60 cm (1 to 2 feet) from the ear being tested, the nurse covers the mouth so that the client is unable to read lips. After exhaling fully, the nurse first whispers softly toward the unoccluded ear, reciting random numbers with equally accented syllables, such as *nine-four-ten*. If necessary, the nurse gradually increases voice intensity until the client correctly repeats the numbers. The other ear is then tested for comparison. Seidel and others (1999) report that clients normally hear numbers clearly when whispered, responding correctly at least 50% of the time. A ticking watch may also be used to test hearing acuity, but the spoken word allows for more accuracy and control in testing.

If a hearing loss is present, there are tests that can be performed using a tuning fork or audiometry. A tuning fork of 256 to 512 hertz (Hz) is most commonly used. The tuning fork allows for comparison of hearing by bone conduction with that of air conduction. The nurse holds the base of the tuning fork with one hand without touching the tines. The fork should be lightly tapped against the palm of the other hand, setting the fork in vibration (Table 32-16).

NOSE AND SINUSES

The nurse uses inspection and palpation to assess the nose and sinuses. The client sits during the examination. A penlight allows for gross examination of each naris. A more detailed examination requires use of a nasal speculum to inspect the deeper nasal turbinates. A student should not use a speculum unless a qualified practitioner is present. Table 32-17 lists components of the nursing history.

Nose.   When inspecting the external nose, the nurse observes for shape, size, skin, color, and the presence of deformity or inflammation. The nose is normally smooth and symmetric and the same color as the face. Recent trauma may have caused edema and discoloration. If swelling or deformities exist, the nurse gently palpates the ridge and soft tissue of the nose by placing one finger on each side of the nasal arch and gently moving the fingers from the nasal bridge to the tip. The nurse notes any tenderness, masses, or underlying deviations. Nasal structures are usually firm and stable.

Air normally passes freely through the nose as a person breathes. To assess patency of the nares, the nurse places a finger on the side of the client's nose and occludes one naris. The client is asked to breathe with the mouth closed. The examination is repeated for the other naris.

While illuminating the anterior nares, the nurse inspects the mucosa for color, lesions, discharge, swelling, and evidence of bleeding. If discharge is present, gloves should be worn. Normal mucosa is pink and moist without lesions. Pale mucosa with clear discharge indicates allergy. A mucoid discharge indicates rhinitis. A sinus infection results in yellowish or greenish discharge. Habitual use of intranasal cocaine and opioids can cause puffiness and increased vascularity of the nasal mucosa (Friedman and others, 1996). For the client with a nasogastric or nasopharyngeal tube, the nurse routinely checks for local skin breakdown (**excoriation**) of the naris, characterized by redness and sloughing of the skin.

To view the septum and turbinates, the client tips the head back slightly to give the nurse a clear view. The septum is inspected for alignment, perforation, or bleeding. Normally the septum is close to the midline, and thicker anteriorly than posteriorly. The turbinates are covered

Table 32-16 Tuning Fork Tests

Tests and Steps	Rationale
Weber's Test (Lateralization of Sound) Hold fork at its base and tap it lightly against heel of palm. Place base of vibrating fork on midline vertex of client's head or middle of forehead (see illustration below). Ask client if the sound is heard equally in both ears or better in one ear.	Client with normal hearing hears sound equally in both ears or in midline of head. In conduction deafness, sound is heard best in impaired ear. In unilateral sensorineural hearing loss, sound is identified only in normal ear.
Rinne Test (Comparison of Air and Bone Conduction) Place stem of vibrating tuning fork against client's mastoid process (see illustration below, right, top). Begin counting the interval with your watch. Ask client to tell you when the sound is no longer heard; note number of seconds. Quickly place still-vibrating tines 1 to 2 cm (1/2 to 1 inch) from ear canal and ask client to tell you when the sound is no longer heard (see illustration below, right, bottom). Continue counting time the sound is heard by air conduction. Compare number of seconds the sound is heard by bone conduction versus air conduction.	Air-conducted sound should be heard twice as long as bone-conducted sound. In conduction deafness, bone-conducted sound can be heard longer. In sensorineural loss, sound is reduced and heard longer through air.

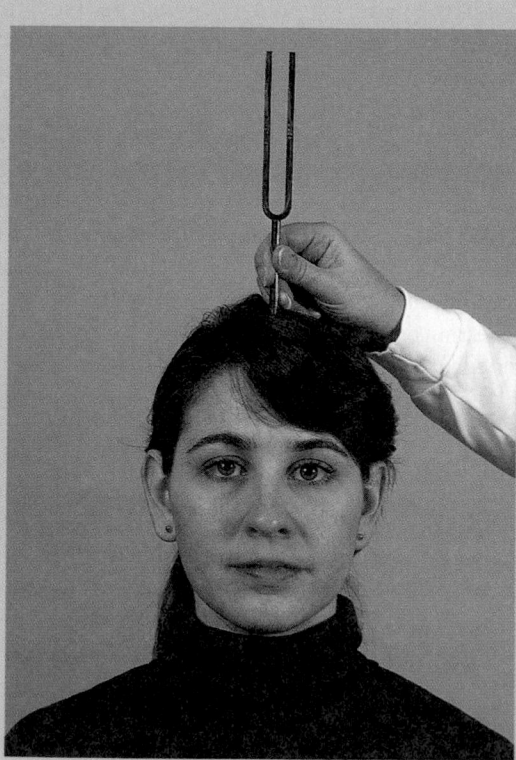

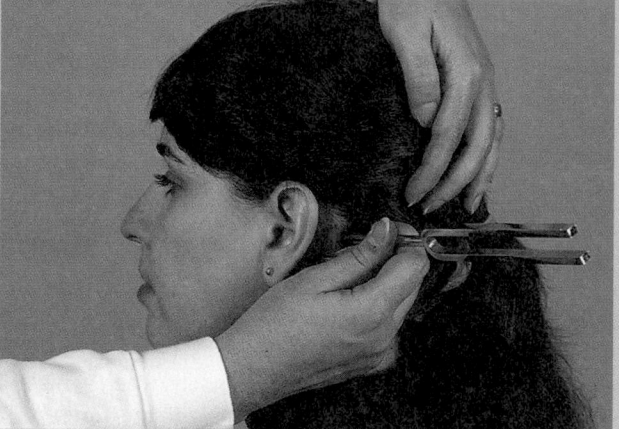

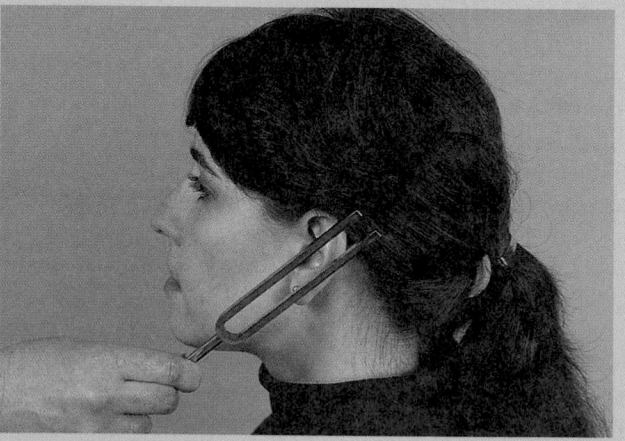

Illustrations from Seidel HM and others: *Mosby's guide to physical examination*, ed 4, St. Louis, 1999, Mosby.

Table 32-17 Nursing History for Nose and Sinus Assessment

Assessment Category	Rationale
Ask if client has had trauma to nose.	Trauma can cause septal deviation and asymmetry of external nose.
Ask if client has history of allergies, nasal discharge, epistaxis (nose bleeds), or postnasal drip.	History is useful in determining source or nature of nasal and sinus drainage.
If there is history of nasal discharge, assess color, amount, odor, duration, and associated symptoms (e.g., sneezing, nasal congestion, obstruction or mouth breathing).	Can help to rule out presence of infection, allergy, or drug use.
Assess for history of nosebleed, including site, frequency, amount of bleeding, treatment, and difficulty stopping bleeding.	Characteristics may reveal trauma, medication use, or excessive dryness as causative factors.
Ask if client uses nasal spray or drops.	Overuse of over-the-counter nasal preparations can cause physical change in mucosa.
Ask if client snores at night or has difficulty breathing.	Difficulty with breathing or snoring may indicate septal deviation or obstruction.

with mucous membranes that warm and moisten inspired air. The mucosa is pink and moist, with clear mucus. A deviated septum can obstruct breathing and interfere with passage of a nasogastric tube. Perforation of the septum can occur after repeated use of intranasal cocaine. The nurse notes any **polyps** (tumorlike growth) or purulent drainage.

Sinuses.   Examination of the sinuses involves palpation. In cases of allergies or infection, the interior of the sinuses become inflamed and swollen. The most effective way to assess for tenderness is by externally palpating the frontal and maxillary facial areas (Figure 32-28). The frontal sinus is palpated by exerting pressure with the thumb up and under the client's eyebrow. Gentle, upward pressure elicits tenderness easily if sinus irritation is present and reveals the severity of sinus irritation. Pressure should not be applied to the eyes. Box 32-16 describes teaching guidelines during nose and sinus assessment.

MOUTH AND PHARYNX

The nurse assesses the mouth and pharynx to detect signs of overall health, determine oral hygiene needs, and develop nursing therapies for clients with dehydration, restricted intake, oral trauma, or oral airway obstruction. To assess the oral cavity, the nurse uses a penlight and tongue depressor or a single gauze square. Gloves should be worn during the examination. The client may sit or lie during the examination. Assessment of the oral cavity can be made during administration of oral hygiene (see Chapter 38). Table 32-18 describes the nursing history for assessment of the mouth and pharynx.

Lips.   The lips are inspected for color, texture, hydration, contour, and lesions. With the client's mouth closed, the nurse views the lips from end to end. Normally they are pink, moist, symmetrical, and smooth (Figure 32-29).

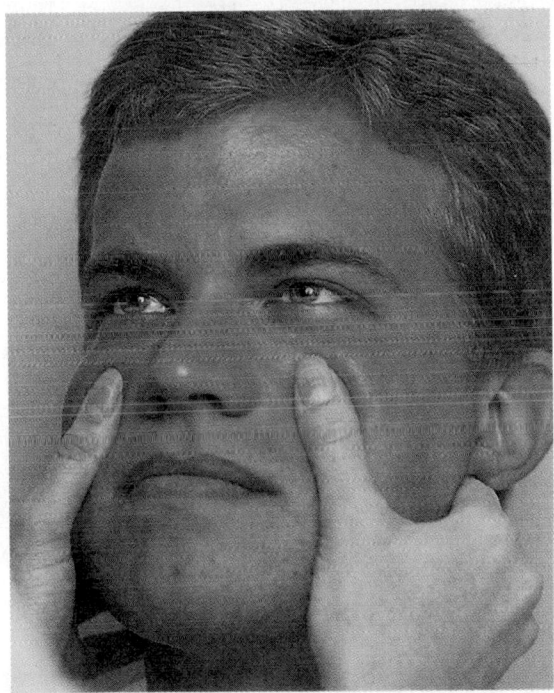

Figure 32-28   Palpation of maxillary sinuses.

Female clients should remove their lipstick before the examination. Pallor of the lips can be caused by anemia, with cyanosis caused by respiratory or cardiovascular problems. Cherry-colored lips may indicate carbon monoxide poisoning. Any lesions such as nodules or ulcerations can be related to infection, irritation, or skin cancer.

Buccal Mucosa, Gums, and Teeth.   The nurse begins inspection by having the client clench the teeth and smile. The maneuver allows assessment of teeth occlusion. The upper molars should rest directly on the lower molars

Client Teaching DURING NOSE AND SINUS ASSESSMENT

Box 32-16

OBJECTIVES

- Client will safely use over-the-counter nasal sprays.
- Parents will take proper measures to stop a child's nosebleed.
- Older adult will take safety precautions with loss of olfaction.

TEACHING STRATEGIES

- Caution client against overuse of over-the-counter nasal sprays, which can lead to "rebound" effect, causing excess nasal congestion.
- Instruct parents on care of a child with nosebleeds: have child sit up and lean forward to avoid aspiration of blood, apply pressure to the anterior nose with the thumb and forefinger as the child breathes through the mouth, and ap-

ply ice or a cold cloth to the bridge of the nose if pressure fails to stop bleeding.

- Instruct older adults to install smoke detectors on each floor of their home.
- Instruct older adults to always check dated labels on food to ensure against spoilage.

EVALUATION

- Have client explain proper use of over-the-counter nasal sprays.
- Have parents demonstrate and describe technique for stopping a nosebleed.
- Inspect client's home during visit and look for smoke detectors. Ask to check some food items in the refrigerator.

Table 32-18 **Nursing History for Mouth and Pharyngeal Assessment**

Assessment Category	Rationale
Determine if client wears dentures or retainers and if they are comfortable.	Dentures must be removed to visualize and palpate gums. Ill-fitting dentures chronically irritate mucosa and gums.
Determine if client has had recent change in appetite or weight.	Symptoms may result from painful mouth conditions or poor hygiene.
Determine if client smokes or chews tobacco.	Tobacco users have greater risk for mouth and throat cancers than nonusers (ACS, 1998).
Review history for alcohol consumption.	Heavy drinkers appear to have greater risk for oral cancer. Effects of alcohol are independent of tobacco use.
Assess dental hygiene practices, including use of fluoride toothpaste, frequency of brushing and flossing, and frequency of dental visits.	Assessment reveals client's need for education and/or financial support. Periodontal disease has a higher prevalence in older adults who have history of high plaque buildup, use tobacco, and visit the dentist infrequently.
Ask if client has pain from chewing or eating. If so, ask if mouth lesions are present, including duration and associated symptoms.	May be associated with broken tooth, tooth grinding, or temporomandibular joint problems. Extra care needed during oral hygiene administration.

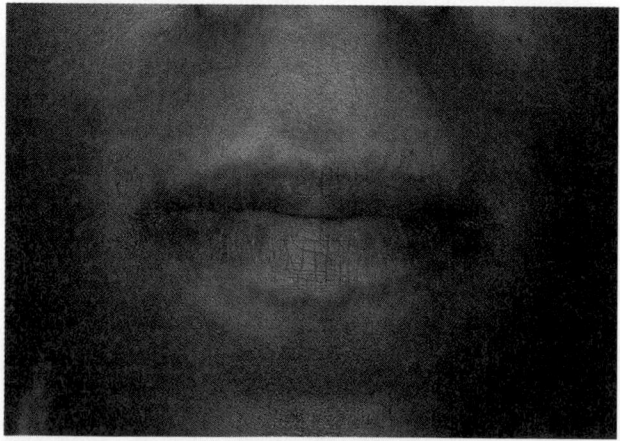

Figure 32-29 The lips are normally pink, symmetrical, smooth, and moist.

with the upper incisors slightly overriding the lower incisors. A symmetrical smile reveals normal facial nerve function.

The quality of dental hygiene is easily determined by inspecting the teeth (Box 32-17). The position and alignment of the teeth are noted. To examine the posterior surface of the teeth, the nurse has the client open the mouth with the lips relaxed. A tongue depressor may be needed to retract the lips and cheeks, especially when viewing the molars. Tartar along the base of the teeth, dental **caries** (cavities), extraction sites, and tooth color should be noted. Normal, healthy teeth are smooth, white, and shiny. A chalky white discoloration of the enamel is an early indication of caries formation. Brown or black discolorations indicate the formation of caries. In the older adult, loose or missing teeth are common because bone

*Data from American Cancer Society: *1999 cancer facts and figures,* New York, 1999, The Society.

Client Teaching DURING MOUTH AND PHARYNGEAL ASSESSMENT   Box 32-17

OBJECTIVES
- Client will practice proper oral hygiene measures and dental care.
- Client will describe warning signs of oral cancer.
- Older adult will maintain normal solid food intake.

TEACHING STRATEGIES
- Discuss proper techniques for oral hygiene, including brushing and flossing (see Chapter 38).
- Explain the early warning signs of oral cancer, including a sore that bleeds easily and does not heal, a lump or thickening, and a red or white patch on the mucosa that persists.* Difficulty chewing or swallowing is a late symptom.

- Encourage regular dental examination every 6 months for children, adults, and older adults.
- Identify older clients who have difficulty in chewing and changes in the teeth. Teach clients to eat soft foods and cut food into small pieces.

EVALUATION
- Ask client to demonstrate brushing.
- Have client identify when to have regular dental checkups.
- Have client identify the warning signs of oral cancer.
- Ask older adult to keep a diet record for 3 days.

---

resorption increases. An older adult's teeth often feel rough when tooth enamel calcifies. Yellow or darkened teeth are also common in the older adult because of the general wear and tear that exposes the darker, underlying dentin.

To view the mucosa and gums, the nurse asks the client to first remove any dental appliance. The nurse views the inner oral mucosa by having the client open and relax the mouth slightly and then gently retracts the client's lower lip away from the teeth (Figure 32-30). This process is repeated for the upper lip. The mucosa is inspected for color, hydration, texture, and lesions such as ulcers, abrasions, or cysts. Normal mucous membrane is pinkish red, smooth, and moist. Small, yellow-white raised lesions commonly seen on the buccal mucosa and lips are Fordyce spots, or ectopic sebaceous glands (Seidel and others, 1999). If lesions are present, the nurse palpates them gently with a gloved hand for tenderness, size, and consistency.

To visualize the buccal mucosa, the nurse asks the client to open the mouth and then gently retracts the cheeks with a tongue depressor or gloved finger covered with gauze (Figure 32-31). The surface of the mucosa must be viewed from right to left and top to bottom. A penlight illuminates the most posterior portion of the mucosa. Normal mucosa is glistening, pink, soft, moist, and smooth. An increase in color or hyperpigmentation is normal in 10% of whites after age 50 and in up to 90% of African-Americans by the same age. For clients with normal pigmentation, the buccal mucosa is a good site to inspect for jaundice and pallor. In older adults the mucosa is normally dry because of reduced salivation. Thick white patches (**leukoplakia**) can be seen in heavy smokers and alcoholics. Leukoplakia should be reported because it can also be a precancerous lesion. The nurse palpates the cheek with one finger along the inner mucosa and the thumb along the outside cheek to check for deep-seated lumps or ulcerations.

While the nurse retracts the cheeks, the gums (gingi-

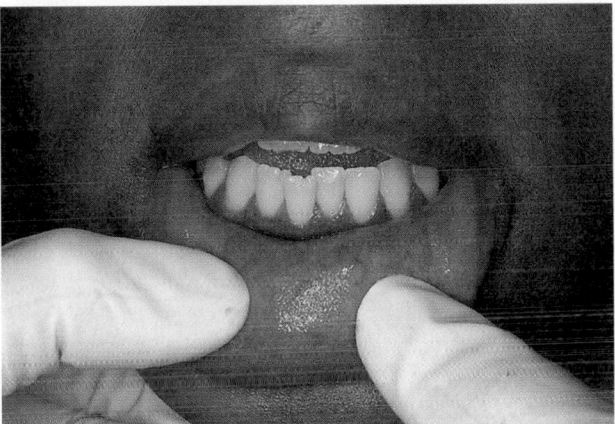

Figure 32-30   Inspection of inner oral mucosa of lower lip.

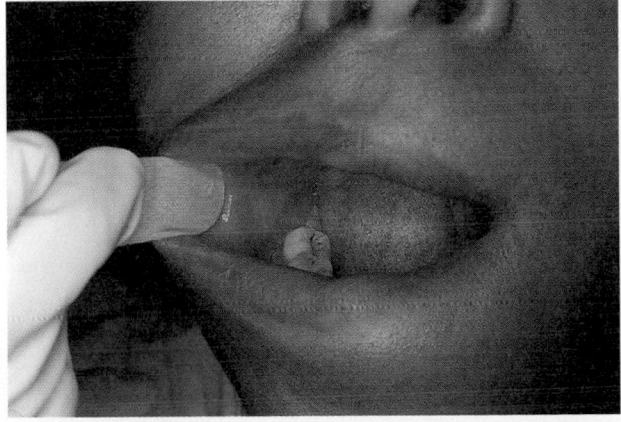

Figure 32-31   Retraction of the buccal mucosa allows for clear visualization.

vae) are inspected for color, edema, retraction, bleeding, and lesions. The gums around the back molars should be viewed because this is a difficult area to reach when cleaning teeth. Healthy gums are pink, smooth, and moist, with a tight margin at each tooth. African-Americans may have patchy pigmentation. In older adults the gums are usually pale. Using gloves, the nurse palpates the gums to assess for lesions, thickening, or masses. There should be no tenderness on palpation. Spongy gums that bleed easily indicate periodontal disease and vitamin C deficiency. If the client has loose or mobile teeth, swollen gums, or pockets containing debris at the tooth margins, periodontal disease or gingivitis can be suspected.

Tongue and Floor of Mouth.

The tongue is carefully inspected on all sides, and the floor of the mouth is checked. The client first relaxes the mouth and sticks the tongue out halfway. The nurse notes any deviation, tremor, or limitation in movement. This tests hypoglossal nerve function. If the client protrudes the tongue too far, the gag reflex may be elicited. When the tongue protrudes, it lies midline. To test for tongue mobility, the nurse asks the client to raise the tongue up and move it from side to side. The tongue should move freely.

Using the penlight for illumination, the nurse examines the tongue for color, size, position, texture, and coatings or lesions. The tongue should be medium or dull red in color, moist, slightly rough on the top surface, and smooth along the lateral margins. The undersurface of the tongue and the floor of the mouth are highly vascular (Figure 32-32). Extra care is taken to inspect these areas, which are common sites for oral cancer lesions. The client lifts the tongue by placing its tip on the palate behind the upper incisors. The nurse looks for color, swelling, and lesions such as nodules or cysts. The ventral surface of the tongue is pink and smooth, with large veins between the frenulum folds.

To palpate the tongue, the nurse explains the procedure and then asks the client to protrude the tongue. The nurse grasps the tip with a gauze square and gently pulls it to one side. With a gloved hand, the nurse palpates the full length of the tongue and the base for any areas of hardening or ulceration. **Varicosities** (swollen, tortuous veins) may be seen. Varicosities rarely cause problems but are common in the older adult.

Palate.

The client should extend the head backward, holding the mouth open so that the nurse can inspect the hard and soft palates for color, shape, texture, and extra bony prominences or defects (Figure 32-33). The hard palate, or roof of the mouth, is located anteriorly. It is whitish and should be dome shaped. The soft palate, best seen while depressing the tongue with a tongue blade, extends posteriorly toward the pharynx. It is normally light pink and smooth. A bony growth, or **exostosis,** between the two palates is common.

Pharynx.

The pharynx can be a site for infection, inflammation, or lesions. Before examining the pharynx, the nurse explains the procedure to the client. The client tips the head back slightly, opens the mouth wide, and says "ah." The nurse places the tip of a tongue depressor on the middle third of the tongue, taking care not to press the lower lip against the teeth. If the tongue depressor is placed too far anteriorly, the posterior part of the tongue mounds up, obstructing the view. The gag reflex is elicited when the tongue depressor touches the posterior tongue.

With a penlight, the nurse inspects the uvula and soft palate (Figure 32-34). Both structures, which are innervated by the tenth cranial (vagus) nerve, should rise centrally as the client says "ah." The nurse also inspects the arch formed by the anterior and posterior pillars, soft palate, and uvula. The tonsils can be viewed in the cavities

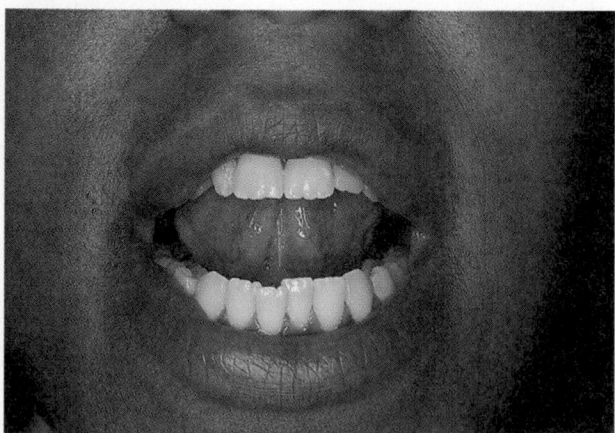

Figure 32-32 The undersurface of the tongue is highly vascular.

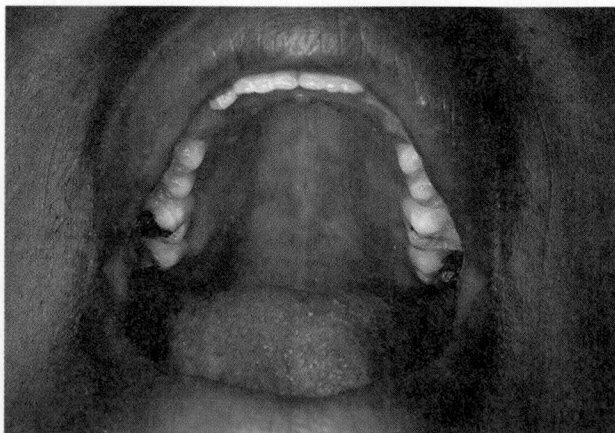

Figure 32-33 The hard palate is located anteriorly in the roof of the mouth.

between the anterior and posterior pillars and are oval, with infoldings of tissue. The posterior pharynx is behind the pillars. The pharyngeal tissues are normally pink and smooth. Edema, ulceration, or inflammation indicates infection or abnormal lesions. Clients with chronic sinus problems frequently exhibit a clear exudate that drains along the wall of the posterior pharynx. Yellow or green exudate indicates infection. A client with a typical sore throat has redness and swelling of the uvula, and tonsillar pillars, as well as the possible presence of yellow exudate.

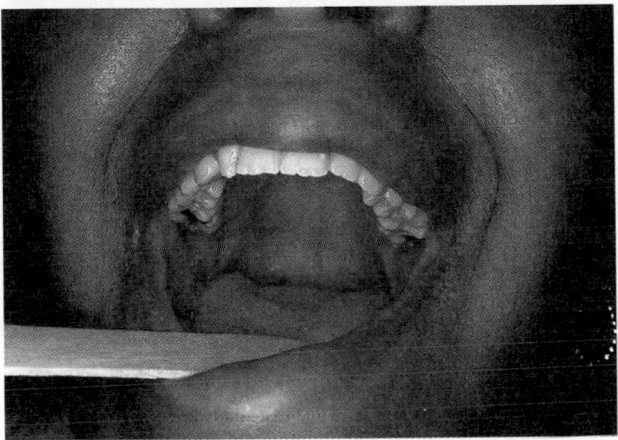

Figure 32-34 A penlight and tongue depressor allow the nurse to visualize the uvula and posterior soft palate.

NECK

The neck muscles, lymph nodes of the head and neck, carotid arteries, jugular veins, thyroid gland, and trachea are located within the neck (Figure 32-35). An examination of the jugular veins and carotid arteries can be deferred until assessment of the vascular system. The nurse inspects and palpates the neck to determine the integrity of the neck structures and to examine the lymphatic system. The lymphatic system is examined region by region during the assessment of other body systems (head and neck, breast, genitalia, and extremities). An abnormality of superficial lymph nodes may reveal an infection or malignancy. Examination of the thyroid gland and trachea also aids in ruling out malignancies. Examination is best performed with the client sitting. The areas of the neck are outlined by the sternocleidomastoid and trapezius muscles, which divide each side of the neck into two triangles. The anterior triangle contains the trachea, thyroid gland, carotid artery, and anterior cervical lymph nodes. The posterior triangle contains the posterior lymph nodes. Table 32-19 reviews the nursing history for the head and neck examination.

Neck Muscles. The nurse begins the examination by inspecting the neck in the usual anatomical position, in slight hyperextension. The nurse inspects for bilateral symmetry of the neck muscles. To test the function of the sternocleidomastoid muscle, the nurse asks the client to flex the neck with the chin to the chest. Then the client hy-

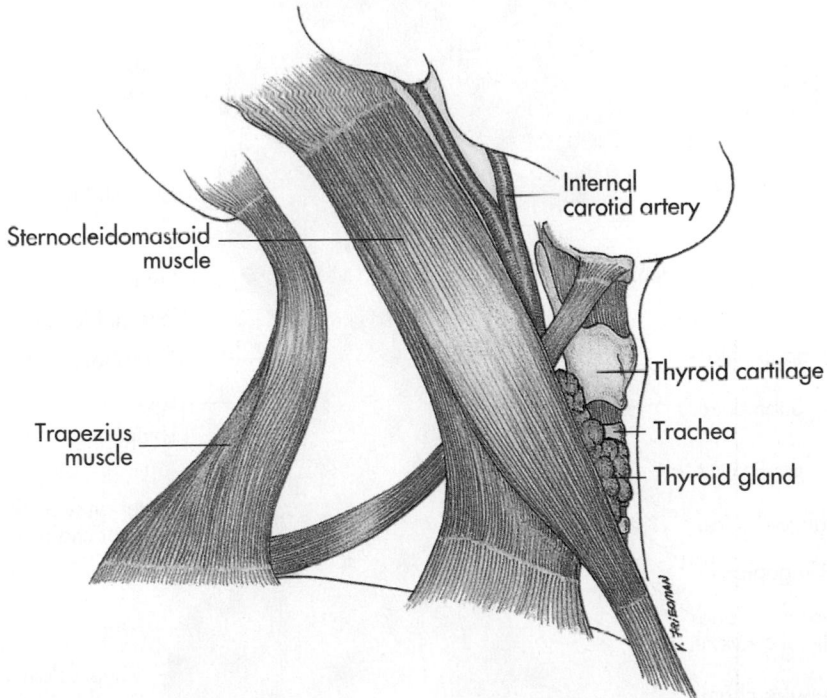

Figure 32-35 Anatomical position of the major neck structures. Note the triangles formed by the sternocleidomastoid muscle, lower jaw, and anterior neck anteriorly and by the sternocleidomastoid muscle, trapezius muscle, and lower neck posteriorly.

Table 32-19 **Nursing History for Neck Assessment**

Assessment Category	Rationale
Assess for history of recent cold or infection.	Colds or infections can cause temporary or permanent lymph node enlargement.
If there is an enlarged lymph node, consider reviewing history of IV drug use, hemophilia, sexual contact with persons infected with HIV, history of blood transfusion, multiple and indiscriminate sexual contacts, or male with homosexual or bisexual activities.	These are risk factors for HIV infection.
Ask if client has had history of neck pain with restriction in movement.	May indicate muscle strain, head injury, local nerve injury, or enlarged or swollen lymph node.
Ask if client has had change in temperature preference (more or less clothing); swelling in neck; change in texture of hair, skin, or nails; or change in emotional stability.	Symptoms indicative of thyroid disease.
Ask if client has history of thyroid problem or takes thyroid medication.	Disease or medications may influence tissue growth of gland.
Review medical history of pneumothorax (collapsed lung) or bronchial tumor.	Conditions place client at risk for tracheal displacement or lateral deviation.

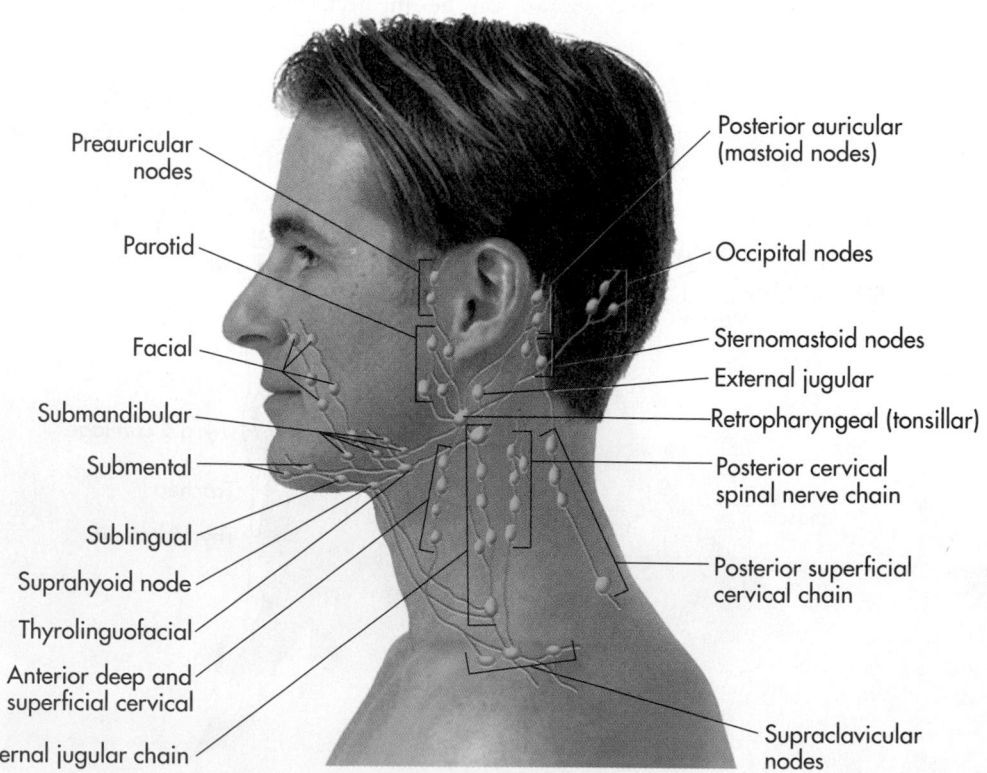

Figure 32-36   Lymphatic drainage system of the head and neck. If the group of nodes is often referred to by another name, the second name appears in parentheses.
From Seidel HM and others: *Mosby's guide to physical examination,* ed 4, St. Louis, 1999, Mosby.

perextends the neck backward so that the nurse can check for trapezius muscle function. Movement of the head sideways so that the ear moves toward the shoulder further tests function of the sternocleidomastoid muscle. The neck should move freely without discomfort or dizziness. Other tests for muscle strength and function can be performed during assessment of the musculoskeletal system.

Lymph Nodes.

An extensive system of lymph nodes collects lymph from the head, ears, nose, cheeks, and lips (Figure 32-36). The immune system protects the body from foreign antigens, removes damaged cells from the circulation, and provides a partial barrier to growth of malignant cells within the body. The nurse should become particularly competent in assessing the lymph nodes when caring for clients with suspected immunoincompetence, which can be linked to allergies, human immunodeficiency virus (HIV) infection, autoimmune disease (e.g., lupus erythematosus), or serious infection.

With the client's chin raised and head tilted slightly, the nurse first inspects the area where lymph nodes are distributed and compares both sides. This position stretches the skin slightly over any possible enlarged nodes. Visible nodes are inspected for edema, erythema, or red streaks. Nodes are not normally visible.

A methodical approach is used to examine the lymph nodes to avoid overlooking any single node or chain. The client relaxes with the neck flexed slightly forward and, if needed, toward the nurse. This maneuver relaxes tissues and muscles. Both sides of the neck are inspected and palpated for comparison. During palpation the nurse faces or stands to the side of the client for easy access to all nodes. Using the pads of the middle three fingers of the hand, the nurse palpates gently in a rotary motion for superficial lymph nodes (Figure 32-37). Each node is checked methodically in the following sequence: occipital nodes at the base of the skull, postauricular nodes over the mastoid, preauricular nodes just in front of the ear, retropharyngeal nodes at the angle of the mandible, submaxillary nodes, and submental nodes in the midline behind the mandibular tip. The nurse tries to detect enlargement and notes the location, size, shape, surface characteristics, consistency, mobility, tenderness, and warmth of the nodes. If the skin is mobile, the nurse moves the skin over the area of the nodes (Seidel and others, 1999). It is important to press underlying tissue in each area and not simply move the fingers over the skin. However, if excessive pressure is applied, small nodes are missed and palpable nodes are obliterated.

To palpate supraclavicular nodes, the nurse asks the client to bend the head forward and relax the shoulders. The nurse may have to hook the index and third finger over the clavicle, lateral to the sternocleidomastoid muscle, to palpate these nodes. The deep cervical nodes can be palpated only with the nurse's fingers hooked around the sternocleidomastoid muscle.

Normally lymph nodes are not easily palpable.

However, small, mobile, nontender nodes are common. Lymph nodes that are large, fixed, inflamed, or tender indicate a problem such as local infection, systemic disease, or neoplasm (Seidel and others, 1999) (Box 32-18). When enlarged nodes are found, the nurse explores adjacent areas and regions drained by the nodes for signs of infection or malignancy. Tenderness is usually a result of inflammation. Noting which nodes are enlarged may help locate the site of an infection. For example, ear infections usually drain to the preauricular or deep cervical nodes. Malignancy is usually associated with nontender, hard, discrete nodes. After a serious infection a node may remain permanently enlarged but may not be tender.

Thyroid Gland.

The thyroid gland lies in the anterior lower neck, in front of and to both sides of the trachea. The gland is fixed to the trachea with the isthmus overlying the trachea and connecting the two irregular, cone-shaped lobes (Figure 32-38). The nurse assesses the gland by inspection, palpation, and auscultation.

The nurse stands in front of the client and inspects the area of the lower neck overlying the thyroid gland for visible masses, symmetry, and any subtle fullness at the base of the neck. Asking the client to hyperextend the neck helps tighten the skin for better visualization. The nurse

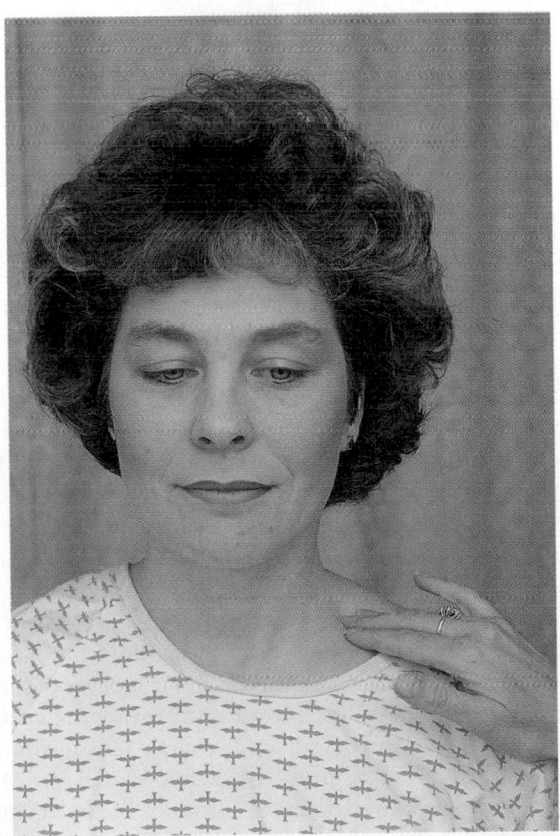

Figure 32-37 Palpation of cervical lymph nodes.

OBJECTIVE
- Client will take proper preventive action if a mass is noted in the neck.

TEACHING STRATEGIES
- Stress importance of regular compliance with medication schedule to clients with thyroid disease.
- Instruct client about the lymph nodes and how infection can commonly cause node tenderness.

- Instruct client to call the physician when an enlarged lump or mass is noted in the neck.
- Teach client risk factors for HIV infection.

EVALUATION
- Have client explain when to notify a physician about a neck mass.

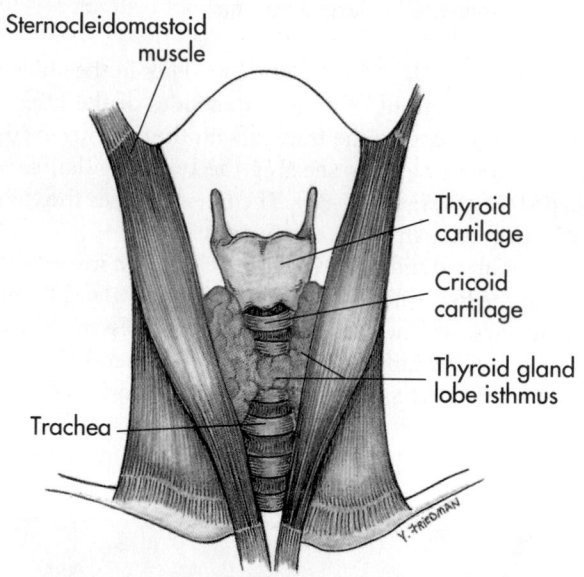

Figure 32-38   Anatomical position of the thyroid gland.

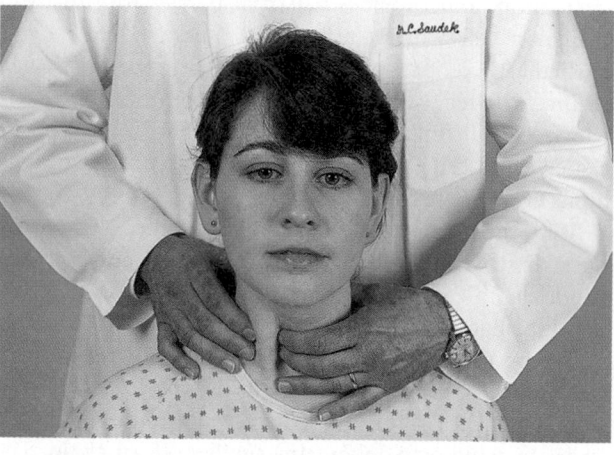

Figure 32-39   Palpation of the right thyroid lobe from behind the client.
From Seidel HM and others: *Mosby's guide to physical examination,* ed 4, St. Louis, 1999, Mosby.

offers the client a glass of water and then has the client swallow while the nurse notes whether there is a bulging of the gland. Normally the thyroid cannot be visualized.

To palpate the gland, the examiner stands in front of or behind the client. Light, gentle palpation is needed to feel any abnormalities. Seidel and others (1999) recommend allowing the fingers to drift over the gland. For both the anterior and posterior approach, the client flexes the neck forward and laterally toward the side being examined to relax the neck muscles. The client holds a cup of water and takes a sip to swallow once instructed by the nurse.

For the posterior approach, the nurse has the client sit with the neck at a comfortable level. Both of the nurse's hands are placed around the neck, with two fingers of each hand on the sides of the trachea just beneath the cricoid cartilage. As the client swallows the nurse feels for movement of the thyroid isthmus. The thyroid should move beneath the fingers when the client swallows. Enlargement of the isthmus as it rises should be noted. To examine each lobe, the nurse has the client swallow while the nurse dis-

places the trachea to the right or left. The nurse then palpates the main body of each lobe (Figure 32-39). During examination of the right lobe, for example, the nurse moves the fingers of the left hand between the trachea and the right sternocleidomastoid muscle. Then the nurse places the fingers of the right hand behind the right sternocleidomastoid muscle and gently presses the hands together to palpate the lobe as the client swallows. The approach is repeated for the left lobe with the hands in the reverse positions. Normally the thyroid gland is small, smooth, and free of nodules. However, in extremely thin individuals the thyroid is more easily palpable. Enlargement is a manifestation of thyroid dysfunction. Masses or nodules may be signs of malignant disease. However, not all nodules are malignant.

The anterior approach requires the client to sit as the nurse stands to the side. Using the pads of the index and middle finger, the nurse palpates the left lobe with the right hand and the right lobe with the left hand as the client swallows. Gentle displacement of the trachea allows palpation of the main body of each thyroid lobe. It helps to move the skin medially over the sternocleidomastoid muscle and to reach under its anterior borders while the fingers stay beneath the cricoid cartilage.

When the gland appears enlarged, the nurse places the bell of the stethoscope over the thyroid. If the gland is enlarged, blood flow through the thyroid arteries increases and causes a fine vibration. The nurse can auscultate the vibration, which is heard as a soft, rushing sound, or bruit.

Carotid Artery and Jugular Vein.
This portion of the examination is described under examination of the vascular system (see later section).

Trachea.
The trachea can be directly palpated and is normally located in the midline of the neck, above the suprasternal notch. Masses in the neck or mediastinum and pulmonary abnormalities can cause displacement laterally. The client may sit or lie down during palpation. The position of the trachea is determined by palpating at the suprasternal notch, slipping the thumb and index fingers to each side. Forceful pressure must not be applied, because this action may elicit a cough.

Thorax and Lungs

Accurate physical assessment of the thorax and lungs requires review of the ventilatory and respiratory functions of the lungs. If the lungs are affected by disease, other body systems will reflect alterations. For example, reduced oxygenation can cause changes in mental alertness because of the brain's sensitivity to lowered oxygen levels. The alert nurse uses the data from all body systems to determine the nature of pulmonary alterations.

Before assessing the thorax and lungs, the nurse must be familiar with the landmarks of the chest (Figure 32-40). These landmarks help the nurse locate findings and use assessment skills correctly. For example, by knowing the position of underlying organs in relation to the landmarks, the nurse can anticipate where to percuss or auscultate the chest wall. The client's nipples, angle of Louis, suprasternal notch, costal angle, clavicles, and vertebrae are key landmarks that provide a series of imaginary lines for sign identification. The lungs and thorax are assessed posteriorly, laterally (on both sides), and anteriorly, with the nurse using landmarks to record localized findings.

During the examination the nurse keeps a mental image of the location of the lobes of the lung and the position of each rib (Figure 32-41). Locating the position of each rib is critical to visualizing the lobe of the lung being assessed. To begin, the nurse locates the angle of Louis at the manubriosternal junction. The angle is a visible and palpable angulation of the sternum and is the point at which the second rib articulates with the sternum. The nurse counts the ribs and intercostal spaces (between the

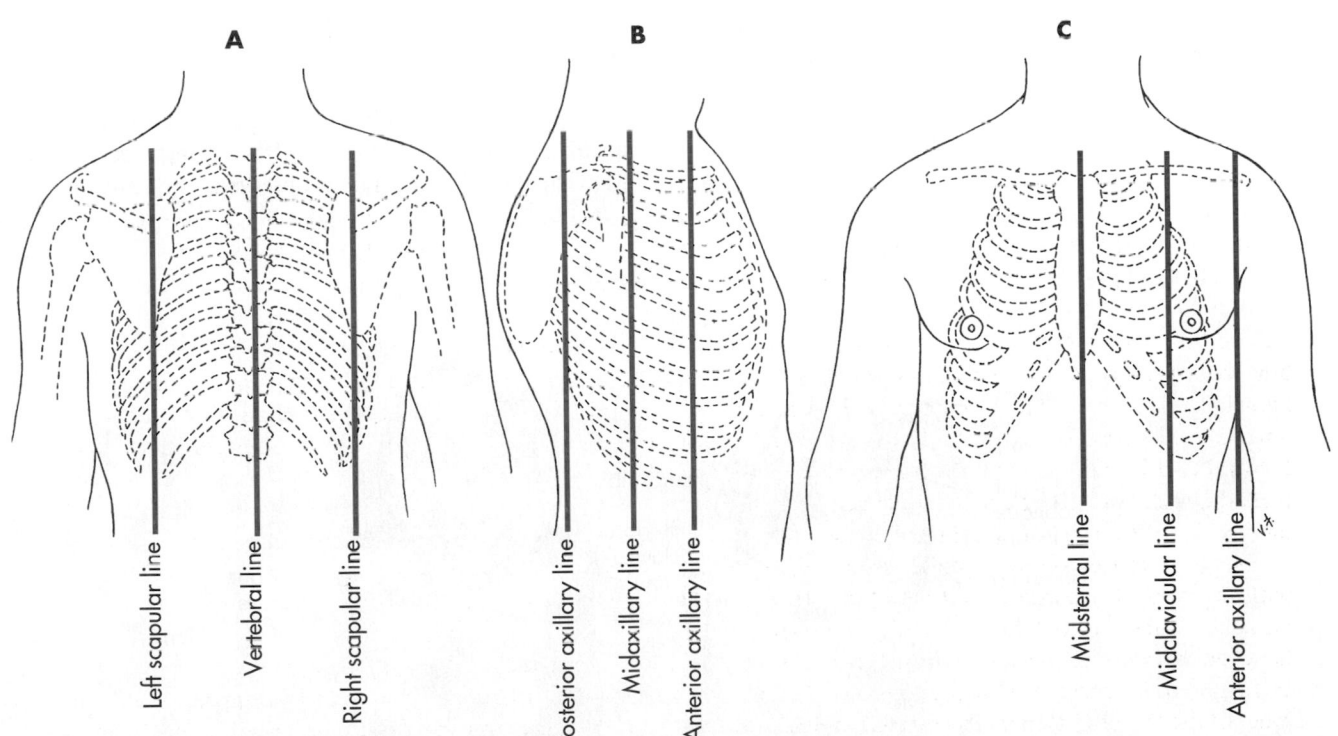

Figure 32-40 Anatomical chest wall landmarks. **A,** Posterior chest landmarks. **B,** Lateral chest landmarks. **C,** Anterior chest landmarks.

ribs) from this point. The number of each intercostal space corresponds with that of the rib just above it. The spinous process of the third thoracic vertebra and the fourth, fifth, and sixth ribs help to locate the lung's lobes laterally. The lower lobes project laterally and anteriorly (Figure 32-42). Posteriorly the tip or inferior margin of the scapula lies approximately at the level of the seventh rib (Figure 32-43). After identifying the seventh rib, the examiner can count upward to locate the third thoracic vertebra and align it with the inner borders of the scapula to locate the posterior lobes.

Examination of the lungs and thorax requires the client to be undressed to the waist. Good lighting is essential. The nurse should assess clients at risk for pulmonary problems, such as the client confined to bed rest or the client with chest pain who cannot fully expand the lungs. The examination begins with the client sitting for assess-

ment of the posterior and lateral chest. For assessment of the anterior chest, the client sits or lies. Table 32-20 reviews the nursing history for lung examination.

POSTERIOR THORAX

The nurse first inspects the shape and symmetry of the client's chest from the back and front. The anteroposterior diameter is noted. The shape of the chest or the client's posture can significantly impair ventilatory movement. Normally the chest contour is symmetrical, with the anteroposterior diameter one third to one half of the transverse, or side-to-side, diameter. Aging and chronic lung disease are characterized by a barrel-shaped chest (anteroposterior diameter equals transverse diameter). Infants have an almost round shape. Abnormal contours are caused by congenital and postural alterations. A client may assume a posture such as leaning over a table or splinting the side of the chest as a result of a breathing problem. Splinting or holding the chest wall as a result of localized pain causes a client to bend toward the side affected. Such a posture impairs ventilatory movement.

Standing at a midline position behind the client, the nurse looks for deformities, the position of the spine, the slope of the ribs, retraction of the intercostal spaces during inspiration, and bulging of the intercostal spaces during expiration. The scapulae are normally symmetrical and closely attached to the thoracic wall. The normal spine is straight without lateral deviation. Posteriorly, the ribs tend to slope across and down. The ribs and intercostal spaces are easier to see in a thin person. Normally no bulging or active movement occurs within the intercostal spaces during breathing. Bulging indicates that the client is using great effort to breathe.

The nurse may also inspect the posterior thorax to determine the rate and rhythm of breathing (see Chapter 31). The thorax as a whole is observed. The entire thorax

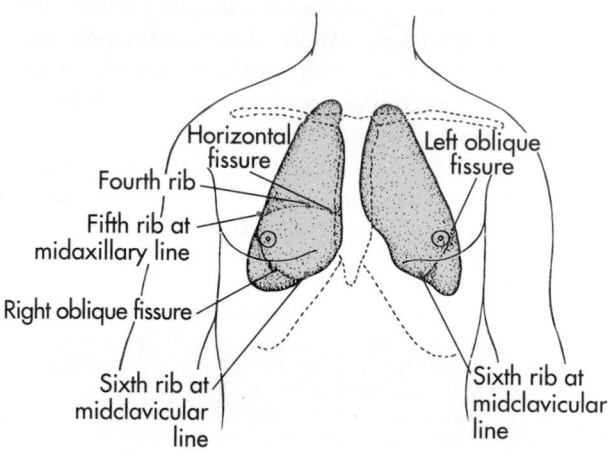

Figure 32-41   Anterior position of lung lobes in relation to anatomical landmarks.

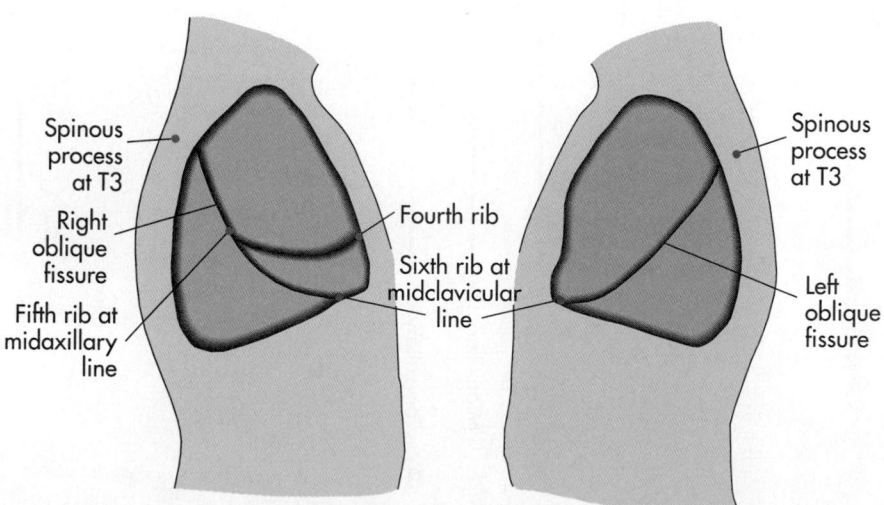

Figure 32-42   Lateral position of lung lobes in relation to anatomical landmarks.

normally expands and relaxes regularly with equality of movement. In healthy adults the normal respiratory rates vary from 12 to 20 respirations per minute.

Palpation of the posterior thorax assesses further characteristics and confirms or supplements assessment findings. The thoracic muscles and skeleton are palpated for lumps, masses, pulsations, and unusual movement. If pain or tenderness is noted, the nurse avoids deep palpation. Fractured rib fragments could be displaced against vital

organs. Normally the chest wall is not tender. If a suspicious mass or swollen area is detected, it is lightly palpated for size, shape, and the typical qualities of a lesion.

To measure chest excursion or depth of breathing, the nurse stands behind the client and places the thumbs along the spinal processes at the tenth rib, with the palms lightly contacting the posterolateral surfaces. The nurse's thumbs should be about 5 cm (2 inches) apart, pointing toward the spine and fingers pointing laterally (Figure 32-44, *A*). The hands are pressed toward the spine so that a small skinfold appears between the thumbs. The nurse does not slide the hands over the skin. The nurse instructs the client to take a deep breath after exhaling. The nurse notes movement of the thumbs (Figure 32-44 *B*). Chest excursion should be symmetrical, separating the thumbs 3 to 5 cm (1¼ to 2 inches). Reduced chest excursion may be caused by pain, postural deformity, or fatigue. In the older adult, chest movement declines because of costal cartilage calcification and respiratory muscle atrophy.

During speech the sound created by the vocal cords is transmitted through the lung to the chest wall. The sound waves create vibrations that can be palpated externally. These vibrations are called **vocal** or **tactile fremitus.** The accumulation of mucus, the collapse of lung tissue, or the presence of lung lesions can block the vibrations from reaching the chest wall.

To palpate for tactile fremitus, the nurse places the ball or lower palm of the hand over symmetrical intercostal

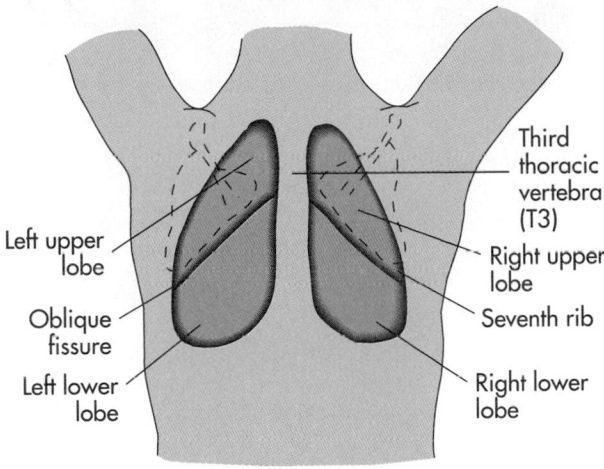

Figure 32-43   Posterior position of lung lobes in relation to anatomical landmarks.

Left upper lobe
Oblique fissure
Left lower lobe
Third thoracic vertebra (T3)
Right upper lobe
Seventh rib
Right lower lobe

Table 32-20   Nursing History for Lung Assessment

Assessment Category	Rationale
Assess history of tobacco or marijuana use, including type of tobacco, duration and amount (pack years = number of years smoking × number of packs per day), age started, and efforts to quit.	Smoking is a risk factor for lung cancer, heart disease, and emphysema or bronchitis. Cigarette smoking accounts for a significant percentage of all cancer deaths.
Ask if client has had a *persistent cough* (productive or nonproductive), *sputum production, chest pain,* shortness of breath, orthopnea, dyspnea during exertion or at rest, poor activity tolerance, or *recurrent attacks of pneumonia or bronchitis.*	Symptoms of respiratory alterations may help nurse localize objective physical findings. (Warning signals for lung cancer are in italic type.)
Determine if client works in environment containing pollutants, (e.g., asbestos, arsenic, coal dust) or requiring exposure to radiation. Does client have exposure to sidestream cigarette smoke?	These risk factors increase chance for various lung diseases.
Review history for known or suspected HIV infection, substance abuse, low income, residence in nursing home, or recent immigration to United States.	These are risk factors for tuberculosis (Haney and others, 1996; Hopkins and Schoener, 1996).
Ask if client has history of persistent cough, hemoptysis, unexplained weight loss, fatigue, night sweats, or fever.	These are risk factors for both tuberculosis and HIV infection.
Does client have history of chronic hoarseness?	Hoarseness may indicate laryngeal disorder or abuse of cocaine or opioids (sniffing).
Assess history of allergies to pollens, dust, or other airborne irritants and to foods, drugs, or chemical substances.	Symptoms such as choking feeling, bronchospasm with respiratory stridor, wheezes on auscultation, and dyspnea may be caused by allergic response.
Review family history for cancer, tuberculosis, allergies, or chronic obstructive pulmonary disease.	Conditions place client at risk for lung disease.

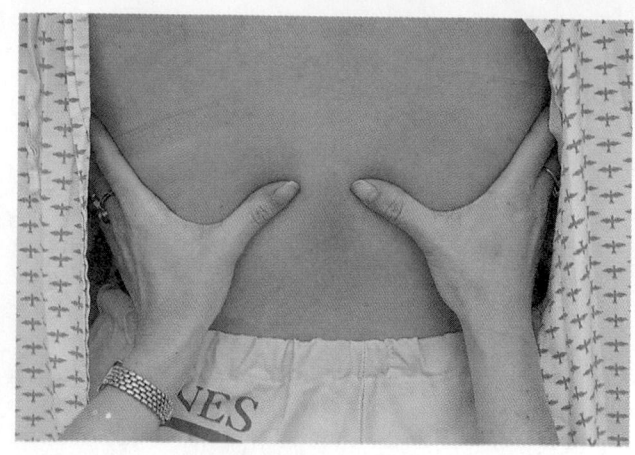
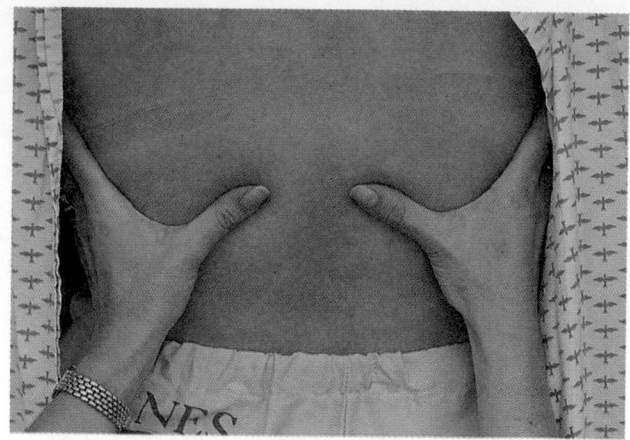

Figure 32-44 **A,** Position of nurse's hands for palpation of posterior thorax excursion. **B,** As the client inhales, the movement of chest excursion separates the nurse's thumbs.

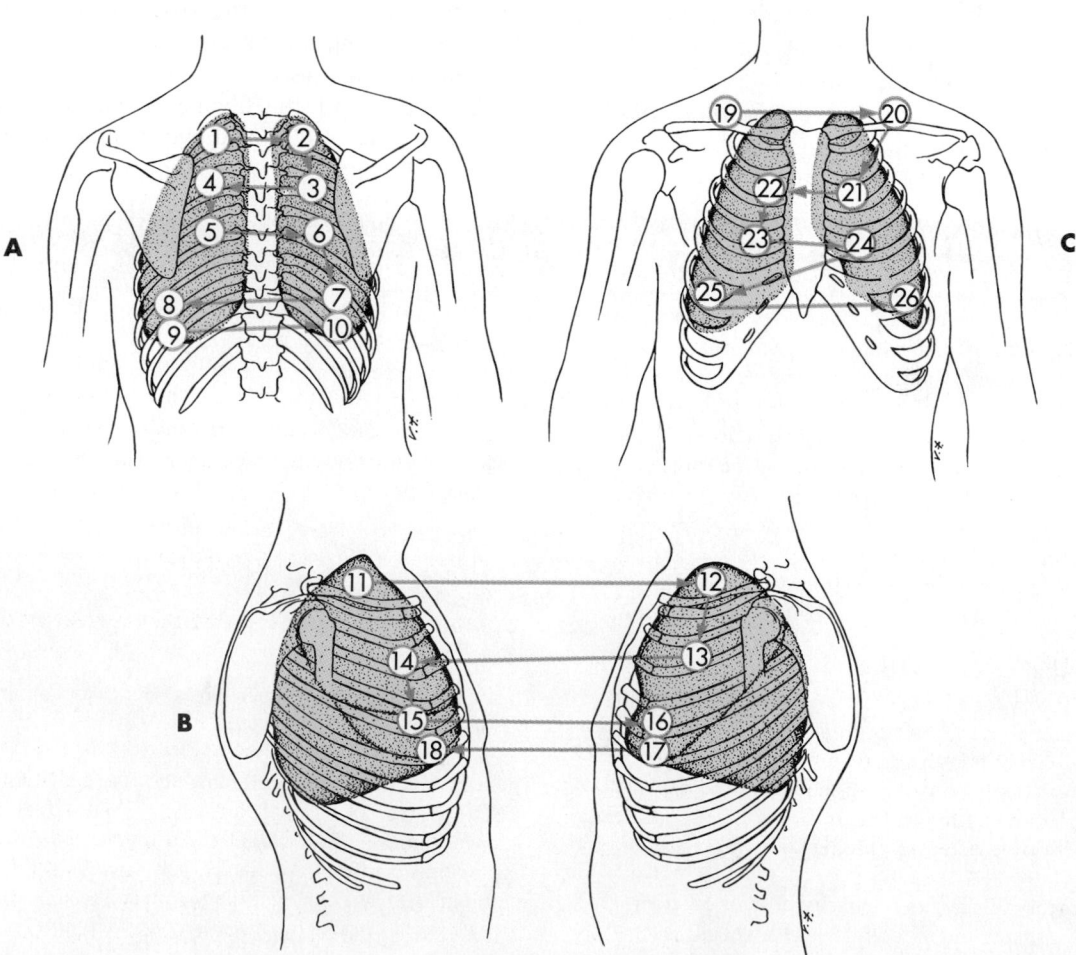

Figure 32-45 **A to C,** The nurse follows a systematic pattern (posterior-lateral-anterior) when comparing fremitus, percussion notes, and auscultation.

spaces, beginning at the lung apex (Figure 32-45, *A*). A firm, light touch is best. The nurse asks the client to say "ninety-nine" or "one-one-one." Normally there is a faint vibration as the client speaks. Both sides of the thorax are compared, moving from top to bottom. Only one hand is used to ensure accuracy. If fremitus is faint, it may be necessary to ask the client to speak in a louder or lower tone of voice. Symmetry of fremitus is normal. Vibrations are strongest at the top, near the level of the tracheal bifurcation. It is easy to assess for tactile fremitus in a crying infant because strong vibrations can be felt through the chest wall.

Percussion of the chest wall is a difficult assessment technique that determines whether underlying lung tissue is filled with air or fluid or is solid. Percussion reaches only 5 to 7 cm (2 to 3 inches) into the chest wall and thus cannot detect deep lesions. The client folds the arms forward across the chest with the head bent forward. This position separates the scapulae further to expose more lung to assessment. Using the indirect technique, the nurse percusses in the intercostal spaces over symmetrical areas of the lungs. Figure 32-45 shows how following a systematic pattern, starting posteriorly and then moving laterally and anteriorly, allows the nurse to compare percussion notes for all lung lobes. Resonance, the sound created by air-filled lungs, is normally heard over the posterior thorax. Percussion over the scapula, ribs, or spine is dull. The chest is normally more resonant in the child than in the adult. A lung mass causes a flat sound. Conditions such as emphysema, asthma, or pneumothorax produce a hyperresonant sound because of hyperinflation of lung tissue. A dull or flat sound may suggest atelectasis, pleural effusion, pneumothorax, or asthma.

Auscultation assesses the movement of air through the tracheobronchial tree and detects mucus or obstructed airways. Normally air flows through the airways in an unobstructed pattern. Recognizing the sounds created by normal airflow allows the nurse to detect sounds caused by obstruction.

In an adult the diaphragm of the stethoscope is placed firmly on the skin, over the posterior chest wall between the ribs (Figure 32-46). The client sits upright (if possible), folds the arms in front of the chest, and keeps the head bent forward while taking slow, deep breaths with the mouth slightly open. It helps to demonstrate for the client. The nurse listens to an entire inspiration and expiration at each position of the stethoscope. If sounds are faint, as in the obese client, the client should be asked to breathe harder and faster. Breath sounds are much louder in children because of the thinness of the chest wall. In children the bell works best because of a child's small chest.

A systematic pattern throughout should be used when comparing the right and left sides (see Figure 32-45, *A*). An inexperienced student may attempt to auscultate all of the left side and then return to the right side. This is in-

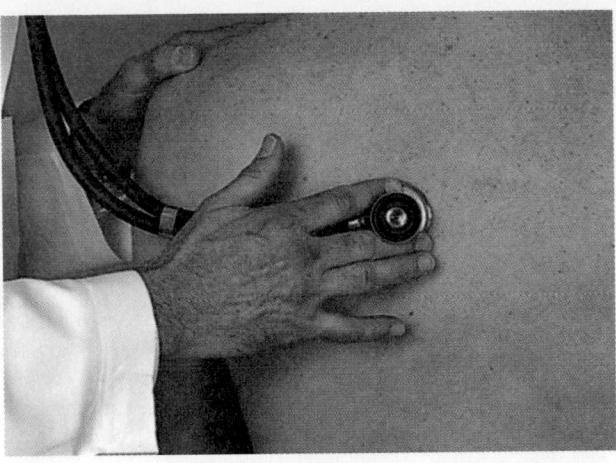

Figure 32-46 In an adult the nurse uses the diaphragm of the stethoscope to auscultate breath sounds.
From Seidel HM and others: *Mosby's guide to physical examination,* ed 4, St. Louis, 1999, Mosby.

correct. The examiner compares lung sounds in one region on one side of the body with sounds in the same region on the opposite side. It is impossible to remember the quality of all sounds noted on one side of the body and then compare them with sounds on the other side.

The nurse auscultates for normal breath sounds and abnormal or **adventitious sounds.** Normal breath sounds differ in character, depending on the area of the lungs being auscultated. Sounds normally heard over the posterior thorax include bronchovesicular and vesicular sounds (Table 32-21).

Abnormal sounds result from air passing through moisture, mucus, or narrowed airways; from alveoli suddenly reinflating; or from an inflammation between the lung's pleural linings. Adventitious or added sounds often occur superimposed over normal sounds. The four types of adventitious sounds are crackles, rhonchi, wheezes, and pleural friction rub. Each sound is caused by a specific entity and is characterized by typical auditory features (Table 32-22). The location and characteristics of the sounds should be noted, as should the absence of breath sounds (found in clients with collapsed or surgically removed lobes).

If the nurse assesses abnormalities in tactile fremitus, percussion, or auscultation, another test is performed for spoken and whispered voice sounds. With the stethoscope placed over the same locations used to assess breath sounds, the client says "ninety-nine" or "eee" in a normal voice tone. Normally the sounds are muffled. If fluid is compressing the lung, vibrations from the client's voice are transmitted to the chest wall and the sounds become clear (**bronchophony**). The nurse then asks the client to whisper "ninety-nine." The whispered voice is usually faint and indistinct. Certain lung abnormalities may cause the

Table 32-21 Normal Breath Sounds

Description	Location	Origin
Vesicular		
Vesicular sounds are soft, breezy, and low pitched. Inspiratory phase is 3 times longer than expiratory phase.	Best heard over lung's periphery (except over scapula)	Created by air moving through smaller airways
Bronchovesicular		
Bronchovesicular sounds are blowing sounds that are medium pitched and of medium intensity. Inspiratory phase is equal to expiratory phase.	Best heard posteriorly between scapulae and anteriorly over bronchioles lateral to sternum at first and second intercostal spaces	Created by air moving through large airways
Bronchial		
Bronchial sounds are loud and high pitched with hollow quality. Expiration lasts longer than inspiration (3:2 ratio).	Best heard over trachea	Created by air moving through trachea close to chest wall

whispered voice to become clear and distinct (**whispered pectoriloquy**).

LATERAL THORAX

The client sits during examination of the lateral chest. Usually the nurse extends the assessment of the posterior thorax to the lateral sides of the chest. The client is asked to raise the arms, which improves access to lateral thoracic structures. The nurse uses all four assessment skills to methodically examine the lateral thorax (see Figure 31-45, *B*). Excursion cannot be assessed laterally. Normally, percussion notes are resonant, and breath sounds are vesicular.

ANTERIOR THORAX

The anterior thorax is inspected for the same features as the posterior thorax. The client sits or lies down with the head elevated. The nurse observes the accessory muscles of breathing: sternocleidomastoid, trapezius, and abdominal muscles. The accessory muscles move little with normal passive breathing. When a client requires effort to breathe as a result of strenuous exercise or disease (e.g., chronic obstructive pulmonary disease), the accessory muscles and abdominal muscles contract (Box 32-19). Some clients produce a grunting sound.

The nurse observes the width of the costal angle. It is usually larger than 90 degrees between the two costal margins. The nurse observes the breathing pattern. Normal breathing is quiet and barely audible near the open mouth. Respiratory rate and rhythm are more often assessed anteriorly (see Chapter 31). A man's respirations are usually diaphragmatic, whereas a woman's are more costal. Accurate assessment occurs as a client breathes passively.

The examiner palpates the anterior thoracic muscles and skeleton for lumps, masses, tenderness, or unusual movement. The sternum and xiphoid are relatively inflexible. To measure chest excursion anteriorly, the nurse uses a technique similar to that for assessing the posterior thorax.

The nurse places the hands over each lateral rib cage, with the thumbs approximately 2.5 cm (2 inches) apart and angled along each costal margin (Figure 32-47, *A*). The thumbs are pushed toward the midline to create a fold of skin between the thumbs. As the client inhales deeply, the thumbs should normally separate approximately 2.5 to 5 cm (1 to 2 inches), with each side expanding equally (Figure 32-47, *B*).

Tactile fremitus is assessed over the chest wall. Anterior findings differ from posterior findings because of the heart and female breast tissue. Fremitus is best felt next to the sternum at the second intercostal space, at the level of the bronchial bifurcation. It is decreased over the heart, lower thorax, and breast tissue. The nurse will not be able to sense vibrations over breast tissue and thus must retract the breasts gently during palpation. If the breasts are large, this portion of the examination may be omitted.

Percussion of the anterior thorax follows a systematic pattern. The nurse must imagine the location of all internal organs anteriorly accessible to examination. The underlying liver, heart, and stomach create percussion notes characteristically different from those of the lung (Figure 32-48). Percussion may be conducted with the client in a sitting or lying position. However, the procedure is easier if the client lies down. The nurse starts above the clavicles and moves across and then down. The female breasts are displaced as needed. The normal lung is resonant. As the

Table 32-22 **Adventitious Breath Sounds**

Sound	Site Auscultated	Cause	Character
Crackles	Are most commonly heard in dependent lobes: right and left lung bases	Random, sudden reinflation of groups of alveoli; disruptive passage of air	Fine crackles are high-pitched fine, short, interrupted crackling sounds heard during end of inspiration, usually not cleared with coughing Medium crackles are lower, more moist sounds heard during middle of inspiration; not cleared with coughing Coarse crackles are loud, bubbly sounds heard during inspiration; not cleared with coughing
Rhonchi (sonorous wheeze)	Are primarily heard over trachea and bronchi; if loud enough, can be heard over most lung fields	Muscular spasm, fluid, or mucus in larger airways, causing turbulence	Are loud, low-pitched, rumbling coarse sounds heard most often during inspiration or expiration; may be cleared by coughing
Wheezes (sibilant wheeze)	Can be heard over all lung fields	High-velocity airflow through severely narrowed bronchus	Are high-pitched, continuous musical sounds like a squeak heard continuously during inspiration or expiration; usually louder on expiration
Pleural friction rub	Is heard over anterior lateral lung field (if client is sitting upright)	Inflamed pleura, parietal pleura rubbing against visceral pleura	Has dry, grating quality heard best during inspiration; does not clear with coughing; heard loudest over lower lateral anterior surface

Data from Basfield-Holland ES: Assessing pulmonary status: it's more than listening to breath sounds, *Nursing 97* 27(8):32, 1997; and Siedel HM and others: *Mosby's guide to physical examination,* ed 4, St. Louis, 1999, Mosby.

examiner proceeds downward, the areas of heart and liver dullness and the tympanic gastric air bubble will be detectable.

Auscultation of the anterior thorax follows the same pattern as percussion (see Figure 32-45, *C*). The client should sit, if possible, to maximize chest expansion. Special attention should be paid to the lower lobes, where mucus commonly gathers. Bronchovesicular and vesicular sounds are heard above and below the clavicles and along the lung periphery. An additional normal breath sound, the bronchial sound, can be heard over the trachea. It is loud, high pitched, and hollow sounding, with expiration lasting longer than inspiration (3:2 ratio).

Client Teaching DURING LUNG ASSESSMENT

OBJECTIVES

- Client will describe warning signs of lung disease.
- Older adult will receive influenza and pneumonia vaccines annually.
- Client with chronic obstructive pulmonary disease (COPD) will clear airways more effectively and report less shortness of breath.

TEACHING STRATEGIES

- Explain risk factors for chronic lung disease and lung cancer, including cigarette smoking, history of smoking for over 20 years, exposure to environmental pollution, and radiation exposure from occupational, medical, and environmental sources. Residential radon exposure may also increase risk especially in cigarette smokers. Exposure to side-stream cigarette smoke increases risk for nonsmokers (ACS, 1999).
- Share brochures on lung cancer from American Cancer Society (ACS) with client and family.

- Discuss warning signs of lung cancer, such as a persistent cough, sputum streaked with blood, chest pains, and recurrent attacks of pneumonia or bronchitis.
- Counsel older adult on benefits from receiving annual influenza and pneumonia vaccinations because of a greater susceptibility to respiratory infection.
- Instruct client with COPD in coughing and pursed-lip breathing exercises.
- Persons at risk for tuberculosis who visit clinics or health care centers should be referred for skin testing.

EVALUATION

- Have client describe risk factors for lung disease and cancer.
- Ask client to identify any known risks for cancer.
- Ask client to name warning signs for cancer.
- In a follow-up visit, review client's immunization record.
- Observe client performing breathing exercises and coughing.

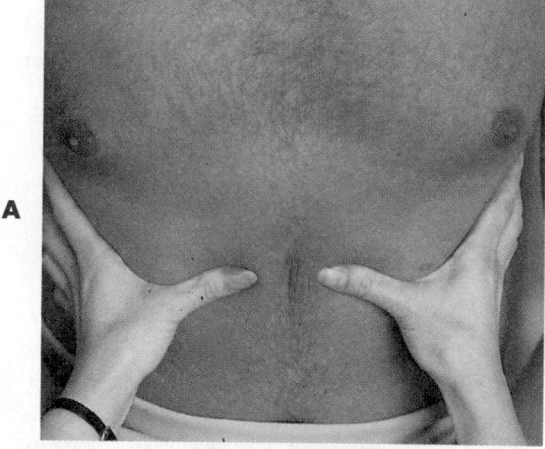

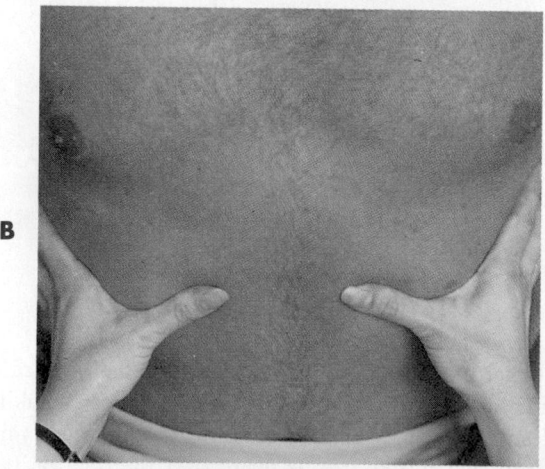

Figure 32-47 **A,** Position of nurse's hands before excursion of the anterior chest wall. **B,** As the client inhales, the nurse's hands normally separate 3 to 5 cm (1½ to 2 inches).

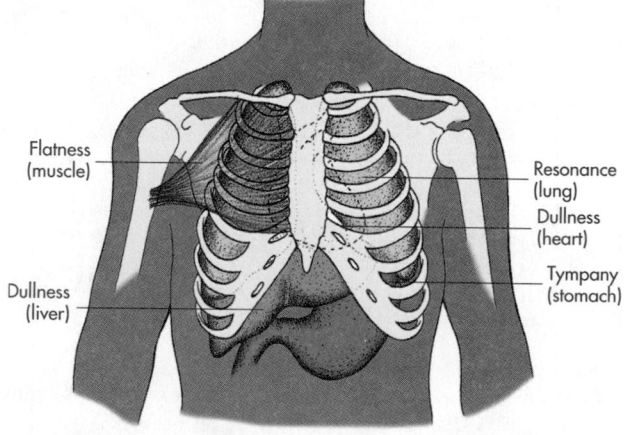

Figure 32-48 Variations in percussion notes in the normal thorax and upper abdomen.

Heart

The assessment of heart function involves a review of signs and symptoms from the nursing history, pulse assessment, and direct examination of the heart. A client who has signs or symptoms of heart (cardiac) problems (e.g., chest pain and irregular heart rate) may be suffering a life-threatening condition requiring immediate attention. In this case the nurse acts quickly and decides on the portions of the examination that are absolutely necessary. When a client's condition is stable, a more thorough assessment can reveal baseline heart function and any risks for heart disease. Abnormal findings require a physician's attention. The nurse performing a cardiac assessment compares findings with those made in the vascular examination (see later section). The nursing history (Table

Table 32-23 Nursing History for Heart Assessment

Assessment Category	Rationale
Determine history of smoking, alcohol intake, use of drugs, exercise habits, and dietary patterns and intake (including fat and sodium intake).	Smoking, alcohol ingestion, cocaine use, lack of regular exercise, and intake of foods high in carbohydrates, fats, and cholesterol are risk factors for cardiovascular disease.
Determine if client is taking medications for cardiovascular function (e.g., antidysrhythmics, antihypertensives) and if client knows their purpose, dosage, and side effects.	Knowledge allows nurse to assess compliance with drug therapies. Medications may affect vital sign values.
Assess for chest pain, palpitations, excess fatigue, cough, dyspnea, leg pain or cramps, edema of feet, cyanosis, fainting, and orthopnea. Ask if symptoms occur at rest or during exercise.	These are key symptoms of heart disease. Cardiovascular function may be adequate during rest but not during exercise.
If client reports chest pain, determine if it is cardiac in nature. Anginal pain is usually a deep pressure or ache that is substernal and diffuse, radiating to one or both arms, neck, or jaw.	Determines nature of pain and need to initiate care immediately.
Determine whether client has a stressful lifestyle. What physical demands or emotional stress exists?	Repeated exposure to stress may increase risk for heart disease.
Assess family history for heart disease, diabetes, high cholesterol levels, hypertension, stroke, or rheumatic heart disease.	Factors increase risk for heart disease.
Ask client about history of heart trouble (e.g., congestive heart failure, congenital heart disease, coronary artery disease, dysrhythmias, murmurs).	Knowledge reveals client's level of understanding of condition. Preexisting condition influences examination techniques used by nurse, as well as findings to expect.
Determine whether client has preexisting diabetes, lung disease, obesity, or hypertension.	These disorders may alter heart function.
Determine whether client drinks excessive amounts of coffee, tea, other caffeine-containing soft drinks, or chocolate.	Caffeine can cause heart dysrhythmias.

32-23) provides data that help the nurse interpret physical findings.

Assessment of cardiac function is performed through the anterior thorax. The nurse forms a mental image of the heart's exact location (Figure 32-49). In the adult it is in the center of the chest (precordium), behind and to the left of the sternum, with a small section of the right atrium extending to the sternum's right. The base of the heart is the upper portion, and the apex is the bottom tip. The surface of the right ventricle composes most of the heart's anterior surface. A section of the left ventricle shapes the left anterior side of the apex. The apex actually touches the anterior chest wall at approximately the fourth to fifth intercostal space just medial to the left midclavicular line. This location is known as the **apical impulse** or **point of maximal impulse (PMI).**

An infant's heart is positioned more horizontally and has a larger diameter compared with that of an adult. The apex of the heart in an infant is at the third or fourth intercostal space, just to the left of the midclavicular line. By the age of 7 a child's PMI is in the same location as the adult's.

In tall, slender persons the heart hangs more vertically and is positioned more centrally. In persons who are

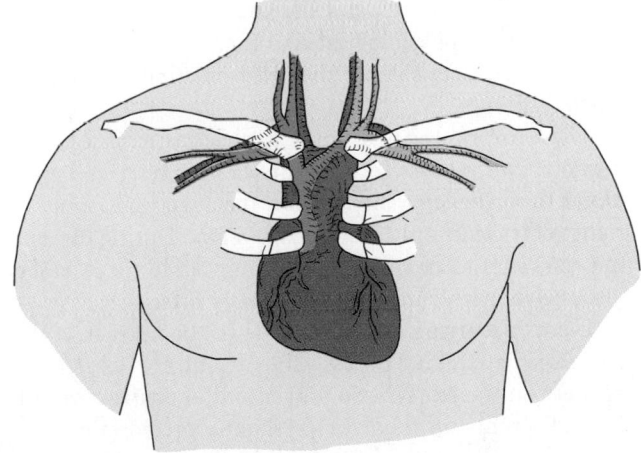

Figure 32-49 Anatomical position of the heart.

stocky and short, the heart tends to lie more to the left and horizontally (Seidel and others, 1999).

To understand the significance of cardiac assessment findings, the nurse must first understand timing in relation to the cardiac cycle (Figure 32-50). The heart nor-

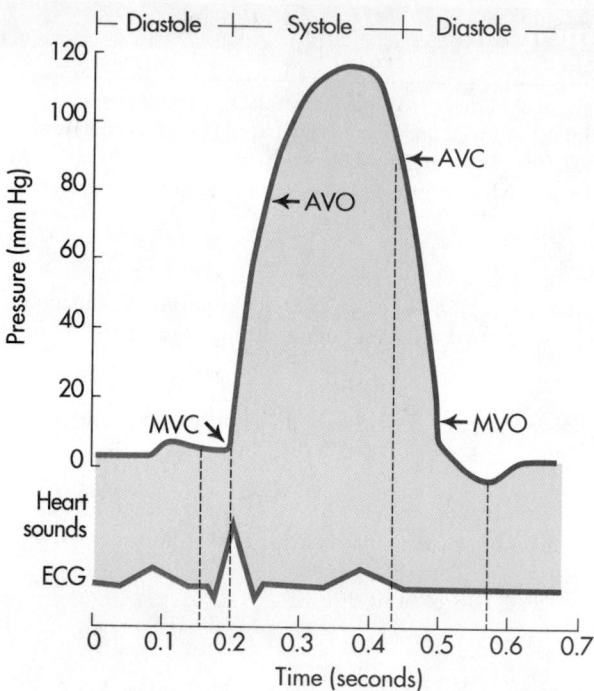

Figure 32-50   Cardiac cycle. *MVC,* Mitral valve closes; *AVO,* aortic valve opens; *AVC,* aortic valve closes; *MVO,* mitral valve opens.

Blood flows into the aorta, elevating aortic pressure. When the ventricle empties, pressure within the chamber falls. To prevent regurgitation from the aorta into the left ventricle, the aortic valve closes, creating the second heart sound (S_2), described as "dub." As ventricular pressure continues to fall, it drops below that of the left atrium. The mitral valve reopens to again allow ventricular filling. The rapid filling of the ventricle may create a third heart sound (S_3), heard more often in children and young adults. An S_3 can also be heard as an abnormality in adults over 30 years of age. When the atria contract to enhance ventricular filling, a fourth heart sound (S_4) is produced. The S_4 is not normally heard in adults but may be heard in healthy older adults, children, and athletes. Because it may also indicate an abnormal condition, it should be reported to a physician.

INSPECTION AND PALPATION

Before beginning the examination, the nurse ensures that the client is relaxed and comfortable. An anxious or uncomfortable client can have mild tachycardia that may lead the nurse to misinterpret the findings. Findings from the examination of other body systems, such as signs of heart failure (crackles in the lungs), influence judgments made during cardiovascular assessment. The nurse must be able not only to successfully examine the client, but also to integrate and interpret findings correctly.

The nurse uses inspection and palpation simultaneously. The examination begins with the client in the supine position or with the upper body elevated 45 degrees because clients with heart disease frequently suffer shortness of breath while lying flat. The nurse stands at the client's right side. The client must not talk, especially when the nurse auscultates heart sounds. Good lighting in the room is essential.

During inspection and palpation the nurse will methodically look for visible pulsations and exaggerated lifts and palpate for the apical impulse and any source of vibrations (thrills). It helps to follow an orderly sequence beginning with assessment of the base of the heart and moving toward the apex. First the nurse inspects the angle of Louis, which lies between the sternal body and manubrium and can be felt as a ridge in the sternum approximately 5 cm (2 inches) below the sternal notch. The nurse can slip the fingers along the angle on each side of the sternum to feel adjacent ribs. The intercostal spaces are just below each rib. The second intercostal space allows identification of the first two anatomical landmarks (Figure 32-51): the second right and left interspace. The third and fourth left interspaces can be found by progressing down along the left side of the sternum, palpating each intercostal space. Deeper palpation is required to feel the spaces in obese clients or in those with well-developed chest muscles. To find the apical area, the nurse locates the fifth intercostal space just to the left of the sternum and moves the fingers laterally, just medial to the left midcla-

mally pumps blood through its four chambers in a methodical, even sequence. Events on the left side occur just before those on the right. As blood flows through each chamber, the valves open and close, the pressures within chambers rise and fall, and the chambers contract. Each event creates a physiological sign that can be detected by an examiner. Both sides of the heart function in a coordinated fashion.

There are two phases to the cardiac cycle: systole and diastole. During systole the ventricles contract and eject blood from the left ventricle into the aorta and from the right ventricle into the pulmonary artery. During diastole the ventricles relax and the atria contract to move blood into the ventricles and fill the coronary arteries.

Events occurring on the left side of the heart have the most dramatic effect on assessment findings. Pressure is greatest on the left side, so longer and louder sounds are created. Events on the left side slightly precede those on the right. When the left ventricle is at rest (diastolic phase), the pressure in the left atrium exceeds that in the ventricle, creating a pressure gradient that moves blood through the opened mitral valve. During ventricular filling, pressure rises in the ventricle to exceed the pressure in the left atrium. Just before the ventricle contracts, the mitral valve closes to prevent regurgitation of blood into the atrium, creating the first heart sound (S_1), often described as "lub." Ventricular pressure builds, causing the aortic valve to open as the ventricle contracts (systolic phase).

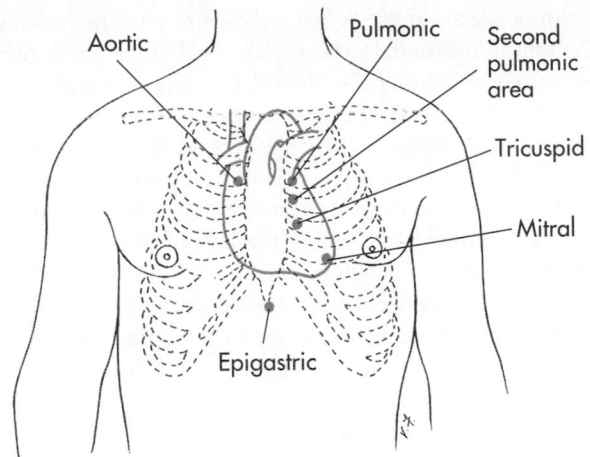

Figure 32-51   Anatomical sites for assessment of cardiac function.

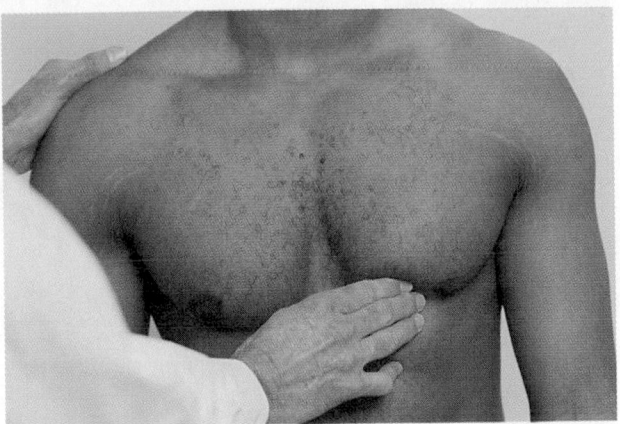

Figure 32-52   Palpation of apical pulse.
From Seidel HM and others: *Mosby's guide to physical examination,* ed 4, St. Louis, 1999, Mosby.

vicular line. Some examiners are able to locate the apical area with the palm of the hand, but others use their fingertips. Normally at the apical impulse there is a light tap felt in an area 1 to 2 cm (½ inch) in diameter at the apex (Figure 32-52). Another landmark is the epigastric area at the tip of the sternum. It is typically used to palpate for aortic abnormalities.

As the nurse locates the six anatomical landmarks of the heart, each area is inspected and palpated. The nurse looks for the appearance of pulsations, viewing each area over the chest at an angle to the side. Normally no pulsations can be seen, except perhaps at the PMI in thin clients or at the epigastric area as a result of abdominal aorta pulsation. Palpation for pulsations is best done using the proximal halves of the four fingers together and then alternating with the ball of the hand. The nurse touches the areas gently to allow movements to lift the hand. Normally no pulsations or vibrations can be felt in the second, third, or fourth intercostal spaces. A vibration is caused by loud murmurs. If pulsations or vibrations are palpated, the nurse times their occurrence in relation to systole or diastole by auscultating heart sounds simultaneously.

If the PMI cannot be found with the client in the supine position, the nurse asks the client to roll onto the left side, which moves the heart closer to the chest wall. The nurse estimates the heart's size by noting the diameter of the PMI and its position relative to the midclavicular line. In cases of serious heart disease, the cardiac muscle enlarges, with the PMI found to the left of the midclavicular line. The PMI may be difficult to find in the older adult because the chest deepens in its anteroposterior diameters. It may also be difficult to locate in a client who is very muscular or overweight. The PMI of an infant can usually be found near the third or fourth intercostal space. It is easy to palpate the child's PMI because of the thin chest wall.

AUSCULTATION

Auscultation of the heart detects normal heart sounds, extra heart sounds, and murmurs. The nursing student should first become skilled in detecting normal heart sounds. These low-intensity sounds created by the closing of the valves are often difficult to hear, especially if breath sounds are noisy. Concentration is needed when detecting heart sounds. To begin auscultation, the nurse eliminates all sources of room noise and explains the procedure to relieve the client's anxiety. The nurse follows a pattern during auscultation, starting at the second right interspace, moving systematically and inching the stethoscope across each of the anatomical sites (see Figure 32-51). It is important to hear heart sounds clearly at each location. Then the sequence is repeated using the bell of the stethoscope. The client may be asked to assume three different positions during the examination (Figure 32-53): sitting up and leaning forward (good position to hear all areas and to hear high-pitched murmurs), supine (good for all areas), and left lateral recumbent (good for all areas and best position to hear low-pitched sounds in diastole).

The nurse usually must lift the female client's left breast to listen better to the chest wall. The nurse learns to identify the first (S_1) and second (S_2) heart sounds. At normal rates, S_1 occurs after the long diastolic pause and preceding the short systolic pause. S_1 is high pitched, dull in quality, and heard best at the apex. If the nurse has difficulty hearing S_1, it can be timed in relation to the carotid pulse. It occurs just before the carotid pulsation. S_2 follows the short systolic pause and precedes the long diastolic pause. It is heard best at the aortic area.

The nurse auscultates for rate and rhythm after both sounds can be heard clearly. Each combination of S_1 and S_2 or "lub-dub" counts as one heartbeat. The nurse counts the rate for 1 minute, listening for the interval between S_1 and S_2, and then the time between S_2 and the next S_1. A

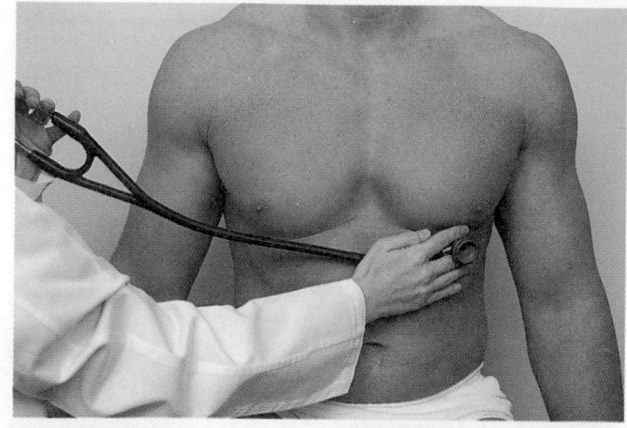

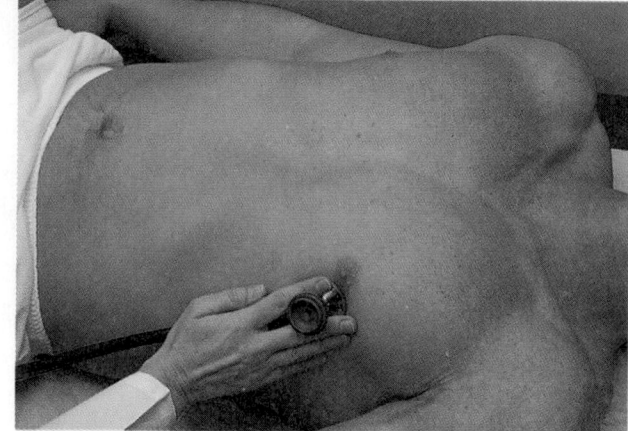

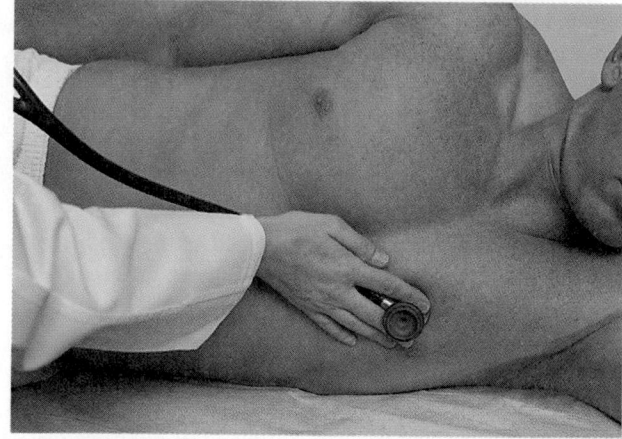

Figure 32-53 Sequence of client positions for heart auscultation. **A,** Sitting, **B,** Supine, **C,** Left lateral recumbent. From Seidel HM and others: *Mosby's guide to physical examination,* ed 4, St. Louis, 1999, Mosby.

regular rhythm involves regular intervals of time between each sequence of beats. There is a distinct silent pause between S_1 and S_2. Failure of the heart to beat at regular successive intervals is a **dysrhythmia.** Some dysrhythmias can be life threatening.

When the heart rhythm is irregular, the nurse compares apical and radial pulse rates simultaneously to determine if a pulse deficit exists. The apical pulse is asculated first and then the radial pulse is immediately palpated (one-

examiner technique). When two examiners are available, the apical and radial rates are assessed at the same time. When a client has a **pulse deficit,** the radial pulse is slower than the apical pulse because ineffective contractions fail to send pulse waves to the periphery. A difference in pulse rates is reported to the physician immediately.

The nurse also learns to assess for extra heart sounds at each auscultatory site. Using the bell of the stethoscope, the nurse listens for low-pitched extra heart sounds such as S_3 and S_4 gallops, clicks, and rubs. The nurse auscultates over all anatomical areas. S_3, or a **ventricular gallop,** occurs just after S_2 at the end of ventricular diastole. It may be caused by a premature rush of blood into a ventricle that is stiff or dilated as a result of heart failure and hypertension. Some examiners describe the combination of S_1, S_2, and S_3 as sounding like "Ken-tuck-ky."

S_4, or an atrial gallop, occurs just before S_1 or ventricular systole. The sound of an S_4 is similar to that of "Tennessee." Physiologically it may be due to an atrial contraction pushing against a ventricle that is not accepting blood because of heart failure or other alterations. One can often hear extra heart sounds more easily with the client lying on the left side and the stethoscope at the apical site.

The final portion of the examination includes assessment for heart murmurs. **Murmurs** are sustained swishing or blowing sounds heard at the beginning, middle, or end of the systolic or diastolic phase. They are caused by increased blood flow through a normal valve, forward flow through a stenotic valve or into a dilated vessel or heart chamber, or backward flow through a valve that fails to close. A murmur can be asymptomatic or a sign of heart disease (Box 32-20). Murmurs are common in children. The nurse keeps the following factors in mind when auscultating to detect murmurs:

- When a murmur is detected, the nurse auscultates the mitral, tricuspid, aortic, and pulmonic valve areas for its place in the cardiac cycle (timing), the place it is heard best (location), radiation, loudness, pitch, and quality.
- If a murmur occurs between S_1 and S_2, it is a systolic murmur. If it occurs between S_2 and the next S_1, it is a diastolic murmur.
- The location of a murmur is not necessarily directly over the valves. With experience, a nurse can learn where each type of murmur is best heard. For example, mitral murmurs are heard best at the apex of the heart.
- To assess for radiation, the nurse listens for a murmur over areas besides where it is heard best. Murmurs can also sometimes be heard over the neck or back.
- Intensity or loudness is related to the rate of blood flow through the heart or the amount of blood regurgitated. In serious murmurs the nurse may feel a thrust or intermittent palpable sensation at the auscultation site. A **thrill** is a continuous palpable sensa-

OBJECTIVES
- Client will know risk factors for heart disease and take appropriate steps to eliminate risks from lifestyle.
- Client with risk for heart disease will seek support from appropriate caregivers.

TEACHING STRATEGIES
- Explain risk factors for heart disease, including high dietary intake of saturated fat or cholesterol, lack of regular aerobic exercise, smoking, excess weight, stressful lifestyle, hypertension, and family history of heart disease.
- Refer client (if appropriate) to resources available for controlling or reducing risks (e.g., nutritional counseling, exercise class, stress reduction programs).
- Explain that research shows clinical benefit from reducing dietary intake of cholesterol and saturated fats. Tell client that about 70% to 75% of saturated fatty acids come from meats, poultry, fish, and dairy products and that the one-step diet recommended by the National Institutes of Health includes an intake of total fat less than 30% of calories, saturated fatty acids less than 10% of calories, and cholesterol less than 300 mg/100 ml (Moore, 1997).

- Encourage client to have regular measurement of total blood cholesterol levels and triglycerides. Desirable levels are 150 to 200 mg/100 ml. More than one cholesterol measurement is needed to assess the blood cholesterol level accurately. Low-density lipoprotein (LDL) cholesterol is the major component of atherosclerotic plaques. Separate measurement of LDL cholesterol is wise in a client with high total blood cholesterol levels. An LDL cholesterol level of 160 mg/100 ml or higher is high risk (Moore, 1997).
- Clients who have known angina may benefit from taking a daily low dose of aspirin. Consult physician before starting therapy.

EVALUATION
- Ask client to identify risk factors for heart disease.
- Have client develop a meal plan low in saturated fat and cholesterol.
- Check client's cholesterol level during follow-up appointments at the clinic or physician's office.

---

tion like the purring of a cat. Intensity is recorded in the following grades:

Grade 1	Barely audible
Grade 2	Audible immediately but faint
Grade 3	Loud, without thrust or thrill
Grade 4	Loud, with thrust or thrill
Grade 5	Very loud, with thrust or thrill; audible with stethoscope only partially applied
Grade 6	Louder, may be heard without stethoscope

- A murmur may be low, medium, or high in pitch, depending on the velocity of blood flow through the valves. A low-pitched murmur is heard best with the bell of the stethoscope. If it is heard best with the diaphragm, a murmur is high pitched.

The quality of a murmur refers to its characteristic pattern and sound. A crescendo murmur starts softly and builds in loudness. A decrescendo murmur starts loudly and then becomes less intense.

Vascular System

Examination of the vascular system includes measurement of the blood pressure (see Chapter 31) and a thorough assessment of the integrity of the peripheral vascular system. Table 32-24 reviews the nursing history data collected before the examination. The nurse may perform portions of the vascular examination during assessment of other body systems. For example, the carotid pulse may be checked after palpation of cervical lymph nodes. As the nurse inspects the skin, signs and symptoms of arterial and venous insufficiency are noted. An experienced nurse integrates vascular assessment with other portions of the examination if it is important to minimize time spent in the total examination.

BLOOD PRESSURE

When auscultating blood pressure, it is important to know that readings between the arms may vary by as much as 10 mm Hg and tend to be higher in the right arm (Seidel and others, 1999). The higher reading is always recorded. Systolic readings that differ by 15 mm Hg or more suggest atherosclerosis or disease of the aorta.

CAROTID ARTERIES

When the left ventricle pumps blood into the aorta, pressure waves are transmitted through the arterial system. Pressure waves are manifested as pulses that are palpable in arteries close to the skin or that lie over bones. The carotid arteries reflect heart function better than peripheral arteries because they are positioned closest to the heart and thus their pressure correlates with that of the aorta.

The carotid arteries supply oxygenated blood to the head and neck (Figure 32-54) and are protected by the overlying sternocleidomastoid muscle. To examine the carotid arteries, the nurse has the client sit or lie supine with the head of the bed elevated 30 degrees. One carotid artery is examined at a time. If both arteries were occluded during palpation, the client could lose consciousness as a

Table 32-24 **Nursing History for Vascular Assessment**

Assessment Category	Rationale
Determine if client experiences leg cramps, numbness or tingling in extremities, sensation of cold hands or feet, pain in legs, or swelling or cyanosis of feet, ankles, or hand.	These signs and symptoms indicate vascular disease.
If client experiences leg pain or cramping in lower extremities, ask if it is relieved or aggravated by walking or standing for long periods or during sleep.	Relationship of symptoms to exercise can clarify whether problem is vascular or musculoskeletal. Pain caused by vascular condition tends to increase with activity. Musculoskeletal pain is not usually relieved when exercise ends.
Ask women if they wear tight-fitting garters or hosiery and sit or lie in bed with legs crossed.	Tight hosiery around lower extremities and crossing legs can impair venous return.
Reconsider previous heart risk factors (e.g., smoking, exercise, nutritional problems).	These predispose client to vascular disease.
Assess medical history for heart disease, hypertension, phlebitis, diabetes, or varicose veins.	Circulatory and vascular disorders influence findings gathered during examination.

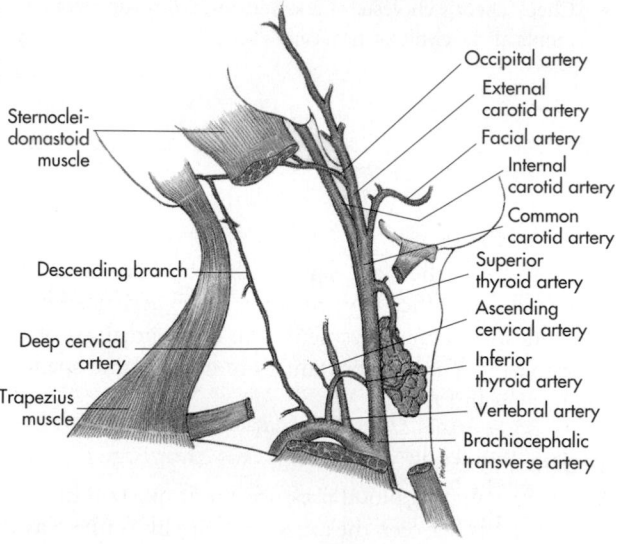

Figure 32-54   Anatomical position of the carotid artery.

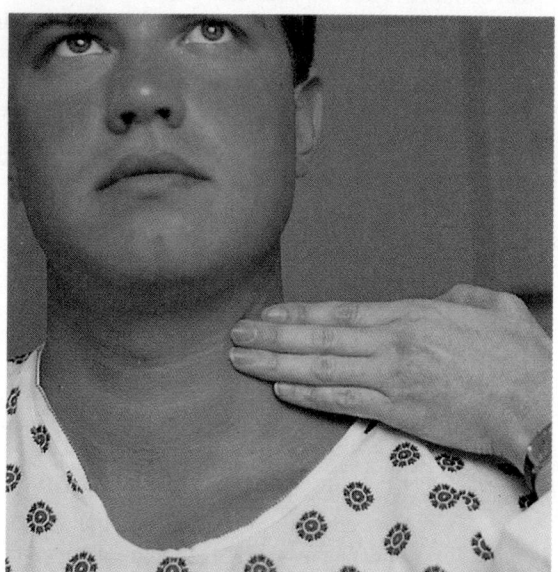

Figure 32-55   Palpation of internal carotid artery along the margin of the sternocleidomastoid muscle.

result of inadequate circulation to the brain. The carotids must not be vigorously palpated or massaged. The carotid sinus is located at the bifurcation of the common carotid arteries in the upper third of the neck. The sinus sends impulses along the vagus nerve. Its stimulation can cause a reflex drop in heart rate and blood pressure, which causes **syncope** or circulatory arrest. This can be a particular problem for older adults.

The neck is first inspected for obvious pulsation of the artery. The client turns the head slightly away from the artery being examined. Sometimes the wave of the pulse can be seen. The carotid is the only site for assessing the quality of a pulse wave. Only an experienced assessor can evaluate the quality of the wave in relation to systole and diastole of the cardiac cycle. An absent pulse wave can indicate arterial **occlusion** (blockage) or **stenosis** (narrowing).

For palpation of the pulse, the client turns the head slightly toward the side being examined. This maneuver relaxes the neck muscles for easier palpation. The nurse slides the tips of the index and middle fingers around the medial edge of the sternocleidomastoid muscle. Gentle palpation avoids occlusion of circulation (Figure 32-55).

The normal carotid pulse is localized rather than diffuse. A strong pulse, the carotid has a thrusting quality. As the client breathes, no change occurs during inspiration or expiration. Rotation of the neck or a shift from a sitting to a supine position does not change the carotid artery's quality. Both carotid arteries should be equal in pulse rate, rhythm, and strength and should be equally elastic.

Diminished or unequal carotid pulsations can indicate **atherosclerosis** or aortic arch disease.

The carotid is the most commonly auscultated pulse. (Others might include the jugular, temporal, femoral, renal, and abdominal arteries.) Auscultation is especially important for middle-age clients, older adults, or clients suspected of having cerebrovascular disease manifested by carotid artery obstruction. When the lumen of a blood vessel is narrowed, its blood flow is disturbed. As blood passes through the narrowed section, a turbulence is created, causing a blowing or swishing sound. The blowing sound is called a **bruit** (pronounced "brew-ee") (Figure 32-56).

The bell of the stethoscope is placed over the carotid artery at the lateral end of the clavicle and the posterior margin of the sternocleidomastoid muscle. The client turns the head slightly away from the side being examined (Figure 32-57). The nurse asks the client to hold the breath for a moment so that breath sounds do not obscure a bruit. Normally no sound is heard during carotid auscultation. If a bruit is heard, the nurse palpates the artery lightly for a thrill (palpable bruit).

JUGULAR VEINS

The most accessible veins are the internal and external jugular veins in the neck. Both veins drain bilaterally from the head and neck into the superior vena cava. The external jugular vein lies superficially and can be seen just above the clavicle. The internal jugular vein lies deeper, along the carotid artery.

It is best to examine the right internal jugular vein because it follows a more direct anatomical path to the right atrium of the heart. The column of blood inside the internal jugular vein serves as a manometer, reflecting pressure in the right atrium. The higher the column, the greater the venous pressure. Raised venous pressure reflects right-sided heart failure.

Normally when a client lies in the supine position, the external jugular vein distends and becomes easily visible. In contrast, the jugular veins normally flatten when the client is in a sitting position. A client with heart disease, however, may have distended jugular veins when sitting.

The jugular veins are inspected to measure venous pressures, which are influenced by blood volume, the capacity of the right atrium to receive blood and send it to the right ventricle, and the ability of the right ventricle to contract and force blood into the pulmonary artery. Any factor resulting in greater blood volume within the venous system results in elevated venous pressure. The nurse assesses venous pressure by using the following steps:

1. Have the client lie supine with the head elevated 30 to 45 degrees (semi-Fowler's position).

2. Be sure the neck and upper thorax are exposed. Use a pillow to align the head. Avoid neck hyperextension or flexion to ensure that the vein is not stretched or kinked (Figure 32-58).

3. Usually pulsations are not evident with the client sitting up. As the client slowly leans back into a supine position, the level of venous pulsations begins to rise above the level of the manubrium as much as 1 or 2 cm as the client reaches a 45-degree angle. Measure venous pressure by measuring the vertical distance

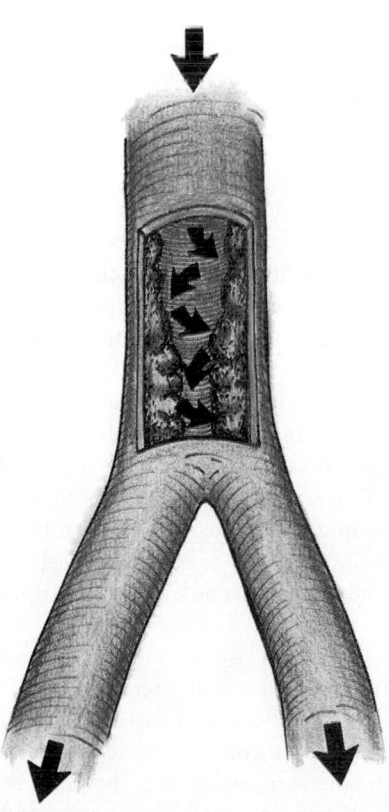

Figure 32-56 Occlusion or narrowing of the carotid artery disrupts normal blood flow. The resultant turbulence creates a sound (bruit) that the nurse can auscultate.

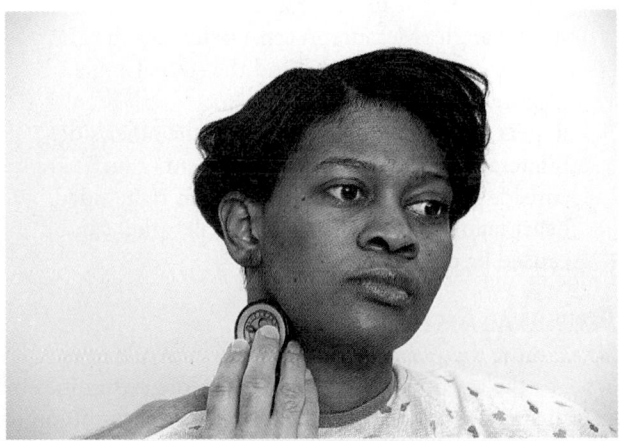

Figure 32-57 Auscultation for carotid artery bruit. From Seidel HM and others: *Mosby's guide to physical examination,* ed 4, St. Louis 1999, Mosby.

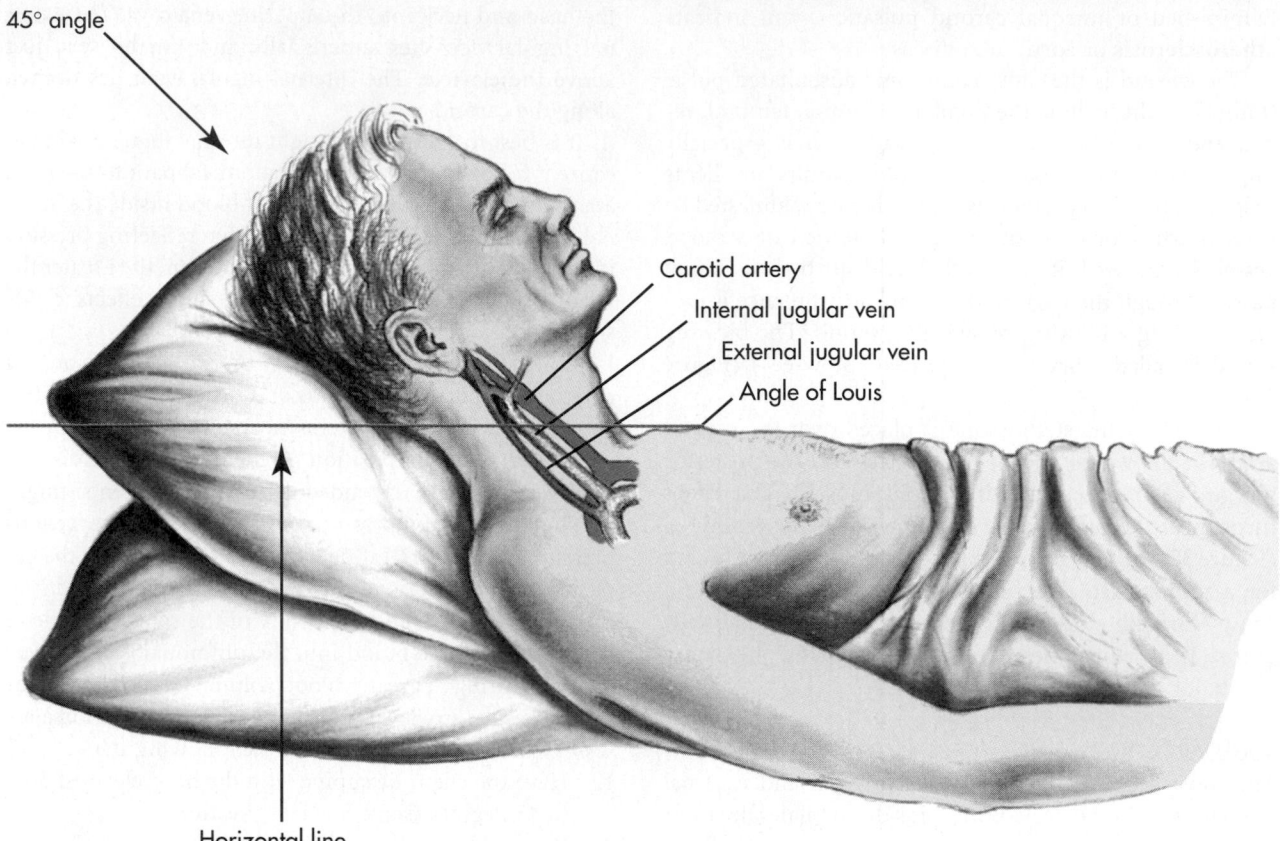

45° angle

Carotid artery
Internal jugular vein
External jugular vein
Angle of Louis

Horizontal line

Figure 32-58   Position of client to assess jugular vein distention.
From Thompson JM and others: *Mosby's manual of clinical nursing,* ed 3, St. Louis, 1993, Mosby.

between the angle of Louis and the highest level of the visible point of the internal jugular vein pulsation.

4. Use two rulers. Line up the bottom edge of a regular ruler with the top of the area of pulsation in the jugular vein. Then take a centimeter ruler and align it perpendicular to the first ruler at the level of the sternal angle. Measure in centimeters the distance between the second ruler and the sternal angle (Figure 32-59).

5. Repeat the same measurement on the other side. Bilateral pressures higher than 2.5 cm (1 inch) are considered elevated and are a sign of right-sided heart failure. One-sided pressure elevation can be caused by obstruction.

PERIPHERAL ARTERIES AND VEINS

To examine the peripheral vascular system, the nurse first assesses the adequacy of blood flow to the extremities by measuring arterial pulses and inspecting the condition of the skin and nails. The integrity of the venous system is also assessed, with attention given to determining whether the client has abnormalities.

A number of factors can impair circulation to the ex-tremities, including altered blood vessel integrity and overlying constriction on vessel walls (Table 32-25). The nurse should anticipate the risk for circulatory impairment (Box 32-21). Some clients, such as older adults and diabetic persons, suffer physical changes in blood vessel walls that increase the risk of perfusion problems.

Peripheral Arteries.   The nurse examines each peripheral artery using the distal pads of the second and third fingers. The thumb may help anchor the brachial and femoral artery. The nurse applies firm pressure but avoids occluding the pulse. When it is difficult to find a pulse, it is helpful to vary pressure and feel all around the pulse site. The nurse must be sure not to palpate his or her own pulse.

Routine vital signs usually include assessment of the rate and rhythm of the radial artery because it is easily accessible. The pulse is counted for either 30 seconds or a full minute, depending on the character of the pulse. With palpation the nurse normally feels the pulse wave at regular intervals. When an interval is interrupted by an early, late, or missed beat, the pulse rhythm is irregular. In emergencies the carotid artery is chosen because it is accessible and most useful in evaluating heart activity. To check local

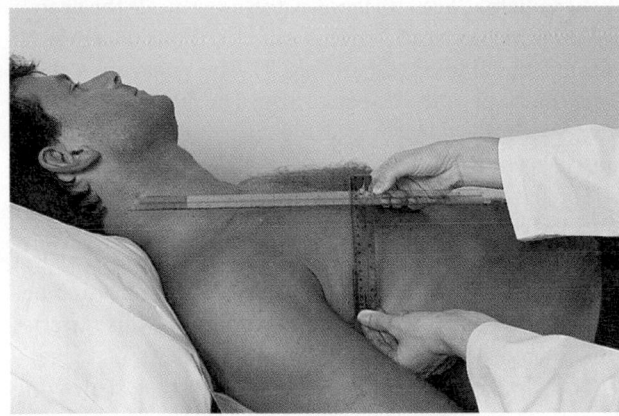

Figure 32-59   Measuring jugular venous pressure.
From Seidel HM and others: *Mosby's guide to physical examination,* ed 4, St. Louis, 1999, Mosby.

	Indicators for Assessing
Table 32-25	**Local Blood Flow**

Indicator	Rationale
Systemic diseases (e.g., arteriosclerosis, atherosclerosis, diabetes)	Diseases result in changes in integrity of walls of arteries and smaller blood vessels.
Coagulation disorders (e.g., thrombosis, embolus)	Blood clot causes mechanical obstruction to blood flow.
Local trauma or surgery (e.g., contusion, fracture, vascular surgery)	Direct manipulation of vessels or localized edema impairs blood flow.
Application of constricting devices (e.g., casts, dressings, elastic bandages, restraints)	Constriction causes tourniquet effect, impairing blood flow to areas below site of constriction.

Client Teaching DURING VASCULAR ASSESSMENT   Box 32-21

OBJECTIVES
- Client will know normal blood pressure range for age and compare it with own blood pressure readings to identify normalcy of blood pressure.
- Client with vascular insufficiency will avoid activities that worsen circulatory status.

TEACHING STRATEGIES
- Tell client the blood pressure reading. Explain the normal reading for the client's age. Discuss implications of abnormalities.
- Instruct client with risk or evidence of vascular insufficiency in the lower extremities to avoid tight clothing over the lower body or legs, to avoid sitting or standing for long periods, to walk regularly, and to elevate feet when sitting.

- Advise client to avoid cigarette smoking because nicotine causes vasoconstriction.
- Identify older adult with hypertension who may benefit from regular monitoring of blood pressure (daily, weekly, or monthly). Teach client how to use home monitoring kits (see Chapter 31).

EVALUATION
- Ask client to identify if blood pressure reading is within normal limits for age.
- Have client with vascular insufficiency describe precautions to take to avoid further circulatory deficiency.
- Have older adult demonstrate self-monitoring of blood pressure.

---

circulatory status of tissues, the nurse palpates peripheral arteries long enough to note that a pulse is present.

The nurse assesses each peripheral artery for elasticity of the vessel wall, strength, and equality. A systematic technique is useful, starting with the temporal arteries in the head and moving down to the arteries in the upper and lower extremities. The wall of an artery is normally elastic, making it easily palpable. After the artery is depressed, it will spring back to shape when pressure is released. An abnormal artery may be described as hard, inelastic, or calcified.

The strength of a pulse is a measurement of the force at which blood is ejected against the arterial wall. Some examiners use a scale rating from 0 to 4+ for the strength of a pulse (Seidel and others, 1999):

0	Absent, not palpable
1+	Pulse diminished, barely palpable
2+	Easily palpable, normal pulse
3+	Full pulse, increased
4+	Strong, bounding pulse, cannot be obliterated

All peripheral pulses are measured for equality and symmetry. The left radial pulse is compared with that of the right, the left brachial pulse is compared with the left radial, and so on. An inequality may indicate localized obstruction or an abnormally positioned artery.

In the upper extremities the primary artery is the brachial artery, which channels blood to the radial and ulnar arteries of the forearm and hand. If circulation in this artery becomes blocked, the hands will not receive adequate blood flow. If circulation in the radial or ulnar arteries becomes impaired, the hand will still receive adequate perfusion. An interconnection between the radial and ulnar arteries guards against arterial occlusion (Figure 32-60).

The nurse should practice locating pulses on a friend. To locate pulses in the arm and hand, the nurse has the client sit or lie down. The radial pulse is found along the radial side of the forearm, at the wrist. In a thin individual a groove is formed lateral to the flexor tendon of the wrist. The radial pulse can be felt with light palpation in the groove (Figure 32-61). The ulnar pulse is on the opposite side of the wrist and tends to feel less prominent than the radial pulse (Figure 32-62). An examiner palpates the ulnar pulse only when arterial insufficiency to the hand is expected.

The **Allen's test** can be performed to assess collateral circulation. The client makes a fist as the ulnar and radial arteries are compressed simultaneously. The client then opens the hand, and the nurse releases the ulnar artery. The hand should quickly turn pink if the ulnar artery is patent. The test may be repeated by releasing only the radial artery.

To palpate the brachial pulse, the nurse finds the groove between the biceps and triceps muscles above the elbow at the antecubital fossa (Figure 32-63). The artery runs along the medial side of the extended arm. The nurse palpates the artery with the fingertips of the first three fingers in the muscle groove.

The femoral artery is the primary artery in the leg, delivering blood to the popliteal, posterior tibial, and dorsalis pedis arteries (Figure 32-64). It is one of the strongest arteries in an infant or small child. An interconnection between the posterior tibial and dorsalis pedis arteries guards against local arterial occlusion.

The femoral pulse is found best with the client lying down with the inguinal area exposed (Figure 32-65). The femoral artery runs below the inguinal ligament, midway between the symphysis pubis and the anterosuperior iliac spine. Deep palpation may be required to feel the pulse. Bimanual palpation is effective in obese clients. This technique differs from the previous description of bimanual palpation. The nurse places the fingertips of both hands on opposite sides of the pulse site. A pulsatile sensation can be felt as the fingertips are pushed apart by arterial pulsation.

The popliteal pulse is found behind the knee. The client should slightly flex the knee, with the foot resting on the examination table, or assume a prone position with the knee slightly flexed (Figure 32-66). The client is instructed to keep leg muscles relaxed. The nurse palpates with the fingers of both hands deeply into the popliteal fossa, just lateral to the midline. The popliteal pulse is difficult to locate.

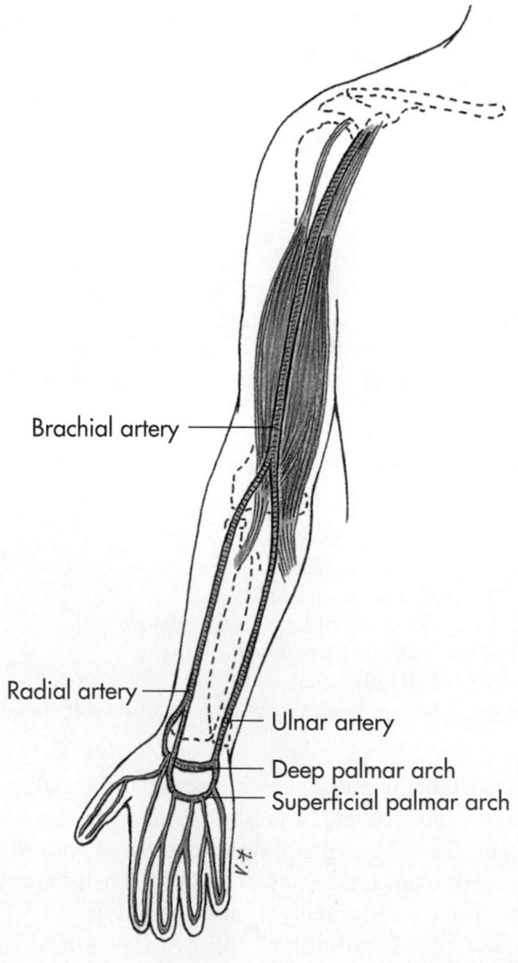

Brachial artery

Radial artery

Ulnar artery
Deep palmar arch
Superficial palmar arch

Figure 32-60 Anatomical positions of brachial, radial, and ulnar arteries.

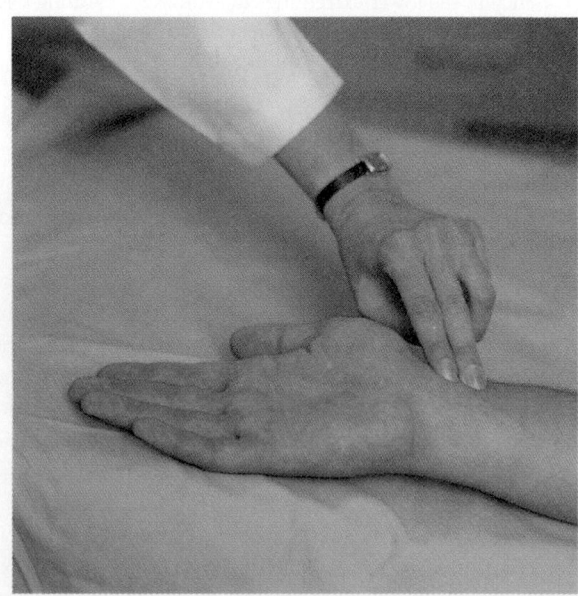

Figure 32-61 Palpation of radial pulse.

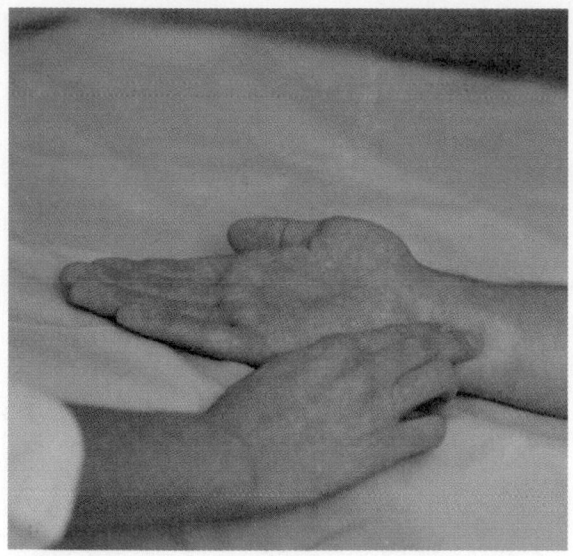

Figure 32-62 Palpation of ulnar pulse.

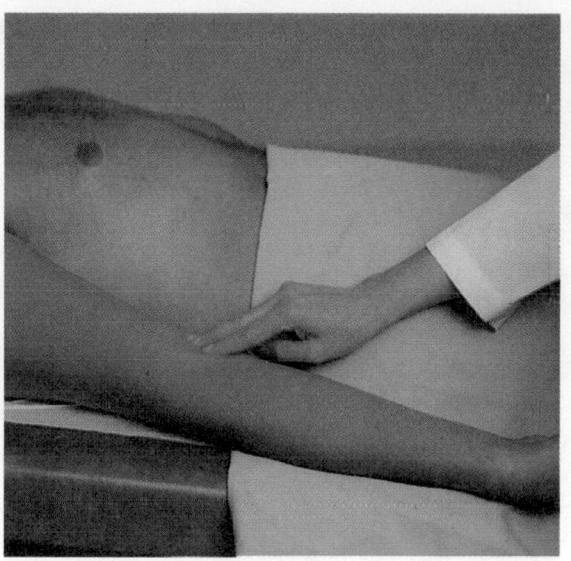

Figure 32-63 Palpation of brachial pulse.

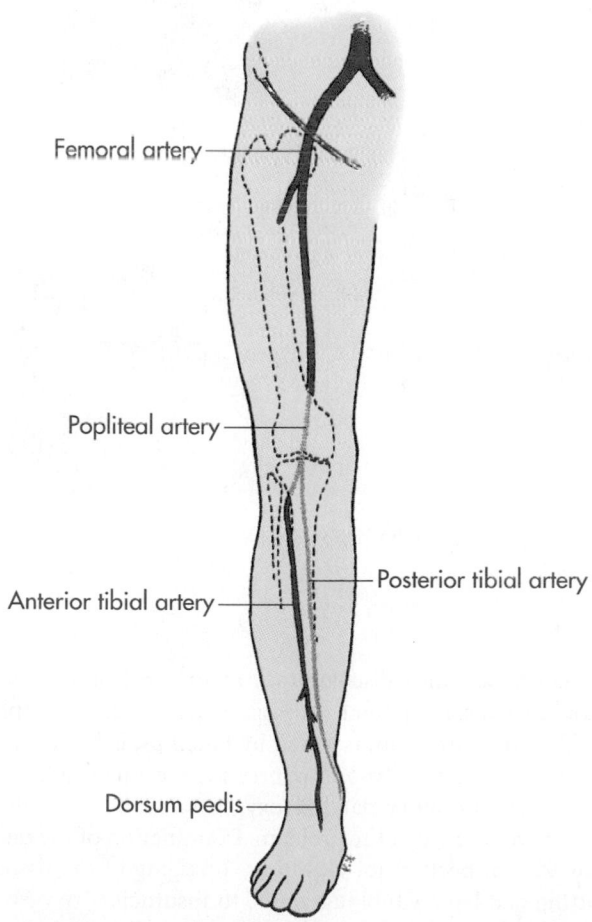

Femoral artery

Popliteal artery

Anterior tibial artery

Posterior tibial artery

Dorsum pedis

Figure 32-64 Anatomical position of femoral, popliteal, dorsalis pedis, and posterior tibial arteries.

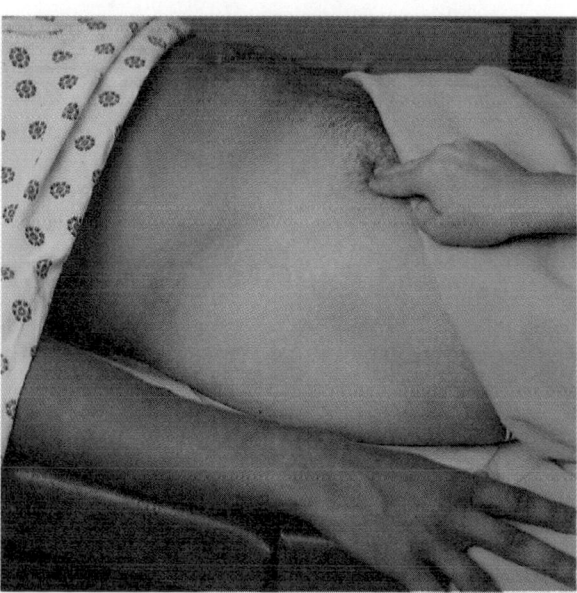

Figure 32-65 Palpation of femoral pulse.

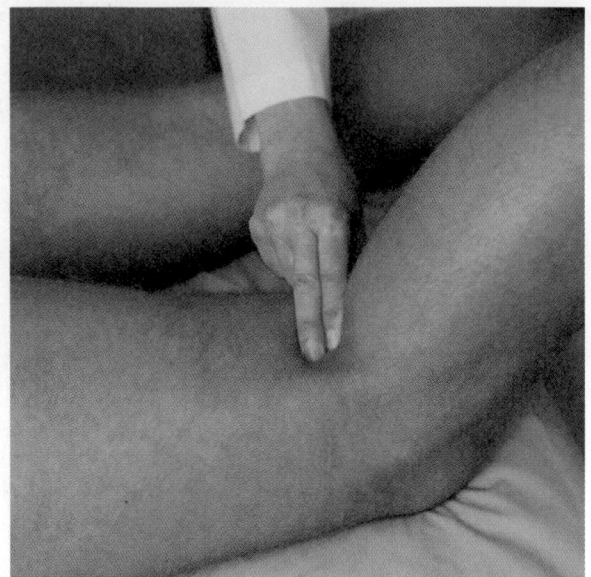

Figure 32-66   Palpation of popliteal pulse.

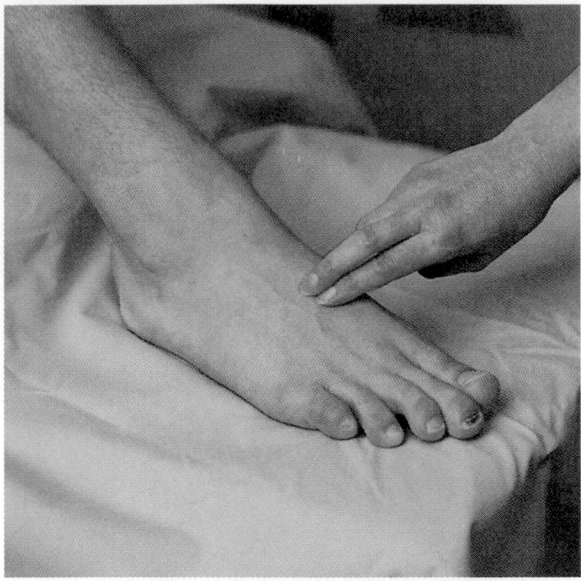

Figure 32-67   Palpation of dorsalis pedis pulse.

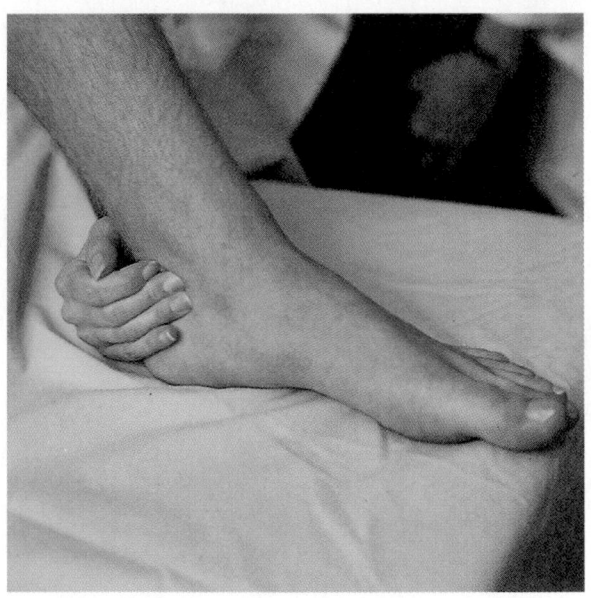

Figure 32-68   Palpation of posterior tibial pulse.

With the client's foot relaxed, the nurse locates the dorsalis pedis pulse. The artery runs along the top of the foot in line with the groove between the extensor tendons of the great toe and first toe (Figure 32-67). Often an examiner finds the pulse by placing the fingertips between the great and first toe and slowly inching up the foot. This pulse may be congenitally absent.

The posterior tibial pulse is found on the inner side of each ankle (Figure 32-68). The nurse places the fingers behind and below the medial malleolus (ankle bone). The artery is easily located with the foot relaxed and slightly extended.

Ultrasound Stethoscopes.   If a nurse cannot palpate a pulse, an ultrasound stethoscope is a useful tool that amplifies the sounds of a pulse wave. Factors that may weaken a pulse or make palpation difficult include obesity, reduction in the heart's stroke volume, diminished blood volume, or arterial obstruction. A thin layer of transmission gel is first applied to the client's skin at the pulse site or directly onto the transducer tip of the probe. The nurse then turns the volume control to "on" and places the tip of the probe at a 45- to 90-degree angle on the skin (Figure 32-69). The nurse moves the probe until a pulsating "whooshing" sound is heard, indicating that arterial blood flow is present.

Tissue Perfusion.   The condition of the skin, mucosa, and nail beds offers useful data about the status of circulatory blood flow. The nurse first examines the face and upper extremities, looking at the color of the skin, mucosa, and nail beds. The presence of cyanosis requires special attention. Central cyanosis, which indicates poor arterial oxygenation, may be due to heart disease. It can be noted by a bluish discoloration of the lips, mouth, and conjunctivae. Peripheral cyanosis, which indicates peripheral vasoconstriction, is noted by blue lips, earlobes, and nail beds. When cyanosis is present, the nurse refers to available laboratory data on oxygen saturation to determine the severity of the problem. Examination of the nails involves inspection for **clubbing,** a bulging of the tissues at the nail base. Clubbing is due to insufficient oxygenation at the periphery resulting from conditions such as chronic emphysema and congenital heart disease.

The nurse inspects the lower extremities for changes in

color, temperature, and condition of the skin indicating either arterial or venous alterations (Table 32-26). This is a good time to ask the client about any history of pain in the legs. If an arterial occlusion is present, the client has signs resulting from an absence of blood flow. Pain will be distal to the occlusion. The three *P*'s—pain, pallor, and pulselessness—characterize an occlusion. Venous congestion causes tissue changes indicating an inadequate circulatory flow back to the heart.

During examination of the lower extremities, the nurse also inspects skin and nail texture; hair distribution on the lower legs, feet, and toes; the venous pattern; and scars, pigmentation, or ulcers. The absence of hair growth over the legs may indicate circulatory insufficiency. The nurse should not be misled by shaven lower legs. Also, many men have less hair around the calves from wearing tight-fitting dress socks. Chronic recurring ulcers of the feet or lower legs are a serious sign of circulatory insufficiency and require a physician's intervention.

Peripheral Veins.

The nurse assesses the status of the peripheral veins by asking the client to assume sitting and standing positions. Assessment includes inspection and palpation for varicosities, peripheral edema, and phlebitis. Varicosities are superficial veins that become dilated, especially when the legs are in a dependent position. They are common in older adults because the veins normally fibrose, dilate, and stretch. They are also common in people who stand for prolonged periods. Varicosities in the anterior or medial part of the thigh and the posterolateral part of the calf are abnormal.

Dependent edema around the area of the feet and ankles can be a sign of venous insufficiency and right-sided heart failure. Dependent edema is common in older adults and persons who spend a lot of time standing (e.g., waitresses, security guards, or nurses). To assess for pitting edema, the nurse uses a thumb to press firmly for 5 seconds and then release over the medial malleolus or the shins. A depression left in the skin indicates edema. The severity of the edema is characterized by grading 1+ through 4+ (Figure 32-70).

Phlebitis is an inflammation of a vein that occurs commonly after trauma to the vessel wall, infection, prolonged immobilization, and prolonged insertion of IV catheters

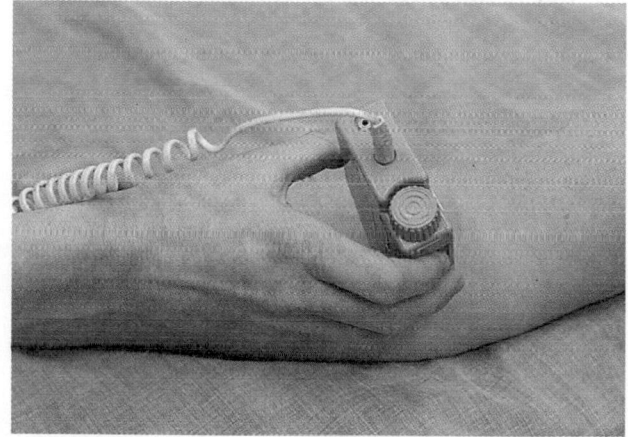

Figure 32-69   Ultrasound stethoscope in position on brachial artery.

Table 32-26	Signs of Venous and Arterial Insufficiency	
Assessment Criterion	Venous	Arterial
Color	Normal or cyanotic	Pale; worsened by elevation of extremity; dusky red when extremity is lowered
Temperature	Normal	Cool (blood flow blocked to extremity)
Pulse	Normal	Decreased or absent
Edema	Often marked	Absent or mild
Skin changes	Brown pigmentation around ankles	Thin, shiny skin; decreased hair growth; thickened nails

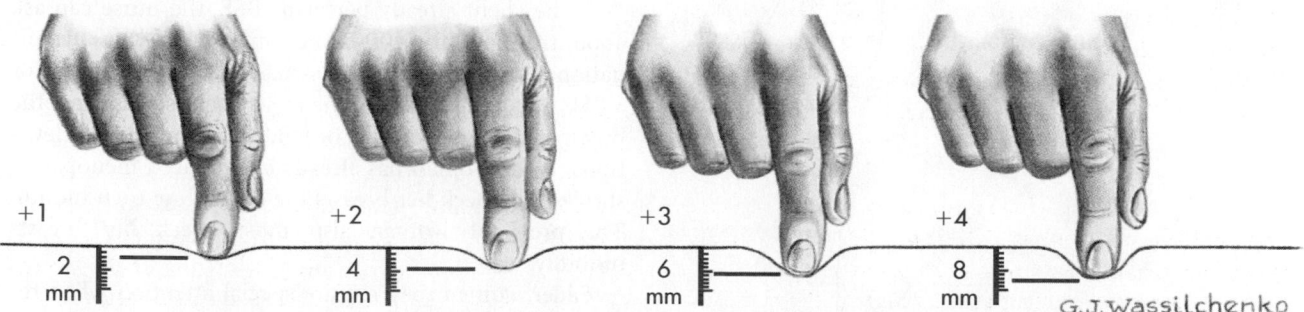

Figure 32-70   Assessing for pitting edema.
From Seidel HM and others: *Mosby's guide to physical examination*, ed 4, St. Louis, 1999, Mosby.

(see Chapter 40). Phlebitis promotes clot formation, a potentially dangerous situation because a clot within a deep vein of the leg can become dislodged and travel through the heart, causing a pulmonary embolus. To assess for phlebitis, the nurse inspects the calves for localized redness, tenderness, and swelling over vein sites. Gentle palpation of calf muscles reveals tenderness and firmness of the muscle. The nurse may also check for Homans' sign by supporting the leg while flexing the foot upward. If phlebitis is present in the lower leg, forceful dorsiflexion of the foot often causes pain in the calf.

LYMPHATIC SYSTEM

Assessment of the lymphatic drainage of the lower extremities is performed during examination of the vascular system. The nurse may also perform this examination just before the female or male genital examination. The legs are drained by superficial and deep nodes, but only the two groups of superficial nodes are palpable. The nurse palpates the area of the superficial inguinal nodes (Figure 32-71), beginning in the groin area and moving down toward the inner thigh. The vertical group of nodes lies close to the upper portion of the great saphenous vein. The horizontal group lies below the inguinal ligament. The nurse uses a firm but gentle pressure when palpating over each lymphatic chain. Multiple nodes are not normally palpable, although a few soft, nontender nodes are not unusual. Enlarged, hardened, tender nodes can reveal potential sites of infection or metastatic disease. An infection site can be identified by drainage collected by the nodes. For example,

the horizontal group drains lymph from the skin of the lower abdominal wall, the external genitalia, the anal canal, and the lower vagina.

Breasts

It is important to examine the breasts of female and male clients. A small amount of glandular tissue, a potential site for the growth of cancer cells, is located in the male breast. In contrast, the majority of the female breast is glandular tissue.

FEMALE BREASTS

Breast cancer was projected to affect an estimated 175,000 women in the United States in 1999 (ACS, 1999). The disease is second to lung cancer as the leading cause of death in women with cancer. Early detection is the key to cure. A major responsibility for nurses is to teach clients health behavior such as breast self-examination (BSE). Studies suggest that a minority of women actually perform BSE. Nurses should know factors that increase the likelihood of a woman performing BSE. Incorporating these interventions into teaching strategies may improve the likelihood of a client detecting breast cancer early. The American Cancer Society (ACS, 1999) recommends the following guidelines for the early detection of breast cancer:

BSE should be performed monthly by women 20 years of age and older.

An examination by a physician should be performed every 3 years from ages 20 to 40, and yearly for women over age 40.

Women with a family history of breast cancer should have a yearly physician's examination.

Asymptomatic women should have a screening mammogram by age 40; women age 40 and over should have a mammogram annually.

For women age 35 with a history of breast cancer, a yearly examination is recommended.

During an examination the nurse explains how to perform a BSE. While assessing the client's breasts, the nurse uses many of the same techniques the client will use in the home (Box 32-22).

If the client already performs BSE, the nurse can ask about the method she uses and times she does the examination in relation to her menstrual cycle. The best time for a BSE is on the last day of the menstrual period, when the breast is no longer swollen or tender from hormone elevations. If the woman has already experienced menopause, she should check her breasts the same time each month. The pregnant woman also must check her breasts monthly.

Older women may require special attention when reviewing the need for regular BSE. Many older women are limited by fixed incomes and thus fail to pursue regular clinical breast examination and mammography. Unfor-

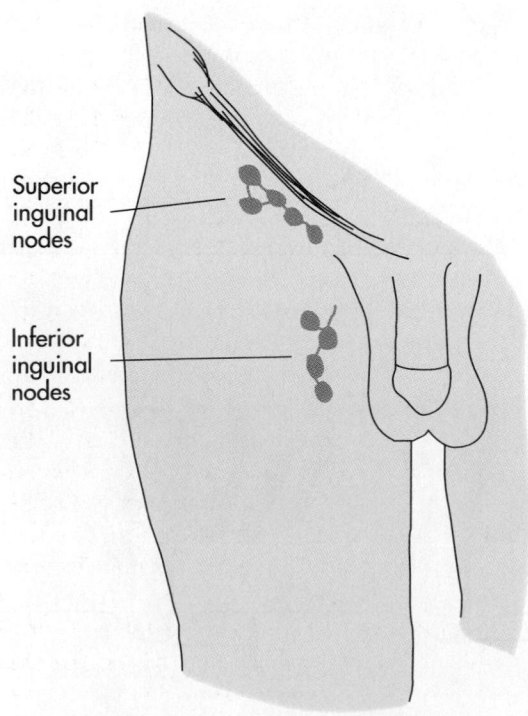

Figure 32-71   Inguinal lymph nodes.

Superior inguinal nodes

Inferior inguinal nodes

Breast Self-Examination

Box 32-22

Breast self-examination (BSE) should be done once a month so that you become familiar with the usual appearance and feel of your breasts. Familiarity makes it easier to notice any changes in the breast from one month to another. Early discovery of a change from what is "normal" is the main idea behind BSE.

If you menstruate, the best time to do BSE is 2 or 3 days after your period ends, when your breasts are least likely to be tender or swollen. If you no longer menstruate, pick a day, such as the first day of the month, to remind yourself it is time to do BSE.

Here is how to do BSE:

1. Stand before a mirror. Inspect both breasts for anything unusual, such as any discharge from the nipples, puckering, dimpling, or scaling of the skin.

The next two steps are designed to emphasize any change in the shape or contour of your breasts. As you do them, you should be able to feel your chest muscles tighten.

2. Watching closely in the mirror, clasp hands behind your head and press hands forward.

3. Next, press hands firmly on hips and bow slightly toward your mirror as you pull your shoulders and elbows forward.

Some women do the next part of the examination in the shower. Fingers glide over soapy skin, making it easy to appreciate the texture underneath.

4. Raise your left arm. Use three or four fingers of your right hand to explore your left breast firmly, carefully, and thoroughly. Beginning at the outer edge, press the flat part of your fingers in small circles, moving the circles slowly around the breast. Gradually work toward the nipple. Be sure to cover the entire breast. Pay special attention to the area between the breast and the armpit, including the armpit itself. Feel for any unusual lump or mass under the skin.

5. Gently squeeze the nipple and look for a discharge. Repeat the exam on your right breast.

6. Steps 4 and 5 should be repeated lying down. Lie flat on your back, left arm over your head and a pillow or folded towel under your left shoulder. This position flattens the breast and makes it easier to examine. Use the same circular motion described earlier.

Repeat on your right breast.

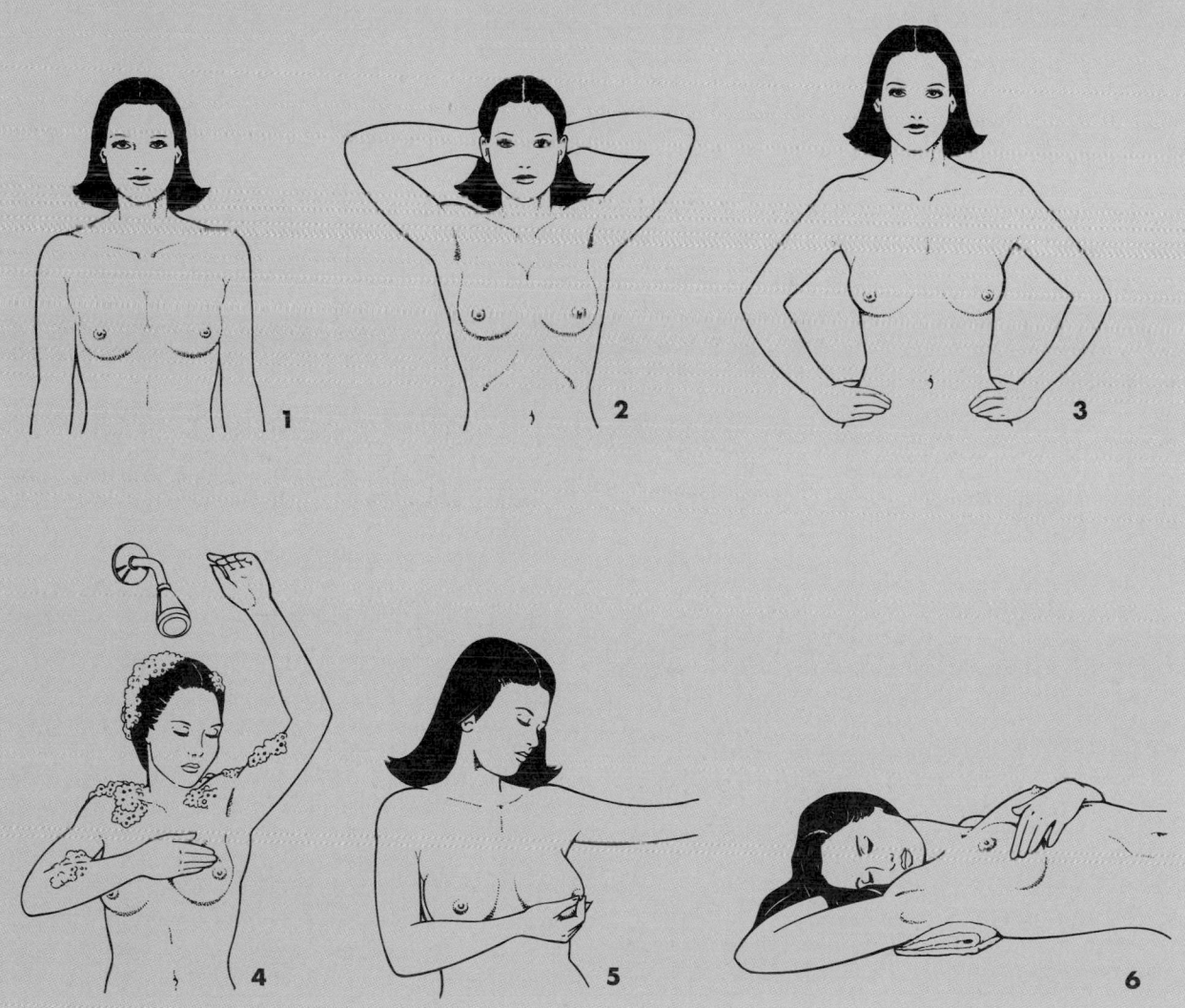

From Seidel HM and others: *Mosby's guide to physical examination,* ed 4, St. Louis, 1999, Mosby.

Table 32-27 **Nursing History for Breast Assessment**

Assessment Category	Rationale
Determine if woman is over age 40; has a personal or family history of breast cancer, early-onset menarche (before age 12), or late-age menopause (after age 50); has never had children or gave birth to first child after age 30; or has not breast-fed.	These are risk factors for breast cancer.
Ask if client (both sexes) has noticed lump, thickening, pain, or tenderness of breast; discharge, distortion, retraction, or scaling of nipple; or change in size of breast.	Potential signs and symptoms of breast cancer allow nurse to focus on specific areas of breast during assessment.
Determine if client is taking oral contraceptives, digitalis, diuretics, steroids, or estrogen hormones intake.	Medications may cause nipple discharge. Hormones and caffeine may cause fibrocystic changes in breast.
Determine client's caffeine intake and intake of foods high in fat.	Breast cancer incidence rates may correlate with fat intake (ACS, 1999).
Ask if client performs monthly BSE. If so, determine time of month she performs examination in relation to menstrual cycle. Have client describe or demonstrate method used.	Nurse's role is to educate client about breast cancer and techniques for BSE.
If client reports a breast mass, ask about length of time since lump was first noted. Does lump come and go, or is it always present? Have there been changes in the lump (e.g., size, relationship to menses), and are there associated symptoms?	Helps to determine nature of mass.

Normal Changes in the Breast During a Woman's Life Span   Box 32-23

PUBERTY (8 TO 20 YEARS)*
Breasts mature in five stages. One breast may grow more rapidly than the other. The ages at which changes occur and rate of developmental progression vary.

Stage 1 (Preadolescent)
- This stage involves elevation of the nipple only.

Stage 2
- The breast and nipple elevate as a small mound, and the areolar diameters enlarge.

Stage 3
- There is further enlargement and elevation of the breast and areola, with no separation of contour.

Stage 4
- The areola and nipple project into the secondary mound above the level of the breast. (May not occur in all girls.)

Stage 5 (Mature Breast)
- Only the nipple projects, and the areola recedes (may vary in some women).

YOUNG ADULTHOOD (20 TO 30 YEARS)
- Breasts reach full (nonpregnant) size. Shape is generally symmetrical. Breasts may be unequal in size.

PREGNANCY
- Breast size gradually enlarges to 2 to 3 times the previous size. Nipples enlarge and may become erect. Areolae darken, and diameters increase. Superficial veins become prominent. A yellowish fluid (colostrum) may be expelled from the nipples.

MENOPAUSE
- Breasts shrink. Tissue becomes softer, sometimes flabby.

OLDER ADULTHOOD†
- Breasts become elongated, pendulous, and flaccid as a result of glandular tissue atrophy. The skin of the breasts tends to wrinkle, appearing loose and flabby.
- Nipples become smaller flatter and lose erectile ability. Nipples may invert because of shrinkage and fibrotic changes.

*Data from Wong DL and others: *Whaley and Wong's nursing care of infants and children,* ed 6, St. Louis, 1999, Mosby.
†Data from Ebersole P, Hess P: *Toward healthy aging,* ed 5, St. Louis, 1998, Mosby.

tunately, many older women ignore changes in their breasts, assuming that they are a part of aging. In addition, physiological factors can affect the ease with which older women can perform a BSE. Musculoskeletal limitations, diminished peripheral sensation, reduced eyesight, and changes in joint range of motion can limit palpation and inspection abilities. The nurse should find resources for older women, including free screening programs. Often family members can be taught to perform examinations.

The client's history (Table 32-27) should alert the nurse to any signs of breast disease and normal developmental changes. Because of its glandular structure, the breast undergoes changes during a woman's life. Knowledge of these changes (Box 32-23) helps the nurse complete an accurate assessment.

Inspection. The client removes the top gown or drape to allow simultaneous visualization of both breasts. The client may stand or sit with her arms hanging loosely at her sides. If possible, the nurse places a mirror in front of the client so that she can see what to look for when performing a BSE. To recognize abnormalities, the client must be familiar with the normal appearance of her breasts. The nurse describes observations or findings in relation to imaginary lines that divide the breast into four quadrants and a tail. The lines cross at the center of the nipple. Each tail extends outward from the upper outer quadrant (Figure 32-72).

The breasts are inspected for size and symmetry. The breasts usually extend from the third to the sixth ribs, with the nipple at the level of the fourth intercostal space. One breast is commonly larger than the other. However, a dif-

ference in size may be caused by inflammation or a mass. As the woman becomes older, the ligaments supporting the breast tissue weaken, causing the breasts to sag and the nipples to lower.

The nurse observes the contour or shape of the breasts and notes masses, flattening, retraction, or dimpling. Breasts vary in shape from convex to pendulous or conical. Retraction or dimpling results from invasion of underlying ligaments by tumors. The ligaments become fibrotic and pull the overlying skin inward toward the tumor. Edema also changes the breasts' contour. To bring out retraction or changes in the shape of breasts, the nurse asks the client to assume three positions: raise arms above the head, press hands against the hips, and extend arms straight ahead while sitting and leaning forward. Each maneuver causes a contraction of the pectoral muscles, which will accentuate retraction.

The overlying skin is carefully inspected for color and venous pattern. Venous patterns are more easily seen in thin clients or pregnant women. The presence of lesions, edema, or inflammation is also noted. The nurse lifts each breast when necessary to observe lower and lateral aspects for color and texture changes. The breasts are the color of neighboring skin, and venous patterns are the same bilaterally. For women with large breasts, the nurse should be sure to look carefully at the undersurface, a common site for redness and excoriation caused by rubbing of skin surfaces.

The nurse inspects the nipple and areola for size, color, shape, discharge, and the direction the nipples point. The normal areolae are round or oval and nearly equal bilaterally. Color ranges from pink to brown. In light-skinned women the areola turns brown during pregnancy and remains dark. In dark-skinned women the areola is brown before pregnancy (Seidel and others, 1999). Normally the nipples point in symmetrical directions, they are everted, and there is no drainage. Their surface may be either smooth or wrinkled. If the nipples are inverted, the nurse asks if this has been a lifetime history. A recent inversion or inward turning of the nipple may indicate an underlying growth. Rashes or ulcerations are not normal on the breast or nipples. Bleeding or discharge from the nipple is noted. Clear yellow discharge 2 days after childbirth is common. While inspecting the breasts, the nurse explains the characteristics observed. The client must be taught the significance of abnormal signs or symptoms.

Palpation. Palpation allows the nurse to determine the condition of underlying breast tissue and lymph nodes. Breast tissue consists of glandular tissue, fibrous supportive ligaments, and fat. Glandular tissue is organized into lobes that end in ducts that open onto the nipple's surface. The largest portion of glandular tissue is in the upper outer quadrant and tail of each breast. Suspensory ligaments connect to skin and fascia underlying the breast to support the breast and maintain its upright position. Fatty tissue is located superficially and to the sides of the breast.

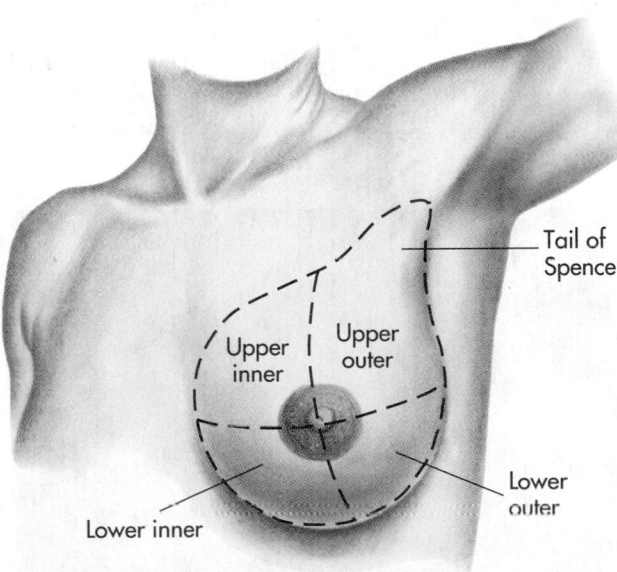

Figure 32-72 Quadrants of the left breast and axillary tail of Spence.
From Seidel HM and others: *Mosby's guide to physical examination,* ed 4, St. Louis, 1999, Mosby.

A large portion of lymph from the breasts drains into axillary lymph nodes. If cancerous lesions **metastasize** (spread), the nodes are commonly involved. The nurse learns the location of supraclavicular, infraclavicular, and axillary nodes (Figure 32-73). The axillary nodes drain lymph from the chest wall, breasts, arms, and hands. A tumor of one breast may involve nodes on the opposite side, as well as those on the same side.

The lymph nodes are best palpated when the client sits, although the examination can be performed with the client supine. Easy access is gained to the axillary nodes with the client's arms at her sides and the muscles relaxed. While facing the client and standing on the side being examined, the nurse supports the client's arm in a slightly flexed position and abducts the arm away from the chest wall. Then the nurse places the free hand against the client's chest wall and high in the axillary hollow. With the fingertips the nurse presses gently down over the surface of the ribs and muscles. The axillary nodes are palpated with the fingertips gently rolling soft tissue (Figure 32-74). Four areas of the axilla are palpated:

1. The edge of the pectoralis major muscle along the anterior axillary line
2. The chest wall in the midaxillary area
3. The upper part of the humerus
4. The anterior edge of the latissimus dorsi muscle along the posterior axillary line

Normally lymph nodes are not palpable. Each area must be assessed carefully because enlarged nodes are easily missed. The nurse notes their number, consistency, mobility, and size. One or two small, soft, nontender nodes may be normal. A palpable node feels like a small mass that may be hard, tender, and immobile. The nurse also palpates along the upper and lower clavicular ridges. The procedure is reversed for the other side.

It may be difficult for the client to learn to palpate for lymph nodes. Lying down with the arm abducted makes the area more accessible. The client is instructed to use her left hand for the right axillary and clavicular areas. The nurse can take the client's fingertips and move them in the proper circular fashion. The client then uses her right hand to palpate for nodes on the left side.

Palpation of breast tissue is best performed with the client lying supine with one arm behind the head (alternating with each breast). The supine position allows the breast tissue to flatten evenly against the chest wall. The client should raise her hand and place it behind the neck to further stretch and position breast tissue evenly (Figure 32-75A). The examiner often places a small pillow or towel under the shoulder blade to further position breast tissue.

The consistency of normal breast tissue varies widely. The breasts of a young client are firm and elastic. In an older client the tissue may feel stringy and nodular. The client's familiarity with the texture of her own breasts is very important. This familiarity is gained through monthly BSE (Box 32-24).

If the client complains of a mass, the nurse examines the opposite breast to ensure an objective comparison of normal and abnormal tissue. The nurse uses the pads of the first three fingers to compress breast tissue gently against the chest wall, noting tissue consistency (Figure 32-75, *B*). Palpation is performed systematically in one of three ways: (1) clockwise or counterclockwise, forming small circles with the fingers along each quadrant and the tail; (2) a back-and-forth technique with the fingers moving up and down each quadrant; or (3) palpating from the center of the breast in a radial fashion, returning to the areola to begin each spoke (Figure 32-76). Whatever approach is used, the nurse must be sure to cover the entire breast and tail, directing attention to any areas of tenderness.

When palpating large, pendulous breasts, the nurse uses a bimanual technique. The inferior portion of the breast is supported in one hand while the nurse uses the

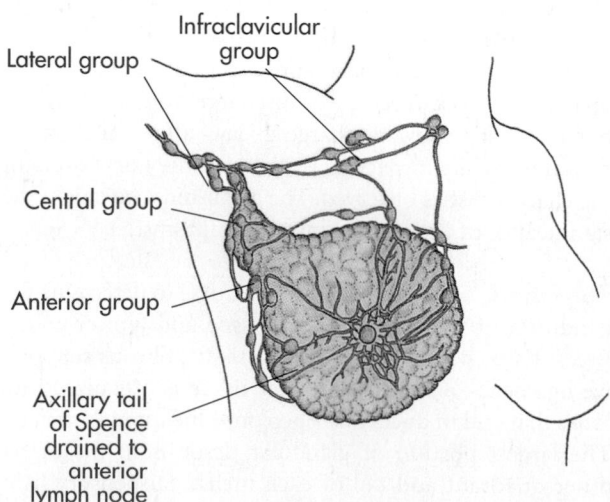

Figure 32-73 Anatomical position of axillary and clavicular lymph nodes.

Infraclavicular group
Lateral group
Central group
Anterior group
Axillary tail of Spence drained to anterior lymph node

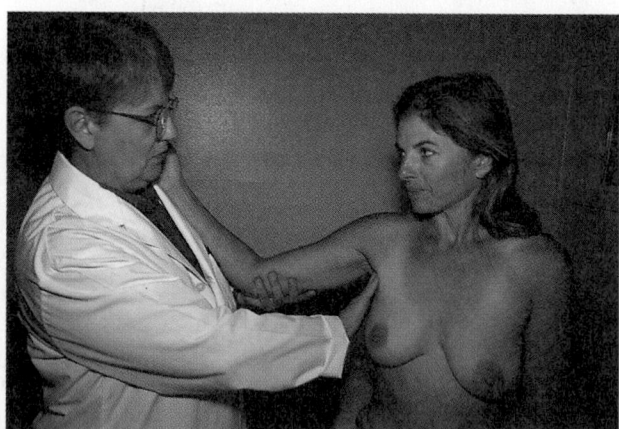

Figure 32-74 The nurse supports the client's arm and palpates axillary lymph nodes.

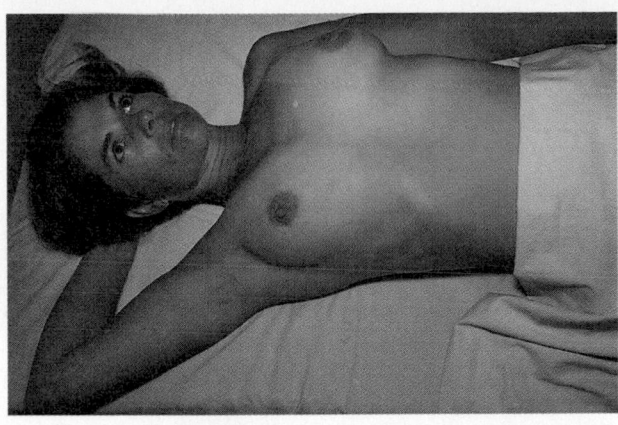

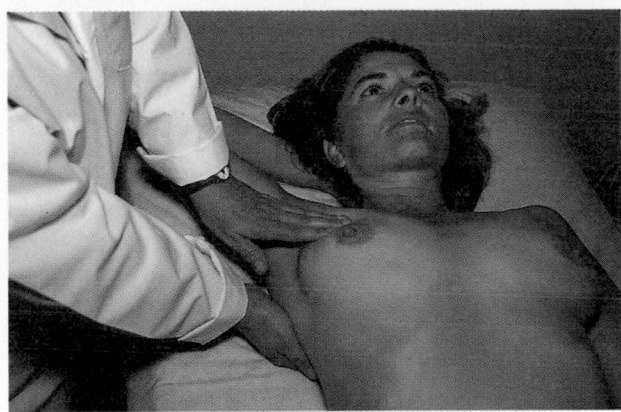

Figure 32-75 **A,** The client lies flat with arm abducted and hand under head to help flatten breast tissue evenly over the chest wall. **B,** The nurse palpates each breast in systemic fashion.

Client Teaching DURING FEMALE BREAST ASSESSMENT | Box 32-24

OBJECTIVES
- Client will perform BSE (see Box 32-22).
- Client will have screening mammography performed at recommended intervals.
- Client will identify signs and symptoms of breast cancer.
- Client will identify signs and symptoms of fibrocystic disease.
- Client will follow a low-fat diet.

TEACHING STRATEGIES
- Have client perform return demonstration of BSE and offer the opportunity to ask questions.
- Explain recommended frequency of mammography and assessment by a health care provider.
- Discuss signs and symptoms of breast cancer.
- Discuss signs and symptoms of fibrocystic disease.
- Inform a woman who is obese or who has a family history of breast cancer that she is at higher risk for the disease

(ACS, 1999). Encourage dietary changes, including limiting meat consumption to well-trimmed, lean beef, pork, or lamb; removing skin from cooked chicken before eating it; selecting tuna and salmon packed in water and not oil; and using low-fat dairy products.
- Encourage client to reduce intake of caffeine and theophyllines. Although this approach is controversial, it may reduce symptoms of fibrocystic disease.

EVALUATION
- Have client demonstrate BSE.
- During follow-up visit, determine whether client has had mammography performed.
- Ask client to explain frequency of mammography.
- Have client describe signs and symptoms of breast cancer compared with fibrocystic disease.

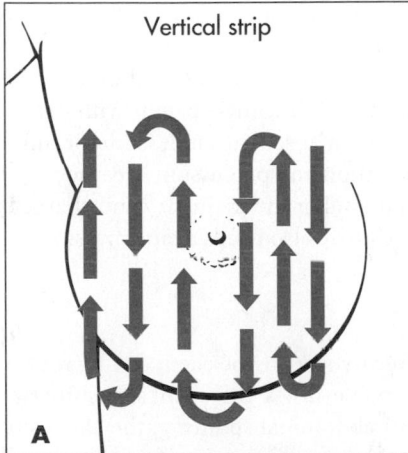

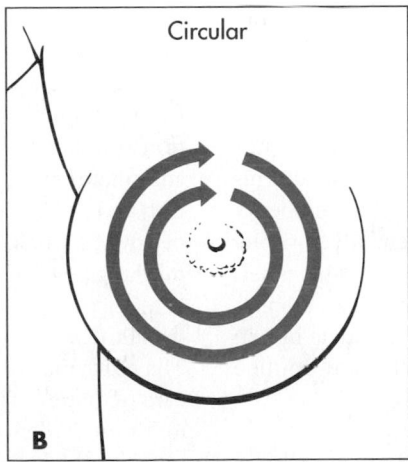

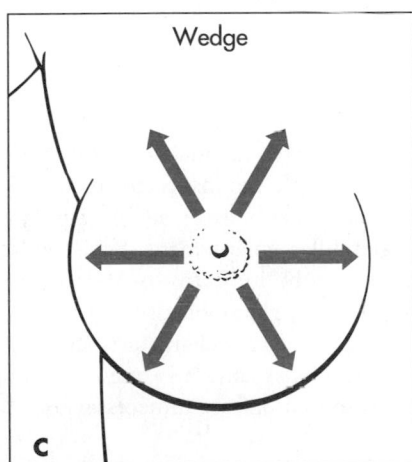

Figure 32-76 Various methods for palpation of the breast. **A,** Palpate from top to bottom in vertical strips. **B,** Palpate in concentric circles. **C,** Palpate out from the center in wedge sections. From Belcher A: *Cancer nursing,* St. Louis, 1993, Mosby.

other hand to palpate breast tissue against the supporting hand.

During palpation the nurse notes the consistency of breast tissue. It normally feels dense, firm, and elastic. In fibrocystic disease, a common problem in women, tissue feels lumpy, but it is found bilaterally. With menopause, breast tissue shrinks and becomes softer. The lobular feel of glandular tissue is normal. The lower edge of each breast may feel firm and hard. This is the normal inframammary ridge and not a tumor. It may be helpful to move the client's hand so that she can feel normal tissue variations. Abnormal masses are palpated to determine the following:

Location in relation to quadrants
Diameter in centimeters
Shape (e.g., round or discoid)
Consistency (soft, firm, or hard)
Tenderness
Mobility
Discreteness (whether boundaries of mass are clear or unclear)

Cancerous lesions are hard, fixed, nontender, and irregular in shape. A common benign condition of the breast is **fibrocystic breast disease.** This condition is characterized by lumpy, painful breasts and sometimes nipple discharge. Symptoms are more apparent during the menstrual period. When palpated, the cysts (lumps) are soft, well differentiated, and movable. Deep cysts may feel hard.

Special attention is given to gently palpating the nipple and areola. The thumb and index finger compress the nipple gently, and the nurse notes any discharge. As the nurse examines the nipple and areola, the nipple may become erect with wrinkling of the areola. These changes are normal.

After the nurse completes the examination, the client can demonstrate self-palpation. Observing the client's technique helps the nurse emphasize the importance of a systematic approach. The client is urged to see her physician if she discovers an abnormal mass during routine monthly BSE. She should also know all of the signs and symptoms of breast cancer.

Male Breasts

Examination of the male breast is relatively easy. The nipple and areola are inspected for nodules, edema, and ulceration. An enlarged male breast may result from obesity or glandular enlargement. Breast enlargement in young males may be indicative of steroid use. Fatty tissue feels soft, whereas glandular tissue is firm. Any masses are palpated for the same characteristics as in the female breast. Because breast cancer in men is relatively rare, routine self-examinations are unnecessary.

Abdomen

The abdominal examination can be complex because of the organs located within and near the abdominal cavity.

A thorough nursing history (Table 32-28) helps the nurse interpret physical signs. The examination includes an assessment of structures of the lower gastrointestinal (GI) tract in addition to the liver, stomach, uterus, ovaries, kidneys, and bladder. Abdominal pain is one of the most common symptoms that clients report when seeking medical care. An accurate assessment requires matching client history data with a careful assessment of the location of physical symptoms.

Landmarks help the nurse map out the abdominal region. The xiphoid process (tip of the sternum) marks the upper boundary of the abdominal region, and the symphysis pubis delineates the lower boundary. By dividing the abdomen into four imaginary quadrants (Figure 32-77, A) the nurse can refer to assessment findings and record them in relation to each quadrant. For example, the nurse may determine that the client is experiencing tenderness over the left lower quadrant (LLQ) with normal bowel sounds present. Posteriorly the kidneys, located from the T12 to L3 vertebrae, are protected by the lower ribs and heavy back muscles (Figure 32-77, B). The costovertebral angle formed by the last rib and vertebral column is a landmark used during kidney palpation.

Clients must be relaxed for abdominal examinations. A tightening of abdominal muscles hinders accuracy with palpation and auscultation. The nurse asks the client to void before beginning. The room should be warm, and the client's upper chest and legs should be draped. The client lies supine or in a dorsal recumbent position with the arms at the sides and knees slightly bent. Small pillows can be placed beneath the knees. If the client places the arms under the head, the abdominal muscles may tighten. The examiner proceeds calmly and slowly, making sure that there is adequate lighting. The abdomen is exposed from just above the xiphoid process down to the symphysis pubis. Warm hands and a warm stethoscope further promote relaxation. Maintaining conversation except during auscultation helps to distract clients. Clients should be asked to report pain and point out tender areas. Tender areas are assessed last.

The order of an abdominal examination differs slightly from previous assessments. The nurse begins with inspection and then follows with auscultation. It is important to auscultate before palpation and percussion because palpation and percussion may alter the frequency and character of bowel sounds. The nurse also needs a tape measure and marking pen.

Inspection

The nurse may be able to observe the client during routine care activities. The nurse notes the client's posture and looks for evidence of abdominal splinting: the client's lying with the knees drawn up or moving restlessly in bed. A client free from abdominal pain will not stoop or splint the abdomen. To inspect the abdomen for abnormal movement or shadows, the nurse stands on the client's

Table 32-28 Nursing History for Abdominal Assessment

Assessment Category	Rationale
If client has abdominal or low back pain, assess character of pain in detail (location, onset, frequency, precipitating factors, aggravating factors, type of pain, severity, course).	Pattern of characteristics of pain helps determine its source.
Carefully observe client's movement and position, including lying still with knees drawn up, moving restlessly to find comfortable position, and lying on one side or sitting with knees drawn to chest.	Positions assumed by client may reveal nature and source of pain, including peritonitis, renal stone, and pancreatitis.
Assess normal bowel habits and stool character; ask if client uses laxatives.	Data compared with physical findings can help identify cause and nature of elimination problems.
Determine if client has had abdominal surgery, trauma, or diagnostic tests of GI tract.	Surgical or traumatic alterations of abdominal organs may cause changes in expected findings (e.g., position of underlying organs). Diagnostic tests may change character of stool.
Assess if client has had recent weight changes or intolerance to diet (e.g., nausea, vomiting, cramping, especially in last 24 hours).	Data may indicate alterations in upper GI tract (stomach or gallbladder) or lower colon.
Assess for difficulty in swallowing, belching, flatulence, bloody emesis (hematemesis), black or tarry stools (melena), heartburn, diarrhea, or constipation.	These characteristic signs and symptoms indicate gastrointestinal alterations.
Ask if client takes antiinflammatory medication (e.g., aspirin, ibuprofen, or steroids) or antibiotics.	Pharmacological agents may cause GI upset or bleeding.
Ask client to locate tender areas.	Nurse assesses painful areas last to minimize discomfort and anxiety.
Inquire about family history of cancer, kidney disease, alcoholism, hypertension, or heart disease.	Data may reveal risk for alterations identifiable during examination.
Determine if female client is pregnant; note last menstrual period.	Pregnancy causes changes in abdominal shape and contour.
Assess client's usual intake of alcohol.	Chronic alcohol ingestion can cause gastrointestinal and liver problems.
Review client's history for the following factors: health care occupation, hemodialysis, IV drug user, household or sexual contact with hepatitis B virus (HBV) carrier, heterosexual person with more than one sex partner in previous 6 months, sexually active homosexual or bisexual male, international traveler in area of high HBV infection rate.	Risk factors for HBV exposure.

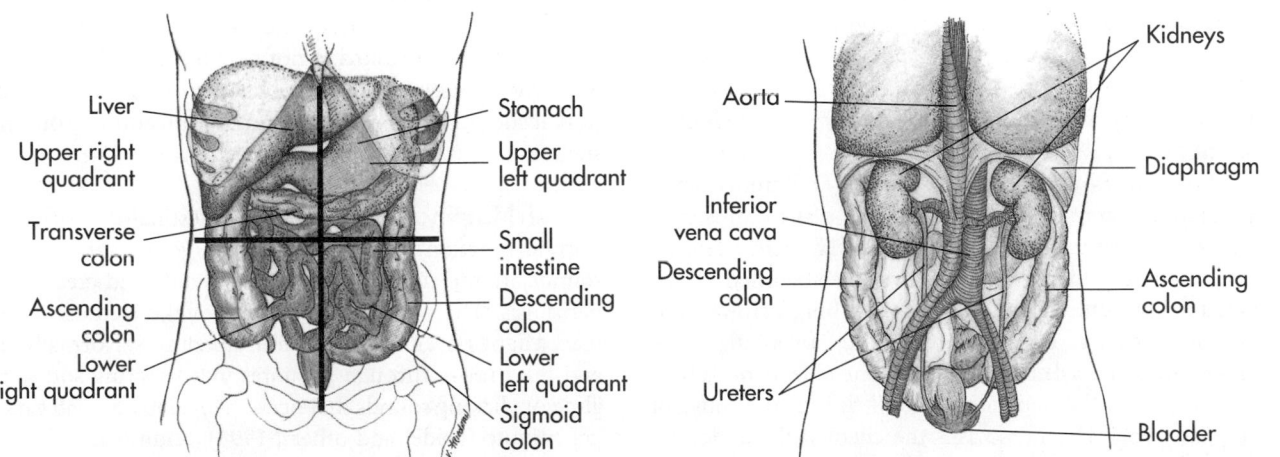

Figure 32-77 **A,** Anterior view of abdomen divided by quadrants. **B,** Posterior view of abdominal sections.

right side and inspects from above the abdomen. By sitting down to look across the abdomen, the nurse assesses contour. The examination light is directed over the abdomen.

Skin.   The nurse inspects the skin over the abdomen for color, scars, venous patterns, lesions, and **striae** (stretch marks). The skin is subject to the same color variations as the rest of the body. Venous patterns are normally faint, except in thin clients. Striae result from stretching of tissue by obesity or pregnancy. An artificial opening may indicate a drainage site resulting from surgery (see Chapter 49) or an ostomy (see Chapters 44 and 45). Scars indicate past trauma or surgery that may have created permanent changes in underlying organ anatomy. Bruising may indicate accidental injury, physical abuse, or a type of bleeding disorder. The nurse should ask if the client self-administers injections (e.g., heparin or insulin). Unexpected findings include generalized color changes such as jaundice or cyanosis. A glistening, taut appearance indicates ascites.

Umbilicus.   When examining the umbilicus, the position; shape; color; and signs of inflammation, discharge, or protruding masses are noted. Normally the umbilicus is a flat or concave hemisphere positioned midway between the xiphoid process and symphysis pubis. The color is the same as that of the surrounding skin. Underlying masses can cause displacement. An everted (pouched-out) umbilicus usually indicates distention. **Hernias** (protrusions of abdominal organs through the muscle wall) cause upward protrusion of the umbilicus. Normally no discharge is emitted from the umbilical area.

Contour and Symmetry.   The nurse inspects for contour, symmetry, and surface motion of the abdomen, noting any masses, bulging, or distention. A flat abdomen forms a horizontal plane from the xiphoid process to the symphysis pubis. A round abdomen protrudes in a convex sphere from the horizontal plane. A concave abdomen appears to sink into the muscular wall. Each of these findings is normal if the abdomen's shape is symmetrical. In older adults there is often an overall increased distribution of adipose tissue. The presence of masses on only one side, or asymmetry, may indicate an underlying pathological condition.

Intestinal gas, a tumor, or fluid in the abdominal cavity may cause **distention** (swelling). When distention is generalized, the entire abdomen protrudes. The skin often appears taut, as if it were stretched over the abdomen. When gas causes distention, the flanks do not bulge. However, if fluid is the source of the problem, the flanks bulge. The client should be asked to roll onto one side. A protuberance forms on the dependent side if fluid is the cause of the distention. The nurse asks the client if the abdomen feels unusually tight. The nurse must be careful not to confuse distention with obesity. In obesity the abdomen is large, rolls of adipose tissue are often present along the flanks, and the client does not complain of tightness in the abdomen. If abdominal distention is expected, the nurse may choose to measure the abdomen's girth by placing a tape measure around the abdomen at the level of the umbilicus. Consecutive measurements will show any increase or decrease in distention. A marking pen is used to indicate where the tape measure was applied.

Enlarged Organs or Masses.   While observing the abdominal contour, the nurse asks the client to take a deep breath and hold it. The contour should remain smooth and symmetrical. This maneuver forces the diaphragm downward and reduces the size of the abdominal cavity. Any enlarged organs in the upper abdominal cavity (e.g., liver or spleen) may descend below the rib cage to cause a bulge. Closer examination can be performed with palpation.

To evaluate the abdominal musculature, the nurse has clients raise their heads. This position causes superficial abdominal wall masses, hernias, and muscle separations to become more apparent.

Movement or Pulsations.   The nurse should remember that a man breathes abdominally and a woman breathes more costally. If the client has severe pain, respiratory movement is diminished, and the client tightens abdominal muscles to guard against the pain. On closer inspection the nurse may see peristaltic movement and aortic pulsation by looking across the abdomen from the side to detect movement. It may take several minutes to see a peristaltic wave. In contrast, aortic pulsations occur with each beat of systole and appear in the midline above the umbilicus (epigastric area).

AUSCULTATION

The nurse changes the usual sequence of assessment skills when auscultating the abdomen for bowel sounds of intestinal motility and for vascular sounds. Auscultation always precedes percussion and palpation during the abdominal assessment because manipulation of the abdomen may alter the frequency and intensity of bowel sounds. Clients are asked to not talk. If a client has a nasogastric or intestinal tube connected to intermittent suction, it should be momentarily turned off. Sound from the suction obscures bowel sounds.

Bowel Motility.   **Peristalsis,** or intestinal motility, is a normal function of the small and large intestine. Bowel sounds are the audible passage of air and fluid created by peristalsis. The warmed diaphragm of the stethoscope is placed lightly over each of the four quadrants. Normally air and fluid move through the intestines, creating soft gurgling or clicking sounds that occur irregularly 5 to 35 times per minute (Seidel and others, 1999). Sounds may last $\frac{1}{2}$ second to several seconds. It normally takes 5 to 20 seconds to hear a bowel sound. However, it may take 5 minutes of continuous listening before it can be determined that bowel sounds are absent. All four quadrants are auscultated to make sure that no sounds are missed. The best time to auscultate is between meals. When the nurse auscultates just after meals or long after the client eats, bowel sounds tend to be increased. Sounds are generally described as normal, audible, absent, hyperactive, or hypoactive. Absent sounds indicate a cessation of gastrointestinal motility that may result from late-stage bowel obstruction, **paralytic ileus,** or **peritonitis.** Hyperactive sounds are loud, "growling" sounds called **borborygmi,** which indicate increased gastrointestinal motility. Inflammation of the bowel, anxiety, diarrhea, bleeding, excessive ingestion of laxatives, and reaction of the intestines to certain foods cause increased motility (Box 32-25).

Vascular Sounds.   The presence of bruits in the abdominal area can reveal aneurysms or stenotic vessels. The nurse uses the stethoscope's bell to auscultate in the epigastric region and each of the four quadrants. Normally there are no vascular sounds over the aorta (midline through the abdomen) or femoral arteries (lower quadrants). Renal artery bruits can be heard by placing the stethoscope over each upper quadrant anteriorly or over the costovertebral angle posteriorly (which can be done when the client sits). A bruit should be reported immediately to a physician.

PERCUSSION

Percussion of the abdomen maps out underlying organs, bone, and masses and helps reveal the presence of air in the stomach and intestines. The beginning student uses this skill in a limited fashion. Practice is needed to ensure accuracy.

Organs and Masses.   The nurse systematically percusses each quadrant to assess areas of tympany and dullness. Potentially painful areas are always percussed last. Tympany usually predominates because of air in the stomach and intestines. A dull percussion note is a medium- to high-pitched short sound heard over solid masses such as the liver, spleen, pancreas, kidneys, and distended bladder. In addition, a dull note may indicate a tumor. When dullness is noted, it may be useful to also use palpation to complete a detailed assessment.

Liver Size.   Percussion allows the nurse to identify borders of the liver to detect organ enlargement. The nurse starts at the right iliac crest and percusses upward along the right midclavicular line. The percussion note changes from tympanic to dull at the liver's lower border, which is usually at the right costal margin. Extension beyond the right costal margin should be reported immediately. The nurse may mark the lower border on the client's abdomen with a water-soluble pencil. The upper border is found by percussing down from the clavicle along the intercostal spaces at the midclavicular line. This time, the note changes from resonant to dull (Figure 32-78). The liver's upper border is usually found in the fifth, sixth, or seventh intercostal space. The distance between the upper and lower liver borders should be 6 to 12 cm (2½ to 5 inches) at the right midclavicular line. Diseases such as **cirrhosis,** cancer, and **hepatitis** cause liver enlargement.

Kidney Tenderness.   With the client sitting or standing erect, the nurse uses direct or indirect percussion to assess for kidney inflammation. With the ulnar surface of the partially closed fist, the nurse percusses posteriorly the

---

Client Teaching DURING ABDOMINAL ASSESSMENT	Box 32-25

OBJECTIVES
- Client will maintain normal bowel elimination.
- Client will achieve pain relief.
- Clients at high risk for HBV will receive immunization.
- Client will identify signs and symptoms of colon cancer.

TEACHING STRATEGIES
- Explain factors that promote bowel elimination, such as diet, regular exercise, limited use of over-the-counter drugs causing constipation, establishment of regular elimination schedule, and a good fluid intake (see Chapter 45). Stress importance for older adults.
- Caution clients about dangers of excessive use of laxatives or enemas.
- If client has acute pain, explain activities or positions to avoid.
- If client has chronic pain, explain measures used for pain relief (e.g., relaxation exercises, positioning) (see Chapter 42).

- If client is a health care worker or has contact with blood or fluids of affected person, encourage client to receive the series of three vaccine doses.
- Instruct client about warning signs of colon cancer, including bleeding from rectum, black or tarry stools, blood in stool, and a change in bowel habits (constipation or diarrhea).

EVALUATION
- Reassess client's bowel elimination pattern and stool character after therapies are started.
- Observe client using pain-relief measures and reassess character of pain.
- During follow-up clinic or office visit, check client's compliance with HBV vaccine schedule.
- Ask client to state signs and symptoms of colon cancer.

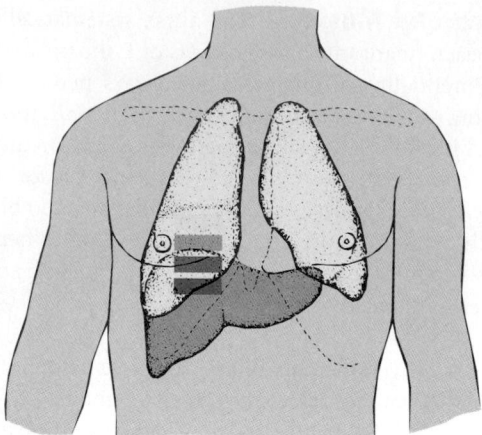

Figure 32-78   To locate the liver's upper border, the nurse percusses downward, noting the change in sound from resonance (lung) to dullness (liver).

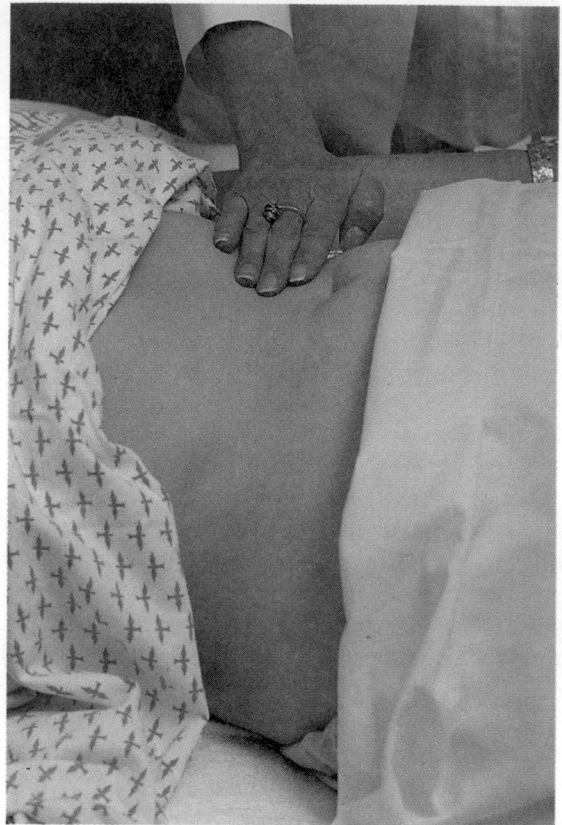

Figure 32-79   Light palpation of abdomen.

costovertebral angle at the scapular line. If the kidneys are inflamed, the client feels tenderness during percussion.

PALPATION

With palpation, nursing students are primarily concerned with detecting areas of abdominal tenderness and noting the quality of abnormal distentions or masses. As students become more skilled, they learn to palpate for specific organs such as the liver. Light and deep palpation are used.

After rubbing the hands together, the nurse uses light palpation over each quadrant. The nurse waits to palpate painful areas last. The nurse lays the palm of the hand with fingers extended and approximated lightly on the abdomen. The nurse keeps the palm and forearm horizontal (Figure 32-79). The pads of the fingertips depress approximately 1.3 cm (½ inch) in a gentle dipping motion. The nurse avoids quick jabs and uses smooth, coordinated movements. If the client is ticklish, it may help to place the client's hand on the abdomen with the nurse's hand on the client's. This continues until the nurse can gradually remove the client's hand.

A systematic palpation of each quadrant assesses for muscular resistance, distention, tenderness, and superficial organs or masses. While palpating, the nurse observes the client's face for signs of discomfort. The abdomen is normally smooth with consistent softness and nontender without masses. The older adult often lacks abdominal tone. If the nurse palpates a sensitive area, guarding or muscle tenseness may occur. If tightening remains after the client is helped to relax, peritonitis, acute **cholecystitis,** or appendicitis may be the cause. A distended bladder is easy to detect with light palpation. Normally the bladder lies below the umbilicus and above the symphysis pubis. The nurse routinely checks for a distended bladder if a client has been unable to void (e.g., because of anesthesia

or sedation) or has been incontinent, or if an indwelling urinary catheter is not draining well.

With experience the nurse can perform deep palpation to delineate abdominal organs and to detect less obvious masses. Short fingernails are needed. It is important for the client to be relaxed as the nurse's hands are depressed approximately 2.5 to 7.5 cm (1 to 3 inches) into the abdomen (Figure 32-80). Deep palpation is never used over a surgical incision or over extremely tender organs. It is also unwise to use palpation on abnormal masses. Deep pressure may cause tenderness in the healthy client over the cecum, sigmoid colon, aorta, and the midline near the xiphoid process (Seidel and others, 1999).

Each quadrant is surveyed systematically. Masses palpated are assessed for size, location, shape, consistency, tenderness, pulsation, and mobility. If tenderness is found, the examiner tests for rebound tenderness by pressing a hand slowly and deeply into the involved area and then letting go quickly. If pain is elicited with the release of the hand, the test is positive. Rebound tenderness occurs in clients with peritoneal irritation such as occurs in appendicitis; **pancreatitis;** or any peritoneal injury causing bile, blood, or enzymes to enter the peritoneal cavity.

Liver.   The liver lies in the right upper quadrant under the rib cage. The nurse uses deep palpation to locate the

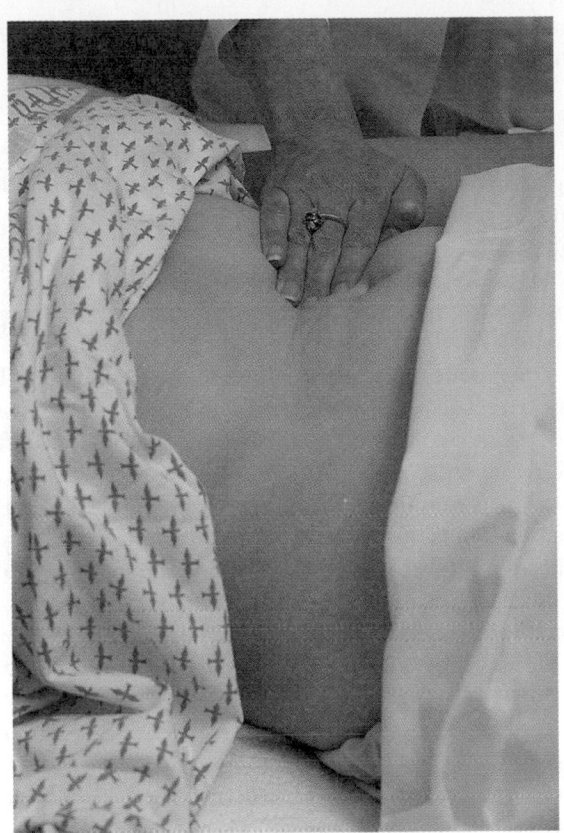

Figure 32-80   Deep palpation of abdomen.

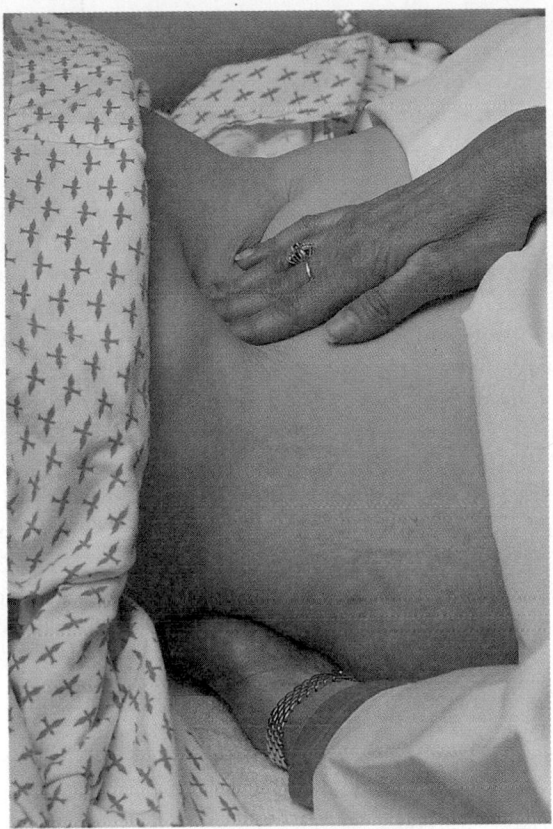

Figure 32-81   The nurse's left hand is placed under the client's posterior thorax at the eleventh and twelfth ribs. The nurse's right hand palpates in and up to feel the liver's edge as the client inhales.

liver's lower edge. This technique detects liver enlargement. To palpate the liver, the nurse places the left hand under the client's right posterior thorax at the eleventh and twelfth ribs and then applies upward pressure. This maneuver makes it easier to feel the liver anteriorly. With the fingers of the right hand pointing toward the right costal margin, the nurse places the hand on the right upper quadrant well below the liver's lower border. As the nurse presses gently in and up (Figure 32-81), the client takes a deep abdominal breath. As the client inhales, the nurse tries to palpate the liver's edge as it descends. A normal liver may not be palpable. However, it is nontender and has a firm, regular, and sharp edge. If the liver is palpable, the nurse traces its edge medially and laterally by repeating the maneuver.

Aortic Pulsation.
To assess aortic pulsation, the nurse palpates with the thumb and forefinger of one hand deeply into the upper abdomen, just left of the midline. Normally a pulsation is transmitted forward. If there is enlargement of the aorta from an **aneurysm** (localized dilation of a vessel wall), the pulsation expands laterally. In obese clients it may be necessary to palpate with both hands, one on each side of the aorta.

Female Genitalia and Reproductive Tract

An examination of the female genitalia can be embarrassing for many women unless the nurse uses a calm and relaxed approach. The gynecological examination is one of the most difficult experiences for adolescents. Cultural background may further add to apprehension. For example, female Mexican-Americans have a strong social value that women do not expose their bodies to men or even to other women. Similarly, Chinese-Americans may believe that the examination of genitalia is offensive. The nurse must provide very thorough explanations as to the reason for the procedure used in the examination. The lithotomy position assumed during the examination is an added source of embarrassment. Comfort is established through correct positioning and draping. Each portion of the examination is explained in advance so that clients can anticipate the nurse's actions. Adolescents may choose to have parents present in the examination room.

The client may require a complete examination of the female reproductive organs, which includes assessment of the external genitalia and a vaginal examination. Most nurses do not perform a vaginal examination until they become nurse practitioners with extensive experience. However, it is important for the nurse to understand the procedure because a physician will require the nurse's assistance. An examination should be part of each woman's preventive health care because uterine cancers have a high incidence rate and ovarian cancer causes more deaths than any other cancer of the female reproductive system (ACS, 1998). Frequently a client will undergo an examination of external genitalia during routine hygiene measures or urinary catheter care.

Adolescents and young adults should be examined because of the growing incidence of sexually transmitted diseases (STDs). The average age of menarche among young girls has declined, and the majority of male and female teenagers are sexually active by age 19 (Wong and others, 1999). As the nurse collects a history (Table 32-29), it is also important to assess the client's level of anxiety. The nurse should ask if the client has ever had a vaginal examination before. Rectal and anal assessment is easily

combined with this examination because the client can assume a lithotomy or dorsal recumbent position.

PREPARATION OF THE CLIENT

If a complete examination will be performed, the following special equipment will be needed: examination table with stirrups, vaginal speculum of correct size, adjustable light source, sink, clean disposable gloves, glass microscopic slides and coverslips, plastic spatula and/or cytobrush, and specimen bottles with fixative spray (hairspray).

Equipment must be ready before the examination begins. The client is asked to empty her bladder so that urine is not accidentally expelled during the examination. Often it is necessary to collect a urine specimen. The client is assisted in assuming the lithotomy position, in bed or on an examination table for an external genitalia assessment, and is assisted into stirrups if a speculum examination is to be performed. The woman stabilizes each foot in a stirrup and then slides her buttocks down to the edge of the examining table. The nurse places a hand at the edge of the table and

Table 32-29 **Nursing History for Female Genitalia and Reproductive Tract Assessment**

Assessment Category	Rationale
Determine if client has had previous illness or surgery involving reproductive organs, including STD.	Illness or surgery can influence appearance and position of organs being examined.
Review menstrual history, including age at menarche, frequency and duration of menstrual cycle, character of flow (e.g., amount, presence of clots), presence of dysmenorrhea (painful menstruation), pelvic pain, dates of last two menstrual periods, and premenstrual symptoms.	This information helps to reveal level of reproductive health, including normalcy of menstrual cycle.
Ask client to describe obstetrical history, including each pregnancy and history of abortions or miscarriages.	Observed physical findings will vary, depending on woman's history of pregnancy.
Ask client to describe current and past contraceptive practices and problems encountered. Determine whether client uses safe sex practices. Discuss risk of STDs and HIV infection.	Use of certain types of contraceptives may influence reproductive health (e.g., sensitivity reaction to spermicidal jelly). Sexual history reveals risk for and understanding of STDs.
Assess if client has signs and symptoms of vaginal discharge, painful or swollen perianal tissues, or genital lesions.	These signs and symptoms indicate STD.
Determine if client has symptoms or history of genitourinary problems, including burning during urination, frequency, urgency, nocturia, hematuria, incontinence, or stress incontinence (see Chapter 44).	Urinary problems may be associated with gynecological disorders, including STDs.
Ask if client has had signs of bleeding outside of normal menstrual period or after menopause or has had unusual vaginal discharge.	These are warning signs for cervical and endometrial cancer.
Determine if client is between ages 40 and 50 and has history of condyloma acuminatum, herpes simplex, or cervical dysplasia; has multiple sex partners; smokes; has had multiple pregnancies; or was young at first intercourse.	These are risk factors for cervical cancer.
Determine if client is between ages 40 and 60 and has history of ovarian dysfunction, breast or endometrial cancer, irradiation of pelvic organs, or endometriosis; has family history of ovarian or breast cancer; or has history of infertility or nulliparity.	These are risk factors for ovarian cancer.
Determine if client is postmenopausal, obese, or infertile; had early menarche (before age 12); had late menopause (after age 50); has history of hypertension, diabetes, or liver disease; or has family history of endometrial, breast, or colon cancer.	These are risk factors for endometrial cancer.

instructs the client to move until touching the hand. The client's arms should be at her sides or folded across the chest to prevent tightening of abdominal muscles.

A woman suffering from pain or deformity of the joints may be unable to assume a lithotomy position. In this situation it may be necessary to have the client abduct only one leg or to have another nurse assist in separating the client's thighs. The side-lying position may also be used with the client on the left side with the right thigh and knee drawn up to her chest.

A square drape or sheet is given to the client. She holds one corner over her sternum, the adjacent corners fall over each knee, and the fourth corner covers the perineum. Once the examination begins, the drape over the perineum is lifted. The male examiner should always have a female attendant present during the examination. A female examiner may prefer to work alone but should have a female attendant if the client is particularly anxious or emotionally unstable.

EXTERNAL GENITALIA

The perineal area must be well illuminated. The nurse gloves both hands to prevent contact with infectious organisms. The perineum is extremely sensitive and tender. The area is not touched suddenly without warning the client. It is best to touch the neighboring thigh first before advancing to the perineum.

To assess sexual maturity, the quantity and distribution of hair growth is noted. A preadolescent has no pubic hair except for fine body hair like that on the abdomen. During adolescence, hair grows along the labia, becoming darker, coarser, and curlier as it spreads over the pubic symphysis. Hair growth eventually forms a triangle over the female perineum and along the medial surfaces of the thighs. Hair growth should not spread up over the abdomen. Hair should be free of nits and lice. The underlying skin should be free of inflammation, irritation, or lesions.

The nurse inspects surface characteristics of the labia majora. The skin of the perineum is smooth, clean, and slightly darker than other skin. The mucous membranes appear dark pink and moist. The labia majora may be gaping or closed and appear dry or moist. They are usually symmetrical. After childbirth the labia majora are separated, causing the labia minora to become more prominent. When a woman reaches menopause, the labia majora become thinned, and with advancing age, they become atrophied. The labia majora are normally without inflammation, edema, lesions, or lacerations.

To inspect the remaining external structures, the nurse gently places the thumb and index finger of the nondominant hand inside the labia minora and retracts the tissues outwardly (Figure 32-82). The nurse should have a firm hold to avoid repeated retraction against the sensitive tissues. The nurse uses the other hand to palpate the labia minora between the thumb and second finger. On inspection, the labia minora are normally thinner than the labia

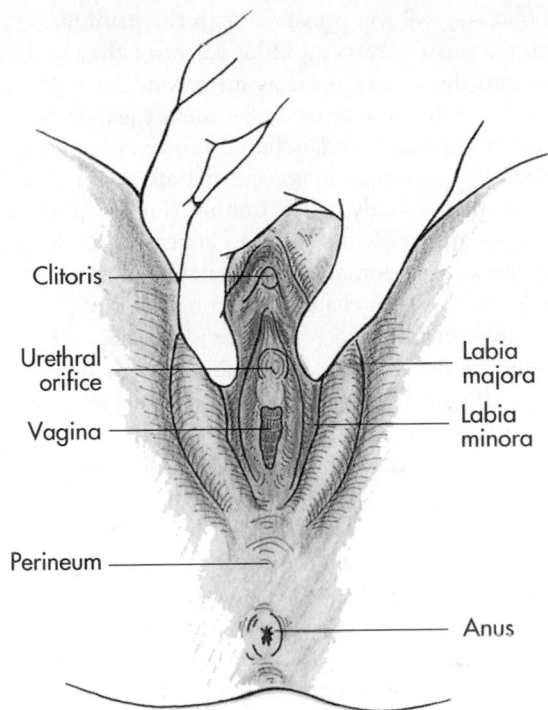

Figure 32-82   Female external genitalia.

majora, and one side may be larger. The tissue should feel soft on palpation and without tenderness. The size of the clitoris is variable. However, it normally is about 2 cm (⅘ inch) or less in length and 0.5 cm (⅕ inch) in width. The nurse looks for atrophy, inflammation, or adhesions. If inflamed, the clitoris will be a bright cherry red. In young women it is a common site for syphilitic lesions, or **chancres**, which appear as small open ulcers that drain serous material. Older women may have malignant changes that result in dry, scaly, nodular lesions.

The urethral orifice is carefully observed for color and position. It is normally intact without inflammation. The urethral meatus is anterior to the vaginal orifice and is pink. At times it is difficult to locate. It may appear as a small slit or pinhole opening just above the vaginal canal. In women who have had several vaginal childbirths, the opening to the vaginal canal often extends upward, interfering with the view of the urethra. The nurse notes any discharge, polyps, or fistulas.

When inspecting the vaginal orifice (introitus), the nurse inspects for inflammation, edema, discoloration, discharge, and lesions. Normally the introitus is a thin, vertical slit or a large orifice. The tissue is moist. The hymen is just inside the introitus. In the virgin the hymen may restrict the opening of the vagina. Only remnants of the hymen remain after sexual intercourse.

With the labia still retracted, the nurse examines Skene's and Bartholin's glands. The client is told that the nurse is going to insert one finger into the client's vagina and that she will feel pressure. With the palm facing upward, the nurse inserts an index finger of the examining hand into the vagina as far as the second joint. Exerting upward pressure, the nurse milks Skene's glands by moving the finger outward. Discharge and tenderness are abnormal. The examination is done on both sides of the urethra and then directly on the urethra (Figure 32-83). The technique may cause discharge to appear. If so, the nurse notes the color, odor, and consistency and obtains a culture. The nurse then changes into a new pair of gloves.

If inflammation and edema are found near the posterior end of the introitus, Bartholin's glands may be infected. The glands cannot normally be palpated. To attempt palpation, the nurse places a thumb and index finger between the labia majora and introitus and palpates one side at a time.

With the gloved index and middle fingers in the vaginal orifice, the nurse asks the client to strain downward as if she were voiding. If the client lacks adequate muscular support, the vaginal walls bulge, blocking the introitus. A portion of the vaginal wall and bladder may prolapse or fall into the orifice anteriorly; this is a **cystocele.** Bulging of the posterior wall may be caused by prolapse of the rectum (**rectocele**). Normally when a client is asked to constrict or close the vaginal orifice, the nurse palpates tension in the muscles. A woman who has undergone vaginal childbirth has less muscle tone than one who has not.

The nurse may also inspect the anus at this time, looking for lesions and hemorrhoids (see section on rectal examination). If the nurse performs only the external examination, the examination gloves are disposed of at this time. The client is then offered perineal hygiene if the skin is soiled with secretions.

Clients who are at risk for contracting an STD should learn to perform a genital self-examination (GSE) (Box 32-26). The purpose is to detect any signs or symptoms of

an STD. Many persons do not know they have an STD, and some STDs can remain undetected for years.

SPECULUM EXAMINATION OF INTERNAL GENITALIA

An examination of the internal genitalia requires much skill and practice. Usually it is performed only by advanced nurse practitioners or nurse-midwives. Beginning students will more than likely only observe the procedure or assist the examiner.

The examination involves use of a plastic or metal speculum. Consisting of two blades and an adjustable thumbscrew, the speculum is inserted into the vagina to assess the internal genitalia for cancerous lesions and other abnormalities. During the examination a **Papanicolaou (Pap)** smear is collected to test for cervical and vaginal cancer.

To assist an examiner, the nurse makes sure that the client is comfortably positioned in the stirrups. A variety of speculum sizes (small, medium, large) should be available so that the examiner may select the appropriate size for the client. The smallest size will fit a virgin. If the woman is sexually active, a medium-sized speculum is best. For women who have had children vaginally, the examiner uses a medium-to-large speculum.

In addition, the nurse will have gloves, specimen slides, and a spatula and/or cytobrush close at hand. Water-soluble lubricant is used only when specimens are not being collected. Most examiners lubricate the speculum with warm water.

Cervix.   The first portion of the examination involves careful insertion of the speculum until the examiner can fully visualize the cervix (Figure 32-84). The examiner sits on a stool facing the client's perineum. The adjustable light is placed over the examiner's shoulder, directed at the examination site. The examiner holds the speculum in the dominant hand and explains the procedure to the client. If the woman has never been examined, two fingers are gently inserted into the vagina to explore for abnormalities. Then with two fingers the examiner presses down on the perineal body just inside the introitus. After checking to be sure that the speculum blades are closed, the examiner introduces the closed speculum obliquely (rotated 50 degrees counterclockwise from the vertical position) past the fingers. The speculum is inserted downward at a 45-degree angle toward the examination table to avoid trauma to the urethra (this maneuver corresponds with the normal downward slope of the vaginal canal). Care is taken to avoid pulling the pubic hair or pinching the labia.

After the wide portions of the blades have passed the introitus, the speculum is rotated so that the blades are horizontal. The blades are opened slowly after full insertion, and the speculum is moved to visualize the cervix. When the cervix is in full view, the blades are locked in the open position. The examiner inspects the cervix for color, appearance of the os or opening, position, size, surface

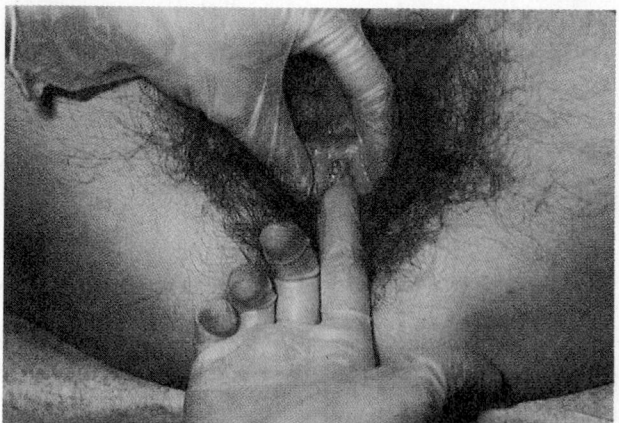

Figure 32-83   Milking the urethra and paraurethral glands.

Client Teaching DURING FEMALE GENITALIA AND REPRODUCTIVE TRACT ASSESSMENT   Box 32-26

OBJECTIVES
- Client will pursue routine gynecological examinations based on her level of risk for cervical cancer.
- Client with an STD will follow safe sexual practices.
- Client will use measures to prevent acquisition and transmission of STDs.

TEACHING STRATEGIES
- Instruct client about purpose and recommended frequency of Pap smears and gynecological examinations. Explain that Pap smears are painless.
- Counsel client with an STD about diagnosis and treatment.
- Instruct on genital self-examination (GSE): Using a mirror, position self in order to examine the area covered by the pubic hair. Spread the hair apart, looking for bumps, sores, or blisters. Also, look for any warts, which may appear as small, bumpy spots and then enlarge to fleshy, cauliflower-like lesions. Next, spread the outer vaginal lips apart and look at the clitoris for bumps, blisters, sores, or warts. Also look at both sides of the inner vaginal lips. The area around the urinary and vaginal opening should be inspected for bumps, blisters, sores, or warts.

- Explain warning signs of STDs: pain or burning on urination, pain in pelvic area, bleeding between menstruation, itchy rash around vagina, and vaginal discharge (different from usual).
- Teach measures to prevent STDs, including preventive measures (e.g., male partner's use of condoms, restricting number of sexual partners, avoiding sex with persons who have several other partners, perineal hygiene measures).
- Tell client with an STD that she must inform sexual partner of the need for an examination.
- Reinforce the importance of perineal hygiene (as appropriate).

EVALUATION
- Ask client to explain when she should routinely have a gynecological examination and Pap smear.
- Have client describe ways to prevent transmission of STDs.
- For client with an STD, determine during follow-up visit if safe sexual practices have been followed (use nonthreatening inquiry).

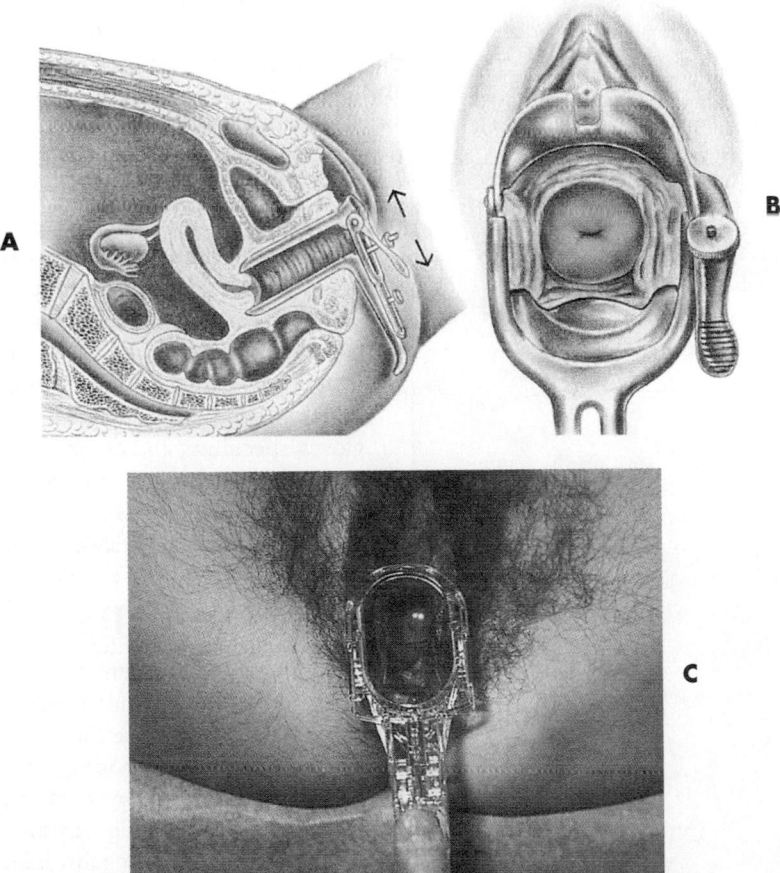

Figure 32-84   **A,** Angle of speculum insertion. **B,** View of cervix. **C,** Vaginal speculum in place with cervix in full view.

characteristics, and discharge. The normal cervix is glistening pink, smooth, and round. Its diameter is 2.5 to 3 cm (about 1 inch) in a young woman and smaller in an older adult. The cervix should be midline and without lesions.

Papanicolaou Smear.   The surface of the cervix at the cervical canal opening is lined with layers of vaginal squamous cells. The cells meet a different group of cells—columnar cells. The columnar cells secrete mucus and line the passageway that leads up into the central cavity of the uterus. The squamous cells have a protective role for the cervix, and the columnar cells have a reproductive role (helping sperm to enter the uterus for fertilization). A Pap smear is a painless screening test for cervical cancer. Specimens are taken from the endocervix and ectocervix (Table 32-30). The test is simple and has no side effects. It should be performed annually with a pelvic examination

in women who are, or have been, sexually active, and in women who have reached the age of 18. After three or more consecutive annual examinations with normal findings, the Pap test may be done less often at the discretion of the physician. Women at high risk for cervical cancer and those over 40 should have annual checkups.

The examiner first collects a sample of the outer cervix or ectocervix. A plastic spatula is rotated 360 degrees against the cervical surface. Once the spatula is withdrawn, the examiner spreads the specimen lightly over a glass slide. The nurse who is assisting sprays the specimen with cytological fixative and labels the slide. The examiner next uses a cytobrush to collect endocervical cells. The cytobrush is inserted into the cervical os and rotated one full turn. The specimen is then spread across the slide by rolling the brush with moderate pressure. The specimen is sprayed again, and the slide is labeled. At the end of the procedure the nurse warns the client that blood spotting is normal for a few hours.

There is also a paintbrush device (Cervex-brush) that can be used to collect both specimens at the same time. It uses flexible plastic bristles, which reportedly cause less blood spotting (Seidel and others, 1999).

Vagina.   Once specimens are collected, the examiner views the vaginal walls as the speculum is slowly withdrawn. As the speculum leaves the cervix, the thumbscrew is loosened, but the blades are kept open with the thumb. During the withdrawal the examiner notes the color, surface characteristics, and secretions. The vaginal walls are normally pink throughout and free from discharge and lesions. The surface should be moist and smooth or rugated. Normal secretions are thin, clear or cloudy, and odorless. Women commonly acquire yeast infections, causing a thick, white, patchy, malodorous, curdlike discharge.

After speculum withdrawal the nurse assists the client to a sitting position and allows the client to dress and perform hygiene. In a hospital setting the client may need assistance with perineal hygiene. The nurse makes sure the gloves, speculum, and other disposable equipment are appropriately discarded in a receptacle. The client is informed that Pap smear results will be available in 3 to 4 days (check agency policy).

Male Genitalia

An examination of the male genitalia includes assessment of the external genitalia (Figure 32-85) and the inguinal ring and canal. Because the incidence of STDs in adolescents and young adults is high, an assessment of the genitalia should be a routine part of any health maintenance examination for this age-group (Box 32-27). The client may be lying or standing for this part of the examination. Inspection and palpation are used. The nurse applies disposable gloves to prevent the chance of cross infection from urethral discharge.

Table 32-30   Methods for Obtaining Pap Smears

Location	Technique
Outer cervix	Use plastic spatula. Place tip of longer arm in os. Rotate spatula, scraping outer surface of cervix. Apply cells to glass slide. Apply fixative solution and label slide.
Endocervical	Use cervical brush (cytobrush). WARNING: Do *not* use on pregnant clients. Gently insert brush through os. Rotate brush 180 to 360 degrees. Apply cells by rolling and twisting brush on glass slide. Apply fixative solution and label slide.

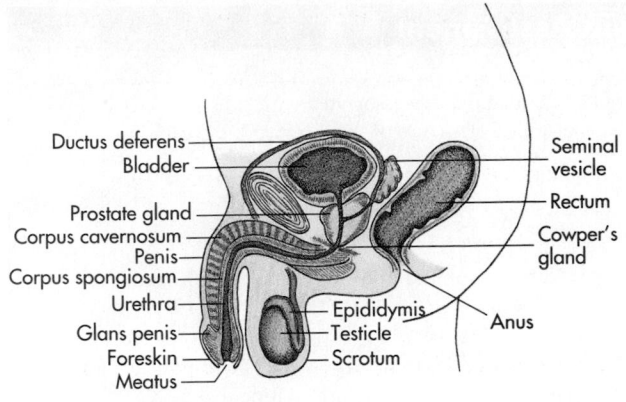

Figure 32-85 External and internal male sex organs.

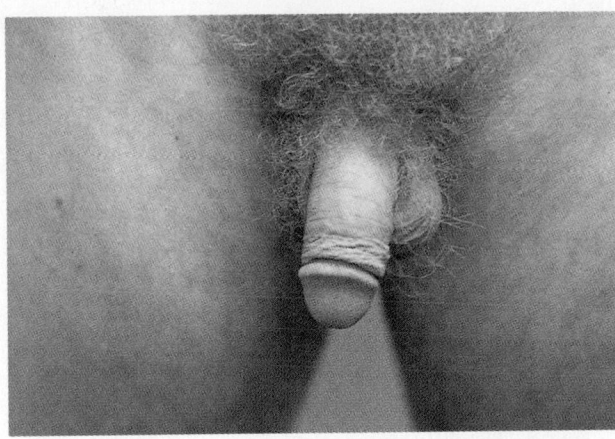

Figure 32-86 Normal male genitalia (circumcised). From Seidel HM and others: *Mosby's guide to physical examination,* ed 4, St. Louis, 1999, Mosby.

The nurse uses a calm and gentle approach to lessen the client's anxiety. Often adolescents and men are fearful of having an erection during the examination. Boys and adolescents may worry about their genitals being normal (Seidel and others, 1999). The nurse should limit discussion of the client's sexual activity during the examination because the client might perceive this as evaluative or judgmental. The client's modesty must be preserved. It may help to provide teaching after the examination. Do not joke or use nonverbal expressions that may convey concern or worry. The genitalia are gently manipulated to avoid causing erection or discomfort. A thorough nursing history (Table 32-31) before the examination ensures that the assessment will be complete.

SEXUAL MATURITY

The nurse begins by assessing the sexual maturity of the client, noting the size and shape of the penis and testes, the color and texture of the scrotal skin, and the character and distribution of pubic hair. The first sign of puberty, an increase in genital and pubic hair development, is variable but generally does not start before 9.5 years of age. During

the preadolescent stage there is no pubic hair except for the fine body hair found on the abdomen. By puberty the pubic hair extends from the base of the penis over the symphysis pubis and becomes coarse and curly. The testes and penis develop, with the scrotal skin darkening and becoming thinner and more wrinkled in texture. The penis slowly lengthens, eventually reaching to the bottom of the scrotum (Figure 32-86). The nurse inspects the skin covering the genitalia for lice, rashes, excoriations, or lesions.

PENIS

The nurse inspects the structures of the penis, including the shaft, corona, prepuce (foreskin), glans, and urethral meatus. The dorsal vein should be apparent on inspection. In uncircumcised males the foreskin is retracted to reveal the glans and urethral meatus. The foreskin should retract easily. A small amount of thick, white secretion between the glans and foreskin is normal. If there is evidence of abnormal discharge, a culture is usually obtained. The urethral meatus is slitlike and should be positioned on the

---

Client Teaching DURING MALE GENITALIA ASSESSMENT   Box 32-27

OBJECTIVES
- Client will describe methods to prevent transmission of STDs.
- Client will perform genital self-examination.
- Client with an STD will follow safe sex practices.

TEACHING STRATEGIES
- Counsel client with an STD about diagnosis and treatment.
- Teach measures to prevent STDs:
  - Use of condoms
  - Avoiding sex with partner who is infected
  - Restricting number of sexual partners

- Avoiding sex with persons who have multiple partners
- Using regular perineal hygiene
- Tell clients with an STD that sexual partners must be informed of the need to have an examination.
- Instruct client on how to perform genital self-examination (see Box 31-28).

EVALUATION
- Ask client to describe methods for treating and preventing STDs.
- During a follow-up visit, determine whether client with an STD has used safe sex practices.

Table 32-31   **Nursing History for Male Genitalia Assessment**

Assessment Category	Rationale
Review normal urinary elimination pattern, including frequency of voiding; history of nocturia; character and volume of urine; daily fluid intake; symptoms of burning, urgency, and frequency; difficulty starting stream; and hematuria (see Chapter 44).	Urinary problems can be directly associated with genitourinary problems because of anatomical structure of men's reproductive and urinary systems.
Assess client's sexual history and use of safe sex habits (multiple partners, infection in partners, failure to use condom).	Sexual history reveals risk for and understanding of STDs and HIV.
Determine if client has had previous surgery or illness involving urinary or reproductive organs, including STD.	Alterations resulting from disease or surgery may be responsible for symptoms or changes in organ structure or function.
Ask if client has noted penile pain or swelling, genital lesions, or urethral discharge.	These signs and symptoms indicate STD.
Determine if client has noticed heaviness or painless enlargement of testis or irregular lumps.	These signs and symptoms are early warning signs for testicular cancer.
If client reports an enlargement in inguinal area, assess if it is intermittent or constant, associated with straining or lifting, and painful, and whether pain is affected by coughing, lifting, or straining at stool.	Signs and symptoms reflect potential inguinal hernia.
Ask if client has difficulty achieving erection or ejaculation; also review whether client is taking diuretics, sedatives, antihypertensives, or tranquilizers.	These medications may influence sexual performance.

ventral surface just millimeters from the tip of the glans. In some congenital conditions the meatus is displaced along the penile shaft. Gentle compression of the glans between the nurse's thumb and index finger opens the urethral meatus to allow inspection for discharge. The opening should be glistening and pink. The meatus is also inspected for lesions, edema, and inflammation.

The glans is carefully checked around its entire circumference for lesions. The area between the foreskin and glans is a common site for venereal lesions. Any lesion is palpated gently to note tenderness, size, consistency, and shape.

The nurse continues to inspect the entire shaft of the penis, including the undersurface, looking for lesions, scars, and edema. The shaft is palpated between the thumb and first two fingers to detect any localized areas of hardness and tenderness. When inspection and palpation of the penis is completed, the foreskin is pulled down to its original position. It is important for any male client to learn to perform a genital self-examination to detect signs or symptoms of an STD. Many people who have an STD do not know it. A self-examination should be a routine part of self-care (Box 32-28).

SCROTUM

The nurse must be particularly cautious when inspecting and palpating the scrotum because the structures lying within the scrotal sac are very sensitive. The scrotum is a saclike structure divided internally into two halves. Each half contains a testicle, epididymis, and the vas deferens, which travels upward into the inguinal ring. Normally the left testicle is lower than the right. The nurse inspects the scrotum's size, shape, and symmetry while observing for lesions or edema. The scrotum is usually more deeply pigmented than the body skin, and the surface is coarse. It is gently lifted to view the posterior surface. The scrotal skin is usually loose. A tightening of the skin may reveal edema. The scrotum's size normally changes with temperature variations as the dartos muscle contracts in cold and relaxes in warm temperatures.

Testicular cancer has become a common solid tumor among young men ages 18 to 34 years. Early detection is critical, and thus clients must learn to perform testicular self-examination (TSE) (see Box 32-28). The nurse can explain the technique while examining the client. The underlying testicles are normally ovoid and approximately 2 to 4 cm ($\frac{4}{5}$ to $1\frac{3}{5}$ inches) in size. The testicles and epididymis are gently palpated between the nurse's thumb and first two fingers. They should be sensitive to gentle compression but not tender, and they should feel smooth, rubbery, and free of nodules. The most common symptoms of testicular cancer are a painless enlargement of one testis and the appearance of a palpable, small, hard lump, about the size of a pea, on the front or side of the testicle.

Male Genital Self-Examination

Box 32-28

All men 15 years and older should perform this examination monthly using the following steps.

GENITAL EXAMINATION

Perform the examination after a warm bath or shower when the scrotal sac is relaxed.

Stand naked in front of a mirror and hold the penis in your hand and examine the head. Pull back the foreskin if uncircumcised.

Inspect and palpate the entire head of the penis in a clockwise motion, looking carefully for any bumps, sores, or blisters.

Look also for any bumpy warts (see illustration).

Look at the opening at the end of the penis for discharge.

Look along the entire shaft of the penis for the same signs.

Be sure to separate pubic hair at the base of the penis and carefully examine the skin underneath.

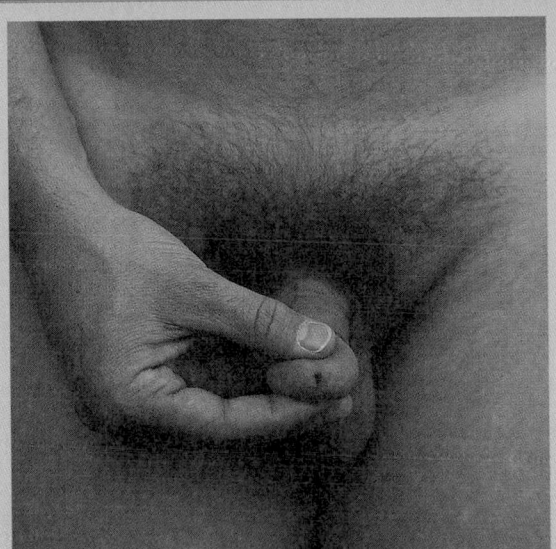

TESTICULAR SELF-EXAMINATION

Look for swelling or lumps in the skin of the scrotum while looking in the mirror.

Use both hands, placing the index and middle fingers under the testicles and the thumb on top (see illustration).

Gently roll the testicle, feeling for lumps, thickening, or a change in consistency (hardening).

Find the epididymis (a cordlike structure on the top and back of the testicle; it is not a lump).

Feel for small, pea-sized lumps on the front and side of the testicle. The lumps are usually painless and are abnormal.

Call your physician if you find a lump.

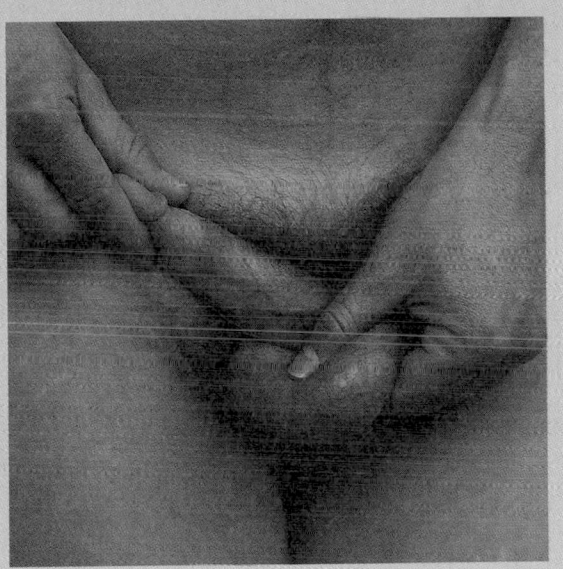

Illustrations from Seidel HM and others: *Mosby's guide to physical examination*, ed 4, St. Louis, 1999, Mosby.

The size, shape, and consistency of the organs are noted. In the older man the testicles decrease in size and are less firm during palpation. The client should be asked about any unusual tenderness. The nurse continues palpating the vas deferens separately as it forms the spermatic cord toward the inguinal ring, noting the presence of nodules or swelling. It normally feels smooth and discrete.

INGUINAL RING AND CANAL

The external inguinal ring provides the opening for the spermatic cord to pass into the inguinal canal. The canal forms a passage through the abdominal wall, a potential site for hernia formation. A hernia is a protrusion of a portion of intestine through the inguinal wall or canal. An intestinal loop may even enter the scrotum. The client stands during this portion of the examination.

During inspection the client is asked to strain or bear down. The maneuver helps make a hernia more visible. The nurse looks for obvious bulging. The nurse next palpates the inguinal ring and canal to be sure a hernia is not present. Standing on the right side of the client, the nurse places the index finger of the examining hand against the scrotal skin low on the right side. Gently the nurse moves the finger toward the inguinal canal with the folds of the scrotal tissue covering the finger. Carrying the index finger upward along the vas deferens into the inguinal canal, the nurse follows the spermatic cord. It is important not to force the finger into the canal. When the finger reaches the farthest point along the canal, the nurse asks the client to cough and strain down. The maneuver is repeated on the left side. As the client strains, no bulging pressure will be felt. A tightening around the finger is normal.

The nurse completes the examination by palpating for inguinal lymph nodes. Small, nontender, mobile horizontal nodes may normally be found. Any abnormality may indicate local or systemic infection or malignant disease.

Rectum and Anus

A good time to perform the rectal examination is after the genital examination. Usually the examination is not performed in young children or adolescents. The examination can detect colorectal cancer in its early stages. In men the rectal examination can also detect prostatic tumors. The nurse collects a thorough history (Table 32-32) to detect the client's risk for bowel or rectal disease or prostatic disease.

The rectal examination can be uncomfortable and embarrassing, so the nurse uses a calm, slow-paced, gentle approach. Explanation of the steps of the procedure helps clients to relax and lessens discomfort during the digital examination. Women can be examined immediately after examination of the genitalia while they are still in a dorsal recumbent position. Otherwise the left lateral side-lying (Sims') position is preferred. Men are best examined by having the client bend over forward with his hips flexed and upper body resting across the examination table. A nonambulatory client can be examined in Sims' position. Clients are draped with only the anal area exposed. The nurse applies disposable gloves for the examination.

INSPECTION

The nurse begins by inspecting the perianal and sacrococcygeal areas. The skin should be smooth and uninterrupted. The nurse looks for lumps, rashes, inflammation, excoriation, and scars. Fungal infection can cause perianal irritation.

Using the nondominant hand, the nurse gently retracts the buttocks apart to inspect the anus. Anal tissues are normally moist and hairless compared with perianal skin. The tissue is coarser and more darkly pigmented. The anus is held closed by the voluntary external muscle sphincter. The nurse inspects anal tissue for skin lesions, external **hemorrhoids** (dilated veins that appear as reddened protrusions), fissures and fistulas, inflammation, rashes, or discoloration. Next, the nurse asks the client to bear down as though having a bowel movement. Any internal hemorrhoids, fistulas, fissures, or polyps will appear at this time. Normally the anal lining is intact.

DIGITAL PALPATION

Some institutions do not permit nurses to perform digital examinations. In institutions where it is permitted, the nursing student should have a qualified examiner present during the first examination.

The nurse lubricates the index finger of the gloved dominant hand. The procedure is explained, and then the client is asked to bear down gently as if having a bowel movement. As the anal sphincter relaxes, the nurse's fingertip is gently slipped into the anal canal in a direction toward the umbilicus. Normally the client feels as though stool is being passed. The nurse never forces digital insertion, so mucosal tissues are not injured.

Table 32-32 **Nursing History for Rectal and Anal Assessment**	
Assessment Category	Rationale
Determine whether client has experienced bleeding from rectum, black or tarry stools (melena), rectal pain, or change in bowel habits (constipation or diarrhea).	These are warning signs of colorectal cancer* or other gastrointestinal alterations.
Determine whether client has personal or family history of colorectal cancer, polyps, or inflammatory bowel disease. Ask if client is over age 40.	These are risk factors for colorectal cancer.*
Assess dietary habits for high-fat intake or deficient fiber content.	Bowel cancer may be linked to dietary intake of fat or insufficient fiber intake.*
Determine whether client has undergone screening for colorectal cancer (digital examination, stool blood slide test, proctosigmoidoscopy).	Undergoing this screening reflects understanding and compliance with preventive health care measures.
Assess medication history for use of laxatives or cathartic medications.	Repeated use can cause diarrhea and eventual loss of intestinal muscle tone.
Assess for use of codeine or iron preparations.	Codeine causes constipation. Iron turns the color of feces black and tarry.
Ask male client if weak or interrupted urine flow, inability to urinate, difficulty in starting or stopping urine flow, polyuria, nocturia, hematuria, or dysuria has been experienced. Does client have continuing pain in lower back, pelvis, or upper thighs?	These are warning signs of prostatic cancer.* Symptoms also can suggest infection or prostate enlargement.

*Data from American Cancer Society: *1999 cancer facts and figures,* New York, 1999, The Society.

Client Teaching DURING RECTAL AND ANAL ASSESSMENT   Box 32-29

OBJECTIVES
- Client will have a regular digital examination performed appropriate to age.
- Client will be able to identify symptoms of colorectal and prostatic cancer.
- Client will follow a diet of increased fiber and reduced fat.

TEACHING STRATEGIES
- Discuss the ACS's guidelines (1999) for early detection of colorectal cancer:
  - Digital rectal examination yearly after age 40
  - Stool blood test (guaiac test) yearly after age 50
  - Proctosigmoidoscopy (flexible): visual inspection of the rectum and lower colon with a hollow, lighted tube, performed by a physician every 3 to 5 years after age 50 on the advice of a physician
  - Warning signs of colorectal cancer (see Table 31-30)
- Discuss dietary planning to reduce fat and increase fiber content.

- Warn client against problems caused by overuse of laxatives, cathartic medications, codeine, or enemas.
- Discuss with male client the ACS's guidelines (1999) for early detection of prostatic cancer:
  - Digital rectal examination performed annually after age 40
  - Annual prostate-specific antigen (PSA) blood test for men age 50 and over
  - Prostate ultrasound testing if either digital rectal examination or PSA test is suspicious
  - Warning signs of prostatic cancer

EVALUATION
- During follow-up visits, determine whether client has had a rectal examination performed.
- Have client explain warning signs of colorectal and prostatic cancer.
- Ask client to describe foods high in fiber and low in fat.

The anal canal is the distal portion of the gastrointestinal tract. The canal extends in a line toward the umbilicus before turning into the mucus-lined rectum. The anus contains a rich supply of sensory nerve fibers. Thus digital manipulation can be painful. At the junction of the anal canal and rectum, the rectum balloons out and turns posteriorly into the hollow of the coccyx and sacrum.

Initially the nurse notes the tone of the anal sphincter as the muscle closes snugly around the finger. After asking the client to tighten the sphincter around the finger, the nurse notes sphincter tone. The sphincter should tighten evenly without discomfort. A weak sphincter may indicate a neurological problem. Acute rectal pain is not normal. Irritation, fissures, inflamed hemorrhoids, or rock-hard constipation can be the source of discomfort.

Beyond the anal canal the nurse palpates each side of the rectal wall for tenderness, irregularities, polyps, masses, or nodules. The wall should feel even and smooth. After the finger is advanced fully, the client is asked to bear down again. High lesions within the rectum will descend against the fingertip (Box 32-29).

In men the nurse turns the hand so that the finger palpates the anterior rectal wall. The client should be warned that he may feel the urge to urinate, but that he will not. The prostate gland is palpable anteriorly as a rounded, heart-shaped structure about 2.5 to 4 cm (1 to 1½ inches) in diameter with less than 1 cm (1 inch) protrusion into the rectum (Figure 32-87). A small medial groove separates the gland into two lateral lobes. The nurse palpates the size, shape, and consistency of the prostate. The gland normally is firm, without bogginess, tenderness, or nodules. Hardness or nodules may indicate the presence of a cancerous lesion. Prostate enlarge-

ment is classified by the amount of projection into the rectum: grade I is 1 to 2 cm protrusion; grade II, 2 to 3 cm; grade III, 3 to 4 cm; grade IV, more than 4 cm (Seidel and others, 1999).

In women it may be possible to palpate the cervix through the anterior rectal wall. It is common to mistake the cervix or an inserted tampon for a rectal tumor.

After palpation is completed, the nurse gently withdraws the finger and observes it for feces. Feces are normally brown. The presence of mucus; blood; or black, tarry stool should be reported. A sample of the feces is tested for occult blood (see Chapter 45). For women suspected of having an STD, a rectal culture may be taken to rule out cross infection from vaginal discharge. The nurse

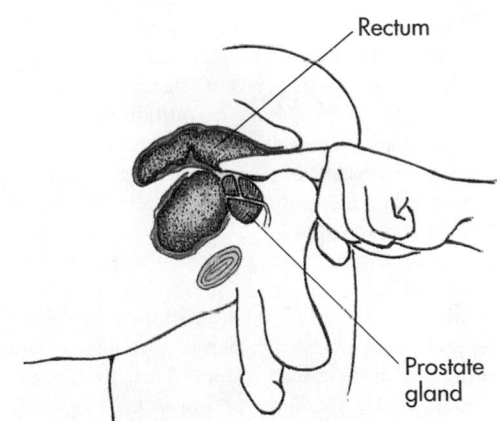

Figure 32-87   Palpation of prostate gland during rectal examination.

cleans the perianal area before continuing to the next part of the examination.

Musculoskeletal System

The nurse can learn to integrate portions of the musculoskeletal assessment when the client walks, moves in bed, or performs any type of physical activity. The assessment of musculoskeletal function focuses on determining range of joint motion, muscle strength and tone, and joint and muscle condition. Assessment of musculoskeletal integrity is especially important when the client reports pain or loss of function in a joint or muscle. Frequently, muscular disorders are manifestations of neurological disease. For this reason, a neurological assessment is often conducted simultaneously.

It is important to review the anatomy of bone and muscle placement and joint structure (see Chapter 46). Joints vary in their degree of mobility. Some, as in the knee, are freely movable. The spinal vertebrae are examples of slightly movable joints.

The examination uses inspection and palpation. The muscles and joints should be exposed and free to move. Depending on the muscle groups assessed, the client assumes a sitting, supine, prone, or standing position. Table 32-33 lists the information gathered in the nursing history.

GENERAL INSPECTION

The nurse observes the client's gait and the anterior, posterior, and lateral aspects of the client's posture as the client walks into and stands in the examination room. When the client is unaware of the nature of the observations, the gait is more natural. Later a more formal test involves having the client walk in a straight line away from the nurse and then return. The nurse looks for foot dragging, limping, shuffling, and the position of the trunk in relation to the legs. Normally the client walks with the arms swinging freely at the sides and the head and face leading the body. An older adult often walks with smaller steps and a wider base of support.

The normal standing posture is an upright stance with parallel alignment of the hips and shoulders (Figure 32-88). There should be an even contour of the shoulders, level scapulae and iliac crests, alignment of the head over the gluteal folds, and symmetry of extremities. Looking sideways at the client, the nurse notes the normal cervical, thoracic, and lumbar curves. The head is held erect. As the client sits, some degree of rounding of the shoulders is normal. Older adults tend to assume a stooped, forward-bent posture with the hips and knees somewhat flexed and arms bent at the elbows, raising the level of the arms (Ebersole and Hess, 1998).

Common postural abnormalities include lordosis, kyphosis, and scoliosis (Figure 32-89). **Kyphosis,** or

Table 32-33 **Nursing History for Musculoskeletal Assessment**	
Assessment Category	Rationale
Determine if client is involved in competitive sports (particularly involving collision and contact), fails to warm up adequately, is in poor physical condition, or had had a rapid growth spurt (adolescents).	These are risk factors for sports injury.
Review client history for heavy alcohol use; cigarette smoking; constant dieting; calcium intake less than 500 mg daily; thin and light body frame; nulliparous status; menopause before age 45; postmenopause status; family history of osteoporosis; or Caucasian, Asian, Native American, or northern European ancestry.	These are risk factors for osteoporosis.
Ask client to describe history of alteration in bone, muscle, or joint function (e.g., recent fall, trauma, lifting of heavy objects, history of bone or joint disease with sudden or gradual onset, location of alteration).	History assists in assessing nature of musculoskeletal problem.
Assess nature and extent of pain, including location, duration, severity, predisposing and aggravating factors, relieving factors, and type.	Alterations in bone, joints, or muscle are frequently accompanied by pain, which has implications for not only comfort but also ability to perform activities of daily living.
Assess client's normal activity pattern, including type of exercise routinely performed.	Provides baseline in assessment.
Determine how alteration influences ability to perform activities of daily living (e.g., bathing, feeding, dressing, toileting, and ambulating) and social functions (e.g., household chores, work, recreation, sexual activities).	Level of nursing care will be determined by extent to which client is able to perform self-care. Type and degree of restriction in continuing social activities influence topics for client education and ability of nurse to identify alternative ways to maintain function.
Assess height loss of woman over age 50 by subtracting current height from recall of maximum adult height.	Measurement may be useful screening tool to predict osteoporosis.

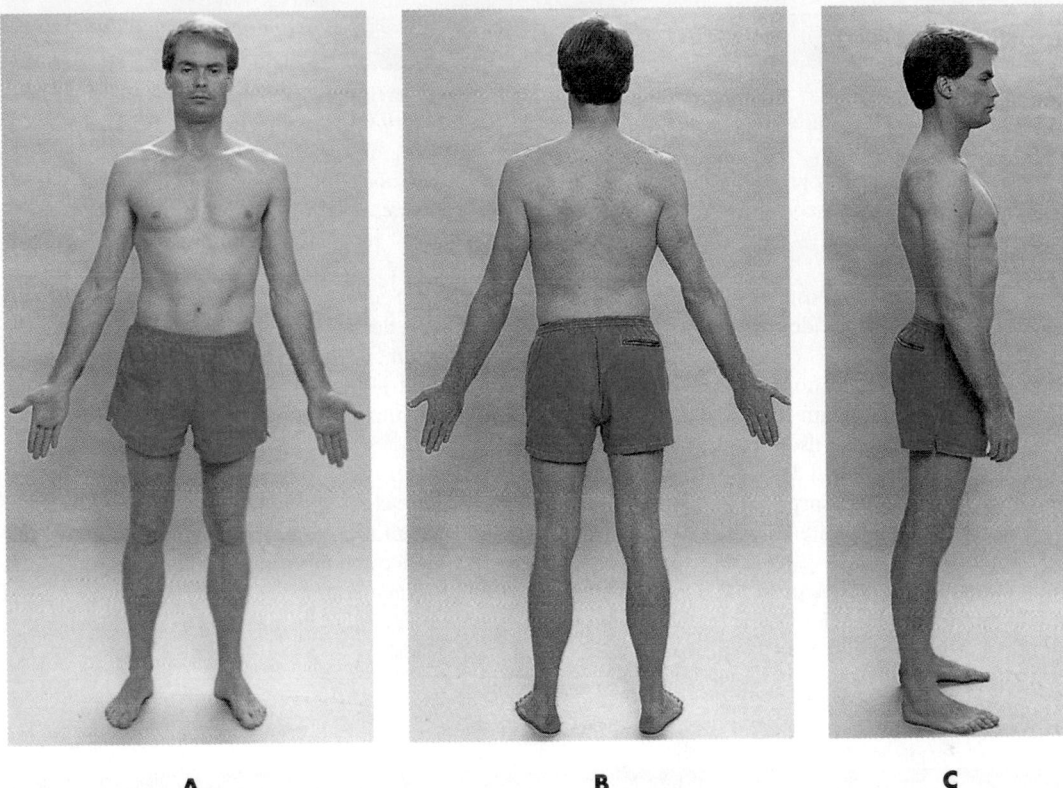

Figure 32-88 Inspection of overall body posture. **A,** Anterior view. **B,** Posterior view. **C,** Lateral view.
From Seidel HM and others: *Mosby's guide to physical examination,* ed 4, St. Louis, 1999, Mosby.

hunchback, is an exaggeration of the posterior curvature of the thoracic spine. This postural abnormality is common in the older adult. **Lordosis,** or swayback, is an increased lumbar curvature. A lateral spinal curvature is called **scoliosis.** Loss of height is frequently the first clinical sign of **osteoporosis,** in which height loss occurs in the trunk as a result of vertebral fracture and collapse (Galsworthy and Wilson, 1996). Although a small amount of height loss is to be expected with aging, if the amount of loss is greater than expected, osteoporosis is likely (Box 32-30). As men and women age, they are more likely to have osteoporotic fractures of the forearms, hips, and vertebrae (Kessenich and Rosen, 1996).

During general inspection the nurse looks at the extremities for overall size, gross deformity, bony enlargement, alignment, and symmetry. There should be bilateral symmetry in length, circumference, alignment, and position, and in the number of skin folds (Seidel and others, 1999). A general review pinpoints areas requiring specialized assessment.

PALPATION

The nurse applies gentle palpation to all bones, joints, and surrounding muscles in a complete examination. In the

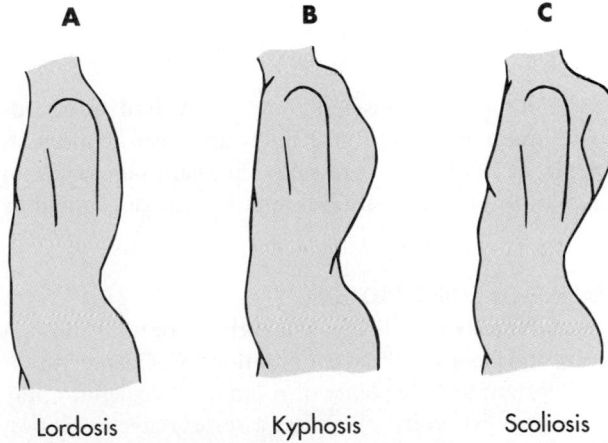

Lordosis   Kyphosis   Scoliosis

Figure 32-89 Common postural abnormalities.
A, Lordosis. **B,** Kyphosis. **C,** Scoliosis.

OBJECTIVES

- Female client will follow measures to prevent or minimize osteoporosis.
- Client will assume proper body posture.
- Client will be able to perform self-care measures.

TEACHING STRATEGIES

- Instruct client about correct postural alignment. Consult with physical therapist to provide client with exercises for improving posture.
- To reduce bone demineralization, instruct older adults about a proper exercise program (e.g., walking) to be followed 3 or more times a week. Also encourage intake of calcium to meet the recommended daily allowance. Increased vitamin D will aid calcium absorption. Recommendations for daily calcium supplements are 1000 mg before and 1500 mg after menopause.
- Explain to clients with low back pain that they can benefit from modification of worker risk factors (e.g., lifting heavy weights, use of protective equipment), regular aerobic exer-

cise, exercises that strengthen the back and increase trunk flexibility, and learning how to lift properly.

- Instruct older adults and those with osteoporosis, on proper body mechanics, as well as range-of-motion and moderate weight-bearing exercises (e.g., swimming and walking) to minimize trauma and subsequent fracture of bones.
- When client is unable to perform self-care, instruct on use of assistive devices (e.g., zippers on clothing instead of buttons; elevation of chairs to minimize bending of knees and hips).
- Instruct older clients to pace activities to compensate for loss in muscle strength.

EVALUATION

- Observe client's posture.
- Ask client to describe therapies for preventing osteoporosis.
- Observe client perform range-of-motion exercises.
- Have client keep log of regular weight-training exercises.
- Ask client or family members to describe client's use of self-care aids.

Table 32-34 Terminology for Normal Range-of-Motion Positions

Term	Range of Motion	Examples of Joints
Flexion	Movement decreasing angle between two adjoining bones; bending of limb	Elbow, fingers, knee
Extension	Movement increasing angle between two adjoining bones	Elbow, knee, fingers
Hyperextension	Movement of body part beyond its normal resting extended position	Head
Pronation	Movement of body part so that front or ventral surface faces downward	Hand, forearm
Supination	Movement of body part so that the front or ventral surface faces upward	Hand, forearm
Abduction	Movement of extremity away from midline of body	Leg, arm, fingers
Adduction	Movement of extremity toward midline of body	Leg, arm, fingers
Internal rotation	Rotation of joint inward	Knee, hip
External rotation	Rotation of joint outward	Knee, hip
Eversion	Turning of body part away from midline	Foot
Inversion	Turning of body part toward midline	Foot
Dorsiflexion	Flexion of toes and foot upward	Foot
Plantar flexion	Bending of toes and foot downward	Foot

case of a focused assessment, only an involved area needs to be examined. The nurse notes any heat, tenderness, edema, or resistance to pressure. The client should feel no discomfort when palpation is applied. Muscles should be firm.

RANGE OF JOINT MOTION

The nurse asks the client to put each major joint through active and passive full range of motion (see Chapter 46). It is important to have plenty of room for the client to fully move each extremity. The nurse assesses range of motion passively by gently supporting and moving the extremities through their range of motion. The nurse must learn the correct terminology for the movements that the joints are

capable of making (Table 32-34) and instruct the client on how to move through each range of motion. It also helps to demonstrate range of motion to the client when possible. The same body parts are compared for equality in movement. Figure 32-90 shows an example of range-of-motion positions for the hand and wrist.

When assessing range of motion, the nurse does not force a joint if there is pain or muscle spasm. The nurse must know the joint's normal range and the extent to which it can be moved. Range of motion should be equal between contralateral joints. Ideally, the normal range is assessed to determine a baseline for assessing later change.

A **goniometer** measures the precise degree of motion in a particular joint and is used mainly in clients who have a

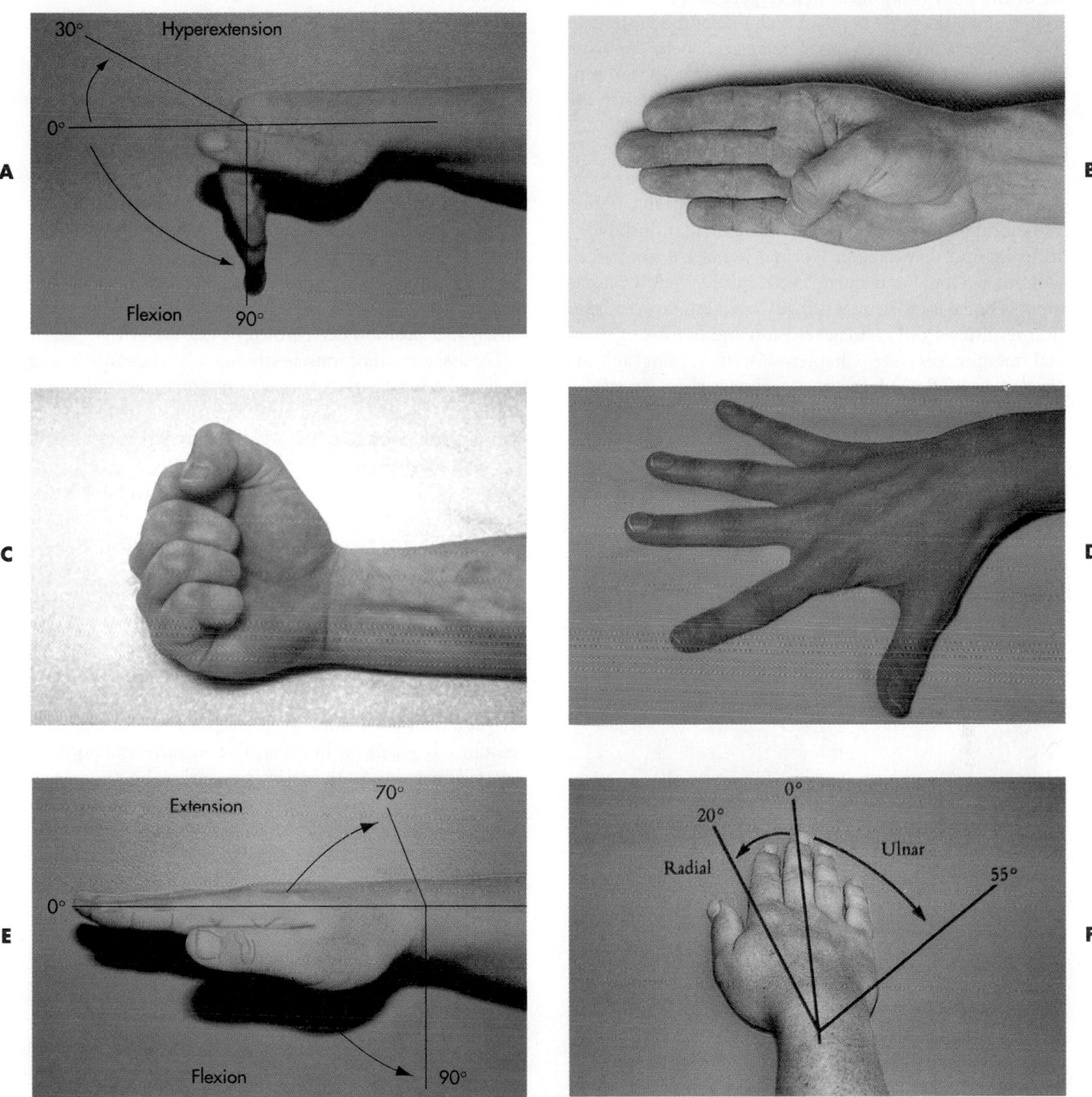

Figure 32-90   Range of motion of the hand and wrist. **A,** Metacarpophalangeal flexion and hyperextension. **B,** Finger flexion: thumb to each fingertip and to the base of the little finger. **C,** Finger flexion, first formation. **D,** Finger abduction. **E,** Wrist flexion and hyperextension. **F,** Wrist radial and ulnar movement.
From Seidel HM and others: *Mosby's guide to physical examination,* ed 4, St. Louis, 1999, Mosby.

suspected reduction in joint movement. The instrument has two flexible arms with a 180-degree protractor in the center. The center of the protractor is positioned at the center of the joint being measured (Figure 32-91). The arms extend along the body parts on each side of the protractor. A measurement is taken of the joint angle before moving the joint. After taking the joint through a full range of motion, the nurse measures the angle again to determine the degree of movement. The reading is compared with the normal degree of joint movement.

When putting each joint through its range of motion, the nurse makes a number of basic observations, noting pain, limited mobility, spastic movement, joint instability, stiffness, and contracture. Normal joints are nontender, without swelling, and move freely. In older adults, joints often become swollen and stiff with reduced range of motion resulting from cartilage erosion and fibrosis of synovial membranes (see Chapter 46). If a joint appears swollen and inflamed, the nurse palpates it for warmth.

MUSCLE TONE AND STRENGTH

The nurse may assess muscle strength and tone during measurement of range of motion. Findings are integrated with those from the neurological assessment. Tone is the slight muscular resistance felt by the examiner as the relaxed extremity is passively moved through its range of motion.

The client is asked to allow an extremity to relax or hang limp. This is often difficult, particularly if the client feels pain in the extremity. The extremity is supported, and each limb is grasped, moving it through the normal range of motion (Figure 32-92). Normal tone causes a mild, even resistance to movement through the entire range.

If a muscle has increased tone, or **hypertonicity,** any sudden passive movement of a joint is met with considerable resistance. Continued movement eventually causes the muscle to relax. A muscle that has little tone (**hypotonicity**) feels flabby. The involved extremity hangs loosely in a position determined by gravity.

For assessment of muscle strength, the client assumes a stable position. The client performs maneuvers demonstrating strength of major muscle groups (Table 32-35). Symmetrical muscle pairs are compared (Table 32-36). The arm on the dominant side is normally stronger than the arm on the nondominant side. In the older adult a loss of muscle mass causes bilateral weakness, but muscle strength remains greater in the dominant arm or leg.

Each muscle group is examined. The nurse asks the client to first flex the muscle to be examined and then to resist when the nurse applies opposing force against that flexion. It is important to not allow the client to move the joint. The nurse gradually increases pressure to a muscle group (e.g., elbow extension). The client resists the pressure applied by the nurse by attempting to move against resistance (e.g., elbow flexion). The client resists until instructed to stop. As the examiner varies the amount of pressure applied, the joint moves. If a weakness is identified, the muscle's size is compared with opposite counterpart by measuring the muscle body's circumference with a

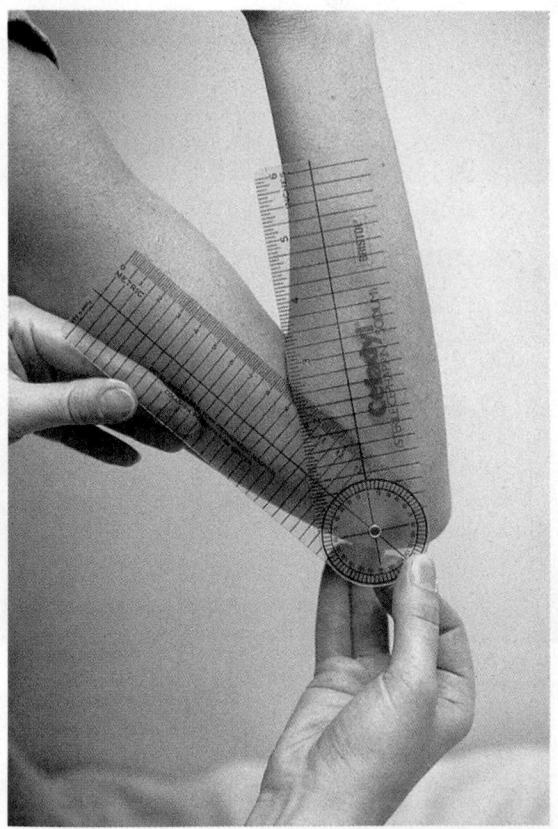

Figure 32-91   After the client flexes the arm, the goniometer measures the degree of joint flexion.
From Seidel HM and others: *Mosby's guide to physical examination,* ed 4, St. Louis, 1999, Mosby.

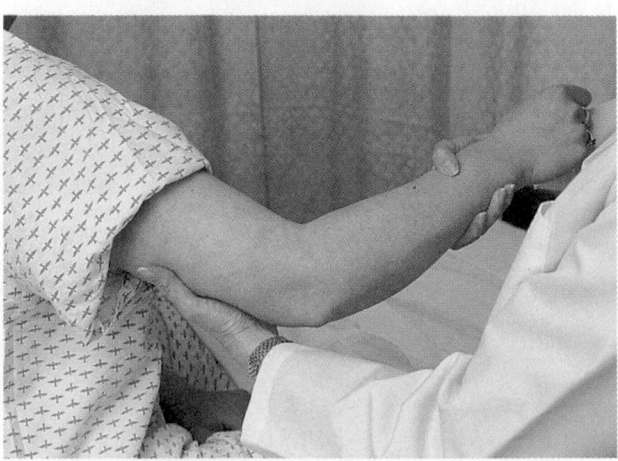

Figure 32-92   The nurse assesses muscle tone.

Table 32-35 Maneuvers to Assess Muscle Strength

Muscle Group	Maneuver
Neck (sternocleidomastoid)	Place hand firmly against client's upper jaw. Ask client to turn head laterally against resistance.
Shoulder (trapezius)	Place hand over midline of client's shoulder, exerting firm pressure. Have client raise shoulders against resistance.
Elbow	
Biceps	Pull down on forearm as client attempts to flex arm.
Triceps	As client's arm is flexed, apply pressure against forearm. Ask client to straighten arm.
Hip	
Quadriceps	When client is sitting, apply downward pressure to thigh. Ask client to raise leg up from table.
Gastrocnemius	Client sits, holding shin of flexed leg. Ask client to straighten leg against resistance.

tape measure. A muscle that has **atrophied** (reduced in size) may feel soft and boggy when palpated.

Neurological System

The neurological system is responsible for many functions, including initiation and coordination of movement, reception and perception of sensory stimuli, organization of thought processes, control of speech, and storage of memory. A close integration exists between the neurological system and all other body systems. For example, urine production relies in part on the adequacy of blood flow to the kidneys, and the size of arterioles supplying the kidneys is under neural control.

An assessment of neurological function can be time consuming. An efficient nurse integrates neurological measurements with other parts of the physical examination. For example, cranial nerve function can be tested during the survey of the head and neck. Mental and emotional status is observed as the nursing history is collected.

Many variables must be considered when deciding the extent of the examination. A client's level of consciousness influences the ability to follow directions. A person's general physical status influences tolerance to assessment. For example, an inability to walk makes a detailed assessment of coordination difficult. The client's chief complaint also helps determine the need for a thorough neurological assessment. If the client complains of headache or a recent loss of function in an extremity, a complete neurological review is needed. Table 32-37 reviews the data collected in the nursing history. For a complete examination, the following special equipment will be needed:

Reading material
Vials containing aromatic substances (e.g., vanilla and coffee)
Opposite tip of cotton swab or tongue blade broken in half
Snellen eye chart
Penlight
Vials containing sugar or salt
Tongue blade
Two test tubes, one filled with hot water and the other with cold water
Cotton balls or cotton-tipped applicators
Tuning fork
Reflex hammer

MENTAL AND EMOTIONAL STATUS

A great deal can be learned about mental capacities and emotional state by simply interacting with a client. A nurse can ask questions throughout an examination to gather data and observe the appropriateness of emotions and ideas. There are special assessment tools designed to assess a client's mental status. Kahn and Goldfarb's mental status questionnaire (MSQ) (1960) is a ten-item instrument and a widely used tool. Folstein, Folstein, and

Table 32-36 Muscle Strength

Muscle Function Level	Scales		
	Grade	% Normal	Lovett Scale
No evidence of contractility	0	0	0 (zero)
Slight contractility, no movement	1	10	T (trace)
Full range of motion, gravity eliminated*	2	25	P (poor)
Full range of motion with gravity	3	50	F (fair)
Full range of motion against gravity, some resistance	4	75	G (good)
Full range of motion against gravity, full resistance	5	100	N (normal)

From Barkauskas VH and others: *Health and physical assessment*, ed 2, St. Louis, 1998, Mosby.
*Passive movement.

Table 32-37 **Nursing History for Neurological Assessment**	
Assessment Category	Rationale
Determine if client is taking analgesics, antipsychotics, antidepressants, or nervous system stimulants.	These medications can alter level of consciousness or cause behavioral changes.
Assess client's use of alcohol, sedative-hypnotics, or recreational drugs.	Abuse can cause tremors, ataxia, and changes in peripheral nerve function.
Determine if client has recent history of seizures/convulsions: clarify sequence of events (aura, fall to ground, motor activity, loss of consciousness); character of any symptoms; and relationship of seizure to time of day, fatigue, or emotional stress.	Seizure activity often originates from central nervous system alteration. Characteristics of seizure help determine its origin.
Screen client for headache, tremors, dizziness, vertigo, numbness or tingling of body part, visual changes, weakness, pain, or changes in speech.	These symptoms frequently originate from alterations in central nervous system or peripheral nervous system function. Identification of specific patterns may aid in diagnosis of pathological condition.
Discuss with spouse, family members, or friends any recent changes in client's behavior (e.g., increased irritability, mood swings, memory loss, change in energy level).	Behavioral changes may result from intracranial pathological states.
Assess client for history of change in vision, hearing, smell, taste, or touch.	Major sensory nerves originate from brainstem. These symptoms may help to localize nature of problem.
If an older client displays sudden acute confusion (delirium), review history for drug toxicity (anticholinergics, diuretics, digoxin, cimetidine, sedatives, antihypertensives, antiarrhythmics), serious infections, metabolic disturbances, heart failure, and severe anemia.	One of the most common mental disorders in older persons. Condition is always potentially reversible (see Box 32-32).
Review past history for head or spinal cord injury, hypertension, or psychiatric disorders.	Factors may cause neurological symptoms or behavioral changes to develop, focusing assessment on possible cause.

McHugh (1975) developed the Mini-Mental State (MMS) to measure orientation and cognitive function (Box 32-31). A maximum score on the MMS is 30. Clients with scores of 21 or less generally reveal cognitive impairment requiring further evaluation.

To ensure an objective assessment, the nurse considers the client's cultural and educational background, values, beliefs, and previous experiences. Such factors influence the client's response to questions. An alteration in mental or emotional status may reflect a disturbance in cerebral functioning. The cerebral cortex controls and integrates intellectual and emotional functioning. Primary brain disorders, medication, and metabolic changes are examples of factors that may change cerebral function.

A common mental disorder affecting older adults is delirium. It is an acute mental disorder characterized by confusion, disorientation, and restlessness. The acute condition is often misdiagnosed as a form of dementia, a more progressive, organic mental disorder such as Alzheimer's disease. Thus the underlying cause of the condition is missed. When it occurs, many nurses and physicians think it is common older adult behavior. Delirium is often overlooked in older adults because of a failure to adequately assess mental status. The condition can fortunately be reversed when correctly assessed. Frequently clients who develop delirium are labeled with sun-

downer's syndrome because the delirium frequently worsens at night. Many practitioners mistake this as being common with old age. The nurse should obtain a good history of the client's behavior before delirium develops so as to recognize the condition early. Family members can usually be a good resource. Box 32-32 summarizes clinical criteria for delirium.

Level of Consciousness.   The level of consciousness exists along a continuum from full awakening, alertness, and cooperation to unresponsiveness to any form of external stimuli. A fully conscious client responds to questions spontaneously. As consciousness lowers, a client may show irritability, a shortened attention span, or an unwillingness to cooperate. To avoid ambiguity in the assessment of the level of consciousness, the Glasgow coma scale (GCS) measures consciousness by an objective numerical scale (Table 32-38). Caution is needed in using the scale with clients who have sensory losses (e.g., vision or hearing). As consciousness deteriorates, a client becomes disoriented to name, time, and place. The nurse asks short, to-the-point questions regarding information that the client knows (e.g., "Tell me your name," "What's the name of this place?" and "What day is this?"). The client's ability to understand and answer questions has a direct effect on the nurse's ability to perform a complete examination.

Folstein's Mini-Mental State   Box 32-31

"MINI-MENTAL STATE"

Maximum
Score

Orientation

5   ( )   What is the (year) (season) (date) (day) (month)?

5   ( )   Where are we: (state) (county) (town) (hospital) (floor).

Registration

3   ( )   Name 3 objects: 1 second to say each. Then ask the patient all 3 after you have said them. Give 1 point for each correct answer. Then repeat them until he learns all 3. Count trials and record.

Attention and Calculation

5   ( )   Serial 7's. 1 point for each correct. Stop after 5 answers. Alternatively spell "world" backwards.

Recall

3   ( )   Ask for the 3 objects repeated above. Give 1 point for each correct.

Language

9   ( )   Name a pencil, and watch (2 points)
           Repeat the following "No ifs, ands or buts" (1 point)
           Follow a 3-stage command:
           "Take a paper in your right hand, fold it in half, and put it on the floor" (3 points)
           Read and obey the following:
           Close Your Eyes (1 point)
           Write a sentence (1 point)
           Copy design (1 point)

_____   Total score

ASSESS level of consciousness along a continuum

Alert   Drowsy   Stupor   Coma

INSTRUCTIONS FOR ADMINISTRATION OF MINI-MENTAL STATE EXAMINATION

Orientation

(1) Ask for the date. Then ask specifically for parts omitted, e.g., "Can you also tell me what season it is?" One point for each correct.

(2) Ask in turn, "Can you tell me the name of this hospital?" (town, county, etc.). One point for each correct.

Registration

Ask the patient if you may test his memory. Then say the names of 3 unrelated objects, clearly and slowly, about 1 second for each. After you have said all 3, ask him to repeat them. This first repetition determines his score (0-3) but keep saying them until he can repeat all 3, up to 6 trials. If he does not eventually learn all 3, recall cannot be meaningfully tested.

Attention and Calculation

Ask the patient to begin with 100 and count backwards by 7. Stop after 5 subtractions (93, 86, 79, 72, 65).

Score the total number of correct answers.

If the patient cannot or will not perform this task, ask him to spell the word "world" backwards. The score is the number of letters in correct order, e.g., dlrow = 5, dlorw = 3.

Recall

Ask the patient if he can recall the 3 words you previously asked him to remember. Score 0-3.

Language

Naming: Show the patient a wrist watch and ask him what it is. Repeat for pencil. Score 0-2.

Repetition: Ask the patient to repeat the sentence after you. Allow only one trial. Score 0 or 1.

3-Stage command: Give the patient a piece of plain blank paper and repeat the command. Score 1 point for each part correctly executed.

Reading: On a blank piece of paper print the sentence "Close your eyes," in letters large enough for the patient to see clearly. Ask him to read it and do what it says. Score 1 point only if he actually closes his eyes.

Writing: Give the patient a blank piece of paper and ask him to write a sentence for you. Do not dictate a sentence; it is to be written spontaneously. It must contain a subject and verb and be sensible. Correct grammar and punctuation are not necessary.

Copying: On a clean sheet of paper, draw intersecting pentagons, each side about 1 inch, and ask him to copy it exactly as it is. All 10 angles must be present and 2 must intersect to score 1 point. Tremor and rotation are ignored.

Estimate the patient's level of sensorium along a continuum, from alert on the left to coma on the right.

From Folstein MF, Folstein S, McHugh PR: Mini-Mental State: a practical method for grading the cognitive state of patients for the clinician, *J Psychiatr Res* 12:189, 1975.

The client must be aroused to full alertness before the assessment can be conducted.

A client may be unable to follow simple commands, such as "Squeeze my finger" or "Move your toes." At this lowered level of consciousness the client often is responsive only to painful stimuli. The nurse tests the client by applying firm pressure with the thumb over the root of the fingernail. The client should withdraw the hand from the painful stimulus. A client with serious neurological impairment exhibits abnormal posturing in response to pain. A flaccid response indicates the absence of muscle tone in the extremities and severe injury to brain tissue.

The GCS allows the nurse to evaluate a client's neurological status over time. The higher the score, the more improved or normal the level of functioning.

Behavior and Appearance.   Behavior, moods, hygiene, grooming, and choice of dress reveal pertinent information about mental status. The nurse must be perceptive of mannerisms and actions during the entire physical as-

Clinical Criteria for Delirium   Box 32-32

Definition: An acute disturbance of consciousness that is accompanied by a change in cognition. It cannot be accounted for by a preexisting or evolving dementia. Delirium develops over a short period of time, usually hours to days, and tends to fluctuate during the course of the day. It is usually a direct physiological consequence of a general medical condition.

There is reduced clarity of awareness of the environment.

Ability to focus, sustain, or shift attention is impaired (questions must be repeated).

Person is easily distracted by irrelevant stimuli.

There is an accompanying change in cognition (memory impairment, disorientation, or language disturbance).

Recent memory is most commonly affected.

Disorientation is usually shown, with client disoriented to time or place.

Language disturbance may involve impaired ability to name objects or ability to write; speech may be rambling.

Perceptual disturbances may include misinterpretations, illusions, or hallucinations.

Modified from American Psychiatric Association: *Diagnostic and statistical manual of mental disorders,* ed 4, Washington, DC, 1994, American Psychiatric Association; and Foreman MD and others: Assessing cognitive function, *Geriatr Nurs* 17(5):228, 1996.

Table 32-38   Glasgow Coma Scale

Action	Response	Score
Eyes open	Spontaneously	(4)
	To speech	3
	To pain	2
	None	1
Best verbal response	Oriented	(5)
	Confused	4
	Inappropriate words	3
	Incomprehensible sounds	2
	None	1
Best motor response	Obeys commands	(6)
	Localized pain	5
	Flexion withdrawal	4
	Abnormal flexion	3
	Abnormal extension	2
	Flaccid	1
	TOTAL SCORE	(15)

sessment. The nurse notes nonverbal, as well as verbal, behavior. Does the client respond appropriately to directions? Does the client's mood vary with no apparent cause? Does the client show concern about appearance? Is the client's hair clean and neatly groomed, and are the nails trim and clean? The client should behave in a manner expressing concern and interest in the examination. The client should make eye contact with the nurse and express appropriate feelings that correspond to the situation. Normally the client will show some degree of personal hygiene.

Choice and fit of clothing may reflect socioeconomic background or personal taste rather than deficiency in self-concept or self-care. The nurse avoids being judgmental and focuses assessment on the appropriateness of clothing for the weather. Older adults may neglect their appearance because of a lack of energy, finances, or reduced vision.

Language.   The ability of an individual to understand spoken or written words and to express the self through writing, words, or gestures is a function of the cerebral cortex. The nurse assesses the client's voice inflection, tone, and manner of speech. The client's voice should have inflections, be clear and strong, and increase in volume appropriately. Speech should be fluent. When communication is clearly ineffective (e.g., omission or addition of letters and words, misuse of words, hesitations), the nurse assesses for **aphasia.** An injury to the cerebral cortex may result in aphasia.

The two types of aphasia are sensory (or receptive) and motor (or expressive). With receptive aphasia a person cannot understand written or verbal speech. With expressive aphasia a person understands written and verbal speech but cannot write or speak appropriately when trying to communicate. A client may suffer a combination of receptive and expressive aphasia, depending on the portion of the cerebral cortex involved. The nurse assesses language capabilities when it is clear that communication with the client is ineffective. Some simple assessment techniques include the following:

Asking the client to name a familiar object to which the nurse points

Asking the client to respond to simple verbal and written commands, such as "Stand up" or "Sit down"

Asking the client to read simple sentences out loud

Normally a client names objects correctly, follows commands, and reads sentences correctly.

INTELLECTUAL FUNCTION

Intellectual function includes memory (recent, immediate, and past), knowledge, abstract thinking, association, and judgment. Each aspect of intellectual function is tested through a specific technique. However, because cultural and educational background influence the ability to respond to test questions, the nurse should not ask questions related to concepts or ideas with which the client is unfamiliar.

Memory.   The nurse assesses immediate recall and recent and remote memory. Often a problem with memory becomes apparent when the nurse takes the nursing history. To assess immediate recall, the nurse has the client repeat a series of numbers (e.g., *7, 4, 1*) in the order they are presented or in reverse order. The nurse gradually increases the number of digits (e.g., *7, 4, 1, 8, 6*) until the client fails to repeat the digits correctly. Normally an individual is able to repeat a series of 5 to 8 digits forward and 4 to 6 digits backward.

The nurse asks if the client's memory can be tested. Then the nurse says clearly and slowly the name of three unrelated objects. After the nurse says all three, the client is asked to repeat each. This is continued until the client is successful. Then, later in the assessment, the nurse asks the client to repeat the three words again. The client should be able to identify the three words. Another test for recent memory involves asking the client to recall events occurring during the same day (e.g., what was eaten for breakfast). Information may need to be validated with a family member.

To assess past memory, the nurse can ask the client to recall his or her mother's maiden name, a birthday, or a special date in history. It is best to ask open-ended questions rather than simple yes/no questions. A client should have immediate recall of such information. With older adults a nurse should not interpret a hearing loss as confusion. Good communication techniques are necessary throughout the examination to ensure that the client clearly understands all directions and testing.

Knowledge.   The nurse can assess knowledge by asking clients what they know about their illnesses or the reason for seeking health care. By assessing knowledge, the nurse determines clients' abilities to learn or understand. If an opportunity to teach exists, the nurse can test mental status by asking for feedback during a follow-up visit.

Abstract Thinking.   Interpreting abstract ideas or concepts reflects the capacity for abstract thinking. A higher level of intellectual functioning is required for an individual to explain such phrases as "A stitch in time saves nine" or "Don't count your chickens before they're hatched." The nurse notes whether the client's explanations are relevant and concrete. The client with altered mentation will likely interpret the phrase literally or merely rephrase the words.

Association.   Another higher level of intellectual functioning involves finding similarities or associations between concepts: a dog is to a beagle as a cat is to a Siamese. The nurse names related concepts and asks the client to identify their associations. Questions should be appropriate to the client's level of intelligence. It is sufficient to use simple concepts.

Judgment.   Judgment requires a comparison and evaluation of facts and ideas to understand their relationships and to form appropriate conclusions. The nurse attempts to measure the ability to make logical decisions. By assessing judgment, the nurse also measures

the ability to organize thought processes. The nurse may choose to ask clients why they decided to seek health care or how they plan to adjust to limitations after returning home. A simpler test would involve asking what clients would do if placed in a situation such as being locked out of their homes or suddenly becoming ill when alone at home.

CRANIAL NERVE FUNCTION

The nurse may assess all 12 cranial nerves or test a single nerve or related group of nerves. A test of the oculomotor nerve measures pupillary response. Assessment of the glossopharyngeal and vagus nerves reveals integrity of the gag reflex. Measurements used to assess the integrity of organs within the head and neck also assess cranial nerve function. For example, the cochlear branch of the eighth cranial nerve is tested during a hearing assessment. The function of the ninth and tenth nerves can be assessed during examination of the pharynx. A dysfunction in any nerve reflects an alteration at some point along the cranial nerve's distribution. Cranial nerve assessment is easy after the nurse is familiar with the nerve's normal functions. To remember the order of the 12 nerves, the nurse can use this simple phrase, "On old Olympus' towering tops, a Finn and German viewed some hops." The first letter of each word in the phrase is the same as the first letter of the names of the cranial nerves (Table 32-39).

SENSORY FUNCTION

The sensory pathways of the central nervous system conduct sensations of pain, temperature, position, vibration, and crude and finely localized touch. Different nerve pathways relay the sensations. For most clients a quick screening of sensory function is sufficient unless there are symptoms of reduced sensation, motor impairment, or paralysis.

Normally a client has sensory responses to all stimuli that are tested. Sensations along the body's surface are felt equally on both sides of the face, trunk, and extremities. A nurse can assess the major sensory nerves by knowing the sensory dermatome zones (Figure 32-93). Some areas of the skin are innervated by specific dorsal root cutaneous nerves. For example, if the nurse notes reduced sensation when checking for light touch along an area of the skin (e.g., the lower neck), the nurse can determine, in general, where a neurological lesion may exist (e.g., fourth cervical spinal cord segment).

All sensory testing is performed with the client's eyes closed so that the client is unable to see when or where a stimulus strikes the skin (Table 32-40). Stimuli are applied in a random, unpredictable order to maintain the client's attention and prevent detection of a predictable pattern. The client is asked to tell the nurse when, what, and where each stimulus is felt. The nurse compares symmetrical areas of the body while applying stimuli to the client's arms, trunk, and legs.

Table 32-39 Cranial Nerve Function and Assessment

Number	Name	Type	Function	Method
I	Olfactory	Sensory	Sense of smell	Ask client to identify different nonirritating aromas such as coffee and vanilla.
II	Optic	Sensory	Visual acuity	Use Snellen chart or ask client to read printed material while wearing glasses.
III	Oculomotor	Motor	Extraocular eye movement	Assess directions of gaze.
			Pupil constriction and dilation	Measure pupillary reaction to light reflex and accommodation.
IV	Trochlear	Motor	Upward and downward movement of eyeball	Assess directions of gaze.
V	Trigeminal	Sensory and motor	Sensory nerve to skin of face	Lightly touch cornea with wisp of cotton. Assess corneal reflex. Measure sensation of light pain and touch across skin of face.
			Motor nerve to muscles of jaw	Palpate temples as client clenches teeth.
VI	Abducens	Motor	Lateral movement of eyeballs	Assess directions of gaze.
VII	Facial	Sensory and motor	Facial expression	As client smiles, frowns, puffs out cheeks, and raises and lowers eyebrows, look for asymmetry.
			Taste	Have client identify salty or sweet taste on front of tongue.
VIII	Auditory	Sensory	Hearing	Assess ability to hear spoken word.
IX	Glossopharyngeal	Sensory and motor	Taste	Ask client to identify sour or sweet taste on back of tongue.
			Ability to swallow	Use tongue blade to elicit gag reflex.
X	Vagus	Sensory and motor	Sensation of pharynx	Ask client to say "ah." Observe movement of palate and pharynx.
			Movement of vocal cords	Assess speech for hoarseness.
XI	Spinal accessory	Motor	Movement of head and shoulders	Ask client to shrug shoulders and turn head against passive resistance.
XII	Hypoglossal	Motor	Position of tongue	Ask client to stick out tongue to midline and move it from side to side.

Client Teaching During Neurological Assessment   Box 32-33

OBJECTIVES
- Client's family will understand relationship of client's behavioral and mental changes to physical status.
- Client with sensory or motor impairment will select safety measures for self-care.
- Older adult will routinely inspect skin for injuries.

TEACHING STRATEGIES
- Explain to family or friends the neurological implications of any behavioral or mental impairment shown by client.
- If client has sensory or motor impairments, explain measures to ensure safety (e.g., use of ambulation aids or safety bars in bathrooms or stairways).

- Teach older adult to plan enough time to complete tasks, because reaction time is slowed.
- Teach older adult to observe skin surfaces for areas of trauma, because perception of pain is reduced.

EVALUATION
- Ask family to discuss client behaviors that result from neurological impairments.
- Have client explain safety measures used to avoid injury from sensory and motor limitations.
- Have older client explain reason for inspecting skin surface routinely.

Table 32-40 **Assessment of Sensory Nerve Function**

Function	Equipment	Method	Precautions
Pain	Broken tongue blade or wooden end of cotton applicator	Ask client to voice when dull or sharp sensation is felt. Alternately apply sharp and blunt ends of tongue blade to skin's surface. Note areas of numbness or increased sensitivity.	Remember that areas where skin is thickened, such as heel or sole of foot, may be less sensitive to pain.

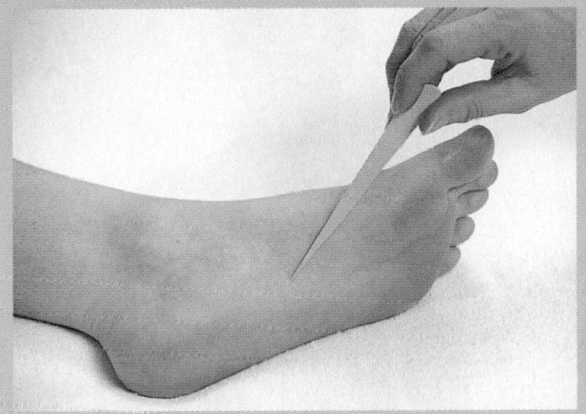 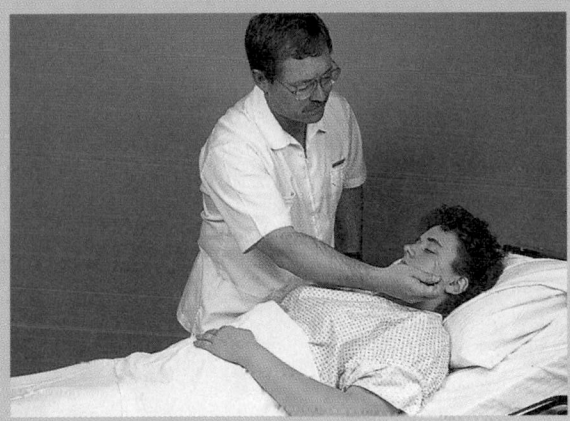

Function	Equipment	Method	Precautions
Temperature	Two test tubes, one filled with hot water and other with cold	Touch skin with tube. Ask client to identify hot or cold sensation.	Omit test if pain sensation is normal.
Light touch	Cotton ball or cotton-tip applicator	Apply light wisp of cotton to different points along skin's surface. Ask client to voice when sensation is felt.	Apply at areas where skin is thin or more sensitive (e.g., face, neck, inner aspect of arms, top of feet and hands).
Vibration	Tuning fork Two broken tongue blades	Apply stem of vibrating fork to distal interphalangeal joint of fingers and interphalangeal joint of great toe, elbow, and wrist. Have client voice when and where vibration is felt.	Be sure client feels vibration and not merely pressure.
Position		Grasp finger or toe, holding it by its sides with thumb and index finger. Alternate moving finger or toe up and down. Ask client to state when finger is up or down. Repeat with toes.	Avoid rubbing adjacent appendages as finger or toe is moved. Do not move joint laterally; return to neutral position before moving again.
Two point discrimination		Lightly apply one or both tongue blade tips simultaneously to the skin's surface. Ask client whether one or two pricks are felt. Find the distance at which client can no longer distinguish two points.	Apply blade tips to same anatomical site (e.g., fingertips, palm of hand, or upper arms). Minimum distance at which client can discriminate two points varies (2 to 8 mm on fingertips).

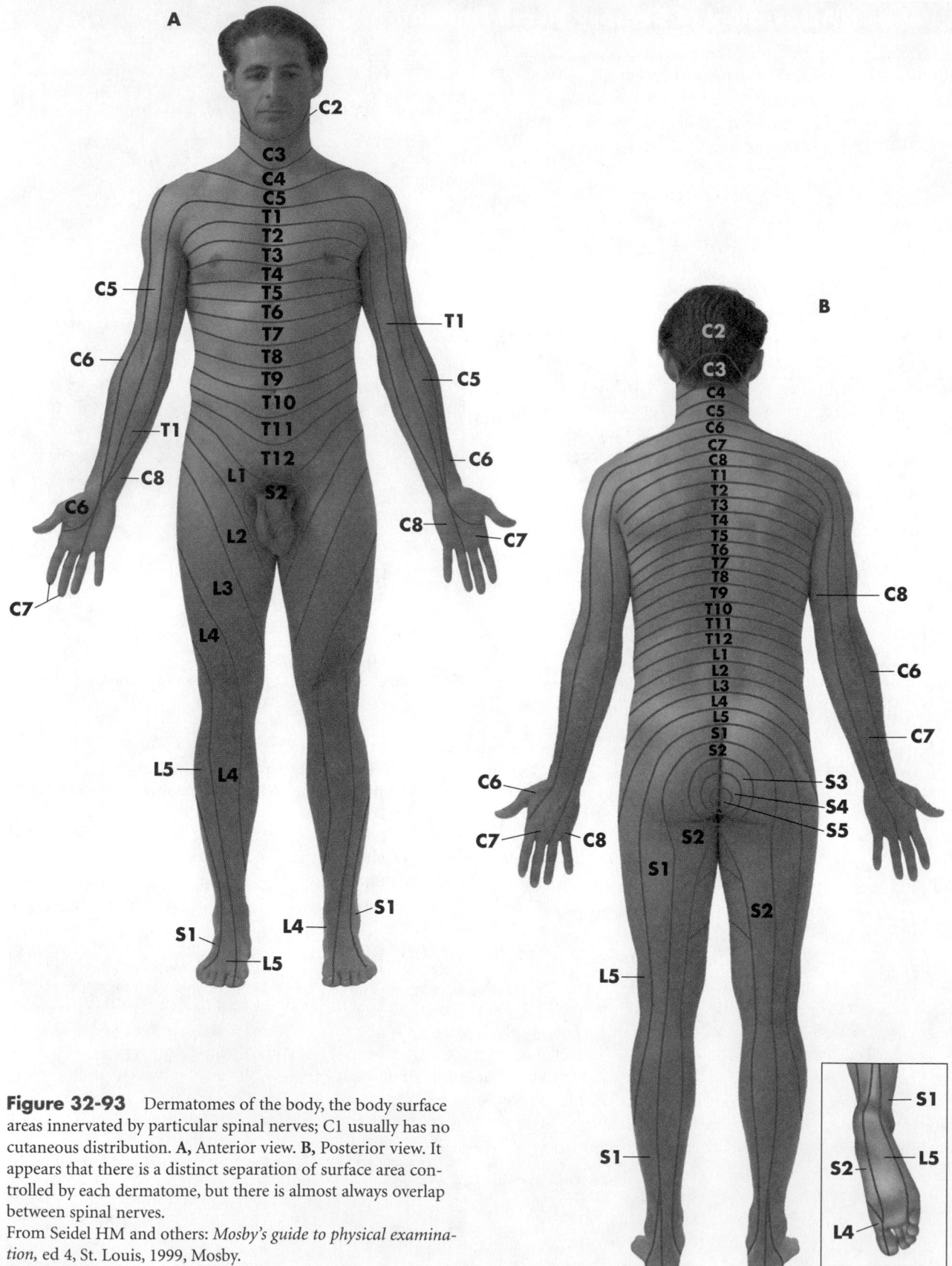

Figure 32-93   Dermatomes of the body, the body surface areas innervated by particular spinal nerves; C1 usually has no cutaneous distribution. **A,** Anterior view. **B,** Posterior view. It appears that there is a distinct separation of surface area controlled by each dermatome, but there is almost always overlap between spinal nerves.

From Seidel HM and others: *Mosby's guide to physical examination,* ed 4, St. Louis, 1999, Mosby.

MOTOR FUNCTION

An assessment of motor function includes the same measurements made during the musculoskeletal examination. In addition, cerebellar function is assessed. The cerebellum coordinates muscular activity by producing smooth, steady, and efficient movements of muscle groups. The maintenance of balance and equilibrium is also a function of the cerebellum. Sensory impulses from the vestibular portion of the inner ear travel to the cerebellum, where impulses are relayed to proper motor nerves to maintain body equilibrium. The cerebellum also controls posture.

Coordination.

It is difficult for the nurse to explain the tests used to measure coordination. To avoid confusion, the nurse demonstrates each maneuver and then has clients repeat it after determining that their mobility is normal and they are physically able to make the necessary movements. The nurse observes the smoothness and balance of movements (Box 32-33). In older adults a slow reaction time may cause movements to be less rhythmical.

To assess fine motor function, the nurse has the client extend the arms out to the sides and touch each forefinger alternately to the nose (first with eyes open, then with eyes closed). Normally the client alternately touches the nose smoothly. Performing rapid, rhythmical, alternating movements demonstrates coordination in the upper extremities. While sitting, the client begins by patting the knees with both hands. Then the client alternately turns up the palm and back of the hands while continuously patting. The maneuver should be done smoothly and regularly with increasing speed.

An additional maneuver for upper extremity coordination involves touching each finger with the thumb of the same hand in rapid sequence. The client moves from the index finger to the little finger and back, with one hand tested at a time. The client's dominant hand is slightly less awkward when performing this movement. Movement should be smooth and in succession.

Lower extremity coordination is tested with the client lying supine, legs extended. The nurse places a hand at the ball of the client's foot. The client taps the nurse's hand with the foot as quickly as possible. Each foot is tested for speed and smoothness. The feet do not move as rapidly or evenly as the hands.

Balance.

The nurse may use one or two of the following tests to assess balance and gross motor function:

  Have the client perform a Romberg test by standing with feet together, arms at the sides, both with eyes open and eyes closed. While protecting the client's safety by standing at the side, observe swaying. Slight swaying is normal. The client normally does not have to break the stance.

  Have the client close the eyes, with arms held straight at the sides, and stand on one foot and then the other. Normally balance is maintained for 5 seconds with slight swaying.

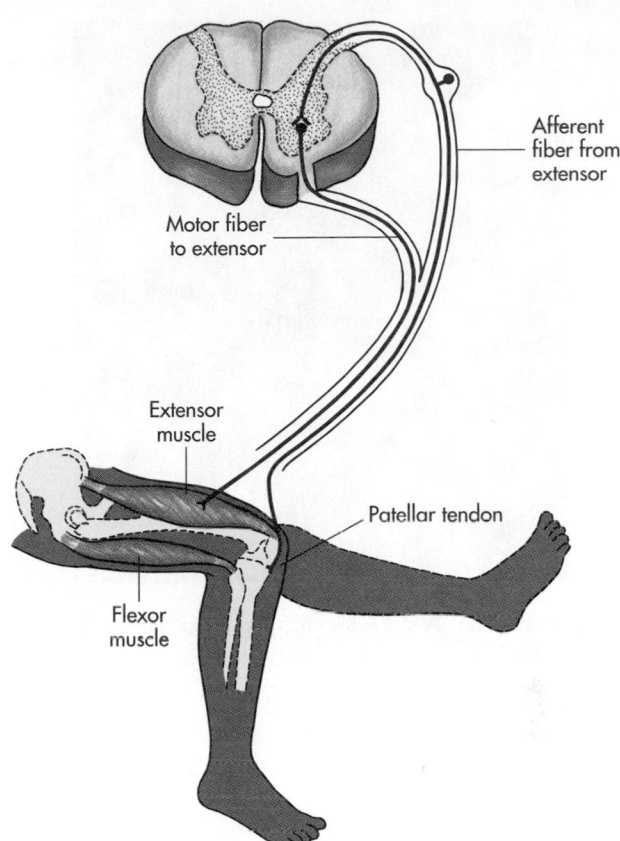

Figure 32-94   Pathway of the reflex arc.

Ask the client to walk a straight line by placing the heel of one foot directly in front of the toes of the other foot.

REFLEXES

Eliciting reflex reactions allows the nurse to assess the integrity of sensory and motor pathways of the reflex arc and specific spinal cord segments. Assessment of reflexes does not determine higher neural center functioning. Figure 32-94 traces the pathway of the reflex arc. Each muscle contains a small sensory unit called a muscle spindle, which controls muscle tone and detects changes in the length of muscle fibers. By tapping a tendon with a reflex hammer, the nurse stretches the muscle and tendon, lengthening the spindle. The spindle sends nerve impulses along afferent nerve pathways to the dorsal horn of the spinal cord segment. Within milliseconds the impulses reach the spinal cord and synapse to travel to the efferent motor neuron in the spinal cord. A motor nerve sends the impulses back to the muscle, causing the reflex response.

The two categories of normal reflexes are deep tendon reflexes, elicited by mildly stretching a muscle and tapping a tendon, and cutaneous reflexes, elicited by stimulating the skin superficially. Reflexes are graded as follows:

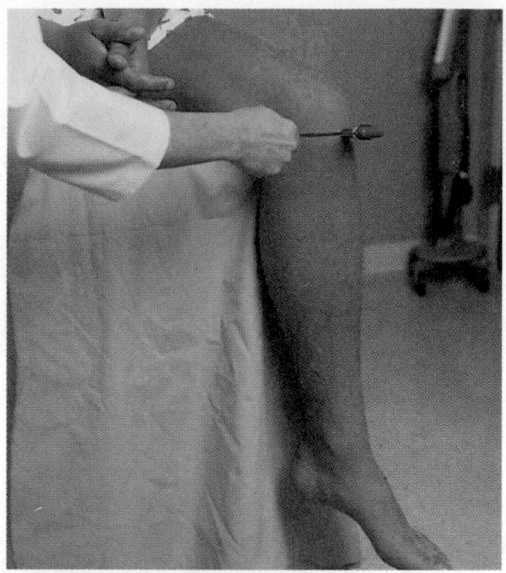

Figure 32-95 Position for eliciting the patellar tendon reflex. The lower leg normally extends.

0   No response
1   Low normal with slight muscle contraction
2+ Normal with visible muscle twitch and movement of the arm or leg
3+ Brisker than normal; may not indicate disease
4+ Hyperactive and very brisk; often associated with spinal cord disorders

When reflexes are being assessed, the client should relax as much as possible to avoid voluntary movement or tensing of muscles. The nurse positions the limbs to slightly stretch the muscle being tested. The reflex hammer is held loosely between the nurse's thumb and fingers so that it can swing freely and tap the tendon briskly (Figure 32-95). The nurse compares the symmetry of the reflex from one side of the body with that of the other side. In the older adult, reflexes are normally slowed. Reflexes can be hyperactive in clients with alcohol, cocaine, or opioid intoxication (Caulker-Burnett, 1994). Practitioners often use stick figures to record reflexes. Table 32-41 summarizes common deep tendon and cutaneous reflexes.

Table 32-41 Assessment of Common Reflexes

Type	Procedure	Normal Reflex
Deep Tendon Reflexes		
Biceps	Flex client's arm up to 45 degrees at elbow with palms down. Place your thumb in antecubital fossa at base of biceps tendon and your fingers over biceps muscle. Strike triceps tendon with reflex hammer.	Flexion of arm at elbow
Triceps	Flex client's arm at elbow, holding arm across chest, or hold upper arm horizontally and allow lower arm to go limp. Strike triceps tendon just above elbow.	Extension at elbow
Patellar	Have client sit with legs hanging freely over side of table or chair or have client lie supine and support knee in a flexed 90-degree position. Briskly tap patellar tendon just below patella.	Extension of lower leg
Achilles	Have client assume same position as for patellar reflex. Slightly dorsiflex client's ankle by grasping toes in palm of your hand. Strike Achilles tendon just above heel at ankle malleolus.	Plantar flexion of foot
Cutaneous Reflexes		
Plantar	Have client lie supine with legs straight and feet relaxed. Take handle end of reflex hammer and stroke lateral aspect of sole from heel to ball of foot, curving across ball of foot toward big toe.	Plantar flexion of all toes
Gluteal	Have client assume side-lying position. Spread buttocks apart and lightly stimulate perineal area with cotton applicator.	Contraction of anal sphincter
Abdominal	Have client stand or lie supine. Stroke abdominal skin with base of cotton applicator over lateral borders of rectus abdominus muscle toward midline. Repeat test in each abdominal quadrant.	Contraction of rectus abdominus muscle with pulling of umbilicus toward stimulated side

After the Examination

The nurse may choose to record findings from the physical assessment during the examination or at the end. Most institutions have special forms that make it easy to record examination data (see Chapter 24). The nurse reviews all findings before assisting the client with dressing, in case there is a need to recheck any information or gather additional data. Physical assessment findings are integrated into the plan of care.

After completing the assessment, the nurse assists the client in dressing, if necessary. The hospitalized client may need a new gown and help in returning to bed and assuming a comfortable position. The client in the home may only need time to dress and join the nurse in the living room or kitchen. When the client is comfortable, it helps to share a summary of the assessment findings. If the findings have revealed serious abnormalities, such as a mass or highly irregular heart rate, the client's physician should be consulted before any findings are revealed. It is the physician's responsibility to make definitive medical diagnoses. The nurse can explain the type of abnormality found and the need for the physician to conduct an additional examination.

The nurse may delegate cleaning the examination area to assistive personnel. Infection-control practices are used in removing materials or instruments soiled with potentially infectious wastes. If the client's bedside was the examination site, the assistant clears away soiled items from the table and makes sure that the bed linen is dry and clean. The client may appreciate a clean gown and the opportunity to wash the face and hands. Afterward, the nurse washes hands.

The nurse checks to make sure that the recording of the assessment is complete. If entry of items into the assessment form was delayed, the nurse records them at this time to avoid forgetting any important information. If entries were made periodically during the examination, they are reviewed for accuracy and thoroughness. Significant findings are communicated to appropriate medical and nursing personnel, either verbally or in the written care plan.

The client often needs a number of ancillary examinations, such as x-ray examinations, laboratory tests, or ultrasonography, after a physical examination. These tests provide additional screening information to rule out the presence of abnormalities and help in the diagnosis of specific abnormalities found during the examination. The nurse explains the purpose of these tests and the sensations that the client can expect.

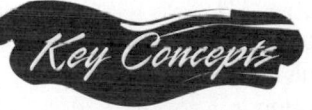

Key Concepts

- Baseline assessment findings reflect the client's functional abilities when the nurse first assesses the client and serve as the basis for comparison with subsequent assessment findings.
- Assessment data are used to make nursing diagnoses, select appropriate nursing interventions, and evaluate the outcomes of nursing care.
- Physical assessment of a child or infant requires the nurse to apply principles of physical growth and development.
- The nurse recognizes that the normal process of aging affects physical findings collected from an older adult.
- Client teaching should be integrated throughout the examination to help clients learn about health promotion and disease prevention.
- The nurse can use time more efficiently by integrating physical assessment with routine nursing care.
- Inspection requires good lighting, full exposure of the body part, and a careful comparison of the part with its counterpart on the opposite side of the body.

- Palpation involves the use of parts of the hand to detect different types of physical characteristics.
- Percussion is the detection of differences in density of underlying tissues by listening to sounds produced while striking the body's surface.
- A good stethoscope should have earpieces that fit snugly, flexible thick-walled tubing of the proper length, and a chestpiece with a bell and diaphragm.
- Through auscultation the nurse assesses the character of sounds created in various body organs.
- A physical examination should be performed only after proper preparation of the environment and equipment and after preparing the client physically and psychologically.
- Throughout the examination the nurse should keep the client warm, comfortable, and informed of each step of the process.
- The client assumes various positions during the physical examination to provide greater accessibility to body parts and to increase accuracy in assessment.

- The nurse uses a systematic approach when conducting a physical assessment.
- A competent examiner learns to combine assessments of different body systems simultaneously.
- Information from the nursing history helps the nurse focus on examining body systems likely to be affected.
- When assessing a seriously ill client, the nurse concentrates on the body systems most likely to be affected.
- Accuracy in assessing the thorax, heart, and abdomen is enhanced by creating a mental image of internal organs in relation to external anatomical landmarks.
- When assessing heart sounds, the nurse imagines events occurring during the cardiac cycle.
- The carotid arteries should never be palpated simultaneously.
- When examining a woman's breasts, the nurse explains the techniques for breast self-examination.
- The abdominal assessment differs from other portions of the examination in that auscultation follows inspection.
- During assessment of the genitalia, the nurse explains the techniques for genital self-examination.
- Assessment of musculoskeletal function can easily be conducted by observing the client ambulating or participating in other active movements.
- The nurse assesses mental and emotional status by interacting with the client throughout the examination.
- At the end of the examination the nurse provides for the client's comfort and then completes a detailed review of physical assessment findings.

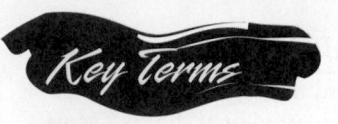

Key Terms

Acromegaly, *p. 752*
Adventitious sounds, *p. 777*
Allen's test, *p. 790*
Alopecia, *p. 749*
Aneurysm, *p. 805*
Aphasia, *p. 824*
Apical impulse, *p. 781*
Arcus senilis, *p. 757*
Atherosclerosis, *p. 787*
Atrophied, *p. 821*
Basal cell carcinoma, *p. 743*
Borborygmi, *p. 803*
Bronchophony, *p. 777*
Bruit, *p. 787*
Caries, *p. 766*
Cerumen, *p. 760*
Chancres, *p. 807*
Cherry angiomas, *p. 746*
Cholecystitis, *p. 804*
Cirrhosis, *p. 803*
Clubbing, *p. 792*
Conjunctivitis, *p. 757*
Cyanosis, *p. 745*
Cystocele, *p. 808*
Dermatitis, *p. 745*
Distention, *p. 802*
Dysrhythmia, *p. 784*
Ectropion, *p. 756*
Eczema, *p. 745*
Edema, *p. 746*
Entropion, *p. 756*
Erythema, *p. 745*
Excoriation, *p. 763*
Exophthalmos, *p. 756*
Exostosis, *p. 768*
Fibrocystic breast disease, *p. 800*
Goniometer, *p. 818*
Hemorrhoids, *p. 814*
Hepatitis, *p. 803*
Hernias, *p. 802*
Hirsutism, *p. 749*
Hydrocephalus, *p. 752*
Hypertonicity, *p. 820*
Hypotonicity, *p. 820*

Indurated, *p. 746*
Integument, *p. 742*
Jaundice, *p. 745*
Kyphosis, *p. 816*
Leukoplakia, *p. 767*
Lordosis, *p. 817*
Melanoma, *p. 742*
Metastasize, *p. 798*
Murmurs, *p. 784*
Nystagmus, *p. 755*
Occlusion, *p. 786*
Ophthalmoscope, *p. 757*
Osteoporosis, *p. 817*
Otoscope, *p. 761*
Ototoxicity, *p. 762*
Pancreatitis, *p. 804*
Papanicolaou (Pap) smear, *p. 808*
Paralytic ileus, *p. 803*
Peristalsis, *p. 802*
Peritonitis, *p. 803*
PERRLA, *p. 757*
Petechiae, *p. 746*
Phlebitis, *p. 793*
Pigmentation, *p. 743*
Point of maximal impulse (PMI), *p. 781*
Polyps, *p. 765*
Ptosis, *p. 756*
Pulse deficit, *p. 784*
Rectocele, *p. 808*
Scoliosis, *p. 817*
Senile keratosis, *p. 746*
Stenosis, *p. 786*
Striae, *p. 802*
Syncope, *p. 786*
Tactile fremitus, *p. 775*
Thrill, *p. 784*
Turgor, *p. 746*
Varicosities, *p. 768*
Ventricular gallop, *p. 784*
Vocal fremitus, *p. 775*
Whispered pectoriloquy, *p. 778*

Critical Thinking Exercises

1. A 32-year-old client entering a neighborhood clinic has the following symptoms: frequent productive cough, fatigue, decreased appetite, and persistent fever. What focused assessment should the nurse conduct?

2. The nurse is performing an abdominal assessment and observes a pulsating midline abdominal mass. What is the nurse's next line of action?

3. A 75-year-old black man is being visited 1 week postoperatively by the home health nurse to assess his peripheral vascular status following a femoral-popliteal bypass graft for arterial insufficiency. What assessment data need to be obtained by the nurse?

4. Develop a teaching plan for a female client (age 40) with a family history of breast cancer who acknowledges that she does not perform a monthly breast self-examination (BSE).

5. What physical examination techniques does the nurse use during assessment of the following clients:

    A. A client suspected of having a head injury

    B. A client with a cast on the lower leg

    C. A client reporting abdominal pain

References

American Cancer Society: *1999 cancer facts and figures,* New York, 1999, The Society.

American Psychiatric Association: *Diagnostic and statistical manual of mental disorders,* ed 4, Washington, DC, 1994, American Psychiatric Association.

Barkauskas VH and others: *Health and physical assessment,* ed 2, St. Louis, 1998, Mosby.

Basfield-Holland ES: Assessing pulmonary status: it's more than listening to breath sounds, *Nursing 97* 27(8):32, 1997.

Benenson AS, editor: *Control of communicable diseases manual,* Washington, DC, 1995, American Public Health Association.

Berlinger JS: Why don't you just leave him? *Nursing 98* 28(4):34, 1998.

Caulker-Burnett I: Primary care screening for substance abuse, *Nurse Pract* 19(6):42, 1994.

Ebersole P, Hess P: *Toward healthy aging,* ed 5, St. Louis, 1998, Mosby.

Folstein MF, Folstein S, McHugh PR: Mini-mental state: a practical method for grading the cognitive state of patients for the clinician, *J Psychiatr Res* 12:82, 1975.

Foreman MD and others: Assessing cognitive function, *Geriatr Nurs* 17(5):228, 1996.

Friedman L and others: *Source book of substance abuse and addiction,* Baltimore, 1996, Williams & Wilkins.

Galsworthy TD, Wilson PL: Osteoporosis: it steals more than bone, *Am J Nurs* 96(6):27, 1996.

Habif TP: *Clinical dermatology: a color guide to diagnosis and therapy,* ed 3, St. Louis, 1996, Mosby.

Haney, PE and others: Tuberculosis makes a comeback, *AORN J* 63(4):705, 1996.

Hardy MA: What can you do about your patient's dry skin, *J Gerontol Nurs* 22(5):10, 1996.

Hopkins ML, Schoener L: Tuberculosis and the elderly living in long-term care facilities, *Geriatr Nurs* 17(1):27, 1996.

Kahn RL and others: Brief objective measures for the determination of mental status of the aged, *Am J Psychiatry* 117:326, 1960.

Kessenich CR, Rosen CJ: Osteoporosis: implications for elderly men, *Geriatr Nurs* 17(4):171, 1996.

Lueckenotte A: *Pocket guide to gerontologic assessment,* ed 3, St. Louis, 1998, Mosby.

Lynch SH: Elder abuse: what to look for, how to intervene, *Am J Nurs* 97(1):27, 1997.

Master S, Terpstra JK: Recognition and diagnosis. In Schnoll SH, Horvatich PK, Terpstra JK, editors: *Prescribing drugs with abuse liability,* Richmond, VA, 1992, DSAM, MCV-VCU.

Moore MC: *Pocket guide to nutritional care,* ed 3, St. Louis, 1997, Mosby.

Pace H, Hoag-Apel CM: Stemming the tide of domestic violence, *Point of View Magazine* 33(3):12, 1996.

Seidel HM and others: *Mosby's guide to physical examination,* ed 4, St. Louis, 1999, Mosby.

Shea CA and others: Breaking through the barriers to domestic violence intervention, *Am J Nurs* 97(6):26, 1997.

Stuart G, Laraia M: *Stuart and Sundeen's principles and practice of psychiatric nursing,* ed 6, St. Louis, 1998, Mosby.

Talbot L, Curtis L: The challenges of assessing skin indicators in people of color, *Home Health Nurse* 14(3), 1996.

Thompson JM and others: *Mosby's manual of clinical nursing,* ed 2, St. Louis, 1989, Mosby.

Thompson JM and others: *Mosby's manual of clinical nursing,* ed 3, St. Louis, 1993, Mosby.

Wong DL and others: *Whaley and Wong's nursing care of infants and children,* ed 6, St. Louis, 1999, Mosby.

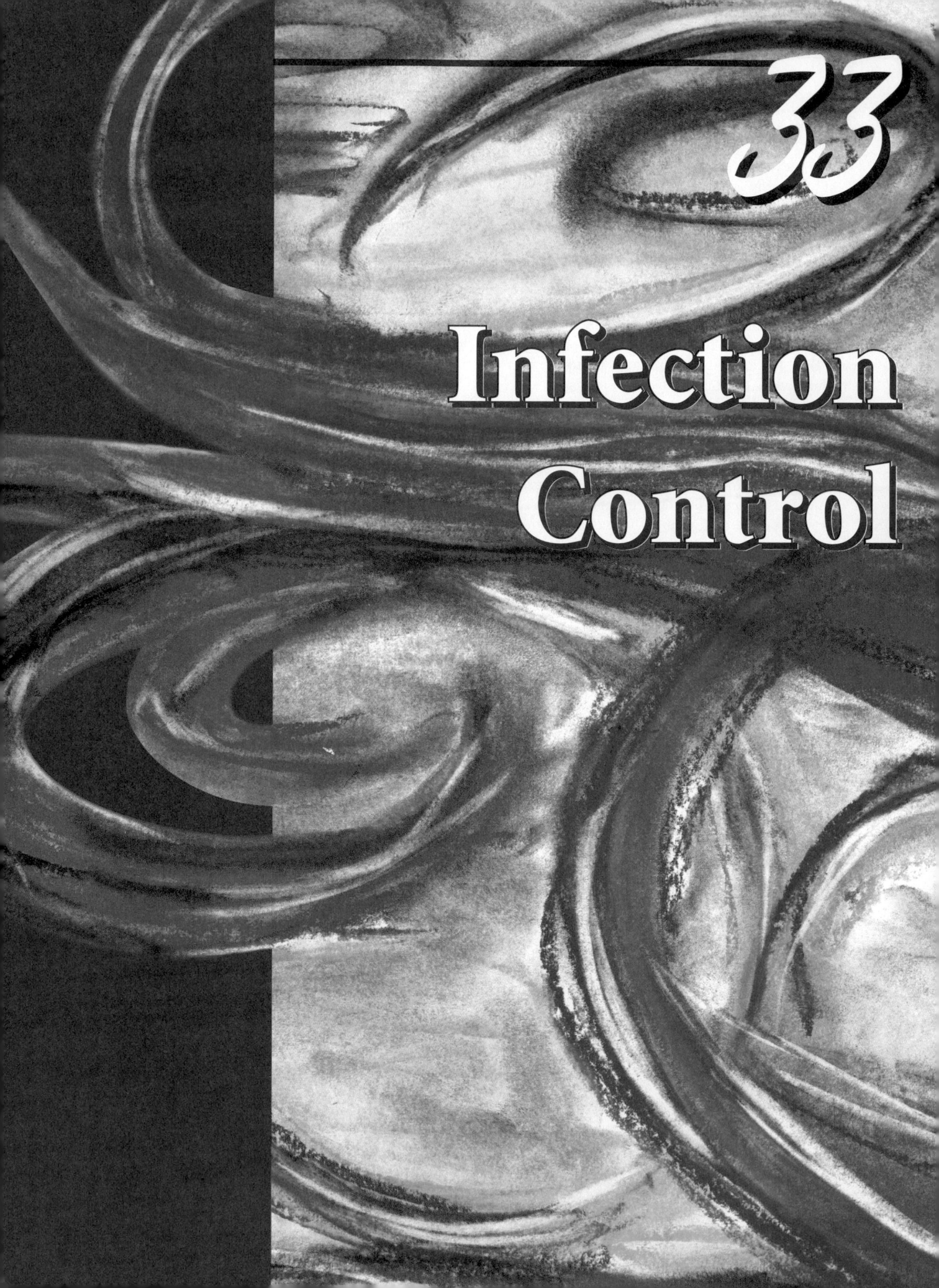

33

Infection Control

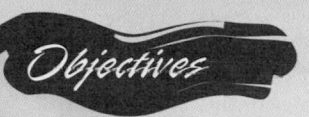
Objectives

Mastery of content in this chapter will enable the student to:

- Define the key terms listed.
- Explain the relationship of the chain of infection to transmission of infection.
- Identify the body's normal defenses against infection.
- Discuss the events in the inflammatory response.
- Explain the difference between cell-mediated and humoral immunity.
- Describe the signs/symptoms of a localized infection and those of a systemic infection.
- Identify clients most at risk for infection.
- Explain conditions that promote the transmission of nosocomial infection.
- Explain the difference between medical and surgical asepsis.
- Give an example for preventing infection for each element of the infection chain.
- Explain the rationale for standard precautions.
- Perform proper procedures for hand washing.
- Explain how infection-control measures may differ in the home versus the hospital.
- Properly don a surgical mask, sterile gown, and sterile gloves.

Good health depends in part on a safe environment. Practices or techniques that control or prevent transmission of infection help to protect clients and health care workers from disease. Clients in all health care settings are at risk for acquiring infections because of lower resistance to infectious **microorganisms**, increased exposure to numbers and types of disease-causing microorganisms, and **invasive** procedures. In acute care or ambulatory care facilities, clients can be exposed to pathogens, some of which may be resistant to most antibiotics. By practicing infection prevention and control techniques, the nurse can avoid spreading microorganisms to clients.

In all settings, clients and their families must be able to recognize sources of infections and be able to institute protective measures. Client teaching should include information concerning infections, modes of transmission, and methods of prevention.

Health care workers can protect themselves from contact with infectious material or exposure to a **communicable** disease by having knowledge of the infectious process and appropriate barrier protection. Diseases such as hepatitis B, acquired immunodeficiency syndrome (AIDS), and tuberculosis have resulted in a greater emphasis on infection-control techniques.

Nature of Infection

An infection is the entry and multiplication of an infectious agent in the tissues of a host. If the infectious agent (**pathogen**) fails to cause injury to cells or tissues, the infection is **asymptomatic**. If the pathogens multiply and cause clinical signs and symptoms, the infection is symptomatic. If the infectious disease can be transmitted directly from one person to another, it is a communicable, or contagious, disease.

CHAIN OF INFECTION

The presence of a pathogen does not mean that an infection will begin. Development of an infection occurs in a cycle that depends on the presence of all of the following elements:

- ℗ An infectious agent or pathogen
- ℝ A reservoir or source for pathogen growth
- Ɛ A portal of exit from the reservoir
- T A mode of transmission
- Ɛ A portal of entry to a host
- H A susceptible host

An infection will develop if this chain remains intact (Figure 33-1). Nurses follow infection prevention and control practices to break the chain so that infection will not develop.

Infectious Agent. Microorganisms include bacteria, viruses, fungi, and protozoa (Table 33-1). Microorganisms on the skin may be resident or transient flora. Resident organisms are considered permanent residents of the skin, where they survive and multiply. Resident organisms are not easily removed by hand washing with plain soaps and detergents unless considerable friction is used. Resident microorganisms in deep skin layers are usually killed only by hand washing with products containing antimicrobial ingredients.

The authors acknowledge the contribution of Mary Dee Miller to this chapter in the previous edition of this text.

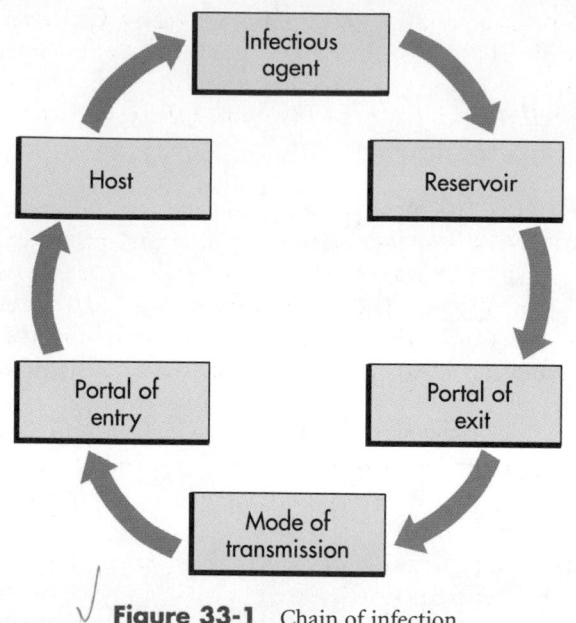

Figure 33-1   Chain of infection.

Transient microorganisms attach to the skin when a person has contact with another person or object during normal activities of living. For example, when a nurse touches a bedpan or a contaminated dressing, transient bacteria adhere to the nurse's skin. The organisms attach loosely to the skin in dirt and grease or under fingernails. These organisms may be readily transmitted unless removed by hand washing (Larson, 1996).

The potential for microorganisms or parasites to cause disease depends on the following factors:
S Sufficient number of organisms
A **Virulence,** or ability to produce disease
E Ability to enter and survive in the host
S Susceptibility of the host

Some resident skin microorganisms are not virulent and may cause only minor skin infections. However, they can cause serious infection when surgery or other invasive procedures allow them to enter deep tissues or when a client is severely **immunocompromised** (impaired immune system).

Table 33-1   Common Pathogens and Some Infections or Diseases They Produce

Organism	Major Reservoir(s)	Major Infections/Diseases
Bacteria		
Escherichia coli	Colon	Gastroenteritis, urinary tract infection
Staphylococcus aureus	Skin, hair, anterior nares	Wound infection, pneumonia, food poisoning, cellulitis
Streptococcus (beta-hemolytic group A) organisms	Oropharynx, skin, perianal area	"Strep throat," rheumatic fever, scarlet fever, impetigo, wound infection
Streptococcus (beta-hemolytic group B) organisms	Adult genitalia	Urinary tract infection, wound infection, postpartum sepsis, neonatal sepsis
Mycobacterium tuberculosis	Droplet nuclei from lungs	Tuberculosis
Neisseria gonorrhoeae	Genitourinary tract, rectum, mouth	Gonorrhea, pelvic inflammatory disease, infectious arthritis, conjunctivitis
Rickettsia rickettsii	Wood tick	Rocky Mountain spotted fever
Staphylococcus epidermidis	Skin	Wound infection, bacteremia, line infection
Viruses		
Hepatitis A virus	Feces	Hepatitis A
Hepatitis B virus	Blood and body fluids	Hepatitis B
Hepatitis C virus	Blood	Hepatitis C
Herpes simplex virus (type I)	Lesions of mouth or skin, saliva, genitalia	Cold sores, aseptic meningitis, sexually transmitted disease, herpetic whitlow
Human immunodeficiency virus (HIV)	Blood, semen, vaginal secretions (also isolated in saliva, tears, urine, and breast milk, but not proved to be sources of transmission)	Acquired immunodeficiency syndrome (AIDS)
Fungi		
Aspergillus organisms	Soil, dust, mouth, skin, colon, genital tract	Aspergillosis, pneumonia, sepsis
Candida albicans	Mouth, skin, colon, genital tract	Candidiasis, pneumonia, sepsis
Protozoa		
Plasmodium falciparum	Blood	Malaria

Reservoir. A reservoir is a place where a pathogen can survive but may or may not multiply. For example, hepatitis A virus survives in shellfish but does not multiply; *Pseudomonas* organisms may survive and multiply in nebulizer reservoirs used in the care of clients with respiratory alterations. The most common reservoir is the human body. A variety of microorganisms live on the skin and within the body cavities, fluids, and discharges. The presence of microorganisms does not always cause a person to be ill. **Carriers** are persons or animals who show no symptoms of illness but who have pathogens on or in their bodies that can be transferred to others. For example, a person can be a carrier of hepatitis B virus without having signs or symptoms of infection. Animals, food, water, insects, and inanimate objects can also be reservoirs for infectious organisms. Shellfish can become contaminated with *Vibrio cholerae,* the bacterium that causes cholera. *Clostridium botulinum* toxin survives in improperly processed foods (e.g., home-canned green beans) to cause botulism. The bacterium *Legionella pneumophila,* which causes Legionnaires' disease, lives in contaminated water and water systems. To thrive, organisms require a proper environment, including food, oxygen, water, appropriate temperature and pH, and light.

Food. Microorganisms require nourishment. Some, such as *Clostridium perfringens,* the microbe that causes gas gangrene, thrive on organic matter. Others, such as *Escherichia coli,* consume undigested foodstuff in the bowel. Carbon dioxide and inorganic material such as soil provide nourishment for other organisms.

Oxygen. **Aerobic** bacteria require oxygen for survival and for multiplication sufficient to cause disease. Aerobic organisms are more commonly the cause of infections in humans, as compared with **anaerobic** organisms. Examples of aerobic organisms are *Staphylococcus aureus* and strains of *Streptococcus* organisms.

Anaerobic bacteria thrive where little or no free oxygen is available. Infections deep within the pleural cavity, in a joint, or in a deep sinus tract are typically caused by anaerobes. Bacteria that cause tetanus, gas gangrene, and botulism are anaerobes.

Water. Most organisms require water or moisture for survival. For example, a favorite place of microorganisms is the moist drainage from a surgical wound. The spirochete that causes syphilis, *Treponema pallidum,* lives only in a moist environment. Some bacteria assume a form, called a spore, that is resistant to drying. These spore-forming bacteria, such as those that cause anthrax, botulism, and tetanus, can live without water.

Temperature. Microorganisms can live only in certain temperature ranges. The ideal temperature for most human pathogens is 35° C (95° F) (Keroack and Rosen-Kotilainen, 1996). However, some can survive temperature extremes that would be fatal to humans. Cold temperatures tend to prevent growth and reproduction of bacteria (**bacteriostasis**). A temperature that destroys bacteria is **bactericidal.**

pH. The acidity of an environment determines the viability of microorganisms. Most microorganisms prefer an environment within a pH range of 5 to 8. Bacteria in particular thrive in urine with an alkaline pH. Most organisms cannot survive the acid environment of the stomach. Acid-reducing medications (e.g., antacids and H_2 blockers) may cause an overgrowth of gastrointestinal organisms, which can contribute to nosocomial pneumonia in a client receiving these medications (Centers for Disease Control and Prevention [CDC], 1997).

Light. Microorganisms thrive in dark environments such as those under dressings and within body cavities. Ultraviolet light may be effective in killing certain forms of bacteria (e.g., *Mycobacterium tuberculosis*).

Portal of Exit. After microorganisms find a site to grow and multiply, they must find a portal of exit if they are to enter another host and cause disease. Microorganisms can exit through a variety of sites, such as the skin and mucous membranes, respiratory tract, urinary tract, gastrointestinal tract, reproductive tract, and blood.

Skin and Mucous Membranes. The skin may be considered a portal of entry because any break in the integrity of the skin and mucous membranes can lead to entry of a pathogen and an infection. Often the body responds to a pathogenic organism with the creation of purulent drainage. For example, *S. aureus* causes a characteristic yellow, creamy drainage, whereas *Pseudomonas aeruginosa* causes a greenish, creamy drainage. This purulent drainage is a potential portal of exit.

Respiratory Tract. Pathogens that infect the respiratory tract, such as *M. tuberculosis,* can be released from the body when an infected person sneezes, coughs, talks, or even breathes. Microorganisms exit through the mouth and nose in normal clients. In clients with artificial airways such as tracheostomy or endotracheal tubes (see Chapter 39), organisms easily exit the respiratory tract through these devices.

Urinary Tract. Normally urine is sterile. However, when a client has a urinary tract infection, microorganisms exit during urination or through urinary diversions such as ileostomies and suprapubic drains (see Chapter 44).

Gastrointestinal Tract. The mouth is one of the most bacterially contaminated sites of the body, although most of the organisms are normal flora—bacteria that normally reside within the body and defend against infection. However, organisms that are normal flora in one person can be pathogens in another. Organisms, for example, exit when a person expectorates saliva. Kissing can also provide a means of exit. Bowel elimination, drainage of bile via surgical wounds or drainage tubes, and escape of gastric contents during vomiting are additional portals of exit.

Reproductive Tract.
Organisms such as *Neisseria gonorrhoeae* and human immunodeficiency virus (HIV) may exit through a man's urethral meatus or a woman's vaginal canal. In the man, semen may be the vehicle of pathogens. Discharge and vaginal fluid from the woman's vaginal canal may carry pathogens.

Blood.
The blood is normally sterile, but in the case of infectious diseases such as hepatitis B or C, it becomes a reservoir for pathogens. A break in the skin allows pathogens to exit the body. Caregivers can easily become exposed unless precautions are taken.

Modes of Transmission.
There are many modes for transmission of microorganisms from the reservoir to the host. Table 33-2 summarizes common modes of transmission. Certain infectious diseases tend to be transmitted more commonly by specific modes. However, the same microorganisms may be transmitted by more than one route. For example, herpes zoster may be spread by the airborne route in droplet nuclei or by direct contact.

Although the major mode of transmission of microorganisms is the hands of the health care worker, almost any object within the environment (e.g., a stethoscope or thermometer) can become a means of transmitting pathogens. All hospital personnel providing direct care (e.g., nurses, physical therapists, and physicians) or performing diagnostic and support services (e.g., laboratory technicians, respiratory therapists, and dietary workers) must follow practices to minimize the spread of infection. Each group follows procedures for handling equipment and supplies used by a client. For example, respiratory therapists wash their hands before working with each client and dispose of soiled therapy equipment in a prescribed man-

Table 33-2 Modes of Transmission

Routes and Means	Examples of Organisms
Contact *gown + gloves*	
Direct	
Person-to-person (fecal, oral) or physical contact between source and susceptible host (e.g., touching client)	Hepatitis A virus, *Shigella, Staphylococcus,* herpes simplex
Indirect	
Personal contact of susceptible host with contaminated inanimate object (e.g., needles or sharp objects, dressings)	Hepatitis B virus, *Staphylococcus,* respiratory syncytial virus (RSV)
Droplet *mask*	
Large particles that travel up to 3 feet and come in contact with susceptible host (e.g., coughing, sneezing, or talking)	Measles virus, influenza virus, rubella virus
Air *neg press room, mask*	
Droplet nuclei, or residue or evaporated droplets suspended in air (e.g., coughing, sneezing) or carried on dust particles	*Mycobacterium tuberculosis* (TB), varicella zoster virus (chickenpox), *Aspergillus*
Vehicles	
Contaminated items	
Water	*Vibrio cholerae*
Drugs, solutions	*Pseudomonas*
Blood	Hepatitis C virus
Food (improperly handled, stored, or cooked, fresh or thawed meats	Salmonella, *Escherichia coli, Clostridium botulinum*
Vector	
External mechanical transfer (flies)	*Vibrio cholerae*
Internal transmission such as parasitic conditions between **vector** and host, such as:	
Mosquito	*Plasmodium falciparum* (malaria)
Louse	*Rickettsia typhi*
Flea	*Yersinia pestis* (plague)

ner. Certain medical devices and diagnostic procedures provide avenues for the spread of pathogens. Invasive procedures such as cystoscopy (visualization of the bladder) facilitate diagnosis of problems but also increase the risk of transmitting infection. Because so many factors can promote the spread of infection to a client, all health care workers must be conscientious in using infection-control practices, such as proper hand washing and ensuring that equipment has been adequately disinfected or sterilized.

Portal of Entry.   Organisms can enter the body through the same routes they use for exiting. For example, when a contaminated needle pierces a client's skin, organisms enter the body. Any obstruction to the flow of urine from a urinary catheter allows organisms to travel up the urethra. Mishandling of sterile bandages over an open wound permits pathogens to enter exposed tissues. Factors that reduce the body's defenses enhance the chances of pathogens entering the body.

Susceptible Host.   Whether a person acquires an infection depends on susceptibility to an infectious agent. **Susceptibility** depends on the individual degree of resistance to a pathogen. Although everyone is constantly in contact with large numbers of microorganisms, an infection will not develop until an individual becomes susceptible to the strength and numbers of microorganisms capable of producing infection. The more virulent an organism, the greater the likelihood of a person's susceptibility. Organisms with greater virulence and resistance to antibiotics are becoming more common in acute care settings. This is believed to be associated with the frequent and sometimes inappropriate use of antibiotics. A person's natural defenses against infection, as well as a number of other factors, influence resistance. A person's resistance to an infectious agent is enhanced by vaccines or by actually contracting the disease.

The Infectious Process

By understanding the chain of infection, the nurse can intervene to prevent infections from developing. When the client acquires an infection, the nurse is able to observe signs and symptoms of infection and take appropriate actions to prevent its spread. Infections follow a progressive course (Box 33-1). The severity of the client's illness depends on the extent of the infection, the **pathogenicity** of the microorganisms, and the susceptibility of the host.

If infection is **localized** (i.e., a wound infection), proper care controls the spread and minimizes the illness. The client may experience localized symptoms such as pain and tenderness at the wound site. An infection that affects the entire body instead of just a single organ or part is **systemic** and can become fatal.

The course of an infection influences the level of nursing care provided. The nurse is responsible for properly

---

Course of Infection by Stage   Box 33-1

INCUBATION PERIOD
- Interval between entrance of pathogen into body and appearance of first symptoms (e.g., chickenpox, 2-3 weeks; common cold, 1-2 days; influenza, 1-3 days; mumps, 18 days)

PRODROMAL STAGE
- Interval from onset of nonspecific signs and symptoms (malaise, low-grade fever, fatigue) to more specific symptoms (During this time, microorganisms grow and multiply, and client is more capable of spreading disease to others.)

ILLNESS STAGE
- Interval when client manifests signs and symptoms specific to type of infection (e.g., common cold manifested by sore throat, sinus congestion, rhinitis; mumps manifested by earache, high fever, parotid and salivary gland swelling)

CONVALESCENCE
- Interval when acute symptoms of infection disappear (Length of recovery depends on severity of infection and client's general state of health; recovery may take several days to months.)

---

administering antibiotics and monitoring the response to drug therapy (see Chapter 34). Supportive therapy includes providing adequate nutrition and rest to bolster defenses against the infectious process. The complexity of care further depends on body systems affected by the infection.

Regardless of whether infection is localized or systemic, the nurse plays a critical role in minimizing its spread. For example, the organism causing a simple wound infection can spread to involve an intravenous (IV) needle insertion site if the nurse uses improper technique during an IV dressing change. Nurses who have breaks in their own skin can also acquire infections from clients if their techniques for controlling infection transmission are inadequate.

DEFENSES AGAINST INFECTION

The body has normal defenses against infection. Normal body flora that reside inside and outside of the body protect a person from several pathogens. Each organ system has defense mechanisms that defend against exposure to infectious microorganisms. The **inflammatory response** is a protective vascular and cellular reaction that neutralizes pathogens and repairs body cells. Normal flora, body system defenses, and inflammation are all nonspecific defenses that protect against microorganisms regardless of prior exposure. The immune system is composed of separate cells and molecules that help the body resist disease. Certain responses of the immune system are nonspecific, whereas others are specific defenses against specific pathogens. If any of the body's defenses fail, an infection can quickly progress to a serious health problem.

Normal Flora.

The body normally contains microorganisms that reside on the surface and deep layers of skin, in the saliva and oral mucosa, and in the gastrointestinal and genitourinary tracts. A person normally excretes trillions of microbes daily through the intestines. The skin also has a large population of resident flora. **Normal flora** do not usually cause disease when residing in their usual area of the body but instead participate in maintaining health.

Normal flora of the large intestine exist in large numbers without causing injury. These bacterial flora compete with disease-producing microorganisms for food. Normal flora also secrete antibacterial substances within the intestine's walls. The skin's normal flora exert a protective action by inhibiting multiplication of organisms landing on the skin. The mouth and pharynx are also protected by flora that impair growth of invading microbes. The mass of normal flora maintains a sensitive balance with other microorganisms to prevent infection. Any factor that disrupts this balance places a person at increased risk for acquiring an infectious disease. For example, the use of **broad-spectrum antibiotics** for the treatment of infection can lead to **suprainfection.** Normal bacterial flora are eliminated, allowing disease-producing microorganisms to multiply.

Body System Defenses.

A number of the body's organ systems have unique defenses against infection (Table 33-3). The skin, respiratory tract, and gastrointestinal tract are easily accessible to microorganisms. Pathogenic organisms easily adhere to the skin's surface, are inhaled into the lungs, or are ingested with food. Each organ system has defense mechanisms physiologically suited to its structure and function. For example, the lungs cannot completely control the entrance of microorganisms. However, the airways are lined with hairlike projections, or cilia, that rhythmically beat to move a blanket of mucus and adherent organisms up to the pharynx to be exhaled. Conditions that impair an organ's specialized defenses increase susceptibility to infection.

Inflammation.

The body's cellular response to injury or infection is inflammation. Inflammation is a protective vascular reaction that delivers fluid, blood products, and nutrients to interstitial tissues in an area of injury. The process neutralizes and eliminates pathogens or dead (**necrotic**) tissues and establishes a means of repairing body cells and tissues. Signs of inflammation may include swelling, redness, heat, pain or tenderness, and loss of function in the affected body part. When inflammation becomes systemic, other signs and symptoms develop, including fever, leukocytosis, malaise, anorexia, nausea, vomiting, and lymph node enlargement.

The inflammatory response may be triggered by physical agents, chemical agents, or microorganisms. Mechanical trauma, temperature extremes, and radiation are examples of physical agents. Chemical agents include external and internal irritants such as harsh poisons or gastric acid. Microorganisms may trigger this response, as previously discussed.

After tissues are injured, a series of well-coordinated events occurs. The inflammatory response includes the following:

1. Vascular and cellular responses
2. Formation of inflammatory **exudate**
3. Tissue repair

Vascular and Cellular Responses.

Acute inflammation is an immediate response to cellular injury. Arterioles supplying the infected or injured area dilate, allowing more blood into the local circulation. The increase in local blood flow causes the characteristic redness of inflammation. The symptom of localized warmth results from a greater volume of blood at the inflammatory site. Local vasodilation delivers blood and white blood cells (WBCs) to injured tissues.

Injury causes tissue necrosis, and as a result the body releases histamine, bradykinin, prostaglandin, and serotonin. These chemical mediators increase the permeability of small blood vessels. Fluid, protein, and cells enter interstitial spaces. Accumulated fluid appears as localized swelling (**edema**).

Another sign of inflammation is pain. The swelling of inflamed tissues increases pressure on nerve endings, causing pain. Chemical substances such as histamine stimulate nerve endings. As a result of physiological changes occurring with inflammation, the involved body part usually undergoes a temporary loss of function. For example, a localized infection of the hand causes the fingers to become swollen, painful, and discolored. Joints may become stiff as a result of swelling, but function of the fingers returns when inflammation subsides.

The cellular response of inflammation involves WBCs arriving at the site. WBCs pass through blood vessels and into the tissues. Through the process of **phagocytosis,** specialized WBCs, called neutrophils and monocytes, ingest and destroy microorganisms or other small particles. As inflammation becomes systemic, other signs and symptoms develop. **Leukocytosis,** or an increase in the number of circulating WBCs, is the body's response to WBCs leaving blood vessels. A serum WBC count is normally 5000 to 10,000/mm^3 but may rise to 15,000 to 20,000/mm^3 and higher during inflammation. Fever is caused by phagocytic release of pyrogens from bacterial cells that cause a rise in the hypothalamic set point (see Chapter 31). Other systemic signs and symptoms include malaise, anorexia, and lymph node enlargement.

Inflammatory Exudate.

Accumulation of fluid and dead tissue cells and WBCs forms an exudate at the site of

Table 33-3   Normal Defense Mechanisms Against Infection

Defense Mechanisms	Action	Factors That May Alter Defense
Skin		
Intact multilayered surface (body's first line of defense against infection)	Provides barrier to microorganisms	Cuts, abrasions, puncture wounds, areas of maceration
Shedding of outer layer of skin cells	Removes organisms that adhere to skin's outer layers	Failure to bathe regularly
Sebum	Contains fatty acid that kills some bacteria	Excessive bathing
Mouth		
Intact multilayered mucosa	Provides mechanical barrier to microorganisms	Lacerations, trauma, extracted teeth
Saliva	Washes away particles containing microorganisms	Poor oral hygiene, dehydration
	Contains microbial inhibitors (e.g., lysozyme)	
Respiratory Tract		
Cilia lining upper airway, coated by mucus	Trap inhaled microbes and sweep them outward in mucus to be expectorated or swallowed	Smoking, high concentration of oxygen and carbon dioxide, decreased humidity, cold air
Macrophages	Engulf and destroy microorganisms that reach lung's alveoli	Smoking
Urinary Tract		
Flushing action of urine flow	Washes away microorganisms on lining of bladder and urethra	Obstruction to normal flow by urinary catheter placement, obstruction from growth or tumor, delayed micturition
Intact multilayered epithelium	Provides barrier to microorganisms	Introduction of urinary catheter, continual movement of catheter in urethra
Gastrointestinal Tract		
Acidity of gastric secretions	Chemically destroys microorganisms incapable of surviving low pH	Administration of antacids
Rapid peristalsis in small intestine	Prevents retention of bacterial contents	Delayed motility resulting from impaction of fecal contents in large bowel or mechanical obstruction by masses
Vagina		
At puberty, normal flora causing vaginal secretions to achieve low pH	Inhibit growth of many microorganisms	Antibiotics and oral contraceptives disrupting normal flora

[Handwritten annotations: "30 ₂ 2nd° Burns Die from mass skin infect"; "mouth Dirtiest part of body"; "Urine is sterile until tract"; "↑ shorter Urethra more susceptible ↑ loca of exit ∴ wipe Front to back"; "HCl"; "Douches excessive alters pH"; "Hypothesis: micro-o Large Intestine → no acid"]

inflammation. Exudate may be **serous** (clear, like plasma), **sanguineous** (containing red blood cells), or **purulent** (containing WBCs and bacteria). Eventually the exudate is cleared away through lymphatic drainage. Platelets and plasma proteins such as fibrinogen form a meshlike matrix at the site of inflammation to prevent its spread.

Tissue Repair.   When there is injury to tissue cells, healing involves the defensive, reconstructive, and maturative stages (see Chapter 47). Damaged cells are eventually replaced with healthy new cells. The new cells undergo a gradual maturation until they take on the same structural characteristics and appearance as the previous cells. If in-

flammation is chronic, tissue defects may fill with fragile **granulation tissue.** Granulation tissue is not as strong as tissue collagen and assumes the form of scar tissue.

Immune Response.   When an invading microorganism enters the body, it is first attacked by monocytes. Remnants of the microorganism then trigger the immune response. The remaining foreign material (**antigen**) causes a series of responses that changes the body's biological makeup so that reactions to future exposures are different from the first reaction. These altered responses are known as **immune responses.** In a normal immune response the antigen is neutralized, destroyed, or eliminated.

Antigens are usually composed of proteins that are not normally found in a person's body. Often antigens exist as part of the structure of a bacterium or virus. After an antigen enters the body, it travels in the blood or lymph and initiates cell-mediated or humoral immunity.

Cell-Mediated Immunity.   There are two classes of lymphocytes: T lymphocytes (CD4T) and B lymphocytes (B cells). T lymphocytes play a major role in cell-mediated immunity. There are antigen receptors on the surface membranes of CD4T lymphocytes. When an antigen meets a cell whose surface receptors fit the antigen, a binding occurs. This binding activates the CD4T lymphocyte to divide rapidly to form sensitized cells. Sensitized CD4T lymphocytes travel to the area of inflammation or injury, bind with antigens, and release chemical compounds called **lymphokines.** The lymphokines attract macrophages and stimulate them to attack antigens. Eventually the antigens are killed. The cell-mediated response is altered by HIV infections which causes AIDS (Figure 33-2).

Humoral Immunity.   Stimulation of B cells triggers the humoral immune response, causing synthesis of immunoglobulins or antibodies that destroy antigens. After a B cell binds with an antigen, it causes formation of plasma and memory B cells. Plasma cells synthesize and secrete large amounts of antibodies, which are proteins normally found in the body that provide general immunity.

Memory B cells prepare the body against future antigen invasion. Thus when an antigen enters the body again, antibodies form more rapidly than during the first exposure, and immunoglobulin levels remain high to attack the antigen.

Antibodies are large protein molecules. There are five classes of antibody **immunoglobulins,** which are identified by the letters *M, G, A, E,* and *D.* Immunoglobulin M (IgM) is the predominant early antibody formed after initial contact with an antigen. This initial contact is the primary immune response, and the presence of IgM denotes current infection. The most abundant circulating antibody is IgG, which is formed after subsequent contacts with antigens or during the secondary immune response, and its presence denotes past infections.

Formation of antibodies is the basis of immunization against disease and can be either a natural or artificially induced event. **Natural immunity** results after having a certain disease, such as measles, and usually lasts a lifetime. **Artificial immunity** follows the receipt of a vaccine, such as tetanus or polio vaccine. The duration is variable and may or may not require a booster vaccine. **Passive immunity** is usually of short duration and is the type that can be obtained transplacentally from mother to child.

Complement.   A **complement** is an inactive protein compound found in blood serum. It is activated when an antigen and antibody bind together. After a complement is activated, a rapid sequence of catalytic activity changes the shape of antigenic cells. The foreign bacteria, for example, assume the shape of a doughnut. The complement actually makes a hole through the antigen's cell membrane. Ions and water enter the cell, causing it to burst. This process is called **cytolysis.**

Interferon.   When certain cells are invaded by viruses, they synthesize the protein interferon. **Interferon** interferes with the ability of viruses to multiply and protects body cells from simultaneous infection with other viruses. Classified as a biological response modifier, interferon also directly inhibits the growth and division of tumor cells (Grimes and Grimes, 1994).

NOSOCOMIAL INFECTIONS

Clients in health care settings may have an increased risk of acquiring infections. **Nosocomial infections** result from delivery of health services in a health care facility. A hospital is one of the most likely places for acquiring an infection because it harbors a high population of virulent strains of microorganisms that may be resistant to antibiotics. The intensive care unit (ICU) is one area in the hospital where the risk of acquiring a nosocomial infection is especially high (Box 33-2). Unfortunately, many nosocomial infections are transmitted by health care workers.

Iatrogenic infections are a type of nosocomial infection resulting from a diagnostic or therapeutic procedure.

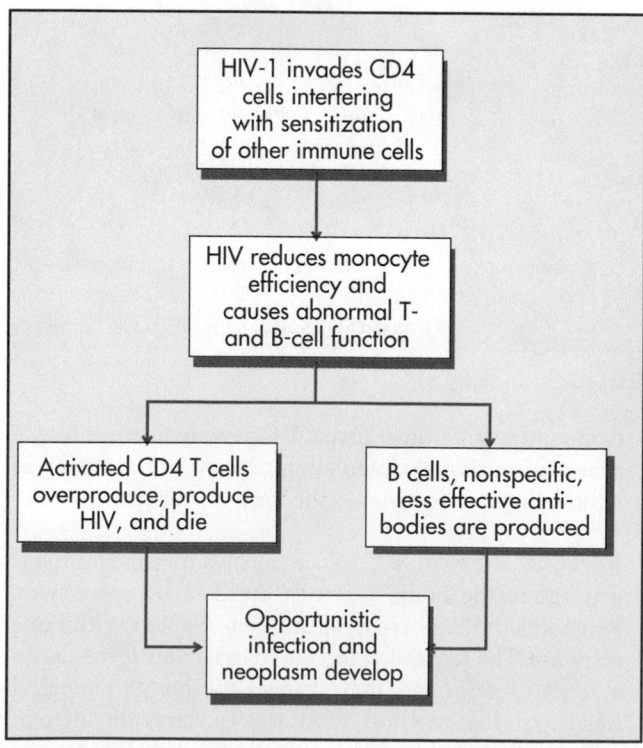

Figure 33-2 Pathologic responses of HIV infection.

A urinary tract infection that develops after catheter insertion is an example of an iatrogenic nosocomial infection. The incidence of nosocomial infections can be reduced if nurses use critical thinking when practicing aseptic techniques. The nurse should always consider the client's risks for infection and anticipate how the approach to care may increase or decrease the chances of infection transmission.

Nosocomial infections may be exogenous or endogenous. An **exogenous infection** arises from microorganisms external to the individual that do not exist as normal flora; examples are *Salmonella* organisms and *Clostridium tetani*. An **endogenous infection** can occur when part of the client's flora becomes altered and an overgrowth results. Examples are infections caused by enterococci, yeasts, and streptococci. When sufficient numbers of microorganisms normally found in one body cavity or lining are transferred to another body site, an endogenous infection develops. For example, transmission of enterococci, normally found in fecal material, from the hands to the skin is a common cause of wound infections. The number of microorganisms needed to cause a nosocomial infection depends on the virulence of the organism, the host's susceptibility, and the site affected.

The number of health care employees having direct contact with a client, the type and number of invasive procedures, the therapy received, and the length of hospitalization influence the risk of infection. Major sites for nosocomial infection include the surgical or traumatic wounds, urinary and respiratory tracts, and bloodstream (Box 33-3).

Nosocomial infections significantly increase costs of health care. Extended stays in health care institutions, increased disability, increased costs of antibiotics, and prolonged recovery times add to the expenses of the client, as well as the expenses of the health care institution and funding bodies (e.g., Medicare). Often, costs for nosocomial infections are not reimbursed; as a result, prevention has a beneficial financial impact and is an important part of managed care.

Risk of Nosocomial Infection in Intensive Care Units   Box 33-2

Nurses working in ICUs should be particularly conscious of aseptic practices. Clients are at risk for infection for the following reasons:

ICU clients are critically ill and often have more underlying disease than other clients.

More invasive devices such as IV or intraarterial lines are used in ICUs.

More invasive procedures are performed in the ICU than in other general care areas.

Often, surgical procedures are performed in the ICU instead of the operating room because of a client's critical condition.

Overuse of broad-spectrum antibiotics causes the formation of resistant microorganisms that later cause infection.

The pace of activities in an ICU can often cause nurses and other health care providers to become less diligent with aseptic technique.

Modified from Crow S: Asepsis: an indispensable part of the patient's care plan, *Crit Care Nurs Q* 11(4):11, 1989.

Sites and Causes for Nosocomial Infections   Box 33-3

URINARY TRACT
Insertion of urinary catheter
Open drainage system
Catheter and tube becoming disconnected
Drainage bag port touching contaminated surface
Improper specimen collection technique
Obstruction or interference with urinary drainage
Urine in catheter or drainage tube being allowed to reenter bladder (reflux)
Improper hand-washing technique
Repeated catheter irrigations with solutions

SURGICAL OR TRAUMATIC WOUNDS
Improper skin preparation (shaving and bathing) before surgery
Improper hand-washing technique
Failure to cleanse skin surface properly
Failure to use aseptic technique during dressing changes
Use of contaminated antiseptic solutions

RESPIRATORY TRACT
Contaminated respiratory therapy equipment
Failure to use aseptic technique while suctioning airway
Improper disposal of mucous secretions
Improper hand-washing technique

BLOODSTREAM
Contamination of IV fluids by tubing or needle changes
Insertion of drug additives to IV fluid
Addition of connecting tube or stopcocks to IV system
Improper care of needle insertion site
Contaminated needles or catheters
Failure to change IV access site when inflammation first appears
Improper technique during administration of multiple blood products
Improper care of peritoneal or hemodialysis shunts
Improper hand-washing technique

The Nursing Process in Infection Control

ASSESSMENT

The nurse assesses the client's defense mechanisms, susceptibility, and knowledge of infections. A review of disease history with the client and family may reveal an exposure to a communicable disease. A thorough review of the client's clinical condition may detect signs and symptoms of infection. An analysis of laboratory findings provides information about a client's defense against infection. By knowing the factors that increase susceptibility or risk for infection, the nurse is better able to plan preventive therapy that includes aseptic techniques. By recognizing early signs and symptoms of infection, the nurse can alert others on the health care team to the potential need for therapy and initiate supportive nursing measures.

Status of Defense Mechanisms.

A review of physical assessment findings and the client's medical condition reveals the status of normal defense mechanisms against infection. For example, any break in the skin or mucosa is a potential site for infection. Similarly, a chronic smoker is at greater risk for acquiring a respiratory tract infection after general surgery because the cilia of the lung are less likely to be active and able to propel retained mucus from the lung's airways. Any reduction in the body's primary or secondary defenses against infection places a client at risk (Box 33-4).

Client Susceptibility.

Many factors influence susceptibility to infection. The nurse gathers information about each factor through the client's and family's history.

Age.

Throughout the life span, susceptibility to infection changes. An infant has immature defenses against infection. Born with only the antibodies provided by the mother, the infant's immune system is incapable of producing the necessary immunoglobulins and WBCs to adequately fight some infections. However, breast-fed infants have greater immunity than bottle-fed infants, because they receive the mother's antibodies through the breast milk. As the child grows, the immune system matures, but the child is still susceptible to organisms that cause the common cold, intestinal infections, and infectious diseases such as mumps and measles if not vaccinated.

The young or middle-age adult has refined defenses against infection. Normal flora, body system defenses, inflammation, and the immune response provide protection against invading microorganisms. Viruses are the most common cause of infectious illness in young or middle-age adults.

Defenses against infection may change with aging (Makris, 1996). The immune response, particularly cell-mediated immunity, declines. Older adults also undergo alterations in the structure and function of the skin, urinary tract, and lungs. For example, the skin loses its turgor and the epithelium thins. As a result, the skin is more easily abraded or torn. This increases the potential for invasion by pathogens (Table 33-4).

Alterations in the immune system may even trigger the aging process. One theory of aging suggests that cells of the immune system, such as lymphocytes, become more diversified with age, and the body undergoes a progressive loss of cellular regulation. When viruses or other antigens and corresponding antibodies lodge in sites such as the kidney and arteries, factors injurious to the tissues are released and deterioration begins. With aging and autoimmune diseases (alterations of the immune system), cellular changes such as depletion of lymphoid tissues occur. The basic mechanism for the aging process is not understood. However, it is known that immunity to infection decreases with advancing age.

Nutritional Status.

When protein intake is inadequate as a result of poor diet or debilitating disease, the rate of protein breakdown exceeds that of tissue synthesis (see Chapter 43). A reduction in the intake of protein and other nutrients such as carbohydrates and fats reduces the body's defenses against infection and impairs wound healing (see Chapter 47).

Clients with illnesses or problems that increase protein requirements are at further risk. These problems include traumatic injury, extensive burns, and conditions causing fever. Clients who have had surgery also require increased protein.

The nurse assesses clients' dietary intakes and abilities to tolerate solid foods. Clients who have difficulty with swallowing, who experience alterations in digestion, or who are too confused or weak to feed themselves are at risk for inadequate dietary intake. A dietitian may be called to assist in calculating the calorie count of foods ingested. In preparation for discharge, the nurse evaluates

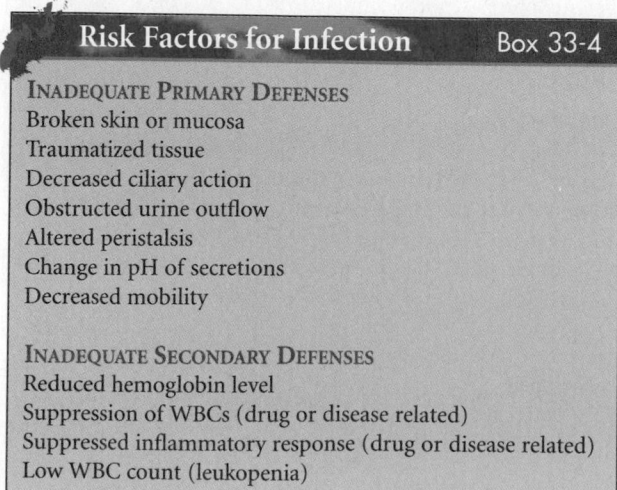

Risk Factors for Infection	Box 33-4

INADEQUATE PRIMARY DEFENSES
Broken skin or mucosa
Traumatized tissue
Decreased ciliary action
Obstructed urine outflow
Altered peristalsis
Change in pH of secretions
Decreased mobility

INADEQUATE SECONDARY DEFENSES
Reduced hemoglobin level
Suppression of WBCs (drug or disease related)
Suppressed inflammatory response (drug or disease related)
Low WBC count (leukopenia)

Table 33-4   Assessing the Risk of Infection in Older Adults

Component	Possible Changes With Age	Outcome
Skin	Thinner dermal and epidermal layers, decreased collagen strength, decreased skin elasticity, decreased sweat	Pressure ulcers
Peripheral nerves	Reduced sensitivity, particularly in clients with history of alcohol abuse, vitamin B_{12} deficiency, and diabetes mellitus	Pressure ulcers, ignored trauma leading to infection
Circulation	Congestive heart failure, calcified mitral and aortic valves	Pneumonia, bacterial endocarditis
Peripheral circulation	More elastic veins, less effective venous valves, blood pooling in lower extremities	Venous stasis ulcers
Mouth	Dehydration, loss of saliva production, functional inability to maintain oral hygiene	Parotid gland infection, peridontal disease, localized abscess, bacteremia
Gastrointestinal tract	Loss of ability to secrete stomach acid in 30% of persons over 70	Salmonella diarrhea
Pulmonary system	Increased colonization of oropharynx, impaired mucociliary clearance, decreased macrophage function, decreased cough reflex	Viral and bacterial pneumonia
Urinary tract	Prostatic hyperplasia, urethral strictures, age-related hormonal changes in vaginal wall, pelvic floor relaxation, ureterocele or cystocele, degeneration of nerves leading to neurogenic bladder, use of tricyclic antidepressants, dehydration	Asymptomatic bacteriuria, cystitis, pyelonephritis
Nutrition	Malnutrition, vitamin deficiency (vitamin A, pyridoxine, and riboflavin), protein and caloric malnutrition	Impaired immune response to infection
Drug therapy	Corticosteroid and cytotoxic drugs	Impaired immune response to infection
Nursing home residency	Exposure to nosocomial infections, including influenza, *Proteus* and *Providencia* organisms with an indwelling catheter, tuberculosis, and wound infections. (Incidence of bacteremia after admission is 50%).	Frequent serious infection, increased risk of pneumonia

Modified from Tideiksaar R: Infections in the elderly. I. Diagnosis and treatment, *Physician Assist* 11(2):17, 1987.

the client's and family's understanding of nutritional needs.

Stress. The body responds to emotional or physical stress by the general adaptation syndrome (see Chapter 30). During the alarm stage, the basal metabolic rate increases as the body uses energy stores. Adrenocorticotropic hormone (ACTH) acts to increase serum glucose levels and decrease unnecessary antiinflammatory responses through the release of cortisone. If stress continues or becomes intense, elevated cortisone levels result in decreased resistance to infection. Continued stress leads to exhaustion, wherein energy stores are depleted and the body has no resistance to invading organisms. The same conditions that increase nutritional requirements, such as surgery or trauma, also increase physiological stress.

Heredity. Certain hereditary conditions impair an individual's response to infection. The client's history of preexisting medical problems should reveal known hereditary disorders. For example, agammaglobulinemia is a rare inherited or acquired disorder characterized by the absence of serum antibodies. The client with this disorder has virtually no ability to initiate defenses because of the inability to form antibodies.

Disease Process. Clients with diseases of the immune system are at particular risk for infection. Leukemia, AIDS, lymphoma, and aplastic anemia are conditions that compromise a host by weakening defenses against infectious organisms. Clients with leukemia, for example, are unable to produce enough WBCs to ward off infection.

Victims of chronic diseases such as diabetes mellitus and multiple sclerosis are also more susceptible to infection because of general debilitation and nutritional impairment. Diseases that impair body system defenses, such as pulmonary emphysema and bronchitis (which impair ciliary action and thicken mucus), cancer (which alters the immune response), and peripheral vascular disease (which reduces blood flow to injured tissues), increase susceptibility to infection. Burn clients have a very high susceptibility to infection because of the damage to skin surfaces. The greater the depth and extent of the burns, the higher the risk for infection.

Medical Therapy.   Some drug and medical therapies compromise immunity to infection. The nurse assesses the client's history to determine whether the client takes medications at home that increase infection susceptibility. A review of therapies received within the health care setting further reveals risks. Adrenal corticosteroids, prescribed for several conditions, are antiinflammatory drugs that cause protein breakdown and impair the inflammatory response against bacteria and other pathogens. Cytotoxic or antineoplastic drugs attack cancer cells but cause side effects of bone marrow depression and normal cell toxicity. With bone marrow depression the body is unable to produce lymphocytes and sufficient WBCs. When normal cells become altered by antineoplastic agents, cellular defenses against infection fail. Cyclosporine and other immunosuppressant drugs, which decrease the body's immune response, are commonly taken by clients who are organ transplant recipients. The immunosuppressants prevent organ and tissue rejection, but they increase susceptibility to infection.

Cancer clients receiving radiotherapy are also at risk for infection. The massive doses of radiation, which destroy cancerous cells, can also depress the bone marrow and destroy normal cells.

Clinical Appearance.

The signs and symptoms of infection may be local or systemic. Localized infections are most common in areas of skin or mucous membrane breakdown, such as surgical and traumatic wounds, pressure ulcers, and mouth lesions. Infections also develop locally in cavities beneath the skin; an example is an abscess.

To assess an area for localized infection, the nurse first inspects the area for redness and swelling caused by inflammation. Because there may be drainage from open lesions or wounds, the nurse wears gloves. Infected drainage may be yellow, green, or brown, depending on the pathogen. The nurse asks the client about pain or tenderness around the site. The client may complain of tightness and pain caused by edema. If the infected area is large enough, movement of a body part may be restricted. Gentle palpation of an infected area usually results in some degree of tenderness.

Systemic infections cause more generalized symptoms than local infection. They usually result in fever, fatigue, and malaise. Lymph nodes that drain the area of infection often become enlarged, swollen, and tender during palpation. For example, an abscess in the peritoneal cavity may cause enlargement of lymph nodes in the groin. An infection of the upper respiratory tract may cause cervical lymph node enlargement. If an infection is serious and widespread, all major lymph nodes may enlarge. Systemic infections commonly cause a loss of appetite, nausea, and vomiting.

Systemic infections may develop after treatment for localized infection has failed. The nurse should be alert for changes in the client's level of activity and responsiveness.

As systemic infections develop, the client may become lethargic and complain of a loss of energy. An elevation in body temperature may lead to episodes of increased heart and respiratory rates. Involvement of major body systems may produce specific signs. For example, a pulmonary infection may result in a productive cough with purulent sputum. A urinary tract infection may result in cloudy, foul-smelling urine.

An infection in older adults may not present with typical signs and symptoms. Often, older adults have advanced infection before it is identified. This is because of their reduced inflammatory and immune responses. Normally, older adults have increased fatigue and diminished pain sensitivity. A reduced or absent fever response may occur from chronic use of aspirin or nonsteroidal antiinflammatory drugs. Atypical symptoms such as confusion, incontinence, or agitation may be the only symptoms of an infectious illness (Makris, 1996). An example is pneumonia, the main complication of influenza. As many as 20% of older adults with pneumonia do not have the typical signs and symptoms of fever, shaking, chills, and rusty productive sputum. The only symptoms may be an increased, unexplained heart rate or generalized fatigue.

Laboratory Data.

A review of laboratory test results may reveal infection (Table 33-5). Laboratory values, however, are not enough to detect infection. Other clinical signs must be assessed. Factors other than infection may alter test values. For example, trauma and physical stress can cause an elevation in the number of neutrophils. A culture result may show growth of an organism in the absence of infection.

Clients With Infection.

A client with infection may have a variety of health problems. The nurse assesses ways that the infection affects the client's and family's needs. These may be physical, psychological, social, or economical. For example, a client with a chronic disease such as AIDS may experience serious psychological problems as a result of self-imposed isolation or rejection by family and friends. Clients or their families may not be able to afford the cost of medical care. The nurse, using a case management approach, determines the client's and family's ability to adjust to the disease and the available resources needed for managing health care challenges (Grimes and Grimes, 1994).

NURSING DIAGNOSIS

During assessment the nurse gathers objective findings, such as an open incision or a reduced caloric intake, and subjective data, such as a client's complaint of tenderness over a surgical wound site. Then the nurse interprets the data carefully, looking for clusters of defining characteristics or risk factors that create a pattern suggesting a specific nursing diagnosis (Box 33-5). It may be nec-

Table 33-5   Laboratory Tests to Screen for Infection

Laboratory Value	Normal (Adult) Values	Indication of Infection
WBC count	5000-10,000/mm³	Increased in acute infection, decreased in certain viral or overwhelming infections
Erythrocyte sedimentation rate	Up to 15 mm/hr for men and 20 mm/hr for women	Elevated in presence of inflammatory process
Iron level	60-90 g/100 ml	Decreased in chronic infection
Cultures of urine and blood	Normally sterile, without microorganism growth	Presence of infectious microorganism growth
Cultures of wound, sputum, and throat	Possible normal flora	Presence of infectious microorganism growth
Differential Count (Percentage of Each Type of WBC)		
Neutrophils	55%-70%	Increased in acute suppurative infection, decreased in overwhelming bacterial infection (older adult)
Lymphocytes	20%-40%	Increased in chronic bacterial and viral infection, decreased in sepsis
Monocytes	2%-8%	Increased in protozoal, rickettsial, and tuberculosis infections
Eosinophils	1%-4%	Increased in parasitic infection
Basophils	0.5%-1%	Normal during infection

NURSING DIAGNOSES   Box 33-5

INFECTION

Body image disturbance
Infection, risk for
Injury, risk for
Nutrition, altered: less than body requirements
Oral mucous membrane, altered
Skin integrity, impaired, risk for
Social isolation
Tissue integrity, impaired

essary for the nurse to validate data (e.g., by inspecting the integrity of a wound more carefully). Likewise, additional data such as laboratory findings may help. The selection of appropriate nursing diagnoses depends on analyzing and organizing data correctly (Box 33-6).

The diagnosis must have the appropriate etiological factor for the nurse to establish an appropriate and well-thought-out plan. For example, minimizing the *risk for infection related to broken skin* requires good hygiene measures and wound care. Minimizing the *risk for infection related to malnutrition* requires good nutritional support and fluid balance.

The nurse may diagnose a risk for infection or make diagnoses that result from the effects of infection on health status. The nurse's success in planning appropriate nursing interventions depends on the accuracy of the diagnosis and the ability to meet the client's needs.

PLANNING

The client's care plan is based on each nursing diagnosis and related factor. The nurse's aim is to develop a plan that sets attainable outcomes so that interventions are purposeful and directed. The nurse caring for the client with the nursing diagnosis of *risk for infection related to broken skin* implements skin care and measures to promote healing. The expected outcomes of "reduction in wound size by 1 cm" and "absence of drainage" set targets for measuring the client's improvement. Once outcomes are met, the goal of "skin intact and without drainage" can be reached. Interventions are selected in collaboration with the client, the family, and others on the health care team. The nurse directs the care in the acute care setting and may involve the dietitian or respiratory therapist in assisting with instruction of procedures that need to be followed after discharge. Common goals of care may include the following:

Preventing exposure to infectious organisms
Controlling or reducing the extent of infection
Maintaining resistance to infection
Educating the client and family about infection control techniques

The nurse establishes priorities for the goals of care. For example, a client has developed an open wound, suffers a debilitating disease such as cancer, and has been unable to tolerate solid foods. The priority of administering therapies that promote wound healing exceeds the goal of educating the client to assume self-care therapies at home. When the client's condition improves, the priorities will change, and client education becomes an essential intervention.

Assessment Activities	Defining Characteristics	Nursing Diagnoses
Check results of laboratory tests.	WBC count 5000/mm³	Risk for infection related to lowered immunity
Review current medications.	Client receiving azathioprine (Imuran), an immunosuppressant	
Identify potential sites of infection.	IV catheter in right forearm, in place for 3 days	
	Foley catheter draining amber-colored urine	
Inspect condition of dependent pressure points.	Area 2 cm in diameter, superficial broken skin over sacrum	Impaired skin integrity related to pressure and exposure to fecal irritants
Observe for skin contamination.	Client incontinent (semiliquid stool)	

The development of a care plan includes infection prevention practices. The nurse may initiate appropriate referrals, such as a dietitian, infection-control professional, or home health care nurse, to collaborate in the client's care. When care is being administered in the home, the nurse plans to be sure the environment promotes good infection-control practices. For example, if a client does not have running water yet requires wound care, even simple hand washing is difficult to achieve. The nurse will bring an antimicrobial solution during visits to ensure adequate hand cleansing. Educating clients and families is also an important aspect of prevention.

IMPLEMENTATION

By recognizing and assessing a client's risk factors and implementing appropriate measures, the nurse can reduce the risk of infection.

Health Promotion. Through critical thinking, the nurse may prevent an infection from developing or spreading by minimizing the numbers and kinds of organisms transmitted to potential infection sites. Eliminating reservoirs of infection, controlling portals of exit and entry, and avoiding actions that transmit microorganisms prevent bacteria from finding a new site in which to grow. Proper use of sterile supplies, barrier protection, and proper hand washing are examples of methods that the nurse may use to control the spread of microorganisms. A final preventive measure is to strengthen a potential host's defenses against infection. Nutritional support, rest, maintenance of physiological protective mechanisms, and recommended immunizations protect a client from invasion by pathogens. Having an infection-control conscience helps the nurse to apply good medical-surgical aseptic practices at the right time and in the right clinical situa-

tion. When a client develops an infection, the nurse continues preventive care so that health care personnel and other clients are not exposed to the infection. Clients with communicable diseases may require isolation precautions that control the environment by forming barriers against transmission of infection.

Acute Care Measures. Treatment of an infectious process includes eliminating the infectious organisms and supporting the client's defenses. To identify the causative organism, the nurse may collect specimens of body fluids or drainage from infected body sites for cultures. When the disease process or causative organism has been identified, the physician prescribes the treatment that is most effective for the situation. The nurse properly administers antibiotics and other treatments, watching for adverse reactions and assessing the progress of the infection.

Systemic infections require measures to prevent complications of fever (see Chapter 31). Maintaining intake of fluids prevents dehydration resulting from diaphoresis. The client's increased metabolic rate requires an adequate nutritional intake. Rest preserves energy for the healing process.

Localized infections often require measures to facilitate removal of debris to promote healing. The nurse applies principles of wound care to remove infected drainage from wound sites and support the integrity of healing wounds. Special dressings can be applied to facilitate removal of infectious drainage and promote healing of wound margins. Drainage tubes may be inserted to remove infected drainage from body cavities. The nurse uses medical and surgical aseptic techniques to manage wounds and ensure correct handling of all drainage or body fluids.

During the course of infection the nurse supports the client's body defense mechanisms. For example, if a client has infectious diarrhea, the nurse must maintain skin integrity to prevent breakdown and the entrance of microorganisms. Other routine hygiene measures such as cleansing the oral cavity and bathing protect the skin and mucous membranes from invasion and overgrowth of microorganisms.

Asepsis. The nurse's efforts to minimize the onset and spread of infection are based on the principles of aseptic technique. **Asepsis** is the absence of pathogenic (disease-producing) microorganisms. Aseptic technique refers to practices that keep a client as free from microorganisms as possible. The two types of aseptic technique are medical and surgical asepsis.

Medical asepsis, or clean technique, includes procedures used to reduce and prevent the spread of microorganisms. Hand washing, using clean gloves to prevent direct contact with blood or body fluids, and cleaning the environment routinely are examples of medical asepsis. Principles of medical asepsis are commonly followed in the home, as in washing hands before preparing food.

After an object becomes unsterile or unclean, it is considered contaminated. In medical asepsis an area or object is considered contaminated if it contains or is suspected of containing pathogens. For example, a used bedpan, the floor, and a wet piece of gauze are contaminated.

The nurse follows certain principles and procedures to prevent infection and control its spread. During daily routine care the nurse uses basic medical aseptic techniques to break the infection chain. Because infections are readily transmissible between clients and caregivers, it may become necessary for the nurse to follow isolation precautions as appropriate.

The nurse is responsible for providing the client with a safe environment. The effectiveness of infection-control practices depends on the nurse's conscientiousness and consistency in using effective aseptic technique. It is easy to forget key procedural steps or, when hurried, to take shortcuts that break aseptic procedures. However, the nurse's failure to be meticulous will place the client at risk for an infection that can seriously impair recovery or lead to death.

Control or Elimination of Infectious Agents. Proper cleansing, disinfection, and sterilization of contaminated objects significantly reduce and often eliminate microorganisms. In health care centers a central supply department disinfects and sterilizes reusable supplies. However, the nurse also may be required to perform these functions. Many principles of cleaning and disinfection also apply to the home.

Cleaning. Cleaning is the removal of all foreign materials, such as soil and organic material, from objects (Rutala and Shafer, 1996). Generally, cleaning involves use of water and mechanical action with or without detergents.

When an object comes in contact with infectious or potentially infectious material, the object is contaminated. If the object is disposable, it is usually discarded unless formal policies and procedures are in place for reprocessing the object. Reusable objects must be cleaned thoroughly before reuse and then either disinfected or sterilized.

When cleaning equipment that is soiled by organic material such as blood, fecal matter, mucus, or pus, the nurse applies a mask and protective eyewear (or a face shield), and waterproof gloves. These barriers provide protection from infectious organisms. A stiff-bristled brush and detergent or soap are needed for cleaning. The following steps ensure that an object is clean:

1. Rinse a contaminated object or article with cold running water to remove organic material. Hot water causes the protein in organic material to coagulate and stick to objects, making removal difficult.
2. After rinsing, wash the object with soap and warm water. Soap or detergent reduces the surface tension of water and emulsifies dirt or remaining material. Few household detergents, however, have disinfectant properties. Rinse the object thoroughly to remove the emulsified dirt.
3. Use a brush to remove dirt or material in grooves or seams. Friction dislodges contaminated material for easy removal. Open any hinged items for cleaning.
4. Rinse the object in warm water.
5. Dry the object and prepare it for disinfection or sterilization if indicated by the intended use of the item.
6. The brush, gloves, and sink in which the equipment is cleaned should be considered contaminated and should be cleaned and dried.

Disinfection and Sterilization. **Disinfection** describes a process that eliminates many or all microorganisms, with the exception of bacterial spores, from inanimate objects (Rutala and Shafer, 1996). This is generally accomplished by the use of a chemical disinfectant or wet pasteurization (used for respiratory therapy equipment). Examples of disinfectants are alcohols, chlorines, glutaraldehydes, and phenols. These chemicals can be caustic and toxic to tissues.

Sterilization is the complete elimination or destruction of all microorganisms, including spores. Steam under pressure, ethylene oxide (ETO) gas, hydrogen peroxide plasma, and chemicals are the most common sterilizing agents.

Whether an item is to be simply cleaned, or cleaned and disinfected or sterilized, depends on the intended use of the item. There are three categories of device classification (Box 33-7). Nurses should be familiar with agency policy and procedures for cleaning, handling, and delivering care items for eventual disinfection and sterilization. Workers especially trained in disinfection and sterilization should perform most of the procedures. Efficacy of the disinfecting or sterilizing method is influenced by the following factors:

Concentration of solution and duration of contact. A weakened concentration or shortened exposure time may lessen effectiveness.

Type and number of pathogens. Certain organisms are killed more easily than others by disruption. The greater the number of pathogens on an object, the longer the required disinfecting time.

Surface areas to treat. All dirty surfaces and areas must be fully exposed to disinfecting and sterilizing agents.

Temperature of the environment. Disinfectants tend to work best at room temperature.

Presence of soap. Soap may cause certain disinfectants to be ineffective. Thorough rinsing of an object is necessary before disinfecting.

Presence of organic materials. Disinfectants can become inactivated unless blood, saliva, pus, or body excretions are washed off.

Table 33-6 lists processes for disinfection and sterilization and their characteristics. Selection of the method for disinfecting or sterilizing an item depends on the intended use of the item and the nature of the item (e.g., some delicate instruments requiring sterilization cannot tolerate steam and must be processed using gas or plasma).

Control or Elimination of Reservoirs.   To control or eliminate reservoir sites for infection, the nurse eliminates or controls sources of body fluids, drainage, or solutions that might harbor microorganisms. The nurse also carefully discards articles that become contaminated with infectious material (Box 33-8). The Occupational Safety and Health Act of 1991 set standards for minimizing oc-

---

Categories for Sterilization, Disinfection, and Cleaning   Box 33-7

CRITICAL ITEMS

Items that enter sterile tissue or the vascular system present a high risk of infection if the items are contaminated with microorganisms, especially bacterial spores. *Critical* items must be *sterile.* Some of these items follow:

Surgical instruments
Intravascular catheters
Urinary catheters
Needles

SEMICRITICAL ITEMS

Items that come in contact with mucous membranes or skin that is not intact also present risks. These objects must be free of all microorganisms (except bacterial spores). *Semicritical items* must be *disinfected* or *sterilized.* Some of these items follow:

Respiratory suction tubing and catheters
Endotracheal tubes
Gastrointestinal endoscopes
Reusable glass thermometers

NONCRITICAL ITEMS

Items that come in contact with intact skin but not mucous membranes must be clean. *Noncritical items* must be *disinfected.* Some of these items follow:

Bedpans
Blood pressure cuffs
Linens
Stethoscopes
Food utensils

Infection Control to Reduce Reservoirs of Infection   Box 33-8

BATHING

Use soap and water to remove drainage, dried secretions, or excess perspiration.

DRESSING CHANGES

Change dressings that become wet and/or soiled (see Chapter 47).

CONTAMINATED ARTICLES

Place tissues, soiled dressings, or soiled linen in moisture-resistant bags for proper disposal.

CONTAMINATED NEEDLES

Place syringes and uncapped hypodermic needles and IV needles in puncture-proof containers, which should be located in client rooms or treatment areas so that exposed, contaminated equipment need not be carried a distance (see Chapter 34).
Do not recap needles or attempt to break them.

BEDSIDE UNIT

Keep table surfaces clean and dry.

BOTTLED SOLUTIONS

Do not leave bottled solutions open for prolonged periods.
Keep solutions tightly capped.
Date bottles when opened and discard according to facility policy.

SURGICAL WOUNDS

Keep drainage tubes and collection bags patent to prevent accumulation of serous fluid under the skin surface.

DRAINAGE BOTTLES AND BAGS

Empty and dispose of drainage suction bottles according to facility policy.
Empty all drainage systems on each shift unless otherwise ordered by a physician.
Never raise a drainage system (e.g., urinary drainage bag) above the level of the site being drained unless it is clamped off.

Table 33-6   Examples of Disinfection and Sterilization Processes

Characteristics	Examples of Use
Moist Heat Moist heat includes steam (moist heat under pressure). When exposed to high pressure, water vapor can attain temperature above boiling point to kill pathogens and spores.	Autoclave is used to sterilize surgical instruments, parenteral solutions, and surgical dressings.
Radiation Ionizing radiation penetrates deeply into objects for effective sterilization and disinfection.	Radiation is used in sterilizing drugs, foods, and other heat-sensitive items.
Chemicals Chemicals are effective disinfectants because they attack all types of microorganisms, act rapidly, work with water, retain no order, are stable in light and heat, are inexpensive, are not harmful to body tissues, do not destroy article being disinfected, and are not inactivated by organic material.	Chemicals are used for disinfection of instruments and equipment such as glass thermometer. Chlorine is useful for disinfecting water and for housekeeping purposes.
Ethylene Oxide Gas This gas destroys spores and microorganisms by altering cells' metabolic processes. Fumes are released within an autoclave-like chamber. Ethylene oxide gas is toxic to humans, and aeration time varies with products.	This gas sterilizes some rubber and plastic items.
Boiling Water Boiling is least expensive for use in home. Bacterial spores and some viruses resist boiling. It is not used in hospitals.	The items (e.g., glass baby bottles) should be boiled for at least 15 minutes.

cupational exposure to blood-borne pathogens or other potentially infectious materials (Occupational Safety and Health Administration [OSHA], 1991). All health care institutions must have guidelines for the disposal of infectious waste according to local and state regulations.

Control of Portals of Exit.   The nurse follows prevention and control practices to minimize or prevent infectious organisms from exiting the body. To control organisms exiting via the respiratory tract, the nurse should avoid talking directly into clients' faces or talking, sneezing, or coughing directly over surgical wounds or sterile dressing fields. The nurse should cover the mouth or nose when sneezing or coughing. The nurse is also responsible for teaching clients to protect others when they sneeze or cough and for providing clients with disposable wipes or tissues to control the spread of microorganisms.

A nurse who has an upper respiratory tract infection and continues to work with clients should wear a mask when working closely with the client and pay special attention to hand washing. The same nurse should refrain from working with clients who are highly susceptible to infection (e.g., an immunosuppressed client or a neonate).

Another way of controlling the exit of microorganisms is through the careful handling of exudate (i.e., urine, feces, emesis, and blood). Contaminated fluids can easily splash while being discarded in toilets or hoppers. The nurse should always wear disposable gloves when handling exudate. Masks, gowns, and protective eyewear are worn if there is a possibility of splashing or contact with any fluids. The nurse appropriately disposes of disposable soiled items in trash bags. Laboratory specimens from all clients are handled as if they were infectious.

Control of Transmission.   Effective control of infection requires a nurse to remain aware of the modes of transmission and ways to control them. In the hospital, home, or extended care facility a client should have a personal set of care items. Sharing bedpans, urinals, bath basins, and eating utensils can easily lead to transmission of infection. Glass thermometers, even when individually used, warrant special care. Because the client's own mucus can become a source for microorganism growth, the glass thermometer is washed in soap and water and dried after each use. Single-use chemical strip thermometers present less risk of infection than glass thermometers. There has been research to suggest that use of electronic thermometers for rectal temperatures can be associated with nosocomial diarrhea (Jernigan and others, 1998). Specifically, the organism *Clostridium difficile* is able to survive on inanimate surfaces such as the thermometer probe. In institutions where nosocomial diarrhea is common, electronic thermometers are not recommended for rectal temperatures. The same electronic thermometer should not be used for clients on contact isolation.

To prevent transmission of microorganisms through indirect contact, soiled items and equipment must be kept from touching the nurse's clothing. A common error is to carry dirty linen in the arms against the uniform. Fluid-resistant linen bags should be used, or soiled linen should be carried with hands held out from the body. Laundry hampers should be replaced before they are overflowing.

Hand Washing. The most important and most basic technique in preventing and controlling transmission of infections is hand washing. **Hand washing** is a vigorous, brief rubbing together of all surfaces of the hands lathered in soap, followed by rinsing under a stream of water (Larson, 1996). The purpose is to remove soil and transient organisms from the hands and to reduce total microbial counts over time.

Contaminated hands are a prime cause of cross infection. For example, a nurse caring for a client who has excessive pulmonary secretions assists the client in expectorating mucus and disposes of the tissues in a bedside container. The client's roommate asks the nurse to open containers of food on the meal tray. The nurse then leaves the client's room to pour a dose of medication that is due in 5 minutes. If the nurse fails to wash hands before opening the containers of food or pouring the medication, organisms from the first client's mucus could easily be transmitted to the roommate's food or to the medication container.

The decision regarding when hand washing should occur depends on the following: the intensity of contact with clients or contaminated objects; the degree or amount of contamination that could occur with that contact; the susceptibility of the client or the health care worker to infection; and the procedure or activity to be performed (Larson, 1996). For example, prolonged and intense contact with a client's wound drainage would require thorough hand washing. Larson (1996) recommends that nurses wash hands in the following situations:

When the hands are visibly soiled

Before and after client contact

After contact with a source of microorganisms (blood or body fluids, mucous membrane, nonintact skin, or inanimate objects that might be contaminated)

Before the performance of invasive procedures such as placement of intravascular catheters or indwelling catheters (antimicrobial soap recommended)

After removing gloves

The Centers for Disease Control and Prevention (CDC) and the U.S. Public Health Service note that washing times of at least 10 to 15 seconds (Larson, 1996) will remove most transient microorganisms from the skin. If the hands are visibly soiled, more time may be needed. Routine hand washing may be performed with plain soap. Plain soap with water can physically remove a certain level of microbes, but antiseptic agents are necessary to kill or inhibit microorganisms and reduce the level still further (Larson, 1996).

Use of antimicrobial soap is encouraged in certain high-risk situations when nurses need to reduce total microbial counts on their hands. These include situations wherein nurses are in contact with clients who are immunosuppressed or have damage to their integumentary system (e.g., wounds or bruises). In addition, an antimicrobial soap should be used before performing an invasive procedure such as care or insertion of an intravascular catheter. There are a number of effective antimicrobial soaps, including chlorhexidine gluconate (CHG), alcohols, and iodophors. Certain antimicrobial soaps can irritate the skin, and the need for antimicrobial soap must be evaluated against the potential for skin irritation (Box 33-9). Skill 33-1 lists the steps for hand washing.

Plain soap with water can be used for general hand washing, but if it is necessary to kill or inhibit microorganisms, such as in a surgical procedure, antiseptic agents should be used (Larson, 1996). Additional alcohol-based solutions are recommended for use in settings where hand-washing facilities are inadequate or inaccessible and hands are not heavily soiled (Larson, 1996). If these solutions are used as a substitute for hand washing, hand washing with soap and water should be performed as soon as possible (OSHA, 1991).

The nurse instructs clients and visitors about the proper technique and times for hand washing. Teaching hand washing is particularly important if health care is to continue at home. Clients should wash their hands before eating or handling food; after handling contaminated equipment, linen, or organic material; and after elimination. Visitors are encouraged to wash their hands before eating or handling food, after coming in contact with infected clients, and after handling contaminated equipment or organic material.

Control of Portals of Entry. Many measures that control the exit of microorganisms likewise control the entrance of pathogens. Maintaining the integrity of skin and mucous membranes reduces the chances of microorganisms reaching a host. The client's skin should be kept well lubricated by using lotion as appropriate. Immobilized and debilitated clients are particularly susceptible to skin breakdown. Clients should not be positioned on tubes or objects that might cause breaks in the skin. Dry, wrinkle-free linen also reduces the chances of skin breakdown. Turning and positioning are needed before a client's skin becomes reddened. Frequent oral hygiene prevents drying of mucous membranes. A water-soluble ointment keeps the client's lips well lubricated.

After elimination, a woman should clean the rectum and perineum by wiping from the urinary meatus toward the rectum. Cleansing in a direction from the least to the

Research HIGHLIGHT
Box 33-9

RESEARCH ABSTRACT

In an observational study of 40 nurses (20 with diagnosed hand irritation and 20 without), nurses with damaged hands did not have higher microbial counts but did have a greater number of colonizing species. Although numbers were small, nurses with damaged hands were significantly more likely to be colonized with *Staphylococcus hominis*. Fifty-nine percent of *S. hominis* isolates from nurses with damaged hands were resistant to methicillin compared with 27% of isolates from those with healthy skin. Twenty percent of nurses with damaged hands were colonized with *Staphylococcus aureus* compared with none of the nurses with normal hands. Nurses with damaged hands were also twice as likely to have gram-negative bacteria, enterococci, and *Candida* organisms present on the hands. Antimicrobial resistance of the coagulase-negative staphylococcal flora (with the exception of *S. hominis*) did not differ between the two groups, nor did a trend toward increasing resistance exist when the data were compared with other studies during the past decade. Skin moisturizers and protectant products were used almost universally by nurses at work; these were primarily products brought from home.

Efforts to improve the condition of the hands are warranted because skin damage can change microbial flora. Such efforts should include assessment or monitoring of hand care practices, formal institutional policy adoption and control of the use of skin-protectant products or lotions, and prudent use of latex gloves or more widespread use of powder-free and nonlatex products.

IMPLICATIONS FOR PRACTICE
- Nurses should regularly assess their hands for skin damage.
- The nurse manager should monitor staff hand-washing and hand care practices, promoting use of institution-supplied hand care lotions and protectants.
- Nurses should monitor their use of latex gloves, using powder-free or nonlatex gloves whenever possible.

REFERENCE
Larson E and others: Changes in bacterial flora associated with skin damage on hands of health care personnel, *Am J Infect Control* 26(5):513, 1998.

Hepatitis B Vaccination and Follow-Up After Exposure
Box 33-10

Health care employers shall make available the hepatitis B vaccine and vaccination series to all employees who may have occupational exposures. Evaluation and follow-up care will be available to all employees who have been exposed.

All medical evaluations and procedures, including the vaccine and vaccination series and evaluation after exposure (prophylaxis), are made available at no cost to at-risk employees.

A confidential written medical evaluation will be available to employees with exposure incidents.

Hepatitis B vaccinations will be made available to employees within 10 working days of assignment.

From Occupational Safety and Health Act of 1991, *Federal Register*, 1991.

the infections most commonly transmitted by contaminated needles. A needle stick should be reported immediately. Health care agencies require the victim of a needle stick to complete an injury report and seek appropriate treatment (Box 33-10).

Another cause for entrance of microorganisms into a host is improper handling and management of urinary catheters and drainage sets (see Chapter 44). The point of connection between a catheter and drainage tube should remain closed and intact. As long as such systems are closed, their contents are considered sterile. Outflow spigots on drainage bags should also remain closed to prevent entrance of bacteria. Movement of the catheter at the urethra should be minimized by stabilizing the catheter with tape to reduce chances of microorganisms ascending the urethra into the bladder. Urine-measuring containers should not be shared between clients.

The nurse may care for clients with closed drainage systems that collect wound drainage, bile, or other body fluids. In each example the site from which a drainage tube exits should remain clear of excess moisture or accumulated drainage. All tubing should remain connected throughout use. Drainage receptacles should only be opened when it is necessary to discard or measure the volume of drainage.

At times the nurse obtains specimens from drainage tubes or inserts needles into IV tubing ports. The nurse disinfects tubes and ports by wiping outward with alcohol or an iodine solution before entering the system. Temporarily placing squares of sterile gauze around the ends of an open drainage tube, such as a urinary catheter, adds further protection against bacteria. However, keeping drainage tubes closed and secure is the best practice.

A final method for reducing the entrance of microorganisms is the technique for cleansing wounds (see Chapter 47). The surgical wound itself is considered to be sterile. To prevent entrance of microorganisms into the wound, the nurse should clean outward from a wound site. When applying an antiseptic or cleaning with soap

most contaminated area helps reduce genitourinary infections. Meticulous and frequent perineal care is especially important in older adult women who wear disposable incontinent pads.

Clients, health care personnel, and even housekeepers are at risk for acquiring infections from accidental needle sticks. After administering an injection or inserting an IV catheter, the nurse should carefully dispose of needles without recapping in a puncture-resistant box (see Chapter 34). A stray needle lying in bed linen or carelessly thrown into a wastebasket is a prime source for exposure to blood-borne pathogens. Hepatitis B and hepatitis C are

Skill 33-1 Hand Washing

Delegation Considerations

Hand washing can be delegated to assistive personnel
- Instruct, assist, and monitor care provider in proper method of hand washing.

- Instruct care provider to inform nurse if any skin irritation from soaps or antimicrobials is encountered.

EQUIPMENT
- Easy-to-reach sink with warm running water
- Antimicrobial or regular soap

- Paper towels or air dryer
- Clean orangewood stick (optional)

STEPS	RATIONALE
1. Inspect surface of hands for breaks or cuts in skin or cuticles. Report and cover lesions before providing client care.	Open cuts or wounds can harbor high concentrations of microorganisms. Agency policy may prevent nurses from caring for high-risk clients. If dermatitis occurs, additional interventions may be needed.
2. Inspect hands for heavy soiling.	Requires lengthier hand washing.
3. Inspect nails for length.	Nails should be short and filed because most microbes on hands come from beneath the fingernails.
4. Assess client's risk for or extent of infection (e.g., WBC count, extent of open wounds, known medical diagnosis).	Use of antimicrobial soaps is encouraged for clients who are immunosuppressed (Larson, 1996).
5. Push wristwatch and long uniform sleeves above wrists. Avoid wearing rings. If worn, remove during washing.	Provides complete access to fingers, hands, wrists. Wearing of rings increases number of microorganisms on hands (Garner, 1996).
6. Stand in front of sink, keeping hands and uniform away from sink surface. (If hands touch sink during hand washing, repeat.)	Inside of sink is a contaminated area. Reaching over sink increases risk of touching edge, which is contaminated.
7. Turn on water. Turn faucet on or push knee pedals laterally or press pedals with foot to regulate flow and temperature (see illustration).	

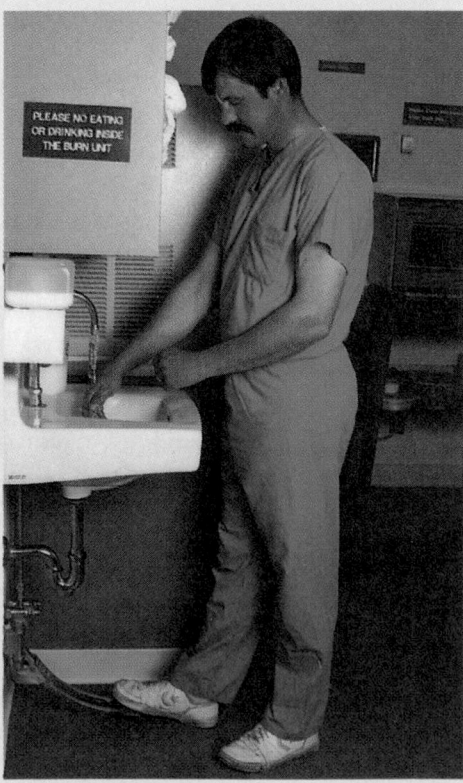

Step 7

STEPS	RATIONALE
8. Avoid splashing water against uniform.	Microorganisms travel and grow in moisture.
9. Regulate flow of water so that temperature is warm.	Warm water removes less of the protective oils than hot water.
10. Wet hands and wrists thoroughly under running water. Keep hands and forearms lower than elbows during washing.	Hands are the most contaminated parts to be washed. Water flows from least to most contaminated area, rinsing microorganisms into the sink.
11. Apply a small amount of soap or antiseptic, lathering thoroughly (see illustration). Soap granules and leaflet preparations may be used.	Use of antiseptic exclusively can be drying to hands and can cause skin irritations. The decision whether to use an antiseptic should depend on the procedure to be performed and the client's immune status.
12. Wash hands using plenty of lather and friction for at least 10 to 15 seconds. Interlace fingers and rub palms and back of hands with circular motion at least 5 times each. Keep fingertips down to facilitate removal of microorganisms.	Soap cleanses by emulsifying fat and oil and lowering surface tension. Friction and rubbing mechanically loosen and remove dirt and transient bacteria. Interlacing fingers and thumbs ensures that all surfaces are cleansed.
13. Areas underlying fingernails are often soiled. Clean them with fingernails of other hand and additional soap or clean orangewood stick.	Area under nails can be highly contaminated, which will increase the risk of infection for the nurse or the client.

Critical Decision Point: Do not tear or cut skin under or around nail.

---

14. Rinse hands and wrists thoroughly, keeping hands down and elbows up (see illustration).	Rinsing mechanically washes away dirt and microorganisms.
15. *Optional:* Repeat steps 5 through 13 and extend period of washing if hands are heavily soiled.	
16. Dry hands thoroughly from fingers to wrists and forearms with paper towel, single-use cloth, or warm air dryer.	Drying from cleanest (fingertips) to least clean (forearms) area avoids contamination. Drying hands prevents chapping and roughened skin.
17. If used, discard paper towel in proper receptacle.	Prevents transfer of microorganisms.
18. Turn off water with foot or knee pedals. To turn off hand faucet, use clean, dry paper towel; avoid touching handles with hands.	Wet towel and hands allow transfer of pathogens by capillary action.

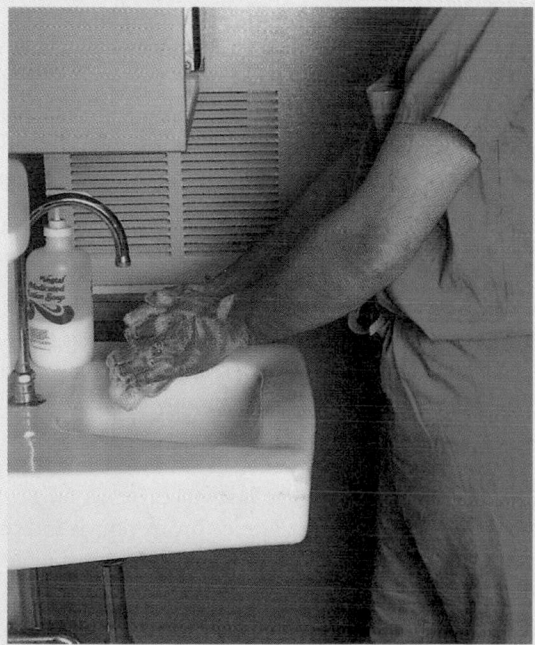

Step 11

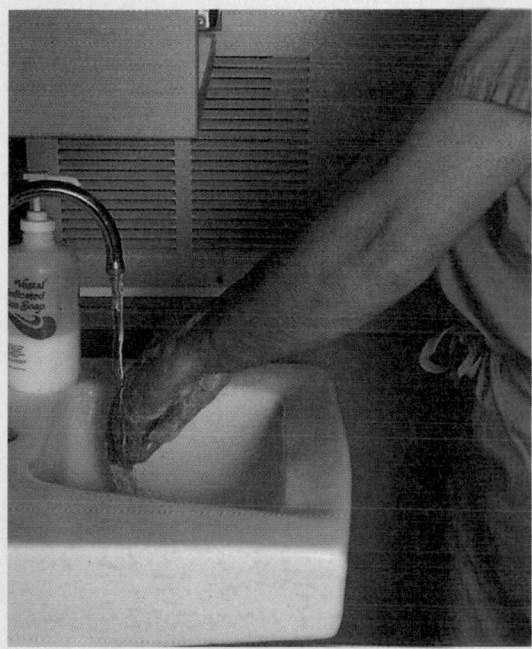

Step 14

STEPS	RATIONALE
19. If hands are dry or chapped, a small amount of lotion or barrier cream can be applied.	Use small, individual-use container of lotion because large, refillable containers have been associated with nosocomial infections.
20. Inspect surfaces of hands for obvious signs of soil or other contaminants.	Determines if hand washing is adequate.
21. Inspect hands for dermatitis or cracked skin.	Indicates complications from excessive hand washing.

Recording and Reporting
- It is not necessary to record or report this procedure.
- Report any dermatitis to employee health and/or infection control per agency policy.

Home Care Considerations
- Evaluate the hand-washing facilities in the home to determine the possibility of contamination, the proximity of the facilities to the client, and available supplies in the area.

- Evaluate the availability of warm running water and soap when conducting home visits and anticipate the need for alternative hand-washing products such as alcohol-based hand rubs and detergent-containing towels.
- Instruct the client and primary caregiver in proper techniques and situations for hand washing.

> ### Infection Control: Protecting the Susceptible Host   Box 33-11
>
> **PROTECTING NORMAL DEFENSE MECHANISMS**
> Regular bathing removes transient microorganisms from the skin's surface. Lubrication helps keep the skin hydrated and intact.
> Regular oral hygiene removes proteins in the saliva that attract microorganisms. Flossing removes tartar and plaque that can cause germ infection.
> Maintenance of adequate fluid intake promotes normal urine formation and a resultant outflow of urine to flush the bladder and urethral lining of microorganisms.
> For physically dependent or immobilized clients, the nurse encourages routine coughing and deep breathing to keep lower airways clear of mucus.
> The nurse encourages proper immunization of children or adult clients who become exposed to certain infectious microorganisms. Children are vaccinated for smallpox, measles, mumps, rubella, and diphtheria. Adults should have tetanus-diphtheria boosters every 10 years. Influenza vaccines are recommended for health care workers. Older adults should regularly receive influenza and pneumococcal vaccines.
>
> **MAINTAINING HEALING PROCESSES**
> The nurse promotes intake of adequate fluids and a well-balanced diet containing essential proteins, vitamins, carbohydrates, and fats. The nurse also uses measures to increase the client's appetite.
> The nurse promotes a client's comfort and sleep so that energy stores are replaced daily.
> The nurse assists the client in learning techniques to reduce stress.

and water, the nurse wipes around the wound edge first and then cleans outward away from the wound. Clean gauze should be used for each revolution around the wound's circumference.

Protection of the Susceptible Host.   A client's resistance to infection improves as the nurse protects normal body defenses against infection. The nurse intervenes to maintain the body's normal reparative processes (Box 33-11). The nurse also protects himself or herself and others through the use of isolation precautions (Box 33-12).

Isolation Precautions.   The risk of transmitting nosocomial infection or infectious disease among clients is high. When a client has a suspected or known infection, health care workers become alerted and follow infection-control practices. However, health care workers may not be aware that clients have infections. The majority of organisms causing nosocomial infections are found in the **colonized** body substances of clients regardless of whether a culture has confirmed infection and a diagnosis has been made (Jackson and Lynch, 1991). Body substances such as feces, saliva, mucus, and wound drainage always contain potentially infectious organisms.

Isolation or barrier precautions include the appropriate use of gowns, gloves, masks, eyewear, and other protective devices or clothing. Barrier protection is indicated for use with all clients because every client has the potential to transmit infection via blood and body fluids, and the risk for infection transmission can be unknown. Because of the increased attention to the prevention of blood-borne pathogens and tuberculosis, the CDC and

Box 33-12 Procedural Guidelines

For Caring for a Client on Isolation Precautions

1. Assess isolation indications (i.e., current laboratory tests or client's history of exposure).
2. Review agency policies and precautions necessary for the specific isolation system and consider care measures to be performed while in client's room.
3. Review nurses' notes or confer with colleagues regarding client's emotional state and adjustment to isolation.
4. Wash hands and prepare all equipment to be taken into client's room.
5. Prepare for entrance into isolation room:
   a. Apply either surgical mask or respirator around mouth and nose. (Type will depend on type of isolation and facility policy.)
   b. Apply eyewear or goggles snugly around face and eyes (when needed).
   c. Apply gown, being sure it covers all outer garments. Pull sleeves down to wrist. Tie securely at neck and waist (see illustration).
   d. Apply disposable gloves (NOTE: Unpowdered, latex-free gloves should be worn if the client or the health care worker has a latex allergy.) If gloves are worn with gown, bring glove cuffs over edge of gown sleeves.

6. Enter client's room. Arrange supplies and equipment. (If equipment will be removed from room for reuse, place on clean paper towel.)
7. Explain purpose of isolation and necessary precautions to client and family. Offer opportunity to ask questions. Assess for evidence of emotional problems that may be caused by being in isolation.
8. Assess vital signs.
   a. If client is infected or colonized with a resistant organism (e.g., vancomycin-resistant enterococcus [VRE], methicillin-resistant *Staphylococcus aureus* [MRSA]), equipment remains in room. Proceed to assess vital signs by routine procedures. Avoid contact of stethoscope or blood pressure cuff with infective material.
   b. If stethoscope is to be reused, clean diaphragm or bell with alcohol. Set aside on clean surface.
   c. Individual or disposable thermometers should be used.
9. Administer medications (see Chapter 34):
   a. Give oral medication in wrapper or cup.
   b. Dispose of wrapper or cup in plastic-lined receptacle.
   c. Administer injection, being sure gloves are worn.
   d. Discard syringe and uncapped needle or sheathed needle into special container.
   e. If gloves are not worn and hands contact contaminated article or body fluids, wash hands immediately.
10. Administer hygiene, encouraging the client to discuss questions or concerns about isolation. Informal teaching can be used at this time.
    a. Avoid allowing gown to become wet.
    b. Remove linen from bed; if excessively soiled, avoid contact with gown. Place in impervious linen bag.
    c. Change gloves and wash hands if they become excessively soiled and further care is necessary.
11. Collect specimens:
    a. Place specimen containers on clean paper towel in client's bathroom.
    b. Follow procedure for collecting specimen of body fluids.
    c. Transfer specimen to container without soiling outside of container. Place container in plastic bag and place label on outside of bag or as per facility policy.

Step 5c

Continued

Box 33-12 **Procedural Guidelines—cont'd**

For Caring for a Client on Isolation Precautions

12. Dispose of linen and trash bags as they become full:
    a. Use sturdy, moisture-resistant single bags to contain soiled articles.
    b. Tie bags securely at top in knot (see illustration).
13. Resupply room as needed.
14. Leave isolation room.
    a. Remove gloves. Remove one glove by grasping cuff and pulling glove inside out over hand. Discard glove. With ungloved hand, tuck finger inside cuff of remaining glove and pull it off, inside out.
    b. Untie *top* mask string and then bottom strings, pull mask away from face and drop into trash receptacle. (Do not touch outer surface of mask.)
    c. Untie waist and neck strings of gown. Allow gown to fall from shoulders. Remove hands from sleeves without touching outside of gown. Hold gown inside at shoulder seams and fold inside out; discard in laundry bag.
    d. Remove eyewear or goggles.
    e. Wash hands minimum of 10 seconds.
    f. Explain to client when you plan to return to room. Ask whether client requires any personal care items, books, or magazines.
    g. Leave room and close door, if necessary. (Door should be closed if client is on airborne precautions.)
    h. All contaminated supplies and equipment should be disposed of in a manner that prevents spread of microorganisms to other persons (see agency policy).

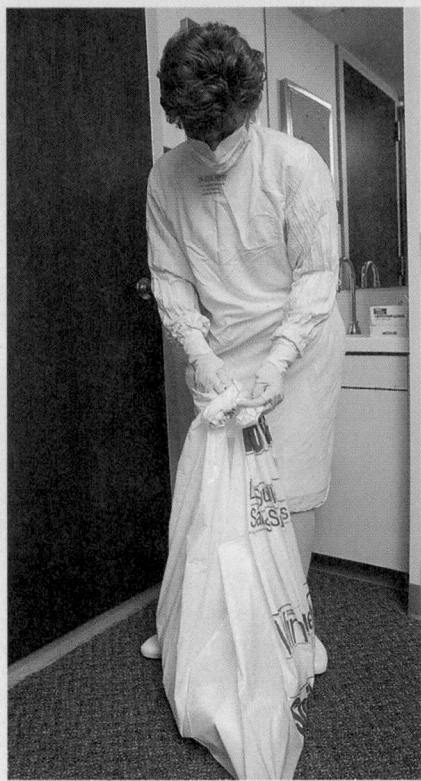

Step 12b

---

the Occupational Safety and Health Administration (OSHA) have stressed the importance of using barrier protection (OSHA, 1991).

The CDC issued new isolation guidelines in 1996 that contain a two-tiered approach (Garner, 1996). The first and most important tier contains precautions designed to care for all clients in any setting regardless of their diagnosis or presumed infectiousness. This guideline is called standard precautions. These precautions apply to (1) blood; (2) all body fluids, secretions, and excretions except sweat regardless of whether they contain blood; (3) nonintact skin; and (4) mucous membranes. These precautions promote hand washing and the use of gloves, masks, eye protection, or gowns, when appropriate, for client contact (Table 33-7).

The second tier uses three transmission categories: airborne, droplet, and contact precautions based on a client's diagnosed infection. These precautions are designed for specific clients with highly transmissible or epidemiologically important pathogens. For example, a client diagnosed with active tuberculosis would require the use of

airborne precautions, using a special mask and ventilated room, in conjunction with standard precautions.

Users of the CDC's isolation guidelines are referred to additional CDC documents to prevent nosocomial aspergillosis and Legionnaires' disease in immunocompromised clients (CDC, 1994) and the spread of vancomycin-resistant organisms (CDC, 1995).

With the increase in numbers of reported cases of tuberculosis (TB) in the United States, the CDC issued guidelines for prevention of transmission of TB in health care facilities in 1990. These and later revisions (CDC, 1994) stress the early identification and treatment of persons with known or suspected TB, facility risk assessment for TB exposures, engineering control, and proper isolation techniques. In addition, OSHA (1999) issued a mandate requiring health care facilities to follow CDC guidelines and required that health care workers be offered free TB skin tests and respiratory protective devices. Airborne precautions are required for TB in addition to the following:

Single-client room maintained under negative pressure

Table 33-7   Centers for Disease Control and Prevention Isolation Guidelines

Standard Precautions (Tier One)

Standard precautions apply to blood, all body fluids, secretions, excretions (except sweat), nonintact skin, and mucous membranes.

Hands are washed between client contacts; after contact with blood, body fluids, secretions, and excretions and after contact with equipment or articles contaminated by them; and immediately after gloves are removed.

Gloves are worn when touching blood, body fluids, secretions, excretions, nonintact skin, mucous membranes, or contaminated items. Gloves should be removed and hands washed between client care.

Masks, eye protection, or face shields are worn if client care activities may generate splashes or sprays of blood or body fluid.

Gowns are worn if soiling of clothing is likely from blood or body fluid. Wash hands after removing gown.

Client care equipment is properly cleaned and reprocessed, and single-use items are discarded.

Contaminated linen is placed in leakproof bag and handled so as to prevent skin and mucous membrane exposure.

All sharp instruments and needles are discarded in a puncture-resistant container. CDC recommends that needles be disposed of uncapped or that a mechanical device be used for recapping.

A private room is unnecessary unless the client's hygiene is unacceptable. Check with an infection-control professional.

Transmission Categories (Tier Two)

Category	Disease	Barrier Protection
Airborne precautions	Droplet nuclei smaller than 5 μm; measles; chickenpox (varicella); disseminated varicella zoster; pulmonary or laryngeal TB	Private room, negative-pressure airflow of at least six exchanges per hour, mask or respiratory protection device
Droplet precautions	Droplets larger than 5 μm; diphtheria (pharyngeal); rubella; streptococcal pharyngitis, pneumonia, or scarlet fever in infants and young children; pertussis; mumps; mycoplasmal pneumonia; meningococcal pneumonia or sepsis; pneumonic plague	Private room or cohort clients; mask
Contact precautions	Direct client or environmental contact; colonization or infection with multidrug-resistant organism; respiratory syncytial virus; shigella and other enteric pathogens; major wound infections; herpes simplex; scabies, varicella zoster (disseminated)	Private room or cohort clients; gloves, gowns

Modified from Garner JS: Guidelines for isolation precautions in hospitals, *Infect Control Hosp Epidemiol* 17(1):54, 1996.

Door kept closed except when entering or exiting the room

Negative pressure monitored daily (using a smoke tube or differential pressure-sensing device)

Minimum of 6 air exchanges per hour in existing facilities and minimum of 12 air exchanges per hour in new-construction facilities

Possible use of ultraviolet germicide irradiation or HEPA filter, which may reduce the number of droplet nuclei

Use of personal respiratory protective devices (masks) capable of filtration of 95% efficiency when entering the isolation room (Figure 33-3)

Ability to qualitatively or quantitatively fit-test masks to obtain a face-seal leakage of $\leq$10%

Use of a mask by the client when out of the room (with the client leaving the room only if necessary)

Regardless of the type of isolation system, the nurse must follow the following basic principles:

The nurse should wash hands thoroughly before entering and leaving the room of a client in isolation.

Contaminated supplies and equipment should be disposed of in a manner that prevents spread of microorganisms to other persons as indicated by the mode of transmission of the organism.

Knowledge of a disease process and the mode of infection transmission should be applied when using protective barriers.

All persons who might be exposed during transport of a client outside the isolation room must be protected.

Psychological Implications of Isolation. When a client requires isolation in a private room, a sense of loneliness may develop because normal social relationships become disrupted. This situation can be psychologically harmful, especially for children.

As a result of the infectious process, client's body images are altered. They may feel unclean, rejected, lonely, or guilty. Infection prevention and control practices further intensify these beliefs of difference or undesirability. Isolation in a private room limits sensory contact. Unless the nurse acts to minimize feelings of psychological and

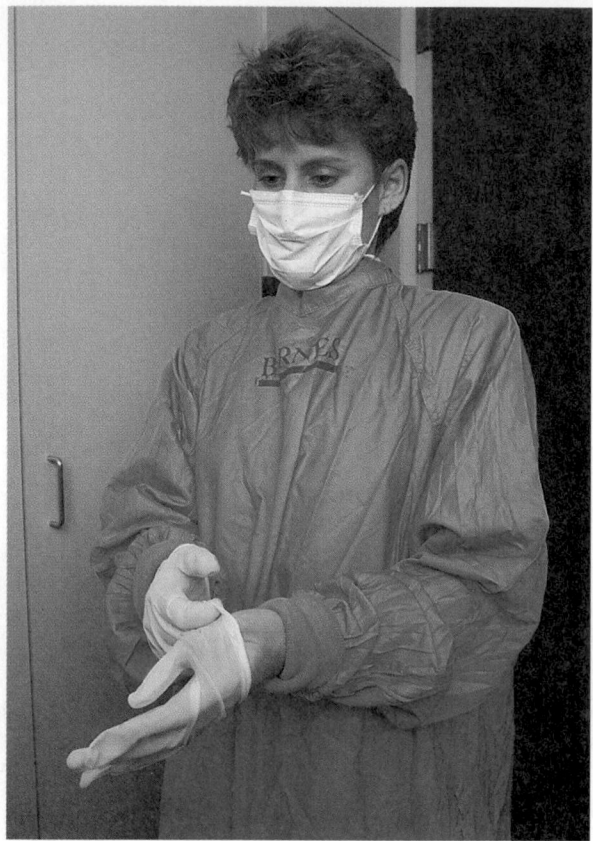

Figure 33-3   Nurse wearing an N-95 respirator.

physical isolation, clients' emotional states can interfere with recovery.

Before isolation measures are instituted, the client and family must understand the nature of the disease or condition, the purposes of isolation, and steps for carrying out specific precautions. If they are able to participate in maintaining infection prevention, the chances of reducing the spread of infection are increased. The client and family should be taught to wash hands and use barrier protection if appropriate. Each procedure should be demonstrated, and the client and family should be given an opportunity for practice. It is also important to explain how infectious organisms can be transmitted so that the client understands the difference between contaminated and clean objects.

The nurse also takes measures to improve the client's sensory stimulation during isolation. The room environment should be clean and pleasant. Drapes or shades should be opened, and excess supplies and equipment removed. The nurse must listen to the client's concerns or interests. If the nurse rushes through care or shows a lack of interest, the client will feel rejected and even more isolated. Mealtime is a particularly good opportunity for conversation. Providing comfort measures such as repositioning, a

back massage, or a tepid sponge bath increases physical stimulation. Depending on the client's condition, the nurse should encourage the client to walk and sit up in a chair. Recreational activities such as board games or cards may be an option to keep the client mentally stimulated.

The nurse must explain to the family the client's risk for depression or loneliness. Visiting family members should be encouraged to avoid expressions or actions that convey revulsion or disgust. The nurse discusses ways to provide meaningful stimulation.

Protective Environment.   Private rooms used for isolation may have negative-pressure airflow to prevent infectious particles from flowing out of the room. There are also special rooms with positive-pressure airflow that are used for highly susceptible clients, such as organ transplant recipients. On the door or wall outside the room, the nurse posts a card listing precautions for the isolation category according to agency policy. The card is a handy reference for health care personnel and visitors and alerts anyone who might enter the room accidentally that special precautions must be followed.

The isolation room or an adjoining anteroom should contain hand-washing, bathing, and toilet facilities. Soap and antiseptic solutions are made available. Personnel and visitors wash their hands before approaching the client's bedside and again before leaving the room. If toilet facilities are unavailable, there are special procedures for handling portable commodes, bedpans, or urinals. Personal protective equipment should be stored in an anteroom between the room and hallway or in a convenient location close to the point of use.

All client care rooms, including those used for isolation, contain an impervious bag for soiled or contaminated linen, as well as a trash container with plastic liners. Impervious receptacles prevent transmission of microorganisms by preventing seepage to and soiling of the outside surface. A disposable rigid container should be available in the room to discard used needles, syringes, and sharp objects.

The nurse must remain aware of infection prevention and control techniques while working with clients in protected environments. The nurse should feel comfortable performing all procedures and yet remain conscious of infection-control principles. Depending on the microorganism and the mode of transmission, the nurse must evaluate what articles or equipment may be taken into an isolation room. For example, the CDC (1995) recommends the dedicated use of articles such as stethoscopes, sphygmomanometers, or rectal thermometers in the isolation room of a client infected or colonized with vancomycin-resistant enterococci (VRE). These devices should not be used on other clients unless they are first adequately cleaned and disinfected. If after bringing any article into the room, the nurse exposes an article to infected material and then touches or removes the article, the risk of transmitting infection to other clients or personnel is increased. Box 33-12 describes the procedures commonly performed in a protective environment.

Personal Protective Equipment.   Personal protective equipment should be readily available for personnel performing client care. The primary reason for gowning is to prevent soiling clothes during contact with the client. Gowns or cover-ups protect health care personnel and visitors from coming in contact with infected material and blood or body fluid. Gowns may also be required for contact precautions, depending on the expected amount of exposure to infectious material. Gowns used for barrier protection are made of a fluid-resistant material and should be changed immediately if damaged or heavily contaminated. Depending on agency policy, isolation gowns can be disposable or reusable.

Isolation gowns usually open at the back and have ties or snaps at the neck and waist to keep the gown closed and secure. Gowns should be long enough to cover all outer garments. Long sleeves with tight-fitting cuffs provide added protection. There is no special technique required for applying clean gowns as long as they are fastened securely. However, the nurse must carefully remove gowns to minimize contamination of the hands and uniform and then discard them after removal.

Masks or masks with face shields should be worn when splashing or spraying of blood or body fluid into the face is anticipated. Masks should also be worn when working with a client on airborne or droplet precautions. The mask protects the nurse from inhaling microorganisms from a client's respiratory tract and prevents transmission of pathogens from the nurse's respiratory tract to the client. The surgical mask protects a wearer from inhaling large-particle aerosols that travel short distances (3 feet) and small-particle droplet nuclei that remain suspended in the air and travel longer distances. At times a client who is susceptible to infection wears a mask to prevent inhalation of pathogens. Clients on droplet or airborne precautions who are transported outside of their rooms should wear masks to protect other clients and personnel.

According to the CDC (1994), masks may prevent transmission of infection by direct contact with mucous membranes. A mask discourages the wearer from touching the eyes, nose, or mouth.

A properly applied mask fits snugly over the mouth and nose so that pathogens and body fluids cannot enter or escape through the sides (Box 33-13). If a person wears glasses, the top edge of the mask fits below the glasses so that they will not cloud over as the person exhales. Talking should be kept to a minimum while wearing a mask to reduce respiratory airflow. A mask that has become moist may not provide a barrier to microorganisms and thus may be ineffective. It should be discarded. A mask should not be reused. Clients and family members should be warned that a mask can cause a sensation of smothering.

Box 33-13   **Procedural Guidelines**

For Donning a Surgical-Type Mask

1. Find top edge of mask (usually has thin metal strip along edge). Pliable metal fits snugly against bridge of nose
2. Hold mask by top two strings or loops. Tie two top ties at top of back of head (see illustration), with ties above ears. (*Alternative:* Slip loops over each ear.)

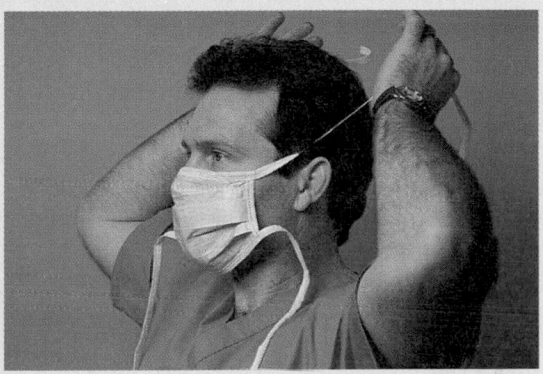

3. Tie two lower ties snugly around neck with mask well under chin (see illustration).

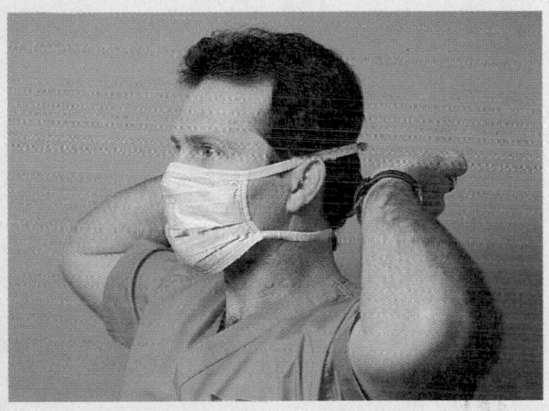

4. Gently pinch upper metal band around bridge of nose.

NOTE: Mask should be changed if wet, moist, or contaminated.

If family members become uncomfortable, they should leave the room and discard the mask.

Special respiratory protective devices or masks are required when caring for a client with known or suspected TB (CDC, 1994; OSHA, 1994). The mask must have a higher filtration rating than the regular surgical mask and be fitted snugly to the wearer's face to prevent leakage around the sides. The nurse should be aware of agency policy regarding the type of respiratory protective device required.

Gloves help to prevent the transmission of pathogens by direct and indirect contact. The CDC (1995) notes that clean, nonsterile gloves should be worn when touching blood, body fluid, secretions, excretions, and contaminated items. Clean gloves should be donned just before touching mucous membranes and nonintact skin. Gloves should be changed between tasks and procedures on the same client after contact with material that may contain a high concentration of microorganisms. Gloves should be removed promptly after use, before touching noncontaminated items and environmental surfaces, and before going to another client. Hands should be washed immediately to avoid transfer of microorganisms to other clients or environments.

When full protective apparel is needed, the nurse first applies a mask and eyewear or goggle (as needed) washes and dries hands, applies a gown, and then applies gloves. Disposable gloves are easily applied and are designed to fit either hand. The glove's thin rubber, however, can be easily torn. The glove cuffs should be pulled up over the wrists or over the cuffs of the gown.

If a break or tear is detected in a glove while providing care, the nurse should change gloves if care is not completed. If the nurse does not plan to have more contact with the client, reapplying gloves is unnecessary.

The nurse should explain the proper use of gloves to the client's family members and emphasize that it is very important to wash hands after removing gloves.

When participating in a procedure that creates droplets or splashing or spraying of blood or other body fluids, a nurse must wear protective eyewear, a mask, or a face shield (Garner, 1996). Examples of such procedures include irrigation of a large abdominal wound or insertion of an arterial catheter in which the nurse assists a physician. Eyewear may be available in the form of plastic glasses or goggles (Figure 33-4). The eyewear should fit snugly around the face so that fluids cannot enter between the face and the glasses.

Specimen Collection. Many laboratory studies may be required when a client is suspected of having an infectious disease. Body fluids and secretions suspected of containing infectious organisms are collected for culture and sensitivity tests. The specimen is placed in a medium that promotes growth of organisms. A laboratory technologist then identifies the microorganisms growing in the culture. Additional test results indicate antibiotics to which the organisms are resistant or sensitive. Sensitivity reports determine the antibiotics used in treatment.

The nurse obtains all culture specimens using disposable gloves and sterile equipment. Collecting fresh material from the site of infection, such as in the case of wound drainage, ensures that the specimen is not contaminated by neighboring microbes. All specimen containers should be sealed tightly to prevent spillage and contamination of the outside of the container. Box 33-14 describes tech-

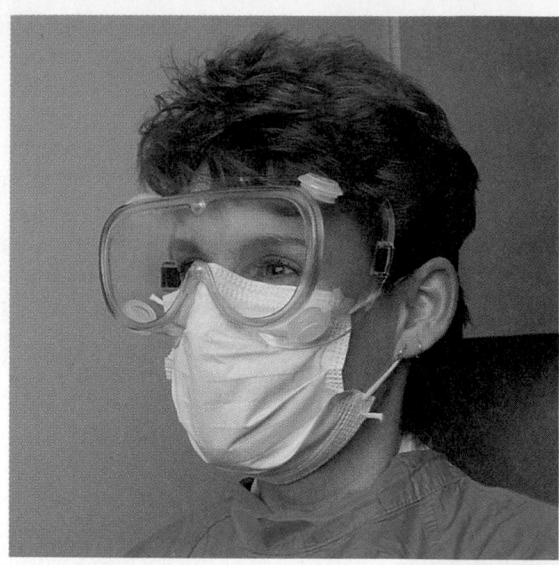

Figure 33-4   Nurse wearing protective goggles and mask.

niques for collecting specimens from the client with a suspected infection.

Bagging Trash or Linen. Nurses use special bagging procedures for removing contaminated items from the client's environment. Bagging contaminated items prevents accidental exposure of personnel and prevents contamination of the surrounding environment.

The CDC recommends a single bag for discarding items if the bag is impervious and sturdy and if the article can be placed in the bag without contaminating the outside of the bag. Soiled linen should be placed in an impervious laundry bag in the client's room (OSHA, 1991).

The CDC recommends double bagging if it is impossible to prevent contamination of the bag's outer surface. Double bagging is not otherwise recommended. Studies have shown that this procedure is not necessary to control infection (Maki and others, 1986; Weinstein and others, 1989). Use of one standard-sized linen bag that is not overfilled, that is tied securely, and that is intact is adequate to prevent infection transmission. The same rule applies to trash bags.

Transporting Clients. Before transferring clients to wheelchairs or stretchers, the nurse gives them clean gowns to serve as robes. Clients infected with organisms transmitted by the airborne route should leave their rooms only for essential purposes, such as diagnostic procedures or surgery. These clients must also wear masks. Personnel transporting these clients should also wear barrier protection as needed.

At times a client being transported may drain body fluids onto a stretcher or wheelchair. When this occurs, the nurse must be sure to have the equipment cleaned after

Specimen Collection Techniques*   Box 33-14

WOUND SPECIMEN

Clean site with sterile water or saline prior to wound specimen collection. Wear gloves and use cotton-tipped swab or syringe to collect as much drainage as possible. Have clean test tube or culture tube on clean paper towel. After swabbing center of wound site, grasp collection tube by holding it with paper towel. Carefully insert swab without touching outside of tube. After securing tube's top, transfer tube into bag for transport and then wash hands.

BLOOD SPECIMEN

Wearing gloves, use syringe and culture media bottles to collect up to 10 ml of blood per culture bottle (check agency policy). After prepping, perform venipuncture at two different sites to decrease likelihood of both specimens being contaminated with skin flora. Place blood culture bottles on bedside table or other surface; swab off bottle tops with alcohol. Inject appropriate amount of blood into each bottle. Remove gloves and transfer specimen into clean, labeled bag for transport. Wash hands.

STOOL SPECIMEN

Wearing gloves, use clean cup with seal top (need not be sterile) and tongue blade to collect small amount of stool, approximately the size of a walnut. Place cup on clean paper towel in client's bathroom. Using tongue blade, collect needed amount of feces from client's bedpan. Transfer feces to cup without touching cup's outside surface. Dispose of tongue blade, and place seal on cup. Transfer specimen into clean bag for transport. Remove gloves and wash hands.

URINE SPECIMEN

Wearing gloves, use syringe and sterile cup to collect 1 to 5 ml of urine. Place cup or tube on clean towel in client's bathroom. If client has a urinary catheter, use syringe to collect specimen. Have client follow procedure to obtain a clean voided specimen (see Chapter 44) if not catheterized. Transfer urine into sterile container by injecting urine from syringe or pouring it from used collection cup. Secure top of container and transfer specimen into clean, labeled bag for transport. Remove gloves and wash hands.

From Pagana KD, Pagana TJ: *Diagnostic testing and nursing implications: a case study approach,* ed 5, St. Louis, 1998, Mosby.
*Agency policies may differ on type of containers and amount of specimen material required.

the client returns to the room. An extra layer of sheets may be used to cover the stretcher or seat of the wheelchair.

Personnel in diagnostic or procedural areas or the operating room should be notified that the client is on isolation precautions. The nurse explains ways that the client can help prevent transmission of infection during transport. A client on respiratory isolation is given tissues and a bag to allow proper disposal of secretions. The nurse records the type of isolation on the client's chart.

Role of the Infection-Control Professional.   Many hospitals employ professionals, most of whom are nurses, who are specially trained in infection prevention and control. These individuals are responsible for advising hospital personnel regarding infection prevention and control and for monitoring infections within the hospital. Duties of an infection-control professional include the following:

   Provide staff education on infection prevention and control.

   Develop and review infection prevention and control policies and procedures.

   Recommend appropriate isolation procedures.

   Screen client records for community-acquired infections that may be reportable to the public health department.

   Consult with employee health departments concerning recommendations to prevent and control the spread of infection among personnel, such as TB testing.

   Gather statistics regarding the **epidemiology** of nosocomial infections.

   Notify the public health department of incidences of communicable diseases within the facility.

   Confer with all hospital departments to investigate unusual events or clusters of infection.

   Educate clients and families.

   Identify infection-control problems with equipment.

   Monitor antibiotic resistant organisms in the institution.

An infection-control professional can be a valuable resource for assisting nurses in controlling nosocomial infections.

Infection Prevention and Control for Hospital Personnel.   Health care workers are continually at risk for exposure to infectious microorganisms. The Occupational Safety and Health Act of 1991 established rules and regulations to protect employees from infectious hazards in the workplace (OSHA, 1991). The OSHA guidelines are incorporated into the policies and procedures of health care institutions. Elements of the OSHA guidelines include the following:

- *Exposure-control plan.* Institutions must have exposure-control plans designed to eliminate or minimize employee exposure. The plan must be accessible to all employees. The plan also describes how to avoid exposure to infectious agents, such as when to use protective equipment.

- *Compliance with standard precautions.* Employees are to follow precautions to prevent contact with blood or other infectious materials during the routine care of clients. Personal protective equipment must be provided at no cost to employees who are at risk for exposure.

- *Housekeeping.* Workplaces are to be maintained in a

clean and sanitary condition. Routine cleaning and decontamination procedures are established.

- *High-risk exposure.* If health care workers have parenteral (needle stick) or mucous membrane exposure to blood or other infectious body fluids, the incident should be reported immediately. Evaluation and appropriate preventive treatment for hepatitis B and HIV infection are critical.

- *Training.* Employers must ensure that all employees with risk of occupational exposure participate in a training program. The program will present the exposure-control plan for the institution and specifically explain the measures to be taken by employees for their safety. Written policies and guidelines must be provided for all personnel with respect to infection prevention and control activities (Joint Commission on Accreditation of Health Care Organizations [JCAHO], 1998).

Client Education.

Often clients must learn to use infection-control practices at home (Box 33-15). Preventive technique becomes almost second nature to the nurse who practices it daily. However, the client is less aware of factors that promote the spread of infection or ways to prevent its transmission. The home environment does not always lend itself to infection prevention. Often a nurse must help a client adapt according to the resources available to maintain hygienic techniques. Generally, clients in a home care setting have a decreased risk of infection because of decreased exposure to resistant organisms such as those found in a hospital and because of fewer invasive procedures.

After clients are at home, nurses determine their compliance with infection-control practices. The nurse educates clients about infection and techniques to prevent or control its spread. Topics the nurse can discuss in a teaching session include the following:

Clients' susceptibility to infection

The chain of infection, with specific reference to means of transmission

Hygienic practices that minimize organism growth and spread, emphasizing hand washing

Preventive health care (e.g., diet, immunizations, and exercise)

Proper methods for handling and storage of food

Family members who are at risk for acquiring infection

Family members caring for such a client must be involved in the teaching plan. The nurse teaches clients and family members a commonsense approach to controlling and preventing infection.

Surgical Asepsis.

Surgical asepsis or sterile technique requires a nurse to use different precautions from those of medical asepsis. Surgical asepsis includes procedures used to eliminate all microorganisms, including pathogens and spores, from an object or area. In surgical asepsis an area or object is considered contaminated if touched by any object that is not sterile. For example, a tear in a surgical glove exposes the outside of the glove to the skin surface, thus contaminating it. The nurse working with a sterile field or with sterile equipment must understand that the slightest break in technique results in contamination (Box 33-16).

Although surgical asepsis is commonly practiced in the operating room, labor and delivery area, and major diagnostic areas, the nurse may also use surgical aseptic techniques at the client's bedside. This includes, for example, inserting IV or urinary catheters, suctioning the tracheobronchial airway, and reapplying sterile dressings. A nurse

---

Client Teaching FOR INFECTION CONTROL   Box 33-15

OBJECTIVE
- Client will assume self-care using proper infection-control techniques.

TEACHING STRATEGIES
- Instruct client about cleaning equipment using soap and water and disinfecting with an appropriate disinfectant.
- Demonstrate proper hand washing, explaining that it should be done before and after all treatments and when infected body fluids are contacted.
- Instruct client about signs and symptoms of wound infection.
- For clients who receive tube feedings at home, explain the importance of preparing enough formula for only 8 hours (commercially prepared) or 4 hours (home prepared). Tell client that contaminated enteral feeding can cause infections. Rinse feeding bag and tubing with mild soap and water daily and dry.

- Instruct client to place contaminated dressings and other disposable items containing infectious body fluids in impervious plastic bags. Place needles in metal containers such as soda cans and tape the openings shut.
- Clean noticeably soiled linen separate from other laundry. Wash in water that is as hot as the fabric will tolerate. Add 1 cup of bleach to detergent. Set dryer temperature as high as fabric will allow.

EVALUATION
- Ask client or family member to describe techniques used to reduce transmission of infection.
- Have client demonstrate select techniques.
- Ask client to explain risks for infection based on the condition.

in an operating room follows a series of steps to maintain sterile technique, including applying a mask, protective eyewear, and a cap; performing a surgical hand scrub; and applying a sterile gown and gloves. In contrast, a nurse performing a dressing change at a client's bedside may only wash hands and apply sterile gloves. (See following section on the principles of surgical asepsis.)

Client Preparation.   Because surgical asepsis requires exact techniques, the nurse must have the client's cooperation. Therefore the nurse must prepare the client before any procedure. Certain clients may fear moving or touching objects during a sterile procedure, whereas others may even try to assist. The nurse explains how a procedure is to be performed and what the client can do to avoid contaminating sterile items, including the following:

Avoid sudden movements of body parts covered by sterile drapes.

Refrain from touching sterile supplies, drapes, or the nurse's gloves and gown.

Avoid coughing, sneezing, or talking over a sterile area. Certain sterile procedures may last an extended time. The nurse assesses the client's needs and anticipates factors that may disrupt a procedure. If a client is in pain, the nurse tries to administer analgesics no more than half an hour before a sterile procedure begins. The nurse allows the client to have elimination needs met. Often clients must assume relatively uncomfortable positions during sterile procedures. The nurse helps the client to assume the most comfortable position possible. Finally, the client's condition may result in actions or events that contaminate a sterile field; for example, a client with a respiratory infection transmits organisms by coughing or breathing. The nurse anticipates such a problem and offers the client a mask.

Principles of Surgical Asepsis.   When beginning a surgically aseptic procedure, the nurse follows certain principles to ensure maintenance of asepsis. Failure to follow these principles places clients at risk for infection. The following principles are important:

1. *A sterile object remains sterile only when touched by another sterile object.* This principle guides the nurse

in placement of sterile objects and how to handle them.

   a. Sterile touching sterile remains sterile; for example, sterile gloves are worn or sterile forceps are used to handle objects on a sterile field.

   b. Sterile touching clean becomes contaminated; for example, if the tip of a syringe or other sterile object touches the surface of a clean disposable glove, the object is contaminated.

   c. Sterile touching contaminated becomes contaminated; for example, when the nurse touches a sterile object with an ungloved hand, the object is contaminated.

   d. Sterile touching questionable is contaminated; for example, when a tear or break in the covering of a sterile object is found, it is discarded regardless of whether the object itself appears untouched.

2. *Only sterile objects may be placed on a sterile field.* All items are properly sterilized before use. Sterile objects are kept in clean, dry storage areas. The package or container holding a sterile object must be intact and dry. A package that is torn, punctured, wet, or open is unsterile.

3. *A sterile object or field out of the range of vision or an object held below a person's waist is contaminated.* Nurses never turn their backs on a sterile tray or leave it unattended. Contamination can occur accidentally by a dangling piece of clothing, falling hair, or an unknowing client touching a sterile object. Any object held below waist level is considered contaminated because it cannot be viewed at all times. Sterile objects should be kept in front with the hands as close together as possible.

4. *A sterile object or field becomes contaminated by prolonged exposure to air.* The nurse avoids activities that may create air currents, such as excessive movements or rearranging linen after a sterile object or field becomes exposed. When sterile packages are being opened, it is important to minimize the number of people walking into the area. Microorganisms also travel by droplet through the air. No one should talk, laugh, sneeze, or cough over a sterile field or when gathering and using sterile equipment. Microorganisms traveling through the air can fall on sterile items or fields if the nurse reaches over the work area. When opening sterile packages, the nurse holds the item or piece of equipment as close as possible to the sterile field without touching the sterile surface. Keeping movement or rearranging of sterile items to a minimum also reduces contamination by air transmission.

5. *When a sterile surface comes in contact with a wet, contaminated surface, the sterile object or field becomes contaminated by capillary action.* If moisture seeps through a sterile package's protective covering, mi-

croorganisms travel to the sterile object. When stored sterile packages become wet, the nurse discards the objects immediately or sends the equipment for resterilization. When working with a sterile field or tray, the nurse may have to pour sterile solutions. Any spill can be a source of contamination unless the object or field rests on a sterile surface that cannot be penetrated by moisture. Urinary catheterization trays contain sterile supplies that rest in a sterile, plastic container. In this example, sterile solutions spilled within the container will not contaminate the catheter or other objects. In contrast, if a nurse places a piece of sterile gauze in its wrapper on a client's bedside table and the table surface is wet, the gauze is considered contaminated.

6. *Fluid flows in the direction of gravity.* A sterile object becomes contaminated if gravity causes a contaminated liquid to flow over the object's surface. To avoid contamination during a surgical hand scrub, the nurse holds the hands above the elbows. This allows water to flow downward without contaminating the nurse's hands and fingers. The principle of water flow by gravity is also the reason for drying from fingers to elbows with hands held up, after the scrub.

7. *The edges of a sterile field or container are considered to be contaminated.* Frequently a nurse places sterile objects on a sterile towel or drape. Because the edge of the drape touches an unsterile surface, such as a table or bed linen, a 2.5-cm (1-inch) border around the drape is considered contaminated. The edges of sterile containers become exposed to air after they are open and are thus contaminated. After a sterile needle is removed from its protective cap or after forceps are removed from a container, the objects must not touch the container's edge. The lip of an opened bottle of solution also becomes contaminated after it is exposed to air. When pouring a sterile liquid, the nurse first pours a small amount of solution and discards it. The solution washes away microorganisms on the bottle lip. Then the nurse pours a second time on the same side to fill a container with the desired amount of solution.

Performing Sterile Procedures.   All of the equipment that will be needed should be assembled before a procedure. Thus the nurse avoids having to leave a sterile area unattended because equipment is missing. A few extra supplies should be available in case objects accidentally become contaminated. Before the sterile procedure, each step should be explained so that the client can cooperate fully. If an object becomes contaminated during the procedure, the nurse should not hesitate to discard it immediately.

Donning and Removing Caps, Masks, and Eyewear. For sterile procedures on a general nursing division, the nurse may wear a surgical mask and eyewear without a cap. Eyewear is worn as a part of standard precautions if there is a risk of fluid or blood splashing into the nurse's eyes. For sterile surgical procedures, the nurse first applies a clean cap that covers all of the hair and then the surgical mask and eyewear. A mask must fit snugly around the face and nose to prevent contamination by droplet nuclei. After a mask is worn for several hours, the area over the mouth and nose often becomes moist. Moisture promotes the spread of microorganisms.

Protective glasses or goggles should fit snugly around the forehead and face to fully protect the eyes. Eyewear needs to be worn only for procedures that create the risk of body fluids splashing into the eyes. Before removing a mask, eyewear, and cap, the nurse removes sterile gloves to prevent contamination of the hair, neck, and facial area. After untying the mask, the nurse holds it by the ties and discards it with the cap. Masks should not be worn hanging from the neck after removal. Eyewear is removed and cleaned later for reuse. After removing all protective wear, the nurse washes hands thoroughly.

Opening Sterile Packages.   Sterile items such as syringes, gauze dressings, or catheters are packaged in paper or plastic containers and are impervious to microorganisms as long as they are dry and intact. Some institutions wrap reusable supplies in a double thickness of paper, linen, or muslin. These packages are permeable to steam and thus allow for steam autoclaving. Sterile items are kept in clean, enclosed storage cabinets and are separated from dirty equipment.

Sterile supplies have chemical tapes indicating that a sterilization process has taken place. The tapes change color during the sterilization process. Failure of the tapes to change color means that the item is not sterile. A sterile supply should never be used if the integrity of the packaging is compromised. Health care facilities may apply the date processed and a lot number to the item after processing ("event-related expiration"), or they may apply an expiration date ("date-related expiration") to the item. With either system it is important for the nurse to check the integrity of the packaging of the item before use.

Before opening a sterile item, the nurse washes hands thoroughly. The nurse inspects the supplies for package integrity and sterility and assembles the supplies in the work area, such as the bedside table or treatment room, before opening packages. A bedside table or countertop provides a large, clean working area for opening items. The work area should be above waist level. Sterile supplies should not be opened in a confined space where a dirty object might fall on or strike them.

Opening a Sterile Item on a Flat Surface.   Sterile packaged items must be opened without contaminating the contents. Commercially packaged items are usually designed so that the nurse only has to tear away or separate the paper or plastic cover. The item is held in one hand

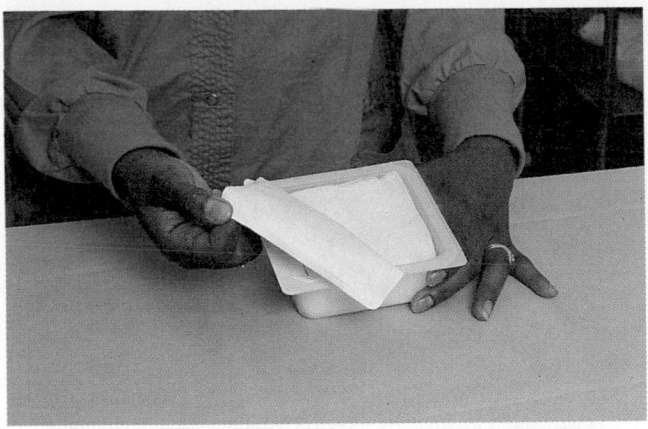

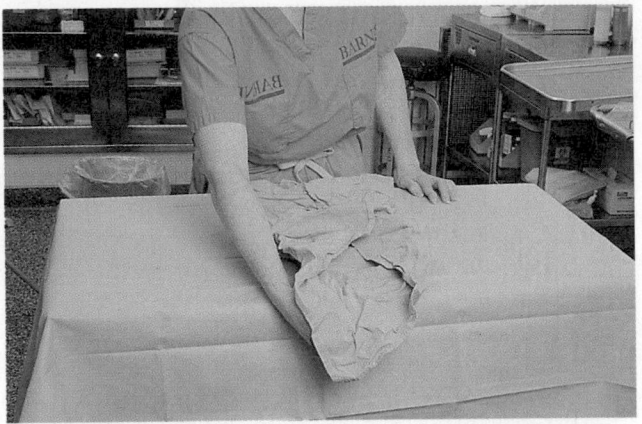
A

Figure 33-5   When opening a commercially packaged sterile item, the nurse tears the wrapper away from the body.

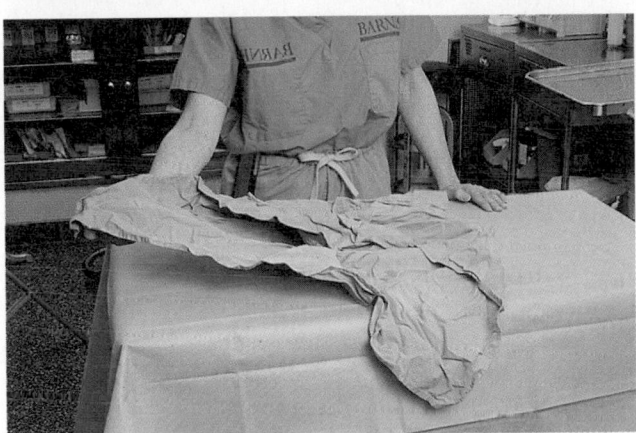
B

while the wrapper is pulled away with the other (Figure 33-5). Care is then taken to keep the inner contents sterile before use. When opening items processed by the facility and packed in paper or linen, the nurse uses the following steps:

1. Place the item flat in the center of the work surface.
2. Remove the sterilization tape or seal.
3. Grasp the outer surface of the tip of the outermost flap.
4. Open the outer flap away from the body, keeping the arm outstretched and away from the sterile field (Figure 33-6, *A*).
5. Grasp the outside surface of the first side flap.
6. Open the side flap, allowing it to lie flat on the table surface. Keep the arm to the side and not over the sterile surface (Figure 33-6, *B*). Do not allow the flaps to spring back over the sterile contents.
7. Grasp the outside surface of the second side flap and allow it to lie flat on the table surface (Figure 33-6, *C*).
8. Grasp the outside surface of the last and innermost flap.
9. Stand away from the sterile package and pull the flap back, allowing it to fall flat on the surface (Figure 33-6, *D*).

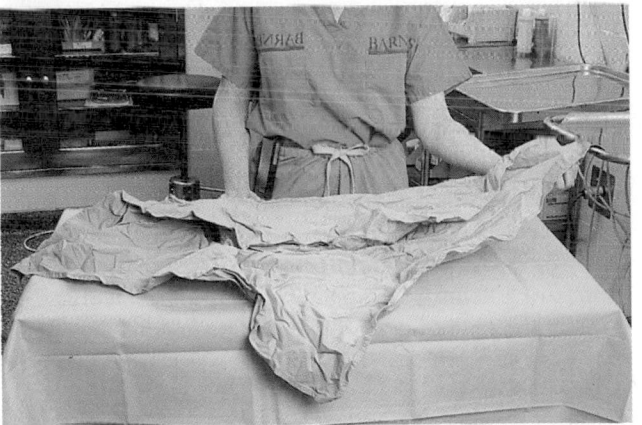
C

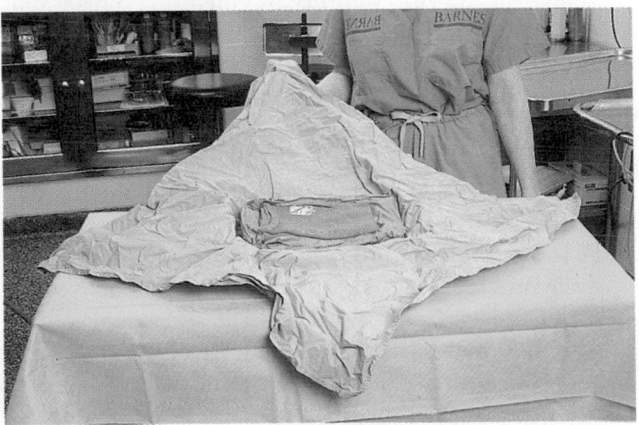
D

Figure 33-6   Opening sterile packaged items on a flat surface. **A,** The nurse opens the top flap away from the body. **B,** The nurse's arm is kept out away from the sterile field while opening a side flap. **C,** The second side flap is opened. **D,** The back flap is opened.

10.   Use the inner surface of the package (except for the 1-inch border around the edges) as a sterile field to add additional sterile items. The 1-inch border can be grasped to maneuver the field on the table surface.

If the sterile supplies are not to be used immediately, the nurse can close the sterile package. In this case the nurse should touch only the wrapper's outside surface. To close a package, the order of unwrapping is reversed, and the nurse does not touch the inside contents or reach over the field.

Opening a Sterile Item While Holding It.   To open small, sterile items, the package is held in the nondominant hand while the top flap is opened and pulled away from the nurse. Using the dominant hand, the nurse carefully opens the sides and top flaps away from the enclosed sterile item in the same order previously mentioned. The nurse opens the item in a hand so that the item can be handed to a person wearing sterile gloves or transferred to a sterile field.

Preparing a Sterile Field.   When performing sterile procedures, the nurse needs a sterile work area that provides room for handling and placing of sterile items. A **sterile field** is an area free of microorganisms and prepared to receive sterile items. The field may be prepared by using the inner surface of a sterile wrapper as the work surface or by using a sterile drape. Skill 33-2 describes preparation of a sterile field. After the surface for the field is created, the nurse adds sterile items by placing them directly on the field or by transferring them with a sterile forceps. When transferring sterile items, the nurse must carefully place objects onto the sterile field. An object that comes in contact with the 1-inch border must be discarded.

The nurse may choose to wear sterile gloves while preparing items on the field. If this is done, the nurse can touch the entire drape, but sterile items must be handed over by an assistant. The nurse's gloves cannot touch the wrappers of sterile items.

Pouring Sterile Solutions.   Often the nurse must pour sterile solutions into sterile containers. A bottle containing a sterile solution is sterile on the inside and contaminated on the outside; the bottle's neck is also contaminated, but the inside of the bottle cap is considered sterile. After a cap or lid is removed, it is held in the hand or placed sterile side (inside) up on a clean surface. This means that the inside of the lid can be seen as it rests on the table surface. A bottle cap or lid should never rest on a sterile surface, even though the inside of the cap is sterile. The outer edge of the cap is unsterile and would contaminate the surface. Likewise, placing a sterile cap down on an unsterile surface increases the chances of the inside of the cap becoming contaminated.

The bottle should be held with its label in the palm of the hand to prevent the possibility of the solution wetting and fading the label. Before pouring the solution into the container, the nurse pours a small amount (1 to 2 ml) into a disposable cap or plastic-lined waste receptacle. The discarded solution cleans the lip of the bottle. The edge of the bottle is kept away from the edge or inside of the receiving container. The nurse pours the solution slowly to avoid splashing the underlying drape or field. The bottle should never be held so high above the container that even slow pouring will cause splashing. The bottle should be held outside the edge of the sterile field.

Surgical Scrub.   Clients undergoing operative procedures are at an increased risk for infection. Nurses working in operating rooms perform surgical hand scrubs to decrease and suppress the growth of skin microorganisms in case of glove tears (Association of Operating Room Nurses [AORN], 1998).

During surgical hand washing, the nurse scrubs from fingertips to elbows with an antiseptic soap before each operation. The optimum duration of the surgical hand scrub is unclear, although research indicates that it may be dependent on the type of antimicrobial product (Pereira and others, 1990; O'Shaughnessy and others, 1991; Hingst and others, 1992). The traditional scrub time in the United States for both the initial and the subsequent scrub has been 5 minutes (Meeker and Rothrock, 1999). Larson (1996) recommends that at least 2 minutes of friction be used for surgical hand washing. The nurse should follow the agency's policy for length of scrub time.

For maximum elimination of bacteria, all jewelry should be removed and the nails should be kept clean and short (AORN, 1998). Artificial nails should not be worn, since they may harbor a greater number of bacteria (Pottinger and others, 1989). Nurses who have active skin infections, open lesions or cuts, or respiratory infections should be excluded from the surgical team. In scrubbing, light friction is effective in removing microorganisms; too much brushing may remove the outer layer of epidermis, thereby exposing bacterial flora in the deeper skin layers (Meeker and Rothrock, 1999). Skill 33-3 describes the steps for surgical scrub.

Applying Sterile Gloves.   Sterile gloves are an additional barrier to bacterial transfer. There are two gloving methods: open and closed. Nurses who work on general nursing divisions use open gloving before procedures such as dressing changes or urinary catheter insertions. The closed gloving method, which is performed after nurses apply sterile gowns, is practiced in operating rooms and special treatment areas. Skills 33-4 and 33-5 review the steps of each gloving technique.

The proper glove size should be selected; the glove should not stretch so tightly that it can easily tear, yet it should be tight enough that objects can be picked up easily.

Text continued on p. 879.

Preparing a Sterile Field   Skill 33-2

Delegation Considerations

Preparing a sterile field requires specialized knowledge regarding surgical asepsis. Delegation is inappropriate unless assistive personnel have received specialized training.

EQUIPMENT
- Sterile drape
- Assorted sterile supplies

STEPS	RATIONALE
1. Prepare sterile field just before planned procedure. Supplies are to be used immediately.	Prevents exposure of sterile field and supplies to air and contamination.
2. Select clean work surface above waist level.	Sterile object held below waist is contaminated.
3. Assemble necessary equipment.	Preparation of equipment in advance prevents break in technique.
4. Check dates or labels on supplies for sterility of equipment.	Equipment stored beyond expiration date is considered unsterile.
5. Wash hands thoroughly.	Prevents transmission of infection.
6. Place pack containing sterile drape on work surface and open as described on p. 867.	Ensures sterility of packaged drape.
7. With fingertips of one hand, pick up folded top edge of sterile drape.	One-inch border around drape is unsterile and may be touched.
8. Gently lift drape up from its outer cover and let it unfold by itself without touching any object. Discard outer cover with your other hand.	If sterile object touches any other nonsterile object, it becomes contaminated.
9. With other hand, grasp adjacent corner of drape and hold it straight up and away from your body (see illustration).	Drape can now be properly placed while using two hands. Drape must be held away from unsterile surfaces.
10. Holding drape, first position and lay bottom half over intended work surface (see illustration).	Prevents nurse from reaching over sterile field.
11. Allow top half of drape to be placed over work surface last (see illustration).	Creates flat, sterile work surface.
12. Grasp 1-inch border around edge to position as needed.	

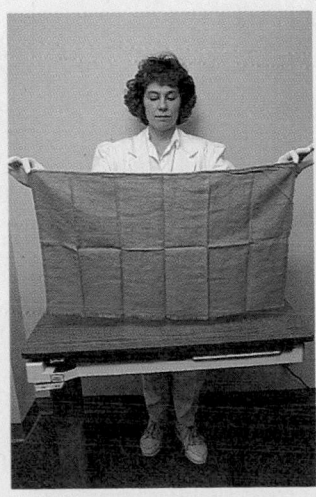   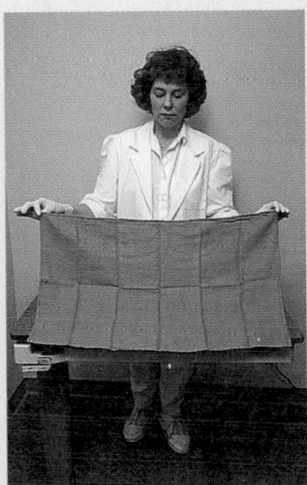   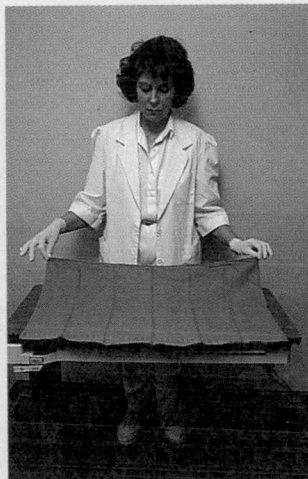

Step 9   **Step 10**   **Step 11**

STEPS	RATIONALE

ADDING STERILE ITEMS

13. Open sterile item (following package directions) while holding outside wrapper in nondominant hand.

Frees dominant hand for unwrapping outer wrapper.

14. Carefully peel wrapper onto nondominant hand.

Item remains sterile. Inner surface of wrapper covers hand, making it sterile.

15. Being sure wrapper does not fall down on sterile field, place item onto field at angle. Do not hold arm over sterile field (see illustration).

Prevents reaching over field and contaminating its surface.

16. Dispose of outer wrapper.

Prevents accidental contamination of sterile field.

17. Perform procedure using sterile technique.

Prevents transmission of infection to client.

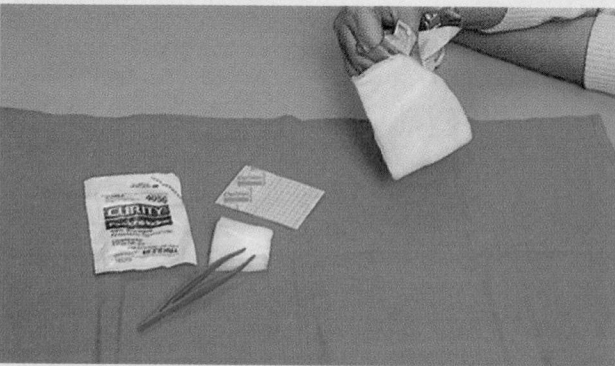

Step 15

Recording and Reporting

* It is not necessary to record or report this procedure.

Surgical Hand Washing: Preparing for Gowning | Skill 33-3

Delegation Considerations

The circulating nurse must always be a registered nurse. The role of the scrub nurse can be delegated to a surgical technologist or licensed practical nurse.

Assistive personnel can help the registered nurse in the circulating role by opening sterile supplies, setting up sterile fields, and running errands under the direction of the registered nurse.

EQUIPMENT

- Deep sink with foot or knee controls for dispensing water and soap (faucets should be high enough for hands and forearms to fit comfortably)
- Antiseptic detergent (nonirritating, broad-spectrum, fast-acting, effective in reducing skin microorganisms, and having a residual effect) (AORN, 1998)

- Surgical scrub brush with plastic nail pick
- Paper mask and cap or hood
- Sterile towel
- Proper scrub attire
- Protective eyewear (glasses or goggles)

STEPS	RATIONALE
1. Consult institutional policy regarding required length of time for hand wash.	Guidelines vary regarding ideal time needed for surgical scrub.
2. Be sure fingernails are short, clean, and healthy. Artificial nails should be removed.	Long nails and chipped or old polish increase number of bacteria residing on nails. Long fingernails can puncture gloves, causing contamination. Artificial nails are known to harbor gram-negative microorganisms and fungus.

Critical Decision Point: Remove nail polish if chipped or worn longer than 4 days because it may harbor microorganisms (AORN, 1998).

3. Inspect hands for presence of abrasions, cuts, or open lesions.	These conditions increase likelihood of more microorganisms residing on skin surfaces.
4. Apply surgical shoe covers, cap or hood, face mask, and protective eyewear.	Mask prevents escape into air of microorganisms that can contaminate hands. Other protective wear prevents exposure to blood and body fluid splashes during the procedure.
5. Turn on water using knee or foot controls and adjust to comfortable temperature.	
6. Wet hands and arms under running lukewarm water and lather with detergent to 5 cm (2 inches) above elbows. (Hands need to be above elbows at all times.)	Water runs by gravity from fingertips to elbows. Hands become cleanest part of upper extremity. Keeping hands elevated allows water to flow from least to most contaminated areas. Washing a wide area reduces risk of contaminating overlying gown that the nurse later applies.
7. Rinse hands and arms thoroughly under running water. **Remember to keep hands above elbows.**	Rinsing removes transient bacteria from fingers, hands, and forearms.
8. Under running water, clean under nails of both hands with nail pick. Discard after use (see illustration, p. 872).	Removes dirt and organic material that harbor large numbers of microorganisms.
9. Wet clean brush and apply antimicrobial detergent. Scrub nails of one hand with 15 strokes. Holding brush perpendicular, scrub palm, each side of thumb and fingers, and posterior side of hand with 10 strokes each. The arm is mentally divided into thirds, and each third is scrubbed 10 times (see illustration, p. 872). Entire scrub should last 5 to 10 minutes. Rinse brush and repeat sequence for other arm. A two-brush method may be substituted. Check agency policy.	Scrubbing loosens resident bacteria that adhere to skin surfaces. Ensures coverage of all surfaces. Scrubbing is performed from cleanest area (hands) to marginal area (upper arms).

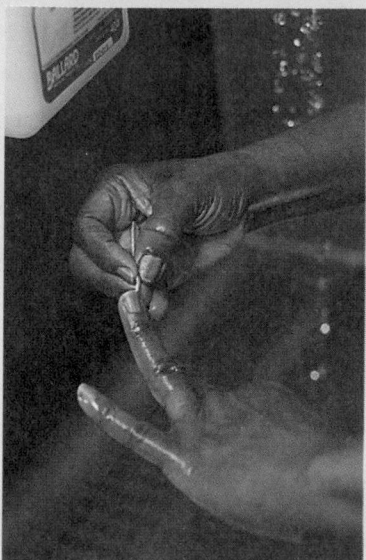

Step 8

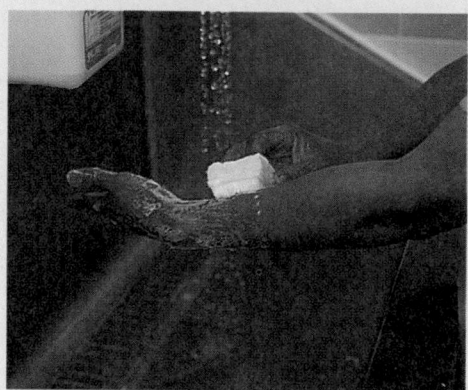

Step 9

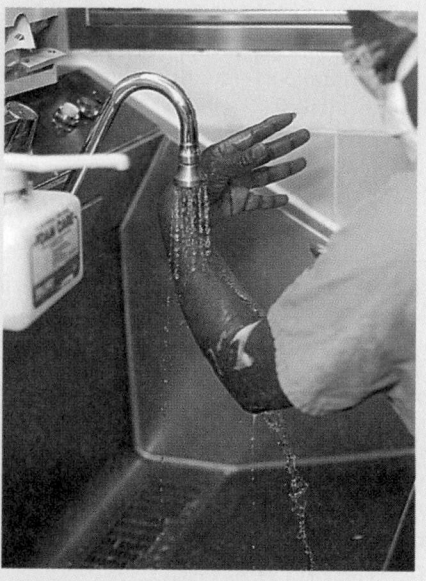

Step 10

10. Discard brush and rinse hands and arms thoroughly (see illustration). Turn off water with foot or knee control and back into room entrance with hands elevated in front of and away from the body.	After touching skin, brush is considered contaminated. Rinsing removes resident bacteria. Prevents accidental contamination.
11. Bending slightly forward at the waist, use a sterile towel to dry one hand thoroughly, moving from fingers to elbow. Dry in a rotating motion. Dry from cleanest to least clean area.	Drying prevents chapping and facilitates donning of gloves. Leaning forward prevents accidental contact of arms with scrub attire.
12. Repeat drying method for other hand by carefully reversing towel or using a new sterile towel.	Prevents accidental contamination.
13. Discard towel.	Prevents accidental contamination.
14. Proceed with sterile gowning (see Skill 33-4).	

Recording and Reporting
- It is not necessary to record or report this procedure.
- Report any dermatitis to employee health or infection control per agency policy.

Applying a Sterile Gown and Performing Closed Gloving   Skill 33-4

Delegation Considerations
The role of the scrub nurse can be delegated to a surgical technician.

EQUIPMENT
- Surgical cap
- Surgical mask
- Eyewear

- Foot covers
- Sterile gown (prepared by circulating nurse)

STEPS	RATIONALE

GOWNING

1. Before entering operating room or treatment area, apply cap, face mask, and eyewear. Foot covers are also required in operating room.

   Prevents hair and air droplet nuclei from contaminating sterile work areas. Eyewear protects mucous membranes of eye. Foot covers are paper or cloth and fit over work shoes.

2. Perform thorough surgical hand wash (see Skill 33-3).

   Removes transient and resident bacteria from fingers, hands, and forearms.

3. Ask circulating nurse to assist by opening sterile pack containing sterile gown (folded inside out).

   Gown's outer surface remains sterile.

4. Have circulating nurse prepare glove package by peeling outer wrapper open while keeping inner contents sterile. Inner glove package is then placed on sterile field created by sterile outer wrapper.

   Keeps gloves sterile and allows nurse who has scrubbed to handle sterile items.

5. Reach down to sterile gown package (see illustration); lift folded gown directly upward and step back away from table (see illustration).

   Provides wide margin of safety, avoiding contamination of gown.

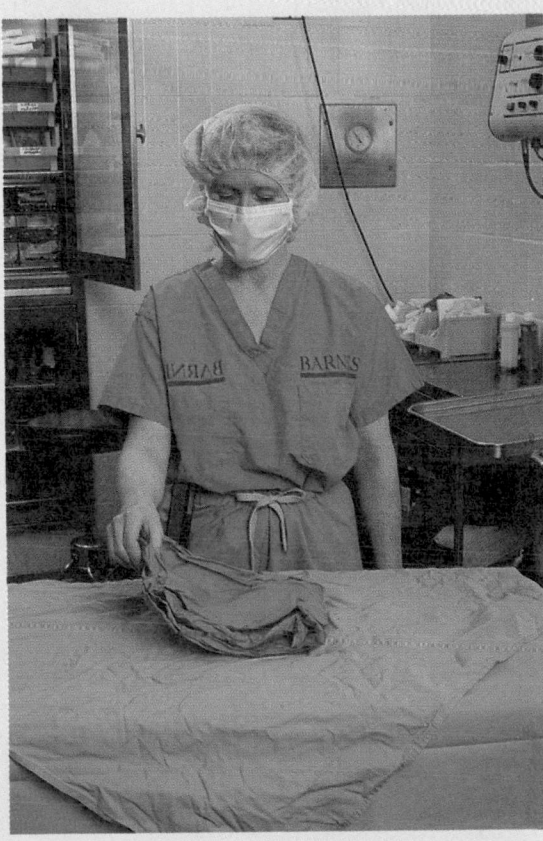
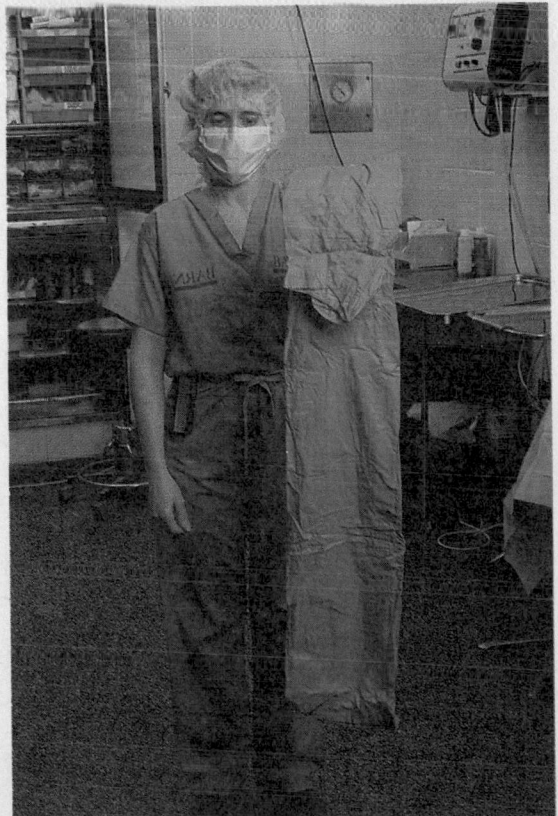

Step 5

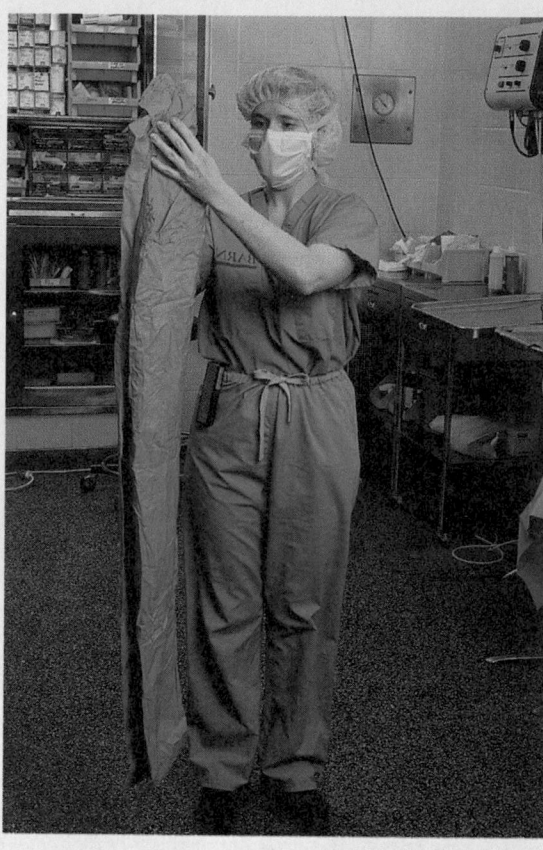

Step 7

STEPS	RATIONALE
6. Holding folded gown, locate neckband. With both hands, grasp inside front of gown just below neckband (see illustration).	Clean hands may touch inside of gown without contaminating outer surface.
7. Allow gown to unfold, keeping inside of gown toward body. Do not touch outside of gown with bare hands (see illustration).	Outside of gown will be sterile surface.
8. With hands at shoulder level, slip both arms into armholes simultaneously (see illustration). Ask circulating nurse to bring gown over shoulders by reaching inside to arm seams. Gown is pulled on, leaving sleeves covering hands (see illustration).	Careful application prevents contamination. Gown covers hands to prepare for closed gloving.
9. Have circulating nurse securely tie back of gown at neck and waist. (If gown is a wraparound style, sterile flap to cover gown is not touched until the nurse has gloved.)	Gown must completely enclose underlying garments.

CLOSED GLOVING

STEPS	RATIONALE
1. With hands covered by gown sleeves, open inner sterile glove package.	Hands remain clean. Sterile gown cuff will touch sterile glove surface.
2. With nondominant hand inside gown cuff, pick up glove for dominant hand by grasping folded cuff.	Sterile gown touches sterile glove.
3. Extend dominant forearm with palm up and place palm of glove against palm of dominant hand. Glove fingers will point toward elbow.	Positions glove for application over cuffed hand, keeping glove sterile.

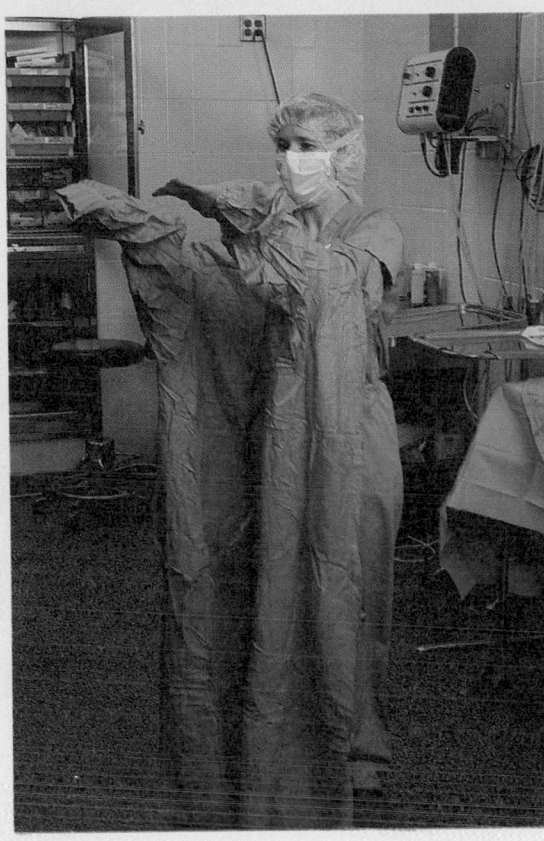 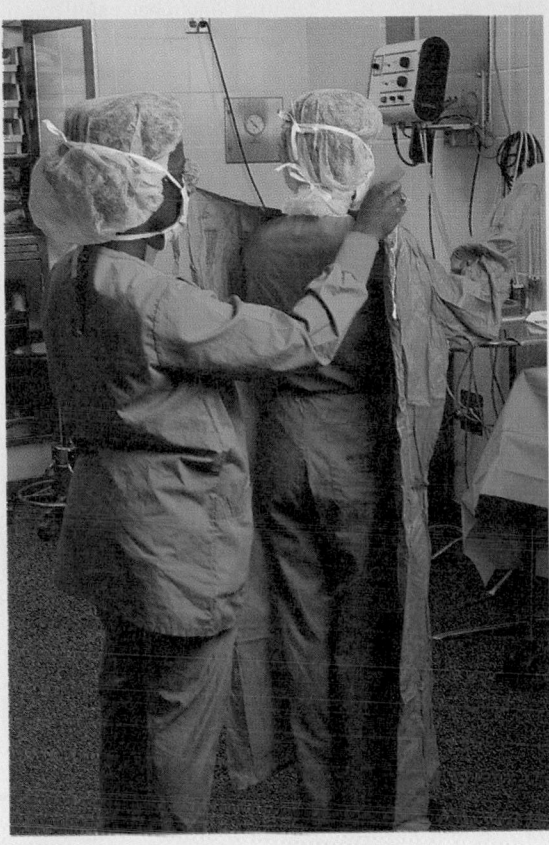

Step 8

4. Grasp back of glove cuff with nondominant hand and turn glove cuff over end of dominant hand and gown cuff (see illustration).

5. Grasp top of glove and underlying gown sleeve with covered nondominant hand. Carefully extend fingers into glove, being sure glove's cuff covers gown's cuff.

Seal created by glove cuff over gown prevents exit of microorganisms over operative sterile field.

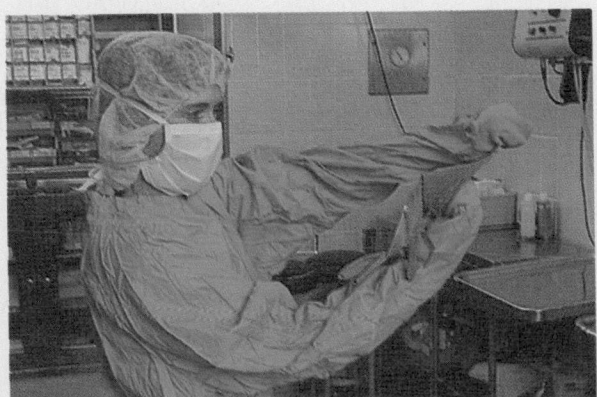

Step 4

STEPS	RATIONALE
6. Glove nondominant hand in same manner, reversing hands (see illustration). Use gloved dominant hand to pull on glove. Keep hand inside sleeve (see illustration).	Sterile touches sterile.
7. Be sure fingers are fully extended into both gloves.	Ensures that nurse has full dexterity while using gloved hand.
8. For wraparound sterile gowns: take gloved hand and release fastener or ties in front of gown.	Front of gown is sterile.
9. Hand tie to sterile team member who stands still. Allowing margin of safety, turn around to the left, covering back with extended gown flap. Take back tie from team member and secure tie to gown.	Contact with team member could contaminate gown and gloves. Gown must enclose undergarments.

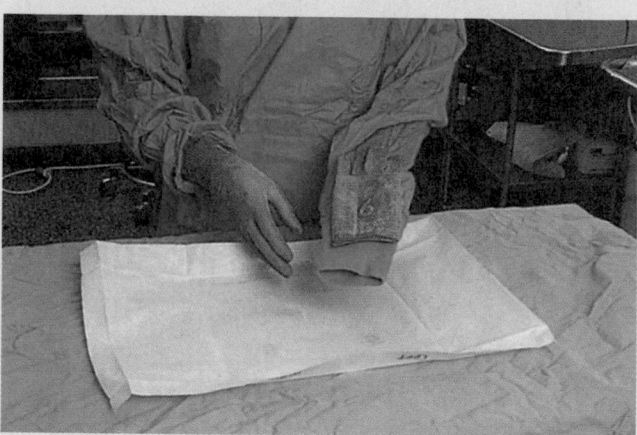 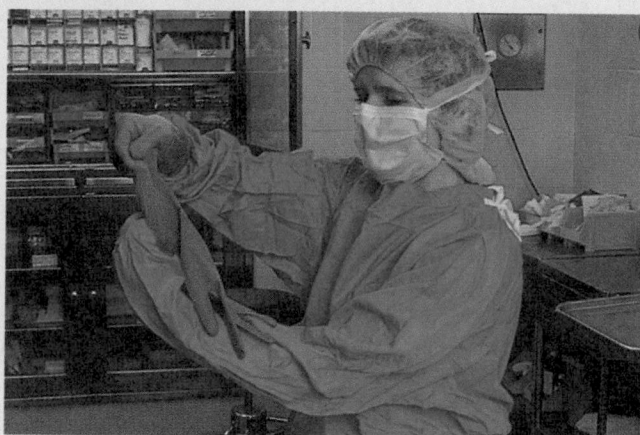

Step 6

Recording and Reporting

- It is not necessary to record or report this procedure.

Open Gloving   Skill 33-5

Delegation Considerations
Delegation of open gloving depends on whether assistive personnel have been instructed and are competent to perform the sterile procedure.

EQUIPMENT
* Sterile gloves (proper size)

STEPS	RATIONALE
1. Perform thorough hand washing.	Removes bacteria from skin surfaces and reduces transmission of infection.
2. Remove outer glove package wrapper by carefully separating and peeling apart sides.	Prevents inner glove package from accidentally opening and touching contaminated objects.
3. Grasp inner package and lay it on clean, flat surface just above waist level. Open package, keeping gloves on wrapper's inside surface (see illustration).	Sterile object held below waist is contaminated. Inner surface of glove package is sterile.

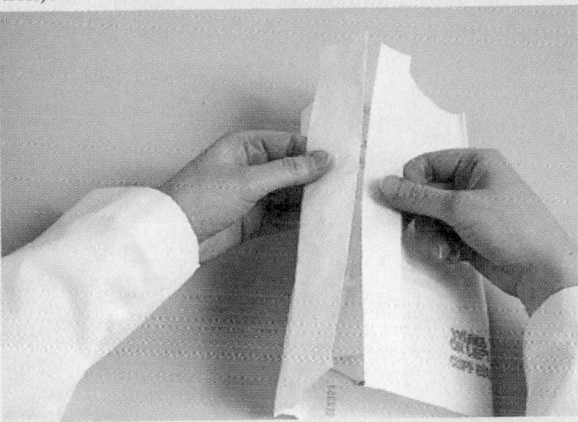

Step 3

4. If gloves are not prepowdered, take packet of powder and apply lightly to hands over sink or wastebasket.	Powder allows gloves to slip on easily. (Some staff members do not use powder for fear of promoting growth of microorganisms.)
5. Identify right and left glove. Each glove has cuff approximately 5 cm (2 inches) wide. Glove dominant hand first.	Proper identification of gloves prevents contamination by improper fit. Gloving of dominant hand first improves dexterity.
6. With thumb and first two fingers of nondominant hand, grasp edge of cuff of glove for dominant hand. Touch only glove's inside surface.	Inner edge of cuff will lie against skin and thus is not sterile.
7. Carefully pull glove over dominant hand, leaving cuff and being sure cuff does not roll up wrist. Be sure thumb and fingers are in proper spaces (see illustration).	If glove's outer surface touches hand or wrist, it is contaminated.

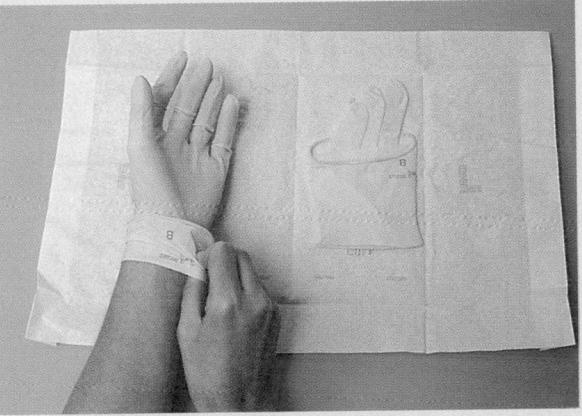

Step 7

STEPS	RATIONALE
8. With gloved dominant hand, slip fingers underneath second glove's cuff (see illustration).	Cuff protects gloved fingers. Sterile touching sterile prevents glove contamination.
9. Carefully pull second glove over nondominant hand. Do not allow fingers and thumb of gloved dominant hand to touch any part of exposed nondominant hand. Keep thumb of dominant hand abducted back (see illustration).	Contact of gloved hand with exposed hand results in contamination.
10. After second glove is on, interlock hands. The cuffs usually fall down after application. Be sure to touch only sterile sides (see illustration).	Ensures smooth fit over fingers.

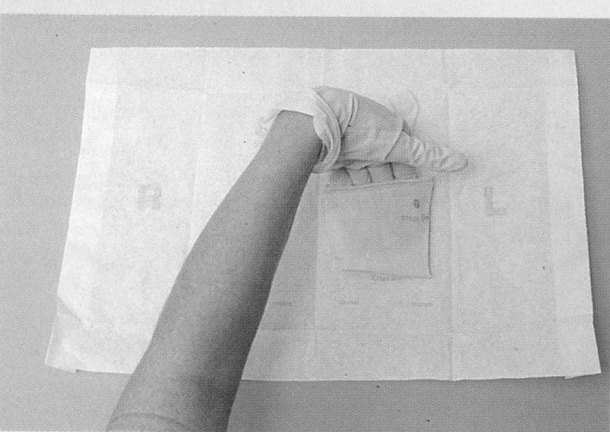

Step 8

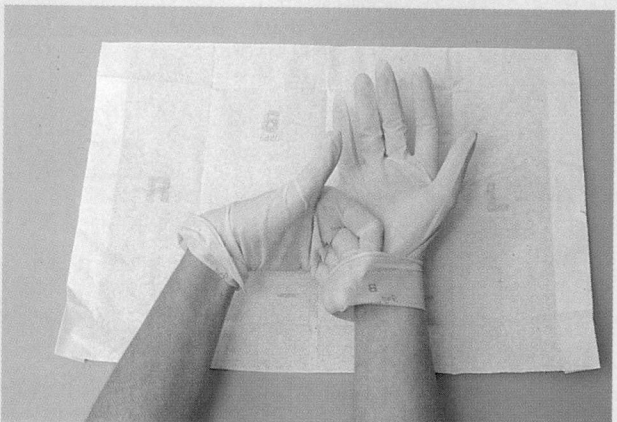

Step 9

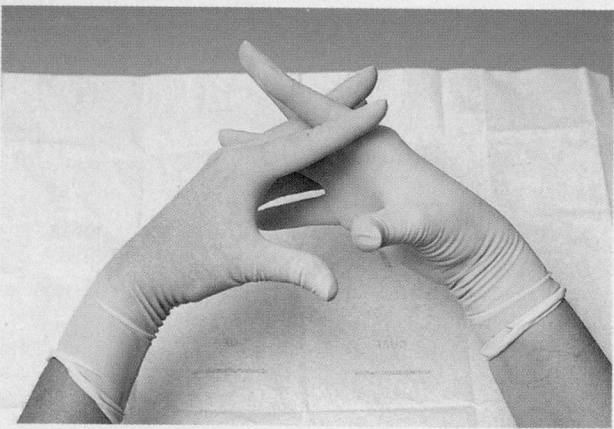

Step 10

GLOVE DISPOSAL

11. Grasp outside of one cuff with other gloved hand; avoid touching wrist.	Minimizes contamination of underlying skin.
12. Pull glove off, turning it inside out. Discard in receptacle.	Outside of glove does not touch skin surface.
13. Take fingers of bare hand and tuck inside remaining glove cuff. Peel glove off, inside out. Discard in receptacle.	

Recording and Reporting

- It is not necessary to record or report this procedure.

Donning a Sterile Gown.   Nurses must wear sterile gowns when assisting at the sterile field in the operating room and delivery room so that sterile objects can be comfortably handled with less risk of contamination. The circulating nurse does not generally wear a sterile gown. The sterile gown acts as a barrier to decrease shedding of microorganisms from skin surfaces into the air and thus prevents wound contamination. Nurses caring for clients with large open wounds or assisting physicians during major invasive procedures (e.g., inserting an arterial catheter) may also wear sterile gowns.

The nurse does not apply a sterile gown until after applying a mask and surgical cap and performing surgical hand washing. The nurse picks up the gown from a sterile pack, or an assistant hands the gown to the nurse. Only a certain portion of the gown—the area from the anterior waist to, but not including, the collar and the anterior surface of the sleeves— is considered sterile. The back of the gown, the area under the arms, the collar, the area below the waist, and the underside of the sleeves are not sterile because the nurse cannot keep these areas in constant view and ensure their sterility. Skill 33-4 reviews the steps for applying a gown.

EVALUATION

The success of the nurse who practices infection-control techniques is measured by determining whether the goals for reducing or preventing infection are achieved. A comparison of the client's response, such as absence of fever or development of wound drainage, with expected outcomes determines the success of nursing interventions (Figure 33-7). Similarly, a determination is made about whether interventions should be revised or eliminated. The ability to correctly assess wounds for healing and the ability to conduct a physical assessment of body systems (see Chapter 32) are important skills in evaluation. The nurse closely monitors clients, especially those at risk, for signs and symptoms of infection. For example, a client who has undergone a surgical procedure is at risk for infection at the surgical site, as well as at other invasive sites, such as the venipuncture site or central line sites. In addition, the client is at risk for a respiratory tract infection as a result of decreased mobility and for a urinary tract infection if an indwelling catheter is present. The nurse closely monitors all invasive and surgical sites for swelling, erythema, or purulent drainage. Breath sounds are monitored for changes, and sputum character is checked for purulence. Laboratory test results are reviewed for leukocytes in the urine, which may indicate a urinary tract infection. The absence of signs or symptoms of infection is the expected outcome of infection prevention and monitoring activities.

The client at risk for infection must understand the measures needed to reduce or prevent microorganism growth and spread. Providing clients or family members the opportunity to discuss infection-control measures or to demonstrate procedures will reveal their ability to comply with therapy. The nurse may determine that clients require new information or that previously instructed information needs reinforcement.

The nurse documents the client's response to therapies for infection control. A clear description of any signs and symptoms of systemic or local infection is necessary to give all nurses a baseline for comparative evaluation. The efficacy of any intervention in reducing infection must also be reported.

SEPSIS WITH NEUTROPENIA

DRG # 416
Target LOS 9 days

	DATE	DATE	DATE
Hosp day	**HOSPITAL DAY 1**	**HOSPITAL DAY 2**	**HOSPITAL DAY 3**
CONSULTS	Notify Radiation Therapy if applicable	Dr. Clements if ordered Social Service Dietician	
TESTS	CBC, SMA 18, Magnesium, Creatinine Blood cultures X 2 sites before antibiotics started Chest Xray Type and Screen	CBC Blood cultures for chills or temp>101 No more than 3 sets in 24 hours	CBC - - - - - - - - - - - - - - - - -> - - - - - - - - - - - - - - - - ->
SPECIMENS	U/A for c&s before antibiotics started Sputum for c&s if productive cough	- - - - - - - - - - - - - - - - ->	- - - - - - - - - - - - - - - - ->
TREATMENTS	O2 at 2L by NC if Hgb<8 Mouth care every 4 hours per protocol	- - - - - - - - - - - - - - - - -> - - - - - - - - - - - - - - - - ->	- - - - - - - - - - - - - - - - -> - - - - - - - - - - - - - - - - ->
VITAL SIGNS	Every 4 hours	- - - - - - - - - - - - - - - - ->	- - - - - - - - - - - - - - - - ->
I & O	Every 8 hours	- - - - - - - - - - - - - - - - ->	- - - - - - - - - - - - - - - - ->
DIET	Neutropenic DAT until WBC>1.5	- - - - - - - - - - - - - - - - ->	- - - - - - - - - - - - - - - - ->
IVs	Fluids as ordered Antibiotics as ordered	Check w/MD re: fluid changes Continue antibiotics as ordered until d/c'd	Continue until d/c'd - - - - - - - - - - - - - - - - ->
MEDS	ID home meds and check with MD Check those that are ordered: ____Tylenol gr X po temp>101 ____Pain PRN ____Sleeper ____Antidiarrhea ____Antiemetic ____Antianxiety	Check those that are ordered: ____Tylenol gr X po temp>101 ____Pain PRN ____Sleeper ____Antidiarrhea ____Antiemetic ____Antianxiety	Check those that are ordered: ____Tylenol gr X po temp>101 ____Pain PRN ____Sleeper ____Antidiarrhea ____Antiemetic ____Antianxiety
ACTIVITY	Up as tolerated	- - - - - - - - - - - - - - - - ->	- - - - - - - - - - - - - - - - ->
MISC	Protective Isolation	- - - - - - - - - - - - - - - - ->	Continue until WBC>1.5
TEACHING	Instruct pt to report any: bleeding, diarrhea, N&V, pain.	Dietician to teach re: neutropenic diet. Mouth Care	Instruct re: personal hygiene
DISCHARGE PLANNING	Evaluate need for d/c planning.	Social services called if appropriate	Determine d/c destination

	Shift	Shift	Shift
Nurse signature	_____/_____	_____/_____	_____/_____
Nurse signature	_____/_____	_____/_____	_____/_____
Nurse signature	_____/_____	_____/_____	_____/_____

Authored by Janie Barnett, RN; Lucy Wallace, LPN

Figure 33-7 First 3 days of 9-day CareMap® for sepsis with neutropenia.
Courtesy Baptist Hospital, Pensacola, Fla, and The Center for Case Management, South Natick, Mass.

SUMMARY
PATIENT PROBLEMS/OUTCOME CRITERIA

Sepsis w/Neutropenia

Target LOS 9 days

Date	Initial	Nsg Diagnosis/Problem	Outcome Criteria/Goal	Date d/c	Initial
		1. Activity intolerance re: disease process.	1. PT will be able to perform own hygeine care by d/c.		
		2. Altered Nutrition re: less than body requirements re: anorexia, illness, dehydration.	2a Patient will be able to eat at least 1/3 of their ordered diets by d/c. 2b Patient will identify at least 3 food items that they find appealing 2c 1500cc po flds q 24 by d/c		
		3. Hyperthermia re: increase in metabolic rate and illness.	3. Pt. will be afebrile by day 5.		
		4. Potential knowledge deficit re: s/s to report neutropenic diet, personal hygiene, activity restrictions	4. Prior to d/c, the pt/s.o. will be able to demonstrate competency and/or verbalize understanding of instructions provided		

Signature

Title

Figure 33-7, cont'd First 3 days of 9-day CareMap® for sepsis with neutropenia.

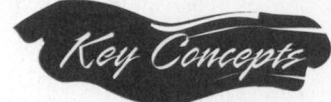

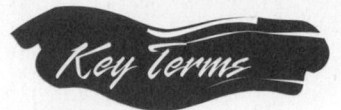

- Hand washing is the most important technique to use in preventing and controlling transmission of infection.
- The potential for microorganisms to cause disease depends on the number of organisms, virulence, ability to enter and survive in a host, and susceptibility of the host.
- Normal body flora helps to resist infection by releasing antibacterial substances and inhibiting multiplication of pathogenic microorganisms.
- The signs of local inflammation and infection are identical.
- An infection can develop as long as the six elements composing the infection chain are uninterrupted.
- Microorganisms are transmitted by direct and indirect contact, by airborne spread, and by vectors and contaminated articles.
- Increasing age, poor nutrition, stress, inherited conditions, chronic disease, and treatments or conditions that compromise the immune response may increase susceptibility to infection.
- The major sites for nosocomial infections include the urinary and respiratory tracts, bloodstream, and surgical or traumatic wounds.
- Invasive procedures, medical therapies, long hospitalization, and contact with health care personnel increase a hospitalized client's risk for acquiring a nosocomial infection.
- Clients within an intensive care unit have a higher risk for infection than clients who are not in this area because of increased exposure to invasive procedures.
- Isolation practices may prevent personnel and clients from acquiring infections and may prevent transmission of microorganisms to other persons.
- Standard precautions use generic barrier techniques when caring for all clients.
- Proper cleansing requires mechanical removal of all foreign material from an object or area.
- A client in isolation is subject to sensory deprivation because of the restricted environment.
- An infection-control professional monitors the incidence of infection within an institution and provides educational and consultative services to maintain infection prevention.
- Surgical asepsis requires more stringent techniques than medical asepsis and is directed at eliminating microorganisms.

   If the skin is broken, or if the nurse performs an invasive procedure into a body cavity normally free of microorganisms, surgical aseptic practices are followed.

Aerobic, *p. 837*
Anaerobic, *p. 837*
Antibodies, *p. 842*
Antigen, *p. 841*
Artificial immunity, *p. 842*
Asepsis, *p. 849*
Asymptomatic, *p. 835*
Bactericidal, *p. 837*
Bacteriostasis, *p. 837*
Broad-spectrum antibiotics, *p. 840*
Carriers, *p. 837*
Colonized, *p. 856*
Communicable, *p. 835*
Complement, *p. 842*
Cytolysis, *p. 842*
Disinfection, *p. 849*
Edema, *p. 840*
Endogenous infection, *p. 843*
Epidemiology, *p. 863*
Exogenous infection, *p. 843*
Exudate, *p. 840*
Granulation tissue, *p. 841*
Hand washing, *p. 852*
Iatrogenic infections, *p. 842*
Immune responses, *p. 841*
Immunocompromised, *p. 836*
Immunoglobulins, *p. 842*

Inflammatory response, *p. 839*
Interferon, *p. 842*
Invasive, *p. 835*
Leukocytosis, *p. 840*
Localized, *p. 839*
Lymphokines, *p. 842*
Medical asepsis, *p. 849*
Microorganisms, *p. 835*
Natural immunity, *p. 842*
Necrotic, *p. 840*
Normal flora, *p. 840*
Nosocomial infections, *p. 842*
Passive immunity, *p. 842*
Pathogenicity, *p. 839*
Pathogen, *p. 835*
Phagocytosis, *p. 840*
Purulent, *p. 841*
Sanguineous, *p. 841*
Serous, *p. 841*
Sterile field, *p. 868*
Sterilization, *p. 849*
Suprainfection, *p. 840*
Surgical asepsis, *p. 864*
Susceptibility, *p. 835*
Systemic, *p. 839*
Vector, *p. 838*
Virulence, *p. 836*

Critical Thinking Exercises

1. Mrs. Jaycock had an indwelling urethral catheter for 1 week. The catheter has now been out for 24 hours. She complains of frequency and pain on urination. Mrs. Jaycock suggests reinsertion of the catheter because of the need to get up frequently. What can frequency or pain on urination be an indication of? Should the catheter be reinserted? Why or why not? Describe at least two independent clinical actions for Mrs. Jaycock.

2. You are caring for Mr. Huang, who has a large, open, and draining abdominal wound. You notice another health care worker changing Mr. Huang's dressing without wearing gloves or using sterile supplies or sterile technique. When you question the health care worker regarding his or her practice, this person says, "Don't worry, the wound is already infected, and the antibiotics and draining will take care of any contaminants." How would you respond to this comment? What would your next steps be in following up on this incident?

3. Ms. Long became ill suddenly with fever, conjunctivitis, and a rash. Her doctor diagnosed measles. Describe the phase of the immune response in which the viral cells are attacked by the body. What class of immunoglobulins would be measured at this time?

4. Mrs. Niles is 83 years of age and lives alone. She has difficulty walking and relies on a church volunteer group to deliver lunches during the week. Her fixed income limits her ability to buy food. Last week, Mrs. Niles's 79-year-old sister died. The two sisters had been very close. As a home health care nurse, explain the factors that might increase Mrs. Niles's risk for infection.

References

Association of Operating Room Nurses: Recommended practices for surgical hand scrubs. In *Standards and recommended practices for perioperative nursing,* Denver, 1998, The Association.

Centers for Disease Control and Prevention: Guideline for preventing the transmission of mycobacterium tuberculosis in health-care facilities, *Federal Register* 59(208):54242, 1994.

Centers for Disease Control and Prevention: Guidelines for prevention of nosocomial pneumonia, *MMWR Morb Mortal Wkly Rep* 46(RR-1):52, 1997.

Centers for Disease Control and Prevention, Hospital Infection Control Practices Advisory Committee: Recommendations for preventing the spread of vancomycin resistance, *Am J Infect Control* 23(2):87, 1995.

Garner JS: Guidelines for isolation precautions in hospitals, *Infect Control Hosp Epidemiol* 17(1):54, 1996.

Grimes D, Grimes R: *AIDS and HIV infections,* St. Louis, 1994, Mosby.

Hingst V and others: Evaluation of the efficacy of surgical hand disinfection following a reduced application time of 3 instead of 5 minutes, *J Hosp Infect* 20:79, 1992.

Jackson M, Lynch P: An attempt to make an issue less murky: a comparison of four systems for isolation precautions, *Infect Control Hosp Epidemiol* 12:448, 1991.

Jernigan JA and others: A randomized crossover study of disposable thermometers for prevention of *Clostridium difficile* and other nosocomial infections, *J Infect Control Hosp Epidemiol* 19(7):494, 1998.

Joint Commission on Accreditation of Health Care Organizations: *Comprehensive accreditation manual for hospitals,* Oakbrook Terrace, Ill, 1998, The Commission.

Keroack MA, Rosen-Kotilainen H: Microbiology/laboratory diagnostics in *APIC infection control and applied epidemiology: principles and practice,* St. Louis, 1996, Mosby.

Larson E: APIC guideline for hand washing and hand antisepsis in health-care settings. In *APIC infection control and applied epidemiology: principles and practice,* St. Louis, 1996, Mosby.

Larson E and others: Changes in bacterial flora associated with skin damage on hands of health care personnel, *Am J Infect Control* 26(5):513, 1998.

Maki DG and others: Double-bagging of items from isolation rooms is unnecessary as an infection control measure: a comparative study of surface contamination with single and double-bagging, *Infect Control* 7(11):535, 1986.

Makris AT: Infections in the elderly. In *APIC infection control and applied epidemiology: principles and practice,* St. Louis, 1996, Mosby.

Meeker MH, Rothrock JC: *Alexander's care of the patient in surgery,* ed 11, St. Louis, 1999, Mosby.

Occupational Safety and Health Administration: Occupational Safety and Health Act of 1991: blood-borne pathogens, *Federal Register* 56(235):64175, 1991.

Occupational Safety and Health Administration: *Occupational exposure to tuberculosis, Federal Register* 64:32447, 1999.

Occupational Safety and Health Administration: Respiratory protection: proposed rule, *Federal Register* 59(219):58884, 1994.

O'Shaughnessy M and others: Given H.F. optimum duration of surgical scrub time, *Br J Surg* 78:685, 1991.

Pagana KD, Pagana TJ: *Diagnostic testing and nursing implications: a case study approach,* ed 5, St. Louis, 1998, Mosby.

Pereira LJ and others: The effect of surgical handwashing routines on the microbial counts of operating room nurses, *Am J Infect Control* 18:354, 1990.

Pottinger J and others: Bacterial carriage by artificial versus natural nails, *Am J Infect Control* 17(6):340, 1989.

Rutala W, Shafer KM: General information on cleaning, disinfection and sterilization. In *APIC infection control and applied epidemiology: principles and practice,* St. Louis, 1996, Mosby.

Weinstein SA and others: Bacterial surface contamination of patient's linen: isolation precautions versus standard care, *Am J Infect Control* 17(5):264, 1989.

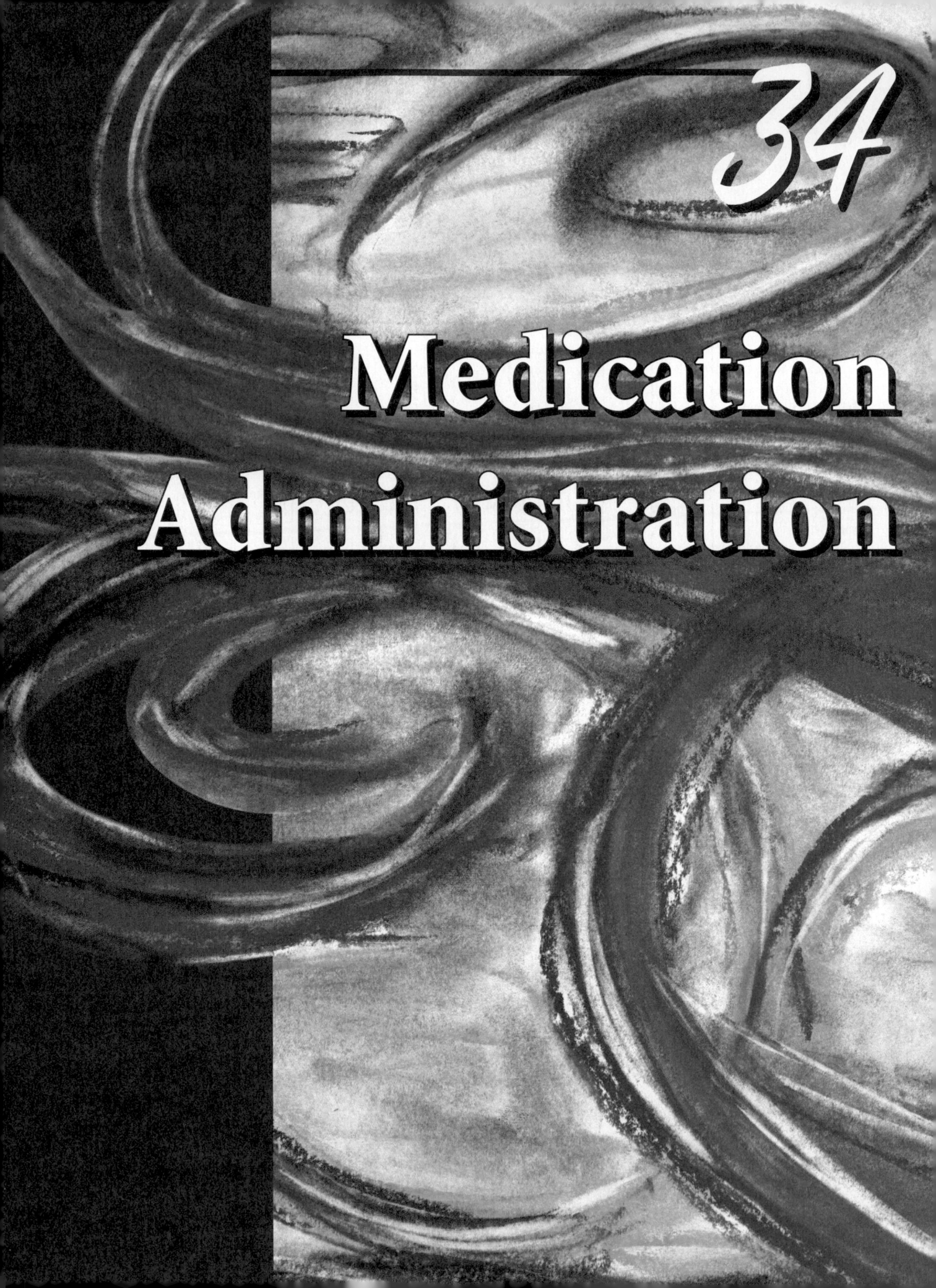

34

Medication Administration

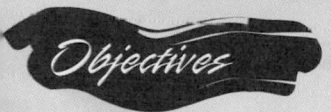

Mastery of content in this chapter will enable the student to:

- Define the key terms listed.
- Discuss the nurse's role and responsibilities in medication administration.
- Describe the physiological mechanisms of medication action, including absorption, distribution, metabolism, and excretion of medications.
- Differentiate among different types of medication actions.
- Discuss developmental factors that influence pharmacokinetics.
- Discuss factors that influence medication actions.
- Discuss methods of educating a client about prescribed medications.
- Describe the roles of the prescriber, pharmacist, and nurse in medication administration.
- Describe factors to consider when choosing routes of medication administration.
- Correctly calculate a prescribed medication dose.
- Discuss factors to include in assessing a client's needs for and response to medication therapy.
- List the five rights of medication administration.
- Correctly prepare and administer subcutaneous, intramuscular, and intradermal injections and intravenous medications; oral and topical skin preparations; eye, ear, and nose drops; vaginal instillations; rectal suppositories; and inhalants.

Clients with acute or chronic alterations in their health use many modalities to help restore or maintain their health. A medication is a substance used in the diagnosis, treatment, cure, relief, or prevention of health alterations. In fact, medications are the primary modality clients associate with restoration of health. No matter where clients receive their health care—hospitals, clinics, or home—the nurse plays an essential role in medication administration, medication teaching, and evaluating clients and the role medications play in restoration or maintenance of their health. The role of the nurse in medication activities is modified based on the setting of the client-nurse interaction.

In the primary care setting, the client often self-administers medications. The nurse is responsible for evaluating the effects of the medications on the client's health status, teaching clients about their medications and their side effects, ensuring client compliance with the medication regimen, and evaluating client technique when the client administers medications that are not given by mouth. In the acute care setting, nurses spend a great deal of time administering medication to clients. The nurse also ensures that clients are adequately prepared to administer their medications when they return to the community. In the home care setting clients usually administer their own medications. When clients cannot administer their own medications, family members or home health aides may be responsible for doing so. The nurse assesses the effect the medications have in restoring or maintaining health and provides continued education to the client, family, or home health care personnel on medication purpose and side effects.

Scientific Knowledge Base

Medications administered to clients are used, almost exclusively, to prevent, diagnose, or treat disease. Because medication administration and evaluation are essential to nursing practice, nurses need to have knowledge about the actions and effects of the medications they deliver to clients. This cannot be done if the nurse does not have an understanding of the life sciences. Moreover, to safely and accurately administer medications to clients nurses must have an understanding of pharmacokinetics (the movement of medications in the human body), growth and development, human anatomy, nutrition, and mathematics. All of the nurse's previous learning is important and is often applied to medication administration. The nursing process provides the framework for nurses to organize their thoughts and actions and is the foundation for medication administration.

PHARMACOLOGICAL CONCEPTS

Drug Names. A medication may have as many as three different names. A medication's chemical name provides an exact description of the medication's composition and molecular structure. Chemical names are rarely used in clinical practice. An example of a chemical name is N-acetyl-para-aminophenol, which is commonly known as Tylenol. The generic or nonproprietary name is given, with United States Adopted Name Council (USAN) approval, by the manufacturer who first develops the medication. Acetaminophen is an example of a generic name. It is the generic name for Tylenol. The generic name becomes the official name that is listed in official publications such as the *United States Pharmacopeia* (*USP*). The trade name, brand name, or proprietary name is the name under which a manufacturer markets a medication. The trade name has the symbol ™, at the upper right of the name, indicating that the manufacturer has trademarked the medication's name (e.g., Panadol, Tempra, and St. Joseph Aspirin for Children).

Manufacturers have chosen names that are easy to pronounce, spell, and remember so that laypersons will recognize trade names. Many companies may produce the same medication, so similarities in trade names can be confusing. Hospitals and clinic pharmacies attempt to consistently dispense medications with the same trade names so nurses can become familiar with them. However, the nurse finds medications under a variety of different nomenclatures or names and must be careful to obtain the exact name and spelling for a particular medication.

Classification.
Nurses learn to categorize medications with similar characteristics by their class. Medication classification indicates the effect of the medication on a body system, the symptoms the medication relieves, or the medication's desired effect. For example, clients who have type 2 diabetes (formerly called non-insulin-dependent diabetes) often take medications to lower their blood sugar level. This class of medication is called oral hypoglycemic agents. Usually each class contains more than one medication that can be prescribed for the type of health problem. For example, there are more than eight different types of oral hypoglycemic agents. The physical and chemical composition of medications within a class may be slightly different. A prescriber chooses a particular oral hypoglycemic medication based on client characteristics, cost, efficacy, dosing frequency, or prescriber experience with the medication.

A medication may also be part of more than one class. For example, aspirin is an analgesic, an antipyretic, and an antiinflammatory medication.

Medication Forms.
Medications are available in a variety of forms, or preparations (Figure 34-1). The form of the medication determines its route of administration. The composition of a medication is designed to enhance its absorption and metabolism. Many medications are made in several forms such as tablets, capsules, elixirs, and suppositories. When administering a medication, the nurse must be certain to use the proper form (Table 34-1).

MEDICATION LEGISLATION AND STANDARDS
Federal Regulations.
The role of the U.S. government in regulation of the pharmaceutical industry is to

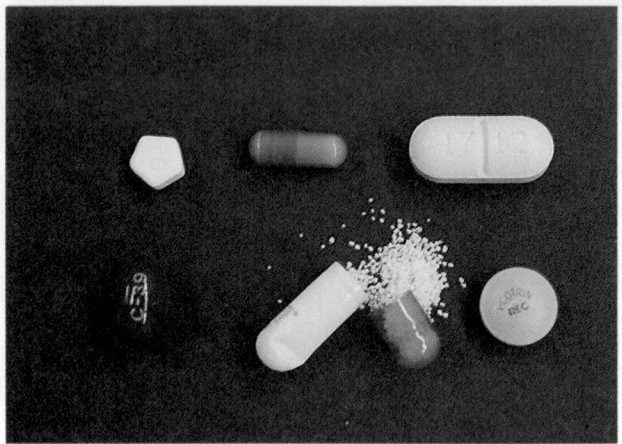

Figure 34-1   Forms of oral medications. *Top row:* Uniquely shaped tablet, capsule, scored tablet. *Bottom row:* Gelatin-coated liquid, extended-release capsule, enteric-coated tablet.

protect the health of the people by ensuring that medications are safe and effective. The first American law to regulate medications was the Pure Food and Drug Act. This law simply requires all medications to be free of impure products. Subsequent legislation (Table 34-2) has set standards related to safety, potency, and efficacy. Enforcement of medication laws rests with the Food and Drug Administration (FDA), which ensures that all medications on the market undergo vigorous review before they are allowed to be dispensed to the public. In 1993 the FDA instituted the MedWatch program. This voluntary program encourages nurses and other health care professionals to report when a medication, product, or medical event causes serious harm to a client. The MedWatch form is available to report such events (Figure 34-2).

Federal medication law has extended and refined controls on medication sales and distribution; medication testing, naming, and labeling; and the regulation of controlled substances. Official publications such as the *USP* and the *National Formulary* set standards for medication strength, quality, purity, packaging, safety, labeling, and dose form. In Canada, the *British Pharmacopoeia* (*BP*) sets similar standards. Table 34-3 list Canadian medication legislation designed to protect consumer.

State and Local Regulation of Medication.
State and locality medication laws must conform to federal legislation. States can also have additional controls, including control of substances not regulated by the federal government. Local governmental bodies also regulate the use of alcohol and tobacco.

Health Care Institutions and Medication Laws.
Health care institutions establish individual policies that must meet federal, state, and local regulations. The size of

Table 34-1 Forms of Medication

Form	Description
Caplet	Solid dosage form for oral use; shaped like capsule and coated for ease of swallowing
Capsule	Solid dosage form for oral use; medication in powder, liquid, or oil form and encased by gelatin shell; capsule colored to aid in product identification
Elixir	Clear fluid containing water and/or alcohol; designed for oral use; usually has sweetener added
Enteric-coated tablet	Tablet for oral use coated with materials that do not dissolve in stomach; coatings dissolve in intestine, where medication is absorbed
Extract	Concentrated medication form made by removing active portion of medication from its other components (e.g., fluid extract is medication made into solution from vegetable source)
Glycerite	Solution of medication combined with glycerin for external use; contains at least 50% glycerin
Intraocular disk	A small, flexible oval consisting of two soft, outer layers and a middle layer containing medication; when moistened by ocular fluid, releases medication for up to 1 week
Liniment	Preparation usually containing alcohol, oil, or soapy emollient that is applied to skin
Lotion	Medication in liquid suspension applied externally to protect skin
Ointment (salve)	Semisolid, externally applied preparation, usually containing one or more medications
Paste	Semisolid preparation, thicker and stiffer than ointment; absorbed through skin more slowly than ointment
Pill	Solid dosage form containing one or more medications, shaped into globules, ovoids, or oblong shapes; true pills rarely used because they have been replaced by tablets
Solution	Liquid preparation that may be used orally, parenterally, or externally; can also be instilled into body organ or cavity (e.g., bladder irrigations); contains water with one or more dissolved compounds; must be sterile for parenteral use
Suppository	Solid dosage form mixed with gelatin and shaped in form of pellet for insertion into body cavity (rectum or vagina); melts when it reaches body temperature, releasing medication for absorption
Suspension	Finely divided drug particles dispersed in liquid medium; when suspension is left standing, particles settle to bottom of container; commonly oral medication and not given intravenously
Syrup	Medication dissolved in concentrated sugar solution; may contain flavoring to make medication more palatable
Tablet	Powdered dosage form compressed into hard disks or cylinders; in addition to primary medication, contains binders (adhesive to allow powder to stick together), disintegrators (to promote tablet dissolution), lubricants (for ease of manufacturing), and fillers (for convenient tablet size)
Tincture	Alcohol or water-alcohol medication solution
Transdermal disk or patch	Medication contained within semipermeable membrane disk or patch, which allows medications to be absorbed through skin slowly over long period
Troche (lozenge)	Flat, round dosage form containing medication, flavoring, sugar, and mucilage; dissolves in mouth to release medication

an institution, the types of services it provides, and the types of professional personnel it employs influence these policies. Institutional policies are often more restrictive than governmental controls. An institution is concerned primarily with preventing health problems resulting from medication use. For example, a common institutional policy is the automatic discontinuation of antibiotic therapy after a set number of days. Although a prescriber may reorder the antibiotic, this policy helps to control unnecessarily prolonged medication therapy.

Medication Regulations and Nursing Practice.

State **Nurse Practice Acts** have the most influence over nursing practice by defining the scope of a nurse's professional functions and responsibilities. In general, most state Nurse Practice Acts are purposefully broad so as not to limit the professional responsibilities of the nurse. For example, most Nurse Practice Acts state that nurses can "execute medical regime prescribed by a licensed physician" (New Jersey Department of Law and Public Safety, 1995). Institutions and agencies may interpret specific actions allowed under the acts, but they cannot modify, expand, or restrict the act's intent. The primary intent of the state Nurse Practice Acts is to protect the public from unskilled, undereducated, and unlicensed personnel.

The nurse is responsible for following legal provisions when administering controlled substances or narcotics (medications that affect the mind and behavior), which are carefully controlled through federal and state guidelines. Violations of the Controlled Substances Act are punishable by fines, imprisonment, and loss of nurse licensure. Hospitals and other health care institutions have policies for the proper storage and distribution of narcotics (Box 34-1).

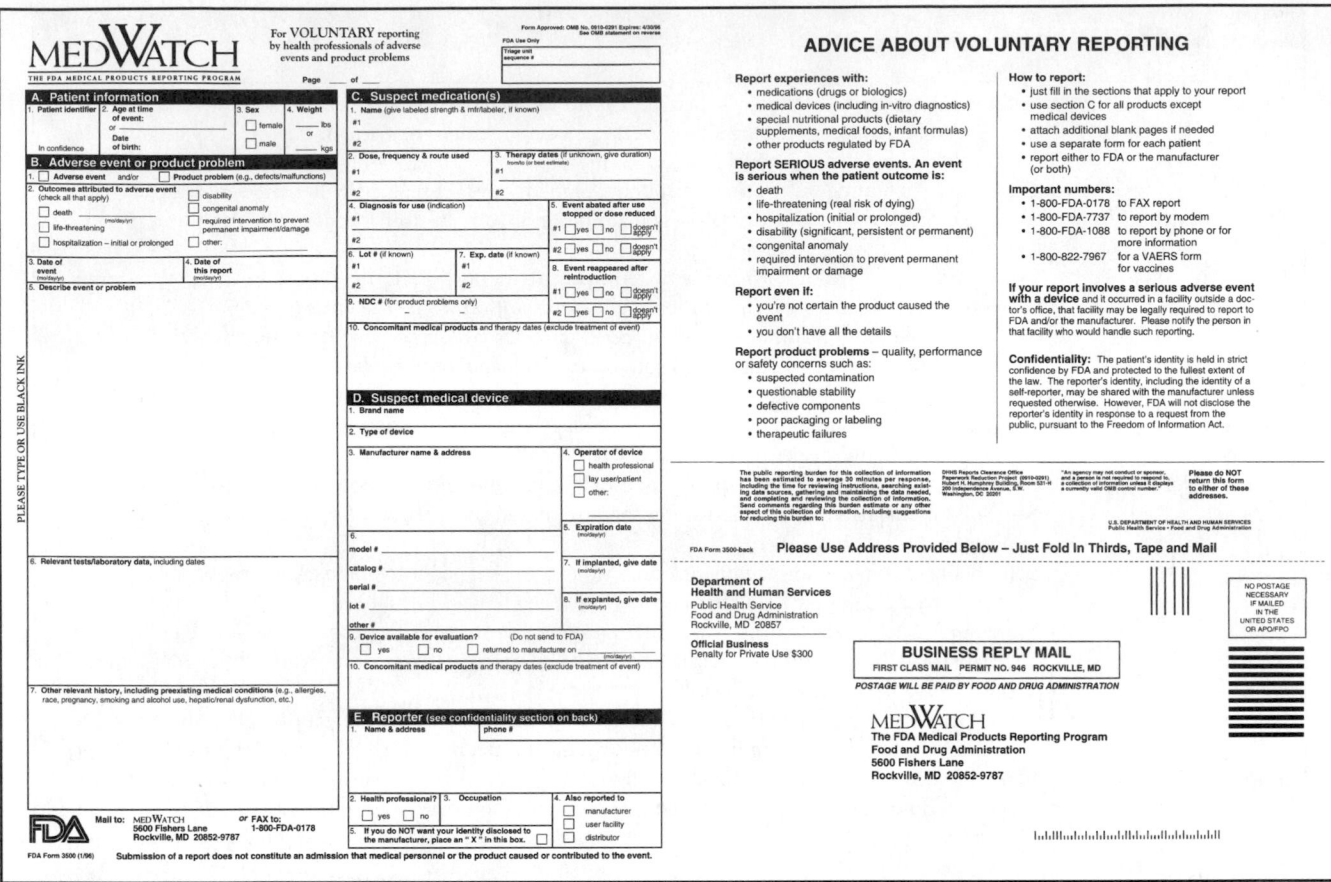

Figure 34-2   MedWatch form. FDA form 3500 (1/96). Courtesy FDA, MedWatch, Rockville, Md.

Table 34-2 **Federal Medication Laws in the United States**		
Date	Title of Law	Provisions
1906	Pure Food and Drug Act	Designated official standards for medications (USP and the National Formulary); specified standards for medication labeling
1912	Sherley Amendment	Prohibited manufacturers from making fraudulent claims about medication efficacy and therapeutic effects
1914	Harrison Narcotic Act	Legally classified medications believed to be habit forming as narcotics; regulated importation, manufacture, sale, and use of narcotic substances
1938	Federal Food, Drug, and Cosmetic Act	Added the Homeopathic Pharmacopeia of the United States as a third medication standard; required that medication preparation be approved as safe by the FDA before marketing; further outlined criteria for medication labeling
1945	Amendment to the Food and Drug Act	Provided for certification of biological products used as medications (e.g., insulin, antibiotics) on batch basis; allowed for direct supervision and inspection of medication production
1952	Durham-Humphrey Amendment	Distinguished between prescription ("legend") and nonprescription medications
1962	Kefauver-Harris Amendment	Authorized FDA to supervise medication production to ensure safety and efficacy and to establish official medication names; specified greater controls on investigational medications
1970	Comprehensive Drug Abuse Prevention and Control Act (Controlled Substances Act)	Set strict controls on manufacture and distribution of controlled medication (possession of controlled substances unlawful without prescription); established government programs to promote prevention and treatment of medication dependence

Table 34-3   Canadian Medication Legislation

Date	Title of Law	Provisions
1908	Proprietary or Patent Medicine Act	Set standards to protect consumers from unsafe and ineffective nonprescription medications
1953	Canadian Food and Drug Act	Prohibited sale of contaminated, unsafe medications and of improperly labeled medications; designated official standards (Pharmacopoeia Internationalis, BP, and Canadian Formulary); defined certain controlled medications; prohibited advertising of prescription and controlled medications to general public; set standards for labeling
1961	Canadian Narcotic Control Act	Restricted sale, possession, and use of narcotics; set guidelines for reporting loss or theft of narcotics; set standards for labeling and record keeping

Guidelines for Safe Narcotic Administration and Control   Box 34-1

Store all narcotics in a locked, secure cabinet or container. (Computerized, locked cabinets are now available.)

Nurses in charge carry a set of keys (or a special computer entry code) for the narcotics cabinet.

During an institution's change of shift, the nurse going off duty counts all narcotics with the nurse coming on duty. Both nurses sign the narcotic record to indicate that the count is correct.

Discrepancies in narcotic counts are reported immediately.

A special inventory record is used each time a narcotic is dispensed.

The record is used to document the client's name, date, time of medication administration, name of medication, dose, and signature of nurse dispensing the medication.

The form provides an accurate ongoing count of narcotics used and remaining.

If only one part of a premeasured dose of a controlled substance is given, a second nurse witnesses disposal of the unused portion and documents such on the record form.

PHARMACOKINETICS AS THE BASIS OF MEDICATION ACTIONS

For medications to be therapeutically useful they must be taken into a client's body, must be absorbed and distributed to cells, tissues, or a specific organ, and must alter its physiological functions. **Pharmacokinetics** is the study of how medications enter the body, reach their site of action, are metabolized, and exit the body. The nurse uses knowledge of pharmacokinetics when timing medication administration, selecting the route of administration, judging the client's risk for alterations in medication action, and observing the client's response.

ABSORPTION

Absorption refers to passage of medication molecules into the blood from its site of administration. Factors that influence medication absorption are the route of administration, ability of the medication to dissolve, blood flow to the site of administration, body surface area, and lipid solubility of medication.

Route of Administration.   Medications can be administered by various routes. Each route has a different rate of absorption. When medications are placed on the skin, absorption is slow due to the physical makeup of the skin. Medications placed on the mucous membranes and respiratory airways are quickly absorbed because these tissues contain many blood vessels. Because orally administered medications must pass through the gastrointestinal tract to be absorbed, the overall rate of absorption may be slowed. Intravenous (IV) **injection** produces the most rapid absorption because this route provides immediate access to the systemic circulation.

Ability of the Medication to Dissolve.   The ability of an oral medication to dissolve depends largely on its form or preparation. Solutions and suspensions already in a liquid state are absorbed more readily than tablets or capsules. Acidic medications pass through the gastric mucosa rapidly. Medications that are basic are not absorbed before reaching the small intestine.

Blood Flow to the Area of Absorption.   When tissue contains many blood vessels, medications are absorbed more rapidly. This occurs because blood is constantly moving in a vessel, allowing for more medication-free blood. This facilitates the passage of blood into the medication.

Body Surface Area.   When a medication is in contact with a large surface area, the medication will be absorbed at a faster rate. This explains why the majority of medications are absorbed in the small intestine rather than the stomach.

Lipid Solubility of a Medication.   Medications that are highly lipid soluble are absorbed more easily. They readily cross the cell membrane because it is made of a lipid layer. Another factor that may affect absorption of medication is whether or not food is in the stomach. Some oral medications are absorbed more easily when administered between meals because food can change the structure of a medication and impair its absorption. Some medications when administered together may interfere with each other so as to impair the absorption of one or both.

Nurses often have knowledge of factors that may alter or impair absorption of the medications that have been prescribed for their clients. This information is based on an understanding of medication pharmacokinetics, the nursing history, and the physical examination and knowledge gained through daily interactions with clients. The nurse uses this knowledge to ensure that all prescribed medications are administered correctly. It may be appropriate for the nurse to administer medications given ½ hour before, ½ hour after, and with meals or withhold medications if absorption is not likely to occur. The nurse consults with and collaborates with the client's prescribers to ensure that the client achieves the therapeutic effect of all medications. Before administering any medication, the nurse should consult pharmacology books or drug references, package inserts, or pharmacists to identify medication-medication **interactions** or medication-nutrient interactions.

DISTRIBUTION

After a medication is absorbed, it is distributed within the body to tissues and organs and ultimately to its specific site of action. The rate and extent of distribution depend on the physical and chemical properties of medications and the physiology of the person taking the medication.

Circulation.

Once a medication enters the bloodstream it is carried throughout the tissues and organs of the body. How fast it reaches the site is dependent on the vascularity of the various tissues and organs. When conditions exist that limit blood flow or intended sites of actions are poorly perfused, the distribution of a medication is inhibited. Consider the client who has a tumor. Solid tumors have a poor blood supply and may not respond to therapy intended to destroy them.

Membrane Permeability.

To be distributed to an organ a medication must pass all of the biologic membranes an organ or tissue has. Some membranes may serve as barriers to the passage of medications. The blood-brain barrier allows only fat-soluble medications to pass into the brain and cerebral spinal fluid. Central nervous system infections require treatment with antibiotics injected directly into the subarachnoid space in the spinal cord. Older clients may experience adverse effects (e.g., confusion) as a result of the change in the permeability of the blood-brain barrier, with easier passage of fat-soluble medications. The placental membrane is a nonselective barrier to medications. Fat soluble and non-fat-soluble agents may cross the placenta and produce fetal deformities, respiratory depression, and, with narcotic abuse, withdrawal symptoms.

Protein Binding.

The degree to which medications bind to serum proteins such as albumin affects medication distribution. Most medications bind to this protein to some extent. When medications bind to albumin, they cannot exert any pharmacological activity. The unbound or "free" medication is the active form of the medication. Older adults have a decrease in albumin in the bloodstream, probably caused by a change in liver function. The same is true for clients with liver disease or malnutrition. Because of the potential for more medication being unbound, the older adult may be at risk for an increase in medication activity or toxicity or both.

METABOLISM

After a medication reaches its site of action, it becomes metabolized into a less active or inactive form that is more easily excreted. **Biotransformation** occurs under the influence of enzymes that **detoxify,** degrade (break down), and remove biologically active chemicals. Most biotransformation occurs within the liver, although the lungs, kidneys, blood, and intestines also metabolize medications. The liver is especially important because its specialized structure oxidizes and transforms many toxic substances. The liver degrades many harmful chemicals before they become distributed to the tissues. If a decrease in liver function occurs, such as with aging or liver disease, a medication may be eliminated more slowly, resulting in an accumulation of the medication. If the organs that metabolize medications are altered, clients are at risk for medication toxicity. For example, a small sedative dose of a barbiturate may cause a client with liver disease to lapse into a hepatic coma.

EXCRETION

After medications are metabolized, they exit the body through the kidneys, liver, bowel, lungs, and exocrine glands. The chemical makeup of a medication determines the organ of excretion. Gaseous and volatile compounds such as nitrous oxide and alcohol exit through the lungs. Deep breathing and coughing (see Chapter 39) help the postoperative client to eliminate anesthetic gases more rapidly. The exocrine glands excrete lipid-soluble medications. When medications exit through sweat glands, the skin may become irritated. The nurse assists the client in good hygiene practices (see Chapter 38) to promote cleanliness and skin integrity.

If a medication is excreted through the mammary glands, there is a risk that a nursing infant will ingest the chemicals. Mothers should check on the safety of any medication used while breast-feeding.

The gastrointestinal tract is another route for medication excretion. Many medications enter the hepatic circulation to be broken down by the liver and excreted into the bile. After chemicals enter the intestines through the biliary tract, the intestines may reabsorb them. Factors that increase peristalsis (e.g., laxatives and enemas) accelerate medication excretion through the feces, whereas factors that slow peristalsis (e.g., inactivity and improper diet) may prolong a medication's effects.

The kidneys are the main organs for medication excretion. Some medications escape extensive metabolism and exit unchanged in the urine. Other medications must undergo biotransformation in the liver before being excreted by the kidney. If renal function declines, a client is at risk for medication toxicity. If the kidney cannot adequately excrete a medication, it may be necessary to reduce the dose. Maintenance of an adequate fluid intake (50 ml/kg/day) promotes proper elimination of medications for the average adult.

Types of Medication Action

Medications vary considerably in the way they act and their types of action. Factors other than characteristics of the medication also influence medication actions. A client may not respond in the same way to each successive dose of a medication. Likewise, the same medication dosage may cause very different responses in different clients. Therefore it is essential for the nurse to understand all the effects that medications can have when taken by or given to clients.

THERAPEUTIC EFFECTS

The **therapeutic effect** is the expected or predictable physiological response a medication causes. Each medication has a desired therapeutic effect for which it is prescribed. For example, nitroglycerin is used to reduce the cardiac workload and increase myocardial oxygen supply. A single medication may have many therapeutic effects. For example, aspirin is an analgesic, antipyretic and antiinflammatory, and it reduces platelet aggregation (clumping). It is important for the nurse to know for which therapeutic effect a medication is prescribed. This will allow the nurse to properly teach the client about the medication's intended effect.

SIDE EFFECTS

Side effects are the unintended, secondary effects a medication predictably will cause. Side effects may be harmless or injurious. If the side effects are serious enough to negate the beneficial effects of a medication's therapeutic action, the prescriber may discontinue the medication. Clients often stop taking medications because of side effects.

ADVERSE EFFECTS

Adverse effects are generally considered severe responses to medication. For example, a client may become comatose when a drug is ingested. When adverse responses to medications occur, the prescriber must discontinue the medication. Some adverse effects are unexpected effects that were not discovered during drug testing. When this situation occurs, health care providers are obligated to report the adverse effect to the FDA (see Figure 34-2).

TOXIC EFFECTS

Toxic effects may develop after prolonged intake of a medication or when a medication accumulates in the blood because of impaired metabolism or excretion. Excess amounts of a medication within the body may have lethal effects, depending on the medication's action. For example, toxic levels of morphine may cause severe respiratory depression and death. Antidotes are available to treat specific types of medication toxicity. For example, Narcan is used to reverse the effects of opioid toxicity.

IDIOSYNCRATIC REACTIONS

Medications may cause unpredictable effects such as an **idiosyncratic reaction** in which a client overreacts or underreacts to a medication or has a reaction different from normal. For example, a child receiving an antihistamine (Benadryl) may become extremely agitated or excited instead of drowsy. It is impossible to assess clients for idiosyncratic responses.

ALLERGIC REACTIONS

Allergic reactions are another unpredictable response to a medication; they make up 5% to 10% of all medication reactions. A client can become sensitized immunologically to the initial dose of a medication. With repeated administration the client develops an allergic response to the medication, its chemical preservatives, or a metabolite. The medication or chemical acts as an antigen, triggering the release of the body's antibodies. A client's **medication allergy** may be mild or severe. Allergic symptoms vary, depending on the individual and the medication. Among the different classes of medications, antibiotics cause a high incidence of allergic reactions. Common, mild allergy symptoms are summarized in Table 34-4. Severe or **anaphylactic reactions** are characterized by sudden constriction of bronchiolar muscles, edema of the pharynx and

Table 34-4 **Mild Allergic Reactions**	
Symptom	Description
Urticaria	Raised, irregularly shaped skin eruptions with varying sizes and shapes; eruptions have reddened margins and pale centers
Rash	Small, raised vesicles that are usually reddened; often distributed over entire body
Pruritus	Itching of skin; accompanies most rashes
Rhinitis	Inflammation of mucous membranes lining nose; causes swelling and clear, watery discharge

larynx, and severe wheezing and shortness of breath. Antihistamines, epinephrine, and bronchodilators may be used to treat anaphylactic reactions.

The client may also become severely hypotensive, necessitating emergency resuscitation measures. A client with a known history of an allergy to a medication should avoid reexposure and wear an identification bracelet or medal (Figure 34-3), which alerts nurses and physicians to the allergy if the client is unconscious when receiving medical care.

MEDICATION INTERACTIONS

When one medication modifies the action of another medication, a **medication interaction** occurs. Medication interactions are common in individuals taking several medications. A medication may potentiate or diminish the action of other medications and may alter the way in which another medication is absorbed, metabolized, or eliminated from the body. When two medications have a **synergistic effect,** or act synergistically, the effect of the two medications combined is greater than the effect of the medications when given separately. For example, alcohol is a central nervous system depressant that has a synergistic effect on antihistamines, antidepressants, barbiturates, and narcotic analgesics.

A medication interaction is not always undesirable. Often a prescriber combines medications to create an interaction that will have a beneficial effect on the client's condition. For example, a client with hypertension (high blood pressure) that cannot be controlled with one medication, typically receives several medications such as diuretics and vasodilators that act together to control the blood pressure.

MEDICATION DOSE RESPONSES

After a nurse administers a medication, it undergoes absorption, distribution, metabolism, and excretion. Except when administered intravenously, medications take time to enter the bloodstream. The quantity and distribution of a medication in different body compartments change constantly. When a medication is prescribed, the goal is a constant blood level within a safe therapeutic range. Repeated doses are required to achieve a constant therapeutic **concentration** of a medication because a portion of a medication is always being excreted. The highest serum concentration (**peak** concentration) of the medication usually occurs just before the last of the medication is absorbed (Clark, Queener, and Karb, 1998). After peaking, the serum medication concentration falls progressively. With intravenous **infusions,** the peak concentration occurs quickly, but the serum level also begins to fall immediately (Figure 34-4).

All medications have a **serum half-life,** which is the time it takes for excretion processes to lower the serum medication concentration by half. To maintain a therapeutic plateau, the client must receive regular fixed doses. For example it has been shown that pain medications are most effective when they are given "around the clock" rather than when the client intermittently complains of pain. In this way an almost constant level of pain medication is maintained. After an initial medication dose the client receives each successive dose when the previous dose reaches its half-life.

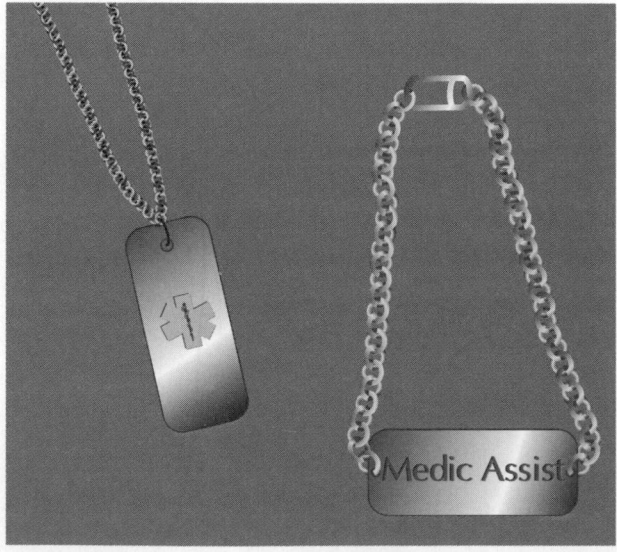

Figure 34-3   Identification bracelet and medal.

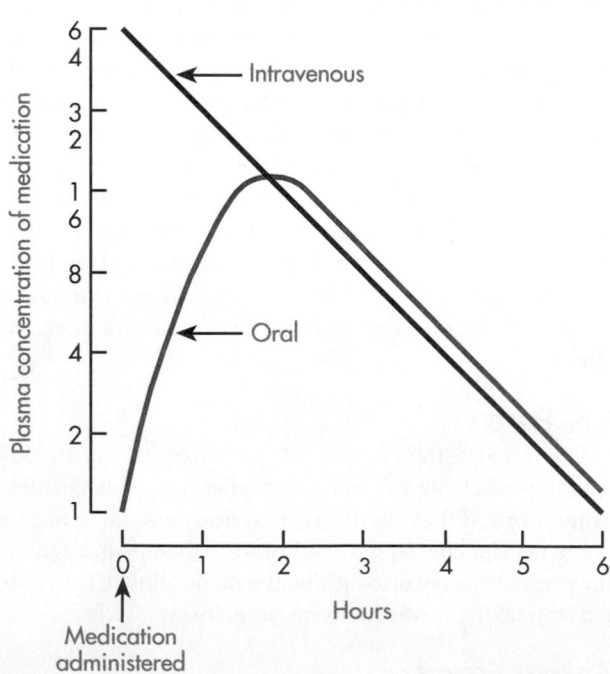

Figure 34-4   Curve showing therapeutic blood levels. From Clark JF, Queener SF, Karb VB: *Pharmacological basis of nursing practice,* ed 6, St. Louis, 1998, Mosby.

The client and nurse must follow regular dosage schedules and adhere to prescribed doses and dosage intervals. Dosage schedules are set by the agency in which the nurse is employed. Table 34-5 lists common dosage schedules used in acute care settings. When teaching clients about dosage schedules the nurse uses language that is familiar to the client. For example, when teaching a client about medication dosing twice a day (bid), the nurse instructs the client to take a medication in the morning and again in the evening. Knowledge of the time intervals of medication action also helps the nurse to anticipate a medication's effect. With this knowledge the nurse can instruct the client when to expect a response. Table 34-6 lists common terms associated with medication actions.

Table 34-5	Common Dosage Administration Schedules
Abbreviation	Meaning
AC, ac	Before meals
ad lib	As desired
BID, bid	Twice a day
h	Hour
HS, hs	Hour of sleep
PC, pc	After meals
prn	Whenever there is a need
qam	Every morning, every am
qd, od	Every day
qh	Every hour
q2h	Every 2 hours
q4h	Every 4 hours
q6h	Every 6 hours
q8h	Every 8 hours
QID, qid	4 times a day
QOD, qod	Every other day
STAT	Give immediately
TID, tid	3 times a day

Table 34-6	Terms Associated With Medication Actions
Term	Meaning
Onset	Time it takes after a medication is administered for it to produce a response
Peak	Time it takes for a medication to reach its highest effective concentration
Trough	Minimum blood serum concentration of medication reached just before the next scheduled dose
Duration	Time during which the medication is present in concentration great enough to produce a response
Plateau	Blood serum concentration of a medication reached and maintained after repeated fixed doses

Routes of Administration

The route prescribed for administering a medication depends on the medication's properties and desired effect and on the client's physical and mental condition (Table 34-7). A nurse collaborates with the physician in determining the best route for a client's medication, as in the following hypothetical situation:

> *The client, Mr. Huels, has progressively worsened physically. His temperature is 39.2° C. He complains of nausea and is unable to tolerate oral fluids. The nurse checks Mr. Huels's order, which reads, "Aspirin 600 mg orally for temperature above 38.5° C." On the basis of the assessment, the nurse believes that because Mr. Huels is nauseated, he will not be able to tolerate an oral dose of aspirin. By consulting the physician, the nurse acquires an order for a rectal suppository instead. A rectal suppository enables the nurse to administer aspirin to decrease fever without increasing client's symptoms of nausea.*

ORAL ROUTES

The oral route is the easiest and the most commonly used. Medications are given by mouth and swallowed with fluid. Oral medications have a slower onset of action and a more prolonged effect than parenteral medications. Clients generally prefer the oral route.

Sublingual Administration. Some medications are designed to be readily absorbed after being placed under the tongue to dissolve (Figure 34-5). A medication given by the **sublingual** route should not be swallowed, or the desired effect will not be achieved. Nitroglycerin is commonly given by sublingual route. The client should not take a drink until the medication is completely dissolved.

Buccal Administration. Administration of a medication by the **buccal** route involves placing the solid medication in the mouth and against the mucous membranes of the cheek until the medication dissolves (Figure 34-6).

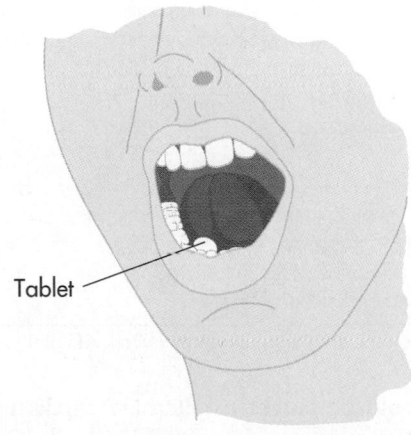

Tablet

Figure 34-5 Sublingual administration of a tablet.

Table 34-7   Factors Influencing Choice of Administration Routes

Advantages	Disadvantages of Contraindications
Oral, Buccal, Sublingual Routes	
Routes are convenient and comfortable for client.	These routes are avoided when client has alterations in gastrointestinal function (e.g., nausea, vomiting), reduced motility (after general anesthesia or bowel inflammation), and surgical resection of portion of gastrointestinal tract.
Routes are economical.	Some medications are destroyed by gastric secretions. Oral administration is contraindicated in clients unable to swallow (e.g., clients with neuromuscular disorders, esophageal strictures, mouth lesions).
Medications may produce local or systemic effects.	Oral medications cannot be given when client has gastric suction and are contraindicated in clients before some tests or surgery.
Routes rarely cause anxiety for client.	Unconscious or confused client is unable or unwilling to swallow or hold medication under tongue.
	Oral medications may irritate lining of gastrointestinal tract, discolor teeth, or have unpleasant taste.
Subcutaneous (SQ), Intramuscular (IM), Intravenous (IV), Intradermal (ID) Routes	
Routes provide means of administration when oral medications are contraindicated.	There is risk of introducing infection, and some medications are expensive. Clients must experience repeated needle sticks. The SQ, IM, and ID routes are avoided in clients with bleeding tendencies.
More rapid absorption occurs than with topical or oral routes.	There is risk of tissue damage with SQ injections.
IV infusion provides medication delivery when client is critically ill or long-term therapy is required. If peripheral perfusion is poor, IV route is preferred over injections.	IM and IV routes are dangerous because of rapid absorption. These routes cause considerable anxiety in many clients, especially children.
Skin	
TOPICAL	
Topical skin applications primarily provide local effect.	Clients with skin abrasions are at risk for rapid medication absorption and systemic effects.
Route is painless.	
Limited side effects occur.	
TRANSDERMAL	
Transdermal applications provide prolonged systemic effects, with limited side effects.	Application leaves oily or pasty substance on skin and may soil clothing.
Mucous Membranes*	
Therapeutic effects are provided by local application to involved sites.	Mucous membranes are highly sensitive to some medication concentrations.
Aqueous solutions are readily absorbed and capable of causing systemic effects.	Insertion of rectal and vaginal medication often causes embarrassment.
Mucous membranes provide route of administration when oral medications are contraindicated.	Client with ruptured eardrum cannot receive irrigations. Rectal suppositories are contraindicated if client has had rectal surgery or if active rectal bleeding is present.
Inhalation	
Inhalation provides rapid relief for local respiratory problems.	Some local agents can cause serious systemic effects.
Route provides easy access for introduction of general anesthetic gases.	

*Includes eyes, ears, nose, vagina, rectum, buccal, and sublingual routes.

Clients should be taught to alternate cheeks with each subsequent dose to avoid mucosal irritation. Clients are also warned not to chew or swallow the medication or to take any liquids with it. A buccal medication acts locally on the mucosa or systemically as it is swallowed in a person's saliva.

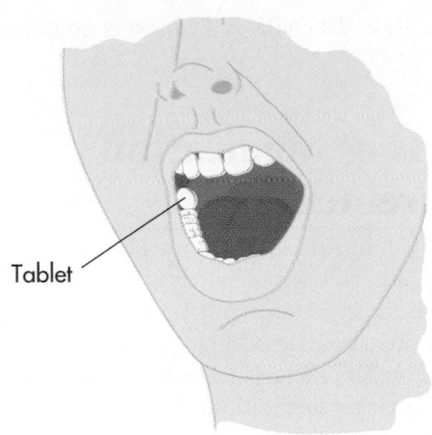

Figure 34-6 Buccal administration of a tablet.

Parenteral Routes

Parenteral administration involves injecting a medication into body tissues. The following are the four major sites of injection:

1. **Subcutaneous (SQ):** Injection into tissues just below the dermis of the skin
2. **Intramuscular (IM):** Injection into a muscle
3. **Intravenous (IV):** Injection into a vein
4. **Intradermal (ID):** Injection into the dermis just under the epidermis

Some medications are administered into body cavities other than the four types listed above. In some institutions nurses may or may not be responsible for the administration of medications through these advanced techniques. Whether or not the nurse actually administers the medication by these routes, the nurse often remains responsible for monitoring the integrity of the system of medication delivery, understanding the therapeutic value of the medication, and evaluating the client's response to the therapy. The following are advanced techniques of medication administration for which the nurse may be responsible.

Epidural. Medications are administered in the epidural space via a catheter, which has been placed by a nurse anesthetist or an anesthesiologist. This technique of medication administration is most commonly used for the administration of analgesia postoperatively (see Chapter 49). Specially trained nurses can administer medications in bolus form (see Skill 34-10) or by continuous infusion.

Intrathecal. Intrathecal medications are administered through a catheter that has been placed into the subarachnoid space or into one of the ventricles of the brain. Intrathecal administration is often associated with long-term medication administration through catheters that have been surgically implanted. In most institutions a physician usually injects medications into intrathecal catheters. However, specially trained nurses may also do this.

Intraosseous. This method of medication administration involves the infusion of medication directly into the bone marrow. It is most commonly used in infants and toddlers who have poor access to their intravascular space. This method is most popular when an emergency arises and IV access is impossible. The physician inserts an intraosseous infusion needle into the bone, usually the tibia, for the administration of medication by the nurse.

Intraperitoneal. Medications are administered into the peritoneal cavity, where they are absorbed into the circulation. Chemotherapeutics and antibiotics are commonly administered in this fashion. One method of dialysis also uses the peritoneal route for the removal of fluid, electrolytes, and waste products. Oncology nurses usually instill chemotherapeutics into the peritoneal cavity. General nurses often initiate and teach clients how to manage peritoneal dialysis.

Intrapleural. Medications are administered through the chest wall and directly into the pleural space. This may be done through an injection or through a chest tube that has been inserted by the physician. Chemotherapeutics are the most common medications administered via this method. Physicians also instill medications that help resolve persistent pleural effusion. This is called pleuradesis. This technique promotes adhesion between the visceral and parietal pleura. Increasingly newer indications of this method of medication delivery are being used. One such indication is for the instillation of analgesic agents through specially designed intrapleural catheters (Martin and Mehery, 1994).

Intraarterial. This method calls for medications to be administered directly into the arteries. Intraarterial infusions are common in clients who have arterial clots. The nurse will manage a continuous infusion of clot-dissolving agents. The nurse must carefully monitor the integrity of this infusion to prevent inadvertent disconnection of the system and subsequent bleeding.

Other methods of medication administration that are usually limited to physician administration are **intracardiac,** injection of a medication directly into cardiac tissue, and **intraarticular,** injection of a medication into a joint.

Topical Administration

Medications applied to the skin and mucous membranes generally have local effects. The topical medication is applied to the skin by painting or spreading it over an area, applying moist dressings, soaking body parts in a solution, or giving medicated baths. Systemic effects can occur if a client's skin is thin, if the medication concentration is high, or if contact with the skin is prolonged.

Some medications (e.g., nitroglycerin, scopolamine, and estrogens) have systemic effects because they are applied topically by a **transdermal disk** or patch. The disk secures the medicated ointment to the skin. These topical applications may be applied for as little as 24 hours or as long as 7 days.

Medications can be applied to mucous membranes in a variety of ways: (1) by directly applying a liquid or ointment (e.g., eye drops, gargling, swabbing the throat); (2) by inserting a medication into a body cavity (e.g., placing a suppository in rectum or vagina or inserting medicated packing into vagina); (3) by instilling fluid into body cavity (e.g., ear drops, nose drops, or bladder and rectal **instillation** [fluid is retained]); (4) by irrigating a body cavity (e.g., flushing eye, ear, vagina, bladder, or rectum with medicated fluid [fluid is not retained]); and (5) by spraying (e.g., instillation into nose and throat).

INHALATION ROUTE

The deeper passages of the respiratory tract provide a large surface area for medication absorption. Medications can be administered through the nasal passages, oral passage, or tubes that have been placed into the client's mouth to the trachea (Figure 34-7). Medications that are administered by the **inhalation** route are readily absorbed and work rapidly because of the rich vascular alveolocapillary network present in the pulmonary tissue. Inhaled medications may have local or systemic effects.

INTRAOCULAR ROUTE

Intraocular medication delivery involves inserting a medication similar to a contact lens into the client's eye. The eye medication disk has two soft outer layers that have medication enclosed in them. The disk is inserted into the client's eye, much like a contact lens. The disk can remain in the client's eye for up to 1 week. Pilocarpine, a medication used to treat glaucoma, is the most common medication disk.

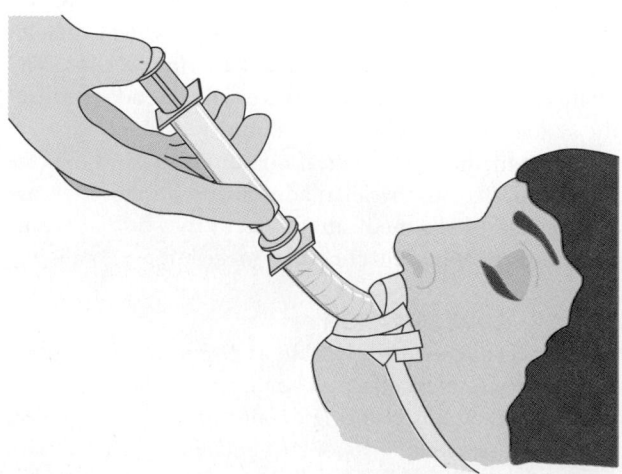

Figure 34-7 Medication being instilled through endotracheal tube.

Systems of Medication Measurement

The proper administration of a medication depends on the nurse's ability to compute medication doses accurately and measure medications correctly. A careless mistake in placing a decimal point or adding a zero to a dose can lead to a fatal error. The nurse is responsible for checking the dose before giving a medication.

The metric, apothecary, and household systems of measurement are used in medication therapy. Most nations, including Canada, use the metric system as their standard of measurement. Although the U.S. Congress has not officially adopted the metric system, most health professionals in the United States use it. Prescriptions to be self-administered are often written in household measures for clients. The apothecary system is rarely used.

METRIC SYSTEM

As a decimal system, the **metric system** is the most logically organized. Metric units can easily be converted and computed through simple multiplication and division. Each basic unit of measurement is organized into units of 10. Multiplying or dividing by 10 forms secondary units. In multiplication, the decimal point moves to the right; in division, the decimal moves to the left. For example:

$$10.0 \text{ mg} \times 10 = 100 \text{ mg}$$
$$10.0 \text{ mg} \div 10 = 1.0 \text{ mg}$$

The basic units of measurement in the metric system are the meter (length), the liter (volume), and the gram (weight). For medication calculations the nurse uses only the volume and weight units. In the metric system, lowercase or capital letters are used to designate basic units:

$$\text{Gram} = \text{g or Gm}$$
$$\text{Liter} = \text{l or L}$$

Lowercase letters are used for abbreviations for other units:

$$\text{Milligram} = \text{mg}$$
$$\text{Milliliter} = \text{ml}$$

A system of Latin prefixes designates subdivision of the basic units: *deci-* (1/10 or 0.1), *centi-* (1/100 or 0.01), and *milli-* (1/1000 or 0.001). Greek prefixes designate multiples of the basic units: *deka-* (10), *hecto-* (100), and *kilo-* (1000). When writing medication doses in metric units, prescribers and nurses use fractions or multiples of a unit. Fractions should be converted to decimal form. A zero is always placed in front of the decimal to prevent error.

500 mg or 0.5 g, *not* ½ g
10 ml or 0.01 L, *not* ¹/₁₀₀ L

HOUSEHOLD MEASUREMENTS

Household units of measure are familiar to most people. The disadvantage of household measures is their inaccuracy. Household utensils such as teaspoons and cups often vary in size. Scales to measure pints or quarts are often not well calibrated. Household measures include drops, teaspoons, tablespoons, and cups for volume and pints and quarts for weight. Although pints and quarts are considered household measures, they are also used in the apothecary system.

The advantage of household measurements is their convenience and familiarity. When the accuracy of a medication dose is not critical, it is safe to use household measures. For example, many over-the-counter medications can safely be measured by this method. Table 34-8 gives common equivalents of metric and household units.

SOLUTIONS

The nurse uses solutions of various concentrations for injections, **irrigations,** and infusions. A **solution** is a given mass of solid substance dissolved in a known volume of fluid or a given volume of liquid dissolved in a known volume of another fluid. When a solid is dissolved in a fluid, the concentration is in units of mass per units of volume (e.g., g/ml, g/L, mg/ml). A concentration of a solution may also be expressed as a percentage. A 10% solution, for example, is 10 g of solid dissolved in 100 ml of solution. A proportion also expresses concentrations. A 1/1000 solution represents a solution containing 1 g of solid in 1000 ml of liquid or 1 ml of liquid mixed with 1000 ml of another liquid.

Clinical Calculations

To administer medications it is essential for the nurse to have an understanding of basic arithmetic to calculate medication doses, mix solutions, and perform a variety of other activities. This skill is important because medications are not always dispensed in the unit of measure in which they are ordered. This occurs because medication companies package and bottle certain standard equivalents. For example, the prescriber may order 250 mg of a medication that is available only in grams. The nurse is responsible for converting available units of volume and weight to the desired doses. Therefore the nurse should be aware of approximate equivalents in all major measurement systems.

Medication administration is not the only function in which nurses use volume and weight conversions. Conversions are used in a variety of nursing activities (Box 34-2).

CONVERSIONS WITHIN ONE SYSTEM

Converting measurements within one system is relatively easy. In the metric system the nurse simply divides or multiplies. To change milligrams to grams, the nurse divides by 1000, moving the decimal 3 points to the left.

$$1000 \text{ mg} = 1 \text{ g}$$
$$350 \text{ mg} = 0.35 \text{ g}$$

To convert liters to milliliters, the nurse multiplies by 1000 or moves the decimal 3 points to the right.

$$1 \text{ L} = 1000 \text{ ml}$$
$$0.25 \text{ L} = 250 \text{ ml}$$

To convert units of measurement within the apothecary or household system, the nurse must consult an equivalent table. For example, when converting fluid ounces to quarts the nurse must first know that 32 ounces is the equivalent of 1 quart. To convert 8 ounces to a quart measurement, for example, the nurse divides 8 by 32 to get the equivalent, ¼ or 0.25 quart.

CONVERSION BETWEEN SYSTEMS

The nurse must frequently determine the proper dose of a medication by converting weights or volumes from one system of measurement to another. Often, metric units

Table 34-8	Equivalents of Measurement	
Metric	**Household**	
1 ml	15 drops (gtt)	
4-5 ml	1 teaspoon (tsp)	
16 ml	1 tablespoon (tbsp)	
30 ml	2 tablespoons (tbsp)	
240 ml	1 cup (c)	
480 ml (approximately 500 ml)	1 pint (pt)	
960 ml (approximately 1 L)	1 quart (qt)	
3840 ml (approximately 4 L)	1 gallon (gal)	

Common Reasons for Measurement Conversions	Box 34-2
Converting fluid ounces to milliliters for measurement of intake and output	
Converting body weight from pounds to kilograms and vice versa	
Converting volume equivalents to calculate IV flow rates and prepare wound irrigation solutions, enemas, or bladder irrigations	

must be converted to equivalent household measures for use at home. To calculate medications, it is necessary to work with units in the same measurement system. Tables of equivalent measurements are available in all health care institutions. The pharmacist is also a good resource.

Before making a conversion, the nurse compares the measurement system available with that ordered. For example, the prescriber orders Robitussin 30 ml. To provide proper instruction to the client, the nurse must convert "ml" to common household measurement. To convert milliliters to tablespoons the nurse must know the equivalent or refer to a table such as Table 34-8.

DOSE CALCULATIONS

There are many formulas that can be used to calculate medication doses. The following basic formula can be applied when preparing solid or liquid forms:

$$\frac{\text{Dose ordered}}{\text{Dose on hand}} \times \frac{\text{Amount on}}{\text{hand}} = \frac{\text{Amount to}}{\text{administer}}$$

The dose ordered is the amount of pure medication the prescriber prescribes. The dose on hand is the weight or volume of medication available in units supplied by the pharmacy; it may be expressed on the medication label as the contents of a tablet or capsule or as the amount of medication dissolved per unit volume of liquid. The amount on hand is the basic unit or quantity of the medication that contains the dose on hand. For solid medications the amount on hand may be one capsule; the amount of liquid on hand may be a milliliter or liter depending on the container. The amount to administer is the actual amount of available medication the nurse will administer. The amount to administer is always expressed in the same unit as the amount on hand.

The following example illustrates how to apply the formula. The prescriber orders the client to receive Demerol 50 mg IM. Thus the dose ordered is 50 mg. The medication is available only in ampules containing 100 mg per milliliter. Thus the dose on hand is 100 mg in an amount on hand of 1 ml. The formula is applied as follows:

$$\frac{50 \text{ mg}}{100 \text{ mg}} \times 1 \text{ ml} = \text{Volume in milliliters to administer}$$

To simplify the $^{50}/_{100}$ fraction, divide numerator and denominator by 50:

$$\frac{1}{2} \times 1 \text{ ml} = \frac{1}{2} \text{ ml to administer}$$

Syringes are calibrated only in decimals. After converting the fraction $\frac{1}{2}$ to 0.5, the nurse can more accurately draw up the correct dose.

Another example demonstrates how the formula applies with solid dose forms. The physician orders 0.125 mg orally (PO) of digoxin. The medication is available in tablets containing 0.25 mg.

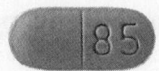

Figure 34-8   Scored medication tablet.
Courtesy Mosby's GenRx 1999.

$$\frac{0.125 \text{ mg}}{0.250 \text{ mg}} \times 1 \text{ tablet} = \text{Tablets to administer}$$

The fraction $^{0.125}/_{0.250}$ equals $\frac{1}{2}$ or 0.5. Therefore,

$$0.5 \times 1 \text{ tablet} = 0.5 \text{ or } \frac{1}{2} \text{ tablet to be administered}$$

Many tablets come with scores or indentations across the center of the tablet (Figure 34-8). A scored tablet is easy to break in half for divided doses. In some institutions pharmacists are responsible for scoring tablets. The potential for giving an incorrect dose is high when the nurse estimates amounts by breaking unscored tablets.

Often, liquid medications come prepared in volumes greater than 1 ml. The formula still applies. For example, the order is "Erythromycin suspension 250 mg PO." The pharmacy delivers 100-ml bottles with the labels stating "5 ml contains 125 mg of erythromycin."

$$\frac{250 \text{ mg}}{125 \text{ mg}} \times 5 \text{ ml} = \text{Volume to administer}$$

The fraction $^{250}/_{125}$ equals 2. Therefore,

$$2 \times 5 \text{ ml} = 10 \text{ ml to administer}$$

Here the nurse ignores the total volume available and instead uses the values noted on the label. If the nurse calculated the dose on the basis of 100 ml available, the following error would occur:

$$\frac{250 \text{ mg}}{125 \text{ mg}} \times 100 \text{ ml} = 200 \text{ ml to administer}$$

On the basis of this calculation the client would receive 20 times the desired dose. The nurse should always double-check calculations or confer with another professional if an answer seems unreasonable (Table 34-9).

PEDIATRIC DOSES

Calculating children's medication doses requires caution. Children are unable to metabolize many medications as readily as adults. The child's body size also requires smaller doses. In most cases, the prescriber will calculate the dose for a child before ordering the medication. However, nurses should be aware of the formulas used to calculate pediatric doses and recheck all doses before administration. Most medication references list the normal ranges for pediatric doses.

The most accurate method of calculating pediatric doses is based on a child's body surface area. Body surface

Table 34-9 Ways to Prevent Medication Administration Errors

Precaution	Rationale
Read medication labels carefully.	Many products come in similar containers, colors, and shapes.
Question administration of multiple tablets or vials for single dose.	Most doses are one or two tablets or capsules or one single-dose vial. Incorrect interpretation of order may result in excessively high dose.
Be aware of medications with similar names.	Many medication names sound alike (e.g., digoxin and digitoxin, Keflex and Keflin, Orinase and Ornade).
Check decimal point.	Some medications come in quantities that are multiples of one another (e.g., Coumadin in 2.5- and 25-mg tables, Thorazine in 30- and 300-mg spansules).
Question abrupt and excessive increases in dosages.	Most dosages are increased gradually so that physician can monitor therapeutic effect and response.
When new or unfamiliar medication is ordered, consult resource.	If prescriber is also unfamiliar with drug, there is greater risk of inaccurate dosages being ordered.
Do not administer medication ordered by nickname or unofficial abbreviation.	Many prescribers refer to commonly ordered medications by nicknames or unofficial abbreviations. If nurse or pharmacist is unfamiliar with name, wrong medication may be dispensed and administered.
Do not attempt to decipher illegible writing.	When in doubt, ask prescriber. Unless nurse questions order that is difficult to read, chance of misinterpretation is great.
Know clients with same last names. Also have clients state their full names. Check name bands carefully.	It is common to have two or more clients with same or similar last names. Special labels on Kardex or medication book can warn of potential problem.
Do not confuse equivalents.	When in a hurry, it may be easy to misread equivalents (e.g., milligram instead of milliliter).

area is estimated on the basis of the child's height and weight. A standard nomogram (e.g., the West nomogram) can be used to for estimation of a child's body surface area (Figure 34-9).

To calculate a pediatric dose the nurse uses the formula below. The formula is a ratio of the child's body surface area compared with the body surface area of an average adult (1.7 square meters, or 1.7 m^2).

$$\text{Child's dose equals: } \frac{\text{Surface area of child}}{1.7 \text{ m}^2} \times \text{Normal adult dose}$$

For example, a prescriber orders ampicillin for a child weighing 12 kg. The normal adult dose for ampicillin is 250 mg. The West nomogram (see Figure 34-9) shows that a child weighing 12 kg has a surface area of 0.54 m^2. Using this information the nurse then can calculate the appropriate child's dose.

$$\text{Child's dose} = \frac{0.54 \text{ m}^2}{1.7 \text{ m}^2} \times 250 \text{ mg}$$

The m^2 units are canceled out.

$$\text{Child's dose} = \frac{0.54}{1.7} \times 250 \text{ mg}$$

$$\frac{0.54}{1.7} = 0.3$$

$$\text{Child's dose} = 0.3 \times 250 \text{ mg} = 75 \text{ mg}$$

Administering Medications

The nurse does not have sole responsibility for medication administration. The prescriber* and pharmacist also help to ensure the right medication gets to the right client. However, the nurse administering medications is accountable for knowing what medications are prescribed, their therapeutic and nontherapeutic effects, and the client's need for medication administration, supervision with administrator, and education about the medication and its effects.

PRESCRIBER'S ROLE

The physician, nurse practitioner, or physician's assistant prescribes the client's medications. The prescriber writes a medication order on a form in the client's medical record, in an order book, on a legal prescription pad, or through a computer terminal. Where allowed, a prescriber may also order a medication by talking directly to the nurse or by telephone. When medications or medical treatments are ordered this way it is called a **verbal order.** When verbal orders are received by the nurse, they should be immediately entered into the client's medical record and signed by the nurse, indicating the time and the name of the prescriber who gave the order. Most institutions require a prescriber's signature within 24 hours after the order is made.

Institutional policies vary regarding the personnel who can take verbal or telephone orders. Generally, nursing

---

*"Prescriber" refers to physician, advanced practice nurse, (e.g., nurse practitioner, clinical nurse specialist), or physician's assistant.

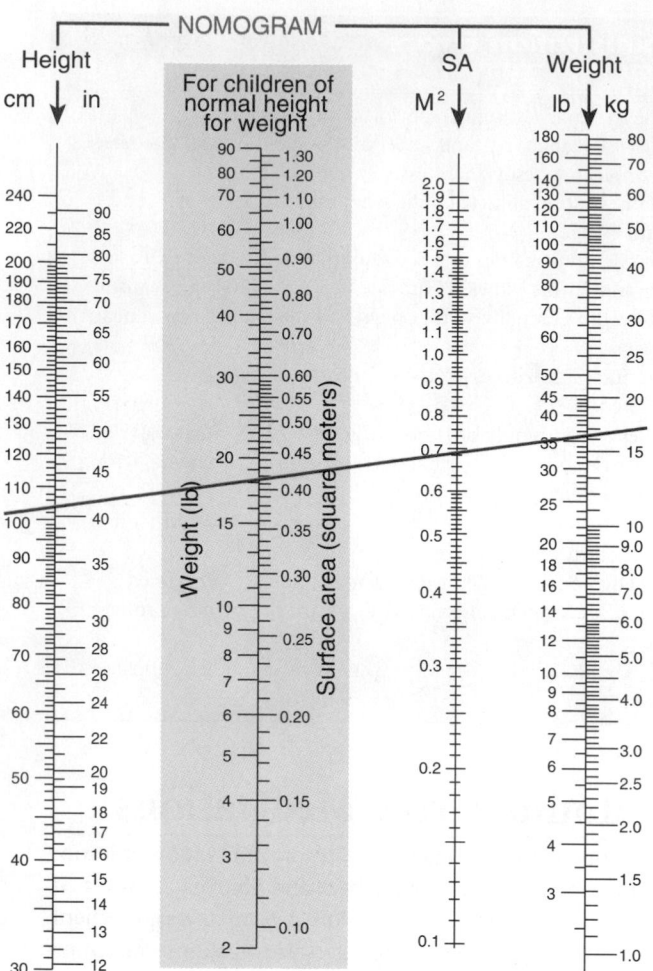

NOMOGRAM

Figure 34-9   West nomogram for estimation of surface areas in children. A straight line is drawn between height and weight. The point where the line crosses the surface area column is the estimated body surface area.
From Behrman RE, Vaughan, VC, editors: *Nelson textbook of pediatrics,* ed 13, Philadelphia, 1987, Saunders; modified from data of Boyd E, by West CD.

students cannot take these types of medication orders. Nursing students should not give any medication without a written medication order. If the technology is available, a prescriber may fax orders to the unit.

Common abbreviations are used when writing orders. The abbreviations indicate dosage frequencies or times, routes of administration, and special information for giving the medication (see Table 34-5).

Types of Orders in Acute Care Agencies.
Four common types of medication orders are based on the frequency and/or urgency of medication administration.

Standing Orders or Routine Medication Orders.
A standing order is carried out until the prescriber cancels

it by another order or until a prescribed number of days elapse. A standing order may indicate a final date or number of treatments or doses. Many institutions have policies for automatically discontinuing standing orders. The following are examples of standing orders: "Tetracycline 500 mg PO q6h" and "Decadron 10 mg qd × 5 days."

prn Orders.   The prescriber may order a medication when a client requires it. This is a prn order. The nurse uses objective and subjective assessment and discretion in determining whether or not the client needs the medication. Often the prescriber sets minimum intervals for the time of administration. This means the medication cannot be given any more often than what is prescribed. Examples of prn orders: "morphine sulfate 2 mg SQ q3-4h prn for incisional pain" and "Maalox 30 ml prn for gastric discomfort." When medications are administered, the nurse documents the assessment made and the time of medication administration. The nurse should make frequent evaluation of the effectiveness of the medication and record findings in the appropriate record.

Single (One-Time) Orders.   A prescriber will often order a medication to be given only once at a specified time. This is common for preoperative medications or medications given before diagnostic examinations, for example, "Versed 25 mg IM on call to OR" and "Valium 10 mg PO at 0900."

STAT Orders.   A STAT order signifies that a single dose of a medication is to be given immediately and only once. STAT orders are often written for emergencies when the client's condition changes suddenly. For example, "Give Apresoline 10 mg IV STAT."

Some conditions change the status of a client's medication orders. For example, surgery automatically cancels all of a client's preoperative medications (see Chapter 49). Because the client's condition changes after surgery, the prescriber must write new orders. When a client is transferred to another health care agency or a different service within a hospital or is discharged, the prescriber should review the medications and write new orders as indicated.

Prescriptions.   The prescriber writes **prescriptions** for clients who are to take medications outside the hospital. The prescription includes more detailed information than a regular order because the client must understand how to take the medication and when to refill the prescription if necessary. The parts of a prescription are included in Figure 34-10.

Pharmacist's Role.   The pharmacist prepares and distributes prescribed medications. Pharmacists may also assess the medication plan and evaluate the client's medication-related needs (American Pharmaceutical Association, 1994). The pharmacist is responsible for filling pre-

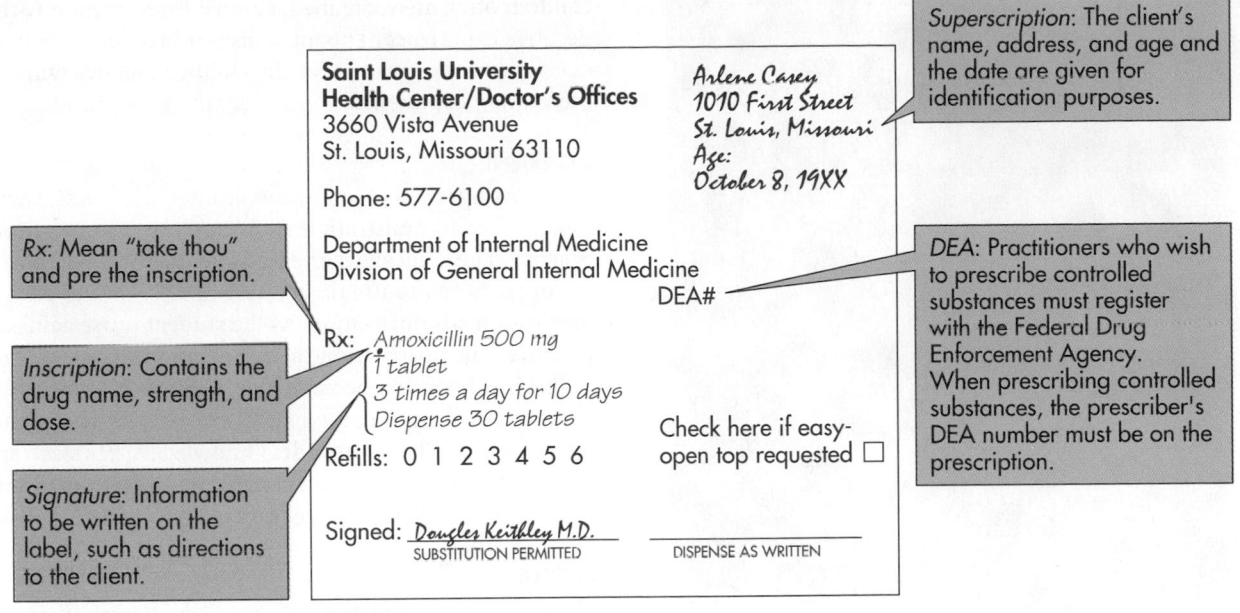

Superscription: The client's name, address, and age and the date are given for identification purposes.

Saint Louis University
Health Center/Doctor's Offices
3660 Vista Avenue
St. Louis, Missouri 63110

Phone: 577-6100

Arlene Carey
1010 First Street
St. Louis, Missouri
Age:
October 8, 19XX

Rx: Mean "take thou" and pre the inscription.

Department of Internal Medicine
Division of General Internal Medicine
                    DEA#

DEA: Practitioners who wish to prescribe controlled substances must register with the Federal Drug Enforcement Agency. When prescribing controlled substances, the prescriber's DEA number must be on the prescription.

Inscription: Contains the drug name, strength, and dose.

Rx: *Amoxicillin 500 mg*
     1 tablet
     3 times a day for 10 days
     Dispense 30 tablets
Refills: 0 1 2 3 4 5 6

Check here if easy-open top requested ☐

Signature: Information to be written on the label, such as directions to the client.

Signed: _Douglas Keithley M.D._ _____
         SUBSTITUTION PERMITTED   DISPENSE AS WRITTEN

Figure 34-10   Example of a medication prescription.
Courtesy Saint Louis University Medical Center, St. Louis, Mo.

scriptions accurately and for being sure that prescriptions are valid. The pharmacist in a health care agency rarely has to mix compounds or solutions, except in the case of IV additive solutions. Most medication companies deliver medications in a form ready for use. Dispensing the correct medication, in the proper dosage and amount, with an accurate label is the pharmacist's main task. The pharmacist can also provide information about medication side effects, toxicity, interactions, and incompatibilities.

Distribution Systems.   Systems for storing and distributing medications vary. Pharmacists provide the medications, but nurses distribute medications to clients. Institutions providing nursing care have a special area for stocking and dispensing medications. Special medication rooms, portable locked carts, computerized medication cabinets, and individual storage units next to clients' rooms are some of the facilities used. Nurses must make sure that storage areas are locked when unattended.

Stock Supply.   With a stock system, medications are available in quantity in larger, multidose containers. This system is time consuming and costly because a nurse must dispense each medication separately for a client. This type of system of medication delivery has been associated with a high rate of medication errors and is not commonly used today (Perini and Vermeulen, 1994).

Unit Dose.   The unit-dose system uses portable carts containing a drawer with a 24-hour supply of medications for each client. The unit dose is the ordered dose of med-

ication the client receives at one time. Each tablet or capsule is wrapped in a foil or paper container. At a designated time each day the pharmacist refills the drawers in the cart with a fresh supply. The cart also contains limited amounts of prn and stock medications for special situations. The unit-dose system is designed to reduce the number of medication errors and saves steps in dispensing medications.

Computer-Controlled Dispensing Systems.   Computer-controlled dispensing systems are used successfully throughout the country (Figure 34-11). They are especially useful for the delivery and control of **narcotics.** Each nurse has a security code allowing access to the system. Then the client's identification number is entered. In these systems the nurse is then allowed to select the desired medication, dosage, and route. The system delivers the medication to the nurse, records it, and charges it to the client.

Nurses may also scan bar codes to identify the client, medication (name, dosage, route), and nurse administering the medication (Abdoo, 1992). This information is then automatically recorded on a computerized database.

NURSE'S ROLE

Since the nurse spends the most time with clients, the nurse is the most appropriate health care worker to administer medications. The administration of medications to clients requires knowledge and a set of skills that is unique to the nurse. The nurse assesses the client's ability to self-administer medications, determines whether a

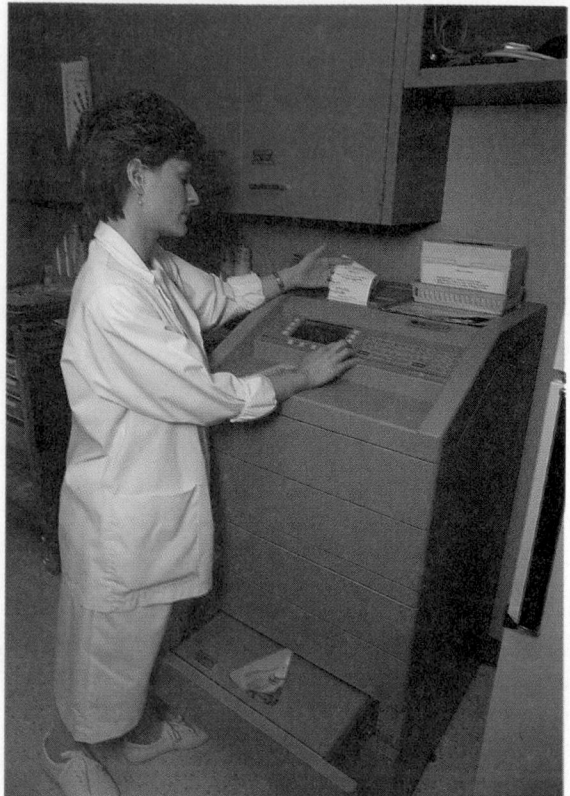

Figure 34-11   Nurse using computer-controlled dispensing system

client should receive a medication at a given time, administers medications correctly, and monitors the effects of prescribed medications. Client and family education about proper medication administration and monitoring is an integral part of the nurse's role. The nurse uses the nursing process to integrate medication therapy into care.

Critical Thinking in Medication Administration

KNOWLEDGE

The nurse uses the knowledge learned from many disciplines when administering medications. It is this knowledge that helps the nurse to understand why a particular medication has been prescribed for a client and how this medication will alter the client's physiology so as to exert a therapeutic effect. For example, in physiology the nurse may have learned that potassium is a major intracellular ion. When clients do not have enough potassium in their body, they may experience signs and symptoms that are associated with hypokalemia, such as muscle fatigue or weakness. Medications may be prescribed that may restore the client's potassium level to normal.

Knowledge about child development may show that

children often associate medication administration with a negative experience. The nurse uses principles from child development to ensure that the child cooperates with the medication experience.

EXPERIENCE

The nursing student often has limited experience with medication administration as it applies to professional practice. The clinical experience provides the student with the opportunity to use the nursing process as it applies to medication administration. As the student nurse gains experiences in medication administration, psychomotor skills ("the how-to") become more refined. However, psychomotor skills represent a small part of medication administration. Client attitudes, knowledge, physical and mental status and responses can make medication administration a complex experience.

ATTITUDES

To administer medication safely to clients certain cognitive skills are essential.

Accountability and Responsibility.   The nurse accepts full responsibility for all actions that are taken; this includes the administration of medications. When a nurse administers a medication to the client, the nurse accepts the responsibility that the medication or the nursing actions in administering it will not harm the client in any way. The nurse does not assume that the medication that is ordered for the client is the correct medication or the correct dose. The nurse could be held accountable for administering an ordered medication that is knowingly inappropriate for the client. Because of this, the nurse should be familiar with the therapeutic effect, usual dosage, laboratory interferences, and side effects of all medications that are administered. The nurse is also responsible for ensuring that clients who will self-administer medications have been properly informed about all aspects of self-administration.

Demonstrating accountability and acting responsibly in professional practice means that the nurse acknowledges when errors in professional practice occur. Most of the errors made by nurses are medication errors. A **medication error** is any event that could cause or lead to a client receiving inappropriate medication therapy or failing to receive appropriate medication therapy (Edgar, Lee, and Cousins, 1994). Most medication errors occur when a nurse fails to follow routine procedures such as checking dose calculations, deciphering illegible handwriting, or administering medications with which the nurse is unfamiliar (see Table 34-9). All medication errors can be linked, in some way, to an inconsistency in adhering to the five rights of medication administration. Hospital medication delivery systems should be designed so that there is a system of checks and balances. This will help to reduce medication errors. Consider this example:

The physician writes an order for a medication. The nurse receives the order and checks for completeness and appropriateness. The nurse may question the order, for example, if the written order is illegible, the dose seems unusually low or high, or the medication seems inappropriate for the client's condition. The order is sent to the pharmacy, where it may be read by a pharmacy technician and may be prepared by the technician. The pharmacist checks the technician's work, that the medication is the appropriate dosage, and for medication interactions and medication allergies. When a medication order seems inappropriate, for example, a medication order written for 2000 mg when the proper dosage calls for 200 mg, the pharmacist may call the nurse for prescriber clarification (or the pharmacist may call the prescriber directly). When the order is appropriate, the medications are sent to the nursing unit. The nurse receives the medication and checks the administration record against what the pharmacy has sent and the prescriber ordered. Before administration, the nurse performs the five rights of medication administration. The nurse allows the client to be the final check by reviewing the name of the medication, the dosage, and why he or she is receiving the medication.

The above example illustrates the important role that nurses play in the prevention of medication errors. The nurse is crucial as the essential link in the prevention of medication errors. Unfortunately, many medication errors are never identified. When an error occurs, it should be acknowledged immediately and reported to the appropriate hospital personnel (e.g., nurse manager and physician). Measures to counteract the effects of the error may be necessary. The nurse is also responsible for completing an incident report describing the nature of the incident. Incident reports assist administrative personnel in identifying hospital system problems that contribute to medication errors.

A nurse may be asked to administer medications about which the nurse has limited knowledge. Critical thinkers admit what they do not know and try to acquire the knowledge needed to safely administer unfamiliar medications. This may mean consulting more expert nurses, a pharmacist, or a medication book.

Institutional policy may place limitations on the nurse's ability to administer certain types of medications, by certain routes, or in certain units of the acute care setting. Most settings have nursing procedure manuals that have policies that define the classes of medications nurses employed by the agency may and may not administer. For example, in most agencies only nurses with specialized training can administer chemotherapeutic medications. Not all prescribers are aware of all of the limitations and may often prescribe these medications. Nurses must recognize these limitations and ensure that the prescriber is informed and that appropriate actions are taken to ensure that the client receives the medications as prescribed and within the time prescribed.

STANDARDS

Standards are those actions that ensure safe nursing practice. To ensure safe medication administration the nurse should be aware of a nursing standard called the five rights of medication administration:

1. The right medication
2. The right dose
3. The right client
4. The right route
5. The right time

Right Medication. When medications are first ordered, the nurse compares the medication recording form or computer orders with the prescriber's written orders. When administering medications, the nurse compares the label of the medication container with the medication form. The nurse does this 3 times: (1) before removing the container from the drawer or shelf, (2) as the amount of medication ordered is removed from the container, and (3) before returning the container to storage. With unit-dose prepackaged medications, the nurse checks the label with the medicine form a third time even though there is no permanent container. Unit-dose medications may be checked before opening at the client's bedside.

Nurses administer only the medications they prepare. If an error occurs, the nurse who administers the medication is responsible for its effects. If a client questions the medication a nurse prepares, it is important not to ignore these concerns. An alert client will know whether a medication is different from those received before. In most cases the client's medication order has been changed; however, the client's questions might reveal an error. The nurse should withhold the medication until the preparation can be rechecked against the prescriber's orders.

Clients who self-administer medications should keep them in their original labeled containers, separate from other medications, to avoid confusion.

The nurse never prepares medications from unmarked containers or containers with illegible labels. If a client refuses a medication, the nurse should discard it rather than return it to the original container. Unit-dose packaged medications can be saved if they are unopened.

Right Dose. The unit-dose system is designed to minimize errors. When a medication must be prepared from a larger volume or strength than needed or when the prescriber orders a system of measurement different from what the pharmacist supplies, the chance of error increases. When performing medication calculations or conversions, the nurse should have another qualified nurse check the calculated doses.

After calculating doses, the nurse prepares the medication using standard measurement devices. Graduated cups, syringes, and scaled droppers can be used to measure medications accurately. At home, clients should use kitchen measuring spoons rather than teaspoons and tablespoons, which vary in volume.

When it is necessary to break a scored tablet, the break should be even. A tablet may be cut in half by using a knife-edge or a cutting device. Tablets that do not break evenly are discarded. The two halves are given in successive doses if the second half was repackaged and labeled.

Often a nurse prepares a tablet by crushing it so that it can be mixed in food. The crushing device should always be cleaned completely before the tablet is crushed. Remnants of previously crushed medications may increase a medication's concentration or result in the client receiving a portion of an unprescribed medication. Crushed medications should be mixed with very small amounts of food or liquid. The client's favorite foods or liquids should not be used because a medication may alter their taste and decrease the client's desire for them.

Right Client.

An important step in administering medications safely is being sure the medication is given to the right client. It is difficult to remember every client's name and face. To identify a client correctly, the nurse checks the medication administration form against the

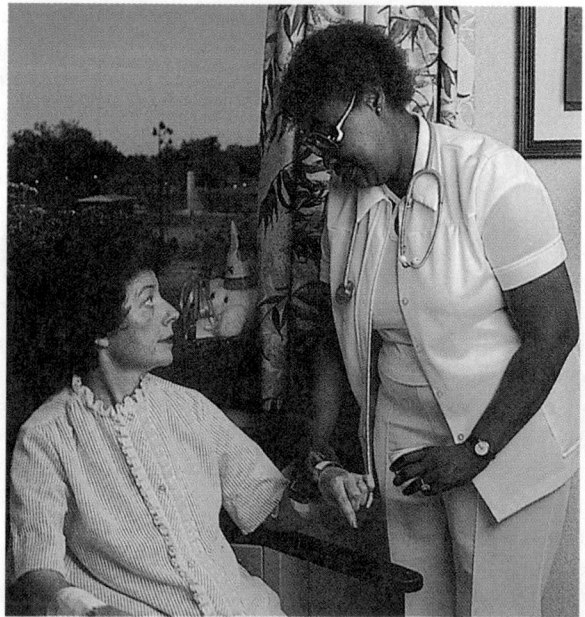

Figure 34-12 Before administering any medications, the nurse checks the client's identification and allergy bracelet.

client's identification bracelet (Figure 34-12) and asks the client to state his or her name.

If an identification bracelet becomes smudged or illegible, or is missing, the nurse must acquire a new one for the client. When asking the client's name, the nurse should not merely speak the name and assume that the client's response indicates that he or she is the right person. Instead, the nurse asks the client to state his or her full name. To avoid making the client feel uneasy, the nurse simply states that the question is routine for giving a medication.

Right Route.

If a prescriber's order does not designate a route of administration, the nurse consults the prescriber. Likewise, if the specified route is not the recommended route, the nurse should alert the prescriber immediately.

When the nurse administers injections, precautions are necessary to ensure that the medications are given correctly. It is also important to prepare injections only from preparations designed for parenteral use. The injection of a liquid designed for oral use can produce local complications, such as a sterile abscess, or fatal systemic effects. Medication companies label parenteral medications for "injectable use only."

Right Time.

The nurse must know why a medication is ordered for certain times of the day and whether the time schedule can be altered. For example, two medications are ordered, one q8h (every 8 hours) and the other tid. (3 times a day). Both medications are to be given 3 times within a 24-hour period. The prescriber intends the q8h medication to be given around the clock to maintain therapeutic blood levels of the medication. In contrast, the tid. medication is given during the waking hours. Each institution has a recommended time schedule for medications ordered at frequent intervals.

The prescriber often gives specific instructions about when to administer a medication. A preoperative medication to be given on call means that the nurse is to administer the medication when the operating room notifies the nursing division. A medication ordered pc (after meals) is to be given within half an hour after a meal, when the client has a full stomach. A STAT medication is to be given immediately.

Medications that must act at certain times are given priority. For example, insulin should be given at a precise interval before a meal. All routinely ordered medications should be given within 30 minutes of the times ordered (30 minutes before or after the prescribed time).

Some medications require the nurse's clinical judgment in determining the proper time for administration. A prn sleeping medication should be administered when the client is prepared for bed or at a time appropriate for maximum benefit. A nurse also uses judgment when administering prn analgesics. For example, the nurse may need to obtain a STAT order from the prescriber if the client requires a medication before the prn interval has elapsed.

At home a client may have to take several medications throughout the day. The nurse helps to plan schedules based on preferred medication intervals and the client's daily schedule. For clients who have difficulty remembering when to take medications, the nurse can make a chart that lists the times when each medication is to be taken or can prepare a special container to hold each timed dose.

Professional standards influence the activities of medication administration. The American Nurses Association's (ANA's) *Standards of Nursing Practice* (see Chapter 19), based on the nursing process, also apply to the activity of medication administration. Other professional nursing standards may apply.

Maintaining Clients' Rights.

In accordance with *A Patient's Bill of Rights* and because of the potential risks related to medication administration, a client has the right to:

Be informed of the medication's name, purpose, action, and potential undesired effects

Refuse a medication regardless of the consequences

Have qualified nurses or physicians assess a medication history, including allergies

Be properly advised of the experimental nature of medication therapy and to give written consent for its use

Receive labeled medications safely without discomfort in accordance with the five rights of medication administration

Receive appropriate supportive therapy in relation to medication therapy

Not receive unnecessary medications

The nurse must be aware of these rights and handle all inquiries by clients and families courteously and professionally. A nurse should not become defensive if a client refuses medication therapy. The nurse must have the necessary knowledge and skill to satisfy the responsibilities of safe and effective medication administration.

Nursing Process and Medication Administration

ASSESSMENT

To determine the need for and potential response to medication therapy, the nurse assesses many factors.

History.

Prior to administering medications the nurse obtains or reviews the client's medical history. A client's medical history may provide indications or contraindications for medication therapy. Disease or illness may place clients at risk for adverse medication effects. For example, if a client has a gastric ulcer, compounds containing aspirin will increase the likelihood of bleeding. Long-term health problems such as diabetes or arthritis, which require medications, suggest to the nurse the type of med-

ications a client is taking. A client's surgical history may indicate use of medications. For example, after a thyroidectomy a client may require hormone replacement.

History of Allergies.

If the client has a history of allergies to medication, the nurse informs other members of the health care team. Food allergies should also be carefully documented because many medications have ingredients also found in food sources. One example is shellfish. If clients are allergic to shellfish, the client may be sensitive to any product containing iodine such as betadine or dyes used in radiological testing. Another example is dye used in food products (e.g., candy, soda). In a hospital, clients wear identification bands listing medications to which they are allergic. All allergies should be noted on the nurse's admission notes, medication records, and physician's history.

Medication Data.

The nurse assesses information about each medication that the client takes, including length of time the medication has been taken, the current dosage, and whether or not the client has experienced adverse effects from the medication. In addition, the nurse reviews medication data, including action, purpose, normal dosages, routes, side effects, and nursing implications for administration and monitoring. Common questions to ask are, Is the smallest possible dose ordered (a question pertinent to older adults)? Can a certain medication interact with other medications being used? Are there special instructions for administering the medication? Often, several resources must be consulted to gather needed information. Pharmacology textbooks, nursing journals, the *Physicians' Desk Reference (PDR)*, medication package inserts, and the pharmacist are valuable resources. The nurse is responsible for knowing as much as possible about each medication given. Many nursing students prepare or purchase cards containing medication data to use as a quick resource.

Diet History.

A diet history reveals normal eating patterns and food preferences. The nurse can then plan the dosage schedule more effectively and advise the client in avoiding foods that may interact with medications.

Client's Perceptual or Coordination Problems.

For a client with perceptual or coordination limitations, self-administration may be difficult. The nurse must assess the client's ability to prepare doses and take medications correctly. If the client is unable to self-administer medications, the nurse may need to assess whether family or friends will be available to assist.

Client's Current Condition.

The ongoing physical or mental status of a client may affect whether a medication is given or how it is administered. The nurse should assess a client carefully before giving any medication. For example, the nurse checks blood pressure before giving an anti-hypertensive. A client who is nauseated may be unable to swallow a tablet. Assessment findings also serve as a baseline in evaluating the effects of medication therapy.

Client's Attitude About Medication Use.   The client's attitude about medications may reveal a level of medication dependence or drug avoidance. Clients may not express their feelings about taking a particular medication, particularly if dependence is a problem. The nurse should observe the client's behavior for evidence of medication dependence or avoidance. The nurse should also be aware that the client's cultural beliefs about Western medicine can interfere with medication compliance (see Chapter 7).

Client's Knowledge and Understanding of Medication Therapy.   The client's knowledge and understanding of medication therapy influence the willingness or ability to follow a medication regimen. Unless a client understands a medication's purpose, the importance of regular dosage schedules and proper administration methods, and the possible side effects, compliance is unlikely. When assessing knowledge of a medication, the nurse asks, What is it for? How is it taken? When is it taken? What side effects have there been? Has the client ever stopped taking doses? Is there anything else the client does not understand and would like to know about the medication? When the client has a history of poor compliance, the nurse should also review resources available for purchase of medications.

Client's Learning Needs.   By assessing the client's level of knowledge about a medication and the resources available to take medications regularly, the nurse determines the need for instruction (see Chapter 23). It may be necessary for the nurse to explain the action and purpose of the medication, expected side effects, correct administration techniques, and ways to help the client to remember the medication regimen. If a client has been placed on a newly prescribed medication, instruction may need to be more involved.

✏ NURSING DIAGNOSIS

Assessment provides data about the client's condition, ability to self-administer medications, and medication use patterns, which can be used to determine actual or potential problems with medication therapy. Certain data are defining characteristics, which when clustered together reveal nursing diagnoses (Box 34-4). For example, a client's admission of missing a dose, evidence that a medication has not reversed symptoms, and evidence that the client has not progressed indicates *noncompliance regarding a medication regimen.* Once the diagnosis is selected, the nurse identifies the related factor. The related factors of in-

adequate resources versus lack of knowledge require different interventions. If the client's noncompliance is related to inadequate finances, the nurse will collaborate with family members, social workers, or community agencies to help a client receive necessary medications. If the related factor is lack of knowledge, the nurse will implement an extensive teaching plan and follow-up.

✏ PLANNING

The nurse organizes care activities to ensure the safe administration of medications. Hurrying to give clients medications can lead to errors. The nurse can also plan to use time during medication administration to teach clients about their medications. It is important to collaborate with the client's family or friends when instruction is given. Family members will often reinforce the importance of medication regimens in the home setting. When clients are hospitalized, it is important for the nurse to not postpone instruction until the day of discharge. In order for the client to understand medications and self-administration guidelines, there must be time for questions and discussion. Early planning is critical.

In the community, the nurse ensures that the client knows where and how to obtain medications. The nurse also ensures that clients know how to read medication labels. Whether a client attempts self-administration or the nurse assumes responsibility for administering medications, the following goals and expected outcomes must be met: (1) the client and family understand medication therapy, (2) the client gains therapeutic effect of the prescribed medications without discomfort or complications, (3) the client has no complications related to the route of administration, and (4) the client safely self-administers medications.

✏ IMPLEMENTATION

Health Promotion.   The nurse, in promoting or maintaining the client's health, identifies factors that may improve or diminish well-being. Health beliefs, personal motivations, socioeconomic factors, and habits (e.g., smoking) can influence the client's compliance with the medication regimen.

Teaching the client and family about the benefit of a medication and the knowledge needed to take it correctly can promote adherence to the regimen and foster independence. Integrating the client's health beliefs and cultural practices into the treatment plan can assist the nurse in establishing a schedule or routine with the client. The nurse may make referrals to community resources if the client is unable to afford, or get out to obtain, necessary medications.

Client and Family Teaching.   Unless a client is properly informed about medications, he or she may take the

NURSING DIAGNOSES Box 34-4
CLIENTS REQUIRING MEDICATION THERAPY

Anxiety
Knowledge deficit regarding a medication regimen
Mobility, impaired physical
Noncompliance regarding a medication regimen
Sensory/perceptual alterations, visual
Swallowing, impaired

medications incorrectly or not at all. The nurse provides information about the purpose of medications and their actions and effects. Many health care institutions offer easy-to-read leaflets on specific types of medications. A client must know how to take a medication properly and the effects if he or she fails to do so. For example, after receiving a prescription for an antibiotic, a client must understand the importance of taking the full prescription. Failure to do this can lead to a worsening of the condition and the development of bacteria resistant to the medication.

Nurses teach proper self-administration of medications to clients who depend on daily injections. The client learns to prepare and administer an injection correctly using aseptic technique. Family members or friends should be taught to give injections in case the client becomes ill or physically unable to handle a syringe. Nurses can provide specially designed equipment such as syringes with enlarged calibrated scales for easier reading or braille-labeled medication vials for clients with visual alterations.

Clients must be aware of the symptoms of medication side effects or toxicity. For example, clients taking anticoagulants learn to notify their primary care providers immediately when signs of bleeding or bruising develop. Family members or friends should be informed of medication side effects such as changes in behavior because they are often the first persons to recognize such effects. Clients are better able to cope with problems caused by medications if they understand how and when to act. All clients should learn the basic guidelines for medication safety. These guidelines ensure the proper use and storage of medications in the home (Box 34-5).

Acute Care.   One rationale for hospitalization may be to have expert nursing observation and documentation of responses to medications (Benner, 1984). When a nurse receives a medication order, several nursing interventions are essential for safe and effective medication administration.

Receiving Medication Orders.   A medication order is required for any medication to be administered by a nurse. Before any other interventions, the nurse ensures that the medication order contains all of the elements in Box 34-6. If the medication order is incomplete, the nurse should inform the prescriber and ensure completeness before carrying out any medication order. Some medication orders can be given verbally or by telephone by the prescriber to the nurse. A verbal order is a medication or treatment order received by the nurse in the presence of the prescriber. Verbal orders are entered into the client's medical record by the registered nurse and transcribed the same way as if the prescriber wrote the order himself or herself. Telephone orders are medication or treatment orders given to the nurse by the prescriber, generally after the nurse updates the prescriber about a change in the client's condition. The nurse follows institutional policy regarding the receiving, recording, and transcription of verbal and telephone orders. Generally the prescriber must sign verbal and telephone orders within 24 hours. *Student nurses are prohibited from receiving verbal and telephone orders.*

Correct Transcription and Communication of Orders.   The nurse or a designated unit secretary writes the prescriber's complete order on the appropriate medication form, called a medication administration record (MAR) (Figure 34-13). The transcribed order includes the client's name, room, and bed number, medication name, dose, frequency, and route of administration. Each time a medication dose is prepared the nurse refers to the medication form. With the unit-dose system, only one transcription is necessary, limiting the opportunity for errors. When transcribing orders, the nurse should be sure that names, dosages, and symbols are legible. The nurse rewrites any smudged or illegible transcriptions.

In some institutions a computer printout lists all currently ordered medications with dosage information.

Client Teaching FOR SAFE MEDICATION ADMINISTRATION   Box 34-5

- Keep each medication in its original labeled container.
- Protect medication from exposure to heat and light, as required.
- Check that labels are legible.
- Discard outdated medications.
- Always finish a prescribed medication unless otherwise instructed, and never save a medication for future illnesses.

- Dispose of medications in a sink or toilet, and never place medications in the trash within reach of children.
- Never give a family member a medication prescribed for another.
- Refrigerate medications that require it.
- Read labels carefully and follow all instructions.
- Notify prescriber of side effects.

Components of Medication Orders   Box 34-6

A medication order is incomplete unless it has the following parts:

Client's full name. The client's full name distinguishes the client from other persons with the same last name.

Date that the order is written. The day, month, year, and time must be included. Designating the time that an order is written helps clarify when certain orders are to stop automatically. If an incident occurs involving a medication error, it is easier to document what happened when this information is available.

Medication name. The prescriber will order a generic or trade-name medication. Correct spelling is essential in preventing confusion with medications with similar spelling.

Dose. The amount or strength of the medication is included.

Route of administration. The prescriber uses common abbreviations for medication routes. Accuracy is important because some medications are administered by more than one route.

Time and frequency of administration. The nurse needs to know when to initiate medication therapy. Orders for multiple doses establish a routine schedule for medication administration.

Signature of physician, nurse practitioner, or physician assistant. Signature makes the order a legal request.

Orders are entered directly into the computer, preventing the need for transcription of orders. The same printout may be used to record medications given.

A registered nurse checks all transcribed orders against the original order for accuracy and thoroughness. If an order seems incorrect or inappropriate, the nurse consults the prescriber. The nurse who gives the wrong medication or an incorrect dose is legally responsible for the error.

Accurate Dose Calculation and Measurement. When measuring liquid medications, the nurse uses standard measuring containers. The procedure for medication measurement is systematic to lessen the chance of error. The nurse calculates each dose when preparing the medication, pays close attention to the process of calculation, and avoids interference from other nursing activities.

Correct Administration. For safe administration, the nurse uses aseptic technique and proper procedures when handling and giving medications. For example, certain medications require the nurse to perform assessments (e.g., assessing heart rate before giving antidysrhythmic medications).

Recording Medication Administration. After administering a medication, the nurse records it immedi-

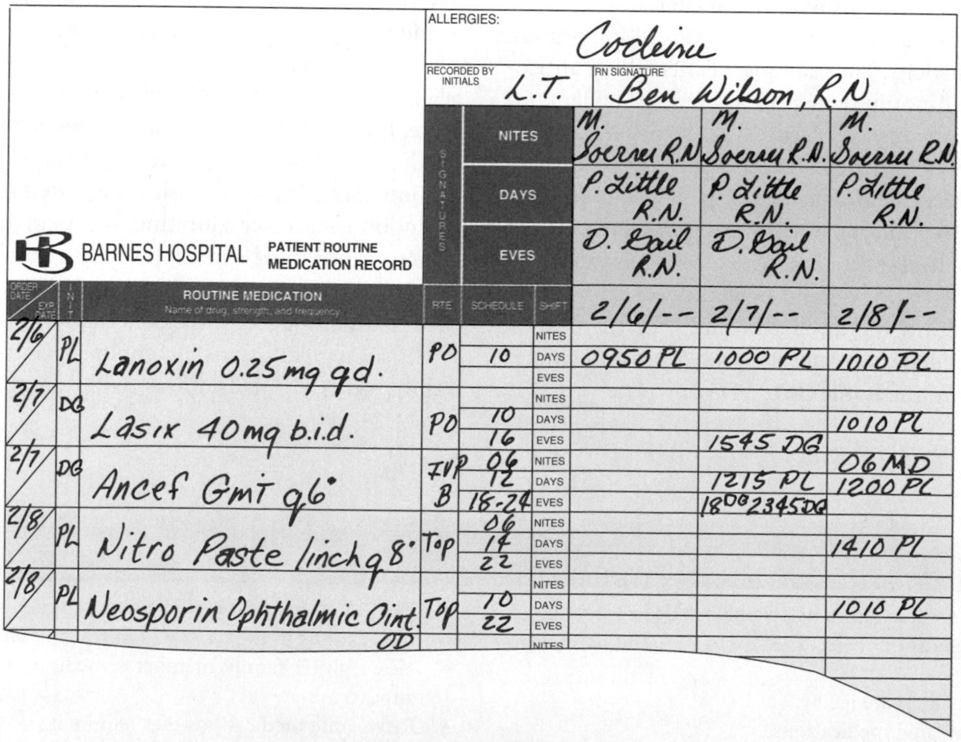

Figure 34-13 Example of medication record.
Courtesy Barnes Hospital, St. Louis, Mo.

ately on the appropriate record form (see Figure 34-13). The nurse never charts a medication before administering it. Recording immediately after administration prevents errors.

The recording of a medication includes the name of the medication, dose, route, and exact time of administration. Often the medication forms are prepared, and the nurse need only record the time. Agency policies may also require that the nurse record the location of an injection.

If a client refuses a medication or is undergoing tests or procedures that result in a missed dose, the nurse explains the reason the medication was not given in the nurse's notes. Some agencies require the nurse to circle the prescribed administration time on the medication record when a dose is missed.

Restorative Care. Because of the numerous types of restorative care settings, medication administration activities vary. Clients with functional limitations may require the nurse to fully administer all medications. In the home health setting the client usually administers his or her own medications. Regardless of the type of medication activity, the nurse remains responsible for instructing clients and families in medication action, administration, and side effects. The nurse is also responsible for monitoring compliance with medication and determines the effectiveness of medications that have been prescribed.

Special Considerations for Administering Medications to Specific Age-Groups. A client's developmental level is a factor in the way nurses administer medications. Knowledge of a client's developmental needs helps the nurse to anticipate responses to medication therapy.

Infants and Children. Children vary in age, weight, surface area, and the ability to absorb, metabolize, and excrete medications. Children's medication doses are lower than those of adults, so special caution is needed when preparing medications for them. Medications are usually not prepared and packaged in standardized dose ranges for children. Preparing an ordered dose from an available amount requires careful calculation (see p. 898).

A child's parents are valuable resources for learning the best way to give a child medications. Sometimes it is less traumatic for the child if a parent gives the medication and the nurse supervises.

All children require special psychological preparation before receiving medications. Supportive care is needed if a child is expected to cooperate. The nurse explains the procedure to a child, using short words and simple language appropriate to the child's level of comprehension. Long explanations may increase a child's anxiety, especially for painful procedures such as an injection. The young child who refuses to cooperate or resists consistently despite explanation and encouragement may re-

quire physical coercion. If so, it is carried out quickly and carefully (Wong, 1998). If it is possible to involve the child, the nurse may have greater success giving a medication. For example, saying "It's time to take your tablet now. Do you want it with water or juice?" allows a child to make a choice. Never give the child the option of not taking a medication. After a medication is given, the nurse praises the child and may even offer a simple reward such as a star or token. Depending on the route of administration, tips exist for effective medication administration for children (Box 34-7).

Older Adults. Older adults also require special consideration during medication administration. In addition to physiological changes of aging (Figure 34-14), behavioral and economic factors influence an older person's use of medications. Ebersole and Hess (1998) describe five behavioral patterns of medication use characteristic of the older client.

Polypharmacy. **Polypharmacy** means that the client is taking many medications, prescribed or not, in an attempt to treat several disorders simultaneously. When this occurs, there is a high risk of medication interactions with

---

Tips for Administering Medications to Children | Box 34-7

ORAL MEDICATIONS

Liquid forms are safer to swallow to avoid aspiration.

Juice, a soft drink, or a frozen juice bar is offered after a medication is swallowed.

Carbonated beverages poured over finely crushed ice reduce nausea.

When mixing medications with palatable flavorings such as syrup or honey, the nurse uses only a small amount. The child may refuse to take all of a larger mixture. The nurse avoids mixing a medication with foods or liquids that the child is taking well because the child may in turn refuse them.

A plastic, disposable syringe is the most accurate device for preparing liquid doses, especially those less than 10 ml. (Cups, teaspoons, and droppers are inaccurate.)

When administering liquid medications, a spoon, plastic cup, or oral syringe (without needle) is useful.

INJECTIONS

The nurse is very careful when selecting IM injection sites. Infants and small children have underdeveloped muscles.

Children can be unpredictable and uncooperative. Someone should be available to restrain a child if needed.

The nurse always awakens a sleeping child before giving an injection.

Distracting the child with conversation or a toy may reduce pain perception.

The nurse gives the injection quickly and does not fight with the child.

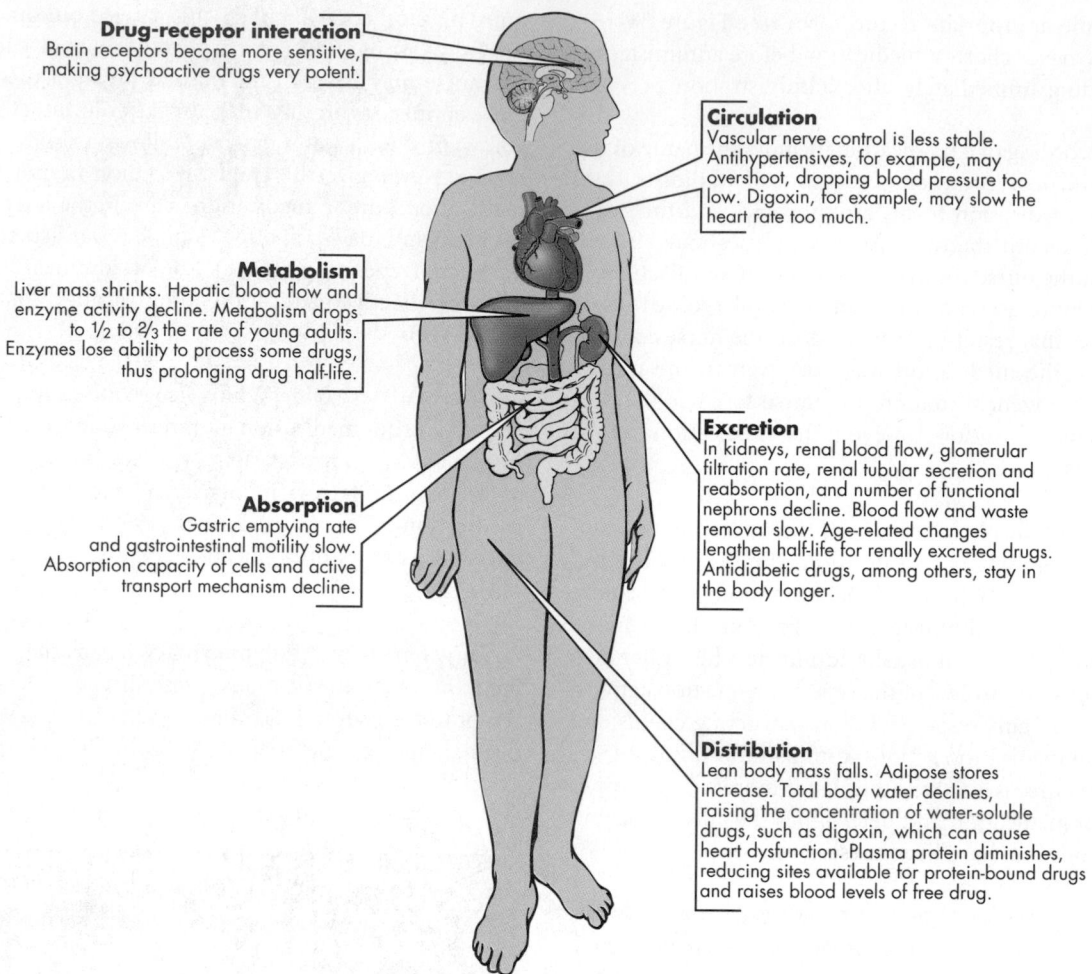

Drug-receptor interaction
Brain receptors become more sensitive, making psychoactive drugs very potent.

Circulation
Vascular nerve control is less stable. Antihypertensives, for example, may overshoot, dropping blood pressure too low. Digoxin, for example, may slow the heart rate too much.

Metabolism
Liver mass shrinks. Hepatic blood flow and enzyme activity decline. Metabolism drops to 1/2 to 2/3 the rate of young adults. Enzymes lose ability to process some drugs, thus prolonging drug half-life.

Absorption
Gastric emptying rate and gastrointestinal motility slow. Absorption capacity of cells and active transport mechanism decline.

Excretion
In kidneys, renal blood flow, glomerular filtration rate, renal tubular secretion and reabsorption, and number of functional nephrons decline. Blood flow and waste removal slow. Age-related changes lengthen half-life for renally excreted drugs. Antidiabetic drugs, among others, stay in the body longer.

Distribution
Lean body mass falls. Adipose stores increase. Total body water declines, raising the concentration of water-soluble drugs, such as digoxin, which can cause heart dysfunction. Plasma protein diminishes, reducing sites available for protein-bound drugs and raises blood levels of free drug.

Figure 34-14   Aging body and drug use.
From Lewis SM and others: *Medical-surgical nursing,* ed 5, St. Louis, 2000, Mosby.

other medications and with foods that the client may eat. There is also an increase risk of the client having an adverse reaction to the medications.

Self-Prescribing of Medications.   A variety of symptoms can be experienced by older adult clients (e.g., pain, constipation, insomnia, and indigestion). All these symptoms are amenable to over-the-counter (OTC) medications. Older adults often attempt to seek relief from the problems by using over-the-counter preparations, folk medicines, and herbs.

Over-The-Counter Medications.   It is known that OTC medications are used by 75% of older adults to relieve symptoms. Many of these OTC preparations have ingredients that, when used inappropriately, may cause undesirable side effects or adverse reactions or may be contraindicated in the client's condition.

Misuse of Medications.   Forms of misuse by older adults include overuse, underuse, erratic use, and contraindicated use.

Noncompliance.   Noncompliance is defined as a deliberate misuse of medication. Of older adults, 75% intentionally do not adhere to their medication regimen by altering the dose either because of ineffectiveness or uncomfortable side effects.

Box 34-8 outlines tips for administering medications to the older client.

EVALUATION

The nurse monitors a client's response to medications on an ongoing basis. This requires that the nurse know the therapeutic action and common side effects of each medication. A change in a client's condition can be

NURSING PRACTICE   Box 34-8

- Space oral medications so that not more than one or two are taken at one time.
- Have client drink a little fluid *before* taking oral medications (to ease swallowing).
- Encourage the client to drink at least 5 to 6 ounces of fluid after taking medications (to ensure that the medications have left the esophagus and are in the stomach and to speed absorption of the medication).
- Do not routinely give analgesics for pain every 4 hours. Because of delayed absorption and distribution and the half-life of the medication, there may be an adverse cumulative effect.
- If the client has difficulty swallowing a large capsule or tablet, ask the physician to substitute a liquid medication if possible (cutting the tablet in half or crushing it and placing it in applesauce or fruit juice may distort the action of some medications, reduce the dose, or cause choking or aspiration of particles of medication or applesauce).
- Teach alternatives to medications, such as the following:
  - Proper diet instead of vitamins
  - Exercise instead of laxatives
  - Bedtime snacks instead of hypnotics
  - Decrease in weight, salt, fats, stress, and smoking and increased exercise instead of hypertensive agents (if approved by the physician)

Modified from Ebersole P, Hess P: *Toward healthy aging: human needs and nursing response,* ed 5, St. Louis, 1998, Mosby.

physiologically related to health status or may result from medications or both. The nurse must be alert for reactions in a client taking several medications. The goal of safe and effective medication administration involves a careful evaluation of technique and the client's response to therapy and ability to assume responsibility for self-care.

To evaluate the effectiveness of nursing interventions when meeting established goals of care, the nurse uses evaluative measures to identify if client outcomes were met. Many different evaluation measures can be used in the context of medication administration: direct observation of behavior or response, rating scales and checklists, and oral questioning. The type of measurement used varies with the action being evaluated, the reading skill and knowledge level of the client, and the client's cognitive and psychomotor ability. The most common type of measurement that the nurse uses is a physiological measure. Examples of physiological measure are blood pressure, heart rate, and visual acuity. Client statements can also be used as evaluative measures. Table 34-10 contains examples of goals, expected outcomes, and corresponding evaluative measures.

Oral Administration

The easiest and most desirable way to administer medications is by mouth (Skill 34-1). Clients usually are able to ingest or self-administer oral medications with a minimum of problems. Most tablets and capsules should be

Text continued on p. 916.

Table 34-10 **Example Evaluation for Client Goals**		
Goal	Expected Outcomes	Evaluative Measure With Example
Client and family understand medication therapy.	Client and family describe information about medication, dosage, schedule, purpose, and adverse effects.	Written measurement: Have client write out medication schedule for a 24-hour period. Oral questioning: Ask client to describe purpose, dosage, and adverse effects of each prescribed medication.
	Client and family identify situations that require medical intervention.	Oral questioning: Have family describe what to do when a client has adverse effects from a medication.
	Client and family demonstrate appropriate administration technique.	Direct observation: Have client demonstrate filling of an insulin syringe and self-injection.
Client safely self-administers medications.	Client follows prescribed treatment regimen.	Anecdotal notes: Have family keep log of client's compliance with therapy for 1 week.
	Client performs techniques correctly.	Direct observation: Observe client instill eye drops.
	Client identifies available resources for obtaining necessary medication.	Oral questioning: Ask family to identify how to contact local pharmacy, community clinic, or American Cancer Society for necessary medications.

Skill 34-1   Administering Oral Medications

Delegation Considerations

Administering medications by the oral route requires problem solving and knowledge application unique to professional nurs-ing. For this procedure delegation to assistive personnel is not appropriate.

EQUIPMENT

- Medication cart or tray
- Disposable medication cups
- Glass of water, juice, or preferred liquid
- Drinking straw

- Pill-crushing or pillating device (optional)
- Paper towels
- MAR or computer printout

STEPS	RATIONALE
1. Assess for any contraindications to client receiving oral medication: Is client able to swallow? Is client suffering from nausea/vomiting? Is client diagnosed as having bowel inflammation or reduced peristalsis? Has client had recent GI surgery? Does client have gastric suction? a. Check the client's swallow, cough, and gag reflexes if in doubt about client's ability to manage oral medications. Withhold medication if swallow, cough, or gag is impaired and notify prescriber.	Alterations in GI function interfere with medication distribution, absorption, and excretion. Clients with GI suction might not receive benefit from the medication because it may be suctioned from the GI tract before it can be absorbed.
2. Assess client's medical history, history of allergies, medication history, and diet history.	These factors can influence how certain medications act. Information also reflects client's need for medications.

Critical Decision Point: Drug allergies should be listed on *each* page of the MAR, on an identification armband, and prominently displayed on the client's medical record.

3. Gather physical examination and laboratory data that may influence medication administration.	Physical examination or laboratory data may contraindicate medication administration.

Critical Decision Point: If contraindications exist, withhold medication and inform prescriber.

4. Assess client's knowledge regarding health and medication use.	Determines client's need for medication education. Also assists in identifying client's adherence to medication therapy at home. Assessment may reveal medication use problems such as medication tolerance. This occurs when a client desires more and more medication to achieve the desired effect. Other medication use problems are noncompliance, abuse, addiction, or dependence.
5. Assess client's preferences for fluids.	Offering fluids during medication administration increases client's fluid intake. Fluids ease swallowing and facilitate absorption from the GI tract. Fluid restrictions must be maintained.
6. Check accuracy and completeness of each MAR or computer printout with prescriber's written medication order. Check client's name, medication name and dose, route of administration, and time for administration.	The order sheet is the most reliable source and only legal record of medications client is to receive.

STEPS	RATIONALE

7. Prepare medications:
   a. Wash hands.

   b. Arrange medication tray and cups in medication preparation area or move medication cart to position outside client's room.

   c. Unlock medicine drawer or cart.

   d. Prepare medication for one client at a time. Keep all pages of MARs or computer printouts for one client together.

   e. Select correct medication from stock supply or unit-dose drawer. Compare label of medication with MAR or computer printout (see illustration).

   f. Calculate medication dose as necessary. Double-check calculation.

   g. To prepare tablets or capsules from a floor stock bottle, pour required number into bottle cap and transfer medication to medication cap. Do not touch medication with fingers. Extra tablets or capsules may be returned to bottle. Medications that need to be broken to administer half the dose can be broken, using a gloved hand, or cut with a pill crushing device (see illustration). Tablets that are to be broken in half must be prescored. Prescored tablets are identified by a manufactured line that transverses the center of the tablet.

Reduces transfer of microorganisms.
Organization of equipment saves time and reduces error.

Medications are safeguarded when locked in cabinet or cart.
Prevents preparation error.

Reading labels and comparing it with transcribed order reduces error.

Double-checking reduces risk of error.

Medications are very expensive; avoid waste.

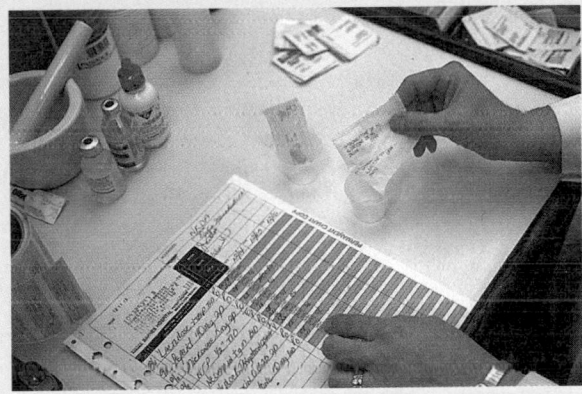

Step 7e

   h. To prepare unit-dose tablets or capsules, place packaged tablet or capsule directly into medicine cup. (Do not remove wrapper; see illustration.)

   i. All tablets or capsules to be given to client at same time may be placed in one medicine cup except for those requiring preadministration assessments (e.g., pulse rate or blood pressure).

Wrapper maintains cleanliness of medications and identifies medication name and dose.

Keeping medications that require preadministration assessments separate from others makes it easier for the nurse to withhold medications as necessary.

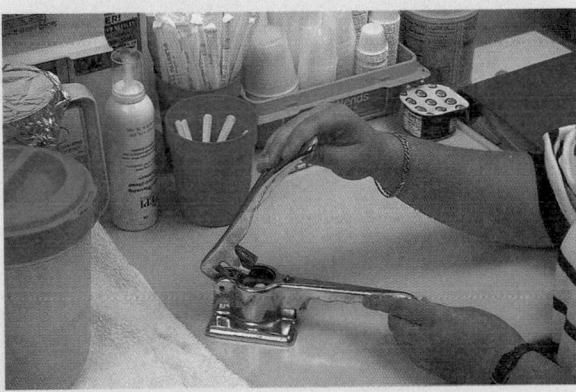

Step 7g

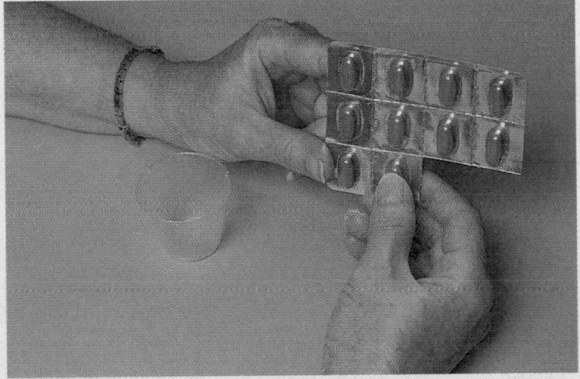

Step 7h

STEPS	RATIONALE
j. If the client has difficulty swallowing, ask physician to substitute with liquid. If liquid medications are not an option, use pill-crushing device such as a mortar and pestle to grind pills. If a pill-crushing device is not available, place tablet between two medication cups and grind with a blunt instrument. Mix ground tablet in small amount of soft food (custard or applesauce.)	Large tablets can be difficult to swallow. Ground tablet mixed with palatable soft food is usually easier to swallow.

Critical Decision Point: Not all medications can be crushed (e.g., capsules, enteric-coated drugs). Consult with pharmacist when in doubt. Choking or aspiration of particles of medication or applesauce can also occur.

k. Prepare liquids:	
(1) Remove bottle cap from container and place cap upside down.	Prevents contamination of inside of cap.
(2) Hold bottle with label against palm of hand while pouring.	Spilled liquid will not soil or fade label.
(3) Hold medication cup at eye level and fill to desired level on scale (see illustration). Scale should be even with fluid level at its surface or base of meniscus, not edges.	Ensures accuracy of measurement.
(4) Discard any excess liquid into sink. Wipe lip and neck of bottle with paper towel.	Prevents contamination of bottle's contents and prevents bottle cap from sticking.
(5) Some liquid medications are in unit-dose containers. Draw up volumes of less than 10 ml in syringe without needle (see illustration).	
l. When preparing narcotics, check narcotic record for previous medication count and compare with supply available.	Controlled substance laws require careful monitoring of dispensed narcotics.
m. Check expiration date on all medications.	Medications used past expiration date may be inactive or harmful to client.
n. Compare MAR or computer printout with prepared medication and container.	Reading label second time reduces error.
o. Return stock containers or unused unit-dose medications to shelf or drawer and read label again.	Third check of label reduces administration errors.
p. Do not leave medications unattended.	Nurse is responsible for safekeeping of drugs.

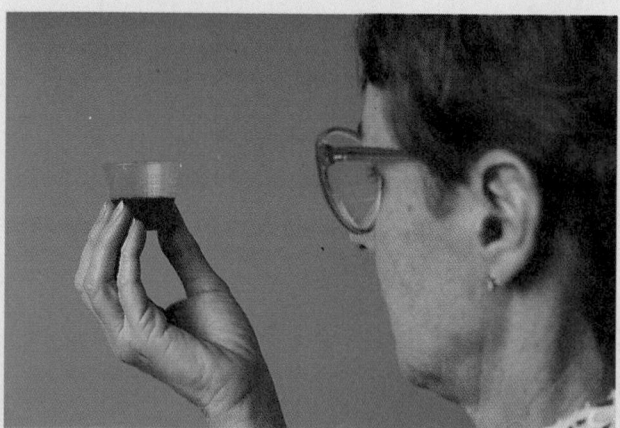

Step 7k(3)

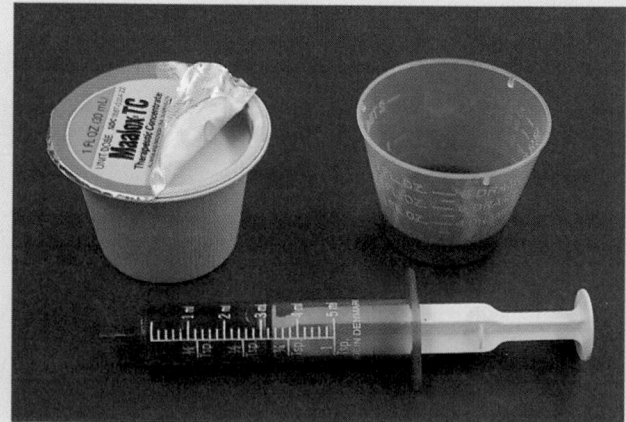

Step 7k(5)

STEPS	RATIONALE
8. Administering medications: a. Take medications to client at correct time.	Medications are administered within 30 minutes before or after prescribed time to ensure intended therapeutic effect. STAT or single-order medications should be given at time ordered.
b. Identify client by comparing name on MAR or computer printout with name on client's identification bracelet. Ask client to state name.	Identification bracelets are made at time of client's admission and are most reliable source of identification. Replace any missing or faded identification bracelets.
c. Explain purpose of each medication and its action to client. Allow client to ask any questions about drugs.	Client has right to be informed, and client's understanding of purpose of each medication improves compliance with medication therapy.
d. Assist client to sitting or side-lying position if sitting is contraindicated.	Sitting position prevents aspiration during swallowing.
e. Administer medications properly: (1) Client may wish to hold solid medications in hand or cup before placing in mouth.	Client can become familiar with medications by seeing each drug.
(2) Offer water or juice to help client swallow medications. Give cold carbonated water if available and not contraindicated.	Choice of fluid promotes client's comfort and can improve fluid intake. Carbonated water helps passage of tablet through esophagus.
(3) For sublingual-administered medications, have client place medication under tongue and allow it to dissolve completely. Caution client against swallowing tablet.	Medication is absorbed through blood vessels of undersurface of tongue. If swallowed, medication is destroyed by gastric juices or so rapidly detoxified by liver that therapeutic blood levels are not attained.
(4) For buccally administered drugs, have client place medication in mouth against mucous membranes of the cheek until it dissolves (see Figure 34-6, p. 895). Avoid administering liquids until buccal medication has dissolved.	Buccal medications act locally on mucosa or systemically as they are swallowed in saliva.
(5) Mix powdered medications with liquids at bedside and give to client to drink.	When prepared in advance, powdered medications may thicken and even harden, making swallowing difficult.
(6) Caution client against chewing or swallowing lozenges.	Medication acts through slow absorption through oral mucosa, not gastric mucosa.
(7) Give effervescent powders and tablets immediately after dissolving.	Effervescence improves unpleasant taste of medication and often relieves GI problems.
f. If client is unable to hold medications, place medication cup to the lips and gently introduce each drug into the mouth, one at a time. Do not rush.	Administering single tablet or capsule eases swallowing and decreases risk of aspiration.
g. If tablet or capsule falls to the floor, discard it and repeat preparation.	Medication is contaminated when it touches floor.
h. Stay until client has completely swallowed each medication. Ask client to open mouth if uncertain whether medication has been swallowed.	Nurse is responsible for ensuring that client receives ordered dosage. If left unattended, client may not take dose or may save medications, causing risk to health.
i. For highly acidic medications (e.g., aspirin), offer client nonfat snack (e.g., crackers) if not contraindicated by client's condition.	Reduces gastric irritation.
j. Assist client in returning to comfortable position.	Maintains client's comfort.
k. Dispose of soiled supplies and wash hands.	Reduces transmission of microorganisms.
9. Return within 30 minutes to evaluate client's response to medications.	Evaluates medication's therapeutic benefit and can detect onset of side effects or allergic reactions.
10. Ask client or family member to identify medication name and explain purpose, action, dosage schedule, and potential side effects of drug.	Determines level of knowledge gained by client and family.
11. Always notify prescriber when the client exhibits a toxic effect or allergic reaction, or with the onset of side effects. Withhold further doses.	Notification alerts prescriber to modify or discontinue medication.

Recording and Reporting
- Record administration of oral medications on MAR, placing nurse's initials or signature.
- Record the reason any drug is withheld and follow agency's policy for proper recording.

Home Care Considerations
- All clients should learn the basic guidelines for medication safety:
  - Keep each medication in its original, labeled container.
  - Be sure labels are legible.

- Discard any outdated medications.
- Always finish a prescribed medication unless otherwise instructed. Never save a medication for future illnesses.
- Dispose of medications by taking them to the pharmacy. Do not place drugs in the trash within reach of children.
- Do not give a family member a medication prescribed for another.
- Refrigerate medications that require it.
- Read labels carefully and follow all instructions.

swallowed and administered with approximately 60 to 100 ml of fluid (as allowed). There may, however, be situations that contraindicate the client's receiving medications by mouth. The primary contraindications to giving oral medications include the presence of gastrointestinal (GI) alterations, the inability of a client to swallow food or fluids, and the use of gastric suction. An important precaution to take when administering any oral preparation is to protect clients from aspiration. Aspiration occurs when food, fluid, or medication intended for gastrointestinal administration inadvertently is administered into the respiratory tract. The nurse protects the client from aspiration by assessing the client's ability to manage oral medications. Box 34-9 provides techniques the nurse can use to protect the client from aspirating. Properly positioning the client is also essential in preventing aspiration. The nurse positions the client in a seated position when administering oral medications, if not contraindicated by a client's condition. The lateral position can also be used when the client's swallow, gag, and cough are intact. A client who has difficulty swallowing should be evaluated by appropriate personnel (e.g., speech therapist) prior to receiving oral preparations.

For clients with nasogastric feeding tubes, liquid medications are preferred, but some tablets can be crushed and capsules opened to mix in a solution for administration (Box 34-10).

Topical Medication Applications

Topical medications are medications that are applied locally, most often to intact skin. They can be in the form of lotions, pastes, or ointments (Table 34-1). They can also be applied to mucous membranes.

SKIN APPLICATIONS

Because many locally applied medications such as lotions, pastes, and ointments can create systemic and local effects, the nurse should apply these medications using gloves and applicators. Sterile technique is used if the client has an open wound.

Skin encrustation and dead tissues harbor microorganisms and block contact of medications with the tissues to be treated. Simply applying new medications over previously applied medications does little to prevent infection or offer therapeutic benefit. Before applying medications, the nurse cleans the skin thoroughly by washing the area gently with soap and water, soaking an involved site, or locally debriding tissue.

Assessments to Protect the Client From Aspiration   Box 34-9

DETERMINE THE CLIENT'S ABILITY TO SWALLOW:
Ask the client to repeat certain sounds that require the same muscle movements as swallowing: "me-me-me" (for the lips); "la-la-la" (for the tongue); "ga-ga-ga" (for the soft palate and pharynx).

Assess the swallowing reflex by having the client slide the tongue backward along the palate.

Position your thumb and index finger on the client's larynx, and ask the client to swallow. Normally the larynx will elevate.

ASSESS THE CLIENT'S COUGH:
See Chapter 39 on proper techniques of coughing.

DETERMINE THE PRESENCE OF A GAG REFLEX:
Assess the gag reflex by stroking the posterior pharyngeal wall with a tongue blade. *Never check the gag reflex in a client who does not exhibit an intact cough or swallow reflex.* To protect the airway the client must have all three: a positive cough, gag, and swallow reflex.

Modified from Gauwitz DG: How to protect the dysphagic stroke patient, *Am J Nurs* 95:34, 1995.

Box 34-10
Guidelines for Giving Medications Through a Nasogastric Tube, J-Tube, G-Tube, or Small-Bore Feeding Tube

Administer medications in a liquid form (suspension, elixir, or solution) when possible to prevent tube obstruction.

Read medication labels carefully before crushing a tablet or opening a capsule.

Do *not* crush buccal or sublingual tablets. (Crushed medications may obstruct small-bore tube. Check agency policy.)

Do not crush enteric-coated or sustained-action medications.

Dissolve crushed tablets and powders in warm water.

Dissolve soft, gelatin capsules in warm water.

Irrigate the tube before and after all medication is given with 50-150 ml of water.

Do not use pigtail vent for irrigation or instillation of fluid.

Avoid giving syrups or medications with a pH of less than 4.

Do not attempt to give whole or undissolved medications.

When applying ointments or pastes, the nurse spreads the medication evenly over the involved surface and covers the area well without applying an overly thick layer. Opaque ointments prevent visualization of underlying skin. Prescribers may order a gauze dressing to be applied over the medication to prevent soiling of clothes and wiping away of the medication. Each type of medication, whether an ointment, lotion, powder, or other type, should be applied a specific way to ensure proper penetration and absorption. The nurse applies lotions and creams by smearing them lightly onto the skin's surface; rubbing may cause irritation. A liniment is applied by rubbing it gently but firmly into the skin. A powder is dusted lightly to cover the affected area with a thin layer. During any application the nurse should assess the skin thoroughly. To record administration, the area applied, name of medication, and condition of skin should be noted.

NASAL INSTILLATION

Clients with nasal sinus alterations may receive medications by spray, drops, or tampons (Skill 34-2). The most commonly administered form of nasal instillation is decongestant spray or drops, used to relieve symptoms of sinus congestion and colds. Clients must be cautioned to avoid abuse of medications because overuse can lead to a rebound effect in which the nasal congestion worsens. When excess decongestant solution is swallowed, serious systemic effects may also develop, especially in children. Saline drops are safer as a decongestant for children than nasal preparations that contain sympathomimetics (e.g., Afrin or Neo-Synephrine).

It is easier to have the client self-administer sprays, since the client can control the spray and inhale as it enters the nasal passages. For clients who use nasal sprays repeatedly, the nurse checks the nares for irritation. Nasal drops are effective in treating sinus infections. The nurse learns the proper way of positioning clients to permit the medication to reach the affected sinus. Severe nosebleeds are usually treated with packing or nasal tampons, which are treated with epinephrine, to reduce blood flow. Usually a physician or advanced practice clinician places nasal tampons.

EYE INSTILLATION

Common medications used by clients are eye drops and ointments, including over-the-counter preparations such as artificial tears and vasoconstrictors (e.g., Visine and Murine). However, many clients receive prescribed **ophthalmic** medications for eye conditions, such as glaucoma, and after cataract extraction. A large percentage of clients receiving eye medications are older adults. Age-related problems, including poor vision, hand tremors, and difficulty grasping or manipulating containers, affect the ease with which the older adult can self-administer eye medications. The nurse instructs clients and family members about the proper techniques for administering eye medications (Skill 34-3). The nurse may determine the client and family's ability to self-administer through a return demonstration of the procedure. Showing clients each step of the procedure for instilling eye drops can improve their compliance. The following principles can be followed when administering eye medications:

- The cornea of the eye is richly supplied with pain fibers and thus very sensitive to anything applied to it. Avoid instilling any form of eye medication directly onto the cornea.
- The risk of transmitting infection from one eye to the other is high. Avoid touching the eyelids or other eye structures with eye droppers or ointment tubes.
- Use eye medication only for the client's affected eye.
- Never allow a client to use another client's eye medications.

Intraocular Administration. Some medications are administered intraocularly. Medications delivered this way resemble a contact lens. The nurse places the medication into the conjunctival sac where it remains in place for up to 1 week. Currently medications such as pilocarpine are administered this way. Experiments are underway to evaluate administering other medications in this manner. The client receiving medications in this way requires teaching about monitoring for adverse reactions to the disk. Clients will also need to be taught how to insert and remove the

Text continued on p. 923.

Skill 34-2 Administering Nasal Instillations

Delegation Considerations

Administration of nasal drops and ointments requires problem solving and knowledge application unique to professional nurs-ing. For this procedure delegation to assistive personnel is not appropriate.

EQUIPMENT

- Prepared medication with clean dropper or spray container
- Facial tissue
- Small pillow (optional)
- Washcloth (optional)

- Disposable gloves (optional, only if client has extensive nasal drainage)
- MAR or computer printout
- Penlight (to inspect nares; if ointment is to be applied to a specific lesion inside the nares)

STEPS	RATIONALE
1. For nasal drops, determine which sinus is affected by referring to medical record.	Affects client's position during drug instillation.
2. Assess client's history of hypertension, heart disease, diabetes mellitus, and hyperthyroidism.	These conditions can contraindicate use of decongestants that stimulate central nervous system (CNS). Side effects of transient hypertension, tachycardia, palpitations, and headache may occur.
3. Identify client; compare name on MAR with client's ID bracelet. Ask client to state name.	Ensures that correct client receives medication.
4. Using a penlight, inspect condition of nose and sinuses. Palpate sinuses for tenderness.	Provides baseline to monitor effects of medication. Presence of discharge interferes with medication absorption.
5. Assess client's knowledge regarding use of nasal instillations and technique for instillation and willingness to learn self-administration.	May necessitate health teaching regarding use of medications. Motivation influences teaching approach.
6. Explain procedure to client regarding positioning and sensations to expect, such as burning or stinging of mucosa or choking sensation as medication trickles into throat.	Helps client anticipate experience of procedure to reduce anxiety.
7. Wash hands. Arrange supplies and medications at bedside.	Reduces transmission of microorganisms; ensures smooth, orderly procedure.
8. Instruct client to clear or blow nose gently unless contraindicated (e.g., risk of increased intracranial pressure or nosebleeds).	Removes mucus and secretions that can block distribution of medication.
9. Administer nasal drops:	
a. Assist client to supine position.	Position provides access to nasal passages.
b. Position head properly:	
(1) For access to posterior pharynx, tilt client's head backward.	
(2) For access to ethmoid or sphenoid sinus, tilt head back over edge of bed or place small pillow under client's shoulder and tilt head back (see illustration).	
(3) For access to frontal and maxillary sinus, tilt head back over edge of bed or pillow with head turned toward side to be treated (see illustration).	Position allows medication to drain into affected sinus.
c. Support client's head with nondominant hand.	Prevents straining of neck muscles.
d. Instruct client to breathe through mouth.	Mouth breathing reduces chance of aspirating nasal drops into trachea and lungs.
e. Hold dropper 1 cm (1/2 in) above nares and instill prescribed number of drops toward midline of ethmoid bone.	Avoids contamination of dropper. Instilling toward ethmoid bone facilitates distribution of medication over nasal mucosa.
f. Have client remain in supine position 5 min.	Prevents premature loss of medication through nares.
g. Offer facial tissue to blot runny nose, but caution client against blowing nose for several minutes.	Allows maximal amount of medication to be absorbed.

STEPS	RATIONALE
10. Assist client to a comfortable position after medication is absorbed.	Restores comfort.
11. Dispose of soiled supplies in proper container and wash hands.	Maintains neat, orderly environment. Reduces spread of microorganisms.
12. Observe client for onset of side effects 15 to 30 min after administration.	Drugs absorbed through mucosa can cause systemic reaction.
13. Ask if client is able to breathe through nose after decongestant administration. May be necessary to have client occlude one nostril at a time and breathe deeply.	Determines effectiveness of decongestant medication.
14. Reinspect condition of nasal passages between instillations.	Condition of mucosa reveals response to medication.
15. Ask client to review risks of overuse of decongestants and methods for administration.	Feedback ensures that client can self-administer medications properly.
16. Have client demonstrate self-medication.	Feedback demonstrates learning.

Recording and Reporting

- Record medication name, concentration, number of drops, nostril into which medication was instilled, and time of administration on MAR.
- Record client's response in nurses' notes.
- Report any unusual systemic effects to nurse in charge or physician.

Home Care Considerations

- Instruct client to expect timely resolution of problems. Instruct client on signs to observe of persistent or worsening problem. Clear nasal discharge indicates sinus problem. Yellow or greenish discharge indicates infection.
- Use OTC nasal sprays or nose drops for only one illness; bottles become easily contaminated with bacteria.
- Instruct clients that each family member should have a different dropper or spray applicator. Applicators should be washed or rinsed after each use.

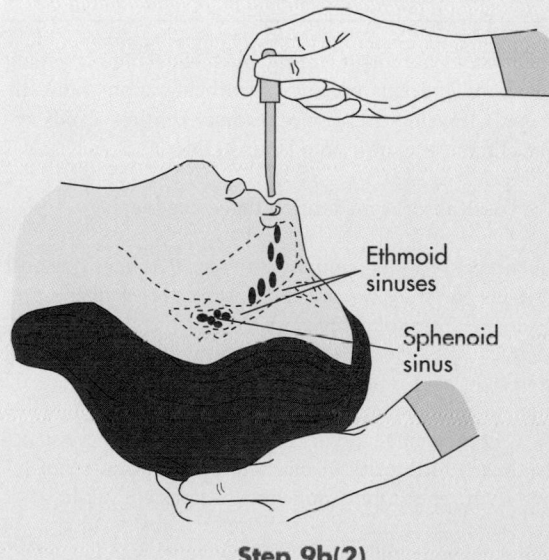

Ethmoid sinuses

Sphenoid sinus

Step 9b(2)

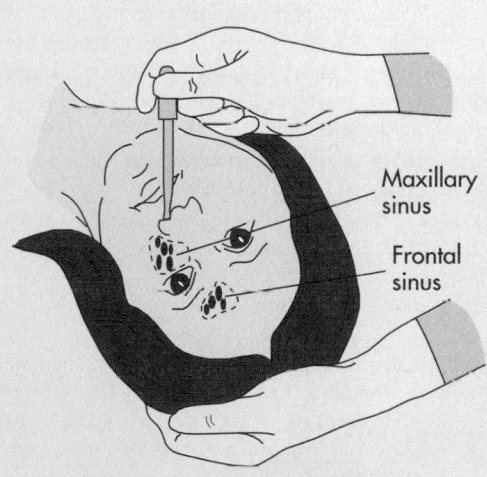

Maxillary sinus

Frontal sinus

Step 9b(3)

Skill 34-3 Administering Ophthalmic Medications

Delegation Considerations

Administration of eye drops and ointments requires problem solving and knowledge application unique to professional nurs-

ing. For this procedure delegation to assistive personnel is not appropriate.

EQUIPMENT
- Medication bottle with sterile eye dropper or ointment tube
- Medicated intraocular disk
- Cotton ball or tissue
- Washbasin filled with warm water and washcloth

- Eye patch and tape (optional)
- Disposable gloves
- MAR or computer printout

STEPS	RATIONALE
1. Review prescriber's medication order for number of drops (if a liquid) and eye (right = O.D.; left = O.S.; both = O.U.) to receive medication.	Ensures correct administration of medication.
2. Identify client. Compare name on MAR with client ID band. Ask client to state name.	Ensures that correct client receives medication.
3. Assess condition of external eye structures. (May also be done just before drug instillation.)	Provides baseline to later determine if local response to medications occurs. Also indicates need to clean eye before medication application.
4. Determine whether client has any known allergies to eye medications. Also ask if client has allergy to latex.	Protects client from risk of allergic medication response. Will require use of nonlatex gloves.
5. Determine whether client has any symptoms of visual alterations.	Certain eye medications act to either lessen or increase these symptoms. Nurse must be able to recognize change in client's condition.
6. Assess client's level of consciousness and ability to follow directions.	If client becomes restless or combative during procedure, a greater risk of accidental eye injury exists.
7. Assess client's knowledge regarding medication therapy and desire to self-administer medication.	Client's level of understanding may indicate need for health teaching. Motivation influences teaching approach.
8. Assess client's ability to manipulate and hold dropper.	Reflects client's ability to learn to self-administer medication.
9. Explain procedure to client.	Relieves anxiety about medication being instilled into eye.
10. Wash hands and arrange supplies at bedside; apply disposable gloves.	Reduces transmission of microorganisms; ensures a smooth, orderly procedure.
11. Ask client to lie supine or sit back in chair with head slightly hyperextended.	Position provides easy access to eye for medication instillation and minimizes drainage of medication through tear duct.

Critical Decision Point: Do not hyperextend the neck of a client with cervical spine injury.

12. If crusts or drainage are present along eyelid margins or inner canthus, gently wash away. Soak any crusts that are dried and difficult to remove by applying damp washcloth or cotton ball over eye for a few minutes. Always wipe clean from inner to outer canthus.	Crusts or drainage harbors microorganisms. Soaking allows easy removal and prevents pressure from being applied directly over eye. Cleansing from inner to outer canthus avoids entrance of microorganism into lacrimal duct.
13. Hold cotton ball or clean tissue in nondominant hand on client's cheekbone just below lower eyelid.	Cotton or tissue absorbs medication that escapes eye.
14. With tissue or cotton resting below lower lid, gently press downward with thumb or forefinger against bony orbit.	Technique exposes lower conjunctival sac. Retraction against bony orbit prevents pressure and trauma to eyeball and prevents fingers from touching eye.
15. Ask client to look at ceiling and explain steps to client.	Action retracts sensitive cornea up and away from conjunctival sac and reduces stimulation of blink reflex.
A. **Instill eye drops:**	
(1) With dominant hand resting on client's forehead, hold filled medication eye dropper or ophthalamic solution approximately 1 to 2 cm (½ to ¾ in) above conjunctival sac (see illustration).	Helps prevent accidental contact of eye dropper with eye structures, thus reducing risk of injury to eye and transfer of infection to dropper. Ophthalmic medications are sterile.

STEPS	RATIONALE
(2) Drop prescribed number of medication drops into conjunctival sac.	Conjunctival sac normally holds 1 or 2 drops. Provides even distribution of medication across eye.
(3) If client blinks or closes eye or if drops land on outer lid margins, repeat procedure.	Therapeutic effect of drug is obtained only when drops enter conjunctival sac.
(4) After instilling drops, ask client to close eye gently.	Helps to distribute medication. Squinting or squeezing of eyelids forces medication from conjunctival sac.
(5) When administering medications that cause systemic effects, apply gentle pressure with your finger and clean tissue on the client's naso-lacrimal duct for 30 to 60 sec.	Prevents overflow of medication into nasal and pharyngeal passages. Prevents absorption into systemic circulation.
B. **Instill eye ointment:**	
(1) Holding ointment applicator above lower lid margin, apply thin stream of ointment evenly along inner edge of lower eyelid on conjunctiva (see illustration) from the inner canthus to outer canthus.	Distributes medication evenly across eye and lid margin.
(2) Have client close eye and rub lid lightly in circular motion with cotton ball, if rubbing is not contraindicated.	Further distributes medication without traumatizing eye.

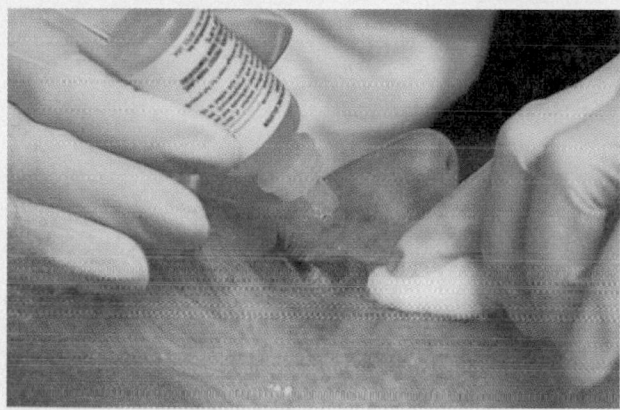

Step 15A(1)

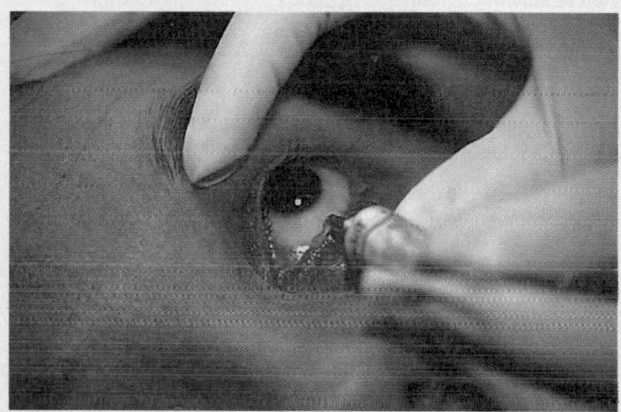

Step 15B(1)

C. **Intraocular disk**	
(1) Application:	
a. Open package containing the disk. Gently press your fingertip against the disk so that it adheres to your finger. Position the convex side of the disk on your fingertip (see illustration).	Allows nurse to inspect disk for damage or deformity.
b. With your other hand, gently pull the client's lower eyelid away from the eye. Ask client to look up.	Prepares conjunctival sac for receiving medicated disk.
c. Place the disk in the conjunctival sac, so that it floats on the sclera between the iris and lower eyelid (see illustration).	Ensures delivery of medication.
d. Pull the client's lower eyelid out and over the disk (see illustration).	Ensures accurate medication delivery.

Critical Decision Point: You should not be able to see the disk at this time. Repeat Step 15C(1)d if you can see the disk.

STEPS   **RATIONALE**

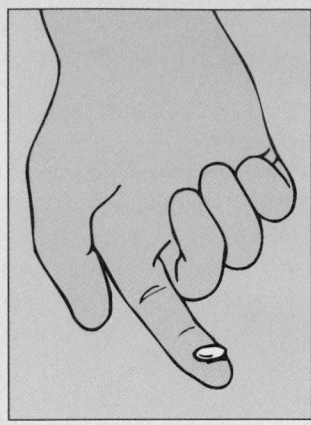   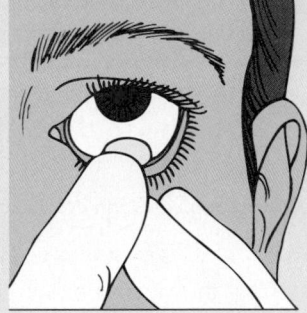   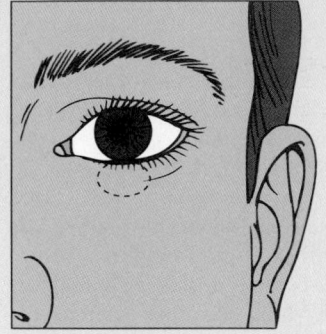   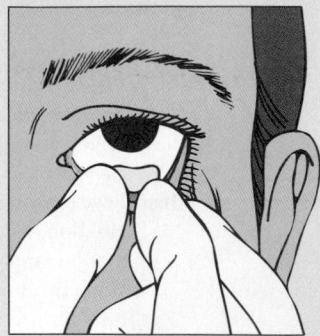

    Step 15C(1)a   Step 15C(1)c   Step 15C(1)d   Step 15C(2)d

(2) Removal:
    a. Wash hands and apply gloves.
    b. Explain procedure to client.
    c. Gently pull on the client's lower eyelid to expose the disk.
    d. Using your forefinger and thumb of your opposite hand, pinch the disk and lift it out of the client's eye (see illustration).

16. If excess medication is on eyelid, gently wipe it from inner to outer canthus.   Promotes comfort and prevents trauma to eye.

17. If client had eye patch, apply clean one by placing it over affected eye so entire eye is covered. Tape securely without applying pressure to eye.   Clean eye patch reduces chance of infection.

18. Remove gloves, dispose of soiled supplies in proper receptacle, and wash hands.   Maintains neat environment at bedside and reduces transmission of microorganisms.

19. Note client's response to instillation; ask if any discomfort was felt.   Determines if procedure was performed correctly and safely.

20. Observe response to medication by assessing visual changes and noting any side effects.   Evaluates effects of medication.

21. Ask client to discuss medication's purpose, action, side effects, and technique of administration.   Determines client's level of understanding.

22. Have client demonstrate self-administration of next dose.   Provides feedback regarding competency with skill.

Recording and Reporting
- Record medication, concentration, number of drops, time of administration, and eye (left, right, or both) that received medication on MAR.
- Record appearance of eye in nurses' notes.

Home Care Considerations
- If eye drops are stored in refrigerator, rewarm to room temperature before administering.
- Many clients lack confidence in their ability to instill drops without supervision. The nurse teaches others, such as a family member, to instill drops into the client's eye.

disk. Skill 34-3 reviews the steps the nurse uses for administering an intraocular disk.

EAR INSTILLATION

Internal ear structures are very sensitive to temperature extremes. Failure to instill ear drops or irrigating fluid at room temperature may cause vertigo (severe dizziness) or nausea. Although the structures of the outer ear are not sterile, it is wise to use sterile drops and solutions in case the eardrum is ruptured. The entrance of nonsterile solutions into middle ear structures could result in infection. With ear drainage, the nurse should assess to be sure the client does not have a ruptured eardrum. A nurse should never occlude the ear canal with the dropper or irrigating syringe. Forcing medication into an occluded ear canal creates pressure that may injure the eardrum. Box 34-11 reviews guidelines for administering ear drops.

External ear structures of children differ from those of adults. When instilling drops or irrigating solutions, the nurse must straighten the ear canal. In infants and young children the nurse straightens the cartilaginous canal by grasping the auricle of the ear and pulling it gently down and backward. In adults the ear canal is longer and composed of underlying bone and is straightened by pulling the auricle upward and outward. Failure to straighten the canal properly may prevent medicinal solutions from reaching the deeper external ear structures.

VAGINAL INSTILLATION

Vaginal medications are available as suppositories, foam, jellies, or creams. Suppositories come individually packaged in foil wrappers. Storage in a refrigerator prevents the solid, oval-shaped suppositories from melting. After a suppository is inserted into the vaginal cavity, body temperature causes it to melt and be distributed and absorbed. Foam, jellies, and creams are administered with an applicator inserter (Skill 34-4). A suppository is given with a gloved hand in accordance with standard precautions (see Chapter 33). Clients often prefer administering their own vaginal medications and should be given privacy. After instillation of the medication, a client may wish to wear a perineal pad to collect drainage. Because vaginal medications are often given to treat infection, discharge may be foul smelling. Aseptic technique should be followed, and the client should be offered frequent opportunities to maintain perineal hygiene (see Chapter 38).

RECTAL INSTILLATION

Rectal suppositories are thinner and more bullet shaped than vaginal suppositories. The rounded end prevents anal trauma during insertion. Rectal suppositories contain medications that exert local effects such as promoting defecation or systemic effects such as reducing nausea. Rectal suppositories are stored in the refrigerator until administered.

Procedural Guidelines for Administering Ear Medications   Box 34-11

EAR DROPS

1. Have client assume side-lying position (if not contraindicated by client's condition) with ear to be treated facing up, or client may sit in chair or at the bedside.
2. Straighten ear canal by pulling auricle down and back (children) or upward and outward (adult).
3. Instill prescribed drops holding dropper 1 cm (½ in) above ear canal (see illustration).
4. Ask client to remain in side-lying position 2 to 3 min. Apply gentle massage or pressure to tragus of ear with finger unless contraindicated due to pain.
5. At times the prescriber orders insertion of portion of cotton ball into outermost part of canal. Do not press cotton into canal. Remove cotton after 15 min.

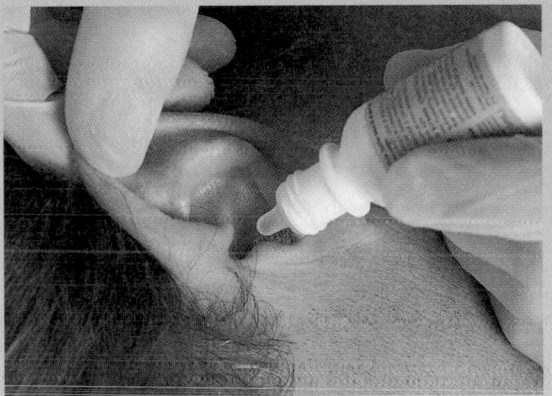

EAR IRRIGATIONS

1. Assess the tympanic membrane or review medical record for history of eardrum perforation, which would contraindicate ear irrigation.
2. Assist client to assume sitting or lying position with head tilted or turned toward affected ear. Place towel under client's head and shoulder and have client hold basin under affected ear.
3. Fill irrigating syringe with solution (approximately 50 ml).
4. Gently grasp auricle and straighten ear canal by pulling it down and back (children) or upward and outward (adult).
5. Slowly instill irrigating solution by holding tip of syringe 1 cm (½ in) above opening of ear canal. Allow fluid to drain out during instillation. Continue until canal is cleansed or all solution is used.

During administration, the nurse must place the suppository past the internal anal sphincter and against the rectal mucosa (Skill 34-5). Otherwise the suppository may be expelled before it can dissolve and be absorbed into the mucosa. With practice a nurse learns to recognize the sensation of the sphincter relaxing around the finger. The

Text continued on p. 927.

Skill 34-4 Administering Vaginal Medications

Delegation Considerations

Administering medications by the vaginal route requires problem solving and knowledge application unique to professional nursing. For this procedure delegation to assistive personnel is not appropriate.

EQUIPMENT

- Vaginal creams, foam, jelly, or suppositories, or irrigating solutions
- Applicators
- Disposable gloves
- Tissues
- Paper towel
- Perineal pad
- Drape
- Water-soluble lubricants
- Bedpan
- Irrigation or douche container
- MAR or computer printout

STEPS	RATIONALE
1. Review physician's order, including client's name, medication name, form (cream or suppository), route, dosage, and time of administration.	Ensures safe and correct administration of medication.
2. Wash hands.	Reduces transfer of microorganisms.

Critical Decision Point: Rectal and vaginal suppositories may be stored near one another in the refrigerator. Vaginal suppositories are larger and more oval.

STEPS	RATIONALE
3. Identify client; compare name on MAR with identification bracelet and asking name.	Ensures that correct client receives medication.
4. Inspect condition of external genitalia and vaginal canal (see Chapter 32).	Findings provide baseline to monitor effect of medication.
5. Assess client's ability to manipulate applicator or suppository and to position self to insert medication.	Mobility restriction indicates level of assistance required from nurse.
6. Explain procedure to client. Be specific if client plans to self-administer medication.	Promotes understanding. Will enable client to self-administer medication if physically able.
7. Arrange supplies at bedside.	Ensures smooth procedure.
8. Close room curtain or door.	Provides privacy.
9. Assist client to lie in dorsal recumbent position.	Provides easy access to and good exposure of vaginal canal. Also allows suppository to dissolve without escaping through orifice.
10. Keep abdomen and lower extremities draped.	Minimizes embarrassment.
11. Apply disposable gloves.	Prevents transmission of microorganisms between nurse and client.
12. Be sure vaginal orifice is well illuminated by room light or gooseneck lamp.	Proper insertion requires visualization of external genitalia.
13. Insert suppository with gloved hand:	
a. Remove suppository from foil wrapper and apply liberal amount of petroleum jelly to smooth or rounded end. Lubricate gloved index finger of dominant hand.	Lubrication reduces friction against mucosal surfaces during insertion.
b. With nondominant gloved hand, gently retract labial folds.	Exposes vaginal orifice.
c. Insert rounded end of suppository along posterior wall of vaginal canal entire length of finger (7.5 to 10 cm or 3 to 4 in) (see the illustration).	Proper placement ensures equal distribution of medication along walls of vaginal cavity.
d. Withdraw finger and wipe away remaining lubricant from around orifice and labia.	Maintains comfort.

STEPS	RATIONALE
14. Apply cream or foam: a. Fill cream or foam applicator following package directions.	Dose is prescribed by volume in applicator.
b. With nondominant gloved hand, gently retract labial folds.	Exposes vaginal orifice.
c. With dominant gloved hand, insert applicator approximately 5 to 7.5 cm (2 to 3 in). Push applicator plunger to deposit medication into vagina (see illustration).	Allows equal distribution of medication along vaginal walls.
d. Withdraw applicator and place on paper towel. Wipe off residual cream from labia or vaginal orifice.	Residual cream on applicator may contain microorganisms.
15. Remove gloves by pulling them inside out and discard in appropriate receptacle. Wash hands.	Reduces transfer of microorganisms.
16. Instruct client to remain on back for at least 10 min.	Medication will be distributed and absorbed evenly throughout vaginal cavity and not be lost through orifice.
17. If applicator is used, wash with soap and warm water, rinse, and store for future use.	Vaginal cavity is not sterile. Soap and water assist in removal of bacteria and residual cream.
18. Offer client perineal pad when she resumes ambulation.	Prevents vaginal discharge from spreading to clothing.
19. Inspect appearance of discharge of vaginal canal and condition of external genitalia between applications.	Evaluates whether vaginal medication effectively reduced irritation or inflammation of tissues.

Recording and Reporting

- Record medication name, dose, route, and time of administration on MAR.
- Record character of discharge on nurses' notes.

Home Care Considerations

- Suppositories should be kept refrigerated but in a container away from children.

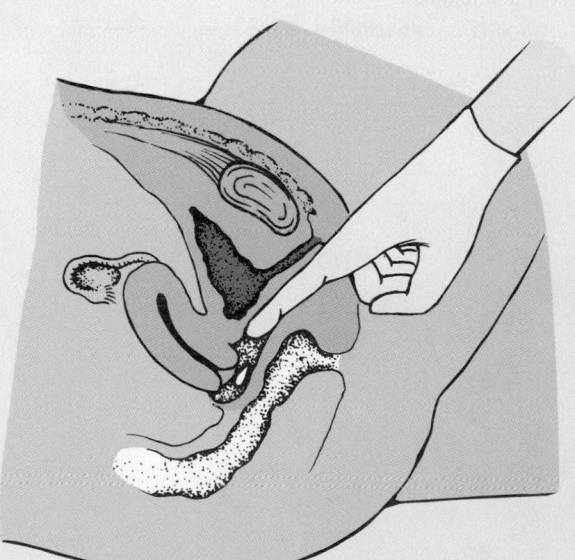

Step 13c

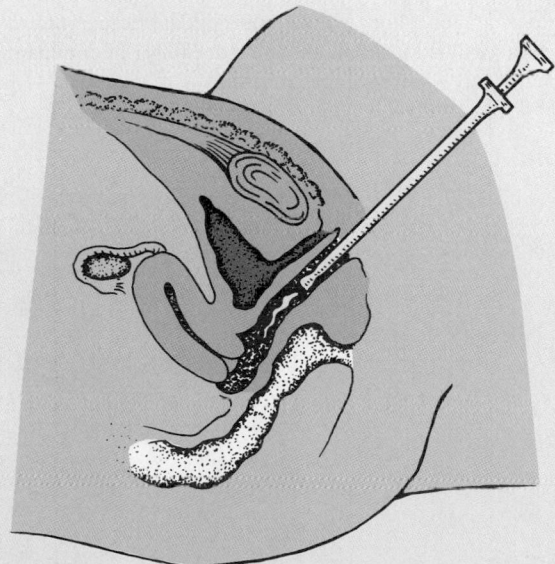

Step 14c

Skill 34-5   Administering Rectal Suppositories

Delegation Considerations

Administering medications by the rectal route requires problem solving and knowledge application unique to professional nurs-

ing. For this procedure delegation to assistive personnel is not appropriate.

EQUIPMENT
- Rectal suppository
- Lubricating jelly (water soluble)
- Disposable gloves

- Tissue
- Drape
- MAR or computer printout

STEPS	RATIONALE
1. Review prescriber's order, including client's name, medication name, form, route, and time of administration.	Ensures safe and correct administration of medication.
2. Review medical record for rectal surgery or bleeding.	Conditions contraindicate use of suppository.
3. Wash hands.	Reduces transfer of microorganisms.
4. Apply disposable gloves.	Prevents contact with infected fecal material.
5. Identify client; check name on MAR with client's identification bracelet and ask client's name.	Ensures that correct client receives medication.
6. Explain procedure. Be specific if client wishes to self-administer medication.	Promotes understanding and cooperation. Will enable client to self-administer medication if physically able.
7. Arrange supplies at bedside.	Ensures smooth procedure.
8. Close room curtain or door.	Maintains privacy and minimizes embarrassment.
9. Assist client in assuming Sims' position. Keep client draped with only anal area exposed.	Exposes anus and helps client relax external anal sphincter. Maintains privacy and facilitates relaxation.
10. Examine condition of anus externally and palpate rectal walls as needed (see Chapter 32). If gloves become soiled, dispose of them by turning them inside out and placing them in proper receptacle.	Determines presence of active rectal bleeding. Palpation determines whether rectum is filled with feces, which may interfere with suppository placement. Reduces transmission of infection.

Critical Decision Point: Generally, rectal suppository is contraindicated in the presence of active rectal bleeding. Unless suppository is for constipation, placing medication in a rectum filled with feces may be poorly absorbed or prematurely expelled with defecation.

11. Apply disposable gloves (if previous gloves were discarded).	Minimizes contact with fecal material and reduces transmission of microorganisms.
12. Remove suppository from wrapper and lubricate rounded end (see illustration). Lubricate index finger of dominant hand with a water-soluble lubricant.	Lubrication reduces friction as suppository enters rectal canal.

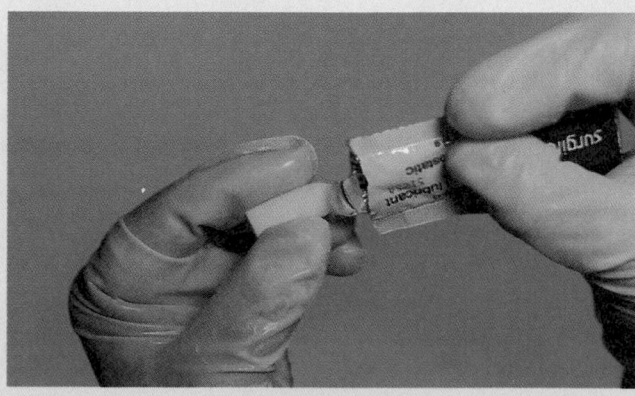

Step 12

STEPS	RATIONALE
13. Ask client to take slow deep breaths through mouth and relax anal sphincter.	Forcing suppository through constricted sphincter causes pain.
14. Retract buttocks with nondominant hand. Insert suppository gently through anus, past internal sphincter and against rectal wall, 10 cm (4 in) in adults, 5 cm (2 in) in children and infants. May need to apply gentle pressure to hold buttocks together momentarily.	Suppository must be placed against rectal mucosa for eventual absorption and therapeutic action.
15. Withdraw finger and wipe anal area with tissue.	Provides comfort.
16. Discard gloves by turning them inside out, and dispose of them in appropriate receptacle.	Reduces transfer of microorganisms.
17. Ask client to remain flat or on side for 5 min.	Prevents expulsion of suppository.
18. If suppository contains laxative or fecal softener, place call light within reach.	Provides client with sense of control over elimination. Allows client to obtain assistance to bedpan or toilet.
19. Wash hands.	Reduces risk of transfer of infection.
20. Return within 5 min to determine whether suppository was expelled.	Reinsertion may be necessary.
21. Observe for effects of suppository (e.g., bowel movement, relief of nausea) 30 min after administration.	Evaluates effectiveness of medication and relief of client's symptoms.

Recording and Reporting
- Report occurrence of rectal bleeding to physician.

suppository should not be forced into a mass of fecal material. It may be necessary to clear the rectum with a small cleansing enema before a suppository can be inserted.

Administering Medications by Inhalation

Medications administered with handheld inhalers are dispersed through an aerosol spray, mist, or powder that penetrates lung airways. The alveolocapillary network absorbs medications rapidly. **Metered-dose inhalers (MDIs)** are usually designed to produce local effects such as bronchodilatation. However, some medications can create serious systemic side effects.

Clients who receive medications by inhalation frequently suffer chronic respiratory disease such as chronic asthma, emphysema, or bronchitis. Medications given by inhalation provide these clients with control of airway obstruction, and because these clients depend on medications for disease control, they must learn about them and ways to administer them safely (Skill 34-6).

A metered-dose inhaler delivers a measured dose of medication with each push of a canister. Approximately 5 to 10 pounds of pressure must be used to activate the aerosol. This is important for the nurse to know because hand strength diminishes with age and from the effects of chronic respiratory disease. The nurse evaluates whether clients have enough hand strength to use the MDI appropriately (Skill 34-6).

Administering Medications by Irrigations

Medications may be used to irrigate or wash out a body cavity and are delivered through a stream of solution. Irrigations most commonly use sterile water, saline, or antiseptic solutions on the eye, ear, throat, vagina, and urinary tract. If there is a break in the skin or mucosa, the nurse uses aseptic technique. When the cavity to be irrigated is not sterile, as in the case of the ear canal (see Box 34-11) or vagina, clean technique is acceptable. In health care settings, however, use sterile solutions. Irrigations can cleanse an area, instill a medication, or apply hot or cold to injured tissue.

Parenteral Administration of Medications

Parenteral administration of medications is the administration of medications by injection. When medications are administered this way, it is an invasive procedure that must be performed using aseptic techniques (Box 34-12). After a needle pierces the skin, there is risk of infection. Each type of injection requires certain skills to ensure that the medication reaches the proper location. The effects of a parenterally administered medication can develop rapidly, depending on the rate of medication absorption. The nurse closely observes the client's response.

Skill 34-6   Using Metered-Dose Inhalers

Delegation Considerations

Administering MDI and supervising clients who self-administer MDIs require problem solving and knowledge application unique to professional nursing. Delegation to assistive personnel is not appropriate.

EQUIPMENT

- MDI with medication canister
- Aerochamber (optional)
- Facial tissues (optional)

- Washbasin or sink with warm water
- Paper towel
- MAR or computer printout

STEPS	RATIONALE
1. Review prescriber's order, including client's name, medication name, number of inhalations.	Ensures safe and correct administration of medication.
2. Identify client, compare name on MAR with client's ID bracelet, and ask client's name.	Ensures that correct client receives medication.
3. Assess client's ability to hold, manipulate, and depress canister and inhaler.	Any impairment of grasp or presence of hand tremors interferes with client's ability to depress canister within inhaler.
4. Assess client's readiness to learn: client asks questions about medication, disease, or complications; requests education in use of inhaler; is mentally alert; participates in own care.	Affects client's ability to understand explanations and actively participate in teaching process.
5. Assess client's ability to learn: client should not be fatigued, in pain, or in respiratory distress; assess level of understanding of technical vocabulary terms.	Mental or physical limitations affect client's ability to learn and methods nurse uses for instruction.
6. Assess client's knowledge and understanding of disease and purpose and action of prescribed medications.	Knowledge of disease is essential for client to realistically understand use of inhaler.
7. Assess medication schedule and number of inhalations prescribed for each dose.	Influences explanations nurse provides for use of inhaler.
8. If previously instructed in self-administration of inhaled medicine, assess client's technique in using an inhaler.	Nurse's instruction may require only simple reinforcement, depending on client's level of dexterity.
9. Instruct client in comfortable environment by sitting in chair in hospital room or sitting at kitchen table in home.	Client will be more likely to remain receptive of nurse's explanations.
10. Provide adequate time for teaching session.	Prevents interruptions. Instruction should occur when client is receptive.
11. Wash hands and arrange equipment needed.	Reduces transfer of microorganisms and saves time.
12. Allow client opportunity to manipulate inhaler, canister, and spacer device. Explain and demonstrate how canister fits into inhaler.	Client must be familiar with how to use equipment.
13. Explain what metered dose is, and warn client about overuse of inhaler, including medication side effects.	Client must not arbitrarily administer excessive inhalations because of risk of serious side effects. If medication is given in recommended doses, side effects are uncommon.
14. Explain steps for administering inhaled dose of medication (demonstrate steps when possible):	Use of simple, step-by-step explanations allows client to ask questions at any point during procedure.
a. Remove mouthpiece cover from inhaler.	
b. Shake inhaler well.	Ensures fine particles are aerosolized.
c. Have client take a deep breath and exhale.	Prepares the client's airway to receive the medication.
d. Instruct the client to position the inhaler in one of two ways.	
(1) Open lips and place inhaler in mouth with opening toward back of throat (see illustration).	
(2) Position the device 1 to 2 in from the mouth (see illustration).	Directs aerosol spray toward airway. Positioning the mouthpiece 1 to 2 in from the mouth is considered the best way to deliver the medication.
e. With the inhaler properly positioned, have client hold inhaler with thumb at the mouthpiece and the index finger and middle finger at the top. This is called a three-point or lateral hand position.	MDIs work best when clients use a three-point or lateral hand position to activate canisters (Statz, 1984).

STEPS	RATIONALE
f. Instruct client to tilt head back slightly, inhale slowly and deeply through mouth, and depress medication canister fully.	Medication is distributed to airways during inhalation. Inhalation through mouth rather than nose draws medication more effectively into airways.
g. Hold breath for approximately 10 sec.	Allows tiny drops of aerosol spray to reach deeper branches of airways.
h. Exhale through pursed lips.	Keeps small airways open during exhalation.
15. Explain steps to administer inhaled dose of medication using a spacer such as an Aerochamber (demonstrate when possible):	
a. Remove mouthpiece cover from MDI and mouthpiece of Aerochamber.	Inhaler fits into end of Aerochamber.
b. Insert MDI into end of Aerochamber.	Aerochamber is a spacer that traps medication released from the MDI; the client then inhales the drug from the device. These devices deposit up to 80% more medication in the lungs rather than in the oropharynx (Weixler, 1994).
c. Shake inhaler well.	Ensures fine particles are aerosolized.
d. Place Aerochamber mouthpiece in mouth and close lips. Do not insert beyond raised lip on mouthpiece. Avoid covering small exhalation slots with the lips (see illustration).	Medication should not escape through mouth.
e. Breathe normally through Aerochamber mouthpiece.	Allows client to relax before delivering medication.
f. Depress medication canister, spraying one puff into Aerochamber.	Emits spray that allows finer particles to be inhaled. Large droplets are retained in Aerochamber.
g. Breathe in slowly and fully (for 5 sec).	Ensures particles of medication are distributed to deeper airways.
h. Hold full breath for 5 to 10 sec.	Ensures full medication distribution.
16. Instruct client to wait 2 to 5 min between inhalations or as ordered by prescriber.	Medications must be inhaled sequentially. First inhalation opens airways and reduces inflammation. Second or third inhalation penetrates deeper airways.
17. Instruct client against repeating inhalations before next scheduled dose.	Medications are prescribed at intervals during day to provide constant drug levels and minimize side effects. Beta-adrenergic MDIs are used either on an "as needed" basis or regularly every 4 to 6 hr.
18. Explain that client may feel gagging sensation in throat caused by droplets of medication on pharynx or tongue.	Results when inhalant is sprayed and inhaled incorrectly.
19. Instruct client in removing medication canister and cleaning inhaler in warm water.	Accumulation of spray around mouthpiece can interfere with proper distribution during use.
20. Ask if client has any questions.	Clarifies misconceptions or misunderstanding.

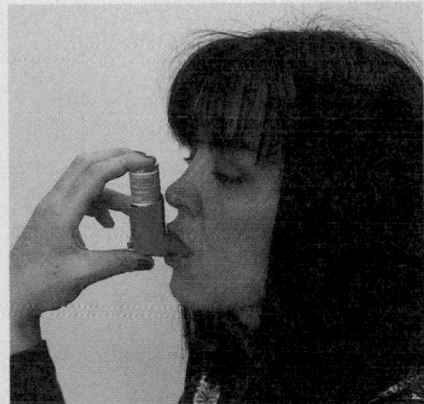

Step 14d(1)

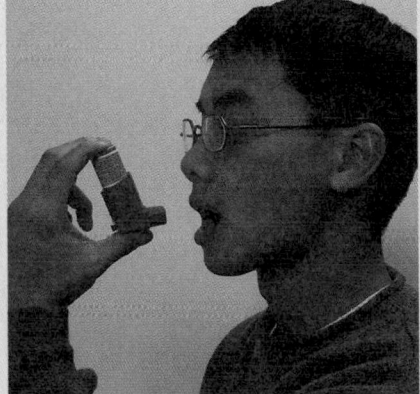

Step 14d(2)

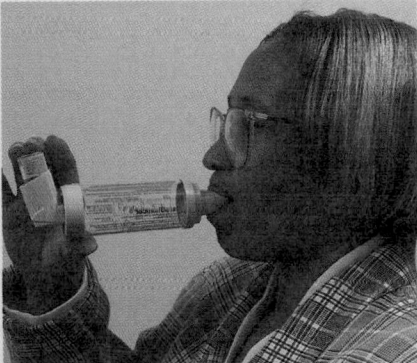

Step 15d

STEPS	RATIONALE
21. Have client explain and demonstrate steps in use of inhaler.	Return demonstration provides feedback for measuring client's learning.
22. Ask client to explain medication schedule.	Improves likelihood of compliance with therapy.
23. Ask client to describe side effects of medication and criteria for calling prescriber.	Will allow client to recognize signs of overuse and need to seek medical support when medications are ineffective.
24. After medication instillation, assess client's respirations and auscultate lungs.	Determines status of breathing pattern and adequacy of ventilation.

Recording and Reporting

- Document in nurses' notes what skills were taught and client's ability to perform skills.
- Record time when client used MDI (amount of puffs).
- Report any undesirable effects from medication.

Home Care Considerations

- Teach clients how to determine fullness of canisters, using displacement in water (see illustration).

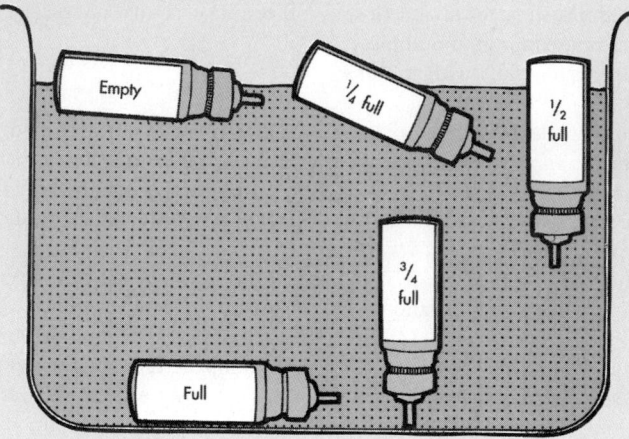

EQUIPMENT

A variety of syringes and needles are available, each designed to deliver a certain volume of a medication to a specific type of tissue. The nurse uses judgment when determining the syringe or needle that will be most effective.

Syringes.   Syringes consist of a cylindrical barrel with a tip designed to fit the hub of a hypodermic needle and a close-fitting plunger. Syringes, in general, are classified as being Luer-lok or non-Luer-lok. This nomenclature is based on the design of the syringe's tip. Luer-lok syringes (Figure 34-15, *A*) require special needles, which are twisted onto the tip and lock themselves in place. This design prevents the inadvertent removal of the needle. Non-Luer-lok syringes (Figure 34-15, *B-D*) require needles that slip onto the tip. Most health care institutions use disposable, single-use plastic syringes, which are inexpensive and easy to manipulate.

Preventing Infection During an Injection
Box 34-12

To prevent contamination of solution, draw medication from ampule quickly. Do not allow it to stand open.

To prevent needle contamination, avoid letting needle touch contaminated surface (e.g., outer edges of ampule or vial, outer surface of needle cap, nurse's hands, countertop, table surface).

To prevent syringe contamination, avoid touching length of plunger or inner part of barrel. Keep tip of syringe covered with cap or needle.

To prepare skin, wash skin soiled with dirt, drainage, or feces with soap and water and dry. Use friction and a circular motion while cleaning with an antiseptic swab. Swab from center of site, and move outward in a 2-inch radius.

The nurse fills a syringe by aspiration, pulling the plunger outward while the needle tip remains immersed in the prepared solution. The nurse may handle the outside of the syringe barrel and the handle of the plunger. To maintain sterility, the nurse avoids letting any unsterile object touch the tip or inside of the barrel, the hub, the shaft of the plunger, or the needle (Figure 34-16).

Syringes come in a number of sizes, from 0.5 to 60 ml. It is unusual to use a syringe larger than 5 ml for an SQ or IM injection. A 2- to 3-ml syringe is usually adequate. A larger volume creates discomfort. The nurse uses large syringes to administer certain intravenous medications, add medications to intravenous solutions, and irrigate wounds or drainage tubes. A 2.5- or 3-ml hypodermic syringe often comes prepackaged with a needle attached. However, the nurse may change needle sizes. The hypodermic has two scales along the barrel; one is divided into minims and the other into tenths of a milliliter.

Insulin syringes (see Figure 34-15, C and D) are available in sizes that hold 0.3 to 1 ml and are calibrated in units. Each milliliter of solution contains 100 units of insulin. Insulin syringes that hold 0.3 ml are known as low-dose syringes (30 units per 0.3 ml). Most insulin syringes are U-100s, designed for use with U-100 strength insulin.

The tuberculin syringe (see Figure 34-15, B) has a long, thin barrel with a pre-attached thin needle. The syringe is calibrated in sixteenths of a minim and hundredths of a milliliter and has a capacity of 1 ml. The nurse uses a tuberculin syringe to prepare small amounts of medications. A tuberculin syringe is also useful when preparing small precise doses for infants or young children.

Needles.
Needles come packaged in individual sheaths to allow flexibility in choosing the right needle for a client. Some needles are preattached to standard-sized syringes. Most needles are made of stainless steel and are disposable.

The needle has three parts: the hub, which fits onto the tip of a syringe; the shaft, which connects to the hub; and the bevel, or slanted tip (see Figure 34-16). The tip of a needle or the bevel is always slanted. The bevel creates a narrow slit when injected into tissue and quickly closes when the needle is removed to prevent leakage of medication, blood, or serum. A short beveled tip is best for intravenous injections because it is not easily occluded against the inside of a blood vessel wall. Long beveled tips are sharper and narrower, which minimizes discomfort when entering tissue used for subcutaneous or intramuscular injections.

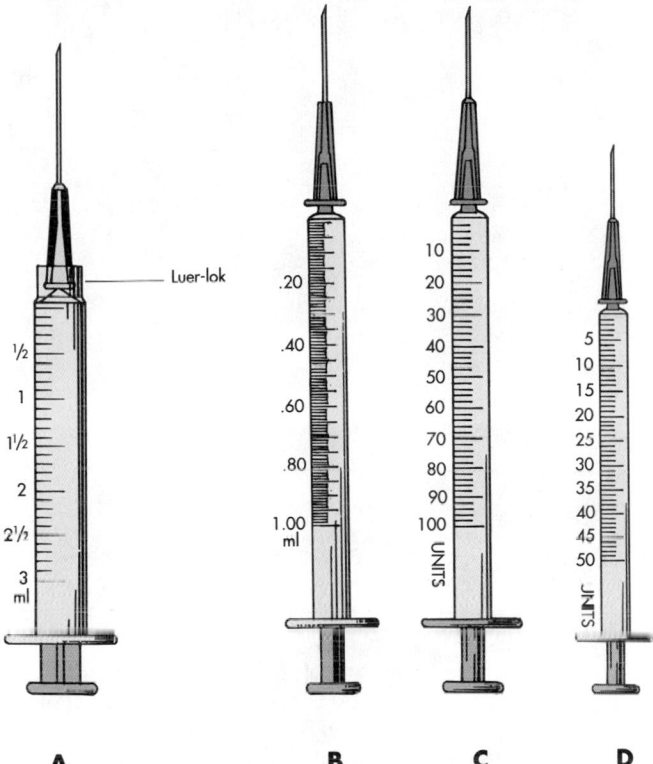

A   **B**   **C**   **D**

Figure 34-15 Types of syringes. **A,** Luer-lok syringe marked in 0.1 (tenths). **B,** Tuberculin syringe marked in 0.01 (hundredths) for doses of less than 1 ml. **C,** Insulin syringe marked in units (100). **D,** Insulin syringe marked in units (50).

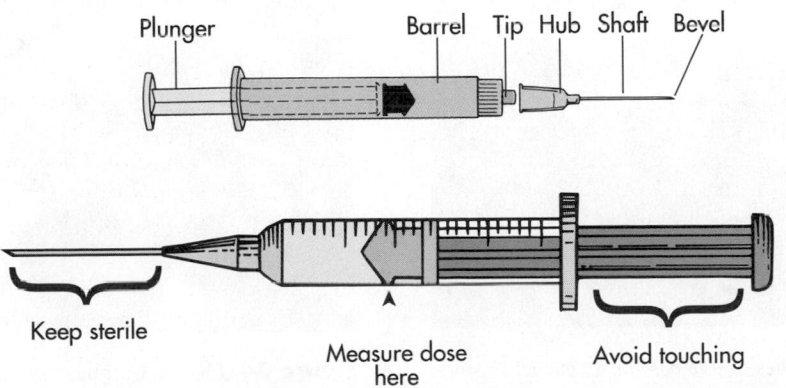

Figure 34-16 Parts of a syringe.

Needles vary in length from ¼ to 3 inches (Figure 34-17). The nurse chooses the needle length according to the client's size and weight and the type of tissue into which the medication is to be injected. A child or slender adult generally requires a shorter needle. The nurse uses longer needles (1 to 1½ inches) for intramuscular injections and a shorter needle (⅜ to ⅝ inch) for subcutaneous injections.

The smaller the needle gauge, the larger the needle diameter (see Figure 34-17). The selection of a gauge depends on the viscosity of fluid to be injected or infused. An intramuscular injection usually requires a 19- to 23-gauge needle, depending on the viscosity of the medication. Subcutaneous injections require smaller-diameter needles such as a 25-gauge needle. A 26-gauge needle is used for an intradermal injection.

Disposable Injection Units.
Disposable, single-dose, prefilled syringes are available for some medications. The nurse must be careful to check the medication and concentration because all prefilled syringes appear very similar. With these syringes the nurse does not have to prepare medication doses, except perhaps to expel portions of unneeded medications.

The Tubex and Carpuject injection systems include reusable plastic mechanisms that hold prefilled, disposable, sterile cartridge-needle units (Figure 34-18). The nurse slips the cartridge into the syringe, secures it (following package directions), and checks for air bubbles in the syringe. The nurse advances the plunger to expel excess medication as in a regular syringe. A new type of injection system involves screwing a plungerlike device into the end of a prefilled vial containing a needle. After the medication is given the entire unit is disposed of in a receptacle. This design reduces the risk of needle-stick injuries.

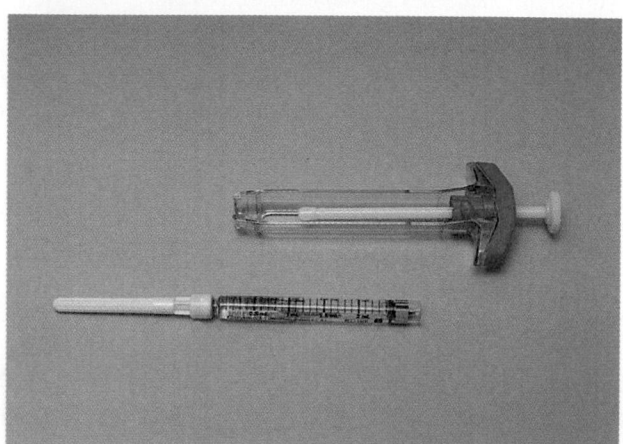

A

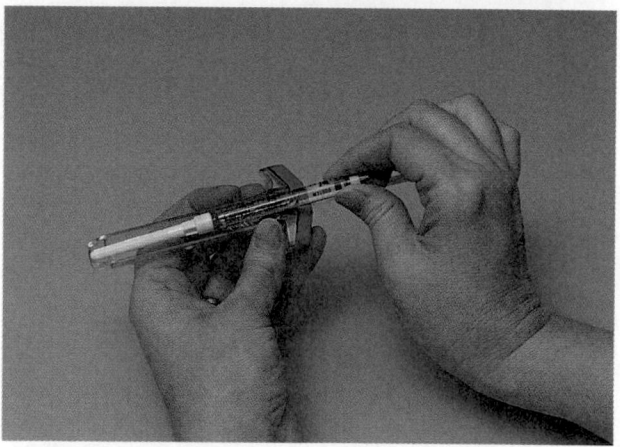

B

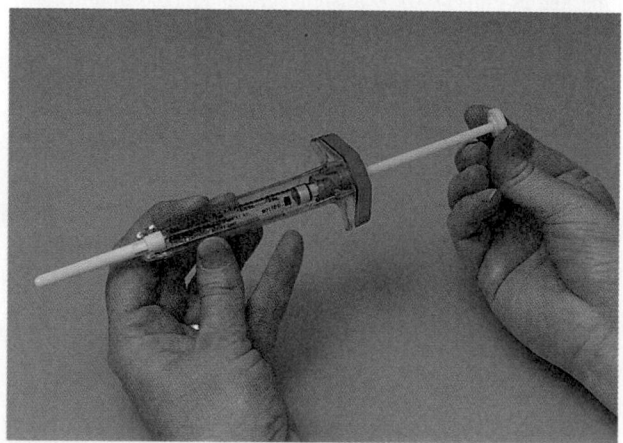

C

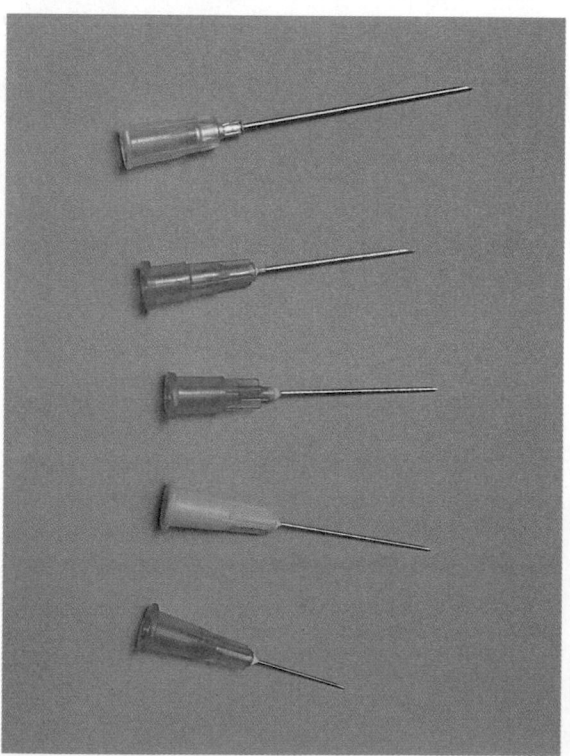

Figure 34-17   Needles. *Top to bottom:* 19 gauge, 1½-inch length; 20 gauge, 1-inch length; 21 gauge, 1-inch length; 23 gauge, 1-inch length; and 25 gauge, ⅝-inch length.

Figure 34-18   **A,** Carpuject syringe and prefilled sterile cartridge with needle. **B,** Assembling the Carpuject. **C,** Cartridge locks at needle end; plunger screws into opposite end.

PREPARING AN INJECTION FROM AN AMPULE

Ampules contain single doses of medication in a liquid. Ampules arc available in several sizes, from 1 ml to 10 ml or more (Figure 34-19, *A*). An ampule is made of glass with a constricted neck that must be snapped off to allow access to the medication. A colored ring around the neck indicates where the ampule is prescored to be broken easily. Aspiration of the medication into a syringe occurs easily (Skill 34-7) and may be completed with a filter needle (if required by institutional policy).

PREPARING AN INJECTION FROM A VIAL

A vial is a single-dose or multidose container with a rubber seal at the top (see Figure 34-19, *B*). A metal cap protects the seal until it is ready for use (see Box 34-13). Vials contain liquid or dry forms of medications. Medications that are unstable in solution are packaged dry. The vial label specifies the solvent or diluent used to dissolve the medication and the amount of diluent needed to prepare a desired medication concentration. Normal saline and sterile distilled water are solutions commonly used to dissolve medications.

Unlike the ampule, the vial is a closed system, and air must be injected into it to permit easy withdrawal of the

Text continued on p. 937.

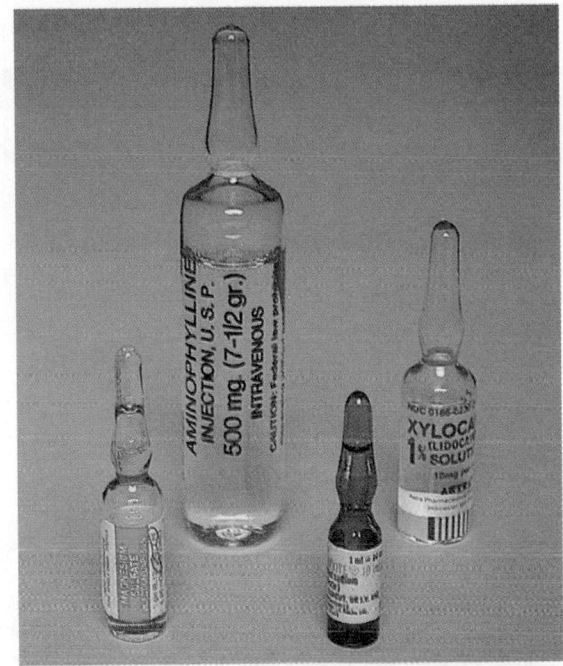

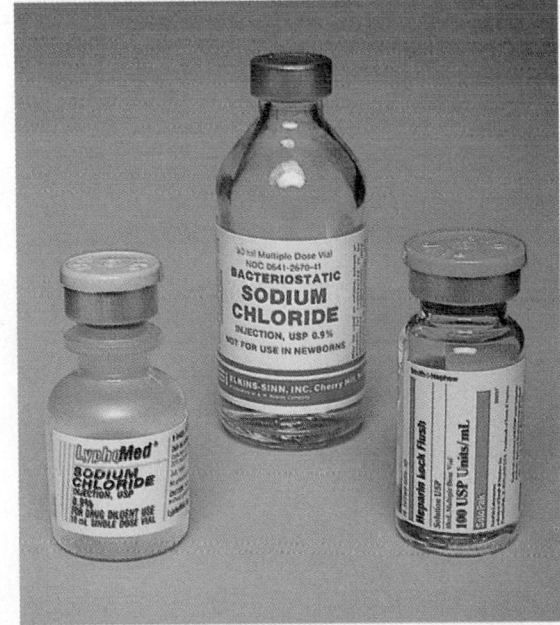

Figure 34-19   **A,** Medication in ampules. **B,** Medication in vials.

| *Research* HIGHLIGHT | Box 34-13 |

RESEARCH ABSTRACT

The purpose of this study was to determine the necessity of alcohol disinfection of the rubber stopper after removing the cap on a single-dose vial and to compare the efficacy of different methods of stopper disinfection before needle penetration on the multiple-dose vials. Controversy exists about whether disinfection of the rubber stopper is necessary before initial needle aspiration of fluid from single-dose vials. The researchers surveyed nurses and found variability in whether they disinfected the stopper of single-dose vials before needle aspiration. On multiple-dose vials, two disinfection techniques arc used before needle penetration. These methods include swabbing the stopper with alcohol only or with povidone-iodine and alcohol. The researchers cultured 5 rubber stoppers of single-dose vials from 20 plastic-wrapped packages (n = 100). They also cultured 87 multiple-dose vials that had been previously opened and had been routinely used. Of the single dose vials 99% of the vial stopper surfaces were sterile. One culture returned positive, and this was thought to be due to air contamination during the culturing procedure. Of the multiple-dose vials using povidone-iodine and alcohol, 95% of the vials were sterile. Of the multiple-dose vials using the alcohol-only technique, all 100 of the surface cultures were sterile. The authors concluded that it is unnecessary to wipe the stopper surface of a single-dose vial after removing the cap. For multiple-dose vials the authors concluded that alcohol swab before disinfection is sufficient.

IMPLICATIONS FOR PRACTICE

• This time-honored nursing practice has been passed on without scientific justification. This study provides a scientific rationale for this procedure.

• Although the savings realized by the change in procedure may be minimal, all levels of practice must be examined for their potential benefit.

REFERENCE

Buckley T, Dudley S, Donowitz L: Defining unnecessary disinfection procedures for single-dose and multiple dose vials, *Am J Crit Care* 3(6):448, 1994.

Skill 34-7　Preparing Injections

Delegation Considerations

Preparing injections from ampules and vials requires problem solving and knowledge application unique to professional nursing. For this procedure delegation to assistive personnel is not appropriate.

EQUIPMENT

- **Medication in an ampule**
  - Syringe and two needles (filter needle optional)
  - Small gauze pad or alcohol swab
- **Medication in a vial**
  - Syringe and two needles (filter needle optional)

- Small gauze pad or alcohol swab
- Diluent (e.g., normal saline or sterile water) (optional)
- **Both**
  - MAR or computer printout

STEPS	RATIONALE
SRs **1.** Review order, including name and medication name, dose, route of administration, and time of administration.	Ensures correct administration of medication.
2. Review pertinent information related to medication, including action, purpose, side effects, and nursing implications.	Allows nurse to administer medication properly and to monitor client's response.
3. Check date of expiration for medication vial or ampule.	Medication potency may increase or decrease when outdated.
4. Assess client's body build, muscle size, and weight.	Determines type and size of syringe and needles for injection.
5. Wash hands.	Reduces transmission of microorganisms.
6. Prepare medication.	
A.　**Ampule preparation**	
(1)　Tap top of ampule lightly and quickly with finger until fluid moves from neck of ampule (see illustration).	Dislodges any fluid that collects above neck of ampule. All solution moves into lower chamber.
(2)　Place small gauze pad around neck of ampule.	Placing pad around neck of ampule protects nurse's fingers from trauma as glass tip is broken off.
(3)　Snap neck of ampule quickly and firmly away from hands (see illustration).	Protects nurse's fingers and face from shattering glass.
(4)　Draw up medication quickly.	System is open to airborne contaminants.
(5)　Hold ampule upside down, or set it on a flat surface. Insert syringe or filter needle (see agency policy) into center of ampule opening. Do not allow needle tip or shaft to touch rim of ampule.	Broken rim of ampule is considered contaminated. When ampule is inverted, solution does dribble out if needle tip or shaft touches rim of ampule.

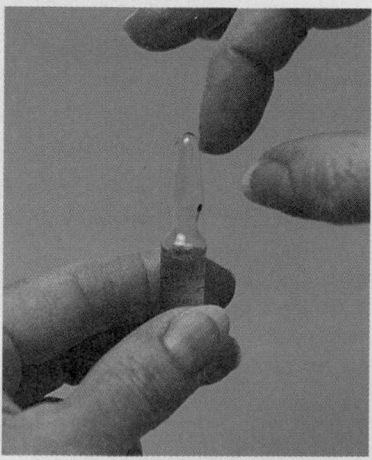

Step 6A(1)

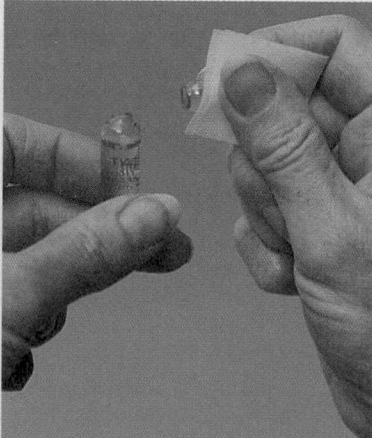

Step 6A(3)

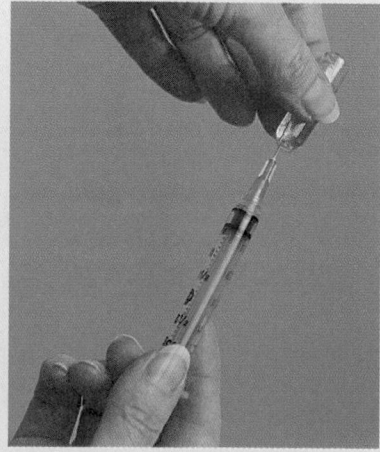

Step 6A(6)

(6) Aspirate medication into syringe by gently pulling back on plunger (see illustration).

Withdrawal of plunger creates negative pressure within syringe barrel, which pulls fluid into syringe.

(7) Keep needle tip under surface of liquid. Tip ampule to bring all fluid within reach of the needle.

Prevents aspiration of air bubbles.

(8) If air bubbles are aspirated, do not expel air into ampule.

Air pressure may force fluid out of ampule and medication will be lost.

(9) To expel excess air bubbles, remove needle from ampule. Hold syringe with needle pointing up. Tap side of syringe to cause bubbles to rise toward needle. Draw back slightly on plunger, and then push plunger upward to eject air. Do not eject fluid.

Withdrawing plunger too far will remove it from barrel. Holding syringe vertically allows fluid to settle in bottom of barrel. Pulling back on plunger allows fluid within needle to enter barrel so fluid is not expelled. Air at top of barrel and within needle is then expelled.

(10) If syringe contains excess fluid, use sink for disposal. Hold syringe vertically with needle tip up and slanted slightly toward sink. Slowly eject excess fluid into sink. Recheck fluid level in syringe by holding it vertically.

Medication is safely dispersed into sink. Position of needle allows medication to be expelled without flowing down needle shaft. Rechecking fluid level ensures proper dose.

(11) Cover needle with its safety sheath or cap. Change needle on syringe or use filter needle if you suspect medication is on needle shaft.

Prevents contamination of needle. New needle prevents tracking medication through skin and SQ tissues.

B. **Vial containing a solution**

(1) Remove cap covering top of unused vial to expose sterile rubber seal, keeping rubber seal sterile. If a multidose vial that has been used before is being used again, firmly and briskly wipe surface of rubber seal with alcohol swab and allow it to dry.

Vial comes packaged with cap to prevent contamination of rubber seal. Cap cannot be replaced after seal removal. Allowing alcohol to dry prevents needle from being coated with alcohol and mixing with medication.

(2) Pick up syringe and remove needle cap. Pull back on plunger to draw amount of air into syringe equivalent to volume of medication to be aspirated from vial.

Air must first be injected into vial to prevent buildup of negative pressure in vial when aspirating medication.

(3) With vial on flat surface, insert tip of needle with beveled tip entering first through center of rubber seal (see illustration). Apply pressure to tip of needle during insertion.

Center of seal is thinner and easier to penetrate. Injecting beveled tip first and using firm pressure prevent coring of rubber seal, which could enter vial or needle.

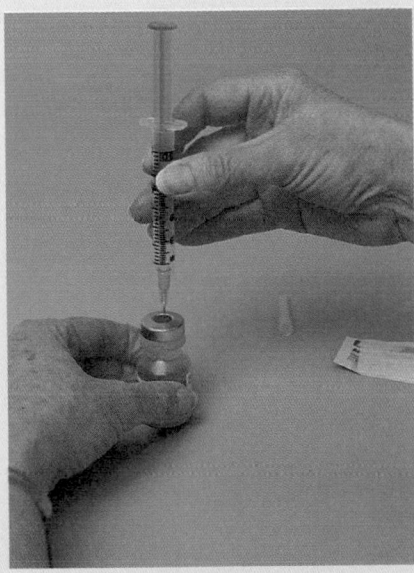

Step 6B(3)

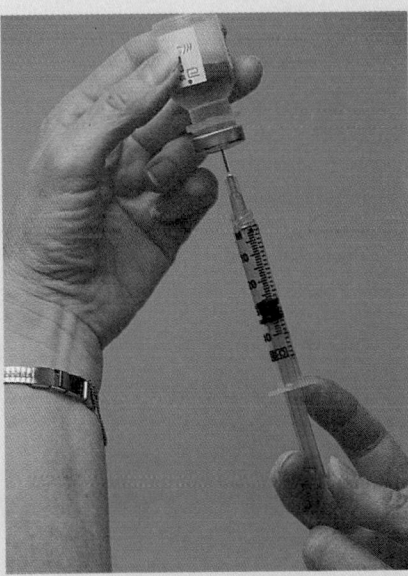

Step 6B(5)

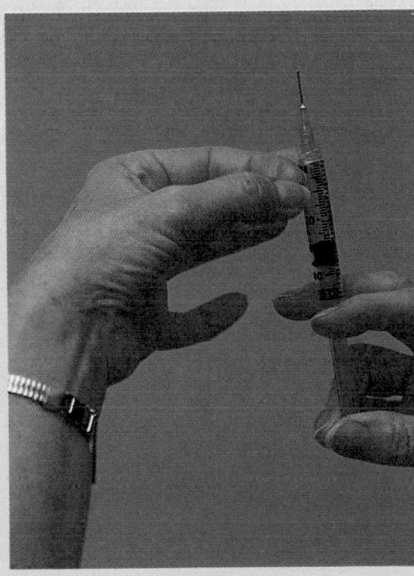

Step 6B(10)

STEPS	RATIONALE
(4) Inject air into the vial's airspace, holding on to plunger. Hold plunger with firm pressure; plunger may be forced backward by air pressure within the vial.	Air must be injected before aspirating fluid. Injecting into vial's airspace prevents formation of bubbles and inaccuracy in dose.
(5) Invert vial while keeping firm hold on syringe and plunger (see illustration). Hold vial between thumb and middle fingers of nondominant hand. Grasp end of syringe barrel and plunger with thumb and forefinger of dominant hand to counteract pressure in vial.	Inverting vial allows fluid to settle in lower half of container. Position of hands prevents forceful movement of plunger and permits easy manipulation of syringe.
(6) Keep tip of needle below fluid level.	Prevents aspiration of air.
(7) Allow air pressure from the vial to fill syringe gradually with medication. If necessary, pull back slightly on plunger to obtain correct amount of solution.	Positive pressure within vial forces fluid into syringe (unless vial has been used several times).
(8) When desired volume has been obtained, position needle into vial's airspace; tap side of syringe barrel carefully to dislodge any air bubbles. Eject any air remaining at top of syringe into vial.	Forcefully striking barrel while needle is inserted in vial may bend needle. Accumulation of air displaces medication and causes dose errors.
(9) Remove needle from vial by pulling back on barrel of syringe.	Pulling plunger rather than barrel causes plunger to separate from barrel, resulting in loss of medication.
(10) Hold syringe at eye level, at 90-degree angle, to ensure correct volume and absence of air bubbles. Remove any remaining air by tapping barrel to dislodge any air bubbles (see illustration, p. 934). Draw back slightly on plunger; then push plunger upward to eject air. Do not eject fluid.	Holding syringe vertically allows fluid to settle in bottom of barrel. Pulling back on plunger allows fluid within needle to enter barrel so fluid is not expelled. Air at top of barrel and within needle is then expelled.
(11) If medication is to be injected into client's tissue, change needle to appropriate gauge and length according to route of medication.	Inserting needle through a rubber stopper may dull beveled tip. New needle is sharper. Because no fluid is along shaft, needle will not track medication through tissues.
(12) For multidose vial, make label that includes date of mixing, concentration of medication per milliliter, and nurse's initials.	Ensures that future doses will be prepared correctly. Some medications must be discarded after certain number of days after mixing of vial.
C. **Vial containing a powder (reconstituting medications)**	
(1) Remove cap covering vial of powdered medication and cap covering vial of proper diluent.	Cap prevents contamination of rubber seal.
(2) Draw up diluent into syringe following Steps 5B(2) through 5B(10).	Prepares diluent for injection into vial containing powdered medication.
(3) Insert tip of needle through center of rubber seal of vial of powdered medication. Inject diluent into vial. Remove needle.	Diluent begins to dissolve and reconstitute medication.
(4) Mix medication thoroughly. Roll in palms. Do not shake.	Ensures proper dispersal of medication throughout solution. Shaking produces bubbles.
(5) Reconstituted medication in vial is ready to be drawn into new syringe. Read label carefully to determine dose after reconstitution.	Once diluent has been added, concentration of medication (mg/ml) determines dose to be given.
7. Dispose of soiled supplies. Place broken ampule and/or used vials and used needle in puncture-proof and leakproof container. Clean work area and wash hands.	Proper disposal of glass and needle prevents accidental injury to staff. Controls transmission of infection.

solution. Failure to inject air when withdrawing creates a vacuum within the vial that makes withdrawal difficult (see Skill 34-7).

To prepare a powdered medication, the nurse draws up the amount of diluent or solvent recommended on the vial's label. The nurse injects the diluent into the vial in the same manner as injecting air into the vial. Most powdered medications dissolve easily, but it may be necessary to withdraw the needle to mix the contents thoroughly. Gently rolling the vial between the hands will dissolve the powdered medication. The needle is reinserted to draw up the dissolved medication. After mixing multidose vials the nurse makes a label that includes the date and time of mixing and the concentration of medication per milliliter. Multidose vials may require refrigeration after the contents are reconstituted.

MIXING MEDICATIONS

If two medications are compatible, it is possible to mix them in one injection if the total dose is within accepted limits. A client will not have to receive more than one injec-tion at a time. Most nursing units have charts that list common compatible medications. If there is any uncertainty about medication compatibilities, consult a pharmacist.

Mixing Medications From Two Vials.   The nurse applies these principles when mixing medications from two vials:

Do not contaminate one medication with another.
Ensure the final dose is accurate.
Maintain aseptic technique.

Only one syringe is needed to mix medications from two vials (Figure 34-20). The nurse takes a syringe with a needle attached and aspirates the volume of air equivalent to the first medication's dose (vial A). The nurse injects the air into vial A, making sure the needle does not touch the solution. The nurse withdraws the needle, aspirates air equivalent to the second medication's dose (vial B), and then injects the volume of air into vial B. The nurse immediately withdraws the medication from vial B into the syringe. At this point the medication from vial A has not contaminated vial B. The nurse applies a new sterile nee-

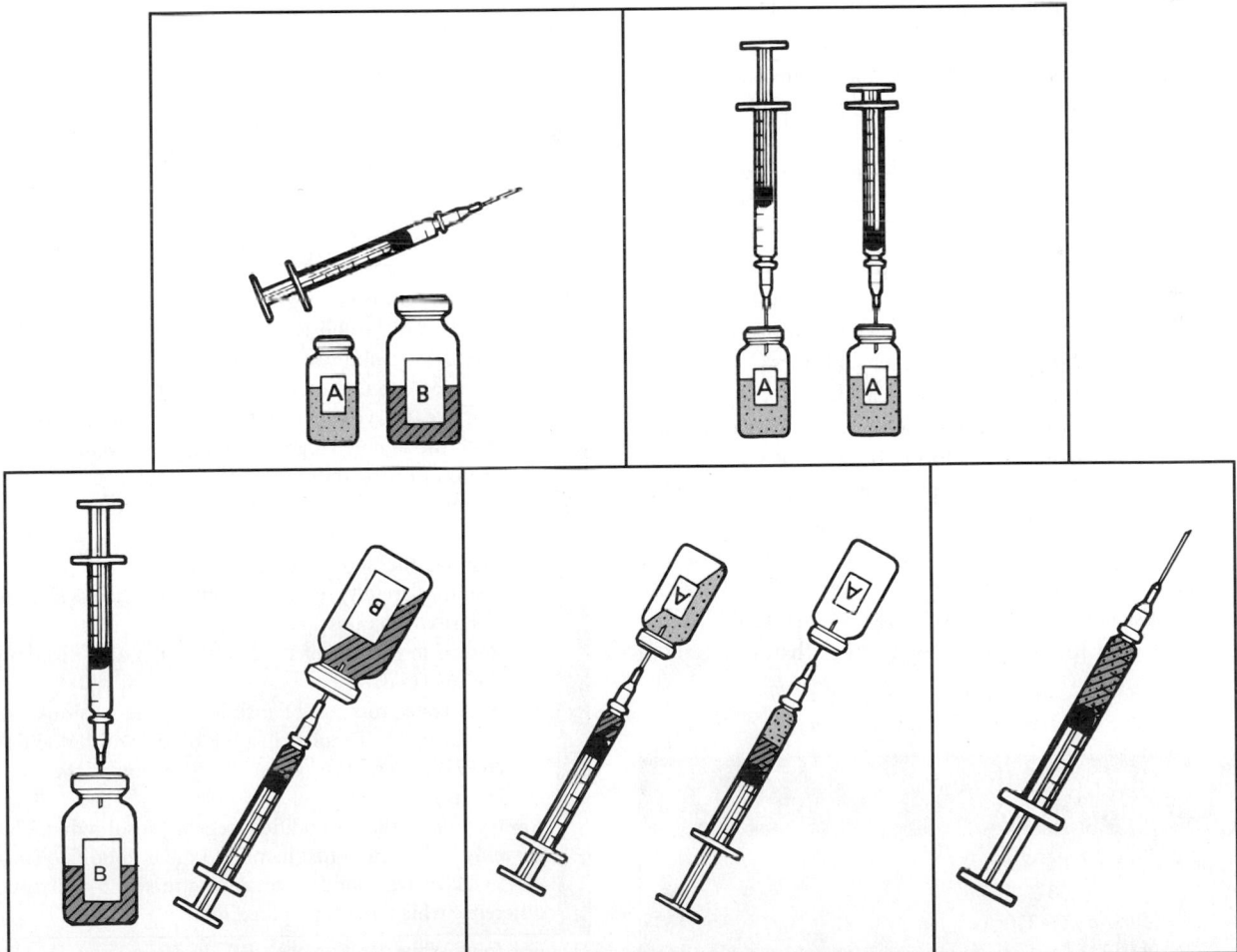

Figure 34-20   Steps in mixing medications from two vials.

dle to the syringe and inserts it into vial A, being careful not to push the plunger and expel the medication within the syringe into the vial. The nurse then withdraws the desired amount of medication from vial A into the syringe. If a vial has excess positive pressure, the plunger may move before the nurse is ready, causing an accidental withdrawal of too much of the medication. After withdrawing the necessary amount, the nurse withdraws the needle and applies a new needle.

Mixing Medications From One Vial and One Ampule.
Mixing medications from a vial and an ampule is simple because it is not necessary to add air to withdraw medication from an ampule. The nurse prepares medication from the vial first and then, using the same syringe and needle, withdraws medication from the ampule. This technique prevents contamination of the solution in the vial and the needle.

INSULIN PREPARATION
Insulin is the hormone used to treat diabetes. It must be administered by injection because it is a protein and therefore would be broken down and destroyed in the gastrointestinal tract. Most clients with diabetes requiring insulin learn to self-administer injections. In the United States and Canada, the medication is available in 100 units (U) per milliliter of solution. When preparing insulin, the correct syringe must be used. A 100-unit scaled syringe is used to prepare 100-unit insulin.

Insulin is classified by rate of action, including rapid, intermediate, and long acting. Each type has a different onset, peak, and duration of action. A client with diabetes may require more than one type of insulin. For example, by receiving a rapid-acting (regular) and an intermediate-acting (NPH) insulin, a client receives more sustained control of blood glucose levels over 24 hours.

Regular insulin is a clear solution that acts rapidly and can be given either subcutaneously or intravenously. Other types of insulin are cloudy because of the addition of a protein, which slows absorption. These slower-acting insulins can be given only subcutaneously.

Insulin is ordered by specific dose at select times or by a sliding scale. A sliding scale dictates a certain dose based on the client's blood glucose level (Box 34-14). Only regular insulin is used for sliding scales. If more than one type of

insulin is required to manage the client's diabetes, the nurse can mix two different types of insulin into one syringe (Box 34-15) using the steps demonstrated in Figure 34-20. This minimizes the discomfort to the client associated with multiple injections. The mixing of insulins, however, is rarely performed today because stable premixed insulins (70% NPH and 30% regular or 50% of each) are available.

Before withdrawing insulin from a vial, the vial should be rotated at least 1 minute between both hands. This resuspends the modified insulin preparations and helps to warm the medication. The nurse should not shake insulin vials. Shaking causes bubbles to form, which take up space and alters the dose.

ADMINISTERING INJECTIONS
Each injection route is unique in regard to the type of tissues into which the medication is injected. The character-

Text continued on p. 942.

Box 34-15   Procedural Guidelines

For Mixing Two Kinds of Insulin in One Syringe

1. Lente insulins (Semilente, Lente, Ultralente) may be mixed with each other, in any ratio.
2. Regular insulin may be mixed with any ratio.
3. Mixing of regular and Lente insulin is not recommended except for clients already adequately controlled on such a mixture. This is caused by the binding of Lente insulin with regular insulin, delaying onset of action.

To prepare insulin from two vials, the nurse or client follows these steps:

1. With an insulin syringe and needle, inject air, equal to the dose of insulin to be withdrawn, into the vial of modified insulin (cloudy vial). Do not touch the tip of the needle to the solution.
2. Remove the syringe from the vial of modified insulin.
3. With the same syringe, inject air, equal to the dose of insulin to be withdrawn, into the vial of unmodified (regular) insulin (clear vial). Then withdraw the correct dose.
4. Remove the syringe from the unmodified (regular) insulin. Carefully remove air bubbles in the syringe to ensure correct dose.
5. Return to the vial of modified insulin and withdraw the correct dose.
6. Administer mixture of insulins within 5 minutes of preparing it. Regular insulin binds with modified (NPH) insulin, thus reducing the action of the regular insulin.

Always prepare the unmodified (regular) insulin first. This prevents adding modified insulin to the unmodified (regular) vial. If two modified forms are mixed, it makes no difference which vial is prepared first.

Modified from White JR, Campbell RK. In Haire-Joshu D, editor: *Management of diabetes mellitus: perspectives of care across the life span*, ed 2, St. Louis, 1996, Mosby.

Example of Sliding Scale Insulin Order   Box 34-14

Give regular insulin SQ:
2 U for glucose 200-240
4 U for glucose 241-250
6 U for glucose 251-300
For glucose ≥300, call physician

Administering Injections | Skill 34-8

Delegation Considerations
Administering injections requires problem solving and knowledge application unique to professional nursing. For this procedure delegation to assistive personnel is not appropriate.

EQUIPMENT
- Proper size syringe and needle:
  - SQ: Syringe (1 to 3 ml) and needle (27 to 25 gauge, $\frac{3}{8}$ to $\frac{5}{8}$ in)
  - IM: Syringe 2 to 3 ml for adult, 0.5 to 1 ml for infants and small children. Two needles: 21 to 23 gauge, 1 to $1\frac{1}{2}$ in for adults; 1 in for children
- ID: 1-ml tuberculin syringe with preattached 26- or 27-gauge needle
- Small gauze pad and/or alcohol swab
- Vial or ampule of medication or skin test solution
- Disposable gloves
- MAR or computer printout

STEPS	RATIONALE
FOR ALL INJECTIONS	
1. Review prescriber's medication order for client's name, medication name, dose, time, and route of administration.	Ensures safe and correct administration of medication.
2. Assess client's history of allergies and know substances client is allergic to and normal allergic reaction.	Certain substances have similar compositions; nurse should not administer any substance to which client is known to be allergic.
3. Observe verbal and nonverbal responses toward receiving injection.	Injections can be painful. Clients may have anxiety, which can increase pain.
4. Assess for contraindications.	
A. **For subcutaneous injections** Assess for factors such as circulatory shock or reduced local tissue perfusion. Assess adequacy of client's adipose tissue.	Reduced tissue perfusion interferes with medication absorption and distribution. Physiological changes of aging or client illness may influence the amount of SQ tissue a client possesses. This influences methods for administering injections.
B. **For intramuscular injections** Assess for factors such as muscle atrophy, reduced blood flow, or circulatory shock.	Atrophied muscle absorbs medication poorly. Factors interfering with blood flow to muscles impair medication absorption.
5. Prepare correct medication dose from ampule or vial (see Skill 34-7). Check carefully. Be sure all air is expelled.	Ensures that medication is sterile. Preparation techniques differ for ampule and vial.
6. Identify client; check identification bracelet with MAR and ask client's name.	Ensures correct client receives ordered medication.
7. Explain steps of procedure and tell client injection will cause a slight burning or sting.	Helps minimize client's anxiety.
8. Close room curtain or door.	Provides privacy.
9. Wash hands thoroughly; apply disposable gloves.	Reduces transfer of microorganisms.
10. Keep sheet or gown draped over body parts not requiring exposure.	Proper selection of injection site may require exposure of body parts.
11. Select appropriate injection site. Inspect skin surface over sites for bruises, inflammation, or edema.	
a. SQ: Palpate sites for masses or tenderness. Avoid these areas. For daily insulin, rotate site daily. Be sure needle is correct size by grasping skinfold at site with thumb and forefinger. Measure fold from top to bottom. Needle should be one-half length.	
b. IM: Note integrity and size of muscle and palpate for tenderness or hardness. Avoid these areas. If injections are given frequently, rotate sites.	
c. ID: Note lesions or discolorations of forearm. Select site three to four fingerwidths below antecubital space and a handwidth above wrist.	

STEPS	RATIONALE

Critical Decision Point: Injection sites should be free of abnormalities that may interfere with medication absorption. Site used repeatedly can become hardened from lipohypertrophy (increased growth in fatty tissue). An ID site should be clear so that results of skin test can be seen and interpreted correctly. Do not use an area that is bruised or has signs associated with infection.

STEPS	RATIONALE
12. Assist client to comfortable position:	
a. SQ: Have client relax arm, leg, or abdomen, depending on site chosen for injection.	Relaxation of site minimizes discomfort.
b. IM: Have client lie flat, on side, or prone, depending on site chosen.	Reduces strain on muscle and minimizes discomfort of injections.
c. ID: Have client extend elbow and support it and forearm on flat surface.	Stabilizes injection site for easiest accessibility.
d. Talk with client about subject of interest.	Distraction reduces anxiety.

Critical Decision Point: Ensure that client's position is not contraindicated by medical condition.

STEPS	RATIONALE
13. Relocate site using anatomical landmarks.	Injection into correct anatomical site prevents injury to nerves, bones, and blood vessels.
14. Cleanse site with an antiseptic swab. Apply swab at center of the site and rotate outward in a circular direction for about 5 cm (2 in) (see illustration).	Mechanical action of swab removes secretions containing microorganisms.
15. Hold swab or gauze between third and fourth fingers of nondominant hand.	Gauze or swab remains readily accessible when needle is withdrawn.
16. Remove needle cap or sheath from needle by pulling it straight off.	Preventing needle from touching sides of cap prevents contamination.
17. Hold syringe between thumb and forefinger of dominant hand	
a. SQ: Hold as dart, palm down (see illustration) or hold syringe across tops of fingertips.	Quick, smooth injection requires proper manipulation of syringe parts.
b. IM: Hold as dart, palm down.	
c. ID: Hold bevel of needle pointing up.	With bevel up, medication is less likely to be deposited into tissues below dermis.
18. Administer injection:	
A. **Subcutaneous**	
(1) For average-size client, spread skin tightly across injection site or pinch skin with nondominant hand.	Needle penetrates tight skin easier than loose skin. Pinching skin elevates SQ tissue and may desensitize area.
(2) Inject needle quickly and firmly at 45- to 90-degree angle. Then release skin, if pinched.	Quick, firm insertion minimizes discomfort. (Injecting medication into compressed tissue irritates nerve fibers.)
(3) For obese client, pinch skin at site and inject needle at 90-degree angle below tissue fold.	Obese clients have fatty layer of tissue above SQ layer.
(4) After needle enters site, grasp lower end of syringe barrel with nondominant hand. Move dominant hand to end of plunger. Avoid moving syringe. Do not aspirate medication	Movement of syringe may displace needle and cause discomfort.
(5) Inject medication slowly.	

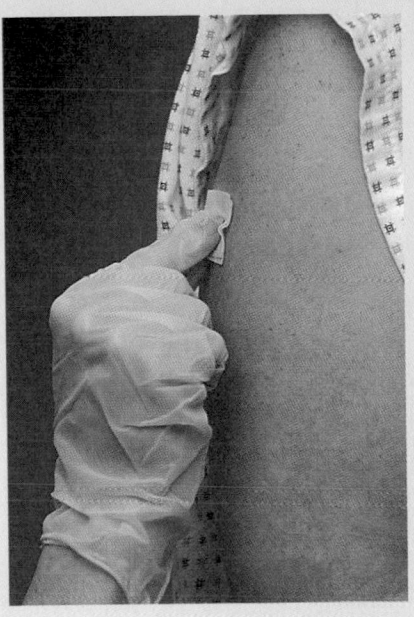

Step 14

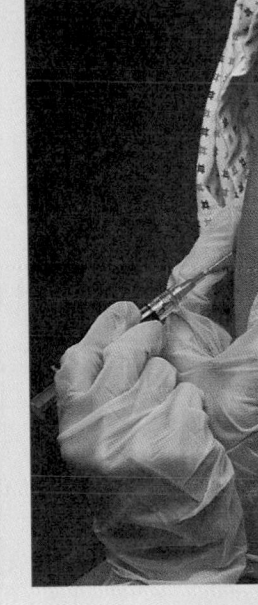

Step 17a

B. **Intramuscular:**
   (1) Position nondominant hand at proper anatomical landmarks and pull skin down to administer in a Z-track.

   (2) If client's muscle mass is small, grasp body of muscle between thumb and fingers.

   (3) Insert needle quickly at 90-degree angle into muscle. Aspirate as in Step 18A(4).

Speeds insertion and reduces discomfort. Creates zigzag path through tissues that seals needle track to avoid tracking of medication.

Ensures that medication reaches muscle mass.

Critical Decision Point: If blood appears in syringe, remove needle and dispose of medication and syringe properly. Repeat preparation procedure.

   (4) Inject medication slowly.

   (5) Wait 10 sec. Then smoothly and steadily withdraw needle and release skin.

Slow injection reduces pain and tissue trauma (Beyea and Nicoll, 1996).

Support of tissues around infection site minimizes discomfort during needle withdrawal. Some advocate use of dry gauze to minimize client discomfort associated with alcohol on nonintact skin.

C. **Intradermal**
   (1) With nondominant hand, stretch skin over site with forefinger or thumb.

   (2) With needle almost against client's skin, insert it slowly at a 5- to 15-degree angle until resistance is felt. Then advance needle through epidermis to approximately 3 mm (⅛ in) below skin surface. Needle tip can be seen through skin.

   (3) Inject medication slowly. Normally, resistance is felt. If not, needle is too deep; remove and begin again.

Needle pierces tight skin more easily.

Ensures needle tip is in dermis.

Slow injection minimizes discomfort at site. Dermal layer is tight and does not expand easily when solution is injected.

STEPS	RATIONALE

(4) While injecting medication, notice that small bleb approximately 6 mm (¼ in) resembling mosquito bite appears on skin's surface (see illustration).

Bleb indicates medication is deposited in dermis.

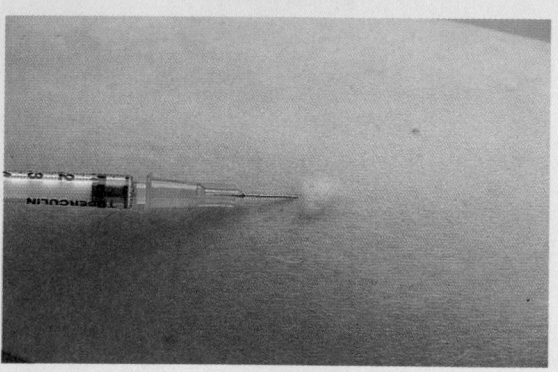

Step 18C(4)

19. Withdraw needle while applying alcohol swab or gauze gently over site. Support of tissue around injection site minimizes discomfort during needle withdrawal.

Some advocate the use of dry gauze to minimize client discomfort associated with alcohol on nonintact skin.

20. Do not massage site after SQ injection of heparin or insulin or after IM or ID injection. Apply bandage over ID site.

Massage of site after heparin injection may cause bleeding; massage after insulin injection may increase absorption of insulin. Massage of IM site may cause underlying tissue damage. Massage of ID site may disperse medication into underlying tissue layers and alter test results.

21. Assist client to comfortable position.

Gives client sense of well-being.

22. Discard uncapped needle or needle enclosed in safety shield and attached syringe into puncture and leakproof receptacle. When nurse is unable to leave client's bedside, a one-handed technique can be used to recap a needle.

Needles should not be recapped before disposal. Safety shields prevent needle-stick injuries.

23. Remove disposable gloves and wash hands.

Reduces transmission of microorganisms.

24. Stay with client 3 to 5 min and observe for any allergic reactions.

Severe anaphylactic reaction is characterized by dyspnea, wheezing, and circulatory collapse.

25. Return to room and ask if client feels any acute pain, burning, numbness, or tingling at injection site.

Continued discomfort may indicate injury to underlying bones or nerves.

26. Inspect site, noting any bruising or induration.

Bruising or induration indicates complication associated with injection. Notify nurse in charge or physician. Provide warm compress to site.

27. Return to evaluate client's response to medication in 10 to 30 min. IM medications absorb quickly; undesired effects may also develop rapidly.

Nurse's observations determine efficacy of medication action.

28. Ask client to explain purpose and effects of medication.

Evaluates client's understanding of information taught.

29. *For ID injections,* use skin pencil and draw circle around perimeter of injection site. Read site within 48 to 72 hr of injection.

Site must be read at various intervals to determine test results. Pencil mark makes site easy to find.

Recording and Reporting

- Chart medication dose, route, site, time, and date given in medication record.
- Report any undesirable effects from medication to nurse in charge or physician.
- Record client's response to medications in nurses' notes.

Home Care Considerations

- Clients with hypertrophy of the skin from repeated insulin injections (common with beef or pork formulations) should be taught not to use the site for 6 months.

istics of the tissues influence the rate of medication absorption and thus the onset of medication action. Before injecting a medication the nurse should know the volume of the medication to administer, the medication's characteristics and viscosity, and the location of anatomical structures underlying injection sites (Skill 34-8).

A nurse's inability to administer injections correctly can have negative consequences. Failure to select an injection site in relation to anatomical landmarks can result in nerve or bone damage during needle insertion. Inability to maintain stability of the needle and syringe unit could result in pain for the client and possibly tissue damage. If the nurse fails to aspirate the syringe before injecting a medication, the medication may accidentally be injected directly into an artery or vein. Injecting too large a volume of medication for the site selected causes extreme pain and may result in local tissue damage.

Many clients, particularly children, fear injections. Clients with serious or chronic illness often are given several injections daily. The nurse may be able to minimize the client's discomfort in the following ways:

Using a sharp-beveled needle in the smallest suitable
    length and gauge

Positioning the client as comfortably as possible to reduce muscular tension

Selecting the proper injection site, using anatomical landmarks

Diverting the client's attention from the injection through conversation

Inserting the needle quickly and smoothly to minimize tissue pulling

Holding the syringe steady while the needle remains in tissues

Injecting the medication slowly and steadily

Subcutaneous Injections.   Subcutaneous injections involve placing medications into the loose connective tissue under the dermis (see Skill 34-8). Because subcutaneous tissue is not as richly supplied with blood as the muscles, medication absorption is somewhat slower than with intramuscular injections. However, medications are absorbed completely if the client's circulatory status is normal. Because subcutaneous tissue contains pain receptors, the client may experience some discomfort.

The best subcutaneous injection sites include the outer posterior aspect of the upper arms, the abdomen from below the costal margins to the iliac crests, and the anterior aspects of the thighs (Figure 34-21). The site most frequently recommended for heparin injections is the abdomen (Figure 34-22). Other sites include the scapular areas of the upper back and the upper ventral or dorsal gluteal areas. The injection site chosen should be free of skin lesions, bony prominences, and large underlying muscles or nerves. Clients with diabetes should practice intrasite rotation of insulin injections.

Use of the same part of the body for a sequence of injections provides more consistency in the absorption of the insulin. For example, if the morning insulin is injected into the client's arm, then a subsequent injection should

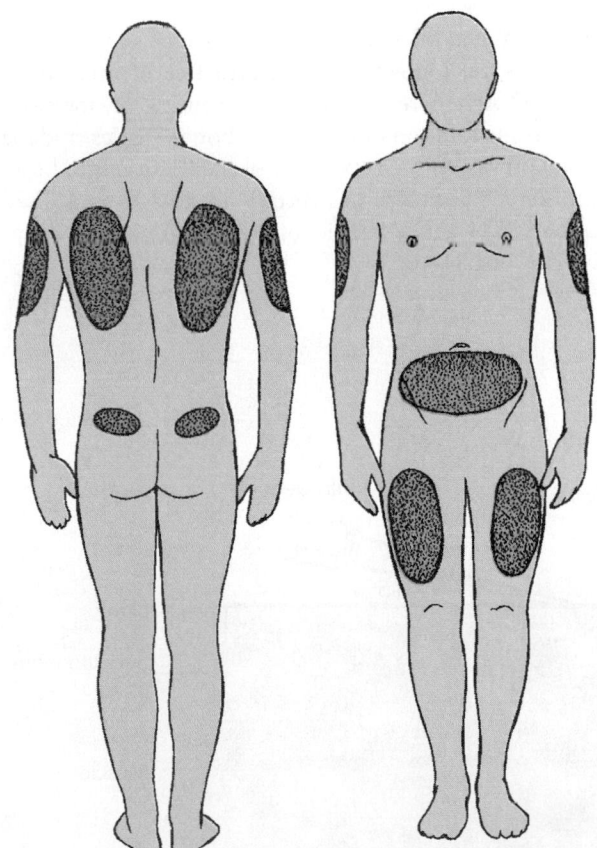

Figure 34-21   Sites recommended for subcutaneous injections

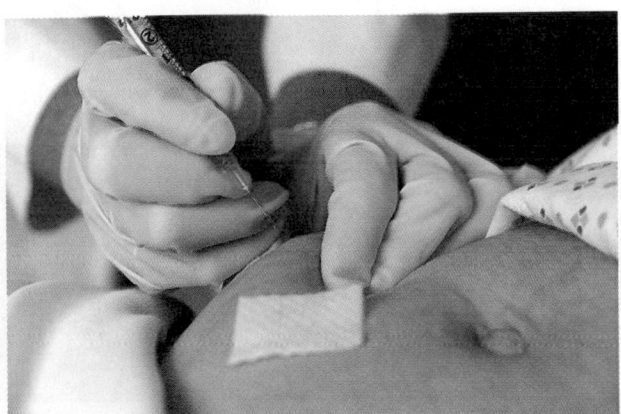

Figure 34-22   Giving SQ heparin in the abdomen.

also be given in the arm. The injections are to be given at least an inch away from the previous site. No injection site should be used again for at least 1 month.

Only small doses (0.5 to 1 ml) of water-soluble medications should be given subcutaneously because the tissue is sensitive to irritating solutions and large volumes of medications. Collection of medications within the tissues can cause sterile abscesses, which appear as hardened, painful lumps under the skin.

A client's body weight indicates the depth of the subcutaneous layer. Therefore the nurse must choose the needle length and angle of insertion based on weight. Generally a 25-gauge ⅝-inch needle inserted at a 45-degree angle (Figure 34-23) or a ½-inch needle inserted at a 90-degree angle deposits medications into the subcutaneous tissue of a normal-size client. A child may require only a ½-inch needle. If the client is obese, the nurse often pinches the tissue and uses a needle long enough to insert through fatty tissue at the base of the skinfold. The preferred needle length is one half the width of the skinfold. With this method the angle of insertion may be between 45 and 90 degrees. Thin clients may have insufficient tissue for subcutaneous injections. The upper abdomen is the best site for injection with this client.

Insulin syringes generally come with 26- to 29-gauge needles. To ensure the insulin reaches the subcutaneous tissue, the nurse follows this rule: If 2 inches of tissue can be grasped, the needle should be inserted at a 90-degree angle; if 1 inch of tissue can be grasped, the needle should be inserted at a 45-degree angle.

Intramuscular Injections.   The intramuscular route provides faster medication absorption than the subcutaneous because of a muscle's greater vascularity. There is less danger of causing tissue damage when medications enter deep muscle, but the risk of inadvertently injecting medications directly into blood vessels exists. The nurse uses a longer and heavier-gauge needle to pass through subcutaneous tissue and penetrate deep muscle tissue (see Skill 34-8). Weight and the amount of adipose tissue can influence needle size selection. For example, an obese client may require a needle 3 inches long, and a thin client may only require a ½- to 1-inch needle.

The angle of insertion for an intramuscular injection is 90 degrees (see Figure 34-23). Muscle is less sensitive to irritating and viscous medications. A normal, well-developed client can tolerate 3 ml of medication into a larger muscle without severe muscle discomfort. A larger volume of medication is unlikely to be absorbed properly. Children, older adults, and thin clients can tolerate only 2 ml of an intramuscular injection. Wong (1998) recommends giving no more than 1 ml to small children and older infants.

The nurse assesses the integrity of a muscle before giving an injection. The muscle should be free of tenderness. Repeated injections in the same muscle can cause severe discomfort. With the client relaxed, the nurse can palpate the muscle to rule out any hardened lesions. The nurse can minimize discomfort during an injection by helping the client assume a position that will help reduce muscle strain.

Sites.   When selecting an intramuscular site, the nurse considers the following: Is the area free of infection or necrosis? Are there local areas of bruising or abrasions? What is the location of underlying bones, nerves, and major blood vessels? What volume of medication is to be administered? Each site has certain advantages and disadvantages. The characteristics of each intramuscular site are listed in Box 34-16.

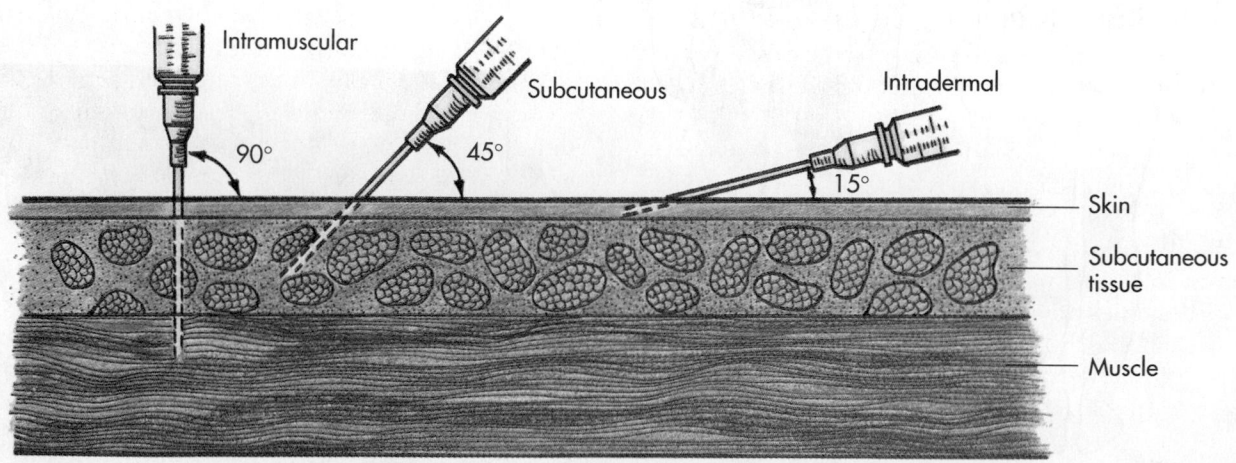

Figure 34-23   Comparison of angles of insertion for intramuscular (90 degrees), subcutaneous (45 degrees), and intradermal (15 degrees) injections.

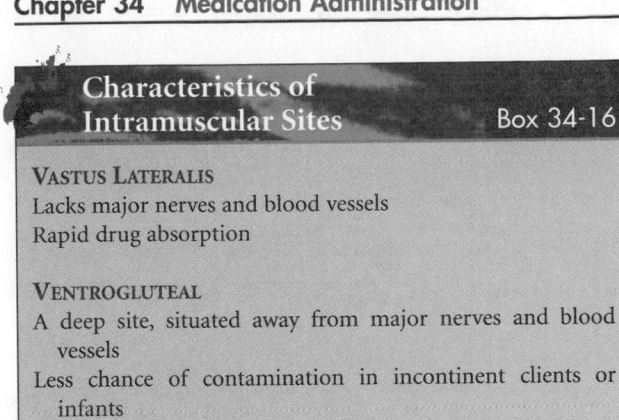

Characteristics of Intramuscular Sites Box 34-16

VASTUS LATERALIS
Lacks major nerves and blood vessels
Rapid drug absorption

VENTROGLUTEAL
A deep site, situated away from major nerves and blood vessels
Less chance of contamination in incontinent clients or infants
Easily identified by any prominent bony landmark

DELTOID
Easily accessible but muscle not well developed in most clients
Used for small amounts of medications
Not used in infants or children with underdeveloped muscles
Potential for injury to radial and ulnar nerves or brachial artery

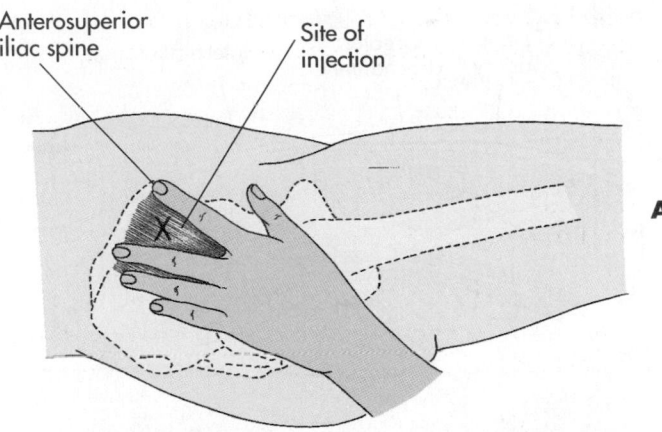

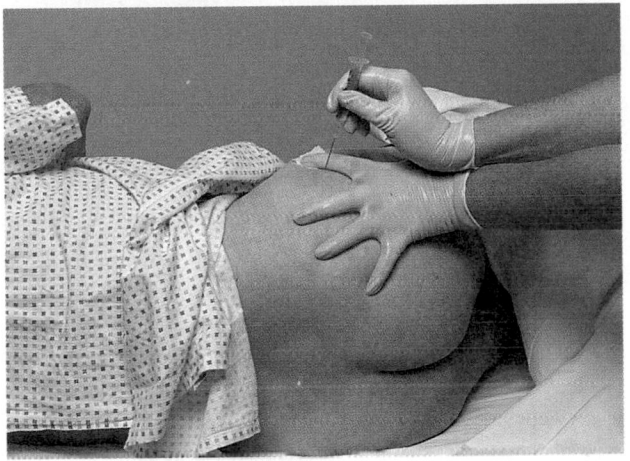

Figure 34-24 **A,** Landmarks for ventrogluteal site. **B,** Locating IM injection for ventrogluteal site.

Ventrogluteal. The ventrogluteal muscle involves the gluteus medius and minimus, is situated deep and away from major nerves and blood vessels, and is a safe site for all clients. Research has shown that injuries such as fibrosis, nerve damage, abscess, tissue necrosis, muscle contraction, gangrene, and pain have been associated with all the common IM sites except the ventrogluteal site. *The ventrogluteal site is the preferred injection site for adults and anyone over 7 months old.* (Beyea and Nicoll, 1996).

The nurse locates the muscle by placing the heel of the hand over the greater trochanter of the client's hip with the wrist perpendicular to the femur. The right hand is used for the left hip, and the left hand is used for the right hip. The nurse points the thumb toward the client's groin and fingers toward the client's head, points the index finger to the anterosuperior iliac spine, and extends the middle finger back along the iliac crest toward the buttock. The index finger, the middle finger, and the iliac crest form a V-shaped triangle, and the injection site is the center of the triangle (Figure 34-24, *A* and *B*). The client may lie on his or her side or back. Flexing of the knee and hip helps the client relax this muscle.

Vastus Lateralis. The vastus lateralis muscle is another injection site used in the adult client. The muscle is thick and well developed, is located on the anterior lateral aspect of the thigh, and extends in an adult from a handbreadth above the knee to a handbreadth below the greater trochanter of the femur (Figure 34-25). The middle third of the muscle is the suggested site for injection. The width of the muscle usually extends from the midline of the thigh to the midline of the thigh's outer side. With young children or cachectic clients, it helps to grasp the

body of the muscle during injection to be sure that the medication is deposited in muscle tissue. To help relax the muscle, the nurse asks the client to lie flat with the knee slightly flexed or in a sitting position.

Dorsogluteal. The dorsogluteal muscle has been a traditional site for intramuscular injections; however, a risk exists of striking the underlying sciatic nerve or major blood vessels (Beyea & Nicoll, 1995). Insertion of a needle into the sciatic nerve can cause permanent or partial paralysis of the involved leg. In clients with flabby, sagging tissues the site is difficult to locate. This site is not being recommended for use in this text.

Deltoid. Although the deltoid site is easily accessible, the muscle is not well developed in many adults. The radial and ulnar nerves and brachial artery lie within the upper arm along the humerus (Figure 34-26, *A*). The nurse should use this site only for small medication volumes or when other sites are inaccessible because of dressings or casts.

To locate the deltoid muscle, the nurse fully exposes the client's upper arm and shoulder. A tight-fitting sleeve

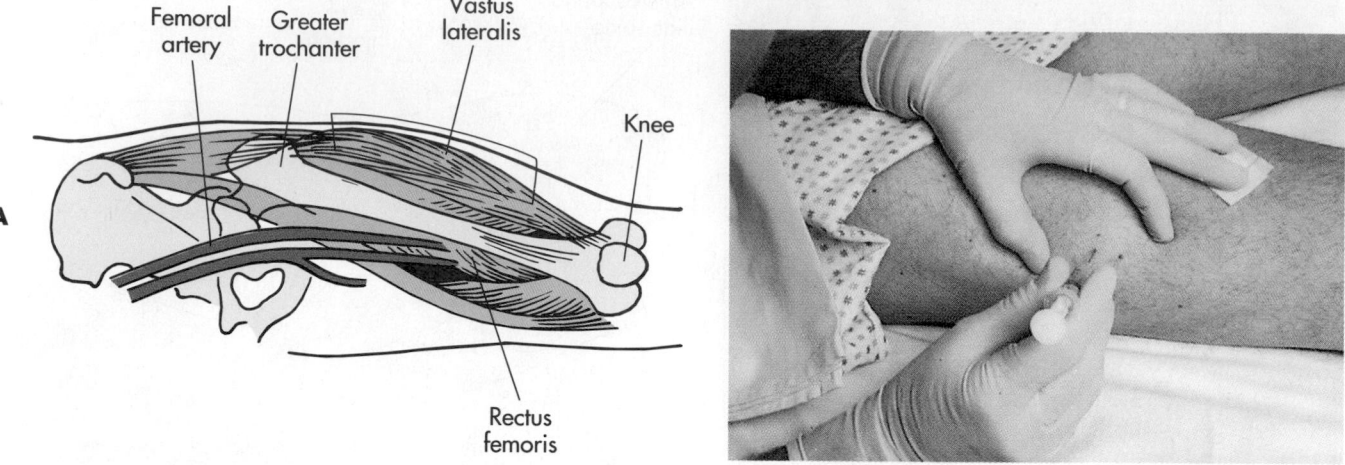

Figure 34-25 **A,** Landmarks for vastus lateralis site. **B,** Giving IM injection in vastus lateralis site.

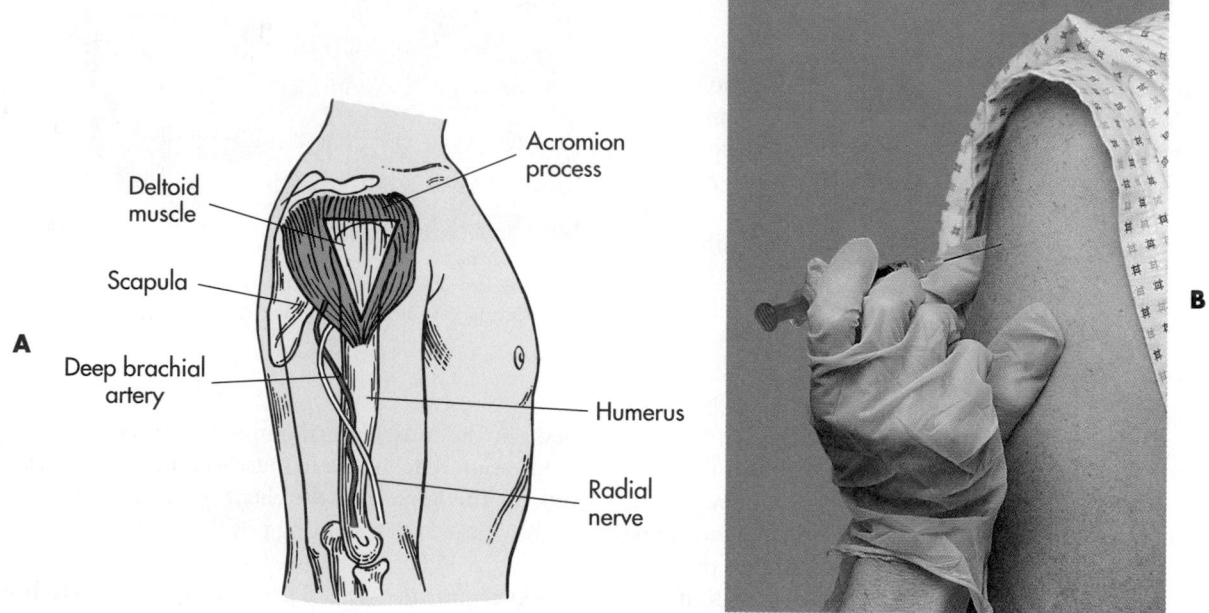

Figure 34-26 **A,** Landmarks for deltoid site. **B,** Giving IM injection in deltoid muscle.

should not be rolled up. The nurse has the client relax the arm at the side and flex the elbow. The client may sit, stand, or lie down (Figure 34-26, *B*). The nurse palpates the lower edge of the acromion process, which forms the base of a triangle in line with the midpoint of the lateral aspect of the upper arm. The injection site is in the center of the triangle, about 2.5 to 5 cm (1 to 2 inches) below the acromion process. The nurse may also locate the site by placing four fingers across the deltoid muscle, with the top finger along the acromion process. The injection site is then three fingerwidths below the acromion process.

Special Techniques in IM Injections

Air-Lock Technique. Intramuscular injections using the air-lock technique are less irritating to subcutaneous tissues during needle withdrawal. When a small volume of air is injected behind a bolus of medication, the air clears the needle of medication, preventing tracking of the medication through subcutaneous tissues. This technique is recommended in the medication information insert of only a few medications. Examples include interferon, Wyeth's vaccines prepared with aluminum adjuvant, diphtheria and tetanus toxoid, and the pertussis vaccine.

After preparing the proper dose, the nurse draws up 0.2 ml of air. The needle then must be injected downward at a 90-degree angle so that the air rises to the top of the medication toward the plunger. As the nurse injects the medication into the muscle, the air follows the medication, creating an air lock (Figure 34-27). If the nurse administers the medication with the needle at an angle less than 90 degrees, the air collects along the barrel of the syringe and enters the muscle too soon. Medication can then easily leak back into subcutaneous tissues.

Z-Track Method.   It is recommended that when administering IM injections the **Z-track method** be used to minimize irritation by sealing the medication in muscle tissue. The nurse selects an IM site, preferably in larger, deeper muscles such as the ventrogluteal muscle. A new needle must be applied to the syringe after preparing the medication so that no solutions remains on the outside needle shaft. After preparing the site with an antiseptic swab, the nurse pulls the overlying skin and subcutaneous tissues approximately 2.5 to 3.5 cm (1 to 1½ inches) laterally to the side. Holding the skin taut with the nondominant hand, the nurse injects the needle deep into the muscle. With practice the nurse learns to hold the syringe and aspirate with one hand. The nurse injects the medication slowly if there is no blood return on aspiration. The needle remains inserted for 10 seconds to allow the medication to disperse evenly. The nurse then releases the skin after withdrawing the needle. This leaves a zigzag path that seals the needle track where tissue planes slide across each other (Figure 34-28). The medication cannot escape from the muscle tissue.

Intradermal Injections.   The nurse typically gives intradermal injections for skin testing (e.g., tuberculin screening and allergy tests). Because these medications are potent, they are injected into the dermis, where blood supply is reduced and medication absorption occurs slowly. A client may have a severe anaphylactic reaction if the medications enter the circulation too rapidly.

Skin testing requires that the nurse be able to clearly see the injection sites for changes in color and tissue integrity. Intradermal sites should be lightly pigmented, free of lesions, and relatively hairless. The inner forearm and upper back are ideal locations.

The nurse uses a tuberculin or small hypodermic syringe for skin testing. The angle of insertion for an intradermal injection is 5 to 15 degrees (see Figure 34-23). As the nurse injects the medication, a small bleb resembling a mosquito bite should appear on the skin's surface (see Skill 34-8). If a bleb does not appear or if the site bleeds after needle withdrawal, there is a good chance the medication entered subcutaneous tissues. In this case, test results will not be valid.

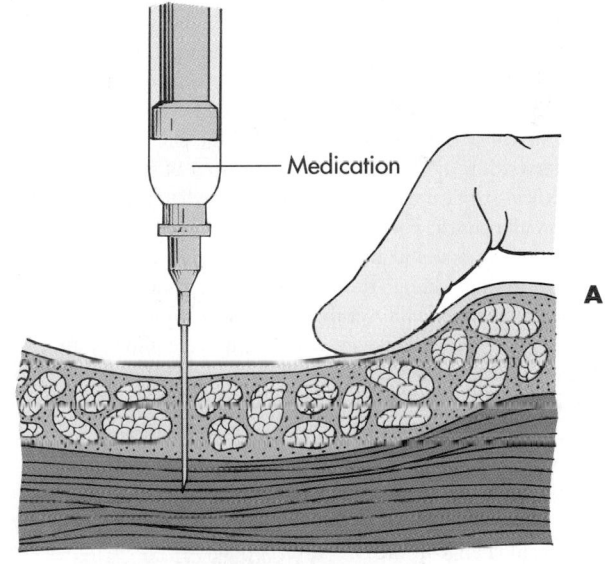

During injection

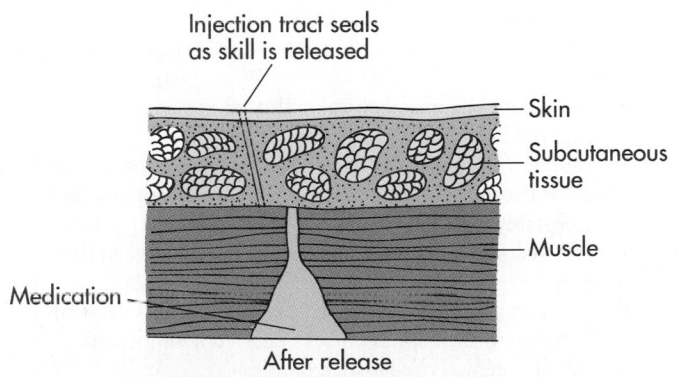

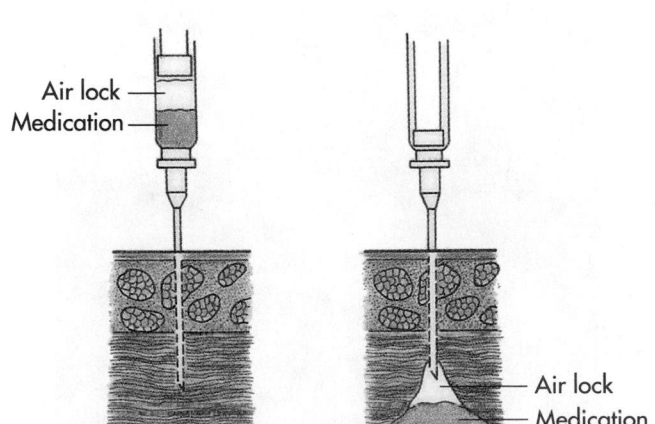

Figure 34-27   Administering IM injection by the air-lock technique prevents tracking of caustic medications through SQ tissue.

Figure 34-28   **A,** Pull on overlying skin during IM injection moves tissue to prevent later tracking. **B,** The Z-track left after injection prevents the deposit of medication through sensitive tissue.

Safety in Administering Medications by Injection

Needleless Devices. Approximately 1 million accidental needle sticks and sharps injuries occur annually in health care settings (Jagger, 1992). These injuries commonly occur when nurses forget and recap needles, mishandle intravenous lines and needles, or contact stray needles left at a client's bedside (Box 34-17). The risk of exposure of health care workers to blood-borne pathogens has led to the development of "needleless devices" or special needle safety devices.

Special syringes are designed with a sheath or guard that covers the needle after it is withdrawn from the skin (Figure 34-29). The needle is immediately covered, eliminating the chance for a needle-stick injury. The syringe and sheath are disposed of together in a receptacle. The Centers for Disease Control and Prevention (CDC) and Occupational Safety and Health Administration (OSHA) have recommended use of "needleless" devices to reduce the risk to health care workers of needle sticks and sharps injuries (Owens-Schwab and Fraser, 1993).

Needles and other instruments considered "sharps" are always disposed of into clearly marked, appropriate containers (Figure 34-30). Containers should be puncture proof and leakproof. A needle should never be forced by anyone into a full needle disposable receptacle. Used needles and syringes are never placed in any wastebasket, in the nurse's pocket, on a client's meal tray, or at the client's bedside.

One-Handed Needle Recapping Technique. In administering injections it may be necessary, for client safety reasons, to recap a contaminated needle. For example, the nurse may be assisting with emergency measures at the bedside and cannot reach a disposable container. If a com-

Research HIGHLIGHT	Box 34-17

RESEARCH ABSTRACT

The researchers compared the proportion of recapped needles, found in disposable boxes on two different types of hospital units, both before and after an intervention. The number of recapped needles (which should not be found) would be an indicator of needle-stick injury risk. The first type of hospital unit was a medical-surgical unit that had existing mounted in-bathroom needle disposal boxes, and the second type was an intensive care unit that had unmounted needle disposal boxes in the room but not necessarily near the client's bedside. The intervention by the researchers consisted of installing, in the medical-surgical unit only, mounted needle disposal boxes on the wall near the client's bed. There was no change in the location of the boxes in the intensive care unit. However, the researchers did change the type of needle disposal unit. Before the intervention, the recapping rates in the medical-surgical units and in the intensive care units were similar, approximately 32% to 34%. Following the intervention (placing the disposal boxes mounted on the wall near the client's bedside), the proportion of recapped needles was significantly reduced, down to 18% to 27%, in the disposal containers adjacent to the bedsides in medical-surgical units. In the intensive care units, which merely had a brand of box changed, there was no significant change in the rate of recapping.

IMPLICATIONS FOR PRACTICE

- An environmental change alone is an effective means of altering the risk to health care workers for needle-stick injuries.
- Environmental changes may also create a behavioral change in hospital workers.
- Despite improvements in needle disposal systems, needle-sticks to health care workers continue to occur at unacceptably high rates.
- Easy access to protective equipment may improve utilization.
- The disposal system appeared to pose no greater risk of infection to clients, and nurses preferred it for its reduced risk of potential needle-stick injuries.

REFERENCE

Mafofsky D, Cone JE: *Infect Control Hosp Epidemiol* 14(3):140, 1993.

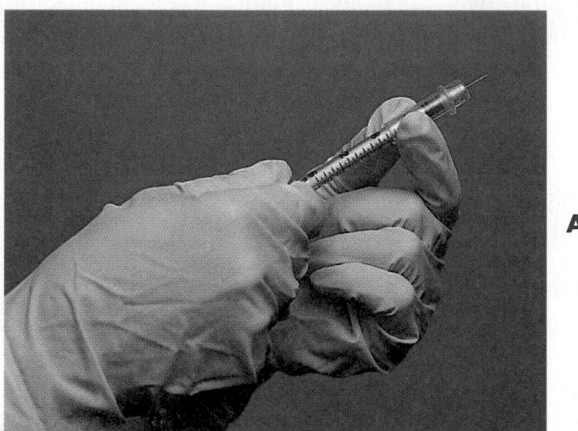

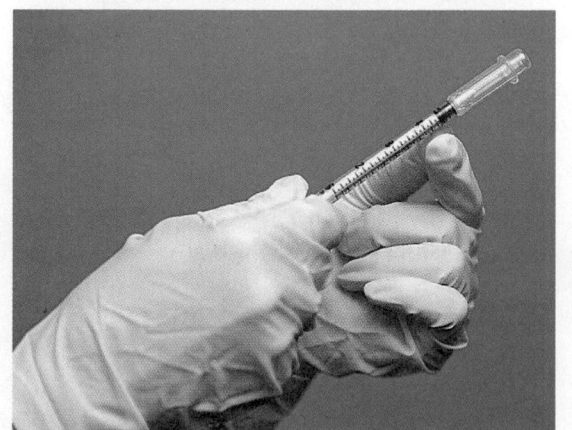

Figure 34-29 Needle with plastic guard to prevent needle sticks. **A,** Position of guard before injection. **B,** After injection the guard locks in place, covering the needle.

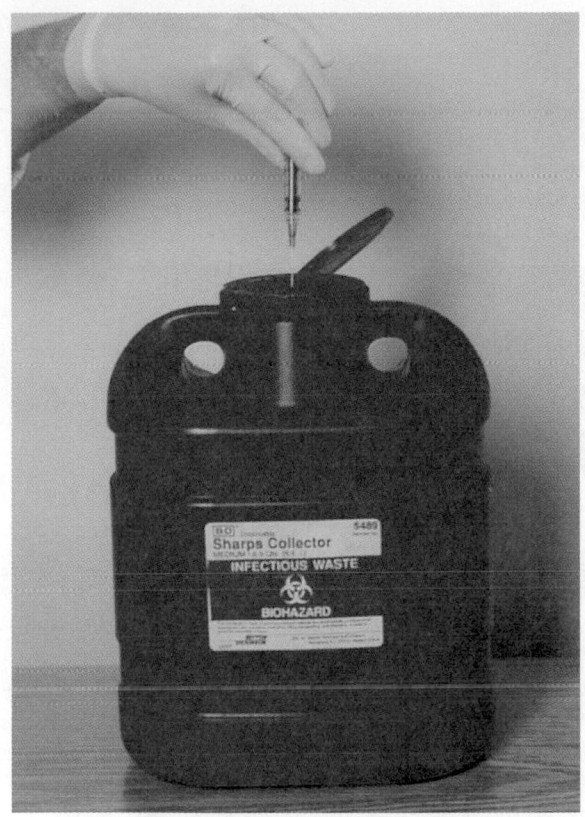

Figure 34-30   Sharps disposal using only hand.

mercially made recapping device is not available, then the nurse should use the one-handed needle recapping technique that is described in Box 34-18.

INTRAVENOUS ADMINISTRATION

The nurse administers medications intravenously by the following methods:

1. As mixtures within large volumes of IV fluids
2. By injection of a bolus, or small volume, of medication through an existing intravenous infusion line or intermittent venous access (heparin or medication lock)
3. By "piggyback" infusion of a solution containing the prescribed medication and a small volume of IV fluid through an existing IV line.

In all three methods the client has either an existing IV infusion line or an IV access site such as an intermittent infusion (sometime called a heparin or medication lock). In most institutions, policies and procedures list persons who may give IV medications and the situations in which they may be given. These policies are based on the medication, capability and availability of staff, and type of monitoring equipment available.

Chapter 40 describes the technique for performing venipuncture and establishing continuous IV fluid infusions. Medication administration is only one reason for

supplying IV fluids. Intravenous fluid therapy is used primarily for fluid replacement in clients unable to take oral fluids and as a means of supplying electrolytes and nutrients.

When using any method of IV medication administration, the nurse must observe clients closely for symptoms of adverse reactions. After a medication enters the bloodstream, it begins to act immediately, and there is no way to stop its action. Thus the nurse takes special care to avoid errors in dose calculation and preparation. The nurse should double-check the five rights of safe medication administration and know the desired action and side effects. If the medication has an antidote, it must be available during administration. When administering potent medications, the nurse assesses vital signs before, during, and after infusion.

Administering medications by the IV route has advantages. Often the nurse uses the IV route in emergencies when a fast-acting medication must be delivered quickly. The IV route is also best when it is necessary to establish constant therapeutic blood levels. Some medications are highly alkaline and irritating to muscle and subcutaneous tissue. These medications cause less discomfort when given intravenously.

Large-Volume Infusions.   Of the three methods of administering IV medications, mixing medications in large volumes of fluids is the safest and easiest. Medications are diluted in large volumes (500 ml or 1000 ml) of compatible IV fluids such as normal saline or lactated Ringer's solution (Skill 34-9). In most institutions the pharmacist adds medications to the primary container of IV solution to ensure asepsis. Because the medication is not in a concentrated form, the risk of side effects or fatal reactions is minimal when infused over the prescribed time frame. Vitamins and potassium chloride are two types of medications commonly added to IV fluids. However, there is a danger with continuous infusion: if the IV fluid is infused too rapidly, the client may suffer circulatory fluid overload.

Intravenous Bolus.   An IV bolus involves introducing a concentrated dose of a medication directly into the systemic circulation (Skill 34-10). Because a bolus requires only a small amount of fluid to deliver the medication, it is an advantage when the amount of fluid the client can take is restricted. The IV bolus, or "push", is the most dangerous method for administering medications because there is no time to correct errors. In addition, a bolus may cause direct irritation to the lining of blood vessels. Before administering a bolus the nurse confirms placement of the IV line. This involves obtaining a blood return through the IV catheter or needle. The inability to obtain a blood return suggests that the needle or catheter is in the client's tissues or resting against the vein wall. A medication should never be given intravenously if the insertion site appears puffy or

Box 34-18 **Procedural Guidelines**

For One-Handed Needle Recapping Technique

Needles should never be recapped. Use this procedure only when a sharps disposal box is unavailable and you cannot leave the client's room. Needle-stick injuries place the health care worker at risk for blood-borne pathogens. After using a needle, the health care worker should dispose of the sharp in the nearest designated container.

1. Before giving the injection, place the needle cover on a solid, immovable object such as the rim of a bedside table. The open end of the cap should face the nurse and be within reach of the nurse's dominant, or injection, hand.
2. Give the injection.
3. Place the tip of the needle at the entrance of the cap. *Gently* slide the needle into the needle cover (see illustrations).
4. Once the needle is inside the cover, use the object's resistance to completely cover the needle (see illustration).
5. Dispose of the needle at the first opportunity.
6. Wash hands.

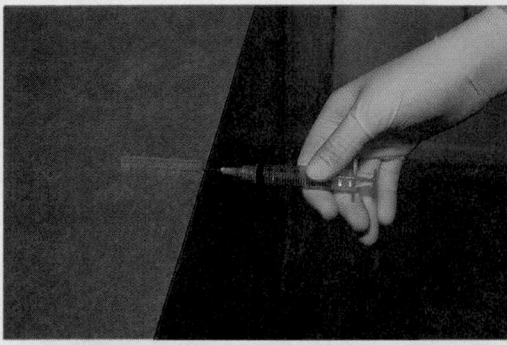

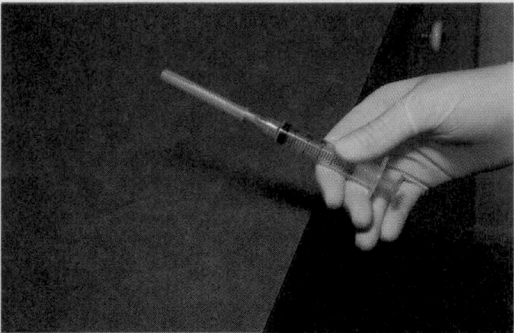

Step 3

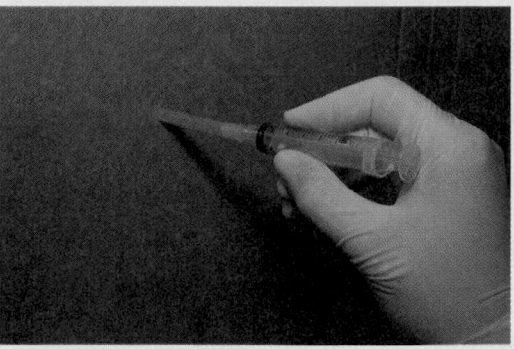

Step 4

edematous or the IV fluid cannot flow at the proper rate. Accidental injection of a medication into the tissues around a vein can cause pain, sloughing of tissues, and abscesses, depending on the medication's composition.

The rate of administration of an IV bolus medication is usually determined by the amount of medication that can be given each minute. The nurse should look up each medication to determine the recommended concentration and rate of administration. The purpose for which a medication is prescribed and any potential adverse effects related to the rate or route of administration must be considered when a nurse gives a medication IV push.

Volume-Controlled Infusions.   Another way of administering IV medications is through small amounts (50 to 100 ml) of compatible IV fluids. The fluid is within a

Text continued on p. 959.

Adding Medications to Intravenous Fluid Containers | Skill 34-9

Delegation Considerations
Adding medications to IV fluid containers requires problem solving and knowledge application unique to professional nursing. For this procedure delegation to assistive personnel is not appropriate. (In some institutions the pharmacist may add medications to primary containers of IV solutions to ensure asepsis.)

EQUIPMENT
- Vial or ampule of prescribed medication
- Syringe of appropriate size (5 to 20 ml)
- Sterile needle (1 to 1½ in, 19 to 21 gauge) with special filters (optional)
- Correct diluent (e.g., sterile water, normal saline)
- Sterile IV fluid container (bag or bottle, 50 to 1000 ml in volume)
- Alcohol or antiseptic swab
- Label to attach to IV bag or bottle
- MAR or computer printout

STEPS	RATIONALE
1. Check prescriber's order to determine type of IV solution to use and type of medication and dosage.	Client's overall physical condition dictates type of IV solution used. Ensures safe and accurate medication administration.
2. Collect information necessary to administer drug safely, including action, purpose, side effects, normal dose, time of peak onset, and nursing implications.	Allows nurse to give medication safely and to monitor client's response to therapy.
3. When more than one medication is to be added to IV solution, assess for compatibility of medications.	Medications often are incompatible when mixed together. Chemical reactions that occur result in clouding or crystallization of IV fluids. Check hospital policy for approved medication compatibility list.
4. Assess client's systemic fluid balance, as reflected by skin hydration and turgor, body weight, pulse, and blood pressure.	Danger of continuous IV infusions is that fluids may infuse too rapidly, causing circulatory overload.
5. Assess client's history of medication allergies.	IV administration of medications causes rapid effects. Allergic response can be immediate.
6. Assess IV insertion site for signs of infiltration or phlebitis (see Chapter 40).	An intact, properly functioning site ensures medication is given safely.
7. Wash hands thoroughly.	Reduces transfer of microorganisms.
8. Assemble supplies in medication room.	Ensures procedure will be orderly, with less likelihood of contaminating supplies.
9. Prepare prescribed medication from vial or ampule (see Skill 34-7).	Ensures accurate delivery of medication.
10. Identify client by reading identification band and asking name. Compare with medication ticket.	Ensures correct client receives medication.
11. Assess client's understanding of purpose of medication therapy.	May reveal need for education.
12. Add medication to new container (usually done in medication room or at medication cart): a. *Solution in a bag:* Locate medication injection port on plastic IV solution bag. Port has small rubber stopper at end. Do not select port for the IV tubing insertion or air vent.	Medication injection port is self-sealing to prevent introduction of microorganisms after repeated use.

STEPS	RATIONALE
b. *Solution in a bottle:* Locate injection site on IV solution bottle, which is often covered by a metal or plastic cap.	Accidental injection of medication through main tubing port or air vent can alter pressure within bottle and cause fluid leaks through air vent. Cap seals bottle to maintain its sterility.
c. Wipe off port or injection site with alcohol or antiseptic swab (see illustration).	Reduces risk of introducing microorganisms into bag during needle insertion.
d. Remove needle cap or sheath from syringe and insert needle of syringe or needleless device through center of injection port or site; inject medication (see illustration).	Injection of needle into sides of port may produce leak and lead to fluid contamination.
e. Withdraw syringe from bag or bottle.	Open tubing port in bottle provides direct route for microorganisms to enter solution. Bags have self-sealing port.
f. Mix medication and IV solution by holding bag or bottle and turning it gently end to end.	Allows even distribution of medication.
g. Complete medication label with name and dose of medication, date, time, and nurse's initials. Stick it on bottle or bag. *Optional (check agency policy): Apply a flow strip that identifies the time the solution was hung and intervals indicating fluid levels (see illustration).* Spike bag or bottle with IV tubing.	Label can be easily read during infusion of solution. Informs nurses and physicians of contents of bag or bottle.

Critical Decision Point: Do not use felt-tip markers on plastic surfaces. The ink can penetrate the plastic and leak into the IV solution.

---

13. Bring assembled items to client's bedside.   Ensures correct client receives ordered medication.

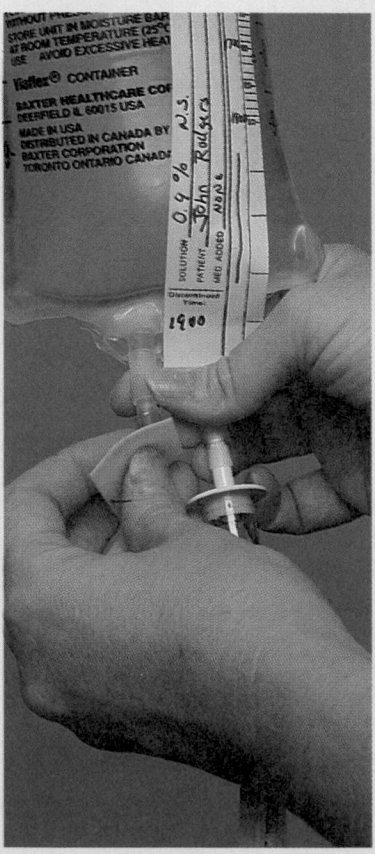

Step 12b

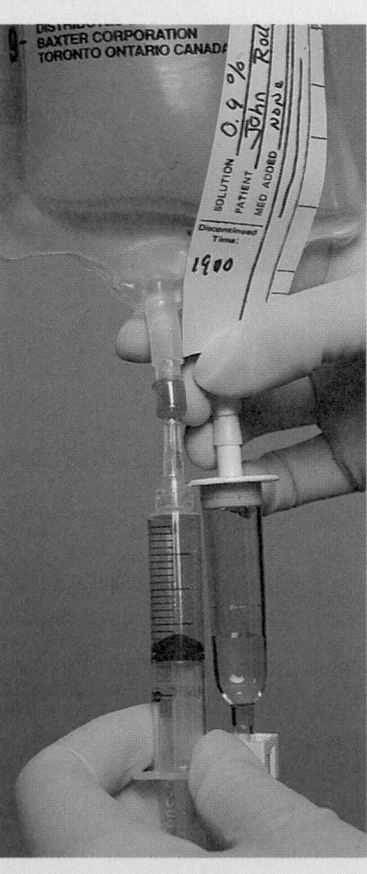

Step 12d

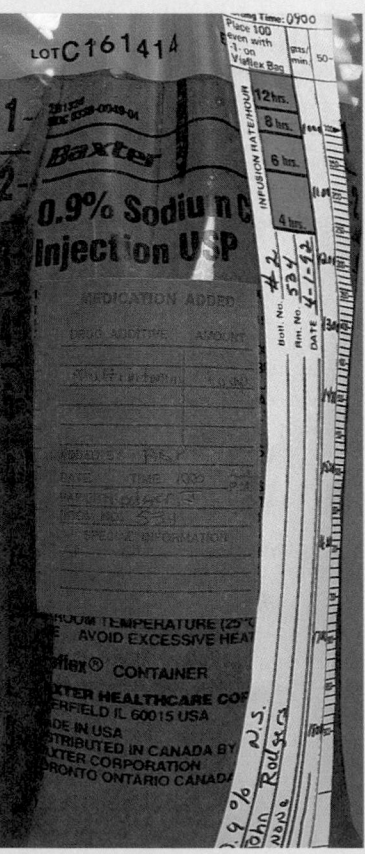

Step 12g

STEPS	RATIONALE
14. Prepare client by explaining that medication is to be given through existing IV line or one to be started. Explain that no discomfort should be felt during medication infusion. Encourage client to report symptoms of discomfort.	Most IV medications do not cause discomfort when diluted. However, potassium chloride can be irritating. Pain at insertion site may be early indication of infiltration.
15. Regulate infusion at ordered rate.	Prevents rapid infusion of fluid.
16. Add medication to existing container:	
a. Prepare vented IV bottle or plastic bag:	
(1) Check volume of solution remaining in bottle or bag.	Proper minimal volume is needed to dilute medication adequately.
(2) Close off IV infusion clamp.	Prevents medication from directly entering circulation as it is injected into bag or bottle.
(3) Wipe off medication port with an alcohol or antiseptic swab.	Mechanically removes microorganisms that could enter container during needle insertion.
(4) Insert syringe needle or needleless device through injection port and inject medication.	Injection port is self-sealing and prevents fluid leaks.
(5) Lower bag or bottle from IV pole and gently mix. Rehang bag.	Ensures medication is evenly distributed.
b. Complete medication label and stick it to bag or bottle.	Informs nurses and physicians of contents of bag or bottle.
c. Regulate infusion to desired rate.	Prevents rapid infusion of fluid.
17. Properly dispose of equipment and supplies. Do not cap needle of syringe. Specially sheathed needles are discarded as a unit with needle covered.	Proper disposal of needle prevents injury to nurse and client. Capping of needles increases risk of needle-stick injuries.
18. Wash hands.	Reduces transmission of microorganisms.
19. Observe client for signs or symptoms of medication reaction.	IV medications can cause rapid effects.
20. Observe for signs and symptoms of fluid volume excess.	Rapid uncontrolled infusion can cause circulatory overload.
21. Periodically return to client's room to assess IV insertion site and rate of infusion.	Over time IV site may become infiltrated or needle malpositioned. Flow rate may change according to client's position or volume left in container.
22. Observe for signs or symptoms of IV infiltration.	Infiltrated medications can injure tissue.

Recording and Reporting

- Record solution and medication added to parenteral fluid on appropriate form.
- Report any side effects to nurse in charge or physician.

| Skill 34-10 | **Administering Medications by Intravenous Bolus** |

Delegation Considerations

Administering medications by intravenous bolus requires problem solving and knowledge application unique to professional

nursing. For this procedure delegation to assistive personnel is not appropriate.

EQUIPMENT

- IV Push (Existing Line)
  - Disposable gloves
  - Medication in vial or ampule
  - Syringe (3-5 ml)
  - Needleless device or sterile needles (21 and 25 gauge) (optional)
  - Antiseptic swab
  - Watch with second hand or digital readout.
  - MAR or computer printout
- IV Push (IV Lock)
  - Disposable gloves

- Medication in vial or ampule
- Syringe (1-5 ml)
- Vial of appropriate flush solution (saline most common, but heparin may also be used; if heparin is used, most common concentration is 10 to 100 units; check agency policy)
- Needleless device or sterile needles (21 and 25 gauge)
- Antiseptic swab
- Watch with second hand or digital readout
- MAR or computer printout

STEPS	RATIONALE
1. Check the prescriber's order for type of medication to be administered, dosage, and route.	This ensures safe and accurate medication administration.
2. Assess IV or heparin (saline) lock insertion site for signs of infiltration or phlebitis (see Chapter 40)	Confirming the placement of the IV catheter and the integrity of the surrounding tissue ensures that the medication is administered safely.
3. If medication is to be pushed into an IV line, assess the patency of the line by noting infusion rate.	The IV line must be patent, and fluids must infuse easily for medication to reach venous circulation effectively.
4. Prepare ordered medication from vial or ampule (see Procedure 34-7). Read package directions carefully for proper IV dilution of medications.	
5. After drawing up medications, apply a small-gauge needle to the syringe.	Used to insert through IV line with needle system only.
6. Wash hands. Apply gloves.	Reduces transmission of infection. During IV bolus administration, risk of blood exposure is low. However, nurse may manipulate IV dressing or expose site while completing other activities. Gloves reduce exposure.
7. Check client's identification by looking at identification bracelet and asking name.	Ensures that medication is administered to correct client.
8. Administer medications by IV push (existing line):	
a. Select injection port of IV tubing closest to client. (Circle on port may indicate site for needle insertion.) If add-on 0.22 μ filter is used, give medication below filter next to client.	Allows for easier fluid aspiration to obtain blood return. Injection ports are self-sealing and will not leak.
b. Clean off injection port with antiseptic swab. Allow to dry.	Prevents introduction of microorganisms during needle insertion.
c. Connect syringe to IV line.	
(1) Needle system	
(a) Insert small-gauge needle of syringe containing prepared drug through center of injection port (see illustration).	Prevents damage to port's diaphragm and subsequent leakage.
(2) Needleless system	
(a) Remove cap of needleless injection port. Connect tip of syringe directly (see illustration).	
d. Occlude IV line by pinching tubing just above injection port (see illustration). Pull back gently on syringe's plunger to aspirate blood return.	Final check that medication is being delivered into the bloodstream.

STEPS	RATIONALE

e. After noting blood return, continue to occlude tubing and inject medication slowly over several minutes (read directions on medication package). Use watch to time administration (see illustration).

Ensures safe medication infusion. Rapid injection of IV medication can prove fatal.

f. After injecting medication, release tubing, withdraw syringe, and recheck fluid infusion rate.

Injection of bolus may alter rate of fluid infusion. Rapid fluid infusion can cause circulatory overload.

g. If using a needleless system, replace injection port cap with new sterile cap.

9. Administering medications by IV push (IV lock or a needleless system)
   A. **Flush solutions**
      (1) Flushing with heparin
         (a) Prepare syringe with 1 ml of heparin flush solution
         (b) Prepare 2 syringes with 1 ml of normal saline
      (2) Flushing with saline only
         (a) Prepare 2 syringes with 1 ml of normal saline each

Flush solution keeps heparin lock patent after medication is administered.

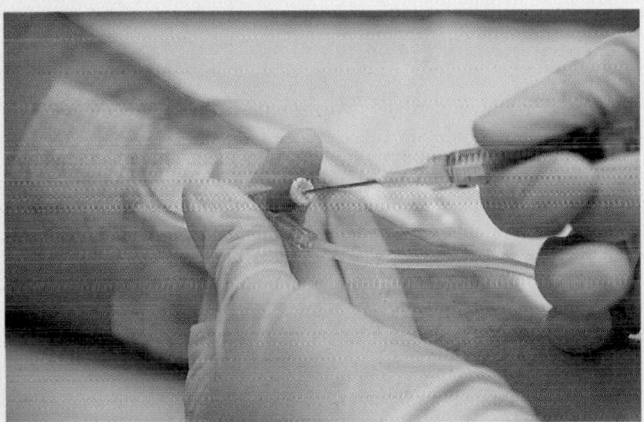

Step 8c(1)(a)

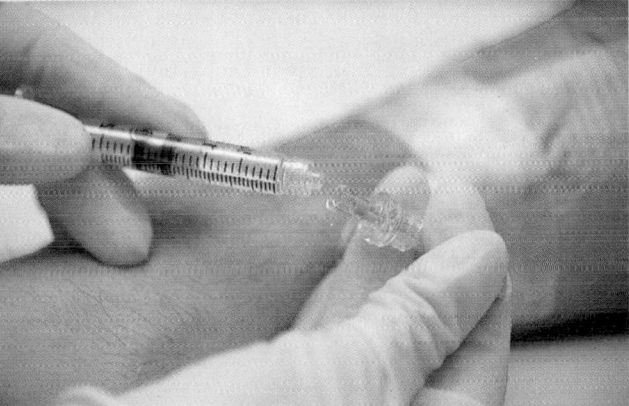

Step 8c(2)(a)

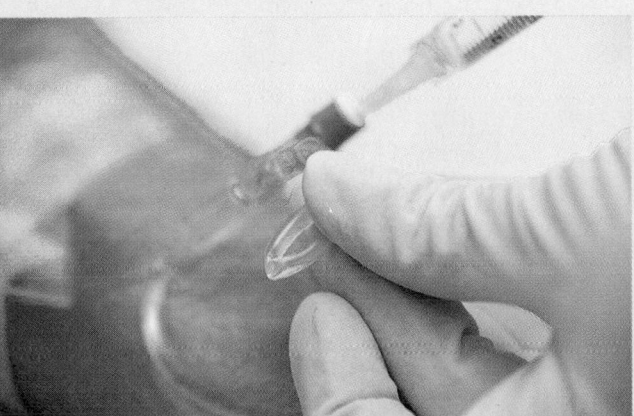

Step 8d

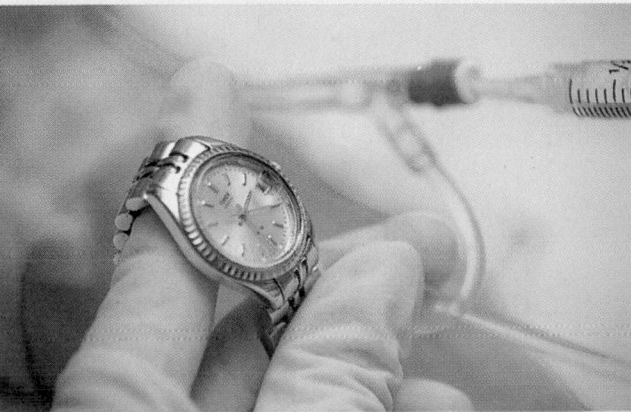

Step 8e

STEPS	RATIONALE
B. **IV lock**	
(1) Clean lock's rubber diaphragm with antiseptic swab.	Prevents introduction of microorganisms during needle insertion.
(2) Insert needle of syringe containing normal saline through center of diaphragm.	
(3) Pull back gently on syringe plunger and look for blood return.	Determines whether IV needle or catheter is positioned in vein.

Critical Decision Point: At times a heparin lock will not yield a blood return even though the lock is patent.

---

(4) Flush reservoir with 1 ml saline by pushing slowly on plunger.	Clears needle and reservoir of blood.

Critical Decision Point: Observe closely the area of skin above the IV catheter. Note any puffiness or swelling as the reservoir is flushed, which could indicate infiltration into the vein, requiring removal of the catheter.

---

(5) Remove needle and saline-filled syringe.	
(6) Clean lock's diaphragm with antiseptic swab.	Prevents transmission of infection.
(7) Insert needle of syringe containing prepared medication through center of diaphragm (see illustration).	Using center of diaphragm prevents leakage.
(8) Inject medication bolus slowly over several minutes. (Each medication has recommended rate for bolus administration. Check package directions.) Use watch to time administration.	Rapid injection of IV medication can result in death.
(9) After administering bolus, withdraw syringe.	
(10) Clean lock's diaphragm with antiseptic swab.	Prevents transmission of microorganisms.
(11) Repeat injection of 1 ml of normal saline.	Flushes reservoir and needle of medication.
(12) *Heparin flush:* Insert needle of syringe containing heparin through diaphragm. Inject heparin slowly, and remove syringe.	Maintains patency of needle by inhibiting clot formation.

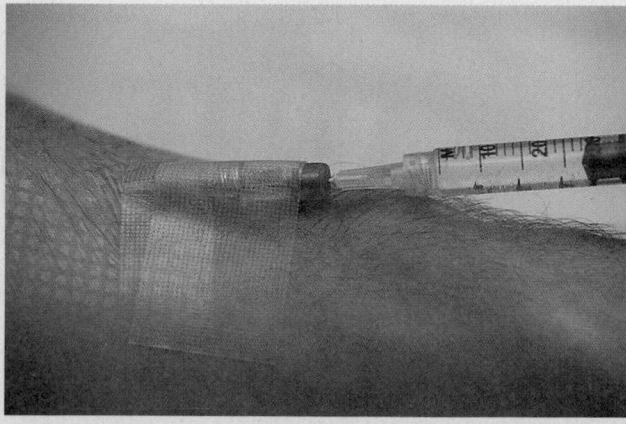

Step 9B(7)

STEPS	RATIONALE

C. **IV needleless valve cap**

    (1) Remove protective cap from needleless port.

    (2) Insert syringe containing normal saline into the valve.

    (3) Flush reservoir with 1 ml saline by pushing slowly on plunger.   *Clears reservoir of any blood.*

    (4) Remove the syringe.

    (5) Insert syringe containing prepared medication into the valve.

    (6) Inject medication slowly over several minutes. Follow precautions in Step 9B(8) (see illustration on p. 956).   *Rapid injection of IV drug can result in death.*

    (7) After administering bolus, withdraw syringe.

    (8) Repeat injection of 1 ml of normal saline.

    (9) See Step 9B(12).

    (10) Replace sterile cap over valve.

10. Administer medications by IV push epidural route (given by specially trained nurses only)

  a. Check prescriber's order for type of medication to be administered and dosage.   *Ensures safe and accurate medication administration. Narcotics, such as morphine or fentanyl, are the only medications administered by the epidural route.*

  b. Prepare equipment and supplies:

    (1) Preservative-free medication in vial or ampule   *Preservative-free medications are used because preservative may be neurotoxic and cause severe spinal cord injury.*

    (2) Syringe (3 ml)   *Used for catheter aspiration.*

    (3) Syringe (5 ml or larger)   *Used for administering narcotic. A large syringe lessens the force of fluid as it exits catheter. This reduces pain that can occur because of the forward pressure of the solution against nerve roots in the epidural space (Wild and Coyne, 1992).*

    (4) Large-gauge needle (19 to 21 gauge)   *Used to aspirate medication from vial or ampule.*

    (5) Two small-gauge needles (23 to 25 gauge)   *Used to verify catheter placement and to inject medication into epidural catheter.*

    (6) Preservative-free normal saline

    (7) Povidone-iodine swabs

    (8) Sterile gauze

    (9) Disposable gloves

  c. Using a 5-ml syringe or larger, draw up the narcotic. *Verify hospital policy if filter needle is required when aspirating medication from ampule.*   *See Skill 34-7.*

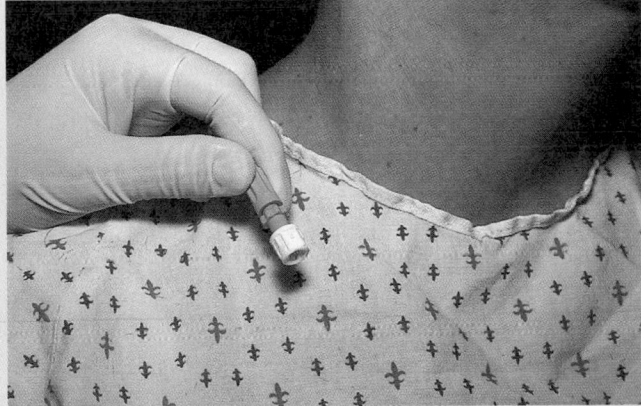 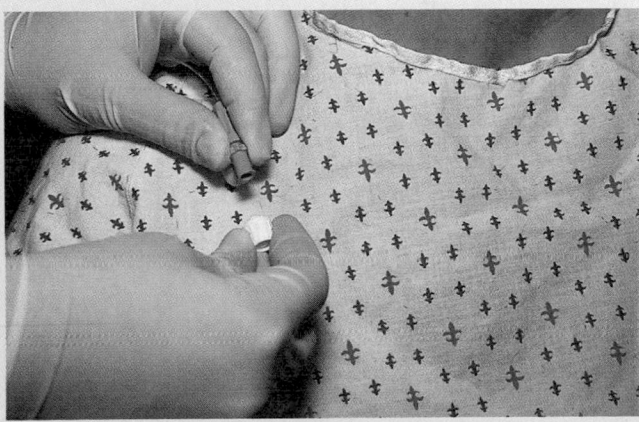

Step 10f

STEPS	RATIONALE
d. Check client's identification by looking at identification bracelet and asking name.	Ensures that the correct medication is administered to correct client.
e. Assets client's sedation using standardized scale.	Oversedation may lead to respiratory depression and death.
f. Remove protective cap from needleless port. Swab the client's injection cap with povidone-iodine. Swab cap with sterile gauze (see illustrations).	Prevents the transmission of microorganisms into the epidural space. Swabbing with gauze prevents the injection of povidone-iodine into epidural space.
g. Using 3-ml syringe, insert the syringe into the needleless port and aspirate. If more than 1 ml of clear fluid or bloody fluid is aspirated, terminate procedure and notify the nurse anesthetist or anesthesiologist (*do not reinject aspirate*). If less than 1/2 ml fluid returns, continue with procedure (see illustration).	More than 1 ml of clear fluid indicates that catheter may be in intrathecal space. A bloody return indicates that the catheter may have punctured an epidural vein.
h. Insert medication syringe into needleless port. Inject drug slowly and steadily. Reduce rate of injection if client complains of pain.	See Step 9c(6).
11. Dispose of equipment properly.	Reduces accidental needle-sticks.
12. Remove and dispose of gloves. Wash hands.	Reduces the transmission of microorganisms.
13. Observe client closely for adverse reaction as drug is administered and for several minutes thereafter.	IV medications act rapidly.
14. Record drug, dose, route and time administered on medication form (Figure 34-13).	

Recording and Reporting

- Record medication, dose, time, and route on appropriate form.
- Report any side effects immediately to physician, because they could be life threatening.

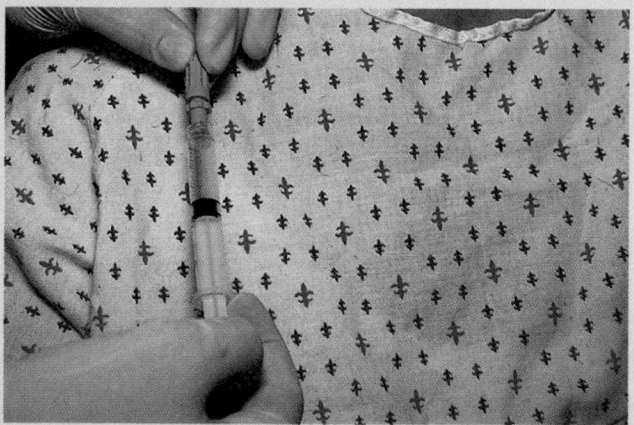

Step 10g

secondary fluid container separate from the primary fluid bag. The container connects directly to the primary IV line or to separate tubing that inserts into the primary line. Three types of containers are volume control administration sets (e.g., Volutrol or Pediatrol), piggyback and/or tandem set, and miniinfusors. Using volume-controlled infusions has several advantages:

Reduces risk of rapid-dose infusion by IV push. Medications are diluted and infused over longer time intervals (e.g., 30 to 60 minutes)

Allows for administration of medications (e.g., antibiotics) that are stable for a limited time in solution

Allows for control of IV fluid intake

Piggyback. A piggyback is a small (25 to 100 ml) IV bag or bottle connected to short tubing lines that connects to the *upper* Y-port of a primary infusion line or to an intermittent venous access (Figure 34-31). The piggyback tubing is a microdrip or macrodrip system (Chapter 40). The set is called a piggyback because the small bag or bottle is set higher than the primary infusion bag or bottle. In the piggyback setup the main line does not infuse when the piggybacked medication is infusing. The port of the primary IV line contains a back-check valve that automatically stops flow of the primary infusion once the piggyback infusion flows. After the piggyback solution infuses and the solution within the tubing falls below the level of the primary infusion drip chamber, the back-check valve opens and the primary infusion again flows.

Tandem. A tandem setup is a small (25 to 100 ml) IV bag or bottle connected to a short tubing line to the *lower* Y-port of a primary infusion line or to an intermittent venous access. The tandem set is placed at the same height as the primary infusion bag or bottle. In the tandem setup the tandem and the main line infuse simultaneously. The nurse must monitor the tandem setup closely. If the tandem setup is not immediately clamped when the medication is infused, the IV solution from the primary line will back up into the tandem line.

Volume-Control Administration. Volume-control administration (Volutrol, Buretrol, Pediatrol) sets are small (50 to 150 ml) containers that attach just below the primary infusion bag or bottle. The set is attached and filled in a manner similar to that used with a regular IV infusion. However, the priming filling of the set is different, depending on the type of filter (floating valve or membrane) within the set. Follow package directions for priming sets (see Chapter 40).

Miniinfusor Pump. The miniinfusor pump is battery operated and allows medications to be given in very small amounts of fluid (5 to 60 ml) within controlled infusion times using standard syringes (Skill 34-11).

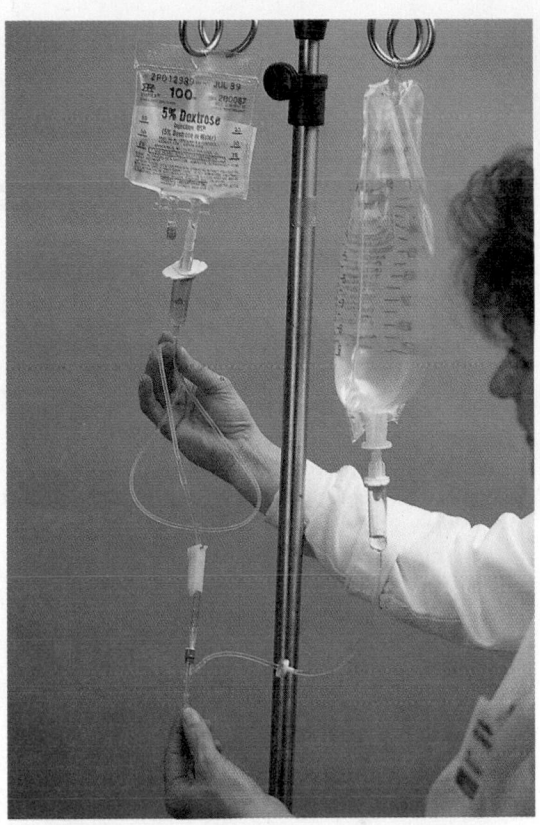

Figure 34-31 Tandem/piggyback setup.

Intermittent Venous Access. An intermittent venous access (commonly called a heparin lock or medication lock) is an IV catheter with a small "well" or chamber covered by a rubber diaphragm or a specially designed red cap (Figure 34-32, p. 964). Special rubber-seal injection caps serve as wells and can be inserted into most IV catheters (see Chapter 40). Advantages to intermittent venous access include the following:

Cost savings resulting from the omission of continuous IV therapy

Convenience to the nurse by eliminating constant monitoring of flow rates

Increased mobility, safety, and comfort for the client

After an IV bolus or piggyback medication has been administered through an intermittent venous access, the access must be flushed with a solution to keep it patent. Traditionally heparin had been used. It is now widely accepted that normal saline is as effective as heparin as a flush solution for peripheral catheters (Shoaf and Oliver, 1992).

Normally, checking for a blood return in an IV lock before bolus administration is unnecessary. However, if the needle site becomes puffy or the client complains of discomfort, the well must be aspirated for a blood return.

Text continued on p. 964.

Administering Intravenous Medications by Piggyback, Intermittent Intravenous Infusion Sets, and Miniinfusion Pumps

Skill 34-11

Delegation Considerations

Administering medications by IV fluid by piggyback, intermittent intravenous infusion sets, and miniinfusion pumps requires problem solving and knowledge application unique to professional nursing. For this procedure delegation is not appropriate.

EQUIPMENT

- **Piggyback, Tandem, or Miniinfusion Pump**
  - Gloves (for connecting IV tubing)
  - Medication prepared in 5- to 150-ml labeled infusion bag or syringe
  - Short microdrip or macrodrip tubing set for piggyback (may have needleless system attachment)
  - Needleless device
  - Needles (21 or 23 gauge, only if stopcocks or other needleless methods are not available)
  - Stopcocks
  - Miniinfusion pump
  - Adhesive tape (optional)

- Antiseptic swab
- IV pole or rack
- MAR or computer printout
- **Volume-Control Administration Set**
  - Gloves (for connecting IV tubing)
  - Volutrol or Buretrol
  - Infusion tubing (may have needleless system attachment)
  - Syringe (5 to 20 ml)
  - Vial or ampule of ordered medication
  - Medication label
  - MAR or computer printout

STEPS	RATIONALE
1. Check prescriber's order to determine type of IV solution to be used, type of medication, dose, route, and time of administration.	Client's overall physical condition dictates type of IV solution used. Ensures safe and accurate medication administration.
2. Collect information necessary to administer medication safely, including action, purpose, side effects, normal dose, time of peak onset, and nursing implications.	Allows nurse to give medication safely and to monitor client's response to therapy.
3. Assess patency of client's existing IV infusion line by noting infusion rate of main IV line.	IV line must be patent and fluids must infuse easily for medication to reach venous circulation effectively.
4. Assess IV insertion site for signs of infiltration or phlebitis: redness, pallor, swelling, tenderness on palpation.	Confirmation of placement of IV needle or catheter and integrity of surrounding tissues ensures medication is administered safely.
5. Assess client's history of medication allergies.	Effects of medications can develop rapidly after IV infusion. Nurse should be aware of clients at risk.
6. Assemble supplies at bedside. Prepare client by informing client that medication will be given through IV equipment.	Medication preparation usually is not required. Nurse may assemble infusion tubing and bag of medication in medication room or client's room.
	Allows client to understand procedure and minimizes anxiety.
7. Wash hands and apply gloves.	Reduces transmission of infection. During handling of IV tubing there is some risk of blood exposure.
8. Check client's identification by looking at identification bracelet and asking client's name.	Ensures medication is administered to correct client.
9. Assess client's understanding of purpose of medication therapy.	May reveal need for education.
10. Explain purpose of medication and side effects to client and explain that medication is to be given through existing IV line. Encourage client to report symptoms of discomfort at site.	Keeps client informed of planned therapies.

11. Administer infusion:
  A. **Piggyback or tandem infusion**
    (1) Connect infusion tubing to medication bag (see Chapter 40). Allow solution to fill tubing by opening regulator flow clamp.

    Infusion tubing should be filled with solution and free of air bubbles to prevent air embolus.

    (2) Hang piggyback medication bag above level of primary fluid bag. (Hook may be used to lower main bag.) Hang tandem infusion at same level as primary fluid bag (see illustration).

    Height of fluid bag affects rate of flow to client.

    (3) Connect tubing of piggyback or tandem infusion to appropriate connector on primary infusion line:
      (a) *Stopcock:* Wipe off stopcock port with alcohol swab and connect tubing. Turn stopcock to open position.

      Stopcock eliminates need for needle.

      (b) *Needleless system:* Wipe off needleless port, and insert tip of piggyback or tandem infusion tubing (see illustrations).

      The CDC strongly recommends needleless connections to prevent accidental needle-stick injuries. Establishes route for IV medication to enter main IV line.

      (c) *Tubing port:* Connect sterile needle to end of piggyback or tandem infusion tubing, remove cap, cleanse injection port on main IV line, and insert needle through center of port.

      Prevents introduction of microorganisms during needle insertion.

    (4) Regulate flow rate of medication solution by adjusting regulator clamp. (Usually medication should infuse within 20 to 90 min.)

    Provides slow, intermittent infusion of medication in 20 to 90 min; maintains therapeutic blood levels.

    (5) After medication has infused, check flow regulator on primary infusion. Back-check valve on piggyback stops flow of the primary infusion until second medication infuses. The tandem and primary infusions flow together until the tandem set empties. The primary infusion should automatically begin to flow after the piggyback or tandem solution is empty.

    Valve prevents backup of medication into main infusion line. Checking flow rate ensures proper administration of IV fluids.

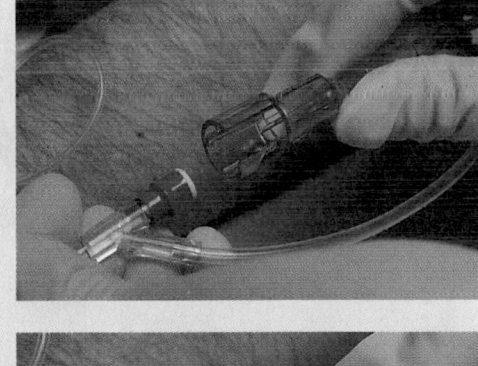

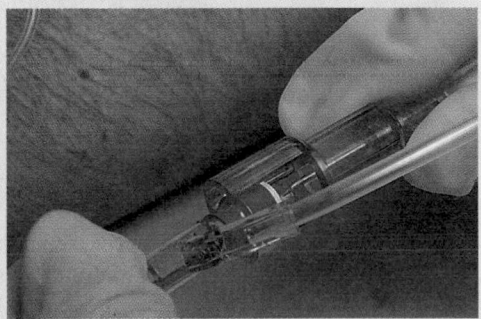

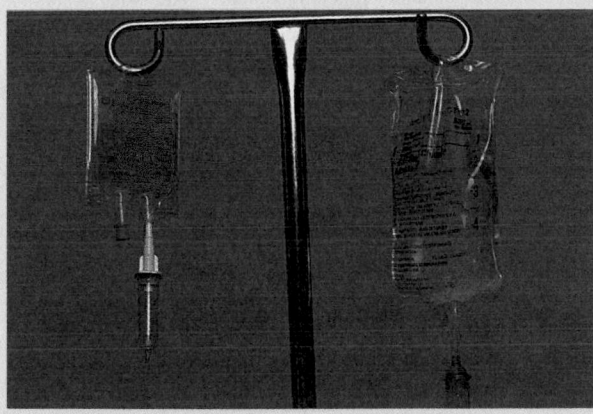

Step 11A(2)

Step 11A(3)(b)

STEPS	RATIONALE
(6) Regulate main infusion line to desired rate, if necessary.	Infusion of piggyback may interfere with the main line infusion rate.
(7) Leave secondary bag and tubing in place for future medication administration or discard in appropriate containers.	Establishment of secondary line produces route for microorganisms to enter main line. Repeated changes in tubing increase risk of infection transmission (check agency policy).
B. **Volume-control administration set (e.g., Volutrol)**	
(1) Assemble supplies in medication room.	Controls risk of contaminating IV solution.
(2) Prepare medication from vial or ampule (see Skill 34-7).	Ensures medication is sterile.
(3) Explain procedure to client. Encourage client to report symptoms of discomfort at site.	Keeps client informed of planned therapies.
(4) Fill Volutrol with desired amount of fluid (50 to 100 ml) by opening clamp between Volutrol and main IV bag (see illustration).	Small volume of fluid dilutes IV medication and reduces risk of too-rapid infusion.
(5) Close clamp and check to be sure clamp on air vent of Volutrol chamber is open.	Prevents additional leakage of fluid into Volutrol. Air vent allows fluid in Volutrol to exit at regulated rate.
(6) Clean injection port on top of Volutrol with antiseptic swab.	Prevents introduction of microorganisms during needle insertion.
(7) Remove needle cap or sheath and insert syringe needle through port, then inject medication (see illustration). Gently rotate Volutrol between hands.	Rotating mixes medication with solution in Volutrol to ensure equal distribution.
(8) Regulate IV infusion rate to allow medication to infuse in 30 to 90 min.	For optimal therapeutic effect, medication should infuse in prescribed time interval.

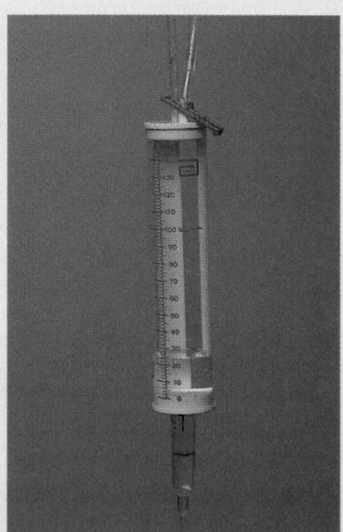

Step 11B(4)

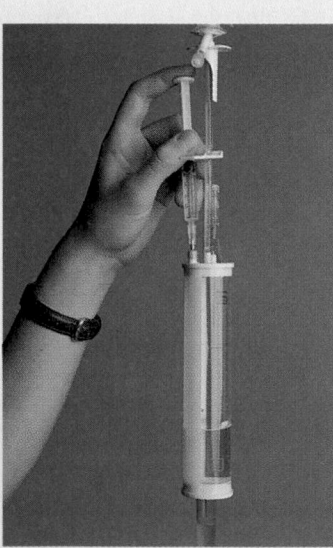

Step 11B(7)

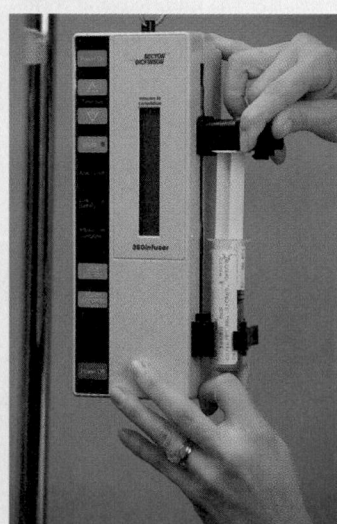

Step 11C(3)

STEPS	RATIONALE
(9) Label Volutrol with name of medication, dosage, total volume including diluent, and time of administration.	Alerts nurses to medication being infused. Prevents other medications from being added to Volutrol.
(10) Dispose of uncapped needle or needle enclosed in safety shield and syringe in proper container.	Prevents accidental needle sticks.

C. Miniinfusor administration

STEPS	RATIONALE
(1) Connect prefilled syringe to miniinfusion tubing.	Special tubing designed to fit syringe delivers medication to main IV line.
(2) Carefully apply pressure to syringe plunger, allowing tubing to fill with medication.	Ensures tubing is free of air bubbles to prevent air embolus.
(3) Place syringe into miniinfusor pump (follow product directions). Be sure syringe is secure (see illustration).	
(4) Connect miniinfusion tubing to main IV line.	
(a) *Stopcock:* Wipe off stopcock port with alcohol swab and connect tubing. Turn stopcock to open position.	Stopcock reduces risk of needle-stick injuries.
(b) *Needleless system:* Wipe off needleless port and insert tip of miniinfusor tubing.	Needleless system reduces risk of needle-stick injuries.
(c) *Tubing port:* Connect sterile needle to miniinfusion tubing, remove cap, cleanse injection port on main IV line, and insert needle through center of port.	Cleansing reduces transmission of microorganisms.
(5) Explain purpose of medication and side effects to client and explain that medication is to be given through existing IV line. Ask client to report symptoms of discomfort at site.	Informs client of planned therapies.
(6) Hang infusion pump with syringe on IV pole alongside main IV bag. Press button on pump to begin infusion. *Optional: Set alarm.*	Pump automatically delivers medication at safe, constant rate based on volume in syringe. (Alarm is used if medication is delivered into heparin/saline lock.)
(7) After medication has infused, check flow regulator on primary infusion. The infusion should automatically begin to flow once the pump stops. Regulate main infusion line to desired rate as needed. (NOTE: If stopcock is used, turn off miniinfusion line.)	Maintains patency of primary IV line.
(8) Remove disposable gloves. Wash hands.	Reduces transmission of infection.
12. Observe client for signs of adverse reactions.	IV medications act rapidly.
13. During 20 to 90 min of infusion, periodically check infusion rate and condition of IV site.	IV must remain patent for proper medication administration. Development of infiltration necessitates discontinuing infusion.
14. Ask client to explain purpose and side effects of medication.	Evaluates client's understanding of instruction.

Recording and Reporting

- Record medication, dose, route, and time administered on MAR or computer printout.
- Record volume of fluid in medication bag or Volutrol on intake and output form.
- Report any adverse reactions to nurse in charge or physician.

Home Care Considerations

- Ensure that all needles contaminated by blood are disposed of in puncture-resistant containers (e.g., coffee can).
- Piggyback tubing and intravenous container should be disposed of in nonpuncture container or according to agency policy.

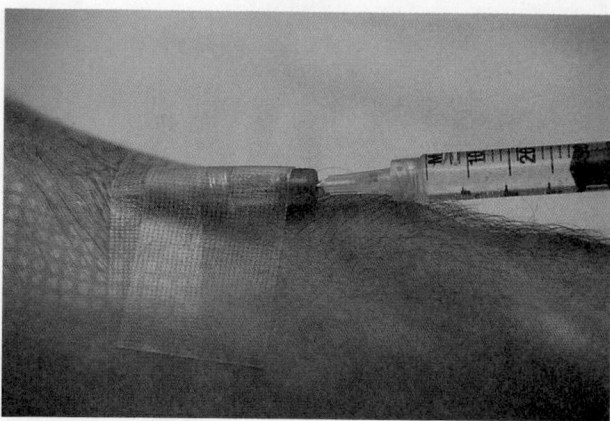

Figure 34-32 Intermittent lock covered with a rubber diaphragm. Requires a needle to flush.

ADMINISTRATION OF INTRAVENOUS THERAPY IN THE HOME

Sometimes clients may be discharged from an acute care setting and continue to receive intravenous therapy in the home setting. Medications such as antibiotics, chemotherapy, total parenteral nutrition, pain medications, and blood transfusions may be given in the home. Most clients who have home intravenous therapy will have a central venous catheter inserted prior to discharge (see Chapter 40). In addition, clients who need to receive intravenous therapy in the home have home care nurses who assist in the management of the intravenous therapy.

However, clients and their families need to be carefully assessed as to their ability to manage this therapy at home. There needs to be instruction on intravenous care management while the client is still in the hospital. Clients and families need to be taught how to recognize problems and what to do when these problems occur. It is important for the family to recognize signs of infection and complications and to know that when these occur the home care nurse or physician must be notified. In addition, clients and their families need information regarding maintenance of intravenous administration equipment, including the infusion pump.

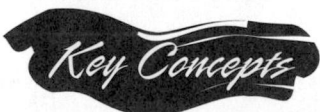

Key Concepts

- Learning medication classifications improves understanding of nursing implications for administering medications with similar characteristics.
- Federal medication legislation regulates the production, distribution, prescription, and administration of medications.
- All controlled substances are handled according to strict procedures that account for each medication.
- The nurse applies understanding of the physiology of medication action when timing administration, selecting routes, initiating actions to promote medication efficacy, and observing responses to medications.
- The older adult's body undergoes structural and functional changes that alter medication actions and influence the manner in which nurses provide medication therapy.
- Children's medication doses are computed on the basis of body surface area or weight.
- Medications given parenterally are absorbed more quickly than medications administered by other routes.
- Each medication order should include the client's name, the order date, the medication name, dosage,

route and time of administration, and the prescriber's signature.
- A medication history reveals allergies, medications a client is taking, and the client's compliance with therapy.
- The nursing process should be used when administering medication.
- The five rights of medication administration ensure accurate preparation and administration of medication doses.
- The five rights of medications administration are the right medication, right dose, right client, right route, right time.
- Nurses administer only medications they prepare, and prepared medications are never left unattended.
- Medications should be charted immediately after administration.
- A nurse uses clinical judgment in determining the best time to administer prn medications.
- The nurse reports a medication error immediately.
- When preparing medications, the nurse checks the medication container label against the medication administration record or computer printout 3 times.

- Air locks prevent tracking of medication through subcutaneous tissues and localize the medication in muscle tissue.
- The Z-track method for intramuscular injections protects subcutaneous tissues from irritating parenteral fluids.
- Failure to select injection sites by anatomical landmarks may lead to tissue, bone, or nerve damage.

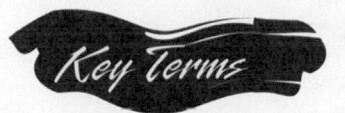

Key Terms

Absorption, *p. 889*
Adverse effects, *p. 891*
Anaphylactic reactions, *p. 891*
Biotransformation, *p. 890*
Buccal, *p. 893*
Concentration, *p. 892*
Detoxify, *p. 890*
Idiosyncratic reaction, *p. 891*
Infusion, *p. 892*
Inhalation, *p. 896*
Injection, *p. 889*
Instillation, *p. 896*
Intraarticular, *p. 895*
Intracardiac, *p. 895*
Intradermal (ID), *p. 895*
Intramuscular (IM), *p. 895*
Intraocular, *p. 917*
Intravenous (IV), *p. 895*
Irrigation, *p. 897*
Medication allergy, *p. 891*
Medication error, *p. 902*
Medication interaction, *p. 892*

Metered dose inhaler (MDI), *p. 927*
Metric system, *p. 896*
Narcotics, *p. 901*
Nurse Practice Acts, *p. 887*
Ophthalmic, *p. 917*
Parenteral administration, *p. 895*
Peak, *p. 892*
Pharmacokinetics, *p. 889*
Polypharmacy, *p. 909*
Prescriptions, *p. 900*
Serum half-life, *p. 892*
Side effects, *p. 891*
Solution, *p. 897*
Subcutaneous (SQ), *p. 895*
Sublingual, *p. 893*
Synergistic effect, *p. 892*
Therapeutic effects, *p. 891*
Toxic effects, *p. 891*
Transdermal disk, *p. 896*
Verbal order, *p. 899*
Z-track method, *p. 947*

Critical Thinking Exercises

1. You are the nurse in charge of a medical unit. A new nurse tells you that there are too many medications to administer to the clients under her care and that she would never be able to administer all of the medications on time. As the charge nurse on this unit, how would you intervene in this situation? What would you tell this new nurse?

2. You are preparing to administer an anticoagulant medication (Coumadin) to a client. When you review the medication with the client, he tells you that the color of the "blood thinner" (Coumadin) does not look like the one he takes at home. How would you respond to this client?

3. You receive a computerized medical order for a medication with which you are very familiar. However, it does not seem clear to you why this medication was ordered for your patient as she does not have a condition for which this medication is commonly used. How would you proceed in this case?

4. Your client is receiving insulin at home and has run out of syringes. You have some 1-ml tuberculin syringes on hand. The client needs to receive 18 units of NPH and 4 units of regular insulin. How would you draw this up? How many tenths of a milliliter of each insulin would you draw up?

References

Abdoo YM: Designing a patient care medication and recording system that uses bar code technology, *Comput Nurs* 10(3):116, 1992.

American Pharmaceutical Association: Summary of the final report of the scope of pharmacy practice project, *Am J Hosp Pharm* 51:2179, 1994.

Behrman RE, Vaughan VC, editors: *Nelson textbook of pediatrics,* ed 13, Philadelphia, 1987, WB Saunders; modified from data of Boyd E, by West CD.

Benner P: *From novice to expert: excellence in clinical nursing practice,* Redwood City, Calif, 1984, Addison-Wesley.

Beyea SC, Nicoll LH: Administration of medication via the intramuscular route: an integrative review of the literature and research-based protocol for the procedure. *Apple Nurse Res* 8(1):23, 1995.

Beyea SC, Nicoll LH: Back to basics: administering IM injections the right way, *Am J Nurs* 96(1):34, 1996.

Buckley T, Dudley S, Donowitz L: Defining unnecessary disinfection procedures for single-dose and multiple dose vials, *Am J Crit Care* 3(6):448, 1994.

Clark JF, Queener SF, Karb VB: *Pharmacologic basis of nursing practice,* ed 6, St. Louis, 1998, Mosby.

Ebersole P, Hess P: *Toward healthy aging: human needs and nursing response,* ed 5, St. Louis, 1998, Mosby.

Edgar TA, Lee DS, Cousins DD: Experience with a national medication error reporting program, *Am J Hosp Pharm* 51:1335, 1994.

Jagger J: *Preventable needlesticks, preventable HIV infection, preventable deaths among health care workers.* Testimony before Rep. Ron Wyden Hearings in Washington, DC, 1992.

Mafofsky D, Cone JE: *Infection Control Hosp Epidemol* 14(3):140, 1993.

Martin M, Mehery D: Intrapleural analgesia: a new technique, *Crit Care Nurs* 14(5):31, 1994.

New Jersey Department of Law and Public Safety, Division of Consumer Affairs: Statutes (N.J.S.A. 45:11-23 et seq.) and Regulations (N.J.A.C. 13:37) Board of Nursing, 1995.

Owens-Schwab E, Fraser VJ: Needles and needle protection devices; a second look at efficacy and selection, *Infect Control Hosp Epidemiol* 14(11):657, 1993.

Perini V, Vermeulen LC: Comparison of automated medication-management systems, *Am J Hosp Pharm* 51:1883, 1994.

Shoaf J, Oliver S: Efficacy of normal saline injection with and without heparin for maintaining intermittent intravenous site, *Appl Nurs Res* 5(1):9, 1992.

Statz E: Hand strength and metered dose inhalers, *Am J Nurs* 84:80, 1984.

Weixler D: Correcting metered-dose inhaler misuse, *Nursing* 24(7):62, 1994.

White JR, Campbell RK. In Haire-Joshu D, editor: *Management of diabetes mellitus: perspectives of care across the life span,* ed 2, St. Louis, 1996, Mosby.

Wild L, Coyne C: Basics and beyond: epidural analgesia, *AJN,* 92(4)26, 1992.

Wong DL: *Whaley and Wong's nursing care of infants and children,* ed 5, St. Louis, 1998, Mosby.

35

Complementary and Alternative Therapies

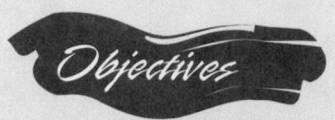

Objectives

Mastery of content in this chapter will enable the student to:

- Define the key terms listed.
- Differentiate between complementary and alternative therapies.
- Describe the clinical applications of relaxation therapies.
- Discuss the relaxation response and its effect on somatic ailments.
- Describe the purpose and principles of biofeedback.
- Identify the principles and effectiveness of imagery, meditation, and hypnotherapy.
- Describe the methods of and the psychophysiologic responses to therapeutic touch.
- Explain the scope of practice of chiropractic therapy.
- Discuss the principles and applications of acupuncture.
- Describe safe and unsafe herbal therapies.

The general health of North American people has steadily improved over the course of the last century as evidenced by lower mortality rates and increased life expectancies. Changes in science and medicine have provided the knowledge and technology that have successfully altered the course of many illnesses. Despite the success of **allopathic medicine** (traditional Western medicine), many conditions such as arthritis, chronic back pain, gastrointestinal problems, allergies, headache, and insomnia have been difficult to treat, and more clients are exploring alternative methods to relieve their symptom distress (Eisenberg and others, 1993). It is estimated that up to 75% of clients seek care from their primary care practitioners for stress, pain, and health conditions for which there are no known causes or cures (Taylor, Lee, and Young, 1997). While allopathic medicine is quite effective in treating numerous physical ailments (e.g., bacterial infections, structural abnormalities, acute emergencies), it is in general less effective in preventing disease, decreasing stress-induced illnesses, managing chronic disease, and caring for the emotional and spiritual needs of individuals.

The number of clients seeking unconventional treatments has risen considerably. In part this increase is due to (1) the perception that the treatments offered by the medical profession do not provide relief for a variety of common illnesses, (2) the increasing interest of clients in becoming more educated about their health and the need to take a more active role in their treatment, and (3) the increased number of articles in journals (Alternative Medicine, 1992) such as *Annals of Behavioral Medicine, Alternative Therapies in Health and Medicine,* and the *Journal of Alternative and Complementary Medicine,* (4) programs seen on television such as Bill Moyers's "Healing and the Mind (Alternative Medicine, 1992)," and (5) the attraction to a holistic approach to health care that

incorporates the mind, body, and spirit (Astin and others, 1999).

Unconventional therapies are frequently referred to as either complementary or alternative medicine (CAM) therapies. **Complementary therapies** are those therapies used in addition to conventional treatment recommended by the person's health care provider. As the name implies, complementary therapies complement the conventional treatment. Many of the complementary therapies such as acupuncture contain diagnostic and therapeutic methods specific to their field, whereas others such as guided imagery are clearly adjunctive in nature. Complementary therapies include relaxation, exercise, massage (Figure 35-1), reflexology, prayer, biofeedback, hypnotherapy, shamanism, creative therapies including art, music, or dance therapy (Figure 35-2), acupuncture and Chinese medicine, Ayurveda and Unani medicine, meditation, chiropractic therapy, osteopathy, herbalism, and homeopathy (Fulder, 1998).

Alternative therapies, on the other hand, may include the same interventions as complementary therapies but frequently become the primary treatment modality that replaces allopathic medical care. Both complementary and alternative therapies vary in the degree to which they are compatible with allopathic medicine. For example, chiropractic and Feldenkrais practitioners frequently use diagnostic terminology and methods similar to those utilized by allopathic practitioners. They base interventions on conventional pathophysiology, anatomy, and kinesiology but at the same time, explore mind-body connections that

---

Content contained in this chapter has been previously published in Caudell KA: Complementary and alternative therapies. In Lewis SM, Heitkemper MM, editors: *Medical-surgical nursing: assessment and management of clinical problems,* ed 5, St. Louis, 2000, Mosby.

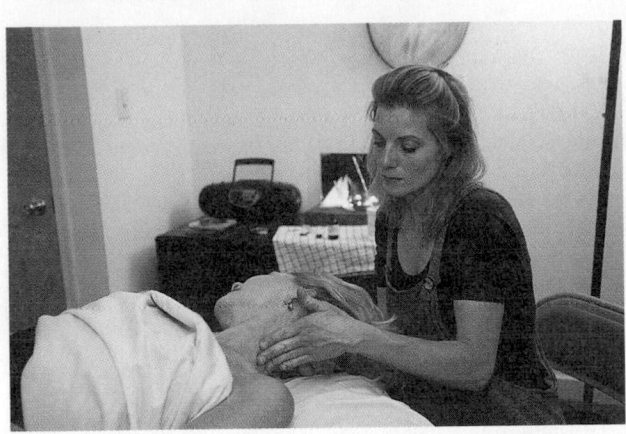

Figure 35-1 Massage therapy can be effectively used to relieve tension.

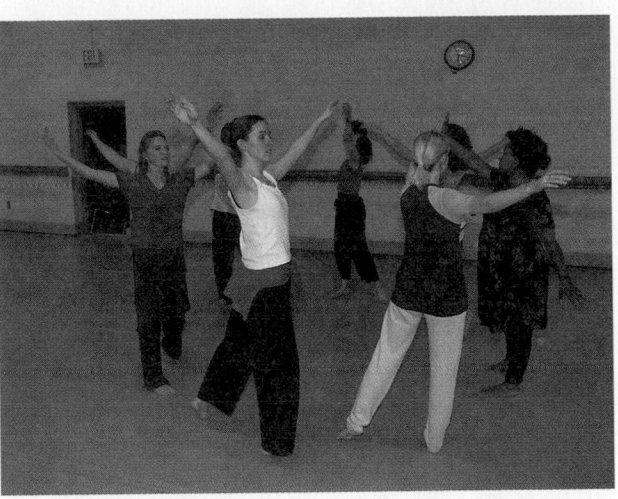

Figure 35-2 Young adults participating in dance therapy.

may drive the physiological condition (Fulder, 1998). Some alternative therapies are not supported by scientific data, such as shark cartilage and coffee enemas. Types of complementary and alternative therapies are presented in Table 35-1.

Between one third and one half of the population in the United States uses one or more forms of CAM (Taylor, Lee, and Young, 1997). Furthermore, extrapolations of data from a recent survey suggest a 47.3% increase in the number of visits to alternative medicine practitioners. This exceeds the number of visits to allopathic practitioners (Eisenberg and others, 1998). Between 1986 and 1991 there was a 70% increase in people in the United Kingdom using complementary medicine, and similar increases have been observed in Holland and France (Alternative Medicine, 1992). Because of this increased interest and use of CAM, many institutions, including some mainstream medical schools, are establishing training programs that incorporate CAM philosophy and content into the curriculum. As of July, 1998, 100 educational programs or courses in complementary and alternative medicine were available for physicians at 65 universities in the United States (Bhattacharya, 1998). **Integrative medical programs** are being developed that allow health care consumers the opportunity to be treated by a team of providers consisting of both allopathic and complementary practitioners. Furthermore, an increasing number of insurance companies are now covering costs for certain types of CAM therapies such as herbal therapy, biofeedback, chiropractic medicine, megavitamin therapy, and acupuncture (Taylor, Lee, and Young, 1997). However, this increase in insurance coverage is not proportionate to the increases in CAM therapy utilization. Many clients continue to pay out-of-pocket for a number of these therapies, including the more conventional therapies such as chiropractic and acupuncture. This may explain why the demographic characteristics of persons seeking CAM therapies typically include those who are professional, well educated, and from a higher socioeconomic standing.

The interest in CAM is also evident in the increased number of articles about it in respected medical journals and the development of several journals that specifically focus on complementary and alternative medicine. The Office of Alternative Medicine (now the National Center for Complementary and Alternative Medicine) was established in 1992 as a part of the National Institutes of Health (Alternative Medicine, 1992). The goals of this office are to facilitate the evaluation of alternative medical treatment modalities, specifically acting as a clearinghouse to disseminate information to the public, media, and professionals and supporting, coordinating, and conducting research and research training in the area of alternative medicine (Alternative Medicine, 1992).

This chapter will discuss several types of complementary and alternative medicine therapies. The therapies are organized into the biobehavioral therapies, which include relaxation therapy, imagery, biofeedback, hypnotherapy, and meditation; manual therapies, which include therapeutic touch and chiropractic therapy; traditional and ethnomedicine therapies, which include traditional Chinese medicine; and herbal therapies. A description, clinical applications, and limitations of each therapy will be presented.

Biobehavioral Therapies

Biobehavioral therapy is designed to teach individuals ways in which to change their behavior to alter physical responses to stress and improve symptoms such as muscle tension, gastrointestinal discomfort, pain, or sleep disturbances. One of the principles of biobehavioral therapy is that the individual becomes actively involved in the treatment. Individuals achieve better responses if they practice

Table 35-1   Complementary and Alternative Therapies

Types	Definitions
Traditional and Ethnomedicine Therapies	
Acupuncture	A traditional Chinese method of producing analgesia or altering the function of a body system by inserting thin needles along a series of lines or channels, called meridians. Direct needle manipulation of energetic meridians influences deeper internal organs.
Ayurveda	Traditional Hindu system of medicine practiced in India since the first century AD. Combination of remedies such as herbs, purgative, and rubbing oils used in treating disease.
Homeopathic medicine	System of medical treatments based on the theory that certain diseases can be cured by giving small doses of drugs that in a healthy person would produce symptoms like those of the disease. Remedies or medicines are made from naturally occurring plant, animal, or mineral substances.
Latin American practices	*Curanderismo* medical system that includes a humoral model for classifying food, activity, drugs, and illnesses and a series of folk illnesses.
Native American practices	Therapies include sweating and purging, herbal remedies, and shamanic healing (healer makes contact with spirits to ask their direction in bringing healing to people).
Naturopathic medicine	System of therapeutics based on natural foods, light, warmth, massage, fresh air, regular exercise, and avoidance of medications. Recognition of inherent healing ability of the body. Treatments integrate traditional natural therapies with modern diagnostic science; includes botanical medicine.
Traditional Chinese (Oriental) medicine	Set of systematic techniques and methods including acupuncture, herbal medicines, massage, acupressure, moxibustion, Qigong, and oriental massage. Fundamental concepts embedded in Taoism, Confucianism, and Buddhism.
Bioelectromagnetic Applications	
Electroacupuncture	Electrical stimulation via acupuncture needles to enhance or replace manual needles. Technique has been used to treat chemotherapy-induced symptom distress, renal colic, postoperative pain, and induce uterine contractions in postterm pregnancy.
Electromagnetic fields	Use of relatively large levels of electrical and magnetic energy. Therapy used to promote healing of bone fractures and for nerve stimulation, wound healing, treatment of osteoarthritis, tissue regeneration, immune system stimulation, and neuroendocrine modulation.
Diet Therapies	
Gerson therapy	Integrated set of treatments that includes primarily raw vegetables and fruit; salt, fat, and protein restriction; potassium and thyroid supplementation; and coffee enemas.
Kelly regimen	Dietary program that includes carrot juice, vegetarian diet, coffee enemas, and pancreatic enzymes. Used in cancer treatment.
Macrobiotic diet	Predominantly a vegan diet (no animal products except fish). Initially used in the management of a variety of cancers. Emphasis placed on whole cereal grains, vegetables, and unprocessed foods.
Orthomolecular medicine (megavitamin)	Increased intake of nutrients such as vitamin C and beta-carotene. Diet used in treatment of cancer, schizophrenia, and certain chronic diseases such as hypercholesterolemia and coronary artery disease.
Herbal Medicine	
European phytomedicines	Products developed under strict quality control in sophisticated pharmaceutical factories, packaged professionally in tablets or capsules. Examples of well-studied herbal medicines include gingko biloba, milk thistle, and bilberry. Herbs have a wide variety of uses (see Table 35-8).

Table 35-1   Complementary and Alternative Therapies—cont'd

Types	Definitions
Herbal Medicine—cont'd	
Traditional Chinese herbal remedies	Over 50,000 medicinal plant species, many of which have been studied extensively. Herbs considered the backbone of medicine. Examples include *Panax ginseng* (ginseng root) for treatment of asthma and stomach disorders, lowering stress, reducing hypoxia, improving cardiac performance, and inhibiting platelet aggregation; fresh ginger rhizome for treatment of acute dysentery and acute orchitis; Chinese foxglove root for treatment of hepatitis and rheumatoid arthritis.
Ayurvedic herbs	Herbs used for over 2000 years. Examples include *Eclipta alba* for the treatment of liver cirrhosis and infectious hepatitis; *Commophora mukul* for reducing serum cholesterol; *Picrorhiza kurroa* for fever and dyspepsia; and *Curcuma longa* (tumeric) for healing chronic ulcers and scabies.
Manual Healing Therapies	
Acupressure	Therapeutic technique of applying digital pressure in a specified way on designated points on the body to relieve pain, produce analgesia, or regulate a body function.
Chiropractic medicine	System of therapy based on establishment of good self-image through awareness and correction of body movements. Application of the knowledge of the relationship between structure and function to diagnose and treat structural dysfunctions that affect the nervous system. Treatment frequently involves manipulation of the spinal column and may also include physiotherapy and diet therapy.
Feldenkrais method	Alternative therapy based on establishment of good self-image through awareness and correction of body movements. Technique integrates the understanding of the physics of the body's movement patterns with an awareness of the way people learn to move, behave, and interact.
Qigong	Technique that incorporates breath, movement, and meditation to cleanse, strengthen, and circulate vital life energy and blood. Therapy used to stimulate immune system and maintain external and internal balance.
Massage therapy	Manipulation of soft tissue through stroking, rubbing, or kneading to increase circulation, improve muscle tone, and relax client.
Osteopathy	Therapeutic approach that uses all forms of medical diagnosis and therapy but places greater emphasis on the influence of the relationship between the organs and musculoskeletal system than conventional medicine.
Reiki therapy	Therapy derived from ancient Buddhist practices in which practitioner places hands on or above a body area and transfers "universal life energy" to the patient. This energy provides strength, harmony, and balance to treat health disturbances.
Rolfing (structural integration)	Technique of deep massage intended to realign the body by altering the length and tone of myofascial tissue. Basis of practice is the belief that misalignment of myofascial tissue may have detrimental effect on person's energy level, self-image, muscular efficiency, and general health.
Biobehavioral Therapies	
Art therapy	Use of art to reconcile emotional conflicts, foster self-awareness, and express clients' unspoken and frequently unconscious concerns about their disease.
Biofeedback	A process providing a person with visual or auditory information about autonomic physiologic functions of the body, such as muscle tension, skin temperature, and brain wave activity, through the use of instruments. Used for treatment of anxiety disorders, Raynaud's disease, hypertension, and temporomandibular joint dysfunction.
Dance therapy	Intimate and powerful medium for therapy because it is a direct expression of the mind and body. Therapy used to treat persons with social, emotional, cognitive, or physical problems.

Continued

Table 35-1	**Complementary and Alternative Therapies**—cont'd
Types	Definitions
Biobehavioral Therapies—cont'd	
Imagery	Formation of mental concepts, figures, and ideas applied therapeutically to decrease anxiety. Mental process and a variety of procedures to encourage changes in attitudes, behavior, or physiologic reactions.
Guided imagery	Therapeutic technique used for relieving pain on discomfort in which the person is encouraged to concentrate on an image that helps relieve pain or discomfort.
Hypnotherapy	Induction of trance states and therapeutic suggestion for treatment of paralysis, headaches, joint pains, addictions, pain control, and phobias.
Meditation	Self-directed practice for relaxing the body and calming the mind. State of consciousness in which individual eliminates environmental stimuli from awareness, producing a state of relaxation and stress relief.
Music therapy	Use of music to address physical, psychological, cognitive, and social needs of individuals with disabilities and illnesses. Therapy used to improve physical movement for people with impaired movement, improve communication in people with communication disorders, develop emotional expression for people with mental health problems, evoke memories for persons with memory impairment, and distract people who are in pain or having painful treatments or chemotherapy.
Prayer therapies	Variety of techniques used in multiple cultures that incorporate caring, compassion, love, or empathy with the target of prayer.
Psychotherapy	Treatment of emotional and mental disorders by psychological techniques.
Relaxation techniques	Variety of techniques that may be used to elicit the relaxation response, a protective mechanism against stress that decreases heart rate, lowers metabolism, decreases respiratory rate, and decreases muscle tension.
Yoga	Discipline that focuses on the body's musculature, posture, breathing mechanisms, and consciousness. Goal of yoga is attainment of physical and mental well-being through mastery of body achieved through exercise, holding of postures, proper breathing, and meditation.
Pharmacological and Biological Treatments	
Antioxidizing agents	Use of vitamins A, E, and beta-carotene to treat and prevent a variety of disorders.
Cartilage products	Cartilage preparations from a variety of animals and fish used to treat several skin disorders, accelerate wound healing, and provide antiinflammatory effect.
Chelation therapy	Use of ethylenediaminetetraacetic acid to remove toxic metals and substances from the body.

the techniques or exercises daily. Another major principle in biobehavioral therapy is that the individual commits to implementing and maintaining the therapy until a desired outcome is achieved. Types of biobehavioral therapies include relaxation, imagery, biofeedback, hypnosis, and meditation (Table 35-1).

RELAXATION THERAPY

People are exposed to stressful situations in everyday life that evoke the **stress response.** A basic core of integrated neuroendocrine processes that support the fight-or-flight response occurs when an individual is exposed to an acute stressor. These responses are initiated in the hypothalamus during which the hypothalamic efferent neurons stimulate the adrenal medulla to secrete catecholamines and the sympathetic postganglionic neurons to secrete norepinephrine.

At the same time, neurosecretory cells discharge neuropeptides such as corticotropin-releasing factor (CRF), which travel via the hypophyseal portal system to the anterior pituitary, where they modulate the release of pituitary hormones such as adrenocorticotropic hormone (ACTH). These hormones then affect the activity of other organs. For example, ACTH stimulates the adrenal cortex to secrete cortisol and other related hormones (Carlson, 1994).

Chronic stress, on the other hand, has been defined as "demands, threats, perceived harm or loss, or responses that persist for long periods of time" (Baum, 1990). Responses to chronic stressors frequently are different than those to acute stressors in that the response is more subdued. Pulse rates and blood pressure tend to be lower. Individuals may eventually habituate to the stressor and adapt by suppressing their responses.

Others suggest that individuals may not adapt to chronic stressors. Individuals may experience continued muscle tension. If the person does not learn how to reduce the muscle tension, a condition of chronic overtension and continued hyperactivity of the autonomic nervous system may occur, leading to pathophysiological changes in the endocrine, cardiovascular, and immune systems (Miller, 1989; Rabin and others, 1994).

Relaxation is the state of generalized decreased cognitive, physiological, and/or behavioral arousal. Relaxation is also defined as arousal reduction. The process of relaxation elongates the muscle fibers, reduces the neural impulses sent to the brain, and thus decreases the activity of brain as well as other body systems. The relaxation response is characterized by decreased heart and respiratory rates, blood pressure, oxygen consumption, and increased alpha brain activity and peripheral skin temperature. The relaxation response can be obtained through a variety of techniques that incorporate a repetitive mental focus and the adoption of a calm, peaceful attitude (Benson, Beary, and Carol, 1974). Teaching strategies for relaxation exercises are listed in Box 35-1.

Relaxation involves the cognitive skills that people develop during relaxation training that help them reduce the negative ways in which they respond to situations within their environment. The cognitive skills include focusing (the ability to identify, differentiate, maintain attention on, and return attention to simple stimuli for an extended period), passivity (the ability to stop unnecessary goal-directed and analytic activity), and receptivity (the ability to tolerate and accept experiences that may be uncertain, unfamiliar, or paradoxical) (Smith and others, 1996). In addition, the individual experiences cognitive restructuring during which negative thoughts are replaced with positive ones (Syrjala and others, 1995). The long-term goal of relaxation therapy is for the person to continually monitor himself or herself for indicators of tension and to consciously let go and release the tension contained in various body parts.

Progressive relaxation training helps to teach the individual how to effectively rest and reduce tension in the body. One initially learns to detect subtle localized sensations of muscle tension in one muscle group (e.g., the forearm muscle). Using the method of diminishing tensions, the individual learns to differentiate between high-intensity tension (strong fist clenching) and very subtle tension (Good, 1996). This activity is then practiced using multiple muscle groups. One active progressive relaxation technique involves the use of slow, deep abdominal breathing while tightening and relaxing an ordered succession of muscle groups. The practitioner may elect to begin with the muscles in the face, followed by those in the arms, hands, abdomen, legs, and feet.

Another important component of progressive relaxation is reducing cognitive or mental activity by having the person focus on muscle contraction and relaxation. If cognitive activities correspond with muscle activity (and energy expenditure), then by reducing the muscle tension through relaxation techniques, positive cognitive activities and emotions can be increased (Snyder, 1998).

Passive relaxation involves teaching the individual to relax individual muscle groups passively (i.e., without actively contracting the muscles). One passive relaxation technique incorporates slow, abdominal breathing exercises in addition to the person imagining warmth and relaxation flowing through specific muscle groups while letting go of muscle tension during expiration. Passive relaxation is useful for persons for whom the effort and energy expenditure of active muscle contracting leads to discomfort or exhaustion.

Clinical Applications of Relaxation Therapy.

Relaxation techniques are effective in lowering heart rate and blood pressure, decreasing muscle tension, improving well-being, and reducing symptom distress in persons experiencing a variety of situations (e.g., complications from medical treatment or disease, grieving the loss of a significant other). The type of relaxation intervention should be matched to the individual's functional status, the energy expenditure of the relaxation technique, and the motivation of the individual for frequent practice.

Relaxation, alone or in combination with deep breathing, imagery, yoga (Figure 35-3), and music has been shown to reduce pain (Syrjala and others, 1995), including headache, postoperative pain, labor, and chronic low back pain (Syrjala and others, 1995; Good, 1996; Snyder, 1998); improve emotional well-being (McCain and others, 1996) and immune function (Houlding, McCarkle, and Lowery, 1993; Van Rood and others, 1993) reduce heart rate and blood pressure; and reduce cancer treatment-related nausea and vomiting in a number of client populations (Burish and others, 1987; Carey and Burish, 1987; Burish, Snyder, and Jenkins, 1991; Holland and others, 1991).

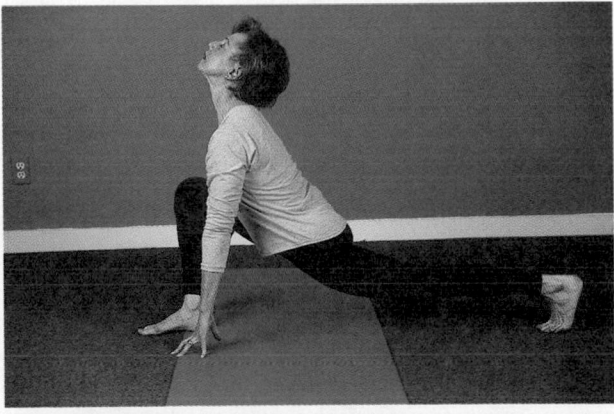

Figure 35-3 Yoga is a discipline that focuses on muscles, posture, breathing, and consciousness.

Relaxation Strategies   Box 35-1

RHYTHMIC BREATHING*
1. Provide a quiet environment.
2. Help the client get comfortable by elevating the legs with the knees bent (relaxing the leg, back, and abdominal muscles)
3. Instruct the client to close eyes and to breathe in and out slowly, saying, "Breathe in, 2, 3, 4; breath out, 2, 3, 4."
4. Once rhythmic breathing is established, instruct client to listen to your voice, and with a low and steady voice, instruct client to do the following:

    Breathe in and out slowly and deeply.

    Try to breathe from the abdomen.

    Feel more relaxed with each exhalation.

    Try to identify your own special feeling of relaxation (e.g., light and weightless or very heavy).

    While you are breathing, let your imagination take you to a place you remember as peaceful and pleasant; look around, listen to the sounds, feel the air, notice the smells.

    When you are ready to end this relaxation exercise, count silently from 1 to 3; on 1, move your lower body; on 2, move your upper body; on 3, breathe in deeply, open your eyes, and while breathing out slowly, say silently, "I am relaxed and alert." Stretch as if just waking up.

PROGRESSIVE RELAXATION
1. Follow steps 1, 2, and 3 of rhythmic breathing.
2. Once the client is breathing slowly and comfortably, instruct client to tighten and relax an ordered succession of muscle groups, tensing them and then relaxing them, while feeling each part relax.
3. Instruct client to tense and then relax the calves, knees, and so on.

RELAXATION BY SENSORY PACING
1. Follow steps 1 and 2 of rhythmic breathing.
2. Instruct client to slowly repeat and finish either in a low voice or to self each of the following sentences:

    Now I am aware of seeing . . .

    Now I am aware of feeling . . .

    Now I am aware of hearing . . .

    Instruct client to repeat and complete each sentence 4 times, then 3 times, then twice, and finally once.
3. Instruct client to allow the eyes to close when they feel heavy.

RELAXATION BY COLOR EXCHANGE
1. Follow steps 1, 2, and 3 of rhythmic breathing.
2. Instruct client to notice any tension, tightness, aches, or pains in the body and to give that sensation the first color that comes to mind.
3. Instruct client to breathe in pure white light from the universe and send the light to the tense or painful place in the body, letting the white light surround the color of the discomfort.
4. Instruct client to exhale the color of the discomfort and let the white light take its place.
5. Instruct client to continue breathing in the white light and exhaling the color of the discomfort, allowing the white light to fill the entire body and bring about a sense of peace, well-being, and energy.

MODIFIED AUTOGENIC RELAXATION
1. Follow steps 1, 2, and 3 of rhythmic breathing.
2. Instruct client to repeat each of the following phrases to self 4 times, saying the first part of the phrases while breathing in for 2 to 3 seconds, holding the breath for 2 to 3 seconds, then saying the last part of the phrases while breathing out for 2 to 3 seconds:

Breathing in	Breathing out
I am	relaxed.
My arm and legs	are heavy and warm.
My heartbeat	is calm and regular.
My breathing	is free and easy.
My abdomen	is loose and warm.
My forehead	is cool.
My mind	is quiet and still.

RELAXING WITH MUSIC
1. Provide client with a tape recorder and headset.
2. Ask client to select a favorite cassette of slow, quiet music.
3. Instruct client to get into a comfortable position (either sitting or lying down but with arms and legs uncrossed) and to close eyes and listen to the music through the headset.
4. Instruct client to imagine floating or drifting with the music while listening.

*In conditioning of a relaxation response, a "signal breath" involving deep inhalation through the nose and forceful exhalation through the mouth is the key. The signal breath precedes and follows each run through the exercise.

More well-controlled studies are needed to validate the effects of relaxation therapy. For example, other variables or activities that may also lead to reduced physiological activity and pain level should be controlled in studies to determine if the improved response is due to the relaxation therapy alone. Such variables may include a healthy support network, a positive attitude including humor, and other behavioral therapies such as yoga and tai chi.

Relaxation is a very valuable technique because it enables individuals to exert some control over their lives. Persons may experience a decreased feeling of helplessness and a more positive psychological state overall, which helps them to have a less negative view of their situation.

Limitations of Relaxation Therapy. Individuals undergoing relaxation training have reported fearing loss of control, feeling like they are floating, and experiencing relaxation-induced anxiety related to these feelings. During relaxation training, individuals are taught to differentiate between low and high levels of muscle tension. During the first months of training sessions, when the person is learning how to focus on body sensations and tensions, there have been reports of increased sensitivity in detecting muscle tension. Usually these feelings are minor and resolve as the person continues with the relaxation training (McGuigan, 1993). However, nurses must be aware that on occasion some relaxation techniques may result in continued intensification of symptoms or the development of altogether new symptoms (Carlson and Nitz, 1991).

Another physiological event that occasionally occurs early in relaxation training is the "predormescent start," in which the trunk and limbs of the individual jerk during the process of falling asleep. This muscle spasm is seen in people who have been very tense during the day or who are experiencing major traumatic events. It will usually disappear as the relaxation training progresses (Carlson and Nitz, 1991).

An important consideration when choosing the type of relaxation technique is the physiological and psychological status of the individual. Clients with advanced disease such as cancer may seek relaxation training to reduce their stress response. However, techniques such as active progressive relaxation training require a moderate expenditure of energy, which can amplify a person's existing fatigue and limit the person's ability to complete individual relaxation sessions and practice. Therefore, active progressive relaxation would not be appropriate for clients with advanced disease or those who have decreased energy reserves. Passive relaxation or guided imagery is more appropriate for these individuals (Lewith, Kenyon, and Lewis, 1996).

Regularly practiced progressive muscle relaxation resulting in a prolonged increased relaxed state has also been found to potentiate the effects of some medications, leading to toxic levels. A lowered dose of the medication may be necessary (Snyder, 1998).

IMAGERY

Imagery or visualization techniques use the conscious mind to create mental images to evoke physical changes in the body, improve perceived well-being, and/or enhance self-awareness. Frequently imagery is combined with some form of relaxation training to facilitate the effect of the relaxation technique. Imagery can be self-directed, in which the individuals create their own mental images, or can be guided, during which a practitioner leads the individual through a particular scenario (Lewith, Kenyon, and Lewis, 1996; Post-White, 1998). For example, the client may be directed to begin slow, abdominal breathing while focusing on the rhythm of breathing. The client is then instructed to visualize ocean waves coming to shore with

each inspiration, then receding with each expiration. Next the client is instructed to take notice of the smells, sounds, and temperatures that he or she is experiencing. As the imagery session progresses, the client may be instructed to visualize warmth entering the body during inspiration and tension leaving the body during expiration. Imagery scenarios should be individualized for each client and/or left up to the client to develop.

Imagery can evoke powerful psychophysiological responses such as alterations in immune function (Norris and Fahrion, 1993). Many imagery techniques involve visual imagery, but they can also include the auditory, proprioceptive, gustatory, and olfactory senses. An example of this involves visualizing a lemon being sliced in half and squeezing the lemon juice under the tongue. This visualization has been observed to produce increased salivation as effectively as the actual event. People typically respond to their environment according to the way they perceive it as well as by their own visualizations and expectancies. Therefore individuals can learn to regulate themselves by selecting appropriate visualizations and expectations (Norris and Fahrion, 1993).

Creative visualization is one form of self-directed imagery that is based on the principle of mind-body connectivity (i.e., every mental image leads to physical or emotional changes) (Patel, 1993). The steps of creative visualization are listed in Box 35-2.

Clinical Applications of Imagery.

Imagery has applications in a number of client populations. Imagery has been used to visualize cancer cells being destroyed by cells of the immune system, control or relieve pain, and achieve calmness and serenity. It has also been used in the treatment of chronic conditions such as asthma, hypertension, functional urinary disorders, menstrual and premenstrual syndromes, gastrointestinal disorders such as irritable

---

Four Basic Steps of Creative Visualization   Box 35-2

1. Set goals that can be accomplished, because confidence and increased self-esteem are achieved through success.
2. The created image must be clear. Although it may be difficult to develop a visual image, if the goals of the imagery are viewed with clear thoughts and in the present tense, the individual may be more successful in creating an effective image.
3. Frequently visualize the image. This visualization should be done during relaxing states as well as throughout the day, but particularly before bedtime or upon wakening, when the person's mind usually is more relaxed.
4. While focusing on the image, repeat encouraging statements, such as positive affirmations. Alleviate any doubts about one's ability to achieve one's goals.

bowel syndrome and ulcerative colitis, and rheumatoid arthritis (Lewith, Kenyon, and Lewis, 1996).

Limitations of Imagery.
Imagery, for the most part, is a behavioral intervention that has few side effects. However, it is probably one of the least clearly defined interventions and can range from being highly structured to consisting of spontaneous daydreams by the individual (Smith and others, 1996).

BIOFEEDBACK

Biofeedback techniques are frequently used in addition to relaxation interventions to assist individuals in learning how to control specific autonomic nervous system responses. **Biofeedback** is a group of therapeutic procedures that use electronic or electromechanical instruments to measure, process, and provide information to persons about their neuromuscular and autonomic nervous system activity (Figure 35-4). The information, or feedback, is given in the form of analog or binary (a continuously varying variable such as temperature corresponds with another value such as voltage) and auditory and/or visual feedback signals. For example, clients may hear a sound if their pulse rate or blood pressure increases out of the therapeutic zone. Practitioners, usually credentialed in biofeedback, help persons develop greater awareness and resulting voluntary control over their physiological responses, of which they are otherwise unaware (Olson, 1987).

Biofeedback is considered an addendum to more traditional relaxation programs because it can immediately demonstrate to the client his or her ability to control some

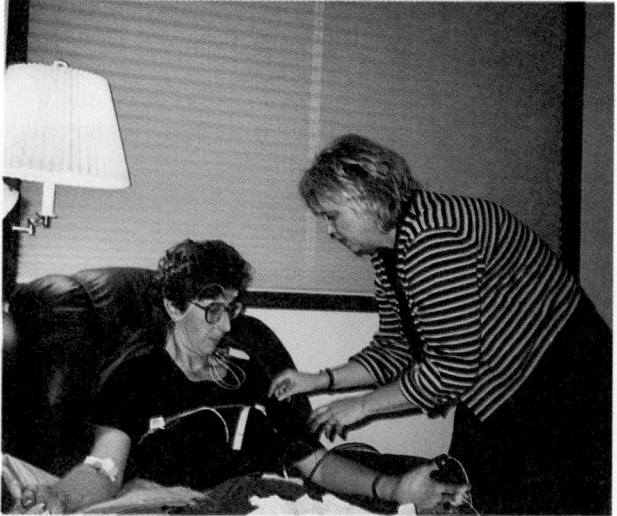

Figure 35-4   Biofeedback monitoring. Electrodes are placed on the frontalis and trapezius muscles as well as the fingers of the left hand. Pneumograph measurements are also made.

physiological responses. It can also help the individual focus on and monitor specific body parts. By providing immediate feedback in terms of what stress relaxation behaviors work most effectively, it helps the client control physiological functions that are most difficult for him or her to control. Eventually the client will be able to notice positive physiological changes without the need for instrument feedback. Finally, biofeedback demonstrates to the client the relationship between thoughts, feelings, and physiological responses (Adler and Adler, 1989).

Clinical Applications of Biofeedback.
Biofeedback has application in a number of situations (Table 35-2). Stroke clients who experience injury to the brain often find that the recovery of their muscle groups occurs at different rates. During the period of inactivity in some muscles, the client may learn to not use muscles that are temporarily paralyzed. When the muscle paralysis decreases over time, the client may not know how to use the muscle in the correct manner. Biofeedback assists in this muscle rehabilitation because it provides the client with information about how much muscle tension is generated when the client attempts to contract a specific muscle group. With continued practice using these muscle groups and the feedback, the client is able to see progress and avoid discouragement. Furthermore, even if the muscle has atrophied, clients can learn exercises to strengthen the muscle, thus achieving a return of function (Miller, 1989).

Biofeedback therapy is also used to treat Raynaud's disease, a disorder in which individuals experience intermittent episodes of ischemia in the extremities of the body. This disorder appears to be mediated by exposure to cold or stress. There appears to be a relationship between decreased peripheral skin temperature and increased affective states such as fear (Turk and others, 1996).

Biofeedback can also be used in **autogenic training,** during which clients are taught to relax and warm their hands or feet, usually the nondominant side initially. The client is directed to repeat the phrase "My left hand is feeling warm and heavy." Biofeedback is used to provide immediate information to the client regarding the effectiveness of the relaxation/autogenic training. This technique has been effectively used to increase skin temperature. Furthermore, temperature differences can be observed from one side of the body to the other, indicating that the individual is learning to control the body's response (Cleeland, 1989).

One of the most critical components of any behavioral program is adherence to the treatment regime (Sedlacek, 1989). Clients who are compliant with appointments, practice times, and goal setting and basically take responsibility for their treatment tend to be the most successful.

When investigating the effectiveness of an intervention in a population of clients, it is important to be aware of differences in responses between genders. For example, on the average males have higher baseline skin temperature

Table 35-2 Types of Biofeedback for Specific Health Problems

Health Problem	Type of Feedback	Outcome	Reference
Anxiety	Electromyogram (EMG)	↓ Anxiety, heart rate, blood pressure ↑ Skin temperature	Taylor, 1995
Fecal incontinence	Double-balloon devices to measure pressure	↓ Incontinence	Ko and others, 1997
Gastrointestinal motility disorders (reflux)	Motility recordings using open-tipped catheters	Learned contraction of lower esophageal sphincter, ↓ reflux	Soykan and others, 1995
Migraine headaches	Electroencephalogram (EEG)	EEG: small to moderate ↓ in headache	Lewis and Solomon, 1995
Parkinsonian symptoms	EMG	Facial muscle relaxed ↓ Hand tremor spike amplitudes	Cleeland, 1989
Raynaud's disease	Autogenic training, peripheral skin temperature, EMG, breathing	↑ Skin temperature ↑ Feeling of warmth ↓ Vasospasm	Miller and Morgan, 1993
Speech-language pathologic condition	EMG	↓ Stuttering Improvement of voice quality	Blood, 1995 McGillivray, Proctor-Williams and McLister, 1994
Supraventricular arrhythmias	Electrocardiogram (ECG) amplifier	Heart rates controlled and lowered	Schaldach, 1995
Tension headaches	EMG	↓ Headaches	Arena and others, 1995
Temporomandibular joint dysfunction	EMG	↓ Jaw tension, ↓ pain	Turk and others, 1996

levels than females and can, during autogenic sessions, increase their skin temperature higher than females. It is also important to note that physiological responses may not correspond with reported anxiety and that women frequently report higher levels of psychological distress than do men (McGrady, 1996). Furthermore, if the goal of the intervention is to elevate skin temperature, for example, a small or insignificant response would be expected if the beginning temperature was elevated.

Limitations of Biofeedback.

Although biofeedback has demonstrated effectiveness in a number of client populations, several precautions should be discussed. During relaxation therapy and/or biofeedback sessions repressed emotions or feelings may be uncovered that clients cannot cope with by themselves. For this reason, it is recommended that practitioners who offer biofeedback should either be trained in more traditional psychological methods or have qualified professionals available for referral. Although biofeedback may be indicated in the treatment of psychosomatic disorders such as phobias, insomnia, or cardiac neurosis, it is not recommended for individuals who have bipolar disease or psychosis such as schizophrenia (Roberts and McGrady, 1996).

HYPNOTHERAPY

Hypnotherapy did not gain medical approval until the middle of the twentieth century, when both the British Medical Association and the American Medical Association approved its use for certain medical problems. *Hypnosis* is defined as a trancelike state of heightened susceptibility. The purpose of hypnosis is to induce a hypnotic state during which posthypnotic suggestions are implanted (Lewith, Kenyon, and Lewis, 1996). These suggestions usually relate to a change in behavior desired by the client. Three levels of **trance** have been identified (Box 35-3).

Hypnosis is a process whereby the individual relaxes followed by a shift in focus of the conscious mind from the external environment to ideas suggested by either the practitioner or the individual (self-hypnosis). The success of hypnotherapy depends on the extent to which individuals can retain a suggestion in a wakeful state. In general,

---

Three Levels of Hypnotic Trance   Box 35-3

1. *Light trance:* The person's eyes are closed; the person is deeply relaxed and accepts suggestions.
2. *Medium trance:* Physiological processes are decreased, and there is partial sensitivity to pain with total cessation of allergic reactions.
3. *Deep trance:* Total anesthesia can occur; the eyes are open, and most posthypnotic suggestions are successful.

hypnosis sessions usually last from 60 to 90 minutes, and between 6 and 12 sessions are needed for results to occur (Adler and Adler, 1989).

Many physiological and psychological responses have been observed during hypnotic trances, depending on the emotion introduced to the person. Tachycardia frequently occurs during the initial stage of the trance. Decreases in cortisol, respiratory rate, sensitivity to pain, temperature, pressure, or touch have been observed in deeper hypnotic states. Changes in senses can occur depending on the suggestion. In addition to these physiological changes, hypnosis can change thought processes, produce feelings of relaxation and calmness, or enhance certain emotional states. For example, a pessimistic person may be given the suggestion of focusing on feelings of optimism (DeBetz and Sunnen, 1985).

Clinical Applications of Hypnosis.

Hypnosis has been used to treat asthmatic clients, particularly children with asthma because they tend to have a greater ability to be hypnotized, resulting in a better response to treatment (Adler and Adler, 1989). Hypnosis also has been used to reduce examination stress (Lewith and Watkins, 1996), facilitate smoking cessation, induce deep relaxation, manage chronic pain for a variety of illnesses, treat irritable bowel syndrome, and relieve symptoms of fibromyalgia (Lewith, Kenyon, and Lewis, 1996).

Limitations of Hypnosis.

The success of hypnotherapy is dependent on the ability of the individual to become hypnotized. The World Health Organization proposes that 90% of the general population can be hypnotized to some extent. The degree of response relates to the suggestibility of the individual to enter the hypnotic state. The World Health Organization also recommends that hypnosis not be used as a treatment for psychosis, organic psychiatric conditions, or antisocial personality disorders. Another potential limitation to hypnosis is that clients may have negative expectations or fears regarding hypnosis such as undesirable outcomes. Irregularities in heart rhythm and increased respiratory rate have been observed when thoughts of fear or anger are introduced. Patients also have reported numbness, tingling, itching, coldness or warmth, and burning sensations (Lewith, Kenyon, and Lewis, 1996).

MEDITATION

Meditation is any activity that limits stimulus input by directing attention to a single unchanging or repetitive stimulus (Whitehouse and others, 1996). Many different forms of meditation have been used by a number of societies to alter consciousness and evoke beneficial responses. Transcendental meditation (TM), mindfulness meditation, Chinese Tao, *gnyana* yoga, Japanese Zen, Buddhist meditation, Christian prayer, and Moslem Sufism are all methods of meditation. Clinically standardized meditation is a technique that was developed with specific clinical objectives in mind. The individual chooses a sound or creates one, then repeats the sound mentally. Respiratory one method is another clinical meditation that also requires the individual to repeat a sound but while doing so links the repetition of the sound with breathing (Whitehouse and others, 1996). Regardless of the type of meditation used, they all evoke a restful state, lower oxygen consumption, a reduction in respiratory and heart rates, and subjective reports of reduced anxiety (Figure 35-5).

Clinical Applications of Meditation.

There are many indications for meditation (Box 35-4). There is some evidence that meditation improves stress-related illnesses and breathing patterns in asthmatics, lowers blood pressure in hypertensive clients and blood glucose levels in diabetics, reduces anxiety in some individuals, decreases episodes of angina pectoris, lowers cholesterol in hypercholesterolemic clients, improves sleep-onset insomnia and stuttering, decreases the central nervous system reactivity, and indirectly reduces the incidence of dental caries by lowering salivary bacteria (Whitehouse and others, 1996). Meditation has also increased productivity, improved mood, increased sense of identity, and lowered irritability (Whitehouse and others, 1996).

Although health care professionals and researchers have attempted to determine which type of person is a candidate for meditative therapy, the data are inconclusive at this point. Other considerations for the appropriateness of meditation include the degree of self-discipline of the person. Meditation can be easily learned and does not require memorization or particular procedures. It actually requires less self-discipline than most other behavioral therapies. Another consideration involves the self-reinforcing properties that meditation offers. Meditation can induce a peaceful, drifting mental state that is unusually pleasurable and provides an incentive for individuals to continue.

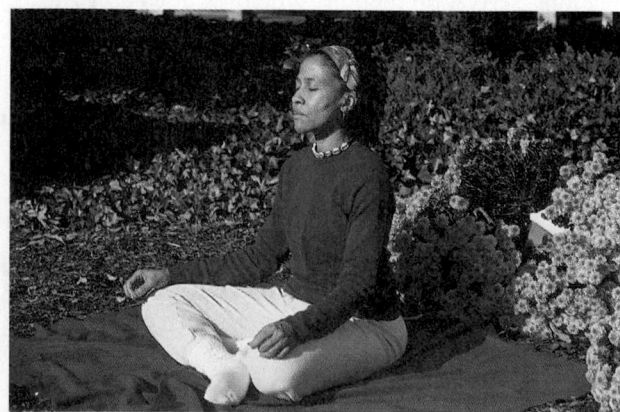

Figure 35-5 Meditation can be used to relax the body and calm the mind.

Anxiety or tension states
Chronic bereavement
Chronic fatigue syndrome
Chronic pain
Drug abuse (alcohol or tobacco)
Hypertension
Irritability
Low self-esteem or self-blame
Mild depression
Psychophysiological disorders
Sleep disorders

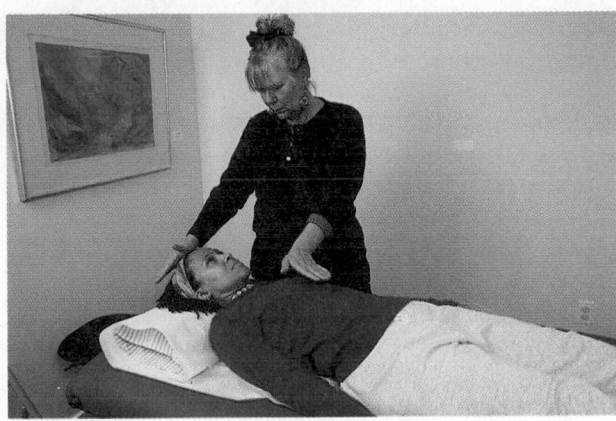

Figure 35-6 In therapeutic touch the practitioner directs the practitioner's own interpersonal energy to help or heal another.

Limitations of Meditation.

Although meditation has demonstrated improvement in a variety of physiological and psychological ailments, it may be contraindicated in some people. For example, a person who has a strong fear of losing control may perceive meditation as a form of mind control and thus may be resistant to learning the technique. Some individuals may also be hypersensitive to meditation and require a much shorter session than the average 15- to 20-minute session.

Overmeditation should also be avoided. The individual who overmeditates may experience the release of emotional material that may be difficult for the person to cope with. Also, overmeditation in an individual with a history of psychoses may precipitate psychotic episodes.

Meditation may also augment the effects of certain drugs. For example, individuals taking antihypertensive medications or thyroid-regulating, antidepressive, or antianxiety medications should be monitored. Prolonged practice of meditation techniques may, in some instances, lead to the reduced need for certain medications such as antihypertensive medications. Whatever the case, individuals learning meditation should be monitored closely for physiological changes with respect to their medications, and adjustment of the medication may be needed (Carrington, 1993; Whitehouse and others, 1996).

Manual Healing Therapies

Manual healing therapies (see Table 35-1) are based on the theory that energy systems in the body need to be balanced in an effort to enhance healing. A number of manual healing therapies originated from ancient Chinese healing disciplines such as Qigong. In Qigong, trained practitioners learn to emit vital energy of the body, or *qi*, for the purpose of healing another person (Sheng-han, 1994; Sancier, 1996).

THERAPEUTIC TOUCH

A more contemporary manual healing therapy is **therapeutic touch** (Krieger, 1979). Although the philosophical and religious assumptions of therapeutic touch are different from those of Qigong and other Eastern healing modalities, therapeutic touch is similar to Qigong in that it involves trained health care professionals who attempt to direct their excess energies in an intentional and motivated manner toward those of the client.

Therapeutic touch is a natural human potential that consists of placing the practitioner's hands either on or close to the body of a person (Figure 35-6). The process of therapeutic touch involves the practitioner scanning the body of the client and diagnosing areas of accumulated tensions. The practitioner then attempts to redirect these energies to bring the person back into energy balance similar to that of the practitioner (Krieger, 1975, 1979). Therapeutic touch consists of five phases: centering, assessment, unruffling, treatment, and evaluation. Centering is the process whereby the practitioner becomes aware and fully present during the entire treatment. The next phase involves the assessment of the client, in which the practitioner moves his or her hands (roughly 2 to 6 inches from the body) in a rhythmic and symmetric movement from the head to the toes. During this phase the practitioner notices the quality of **energy flow** and detects accumulations of energy. The physiological indicators of energy imbalance are perceived as feelings of congestion, pressure, warmth, coolness, blockage, pulling or drawing, or static or tingling (Krieger, 1975). During the third phase, the practitioner unruffles the energy flow or facilitates the symmetrical and rhythmical flow of energy through the body. This technique is accomplished by long downward strokes over the energy field located over the entire body. During the actual treatment the practitioner directs and modulates the energy, attempting to rebalance the energy flow. This remodulation of energy is achieved either by the practitioner touching the body or maintaining the hands in a position a few inches away from the body. The final phase consists of an evaluation of the client and a reassessment of the energy field. If a rebalance has occurred, the practitioner detects a more symmetric, freely flowing energy field (Krieger, 1979).

Clinical Applications of Therapeutic Touch.

Some of the earliest studies found that therapeutic touch was able to increase hemoglobin (Hb) levels in several clients (Krieger, 1975, 1979). Other studies have found that therapeutic touch was effective in reducing anxiety levels in hospitalized clients with cardiovascular disease, reducing headache pain, and improving mood in bereaved adults (Krieger, 1975, 1979) (Table 35-3). Anecdotal clinical reports have also suggested that therapeutic touch is useful in facilitating healing of traumatic injuries such as sprains, fractures, burns, and wounds; managing suicidal tendencies; reducing chemotherapy-related nausea and vomiting; and facilitating recovery from incest and abuse (Mulloney and Wells-Federman, 1996).

Limitations of Therapeutic Touch.

Although some studies have demonstrated that therapeutic touch produced positive outcomes, others have not. Suggestions for this lack of response include an absence of eye and facial contact during the therapeutic session and too brief of a session. Therapeutic touch may be contraindicated in certain client populations. For example, persons who are sensitive to human interaction and touch (e.g., those who have been physically abused or have psychiatric disorders) may misinterpret the intent of the treatment and may feel threatened and anxious by the treatment. Other clients who are sensitive to energy repatterning may also need to avoid therapeutic touch. These include premature infants, newborns, children, pregnant women, older or debilitated people, or those in critical, unstable conditions (Mulloney and Wells-Federman, 1996). This is clinical advice based on theory and not research that has demonstrated negative outcomes or increased risk.

CHIROPRACTIC THERAPY

Chiropractic therapy, a manual healing art, was developed in 1895 in Iowa. Of the independently practicing health professions, it is the third largest in the Western world (Leach, 1986). The central tenet of the chiropractic profession is intervertebral manipulation that is characterized by short-lever, specific, high-velocity, controlled forceful thrusts directed at certain joints by the practitioner using his or her hand or an instrument. **Manipulation** is defined as the forceful passive movement of a joint beyond its active limit of motion (Leach, 1986). Chiropractic practice does not typically include drug therapy or surgery.

Spinal manipulation received an endorsement from the U.S. Department of Health and Human Service's Agency for Health Care Policy and Research in 1994. The agency developed guidelines that concluded "spinal manual therapy provides relief of symptomatic discomfort as well as functional improvement." The basic principles of chiropractic therapy incorporate the idea that human beings have an innate healing potential, and the goal of healing professions is to access this potential. Drug therapy may compromise the body's natural healing ability, and because of this, natural, nonpharmaceutical therapies should be the first line of treatment. Finally, both a natural diet and regular exercise are critical components for the body to function properly (Redwood, 1996).

Clinical Applications of Chiropractic Therapy.

The basic goals of chiropractic therapy focus on restoring the structural and functional imbalances that may result in pain. It is believed that structure and function coexist with one another and that alterations or distortions in structure can ultimately lead to abnormalities in function. One of the major structural distortions that chiropractors treat is vertebral subluxation, in which the motion of the joints is decreased due to slight changes in the position of the articulating bones and subjective symptoms such as pain (Redwood, 1996). A more severe form of subluxation, called fixation, exists when joint motion is restricted.

Chiropractic interventions are used to treat not only musculoskeletal abnormalities, but headaches, dysmenorrhea, blood pressure, vertigo, tinnitus, and visual disorders. In one study chiropractic therapy has also been shown to increase the activity of polymorphonuclear cells and monocytes (Brennan and others, 1992).

Limitations of Chiropractic Therapy.

Several diseases or joint conditions should not be treated with manipulation. If a malignancy is suspected or determined through diagnostic testing, the client should be referred to

Table 35-3 **Effects of Therapeutic Touch on Outcome Variables**			
Outcome Variable	Population	Findings	Reference
Hemoglobin (Hb)	Ill people	↓ Hb	Krieger, 1975, 1979
Anxiety	Cardiovascular clients	↓ Anxiety	Heidt, 1980
			Quinn, 1984
Tension headache pain	Outpatient adults	↓ Headache	Keller and Bzdek, 1986
Anxiety and mood	Therapeutic touch practitioners	↑ Positive mood	Quinn and Strelkauskas, 1993
	Bereaved adults	↓ Negative mood	
		↓ Anxiety	

Table 35-4 **Three Causes of Disease According to Traditional Chinese Medicine**	
Cause of Disease	Influences
External causes, or "the six evils"	Wind, cold, fire, damp, summer heat, dryness
Internal causes, or internal damage by seven effects	Joy, anger, anxiety, thought, sorrow, fear, fright
Nonexternal, noninternal causes	Dietary irregularities, excessive sexual activity, taxation fatigue, trauma, parasites

a medical physician for further evaluation and treatment. Bone and joint infections also require pharmaceutical or surgical intervention, and the structural integrity of the bone may be compromised if excessive force is used. Contraindications for chiropractic therapy include acute myelopathy, fractures, dislocations, and rheumatoid arthropathies.

Traditional and Ethnomedicine Therapies

TRADITIONAL CHINESE MEDICINE

Traditional Chinese medicine (TCM) comprises several healing modalities, including herbs, acupuncture, moxibustion, diet, exercise, and meditation. TCM is several thousand years old and has its roots in Taoism. There are several major concepts that constitute Chinese medicine. The most important of these is the concept of **yin and yang,** which represent opposing yet complementary phenomena that exist in a state of dynamic equilibrium. Examples are night/day, hot/cold, and shady/sunny. Yin represents shade, cold, and inhibition, whereas yang represents fire, light, and excitement. Yin also represents the inner part of the body, specifically the viscera, liver, heart, spleen, lung, and kidney, whereas yang represents the outer part, specifically the bowels, stomach, and bladder. When there is an imbalance in these two paired opposites, then it is thought that disease occurs (Ergil, 1996).

Qi is defined as the vital energy of the human body. Disease is classified into three major categories: external causes, internal causes, and neither internal nor external causes (Table 35-4). Regardless of the cause, it is thought that yin and yang go out of balance, thus altering the movement of *qi*. The body consists of several forms of this energy that directly influence physiological functions of the body and help to maintain homeostasis (Table 35-5).

Channels of energy run in regular patterns through the body and over its surface. These channels, called **meridians,** are like rivers flowing through the body. An obstruction in the movement of these energy rivers is like a dam that backs up the flow in one part of the body and restricts it in others. Any obstruction and blockages or deficiencies of energy would eventually lead to disease. Evaluations have been done to identify and systematize the meridians or channels through which *qi* flows. Twelve primary and eight secondary or extra channels have been identified. Located

Table 35-5 **Types of Qi**	
Type	Function
Ying qi (construction *qi*)	Supports and nourishes the body
Wei qi (defense *qi*)	Protects and warms the body
Jing qi (channel *qi*)	Flows in the channels (felt during acupuncture)
Zang qi (organ *qi*)	Flows in the organs (physiological function of the organs)
Zong qi (ancestral *qi*)	Responsible for respiration and circulation

along the channels are **acupoints,** or holes through which *qi* can be influenced by the insertion of needles, a process known as **acupuncture.**

Another important component of Chinese medicine involves five elements. The five elements consist of earth, metal, water, wood, and fire. Various health phenomena are organized according to these phases and interact with each other (Brennan and others, 1992).

In Chinese medicine outward manifestations are reflective of the internal environment. There are two primary areas that are assessed in Chinese medicine: the tongue and several pulses. The color, shape, and coating of the tongue are reflective of the general condition of the internal organs. The pulses provide information about the condition and balance of *qi*, blood, ying and yang, and the internal organs (Lewith, Kenyon, and Lewis, 1996).

ACUPUNCTURE

Acupuncture is a method of stimulating certain points (acupoints) on the body by the insertion of special needles to modify the perception of pain, normalize physiological functions, or treat or prevent disease (Figure 35-7) (Lewith, Kenyon, and Lewis, 1996). Acupuncture is used to regulate the flow of *qi*. According to Chinese traditional medicine, acupuncture needles unblock the obstruction of energy and reestablish the flow of *qi* through the meridians, thereby stimulating and activating the body's self-healing mechanism.

There are several types of acupuncture. Auricular acupuncture is based on the perspective that regions of the body are parallel to sites on the ear. Auricular acupuncture is frequently indicated for conditions that are painful and acute, such as renal colic. The therapeutic effect from this

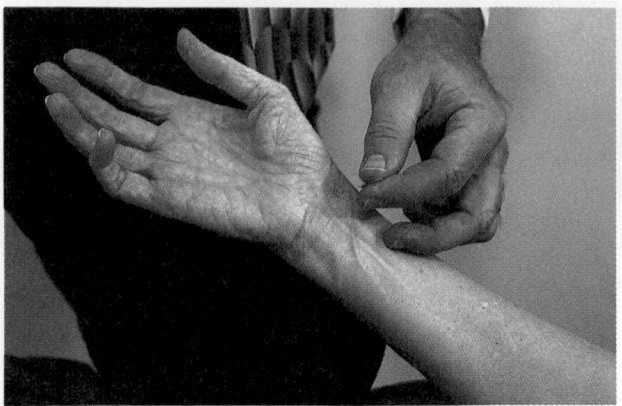

Figure 35-7   Acupuncture.

method is usually quick, but the duration is not as long as body acupuncture. For this reason, occasionally semipermanent needles may be left in the tissue until the treatment is terminated. Electroacupuncture is another type of acupuncture in which electrical currents are applied to the needles. Different frequencies of electrical stimulation result in the release of different neuropeptides within the central nervous system (Ulett, 1996).

Clinical Applications of Acupuncture.
Acupuncture is the primary treatment modality used by physicians of Chinese medicine. Many allopathic physicians and health care professionals are also being trained and certified in acupuncture. Many states now have regulations and licensure requirements to practice as an acupuncturist.

The most common problems for which acupuncture is used include low back pain, myofascial pain, simple and migraine headaches, sciatica, shoulder pain, tennis elbow, osteoarthritis, whiplash, and musculoskeletal sprains. Other problems that have been successively treated include sinusitis, gastrointestinal disorders, perimenstrual symptoms, neurological disorders, chronic pulmonary diseases (including asthma), hypertension, smoking and other addictions, and clinical depression (Ulett, 1996; Diehl and others, 1997).

Limitations of Acupuncture.
Acupuncture is considered a safe therapy when the practitioner has been appropriately trained and uses sterilized needles. Although complications have been noted, they are rare if appropriate steps are taken to ensure the safety of the equipment and the client. These complications include infections resulting from inadequately sterilized needles or those that are left in place for an extended length of time, broken needles, puncture of an internal organ, bleeding, fainting, seizures, miscarriage, and posttreatment drowsiness (Lewith, Kenyon, and Lewis, 1996). To prevent fainting, it is recommended that clients be treated lying down. For

clients who become drowsy after treatment, care should be taken to ensure their safe return home.

Acupuncture should be used with caution in pregnant clients and those who have a history of seizures, are carriers of hepatitis, or are infected with human immunosuppressive virus (HIV). Treatment is contraindicated in persons who have bleeding disorders, thrombocytopenia, or skin infections. The semipermanent needles should not be used with persons who have valvular heart disease because of the increased risk of infection. Electroacupuncture should be avoided in persons with a pacemaker and those who have cardiac arrhythmias, epilepsy, or are pregnant (Lewith, Kenyon, and Lewis, 1996).

Herbal Therapies

It is estimated that approximately 25,000 plant species are used medicinally throughout the world. It is the oldest form of medicine known to man, and archeologic evidence suggests that herbal remedies were used 60,000 years ago by Neanderthals. Use of **herbal therapy** gained widespread popularity in many countries as early as 3000 BC but began to decline with the development of modern scientific medicine in the early eighteenth century. However, because approximately 80% of the world's population live in developing countries, herbal medicine constitutes a prominent part of health care in these countries. Furthermore, a resurgence in interest has developed in countries whose health care is dominated by allopathic medicine. The increase in herbal medicine has occurred because of a growing concern by the general public about the complications and limitations of modern scientific medicine and consumer interest in "natural" foods (Lewith, Kenyon, and Lewis, 1996).

The federal Food, Drug, and Cosmetic Act mandates that all drugs have to be proven safe and effective before being sold to the public. Because herbal medicines have not undergone the same rigorous research as have pharmaceuticals, the majority have not received approval for use as drugs. For this reason many herbal medicines are sold as foods or food supplements in health food stores and through private companies. The Dietary Supplement Health and Education Act passed in 1994 now allows for herbs to be sold as dietary supplements as long as there are no health claims written on their labels (Tyler, 1996).

Herbal substances used in Chinese medicine are taken from plants, animals, or minerals, whereas those used in Western herbal medicine are prepared primarily from plant materials. The active ingredients are "packaged" in tinctures or extracts, elixirs, syrups, capsules, pills, tablets, lozenges, powders, ointments or creams, drops, and suppositories. Many people tend to think that because herbs are natural plants they will not cause harm or side effects. Many herbs are also sold with claims that they can "cure" certain ailments, such as pau d'arco for curing cancer, when their efficacy has not been determined through clinical trials. Herbs are generally classified as beneficial, harmful, or neutral, in which case they have no effects on the specific ailment.

The philosophy of herbal therapy is also different from that of conventional drug therapy. The goal of herbal therapy is to restore balance within the individual by facilitating the person's self-healing ability. Drug therapy, on the other hand, is aimed at the treatment of specific diseases or symptoms. Herbal therapy is also prescribed on an individual basis with unique herbal concoctions tailored for each person.

CLINICAL APPLICATIONS OF HERBAL THERAPY

A number of herbs have been determined to be safe and effective for a variety of conditions (Table 35-6). Milk thistle, for example, has been observed to be effective in treating a number of liver and gallbladder conditions. It is thought to protect the liver through its antioxidant properties and by facilitating regeneration of liver cells. St. John's Wort has effectiveness as a mild antidepressant and mild sedative. Hypericin and pseudohypericin, major constituents of the drug, have also been shown to have potent action against viruses. Clinical trials investigating the effectiveness of St. John's Wort against acquired immunodeficiency syndrome have begun (Tyler, 1996).

LIMITATIONS OF HERBAL THERAPY

While herbal medicine has shown to provide beneficial effects for a variety of conditions, a number of problems may exist. When herbal medicines are developed, concentrations of the active ingredients have been found to vary considerably. Contamination with other herbs or chemicals, including pesticides and heavy metals, may also occur. Not all companies follow strict quality control and manufacturing guidelines, which set standards for acceptable levels of pesticides, residual solvents, bacterial levels, and heavy metals (Lewith, Kenyon, and Lewis, 1996). For this reason, herbal medicine should be purchased only from reputable manufacturers. In addition, labels on herbal products should contain the scientific name of the botanical, the name and address of the actual manufacturer, a batch or lot number, the date of manufacture, and the expiration date (Diehl and others, 1997). Some herbs have also been found to contain very toxic products and can cause cancer. Comfrey, for example, has been used for its wound-healing properties. However, various species of comfrey contain certain pyrrolizidine alkaloids that are highly carcinogenic. Comfrey has been shown to produce liver cancer in small animals and fatal venoocclusive disease in humans. For this reason comfrey should not be used internally and, as a poultice, only on intact skin (Diehl and others, 1997). Other unsafe herbs are listed in Table 35-7.

Despite the increased use of herbal products, there has not been a parallel increase in reports of toxicity. Nonetheless, herbal products should be used with caution

in pregnant women, nursing mothers, infants or young children, or older adults with liver or cardiovascular disease (Diehl and others, 1997).

Nursing Role in Complementary and Alternative Therapies

The interest in CAM therapies has increased significantly in the past 15 years. The majority of people using and seeking information about complementary and alternative therapies are well educated and have a strong desire to actively participate in the decision making about their health care. This increased interest comes not only from health care consumers, but also allopathic physicians who have increasing concerns that current Western medicine is not meeting the needs of their clients. Many allopathic physicians do not refer their clients for CAM therapies because they are not familiar with the therapies and have had little, if any, education and training in complementary and alternative medicine. Many physicians have reservations about CAM therapies because they have not been appropriately tested in clinical trials in which other factors that may influence the outcomes are strictly controlled.

In North America and the United Kingdom many professional groups are exploring the use of CAM and facilitating and monitoring research being conducted in this area. Proposals put forth by several of the these groups include assessing the need of the public for CAM therapies, incorporating CAM educational components in the curriculum for all health care programs, providing appropriate information to the public, and encouraging and facilitating communication between CAM practitioners and allopathic physicians so each can be open to the other's approaches and values (Foundation of Integrated Medicine, 1997). For example, if CAM therapies are to be accepted and incorporated into Western medicine as a more integrative medical approach, practitioners of CAM should realize the advantages of their therapies' being researched more rigorously. On the other hand, allopathic physicians and more conventional practitioners should also begin to understand the benefits of therapies that encourage active participation by their clients in preventing illness or managing chronic illness rather than relying solely on surgery or drugs.

Integrative medicine, a health care strategy that is gaining popularity, involves a multiple-practitioner treatment group in which a client seeks care simultaneously from more than one type of practitioner. The clients are given the option to choose the kind of practitioner they feel would benefit their particular health problem. Clients who may benefit from these groups are those who have chronic health problems that have historically been difficult to treat using traditional allopathic medicine, such as fi-

Table 35-6 Safe or Effective Herbs Determined by Non-U.S. Regulatory Authorities

Common Name	Effects	Examples of Uses
Aloe	Antiinflammatory	Minor burns
	Acceleration of wound healing	Wound healing
	Alkalinization of digestive juices	Gastrointestinal disorders
Astralagus	Stimulant of immune system	Cancer
Bilberry	Improvement of microcirculation in eyes	Myopia
	Mild antiinflammatory	
Cat's claw	Stimulant of immune system	Cancer
	Antioxidant	Gastrointestinal disorders
	Antiinflammatory	Hypertension
	Lowering of blood pressure	Infections
Chamomile	Antiinflammatory	Inflammatory diseases of gastrointestinal and upper respiratory tracts
	Antispasmodic	
	Antiinfective	Inflammation of skin and mucous membranes
		Gastrointestinal spasms
Dong quai	Antispasmodic	Menstrual cramps
	Vasodilation	Premenstrual syndrome
	Balancing effects of estrogen	Menstrual irregularities
	Mild sedative effect	Hot flashes
		Vaginal dryness
Echinacea	Stimulant of immune system	Upper respiratory tract infections
	Antiinflammatory	Allergic rhinitis
	Antibacterial	Wound healing
Feverfew	Antiinflammatory	Arthritis
	Inhibition of serotonin and prostaglandins	
	Vasodilator	
Garlic	Lowering of lipids	Elevated cholesterol levels
	Inhibition of platelet aggregation	Hypertension
	Antibacterial	Diabetes
Ginger	Antiemetic	Nausea and vomiting
		Motion sickness
Gingko biloba	Memory improvement	Alzheimer's disease
	Increasing blood flow	Dementia
	Antioxidant	Eye disease
	Increased metabolism efficiency	Heart disease
		Poor circulation
		Varicose veins
		Anxiety
		Age-related diseases
Ginseng	Increased physical endurance	Fatigue
	Balancing of body	Headaches
	Resistance to stress	Decreased libido
Goldenseal	Antiinflammatory	Infections of gastrointestinal and respiratory tracts
	Antibacterial	Gallbladder inflammation
	Laxative	Cirrhosis of liver
Hawthorn	Increased oxygen utilization by heart	Angina
	Lowering of cholesterol	Coronary artery disease
	Peripheral vasodilator	
Milk thistle	Stimulation of production of new liver cells	Liver disease
	Protection of liver from damage	
St. John's Wort (hypericum)	Inhibition of monoamine oxidase (MAO) and serotonin reuptake	Mild to moderate depression
		Wound healing
	Antiviral	Viral infections
	Antibacterial	
	Warning: Avoid foods containing tyramine, such as aged cheese, red wine	
Saw palmetto	Prevention of conversion of testosterone to dihydrotestosterone (needed for prostate cell multiplication)	Benign prostatic hyperplasia
		Urinary problems
Valerian	Minor tranquilizer	Sleep disorders
	Central nervous system depression	Restlessness

Table 35-7 Unsafe Herbs

Common Name	Effects	Comments
Borage	Diuretic Antidiarrheal	Contains toxic pyrrolizidine alkaloids
Calamus	Fever Digestive aid	Contains varying amounts of carcinogenic *cis*-isoasarone Indian-type most toxic North American–type nontoxic
Chaparral	Anticancer	No proven efficacy May induce severe liver toxicity
Coltsfoot	Antitussive Demulcent	Contains carcinogenic pyrrolizidine alkaloids
Comfrey	Wound healing	Contains large number of toxic pyrrolizidine alkaloids May induce venoocclusive disease
Ephedra (*ma huang*)	Central nervous system stimulant Anorectic Bronchodilator Cardiac stimulation	Unsafe for people with hypertension, diabetes, or thyroid disease Avoid consumption with caffeine
Germander	Anorectic	Causes hepatotoxicity because of diterpenoid derivatives
Life root	Menstrual flow stimulant	Hepatotoxic Contains toxic pyrrolizidine alkaloids
Pokeroot	Antirheumatic Anticancer	May be fatal in children
Sassafras	Stimulant Antispasmodic Antirheumatic	Volatile oil Contains carcinogenic safrole

bromyalgia or chronic fatigue syndrome. This represents a pluralistic and truly complementary health care system in which both alternative and allopathic practitioners work side-by-side to improve the well-being of their clients. Although this is not reality in the majority of settings, this approach of open communication and practice between allopathic and alternative practitioners could potentially benefit a large number of patients.

The integrative medicine approach is consistent with the holistic approach nurses are taught to practice. Nurses have the potential for becoming essential participants in this type of health care philosophy. Many nurses already practice forms of CAM by offering relaxation, imagery, massage, and therapeutic touch to their clients (Figure 35-8). Nurses should be knowledgeable of CAM therapies to make appropriate recommendations to allopathic primary care providers about which therapies may be useful for clients. Nurses should also be able to provide advice to clients regarding when to seek conventional therapy or CAM therapy. For example, if a client complains of right lower abdominal pain, nausea, and vomiting, the nurse should be suspicious of appendicitis and recommend that the client be assessed by an allopathic physician. However, if the client has a chronic gastrointestinal disorder and has been diagnosed with irritable bowel syndrome, the client may benefit from relaxation and herbal therapy. Nurses need to be aware of their state Nurse Practice Acts with regard to com-

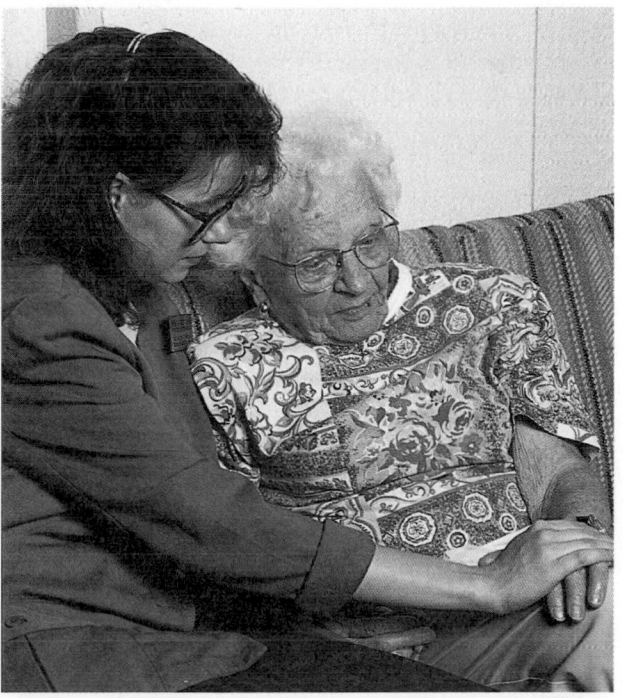

Figure 35-8 The nurse encourages the client to use imagery to relax and relieve pain

plementary therapies and practice accordingly within the scope of these laws.

Nurses work very closely with their clients and are in the unique position of becoming familiar with the client's religious and cultural viewpoints and existential issues. Nurses may be able to determine which CAM therapies would be more appropriately aligned with these beliefs and offer recommendations accordingly.

Client interest and participation in CAM therapies is increasing. Therefore, it is important for nurses to be knowledgeable of the multiple CAM therapies available and the use of these therapies by their clients. It is also important for nurses to keep abreast of the current research being done in this area to provide accurate information, not only to the clients, but to other health care professionals. Many studies related to CAM therapies have involved small numbers of subjects and were not well controlled. More studies are needed to validate the effectiveness of CAM therapies.

Key Concepts

- Alternative and complementary therapies can be the same, depending on whether the therapy is a primary treatment or treatment in addition to the Western medicine treatment.
- Integrative medical programs utilize a multidisciplinary (both allopathic and complementary) treatment approach providing holistic care to clients.
- The stress response is an adaptive response allowing individuals to react appropriately to stressful situations.
- A chronic stress response may be maladaptive, leading to chronic muscle tension, mood changes, and immune changes.
- Relaxation is a beneficial state characterized by lowered pulse rates, respiratory rates, blood pressure and muscle tension and improved mood states.
- Biobehavioral therapies require commitment and regular involvement by the client to be most effective and have prolonged beneficial outcomes.
- Biobehavioral therapies should appropriately be chosen according to the person's functional status, belief or religious perspectives, access to health care, and insurance coverage.
- Some biobehavioral therapies may alter physiological responses such that routine medication doses may need changing.
- Imagery is usually visual but can also involve the auditory, proprioceptive, gustatory, and olfactory senses.
- Many complementary and alternative therapies lack a scientific basis but are thought to be effective based on observed positive outcomes in a number of clients.
- Herbal therapies are not necessarily safe because they are derived from plants. Note the potentially toxic plant-derived chemotherapy agents vincristine and Taxol.

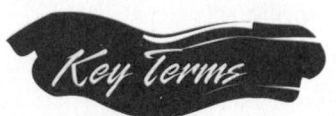

Key Terms

Acupoints, *p. 981*
Acupuncture, *p. 981*
Allopathic medicine, *p. 968*
Alternative therapies, *p. 968*
Autogenic training, *p. 976*
Biofeedback, *p. 976*
Chiropractic therapy, *p. 980*
Complementary therapies, *p. 968*
Creative visualization, *p. 975*
Energy flow, *p. 979*
Herbal therapy, *p. 982*
Hypnotherapy, *p. 977*
Imagery, *p. 975*
Integrative medical programs, *p. 969*

Manipulation, *p. 980*
Manual healing therapy, *p. 979*
Meditation, *p. 978*
Meridians, *p. 981*
Passive relaxation, *p. 973*
Progressive relaxation, *p. 973*
Qi, p. 981
Relaxation, *p. 973*
Stress response, *p. 972*
Therapeutic touch, *p. 979*
Traditional Chinese therapy, *p. 981*
Trance, *p. 977*
Yin and yang, *p. 981*

Critical Thinking Exercises

Client Profile: Jane, a 21-year-old college student, was seen in the student health center for increasing episodes of abdominal fullness and discomfort with alternating diarrhea and constipation. She reports that she was diagnosed with irritable bowel syndrome several years ago and was told to eat more fiber. Nothing has seemed to be effective in reducing her abdominal distress. She is taking a heavy course load this semester and has to work 20 hours each week for her work-study contract. She eats mainly fast food and drinks several colas daily.

1. Explain the psychological stressors that may be contributing to Jane's abdominal discomfort.
2. Describe how her current diet may be affecting her both physiologically and psychologically.
3. What complementary and alternative therapy(ies) would be appropriate for Jane?
4. How would you recommend complementary therapies to her physician? What arguments could you use to support their use?

References

Adler C, Adler S: Biofeedback and psychosomatic disorders. In Basmajian JV, editor: *Biofeedback: principles and practice for clinicians,* ed 3, Baltimore, 1989, Williams & Wilkins.

Adler C, Adler S: Strategies in general psychiatry. In Basmajian JV, editor: *Biofeedback: principles and practice for clinicians,* ed 3, Baltimore, 1989, Williams & Wilkins.

Alternative medicine: expanding medical horizons. Workshop on alternative medicine, Chantilly, Va, Sept 14-16, 1992, Rockville, Md, US Government Printing Office.

Arena J and others: A comparison of frontal electromyographic biofeedback training, trapezius electromyographic biofeedback training, and progressive muscle relaxation therapy in the treatment of tension headache, *Headache* 35:411, 1995.

Astin J and others: The construct of control in mind-body medicine: implications for healthcare, *Altern Ther Health Med* 5:42, 1999.

Baum A: Stress, intrusive imagery, and chronic distress, *Health Psychol* 2:653, 1990.

Benson H, Beary J, Carol M: The relaxation response, *Psychiatry* 37:37, 1974.

Bhattacharya B: MD programs in the United States with complementary and alternative medicine education: an ongoing listing, *J Altern Complement Med* 4:325, 1998.

Blood G: A behavioral-cognitive therapy program for adults who stutter: computers and counseling, *J Commun Dis* 28:165, 1995.

Brennan P and others: Enhanced phagocytic cell respiratory burst induced by spinal manipulation: potential role of substance P, *J Manipulative Physiol Ther* 14:399, 1992.

Burish, T, Snyder S, Jenkins R: Preparing patients for cancer chemotherapy: effect of coping preparation and relaxation interventions, *J Consult Clin Psychol* 59:518, 1991.

Burish T and others: Conditioned side effects induced by cancer chemotherapy: prevention through behavioral treatment, *J Consult Clin Psychol* 55:42, 1987.

Carey M, Burish T: Providing relaxation training to cancer chemotherapy patients: a comparison of three delivery techniques, *J Consult Clin Psychol* 55:732, 1987.

Carlson C, Nitz A: Negative side effects of self-regulation training: relaxation and the role of the professional in service delivery, *Biofeedback Self Regul* 16:191, 1991.

Carlson N: Emotion and stress. In Carlson N, editor: *Physiology of behavior,* ed 5, Boston, 1994, Allyn & Bacon.

Carrington P: Modern forms of meditation. In Lehrer PM, Woolfolk RL, editors: *Principles and practice of stress management,* ed 2, New York, 1993, Guilford Press.

Cleeland C: Biofeedback and other behavioral techniques in the treatment of disorders of voluntary movement. In Basmajian JV, editor: *Biofeedback: principles and practice for clinicians,* ed 3, Baltimore, 1989, Williams & Wilkins.

DeBetz B, Sunnen G: *A primer of clinical hypnosis,* Littleton, Mass, 1985, PSG.

Diehl D and others: Use of acupuncture by American physicians, *J Altern Complement Med* 3:119, 1997.

Eisenberg D and others: Unconventional medicine in the United States: prevalence, costs, and patterns of use, *N Engl J Med* 328:246, 1993.

Eisenberg D and others: Trends in alternative medicine use in the United States, 1990-1997, *JAMA* 280:1569, 1998.

Ergil K: China's traditional medicine. In Micozzi MS, editor: *Fundamentals of complementary and alternative therapy,* New York, 1996, Churchill Livingstone.

Foundation of integrated medicine, Steering Committee for Prince of Wale's Initiative on Integrated Medicine, 1997.

Fulder S: The basic concepts of alternative medicine and their impact on our views of health, *J Altern Complement Med* 4:147, 1998.

Good M: Effects of relaxation and music on postoperative pain: a review, *J Adv Nur* 24:905, 1996.

Heidt P: Effect of therapeutic touch on anxiety level of hospitalized patients, *Nurs Res* 30:32, 1980.

Holland J and others: A randomized clinical trial of alprazolam versus progressive muscle relaxation in cancer patients with anxiety and depressive symptoms, *J Clin Oncol* 9:1004, 1991.

Houlding A, McCarkle R, Lowery B: Relaxation training and psychoimmunological status of bereaved spouses, *Cancer Nurs* 16:47, 1993.

Keller E, Bzdek V: Effects of therapeutic touch on tension headache pain, *Nurs Res* 35:101, 1986.

Ko C and others: Biofeedback is effective therapy for fecal incontinence and constipation, *Arch Surg* 132:829, 1997.

Krieger D: Therapeutic touch: the imprimatur of nursing, *Am J Nurs* 75:784, 1975.

Krieger D: Searching for evidence of physiological change, *Am J Nurs* 79:660, 1979.

Leach R: Manipulation terminology in the chiropractic, osteopathic, and medical literature. In Leach R, editor: *The chiropractic theories,* Baltimore, 1986, Williams & Wilkins.

Lewis T, Solomon G: Advances in migraine management, *Cleve Clin J Med* 62:148, 1995.

Lewith G, Kenyon J, Lewis P, editors: *Complementary medicine: an integrated approach,* Oxford, 1996, Oxford University Press.

Lewith G, Watkins A: Unconventional therapies in asthma: an overview, *Allergy* 51:761, 1996.

McCain N and others: The influence of stress management training in HIV disease, *Nurs Res* 45:246, 1996.

McGillivray R, Proctor-Williams K, McLister B: Simple biofeedback device to reduce excessive vocal intensity, *Med Biol Eng* 32:348, 1994.

McGrady A: Good news-bad press: applied psychophysiology in cardiovascular disorders, *Biofeedback Self Regul* 21:335, 1996.

McGuigan F: Progressive relaxation: origins, principles, and clinical applications. In Lehrer P, Woolfolk R, editors: *Principles and practice of stress management,* ed 2, New York, 1993, Guilford Press.

Miller L, Morgan R: Vasospastic disorders: etiology, recognition, and treatment, *Hand Clin* 9:171, 1993.

Miller N: Biomedical foundations for biofeedback as a part of behavioral medicine. In Basmajian JV, editor: *Biofeedback: principles and practice for clinicians,* ed 3, Baltimore, 1989, Williams & Wilkins.

Mulloney S, Wells-Federman C: Therapeutic touch: a healing modality, *J Cardiovasc Nurs* 10:27, 1996.

Norris P, Fahrion S: Autogenic biofeedback in psychophysiological therapy and stress management. In Lehrer P, Woolfolk R, editors: *Principles and practice of stress management,* ed 2, New York, 1993, Guilford Press.

Olson R: Definitions of biofeedback. In Schwartz MS and others, editors: *Biofeedback: a practitioner's guide,* New York, 1987, Guilford Press.

Patel C: Yoga-based therapy. In Lehrer P, Woolfolk R, editors: *Principles and practice of stress management,* ed 2, New York, 1993, Guilford Press.

Post-White J: Imagery. In Snyder M, Lindquist R, editors: *Complementary/alternative therapies in nursing,* ed 3, New York, 1998, Springer.

Quinn J: Therapeutic touch an energy exchange: testing the theory, *ANS Adv Nurs Sci* 6:42, 1984.

Quinn J, Strelkauskas A: Psychoimmunologic effects of therapeutic touch on practitioners and recently bereaved recipients: a pilot study, *ANS Adv Nurs Sci* 15:13, 1993.

Rabin B and others: Mechanistic aspects of stressor-induced immune alteration. In Glaser R, Kiecolt-Glaser J, editors: *Human stress and immunity,* San Diego, 1994, Academic Press.

Redwood D: Chiropractic. In Micozzi MS, editor: *Fundamentals of complementary and alternative therapy,* New York, 1996, Churchill Livingstone.

Roberts G, McGrady A: Racial and gender effects on the relaxation response: implications for the development of hypertension, *Biofeedback Self-Regul* 21:51, 1996.

Sancier K: Medical applications of qigong, *Altern Ther Health Med* 2:40, 1996.

Schaldach M: New aspects in electrostimulation of the heart, *Med Prog Technol* 21:1, 1995.

Sedlacek K: Biofeedback treatment of primary Raynaud's disease. In Basmajian JV, editor: *Biofeedback: principles and practice for clinicians,* ed 3, Baltimore, 1989, Williams & Wilkins.

Sheng-han X: Psychophysiological reactions associated with qigong therapy, *Chin Med J* 107:230, 1994.

Smith J and others: Relaxation: mapping an uncharted world, *Biofeedback Self Regul* 21:63, 1996.

Snyder M: Progressive muscle relaxation. In Synder M, Lindquist R, editors. *Complementary/alternative therapies in nursing,* ed 3, New York, 1998, Springer.

Soykan I and others: The rumination syndrome: clinical and manometric profile, therapy, and long-term outcome, *Dig Dis Sci* 41:1866, 1995.

Syrjala K and others: Relaxation and imagery and cognitive-behavioral training reduce pain during cancer treatment: a controlled clinical trial, *Pain* 63:189, 1995.

Taylor D: Effects of a behavioral stress-management program on anxiety, mood, self-esteem, and T-cell count in HIV positive men, *Psychol Rep* 76:451, 1995.

Taylor E, Lee C, Young J: Bringing mind-body medicine into the mainstream, *Hosp Pract* 32:183, 1997.

Turk D and others: Dysfunctional patients with temporomandibular disorders: evaluating the efficacy of a tailored treatment protocol, *J Consult Clin Psychol* 64:139, 1996.

Tyler V: What pharmacists should know about herbal remedies, *J Am Phar Assoc* NS36:29, 1996.

Ulett G: Conditioned healing with electroacupuncture, *Altern Ther Health Med* 2:56, 1996.

Van Rood Y and others: The effects of stress and relaxation on the in vitro immune response in man: a meta-analytic study, *J Behav Med* 16:163, 1993.

Whitehouse WG and others: Psychological and immune effects of self-hypnosis training for stress management throughout the first semester of medical school, *Psychosom Med* 58:249, 1996.

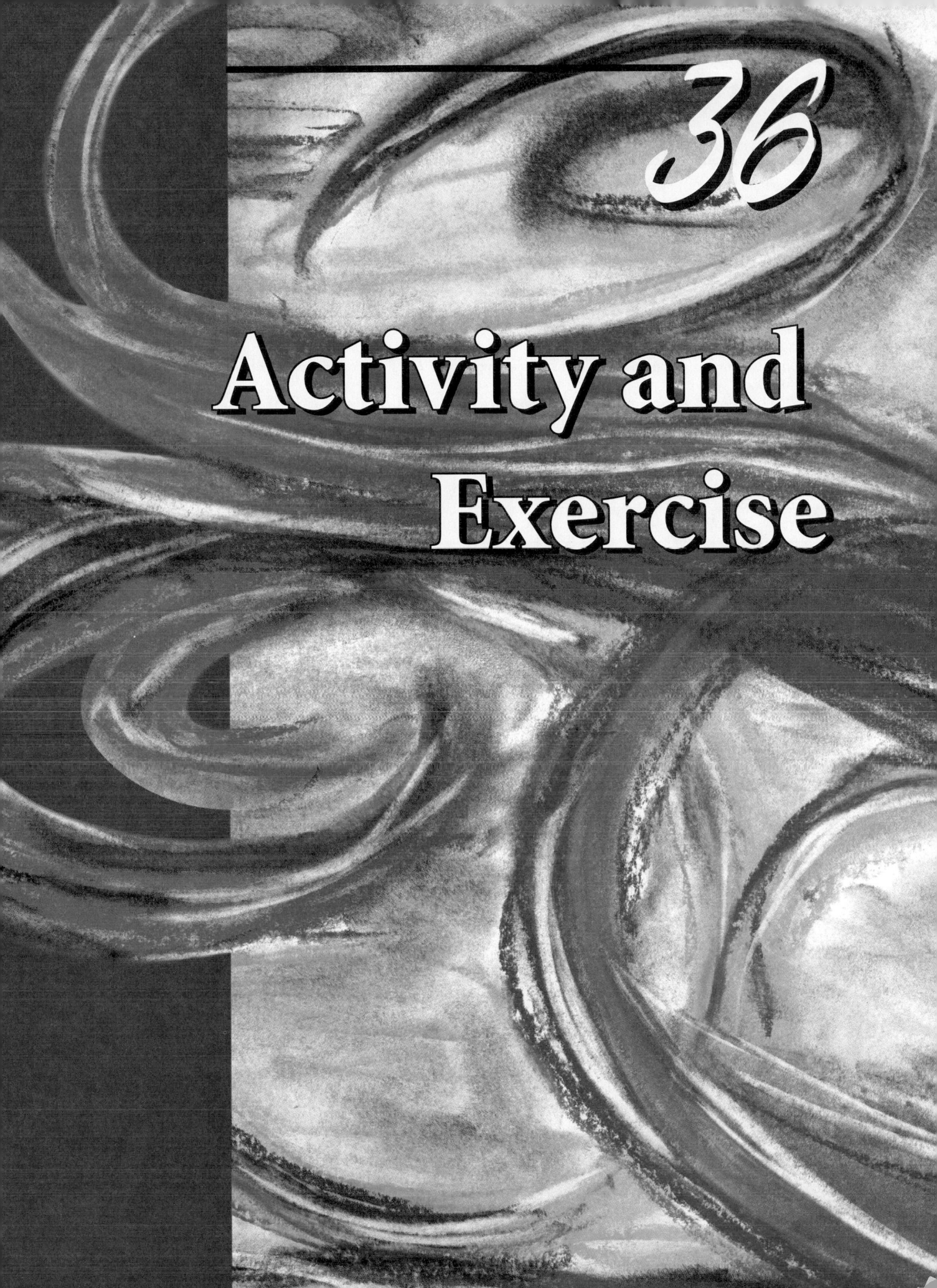

36

Activity and Exercise

Mastery of content in this chapter will enable the student to:

- Define the key terms listed.
- Describe the role of the musculoskeletal and nervous systems in the regulation of movement.
- Discuss physiological and pathological influences on body alignment and joint mobility.
- Describe how exercise and activity benefit physiological and psychological functioning.
- Describe the benefits of implementing an exercise program for the purpose of health promotion.
- Describe the benefits of implementing exercise and activity during the acute, restorative, and continuing care of clients.
- Describe important factors to consider when planning an exercise program for clients across the life span and for those with specific chronic illnesses.
- Assess clients for impaired mobility and activity intolerance.
- Formulate nursing diagnoses for clients experiencing problems with impaired mobility and activity intolerance.
- Write a nursing care plan for a client with impaired mobility and activity intolerance.
- Describe the interventions for maintaining activity tolerance and mobility during the acute, restorative, and continuing care of clients.
- Evaluate the nursing care plan for maintaining activity and exercise for clients across the life span and with specific chronic illnesses.

The actions of walking, turning, lifting, and carrying are essential components in the provision of nursing care. Such activities require muscle exertion by the nurse. To reduce the risk of injury to the client or nurse, the nurse must know and practice proper **body mechanics.** This includes knowledge of the actions of various muscle groups, understanding of the factors involved in the coordination of body movement, and familiarity with the integrated functioning of the skeletal, muscular, and nervous systems.

In addition, nurses must promote activity and **exercise** because of the beneficial impact on wellness, prevention of illness, and restoration of optimal functioning. A program of regular physical activity and exercise has the potential to enhance all aspects of a client's biopsychosocial and spiritual model of health (Box 36-1). This chapter provides the student with knowledge of exercise and activity as it relates to health promotion, the acute phase of illness, and the restorative and continuing care of clients. Nursing strategies are included to help plan an individualized exercise and activity program for a variety of clients with specific disease entities and needs.

Scientific Knowledge Base

Activity and exercise are important to all individuals' well-being. The nurse is able to provide a more individualized approach to care by knowing the physiology and regulation of body mechanics, exercise, and activity.

OVERVIEW OF BODY MECHANICS, EXERCISE, AND ACTIVITY

The coordinated efforts of the musculoskeletal and nervous systems to maintain balance, **posture,** and body alignment during lifting, bending, moving, and performing **activities of daily living** (ADLs) provide the foundation for body mechanics. The proper implementation of these activities reduces the risk of injury to the musculoskeletal system and facilitates body movements, allowing physical **mobility** without muscle strain and excessive use of muscle energy.

Body Alignment.   Body alignment refers to the relationship of one body part to another body part along a horizontal or vertical line. Correct alignment reduces strain on musculoskeletal structures, maintains adequate **muscle tone,** and contributes to balance.

Body Balance.   Body balance is achieved when a relatively low **center of gravity** is balanced over a wide, stable base of support and a vertical line falls from the center of gravity through the base of support. The base of support is the foundation. When the vertical line from the center of gravity does not fall through the base of support, the body loses balance. Body balance is also enhanced by proper posture, or the body position that most favors function, requires the least muscular work to maintain, and places the least strain on muscles, ligaments, and bones (Thibodeau and Patton, 1999).

The authors acknowledge the contributions of Jana Weindel Dees to this chapter in the previous edition of this text.

The Gift of Exercise
Box 36-1

The other day I was looking for a gift to give to a friend. This friend is very important to me and I want her to be around for a long time; I want her to live a long and healthy life. I thought how great it would be if I could give her a gift that would improve the quality of her life.

So I sat down and made a list of what I would look for in this special gift:

It would help her to be stronger, firmer, leaner, more flexible, and energetic.

It would help lower her risk of dying from heart disease, help lower blood pressure and improve lipid profile, control blood glucose level, fight obesity, and help her to age more gracefully.

It would help improve immune function, concentration and task performance, and the quality of sleep.

It would help reduce stress, improve mood, enhance self-esteem, and increase optimism and confidence.

It would help to increase self-awareness and control over choices in her life.

It would be fun but also challenging.

It would allow for socialization but also time alone, depending on her needs.

It would come in all different modes and styles and adapt to various environments and weather conditions.

Finally, it would have a good *Consumer Reports* rating, supported by scientific data from reputable sources.

After completing my list, I realized that the only gift that meets all the criteria is the gift of exercise. Have a happy and healthy life, my friend.

From Huddleston JS: Exercise. In Edelman CL, Mandle CL editors: *Health promotion throughout the lifespan*, ed 4, St. Louis, 1998, Mosby.

The nurse maintains proper body alignment and posture by using two simple techniques. First, the base of support can easily be widened by separating the feet to a comfortable distance. Second, balance is increased by bringing the center of gravity closer to the base of support. This is achieved by bending the knees and flexing the hips until the person is squatting and still maintaining proper back alignment by keeping the trunk erect. The nervous system is responsible for muscle tone and regulates and coordinates the amount of pull exerted by the individual muscles (Thibodeau and Patton, 1999).

Coordinated Body Movement. Coordinated body movement is a result of weight, center of gravity, and balance. Weight is the force exerted on a body by gravity. When an object is lifted, the lifter must overcome the object's weight and be aware of its center of gravity. In symmetrical objects the center of gravity is located at the exact center of the object. The force of weight is always directed downward. An object that is unbalanced has its center of gravity away from the midline and falls without support. Because people are not geometrically perfect, their centers of gravity are usually at 55% to 57% of standing height and are located in the midline. Like unbalanced objects, clients who fail to maintain a balance with their center of gravity are unsteady, which places them at risk for falling. Nurses must be able to identify such clients and intervene in such a way that safety is maintained.

Friction. **Friction** is a force that occurs in a direction to oppose movement. As the nurse turns, transfers, or moves a client up in bed, friction must be overcome. A nurse can reduce friction by following some basic principles. The greater the surface area of the object to be moved, the greater the friction. If a client is unable to assist in moving up in bed, the client's arms should be placed across the chest. This decreases surface area and reduces friction.

A passive or immobilized client produces greater friction to movement (see Chapter 46). Thus when possible, the nurse should use some of the client's strength and mobility when lifting, transferring, or moving the client up in bed. This can be done by explaining the procedure and telling the client when to move. For instance, friction is decreased if the client can bend his or her knees as the nurse assists him or her in moving up in the bed.

Friction can also be reduced by lifting rather than pushing a client. Lifting has an upward component and decreases the pressure between the client and the bed or the chair. The use of a lift sheet reduces friction because the client is more easily moved along the bed's surface.

Exercise and Activity. Exercise is physical activity for the purpose of conditioning the body, improving health, and maintaining fitness, or it may be used as a therapeutic measure. The exercise program chosen and developed for a client depends heavily on the individual's **activity tolerance,** or the kind and amount of exercise or activity that the person is able to perform. Physiological, emotional, and developmental factors influence the client's activity tolerance.

A program of regular physical activity and exercise promotes physical and psychological health. An active lifestyle is important for maintaining and promoting health; it is also an essential treatment modality for chronic illnesses. A program of regular physical activity and exercise enhances functioning of all body systems, including cardiopulmonary functioning (endurance), musculoskeletal fitness (flexibility and bone integrity), weight control and maintenance (body image), and psychological well-being.

The best program of physical activity includes a combination of exercises that produce different physiological and psychological benefits. Isotonic, isometric, and resistive isometric are three categories of exercise classified according to the type of muscle contraction involved. Isotonic exercises cause muscle contraction and change in muscle length (**isotonic contraction**). Examples of isotonic exercises are walking, swimming, dance aerobics, jogging, bicycling, and moving arms and legs with light resistance. The benefits of isotonic exercises are increased circulation and respiratory functioning; increased osteoblastic activity (activity by bone-forming cells), thus combating osteoporosis; and increased muscle tone, mass, and strength.

Isometric exercises involve tightening or tensing of muscles without moving body parts (**isometric contraction**). Examples of isometric exercises are quadriceps set exercises and contraction of the gluteal muscles. This form of exercise is ideal for clients who are unable to tolerate an increase in activity that is expected during isotonic exercises. Isometric exercises are easily accomplished by an immobilized client in bed. The benefits are increased muscle mass, tone, and strength, thus decreasing the potential for muscle wasting; increased circulation to the involved body part; and increased osteoblastic activity.

Isometric exercises may also be resistive. Resistive isometric exercises are those in which the individual contracts the muscle while pushing against a stationary object or resisting the movement of an object (Borgman-Gainer, 1996). A gradual increase in the amount of resistance and length of time that the muscle contraction is held will increase muscle strength and endurance (Topp, Mikesky, and Bawel, 1994). Examples of resistive isometric exercises are push-ups, pushing against a **footboard** to move up in bed, and hip lifting. In hip lifting, the client, who is in a sitting position, pushes with the hands against a surface such as the seat of a chair and raises the hips. Resistive isometric exercises help to promote muscle strength and provide sufficient stress against bone to promote osteoblastic activity.

REGULATION OF MOVEMENT

Coordinated body movement involves the integrated functioning of the skeletal, muscular, and nervous systems. Because these three systems cooperate so closely in mechanical support of the body, they are often considered as a single functional unit.

Skeletal System.

Bones perform five functions in the body: support, protection, movement, mineral storage, and hematopoiesis (blood cell formation). In the discussion of body mechanics two of these functions—support and movement—are most important (see Chapter 46). In support, bones serve as the framework and contribute to the shape, alignment, and positioning of the body parts. In movement, bones together with their joints constitute levers for muscle attachment. As muscles contract and shorten, they pull on bones, producing joint movement (Thibodeau and Patton, 1999).

Joints.

An articulation, or **joint,** is the connection between bones. Each joint is classified according to its structure and degree of mobility. On the basis of connective structures, joints are classified as fibrous, cartilaginous, or synovial (McCance and Huether, 1998). **Fibrous joints** fit closely together and are fixed, permitting little, if any, movement. **Cartilaginous joints** have little movement but are elastic and use cartilage to unite separate body surfaces. **Synovial joints,** or true joints, are freely movable and are the most mobile, numerous, and anatomically complex of the body's joint's.

Ligaments, Tendons, and Cartilage.

Ligament, tendons, and joints are structures that support the skeletal system (see Chapter 46). **Ligaments** are white, shiny, flexible bands of fibrous tissue that bind joints and connect bones and cartilage. Ligaments are elastic and aid joint flexibility and support. In some areas of the body, ligaments also have a protective function. **Tendons** are white, glistening, fibrous bands of tissue that connect muscle to bone. **Cartilage** is nonvascular, supporting connective tissue with the flexibility of a firm, plastic material. The gristlelike nature of cartilage permits it to sustain weight and serve as a shock absorber between articulating bones.

Skeletal Muscle.

When we walk, talk, run, breathe, or participate in physical activity, we do so by the contraction of skeletal muscles. There are over 600 skeletal muscles in the body. In addition to facilitating movement, these muscles determine the form and contour of our bodies. Most of our muscles span at least one joint and attach to both articulating bones. When contraction occurs, one bone is fixed while the other moves. The origin is the point of attachment that remains still; the insertion is the point that moves when the muscle contracts (Thibodeau and Patton, 1999).

Muscles Concerned With Movement. The muscles of movement are located near the skeletal region, where movement is caused by a lever system (Thibodeau and Patton, 1999). The lever system makes the work of moving a weight or load easier. It occurs when specific bones, such as the humerus, ulna, and radius, and the associated joints, such as the elbow, act as a lever. Thus the force applied to one end of the bone to lift a weight at another point tends to rotate the bone in the direction opposite that of the applied force. Muscles that attach to bones of leverage provide the necessary strength to move the object.

Muscles Concerned With Posture. Gravity pulls on parts of the body all the time; the only way the body can be held in position is for muscles to exert pull on bones in the opposite direction. Muscles accomplish this counterforce by maintaining a low level of sustained contraction. Poor posture places more work on muscles to counteract the force of gravity. This leads to fatigue and can eventually interfere with bodily functions and cause deformities.

Muscle Groups. The antagonistic, synergistic, and antigravity muscle groups are coordinated by the nervous system and maintain posture and initiate movement. **Antagonistic muscles** bring about movement at the joint. During movement the active mover muscle contracts while its antagonist relaxes. For example, during flexion of the arm the active mover, the biceps brachii, contracts and its antagonist, the triceps brachii, relaxes. During extension of the arm the active mover, now the triceps brachii, contracts and the new antagonist, the biceps brachii, relaxes.

Synergistic muscles contract to accomplish the same movement. When the arm is flexed, the strength of the contraction of the biceps brachii is increased by contraction of the synergistic muscle, the brachialis. Thus with synergistic muscle activity there are now two active movers—the biceps brachii and the brachialis—which contract while the antagonistic muscle, the triceps brachii, relaxes.

Antigravity muscles are involved with joint stabilization. These muscles continuously oppose the effect of gravity on the body and permit a person to maintain an upright or sitting posture. In an adult the antigravity muscles are the extensors of the leg, the gluteus maximus, the quadriceps femoris, the soleus muscles, and the muscles of the back.

Skeletal muscles support posture and carry out voluntary movement. The muscles are attached to the skeleton by tendons, which provide strength and permit motion. The movement of the extremities is voluntary and requires coordination from the nervous system.

Nervous System.   Movement and posture are regulated by the nervous system. The major voluntary motor area, located in the cerebral cortex, is the precentral gyrus, or motor strip. A majority of motor fibers descend from the motor strip and cross at the level of the medulla. Thus the motor fibers from the right motor strip initiate voluntary movement for the left side of the body, and motor fibers from the left motor strip initiate voluntary movement for the right side of the body.

Transmission of the impulse from the nervous system to the musculoskeletal system is an electrochemical event and requires a neurotransmitter. Basically, neurotransmitters are chemicals (e.g., acetylcholine) that transfer the electric impulse from the nerve across the myoneural junction to stimulate the muscle, causing movement.

Movement can be impaired by disorders that alter neurotransmitter production, transfer from the neurotransmitter to the muscle, or activation of muscle activity.

Proprioception.   **Proprioception** is the awareness of the position of the body and its parts (McCance and Huether, 1998). Proprioception is monitored by proprioceptors located on nerve endings in muscles, tendons, and joints. Posture is regulated by the nervous system and requires coordination of proprioception and balance. As a person carries out ADLs, proprioceptors monitor muscle activity and body position. For example, the proprioceptors on the soles of the feet contribute to correct posture while standing or walking. In standing, pressure is contin-

uous on the bottom of the feet. The proprioceptors monitor the pressure, communicating this information through the nervous system to the antigravity muscles. The standing person remains upright until deciding to change position. As a person walks, the proprioceptors on the bottom of the feet monitor pressure changes. Thus when the bottom of the moving foot comes in contact with the walking surface, the individual automatically moves the stationary foot forward. The proprioceptors allow people to walk without having to watch their feet.

Balance.   When standing, running, lifting, or performing ADLs, a person must have adequate balance. Balance is controlled by the nervous system, specifically by the cerebellum and the inner ear. The major function of the cerebellum is to coordinate all voluntary movement, particularly highly skilled movements, such as those required in skiing.

Within the inner ear are the semicircular canals, three fluid-filled structures that assist in maintaining balance. Fluid within the canals has a certain inertia, and when the head is suddenly rotated in one direction, the fluid remains stationary for a moment, whereas the canal turns with the head. This allows a person to change position suddenly without losing balance.

PRINCIPLES OF BODY MECHANICS

Using principles of body mechanics during routine activities also prevents injury. The nurse teaches colleagues and clients' families to lift, transfer, or position clients properly. A nurse who is teaching a client's family to transfer the client from bed to chair can increase and reinforce the family's knowledge by consistently demonstrating proper body mechanics.

Whether the nurse is moving an immobilized client, assisting a client from the bed to the chair, or teaching a client to carry out ADLs efficiently, knowledge of basic principles of body mechanics is crucial. The nurse also incorporates knowledge of physiological and pathological influences on body alignment and mobility (Box 36-2).

Pathological Influences on Body Mechanics. Many pathological conditions affect body alignment and mobility. These conditions include congenital defects; disorders of bones, joints, and muscles, central nervous system damage, and musculoskeletal trauma.

Congenital Defects.   Congenital abnormalities affect the efficiency of the musculoskeletal system in regard to alignment, balance, and appearance. Osteogenesis imperfecta is an inherited disorder that affects bone. Bones are porous, short, bowed, and deformed; as a result, children experience curvature of the spine and shortness of stature. Scoliosis is a structural curvature of the spine associated with vertebral rotation. Muscles, ligaments, and other soft tissues become shortened. Balance and mobility are af-

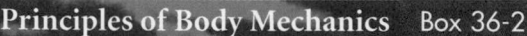

Principles of Body Mechanics   Box 36-2

The wider the base of support, the greater the stability of the nurse.

The lower the center of gravity, the greater the stability of the nurse.

The equilibrium of an object is maintained as long as the line of gravity passes through its base of support.

Facing the direction of movement prevents abnormal twisting of the spine.

Dividing balanced activity between arms and legs reduces the risk of back injury.

Leverage, rolling, turning, or pivoting requires less work than lifting.

When friction is reduced between the object to be moved and the surface on which it is moved, less force is required to move it.

Reducing the force of work reduces the risk of injury.

Maintaining good body mechanics reduces fatigue of the muscle groups.

Alternating periods of rest and activity helps to reduce fatigue.

---

fected in proportion to the severity of abnormal spinal curvatures (McCance and Huether, 1998).

Disorders of Bones, Joints, and Muscles.

Osteoporosis is a well-known and well-publicized disorder of aging in which the density or mass of bone is reduced. The bone remains biochemically normal but has difficulty maintaining integrity and support. The cause is uncertain, and theories vary from hormonal imbalances to insufficient intake of nutrients (McCance and Huether, 1998).

Osteomalacia is a metabolic disease characterized by inadequate and delayed mineralization, resulting in compact and spongy bone. Mineral calcification and deposition do not occur. Replaced bone consists of soft material rather than rigid bone.

Joint mobility can be altered by inflammatory and noninflammatory joint diseases and by articular disruption. Inflammatory joint disease (e.g., arthritis) is characterized by inflammation or destruction of the synovial membrane and articular cartilage, and by systemic signs of inflammation. Noninflammatory diseases have none of these characteristics, and the synovial fluid is normal (McCance and Huether, 1998). Joint degeneration, which can occur with inflammatory and noninflammatory disease, is marked by changes in articular cartilage combined with overgrowth of bone at the articular ends. Degenerative changes commonly affect weight-bearing joints.

Articular disruption may be as mild as a sprain or as severe as dislocation. Articular disruption involves trauma to the articular capsules, such as a tear in a sprain or a separation in a dislocation. Articular disruption usually re-

sults from trauma but can also be congenital, as with congenital hip dysplasia.

Central Nervous System Damage.

Damage to any component of the central nervous system that regulates voluntary movement results in impaired body alignment and mobility. For example, the motor strip in the cerebrum can be damaged by trauma from a head injury. The amount of voluntary motor impairment is directly related to the amount of destruction of the motor strip. A client with a right-sided cerebral hemorrhage and damage to the right motor strip may have left-sided hemiplegia. However, a client with a right-sided head injury may only have cerebral edema (but not destruction) of the motor strip. With extensive physical therapy, voluntary movement gradually returns to the left side.

Musculoskeletal Trauma.

Musculoskeletal trauma can result in bruises, contusions, sprains, and fractures. A fracture is a disruption of bone tissue continuity. Fractures most commonly result from direct external trauma. They can also occur because of some deformity of the bone, as with pathological fractures of osteoporosis (see Chapter 46).

Nursing Knowledge Base

This section is concerned with knowledge from areas of nursing practice that enable the nurse to meet the holistic needs of the client. Developmental changes, behavioral aspects, family and social support, cultural and ethnic origin, and environmental issues are important aspects of an individual and must be incorporated into the plan of care whether the client is seeking health promotion, acute care, or restorative and continuing care.

DEVELOPMENTAL CHANGES

Throughout the life span the body's appearance and functioning undergo change. The greatest change and impact on the maturational process is observed in childhood and old age.

Infants.

The newborn infant's spine is flexed and lacks the anteroposterior curves of the adult. The first spinal curve occurs when the infant extends the neck from the prone position. As growth and stability increase, the thoracic spine straightens, and the lumbar spinal curve appears, which allows sitting and standing. The infant's musculoskeletal system is flexible. The extremities are flexed, and joints have complete **range of motion (ROM)**. As the newborn matures, the musculoskeletal system becomes stronger, and the infant is able to resist movement and reach out and grasp objects (see Chapter 10). As the baby grows, musculoskeletal development permits support of weight for standing and walking. Posture is awkward because the head and upper trunk are carried forward.

Because body weight is not evenly distributed along a line of gravity, posture is off balance, and falls occur often.

Toddlers.

The toddler's posture is awkward because of the slight swayback and protruding abdomen. As the child walks, the legs and feet are usually far apart and the feet are slightly everted. Toward the end of toddlerhood, posture appears less awkward, curves in the cervical and lumbar vertebrae are accentuated, and foot eversion disappears.

Preschool Through Adolescence.

By the third year the body is slimmer, taller, and better balanced. Abdominal protrusion is decreased, the feet are not as far apart, and the arms and legs have increased in length. The child appears more coordinated. From the third year through the beginning of adolescence, the musculoskeletal system continues to grow and develop. Long bones in the arms and legs grow. Greater coordination enables the child to perform tasks that require fine motor skills (see Chapter 10).

The period of adolescence is usually initiated by a tremendous growth spurt. Growth is frequently uneven. As a result, the adolescent may appear awkward and uncoordinated. Adolescent girls usually grow and develop earlier than boys. Hips widen, and fat is deposited in the upper arms, thighs, and buttocks. The adolescent boy's changes in shape are usually a result of long-bone growth and increased muscle mass. Legs become longer, and hips become narrower. Muscular development increases in the chest, arms, shoulders, and upper legs (see Chapter 10).

Young to Middle Adults.

An adult who has correct posture and body alignment feels good, looks good, and generally appears self-confident. The healthy adult also has the necessary musculoskeletal development and coordination to carry out ADLs (see Chapter 11). Normal changes in posture and body alignment in adulthood occur mainly in pregnant women. These changes result from the body's adaptive response to weight gain and the growing fetus. The center of gravity shifts toward the anterior. The pregnant woman leans back and is slightly swaybacked. She may complain of back pain.

Older Adults.

A progressive loss of total bone mass occurs with the older adult. Some of the possible causes of this loss include physical inactivity, hormonal changes, and increased osteoclastic activity (activity by cells responsible for bone tissue absorption). The effect of bone loss is weaker bones, causing vertebrae to be softer and long shaft bones to be less resistant to bending.

In addition, older adults may walk more slowly and appear less coordinated. They may also take smaller steps, keeping their feet closer together, which decreases the base of support. Thus body balance is unstable, and they are at greater risk for falls and injuries (see Chapter 12).

BEHAVIORAL ASPECTS

Clients are more likely to incorporate an exercise program into their daily lives if this is supported and assisted by nurses, physicians, and other members of the health care team. The nurse should take into consideration the client's knowledge of exercise and activity, barriers to a program of exercise and physical activity, and current exercise habits. Clients are more open to developing an exercise program if they are at the stage of readiness to change their behavior (Prochaska, Norcross, and DiClemente, 1994). Information on the benefits of regular exercise may be helpful in the client who is not at the stage of readiness to act. Clients' decisions to change behavior and include a daily exercise routine in their lives may occur gradually with repeated information that is individualized to their needs and lifestyle (Box 36-3). Once the client has reached the stage of readiness, the nurse must develop in collaboration with the client an exercise program that is customized to fit his or her needs; the nurse then provides continued follow-up support and assistance until the exercise program becomes a daily routine.

ENVIRONMENTAL ISSUES

Work Site.

A common barrier for many clients is the lack of time that is needed to engage in a daily exercise program. Work sites have the potential to help their employees overcome the obstacle of time constraints by offering opportunities, reminders, and rewards for those committed to physical fitness (National Institutes of Health [NIH], 1996). Opportunities such as an indoor

---

General Guidelines for Initiating and Maintaining an Exercise Program   **Box 36-3**

The client will most likely initiate and maintain an exercise program if the individual:
Perceives a net benefit
Chooses an enjoyable activity
Feels competent doing the activity
Feels safe doing the activity
Can easily access the activity on a regular basis
Can fit the activity into the daily schedule
Feels that the activity does not generate financial or social costs that he or she is unwilling to bear
Experiences a minimum of negative consequences such as injury, loss of time, negative peer pressure, and problems with self-identity
Is able to successfully address issues of competing time demands
Recognizes the need to balance the use of labor-saving devices and sedentary activities with activities that involve a higher level of physical exertion

From National Institutes of Health Consensus Development Panel on Physical Activity and Cardiovascular Health: Physical activity and cardiovascular health, *JAMA* 276(3):241, 1996.

walking track and exercise equipment room could be made available free of charge to employees and their families. Reminders such as signs could be used to encourage employees to use the stairs instead of elevators. Rewards such as free parking or discounted parking fees could be given to employees who park in distant lots and walk (NIH, 1996).

Schools. It has become increasingly clear that children are becoming less active and spending more time playing video games and watching television, with the result being an increase in childhood obesity (U.S. Department of Health and Human Services [USDHHS], 1995). Children and adolescents spend a great deal of their time in school. However, the number of students involved in daily school physical education decreased from 42% in 1991 to 25% in 1995 (USDHHS, 1996). Schools can be an excellent facilitator of physical fitness and exercise. Strategies for physical activity incorporated early into a child's daily routine could provide a foundation for lifetime commitment to exercise and physical fitness. The NIH Consensus Development Panel (1996) recommends that all schools provide physical activity programs that are appropriate for children of all skill levels and not limited to competitive sports or physical education classes, that appeal to both girls and boys, as well as to children from diverse backgrounds; and that are offered on a daily basis.

Community. The community's support of physical fitness can be instrumental in promoting the health of its members. Examples of community involvement to promote physical fitness is the provision of walking tracks in community parks and physical fitness classes offered by trained professionals in exercise and physical fitness. This may be a difficult task because of cost restraints. However, success in implementing physical fitness programs is dependent on a collaborative effort from public health agencies, parks and recreational associations, state and local government agencies, health care agencies, and the members of the community (Pate and others, 1995).

CULTURAL AND ETHNIC INFLUENCES

Exercise and physical fitness is beneficial to all people. However, there is less physical activity and exercise among ethnic minority populations than among white Americans (Pate and others, 1995). When developing a physical fitness program for culturally diverse populations, the nurse must consider what motivates and what is deemed appropriate and enjoyable. The nurse must also have knowledge of what specific disease entities are associated with different cultural and ethnic origins. For example, hypertension is more prevalent in African-Americans. The use of blood pressure monitoring over the course of an exercise program could be a motivational tool for this population. The African-American client may see his or her blood pressure decrease as a result of weight loss and cardiovascular fit-

ness, thus reinforcement and positive feedback would be provided that would support a daily routine of exercise and at the same time decrease the risk of hypertension and stroke (Box 36-4).

FAMILY AND SOCIAL SUPPORT

Social support can be used as a motivational tool to encourage and promote exercise and physical fitness. The client can engage a friend or significant other to participate in a "buddy system" whereby they walk together each day at a specified time. This companionship provides for socialization and increases the enjoyment for some clients, who may begin a lifelong commitment to physical fitness. Parents can support their children in sports and physical activity by providing encouragement, praise, and transportation (NIH, 1996). In addition, parents can include their children in family outings that include such activities as bicycling or a basketball game in the neighborhood schoolyard.

Cultural ASPECTS OF CARE   Box 36-4

In the United States, African-Americans have a disproportionate number of poor, unemployed, and disadvantaged individuals who lack access to the health care system (Huddleston, 1998). The methods to ensure and promote exercise in African-Americans need to be tailored to include the belief systems and lifestyles of the African-American population. Barriers to participating in a regular exercise program include the prohibitive cost of membership at health and fitness centers, the lack of safety in inner-city neighborhoods that prohibits walking or jogging as a form of exercise, lack of motivation, and lack of support from family and friends to participate in exercise (Graham and Pohlman, 1994).

By addressing these barriers and incorporating the suggestions of a group of inner-city African-Americans, a successful, inexpensive exercise program was developed. African-Americans tend to have well-organized churches that are a major influence in their daily lives. Churches are natural gathering places and can be used to promote and facilitate health promotion activities. Graham and Pohlman (1994) used this knowledge to motivate a group of inner-city African-Americans to participate in an exercise program by using the church as a meeting place for the exercise program. The members in the group chose step aerobics as a means of meeting their goal of cardiovascular fitness. Steps for this type of exercise can cost about $50 to $80. They reduced the cost to $8 by having a volunteer from the church build the steps. To motivate the group further, the choice of music was left up to the group, and a Christian music tape was chosen. Educating a member of the congregation to lead the exercise sessions helped to maintain and continue the exercise program past the original 10-week session. The success of this intervention for this group of African-Americans depended heavily on the nurse's ability to incorporate the knowledge of cultural diversity and allow the participants to take an active role in health promotion activities.

Critical Thinking and Application of Exercise and Activity

Successful critical thinking requires a synthesis of knowledge, experience, information gathering from clients, critical thinking attitudes, and intellectual and professional standards. Clinical judgments require the nurse to anticipate the information necessary, analyze the data, and make decisions regarding client care. Critical thinking is always changing. During assessment (Figure 36-1) the nurse must consider all of the elements that build toward making appropriate nursing diagnoses.

To understand activity tolerance and physical fitness and the impact on the client, the nurse must integrate knowledge from nursing and other disciplines, previous experiences, and information gathered from clients. As the nurse begins the process of problem solving for client care, a variety of concepts must be considered and woven together to provide the best outcome for the client. Knowledge of the musculoskeletal system and health alterations that create problems for the client in the area of activity, exercise, and body mechanics lays the foundation for planning and decision making. The use of professional standards, such as those developed by the American College of Sports Medicine (ACSM, 1995), provides valuable guidelines for exercise and physical fitness. The

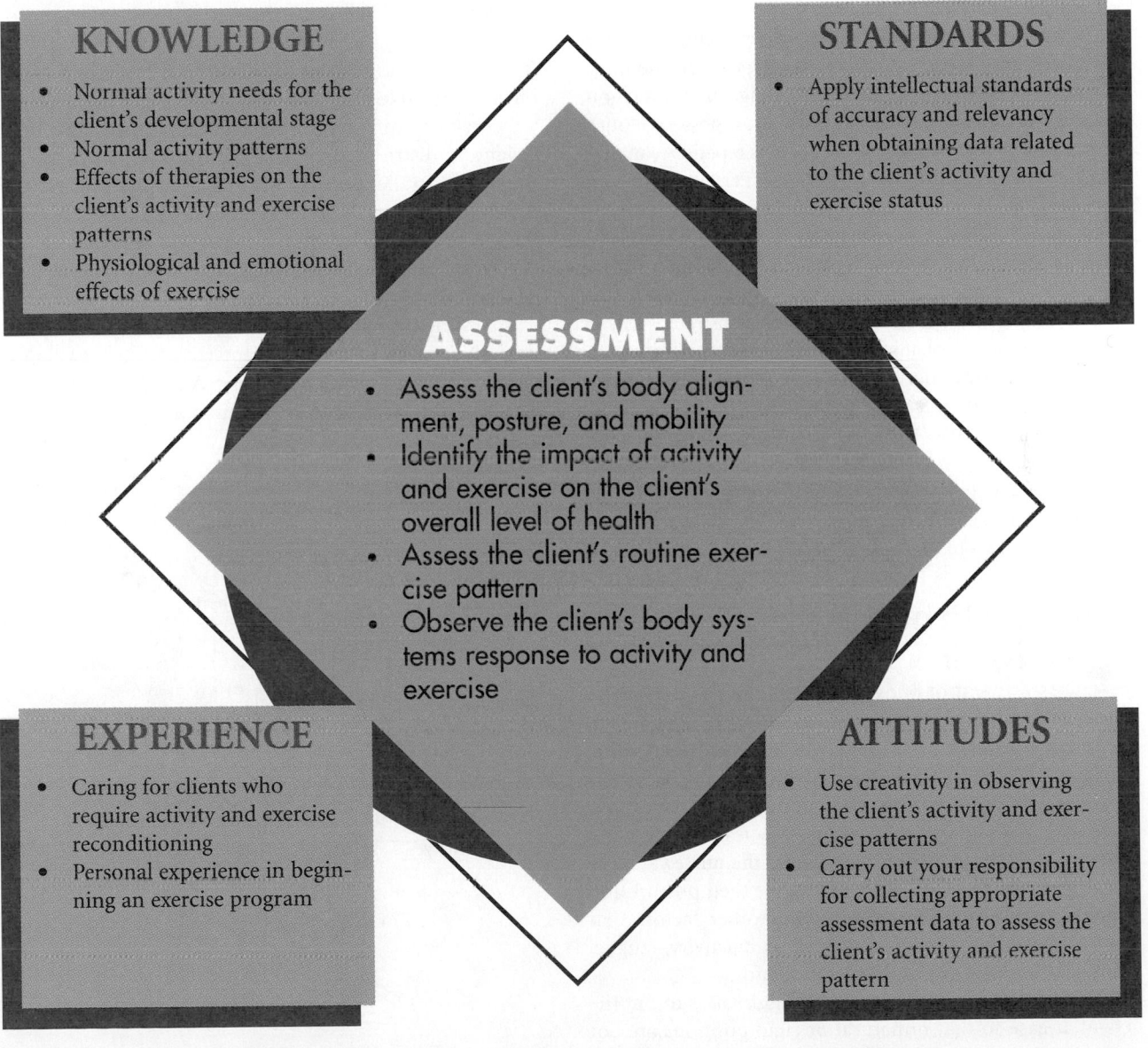

KNOWLEDGE

- Normal activity needs for the client's developmental stage
- Normal activity patterns
- Effects of therapies on the client's activity and exercise patterns
- Physiological and emotional effects of exercise

STANDARDS

- Apply intellectual standards of accuracy and relevancy when obtaining data related to the client's activity and exercise status

ASSESSMENT

- Assess the client's body alignment, posture, and mobility
- Identify the impact of activity and exercise on the client's overall level of health
- Assess the client's routine exercise pattern
- Observe the client's body systems response to activity and exercise

EXPERIENCE

- Caring for clients who require activity and exercise reconditioning
- Personal experience in beginning an exercise program

ATTITUDES

- Use creativity in observing the client's activity and exercise patterns
- Carry out your responsibility for collecting appropriate assessment data to assess the client's activity and exercise pattern

Figure 36-1 *Synthesis Model for Activity and Exercise Assessment Phase.*

nurse's experiences and critical thinking attitude affect the problem-solving approach with clients and must be reevaluated with each new client.

Any acquired or congenital condition that affects the structure of the musculoskeletal or nervous system impairs to some degree activity, body alignment, or joint mobility. The impairment can be temporary, such as casting of an extremity, or permanent, as in contractures. For clients with limited ROM or mobility, the nursing care plan should include interventions that maintain the present level of alignment and joint mobility and increase the level of motor function.

The nurse must remember that clients may have the capacity for recovery in spite of the loss of some physical function. Restoration of functioning begins early in the care of clients experiencing disruption in their ability to perform self-care. Encouragement, support, commitment, and perseverance are important attitudes in critical thinking for these clients.

When intervening with clients experiencing problems with body mechanics and who may depend on the nurse for assistance with positioning, turning, or ambulation, perseverance is one attitude the nurse must possess. Hourly responsibility for turning often becomes repetitive, and the nurse may lose sight of its importance. Perseverance is especially important in the delegation of these activities to unlicensed health care providers or family members. Making certain that the task is performed and is performed correctly is an essential nursing function.

Another attitude for the nurse to demonstrate is one of creativity. Since problems with activity and mobility are often prolonged, the more creative the nurse's approach for improving activity tolerance and mobility skills, the greater the chance of success. This is especially important with children. Children enjoy receiving rewards for any accomplishment. When a child makes strides toward greater mobility the nurse can make it a game by giving the child stickers in and pretty colors to symbolize successes.

Nursing Process

ASSESSMENT

Assessment of body alignment and posture can be carried out with the client standing, sitting, or lying down. Through assessment the nurse will be able to determine normal physiological changes in growth and development; deviations related to poor posture, trauma, muscle damage, or nerve dysfunction; and any learning needs of clients. In addition, during assessment the nurse can provide opportunities for clients to observe their posture and obtain important information about other factors that contribute to poor alignment, such as inactivity, fatigue, malnutrition, and psychological problems.

The first step in assessing body alignment is to put the client at ease so that unnatural or rigid positions are not assumed. When assessing body alignment of an immobi-

lized or unconscious client, pillows and positioning supports should be removed from the bed if not contraindicated, and the client placed in the supine position.

Standing.   Assessment for the standing client includes the following: the head is erect and midline; body parts are symmetrical; the spine should be straight with normal curvatures (cervical concave, thoracic convex, lumbar concave); the abdomen is comfortably tucked; the knees should be in a straight line between the hips and ankles and slightly flexed; the feet should be flat on the floor and pointed directly forward and slightly apart to maintain a wide base of support; and the arms should hang comfortably at the sides (Figure 36-2). The client's center of gravity is in the midline, and the line of gravity is from the middle of the forehead to a midpoint between the feet. Laterally, the line of gravity runs vertically from the middle of the skull to the posterior third of the foot (Thompson and Wilson, 1996).

Sitting.   Assessment of the client in the sitting position includes the following: the head is erect, and the neck and vertebral column are in straight alignment; the body weight is distributed on the buttocks and thighs; the thighs are parallel and in a horizontal plane (be careful to avoid pressure on the popliteal nerve and blood supply); the feet are supported on the floor; and the forearms are supported on the armrest, in the lap, or on a table in front of the chair.

Assessment of alignment in the sitting position is particularly important for the client with muscle weakness, muscle paralysis, or nerve damage. A client with these alterations has diminished sensation in affected areas and is

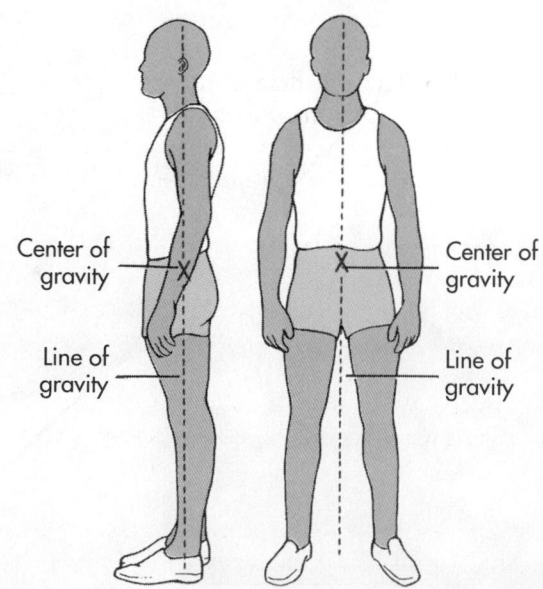

Figure 36-2   Correct body alignment when standing.

unable to perceive pressure or decreased circulation. Proper sitting alignment reduces the risk of musculoskeletal system damage in such a client.

Recumbent Position.   Assessment of the client in the recumbent position requires that the client be placed in the lateral position with all but one pillow and all positioning supports removed from the bed. The vertebrae should be in straight alignment without observable curves. This assessment provides baseline data concerning the client's body alignment.

Conditions that create a risk of damage to the musculoskeletal system when lying down include impaired mobility (e.g., traction), decreased sensation (e.g., hemiparesis from a stroke), impaired circulation (e.g., diabetes), and lack of voluntary muscle control (e.g., spinal cord injuries).

When a client is unable to change position voluntarily, the nurse assesses the position of body parts while the client is lying down. The vertebrae should be in straight alignment without any observable curves. The extremities should be in alignment and not crossed over one another. The head and neck should be aligned without excessive flexion or extension.

Mobility.   Assessment of mobility enables the nurse to determine the client's coordination and balance while walking, the ability to carry out ADLs, and the ability to participate in an exercise program. The assessment of **mobility** has three components: range of joint motion, **gait**, and exercise.

Range of Motion.   Assessing ROM is one of the first assessment techniques used to determine the degree of damage or injury to a joint (see Chapter 46). The nurse assesses ROM to collect data to answer questions about joint stiffness, swelling, pain, limited movement, and unequal movement. Limited range of motion may indicate inflammation such as arthritis, fluid in the joint, altered nerve supply, or contractures. Increased mobility (beyond normal) of a joint may indicate connective tissue disorders, ligament tears, or possible joint fractures.

Gait.   Gait is the manner or style of walking, including rhythm, cadence, and speed. Assessing gait allows the nurse to draw conclusions about balance, posture, and the ability to walk without assistance. The nurse should note conformity; a regular, smooth rhythm; symmetry in the length of leg swing; smooth swaying related to the gait phase; and a smooth, symmetrical arm swing (Thompson and Wilson, 1996).

Exercise.   Exercise is physical activity for conditioning the body, improving health, maintaining fitness, or providing therapy for correcting a deformity or restoring the overall body to a maximal state of health. When a person

exercises, physiological changes occur in body systems (Box 36-5).

The nurse determines how much the client regularly exercises. What type of exercise does the client prefer? How many times per week? How long does the client exercise at any given time?

Activity Tolerance.   Activity tolerance is the kind and amount of exercise or activity a person is able to perform. Assessment of activity tolerance is necessary when planning physical activity for health promotion and for clients with acute or chronic illness. This assessment provides the nurse with baseline data about the client's activity patterns and assists in determining which factors (physical, psy-

---

Effects of Exercise   Box 36-5

CARDIOVASCULAR SYSTEM
Increased cardiac output
Improved myocardial contraction, thereby strengthening cardiac muscle
Decreased resting heart rate
Improved venous return

PULMONARY SYSTEM
Increased respiratory rate and depth followed by a quicker return to resting state
Improved alveolar ventilation
Decreased work of breathing
Improved diaphragmatic excursion

METABOLIC SYSTEM
Increased basal metabolic rate
Increased use of glucose and fatty acids
Increased triglyceride breakdown
Increased gastric motility
Increased production of body heat

MUSCULOSKELETAL SYSTEM
Improved muscle tone
Increased joint mobility
Improved muscle tolerance to physical exercise
Possible increase in muscle mass
Reduced bone loss

ACTIVITY TOLERANCE
Improved tolerance
Decreased fatigue

PSYCHOSOCIAL FACTORS
Improved tolerance to stress
Reports of "feeling better"
Reports of decrease in illness (e.g., colds, influenza)

Data from Huether SE, McCance KL: *Understanding pathophysiology,* St. Louis, 1996, Mosby; and Hoeman SP: *Rehabilitation nursing: process and application,* St. Louis, 1996, Mosby.

chological, or motivational) are affecting activity tolerance (Ackley and Ladwig, 1997). Box 36-6 lists factors affecting activity tolerance.

Client Expectations.

In assessing the client's expectations concerning activity and exercise, the nurse will first need insight into the client's perception of what is normal or acceptable in regard to physical fitness. For example, one of the factors affecting physical activity is freedom from pain. If exercising is painful or tiresome to the client, compliance and commitment to the desired interventions may be lacking. Clients may be content with their present physical activity and fitness and may not perceive a need for improvement. Unless there is a real threat to health maintenance, forcing the client to accept the nurse's perspective is a breach of standards of care.

NURSING DIAGNOSIS

Assessment of the client's activity tolerance, physical fitness, body alignment, and joint mobility provides related clusters of data or defining characteristics that lead the nurse to identify nursing diagnoses (Box 36-7). The nurse must be accurate identifying diagnoses. For exam-

ple, a client who reports being tired or weakened could be potentially diagnosed as having activity intolerance or fatigue. Further review of assessed defining characteristics (e.g., abnormal heart rate or dyspnea) can lead to the definitive diagnosis (activity intolerance).

When activity and exercise are problems for a client, nursing diagnoses often focus on the individual's ability to move. The diagnostic label should direct nursing interventions. This requires the correct selection of the related factors. For example, activity intolerance related to excess weight gain and lack of cardiovascular fitness will require very different interventions if the related factor is prolonged bedrest. Box 36-8 provides an example of how the diagnostic process leads to accurate diagnosis selection.

PLANNING

During planning the nurse again synthesizes information from multiple resources (Figure 36-3). Critical thinking ensures that the client's plan of care integrates all that the nurse knows about the individual, as well as key critical thinking elements. Professional standards are especially important to consider when the nurse develops a plan of care. These standards often establish scientifically proven guidelines for selecting effective nursing interventions.

Once the nursing diagnoses have been defined, the nurse and client set goals and expected outcomes to direct interventions. The plan should include consideration of any risks for injury to the client. It should also take into consideration preexisting health concerns. It is especially important to have knowledge of the client's home environment when planning therapies to maintain or improve activity, body alignment, and mobility. The client's family should be included in the care plan. For some clients with alterations in joint mobility, family members may be the providers of care.

Planning also involves an understanding of the client's need to maintain motor function and independence. Collaboration with other members of the health care team (e.g., physical or occupational therapists) will be especially important for these clients. Long-term rehabilitation may

---

Factors Influencing Activity Tolerance
Box 36-6

PHYSIOLOGICAL FACTORS
Skeletal abnormalities
Muscular impairments
Endocrine or metabolic illnesses (e.g., diabetes mellitus or thyroid disease)
Hypoxemia
Decreased cardiac function
Decreased endurance
Impaired physical stability
Pain
Sleep pattern disturbance
Prior exercise patterns
Infectious processes and fever

EMOTIONAL FACTORS
Anxiety
Depression
Chemical addictions
Motivation

DEVELOPMENTAL FACTORS
Age
Sex

PREGNANCY
Physical growth and development of muscle and skeletal support

Modified from Phipps WJ, Sands JK, and Marek JF: *Medical-surgical nursing: concepts and clinical practice,* ed 6, St. Louis, 1999, Mosby.

NURSING DIAGNOSES   Box 36-7

IMPAIRED MOBILITY AND IMPROPER BODY MECHANICS

Activity intolerance
Body image disturbance
Coping, ineffective individual
Gas exchange, impaired
Injury, risk for
Mobility, impaired physical
Nutrition, altered: more than body requirements
Pain
Skin integrity, impaired

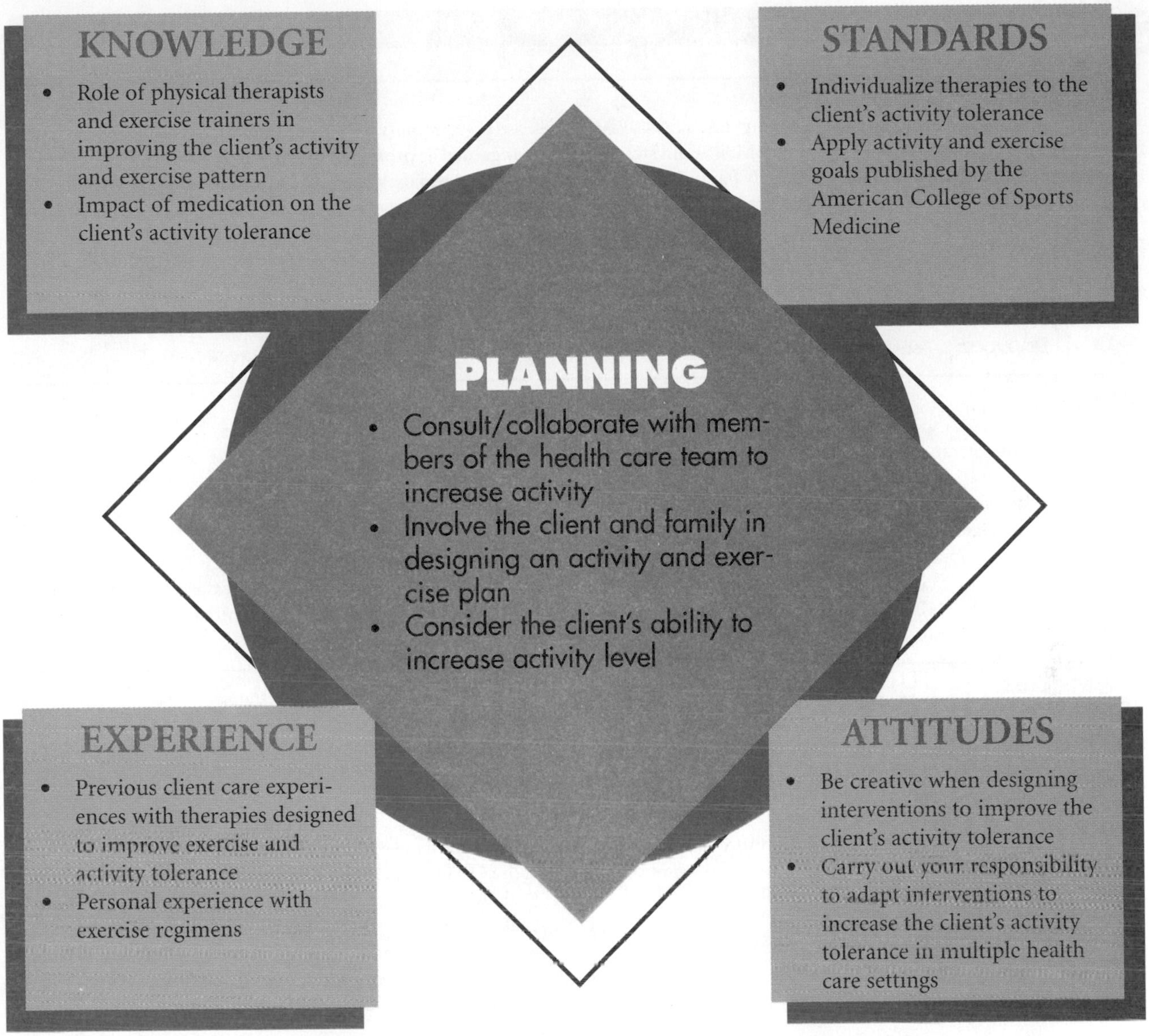

KNOWLEDGE

- Role of physical therapists and exercise trainers in improving the client's activity and exercise pattern
- Impact of medication on the client's activity tolerance

STANDARDS

- Individualize therapies to the client's activity tolerance
- Apply activity and exercise goals published by the American College of Sports Medicine

PLANNING

- Consult/collaborate with members of the health care team to increase activity
- Involve the client and family in designing an activity and exercise plan
- Consider the client's ability to increase activity level

EXPERIENCE

- Previous client care experiences with therapies designed to improve exercise and activity tolerance
- Personal experience with exercise regimens

ATTITUDES

- Be creative when designing interventions to improve the client's activity tolerance
- Carry out your responsibility to adapt interventions to increase the client's activity tolerance in multiple health care settings

Figure 36-3   *Synthesis Model for Activity and Exercise Planning Phase.*

be necessary. The nurse individualizes a plan of care directed at meeting the actual or potential needs of the client (see care plan).

IMPLEMENTATION

Health Promotion Activities. A sedentary lifestyle contributes to the development of health-related problems. Nurses promote health by encouraging clients to engage in a regular exercise program (Box 36-9). A holistic approach is taken to develop and implement a plan to enhance the client's overall physical fitness. The recommendations for physical activity and fitness should be discussed with the client, and a program of exercise designed in collaboration with the client (Box 36-10).

Before starting an exercise program, clients should calculate their maximum heart rate (MHR) by subtracting their current age in years from 220 and then obtain their target heart rate by taking 60% to 90% of the maximum. No matter what exercise prescription is implemented for the client, a warm-up and cool-down period must be included in the program (ACSM, 1995). The warm-up period usually lasts about 5 to 10 minutes and may include stretching, calisthenics, and/or the aerobic activity performed at a lower intensity. The warm-up activity prepares the body and decreases the potential for injury. The cool-down period follows the exercise routine and usually lasts about 5 to 10 minutes. The cool-down period allows the body to readjust gradually to baseline functioning and provides an opportunity to combine movement such as

SAMPLE NURSING CARE PLAN

ACTIVITY AND EXERCISE

ASSESSMENT*

Mrs. Swain is a 38-year-old housewife. She attends a cardiovascular disease prevention (CDP) program prescribed by her physician and conducted by Mary, a registered nurse. Mrs. Swain states that she has **gained approximately 50 pounds since the birth of her last child.** She complains of **becoming easily fatigued and lacks the energy to keep up with household chores.** She states that she eats in response to her feelings of stress caused by the demands of child care and her mother's need for 24-hour care after experiencing a stroke. She states that she **does not participate in a regular exercise program.** When Mary questions her about her social activities, Mrs. Swain states, **"I feel so fat, I just don't want to go out anymore."** Mary performs a baseline assessment: height: 5 feet 3 inches (160 cm); weight 225 pounds (102 kg); blood pressure: **140/88; pulse: 96 (radial, at rest).**

*Defining characteristics are shown in bold type.

NURSING DIAGNOSIS: Activity intolerance related to excessive weight gain and lack of cardiovascular fitness.

PLANNING

GOALS
Client's activity tolerance will improve.

Client will develop a plan of exercise incorporating isotonic and isometric exercises.

Client's cardiopulmonary response to exercise will improve.

EXPECTED OUTCOMES
Client will discuss the physiological and psychological effects of exercise.

Client will perform and record regular exercise 3 to 4 times over the next week.

Client's resting diastolic blood pressure will be below 84 mm Hg. Client's resting systolic blood pressure will be below 130 mm Hg. Client's resting heart rate will range between 75 and 85 beats per minute.

INTERVENTIONS†

Exercise Promotion

- Teach client about the physiological and psychological benefits of a regular exercise program.

- Teach client to exhale while exerting effort during isometric exercises.

Exercise Promotion: Strength Training

- Develop a plan of exercise with the client, such as 2 to 3 miles of brisk walking and quadricep, bicep, and gluteal muscle isometric exercises 3 to 4 times per week.

- Teach client to use an exercise log and to record the day, time, duration, and responses (pulse, feelings, shortness of breath, daily weight).
- Set up weekly meetings with the client for follow-up and review of the exercise log.

RATIONALE

Physical activity and exercise protect against the development of cardiovascular disease (CVD) and decreases other risk factors associated with CVD, such as obesity, hypertension, and hyperlipidemia (Kelly and McClellan, 1994; NIH, 1996).

Clients should exhale while exerting effort during isometric exercises. Many persons hold their breath when exerting effort (Valsalva maneuver). This increases intrathoracic pressure, causing decreased venous return to the heart. When breath is released, intrathoracic pressure decreases, causing a large surge of blood to return to the heart and increase the cardiac workload (Borgman-Gainer, 1996; Griego and House-Fancher, 1996).

Walking 2 miles briskly, preferably every day, will achieve the health benefits of exercise (Pate and others, 1995). Cross training (combination of exercise activities) provides variety to combat boredom and increases potential for total-body conditioning (Huddleston, 1998).

Keeping a log may increase compliance (Kim, McFarland, and McLane, 1997).

Clients are more likely to increase physical activity and remain compliant with an exercise program if they are counseled by a health care professional (Huddleston, 1998).

†Intervention Classification labels from McCloskey JC, Bulechek GM: *Nursing interventions classification (NIC)*, ed 3, St. Louis, 2000, Mosby.

EVALUATION

Observe client's ability to perform exercises.

Record blood pressure and pulse (radial, at rest).

Ask client if exercise is helping to lower stress level.

Ask client about improved feelings of well-being and increased social interaction.

Review client's exercise log at each visit.

SAMPLE NURSING DIAGNOSTIC PROCESS

Box 36-8

ACTIVITY INTOLERANCE

Assessment Activities	Defining Characteristics	Nursing Diagnosis
Ask client about perception of effects of exercise.	Client's report of fatigue or weakness during or after exercise	Activity intolerance related to sedentary lifestyle
Measure pulse and blood pressure before and after exercise.	Abnormal heart rate and blood pressure in response to exercise	
Observe client's respirations.	Dyspnea, abnormal respiratory maneuvers Prolonged recovery time for client's preexercise pulse, blood pressure, and respiratory rate to return to baseline	

Box 36-9 Procedural Guidelines

For Helping Clients to Exercise

1. Be aware of any medical limitations (e.g., weight-bearing status, untreated fracture, cardiovascular disease).
2. Teach clients breathing skills to help reduce anxiety and to fully oxygenate tissues and expand lungs.
3. Always know the client's limitations.
4. Do not force a muscle or a joint during exercise.
5. Let each client move at his or her own pace.
6. Posture, body alignment, and good body mechanics should be maintained during exercise.
7. Monitor vital signs before, during, and after exercise.
8. Stop exercising if the client has pain, shortness of breath, or a change in vital signs.
9. Clients should wear shoes and comfortable clothing.
10. Know what the client's mobility skills were before hospitalization.
11. Keep a record of the client's progress and provide feedback as the client exercises.

Recommendations for Exercise

Box 36-10

Adults should accumulate 30 minutes or more a day of moderate-intensity (brisk) physical activity on most (or all) days of the week for a weekly total of 3 to 4 hours.

The activity does not have to be continuous; benefits can be realized with short bouts of activity (10 minutes minimum) over the course of the day.

This amount of activity will expend about 150 to 200 calories per day (the equivalent of walking 2 miles briskly) or 1000 to 1400 calories per week.

All types of activity can be applied to the daily total (e.g., raking leaves, dancing, gardening).

Lower-intensity activities should be done more often, for longer periods of time, or both. More vigorous activities should be done for shorter periods of time or less frequently.

Data from Pate RR and others: Physical activity and public health: a recommendation from the Centers for Disease Control and Prevention and the American College of Sports Medicine, *JAMA* 273(5):402, 1995; and Huddleston JS: Exercise. In Edelman CL, Mandle CL, editors: *Health promotion throughout the lifespan,* ed 4, St. Louis, 1998, Mosby.

---

stretching with relaxation-enhancing mind-body awareness (ACSM, 1995; Huddleston, 1998).

Many clients find it difficult to incorporate an exercise program into their daily lives because of time constraints. For these clients it is beneficial to reinforce that many ADLs can be used to accumulate the recommended 30 minutes or more per day of moderate-intensity physical activity (Box 36-11).

Other clients may benefit from a prescribed exercise and physical fitness program carefully designed to meet their needs and expectations. An exercise prescription may incorporate a combination of aerobic exercise, stretching and flexibility exercises, and resistance training. Aerobic exercise includes such activities as walking, running, bicycling, aerobic dance, jumping rope, cross-country skiing, and raquetball. Recommended frequency of aerobic exer-

cise is 3 to 5 times per week or every other day. Cross training is recommended for the client who prefers to exercise everyday. For example, the client may run one day and do hatha yoga the next day.

Stretching and flexibility exercises include active ROM that allows for stretching of all muscle groups and joints. This form of exercise is ideal for warm-up and cool-down periods. Benefits include increased flexibility, improved circulation and posture, and an opportunity for relaxation.

Resistance training increases muscle strength and endurance and is associated with improved performance of daily activities and avoidance of injuries and disability (Pate and others, 1995). People lose about ½ pound of muscle mass per year from lack of use (Huddleston, 1998). Formal resistance training includes weight training, but

Incorporating Active Exercise into Activities of Daily Living   Box 36-11

Nodding head "yes" exercises *neck* (flexion and extension).

Shaking head "no" exercises *neck* (rotation).

Moving right ear to right shoulder exercises *neck* (lateral flexion).

Moving left ear to left shoulder exercises *neck* (lateral flexion).

Reaching to turn on overhead light exercises *shoulder* (flexion).

Reaching to bedside stand for book exercises *shoulder* (abduction).

Scratching back exercises *shoulder* (extension and internal rotation).

Rotating shoulders toward chest exercises *shoulder* (scapular protraction).

Rotating shoulders toward back exercises *shoulder* (scapular retraction).

Eating, bathing, shaving, and grooming exercise *elbow* (flexion, extension).

All activities requiring fine motor coordination, such as writing and eating, exercise *fingers* and *thumb* (flexion, extension, abduction, adduction, opposition).

Walking exercises *hip* (flexion, extension).

Rolling toes inward exercises *hip* (internal rotation).

Rolling toes outward exercises *hip* (external rotation).

Walking exercises *knee* (flexion, extension).

Walking exercises *ankle* (dorsiflexion, plantar flexion).

Pointing toe toward head of bed exercises *ankle* (dorsiflexion).

Pointing toe toward foot of bed exercises *ankle* (plantar flexion).

Walking exercises *toes* (extension).

Wiggling toes exercises *toes* (abduction, adduction).

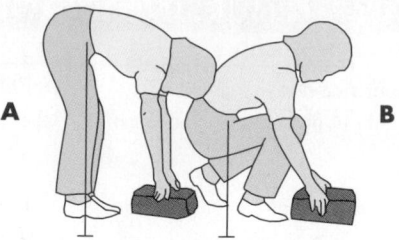

Figure 36-4   Incorrect (**A**) and correct (**B**) body position for lifting.

1. Tighten stomach muscles and tuck pelvis; this provides balance and protects the back.
2. Bend at the knees; this helps to maintain the nurse's center of gravity and lets the strong muscles of the legs do the lifting (Figure 36-4).
3. Keep the weight to be lifted as close to the body as possible; this action places the weight in the same plane as the lifter and close to the center of gravity for balance.
4. Maintain the trunk erect and the knees bent so that multiple muscle groups work together in a synchronized manner (Gassett and others, 1996).
5. Avoid twisting. Twisting can overload your spine and lead to serious injury.

The best height for lifting vertically is approximately 2 feet off the ground and close to the lifter's center of gravity (Gassett and others, 1996).

To reach an object overhead the nurse should do the following:

1. Use a safe, stable step stool or ladder for elevation. Avoid standing on tiptoe with the feet together. This decreases the base of support, elevates the center of gravity, and decreases balance.
2. Stand as close to the shelf as possible. This decreases the amount of time the nurse must support the weight of the object with the arms.
3. Transfer the weight of the object from the shelf to the arms and over the base of support. This maintains the nurse's base of support and aligns the weight of the object close to the nurse's center of gravity.

the same benefits can be obtained by performing ADLs such as pushing a vacuum cleaner, raking leaves, shoveling snow, and kneading bread. Some clients may use weight training to bulk up their muscles. However, the purpose of weight training from a health perspective is to develop tone and strength and to stimulate and maintain healthy bone (Huddleston, 1998).

Body Mechanics.   In recent years the rate of injuries in occupational settings has increased dramatically. Half of all back pain is associated with manual lifting tasks (Gassett and others, 1996). The most common back injury is strain on the lumbar muscle group, which includes the muscles around the lumbar vertebrae. Injury to these areas affects the ability to bend forward, backward, and from side to side. The ability to rotate the hips and lower back is also decreased. To protect the client and the nurse, proper body mechanics must be learned and mastered (Table 36-1).

Lifting Techniques.   Before lifting, the nurse should assess the weight to be lifted and what assistance, if any, is needed. If help is needed, the nurse should assess if a second person is adequate or if mechanical assistance is needed. Once the amount of needed assistance is determined, these steps are followed:

Acute Care.   Hospitalized clients can be encouraged to do stretching and isometric exercises, active ROM exercises, and low-intensity walking, depending on their condition. The nurse is responsible for maintaining musculoskeletal function by implementing passive ROM in those clients who are unable to perform physical activity for themselves.

Musculoskeletal System.   The musculoskeletal system can be maintained during the acute care of the client by encouraging the use of stretching and isometric-type

Table 36-1   Body Mechanics for Health Care Workers

Action	Rationale
When planning to move a client, arrange for adequate help. Use mechanical aids if help is unavailable.	Two workers lifting together divide the workload by 50%.
Encourage client to assist as much as possible.	This promotes client's independence and strength while minimizing workload.
Keep back, neck, pelvis, and feet aligned. Avoid twisting.	Reduces risk of injury to lumbar vertebrae and muscle groups. Twisting increases risk of injury.
Flex knees; keep feet wide apart.	A broad base of support increases stability.
Position self close to client (or object being lifted).	The force is minimized. Ten pounds at waist height close to body is equal to 100 pounds at arms' length.
Use arms and legs (not back).	The leg muscles are stronger, larger muscles capable of greater work without injury.
Slide client toward yourself using a pull sheet.	Sliding requires less effort than lifting. Pull sheet minimizes shearing forces, which can damage client's skin.
Set (tighten) abdominal and gluteal muscles in preparation for move.	Preparing muscles for the load minimizes strain and stabilizes the trunk.
Person with the heaviest load coordinates efforts of the team involved by counting to three.	Simultaneous lifting minimizes the load for any one lifter.

exercises. Review of the client's chart and collaboration with the physician is undertaken to alert the nurse to any possible contraindications before initiating isometric exercises. An isometric exercise program is designed for the specific needs of a client. For example, an exercise program may be implemented that includes biceps and triceps isometric exercises to prepare the client for crutch walking. The nurse needs to tell the client to stop the activity if pain, fatigue, or discomfort is experienced, and reinforce this as necessary.

Generally, the muscle group is tightened (contracted) for 8 seconds and then completely relaxed for several seconds (Borgman-Gainer, 1996). Repetitions are gradually increased for each muscle group until the isometric exercise can be repeated 8 to 10 times. Clients should be instructed to perform the exercises slowly and increase repetitions as their physical condition improves. Muscle groups (quadriceps and gluteal) used for walking should be exercised isometrically 4 times per day until the client is ambulatory.

The following isometric exercises can be used alone or in combination, depending on the client's condition and needs:

- *Quadriceps:* The client is in a supine recumbent position. Instruct the client to press the back of the knee against the mattress while trying to lift the heel of the foot from the bed. Hold for 8 seconds, relax completely, and repeat as tolerated. This exercise strengthens and maintains large muscles of the thigh (quadriceps) that will enable the client to ambulate and get out of a chair.
- *Gluteal muscle:* The client is in a recumbent position. Instruct the client to squeeze the buttocks together.

Hold for 8 seconds, relax completely, and repeat as tolerated. This exercise improves and contributes to balance while sitting.

- *Abdominal muscle:* Instruct the client to pull the abdominal muscles in as tightly as possible. Hold for 8 seconds, release the muscles gradually, and repeat as tolerated. This exercise improves trunk stability.
- *Foot muscles:* Instruct the client to move the foot in a circle in all directions and flex the foot toward and away from the knee. This exercise increases muscle activity in the leg and thereby promotes circulation and venous return to the heart.
- *Hand muscles:* Instruct the client to grip a spherical object (tennis or sponge ball) with the entire hand 5 to 10 times, then dig each fingertip, one at a time, into the ball 5 to 10 times each. This exercise strengthens the grip to hold onto crutches or a walker more effectively.
- *Biceps:* Instruct the client to raise the arms to shoulder height and interlock the fingertips of both hands. Tell the client to pull the hands apart using the arm muscles and hold for 8 seconds, relax, and repeat. This exercise strengthens the biceps muscles, which is necessary if the client requires an assistive ambulatory device such as a walker.
- *Triceps:* Instruct the client to raise the arms to shoulder height, make a fist with one hand, and place the fist against the palm of the opposite hand. Tell the client to push the fist into the palm of the opposite hand as hard as possible for 8 seconds, relax, and repeat. This exercise promotes strength in the triceps muscles, which is necessary for transfer techniques and the use of crutches and walkers.

Joint Mobility. The easiest intervention to maintain or improve joint mobility for clients and one that can be coordinated with other activities is the use of ROM exercises (see Chapter 46). In active ROM exercises, the client is able to move his or her joints. The nurse moves each joint in passive ROM exercises in clients who are unable to perform these exercises themselves. The use of these exercises enables the nurse to systematically assess and improve the client's joint mobility.

Joints that are not moved periodically can develop contractures, a permanent shortening of a muscle followed by the eventual shortening of associated ligaments and tendons. Over time, the joint may become fixed in one position and the client loses normal use of the joint. For the client who does not have voluntary motor control, passive ROM exercises are the exercises of choice.

The older adult has a decline in physical activity and changes in joints that may predispose the client to problems with mobility, and joint flexibility may be limited. The nurse can recommend approaches to help older adults use proper body mechanics and prevent injury (Box 36-12).

Mechanical devices are available for specific joints, which place these joints through continuous passive ROM (CPM). These CPM machines are used postoperatively to place joints through a selective repetitive range of motion. The machine can be set to certain degrees of joint mobility with increasing joint mobility or flexion as the goal. The most common clients who use the CPM machine are those who have undergone some form of total joint replacement surgery (see Chapter 46).

NURSING PRACTICE   **Box 36-12**

- Encourage the older client to avoid prolonged sitting, to get up and stretch. Frequent stretching decreases joint contractures.
- Be sure that the client maintains proper body alignment when sitting. Proper alignment minimizes joint and muscle stress.
- Teach clients how to use stronger joints or larger muscle groups for tasks such as manipulating spray cans or container lids. Efficient distribution of the workload decreases joint stress and pain.
- Some studies have demonstrated that nonstrenuous exercise (such as active ROM) may improve memory or the ability to recall for up to 30 minutes or more (Dawe and Moore-Orr, 1995).
- Provide resources for planned exercise programs. Proper exercise activities slow further bone loss and prevent fractures in the older adult with osteoporosis (Barry and Eathorne, 1994).
- It is never too late to begin an exercise program (Huddleston, 1998). Consult a health care provider before beginning an exercise program, particularly in the presence of heart or lung disease and other chronic illnesses.

Unless contraindicated, the nursing care plan should include exercising each joint through as nearly a full ROM as possible. Passive ROM exercises should be initiated as soon as the client loses the ability to move the extremity or joint. The following guidelines apply to the use of ROM exercises:

Provide explanation to the client; this elicits cooperation and assistance.

Start slowly; movements should be smooth and easy.

Flexion of the joint can continue until slight resistance is felt; do not move a joint to the point of pain; avoid hyperextending the joint.

Work from distal joints to proximal joints on one extremity at a time.

Provide support for joints distal to the joint being manipulated.

Assess the client closely for signs of generalized fatigue.

When exercises are completed, make certain to leave joints in correct alignment position.

Chapter 46 details ROM exercises for each area and illustrates the motion of each joint.

Walking. Joint mobility is also increased by walking. Distances walked should be measured in feet or yards instead of charting "ambulated to nurses' station and back."

In the normal walking posture the head is erect; the cervical, thoracic, and lumbar vertebrae are aligned; the hips and knees have appropriate flexion; and the arms swing freely in alternation with the legs. Illness or trauma can reduce activity tolerance, resulting in the need for assistance with walking or the use of mechanical devices such as crutches, canes, or walkers.

Helping a Client to Walk. Helping a client to walk requires preparation. The nurse assesses the client's activity tolerance, strength, coordination, and balance to determine the type of assistance needed. The nurse should also assess the client's orientation and determine if there are any signs of distress. This would preclude attempts at ambulation.

The nurse evaluates the environment for safety before ambulation; this includes the removal of obstacles, a clean and dry floor, and the establishment of rest points should the client's activity tolerance become less than expected. The client should also wear supportive, nonslipping shoes. Resting points should be established in the event that the client's activity tolerance is less than was estimated or the client becomes dizzy.

When preparing a client for ambulation, dangling is an important technique. The client should be assisted to a position of sitting at the side of the bed and should rest for 1 to 2 minutes before standing. The longer the period of inactivity, or **immobility,** the greater the physiological changes (see Chapter 46). This is especially true regarding changes in circulation. When the client has been lying flat for extended periods, blood pressure may drop when the client stands. Dangling helps to prevent this. After standing, the client should remain stationary for a minute or two before moving. If the client becomes dizzy, the bed is still nearby and the nurse can quickly ease him or her back to bed.

Several methods are used for assisting a client with ambulation. The nurse should provide support at the waist so that the client's center of gravity remains midline. This can be achieved when the nurse places both hands at the client's waist or uses a gait belt. A gait belt is a leather belt that encircles the client's waist and has handles attached for the nurse to hold while the client ambulates. Clients should not lean to one side, because then their center of gravity is no longer midline, which distorts their balance and increases their risk of falling.

The client who appears unsteady or complains of dizziness should be returned to the closest bed or a chair. If the client has a syncopal episode or begins to fall, the nurse should assume a wide base of support with one foot in front of the other, thus supporting the client's body weight. The nurse gently lowers the client to the floor, protecting the client's head. During the next ambulation attempt the nurse should proceed more slowly, monitoring for complaints of dizziness, as well as the client's blood pressure, before, during, and after ambulation. Although lowering a client to the floor is not difficult, the student should practice this technique with a friend or classmate before attempting it in a clinical setting (Figure 36-5).

Clients with **hemiplegia** (one-sided paralysis) or **hemiparesis** (one-sided weakness) need assistance in ambulating. The nurse stands by the client's affected side and supports the client by holding one arm around the client's waist and the other arm around the inferior aspect of the client's upper arm so that the nurse's hand is supporting the client's axilla. The client's unaffected arm is left free to enable the client to assist. Providing support by holding the client's arm is incorrect because if the client should experience syncope or fall, the nurse cannot easily support the weight and lower the client to the floor. In addition, if the client falls with the nurse holding the arm, the shoulder joint may be dislocated.

A nurse who has even the slightest doubt about his or her strength and ability to ambulate a client alone should request help. The two-nurse method helps to distribute the client's weight evenly. The two nurses stand on either side of the client. Each nurse's near arm is around the client's waist, and the other arm is around the inferior aspect of the client's arm so that the hands of both nurses are supporting the client's axillae.

Restorative and Continuing Care.

Restorative and continuing care involving activity and exercise involves implementing strategies to assist the client in ADLs after the client's need for acute care is no longer warranted. The nurse, in collaboration with other health care profession-

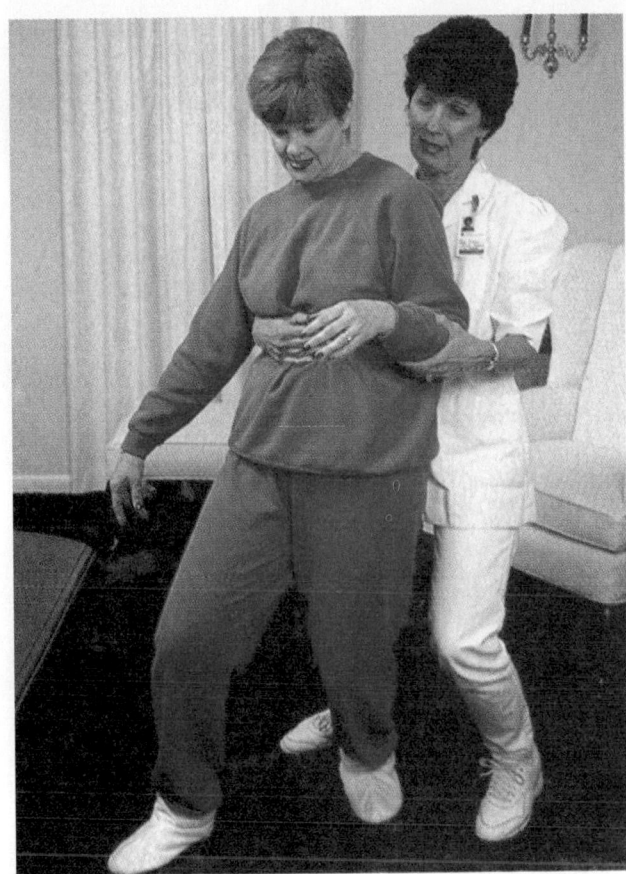

Figure 36-5   Ease the client down to the floor by bending your knees, keeping your back straight.
From Birchenall JM, Streight ME: *Mosby's textbook for the home care aide,* St. Louis, 1997, Mosby.

als such as physical therapists, promotes activity and exercise by teaching the use of canes, walkers, or crutches, depending on the assistive device most appropriate for the client's condition. Restorative and continuing care includes activities and exercises that restore and promote optimal functioning in clients with specific chronic illnesses, such as coronary heart disease (CHD), hypertension, chronic obstructive pulmonary disease (COPD), and diabetes mellitus.

Assistive Devices for Walking.

Walkers are extremely light, movable devices that are about waist high and made of metal tubing (Figure 36-6). They have four widely placed, sturdy legs. The client holds the handgrips on the upper bars, takes a step, moves the walker forward, and takes another step.

Canes.   Canes are lightweight, easily movable devices that are about waist high and made of wood or metal. Two common types of canes are the single straight-legged cane and the quad cane. The single straight-legged cane is more

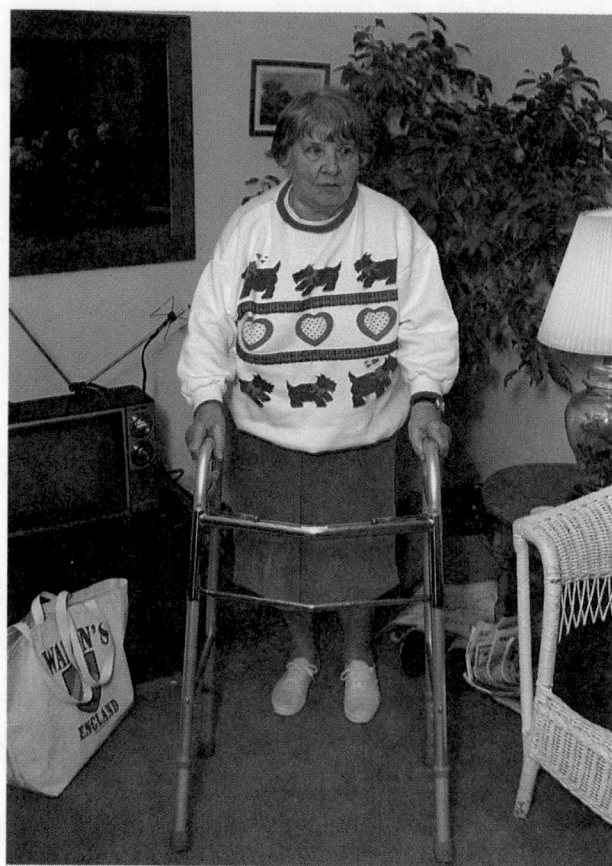

Figure 36-6 Client using a walker.

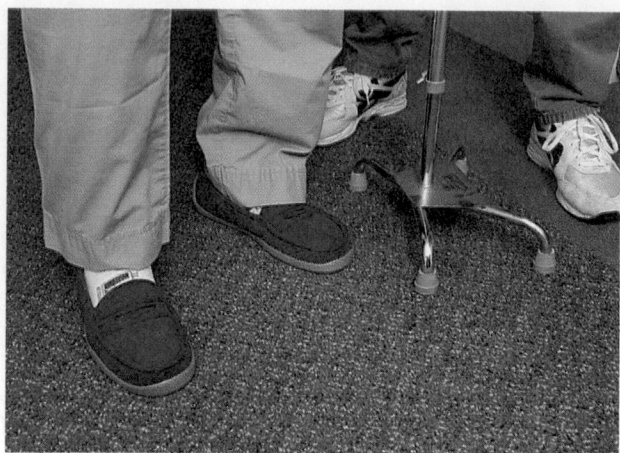

Figure 36-7 Quad cane.

common and is used to support and balance a client with decreased leg strength. This cane should be kept on the stronger side of the body. For maximum support when walking, the client places the cane forward 15 to 25 cm (6 to 10 inches), keeping body weight on both legs. The weaker leg is moved forward to the cane so that body weight is divided between the cane and the stronger leg. The stronger leg is then advanced past the cane so that the weaker leg and the body weight are supported by the cane and weaker leg. During walking, the client continually repeats these three steps. The client must be taught that two points of support, such as both feet or one foot and the cane, are present at all times.

The quad cane provides the most support and is used when there is partial or complete leg paralysis or some hemiplegia (Figure 36-7). The same three steps that are used with the straight-legged cane are taught to the client.

Crutches.   Crutches are often needed to increase mobility. The nurse begins crutch instruction with guidelines for safe use (Box 36-13). The use of crutches may be temporary, such as after ligament damage to the knee. However, crutches may be needed permanently by a client with paralysis of the lower extremities. A crutch is a wooden or metal staff. The two types of crutches are the

double adjustable Lofstrand, or forearm, crutch (Figure 36-8) and the axillary wooden or metal crutch. The forearm crutch has a handgrip and a metal band that fits around the client's forearm. The metal band and the handgrip are adjusted to fit the client's height. The axillary crutch has a padded curved surface at the top, which fits under the axilla. A handgrip in the form of a crossbar is held at the level of the palms to support the body. It is important that crutches be measured for the appropriate length and that clients be taught to use their crutches safely, to achieve a stable gait, to ascend and descend stairs, and to rise from a sitting position.

Measuring for Crutches.   The axillary crutch is the more common crutch used. Measurements include the client's height, the angle of elbow flexion, and the distance between the crutch pad and the axilla. When crutches are fitted, the length of the crutch should be from three to four fingerwidths from the axilla to a point 15 cm (6 inches) lateral to the client's heel (Hoeman, 1996) (Figure 36-9).

The handgrips should be positioned so that the client's body weight is not supported by the axillae. Pressure on the axillae increases risk to underlying nerves, which could result in partial paralysis of the arm. Correct position of the handgrips is determined with the client upright, supporting weight by the handgrips with the elbows slightly flexed (20 to 25 degrees). Elbow flexion may be verified with a goniometer (Figure 36-10). When the height and placement of the handgrips have been determined, the nurse should again verify that the distance between the crutch pad and the client's axilla is three to four fingerwidths (Figure 36-11).

Crutch Gait.   The **crutch gait** is assumed by alternately bearing weight on one or both legs and on the crutches. The gait selected by the physician is determined by assessing the client's physical and functional abilities

---

Client Teaching FOR CRUTCH SAFETY   Box 36-13

OBJECTIVE
- Client will state and demonstrate safe crutch walking.

TEACHING STRATEGIES
- Teach client with axillary crutches about the dangers of pressure on the axillae, which occurs when leaning on the crutches to support body weight.
- Explain why client must use crutches that were measured for him or her.
- Show client how to routinely inspect crutch tips. Rubber tips should be securely attached to the crutches. When tips are worn, they should be replaced. Rubber crutch tips increase surface friction and help prevent slipping.
- Explain that the crutch tips should remain dry. Water decreases surface friction and increases the risk of slipping.

- Show client how to dry the crutch tips if they become wet; client may use paper or cloth towels.
- Show client how to inspect the structure of the crutches. Cracks in a wooden crutch decrease its ability to support weight. Bends in aluminum crutches can alter body alignment.
- Provide client with a list of medical supply companies in the community for obtaining repairs, new rubber tips, handgrips, and crutch pads.
- Instruct client to have spare crutches and tips readily available.

EVALUATION
- Client states and demonstrates principles of crutch safety.

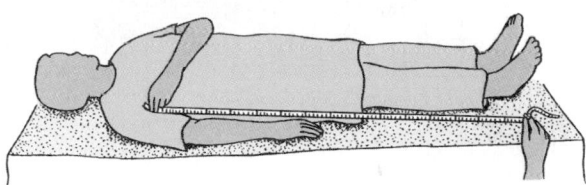

Figure 36-9   Measuring crutch length.

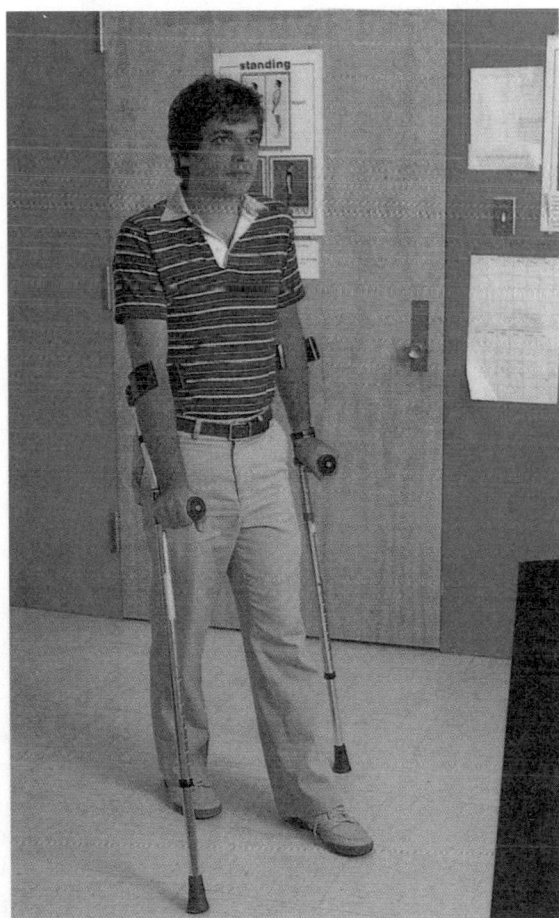

Figure 36-8   Double adjustable Lofstrand, or forearm, crutch.

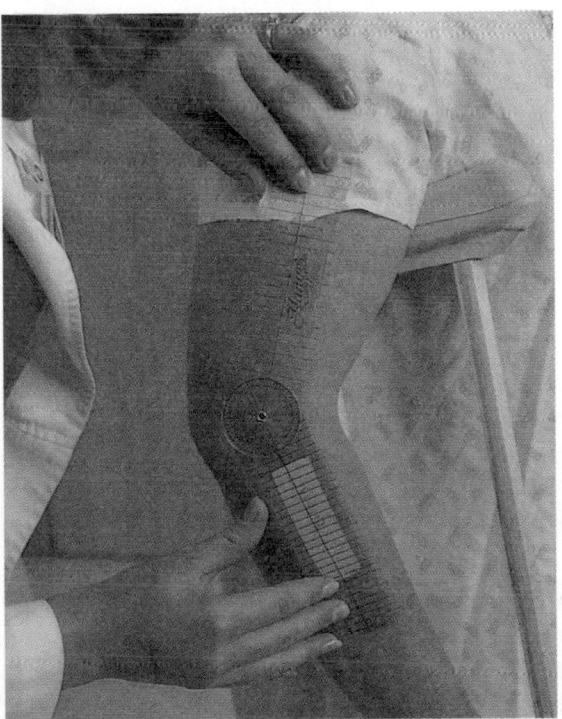

Figure 36-10   Using the goniometer to verify correct degree of elbow flexion for crutch use.

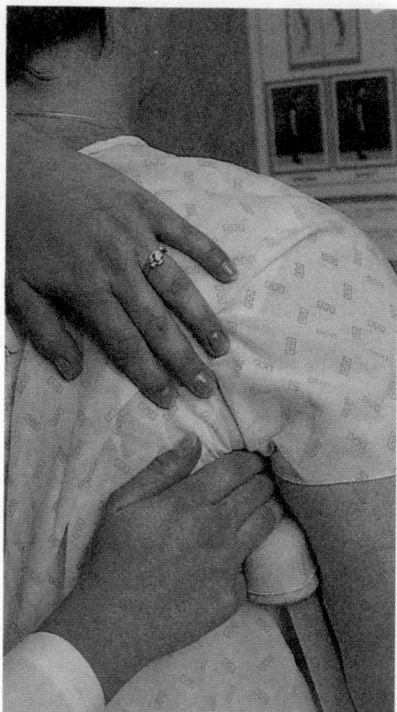

Figure 36-11 Verifying correct distance between crutch pads and axilla.

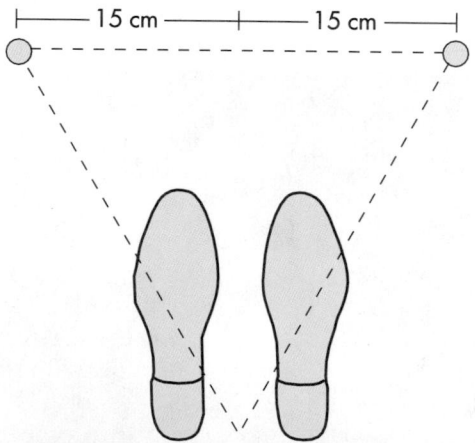

Figure 36-12 Tripod position, basic crutch stance.

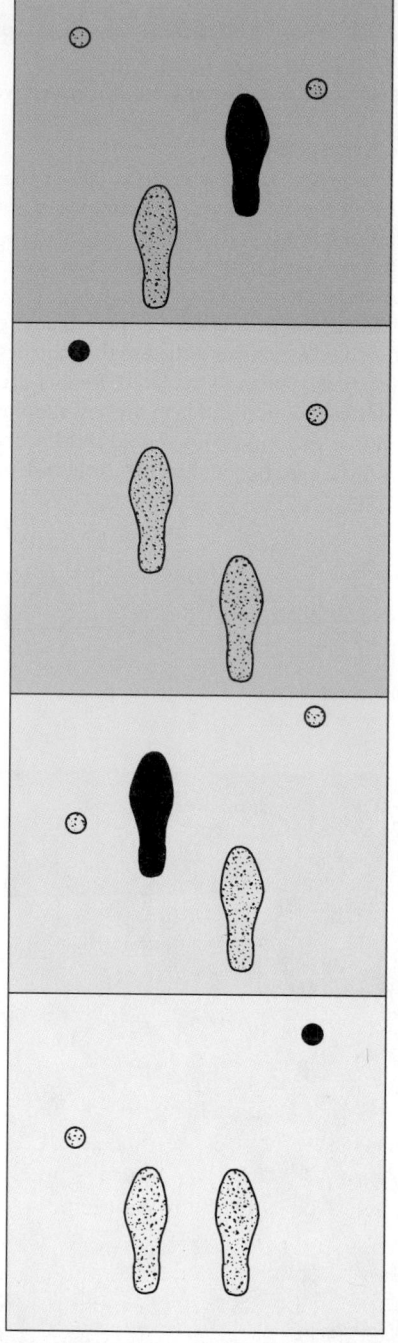

Figure 36-13 Four-point alternating gait. Solid feet and crutch tips show foot and crutch tip moved in each of the four phases. (Read from bottom to top.)

and the disease or injury that resulted in the need for crutches. This section summarizes the basic crutch stance and the four standard gaits: four-point alternating gait, three-point alternating gait, two-point gait, and swing-through gait.

The basic crutch stance is the tripod position, formed when the crutches are placed 15 cm (6 inches) in front of and 15 cm to the side of each foot (Figure 36-12). This position improves the client's balance by providing a wider base of support. The body alignment of the client in the tripod position includes an erect head and neck, straight vertebrae, and extended hips and knees. No weight should be borne by the axillae. The tripod position is assumed before crutch walking.

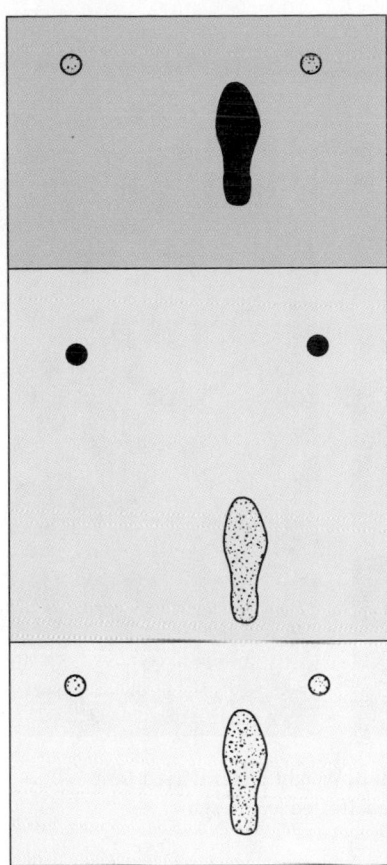

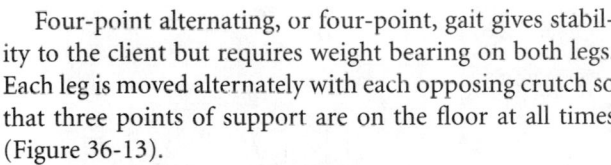

Figure 36-14 Three-point gait with weight borne on unaffected leg. Solid foot and crutch tips show weight-bearing in each phase. (Read from bottom to top.)

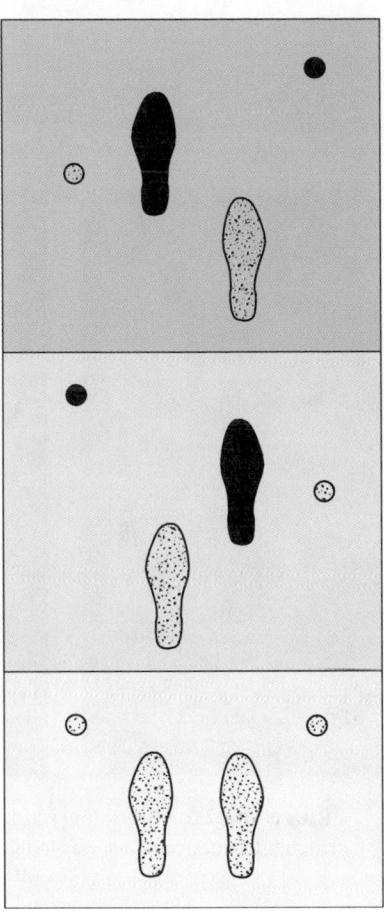

Figure 36-15 Two-point gait with weight borne partially on each foot and each crutch advancing with opposing leg. Solid areas indicate leg and crutch tips bearing weight. (Read from bottom to top.)

Four-point alternating, or four-point, gait gives stability to the client but requires weight bearing on both legs. Each leg is moved alternately with each opposing crutch so that three points of support are on the floor at all times (Figure 36-13).

Three-point alternating, or three-point, gait requires the client to bear all of the weight on one foot. In a three-point gait, weight is borne on both crutches and then on the uninvolved leg, and the sequence is repeated (Figure 36-14). The affected leg does not touch the ground during the early phase of the three-point gait. Gradually the client progresses to touchdown and full weight bearing on the affected leg.

The two-point gait requires at least partial weight bearing on each foot (Figure 36-15). The client moves a crutch at the same time as the opposing leg, so that the crutch movements are similar to arm motion during normal walking.

The swing-through, or swing-through gait, is frequently used by paraplegics who wear weight-supporting braces on their legs. With weight placed on the supported legs, the client places the crutches one stride in front and then swings to or through the crutches while they support the client's weight.

Crutch Walking on Stairs. When ascending stairs on crutches, the client usually uses a modified three-point gait (Figure 36-16). The client stands at the bottom of the stairs and transfers body weight to the crutches. The unaffected leg is advanced between the crutches to the stairs. The client then shifts weight from the crutches to the unaffected leg. Finally, the client aligns both crutches on the stairs. This sequence is repeated until the client reaches the top of the stairs.

To descend the stairs (Figure 36-17), a three-phase sequence is also used. The client transfers body weight to the unaffected leg. The crutches are placed on the stairs, and the client begins to transfer body weight to the crutches, moving the affected leg forward. Finally, the unaffected leg is moved to the stairs with the crutches. Again, the client repeats the sequence until reaching the bottom of the stairs.

Because in most cases clients will need to use crutches for some time, they should be adequately taught to use

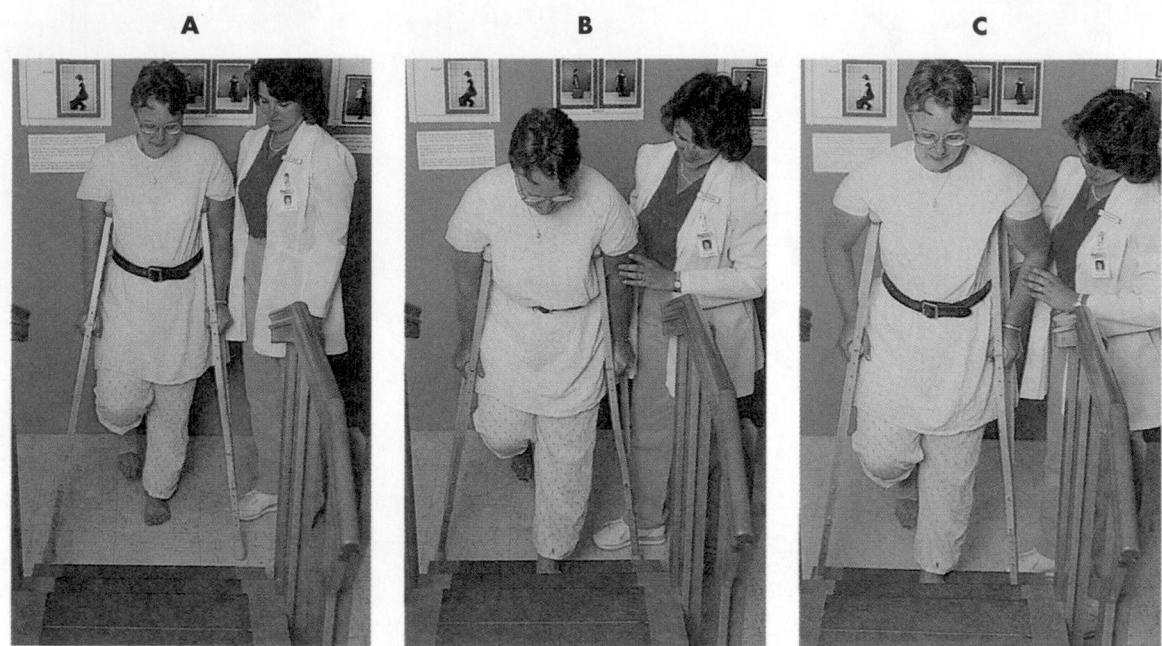

Figure 36-16   Ascending stairs. **A,** Weight is placed on crutch. **B,** Weight is transferred from crutches to unaffected leg on stairs. **C,** Crutches are aligned with unaffected leg on stairs.

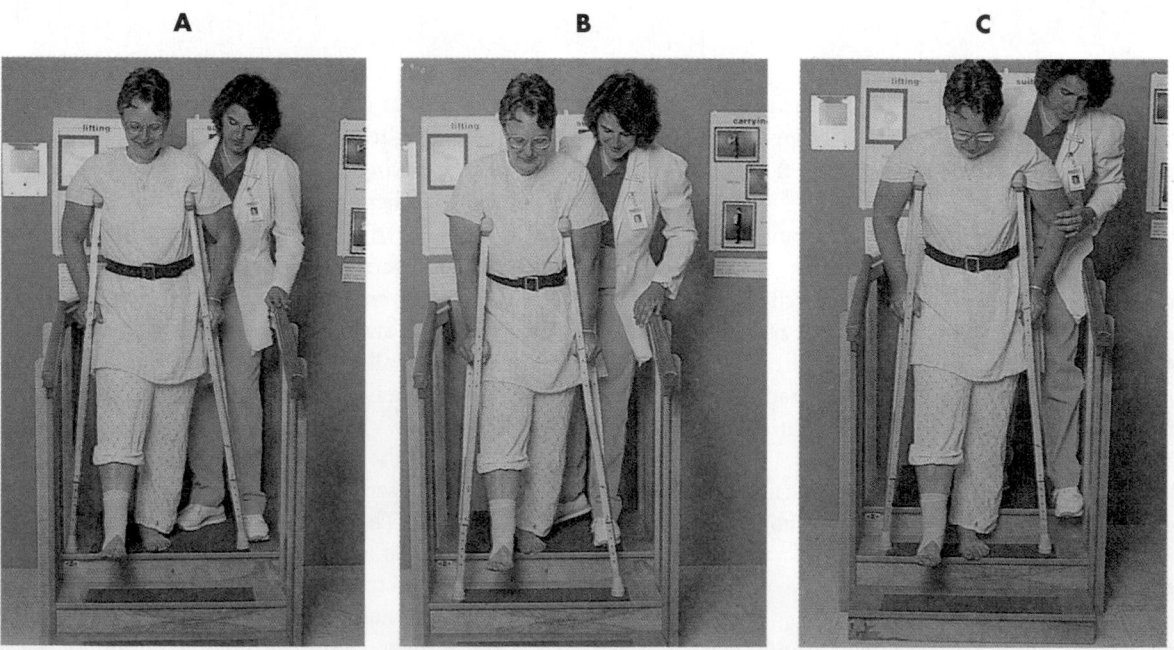

Figure 36-17   Descending stairs. **A,** Body weight is on unaffected leg. **B,** Body weight is transferred to crutches. **C,** Unaffected leg is aligned on stairs with crutches.

crutches on stairs before discharge. This instruction applies to all crutch-dependent clients, not only those who have stairs in their homes.

Sitting in a Chair With Crutches. As with crutch walking and crutch walking up and down stairs, the procedure for sitting in a chair involves phases and requires the client to transfer weight (Figure 36-18). First, the client gets positioned at the center front of the chair with the posterior aspect of the legs touching the chair. Then the client holds both crutches in the hand opposite the affected leg. If both legs are affected, as with a paraplegic who wears weight-supporting braces, the crutches are held in the hand on the client's stronger side. With both crutches in one hand, the client supports body weight on the unaffected leg and the crutches. While still holding the crutches, the client grasps the arm of the chair with the remaining hand and lowers the body into the chair. To stand, the procedure is reversed, and the client, when fully erect, should assume the tripod position before beginning to walk.

The nurse is also involved in implementing a plan of care designed to increase activity and exercise in clients with specific disease conditions and chronic illnesses such as CHD, hypertension, COPD, and diabetes mellitus.

Coronary Heart Disease. Activity and exercise have been shown to play a role in secondary prevention or recurrence of CHD. Cardiac rehabilitation is becoming an integral part of comprehensive care of clients who have been diagnosed with CHD. Nurses are involved in many aspects of cardiac rehabilitation and may assist clients in developing a program of exercise that fits their needs and level of functioning. Increased physical activity appears to benefit individuals with myocardial infarction (MI), angina pectoris, or congestive heart failure, as well as clients who have had a coronary artery bypass graft (CABG) or percutaneous transluminal coronary angioplasty (PTCA). Clients with CHD benefit from exercise and activity in terms of reduced mortality and morbidity, improved quality of life, improved left ventricular function, increased functional capacity, and psychological well-being (NIH, 1996; Thompson and Bowman, 1998).

Hypertension. Studies have supported the role of exercise in the reduction of systolic and diastolic blood pressure readings (Kelly and McClellan, 1994). Low- to moderate-intensity aerobic exercise (brisk walking, bicycling) appears to be the most effective in lowering blood pressure, whereas weight-training and high-intensity aerobics seem to have minimal benefits (Huddleston, 1998).

Chronic Obstructive Pulmonary Disease. Pulmonary rehabilitation is a beneficial therapeutic tool in helping clients reach an optimal level of functioning (Box 36-14). Some clients are fearful of participating in exercise

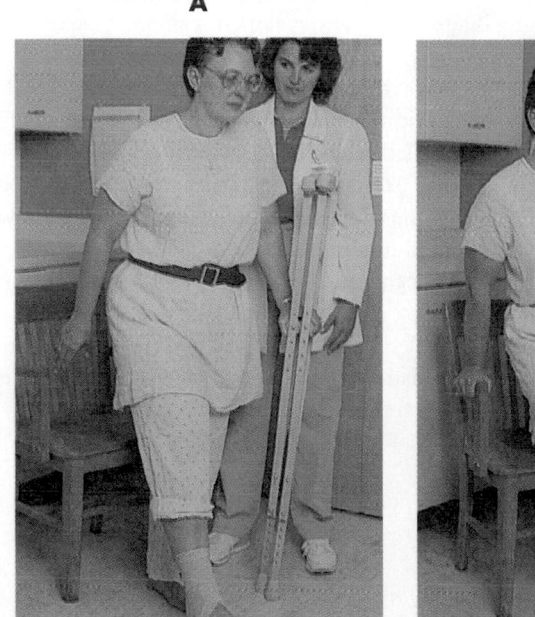
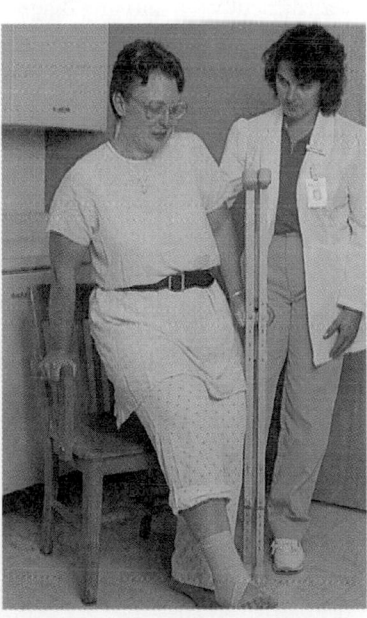
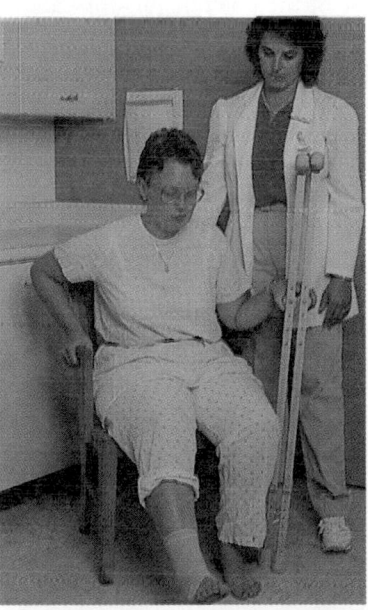

Figure 36-18 Sitting in a chair. **A,** Both crutches are held by one hand. Client transfers weight to crutches and unaffected leg. **B,** Client grasps arm of chair with free hand and begins to lower herself into chair. **C,** Client completely lowers herself into chair.

Research HIGHLIGHT   **Box 36-14**

RESEARCH

The purpose of this study was to determine the effect of attendance at an outpatient pulmonary rehabilitation (OPR) program on changes in self-efficacy, perception of dyspnea, and exercise endurance in clients with chronic obstructive pulmonary disease (COPD). Sixty clients with a diagnosis of COPD were included in the study. Subjects ranged in age from 35 to 82.

The intervention consisted of an educational component and exercise training. Outcome measures were scores on the COPD Self-Efficacy Scale (CSES), the Dyspnea Scale, and distance walked recorded in feet on the 12-minute walking-distance test (12 MD).

Conclusions indicated that self-efficacy, perception of dyspnea, and exercise endurance significantly improved after completion of an outpatient pulmonary rehabilitation program.

IMPLICATIONS FOR PRACTICE

- Before initiating exercise, clients should consult their primary care provider.
- Encouraging clients with chronic illnesses to exercise has the potential to maintain and improve activity tolerance.
- Activity and exercise may potentially increase self-confidence in clients with COPD to manage and control perceptions of dyspnea.

REFERENCE

Scherer YK, Schmieder LE: The effect of a pulmonary rehabilitation program on self-efficacy, perception of dyspnea, and physical endurance, *Heart Lung* 26(1):15, 1997.

---

because of the potential of worsening dyspnea (difficulty breathing). This aversion to physical activity sets up a progressive deconditioning in which minimal physical exertion results in dyspnea. Pulmonary rehabilitation provides a safe environment with nurses and other health care professionals monitoring the progress of the client, thus providing encouragement and support to increase activity and exercise.

Diabetes Mellitus. Along with diet, glucose monitoring, and medication, exercise is an important component in the care of clients with diabetes mellitus. Individuals with type 1 diabetes are encouraged to exercise because it leads to improved cardiovascular fitness and psychological well-being. The nurse instructs the diabetic with type 1 diabetes about certain risks and precautions regarding exercise. Instruction should include the need for a preexercise physical examination and precautions to monitor blood glucose immediately before and after exercise, to avoid injecting insulin into muscles that will be active during exercise, to perform low- to moderate-intensity exercises, to carry a concentrated form of carbohydrates (sugar packets, hard candy), and to wear a medical-alert bracelet. The client with type 2 diabetes who decides to participate in a regular program of exercise should have a preexercise physical examination, include low-intensity warm-up and cool-down exercises, include aerobic exercise at 50% to 75% of maximal oxygen uptake, and exercise for 20 to 45 minutes 3 days per week (American Diabetes Association, 1997).

✂ EVALUATION

Client Care. For activity and exercise, the effectiveness of nursing interventions is measured by the success of meeting the client's expected outcomes and goals of care. The client is the only one who will know the effectiveness and benefits of activity and exercise (Figure 36-19). To evaluate the effectiveness of nursing interventions to enhance activity and exercise, comparisons are made with baseline measures that include pulse, blood pressure, strength, endurance, and psychological well-being. Actual outcomes are compared with expected outcomes to determine the client's health status and progression. Continuous evaluation allows the nurse to determine whether new or revised therapies are required and if new nursing diagnoses have developed.

Client Expectations. For the nurse to evaluate the client's perception of the interventions, the nurse must first have knowledge of the client's expectations concerning activity and exercise. What is acceptable or anticipated on the part of the nurse may be vastly different from what the client and family members anticipate or can accept. It is important for the nurse to ask the client if his or her expectations of care have been met. Working closely with the client will enable the nurse to redefine those expectations that can be realistically met within the limits of the client's conditions and treatment.

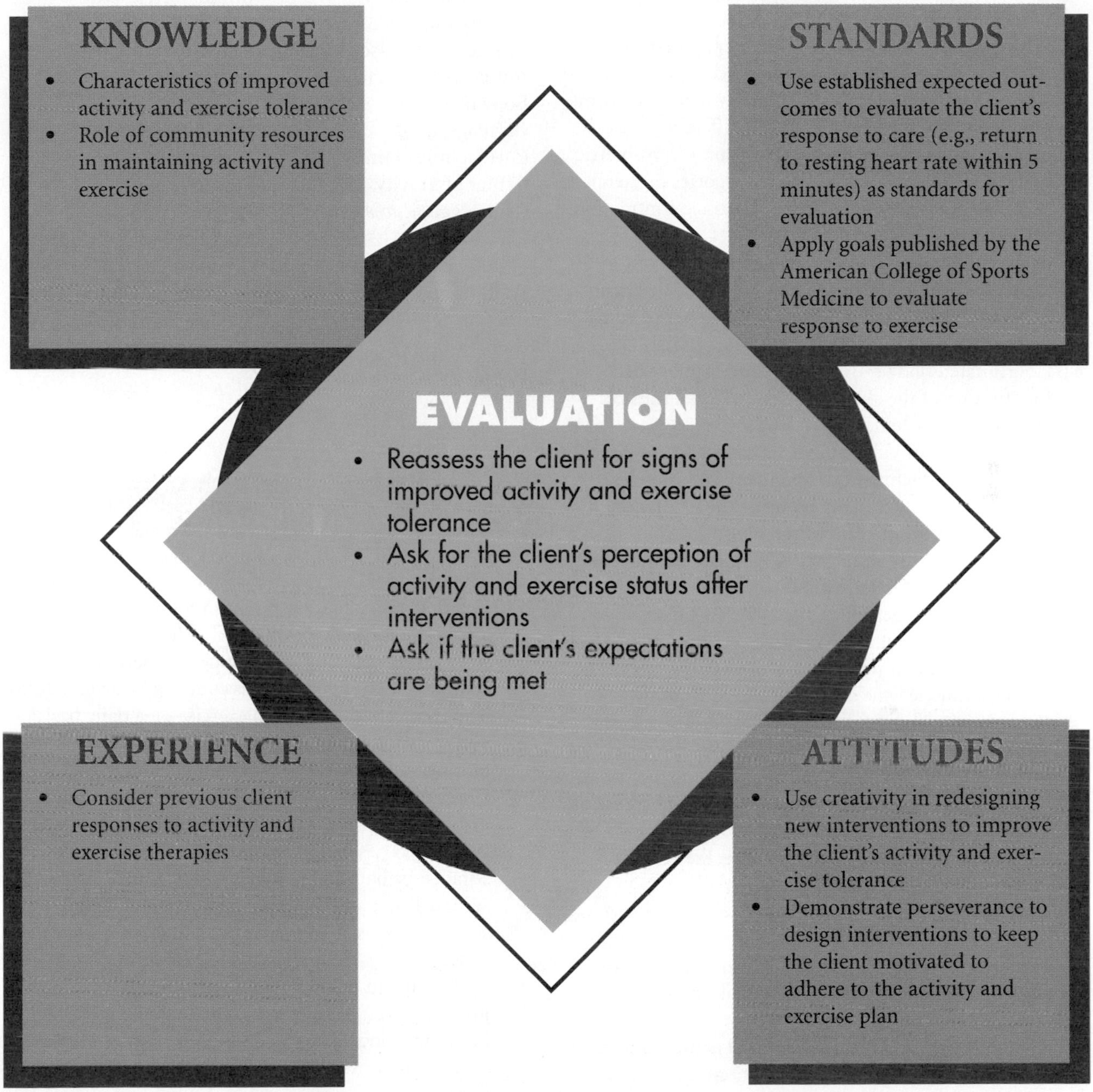

KNOWLEDGE

- Characteristics of improved activity and exercise tolerance
- Role of community resources in maintaining activity and exercise

STANDARDS

- Use established expected outcomes to evaluate the client's response to care (e.g., return to resting heart rate within 5 minutes) as standards for evaluation
- Apply goals published by the American College of Sports Medicine to evaluate response to exercise

EVALUATION

- Reassess the client for signs of improved activity and exercise tolerance
- Ask for the client's perception of activity and exercise status after interventions
- Ask if the client's expectations are being met

EXPERIENCE

- Consider previous client responses to activity and exercise therapies

ATTITUDES

- Use creativity in redesigning new interventions to improve the client's activity and exercise tolerance
- Demonstrate perseverance to design interventions to keep the client motivated to adhere to the activity and exercise plan

Figure 36-19   *Synthesis Model for Activity and Exercise Evaluation Phase.*

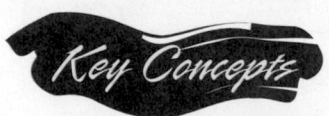

Key Concepts

- Exercise is physical activity for the purpose of conditioning the body, improving health, and maintaining fitness, or it may be used as a therapeutic measure.
- Activity tolerance is the kind and amount of exercise or work that a person is able to perform. Physiological, emotional, and developmental factors influence the client's activity tolerance.
- The best program of physical activity includes a combination of exercises that produce different physiological and psychological benefits. Isotonic, isometric, and resistive isometric are three categories of exercise classified according to the type of muscle contraction involved.
- Body mechanics are the coordinated efforts of the musculoskeletal and nervous systems as the person moves, lifts, bends, stands, sits, lies down, and completes daily activities.
- Coordinated body movement requires integrated functioning of the skeletal system, skeletal muscles, and nervous system.
- The skeleton provides bony support structure for movement, attachment of ligaments and muscles, protection of vital organs, some of the regulation of calcium, and production of red blood cells.
- Muscles primarily associated with movement are located near the skeletal region, where movement results from leverage, which is characteristic of movements of the upper extremities.
- Coordination and regulation of muscle groups depend on muscle tone and activity of antagonistic, synergistic, and antigravity muscles.
- Balance is assisted through nervous system control in the cerebellum and inner ear function.
- Body balance is achieved when there is a wide base of support, the center of gravity falls within the base of support, and a vertical line falls from the center of gravity through the base of support.
- Developmental changes, behavioral aspects, environmental issues, cultural and ethnic origin, and family and social support influence the client's perception and motivation to engage in physical activity and exercise.
- Ability to engage in normal physical activity and exercise depends on intact and functioning nervous and musculoskeletal systems.
- The nurse uses the nursing process to provide care for clients who are experiencing or are at risk for activity intolerance and impaired physical mobility.
- After identifying nursing diagnoses, the nurse plans and implements interventions to increase activity and exercise in collaboration with the client when possible.
- Range-of-motion exercises include one or all of the body joints.
- Mechanical devices to promote walking include canes, walkers, and crutches.

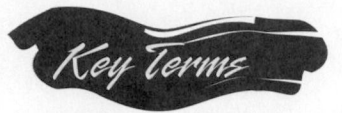

Key Terms

Activities of daily living (ADLs), p. 990
Activity tolerance, p. 991
Antagonistic muscles, p. 992
Antigravity muscles, p. 993
Body mechanics, p. 990
Cartilage, p. 992
Cartilaginous joints, p. 992
Center of gravity, p. 990
Crutch gait, p. 1008
Exercise, p. 990
Fibrous joints, p. 992
Footboard, p. 992
Friction, p. 991
Gait, p. 999
Hemiparesis, p. 1007
Hemiplegia, p. 1007
Immobility, p. 1006
Isometric contraction, p. 992
Isotonic contraction, p. 991
Joint, p. 992
Ligaments, p. 992
Mobility, p. 999
Muscle tone, p. 990
Posture, p. 990
Proprioception, p. 993
Range of motion (ROM), p. 994
Synergistic muscles, p. 993
Synovial joints, p. 992
Tendons, p. 992

Critical Thinking Exercises

1. Mr. Schmidt is a 65-year-old man who has enrolled in a cardiac rehabilitation program following a coronary artery bypass graft (CABG). What factors do you consider in developing an exercise program for Mr. Schmidt? What interventions could be incorporated to help motivate this client to exercise on a daily basis?

2. You're caring for an 81-year-old woman in her home. She sustained a fracture of the left femur and must use crutches for 1 week until her follow-up visit at the orthopedic clinic. You notice that she has not bathed or combed her hair. When you ask her if she needs assistance in bathing, she states, "My shower is on the second floor, and I'm afraid to go up and down the stairs." What is a priority nursing intervention at this time?

3. A 30-year-old woman has sustained a spinal cord injury. The client is to be maintained on bed rest. She is becoming increasingly depressed and withdrawn. What actions are important at this point in the client's care?

4. You have been asked to develop an exercise program for a support group for clients with type I diabetes. List some of the precautions and guidelines when developing an exercise prescription specific for persons with type I diabetes. What are some of the factors to consider when planning this program?

References

Ackley BJ, Ladwig GB: *Nursing diagnosis handbook: a guide to planning care,* ed 3, St. Louis, 1997, Mosby.

American College of Sports Medicine: *Guidelines for exercise testing and prescription,* ed 5, Media, Pa, 1995, Williams & Wilkins.

American Diabetes Association: Diabetes and exercise: position statement, *Diabetes Care* 20(suppl 1):S51, 1997.

Barry HC, Eathorne SW: Exercise and aging, *Med Clin North Am* 78(2):357, 1994.

Birchenall JM, Streight ME: *Mosby's textbook for the home care aide,* St. Louis, 1997, Mosby.

Borgman-Gainer M: Independent function: movement and mobility. In Hoeman SP, editor: *Rehabilitation nursing: process and application,* ed 2, St. Louis, 1996, Mosby.

Dawe D, Moore-Orr R: Low-intensity, range of motion exercise: invaluable nursing care for elderly patients, *J Adv Nurs* 21(4):675, 1995.

Gassett RS and others: Ergonomics and body mechanics in the work place, *Nurs Clin North Am* 274(10):861, 1996.

Graham MC, Pohlman RL: Innovations in family and community health, *Fam Community Health* 17(3):80, 1994.

Griego L, House-Fancher M: Coronary artery disease. In Lewis S, Collier I, Heitkemper M, editors: *Medical-surgical nursing: assessment and management of clinical problems,* ed 4, St. Louis, 1996, Mosby.

Hoeman SP: *Rehabilitation nursing: process and application,* St. Louis, 1996, Mosby.

Huddleston JS: Exercise. In Edelman CL, Mandle CL, editors: *Health promotion throughout the lifespan,* ed 4, St. Louis, 1998, Mosby.

Huether SE, McCance KL: *Understanding pathophysiology,* St. Louis, 1996, Mosby.

Kelly G, McClellan P: Anti-hypertensive effects of aerobic exercise: a brief meta-analytic review of randomized controlled trials, *Am J Hypertens* 7:115, 1994.

Kim MJ, McFarland GK, McLane AM: *Pocket guide to nursing diagnoses,* ed 7, St. Louis, 1997, Mosby.

McCance KL, Huether SE: *Pathophysiology: the biologic basis for disease in adults and children,* ed 3, St. Louis, 1998, Mosby.

National Institutes of Health Consensus Development Panel on Physical Activity and Cardiovascular Health: Physical activity and cardiovascular health, *JAMA* 276(3):241, 1996.

Pate RR and others: Physical activity and public health: a recommendation from the Centers for Disease Control and Prevention and the American College of Sports Medicine, *JAMA* 273(5):402, 1995.

Phipps WJ, Sands JK, Marek JF: *Medical-surgical nursing: concepts and clinical practice,* ed 6, St. Louis, 1999, Mosby.

Prochaska JO, Norcross JC, DiClemente CC: *Changing for good,* New York, 1994, William Morrow.

Scherer YK, Schmieder LE: The effect of a pulmonary rehabilitation program on self-efficacy, perception of dyspnea, and physical endurance, *Heart Lung* 26(1):15, 1997.

Thibodeau GA, Patton KT: *Anatomy and physiology,* ed 4, St. Louis, 1999, Mosby.

Thompson DR, Bowman GS: Evidence for the effectiveness of cardiac rehabilitation, *Intensive Crit Care Nurs* 14:38, 1998.

Thompson JM, Wilson SF: *Health assessment for nursing practice,* St. Louis, 1996, Mosby.

Topp R, Mikesky A, Bawel K: Developing a strength training program for older adults: planning, programming, and potential outcomes, *Rehabil Nurs* 19(5):266, 1994.

U.S. Department of Health and Human Services: *Healthy people 2000: mid-course review and 1995 revisions,* Washington, DC, 1995, U.S. Department of Health and Human Services: Public Health Service.

U.S. Department of Health and Human Services: *Physical activity and health: a report of the Surgeon General,* Atlanta, 1996, U.S. Department of Health and Human Services, Centers for Disease Control and Prevention, National Center for Chronic Disease Prevention and Health Promotion.

37

Safety

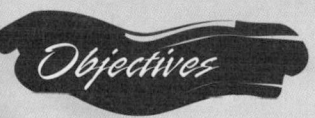
Mastery of content in this chapter will enable the student to:

- Define the key terms listed.
- Describe how unmet basic physiological needs of oxygen, fluids, nutrition, and temperature can threaten clients' safety.
- Discuss the specific risks to safety related to developmental age.
- Describe the four categories of risks in a health care agency.
- Describe assessment activities designed to identify clients' physical, psychosocial, and cognitive status as it pertains to their safety status.
- State nursing diagnoses associated with risks to safety.
- Develop care plans for clients whose safety is threatened.
- Describe nursing interventions specific to clients' age for reducing risk of falls, fires, poisonings, and electrical hazards.
- Describe methods to evaluate interventions designed to maintain or promote safety.

Safety, often defined as freedom from psychological and physical injury, is a basic human need that must be met. Health care, provided in a safe manner, and a safe community environment are essential for a client's survival and well-being. The nurse, incorporating critical thinking skills when using the nursing process, is responsible for assessing the client and the environment for hazards that threaten safety, as well as planning and intervening appropriately to maintain a safe environment. By doing this, the nurse is not only a provider of safe acute, restorative, and continuing care, but also an active participant in health promotion.

Scientific Knowledge Base

ENVIRONMENTAL SAFETY

A client's **environment** includes all of the many physical and psychosocial factors that influence or affect the life and survival of that client. This broad definition of environment incorporates all of the settings in which the nurse and client interact (e.g., the home, community center, school, clinic, hospital, and long-term care facility). Safety in these settings reduces the incidence of illness and injury, shortens the length of treatment and/or hospitalization, improves or maintains a client's functional status, and increases the client's sense of well-being. A safe environment affords protection to the staff as well, allowing them to function at an optimal level. A safe environment is an environment in which basic needs are met, physical hazards are reduced, transmission of pathogens is reduced, sanitation is maintained, and pollution is controlled.

Basic Needs. Physiological needs, including the need for sufficient oxygen, nutrition, and optimum temperature and humidity, influence a person's safety.

Oxygen. The nurse must be aware of factors in a client's environment that decrease the amount of available oxygen. A common environmental hazard in the home is an improperly functioning heating system. A furnace that is not properly vented or a car left running inside a closed garage may introduce carbon monoxide into the environment. **Carbon monoxide** is a colorless, odorless, poisonous gas produced by the combustion of carbon or organic fuels. Carbon monoxide binds strongly with hemoglobin, preventing the formation of oxyhemoglobin and thus reducing the supply of oxygen delivered to tissues (see Chapter 39). Low concentrations can cause nausea, dizziness, headache, and fatigue. Higher concentrations can be fatal (Air Pollution Fact Sheet, 1998). Seasonal inspections of heating systems and appliances should be done in private homes, as well as in institutions. Carbon monoxide detectors (Figure 37-1) are available for home or institutional use at a reasonable cost.

Nutrition. Meeting nutritional needs adequately and safely requires environmental controls and knowledge. In the home the client needs a refrigerator with a freezer compartment to keep perishable foods fresh. An adequate, clean water supply is needed for drinking and to wash fresh produce and dishes. Provisions for garbage collection are necessary to maintain sanitary conditions.

Foods that are inadequately prepared or stored, or that are subject to unsanitary conditions, increase the client's risk for infections and food poisoning. Bacterial food infections result from eating food contaminated by bacteria

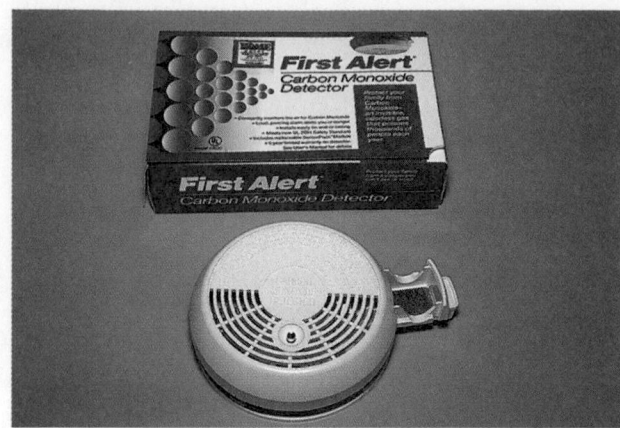

Figure 37-1   Carbon monoxide detector.

such as *Escherichia coli*, or *Salmonella, Shigella,* or *Listeria* organisms. **Food poisoning** is caused by ingestion of bacterial toxins produced in food; staphylococcal and clostridial bacteria are the most common causes. Although most food-borne diseases are bacterial, the hepatitis A virus is spread by fecal contamination of food, water, or milk (Williams, 1997).

For illnesses caused by bacterial contamination, the onset of symptoms may be very rapid or may take a week or longer. The incubation period for hepatitis A is from 2 to 6 weeks (Pagana and Pagana, 1998). In general, assessments for suspected food infections or poisoning encompass obtaining a client's history, including a detailed dietary assessment for the past week; conducting an examination of gastrointestinal (GI) and central nervous system (CNS) function; observing for a fever; and analyzing cultures of feces and vomitus. Suspected food and water sources are also studied. Preventive measures include thorough hand washing before handling food, adequate cooking, and proper storage and refrigeration of perishable foods.

To protect consumers, commercially processed and packaged foods are subject to **Food and Drug Administration (FDA)** regulations. The FDA is a federal agency responsible for the enforcement of federal regulations regarding the manufacture, processing, and distribution of foods, drugs, and cosmetics to protect consumers against the sale of impure or dangerous substances.

Temperature and Humidity.   The comfort zone for environmental temperature varies among individuals, but the usual comfort range is between 18.3° and 23.9° C (65° and 75° F). Temperature extremes that frequently occur during the winter and summer affect not only comfort and productivity, but also safety.

Exposure to severe cold for prolonged periods causes frostbite and accidental hypothermia. Frostbite occurs when a surface area of the skin freezes as a result of exposure to extremely cold temperatures. **Hypothermia** occurs when the core body temperature is 35° C (95° F) or below. Older adults, the young, clients with cardiovascular conditions, clients who have ingested drugs or alcohol in excess, and the homeless are at high risk for hypothermia. A faint, irregular heart rate; slow and shallow respirations; pallor; and mild shivering may be observed. Death may ensue if the condition is not corrected.

Exposure to extreme heat can result in heatstroke or heat exhaustion. Chronically ill clients, older adults, and infants are at greatest risk for injury from extreme heat. Heat exhaustion is manifested by diaphoresis, hypotension, changes in mental status, muscle cramps, and nausea. Heatstroke is a life-threatening condition with severe changes in mental status, including coma; **hyperthermia** with hot, dry skin; and rectal temperatures in excess of 40.5° C (105° F).

The relative humidity of the air in the environment may affect the client's health and safety. **Relative humidity** is the amount of water vapor in the air compared with the maximum amount of water vapor that the air could contain at the same temperature. The comfort zone for humidity varies from person to person, but most people are comfortable when the humidity is between 60% and 70%.

When the relative humidity is high, the skin's moisture evaporates slowly. Thus during hot, humid weather, people feel uncomfortably hot and sticky. If the relative humidity is low, the skin's moisture evaporates quickly. This is why people feel cooler and more comfortable when the temperature is 32.2° C (90° F) with a relative humidity of 30% than when the temperature is 32.2° C (90° F) with a relative humidity of 85%.

Increasing the environmental humidity can have therapeutic benefits. Children and adults with upper respiratory tract infections may experience some improvement in their symptoms when a humidifier is placed in the room while they sleep. Increasing the relative humidity of inhaled air liquefies secretions and improves breathing. It is important to follow the manufacturer's directions regarding the cleaning and maintenance of home humidifiers to reduce the contamination of the water.

Physical Hazards.   Physical hazards in the community and health care settings place clients at risk for accidental injury and death. Motor vehicle accidents are the leading cause of unintentional death, followed by falls, poisonings, drownings, fires, and burns. More than half of the falls occurred in the home, and almost 4 out of 5 involved a person 65 years of age or older (Accident Facts, 1998). Falls are the most common cause of hospital admissions for trauma for older clients. Among people over age 65, falls account for 87% of all fractures and are the second leading cause of spinal cord and brain injury (Unintentional Injury Fact Sheet, 1997). Many physical hazards, especially those contributing to falls, can be minimized through adequate lighting, reduction of obstacles,

Home Hazard Assessment   Box 37-1

HOME EXTERIOR

Are sidewalks uneven?
Are steps in good repair?
Do steps have securely fastened handrails?
Is there adequate lighting?
Is outdoor furniture sturdy?

HOME INTERIOR

Do all rooms, stairways and halls have adequate, nonglare lighting?
Are night-lights available?
Are area rugs secured?
Are wooden floors nonslippery?
Is furniture placed appropriately to permit mobility?
Is furniture sturdy enough to provide support for getting up and down?
Are temperature and humidity within normal range?
Are there any steps or thresholds that may pose a hazard?
Are step edges clearly marked with colored tape?
Are handrails available and secure?
In homes with young children, are window guards installed?
Can all doors and windows with security gates and locks be opened from the inside without a key?

KITCHEN

Are hand-washing facilities available?
Is the pilot light on for the gas stove?
Are the stove top and oven clean?
Are the dials on the stove readable?
Are storage areas within easy reach?
Are fluids such as cleaners and bleach in original containers and stored properly?
Is the water temperature within normal range?
Are there clean areas for food storage and preparation?
Is refrigeration adequate? Are the refrigerator and freezer temperatures correct?

BATHROOM

Are hand-washing facilities available?
Are there skidproof strips or surfaces in the tub or shower?
Are bath mats secured?
Does the client need grab bars near the bathtub and toilet?
Does the client need an elevated toilet seat?
Is the medicine cabinet well lighted?
Are medications in their original containers?
Are medication containers child resistant if children live in the home or visit?
Have outdated medications been discarded?

BEDROOM

Are beds of adequate height to allow getting on and off easily?
Is day and night lighting adequate?
Are floor coverings nonskid?
Does the client have a telephone nearby?
Are emergency numbers visible near the telephone?

ELECTRICAL AND FIRE HAZARDS

Are smoke and carbon monoxide detectors installed?
Are the batteries for all detectors tested every month and changed twice a year?
Have furnaces, chimneys, and stoves been checked for proper ventilation?
Are extension cords in good condition and used appropriately?
Are appliances in good working order?
Are electrical appliances located away from water sources?
Is there a fire extinguisher near the cooking area?
Are combustible items such as oil-based paints, gasoline, and oily rags being stored in a garage and/or basement?
Are flashlights available?
Is there a first aid kit available to the adult members of the household?
Does everyone in the family have easy access to emergency phone numbers?

Data from Tideiksaar R: Home safe home: practical tips for fall-proofing, *Geriatr Nurs* 11(6):280, 1989; Ebersole P, Hess P: *Toward healthy aging*, ed 5, St. Louis, 1998, Mosby.

control of bathroom hazards, and security measures. Box 37-1 provides a sample home hazard assessment.

Lighting.   Adequate lighting reduces physical hazards by illuminating areas in which the client moves and works. Outside the home, there should be adequate lighting on all walkways. Outdoor lighting also helps protect the home and its inhabitants from crime. Well-lighted garages, walkways, and doorways discourage intruders from entering the premises or hiding in shadows.

Inside the house, halls, staircases, and individual rooms should be adequately lighted so that residents can safely carry out activities of daily living. Night-lights in dark halls, bathrooms, and the rooms of children and older adults help maintain safety by reducing the risk of falls. A night-light in a guest room can help orient an overnight guest who needs to get up in the middle of the night.

Artificial lighting should be soft and nonglaring, because glare is a major problem for older adults (Ebersole and Hess, 1998).

Obstacles.   Injuries in the home frequently result from tripping over or coming into contact with common household objects, including doormats, small rugs on the stairs and floor, wet spots on the floor, and clutter on bedside tables, closet shelves, the top of the refrigerator, and bookshelves. The risk of falls from obstacles is present for all age-groups; however, it is greatest for older adults. Falls are usually a result of a combination of intrinsic risk factors (e.g., illness, drug therapy, or alcohol use) and extrinsic or environmental factors. In some cases an obstacle or extrinsic factor may be the only cause of a fall. Intrinsic factors may be difficult to modify or eliminate, but extrinsic ones are usually not.

To reduce the risk of injury, all obstacles should be removed from halls and other heavily traveled areas. Necessary objects such as clocks, glasses, tissues, or medications should remain on bedside tables within reach of the client but out of the reach of children in the home. Care should also be taken to ensure that end tables are secure and have stable, straight legs. Nonessential items should be placed in drawers to eliminate clutter. If small area rugs are used, they should be secured with a nonslip pad or skid-resistant adhesive strips. Any carpeting on the stairs should be secured with carpet tacks.

Bathroom Hazards.   Accidents such as falls, burns, and poisoning frequently occur in the bathroom. Secure, easily seen grab bars and nonslip, colored adhesive tape on the bottom of the tub are useful in reducing falls in the bathtub. A raised toilet seat with armrests and nonslip strips on the floor in front of the toilet are also helpful (Tideiksaar, 1989). Lowering the thermostat setting on the water heater reduces the risk of scalding. In the medicine cabinet, medications should be clearly marked and out of the reach of children. Child-resistant caps should be on all medication containers when there are children living in the home or visiting the home. Medication not in use or out-of-date should be discarded by flushing it down the toilet.

Security.   Home fires are a major cause of death and injury. According to the National Fire Protection Association, approximately 4000 people in the United States are killed and 15,000 to 20,000 are injured in home fires each year. The leading cause of fire deaths is careless smoking, and most fire deaths occur between the hours of 11 PM and 8 AM. Cooking equipment and appliances, particularly stoves, are the main items involved in home fires and fire injuries. Smoke detectors (Figure 37-2), along with carbon monoxide detectors, should be placed strategically throughout the home. Multipurpose fire extinguishers should be installed near the kitchen and any workshop areas.

Homes should be inspected for lead. Although lead has not been used in house paint or plumbing materials since the U.S. Consumer Product Safety Commission banned it in 1978, older homes continue to contain high lead levels. Soil and water systems may also be contaminated. Poisoning may occur from swallowing or inhaling lead. Children under the age of 6 and pregnant women are at the greatest risk for poisoning (Lead Poisoning, 1997-1998).

Clients need to take precautions to secure their homes from intruders. When assessing the home for safety, the client should evaluate doors and windows for the presence and quality of locks. Clients should be encouraged to join block associations and work closely with law enforcement personnel to reduce crime in their neighborhoods.

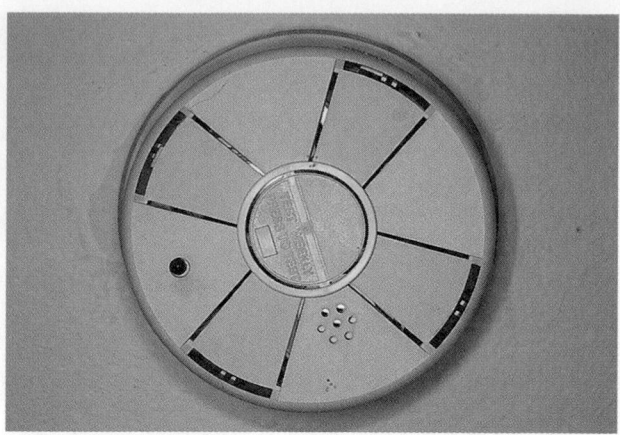

Figure 37-2   Smoke and fire detector.

Transmission of Pathogens.   A **pathogen** is any microorganism capable of producing an illness. One of the most effective methods for limiting the transmission of pathogens is the medical aseptic practice of hand washing (see Chapter 33). Clients must be instructed in proper hand-washing technique and encouraged to use it frequently in the home and hospital.

The transmission of disease from person to person can also be reduced, and in some cases prevented, by immunization. **Immunization** is the process by which resistance to an infectious disease is produced or augmented. Active immunity is acquired by injecting a small amount of attenuated (weakened) or dead organisms or modified toxins from the organism (toxoids) into the body. Passive immunity occurs when antibodies produced by other persons or animals can be introduced into a person's bloodstream for protection against a pathogen.

The human immunodeficiency virus (HIV)—the pathogen that causes acquired immunodeficiency syndrome (AIDS)—and the hepatitis B virus are transmitted through blood and other body fluids. Drug abusers frequently share syringes and needles, which increases the risk of acquiring these viruses. Safe sexual practices, including the correct use of condoms and engaging in monogamous relationships, reduce the risk for both of these diseases, as well as for other sexually transmitted diseases (STDs). Nurses use standard precautions when caring for all clients to protect themselves from contact with blood and body fluids (see Chapter 33).

The transmission of disease is also controlled by adequate disposal of human waste through proper construction and repair of sewers and drains. Insect and rodent control is also necessary to reduce the transmission of disease.

Pollution.   A healthy environment is free of pollution. A **pollutant** is a harmful chemical or waste material discharged into the water, soil, or air. People commonly think of pollution only in terms of air, land, or water pollution, but excessive noise can also be a form of pollution that presents health risks.

Air pollution is the contamination of the atmosphere with a harmful chemical. Prolonged exposure to air pollution increases the risk of pulmonary disease. In urban areas, industrial waste and vehicle exhaust are common contributors to air pollution. In the home, school, or workplace, cigarette smoke is the primary cause of air pollution. **Land pollution** of soil can be caused by improper disposal of radioactive and bioactive waste products (e.g., dioxin).

Water pollution is the contamination of lakes, rivers, and streams, usually by industrial pollutants. Water treatment facilities filter harmful contaminants from the water, but these systems may contain flaws. If water becomes contaminated, the public is notified to boil water used for drinking and cooking. Flooding frequently causes damage to water treatment stations and also requires the boiling of drinking and cooking water.

Noise pollution occurs when the noise level in an environment becomes uncomfortable to the inhabitants of the environment. Noise levels are measured in units of sound intensity called decibels. Tolerance for noise varies from individual to individual and is influenced by health status. Irreversible hearing loss may result from constant exposure to high sound intensity. Clients working in environments with high noise levels need to wear protective devices to reduce hearing loss (Figure 37-3). Adolescents should limit their exposure to intense noise such as that found at rock concerts.

A health care facility can also be polluted by noise. The sounds of machines, people talking, and intercoms and paging systems can create increased noise levels. Even when the noise level is not high enough to affect hearing acuity, it may produce a syndrome called sensory overload. Sensory overload is a marked increase in the intensity of auditory and visual stimuli. It disrupts processing of information, and the client no longer perceives the environment in a meaningful way (see Chapter 48).

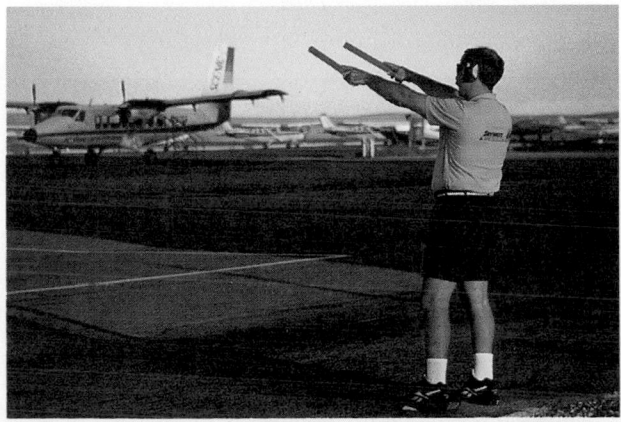

Figure 37-3   Protective device to reduce hearing loss.

Nursing Knowledge Base

Nurses, in addition to being knowledgeable about the environment, must be familiar with a client's developmental level; mobility, sensory, and cognitive status; lifestyle choices; and knowledge of common safety precautions. They must also be aware of the special risks to safety that are found in agency settings.

RISKS AT DEVELOPMENTAL STAGES
Threats to safety are influenced by clients' developmental stage, lifestyle, mobility status, sensory impairments, and safety awareness.

Infant, Toddler, and Preschooler.   Injuries are the leading cause of death in children over age 1 and cause more death and disabilities than do all diseases combined (Wong and others, 1999). The nature of the injury sustained is closely related to normal growth and development. For example, the incidence of lead poisoning is highest in late infancy and toddlerhood because of the increased level of oral activity and the growing ability to explore the environment. Accidents involving children are largely preventable, but parents need to be aware of specific dangers at each stage of growth and development. Accident prevention thus requires health education for parents and the removal of dangers whenever possible.

School-Age Child.   When a child enters school, the environment expands to include the school, transportation to and from school, school friends, and after-school activities. Through discussions with examples, parents, teachers, and nurses must instruct the child in safe practices to follow at school or play.

Because school-age children are participating in more activities outside their home and neighborhood environments, they are at greater risk of injury from strangers. Therefore the child should be warned repeatedly not to accept candy, food, gifts, or rides from strangers. In addition, a child needs to know what to do if a stranger approaches. Frequently neighborhoods have a "block home" or "safe house." In these homes the owner ensures that an adult is home during the times when children are walking to and from school. If a stranger approaches a child, the child can run to that home, and the adult will protect the child and call the proper authorities. Nurses can work with school systems or neighborhoods to initiate such a system to protect children.

Sports safety is stressed in school sports, but parents and health professionals can reinforce these safety tips by insisting that children wear protective gear while participating in sports. For example, schools provide hard batting helmets for baseball games, and parents should also provide this equipment when children are playing baseball in their own backyards.

Bicycle-related injuries are a major cause of death and disability among children. Bikes should be in good working order and be the proper size for the child. The child should be taught the rules of the road and cautioned not to engage in dangerous stunts or activities while bike riding. A properly fitted helmet should be worn. Since most fatalities from bicycle accidents are related to head injuries, many states are implementing laws requiring bicycle helmets (Figure 37-4).

Adolescent.

As children enter adolescence, they develop greater independence and begin to develop a sense of identity and their own values. In addition, adolescents begin to separate emotionally from their families, and peers generally have a stronger influence.

The struggle toward identity may cause the teenager to experience shyness, fear, and anxiety, with resulting dysfunction at home or school. In an attempt to relieve the tensions associated with the physical and psychosocial changes, as well as peer pressures, adolescents may begin smoking and using drugs. In addition to the health risks posed by nicotine and other drugs, the ingestion of drugs, including alcohol, increases the incidence of accidents such as drowning and motor vehicle accidents.

When adolescents learn to drive, their environment expands and so does their potential for injury. The young driver must be taught to comply with rules and regulations regarding use of a car. Common rules include proper use of seat belts and abstinence from alcohol and other drugs.

Because adolescence is a time when mature sexual physical characteristics develop, adolescents may begin to have physical relationships with others. They need prompt, accurate instruction about abstinence and/or safe sexual practices and birth control.

Adult.

The threats to an adult's safety are frequently related to lifestyle habits. For example, the client who uses alcohol excessively is at greater risk for motor vehicle accidents. The long-term smoker has a greater risk of cardiovascular or pulmonary disease as a result of the inhalation of smoke into the lungs and the effect of nicotine on the circulatory system. Likewise, the adult experiencing a high level of stress is more likely to have an accident or illness such as headaches, GI disorders, and infections (see Chapter 30).

Older Adult.

The physiological changes that occur during the aging process increase the client's risk for falls and other types of accidents such as burns and car accidents (Box 37-2). Older clients are more likely to fall in the bedroom, bathroom, and kitchen, and outside as a result of ice on walkways or obstacles in the garden. Inside falls most often occur while transferring from beds, chairs, and toilets; getting into or out of bathtubs; tripping over carpet edges or doorway thresholds; slipping on wet surfaces; and descending stairs (Tideiksaar, 1989).

• • •

Unfortunately, clients throughout all developmental stages may be subject to abuse. Child abuse, domestic violence, and abuse of older adults are serious threats to safety. These topics are discussed in Chapters 10 through 12.

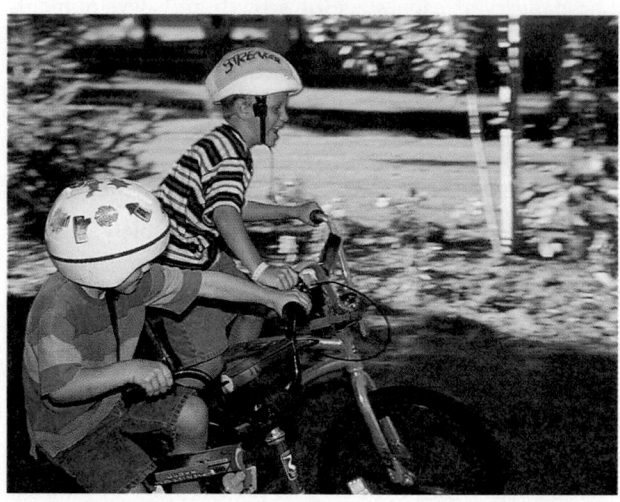

Figure 37-4   Proper bicycle safety equipment for school-age child.

Physical Assessment Findings in the Older Adult That Increase the Risk of Accidents	Box 37-2

MUSCULOSKELETAL CHANGES
Muscle strength and function decrease, joints become less mobile, posture changes (some kyphosis is common), and range of motion is limited.

NERVOUS SYSTEM CHANGES
All voluntary or automatic reflexes slow to some extent, ability to respond to multiple stimuli decreases, and kinesthetic sense is less efficient.

SENSORY CHANGES
Peripheral vision and lens accommodation decrease, lens may develop opacity (cataracts), stimuli threshold for light touch and pain increases, transmission of hot and cold impulses is delayed, and hearing is impaired as high-frequency tones become less perceptible.

GENITOURINARY CHANGES
Nocturia and occurrences of incontinence increase.

Modified from Ebersole P, Hess P: *Toward healthy aging,* ed 5, St. Louis, 1998, Mosby.

INDIVIDUAL RISK FACTORS

Other risk factors posing threats to safety include lifestyle, impaired mobility, sensory or communication impairment, and lack of safety awareness.

Lifestyle.   Lifestyle can increase safety risks. People who drive or operate machinery while under the influence of chemical substances, who work at inherently dangerous jobs, or who are risk takers are at greater risk of injury. In addition, people experiencing stress, anxiety, fatigue, or alcohol or drug withdrawal, or those taking prescribed medications may be more accident prone. Because of these factors, clients may be too preoccupied to notice the source of potential accidents, such as cluttered stairs or a stop sign.

Impaired Mobility.   Impaired mobility due to muscle weakness, paralysis, or poor coordination or balance is a major factor in client falls. Immobilization predisposes the client to additional physiological and emotional hazards, which in turn can further restrict mobility and independence (see Chapter 36).

Sensory or Communication Impairment.   Clients with visual, hearing, tactile, or communication impairment, such as aphasia or a language barrier, are at greater risk for injury. Such clients may not be able to perceive a potential danger or express their need for assistance (see Chapter 48).

Lack of Safety Awareness.   Some clients are unaware of safety precautions, such as keeping medicine away from children or reading the expiration date on food products. A complete nursing assessment, including a home inspection (see Box 37-1), should help the nurse identify the client's level of knowledge regarding home safety so that deficiencies can be corrected with an individualized nursing care plan.

RISKS IN THE HEALTH CARE AGENCY

The issues related to environmental safety in terms of basic needs, reduction of physical hazards, reduction of transmission of pathogens, and pollution control apply to the health care agency, as well as to the client's home and community. However, there are specific risks in health care agencies that must also be addressed.

The types of risks to a client's safety within the health care environment are falls, client-inherent accidents, procedure-related accidents, and equipment-related accidents. The nurse must assess for these four potential problem areas and, considering the developmental level of the client, take steps to prevent or minimize accidents in the agency.

An accident necessitates the filing of an incident report, a confidential document that completely describes any client accident occurring on the premises of a health care agency (see Chapter 24). It documents the accident, client assessment, and interventions carried out for the client. In addition to completing the incident report, the nurse must objectively document the incident in the client's medical record.

Falls.   Falls account for up to 90% of all reported incidences in hospitals. The risk for falling is significantly higher in older clients. In addition to age, a history of previous falls, gait, balance and mobility problems, postural hypotension, sensory impairment, urinary and bladder dysfunction, and certain medical diagnostic categories (e.g., cancer and cardiovascular, neurological, and cerebrovascular diseases) increase the risk. Drug use and drug interactions are also implicated in falls (Box 37-3). In older clients the fear of falling may be so great that they significantly reduce their activities (Ebersole and Hess, 1998).

Client-Inherent Accidents.   Client-inherent accidents are accidents (other than falls) in which the client is the primary factor. Examples of client-inherent accidents are self-inflicted cuts, injuries, and burns; ingestion or injection of foreign substances; self-mutilation or fire setting; and pinching fingers in drawers or doors.

A client-inherent accident may occur as a result of a seizure. A **seizure** is a hyperexcitation and disorderly discharge of neurons in the brain leading to a sudden, violent, involuntary series of muscle contractions that may be paroxysmal and episodic, as in a seizure disorder, or transient and acute, such as following a head injury. A generalized tonic-clonic, or grand mal, seizure lasts approximately 2 minutes (no longer than 5) and is characterized by a cry, loss of consciousness with falling, tonicity (rigidity), clonicity (jerking), and incontinence (Beare and Meyers, 1998). Before a convulsive episode, a few clients may report an aura, which serves as a warning or sense that a seizure is about to occur. An aura may be a bright light, smell, or taste. During the seizure activity the client may have shallow breathing, cyanosis, and possibly loss of bladder and bowel control. Following the seizure there is a postictal phase during which the client may have amnesia or confusion and may fall into a deep sleep.

Continuous seizures that last 15 minutes or a series of seizures over a 20- to 30-minute period in which the client does not regain consciousness between attacks is status epilepticus. This condition is a medical emergency and requires intensive monitoring and treatment. It is important that the nurse observe the client carefully before, during, and after the seizure so that the episode can be documented accurately (Beare and Meyers, 1998).

Procedure-Related Accidents.   Procedure-related accidents occur during therapy. They include medication and fluid administration errors, improper application of external devices, and accidents related to improper performance of procedures (e.g., Foley catheter insertion).

RISK Assessment Tool for Fall Prevention

Box 37-3

TOOL 1: RISK ASSESSMENT TOOL FOR FALLS
Directions: Place a check mark in front of elements that apply to your client. The decision as to whether a client is at risk for falls is based on your nursing judgment.
Guideline: A client with a check next to an item with an asterisk (*) or four or more of the other items would be identified as at risk for falls.

General Data
___   Over 60 years of age
___   History of falls before admission*
___   History of smoking, alcohol, drug use
___   Perioperative status

Physical Condition
___   Vertigo
___   Unsteady gait
___   Problems affecting weight-bearing joints
___   Weakness
___   Paresis/paralysis
___   Seizure disorder
___   Impaired vision
___   Impaired hearing
___   Slow reaction times
___   Diarrhea
___   Urinary frequency, urgency, nocturia

Mental Status
___   Lethargic
___   Confused or disoriented
___   Inability to understand or follow directions

Medications
___   Diuretics
___   Hypotensive or central nervous system depressants (e.g., narcotics, sedatives, psychotropics, hypnotics, tranquilizers, antihypertensives, antidepressants)
___   Medication that increases gastrointestinal motility (e.g., laxatives)
___   Effect of drug interactions

Ambulatory Devices Used
___   Cane
___   Crutches
___   Walker
___   Wheelchair
___   Geriatric (geri) chair
___   Braces

TOOL 2: REASSESSMENT IS SAFE "KARE" (RISK) TOOL
Directions: Place a check mark in front of any element that applies to your client. A client who has a check mark in front of any of the first four elements would be identified as at risk for falls. In addition, when a high-risk client has a check mark in front of the element "use of a wheelchair," the client is considered to be at greater risk for falls.
___   Unsteady gait/dizziness/imbalance
___   Impaired memory or judgment
___   Weakness
___   History of falls
___   Use of a wheelchair

From Brians LK and others: The development of the RISK tool for fall prevention, *Rehabil Nurs* 16(2):67, 1991.

The nurse can prevent many procedure-related accidents. For example, strictly following the procedure for administering medications will prevent medication errors. Proper administration of intravenous (IV) fluids prevents fluid overload or deficit. The potential for infection is reduced when surgical asepsis is used for sterile dressing changes or any invasive procedure, such as insertion of a Foley catheter. Finally, correct use of body mechanics and transfer techniques reduces the risk of injuries when moving and lifting clients.

Equipment-Related Accidents.   Equipment-related accidents result from the malfunction, disrepair, or misuse of equipment or from an electrical hazard. To avoid injury, the nurse should not operate monitoring or therapy equipment without instruction.

A checklist should be used to assess potential electrical hazards to reduce the risk of electrical fires, electrocution, or injury from faulty equipment (see Box 37-1). In health care settings the engineering staff make regular safety checks of equipment.

Critical Thinking Synthesis

Successful critical thinking requires a synthesis of knowledge, experience, information gathered from clients, critical thinking attitudes, and intellectual and professional standards. Clinical judgments require the nurse to anticipate the necessary information, analyze the data, and make decisions regarding client care. Critical thinking is always changing. During assessment (Figure 37-5) the nurse must consider all critical thinking elements, as well as information about the specific client, to make appropriate nursing diagnoses.

In the case of safety the nurse integrates knowledge from nursing and other scientific disciplines, previous experiences in caring for clients who had an injury or were at risk, critical thinking attitudes such as perseverance, and any standards of practice that are applicable. For example, the American Nurses Association (ANA) standards for nursing practice address the nurse's responsibility in maintaining client safety. The Joint Commission for Accreditation of Healthcare Organizations (JCAHO) also provides standards for safety (e.g., in the administration of

KNOWLEDGE

- Basic human needs
- Potential risks to client safety from physical hazards, lifestyle, risks associated with health care environment, and environmental risks
- Influence of developmental stage on safety needs
- Influence of illness/medications on client safety

STANDARDS

- Apply intellectual standards of accuracy, significance, and completeness when assessing for threats to the client's safety
- Apply ANA standards for nursing practice
- Apply practice standards (e.g., fall prevention protocols)

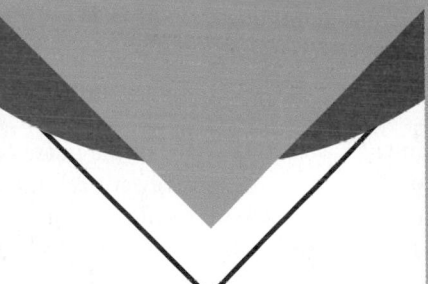

ASSESSMENT

- Identify actual and potential threats to the client's safety
- Determine impact of the underlying illness on the client's safety
- Identify the presence of risks for the client's developmental stage

EXPERIENCE

- Caring for clients whose mobility or sensory impairments increase threats to safety
- Personal experience in caring for younger siblings or children

ATTITUDES

- Demonstrate perseverance when necessary to identify all safety threats
- Be responsible for collecting unbiased, accurate data regarding threats to the client's safety
- Show discipline in conducting a thorough review of the client's home environment

Figure 37-5   *Synthesis Model for Safety Assessment Phase.*

medications, use of restraints, and use of medical devices). All of this information and experience is referred to by the nurse as he or she conducts a detailed assessment of a specific client. For example, while assessing a specific client's home environment, the nurse will consider knowledge regarding typical locations within the home where dangers commonly exist. If a client has a visual impairment, the nurse will apply previous experiences in caring for clients with visual changes to anticipate how to thoroughly assess the client's needs. Critical thinking directs the nurse to anticipate what needs to be assessed and how to make conclusions about available data.

Safety and the Nursing Process

ASSESSMENT

To conduct a thorough client assessment, the nurse considers possible threats to the client's safety, including the client's immediate environment, as well as any individual risk factors. When caring for a client in the home, a home hazard assessment is necessary (see Box 37-1). The nurse should walk through the home with the client and discuss how the client normally conducts daily activities. Getting a sense of the client's routines helps the nurse recognize hazards that are not as obvious. For example, if a client typically uses certain items in a kitchen that require the client to use a footstool, the nurse can anticipate the need to assess risks for falls. Including the family in the assessment may also help reveal hazards or risks.

When the client is cared for within a health care facility, the nurse must determine if any hazards exist in the immediate care environment. Does the placement of equipment or furniture pose barriers when the client attempts to ambulate? Does positioning of the client's bed allow the client to reach items on a bedside table or stand? In what way are self-care items in a bathroom arranged for accessibility? The nurse also collaborates with clinical engineering staff to make sure that equipment has been assessed to ensure proper function and condition.

A nursing history will include data about the client's level of wellness to determine if any underlying conditions exist that pose threats to safety. For example, the nurse will give special attention to assessing the client's gait, muscle strength and coordination, balance, and vision. A review of the client's developmental status must be considered as assessment information is analyzed. The nurse will also review if the client is taking any medications or undergoing any procedures that pose risks. For example, use of diuretics increases the frequency of voiding and may result in the client having to use toilet facilities more often. Falls often occur with clients who must get out of bed quickly because of urinary urgency. An example of a procedure that may pose risks is use of an electric aquathermia pad (see Chapter 47).

Client Expectations.   Clients generally expect to be safe in their home and in the health care setting. However, there are times when a client's view of what is safe does not agree with that of the nurse. For this reason, any assessment must include the client's understanding of his or her perception of risk factors. This will be important later as the nurse attempts to make changes in the client's environment. Clients usually do not purposefully put themselves in jeopardy. When clients are uninformed or inexperienced, threats to their safety can occur. Clients must always be consulted on ways to reduce hazards in their environment.

NURSING DIAGNOSIS

After completing an assessment of the client's safety status, the nurse reviews any clusters of data showing patterns suggesting that safety is threatened. Identification of defining characteristics from the data direct the nurse in identifying appropriate nursing diagnoses (Box 37-4). The diagnostic process requires accurate recognition of defining characteristics, as well as the related factors (Box 37-5).

The related factor becomes the basis for selecting nursing therapies. For example, *risk for injury related to impaired mobility* and *risk for injury related to barriers in the home environment* require different nursing interventions. The client with altered mobility may require ambulatory aids and physical therapy. When the related factor is barriers in the home, the nurse intervenes to make changes that will create a safer environment. At times, as in the example in Box 37-5, multiple related factors may apply.

PLANNING

During planning the nurse critically synthesizes information from multiple sources (Figure 37-6). Critical thinking ensures that the client's plan of care integrates all that the nurse has learned about the client, as well as the key critical thinking elements. For example, the nurse will reflect on knowledge regarding the services other disciplines (e.g., occupational therapy) can provide in helping

NURSING DIAGNOSES   Box 37-4
CLIENTS WITH SAFETY RISKS

Body temperature, altered, risk for	Sensory/perceptual alterations
Home maintenance management, impaired	Suffocation, risk for
Injury, risk for	Thought processes, altered
Knowledge deficit	Trauma, risk for
Poisoning, risk for	

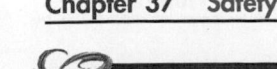

SAMPLE NURSING DIAGNOSTIC PROCESS

Box 37-5

RISK FOR INJURY

Assessment Activities	Defining Characteristics	Nursing Diagnosis
Observe client's mobility.	Uncoordinated gait	Risk for injury related to impaired
	Poor posture	mobility, decreased vision, poorly
Ask client about visual acuity.	Reports difficulty seeing at night	lighted home, and cluttered envi-
	Reports "tripping" over rugs and fur-	ronment
	niture	
Complete a home hazard appraisal.	Poorly lighted home	
	Rooms filled with small items	
	Excessive amount of furniture for size	
	of room	
	Rugs not secure	

clients return to their home environments safely. The nurse will also reflect on any previous experience whereby a client benefitted from safety interventions. Such experience helps the nurse adapt approaches with a new client. Applying critical thinking attitudes such as creativity helps the nurse and client collaborate in planning interventions that are relevant and most useful, particularly when changes are made in the home environment. Planning and goal setting need to be done with the client, family, and other members of the health care team (see care plan on p. 1031). Expected outcomes must be measurable and realistic. The following are common goals that focus on the client's need for safety:

Modifiable hazards will be reduced in the home environment.

Client will identify and avoid risks within the home and community.

Client will remain free of injuries.

The client who is an active participant in reducing threats to safety will be more alert to potential hazards. Clients need to learn how to identify and select resources within their community that enhance safety (e.g., neighborhood block homes, local police departments, and neighbors willing to check on a client's well-being).

The overall goal for a client with a threat to safety is remaining free from injury. Nursing interventions are designed to provide safe and efficient care. The nurse plans individualized interventions based on the severity of risk factors and the client's developmental stage, level of health, lifestyle, and culture (Box 37-6). Collaboration with other disciplines such as occupational and physical therapy may become an important part of the nurse's plan of care. Planning also involves an understanding of the client's need to maintain independence within physical and cognitive capabilities. The nurse and client collaborate to establish ways of maintaining the client's active involvement within the home and health care environment. Education of the client and family is also an important intervention to reduce safety risks over the long term.

IMPLEMENTATION

Nursing interventions are directed toward maintaining the client's safety in all types of settings. Nursing measures for providing a safe environment include health promotion, developmental interventions, and environmental interventions. Each of these areas of implementation is appropriate for acute and restorative care settings.

Health Promotion. To promote an individual's health, it is necessary for the individual to be in a safe environment and to practice a lifestyle that minimizes risk of injury. Edelman and Mandle (1998) describe passive and active strategies aimed at health promotion. Passive strategies are implemented through public health and government legislative interventions (e.g., sanitation and clean water laws) (see Chapter 3). Active strategies are those in which the individual is actively involved through changes in lifestyle (e.g., wearing seat belts or installing outdoor lighting) and participation in wellness programs.

The nurse participates by supporting legislation and working in community-based settings. Because environmental and community values have the greatest influence on health promotion, community and home health nurses can assess and recommend safety measures in the home, school, neighborhood, and workplace.

Developmental Interventions

Infant, Toddler, and Preschooler. Infants, toddlers, and preschoolers depend on adults to protect them from injury. Growing children are curious and completely trusting of their environment and do not perceive themselves to be in danger. Nurses are frequently in a position to educate parents or guardians about reducing risks of injuries for young children (see Chapter 10). Nurses working in prenatal and postpartum settings can easily incorporate safety into the care plan of the childbearing family. Community health nurses can assess the home and show parents how to promote safety in their homes (Table 37-1, p. 1032, and Figures 37-7 and 37-8, p. 1034).

KNOWLEDGE

- Role of community resources in safety promotion
- Safety risks posed in use of home care therapies (e.g., home oxygenation, IV therapy)

STANDARDS

- Establish interventions individualized to the client's safety needs
- Apply ANA standards of providing intervention in a safe and appropriate manner
- Apply ANA code of ethics to safeguard the client from incompetent or unethical care

PLANNING

- Select nursing interventions to promote safety according to the client's developmental and health care needs
- Consult with occupational and physical therapists for assistive devices
- Select interventions that will improve the safety of the client's home environment

EXPERIENCE

- Previous client responses to planned nursing therapies to improve safety (e.g., what worked and what did not work)

ATTITUDES

- Use creativity to assist in designing interventions suited to client needs and available resources
- Take risks to implement interventions that explore new resources or use current resources in new ways

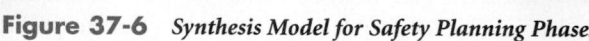

Figure 37-6   *Synthesis Model for Safety Planning Phase.*

SAMPLE NURSING CARE PLAN

RISK FOR INJURY

ASSESSMENT*

Mr. Key, a visiting nurse, is seeing Ms. Cohen, an 85-year-old woman, at home. The client has been recovering from a mild stroke. On physical examination, Mr. Key finds Ms. Cohen's blood pressure to be 122/78 with a pulse of 84 and regular. Ms. Cohen lives alone but receives regular assistance from her daughter, a schoolteacher. Her son also lives in town and helps when needed. Ms. Cohen has a **marked kyphosis** and an **uncoordinated, hesitant gait.** She also has a **slight weakness of her left arm and leg** as a result of her stroke. Mr. Key's assessment also reveals that Ms. Cohen has **trouble reading and seeing objects at a distance.** Her last eye examination was 18 months ago, when she received a prescription for glasses. Although she has no history of falling, she notes that since returning home from the hospital, "**I bump into things, and I am so afraid I am going to fall.**" She shows Mr. Key the **bruises on her left leg and thigh.** As Mr. Key completes a home hazard assessment, he finds Ms. Cohen's home **cluttered with furniture and small objects,** such as planters and magazines. **Cabinets in the kitchen are in disarray and full of breakable items that could fall out. Several throw rugs are seen throughout the house. The bathroom is poorly lighted and does not have safety strips in the tub or grab bars.**

*Defining characteristics are shown in bold type.

NURSING DIAGNOSIS: Risk for injury related to impaired mobility, decreased visual acuity, and physical environmental hazards.

PLANNING

GOAL	EXPECTED OUTCOMES
Home will be free of hazards within 1 week.	Modifiable hazards will be reduced in the home within 1 week.
Client and family will be knowledgeable of potential hazards for Ms. Cohen's age-group within 1 week.	Client and daughter will identify risks and the steps to avoid them in the home at the conclusion of a teaching session.
Client will express greater sense of feeling safe from falls in 1 month.	Client will be able to see objects at a distance clearly while wearing glasses.
Client will be free of injury.	Client will be able to ambulate unencumbered throughout the home within 2 weeks.

INTERVENTIONS†

Fall Prevention

- Review findings from home hazard assessment with client and daughter.

- Establish a list of priorities to modify and have son assist in installing bathroom safety devices (grab bars and nonskid strips).
- Install lighting (75-watt bulbs, nonglare) throughout the home. Have son install blinds over kitchen windows.

- Discuss with client and daughter the normal changes of aging, effects of recent stroke, associated risks for injury, and how to reduce risks.
- Encourage daughter to schedule vision testing for new prescription within 2 to 4 weeks.
- Refer to a physical therapist to assess need for assistive devices for kyphosis, left-sided weakness, and gait.

RATIONALE

Fall risks for homebound older adults include visual disturbances, unsteady gait, and postural changes (Lueckenotte, 1996). Evaluation of home hazards will highlight extrinsic factors that may lead to falls (Tideiksaar, 1989).

Modification of environment reduces fall rates (Shepherd and others, 1992).

With aging, the pupil loses the ability to adjust to light, causing sensitivity to glare. Glare can prevent an individual from seeing a walking path clearly.

Fear of falling is associated with an older adult's frailty (Arfken and others, 1994). Education regarding hazards has reduced fear of falling (Walker and Howland, 1991).

Enhanced sensory function reduces incidence of falls (Ebersole and Hess, 1998).

Exercise often improves gait, balance, and flexibility (Ebersole and Hess, 1998). Modifying gait problems by increasing lower extremity strength reduces fall risk (Shepherd and others, 1992).

†Intervention Classification labels from McCloskey JC, Bulechek GM: *Nursing interventions classification (NIC),* ed 3, St. Louis, 2000, Mosby.

EVALUATION

Schedule 1-week follow-up visit and inspect client's home for hazards.
Ask client and daughter to identify normal changes of aging and associated risks for injury.
During a follow-up visit observe whether client is wearing new glasses for reading and distance.
Observe client ambulating throughout the home using an assistive device.

Cultural ASPECTS OF CARE   Box 37-6

Cultural phenomena affecting health and safety include personal space, territoriality, communication, and environmental control (Giger and Davidhizar, 1999). While conducting a home assessment for risks to safety, the nurse must realize that he or she has entered the client's territory and that the client's attitude toward his or her residence and belongings must be appreciated. For example, clients from western Europe and the British Isles are considered aloof and distant in terms of space. It may be very difficult for them to have an outsider in their home who is suggesting changes with regard to their personal belongings to reduce physical hazards.

It is particularly difficult to determine a client's attitude toward his or her home when another language is spoken. The nurse should use an interpreter or engage the client's family to interpret if available. Attentiveness to the client's nonverbal communication becomes extremely important as the nurse assesses the home.

Another culturally sensitive issue is the client's sense of environmental control. The nurse must be aware of health beliefs and practices that will affect the outcome of interventions. For example, reliance on family and religious organizations, as opposed to community resources, may affect the client's compliance with nursing interventions and referrals.

Table 37-1   **Interventions to Promote Safety for Children and Adolescents**

Intervention	Rationale
Infants and Toddlers	
Have infants sleep on their backs or sides. Teach parents the slogan "back to sleep."	Sleeping on the stomach with the mouth and nose in close proximity to the mattress is associated with sudden infant death syndrome (SIDS).
Do not fill cribs with pillows, large stuffed toys, or comforters. Sheets should fit snugly.	Infants may become entwined in sheets and other bedding and suffocate.
Pacifiers should not be attached to string or ribbon and placed around a child's neck.	Choking may occur.
All instructions for preparing and storing formula must be followed.	Proper formula preparation and storage prevents contamination. A formula may come in a concentrated form, or it may already be diluted and ready to use. Following directions ensures proper concentration of the formula. Undiluted formula can cause fluid and electrolyte disturbances; very diluted formula will not provide sufficient nutrients.
Use large, soft toys without small parts, such as buttons.	Small parts can become dislodged, and choking and aspiration may occur.
Playpens with mesh sides should not be left with a side down; spaces between crib slats should be less than 2⅜ inches (6 cm) apart.	A child's head may become wedged in the lowered mesh side or in-between crib slats, and asphyxiation may occur.
Never leave crib sides down or leave babies unattended on changing tables or in infant seats, walkers, swings, strollers, or highchairs.	Infants and toddlers can roll or move and fall from changing tables or out of accessories such as infant seats or walkers.
Discontinue using accessories such as infant seats, walkers, and swings when the child becomes too active, physically too big, and/or according to the manufacturer's directions.	When physically active or too big, the child can fall out of or tip over these accessories and suffer an injury.
Never leave a child alone in the bathroom, tub, or near any water source (e.g., pool).	Accidental drowning may occur.
Baby-proof the home, removing small or sharp objects and toxic or poisonous substances, including plants.	Babies explore their world with their hands and mouth. Choking and poisoning may occur.
Remove plastic bags from the cleaners or grocery from the home.	Suffocation may occur if plastic covers the nose and mouth.
Electrical outlets should have covers (see Figure 37-7).	Crawling babies may insert objects into outlets and experience an electrical shock.
Window guards should be on all windows.	This prevents children from falling out of windows.
Install keyless locks (e.g., deadbolts) on doors above a child's reach, even when they are standing on a chair.	This prevents a toddler from leaving the house and wandering off. Death from exposure, car accidents, and drowning may occur. Keyless locks allow for rapid exit in case of fire.

Modified from Wong DL and others: *Whaley and Wong's nursing care of infants and children,* ed 6, St. Louis, 1999, Mosby.

Continued

Table 37-1   Interventions to Promote Safety for Children and Adolescents—cont'd

Intervention	Rationale
Children under 4 years of age should always be in an age/weight-appropriate car seat that has been installed according to the manufacturer's instructions. In cars with passenger-side air bags, children under 12 should be in back seats. All passengers should have seat belts on.	In case of a sudden stop or crash, an unrestrained child may suffer severe head injuries and death.
Caregivers should learn CPR and the Heimlich maneuver.	Caregivers should be prepared to intervene in acute emergencies, such as choking.
Preschoolers	
Teach children to swim at an early age, but always provide supervision near water.	Learning to swim is a useful skill that may someday save a child's life. However, all children need constant supervision near water.
Teach children how to cross streets and walk in parking lots. Instruct them to never run out after a ball or toy.	Pedestrian accidents involving young children are common.
Teach children not to talk to, go with, or accept any item from a stranger.	This reduces the risk of injury and stranger abduction.
Teach children basic physical safety rules, such as proper use of safety scissors, never running with an object in their mouth or hand, and never attempting to use the stove or oven unassisted.	Risk of injury is lowered if children are taught basic safety procedures.
Teach children not to eat items found in the street or grass.	Poisoning may occur.
Remove doors from unused refrigerators and freezers. Instruct children not to play or hide in a car trunk or unused appliances.	If a child cannot freely exit from appliances and car trunks, asphyxiation may occur.
School-Age Children	
Teach children the safe use of equipment for play and work.	The child needs to learn the safe, appropriate use of implements to avoid injury.
Teach children proper bicycle safety, including use of helmet and rules of the road.	This may reduce injuries from falling off a bike or being hit by a car.
Teach children proper techniques for specific sports, as well as the need to wear proper safety gear.	Using proper sports techniques, correct equipment, and protective gear prevents injuries.
Teach children not to operate electrical equipment while unsupervised.	If an electrical mishap were to occur, no one would be available to help.
Children should never have access to firearms or other weapons.	Children are often fascinated by firearms and weapons and may attempt to play with them.
Adolescents	
Encourage enrollment in driver's education classes.	Many injuries in this age-group are related to motor vehicle accidents.
Provide information about the effects of using alcohol and drugs.	Adolescents are prone to risk-taking behaviors and are subject to peer pressures.
Provide sex education, emphasizing safe sex practices, including abstinence.	Many adolescents begin sexual relationships. Pregnancy and sexually transmitted diseases may result.
Refer adolescents to community and school-sponsored activities.	The adolescent needs to socialize with peers, yet needs some supervision.
Encourage mentoring relationships between adults and adolescents.	Adolescents are in need of role models after which they can pattern their behavior.

School-Age Child. School-age children increasingly explore their environment (see Chapter 10). They have friends outside their immediate neighborhood, and they become more active in school, church, and community activities. The school-age child needs specific teaching regarding safety in school and at play (see Figure 37-4). See Table 37-1 for nursing interventions to help guide the parent in providing for the safety of the school-age child.

Adolescent. Risks to the safety of adolescents involve many factors outside the home environment, particularly their almost constant involvement with members of their peer group (see Chapter 10). Adults serve as role models for adolescents and, through providing examples, setting expectations, and providing education, can help adolescents minimize risks to their safety. This age-group has a high incidence of suicide because of feelings of decreased

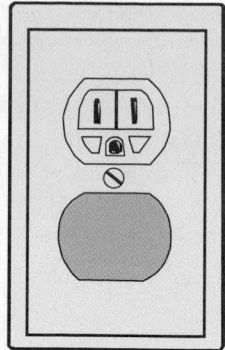

Figure 37-7   Safety covers for electrical outlets.

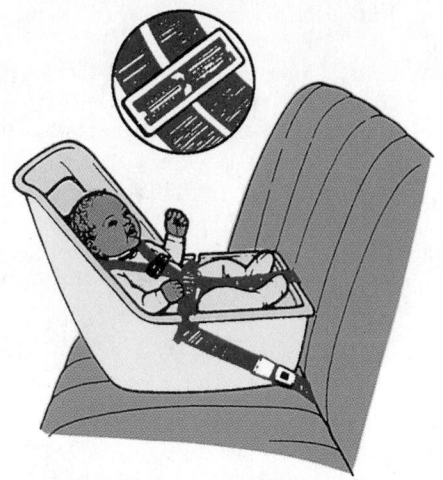

Figure 37-8   Infant car seat.

self-worth and hopelessness. The nurse must be aware of the risks posed at this time and be prepared to teach adolescents and their parents measures to prevent accidents and injury (see Table 37-1).

Adult.   Risks to young and middle-age adults frequently result from lifestyle factors such as child rearing, high stress levels, inadequate nutrition, use of firearms, excessive alcohol intake, and substance abuse (see Chapter 11). In this fast-paced society there also appears to be more expression of anger, which can quickly precipitate accidents (e.g., "road rage"). Adults need to have the opportunity to discuss the choices they have made in their lifestyle and the types of threats to safety that exist. Given information about threats to their well-being, adults may make necessary modifications in lifestyle practices. Useful resources are stress management centers (see Chapter 30) and health promotion activities, which can be found in many community service programs and hospitals. In addition, neighborhood centers, community clinics, and outpatient clinics are equipped to assist adults in modifying lifestyle habits (e.g., smoking, overeating, lack of exercise, and alcoholism) that present risks to health.

Older Adult.   Nursing interventions for older adults are designed to reduce the risk of falls and other accidents and to compensate for the physiological changes of aging (Box 37-7). Most injuries to older adults involve falls, automobile accidents, and burns (Ebersole and Hess, 1998). Advancing age and the concurrent physiological changes in vision, hearing, mobility, reflexes, circulation, and the ability to make quick judgments all predispose older adults to falls (see Chapter 12). Steinmetz and Hobson (1994) reported mental status change and mobility deficit as the most frequent risk factors for falls. Certain disease states common to older adults, such as arthritis or cerebrovascular accidents, increase chances of injury. In addition, the effects of many medications, such as sedatives, diuretics, and laxatives, given to older adults make falls more likely.

Older adults are more likely to have automobile accidents because of three specific physiological changes. First, changes in visual acuity, depth perception, and poor peripheral vision prevent the client from quickly observing situations in which an accident is likely to occur. Second, decreased hearing acuity alters the older client's ability to hear emergency vehicle sirens or car and truck horns. Third, because of decreased nervous system response, older adults may be unable to react as quickly as they once could to avoid an accident (Ebersole and Hess, 1998). A decline in these skills may account for the most common types of accidents, including right-of-way and turning accidents. The nurse can educate clients regarding safe driving tips (e.g., driving shorter distances or only in daylight, using side and rearview mirrors carefully, and looking behind them toward their "blind spot" before changing lanes). If hearing is a problem, the client might try to keep a window rolled down while driving or reduce the volume of the radio or CD or cassette player. Eventually, counseling may be necessary to help clients make the decision of when to stop driving. At that time the nurse should help locate resources in the community that provide transportation.

Burns and scalds are also more apt to occur with older people because they may forget and leave hot water running or become confused when turning the dials on a stove or other heating appliance. Nursing measures for preventing burns are designed to minimize the risk from impaired vision. Hot water faucets and dials can be color coded to make it easier for the adult to know what has been turned on. Recommending a reduction in temperature of the water heater can also be very beneficial.

Older adults love to walk. Pedestrian accidents can be reduced for older adults and for all other age-groups by persuading people to wear reflectors on garments when walking at night; to stand on the sidewalk and not in the street when waiting to cross a street; to always cross at corners and not in the middle of the block (particularly if the street is a major one); to cross with the traffic light and not against it; and to look left, right, and left again before entering the street or crosswalk.

- The older adult experiences alterations in vision and hearing. The nurse should encourage yearly vision and hearing examinations and frequent cleansing of glasses and hearing aids as a means of preventing falls and burns. Driving may need to be restricted to daylight hours or suspended.
- Range of motion, flexibility, and strength are decreased. The nurse should encourage supervised exercise classes for older adults and teach them to seek assistance with household tasks as needed. Safety features, such as grab bars in the bathroom, may be needed.
- Reflexes are slowed, and the ability to respond to multiple stimuli is reduced. The nurse should provide adequate, meaningful stimuli but prevent sensory overload.
- Nocturia and incontinence are more frequent in older adults. The nurse should institute a toileting schedule for the client. Diuretics should be given in the morning. Assistance should be provided, along with adequate lighting, to clients who need to go to the bathroom at night.
- Memory may be impaired. Clients should use medication organizers, which can be purchased at any drugstore at a very reasonable cost. These dispensers can be filled once a week with the proper medications to be taken at a specific time during the day (see Figure 37-14).

Environmental Interventions.   Nursing interventions directed at eliminating environmental threats include general preventive measures such as meeting basic needs, reducing physical hazards, and reducing pathogen transmission. They also deal with specific safety concerns.

General Preventive Measures.   Nurses can contribute to a safer environment by helping the client meet basic needs related to oxygen, nutrition, temperature, and humidity. To ensure that oxygen availability is not threatened, the nurse might recommend that the client be sure to periodically have the furnace inspected for proper functioning. To achieve a comfortable level of humidity in the home, the client might attach a humidifier to the furnace or, in the case of clients who have upper respiratory tract infections, use a room humidifier where the client sleeps. The nurse can teach basic techniques for food handling (e.g., hand washing, checking for spoilage) and preparation (e.g., keeping food refrigerated before serving) so that nutritional needs are met safely. Client education for older adults or clients who enjoy outdoor activities should include ways to prevent and treat frostbite, hypothermia, heatstroke, and heat exhaustion (see Chapter 31).

Adequate lighting and security measures in and around the home, including the use of night-lights, exterior lighting, and locks on windows and doors, enable clients to reduce the risk of injury from crime. The local police department and community organizations often have safety classes available for residents to learn how to take precautions to minimize the chance of becoming involved in a crime. For example, some useful tips include always parking the car near a bright light or busy public area, carrying a whistle attached to the car keys, keeping car doors locked while driving, and always paying attention while driving to notice if anyone starts to follow the car.

To prevent the transmission of pathogens, nurses can teach aseptic practices. Medical asepsis, which includes hand washing and environmental cleanliness, reduces the transfer of organisms (see Chapter 33). Clients and family members need to learn thorough hand washing and when to use it (e.g., before and after caring for a family member, before food preparation, before preparing a medication for a family member, and after contacting any body fluids). When clients require dressing changes or the use of syringes and needles, families should be shown how to properly dispose of contaminated items in the home.

Specific Safety Concerns.   The nurse takes measures to help clients avoid falls, injuries from use of restraints and side rails, fires, poisoning, and electrical hazards. Special precautions are necessary to prevent injury in clients susceptible to having seizures. Radiation injuries are also a specific safety concern.

Falls.   Modifications in the home and health care environment can easily reduce the risk of falls (Table 37-2). A heavy or debilitated client in a bed or wheelchair or on a toilet should be properly supported and secured. Side rails are necessary unless a client is able to freely and easily ambulate independently. Safety bars on toilets, locks on beds and wheelchairs, and call bells are additional safety features found in health care settings (Figures 37-9 and 37-10). Excess furniture and equipment should be removed, and a weakened client should wear rubber-soled shoes or slippers for walking or transferring. The nurse should also encourage clients to remove clutter from halls, stairs, and traffic areas. When clients use assistive aids such as canes, crutches, or walkers, it is important to routinely check the condition of rubber tips and the integrity of the aid.

Restraints.   A physical **restraint** is a device used to immobilize a client or extremity and that restricts the freedom of movement or normal access to a person's body. Restraints were commonly used in the past to limit activity of clients who were confused, combative, or at high risk for falling when unattended. An overbed table placed in front of a client who has difficulty rising from a chair is an example of a restraint. Typical extremity restraints include belts or soft cloth ties.

Whenever a client is restrained, there is a natural tendency for the client to try to remove the restraint. When

Table 37-2 **Measures to Prevent Falls by Older Adults**	
Measure	Rationale
Stairs	
Install treads with uniform depth of 9 inches (22.5 cm) and 9-inch risers (vertical face of steps).	If stairs are of uniform size, older adults do not have to continually adjust vision.
Install uniform-textured or plain-colored surfaces on each tread, and mark edge of tread with contrasting color.	Uniform textures or color help to decrease vertigo. Marking edge of tread provides obvious visual clue to end of stair.
Ensure proper lighting of each tread. Block sun or light-bulb glare with translucent shades or screen, or use lower-wattage bulbs.	Older adults' vision is unable to adjust quickly to changes in lighting.
Ensure adequate head room so that users do not have to duck to negotiate stairs.	Sudden changes in head position may result in dizziness.
Remove protruding objects from staircase walls.	Decreased peripheral vision may prevent client from seeing object.
Maintain outdoor walkways and stairs in good condition and free of holes, cracks, and splinters.	Decreased visual acuity can prevent client from seeing any structural defect.
Handrails	
Install smooth but slip-resistant handrail at least 2 inches (5 cm) from wall.	Two-inch distance allows client to grasp handrail firmly for support.
Secure handrail firmly so that user's weight is supported, especially at bottom and top of stairway.	Older adults have greatest risk of falling at top and bottom of stairs, because center of gravity is being shifted and balance is unstable.
Install grab rails in bathroom near toilet and tub.	This enables client to have support while rising from sitting to standing position.
Floor Coverings	
Ensure that clients wear properly fitting shoes or slippers with nonskid surface.	Reduces chances of slipping.
Secure all carpeting, mats, and tile; place nonskid backing under small rugs.	Sudden slip may cause dizziness and inability to regain balance.
Orientation	
Place disoriented clients in room near nurses' station.	Provides for more frequent observation on the part of nursing staff.
Maintain close supervision of confused clients.	Confused clients often attempt to wander out of bed or room.

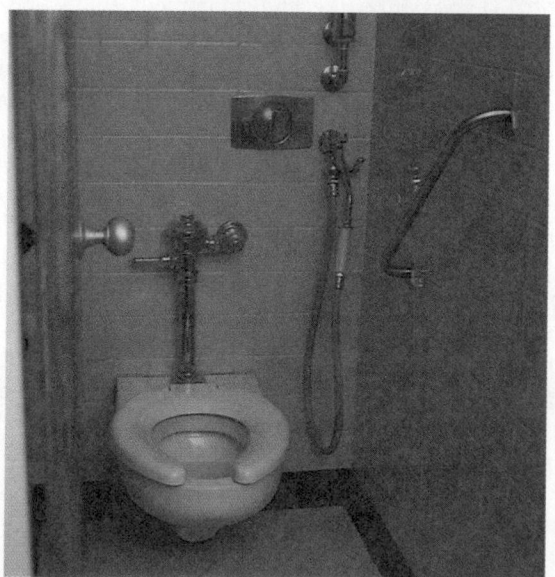

Figure 37-9   Safety bars around toilets and showers.

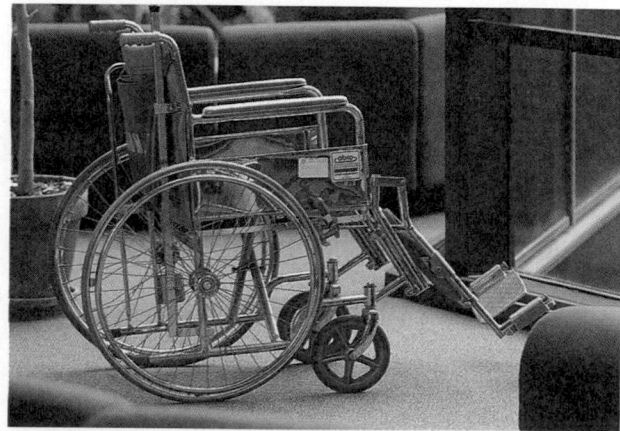

Figure 37-10   Safety locks on wheelchairs.

this occurs, client injury is common. Although almost all types of restraints have been implicated in client deaths, the majority of these deaths have been associated with suffocation using the vest or jacket type of restraint (Weick, 1992). The immobility imposed by restraining a client can lead to pressure ulcer formation, hypostatic pneumonia, constipation, urinary and fecal incontinence, and urinary retention (see Chapter 46). Contractures, nerve damage, and circulatory impairment are also potential hazards. Loss of self-esteem, humiliation, fear, and anger can also result.

Because of the risk of injury from restraints, current legislation has reduced the use of restraints in nursing homes and extended care facilities (National Citizens' Coalition for Nursing Home Reform). In addition, the JCAHO (1999) enforces standards for the safe use of restraints in inpatient settings. The Omnibus Budget Reconciliation Act (OBRA) of 1987 defines clients' rights and choices regarding use of restraints. Under these guidelines, reasons for use of physical restraint are to be clearly stated. The use of restraints must be part of the client's medical treatment, all less restrictive interventions must be tried first, other disciplines must be used, and supporting documentation must be provided (Health Care Financing Administration, 1990).

The impetus is for health care organizations to move to more restraint-free environments. Restraints do not prevent falls or injury. In fact, it has been shown that clients incur less severe injuries if left unrestrained. Research has shown that a multidisciplinary approach that conducts individualized assessments and develops structured treatment plans can reduce the number of falls in nursing homes (Box 37-8). If possible, nurses should use alternative interventions instead of restraints (Box 37-9).

The use of restraints involves a psychological adjustment for the client and family. If restraints must be used, the nurse assists family members and clients by explaining their purpose and precautions taken to avoid injury.

Research HIGHLIGHT Box 37-8

RESEARCH ABSTRACT

This article describes a randomized trial of a multidisciplinary consultation service to reduce falls and associated injuries in high-risk nursing home residents. Individual client assessments, along with specific safety recommendations related to environmental and personal safety, wheelchair use, psychotropic drug use, transferring clients, and ambulation, were made.

Individual assessments led to the development of structured, individual treatment plans for clients. In the area of environmental and personal safety, potential hazards (e.g., problems concerning the bed, floor surfaces, clutter, lighting, accessibility of objects, bathroom equipment, foot care, and footwear) were brought to the staff's attention and corrected. Wheelchair maintenance and safety features, as well as the client's posture and use of the chair, were analyzed. Corrective measures and teaching were done when indicated. Staff and clients were observed during transfer and ambulation. Observations were used to formulate instructions for the residents and staff.

The results showed that the mean proportion of recurrent fallers in the intervention facilities was 19.1% lower than in the control facilities. The authors conclude that the high rate of falls and related injuries in nursing homes should not be viewed as inevitable. The rate of falls can be substantially reduced through structured safety programs.

IMPLICATIONS FOR PRACTICE

- Individual client assessment and plans are essential for the success of any fall prevention program.
- Frequent, periodic self-assessments of all facilities, including long-term care facilities, are necessary to ensure continued safety.
- Nurses must review their usual practices (e.g., transfer and ambulation activities) for safety aspects that can be improved through staff development.

REFERENCE

Ray W and others: A randomized trial of a consultation service to reduce falls in nursing homes, *JAMA* 278(7):557, 1997.

Alternatives to Restraints   Box 37-9

Orient clients and families to surroundings; explain all procedures and treatments to them.

Encourage family and friends to stay, or use sitters for clients who need supervision.

Assign confused or disoriented clients to rooms near the nurses' station. Observe these clients frequently.

Provide appropriate visual and auditory stimuli (e.g., family pictures, clock, radio).

Eliminate bothersome treatments as soon as possible. For example, discontinue tube feedings and begin oral feedings as quickly as allowed by the client's condition.

Use relaxation techniques (e.g., massage).

Institute exercise and ambulation schedules as allowed by the client's condition.

Maintain toileting routines.

Consult with physical and occupational therapists to enhance clients' abilities to carry out activities of daily living.

Evaluate all medications clients are receiving to determine if the medication is having the desired therapeutic effect.

Conduct ongoing assessment and evaluation of clients' care and their ongoing response to care.

Modified from Stolley J: Freeing your patients from restraints, *Am J Nurs* 95(2):27, 1995.

Nursing homes must obtain informed consent from family members before using restraints. For legal purposes, the nurse must know agency policy and procedures for appropriate use and monitoring of restraints. Institutions require a physician's order that states the type of restraint, specific client behaviors for which restraints are to be used, and a limited time frame. These orders should be renewed within a specific time frame according to the agency's policy (usually 24 hours). Restraints are not to be ordered prn (as needed). Assessment of clients who are restrained must be ongoing. Proper documentation, including the behaviors that necessitated the application of restraints, the procedure used in restraining, the condition of the body part restrained (e.g., circulation to hand), and the evaluation of the client response, is essential. Clients periodically have their restraints removed, and the nurse assesses them to determine if the restraints continue to be needed.

Skill 37-1 includes guidelines for the proper use and application of restraints. Use of restraints must meet the following objectives:

Reduce the risk of client injury from falls.

Prevent interruption of therapy such as traction, IV infusions, nasogastric tube feeding, or Foley catheterization.

Prevent the confused or combative client from removing life support equipment.

Reduce the risk of injury to others by the client.

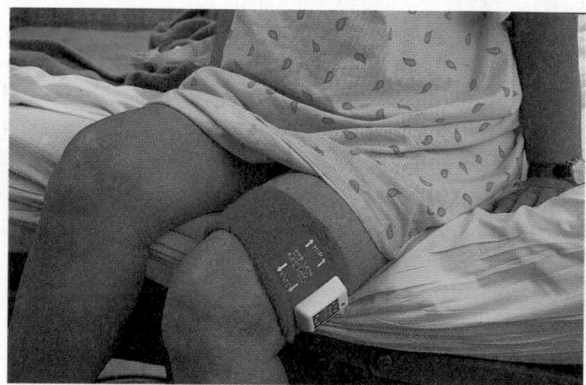

Figure 37-11   Client wearing an Ambularm device.

In keeping with current trends toward health promotion, improved assessment techniques and modifications of the environment are offered as alternatives to restraints. A device known as the **Ambularm** is worn on the leg and signals when the leg is in a dependent position, such as over the side rail or on the floor (Figure 37-11). The device is used for clients who climb out of bed unassisted and are in danger of falling. There are also devices that can be placed on clients' mattresses or attached to the client's nightgown or chair that sound an alarm when triggered. The devices allow a zone of free movement. When the safe zone is exceeded, an alarm sounds. The alarm can be designed to signal at the central nurses' station so that staff are alerted quickly when a client is up and out of bed.

Text continued on p. 1044.

Applying Restraints   Skill 37-1

Delegation Considerations

Use of restraints is an intervention with elements that *can* be delegated and elements that *cannot* be delegated. Elements that *cannot* be delegated because they require problem solving and knowledge application unique to professional nursing include the following:

- Assessment of safety needs
- Selection of appropriate interventions
- Evaluation of effectiveness of restraint
- Ongoing assessment to prevent complications of restraint use

Elements that *can* be delegated to assistive personnel include the following:

- Instruct care provider to inform the nurse if any skin excoriation is present under or around restraint location.
- Instruct care provider in proper way to remove and reapply restraint to provide skin care and allow supervised movement.

EQUIPMENT

- Proper restraint
- Padding

STEPS	RATIONALE
1. Assess whether client needs a restraint.	Restraints are used when other measures have failed to prevent interruption of therapy such as traction, IV infusions, or nasogastric tube feedings; to prevent a confused or combative client from self-injury by falling out of bed or a wheelchair; to prevent a client from removing a Foley catheter, surgical drain, or life support equipment; and to reduce risk of injury to others by the client.
2. Review agency policies regarding restraints. Check physician's order for purpose of restraint and type and duration of restraint.	A physician's order is necessary to apply restraints and should be renewed every 24 hours. The least restrictive type of restraint should be ordered. Because restraints limit the client's ability to move freely, the nurse must make clinical judgments appropriate to the client's condition and agency policy. If the nurse restrains a client in an emergency situation, a physician's order should be obtained as soon as possible.
3. Review manufacturer's instructions before entering client's room.	The nurse should be familiar with all devices used for client care and protection. Incorrect application of a restraining device may result in client injury or death.
4. Inspect area where restraint is to be placed. Assess condition of skin underlying area on which restraint is to be applied.	Restraints may compress and interfere with functioning of devices or tubes. Provides baseline assessment data regarding skin integrity. Provides nursing personnel with an objective measure for subsequent skin assessment.
5. Explain to client and family the need for the restraint. Attempt to obtain consent.	Helps minimize client anxiety during application of the device and helps minimize family concern during maintenance of restraint.
6. Place client in proper body alignment.	Proper body alignment should be maintained to prevent contractures and neurovascular injury.
7. Pad skin and bony prominences before applying restraints.	Padding reduces friction and pressure to skin and underlying tissue.
8. Apply appropriate restraint, making sure it is not over an IV line or other device (e.g., dialysis shunt).	IV lines and other therapeutic devices may become occluded.
A. **Jacket (vest or Posey) restraint:** Vestlike garment. Front and back of garment should be labeled as such (see illustration). Apply over clothing or hospital gown.	Restrains client while lying or reclining in bed and while sitting in chair or wheelchair. Proper application prevents suffocation or choking. Clothing or gown prevents friction against skin.
B. **Belt restraint:** Device that secures client to bed or stretcher. Avoid placing belt too tightly across client's chest or abdomen (see illustration).	Restrains center of gravity and prevents client from rolling off stretcher or sitting up while on stretcher or from falling out of bed. Tight application may interfere with ventilation.

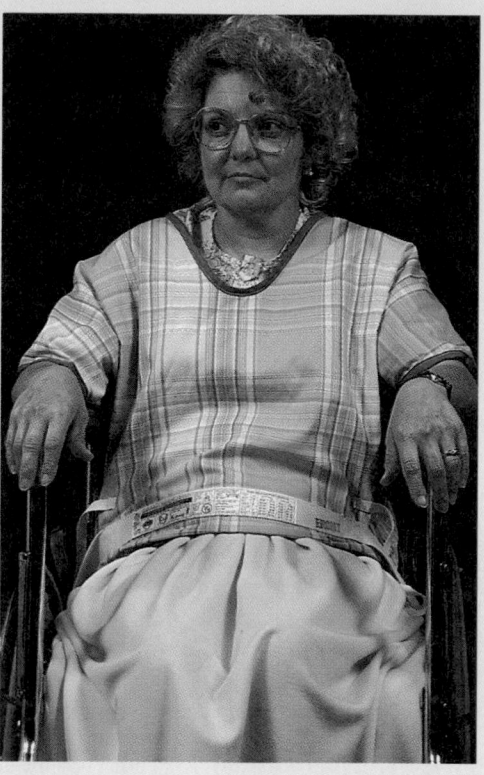

Step 8A

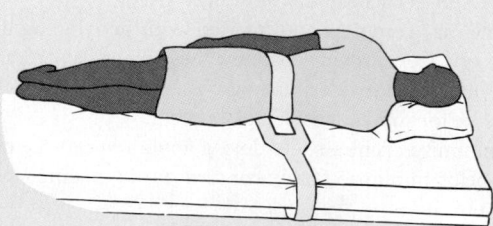

Step 8B

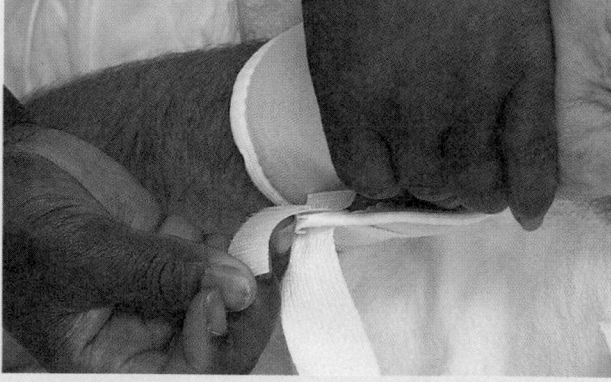

Step 8C

C. **Extremity (ankle or wrist) restraint:** Restraint designed to immobilize one or all extremities. Commercially available limb restraints are composed of sheepskin with foam padding (see illustration).

Maintains immobilization of extremity to protect client from injury from fall or accidental removal of therapeutic device (e.g., IV tube or Foley catheter).

STEPS	RATIONALE

D. **Mitten restraint:** Thumbless mitten device to restrain client's hands (see illustration).

Prevents clients from dislodging invasive equipment, removing dressings, or scratching, yet allows greater movement than a wrist restraint.

E. **Elbow restraint:** Piece of fabric with slots in which tongue blades are placed so that elbow joint remains rigid (see illustration).

Used with infants and children to prevent elbow flexion (e.g., when an IV line is in place).

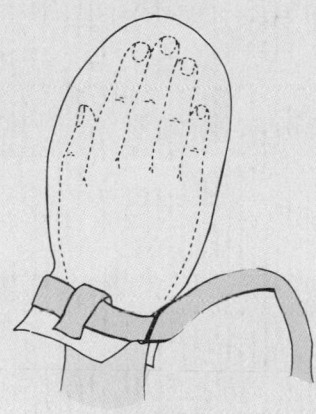

Step 8D

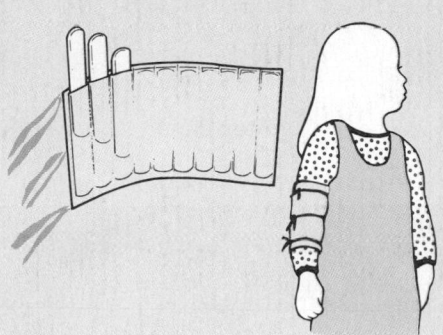

Step 8E

F. **Mummy restraint:** Blanket or sheet that is opened on bed or crib with one corner folded toward center. Child is placed on blanket with shoulders at fold and with feet toward opposite corner (see illustration for Step 8F-1). With child's right arm straight down or secured against body, right side of blanket is pulled firmly across right shoulder and chest and secured beneath left side of body (see illustration for Step 8F-2). Left arm is placed straight against body or secured, and left side of blanket is brought across shoulder and chest and locked beneath child's body on right side (see illustration for Step 8F-3). Lower corner is folded and brought over body and tucked or fastened securely with safety pins (see illustration for Step 8F-4).

Maintains short-term restraint of small child or infant for examination or treatment involving head and neck. Effectively controls movement of torso and extremities.

9. Attach restraints to bed frame, which moves when the head of bed is raised or lowered (see illustration).

Client may be injured if restraint is secured to side rail and it is lowered.

Critical Decision Point: Do not attach to side rails.

---

10. When client is in a chair, a jacket restraint should be secured by placing ties under armrests and securing at the back of chair (see illustration for Step 10).

Prevents client from sliding restraint ties up the back of the chair.

Critical Decision Point: If ties are not under armrests, clients may be able to slide ties up the back of the chair and free themselves.

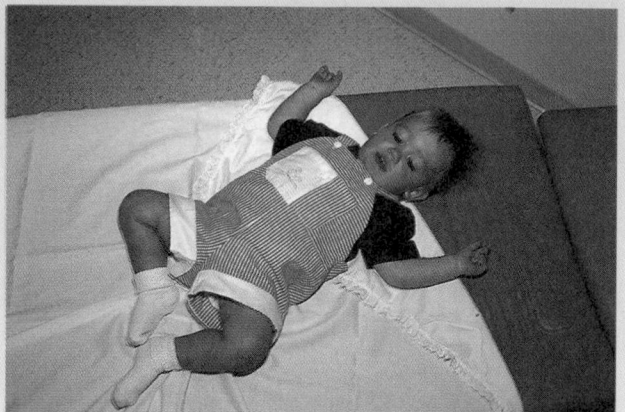

Step 8F-1

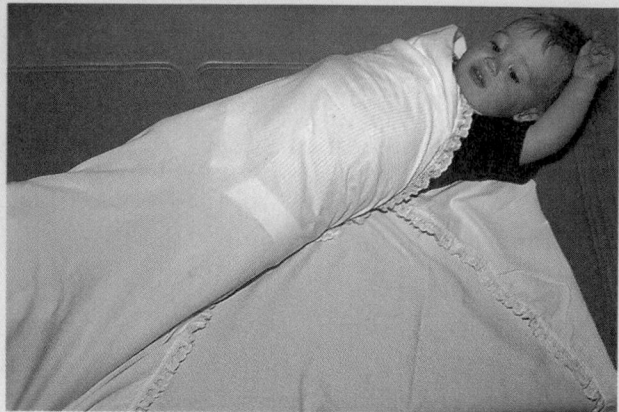

Step 8F-2

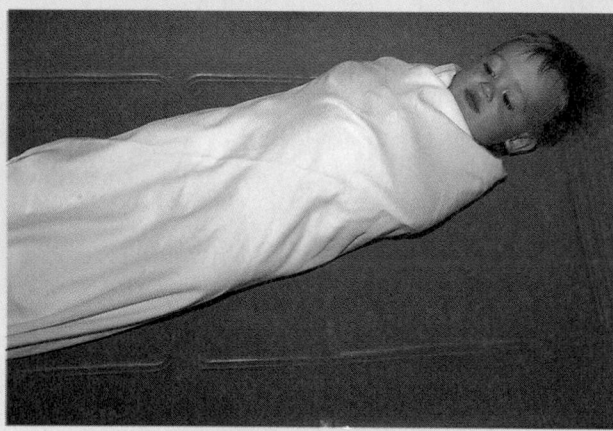

Step 8F-3

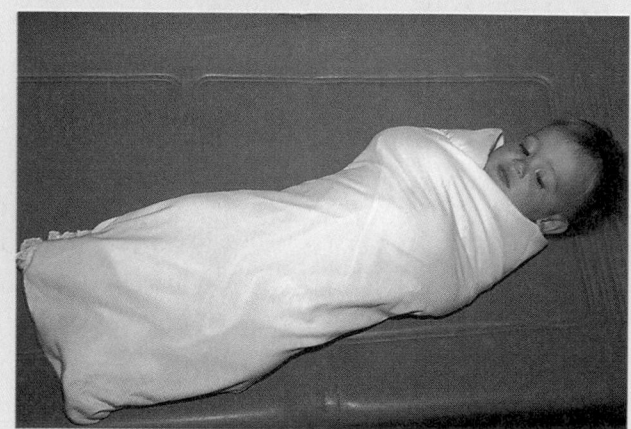

Step 8F-4

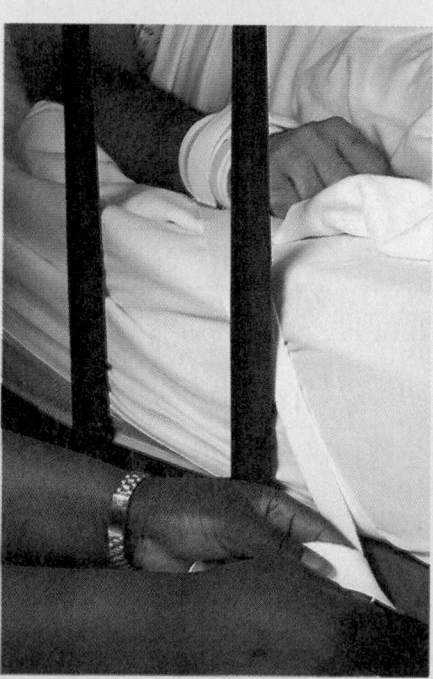

Step 9

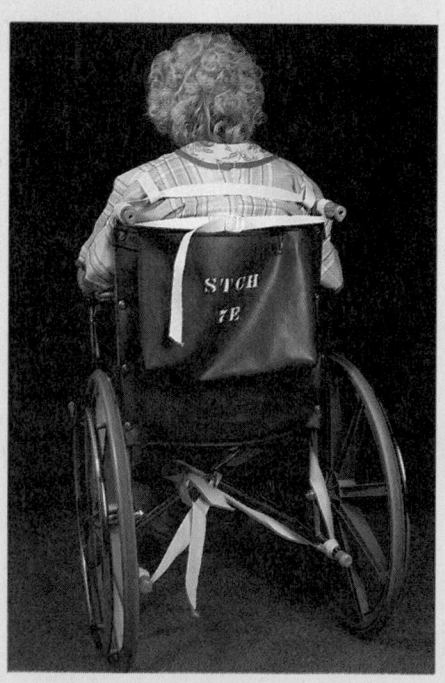

Step 10

STEPS	RATIONALE
11. Secure restraints with a quick-release tie (see illustration).	Allows for quick release in an emergency.
12. Insert two fingers under the secured restraint (see illustration).	A tight restraint may cause contriction and impede circulation. Checking for constriction prevents neurovascular injury.

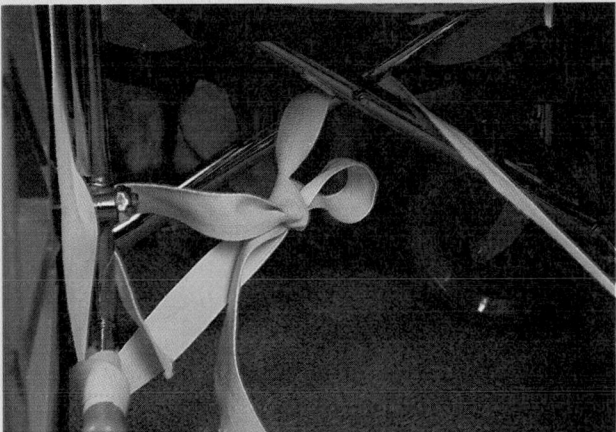

Step 11

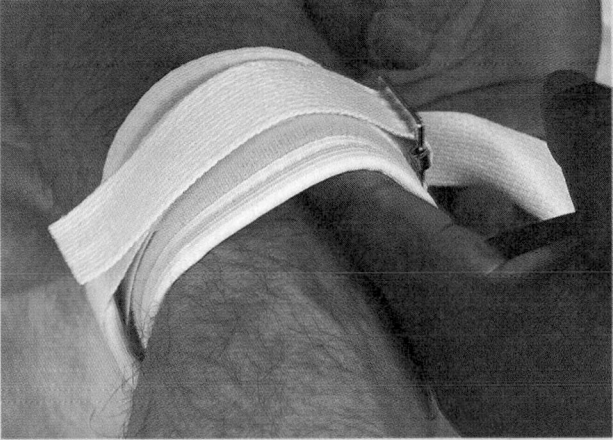

Step 12

13. Every 30 minutes, proper placement of restraint and skin integrity, pulses, temperature, color, and sensation of restrained body part should be assessed.	Frequent assessment prevents complications, such as suffocation, skin breakdown, and impaired circulation.
14. Restraints should be removed for 30 minutes every 2 hours. If client is violent and noncompliant, remove one restraint at a time and/or have staff assistance while removing restraints. Client should not be left unattended at this time.	Provides opportunity to change client's position and perform full range of motion (ROM).
15. Secure call bell or intercom system within reach.	Allows client, family, or caregiver to obtain assistance quickly.
16. Leave bed or chair with wheels locked. Bed should be in lowest position.	Locked wheels prevent bed or chair from moving if client attempts to get out. If client falls when bed is in lowest position, the chances of injury are reduced.
17. Inspect client for any injury, including all hazards of immobility, while restraints are in use.	Client should be free of injury and not exhibit any signs of immobility complications. Use of restraints should be seen as a temporary measure and discontinued as soon as possible (Stolley, 1995).
18. Observe IV catheters and urinary catheters to ensure that they are positioned correctly and that therapy remains uninterrupted.	
19. Provide appropriate sensory stimulation and reorient client as needed.	Use of restraints can further increase disorientation.

Recording and Reporting

- Record client behaviors that place client at risk for injury, type of restraint applied, time restraints were applied, and client's behavior after restraints were applied.
- Document specific assessments related to ventilation, skin integrity, musculoskeletal system, and peripheral vascular integrity.
- Describe client's response when restraints were removed.
- Describe alternatives to restraints that were employed and client's response.

Home Care Considerations

- Plan care with family. If possible, use of an Ambularm may free client from physical restraints.
- Instruct family (or other caregiver) in use of alternatives to restraints (see Box 37-9).
- If physical restraints are necessary, instruct family (or other caregiver) in proper application and observation of possible complications related to restraint use. Also inform caregiver whom to contact if any abnormal findings occur.
- A client who needs to be restrained in bed should have a hospital bed and will require constant supervision in the home.

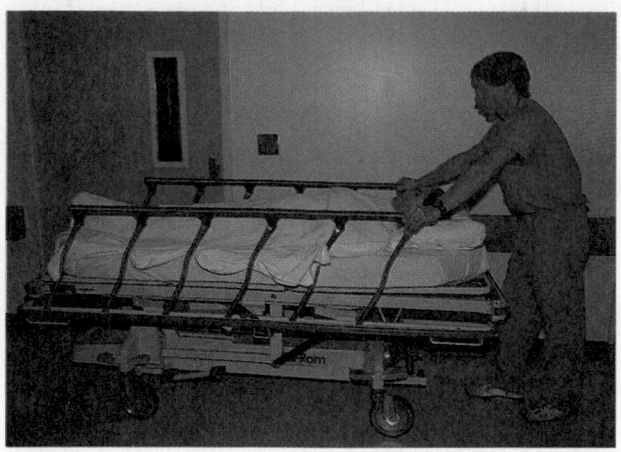

Figure 37-12   Side rails in the *up* position on a stretcher.

Side Rails.   Side rails may help to increase a client's mobility and/or stability when in bed or when moving from bed to chair. Side rails also help prevent the unconscious client from falling out of bed or from a stretcher (Figure 37-12). When side rails restrict a person's mobility, they may be considered a restraint. The use of side rails alone for a disoriented client may cause more confusion and further injury. A confused client who is determined to get out of bed attempts to climb over the side rail or climbs out at the foot of the bed. Either attempt usually results in a fall. Nursing interventions to reduce a client's confusion should first focus on the cause of the confusion. Frequently nurses mistake a client's attempt to explore his or her environment or to self-toilet as confusion. A thorough assessment is essential. Whenever side rails are used, the bed should be maintained in the lowest position possible.

Fires.   A fire is always possible in the home or hospital. Accidental home fires typically result from smoking in bed, placing cigarettes in trash cans, grease fires, or electrical fires resulting from faulty wiring or appliances. Institutional fires typically result from an electrical or anesthetic-related fire, since few institutions now allow clients to smoke in their rooms.

The interventions described here are directed toward fires occurring in health care agencies, but the same principles apply for fires in the home (Box 37-10). Homes should be equipped with smoke and fire alarms. It is important to have a plan of action in the event of fire. All clients, even young children, should be familiar with the phrase "stop, drop and roll," which describes the actions to be followed when a client's clothing and skin are burning.

If a fire occurs in a health care agency, the nurse protects clients from immediate injury, reports the exact location of the fire, and contains the fire and extinguishes it if possible. All personnel are mobilized to evacuate clients.

Clients who are close to the fire, regardless of its size, are at risk of injury and should be moved to another area. If a client is receiving oxygen but not life support, the nurse discontinues the oxygen, which is combustible and can fuel an existing fire. If the client is on life support, the nurse may need to maintain the client's respiratory status manually with an Ambu-bag (see Chapter 39) until the client is moved away from the fire. Ambulatory clients can be directed to walk by themselves to a safe area and in some cases may be able to assist in moving clients in wheelchairs. Bedridden clients are generally moved from the scene of a fire by a stretcher, their bed, or a wheelchair. If none of these methods is appropriate, clients must be carried from the area. If a client must be carried, the nurse should be careful not to overextend physical limits for lifting because injury to the nurse can result in further injury to the client. If fire department personnel are on the scene, they can help evacuate the clients.

After a fire has been reported and clients are out of danger, nurses and other personnel must take measures to contain or put out the fire, such as closing doors and windows, placing wet towels along the base of doors, turning off oxygen and electrical equipment, and using a fire extinguisher. Fire extinguishers are categorized as type A, used for ordinary combustibles (e.g., wood, cloth, paper, and many plastic items); type B, used for flammable liquids (e.g., gasoline, oil, grease, tar, and oil-based paint); and type C, used for electrical equipment. The correct use of an extinguisher is discussed in Box 37-11 and demonstrated in Figure 37-13.

The best intervention is to prevent fires. Nursing measures include complying with the agency's smoking policies and keeping combustible materials away from heat sources. Some agencies have fire doors that are held open by magnets and close automatically when a fire alarm sounds. It is important to keep equipment away from these doors.

Client Teaching FOR CORRECT USE OF A FIRE EXTINGUISHER IN THE HOME — Box 37-11

OBJECTIVES
- Client will correctly place the extinguisher in the home.
- Client will describe when it is appropriate to use a home fire extinguisher.
- Client will demonstrate the correct technique when using a fire extinguisher.
- Client will state when fire extinguishers need to be replaced.

TEACHING STRATEGIES
- Discuss correct placement of the extinguisher. It is recommended that one be placed on each level of the home, near an exit, in clear view, away from stoves and heating appliances, and above the reach of small children. The instructions should be read when the extinguisher is purchased and kept available for periodic review.
- Describe the steps to take before using the extinguisher. Attempt to fight the fire only when all occupants have left the home, the fire department has been called, the fire is confined to a small area, there is an exit route readily available, the extinguisher is the right type for the fire (see p. 1044 for a discussion of the types of extinguishers), and the client knows how to use the extinguisher.
- Instruct the client to memorize the mnemonic PASS: *P*ull the pin to unlock handle, *A*im low at the base of the fire, *S*queeze the handles, and *S*weep the unit from side to side (see Figure 37-13).

EVALUATION
- Client can correctly place an extinguisher in the home.
- Client correctly lists the steps to take before attempting to use an extinguisher.
- Client demonstrates correct use of the extinguisher while reciting the instructions with the mnemonic PASS (see Figure 37-13).

Modified from *Fire extinguisher fact sheet*, Washington, DC, 1997, National Safety Council.

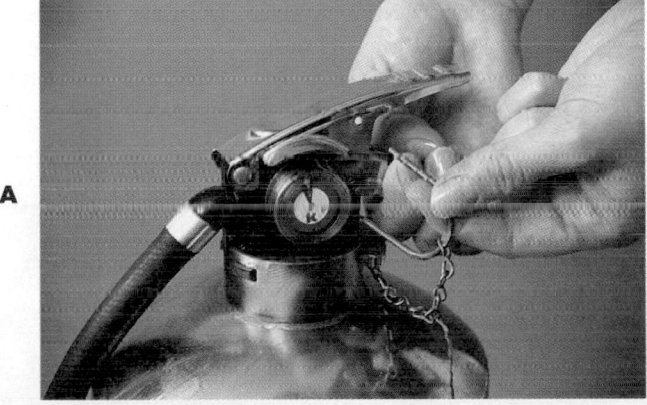

A

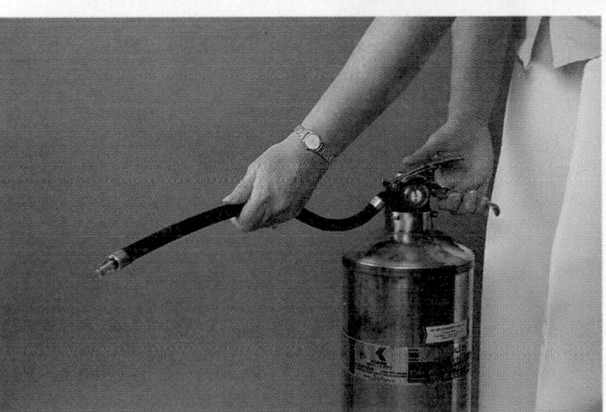

B

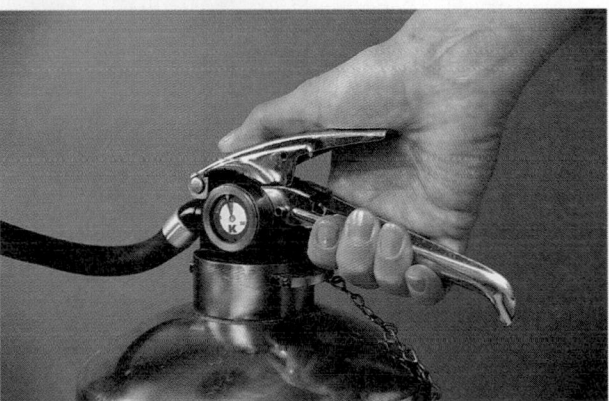

C

Figure 37-13 **A,** *Pull the pin.* **B,** *Aim at the base of the fire.* **C,** *Squeeze the handles. Sweep from side to side to coat the area evenly.*
Modified from Sorrentino SA: *Mosby's assisting with patient care,* St. Louis, 1999, Mosby.

Poisoning. A **poison** is any substance that impairs health or destroys life when ingested, inhaled, or otherwise absorbed by the body. Specific antidotes or treatments are available for only some types of poisons. The capacity of body tissue to recover from the poison determines the reversibility of the effect. Poisons can impair the respiratory, circulatory, central nervous, hepatic, GI, and renal systems of the body.

The toddler, preschooler, young school-age child, and older adult must be protected from accidental poisoning. Using child-resistant caps, placing medications and cleaning fluids and powders out of the reach of children, leaving potentially poisonous materials in original containers, and removing poisonous plants from the home prevent accidental ingestion of poisonous materials. McKenry and Salerno (1998) note that poisoning can result from swallowing miniature button or disk batteries commonly found in games, cameras, calculators, and watches. In older adults, diminished eyesight and impaired memory may result in accidental ingestion of poisonous substances or in accidental overdose of prescribed medications. To prevent medication errors on the part of clients in the home, the nurse should recommend the use of medication organizers that are filled once a week by the client and/or family. These organizers have the day and time on each box, so the client knows when and what to take at any given time (Figure 37-14). This is particularly useful for clients who may forget whether they have taken their medications.

Guidelines for intervening in accidental poisoning should be adhered to. The Poison Control Center phone number should be visible on the telephone itself in homes with young children. In all cases of suspected poisoning, this number should be called immediately (Box 37-12).

Electrical Hazards. Electrical equipment must be maintained in good working order and should be **grounded.** The third (longer) prong in an electrical plug is the ground (Figure 37-15). Theoretically, the ground prong carries any stray electrical current back to the ground, hence its name. The other two prongs carry the power to the piece of electrical equipment. Improperly grounded or malfunctioning electrical equipment increases the risk of electrical injury and fire. Educating both the client and the family can reduce the risk for electrical hazards in the home environment (Box 37-13).

If a client receives an electrical shock, the nurse should immediately determine whether the client has a pulse. If the client has no pulse, cardiopulmonary resuscitation (CPR) should be initiated and emergency personnel should be notified (see Chapter 39). If the client has a pulse and remains alert and oriented, the nurse should quickly obtain vital signs and assess the skin for signs of thermal injury. The client's physician must be notified. If an electrical shock occurs in the home, the nurse follows the same procedure but has the client go to the emergency department and then notifies the client's physician.

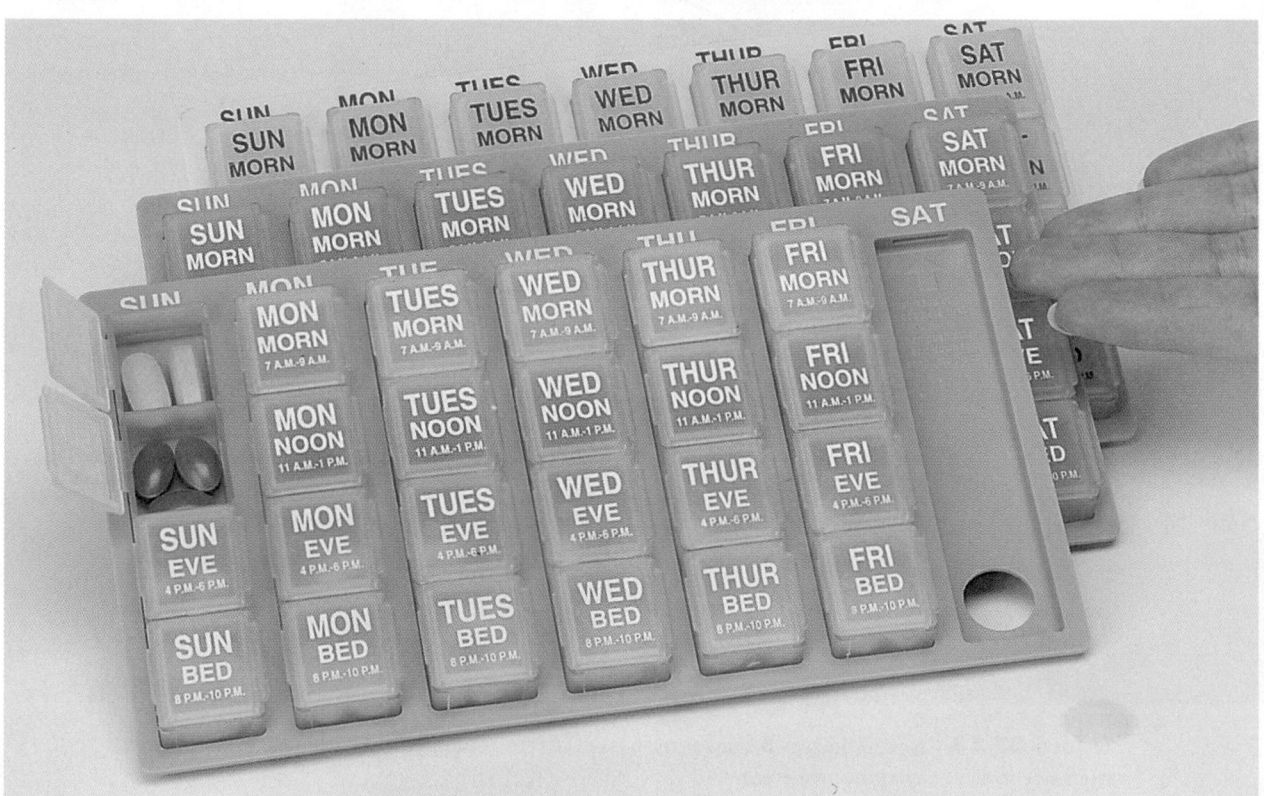

Figure 37-14 One-Day-At-A-Time.
Courtesy Apothecary Products, Inc., Burnsville, Minnesota.

Box 37-12 **Procedural Guidelines**

For Interventions in Accidental Poisoning

1. Assess for airway patency, breathing, and circulation (ABCs) in all clients in whom accidental poisoning is suspected.
2. Remove any visible materials from areas such as the mouth and eyes to terminate exposure.
3. Identify the type and amount of substance ingested, if possible. This may help to determine the antidote.
4. Call the Poison Control Center before attempting interventions.
5. If instructed to induce vomiting, give ipecac syrup, an emetic (Skidmore-Roth, 1998). All households with young children should have ipecac syrup on hand.
    a. Infants (up to 12 months): 5-10 ml of ipecac syrup, then 100-200 ml of water; may repeat if necessary.
    b. Children (1 to 12 years): 1 tablespoon (15 ml) of ipecac syrup, then 200-300 ml of water; may repeat once in 30 minutes.
    c. Adults: 2 tablespoons (15-30 ml) of ipecac syrup, then 200-300 ml of water; may repeat once in 30 minutes.
6. If directed, save vomitus for laboratory analysis, which may assist with further treatment.
7. Position the victim with the head to the side to prevent aspiration of vomitus and assist in keeping the airway open.
8. Never induce vomiting in an unconscious victim or in a client experiencing convulsions, since aspiration may occur.
9. Never induce vomiting if any of the following substances have been ingested: household cleaners, grease or petroleum products, or furniture polish. Vomiting may increase internal burns.
10. If instructed to take the victim to the emergency department, call an ambulance. Emergency equipment may be needed en route.

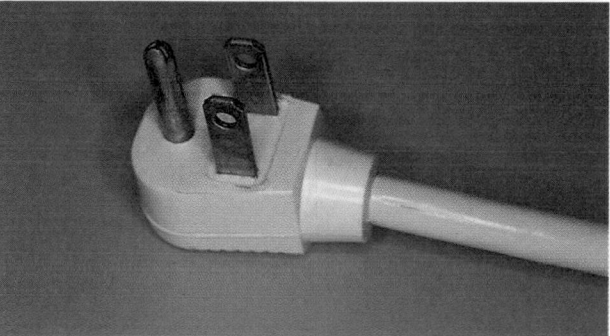

Figure 37-15 Three-pronged grounded plug.

Client Teaching

FOR PREVENTION OF ELECTRICAL HAZARDS Box 37-13

OBJECTIVE
- Client will recognize electrical hazards in the home and eliminate them.

TEACHING STRATEGIES
- Discuss grounding appliances and other equipment.
- Provide examples of common hazards: frayed cords, damaged equipment, and overloaded outlets.
- Discuss guidelines to prevent electrical shocks:
    - Use extension cords only when necessary and use electrical tape to secure the cord to the floor where it will not be stepped on.
    - Do not run wires under carpeting.
    - Grasp the plug, not the cord, when unplugging items.
    - Keep electrical items away from water.
    - Do not operate unfamiliar equipment.
    - Disconnect items before cleaning.

EVALUATION
- Have client list electrical hazards existing in the home.
- Review steps the client will take to eliminate these hazards.
- Check the home after the client has had an opportunity to eliminate hazards.

Seizures. Clients who have experienced some form of neurological injury or metabolic disturbance are at risk for a seizure. A seizure involves a hyperexcitation of neurons in the brain leading to a sudden, violent, involuntary series of contractions of a group of muscles. The client often loses consciousness. **Seizure precautions** encompass all nursing interventions to protect the client from traumatic injury, positioning for adequate ventilation and drainage of oral secretions, and providing privacy and support following the seizure (Skill 37-2).

During a seizure a client's jaw muscles can become tense. It has been found that significant injury to the client's oral cavity is rare, even during the most violent seizures. Injury may instead occur from a caregiver forcing an object into the client's mouth and from the teeth biting down on a hard object. Soft objects may break in the mouth during a seizure and be aspirated. Therefore the Epilepsy Foundation of America, in its recommendations for seizure first aid, includes avoiding the insertion of objects into the mouth (Seizure Recognition and Observation, 1992). The exception is in the case of **status epilepticus**, a medical emergency whereby a person has continual seizures without interruption. An adequate airway is maintained with an oral airway. Clients experiencing a seizure are never restrained but are placed on seizure precautions and need to be adequately protected from traumatic injury.

Skill 37-2 | Seizure Precautions

Delegation Considerations

Interventions for a client who is experiencing a seizure cannot be delegated. The nurse must constantly assess the client's airway patency, adequacy of breathing, and circulatory status. Clinical judgments must be made quickly, using the elements of critical thinking. Assistive personnel can remain with the nurse during a seizure, to obtain needed supplies and notify other personnel at the nurse's request.

EQUIPMENT

- Oral airway
- Padding for side rails and headboard
- Suction machine, oral suction equipment
- Clean disposable gloves

STEPS	RATIONALE
1. Assess seizure history, noting frequency of seizures, presence of aura, and sequence of events, if known. Assess for medical and surgical conditions that may lead to seizures or exacerbate existing seizure condition. Assess medication history.	This enables the nurse to anticipate onset of seizure activity. Seizure medications must be taken as prescribed and not stopped suddenly, as this may precipitate seizure activity.
2. Inspect client's environment (in a health care agency or in the home) for potential safety hazards if a seizure occurs.	Client's bed should be in its lowest position, with side rails padded and client positioned in side-lying position when possible (see illustration).

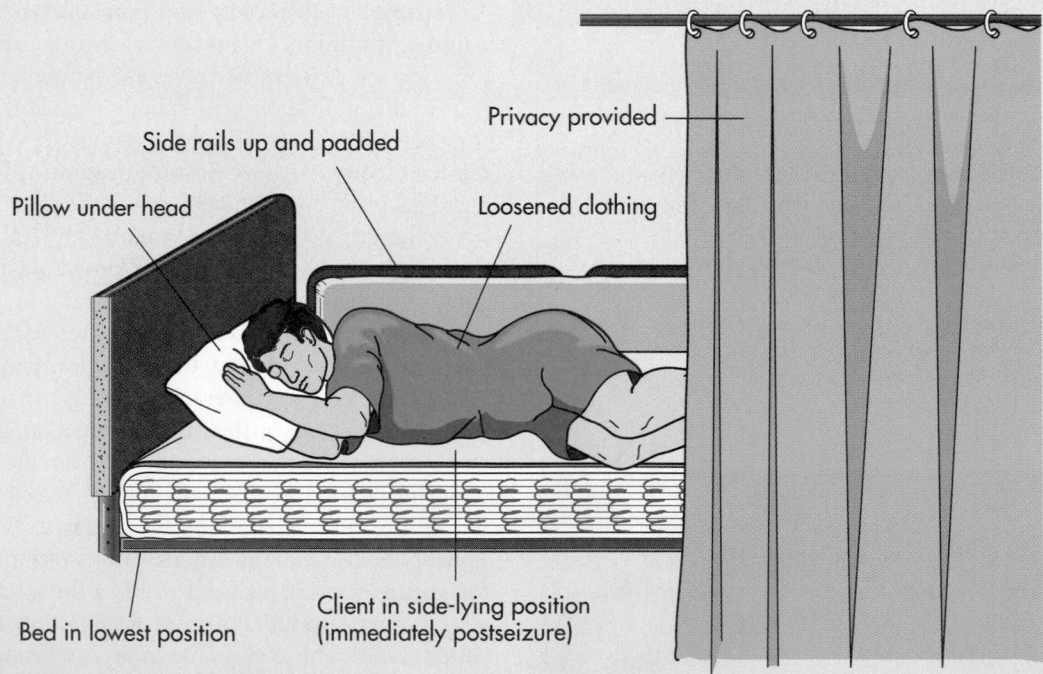

Side rails up and padded

Pillow under head

Privacy provided

Loosened clothing

Bed in lowest position

Client in side-lying position
(immediately postseizure)

Step 2

STEPS	RATIONALE
3. For clients with a history of seizures, an airway (see illustration) suction apparatus, clean gloves, and pillows should be visible in the hospital setting for immediate use.	This ensures prompt, organized intervention.

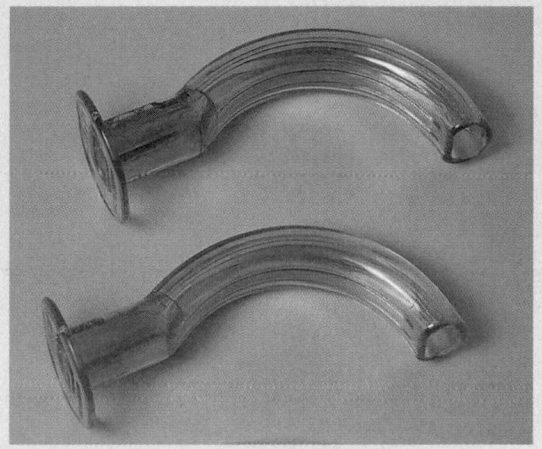

Step 3

STEPS	RATIONALE
4. When a seizure begins, position client safely. If client is standing or sitting at time of seizure, guide client to floor and protect head by cradling in nurse's lap or placing a pillow under head. Clear surrounding area of furniture. If client is in bed, raise side rails, add padding, and put bed in low position.	Protects client from traumatic injury, especially head injury.
5. Provide privacy.	Embarrassment is common after a seizure, especially if the seizure was witnessed by others.
6. If possible, turn client on side, with head flexed slightly forward.	Prevents tongue and dentures from blocking the airway and promotes drainage of secretions, thus reducing risk of aspiration.
7. Do not restrain client. Loosen clothing.	Prevents musculoskeletal injury.
8. Do not place any objects in client's mouth.	

Critical Decision Point: Injury may result from forcible insertion of a hard object. Soft objects may break or come apart and be aspirated. Placing objects in the client's mouth could result in tooth loss, lacerations, stimulation of the gag reflex with vomiting, and aspiration and respiratory distress (Ziemba, 1995).

STEPS	RATIONALE
9. Stay with client, observing the sequence and timing of seizure activity.	Continued observation is necessary to ensure adequate ventilation during and following seizure activity. Accurate, specific observations will assist in documentation, diagnosis, and treatment of the seizure disorder.
10. After the seizure is over, explain what happened and answer client's questions.	Informing clients of the type of seizure activity experienced will assist them in participating knowledgeably in their care.

STATUS EPILEPTICUS

STEPS	RATIONALE
11. For a client experiencing status epilepticus, put on clean gloves and insert an oral airway (see illustration for Step 3) when the jaw is relaxed between seizure activity. Do not place fingers near or in client's mouth.	Prevents transmission of infection. Client is in continual seizure state and requires oral airway to ensure airway patency.
12. Access oxygen and suction equipment. Prepare for IV insertion.	In this emergency client requires adequate airway and IV access.
13. Use pillows/pads to protect client from injuring self.	Traumatic injury will be avoided.

Recording and Reporting

- Record the timing of seizure activity and sequence of events. Record presence of **aura** (if any), level of consciousness, posture, color, movements of extremities, incontinence, and patterns of sleep following the seizure.
- Document client's response and expected or unexpected outcomes.

Home Care Considerations

- Communicate with client and family to identify precipitating factors.
- Teach family to care for the client during a seizure.

- Provide family with guidelines to detect status epilepticus.
- Until a seizure condition is well controlled (usually for at least 1 year), the client should not take a tub bath or engage in activities such as swimming unless a knowledgeable family member is present. Driving may also be restricted during this time.
- Client should wear a medical alert bracelet or tag, have an ID card noting the presence of a seizure disorder and listing the medications taken.
- Referral to a support group or the Epilepsy Foundation of America may be indicated.

Radiation. Radiation is a health hazard in the health care setting and the community. Radiation and radioactive materials are used in the diagnosis and treatment of clients. Hospitals have strict guidelines on the care of clients who are receiving radiation and radioactive materials. The nurse must be familiar with established agency protocols. To reduce the nurse's exposure to radiation, time spent near the source should be limited, the distance from the source should be as great as possible, and shielding devices such as lead aprons should be used. Staff working near radiation will wear devices that can track the accumulative exposure to radiation.

The community may be at risk for radiation exposure because of incorrect disposal and transportation of radioactive waste products. Community health agencies and the Environmental Protection Agency (EPA) have established specific, strict guidelines for the disposal of radioactive waste. If a radioactive leak occurs, these agencies institute measures to prevent exposure of surrounding neighborhoods, to clean up radioactive leaks as quickly as possible, and to ensure that injured parties receive prompt medical care.

EVALUATION

Client Care. The components of critical thinking are applied to the evaluation step of the nursing process (Figure 37-16). The actual care delivered by the health care team is evaluated based on the expected outcomes. If the goals have been met, the nursing interventions can be considered effective and appropriate. If not,

the nurse determines whether new risks to the client have developed or whether previous risks remain. The client and family need to participate to find permanent ways to reduce risks to safety. The nurse continually assesses the client's and family's need for additional support services such as home health care, physical therapy, counseling, and further teaching.

Client Expectations. When the nurse has developed a good relationship with a client and the client feels safe and secure in their relationship, as well as in the environment, the client will most likely demonstrate less anxiety and verbalize satisfaction with the surroundings. The nurse must determine, however, if client expectations have been met. Is the client satisfied with any changes made to the environment? Does the client believe that his or her safety is ensured? If client expectations have not been met, the nurse must reassess not only the client and the environment but also the client's expressed desires.

• • •

A safe environment is essential to promoting, maintaining, and restoring health. Incorporating critical thinking skills in the application of the nursing process, the nurse assesses the client and the environment to determine risk factors for injury; clusters risk factors; formulates a nursing diagnosis; and plans specific interventions, including client education. The expected outcomes include a safe physical environment, a client whose expectations have been met, a client who is knowledgeable about safety factors and precautions, and a client free of injury.

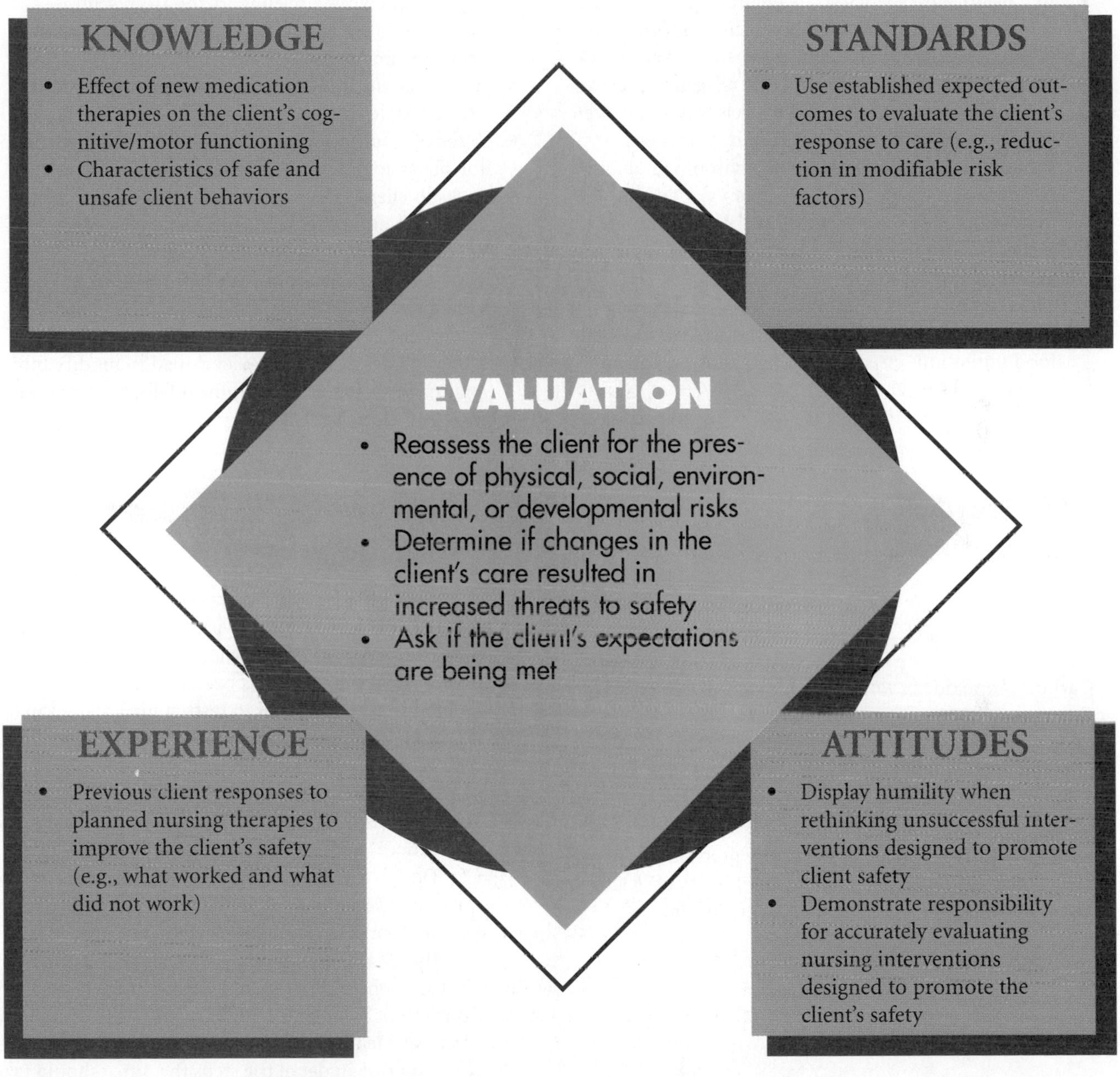

KNOWLEDGE

- Effect of new medication therapies on the client's cognitive/motor functioning
- Characteristics of safe and unsafe client behaviors

STANDARDS

- Use established expected outcomes to evaluate the client's response to care (e.g., reduction in modifiable risk factors)

EVALUATION

- Reassess the client for the presence of physical, social, environmental, or developmental risks
- Determine if changes in the client's care resulted in increased threats to safety
- Ask if the client's expectations are being met

EXPERIENCE

- Previous client responses to planned nursing therapies to improve the client's safety (e.g., what worked and what did not work)

ATTITUDES

- Display humility when rethinking unsuccessful interventions designed to promote client safety
- Demonstrate responsibility for accurately evaluating nursing interventions designed to promote the client's safety

Figure 37-16   *Synthesis Model for Safety Evaluation Phase.*

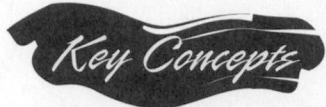

Key Concepts

- In the community a safe environment is one in which basic needs are achievable, physical hazards are reduced, transmission of pathogens is reduced, pollution is controlled, and sanitation is maintained.
- In a health care agency a safe environment is one that minimizes falls, client-inherent accidents, procedure-inherent accidents, and equipment-related accidents.
- A factor that reduces atmospheric oxygen is the presence of high carbon monoxide levels, which may result from an improperly functioning furnace.
- Prolonged exposure to extreme environmental temperatures can cause client injury or even death.
- Reduction of physical hazards in the environment includes providing adequate lighting, decreasing clutter, and securing the home.
- The transmission of pathogens is reduced through medical and surgical asepsis, immunization, adequate food sanitation, insect and rodent control, and appropriate disposal of human waste.

- Children under 5 years of age are at greatest risk for home accidents that may result in severe injury and death.
- The school-age child is at risk for injury at home, at school, and while traveling to and from school.
- Adolescents are at risk for injury from automobile accidents and substance abuse.
- Threats to an adult's safety are frequently associated with lifestyle habits.
- Risks of injury for older clients are directly related to the physiological changes of the aging process.
- Risks to client safety within a health care agency include falls and other client-inherent, procedure-related, and equipment-related accidents.
- Nursing interventions for promoting safety are individualized for developmental stage, lifestyle, and environment.
- Nursing interventions are developed to modify the environment for protection from falls, fires, poisonings, and electrical hazards.

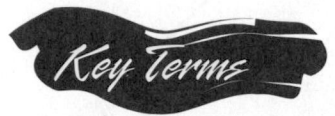

Key Terms

Air pollution, *p. 1023*
Ambularm, *p. 1038*
Aura, *p. 1050*
Carbon monoxide, *p. 1019*
Environment, *p. 1019*
Food and Drug
   Administration (FDA),
   p. 1020
Food poisoning, *p. 1020*
Grounded, *p. 1046*
Hyperthermia, *p. 1020*
Hypothermia, *p. 1020*

Immunization, *p. 1022*
Land pollution, *p. 1023*
Noise pollution, *p. 1023*
Pathogen, *p. 1022*
Poison, *p. 1046*
Pollutant, *p. 1022*
Relative humidity, *p. 1020*
Restraint, *p. 1035*
Seizure, *p. 1025*
Seizure precautions, *p. 1047*
Status epilepticus, *p. 1047*
Water pollution, *p. 1023*

Critical Thinking Exercises

1. Mr. Santiago, who is 88 years old, lives alone. Within the past year he has fallen twice at home, once by tripping over a rug and once when he got up to go to the bathroom at night. He has become increasingly afraid of falling again and tends to restrict his activities in the home. He goes out only when accompanied by a son.
    A. What physical assessment findings would be significant?
    B. What aspects of the environment need to be assessed?
    C. Design specific interventions to ensure the client's safety in his home.
    D. In terms of evaluation, what findings indicate that Mr. Santiago cannot live alone in the house?
2. Mr. Carr, who is 20 years old, comes to the emergency department following a night of drinking and illegal drug use. He is extremely combative with the staff.
    A. Describe in detail the steps the nurse should take to protect Mr. Carr, staff, and other clients.
3. A nurse does health teaching in a senior center. The nurse believes that the clients, who are all ambulatory and in good health, would benefit from exercises to increase their strength, balance, and flexibility.
    A. How should the nurse validate these beliefs?
    B. What benefits would the clients gain from increased strength, balance, and flexibility?
    C. What steps should the nurse take to initiate a program for these clients?

References

Accident facts, Itasca, Ill, 1998, National Safety Council.

Air pollution fact sheet, Washington, DC, 1998, Environmental Health Center, National Safety Council.

Arfken CL and others: The prevalence and correlates of fear of falling in elderly persons living in the community, *Am J Public Health* 84:565, 1994.

Beare P, Meyers J: *Adult health nursing,* ed 3, St. Louis, 1998, Mosby.

Brians LK and others: The development for the RISK tool for fall prevention, *Rehabil Nurs* 16(2):67, 1991.

Ebersole P, Hess P: *Toward healthy aging,* ed 5, St. Louis, 1998, Mosby.

Edelman CL, Mandle CL: *Health promotion throughout the life-span,* ed 4, St. Louis, 1998, Mosby.

Fire extinguisher fact sheet, Washington, DC, 1997, National Safety Council.

Giger JN, Davidhizar RE: *Trancultural nursing intervention,* ed 3, St. Louis, 1999, Mosby.

Health Care Financing Administration: *Federal Register* 54(21):1, 1990.

Joint Commission on Accreditation of Healthcare Organizations: *Accreditation manual for hospitals,* vol 1, standards, Chicago, 1999, The Commission.

Lead poisoning. In *Family safety and health,* Washington, DC, winter 1997-1998, National Safety Council.

Lueckenotte A: *Gerontologic nursing,* St. Louis, 1996, Mosby.

McCloskey JC, Bulechek GM: *Nursing interventions classification (NIC),* ed 3, St. Louis, 2000, Mosby.

McKenry LM, Salerno E: *Pharmacology in nursing,* ed 20, St. Louis, 1998, Mosby.

Pagana KD, Pagana TJ: *Diagnostic and laboratory test reference,* ed 4, St. Louis, 1998, Mosby.

Ray W and others: A randomized trial of a consultation service to reduce falls in nursing homes, *JAMA* 278(7):557, 1997.

Seizure recognition and observation: a guide for allied health professionals, ed 2, Baltimore, Md, 1992, Epilepsy Foundation of America.

Shepherd J and others: Patients presenting to family physicians after a fall: a report from the ambulatory sentinel practice network, *J Fam Pract* 35(1):43, 1992.

Skidmore-Roth L: *Mosby's drug guide for nurses,* ed 3, St. Louis, 1998, Mosby.

Sorrentino SA: *Mosby's assisting with patient care,* St. Louis, 1999, Mosby.

Steinmetz H, Hobson S: Prevention of falls among the community dwelling elderly: an overview, *Phys Occup Ther Geriatr* 12(4):13, 1994.

Stolley J: Freeing your patients from restraints, *Am J Nurs* 95(2):27, 1995.

Tideiksaar R: Home safe home: practical tips for fall-proofing, *Geriatr Nurs* 11(6):280, 1989.

Unintentional injury fact sheet: falls and hip fractures among the elderly, Atlanta, Fall 1997, National Center for Injury Prevention and Control, Centers for Disease Control and Prevention.

Walker J, Howland J: Falls and fear of falling among elderly people living in the community: occupational therapy interventions, *Am J Occup Ther* 45(2):119, 1991.

Weick M: Physical restraints: an FDA update, *Am J Nurs* 92(11):74, 1992.

Williams SR: *Nutrition and diet therapy,* ed 8, St. Louis, 1997, Mosby.

Wong DL and others: *Whaley and Wong's nursing care of infants and children,* ed 6, St. Louis, 1999, Mosby.

Ziemba S: Clinical snapshot: seizures, *Am J Nurs* 95(2):32, 1995.

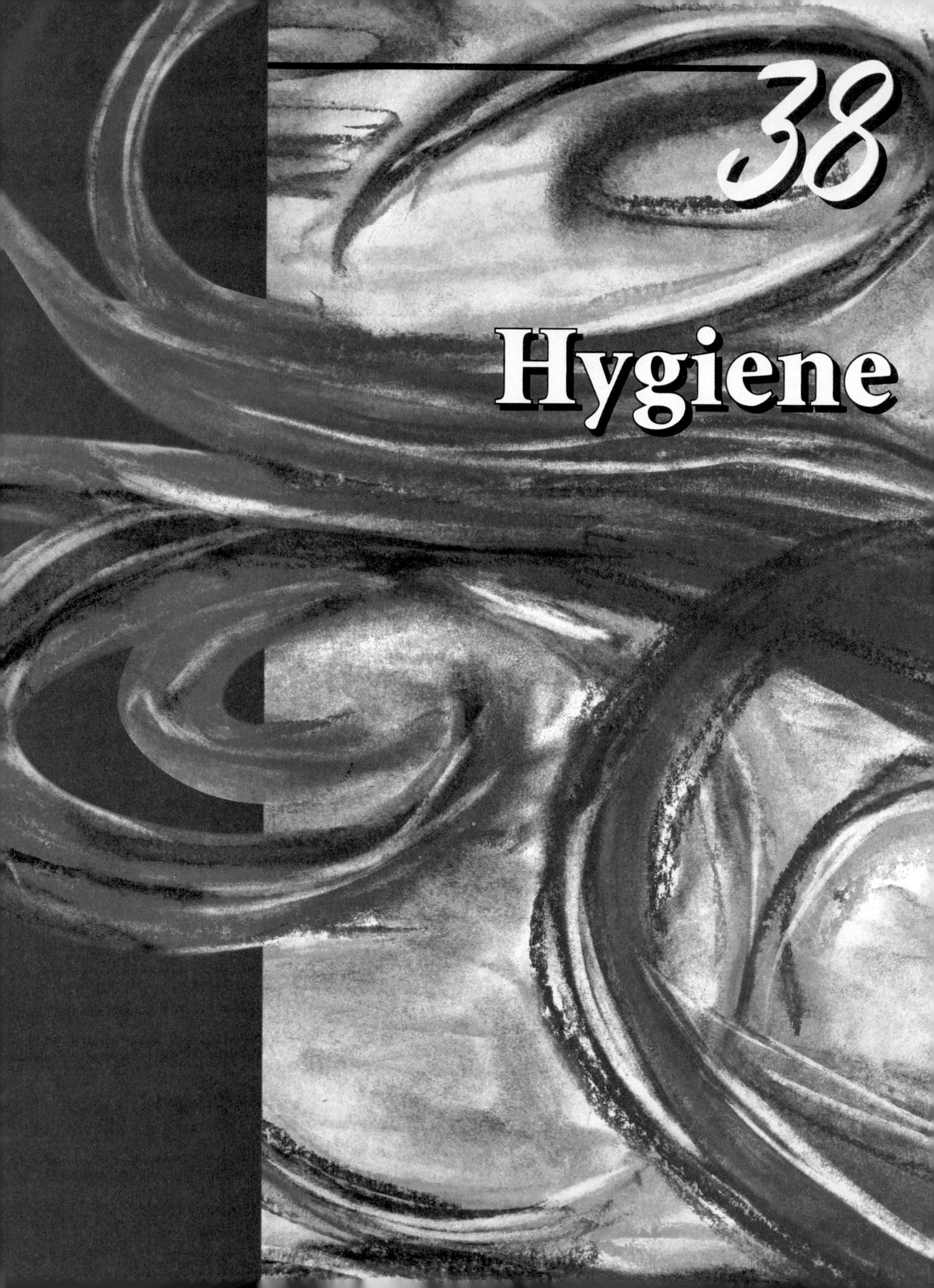

38

Hygiene

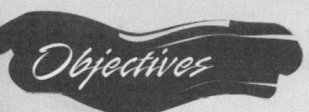

Mastery of content in this chapter will enable the student to:

- Define the key terms listed
- Describe factors that influence personal hygiene practices.
- Discuss the role critical thinking plays in the provision of hygienic care.
- Conduct a comprehensive assessment of a client's total hygiene needs.
- Discuss conditions that place clients at risk for impaired skin integrity.
- Discuss factors that influence the condition of the nails and feet.
- Explain the importance of foot care for the diabetic client.
- Discuss conditions that place clients at risk for impaired oral mucous membranes.
- List common hair and scalp problems and their related interventions.
- Describe how hygiene care for the older adult client may differ from that for the younger client.
- Discuss the different approaches used in maintaining a client's comfort during hygiene care.
- Successfully perform hygiene procedures for the care of the skin, perineum, feet and nails, mouth, eyes, ears, and nose.

Maintenance of personal hygiene is necessary for an individual's comfort, safety, and well-being. Whereas well people are capable of meeting their own hygienic needs, ill or physically challenged people may require assistance. A variety of personal and sociocultural factors influence the client's hygiene practices. The nurse determines a client's ability to perform self-care and provides hygienic care according to the client's needs and preferences. In the home setting, the nurse assists in helping the client and family adapt hygiene techniques and approaches.

Because hygienic care requires close contact with the client, the nurse uses communication skills (see Chapter 22) to promote a caring therapeutic relationship and to use the time with the client for teaching and counseling. The nurse can integrate other nursing activities during hygiene care, including client assessment and interventions such as range-of-motion exercises, application of dressings, or inspection and care of intravenous sites. While providing hygiene the nurse must preserve as much of the client's independence as possible, ensure privacy, convey respect, and foster the client's physical comfort.

Scientific Knowledge Base

Proper hygienic care requires an understanding of the anatomy and physiology of the integument, oral cavity, and the eyes, ears, and nose. While administering hygiene the nurse is able to apply this knowledge in recognizing abnormalities and in taking appropriate action that prevents further injury to sensitive tissues. The skin and mucosa

The authors acknowledge the contribution of Dr. Ann Bernadette Tritak to this chapter in the previous edition of this text.

cells exchange oxygen, nutrients, and fluids with underlying blood vessels. The cells require adequate nutrition, hydration, and circulation to resist injury and disease. Good hygiene techniques promote the normal structure and function of body tissues.

In addition to anatomy and physiology, the nurse applies knowledge of pathophysiology to provide good preventive hygienic care. The nurse learns to recognize those disease states that create changes in the integument, oral cavity, and sensory organs. For example, diabetes mellitus results in chronic vascular changes that impair healing of the skin and mucosa. In the early stages of acquired immunodeficiency syndrome (AIDS), fungal infections of the oral cavity are common. As a result of a stroke, paralysis of the trigeminal nerve eliminates the blink reflex, causing risk of corneal drying. In the presence of conditions such as these, the nurse adapts hygiene practices to anticipate client needs and minimize any injurious effects.

THE SKIN

The skin is an active organ with the functions of protection, secretion, excretion, temperature regulation, and sensation (Table 38-1). The skin has three primary layers: epidermis, dermis, and subcutaneous. The **epidermis** (outer layer) is composed of several thin layers of cells undergoing different stages of maturation. It shields underlying tissue against water loss and injury and prevents entry of disease-producing microorganisms. The innermost layer of the epidermis generates new cells to replace the dead cells that are continuously shed from the skin's outer surface. The epidermis also contains melanocytes, special cells that produce melanin, or dark pigment, of the skin. Bacteria commonly reside on the outer epidermis. These

Table 38-1	**Function of the Skin and Implications for Care**
Function/Description	Implications for Care
Protection Epidermis is relatively impermeable layer that prevents entrance of microorganisms. Although microorganisms reside on skin surface and in hair follicles, relative dryness of skin's surface inhibits bacterial growth. Sebum removes bacteria from hair follicles. Acidic pH of skin further retards bacterial growth.	Weakening of epidermis occurs by scraping or stripping its surface (e.g., use of dry razors, tape removal, or improper turning or positioning techniques). Excessive dryness causes cracks and breaks in skin and mucosa that allow bacteria to enter. Emollients soften skin and prevent moisture loss, soaking of skin improves moisture retention, and hydration of mucosa prevents dryness. However, constant exposure of skin to moisture causes maceration or softening, which interrupts dermal integrity and promotes ulcer formation and bacterial growth. Bed linen and clothing should be kept dry. Misuse of soap, detergents, cosmetics, deodorant, and depilatories can cause chemical irritation. Alkaline soaps neutralize the protective acid condition of skin. Cleansing of skin removes excess oil, sweat, dead skin cells, and dirt that can promote bacterial growth.
Sensation Skin contains sensory organs for touch, pain, heat, cold, and pressure.	Friction should be minimized to avoid loss of stratum corneum, which can result in development of pressure ulcers. Smoothing linen removes sources of mechanical irritation. Removing rings from fingers prevents nurse from accidentally injuring client's skin. Bath water should not be excessively hot or cold.
Temperature Regulation Body temperature is controlled by radiation, evaporation, conduction, and convection.	Factors that interfere with heat loss can alter temperature control. Wet bed linen or gowns interfere with convection and conduction. Excess blankets or bed coverings can interfere with heat loss through radiation and conduction. Coverings can promote heat conservation.
Excretion and Secretion Sweat promotes heat loss by evaporation. Sebum lubricates skin and hair.	Perspiration and oil can harbor microorganisms. Bathing removes excess body secretions, although if excessive it can cause drying of skin.

resident bacteria are normal flora (see Chapter 33) that do not cause disease but instead inhibit the multiplication of disease-causing microorganisms.

The **dermis** is a thicker skin layer containing bundles of collagen and elastic fibers to support the epidermis. Nerve fibers, blood vessels, sweat glands, sebaceous glands, and hair follicles course through the dermal layers. Sebaceous glands secrete sebum, an oily, odorous fluid, into the hair follicles. Sebum lubricates the skin and hair. There are two types of sweat glands: eccrine and apocrine. The **eccrine** glands are distributed throughout the skin. Sweat excreted from the eccrine glands assists in temperature control through evaporation. The **apocrine** glands can be found in the axillary and genital areas. The bacterial decomposition of sweat from these areas is responsible for body odor. In the ears, ceruminous glands secrete **cerumen** (earwax) into the external ear canal. This heavy, oily substance traps foreign material entering the ear.

The subcutaneous tissue layer contains blood vessels, nerves, lymph, and loose connective tissue filled with fat cells. The fatty tissue is a heat insulator for the body. Subcutaneous tissue also supports upper skin layers to withstand stresses and pressure without injury. Very little subcutaneous tissue underlies the oral mucosa.

The skin often reflects a change in physical condition by alterations in color, thickness, texture, turgor, temperature, and hydration (see Chapter 32). As long as the skin remains intact and healthy, its physiological function remains optimal.

THE FEET, HANDS, AND NAILS

The feet and hands are important to physical and emotional health. The structure of the foot is similar to that of the hand, with certain differences that adapt it for supporting weight (Thibodeau and Patton, 1993). The tarsal and metatarsals play the major role in the functioning of the foot as a supporting structure. Any injury or deformity to the foot, including any growths or injuries to the overlying skin, can be painful and thus interfere with a client's normal ability to walk and bear weight. The hand, in contrast to the foot, is constructed largely for manipulation rather than support. A wide range of dexterity exists in the hand because of the wide range of movement between the thumb and fingers. Any condition that interferes with movement of the hand (e.g., superficial or deep pain, joint inflammation) can impair a client's self-help abilities.

The nails are epithelial tissues that grow from the root of the nail bed, located in a groove hidden by the fold of skin called the **cuticle.** The visible part of the nail is the nail body. It has a crescent-shaped white area known as the **lunula.** Under the nail lies a layer of epithelium called the nail bed (Figure 38-1). The abundance of blood vessels in the nail bed creates its pink or light tan appearance (depending on race). Normally the nails grow about 0.5 mm a week with fingernails growing faster than toenails (Thibodeau and Patton, 1993).

THE ORAL CAVITY

The oral cavity is lined with mucous membranes continuous with the skin. The oral or buccal cavity consists of the lips surrounding the opening of the mouth, the cheeks running along the side walls of the cavity, the tongue and its muscles, and the hard and soft palate. The oral mucosa is normally light pink and moist. The floor of the mouth and the undersurface of the tongue are richly supplied with blood vessels. Any type of ulceration or trauma can result in significant bleeding. There are three pairs of salivary glands that secrete about 1 L of saliva a day. The **buccal glands** found in the mucosa lining the cheeks and mouth secrete less than 5% of the total saliva; however, buccal gland secretion maintains the hygiene and comfort of oral tissues. Salivary secretion in the mouth can be impaired through the effects of medications, exposure to radiation, and mouth breathing.

The teeth are the organs of chewing, or **mastication.** They are designed to cut, tear, and grind ingested food so it can be mixed with saliva and swallowed (Thibodeau and Patton, 1993). A normal tooth consists of the crown, neck and root (Figure 38-2). The periodontal membrane lies just below the gum margins, surrounds a tooth, and holds it firmly in place. Healthy teeth appear white, smooth, shiny, and properly aligned.

Difficulty in chewing can develop when surrounding gum tissues become inflamed or infected or when teeth are lost or become loosened. Regular oral hygiene is necessary to maintain the integrity of tooth surfaces and to prevent **gingivitis,** or gum inflammation.

THE HAIR

Hair growth, distribution, and pattern can indicate a person's general health status. Hormonal changes, emotional and physical stress, aging, infection, and certain illnesses can affect hair characteristics. The hair shaft itself is inert and cannot be directly affected by physiological factors. However, changes in its color or condition are caused by hormonal and nutrient deficiencies of the hair follicle. The hair follicle contains live cells and a rich capillary blood supply (Figure 38-3).

THE EYES, EARS, AND NOSE

When nurses provide hygienic care, the eyes, ears, and nose require careful attention. Chapter 32 describes the structure and function of these organs. Cleansing of the sensitive sensory tissues should be done in a way that prevents injury and discomfort for the client.

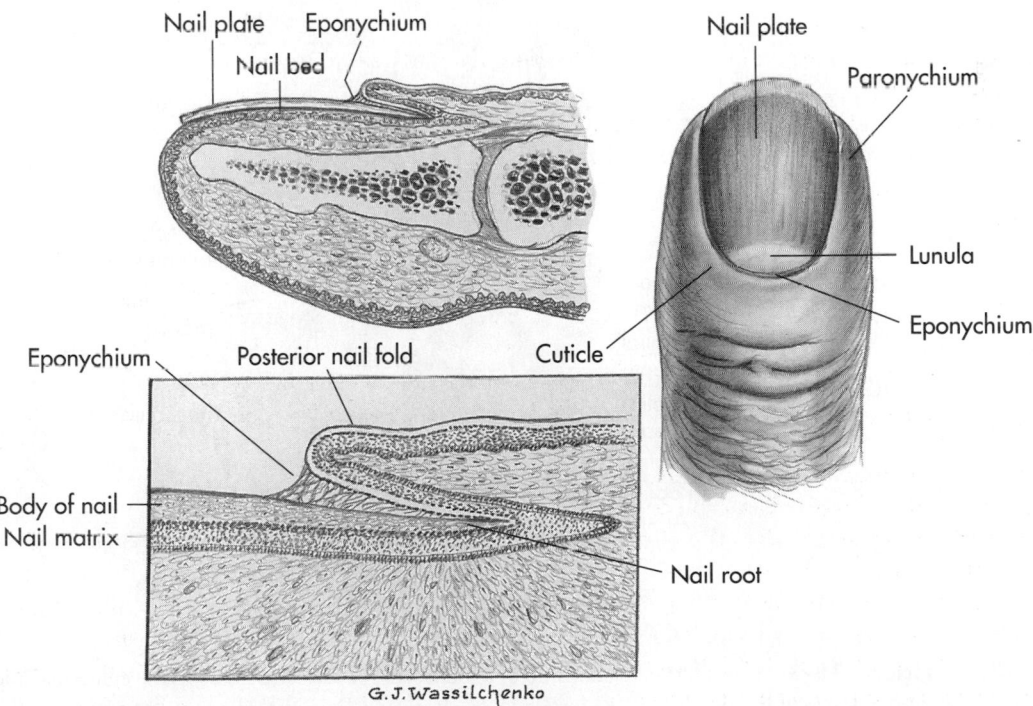

G.J.Wassilchenko

Figure 38-1 Anatomic structure of a normal nail.
From Thompson and others: *Clinical nursing,* ed 4, St. Louis, 1997, Mosby.

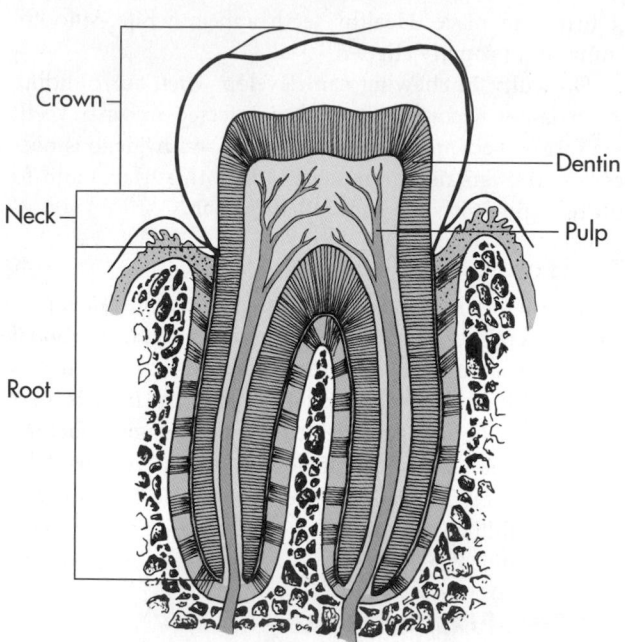

Figure 38-2   A normal tooth.

Nursing Knowledge Base

Nurses view clients' health care needs from a holistic perspective. In the case of hygiene, it is important to consider the knowledge that is available regarding the numerous sociocultural, economic, and developmental factors that influence a client's hygiene. Application of this knowledge base allows the nurse to provide individualized hygienic care.

SOCIAL PRACTICES

Social groups influence hygiene preferences and practices, including the type of hygienic products used and the nature and frequency of personal care. During childhood, hygiene is influenced by family customs. This may include, for example, the frequency of bathing, the time of day bathing is performed, and the type of oral hygiene practiced. As children enter their adolescent years, personal hygiene may be influenced by peer group behavior. Young girls, for example, may become more interested in their personal appearance and begin to wear makeup. During the adult years, involvement with friends and work groups shape the expectations people have about their personal appearance. Older adults' hygiene practices may change because of living conditions and available resources.

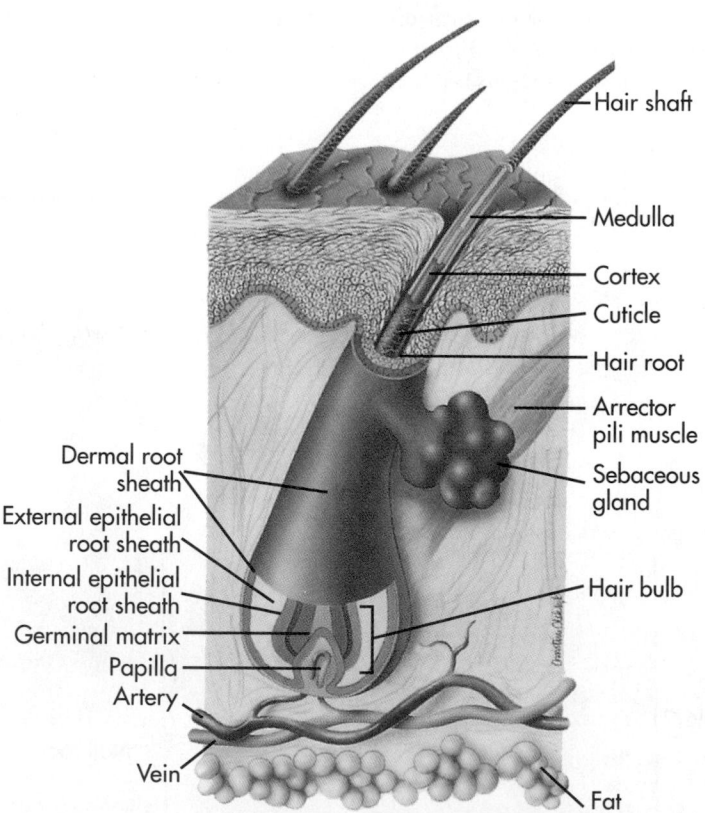

Figure 38-3   Hair follicle, relationship of a follicle and related structures to the epidermal and dermal layers of the skin.
From Thibodeau GA, Patton KT: *Anatomy and physiology,* ed 4, St. Louis, 1999, Mosby.

PERSONAL PREFERENCES

Each client has individual desires and preferences about when to bathe, shave, and perform hair care. Clients select different products according to personal preferences, needs, and financial resources. These desires should assist the nurse in delivering individualized care for the client. In addition, the nurse should also assist the client in developing new hygiene practices when indicated by an illness or condition.

BODY IMAGE

A client's general appearance may reflect the importance hygiene holds for that person. Body image is a person's subjective concept of his or her physical appearance (Chapter 26). These images can change frequently. Body image affects the way in which hygiene is maintained. If a client is neatly groomed, the nurse considers the details of grooming when planning care and consults the client before making decisions about how hygienic care is to be provided. Clients who appear unkempt or uninterested in hygiene may require education about the importance of hygiene. The nurse should be sensitive in considering that the client's economic status may influence his or her ability to regularly maintain hygiene. Culturally, maintaining cleanliness may not hold the same importance for some ethnic groups as it does for others. The nurse must not convey feelings of disapproval when caring for clients whose hygienic practices are different from the nurse's.

When clients undergo surgery, illness, or a change in functional status, body image can change dramatically. For this reason, the nurse will take extra effort to promote the client's hygienic comfort and appearance.

SOCIOECONOMIC STATUS

A person's economic resources influence the type and extent of hygiene practices used. The nurse determines whether clients can afford necessary supplies such as deodorant, shampoo, toothpaste, and cosmetics. When basic care items are not affordable, the nurse will work to find alternatives. It is also important to learn if use of these products is a part of the social habits practiced by the client's social group. For example, not all clients may choose to use deodorant or cosmetics.

When a nurse cares for a client, it is important to learn about the individual's routine adherence to hygiene practices and whether the client values those practices. Health promotion is a process of enabling individuals to increase control over the determinants of their health and thereby improve their health (Stachtchenko and Jenicek, 1990). Thus health promotion represents combining personal choice with social responsibility for health. When clients have the added problem of a lack of socioeconomic resources, it becomes difficult to participate and take a responsible role in health promotion activities such as basic hygiene.

HEALTH BELIEFS AND MOTIVATION

Knowledge about the importance of hygiene and its implications for well-being influences hygiene practices. However, knowledge alone is not enough. The client also must be motivated to maintain self-care. Health motivation is a generalized state of intent that results in behaviors to maintain or improve health (Champion, 1984). Motivation is part of an individual's health beliefs or attitudes that influence health-related behaviors. The classic health belief model (HBM) includes four concepts: perceived susceptibility or likelihood of experiencing a harmful condition, perceived seriousness or threat of the condition, perceived benefit or effectiveness of a behavior in reducing a threat, and perceived barriers or the negative aspects of the behavior (Becker, 1974). Studies have shown that clients' health beliefs predict the likelihood of assuming health promotion behavior (Champion, 1984). In regard to a client's hygiene practices it is important for the nurse to know if a client, for example, perceives being at risk for dental disease, perceives dental disease to be serious, perceives brushing and flossing to be effective in reducing risk, and perceives any negative implications from following recommended hygiene practices. When a client recognizes there is a risk and reasonable action can be taken with no negative consequence, he or she will be more receptive to the nurse's counseling and teaching efforts.

CULTURAL VARIABLES

A client's cultural beliefs and personal values influence hygiene care. People from diverse cultural backgrounds follow different self-care practices (Chapter 7). In North America it is common to bathe or shower daily, whereas in some other cultures it is customary to completely bathe only once a week (Box 38-1).

PHYSICAL CONDITION

The nurse quickly learns that clients with certain types of physical limitations or disabilities often lack the physical energy and dexterity to perform hygienic care. A client in traction or a cast or who has an intravenous line or other device connected to the body will need assistance with

---

Cultural ASPECTS OF CARE   Box 38-1

One culture that considers personal hygiene to be extremely important is that of the East Indian Hindus. A daily bath is part of their religious duty. Bathing after a meal is believed by some Hindus to be injurious. Likewise, a bath that is too hot may injure the eyes. Hot water may be added to cold water, but cold water is not to be added to hot water when one is preparing a bath. Once a bath is completed, the individual carefully dries the body thoroughly with a towel (Jee, 1981; Giger and Davidhizar, 1995).

hygiene. Illnesses that cause pain may limit the dexterity and range of motion needed to perform certain measures. Clients still under the effects of sedation will not have the mental clarity or coordination to perform self-care. Chronic illnesses, such as cardiac disease, cancer, neurological disorders, and certain psychiatric conditions may exhaust or incapacitate a client. A weakened grasp resulting from arthritis, stroke, or muscular disorders can prevent a client from using a toothbrush, washcloth, or comb.

Critical Thinking Synthesis

Because hygienic care is so important for a client to feel comfortable, refreshed, and renewed, the nurse avoids making hygiene care a simple routine. Instead, the nurse synthesizes knowledge, previous experience with clients, critical thinking attitudes, and standards in judging the most effective way to provide effective hygiene. A middle-age woman with abdominal pain who had major surgery only 24 hours ago will require a different approach to hy-

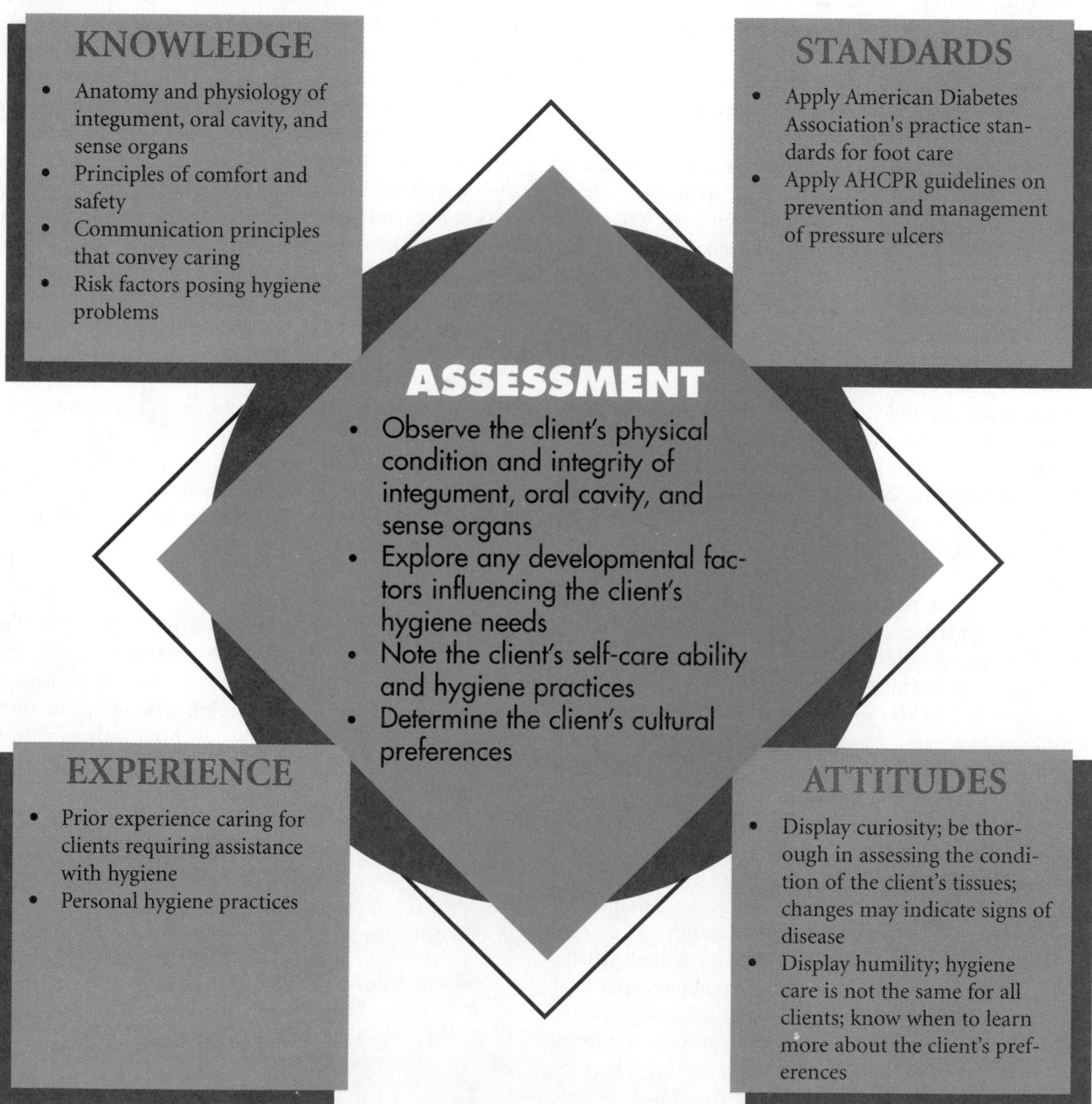

KNOWLEDGE

- Anatomy and physiology of integument, oral cavity, and sense organs
- Principles of comfort and safety
- Communication principles that convey caring
- Risk factors posing hygiene problems

STANDARDS

- Apply American Diabetes Association's practice standards for foot care
- Apply AHCPR guidelines on prevention and management of pressure ulcers

ASSESSMENT

- Observe the client's physical condition and integrity of integument, oral cavity, and sense organs
- Explore any developmental factors influencing the client's hygiene needs
- Note the client's self-care ability and hygiene practices
- Determine the client's cultural preferences

EXPERIENCE

- Prior experience caring for clients requiring assistance with hygiene
- Personal hygiene practices

ATTITUDES

- Display curiosity; be thorough in assessing the condition of the client's tissues; changes may indicate signs of disease
- Display humility; hygiene care is not the same for all clients; know when to learn more about the client's preferences

Figure 38-4   *Synthesis Model for Hygiene Assessment Phase.*

giene than an older adult who has left-sided paralysis. During the nurse's assessment (Figure 38-4) all critical thinking elements are considered in understanding the client's needs and in making appropriate nursing diagnoses. In addition, while hygiene is being administered, the nurse will make important observations (e.g., condition of client's skin, ability of client to move and initiate activities) that are applied when making clinical judgments about the client's overall nursing care.

Nursing Process

ASSESSMENT

Nursing assessment is an ongoing process. The nurse may not assess all body regions before administering hygiene; however, the nurse does routinely assess the client's condition whenever care to the client is given. For example, during oral care the condition of the teeth and mucosa can be inspected. When a client has had a repeated problem (e.g., dry skin, inflamed oral mucosa), then it is important to conduct an assessment before care is administered because variations in technique may be necessary. Hygienic care allows the nurse to make assessment findings for a variety of health care problems and thus helps set health care priorities.

Physical Examination. While assisting a client with personal hygiene, the nurse assesses the integument, oral cavity structures, and the eyes, ears, and nose (Chapter 32). Using the skills of inspection and palpation, the nurse looks for alterations in the integrity and function of tissues. The assessment also reveals the type and extent of hygienic care required. Special attention is given to the characteristics most influenced by hygiene measures. Is the skin dry from too much bathing? Are there calluses of the feet that may benefit from soaking? Is there a coating of the tongue that requires frequent brushing and hydration? Over time, the nurse's assessment provides the baseline for determining whether hygienic measures maintain or improve the client's condition.

Skin. While inspecting the skin, the nurse thoroughly examines its color, texture, thickness, turgor, temperature, and hydration. The skin should be smooth, warm, and supple with good turgor. The nurse pays special attention to the presence and condition of any lesions (see Chapter 32). Certain common skin problems affect how hygiene is administered (Table 38-2). Special care is also given to assess less obvious or difficult-to-reach skin surfaces, such as under the female client's breasts, under the male client's scrotum, or around the female's perineal tissues (see Chapter 44). The nurse who observes skin problems should explain proper skin care to the client and use the time to instruct on specific hygiene techniques.

Certain conditions place clients at risk for impaired skin integrity (Box 38-2). Nurses must be particularly alert when assessing clients with reduced sensation, vascular insufficiency, and immobility. Be sure to assess both extremities and assist in turning a client so that a skin surface can be fully viewed. The development of pressure ulcers is a common complication that can extend hospital stays and threaten the well-being of the long term care client.

Feet and Nails. Assessment of the feet involves a thorough examination of all skin surfaces, including areas between the toes and over the soles of the feet. The heels,

---

Risk Factors for Skin Impairment   Box 38-2

IMMOBILIZATION
When restricted from moving freely, dependent body parts are exposed to pressure, reducing circulation to affected body parts. The nurse should know which clients require assistance to turn and change positions.

REDUCED SENSATION
Clients with paralysis, circulatory insufficiency, or local nerve damage are unable to sense an injury to the skin. During a bath assess the status of sensory nerve function by checking for pain, tactile sensation, and temperature sensation.

NUTRITION AND HYDRATION ALTERATIONS
Clients with limited caloric and protein intake can develop thinner, less elastic skin, with loss of subcutaneous tissue. This can result in impaired or delayed wound healing.

SECRETIONS AND EXCRETIONS ON THE SKIN
Moisture on the skin's surface serves as a medium for bacterial growth and can cause irritation, soften epidermal cells, and lead to skin maceration. Presence of perspiration, urine, watery fecal material, and wound drainage on the skin can result in breakdown and infection.

VASCULAR INSUFFICIENCY
Inadequate arterial supply to tissues and impaired venous return decrease circulation to the extremities. Inadequate blood flow can cause ischemia and breakdown. Risk of infection also exists because delivery of nutrients, oxygen, and white blood cells to injured tissues is inadequate.

EXTERNAL DEVICES
An external device applied to or around the skin exerts pressure or friction on the skin. The nurse assesses all surfaces exposed to casts, cloth restraints, bandages and dressings, tubing, or orthopedic braces.

Table 38-2 Common Skin Problems

Characteristics	Implications	Interventions
Dry Skin		
Flaky, rough texture on exposed areas such as hands, arms, legs, or face	Skin may become infected if epidermal layer is allowed to crack.	Have client bathe less frequently and rinse body of all soap because residue left on skin can cause irritation and breakdown. Add moisture to air through use of humidifier. Increase fluid intake when skin is dry. Use moisturizing cream to aid healing. (Cream forms protective barrier and helps maintain fluid within skin.) Use cream such as Eucerin. Use creams to clean skin that is dry or allergic to soaps and detergents.
Acne		
Inflammatory, papulopustular skin eruption, usually involving bacterial breakdown of sebum; appears on face, neck, shoulders, and back	Infected material within pustule can spread if area is squeezed or picked. Permanent scarring can result.	Wash hair and skin thoroughly each day with hot water and soap to remove oil. Use cosmetics sparingly because oily cosmetics or creams accumulate in pores and tend to make condition worse. Implement dietary restrictions, if necessary. (Foods that aggravate condition should be eliminated from diet.) Inform client that exposure to ultraviolet rays, either from sunshine or heat lamp, may help control acne. (Caution should be used to prevent burning of skin.) Use prescribed topical antibiotics for severe forms of acne.
Hirsutism		
Excessive growth of body and facial hair, especially in women	Hirsutism may cause negative body image by giving women a male appearance.	Use following to remove unwanted hair: depilatories (can cause infection, rashes, dermatitis), shaving (safest method), electrolysis (permanently removes hair by destroying hair follicles), tweezing (lasts only temporarily), bleaching of hair (lasts only temporarily), waxing (can cause ingrown hair).
Skin Rashes		
Skin eruption that may result from overexposure to sun or moisture or from allergic reaction (may be flat or raised, localized or systemic, pruritic or nonpruritic)	If skin is continually scratched, inflammation and infection may occur. Rashes can also cause discomfort.	Wash area thoroughly and apply antiseptic spray or lotion to prevent further itching and aid in healing process. Apply warm or cold soaks to relieve inflammation, if indicated.
Contact Dermatitis		
Inflammation of skin characterized by abrupt onset with erythema, pruritus, pain, and appearance of scaly oozing lesions (seen on face, neck, hands, forearms, and genitalia)	Dermatitis is often difficult to eliminate because person is usually in continual contact with substance causing skin reaction. Substance may be hard to identify.	Avoid causative agents (e.g., cleansers and soaps).
Abrasion		
Scraping or rubbing away of epidermis that may result in localized bleeding and later weeping of serous fluid	Infection occurs easily because of loss of protective skin layer.	Be careful not to scratch client with jewelry or fingernails. Wash abrasions with mild soap and water; dry thoroughly and gently. Observe dressing or bandage for retained moisture because it could increase risk of infection.

soles, and sides of the feet are prone to irritation from poorly fitting shoes. In addition, the nurse inspects the shape and size of toes and shape of the foot. The toes are normally straight and flat. The feet should be in straight alignment with the ankle and tibia. Inspection of the feet for lesions includes noting areas of dryness, inflammation, or cracking.

The nurse assesses the client's gait. Painful foot disorders or decreased sensation can cause limping or an unnatural gait. The nurse asks whether the client has foot discomfort and determines factors that aggravate the pain. Foot problems may result from bone or muscular alterations rather than skin disorders.

Clients with peripheral vascular disease, such as those with diabetes mellitus, should be assessed for the adequacy of circulation to the feet (Chapter 32). Palpation of the dorsalis pedis and posterior tibial pulses indicates whether adequate blood flow is reaching peripheral tissues. Edema and changes in skin color, texture, and temperature can indicate if the client requires special hygienic care.

Persons with diabetes mellitus should also be checked for **neuropathy,** degeneration of the peripheral nerves characterized by a loss of sensation. The nurse assesses the client's sensation to light touch, pinprick, and temperature.

The nurse inspects the condition of the fingernails and toenails, looking for lesions, dryness, inflammation, or cracking (Table 38-3). The nail is surrounded by a cuticle, which slowly grows over the nail and must be regularly pushed back. The skin around the nail beds and cuticles should be smooth and without inflammation. The nurse should ask women whether they frequently polish their nails and use polish remover, because chemicals in these products can cause excessive nail dryness. Disease can change the shape and curvature of the nails (see Chapter 32). Inflammatory lesions and fungus of the nail bed can cause thickened, horny nails, which can separate from the nail bed.

Oral Cavity. Chapter 32 describes in detail the nurse's assessment of the client's lips, teeth, buccal mucosa, gums, palate, and tongue. The nurse inspects all areas carefully for color, hydration, texture, and lesions. Clients who do not follow regular oral hygiene practices may have receding gum tissue, inflamed gums, a coated tongue, discolored teeth (particularly along gum margins), dental caries, missing teeth, and **halitosis** (bad breath). Localized pain is a common symptom of a gum disease and certain tooth disorders. An infection of the mouth may involve organisms such as *Treponema pallidum, Neisseria gonorrhoeae,* and Herpes virus hominis.

It is especially important to examine the oral cavity of clients receiving radiation or chemotherapy. Both treatments can cause serious changes in salivary gland function and mucosal integrity. The nurse's assessment serves as a basis for preventive care for clients as they undergo treatment (Greifzu and others, 1990).

Hair. Before performing hair care, the nurse assesses the condition of the hair and scalp. Normally the hair is clean, shiny, and untangled, and the scalp is clear of lesions. The hair of black-skinned clients is usually thicker, drier, and curlier than that of lighter skinned clients. Table 38-4 summarizes hair and scalp problems the nurse may identify. In the community health and home care settings it is particularly important to inspect the hair for lice so that appropriate hygienic treatment can be provided. If pediculosis capitis (head lice) is suspected, the nurse guards against self-infestations by hand washing and use of gloves or tongue blades to inspect the client's hair. The loss of hair (**alopecia**) can result from the effects of chemotherapy medications, hormonal changes, or improper hair care practices. Clients at risk for scalp problems are those who have experienced head trauma and those who practice poor hygiene.

Eyes, Ears, and Nose. The nurse's examination assesses the condition and function of the eyes, ears, and nose (see Chapter 32). Normally the eyes are free of infection and irritation. The sclerae are visible anteriorly as the white portion of the eye. The conjunctivae (the lining of the eyelids) are clear, pink, and without inflammation. The eyelid margins are in close approximation with the eyeball, and the lashes are turned outward. The lid margins are without inflammation, drainage, or lesions. The eyebrows should be symmetrical.

Another important aspect of an eye examination is to determine if the client wears contact lenses. This is especially significant for clients who enter hospitals or other agencies unresponsive or in a confused state. An undetected lens can cause severe corneal injury when left in place too long.

Assessment of the external ear structures includes inspection of the auricle, external ear canal, and tympanic membrane. While performing hygienic measures, the nurse is most concerned with noting the presence of accumulated cerumen or drainage in the ear canal, local inflammation, or pain.

The nurse inspects the nares for signs of inflammation, discharge, lesions, edema, and deformity. The nasal mucosa is normally pink and clear and has little or no discharge. A clear, watery discharge may be the result of allergies. If clients have any form of tubing exiting the nose (e.g., nasogastric), the nurse should look at the nares surfaces that come in contact with the tubing for tissue sloughing, localized tenderness, inflammation, and bleeding.

Developmental Changes. The normal process of aging influences the condition of body tissues and structures and thus the manner in which hygienic measures are performed.

Skin. The neonate's skin is relatively immature at birth. The epidermis and dermis are loosely bound together and

Table 38-3 Common Foot and Nail Problems

Characteristics	Implications	Interventions
Callus Thickened portion of epidermis consists of mass of horny, keratotic cells. Callus is usually flat, painless, and found on undersurface of foot or on palm of hand. Problem is caused by local friction or pressure.	Condition may cause discomfort when wearing tight shoes.	Nurse advises client to wear gloves when using tools or objects that may create friction on palmar surfaces. Soft-sole shoes with insoles are recommended. Nurse soaks callus in warm water and Epsom salts to soften cell layers. Applications of creams or lotions can reduce reformation. Encourage client to see podiatrist.
Corns Keratosis is caused by friction and pressure from ill-fitting or loose shoes. It is seen mainly on or between toes, over bony prominence. Corn is usually cone shaped, round, and raised. Soft corns are macerated.	Conical shape compresses underlying dermis, making it thin and tender. Pain is aggravated when tight shoes are worn. Tissue can become attached to bone if allowed to grow. Client may suffer alteration in gait resulting from pain.	Surgical removal may be necessary, depending on severity of pain and size of corn. Nurse avoids use of oval corn pads, which increase pressure on toes and reduce circulation. Warm water soaks can soften corns before gentle rubbing with a callus file or pumice stone (consult with physician). Wider and softer shoes are suggested.
Plantar Warts Fungating lesion appears on sole of foot and is caused by papilloma virus.	Warts may be contagious. They are painful and make walking difficult.	Treatment ordered by physician may include applications of salicyclic acid, electrodesiccation (burning with electrical spark), or freezing with solid carbon dioxide.
Athlete's Foot (Tinea Pedis) Athlete's foot is fungal infection of foot; scaliness and cracking of skin occurs between toes and on soles of feet. Small blister containing fluid may appear. Problem is apparently induced by wearing of constricting footwear.	Athlete's foot can spread to other body parts, especially hands. It is contagious and frequently recurs.	Feet should be well ventilated. Drying feet well after bathing and applying powder help prevent infection. Wearing of clean socks or stockings reduces incidence. Physician may order application of griseofulvin, miconazole, or tolnaftate.
Ingrown Nails Toenail or fingernail grows inward into soft tissue around nail. Ingrown nail often results from improper nail trimming.	Ingrown nails can cause localized pain when pressure is applied.	Treatment is frequent hot soaks in antiseptic solution and removal of portion of nail that has grown into skin. Instruct client on proper nail-trimming techniques and refer to podiatrist.
Ram's Horn Nails Ram's horn nails are usually long curved nails.	Attempt by nurse to cut nails may result in damage to nail bed with risk of infection.	Nurse refers client to podiatrist.
Paronychia Inflammation of tissue surrounding nail occurs after hangnail or other injury. It occurs in people who frequently have their hands in water and is common in diabetic clients.	Area can become infected.	Treatment is hot compresses or soaks and local application of antibiotic ointments. Paronychia can be prevented by careful manicuring.
Foot Odors Foot odors are the result of excess perspiration promoting microorganism growth.	Condition may cause discomfort because of excess perspiration.	Frequent washing, use of foot deodorants and powders, and wearing clean footwear prevent or reduce problem.

Table 38-4   Hair and Scalp Problems

Characteristics	Implications	Interventions
Dandruff Scaling of scalp is accompanied by itching. In severe cases, dandruff is found on eyebrows.	Dandruff causes person embarrassment. If dandruff enters eyes, conjunctivis may develop.	Shampoo regularly with medicated shampoo. In severe cases, obtain physician's advice.
Ticks Small, gray-brown parasites burrow into skin and suck blood.	Ticks transmit several diseases to people. Most common are Rocky Mountain spotted fever, tularemia, and Lyme disease.	Do not pull ticks from skin because sucking apparatus remains and may become infected. Suffocate tick by placing a drop of oil or ether on tick or covering it with petrolatum to ease removal.
Pediculosis (Lice) Tiny, grayish-white parasite insects infest mammals.		
Pediculosis Capitis (Head Lice) Parasite is found on scalp attached to hair strands. Eggs look like oval particles, similar to dandruff. Bites or pustules may be observed behind ears and at hairline.	Head lice are difficult to remove and may spread to furniture and other people if not treated.	Thorough combing can remove lice. Physician may recommend shampooing with Kwell shampoo, repeating 12-24 hr later. Certain shampoos can be toxic. Change bed linens. Wash linens in hot water to kill lice.
Pediculosis Corporis (Body Lice) Parasites tend to cling to clothing, so they may not be easily seen. Body lice suck blood and lay eggs on clothing and furniture.	Client itches constantly. Scratches seen on skin may become infected. Hemorrhagic spots may appear on skin where lice are sucking blood.	Bathe or shower thoroughly. After skin is dried, apply recommended pediculocid lotion. After 12-24 hr, take another bath or shower. Bag infested clothing or linen until laundered in hot water. Vacuum rooms thoroughly and throw away bag after completion.
Pediculosis Pubis (Crab Lice) Parasites are found in pubic hair. Crab lice are grayish white with red legs.	Lice may spread through bed linen, clothing, or furniture or between persons via sexual contact.	Shave hair off affected area. Cleanse as for body lice. If lice were sexually transmitted, notify partner.
Hair Loss (Alopecia) Alopecia occurs in all races. Balding patches are seen in periphery of hair line. Hair becomes brittle and broken. Condition is caused by use of hair curlers, hair picks, tight braiding, and use of hot comb.	Patches of uneven hair growth and loss alter client's appearance.	Stop hair-care practices that damage hair.

the skin is very thin. Friction against the skin layers can cause bruising. The nurse must handle the neonate carefully during bathing. Any break in the skin can easily lead to infection.

A toddler's skin layers are more tightly bound together. Thus the child has a greater resistance to infection and skin irritation. However, because of the child's more active play and the absence of established hygienic habits, greater attention is needed from parents and caregivers to provide thorough hygiene and to begin teaching good hygiene habits.

During adolescence the growth and maturation of the integument increases. In girls, estrogen secretion causes the skin to become soft, smooth, and thicker, with increased vascularity. In boys, male hormones produce an increased thickness of the skin with some darkening in color. Sebaceous glands become more active, predisposing adolescents to **acne.** Eccrine and apocrine sweat glands become fully functional during puberty. Adolescents usually begin to use antiperspirants. More frequent bathing and shampooing also become necessary to reduce body odors and eliminate oily hair. Sweating is usually more pronounced in boys.

The condition of the adult's skin depends on hygienic practices and exposure to environmental irritants. Normally the skin is elastic, well hydrated, firm, and smooth. When an adult practices frequent bathing or is exposed to an environment with low humidity, the skin can become very dry and flaky. With age, the skin loses its resiliency and moisture, and sebaceous and sweat glands become less active. The epithelium thins and elastic collagen fibers shrink, making the skin fragile and subject to bruising and breaking. These changes warrant caution when turning and repositioning older adults. Typically the older person's skin is dry and wrinkled. Daily bathing as well as bathing with water that is too hot or soap that is harsh may cause the skin to become excessively dry.

Feet and Nails.

Changes in the infant's feet occur during infancy and early childhood as locomotion and weight bearing progress. At birth the feet are flat because the arches are protected by fat pads on the soles. As the bones in the arches develop, the pads disappear and the feet begin to assume a mature shape (Wong, 1999). The primary reason for shoes is protection. Shoes should retain their fit, be made of durable material with a smooth interior and few construction seams to irritate the skin, and be soft and flexible, especially in the toes. During weight bearing there should be at least the space of half the width of the thumbnail, or 1.25 cm (½ inch), between the end of the longest toe and the shoe (Wong, 1999). Frequent shoe size changes are needed to accommodate the infant's rapidly growing feet. Curled toes when shoes are removed and redness and irritation of the skin on the bottom of the toes indicate the need for a larger shoe size.

As children grow, it continues to be important that they are fitted with a proper shoe size. The more active a child becomes, the greater is the need for sturdy shoes that protect the feet from injury.

During standing, the foot provides body support and absorbs shock. With aging, the feet begin to show signs of wear and tear. This may occur earlier if a person has failed to wear comfortable, supportive footwear. The cushioning layer of fat on the soles of the feet become thin. Years of walking cause the metatarsal bones to spread and ligaments to stretch, which results in wider feet (Gudas, 1992).

Chronic foot problems are a common part of aging. Older adults often have dry feet because of a decrease in sebaceous gland secretion, dehydration of epidermal cells, and poor condition of footwear. Fissures that result in itching frequently develop. One of the most common problems for older adults is foot pain (Lueckenotte, 1996).

Painful feet can be the result of congenital deformities, weak structure, injuries, and diseases such as diabetes, rheumatoid arthritis, or osteoarthritis. Arthritis is generally the cause for changes in the feet after age 55. Additional common problems of the feet include hammer and claw toes (flexion contractures); bunions, corns, and calluses; loss of sensation; and pathological nail conditions (Ostermann, 1990). Fungal infections occur under toenails, causing dirty yellow streaks or total discoloration. The nails can also become opaque, scaly, and hypertrophied. If foot or nail problems stay unresolved, an older adult can easily become disabled. The nurse applies knowledge of typical changes in the feet and nails when anticipating the type of hygiene a client will require.

The Mouth.

At approximately 6 to 8 months of age, infants begin teething (Wong, 1999). The eruption of the deciduous (primary) teeth usually begins with the lower central incisors, followed closely by the upper central incisors (Table 38-5). When the crown of a tooth breaks through the periodontal membrane, some discomfort can be experienced. Drooling, increased finger sucking, or biting on hard objects may be the only signs of discomfort. Other children can become very irritable and have difficulty sleeping and eating. Teething continues to occur until the final molars erupt around 27 to 29 months of age.

The first permanent (secondary) teeth erupt at about 6 years of age (Wong, 1995). Before their appearance they have been developing in the jaw beneath the primary teeth. Meanwhile, the roots of primary teeth are gradually absorbed, so that at the time a deciduous tooth is shed, only the crown remains. The pattern of shedding primary teeth and the eruption of secondary teeth varies widely among children. Many of the difficulties created by crowding of teeth become apparent. Since it is during the school-age years that the permanent teeth erupt, good dental hygiene and regular attention to dental caries are a part of health promotion practices. Children of this age tend to be lax about oral hygiene and are not motivated by improved appearance and odor, as they will be during adolescence. In addition, school-agers prefer sugary candy and sodas for snacks. Parental support is critical for health maintenance.

From adolescence, when all of the permanent teeth are in place, through middle adulthood, the teeth and gums remain healthy if a person follows good eating patterns and good dental care. Avoidance of fermentable carbohydrates and sticky sweets are central to keeping the teeth free of **caries.** Regular brushing and flossing (p. 1094) help to prevent caries and periodontal disease.

As a person grows older there are numerous factors that can result in poor oral care. These include age-related changes of the mouth, chronic disease such as diabetes, physical disabilities involving hand grasp or strength, lack of attention to oral care, and prescribed medications that have oral side effects. Effects of inadequate care include

Table 38-5 Physiological Development of the Mouth

Developmental Level	Changes
Infant	Deciduous teeth begin to erupt at about 6 mo of age. Solid food can be taken in mouth at 5-6 mo. Chewing begins by 6-8 mo.
18 mo-6 yr	Twenty deciduous teeth are present. By age 2, child can begin to brush teeth and learn hygienic practices from parents. Dental caries may become problem if dental hygiene is neglected. By age 6, "baby" teeth begin to fall out and are replaced by permanent teeth.
6-12 yr	Deciduous teeth are replaced by permanent teeth. Permanent teeth are present by age 12 except second and third molars. Definite food preferences become apparent. Dental caries and irregularity in spacing of teeth are significant health problems.
12-18 yr	All permanent teeth are present. Dental hygienic practices tend to improve because of increased awareness of body image.
18-40 yr	Third molars appear. Good oral hygiene and nutrition practices are needed to avoid problems in later years.
Pregnancy	Changes in female sex hormones may exaggerate reaction to irritants in dental plaque, causing gingivitis and increased risk of severe periodontal disease.*
40-65 yr	Although loss of teeth, usually a result of periodontal disease, is declining, about half of people over age 55 have lost some or all of their teeth because of poor oral care. Root caries and oral cancer occur with higher frequency.
65 yr and over	Aging teeth become brittle, drier, and darker in color. Teeth become uneven, jagged, and fractured after years of crushing and grinding. Gums lose vascularity and tissue elasticity, causing dentures to fit poorly. Eating habits often change, and malnutrition may be a problem. Diminished taste sensitivity, thinning of mucosa, and decreased mass and strength of muscles of mastication also occur.

*Data from de Liefde B, Ritchie GR: Evaluation in dental public health in New Zealand, *N Z Dent J* 80:8, 1984.

Table 38-6 Physiological Development of Hair Growth

Age	Condition of Hair
Infancy	Infants may have little or no scalp hair at birth. Scalp hair grows by first year. Fine body hair (lanugo) is present on forehead, cheeks, shoulders, and back.
Childhood	Scalp hair is lustrous, silky, strong, and elastic. Hair of black skinned child is curlier and coarser.
Middle childhood to puberty	Androgenic hormones cause increase in thickening and darkening of scalp hair, growth of hair in axillae and pubic areas in both sexes, and growth of facial hair in boys.
Adolescence	Boys may acquire additional amounts of distribution of body hair, such as on chest. Increase in sebaceous gland activity causes hair to become oily.
Adulthood	Men with genetic tendency develop baldness.
Older adulthood	Axillary and pubic hair diminish in women. Scalp hair becomes thinner and depleted of melanin, causing gray coloring. Older women may develop chin and facial hair because of decreased estrogen production. Men may experience balding or receding hairline.

dental caries and loss of teeth; periodontal disease; systemic infection; and long-term effects on self-esteem, the ability to eat, and the maintenance of relationships (Danielson, 1988). Many elders are **edentulous** and wear complete or partial dentures. It is important for the nurse to learn if older adults wear dentures and the condition of underlying supportive gum tissue.

Hair.   Throughout life, changes in the growth, distribution, and condition of the hair influence the hygiene that a person requires (Table 38-6). As males reach adolescence, shaving becomes a part of routine grooming. Young girls who reach puberty may begin to shave their legs and axillae. With aging, as scalp hair becomes thinner and drier shampooing is usually performed less frequently.

Eyes, Ears, and Nose.   Chapter 48 addresses the changes in hearing, vision, and olfaction as a result of growth and development.

Self-Care Ability.   Clients' self-care abilities determine if assistance is needed in managing activities of daily living, including routine hygiene. The nurse assesses a client's physical and cognitive ability to perform basic hygiene measures. The nurse's assessment must include measurement of a client's muscle strength, flexibility and dexterity, balance, coordination, and activity tolerance necessary in performing activities such as bathing, brushing teeth, and bending over to inspect the feet (Figure 38-5). For example, observing and timing a client's ability to completely brush the front surfaces of all lower front teeth in 30 seconds and noting the client's ability to pick up and use the brush is a way to assess toothbrushing ability (Felder and others, 1994). The degree of assistance needed by a client during hygienic care may also depend on vision, the ability to sit without support, attached equipment, hand grasp, and the range of motion in the client's extremities. Painful conditions of the upper extremities pose special problems. The nurse can assess self-care ability by asking clients to perform activities such as toothbrushing or combing the hair. Observe the client carefully and note not only if the activity is performed correctly, but if the client is able to be thorough and complete the task.

When clients have self-care limitations, part of the nurse's assessment becomes determining if family or friends are available to assist. In addition, the nurse also assesses the home environment and its influence on the client's hygiene practices. Are there barriers in the home that may affect the client's self-care abilities? Water faucets that are too tight to easily adjust, bathtubs with high sides,

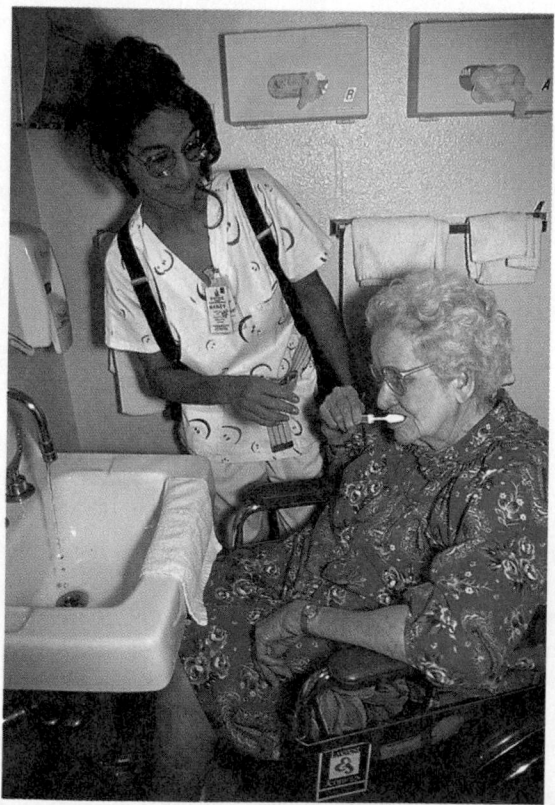

Figure 38-5   The nurse observes client brushing teeth. During such observations the nurse can determine how much assistance the client may need.

and a bathroom too small to fit a chair in front of a sink are a few examples.

Hygienic Practices.   Each client has a preferred routine for how to perform hygiene. The nurse should not assume that all clients typically bathe and groom early each morning after arising from bed. Some clients may only bathe on a weekly basis. In addition, clients vary in the type of hygiene products used and in which hygiene measures they choose to practice. In assessing a client's practices, the nurse may ask a client to describe what is typically done to care for the skin, teeth, hair, and feet. The nurse also observes the client's appearance. For example, dull, tangled, and dirty hair indicates improper care. Unkempt hair may result from lack of interest, depression, lack of grooming resources, or a physical inability to care for the hair. When a client's appearance suggests poor hygiene, the nurse must be sensitive in learning what the causal factors are.

Assessment of hygiene practices reveals the client's preferences for how to perform grooming. For example, a client may choose to groom the hair in a certain style or choose to trim nails in a certain way. When a client has a physical disability, special precautions may be needed to perform grooming without injury. Asking the client to assist or teach the nurse how to perform preferred grooming practices gives the client a greater sense of independence and helps the nurse avoid causing the client any discomfort or injury.

Because of the significant increase in the numbers of older adults and minorities, dental practice is facing new challenges. Data have shown a pattern of untreated dental caries in African-Americans and Mexican-Americans and a prevalence of gingivitis in Spanish-Americans (Ismail and Szpunar, 1990). These patterns suggest either deficient hygiene practices, limited access to dental care resources, or improper hygiene techniques. Helpful questions to use in assessing dental hygiene practices include the following:

How often does the client brush the teeth?

What type of toothbrush, toothpaste, or dentifrice is used?

Does the client have dentures? Partials or bridges? When and how are they cleansed?

Does the client use mouthwash or lemon-glycerine preparations that can cause excess mucosal drying?

Does the client floss? If so, how often?

When was the client's last dental visit? How often are visits to a dentist made? What were the most recent results?

Is the water the client drinks fluoridated?

Cultural Factors.   A client's cultural background is an influential factor when determining hygiene needs. Culture plays a role not only in hygiene practices and preferences but also in sensitivity to personal space (see Chapter 22). For example, some Chinese-Americans may view tasks associated with closeness and touch as being offensive or impolite, whereas Vietnamese-Americans may feel very uneasy during a back rub (Giger and Davidhizar, 1995). The nurse should ask a client what will make him or her feel most comfortable during a bath. Perhaps the client would prefer only a partial instead of a full bath from the nurse, with a family member completing the bathing of more private body parts. The client may also defer part of hygiene. If in the nurse's judgment, hygiene is critical to prevent developing or worsening problems, such as skin breakdown, the nurse must take the time to understand the client's con-

cerns and then offer an explanation that will help the client accept the nurse's intervention.

Clients at Risk for Hygiene Problems. There are clients who present risks that require more attentive and rigorous hygienic care (Table 38-7). These risks result from side effects of medications, a lack of knowledge, an inability to perform hygiene, or a physical condition that potentially injures the skin, integument, or other structures. An immobilized client who has a fever for example, will require more frequent bathing to minimize perspira-

---

Table 38-7 Risk Factors for Hygiene Problems

Risks	Hygiene Implications
Oral Problems	
Clients who are unable to use upper extremities due to paralysis, weakness, or restriction (e.g., cast or dressing)	Client lacks upper extremity strength or dexterity needed to brush teeth (Phipps, 1995).
Dehydration, inability to take fluids or food by mouth (NPO)	Causes excess drying and fragility of mucosa; increases accumulation of secretions on tongue and gums.
Presence of nasogastric or oxygen tubes; mouth breathers	Causes drying of mucosa.
Chemotherapeutic drugs	Drugs kill rapidly multiplying cells, including normal cells lining oral cavity. Ulcers and inflammation can develop.
Lozenges, cough drops, antacids, and chewable vitamins over-the-counter (OTC)	Medications contain large amounts of sugar. Repeated use increases sugar or acid content in mouth.
Radiation therapy to head and neck	Reduces salivary flow and lowers pH of saliva; can lead to stomatitis and tooth decay (Danielson, 1988).
Oral surgery, trauma to mouth, placement of oral airway	Cause trauma to oral cavity with swelling, ulcerations, inflammation and bleeding.
Immunosuppression; alters blood clotting	Predisposes to inflammation and bleeding gums
Diabetes mellitus	Prone to dryness of mouth, gingivitis, periodontal disease, and loss of teeth.
Skin Problems	
Immobilization	Dependent body parts are exposed to pressure from underlying surfaces. The inability to turn or change position increases risk for pressure ulcers.
Reduced sensation due to stroke, spinal cord injury, diabetes, local nerve damage	Client does not receive normal transmission of nerve impulses when excessive heat or cold, pressure, friction, or chemical irritants are applied to skin.
Limited protein or caloric intake and reduced hydration (e.g., fever, burns, gastrointestinal alterations, poorly fitting dentures)	Limited caloric and protein intake predispose to impaired tissue synthesis. Skin becomes thinner, less elastic, and smoother with a loss of subcutaneous tissue. Poor wound healing may result. Reduced hydration impairs skin turgor.
Excessive secretions or excretions on the skin from perspiration, urine, watery fecal material, and wound drainage	Moisture is a medium for bacterial growth and can cause local skin irritation, softening of epidermal cells, and skin maceration.
Presence of external devices (e.g., casts, restraint, bandage, dressing)	Device can exert pressure or friction against skin's surface.
Vascular insufficiency	Arterial blood supply to tissues is inadequate, or venous return is impaired, causing decreased circulation to extremities. Tissue ischemia and breakdown may occur. Risk for infection is high.
Foot Problems	
Client unable to bend over or has reduced visual acuity	Client is unable to fully visualize entire surface of each foot, impairing ability to adequately assess condition of skin and nails.
Eye Care Problems	
Reduced dexterity and hand coordination	Physical limitations create inability to safely insert or remove contact lens.

tion on the skin, and more frequent turning and positioning to reduce the chance of skin breakdown. The nurse anticipates whether a client is predisposed to such risks and follows through with a complete assessment. For example, if a client is receiving chemotherapy there is the risk of the medication destroying normal flora in the mouth, allowing for the overgrowth of opportunistic bacteria. Therefore the oral examination should be more thorough and detailed with the nurse examining all surfaces of the tongue and mucosa. If a client is diaphoretic, the nurse will give special attention to body areas, such as a woman's breasts and perineal area, to check where moisture may collect and irritate skin surfaces. The nurse anticipates problems created by these risks so as to provide appropriate preventive care. The nurse's assessment will include a review of the client's medical and surgical history, medications, and the specific risk factors the client is likely to have.

Special Considerations in Hygiene Assessment.

Depending on the type of hygiene a nurse plans to provide, there are focused assessments that are important to conduct. Before giving foot care, the nurse assesses the type of footwear worn by a client. Children or young adults who frequently fail to wear socks may have excess perspiration that promotes fungal growth. Tight or poorly fitting shoes, socks, garters, or knee-high nylon stockings may cause skin irritation and interfere with circulation to the feet. The nurse also assesses whether clients wear clean footwear daily because repeated use of soiled footwear can lead to infection. If the client has diabetes mellitus or other peripheral vascular disease, it is extremely important that correct footwear be worn. Extrawide and extradeep shoes will accommodate bunions or hammer toes. Cushioned inner soles help redistribute pressure on the metatarsal head. Rocker-bottom shoes help with ambulation (Young and Young, 1994).

A client's eating patterns are important to assess prior to oral care. The presence of any problems may help the nurse to locate abnormalities. The nurse asks a client if any problems are noted with chewing, denture fit, or swallowing. A client may have changed the type of food in the diet as a result of chewing difficulties. The presence of an ulcer or irritation may impair chewing and cause a client to avoid eating. This is common in an older adult with poorly fitting dentures.

If clients wear eyeglasses, contact lenses, artificial eyes, or hearing aids, the nurse assesses the client's knowledge of methods used to care for the aids and the presence of any problems. Box 38-3 outlines factors to assess in clients who use sensory aids. Findings have implications for client education.

Client Expectations.

As is the case in any nursing assessment, it is important to know what a client expects from nursing care. In regard to hygienic care, the client

---

| Assessing a Client's Use of Sensory Aids | Box 38-3 |

EYEGLASSES
Purpose for wearing glasses (e.g., reading, distance, or both)
Methods used to clean glasses
Presence of symptoms (e.g., blurred vision, photophobia, headaches, irritation)

CONTACT LENSES
Type of lens worn
Frequency and duration of time lenses are worn (including sleep time)
Presence of symptoms (e.g., burning, excess tearing, redness, irritation, swelling, sensitivity to light)
Techniques used by the client to cleanse, store, insert, and remove lenses
Use of eye drops or ointments
Use of emergency identification bracelet or card that warns others to remove client's lenses in case of emergency

ARTIFICIAL EYE
Method used to insert and remove eye
Method for cleansing eye
Presence of symptoms (e.g., drainage, inflammation, pain involving the orbit)

HEARING AID
Type of aid worn
Methods used to cleanse aid
Client's ability to change battery and adjust hearing aid volume

---

may simply expect to have hygiene preferences and practices applied in the health care setting. The nurse can learn a client's expectations by asking questions such as, "To make you most comfortable and feel at home, how can I best perform your bath and personal care?" or "How can we help you to care for your teeth, nails, and hair, now that you are back home?"

Learning a client's expectations and applying them in practice is important in establishing a caring relationship. Truly individualizing hygienic care shows the nurse's respect for the client's needs. As the nurse learns what the client expects, this information can be incorporated into goal development (see planning).

NURSING DIAGNOSIS

The nurse's assessment will reveal the condition of the skin, oral cavity, and other tissues, as well as the client's need for and ability to meet personal hygiene needs. The nurse reviews all data gathered, considers previous clients cared for, reviews knowledge pertaining to preexisting conditions, and then looks for clusters of data suggesting a problem trend. For example, an older adult with degenerative arthritis presents to the home health nurse with pain in the joints, weakness, mobility limitations in the dominant hand, and a generally unkempt appearance. Closer review of assessment data reveal defining characteristics of an inability to wash body parts and difficulty turning and regulating a water faucet. The nursing diagnosis of *bathing/hygiene self-care deficit* is supported and becomes part of the nurse's plan of care. The nurse's accurate selection of nursing diagnoses requires critical thinking to identify actual or potential health problems (Box 38-4). Assessment activities must be thorough in revealing all appropriate defining characteristics so that an accurate diagnosis can be made.

Whether a client has an actual alteration (e.g., impaired tissue integrity) or is at risk (e.g., risk for infection) determines the focus of nursing interventions. The client with an actual alteration will require extensive hygienic care, often more thorough that what routine hygiene might involve. For example, if the client has skin breakdown, the nurse must initiate care more frequently to keep existing skin surfaces clean and dry and to eliminate factors such as moisture or drainage that can worsen the condition of the skin. The nurse would also provide care to promote healing of injured skin surfaces (see Chapter 47). If the client is at risk for a problem, the nurse will institute preventive measures. In the case of risk for impaired oral mucous membranes, the nurse will keep the mucosa well hydrated, minimize foods irritating to tissues, and provide cleansing that soothes and reduces tissue inflammation.

The identification of related factors guides the nurse in the selection of nursing interventions. *Altered oral mucous membrane related to malnutrition* and a diagnosis of *altered oral mucous membrane related to chemical trauma*, require very different interventions. When malnutrition is a causal factor, the nurse will obviously confer with a dietitian for appropriate dietary supplements and incorporate client education into the plan. When mucosa are in-

jured as a result of chemical trauma from chemotherapy, techniques for cleansing and hydrating inflamed tissues and eliminating sources of irritation will be the focus of nursing care. Box 38-5 summarizes possible nursing diagnoses that apply to clients in need of hygienic care.

PLANNING

During planning the nurse synthesizes information from multiple resources (Figure 38-6). Critical thinking ensures that the client's plan of care integrates all that the nurse knows about the individual client and key critical thinking elements. Previous experience with other clients can be very useful in knowing how to adapt hygiene techniques for special needs. Professional standards are especially important to consider when the nurse develops a plan of care. These standards often establish scientifically proven guidelines for effective nursing interventions. For example, the American Diabetes Association's clinical practice recommendations for 1999 offer valuable guidelines for preventive foot care in diabetic clients.

The nurse develops an individualized plan of care for each of the client's nursing diagnoses (see care plan). The nurse and client partner together to identify goals and expected outcomes. Goals are established with the client's self-care abilities and resources in mind. Outcomes should be measurable and achievable within client limitations. The nurse works further with the client to then select hygiene measures that are appropriate and realistic.

The client's condition influences the plan for delivering hygiene. A seriously ill client usually needs a daily bath because body secretions accumulate. An older client at home may require a visit from a home health aide to assist with a tub bath. Clients who are normally inactive during the day and have skin that tends to be dry may need to bathe only twice a week. The nurse must plan for necessary assistance for clients who are weakened or possess poor co-

---

SAMPLE NURSING DIAGNOSTIC PROCESS   Box 38-4

HYGIENIC CARE

Assessment Activities	Defining Characteristics	Nursing Diagnoses
Inspect condition of client's perianal and perineal tissues.	Skin is becoming reddened over perianal area.	Risk for impaired skin integrity related to chemical irritation
Observe character of client's loose stools.	Stools are diarrheal in nature, occurring 5 to 6 times daily.	
Note frequency of loose stools.		
Observe client attempt to bathe self either in bed or at bathroom sink. (Note: Be sure positioning does not restrict potential movement.)	Client is unable to wash body or body parts.	Self-care deficit, bathing/hygiene related to upper extremity weakness
Observe client adjust flow of water faucet.	Client is unable to regulate water flow.	
Assess client's upper extremity strength, range of motion, and coordination.	Client has reduced upper extremity movement and strength.	

NURSING DIAGNOSES   Box 38-5
ASSOCIATED WITH HYGIENE PROBLEMS

Dentition, altered
Fatigue
Health maintenance, altered
Infection, risk for
Knowledge deficit about hygiene practices
Mobility, impaired physical
Oral mucous membrane, altered
Powerlessness
Self-care deficit, bathing/hygiene
Self-care deficit, dressing/grooming
Self-esteem disturbance
Skin integrity, impaired
Skin integrity, impaired, risk for
Tissue integrity, impaired
Tissue perfusion, altered peripheral

ordination. For example, a partially paralyzed client who has had difficulty getting out of a tub should have a tub chair, handrails, or extra personnel available for help.

Timing is also important in planning hygiene. Being interrupted in the middle of a bath to go to an x-ray examination can frustrate and embarrass a client. Following extensive diagnostic tests (e.g., a stress test), it may be best to delay hygiene and allow a client to rest. In the home, bathing may be planned to refresh the client before daily activities. The nurse should try to plan hygiene around tests, procedures, and client needs. This can be difficult in a hospital because tests are often not scheduled for specific times.

When a client needs assistance as a result of a self-care limitation, the family becomes a valuable resource to the nurse. Family members can usually assist with hygiene measures but may need guidance in adapting techniques

KNOWLEDGE

- Principles of comfort and safety
- Adult learning principles to apply when educating the client and family
- Services available through community agencies

STANDARDS

- Individualize hygiene care to meet client preferences
- Apply standards of safety and promotion of client dignity

PLANNING

- Involve the client and family in planning and adapting approaches, as well as in hygiene instruction
- Know community resources applicable for the client's needs
- Consider the timing of other care activities when choosing the best time for hygiene care

EXPERIENCE

- Care of previous clients that required adaptation of hygiene approaches

ATTITUDES

- Be creative when adapting approaches to any self-care limitations client might have
- Take responsibility for following standards of good hygiene practice

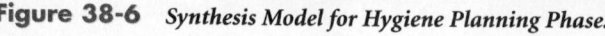

Figure 38-6   *Synthesis Model for Hygiene Planning Phase.*

to fit client limitations. In devising a plan that involves family members, the nurse tries to match the family's schedule of availability with client needs. It is also important to have the family member with whom the client is most comfortable routinely involved.

Various community resources may be needed by the nurse in planning hygienic care. For example, the nurse involved in the care of a homeless client may need to be aware of the location of clothing distribution centers for basic hygiene supplies or a shelter where bathing facilities are avail-

SAMPLE NURSING CARE PLAN

HYGIENIC CARE

ASSESSMENT*

Mrs. Wyatt is a 57-year-old who has had multiple sclerosis for 10 years. She was recently hospitalized for an acute exacerbation of the disease. The nurse, Jeannette, makes the initial home visit for Mrs. Wyatt. Jeannette's assessment reveals Mrs. Wyatt has reduced hearing, requiring Jeannette to speak clearly and to stand so Mrs. Wyatt can see her lip movements. Mrs. Wyatt is married, but her husband, Lon, works full time during the day. Her sister comes over periodically to help with her care and household chores. Mrs. Wyatt **has muscular weakness of both upper extremities,** making it **difficult for her to raise her arms above her shoulders.** She has some foot dragging and ataxia (unsteady gait) so **she bathes in a chair placed in front of the bathroom sink.** Recently her sister has assisted with bathing. With some spasticity in her right dominant arm, Mrs. Wyatt has **difficulty grasping objects.** Jeannette arranged her assessment in the morning to observe Mrs. Wyatt bathe. The **client had increased spasticity while bathing and became very fatigued after only about 5 minutes.** Mrs. Wyatt continues to be very independent in making decisions about her care. She tells Jeannette, "It is important for me to be able to bathe myself."

*Defining characteristics are shown in bold type.

NURSING DIAGNOSIS: Self-care deficit, bathing/hygiene related to muscle spasticity and fatigue.

PLANNING

GOALS	EXPECTED OUTCOMES
Client will be able to perform self-bathing without assistance within 1 month.	Client will experience decreased duration of muscle spasms within 2 weeks. Client will experience less fatigue during bathing activities within 1 month. Client will be able to grasp and manipulate bathing equipment.

INTERVENTIONS†	RATIONALE
Energy Management • Plan bathing at a time when client has most energy.	Will minimize occurrence of fatigue.
Self-Care Assistance • Set up bathing area (with assistance of husband or sister) so that all bathing equipment is at waist level, easy for client to reach.	Easy access to equipment will reduce muscle fatigue.
• Instruct client's sister to encourage client's independence and to intervene only when client is unable to bathe self.	Multiple sclerosis is a degenerative disease that progresses. Clients may have remissions along with exacerbations. An aim in therapy is to keep clients active and as independent as possible (Lewis, Collier, and Heitkemper, 1996).
• Confer with physical or occupational therapist about the appropriateness of assistive devices for client to use during bathing.	Decrements in the ability to perform gross motor function over time indicate need for adaptive devices and a modified environment to assist in control of symptoms and to make activities of daily living easier to perform (Gulick, 1998).
Exercise Promotion: Stretching • Perform stretching exercises prescribed by physical therapy every 6-8 hr.	Relieves spasms and contracted muscles (Lewis, Collier, and Heitkemper, 1996).

†Intervention Classification labels from McCloskey JC, Bulechek GM: *Nursing interventions classification (NIC),* ed 3, St. Louis, 2000, Mosby.

EVALUATION

Assess upper extremities' range of motion for presence of spasticity.

Ask client to report if fatigue is experienced during bathing.

Observe client bathing at bathroom sink.

able. Frequently the nurse will consult with social workers or staff in local area churches and schools to be sure clients have the resources they need to maintain hygiene.

IMPLEMENTATION

Providing hygiene is a very basic part of a client's care. The nurse learns to use caring practices that help to alleviate the client's anxiety and promote comfort and relaxation while performing each hygiene measure. For example, while giving a client a bath and changing a gown, the nurse uses a gentle approach in turning and repositioning. Using a soft, gentle voice while conversing with the client helps to relieve any fears or concerns. For clients suffering symptoms such as pain or nausea, administering symptom relief therapies prior to hygiene will better prepare the client for any procedure.

Another important part of implementation is assisting and preparing clients so that they are able to administer their own hygiene. This includes educating clients on proper hygienic techniques and connecting clients with the community resources necessary to enable them to perform hygienic care. The same clients at risk for hygiene problems are the ones in greatest need of understanding their risks, knowing the implications, and then having the information they need to make choices about when and how hygiene is performed.

Health Promotion.

In primary health care settings, nurses educate and counsel clients and families on proper hygiene techniques. A new mother will need assistance in learning how to bathe her newborn infant. An older adult will need to become informed on the importance of regular ear care to avoid any hearing deficits resulting from accumulated cerumen. The hygiene skills described throughout this chapter provide standards for excellent physical care. When assisting clients, the nurse tries to maintain these standards and incorporate adaptations as needed to the client's lifestyle, living arrangements, and preferences. Tips to help the nurse in educating clients about hygiene include the following:

- Make any instruction relevant. After assessing a client's knowledge, motivation, and health beliefs, provide information that relates to the client's situation and will be most useful in resolving the client's problem. For example, when offering foot care instruction to a client with diabetes mellitus, explain how the circulation to the feet can be impaired and how that poses a risk for poor healing and infection, especially when the skin becomes cut or broken.
- Adapt instruction of any techniques to the client's personal bathing facilities. Not all clients will have the ideal situation that exists in a health care setting (e.g., easily accessible shower or a bedside table to place over a bed). Use what facilities or equipment the client has so that personal care items are easy to reach,

the client's safety is ensured, and the client feels comfortable in performing hygiene. For example, a young mother may have more room and feel that bathing an infant will be safer if she uses her kitchen sink and counter rather than her bathroom sink.

- Be sure to teach the client steps to take to avoid injury. Almost any hygienic procedure can pose risks, (e.g., cutting a nail too close to the skin, failing to adjust the water temperature of the bath, or using tap water for contact lens care). Any instruction must clearly outline safety risks.
- Reinforce infection control practices. Damage to the skin, mucosa, eyes, or other tissues creates an immediate risk for infection. Be sure the client understands the relationship between healthy and intact skin and tissues and the prevention of infection.

The *Healthy People 2000* initiative (see Chapter 1) included recommendations to improve the dental health of the population of the United States. Currently the *Healthy People 2010* objectives are being developed through the cooperation of federal and state health agencies. The goals for oral health in *Healthy People 2000* were to decrease tooth loss caused by tooth decay or periodontal disease for people ages 35 to 44; reduce the number of older adults who have lost their natural teeth; reduce the prevalence of gingivitis; and reduce destructive periodontal disease among individuals ages 35 to 44. The nurse can play a very important role in this effort, particularly when caring for clients in rural settings, clients who are indigent, and older adults.

Acute and Restorative Care.

In health care settings where clients receive direct nursing care, nurses provide a variety of hygiene measures. Box 38-6, p. 1081 describes the different hygiene care schedules commonly found in acute care settings. Times may change because of factors affecting the nurse's organization or scheduling of care such as client preferences, planned diagnostic and treatment procedures, the client's need for more hygiene, or the nurse's work assignment. In extended care facilities and nursing homes, the schedule for hygiene may be less frequent.

Bathing and Skin Care.

Bathing and skin care are a part of total hygiene. The extent of a client's bath and the methods used for bathing depend on the client's physical abilities, health problems, and the degree of hygiene required. If a client is physically dependent or cognitively impaired, more attention must be given by the nurse in providing thorough, preventive skin care.

A **complete bed bath** is for clients who are totally dependent and require total hygiene care (Skill 38-1). It is an activity that can be exhausting for a client, even if the nurse provides all of the care. Turning during a complete bed bath and receiving back care have been shown to increase oxygen consumption in healthy men and women

Text continued on p. 1082.

Bathing a Client   Skill 38-1

Delegation Considerations

Skills of bathing may be delegated to assistive personnel.

- Inform caregiver about early signs of impaired skin integrity, and tell caregiver to have nurse reassess the skin when changes are noted.

- Warn against massaging reddened areas.
- Review type of bath, client's ability to participate, and any safety precautions needed.

EQUIPMENT

- Two washcloths
- Two bath towels
- Bath blanket
- Soap and soap dish

- Toiletry items (deodorant, powder, lotion, cologne)
- Clean hospital gown or client's own pajamas or gown
- Laundry bag
- Disposable gloves (when risk for contacting body fluids)

STEPS	RATIONALE
1. Assess client's tolerance for activity, discomfort level, cognitive ability, and musculoskeletal function.	Determines client's ability to perform self-care and level of assistance required from nurse. Also determines type of bath to administer (e.g., tub bath or partial bed bath).
2. Review orders for specific precautions concerning client's movement or positioning.	Prevents accidental injury to client during bathing activities. Determine level of assistance required by client.
3. Explain procedure, and ask client for suggestions on how to prepare supplies. If partial bath, ask how much of bath client wishes to complete.	Promotes client's cooperation and participation.
3. Adjust room temperature and ventilation, close room doors and windows, and draw room divider curtain.	Warm room that is free of drafts prevents rapid loss of body heat during bathing. Privacy ensures client's mental and physical comfort.
5. Prepare equipment and supplies.	Avoids interrupting procedure or leaving client unattended to retrieve missing equipment.
6. Bathe client.	
A. Complete or partial bed bath	
(1) Offer client bedpan or urinal. Provide towel and washcloth.	Client will feel more comfortable after voiding. Prevents interruption of bath.
(2) Wash hands. If client's skin is soiled with drainage or body secretions, apply disposable gloves. Ensure client is not allergic to latex.	Reduces transmission of microorganisms.
(3) Lower side rail closest to you, and assist client in assuming comfortable position, maintaining body alignment. Bring client toward side closest to nurse. Place hospital bed in high position.	Aids nurse's access to client. Maintains client's comfort throughout procedure. Nurse does not have to reach across bed, thus minimizing strain on back muscles.
(4) Loosen top covers at foot of bed. Place bath blanket over top sheet. Fold and remove top sheet from under blanket. If possible, have client hold bath blanket while withdrawing sheet. Optional: Use top sheet when bath blanket is not available.	Removal of top linens prevents them from becoming soiled or moist during bath. Blanket provides warmth and privacy.
(5) If top sheet is to be reused, fold it for replacement later. If not, dispose in laundry bag, taking care not to allow linen to contact uniform.	Proper disposal prevents transmission of microorganisms.
(6) Remove client's gown or pajamas. If an extremity is injured or has reduced mobility, begin removal from *unaffected* side. If client has intravenous (IV) tube, remove gown from arm *without* IV first; then lower IV container or remove from pump and slide gown covering affected arm over tubing and container. Rehang IV container and check flow rate (see illustrations) or reset pump rate. Do not disconnect tubing.	Provides full exposure of body parts during bathing. Undressing unaffected side first allows easier manipulation of gown over body part with reduced range of motion (ROM).

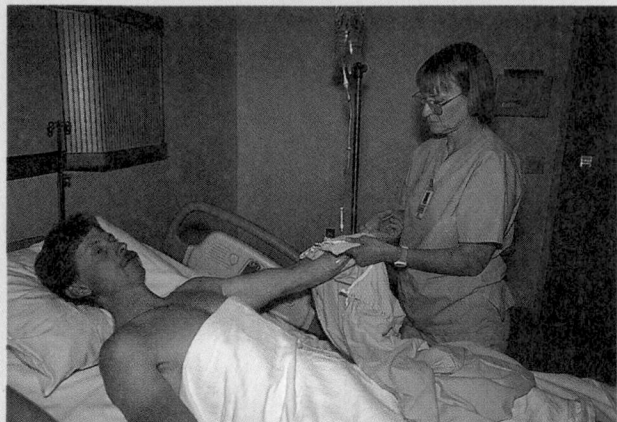
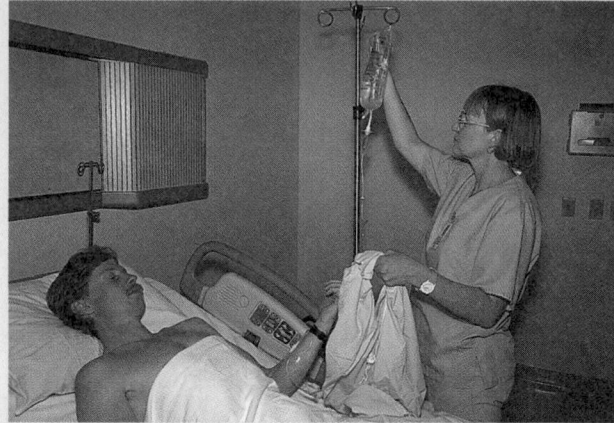
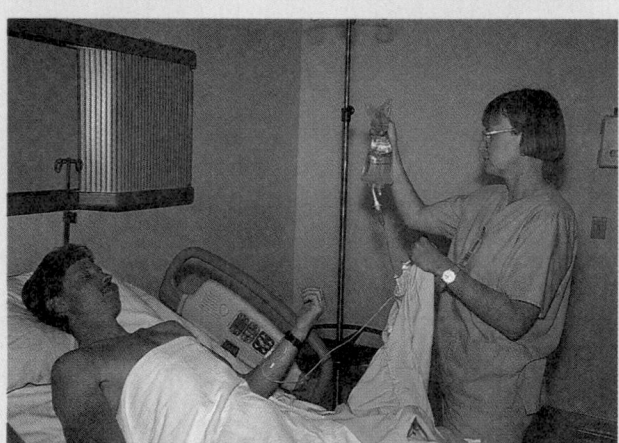
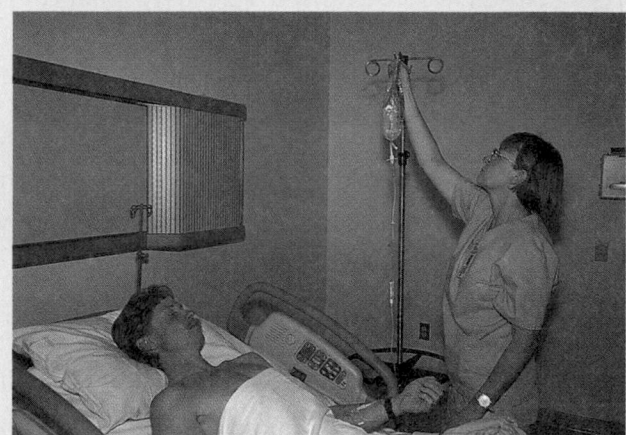

Step 6A(6)

(7)   Pull side rail up. Fill washbasin two thirds full, with warm water. Have client place fingers in water to test temperature tolerance. Place plastic container of bath lotion in bath water to warm, if desired.

Raising side rail maintains client's safety as nurse leaves bedside. Warm water promotes comfort, relaxes muscles, and prevents unnecessary chilling. Testing temperature prevents accidental burns. Bath water warms lotion for application to client's skin.

(8)   Remove pillow if allowed, and raise head of bed 30 to 45 degrees. Place bath towel under client's head. Place second bath towel over client's chest.

Removal of pillow makes it easier to wash client's ears and neck. Placement of towels prevents soiling of bed linen and bath blanket.

(9)   Fold washcloth around fingers of nurse's hand to form mitt (see illustration). Immerse mitt in water and wring thoroughly.

Mitt retains water and heat better than loosely held washcloth; keeps cold edges from brushing against client and prevents splashing.

(10)   Wash client's eyes with plain warm water. Inquire if client is wearing contact lenses. If so, perform eye care as described in Skill 38-7. Use different section of mitt for each eye. Move mitt from inner to outer canthus (see illustration). Soak any crusts on eyelid for 2 to 3 min with damp cloth before attempting removal. Dry eye thoroughly but gently.

Soap irritates eyes. Use of separate sections of mitt reduces infection transmission. Bathing eye from inner to outer canthus prevents secretions from entering nasolacrimal duct. Pressure can cause internal injury.

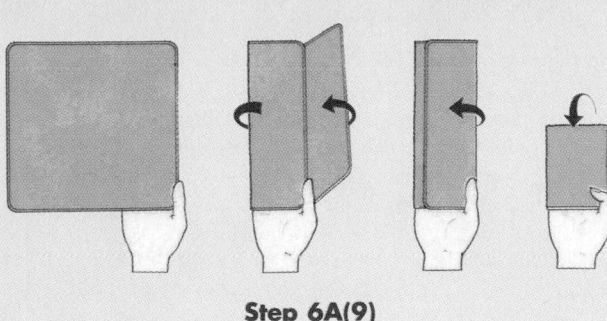

Step 6A(9)

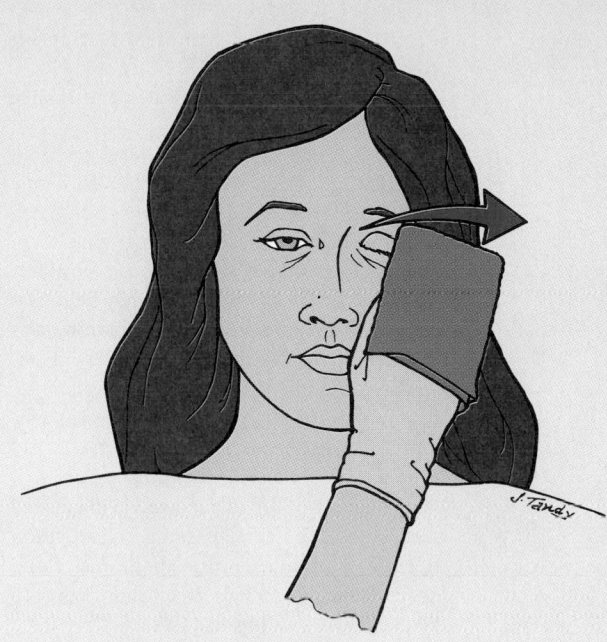

Step 6A(10)

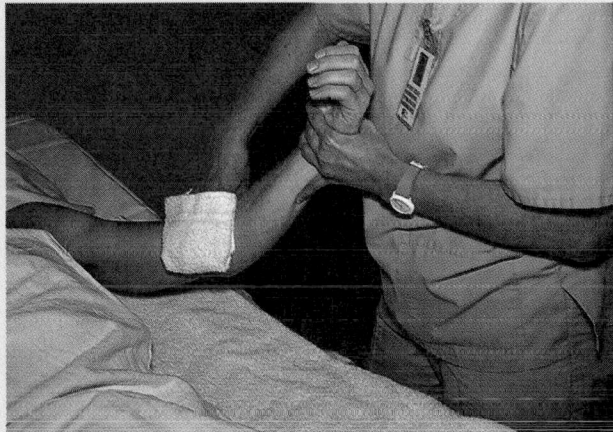

Step 6A(13)

(11) Ask if client prefers to use soap on face. Wash, rinse, and dry well forehead, cheeks, nose, neck, and ears. (Men may wish to shave at this point or after bath.)

Soap tends to dry face, which is exposed to air more than other body parts.

(12) Remove bath blanket from client's arm that is closest to nurse. Place bath towel lengthwise under arm.

Prevents soiling of bed.

(13) Bathe arm with soap and water using long, firm strokes from distal to proximal areas (fingers to axilla). Raise and support arm as needed while thoroughly washing axilla (see illustration).

Soap lowers surface tension and facilitates removal of debris and bacteria when friction is applied during washing. Long, firm strokes stimulate circulation. Movement of arm exposes axilla and exercises joint's normal ROM.

(14) Rinse and dry arm and axilla thoroughly. If client uses deodorant or talcum powder, apply it.

Alkaline residue from soap discourages growth of normal skin bacteria (Barnes, 1987). Excess moisture causes skin maceration or softening. Deodorant controls body odor.

(15) Fold bath towel in half, and lay it on bed beside client. Place basin on towel. Immerse client's hand in water. Allow hand to soak for 3 to 5 min before washing hand and fingernails (see Skill 38-4). Remove basin and dry hand well.

Soaking softens cuticles and calluses of hand, loosens debris beneath nails, and enhances feeling of cleanliness. Thorough drying removes moisture from between fingers.

STEPS	RATIONALE
(16) Raise side rail, and move to other side of bed. Lower side rail, and repeat Steps 12 through 15 for other arm.	
(17) Check temperature of bath water, and change water if necessary.	Warm water maintains client's comfort.
(18) Cover client's chest with bath towel, and fold bath blanket down to umbilicus. With one hand, lift edge of towel away from chest. With mitted hand, bathe chest using long, firm strokes. Take special care to wash skinfolds under female client's breasts. It may be necessary to lift breast upward while bathing underneath it. Keep client's chest covered between wash and rinse periods. Dry well.	Draping prevents unnecessary exposure of body parts. Towel maintains warmth and privacy. Secretions and dirt collect easily in areas of tight skinfolds. Skinfolds are susceptible to excoriation if breasts are pendulous.
(19) Place bath towel lengthwise over chest and abdomen. (Two towels may be needed.) Fold blanket down to just above pubic region.	Prevents chilling and exposure of body parts.
(20) With one hand, lift bath towel. With mitted hand, bathe abdomen, giving special attention to bathing umbilicus and abdominal folds. Stroke from side to side. Keep abdomen covered between washing and rinsing. Dry well.	Moisture and sediment that collect in skinfolds predispose skin to maceration and irritation.
(21) Apply clean gown or pajama top. If one extremity is injured or immobilized, always dress affected side first. This step may be omitted until completion of bath; gown should not become soiled during remainder of bath.	Maintains client's warmth and comfort. Dressing affected side first allows easier manipulation of gown over body part with reduced ROM.
(22) Cover chest and abdomen with top of bath blanket. Expose near leg by folding blanket toward midline. Be sure perineum is draped.	Prevents unnecessary exposure.
(23) Bend client's leg at knee by positioning nurse's arm under leg. While grasping client's heel, elevate leg from mattress slightly, and slide bath towel lengthwise under leg. Ask client to hold foot still. Place bath basin on towel on bed, and secure its position next to foot to be washed.	Towel prevents soiling of bed linen. Support of joint and extremity during lifting prevents strain on musculoskeletal structures. Sudden movement by client could spill bath water. (Omit this step if client is unable to hold leg in basin.)
(24) With one hand supporting lower leg, raise it and slide basin under lifted foot. Make sure foot is firmly placed on bottom of basin. Allow foot to soak while washing leg. If client is unable to hold leg, do not immerse; simply wash with washcloth (see illustration).	Proper positioning of foot prevents pressure being applied from edge of basin against calf. Soaking softens calluses and rough skin.
(25) Unless contraindicated, use long, firm strokes in washing from ankle to knee and from knee to thigh. Dry well.	Promotes venous return.

Critical Decision Point: Clients with history of deep vein thromboses or hypercoagulation disorders should not have their lower extremities washed with long firm strokes.

(26) Cleanse foot, making sure to bathe between toes. Clean and clip nails as needed (see Skill 38-4). Dry well. If skin is dry, apply lotion. Do not massage any reddened area on client's skin.	Secretions and moisture may be present between toes. Lotion helps retain moisture and soften skin.

STEPS | RATIONALE

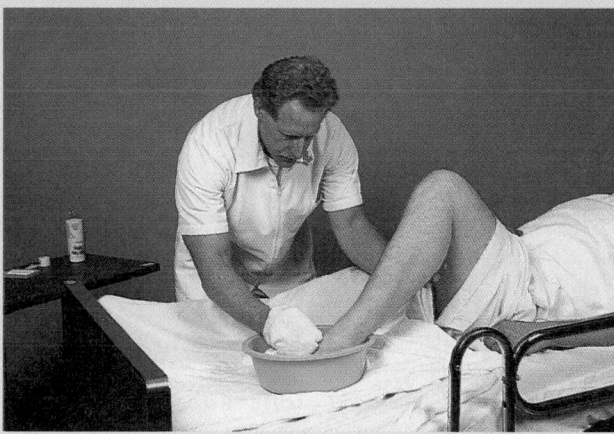

Step 6A(24)

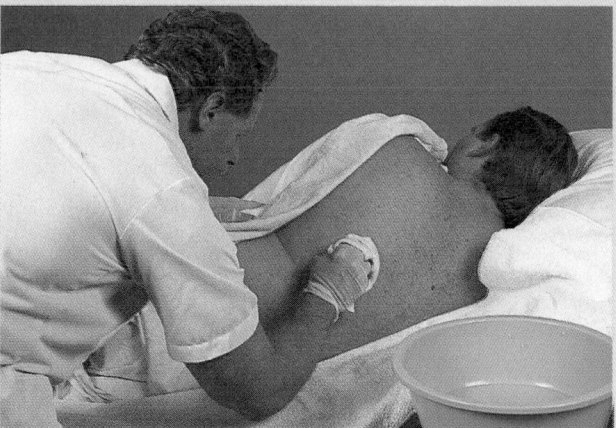

Step 6A(30)

(27) Raise side rail, and move to other side of the bed. Lower side rail, and repeat steps 22 through 26 for other leg and foot.

(28) Cover client with bath blanket, raise side rail for client's safety, and change bath water. — Decreased bath water temperature can cause chilling. Clean water reduces microorganism transmission.

(29) Lower side rail. Assist client in assuming prone or side-lying position (as applicable). Place towel lengthwise along client's side. — Exposes back and buttocks for bathing.

(30) Keep client draped by sliding bath blanket over shoulders and thighs. Wash, rinse, and dry back from neck to buttocks using long, firm strokes (see illustration). Pay special attention to folds of buttocks and anus. Give a back rub (see Skill 38-3). Change bath water. — Maintains warmth, and prevents unnecessary exposure. Skinfolds near buttocks and anus may contain fecal secretions that harbor microorganisms.
Changing water prevents transfer of microorganisms from anal area to genitalia.

(31) Apply disposable gloves if not done previously. — Prevents contact with microorganisms in body secretions.

(32) Assist client in assuming side-lying or supine position. Cover chest and upper extremities with towel and lower extremities with bath blanket. Expose only genitalia. (If client can wash, covering entire body with bath blanket may be preferable.) Wash, rinse, and dry perineum (see Skill 38-2). Pay special attention to skin-folds. Apply water-repellent ointment to area exposed to moisture. — Maintains client's privacy. Clients capable of performing partial bath usually prefer to wash their own genitalia. Water-repellent ointments (e.g., A & D, Pericare) protect skin from moisture.

(33) Dispose of gloves in receptacle. — Prevents transmission of infection.

(34) Apply additional body lotion or oil as desired. — Moisturizing lotion prevents dry, chapped skin.

(35) Assist client in dressing. Comb client's hair. Women may want to apply makeup. — Promotes client's body image.

(36) Make client's bed (see Skill 38-8). — Provides clean environment.

(37) Remove soiled linen, and place in dirty-linen bag. Clean and replace bathing equipment. Replace call light and personal possessions. Leave room as clean and comfortable as possible. — Prevents transmission of infection. Clean environment promotes client's comfort. Keeping call light and articles of care within reach promotes client's safety.

(38) Wash hands. — Reduces transmission of microorganisms.

STEPS	RATIONALE
B. **Tub or whirlpool bath or shower**	
(1) Consider client's condition, and review orders for precautions concerning client's movement or positioning.	Prevents accidental injury to client during bathing.
(2) Check tub or shower for cleanliness. Use cleaning techniques outlined in agency policy. Place rubber mat on tub or shower bottom. Place disposable bath mat or towel on floor in front of tub or shower.	Cleaning prevents transmission of microorganisms. Mats prevent slipping and falling.
(3) Collect all hygienic aids, toiletry items, and linens requested by client. Place within easy reach of tub or shower.	Placing items close at hand prevents possible falls when client reaches for equipment.
(4) Assist client to bathroom if necessary. Have client wear robe and slippers to bathroom.	Assistance prevents accidental falls. Wearing robe and slippers prevents chilling.
(5) Demonstrate how to use call signal for assistance.	Bathrooms are equipped with signaling devices in case client feels faint or weak or needs immediate assistance. Clients prefer privacy during bath if safety is not jeopardized.
(6) Place "occupied" sign on bathroom door.	Maintains client's privacy.
(7) Provide shower seat or tub chair if needed (see illustration). Fill bathtub halfway with warm water. If sensation is normal, ask client to test water, and adjust temperature if water is too warm. Explain which faucet controls hot water. If client is taking shower, turn shower on, and adjust water temperature before client enters shower stall.	Adjusting water temperature prevents accidental burns. Older adults and clients with neurological alterations (e.g., spinal cord injury) are at high risk for burns as a result of reduced sensation. Use of assistive devices facilitates bathing and minimizes physical exertion.
(8) Instruct client to use safety bars when getting in and out of tub or shower. Caution client against use of bath oil in tub water.	Prevents slipping and falling. Oil causes tub surfaces to become slippery.
(9) Instruct client not to remain in tub longer than 20 min. Check on client every 5 min.	Prolonged exposure to warm water may cause vasodilation and pooling of blood, leading to lightheadedness or dizziness.
(10) Return to bathroom when client signals, and knock before entering.	Provides privacy.
(11) For client who is unsteady, drain tub of water before client attempts to get out of it. Place bath towel over client's shoulders. Assist client in getting out of tub as needed, and assist with drying. If client is weak or unstable, have assistive personnel assist.	Prevents accidental falls. Client may become chilled as water drains.

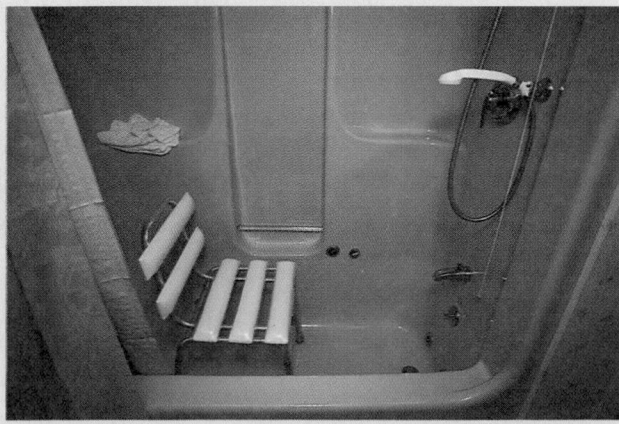

Step 6B(7)

STEPS	RATIONALE
(12) Assist client as needed in donning clean gown or pajamas, slippers, and robe. (In home setting, client may don regular clothing.)	Maintains warmth to prevent chilling.
(13) Assist client to room and comfortable position in bed or chair.	Maintains relaxation gained from bathing.
(14) Clean tub or shower according to agency policy. Whirlpool baths may require special cleansing. Remove soiled linen and place in dirty-linen bag. Discard disposable equipment in proper receptacle. Place "unoccupied" sign on bathroom door. Return supplies to storage area.	Prevents transmission of infection through soiled linen and moisture.
(15) Wash hands.	Reduces transfer of microorganisms.
7. Observe skin, paying particular attention to areas that were previously soiled, reddened, or showed early signs of breakdown.	Techniques used during bathing should leave skin clean and clear.
8. Observe ROM during bath.	Measures joint mobility.
9. Ask client to rate level of comfort.	

Recording and Reporting

- Record bath on flow sheet. Note level of assistance required.
- Record condition of skin and any significant findings (e.g., reddened areas, bruises, nevi, or joint or muscle pain).
- Report evidence of alterations in skin integrity to nurse in charge or physician.

Home Care Considerations

- Assess client's tub and shower area for need for adaptive devices, such as grab bars, shower chair, or handheld shower.

Hygiene Care Schedule in Acute and Long-Term Care Settings   Box 38-6

EARLY MORNING CARE

Nursing personnel on the night shift provide basic hygiene to clients getting ready for breakfast, scheduled tests, or early morning surgery. "AM care" includes offering a bedpan or urinal if the client is not ambulatory, washing the client's hands and face, and assisting with oral care.

MORNING, OR AFTER-BREAKFAST, CARE

In care performed after breakfast, the nurse assists by offering a bedpan or urinal to clients confined to bed; providing a bath or shower; providing oral, foot, nail, and hair care; giving a back rub, changing the client's gown or pajamas; changing the bed linens; and straightening the client's bedside unit and room. This is often referred to as "complete AM care."

AFTERNOON CARE

Hospitalized clients often undergo many exhausting diagnostic tests or procedures in the morning. In rehabilitation centers, clients may participate in physical therapy during the morning. Afternoon hygiene care includes washing the hands and face, assisting with oral care, offering a bedpan or urinal, and straightening bed linen.

EVENING, OR HOUR-BEFORE-SLEEP, CARE

Before bedtime the nurse offers personal hygiene care that helps a client relax to promote sleep. "PM care" may include changing soiled bed linens, gowns, or pajamas; assisting the client in washing the face and hands; providing oral hygiene; giving a back massage; and offering the bedpan or urinal to nonambulatory clients. Some clients may enjoy a beverage such as juice.

Research HIGHLIGHT   **Box 38-7**

RESEARCH ABSTRACT

Before studying the effects nursing interventions have on the oxygen requirements of critically ill clients, Verderber and Gallagher (1994) first investigated healthy men and women. A convenience sample of 30 healthy men and women were randomly assigned to one of three groups. Each group received the nursing interventions of bathing, passive range-of-motion exercises, and turning; however, the order of the interventions differed by group. Each subject's oxygen consumption was measured before (baseline) and during the nursing interventions. The average oxygen consumption for both men and women was significantly higher than baseline during unassisted turning and back care. Men had a significantly higher average oxygen consumption than women. Changes in oxygen consumption were not significant during passive range-of-motion exercises or the anterior portion of the bath. The order of interventions did not have any appreciable effect on oxygen consumption.

IMPLICATIONS FOR PRACTICE

- This study suggests that since turning and back care can increase oxygen consumption in healthy individuals, clients with physical limitations may be at even greater risk.
- Prior to and during bathing activities monitor for changes in client's heart rate and breathing pattern.

REFERENCE

Verderber A, Gallagher KJ: Effects of bathing, passive range-of-motion exercises, and turning on oxygen consumption in healthy men and women, *Am J Crit Care* 3:374, 1994.

(Verderber and Gallagher, 1994) (Box 38-7). The nurse must anticipate and assess whether clients are physically able to tolerate a complete bath. Measuring heart rate before, during, and after the bath provides a measure of the client's physical tolerance. A **partial bed bath** involves bathing only body parts that would cause discomfort or odor if left unbathed. Aging or dependent clients in need of only partial hygiene or self-sufficient bedridden clients unable to reach all body parts receive partial bed baths. Nurses assess carefully to determine that clients can sufficiently bathe other body parts on their own.

When administering either a complete or partial bath, it is important for the nurse to assess of the condition of the skin in determining if soap is necessary or if the client requires daily bathing. Clients with excessively dry skin are predisposed to skin impairment. The nurse may decide to skip a bath for a day or bathe only badly soiled areas. Use of soaps that contain emollients is another option. Lubricating the skin with lotion can also help reduce dryness.

The tub bath or shower can be used to give a more thorough bath than a bed bath. Safety is of primary concern because the surface of a tub or shower stall is slippery. In some agencies, showers are equipped with a chair for clients with weakness or poor balance. Both tubs and showers should be equipped with grab bars for clients to hold on to during entry and exit and maneuvering. Clients vary in how much help they will need. Regardless of the type of bath the client receives, the nurse should use the following guidelines:

- *Provide privacy.* Close the door, or pull room curtains around the bathing area. While bathing the client, expose only the areas being bathed.
- *Maintain safety.* Keep side rails up while away from the client's bedside. (This is critical for dependent and unconscious clients.) Place the call light in the client's reach if leaving the room temporarily.
- *Maintain warmth.* The room should be kept warm because the client is partially uncovered and may easily be chilled. Wet skin causes an excess loss of heat through convection. Control drafts, and keep windows closed. Keep client covered, only exposing the body part being washed during the bath.
- *Promote independence.* Encourage the client to participate in as much of the bathing activities as possible. Offer assistance when needed.
- *Anticipate needs.* Bring a new set of clothing and hygiene products to the bedside or bathroom.

Bag Baths.   An innovative approach to the traditional bed bath was developed because of nurses' concern for clients who are predisposed to dry skin and the risk for infection. When washbasins are not cleaned and dried completely after use, there is the risk of contamination by gram-negative organisms (Gooch, 1989). Successive uses of the basin may cause the client's skin to harbor more gram-negative organisms (Skewes, 1994). The "bag bath" is a specially prepared package containing 10 washcloths that are premoistened in a mixture of water and a non-rinsable cleanser. A bag is warmed in a microwave before use, and then the nurse uses a different cloth for each part of the client's body. In this technique the skin is allowed to air dry, since towel drying removes the emollient that is left behind after the water/cleanser solution evaporates. Staff who have used the bag bath report shorter bathing times and client and nurse satisfaction (Skewes, 1994).

Perineal Care.   **Perineal care** is usually part of the complete bed bath (Skill 38-2). Clients most in need of perineal care are those at greatest risk for acquiring an infection (e.g., uncircumcised males, clients who have indwelling urinary catheters, or clients who are recovering from rectal or genital surgery or childbirth). In addition, women who are having a menstrual period will require good perineal care. A client able to perform self-care should be allowed to do so. Nurses can become embarrassed about providing perineal care, particularly to clients of the opposite sex. Similarly the client usually feels embarrassed. This should not cause the nurse to overlook the client's hygiene needs. It may help to have a nurse of

Perineal Care   Skill 38-2

Delegation Considerations

Skills of perineal care can be delegated to assistive personnel.

- Inform and assist caregiver in proper way to position male and female clients.
- Inform caregiver about proper positioning of indwelling catheter during perineal care.

- Instruct caregiver to inform nurse if any perineal drainage, excoriation, or rash is observed.

EQUIPMENT

- Washbasin
- Soap dish with soap
- Two or three washcloths
- Bath towel
- Bath blanket
- Waterproof pad or bedpan
- Toilet tissue or diaper wipes
- Disposable gloves

Additional supplies are needed when pericare is given other than during a bath:

- Cotton balls or swabs
- A solution bottle or container filled with warm water or prescribed rinsing solution
- Waterproof bag

STEPS	RATIONALE
1. Identify clients at risk for developing infection of genitalia, urinary tract, or reproductive tract (e.g., uncircumcised male, presence of indwelling catheter, fecal incontinence).	Secretions that accumulate on surface of skin surrounding female and male genitalia act as reservoir for infection. Tissues traumatized by surgery or by presence of foreign object provide route for introduction of infectious organisms.
2. Assess client's cognitive and musculoskeletal function.	Determines client's ability to perform self care and determines level of assistance required from nurse.
3. Assess genitalia for signs of inflammation, skin breakdown, or infection (see Chapter 32).	Determines extent of perineal care required by client.
4. Assess client's knowledge of importance of perineal hygiene.	Clients at risk for infection in perineal area may be unaware of importance of cleanliness. Reflects client's need for education.
5. Explain procedure and its purpose to client.	Helps minimize anxiety during procedure that is often embarrassing to nurse and client.
6. Prepare necessary equipment and supplies.	Used when administering a bed bath.
7. Pull curtain around client's bed, or close room door. Assemble supplies at bedside.	Maintains client's privacy and ensures orderly procedure.
8. Raise bed to comfortable working position. Lower side rail, and assist client in assuming side-lying position, placing towel lengthwise along client's side and keeping client covered with bath blanket or top sheet.	Facilitates good body mechanics. Provides easy access to genitalia.
9. Apply disposable gloves.	Eliminates transmission of microorganisms.
10. If fecal material is present, enclose in a fold of underpad or toilet tissue, and remove with disposable wipes or tissue. Cleanse buttocks and anus, washing front to back (see illustration). Cleanse, rinse, and dry area thoroughly. If needed, place an absorbent pad under client's buttocks. Remove and discard underpad, and replace with clean one.	Cleansing reduces transmission of microorganisms from anus to urethra or genitalia.

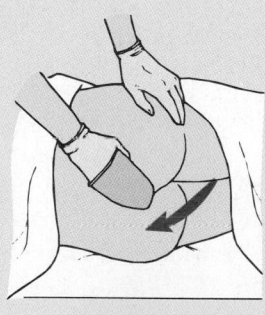

Step 10

STEPS	RATIONALE
11. Change gloves when they are soiled.	
12. Fold top bed linen down toward foot of bed, and raise client's gown above genital area.	Exposes perineal area for easy accessibility.
a. "Diamond" drape client by placing bath blanket with one corner between client's legs, one corner pointing toward each side of bed, and one corner over client's chest. Tuck side corners around client's legs and under hips.	Prevents unnecessary exposure of body parts and maintains client's warmth and comfort during procedure.
b. Raise side rail. Fill washbasin with warm water.	Prevents client from falling. Proper water temperature prevents burns to perineum.
c. Place washbasin and toilet tissue on overbed table. Place washcloths in basin.	Equipment placed within nurse's reach prevents accidental spills.
13. Provide perineal care.	
A. **Female perineal care**	
(1) Assist client to dorsal recumbent position.	Provides easy access to genitalia.
(2) Lower side rail, and help client flex knees and spread legs. Note restrictions or limitations in client's positioning.	Provides full exposure of female genitalia. Minimize degree of abduction in female if position causes pain because of arthritis or reduced joint mobility.
(3) Fold lower corner of bath blanket up between client's legs onto abdomen. Wash and dry client's upper thighs.	Minimizes transmission of microorganisms. Keeping client draped until procedure begins minimizes anxiety. Buildup of perineal secretions can soil surrounding skin surfaces.
(4) Wash labia majora. Use nondominant hand to gently retract labia from thigh; with dominant hand, wash carefully in skinfolds. Wipe in direction from perineum to rectum (front to back). Repeat on opposite side using separate section of washcloth. Rinse and dry area thoroughly.	Skinfolds may contain body secretions that harbor microorganisms. Wiping from perineum to rectum (front to back) reduces chance of transmitting fecal organisms to urinary meatus.
(5) Separate labia with nondominant hand to expose urethral meatus and vaginal orifice. With dominant hand, wash downward from pubic area toward rectum in one smooth stroke (see illustration). Use separate section of cloth for each stroke. Cleanse thoroughly around labia minora, clitoris, and vaginal orifice.	Cleansing method reduces transfer of microorganisms to urinary meatus. (For menstruating women or clients with indwelling urinary catheters, cleanse with cotton balls.)
(6) If client uses bedpan, pour warm water over perineal area. Dry perineal area thoroughly, using front-to-back method.	Rinsing removes soap and microorganisms more effectively than wiping. Retained moisture harbors microorganisms.
(7) Fold lower corner of bath blanket back between client's legs and over perineum. Ask client to lower legs and assume comfortable position.	

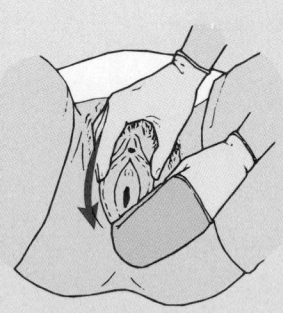

Step 13A(5)

STEPS	RATIONALE

B. **Male perineal care**

(1)   Lower side rails, and assist client to supine position. Note restriction in mobility.

Provides full exposure of male genitalia.

(2)   Fold top half of bath blanket down below the penis. Allow gown to cover chest. Wash and dry client's upper thighs.

Minimizes transmission of microorganisms. Keeping client draped until procedure begins minimizes anxiety. Buildup of perineal secretions can soil surrounding skin surfaces.

Towel prevents moisture from collecting in inguinal area. Gentle but firm handling reduces chance of client having an erection. Secretions capable of harboring microorganisms collect underneath foreskin.

(3)   Gently raise penis, and place bath towel underneath. Gently grasp shaft of penis. If client is uncircumcised, retract foreskin (see illustration). If client has an erection, defer procedure until later.

(4)   Wash tip of penis at urethral meatus first. Using circular motion, cleanse from meatus outward (see illustration). Discard washcloth, and repeat with clean cloth until penis is clean. Rinse and dry gently.

Direction of cleansing moves from area of least contamination to area of most contamination, preventing microorganisms from entering urethra.

(5)   Return foreskin to its natural position.

Tightening of foreskin around shaft of penis can cause local edema and discomfort.

(6)   Wash shaft of penis with gentle but firm downward strokes. Pay special attention to underlying surface of penis. Rinse and dry penis thoroughly. Instruct client to spread legs apart slightly.

Vigorous massage of penis can lead to erection, which can embarrass client and nurse. Underlying surface of penis may have greater accumulation of secretions. Abduction of legs provides easier access to scrotal tissues.

(7)   Gently cleanse scrotum. Lift it carefully, and wash underlying skinfolds. Rinse and dry.

Pressure on scrotal tissues can be painful to client. Secretions collect between skinfolds.

(8)   Fold bath blanket back over client's perineum, and assist client in turning to side-lying position.

Draping promotes comfort and minimizes client's anxiety. Side-lying position provides access to anal area.

14.   If client has had urinary or bowel incontinence, apply thin layer of skin barrier containing petrolatum or zinc oxide over anal and perineal skin.

Protects skin from excess moisture and toxins from urine or stool (Makelbust, 1991).

15.   Remove disposable gloves, and dispose in proper receptacle.

Moisture and body secretions on gloves can harbor microorganisms.

16.   Assist client in assuming a comfortable position, and cover with sheet.

Client's comfort helps to minimize stress of procedure.

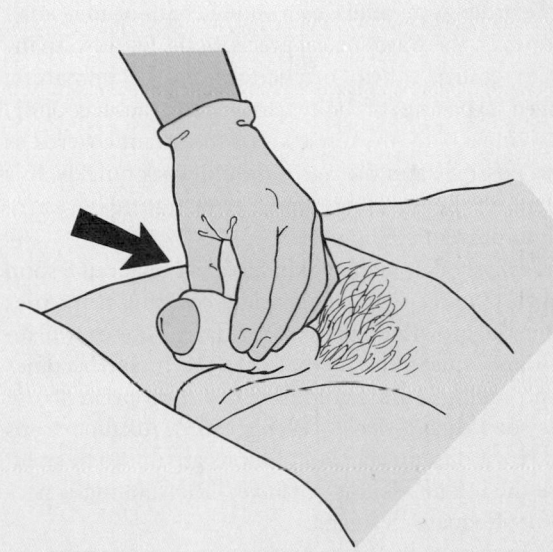

Step 13B(3)

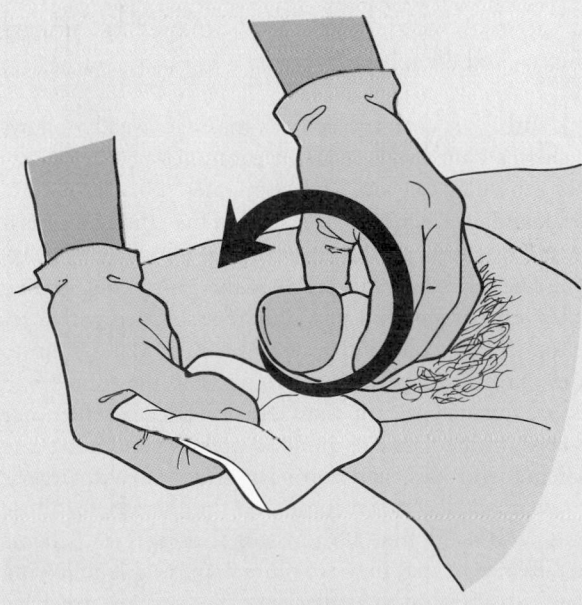

Step 13B(4)

STEPS	RATIONALE
17. Remove bath blanket, and dispose of all soiled bed linen. Return unused equipment to storage area.	Reduces transmission of microorganisms.
18. Inspect surface of external genitalia and surrounding skin after cleansing.	Thick secretions may cover underlying skin lesions or areas of breakdown. Evaluation determines need for additional hygiene.
19. Ask if client feels sense of cleanliness.	Evaluates client's comfort level.
20. Observe for abnormal drainage or discharge from genitalia.	Evaluates presence of infection.

Recording and Reporting

- Record procedure and presence of any abnormal findings (e.g., character and amount of discharge or condition of genitalia).
- Record appearance of suture line, if present.
- Report any break in suture line or presence of abnormalities to nurse in charge or physician.

Home Care Considerations

- For clients who require bathing, assess perineum at every visit because of the risk for infection and skin breakdown. When appropriate, teach caregiver how to make this assessment, and instruct caregiver to do this assessment daily.

the opposite sex present in the room when providing perineal care. A professional, dignified, and sensitive approach can reduce embarrassment and put the client at ease.

If a client performs self-care, various problems such as vaginal and urethral discharge, skin irritation, and unpleasant odors may go unnoticed. The nurse must be alert for complaints of burning during urination or localized soreness, excoriation, or pain in the perineum. The nurse also inspects the client's bed linen for signs of discharge. Clients most at risk for skin breakdown in the perineal area are those with urinary or fecal incontinence, rectal and perineal surgical dressings, indwelling urinary catheters, and the morbidly obese.

Back Rub.   A back rub or back massage usually follows the client's bath (Skill 38-3). It promotes relaxation, relieves muscular tension, and stimulates skin circulation. Labyak and Metzger (1997) evaluated the efficacy of massage and its effects on the physiological measures of relaxation. Their analysis showed that the long, slow, gliding strokes (**effleurage**) of a massage are associated with a reduction in heart rate and respiratory rate. Males seem to achieve greater reductions in systolic and diastolic blood pressure during back rub than females. Because effleurage causes an immediate rise in blood pressure and heart rate in clients who have had coronary artery bypass surgery, the researchers do not recommend the therapy for those clients within the first 48 hours of their surgery. Clients generally report that they are more comfortable following a back rub and find the experience pleasant, regardless of the length of the massage. However, a back rub of 3 min-

utes' duration can actually enhance client comfort and relaxation and thus be very therapeutic (Labyak and Metzger, 1997).

When providing a back rub, the nurse can enhance relaxation by reducing any noise and ensuring the client is comfortable. It is important to ask whether a client would like a back rub, or if the client prefers gentle instead of heavy massage, because some individuals dislike physical contact. The nurse should consult the medical record for any contraindications to a massage (e.g., fractured ribs, burns of the skin, and heart surgery).

Bathing an Infant.   An infant can be bathed in much the same order as an adult, by a sponge bath or in a small tub. However, there are special precautions. Because an infant's temperature control mechanisms are still immature, prolonged exposure of body parts may cause cooling. When giving a bath, the nurse keeps the infant covered as much as possible, and the nurse should work quickly. It is important to be sure the water temperature is warm enough to prevent chilling.

The surface of an infant's skin has a pH of about 5 soon after birth (Wong, 1995). This acidic covering helps prevent bacterial growth on the skin's surface. Thus only plain warm water is used for the bath. As the infant becomes older and soiling is more common, it is appropriate to use a gentle soap such as Dove (Wong, 1995). Alkaline soaps such as Ivory, oils, powder, and lotions are not to be used. Because the infant's skin is sensitive, little rubbing is necessary for adequate cleansing.

The nurse gives the bath in a head-to-toe direction using a clean washcloth. First the nurse washes the face, eyes,

Administering a Back Rub | Skill 38-3

Delegation Considerations

The skill of administering a back rub can be delegated to assistive personnel.

- Registered professional nurse (RN) should assess for any possible contraindication to back rub.

- Inform caregiver to report any change in vital signs or client behavior during back rub.

EQUIPMENT

- Moisturizing lotion or lubricant
- Sphygomomanometer and stethoscope

- Bath towel
- Bath blanket

STEPS	RATIONALE
1. Identify factors or conditions such as rib or vertebral fractures, burns, reddened areas on the skin, or open wounds and status post-coronary artery bypass (CAB), that contraindicate backrub.	Massage of sensitive tissues might lead to further tissue injury. Massaging reddened areas of skin increases breaks in capillaries in underlying tissues (AHCPR, 1992). An increase in heart rate and systolic and diastolic blood pressure occurs in post-CAB (Labyak and Metzger, 1997).
2. Explain procedure and desired position to client. • Determine if client is comfortable with heavy massage stroke.	Helps promote relaxation.
3. Adjust bed to high, comfortable position.	Ensures proper body mechanics and prevents strain on back muscles.
4. Adjust light, temperature, and sound within room.	Environmental distractions can prevent client from relaxing.
5. Lower side rail and help client assume prone or side-lying (Sims') position with back toward you. Close curtain around bed.	Position makes it easier to apply necessary pressure to back muscles. Privacy promotes relaxation.
6. Assess client's heart rate (HR), respiratory rate (RR) and blood pressure.	Three-minute effleurage back rubs result in a decline in HR, RR, systolic and diastolic blood pressure. Assessment establishes baseline (Labyak and Metzger, 1997).
7. Expose client's back, shoulders, upper arms, and buttocks. Cover remainder of body with bath blanket. Lay towel alongside client's back.	Prevents unnecessary exposure of body parts and prevents excess lotion from touching linens.
8. Wash your hands in warm water. Warm lotion in your hands or by placing container under warm water. Place small amount of lotion in hands.	Cold causes muscle tension.
9. Explain to client that lotion will feel cool and wet.	Warning client reduces startled response.
10. Apply hands first to sacral area, massaging in circular motion. Stroke upward from buttocks to shoulders. Massage over scapulae with smooth, firm stroke. Continue in one smooth stroke to upper arms and laterally along sides of back down to iliac crests (see illustration). Do not allow your hands to leave client's skin. Continue massage pattern for at least 3 min.	Gentle, firm pressure applied to all muscle groups promotes relaxation. Continuous contact with skin's surface is soothing and stimulates circulation to tissues.

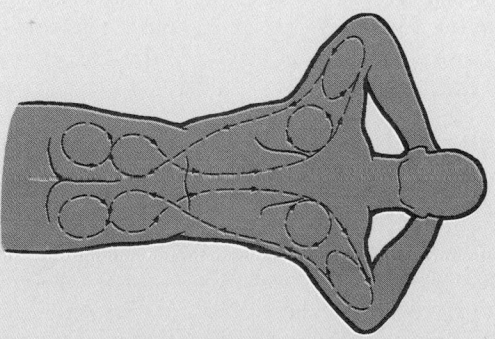

Step 10

STEPS	RATIONALE

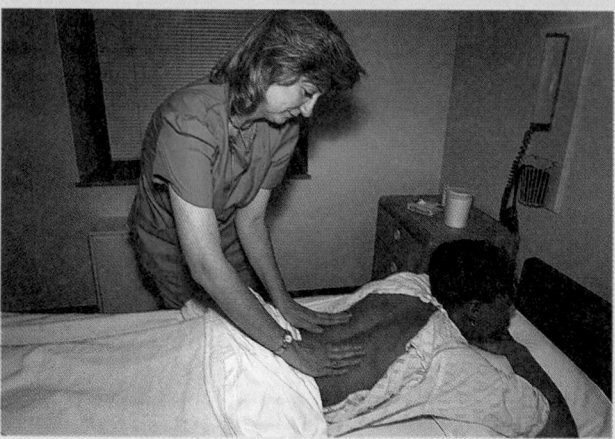 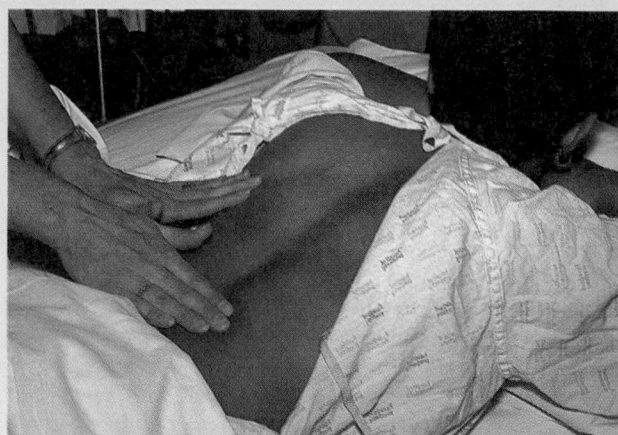

Step 11

11. Knead skin by gently grasping tissue between your thumb and fingers (see illustrations). Knead upward along one side of spine from buttocks to shoulders and around nape of neck. Knead or stroke downward toward sacrum. Repeat along other side of back.

Kneading increases circulation. Motion is soothing and relieving.

12. End massage with long stroking movements for an additional 3 min and tell client you are ending massage.

Long stroking is most soothing.

13. If lying on side, ask client to turn to opposite side, and massage other hip.

14. Wipe excess lubricant from client's back with bath towel. Retie gown or assist with pajamas. Help client to comfortable position. Raise side rails as needed, and open curtain. Lower bed.

Excess lotion can be irritant. Comfortable position enhances back rub's effects.

15. Dispose of soiled towel and wash hands.

Promotes infection control.

16. Ask client about comfort. Note any areas of muscle pain or tension.

Degree of relief gained depends on length of massage, client's ability to relax, and degree of discomfort before massage.

17. Reassess pulse and blood pressure.

Gentle back massage may increase heart rate and systolic blood pressure.

Recording and Reporting
- Record response to massage and condition of skin.

Home Care Considerations
- Massage is an easy technique to teach a family member to promote client's relaxation any time of day.

ears, and scalp before removing the infant's shirt and diaper. The washcloth is used and turned so that a clean part touches the skin with each stroke. The eyes are carefully washed from the inner to the outer canthus. It may be necessary to shampoo the scalp and hair. The infant can be positioned over a small basin, lathering the scalp with a mild soap, and rinsing by pouring water from a small container into a basin. A washcloth can be used to wash and rinse as well. The infant is kept covered during shampooing. A rolled wisp of dampened cotton or the twisted end of the washcloth works well to clean the external ear.

After undressing the infant for the remainder of the bath, the nurse gives special attention to around the neck, where food that has been regurgitated collects, and in skin folds of the axillae and joints. Genitalia of both sexes require careful and gentle cleansing. For a girl, it is important to retract the labia fully to remove the **vernix caseosa** after it has dried. With successive baths the vernix caseosa will disappear. The vulva is cleansed front to back to prevent the spread of infection. In male infants, the nurse washes carefully around the penis and scrotum. To complete the bath, the nurse washes the buttocks and anal area thoroughly of fecal material. After bathing the infant must be completely dried and a diaper reapplied.

Care of the umbilical cord is a special consideration for the newborn. The umbilical stump is a good medium for bacterial growth. Thus sponge baths are given until the cord falls off and the skin heals. Triple dye is used in many agencies to prevent infection. A diaper should be positioned below the cord to avoid wetness and irritation. Daily application of alcohol to the base of the cord aids drying (Wong, 1995).

The nurse also gives special care to infants who have been circumcised. A small amount of bleeding normally occurs from the penis. The physician applies a sterile gauze dressing impregnated with petrolatum around the circumcised area. The nurse may clean the penis periodically with moistened cotton balls until the dressing can be removed permanently (Wong, 1995).

Infants can be given a tub bath after the umbilicus has healed. Supplies are the same as those used in the sponge bath. The face, neck, ears, eyes, and scalp are washed before the infant is undressed and placed in the tub. Lowering the infant slowly into the tub avoids startling. The infant must always be held firmly with one hand (Figure 38-7). The nurse never leaves the child unattended. Body creases are much easier to cleanse and rinse in a tub. After the bath, the nurse wraps the infant completely in a towel and gently pats the infant dry.

In hospitals where there is rooming-in of the infant and mother, the infant's bath is an excellent opportunity to involve the parents in the child's care. The parents can examine the infant's body parts and learn about normal variation in skin characteristics. This is also a good time to stress the importance of safety in terms of water temperature and supervision of the infant.

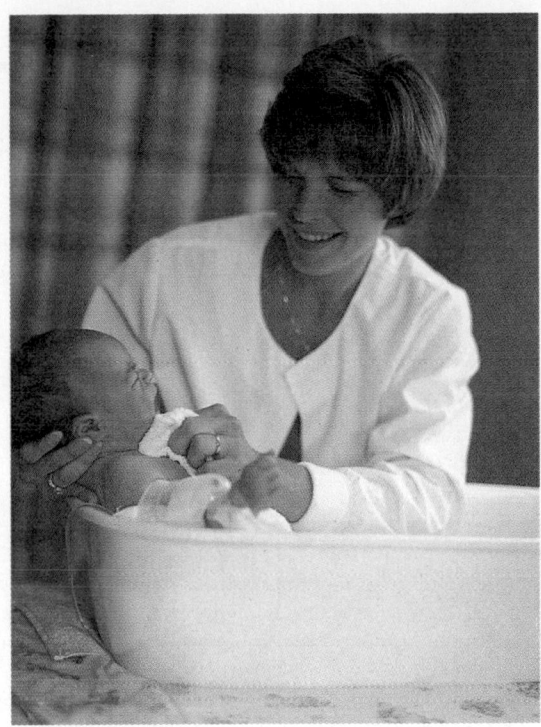

Figure 38-7   Holding infant during tub bath.

Foot and Nail Care.   Foot and nail care should be incorporated into a person's regular hygiene routine. Routine care involves soaking to soften cuticles and layers of horny cells, thorough cleansing, drying, and proper nail trimming. The exception involves clients with diabetes mellitus who do not soak their nails due to the risk of infection. When the nurse administers care, the client may remain in bed or sit in a chair (Skill 38-4).

The nurse takes time during the procedure to teach the client and family proper techniques for cleaning and nail trimming. Measures to prevent infection and promote good circulation should be stressed. Clients learn to protect the feet from injury, keep the feet clean and dry, and wear footwear that fits properly. The nurse instructs clients on the proper way to inspect all surfaces of the feet and hands for lesions, dryness, or signs of infection. It is important for clients to know the appearance of any abnormalities and the importance of reporting these conditions to their caregiver.

A client with diabetes mellitus or peripheral vascular disease is at risk for foot and nail problems as a result of poor peripheral blood supply to the feet. In addition, sensation in the feet can be reduced. These clients are especially at risk for the development of chronic foot ulcers. These lesions typically heal very slowly and once present are difficult to treat. Over time circulation can become compromised enough to cause ischemia and sloughing of tissue. Although ongoing foot care can help prevent toe amputation, studies show that many clients have not learned proper care (Christensen and others, 1991). The American Diabetes

Skill 38-4 Performing Nail and Foot Care

Delegation Considerations

The skill of nail and foot care of the nondiabetic client can be delegated to assistive personnel. If the client is diabetic, this skill should not be delegated.

- Inform and assist caregiver in proper way to use nail clippers.
- Instruct caregiver to report immediately any cuts in skin.

EQUIPMENT

- Washbasin
- Emesis basin
- Washcloth
- Bath or face towel
- Nail clippers
- Orange stick

- Emery board or nail file
- Body lotion
- Disposable bath mat
- Paper towels
- Disposable gloves

STEPS	RATIONALE
1. Inspect all surfaces of fingers, toes, feet, and nails. Pay particular attention to areas of dryness, inflammation, or cracking. Also inspect areas between toes, heels, and soles of feet.	Integrity of feet and nails determines frequency and level of hygiene required. Heels, soles, and sides of feet are prone to irritation from ill-fitting shoes.
2. Assess color and temperature of toes, feet, and fingers. Assess capillary refill of nails. Palpate radial and ulnar pulse of each hand and dorsalis pedis pulse of foot; note character of pulses.	Assesses adequacy of blood flow to extremities. Circulatory alterations may change integrity of nails and increase client's chance of localized infection when break in skin integrity occurs.
3. Observe client's walking gait. Have client walk down hall or walk straight line (if able).	Painful disorders of feet can cause limping or unnatural gait.
4. Ask female clients about whether they use nail polish and polish remover frequently.	Chemicals in these products can cause excessive dryness.
5. Assess type of footwear worn by clients: Are socks worn? Are shoes tight or ill fitting? Are garters or knee-high nylons worn? Is footwear clean?	Types of shoes and footwear may predispose client to foot and nail problems (e.g., infection, areas of friction, ulcerations).
6. Identify client's risk for foot or nail problems:	Certain conditions increase likelihood of foot or nail problems.
a. Older adult	Poor vision, lack of coordination, or inability to bend over contributes to difficulty in performing foot and nail care. Normal physiological changes of aging also result in nail and foot problems.
b. Diabetes mellitus	Vascular changes associated with diabetes mellitus reduce blood flow to peripheral tissues. Break in skin integrity places diabetic at high risk for skin infection.
c. Heart failure, renal disease	Both conditions can increase tissue edema, particularly in dependent areas (e.g., feet). Edema reduces blood flow to neighboring tissues.
d. Cerebrovascular accident, stroke	Presence of residual foot or leg weakness or paralysis results in altered walking patterns. Altered gait pattern causes increased friction and pressure on feet.
7. Assess type of home remedies client uses for existing foot problems:	Certain preparations or applications may cause more injury to soft tissue than initial foot problem.
a. Over-the-counter liquid preparations to remove corns	Liquid preparations can cause burns and ulcerations.
b. Cutting of corns or calluses with razor blade or scissors	Cutting of corns or calluses may result in infection caused by break in skin integrity.
c. Use of oval corn pads	Oval pads may exert pressure on toes, thereby decreasing circulation to surrounding tissues.
d. Application of adhesive tape	Skin of older adult is thin and delicate and prone to tearing when adhesive tape is removed.
8. Assess client's ability to care for nails or feet: visual alterations, fatigue, musculoskeletal weakness.	Determines client's ability to perform self-care and degree of assistance required from nurse.

STEPS	RATIONALE
9. Assess client's knowledge of foot and nail care practices.	Determines client's need for health teaching.
10. Explain procedure to client, including fact that proper soaking requires several minutes.	Client must be willing to place fingers and feet in basins for 10 to 20 min. Client may become anxious or fatigued.

Critical Decision Point: Note: Diabetic clients do not soak hands and feet. Soaking increases risk of infection in diabetic.

11. Obtain physician's order for cutting nails if agency policy requires it.	Client's skin may be accidentally cut. Certain clients are more at risk for infection, depending on their medical condition.
12. Wash hands. Arrange equipment on overbed table.	Easy access to equipment prevents delays.
13. Pull curtain around bed or close room door (if desired).	Maintaining client's privacy reduces anxiety.
14. Assist ambulatory client to sit in bedside chair. Help bedbound client to supine position with head of bed elevated. Place disposable bath mat on floor under client's feet or place towel on mattress.	Sitting in chair facilitates immersing feet in basin. Bath mat protects feet from exposure to soil or debris.
15. Fill washbasin with warm water. Test water temperature.	Warm water softens nails and thickened epidermal cells, reduces inflammation of skin, and promotes local circulation. Proper water temperature prevents burns.
16. Place basin on bath mat or towel, and help client place feet in basin. Place call light within client's reach.	Clients with muscular weakness or tremors may have difficulty positioning feet. Client's safety is maintained.
17. Adjust overbed table to low position, and place it over client's lap. (Client may sit in chair or lie in bed.)	Easy access prevents accidental spills.
18. Fill emesis basin with warm water, and place basin on paper towels on overbed table.	Warm water softens nails and thickened epidermal cells.
19. Instruct client to place fingers in emesis basin and place arms in comfortable position.	Prolonged positioning can cause discomfort unless normal anatomical alignment is maintained.
20. Allow client's feet and fingernails to soak for 10 to 20 min. Rewarm after 10 min.	Softening of corns, calluses, and cuticles ensures easy removal of dead cells and easy manipulation of cuticle.
21. Clean gently under fingernails with orange stick while fingers are immersed (see illustration). Remove emesis basin, and dry fingers thoroughly.	Orange stick removes debris under nails that harbors microorganisms. Thorough drying impedes fungal growth and prevents maceration of tissues.

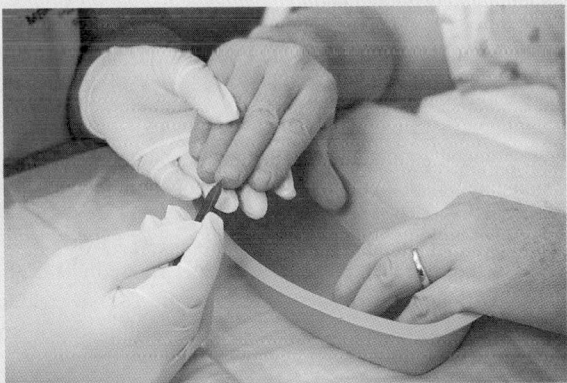

Step 21

22. With nail clippers, clip fingernails straight across and even with tops of fingers (see illustrations on p. 1092). Shape nails with emery board or file. If client has circulatory problems, do not cut nail; file the nail only.	Cutting straight across prevents splitting of nail margins and formation of sharp nail spikes that can irritate lateral nail margins. Filing prevents cutting nail too close to nail bed.
23. Push cuticle back gently with orange stick.	Reduces incidence of inflamed cuticles.
24. Move overbed table away from client.	Provides easier access to feet.
25. Put on disposable gloves, and scrub callused areas of feet with washcloth.	Gloves prevent transmission of fungal infection. Friction removes dead skin layers.

STEPS	RATIONALE

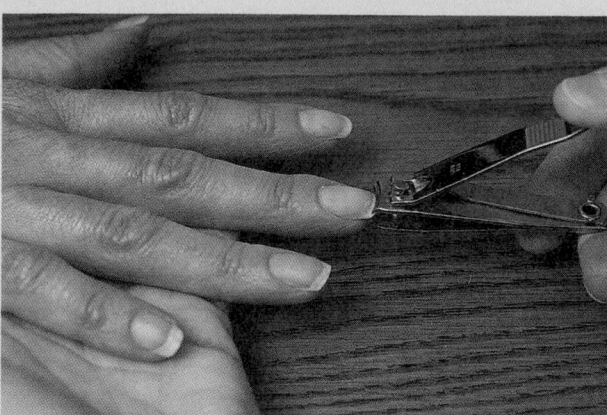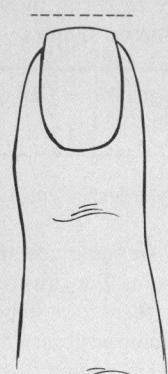

Step 22

26. Clean gently under nails with orange stick. Remove feet from basin, and dry thoroughly.	Removal of debris and excess moisture reduces chances of infection.
27. Clean and trim toenails using procedures in Steps 22 and 23. Do not file corners of toenails.	Shaping corners of toenails may damage tissues.
28. Apply lotion to feet and hands, and assist client back to bed and into comfortable position.	Lotion lubricates dry skin by helping to retain moisture.
29. Remove disposable gloves, and place in receptacle. Clean and return equipment and supplies to proper place. Dispose of soiled linen in hamper. Wash hands.	Reduces transmission of infection.
30. Inspect nails and surrounding skin surfaces after soaking and nail trimming.	Evaluates condition of skin and nails. Allows nurse to note any remaining rough nail edges.
31. Ask client to explain or demonstrate nail care.	Evaluates client's level of learning techniques.
32. Observe client's walk after toenail care.	Evaluates level of comfort and mobility achieved.
33. Record procedure and observations (e.g., breaks in skin, inflammation, ulcerations).	Documents procedure, client's response, and presence of abnormalities requiring additional therapy.
34. Report any breaks in skin or ulcerations to nurse in charge or physician.	These abnormalities can seriously increase client's risk of infection and must be carefully observed.

Recording and Reporting

- Record procedure and observations (e.g., breaks in skin, inflammation, ulcerations).
- Report any breaks in skin or ulcerations to nurse in charge or physician. These are serious in client with peripheral vascular disease and illnesses in which client's circulation is impaired. Special foot care treatments may be needed.

Home Care Considerations

- Alternative therapies: moleskin applied to areas of feet that are under friction is less likely to cause pressure than corn pads; spot adhesive bandages can guard against friction, but they do not have padding to protect against pressure; wrapping small pieces of lamb's wool around toes reduces irritation of soft corns between toes.
- If client is ambulatory, instruct to soak feet in bathtub. When client's mobility is limited, a large basin or pan can be used.

Association (ADA) (1999) identifies the following risk conditions to be associated with an increased risk of amputation: peripheral neuropathy; altered biomechanics; evidence of increased pressure from callus, erythema, or hemorrhage under a callus; limited joint mobility, bony deformity, or severe nail pathologic condition; peripheral vascular disease; a history of ulcers or amputation.

The nurse observes for changes that would indicate peripheral neuropathy or vascular insufficiency (Box 38-8). The client must be given information to understand how circulation directly affects the health and integrity of tissues. The nurse advises clients to use the following guidelines in a routine foot and nail care program:

- Inspect the feet daily, including the tops and soles of the feet, the heels, and the areas between the toes. Use a mirror to help inspect the feet thoroughly or ask a family member to check daily.
- All clients with diabetes mellitus should receive a thorough foot examination at least once a year. People with one or more high-risk foot conditions should be evaluated more frequently. People with neuropathy should have a visual inspection of their feet at every visit with a health care professional (ADA, 1999).
- Wash the feet daily using lukewarm water; **do not soak.** Clients with reduced sensation may want to use a bath thermometer at home to test water temperature. Thoroughly pat the feet dry, and dry well between toes.
- Do not cut corns or calluses or use commercial removers. Consult a physician or podiatrist.
- If the feet perspire, apply an unscented foot powder. Wear shoes with porous uppers.

- If dryness is noted along the feet or between the toes, apply lanolin, baby oil, or even corn oil, and rub gently into the skin.
- File the toenails straight across and square; do not use scissors or clippers. Consult a podiatrist as needed.
- Do not use over-the-counter preparations to treat athlete's foot or ingrown toenails. Consult a physician or podiatrist.
- Avoid wearing elastic stockings, knee-high hose, or constricting garters. Do not cross the legs while sitting. Both impair circulation to the lower extremities.
- Wear clean socks or stockings daily. Change socks twice a day if feet perspire heavily. Socks should be dry and free of holes or darns that might cause pressure.
- Do not walk barefoot.
- Wear properly fitted shoes. The soles of shoes should be flexible and nonslipping. Small amounts of lamb's wool can be used between toes that rub or overlap. Shoes should be sturdy, closed in, and not restrictive to the feet. Clients with increased plantar pressure (e.g., erythema, callus) should use footwear that cushions and redistributes pressure (ADA, 1999). Clients with bony deformity (e.g., bunion or Charcot's joint) may need extrawide or extradeep shoes with cushioned insoles (Young and Young, 1994).
- Do not wear new shoes for an extended time. Wear them for short periods over several days to break them in.
- Exercise regularly to improve circulation to the lower extremities. Walk slowly and elevate, rotate, flex, and extend the feet at the ankles. Dangle the feet over the side of the bed 1 minute, and then extend both legs and hold them parallel to the bed while lying supine for 1 minute, and, finally, rest 1 minute.
- Avoid applying hot-water bottles or heating pads to the feet; use extra coverings instead.
- Minor cuts should be washed immediately and dried thoroughly. Use only mild antiseptics (e.g., Neosporin ointment). Avoid iodine or Mercurochrome. Contact a physician to treat cuts or lacerations.

Generally, any client who requires regular, thorough foot care should have a family member who is able to provide care during times when the client is incapacitated. Clients with visual difficulties, physical constraints preventing movement, or cognitive problems that impair their ability to assess the condition of the feet will need family assistance (ADA, 1999).

Oral Hygiene. Oral hygiene helps to maintain the healthy state of the mouth, teeth, gums and lips. Brushing cleans the teeth of food particles, plaque, and bacteria. It also massages the gums and relieves discomfort resulting from unpleasant odors and tastes. Flossing further helps remove plaque and tartar from between teeth to reduce

---

Objective Signs of Peripheral Neuropathy or Vascular Disease   Box 38-8

PERIPHERAL NEUROPATHY
Muscle wasting of lower extremities
Absence of deep tendon reflexes
Foot deformities
Abnormal gait
Decreased or absent vibratory sensation

VASCULAR INSUFFICIENCY
Decreased hair growth on legs and feet
Absent or decreased pulses
Infection in the foot
Shiny appearance of the skin
Blanching of the skin on elevation

From Harley JR: Preventing diabetic foot disease, *Nurs Pract* 18(10):37, 1993.

gum inflammation and infection. Complete oral hygiene enhances well-being and comfort and stimulates the appetite. Clients also benefit from a proper diet, which excludes foods promoting plaque formation and tooth decay and promotes healthy periodontal structures. The nurse assists clients in maintaining good oral hygiene by teaching the importance of correct techniques and a routine daily schedule. Clients of all ages should be advised to have a dental checkup at least every 6 months. Education about common gum and tooth disorders and methods of prevention can motivate clients to follow good oral hygiene practices. The nurse also assists in performing hygiene for weakened or disabled clients. When clients have variations in oral mucosal integrity, the nurse adapts hygiene techniques to ensure thorough and effective care (Box 38-9).

Brushing and Flossing.   Thorough toothbrushing at least 4 times a day (after meals and at bedtime) is basic to an effective oral hygiene program. A toothbrush should have a straight handle and brush small enough to reach all areas of the mouth. An even, rounded brushing surface with soft, multitufted, nylon bristles is best. Rounded soft bristles stimulate the gums without causing abrasion and bleeding. Older adult clients with reduced dexterity and grip may require an enlarged handle with an easier grip or an electric toothbrush (Felder and others, 1994). One simple way to devise an enlarged brush handle is to pierce a soft rubber ball and push the brush handle through or glue a short piece of plastic tubing around the handle. Clients should know to obtain a new toothbrush every 3 months or following a cold or strep throat to minimize growth of microorganisms on the brush surfaces.

All tooth surfaces should be brushed thoroughly using a fluoride toothpaste. Commercially made foam rubber toothbrushes are useful for clients with sensitive gums. However, swabbing fails to cleanse teeth adequately because plaque accumulates around the base of the teeth. Foam rubber swabs should be used in moderation. Electric toothbrushes can be used, but the nurse working

---

Gerontological NURSING PRACTICE   **Box 38-9**

- Most clients over age 65 are edentulous (without teeth), and those that are present are often diseased or decayed.
- The periodontal membrane weakens, making it more prone to infection.
- Partial plates or dentures may not fit properly, causing pain and discomfort.
- Weaker jaw muscles and a shrinkage of the bony structure of the mouth may increase the work of chewing and lead to increased fatigue when eating.
- There is a decrease in saliva with aging that may cause mucous membranes to become more dry.

Modified from Lueckenotte A: *Gerontologic nursing,* St. Louis, 1996, Mosby.

---

in an agency setting should check for electrical hazards. Lemon-glycerin sponges should not be used because they dry mucous membranes and erode teeth enamel. Moi-Stin is a salivary supplement that improves moisture and texture of the tongue and mucosa (Poland, 1987).

Whether a brush or sponge is used, thorough rinsing after brushing is important to remove dislodged food particles and excess toothpaste. Some people enjoy using mouthwash for its pleasant taste. Used over a long period, however, mouthwash dries mucosa.

When teaching clients about mouth care, the nurse should recommend they do not share toothbrushes with family members or drink directly from a bottle of mouthwash. Cross contamination occurs easily. The use of disclosure tablets or drops to stain the plaque that collects at the gumline can be useful for showing clients how effectively they brush.

The amount of assistance needed by the client when brushing the teeth may vary (Skill 38-5). Many clients can perform their own oral care and should be encouraged to do so. The nurse observes the client to be sure proper techniques are used.

Clients will experience conditions that threaten the integrity of oral mucosa. For example, mucosal changes associated with aging, use of chemotherapeutic drugs, or dehydration require the nurse to adapt oral hygiene approaches. More frequent mouth care and use of antiinfective agents are examples of ways the nurse will revise approaches to meet client needs.

Flossing.   Dental flossing removes plaque and tartar between teeth. Flossing involves inserting waxed or unwaxed dental floss between all tooth surfaces, one at a time. The seesaw motion used to pull floss between teeth removes plaque and tartar from tooth enamel. To prevent bleeding, clients who are receiving chemotherapy or radiation or are on anticoagulant therapy should use unwaxed floss and avoid vigorous flossing near the gumline. If toothpaste is applied to the teeth before flossing, fluoride can come in direct contact with tooth surfaces, aiding in cavity prevention. Flossing once a day is sufficient. Because it is important to clean all teeth surfaces thoroughly, the nurse should not rush to complete flossing. Placing a mirror in front of the client will help the nurse to demonstrate the proper method for holding the floss and cleaning between the teeth.

Clients With Special Needs.   Some clients require special oral hygiene methods because of their level of dependence on the nurse or the presence of oral mucosa problems. Unconscious clients are susceptible to drying of mucous-thickened salivary secretions because they are unable to eat or drink, frequently breathe through the mouth, and often receive oxygen therapy. The unconscious client also cannot swallow salivary secretions that accumulate in the mouth. These secretions often contain

Providing Oral Hygiene | Skill 38-5

Delegation Considerations

Skills of brushing teeth can be delegated to assistive personnel.

- Inform and assist caregiver in proper way to provide tooth-brushing.

- Instruct caregiver in how to recognize impaired integrity of oral mucosa.

EQUIPMENT

- Soft-bristled toothbrush
- Nonabrasive fluoride toothpaste or dentifrice
- Dental floss
- Water glass with cool water
- Normal saline or fluoride mouthwash (optional; follow client's preference)

- Emesis basin
- Face towel
- Paper towels
- Disposable gloves

STEPS	RATIONALE
1. Wash hands and apply disposable gloves.	Reduces transmission of microorganisms.
2. Inspect integrity of lips, teeth, buccal mucosa, gums, palate, and tongue (see Chapter 32).	Determines status of client's oral cavity and extent of need for oral hygiene.

3. Identify presence of common oral problems:
  a. Dental caries—chalky white discoloration of tooth or presence of brown or black discoloration
  b. Gingivitis—inflammation of gums
  c. Periodontitis—receding gum lines, inflammation, gaps between teeth
  d. Halitosis—bad breath
  e. Cheilosis—cracking of lips
  f. Stomatitis—inflammation of the mouth
	Helps determine type of hygiene client requires and information client requires for self-care.

4. Remove gloves and wash hands.	Prevents spread of microorganisms.
5. Assess risk for oral hygiene problems (See Table 38-7).	Certain conditions increase likelihood of impaired oral cavity integrity and need for preventive care.

6. Determine client's oral hygiene practices:
  a. Frequency of toothbrushing and flossing
  b. Type of toothpaste or dentifrice used
  c. Last dental visit
  d. Frequency of dental visits
  e. Type of mouthwash or moistening preparation
	Allows nurse to identify errors in technique, deficiencies in preventive oral hygiene, and client's level of knowledge regarding dental care.
	
	Lemon-glycerin preparations can be detrimental. Glycerin is an astringent that dries and shrinks mucous membranes and gums. Lemon exhausts salivary reflex and can erode tooth enamel (Poland, 1987). Mouthwash provides pleasant aftertaste but can dry mucosa after extended use if it has an alcohol base (Blaney, 1986).

7. Asseses client's ability to grasp and manipulate toothbrush. (For older adult try 30-sec toothbrush assessment).	Determines level of assistance required.
8. Prepare equipment at bedside.	Toothbrush test useful in assessing dexterity and strength.
9. Explain procedure to client and discuss preferences regarding use of hygiene aids.	Some clients feel uncomfortable about having the nurse care for their basic needs. Client involvement with procedure minimizes anxiety.
10. Place paper towels on overbed table, and arrange other equipment within easy reach.	
11. Raise bed to comfortable working position. Raise head of bed (if allowed) and lower side rail. Move client, or help client move closer. Side-lying position can be used.	Raising bed and positioning client prevent nurse from straining muscles. Semi-Fowler's position helps prevent client from choking or aspirating.
12. Place towel over client's chest.	
13. Apply gloves.	Prevents contact with microorganisms or blood in saliva.
14. Apply toothpaste to brush, holding brush over emesis basin. Pour small amount of water over toothpaste.	Moisture aids in distribution of toothpaste over tooth surfaces.

STEPS	RATIONALE
15. Client may assist by brushing. Hold toothbrush bristles at 45-degree angle to gum line (see illustration). Be sure tips of bristles rest against and penetrate under gum line. Brush inner and outer surfaces of upper and lower teeth by brushing from gum to crown of each tooth. Clean biting surfaces of teeth by holding top of bristles parallel with teeth and brushing gently back and forth (see illustration). Brush sides of teeth by moving bristles back and forth (see illustration).	Angle allows brush to reach all tooth surfaces and to clean under gum line where plaque and tartar accumulate. Back-and-forth motion dislodges food particles caught between teeth and along chewing surfaces.
16. Have client hold brush at 45-degree angle and lightly brush over surface and sides of tongue. Avoid initiating gag reflex.	Microorganisms collect and grow on tongue's surface and contribute to bad breath. Gagging may cause aspiration of toothpaste.
17. Allow client to rinse mouth thoroughly by taking several sips of water, swishing water across all tooth surfaces, and spitting into emesis basin.	Irrigation removes food particles.
18. Allow client to gargle to rinse mouth with mouthwash as desired.	Mouthwash leaves pleasant taste in mouth.
19. Assist in wiping client's mouth.	Promotes sense of comfort.
20. Allow client to floss (see illustration).	Reduces tartar on tooth surfaces.
21. Allow client to rinse mouth thoroughly with cool water and spit into emesis basin. Assist in wiping client's mouth.	Irrigation removes plaque and tartar from oral cavity.
22. Assist client to comfortable position, remove emesis basin and bedside table, raise side rail, and lower bed to original position.	Provides for client comfort and safety.
23. Wipe off overbed table, discard soiled linen and paper towels in appropriate containers, remove soiled gloves, and return equipment to proper place.	Proper disposal of soiled equipment prevents spread of infection.
24. Wash hands.	Reduces transmission of microorganisms.
25. Ask client if any area of oral cavity feels uncomfortable or irritated.	Pain indicates more chronic problem.
26. Apply gloves and inspect condition of oral cavity.	Determines effectiveness of hygiene and rinsing.
27. Ask client to describe proper hygiene techniques.	Evaluates client's learning.
28. Observe client brushing.	Evaluates client's ability to use correct technique.

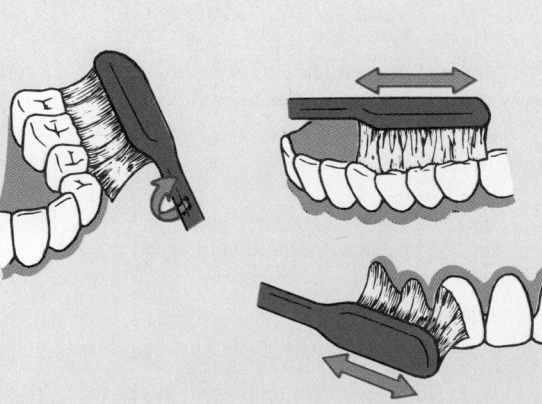

Step 15

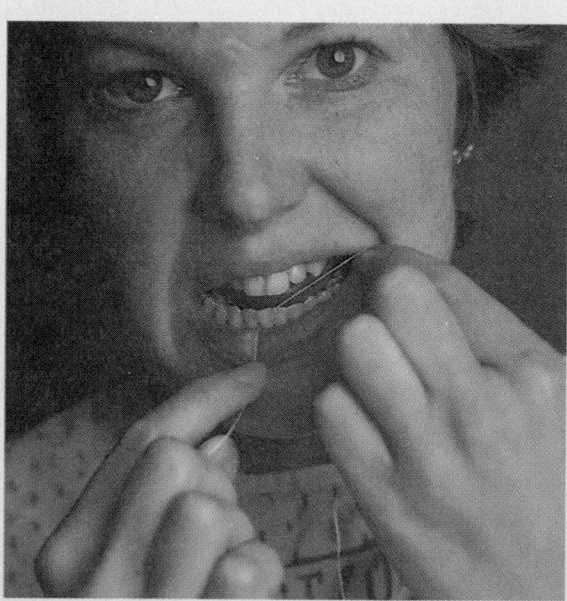

Step 20

Recording and Reporting
- Record procedure on flow sheet. Note condition of oral cavity in nurses' notes.
- Report bleeding or presence of lesions to nurse in charge or physician.

Home Care Considerations
- Assess oral cavity at each visit to determine the effects of medications on the structures of the oral cavity.

gram-negative bacteria that can cause pneumonia if aspirated into the lungs. While providing hygiene to an unconscious client, the nurse must protect the client from choking and aspiration. The safest technique is to have two nurses provide the care. The nurse may delegate assistive personnel to participate. One nurse does the actual cleaning, and the other removes secretions with suction equipment. While cleansing the oral cavity, the nurse should never use fingers to hold the client's mouth open. A human bite is highly contaminated. It may be necessary to perform mouth care at least every 2 hours. The nurse explains the steps of mouth care and the sensations the client will feel. The nurse also tells the client when the procedure is completed (Skill 38-6).

Clients who receive chemotherapy, radiation, or nasogastric tube intubation, or who have an infection of the mouth can suffer from stomatitis. Inflammation of the oral mucosa can cause oral burning, pain, and change in food tolerance. Gentle brushing and flossing are important in preventing bleeding of the gums. Clients should be advised to avoid alcohol and commercial mouthwash and to stop smoking. Normal saline rinses (approximately 30 ml) upon awaking in the morning, after each meal, and at bedtime can effectively clean the oral cavity. The rinses can be increased to every 2 hours if necessary. The physician may order a mild oral analgesic for pain control.

Clients with diabetes mellitus frequently have periodontal disease. Visits to the dentist are needed every 3 to 4 months. All tissues should be handled gently with a minimum of trauma. Clients should learn to follow rigid cleansing schedules, at least 4 times a day.

Denture Care. Clients should be encouraged to clean their dentures on a regular basis to avoid gingival infection and irritation. When clients become disabled, the nurse or family caregiver can assume responsibility for denture care (Box 38-10, p. 1100). Dentures are the client's personal property and need to be handled with care because they can be easily broken. Dentures must be removed at night to give the gums a rest and prevent bacterial buildup. To prevent warping, dentures should be kept covered in water when they are not worn, and they should always be stored in an enclosed, labeled cup with the cup placed in the client's bedside stand. Discourage clients from removing their dentures and placing them on a napkin or tissue because they could be easily thrown away.

Hair and Scalp Care. A person's appearance and feeling of well-being often depend on the way the hair looks and feels. Illness or disability may prevent a client from maintaining daily hair care. An immobilized client's hair soon becomes tangled. Dressings may leave sticky blood or antiseptic solutions on the hair. In the clinic and home care setting, nurses will encounter clients who have head lice. Proper hair care is important to the client's body image. Brushing, combing, and shampooing are basic hygiene measures for all clients.

Brushing and Combing. Frequent brushing helps to keep hair clean and distributes oil evenly along hair shafts. Combing prevents hair from tangling. The client should be encouraged to maintain routine hair care. However, clients with limited mobility or weakness and those who are confused require help. Clients in a hospital or extended care facility appreciate the opportunity to have their hair brushed and combed before being seen by others.

When caring for clients from different cultures, it is important to learn as much as possible from them or their family about preferred hair care practices. For example, the hair of African-Americans tends to be quite dry. Special lanolin conditioners may be used for conditioning. Cultural preferences will also affect how hair is combed and styled.

Long hair can easily become matted after a client is confined to bed, even for a short period. When lacerations or incisions involve the scalp, blood and topical medications can also cause tangling. Frequent brushing and combing keep long hair neatly groomed. Braiding can help to avoid repeated tangles, however braids should be unbraided periodically and hair combed to ensure good hygiene. Braids made too tightly can lead to bald patches. The nurse obtains permission from the client before braiding his or her hair.

To brush hair the nurse parts the hair into two sections and separates each into two more sections. It is easier to brush smaller sections of hair. Brushing from the scalp toward the hair ends minimizes pulling. Moistening the hair with water or alcohol frees tangles for easier combing. The nurse never cuts a client's hair without written consent.

Clients who develop head lice require special considerations in the way combing is performed. The lice are small, about the size of a sesame seed. Bright light or natural sunlight is necessary for the lice to be seen. Thorough

Performing Mouth Care for an Unconscious or Debilitated Client

Skill 38-6

Delegation Considerations

Skills of brushing teeth of an unconscious or debilitated client can be delegated to assistive personnel.

- After RN checks for gag reflex, inform caregiver about proper way to position clients for mouth care.

- Instruct caregiver in how to use the oral suction catheter for clearing oral secretions.
- Instruct caregiver in how to recognize impaired integrity of oral mucosa.

EQUIPMENT

- Antiinfective solution (e.g., diluted hydrogen peroxide) that loosens crusts
- Small soft-bristled toothbrush
- Sponge toothette or tongue blade wrapped in single layer of gauze
- Padded tongue blade
- Face towel
- Paper towels
- Emesis basin
- Water glass with cool water
- Water-soluble lip lubricant
- Small-bulb syringe (optional)
- Suction machine equipment (optional)
- Disposable gloves (three pair)

STEPS	RATIONALE
1. Wash hands. Apply disposable gloves.	Reduces transmission of microorganisms. Gloves prevent contact with microorganisms in blood or saliva.
2. Test for presence of gag reflex by placing tongue blade on back half of tongue. Clients with impaired gag reflex require oral care as well. The nurse determines the type of suction apparatus needed at the bedside to protect the client's airway against aspiration.	Reveals whether client is at risk for aspiration.
3. Inspect condition of oral cavity (see Chapter 32).	Determines condition of oral cavity and need for hygiene.
4. Remove gloves. Wash hands.	Prevents spread of infection.
5. Assess client's risk for oral hygiene problems (see Table 38-7, p. 1069).	Certain conditions increase likelihood of alterations in integrity of oral cavity structures and may require more frequent care.
6. Position client on side (Sims' position) with head turned well toward dependent side and head of bed lowered. Raise side rail.	Allows secretions to drain from mouth instead of collecting in back of pharynx. Prevents aspiration.
7. Explain procedure to client.	Allows debilitated client to anticipate procedure without anxiety. Unconscious client may retain ability to hear.
8. Wash hands and apply disposable gloves.	Reduces transfer of microorganisms.
9. Place paper towels on overbed table and arrange equipment. If needed, turn on suction machine, and connect tubing to suction catheter.	Prevents soiling of table top. Equipment prepared in advance ensures smooth, safe procedure.
10. Pull curtain around bed, or close room door.	Provides privacy.
11. Raise bed to its highest horizontal level; lower side rail.	Use of good body mechanics with bed in high position prevents injury.
12. Position client close to side of bed; turn client's head toward mattress.	Proper positioning of head prevents aspiration.
13. Place towel under client's head and emesis basin under chin.	Prevents soiling of bed linen.
14. Carefully separate upper and lower teeth with padded tongue blade by inserting blade, quickly but gently, between back molars. Insert when client is relaxed, if possible. Do not use force (see illustration). Never use fingers to separate client's teeth.	Prevents client from biting down on nurse's fingers and provides access to oral cavity.

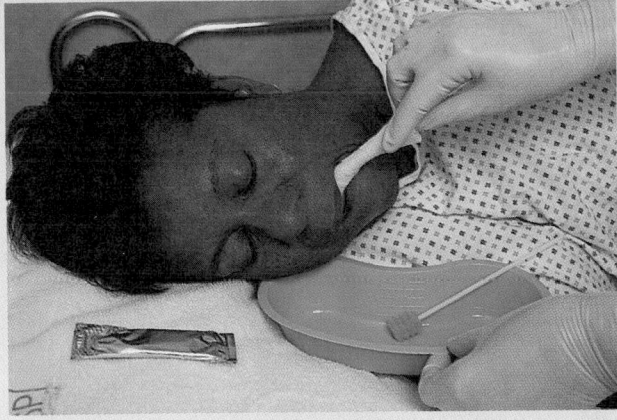

Step 14

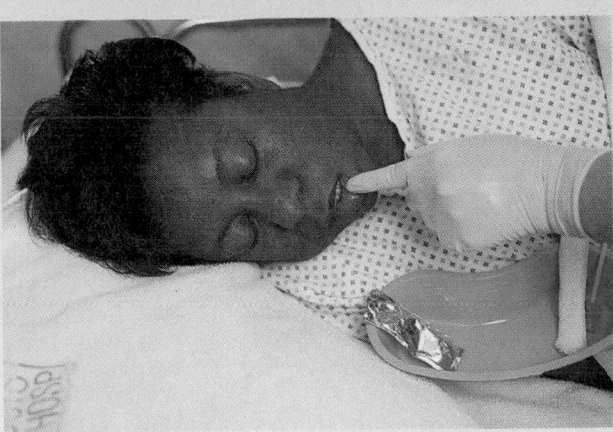

Step 17

15. Clean mouth using brush or sponge toothettes moistened with peroxide and water. Clean chewing and inner tooth surfaces first. Clean outer tooth surfaces. Swab roof of mouth, gums, and inside cheeks. Gently swab or brush tongue but avoid stimulating gag reflex (if present). Moisten clean swab or toothette with water to rinse. (Bulb syringe may also be used to rinse.) Repeat rinse several times.

Brushing action removes food particles between teeth and along chewing surfaces. Swabbing helps remove secretions and crusts from mucosa and moistens mucosa. Repeated rinsing removes peroxide that can be irritating to mucosa.

16. Suction secretions as they accumulate, if necessary.

Suction removes secretions and fluid that can collect in posterior pharynx.

17. Apply thin layer of water-soluble jelly to lips (see illustration).

Lubricates lips to prevent drying and cracking.

18. Inform client that procedure is completed.

Provides meaningful stimulation to unconscious or less responsive client.

19. Remove gloves and dispose in proper receptacle.

Prevents transmission of infection.

20. Reposition client comfortably, raise side rail, and return bed to original position.

Maintains client's comfort and safety.

21. Clean equipment and return to its proper place. Place soiled linen in proper receptacle.

Proper disposal of soiled equipment prevents spread of infection.

22. Wash hands.

Reduces transmission of microorganisms.

23. Apply gloves, and inspect oral cavity.

Determines efficacy of cleansing. Once thick secretions are removed, underlying inflammation or lesions may be revealed.

24. Ask debilitated client if mouth feels clean.

Evaluates level of comfort.

25. Assess client's respirations on an ongoing basis.

Ensures early recognition of aspiration.

Recording and Reporting

- Record procedure, including pertinent observations (e.g., presence of bleeding gums, dry mucosa, ulcerations, crusts on tongue).
- Report any unusual findings to nurse in charge or physician.

Home Care Considerations

- Irrigate cavity with bulb syringe; a gravy baster may be substituted.
- Mouth care should be given at least twice a day. Caregivers can get nonprescription oral care solutions (e.g., carbamide peroxide solutions) at most pharmacies. Have caregivers demonstrate positioning client to prevent aspiration.

| Box 38-10 | **Procedural Guidelines** |

For Cleaning Dentures

Equipment: Soft-bristled toothbrush, denture toothbrush, emesis basin or sink, denture dentifrice or toothpaste, water glass, 4 × 4 inch gauze, washcloth, denture cup, disposable gloves

1. Clean dentures for client during routine mouth care. Dentures need to be cleansed as often as natural teeth.
2. Fill emesis basin with tepid water. (If using sink, place washcloth in bottom of sink, and fill sink with approximately 1 in of water.)
3. Remove dentures: If client is unable to do this independently, don gloves, grasp upper plate at front with thumb and index finger wrapped in gauze, and pull downward. Gently lift lower denture from jaw, and rotate one side downward to remove from client's mouth. Place dentures in emesis basin or sink.
4. Apply dentifrice or toothpaste to denture, and brush surfaces of dentures (see illustration). Hold dentures close to water. Hold brush horizontally, and use back-and-forth motion to cleanse biting surfaces. Use short strokes from top of denture to biting surfaces of teeth to clean outer tooth surface. Hold brush vertically, and use short strokes to clean inner tooth surfaces. Hold brush horizontally, and use back-and-forth motion to clean undersurface of dentures.
5. Rinse dentures thoroughly in tepid water.
6. Return dentures to client, or store in tepid water in denture cup. Keep denture cup inside bedside cabinet.

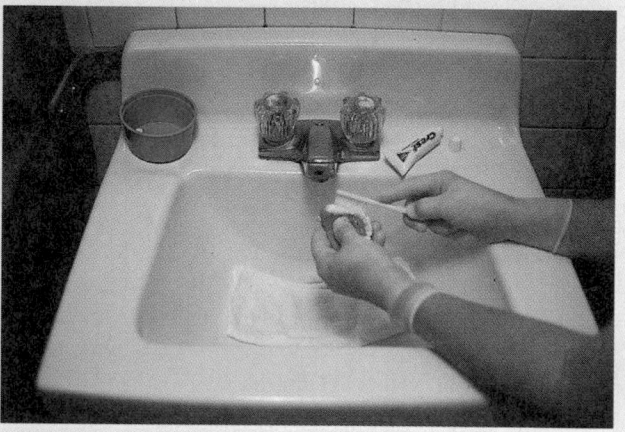

Step 4

---

combing is recommended and may be more effective than use of pediculicidal shampoos, which are often toxic and ineffective against resistant lice. Follow these steps:

Use a grooming comb or hairbrush to remove tangles.

Divide the client's hair in sections and fasten off hair that is not being combed.

Comb out from the scalp to the end of the hair (special combs are available in drug stores).

Dip the comb in a cup of water or use a paper towel to remove lice between each passing.

After combing, look through the hair carefully for attached lice.

Live lice may be caught with a tweezers or comb.

Move to next section of hair after combing thoroughly.

Clean the comb with an old toothbrush and dental floss and boil the comb (if possible).

Instruct family to comb and screen for lice daily.

Shampooing.   Frequency of shampooing depends on a person's daily routines and the condition of the hair. The nurse should remind clients in hospitals or extended care facilities that staying in bed, excess perspiration, or treatments that leave blood or solutions in the hair may require more frequent shampooing. For clients at home, the nurse is challenged to find ways the client can shampoo the hair without causing injury.

If the client is able to take a shower or bath, the hair can usually be shampooed without difficulty. A shower or tub chair may be used for the ambulatory, weight-bearing client who becomes tired or faint. Handheld shower nozzles allow clients to easily wash the hair in the tub or shower. Clients allowed to sit in a chair may choose to be shampooed in front of a sink or over a washbasin. However, bending is limited or contraindicated in certain conditions (e.g., eye surgery or neck injury). In these situations the nurse needs to teach the client the degree of bending allowed.

If a client is unable to sit but can be moved, the nurse may transfer the client to a stretcher for transportation to a sink or shower equipped with a handheld nozzle. Long-term care facilities are commonly equipped with this option. Caution is again needed when the client's head and neck are positioned, particularly in clients with any form of head or neck injury.

If the client is unable to sit in a chair or be transferred to a stretcher, shampooing must be done with the client in bed (Box 38-11). A special shampoo trough can be positioned under the client's head to catch water and suds. After shampooing, clients like having their hair styled and dried. Most health care centers have portable hair dryers. Dry shampoos that reduce the need to wet the client's hair are also available but are not highly effective. In most

Box 38-11 **Procedural Guidelines**

For Shampooing Hair of Bed-Bound Client

Equipment: Bath towels, washcloths, shampoo and hair conditioner (optional), water pitcher, plastic shampoo trough, washbasin, bath blanket, waterproof pad, clean comb and brush, hair dryer (optional)

1. Before washing client's hair, determine that there are no contraindications to this procedure. Certain medical conditions, such as head and neck injuries, spinal cord injuries, and arthritis, could place the client at risk for injury during shampooing because of positioning and manipulation of client's head and neck.

2. Inspect the hair and scalp prior to initiating the procedure. This determines the presence of any conditions that may require the use of special shampoos or treatments (e.g., for dandruff or the removal of dried blood).

3. Place waterproof pad under client's shoulders, neck, and head (see illustration). Position client supine, with head and shoulders at top edge of bed. Place plastic trough under client's head and washbasin at end of trough. Be sure trough spout extends beyond edge of mattress.

4. Place rolled towel under client's neck and bath towel over client's shoulders.

5. Brush and comb client's hair.

6. Obtain warm water.

7. Offer client the option of holding face towel or washcloth over eyes.

8. Slowly pour water from water pitcher over hair until it is completely wet (see illustration). If hair contains matted blood, don gloves, apply peroxide to dissolve clots, and then rinse hair with saline. Apply small amount of shampoo.

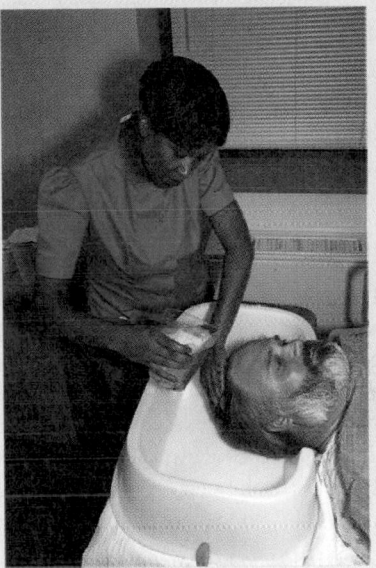

Step 8

9. Work up lather with both hands. Start at hairline, and work toward back of neck. Lift head slightly with one hand to wash back of head. Shampoo sides of head. Massage scalp by applying pressure with fingertips.

10. Rinse hair with water. Make sure water drains into basin. Repeat rinsing until hair is free of soap.

11. Apply conditioner or cream rinse if requested, and rinse hair thoroughly.

12. Wrap client's head in bath towel. Dry client's face with cloth used to protect eyes. Dry off any moisture along neck or shoulders.

13. Dry client's hair and scalp. Use second towel if first becomes saturated.

14. Comb hair to remove tangles, and dry with dryer if desired.

15. Apply oil preparation or conditioning product to hair, if desired by client.

16. Assist client to comfortable position, and complete styling of hair.

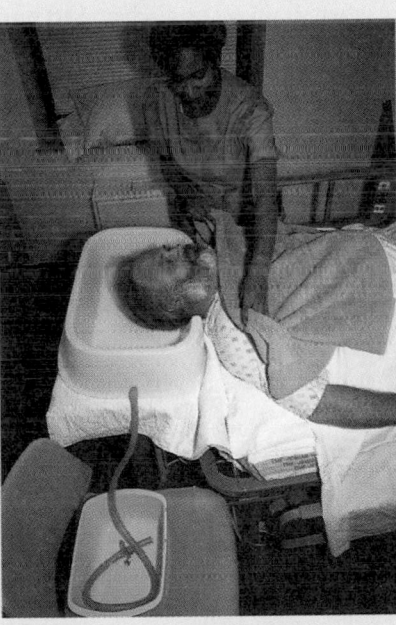

Step 3

agencies a physician's order is necessary for shampooing the dependent client.

When clients are being treated for head lice, the physician will often prescribe a pediculicide shampoo. Have clients consult with the doctor or a pharmacist carefully if they have questions about the toxicity of the shampoo.

Shaving. Shaving facial hair can be done after the bath or shampoo. Women may prefer to shave their legs or axillae while bathing. When assisting a client, the nurse should take care to avoid cutting the client with a razor blade. Clients prone to bleeding (e.g., those receiving anticoagulants or high doses of aspirin or those with low platelet counts) should use an electric razor. Before using an electric razor, the nurse should check for frayed cords or other electrical hazards. Electric razors should be used on only one client because of infection-control considerations.

When a razor blade is used for shaving, the skin must be softened to prevent pulling, scraping, or cuts. For example, placing a warm washcloth over the male client's face for a few seconds, followed by application of shaving cream or a lathering of mild soap, softens the skin. If the client is unable to shave, the nurse may perform the shave. To avoid causing discomfort or razor cuts, the nurse gently pulls the skin taut and uses short, firm razor strokes in the direction the hair grows (see Figure 38-8). Short downward strokes work best to remove hair over the up-

per lip. A client usually can explain to the nurse the best way to move the razor across the skin. In the case of African-Americans, facial hair tends to be curly and can become ingrown unless shaved close to the skin.

Mustache and Beard Care. Clients with mustaches or beards require daily grooming. Keeping these areas clean is important because food particles and mucus can easily collect in the hair. If the client is unable to carry out self-care, the nurse should do so at the client's request. Beards can be gently combed out. A shaggy or unkempt mustache or beard can be trimmed. Shaving off a mustache or beard cannot be performed without the client's consent.

Hair and Scalp Care. To best promote and restore hair and scalp health, clients should be instructed to keep hair clean, combed, and brushed regularly. Clients may also need to know how to check for and remove parasites (see Table 38-4). The nurse should tell clients they need to notify their primary caregiver of changes in the texture and distribution of hair, which may indicate a serious systemic problem.

Care of the Eyes, Ears, and Nose.
Special attention is given to cleansing the eyes, ears, and nose during a routine bath and when drainage or discharge accumulate. This aspect of hygiene not only makes the client more comfortable but also improves sensory reception (Chapter 48). Care focuses on preventing infection and maintaining normal sensory function. In addition, care of the eyes, ears, and nose requires approaches that consider the client's special needs (Box 38-12).

Basic Eye Care. Cleansing the eyes simply involves washing with a clean washcloth moistened in water. Soap may cause burning and irritation (see Skill 38-1). Direct

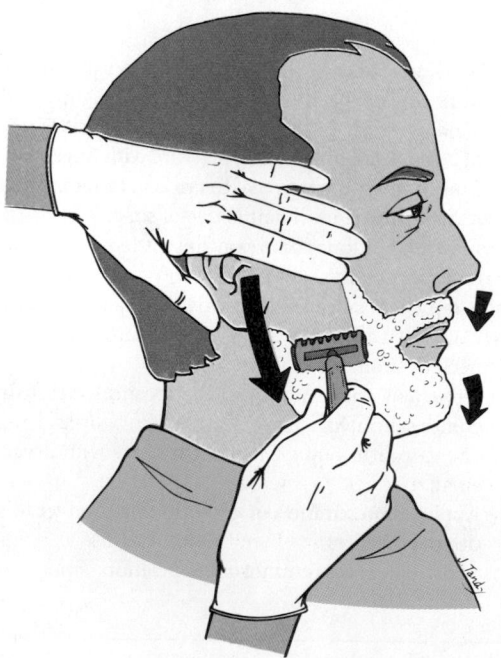

Figure 38-8 Shave in the direction of hair growth. Use longer strokes on the larger areas of the face. Use short strokes around the chin and lips.
From Sorrentino SA: *Assisting with patient care,* St. Louis, 1999, Mosby.

Gerontological NURSING PRACTICE Box 38-12

- Maintaining and improving eyesight are important aspects of an independent and satisfying life for older adults.
  Encourage regular eye examinations.
  Discuss vision changes that occur naturally with aging.
  Describe signs and symptoms of major eye diseases associated with aging.
- 25% to 40% of people 65 years of age and older are hearing impaired (Ney, 1993); speak slowly and articulate carefully. However, do not shout, and do not assume that *all* older clients have difficulty hearing.
- Ear wax tends to be drier in older people, impacts more easily, and takes longer to soften. Complaints of feeling of fullness, itching or ringing, and "blocked hearing" warrant regular assessment (Mahoney, 1993).

pressure should never be applied over the eyeball because it may cause serious injury.

Unconscious clients often require more frequent eye care. Secretions may collect along the lid margins and inner canthus when the blink reflex is absent or when the eye does not totally close. It may be necessary to place an eye patch over the involved eye to prevent corneal drying and irritation. Lubricating eye drops may be given according to the physician's orders.

Eyeglasses. Glasses are made of hardened glass or plastic that is impact resistant to prevent shattering. Nevertheless, because of the cost, the nurse should be careful when cleaning glasses and should protect them from breakage or other damage when they are not worn. Glasses should be put in a case in a drawer of the bedside table when not in use.

Cool water is sufficient for cleaning glass lenses. A soft cloth is best for drying to prevent scratching the lens. Paper towels can scratch a lens. Plastic lenses in particular are scratched easily, and special cleansing solutions and drying tissues are available. Use whatever the client's eye care specialist recommends.

Contact Lenses. A contact lens is a small, round, transparent, and sometimes colored disk that fits directly over the cornea of the eye. Contact lenses are designed specifically to correct refractive errors of the eye or abnormalities in the cornea's shape. They are relatively easy to apply and remove.

There are three basic types of contact lenses: rigid (hard), soft, and rigid gas permeable (RGP), also known as oxygen permeable. They differ in size, material, and amount of oxygen flow they permit to the eye's surface. For example, the rigid lenses ride on the tear film layer of the cornea and are held in place by surface tension. The tear film moves under and over the lens during blinking to provide oxygen to the cornea. Soft lenses cover the entire cornea and a small rim of the sclera. They do not ride on the corneal tear film. The cornea receives oxygen through the soft lens, which is oxygen permeable. Rigid glass permeable lenses are made of plastic that allows oxygen to pass through to the cornea. All three lenses are available as clear (untinted) or tinted.

Contact lenses are also available as daily wear, extended wear, and disposable. In terms of a client's hygiene care it is important to know that all lenses must be removed periodically to prevent ocular infection and corneal ulcers or abrasions. Common infectious agents are *Pseudomonas aeruginosa* and staphylococci. Client education must include a discussion of proper lens care techniques (Box 38-13). Daily-wear lenses should be removed overnight for cleaning and disinfection and should not be worn for more than 10 to 14 hours daily (Cohen and Krachmer, 1992). It is recommended that all extended-wear lenses be worn no longer than six consecutive nights without cleaning and disinfecting (Johnson & Johnson Vision Products, 1994). Disposable lenses are available for daily wear and extended wear and are usually replaced every 1 to 2 weeks. Pain, tearing, discomfort, and redness of the conjunctivae

---

Client Teaching FOR CONTACT LENS CARE   Box 38-13

OBJECTIVES
- Client will be able to identify warning signs of corneal irritation and eye infection.
- Client will be able to clean and care for contact lenses correctly.

TEACHING STRATEGIES
- Encourage client to see a vision care specialist (**ophthalmologist** or **optometrist**) regularly: every 3 to 5 years before age 40, every 2 years after age 40, and yearly after age 65.
- Plastic lenses scratch easily. Special cleaning solutions and drying tissues are recommended.
- Never use fingernail on lens to remove dirt or debris that does not loosen during washing.
- Follow recommendations of lens manufacturer or eye care practitioner when cleaning and disinfecting lenses.
- Encourage client to remember the mnemonic RSVP: *Redness, Sensitivity, Vision problems,* and *Pain.* If one of these problems occurs, remove contact lenses immediately. If problems continue, contact vision care specialist (Lewis, Collier, and Heitkemper, 1996).
- Lenses become very slippery once cleaning solution is applied.

- If lens is dropped on a hard surface, moisten finger with cleaning or wetting solution and gently touch lens to pick it up. Then clean, rinse, and disinfect lens.
- Lens should be kept moist or wet when not worn.
- Use fresh solution daily when storing and disinfecting lenses.
- Do not wipe lens with tissue or towel.
- Thoroughly wash and rinse lens storage case on a daily basis. Clean periodically with soap or liquid detergent; rinse thoroughly with warm water and air dry.
- To avoid mix-up, always start with the same lens when removing or inserting lenses.
- Disposable or planned replacement lenses should be thrown away after prescribed wearing period.

EVALUATION
- Have client identify warning signs of corneal irritation and eye infection.
- Ask client to describe methods of contact lens care that can lead to infection.
- Ask client to describe techniques to use in cleaning and storing contact lens.

may be symptoms of lens overwear. Persistence of symptoms even after lens removal is abnormal, however, and may indicate serious ocular damage.

As contact lenses are worn, they accumulate secretions and foreign matter. This material deteriorates and then irritates the eye, causing distorted vision and risk for infection. Once removed, contact lenses should be cleaned and thoroughly disinfected. Clients should be cautioned to never use saliva, homemade saline, or tap water when cleaning lenses as these solutions may contain microorganisms that can cause serious infection. Skill 38-7 reviews steps for contact lens removal, cleansing, and reinsertion.

Artificial Eyes.   Clients with artificial eyes have had an **enucleation** of an entire eyeball as a result of tumor growth, severe infection, or eye trauma. Some artificial eyes are permanently implanted. Others can be removed for routine cleaning. Clients with artificial eyes usually prefer to care for their own eyes. The nurse should respect the client's wishes and help by assembling needed equipment.

Clients may at times require assistance in prosthesis removal and cleansing. To remove an artificial eye, the nurse retracts the lower eyelid and exerts slight pressure just below the eye (Figure 38-9). This action causes the artificial

eye to rise from the socket because the suction holding the eye in place has been broken. The nurse may also use a small, rubber bulb syringe or medicine dropper bulb to create a suction effect. The suction created by placing the bulb tip directly over the eye and squeezing lifts the eye from the socket.

The artificial eye is usually made of glass or plastic. Warm normal saline cleanses the prosthesis effectively. The nurse also cleanses the edges of the eye socket and surrounding tissues with soft gauze moistened in saline or clean tap water. Signs of infection should be reported immediately because bacteria can spread to the neighboring eye, underlying sinuses, or even underlying brain tissue. To reinsert the eye, the nurse retracts the upper and lower lids and gently slips the eye into the socket, fitting it neatly under the upper eyelid. An artificial eye may be stored in a labeled container filled with tap water or saline.

Ear Care.   Routine ear care involves cleansing the ear with the end of a moistened washcloth, rotated gently into the ear canal. When cerumen is visible, gentle, downward retraction at the entrance of the ear canal may cause the wax to loosen and slip out. The nurse warns clients never to use sharp objects such as bobby pins or paper clips to remove ear wax. The use of such objects can traumatize the ear canal and rupture the tympanic membrane. Use of cotton-tipped applicators should also be avoided because they can cause ear wax to become impacted within the canal.

Children and older adults commonly have impacted cerumen. Excessive or impacted cerumen can usually be removed only by irrigation. If a client has a history of a perforated eardrum or if perforation is discovered during assessment, the procedure is contraindicated. The procedure first involves instilling three drops of glycerine at bedtime to soften the wax, and three drops of hydrogen peroxide twice a day to loosen the wax (Phipps and others, 1995). Then the instillation of approximately 250 ml of warm water (37° C, or 98.6° F) into the ear canal mechanically washes away loosened wax. Cold or hot water causes nausea or vomiting.

The client may sit or lie on his or her side with the affected ear up. The nurse places a small curved basin under the affected ear to catch the irrigating solution. A Water Pik (set on No. 2 setting) or a bulb irrigating syringe can be used to irrigate the ear canal. The tip of the syringe or Water Pik should not occlude the canal to avoid exerting pressure against the tympanic membrane. Gentle irrigation directed at the top of the canal loosens the cerumen from the sides of the canal. After the canal is clear, the nurse wipes off any moisture from the ear and inspects the canal for remaining cerumen.

Hearing Aid Care.   Chapter 48 discusses the need for and use of hearing aids. Hearing aids are instruments made up of miniature parts working together as a system

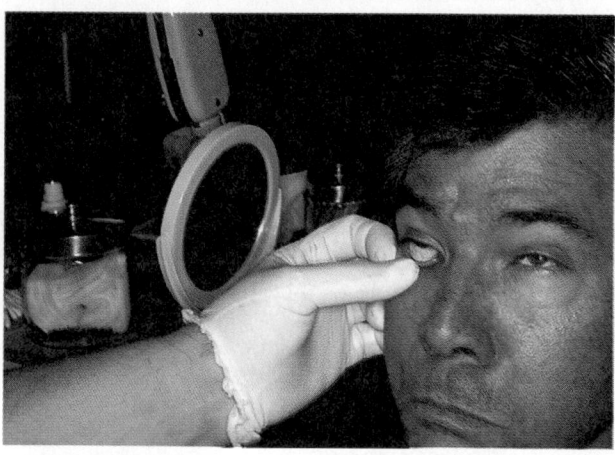

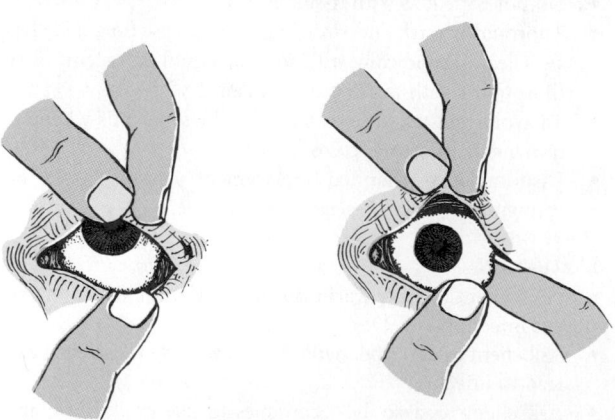

Figure 38-9   Removal of prosthetic eye.

Caring for the Client With Contact Lenses   Skill 38-7

Delegation Considerations
The skills of caring for eye prostheses can be delegated to assistive personnel.
- Inform and assist caregiver in proper way to care for eye prostheses.

- Stress to caregiver that careful handling of these devices is of utmost importance to prevent physical injury to the client and damage to the devices.
- Inform caregiver of types of findings to report (e.g., eye pain, eye socket drainage).

EQUIPMENT
- Clean lens storage container
- Bath towel
- Suction cup (optional)
- Sterile saline solution
- Sterile lens cleaning solution
- Sterile lens rinsing solution

- Sterile lens disinfectant
- Sterile enzyme solution (depends on care regimen)
- Sterile wetting solution (depends on care regimen)
- Cotton ball or cotton-tipped applicator
- Emesis basin
- Disposable gloves

STEPS	RATIONALE
1. Place towel just below client's face.	Catches lens if one should accidentally fall from eye.
2. Stand at client's side. Inspect eye, or ask client if contact lens is in place. Unconscious or confused clients should be carefully assessed; lenses are often difficult to assess if clear (untinted).	Lenses are generally comfortable to wear, and client may forget they are in place. Prolonged wear may cause injury to eye.
3. Ask if client feels any eye discomfort, and assess length of time client normally wears lenses.	Scratched lens can cause corneal irritation and abrasion. Accumulation of dust or debris between lens and cornea causes irritation. Continuous wearing of certain types of lenses can irritate cornea.
4. Ask if client is able to manipulate and hold contact lens.	Determines level of assistance required in care.
5. Assess client for any unusual visual signs/symptoms (reduced visual acuity, blurred vision, pain photophobia).	May indicate underlying visual alteration or need to change lens prescription. A reduction in visual acuity calls for referral.
6. Assess types of medications prescribed for client: sedatives, hypnotics, muscle relaxants, antihistamines, anticholinergics, and antidepressants.	Sedatives, hypnotics, and muscle relaxants reduce blink reflex and thus reduce lubrication of cornea. Antihistamines, anticholinergics, and antidepressants can reduce tear production.
7. After lenses are removed (see Step 11), inspect eye for signs of corneal irritation (e.g., redness, pain, swelling of eyelids and conjunctivae, discharge, and excess tearing). If pain persists or worsens after removal of lenses, an immediate referral to the ophthalmologist should be made.	Signs/symptoms indicate corneal irritation or abrasion. Severe pain may indicate corneal epithelium disruption or infection (Cohen and Krachmer, 1992).
8. Discuss procedure with client.	Client can assist in planning by explaining technique that may aid removal and insertion. Client may be anxious as nurse retracts eyelids and manipulates lenses.
9. Have client assume supine or sitting position in bed or chair.	Provides easy access for nurse while retracting eyelids and manipulating lenses.
10. Assemble supplies at bedside.	Provides easy access to supplies.
11. Remove lenses.	
A. **Soft lenses**	
(1) Wash hands. Apply disposable gloves if there are cuts, scratches, or dermatological lesions on nurse's hands.	Reduces transmission of microorganisms.
(2) Add a few drops of sterile saline solution to client's eye.	Lubricates eye to facilitate lens removal.
(3) Tell client to look straight ahead.	Eases tipping of lens during removal.
(4) Using middle finger, retract lower eyelid.	Exposes lower edge of lens.
(5) With pad of index finger of same hand, slide lens off cornea onto white of eye.	Positions lens for easy grasping. Use of finger pad (rather than fingernail) prevents injury to cornea and damage to lens.
(6) Pull upper eyelid down gently with thumb of other hand, and compress lens slightly between thumb and index finger.	Causes soft lens to double up. Air enters underneath lens to release suction.

STEPS	RATIONALE
(7) Gently pinch lens, and lift out.	Protects lens from damage. Avoid allowing lens edges to stick together. Soft lenses can be easily torn.
(8) Clean and rinse lens. Place lens in proper storage case compartment: *R* for right lens and *L* for left lens (see illustration).	Ensures proper lens will be reinserted into correct eye. Proper storage prevents cracking or tearing.
(a) After removing one lens from case, apply one or two drops of cleaning solution to lens in palm of hand (use cleanser recommended by lens manufacturer or eye care practitioner).	Removes tear components, including mucus, lipids, and proteins that collect on lens.
(b) Rub lens gently but thoroughly on both sides for 20 to 30 sec. Use index finger (soft lenses) or little finger or cotton-tipped applicator soaked with cleaning solution (rigid lenses) to clean inside lens. Be careful not to turn lens wrong side out or touch or scratch lens with fingernail.	It is easier to manipulate and clean lens using fingertips. Cleans microorganisms from all surfaces.
(c) Holding lens over emesis basin, rinse thoroughly with manufacturer-recommended rinsing solution (soft lenses) or cold tap water (rigid lenses).	Removes debris and cleaning solution from lens surface. Rinsing methods and solutions differ for each type of lens.
(d) Place lens in proper storage case compartment and fill with storage solution recommended by manufacturer or eye care practitioner.	Disinfects lens, removes residue, enhances wetability of lens, and prevents scratches to lens that can be caused by a dry case.
(9) Repeat Steps (2) through (8) for other lens. Secure cover over storage case. Label with client's name and room number.	Proper storage prevents damage to or loss of lenses.
(10) Dispose of towel, remove gloves, and wash hands.	Reduces transmission of infection.

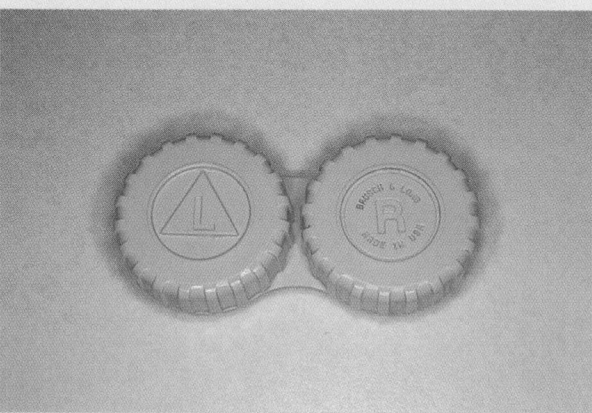

Step 11A(8)

STEPS	RATIONALE

B. **Rigid lenses**

(1) Wash hands, and apply gloves if needed. — Reduces transmission of microorganisms.

(2) Be sure lens is positioned directly over cornea. If lens is not positioned directly over cornea, have client close eyelids, place index and middle fingers of one hand on eyelid just beside the lens and beneath it, and gently but firmly massage lens back into place. — Correct position of lens allows easy removal from eye.

(3) Place index finger on outer corner of client's eye, and draw skin gently back toward ear. — Tightens eyelid against eyeball.

(4) Tell client to blink. Do not release pressure on eyelid until blink is completed. — Maneuver should cause lens to dislodge and pop out. Lid margins must clear top and bottom of lens until the blink.

(5) If lens fails to pop out, gently retract eyelid beyond edges of lens. Press lower eyelid gently against lower edge of lens. — Pressure causes upper edge of lens to tip forward.

(6) Allow both eyelids to close slightly, and grasp lens as it rises from eye. Cup lens in hand. — Maneuver causes lens to slide off easily. Protects lens from breakage.

(7) A lens suction cup can be used to remove lenses from the eyes of confused or unconscious clients. Gently apply suction cup to lens surface, and lift out.

(8) Clean and rinse lens (see Step 11A[8]). Place lens in proper storage case compartment: *R* for right lens and *L* for left lens. Center lens in storage case, convex side down. — Both lenses may not have the same prescription. Proper storage prevents breaking, scratching, chipping, and discoloration.

(9) Repeat Steps (2) through (8) for other lens. Secure cover over storage case. Label with client's name and room number. — Proper storage prevents damage to or loss of lenses.

(10) Dispose of towel, remove gloves, and wash hands. — Reduces spread of infection and keeps client's environment neat.

12. Insert Lenses

A. **Soft lenses**

(1) Remove right lens from storage case and rinse with recommended rinsing solution; inspect lens for foreign materials, tears, or other damage.

(2) Check that lens is not inverted (inside out). Apply wetting agent (sterile saline). — Soft lens is inverted if the edge has a lip; it is in proper position if curve is even from base to rim.

(3) Using middle or index finger of opposite hand, retract upper lid until iris is exposed.

(4) Use middle finger of the hand holding lens to pull down lower lid.

(5) Tell client to look straight ahead; gently place lens directly on cornea; release lids slowly, starting with lower lid.

(6) Tell client to close eyes slowly and roll them toward lens if not on the cornea.

(7) Tell client to blink a few times.

(8) Ask client to open eyes. Check for blurred vision or discomfort. — Ensures lens is centered, free of trapped air, and comfortable.

(9) Repeat Steps (1) to (8) for left eye.

(10) Discard used solution in the storage case.

(11) Wash lens case with soap and a scrubber. Rinse case in sterile saline or a known disinfectant. Store dry. — Prevents multiplication of amoeba and bacteria (Martin and Barr, 1997).

STEPS	RATIONALE

B. **Rigid lenses**

(1) Remove right lens from storage case; attempt to lift lens straight up (see illustration).

(2) Rinse with recommended rinsing solution; inspect lens for foreign material or chips.

(3) Wet lens on both sides, using prescribed wetting solution.

(4) Place right lens concave side up on tip of index finger of dominant hand (see illustration).

(5) Instruct client to look straight ahead while retracting both upper and lower lids; place lens gently over center of cornea (see illustration).

(6) Ask client to close eyes briefly and avoid blinking.

(7) Ask client to open eyes. Check for blurred vision or discomfort.

(8) Repeat Steps (1) to (7) for left eye.

(9) Discard used solution. See Step 12A(11) for case cleansing.

Sliding lens out of case can cause scratches on the surface.

Hot water causes lens to warp.

Inner surface of lens should face up so that it is applied against cornea.

Helps to secure position of lens.

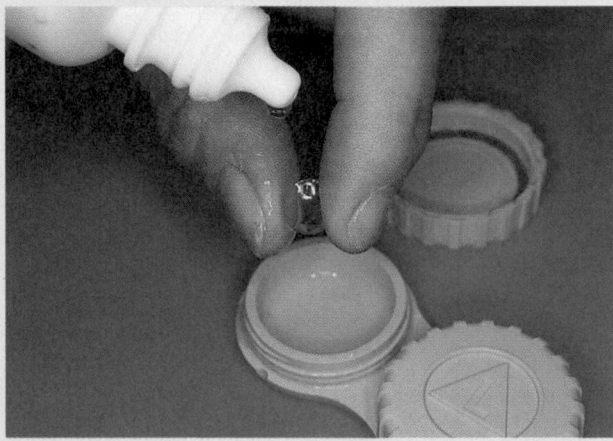

Step 12B(1)

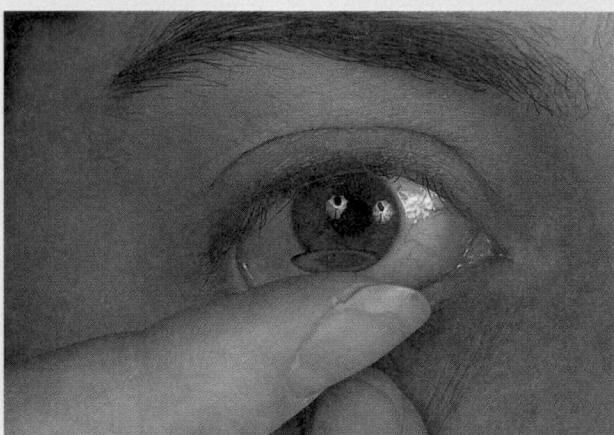

Step 12B(4)

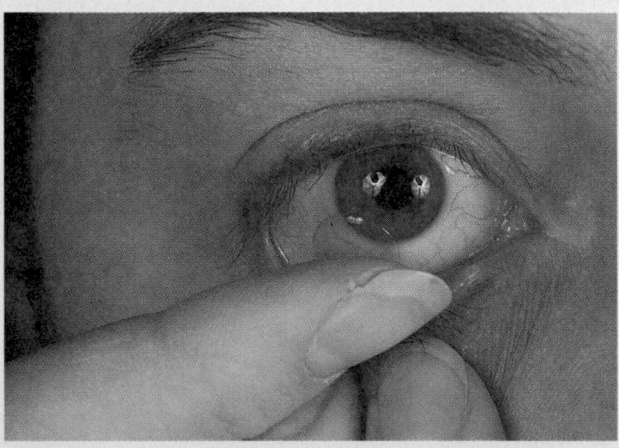

Step 12B(5)

STEPS	RATIONALE
13. Ask client if lens feels comfortable after removal and rein-sertion of lenses.	Determines if any debris is caught between lens and cornea. Lens should be removed if client experiences discomfort.
14. Inspect eye (over time) for signs of ocular infection.	
15. Assess client's visual acuity (see Chapter 32).	Determines improvement in visual perception.
16. Observe client for signs of eye injury.	

Recording and Reporting

- Record or report any signs/symptoms of visual alterations or corneal irritation noted during procedure.
- Record on nursing care plan or Kardex times of lens insertion and removal if client is going to surgery or special procedure.

Home Care Considerations

- Clients must be taught not to wear lenses in presence of noxious or irritating vapors or fumes because these irritants can cause damage to lens surface.

to amplify sound in a controlled manner. The aid receives normal low-intensity sound inputs and delivers them to the client's ear as louder outputs. The new class of hearing aids can reduce background noise interference. Computer chips placed in the aids allow for fine adjustments to the specific client's hearing needs. Hearing aids are used by both hard-of-hearing (slight or moderate hearing loss) and deaf persons (severe or prolonged hearing loss).

There are three popular types of hearing aids. An in-the-canal (ITC) aid is the newest, smallest, and least visible and fits entirely in the ear canal. It has cosmetic appeal, is easy to manipulate and place in the ear, does not interfere with wearing eyeglasses or using the telephone, and can be worn during most physical exercise. However, it requires adequate ear diameter and depth for proper fit. It does not accomodate progressive hearing loss, and it requires manual dexterity to operate, insert, remove, and change batteries. Also, cerumen tends to plug this model more than the others.

An in-the-ear (ITE, or intraaural) aid (see Figure 38-10, *A*) fits into the external auditory canal and allows for more fine tuning. It is more powerful and stronger and therefore is useful for a wider range of hearing loss than the ITC aid. It is easy to position and adjust and does not interfere with eyeglass wearing. It is, however, more noticeable than the ITC aid and is not recommended for persons with moisture or skin problems in the ear canal.

A behind-the-ear (BTE, or postaural) aid (see Figure 38-10, *B*) hooks around and behind the ear and is connected by a short, clear, hollow plastic tube to an ear mold inserted into the external auditory canal. It allows for fine tuning. It is the largest of the three aids and is useful for clients with rapidly progressive hearing loss or manual dexterity difficulties or those who find partial ear occlusion intolerable. Disadvantages are that it is more visible and may interfere with wearing eyeglasses and using a

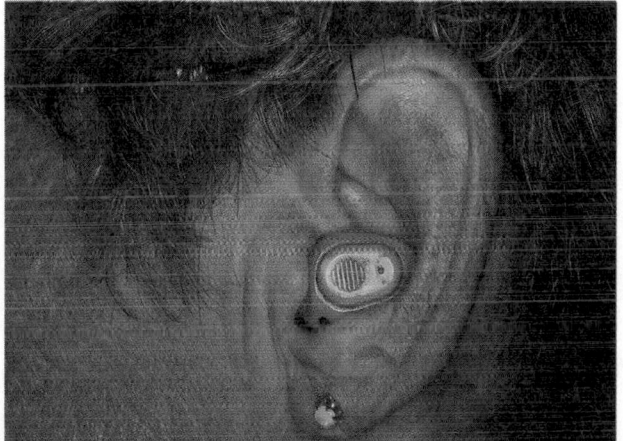

A

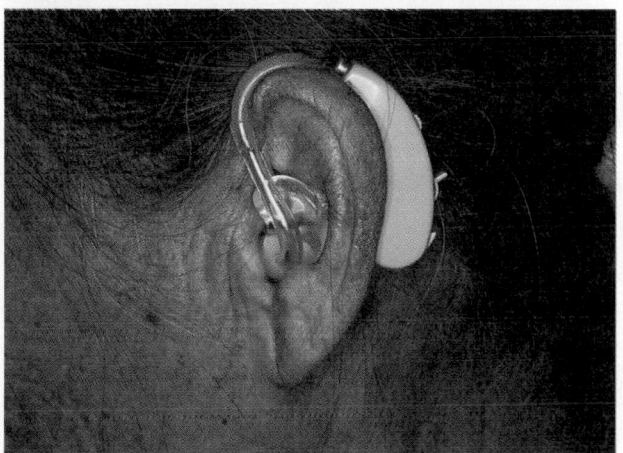

B

Figure 38-10 Two common types of hearing aids. **A,** In the ear. **B,** Behind the ear.

Care and Use of Hearing Aids   Box 38-14

Initially wear a hearing aid 15 to 20 minutes; then gradually increase time until 10 to 12 hours.

Once inserted, turn the aid slowly to one-third to one-half volume.

A whistling sound indicates incorrect ear mold insertion.

Adjust volume to a comfortable level for talking at a distance of 1 yard.

Do not wear aid under heat lamps; a hair dryer; or in very wet, cold weather.

Batteries last 1 week with daily wearing of 10 to 12 hours.

Remove or disconnect battery when not in use.

Replace ear molds every 2 or 3 years.

- Routinely check battery compartment: Is it clean? Are batteries inserted properly? Is compartment shut all the way?
- Dials on hearing aid should be clean and easy to rotate, creating no static during adjusting.
- Routinely check cord or tubing (depending on type of aid) for cracking, fraying, and poor connections.

Modified from Ebersole P, Hess P: *Toward healthy aging*, ed 4, St. Louis, 1995, Mosby, and Lueckenotte AG: *Gerontologic nursing*, St. Louis, 1996, Mosby.

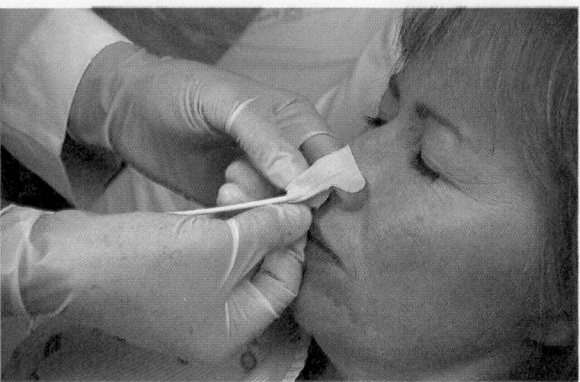

Figure 38-11   Applying new tape over feeding tube.

phone, and it is more difficult to keep in place during physical exercise. Box 38-14 reviews guidelines for the care and cleaning of a hearing aid.

Nasal Care.   The client can usually remove secretions from the nose by gently blowing into a soft tissue. The nurse cautions the client against harsh blowing that creates pressure capable of injuring the eardrum, nasal mucosa, and even sensitive eye structures. Bleeding from the nares is a sign of harsh blowing.

If the client is unable to remove nasal secretions, the nurse assists by using a wet washcloth or a cotton-tipped applicator moistened in water or saline. The applicator should never be inserted beyond the length of the cotton tip. Excessive nasal secretions can also be removed by gentle suctioning.

When clients have nasogastric, feeding, or endotracheal tubes inserted through the nose, the nurse should change the tape anchoring the tube at least once a day. When tape becomes moist from nasal secretions, the skin and mucosa can easily become macerated. Friction from a tube can cause tissue sloughing. After carefully removing the tape, the nurse maintains hold of the tubing and thoroughly cleanses and dries the nasal surface. The nurse should know how to tape tubing correctly to minimize tension or friction on the nares. In the case of a feeding tube the nurse can apply a light film of tincture of benzoin on the nose to make it "tacky." A tube fixation device consisting of a shaped adhesive patch is then applied to the nose and around both sides of the tubing (Figure 38-11). Another option is to take a 2-inch-long piece of hypoallergenic tape and split one end about halfway down

the tape. Place the intact end over the bridge of the client's nose. Then wrap each of the strips around the tube as it exits the nose. When sloughing of nasal tissue occurs, it may be necessary for the nurse to remove the tube and insert one through the other nares, pending a physician's order.

Client's Room Environment.   Attempting to make a client's room as comfortable as the home is one of the nurse's priorities. The client's room should be comfortable, safe, and large enough to allow the client and visitors to move about freely. The nurse can control room temperature, ventilation, noise, and odors to create a more comfortable environment. Keeping the room neat and orderly also contributes to the client's sense of well-being.

Maintaining Comfort.   The nature of what constitutes a comfortable environment depends on the client's age, severity of illness, and level of normal daily activity. Depending on the client's age and physical condition, the room temperature should be maintained between 20° and 23° C (68° and 74° F). Infants, older adults, and the acutely ill may need a warmer room. However, certain ill clients benefit from cooler room temperatures to lower the body's metabolic demands.

A good ventilation system keeps stale air and odors from lingering in the room. The nurse must protect the acutely ill, infants, and older adults from drafts by ensuring they are adequately dressed and covered with a lightweight blanket.

Good ventilation also reduces lingering odors caused by draining wounds, vomitus, bowel movements, and unemptied urinals. Room deodorizers can help remove many unpleasant odors but should be used with discretion in consideration of the client's possible embarrassment. Nurses should always empty and rinse bedpans or urinals promptly. Thorough hygiene measures are the best way to control body or breath odors. Most health care institutions now prohibit smoking. Before using room deodorizers the nurse should determine that the client is not allergic to or sensitive to the deodorizer itself.

Ill clients seem to be more sensitive to common hospital noises (e.g., intravenous pump alarms, suction apparatus, or stretchers exiting an elevator). Until the client is familiar with hospital noises, the nurse should try to control the noise level. This can also help the client gain necessary sleep. The nurse also explains the source of any unfamiliar noise to the client and family members.

Proper lighting is necessary for everyone's safety and comfort. A brightly lit room is usually stimulating, but a darkened room is best for rest and sleep. Room lighting can be adjusted by closing or opening drapes, regulating overbed and floor lights, and closing or opening room doors. When entering a client's room at night, refrain from abruptly turning on an overhead light unless necessary.

Room Equipment.
A typical hospital room contains the following basic pieces of furniture: overbed table, bedside stand, chairs, lamp, and bed (Figure 38-12). Long-term care and rehabilitation facilities may have similar equipment. The overbed table rolls on wheels and can be adjusted to various heights over the bed or a chair. Usually two storage areas are under the tabletop. The table provides ideal working space for the nurse performing procedures. It also provides a surface on which to place meal trays, toiletry items, and objects frequently used by the client. The bedpan and urinal should not be placed on the overbed table. The bedside stand is used to store the client's personal possessions and hygiene equipment. The telephone, water pitcher, and drinking cup are commonly found on a bedside stand.

Most hospital rooms contain an armless straight-backed chair and an upholstered lounge chair with arms. The lounge chair is used by the client and visitors and is usually placed at the foot of the bed or beside it. Straight-backed chairs are convenient when temporarily transferring the client from the bed, such as during bed making.

Each room usually has an overbed light and a floor or table lamp. Movable lights that extend over the bed from the wall should be positioned for easy reach but moved aside when not in use. Gooseneck or special examination lights are portable standing lights used to provide extra light during bedside procedures.

Other equipment usually found in a client's room includes a call light, a television set, a blood pressure gauge, oxygen and vacuum wall outlets, and personal care items. Special equipment designed for comfort or positioning clients includes footboards and foot boots (Figure 38-13), special mattresses (see Chapter 47), and bed boards.

Beds.
Seriously ill clients may remain in bed for a long time. Because a bed is the piece of equipment used

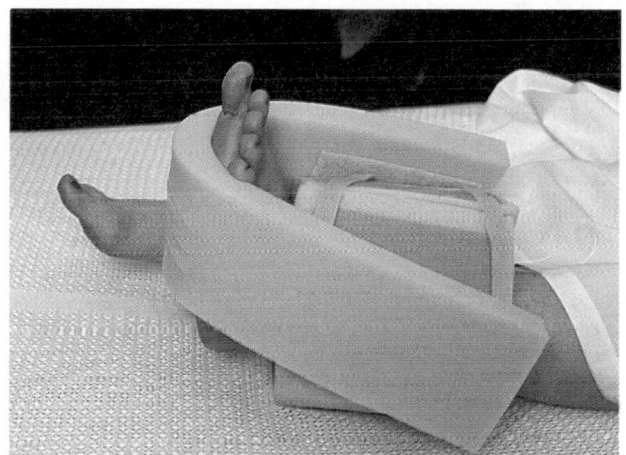

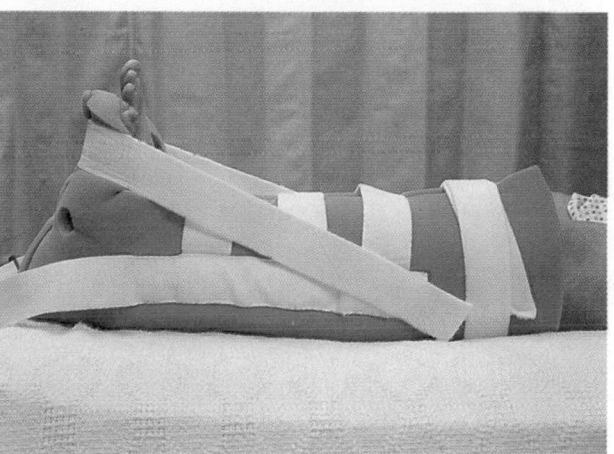

Figure 38-13 **A,** Foot boot. **B,** Foot boot with lower leg extension.

Figure 38-12 Typical hospital room.

most by a hospitalized client, it should be designed for comfort, safety, and adaptability for changing positions.

The typical hospital bed has a firm mattress on a metal frame that can be raised and lowered horizontally. More and more hospitals are converting the standard hospital bed to one in which the mattress surface can be electronically adjusted for client comfort. Different bed positions are used to promote client comfort, minimize symptoms, promote lung expansion, and to improve access during certain procedures (Table 38-8).

The position of a bed is usually changed by electrical controls incorporated into the client's call light and in a panel on the side or foot of the bed (Figure 38-14). It is important for the nurse to become familiar with use of the bed controls. Ease in raising and lowering a bed and in changing position of the head and foot eliminates undue musculoskeletal strain on the nurse. Nurses should instruct clients on the proper use of controls and caution them against raising the bed to a position that might cause harm.

Beds contain safety features such as locks on the wheels or casters. Wheels should be locked when the bed is sta-tionary to prevent accidental movement. Side rails protect clients from accidental falls. The headboard can be removed from most beds. This is important when the medical team must have easy access to the head, such as during cardiopulmonary resuscitation.

Bed Making.   A client's bed should be kept clean and comfortable. This requires frequent inspections to be sure linen is clean, dry, and free of wrinkles. When clients are diaphoretic, have draining wounds, or are incontinent, the nurse should check frequently for soiled linen.

The nurse usually makes a bed in the morning after the client's bath or while the client is bathing in a shower, sitting in a chair eating, or out of the room for procedures or tests. Throughout the day the nurse straightens linen that becomes loose or wrinkled. The bed linen should also be checked for food particles after meals and for wetness or soiling. Linen that becomes soiled or wet should be changed.

When changing bed linen, the nurse follows principles of medical asepsis by keeping soiled linen away from the uniform (Figure 38-15). Soiled linen is placed in special linen bags before discarding in a hamper. To avoid air cur-

Table 38-8 Common Bed Positions

Position	Description	Uses
Fowler's	Head of bed raised to angle of 45 degrees or more; semisitting position; foot of bed may also be raised at knee	Is preferred while client eats Is used during nasogastric tube insertion and nasotracheal suction Promotes lung expansion
Semi-Fowler's	Head of bed raised approximately 30 degrees; inclination less than Fowler's position; foot of bed may also be raised at knee	Promotes lung expansion Used when clients receive gastric feedings to reduce regurgitation and risk of aspiration
Trendelenburg's	Entire bed frame tilted with head of bed down	Is used for postural drainage Facilitates venous return in clients with poor peripheral perfusion
Reverse Trendelenburg's	Entire bed frame tilted with foot of bed down	Is used infrequently Promotes gastric emptying Prevents esophageal reflux
Flat	Entire bed frame horizontally parallel with floor	Is used for clients with vertebral injuries and in cervical traction Is used for clients who are hypotensive Is generally preferred by clients for sleeping

rents, which can spread microorganisms, the nurse never fans linen. To avoid transmitting infection, the nurse should not place soiled linen on the floor. If clean linen touches the floor, it is immediately discarded.

During bed making, the nurse must use proper body mechanics (Chapter 36). The bed should always be raised to its highest position before changing linen so that the nurse does not have to bend or stretch over the mattress. The nurse also moves back and forth to opposite sides of the bed while applying new linen. Body mechanics also become important when turning or repositioning the client in bed.

When clients are confined to bed, the nurse organizes bed-making activities to conserve time and energy (Skill 38-8). The client's privacy, comfort, and safety are all important when making a bed. Using side rails, keeping call lights within the client's reach, and maintaining the proper bed position help promote comfort and safety. After making a bed, the nurse always returns it to the lowest horizontal position to prevent accidental falls should the client get in and out of the bed alone.

When possible the nurse should make the bed while it is unoccupied (Box 38-15, p. 1120). The nurse uses judgment in regard to when is the best time to have the client sit up in a chair while the bed is made. When making an unoccupied bed, the nurse follows the same basic principles as for occupied bed making.

An unoccupied bed can be open or closed. In an open bed, the top covers are folded back so that a client can easily get into bed. In a closed bed, the top sheet, blanket, and bedspread are drawn up to the head of the mattress and under the pillows. A closed bed is prepared in a hospital room before a new client is admitted to that room. A surgical, recovery, or postoperative bed is a modified version of the open bed. The top bed linen is arranged for easy transfer of the client from a stretcher to the bed. The top sheets and spread are not tucked or mitered at the corners. Instead, the top sheets are folded to one side or fanfolded to the bottom third of the bed (Figure 38-16). This makes it easier to transfer the client into the bed.

Linens. In any health care agency, it is important to have an adequate supply of linen to care appropriately for clients. Many agencies have what are called "nurse servers" either within or just outside a client's room where a daily supply of linen is stored. Because of the importance of cost control in health care, it is important to not bring excess linen into a client's room. Once the linen is brought into a client's room, if unused, it must be discarded for laundering. This can increase an agency's costs. Excess linen lying around a client's room creates clutter and obstacles for client care activities.

Before bed making, it is important to collect necessary bed linens and the client's personal items. In this way the nurse will have all equipment accessible to prepare the bed and room. Linens are pressed and folded to prevent the spread of microorganisms and to make bed making easier.

Text continued on p. 1120.

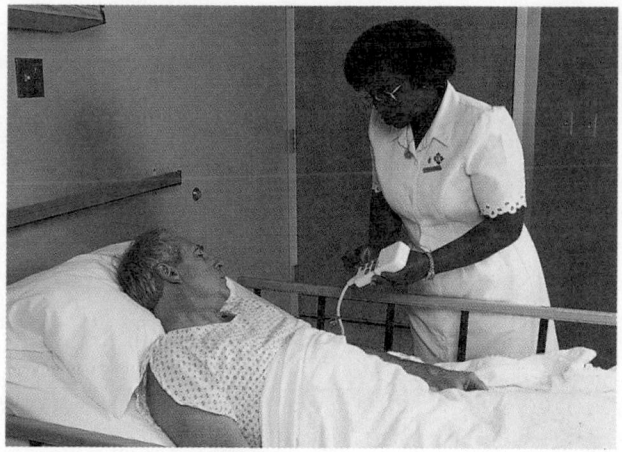

Figure 38-14 Nurse instructing client in use of call light and bed controls.

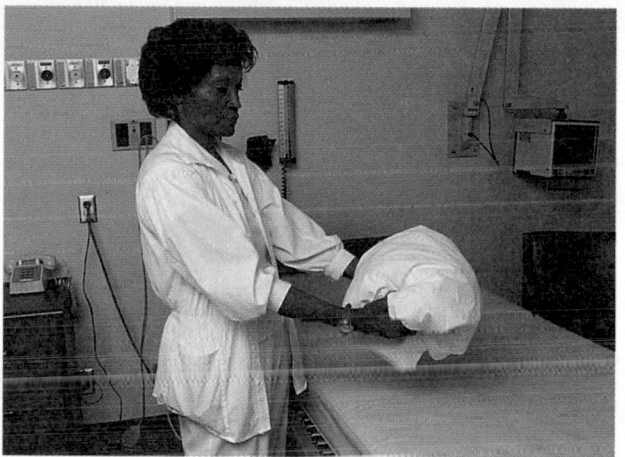

Figure 38-15 Holding linen away from the uniform prevents contact with microorganisms.

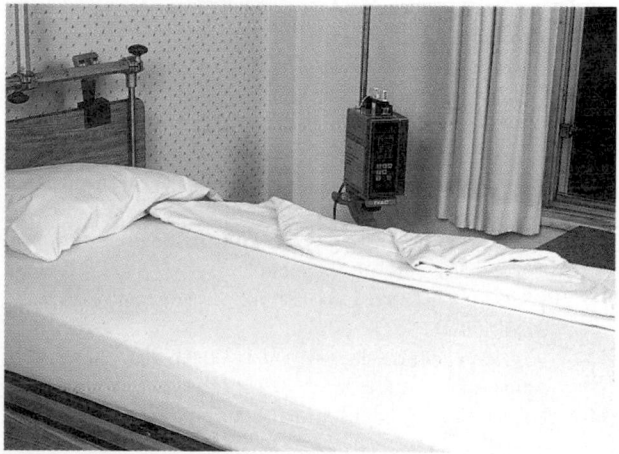

Figure 38-16 Surgical or recovery bed.

Skill 38-8   Making an Occupied Bed

Delegation Considerations

The skill of making an occupied bed can be delegated to assistive personnel.

- Inform caregiver how to properly position clients during occupied bed-making procedure.
- Tell caregiver what to do if wound drainage, dressing material, drainage tubes, or intravenous (IV) tubing becomes dislodged or is found in the linens.

- Instruct caregiver on what to do if client becomes fatigued.
- Stress safety procedures, for example, location of call system for easy access in the event that staff assistance is needed.
- Instruct caregiver to report any changes in client's level of consciousness, breathing patterns, level of pain, or dizziness.

EQUIPMENT

- Linen bag(s)
- Mattress pad (needs to be changed only when soiled)
- Bottom sheet (flat or fitted)
- Drawsheet
- Top sheet
- Blanket

- Bedspread
- Waterproof pads and/or bath blankets (optional)
- Pillowcases
- Bedside chair or table
- Disposable gloves (optional)

STEPS	RATIONALE
1. Determine if client is incontinent or has excess drainage on bed linen.	Determines need for protective waterproof pads or extra bath blankets on bed.
2. Check chart for orders or specific precautions for movement and positioning.	Ensures safety and use of proper body mechanics for nurse and client.
3. Explain procedure to client, noting that client will be asked to turn on side to roll over linen.	Minimizes anxiety and promotes cooperation.
4. Prepare needed equipment and supplies.	
5. Wash hands.	Minimizes spread of infection.
6. Assemble and arrange equipment on bedside chair or table. Remove unnecessary equipment.	Provides for smooth procedure and ensures comfort.
7. Draw room curtain around bed or close door.	Maintains privacy, thus promoting emotional and physical comfort.
8. Lower side rail on near side of bed. Remove call light.	Provides easy access to bed and linen.
9. Adjust bed height to comfortable working position.	Minimizes strain on nurse's back. It is easier to remove and apply linen evenly to bed in flat position.
10. Loosen top linen sheet at foot of bed.	Makes linen easier to remove.
11. Remove bedspread and blanket separately by folding them into squares and placing them in linen bag (if not to be reused). Do not allow linen to contact uniform. Do not fan or shake linen.	Reduces transmission of microorganisms.
12. If blanket and spread are to be reused, fold by bringing top and bottom edges together. Fold into neat squares and place folded linen over back of chair.	Facilitates replacement and prevents wrinkling.
13. Cover client with bath blanket in following manner. Unfold bath blanket over top sheet. Ask client to hold top edge of bath blanket. If client is unable to help, tuck top of bath blanket under shoulder. Grasp top sheet under bath blanket at client's shoulders, and bring sheet down to foot of bed. Remove sheet, and discard it in linen bag. Optional: Client may be covered with loosened top sheet if bath blanket is not available.	Bath blanket provides warmth and keeps body parts covered during linen removal.
14. With assistance from another nurse, slide mattress toward head of bed.	If mattress slides toward foot of bed when head of bed is raised, it is difficult to tuck linen and is uncomfortable for client.
15. Position client on the side on far side of bed, facing away. Adjust pillow under head. Be sure farthest side rail is up.	Provides space for placement of clean linen. Side rail ensures safety.
16. Loosen bottom linens, moving from head to foot of bed.	

STEPS	RATIONALE
17. Fanfold first drawsheet and then bottom sheet toward client (see illustration). Tuck edges of linen just under buttocks, back, and shoulders. Do not fanfold mattress pad if it is to be reused.	Provides maximum work space for placing clean linen. Later, when client turns to other side, soiled linen can be easily removed.
18. Wipe off moisture on mattress with towel and appropriate disinfectant.	Reduces transmission of microorganisms.
19. Apply clean linen to exposed half of bed:	
a. Place clean mattress pad on bed by folding it lengthwise with center crease in middle of bed. Fanfold top layer over mattress. (If pad is reused, simply smooth out wrinkles.)	Applying linen over bed in successive layers minimizes energy and time nurse uses in bed making.
b. Unfold bottom sheet lengthwise so center crease is situated lengthwise along center of bed. Fanfold sheet's top layer toward center of bed alongside client (see illustration). Smooth bottom layer of sheet over mattress, and bring edge over near side. Allow sheet's edge to hang about 25 cm (10 in) over mattress edge. Lower hem of bottom sheet should lie seam down and even with bottom edge of mattress.	Proper positioning of linen on one side ensures that adequate linen will be available to cover opposite side of bed. Keeping seam edges down eliminates irritation to client's skin.
20. Miter bottom sheet at head of bed:	Mitered corner cannot be loosened easily, even if client moves about frequently in bed.
a. Face head of bed diagonally. Place hand away from head of bed under top corner of mattress, near mattress edge, and lift.	

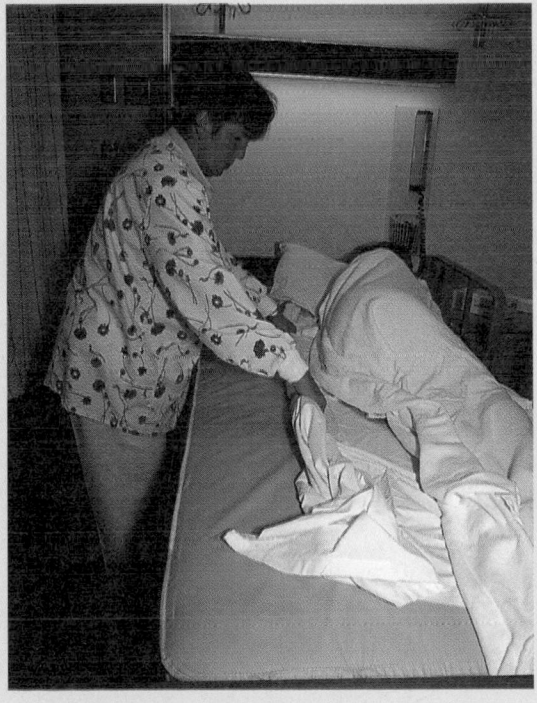

Step 17

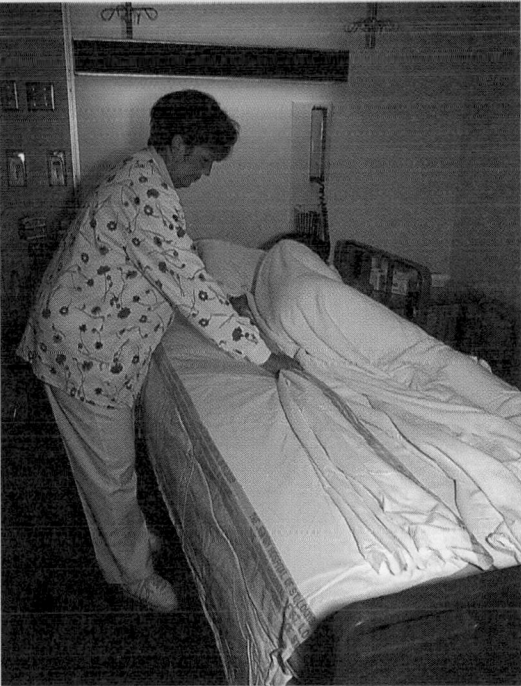

Step 19b

STEPS	RATIONALE

b. With other hand, tuck top edge of bottom sheet smoothly under mattress so side edges of sheet above and below mattress would meet if brought together.

c. Face side of bed, and pick up top edge of sheet at approximately 45 cm (18 in) down from top of mattress (see illustration).

d. Lift sheet, and lay it on top of mattress to form neat triangular fold, with lower base of triangle even with mattress side edge (see illustration).

e. Tuck lower edge of sheet, which is hanging free below mattress, under mattress (see illustration). Tuck with palms down without pulling triangular fold.

f. Hold portion of sheet covering side edge of mattress in place with one hand. With other hand, pick up top of triangular linen fold, and bring it down over side of mattress. Tuck this portion of sheet under mattress (see illustrations).

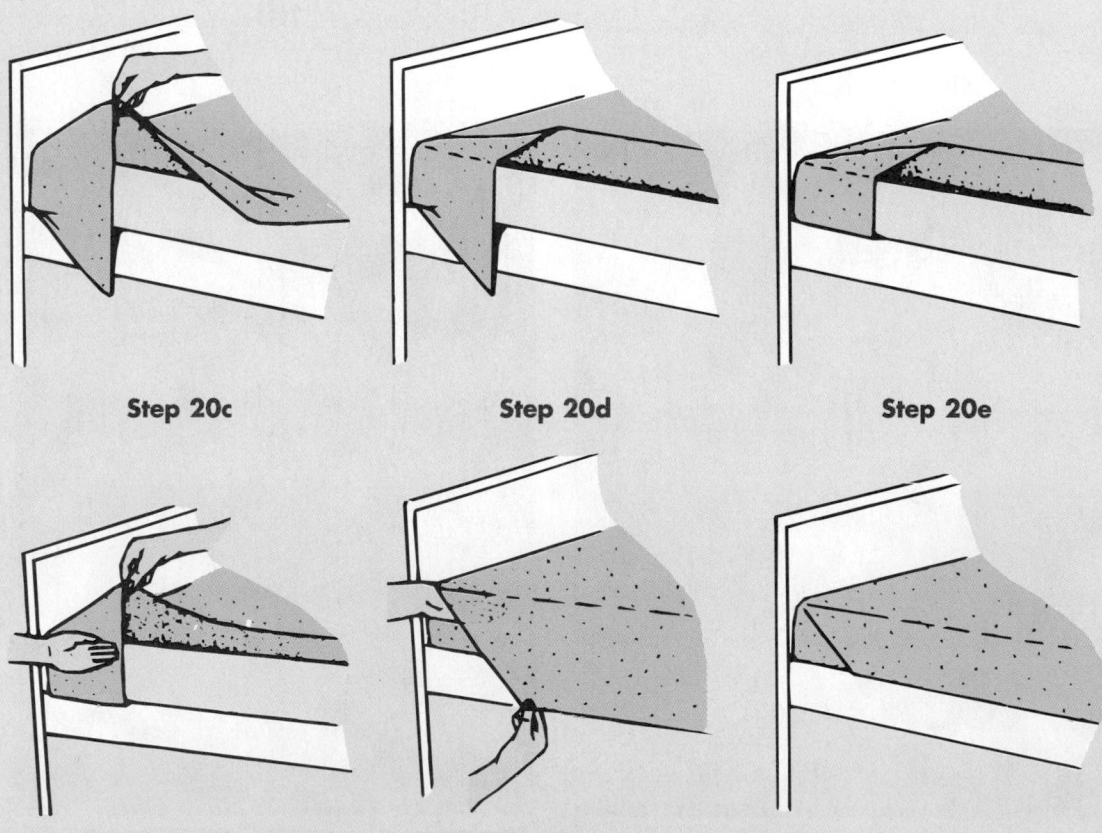

Step 20c   **Step 20d**   **Step 20e**

Step 20f

STEPS	RATIONALE
21. Tuck remaining portion of sheet under mattress, moving toward foot of bed. Keep linen smooth.	Folds of linen are source of irritation.
22. Optional: Open drawsheet so it unfolds in half. Lay center fold along middle of bed lengthwise, and position sheet so it will be under buttocks and torso (see illustration). Fanfold top layer toward client with edge alongside back. Smooth bottom layer out over mattress and tuck excess edge under mattress (keep palms down).	Drawsheet is used to lift and reposition client. Placement distributes most of body weight over sheet.
23. Place waterproof pad over drawsheet with center fold against client's side. Fanfold far half toward client.	Used to protect bed linen from soiling.
24. Raise side rail on working side, and go to other side.	Maintains safety.
25. Lower side rail. Assist client to roll slowly onto other side, over folds of linen (see illustration).	Exposes opposite side of bed for removal of soiled linen and placement of clean linen.
26. Loosen edge of soiled linen from underneath mattress.	Makes linen easier to remove.
27. Without allowing dirty linen to touch uniform, remove soiled linen by folding it into a bundle or square, with soiled side turned in. Discard it in linen bag.	Reduces transmission of microorganisms.
28. Spread clean, fanfolded linen smoothly over edge of mattress from head to foot of bed (see illustration).	Smooth linen will not irritate client's skin.
29. Assist client in rolling back into supine position. Reposition pillow.	Client's comfort is maintained.
30. Miter top corner of bottom sheet (see Step 20). When tucking corner, be sure sheet is smooth and free of wrinkles.	Wrinkles and folds can cause mechanical irritation to skin.
31. Facing side of bed, grasp remaining edge of bottom sheet, keep back straight, and pull as excess linen is tucked under mattress. Proceed from head to foot of bed. (Avoid lifting mattress during tucking to ensure fit.)	Proper use of body mechanics while tucking linen prevents injury to nurse.

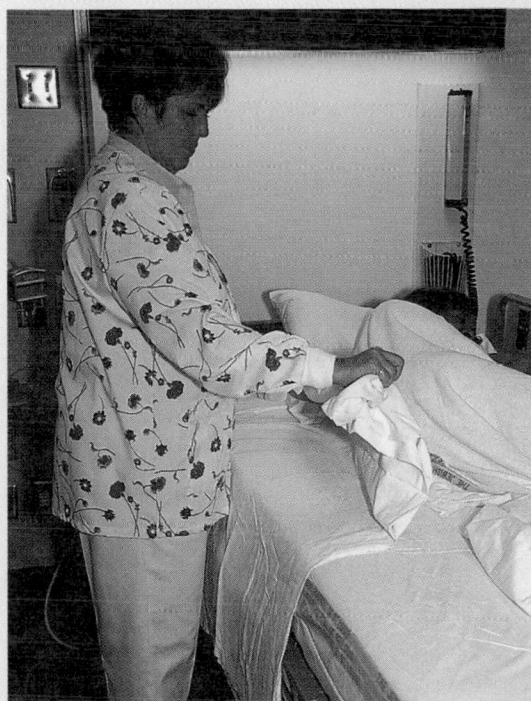

Step 22

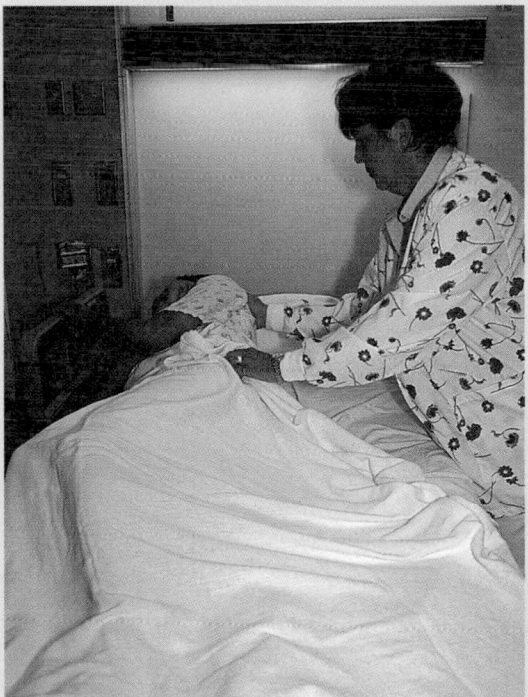

Step 25

STEPS	RATIONALE
32. Smooth fanfolded drawsheet over bottom sheet. Grasp edge of sheet with palms down, lean back, and tuck sheet under mattress. Tuck from middle to top and to bottom.	Tucking first at top or bottom may pull sheet sideways, causing poor fit.
33. Place top sheet over client with center fold lengthwise down middle of bed. Open sheet from head to foot, and unfold it over client (see illustration).	Sheet should be equally distributed over bed by correctly positioning center fold.
34. Without allowing dirty linen to touch uniform, ask client to hold clean top sheet, or tuck sheet around shoulders. Remove bath blanket, and discard it into linen bag.	Sheet prevents exposure of body parts. Having client hold sheet encourages participation in care.
35. Place blanket on bed, unfolding it so that crease runs lengthwise along middle of bed. Unfold blanket to cover client. Top edge should be parallel with edge of top sheet and 15 to 20 cm (6 to 8 in) down from top sheet's edge.	Blanket should be placed to cover client completely and provide adequate warmth.
36. Place spread over bed according to Step 35. Be sure top edge of spread extends about 2.5 cm (1 in) above blanket's edge. Tuck top edge of spread over and under top edge of blanket.	Spread gives bed neat appearance and provides extra warmth.
37. Make cuff by turning edge of top sheet down over top edge of blanket and spread.	Smooth cuff protects client's face from rubbing against blanket or spread.
38. Standing on one side at foot of bed, lift mattress corner slightly with one hand, and tuck top linens under mattress. Top sheet and blanket are tucked under together. Be sure linens are loose enough to allow for movement of client's feet. (Horizontal toe pleat may be made (see illustration).	Tucking all top linens together makes neat-appearing bed. Pressure sores can develop on client's toes and heels from feet rubbing between tight-fitting bed sheets.

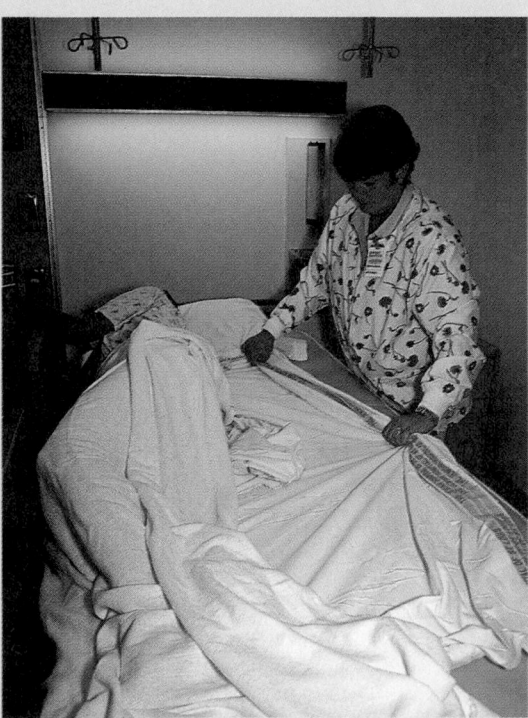

Step 28

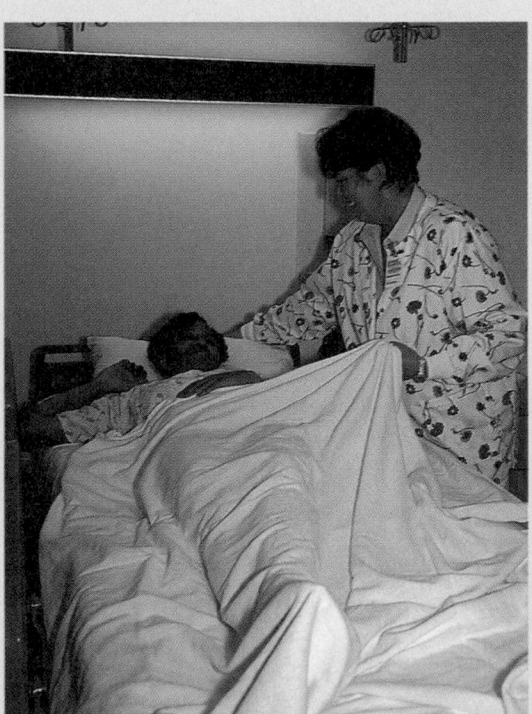

Step 33

STEPS	RATIONALE

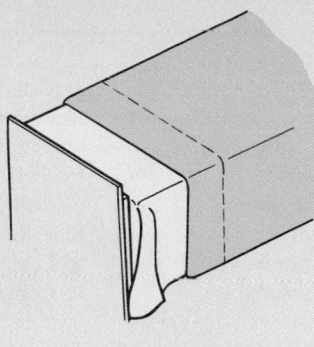

Step 38

39. Make modified mitered corner with top sheet, blanket, and spread:

    a. Pick up side edge of top sheet, blanket, and spread approximately 45 cm (18 in) up from foot of mattress. Lift linens to form triangular fold, and lay it on bed. — Modified mitered corner secures top linen but keeps an even edge of blanket and top sheet draped over mattress.

    b. Tuck lower edge of sheet, which is hanging free below mattress, under mattress. Do not pull triangular fold.

    c. Pick up triangular fold, and bring it down over mattress while holding linen in place along side of mattress. Do not tuck tip of triangle.

40. Raise side rail. Make other side of bed; spread sheet, blanket, and bedspread out evenly; fold top edge of spread over blanket, and make cuff with top sheet (see Step 37); make modified corner at foot of bed (see Step 39). — Side rail protects client from accidental falls.

41. Change pillowcase:

    a. Have client raise head. While supporting neck with one hand, remove pillow. — Prevents injury during flexion and extension of neck.

    b. Remove soiled case and discard in linen bag.

    c. Grasp clean pillowcase at center of closed end. Gather case, turning it inside out over hand holding it. With same hand pick up middle of one end of pillow. Pull pillowcase down over pillow with other hand and be sure pillow corners fit evenly in corners of pillowcase. — Method makes it easy to slide pillowcase over pillow. Poorly fitting case constricts fluffing and expansion of pillow.

42. Support client's head under neck, and place pillow under head. — Prevents hyperextension of neck muscles.

43. Place call light within client's reach; return bed to comfortable position. — Ensures safety and comfort.

44. Open room curtains. Rearrange furniture. Place personal items within easy reach on overbed table or bedside stand. Return bed to comfortable height. — Promotes sense of well-being.

45. Discard dirty linen in linen hamper or chute; wash hands. — Prevents transmission of microorganisms.

Recording and Reporting

- Bed making need not be documented. Record the client's vital signs and symptoms only if there are changes.

Home Care Considerations

- Assess the primary caregiver's ability to safely make an occupied bed.
- Assess the home laundry facilities to plan for the frequency with which the linen can be laundered.
- Assess the amount of linen in the home for the anticipated amount of linen changes needed.

Box 38-15 **Procedural Guidelines**

For Making an Unoccupied Bed

Equipment: Linen bag, mattress pad (change only when soiled), bottom sheet (flat or fitted), drawsheet (optional), top sheet, blanket, bedspread, waterproof pads (optional), pillowcases, bedside chair or table, disposable gloves (if linen is soiled), washcloth, and antiseptic cleanser.

1. Determine if client has been incontinent or if excess drainage is on linen. Gloves will be necessary.
2. Assess activity orders or restrictions in mobility in planning if client can get out of bed for procedure. Assist to bedside chair or recliner.
3. Lower side rails on both sides of bed and raise bed to comfortable working position.
4. Remove soiled linen and place in laundry bag. Avoid shaking or fanning linen.
5. Reposition mattress and wipe off any moisture using a washcloth moistened in antiseptic solution. Dry thoroughly.
6. Apply all bottom linen on one side of bed before moving to opposite side.
7. Be sure fitted sheet is placed smoothly over mattress. To apply a flat unfitted sheet, allow about 25 cm (10 in) to hang over mattress edge. Lower hem of sheet should lie seam down, even with bottom edge of mattress. Pull remaining top portion of sheet over top edge of mattress.
8. While standing at head of bed, miter top corner of bottom sheet (see Skill 38-8, Step 20).
9. Tuck remaining portion of unfitted sheet under mattress.
10. Optional: Apply drawsheet, laying center fold along middle of bed lengthwise. Smooth drawsheet over mattress and tuck excess edge under mattress, keeping palms down.
11. Move to opposite side of bed and spread bottom sheet smoothly over edge of mattress from head to foot of bed.
12. Apply fitted sheet smoothly over each mattress corner. For an unfitted sheet, miter top corner of bottom sheet (see Step 8) making sure corner is taut.
13. Grasp remaining edge of unfitted bottom sheet and tuck tightly under mattress while moving from head to foot of bed. Smooth folded drawsheet over bottom sheet and tuck under mattress, first at middle, then at top, and then at bottom.

14. If needed, apply waterproof pad over bottom sheet or drawsheet.
15. Place top sheet over bed with vertical center fold lengthwise down middle of bed. Open sheet out from head to foot, being sure top edge of sheet is even with top edge of mattress.
16. Make horizontal toe pleat: stand at foot of bed and fan fold in sheet 5 to 10 cm (2 to 4 in) across bed. Pull sheet up from bottom to make fold approximately 15 cm (6 in) from bottom edge of mattress (see Skill 38-8, Step 38).
17. Tuck in remaining portion of sheet under foot of mattress. Then place blanket over bed with top edge parallel to top edge of sheet and 15 to 20 cm (6 to 8 in) down from edge of sheet. (Optional: Apply additional spread over bed.)
18. Make cuff by turning edge of top sheet down over top edge of blanket and spread.
19. Standing on one side at foot of bed, lift mattress corner slightly with one hand, and with other hand tuck top sheet, blanket, and spread under mattress. Be sure toe pleats are not pulled out.
20. Make modified mitered corner with top sheet, blanket, and spread. After triangular fold is made, do not tuck tip of triangle (see illustration).

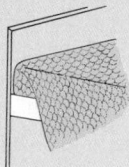

Step 20

21. Go to other side of bed. Spread sheet, blanket, and spread out evenly. Make cuff with top sheet and blanket. Make modified corner at foot of bed.
22. Apply clean pillowcase.
23. Place call light within client's reach on bed rail or pillow and return bed to height allowing for client transfer. Assist client to bed.
24. Arrange client's room. Remove and discard supplies. Wash hands.

When fitted sheets are not available, flat sheets usually are pressed with a center crease to be placed down the center of the bed. The linens unfold easily to the sides, with creases often fitting over the mattress edge. A complete linen change is not always necessary. The nurse may reuse the mattress pad, sheet, blanket, and bed spread for the same client if they are not wet or soiled.

Disposal of linen must be done to minimize the spread of infection (Chapter 33). Agency policies provide guidelines for the proper way to bag and dispose of soiled linen.

After a client is discharged, all bed linen is sent to the laundry, the mattress and bed are cleansed by housekeeping staff, and new bed linen is applied.

✎ EVALUATION

Client Care. Evaluation of hygiene measures occurs both during and after each particular skill. For example, as the nurse bathes a client, close inspection of the skin reveals if drainage or other soiling is effectively removed from the skin's surface. Once the bath is completed the nurse will ask if the client's comfort and relaxation have improved. When evaluating for the effectiveness of hygiene measures, the nurse observes for changes in the client's behavior. Does the client assume a more relaxed position? Is the client free of body odor? Is the client able to fall asleep? Does the client's facial expression convey a sense of comfort?

Frequently it takes time for hygienic care to result in an improvement in the client's condition. The presence of oral lesions, a scalp infestation, or skin excoriation will often require repeated measures and a combination of nursing interventions. The nurse will evaluate for improvement in the client's condition over time and determine if existing therapies are effective.

Throughout evaluation the nurse considers the goals of care and evaluates whether expected outcomes are achieved. A critical thinking approach ensures that the nurse considers all factors when evaluating the client's care (Figure 38-17). The nurse's knowledge base and experience provide important perspectives when the nurse analyzes observations made about a client. For example, if the nurse has seen how dehydration of the oral mucosa clears with repeated hygiene, this helps in recognizing when another client's progress is slow. The standards for evaluation are the expected outcomes established in the planning stage of the client's care. If outcomes are not met, the care plan may need to be revised. The nurse continues to apply critical thinking attitudes when considering all evaluation findings.

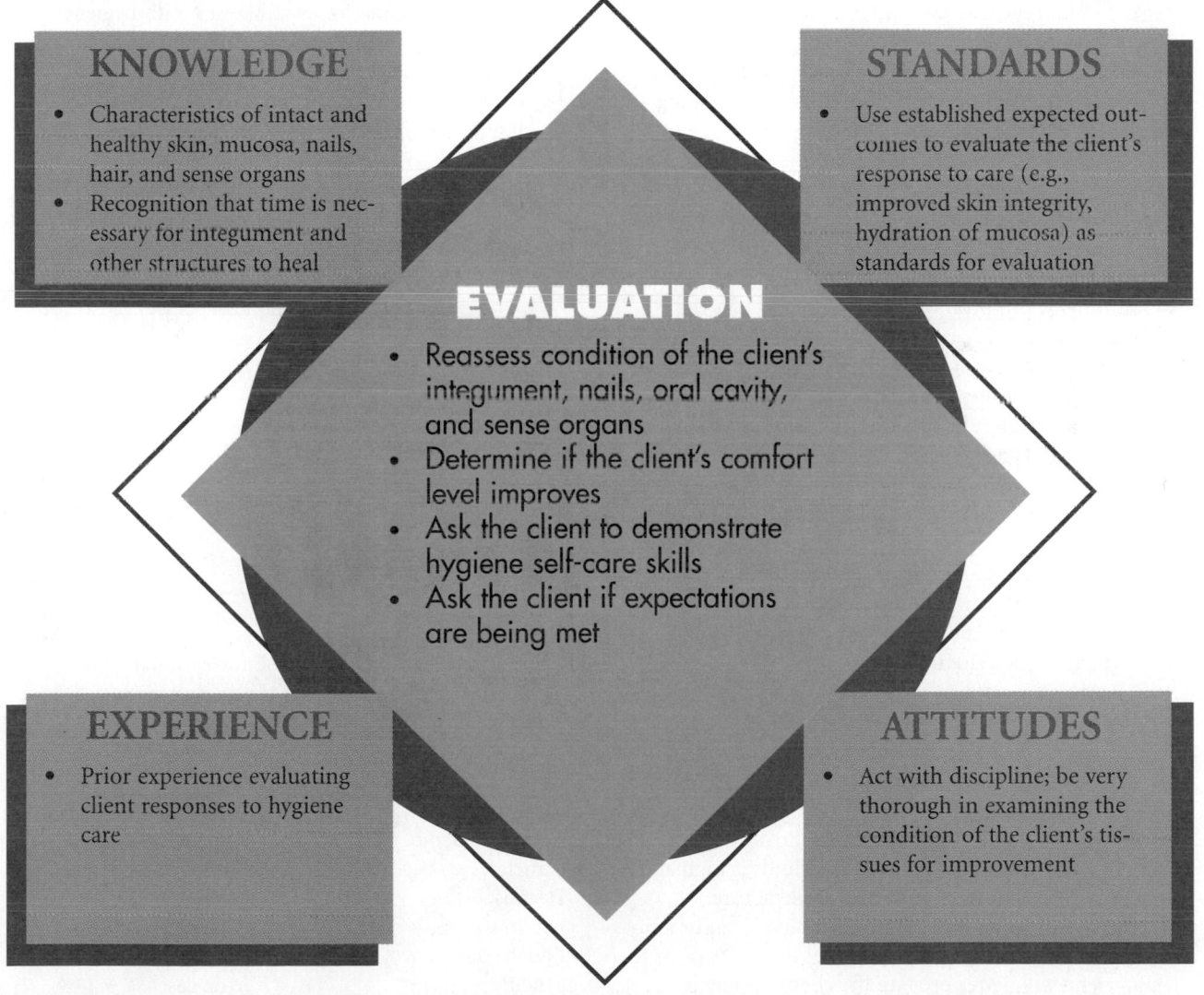

Figure 38-17 *Synthesis Model for the Evaluation Phase.*

Client Expectations.   The final portion of the evaluation considers whether or not the client's expectations were met through hygienic care. The nurse might ask: Do you feel your bath and back rub helped to make you comfortable? Are there ways you feel we can do a better job with your foot care? What further measures do you think are necessary to keep your mouth clean and refreshed?

The client's expectations are important guidelines in determining client satisfaction. The nurse must feel comfortable in addressing the client's concerns and expectations. A caring approach can help in facilitating discussion of these issues.

Key Concepts

- The nurse determines a client's ability to perform self-care and provides hygienic care according to the client's needs and preferences
- During hygiene, the nurse integrates other activities such as physical assessment, wound care, and range-of-motion exercises.
- While providing daily hygiene needs, the nurse uses teaching and communication skills in developing a caring relationship with the client.
- Proper hygienic care requires an understanding of anatomy and physiology.
- Various sociocultural, economic, and developmental factors influence clients' hygiene practices.
- Clients' health beliefs predict the likelihood of assuming health promotion behavior, such as the maintenance of good hygiene.
- The nurse may not assess all body regions before administering hygiene; however, the nurse does routinely assess the client's condition whenever care to the client is given.
- Clients with reduced sensation, vascular insufficiency, and immobility are at greater risk for impaired skin integrity.
- The nurse assesses a client's physical and cognitive ability to perform basic hygiene measures, including muscle strength, flexibility and dexterity, balance, coordination, activity tolerance, and ability to attend.
- The nurse maintains a client's privacy, comfort, and safety when providing hygienic care.
- Culture plays a role not only in hygiene practices and preferences but also in sensitivity to a client's personal space.
- Gloves should be worn by nurses during hygiene care when the risk of contacting body fluids is high and should always be worn during perineal care.
- For clients suffering symptoms such as pain or nausea, administering symptom relief therapies prior to hygiene will better prepare the client for any procedure.

- Clients with diabetes mellitus require special nail and foot care.
- When administering oral care to unconscious clients, the nurse takes measures to prevent aspiration.
- Family members can usually assist with hygiene measures but may need guidance in adapting techniques to fit client limitations.
- The techniques used in the care of contact lenses are designed to prevent corneal injury.
- The client's room should be comfortable, safe, and large enough to allow the client and visitors to move about freely.
- Evaluation of hygiene care is based on the client's sense of comfort, relaxation, well-being, and understanding of hygiene techniques.

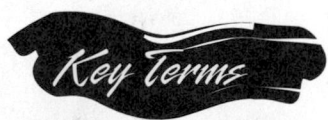

Key Terms

Acne, *p. 1066*

Alopecia, *p. 1063*

Apocrine, *p. 1056*

Buccal glands, *p. 1057*

Caries, *p. 1066*

Cerumen, *p. 1056*

Complete bed bath, *p. 1074*

Cuticle, *p. 1057*

Dermis, *p. 1056*

Eccrine, *p. 1056*

Edentulous, *p. 1067*

Effleurage, *p. 1086*

Enucleation, *p. 1104*

Epidermis, *p. 1055*

Gingivitis, *p. 1057*

Halitosis, *p. 1063*

Lunula, *p. 1057*

Mastication, *p. 1057*

Neuropathy, *p. 1063*

Ophthalmologist, *p. 1103*

Optometrist, *p. 1103*

Partial bed bath, *p. 1082*

Perineal care, *p. 1082*

Vernix caseosa, *p. 1089*

Critical Thinking Exercises

1. Mrs. Truman is a 62-year-old female being seen in the internal medicine clinic during her followup appointment for management of her diabetes mellitus. During the nurse's conversation with Mrs. Truman, the client says, "You know, last week I found a sore on my left foot; I didn't even know it was there." What type of assessment should the nurse conduct for Mrs. Truman, and what might be the implications of her findings?

2. Mr. Wilkes is a 54-year-old client with advanced stages of lung cancer. The tumor has spread to the bone, causing Mr. Wilkes considerable pain and predisposing him to pathologic fractures (fractures that result when bone is weakened by tumor growth). The client has been experiencing a high fever almost on a daily basis. What considerations might you give in anticipating Mr. Wilkes's hygiene needs?

3. Peter Nixon is an 18-year-old admitted to the neurosurgical intensive care unit following a head injury. Peter is currently unconscious, responsive only to painful stimulus. What assessment is critical for the nurse to perform prior to providing oral hygiene?

References

Agency for Health Care Policy and Research: *Pressure ulcers in adults: prediction and prevention*, pub nos. 92-0047, 92-0050, Rockville, MD, 1992, U.S. Dept of Health and Human Services, Public Health Service.

American Diabetes Association: Position statement on preventive foot care in people with diabetes: clinical practice recommendations 1999, *Diabetes Care* 22 (suppl 1) 1999.

Barnes SH: Patient and family education for the patient with a pressure necrosis, *Nurs Clin North Am* 22:463, 1987.

Becker MH: The health belief model and personal health behavior, *Health Educ Monogr* 2:324, 1974.

Blaney GM: Mouth care: basic and essential, *Geriatr Nurs* 7:242, 1986.

Champion VL: Instrument development for health belief model constructs, *Adv Nurs Sci* 6(3):73, 1984.

Christensen MH and others: How to care for the diabetic foot, *Am J Nurs* 91(3):50, 1991.

Cohen E, Krachmer J: Red eyes and contact lenses, *Patient Care* 26(9):143, 1992.

Danielson LH: Oral care and older adults, *J Gerontol Nurs* 7:242, 1988.

de Liefde B, Ritchie GR: Evaluation in dental public health in New Zealand, *N Z Dent J* 80:8, 1984.

Ebersole P, Hess P: *Toward healthy aging*, ed 4, St. Louis, 1995, Mosby.

Felder R and others: Dexterity testing as a prediction of oral care ability, *J Am Geriatr* 42(10):1081, 1994.

Giger JN, Davidhizar RE: *Transcultural nursing: assessment and intervention*, ed 2, St. Louis, 1995, Mosby.

Gooch J: Skin hygiene, *Prof Nurse* 5(1):13, 1989.

Greifzu S and others: Oral care is part of cancer care, *RN* 53:43, 1990.

Gudas J: Foot problems. In Calkins E, Ford B, Katz R, editors: *Practice of geriatrics*, Philadelphia, 1992, WB Saunders.

Gulick EE: Symptom and activities of daily living trajectory in multiple sclerosis: a ten year study, *Nurs Res* 47(3):137, 1998.

Harley JR: Preventing diabetic foot disease, *Nurs Pract* 18(10):37, 1993.

Ismail AI, Szpunar SM: The prevalence of total tooth loss, dental caries and periodontal disease among Mexican Americans, Cuban Americans, and Puerto Ricans: finding from HHANES 1982-1984, *Am J Public Health* 80(suppl):66, 1990.

Jee HH: Aryan medical science: a short history, Delhi, India, 1981, Maharaja of Gundal.

Johnson & Johnson Vision Products: *Your guide to healthy contact lens wear*, New Brunswick, NJ, 1994, Johnson & Johnson.

Labyak SE, Metzger BL: The effects of effleurage backrub on the physiological components of relaxation: a meta-analysis, *Nurs Res* 46:59, 1997.

Lewis S, Collier I, Heitkemper M: *Medical-surgical nursing: assessment and management of clinical problems*, ed 4, St. Louis, 1996, Mosby.

Lueckenotte AG: *Gerontologic nursing*, St. Louis, 1996, Mosby.

Mahoney DF: Cerumem impaction: prevalance and detection in nursing homes, *J Gerontol Nurse* 54(12):56, 1993.

Makelbust J: Pressure ulcer update, *RN* 41(12):56, 1991.

Martin S, Barr O: Preventing complications in people who wear contact lenses, *Br J Nurs* 6(11):614, 1997.

McCloskey JC, Bulechek GM: *Nursing interventions classification (NIC)*, ed 3, St. Louis, 2000, Mosby.

Ney DF: Cerumem impaction, ear hygiene practices, and hearing acuity, *Geriatr Nurse* 14(2):70, 1993.

Ostermann HM, Stock EM: The aging foot, *Orthop Nurs* 9:43, 1990.

Phipps W and others: *Medical-surgical nursing concepts and clinical practice*, ed 5, St. Louis, 1995, Mosby.

Poland JM: Comparing Moi-Stin to lemon glycerin swabs, *Am J Nurs* 87:422, 1987.

Skewes SM: No more bed baths! *RN* 57:34, 1994.

Sorrentino SA: *Assisting with patient care*, St. Louis, 1999, Mosby.

Stachtchenko S, Jenicek M: Conceptual differences between prevention and health promotion: research implications for community health programs, *Can J Public Health* 81:53, 1990.

Thibodeau GA, Patton KT: *Anatomy and physiology*, ed 2, St. Louis, 1993, Mosby.

Thompson and others: *Clinical nursing*, ed 4, St. Louis, Mosby.

Verderber A, Gallagher KJ: Effects of bathing, passive range-of-motion exercises, and turning on oxygen consumption in health men and women, *Am J Crit Care* 3:374, 1994.

Wong DL: Wong & Whaley's *Clinical manual of pediatric nursing*, ed 5, St. Louis, 1999, Mosby.

Young M, Young C: Footwork, *Nurs Times* 90(7):70, 1994.

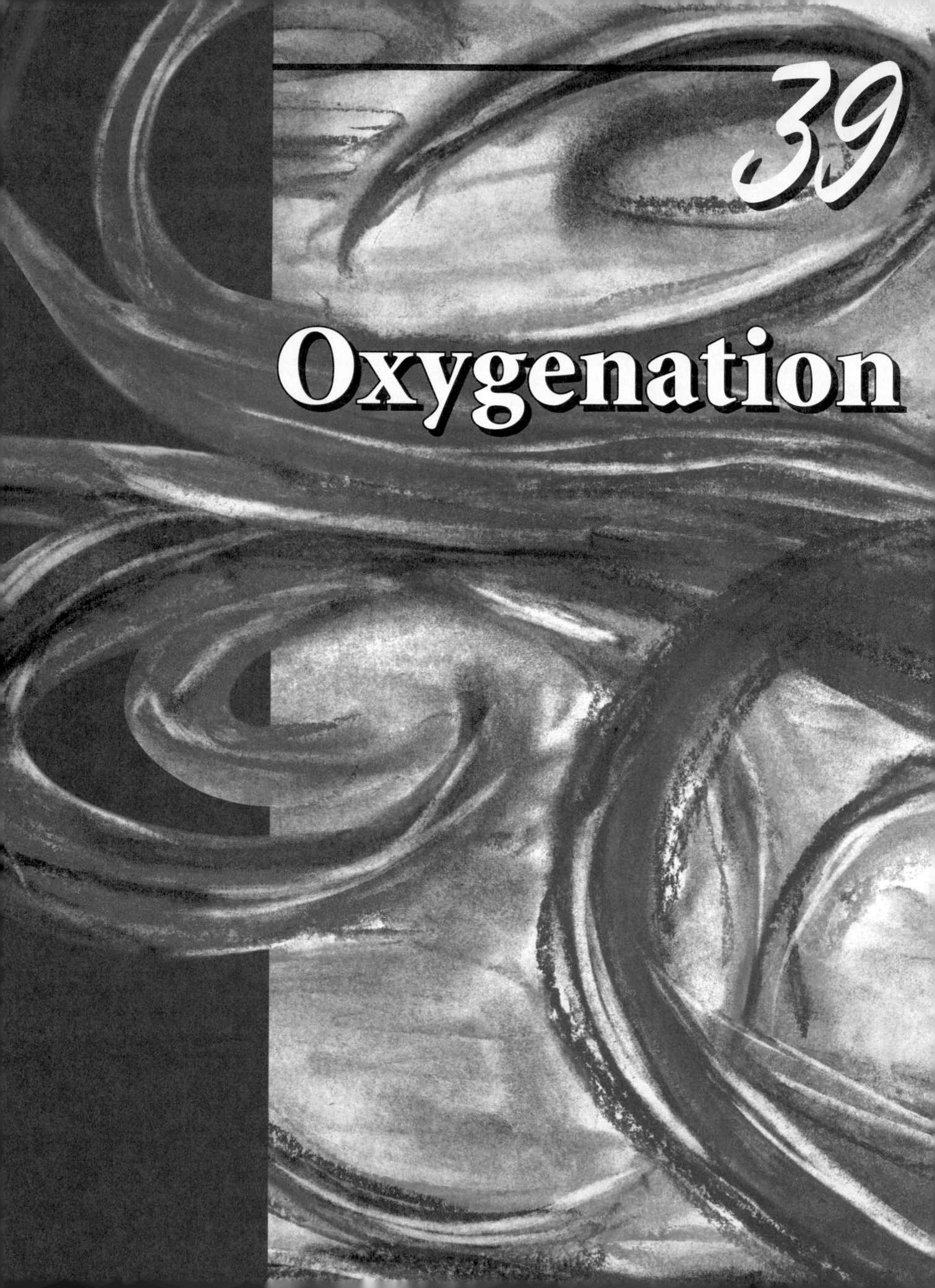

39

Oxygenation

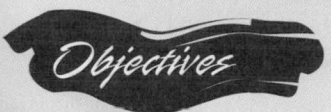

Objectives

Mastery of content in this chapter will enable the student to:

- Define the key terms listed.
- Describe the structure and function of the cardiopulmonary system.
- Identify physiological processes of cardiac output, myocardial blood flow, and coronary artery circulation.
- Diagram the electrical conduction system of the heart.
- Describe the relationship of cardiac output, preload, afterload, contractility, and heart rate.
- Identify physiological processes involved in ventilation, perfusion, and exchange of respiratory gases.
- Describe neural and chemical regulation of respiration.
- Describe the impact of a client's level of health, age, lifestyle, and environment on tissue oxygenation.
- Identify and describe clinical outcomes as a result of disturbances in conduction, altered cardiac output, impaired valvular function, myocardial ischemia, and impaired tissue perfusion.
- Identify and describe clinical outcomes of hyperventilation, hypoventilation, and hypoxemia.
- Identify nursing care interventions in the primary care, acute care, and restorative and continuing care settings that promote oxygenation.

Scientific Knowledge Base

Oxygen is required to sustain life. The cardiac and respiratory systems function to supply the body's oxygen demands. Cardiopulmonary physiology involves delivery of deoxygenated blood to the right side of the heart and to the pulmonary circulation and oxygenated blood from the lungs to the left side of the heart and the tissues. Blood is oxygenated through the mechanisms of ventilation, perfusion, and transport of respiratory gases. Neural and chemical regulators control the rate and depth of respiration in response to changing tissue oxygen demands.

CARDIOVASCULAR PHYSIOLOGY

The function of the cardiac system is to deliver oxygen, nutrients, and other substances to the tissues and to remove the waste products of cellular metabolism through the cardiac pump, the circulatory vascular system, and the integration of other systems (e.g., respiratory, digestive, and renal) (McCance and Huether, 1998).

Structure and Function. The right ventricle pumps blood through the pulmonary circulation while the left ventricle pumps blood to the systemic circulation, supplying oxygen and nutrients to the tissues and removing wastes from the body (Figures 39-1 and 39-2). The circulatory system exchanges respiratory gases, nutrients, and waste products between the blood and the tissues.

Myocardial Pump. The pumping action of the heart is essential to maintenance of oxygen delivery. Decreased pump effectiveness, as in coronary artery disease (CAD) and cardiomyopathic conditions, results in a diminished stroke volume—the volume of blood ejected from the ventricles. Hemorrhage and dehydration decrease pump effectiveness by reducing the circulating blood volume, thereby decreasing the amount of blood ejected from the ventricles.

The chambers of the heart fill during diastole and empty during systole. The effectiveness of the diastolic and systolic events of the cardiac cycle can be assessed by monitoring the client's blood pressure (see Chapter 31). The myocardial fibers have contractile properties that enable them to stretch during filling. In a healthy heart this stretch is proportionally related to the strength of contraction. As the myocardium stretches, the strength of the subsequent contraction increases; this is known as the Frank-Starling (Starling's) law of the heart. In the diseased heart, Starling's law does not apply because the stretch of the myocardium is beyond the heart's physiological limits. The subsequent contractile response results in insufficient ventricular ejection (volume), and blood begins to "back up" in the pulmonary (left heart failure) or systemic circulation (right heart failure).

Myocardial Blood Flow. To maintain adequate blood flow to the pulmonary and systemic circulation, myocardial blood flow must supply sufficient oxygen and nutrients to the myocardium itself. Blood flow through the heart is unidirectional. There are four heart valves that ensure this forward blood flow (Figure 39-3). During ventricular diastole the atrioventricular (mitral and tricuspid) valves open and blood flows from the higher-pressure atria into the relaxed ventricles. Once the ventricles are filled, the atrioventricular valves close, this represents S_1,

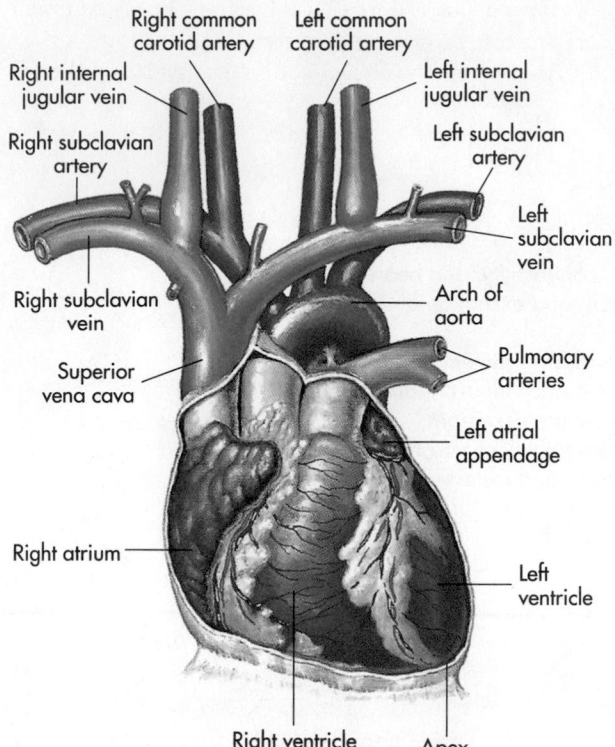

Figure 39-1   Diagram showing serially connected pulmonary and systemic circulation. Right heart chambers propel unoxygenated blood through the pulmonary circulation; left heart chambers propel oxygenated blood through the systemic circulation.
From Canobbio MM: *Cardiovascular disorders,* St. Louis, 1990, Mosby.

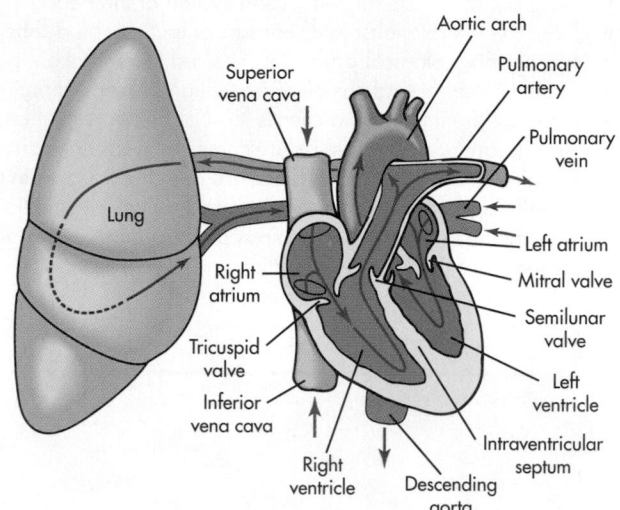

Figure 39-2   Schematic representation of blood flow through the heart. Arrows indicate direction of flow.
From Lewis SM and others: *Medical-surgical nursing: assessment and management of clinical problems,* ed 5, St. Louis, 2000, Mosby.

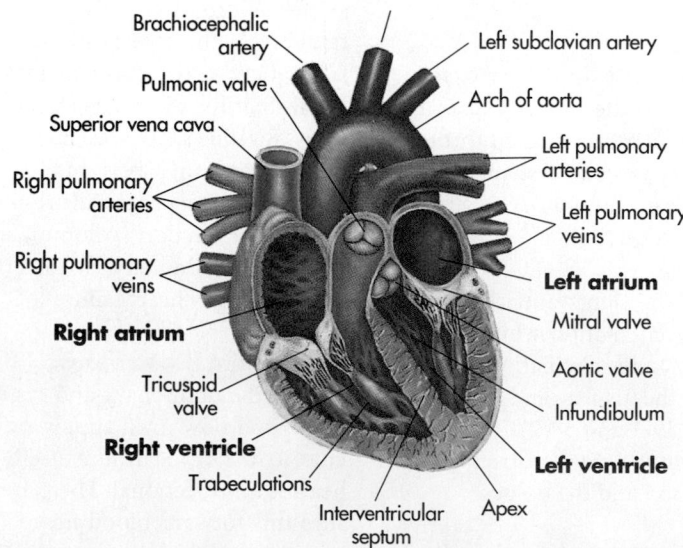

Figure 39-3   Cross-sectional view of the heart showing atrium, ventricles, and valves.
Modified from Canobbio MM: *Cardiovascular disorders,* St. Louis, 1990, Mosby.

or the first heart sound. After ventricular filling, the systolic phase begins. As the systolic intraventricular pressure rises, the atrioventricular valves close, preventing the backflow of blood into the atria, and ventricular contraction begins. During the systolic phase, ventricular pressure rises, causing the semilunar (aortic and pulmonic) valves to open. As the ventricles eject blood, the intraventricular pressure falls and the semilunar valves close, thus preventing the backflow of blood from the aorta and pulmonary artery into the ventricles. Closure of aortic and pulmonic valves represents S_2, or the second heart sound. Clients

with valvular disease may have backflow or regurgitation of blood through the incompetent valve, causing a murmur that is heard on auscultation (see Chapter 32).

Coronary Artery Circulation.   Blood in the atria and ventricles does not supply oxygen and nutrients to the myocardium itself. The coronary circulation is the branch of the systemic circulation that supplies the myocardium with oxygen and nutrients and removes waste. The coronary arteries fill during ventricular diastole (McCance and Huether, 1998). The right and left coronary arteries arise from the aorta just above and behind the aortic valve through openings called the coronary ostia (coronary openings). The left coronary artery, the most abundant blood supply, feeds the left ventricular myocardium, which is more muscular and does most of the heart's work (Figure 39-4) (Box 39-1).

Systemic Circulation.   The arteries and veins of the systemic circulation deliver nutrients and oxygen to and remove waste from the tissues. Oxygenated blood flows from the left ventricle by way of the aorta and into large systemic arteries. These arteries branch into smaller arteries, into arterioles, and finally into the smallest vessels, the capillaries. At the capillary level the exchange of respiratory gases, nutrients, and wastes occurs, and the tissues are oxygenated. The waste products exit the capillary network by way of the venules that join to form veins. These veins form larger veins, which carry deoxygenated blood to the right side of the heart, where it is returned to pulmonary circulation.

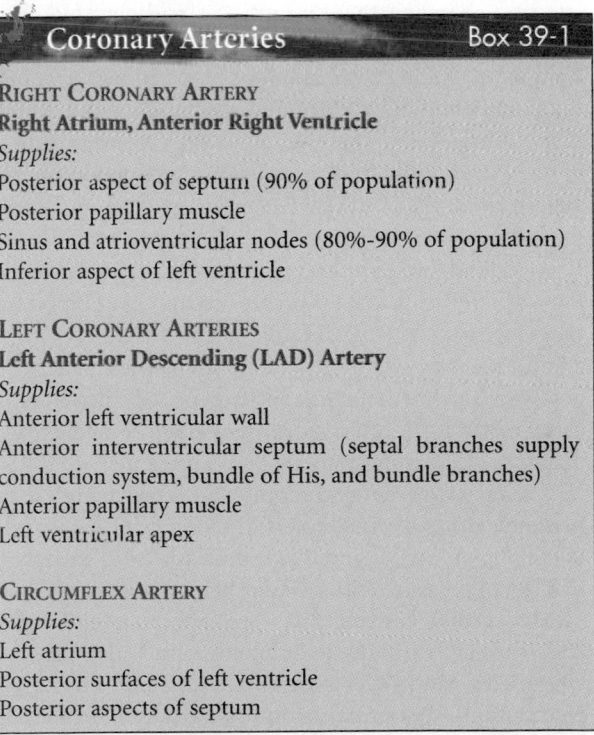

Figure 39-4   Coronary arteries and veins.
From Lewis SM and others: *Medical-surgical nursing: assessment and management of clinical problems,* ed 5, St. Louis, 2000, Mosby.

Coronary Arteries   Box 39-1

RIGHT CORONARY ARTERY
Right Atrium, Anterior Right Ventricle
Supplies:
Posterior aspect of septum (90% of population)
Posterior papillary muscle
Sinus and atrioventricular nodes (80%-90% of population)
Inferior aspect of left ventricle

LEFT CORONARY ARTERIES
Left Anterior Descending (LAD) Artery
Supplies:
Anterior left ventricular wall
Anterior interventricular septum (septal branches supply conduction system, bundle of His, and bundle branches)
Anterior papillary muscle
Left ventricular apex

CIRCUMFLEX ARTERY
Supplies:
Left atrium
Posterior surfaces of left ventricle
Posterior aspects of septum

From Canobbio MM: *Cardiovascular disorders,* St. Louis, 1990, Mosby.

Blood Flow Regulation. The amount of blood ejected from the left ventricle each minute is the **cardiac output.** The normal cardiac output is 4 to 6 L/min in the healthy 150-pound (70-kg) adult at rest. The circulating volume of blood changes according to the oxygen and metabolic needs of the body. For example, during exercise, pregnancy, and fever, the cardiac output increases, but during sleep it decreases. Cardiac output is represented by the following formula:

$$\text{Cardiac output (CO)} = \text{Stroke volume (SV)} \times \text{Heart rate (HR)}$$

Cardiac output in the older adult may be affected by increased arterial wall tension and moderate myocardial hypertrophy due to an increased systolic blood pressure.

Cardiac index (CI) is the adequacy of the cardiac output for an individual. It takes into account the body surface area (BSA) of the client. The CI is determined by dividing the cardiac output by the BSA. The normal range is 2.5 to 4 L/min/m^3. Both cardiac output and the CI are measured with invasive pulmonary artery catheters.

Stroke volume is the amount of blood ejected from the left ventricle with each contraction. It can be affected by the amount of blood in the left ventricle at the end of diastole (preload), the resistance to left ventricular ejection (afterload), and myocardial contractility.

Preload is essentially the end-diastolic volume. As the ventricles fill, they stretch. The greater the stretch on the ventricle, the greater the contraction and the greater the stroke volume (Starling's law). In clinical situations the preload and subsequent stroke volume can be manipulated by changing the amount of circulating blood volume. For example, in the client with hemorrhagic shock, fluid therapy and replacement of blood increases volume, thus increasing the preload and cardiac output. If volume is not replaced, preload decreases, the cardiac output decreases, and ultimately the venous return to the right atrium decreases, further decreasing preload and cardiac output.

Afterload is the resistance to left ventricular ejection: the work the heart must overcome to fully eject blood from the left ventricle. The diastolic aortic pressure is a good clinical measure of afterload. In a client with an acute hypertensive crisis, the afterload is increased, increasing the cardiac workload. Afterload in this situation can be manipulated by decreasing systemic blood pressure.

The measurement and monitoring of cardiopulmonary hemodynamics is usually performed in critical care units. Some step-down or special care units may also have the capability to measure and monitor hemodynamics.

Myocardial contractility also affects stroke volume and cardiac output. Poor contraction decreases the amount of blood ejected by the ventricles during each contraction. Myocardial contractility can be increased by drugs that increase the force of contraction, such as digi-

talis preparations, epinephrine, and sympathomimetic drugs (drugs that mimic the effects of the sympathetic nervous system). Injury to the myocardial muscle, such as an acute myocardial infarction (AMI) can cause a decrease in myocardial contractility. The myocardium of the older adult is more rigid and slower in recovering its contractility (Lueckenotte, 2000).

Heart rate affects blood flow because of the interaction between rate and diastolic filling time. With a sustained heart rate greater than 160 beats per minute, diastolic filling time decreases, decreasing stroke volume and cardiac output. The heart rate of the older adult is slow to increase under stress. The stroke volume may increase to increase the cardiac output and blood pressure (Lueckenotte, 2000).

Conduction System. The rhythmic relaxation and contraction of the atria and ventricles depend on continuous, organized transmission of electrical impulses. These impulses are generated and transmitted by way of the cardiac conduction system (Figure 39-5).

The heart's conduction system generates the necessary action potentials that conduct the impulses required to initiate the electrical chain of events resulting in the heartbeat. The autonomic nervous system influences the rate of impulse generation, as well as the speed of transmission through the conductive pathway and the strength of atrial and ventricular contractions. Sympathetic nerve fibers, which increase the rate of impulse generation and the

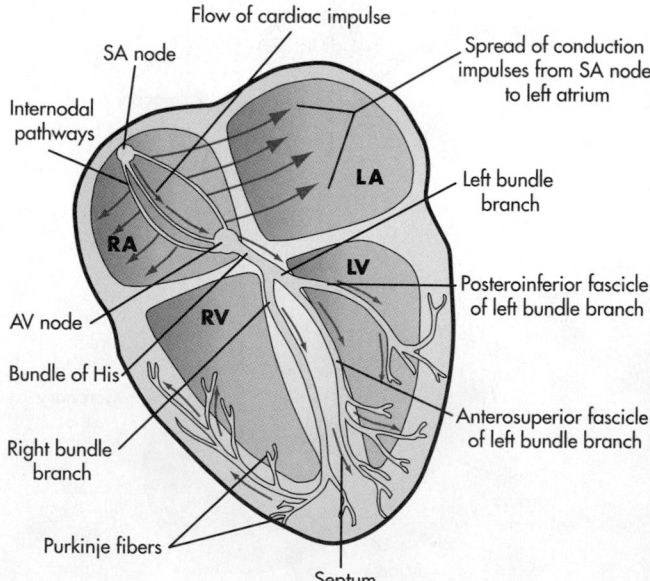

Figure 39-5 Conduction system of the heart. *LA*, left atrium; *LV*, left ventricle; *RA*, right atrium; *RV*, right ventricle; *SA*, sinoatrial; *AV*, atrioventricular.
From Lewis SM and others: *Medical-surgical nursing: assessment and management of clinical problems,* ed 5, St. Louis, 2000, Mosby.

speed of impulse transmission, innervate all parts of the atria and ventricles. Parasympathetic fibers from the vagus nerve, which decrease this rate, also innervate these parts, as well as the sinoatrial and atrioventricular nodes (McCance and Huether, 1998).

The conduction system originates with the **sinoatrial (SA) node,** the "pacemaker" of the heart. The SA node is in the right atrium next to the entrance of the superior vena cava (McCance and Huether, 1998). Impulses are initiated at the SA node at an intrinsic rate of 60 to 100 beats per minute. The resting adult rate is approximately 75 beats per minute.

The electrical impulses are then transmitted through the atria along intraatrial pathways to the **atrioventricular (AV) node.** The AV node mediates impulses between the atria and the ventricles. The intrinsic rate of the normal AV node is 40 to 60 beats per minute. The AV node assists atrial emptying by delaying the impulse before transmitting it through the **bundle of His** and the ventricular **Purkinje network.** The intrinsic rate of the bundle of His and the ventricular Purkinje network is 20 to 40 beats per minute.

An **electrocardiogram (ECG)** reflects the electrical activity of the conduction system. An ECG monitors the regularity and path of the electrical impulse through the conduction system; however, it does not reflect muscular work of the heart. The normal sequence on the ECG is called **normal sinus rhythm (NSR)** (Figure 39-6).

NSR implies that the impulse originates at the SA node and follows the normal sequence through the conduction system. The P wave represents the electrical conduction through both atria. Atrial contraction follows the P wave. The PR interval represents the impulse travel time through the AV node, through the bundle of His, and to the Purkinje fibers. The normal length for the PR interval is 0.12 to 0.20 second. An increase in the time, >0.20 second, indicates that there is a block in the impulse transmission though the AV node, whereas a decrease, <0.12 second, indicates the initiation of the electrical impulse from a source other than the SA node.

The QRS complex indicates that the electrical impulse has traveled through the ventricles. Normal QRS duration is 0.06 to 0.12 second. An increase in QRS duration indicates a delay in conduction time through the ventricles. Ventricular contraction usually follows the QRS complex.

The QT interval represents the time needed for ventricular depolarization and repolarization. The normal QT interval is 0.12 to 0.42 second. Changes in electrolyte values, such as hypocalcemia, or therapy with drugs such as quinidine, disopyramide, amiodarone, and theophylline (Theo-Dur) can increase the QT interval. Shortening of the QT interval occurs with digitalis therapy, hyperkalemia, and hypercalcemia.

RESPIRATORY PHYSIOLOGY

Most cells in the body obtain their energy from chemical reactions involving oxygen and the elimination of carbon dioxide. The exchange of respiratory gases occurs between environmental air and the blood (Figure 39-7). There are three steps in the process of oxygenation: ventilation, perfusion, and diffusion (McCance and Huether, 1998). For the exchange of respiratory gases to occur, the organs, nerves, and muscles of respiration must be intact and the central nervous system able to regulate the respiratory cycle.

Structure and Function. Respiration can be altered by conditions or diseases that change the structure and function of the lung. The respiratory muscles, pleural space, lungs, and alveoli (Figure 39-8) are essential for ventilation, perfusion, and exchange of respiratory gases (Box 39-2).

Ventilation is the process of moving gases into and out of the lungs. Ventilation requires coordination of the muscular and elastic properties of the lung and thorax, as well

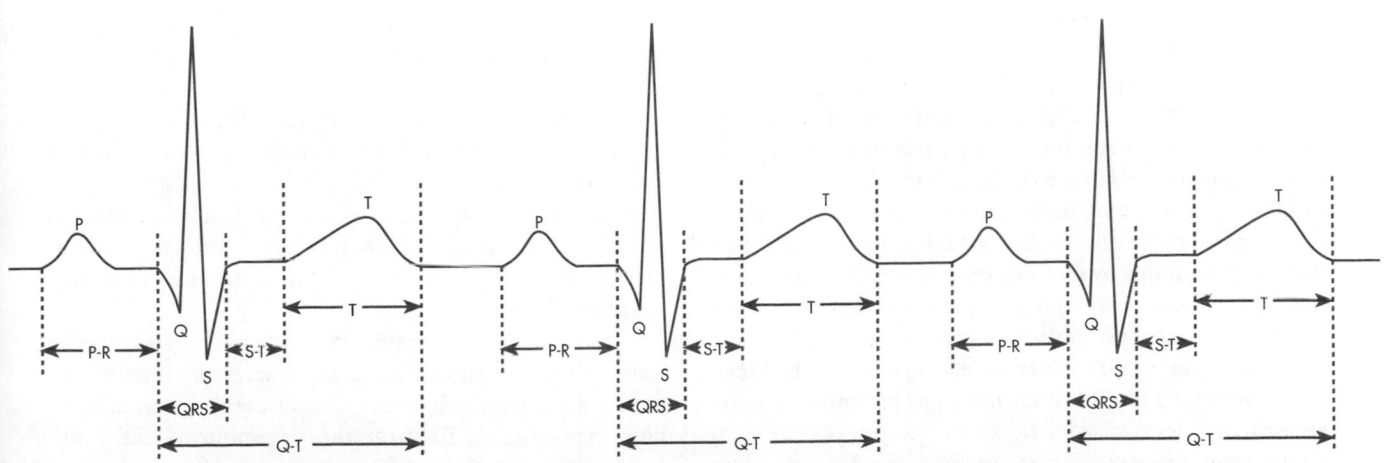

Figure 39-6 Normal ECG waveform.

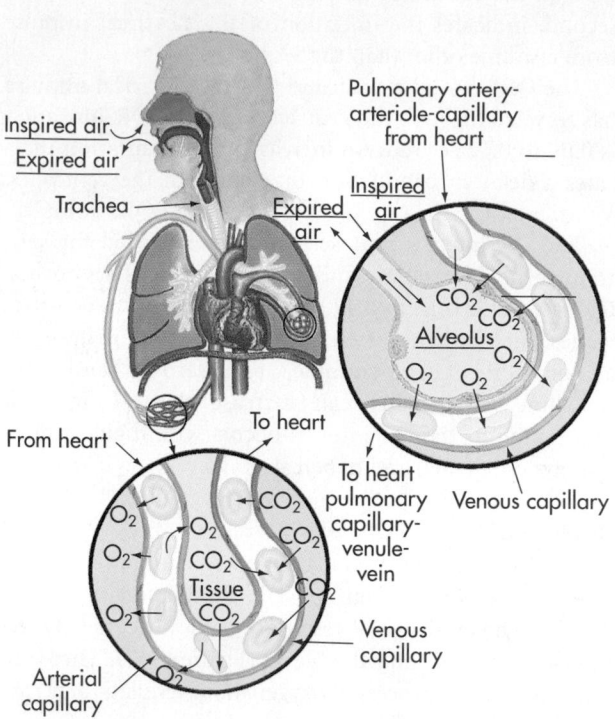

Figure 39-7 Structures of the pulmonary system. The circle denotes the alveoli.
Modified from Wilson SF, Thompson JM: *Respiratory disorders*, St. Louis, 1990, Mosby.

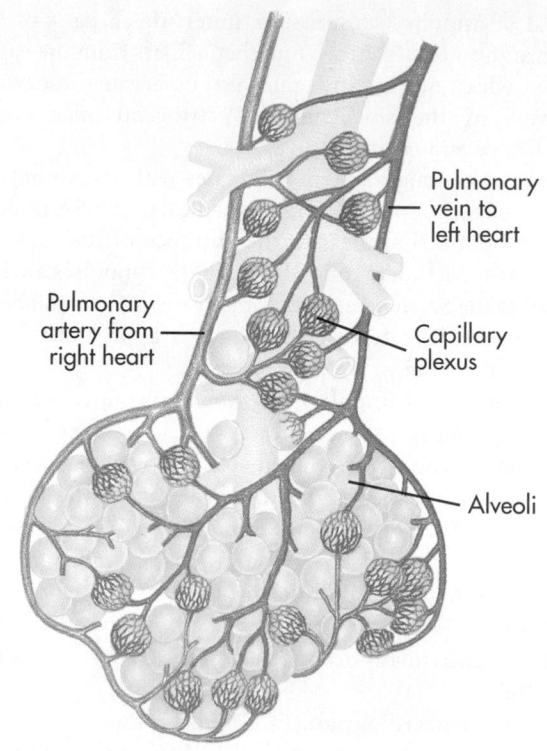

Figure 39-8 Alveoli at the terminal end of the lower airway.
From Thompson J and others: *Mosby's manual of clinical nursing*, ed 3, St. Louis, 1993, Mosby.

as intact innervation. The major inspiratory muscle of respiration is the diaphragm. It is innervated by the phrenic nerve, which exits the spinal cord at the fourth cervical vertebra.

Work of Breathing. Breathing is the effort required for expanding and contracting the lungs. The work of breathing is determined by the degree of compliance of the lungs, airway resistance, presence of active expiration, and use of accessory muscles of respiration.

Inspiration is an active process, stimulated by chemical receptors in the aorta. Expiration is a passive process that depends on the elastic recoil properties of the lungs, requiring little or no muscle work. Elastic recoil is produced by elastic fibers in lung tissue and by surface tension in the fluid film lining the alveoli. Surfactant is the chemical produced in the lungs by alveolar type 2 cells that maintains the surface tension of the alveoli and keeps them from collapsing. Clients with advanced chronic obstructive pulmonary disease (COPD) lose the elastic recoil of the lungs and thorax. As a result, the client's work of breathing is increased.

Accessory muscles of respiration can increase lung volume during inspiration. Clients with COPD, especially

emphysema, frequently use these muscles to increase lung volume. Prolonged use of the accessory muscles of respiration does not promote effective ventilation and causes fatigue. During assessment the nurse may observe elevation of the client's clavicles during inspiration.

Compliance is the ability of the lungs to distend or to expand in response to increased intraalveolar pressure. Compliance is decreased in diseases such as pulmonary edema, interstitial and pleural fibrosis, and congenital or traumatic structural abnormalities such as kyphosis or fractured ribs.

Airway resistance is the pressure difference between the mouth and the alveoli in relation to the rate of flow of inspired gas. Airway resistance can be increased by an airway obstruction, small airway disease (such as asthma), and tracheal edema. When resistance is increased, the amount of air traveling through the anatomical airways is decreased.

Decreased lung compliance, increased airway resistance, active expiration, or the use of accessory muscles increases the work of breathing, resulting in increased energy expenditure. To meet this expenditure, the body increases its metabolic rate, and the need for oxygen, as well as for the elimination of carbon dioxide, increases.

Major Anatomical Structures of the Thorax and Their Functions
Box 39-2

INSPIRATORY MUSCLES

Diaphragm

Contraction causes the diaphragm to descend, creating a negative pleural pressure and increasing the vertical dimension of the lungs, which contributes to inflation of the lungs. The increase in vertical dimension and the decrease in intrapulmonary pressure (negative with respect to atmospheric pressure) cause air to enter the lungs.

External Intercostal Muscles

Contraction elevates the anterior ends of the ribs, causing them to move upward and outward. This increases the anteroposterior dimension of the thorax.

Accessory Muscles

Accessory muscles include the scalene, sternocleidomastoid, and trapezius muscles. Contraction elevates the first two ribs and the sternum.

EXPIRATORY MUSCLES

Internal Intercostal Muscles

Contraction pulls the ribs down and in, thereby decreasing the anteroposterior diameter of the thorax.

Abdominal Respiratory Muscles

Abdominal respiratory muscles include the rectus, transverse abdominis, internal oblique, and external oblique muscles. Contraction depresses the lower ribs, forces the diaphragm up, and decreases the vertical dimension of the thoracic cavity.

PLEURAL SPACE

The pleural space is a potential space that is only a thin film of liquid lying between the outer layer of the lung (visceral pleura) and the inner layer of the chest cavity (parietal pleura). It permits a smooth, gliding movement of the lungs along the chest wall. Normally air is not present in the pleural space.

LUNGS

Left (Two Lobes) and Right (Three Lobes)

The lungs transfer oxygen from the atmosphere into the alveoli and carbon dioxide from the alveoli to the lungs to be excreted as a waste product. They also filter toxic material from circulation and metabolize compounds such as angiotensin I, bradykinin, and prostaglandins.

Alveoli

Alveoli transfer oxygen and carbon dioxide to and from the blood through the alveolar membrane. These tiny air sacs expand during inspiration, greatly increasing the surface area over which exchange of gases occurs.

This sequence is a vicious cycle for a client with impaired ventilation, causing further deterioration of respiratory status and the ability to oxygenate adequately.

Lung Volumes and Capacities.   Spirometry is used to measure the volume of air entering or leaving the lungs. Variations in lung volumes may be associated with health states such as pregnancy, exercise, obesity, or obstructive and restrictive conditions of the lungs. The amount of surfactant, degree of compliance, and strength of respiratory muscles can affect pressures and volumes within the lungs.

Lung capacities are made up of two or more lung volumes. For example, the total lung capacity is the sum of the tidal volume and the inspiratory and expiratory reserve volume. The total lung capacity is the sum of the tidal volume, the inspiratory reserve volume, the expiratory reserve volume, and the reserve volume (see pulmonary function tests, p. 1150.)

Gases are moved into and out of the lungs through pressure changes (Figure 39-9). Intrapleural pressure is negative or less than atmospheric pressure, which is 760 mm Hg at sea level. For air to flow into the lungs, intrapleural pressure must become more negative, setting up a pressure gradient between the atmosphere and the alveoli.

Pulmonary Circulation.   The primary function of the pulmonary circulation is to move blood to and from the alveolocapillary membrane for gas exchange to occur. The pulmonary circulation is a reservoir for blood so that the lung can increase its blood volume without large increases in pulmonary artery or venous pressures. The pulmonary circulation also acts as a filter, removing small thrombi before they can reach vital organs.

The pulmonary circulation begins at the pulmonary artery, which receives poorly oxygenated mixed venous blood from the right ventricle. Blood flow through this system depends on the pumping ability of the right ventricle, which has an output of approximately 4 to 6 L/min. The flow continues from the pulmonary artery through the pulmonary arterioles to the pulmonary capillaries, where blood comes in contact with the alveolocapillary membrane and the exchange of respiratory gases occurs. The oxygen-rich blood then circulates through the pulmonary venules and pulmonary veins, returning to the left atrium.

Pressure and resistance within the pulmonary circulatory system is lower than that within the systemic circulatory system. The normal pulmonary artery systolic pressure is 20 to 30 mm Hg, the diastolic pressure is less than

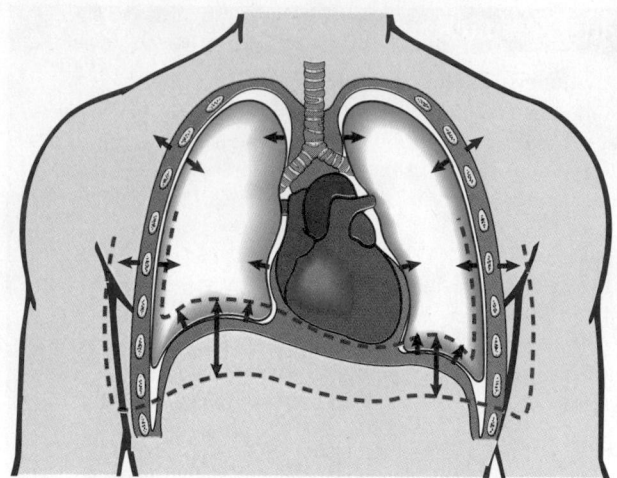

Figure 39-9   Frontal section of chest showing movement of the lung and chest wall during inspiration and expiration. During inspiration the inspiratory muscles contract and the chest expands. Alveolar pressure becomes subatmospheric with respect to pressure at the airway opening, and air flows into the lungs. During expiration the inspiratory muscles relax. Recoil of the lung causes alveolar pressure to exceed pressure at the airway opening and air to flow out of the lungs. Single arrows show excursion of the lungs and chest wall. Double arrows show movement of the lung bases.
From Lewis SM and others: *Medical-surgical nursing: assessment and management of clinical problems,* ed 5, St. Louis, 2000, Mosby.

12 mm Hg, and the mean pressure is less than 20 mm Hg. The walls of the pulmonary vessels are thinner and contain less smooth muscle. The lung accepts the total cardiac output from the right ventricle and, except in cases of alveolar hypoxia or cor pulmonale, does not direct blood flow from one region to another.

Respiratory Gas Exchange.   Respiratory gases are exchanged in the alveoli and the capillaries of the body tissues. Oxygen is transferred from the lungs to the blood, and carbon dioxide is transferred from the blood to the alveoli to be exhaled as a waste product. At the tissue level, oxygen is transferred from the blood to tissues, and carbon dioxide is transferred from tissues to the blood to return to the alveoli and be exhaled. This transfer is dependent on the process of diffusion.

    Diffusion is the movement of molecules from an area of higher concentration to an area of lower concentration. Diffusion of respiratory gases occurs at the alveolocapillary membrane, and the rate of diffusion can be affected by the thickness of the membrane. Increased thickness of the membrane impedes diffusion because gases take longer to transfer across. Clients with pulmonary edema,

pulmonary infiltrates, or a pulmonary effusion have an increased thickness of the alveolocapillary membrane, resulting in slowed diffusion, slowed exchange of respiratory gases, and impaired delivery of oxygen to tissues. The surface area of the membrane can be altered as a result of a chronic disease (e.g., emphysema), an acute disease (e.g., pneumothorax), or a surgical process (e.g., lobectomy). The alveolocapillary membrane can be destroyed or may thicken, changing the rate of diffusion. When fewer alveoli are functioning, the surface area is decreased.

Oxygen Transport.   The oxygen transport system consists of the lungs and cardiovascular system. Delivery depends on the amount of oxygen entering the lungs (ventilation), blood flow to the lungs and tissues (perfusion), rate of diffusion, and oxygen-carrying capacity. The capacity of the blood to carry oxygen is influenced by the amount of dissolved oxygen in the plasma, amount of hemoglobin, and tendency of hemoglobin to bind with oxygen. Only a relatively small amount of required oxygen, less than 1%, is dissolved in the plasma (Lewis and others, 2000). Most oxygen is transported by hemoglobin, which serves as a carrier for oxygen and carbon dioxide. The hemoglobin molecule combines with oxygen to form oxyhemoglobin. The formation of oxyhemoglobin is easily reversible, allowing hemoglobin and oxygen to dissociate, which frees oxygen to enter tissues.

Carbon Dioxide Transport.   Carbon dioxide diffuses into red blood cells and is rapidly hydrated into carbonic acid (H_2CO_3) because of the presence of carbonic anhydrase. The carbonic acid then dissociates into hydrogen (H^+) and bicarbonate (HCO_3^-) ions. The hydrogen ion is buffered by hemoglobin, and the HCO_3^- diffuses into the plasma (see Chapter 40). In addition, some of the carbon dioxide in red blood cells reacts with amino acid groups, forming carbamino compounds. This reaction can occur rapidly without the presence of an enzyme. Reduced hemoglobin (deoxyhemoglobin) can combine with carbon dioxide more easily than oxyhemoglobin, and therefore venous blood transports the majority of carbon dioxide.

Regulation of Respiration.   Regulation of respiration is necessary to ensure sufficient oxygen intake and carbon dioxide elimination to meet the body's demands (e.g., during exercise, infection, or pregnancy). Neural and chemical regulators control the process of respiration. Neural regulation includes the central nervous system control of respiratory rate, depth, and rhythm. Chemical regulation involves the influence of chemicals such as carbon dioxide and hydrogen ions on the rate and depth of respiration (Box 39-3).

FACTORS AFFECTING OXYGENATION
Adequacy of circulation, ventilation, perfusion, and transport of respiratory gases to the tissues is influenced by

Neural and Chemical Regulation of Respiration   Box 39-3

NEURAL REGULATION
Maintains rhythm and depth of respiration and balance between inspiration and expiration.

Cerebral Cortex
Voluntary control of respiration delivers impulses to the respiratory motor neurons by way of the spinal cord; accommodates speaking, eating, and swimming.

Medulla Oblongata
Automatic control of respiration occurs continuously.

CHEMICAL REGULATION
Maintains appropriate rate and depth of respirations based on changes in the blood's carbon dioxide (CO_2), oxygen (O_2), and hydrogen ion (H^+) concentration.

Chemoreceptors
Located in the medulla, aortic body, and carotid body. Changes in chemical content of O_2, CO_2, and H^+ stimulate chemoreceptors, which in turn stimulate neural regulators to adjust the rate and depth of ventilation to maintain normal arterial blood gas levels. Chemical regulation can occur during physical exercise and in some illnesses. It is a short-term adaptive mechanism.

Table 39-1 Physiological Processes Affecting Oxygenation

Process	Effect on Oxygenation
Anemia	Decreases oxygen-carrying capacity of blood
Toxic inhalant	Decreases oxygen-carrying capacity of blood
Airway obstruction	Limits delivery of inspired oxygen to alveoli
High altitude	Atmospheric oxygen concentration is lower and inspiratory oxygen concentration decreases
Fever	Increases metabolic rate and tissue oxygen demand
Decreased chest wall motion (e.g., from musculoskeletal impairments)	Prevents lowering of diaphragm and reduces anteroposterior diameter of thorax on inspiration, reducing volume of air inspired

four types of factors: (1) physiological, (2) developmental, (3) behavioral, and (4) environmental.

Physiological Factors. Any condition that affects cardiopulmonary functioning directly affects the body's ability to meet oxygen demands. The general classifications of cardiac disorders include disturbances in conduction, impaired valvular function, myocardial hypoxia, cardiomyopathic conditions, and peripheral tissue hypoxia. Respiratory disorders include hyperventilation, hypoventilation, and hypoxia.

Other physiological processes affecting a client's oxygenation include alterations that affect the oxygen-carrying capacity of blood, such as the anemias; increases in the body's metabolic demands, such as pregnancy or fever and infection; and alterations that affect the client's chest wall movement or the central nervous system (Table 39-1).

Decreased Oxygen-Carrying Capacity. Hemoglobin carries 99% of the diffused oxygen to tissues (Lewis and others, 2000). Anemia and inhalation of toxic substances decreases the oxygen-carrying capacity of blood by reducing the amount of available hemoglobin to transport oxygen. Anemia, a lower than normal hemoglobin level, is a result of decreased hemoglobin production, increased red blood cell destruction, and/or blood loss. Clients will have complaints of fatigue, decreased activity tolerance, and increased breathlessness, as well as pallor (especially seen in the conjunctiva of the eye) and an increased heart rate.

Carbon monoxide is the most common toxic inhalant that decreases the oxygen-carrying capacity of blood. The affinity for hemoglobin to bind with carbon monoxide is greater than 200 times its affinity to bind with oxygen, creating a functional anemia. Because of the bond's strength, carbon monoxide is not easily dissociated from hemoglobin, making the hemoglobin unavailable for oxygen transport.

Decreased Inspired Oxygen Concentration. When the concentration of inspired oxygen declines, the oxygen-carrying capacity of the blood is decreased. Decreases in the fraction of inspired oxygen concentration (F_IO_2) can be caused by an upper or lower airway obstruction limiting delivery of inspired oxygen to alveoli; decreased environmental oxygen, such as at high altitudes; or decreased inspiration as a result of an incorrect oxygen concentration setting on respiratory therapy equipment.

Hypovolemia. Conditions such as shock and severe dehydration resulting from extracellular fluid loss and reduced circulating blood volume cause **hypovolemia.** With a significant fluid loss, the body tries to adapt by increasing the heart rate and peripheral vasoconstriction to increase the volume of blood returned to the heart and, in turn, increase the cardiac output.

Increased Metabolic Rate. Increases in metabolic activity result in an increased oxygen demand. When body systems are unable to meet this increased demand, the level of oxygenation declines. An increased metabolic rate is a normal physiological response to pregnancy, wound healing, and exercise because the body is building tissue. Most people can meet the increased oxygen demand and do not display signs of oxygen deprivation. Fever increases the tissues' need for oxygen, and as a result, carbon dioxide production also increases. If the febrile state persists, the metabolic rate remains high and the body begins to break down protein stores, resulting in muscle wasting and decreased muscle mass. Respiratory muscles such as the diaphragm and intracostal muscles are also wasted. The body attempts to adapt to the increased carbon dioxide levels by increasing the rate and depth of respiration. The client's work of breathing increases, and the client will eventually display signs and symptoms of hypoxemia. Those clients with pulmonary diseases are at greater risk for hypoxemia and hypercapnia. Assessment findings include an increased rate and depth of respiration, use of the accessory muscles of respiration, pursed-lip breathing, and decreased activity tolerance.

Conditions Affecting Chest Wall Movement.

Any condition that reduces chest wall movement can result in decreased ventilation. If the diaphragm cannot fully descend with breathing, the volume of inspired air decreases and less oxygen is delivered to the alveoli and subsequently to tissues.

Pregnancy. As the fetus grows during pregnancy, the greater size of the uterus pushes abdominal contents upward against the diaphragm. In the last trimester of pregnancy the inspiratory capacity declines, resulting in dyspnea on exertion and increased fatigue.

Obesity. Obese clients have reduced lung volumes from the heavy lower thorax and abdomen, particularly when in the recumbent and supine positions. Obese clients have a reduction in compliance as a result of encroachment of the abdomen into the chest, increased work of breathing, and decreased lung volumes, and they may have fatigue and carbon dioxide retention. In some clients an obesity-hypoventilation syndrome develops in which oxygenation is decreased and carbon dioxide is retained, resulting in daytime sleepiness. Obese clients may also develop obstructive sleep apnea. This is characterized by excessive daytime somnolence, and loud snoring and periods of apnea when sleeping. The obese client is also susceptible to pneumonia after an upper respiratory tract infection because the lungs cannot fully expand and pulmonary secretions are not mobilized in the lower lobes.

Musculoskeletal Abnormalities. Musculoskeletal impairments in the thoracic region reduce oxygenation. Such impairments may result from abnormal structural configurations, trauma, muscular diseases, and diseases of the central nervous system. Abnormal structural configurations impairing oxygenation include those that affect the rib cage, such as pectus excavatum, and those that affect the vertebral column, such as kyphosis.

Trauma. The person with multiple rib fractures can develop a flail chest, a condition in which fractures cause instability in part of the chest wall. The unstable chest wall allows the lung underlying the injured area to contract on inspiration and bulge on expiration, resulting in hypoxia. Chest wall or upper abdominal incisions may also decrease chest wall movement as the client uses shallow respirations to minimize chest wall movement to avoid pain. Excessive or high doses of narcotic analgesics may depress the respiratory center, further decreasing respiratory rate and chest wall expansion.

Neuromuscular Diseases. Diseases such as muscular dystrophy affect oxygenation of tissues by decreasing the client's ability to expand and contract the chest wall. Ventilation is impaired, and atelectasis, hypercapnia, and hypoxemia can occur. Myasthenia gravis, Guillain-Barré syndrome, and poliomyelitis affect respiratory functioning and result in hypoventilation. Myasthenia gravis interferes with normal transmission of impulses from nerves to muscles, involving the whole body, including muscles of respiration. Guillain-Barré syndrome and poliomyelitis cause inflammation and paralysis of muscle groups. Guillain-Barré syndrome usually results in an ascending pattern of paralysis. Respiratory muscles become paralyzed as paralysis ascends to the thoracic region. Poliomyelitis may lead to general or local paralysis. Both may reverse, but poliomyelitis usually results in more residual paralysis.

Central Nervous System Alterations. Diseases or trauma involving the medulla oblongata and spinal cord may result in impaired respiration. When the medulla oblongata is affected, neural regulation of respiration is damaged and abnormal breathing patterns may develop. If the phrenic nerve is damaged, the diaphragm may not descend, thus reducing inspiratory lung volumes and causing hypoxemia. Cervical trauma at C3 to C5 can result in paralysis of the phrenic nerve. Spinal cord trauma below the fifth cervical vertebra usually leaves the phrenic nerve intact but damages nerves that innervate the intercostal muscles, preventing anteroposterior chest expansion.

Influences of Chronic Disease. Oxygenation can be decreased as a direct consequence of chronic disease. It can also be decreased as a secondary effect, as with anemia. The physiological response to chronic hypoxemia is the development of a secondary polycythemia. This adaptive response is the body's attempt to increase the amount of circulating hemoglobin to increase the available oxygen-binding sites.

ALTERATIONS IN CARDIAC FUNCTIONING

Illnesses and conditions that affect cardiac rhythm, strength of contraction, blood flow through the chambers, myocardial blood flow, and peripheral circulation cause alterations in cardiac functioning.

Disturbances in Conduction.

Some disturbances in conduction are a result of electrical impulses that do not originate from the SA node. These rhythm disturbances are called **dysrhythmias,** meaning a deviation from the normal sinus heart rhythm (Table 39-2). Dysrhythmias may occur as a primary conduction disturbance; as a response to ischemia, valvular abnormality, anxiety, or drug toxicity; as a result of caffeine, alcohol, or tobacco use; or as a complication of acid-base or electrolyte imbalance (see Chapter 40).

Dysrhythmias are classified by cardiac response and site of impulse origin. Cardiac response can be either tachycardiac (greater than 100 beats per minute), bradycardiac (less than 60 beats per minute), a premature (early) beat, or a blocked (delayed or absent) beat. Tachydysrhythmias and bradydysrhythmias can lower cardiac output and blood pressure. Tachydysrhythmias reduce cardiac output by decreasing diastolic filling time. Bradydysrhythmias lower cardiac output because of the decreased heart rate.

Abnormal impulses originating above the ventricles are referred to as supraventricular dysrhythmias. The abnormality on the waveform is the configuration and placement of the P wave. Ventricular conduction usually remains normal, and a normal QRS complex is observed. Junctional dysrhythmias represent an abnormal site of impulse conduction above or below the AV node. The P wave can occur before, during, or after the QRS complexes and is often inverted if visible. Because the beat originates above the ventricle, ventricular conduction and the QRS complex are usually normal.

Ventricular dysrhythmias represent an ectopic site of impulse formation within the ventricles. The configuration of the QRS complex is usually widened and bizarre. P waves may or may not be present; often they are buried in the QRS complex. Ventricular tachycardia and ventricular fibrillation are life-threatening rhythms that require immediate intervention. Ventricular tachycardia is considered a life-threatening dysrhythmia because of the decreased cardiac output and the potential to deteriorate into ventricular fibrillation (Lewis and others, 2000).

Altered Cardiac Output.

Failure of the myocardium to eject sufficient volume to the systemic and pulmonary circulations can result in heart failure. Failure of the myocardial pump results from primary coronary artery disease, cardiomyopathic conditions, valvular disorders, and pulmonary disease.

Table 39-2 Common Basic Cardiac Dysrhythmias

Rhythm Characteristics	Etiology	Clinical Significance	Management
Sinus Tachycardia Regular rhythm, rate 100-180 beats/min (higher in infants), normal P wave, normal QRS complex	Rate increase may be normal response to exercise, emotion, or stressors such as pain, fever, pump failure, hyperthyroidism, and certain drugs (e.g., caffeine, nitrates, atropine, epinephrine, isoproterenol, nicotine)	May have hemodynamic consequence in client with damaged heart that is unable to sustain increased workloads (increased myocardial oxygen consumption) brought on by persistent increases in heart rate	Correct underlying factors, remove offending drugs

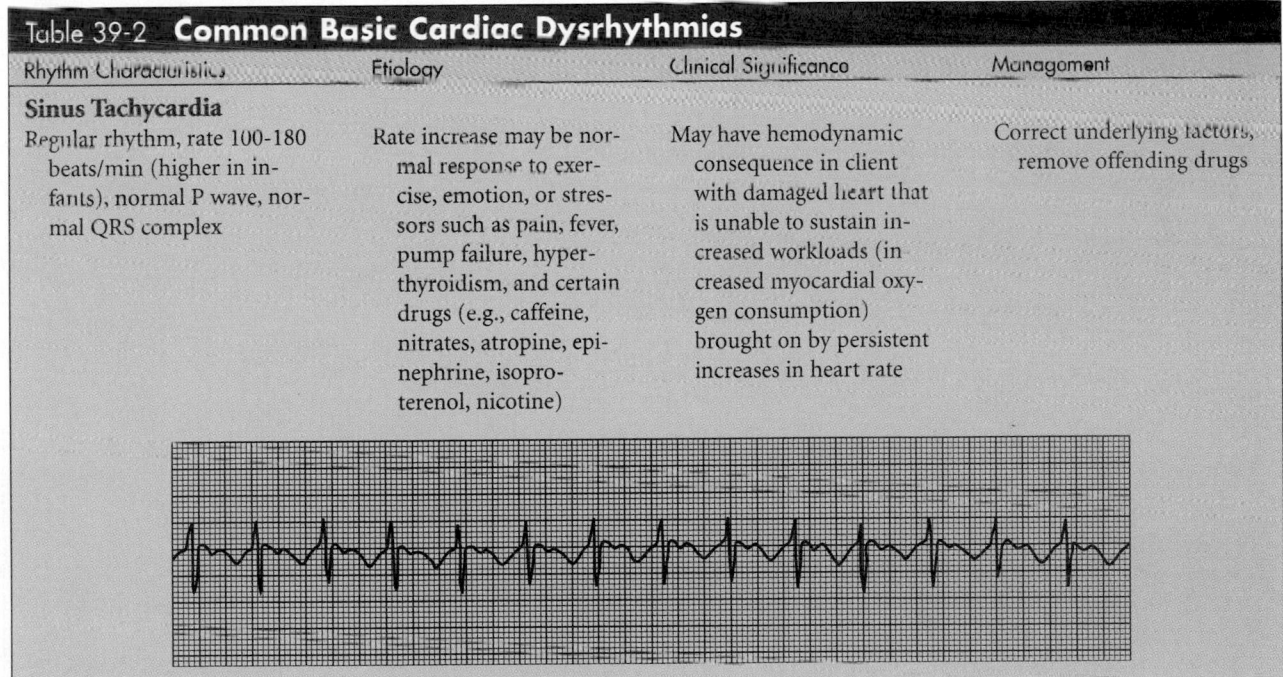

Modified from Canobbio MM: *Cardiovascular disorders,* St. Louis, 1990, Mosby.

PSVT management: Vagal stimulation such as carotid sinus massage or Valsava maneuver to decrease ventricular response with medication to block AV conduction; adenosine 6 mg IV over 1-3 seconds; adenosine 12 mg IV over 1-3 seconds; assess complex width; narrow-check blood pressure, normal verapamil 2.5-5 mg IV; if blood pressure low or unstable, proceed to synchronized cardioversion; wide complex, lidocaine 1-1.5 mg/kg IV push, procainamide 20-30 mg/min; synchronized cardioversion if resistant to drug therapy (ECC, 1992).

Sinus bradycardia management: Correct underlying causes. If symptomatic, (e.g., hypotension, chest pain, decreased level of consciousness, shortness of breath), administer atropine 0.04 mg/kg IV; transcutaneous pacing if available; dopamine 5-20 μg/kg/min; epinephrine 2-10 μg/min; temporary transvenous pacemaker if resistant to drug therapy (ECC, 1992).

Continued

Table 39-2 Common Basic Cardiac Dysrhythmias—cont'd

Rhythm Characteristics	Etiology	Clinical Significance	Management
Sinus Bradycardia Regular rhythm, rate less than 60 beats/min, normal P wave, normal PR interval, normal QRS complex	Rate decrease may be normal response to sleep or in well-conditioned athlete; abnormal drops in rate may be caused by diminished blood flow to SA node, vagal stimulation, hypothyroidism, increased intracranial pressure, or pharmacological agents (e.g., digoxin, propranolol, quidinine, procainamide)	No clinical significance unless associated with signs and symptoms of reduced cardiac output such as dizziness or syncope or presence of chest pain	Symptomatic bradycardia (hypotension with decreased cardiac output) is treated with atropine; pacemaker may be required

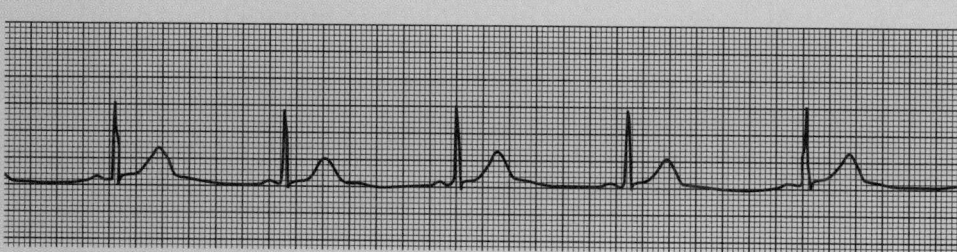

Rhythm Characteristics	Etiology	Clinical Significance	Management
Sinus Dysrhythmia Irregular rhythm; possibly phasic with respiration, slowing during inspiration and increasing with expiration; rate of 60-100 beats/min; normal P wave; normal PR interval; normal QRS complex	Sinus rhythm with cyclic variation caused by vagal impulses that influence rhythm during respiration; occurs commonly in children, young adults, and older adults; usually disappears as heart rate increases	No clinical significance unless heart rate decreases and symptoms of dizziness occur with decreased rate	None indicated unless heart rate decreases and symptoms occur

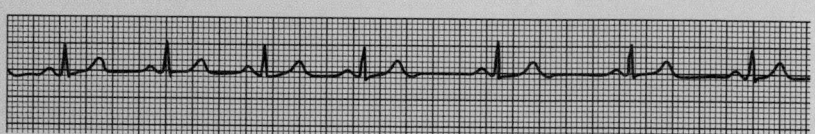

Rhythm Characteristics	Etiology	Clinical Significance	Management
Paroxysmal Supraventricular Tachycardia (PSVT) Sudden, rapid onset of tachycardia with stimulus originating above AV node; regular rhythm; rate 150-250 beats/min; P wave uniform, possibly buried in preceding T wave; PR interval variable, often difficult to measure; normal QRS complex	May begin and end spontaneously or be precipitated by excitement, fatigue, caffeine, smoking, or alcohol use	Usually no significant impairment; client complains of palpitations and shortness of breath; if persistent or occurring in client with preexisting organic heart disease, may cause decrease in cardiac output and/or blood pressure, resulting in pump failure or shock	Vagal stimulation by carotid sinus massage or Valsalva maneuver, adenosine, diltiazem, digitalis, or beta-adrenergic blockers

Modified from Canobbio MM: *Cardiovascular disorders*, St. Louis, 1990, Mosby. For footnote see p. 135.

Table 39-2   Common Basic Cardiac Dysrhythmias—cont'd

Rhythm Characteristics	Etiology	Clinical Significance	Management

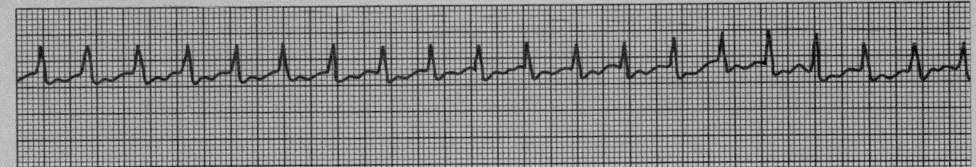

Premature Ventricular Contractions (PVCs)

Rhythm Characteristics	Etiology	Clinical Significance	Management
Irregular rhythm with ectopic beats followed by full compensatory pause; rate normal or increased, depending on number of ectopic beats; P wave absent in ectopic beat; PR interval absent; QRS complex widened and distorted; T wave in opposition to R wave	Caused by irritable focus within ventricle, commonly associated with myocardial infarction; other causes include hypoxia, hypocalcemia, acidosis	PVCs occurring frequently (more than 6/min) or in pairs, indicating increased ventricular irritability	Suppress PVCs; if PVCs are frequent, administer intravenous bolus of lidocaine 1-1.5 mg/kg IV push followed by continuous IV infusion; administer additional antiarrhythmic agents as needed; treat underlying cause

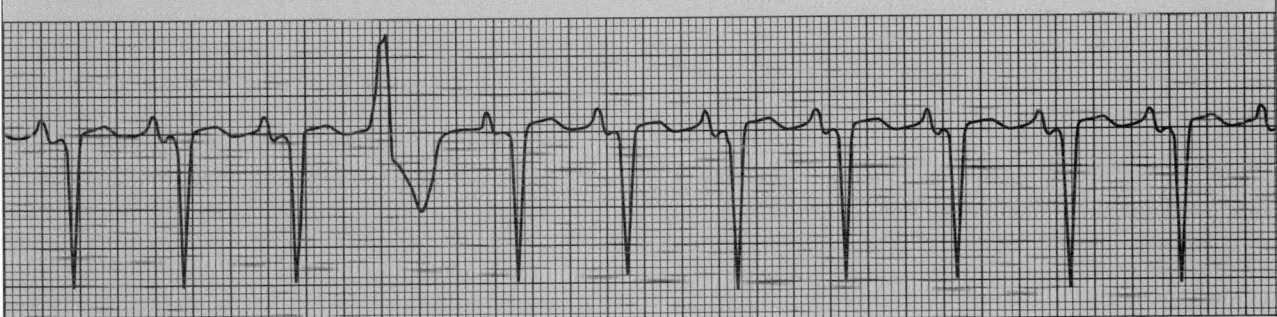

Ventricular Tachycardia

Rhythm Characteristics	Etiology	Clinical Significance	Management
Rhythm slightly irregular, rate 100-200 beats/min, P wave absent, PR interval absent, QRS complex wide and bizarre, >0.12 second	Caused by irritable ventricular foci firing repetitively, commonly caused by myocardial infarction	Often a forerunner of ventricular fibrillation; if condition is persistent and rapid, causes decreased cardiac output because of decreased ventricular filling time	Most episodes terminate abruptly without treatment; administer lidocaine bolus 1-1.5 mg/kg IV followed by continuous IV drip; perform cardiac defibrillation if indicated

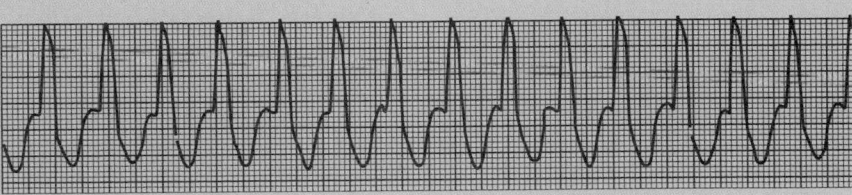

Left-Sided Heart Failure.   **Left-sided heart failure** is an abnormal condition characterized by impaired functioning of the left ventricle due to elevated pressures and pulmonary congestion. If left ventricular failure is significant, the amount of blood ejected from the left ventricle drops greatly, resulting in decreased cardiac output. Assessment findings may include decreased activity tolerance, breathlessness, dizziness, and confusion as a result of tissue hypoxia from the diminished cardiac output. As the left ventricle continues to fail, blood begins to pool in the pulmonary circulation, causing pulmonary congestion. Clinical findings include crackles on auscultation, hypoxia, shortness of breath on exertion and often at rest, cough, and paroxysmal nocturnal dyspnea.

Right-Sided Heart Failure.   **Right-sided heart failure** results from impaired functioning of the right ventricle characterized by venous congestion in the systemic circulation. Right-sided heart failure more commonly results from pulmonary disease or as a result of long-term left-sided failure. The primary pathological factor in right-sided failure is elevated pulmonary vascular resistance (PVR). As the PVR continues to rise, the right ventricle must generate more work, and the oxygen demand of the heart increases. As the failure continues, the amount of blood ejected from the right ventricle declines, and blood begins to "back up" in the systemic circulation. Clinically the client has weight gain, distended neck veins, hepatomegaly and splenomegaly, and dependent peripheral edema.

Impaired Valvular Function.   **Valvular heart disease** is an acquired or congenital disorder of a cardiac valve characterized by stenosis and obstructed blood flow or valvular degeneration and regurgitation of blood. When stenosis occurs in the semilunar valves (aortic and pulmonic valves), the adjacent ventricles must work harder to move the ventricular volume beyond the stenotic valve. Over time the stenosis can cause the ventricle to hypertrophy (enlarge), and if the condition is untreated, left- or right-sided heart failure can occur. If stenosis occurs in the atrioventricular valves (mitral and tricuspid valves), the atrial pressure rises, causing the atria to hypertrophy. When regurgitation occurs, there is a backflow of blood into an adjacent chamber. For example, in mitral regurgitation the mitral leaflets do not close completely. When the ventricle contracts, blood escapes back into the atria, causing a murmur, or "whooshing" sound (see Chapter 32).

Myocardial Ischemia.   **Myocardial ischemia** results when the supply of blood to the myocardium from the coronary arteries is insufficient to meet the oxygen demands of the organ. Two common manifestations of this ischemia are angina pectoris and myocardial infarction.

Angina.   **Angina pectoris** is usually a transient imbalance between myocardial oxygen supply and demand. The condition results in chest pain that is aching, sharp, tingling, or burning, or that feels like pressure. The chest pain may be left sided or substernal and may radiate to the left or both arms, and to the jaw, neck, and back. In some clients anginal pain may not radiate. The pain can last from 1 to 15 minutes. Clients report that pain is often precipitated by activities that increase myocardial oxygen demand (e.g., exercise, anxiety, or stress). The pain is usually relieved with rest and coronary vasodilators, the most common being a nitroglycerin preparation.

Myocardial Infarction.   **Myocardial infarction** results from sudden decreases in coronary blood flow or an increase in myocardial oxygen demand without adequate coronary perfusion. Infarction occurs because of ischemia (which is reversible) and necrosis (which is not reversible) of myocardial tissue.

Chest pain associated with myocardial infarction in men is usually described as crushing, squeezing, or stabbing. The pain may be retrosternal and left precordial, and it may radiate down the left arm to the neck, jaws, teeth, epigastric area, and back. The pain occurs at rest or exertion, lasts more than 30 minutes, and is unrelieved by rest, position change, or sublingual nitroglycerin administration.

Current research indicates that there is a significant difference between men and women in relation to coronary artery disease. It is known that women do not present the same type of symptoms as men (Jensen and King, 1997). The most common initial symptom in women is angina. Women tend to have fewer Q waves and ST segment changes with chest pain when compared with men (Jensen and King, 1997). Estrogen replacement in healthy postmenopausal women may reduce and prevent coronary artery disease. Additional risk factors for coronary artery disease in women include menopause and hormonal contraceptives, such as birth control pills. The initial signs and symptoms in women may be more atypical, including epigastric pain, shortness of breath, variant angina, and vasospasm (Jensen and King, 1997).

ALTERATIONS IN RESPIRATORY FUNCTIONING

Illnesses and conditions that affect ventilation or oxygen transport cause alterations in respiratory functioning. The three primary alterations are hyperventilation, hypoventilation, and hypoxia.

Hyperventilation.   The goal of ventilation is to produce a normal arterial carbon dioxide tension ($PaCO_2$) between 35 and 45 mm Hg and maintain a normal arterial oxygen tension (PaO_2) between 95 and 100 mm Hg. Hyperventilation and hypoventilation refer to alveolar ventilation and not to the client's respiratory rate.

Arterial oxygen levels can be monitored using a noninvasive oxygen saturation monitor. The normal range is 95% to 100%.

Hyperventilation is a state of ventilation in excess of

that required to eliminate the normal venous carbon dioxide produced by cellular metabolism. Anxiety, infections, drugs, or an acid-base imbalance can induce hyperventilation, as well as hypoxia associated with pulmonary embolus or shock. Acute anxiety can lead to hyperventilation and may cause loss of consciousness from excess carbon dioxide exhalation. Fever can cause hyperventilation. For each increase of 1° F, there is a 7% increase in the metabolic rate, thereby increasing carbon dioxide production. The clinical response is an increased rate and depth of respiration.

Hyperventilation may also be chemically induced. Salicylate (aspirin) poisoning causes excessive stimulation of the respiratory center as the body's attempt to compensate for excess carbon dioxide. Amphetamines also increase ventilation by raising carbon dioxide production. Hyperventilation can also occur as the body tries to compensate for metabolic acidosis by producing a respiratory alkalosis. For example, the diabetic client who has gone into diabetic ketoacidosis is producing large amounts of metabolic acids. The respiratory system tries to correct the acid-base balance by overbreathing. Ventilation increases to reduce the amount of carbon dioxide available to form carbonic acid (see Chapter 40).

Alveolar hyperventilation produces many signs and symptoms that can be assessed (Box 39-4). Hemoglobin does not release oxygen to tissues as readily, and tissue hypoxia results. As symptoms worsen, the client may become more agitated, which further increases the respiratory rate and can result in respiratory alkalosis.

Hypoventilation.   **Hypoventilation** occurs when alveolar ventilation is inadequate to meet the body's oxygen demand or to eliminate sufficient carbon dioxide. As alveolar ventilation decreases, $PaCO_2$ is elevated. Severe atelectasis can produce hypoventilation. **Atelectasis** is a collapse of the alveoli that prevents normal respiratory exchange of oxygen and carbon dioxide. As alveoli collapse, less of the lung can be ventilated and hypoventilation occurs.

In clients with COPD, the inappropriate administration of excessive oxygen can result in hypoventilation. These clients have adapted to a high carbon dioxide level, and their carbon dioxide–sensitive chemoreceptors are essentially not functioning. Their stimulus to breathe is a decreased PaO_2. If excessive oxygen is administered, the oxygen requirement is satisfied and the stimulus to breathe is negated. High concentrations of oxygen (e.g., greater than 24% to 28% [1 to 3 L/min]) prevent the PaO_2 from falling and obliterate the stimulus to breathe, resulting in hypoventilation. The excessive retention of carbon dioxide may lead to respiratory arrest.

Signs and symptoms of hypoventilation are presented in Box 39-4. If untreated, the client's status can rapidly decline. Convulsions, unconsciousness, and death can result. Treatment for hyperventilation and hypoventilation requires improving tissue oxygenation, restoring ventilatory function, and treating the underlying cause and achieving acid-base balance.

Hypoxia.   **Hypoxia** is inadequate tissue oxygenation at the cellular level. This can result from a deficiency in oxygen delivery or oxygen utilization at the cellular level. Hypoxia can be caused by (1) a decreased hemoglobin level and lowered oxygen-carrying capacity of the blood; (2) a diminished concentration of inspired oxygen, which

Differentiating Alveolar Hyperventilation from Hypoventilation   Box 39-4

	Hyperventilation	Hypoventilation
MENTAL STATUS	Disorientation Light-headedness Dizziness	Disorientation Lethargy Dizziness Headache Decreased ability to follow instructions Convulsions Coma
CARDIOVASCULAR SIGNS AND SYMPTOMS	Tachycardia Chest pain Shortness of breath	Dysrhythmias Cardiac arrest
NEUROLOGICAL SIGNS AND SYMPTOMS	Blurred vision Paresthesias Extremity and circumoral numbness Carpopedal spasm (tetany) Tinnitus	
OTHER	Acid-base imbalances and electrolyte imbalances	Acid-base and electrolyte imbalances

may occur at high altitudes; (3) the inability of the tissues to extract oxygen from the blood, as with cyanide poisoning; (4) decreased diffusion of oxygen from the alveoli to the blood, as in pneumonia; (5) poor tissue perfusion with oxygenated blood, as with shock; and (6) impaired ventilation, as with multiple rib fractures or chest trauma.

The clinical signs and symptoms of hypoxia include apprehension, restlessness, inability to concentrate, declining level of consciousness, dizziness, and behavioral changes (Box 39-5). The client with hypoxia is unable to lie down and appears fatigued and agitated. Vital sign changes include an increased pulse rate and increased rate and depth of respiration. The client with a narcotic overdose, such as a heroin overdose, may display signs of hypoventilation. During early stages of hypoxia the blood pressure is elevated unless the condition is caused by shock. As the hypoxia worsens, the respiratory rate may decline as a result of respiratory muscle fatigue.

Cyanosis, blue discoloration of the skin and mucous membranes caused by the presence of desaturated hemoglobin in capillaries, is a late sign of hypoxia. The presence or absence of cyanosis is not a reliable measure of oxygenation status. Central cyanosis, observed in the tongue, soft palate, and conjunctiva of the eye, where blood flow is high, indicates hypoxemia. Peripheral cyanosis, seen in the extremities, nail beds, and earlobes, is often a result of vasoconstriction and stagnant blood flow. Hypoxia is a life-threatening condition. Untreated, it can produce cardiac dysrhythmias that result in death. Hypoxia is managed by administration of oxygen and treatment of the underlying cause, such as airway obstruction.

Signs and Symptoms of Hypoxia   Box 39-5

Restlessness
Apprehension, anxiety
Disorientation
Decreased ability to concentrate
Decreased level of consciousness
Increased fatigue
Dizziness
Behavioral changes
Increased pulse rate
Increased rate and depth of respiration
Elevated blood pressure
Cardiac dysrhythmias
Pallor
Cyanosis
Clubbing
Dyspnea
Hypoventilation

Nursing Knowledge Base

DEVELOPMENTAL FACTORS

The developmental stage of the client and the normal aging process can affect tissue oxygenation.

Premature Infants.   Premature infants are at risk for hyaline membrane disease, which is caused by a surfactant deficiency. The surfactant-synthesizing ability of the lungs develops late in pregnancy, about the seventh month, and may therefore be lacking in preterm infants.

Infants and Toddlers.   Infants and toddlers are at risk for upper respiratory tract infections as a result of frequent exposure to other children and exposure to secondhand smoke. In addition, during the teething process some infants develop nasal congestion, which encourages bacterial growth and increases the potential for respiratory tract infection. Upper respiratory tract infections are usually not dangerous, and infants or toddlers recover with little difficulty. Common airway infections are nasopharyngitis (e.g., rhinoviruses, respiratory syncytial virus, and adenovirus), pharyngitis (e.g., viral and beta-hemolytic streptococci), *Hemophilus influenzae* infection, and tonsillitis. Airway obstruction can also occur with aspirated foreign objects, such as food, buttons, and candy.

School-Age Children and Adolescents.   School-age children and adolescents are exposed to respiratory infections and respiratory risk factors such as secondhand smoke and cigarette smoking. A healthy child usually does not have adverse pulmonary effects from respiratory infections. A person who starts smoking in adolescence and continues to smoke into middle age, however, has an increased risk for cardiopulmonary disease and lung cancer.

Young and Middle-Age Adults.   Young and middle-age adults are exposed to multiple cardiopulmonary risk factors: an unhealthy diet, lack of exercise, stress, drugs, and smoking. Reducing these modifiable factors may decrease the client's risk for cardiac or pulmonary diseases. This is also the time when lifelong habits and lifestyles are established. It is important to help these clients make good choices and informed decisions about the rest of their lives and their health care practices.

Older Adults.   The cardiac and respiratory systems undergo changes throughout the aging process. In the arterial system atherosclerotic plaques develop and the systemic blood pressure may rise. Chest wall compliance is decreased in the older client as a result of osteoporosis and calcification of the costal cartilages. The respiratory muscles weaken, and the pulmonary vascular circulation becomes less distensible (Box 39-6). The trachea and large bronchi become enlarged from calcification of the airways, and alveoli enlarge, decreasing the surface area available for gas exchange. In addition, the number of functional cilia is reduced. Decreased ciliary action and effectiveness of cough mechanisms put the older adult at increased risk for respiratory infections (Lueckenotte, 2000). Ventilation and transfer of respiratory gases decline with age. Osteoporotic changes of the thoracic cage and kyphosis of the vertebrae occur normally with aging (Lueckenotte, 1998). With these changes the lungs are unable to expand fully, leading to lower oxygenation levels (Table 39-3).

Gerontological NURSING PRACTICE   Box 39-6

- Older adults generally have a respiratory rate between 16 and 25 breaths per minute. Because they depend on changes in intraabdominal pressure, positioning can greatly affect their breathing pattern. Position the client to maximize ventilation. Positions such as semi-Fowler's and high-Fowler's provide the best ventilation. The older client should be encouraged to sit up in the chair to promote good lung expansion.
- Frequent, smaller meals and fewer bloating and gas-producing foods will help prevent an overdistended abdomen and reduce pressure on the diaphragm.

LIFESTYLE FACTORS

Lifestyle factors that influence cardiopulmonary functioning include nutrition, exercise, cigarette smoking, substance abuse, and stress (Box 39-7).

Nutrition.   Nutrition affects cardiopulmonary function in several ways. Severe obesity decreases lung expansion, and the increased body weight increases oxygen demands to meet metabolic needs. The malnourished client may experience respiratory muscle wasting, resulting in decreased muscle strength and respiratory excursion. Cough efficiency is reduced secondary to respiratory muscle weakness, putting the client at risk for retention of pulmonary secretions. Diets high in fat increase cholesterol and atherogenesis in the coronary arteries.

Clients who are obese and/or malnourished are at risk for anemia. Diets high in carbohydrates may play a role in increasing the carbon dioxide load for clients with carbon dioxide retention. As carbohydrates are metabolized, an increased load of carbon dioxide is created and excreted via the lungs.

Dietary restriction of sodium has been shown to be beneficial in reducing antihypertensive medication requirements and may cause left ventricular hypertrophy to regress (Joint National Committee [JNC], 1997). Diets

---

Table 39-3   **Changes in the Aging Lung**

Function	Pathophysiological Change	Key Clinical Findings
Breathing mechanics	Decreased chest wall compliance	Decreased vital capacity
	Loss of elastic recoil	Increased reserve volume
	Decreased respiratory muscle mass and strength	Decreased expiratory flow rates
Oxygenation	Increased ventilation/perfusion mismatch	
	Decreased cardiac output	Decreased PaO_2
	Decreased mixed venous oxygen	Increased alveolar-arterial oxygen gradient
	Increased physiological dead space	Decreased cardiac output
	Decreased alveolar surface area	
	Decreased carbon dioxide diffusion capacity	
Ventilation control and breathing pattern	Decreased responsiveness of central and peripheral chemoreceptors to hypoxemia and hypercapnia	Decreased tidal volume
		Increased respiratory rate
		Increased minute ventilation
Lung defense mechanisms	Decreased number of cilia and effectiveness of the mucociliary clearance	Decreased airway clearance
	Diminished cough reflex	Increased risk for infection
	Decreased humoral and cellular immunity	Increased risk of aspiration
	Decreased IgA production	
Sleep and breathing	Decreased ventilatory drive	Increased risk of apnea, hypopnea, and arterial oxygen desaturation during sleep
	Decreased tone of upper airway muscles	
	Decreased arousal	Increased risk of aspiration
		Snoring
		Obstructive sleep apnea
Exercise capacity	Muscle deconditioning and efficiency	Decreased maximum oxygen consumption
	Decreased muscle mass	Breathlessness at low exercise levels
	Decreased reserves	

Modified from Pierson DJ: Effects of aging on the respiratory system. In Pierson DJ, Kacmarek RM, editors: *Foundations of respiratory care,* New York, 1992, Churchill Livingstone.

Cardioplumonary Health Promotion*   Box 39-7

Maintain ideal body weight.
Eat a low-fat, low-salt, calorie-appropriate diet.
Engage in regular aerobic exercise.
Be smoke free.
Monitor blood pressure.
Monitor cholesterol and triglyceride levels.
Get an annual influenza vaccine if at risk for the development of influenza.
Get a pneumococcal vaccine if appropriate.
Cover the mouth and nose when coughing or sneezing.
Avoid secondhand smoke and other pollutants.
Use a filter mask when exposed to occupational hazards.
Use stress reduction techniques.
Reduce exposure to secondary infections.

*Target population: young to older adults.

Research **HIGHLIGHT**   Box 39-8

RESEARCH ABSTRACT

Sixteen subjects ages 60 to 72 years who did not routinely exercise and who had no evidence of cardiopulmonary disease or history of smoking were enrolled in the study. Subjects completed a timed 440 yard (400 meter) walking test, walking as fast as they could while remaining comfortable. Subjects then completed surveys about perceived frustration, tension, and coping ability related to stress. All subjects engaged in a supervised exercise program 3 days a week for 50 to 60 minutes each session, working out at 50% to 60% of their individual predicted maximal heart rate reserves.

All subjects increased their walking capacity. Of the 14 subjects who completed the study, 12 showed a reduction in the incidence of respiratory tract infections and related symptoms. Eleven of the subjects improved their scores on the stress survey, reporting less self-perceived stress.

IMPLICATIONS FOR PRACTICE

- Aerobic activity may produce a buffering effect against stress; nurses should encourage clients to exercise within their capacity.
- The secondary benefits of exercise include improved cardiovascular function, improved musculoskeletal strength, endurance, improved joint flexibility, and reduced incidence of respiratory infections and related symptoms. Nurses should educate their clients about the benefits of regular exercise and help them develop a plan for health promotion.

REFERENCE

Karper WB, Boshen MB: Effects of exercise on acute respiratory tract infections and related symptoms, *Geriatr Nurs* 14(1):15, 1993.

high in potassium may prevent hypertension and help improve control in clients with hypertension. A 2000-calorie diet high in fiber, potassium, calcium, and magnesium; made up of fruits, vegetables, and low-fat dairy foods; and low in saturated and total fat is recommended to help prevent and reduce the effects of hypertension (JNC, 1997).

Exercise.   Exercise increases the body's metabolic activity and oxygen demand. The rate and depth of respiration increase, enabling the person to inhale more oxygen and exhale excess carbon dioxide. A physical exercise program has many benefits (see Chapter 36). People who exercise 3 to 4 times per week for 20 to 40 minutes have a lower pulse rate, blood pressure, decreased cholesterol level, increased blood flow, and greater oxygen extraction by working muscles (Box 39-8). Fully conditioned people can increase oxygen consumption by 10% to 20% because of increased cardiac output and increased efficiency of the myocardial muscle (JNC, 1997).

Cigarette Smoking.   Cigarette smoking is associated with a number of diseases, including heart disease, chronic obstructive lung disease, and lung cancer. Cigarette smoking can worsen peripheral vascular and coronary artery diseases (JNC, 1997). Inhaled nicotine causes vasoconstriction of peripheral and coronary blood vessels, increasing blood pressure and decreasing blood flow to peripheral vessels. The risk of lung cancer is 10 times greater for a person who smokes than for a nonsmoker. Exposure to secondhand smoke increases the risk of lung cancer in the nonsmoker. The number of female smokers has increased substantially over the past 30 years, resulting in a tenfold increase in the number of women diagnosed with lung cancer. Only recently has the rate of increase among women begun to slow (American Cancer Society [ACS], 1998). Women who take birth control pills

and smoke cigarettes are at increased risk for cardiovascular problems such as thrombophlebitis and pulmonary emboli. The 5-year survival rate for all clients with lung cancer is only 14%, regardless of the diagnosis (ACS, 1998). Frequently lung cancer is diagnosed only when it has reached an advanced stage. If lung cancer is detected when the disease is still localized, the survival rate is 49% (ACS, 1998). Only 15% of lung cancers are diagnosed when the disease is still localized (ACS, 1998).

Substance Abuse.   Excessive use of alcohol and other drugs can impair tissue oxygenation in two ways. First, the person who chronically abuses substances often has a poor nutritional intake. With the resultant decrease in intake of iron-rich foods, hemoglobin production declines. Second, excessive use of alcohol and certain other drugs can depress the respiratory center, reducing the rate and depth of respiration and the amount of inhaled oxygen. Substance abuse by either smoking or inhaling, such as crack cocaine or inhaling fumes from paint or glue cans, causes direct injury to lung tissue that can lead to permanent lung damage and impaired oxygenation.

ENVIRONMENTAL FACTORS

The environment can also influence oxygenation. The incidence of pulmonary disease is higher in smoggy, urban areas than in rural areas. In addition, the client's workplace may increase the risk for pulmonary disease. Occupational pollutants include asbestos, talcum powder, dust, and airborne fibers. For example, farm workers in dry regions of the southwestern United States are at risk for coccidioidomycosis, a fungal disease caused by inhalation of spores of the airborne bacterium *Coccidioides immitis.* Asbestosis is an occupational lung disease that develops after exposure to asbestos. The lung in asbestosis is characterized by diffuse interstitial fibrosis, creating a restrictive lung disease. It can also cause pleural mesotheliomas and pleural plaques. Clients at risk for developing asbestosis include those working with textiles, fireproofing, or milling, or in the production of paints, plastics, or some prefabricated construction. Clients exposed to asbestos who also smoke are at increased risk of developing lung cancer.

STRESS/ANXIETY

A continuous state of stress or severe anxiety increases the body's metabolic rate and the oxygen demand. The body responds to anxiety and other stresses with an increased rate and depth of respiration. Most people can adapt, but some, particularly those with chronic illnesses or acute life-threatening illnesses such as a myocardial infarction, cannot tolerate the oxygen demands associated with anxiety.

Critical Thinking Synthesis

Successful critical thinking requires a synthesis of knowledge, experience, information gathered from clients, critical thinking attitudes, and intellectual and professional standards. Clinical judgments require the nurse to anticipate the information necessary, analyze the data, and make decisions regarding the client area. Critical thinking is always changing. During assessment the nurse must consider all elements that build toward making an appropriate nursing diagnosis (Figure 39-10).

To understand the oxygen demands of a client and the ability of the client's body to meet those demands, the nurse integrates knowledge from nursing and other disciplines, previous experiences, and information gathered from clients. The nurse must consider current and future oxygenation demands, plan for change in client status, and develop a plan that can change with the changing demands of the client. The use of professional standards, such as those developed by the Agency for Health Care Policy and Research (AHCPR), the Respiratory Nursing Society (RNS), the American Heart Association (AHA), the American Lung Association (ALA), the American

Thoracic Society (ATS), and the American Nurses Association (ANA), provide valuable guidelines for care and management of clients with altered oxygenation.

Nursing Process

ASSESSMENT

The nursing assessment of a client's cardiopulmonary functioning should include data collected from the following areas:

Nursing history of the client's normal and present cardiopulmonary function, past impairments in circulatory or respiratory functioning, and measures that the client may use to optimize oxygenation

Physical examination of the client's cardiopulmonary status, including inspection, palpation, percussion, and auscultation

Review of laboratory and diagnostic test results, including a complete blood count, ECG, pulmonary function test, sputum, and oxygenation such as arterial blood gas tests or pulse oximetry

Nursing History.   The nursing history should focus on the client's ability to meet oxygen needs. The nursing history for cardiac function includes pain and characteristics of pain, dyspnea, fatigue, peripheral circulation, cardiac risk factors, and the presence of past or concurrent cardiac conditions. The nursing history for respiratory function includes the presence of a cough, shortness of breath, wheezing, pain, environmental exposures, frequency of respiratory tract infections, pulmonary risk factors, past respiratory problems, current medication use, and smoking history or secondhand smoke exposure.

Fatigue.   Fatigue is a subjective sensation in which the client reports a loss of endurance. Fatigue in the client with cardiopulmonary alterations is often an early sign of a worsening of the chronic underlying process. To provide an objective measure of fatigue, the client may be asked to rate the fatigue on a scale of 1 to 10, with 10 being the worst level of fatigue and 1 representing no fatigue.

Dyspnea.   **Dyspnea** is a clinical sign of hypoxia and manifests as breathlessness. It is the subjective sensation of difficult or uncomfortable breathing. Physiological dyspnea is shortness of breath associated with exercise or excitement. Pathological dyspnea is the inability to catch a breath without relation to activity or exercise.

Dyspnea can be associated with clinical signs such as exaggerated respiratory effort, use of the accessory muscles of respiration, nasal flaring, and marked increases in the rate and depth of respirations. The use of a visual analog scale can help clients to make an objective assessment of their dyspnea (Figure 39-11). This allows the nurse and client to determine if specific nursing interventions are having an effect on the client's dyspnea. The visual analog

KNOWLEDGE

- Cardiac and respiratory anatomy and physiology
- Cardiopulmonary patho-physiology
- Clinical signs and symptoms of altered oxygenation
- Developmental factors affecting oxygenation
- Impact of lifestyle
- Environmental impact

STANDARDS

- Apply intellectual standards of clarity, precision, specificity, and accuracy when obtaining a health history for the client with cardiopulmonary alterations

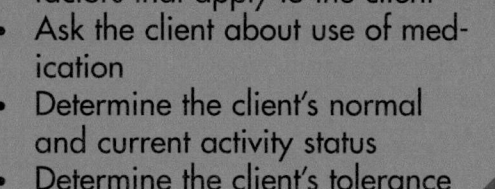

ASSESSMENT

- Identify recurring and present signs and symptoms associated with the client's impaired oxygenation
- Determine the presence of risk factors that apply to the client
- Ask the client about use of medication
- Determine the client's normal and current activity status
- Determine the client's tolerance to activity

EXPERIENCE

- Caring for clients with impaired oxygenation, activity intolerance, and respiratory infections
- Observations of changes in client respiratory patterns made during poor air quality days
- Personal experience with how a change in altitudes or physical conditioning affects respiratory patterns
- Personal experience with respiratory infections or cardiopulmonary alterations

ATTITUDES

- Carry out the responsibility of obtaining correct information about the client
- Display confidence in assessing the client's management of illness

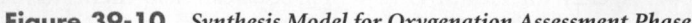

Figure 39-10   *Synthesis Model for Oxygenation Assessment Phase.*

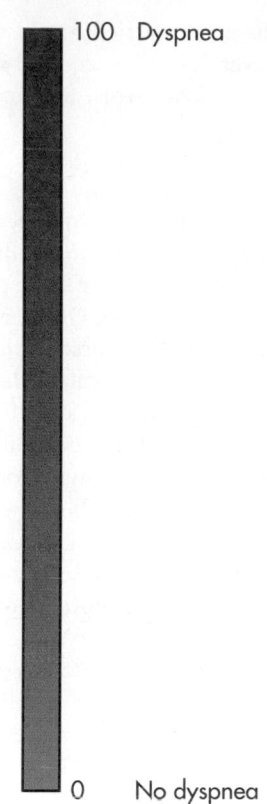

100   Dyspnea

0   No dyspnea

Figure 39-11   Visual analog scale.

Box 39-9

Sputum Characteristics

COLOR
Clear
White
Yellow
Green
Brown
Red
Streaked with blood

CHANGES IN COLOR
Same color throughout the day
Clearing with coughing
Progressively darker

ODOR
None
Foul

QUALITY
Same as usual
Increased
Decreased

CONSISTENCY
Frothy
Watery
Tenacious, thick

PRESENCE OF BLOOD
Occasional
Early morning
Bright or dark red
Blood tinged

scale is a 100 mm vertical line with 0 equated with no dyspnea and the 100-mm marker equated with the worst breathlessness the client has experienced. Studies have validated the use of the visual analog scale to evaluate a client's dyspnea in the clinical setting.

The nursing history of dyspnea includes the circumstances under which it occurred, such as with exertion, stress, or respiratory tract infection. The nurse also determines whether the client's perception of dyspnea affects the ability to lie flat. **Orthopnea** is an abnormal condition in which the person must use multiple pillows when lying down or must sit with the arms elevated and leaning forward to breathe. The number of pillows required for sleeping, such as two- or three-pillow orthopnea, usually quantifies the presence of orthopnea.

Cough.   **Cough** is a sudden, audible expulsion of air from the lungs. The person breathes in, the glottis is partially closed, and the accessory muscles of expiration contract to expel the air forcibly. Coughing is a protective reflex to clear the trachea, bronchi, and lungs of irritants and secretions. The carina, the point of bifurcation of the right and left mainstem bronchus, is the most sensitive area for cough production. A cough is difficult to evaluate, and almost everyone has periods of coughing. Clients with a chronic cough tend to deny, underestimate, or minimize

their coughing, often because they are so accustomed to it that they are unaware of how frequently it occurs.

Coughing is classified according to the time when the client most frequently coughs. Clients with chronic sinusitis may cough only in the early morning or immediately after rising from sleep. This clears the airway of mucus resulting from sinus drainage. Clients with chronic bronchitis generally produce sputum all day, although greater amounts are produced after rising from a semirecumbent or flat position. This is a result of the dependent accumulation of sputum in the airways and is associated with reduced mobility (see Chapter 36). Once the nurse determines that the client has a cough, it must be identified as productive or nonproductive and its frequency must be assessed. A **productive cough** results in sputum production, material coughed up from the lungs that may be swallowed or expectorated. Sputum contains mucus, cellular debris, and microorganisms, and it may contain pus or blood. The nurse must collect data about the type and quantity of sputum (Box 39-9). The client is instructed to try to produce some sputum, being careful not to simply clear the throat to produce a sample of saliva. The nurse then inspects it for color, consistency, odor, and amount.

If **hemoptysis** (bloody sputum) is reported, the nurse determines if it is associated with coughing and bleeding from the upper respiratory tract, from sinus drainage, or from the gastrointestinal tract (**hematemesis**). In addition, the hemoptysis should be described according to amount, color, and duration and whether it is mixed with sputum. When a client reports bloody or blood-tinged sputum, diagnostic tests, such as examination of sputum specimens, chest x-ray examinations, bronchoscopy, and other x-ray studies, should be performed.

Wheezing.   **Wheezing** is characterized by a high-pitched musical sound caused by high-velocity movement of air through a narrowed airway. Wheezing may be associated with asthma, acute bronchitis, or pneumonia. Wheezing can occur on inspiration, expiration, or both. The nurse should determine any precipitating factors, such as respiratory infection, allergens, exercise, or stress.

Pain.   The presence of chest pain needs to be thoroughly evaluated with regard to location, duration, radiation, and frequency. Cardiac pain does not occur with respiratory variations and is most often on the left side of the chest and radiates to the left arm in men. Chest pain in women is much less definitive and may be a sensation of choking, breathlessness, or pain that radiates through to the back. Pericardial pain resulting from an inflammation of the pericardial sac is usually nonradiating and may occur with inspiration.

Pleuritic chest pain is peripheral and may radiate to the scapular regions. It is worsened by inspiratory maneuvers, such as coughing, yawning, and sighing. Pleuritic pain is often caused from an inflammation or infection in the pleural space and is described as knifelike, lasting from a minute to hours and always in association with inspiration.

Musculoskeletal pain may be present following exercise, rib trauma, and prolonged coughing episodes. This pain is also aggravated by inspiratory movements and may easily be confused with pleuritic chest pain.

Environmental   or   Geographical   Exposures.
Environmental exposure to many inhaled substances is closely linked with respiratory disease. The nurse should investigate exposures in the client's home and workplace. The most common environmental exposures in the home are cigarette smoke, carbon monoxide, and radon. The nurse should determine whether a client who is a non-smoker is passively exposed to smoke. Carbon monoxide poisoning can result from a blocked furnace flue or fireplace. The client may have vague complaints of general malaise, flulike symptoms, and excessive sleepiness. Clients are particularly at risk in the late fall when they turn the heat on or begin to use the fireplace again. Radon gas, a radioactive substance, enters homes through the ground. When homes are underventilated, this gas is not able to escape into the atmosphere and becomes trapped in the home.

An employment history is obtained to assess exposure to substances such as asbestos, coal, cotton fibers, fumes, or chemical inhalants. This is particularly important with middle-age and older adults, who may have worked in places without regulations to protect workers from carcinogens, such as asbestos.

Exposure to substances may occur during travel. Schistosomiasis can be acquired in Asia, Africa, the Caribbean, and South America. This is infection of a human with a species of fluke found in fresh water that has been contaminated by human feces. Coccidioidomycosis is a fungal disease caused by inhalation of *Coccidioides im-*

mitis, a windborne spore carried on dust particles. Also known as valley fever, it can be acquired in southwestern desert regions, at chicken farms, and in the Ohio and Mississippi river valleys.

Respiratory Infections.   A nursing history should contain information about the client's frequency and duration of respiratory tract infections. Although everyone occasionally experiences a cold, for some people it can result in bronchitis or pneumonia. On average, clients will have four colds per year. The nurse should determine if the client has had a pneumococcal or flu vaccine in the past and should also ask about any known exposure to tuberculosis and the results of the tuberculin skin test.

The client's risk for human immunodeficiency virus (HIV) infection is determined. Clients with a history of intravenous (IV) drug use and multiple unprotected sexual partners are at risk of developing HIV infection. Clients may not display any symptoms of HIV infection until they present with *Pneumocystis carinii* (PCP) or *Mycoplasma* pneumonia. Presentation with PCP or *Mycoplasma* pneumonia indicates a significant depression of the client's immune system and progression to acquired immunodeficiency syndrome (AIDS).

Risk Factors.   The nurse must also investigate familial and environmental risk factors, such as a family history of lung cancer or cardiovascular disease. Documentation should include which blood relatives have had the disease and their present level of health or age at time of death. Other family risk factors include the presence of infectious diseases, particularly tuberculosis. The nurse should determine who in the client's household has been infected and the status of treatment.

Medications.   The last component of the nursing history should describe medications the client is using. These include prescribed, over-the-counter, folk medicine, herbal medicines, alternative therapies, and illicit drugs and substances. Such medications may have adverse effects by themselves or because of interactions with other drugs. A person using a prescribed bronchodilator drug, for example, may decide that using an over-the-counter inhalant as well will be beneficial. Many of these contain ephedrine or *ma huag,* a natural ephedrine, which acts like epinephrine. This product may react with the prescribed medication by potentiating or decreasing the effect of the prescribed medication.

As with all medication, the nurse assesses the client's knowledge and ability to use the five rights of medication administration (see Chapter 34). Of particular importance is the nurse's assessment of the client's understanding of potential side effects of the medications. Clients should be able to recognize adverse reactions and be aware of the dangers in combining prescribed medications with over-the-counter drugs.

When clients are prescribed drugs for which toxic levels can be monitored by blood analyses, the nurse needs to review these laboratory values. Common drugs that can be monitored include theophylline preparations (theophylline levels), digitalis preparations (digitalis levels), anticoagulants such as warfarin (Coumadin) (international normalized ratio [INR] level), and phenobarbital (phenobarbital levels). Toxic effects of these medications can impair cardiopulmonary functioning. Illicit drugs, particularly parenterally administered narcotics, which are often diluted with talcum powder, can cause pulmonary disorders resulting from the irritant effect of the powder on lung tissues.

Physical Examination. The physical examination performed to assess the client's level of tissue oxygenation includes evaluation of the entire cardiopulmonary system. Inspection, palpation, auscultation, and percussion techniques are used (see Chapter 32).

Inspection. Using inspection techniques, the nurse performs a head-to-toe observation of the client for skin and mucous membrane color, general appearance, level of consciousness, adequacy of systemic circulation, breathing patterns, and chest wall movement (Tables 39-4 to 39-6). Breathing patterns are obtained with a plethysmograph, which is usually reserved for use in critical care areas. Any abnormalities should be investigated during palpation, percussion, and auscultation.

Inspection includes observations of the nails for clubbing. Clubbed nails, obliteration of the normal angle between the base of the nail and the skin, is seen in clients with prolonged oxygen deficiency, endocarditis, and congenital heart defects.

Palpation. Palpation of the chest provides assessment data in several areas. It documents the type and amount of thoracic excursion, elicits any areas of tenderness, and can identify tactile fremitus, thrills, heaves, and the cardiac

Table 39-4 Inspection of Cardiopulmonary Status

Abnormality	Cause
Eyes	
Xanthelasma (yellow lipid lesions on eyelids)	Hyperlipidemia
Corneal arcus (whitish opaque ring around junction of cornea and sclera)	Hyperlipidemia in young to middle adults, normal finding in older adults with arcus senilis
Pale conjunctivae	Anemia
Cyanotic conjunctivae	Hypoxemia
Petechiae on conjunctivae	Fat embolus or bacterial endocarditis
Mouth and Lips	
Cyanotic mucous membranes	Decreased oxygenation (hypoxia)
Pursed-lip breathing	Associated with chronic lung disease
Neck Veins	
Distention	Associated with right-sided heart failure
Nose	
Flaring nares	Air hunger, dyspnea
Chest	
Retractions	Increased work of breathing, dyspnea
Asymmetry	Chest wall injury
Skin	
Peripheral cyanosis	Vasoconstriction and diminished blood flow
Central cyanosis	Hypoxemia
Decreased skin turgor	Dehydration (normal finding in older adults as a result of decreased skin elasticity)
Dependent edema	Associated with right- and left-sided heart failure
Periorbital edema	Associated with kidney disease
Fingertips and Nail Beds	
Cyanosis	Decreased cardiac output or hypoxia
Splinter hemorrhages	Bacterial endocarditis
Clubbing	Chronic hypoxemia

Table 39-5	**Respiratory Pattern**	
Type Pattern	Rate (Breaths per Minute)	Clinical Significance
Eupnea	16-20	Normal

Tachypnea	>35	Respiratory failure Response to fever Anxiety Shortness of breath Respiratory infection

Bradypnea	<10	Sleep Respiratory depression Drug overdose Central nervous system (CNS) lesion

Apnea	Periods of no respiration lasting >15 seconds	May be intermittent, such as in sleep apnea Respiratory arrest

Hypernea	16-20	Can result from anxiety or response to pain Can cause marked respiratory alkalosis, paresthesia, tetany, confusion

Kussmaul's	Usually >35, may be slow or normal	Tachypnea pattern associated with diabetic ketoacidosis, metabolic acidosis, or renal failure

Cheyne-Stokes	Variable	Increasing and decreasing pattern caused by alterations in acid-base status; underlying metabolic problem or neurocerebral insult

Biot's	Variable	Periods of apnea and shallow breathing caused by CNS disorder; found in some healthy clients

Apneustic	Increased	Increased inspiratory time with short grunting expiratory time; seen in CNS lesions of the respiratory center

From Weilitz PB: *Pocket guide to respiratory care*, St. Louis, 1991, Mosby.

point of maximal impulse (PMI). Palpation also allows the nurse to feel for abnormal masses or lumps in the axilla and breast tissue. Palpation of the extremities provides data about the peripheral circulation, the presence and quality of peripheral pulses, skin temperature, color, and capillary refill (see Chapter 32).

Palpation should also include the feet and legs to assess the presence or absence of peripheral edema. Clients with alterations in their cardiac function, such as those with congestive heart failure or hypertension, often have pedal or lower extremity edema. Edema is graded from 1+ to 4+, depending on the depth of visible indentation after firm application of a finger.

Palpation of the pulses in the neck and extremities is performed to assess arterial blood flow. A scale of 0 (absent pulse) to 3+ (full, bounding pulse) is used to describe what is palpated. The normal pulse is graded at 2+, and a weak, thready pulse is graded as 1+.

Percussion.   Percussion allows the nurse to detect the presence of abnormal fluid or air in the lungs. It is also used to determine diaphragmatic excursion (see Chapter 32).

Auscultation.   Auscultation enables the nurse to identify normal and abnormal heart and lung sounds (see Chapter 32). Auscultation of the cardiovascular system should include assessment for normal S_1 and S_2 sounds, the presence of abnormal S_3 and S_4 sounds (gallops), and murmurs or rubs. The examiner must identify the location, radiation, intensity, pitch, and quality of a murmur. Auscultation is also used to identify a bruit over the carotid arteries, abdominal aorta, and femoral arteries.

Auscultation of lung sounds involves listening for movement of air throughout all lung fields: anterior, posterior, and lateral. Adventitious breath sounds occur with collapse of a lung segment, fluid in a lung segment, or narrowing or obstruction of an airway. Auscultation also evaluates the client's response to interventions for improving the respiratory status.

Diagnostic Tests
Cardiac Conduction Tests.   Tests used to determine the cardiac conduction of the heart include ECG, Holter monitor, exercise stress test, and electrophysiological studies.

Electrocardiogram.   The ECG produces a graphic recording of the heart's electrical activity, detecting transmission of impulses and the electrical position of the heart (the axis).

Holter Monitor.   The **Holter monitor** is a portable device that records the heart's electrical activity and produces a continuous ECG tracing over a specified period, such as 12 hours or longer. The Holter monitor allows clients to continue with their normal activities while

Table 39-6 **Assessment of Abnormal Chest Wall Movement**	
Abnormality	Cause
Retraction—sinking in of soft tissues of chest between and around cartilaginous and bony ribs, such as intercostal space, intraclavicular space, and trachea, and substernally* worsening with need for increased inspiratory effort	Any condition that causes increased inspiratory effort (e.g., airway obstruction, asthma, tracheobronchitis)
Paradoxical breathing—asynchronous breathing; chest contraction during inspiration and expansion during expiration	Flail chest resulting from rib fractures due to chest trauma or CPR
Increased anteroposterior diameter	Emphysema, chronic obstructive pulmonary disease, advancing age

*Infants can experience sternal and substernal retractions with only slight inspiratory effort because of chest pliability.

recording the heart's electrical activity. Clients keep a diary of activity, noting when they experience rapid heartbeats or periods of dizziness. Correlation between activities and abnormal electrical activity can then be determined.

Exercise Stress Test. **Exercise stress tests** are used to evaluate the cardiac response to physical stress. These provide information on myocardial response to increased oxygen requirements and determine the adequacy of coronary blood flow. Heart rate, electrical activity, and cardiac recovery time are reflected in the ECG tracing. In addition, data about the client's blood pressure, presence of chest pain, changes in respiration, color, and rate of muscular fatigue are monitored. There are more false-positive findings in women. Therefore it is not a valuable tool for evaluation of cardiac response in women.

Thallium Stress Test. Thallium imaging involves IV injection of thallium-201, a potassium analogue that accumulates in the heart in proportion to blood flow. Stress testing determines whether coronary blood flow changes with increased activity (treadmill exercises).

Electrophysiological Studies. An **electrophysiological study (EPS)** is an invasive measure of electrical activity. An electrode catheter is inserted into the right atrium, usually via the femoral vein. Electrical stimulation is then delivered through the catheter while the ECG monitors and computers record the heart's electrical response to the stimulus. Specific dysrhythmias can also be induced to determine the pathways through the heart, provide more specific information about difficult-to-treat dysrhythmias, and assess the adequacy of antidysrhythmic medication.

Myocardial Contraction and Blood Flow Studies. Echocardiography, scintigraphy, cardiac catheterization, and angiography are used to determine myocardial contraction and blood flow.

Echocardiography. **Echocardiography** is a noninvasive measure to evaluate the internal structures of the heart and heart wall motion. Sonar (radar) technology is used to measure ultrasonic waves and translate them into formed images. The echocardiogram graphically demonstrates overall cardiac performance.

Scintigraphy. **Scintigraphy,** or radionuclide angiography, is a noninvasive imaging technique. Radioisotopes are used to evaluate cardiac structures, myocardial perfusion, and contractility.

Cardiac Catheterization and Angiography. **Cardiac catheterization** and **angiography** are invasive procedures used to visualize cardiac chambers, valves, the great vessels, and coronary arteries and to measure pressure and volumes within the four chambers. The procedures require insertion of a catheter into the heart via a percutaneous venous puncture. Contrast material is injected through the catheter, and fluoroscopic pictures are obtained. Both right- and left-sided catheterization can be performed.

Diagnostic cardiac catheterization is usually done as an outpatient procedure. If there are no complications from the procedure, the client may go home within 6 to 8 hours. Some clients may need to stay overnight for observation. Other clients may be taken directly to the operating room if the catheterization reveals significant, life-threatening coronary artery disease and/or blockage. Complications associated with the cardiac catheterization procedure include dysrhythmias, bleeding at the puncture site, hematoma, and stroke.

Ventilation and Oxygenation Studies. Pulmonary function tests, peak expiratory flow rates, arterial blood gas tests, oximetry, and complete blood counts are used to assess the adequacy of ventilation and oxygenation.

Pulmonary Function Tests. **Pulmonary function tests** determine the ability of the lungs to efficiently exchange oxygen and carbon dioxide. Basic ventilation studies are performed with a spirometer and recording device as the client breathes through a mouthpiece into a con-

Table 39-7   Pulmonary Function Measurements

Description	Average Value	Clinical Significance
Tidal Volume (V$_T$)		
Volume of air (ml) inhaled or exhaled per breath	5-10 ml/kg	Decreased in restrictive lung disease and older client
Residual Volume (RV)		
Volume of air (ml) left in lungs after a maximal exhalation	1200 ml	Increased in clients with chronic obstructive pulmonary disease (COPD) and older clients as a result of changes in elastic recoil of the lungs, chest wall compliance, and decreased respiratory muscle mass and strength
Functional Residual Capacity (FRC)		
Volume of air (ml) left in lungs after a normal exhalation	2400 ml	Increased in clients with obstructive lung disease and older clients as a result of changes in chest wall compliance, and elastic recoil of the lungs, and decreased respiratory muscle mass and strength
Vital Capacity (VC)		
Volume of air (ml) exhaled after a maximal inhalation	4800 ml	Decreased in association with decreased flow rates found in pulmonary edema, atelectasis, and changes associated with aging, such as decreased respiratory muscle strength and chest wall compliance
Total Lung Capacity (TLC)		
Total volume of air (ml) in lungs following a maximal inhalation	6000 ml	Decreased in restrictive lung disease; increased in obstructive lung disease

necting tube. For example, measurements can include tidal volume (V$_T$), inspiratory reserve volume (IRV), residual volume (RV), and functional residual capacity (FRC) (Table 39-7). Pulmonary functions are variable by ethnic group (Box 39-10).

Pulmonary function tests are usually performed in a pulmonary function laboratory. A nose clip prevents air from being inhaled or exhaled through the nose. The client breathes through a mouthpiece attached to a spirometer for measuring lung volume. The client is asked at certain times in the test to inhale or exhale as much air as possible. The client's cooperation is critical to ensure accurate results.

Peak Expiratory Flow Rate. The **peak expiratory flow rate (PEFR)** is the point of highest flow during maximal expiration. The PEFR reflects changes in large airway sizes and correlates well with the FEV$_1$. The peak expiratory flow meter is a handheld instrument that allows clients with asthma to monitor their disease. All clients with asthma should monitor their PEFR, just as clients with diabetes monitor their blood glucose level.

Arterial Blood Gas Tests. Arterial blood gas (ABG) measurement is performed in conjunction with pul-

monary function tests to determine the hydrogen ion concentration, partial pressure of carbon dioxide and oxygen concentration, and oxyhemoglobin saturation. ABG tests provide information about diffusion of gas across the alveolocapillary membrane and adequacy of tissue oxygenation (Chapter 40).

Oximetry. Continuous measurements of capillary oxygen saturation are available with cutaneous **oximetry** (Skill 39-1). Oxygen saturation is the percentage of hemoglobin saturated with oxygen. Transcutaneous oximeter measurements have the advantages of being easy to use, noninvasive, and readily available. Clients with ventilation/perfusion abnormalities such as pneumonia, emphysema, chronic bronchitis, asthma, pulmonary embolism, or congestive heart failure are ideal candidates for pulse oximetry. The most common oximetry is done with the pulse oximeter, which displays the amplitude of the pulse with the oxygen saturation reading. The nurse usually attaches a noninvasive sensor to the client's finger, toe, or bridge of the nose to monitor capillary blood oxygen saturation. The nasal probe is recommended in low perfusion states because the blood flow in the nasal septum anterior ethmoid artery remains greater than peripheral flow in compromised flow states. Continuous monitoring of

Pulmonary functions vary between cultures as a result of the variation in chest size. Whites have the largest chest volumes, followed by African-Americans, Asian-Americans, and Native Americans. The variations in the chest size affect the forced expiratory volume (FEV$_1$), forced vital capacity (FVC), and the FEV$_1$/FVC ratio.

	FEV$_1$ (L)	FVC (L)	FEV$_1$/FVC (%)
White	3.22	4.3	74.4
African-American	2.85	3.7	76.7
Asian-American	2.53	3.27	77.0
Native American	2.53	3.27	77.0

Modified from Lueckenotte: *Gerontologic nursing,* ed 2, St. Louis, 2000, Mosby.

oxygen saturation is useful in assessing sleep disorders, exercise tolerance, weaning from mechanical ventilation, and transient decreases in oxygen saturation.

The accuracy of the pulse oximetry value is directly related to the perfusion of the probe area. Clients with poor tissue perfusion caused by shock, hypothermia, or peripheral vascular diseases may not have reliable oximetry measures. The accuracy of the pulse oximetry is decreased when the systolic blood pressure is less than 90 mm Hg. The nasal probe is recommended in low perfusion states because the blood flow in the nasal septum anterior ethmoid artery remains greater than peripheral flow in compromised flow states.

Spot-check oximetry readings have little clinical value. Trends over time provide the best information about the client's oxygenation.

Blood Studies

Complete Blood Count.   A complete blood count (CBC) determines the number and type of red and white blood cells per cubic millimeter of blood. The assistive personnel or nurse obtains a venous blood sample by performing a venipuncture. Normal values for a CBC vary with age and gender.

The CBC measures the hemoglobin level within the red blood cells (erythrocytes). A deficiency in red blood cells decreases the blood's oxygen-carrying capacity because there are fewer hemoglobin molecules available to carry oxygen to tissues. When the number of red blood cells is increased, such as with polycythemia in chronic lung conditions and cyanotic heart conditions, the oxygen-carrying capacity of the blood is increased. However, increased red blood cells increase blood viscosity and the client's risk for thrombus formation.

Cardiac Enzymes.   Cardiac enzymes are used to diagnose acute myocardial infarcts. Creatine phosphokinase (CK) and MB-CK (isoenzyme portion of the CK specific for myocardial damage) are used routinely because they are highly sensitive, specific, and cost-effective (Alexander and others, 1999). Within 12 to 16 hours of the onset of symptoms, the MB-CK is elevated. Maximal levels are reached within 14 to 36 hours, with levels returning to normal after 48 to 72 hours (Alexander and others, 1999). MB-CK >10 to 13 units/L, a serial MB-CK with >50% increase between two samples 4 hours apart, or a single MB-CK elevation >twofold is diagnostic for an acute myocardial infarction (Alexander and others, 1999).

Another marker of myocardial damage is the plasma cardiac troponin I. Within 12 to 16 hours the troponin I level is elevated. Maximal levels are reached within 24 to 36 hours. For clients admitted for evaluation 48 to 72 hours after the onset of symptoms, the troponin I level is the preferred diagnostic marker (Alexander and others, 1999). Troponin I levels remain elevated for 10 to 14 days.

Serum Electrolytes.   It is important to monitor the serum electrolytes of clients receiving diuretic therapy for hypertension and congestive heart failure. The potassium (K$^+$) level should be between 3.5 and 5 mmol/L. Clients receiving diuretic therapy are at risk for hypokalemia. Clients taking diuretics are usually monitored within 4 weeks of initiation of therapy and then every 6 to 12 months.

The nurse should also be alert for hyperkalemia (elevated potassium) in clients receiving angiotensin-converting enzyme (ACE) inhibitors. These medications include lisinopril (Zestril), captopril (Capoten), ramipril (Altace), quinapril (Accupril), enalapril (Vasotec), fosinopril (Monopril), and moexipril (Univasc). ACE inhibitors are used for clients with congestive heart failure or left ventricular dysfunction following acute myocardial infarction, and to treat systemic hypertension.

Cholesterol.   Clients with risk factors for coronary artery disease need to have their cholesterol, low-density lipoprotein (LDL) cholesterol, high-density lipoprotein (HDL) cholesterol, and triglyceride levels measured and monitored. A fasting cholesterol and triglyceride level should be less than 200 mg/100 ml. LDL cholesterol (bad cholesterol) should be <130 mg/100 ml, and HDL cholesterol (good cholesterol) should be >35 mg/100 ml.

Factors such as cigarette smoking, obesity, lack of regular exercise, beta-adrenergic blocking agents, genetic disorders of HDL metabolism, hypertriglyceridemia, and type 2 diabetes contribute to low-HDL cholesterol. High-LDL cholesterol (hypercholesterolemia) is caused by excessive intake of saturated fatty acids, dietary cholesterol intake, and obesity. Familial hypercholesterolemia and hyperlipidemia are also contributing factors, as well as hypothyroidism, nephrotic syndrome, and diabetes mellitus. Obesity, excessive alcohol intake, diabetes mellitus, beta-adrenergic blocking agents, and familial hypertriglyceridemia cause hypertriglyceridemia.

Skill 39-1   Pulse Oximetry

Delegation Considerations

The skill of oxygenation saturation measurement can be delegated to assistive personnel.

- Inform care provider of the appropriate sensor site for measurement.

- Instruct care provider regarding unexpected outcomes associated with the pulse oximeter and the need to inform the nurse if any occur.

EQUIPMENT

- Pulse oximeter
- Sensor probe

- Continuous printout (optional)

Type of Sensor	Client's Weight
Adhesive neonatal	less than 3 kg (6.6 lb)
Adhesive infant	1-20 kg (2.2-44 lb)
Adhesive pediatric	10-50 kg (22-110 lb)
Adhesive adult	30 kg (66 lb) or greater
Adhesive adult nasal	50 kg (110 lb) or greater
Finger clip	40 kg (88 lb) or greater

STEPS	RATIONALE
1. Explain purpose of procedure to client and family.	Ensures client and family understanding and increases compliance.
2. Wash hands.	Reduces transmission of microorganisms.
3. Select appropriate area to apply sensor based on peripheral circulation and extremity temperature.	Peripheral vasoconstriction alters oxygen saturation.
a. Determine adequacy of peripheral circulation by assessing capillary refill (toe and finger sites).	
b. Do not use adhesive adult nasal sensor if client has large-bore nasogastric tube or nasoendotracheal tube (nose).	Interferes with oxygen saturation readings because of poor peripheral circulation and excessive equipment or dressings.
c. Determine use of vasoactive drugs.	
d. Align photoelectron and light-emitting diode.	Permits transmission of light. Alignment ensures accurate oxygen saturation readings.

Critical Decision Point: Do not attach probe to an area that is edematous or has compromised skin integrity, to fingers or toes that are hypothermic, or where there is peripheral vascular disease.

4. Prepare selected site:	Body oils, nail polish, and artificial nails interfere with transmission of light through nail, tissue, venous and arterial blood, and skin pigmentation (Sonnesso, 1991).
a. Remove nail polish and artificial nails.	
b. Remove earrings.	
c. Wash selected site, wipe with alcohol, and air dry.	
5. Attach sensor probe to appropriate site.	
6. Instruct client to breathe normally.	Prevents large fluctuations in minute ventilation and possible changes in oxygen saturation.
7. Attach pulse oximeter sensor to client cable.	
a. Turn machine on.	
b. Listen for audible beep.	Senses with each pulse and indicates how well oximeter monitors pulse.
c. Observe waveform for bar of light.	Light or waveform fluctuates with each pulsation and reflects pulse strength. Poor light or small waveform usually indicates that signal is too weak to give accurate oxygen saturation reading.

Critical Decision Point: Check client's radial or apical rate with the pulse oximeter rate. If differences exist, reevaluate placement of the probe.

STEPS	RATIONALE
8. Ensure that alarm limits for *both* high and low oxygen saturation and high and low pulse are set according to physician's order and *turned on*.	Manufacturers preset limits, and adjustments can be made according to client's underlying physical condition, therapy, and risks (Sonnesso, 1991).
	Provides an audible and visual signal that high or low limits have been exceeded.
9. Read saturation level as ordered and while performing nursing interventions.	Documents oxygen saturation levels at rest, with activity such as ambulation, during procedure such as suctioning, and with changes in physical condition.
10. Move a finger sensor every 4 hours and a spring-tension sensor every 2 hours (see illustration).	Allows nurse to assess for and prevent impaired skin integrity caused by pressure from sensor.

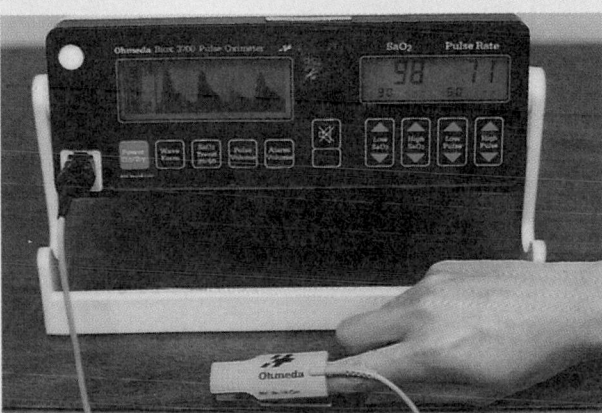

Step 10

11. Record in nurse's notes client's use of continuous pulse oximetry and record oxygen saturation.	Documents use of equipment for third-party payers, documents oxygen saturation.
12. Correlate oxygen saturation value with arterial blood gas measurements if available.	Documents reliability of oximeter.
13. Report oxygen saturation and response to changes in therapy to oncoming shift.	Provides oncoming nurse with baseline information and response to therapy.

Recording and Reporting
- Record pulse rate and oxygen saturation measure in medical record.
- Record client and family education provided about pulse oximetry.
- Report oxygen saturation and response to changes in therapy to oncoming shift.

Home Care Considerations
- Pulse oximetry is used in home care to noninvasively monitor oxygen therapy and changes in oxygen therapy.

Visualizing Structures of the Respiratory System.
Chest x-ray examination, bronchoscopy, and lung scans are used to visualize structures of the respiratory system.

Chest X-Ray Examination.   A chest x-ray examination consists of a radiograph of the thorax that allows the physician and nurse to observe the lung fields for fluid (i.e., occurs with pneumonia), masses (i.e., lung cancer), fractures (i.e., rib and clavicular fractures), and other abnormal processes (i.e., tuberculosis). Usually posteroanterior and lateral films are taken to adequately visualize all of the lung fields.

Bronchoscopy.   **Bronchoscopy** is visual examination of the tracheobronchial tree through a narrow, flexible fiberoptic bronchoscope. Bronchoscopy is performed to obtain biopsy and fluid or sputum samples and to remove mucous plugs or foreign bodies that have become lodged in the airways.

The client is usually kept NPO before bronchoscopy. The nurse may assist in the procedure by administering medications such as a sedative or atropine to reduce oral secretions, or by assisting with obtaining and labeling bronchial specimens. The nurse continues to observe and monitor the client after the procedure for signs and symptoms of respiratory distress, hemoptysis, or hypoxia. Before beginning oral fluids, the nurse assesses that the client's gag and swallow reflex is intact.

Lung Scan.   The most common lung scan is the computed tomography (CT) scan. CT scanning combines radiographic and computer technology. X-ray beams pass through a section or plane of the thorax from different angles, and the computer calculates tissue absorption and displays a printout and scan picture of the tissues, showing densities of various intrathoracic structures. A CT scan can identify abnormal masses by size and location but cannot identify tissue types, which requires a biopsy.

Determining Abnormal Cells or Infection in the Respiratory Tract.

Tests to determine whether there are abnormal cells or infection in the respiratory tract include throat cultures, sputum specimens, skin testing, and thoracentesis.

Throat Cultures.   A throat culture sample is obtained by swabbing the oropharynx and tonsillar regions with a sterile swab. The throat culture determines the presence of pathogenic microorganisms. If sensitivity is ordered, the antibiotics to which the microorganisms are resistant and those to which they are sensitive can also be determined.

When obtaining a throat culture, the nurse inserts the swab into the pharyngeal region and passes it along reddened areas and areas of exudate. Some clients have an active gag reflex, making it difficult to obtain the specimen. The reflex may be less active if the client is sitting straight and leaning forward slightly. The client may be able to control gagging if informed that the procedure will take only a few seconds.

Sputum Specimens.   Sputum specimens are obtained to identify the type of organism growing in the sputum. A sputum culture and sensitivity (C and S) identifies a specific microorganism and its drug resistance and sensitivities. A sputum specimen may also be obtained to screen for the presence of acid-fast bacillus (AFB). The AFB specimen is obtained on 3 consecutive days in the early morning. Sputum for cytology is a sputum specimen obtained to identify abnormal lung cancer by cell type. It involves a serial collection of three early-morning specimens.

The nurse must teach the client to cough effectively so that the sputum specimen consists of mucus from deep in

the bronchus and not saliva. The collection of the specimen may be delegated to assistive personnel; however, teaching the client the coughing techniques is the responsibility of the nurse. The color, consistency, amount, and odor of the sputum are recorded, and the date and time the specimen was sent to a specific laboratory for analysis is documented.

Skin Testing.   Skin testing enables the clinician to determine the presence of bacterial, fungal, or viral pulmonary diseases. The antigen is injected intradermally (see Chapter 34); the injection site may be circled, and the client is instructed not to wash it off. This procedure enables the clinician to evaluate the response. Tuberculin skin tests are read at 48 hours. Positive results are based on the size of the induration. An induration is a palpable, elevated, hardened area around the client's injection site. It is caused by edema and inflammation from the antigen-antibody reaction. The induration is measured in millimeters. Reddened flat areas are not positive reactions and should not be measured. TB testing in older adults is less reliable (see Box 39-11).

Thoracentesis.   Thoracentesis is surgical perforation of the chest wall and pleural space with a needle to aspirate fluid for diagnostic or therapeutic purposes or to remove a specimen for biopsy. The procedure is performed with aseptic technique using a local anesthetic. The client usually sits upright with the anterior thorax supported by pillows or an over-the-bed table (Figure 39-12).

Whether this procedure is painful depends on the client's tolerance for pain (see Chapter 42). The nurse can reduce the client's anxiety by explaining the procedure and telling the client what to expect. The client must understand the importance of holding the breath as requested and of not coughing during the procedure. Sudden movements may result in lung puncture by the thoracentesis needle. The client is instructed to notify the physician be-

---

Gerontological **NURSING PRACTICE   Box 39-11**

- The tuberculin skin test is an unreliable indicator of tuberculosis in older clients. They frequently display false-positive or false-negative skin test reactions. Older clients are at an increased risk for reactivation of dormant organisms that have been present for decades as a result of age-related changes in the immune system.
- The standard 5-TU Mantoux test is given and repeated or repeated with the 250-TU strength to create a booster effect. If the older client has a positive reaction, a complete history is necessary to determine any risk factors. Weight loss, night sweats, hemoptysis, and fatigue are signs and symptoms that should alert the nurse to possible tuberculosis. Early-morning sputum for AFB and a chest x-ray film are usually indicated.

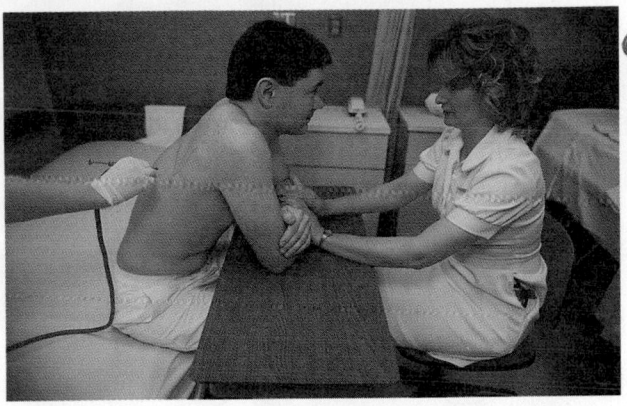

Figure 39-12 Position for thoracentesis.
From Wilson SF, Thompson JM: *Respiratory disorders*, St. Louis, 1990, Mosby.

NURSING DIAGNOSES Box 39-12
CARDIOPULMONARY DYSFUNCTION

Activity intolerance
Airway clearance, ineffective
Anxiety
Breathing pattern, ineffective
Cardiac output, decreased
Coping, ineffective individual
Fear
Gas exchange, impaired
Health maintenance, altered
Infection, risk for
Knowledge deficit (specify)
Tissue perfusion, altered (cardiopulmonary)
Ventilation, inability to sustain spontaneous

fore coughing or sneezing, so that the needle can be withdrawn.

After the procedure the nurse monitors the client for signs of pneumothorax: sudden shortness of breath, tracheal deviation, oxygen desaturation, and anxiety. The development of a pneumothorax following thoracentesis is an emergency. This type of pneumothorax is known as a *tension pneumothorax* and can result in cardiopulmonary arrest if it is not treated promptly.

Client Expectations. The nurse should ask clients what they expect with regard to their care. This includes asking clients what they expect from the encounter and what their priority is for management of their health. It also includes involving clients in the decision-making process about what will happen to them. For example, planning a smoking cessation or weight reduction program for a client who is not ready for the change will be frustrating for both the client and the nurse. Short-term realistic goals should be established that build to a larger goal. For example, reducing the fat in the client's diet may start out with replacing food such as whole milk with 2% milk and gradually introducing skim milk. A plan for adding exercise to the client's lifestyle may start with a commitment to exercise once a week for 20 minutes, or the client may commit to a weight reduction plan of 5 pounds per month.

It is important to remember that the goals and expectations of the nurse may not always coincide with those of the client. By addressing the client's concerns and expectations, the nurse will establish a relationship that can address other health care goals and expected outcomes.

NURSING DIAGNOSIS
Clients with an altered level of oxygenation can have nursing diagnoses that are primarily from a cardiovascular or pulmonary origin (Box 39-12). Each nursing diagnosis is based on specific defining characteristics and the related etiology. The nurse uses the information gathered in the nursing assessment to identify and cluster the defining characteristics. The clustered defining characteristics support the nursing diagnosis (Box 39-13).

PLANNING
During planning the nurse again synthesizes information from multiple resources (Figure 39-13). Critical thinking ensures that the client's plan of care integrates all that the nurse knows about the individual, as well as key critical thinking elements. Professional standards are especially important to consider when the nurse develops a plan of care. These standards often establish scientifically proven guidelines for selecting effective nursing interventions.

The nurse develops an individualized plan of care for each nursing diagnosis. The nurse and client set realistic expectations for care. Goals are to be individualized and realistic with measurable outcomes.

Clients with impaired oxygenation require a nursing care plan directed toward meeting the actual or potential oxygenation needs of the client (see care plan). Individual outcomes are derived from client-centered needs. The nurse identifies specific outcomes of nursing care and identifies the appropriate interventions necessary to achieve the desired outcome. The plan includes one or more of the following client-centered outcomes (Johnson, Maas, and Moorhead, 2000):

The client maintains a patent airway.
The client achieves and maintains adequate gas exchange and ventilation.
The client achieves and maintains stable vital signs.
The client achieves and maintains adequate electrolyte and acid-base balance.
The client achieves maintenance and promotion of lung expansion.
The client mobilizes pulmonary secretions.

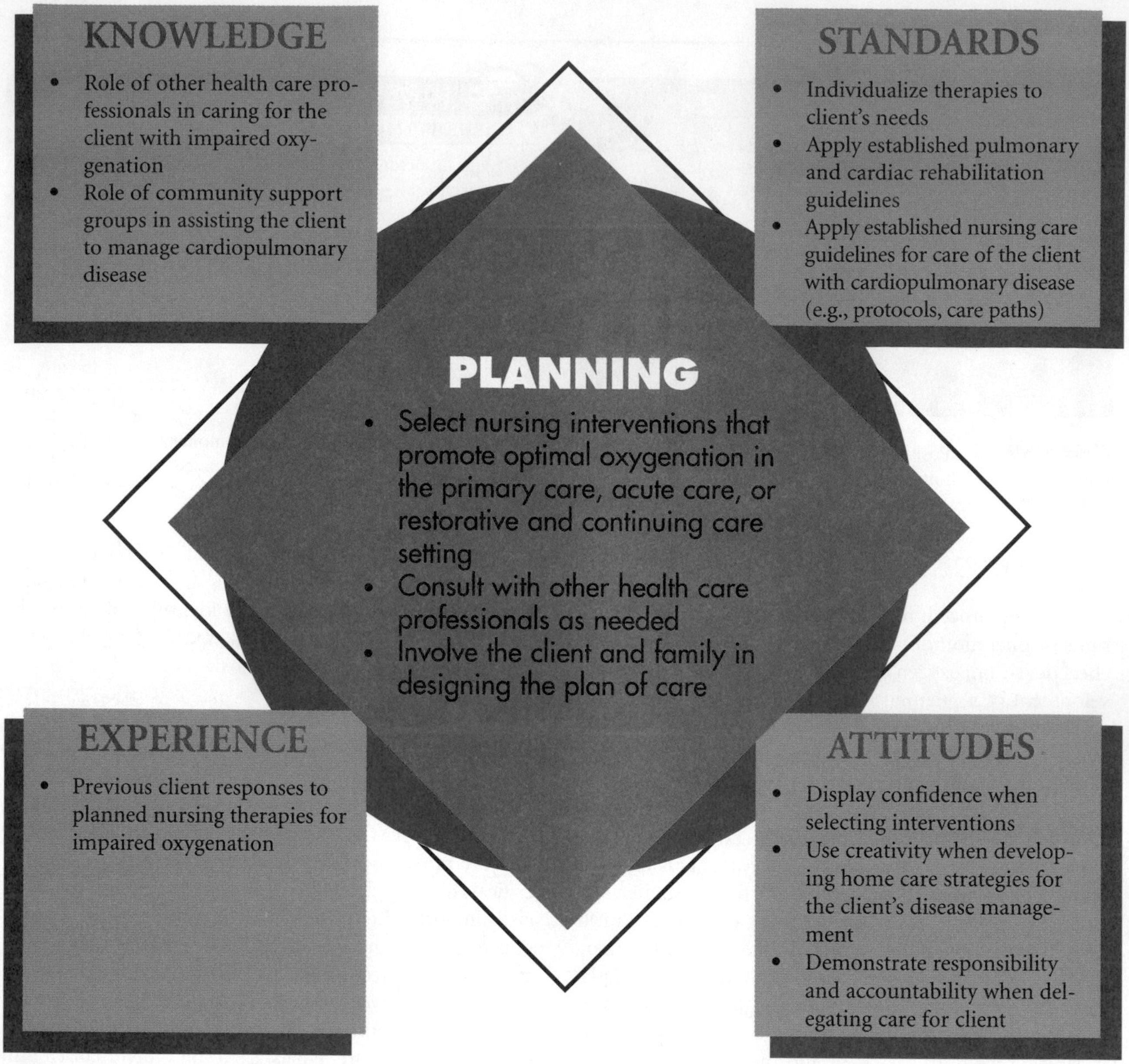

KNOWLEDGE

- Role of other health care professionals in caring for the client with impaired oxygenation
- Role of community support groups in assisting the client to manage cardiopulmonary disease

STANDARDS

- Individualize therapies to client's needs
- Apply established pulmonary and cardiac rehabilitation guidelines
- Apply established nursing care guidelines for care of the client with cardiopulmonary disease (e.g., protocols, care paths)

PLANNING

- Select nursing interventions that promote optimal oxygenation in the primary care, acute care, or restorative and continuing care setting
- Consult with other health care professionals as needed
- Involve the client and family in designing the plan of care

EXPERIENCE

- Previous client responses to planned nursing therapies for impaired oxygenation

ATTITUDES

- Display confidence when selecting interventions
- Use creativity when developing home care strategies for the client's disease management
- Demonstrate responsibility and accountability when delegating care for client

Figure 39-13 *Synthesis Model of Oxygenation Planning Phase.*

SAMPLE NURSING DIAGNOSTIC PROCESS

Box 39-13

CARDIOPULMONARY DYSFUNCTION

Assessment Activities	Defining Characteristics	Nursing Diagnosis
Observe client while breathing.	Dyspnea	Ineffective airway clearance related to thickened pulmonary secretions.
	Tachypnea	
	Use of accessory muscles	
	Nasal flaring	
	Diaphoresis	
Inspect client's skin and mucous membranes.	Cyanotic nail beds	
	Circumoral cyanosis	
	Pale mucous membranes	
Auscultate lung fields.	Lower lobe crackles	
	Inspiratory wheezes throughout fields	
Observe cough and inspect sputum.	Poor cough	
	Client tires trying to produce sputum	
	Thick, yellow sputum	

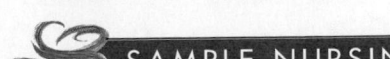

SAMPLE NURSING CARE PLAN

RESPIRATORY ALTERATIONS

ASSESSMENT*

Mr. Edwards, an older adult with a history of COPD, comes to the primary care office with complaints of **coughing.** He states that he has been **coughing for about a week,** and his ribs are getting sore. He denies sputum production and states that there is nothing to cough up. He notes that his mouth is dry, however, and he has had **increased fatigue** over the past week. He continues to **smoke 2 to 3 cigarettes** a day, an improvement from his previous 10 to 15 per day. His skin and mucous membranes are dry. Lung sounds reveal **rhonchus** in the upper lobes. The lower lobes are clear. He is **unable to produce a sputum sample** for evaluation.

*Defining characteristics are shown in bold type.

NURSING DIAGNOSIS: Ineffective airway clearance related to retained secretions.

PLANNING	**EXPECTED OUTCOMES**
GOALS	Lung sounds will be normal in 48 hours.
Client will be able to effectively clear secretions.	Sputum will be thin, white, and watery.
	Respiratory rate will be within 20 to 24 breaths per minute in 48 hours.
	Client will be able to clear airway by coughing.

INTERVENTIONS†	**RATIONALE**
Airway Management	
• Increase fluids to 1000 ml in 24 hours if not contraindicated by cardiovascular disease (Lewis and others, 2000).	Fluids help to liquefy secretions and promote ease of removal.
• Have client deep breathe and cough every 2 hours 4 to 5 times (Lewis and others, 2000).	Retained secretions predisposes client to atelectasis and pneumonia.
• Consider chest physiotherapy (CPT) if there is evidence of infiltrates on chest X-ray film.	Standards for CPT include sputum production greater than 30 ml/day or infiltrates on chest X-ray film (AARC, 1991).

†Intervention Classification labels from McCloskey JC, Bulechek GM: *Nursing interventions classification (NIC),* ed 3, St. Louis, 2000, Mosby.

EVALUATION

Observe client's ability to deep breathe and cough effectively.
Auscultate for adventitious lung sounds.
Assess client's level of hydration and respiratory rate.
Observe appearance of sputum.

Tissue oxygenation is maintained or improved.

The client will be able to increase endurance for activities of daily living.

The client's level of health, age, lifestyle, and environmental risks affect the level of tissue oxygenation. Clients with severe impairments in oxygenation frequently require nursing interventions in multiple areas. A critical pathway or clinical practice guideline can provide a multidisciplinary template for care (Figure 39-14).

IMPLEMENTATION

Nursing interventions for promoting and maintaining adequate oxygenation are included in the domain of nursing: administering and monitoring therapeutic interventions and regimens (Benner, 1984). These include independent nursing actions such as health promotion and prevention behaviors, positioning, and coughing techniques, and interdependent or dependent interventions such as oxygen therapy, lung inflation techniques, hydration, medications, and chest physiotherapy.

Health Promotion.   Maintaining the client's optimal level of health is important in reducing the number and/or severity of respiratory symptoms. Prevention of respiratory infections is foremost in maintaining optimal health. The nurse practices in the teaching-coaching function domain (Benner, 1984) to provide cardiopulmonary-related health information (Boxes 39-14 and 39-15).

Influenza and Pneumococcal Vaccine.   Annual influenza vaccines are recommended for older clients and clients with chronic illnesses. This includes clients older than 65 years of age; clients of any age with chronic disease of the heart, lung or kidneys; clients with diabetes; and clients with immunosuppression or severe forms of anemia (Advisory Committee on Immunization Practices [ACIP], 1997). The vaccine is also recommended for peo-

Admitting Diagnosis: COPD Sub-Acute Stay
DRG# _____
Target LOS _____

Summary of Acute Stay	Hosp. day	SUB-ACUTE DAY 1	SUB-ACUTE DAY 3	SUB-ACUTE DAY 6
		DATE:	DATE:	DATE:
Consults done: _____ date: _____ _____ date: _____	CONSULTS	Interdisciplinary discharge planning team (to include Pulmonary Rehab, PT, OT, Dietary, Social Worker, Case Manager)	Notify dietician via HIS if patient is consuming less than 1/2 meals.	
Most recent results: ABG's _____ date: _____ CXR _____ date: _____ Serum Theo _____ date: _____ Pulse ox _____ date: _____ Other _____ date: _____	TESTS	Daily pulse oximetry to evaluate & determine pt's O2 needs at rest and exertion. Target O2 sat. >/= 90%. ABG's prn, Serum theophylline level after any changes in dosage.	Daily pulse oximetry to evaluate/determine pt's O2 needs at rest and exertion. Target O2 sat. >/= 90%. ABG's prn, Serum theophylline level after any changes in dosage.	ABG's prn Serum theophylline level after any changes in dosage ABG's and theophylline level prior to discharge
Specimen results: Sputum _____ date: _____ Urine _____ date: _____	SPECIMENS			
Treatment Regime: Most current Oxygen: _____ Most current resp tx orders: _____ _____ _____	TREATMENTS	Oxygen at _____ Titrate oxygen to 90% saturation Nebulized bronchodilator/respiratory tx as ordered, controlled coughing after tx	Oxygen at _____ Titrate oxygen to 90% saturation Nebulized bronchodilator/respiratory tx as ordered, controlled coughing after tx	Oxygen at _____ Titrate oxygen to 90% saturation Nebulized bronchodilator/respiratory tx as ordered, controlled coughing after tx
	VITAL SIGNS	Every 8 hours	Every 8 hours	Every 8 hours
Vital sign range: Temp _____ Resp _____ Pulse _____ B/P _____	I & O	Every 8 hours if receiving IV fluid Daily weights if on IV fluids, otherwise weights weekly	Every 8 hours if receiving IV fluid Daily weights if on IV fluids, otherwise weights weekly	Weeky weights
Diet tolerance:	DIET	DAT specify _____ Small frequent meals if indicated Encourage po fluids unless contraindicated Offer supplements — Pulmocare or milkshakes	DAT specify _____ Small frequent meals if indicated Encourage po fluids unless contraindicated Offer supplements — Pulmocare or milkshakes	DAT specify _____ Small frequent meals if indicated Encourage po fluids unless contraindicated Offer supplements — Pulmocare or milkshakes
	IVs			
Activity tolerance:	MEDS	Bronchodilators, antibiotics, steroids, expectorants, as ordered Avoid narcotics, sedatives, tranquilizers, antiemitcs, antihistamines, & hypnotics	Bronchodilators, antibiotics, steroids, expectorants, as ordered Avoid narcotics, sedatives, tranquilizers, antiemitcs, antihistamines, & hypnotics	Bronchodilators, antibiotics, steroids, expectorants, as ordered Avoid narcotics, sedatives, tranquilizers, antiemitcs, antihistamines, & hypnotics If unresponsibe to relax. techniques, consider selective anxioletics/antidepressant
Sleep pattern:	ACTIVITY	Encourage pursed-lip breathing Ambulate TID with pulse oximeter — gradually increase activity as tolerated Schedule care activities to allow for rest HOB ↑ 45 degrees; may decrease as patient condition allows Provide pillows for propping Keep overbed table in reach	Encourage pursed-lip breathing Ambulate TID with pulse oximeter — gradually increase activity as tolerated Schedule care activities to allow for rest Provide pillows for propping Keep overbed table in reach HOB ↑ 45 degrees; may decrease as patient condition allows When off oxygen, encourage self-reliant activities	Encourage pursed-lip breathing Ambulate TID with pulse oximeter Gradually ↑ activity as tolerated Schedule care activities to allow for rest Provide pillows for propping Keep overbed table in reach When off oxygen, encourage self-reliant activities
Assessment status: Resp: Anxiety level: Mental status:	NURSING ASSESSMENT	Check resp. rate, pattern, breath sounds, color/amt. of sputum, dietary intake, activity tolerance, sleep pattern, anxiety level, comprehension of teaching, mental status, tremor, asterixis & V.S. changes	Check resp. rate, pattern, breath sounds, color/amt. of sputum, dietary intake, activity tolerance, sleep pattern, anxiety level, comprehension of teaching, mental status, tremor, asterixis & V.S. changes	Resp. rate, pattern, breath sounds, color/amt. of sputum, dietary intake, activity tolerance, sleep pattern, anxiety level, comprehension of teaching, mental status, tremor, asterixis, & vital sign changes
Other: Comprehension of teaching:	TEACHING	Assessment/orientation	Begin phase I of teaching; Continue through phases according to patient's understanding	Continue instruction according to patient's understanding
Current D/C plan:	DISCHARGE PLANNING	Notify PT, OT, ST for screening Notify Social Worker of admission if pt is a short stay Assess need for home health care, nsg. home placement, outpatient pulmonary rehab. Discharge plan is to:		If home health care is to follow, call HHC for resp. therapist or other representative to visit prior to D/C Consider and make referrals to community resources as indicated

Nurse signature _____ Shift ____/____   _____ ____/____   _____ ____/____
Nurse signature _____ ____/____   _____ ____/____   _____ ____/____
Nurse signature _____ ____/____   _____ ____/____   _____ ____/____

Figure 39-14   Portion of CareMap® for chronic obstructive pulmonary disease (COPD), suba-cute stay.
Courtesy Baptist Hospital, Pensacola, Fla., and the Center for Case Management, South Natick, Mass.

ple in close or frequent contact with anyone in the high-risk groups. The vaccine has been shown to be 70% to 90% effective in healthy young adults. The vaccine is most effective in reducing the severity of illness and the risk of serious complications and death. Studies have shown a 70% reduction in the number of older adults requiring hospitalization for pneumonia and an 85% reduction in mortality for those not in nursing homes (ACIP, 1997).

Influenza in the United States occurs from November until April. The incidence is usually very low until December and peaks between January and March. Vaccines should be given between September and mid-November. It takes about 1 to 2 weeks after vaccination for antibody development and protection (ACIP, 1997).

The value of vaccination of immunocompromised clients is not completely understood. HIV-positive clients may receive the flu vaccine; however, they may require a second vaccine to gain protection (ACIP, 1997). Persons who should not be vaccinated include those with a known hypersensitivity to eggs or other components of the vac-

TEACHING OUTLINE

Patient Name _____

Room Number _____

Diagnosis _____ COPD — Sub-Acute Stay _____

	Responsible	Date	Signature
1. **Assessment/Orientation:** Review CareMap with pt/family. Re-evaluate learning needs: current knowledge, med compliance, level of anxiety, support systems, and understanding of instruction provided in acute care. Provide instruction books, "Rising to the Challenge of Managing Lung Disease" and "Occupational Therapy COPD Program". Explain self report scale, provide relaxation tape, review pt's perception of stressful events.	Respiratory and/or Nsg. Day 1		
2. **PHASE I: Disease Process, Treatment/Exercise, and Preventing Infection:** Define COPD, review normal anatomy and physiology of the pulmonary system. Review COPD type appropriate to patient (pg. 4–14). Emphasize need to stop smoking if indicated (pg. 15). Inform patient of Health Management Services classes, "Freedom from Smoking" (434–4747). Describe all components of treatment, from pursed lip breathing & diaphramatic/abdominal breathing (pg. 16–18). Review benefits of exercise, precautions, rehab, upper and lower body stretches (pg. 19–21). Emphasize handwashing, annual vaccine, avoidance of people with colds/flu.	Respiratory Therapy/Nsg. Day 2		
Review Section A, OT Booklet, Intro to COPD and Related Effects on your Body and your Surroundings.	Occupational Therapy Day 2		
3. **PHASE II: Medications/Oxygen/Aerosol Therapy, Managing Mucus:** Review and highlight medications specific to patient, emphasize medication guidelines (pg. 23–29). Review oxygen therapy and guidelines if indicated (pg. 30–31). Review MDI/nebulizer use as instructed regimen. Review guidelines (pg. 32–34). Revi~~ controlled coug~~	Respiratory Therapy/Nsg		

SUMMARY
PATIENT PROBLEMS/OUTCOME CRITERIA

Admitting Diagnosis _____ COPD — Sub-Acute _____   Target LOS _____

Date	Initial	Patient Problem	Outcome Criteria/Goal	Date d/c	Initial
		1. Ineffective airway clearance and impaired gas exchange r/t excessive secretions, ineffective cough & disease process	By discharge the patient will: 1. Re-establish usual compensated baseline of $PaCO_2$ and PO_2. 2. Demonstrate effective cough. 3. Return of baseline breath sounds.		
		2. Anxiety r/t dyspnea	By discharge the patient will: 1. Be free of signs/symptoms of anxiety. 2. Demonstrate use of accessory muscles appropriate to activity level.		
		3. Alteration in nutrition: less than body requirements r/t reduced appetite, decreased energy levels, and dyspnea	By discharge the patient will: 1. Be consuming at least 3/4 of meals. 2. Verbalize strategies for adequate caloric intake.		
		4. Activity intolerance r/t fatigue and dyspnea	By discharge the patient will: 1. Be able to ~~perform oxy~~		

Figure 39-14, cont'd   Portion of CareMap® for chronic obstructive pulmonary disease (COPD), subacute stay.

Client Teaching FOR CARDIOVASCULAR DISEASE   Box 39-14

OBJECTIVES
- Client will be able to verbalize risk factors associated with cardiovascular disease.
- Client will be able to demonstrate health promotion behaviors.

TEACHING STRATEGIES
- Teach risk factors that cannot be changed and those that can, such as smoking, high blood pressure, and blood cholesterol levels.
- Educate client about other risk factors for cardiovascular disease, such as diabetes, obesity, physical inactivity, stress, oral contraceptives, and alcohol.
- Educate client about the importance of regular blood pressure monitoring and adherence to a medication regimen.
- Educate client about the importance of blood cholesterol monitoring and maintaining a fasting total cholesterol and triglyceride level less than 200 mg/100 ml.
- Educate client about low-fat, low-salt, and calorie-appropriate diets. Provide sample menus.
- Discuss strategies for stress reduction, such as realistic goal setting, relaxation techniques, exercise, proper diet, and rest.
- Educate client about the benefits of exercising for 20 to 30 minutes 3 to 4 times per week to help reduce weight and help lower blood pressure.
- Set realistic goals with the client for follow-up for blood pressure monitoring.
- Determine cultural, religious, or economic issues that may interfere with client's ability to complete the plan of care.
- Determine age-related issues that may prevent client from achieving the goals.

EVALUATION
- Have client verbalize his or her risk factors for cardiovascular disease.
- Ask client to verbalize what he or she will do to achieve some balance in his or her life and reduce stress.
- Client can list his or her medications, use, and dosage, and reports that he or she had been taking the medication as prescribed.
- Obtain client's weight, pedal edema, and blood pressure.
- Monitor serum cholesterol (total, high- and low-density lipids) and triglyceride levels.
- Client returns for follow-up as scheduled.

Modified from *Mosby's patient teaching guides,* St. Louis, 1998, Mosby.

Client Teaching FOR RESPIRATORY DISEASE   Box 39-15

OBJECTIVES
- Client will be able to verbalize risk factors associated with respiratory disease.
- Client will be able to demonstrate health promotion behaviors.

TEACHING STRATEGIES
- Teach risk factors that cannot be changed and those that the client has control over, such as smoking.
- Educate client about other risk factors, such as exposure to secondhand smoke, repeated respiratory infections, exposure to allergens, and secondary infections.
- Educate client about the importance of smoking cessation. Review current programs and medications available to assist the client.
- Educate client about the importance of monitoring pollution levels and "bad air" days to reduce exposure.
- Discuss the need to avoid secondhand smoke.
- Discuss strategies to avoid or control secondary infection exposure during the influenza season.
- Discuss importance of pneumococcal vaccine and an annual influenza vaccine.
- Educate client about covering the mouth and nose when going out into cold air and limiting exposure time.
- Educate client about the importance of taking medications as prescribed.
- Teach and have client return-demonstrate proper technique and sequencing of metered dose inhalers, including the use of spacers.
- Educate client with asthma about importance of monitoring the peak expiratory flow rate (PEFR).
- Teach and have client return-demonstrate proper use of the peak expiratory flow meter.
- Have client demonstrate proper coughing and sneezing techniques.
- Plan realistic follow-up care with client.
- Determine cultural, religious, or economic issues that may interfere with client's ability to complete the plan of care.
- Determine age-related issues that may prevent client from achieving the goals.

EVALUATION
- Have client verbalize his or her medication regimen, including the purpose and dosage.
- Client is no longer smoking.
- Client covers the mouth and nose when sneezing and coughing.
- Client is able to list his or her medications, dosage, and purpose, and reports that he or she has been taking medications as prescribed.
- Client gets an annual influenza vaccine and a pneumococcal vaccine as appropriate.
- Client is able to demonstrate proper use of metered dose inhalers and spacer use.
- Client is able to demonstrate proper use of the peak expiratory flow meter.
- Review client's record of PEFRs.
- Client returns for follow-up as scheduled.

Modified from *Mosby's patient teaching guides,* St. Louis, 1998, Mosby.

cine and adults with an acute febrile illness (APIC, 1997). The vaccines are formulated annually based on worldwide surveillance data.

Pneumococcal vaccine is recommended for clients at increased risk of developing pneumonia, those with chronic illnesses or immunosuppression (such as HIV/AIDS), those living in special environments such as nursing homes or the American Indian population, and clients over the age of 65. HIV-positive clients can also receive the pneumococcal vaccination. Studies have shown declining antibody levels to certain antigens 5 to 10 years after vaccination. Revaccination has been recommended for clients vaccinated before 1983, because of reformulation of the vaccine from a 14-valent to a 23-valent pneumococcal vaccine in 1983. Both the influenza vaccine and pneumococcal vaccine can be used in pregnant women.

There are no contraindications to the pneumococcal vaccine (APIC, 1997), and influenza vaccine can be given after the first trimester (APIC, 1997). However, in all cases it is important to consult the client's obstetrician before administering either vaccine.

Environmental Pollutants. Avoiding exposure to secondhand smoke is essential to maintaining optimal cardiopulmonary function. Most businesses and restaurants now ban smoking or have separate areas designated as smoking areas. If clients are exposed to secondhand smoke in their home environments, counseling and support may be necessary to assist the smoker in successful smoking cessation or alterations in behavior patterns, such as smoking outside.

Exposure to chemicals and pollutants in the work environment must also be considered. Clients such as farmers, painters, carpenters, and others benefit from the use of particulate filter masks to reduce inhalation of particles.

Healthy Lifestyle Behavior. Identification and elimination of risk factors for cardiopulmonary disease is an important part of primary care. Clients are encouraged to eat a healthy low-fat, high-fiber diet; monitor their cholesterol level, triglyceride level, and HDL/LDL ratio; reduce stress; exercise; and maintain a body weight in proportion to their height. Elimination of cigarette and other tobacco, reduction of pollutants, monitoring of air quality, and adequate hydration are additional healthy behaviors. Clients should be encouraged to examine their habits and make changes to achieve their goals.

Exercise is a key factor in promoting and maintaining a healthy heart and lungs. Clients should be encouraged to exercise 3 to 4 times a week for 20 to 30 minutes. Aerobic exercise is necessary to improve lung function, strengthen muscles, and achieve the desired outcome. Walking is one of the most efficient ways to achieve a good aerobic workout. Many shopping malls have programs that allow people to enter the mall before the shops open and use the enclosed area for walking. Some even have measured the distances to help clients plan their activity and measure their progress. Clients should be taught how to take their pulse and pace themselves. It is better to walk 15 minutes every day than to walk to exhaustion to achieve a goal. Clients should plan a time interval and walk for the designated time. Gradually they will notice that the distance increases as their endurance and fitness improve.

Clients with cardiopulmonary alterations need to minimize their risk for infection, especially during the winter months. Clients are taught to avoid large, crowed places, keep their mouth and nose covered, and be sure to dress warmly, including a scarf, hat, and gloves. This is especially important during the peak of the influenza season.

Clients with known cardiac disease and those with multiple risk factors should be cautioned to avoid exertion in cold weather. Shoveling snow is especially risky and has been known to precipitate a cardiac event in many clients. Other activities such as hanging holiday lights and decorations in the extreme cold can precipitate chest pain and bronchospasm. Clients are advised to avoid alcohol, since it blunts the respiratory drive when used in excess and may contribute to exposure to the cold by making the client feel warm when the client is really not protected.

Clients should also be taught to plan for the hot summer months. Activities should be limited to early in the day or late in the evening, when temperatures are lower. Care should be taken to maintain adequate hydration and sodium intake, especially in those clients who are taking diuretics. Caffeinated and alcoholic beverages should be limited or avoided completely, since they act as diuretics and can contribute to dehydration.

Acute Care. Clients with acute pulmonary illnesses require nursing interventions directed toward halting the pathological process, as with a respiratory tract infection; shorten the duration and severity of the illness, such as hospitalization with pneumonia; and prevent complications from the illness or treatments, such as nosocomial infection resulting from invasive procedures.

Dyspnea Management. Dyspnea is difficult to quantify and to treat. Treatment modalities need to be individualized for each client, and more than one therapy is usually implemented (Box 39-16). The underlying process that causes or worsens dyspnea must be treated and stabilized initially, then four additional therapies—pharmacological measures, oxygen therapy, physical techniques, and psychosocial techniques—are implemented. Pharmacological agents may include bronchodilators, steroids, mucolytics, and low-dose antianxiety medications. Oxygen therapy can reduce dyspnea associated with exercise. Physical techniques, such as cardiopulmonary reconditioning, breathing techniques, and cough control, can help to reduce dyspnea. Relaxation techniques, biofeedback, and meditation are physiosocial measures that can lessen the sensation of dyspnea.

RESEARCH HIGHLIGHT   Box 39-16

RESEARCH ABSTRACT

Clients with dyspnea were studied to determine if the use of a taped relaxation message would reduce their breathlessness. Twenty-six adult clients with COPD with dyspnea were randomly assigned to two groups. The treatment group was taught relaxation using a prerecorded tape, whereas the control group was instructed to sit quietly. Skin temperature, heart rate, and respiratory rate were recorded for a total of four weekly sessions. Anxiety, dyspnea, and airway obstruction were measured at the start and end of the study. The relaxation group achieved the study relaxation criteria and reduced their dyspnea, anxiety, and airway obstruction. The control group remained the same or became worse.

IMPLICATIONS FOR PRACTICE

- Alternative methods to relieve dyspnea have been shown to be effective.
- There is a connection between the psychological response and the physiological response of dyspnea.
- Relaxation techniques are appropriate alternative methodologies for controlling breathlessness.
- A nursing care plan for a client experiencing dyspnea should include a component of relaxation.

REFERENCE

Gift AG, Moore T, Soeken K: Relaxation to reduce dyspnea and anxiety in COPD patients, *Nurs Res* 41(4):242, 1992.

Airway Maintenance.   The airway is patent when the trachea, bronchi, and large airways are free from obstructions. Airway maintenance requires adequate hydration to prevent thick, tenacious secretions; proper coughing techniques to remove secretions and keep the airway open; and a variety of interventions to assist the client with alterations in airway clearance, such as suctioning, chest physiotherapy, and nebulizer therapy.

Mobilization of Pulmonary Secretions.   The ability of a client to mobilize pulmonary secretions may make the difference between a short-term illness and a long recovery involving complications. Nursing interventions that promote mobilization of pulmonary secretions assist the client in achieving and maintaining a clear airway and help promote lung expansion and gas exchange.

Hydration.   Maintenance of adequate systemic hydration keeps mucociliary clearance normal. In clients with adequate hydration, pulmonary secretions are thin, white, watery, and easily removable with minimal coughing. Excessive coughing to clear thick, tenacious secretions is fatiguing and energy depleting. The best way to maintain thin secretions is to provide a fluid intake of 1500 to 2000 ml/day unless contraindicated by cardiac status. The color, consistency, and ease of secretion expectoration can determine adequacy of hydration.

Humidification.   **Humidification** is the process of adding water to gas. Temperature is the most important factor affecting the amount of water vapor a gas can hold. The percentage of water in the gas in relation to its capacity for water is the relative humidity. Air or oxygen with a high relative humidity keeps the airways moist and helps loosen and mobilize pulmonary secretions. Humidification is necessary for clients receiving oxygen therapy at greater than 4 L/min. Bubbling oxygen through water can add humidity to the oxygen delivered to the upper airways, as with a nasal catheter, nasal cannula, or face mask. The humidity tent is used for infants and children with illnesses such as croup and tracheitis to liquefy secretions and help reduce fever. The nebulizer at the top of the humidity tent must remain filled with water to prevent nonhumidified air or oxygen from entering the tent. Air in the humidity tent can become cool and fall below 20° C (68° F), causing the child to become chilled. The nurse monitors the child's body temperature, as well as respiratory status. Children in humidity tents require frequent changes of clothing and bed linen to remain warm and dry.

Nebulization.   **Nebulization** is a process of adding moisture or medications to inspired air by mixing particles of varying sizes with the air. A nebulizer uses the aerosol principle to suspend a maximum number of water drops or particles of the desired size in inspired air. The moisture added to the respiratory system through nebulization improves clearance of pulmonary secretions. Nebulization is often used for administration of bronchodilators and mucolytic agents.

When the thin layer of fluid that supports the mucous layer over the cilia is allowed to dry, the cilia are damaged and cannot adequately clear the airway. Humidification through nebulization enhances mucociliary clearance, the body's natural mechanism for removing mucus and cellular debris from the respiratory tract.

The major types of nebulizers are the jet-aerosol nebulizer and the ultrasonic nebulizer. A jet-aerosol nebulizer uses gas under pressure, and the ultrasonic nebulizer uses high-frequency vibrations to break up the water or medication into fine drops or particles. When inspired with air or administered oxygen, the drops of particles are then deposited throughout the tracheobronchial tree.

Coughing Techniques.   Coughing is effective for maintaining a patent airway. Coughing permits the client to remove secretions from both the upper and lower airways. The normal series of events in the cough mechanism are deep inhalation, closure of the glottis, active contraction of the expiratory muscles, and glottis opening. Deep inhalation increases the lung volume and airway diameter, allowing the air to pass through partially obstructing mucous plugs or other foreign matter. Contraction of the expiratory muscles against the closed glottis causes a high intrathoracic pressure to develop. When the glottis opens, a large flow of air is expelled at a high speed, providing momentum for mucus to move to the upper airways, where it can be expectorated or swallowed.

The effectiveness of coughing is evaluated by sputum expectoration, the client's report of swallowed sputum, or clearing of adventitious sounds by auscultation. Clients with chronic pulmonary diseases, upper respiratory tract infections, and lower respiratory tract infections should be encouraged to deep breathe and cough at least every 2 hours while awake. Clients with a large amount of sputum should be encouraged to cough every hour while awake and every 2 to 3 hours while asleep until the acute phase of mucus production has ended. Coughing techniques include deep breathing and coughing for the post-operative client, cascade, huff, and quad coughing.

With the *cascade cough*, the client takes a slow, deep breath and holds it for 2 seconds while contracting expiratory muscles. Then the client opens the mouth and performs a series of coughs throughout exhalation, thereby coughing at progressively lowered lung volumes. This technique promotes airway clearance and a patent airway in clients with large volumes of sputum.

The *huff cough* stimulates a natural cough reflex and is generally effective only for clearing central airways. While exhaling, the client opens the glottis by saying the word *huff*. With practice the client inhales more air and may be able to progress to the cascade cough.

The *quad cough* technique is used for clients without abdominal muscle control, such as those with spinal cord injuries. While the client breathes out with a maximal expiratory effort, the client or nurse pushes inward and upward on the abdominal muscles toward the diaphragm, causing the cough.

Chest Physiotherapy. **Chest physiotherapy (CPT)** is a group of therapies used in combination to mobilize pulmonary secretions (Box 39-17). These therapies include postural drainage, chest percussion, and vibration. Chest physiotherapy should be followed by productive coughing and suctioning of the client who has a decreased ability to cough. Chest physiotherapy is recommended for clients who produce greater than 30 cc of sputum per day or have evidence of atelectasis by chest x-ray examination (American Association of Respiratory Care [AARC] 1991). This procedure can be safely used with infants and young children; however, conditions and diseases unique to children may at times contraindicate this procedure.

Chest percussion involves striking the chest wall over the area being drained. The hand is positioned so that the fingers and thumb touch and the hand is cupped (Figure 39-15). Percussion on the surface of the chest wall sends waves of varying amplitude and frequency through the chest, changing the consistency and location of the sputum. Chest percussion is performed by alternating hand motion against the chest wall (Figure 39-16). Percussion is performed over a single layer of clothing, not over buttons, snaps, or zippers. The single layer of clothing prevents slapping the client's skin. Thicker or multiple layers of material dampen the vibrations.

Percussion is contraindicated in clients with bleeding disorders, osteoporosis, or fractured ribs. Caution should be taken to percuss the lung fields and not the scapular regions, or trauma may occur to the skin and underlying musculoskeletal structures.

Vibration is a fine, shaking pressure applied to the chest wall only during exhalation. This technique is

---

Guidelines for Chest Physiotherapy

Box 39-17

Nursing care and selection of chest physiotherapy (CPT) skills are based on specific assessment findings. The following guidelines help the nurse in physical assessment and subsequent decision making:

- Know the client's normal range of vital signs. Conditions such as atelectasis and pneumonia requiring CPT can affect vital signs. The degree of change is related to the level of hypoxia, overall cardiopulmonary status, and tolerance to activity.
- Know the client's medications. Certain medications, particularly diuretics and antihypertensives, cause fluid and hemodynamic changes. These may decrease the client's tolerance to the positional changes of postural drainage. Steroid medications increase the client's risk of pathological rib fractures and often contraindicate rib shaking.
- Know the client's medical history. Certain conditions such as increased intracranial pressure, spinal cord injuries, and abdominal aneurysm resection contraindicate the positional changes of postural drainage. Thoracic trauma or surgery may also contraindicate percussion, vibration, and rib shaking.
- Know the client's level of cognitive function. Participation in controlled coughing techniques requires the client to follow instructions. Congenital or acquired cognitive limitations may alter the client's ability to learn and participate in these techniques.
- Be aware of the client's exercise tolerance. CPT maneuvers are fatiguing. When the client is not used to physical activity, initial tolerance to the maneuvers may be decreased. However, with gradual increases in activity and planned CPT, client tolerance for the procedure improves.

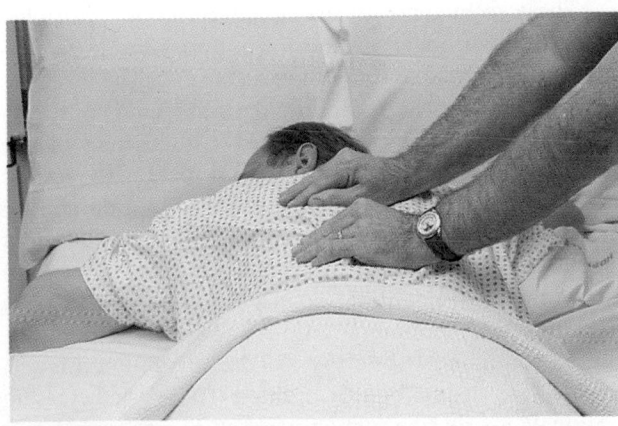

Figure 39-15 Hand position for chest wall percussion during physiotherapy.

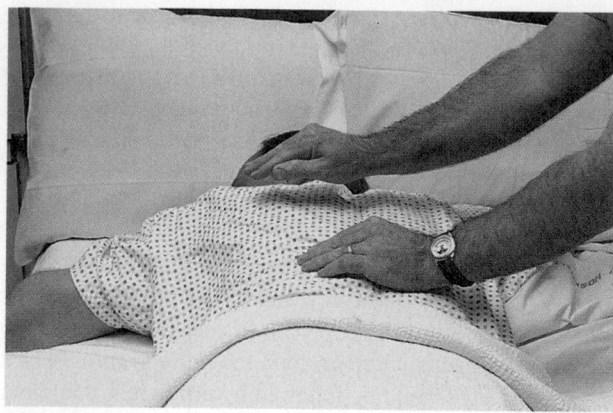

Figure 39-16 Chest wall percussion, alternating hand clapping against the client's chest wall.

thought to increase the velocity and turbulence of exhaled air, facilitating secretion removal. Vibration increases the exhalation of trapped air and may shake mucus loose and induce a cough.

Postural drainage is the use of positioning techniques that draw secretions from specific segments of the lungs and bronchi into the trachea. Coughing or suctioning normally removes secretions from the trachea. The procedure for postural drainage can include most lung segments (Table 39-8). Because clients may not require postural drainage of all lung segments, the procedure is based on clinical assessment findings. For example, clients with left lower lobe atelectasis may require postural drainage of only the affected region, whereas a child with cystic fibrosis may require postural drainage of all lung segments.

Suctioning Techniques.

When a client is unable to clear respiratory tract secretions with coughing, the nurse must use suctioning to clear the airways. The suctioning techniques include oropharyngeal and nasopharyngeal suctioning, orotracheal and nasotracheal suctioning, and suctioning an artificial airway.

These techniques are based on common principles. Because the oropharynx and trachea are considered sterile, sterile technique is used for suctioning. The mouth is considered clean, and therefore the suctioning of oral secretions should be performed after suctioning of the oropharynx and trachea. Each type of suctioning requires the use of a rounded-tipped catheter with a number of side holes at the distal end of the catheter. Frequency of suctioning is determined by client assessment and need. If secretions are identified by inspection or auscultation techniques, suctioning is required. Sputum is not produced continuously or every 1 or 2 hours but occurs as a response to a pathological condition. Therefore there is no rationale for routine suctioning of all clients every 1 to 2 hours. In addition, suctioning reduces the amount of the

available dead space in the oropharynx and trachea, often resulting in significant desaturation of the client. The nurse must be careful to monitor the client to ensure adequate oxygenation. Too frequent suctioning can put the client at risk for development of hypoxemia, hypotension, arrythmias, and possible trauma to the mucosa of the lungs.

Oropharyngeal and Nasopharyngeal Suctioning. The oropharynx extends behind the mouth from the soft palate above the level of the hyoid bone and contains the tonsils. The nasopharynx is located behind the nose and extends to the level of the soft palate. Oropharyngeal or nasopharyngeal suctioning is used when the client is able to cough effectively but is unable to clear secretions by expectorating or swallowing. The suction procedure is used after the client has coughed (Skill 39-2). As the amount of pulmonary secretions is reduced and the client is less fatigued, the client may be able to expectorate or swallow the mucus and suctioning is no longer required.

Orotracheal and Nasotracheal Suctioning. Orotracheal or nasotracheal suctioning is necessary when the client with pulmonary secretions is unable to manage secretions by coughing and does not have an artificial airway present (see Skill 39-2). A catheter is passed through the mouth or nose into the trachea. The nose is the preferred route because stimulation of the gag reflex is minimal. The procedure is similar to nasopharyngeal suctioning, but the catheter tip is moved farther into the client's trachea. The entire procedure from catheter passage to its removal should be done quickly, lasting no longer than 15 seconds. Unless in respiratory distress, the client should be allowed to rest between passes of the catheter. If the client is using supplemental oxygen, the oxygen cannula or mask should be replaced during rest periods.

Tracheal Suctioning. Tracheal suctioning is accomplished through an artificial airway such as an endotracheal tube or tracheostomy tube. The suction catheter should be no greater than one half the size of the internal diameter of the artificial airway. Secretion removal should be as atraumatic as possible. To avoid trauma to the mucosa of the lung, suction pressure should never be applied while inserting the catheter and suction pressure should be maintained between 120 and 180 mm Hg. Suction is applied intermittently as the catheter is withdrawn. Rotating the catheter will enhance removal of secretions that have adhered to the sides of the endotracheal tube. The nurse should wear a mask and goggles and may need to wear a barrier gown to prevent splashes with body fluids.

The two current methods of suctioning are the open and closed methods. Open suctioning involves a sterile catheter that is opened at the time of suctioning. The nurse wears sterile gloves to perform the suction proce-

Table 39-8   Positions for Postural Drainage

Lung Segment	Position of Client	Lung Segment	Position of Client
Adult			
Bilateral	High-Fowler's position	Right middle lobe— posterior segment	Prone with thorax and abdomen elevated
Apical segments Right upper lobe— anterior segment	Sitting on side of bed	Both lower lobes— anterior segments	Supine in Trendelenburg's position
Left upper lobe— anterior segment	Supine with head elevated	Left lower lobe— lateral segment	
Right upper lobe— posterior segment	Side lying with right side of chest elevated on pillows	Right lower lobe— lateral segment	
Left upper lobe— posterior segment	Side lying with left side of chest elevated on pillows	Right lower lobe— posterior segment	
Right middle lobe— anterior segment	Three-fourths supine position with dependent lung in Trendelenburg's position	Both lower lobes— posterior segments	Prone in Trendelenburg's position

Continued

Lung Segment	Position of Client	Lung Segment	Position of Client
Child			
Bilateral—apical segments	Sitting on nurse's lap, leaning slightly forward, flexed over pillow	Bilateral lobes—anterior segments	Lying supine on nurse's lap, back supported with pillow
Bilateral—middle anterior segments	Sitting on nurse's lap, leaning against nurse		

Table 39-8 **Positions for Postural Drainage**—cont'd

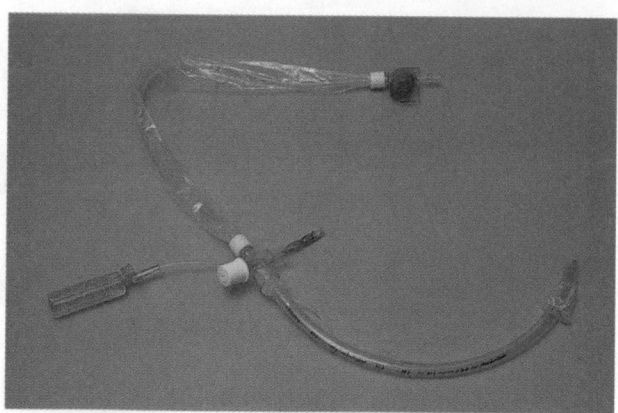

Figure 39-17   Ballard trach care, closed suction.

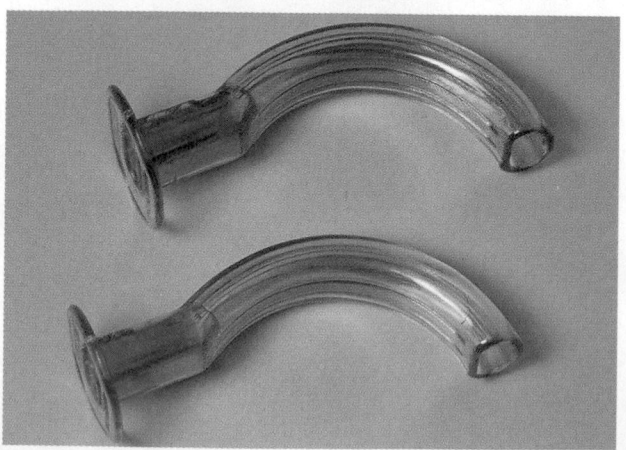

Figure 39-18   Artificial oral airways.

dure. Closed suctioning involves a multiple-use suction catheter that is encased in a plastic sheath (Figure 39-17). Although intended for 24-hour use, research studies have shown that the catheter is safe to use for extended periods of time (Kollef and others, 1997). Closed suctioning is most often used on clients who require mechanical ventilation to support their respiratory efforts, because it permits continuous delivery of oxygen while suction is performed, thus reducing the risk of oxygen desaturation. Although sterile gloves are not used in this procedure, nonsterile gloves are recommended to prevent splashes with body fluids.

Artificial Airways.   An artificial airway is indicated for clients with decreased level of consciousness or airway obstruction and to aide in removal of tracheobronchial secretions.

Oral Airway.   The oral airway, the simplest type of artificial airway, prevents obstruction of the trachea by displacement of the tongue into the oropharynx (Figure 39-18). The oral airway extends from the teeth to the oropharynx, maintaining the tongue in the normal position. The correct-size airway must be used. Proper oral airway size is determined by measuring the distance from the corner of the mouth to the angle of the jaw just below the ear. The length is equal to the distance from the flange of the airway to the tip. If the airway is too small, the tongue is not held in the anterior portion of the mouth; if the airway is too large, it may force the tongue toward the epiglottis and obstruct the airway.

Suctioning   Skill 39-2

Delegation Considerations

This skill requires problem solving and knowledge application unique to a professional nurse. For this skill, delegation is inappropriate.

EQUIPMENT

- Appropriate-size suction catheter (smallest diameter that will remove secretions effectively) or Yankauer catheter (oral suction)
- Small Y adapter (if catheter does not have a suction-control port)
- Water-soluble lubricant
- Two sterile gloves or one sterile and one nonsterile glove

- Sterile basin
- Sterile normal saline solution or water (about 100 ml)
- Clean towel or paper drape
- Portable or wall suction
- Connecting tube (6 feet)
- Nasal or oral airway (if indicated)
- Mask or face shield

STEPS	RATIONALE
1. Assess signs and symptoms of upper and lower airway obstruction requiring nasotracheal or orotracheal suctioning, including respiratory rate or adventitious sounds, nasal secretions, drooling, gastric secretions or vomitus in mouth. Assess signs and symptoms associated with hypoxia and hypercapnia: apprehension, anxiety, decreased ability to concentrate, lethargy, decreased level of consciousness (especially acute), increased fatigue, dizziness, behavioral changes (especially irritability), increased pulse rate or rate of breathing, decreased depth of breathing, elevated blood pressure, cardiac dysrhythmias, pallor, cyanosis, and dyspnea.	Physical signs and symptoms result from decreased oxygen to tissues as well as pooling of secretions in upper and lower airways.
2. Determine factors that normally influence upper or lower airway functioning.	
a. Fluid status	Fluid overload may increase amount of secretions. Dehydration promotes thicker secretions.
b. Lack of humidity	The environment influences secretion formation and gas exchange, necessitating airway suctioning when client cannot clear secretions effectively.
c. Infection	Clients with respiratory infections are prone to increased secretions that are thicker and sometimes more difficult to expectorate.
d. Anatomy	Abnormal anatomy can impair normal drainage of secretions. For example, nasal swelling, a deviated septum, or facial fractures may impair nasal drainage. Tumors in or around the lower airway may impair secretion removal by occluding or externally compressing the lumen of the airway.
3. Assess client's understanding of procedure.	Reveals need for client instruction and encourages cooperation.
4. Obtain physician's order if indicated by agency policy.	Some institutions require a physician's order for tracheal suctioning.
5. Explain to client how procedure will help clear airway and relieve breathing problems and that temporary coughing, sneezing, gagging, or shortness of breath is normal. Encourage client to cough out secretions. Practice coughing, if able. Splint surgical incisions, if necessary.	Encourages cooperation and minimizes risks, anxiety, and pain.
6. Help client to assume position comfortable for nurse and client (usually semi-Fowler's or sitting upright with head hyperextended, unless contraindicated).	Reduces stimulation of gag reflex, promotes client comfort and secretion drainage, and prevents aspiration and nurse strain. Hyperextension facilitates insertion of catheter into trachea.
7. Place towel across client's chest.	Reduces transmission of microorganisms by protecting gown from secretions.
8. Wash hands, and apply face shield if splashing is likely.	Reduces transmission of microorganisms.

STEPS	RATIONALE
9. Connect one end of connecting tubing to suction machine and place other end in convenient location near client. Turn suction device on and set vacuum regulator to appropriate negative pressure.	Excessive negative pressure damages nasopharyngeal and tracheal mucosa and can induce greater hypoxia.
10. If indicated, increase supplemental oxygen therapy to 100% or as ordered by physician. Encourage client's deep breathing.	These measures reduce suction-induced hypoxemia.
11. Prepare suction catheter:	
a. Open suction kit or catheter with use of aseptic technique. If sterile drape is available, place it across client's chest or on the overbed table. Do not allow the suction catheter to touch any nonsterile surfaces.	Maintains asepsis and reduces transmission of microorganisms.
b. Unwrap or open sterile basin and place on bedside table. Be careful not to touch inside of basin. Fill with about 100 ml of sterile normal saline solution or water.	Saline or water is used to clean tubing after each suction pass.
c. Open lubricant. Squeeze small amount onto open sterile catheter package without touching package.	Prepares lubricant while maintaining sterility. Water-soluble lubricants is used to avoid lipoid aspiration pneumonia.
12. Apply sterile glove to each hand, or apply nonsterile glove to nondominant hand and sterile glove to dominant hand.	Reduces transmission of microorganisms and allows nurse to maintain sterility of suction catheter.
13. Pick up Yankauer or suction catheter with dominant hand without touching nonsterile surfaces. Pick up connecting tubing with nondominant hand. Secure catheter to tubing (see illustration).	Maintains catheter sterility. Connects catheter to suction.
14. Suction small amount of normal saline solution from basin.	Ensures equipment function. Lubricates internal catheter and tubing.
15. Coat distal 6 to 8 cm (2 to 3 inches) of catheter with water-soluble lubricant. Do not lubricate Yankauer catheter.	Lubricates catheter for easier insertion.
16. Suction airway.	
A. Oropharyngeal	
(1) Insert catheter or Yankauer into mouth along gum line to pharynx. Move around mouth until secretions are cleared (see illustration). Encourage client to cough. Replace oxygen mask.	Catheter provides continuous suction. Take care not to allow suction tip to invaginate oral mucosal surfaces. Coughing moves secretions from lower airway into mouth and upper airway.

Critical Decision Point: Be careful not to dislodge any oral tubing or tubing in posterior pharynx, such as nasogastric tubes.

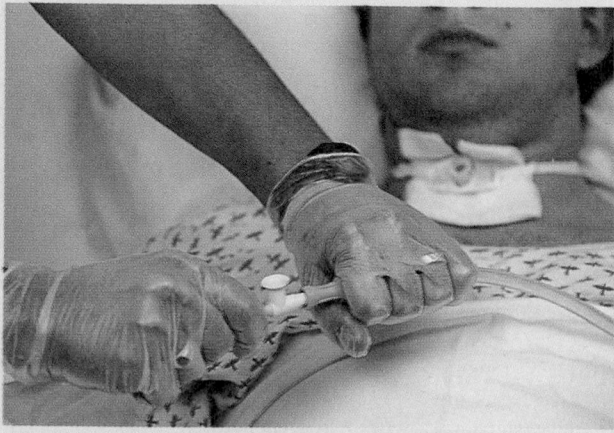

Step 13

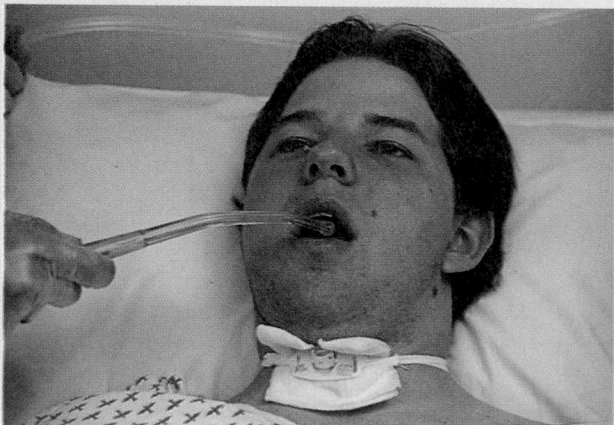

Step 16A (1)

STEPS	RATIONALE

(2) Rinse catheter with water in cup or basin until connecting tubing is cleared of secretions. Turn off suction. May need to wash face if secretions are present on client's skin.

B. **Nasopharyngeal and nasotracheal**

(1) Remove oxygen delivery device, if applicable, with nondominant hand. Without applying suction and using dominant thumb and forefinger, gently but quickly insert catheter into naris during inhalation with slight downward slant or through mouth. Do not force through naris (see illustration).

Rinses catheter and reduces probability of transmission of microorganisms. Clean suction tubing enhances delivery of set suction pressure. Prevents skin breakdown.

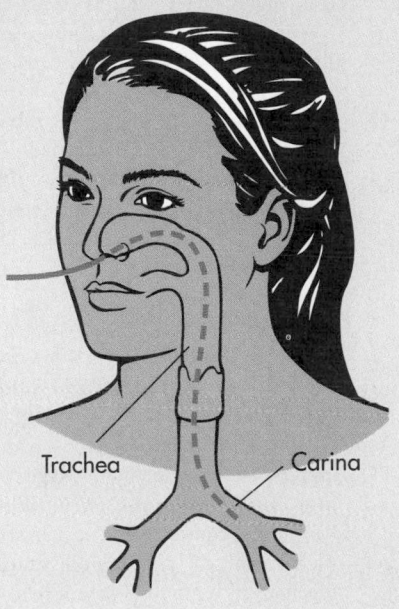

Trachea   Carina

Step 16B (1)

Critical Decision Point: Be sure to insert catheter during client inhalation, especially if inserting catheter into trachea, because epiglottis is open. Do not insert during swallowing, or catheter will most likely enter esophagus. *NEVER* APPLY SUCTION DURING INSERTION.

(a) *Nasopharyngeal suctioning:* In adults, insert catheter about 16 cm; in older children, 8 to 12 cm (3 to 5 inches); in infants and young children, 4 to 8 cm (2 to 3 inches). Rule of thumb is to insert catheter distance from tip of nose (or mouth) to base of earlobe.

(b) *Nasotracheal suctioning:* In adults, insert catheter about 20 cm; in older children, 14 to 20 cm (5.5 to 8 inches); in young children and infants, 8 to 14 cm (3 to 5.5 inches).

(c) *Positioning:* In some instances turning client's head to right helps nurse suction left mainstem bronchus; turning head to left helps nurse suction right mainstem bronchus.

   If resistance is felt after insertion of catheter for maximum recommended distance, catheter has probably hit carina. Pull catheter back 1 cm before applying suction.

Application of suction pressure while introducing catheter into trachea increases risk of damage to mucosa and increases risk of hypoxia because of removal of entrained oxygen present in airways. Epiglottis is open on inspiration and facilitates insertion into trachea. Client should cough. If client gags or becomes nauseated, catheter is most likely in esophagus and must be removed.

Critical Decision Point: Use nasal approach and perform tracheal suctioning before pharyngeal suctioning whenever possible. The mouth and pharynx contain more bacteria than the trachea does. If copious oral secretions are present before beginning the procedure, suction mouth with Yankauer suction device.

STEPS	RATIONALE
(2) Apply intermittent suction for up to 10 to 15 seconds by placing and releasing nondominant thumb over vent of catheter and slowly withdrawing catheter while rotating it back and forth between dominant thumb and forefinger. Encourage client to cough. Replace oxygen device, if applicable.	Intermittent suction and rotation of catheter prevent injury to mucosa. If catheter "grabs" mucosa, remove thumb to release suction. Suctioning longer than 10 seconds can cause cardiopulmonary compromise, usually from hypoxemia or vagal overload.
(3) Rinse catheter and connecting tubing with normal saline or water until cleared.	Removes secretions from catheter. Secretions that remain in suction catheter or connecting tubing decrease suctioning efficiency.
(4) Assess for need to repeat suctioning procedure. Allow adequate time between suction passes for ventilation and oxygenation. Ask client to deep breathe and cough.	Observe for alterations in cardiopulmonary status. Suctioning can induce hypoxemia, dysrhythmias, laryngospasm, and bronchospasm. Deep breathing reventilates and reoxygenates alveoli. Repeated passes clear the airway of excessive secretions but can also remove oxygen and may induce laryngospasm.
(5) When pharynx and trachea are sufficiently cleared of secretions, perform oropharyngeal suctioning to clear mouth of secretions. Do not suction nose again after suctioning mouth.	Removes upper airway secretions. More microorganisms are generally present in mouth.
C. Endotracheal or tracheal tube	
(1) Hyperinflate and/or hyperoxygenate client before suctioning, using manual resuscitation Ambu-bag connected to oxygen source or sigh mechanism on mechanical ventilator. Some mechanical ventilators have a button that when pushed delivers 100% oxygen for a few minutes and then resets to the previous value.	Hyperinflation decreases atelectasis caused by negative pressure of suctioning. Preoxygenation converts large proportion of resident lung gas to 100% oxygen to offset amount used in metabolic consumption while ventilator or oxygenation is interrupted, as well as to offset volume lost during suction procedure.
(2) Open swivel adapter or if necessary remove oxygen or humidity delivery device with nondominant hand.	Exposes artificial airway.
(3) Without applying suction, gently but quickly insert catheter using dominant thumb and forefinger into artificial airway (best to time catheter insertion with inspiration) until resistance is met or client coughs; then pull back 1 cm ($\frac{1}{2}$ inch).	Application of suction pressure while introducing catheter into trachea increases risk of damage to tracheal mucosa, as well as increased hypoxia related to removal of entrained oxygen present in airways. Pulling back stimulates cough and removes catheter from mucosal wall.
(4) Apply intermittent suction by placing and releasing nondominant thumb over vent of catheter; slowly withdraw catheter while rotating it back and forth between dominant thumb and forefinger. Encourage client to cough. Watch for respiratory distress.	Intermittent suction and rotation of catheter prevent injury to tracheal mucosal lining. If catheter "grabs" mucosa, remove thumb to release suction.

Critical Decision Point: If client develops respiratory distress during the suction procedure, immediately withdraw catheter and supply additional oxygen and breaths as needed. Oxygen can be administered directly through the catheter in an emergency. Disconnect suction and attach oxygen at prescribed flow rate through the catheter.

STEPS	RATIONALE
(5) Close swivel adapter or replace oxygen delivery device. Encourage client to deep breathe, if able. Some clients respond well to several manual breaths from the mechanical ventilator or Ambu-bag.	Reoxygenates and reexpands alveoli. Suctioning can cause hypoxemia and atelectasis.
(6) Rinse catheter and connecting tubing with normal saline until clear. Use continuous suction.	Removes catheter secretions. Secretions left in tubing decrease suction and provide environment for microorganism growth. Secretions left in connecting tube decrease suctioning efficiency.

STEPS	RATIONALE
(7) Assess client's cardiopulmonary status for secretion clearance and complications. Repeat Steps (1) through (7) once or twice more to clear secretions. Allow adequate time (at least 1 full minute) between suction passes for ventilation and reoxygenation.	Suctioning can induce dysrhythmias, hypoxia, and bronchospasm and impair cerebral circulation or adversely affect hemodynamics. Repeated passes with suction catheter clear airway of excessive secretions and promote improved oxygenation.
(8) Perform nasopharyngeal and oropharyngeal suctioning. After nasopharyngeal and oropharyngeal suctioning is performed, catheter is contaminated; do not reinsert into endotracheal or tracheostomy tube.	Removes upper airway secretions.
17. When suctioning is completed, roll catheter around fingers of dominant hand. Pull glove off inside out so that catheter remains coiled in glove. Pull off other glove over first glove in same way to seal in contaminants. Discard in appropriate receptacle. Turn off suction device.	Reduces transmission of microorganisms.
18. Remove towel, place in laundry or appropriate receptacle, and reposition client. (Nurse may need to wear clean gloves for personal care.)	Reduces transmission of microorganisms. Promotes comfort.
19. If indicated, readjust oxygen to original level because client's blood oxygen level should have returned to baseline.	Prevents absorption atelectasis and oxygen toxicity while allowing client time to reoxygenate blood.
20. Reposition client as indicated by condition. Nurse may need to reapply clean gloves for client's personal care.	Promotes comfort. Sims' position encourages drainage and reduces risk of aspiration.
21. Discard remainder of normal saline into appropriate receptacle. If basin is disposable, discard into appropriate receptacle. If basin is reusable, rinse and place in soiled utility room.	
22. Remove and discard face shield, and wash hands.	Reduces transmission of microorganisms.
23. Place unopened suction kit on suction machine or at head of bed according to institution preference.	Provides immediate access to suction catheter.
24. Compare client's respiratory assessments before and after suctioning.	Identifies physiological effects of suction procedure to restore airway patency.
25. Ask client if breathing is easier and if congestion is decreased.	Provides subjective confirmation that airway obstruction is relieved with suctioning procedure.
26. Observe airway secretions.	Provides data to document presence or absence of respiratory tract infection.

Recording and Reporting

- Record amount, consistency, color, and odor of secretions and client's response to procedure; document client's presuctioning and postsuctioning respiratory status.

Home Care Considerations

- Normal saline may be made at home by adding 2 teaspoons of table salt to 1 quart of boiled water. Store in jar that has been sterilized (i.e., boiled). Several quart or pint jars can be processed at one time if prepared with home canning equipment.

The airway is inserted by turning the curve of the airway toward the cheek and placing it over the tongue. When the airway is in the oropharynx, the nurse turns it so that the opening points downward. Correctly placed, the airway moves the tongue forward away from the oropharynx and the flange, the flat portion of the airway, rests against the client's teeth. Incorrect insertion merely forces the tongue back into the oropharynx.

Tracheal Airway.   Tracheal airways include endotracheal, nasotracheal, and tracheal tubes. These allow easy access to the client's trachea for deep tracheal suctioning. Because of the presence of the artificial airway, the client no longer has normal humidification of the tracheal mucosa. The nurse should collaborate with the respiratory therapist to ensure that humidity is being supplied to the airway through nebulization or with the oxygen delivery system. This humidification is protective and helps reduce the risk of airway plugging.

Maintenance or Promotion of Lung Expansion.
Nursing interventions to maintain or promote lung expansion include noninvasive techniques. This includes positioning, procedures using equipment such as incentive spirometry, and invasive procedures such as management of a chest tube.

Positioning. In the healthy, completely mobile person, adequate ventilation and oxygenation are maintained by frequent position changes during daily activities. However, when a person's illness or injury restricts mobility, there is an increased risk for respiratory impairment. Frequent changes of position are simple and cost-effective methods for reducing the risks of stasis of pulmonary secretions and decreased chest wall expansion.

The most effective position for client with cardiopulmonary diseases is the 45-degree semi-Fowler's position, using gravity to assist in lung expansion and reduce pressure from the abdomen on the diaphragm. When the client uses this position, the nurse needs to ensure that the client does not slide down in bed, which could reduce lung expansion. A client with unilateral lung disease, such as pneumothorax, atelectasis, pneumonia, thoracotomy, and multiple trauma affecting one lung, should be positioned with the "good lung down." This promotes better perfusion of the healthy lung, improving oxygenation. In the presence of pulmonary abscess or hemorrhage, the client should be placed with the affected lung down to prevent drainage toward the healthy lung.

Incentive Spirometry. **Incentive spirometry** is a method of encouraging voluntary deep breathing by providing visual feedback to clients about inspiratory volume. Incentive spirometry is used to promote deep breathing to prevent or treat atelectasis in the postoperative client. Studies have shown no respiratory benefit to postoperative incentive spirometry when compared with deep breathing and early ambulation (Bell, 1993).

Flow-oriented incentive spirometers consist of one or more plastic chambers that contain freely moving colored balls. The client inhales slowly and with an even flow to elevate the balls and to keep them floating as long as possible to ensure a maximally sustained inhalation.

Volume-oriented incentive spirometry devices have a bellows that is raised to a predetermined volume by an inhaled breath (Figure 39-19). An achievement light or counter is used to provide feedback. Some devices are constructed so that the light will not turn on unless the bellows is held at a minimum desired volume for a specified period to enhance lung expansion.

Incentive spirometry encourages clients to breathe to their normal inspiratory capacities. A postoperative inspiratory capacity one half to three fourths of the preopera-

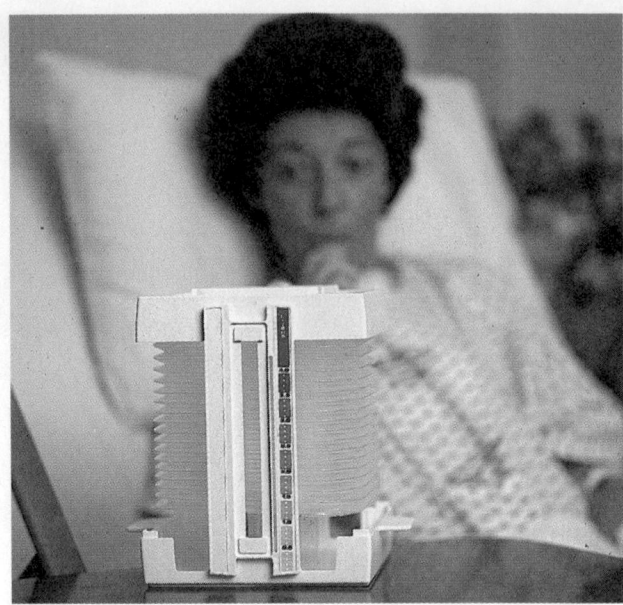

Figure 39-19 Volume-oriented spirometer.

tive volume is acceptable because of postoperative pain. Administration of pain medications before incentive spirometry will help the client achieve deep breathing by reducing pain and splinting (see Chapter 49).

Chest Tubes. Chest tubes are inserted to remove air and fluids from the pleural space, to prevent air or fluid from reentering the pleural space, and to reestablish normal intrapleural and intrapulmonic pressures. A **chest tube** is a catheter inserted through the thorax to remove fluid or air. Chest tubes are used after chest surgery and chest trauma and for pneumothorax or hemothorax to promote lung reexpansion (Skill 39-3).

A **pneumothorax** is a collection of air in the pleural space. The loss of negative intrapleural pressure causes the lung to collapse. There are a variety of mechanisms for a pneumothorax. It may occur spontaneously or as a result of chest trauma, such as a stabbing or the chest striking the steering wheel in an automobile accident. A pneumothorax may result from the rupture of an emphysematous bleb on the surface of the lung (a large bulla resulting from the destruction caused by emphysema) or from an invasive procedure, such as insertion of a subclavian IV line.

A client with a pneumothorax usually feels pain as atmospheric air irritates the parietal pleura. The pain may be sharp and pleuritic. Dyspnea is common and worsens as the size of the pneumothorax increases.

A **hemothorax** is an accumulation of blood and fluid in the pleural cavity between the parietal and visceral pleurae, usually as a result of trauma. It produces a coun-

Care of Clients With Chest Tubes   Skill 39-3

Delegation Considerations

This skill requires problem solving and knowledge application unique to a professional nurse and should not be delegated. Assistive personnel may help with positioning.

- Inform and assist care provider in the proper positioning of a client with chest tubes to facilitate drainage.

- Explain to care provider what is the appropriate setup of drainage equipment for the type of system to be used.
- Instruct care provider to inform nurse of any changes in the vital signs, chest tube drainage, or excessive bubbling in water-seal chamber.

EQUIPMENT

- Chest drainage system (bottles or disposable system)
- Suction source and setup (wall canister or portable)
- Nonsterile gloves
- Sterile irrigation saline or sterile water (500-ml bottle)

- Tape (2-inch width)
- Sterile gauze sponges
- Two shodded hemostats

STEPS	RATIONALE
1. Assess client for respiratory distress and chest pain, breath sounds over affected lung area, and stable vital signs (see Chapter 31).	Signs and symptoms reflect improvement in respiratory distress and chest pain after insertion of chest tube.
2. Observe for increased respiratory distress.	Signs and symptoms of increased respiratory distress and/or chest pain, decrease in breath sounds over the affected and nonaffected lungs, marked cyanosis, asymmetrical chest movements, presence of subcutaneous emphysema around tube insertion site or neck, hypotension, and tachycardia. Notify physician immediately.
3. Observe: a. Chest tube dressing. b. Tubing for kinks, dependent loops, or clots. c. Chest drainage system, which should be upright and below level of tube insertion.	Ensures that tubing is patent. Maintains a patent, freely draining system, preventing fluid accumulation in chest cavity. System must be in this position to function properly.
4. Provide two shodded hemostats for each chest tube, attached to top of client's bed with adhesive tape. Chest tubes are only clamped under specific circumstances: a. To assess air leak. b. To quickly empty or change collection bottle or chamber; performed by nurse who has received training in procedure. c. To change disposable systems; have new system ready to be connected before clamping tube so that transfer can be rapid and drainage system reestablished. d. To change a broken water-seal bottle in the event that no sterile solution container is available. e. To assess if client is ready to have chest tube removed (which is done by physician's order); the nurse must monitor client for recreation of pneumothorax.	Shodded hemostats have a covering to prevent hemostat from penetrating chest tube.
5. Position client. a. Semi-Fowler's position to evacuate air (pneumothorax). b. High-Fowler's position to drain fluid (hemothorax).	Permits optimal drainage of fluid and/or air. Air rises to highest point in chest. Pneumothorax tubes are usually placed on anterior aspect at midclavicular line, second or third intercostal space. Permits optimal drainage of fluid. Posterior tubes are placed on midaxillary line, eighth or ninth intercostal space.
6. Maintain tube connection between chest and drainage tubes intact and taped. a. Water-seal vent must be without occlusion. b. Suction-control chamber vent must be without occlusion when suction is used.	Secures chest tube to drainage system and reduces risk of air leak causing breaks in airtight system. Permits displaced air to pass into atmosphere. Provides safety factor of releasing excess negative pressure into atmosphere.

STEPS	RATIONALE
7. Coil excess tubing on mattress next to client. Secure with rubber band and safety pin or system's clamp.	Prevents excess tubing from hanging over edge of mattress in dependent loop. Drainage could collect in loop and occlude drainage system.
8. Adjust tubing to hang in straight line from top of mattress to drainage chamber. If chest tube is draining fluid, indicate time (e.g., 0900) that drainage was begun on drainage bottle's adhesive tape or on write-on surface of disposable commercial system.	Provides a baseline for continuous assessment of type and quality of drainage.

9. Strip or milk chest tube only if indicated:
   a. Postoperative mediastinal chest tubes are manipulated if nursing assessment indicates obstruction of drainage secondary to clots or debris in tubing.
   b. Postoperative assessment is done every 15 minutes for the first 2 hours. This assessment interval then changes based on client's status.
	Stripping is controversial and should be performed only if hospital policy permits it and there is a physician's order. Stripping creates a high degree of negative pressure and has potential of pulling lung tissue or pleura into drainage holes of chest tube.

Critical Decision Point: Review agency policy before milking or stripping chest tubes.

STEPS	RATIONALE
10. Wash hands.	Reduces transmission of infection.
11. Observe: a. Chest tube dressing, tubing, and chest tube drainage system, which should be upright and below level of tube insertion.	Ensures that tube is patent, and notes any drainage. Maintains tubing free of kinks and dependent loops. Note presence of clots or debris in tubing.
b. Water seal for fluctuations with client's inspiration and expiration.	Fluid should rise in water seal with inspiration and fall with expiration, indicating that system is functioning properly.
c. Bubbling in water-seal bottle or chamber (see Table 39-9).	When system is initially connected to client, bubbles are expected in chamber from air that was present in system and in client's intrapleural space. After a short period, bubbling will stop. Fluid will continue to fluctuate in water seal on inspiration and expiration until lung is reexpanded or system becomes occluded.
d. Type and amount of fluid drainage. Nurse should note color and amount of drainage, client's vital signs, and skin color.	Sudden gush of drainage may be retained blood and not active bleeding. Increase in drainage can be result of client position.
(1) Less than 50 to 300 ml/hr immediately postoperative in mediastinal chest tube; approximately 500 ml in first 24 hours; dark red drainage is expected early in postoperative period, turning serous with time.	Reexpansion of lungs forces drainage into tube. Coughing can also cause large gushes of drainage.
(2) Between 100 and 300 ml of fluid may drain in posterior chest tube during first 2 hours after insertion; rate will decrease after 2 hours; 500 to 1000 ml can be expected in first 24 hours; drainage will be grossly bloody during first several hours after surgery and then change to serous.	Excessive amounts and/or continued presence of frank, bloody drainage after first several hours of surgery should be reported to physician, along with client's vital signs and respiratory status.
e. Bubbling in the suction-control chamber (when suction is being used) (see Table 39-9).	Suction-control chamber has constant, gentle bubbling. Tubing to suction source should be free of obstruction, and suction source should be turned on to appropriate setting.

Recording and Reporting
- Record in nurse's notes patency of chest tubes, presence of drainage, presence of fluctuations, client's vital signs, chest dressing status, type of suction, and level of comfort.

Home Care Considerations
- If client goes home with chest tube (i.e., empyema), teach client and family to care for chest tube and drainage bottle.

terpressure and prevents the lung from full expansion. A hemothorax can also be caused by rupture of small blood vessels from inflammatory processes, such as pneumonia or tuberculosis. In addition to pain and dyspnea, signs and symptoms of shock can develop if blood loss is severe.

The one-bottle system is the simplest closed drainage system because the single bottle serves as a collector and a water seal (Figure 39-20, *A*). During normal respiration the fluid should ascend with inspiration and descend with expiration. The one-bottle system is used for smaller amounts of drainage, such as an empyema. An empyema is a collection of infected fluid or pus in the pleural space.

A two-bottle system permits the liquid to flow into the collection bottle as air flows into the water-seal bottle (Figure 39-20, *B*). Fluctuations in the water-seal tube are still anticipated. The two-bottle system allows for more accurate measurement of chest drainage and is used when larger amounts of drainage are expected.

A three-bottle system is used to evacuate any volume of air or fluid with controlled suction (Figure 39-20, *C*). The suction-control bottle contains a long tube, submerged under water, and vented to the atmosphere. There are two short tubes: one tube connects bottles two and three, and the second tube is connected to an external suction source. The suction pressure causes gentle, continuous bubbling in bottle three. Suction pressure is measured in centimeters of water and is equated with the length of the long tube submerged in water. Usually 15 to 20 cm of water is used for adults. This means that the long tube is submerged in 15 to 20 cm of water. Children require lesser amounts of pressure.

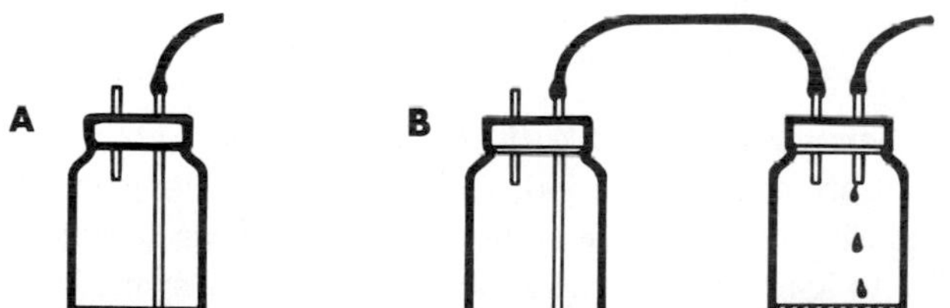

The disposable systems, such as a Thora-Sene III or Pleur-Evac chest drainage system (Dekental), are a one-piece molded plastic unit that duplicates the three-bottle system (Figure 39-21). The disposable units appear to be the system of choice because they are cost-effective and some facilitate autotransfusion, a common practice in open-heart surgeries. Knowledge of the basics of chest tube management and troubleshooting maneuvers reduces the client's risk of complications (Table 39-9).

Special Considerations. Clamping chest tubes is contraindicated when the client is ambulating or being transported. The nurse should handle the chest drainage unit or bottles carefully and maintain the drainage device below the client's chest. If the tubing disconnects from the bottles, the nurse should instruct the client to exhale as much as possible and to cough. This maneuver rids the pleural space of as much air as possible. The nurse needs to cleanse the tips of the tubing and reconnect them to the bottles quickly. If the chest bottle breaks, the end of the tubing can be quickly submerged in a container of sterile water to reestablish the seal. Clamping the chest tube may result in a tension pneumothorax, which is a life-threatening event.

Removal of chest tubes requires client preparation. Clients report sensations during chest tube removal. The

Figure 39-20   Chest tube drainage. **A,** One-bottle system. **B,** Two-bottle system. **C,** Three-bottle system with suction.

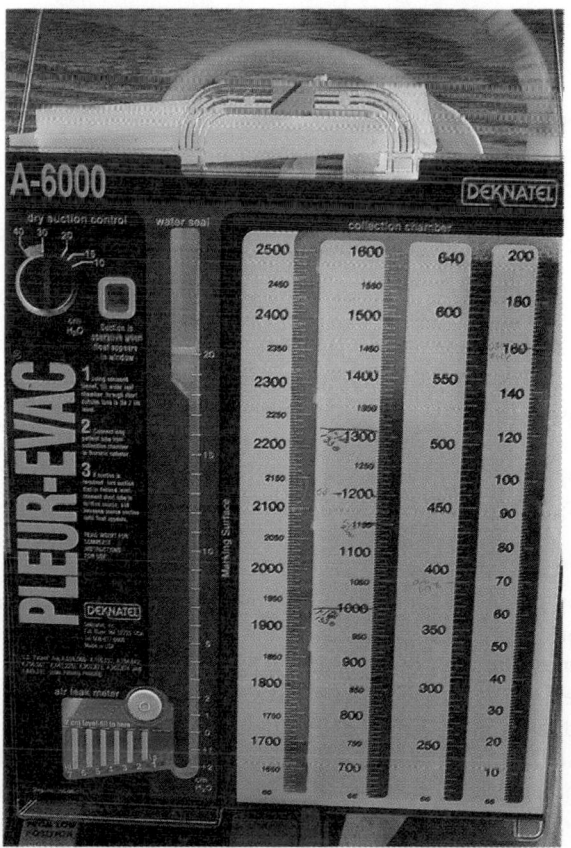

Figure 39-21   Disposable, commercial chest drainage system.

Table 39-9 **Problem Solving With Chest Tubes**

Problem	Solution
Air leak is present.	Locate leak.
Continuous bubbling is seen in water-seal bottle/chamber, indicating that leak is between client and water seal.	Tighten loose connections between client and water seal. Loose connections cause air to enter system. Leaks are corrected when constant bubbling stops.
Bubbling continues, indicating that air leak has not been corrected.	Cross-clamp chest tube close to client's chest. If bubbling stops, air leak is inside client's thorax or at chest tube insertion site. *Unclamp tube and notify physician immediately.* Reinforce chest dressing. Leaving chest tube clamped causes a tension pneumothorax and mediastinal shift.
Bubbling continues, indicating that leak is not in client's chest or at insertion site.	Gradually move clamps down drainage tubing away from client and toward suction-control chamber, moving one clamp at a time. When bubbling stops, leak is in section of tubing or connection distal to clamp. Replace tubing or secure connection and release clamp.
Bubbling continues, indicating that leak is not in tubing.	Leak is in drainage system. Change drainage system.
Tension pneumothorax is present.	Determine that chest tubes are not clamped, kinked, or occluded. Obstructed chest tubes trap air in intrapleural space when air leak originates within client.
Severe respiratory distress	
Chest pain	
Absence of breath sounds on affected side	Notify physician immediately.
Hyperresonance on affected side	Prepare immediately for another chest tube insertion; obtain a flutter (Heimlich) valve or large-gauge needle for short-term emergency release of air in intrapleural space; have emergency equipment (e.g., oxygen and code cart) near client.
Mediastinal shift to unaffected side	
Tracheal shift to unaffected side	
Hypotension	
Tachycardia	
Dependent loops of drainage tubing have trapped fluid.	Drain tubing contents into drainage bottle. Coil excess tubing on mattress and secure in place.
Water seal is disconnected.	Connect water seal and tape connection.
Water-seal bottle is broken.	Insert distal end of water-seal tube into sterile solution so that tip is 2 cm below surface and set up new water-seal bottle. If no sterile solution is available, double-clamp chest tube while preparing new bottle.
Water-seal tube is no longer submerged in sterile fluid.	Add sterile solution to water-seal bottle until distal tip is 2 cm under surface or set water-seal bottle upright so that tip is submerged.

most frequent sensations include burning, pain, and a pulling sensation.

Maintenance and Promotion of Oxygenation.
Promotion of lung expansion, mobilization of secretions, and maintenance of a patent airway assists the client in meeting oxygenation needs. Some clients, however, also require oxygen therapy to keep a healthy level of tissue oxygenation.

Goals of Oxygen Therapy. The goal of oxygen therapy is to prevent or relieve hypoxia. Any client with impaired tissue oxygenation can benefit from controlled oxygen administration. Oxygen is not a substitute for other treatment, however, and should be used only when indicated. Oxygen should be treated as a drug. It is expensive and has dangerous side effects. As with any drug, the dosage or concentration of oxygen should be continuously monitored. The nurse should routinely check the physician's orders to verify that the client is receiving the prescribed oxygen concentration. The five rights of medica-

tion administration also pertain to oxygen administration (see Chapter 34).

Safety Precautions With Oxygen Therapy. Oxygen is a highly combustible gas. Although it will not spontaneously burn or cause an explosion, it can easily cause a fire to ignite in a client's room if it contacts a spark from an open flame or electrical equipment. Oxygen in high concentrations has a great combustion potential and readily fuels fire. With increasing use of home oxygen therapy, clients and health care professionals must be aware of the dangers of combustion. The nurse should promote safety by using the following measures:

"No smoking" signs should be placed on the client's room door and over the bed. The client, visitors and roommates, and all personnel should be informed that smoking is not permitted in areas where oxygen is in use.

The nurse determines that all electrical equipment in the room is functioning correctly and is properly grounded (see Chapter 37). An electrical spark in the presence of oxygen can result in a serious fire. The nurse should know the fire procedures and the location of the closest fire extinguisher.

The nurse should always check the oxygen level of portable tanks before transporting to ensure that there is enough oxygen remaining in the tank.

Supply of Oxygen. Oxygen is supplied to the client's bedside either by oxygen tanks or through a permanent wall-piped system. Oxygen tanks are transported on wide-based carriers that allow the tank to be placed upright at the bedside. Regulators are used to control the amount of oxygen delivered. One common type is an upright flow meter with a flow adjustment valve at the top. A second type is a cylinder indicator with a flow adjustment handle.

In the hospital or home, oxygen tanks are delivered with the regulator in place. In the hospital the respiratory care department usually connects the regulator to the oxygen source. Home care vendors are usually responsible for connecting the oxygen tank to the regulator for home use.

Methods of Oxygen Delivery. Oxygen can be delivered to the client by nasal cannula, nasal catheter, face mask, or mechanical ventilator.

Nasal Cannula. A **nasal cannula** is a simple, comfortable device (Skill 39-4). The two cannulas, about 1.5 cm (½ inch) long, protrude from the center of a disposable tube and are inserted into the nares. Oxygen is delivered via the cannulas with a flow rate of up to 6 L/min. Flow rates greater than 4 L/min are not often used because of the drying effect on the mucosa and the relatively little increase in delivered oxygen concentration. The nurse must know what flow rate produces a given percentage of inspired oxygen concentration (F_IO_2) (Table 39-10). The nurse must also be alert for skin breakdown over the ears and in the nares from too tight an application of the nasal cannula.

Nasal Catheter. Nasal catheters are used infrequently, but they are not obsolete. The procedure involves inserting an oxygen catheter into the nose to the nasopharynx. Because securing the catheter can cause pressure on the nostril, the catheter must be changed at least every 8 hours and inserted into the other nostril. For this reason, the nasal catheter is a less desirable method because the client may have pain when the catheter is passed into the nasopharynx and because trauma can occur to the nasal mucosa.

Transtracheal Oxygen. **Transtracheal oxygen (TTO)** is a method of oxygen delivery for clients with chronic lung diseases in which a small, IV-size catheter is inserted directly into the trachea through a surgical tract in the lower neck and oxygen is delivered directly into the trachea.

The advantages of TTO are the following: (1) no oxygen is lost to the atmosphere; (2) clients achieve adequate oxygenation at lower flow rates, making oxygen delivery more efficient, less expensive, and with fewer side effects;

Table 39-10 Approximate F_IO_2 With Different Delivery Devices

Liter Flow (L/min)	Approximate Percent F_IO_2	Delivery Device
1	24	Nasal cannula
2	24	Venturi mask
	28	Nasal cannula
3	28	Venturi mask
	32	Nasal cannula
4	30	Venturi mask
	36	Nasal cannula
5	40	Nasal cannula
5-6	40	Face mask
6	35	Venturi mask
	44	Nasal cannula
6-7	50	Face mask
7-8	60	Face mask
8	40	Venturi mask
10	50	Venturi mask
14	55	Venturi mask

and (3) clients are more likely to use oxygen because of the mobility, comfort, and cosmetic improvement.

Once the tracheal stoma is healed, the client is taught to remove and irrigate the catheter with normal saline at least 3 times a day to maintain catheter patency. The final oxygen flow rate, usually less than 4 L/min, is delivered through an 8 Fr catheter through the mature tract.

Oxygen Masks. An oxygen mask is a device used to administer oxygen, humidity, or heated humidity. It is shaped to fit snugly over the mouth and nose and is secured in place with a strap. There are two primary types of oxygen masks: those delivering low concentrations of oxygen and those delivering high concentrations.

The simple face mask (Figure 39-23, p. 1178) is used for short-term oxygen therapy. It fits loosely and delivers oxygen concentrations from 30% to 60%. The mask is contraindicated for clients with carbon dioxide retention because retention can be worsened.

A plastic face mask with a reservoir bag (Figure 39-24, p. 1180) and a Venturi mask (Figure 39-25, p. 1178) are capable of delivering higher concentrations of oxygen. When used as a nonrebreather, the plastic face mask with a reservoir bag can deliver from 80% to 90% oxygen (70% when used as a rebreather) with a flow rate of 10 L/min. This oxygen mask maintains a high-concentration oxygen supply in the reservoir bag.

The nurse should frequently inspect the bag to make sure it is inflated. If it is deflated, the client may be breathing large amounts of exhaled carbon dioxide.

The Venturi mask can be used to deliver oxygen concentrations of 24% to 55% with oxygen flow rates of 2 to 14 L/min, depending on which flow-control meter is selected (Table 39-10).

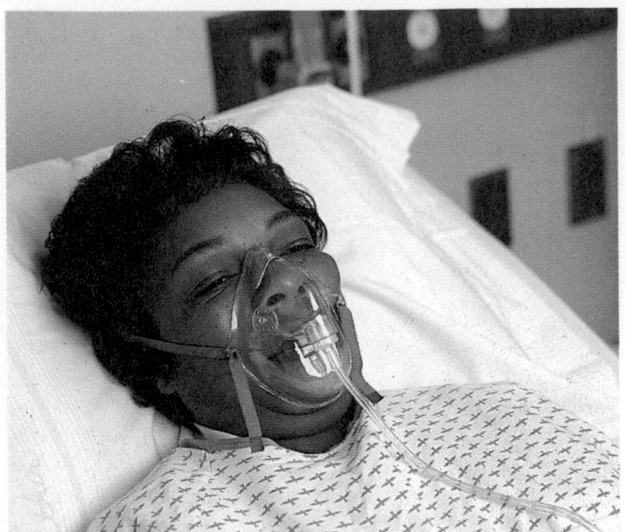

Figure 39-23   Simple face mask.

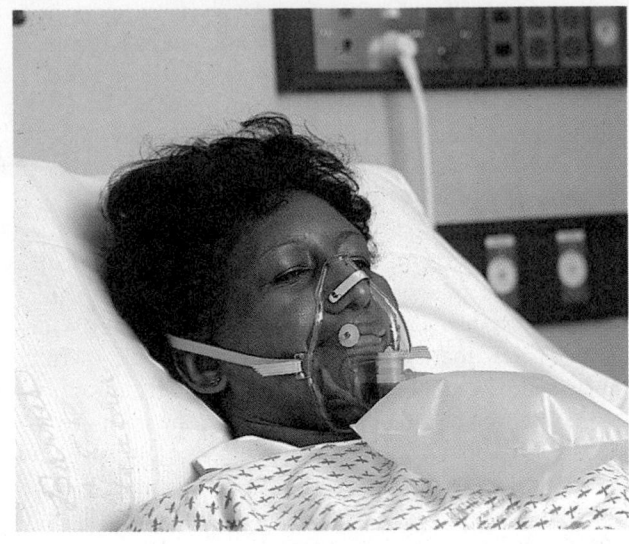

Figure 39-24   Plastic face mask with reservoir bag.

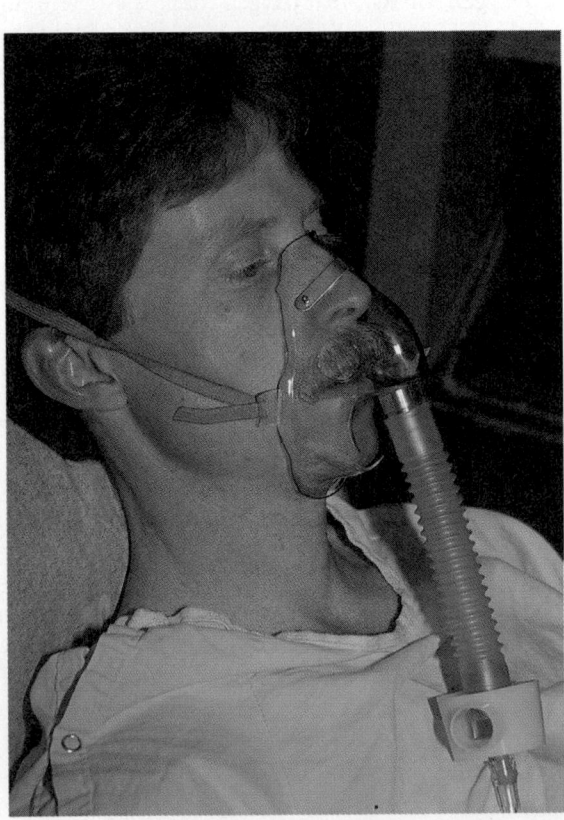

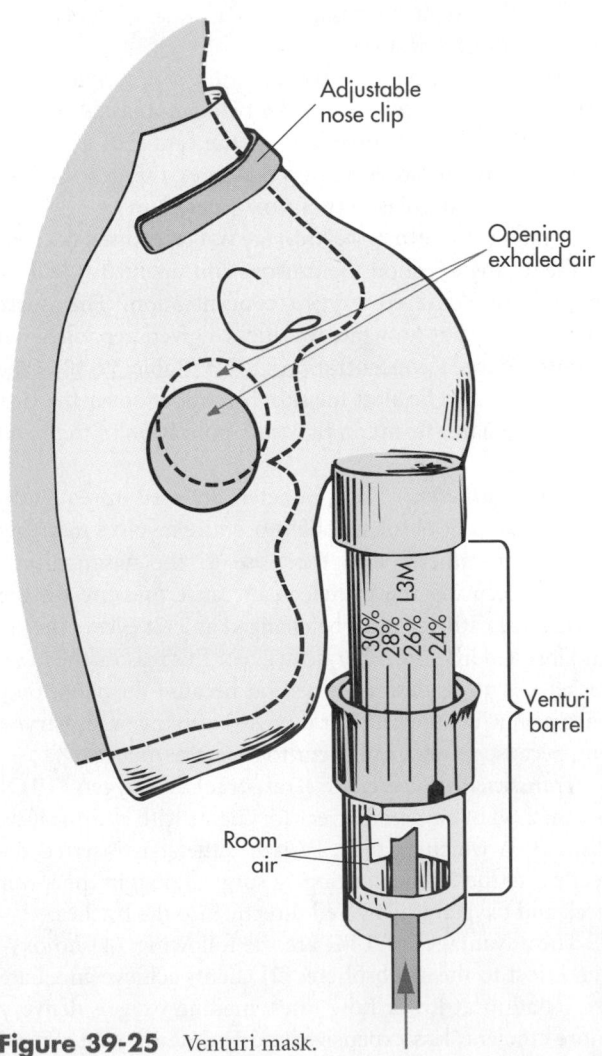

Figure 39-25   Venturi mask.

Applying a Nasal Cannula or Oxygen Mask Skill 39-4

Delegation Considerations
This skill can be delegated to appropriately trained assistive personnel. The nurse is responsible for assessing and checking the device setup and the client.

• Inform and assist care provider in the proper way to set up and apply the nasal cannula or oxygen mask.

• Instruct caregiver regarding unexpected outcomes associated with the oxygen delivery device and the need to inform the nurse if any occur.

EQUIPMENT
• Nasal cannula or oxygen mask
• Oxygen tubing (Figure 39-22)
• Humidifier, if indicated
• Sterile water for humidification, if indicated
• Oxygen source
• Oxygen flowmeter
• Appropriate room signs

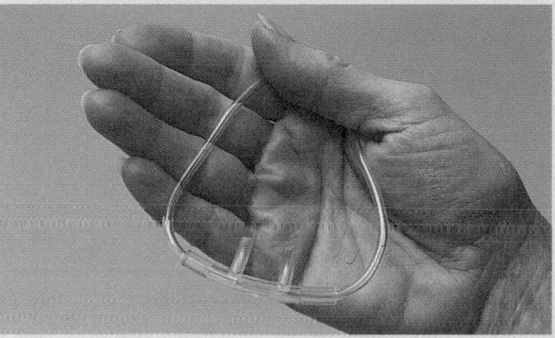

Figure 39-22   Simple face mask.

STEPS	RATIONALE
1. Inspect client for signs and symptoms associated with hypoxia and presence of airway secretions.	Left untreated, hypoxia can produce cardiac dysrhythmias and death. Presence of airway secretions decreases effectiveness of oxygen delivery.

Critical Decision Point: Clients with sudden changes in their vital signs, level of consciousness, or behavior may be experiencing profound hypoxia. Clients who demonstrate subtle changes over time may have worsening of a chronic or existing condition or a new medical condition.

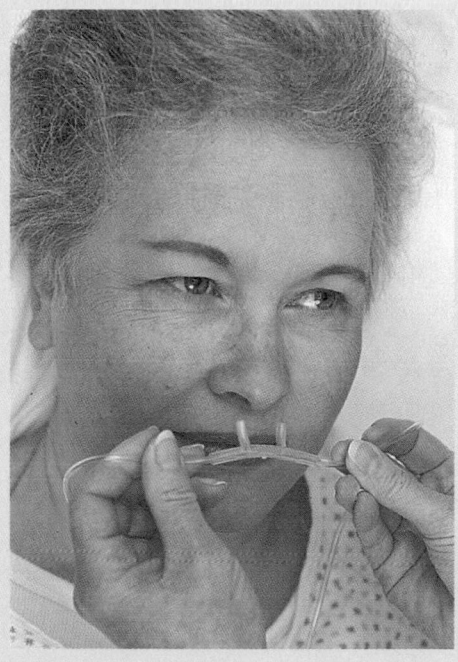

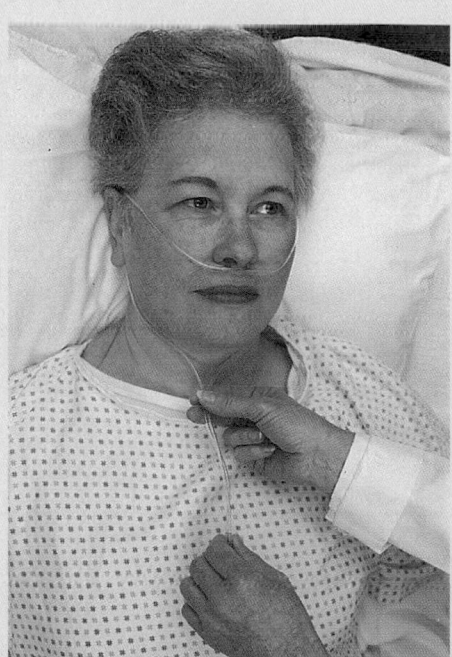

Step 5

STEPS	RATIONALE
2. Explain to client and family what procedure entails and purpose of oxygen therapy.	Decreases client's anxiety, which reduces oxygen consumption and increases client cooperation.
3. Wash hands.	Reduces transmission of infection.
4. Attach nasal cannula to oxygen tubing and attach to humidified oxygen source adjusted to prescribed flow rate.	Prevents drying of nasal and oral mucous membranes and airway secretions.
5. Place tips of cannula into client's nares (see illustration) and adjust elastic headband or plastic slide until cannula fits snugly and comfortably (see illustration).	Directs flow of oxygen into client's upper respiratory tract. Client is more likely to keep cannula in place if it fits comfortably.
6. Maintain sufficient slack on oxygen tubing and secure to client's clothes.	Allows client to turn head without dislodging cannula and reduces pressure on tips of nares.
7. Check cannula every 8 hours and keep humidification jar filled at all times.	Ensures patency of cannula and oxygen flow. Prevents inhalation of dehumidified oxygen.
8. Observe client's nares and superior surface of both ears for skin breakdown.	Oxygen therapy can cause drying of nasal mucosa. Pressure on ears from cannula tubing or elastic can cause skin irritation.
9. Check oxygen flow rate and physician's orders every 8 hours (see illustration).	Ensures delivery of prescribed oxygen flow rate and patency of cannula.
10. Wash hands.	Reduces transmission of microorganisms.
11. Inspect client for relief of symptoms associated with hypoxia.	Indicates that hypoxia is corrected or reduced.

Critical Decision Point: Note if current oxygen therapy is meeting client's oxygenation needs. Determine what factors have changed, resulting in new assessment findings.

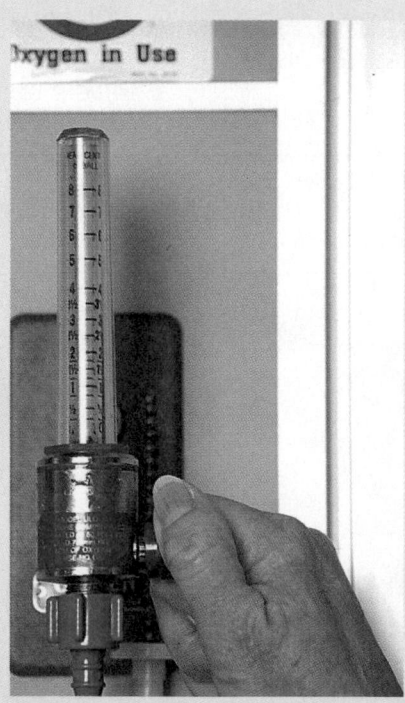

Step 10

Recording and Reporting
- Document oxygen delivery device and liter flow in medical record.
- Document client and family education.
- Report oxygen delivery device, liter flow, and response to changes in therapy to oncoming shift.

Home Care Considerations
- If client is to have home oxygen therapy, teach client and family how to use the oxygen equipment and properly apply the oxygen delivery device (see Skill 39-5).

Home Oxygen Therapy. Indications for home oxygen therapy include an arterial partial pressure (PaO_2) of 55 mm Hg or less or an arterial oxygen saturation (SaO_2) of 88% or less on room air at rest, on exertion, or with exercise. Clients with a PaO_2 from 56 to 59 mm Hg may also receive oxygen if there is also evidence of cor pulmonale, pulmonary hypertension, erythrocytosis, central nervous system dysfunction, impaired mental status, or increasing hypoxemia with exertion.

When home oxygen is required, it is usually delivered by nasal cannula. When a client has a permanent tracheostomy, however, a T tube or tracheostomy collar is necessary. Three types of oxygen are used: compressed oxygen, liquid oxygen, and oxygen concentrators. The advantages and disadvantages (Table 39-11) of each type are assessed, along with the client's needs and community resources, before placing a certain delivery system in the home. In the home the major consideration is the oxygen delivery source.

Clients requiring home oxygen need extensive teaching to be able to continue oxygen therapy at home efficiently and safely (Skill 39-5). This includes oxygen safety, regulation of the amount of oxygen, and how to use the prescribed home oxygen delivery system. The nurse coordinates the efforts of the client and family, home care nurse, home respiratory therapist, and home oxygen equipment vendor. The social worker usually assists with arranging for the home care nurse and oxygen vendor. The nurse must assist the client and family in learning about home oxygen and ensure their ability to maintain the oxygen delivery system.

Restoration of Cardiopulmonary Functioning. If a client's hypoxia is severe and prolonged, cardiac arrest may result. A cardiac arrest is a sudden cessation of cardiac output and circulation. When this occurs, oxygen is not delivered to tissues, carbon dioxide is not transported from tissues, tissue metabolism becomes anaerobic, and metabolic and respiratory acidosis occur. Permanent heart, brain, and other tissue damage occurs within 4 to 6 minutes.

Cardiopulmonary Resuscitation. Cardiac arrest is characterized by an absence of pulse and respiration. If the nurse determines that the client has cardiac arrest, **cardiopulmonary resuscitation (CPR)** must be initiated. CPR is a basic emergency procedure of artificial respiration and manual external cardiac massage (Skill 39-6). Most nursing students are required to have successfully completed a CPR course before their clinical experiences.

The "ABCs" of cardiopulmonary resuscitation are to establish an *Airway*, initiate *Breathing*, and maintain *Circulation*. When an airway cannot be established, the nurse must reassess proper head position and assess for airway obstruction. There is no clinical benefit to cardiac compressions if an airway cannot be established. The purpose of CPR is to circulate oxygenated blood to the brain to prevent permanent tissue damage (AHA, 1994).

Restorative and Continuing Care. Restorative and continuing care may emphasize cardiopulmonary reconditioning as a structured rehabilitation program. **Cardiopulmonary rehabilitation** is actively helping the client to

Table 39-11 Home Oxygen Systems

Primary Use	Advantages	Disadvantages
Compressed Gas Cylinders Intermittent therapy, such as for exercise or sleep only	100% oxygen, relatively inexpensive, no loss of gas during storage, relatively portable, delivery of up to 15 L/min	Bulky, possibly unsightly, frequent refilling necessary with continuous use
Liquid Oxygen Systems High liter flows and active clients	100% oxygen, conveniently portable, portable units refilled at home, delivery of up to 6 L/min	Usually weekly delivery necessary for refill, evaporates if not used, potential for frostbite at connections and if liquid is spilled
Concentrators Moderate liter flows and clients with limited mobility inside or outside home	Fixed monthly cost, minimal interruption of household by supplier, no refills of "main tank," most units with delivery of up to 4 or 5 L/min	Oxygen concentration decreases as liter flow increases (usually 85% to 90%), power supply necessary, electric bill increase of $15 to $20 a month, second system for portability necessary (usually gas cylinders)

Modified from Dettenmeier PA: *Pulmonary nursing care*, St. Louis, 1992, Mosby.

Skill 39-5 Using Home Liquid Oxygen Equipment

Delegation Considerations

This skill can be delegated to appropriately trained assistive personnel. The nurse is responsible for assessing and checking the device setup and the client.

- Inform and assist care provider in the proper way to set up and use home oxygen equipment.

- Instruct care provider regarding unexpected outcomes associated with use of home oxygen and the need to inform the nurse if any occur.

EQUIPMENT

- Nasal cannula equipment (see Skill 39-4)

- Primary and portable liquid oxygen source for ambulation (see Figure 39-26)

STEPS	RATIONALE
1. Assess: a. Client for need for home oxygen therapy.	Candidates for home oxygen have a PaO_2 ≤55 mm Hg or oxygen saturation of 88% on room air, or PaO_2 of 55 to 59 mm Hg or oxygen saturation of 86% to 89% with evidence of right heart failure, cor pulmonale, or polycythemia.
b. Client's or family's ability to use oxygen equipment properly, or for appropriate use of oxygen equipment in home setting.	Physical or cognitive impairments may require instructing family members or significant others on how to operate home oxygen equipment.
c. Client's and family's ability to observe for signs and symptoms of hypoxia: apprehension, anxiety, decreased ability to concentrate, decreased level of consciousness, increased fatigue, dizziness, behavioral changes, increased pulse, increased respiratory rate, pallor, or cyanosis of the mucous membranes.	Hypoxia can occur at home despite use of oxygen therapy. It can be caused by worsening of client's physical condition or another underlying condition, such as a change in the respiratory status.
2. Explain procedure to client and family.	Reinforces information given to client and family; allows opportunity to ask questions.
3. Wash hands.	Reduces transmission of infection.
4. Demonstrate steps for preparation and completion of oxygen therapy.	Teaches psychomotor skill and enables client to ask questions.
5. Prepare primary and portable oxygen a. Place primary oxygen source in clutter-free environment.	Primary oxygen source replaces compressed oxygen cylinders.

Critical Decision Point: Check oxygen levels in the primary and portable sources to ensure that there is an adequate supply, especially when leaving the home.

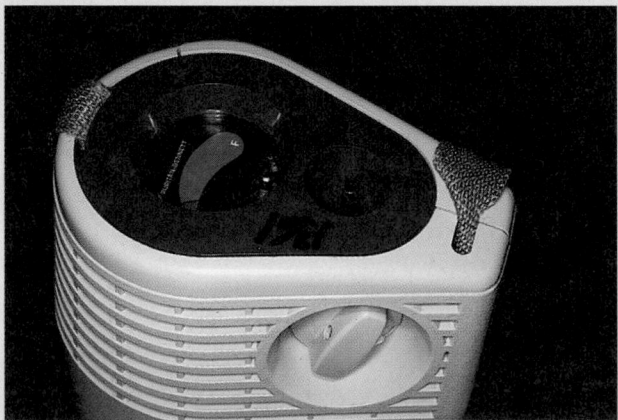 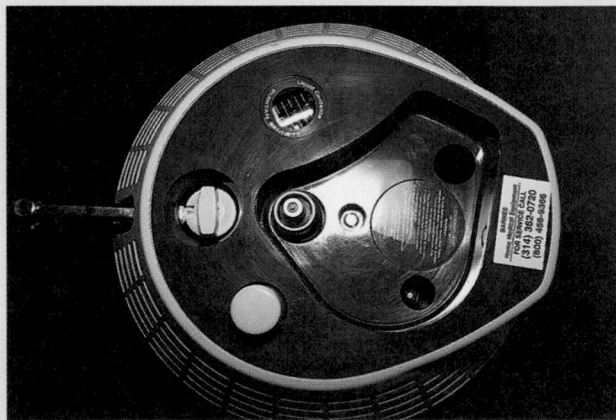

Step 5b

STEPS	RATIONALE
b. Check oxygen levels of both sources by reading gauge on top (see illustrations).	Ensures adequate amount of oxygen available for use and timely refills of primary source.
c. Refill portable source by placing on top of primary source and pressing down firmly. Check oxygen gauge to determine fullness of portable source (see illustration).	Provides secure connection and prevents leakage of oxygen into room. If not seated securely, the cold liquid oxygen will leak out, creating a snowlike precipitate.
d. Select prescribed rate.	Ensures delivery of prescribed amount of oxygen.
e. Connect nasal cannula and oxygen tubing to oxygen source.	Connects oxygen source to delivery method.
6. Have client and family perform each step with guidance from the nurse.	Allows nurse to correct for errors in technique and discuss their implications.

Critical Decision Point: Discuss signs and symptoms of respiratory tract infection: fever; increased sputum production; change in color, consistency or smell of sputum; difficulty clearing secretions or shortness of breath.

Recording and Reporting

• Record client's and family's ability to safely use the home oxygen equipment.

• If multiple care providers are in the home, report the type of equipment, client's and family's understanding, and any concerns to the additional providers.

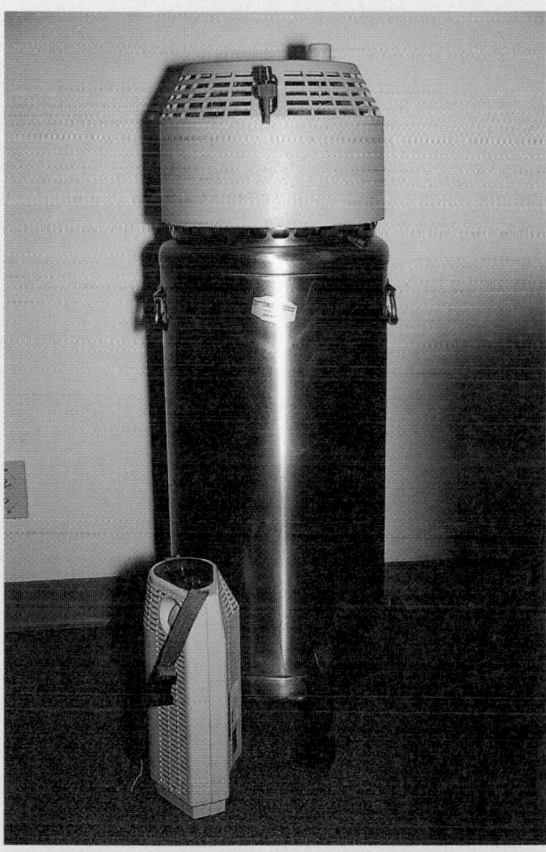

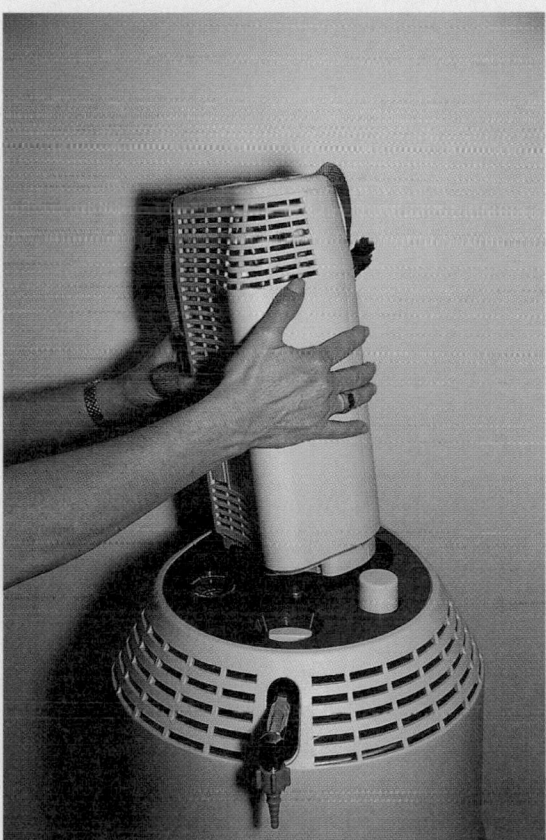

Figure 39-26   Primary and portable liquid oxygen source for ambulation.

Step 5c

Skill 39-6   Cardiopulmonary Resuscitation

Delegation Considerations

This skill of cardiopulmonary resuscitation (CPR) can be performed by trained assistive personnel.

- Caution care provider to make certain the client is indeed pulseless before initiating chest compressions.

- Review procedures for opening the airway if the client has any risk for cervical neck trauma.
- Caution care provider regarding differences between infants, children, and adults.

EQUIPMENT

- Ambu-bag, if available
- CPR pocket mask or barrier device, if available
- Chest compression board, if available

- Gloves, if available
- Resuscitation cart, if available
- Face shield, if available

STEPS	RATIONALE
1. Determine if client is unconscious by shaking client and shouting, "Are you OK?"	Confirms that client is unconscious as opposed to intoxicated, sleeping, or hearing impaired.
2. Activate emergency medical services. Know telephone numbers for access of emergency services, both in the community and in the hospital.	The majority of adult victims are in ventricular fibrillation and need defibrillation and antidysrhythmic drugs as soon as possible.
3. Determine breathlessness and carotid or brachial (use with infants) pulse.	Presence of pulse and respirations contraindicates initiation of CPR.
4. Place victim on hard surface such as floor, ground, or backboard. Victim must be flat. If necessary, logroll victim to flat, supine position using spine precautions.	External compression of heart is facilitated. Heart is compressed between sternum and spinal vertebrae, which must be on a hard and firm surface.
5. Assume correct and comfortable position.	Nurse may be administering CPR for extended period, particularly in community setting. Correct, comfortable position decreases skeletal muscle fatigue and promotes more effective compressions.
A. **One-person rescue** (1) Position to face victim, on knees, parallel to victim's sternum.	Allows rescuer to quickly move back and forth from victim's mouth to sternum.
B. **Two-person rescue** (1) One person faces victim, kneeling parallel to victim's head. Second person moves to opposite side and faces victim, kneeling parallel to victim's sternum.	Allows one rescuer to maintain breathing while other maintains circulation, without getting in each other's way.
6. If available, apply gloves and face shield.	Reduces transmission of microorganisms.
7. Open airway: a. If no head or neck trauma, use head tilt-chin lift method (AHA, 1994) (see illustration).	The tongue is the most common cause of airway obstruction in an unconscious client. Airway obstruction from the tongue is relieved. If necessary, remove foreign body.

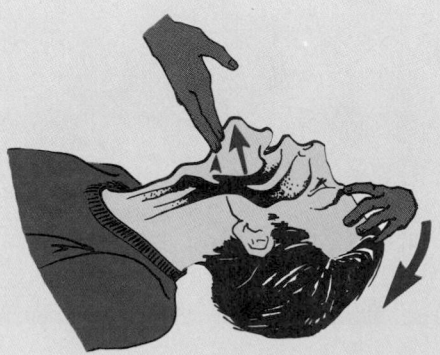

Step 7a

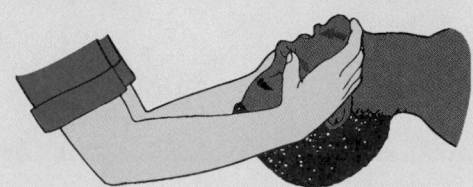

Step 7b

STEPS	RATIONALE
b. Jaw thrust maneuver (see illustration) can be used by health professionals but is not taught to general public. Grasp angles of victim's lower jaw and lift with both hands, displacing mandible forward while tilting head backward.	When head and/or neck trauma is suspected, this maneuver opens the airway while maintaining proper head and neck alignment, thus reducing the risk further damage to the neck.
8. If readily available, insert oral airway.	Maintains tongue on anterior floor of mouth and prevents obstruction of posterior airway by tongue.
9. If victim does not resume breathing, administer artificial respiration.	Airtight seal is formed, and air is prevented from escaping through nose.
A. **Mouth-to-mouth**	
Adult	
(1) Pinch victim's nose with thumb and index fingers, and occlude mouth with nurse's mouth or use CPR pocket mask. Maintain head tilt-chin lift while administering breaths so air enters lungs and not stomach. Blow two slow, full breaths into victim's mouth (each breath should take 0.5 to 2 seconds); allow victim to exhale between breaths. Continue giving 12 breaths per minute (AHA, 1994).	Hyperventilation is promoted and assists in maintaining adequate blood oxygen levels. In most adults this volume is 800 to 1200 ml and is sufficient to make the chest rise.
Child	
(2) Place nurse's mouth over child's mouth (see illustration) or use CPR pocket mask. For mouth-to-mouth resuscitation of child, administer two slow breaths lasting 1 to 1½ seconds with a pause between. Continue giving 20 breaths per minute (AHA, 1994).	Airtight seal is formed, and air is prevented from escaping from nose.
Infant	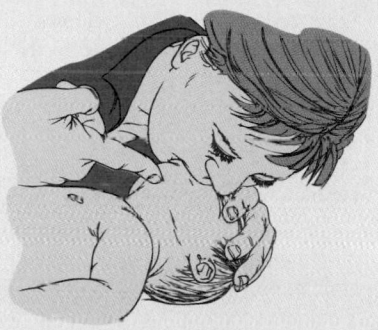
(3) Because an infant's air passages are smaller and resistance to flow is quite high, making recommendations about the force or volume of the rescue breaths is difficult. Place nurse's mouth over infant's nose and mouth. However, three factors should be remembered: (1) rescue breaths are the single most important maneuver in assisting a nonbreathing child, (2) an appropriate volume is one that makes the chest rise and fall, and (3) slow breaths provide an adequate volume at the lowest possible pressure, thereby reducing the risk of gastric distention.	**Step 9A(2)**
B. **Mouth-to-nose**	
(1) Keep victim's head tilted with one hand on forehead. Use other hand to lift jaw and close mouth. Seal nurse's lips around victim's nose and blow. Allow passive exhalation.	In some victims (those whose mouths cannot be opened or whose jaws or mouths are seriously injured) mouth-to-nose ventilation can be more effective.

Critical Decision Point: It may be necessary to open victim's mouth on occasion to allow trapped exhaled air to escape.

1186   Unit 7   Basic Human Needs

STEPS	RATIONALE

C. **Ambu-bag**
   Adult and child
   (1) For Ambu-bag resuscitation use proper-size face mask and apply it under chin, up and over victim's mouth and nose.

Airtight seal is formed; as bag is compressed, oxygen enters client.

10. Observe for rise and fall of chest wall with each respiration (see illustration). Listen for air escaping during exhalation, and feel for flow of air. If lungs do not inflate, reposition head and neck and check for visible airway obstruction, such as vomitus.

Repositioning ensures that airway is properly opened and that artificial respirations are entering lungs.

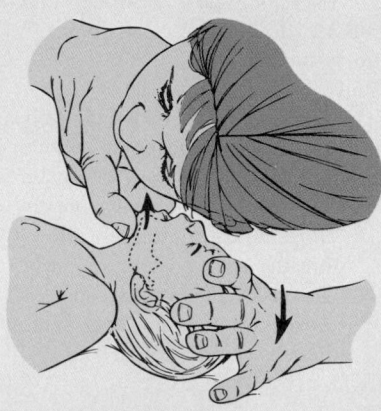

Step 10

11. Suction secretions if necessary, or turn victim's head to one side, unless contraindicated.
12. Check for presence of carotid (adults) or brachial (infants) pulse after restoring breathing.
13. If pulse is absent, initiate chest compressions:
    a. Assume correct hand position:

Suctioning prevents airway obstruction. Turning client's head to one side allows gravity to drain secretions.
Carotid artery pulse is the most easily accessible and persists when other peripheral pulses are no longer palpable.

   Adult
   (1) Place hands 1 to 2 cm above xiphoid process on sternum (see illustration). Keep hands parallel to chest and fingers above chest. Interlocking fingers is helpful. Keep fingers off of chest wall. Extend arms and lock elbows. Maintain arms straight and shoulders directly over victim's sternum.

Places hands and fingers over heart in proper position. Prevents xiphoid process and rib fracture, which can further compromise cardiopulmonary status.

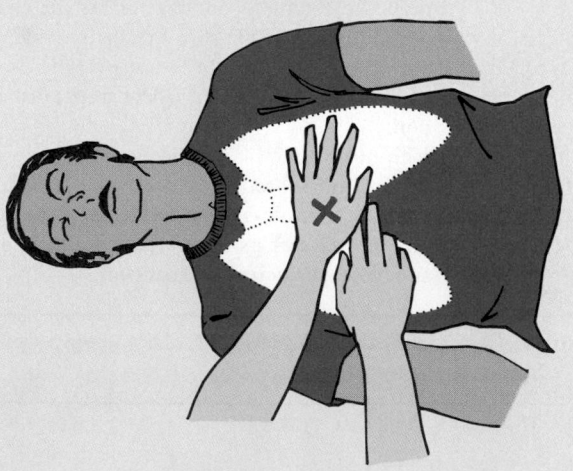

Step 13a (1)

STEPS	RATIONALE

Critical Decision Point: It is critical to keep hands off of the xiphoid process by marking that area with two fingers of one hand and then placing the heel of the other hand next to them. The hand marking the xiphoid process can then be moved and placed on top of the other hand.

Child
(2) Place heel of one hand 1 to 2 cm above xiphoid process (see illustration). Maintain head tilt with other hand, if possible, to maintain patent airway.

Infant
(3) Place index and middle fingers of one hand on sternum above xiphoid process. Fingers should be 1 cm below nipple line and perpendicular to sternum and not slanted (see illustration).

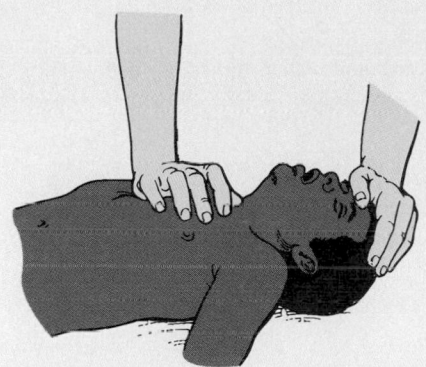

Step 13a(2)

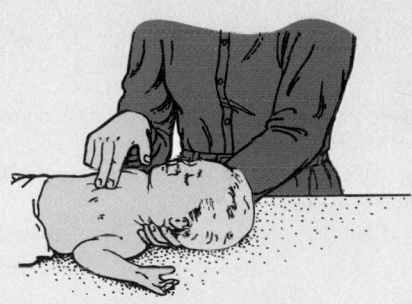

Step 13a(3)

b. Compress sternum to proper depth from shoulders and then release pressure, maintaining contact with skin to ensure ongoing proper placement of hands. Do not rock, but transmit weight vertically down.
   (1) Adult and adolescent: 4 to 5 cm (1½ to 2 inches) (see illustration).
   (2) Older child: 3 to 4 cm (1 to 1½ inches).
   (3) Toddler and preschooler: 2 to 4 cm (¾ to 1½ inches).
   (4) Infant: 1 to 2 cm (½ to 1 inch).

Compression occurs only on sternum and is meant squeeze the heart between the sternum and spin. Pressure necessary for external compression is created by nurse's upper arm muscle strength and upper body. When compression is released, the heart fills.

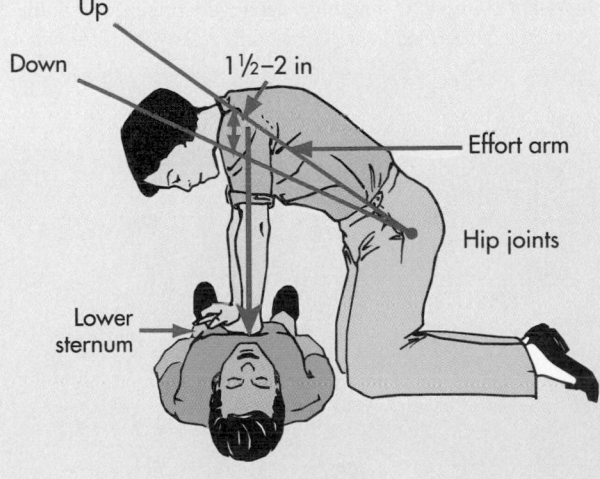

Step 13b(1)

STEPS	RATIONALE
c. Maintain proper rate of compression: (1) Adult and adolescent: 80 to 100/min (count "one 1000; two 1000"). (2) Older child: 100/min. (3) Child: 100/min. (4) Infant: at least 100/min.	Proper number of compressions per minute should delivered to ensure adequate cardiac output.

Critical Decision Point: Ratio of compressions to breaths for two rescuers is 5 to 1; for one rescuer, the ratio is 15 to 2.

STEPS	RATIONALE
d. Continue mouth-to-mouth or Ambu-bag ventilations. (1) Adult and adolescent: every 5 seconds (12/min). (2) Older child: every 4 seconds (15/min). (3) Child: every 3 seconds (20/min). (4) Infant and toddler: every 3 seconds (20/min).	Promotes adequate ventilations to excrete waste gas and supply oxygen.
14. Palpate for carotid or brachial pulse with each external chest compression for first full minute (two-person rescue). If carotid pulse is not palpable, compressions are not strong enough or hand position is incorrect.	Assessment of pulse validates that adequate stroke volume is achieved with each compression.
15. Continue CPR until relieved, until victim regains spontaneous pulse and respirations, until rescuer is exhausted and unable to perform CPR effectively, or until physician discontinues CPR.	Artificial cardiopulmonary function is maintained.
16. Remove and discard into appropriate receptacle: gloves, face shield, and pocket mask.	Reduces transmission of microorganisms.
17. Assess carotid pulse at 5-minute intervals following first minute of CPR.	Documents adequacy of external cardiac compressions.
18. CPR is not interrupted for more than 5 seconds.	Maintain adequacy of oxygenation and circulation.

Recording and Reporting

- Immediately report arrest, indicating exact location of victim. In hospital setting, follow hospital policy.
  In community setting, dial 911 or other emergency number.
- Record in nurse's notes and appropriate code sheet onset of arrest, medication, and other treatments given, procedures performed, and victim's response.

Home Care Considerations

- Assess home environment to determine presence of a suitable backboard and client's room to determine if there is sufficient room to pull client to the floor, if necessary, to perform CPR.
- A mouthpiece for CPR should be kept handy during all home health visits, and family should be advised to obtain mouthpieces when appropriate.
- If client is at high risk for cardiopulmonary arrest, family or caregivers should be instructed and certified in CPR.
- Client and family should keep emergency numbers taped to the phone. These numbers may include fire department, ambulance, hospital, and physician. Instruct client and family on whom to call.

achieve and maintain an optimal level of health through controlled physical exercise, nutrition counseling, relaxation and stress management techniques, prescribed medications and oxygen, and compliance. As physical reconditioning occurs, the client's complaints of dyspnea, chest pain, fatigue, and activity intolerance should decrease. The client's anxiety, depression, or somatic concerns also often decrease. The client and the rehabilitation team define goals of rehabilitation.

Respiratory Muscle Training. Respiratory muscle training improves muscle strength and endurance, resulting in improved activity tolerance. Respiratory muscle training may prevent respiratory failure in clients with COPD.

One method for respiratory muscle training is the **incentive spirometer resistive breathing device (ISRBD).** Resistive breathing is achieved by placing a resistive breathing device into a volume-dependent incentive spirometer. Muscle training is achieved when the client uses the ISRBD on a scheduled routine (e.g., twice a day for 15 minutes or 4 times a day for 15 minutes).

Breathing Exercises. Breathing exercises include techniques to improve ventilation and oxygenation. The three basic techniques are deep breathing and coughing exercises, pursed-lip breathing, and diaphragmatic breathing. Deep breathing and coughing exercises are routine interventions for postoperative clients (see Chapter 49).

Pursed-Lip Breathing. **Pursed-lip breathing** involves deep inspiration and prolonged expiration through pursed lips to prevent alveolar collapse. While sitting up, the client is instructed to take a deep breath and to exhale slowly through pursed lips, as if blowing through a straw. The nurse can also have the client blow through a straw into a glass of water to learn the technique. Clients need to gain control of the exhalation phase so that it is longer than inhalation. The client is usually able to perfect this technique by counting the inhalation time and gradually increasing the count during exhalation. In studies using pulse oximetry as a feedback tool, clients have been able to demonstrate an increase in their arterial oxygen saturation during pursed-lip breathing.

Diaphragmatic Breathing. **Diaphragmatic breathing** is more difficult and requires the client to relax intercostal and accessory respiratory muscles while taking deep inspirations. The client concentrates on expanding the diaphragm during controlled inspiration, and is taught to place one hand flat below the breastbone above the waist and the other hand 2 to 3 cm below the first hand. The client is asked to inhale while the lower hand moves outward during inspiration. The client observes for inward movement as the diaphragm ascends. These exercises are initially taught with the client in the supine position and then practiced while the client sits and stands. The exercise is often used with the pursed-lip breathing technique.

Diaphragmatic breathing is also useful for clients with pulmonary disease, for postoperative clients, and for women in labor to promote relaxation and provide pain control. The exercise improves efficiency of breathing by decreasing air trapping and reducing the work of breathing.

EVALUATION

Nursing interventions and therapies are evaluated by comparing the client's progress with the goals and expected outcomes of the nursing care plan. Client care evaluates the actual care given to the client by the health care team based on the expected outcomes (Figure 39-27). Client expectations evaluate the care from the client's perspective.

Client Care. The client is the only one who can evaluate his or her degree of breathlessness. The client should be asked to rate his or her breathlessness on a scale of 1 to 10, with 1 being no shortness of breath and 10 being severe shortness of breath (see Figure 39-11, p. 1145). Evaluation of arterial blood gases, pulmonary function tests, vital signs, ECG tracings, and physical assessment data provide the nurse with objective measurement of the success of therapies and treatments. Outcomes are compared with expected outcomes to determine the client's health status. Continuous evaluation allows the nurse to determine whether new or revised therapies are required and if new nursing diagnoses have developed and require a new plan of care. When nursing measures directed to improve oxygenation are unsuccessful, the nurse must immediately modify the nursing care plan. The nurse should not hesitate to notify the physician about a client's deteriorating oxygenation status. Prompt notification can avoid an emergency situation or even the need for CPR. Continuous evaluation allows the nurse to determine whether new or revised therapies are required and if new nursing diagnoses have developed and require a new plan of care.

Client Expectations. If the nurse has successfully developed a good relationship with a client, the client will be more willing to share his or her satisfaction. It is important for the nurse to ask the client if his or her expectations of care have been met. For example, the nurse can ask the client, "Do you feel like you will be able to use the breathing techniques we have practiced at home?" If the client states that he or she does not think this will work at home, then the client's expectations for care management have not been met. The nurse should ask the client whether all of his or her questions and needs have been met. If not, the nurse needs to spend more time understanding what the client wants and needs to meet his or her expectations. Working closely with the client will enable the nurse to redefine those client expectations that can be realistically met within the limitations of the client's condition and treatment.

KNOWLEDGE

- Characteristics of adequate oxygenation status

STANDARDS

- Use established expected outcomes to evaluate the client's response to care (e.g., pulse oximetry remains above 92%, respiratory rate remains between 20 and 24 breaths per minute)
- Apply intellectual standards of clarity, precision, specificity, and accuracy when evaluating outcomes of care

EVALUATION

- Reassess signs and symptoms of the client's oxygenation status after nursing interventions
- Ask for the client's perception of oxygenation after interventions
- Ask if the client's expectations are being met

EXPERIENCE

- Previous client responses to planned nursing therapies for impaired oxygenation

ATTITUDES

- Demonstrate perseverance when an intervention is unsuccessful and must be revised
- Use discipline to reassess and evaluate the client's signs and symptoms to determine the true success of interventions

Figure 39-27 *Synthesis Model for Oxygenation Evaluation Phase.*

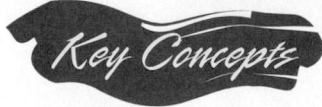

Key Concepts

- The primary function of the heart is to deliver deoxygenated blood to the lungs for oxygenation and to deliver oxygen and nutrients to the tissues.
- Preload, afterload, contractility, and heart rate alter cardiac output.
- Cardiac dysrhythmias are classified by cardiac activity and site of impulse origin.
- The primary function of the lungs is to transfer oxygen from the atmosphere into the alveoli and to transfer carbon dioxide out of the body as a waste product.

- Ventilation is the process of providing adequate oxygenation from the alveoli to the blood.
- Compliance, or the ability of the lungs to expand and contract, depends on the function of musculoskeletal and neurological systems and on other physiological factors.
- The process of inspiration (active process) and expiration (passive process) is caused by changes in intrapleural and intraalveolar pressures and lung volumes.
- Respiration is controlled by the central nervous system and by chemicals within the blood.
- Decreased hemoglobin levels alter the client's ability to transport oxygen.
- Impaired chest wall movement reduces the level of tissue oxygenation.
- Hyperventilation is a respiratory rate greater than that required to maintain normal levels of carbon dioxide.
- Hypoventilation causes carbon dioxide retention.
- Hypoxia occurs if the amount of oxygen delivered to tissues is too low.
- The nursing assessment includes information about the client's cough, dyspnea, fatigue, wheezing, chest pain, environmental exposures, respiratory infection, cardiopulmonary risk factors, use of medications, and physical functioning.
- Diagnostic and laboratory tests may be needed to complete the database for a client with decreased oxygenation.
- Pursed-lip breathing is an effective intervention to control breathing and increase oxygenation.
- Breathing exercises improve ventilation, oxygenation, and sensations of dyspnea.
- Relaxation techniques and imagery are valuable interventions in controlling dyspnea and anxiety in clients with chronic obstructive pulmonary disease.
- Nebulization delivers small drops of water or particles of medication to the airways.
- Chest physiotherapy includes postural drainage, percussion, and vibration to mobilize pulmonary secretions.
- Coughing and suctioning techniques are used to maintain a patent airway.
- Oxygen therapy is used to improve levels of tissue oxygenation and is delivered by a nasal cannula, nasal catheter, or oxygen mask.
- Cardiac arrest requires the use of cardiopulmonary resuscitation.

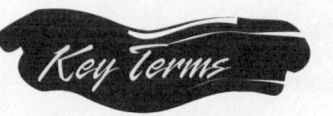

Key Terms

Accessory muscles, *p. 1130*
Afterload, *p. 1128*
Airway resistance, *p. 1130*
Angina pectoris, *p. 1138*
Angiography, *p. 1149*
Atelectasis, *p. 1139*
Atrioventricular (AV) node, *p. 1129*
Bronchoscopy, *p. 1153*
Bundle of His, *p. 1129*
Cardiac catheterization, *p. 1149*
Cardiac index (CI), *p. 1128*
Cardiac output, *p. 1128*
Cardiopulmonary rehabilitation, *p. 1181*
Cardiopulmonary resuscitation (CPR), *p. 1181*
Chest percussion, *p. 1163*
Chest physiotherapy (CPT), *p. 1163*
Chest tube, *p. 1172*
Compliance, *p. 1130*
Cough, *p. 1145*
Cyanosis, *p. 1140*
Diaphragmatic breathing, *p. 1189*
Diffusion, *p. 1132*
Dyspnea, *p. 1143*
Dysrhythmias, *p. 1135*
Echocardiography, *p. 1149*
Electrocardiogram (ECG), *p. 1129*
Electrophysiological study (EPS), *p. 1149*
Exercise stress tests, *p. 1149*
Hematemesis, *p. 1145*
Hemoptysis, *p. 1145*
Hemothorax, *p. 1172*
Holter monitor, *p. 1148*
Humidification, *p. 1162*
Hyperventilation, *p. 1138*
Hypoventilation, *p. 1139*

Hypovolemia, *p. 1133*
Hypoxia, *p. 1139*
Incentive spirometer resistive breathing device (ISRBD), *p. 1189*
Incentive spirometry, *p. 1172*
Left-sided heart failure, *p. 1138*
Myocardial contractility, *p. 1128*
Myocardial infarction, *p. 1138*
Myocardial ischemia, *p. 1138*
Nasal cannula, *p. 1177*
Nebulization, *p. 1162*
Normal sinus rhythm (NSR), *p. 1129*
Orthopnea, *p. 1145*
Oximetry, *p. 1150*
Peak expiratory flow rate (PEFR), *p. 1150*
Pneumothorax, *p. 1172*
Postural drainage, *p. 1164*
Preload, *p. 1128*
Productive cough, *p. 1145*
Pulmonary function tests, *p. 1149*
Purkinje network, *p. 1129*
Pursed-lip breathing, *p. 1189*
Right-sided heart failure, *p. 1138*
Scintigraphy, *p. 1149*
Sinoatrial (SA) node, *p. 1129*
Stroke volume, *p. 1128*
Thoracentesis, *p. 1154*
Transtracheal oxygen (TTO) *p. 1177*
Valvular heart disease, *p. 1138*
Ventilation, *p. 1129*
Vibration, *p. 1163*
Wheezing, *p. 1145*

Critical Thinking Exercises

1. Ms. Wanda Johnson is a 56-year-old postmenopausal woman with a history of hypertension. What would you include in the teaching portion of her plan of care?

2. Mr. Jose Martinez has recently immigrated to the United States from his homeland of Cuba to join his family. He comes to the primary care office to establish a health care provider and because he has been increasingly fatigued, has had a persistent cough, and has been losing weight. What questions would be important to ask when completing the health history interview?

3. Mrs. Amanda Miller, age 45, has been admitted to the hospital with community-acquired pneumonia. She has a productive cough, fever, chills, crackles and wheezes on auscultation of her chest, and a heart rate of 104 beats per minute. What nursing diagnosis would you consider for this client?

4. Mr. Chen Lee, age 72, has been having chest pain, shortness of breath, and pain down his left arm for about 2 hours. He comes to the emergency department for care. What nursing diagnosis would be appropriate for this client?

References

Advisory Committee on Immunization Practices: Recommendations for the prevention and control of influenza, *MMWR Morb Mortal Wkly Rep* 46(RR-9), 1997.

Alexander RW and others, editors: *Hurst's the heart: arteries and veins: companion handbook,* New York, 1999, McGraw-Hill.

American Association of Respiratory Care: AARC clinical practice guidelines, postural drainage therapy, *Respir Care* 36(12):1418, 1991.

American Cancer Society: *Cancer facts and figures—1998,* Atlanta, 1998, The Society.

American Heart Association: *Basic life support for health care providers,* Dallas, 1994, The Association.

Bell DA: Do incentive spirometers reduce the rate of postoperative complications? *Perspect Respir Nurs* 4(3):1, 1993.

Benner P: *From novice to expert,* Philadelphia, 1984, Addison-Wesley.

Canobbio MM: *Cardiovascular disorders,* St. Louis, 1990, Mosby.

Dettenmeier PA: *Pulmonary nursing care,* St. Louis, 1992, Mosby.

Emergency Cardiac Care (ECC) Committee and Subcommittee, American Heart Association: Guidelines for cardiopulmonary resuscitation and emergency cardiac care, *JAMA* 268:217, 1992.

Gift AG, Moore T, Soeken K: Relaxation to reduce dyspnea and anxiety in COPD patients, *Nurs Res* 41(4):242, 1992.

Jensen K, King KM: Women and heart disease: the issues, *Crit Care Nurs* 17(2):45, 1997.

Johnson M, Maas M, Moorhead S: *Nursing outcomes classification (NOC)* ed 2, St. Louis, 2000, Mosby.

Joint National Committee on Prevention, Detection, Evaluation and Treatment of High Blood Pressure: The sixth report of the Joint National Committee on Prevention, Detection, Evaluation and Treatment of High Blood Pressure (JNC VI), *Arch Intern Med* 157:2413, 1997.

Karper WB, Boshen MB: Effects of exercise on acute respiratory tract infections and related symptoms, *Geriatr Nurs* 14(1):15, 1993.

Kollef MH and others: Mechanical ventilation with or without daily changes of in-line suction catheters, *Am J Respir Crit Care Med* 156:466, 1997.

Lewis SM and others: *Medical-surgical nursing: assessment and management of clinical problems,* ed 5, St. Louis, 2000, Mosby.

Lueckenotte AG: *Pocket guide to gerontologic assessment,* ed 3, St. Louis, 1998, Mosby.

Lueckenotte AG: *Gerontologic nursing,* ed 2, St. Louis, 2000, Mosby.

McCance KL, Huether SE: *Pathophysiology: the biologic basis for disease in adults and children,* ed 3, St. Louis, 1998, Mosby.

McCloskey JC, Bulechek GM: *Nursing interventions classification (NIC),* ed 3, St. Louis, 2000, Mosby.

Mosby's patient teaching guides, St. Louis, 1998, Mosby.

Pierson DJ: Effects of aging on the respiratory system. In Pierson DJ, Kacmarek RM, editors: *Foundations of respiratory care,* New York, 1992, Churchill Livingstone.

Respiratory Nursing Society and American Nurses Association: *Standards and scope of respiratory nursing practice,* Washington, DC, 1994, American Nurses Publishing.

Sonnesso G: Are you ready to use pulse oximetry? *Nurs 91* 21(8):60, 1991.

Thompson J and others: *Mosby's manual of clinical nursing,* ed 3, St. Louis, 1993, Mosby.

Weilitz PB: *Pocket guide to respiratory care,* St. Louis, 1991, Mosby.

Wilson SF, Thompson JM: *Respiratory disorders,* St. Louis, 1990, Mosby.

40

Fluid, Electrolyte, and Acid-Base Balances

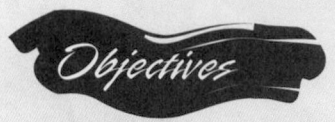

Mastery of content in this chapter will enable the student to:

- Define the key terms listed.
- Describe the distribution, composition, movement, and regulation of body fluids.
- Describe the regulation and movement of sodium, potassium, calcium, magnesium, chloride, bicarbonate, and phosphate.
- Describe the processes involved in acid-base balance.
- Describe common disturbances in fluid, electrolyte, and acid-base balances.
- Identify the variables affecting normal fluid, electrolyte, and acid-base balances.
- Discuss the clinical assessment for a client for fluid, electrolyte, and acid-base balances.
- Describe laboratory studies associated with fluid, electrolyte, and acid-base imbalances.
- List and discuss nursing interventions for clients with fluid, electrolyte, and acid-base imbalances.
- Discuss purpose, procedure, and maintenance of intravenous therapy.
- Calculate intravenous flow rate.
- Measure and record fluid intake and output.
- Demonstrate how to change intravenous solutions, tubing, and dressings and how to discontinue an infusion.
- Discuss the complications of intravenous therapy.
- Discuss the procedure for administering a blood transfusion and nursing actions for a transfusion reaction.

Fluid, electrolyte, and acid-base balances within the body are necessary to maintain health and function in all body systems. These balances are maintained by the intake and output of water and electrolytes and regulation by the renal and pulmonary systems. Imbalances may result from many factors, including illnesses, altered fluid intake, or prolonged episodes of vomiting or diarrhea. Acid-base balance is necessary for many physiological processes, and imbalances can alter respiration, metabolism, and the function of the central nervous system. Knowledge and understanding of the mechanisms that contribute to fluid, electrolyte, and acid-base imbalances are essential (Beare and Myers, 1998).

Scientific Knowledge Base

Water is the largest single component of the body; 60% of the average adult's weight is fluid. A healthy, mobile, well-oriented adult can usually maintain normal fluid, electrolyte, and acid-base balances because of the body's adaptive physiological mechanisms.

DISTRIBUTION OF BODY FLUIDS

Body fluids are distributed in two distinct compartments, one containing **intracellular fluids** and the other **extracellular fluids** (Table 40-1). Intracellular fluid (ICF) comprises all fluid within body cells. This fluid contains dissolved solutes essential to fluid and electrolyte balance and metabolism. In adults, approximately 40% of body weight

is ICF (Beare and Myers, 1998). Many of the solutes in the intracellular fluid compartment are the same as those located in the extracellular fluid space. However, the proportion of the substances is different. For example, a larger proportion of potassium exists in intracellular fluids than in extracellular fluids.

Extracellular fluid (ECF) is all the fluid outside a cell, which is divided into two smaller compartments: **interstitial fluid** and **intravascular fluid.** Interstitial fluid is the fluid between the cells and outside the blood vessels, whereas intravascular fluid is blood plasma. Other extracellular fluids are the lymph, transcellular, and organ fluids (McCance and Huether, 1998). Extracellular fluid makes up about 20% of the total body weight.

COMPOSITION OF BODY FLUIDS

As water moves through the compartments of the body, it contains substances that are sometimes called minerals or salts but are technically known as **electrolytes** (Christensen and Kockrow, 1998). An electrolyte is an element or compound that, when melted or dissolved in water or another solvent, separates into **ions** and is able to carry an electrical current. Positively charged electrolytes are **cations.** Negatively charged electrolytes are **anions.** Although the accumulation of electrolytes differs in ICF and ECF, the to-

The authors acknowledge the contribution of Susan Hauser Jefferies to this chapter in the previous edition of this text.

Table 40-1	Electrolyte Distribution in Body Fluid	
Electrolytes	Extracellular (mEq/L)	Intracellular (mEq/L)
Sodium (Na$^+$)	135-154	15-20
Potassium (K$^+$)	3.5-5	150-155
Calcium (Ca^{2+})	4.5-5.5	1-2
Bicarbonate (HCO$_3^-$)	25-27	10-12
Chloride (Cl$^-$)	98-106	1-4
Magnesium (Mg^{2+})	4.5-5.5	27-29
Phosphate (PO$_4^{3-}$)	1.7-4.6	100-104

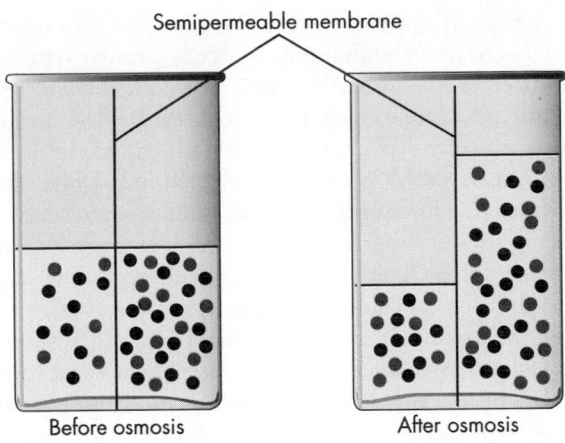

Figure 40-1   Osmosis through a semipermeable membrane.
From Lewis SM, Collier IC, Heitkemper M: *Medical-surgical nursing: assessment and management of clinical problems*, ed 4, St. Louis, 1996, Mosby.

tal number of anions and cations in each fluid compartment should be the same.

Electrolytes are vital to many body functions. The value **milliequivalents per liter (mEq/L)** represents the number of grams of the specific electrolyte **(solute)** dissolved in a liter of plasma **(solution).** The solution in which a solute is dissolved is called a **solvent** (Weldy, 1996).

Minerals, which are ingested as compounds, are usually referred to by the name of a metal, nonmetal, radical, or phosphate rather than by the name of the compound of which they are a part. They are constituents of all body tissues and fluids and are important in maintaining physiological processes. Minerals also act as catalysts in nerve response, muscle contraction, and metabolism of nutrients in foods. In addition, they regulate electrolyte balance and hormone production and strengthen skeletal structures. Examples of minerals include iron and zinc.

Cells are the functional basic units of all living tissue. Examples of cells within body fluids are the red blood cell (RBC) and the white blood cell (WBC).

MOVEMENT OF BODY FLUIDS

Fluids and electrolytes constantly shift from compartment to compartment to facilitate body processes such as tissue oxygenation, acid-base balance, and urine formation. Because cell membranes separating the body fluid compartments are selectively permeable, water can pass through them easily. However, most ions and molecules pass through them more slowly. Fluids and solutes move across these membranes by four processes: osmosis, diffusion, filtration, and active transport.

Osmosis involves the movement of a pure solvent, such as water, through a semipermeable membrane from an area of lesser solute concentration to an area of greater solute concentration (Figure 40-1). The membrane is permeable to the solvent, but it is impermeable to the solute. The rate of osmosis depends on the concentration of the solutes in the solution, the temperature of the solution, the electrical charges of the solutes, and the differences between the osmotic pressures exerted by the solutions. The concentration of a solution is measured in **osmols,** which

reflect the amount of a substance in solution in the form of molecules, ions, or both. Boiling a hot dog is an example of osmosis. The concentration of molecules inside the hot dog is greater than in water. The water passes through the hot dog skin, a semipermeable membrane, in an attempt to equalize the number of molecules on both sides of the membrane. Finally, when the hot dog can no longer hold any water, the skin ruptures (Christensen and Kockrow, 1995).

Osmotic pressure is the drawing power for water and depends on the number of molecules in solution. A solution with a high solute concentration has a high osmotic pressure and draws water into itself. If the concentration of the solute is greater on one side of the semipermeable membrane, the rate of osmosis is quicker, and a more rapid transfer of solvent across the membrane occurs. This continues until an equilibrium is reached. The osmotic pressure of a solution is called its **osmolarity,** which is expressed in osmols, or milliosmols per kilogram (mOsm/kg) of the solution. The normal serum osmolarity is 280 to 295 mOsm/kg. Osmolarity is the measure used to evaluate serum and urine in clinical practice. Changes in extracellular osmolarity may result in changes in both ECF and ICF volume.

Solutions are classified as **hypertonic, isotonic,** or **hypotonic.** A solution with the same osmolarity as blood plasma is called isotonic. A hypertonic solution (a solution of higher osmotic pressure) pulls fluid from cells; an isotonic solution (a solution of same osmotic pressure) expands the body's fluid volume without causing a fluid shift from one compartment to another; and a hypotonic solution (a solution of lower osmotic pressure) moves fluid into the cells, causing them to enlarge. Each of these actions occurs through osmosis.

The osmotic pressure of the blood is affected by plasma proteins, especially albumin, a serum protein naturally produced by the body. Albumin exerts **colloid osmotic** or **oncotic pressure,** which tends to keep fluid in the intravascular compartment. At the venous end of capillaries, this oncotic pressure and decreased venous **hydrostatic pressure** (the force of the fluid pressure outward against a surface) draws water and waste products back into the capillaries to be filtered through the kidneys. At the arterial end of the capillary, the hydrostatic pressure is greater than the colloid pressure, causing fluid and diffusible solutes to move out of the capillary into the interstitial space. The excess fluid and solutes remaining in the interstitial space are returned to the intravascular compartment by the lymph channels (Weldy, 1996).

Diffusion is the movement of a solute (gas or substance) in a solution across a semipermeable membrane from an area of higher concentration to an area of lower concentration (Figure 40-2). The result is an even distribution of the solute in a solution. For example, when you pour a small amount of cream into a cup of black coffee, the cream left unmixed will diffuse through the whole cup of coffee (Weldy, 1996). A physiological example is the movement of oxygen and carbon dioxide between the alveoli and blood vessels in the lungs. The difference between the two concentrations is known as a **concentration gradient.**

Filtration is the process by which water and diffusable substances move together in response to fluid pressure. This process is active in capillary beds, where hydrostatic pressure differences determine the movement of water (Figure 40-3). When there is increased hydrostatic pressure on the venous side of the capillary bed, as occurs in congestive heart failure (CHF), the normal movement of water from the interstitial space into the intravascular

space by filtration is reversed, resulting in an accumulation of excess fluid in the interstitial space, known as **edema.**

Unlike diffusion, osmosis, and filtration, **active transport** requires metabolic activity and expenditure of energy to move materials across cell membranes. This allows cells to admit larger molecules than they would otherwise be able to admit or to move molecules from areas of lesser concentration to areas of greater concentration "uphill" (Figure 40-4). Examples of active transport are the sodium and potassium pump. Sodium is pumped out of the cell and potassium is pumped in, against the concentration gradient. This process makes it possible to keep a higher concentration of potassium in the ICF and a higher concentration of sodium in the ECF.

Active transport is enhanced by carrier molecules within a cell that bind themselves to incoming molecules. For example, glucose is able to enter cells after it binds with the transport vehicle insulin. Active transport is the mechanism by which cells absorb glucose and other substances to carry out metabolic activities.

REGULATION OF BODY FLUIDS

Body fluids are regulated by fluid intake, hormonal controls, and fluid output. This physiological balance is termed **homeostasis** (Horne and others, 1997). In health, the body is able to respond to disturbances in fluids and electrolytes to prevent or repair damage.

Fluid Intake. Fluid intake is regulated primarily through the thirst mechanism. The thirst-control center is located within the hypothalamus in the brain. Thirst is the conscious desire for water and is one of the major factors that determines fluid intake (Weldy, 1996). The **osmoreceptors** continually monitor the serum osmotic pressure, and when osmolality increases, the hypothalamus is stimulated. Eating potato chips is an example; the salt on the chips increases the osmotic pressure of the body fluids and stimulates the thirst mechanism (Beare and Myers, 1998). Increased plasma osmolality can occur with any condition that interferes with the oral ingestion of fluids, or it can occur with the intake of hypertonic fluids. The hypothalamus will also be stimulated when excess fluid is lost and **hypovolemia** occurs, as in excessive vomiting and hemorrhage. In addition, the stimulation of the renin-angiotensin-aldosterone mechanism, potassium depletion, psychological factors, and oropharyngeal dryness initiate the sensation of thirst (Figure 40-5).

The average adult's intake is about 2200 to 2700 ml per day; oral intake accounts for 1100 to 1400 ml, solid foods about 800 to 1000 ml, and oxidative metabolism 300 ml daily (Horne and others, 1997). Water oxidation (oxidative metabolism) is the by-product of cellular metabolism of ingested solid foods. Fluid intake requires an alert state. Infants, clients with neurological or psychological problems, and some older adults who are unable to per-

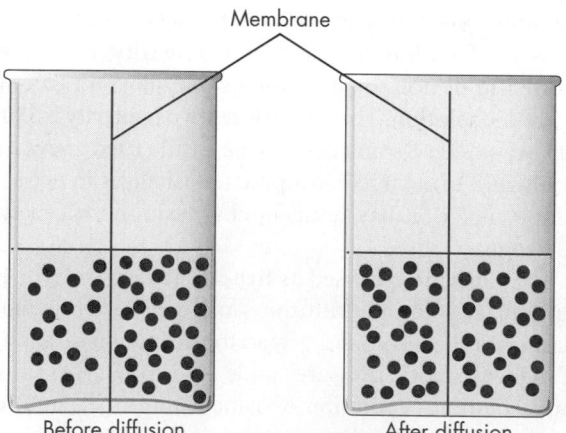

Membrane

Before diffusion   After diffusion

Figure 40-2 Diffusion across a semipermeable membrane. From Lewis SM, Collier IC, Heitkemper M: *Medical-surgical nursing: assessment and management of clinical problems,* ed 4, St. Louis, 1996, Mosby.

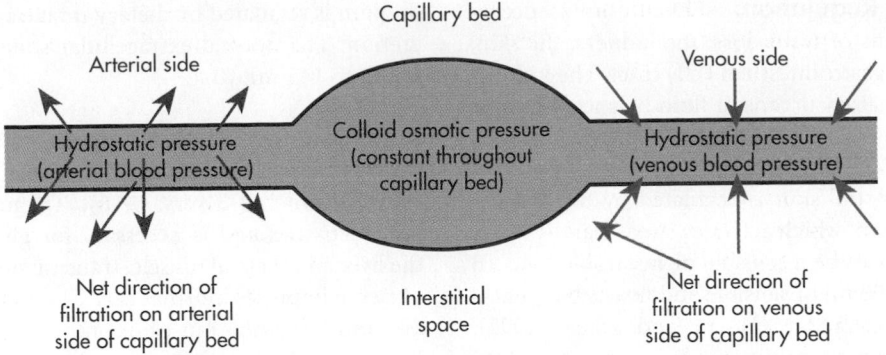

Figure 40-3 An example of filtration and hydrostatic pressure.

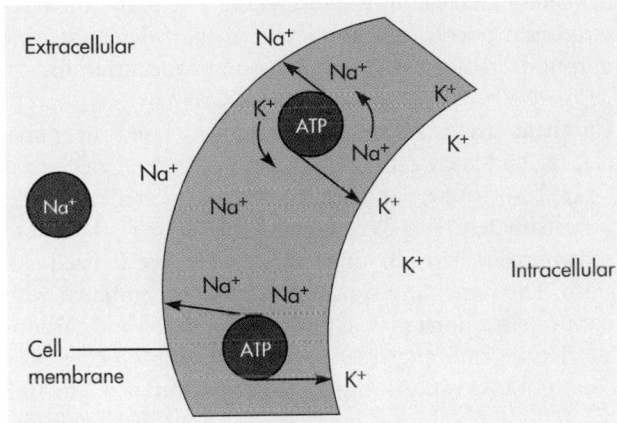

Figure 40-4 The sodium-potassium pump. As sodium diffuses into the cell and potassium out of the cell, active transport delivers sodium back to the extracellular compartment and potassium to the intracellular compartment.
From Lewis SM, Collier IC, Heitkemper M: *Medical-surgical nursing: assessment and management of clinical problems,* ed 4, St. Louis, 1996, Mosby.

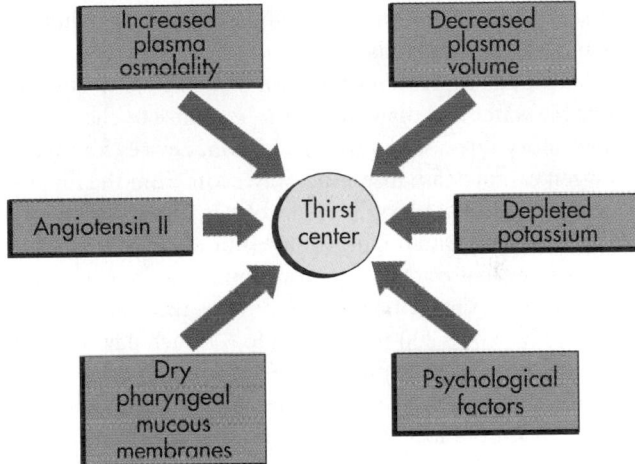

Figure 40-5 Stimuli affecting the thirst mechanism.

ceive or respond to the thirst mechanism are at risk for **dehydration.**

Hormonal Regulation. Hormones regulate fluid intake through various mechanisms. **Antidiuretic hormone (ADH)** is stored in the posterior pituitary gland and is released in response to changes in blood **osmolarity.** The osmoreceptors in the hypothalamus are stimulated when there is an increase in the osmolarity to release the hormone ADH. The ADH works directly on the renal tubules and collecting ducts to make them more permeable to water. This in turn causes water to return to the systemic circulation, which dilutes the blood and decreases its osmolarity. As the body attempts to compensate, the client will experience a decrease in urinary output temporarily. When the blood has been sufficiently diluted, the osmoreceptors stop the release of ADH and urinary output is restored.

Aldosterone is released by the adrenal cortex in response to increased plasma potassium levels or as a part of the renin-angiotensin-aldosterone mechanism to counteract hypovolemia. It acts on the distal portion of the renal tubule to increase the reabsorption (saving) of sodium and the secretion and excretion of potassium and hydrogen. Because sodium retention leads to water retention, the release of aldosterone acts as a volume regulator (Horne and others, 1997).

Renin, a proteolytic enzyme secreted by the kidneys, responds to decreased renal perfusion secondary to a decrease in extracellular volume. Renin acts to produce **angiotensin** I, which causes some vasoconstriction. However, angiotensin I almost immediately becomes reduced by an enzyme that converts angiotensin I into angiotensin II. Angiotensin II then causes massive selective vasoconstriction of many blood vessels and relocates and increases the blood flow to the kidney, improving renal perfusion. Angiotensin II also stimulates the release of aldosterone when the sodium concentration is low (Weldy, 1996).

Fluid Output Regulation. Fluid output occurs through four organs of water loss: the kidneys, the skin, the lungs, and the gastrointestinal (GI) tract. The kidneys are the major regulatory organs of fluid balance. They receive approximately 180 L of plasma to filter each day and produce 1200 to 1500 ml of urine (Table 40-2).

Water loss from the skin is regulated by the sympathetic nervous system, which activates sweat glands. Water loss from the skin can be a sensible or insensible loss. An average of 500 to 600 ml of sensible and insensible fluid is lost via the skin each day (Horne and others, 1997). **Insensible water loss** is continuous and is not perceived by the person but can increase significantly with fever or burns (Horne and others, 1997). **Sensible water loss** occurs through excess perspiration and can be perceived by the client or by the nurse through inspection. The amount of sensible perspiration is directly related to the stimulation of the sweat glands.

The lungs expire about 400 ml of water daily. This insensible water loss may increase in response to changes in respiratory rate and depth. In addition, devices for giving oxygen can increase insensible water loss from the lungs.

The GI tract plays a vital role in fluid regulation. Approximately 3 to 6 L of isotonic fluid is moved into the gastrointestinal tract and then returns again to the extracellular fluid. Under normal conditions, the average adult loses only 100 to 200 ml of the 3 to 6 L each day through feces. However, in the presence of a disease process, for example, diarrhea, the GI tract may become a site of a large amount of fluid loss. This loss may have a significant impact on maintaining normal fluid regulation.

REGULATION OF ELECTROLYTES

Cations. Major cations within the body fluids include sodium (Na^+), potassium (K^+), calcium (Ca^{2+}), and magnesium (Mg^{2+}). Cations interchange when one cation leaves the cell and is replaced by another. This occurs because cells tend to maintain electrical neutrality.

Sodium Regulation. Sodium is the most abundant cation (90%) in ECF. Sodium ions are the major contributors to maintaining water balance through their effect on serum osmolality, nerve impulse transmission, regulation of acid-base balance, and participation in cellular chemical reactions (McCance and Huether, 1998).

Table 40-2	Adult Average Daily Fluid Gains and Losses		
Fluid Gains	(ml)	Fluid Losses	(ml)
Oral fluids	1100-1400	Kidneys	1200-1500
Solid foods	800-1000	Skin	500-600
Metabolism	300	Lungs	400
		Gastrointestinal	100-200
TOTAL GAINS	2200-2700	TOTAL LOSSES	2200-2700

Sodium is regulated by dietary intake and aldosterone secretion. The normal extracellular sodium concentration is 135 to 145 mEq/L.

Potassium Regulation. Potassium is the major electrolyte and principle cation in the intracellular compartment (Beare and Myers, 1998). It regulates many metabolic activities and is necessary for glycogen deposits in the liver and skeletal muscle, transmission and conduction of nerve impulses, normal cardiac conduction, and skeletal and smooth muscle contraction (McCance and Huether, 1998). A relatively small amount (approximately 2%) of potassium is located within the ECF (Horne and others, 1997). The normal range for serum potassium concentrations is 3.5 to 5 mEq/L. Potassium is regulated by dietary intake and renal excretion. The body conserves potassium poorly, so any condition that increases urine output decreases the serum potassium concentration.

Calcium Regulation. Calcium is stored in bone, plasma, and body cells. Ninety-nine percent of calcium is located in bone, and only 1% is located in ECF. Approximately 50% of calcium in the plasma is bound to protein, primarily albumin, and 40% is free ionized calcium. The remaining small percentage is combined with nonprotein anions such as phosphate, citrate, and carbonate (Horne and others, 1997). Normal serum ionized calcium is 4 to 5 mEq/L. Normal total calcium is 8.5 to 10.5 mg/100 ml. Calcium is necessary for bone and teeth formation, blood clotting, hormone secretion, cell membrane integrity, cardiac conduction, transmission of nerve impulses, and muscle contraction.

Magnesium Regulation. Magnesium is essential for enzyme activities, neurochemical activities, and cardiac and skeletal muscle excitability. Plasma concentrations of magnesium range from 1.5 to 2.5 mEq/L. Serum magnesium is regulated by dietary intake, renal mechanisms, and actions of the parathyroid hormone (PTH). About 50% to 60% of body magnesium is contained within the bone, and only 1% is contained within the ECF compartment; the rest is located inside the cell (Beare and Myers, 1998).

Anions. The three major anions of body fluids are chloride (Cl^-), bicarbonate (HCO_3^-), and phosphate (PO_4^{3-}) ions.

Chloride Regulation. Chloride is the major anion in ECF. The transport of chloride follows sodium. Normal concentrations of chloride range from 95 to 108 mEq/L. Serum chloride is regulated by dietary intake and the kidneys. A person with normal renal function who has a high chloride intake will excrete a higher amount of urine chloride.

Bicarbonate Regulation. Bicarbonate is the major chemical base buffer within the body. The bicarbonate ion is found in ECF and ICF. The bicarbonate ion is an essential component of the carbonic acid-bicarbonate buffering system essential to acid-base balance. The kidneys regulate bicarbonate. Normal arterial bicarbonate levels range between 22 and 26 mEq/L; venous bicarbonate is measured as carbon dioxide content, and the normal value is 24 to 30 mEq/L.

Phosphorus-Phosphate Regulation. Nearly all the phosphorus in the body exists in the form of phosphate (PO_4^{3-}), and the terms phosphorus and phosphate often are used interchangeably (Horne and others, 1997). Phosphate is a buffer anion found primarily in ICF, with a small amount found in ECF. It assists in acid-base regulation. Phosphate and calcium help to develop and maintain bones and teeth. Calcium and phosphate are inversely proportional; if one rises, the other falls. Phosphate also promotes normal neuromuscular action and participates in carbohydrate metabolism. Phosphate is normally absorbed through the GI tract. It is regulated by dietary intake, renal excretion, intestinal absorption, and PTH. The normal serum level is 2.5 to 4.5 mg/100 ml.

REGULATION OF ACID-BASE BALANCE

For optimal functioning of the cells, metabolic processes maintain a steady balance between acids and bases. Arterial pH is an indirect measurement of hydrogen ion (H^+) concentration (i.e., the greater the concentration, the more acidic the solution and the lower the pH; the lower the concentration, the more alkaline the solution and the higher the pH). The pH is also a reflection of the balance between carbon dioxide (CO_2), which is regulated by the lungs, and bicarbonate (HCO_3^-), a base regulated by the kidneys (Horne and others, 1997). Acid-base balance exists when the net rate at which the body produces acids or bases equals the rate at which acids or bases are excreted. This balance results in a stable concentration of hydrogen ions in body fluids that is expressed as the pH value. Normal hydrogen ion level is necessary to maintain cell membrane integrity and the speed of cellular enzymatic actions. The pH is a scale for measuring the acidity or alkalinity of a fluid. A pH value of 7 is neutral, below 7 is acid, and above 7 is alkaline. Normal values in arterial blood range from 7.35 to 7.45. The three general types of acid-base regulators in the body are chemical, biological, and physiological buffering systems. A **buffer** is a substance or a group of substances that can absorb or release H^+ to correct an acid-base imbalance.

Chemical Regulation. The largest chemical buffer in ECF is the carbonic acid and bicarbonate buffer system (Figure 40-6). This system can be expressed as the following:

$$CO_2 \;+\; H_2O \;\rightleftharpoons\; H_2CO_3 \;\rightleftharpoons\; H^+ \;+\; HCO_3^-$$

Carbon + Water ⇌ Carbonic ⇌ Hydrogen + Bicarbonate
dioxide   acid   ion

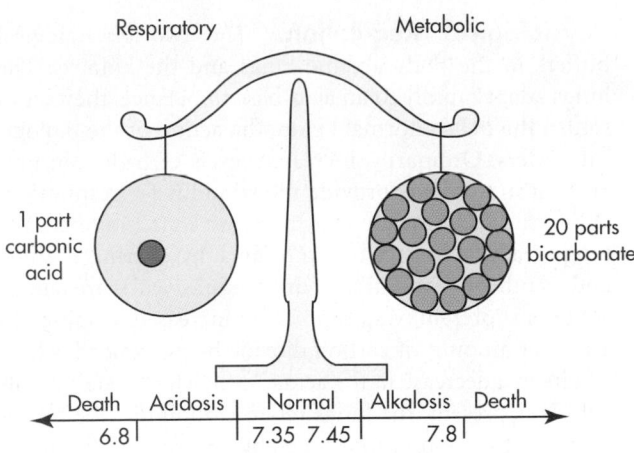

Figure 40-6 Carbonic acid-bicarbonate ratio and pH.

The carbonic acid-bicarbonate buffer system is the first buffering system to react to change in the pH of ECF, and it reacts within seconds. The equation demonstrates how hydrogen ions (H^+) and carbon dioxide (CO_2) concentrations are directly related to each other, in that an increase in one causes an increase in the other. Whenever carbon dioxide is made to increase, there is an increase in hydrogen ions produced, and whenever hydrogen ions are produced, there is more carbon dioxide produced (Ignatavicius, Workman, and Mishler, 1999). Remember, the excretion of carbon dioxide resulting from metabolism is controlled primarily by the lungs, and the excretion of hydrogen and bicarbonate ions is controlled by the kidneys.

Biological Regulation. Biological buffering occurs when hydrogen ions are absorbed or released by cells. Biological buffering occurs after chemical buffering and takes 2 to 4 hours. The hydrogen ion has a positive charge and must be exchanged with another positively charged ion, frequently potassium (K^+). In conditions with excess acid, a hydrogen ion enters the cell and a potassium ion leaves the cell and enters the ECF, thus causing an elevated serum potassium. An example is the release of fatty acids that occurs with diabetic ketoacidosis and starvation. A second biological buffer is the hemoglobin-oxyhemoglobin system. Carbon dioxide diffuses into the RBC and forms carbonic acid. The carbonic acid dissociates into hydrogen and bicarbonate ions. The hydrogen ions attach to hemoglobin, and the bicarbonate ion becomes available for buffering by exchanging with extracellular chloride (Kokko and Tannen, 1990).

Another biological buffer is the chloride shift within RBCs. When blood is oxygenated in the lungs, bicarbonate diffuses into the cells and chloride travels from the hemoglobin to the plasma to maintain electrical neutrality. The reverse occurs when carbon dioxide moves into the red cell in tissue capillary beds. This process is referred to as the chloride shift and is a reciprocal exchange between these anions (Groer and Shekleton, 1989).

Physiological Regulation. The two physiological buffers in the body are the lungs and the kidneys. The lungs adapt rapidly to an acid-base imbalance; they act to return the pH to normal before the action of the biological buffers. Ordinarily, increased levels of hydrogen ions and carbon dioxide provide the stimulus for respiration. When the concentration of hydrogen ions is altered, the lungs react to correct the imbalance by altering the rate and depth of respiration. For example, when metabolic acidosis is present, respirations are increased, resulting in a greater amount of carbon dioxide being exhaled, which results in a decrease in the acidic level; when metabolic alkalosis is present, the lungs retain carbon dioxide by decreasing the respirations, thereby increasing the acidic level (Beare and Myers, 1998).

The kidneys take from a few hours to several days to regulate acid-base imbalance. They reabsorb bicarbonate in cases of acid excess and excrete it in cases of acid deficit. In addition, the kidneys use a phosphate ion (PO_4^{3-}) to excrete hydrogen ions by forming phosphoric acid (H_3PO_4); sulfuric acid (H_2SO_4) may also be excreted. Finally, the kidneys use the ammonia mechanism to regulate acid-base balance. In this mechanism certain amino acids are chemically changed within the renal tubules into ammonia, which in the presence of hydrogen ions forms ammonium and is excreted in the urine, hence releasing hydrogen ions from the body (Beare and Myers, 1998).

DISTURBANCES IN ELECTROLYTE, FLUID, AND ACID-BASE BALANCES

Disturbances in electrolyte, fluid, or acid-base balances seldom occur alone and can disrupt normal body processes. When there is a loss of body fluids because of burns, illnesses, or trauma, the client is also at risk for electrolyte imbalances. In addition, some untreated electrolyte imbalances (e.g., potassium loss) result in acid-base disturbances.

Electrolyte Imbalances

Sodium Imbalances. Hyponatremia is a lower-than-normal concentration of sodium in the blood (serum), which can occur with a net sodium loss or net water excess (Table 40-3). It occurs frequently in seriously ill clients. Clinical indicators and treatment depend on the cause of hyponatremia and whether it is associated with a normal, decreased, or increased ECF volume (Horne and others, 1997). The usual situation is a loss of sodium without a loss of fluid, and this results in a decrease in the osmolality of ECF. The body initially adapts by reducing water excretion and thus sodium excretion to maintain serum osmolality at near normal levels. As the sodium loss continues, the body continues to preserve the blood and interstitial (tissue) volume. As a result, the sodium in ECF becomes diluted.

Hypernatremia is a greater-than-normal concentration of sodium in ECF that can be caused by excess water loss or an overall sodium excess (see Table 40-3). When the cause of hypernatremia is an increased aldosterone secretion, sodium is retained and potassium is excreted. When hypernatremia occurs, the body attempts to conserve as much water as possible through renal reabsorption.

Potassium Imbalances. Hypokalemia is one of the most common electrolyte imbalances, in which an inadequate amount of potassium circulates in ECF (see Table 40-3). When severe, hypokalemia can affect cardiac conduction and function. Because the normal amount of serum potassium is so small, there is little tolerance for fluctuations. The most common cause of hypokalemia is the use of potassium-wasting diuretics such as thiazide and loop diuretics.

Hyperkalemia is a greater-than-normal amount of potassium in the blood. Severe hyperkalemia produces marked cardiac conduction abnormalities (see Table 40-3). The primary cause of hyperkalemia is renal failure, because any decrease in renal function diminishes the amount of potassium the kidney can excrete.

Calcium Imbalances. Hypocalcemia represents a drop in serum and/or ionized calcium. It can result from several illnesses, some of which directly affect the thyroid and parathyroid glands (see Table 40-3). Another cause is renal insufficiency (in which the kidneys' inability to excrete phosphorus causes the phosphorus level to rise and the calcium level to decline). Signs and symptoms can be related to a diminished function of the neuromuscular, cardiac, and renal systems.

Hypercalcemia is an increase in the total serum concentration of calcium and/or ionized calcium. Hypercalcemia is frequently a symptom of an underlying disease resulting in excess bone resorption with release of calcium.

Magnesium Imbalances. Disturbances in magnesium levels are summarized in Table 40-3. Symptoms are the result of changes in neuromuscular excitability. Hypomagnesemia, a drop in serum magnesium, occurs with malnutrition and with malabsorption disorders, and signs and symptoms are directly related to the neuromuscular system. Hypermagnesemia is an increase in serum magnesium levels. It depresses skeletal muscles and nerve function. The depression of acetylcholine leads to a sedative effect, which can lead to bradycardia, ECG changes, cardiac arrhythmias, and decreased respiratory rate and depth (Beare and Myers, 1998).

Chloride Imbalances. Hypochloremia occurs when the serum chloride level falls below normal. Vomiting or prolonged and excessive nasogastric or fistula drainage can result in hypochloremia because of the loss of hydrochloric acid. The use of loop and thiazide diuretics also results in increased chloride loss as sodium is excreted. When serum chloride levels fall, metabolic alkalosis results

Table 40-3   Electrolyte Imbalances

Causes	Signs and Symptoms
Hyponatremia Kidney disease resulting in salt wasting Adrenal insufficiency GI losses Increased sweating Use of diuretics, especially when combined with low-sodium diet Psychogenic polydipsia Syndrome of inappropriate ADH (SIADH)	*Physical examination:* apprehension, personality change, postural hypotension, postural dizziness, abdominal cramping, nausea and vomiting, diarrhea, tachycardia, convulsions and coma, and fingerprints remaining on sternum after palpation *Laboratory findings:* serum sodium level <135 mEq/L, serum osmolality <280 mOsm/kg, and urine specific gravity <1.010 (if not caused by SIADH)
Hypernatremia Ingestion of large amounts of concentrated salt solutions Iatrogenic administration of hypertonic saline solution parenterally Excess aldosterone secretion Diabetes insipidus Increased sensible and insensible water loss Water deprivation	*Physical examination:* thirst, dry and flushed skin, dry and sticky tongue and mucous membranes, fever, agitation, convulsions, restlessness, and irritability *Laboratory findings:* serum sodium levels >145 mEq/L, serum osmolality >295 mOsm/kg, and urine specific gravity >1.030 (if not caused by diabetes insipidus)
Hypokalemia Use of potassium-wasting diuretics Diarrhea, vomiting, or other GI losses Alkalosis Excess aldosterone secretion Polyuria Extreme sweating Excessive use of potassium-free intravenous (IV) solutions Treatment of diabetic ketoacidosis with insulin	*Physical examination:* weakness and fatigue, decreased muscle tone, intestinal distention, decreased bowel sounds, ventricular dysrhythmias, paresthesias and weak, irregular pulse *Laboratory findings:* serum potassium level <3.5 mEq/L and electrocardiogram (ECG) abnormalities (e.g., ventricular dysrhythmias)*
Hyperkalemia Renal failure Fluid volume deficit Massive cellular damage such as from burns and trauma Iatrogenic administration of large amounts of potassium intravenously Adrenal insufficiency Acidosis, especially diabetic ketoacidosis Rapid infusion of stored blood Use of potassium-sparing diuretics	*Physical examination:* anxiety, dysrhythmias, paresthesia, weakness, abdominal cramps, and diarrhea *Laboratory findings:* serum potassium level >5.3 mEq/L and ECG abnormalities (bradycardia, heart block, dysrhythmias); eventually QRS pattern widens and cardiac arrest occurs*
Hypocalcemia Rapid administration of blood transfusions containing citrate Hypoalbuminemia Hypoparathyroidism Vitamin D deficiency Pancreatitis Alkalosis	*Physical examination:* numbness and tingling of fingers and circumoral region, hyperactive reflexes, positive Trousseau's sign (carpopedal spasm with hypoxia), positive Chvostek's sign (contraction of facial muscles when facial nerve is tapped), tetany, muscle cramps, and pathological fractures (chronic hypocalcemia) *Laboratory findings:* serum calcium level <4.0 mEq/L or 8.5 mg/100 ml and ECG abnormalities

*Data from Horne MM and others: *Mosby's pocket guide series: fluid, electrolyte, and acid-base balance,* ed 3, St. Louis, 1997, Mosby.

Continued

Table 40-3 **Electrolyte Imbalances**—cont'd	
Causes	Signs and Symptoms
Hypercalcemia	
Hyperparathyroidism	*Physical examination:* anorexia, nausea and vomiting, weakness, lethargy, low back pain (from kidney stones), decreased level of consciousness, personality changes, and cardiac arrest
Malignant neoplastic disease	
Paget's disease	
Osteoporosis	*Laboratory findings:* serum calcium level >5 mEq/L or 10.5 mg/100 ml; x-ray examination showing generalized osteoporosis, widespread bone cavitation, radiopaque urinary stones; and elevated blood urea nitrogen (BUN) level >25 mg/100 ml and elevated creatinine level >1.5 mg/100 ml caused by fluid volume deficit (FVD) or renal damage caused by urolithiasis; ECG abnormalities
Prolonged immobilization	
Acidosis	
Hypomagnesemia	
Inadequate intake: malnutrition and alcoholism	*Physical examination:* muscular tremors, hyperactive deep tendon reflexes, confusion and disorientation, dysrhythmias, and positive Chvostek's sign and Trousseau's sign
Inadequate absorption: diarrhea, vomiting, nasogastric drainage, fistulas; diseases of small intestine	
Excessive loss resulting from thiazide diuretics	*Laboratory findings:* serum magnesium level <1.5 mEq/L
Aldosterone excess	
Polyuria	
Hypermagnesemia	
Renal failure	*Physical examination:* physical findings that are more frequent in acute elevations in magnesium levels: hypoactive deep tendon reflexes, decreased depth and rate of respirations, hypotension, and flushing
Excess oral or parenteral intake of magnesium	
	Laboratory findings: serum magnesium level >2.5 mEq/L

*Data from Horne MM and others: *Mosby's pocket guide series: fluid, electrolyte, and acid-base balance,* ed 3, St. Louis, 1997, Mosby.

as the body adapts by increasing reabsorption of the bicarbonate ion to maintain electrical neutrality.

Hyperchloremia occurs when the serum chloride level rises above normal, which usually occurs when the serum bicarbonate value falls or sodium level rises. Hypochloremia and hyperchloremia rarely occur as single disease processes but are commonly associated with acid-base imbalance. There is no single set of symptoms associated with these two alterations.

Fluid Disturbances. The basic types of fluid imbalances are isotonic and osmolar. Isotonic deficit and excess exist when water and electrolytes are gained or lost in equal proportions. In contrast, osmolar imbalances are losses or excesses of only water so that the concentration (osmolality) of the serum is affected. Table 40-4 lists the causes and symptoms of common disturbances.

Acid-Base Balance. Arterial blood gas (ABG) analysis is the best way to evaluate acid-base balance. Measurement of ABGs, involves analysis of six components. Deviation from a normal value will indicate that the client is experiencing an acid-base imbalance. These six components are pH, $PaCO_2$, PaO_2, oxygen saturation, base excess, and HCO_3^-.

pH. pH measures hydrogen ion (H^+) concentration in the body fluids. Even a slight change can be potentially life threatening. An increase in concentration of H^+ makes a solution more acidic; a decrease makes the solution more alkaline. Normal pH value is 7.35 to 7.45 (acidic is <7.35, and alkalotic is >7.45).

$PaCO_2$. $PaCO_2$ is the partial pressure of carbon dioxide in arterial blood and is a reflection of the depth of pulmonary ventilation. The normal range is 35 to 45 mm Hg. When the $PaCO_2$ is less than 35 mm Hg, it is an indication that hyperventilation has occurred. As rate and depth of respiration increase, more carbon dioxide is exhaled and the carbon dioxide concentration decreases. When the $PACO_2$ is more than 45 mm Hg, hypoventilation has occurred. As rate and depth of respiration decrease, less carbon dioxide is exhaled and more is retained, increasing the concentration of carbon dioxide.

PaO_2. PaO_2 is the partial pressure of oxygen in arterial blood. It has no primary role in acid-base regulation if it is within normal limits. A PaO_2 less than 60 mm Hg can lead to anaerobic metabolism, resulting in lactic acid production and metabolic acidosis. There is a normal decline in PaO_2 in older adults. Hypoxemia also may cause hyperventilation, resulting in respiratory alkalosis (Horne and others, 1997). Normal range is 80 to 100 mm Hg.

Oxygen Saturation. Saturation is the point at which hemoglobin is saturated by oxygen (O_2). When a client is

Table 40-4   **Fluid Disturbances**

Causes	Signs and Symptoms
Isotonic Imbalances	
FLUID VOLUME DEFICIT (FVD)—WATER AND ELECTROLYTES LOST IN EQUAL OR ISOTONIC PROPORTIONS	
Losses from the GI system, such as from diarrhea, vomiting, or drainage from fistulas or tubes	*Physical examination:* postural hypotension, tachycardia, dry mucous membranes, poor skin turgor, thirst, confusion, rapid weight loss, slow vein filling, lethargy, oliguria, weak pulse
Loss of plasma or whole blood, such as with burns or hemorrhage	*Laboratory findings:* urine specific gravity >1.025, increased hematocrit level >50%, and increased BUN level >25 mg/100 ml (hemoconcentration)
Excessive perspiration	
Fever	
Decreased oral intake of fluids	
Use of diuretics	
FLUID VOLUME EXCESS (FVE)—WATER AND SODIUM RETAINED IN ISOTONIC PROPORTIONS	
Congestive heart failure	*Physical examination:* rapid weight gain, edema (especially in dependent areas), hypertension, polyuria (if renal mechanisms are normal), neck vein distention, increased venous pressure, crackles in lungs
Renal failure	
Cirrhosis of the liver	*Laboratory findings:* decreased hematocrit level <38% and decreased BUN level <10 mg/100 ml (hemodilution)
Increased serum aldosterone and steroid levels	
Excessive sodium intake or administration	
Osmolar Imbalances	
HYPEROSMOLAR IMBALANCE—DEHYDRATION	
Diabetes insipidus	*Physical examination:* dry and sticky mucous membranes, flushed and dry skin, thirst, elevated body temperature, irritability, convulsions, coma
Interruption of neurologically driven thirst drive	
Diabetic ketoacidosis	*Laboratory findings:* increased serum sodium level >145 mEq/L and increased serum osmolality >295 mOsm/kg
Osmotic diuresis	
Administration of hypertonic parenteral fluids or tube feeding formulas	
HYPOOSMOLAR IMBALANCE—WATER EXCESS	
SIADH	*Physical examination:* decreased level of consciousness, convulsions, coma
Excess water intake	*Laboratory findings:* decreased serum sodium level <135 mEq/L and decreased serum osmolality <280 mOsm/kg

hypoxic and uses up readily available oxygen, the reserve oxygen (oxygen attached to hemoglobin) is drawn upon to provide oxygen to the tissues (Ignatavicius, Workman, and Mishler, 1999). Oxygen can be affected by changes in temperature, pH, and $PaCO_2$. When the PaO_2 falls below 60 mm Hg, there is a large drop in saturation (Horne and others, 1997). Normal range is 95% to 99%.

Base Excess. Base excess is the amount of blood buffer (hemoglobin and bicarbonate) that exists. A high value indicates alkalosis and can result from the ingestion of large amounts of sodium bicarbonate solutions (some antacids), citrate excess with rapid blood transfusions, or intravenous infusion of sodium bicarbonate to correct ketoacidosis. A low value indicates acidosis and is usually the result of the elimination of too many bicarbonate ions. An example is diarrhea, where the increased intestinal motility that accompanies diarrhea forces the bicarbonate-containing fluid to be lost instead of being absorbed (Ignatavicius, Workman, and Mishler, 1999). The normal range is ±2.

Bicarbonate. Serum bicarbonate (HCO_3^-) is the major renal component of acid-base balance and is excreted and

reproduced by the kidneys to maintain a normal acid-base environment. It is the principal buffer of the extracellular fluids of the body, and once bicarbonate is in the ECF, it is maintained at a concentration of 20 times that of the fluid concentration of carbonic acid (Ignatavicius, Workman, and Mishler, 1999). The normal range is 22 to 26 mEq/L. Less than 24 mEq/L usually indicates metabolic acidosis, more than 28 mEq/L indicates metabolic alkalosis.

Types of Acid-Base Imbalances. The four primary types of acid-base imbalance are respiratory acidosis, respiratory alkalosis, metabolic acidosis, and metabolic alkalosis (Table 40-5).

Respiratory Acidosis. **Respiratory acidosis** is marked by an increased arterial carbon dioxide concentration ($PaCO_2$), excess carbonic acid (H_2CO_3), and an increased hydrogen ion concentration (decreased pH). With respiratory acidosis, the cerebrospinal fluid and brain cells become acidic, causing neurological changes. Hypoxemia occurs because of respiratory depression, resulting in further neurological impairment. Electrolyte changes such as hyperkalemia and hypercalcemia may accompany the acidosis.

Table 40-5 Acid-Base Imbalances

Causes	Signs and Symptoms
Respiratory Acidosis	
HYPOVENTILATION RESULTING FROM PRIMARY RESPIRATORY PROBLEMS	
Atelectasis (obstruction of small airways often caused by retained mucus)	*Physical examination:* confusion, dizziness, lethargy, headache, ventricular dysrhythmias, warm and flushed skin, muscular twitching, convulsions, and coma
Pneumonia	*Laboratory findings:* arterial blood gas alterations: pH <7.35, partial pressure of carbon dioxide in arterial blood ($PaCO_2$) >45 mm Hg, arterial partial pressure of oxygen (PaO_2) <80 mm Hg, and bicarbonate level normal (if uncompensated) or >26 mEq/L (if compensated)
Cystic fibrosis	
Respiratory failure	
Airway obstruction	
Chest wall injury	
HYPOVENTILATION RESULTING FROM FACTORS OUTSIDE OF THE RESPIRATORY SYSTEM	
Drug overdose with a respiratory depressant	
Paralysis of respiratory muscles caused by various neurological alterations	
Head injury	
Obesity	
Respiratory Alkalosis	
HYPERVENTILATION RESULTING FROM PRIMARY RESPIRATORY PROBLEMS	
Asthma	*Physical examination:* dizziness, confusion, dysrhythmias, tachypnea, numbness and tingling of extremities, convulsions, and coma
Pneumonia	*Laboratory findings:* arterial blood gas alterations: pH >7.45, $PaCO_2$ <35 mm Hg, PaO_2 normal, and bicarbonate level normal (if short lived or uncompensated) or <22 mEq/L (if compensated)
Inappropriate mechanical ventilator settings	
HYPERVENTILATION RESULTING FROM FACTORS OUTSIDE OF THE RESPIRATORY SYSTEM	
Anxiety	
Hypermetabolic states	
Disorders of the central nervous system (head injuries, infections)	
Salicylate overdose	
Metabolic Acidosis	
HIGH ANION GAP	*Physical examination:* headache, lethargy, confusion, dysrhythmias, tachypnea with deep respirations, abdominal cramps, and flushed skin
Starvation	*Laboratory findings:* arterial blood gas alterations: pH <7.35, $PaCO_2$ normal (if uncompensated) or <35 mm Hg (if compensated), PaO_2 normal or increased (with rapid, deep respirations), bicarbonate level <22 mEq/L, and oxygen saturation normal
Diabetic ketoacidosis	
Renal failure	
Lactic acidosis from heavy exercise	
Use of drugs (methanol, ethanol, formic acid, paraldehyde, aspirin)	
NORMAL ANION GAP	
Renal tubular acidosis	
Diarrhea	
Metabolic Alkalosis	*Physical examination:* dizziness; dysrhythmias; numbness and tingling of fingers, toes, and circumoral region; muscle cramps; tetany
Excessive vomiting	*Laboratory findings:* arterial blood gas alterations: pH >7.45, $PaCO_2$ normal (if uncompensated) or >45 mm Hg (if compensated), PaO_2 normal, and bicarbonate level >26 mEq/L
Prolonged gastric suctioning	
Hypokalemia or hypercalcemia	
Excess aldosterone	
Use of drugs (steroids, sodium bicarbonate, diuretics)	

Respiratory Alkalosis.   **Respiratory alkalosis** is marked by decreased $PaCO_2$ and increased pH. Like respiratory acidosis, respiratory alkalosis can begin outside the respiratory system (e.g., anxiety with hyperventilation) or within the respiratory system (e.g., initial phase of an asthma attack).

Metabolic Acidosis.   **Metabolic acidosis** results because of the high acid content of the blood, which also causes a loss of sodium bicarbonate, the alkaline half of the carbonate buffer system (Weldy, 1996). In an attempt to identify the cause of the metabolic acidosis, an analysis of serum electrolytes to detect an anion gap may be helpful. An **anion gap** reflects unmeasurable anions present in plasma and is calculated by subtracting the sum of chloride and bicarbonate from the amount of plasma sodium concentration (Table 40-6) (Horne and others, 1997).

Metabolic Alkalosis.   **Metabolic alkalosis** is marked by the heavy loss of acid from the body or by increased levels of bicarbonate. The most common causes are vomiting and gastric suction. Other causes include the overcorrection of metabolic acidosis, potassium deficiency, hyperaldosteronism, and the use of thiazide therapy that causes an increase of renal excreted acid (Beare and Myers, 1998).

Nursing Knowledge Base

Fluid and electrolyte imbalances may affect anyone regardless of age, sex, color, or religious beliefs. Infants, severely ill adults, disoriented or immobile clients, and older adults are frequently at greater risk because of their inability to respond independently to the early warnings of an impending problem. Over time, the body's adaptive compensatory mechanisms can no longer maintain fluid and electrolyte or acid-base balance adequately, and the client's health becomes compromised. The severity and long-term effects on the client's health will influence a client's ability to return to a state of optimal functioning. Prolonged or severe compromises may lead to irreversible chronic health problems that not only may change the lifestyle of the client but also may have an impact on the caregiver(s), guardians, parents, families, and/or friends (Box 40-1).

Critical Thinking Synthesis

Successful critical thinking requires a synthesis of knowledge, experience, information gathered from clients, critical thinking attitudes, and intellectual and professional standards. Clinical judgments require the nurse to anticipate the information necessary, to analyze the data, and to make decisions regarding client care. Critical thinking is always changing. During assessment (Figure 40-7) the nurse must consider all critical thinking elements, as well as data about the specific client, to make appropriate nursing diagnoses.

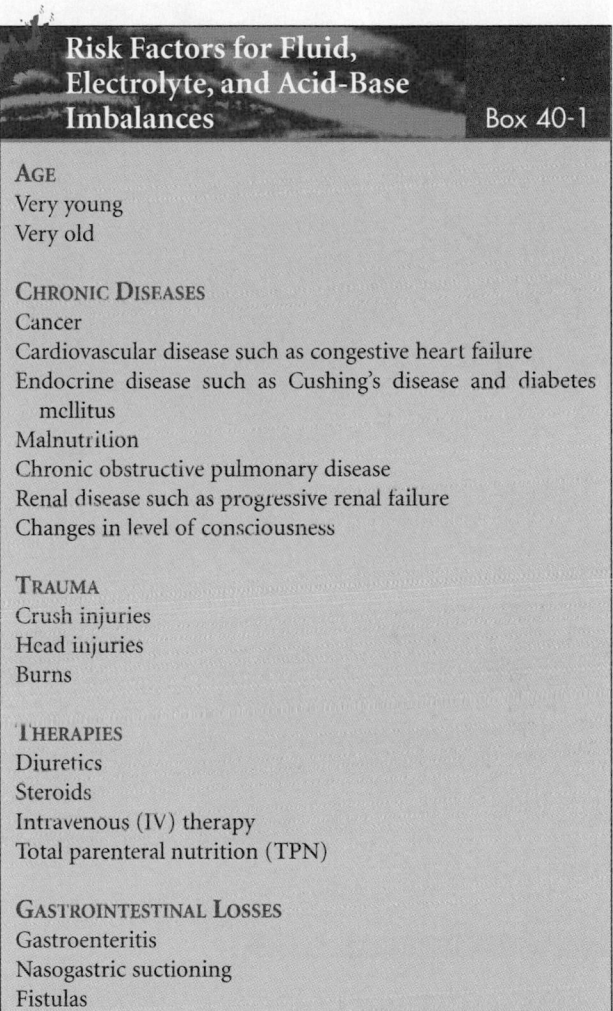

Risk Factors for Fluid, Electrolyte, and Acid-Base Imbalances   Box 40-1

AGE
Very young
Very old

CHRONIC DISEASES
Cancer
Cardiovascular disease such as congestive heart failure
Endocrine disease such as Cushing's disease and diabetes mellitus
Malnutrition
Chronic obstructive pulmonary disease
Renal disease such as progressive renal failure
Changes in level of consciousness

TRAUMA
Crush injuries
Head injuries
Burns

THERAPIES
Diuretics
Steroids
Intravenous (IV) therapy
Total parenteral nutrition (TPN)

GASTROINTESTINAL LOSSES
Gastroenteritis
Nasogastric suctioning
Fistulas

Table 40-6	**Anion Gap**	
Anion Gap Type	Values	Causes
Normal anion gap	12 ($\pm$2) mEq/L	Diarrhea, renal tubular acidosis, or pancreatic fistula causing a direct loss of HCO_3^-; addition of chloride-containing acids
Increased anion gap	>14 mEq/L	Lactic acidosis, uremia, diabetic ketoacidosis (DKA), or salicylate and methanol toxicity, resulting in accumulation of nonvolatile acids with decrease in HCO_3^-

From Horne MM and others: *Mosby's pocket guide series: fluid, electrolyte, and acid-base balance,* ed 3, St. Louis, 1997, Mosby.

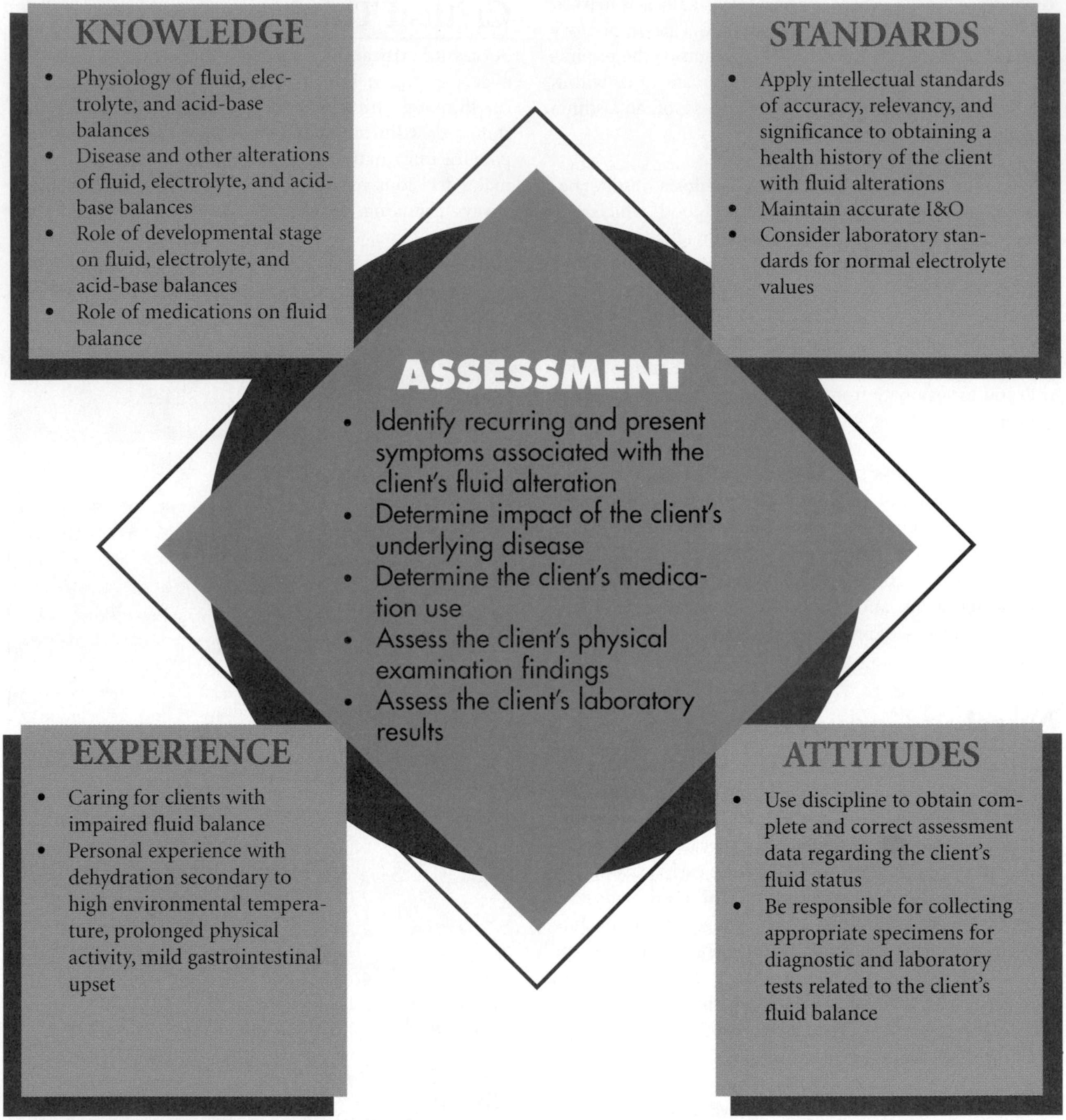

KNOWLEDGE

- Physiology of fluid, electrolyte, and acid-base balances
- Disease and other alterations of fluid, electrolyte, and acid-base balances
- Role of developmental stage on fluid, electrolyte, and acid-base balances
- Role of medications on fluid balance

STANDARDS

- Apply intellectual standards of accuracy, relevancy, and significance to obtaining a health history of the client with fluid alterations
- Maintain accurate I&O
- Consider laboratory standards for normal electrolyte values

ASSESSMENT

- Identify recurring and present symptoms associated with the client's fluid alteration
- Determine impact of the client's underlying disease
- Determine the client's medication use
- Assess the client's physical examination findings
- Assess the client's laboratory results

EXPERIENCE

- Caring for clients with impaired fluid balance
- Personal experience with dehydration secondary to high environmental temperature, prolonged physical activity, mild gastrointestinal upset

ATTITUDES

- Use discipline to obtain complete and correct assessment data regarding the client's fluid status
- Be responsible for collecting appropriate specimens for diagnostic and laboratory tests related to the client's fluid balance

Figure 40-7 *Synthesis Model for Fluid, Electrolyte, and Acid-Base Balances Assessment Phase.*

In the case of fluid, electrolyte, and acid-base balance, the nurse must integrate knowledge of physiology, pathophysiology, and pharmacology, as well as previous experiences and information gathered from clients. Critical analysis of data enables the nurse to understand how fluid, electrolyte, and acid-base imbalances affect the client and family. In addition, the use of critical thinking attitudes such as discipline and integrity is needed to correctly identify diagnoses and then plan successful interventions. The use of professional standards, such as those developed by the clinical laboratory for electrolyte values, provides valuable guidelines for comprehensive assessment.

Nursing Process

ASSESSMENT

The nurse understands the importance of fluid, electrolyte, and acid-base balances to homeostasis dynamics. By gathering assessment data through a history and physical examination, the nurse will identify clients at risk and then identify all appropriate nursing diagnoses.

Nursing History.   The nursing assessment begins with a client history, which is designed to reveal any risk factors or preexisting conditions that may cause or contribute to a disturbance of fluid, electrolyte, and acid-base balances. The nurse will explore with the client any factors that may cause a disturbance and integrate the information with knowledge of fluid volume regulation, electrolyte concentration, and acid-base regulation.

Age.   The nurse first considers the client's age. An infant's proportion of total body water is greater that that of children or adults. Infants are not protected from fluid loss because they ingest and excrete a relatively greater daily water volume than adults (Horne and others, 1997). Therefore they are at a greater risk for **fluid volume deficits (FVDs)** and hyperosmolar imbalance because body water loss is proportionately greater per kilogram of weight.

Children ages 2 through 12 have less stable regulatory responses to imbalance, and in childhood illnesses they tend to operate within a more narrow range with less tolerance for large changes. Children frequently respond to illnesses with fevers of higher temperatures and longer duration than those of adults. At any age, fever in childhood can increase the rate of insensible water loss.

Adolescents have increased metabolic processes and increased water production because of the major rapid changes that occur in the anatomical and physiological process. Changes in fluid balance are greater in adolescent girls because of hormonal changes associated with the menstrual cycle.

Older adults experience a number of age-related changes that can affect fluid, and electrolyte, and acid-base balances. The kidneys have a decrease in glomerular filtration rate and in the number of filtering nephrons (Lueckenotte, 1996). These changes can mean that in the presence of sodium depletion or overload the older adult may be unable to maintain homeostasis and the imbalance is instead worsened. In addition, older adults are at risk for decreased excretion of medications, which can lead to imbalances causing metabolic or respiratory acidosis, FVD, and hyperosmolar imbalance, hyponatremia, and hypernatremia (Horne and others, 1997). The changes in lung function that accompany aging can lead to respiratory acidosis and the inability to compensate for metabolic acidosis. Therefore the older adult who has any condition that involves renal function, fluid and electrolyte balance, or plasma volume and osmolality is more likely to experience more serious consequences (Beare and Myers, 1998).

Acute Illness.   Recent surgery, head and chest trauma, shock, and second- or third-degree burns are conditions that place clients at high risk for fluid, electrolyte, and acid-base alterations. Additionally, the client continues to be at risk during the acute phase until the underlying process is resolved. For example, the stress response of surgery may cause fluid-balance changes in the second to fifth postoperative day, when aldosterone, glucocorticoids, and ADH are increasingly secreted, causing sodium and chloride retention, potassium excretion, and decreased urinary output.

Surgery.   The more extensive the surgery and fluid loss during the surgical procedure, the greater the body's response to the surgical trauma. In addition, after surgery clients can exhibit many acid-base changes. The client who is reluctant to breathe deeply and cough may develop respiratory acidosis due to retained $PaCO_2$. The client with nasogastric suction may develop metabolic alkalosis due to the loss of gastric acid, fluids, and electrolytes.

Burns.   The greater the body surface burned, the greater the fluid loss. The burned client loses body fluids by one of five routes. First, plasma leaves the intravascular space and becomes trapped edema. This is also called the plasma-to-interstitial fluid shift. It is accompanied by a loss of serum proteins. Second, plasma and interstitial fluids are lost as burn exudate. Third, water vapor and heat are lost in proportion to the amount of skin that is burned away. Fourth, blood leaks from damaged capillaries, adding to the intravascular fluid volume loss. Last, sodium and water shift into the cells, further compromising extracellular fluid volume (Long and others, 1993).

Respiratory Disorders.   Many alterations in respiratory function predispose the client to respiratory acidosis. For example, the changes involved in pneumonia, sedative overdose, and exacerbated chronic airflow limitation interfere with the elimination of carbon dioxide as the client retains carbon dioxide during hypoventalation. As the carbon dioxide continues to build up in the bloodstream, the body's compensatory mechanisms can no longer adapt and the pH decreases. Likewise, hyperventilation that occurs with such conditions as fever or anxiety causes the client to experience respiratory alkalosis by blowing off too much carbon dioxide with the increased respiratory rate.

Head Injury.   Head injury can result in cerebral edema. Occasionally this edema creates pressure on the pituitary gland, and as a result, ADH secretion is changed. Two alterations can occur. Diabetes insipidus occurs when too little ADH is secreted and the client excretes large volumes of diluted urine with a low specific gravity. The second alteration is syndrome of inappropriate antidiuretic hormone (SIADH), in which there is continued inappropriate secretion of ADH. This results in water intoxication characterized by fluid volume expansion and hyponatremia, and hypotonicity of fluids as a result of high urine osmolality and low serum osmolality (Beare and Myer, 1998).

Chronic Illness.   Chronic disease (e.g., cancer, CHF, renal disease) comprises a variety of conditions that can create fluid, electrolyte, and acid-base imbalances. In the presence of chronic disease the nurse must review the normal course of such conditions to understand how fluid, electrolyte, and acid-base status may be affected.

Cancer.   The types of fluid and electrolyte imbalances that are observed in a client with cancer depends on the type and progression of the cancer. All electrolyte imbalances can occur in the client with cancer and are caused by anatomical distortion and functional impairment from tumor growth and tumor-caused metabolic and endocrine abnormality. In addition, clients with cancer are at risk for fluid and electrolyte imbalances related to the side effects (e.g., diarrhea and anorexia) of their chemotherapeutic and radiological treatments.

Cardiovascular Disease.   In the client with cardiovascular disease a diminished cardiac output reduce kidney perfusion, causing the client to experience a decrease in urinary output. The client will retain sodium and water, resulting in circulatory overload, and run the risk of developing pulmonary edema. Fluid and electrolyte imbalances associated with heart disease can be controlled for a time with medications and fluid and sodium restrictions. The goal of fluid reduction is to decrease the workload of the left ventricle by reducing the excess circulating fluid volume.

Renal Disorders.   Kidney disease alters fluid and electrolyte balance by the abnormal retention of sodium, chloride, potassium, and water in the extracellular compartment. The plasma levels of metabolic waste products such as blood urea nitrogen (BUN) and creatinine are elevated because the kidneys are unable to filter and excrete the waste products of cellular metabolism. This elevation is toxic to cellular processes. Metabolic acidosis results when hydrogen ions are retained due to decreased renal function. Because of the renal disorder, the usual renal compensatory mechanisms such as bicarbonate reabsorption are not available, so the body's ability to restore normal acid-base balance is limited.

The severity of fluid and electrolyte imbalance is proportional to the degree of renal failure. Occasionally, acute renal failure-induced shock or a decrease in extracellular fluid may be reversible. Although chronic renal failure is progressive, the client may be treated successfully with dietary control of protein and salt intake, diuretic medications, and fluid restrictions.

Gastrointestinal Disturbances.   Gastroenteritis and nasogastric suctioning result in a loss of fluid, potassium,

and chloride ions. Hydrogen ions are also lost, causing a disturbance in acid-base balance. Timely education of infant and child caregivers is necessary to prevent dehydration when the infant or child is experiencing diarrhea. Gastrointestinal fistulas can also result in a loss of potassium, resulting in an increased risk for hypokalemia. The loss of potassium increases the risk for acid-base disturbances as well.

Regardless of the presence of any disease process, the nurse must determine how long the client has suffered from that disease and the type of treatment currently being administered. In addition to chronic health problems, the nurse determines if the client has a history of new onset acute illnesses such as diarrhea, vomiting, colostomy, nasogastric suctioning, or intestinal drainage. Any condition that results in the loss of GI fluids predisposes the client to dehydration and a variety of electrolyte disturbances.

Environmental Factors.   The nurse should also include certain environmental factors in the nursing history. Clients who have participated in vigorous exercise or who have become exposed to temperature extremes may have clinical signs of fluid and electrolyte alterations. Exposure to environmental temperatures exceeding 28° to 30° C (82.4° to 86° F) results in excessive sweating with weight loss. A body weight loss over 7% decreases the ability of the cooling mechanism to conserve water. Loss of fluid from sweating varies and can reach a maximal rate of 2 L/hour (Ignatavicius, Workman, and Mishler, 1999). Inadequate fluid replacement can lead to fluid volume disturbances.

Diet.   A client's current dietary history is an important component of nursing assessment. Dietary intake of fluids, salt, potassium, calcium, magnesium, and necessary carbohydrates, fats, and protein helps maintain normal fluid, electrolyte, and acid-base status. Recent changes in appetite or the ability to chew and swallow can affect nutritional status and fluid hydration. When nutritional intake is inadequate, the body tries to preserve its protein stores by breaking down glycogen and fat stores. When excess free fatty acids are released, metabolic acidosis can occur because the liver converts free fatty acids to ketone, a strong acid. However, after those resources are depleted, the body begins to destroy protein stores. When serum protein levels drop below normal, hypoalbuminemia results. In hypoalbuminemia the serum colloid osmotic pressure is decreased, and fluid shifts from the circulating blood volume and enters the interstitial fluid space in the peritoneal cavity. Additionally, dieting can lead to acidosis, because rapid water loss can lead to osmolar fluid imbalance.

Lifestyle.   Lifestyle factors should also be included in the nurse's history. If a client already has preexisting medical risks, such as a history of smoking or alcohol consumption, they can further impair the client's ability to adapt to fluid, electrolyte, and acid-base alterations. For example, the consistent use of alcohol and tobacco use can ultimately cause respiratory depression, which can result in respiratory acidosis and alteration in maintaining adequate fluid and electrolyte balance.

Medication.   A final category to include in the nurse's assessment is a history of medication use (Box 40-2). If the assessment reveals a medication that is likely to cause an electrolyte or acid-base disorder, the nurse will also closely examine laboratory values. In addition, the nurse will assess the client's knowledge of side effects and adherence to medication schedules and the client's knowledge of the potential side effects of over-the-counter medications on fluid, electrolyte, and acid-base balances (Beare and Myers, 1998).

Physical Assessment.   A thorough examination is necessary, because fluid and electrolyte imbalances or acid-base disturbances can affect all body systems. While examining each system, the nurse carefully considers the signs and symptoms to expect as a result of any imbalance. For example, an examination of the oral cavity will likely reveal signs of dehydration if the nurse suspects the client is experiencing a fluid loss. Table 40-7 summarizes possible physical findings for clients with fluid, electrolyte, and acid-base imbalances.

Measuring Fluid Intake and Output.   Measuring and recording all liquid intake and output (I&O) during a 24-hour period is an important part of the client's assessment database for fluid and electrolyte balance. It is important to note trends in the I&O (e.g., a gradually decreasing urine output can indicate that the body is trying to adapt to an FVD or hyperosmolar fluid imbalance). Accurate I&O measurements identify both clients at risk

for and clients who are experiencing fluid, electrolyte, and acid-base disturbances.

For clients in health care settings, the nurse neither needs to nor should wait for a physician's order to begin I&O measurements. Generally I&O is routinely measured for clients after surgery, clients whose conditions are unstable, clients who have a temperature elevation, clients whose fluids are restricted, or clients who are receiving diuretic or intravenous (IV) therapy. The nurse also measures I&O for clients with chronic cardiopulmonary or renal illnesses and clients whose health status has deteriorated.

Oral intake includes all liquids taken by mouth, such as gelatin, ice cream, soup, juice, and water. Liquid intake also includes fluids given through nasogastric or jejunostomy feeding tubes (see Chapter 43), liquids given as IV fluids (including both continuous infusions and intermittent IV piggybacks), and blood or its components. Output includes urine, diarrhea, vomitus, gastric suction, and drainage from postsurgical wounds or other tubes (see Chapter 49).

Ambulatory clients' urinary output is recorded after each trip to the bathroom. These clients are instructed to save their urine in a container so that the nurse can record the amount, or clients may be instructed to measure and record their own output. When a client has an indwelling Foley catheter, drainage tube, or suction, that output is recorded at the end of each nursing shift or more frequently (e.g., every hour) as the client's condition requires. The nurse should measure, not estimate, I&O.

In the hospital, forms for recording I&O are attached to the bedside chart or room door (see Figure 40-8, p. 1212). The 24-hour total is calculated at midnight or 6 AM, depending on agency policy. Taking I&O measurements is a procedure requiring help from the client and family. The nurse explains the reasons that measurements are needed and instructs the client and family to not empty any container with voided fluid but to ask the nurse to do so. A client using a toilet should be instructed to use a calibrated insert, which attaches to the rim of the toilet bowl (see Figure 40-9, p. 1213). After each urination the client notifies the nurse, who measures, records, and empties the urine and rinses the insert. Occasionally, clients may also be instructed to measure and record their own output. It is important for the client to have good vision and motor skills to ensure accuracy.

Occasionally clients receive a specific amount of a liquid medication every 1 to 2 hours. A client receiving tube feedings may receive numerous liquid medications, and water may be used to flush the tube of the medications. Over a 24-hour period, these liquids can amount to significant intake and should always be recorded on the I&O record.

Recording I&O is essential for obtaining an accurate database. This information helps maintain an ongoing evaluation of the client's hydration status to prevent severe imbalances. I&O recording can be delegated to assistive personnel. The nurse is responsible to make sure staff members can correctly measure and calculate I&O and are

---

Medications That Cause Fluid, Electrolyte, and Acid-Base Disturbances   Box 40-2

Diuretics—metabolic alkalosis, hyperkalemia, and hypokalemia

Steroids—metabolic alkalosis

Potassium supplements—GI disturbances, including intestinal and gastric ulcers and diarrhea

Respiratory center depressants such as narcotic analgesics—decreased rate and depth of respirations, resulting in respiratory acidosis

Antibiotics—nephrotoxicity (e.g., vancomycin, methicillin, aminoglycosides); hyperkalemia and/or hypernatremia (e.g., azlocillin, carbenicillin, piperacillin, ticarcillin, Unasyn)*

Calcium carbonate (Tums)—mild metabolic alkalosis with nausea and vomiting*

Magnesium hydroxide (Milk of Magnesia)—hypokalemia*

*Data from McKenry LM, Salerno E: *Mosby's pharmacology in nursing*, ed 19, St. Louis, 1998, Mosby.

Table 40-7 Physical and Behavioral Nursing Assessment for Fluid, Electrolyte, and Acid-Base Imbalances

Assessment	Imbalance
Weight Changes	
2%-5% loss	Mild FVD*
5%-10% loss	Moderate FVD*
10%-15% loss	Severe FVD*
15%-20% loss	Death*
2% gain	Mild fluid volume excess (FVE)
5% gain	Moderate FVE
8% gain	Severe FVE
Head	
History:	
Headache	FVD,* metabolic or respiratory acidosis, metabolic alkalosis
Dizziness	FVD,* respiratory acidosis or alkalosis, hyponatremia
Observation:	
Irritability	Metabolic or respiratory alkalosis, hyperosmolar imbalance, hypernatremia, hypokalemia
Lethargy	FVD,* metabolic acidosis or alkalosis, respiratory acidosis, hypercalcemia
Confusion, disorientation	FVD,* hypomagnesemia, metabolic acidosis, hypokalemia
EYES	
Inspection:	
Sunken, dry conjunctivae, decreased or absent tearing	FVD
Periorbital edema, papilledema	FVE
History:	
Blurred vision	FVE
THROAT AND MOUTH	
Inspection:	
Sticky, dry mucous membranes, dry cracked lips, decreased salivation	FVD, hypernatremia
Longitudinal tongue furrows	
Cardiovascular System	
Inspection:	
Flat neck veins	FVD
Distended neck veins	FVE
Dependent body parts: legs, sacrum, back	
Slow venous filling	FVD*
Palpation:	
Edema (dependent body parts: back, sacrum, legs)	FVE*
Dysrhythmias (also noted as ECG changes)	Metabolic acidosis, respiratory alkalosis and acidosis, potassium imbalance, hypomagnesemia
Increased pulse rate	Metabolic alkalosis, respiratory acidosis, hyponatremia, FVD, hypomagnesemia
Decreased pulse rate	Metabolic alkalosis, hypokalemia
Weak pulse	FVD, hypokalemia
Decreased capillary filling	FVD
Bounding pulse	FVE
Auscultation:	
Blood pressure low or without orthostatic changes	FVD, hyponatremia, hyperkalemia, hypermagnesemia
Third heart sound	FVE
Hypertension	FVE

*Data from Horne MM and others: *Mosby's pocket guide series: fluid, electrolyte, and acid-base balance,* ed 3, St. Louis, 1997, Mosby.

Table 40-7	**Physical and Behavioral Nursing Assessment for Fluid, Electrolyte, and Acid-Base Imbalances**—cont'd
Assessment	Imbalance

Respiratory System

Inspection:

Increased rate	FVE, respiratory alkalosis, metabolic acidosis
Dyspnea	FVE

Auscultation:

Crackles	FVE

Gastrointestinal System

History:

Anorexia	Metabolic acidosis
Abdominal cramps	Metabolic acidosis

Inspection:

Sunken abdomen	FVD
Distended abdomen	Third-space syndrome
Vomiting	FVD, hypercalcemia, hyponatremia
Diarrhea	Hyponatremia

Auscultation:

Hyperperistalsis with diarrhea, or hypoperistalsis	FVD, hypokalemia

Renal System

Inspection:

Oliguria or anuria	FVD, FVE
Diuresis (if kidneys are normal)	FVE
Increased urine specific gravity	FVD

Neuromuscular System

Inspection:

Numbness, tingling	Metabolic alkalosis, hypocalcemia, potassium imbalances
Muscle cramps, tetany	Hypocalcemia, metabolic or respiratory alkalosis
Coma	Hyperosmolar or hypoosmolar imbalances, hyponatremia
Tremors	Respiratory acidosis, hypomagnesemia

Palpation:

Hypotonicity	Hypokalemia, hypercalcemia*
Hypertonicity	Hypocalcemia, hypomagnesemia, metabolic alkalosis

Percussion:

Decreased or absent deep tendon reflexes	Hypercalcemia, hypermagnesemia
Increased or hyperactive deep tendon reflexes	Hypocalcemia, hypomagnesemia

Skin

Body temperature:

Increased	Hypernatremia, hyperosmolar imbalance, metabolic acidosis
Decreased	FVD

Inspection:

Dry, flushed	FVD, hypernatremia, metabolic acidosis

Palpation:

Inelastic skin turgor, cold, clammy skin	FVD

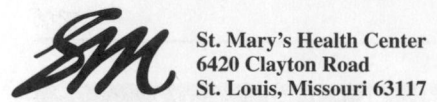

St. Mary's Health Center
6420 Clayton Road
St. Louis, Missouri 63117

PATIENT LABEL

INTAKE AND OUTPUT SUMMARY

	DATE 6-10-XX	2200 – 0600	0600 – 1400	1400 – 2200	24 Hr.	
INTAKE	P.O. Intake	120	800	650	1570	TOTAL INTAKE
	Tube Feedings					
	Hyperalimentation					
	I.V. Primary					
	I.V.P.B.	50		50	100	1670
	Blood/Blood Products					
OUTPUT	Urine	325	700	500	1525	TOTAL OUTPUT
	Emesis					
	G.I. Suction					
	Drainage	50	75	30	155	1855
	Chest tube	75	50	50	175	

	DATE	2200 – 0600	0600 – 1400	1400 – 2200	24 Hr.	
INTAKE	P.O. Intake					TOTAL INTAKE
	Tube Feedings					
	Hyperalimentation					
	I.V. Primary					
	I.V.P.B.					
	Blood/Blood Products					
OUTPUT	Urine					TOTAL OUTPUT
	Emesis					
	G.I. Suction					
	Drainage					

	DATE	2200 – 0600	0600 – 1400	1400 – 2200	24 Hr.	
INTAKE	P.O. Intake					TOTAL INTAKE
	Tube Feedings					
	Hyperalimentation					
	I.V. Primary					
	I.V.P.B.					
	Blood/Blood Products					
OUTPUT	Urine					TOTAL OUTPUT
	Emesis					
	G.I. Suction					
	Drainage					

	DATE	2200 – 0600	0600 – 1400	1400 – 2200	24 Hr.	
INTAKE	P.O. Intake					TOTAL INTAKE
	Tube Feedings					
	Hyperalimentation					
	I.V. Primary					
	I.V.P.B.					
	Blood/Blood Products					
OUTPUT	Urine					TOTAL OUTPUT
	Emesis					
	G.I. Suction					
	Drainage					

Figure 40-8   Twenty-four-hour intake and output record.
Courtesy St. Mary's Health Center, St. Louis, Mo.

members can correctly measure and calculate I&O and are aware of the need to be accurate and timely.

Laboratory Studies.

The nurse reviews laboratory tests to obtain further objective data about fluid, electrolyte, and acid-base balances (Box 40-3). These tests include serum and urinary electrolyte levels, hematocrit, blood creatinine level, BUN levels, urine specific gravity, and ABG readings. Serum electrolyte levels are measured to determine the hydration status, the electrolyte concentration of the blood plasma, and acid-base balance. The frequency with which these electrolyte levels are measured depends on the severity of the client's illness. Serum electrolyte tests are routinely performed on any client entering a hospital to screen for alterations and to serve as a baseline for future comparisons.

The complete blood count (CBC) is a determination of the number and type of red and white blood cells per cubic millimeter of blood. When the client does not have anemia, the hematocrit can be an indication of the hydration status of the client. The hematocrit will increase (become more concentrated) in situations where fluid is lost, whereas it will decrease in situations in which fluid is excessively retained in the vascular space.

Blood creatinine levels are useful in measuring kidney function. Creatinine is a normal by-product of muscle metabolism and is excreted by the kidneys at fairly constant levels, regardless of factors such as fluid intake, diet, or exercise. Therefore it provides a measure of renal function that is relatively independent of the hydration status of the client or the client's dietary intake. An increased value indicates renal disease since no other pathological condition would result in an elevation. Generally 50% of renal function is lost before there is an increase in the serum creatinine level (Ignataviscius, Workman, and Mishler, 1999). A decreased level may reflect a loss of muscle mass. The normal serum creatinine level is 0.5 to 1.2 mg/100 ml.

Blood urea nitrogen is the amount of nitrogenous substance present in the blood as urea. It is a rough indicator of kidney function because other factors may influence the BUN level. An elevation in the BUN level may not indicate renal dysfunction. In fact, rapid cell destruction from an infection or steroidal therapy may produce an elevation. Therefore the BUN level is not the most reliable indicator of renal disease. A decreased BUN level may indicate malnutrition or hepatic damage. The normal serum BUN level is 10 to 20 mg/100 ml.

BUN: creatinine ratio may be a better indicator of renal function. The normal ratio is 10:1. When there is an intravascular fluid volume deficit, the BUN level rises more rapidly than the creatinine level, causing an increase in the ratio. An increase in both the BUN and the creatinine level is usually an indicator of renal dysfunction.

Serum osmolality measures the concentration of the plasma. The osmolality will decrease when the client is experiencing hypoosmolar fluid imbalance (water excess) or hyponatremia. Decreased serum osmolality results in the movement of fluid into body cells (cellular edema) by osmosis. The osmolality will increase with a hyperosmolar fluid imbalance (water deficit) or hypernatremia or other gains of solutes such as glucose. This will result in the movement of fluid out of body cells into the interstitial space (cellular shrinkage). Both cellular edema and shrinkage will disrupt normal cell processes.

The urine specific gravity test measures the urine's degree of concentration and evaluates the kidney's ability to conserve or excrete water. The specific gravity, measured at the bedside using a urinometer, normally ranges between 1.010 and 1.025.

Arterial blood gas analysis provides information on the status of acid-base balance and the effectiveness of ventilatory function in providing normal oxygen-carbon dioxide exchange. The nurse should understand that an

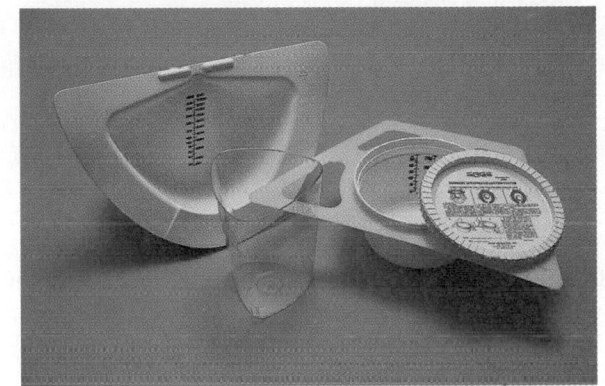

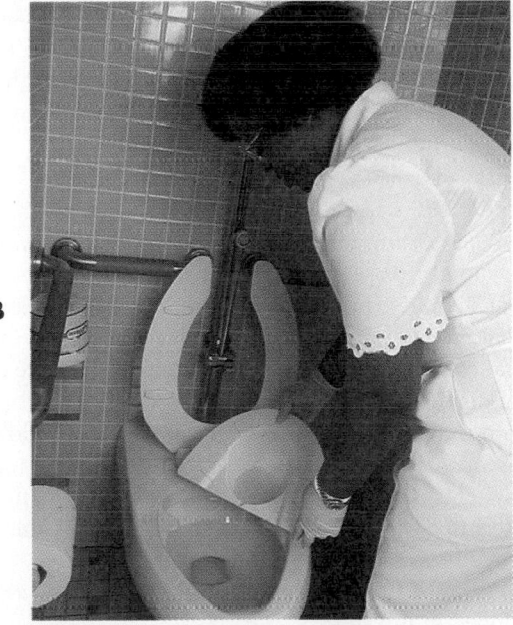

Figure 40-9   **A,** Graduated measuring containers. Clockwise from left to right: "hat" receptacle, specipan, and graduated measuring container. **B,** Emptying collected urine.

Laboratory Data for Fluid, Electrolyte, and Acid-Base Imbalances   Box 40-3

FLUID AND ELECTROLYTES

Altered concentrations of sodium, potassium, magnesium, calcium, phosphates, chloride, and bicarbonate (venous CO_2 contentions)

Increase in hematocrit, BUN, sodium, and osmolality in serum (related to loss of ECF fluid or gain of solutes)

Decrease in hematocrit, BUN, sodium, and osmolality in serum (related to gain of ECF fluid or loss of solutes)

Concentrated urine demonstrated by urine specific gravity >1.030

Dilute urine demonstrated by a specific gravity <1.012

METABOLIC ALKALOSIS

pH >7.45

$PaCO_2$ normal or >45 mm Hg if lungs are compensating

PaO_2 normal

O_2 saturation (SaO_2) normal

HCO_3^- >26 mEq/L

K^+<3.5 mEq/L

METABOLIC ACIDOSIS

pH <7.35

$PaCO_2$ normal or <35 mm Hg if lungs are compensating

METABOLIC ACIDOSIS—continued

PaO_2 normal

SaO_2 normal

HCO_3^- <22 mEq/L

K^+ >5.3 mEq/L

K^+ <3.5 mEq/L

RESPIRATORY ALKALOSIS

pH >7.45

$PaCO_2$ <35 mm Hg

PaO_2 normal

SaO_2 normal

HCO_3^- normal

K^+ <3.5 mEq/L

RESPIRATORY ACIDOSIS

pH <7.35

$PaCO_2$ >45 mm Hg

PaO_2 normal or <80 mm Hg, depending on cause of acidosis

SaO_2 normal or <95%, depending on cause of acidosis

HCO_3^- normal if early respiratory acidosis or >26 mEq/L if kidneys are compensating

K^+ >5.3 mEq/L

ABG result gets evaluated in the following systematic approach.

First, the pH is examined; less than 7.35 is considered acidic, and greater than 7.45 is considered alkalotic. The second step is to check the $PaCO_2$ to assess the respiratory parameter. The pH and $PaCO_2$ should move in opposite directions (e.g., as pH increases, the $PaCO_2$, should decrease). If the $PaCO_2$ increases, it is indicative that CO_2 is being retained. A high $PaCO_2$ indicates respiratory acidosis. Respiratory alkalosis would then occur when the $PaCO_2$ decreases because CO_2 is being exhaled. Normal $PaCO_2$ is 32 to 45 mm Hg. When the pH is abnormal, either in acidosis or alkalosis, and the $PaCO_2$ is within normal limits, a metabolic condition must be considered.

The bicarbonate (HCO_3^-) is then evaluated. Normal HCO_3^- is 20 to 26 mEq/L. The pH and HCO_3^- should move in the same direction. A decreased bicarbonate level with a decreased pH and a normal $PaCO_2$ indicates the acidosis is metabolic. Likewise, an increasing pH with an increased bicarbonate level and a normal $PaCO_2$ will indicate that the alkalosis is metabolic. If the $PACO_2$ and the HCO_3^- are both abnormal, than the value that corresponds more closely to the pH is examined. The value that more closely corresponds to the pH and deviates more from the norm usually points to the primary disturbance responsible for altering the pH.

Client Expectations.   Often a fluid, electrolyte, or acid-base disturbance is so serious or acute that the client's

condition prevents a review of his or her expectations. However, if a client is alert enough to discuss care with the nurse, a review of expectations may reveal short-term needs (e.g., provision of comfort from nausea) or long-term needs (e.g., understanding how to prevent alterations from occurring in the future). The client must be able to understand the implications of fluid, electrolyte, or acid-base changes to be able to express expectations of care. The client's trust in the nurse is strengthened through the nurse's competent response to sudden changes in the client's condition.

NURSING DIAGNOSIS

When caring for clients with suspected fluid, electrolyte, and acid-base imbalances, it is particularly important that the nurse be skilled in using critical thinking to formulate nursing diagnoses (Box 40-4). The assessment data that establish the risk for or the actual presence of a nursing diagnosis in these areas may be subtle, and patterns and trends emerge only when the nurse consciously assesses for them. The nurse must keep in mind that many body systems may be involved. Clustering of defining characteristics will lead the nurse to selection of the appropriate diagnoses.

For example, the nursing diagnosis *fluid volume deficit* is developed in Box 40-5.

An important part of formulating nursing diagnoses is identifying the relevant causative or related factor. The nursing interventions that are chosen must treat or modify the related factor for the diagnosis to be resolved. *Fluid volume deficit related to loss of gastrointestinal fluids via vomiting* will require therapies different to a degree from therapies needed for *fluid volume deficit related to elevated body temperature.*

PLANNING

During the planning process the nurse again critically thinks, synthesizing information from multiple resources (Figure 40-10). Critical thinking ensures that the

client's plan of care integrates both the nurse's scientific and nursing knowledge, as well as all the knowledge the nurse has gathered about the individual client. Professional standards are especially important to consider when the nurse develops a plan of care. These standards often establish scientifically proven guidelines for selecting effective nursing interventions. For example, the Intravenous Nurses Society standards of practice should be applied when intravenous therapy becomes a part of the plan. The nurse develops an individual plan of care for each of the nursing diagnoses (see care plan, p. 1217). The nurse and client set realistic expectations for care. Goals are to be individualized and realistic with measurable outcomes.

The client's clinical condition will determine which of the diagnoses takes the greatest priority. Many nursing diagnoses in the area of fluid, electrolyte, and acid-base balances are of highest priority, because the consequences for the client can be serious or even life threatening. Consultation with the client's physician may assist in setting realistic time frames for the goals of care, particularly when the client's physiological status is unstable. During planning the nurse collaborates as much as possible with the client and family and other members of the interdisciplinary health care team such as IV therapy and pharmacy. The family can be particularly helpful in identifying subtle changes in a client's behavior associated with any imbalances (e.g., anxiety, confusion, irritability). The nurse also incorporates client preferences and resources into the plan of care.

For those clients with acute disturbances, discharge planning must begin early. In the hospital the nurse antic-

---

NURSING DIAGNOSES Box 40-4

CLIENTS WITH FLUID, ELECTROLYTE, AND ACID-BASE ALTERATIONS

Body temperature, altered, risk for
Breathing pattern, ineffective
Cardiac output, decreased
Fluid volume deficit
Fluid volume deficit, risk for
Fluid volume excess
Gas exchange, impaired
Knowledge deficit regarding disease management
Management of therapeutic regimen, individuals: ineffective
Mobility, impaired
Oral mucous membrane, altered
Skin integrity, impaired
Skin integrity, impaired, risk for
Tissue integrity, impaired
Tissue perfusion, altered, peripheral

SAMPLE NURSING DIAGNOSTIC PROCESS Box 40-5

FLUID, ELECTROLYTE, AND ACID-BASE DISTURBANCES

Assessment Activities	Defining Characteristics	Nursing Diagnosis
Assess blood pressure and pulse.	Client is hypotensive with increased heart rate.	Fluid volume deficit related to loss of gastrointestinal fluids via vomiting
Obtain daily weight measurements.	Client experiences sudden weight loss.	
Observe volume of urine output related to intake and specific gravity.	Decreased volume of output in comparison to intake; increased urine specific gravity is present.	
Palpate skin turgor.	Inelastic skin turgor noted.	
Ask if client is thirsty or weak.	Client verbalizes thirst and weakness.	
Inspect mucous membranes for degree of moisture.	Dry mucous membranes are noted.	
Observe for abnormal losses of fluids.	Client is vomiting.	
Assess client's tolerance to changing from lying to sitting position.	Client complains of dizziness when changing position.	

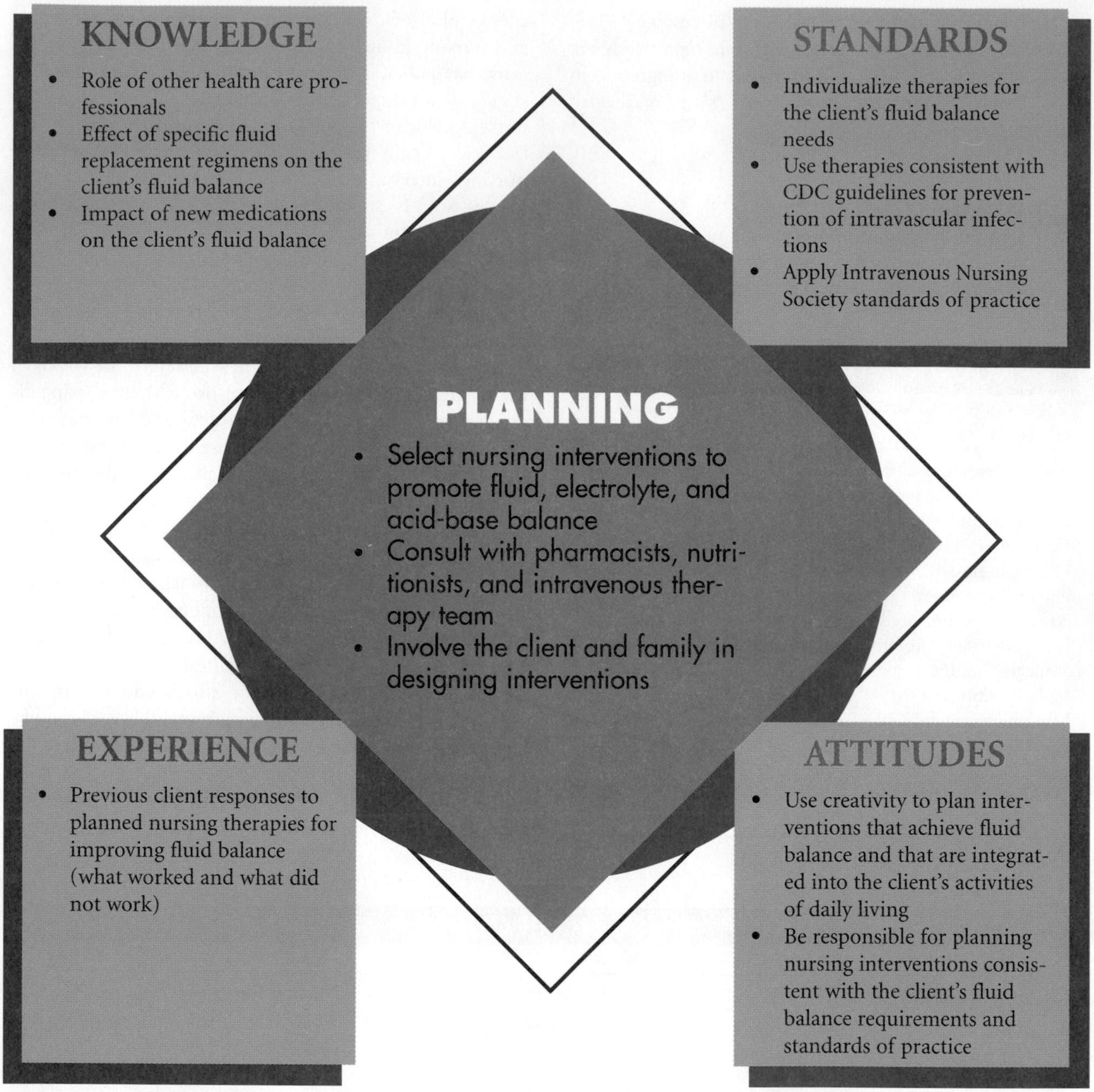

KNOWLEDGE

- Role of other health care professionals
- Effect of specific fluid replacement regimens on the client's fluid balance
- Impact of new medications on the client's fluid balance

STANDARDS

- Individualize therapies for the client's fluid balance needs
- Use therapies consistent with CDC guidelines for prevention of intravascular infections
- Apply Intravenous Nursing Society standards of practice

PLANNING

- Select nursing interventions to promote fluid, electrolyte, and acid-base balance
- Consult with pharmacists, nutritionists, and intravenous therapy team
- Involve the client and family in designing interventions

EXPERIENCE

- Previous client responses to planned nursing therapies for improving fluid balance (what worked and what did not work)

ATTITUDES

- Use creativity to plan interventions that achieve fluid balance and that are integrated into the client's activities of daily living
- Be responsible for planning nursing interventions consistent with the client's fluid balance requirements and standards of practice

Figure 40-10   *Synthesis Model for Fluid, Electrolyte, and Acid-Base Balances Planning Phase.*

ipates the needs of the client and family and collaborates with the other members of the health care team to ensure that care can continue in the home or long-term care setting with few disruptions. For example, for the client who is discharged on IV therapy the nurse must determine the knowledge and skills of the family member or friend who is to assume caregiving responsibilities and make a referral to home IV therapy as soon as possible. The nurse also collaborates closely with other members of the health care team, such as the physician, dietician, and pharmacist. The dietitian can be a valuable resource in recommending food sources to either increase or reduce intake of certain electrolytes. Chapter 43 describes various therapeutic diets (e.g., low sodium). The pharmacist can assist the nurse and physician in identifying medications or combinations of medications likely to cause electrolyte or acid-base disturbances. Furthermore, the pharmacist can offer information regarding client education on side effects to anticipate for those drugs prescribed to the client. The physician will direct the treatment of any fluid, electrolyte, or acid-base alteration.

SAMPLE NURSING CARE PLAN

FLUID AND ELECTROLYTE ALTERATIONS

ASSESSMENT*

Mrs. Hilda Bottomley is a 72-year-old seen by her physician this morning with complaints of **productive cough, chills, malaise, anorexia, a temperature of 36.7° C (101° F), and body aches.** She reported a history of **congestion for the last 2 weeks** and has noted that her **secretions are now thick and yellow-greenish.** She admits that she has not felt like eating and drinking much lately. After an outpatient chest x-ray, Mrs. Bottomley has been admitted for respiratory toileting and IV antibiotic and fluid therapy. On admission her **vital signs are within normal limits except for a temperature of 36.6° C (100.8° F), an increased respiratory rate from 16 to 28 with activity, and rhonchi breath sounds. Arterial blood gas results indicate a mild respiratory acidosis, and the chest x-ray revealed a left lower lobe pneumonia.** The physician orders O_2 at 4 L/min with humidification, respiratory treatments, fluids by mouth and IV, pulse oximetry, and activity with assistance.

*Defining characteristics are shown in bold type.

NURSING DIAGNOSIS:
Ineffective airway clearance related to increased mucus in response to airway infection and manifested by mild respiratory acidosis; Risk for fluid volume deficit related to reduced fluid intake.

PLANNING

GOALS	EXPECTED OUTCOMES
Client's airway will be free from secretions with normal ABG levels by discharge.	ABG levels will be within normal limits in 24 hours.
	Respiratory rate will be within normal limits with activity in 24 hours.
	Temperature will be within normal limits in 24 hours.
	Breath sounds will be clear on auscultation.
	Mucus will become thin and clear in 48 hours.
Client's fluid volume will remain within normal limits.	Urine output will equal intake.
	Mucous membranes will remain moist.
	Vital signs will remain within normal limits.

INTERVENTIONS†

Airway Maintenance

INTERVENTIONS	RATIONALE
• Schedule coughing and deep breathing exercises every 2 hours while awake.	Cough control exercises and deep breathing promote pulmonary secretion clearance (Ciesla, 1996, Carlson-Catalano and others, 1998).
• Administer chest physiotherapy every 4 hours while awake to affected regions of the lung.	Chest physiotherapy, breathing exercises, cough techniques, along with ambulating the client, are effective in promoting airway clearance (Ciesla, 1996).
• Ambulate client once every 8 hours and encourage client to get out of bed into chair often.	
• Provide client with an additional 16 ounces of noncaffeinated oral fluids every 8 hours.	Increased fluid intake helps to liquefy pulmonary secretions and in turn facilitate productive coughing (Carson-Catalano and others, 1998).

†Intervention Classification labels from McCloskey JC, Bulechek GM: *Nursing interventions classification (NIC)*, ed 3, St. Louis, 2000, Mosby.

EVALUATION

Monitor ABG levels, vital signs, I&O, and O_2 saturation levels.
Auscultate breath sounds.
Evaluate effectiveness of coughing and deep breathing exercises.
Identify methods to provide for adequate rest.

IMPLEMENTATION

Health Promotion. Health promotion activities in the area of fluid, electrolyte, and acid-base imbalances focus primarily on client teaching. Clients and caregivers need to recognize risk factors for these imbalances and implement appropriate preventive measures. For example, parents of infants need to understand that GI losses can quickly lead to serious imbalances; therefore when vomiting or diarrhea occur in the infant, the parent needs to recognize the risk and promptly seek health care to restore normal balance. Even the healthy adult is at risk for developing imbalances when subjected to elevated environmental temperatures. Nurses need to advise them to supplement the fluid loss from perspiration by increasing oral fluids such as water, maintaining adequate environmental ventilation, and refraining from excessive activity during this period of time.

Sometimes it is difficult to separate the effects of age-related changes from changes associated with disease processes. For an example, any older adult who has a chronic condition involving renal or respiratory function is more likely to suffer serious consequences when an acute disease process occurs (Beare and Myers, 1998).

All clients with a chronic health alteration are at risk for developing changes in their fluid, electrolyte, and acid-base balances. They need to understand their own risk factors and the measures to be taken to avoid imbalances. For example, clients with renal failure must avoid excess intake of fluid, sodium, potassium, and phosphorus. Through diet education these clients learn the types of foods to avoid and the suitable volume of fluid they are permitted daily (see Chapter 43). Clients with chronic health diseases need to be made aware of early signs and symptoms of fluid, electrolyte, and acid-base imbalances. A client with heart disease should be instructed to obtain an accurate body weight each day at the approximate same time and to inform the physician of significant changes of weight from one day to another. Increase in weight, shortness of breath, orthopnea, and dependent edema are all associated with fluid retention.

Acute Care.
Although fluid, electrolyte, and/or acid-base imbalance can occur in all settings, changes in the acute care delivery system place more demanding expectations on the nurse. Today the nurse must manage the client's complex medical care in a shorter span of time while being expected to perform more difficult technological skills.

Daily Weights and Intake and Output Measurement.
When implementing specific measures to increase or decrease fluid, two nursing interventions are necessary: daily weight and I&O measurements. Clients with fluid and electrolyte alterations should be weighed daily. Daily weights are the single most important indicator of fluid status (Horne and others, 1997). Weight should be determined at the same time each day with the same scale after the client voids. The scale should be calibrated each day or routinely. The client should wear the same clothes or clothes that weigh the same; if a bed scale is used, the same number of sheets should be used on the scale with each weighing.

I&O records provide additional information about fluid balance (see section on assessment). I&O measurements, when examined for trends, can indicate whether excess fluid volume is excreted in the form of urine or whether excretion of fluids through the kidneys has diminished. The I&O is not as accurate as daily weights in assessing daily fluid balance unless it has been measured strictly and precisely.

Enteral Replacement of Fluids.
Oral replacement of fluids and electrolytes is appropriate as long as the client is not so physiologically unstable that oral fluids cannot be replaced rapidly. Oral replacement of fluids is contraindicated when the client is vomiting, has a mechanical obstruction of the GI tract, is at risk for aspiration, or has impaired swallowing. Clients unable to tolerate solid foods may still be able to ingest fluids.

When replacing fluids by mouth in a client with a fluid deficit, it is wise to choose fluids with adequate calories and electrolyte content (e.g., fruit juices, gelatin, and replacements like Pedialyte and Gastrolyte). However, it is important to remember that liquids containing lactose, caffeine, or low-sodium content may not be appropriate when the client has diarrhea.

A feeding tube may be appropriate when the client's GI tract is healthy but the client cannot ingest fluids (e.g., after oral surgery or with impaired swallowing). Fluids can also be replaced through a gastrostomy or jejunostomy feeding tube, or they can be administered via a small-bore nasogastric feeding tube.

Restriction of Fluids.
Clients who retain fluids and have **fluid volume excess (FVE)** require restricted fluid intake. Fluid restriction is often difficult for clients, particularly if they take drugs that dry the oral mucous membranes or if they breathe through the mouth and experience the sensation of thirst. The nurse should explain the reason fluids are restricted. In addition, the client needs to know the amount of fluid permitted orally and should understand that ice chips, gelatin, and ice cream are considered fluid. The client should help to decide the amount of fluid with each meal, between meals, before bed, and with medications. Frequently clients on fluid restriction can swallow a number of pills with as little as 1 ounce (30 ml) of liquid.

A good rule of thumb for fluid restrictions is to allow half of the allotted total oral fluids between 7 AM and 3 PM, the period when clients usually are more active, receive two meals, and take most of their oral medications. Clients on fluid restriction require mouth care frequently to moisten mucous membranes, decrease the chance of mucosal drying and cracking, and maintain comfort (see Chapter 38).

Parenteral Replacement of Fluids and Electrolytes.
Fluid and electrolytes may be replaced through infusion directly into the blood rather than via the digestive system. Parenteral replacement includes total parenteral nutrition (TPN), IV fluid and electrolyte therapy (**crystalloids**), and blood and blood component (**colloids**) administration.

With increasing risk to health care workers for transmission of the human immunodeficiency virus (HIV), the cause of acquired immunodeficiency syndrome (AIDS), hepatitis B virus (HBV), and other infectious diseases, standard precautions must be practiced when administering parenteral fluids (see Chapter 33).

Vascular Access Devices. **Vascular access devices** are catheters, cannulas, or infusion ports designed for long-term repeated access to the vascular system. These devices are more effective than peripherally placed catheters for administering medications and solutions that are irritating to veins and for the delivery of long-term IV therapy. Increased use of central venous catheters and implanted infusion ports (Figure 40-11) requires nurses to be educated in the care of these devices.

Total Parenteral Nutrition. **Total parenteral nutrition** is a nutritionally adequate hypertonic solution consisting of glucose and other nutrients and electrolytes given through an indwelling peripheral or central IV catheter. Chapter 43 reviews principles and guidelines for TPN administration, which is used as an intervention in severe cases of malnutrition.

Intravenous Therapy (Crystalloids). The goal of IV fluid administration is to correct or prevent fluid and electrolyte disturbances. It allows for direct access to the vascular system, permitting the infusion of continuous fluids over a period of time. Intravenous fluid therapy must be continuously regulated because of continual changes in the client's fluid and electrolyte balance.

When IV fluid administration is required, the nurse must know the correct ordered solution, the equipment needed, the procedures required to initiate an infusion, how to regulate the infusion rate and maintain the system, how to identify and correct problems, and how to discontinue the infusion if necessary.

Administration of Intravenous Therapy

Types of Solutions. Many prepared IV solutions are available for use (Table 40-8). Intravenous solutions fall into the following categories: isotonic, hypotonic, and hypertonic. Isotonic solutions are those that have the same effective osmolality as body fluids. Hypotonic solutions are those that have an effective osmolality less than body fluids. Hypertonic solutions are those that have an effec-

tive osmolality greater than body fluids (Horne and others, 1997).

In general, isotonic fluids are used most commonly for extracellular volume replacement (e.g., FVD after prolonged vomiting). The decision to use a hypotonic or hypertonic solution is based on the specific fluid and electrolyte imbalance. For example, the client with a hypertonic fluid imbalance will generally receive a hypotonic IV to dilute the ECF and rehydrate the cells. All IV fluids should be given carefully, especially hypertonic solutions, because these pull fluid into the vascular space by osmosis, resulting in an increased vascular volume that can lead to pulmonary edema, particularly in clients with heart or renal failure. Certain additives, most commonly vitamins and potassium chloride (KCl), are frequently added to IV solutions. *However, under no circumstances can potassium chloride (KCl) be given IV push. A direct IV infusion of KCl is fatal.*

If an IV is to have additives added, a physician's order must be obtained that includes the required additives, for

Table 40-8	**Intravenous Solutions**	
Solution	Concentration	Other Names
Dextrose in Water Solutions		
Dextrose 5% in water*	Isotonic	D₅W
Dextrose 10% in water	Hypertonic	D₁₀W
Saline Solutions		
0.45% sodium chloride (half normal saline)	Hypotonic	½ NS 0.45% NS
0.9% sodium chloride† (normal saline)	Isotonic	NS 0.9% NS 0.9% NaCl
3%-5% sodium chloride	Hypertonic	3%-5% NS 3%-5% NaCl
Dextrose in Saline Solutions		
Dextrose 5% in 0.9% sodium chloride	Hypertonic	D₅0.9% NaCl D₅0.9% NS D₅NS
Dextrose 5% in 0.45% NaCl sodium chloride	Hypertonic	D₅0.45% NaCl D₅0.45% NS D₅½ NS
Multiple Electrolyte Solutions		
Lactated Ringer's‡	Isotonic	LR
Dextrose 5% in Lactated Ringer's	Hypertonic	D₅LR

*Dextrose is quickly metabolized, leaving free water to be distributed evenly in all fluid compartments (Horne and others, 1997).
†Although it is isotonic because the total concentration of electrolytes equals plasma concentration, it contains 154 mEq of both sodium and chloride, which is a higher concentration of these electrolytes than is found in the plasma, which can cause FVE (Metheny, 1996).
‡Contains sodium, potassium, calcium, chloride, and lactate.

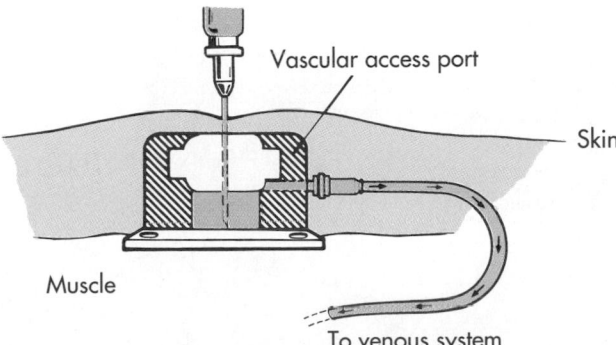

Figure 40-11 Example of an implantable vascular access device.

example, Bottle 1: 1000 ml D5 1/2 NS with 20 mEq KCl at 125 ml/hour.

Clients with normal renal function who are receiving nothing by mouth should have potassium added to IV solutions. The body cannot conserve potassium, and even when the serum level falls, the kidneys continue to excrete potassium. If there is no potassium intake orally or parenterally, hypokalemia can develop quickly. Conversely, the nurse should verify that the client has adequate urine output before administering an IV solution containing potassium, because hyperkalemia can quickly develop.

Equipment.   Correct selection and preparation of IV equipment assists in safe and quick placement of an IV line. Because fluids are instilled into the bloodstream, sterile technique is necessary; the nurse must therefore have all equipment organized and at the bedside. The nurse who must leave the bedside to obtain another piece of equipment will need to start the procedure over again. Intravenous equipment includes needles or catheters, tourniquet, gloves, dressings, solution containers, various types of tubing, and IV pumps or volume control devices. Injectable medications such as antibiotics may be added to a small IV solution bag and "piggybacked" into the main line to be administered over a 30- to 60-minute period (see Chapter 34). The type and amount of solution depend on the medication added and the client's physiological status. Different types of tubing are used to administer medications or IV fluids. A solution given rapidly needs to be infused with macrodrip tubing, which delivers large drops (standard drop size is 10 or 15 gtt/ml depending on the manufacturer) so that a rapid rate can be maintained. In contrast, microdrip tubing provides a standard drop size of 60 gtt/ml. Microdrip tubing is used to allow

precise regulation of IV fluids even at slow rates. In addition, clients may require IV extension tubing to increase mobility or to facilitate changes in position. Intravenous pumps or volume control devices are used with children, with clients with renal or cardiac failure, or with critically ill clients to prevent sudden uncontrolled fluid administration.

Initiating the Intravenous Line.   After the equipment is collected at the bedside, the nurse prepares to place the IV line by assessing the client for a venipuncture site (Skill 40-1). Common IV puncture sites include the hand and the arm (Figure 40-12). The use of the foot for an IV site is common with children but is avoided in the adult because of the danger of thrombophlebitis (Pearson, 1996). The nurse assessing the client for potential venipuncture sites for IV infusion should consider conditions and contraindications that exclude certain sites. Because the very young and older adults have fragile veins, the nurse should avoid sites easily moved or bumped such as the dorsal surface of the hand (Box 40-6, p. 1228). Venipuncture is contraindicated in a site that has signs of infection, infiltration, or thrombosis. An infected site is red, tender, swollen, and possibly warm to the touch. Exudate may be present. An infected site is not used because of the danger of introducing bacteria from the skin surface into the bloodstream. Avoid using an extremity with a vascular (dialysis) graft/fistula or on the side of a mastectomy. Place IVs at the most distal point when possible. Using a distal site first allows for the use of proximal sites later if the client would need a venipuncture site change.

A **venipuncture** is a technique in which a vein is punctured through the skin by a sharp rigid stylet (e.g., butterfly needle or metal needle), a partially covered plastic

Text continued on p. 1233.

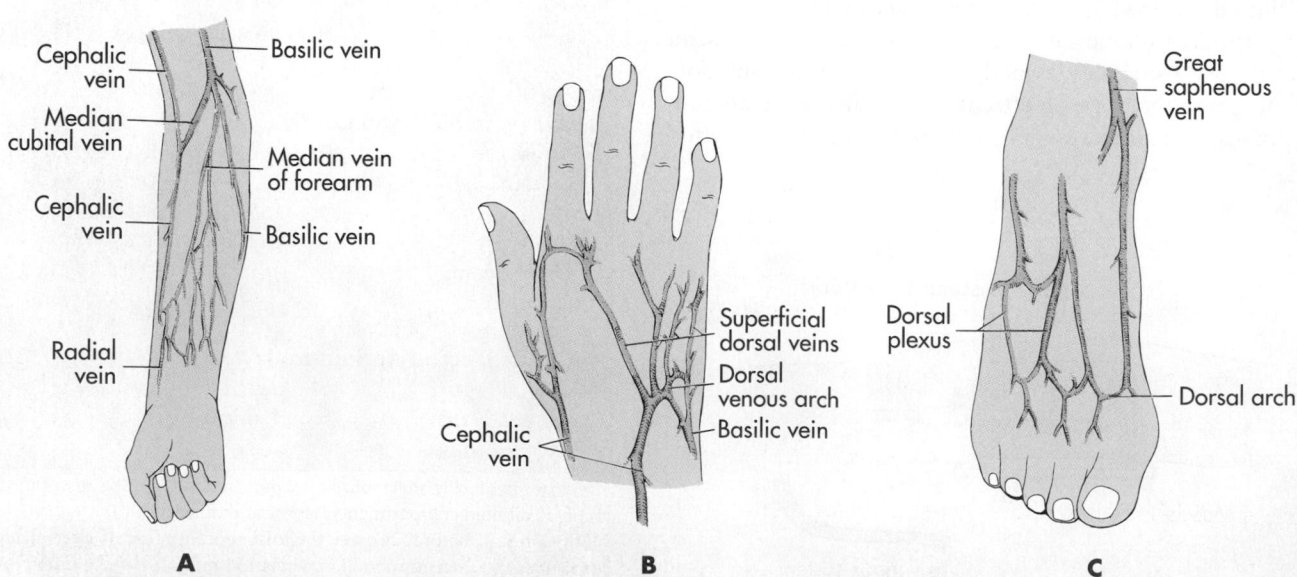

Figure 40-12   Common IV sites. **A,** Inner arm. **B,** Dorsal surface of hand. **C,** Dorsal surface of foot (used only for children).

Initiating a Peripheral Intravenous Infusion   Skill 40-1

Delegation Considerations

The skill of initiating IV therapy requires problem solving and knowledge application unique to professional nursing. For this procedure delegation is not appropriate.

EQUIPMENT

- Correct IV solution (with time tape attached)
- Proper catheter for venipuncture (gauge will vary with client's body size and reason for IV fluid administration)
- **For IV fluid infusion**
  - Administration set (choice depends on type of solution and rate of administration; infants and children require microdrip tubing, which provides 60 gtt/ml)
  - 0.22 μm filter (if required by agency policy or if particulate matter is likely)
  - Extension tubing (used when a longer IV line is necessary)
  - Alcohol and povidone-iodine cleaning swabs or sticks
  - Disposable gloves
  - Tourniquet (can be a source of contamination; use a single-use product)
  - Arm board, if needed (used to maintain wrist or elbow joint position when over-the-needle catheter [ONC] is placed close to or over a joint; will help prevent infiltration of IV)
  - Nonallergenic tape
  - Towel (to place under client's hand or arm)

- IV pole, rolling or ceiling mounted
- Special client gown with snaps at shoulder seams (makes removal with IV tubing easier), if available
- Needle disposal container (also called sharps container)
- Optional: IV kit
  Some agencies use an IV start kit, which contains a sterile drape to place under the client's arm, cleansing and antiseptic preparations, dressings, and a small roll of sterile, precut tape
- **Gauze dressing only**
  - 2 × 2 or 4 × 4 sterile gauze sponge
- **Transparent dressing**
  - Transparent dressing
- **For heparin or normal saline lock**
  - Injection cap (also called IV plug)
  - IV loop or short piece of extension tubing, if necessary
  - 1 to 3 ml of normal saline or heparin flush (10 to 100 U/ml as ordered)
  - Syringes and 25-gauge needles

STEPS	RATIONALE
1. Review physician's order for type and amount of IV fluid, rate of fluid administration, and purpose of infusion. In addition, nurse follows five rights for administration of medications (see Chapter 34).	An order requesting the initiation of a peripheral IV access and administration of an IV solution must be made by a physician before the implementation of this procedure. Assists in selection of appropriate access device.
2. Observe for signs and symptoms indicating fluid or electrolyte imbalances (e.g., decrease in body weight, blood pressure changes, tachycardia, inelastic skin turgor).	Provides baseline data for later evaluation of change in fluid and electrolyte status.
3. Assess client's previous or perceived experience with IV therapy and arm placement preference.	Determines level of emotional support and instruction necessary.
4. Determine if client is to undergo any planned surgeries or is to receive blood infusion later.	Allows nurse to place an adequate-size catheter (i.e., 18 or 16 gauge for surgery) and avoids placement in an area that will interfere with medical procedures.
5. Assess laboratory data and client's history of allergies.	May reveal information that affects insertion of devices, such as fluid volume deficit or allergy to iodine, adhesive, or latex.
6. Assess for the following risk factors: child or older adult, presence of heart failure or renal failure, or low platelet count.	Persons at extremes in age develop fluid imbalances more rapidly because they have proportionately larger ECF volume; persons with heart failure may require fluid restriction and cannot adapt to sudden increases in vascular volume, and persons with renal failure cannot eliminate excess ECF. A low platelet count predisposes clients to bleeding at IV site.
7. Prepare client and family by explaining the procedure, its purpose, and what is expected of client.	Decreases anxiety and promotes cooperation.
8. Assist client to comfortable sitting or supine position.	
9. Wash hands.	Reduces transmission of microorganisms.
10. Organize equipment on clean clutter-free bedside stand or overbed table.	Reduces risk of contamination and accidents.

STEPS	RATIONALE
11. Change client's gown to the more easily removed gown with snaps at the shoulder, if available.	Use of a special IV gown facilitates safe removal of the gown.
12. Open sterile packages using sterile aseptic technique.	Maintains sterility of equipment and reduces spread of microorganisms.
13. Check IV solution, using five rights of drug administration (see Chapter 34). Make sure prescribed additives, such as potassium and vitamins, have been added. Check solution for color, clarity, and expiration date. Check bag for leaks, which is best if done before reaching the bedside.	IV solutions are medications and should be carefully checked to reduce risk of error. Solutions that are discolored, contain particles, or are expired are not to be used. Leaky bags present an opportunity for infection and must not be used.
14. Open infusion set, maintaining sterility of both ends of tubing. Many sets allow for priming of tubing without removal of end cap.	Prevent bacteria from entering infusion equipment and blood-stream.
15. Place roller clamp about 2 to 5 cm (1 to 2 in) below drip chamber and move roller clamp to "off" position (see illustrations).	Close proximity of roller clamp to drip chamber allows more accurate regulation of flow rate. Moving clamp to "off" prevents accidental spillage of fluid.
16. Remove protective sheath over IV tubing port on plastic IV solution bag (see illustration). For bottled IV solution, remove metal cap and metal and rubber disks beneath cap.	Provides access for insertion of infusion tubing into solution.
17. Insert infusion set into fluid bag or bottle. Remove protector cap from tubing insertion spike (keeping spike sterile), and insert spike into opening of IV bag (see illustration). Cleanse rubber stopper on bottled solution with antiseptic, and insert spike into black rubber stopper of IV bottle.	Prevents contamination of solution from contaminated insertion spike.
18. Prime infusion tubing by filling with IV solution. Compress drip chamber and release, allowing it to fill one-third to one-half full.	Creates suction effects; fluid enters drip chamber to prevent air from entering tubing.
19. Remove tubing protector cap (some tubing can be primed without removal) and slowly release roller clamp to allow fluid to travel from drip chamber through tubing to needle adapter. Return roller clamp to "off" position after tubing is primed (filled with IV fluid).	Slow fill of tubing decreases turbulence and chance of bubble formation. Removes air from tubing and permits tubing to fill with solution. Closing the clamp prevents accidental loss of fluid.

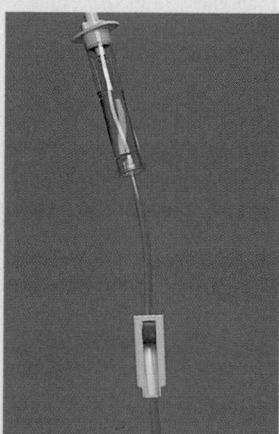
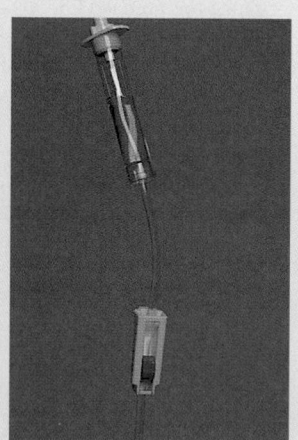

Step 15

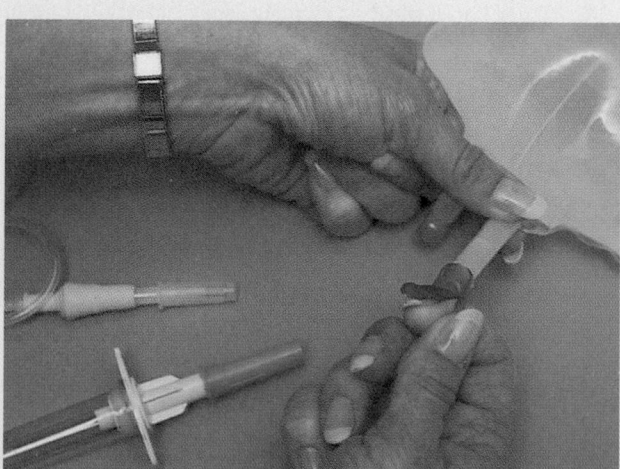

Step 16

STEPS	RATIONALE
20. Be certain tubing is clear of air and air bubbles. To remove small air bubbles, firmly tap IV tubing where air bubbles are located. Check entire length of tubing to ensure that all air bubbles are removed (see illustration).	Large air bubbles can act as emboli.
21. Replace tubing cap protector on end of tubing.	Maintains system sterility.
22. Optional: Prepare heparin or normal saline lock for infusion. If a loop or short extension tubing is needed because of an awkward IV site placement, use sterile technique to connect the IV plug to the loop or short extension tubing. Inject 1 to 3 ml normal saline through the plug and through the loop or short extension tubing.	Removes air to prevent introduction into the vein. Do the same with the saline plug.
23. Apply disposable gloves.	Reduces transmission of microorganisms.
24. Identify accessible vein for IV placement. Apply tourniquet 4 to 6 in (10 to 15 cm) above the proposed insertion site (see illustration). Check for presence of radial pulse. OPTION: Apply blood pressure cuff instead of tourniquet. Inflate to a level just below client's normal diastolic pressure. Maintain inflation at that pressure until venipuncture is completed.	Tourniquet should be tight enough to impede venous return but *not* occlude arterial flow.

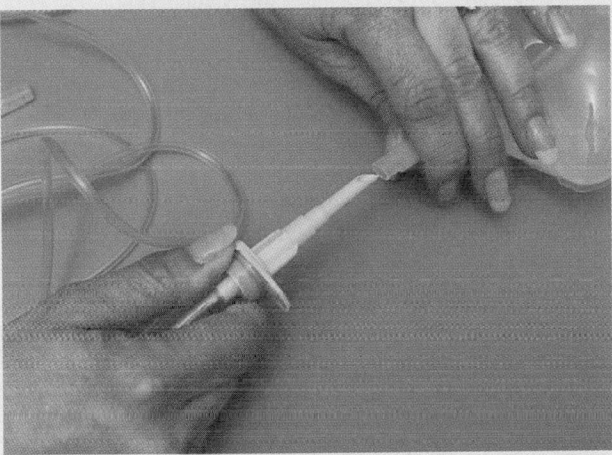

Step 17

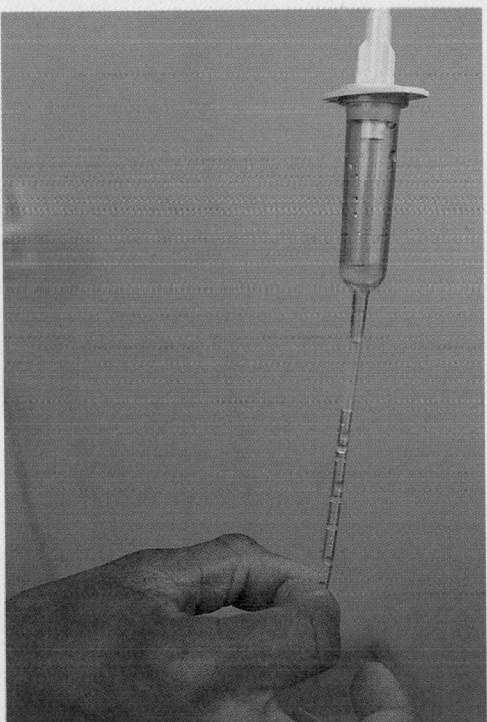

Step 20

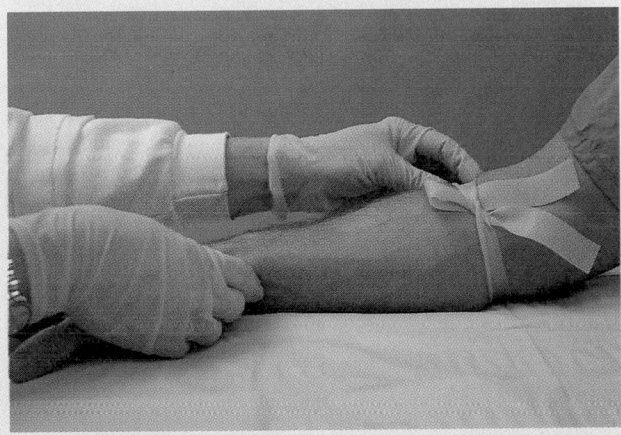

Step 24

STEPS	RATIONALE

25. Select the vein.

   a. Use the most distal site in the nondominant arm, if possible.

   b. Avoid areas that are painful to palpation.

   c. Select a vein large enough for catheter placement.

   d. Choose a site that will not interfere with client's activities of daily living (ADLs) or planned procedures.

   e. Palpate the vein by pressing downward and noting the resilient, soft, bouncy feeling as the pressure is released. Always use the same finger to palpate.

   f. Promote venous distention by instructing the client to open and close the fist several times, lowering the client's arm in a dependent position, rubbing or stroking the client's arm from distal to proximal below proposed site.

   g. Avoid sites distal to previous venipuncture site, sclerosed or hardened cordlike veins, infiltrated site or phlebotic vessels, bruised areas, and areas of venous valves or bifurcation.

   h. Avoid fragile dorsal veins in older adult clients and vessels in an extremity with compromised circulation (e.g., in cases of mastectomy, dialysis graft or paralysis).

26. Release tourniquet temporarily and carefully. Clip arm hair with scissors (if necessary). Do not shave area.

27. (If area of insertion appears to need cleansing, use soap and water first.) Then cleanse insertion site using firm, circular motion (middle to outward) with povidone-iodine solution; refrain from touching the cleansed site; allow the site to dry for at least 2 minutes. If the client is allergic to iodine, use 70% alcohol and allow to dry for 60 seconds (see illustration).

Venipuncture should be performed distal to proximal, which increases the availability of other sites for future IV therapy.

Prevents interruption of venous flow while allowing adequate blood flow around the catheter.

Use of the same finger causes a development of sensitivity to better assess the vein condition (Perucca, 1993).

Such sites cause infiltration of newly placed IV line and excessive vessel damage.

Venous alterations can increase risk of complications (e.g., infiltration and decreased catheter dwell time).

Hair impedes venipuncture or adherence of dressing. Shaving can cause microabrasions and predispose client to infection.

Povidone-iodine is a topical antiinfective that reduces skin surface bacteria; touching the cleansed area would introduce organisms from the nurse's hand to the site. Povidone-iodine must dry to be effective in reducing microbial counts (Baranowski, 1993).

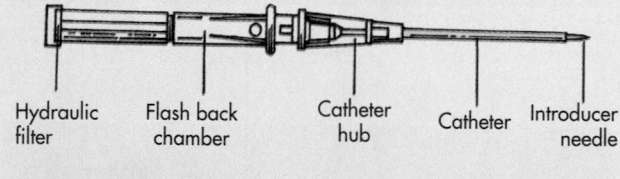

Hydraulic   Flash back   Catheter   Catheter   Introducer
filter   chamber   hub   needle

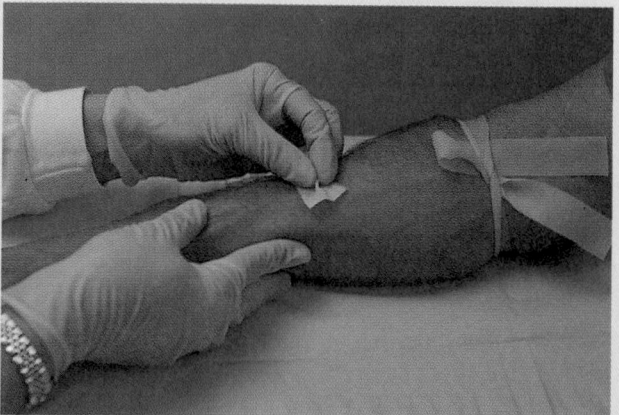

Step 27

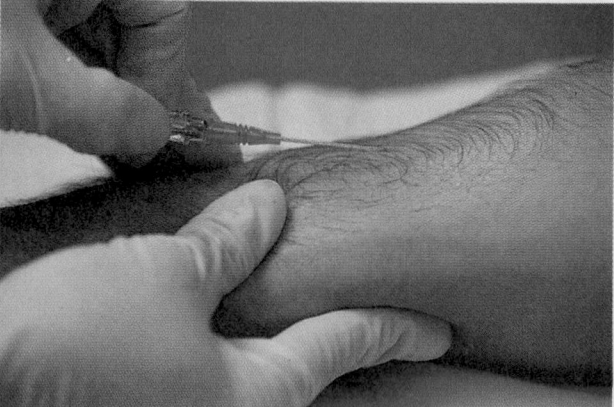

Step 28B

STEPS	RATIONALE
28. Perform venipuncture. Anchor vein by placing thumb over vein and by stretching the skin against the direction of insertion 5 to 7.5 cm (2 to 3 in) distal to the site. A. **Butterfly needle:** Hold needle at 20- to 30-degree angle with bevel up slightly distal to actual site of venipuncture. B. **ONC:** Insert ONC (see illustration) with bevel up at 20- to 30-degree angle slightly distal to actual site of venipuncture in the direction of the vein. C. **Needleless IV catheter safety device:** Insert using same position as for ONC.	Places needle parallel to vein. When vein is punctured, risk of puncturing posterior vein wall is reduced.

Critical Decision Point: No more than three attempts at inserting an IV should be made by a single nurse (check agency policy).

29. Look for blood return through tubing of butterfly needle or flashback chamber of ONC, indicating that needle has entered vein (see illustration). Lower needle until almost flush with skin. Advance butterfly needle until hub rests at venipuncture site. Advance ONC catheter ¼ in into vein and then loosen stylet. Advance catheter into vein until hub rests at venipuncture site (see illustration). Do not reinsert the stylet once it is loosened. (If available, advance the safety device by using push-off tab to thread the catheter.)	Increased venous pressure from tourniquet increases backflow of blood into catheter or tubing. Reinsertion of the stylet can cause catheter breakage in the vein.
30. Stabilize the catheter with one hand by placing pressure on the hub or on the vein above the insertion site. Release tourniquet and remove stylet from ONC. Do not recap the stylet. For a safety device, slide the catheter off the stylet while gliding the protective guard over the stylet. A click indicates the device is locked over the stylet.	Permits venous flow, reduces backflow of blood, and allows connection with administration set.
31. Quickly connect needle adapter of administration set or heparin lock to hub of ONC or butterfly tubing. Do not touch point of entry of needle adapter.	Prompt connection of infusion set maintains patency of vein. Maintains sterility.
32. Bloodless method: Hold pressure over tip of inserted catheter with your thumb; with your index finger and thumb remove cap and attach tubing to catheter hub (see illustration, p. 1226).	Prevents risk of exposure to blood.

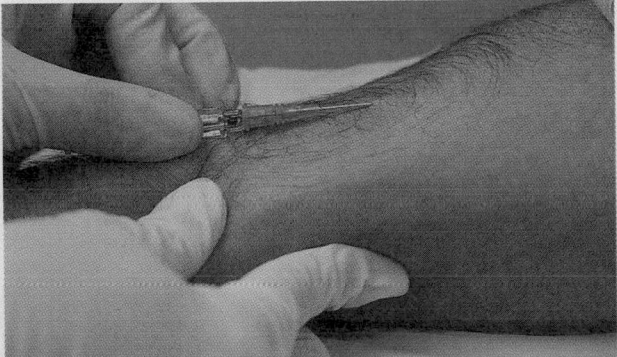
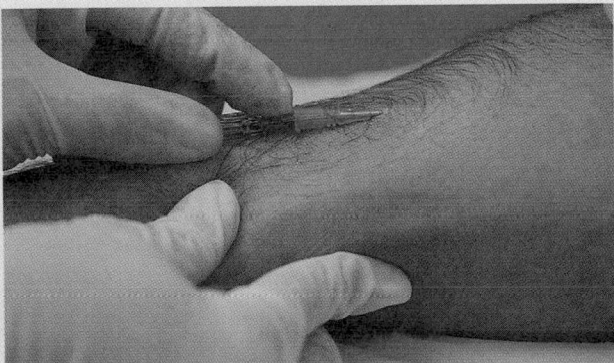

Step 29

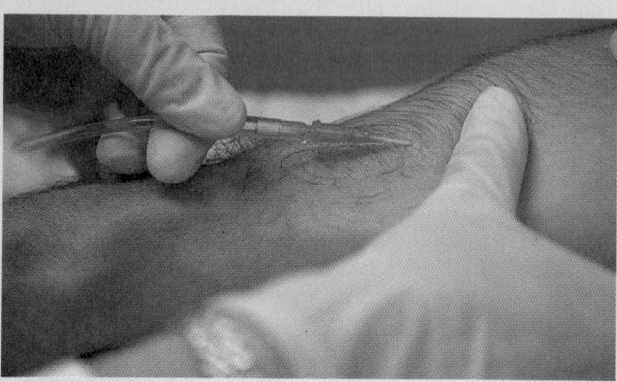

Step 32

33. Release roller clamp slowly to begin infusion at a rate to maintain patency of IV line (not necessary with a heparin lock).	Permits venous flow and prevents clotting of vein and obstruction of flow of IV solution.

Critical Decision Point: Be sure to calculate rate so as not to infuse IV solution too rapidly or too slowly.

---

34. Tape or secure catheter.
   A. **If applying a gauze dressing**
      (1) Tape the IV catheter. Place narrow piece (½ in) of tape under hub of catheter with adhesive side up and cross tape over hub (see illustration).
      (2) Place tape only on the catheter, *never* over the insertion site. Secure the site to allow easy visual inspection and early recognition of infiltration and phlebitis. Avoid applying tape around the extremity.
   B. **If applying transparent dressing,** secure catheter with nondominant hand while preparing to apply dressing.

Securing the catheter and tubing prevents movement and tension on the device, reducing mechanical irritation and possible phlebitis or infection.

Taping around extremity could result in a "tourniquet effect" and impede venous return.

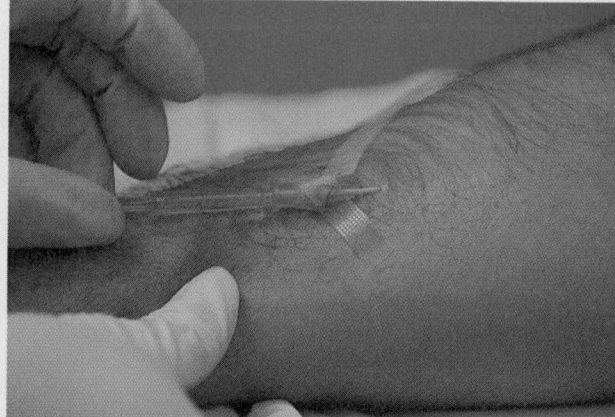

Step 34A(1)

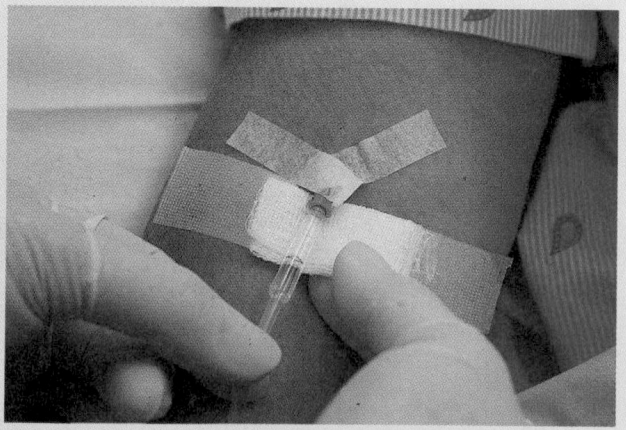

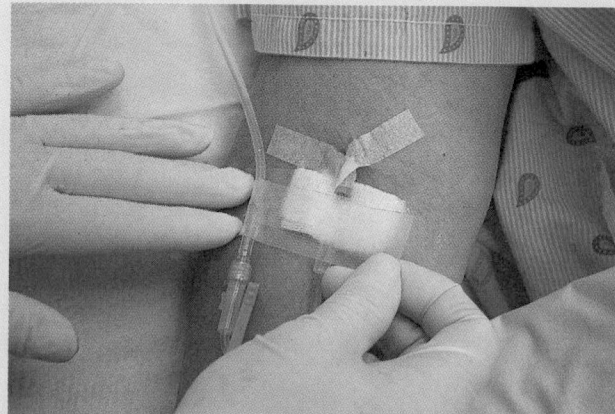

Step 35A(1)

STEPS	RATIONALE

35. Apply sterile dressing over site.

  A. **Sterile gauze dressing**

    (1) Fold a 2 × 2 gauze in half and cover with a 1-in-wide tape extending about an inch from each side. Place under the tubing/catheter hub junction. Curl a loop of tubing alongside the arm and place a second piece of tape directly over the padded 2 × 2, securing tubing in two places. (see illustrations).

Tape on top of tape makes it easier to access hub/tubing junction. Securing loop of tubing reduces risk of dislodging catheter from accidental pull.

    (2) Place another 2 × 2 gauze pad over venipuncture site and catheter hub. Secure all edges with tape. Do not cover connection between IV tubing and catheter hub.

  B. **Transparent dressing**

    (1) Carefully remove adherent backing. Apply one edge of dressing and then gently smooth remaining dressing over site, leaving end of catheter hub uncovered (see illustrations).

    (2) Follow step 35A(1).

36. For *IV fluid administration* adjust flow rate to correct drops per minute (Skill 40-2).

Maintains correct rate of flow for IV solution. Flow can fluctuate, so it must be checked at intervals.

  A. **Heparin lock.** Flush with 1 to 3 ml of heparin (10 to 100 U/ml).

  B. **Saline lock.** Flush with 1 to 3 ml of sterile normal saline.

Maintains patency of IV catheter.

37. Write date and time, gauge size and size of catheter, and placement of IV line and dressing.

Documents when IV was inserted and when subsequent dressing changes are needed.

38. Dispose of used needles in appropriate sharps container. Discard supplies. Remove gloves and wash hands.

Reduces transmission of microorganisms and protects staff from injury.

39. Observe client every hour to determine if fluid is infusing correctly.

  a. Check if correct amount of solution is infused as prescribed by looking at time tape.

  b. Count flow rate.

  c. Check patency of IV catheter or needle: briefly compress cannulated vein proximal to site. Observe for slowing or cessation of IV rate.

Compression results in mechanical obstruction of vein. When IV catheter is patent, compression results in slowing or cessation of flow rate. No change in flow rate may indicate infiltration.

  d. Also observe client during compression of vessel for signs of discomfort.

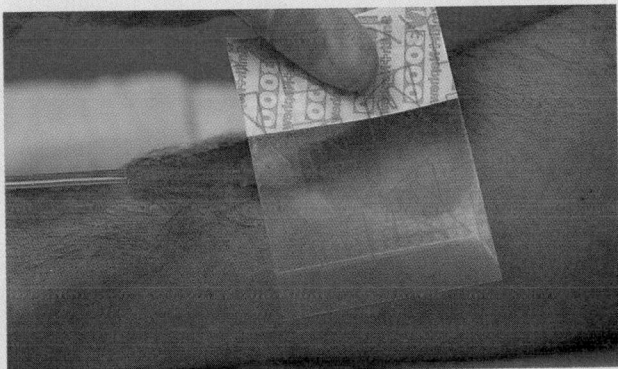
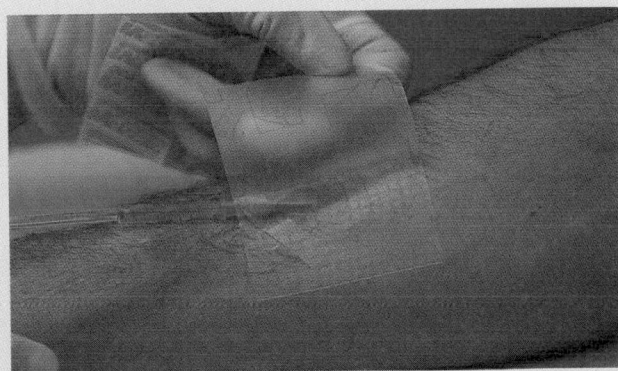

Step 35B(1)

STEPS	RATIONALE
e. Inspect insertion site for absence of infiltration, phlebitis, or inflammation (Table 40-9)	Provides continuous evaluation of type and amount of fluid delivered to client. Hourly inspection prevents accidental fluid overload or inadequate infusion rate and identifies early incidence of vein inflammation or tissue damage.
40. Observe client every hour to determine response to therapy (i.e., measure vital signs, conduct postprocedure assessments).	IV fluids and additives are given to maintain or restore fluid and electrolyte balance. They can also cause unexpected effects, which can be serious.

Recording and Reporting

- Record in nurses' notes number of attempts for insertion, type of fluid, insertion site by vessel, flow rate, size and type of catheter or needle, and when infusion was begun. A special parenteral therapy flow sheet may be used.
- Record client's response to IV fluid, amount infused, and integrity and patency of system every 4 hours or according to agency policy.
- Report to oncoming nursing staff: type of fluid, flow rate, status of venipuncture site, amount of fluid remaining in present solution, expected time to hang next IV bag or bottle, and any side effects.

Home Care Considerations

See Box 40-8 (p. 1219).

- Teach caregiver to apply pressure with sterile gauze if catheter falls out and, if client is on anticoagulant therapy, to tape several pieces of sterile gauze in place for at least 20 min or until bleeding stops.
- Teach client and caregiver to perform tub bath without getting IV tubing wet and to unplug pump first if one is used. For showering, the client must insert hand and forearm into a plastic bag. Tape bag in place to ensure that IV site is completely covered.
- Teach client and family to monitor I&O using household measuring devices.

Table 40-9   Phlebitis Scale

Grade	Clinical Criteria
0	No symptoms
1	Erythema at access site with or without pain
2	Pain at access site with erythema and/or edema
3	Pain at access site with erythema and/or edema Streak formation Palpable venous cord
4	Pain at access site with erythema and/or edema Streak formation Palpable venous cord >1 inch in length Purulent drainage

From Intravenous Nurses Society: Infusion nursing standards of practice, *J Intraven Nurs* 23(65):556, 2000.

NURSING PRACTICE   Box 40-6

- In older clients, use the smallest gauge catheter or needle possible (e.g., 24 to 26 gauge). This is less traumatizing to the vein and allows better blood flow to provide increased hemodilution of the IV fluids or medications. This gauge can be used for hourly flow rates of 75 to 100 ml/hr.
- Avoid the back of the older adult's hand or the dominant arm for venipuncture because these sites greatly interfere with the older adult's independence.
- If the older adult has fragile skin and veins, use minimal tourniquet pressure.
- When the older adult has lost subcutaneous tissue, the veins lose stability and will roll away from the needle. To stabilize the vein, apply traction to the skin below the projected insertion site.
- Using an angle of 5 to 15 degrees on insertion is helpful because the older adult's veins are more superficial.
- In the older person with fragile skin, prevent skin tears by minimizing the amount of tape used.

Modified from Coulter K: Intravenous therapy for the elder patient: implications for the intravenous nurse, *J Intraven Nurs* 15(suppl):S18, 1992.

Regulating Intravenous Flow Rate | Skill 40-2

Delegation Considerations

The skill of regulating IV therapy requires problem solving and knowledge application unique to professional nursing. For this procedure delegation is not appropriate.

EQUIPMENT

- Watch with second hand
- Paper and pencil

- IV infusion pump (optional)
- Volume control device (optional)

STEPS	RATIONALE
1. Observe for patency of IV line and needle or catheter:	For fluid to infuse at proper rate, IV line and needle must be free of kinks, knots, and clots.
a. Open drip regulator and observe for rapid flow of fluid from solution into drip chamber, then close drip regulator to prescribed rate.	Rapid flow of fluid into drip chamber indicates patency of IV line. Closing drip chamber to prescribed rate prevents fluid overload.
b. Compress cannulated vein slightly proximal to the end of the catheter and observe the drip chamber.	Cessation of drops from drip chamber indicates catheter or needle is in vein. If fluid continues to drip, infiltration may be present and further assessment is needed.
2. Check client's medical record for correct solution, additives, and time of infusion. Usual order includes solution for 24 hours, usually divided into 2 or 3 L. Occasionally, IV order contains only 1 L to keep vein open (KVO). Record also shows time over which each liter is to infuse.	Five rights of drug administration ensure correct fluids are given to correct client.
3. Check client's knowledge of how positioning of the IV site affects flow rate.	Fosters client participation in maintaining most effective position of arm with IV equipment.
4. Verify with client how venipuncture site feels (e.g., determine if there is pain or burning).	Pain or burning may be early indication of phlebitis. Includes client in decision making.
5. Have paper and pencil to calculate flow rate.	The beginning student is unfamiliar with IV fluid rates and should use mathematical calculations to obtain correct rate.

6. Know calibration (drop factor) in drops per milliliter (gtt/ml) of infusion set:
  A. **Microdrip:** 60 gtt/ml
  B. **Macrodrip:** (Metheny, 1992):
      Abbott: 15 gtt/ml
      Travenol: 10 gtt/ml
      McGaw: 15 gtt/ml
	Microdrip tubing, also called pediatric tubing, universally delivers 60 gtt/ml and is used when small or very precise volumes are to be infused. However, there are different commercial parenteral administration sets for macrodrip tubing. Macrodrip tubing should be used when large quantities or fast rates are necessary.

Critical Decision Point: Know which company's infusion set your agency uses.

---

7. Select one of the following formulas to calculate flow rate after determining ml/hr:
  ml/hr = total infusion (ml)/hour of infusion
  (a) ml/hr/60 minutes = ml/minute
  (b) Drop factor × ml/minute = Drops/minute
                OR
  ml/hr × Drop factor/60 minutes = Drops/minute
	Once hourly rate has been determined, these formulas give correct flow rate.

8. Read physician's orders and follow five rights for correct solution and proper additives.
    IV fluids are usually ordered for 24-hour period, indicating how long each liter of fluid should run; for example, IV order for client is:
      Bottle 1: 1000 ml D_5W with 20 mEq KCl to run 8 hr
      Bottle 2: 1000 ml D_5W with 20 mEq KCl to run 8 hr
      Bottle 3: 1000 ml D_5W with 20 mEq KCl to run 8 hr
      Total 24-hour IV intake: 3000 ml
	IV fluids are medications; following five rights decreases chance of medication error.
	
	Determines volume of fluid that should infuse hourly.

STEPS	RATIONALE
9. Determine hourly rate by dividing volume by hours; for example: 1000 ml/8 = 125 ml/hr *or* if 3 L is ordered for 24 hr 3000 ml/24 hr = 125 ml/hr	Provides even infusion of fluid over prescribed hourly rate.
10. Place adhesive or fluid indicator tape on IV bottle or bag next to volume markings (see illustration).	Time taping IV bag gives nurse visual cue as to whether fluids are being administered over correct period of time. Time tapes should be used for all IV infusions, including those on therapies infused via electronic infusion devices.

Critical Decision Point: Do not use felt-tip pens or permanent markers on IV bags, because ink could contaminate the solution (Millam, 1992).

11. After hourly rate has been determined, calculate minute rate based on drop factor of infusion set. Microdrip infusion set has a drop factor of 60 gtt/ml. Regular drip or macrodrip infusion set used in this example has drop factor of 15 gtt/ml.
 	
Using formula, calculate minute flow rates: Bottle 1:1000 ml with 20 mEq KCl
 	
A. Microdrip
125 ml × 60 gtt/ml/60 minutes =
        7500 gtt/60 minutes = 125 gtt/minute
 	
B. Macrodrip
125 ml × 15 gtt/ml/60 minutes =
        31 to 32 gtt/minute
Volume is multiplied by drop factor and the product is divided by time (in minutes).
	Allows nurse to calculate minute flow rate based on this formula:
	
	Total volume × Drop factor/infusion time in minutes
	
	When using microdrip, ml/hr always equals gtt/min.

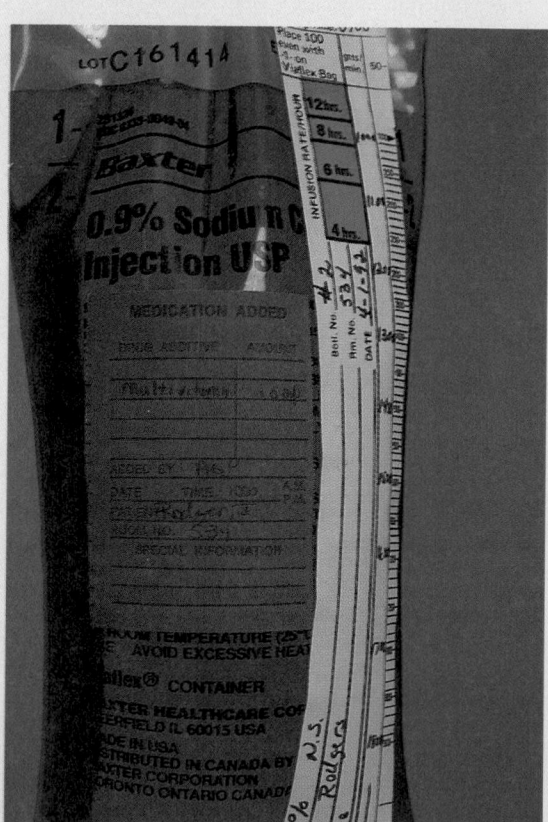

Step 10

STEPS	**RATIONALE**
12. Time flow rate by counting drops in drip chamber for 1 min by watch, then adjust roller clamp to increase or decrease rate of infusion (see illustration).	Determines if fluids are administered too slowly or too fast.
13. Follow this procedure for infusion controller or pump:	
a. Place electonic eye on drip chamber below origin of drop and above fluid level in chamber, or consult manufacturer's directions for setup of the infusion (see illustration). If a controller is used, ensure that IV bag is 36 in above the IV site.	The electronic eye counts the number of drops flowing from administration set to ensure that proper rate infuses. IV controller works by gravity.
b. IV infusion tubing is placed within ridges of control box in direction of flow (i.e., portion of tubing nearest IV bag at top and portion of tubing nearest client at bottom) or consult manufacturer's directions for use of pump (see illustration). Required drops per minute or volume per hour are selected, door to control chamber is closed, power button is turned on, and start button is pressed.	Infusion pumps move fluid by compressing and milking IV tubing, thus propelling fluid through tubing.

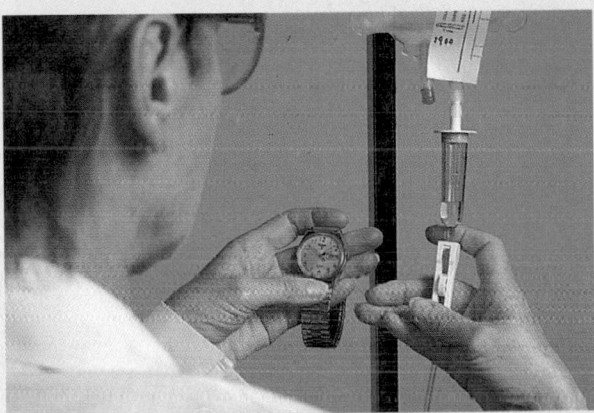

Step 12

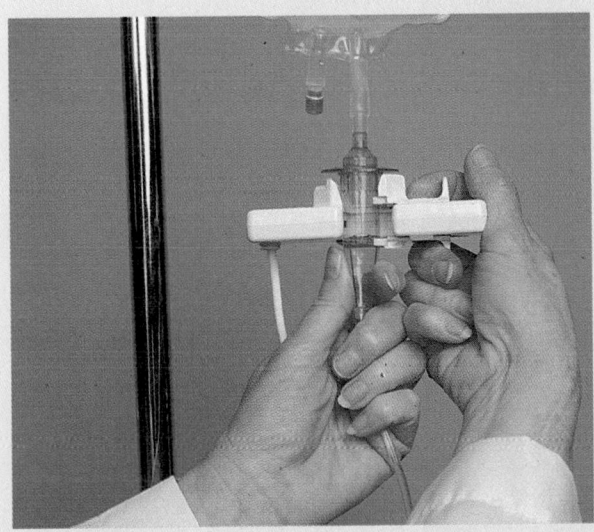

Step 13a

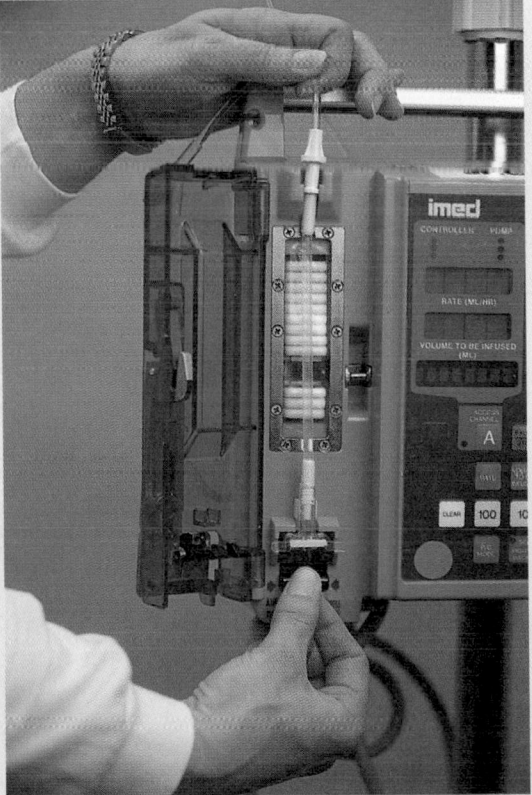

Step 13b

| STEPS | RATIONALE |

Critical Decision Point: Special infusion tubing is required for some pumps (check agency policy).

   c. Drip regulator must be open while infusion controller or pump is in use.

   d. Monitor infusion rates and IV site for infiltration according to agency policy.

        Infusion controllers or pumps are not infallible and do not replace frequent, accurate nursing assessments. Infusion pumps may continue to infuse IV fluids after an infiltration has begun.

   e. Assess patency and integrity of system when alarm sounds.

        Alarm indicates that electronic eye has not noted precise number of drops from drip chamber, or there is an empty solution bag or bottle, kink in tubing, closed drip regulator, infiltrated or clotted needle, and/or air in the tubing.

14. Follow this procedure for volume control device:

   a. Place volume control device between IV bag and insertion spike of infusion set (see illustration).

        Reduces risk of sudden increase in fluid volume.

   b. Place 2 hours' allotment of fluid into device.

        Prevents IV line from running dry if nurse does not return in exactly 60 min. In addition, if there is accidental increase in flow rate, client receives at most only a 2-hr allotment of fluid.

   c. Assess system at least hourly; add fluid to volume control device. Regulate flow rate.

        Maintains patency of system.

15. Observe client for signs of overhydration or dehydration to determine response to therapy and restoration of fluid and electrolyte balance.

        Signs and symptoms of dehydration or overhydration warrant changing rate of fluid infused.

16. Evaluate for signs of infiltration: inflammation at site, clot in catheter, kink or knot in infusion tubing.

        Prevents decrease or cessation of flow rate.

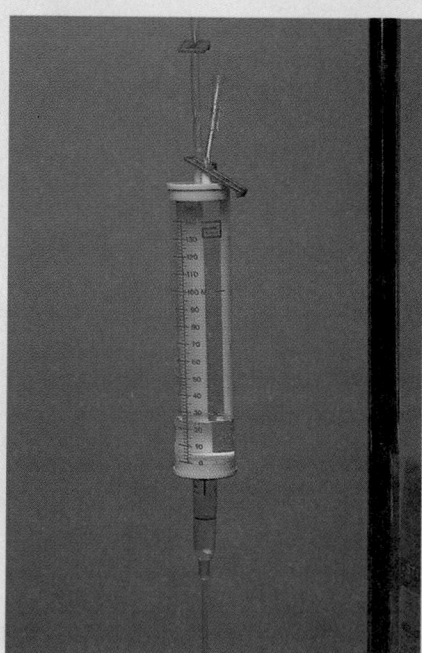

Step 14a

Recording and Reporting

- Record name of solution, rate of infusion, drops/min, and ml/hr in nurses' notes every 4 hours or according to agency policy.
- Immediately record in nurses' notes any new IV fluid rates.
- Document use of any EID or controlling device and number on that device.
- At change of shift or when leaving on break, report rate of infusion to nurse in charge or next nurse assigned to care for client.

Home Care Considerations

- Ensure that client is able and willing to operate the EID (if applicable) and administer IV therapy or that there is a reliable caregiver or nursing support personnel at home to provide this IV therapy care.
- Teach client and primary caregiver to time drops per minute using watch with second hand.

catheter (over-the-needle catheter [ONC]), or a needle attached to a syringe. Large catheters placed into a central vein such as the subclavian vein are used to deliver large volumes of fluids and TPN or to administer irritating medications. Although these central line catheters are inserted by physicians, nurses are responsible for maintaining them. When veins are fragile or collapse, venipuncture may become extremely difficult, but it may be a life-saving measure as well. For these difficult clients, venipuncture should be performed by an experienced practitioner. The general purposes of venipuncture are to collect a blood specimen, to instill a medication, to start an IV infusion, or to inject a radiopaque or radioactive tracer for special examinations. Skill 40-1 describes venipuncture for IV fluid infusion.

Regulating the Infusion Flow Rate. After the IV infusion is secured and the line is patent, the nurse must regulate the rate of infusion according to the physician's orders (Skill 40-2). An infusion rate that is too slow can lead to further cardiovascular and circulatory collapse in a critically ill client who has FVD or hyperosmolar imbalance or who is in shock. An IV that is running too slowly can also become clotted off more easily. An infusion rate that is too rapid can result in FVE. The nurse calculates the infusion rate to prevent too-slow or too-rapid administration of the IV fluids. The minimal rate used to keep a vein open and patent is about 10 to 15 ml/hr using a microdrip infusion. Many electronic infusion devices record the volume of the fluid infused. An **infusion pump** is designed to deliver a measured amount of fluid over a period of time (e.g., milliliters per hour). The pump has a drop sensor, and an alarm that will sound if drops are not detected at the appropriate rate. There are also alarms to alert the nurse to increased system pressure that can occur with an infiltration (IV fluid seeping into the tissue instead of the vascular space).

A second type of infusion device is an IV controller (e.g., Dial-A-Flow) that delivers fluids with the aid of gravity; IV controllers deliver fluids based on a determination of milliliters per hour. The rate of infusion with an IV controller depends on the height of the IV fluid container, IV tubing size, and fluid viscosity. The IV controller is less precise than the IV pump in delivering IV fluids with precision. With either device, the client requires close monitoring to verify the correct infusion of the IV solution and to detect the occurrence of any complication. Patency of the IV needle or catheter means that there are no clots at the tip of the needle or catheter and that the catheter or needle tip is not against the vein wall. A blocked catheter or needle can affect the rate of infusion of the IV fluids. IV flow rates can also be affected by the patency of the IV needle or catheter, infiltration, a knot or kink in the tubing, the height of the solution, and the position of the client's extremity. The nurse can assess patency by lowering the IV bag below the level of the IV insertion site and observing for a blood return. If no blood return occurs and fluid does not flow easily from the drip chamber when the roller clamp is opened, several problems may exist: a too-tight IV dressing may be impeding the flow, a clot may be occluding the cannula of the IV catheter, or the catheter tip may be occluded against the wall of the vein. The tubing and area around the insertion site should be inspected for anything that could obstruct the flow of IV fluids. A knot or kink in the tubing can decrease the flow rate. Occasionally the tubing is kinked under a dressing, which requires the nurse to remove the dressing to locate the problem. The flow rate frequently resumes after the tubing is straightened. The client may also occlude the tubing by lying or sitting on it. The height of the IV bag can also affect flow rates. Raising the bag usually increases the rate because of increased hydrostatic pressure.

The position of the extremity, particularly at the wrist or elbow, can decrease flow rates. Occasionally the use of an arm board helps to keep the joint extended (Figure 40-13). The arm board also provides some protection to the IV site and tubing. Sometimes it is more comfortable for the client to have an infusion started in a new location rather than dealing with a site that causes problems. However, before discontinuing the infusion hampered by an extremity position, the nurse should start the infusion in another site to verify that the client has other accessible veins.

An infiltration may be present when the insertion site becomes cool, clammy, swollen, and in some cases painful. An infiltration occurs when the needle or catheter has dislodged from the vein and is in the subcutaneous space. When an infiltration occurs, the IV line must be discontinued and a new line inserted. Factors that alter IV flow rates can occur with any client at any time. When caring for a client with an infusion, the nurse should assess the site and the infusion rate at least every hour.

Children, older adults, clients with severe head trauma, and clients susceptible to volume overload must be protected from sudden increases in infusion volumes. The nurse needs to understand that when certain IV controller devices are opened, the IV fluid will infuse rapidly. If this is not controlled, an excessive amount of solution can infuse. Sudden increases can occur accidentally. For example, a restless client may loosen the roller clamp with a sudden movement and increase the flow rate, or the flow rate may be accidentally increased if the client ambulates. A sudden increase in IV infusion rate causes a rapid increase in vascular volume, which can make the client critically ill or even cause death. Volume control devices, such as a Volutrol buret, can prevent sudden excessive increases in the volume of IV solution infused.

Maintaining the System. After the IV line is in place and the flow rate is regulated, the nurse must maintain the system. The nurse keeps in mind agency policy regarding the maintenance of IV lines. Line maintenance is achieved by (1) keeping the system sterile; (2) changing solutions, tubing, and site dressings; and (3) assisting the client with self-care activities so as to not disrupt the system.

The nurse plays an important role in maintaining the integrity of an IV to prevent infection from developing. Figure 40-14 demonstrates the potential sites for contamination of an intravascular device. The client's microflora and contamination by insertion are initially controlled for in the procedure for IV insertion. However, the other factors are controlled through conscientious use of infection-control principles. This begins with the use of thorough hand washing before and after the nurse handles any component of the IV system.

The integrity of the IV system must always be maintained. The nurse never disconnects tubing because it becomes tangled or because it might be more convenient in positioning or moving a client or applying a gown. If a client needs more room to maneuver, extension tubing can be added to an IV line. Stopcocks are available for connecting more than one IV solution to a single IV site. An IV tubing should be inserted into each port of a stopcock;

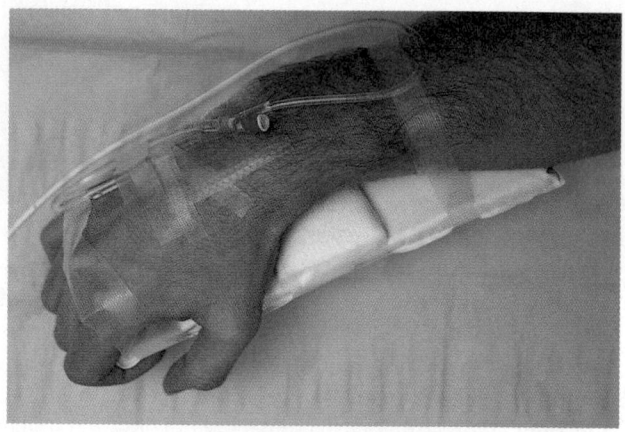

Figure 40-13   IV arm board.

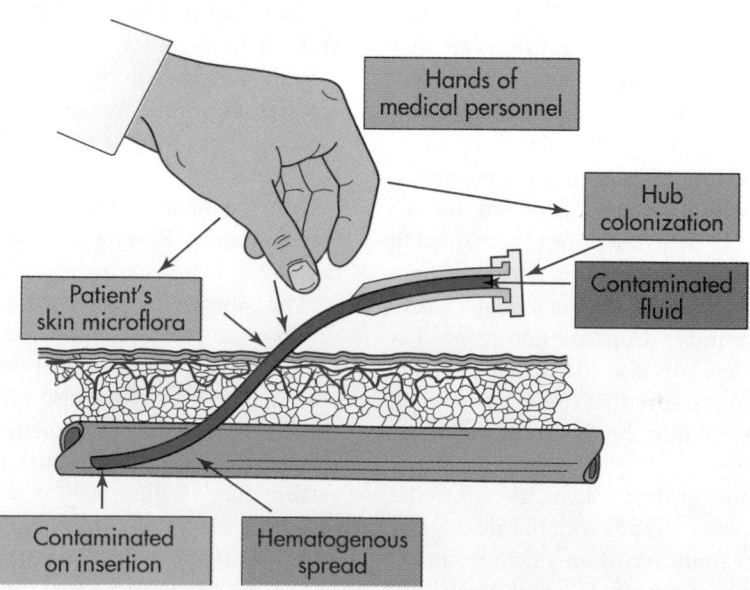

Figure 40-14   Potential sites for contamination of an intravascular device.

otherwise the port should be plugged with a sterile cap. Do not allow a port to remain exposed to air.

Intravenous tubing also contains injection ports through which needles can be inserted for medication injections. An injection port must be cleaned thoroughly with 70% alcohol or povidone-iodine solution before accessing the system (Pearson, 1996).

Clients receiving IV therapy over several days will require frequent changing of solutions. It is important for the nurse to organize tasks so that this can be done in plenty of time before the solution runs out and possibly becomes clotted. The Centers for Disease Control and Prevention (CDC) (Pearson, 1996) has no recommendation for the hang time of IV fluids; however, the nurse should refer to agency policy. Skill 40-3 reviews steps for changing IV solutions.

Intravenous tubing administration sets can remain sterile for 72 hours (Pearson, 1996). The exception is tubing containing blood, blood products, and lipid emulsions, which are more likely to promote bacterial growth. Agency policy may require more frequent tubing changes. It is easier to change tubing when a new IV bag or bottle is being hung. To prevent entry of bacteria into the bloodstream, sterility must be maintained during tubing and solution changes.

The dressings over IV sites are applied to reduce the entrance of bacteria into the insertion site. The two forms of dressings are gauze and transparent. Transparent dressings reliably secure the IV device, allow continuous visual inspection of the IV site, become less easily soiled or moistened, and require less frequent changes than standard gauze (Pearson, 1996). Either form of dressing must be changed when the IV device is removed or replaced or when the dressing becomes damp, loosened, or soiled (Pearson, 1996). Agency policy may require IV dressings to be routinely changed within a certain time frame (e.g., 48 to 72 hours) (Skill 40-4).

To prevent the accidental disruption of an IV system, the nurse may need to assist the client with hygiene, comfort measures, meals, and ambulation. Because a client with an infusion in the arm finds it difficult to meet hygiene needs, the nurse should help with bathing and changing gowns. It helps to use a gown specifically made with snaps along the top sleeve seam to facilitate changing the gown without disturbing the venipuncture site. Regular gowns are changed by following these six steps for maximum arm mobility and speed:

1. Remove the sleeve of the gown from the arm without the IV, maintaining the client's privacy.
2. Remove the sleeve of the gown from the arm with the IV.
3. Remove the IV bottle or bag from its stand and pass it and the tubing through the sleeve. (If this involves removing the tubing from an IV pump, use the roller clamp to slow the infusion to prevent the accidental infusion of a large volume of solution or medication).

4. Place the IV bottle or bag and tubing through the sleeve of the clean gown and hang it on its stand. (If the IV is connected to a pump, reassemble and open the roller clamp. Turn the pump on.)
5. Place the arm with the IV through the gown sleeve.
6. Place the arm without the IV through the gown sleeve. (Breaking the integrity of an IV line to change a gown leads to contamination.)

The client with an arm or a hand infusion is able to walk, unless contraindicated. A walking IV pole (a standard IV pole with wheels) is needed. The nurse helps the client get out of bed and places the pole next to the involved arm. The client is instructed to hold on to the pole with the involved hand and to push it while walking. The nurse should assess the equipment to make sure that the IV bag is at the proper height, that there is no tension on the tubing, and that the flow rate is correct. The nurse should instruct the client to report any blood in the tubing, a stoppage in the flow, or increased discomfort. Intravenous catheters and drugs, especially antibiotics and potassium, can cause discomfort and burning sensations at the IV site. Clients must be reassured that occasional discomfort is normal. Sometimes discomfort is relieved by repositioning the extremity, but occasionally it is necessary to start a new IV line in a larger vein.

Complications of Intravenous Therapy. An **infiltration** occurs when IV fluids enter the subcutaneous space around the venipuncture site. This is manifested as swelling (from increased tissue fluid) and pallor (caused by decreased circulation) around the venipuncture site. Fluid may be flowing through the IV line at a decreased rate or may have stopped flowing. Pain may also be present and usually results from edema and increases proportionately as the infiltration continues.

When infiltration occurs, the infusion must be discontinued and, if IV therapy is still necessary, the catheter or needle is reinserted into another extremity. To reduce discomfort, the nurse raises the extremity, which promotes venous drainage. To help decrease the edema, the nurse wraps the extremity in a warm towel for 20 minutes while keeping it elevated on a pillow. This promotes venous return, increases circulation, and reduces pain and edema.

Phlebitis is an inflammation of the vein. Selected risk factors for phlebitis include the type of catheter material, chemical irritation of additives and drugs given intravenously (e.g., antibiotics), and the anatomical position of the catheter. Signs and symptoms include pain, increased skin temperature over the vein, and, in some instances, redness traveling along the path of the vein. Dehydration may also be a contributing factor because of the increase in blood viscosity (Beare and Myers, 1998).

When phlebitis develops, the IV line must be discontinued and a new line inserted in another vein. Warm, moist heat on the site of phlebitis can offer some relief to the client (see Chapter 47). Phlebitis can be dangerous, be-

Text continued on p. 1239.

Skill 40-3 Changing Intravenous Solution and Infusion Tubing

Delegation Considerations

The skill of changing IV solutions and tubing requires problem solving and knowledge application unique to professional nursing. For this procedure delegation is not appropriate.

EQUIPMENT

- **IV infusion**
  - Bottle/bag of IV solution as ordered by physician
  - Time tape
  - Infusion tubing
  - 0.22 mμ filter and extension tubing (if necessary)
- **Heparin flush**
  - Injection cap, loop, or short extension tubing (if necessary)

- **Normal saline flush**
  - Syringes
  - 2 sterile 2 × 2 gauze pads
  - Tape
  - Disposable nonsterile gloves

STEPS	RATIONALE
CHANGING IV SOLUTION	
1. Check physician's orders.	Ensures that correct solution will be used.
2. If order is written for keep vein open (KVO) or to keep open (TKO), note date and time when solution was last changed.	A hang time is no longer recommended by the CDC (Pearson, 1996) to ensure sterility of solutions in bag or bottle. Refer to agency policy.
3. Determine the compatibility of all IV fluids and additives by consulting appropriate literature or the pharmacy.	Incompatibilities can cause physical, chemical, and therapeutic client changes.
4. Determine client's understanding of need for continued IV therapy.	Reveals need for client instruction.
5. Assess patency of current IV access site.	If patency is not verified, a new IV access site may be needed. Notify physician.
6. Have next solution prepared at least 1 hr before needed. If prepared in pharmacy, be sure it has been delivered to the client's hospital unit. Check that solution is correct and properly labeled. Check solution expiration date.	Adequate planning reduces risk of clot formation in vein caused by empty IV bag. Checking prevents medication error.
7. Prepare to change solution when less than 50 ml of fluid remains in bottle or bag.	Prevents air from entering tubing and vein from clotting from lack of flow.
8. Prepare client and family by explaining the procedure, its purpose, and what is expected of client.	Decreases anxiety and promotes cooperation.
9. Be sure drip chamber is at least half full.	Provides fluid to vein while bag is changed.
10. Wash hands.	Reduces transmission of microorganisms.
11. Prepare new solution for changing. If using plastic bag, remove protective cover from IV tubing port. If using glass bottle, remove metal cap and metal and rubber disks.	Permits quick, smooth, and organized change from old to new solution.
12. Move roller clamp to stop flow rate.	Prevents solution remaining in drip chamber from emptying while changing solutions.
13. Remove old IV fluid container from IV pole.	Brings work to nurse's eye level.
14. Quickly remove spike from old solution bag or bottle and, without touching tip, insert spike into new bag or bottle.	Reduces risk of solution in drip chamber running dry and maintains sterility.

Critical Decision Point: If spike is contaminated, a new IV tubing set is required.

15. Hang new bag or bottle of solution.	Gravity assists with delivery of fluid into drip chamber.

STEPS	RATIONALE
16. Check for air in tubing. If bubbles form, they can be removed by closing the roller clamp, stretching the tubing downward, and tapping the tubing with the finger (the bubbles rise in the fluid to the drip chamber). For a larger amount of air, insert a needle and syringe into a port below the air and aspirate the air into the syringe. Swab port with alcohol and allow to dry before inserting needle into port. Reduce air in tubing by priming slowly instead of allowing a wide-open flow.	Reduces risk of air embolus. Use of an air-eliminating filter also reduces this risk.
17. Make sure drip chamber is one-third to one-half full. If the drip chamber is too full, pinch off tubing below the drip chamber, invert the container, squeeze the drip chamber, hang up the bottle, and release the tubing.	Reduces risk of air entering tubing.
18. Regulate flow to prescribed rate.	Maintains measures to restore fluid balance and deliver IV fluid as ordered.
19. Observe client for signs of overhydration or dehydration to determine response to IV fluid therapy.	Provides ongoing evaluation of client's fluid and electrolyte status.
20. Observe IV system for patency and development of complications (e.g., infiltration or phlebitis).	Provides ongoing evaluation of IV system.

CHANGING IV TUBING

STEPS	RATIONALE
21. Determine when new infusion set is needed:	
a. Agency policy will indicate frequency of routine change for IV administration sets and heparin flushes.	The CDC (Pearson, 1996) recommends tubing change no more often than 72-hour intervals.
b. Puncture of infusion tubing.	Punctured tubing results in fluid leakage and bacterial contamination.
c. Contamination of tubing.	Contamination of tubing allows entry of bacteria into client's bloodstream.
22. Observe for occlusions in existing tubing. Such occlusions can occur after infusion of packed red cells, whole blood, albumin, or other blood components.	Whole blood or blood component product can occlude or partially occlude tubing, because viscous solutions adhere to walls of tubing and decrease the size of the lumen.
23. Prepare client and family by explaining the procedure, its purpose, and what is expected of client.	Decreases anxiety, promotes cooperation, and prevents sudden movement of extremity, which could dislodge IV needle or catheter.
24. Wash hands.	Reduces transmission of microorganisms.
25. Open new infusion set, keeping protective coverings over infusion spike and connector and connector site for butterfly needle or IV catheter.	Provides nurse with ready access to new infusion set and maintains sterility of infusion set.
26. Apply nonsterile, disposable gloves.	Reduces risk of exposure to HIV, hepatitis, and other blood-borne bacteria (CDC, 1987; Garner, 1996).
27. If needle or catheter hub is not visible, remove IV dressing. Do not remove tape securing needle or catheter to skin.	Needle hub must be accessible to provide smooth transition when removing old and inserting new tubing.
28. For IV infusion:	
a. Move roller clamp on new IV tubing to "off" position.	Prevents spillage of solution after bag or bottle is spiked.
b. Slow rate of infusion by regulating drip rate on old tubing. Be sure rate is at KVO rate.	Prevents complete infusion of solution that remains in tubing, which can increase risk of occlusion of IV catheter or needle.
c. With old tubing in place, compress drip chamber and fill chamber.	Provides surplus of fluid in drip chamber so there is enough fluid to maintain IV patency while changing tubing.
d. Remove old tubing from solution and hang or tape drip chamber on IV pole 36 in above IV site.	Allows fluid to continue to flow through IV catheter while nurse is preparing new tubing.
e. Place insertion spike of new tubing into old solution bag opening and hang solution bag on IV pole.	Permits flow of fluid from solution into new infusion tubing.
f. Compress and release drip chamber on new tubing; slowly fill drip chamber one-third to one-half full.	Allows drip chamber to fill and promotes rapid, smooth flow of solution through new tubing.
g. Slowly open roller clamp, remove protective cap from needle adapter (if necessary), and flush tubing with solution. Replace cap.	Removes air from tubing and replaces it with fluid.
h. Turn roller clamp on old tubing to "off" position.	Prevents spillage of fluid as tubing is removed from needle hub.

STEPS	RATIONALE
29. For heparin lock:	
a. If a loop or short extension tubing is needed because of an awkward IV site placement, use sterile technique to connect the new injection cap to the loop or tubing.	
b. Swab injection cap with alcohol. Insert syringe with 1 to 3 ml saline and inject through the injection cap into the loop or short extension tubing.	Removes air to prevent introduction into the vein.
30. Stabilize hub of catheter or needle and apply pressure over vein just above insertion site. Gently pull out old tubing (see illustration). Maintain stability of hub and quickly insert needle adapter of new tubing or heparin lock into hub (see illustrations).	Prevents accidental displacement of catheter or needle. Prevents clot formation in catheter or needle and backflow of blood.
31. Open roller clamp on new tubing. Allow solution to run rapidly for 30 to 60 seconds.	Permits IV solution to enter catheter to prevent catheter occlusion.
32. Regulate IV drip according to physician's orders and monitor rate hourly (see illustration).	Maintains infusion flow at prescribed rate.
33. If necessary, apply new dressing.	Reduces risk of bacterial infection from skin.
34. Discard old tubing in proper container.	Reduces accidental transmission of microorganisms.
35. Remove and dispose of gloves. Wash hands.	Reduces transmission of microorganisms.
36. Evaluate flow rate and observe connection site for leakage	Maintains prescribed rate of flow of IV fluid and determines if fit is secure.

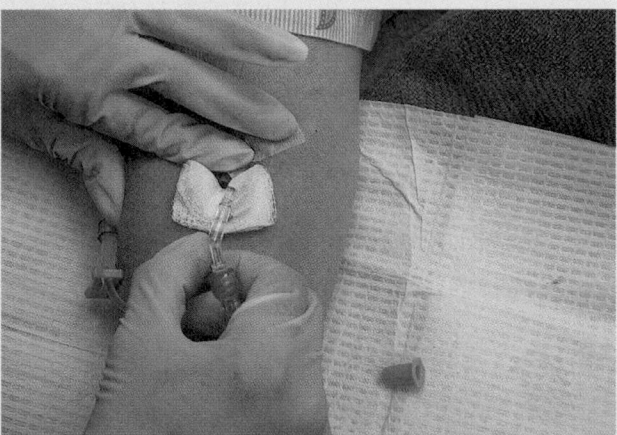

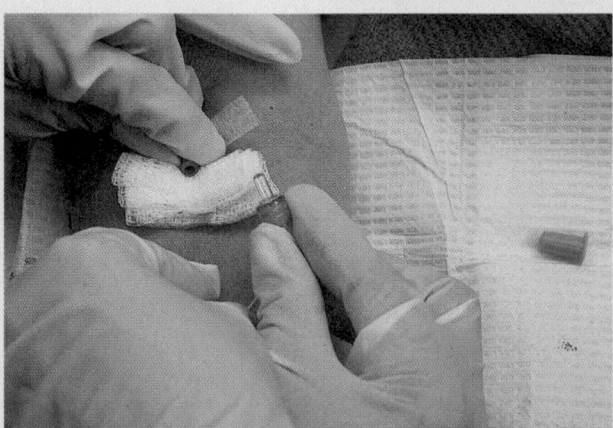

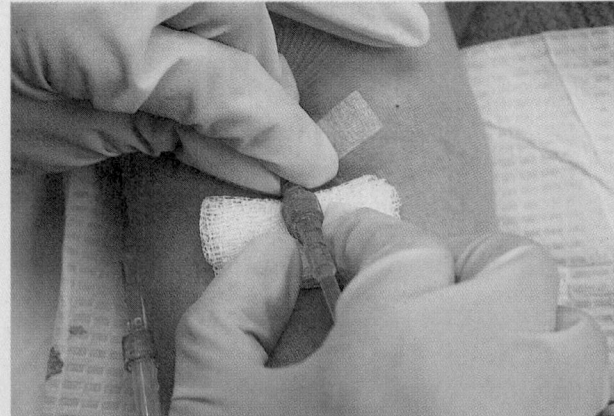

Step 30

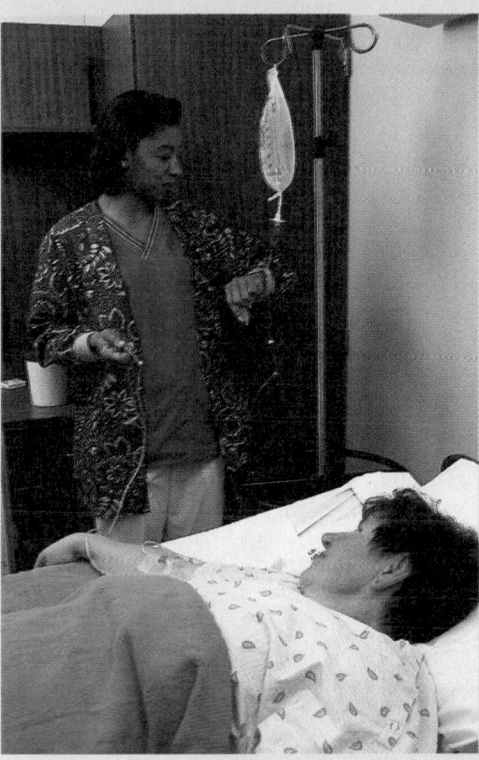

Step 32

Recording and Reporting
- Record changing of tubing and solution on client's record. A special parenteral therapy flow sheet may be used.
- Place a piece of tape or preprinted label with the date and time of tubing change and attach to tubing below the level of drip chamber.

Home Care Considerations
- Emphasize to client and family the importance of changing solutions when IV tubing still contains fluid.

---

cause blood clots (thrombophlebitis) can occur and in some cases may result in emboli. Phlebitis is prevented by the routine removal and rotation of IV sites. The CDC (Pearson, 1996) recommends replacing peripheral venous catheters and rotating sites every 48 to 72 hours.

Fluid volume excess occurs when the client has received a too-rapid administration of IV solutions. The assessment findings include shortness of breath, crackles in the lungs, and tachycardia. The nurse should slow the rate of infusion, notify the physician, raise the head of the bed, and monitor vital signs.

Bleeding can occur around the venipuncture site during the infusion or through the catheter needle or tubing if these become inadvertently disconnected. Bleeding is common in clients who have received heparin or who have a bleeding disorder (e.g., leukemia or thrombocytopenia). If bleeding occurs around the venipuncture site and the catheter is within the vein, a pressure dressing may be applied over the site to control the bleeding. Bleeding from a vein is usually a slow, continuous seepage and is not serious.

Discontinuing Intravenous Infusions.   Discontinuing an infusion is necessary after the prescribed amount of fluid has been infused, when an infiltration occurs, if phlebitis is present, or if the infusion catheter or needle develops a clot at its tip. The nurse discontinuing an infusion first applies disposable gloves and then removes the tape and dressing in the same manner as for the daily infusion dressing changes. The nurse then moves the roller clamp to the "off"/closed position to prevent spillage of IV fluid. The nurse places a sterile 2 × 2 gauze pad over the

Skill 40-4   Changing a Peripheral Intravenous Dressing

Delegation Considerations

The skill of changing a peripheral IV dressing requires problem solving and knowledge application unique to professional nursing. For this procedure delegation is not appropriate.

EQUIPMENT

- Povidone-iodine swab stick
- Alcohol swab stick
- Adhesive remover (if needed)
- Strips of nonallergenic tape
- Disposable gloves

- **For gauze dressing**
  - Sterile 2 × 2 gauze pad
    OR
  - Sterile 4 × 4 gauze pad
- **For transparent dressing**
  - Sterile transparent dressing

STEPS	RATIONALE
1. Determine when dressing was last changed. Many institutions require nurse to write date and time on dressing and date the device was first placed.	Provides information regarding length of time present dressing has been in place. In addition, nurse is able to plan for dressing change.
2. Observe present dressing for moisture and intactness.	Moisture is a medium for bacterial growth and renders dressing contaminated.
3. Observe IV system for proper functioning or complications: kinks in infusion tubing or IV catheter. Palpate the catheter site through the intact dressing for inflammation or subjective complaints of pain or burning.	Unexplained decrease in flow rate requires the nurse to investigate placement and patency of the IV catheter. Pain can be associated with both phlebitis and infiltration.
4. Inspect exposed catheter site for swelling or infiltration.	Indicates fluid infusing into surrounding tissues. Will require removal of IV catheter.
5. Assess client's understanding of need for continued IV infusion.	Determines need for client instruction.
6. Explain procedure and purpose to client and family. Explain that affected extremity must be held still and how long procedure will take.	Decreases anxiety, promotes cooperation, and gives client time frame around which personal activities can be planned.
7. Wash hands. Apply disposable gloves.	Reduces transmission of microorganisms.
8. Remove tape, gauze, and/or transparent dressing from old dressing one layer at a time, leaving tape that secures IV needle or catheter in place. Be cautious if catheter tubing becomes tangled between two layers of dressing. When removing transparent dressing, hold catheter hub and tubing with nondominant hand.	Prevents accidental displacement of catheter or needle.
9. Observe insertion site for signs and/or symptoms of infection, namely redness, swelling, and exudate.	
10. If infiltration, phlebitis, or clot occurs or if ordered by physician, discontinue infusion (see p. 1239).	
11. If IV is infusing properly, gently remove any tape securing needle or catheter. Stabilize needle or catheter with one hand. Use adhesive remover to cleanse skin and remove adhesive residue, if needed.	Exposes venipuncture site. Stabilization prevents accidental displacement of catheter or needle. Adhesive residue decreases ability of new tape to adhere tightly to skin.
12. Keep one finger over catheter at all times until tape or dressing is replaced.	Prevents decannulation from vein.
13. Using circular motion, cleanse peripheral IV insertion site with alcohol, then povidone-iodine solution starting at insertion site and working outward creating concentric circles (see illustration). Allow each solution to dry for 2 minutes.	Circular motion prevents cross contamination from skin bacteria near venipuncture site. Povidone-iodine is a topical anti-infective that reduces skin surface bacteria; the solution must be dry to be effective in reducing microbial counts (Baranowski, 1993).

Critical Decision Point: Do not tape over connection of access tubing or port to IV catheter.

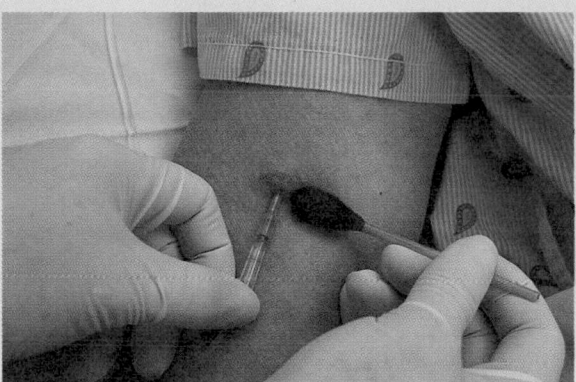

Step 13

14. Apply new transparent or gauze dressing (See Skill 40-1, Steps 34 and 35).	Ensures protection of IV site and reduces chance of infection.
15. Remove and discard gloves.	
16. Anchor IV tubing with additional pieces of tape. When using polyurethane dressing, minimize the tape placed over dressing.	Prevents accidental displacement of IV needle or catheter or separation of IV tubing from needle adapter.
17. Place date and time of dressing change and size and gauge of catheter directly on dressing.	Documents dressing change.
18. Discard equipment and wash hands.	Reduces transmission of microorganisms.
19. Observe functioning and patency of IV system in response to changing dressing.	Validates that IV is patent and functioning correctly.
20. Monitor client's body temperature.	Elevated temperature indicates an infection that may be associated with bacterial contamination of the venipuncture site.

Recording and Reporting

- Record appearance of IV site, type of dressing, and status of IV fluid infusion.

- A special parenteral fluid flow sheet may be used for recording.

---

venipuncture site and, using the other hand, withdraws the catheter needle by pulling straight back away from the puncture site (Figure 40-15). If necessary, alcohol or soap and water can be used to remove dried blood or other drainage from around the site. Alcohol is not used on the IV site, because it can cause stinging and prolongs bleeding (Phillips, 1993). The nurse elevates the extremity and applies pressure to the site for 1 to 2 minutes to control bleeding and prevent hematoma formation. Clients who have received heparin require longer pressure because of the action of heparin on blood-clotting mechanisms. If needed, the nurse applies a bandage over a sterile cotton ball or applies a larger sterile dressing over the venipuncture site. The nurse records the amount of fluid infused and the time of the discontinuation.

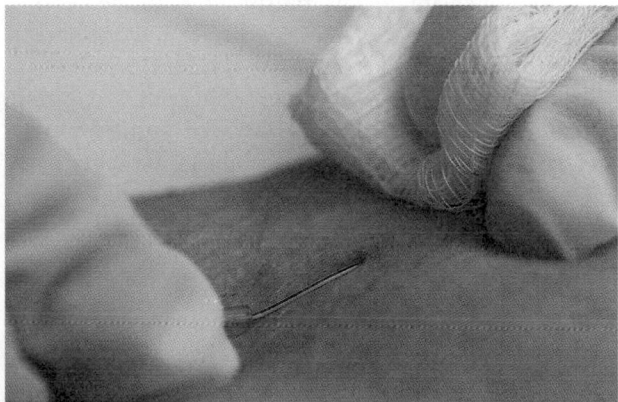

Figure 40-15   IV catheter is removed slowly, keeping catheter parallel to vein.

Blood Replacement (Colloids).   Blood replacement or transfusion is the IV administration of whole blood or a component such as plasma, packed RBCs, or platelets. The objectives for blood transfusions include (1) to increase circulating blood volume after surgery, trauma, or hemorrhage; (2) to increase the number of RBCs and to maintain hemoglobin levels in clients with severe anemia; and (3) to provide selected cellular components as replacement therapy (e.g., clotting factors, platelets, albumin).

Blood Groups and Types.   The most important grouping for transfusion purposes is the ABO system, which includes A, B, 0, and AB blood types. The determination of blood groups is based on the presence or absence of A and B red cell antigens. Individuals with A antigens, B antigens, or no antigens belong to groups A, B, and 0 respectively. The person with A and B antigens has AB blood. Individuals with type A blood naturally produce anti-B antibodies in their plasma. Similarly, type B individuals naturally produce anti-A antibodies. A type 0 individual has neither type A nor type B antigen and thus is considered a universal blood donor. A type AB individual produces neither antibody, which is why a type AB individual, can be a universal recipient and receive any type of blood. If blood that is mismatched with the client's blood is transfused, a **transfusion reaction** occurs. The transfusion reaction is an antigen-antibody reaction and can range from a mild response to severe anaphylactic shock, which can be life threatening.

Another consideration when matching for blood transfusions is the Rh factor, which is an antigenic substance in the erythrocytes of most people. A person with the factor is Rh positive, and a person without it is Rh negative.

Autologous Transfusion.   **Autologous transfusion** or autotransfusion is the collection of a client's own blood. The blood for an autologous transfusion can be obtained by preoperative donation up to 5 weeks before the planned surgery (e.g., heart, orthopedic, plastic, gynecological). The client can donate 1 to 5 units of his or her own blood depending on the type of surgery and the ability of the client to maintain an acceptable hematocrit. The blood will be tested for HIV and HBV. Another way to collect blood for an autologous transfusion is during perioperative blood salvage (e.g., during vascular and orthopedic surgery, organ transplant surgery, and traumatic injuries). The blood that has been salvaged is then reinfused during the surgery. Blood can also be salvaged postoperatively from mediastinal and chest-tube drainage and after joint and spinal surgery. Autologous transfusions are safer for the client because they decrease the risk of complications such as mismatched blood and exposure to blood-borne infectious agents.

Blood Transfusions.   Transfusing blood or blood components is a nursing procedure. The nurse is responsible for assessment before, during, and after the transfusion and for regulation of the transfusion. Assessment is critical because of the risk of allergic reactions.

If the client has an IV line in place, the nurse should assess the venipuncture site for signs of infection or infiltration. The nurse should also determine whether the venipuncture was performed with an 18- or 19-gauge catheter. The large catheter is needed because blood is thicker and stickier than IV fluids. The nurse should determine that the IV catheter is patent and functioning properly. The tubing for blood administration has an in-line filter (Figure 40-16). The tubing should be filled with 0.9% normal saline to prevent **hemolysis,** or breakdown of RBCs.

Pretransfusion assessment also includes obtaining information from the client. The nurse asks whether the client knows the reason for the blood transfusion and whether the client has ever had a previous transfusion or transfusion reaction. A client who has had a transfusion reaction is usually at no greater risk for a reaction with a subsequent transfusion. However, the client may be anxious about the transfusion, requiring nursing intervention. Before giving a transfusion, the nurse explains the procedure and instructs the client to report any side effects (e.g., chills, dizziness, fever) once the transfusion begins. The nurse also checks to be sure the client has signed an informed consent.

Because of the danger of transfusion reactions, it is very important to use specific precautions in administering blood or blood products. The nurse must obtain the client's baseline vital signs before the transfusion begins. This data will allow the nurse to determine when changes in vital signs occur, which can indicate that a transfusion

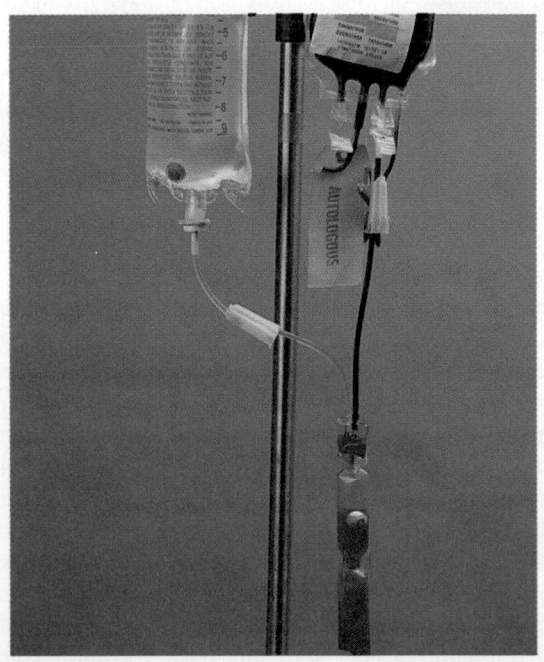

Figure 40-16   Tubing for blood administration has an in-line filter.

reaction is developing. To ensure that the right client receives the correct type of blood or blood product, a thorough procedure is used to check the identity of the blood products, the client, and the compatibility of the blood and the client. The nurse, although not involved in the blood labeling process, is responsible for determining that the blood delivered to the client corresponds to the client's blood type listed in the medical record. Two registered nurses or one registered nurse and a licensed practical nurse (see agency policy) must together check the label on the blood product against the client's identification number, blood group, and complete name. If even a minor discrepancy exists, the blood should not be given and the blood bank should be notified immediately.

Initiation of a transfusion begins slowly to allow for the early detection of a transfusion reaction. The nurse maintains the infusion rate, monitors for side effects, assesses vital signs, and promptly records all findings. The nurse usually stays with the client during the first 15 minutes, the time when a reaction is most likely to occur. The nurse will continue to monitor the client and obtain vital signs periodically during the transfusion as directed by agency policy. If a transfusion reaction is anticipated or suspected, the nurse will obtain vital signs more frequently (Table 40-10).

The rate of transfusion is usually specified in the physician's orders. Ideally a unit of whole blood or packed RBCs is transfused in 2 hours. This time can be lengthened to 4 hours if the client is at risk for FVE. Beyond 4 hours there is a risk of the blood becoming contaminated.

When clients have a severe blood loss such as with hemorrhage, they may receive rapid transfusions through a central venous catheter. A blood-warming device is often necessary, because the tip of the central venous catheter lies in the superior vena cava, above the right atrium. Rapid administration of cold blood can result in cardiac dysrhythmia (LaRocca and Otto, 1989).

Transfusion Reactions.   A transfusion reaction is a systemic response by the body to incompatible blood. Causes include red cell incompatibility or allergic sensitivity to the components of the transfused blood or to the potassium or citrate preservative in the blood. Blood transfusion can also result in the transmission of infectious disease. Several types of acute reactions can result from blood transfusions (see Table 40-10).

A second category of reactions includes diseases transmitted by infected blood donors who are asymptomatic. Diseases transmitted through transfusions are malaria, hepatitis, and AIDS. Because all units of blood collected must undergo serological testing and screening for HIV and HBV, the risk of acquiring blood-borne infections from blood transfusions is reduced.

Circulatory overload is a risk when a client receives massive whole blood or packed RBC transfusions for massive hemorrhagic shock or when a client with normal blood volume receives blood. Clients particularly at risk

for circulatory overload are older adults and those with cardiopulmonary diseases.

Blood transfusion reactions are life threatening, but prompt nursing intervention can maintain the client's physiological stability.

- If a blood reaction is suspected, the nurse *stops the transfusion immediately.*
- The nurse keeps the IV line open by "piggybacking" 0.9% normal saline directly into the IV line and running the saline.
- The nurse should not turn off the blood and simply turn on the 0.9% normal saline that is connected to the Y-tubing infusion set. This would cause blood remaining in the Y-tubing to infuse into the client. Even a small amount of mismatched blood can cause a major reaction.
- The nurse has the physician notified immediately.
- The nurse remains with the client, observing signs and symptoms and monitoring vital signs as often as every 5 minutes.
- The nurse prepares to administer emergency drugs such as antihistamines, vasopressors, fluids, and steroids as per physician order.
- The nurse prepares to perform cardiopulmonary resuscitation.
- The nurse obtains a urine specimen and sends it to the laboratory.
- The blood container, tubing, attached labels, and transfusion record are saved and returned to the laboratory.

Interventions for Acid-Base Imbalances.   Nursing interventions to promote acid-base balance support prescribed medical therapies and are aimed at reversing the acid-base imbalance that exists. Such imbalances can be life threatening and require rapid correction. The nurse must maintain a functional IV line and frequently check the physician's orders for new medications or fluids. Prescribed drugs, such as insulin or sodium bicarbonate, and fluid and electrolyte replacement should be given promptly. Chapter 39 reviews appropriate therapies for clients with respiratory acidosis.

The nurse also monitors clients closely for changes in acid-base balance. Clients with acid-base disturbances usually require repeated ABG analysis. This procedure provides arterial blood samples for analysis of hydrogen ion concentration.

Arterial Blood Gases.   Determination of ABG levels requires the removal of a sample of blood from an artery to assess the client's acid-base status and the adequacy of ventilation and oxygenation. Arterial blood is drawn from a peripheral artery (usually the radial) or from an arterial line inserted by a physician. In some agencies, nurses are responsible for radial artery punctures. Beginning nursing students do not draw arterial samples but frequently assist

Table 40-10 Acute Transfusion Reactions

Reaction	Cause	Clinical Manifestations	Management	Prevention
Acute hemolytic	Infusion of ABO-incompatible whole blood, RBCs, or components containing 10 ml or more of RBCs. Antibodies in the recipient's plasma attach to antigens on transfused RBCs causing RBC destruction.	Chills, fever, low back pain, flushing, tachycardia, tachypnea, hypotension, vascular collapse, hemoglobinuria, hemoglobinemia, bleeding, acute renal failure, shock, cardiac arrest, death.	Stop transfusion. Treat shock, if present. Draw blood samples for serologic testing slowly to avoid hemolysis from the procedure. Send urine specimen to the laboratory. Maintain BP with IV colloid solutions. Give diuretics as prescribed to maintain urine flow. Insert indwelling catheter or measure voided amounts to monitor hourly urine output. Dialysis may be required if renal failure occurs. Do not transfuse additional RBC-containing components until transfusion service has provided newly crossmatched units.	Meticulously verify and document client identification from sample collection to component infusion.
Febrile, non-hemolytic (most common)	Sensitization to donor white blood cells, platelets or plasma proteins.	Sudden chills and fever (rise in temperature of greater than 1°C), headache, flushing, anxiety, muscle pain.	Give antipyretics as prescribed—avoid aspirin in thrombocytopenic patients. **Do not restart transfusion.**	Consider leukocyte-poor blood products (filtered, washed, or frozen).
Mild allergic	Sensitivity to foreign plasma proteins.	Flushing, itching, urticaria (hives).	Give antihistamine as directed. If symptoms are mild and transient, transfusion may be restarted slowly. Do not restart transfusion if fever or pulmonary symptoms develop.	Treat prophylactically with antihistamines.
Anaphylactic	Infusion of IgA proteins to IgA-deficient recipient who has developed IgA antibody.	Anxiety, urticaria, wheezing, progressing to cyanosis, shock, possible cardiac arrest.	Initiate CPR, if indicated. Have epinephrine ready for injection (0.4 ml of a 1:1000 solution subcutaneously or 0.1 ml of 1:1000 solution diluted to 10 ml with saline for IV use). **Do not restart transfusion.**	Transfuse extensively washed RBC products, from which all plasma has been removed. Alternatively, use blood from IgA-deficient donor.

From National Blood Resource Education Programs: *Transfusion therapy guidelines for nurses,* NIH Pub No. 90-2668a, September 1990. *ABO,* Blood group consisting of groups A, AB, B, and O; *RBCs,* red blood cells; *BP,* blood pressure; *IV,* intravenous; *IgA,* immunoglobulin A; *CPR;* cardiopulmonary resuscitation.

Table 40-10 **Acute Transfusion Reactions**—cont'd				
Reaction	Cause	Clinical Manifestations	Management	Prevention
Circulatory overload	Fluid administered faster than the circulation can accommodate.	Cough, dyspnea, pulmonary congestion (rales), headache, hypertension, tachycardia, distended neck veins.	Place client upright with feet in dependent position. Administer prescribed diuretics, oxygen, morphine. Phlebotomy may be indicated.	Adjust transfusion volume and flow rate based on client size and clinical status. Have transfusion service divide unit into smaller aliquots for better spacing of fluid input.
Sepsis	Transfusion of contaminated blood components.	Rapid onset of chills, high fever, vomiting, diarrhea, and marked hypotension and shock.	Obtain culture of client's blood and send bag with remaining blood to transfusion service for further study. Treat septicemia as directed—antibiotics, IV fluids, vasopressors, steroids.	Collect, process, store, and transfuse blood products according to blood banking standards and infuse within 4 hr of starting time.

in the sampling process and care for the client after the procedure. After the specimen is obtained, care is taken to prevent air from entering the syringe because this will affect the blood gas analysis. To reduce metabolism of cells, the syringe is submerged in crushed ice and transported immediately to the laboratory. The nurse applies pressure to the puncture site for at least 5 minutes to reduce the risk of hematoma formation. The nurse might also reassess the radial pulse after pressure has been removed.

Restorative Care.   After experiencing acute alterations in fluid, electrolyte, or acid-base balance, clients often require ongoing maintenance to prevent a recurrence of health alterations. Older adults and the chronically ill require special considerations to prevent complications from developing (Box 40-7).

Home Intravenous Therapy.   Intravenous therapy is often continued in the home setting for clients requiring long-term hydration, parenteral nutrition (see Chapter 43), or long-term medication administration. The client must have a family member who can be available if the client suddenly cannot manage the IV or if a problem develops. A home IV therapy nurse will work closely with the client to ensure that a sterile IV system is maintained and that complications can be avoided or recognized promptly. Box 40-8 summarizes client education guidelines for home IV therapy.

Nutritional Support.   Most clients who have had electrolyte disorders or metabolic acid-base disturbances require ongoing nutritional support. Depending on the type

of disorder, fluid or food intake may be encouraged or restricted (see Chapter 43). The client needs a nutritionally well-balanced diet. If clients are still responsible for preparing their own meals, they should learn to look at the lists of the nutrient content of foods and to read the labels of commercially prepared foods.

Medication Safety.   Numerous drugs contain components or create potential side effects that can alter fluid and electrolyte balance. Clients with chronic disease who are receiving multiple medications and those with renal or liver disorders are at significant risk for alterations to develop. Once clients return to a restorative care setting, whether in the home, long-term care, or a nursing home, drug safety becomes very important. Client and family education is essential to provide information on knowing what is contained in a drug and what side effects to observe for. The nurse should review all medications with clients and encourage them to consult with their local pharmacist, especially if they try a new over-the-counter medication.

EVALUATION

Client Care.   The evaluation of a client's clinical status is especially important if an acute fluid and electrolyte or acid-base disturbance exists. The client's condition can change very quickly, and the nurse must be able to recognize the signs and symptoms of impending problems. To do this well, the nurse integrates what he or she knows about the health alterations, the effects of medications and fluids, and the client's presenting clinical status

Research HIGHLIGHT   Box 40-7

RESEARCH ABSTRACT

Inadequate water intake frequently contributes to a number of health problems, such as confusion, dehydration, and constipation for elderly individuals. This study examined 99 nursing home residents from one urban nursing home in Utah and two rural skilled nursing homes in South Dakota. The residents were monitored during two 24-hour periods, and their food and fluid intake along with ingestion behaviors and function were recorded. Participation in this study required that the subjects were not on a fluid restriction or receiving tube feedings and were at least 70 years or older. After an initial chart review each resident's height, weight, and urine output were documented and a data recording instrument developed by the investigator monitored and recorded each resident's intake. This study found that the fluid intake of the 99 nursing home residents was less than 100% of the standard water requirement and inadequate. In addition the researcher identified that nursing residents who experienced an inadequate water intake were older, more independent, had an intact speech pattern, did not experience any drooling, had fewer ingestion sessions per day, were semidependent with eating, and had an inadequate nutrient intake.

IMPLICATIONS FOR PRACTICE

- Continued research is needed to determine what an appropriate standard water intake for the elderly is.
- Nurses need to understand and implement preventive interventions for residents with an inadequate water intake or for any client who is at risk.
- Nurses need to be aware of the potential risks associated with older adult inadequate water intake and its effect on fluid and electrolyte balance.

REFERENCE

Meyer-Gaspar P: Water intake of nursing home residents, *J Gerontol Nurs* 25(4):23, 1999.

(Figure 40-17). The nurse will perform evaluative measures and determine if changes have occurred from the last client assessment. For example, if the nurse's assessment of a client's hypokalemia is showing signs of improvement, the physical signs and symptoms of hypokalemia should begin to disappear or lessen in intensity. The client's heart rhythm becomes more regular and normal bowel function returns.

For clients with less acute alterations evaluation likely occurs over a longer period of time. In this situation the nurse's evaluation may be focused more on behavioral changes (e.g., the client's ability to follow dietary restrictions and medication schedules). The family's ability to anticipate alterations and prevent problems from recurring is also an important element of evaluation.

The client's level of progress determines whether the nurse needs to continue or revise the plan of care. If goals are not met as a result of the failure to meet expected outcomes, the nurse may need to consult with a physician and discuss additional methods such as increasing the frequency of an intervention (e.g., provide more fluids to a dehydrated client), introducing a new therapy (e.g., initiate insertion of an IV), or discontinuing a particular therapy. Once outcomes have been met, the nurse can resolve the nursing diagnosis and focus on other priorities.

Client Expectations. The nurse routinely reviews with the client his or her success in meeting the client's expectations of care. "Tell me if I have helped you feel more comfortable" is a question that the nurse might raise if the client's expectations revolve around comfort and symptom management. If the client's concerns involve having a better understanding of a chronic problem, the nurse's evaluation might focus on the client's satisfaction with educational offerings. Often the client's level of satisfaction with care also depends on the nurse's success in involving family and friends. If the client has concerns about returning home or to a different care setting, it will be important to evaluate if the client feels prepared for the transition from acute care.

Client Teaching FOR HOME INTRAVENOUS THERAPY   Box 40-8

- Explain to client and caregiver the importance of IV therapy in maintaining hydration and access for the delivery of medications.
- Emphasize the risks involved when the IV system is not kept sterile.
- Be sure the client and/or caregiver is able to manipulate the required equipment.
- Instruct client or caregiver in how to change IV solutions, tubing, and dressing when they become soiled or dislodged. (NOTE: The home health nurse may be able to visit frequently enough to perform scheduled tubing and dressing changes.)

- Instruct client and caregiver about signs and symptoms of infiltration, phlebitis, and infection and to notify the home health nurse immediately.
- Instruct client and caregiver to notify the home health nurse if the infusion slows or stops or if blood is seen in the tubing.
- Teach client with caregiver's assistance how to ambulate, perform hygiene, and participate in other activities of daily living without dislodging or disconnecting catheter and tubing.

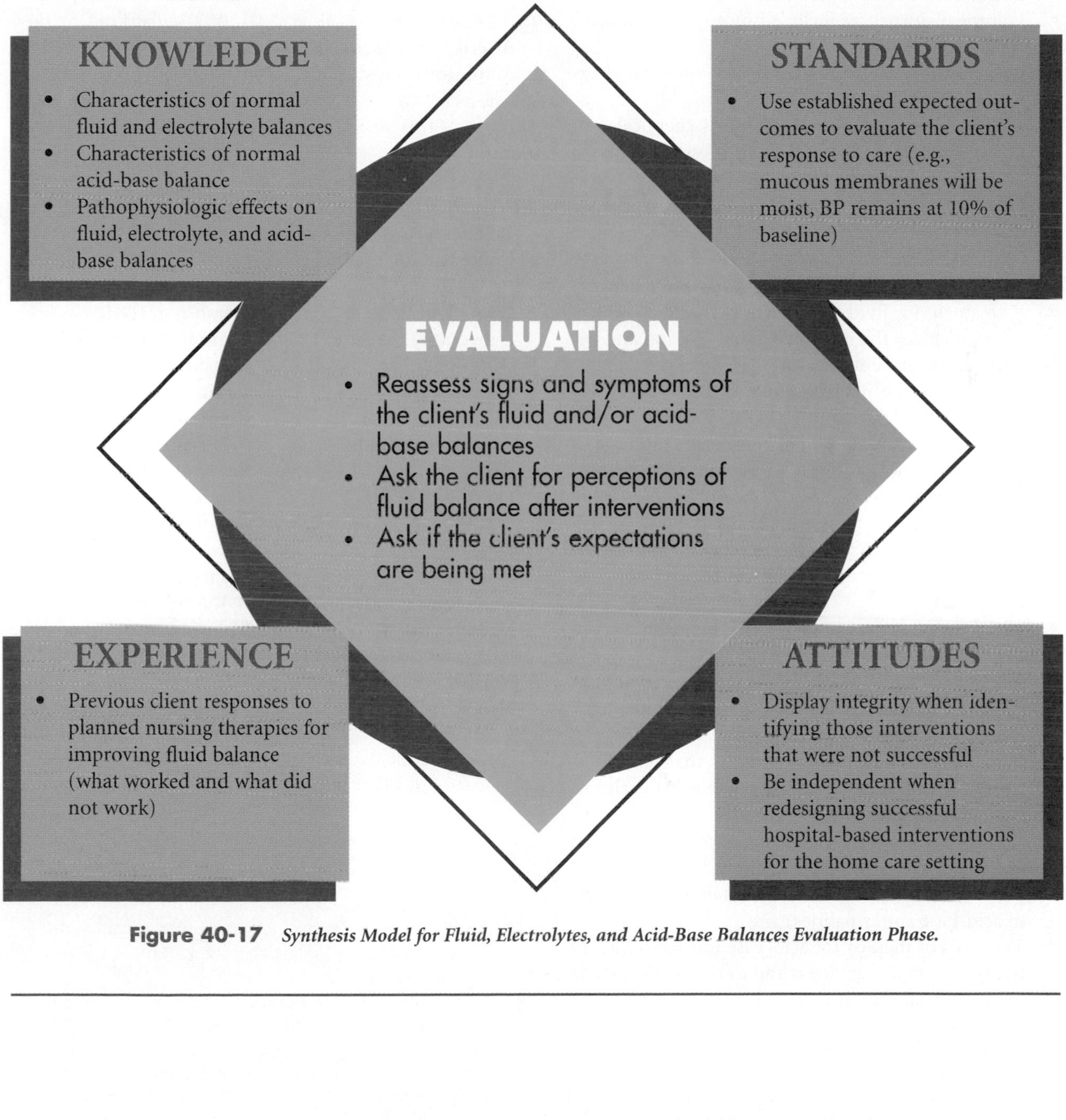

KNOWLEDGE

- Characteristics of normal fluid and electrolyte balances
- Characteristics of normal acid-base balance
- Pathophysiologic effects on fluid, electrolyte, and acid-base balances

STANDARDS

- Use established expected outcomes to evaluate the client's response to care (e.g., mucous membranes will be moist, BP remains at 10% of baseline)

EVALUATION

- Reassess signs and symptoms of the client's fluid and/or acid-base balances
- Ask the client for perceptions of fluid balance after interventions
- Ask if the client's expectations are being met

EXPERIENCE

- Previous client responses to planned nursing therapies for improving fluid balance (what worked and what did not work)

ATTITUDES

- Display integrity when identifying those interventions that were not successful
- Be independent when redesigning successful hospital-based interventions for the home care setting

Figure 40-17   *Synthesis Model for Fluid, Electrolytes, and Acid-Base Balances Evaluation Phase.*

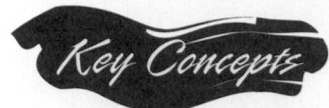

Key Concepts

- Body fluids are distributed in ECF and ICF compartments.
- Body fluids are composed of electrolytes, minerals, cells, and water.
- Body fluids are regulated through fluid intake, output, and hormonal regulation.
- Volume disturbances include isotonic and osmolar deficits and excesses.
- Electrolytes are regulated by dietary intake and hormonal controls.
- Acid-base imbalances are buffered by chemical, biological, and physiological buffering, especially the lungs and kidneys.
- Chronic and serious illnesses increase the risk of fluid, electrolyte, and acid-base imbalances.
- Clients who are very young or very old are at greater risk for fluid, electrolyte, and acid-base imbalances.
- Assessment for fluid, electrolyte, and acid-base alterations includes the nursing history, physical and behavioral assessment, measurements of I&O, daily weights, and specific laboratory data.
- Osmolar imbalances and FVD can be corrected by enteral or parenteral administration of fluid.
- Common complications of IV therapy include infiltration, phlebitis, infection, FVE, and bleeding at the infusion site.
- Blood transfusions are given to replace fluid volume loss from hemorrhage, treat anemia, or replace coagulation factors.
- Blood transfusions can be donor, autologous, or obtained through perioperative salvage.
- Administration of blood or blood products requires the nurse to follow a specific procedure to identify transfusion reactions quickly.
- In addition to transfusion reactions, the risks of transfusion also include hyperkalemia, hypocalcemia, FVE, and infection.
- Treatment for electrolyte disturbances include dietary and pharmacological interventions.
- The body's chemical buffering system responds first to acid-base abnormalities.
- The goals of therapy for acid-base imbalances are to treat the underlying illness and to restore the arterial pH to normal.

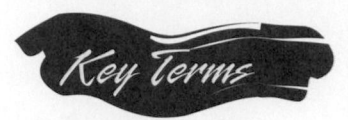

Key Terms

Active transport, *p. 1196*
Aldosterone, *p. 1197*
Angiotensin, *p. 1197*
Anion gap, *p. 1205*
Anions, *p. 1194*
Antidiuretic hormone (ADH), *p. 1197*
Arterial blood gas, *p. 1213*
Autologous transfusion, *p. 1242*
Buffer, *p. 1199*
Cations, *p. 1194*
Colloid osmotic pressure, *p. 1196*
Colloids, *p. 1218*
Concentration gradient, *p. 1196*
Crystalloids, *p. 1218*
Dehydration, *p. 1197*
Diffusion, *p. 1196*
Edema, *p. 1196*
Electrolyte, *p. 1194*
Extracellular fluids, *p. 1194*
Filtration, *p. 1196*
Fluid volume deficit (FVD), *p. 1207*
Fluid volume excess (FVE), *p. 1218*
Hemolysis, *p. 1242*
Homeostasis, *p. 1196*
Hydrostatic pressure, *p. 1196*
Hypertonic, *p. 1195*
Hypotonic, *p. 1195*

Hypovolemia, *p. 1196*
Infiltration, *p. 1235*
Infusion pump, *p. 1233*
Insensible water loss, *p. 1198*
Interstitial fluid, *p. 1194*
Intracellular fluids, *p. 1194*
Intravascular fluid, *p. 1194*
Ions, *p. 1194*
Isotonic, *p. 1195*
Metabolic acidosis, *p. 1205*
Metabolic alkalosis, *p. 1205*
Milliequivalents per liter (mEq/L), *p. 1195*
Oncotic pressure, *p. 1196*
Osmolarity, *p. 1195*
Osmols, *p. 1195*
Osmoreceptors, *p. 1196*
Osmosis, *p. 1195*
Osmotic pressure, *p. 1195*
Phlebitis, *p. 1235*
Renin, *p. 1197*
Respiratory acidosis, *p. 1203*
Respiratory alkalosis, *p. 1205*
Sensible water loss, *p. 1198*
Solute, *p. 1195*
Solution, *p. 1195*
Solvent, *p. 1195*
Total parenteral nutrition, *p. 1218*
Transfusion reaction, *p. 1242*
Vascular access devices, *p. 1219*
Venipuncture, *p. 1220*

Critical Thinking Exercises

1. Mrs. Emanuele is an 81-year-old admitted to the hospital with a 3-day history of vomiting and diarrhea. She has had only ice chips since the first episode of vomiting and is now complaining of malaise, cramping muscles, and a temperature of 101° F. Which laboratory findings would you expect to be abnormal based on her complaints? What interventions would you expect the physician to order?

2. Alexandra is the nurse assigned to Mrs. Emanuele. What nursing measures should she employ to make her comfortable and why? Will Alexandra need to provide for Mrs. Emanuele's safety? If so, how might she do this?

3. Caroline has just received a new client on her unit who is to receive 1 unit of RBCs with in the next hour. What nursing actions are necessary before administering blood? What are the signs and symptoms of a transfusion reaction? Can Caroline delegate the administration of blood to a licensed practical nurse or a nursing assistant on her team?

4. Bob is caring for a 52-year-old man who has been seen in the emergency department after being involved in a motor vehicle accident. He is complaining of difficulty breathing and a respiratory rate of 40 breaths per minute. Bob's client is transferred to the intensive care unit, intubated, and placed on a ventilator. After the client leaves, a nursing student asks Bob to interpret his client's last ABG results: pH, 7.30; PaO_2, 70; $PaCO_2$, 50; HCO_3, 24. What interpretation will Bob give to the student nurse? What is the relationship between the ABG results and the client being intubated and ventilated?

5. Jane is the nurse caring for Betty, a 59-year-old who has just had a total knee replacement. The physician has ordered Ancef 1 gm in 50 ml to run over 30 minutes IV piggyback tid. Betty has a continuous infusion of Ringer's lactate at 75 ml/hr in the left forearm. What type of tubing will Jane use to administer the IV piggyback medication? Calculate the drops per minute of the piggyback using both microtubing (60 drops/ml) and macrotubing (15 drops/ml).

References

Baranowski L: Central venous access device: current technologies, users, and management strategies, *J Intraven Nurs* 16(3):167, 1993.

Beare PG, Myers JL: *Adult health nursing,* ed 3, St. Louis, 1998, Mosby.

Carlson-Catalano J and others: Clinical validation of ineffective breathing pattern, ineffective airway clearance, and impaired gas exchange, *Image J Nurs Sch* 30(3):243, 1998.

Centers for Disease Control: Recommendations for prevention of HIV transmission in health care settings, *MMWR Morb Mortal Wkly Rep* 36 (suppl 25):35, 1987.

Christensen B, Kockrow E: *Foundations of nursing,* ed 3, St. Louis, 1998, Mosby.

Ciesla ND: Chest physical therapy for patients in the intensive care unit, *Phys Ther* 76(6):609, 1996.

Coulter, K: Intravenous therapy for the elder patient: implications for the intravenous nurse, *J Intraven Nurs* 15(suppl): S18, 1992.

Garner J: Guidelines for isolation precautions in hospitals, *Infect Control Hosp Epidemiol* 17(1):53, 1996.

Groer MW, Shekleton ME: *Basic pathophysiology: a holistic approach,* St. Louis, 1989, Mosby.

Horne MM and others: *Mosby's pocket guide series: fluid, electrolyte, and acid-base balance,* ed 3, St. Louis, 1997, Mosby.

Ignatavicius D, Workman MJ, Mishler MA: *Medical-surgical nursing,* ed 3, Philadelphia, 1999, WB Saunders.

Intravenous Nurses Society: Intravenous nursing standards of practice, *J Intraven Nurs* 21(15):535, 1998.

Kokko JP, Tannen RL: *Fluids and electrolytes,* Philadelphia, 1990, WB Saunders.

LaRocca JC, Otto SE: *Pocket guide to intravenous therapy,* ed 3, St. Louis, 1997, Mosby.

Lewis SM, Collier IC, Heitkemper M: *Medical-surgical nursing: assessment and management of clinical problems,* ed 4, St. Louis, 1996, Mosby.

Lewis SM, Collier IC, Heitkemper M: *Medical-surgical nursing: assessment and management of clinical problems,* ed 5, St. Louis, 1999, Mosby.

Long B and others: *Medical-surgical nursing: A nursing process approach,* ed 3, St. Louis, 1993, Mosby.

Lueckenotte A: *Gerontologic nursing,* St. Louis, 1996, Mosby.

McCance KL, Huether SE: *Pathophysiology: the biologic basis for disease in adults and children,* ed 3, St. Louis, 1998, Mosby.

McCloskey JC, Bulechek GM: *Nursing interventions classification (NIC),* ed. 3, St. Louis, 2000, Mosby.

McKenry LM, Salerno E: *Mosby's pharmacology in nursing,* ed 20, St. Louis, 1998, Mosby.

Metheny NM: *Fluid and electrolyte balance: nursing considerations,* ed 4, Philadelphia, 1996, JB Lippincott.

Meyer-Gaspar P: Water intake of nursing home residents, *J Gerontol Nurs* 25(4):23, 1999.

Millam DA: Starting IVs: how to develop your venipuncture experience, *Nursing* 22(9):33, 1992.

National Blood Resource Education Programs: *Transfusion therapy guidelines for nurses,* NIH Pub No. 90-2668a, September 1990.

Pearson ML: Hospital infection control practices: advisory committee guideline for prevention of intravascular device-related infections, *Infect Control Hosp Epidemiol* 17(7):438, 1996.

Perucca R, Micek J: Treatment of infusion related phlebitis: review and nursing protocol, *J Intraven Nurs* 16:5, 286, 1993.

Phillips LD: *Manual of IV therapeutics,* Philadelphia, 1993, FA Davis.

Weldy NJ: *Body fluids and electrolytes: a programmed presentation,* ed 7, St. Louis, 1996, Mosby.

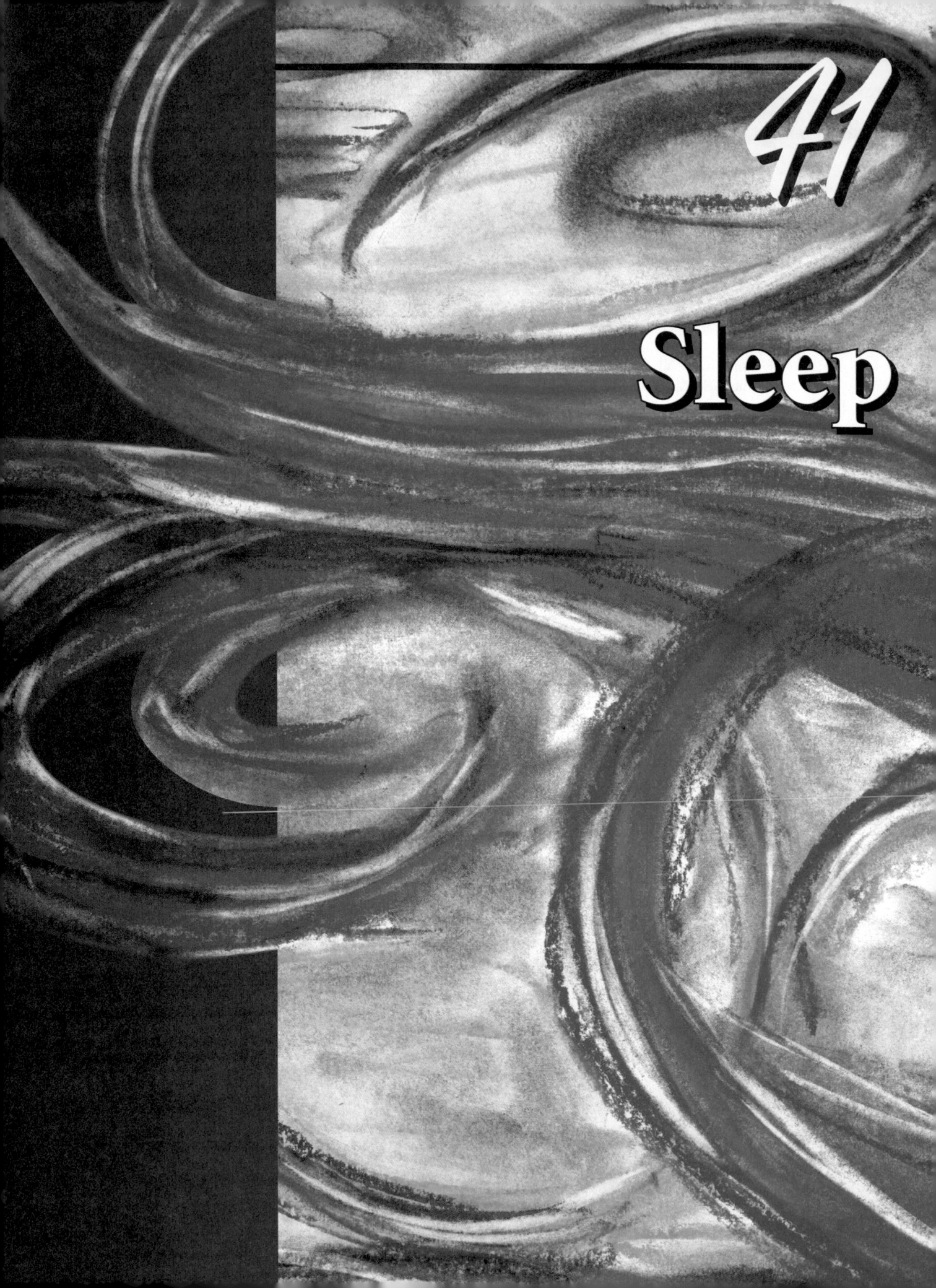

41

Sleep

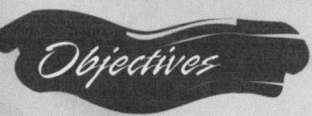
Objectives

Mastery of content in this chapter will enable the student to:

- Define the key terms listed.
- Compare the characteristics of rest and sleep.
- Explain the effect the 24-hour sleep-wake cycle has on biological function.
- Discuss mechanisms that regulate sleep.
- Describe the stages of a normal sleep cycle.
- Explain the functions of sleep.
- Compare and contrast the sleep requirements of different age groups.
- Identify factors that normally promote and disrupt sleep.
- Discuss characteristics of common sleep disorders.
- Conduct a sleep history for a client.
- Identify nursing diagnoses appropriate for clients with sleep alterations.
- Identify nursing interventions designed to promote normal sleep cycles for clients of all ages.
- Describe ways to evaluate sleep therapies.

Proper rest and sleep are as important to good health as good nutrition and adequate exercise. Individuals need different amounts of sleep and rest. Physical and emotional health depend on the ability to fulfill these basic human needs. Without proper amounts of rest and sleep, the ability to concentrate, make judgments, and participate in daily activities decreases and irritability increases.

Identifying and treating clients' sleep pattern disturbances is an important goal for a nurse. To help clients' a nurse must understand the nature of sleep, the factors influencing it, and the clients' sleep habits. Clients require an individualized approach based on their personal habits and pattern of sleep, as well as the inparticular problem influencing sleep. Nursing interventions can be effective in resolving short- and long-term sleep disturbances.

One theory about the function of sleep is that it is associated with healing and restoration (Evans and French, 1995; McCance and Huether, 1998). Achieving the best possible sleep quality is important for the promotion of good health as well as the recovery of ill individuals. Nurses care for clients who often have preexisting sleep disturbances and for clients who develop sleep problems as a result of illness or hospitalization. Sometimes clients seek health care because they have a sleep problem that may have gone unnoticed for many years. Ill clients often require more sleep and rest than healthy clients. However, the nature of illness may prevent clients from gaining adequate rest and sleep. The institutional environment of a hospital or long-term care facility and the activities of health care personnel make sleep difficult.

The authors acknowledge the contribution of Sharon Merritt to this chapter in the previous edition of this text.

Scientific Knowledge Base

PHYSIOLOGY OF SLEEP

Sleep is a cyclical physiological process that alternates with longer periods of wakefulness. The sleep-wake cycle influences and regulates physiological function and behavioral responses.

Circadian Rhythms. People experience cyclical rhythms as part of their everyday life. The most familiar rhythm is the 24-hour, day-night cycle known as the diurnal or **circadian rhythm** (derived from Latin: *circa*, "about," and *dies*, "day"). A woman's menstrual cycle is an infradian rhythm, one that occurs in a cycle longer than 24 hours. Biological cycles lasting less than 24 hours are called ultradian rhythms. Circadian rhythms influence the pattern of major biological and behavioral functions. The fluctuation and predictability of body temperature, heart rate, blood pressure, hormone secretion, sensory acuity, and mood depend on the maintenance of the 24-hour circadian cycle.

Circadian rhythms, including daily sleep-wake cycles, are affected by light and temperature and external factors such as social activities and work routines. All persons have **biological clocks** that synchronize their sleep cycles. Some people can fall asleep at 8 PM, whereas others go to bed at midnight or early in the morning. Different people also function best at different times of the day. Horne and Ostberg (1976) described two groups of people, morning and evening types. The morning person prefers to go to bed and get up early, performing best in the morning. The evening person prefers to go to bed and get up later, functioning best in the evenings.

Hospitals or extended care facilities usually do not adapt care to an individual's sleep-wake cycle preferences. Typical routines cause interruptions in sleep or prevent clients from falling asleep at their usual time. If a person's sleep-wake cycle is altered significantly, a poor quality of sleep can result. Reversals in the sleep-wake cycle such as falling asleep during the day (or vice versa for people who work nights) can indicate a serious illness. Anxiety, restlessness, irritability, and impaired judgment are common symptoms of disturbances in the sleep cycle.

The biological rhythm of sleep frequently becomes synchronized with other body functions. Changes in body temperature, for example, correlate with sleep patterns. Normally, body temperature peaks in the afternoon, decreases gradually, and then drops sharply after a person falls asleep. When the sleep-wake cycle becomes disrupted (e.g., by working rotating shifts), other physiological functions may change as well. For example, the person may experience a decreased appetite and lose weight. Failure to maintain the individual's usual sleep-wake cycle can adversely influence the client's overall health.

Sleep Regulation.

Sleep involves a sequence of physiological states maintained by highly integrated central nervous system (CNS) activity that is associated with changes in the peripheral nervous, endocrine, cardiovascular, respiratory, and muscular systems (McCance and Huether, 1998). Each sequence can be identified by specific physiological responses and patterns of brain activity. Instruments such as the electroencephalogram (EEG), which measures electrical activity in the cerebral cortex, the electromyogram (EMG), which measure muscle tone, and the electrooculogram (EOG), which measures eye movements, provide information about some structural physiological aspects of sleep.

Current theory indicates sleep is thought to be an active inhibitory process (Guyton and Hall, 1997). The control and regulation of sleep may depend on the interrelationship between two cerebral mechanisms that intermittently activate and suppress the brain's higher centers to control sleep and wakefulness. One mechanism causes wakefulness, whereas the other causes sleep.

The **reticular activating system (RAS)** is located in the upper brain stem. It is believed to contain special cells that maintain alertness and wakefulness. The RAS receives visual, auditory, pain, and tactile sensory stimuli. Activity from the cerebral cortex (e.g., emotions or thought processes) also stimulates the RAS. Wakefulness results from neurons in the RAS that release catecholamines such as norepinephrine (Sleep Research Society, 1993).

Sleep may be produced by the release of serotonin from specialized cells in the raphe sleep system of the pons and medulla. This area of the brain is also called the **bulbar synchronizing region (BSR)**. Whether a person remains awake or falls asleep depends on a balance of impulses received from higher centers (e.g., thoughts), peripheral sensory receptors (e.g., sound or light stimuli), and the limbic system (emotions) (Figure 41-1).

As people try to fall asleep, they close their eyes and assume relaxed positions. Stimuli to the RAS decline. If the room is dark and quiet, activation of the RAS further declines. At some point the BSR takes over, causing sleep.

Stages of Sleep.

EEG, EMG, and EOG electrical signals show that different levels of brain, muscle, and eye activity are associated with different stages of sleep (Sleep Research Society, 1993). Normal sleep involves two phases: **nonrapid eye movement (NREM) sleep** and **rapid eye movement (REM) sleep** (Box 41-1). During NREM a sleeper progresses through four stages during a typical 90-minute sleep cycle. The quality of sleep from stage 1 through stage 4 becomes increasingly deep. Lighter sleep is characteristic of stages 1 and 2, and a person is more easily arousable. Stages 3 and 4 involve a deeper sleep, called slow-wave sleep, from which a person is more difficult to arouse. Rapid eye movement sleep is the phase at the end of each 90-minute sleep cycle.

Memory consolidation (Karni and others, 1994) and psychological restoration may occur at this time. Different factors may promote or interfere with various stages of the sleep cycle. The nurse chooses therapies that foster sleep or attempts to eliminate factors that can disrupt it.

Sleep Cycle.

Normally in an adult the routine sleep pattern begins with a presleep period during which the person is aware only of a gradually developing sleepiness. This period normally lasts 10 to 30 minutes, but if a per-

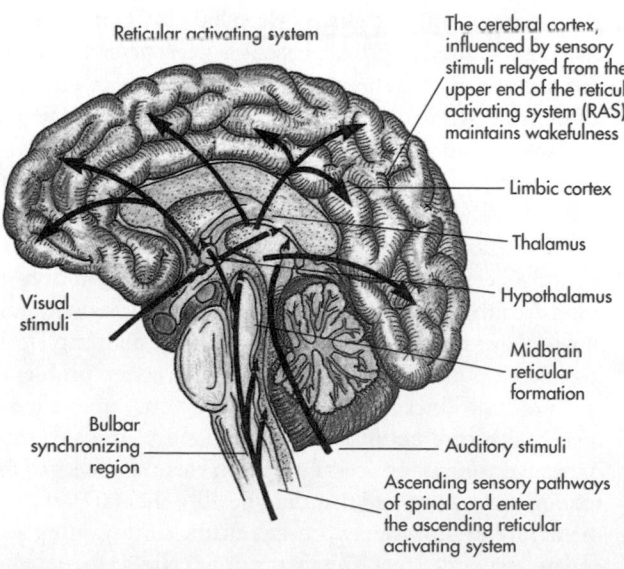

Figure 41-1 RAS and BSR control sensory input, intermittently activating and suppressing the brain's higher centers to control sleep and wakefulness.

Box 41-1

Stages of the Sleep Cycle

STAGE 1: NREM

Includes lightest level of sleep.

Stage lasts a few minutes.

Decreased physiological activity begins with gradual fall in vital signs and metabolism.

Person is easily aroused by sensory stimuli such as noise.

Awakened, person feels as though daydreaming has occurred.

STAGE 2: NREM

Period of sound sleep.

Relaxation progresses.

Arousal is still relatively easy.

Stage lasts 10 to 20 minutes.

Body functions continue to slow.

STAGE 3: NREM

Involves initial stages of deep sleep.

Sleeper is difficult to arouse and rarely moves.

Muscles are completely relaxed.

Vital signs decline but remain regular.

Stage lasts 15 to 30 minutes.

STAGE 4: NREM

Deepest stage of sleep.

Very difficult to arouse sleeper.

If sleep loss has occurred, sleeper will spend considerable portion of night in this stage.

Vital signs are significantly lower than during waking hours.

Stage lasts approximately 15 to 30 minutes.

Sleepwalking and enuresis may occur.

REM SLEEP

Vivid, full-color dreaming may occur.

Less vivid dreaming may occur in other stages.

Stage usually begins about 90 minutes after sleep has begun.

Typified by autonomic response of rapidly moving eyes, fluctuating heart and respiratory rates, and increased or fluctuating blood pressure.

Loss of skeletal muscle tone occurs.

Gastric secretions increase.

Very difficult to arouse sleeper.

Duration of REM sleep increases with each cycle and averages 20 minutes.

---

son has difficulty falling asleep, it may last an hour or more.

Once asleep, the person usually passes through four to six complete sleep cycles per night, each consisting of four stages of NREM sleep and a period of REM sleep (McCance and Huether, 1998). The cyclical pattern usually progresses from stage 1 through stage 4 of NREM, followed by a reversal from stage 4 to 3 to 2, ending with a period of REM sleep (Figure 41-2). A person usually reaches REM sleep about 90 minutes into the sleep cycle.

With each successive cycle, stages 3 and 4 shorten, and the period of REM lengthens. REM sleep may last up to 60 minutes during the last sleep cycle. Not all people progress consistently through the usual stages of sleep. For example, a sleeper may fluctuate for short intervals between NREM stages 2, 3, and 4 before entering REM stage. The amount of time spent in each stage varies over the life span (Figure 41-3). Shifts from stage to stage tend to accompany body movements, and shifts to light sleep tend to occur suddenly, whereas shifts to deep sleep tend to be gradual (Closs, 1988). The number of sleep cycles depends on the total amount of time that the client spends sleeping.

FUNCTIONS OF SLEEP

The purpose of sleep remains unclear (Hodgson, 1991). Sleep is believed to contribute to physiological and psychological restoration (Anch and others, 1988; McCance and Huether, 1998). According to one theory, sleep is a time of restoration and preparation for the next period of wakefulness. During NREM sleep, biological functions slow. A healthy adult's normal heart rate throughout the day averages 70 to 80 beats per minute or less if the indi-

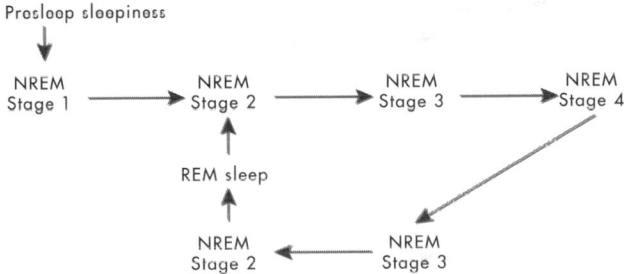

Figure 41-2 The stages of the adult sleep cycle.

vidual is in excellent physical condition. However, during sleep the heart rate falls to 60 beats per minute or less. This means that the heart beats 10 to 20 fewer times in each minute during sleep or 60 to 120 fewer times in each hour. Clearly, restful sleep may be beneficial in preserving cardiac function. Other biological functions decreased during sleep are respirations, blood pressure, and muscle tone (McCance and Huether, 1998).

Sleep appears to be needed to routinely restore biological processes. During deep slow-wave (NREM stage 4) sleep, the body releases human growth hormone for the repair and renewal of epithelial and specialized cells such as brain cells (Born, Muth, and Fehm, 1988; McCance and Huether, 1998). However, Horne (1983) also argues that the usual role of growth hormone as a promoter of protein synthesis is limited because its release is unrelated to blood glucose levels and amino acids. Other studies have shown that protein synthesis and cell division for renewal of tissues such as the skin, bone marrow, gastric mucosa,

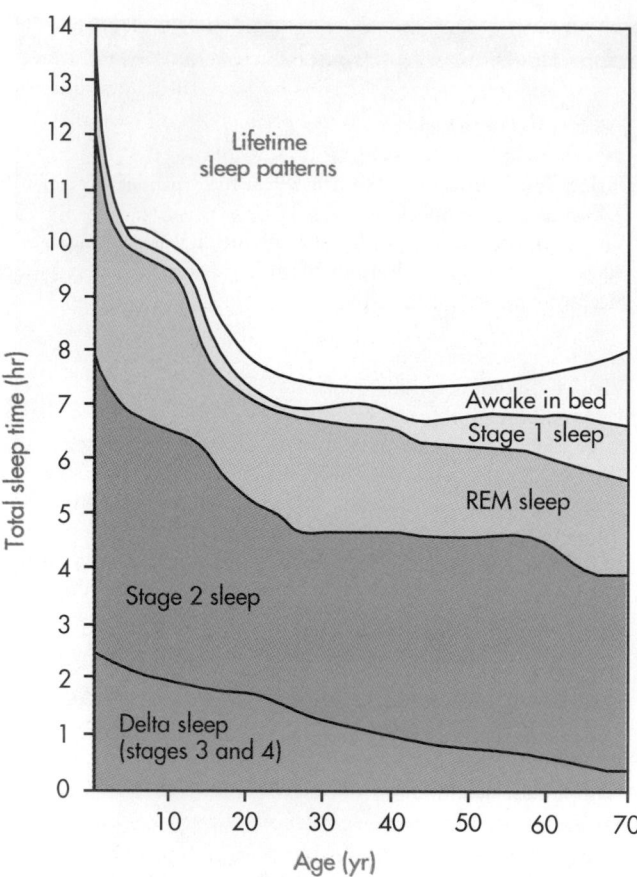

Figure 41-3 Distribution of sleep stages over the life span. From Berman and others: Sleep disorders: take them seriously, *Patient Care* 24:85, 1990.

or brain occur during rest and sleep (Oswald, 1984). NREM sleep may be especially important in children, who experience more stage 4 sleep.

Another theory about the purpose of sleep is that the body conserves energy during sleep. The skeletal muscles relax progressively, and the absence of muscular contraction preserves chemical energy for cellular processes. Lowering of the basal metabolic rate further conserves the body's energy supply (Anch and others, 1988).

REM sleep appears to be important for cognitive restoration. REM sleep is associated with changes in cerebral blood flow, increased cortical activity, increased oxygen consumption, and epinephrine release. This association may assist with memory storage and learning. During sleep, the brain filters stored information about the day's activities.

The benefits of sleep on behavior often go unnoticed until a person develops a problem resulting from sleep deprivation. A loss of REM sleep can lead to feelings of confusion and suspicion. No clear cause-and-effect relationship exists between sleep loss and a specific body dysfunction (Webster and Thompson, 1986). However, various body functions (e.g., mood, motor performance,

memory, and equilibrium) can be altered when prolonged sleep loss occurs (Pilcher and Huffcutt, 1996). Alterations in the natural and cellular immune function also occur with moderate to severe sleep deprivation (Irwin and others, 1996). Some of the more recent industrial accidents, such as the nuclear accident in Chernobyl, have been attributed to human error associated with sleep deprivation. Traffic, home, and work-related accidents caused by falling asleep have been estimated to cost billions of dollars a year in the United States (Coren, 1996; National Sleep Foundation, 1998a). Because of concern over an increased incidence of automobile accidents, some states in the United States have implemented guidelines regulating the driving privileges of people with disorders that cause excessive sleepiness, which can affect driving performance (Pakola, Dinges, and Pack, 1995).

Dreams. Although dreams occur during both NREM and REM sleep, the dreams of REM sleep are more vivid and elaborate and are believed to be functionally important to the consolidation of long-term memory. REM dreams may progress in content throughout the night from dreams about current events to emotional dreams of childhood or the past. Personality can influence the quality of dreams; for example, a creative person may have creative dreams, and a depressed person may dream of helplessness.

Most people dream about immediate concerns such as an argument with a spouse, plans for a wedding, or worries over work. Sometimes a person is unaware of fears represented in bizarre dreams. People with graduate-level education related to the field of psychology may attempt to analyze the symbolic nature of dreams. For example, an apple may represent a forbidden object, or a lion may symbolize rage. The ability to describe a dream and interpret its significance may help resolve personal concerns or fears.

Another theory suggests that dreams erase certain fantasies or nonsensical memories. Since most dreams are forgotten, many people have little dream recall and do not believe they dream at all. To remember a dream, a person must consciously think about it on awakening. People who recall dreams vividly usually awake just after a period of REM sleep.

PHYSICAL ILLNESS

Any illness that causes pain, physical discomfort (e.g., difficulty breathing), or mood problems, such as anxiety or depression, can result in sleep problems. Persons with such alterations may have trouble falling or staying asleep. Illnesses also may force clients to sleep in positions to which they are unaccustomed. For example, assuming an awkward position when an arm or leg has been immobilized in traction can interfere with sleep.

Respiratory disease often interferes with sleep. Clients with chronic lung disease such as emphysema are short of breath and frequently cannot sleep without two or three pillows to raise their heads. Asthma, bronchitis, and allergic rhinitis alter the rhythm of breathing and disturb sleep. A person with a common cold has nasal congestion, sinus drainage, and a sore throat, which impair breathing and the ability to relax.

Coronary heart disease often is characterized by episodes of sudden chest pain and irregular heart rates. Clients with this disease often experience frequent awakenings and stage changes during sleep (i.e., frequent shifts from stages 3 and 4 to lighter stage 2 sleep) and significant alterations in all stages of sleep, for example, suppressed REM sleep (Landis, 1988). Hypertension often causes early morning awakening and fatigue. Hypothyroidism decreases stage 4 sleep, whereas hyperthyroidism causes persons to take more time to fall asleep.

Nocturia, or urination during the night, disrupts sleep and the sleep cycle. This condition is most common in older people with reduced bladder tone or persons with cardiac disease, diabetes, urethritis, or prostatic disease. After a person awakens repeatedly to urinate, returning to sleep may be difficult.

Older adults often experience restless legs syndrome (RLS), which occurs prior to sleep onset. People experience recurrent, rhythmical movements of the feet and legs. An itching sensation is felt deep in the muscles. Relief comes only from moving the legs, which prevents relaxation and subsequent sleep. Depending on how severely sleep is disrupted, RLS may be a relatively benign condition. Restless legs syndrome has been found to be associated with lower levels of iron (Sun and others, 1998). In contrast, people who have severe leg cramps during the night may have a problem with arterial circulation.

Persons with peptic ulcer disease often awaken in the middle of the night. Research results demonstrating a relationship between gastric acid secretion and stages of sleep are conflicting. One consistent finding is that persons with duodenal ulcers fail to suppress acid secretion in the first 2 hours of sleep (Orr, 1994).

SLEEP DISORDERS

Sleep disorders are conditions that, if untreated, generally cause disturbed nighttime sleep that results in one of three problems: insomnia, abnormal movements or sensation during sleep or when awakening at night, or excessive daytime sleepiness (Naylor and Aldrich, 1994). Many adults in the United States have significant sleep debt from inadequacies in either the quantity or quality of their nighttime sleep and experience **hypersomnolence** on a daily basis (National Commission on Sleep Disorders Research, 1993).

Sleep disorders have been classified into four major categories (Thorpy, 1994) (Box 41-2). The **dyssomnias** are primary disorders that have their origin in different body systems and are subdivided into three major groups. The intrinsic sleep disorders include disorders of initiating and maintaining sleep, that is, various forms of insomnia and disorders of excessive sleepiness such as narcolepsy and obstructive sleep apnea. Extrinsic sleep disorders develop from external factors, which if removed, lead to resolution of the sleep disorder. The circadian rhythm sleep disorders arise from a misalignment between the timing of sleep and what is desired by the individual or is a societal norm. The **parasomnias** are undesirable behaviors that occur predominantly during sleep: arousal disorders, partial arousals, or disorders during transitions in the sleep cycle or from sleep to wakefulness. Many medical and psychiatric sleep disorders are associated with sleep and wake disturbances. These sleep disturbances are divided into those associated with psychiatric, neurological, or other medical specialty disorders. The proposed sleep disorders are newly described disturbances for which inadequate information currently exists to substantiate their existence.

Sleep laboratory studies such as a nighttime **polysomnogram** (PSG) and the Multiple Sleep Latency Test (MSLT) are often used to diagnose a sleep disorder (Carskadon, 1994). A polysomnogram involves the use of EEG, EMG, and EOG to monitor stages of sleep and wakefulness during nighttime sleep. The MSLT provides objective information about sleepiness and selected aspects of sleep structure by measuring how rapidly individuals fall asleep during at least four napping opportunities spread throughout the day. Sleep-onset REM episodes are also noted since this abnormality is associated with several sleep disorders.

Insomnia.   **Insomnia** is a symptom experienced by clients who have chronic difficulty falling asleep, frequent awakenings from sleep, and/or a short sleep or nonrestorative sleep (Zorick, 1994). The insomniac complains of excessive daytime sleepiness as well as insufficient quantity and quality of sleep. Frequently, however, the client gets more sleep than is realized. Insomnia may signal an underlying physical or psychological disorder. Insomnia occurs more frequently in women (Rogers, 1997a).

People may experience transient insomnia as a result of situational stresses such as family, work, or school problems; jet lag; illness; or loss of a loved one. Insomnia may recur, but between episodes the client is able to sleep well. However, a temporary case of insomnia due to a stressful situation can lead to chronic difficulty in obtaining sufficient sleep, perhaps due to the worry and anxiety that develops about obtaining adequate sleep.

Insomnia is often associated with poor **sleep hygiene,** or habits and practices the client uses that are associated with sleep. If the condition continues, the fear of not being able to sleep can be enough to cause wakefulness. During the day, persons with chronic insomnia may feel sleepy, fatigued, depressed, and anxious.

Because there are many causes of insomnia, management involves several approaches (Walsh, Hartman, and

Classification of Sleep Disorders

Box 41-2

DYSSOMNIAS

Intrinsic Sleep Disorders
Psychophysiological insomnia
Narcolepsy
Periodic limb movement disorder
Sleep apnea syndromes

Extrinsic Sleep Disorders
Inadequate sleep hygiene
Insufficient sleep syndrome
Hypnotic-dependent sleep disorders
Alcohol-dependent sleep disorders

Circadian Rhythm Sleep Disorders
Time-zone change (jet lag) syndrome
Shift-work sleep disorder
Delayed sleep phase syndrome

PARASOMNIAS
Arousal Disorders
Sleepwalking
Sleep terrors

Sleep-Wake Transition Disorders
Sleeptalking
Sleep starts
Nocturnal leg cramps

Parasomnias Usually Associated With REM Sleep
Nightmares
REM sleep behavior disorder
Sleep paralysis

Other Parasomnias
Sleep bruxism (teeth grinding)
Sleep enuresis (bed-wetting)
Sudden infant death syndrome

SLEEP DISORDERS ASSOCIATED WITH MEDICAL-PSYCHIATRIC DISORDERS
Associated With Psychiatric Disorders
Mood disorders
Anxiety disorders
Psychoses
Alcoholism

Associated With Neurological Disorders
Dementia
Parkinsonism
Central degenerative disorders

Associated With Other Medical Disorders
Nocturnal cardiac ischemia
Chronic obstructive pulmonary disease
Peptic ulcer disease

PROPOSED SLEEP DISORDERS
Menstruation-associated sleep disorders
Sleep choking syndrome
Pregnancy-associated sleep disorders

Modified from American Sleep Disorders Association: *The international classification of sleep disorders: diagnostic and coding manual,* Rochester, NY, 1990, Allen Press.

Kowall, 1994). As appropriate, it is important to treat underlying emotional or medical problems that may be causing this nighttime sleep problem. Treatment can also be symptomatic, including improved sleep hygiene measures, biofeedback, cognitive techniques, and relaxation techniques. When insomnia develops secondary to inappropriate health behaviors, treatment is directed at changing these behaviors. For example, in drug-dependence insomnia the client is unable to fall asleep because of excessive use of hypnotic medications. This client usually benefits from a gradual withdrawal of the hypnotics.

Sleep Apnea. **Sleep apnea** is a disorder characterized by the lack of airflow through the nose and mouth for periods of 10 seconds or longer during sleep. There are three types of sleep apnea: central, obstructive, and mixed apnea, which has both a central and an obstructive component.

The most common form, obstructive sleep apnea (OSA), occurs when muscles or structures of the oral cavity or throat relax during sleep. The upper airway becomes

partially or completely blocked, and nasal airflow is diminished (hypopnea) or stopped (apnea) for as long as 30 seconds (Guilleminault, 1994). The person still attempts to breathe because chest and abdominal movement continue, which often results in loud snoring and snorting sounds. When breathing is partially or completely diminished, each successive diaphragmatic movement becomes stronger until the obstruction is relieved. Structural abnormalities such as a deviated septum, nasal polyps, certain jaw configurations, or enlarged tonsils predispose a client to obstructive apnea. The effort to breathe during sleep results in arousals from deep sleep often to the stage 2 cycle. In severe cases, hundreds of hypopnea/apnea episodes can occur every hour, resulting in severe interference with deep sleep. **Excessive daytime sleepiness (EDS)** is the most common complaint of people with OSA. Persons with severe OSA may report taking daytime naps and experiencing a disruption in their daily activities because of sleepiness (Rosenthal and others, 1997). The National Commission on Sleep Disorders Research (1993) estimated that 18 million people in the United States meet the diagnostic criteria for OSA.

Obstructive apnea causes a serious decline in arterial oxygen level. Clients are at risk for cardiac dysrhythmia, right heart failure, pulmonary hypertension, anginal attacks, stroke, and hypertension. Middle-aged men are usually thought to be more frequently affected, particularly when they are obese (Rogers, 1997a). However, evidence is accumulating that postmenopausal women also commonly experience obstructive sleep apnea that is strongly related to hypertension (Gislason and others, 1993). Some researchers believe that sleep apneas are a cause for many of the naturally occurring or otherwise unexplained deaths that occur between 1 and 6 AM (Berman and others, 1990).

Central sleep apnea (CSA) involves dysfunction in the brain's respiratory control center. The impulse to breathe temporarily fails, and nasal airflow and chest wall movement cease. The oxygen saturation of the blood falls. The condition is seen in clients with brain stem injury, muscular dystrophy, and encephalitis and people who breathe normally during the day. Less than 10% of sleep apnea is predominantly central in origin. People with CSA tend to awaken during sleep and therefore complain of insomnia and excessive daytime sleepiness (EDS). Mild and intermittent snoring is also present.

The client with sleep apnea is often significantly deprived of deep sleep. In addition to complaints of excessive daytime sleepiness, sleep attacks, fatigue, morning headaches, and decreased sex drive are common (White, 1994). Treatment includes therapy for underlying cardiac or respiratory complications and emotional problems that arise as a result of the symptoms of this disorder. Sleep hygiene and a weight-loss program may help. One of the most effective therapies is use of a nasal continuous positive airway pressure (CPAP) device at night, which requires a client to wear a mask over the nose. Room air is delivered through the mask at a high pressure. The air pressure prevents airway collapse. The CPAP device is portable and effective particularly for obstructive apnea. In cases of severe sleep apnea the tonsils, uvula, or portions of the soft palate may be surgically removed. Success with surgical procedures is variable.

Narcolepsy.
Narcolepsy is a dysfunction of mechanisms that regulate the sleep and wake states. Excessive daytime sleepiness is the most common complaint associated with this disorder. During the day a person may suddenly feel an overwhelming wave of sleepiness and fall asleep; REM sleep can occur within 15 minutes of falling asleep. **Cataplexy,** or sudden muscle weakness during intense emotions such as anger, sadness, or laughter, may occur at any time during the day. If the cataplectic attack is severe, the client may lose voluntary muscle control and fall to the floor. A person with narcolepsy may have vivid dreams that occur as the person is falling asleep that are

difficult to distinguish from reality (called hypnagogic hallucinations). Sleep paralysis, or the feeling of being unable to move or talk just before waking or falling asleep, is another symptom (Cohen, Nehring, Cloninger, 1996). Some studies show a genetic link for narcolepsy (Mitler and others, 1990; Aldrich, 1992).

A significant problem for the person with narcolepsy is that the individual falls asleep uncontrollably at inappropriate times. Unless this disorder is understood, a sleep attack can easily be mistaken for laziness, lack of interest in activities, or drunkenness. Typically, the symptoms first begin to arise in adolescence and may be confused with the excessive daytime sleepiness that is thought to commonly occur in teens. Narcoleptics are treated with stimulants that may only partially increase wakefulness and reduce sleep attacks, and medications that suppress cataplexy and the other REM-related symptoms. Brief daytime naps no longer than 20 minutes may help reduce subjective feelings of sleepiness. Other management methods that have been reported as helpful are following a regular exercise program, eating light meals high in protein, practicing deep breathing, chewing gum, and taking vitamins (Cohen, Nehring, Cloninger, 1996). Factors that increase a narcoleptic client's drowsiness should be avoided (e.g., alcohol, heavy meals, exhausting activities, long-distance driving, long periods of sitting, hot stuffy rooms).

Sleep Deprivation.
Sleep deprivation is a problem many clients experience as a result of the dyssomnia. Causes may include illness (e.g., fever, difficulty breathing, or pain), emotional stress, medications, environmental disturbances (e.g., frequent nursing care), and variability in the timing of sleep due to shift work. Physicians and nurses may be particularly prone to sleep deprivation due to long work schedules and rotating shifts. Gold and others (1992) found that nurses who worked rotating shifts reported sleeping fewer hours and were significantly more likely to report accidents or errors compared with nurses who worked a straight day or evening shift.

Hospitalization, especially in intensive care units, makes clients particularly vulnerable to the extrinsic and circadian sleep disorders (Wood, 1992). Sleep deprivation involves decreases in the quantity and quality of sleep and inconsistency in the timing of sleep. When sleep becomes interrupted or fragmented, changes in the normal sequencing of the sleep cycles occur. A cumulative sleep deprivation develops.

A person's response to sleep deprivation is highly variable. Clients may experience a variety of physiological and psychological symptoms (Box 41-3). The severity of symptoms is often related to the duration of sleep deprivation. The most effective treatment for sleep deprivation is elimination or correction of factors that disrupt the sleep pattern. Nurses can play an important role in identifying treatable sleep deprivation problems.

Sleep Deprivation Symptoms   Box 41-3

PHYSIOLOGICAL SYMPTOMS
Ptosis, blurred vision
Fine motor clumsiness
Decreased reflexes
Slowed response time
Decreased reasoning and judgment
Decreased auditory and visual alertness
Cardiac arrhythmias

PSYCHOLOGICAL SYMPTOMS
Confusion and disorientation
Increased sensitivity to pain
Irritable, withdrawn, apathetic
Excessive sleepiness
Agitation
Hyperactivity
Decreased motivation

Parasomnias.   The parasomnias are sleep problems that are more common in children than in adults. Sudden infant death syndrome (SIDS) is hypothesized to be related to apnea, hypoxia, and cardiac arrhythmias caused by abnormalities in the autonomic nervous system that are manifested during sleep (Gillis and Flemons, 1994). Currently, the American Academy of Pediatrics recommends that apparently healthy infants be placed in the side lying or supine positions during sleep because of an association between the prone position and the occurrence of SIDS (Kattwinkel, Brooks, Myerberg, 1992).

Parasomnias that occur among older children include somnambulism (sleepwalking), night terrors, nightmares, nocturnal enuresis (bed-wetting), and tooth grinding (bruxism) (Wong, 1998). When adults have these problems, it may indicate more serious disorders. Specific treatment for these disorders varies. However, in all cases it is important to support clients and maintain their safety. For example, sleepwalkers are unaware of their surroundings and are slow to react. Thus the risk of falls is great. A nurse should not startle sleepwalkers but instead gently awaken them and lead them back to bed.

Nursing Knowledge Base

SLEEP AND REST

When people are at **rest** they usually feel mentally relaxed, free from anxiety, and physically calm. Rest does not imply inactivity, although everyone often thinks of it as settling down in a comfortable chair or lying in bed. When people are at rest they are in a state of mental, physical, and spiritual activity that leaves them feeling refreshed, rejuvenated, and ready to resume the activities of the day

(Mornhinweg and Voignier, 1996). All persons have their own habits for obtaining rest and can find ways to adjust as well as possible to new environments or conditions that affect the ability to rest. Rest may be gained from reading a book, practicing a relaxation exercise, listening to music, taking a long walk, or sitting quietly (Mornhinweg and Voignier, 1996).

Nurses frequently care for clients on bed rest in a variety of health care settings. This treatment confines clients to bed to reduce physical and psychological demands on the body. Such people do not necessarily feel rested. They still may have emotional worries that prevent complete relaxation. For example, concern over physical limitations or a fear of being unable to return to their usual lifestyle may cause such clients to feel stressed and unable to relax.

Sleep is a recurrent, altered state of consciousness that occurs for sustained periods. When people obtain proper sleep, they feel that their energy has been restored. Some sleep experts believe that these feelings of energy restoration imply that sleep provides time for the repair and recovery of body systems for the next period of wakefulness.

The usual rest and sleep patterns of persons entering a hospital or other health care facility can easily be affected by illness or unfamiliar health care routines. The extent of change in usual sleep and rest patterns depends on the client's physiological and psychological states and the physical environment, such as background noise and the work patterns of caregivers. The nurse must always be aware of the client's need for rest. A lack of rest for long periods can cause illness or worsening of existing illness. The nurse can help clients learn the importance of rest and ways to promote it at home or in the health care environment.

NORMAL SLEEP REQUIREMENTS AND PATTERNS

Sleep duration and quality vary among persons of all age groups. One person may feel adequately rested with 4 hours of sleep, whereas another requires 10 hours.

Neonates.   The neonate up to the age of 3 months averages about 16 hours of sleep a day. The sleep cycle is generally 40 to 50 minutes with wakening occurring after one to two sleep cycles (Renaud, 1996). The infant born of an unmedicated mother enters the world in a state of wakefulness. Eyes are wide open, and sucking is vigorous. After about an hour the newborn becomes quiet and less responsive to internal and external stimuli. A period of sleep lasting a few minutes up to 2 to 4 hours follows (Wong, 1995). The infant then awakens again and often becomes overly responsive to stimuli. Hunger, pain, cold, or other stimuli frequently cause crying. For the first week the neonate sleeps almost constantly. Approximately 50% of this sleep is REM sleep, which stimulates the higher brain centers. This is thought to be essential for development because the neonate is not awake long enough for significant external stimulation.

Infants. Infants usually develop a nighttime pattern of sleep by 3 months of age. The infant may take several naps during the day but usually sleeps an average of 8 to 10 hours during the night for a total daily sleep time of 15 hours. About 30% of sleep time is spent in the REM cycle. Awakening commonly occurs early in the morning, although it is not unusual for an infant to awaken during the night. If awakening during the night becomes routine, the problem may be with diet because hunger frequently awakens the child. A breast-fed infant usually sleeps for shorter periods, with more frequent awakenings, than a bottle-fed infant (Wong, 1998). A large infant sleeps longer than a smaller one because of greater stomach capacity. Compared with older children, active (REM) sleep makes up a larger proportion of sleep. In contrast with newborns in whom sleep and wakefulness alternate throughout a 24-hour period, by 3 months of age the longest sleep period appears at night.

Toddlers. By the age of 2, children usually sleep through the night and take daily naps. Total sleep averages 12 hours a day. Children after 3 years of age often give up daytime naps (Wong, 1998). It is common for toddlers to awaken during the night. The percentage of REM sleep continues to fall. During this period the toddler may be unwilling to go to bed at night. This unwillingness may be due to a need for autonomy or a fear of separation from their parents. Toddlers have a need to explore and satisfy their curiosity, which may explain why some of them try to delay bedtime.

Preschoolers. On average a preschooler sleeps about 12 hours a night (about 20% is REM). By the age of 5, the preschooler rarely takes daytime naps except in cultures where a siesta is the custom (Wong, 1998). The preschooler usually has difficulty relaxing or quieting down after long, active days. A preschooler also has problems with bedtime fears, waking during the night, or nightmares. Parents are most successful in getting a preschooler to bed by establishing a consistent ritual that includes some quiet time activity before bedtime. Ordinarily experts do not recommend that a child be allowed to sleep with parents. However, in some cultures sharing a bed or room with parents is an accepted sleeping practice. Partial wakening followed by normal return to sleep may be seen (Wong, 1998). In the waking period, the child may exhibit brief crying, walking around, unintelligible speech, sleepwalking or bed-wetting. Partial wakening can also occur in school-age children.

School-Age Children. The amount of sleep needed during the school years is individualized because of varying states of activity and levels of health. The school-age child enters a wakeful time in life and usually does not require a nap (Ferber, 1995). A 6-year-old averages 11 to 12 hours of sleep nightly, whereas an 11-year-old sleeps about 9 to 10 hours (Wong, 1998). The 6- or 7-year-old can usually be persuaded to go to bed by encouraging quiet activities. The older child often resists sleeping because of an unawareness of fatigue or a need to be independent. A school-age child will be tired the following day if allowed to stay up later than usual. An older child may seek a later bedtime as a symbol of dominance over a younger child. Parents are usually successful in getting the older child to bed by using a firm, consistent approach. The older school-age child may be allowed to go to bed later, but such a privilege may be dependent on the child going to bed promptly without complaints. Excessive daytime sleepiness in not normal in this age group and should be investigated further (Ferber, 1995).

Adolescents. Typically, teenagers get about 7½ hours of sleep per night (Carskadon, 1990). At a time when sleep needs actually increase, the typical adolescent is subject to a number of changes that often reduce the time spent sleeping (Dahl and Carskadon, 1995). Usually parents are no longer involved in setting a specific bedtime. School demands, after-school social activities, and part-time jobs may result in compressed time available for sleep. Teens go to bed later and rise earlier during the high school years. A common societal expectation is that adolescents require less sleep than preadolescents. However, laboratory data indicate that adolescents may have a physiological need for more sleep when compared with preadolescents (Dahl and Carskadon, 1995). Because of lifestyle demands that shorten the time available for sleep and probable physiological need, teens often experience EDS. In middle adolescents, sleep disturbance and sleep effectiveness are positively related to health status (Mahon, 1995). Performance in school, vulnerability to accidents, and behavior and mood problems can be the result of EDS due to insufficient sleep. Parents, teachers, and teens themselves often lack knowledge about what is proper sleep. All may need education in order to improve what can be a significant health problem for teens.

Young Adults. Most young adults average 6 to 8½ hours of sleep a night, but this can vary. Young adults rarely take regular naps. Approximately 20% of sleep time is spent in REM sleep, which remains consistent throughout life. Healthy young adults require adequate sleep to participate in the busy activities that fill their days. However, it is common for lifestyle demands to interrupt usual sleep patterns. The stresses of jobs, family relationships, and social activities may lead to insomnia (i.e., difficulties initiating and/or maintaining sleep) and the use of medication for sleep. Long-term use of such medications can disrupt sleep patterns and make the insomnia problem worse. Daytime sleepiness contributes to an increased number of accidents, decreased productivity, and interpersonal problems in this age group. Full-time employment and single marital status are the most common risk factors for sleep problems in this age group (Breslau and others, 1997). Pregnancy increases the need for sleep and rest. Insomnia is a common problem during the third trimester of pregnancy (Bobak, Lowdermilk, and Jensen, 1995).

Middle Adults.
During middle adulthood the total time spent sleeping at night begins to decline. The amount of stage 4 sleep begins to fall, a decline that continues with advancing age. Sleep disturbances are often initially diagnosed among people in this age range even when the symptoms of a disorder have been present for several years. Insomnia is particularly common, probably because of the changes and stresses of middle age. Sleep disturbances can be caused by anxiety, depression, or certain physical ailments. Women experiencing menopausal symptoms may have insomnia. Members of this age group may rely on sleeping medications (Johnson and others, 1998).

Older Adults.
The total amount of sleep does not change as age increases. However, the quality of sleep appears to deteriorate for many older adults, which results in decreased reports of feeling rested (Beck-Little and Weinrich, 1998). Episodes of REM sleep tend to shorten. There is a progressive decrease in stages 3 and 4 NREM sleep; some older adults have almost no stage 4, or deep sleep. An older adult awakens more often during the night, and it may take more time for an older adult to fall asleep. However, older adults who adapt successfully to the physiological and psychosocial changes in aging are more likely to preserve REM sleep and continuity in the sleep cycle that is similar to younger adults (Reynolds and others, 1993).

Variability in the sleep behaviors of older adults is common. Complaints about difficulties with nighttime sleep frequently occur among older adults, often resulting from the presence of another chronic illness. For example, an older adult with arthritis may have difficulty sleeping because of painful joints. The tendency to nap seems to increase progressively with age. The increase in daytime napping may occur because of the frequent wakenings experienced at night. Compared with the amount of time spent in bed, the time spent sleeping may be decreased by an hour or more (Evans and Rogers, 1994). The changes in an older person's sleep pattern may be due to changes in the CNS that affect the regulation of sleep. Sensory impairment, which is common with aging, may reduce an older person's sensitivity to time cues that maintain circadian rhythms.

FACTORS AFFECTING SLEEP
A number of factors affect the quantity and quality of sleep. Often a single factor may not be the only cause for a sleep problem. Physiological, psychological, and environmental factors can alter the quality and quantity of sleep.

Drugs and Substances.
Sleepiness and sleep deprivation are common side effects of commonly prescribed medications (Box 41-4). These medications alter sleep and impair daytime alertness, which can be problematic for individuals (Nicholson, Bradley, and Pascoe, 1994; McKenry and Salerno, 1998). Medications prescribed for sleep may cause more problems than benefits. Older adults often take a variety of drugs to control or treat chronic illness, and the combined effects of several drugs can seriously disrupt sleep. L-Tryptophan, a natural protein found in foods such as milk, cheese, and meats, may help a person sleep.

Lifestyle.
A person's daily routine may influence sleep patterns. An individual working a rotating shift (e.g., 2 weeks of days followed by a week of nights) often has difficulty adjusting to the altered sleep schedule. The body's internal clock might be set at 11 PM, but the work schedule forces sleep at 9 AM instead. The individual may be able to sleep only 3 or 4 hours because the body's clock perceives that it is time to be awake and active. Difficulties with maintaining alertness during work time can result in decreased and even hazardous performance. After several weeks of working a night shift a person's biological clock usually does adjust. Other alterations in routines that can disrupt sleep patterns include performing unaccustomed heavy work, engaging in late-night social activities, and changing evening mealtime.

Usual Sleep Patterns and Excessive Daytime Sleepiness.
In the past century the amount of sleep obtained nightly by U.S. citizens has decreased over 20% (National Sleep Foundation, 1998b), indicating that many Americans are sleep deprived and experience excessive sleepiness during the day. EDS often results in impairment of waking function, poor work or school performance, accidents while driving or using equipment, and behavioral or emotional problems. Feelings of sleepiness are usually most intense upon awakening from, or right before going to, sleep, and about 12 hours after the midsleep period.

Sleepiness becomes pathological when it occurs at times when individuals need or want to be awake. People who experience temporary sleep deprivation as a result of an active social evening or lengthened work schedule usually feel sleepy the next day. However, they may be able to overcome these feelings even though they have difficulty performing tasks and remaining attentive. Chronic lack of sleep is much more serious than temporary sleep deprivation and can cause serious alterations in the ability to perform daily functions. EDS tends to be most difficult to overcome during sedentary tasks. For example, single-vehicle accidents related to a driver falling asleep at the wheel occur most often between midnight and 6 AM due to

Drugs and Their Effects on Sleep

Box 41-4

HYPNOTICS
Interfere with reaching deeper sleep stages
Provide only temporary (1 week) increase in quantity of sleep
Eventually cause "hangover" during day: excess drowsiness, confusion, decreased energy
May worsen sleep apnea in older adults

DIURETICS
Cause nocturia

ANTIDEPRESSANTS AND STIMULANTS
Suppress REM sleep
Decrease total sleep time

ALCOHOL
Speeds onset of sleep
Disrupts REM sleep
Awakens person during night and causes difficulty returning to sleep

CAFFEINE
Prevents person from falling asleep
May cause person to awaken during night
Adrenergic

BETA-ADRENERGIC BLOCKERS
Cause nightmares
Cause insomnia
Cause awakening from sleep

BENZODIAZEPINES
Increase sleep time
Increase daytime sleepiness

NARCOTICS
Suppress REM sleep
Cause increased daytime drowsiness

ANTICONVULSANTS
Decrease REM sleep time
May cause daytime drowsiness

the sleepiness that can occur when people are awake during what is their normal period of sleep (Leger, 1994; National Sleep Foundation, 1998b).

Emotional Stress.   Worry over personal problems or situations can disrupt sleep. Emotional stress causes a person to be tense and often leads to frustration when sleep does not come. Stress may also cause a person to try too hard to fall asleep, to awaken frequently during the sleep cycle, or to oversleep. Continued stress may cause poor sleep habits.

Older clients frequently experience losses that lead to emotional stress such as retirement, physical impairment, or the death of a loved one. Older adults and other individuals who experience depressive mood problems often experience delays in falling asleep, earlier appearance of REM sleep, frequent awakening, increased total bed time, feelings of sleeping poorly, and early awakening (Beck-Little and Weinrich, 1998).

Environment.   The physical environment in which a person sleeps has a significant influence on the ability to fall and remain sleep. Good ventilation is essential for restful sleep. The size, firmness, and position of the bed can affect the quality of sleep. Hospital beds are often smaller and harder than those at home. If a person usually sleeps with another individual, sleeping alone can cause wakefulness. On the other hand, sleeping with a restless or snoring bed partner can also disrupt sleep.

Sound also influences sleep. The level of noise needed to awaken people depends on the stage of sleep (Webster and Thompson, 1986). Low noises are more likely to arouse a person from stage 1 sleep, whereas louder noises awaken people in stage 3 or 4 sleep. Some persons require silence to fall asleep, whereas others prefer background noise such as soft music or television.

In hospitals and other in-patient facilities, noise creates a problem for clients. Noise in hospitals is usually new or strange. Thus clients are prone to awaken. This problem is greatest the first night of hospitalization, when clients often experience increased total wake time, increased awakenings, and decreased REM sleep and total sleep time (Agnew and others, 1966). The level of noise in hospitals can be very loud. Normal conversation measures about 50 decibels. Hilton (1987) found that an intravenous controller-alarm created noise at 44 to 80 decibels, a flushing toilet at 44 to 76 decibels, and paper ripping at 41 to 81 decibels. Sound becomes noise at 35 to 40 decibels. People-induced noises (e.g., nursing activities) are sources of increased sound levels. Intensive care units are sources for high noise levels (Box 41-5). Close proximity of clients, noise from confused and ill clients, the ringing of alarm systems and telephones, and disturbances caused by emergencies make the environment unpleasant. Noise is related to subjective quality of sleep. Persons exposed to coronary care unit sound levels reported poorer quality of sleep as evidenced by taking more time to fall asleep, less time sleeping, and more awakenings (Topf, Bookman, and Arand, 1996).

Light levels may affect the ability to fall asleep. Some clients may prefer a dark room, whereas others, such as

Research HIGHLIGHT   **Box 41-5**

RESEARCH ABSTRACT

Sleep disturbances often occur in clients following cardiac surgery in the intensive care unit and after transfer to a general nursing unit. The client's perception of factors that disturb sleep is important when planning care to promote sleep. One hundred two clients recovering from cardiac surgery in an acute care hospital in the Northwest were studied. The clients responded to the Factors Influencing Sleep Questionnaire, which was administered verbally. Demographic and surgical information were also collected. The results showed that women identified more factors as being disturbing to their sleep than men. The factors identified most frequently as being disruptive to sleep were pain, the inability to get comfortable, procedures done to the client, the ventilation system, and the inability to perform one's own bedtime ritual. Other factors that were moderately disruptive were anxiety, nurses' interruptions, talking in the halls or at the nurses' station, and equipment. These factors were identified as disruptive to sleep in both the intensive care unit and after transfer to a general floor.

IMPLICATIONS FOR PRACTICE

- Nurses should medicate clients regularly with narcotics after surgery to alleviate pain.
- If possible, nurses should allow clients to perform their usual bedtime sleep rituals while in the hospital.
- Nurses should attempt to keep client interruptions and noise in the hallways to a minimum.
- Nurses should schedule needed procedures for clients earlier in the day, not right before bedtime.
- Clients should have periods of uninterrupted rest after surgery.
- Nurses should attempt to control environmental temperature so that client rooms are comfortable.
- Nurses should spend time talking to the client to reduce anxiety.

REFERENCE

Simpson T, Lee ER, Cameron C: Patients' perceptions of environmental factors that disturb sleep after cardiac surgery, *Am J Crit Care* 5(3):173, 1996.

children or older adults, may prefer keeping a soft light on during sleep. Clients also may have trouble sleeping based on the temperature of a room. A room that is too warm or too cold often causes a client to become restless.

Exercise and Fatigue.   A person who is moderately fatigued usually achieves restful sleep, especially if the fatigue is the result of enjoyable work or exercise. Exercising 2 hours or more before bedtime allows the body to cool down and maintains a state of fatigue that promotes relaxation. However, excess fatigue resulting from exhausting or stressful work can make falling asleep difficult. This can be a common problem for grade school children and adolescents.

Food and Caloric Intake.   People sleep better when they are healthy, so following good eating habits is important for proper health and sleep (Hauri and Linde, 1990). Eating a large, heavy, and/or spicy meal at night may result in indigestion that interferes with sleep. Caffeine and alcohol consumed in the evening have insomnia-producing effects. A drastic reduction or avoidance of these substances is an important strategy that people can use to improve sleep. Food allergies may cause insomnia. In infants, nighttime waking and crying or colic may be caused by a milk allergy requiring that breast milk or a nonmilk formula be used. Besides milk, other foods that often result in an insomnia-producing allergy among both children and adults include corn, wheat, nuts, chocolate, eggs, seafood, red and yellow food dyes, and yeast (Hauri and Linde, 1990). Restoration of normal sleep may take up to 2 weeks when the particular food that is causing the difficulty has been eliminated from the diet.

Weight loss or gain influences sleep patterns. When a person gains weight, sleep periods become longer with fewer interruptions. Weight loss can cause short and fragmented sleep. Certain sleep disorders may be the result of the semistarvation diets popular in a weight-conscious society.

Critical Thinking Synthesis

Successful critical thinking requires a synthesis of knowledge, experience, information gathered from clients, critical thinking attitudes, and intellectual and professional standards. Clinical judgments require the nurse to anticipate the information necessary, analyze the data, and make decisions regarding client care. Critical thinking is always changing. During assessment (Figure 41-4), the nurse must consider all elements that build toward making appropriate nursing diagnoses.

In the case of sleep, the nurse integrates knowledge from nursing and other disciplines, previous experiences, and information gathered from clients to understand the client's sleep problem and its effect on the client and family. In addition, the use of critical thinking attitudes such as perseverance, confidence, and discipline are needed to find a plan of care to provide successful management of the sleep problem. The use of professional standards, such as the *Standards of Clinical Nursing Practice* (American Nurses' Association, 1991) and the "Nursing Standard-of-Practice Protocol: Sleep Disturbances in Elderly Patients" (Foreman and Wykle, 1995) provide valuable guidelines for the nurse to assess and address the needs of clients with sleep disorders. The protocol was developed for hospital nurses to use to prevent or manage sleep problems in older hospitalized adults. The project was part of the John A. Hartford Foundation's Nurses Improving Care of Hospitalized Elderly (NICHE) Project (Foreman and Wykle, 1995).

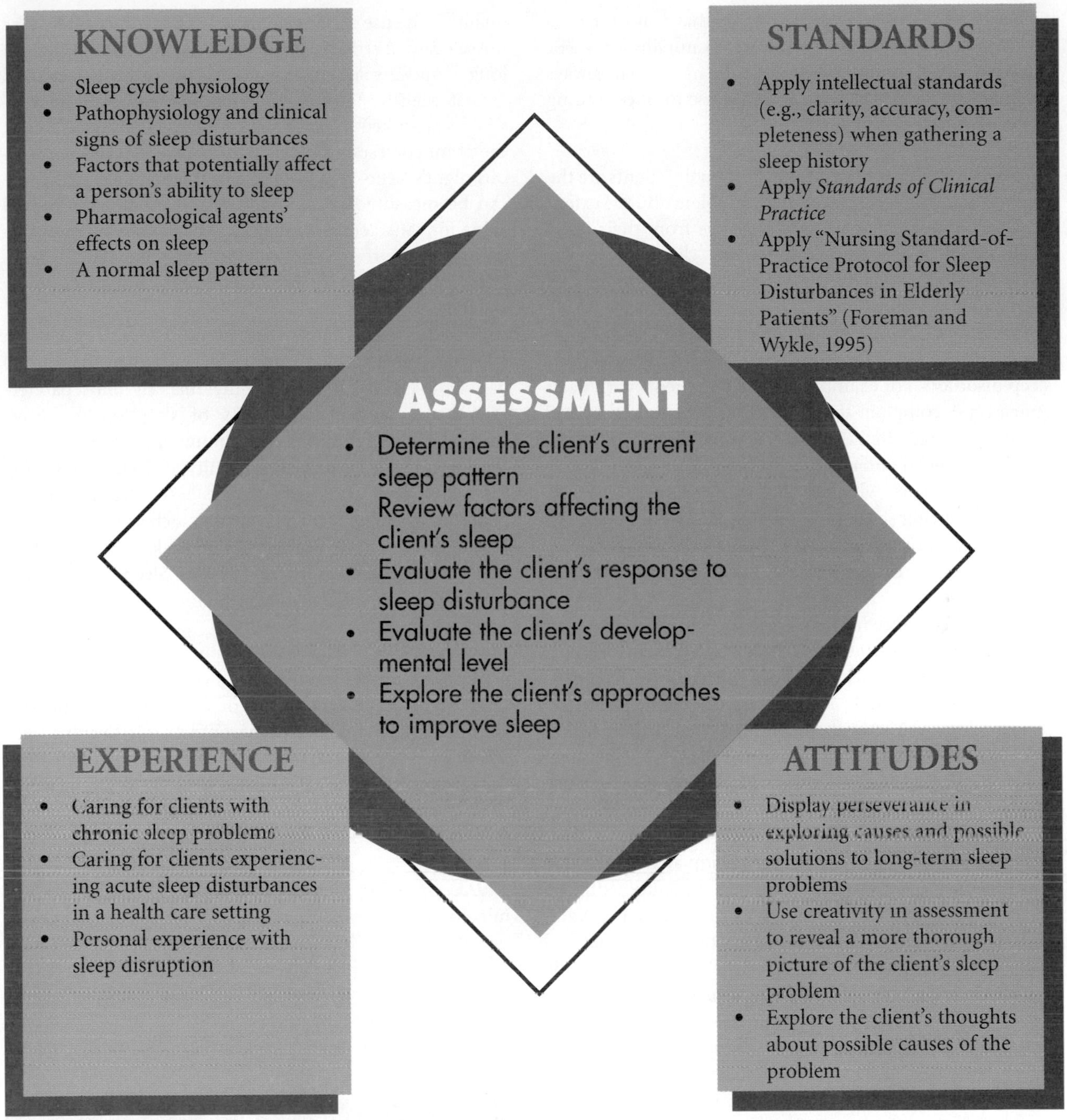

KNOWLEDGE

- Sleep cycle physiology
- Pathophysiology and clinical signs of sleep disturbances
- Factors that potentially affect a person's ability to sleep
- Pharmacological agents' effects on sleep
- A normal sleep pattern

STANDARDS

- Apply intellectual standards (e.g., clarity, accuracy, completeness) when gathering a sleep history
- Apply *Standards of Clinical Practice*
- Apply "Nursing Standard-of-Practice Protocol for Sleep Disturbances in Elderly Patients" (Foreman and Wykle, 1995)

ASSESSMENT

- Determine the client's current sleep pattern
- Review factors affecting the client's sleep
- Evaluate the client's response to sleep disturbance
- Evaluate the client's developmental level
- Explore the client's approaches to improve sleep

EXPERIENCE

- Caring for clients with chronic sleep problems
- Caring for clients experiencing acute sleep disturbances in a health care setting
- Personal experience with sleep disruption

ATTITUDES

- Display perseverance in exploring causes and possible solutions to long-term sleep problems
- Use creativity in assessment to reveal a more thorough picture of the client's sleep problem
- Explore the client's thoughts about possible causes of the problem

Figure 41-4 *Synthesis Model for Sleep Assessment Phase.*

Nursing Process

ASSESSMENT

To promote a normal restful sleep for clients, the nurse assesses their sleep patterns using the nursing history to gather information about factors that usually influence sleep. If the client perceives that sleep is adequate, the nursing history can be brief.

Sleep is a subjective experience. Only the client can report whether or not it is sufficient and restful. If the client is satisfied with the quantity and quality of sleep received, it may be considered normal. If a client admits to or the nurse suspects a sleep problem, a more detailed history is needed.

Sleep Assessment. Most persons can provide a reasonably accurate estimate of their sleep patterns, particularly if any changes have occurred. Assessment is aimed at understanding the characteristics of any sleep problem and the client's usual sleep habits so that ways for promoting sleep can be incorporated into nursing care. For example, if the nursing history reveals that a client always reads before falling asleep, it makes sense to offer reading material at bedtime.

Sources for Sleep Assessment.   Usually clients are the best resource for describing a sleep problem and the extent to which a problem represents a change from their usual sleep and waking patterns. Often the client knows the cause for sleep problems, such as a noisy environment or worry over a relationship.

Additionally, bed partners can provide information on the client's patterns that may reveal the nature of certain sleep disorders. For example, partners of clients with sleep apnea often complain that their sleep is disturbed by the client's snoring. Often the partners must sleep in different beds or rooms to obtain adequate sleep. The nurse should ask bed partners whether the clients have pauses of breathing during sleep and how frequently the apneic attacks occur. Some partners mention becoming fearful when clients apparently stop breathing for periods during sleep.

When caring for children, it can be helpful to ask older children to tell you about their sleep problem (Ferber, 1995). The nurse also seeks information about sleep patterns from parents since they are usually a good source of information about how their child is having trouble sleeping. Some parents may not realize that there is a wide variability in the sleeping patterns of infants and may need reassurance if their infant seems to sleep less than others but is otherwise healthy and thriving (Parkinson, 1994). Hunger, excessive warmth, and separation anxiety are factors that may contribute to an infant's difficulty with going to sleep or frequent wakenings during the night. Older children often are able to relate fears or worries that inhibit their ability to fall asleep. If children frequently awaken in the middle of bad dreams, parents can identify the problem but perhaps do not understand the meanings of the dreams. Parents can also describe the typical behavior patterns that foster or impair sleep. For example, excessive stimulation from active play or visiting friends may predictably impair sleep. With chronic sleep problems, parents can relate the duration of the problem, its progression, and children's responses. Parents of infants may need to keep a 24-hour log of their infant's waking and sleeping behavior for several days to determine what may be causing the problem. The infant's eating pattern and sleeping environment also need to be described since these may influence sleeping behavior.

Tools for Assessment of Sleep.   Subjective reports of sleep have been shown to be reliable and valid measures of sleep (Closs, 1988; Richardson, 1997). There are several subjective sleep assessment tools that are easy and quick to administer. One effective, brief method for assessing sleep

quality is the use of a visual analog scale (Closs, 1988). The nurse draws a straight horizontal line 100 mm (4 inches) long. Opposing statements such as "best night's sleep" and "worst night's sleep" are at opposite ends of the line. Clients are asked to place a mark on the horizontal line at the point corresponding to their perceptions of the previous night's sleep. The distances of the mark along the line can be measured in millimeters and offers a numerical value for satisfaction with sleep. The scale can be repeatedly administered to show change over time. Such a scale is useful to assess an individual client, not to compare clients.

Another brief subjective method to assess sleep is a 0 to 10 sleep rating scale similar to the concept of the 0 to 10 pain scale (Richards, 1996). Individuals should separately rate their quantity and quality of sleep on the scale. Instruct clients to indicate with a number between 0 and 10 their sleep quantity then their quality of sleep with 0 being the worst sleep and 10 being the best sleep. Additional paper-and-pencil tools are available, such as the St. Mary's Hospital Sleep Questionnaire, the Baekeland-Hoy Sleep Log, and the Verran-Snyder-Halpern Sleep Scale (Leigh and others, 1988; Richardson, 1997).

Sleep History.   Clients may report that they enjoy adequate sleep. In this situation the sleep history can be brief (Box 41-6). A determination of usual bedtime, normal bedtime rituals, preferred environment for sleeping, and what time the client usually rises gives the nurse information for planning care conducive to sleep. When suspecting a sleep problem, the nurse assesses the quality and characteristics of sleep in greater depth.

Description of Sleeping Problems.   When a client admits to or the nurse suspects a sleep problem, the nursing history must be detailed so that therapeutic care can be provided. Open-ended questions help a client to describe a

---

Components of a Sleep History   Box 41-6

Description of client's sleep problem
Usual sleep pattern prior to sleep problem
Recent changes in sleep pattern
Bedtime routines and sleeping environment
Use of sleep and other prescription medications and over-the-counter drugs
Pattern of dietary intake and amount of substances (e.g., alcohol) that influence sleep
Symptoms experienced during waking hours
Concurrent physical illness
Recent life events
Current emotional and mental status

problem more fully. A general description of the problem followed by more focused questions usually reveals specific characteristics that can be used in planning therapies.

To begin, the nurse needs to understand the nature of the sleep problem, its signs and symptoms, its onset and duration, its severity, any predisposing factors or causes, and the overall effect on the client. Assessment questions might include the following:

- *Nature of the problem:* Tell me what type of problem you have with your sleep. Tell me why you think your sleep is inadequate. Describe for me a recent typical night's sleep. How is this sleep different from what you are used to?
- *Signs and symptoms:* Do you have difficulty falling asleep, staying asleep, or waking up? Have you been told that you snore loudly? Do you have headaches when awakening? Does your child awaken from nightmares?
- *Onset and duration:* When did you notice the problem? How long has this problem lasted?
- *Severity:* How long does it take you to fall asleep? How often during the week do you have trouble falling asleep? Tell me how many hours of sleep a night you got this week; compare that to what is usual for you. What do you do when you awaken during the night or too early in the morning?

- *Predisposing factors:* Tell me what you do just before going to bed. Have you recently had any changes at work or at home? How is your mood, and have you noticed any changes recently? What medications or recreational drugs do you take on a regular basis? Are you taking any new prescription or over-the-counter medications? How long have you been taking medications? Do you eat food (e.g., spicy or greasy foods) or drink substances (e.g., alcohol or caffeinated beverages) that could be interfering with your sleep? Do you have a physical illness that might be interfering with your sleep? Does anyone in your family have a history of sleep problems?
- *Effect on client:* How has the loss of sleep affected you? (Ask a spouse or friend: Have you noticed any changes in behavior since the sleep problem started?) Do you feel excessively sleepy, irritable, or have trouble concentrating during waking hours? Do you have trouble staying awake or have you fallen asleep at inappropriate times, for example, while driving, sitting quietly in a meeting, or watching TV?

Proper questioning helps the nurse determine the type of sleep disturbance and the nature of the problem. Table 41-1 gives examples of additional questions for the nurse to ask the client when specific sleep disorders are suspected.

Table 41-1 Questions to Ask to Assess for Sleep Disorders

Assessment Questions	Rationale
Insomnia How easily do you fall asleep? Do you fall asleep and have difficulty staying asleep? How many times do you awaken? Do you awaken early from sleep? What time do you awaken for good? What causes you to awaken early? What do you do to prepare for sleep? To improve your sleep? What do you think about as you try to fall asleep? How often do you have trouble sleeping?	Determine nature and severity of insomnia. Help in selection of sleep therapies.
Sleep Apnea Do you snore loudly? Has anyone ever told you that you often stop breathing for short periods during sleep? (Spouse or bed partner/roommate may report this). Do you experience headaches after awakening? Do you have difficulty staying awake during the day? Does anyone else in your family snore loudly or stop breathing during sleep?	Reveal presence of sleep apnea and severity of condition.
Narcolepsy Are you tired during the day? Do you fall asleep at inopportune times? (Friends or relatives may report this.) Do you have episodes of losing muscle control or falling to the floor? Have you ever had the feeling of being unable to move or talk just before falling asleep? Do you have vivid lifelike dreams when going to sleep or waking up?	Help diagnose narcolepsy and influence on daily activities.

As an adjunct to the sleep history, a client and bed partner may be asked to keep a sleep-wake log for 1 to 4 weeks (Beck-Little and Weinrich, 1998). The sleep-wake log is completed daily to provide information on day-to-day variations in sleep-wake patterns over extended periods. Entries in the log often include 24-hour information about various waking and sleeping health behaviors such as physical activities, mealtimes, type and amount of intake (alcohol and caffeine), time and length of daytime naps, evening and bedtime routines, the time the client tries to fall asleep, nighttime awakenings, and the time of morning awakening. A partner can help record the estimated times the client falls asleep or awakens. Although the log is helpful, the client must be motivated to participate in its completion. Ordinarily it is not used with acutely ill clients who have short hospital stays.

Usual Sleep Pattern.   Normal sleep is difficult to define because individuals vary in the quantity and quality of sleep that they perceive as adequate for them. It is important, however, to have clients describe their usual sleep pattern to determine the significance of the changes being created by a sleep disorder. Knowing a client's usual, preferred sleep pattern allows a nurse to try to match sleeping conditions in a health care setting with those in the home. To determine the client's sleep pattern the nurse asks the following questions:

1.   What time do you usually get in bed each night?
2.   What time do you usually fall asleep? Do you do anything special to help you fall asleep?
3.   How many times do you awaken at night? Why?
4.   What time do you typically wake up in the morning?
5.   What time do you get out of bed for good once you have awakened?
6.   What is the average number of hours you sleep each night?

The nurse compares these data with the predominant pattern usually found for other clients of the same age. Based on this comparison, the nurse begins to assess for identifiable patterns such as insomnia.

Clients with sleep problems may show patterns drastically different from their usual one, or the change may be relatively minor. Hospitalized clients usually need or want more sleep as a result of illness. However, some may require less sleep because they are less active. Clients who are ill may think that it is important to try to sleep more than what is usual for them, eventually making sleeping difficult.

Physical Illness.   The nurse determines whether the client has any preexisting health problems that might interfere with sleep. A history of psychiatric problems may also make a difference. For example, a manic-depressive client sleeps more when depressed than when manic. A depressed client often experiences an inadequate amount of sleep that is fragmented. Chronic diseases such as chronic obstructive pulmonary disease and painful disorders such as arthritis interfere with sleep. The nurse also assesses the client's medication history, including a description of over-the-counter and prescribed drugs. If a client takes medications to aid sleep, the nurse gathers information about the type and amount of medication that is being used. The nurse may also assess daily caffeine intake.

If the client has recently undergone surgery, the nurse can expect the client to experience some disturbance in sleep. The effect on sleep depends on the severity of pain experienced after surgery (Closs, 1992). Clients may awaken frequently during the first night after surgery and receive little deep or REM sleep. Depending on the type of surgery, it may take several days for a normal sleep cycle to return.

Current Life Events.   The nurse learns whether the client is experiencing any changes in lifestyle that may be disrupting sleep. A person's occupation may offer a clue to the nature of the sleep problem. Changes in job responsibilities, rotating shifts, or long hours can contribute to a sleep disturbance. Questions about social activities, recent travel, or mealtime schedules help clarify the sleep assessment.

Emotional and Mental Status.   If a client is anxious, excitable, or angry, mental preoccupations can seriously disrupt sleep. The client may be experiencing emotional stress related to illness or situational crises such as loss of job or a loved one. Thus the client's emotions may affect the ability to sleep. Clients with psychiatric disorders may need mild sedation for adequate rest. The nurse assesses the effectiveness of the medication and its effect on daytime function.

Bedtime Routines.   The nurse asks what the client does to prepare for sleep. For example, the client may drink a glass of milk, take a sleeping pill, eat a snack, or watch television. The nurse assesses habits that are beneficial compared with those that have been found to disturb sleep. Not all clients are alike. Watching television may promote sleep for one person, whereas another individual may be stimulated to stay awake while watching TV. Sometimes pointing out that a particular habit may be interfering with sleep can help clients to find ways to change or eliminate habits that may be disrupting sleep.

The nurse should pay special attention to a child's bedtime rituals. The parents can report whether it is necessary, for example, to read the child a bedtime story, rock the child to sleep, or engage in quiet play. Some young children need a special blanket or stuffed animal when going to sleep.

Bedtime Environment.   The nurse asks the client to describe preferred bedroom conditions. The bedroom may be dark or light, and the door to the room may be open or closed. The client may listen to the radio or watch television, or prefer a quiet environment. The nurse also observes the bed and mattress for preferred type (e.g., soft). In addition, a child may require the company of a parent to fall asleep. The nurse may learn that changes in the home or institutional environment may be necessary to promote sleep. In a health care environment there may be environmental distractions that can interfere with sleep such as a roommate's television, an electronic monitor in the hallway, a noisy nurses' station, or another client who cries out at night. The nurse identifies factors that can be reduced or controlled.

NURSING DIAGNOSES Box 41-7
CLIENTS WITH SLEEP DISTURBANCES

Anxiety
Breathing pattern, ineffective
Confusion, acute
Coping, ineffective family
Coping, ineffective individual
Fatigue
Protection, altered
Sensory/perceptual alteration
Sleep pattern disturbance: insomnia, sleep apnea

Behaviors of Sleep Deprivation. Some clients may be unaware of how their sleep problems are affecting their behavior. The nurse observes for behaviors such as irritability, disorientation (similar to a drunken state), frequent yawning, and slurred speech. If sleep deprivation has lasted a long time, psychotic behavior such as delusions and paranoia may develop. For example, a client may report seeing strange objects or colors in the room. The client may act afraid when the nurse enters the room.

Clients hospitalized in intensive care units (ICUs) for extended time may show the "ICU syndrome" of sleep deprivation (Thelan and others, 1998). Constant environmental stimuli within the ICU, such as strange noises from equipment, the frequent monitoring and care given by nurses, and ever-present lights, confuse clients. Repeated environmental stimuli and the client's poor physical status lead to sleep deprivation (Richards and Barnsfather, 1988).

Client Expectations. A poor night's sleep for a client often starts a vicious cycle of anticipatory anxiety, with fear that sleep will again be disturbed, which then causes another night of disrupted sleep (Appling, 1997). The nurse must use a skilled and caring approach to assess the client's sleep needs. A caring nurse is one perceived to tailor care to the individual's needs. The nurse should always ask clients what they expect regarding sleep. This includes asking clients what interventions they currently use and how successful the interventions are. The nurse also asks clients what other interventions to promote sleep they prefer and how they might be implemented. It is important to understand clients' expectations regarding their sleep pattern. When clients ask the nurse for assistance because of sleep disturbances, they typically expect the nurse to respond promptly to assist them in improving their quantity and quality of sleep.

NURSING DIAGNOSIS

Assessment reveals clusters of data that include defining characteristics for a sleep problem that results from disturbed sleep (Ackley and Ladwig, 1997). If a sleep pattern disturbance is identified, the nurse specifies the condition (Box 41-7) (Kim, McFarland, and McLane,

1997). By specifying the nature of a sleep disturbance, the nurse can design more effective interventions. For example, the nurse uses different therapies for clients who are unable to fall asleep than for those with sleep apnea. Box 41-8 demonstrates how to use nursing assessment activities to identify and cluster defining characteristics to make an accurate nursing diagnosis.

Assessment should also identify the related factor or probable cause of the sleep disturbance, such as a noisy environment, a high intake of caffeinated beverages in the evening, or stress involving a marital relationship. These causes become the focus of interventions for minimizing or eliminating the problem. For example, if a client is experiencing insomnia as a result of a noisy health care environment, the nurse could offer some basic recommendations for helping sleep such as controlling the noise of hospital equipment, reducing interruptions, or keeping doors closed. If the insomnia is related to worry over a threatened marital separation, the nurse's actions involve introduction of coping strategies and creation of an environment for sleep. If the probable cause or related factors are incorrectly defined, the client may not benefit from care.

Sleep problems may affect clients in other ways. For example, a nurse may find that a client with sleep apnea has problems with a spouse who is tired and frustrated over the client's snoring. In addition, the spouse is concerned that the client is breathing improperly and thus is in danger. The nursing diagnosis of *ineffective family coping* indicates that the nurse must provide support to the client and spouse so that they can understand sleep apnea and obtain the medical treatment needed.

PLANNING

During planning the nurse again synthesizes information from multiple resources (Figure 41-5). Critical thinking ensures that the client's plan of care integrates all that the nurse knows about the individual as well as key critical thinking elements. Professional standards are especially important to consider when the nurse develops a

SAMPLE NURSING DIAGNOSTIC PROCESS   Box 41-8

SLEEP DISTURBANCES

Assessment Activities	Defining Characteristics	Nursing Diagnosis
Ask client to explain nature of sleep problem.	Client reports difficulty in falling asleep, taking up to an hour. Client reports awakening two to three times nightly, with difficulty returning to sleep.	Sleep pattern disturbance, difficulty falling and/or remaining asleep related to worry over job loss
Observe client's behavior and ask bed partner if behavior changes have been noted.	Client admits to not feeling well rested. Spouse describes episodes of client being lethargic and irritable.	
Determine if client has had recent lifestyle changes.	Spouse reports client recently lost job, has concern over finding new position.	

plan of care. These standards often establish scientifically proven guidelines for selecting effective nursing interventions. For example, the "Nursing Standard-of-Practice Protocol: Sleep Disturbances in Elderly Patients" (Foreman and Wykle, 1995) recommends individualized nursing interventions that maintain and support the client's normal sleep pattern and bedtime routine or ritual.

The nurse develops an individualized plan of care for each nursing diagnosis (see care plan, p. 1270). The nurse and client set realistic expectations for care. Goals are to be individualized and realistic with measurable outcomes (e.g., achieving a sleep pattern normal for the client).

It is important for the plan of care to include strategies that are appropriate for the client's living environment and lifestyle. An effective plan includes outcomes established over a realistic time that focus on the goal of improving the quantity and quality of sleep in the home. This type of plan may require many weeks to accomplish. The nurse partners closely with the client and significant others to ensure that any therapies, such as a change in the sleep schedule or changes to the bedroom environment, are realistic and achievable.

In a health care setting the nurse plans treatments or routines so that the client will be able to rest. For example, in the intensive care unit, nurses check available electronic monitors to track trends in vital signs without awakening a client each hour. Other staff members should be aware of the care plan so that they can cluster activities at certain times to reduce awakenings. In a nursing home the focus of the plan may involve better planning of rest periods around the activities of the other residents. Often the schedule of one roommate may not coincide with that of another.

The nature of the sleep disturbance determines whether referrals to additional health care providers are necessary. For example, if a sleep problem is related to a situational crisis or emotional problem, the nurse may refer the client to a psychiatric clinical nurse specialist or clinical psychologist for counseling. When chronic insomnia is the prob-

lem, a medical referral or referral to a sleep center may be beneficial. If the nurse works in an in-patient setting and the client is to receive a referral for continued care after discharge, offering information about the sleep problem will be useful to the home health care nurse.

The success of sleep therapy depends on an approach that fits the client's lifestyle and the nature of the sleep disorder. The goals of any care plan for a client needing sleep or rest include the following:

The client obtains a sense of restfulness and renewed energy following sleep.

The client establishes a healthy sleep pattern.

The client understands factors that promote or disrupt sleep.

The client assumes self-care behaviors to eliminate factors contributing to the sleep disturbance.

IMPLEMENTATION

Nursing interventions designed to improve the quality of a person's rest and sleep are largely focused on health promotion. Clients need adequate sleep and rest to maintain active and productive lifestyles. During times of illness, rest and sleep promotion is important for recovery. Nursing care in an acute care, restorative care, or continuing care setting differs from that provided in a client's home. The primary differences are in the environment and the nurse's ability to support normal rest and sleep habits. The client's age also influences the types of therapies that are most effective. Box 41-9 provides principles for promoting sleep in older clients. Despite the cause or related factors for sleep problems, the nurse performs specific interventions that promote normal sleep patterns.

Health Promotion.   Many factors affect the ability to gain adequate rest and sleep. In community health and home settings the nurse helps clients develop behaviors conducive to rest and relaxation. This may include suggesting changes in the environment or certain lifestyle habits. To develop good sleep habits at home, clients and

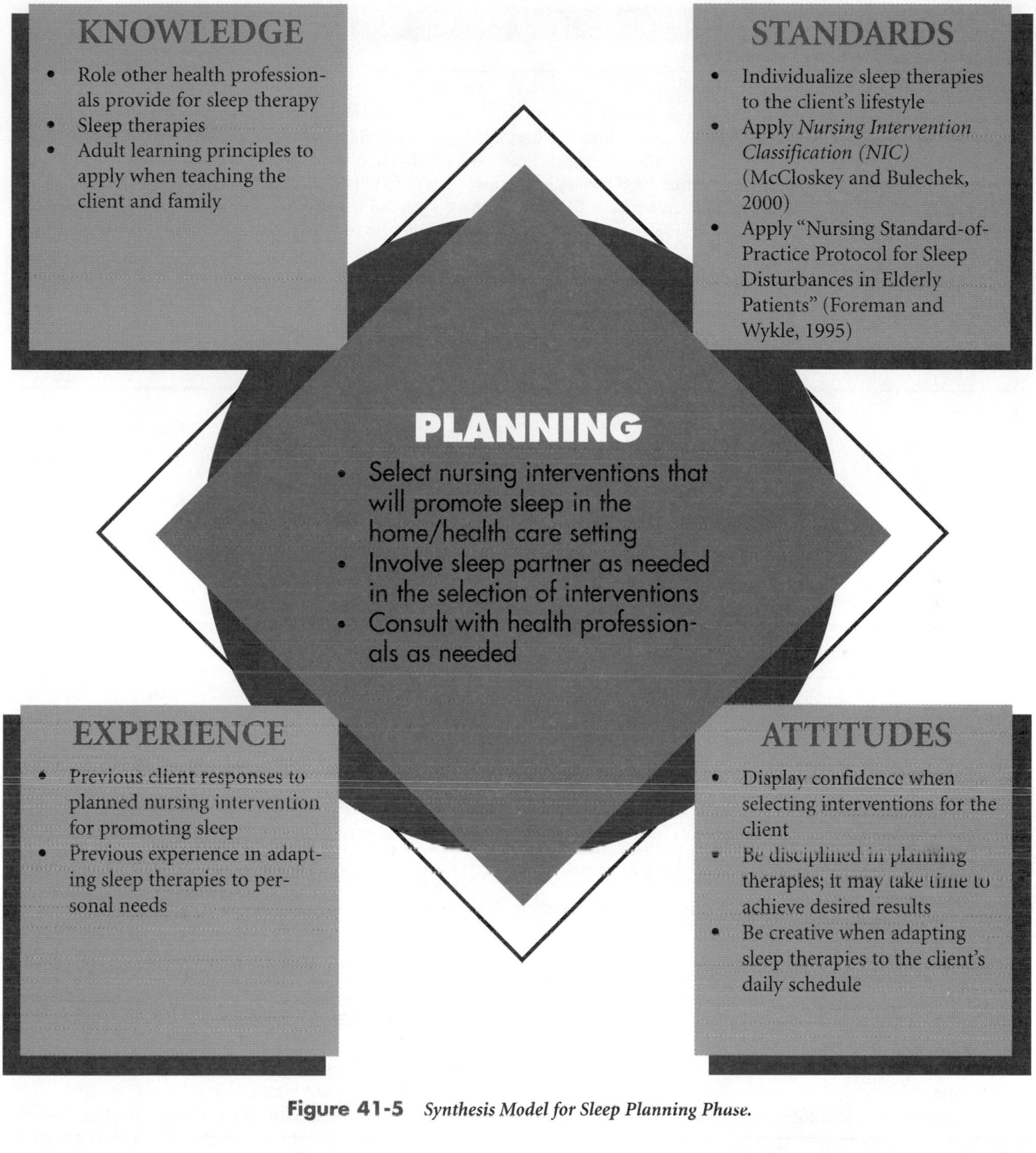

KNOWLEDGE

- Role other health professionals provide for sleep therapy
- Sleep therapies
- Adult learning principles to apply when teaching the client and family

STANDARDS

- Individualize sleep therapies to the client's lifestyle
- Apply *Nursing Intervention Classification (NIC)* (McCloskey and Bulechek, 2000)
- Apply "Nursing Standard-of-Practice Protocol for Sleep Disturbances in Elderly Patients" (Foreman and Wykle, 1995)

PLANNING

- Select nursing interventions that will promote sleep in the home/health care setting
- Involve sleep partner as needed in the selection of interventions
- Consult with health professionals as needed

EXPERIENCE

- Previous client responses to planned nursing intervention for promoting sleep
- Previous experience in adapting sleep therapies to personal needs

ATTITUDES

- Display confidence when selecting interventions for the client
- Be disciplined in planning therapies; it may take time to achieve desired results
- Be creative when adapting sleep therapies to the client's daily schedule

Figure 41-5   *Synthesis Model for Sleep Planning Phase.*

their bed partners should learn techniques that promote sleep and conditions that interfere with sleep (Zarcone, 1994) (Box 41-10). Parents should also learn how to promote good sleep habits for their children. Clients benefit most from instructions based on information about their homes and lifestyles. Similarly, they will more likely apply information that is useful and valued.

Environmental Controls.   All clients require a sleeping environment with a comfortable room temperature and proper ventilation, minimal sources of noise, a comfortable bed, and proper lighting (McCloskey and Bulechek, 2000). Infants sleep best when the room temperature is 18° C to 21° C (64.4° F to 69.8° F) at night. Cribs should be positioned away from open windows or drafts. The infant is covered with a light, warm blanket. Children and adults vary more in regard to comfortable room temperature. Some prefer to sleep without covers. Older adults often require extra blankets or covers. Many older clients sleep wearing socks.

SAMPLE NURSING CARE PLAN

SLEEP ALTERATIONS

ASSESSMENT*

Julie Arnold, a 42-year-old attorney, is the first client of the morning at the neighborhood health clinic where you work. When you ask her how she is doing, she **tells you she is having difficulty sleeping.** She tells you this **started several days** after she began **feeling pressured at work** to complete an important case. On further questioning you find out she is **going to bed between 12 and 1 am,** which is **2 hours later than her normal bedtime** and it **takes her almost an hour to fall asleep.** Julie normally gets 7 hours of sleep a night. Because she is having trouble falling asleep, Julie has **been drinking a glass of wine before bedtime.** She has **2 to 3 cups of coffee after dinner** to stay awake while **working on her case before bedtime.** Julie also reports that she **wakes up at least once during the night.** Julie states, "**I feel tired when I wake up, and sometimes I have trouble concentrating** in the afternoon at work. I have stopped my routine of walking a mile a day." As you observe Julie, you notice she has **dark circles under her eyes, shifts her position in the chair multiple times,** and **yawns frequently.** Julie also says she seems to **have less patience** with her children at home.

*****Defining characteristics** are shown in bold type.

NURSING DIAGNOSIS: Sleep pattern disturbance related to psychological stress from job pressures

PLANNING

GOALS

Client will achieve an improved sense of adequate sleep within 2 weeks.

Client will achieve a more normal sleep pattern within 2 weeks.

EXPECTED OUTCOMES

Client will report waking up less frequently during the night and feeling rested within 2 weeks.

Client will verbalize adherence to a regular bedtime routine within 1 week.

Client will fall asleep within 30 minutes of going to bed within 2 weeks.

Client will report sleeping 7 hours nightly within 2 weeks.

INTERVENTIONS†

Sleep Enhancement

- Encourage client to establish a bedtime routine and a regular sleep pattern.
- Instruct client to limit caffeine, nicotine, and alcohol before bedtime.

- Assist client to identify ways to eliminate stressful concerns about work before bedtime (e.g., taking time before actual sleep time to read a light novel).
- Adjust environment, have client control noise, temperature, and light in the bedroom.

Exercise Promotion

- Encourage client to reinstitute walking routinely during the day, but not 2 to 3 hours before bedtime.

Simple Relaxation Therapy

- Instruct client on how to perform muscle relaxation before bedtime.

RATIONALE

Maintaining a consistent schedule helps induce sleep (Appling, 1997).

Caffeine and nicotine are stimulants and cause difficulty in falling asleep. Alcohol lightens and fragments sleep (Rogers, 1997b).

Excess worry and intense activities before bedtime may stimulate client and prevent sleep (Rogers, 1997b).

This develops an environment conducive to sleep (Appling, 1997).

Exercise can increase activity levels and the need for sleep. Exercise just prior to bedtime is a stimulant that prevents sleep (Rogers, 1997b).

Relaxation therapy can help reduce anxiety, which interferes with sleep (Hyman and others, 1989).

†Intervention Classification labels from McCloskey JC, Bulechek GM, editors: *Nursing interventions classification (NIC),* ed 3, St. Louis, 2000, Mosby.

EVALUATION

Ask if client is successful in falling and staying asleep.

Ask client to describe waking behaviors at work or home during the day.

Observe the waking nonverbal expressions and behavior of client.

NURSING PRACTICE   **Box 41-9**

Promoting Sleep

SLEEP-WAKE PATTERN
- Maintain a regular bedtime and wake-up schedule (Richards, 1996).
- Eliminate naps unless they are a routine part of the schedule.
- If naps are used, limit to 20 minutes or less twice a day.
- Go to bed when sleepy.
- Use relaxation techniques to promote sleep.
- If unable to sleep in 15 to 30 minutes, get out of bed.

ENVIRONMENT
- Sleep where you sleep best.
- Keep noise to minimum; use soft music to mask noise if necessary.
- Use night-light and keep path to bathroom free of obstacles.
- Set room temperature to preference; use socks to promote warmth.

MEDICATIONS
- Use sedatives and hypnotics as last resort and then only short-term if absolutely necessary (Foreman and Wykle, 1995).
- Adjust medications being taken for other conditions and look for drug interactions that may cause insomnia or EDS.

DIET
- Limit alcohol, caffeine, and nicotine in late afternoon and evening (Ancoli-Israel, 1997).
- Consume carbohydrates or milk as a light snack before bedtime.
- Decrease fluids 2 to 4 hours before sleep (Ancoli-Israel, 1997).

PHYSIOLOGICAL/ILLNESS FACTORS
- Elevate head of bed and provide extra pillows as preferred.
- Use analgesics 30 minutes before bed to ease aches and pains (Foreman and Wykle, 1995).
- Use therapeutics to control symptoms of chronic conditions as prescribed (Beck-Little and Weinrich, 1998).

Client Teaching FOR SLEEP HYGIENE HABITS   **Box 41-10**

OBJECTIVE
- Client will follow proper sleep hygiene habits at home.

TEACHING STRATEGIES
- Instruct client to try to exercise daily, preferably in morning or afternoon, and to avoid vigorous exercise in the evening within 3 hours of bedtime.
- Caution client against sleeping long hours during weekends or holidays to prevent disturbance of normal sleep-wake cycle.
- Explain that if possible, the bedroom should not be used for intensive studying, snacking, TV watching, or other nonsleep activity, besides sex.
- Explain that client should try to avoid worrisome thinking when going to bed and should use relaxation exercises.
- Advise to get out of bed and do some quiet activity until feeling sleepy enough to go back to bed if client does not fall asleep within 30 minutes of going to bed.

- Recommend client limit caffeine to morning coffee and limit alcohol intake (more than 1 to 2 drinks a day can interrupt sleep cycle).
- Ask client to examine environment: keep room dark, well ventilated, quiet, and at a comfortable temperature. Instruct that use of earplugs and eyeshades may be helpful.
- Instruct client to avoid heavy meals for 3 hours before bedtime; a light snack may help.

EVALUATION
- Have client complete sleep-wake log for 1 week, and compare it with previous sleep-wake log.
- Ask client to periodically complete visual analog or sleep rating scale for perceptions of quality of sleep.

Distracting noise needs to be eliminated so that the bedroom is as quiet as possible. In the home the television, telephone, or the intermittent chiming of a clock may disrupt a client's sleep. The family becomes an important part of the nurse's approach, especially if there are several family members, all with different schedules for going to sleep. At home it may require the cooperation of several people living with the client to reduce noise. It is also important to remember that some clients are used to sleeping with familiar inside noises, such as the hum of a fan.

A bed and mattress should provide support and comfortable firmness. Bed boards can be placed under mattresses to add support. Sometimes extra pillows are important to help a person position comfortably in bed. The position of the bed in the room may also make a difference for some clients.

Infants' beds must be safe. To reduce the chance of suffocation, pillows, stuffed toys, or the ends of loose blankets should not be placed in cribs. Loose-fitting plastic mattress covers should not be used because infants might pull them over their faces and suffocate. Infants are usually placed on their back to prevent suffocation or on their sides to prevent aspiration of stomach contents.

For any client prone to confusion or falls, safety is critical. In the home a small night-light might assist the client in orienting to the room environment before arising to go to the bathroom. Beds set lower to the floor may lessen the chance of a person falling when first standing. Clutter and throw rugs should always be removed from the path a client uses to walk from the bed to the bathroom. If a client needs assistance in ambulating from a bed to the bathroom, a small bell at the bedside can be used to call family members.

Clients vary in regard to the amount of light that they prefer at night. Infants and older adults sleep best in softly lit rooms. Light should not shine directly on their eyes. Small table lamps prevent total darkness. For older adults this reduces the chance of confusion and prevents falls en route to the bathroom. If streetlights shine through windows or when clients nap during the day, heavy shades, drapes, or slatted blinds are helpful.

Promoting Bedtime Routines.

Bedtime routines relax clients in preparation for sleep (McCloskey and Bulechek, 2000). It is always important for persons to go to sleep when they feel fatigued or sleepy. Going to bed while fully awake and thinking about other things can cause insomnia and interfere with the bed as a stimulus for sleep.

Newborns and infants sleep through so much of the day that a specific routine is hardly necessary. However, quieting activities, such as holding them snugly in blankets, singing or talking softly, and gentle rocking, help infants fall asleep.

A bedtime routine (e.g., same hour for bedtime, snack or quiet activity) used consistently helps young children avoid delaying sleep. Toddlers and preschoolers may be too excited and full of energy to go to bed. Patterns of preparing for bedtime need to be reinforced. Reading stories, allowing children to sit in a parent's lap while listening to music, or listening to a prayer are routines that can be associated with preparing for bed. Quiet activities such as coloring and reading work well with school-age children.

Adults need to avoid excessive mental stimulation just before bedtime. Reading a light novel, watching a relaxing television program, or listening to music helps a person relax. Relaxation exercises can be useful at bedtime. Slow, deep breathing for 1 or 2 minutes induces calm (see Chapter 42). Rhythmic contraction and relaxation of muscles alleviates tension and prepares the body for rest (Hoch and Reynolds, 1986). Guided imagery and praying may also promote sleep.

At home a client should not try to finish office work or resolve family problems before bedtime. The bedroom should not be used as a place to work and should always be associated with sleep. Working toward a consistent time

for sleep and wakening helps most clients gain a healthy sleep pattern and strengthens the rhythm of the sleep-wake cycle.

Promoting Comfort.

People fall asleep only after feeling comfortable and relaxed (McCloskey and Bulechek, 2000). Minor irritants can keep clients awake. Soft cotton nightclothes keep infants or small children warm and comfortable. Clients should be instructed to wear loose-fitting nightwear. An extra blanket may be all that is needed to prevent a person from feeling chilled and being unable to fall asleep. Clients should void before retiring so they are not kept awake by a full bladder.

Establishing Periods of Rest and Sleep.

In the home it may help to encourage clients to stay physically active during the day so that they are more likely to sleep at night. Increasing daytime activity lessens problems with falling asleep. Rigorous exercise should always be planned at least several hours before bedtime.

Although older adults get less deep nighttime sleep, some often take short naps during the day (Bliwise, 1993). This change in pattern associated with aging may not represent a decrease in need for sleep but a redistribution of sleeping behavior during a 24-hour period. Naps should be taken at the same time each day to maintain a consistent schedule.

In the home setting the nurse frequently cares for clients with chronic debilitating disease. The nursing care plan might include having clients set aside afternoons for rest to promote optimal health. The nurse helps adjust medication schedules, instructs clients to regularly void before rest periods, and suggests unplugging the telephone so that rest periods are uninterrupted. Box 41-11 lists conditions needed to promote rest.

Stress Reduction.

The inability to sleep because of emotional stress can also make a person feel irritable and tense. When clients feel emotionally upset, they should be encouraged to try not to force sleep. Otherwise, insomnia frequently develops, and soon bedtime is associated with the inability to relax. A client who has difficulty falling asleep can be helped by getting up and pursuing a relaxing activity, such as sewing or reading, rather than staying in bed and thinking about sleep.

Preschoolers have bedtime fears (fear of the dark or strange noises), awaken during the night, or have nightmares. After nightmares, the parent should enter the child's room immediately and talk to them briefly about fears to provide a cooling-down period. One approach is to comfort children and leave them in their own beds so that their fears are not used as excuses to delay bedtime. Keeping a light on in the room may also help. Cultural tradition may cause families to approach sleep practices differently (Box 41-12). The nurse should respect those that differ from traditional recommendations.

Conditions for Proper Rest   Box 41-11

PHYSICAL COMFORT

Eliminate sources of physical irritation.

Control sources of pain.

Control room temperature.

Maintain proper anatomical alignment or positioning.

Remove environmental distractions.

Provide adequate ventilation.

FREEDOM FROM WORRY

Have knowledge needed to understand health problems and implications.

Make own decisions.

Participate in personal health care.

Practice restful activities regularly.

Know that the environment is safe.

SUFFICIENT SLEEP

Obtain hours of sleep needed to feel refreshed.

Follow good sleep hygiene habits.

Cultural ASPECTS OF CARE   Box 41-12

Practices and patterns of sleep and rest vary among cultures. These patterns are generally established in infancy or childhood and are reinforced throughout the life span (Leininger, 1995). Traditionally experts recommend having infants and children sleep in their own beds (Lozoff, 1995). Co-sleeping, in which children are allowed to sleep with parents or siblings, is a more common practice among African-American, Hispanic, Italian, Asian, and American Samoan families (Andrews and Boyle, 1995; Lozoff, 1995). The type of bed for a child may also vary. Some Native American tribes use a cradle board for infants whereas American Samoan infants sleep on a pandanus mat covered with a blanket (Andrews and Boyle, 1995). These approaches lessen the child's anxiety and create a strong sense of security.

Control of Noise in the Hospital   Box 41-13

Close doors to client's room when possible.

Keep doors to work areas on unit closed when in use.

Reduce volume of nearby telephone and paging equipment.

Wear rubber-soled shoes. Avoid clogs.

Turn off bedside oxygen and other equipment that is not in use.

Turn down alarms and beeps on bedside monitoring equipment.

Turn off room TV and radio unless client prefers soft music.

Avoid abrupt loud noise such as flushing a toilet or moving a bed.

Keep necessary conversations at low levels, particularly at night.

Conduct conversations and reports in a private area away from client rooms.

Bedtime Snacks. Some persons enjoy bedtime snacks, whereas others cannot sleep after eating. A dairy product snack such as warm milk or cocoa that contains L-tryptophan may be helpful in promoting sleep. A full meal before bedtime can often cause gastrointestinal upset and interfere with the ability to fall asleep.

Nurses should encourage clients to try to refrain from drinking or ingesting caffeine before bedtime. Coffee, tea, cola, and chocolate act as stimulants, causing a person to stay awake or awaken throughout the night. Alcohol can interrupt sleep cycles and reduce the amount of deep sleep. Coffee, tea, colas, and alcohol act as diuretics and may cause a person to awaken in the night to void.

Infants require special measures to minimize nighttime awakenings for feeding. It is common for children to have a need for middle-of-the-night bottle- or breast-feeding. Wong (1998) recommends offering the last feeding as late as possible. Infants should not be given bottles in bed.

Pharmacological Approaches. The use of nonprescription sleeping medications is not advisable. Clients should learn the risks of such drugs, especially that, over the long term, these drugs can lead to further sleep disruption even when they initially seemed to be effective (see p. 1275). The nurse can help clients use behavioral and proper sleep hygiene measures to establish sleep patterns that do not require the use of drugs.

Acute Care. Clients in an acute care setting have their normal rest and sleep routine disrupted, which generally leads to sleep problems. In this setting the nursing interventions focus on controlling factors in the environment that disrupt sleep, relieving physiological or psychological disruptions to sleep, and providing for uninterrupted rest and sleep periods for the client.

Environmental Controls. In a hospital the nurse can control the environment in several ways. Nurses should close the curtains between clients in semiprivate rooms. Lights on a hospital nursing unit can be dimmed at night. One of the biggest problems for clients in the hospital is noise. Important ways to reduce noise are to conduct conversations and reports in a private area away from client rooms and to keep necessary conversations to a minimum, especially at night. Additional ways to control noise in the hospital can be found in Box 41-13.

Promoting Comfort. Compared with beds at home, hospital beds are often harder and of a different height, length, or width. Keeping beds clean and dry and in a comfortable position may help clients relax. Some clients suffer painful illnesses requiring special comfort measures such as application of dry or moist heat, use of supportive dressings or splints, and proper positioning before retiring (Figure 41-6).

Establishing Periods of Rest and Sleep.   In a hospital or extended care setting it is difficult to provide clients with the time needed to rest and sleep. However, the nurse plans care to avoid awakening clients for nonessential tasks. The nurse can help by scheduling assessments, treatments, procedures, and routines for times when clients are awake. For example, if a client's physical condition has been stable, the nurse should avoid awakening the client to check vital signs. Rest can be promoted by allowing clients to determine the timing and methods of delivery of basic care measures. Baths and routine hygiene measures should not be given during the night for nursing convenience. Blood should be drawn at a time when the client is awake. Unless maintaining a drug's therapeutic blood level is essential, medications should be given during waking hours. The nurse should work with the radiology department and other support services to schedule diagnostic studies and therapies at intervals that allow clients time for rest.

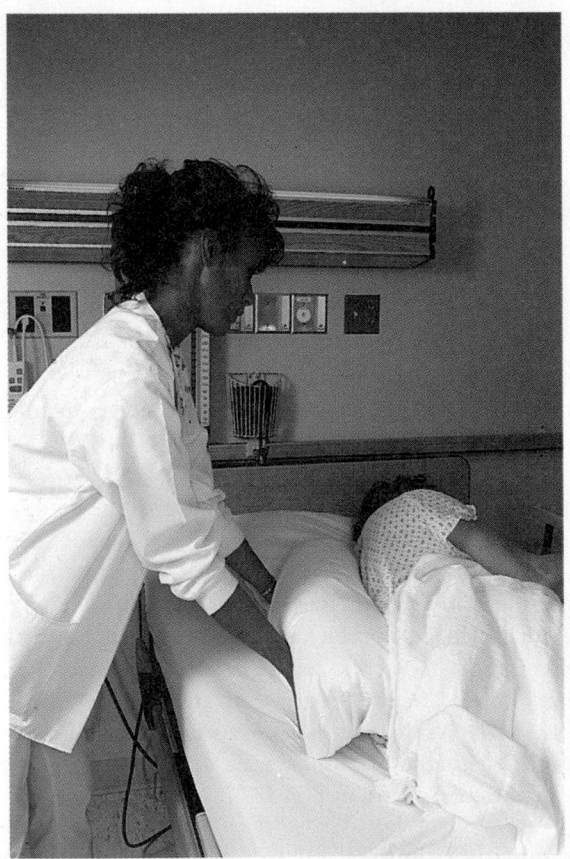

Figure 41-6   Client position for sleep.

When the client's condition demands more frequent monitoring, the nurse can plan activities to allow extended rest periods. The nurse can instruct assistive personnel on the coordination of client care to reduce client disturbances. This means planning activities so that instead of a nurse or other personnel returning to the room every few minutes, the client may have up to an hour or more to rest quietly. For example, if a client needs frequent dressing changes, is receiving intravenous therapy, and has drainage tubes from several sites, the nurse should not make a separate trip into the room to check each problem. Instead the nurse should use a single visit to change the dressing, regulate the intravenous system, and empty the drainage tubes. The nurse can become the client's advocate for promoting optimal sleep. This may mean becoming a gatekeeper by postponing or rescheduling visits by family, asking consultants to reschedule visits, or questioning the frequency of certain procedures.

Stress Reduction.   Clients who are hospitalized for extensive diagnostic testing may have difficulty resting or sleeping because of uncertainty about their state of health. Giving clients control over their health care minimizes uncertainty and anxiety. Providing information about the purpose of procedures and routines and answering questions may give clients the peace of mind needed to rest or fall asleep. A nurse on the night shift should take time to sit and talk with clients unable to sleep. This helps the nurse determine the factors keeping clients awake. Back rubs can also be used to help clients relax more thoroughly. If a sedative is indicated, the nurse confers with the physician to be sure that the lowest dosage is used initially. Discontinuing a sedative as soon as possible prevents a dependence that can seriously disrupt the normal sleep cycle. Older adults can be vulnerable to the side effects of sedatives, hypnotics, or analgesics because the medications are metabolized slowly.

Restorative or Continuing Care.   The nursing interventions that are implemented in the acute care setting can also be used in the restorative or continuing care environment. Controlling the environment, especially noise, establishing periods of rest and sleep, and promoting comfort are important considerations. Nursing interventions related to stress reduction and controlling physiological disturbances are also implemented in these settings.

Promoting Comfort.   Providing for personal hygiene improves a client's sense of comfort. A warm bath or shower before bedtime can be relaxing. Clients restricted to bed should be offered the opportunity to void and wash their face and hands. Toothbrushing and care of dentures also help to prepare the client for sleep. The nurse can recommend and use several additional measures to promote comfort in these clients (Box 41-14).

Controlling Physiological Disturbances. For clients with physical illness, the nurse can help control symptoms that disrupt sleep. For example, a client with respiratory abnormalities should sleep with two pillows or in a semisitting position to ease the effort to breathe. The client may benefit from taking prescribed bronchodilators before sleep to prevent airway obstruction. A client with a hiatal hernia also needs special care. After meals the client may experience a burning sensation as a result of gastric reflux. To prevent sleep disturbances, the client should eat a small meal several hours before bedtime and sleep in a semisitting position. Clients with pain, nausea, or other recurrent symptoms should receive any symptom-relieving medication timed so that the drug takes effect at bedtime.

Pharmacological Approaches. The liberal use of drugs to manage symptoms is quite common in American culture. There are drugs commonly used that are associated with insomnia. Central nervous system stimulants such as amphetamines, caffeine, nicotine, terbutaline, theophylline, and pemoline should be used sparingly and under medical management (McKenry and Salerno, 1998). In addition, withdrawal from CNS depressants such as alcohol, barbiturates, tricyclic antidepressants (amitriptyline, imipramine, and doxepin), and triazolam can cause insomnia and must be managed carefully.

Medications used to induce sleep are called **hypnotics. Sedatives** are medications that produce a calming or soothing effect (McKenry and Salerno, 1998). Hypnotics and sedatives as sleep medications can help if used correctly. A client who takes sleep medications should know about their proper use as well as the risks and possible side effects. However, long-term use of antianxiety, sedative, or hypnotic agents can disrupt sleep and lead to more serious problems. One group of drugs considered to be relatively safe are the benzodiazepines (Table 41-2). The benzodiazepines cause relaxation, antianxiety, and hypnotic effects by facilitating the action of neurons in the CNS that suppress responsiveness to stimulation, therefore decreasing levels of arousal (Trevor and Way, 1995). These medications do not cause general CNS depression as sedatives or hypnotics do. Physicians prescribe this group of drugs because antianxiety effects occur at safe, nontoxic doses.

The benzodiazepines are used cautiously with children under 12 years of age and are contraindicated in infants under 6 months. Pregnant clients should avoid benzodiazepines because their use is associated with risk of congenital anomalies. Nursing mothers should not receive the drugs because they are excreted in breast milk. Older adults are susceptible to side effects of any antianxiety or sedative agent because of physiological changes in metabolism. Short-acting benzodiazepines such as oxazepam or lorazepam are usually recommended. Initial doses should be small, and increments are added gradually, based on client response, for a limited period of time. Nurses should warn clients not to take more than the prescribed dose, especially if the medication seems to become less effective after initial use. If older clients who were recently continent, ambulatory, and alert become incontinent,

---

Comfort Measures in Restorative Care   Box 41-14

Administer hygiene measures for clients on bed rest.

Encourage client to wear loose-fitting nightwear.

Remove or change any irritants against the client's skin such as moist dressings or drainage tubing.

Position and support dependent body parts to protect pressure points and aid muscle relaxation.

Provide caps and socks for older clients and those prone to cold.

Encourage client to void before going to sleep.

Administer analgesics or sedatives about 30 minutes before bedtime.

Offer a massage just before client goes to sleep.

Table 41-2   **Pharmacology of Antiinsomnia Agents**

Generic Name	Trade Name	Onset of Action (in Minutes)	Oral Dosage* (mg)	Indications
Alprazolam	Xanax	15-60	0.25-0.5 (3 times/day)	Anxiety
Diazepam	Valium	15-45	5-10 at bedtime	Sleep disorder
Flurazepam	Dalmane Apo-Flurazepam	15-45	15-30 at bedtime	Sleep disorder
Lorazepam	Ativan Apo-Lorazepam	15-60	2-4 at bedtime	Anxiety, sleep disorder
Oxazepam	Serax Zapex	45-90	10-30 (3-4 times/day)	Anxiety
Temazepam	Restoril	25-27	15-30 at bedtime	Sleep disorder
Triazolam	Halcion	15-30	0.125-0.25 at bedtime	Sleep disorder
Zolpidem	Ambien	15-45	5-10 at bedtime	Sleep disorder

*Dosage may be reduced in older adult clients.

confused, and/or demonstrate impaired mobility, the use of benzodiazepines should be considered as a possible cause.

Regular use of any sleep medication can lead to tolerance and withdrawal. Rebound insomnia can occur after stopping the medication. Immediately administering a sleeping medication when a hospitalized client complains of being unable to sleep may be doing the client more harm than good. Alternative approaches to promote sleep must be considered. Routine monitoring of client response to sleeping medications is important.

EVALUATION

Client Care. With regard to problems with sleep, the client is the source for evaluating outcomes.

Each client has a unique need for sleep and rest. The client is the only who will know if sleep problems are improved and which interventions or therapies are most successful in promoting sleep (Figure 41-7). To evaluate the effectiveness of nursing interventions, the nurse makes comparisons with baseline sleep assessment data to evaluate if sleep has improved.

The nurse determines whether expected outcomes have been met. Evaluative measures may be used shortly after a therapy has been tried (e.g., observing whether a client falls asleep after reducing noise and darkening a room). Other evaluative measures may be used after a client awakens from sleep (e.g., asking a client to describe the number of awakenings during the previous night). The client and bed partner can usually provide accurate evaluative information. Over longer periods, the nurse may use

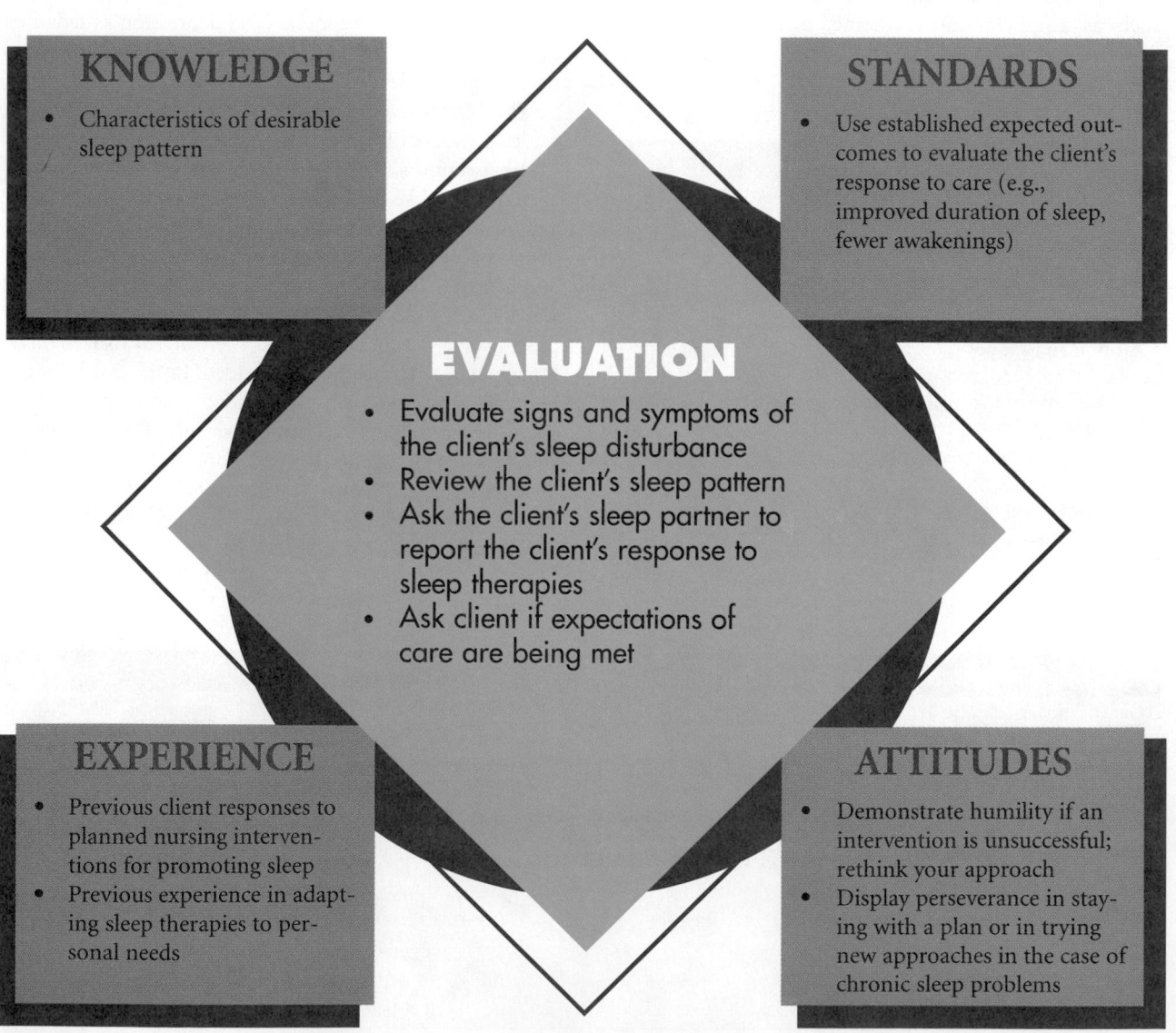

KNOWLEDGE
- Characteristics of desirable sleep pattern

STANDARDS
- Use established expected outcomes to evaluate the client's response to care (e.g., improved duration of sleep, fewer awakenings)

EVALUATION
- Evaluate signs and symptoms of the client's sleep disturbance
- Review the client's sleep pattern
- Ask the client's sleep partner to report the client's response to sleep therapies
- Ask client if expectations of care are being met

EXPERIENCE
- Previous client responses to planned nursing interventions for promoting sleep
- Previous experience in adapting sleep therapies to personal needs

ATTITUDES
- Demonstrate humility if an intervention is unsuccessful; rethink your approach
- Display perseverance in staying with a plan or in trying new approaches in the case of chronic sleep problems

Figure 41-7 *Synthesis Model for Sleep Evaluation Phase.*

assessment tools such as the visual analog scale or sleep rating scale to determine whether sleep has progressively improved or changed.

The nurse also assesses the level of understanding that clients or family members gain after receiving instruction on sleep habits. Compliance with these practices may best be measured during a home visit, when the environment can be observed. When expected outcomes are not met, the nurse revises the nursing measures or expected outcomes based on the client's needs or preferences.

Client Expectations.   If the nurse has successfully developed a good relationship with a client and has developed a therapeutic plan of care, subtle behaviors often indicate the level of the client's satisfaction. The nurse may note the absence of signs of sleep problems, such as lethargy, frequent yawning or position changes, in the client. It is important for the nurse to ask the client if his or her sleep needs have been met. For example, ask the client, "Are you feeling more rested?" or "Can you tell me if you feel we have done all we can to help improve your sleep?" If the client's expectations have not been met, the nurse needs to spend more time trying to understand the client's needs and preferences. Working closely with the client and bed partner will enable the nurse to redefine those expectations that can be realistically met within the limits of the client's condition and treatment. The nurse is effective in promoting rest and sleep if the client's goals and expectations are met.

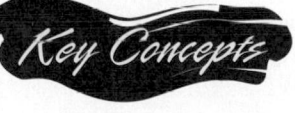

Key Concepts

- Rest is not inactivity but a feeling of physical calm and freedom from worry.
- Sleep is believed to provide physiological and psychological restoration.
- The 24-hour sleep-wake cycle is a circadian rhythm that influences physiological function and behavior.
- The control and regulation of sleep depends on a balance between regulators within the central nervous system.
- During a typical night's sleep a person passes through four to six complete sleep cycles. Each sleep cycle contains three NREM stages of sleep and a period of REM sleep.
- The number of hours of sleep needed by each person to feel rested is variable.
- Neonates, infants, children, and adolescents require more sleep than adults.
- Symptoms of various diseases may disrupt sleep.
- The most common type of sleep disorder is insomnia, which is characterized by the inability to fall asleep, remain asleep during the night, or go back to sleep after awakening earlier than is desired.
- The hectic pace of a person's lifestyle, emotional and psychological stress, and alcohol ingestion can disrupt the sleep pattern.
- Only a client can report whether sleep is restful.

- If a client's sleep is adequate, the nurse assesses the client's usual bedtime, normal bedtime ritual, the preferred environment for sleeping, and usual preferred rising time.
- When a client has a sleep problem, the nurse conducts a complete sleep history. Diagnosing sleep problems depends on identifying factors that impair sleep.
- When planning interventions to promote sleep, the nurse should consider the usual characteristics of the client's home environment and normal-lifestyle.
- A regular bedtime routine of relaxing activities prepares a person physically and mentally for sleep.
- An environment with a darkened room, reduced noise, comfortable bed, and good ventilation promotes sleep.
- One of the most important nursing interventions for promoting sleep in the hospitalized client is establishing periods for uninterrupted sleep and rest.
- Noise is one of the most common causes of sleep disturbances in the hospitalized client. The nurse should implement noise-reducing interventions to promote sleep.
- Pain or other disease symptom control is essential to promote the ability to sleep.
- Long-term use of sleeping pills may lead to difficulty in initiating and maintaining sleep.

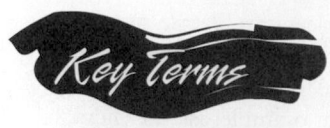
Key Terms

Biological clocks, *p. 1251*

Bulbar synchronizing region (BSR), *p. 1252*

Cataplexy, *p. 1257*

Circadian rhythm, *p. 1251*

Dyssomnias, *p. 1255*

Excessive daytime sleepiness (EDS), *p. 1256*

Hypersomnolence, *p. 1255*

Hypnotics, *p. 1275*

Insomnia, *p. 1255*

Narcolepsy, *p. 1257*

Nocturia, *p. 1255*

Nonrapid eye movement (NREM) sleep, *p. 1252*

Parasomnia, *p. 1255*

Polysomnogram, *p. 1255*

Rapid eye movement (REM) sleep, *p. 1252*

Rest, *p. 1258*

Reticular activating system (RAS), *p. 1252*

Sedatives, *p. 1275*

Sleep, *p. 1251*

Sleep apnea, *p. 1256*

Sleep deprivation, *p. 1257*

Sleep hygiene, *p. 1255*

Critical Thinking Exercises

1. Mrs. Davis, age 66, visits the community clinic for her annual checkup. She tells you as the nurse that she is having trouble sleeping at night because her husband is restless and snores. What assessment data is appropriate to gather regarding this situation?

2. As a nurse you are asked to help develop a health promotion brochure for senior citizens that includes information on how to promote sleep. The brochure will be available in clinics and senior centers. What general information should be included in the brochure for sleep enhancement in this group?

3. Mr. Walker, age 55, is recovering on your unit from heart surgery. You find him awake at 2 AM as you make rounds, and he tells you he has been having trouble sleeping since surgery 3 days ago. Develop a plan of care for Mr. Walker to promote sleep for him while he is in the hospital.

References

Ackley BJ, Ladwig GB: *Nursing diagnosis handbook: a guide to planning care,* ed 3, St. Louis, 1997, Mosby.

Agnew HW and others: The first night effect: an EEG study of sleep, *Psychophysiology* 2:263, 1966.

Aldrich MS: Narcolepsy, *Neurology* 42(Suppl 6):34, 1992.

American Nurses Association: Standards of clinical nursing practice, Washington, DC, 1991, The Association.

American Sleep Disorders Association: *The international classification of sleep disorders: diagnostic and coding manual,* Rochester, NY, 1990, Allen Press.

Anch AM and others: *Sleep: a scientific perspective,* Englewood Cliffs, NJ, 1988, Prentice-Hall.

Ancoli-Israel S: Sleep problems in older adults: putting myths to bed, *Geriatrics,* 52(1):20, 1997.

Andrews MM, Boyle JS: *Transcultural concepts in nursing care,* Philadelphia, 1995, Lippincott.

Appling SE: Sleep: linking research to improved outcomes, *Medsurg Nurs* 6(3):159, 1997.

Beck-Little R, Weinrich SP: Assessment and management of sleep disorders in the elderly, *J Gerontol Nurs,* 24(4):14, 1998.

Berman TM and others: Sleep disorders: take them seriously, *Patient Care* 24:85, 1990.

Bliwise DL: Sleep in normal aging and dementia, *Sleep* 16(1):40, 1993.

Bobak IM, Lowdermilk DL, Jensen MD: *Maternity nursing,* ed 4, St. Louis, 1995, Mosby.

Born J, Muth S, Fehm HL: The significance of sleep onset and slow wave sleep for nocturnal release of growth hormone (GH) and cortisol, *Psychoneuroendocrinology* 13:233, 1988.

Breslau N and others: Daytime sleepiness: an epidemiological study of young adults, *Am J Public Health* 87(10):1649, 1997.

Carskadon MA: Patterns of sleep and sleepiness in adolescents, *Pediatrician* 17:5, 1990.

Carskadon MA: Measuring daytime sleepiness. In Kryger MH, Roth T, Dement WC, editors: *Principles and practice of sleep medicine,* ed 2, Philadelphia, 1994, WB Saunders.

Closs SJ: Assessment of sleep in hospital patients: a review of methods, *J Adv Nurs* 13:501, 1988.

Closs SJ: Post-operative patient's views of sleep, pain and recovery, *J Clin Nurs* 1(2):83, 1992.

Cohen FL, Nehring WM, Cloninger L: Symptom description and management in narcolepsy, *Holist Nurs Pract* 10(4):44, 1996.

Coren S: Daylight savings time and traffic accidents, *N Engl J Med,* 334(14):924, 1996.

Dahl RE, Carskadon MA: Sleep and its disorders in adolescence. In Ferber E, Kryger M, editors: *Principles and practice of sleep medicine in the child,* Philadelphia, 1995, WB Saunders.

Evans BD, Rogers AE: 24-hour sleep/wake patterns in healthy elderly persons, *Appl Nurs Res* 7(2):75, 1994.

Evans JC, French DG: Sleep and healing in intensive care settings, *Dimen Crit Care Nurs* 14(4):189, 1995.

Ferber R: Assessment of sleep disorders in the child. In Ferber R, Kryger M, editors: *Principles and practice of sleep medicine in the child,* Philadelphia, 1995, WB Saunders.

Foreman MD, Wykle M: Nursing standard-of-practice protocol: sleep disturbances in elderly patients, *Geriatr Nurs* 16(3):238, 1995.

Gillis AM, Flemons WW: Cardiac arrhythmias during sleep. In Kryger MH, Roth T, Dement WC, editors: *Principles and practice of sleep medicine,* ed 2, Philadelphia, 1994, WB Saunders.

Gislason R and others: Snoring, hypertension and the sleep apnea syndrome: an epidemiologic survey of middle-aged women, *Chest* 103(4):1147, 1993.

Gold DR and others: Rotating shift work, sleep, and accidents related to sleepiness in hospital nurses, *Am J Public Health* 82(7):1011, 1992.

Guilleminault C: Clinical features and evaluation of obstructive apnea. In Kryger MH, Roth T, Dement WC, editors, *Principles and practice of sleep medicine,* ed 2, Philadelphia, 1994, WB Saunders.

Guyton AC, Hall JE: *Human physiology and mechanisms of disease,* ed 6, Philadelphia, 1997, WB Saunders.

Hauri P, Linde S: *No more sleepless nights,* New York, 1990, Wiley.

Hilton A: The hospital racket: how noisy is your unit? *Am J Nurs* 87:59, 1987.

Hoch C, Reynolds C III: Sleep disturbances and what to do about them, *Geriatr Nurs* 7:24, 1986.

Hodgson LA: Why do we need sleep: relating theory to nursing practice, *J Adv Nurs* 16:1503, 1991.

Horne JA: Human sleep and tissue restitution: some qualifications and doubts, *Clin Sci* 65:569, 1983.

Horne JA, Ostberg O: A self-assessment questionnaire to determine morningness-eveningness in human circadian rhythms, *Int J Chronobiol* 4:97, 1976.

Hyman RB and others: The effects of relaxation training on clinical symptoms: a meta-analysis, *Nurs Res* 38:216, 1989.

Irwin M and others: Partial night sleep deprivation reduces natural killer and cellular immune responses, *FASEB J* 10(5):643, 1996.

Johnson EO and others: Epidemiology of alcohol and medication as aids to sleep in early adulthood, *Sleep* 21(2):178, 1998.

Karni A and others: Dependence on REM sleep of overnight improvement of a perceptual skill, *Science* 265:679, 1994.

Kattwinkel J, Brooks J, Myerberg D: Positioning and SIDS: American Academy of Pediatrics task force on infant positioning and SIDS, *Pediatrics* 89:1120, 1992.

Kim MJ, McFarland GK, McLane AM: *Pocket guide to nursing diagnosis,* ed 7, St. Louis, 1997, Mosby.

Landis CA: Arrhythmias and sleep pattern disturbances in cardiac patients, *Prog Cardiovasc Nurs* 3:73, 1988.

Leger D: The cost of sleep-related accidents: a report for the National Commission on Sleep Disorders Research, *Sleep* 17(1):84, 1994.

Leigh TJ and others: Factor analysis of the St. Mary's Hospital Sleep Questionnaire, Sleep 11(5):448, 1988.

Leininger M: *Transcultural nursing: concepts, theories, research and practice,* ed 2, New York, 1995, McGraw-Hill.

Lozoff B: Culture and family: influences on childhood sleep practices and problems. In Ferber R, Kryger M, editors: *Principles and practice of sleep medicine in the child,* Philadelphia, 1995, WB Saunders.

Mahon NE: The contributions of sleep to perceived health status during adolescence, *Pub Health Nurs* 12(2):127, 1995.

McCance KL, Huether SE: *Pathophysiology: the biologic basis for disease in adults and children,* ed 3, St. Louis, 1998, Mosby.

McCloskey JC, Bulechek GM, editors: *Nursing interventions classification (NIC),* ed 3, St. Louis, 2000, Mosby.

McKenry LM, Salerno E: *Mosby's pharmacology in nursing,* ed 20, St. Louis, 1998, Mosby.

Mitler MM and others: Narcolepsy, *J Clin Neurophysiol* 7(1):93, 1990.

Mornhinweg GC, Voignier RR: Rest, *Holist Nurs Pract* 10(4):54, 1996.

National Commission on Sleep Disorders Research: *Wake up America: a national sleep alert,* vol 3, Washington, DC, 1993, U.S. Government Printing Office.

National Sleep Foundation: *Facts about drowsy driving,* http://www.sleepfoundation.org/activities/daafacts.html, 1998a.

National Sleep Foundation: *The nature of sleep,* http://www.sleepfoundation.org/publications/nos.html, 1998b.

Naylor MW, Aldrich MS: Approach to the patient with disordered sleep. In Kryger MH, Roth T, Dement WC, editors: *Principles and practice of sleep medicine,* ed 2, Philadelphia, 1994, WB Saunders.

Nicholson AN, Bradley CM, Pascoe PA: Medications: effect on sleep and wakefulness. In Kryger MH, Roth T, Dement WC, editors: *Principles and practice of sleep medicine,* ed 2, Philadelphia, 1994, WB Saunders.

Orr WC: Gastrointestinal physiology. In Kryger MH, Roth T, Dement WC, editors: *Principles and practice of sleep medicine,* ed 2, Philadelphia, 1994, WB Saunders.

Oswald I: Good, poor, and disordered sleep. In Priest RG, editor: *Sleep: an international monograph,* London, 1984, Update Books.

Pakola SJ, Dinges, DF, Pack AI: Driving and sleepiness: review of regulations and guidelines for commercial and noncommercial drivers with sleep apnea and narcolepsy, *Sleep* 18(9):787, 1995.

Parkinson D: Strategies for helping parents: overcoming sleep problems in babies and toddlers, *Prof Care Mother Child* 4:215, 1994.

Pilcher JJ, Huffcutt AI: Effects of sleep deprivation on performance: a meta-analysis, *Sleep* 19(4):318, 1996.

Renaud MT: Neonatal sleep patterns: implications for nursing, *Holist Nurs Pract* 10(4):27, 1996.

Reynolds CF and others: REM sleep in successful, usual, and pathological aging: the Pittsburgh experience 1980-1993, *J Sleep Res* 2:203, 1993.

Richards KC: Sleep promotion, *Crit Care Nurs Clin North Am* 8(1):39, 1996.

Richards KC, Barnsfather L: A description of night sleep patterns in the critical care unit, *Heart Lung* 18(1):35, 1988.

Richardson SJ: A comparison of tools for assessment of sleep pattern disturbance in critically ill adults, *Dimens Crit Care Nurs* 16(5):226, 1997.

Rogers AE: Nursing management of sleep disorders. I. Assessment, *ANNA J* 24(6):666, 1997a.

Rogers AE: Nursing management of sleep disorders. II. Behavioral interventions, *ANNA J* 24(6):672, 1997b.

Rosenthal L and others: The sleep/wake habits of patients diagnosed as having obstructive sleep apnea, *Chest* 111:1494, 1997.

Simpson T, Lee ER, Cameron C: Patients' perceptions of environmental factors that disturb sleep after cardiac surgery, *Am J Crit Care* 5(3):173, 1996.

Sleep Research Society: *Brain mechanisms of sleep and wakefulness: basics of sleep behavior,* Rochester, Minn, 1993, UCLA & Sleep Research Society.

Sun ER and others: Iron and the restless leg syndrome, *Sleep* 21(4):371, 1998.

Thelan LA and others: *Critical care nursing: diagnoses and management,* ed 3, St. Louis, 1998, Mosby.

Thorpy M: Classification of sleep disorders. In Chokroverty S, editor: *Sleep disorders medicine: basic science, technical considerations and clinical aspects,* Boston, 1994, Butterworth-Heineman.

Topf M, Bookman M, Arand D: Effects of critical care noise on the subjective quality of sleep, *J Adv Nurs* 24:545, 1996.

Trevor AJ, Way WL: Sedative-hypnotic drugs. In Katzung BG, editor: *Basic and clinical pharmacology,* ed 6, Norwalk, Conn, 1995, Appleton & Lange.

Walsh JK, Hartman PG, Kowall JP: Insomnia. In Chokroverty S, editor: *Sleep disorders medicine: basic science, technical considerations and clinical aspects,* Boston, 1994, Butterworth-Heineman.

Webster RA, Thompson DR: Sleep in hospital, *J Adv Nurs* 11:447, 1986.

White DP: Central sleep apnea. In Kryger MH, Roth T, Dement WC, editors: *Principles and practice of sleep medicine,* ed 2, Philadelphia, 1994, WB Saunders.

Wong DL: Whaley and Wong's nursing care of infants and children, ed 6, St. Louis, 1998, Mosby.

Wood AM: A review of literature relating to sleep in hospitals with emphasis on the sleep of the ICU patient, *Inten Crit Care Nurs* 9:129, 1992.

Zarcone VP: Sleep hygiene. In Kryger MH, Roth T, Dement WC, editors: *Principles and practice of sleep medicine,* ed 2, Philadelphia, 1994, WB Saunders.

Zorick F: Insomnia. In Kryger MH, Roth T, Dement WC, editors: *Principles and practice of sleep medicine,* ed 2, Philadelphia, 1994, WB Saunders.

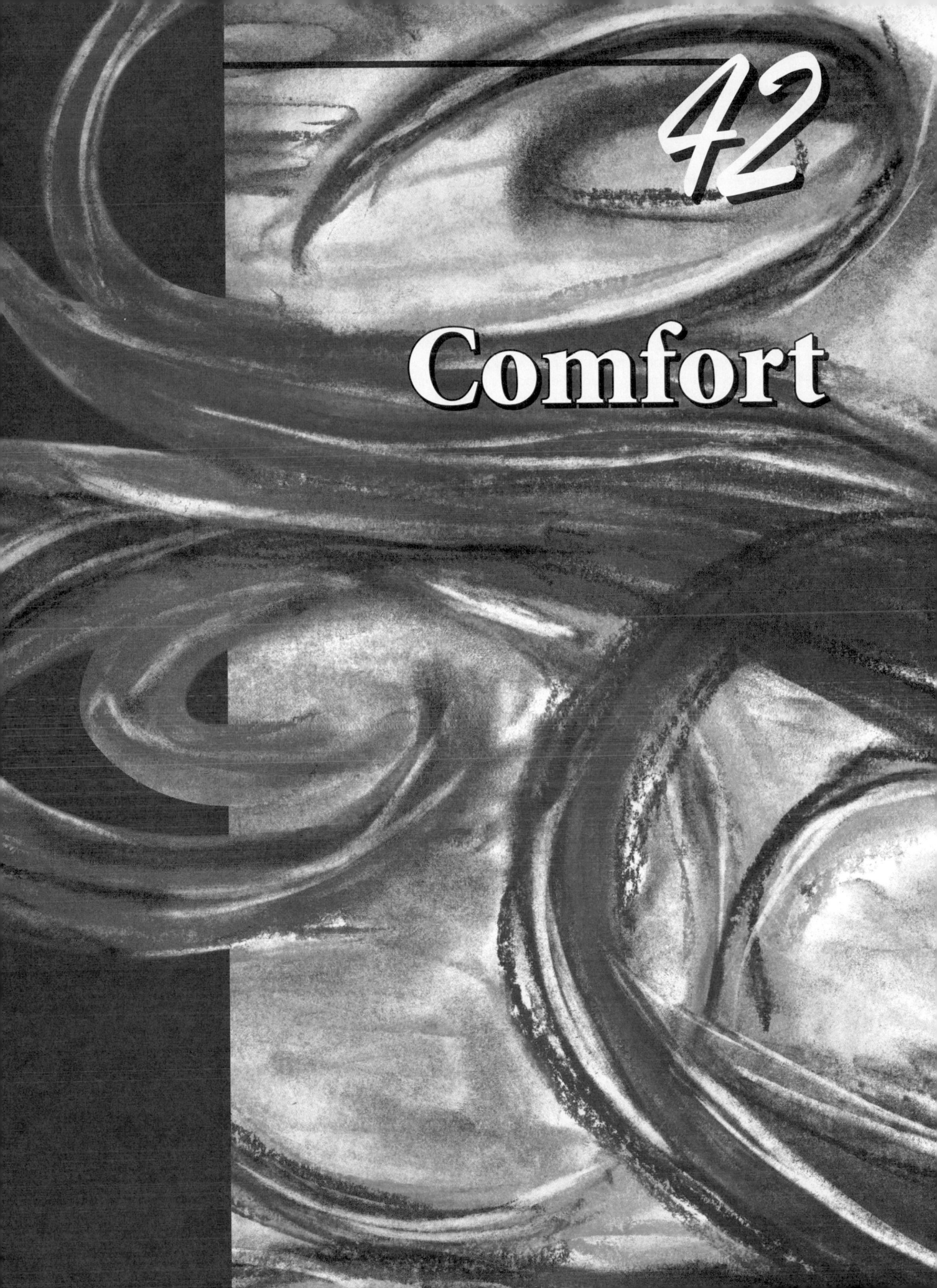

42

Comfort

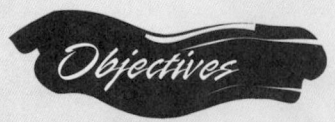

Mastery of content in this chapter will enable the student to:

- Define the key terms listed.
- Discuss common misconceptions about pain.
- Describe the physiology of pain.
- Identify components of the pain experience.
- Explain how the physiology of pain relates to selecting interventions for pain relief.
- Describe the components of pain assessment.
- Perform an assessment of a client experiencing pain.
- Explain how cultural factors influence the pain experience.
- Describe the appropriate nursing diagnoses, outcomes, and interventions for a client with pain.
- Describe guidelines for selecting and individualizing pain interventions.
- Explain the various pharmacological approaches to treating pain.
- Describe applications for use of nonpharmacological pain interventions.
- Discuss nursing implications for administering analgesics.
- Evaluate a client's response to pain interventions.

Everyone has experienced some type or degree of pain. It is the most common reason why people seek health care. Despite being one of the most commonly occurring symptoms in the medical world, pain is one of the least understood. A person in pain feels distress or suffering and seeks relief. The nurse uses a variety of interventions to bring relief or to restore comfort. However, the nurse cannot see or feel the client's pain. Pain is subjective; no two persons experience pain in the same way, and no two painful events create identical responses or feelings in a person. The International Association for the Study of Pain (IASP, 1979) defined pain as "an unpleasant, subjective sensory and emotional experience associated with actual or potential tissue damage, or described in terms of such damage." Pain can be a major factor inhibiting the ability and willingness to recover from illness.

Nurses care for clients in many settings and situations in which interventions are provided to promote comfort. Comfort is a concept central to the art of nursing. As Donahue (1989) summarized, "Through comfort and comfort measures . . . nurses provide strength, hope, solace, support, encouragement, and assistance." A variety of nursing theorists refer to comfort as a basic client need for which nursing care is delivered.

The concept of comfort is as subjective as that of pain. Each individual has physiological, social, spiritual, psychological, and cultural characteristics that influence how comfort is interpreted and experienced. Kolcaba (1992) defined comfort in a manner consistent with clients' subjective experiences. She defines comfort as the state of having met basic human needs for ease (contentment that

promotes routine performance), relief (need being met), and transcendence (state in which one rises above problems or pain).

The context of comfort is the umbrella under which pain and pain management options are viewed. Since the experience of pain is dynamic, the nurse has a responsibility to understand the pain experience. The nurse, client, family, and members of the health care team must collaborate to find the most effective approach to pain control. According to McCaffery (1979), "Pain is whatever the experiencing person says it is, existing whenever he says it does." Nurses are ethically responsible for managing pain and relieving suffering. Effective pain management not only reduces physical discomfort, but also promotes earlier mobilization and return to work, fewer clinic visits, shortened hospital stays, and reduced health care costs.

Scientific Knowledge Base

Recorded history allows us to see that pain has been an integral component of the human experience. By viewing pain as a punishment for wrongdoing, as a tribulation, or as a warning of physical ills, we have sought to explain what is the thing that we call pain. In the latter part of this century there has been renewed interest in researching pain. In this chapter the current knowledge of the nature of pain and its management is explored.

NATURE OF PAIN

Pain is much more than a single sensation caused by a specific stimulus. Pain is subjective and highly individualized.

The stimulus for pain can be physical and/or mental in nature, whereby damage may be to actual tissues or to a person's ego (Mahon, 1994). Pain is tiring and demands a person's energy. It can interfere with personal relationships and influence the meaning of life. Pain cannot be objectively measured, such as with an x-ray film or blood test. Although certain types of pain create predictable signs and symptoms, often the nurse can only assess pain by relying on the client's words and behavior. Only the client knows whether pain is present and what the experience is like. It is not the responsibility of clients to prove that they are in pain; it is the nurses' responsibility to believe them.

Pain is a protective physiological mechanism. When felt, pain changes how a person behaves. For example, a person with a sprained ankle avoids bearing full weight on the foot to prevent further injury. A client with a history of chest pain learns to stop all activity when pain develops. Careful techniques must be used to assess for injury, such as in the case of a burned hand or a bruised chest wall. Clients who are unable to feel sensations, such as after spinal cord injury or stroke, are unaware of pain-inducing injuries. In these cases the nurse must anticipate what sources of injury the client might have and learn to closely monitor physiological changes, such as in vital signs. Pain is a leading cause of disability. As the average life span increases, more people have chronic disease in which pain is a common symptom.

Nurses care for clients with pain on a daily basis. Therefore just as it is necessary to monitor vital signs so, too, can pain be considered an important routine assessment, along with temperature, pulse, respirations, and blood pressure. In some institutions pain is treated as the fifth vital sign.

PHYSIOLOGY OF PAIN

Pain is often difficult to precisely categorize. However, the literature does speak of three types of pain: acute, chronic (often called chronic nonmalignant or chronic benign), and cancer pain (McCaffery and Pasero, 1999). The pain that nurses most often observe in clients falls into one or some combination of these types. Another way to categorize pain is to speak to the pathophysiology of the pain: nociceptive pain (either somatic or visceral) or neuropathic pain (Table 42-1).

There are four processes of nociceptive pain: transduction, transmission, perception and modulation (McCaffery and Pasero, 1999). A client in pain cannot discriminate among the processes. However, understanding each process helps the nurse recognize factors that can cause

Table 42-1 Classification of Pain by Inferred Pathology

Nociceptive Pain	Neuropathic Pain
I. *Nociceptive pain:* Normal processing of stimuli that damages normal tissues or has the potential to do so if prolonged; usually responsive to nonopioids and/or opioids.	II. *Neuropathic pain:* Abnormal processing of sensory input by the peripheral or central nervous system; treatment usually includes adjuvant analgesics.
A. Somatic pain. Arises from bone, joint, muscle, skin, or connective tissue. It is usually aching or throbbing in quality and is well localized.	A. Centrally generated pain 1. Deafferentation pain. Injury to either the peripheral or central nervous system. *Examples:* Phantom pain may reflect injury to the peripheral nervous system; burning pain below the level of a spinal cord lesion reflects injury to the central nervous system.

B. Visceral pain: Arises from visceral organs, such as the gastrointestinal tract and pancreas. This may be subdivided:
    1. Tumor involvement of the organ capsule that causes aching and fairly well localized pain.
    2. Obstruction of hollow viscus, which causes intermittent cramping and poorly localized pain.
	2. Sympathetically maintained pain. Associated with dysregulation of the autonomic nervous system. *Examples:* May include some of the pain associated with reflex sympathetic dystrophy/causalgia (complex regional pain syndrome, type I, type II).
	  B. Peripherally generated pain
	    1. Painful polyneuropathies. Pain is felt along the distribution of many peripheral nerves. *Examples:* diabetic neuropathy, alcohol-nutritional neuropathy, and those associated with Guillain-Barré syndrome.
	    2. Painful mononeuropathies. Usually associated with a known peripheral nerve injury, and pain is felt at least partly along the distribution of the damaged nerve. *Examples:* Nerve root compression, nerve entrapment, trigeminal neuralgia.

Modified from McCaffery M, Pasero C: *Pain: clinical manual,* ed 2, St. Louis, 1999, Mosby; data from Max MB, Portenoy RK: Methodological challenges for clinical trials of cancer pain treatments. In Chapman CR, Foley KM, editors: *Current and emerging issues in cancer pain: research and practice,* New York, 1993, Raven Press; and Portenoy RK: Neuropathic pain. In Portenoy RK, Kanner RM, editors: *Pain management: theory and practice,* Philadelphia, 1996, FA Davis.

pain, symptoms that accompany pain, and the rationale and actions of select therapies.

Transduction begins in the periphery when a pain-producing stimulus sends an impulse across a peripheral nerve fiber. The pain fiber enters the spinal cord and travels one of several routes until ending within the gray matter of the spinal cord. There the pain message either interacts with inhibitory nerve cells, preventing the pain stimulus from reaching the brain, or is transmitted uninhibited through the thalamus to the cerebral cortex. Once a pain stimulus reaches the cerebral cortex, the brain interprets the quality of the pain and processes information from past experience, knowledge, and cultural associations in the perception of the pain, causing a physical or behavioral response from the client (Salerno and Willens, 1996).

All cellular damage caused by thermal, mechanical, or chemical stimuli results in the release of pain-producing substances (Table 42-2). When there is an exposure to hot or cold, pressure, or friction, there is a release of **neurotransmitter** substances such as bradykinin, potassium, serotonin, histamine, and substance P. These pain-producing substances surround the pain fibers in the extracellular fluid, creating the spread of the pain message and causing an inflammatory response (Paice, 1994).

Nerve impulses resulting from the painful stimulus travel along afferent peripheral nerve fibers. Two types of peripheral nerve fibers conduct painful stimuli: the fast, myelinated A-delta fibers and the very small, slow, unmyelinated C fibers. The A fibers send sharp, localized, and distinct sensations that localize the source of the pain and detect its intensity. The C fibers relay impulses that are poorly localized, burning, and persistent (McCance and Heuther, 1998). For example, after stepping on a nail, a person initially feels a sharp, localized pain, which is a result of A-fiber transmission. Within a few seconds, the pain becomes more diffuse and widespread, until the whole foot aches because of C-fiber innervation. The C fibers remain exposed to the chemicals released when cells are damaged.

When A-delta and C fibers transmit impulses from peripheral nerve fibers, biochemical mediators that activate or sensitize the pain response are released. For example, potassium and **prostaglandins** are released when local cells are damaged. Transmission of the pain stimulus continues along the afferent nerve fibers until they end in the dorsal horn of the spinal cord. Within the dorsal horn, neurotransmitters such as substance P are released, causing a synaptic transmission from the afferent (sensory) peripheral nerve to spinothalamic tract nerves (Paice, 1991) (Figure 42-1). This allows the pain impulse to be transmitted further within the central nervous system. Pain stimuli continue to travel through nerve fibers in the spinothalamic tracts that cross to the opposite side of the spinal cord. Pain impulses then travel up the spinal cord. Figure 42-2 shows the normal pain reception pathway. After the pain impulse ascends the spinal cord, information is transmitted quickly to higher centers in the brain, including the reticular formation, limbic system, thalamus, and somatosensory and association cortex.

A protective reflex response also occurs with pain reception (Figure 42-3). A-delta fibers send sensory impulses to the spinal cord, where they synapse with spinal

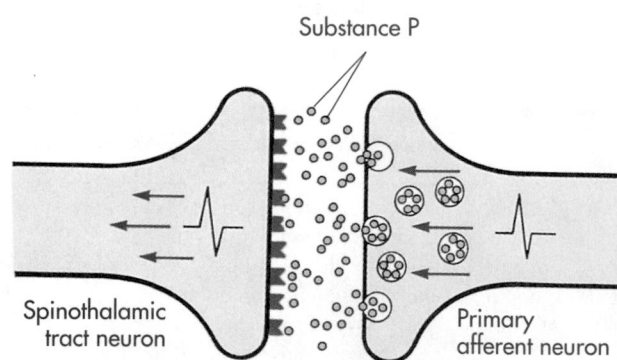

Figure 42-1 Substance P and other neurotransmitters are released from primary afferent fibers that terminate in the dorsal horn of the spinal cord.
From Paice JA: Unraveling the mystery of pain, *Oncol Nurs Forum* 18(5):843, 1991.

Table 42-2 Examples of Physical Sources of Pain

Type of Stimulus	Source	Pathophysiological Process
Mechanical	Alteration in body fluids	Edema distending body tissues
	Duct distention	Overstretching of duct's narrow lumen (e.g., passage of kidney stone through ureter)
Biological	Space-occupying lesion (tumor)	Irritation of peripheral nerves by growth of lesion within confined space
Chemical	Perforated visceral organ	Chemical irritation by secretions on sensitive nerve endings (e.g., ruptured appendix, duodenal ulcer)
Thermal	Burn (heat or extreme cold)	Inflammation or loss of superficial layers of epidermis, causing increased sensitivity of nerve endings
Physical	Burn	Skin layers burned with muscle and subcutaneous tissue injury, causing injury to nerve endings

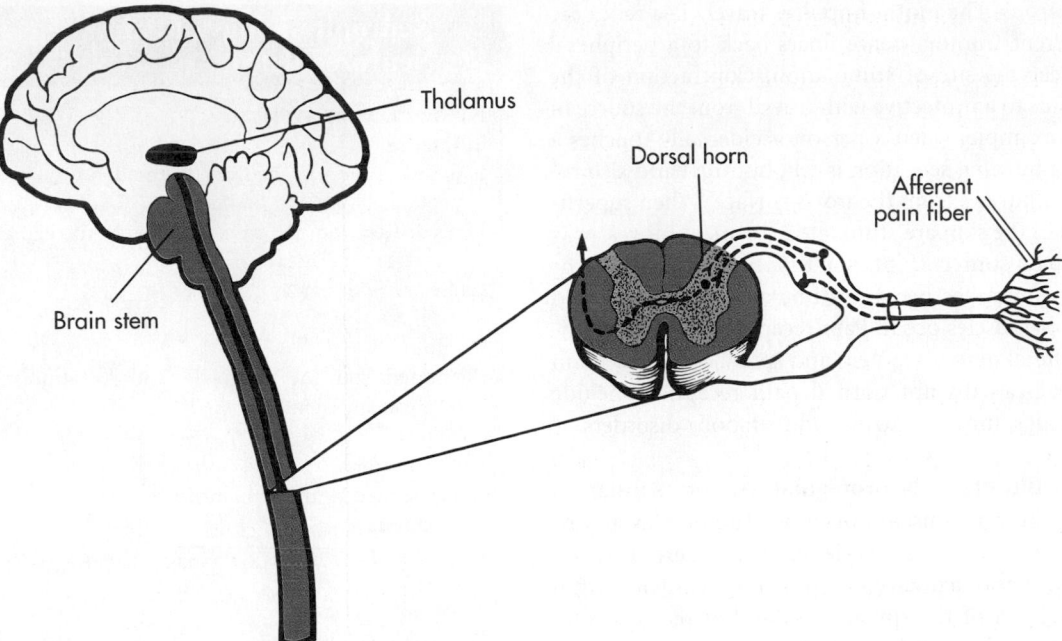

Figure 42-2 Pain reception pathway. Pain is transmitted from primary afferent fibers to the dorsal horn of the spinal cord. The fibers synapse with spinothalamic tract neurons, which cross over and then ascend the spinal cord to the thalamus.

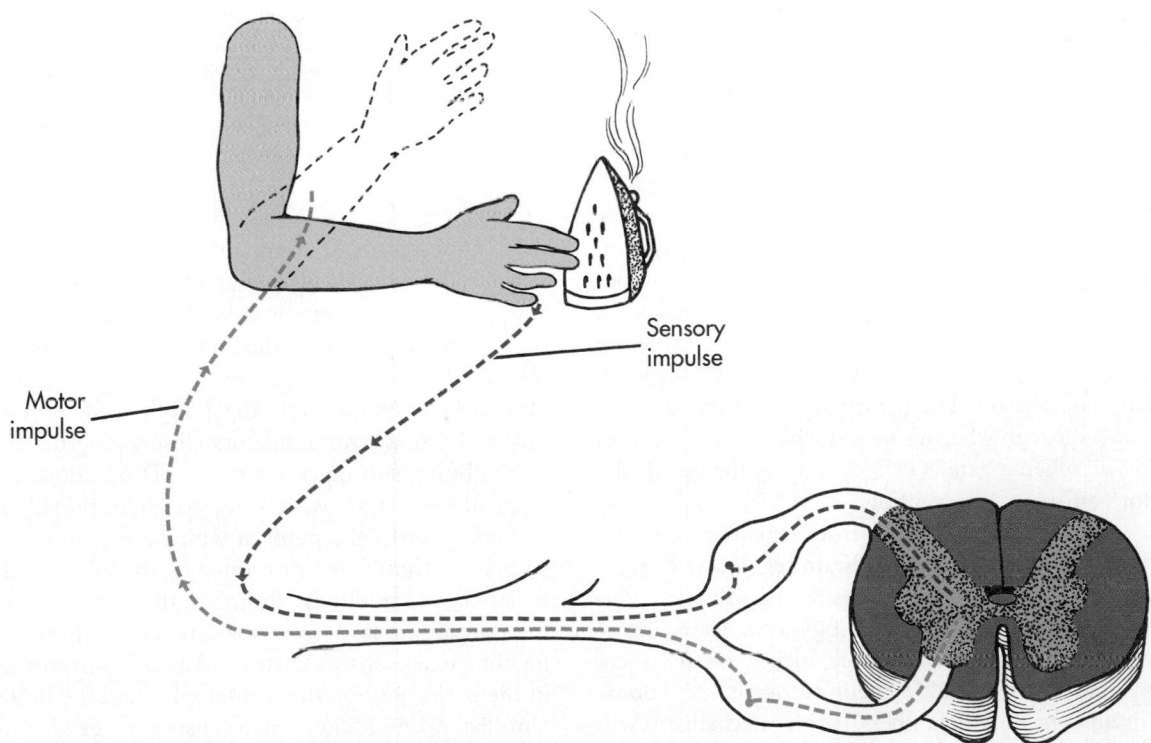

Figure 42-3 Protective reflex to pain stimulus.

motor neurons. The motor impulses travel via a reflex arc along efferent (motor) nerve fibers back to a peripheral muscle near the site of stimulation. Contraction of the muscle leads to a protective withdrawal from the source of pain. For example, when a person accidentally touches a hot iron, a burning sensation is felt, but the hand also reflexively withdraws from the iron's surface. When superficial fibers in the skin are stimulated, a person moves away from the pain source. If internal tissues such as muscle or mucous membranes become stimulated, tightening and guarding of muscles occur. Pain reception requires an intact peripheral nervous system and spinal cord. Common factors that can disrupt normal pain reception include trauma, drugs, tumor growth, and metabolic disorders.

Neuroregulators.

Neuroregulators, or substances that affect the **transmission** of nerve stimuli, play an important role in the pain experience. These substances are found at the site of a **nociceptor**, at nerve terminals within the dorsal horn of the spinal cord, and at receptor sites within the spinothalamic tract. Neuroregulators are divided into two groups: neurotransmitters and neuromodulators (Box 42-1). Neurotransmitters such as substance P send electrical impulses across the synaptic cleft between two nerve fibers. They are excitatory or inhibitory. Neuromodulators modify neuron activity and adjust or vary the transmission of pain stimuli, without directly transferring a nerve signal through a synapse. They are believed to act indirectly by increasing and decreasing the effects of particular neurotransmitters. Endorphins are an example of a neuromodulator. Pharmacological therapy for pain is largely based on the influence that select medications have on neuroregulators.

Gate-Control Theory of Pain.

Researchers know that there is no specific pain center in the nervous system. Melzack and Wall's gate-control theory (1965) suggests that pain impulses can be regulated or even blocked by gating mechanisms along the central nervous system. Gating mechanisms can be found in substantia gelatinosa cells within the dorsal horn of the spinal cord, thalamus, and limbic system. By understanding what can influence these gates, nurses can gain a useful conceptual framework for pain management. The theory suggests that pain impulses pass through when a gate is open and that impulses are blocked when a gate is closed. Closing the gate is the basis for pain-relief interventions.

A balance of activity from sensory neurons and descending control fibers from the brain regulate the gating process. The A-delta and C neurons release substance P to transmit impulses through the gating mechanisms. In addition, there are mechanoreceptor, thicker, faster A-beta neurons that release inhibiting neurotransmitters. If dominant input is from A-beta fibers, gating mechanisms will close. It is believed that this action can be seen when a nurse gives a gentle back rub. The massage stimulates

---

Neurophysiology of Pain: Neuroregulators   Box 42-1

NEUROTRANSMITTERS

Substance P
Is found in the pain neurons of the dorsal horn (excitatory peptide)
Is needed to transmit pain impulses from the periphery to higher brain centers
Causes vasodilation and edema

Serotonin
Is released from the brain stem and dorsal horn to inhibit pain transmission

Prostaglandins
Are generated from the breakdown of phospholipids in cell membranes
Are believed to increase sensitivity to pain

NEUROMODULATORS

Endorphins and Dynorphins
Are the body's natural supply of morphine-like substances
Are activated by stress and pain
Are located within the brain, spinal cord, and gastrointestinal tract
Cause analgesia when they attach to opiate receptors in the brain
Are present in higher levels in people who have less pain than others with a similar injury

Bradykinin
Is released from plasma that leaks from surrounding blood vessels at the site of tissue injury
Binds to receptors on peripheral nerves, increasing pain stimuli
Binds to cells that cause the chain reaction producing prostaglandins

---

mechanoreceptors. If dominant input is from A-delta and C fibers, the gates likely open and the client perceives pain. Even if pain impulses flow to the brain, there may be higher cortical centers in the brain to modify pain perception. Descending neural pathways release endogenous opiates such as endorphins, the body's own natural pain killers. These neuromodulators close gating mechanisms by inhibiting substance P's release. Distraction, counseling, and exercise are ways to release endorphins.

Perception is the point at which a person is aware of pain. Pain stimuli are transmitted up the spinal cord to the thalamus and midbrain. From the thalamus, fibers transmit the pain message to various areas of the brain, including the somatosensory cortex and association cortex (both in the parietal lobe), the frontal lobe, and the limbic system (Paice, 1991). The somatosensory cortex identifies the location and intensity of pain, and the association cortex determines how we feel about the pain. There are cells within the limbic system that are believed to control emotion, particularly anxiety. Thus the limbic system may play an active role in processing the emotional reaction to pain. After nerve transmission ends within the higher brain centers, a person perceives the sensation of pain.

As a person becomes aware of pain, a complex reaction unfolds. Psychological and cognitive factors interact with neurophysiological ones in the perception of pain. Perception gives awareness and meaning to pain so that a person can then react. The reaction to pain is the physiological and behavioral responses that occur after pain is perceived.

Physiological Responses.

As pain impulses ascend the spinal cord toward the brain stem and thalamus, the autonomic nervous system becomes stimulated as part of the stress response. Pain of low to moderate intensity and superficial pain elicit the fight-or-flight reaction of the general adaptation syndrome (see Chapter 30). Stimulation of the sympathetic branch of the autonomic nervous system results in physiological responses (Table 42-3). If the pain is continuous, severe, or deep, typically involving the visceral organs (e.g., with a myocardial infarction or colic from gallbladder or renal stones), the parasympathetic nervous system goes into action. Sustained physiological responses to pain could cause serious harm to an individual. Except in cases of severe traumatic pain, which may send a person into shock, most people reach a level of adaptation in which physical signs return to normal. Thus a client in pain will not always have physical signs.

Behavioral Responses.

Once pain is experienced, there begins a cycle of events that if left untreated or unrelieved can significantly alter the quality of a person's life. Mahon (1994) notes that pain can have a dominating nature, interfering with the ability to relate and care for oneself. This component of pain reaction helps to explain why the management of pain can be such a challenge.

Pain threatens physical and psychological well-being. Clients may choose not to express pain if they believe such expression would inconvenience others or signal loss of self-control. Some clients will endure severe pain without assistance. Often a nurse must encourage such a client to accept pain-relieving measures so that activity or nutritional intake is not seriously curtailed. In contrast, other clients may seek relief before pain even occurs. For example, a client may request an aspirin in anticipation of a headache. The client's ability to tolerate pain significantly influences the nurse's perceptions of the degree of the discomfort. Often the nurse is more willing to attend to the client whose endurance of pain seems high.

Typical body movements and facial expressions that indicate pain include clenching the teeth, holding the painful part, bent posture, and grimaces. A client may cry or moan, be restless, or make frequent requests of the nurse. The nurse soon learns to recognize patterns of behavior that reflect pain. However, lack of pain expression, as in the case of a confused client, does not necessarily mean that the client is not experiencing pain (McCaffery and Pasero, 1999). The nurse needs to help the client communicate the pain response effectively.

Along with transmission of pain stimuli, the body is able

Table 42-3 Physiological Reactions to Pain

Response	Cause or Effect
Sympathetic Stimulation*	
Dilation of bronchial tubes and increased respiratory rate	Provides increased oxygen intake
Increased heart rate	Provides increased oxygen transport
Peripheral vasoconstriction (pallor, elevation in blood pressure)	Elevates blood pressure with shift of blood supply from periphery and viscera to skeletal muscles and brain
Increased blood glucose level	Provides additional energy
Diaphoresis	Controls body temperature during stress
Increased muscle tension	Prepares muscles for action
Dilation of pupils	Affords better vision
Decreased gastrointestinal motility	Frees energy for more immediate activity
Parasympathetic Stimulation†	
Pallor	Causes blood supply to shift away from periphery
Muscle tension	Results from fatigue
Decreased heart rate and blood pressure	Results from vagal stimulation
Rapid, irregular breathing	Causes body defenses to fail under prolonged stress of pain
Nausea and vomiting	Causes return of gastrointestinal function
Weakness or exhaustion	Results from expenditure of physical energy

*Pain of low to moderate intensity and superficial pain.
†Severe or deep pain.

to adjust or vary pain perception. There are nerve fibers in the spinothalamic tract that end in the midbrain, stimulating regions to send stimuli back down to the dorsal horn of the spinal cord (Paice, 1991). These fibers are called the descending pain system, which acts by releasing neuroregulators that inhibit transmission of painful stimuli.

The process of inhibiting or changing pain impulses is called **modulation,** the final processes in nociception. During modulation, neurons that originate in the brain stem descend to the dorsal horn of the spinal cord. These neurons release substances such as serotonin, norepinephrine, and endogenous opiates (endorphins and enkephalins) that work to inhibit the transmission of pain and help produce an analgesic effect (McCaffery and Pasero, 1999).

Stress, excessive exercise, and other factors increase the release of endorphins, raising an individual's pain threshold (McCance and Huether, 1998). Because the amount of circulating substances vary with every individual, the response to pain will be different. For example, an individual in an automobile accident may help rescue passengers, getting them to safety before realizing he has a fracture of the forearm.

TYPES OF PAIN
Acute Pain.
Everyone experiences some level of pain throughout the day. Common examples include the ache of overexercised muscles, the burning discomfort from eye strain, and pressure from sitting in one position for too long. These minor discomforts rarely cause a person to seek health care. However, some episodes of acute, chronic, and cancer pain can be distressing to a client, causing the client to seek health care. **Acute pain** follows acute injury, disease, or surgical intervention and has a rapid onset, varying in intensity (mild to severe) and lasting for a brief time, usually less than 6 months (National Institutes of Health [NIH], 1986). It eventually resolves with or without treatment after a damaged area heals.

The fact that acute pain has a predictable ending (healing) and an identifiable cause usually results in a willingness by health team members to treat acute pain aggressively. However, conflict between nurse and client may arise if the nurse does not provide quick relief.

Acute pain seriously threatens a client's recovery and should be one of the priorities in the client's care. For example, acute postoperative pain hampers the client's ability to become active and increases the risk of complications from immobility (see Chapter 36). Rehabilitation may be delayed and hospitalization may be prolonged if acute pain is not controlled. There cannot be physical or psychological progress as long as acute pain persists, because the client focuses all interests on pain relief. The nurse's efforts at teaching and motivating the client toward self-care will often be useless. After pain is relieved, the client and health care team can direct full attention toward recovery.

Chronic Pain.
There are many labels given to pain that is prolonged, varies in intensity, and lasts longer than 6 months. The terms *chronic, chronic nonmalignant,* and *chronic benign* are all found in the literature. Examples of **chronic nonmalignant pain** include arthritis, low back pain, myofascial pain, headache, and peripheral neuropathy (McCaffery and Pasero, 1999). These pains are due to non-life-threatening causes, and frequently the cause is unknown. An injured area may have healed long ago, yet the pain is ongoing and may not respond to treatment.

Health care workers are usually less willing to treat chronic nonmalignant pain as aggressively as acute pain. The unpredictability of chronic nonmalignant pain frustrates the client, frequently leading to psychological depression. Chronic nonmalignant pain is a major cause of psychological and physical disability, leading to problems such as loss of a job, inability to perform simple daily activities, sexual dysfunction, and social isolation from family and friends.

The person with chronic nonmalignant pain often does not show overt symptoms and does not adapt to the pain; rather, the person seems to suffer more with time because of physical and mental exhaustion. Chronic nonmalignant pain creates the insecurity of never knowing how one will feel from day to day. Symptoms of chronic pain include fatigue, insomnia, anorexia, weight loss, depression, hopelessness, and anger.

The life of a person with chronic nonmalignant pain can be tragic. Often the person consults many physicians and therefore accumulates various medications and interventions. However, taking several medications may result in undesirable side effects. Physicians and other health care providers in multidisciplinary pain clinics can offer interventions in addition to pharmacological remedies, such as exercise and biofeedback, that assist in chronic pain management.

Caring for the client with chronic nonmalignant pain can be challenging. The nurse should not become frustrated when relief measures fail. Likewise, the nurse should not offer false hope for a cure.

Cancer Pain.
Cancer pain is pain that may be due to tumor progression and its related pathology, invasive procedures, toxicities of treatment, infection, and physical limitation (Foley, 1979). Not all clients with cancer will experience pain. But for those who do, the Agency for Health Care Policy and Research (AHCPR) reports that up to 90% can have their pain managed with relatively simple means (Jacox and others, 1994).

Cancer pain can be chronic and/or acute; nociceptive and/or neuropathic. It can be at the actual site of the tumor or distant to the site, which is called referred pain. A new report of pain by a client with existing pain needs to be investigated.

Although the need for treatment of cancer pain has become more visible, the issue of under management continues. In a study conducted in a hospice setting, of those clients with pain, 42% stated they had pain-relief scores of 5 or less on a scale of 1 to 10 (1 being no relief and 10 being complete relief) (McMillan, 1996).

Nursing Knowledge Base

The history of nursing emphasizes the unique role that nurses have in caring for clients. The nurse sees clients in their most vulnerable state and can view the impact that pain has on many aspects of the client's life. It is often the nurse to whom clients confess their dreaded fears about pain and its meaning. The trust given to the nurse by clients is predicated on the assumption that the nurse will view their pain experience in the context of all that is happening in their life and apply the knowledge the nurse had gained to help them manage. In this section factors that influence pain are explored.

KNOWLEDGE, ATTITUDES, AND BELIEFS

Health care personnel often have attitudes regarding clients in pain. Unless clients have objective signs of pain, a nurse may not believe that they are uncomfortable. These attitudes about pain are caused in part by the traditional medical model of illness. This model suggests that physical problems result from physical causes. Thus pain is viewed as a physical response to organic dysfunction. When no obvious source of pain can be found (e.g., the client with chronic low back pain or neuropathies), nurses, as well as physicians, may stereotype pain sufferers as complainers or difficult clients (Box 42-2).

Ryan, Vortherms, and Ward (1994) studied the attitudes of nurses toward management of cancer pain. Their study compared oncology nurses with nurses working in long-term care facilities, where a large number of clients with cancer are eventually cared for. Their study showed a reluctance on the part of nurses from both groups to administer opioids, a reluctance on the part of clients to take opioids, and inadequate staff knowledge of pain management (Mahon, 1994). In a study by Clarke and others (1996), inadequate pain assessment and treatment in clients who report pain was a result of ineffective pain management education.

The extent to which nurses make assumptions about clients in pain seriously limits their ability to offer pain relief. Unfortunately, all people are influenced by biases based on their culture, education, and experience. Too often, nurses allow misconceptions about pain (Box 42-3) to affect their willingness to intervene. Many nurses even avoid acknowledging a client's pain because of their own fear and denial.

To help a client gain comfort or relief, the nurse must view the experience through the client's eyes. Pain is tiring and demands energy from the person experiencing it (Mahon, 1994). It interferes with relationships and the individual's ability to maintain self-care. Acknowledging

Research HIGHLIGHT   Box 42-2

RESEARCH ABSTRACT

Three hundred thirty-nine nursing home residents participated in a study to determine differences in the prescription and administration of analgesics between cognitively impaired residents and residents not described as cognitively impaired. Forty-five percent of the population were labeled as cognitively impaired by either medical diagnosis or meeting criteria using a five-dimension behavioral tool. Fifty-five percent of the residents had a painful diagnosis at the time of the study. Musculoskeletal disorders such as arthritis and osteoporosis were the most common painful conditions. The results show that residents were more likely to have analgesics prescribed if they experienced more acute pain (e.g., diverticulitis, pancreatitis). Cognitively impaired residents had less medication prescribed and administered. Those cognitively impaired residents who were disoriented, withdrawn, or functionally impaired were even less likely to have analgesics administered.

IMPLICATIONS FOR PRACTICE
- Physicians are less likely to prescribe analgesics in the face of chronic pain.
- Physicians are less likely to prescribe analgesics for cognitively impaired older adults.
- Nurses who are responsible for the administration of medication must be aware that cognitively impaired clients with painful conditions need careful assessment to determine the presence of pain.

REFERENCE

Horgas AL, Tpai PF: Analgesic prescription and use in cognitively impaired nursing home residents, *Nurs Res* 47(4):235, 1998.

personal prejudices or misconceptions helps the nurse address the client's problem more professionally. The nurse who becomes an active, knowledgeable observer of a client in pain will make a more objective analysis of the pain experience. The client makes the diagnosis that pain is present, and the nurse works to apply techniques and skills that ultimately give relief.

FACTORS INFLUENCING PAIN

Because pain is complex, numerous factors influence an individual's pain experience. The nurse considers all factors that affect the client in pain. This is necessary to ensure a holistic approach to the assessment and care of the client in pain.

Age.   Age is an important variable that influences pain, particularly in infants and older adults. Developmental differences found among these age-groups can influence how children and older adults react to pain. Young children have difficulty understanding pain and the procedures

Common Biases and Misconceptions About Pain
Box 42-3

The following statements are *false*:

Drug abusers and alcoholics overreact to discomforts.

Clients with minor illnesses have less pain than those with severe physical alteration.

Administering analgesics regularly will lead to drug addiction.

The amount of tissue damage in an injury can accurately indicate pain intensity.

Health care personnel are the best authorities on the nature of a client's pain.

Psychogenic pain is not real.

Chronic pain is psychological.

Clients should expect to have pain in a hospital.

Clients who cannot speak do not feel pain.

nurses administer that may cause pain. Young children who have not developed full vocabularies also have difficulty verbally describing and expressing pain to parents or caregivers. Cognitively, toddlers and preschoolers are unable to recall explanations about pain or associate pain with experiences that can occur in various situations. With these developmental considerations in mind, the nurse must adapt approaches for assessing a child's pain (including what to ask and the behaviors to observe for) and how to prepare a child for a painful medical procedure.

Because an older adult has lived longer, there is a greater likelihood of having developed a pathological condition that may be accompanied by pain, but pain is not an inevitable part of aging. Once an older client suffers pain, there can be serious impairment of functional status. Mobility, activities of daily living, social activities outside the home, and activity tolerance can all be reduced. The presence of pain in an older adult requires aggressive assessment, diagnosis, and management.

The ability of older clients to interpret pain can be complicated by the presence of multiple diseases with vague symptoms that may affect similar parts of the body. When older clients have more than one source of pain, a nurse must make detailed assessments. The manifestations of different diseases can cause an atypical presentation of painful conditions. In other words, different diseases can cause similar symptoms. For example, chest pain does not always indicate a heart attack; it may be a symptom of arthritis of the spine or of an abdominal disorder. Not all older adults experience cognitive impairment. However, when an older adult experience confusion, recalling pain experiences and providing detailed explanations is difficult. It is important to recognize that there are misconceptions about pain management in the very young and in the elderly that need to be addressed before nurses can adequately intervene in a client's pain (Tables 42-4 and 42-5).

Gender.   Generally, men and women do not differ significantly in their responses to pain (Gil, 1990). It is doubtful whether gender alone is a factor in the expression of pain. There are cultural influences on gender (e.g., deeming it appropriate for a little boy to be brave and not cry, whereas a little girl in the same situation is allowed to cry). Pain tolerance has been the subject of research involving men and women. However, tolerance to pain is influenced by biochemical factors and is unique to each individual, regardless of gender. In a review article by Vallerand (1995), it was apparent that health care providers were influenced in their choice of medications by the gender of the client. Nurses need to be cognizant of their own biases when managing pain.

Culture.   Cultural beliefs and values affect how individuals deal with pain. Individuals learn what is expected and accepted by their culture; this includes how to react to pain (Calvillo and Flaskerud, 1991). Health care providers often assume that their ways and beliefs are equal to those of others. Thus they try to presume how clients will respond to pain. There are different meanings and attitudes associated with pain across various cultural groups. An understanding of the cultural meaning of pain helps the nurse to design relevant care for people with pain.

How people express pain is another cultural trait. Some cultures believe it is natural to be demonstrative about pain. Others tend to be more introvertive. In addition, it is also important to know to what extent a member of a particular culture has assimilated into American society. For example, if several generations of a Hispanic client's family have lived in the United States, the influence of the Spanish culture may be limited. In contrast, a client who has just recently come to the United States and who embraces the cultural norms of his or her ethnic group may have very different attitudes than an Anglo-Saxon American.

Knowing that cultural differences exist is not enough in the treatment of pain. Nurses must explore the impact of those differences and include cultural patterns and beliefs into the plan of care (Box 42-4). The nurse, the client, and the family must work together to facilitate communication about the assessment and management of pain. Finding a common assessment tool and communicating that tool to other health care providers is imperative.

Meaning of Pain.   The meaning that a person associates with pain affects the experience of pain and how one adapts to it. This can be closely associated with the person's cultural background. A person will perceive pain differently if it suggests a threat, loss, punishment, or challenge. For example, a woman in labor will perceive pain differently than a woman with a history of cancer who is experiencing a new pain and fearing recurrence. The degree and quality of pain perceived by a client are related to the meaning of pain.

Table 42-4 **Pain in Infants**

Misconception	Correction
Infants are incapable of feeling pain.	Infants have the anatomical and functional requirements for pain processing by mid to late gestation (Anand, 1993).
Infants are less sensitive to pain than older children and adults.	Term neonates have the same sensitivity to pain as older infants and children. Preterm neonates may have a greater sensitivity to pain than term neonates or older children (Anand, 1995).
Infants are incapable of expressing pain.	Although infants cannot verbalize pain, they respond with behavioral cues and physiological indicators that can be observed by others (Anand and Craig, 1996).
Infants must learn about pain from previous painful experiences.	Pain requires no prior experience; it need not be learned from earlier painful experience. Pain is present with the first insult (Anand and Craig, 1996).
Pain cannot be accurately assessed in infants.	Behavioral cues (i.e., facial expressions, cry, body movements) and physiological indicators of pain can be reliably and validly assessed either alone (univariate approach) or in combination (multivariate approach). The most valid univariate approach is facial expression (Craig, 1998). The most valid multivariate approach is through the use of a composite pain measure (Stevens, 1998).
Infants are incapable of remembering pain.	Early exposure to noxious stimuli may have an effect on the infant's future responses to painful events (Grunau, Whitfield, and Petrie, 1994; Grunau and others, 1994; Taddio and others, 1995; Taddio and others, 1997).
Analgesics and anesthetics cannot be safely given to infants and neonates because of their immature capacity to metabolize and eliminate drugs and their sensitivity to opioid-induced respiratory depression.	Infants older than 1 month of age metabolize drugs in the same manner as older infants and children. Careful selection of the agent, dosage, administration route and time, and frequent monitoring for desired and undesired effects, and drug titration and weaning can minimize the adverse effects of opioids and nonopioids for pain management in neonates (Stevens, 1997; Yaster and others, 1997).

From McCaffery M, Pasero C: *Pain: clinical manual*, ed 2, St. Louis, 1999, Mosby.

Attention. The degree to which a client focuses attention on pain can influence pain perception. Increased attention has been associated with increased pain, whereas distraction has been associated with a diminished pain response (Gil, 1990). This concept is one that nurses apply in various pain-relief interventions such as relaxation, guided imagery, and massage. By focusing a client's attention and concentration on other stimuli, the nurse places pain on the periphery of awareness.

Anxiety. The relationship between pain and anxiety is complex. Anxiety often increases the perception of pain, but pain may also cause feelings of anxiety. It is difficult to separate the two sensations. Paice (1991) reported evidence that painful stimuli activate the portion of the limbic system believed to control emotion, particularly anxiety. The limbic system may process the emotional reaction to pain, aggravating or relieving it.

Critically ill or injured clients, who often perceive a lack of control over their environment and care, may have high anxiety levels. This anxiety, if it has gone unnoticed in the high-tech environment of an intensive care unit (ICU), can lead to serious pain management problems. The challenge is to relieve the pain in a client who is anxious in any setting (long-term care, acute care, or home care). Although

Cultural ASPECTS OF CARE | Box 42-4

For the Mexican-American, pain is associated with suffering and a sense of loss. One's obligation as a person and as a member of a family is to bear the burden of the pain. This attitude reflects an acceptance of pain as a measure of the human condition. Mexican-Americans tend to be stoic in their response to pain. In assessing pain, the nurse must be cued into not necessarily what clients say, but into what they do not say. Withdrawing, going to bed, or trying to hide might indicate pain (Villarruel, 1995).

Chinese-American clients are known to tell their family and physician how they feel rather than report pain to their nurse. A strong bond of trust must form between the client and the nurse before pain is discussed freely (Walker and others, 1995). First-generation Chinese-Americans often delegate to a family member, often male, the gatekeeper role in relation to information to be exchanged between the client and health care providers. This can frustrate the nurse, who benefits from knowing subtle changes in a client's condition as soon as possible.

Table 42-5 Pain Management in Older Adults

Misconception	Correction
Pain is a natural outcome of growing old.	It is true that older adults are at greater risk (as much as twofold) than younger adults for many painful conditions; however, pain is not an inevitable result of aging.
Pain perception, or sensitivity, decreases with age.	This assumption is unsafe. Although there is evidence that emotional suffering specifically related to pain may be less in older than in younger clients, no scientific basis exists for the assertion that a decrease in perception of pain occurs with age or that age dulls sensitivity to pain. Assessment and intervention for pain in older adults should begin with the assumption that all neurophysiological processes involved in nociception are unaltered by age.
If the older client does not report pain, he or she does not have pain.	Older clients commonly underreport pain. Reasons include expecting to have pain with increasing age; not wanting to alarm loved ones; being fearful of losing their independence; not wanting to distract, anger, or bother caregivers; and believing caregivers know they have pain and are doing all that can be done to relieve it. The absence of a report of pain does not mean the absence of pain.
If an older client appears to be occupied, asleep, or otherwise distracted from pain, he or she does not have pain.	Older clients often believe it is unacceptable to show pain and have learned to use a variety of ways to cope with it instead (e.g., many clients use distraction successfully for short periods of time). Sleeping may be a coping strategy or indicate exhaustion, not pain relief. Assumptions about the presence or absence of pain cannot be made solely on the basis of a client's behavior.
The potential side effects of opioids make them too dangerous to use to relieve pain in older adults.	Opioids may be used safely in older adults. Although the opioid-naïve older adult may be more sensitive to opioids, this does not justify withholding the use of them in the management of pain in this population. The key to use of opioids in the older adult is to "start low and go slow." Potentially dangerous opioid-induced side effects can be prevented with slow titration; regular, frequent monitoring and assessment of the client's response; and adjustment of dose and interval between doses when side effects are detected. If necessary, clinically significant respiratory depression can be reversed by an opioid antagonist drug.
Clients with Alzheimer's disease and others with cognitive impairment do not feel pain, and their reports of pain are most likely invalid.	No evidence exists that cognitively impaired older adults experience less pain or that their reports of pain are less valid than those of individuals with intact cognitive function. It is probable that clients with dementia, progressive deficits of cognition, apraxias, and agnosia, particularly those in long-term care facilities, suffer significant unrelieved pain and discomfort. Assessment of pain in these clients is challenging but possible. The best approach is to accept the client's report of pain and treat the pain as it would be treated in an individual with intact cognitive function.
Older clients report more pain as they age.	Even though older clients experience a higher incidence of painful conditions, such as arthritis, osteoporosis, peripheral vascular disease, and cancer, than younger clients, studies have shown that they underreport pain. Many elderly clients grew up valuing the ability to "grin and bear it," and, unfortunately, have been heavily influenced by the "Just Say No" to drugs campaign.

Modified from McCaffery M, Pasero C: *Pain: clinical manual,* St. Louis, 1999, Mosby; data from Butler RN, Gastel B: Care of the aged: perspectives on pain and discomfort. In Ng LK, Bonica J, editors: *Pain, discomfort and humanitarian care,* New York, 1980, Elsevier; Harkins SW, Price DD: Assessment of pain in the elderly. In Turk DC, Melzack R, editors: *The handbook of pain assessment,* New York, 1992, Guilford Press; Harkins SW, Price DD: Are there special needs for pain assessment in the elderly? *APS Bull* 3:1, January/February 1993; and Harkins SW and others: Geriatric pain. In Wall PD, Melzack R, editors: *Textbook of pain,* London, 1994, Churchill Livingstone.

pharmacological and nonpharmacological approaches to the management of anxiety are appropriate, anxiolytic medications should not be a substitute for analgesia.

Fatigue.   Fatigue heightens the perception of pain. The sense of exhaustion intensifies pain and decreases coping abilities. This can be a common problem with any person experiencing a long-term illness or who has fatigue as a result of treatment. If fatigue occurs along with sleeplessness, the perception of pain may be even greater. Pain is often experienced less after a restful sleep than at the end of a long day.

Previous Experience.   Each person learns from painful experiences. Previous experience does not necessarily mean that a person will accept pain more easily in the future. If a person has had frequent episodes of pain without relief or has had bouts of severe pain, anxiety or even fear may recur. In contrast, if a person has had repeated experiences with the same type of pain but the pain has been successfully relieved, it becomes easier to interpret the pain sensation. As a result, the client is better prepared to take necessary actions to relieve the pain.

When a client has had no experience with pain, the first perception of it can impair the ability to cope. For example, after abdominal surgery, it is common for a client to experience severe incisional pain for several days. Unless the client is aware of this, the onset of pain may be viewed as a serious complication. Rather than participate actively in postoperative breathing exercises (see Chapter 49), the client may lie immobile in bed and maintain shallow breathing because of fear that something has gone wrong. The nurse should prepare the client with a clear explanation of the type of pain that will be experienced and methods to reduce it.

Coping Style.   The experience of pain can be lonely. When clients experience pain in health care settings such as hospitals, the loneliness can be unbearable. Coping style influences the ability to deal with pain. Persons with internal loci of control perceive themselves as having personal control over their environments and the outcome of events, such as pain (Gil, 1990). In contrast, persons with external loci of control perceive other factors in their environments, such as nurses, as being responsible for the outcome of events. This concept is applied in the use of patient-controlled analgesia (PCA). Clients who are able to self-administer small doses of intravenous (IV) pain medication during an acute episode successfully achieve pain control more quickly than those who rely on nurses to administer intermittent doses of pain medications.

Pain may cause partial or total disability. Clients often find various ways to cope with the physical and psychological effects of pain. It is important to understand a client's coping resources during a painful experience. These resources, such as communicating with a supportive family, exercise, or singing, can be used in the nurse's plan of care to support the client and offer a degree of pain relief.

Family and Social Support.   Another factor that can significantly affect pain response is the presence and attitudes of significant others. People in pain often depend on family members or close friends for support, assistance, or protection. Although pain still exists, the presence of a loved one can minimize loneliness and fear. An absence of family or friends can often make the pain experience more stressful. The presence of parents is especially important for children experiencing pain.

Critical Thinking Synthesis

Successful critical thinking requires a syntheses of knowledge, experience, information gathered from clients, critical thinking attitudes, and intellectual and professional standards. Clinical judgments require that the nurse anticipate what information is needed, analyze the data, and make decisions regarding client care. Critical thinking is always changing. During assessment the nurse must consider all elements that build toward making appropriate nursing diagnoses.

In the case of comfort, knowledge of pain physiology and the many factors that influence pain place the nurse in a better situation to anticipate ways to manage a client's pain. Previous experience in caring for clients with pain sharpens the nurse's assessment skills and ability to choose effective therapies. Critical thinking attitudes and intellectual standards ensure the aggressive assessment, creative planning, and diligent evaluation that are needed on the part of the nurse for the client to obtain an acceptable level of comfort.

Nursing Process and Pain

Nurses need to approach pain management systematically to understand a client's pain and to provide appropriate intervention. Successful management of pain depends on establishing a relationship of trust between the health care provider, client, and family. Pain management extends beyond pain relief, encompassing the client's quality of life and ability to work productively, to enjoy recreation, and to function normally in the family and society (Jacox and others, 1994).

ASSESSMENT

Establishing a nursing diagnosis, deciding on appropriate interventions, and evaluating the client's response (outcomes) of the interventions are contingent on the fundamental activity of a factual, timely, accurate pain assessment (Figure 42-4). The core of this complex activity is the exploration of the pain experience through the eyes of the client.

KNOWLEDGE

- Physiology of pain
- Factors that potentially increase or decrease responses to pain
- Pathophysiology of conditions causing pain
- Awareness of biases affecting pain assessment and treatment
- Cultural variations in how pain is expressed
- Knowledge of nonverbal communication

STANDARDS

- Refer to AHCPR guidelines for acute pain management
- Apply intellectual standards (e.g., clarity, specificity, accuracy, and completeness when gathering assessment)
- Apply relevance when letting the client explore the pain experience

ASSESSMENT

- Determine the client's perspective of pain including history of pain; its meaning; and physical, emotional, and social effects
- Measure objectively the characteristics of the client's pain
- Review potential factors affecting the client's pain

EXPERIENCE

- Caring for clients with acute, chronic, and cancer pain
- Caring for clients who experienced pain as a result of a health care therapy
- Personal experience with pain

ATTITUDES

- Persevere in exploring causes and possible solutions for chronic pain
- Display confidence when assessing pain to relieve the client's anxiety
- Display integrity and fairness to prevent prejudice from affecting assessment

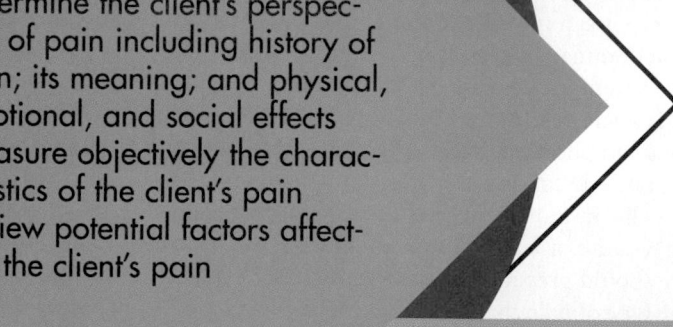

Figure 42-4 *Synthesis Model for Comfort Assessment Phase.*

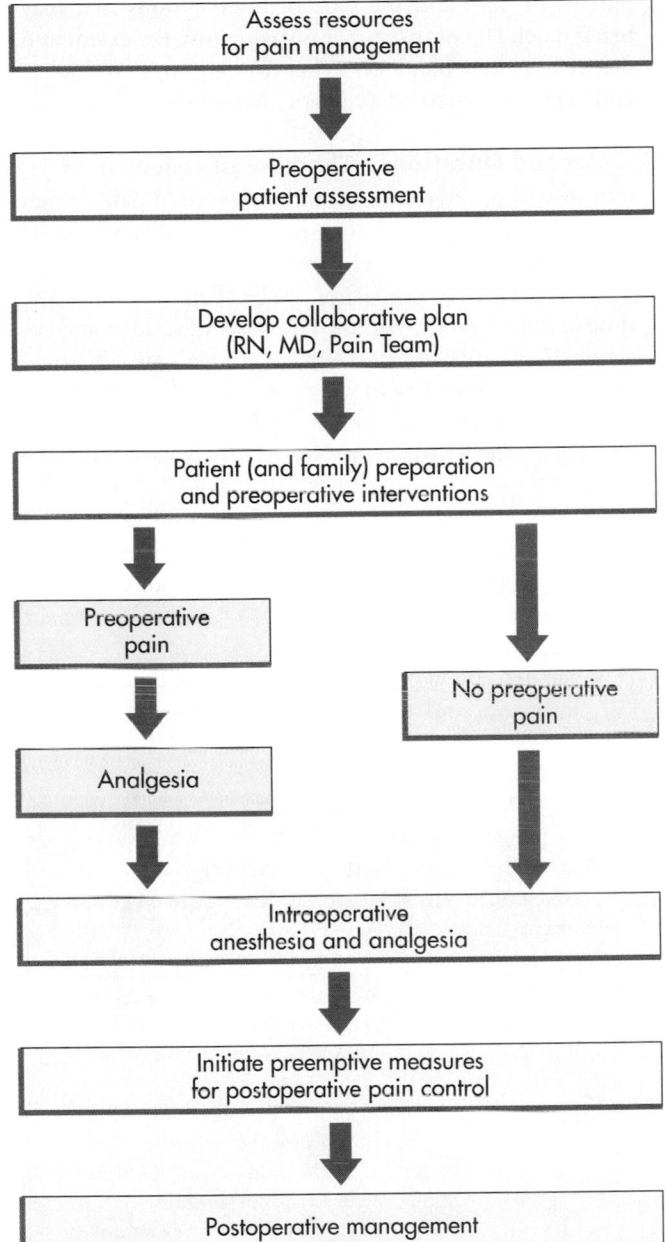

Figure 42-5   Pain treatment flow chart: preoperative and intraoperative phases.
From Agency for Health Care Policy and Research, Acute Pain Management Guideline Panel: *Acute pain management: operative or medical procedures and trauma,* Clinical Practice Guideline, AHCPR Pub No. 92-0032, Rockville, Md, 1992, Agency for Health Care Policy and Research, Public Health Service, U.S. Department of Health and Human Services.

AHCPR has established specific guidelines for assessing clients with acute and cancer pain. The focus is on planning successful pain management interventions before pain is experienced. Because it involves a collaborative approach, the AHCPR pain treatment flow chart (Figure 42-5) offers a useful conceptual approach to the control of acute pain. Clients must understand that informed reporting of pain is valuable and necessary if the health care team is to manage pain effectively.

When assessing pain, the nurse must be sensitive to the client's level of discomfort. In addition, the nurse must ask the client at what level will the discomfort not interfere with his or her functional ability. For example, the nurse caring for a client with pain should ask, "What is an acceptable level of pain for you?" The client might answer that a level 2 pain (on a scale of 0 to 10, with 0 being no pain and 10 being excruciating) is "manageable." The nurse then focuses efforts on getting the pain decreased to at least that level. If pain is acute or severe, it is unlikely that the client can provide a detailed description of the entire experience. During an episode of acute pain the nurse primarily assesses the location, severity, and quality of the pain. A more thorough pain assessment can occur when the client has been made more comfortable.

For clients with chronic pain, assessment may best be focused on affective, cognitive, and behavioral dimensions of the pain experience and on its history and context (NIH, 1986; McGuire, 1992). In the case of chronic nonmalignant pain, assessment should include the level of function, because it may not be possible to achieve complete pain relief. In the home care setting, family members may become the assessors of pain. Using the *ABCs* of pain management is an effective way to manage pain (Box 42-5).

Routine Clinical Approach to Pain Assessment and Management: *ABCDE*   Box 42-5

A   *Ask about pain regularly.*
    Assess pain systematically.
B   *Believe the client and family in their report of pain and what relieves it.*
C   *Choose pain control options appropriate for the client, family, and setting.*
D   *Deliver interventions in a timely, logical, and coordinated fashion.*
E   *Empower clients and their families.*
    Enable them to control their course to the greatest extent possible.

From Jacox A and others: *Management of cancer pain,* Clinical Practice Guideline No. 9, AHCPR Publication No. 94-0592, Rockville, Md, 1994, Agency for Health Care Policy and Research, Public Health Service, U.S. Department of Health and Human Services.

The nurse should be aware of possible errors in pain assessment (Box 42-6). Using the right tools and methods can help to avoid errors and to ensure that the right pain interventions are chosen.

Client's Expression of Pain.
Many clients fail to report or discuss discomfort, at the same time, many nurses believe that clients will report pain if they have it. In addition, if clients sense that the nurse doubts that pain exists, they will share little information about their pain experience or will minimize their report. It is imperative that the nurse set the stage for the relationship that allows for open communication about pain. Simple measures such as sitting when talking to clients about pain lets clients know that the nurse has the time and the interest to assess their pain.

The nurse should learn the verbal and nonverbal ways that clients communicate discomfort. Grimacing, splinting a body part, and unusual posturing are examples of nonverbal expressions of pain. Clients unable to communicate effectively often require special attention during assessment. Children, persons who are developmentally delayed, clients who are psychotic, the critically ill, clients with dementia, and clients who do not speak English all require different approaches. Children's verbal statements are most important (Wong and others, 1999). Young children may not know what the word *pain* means, and therefore assessment may require the nurse to use words such as *owie*, *boo-boo*, or *hurt*. Cognitively impaired clients might require simple assessment approaches involving close observation of behavior changes. A critically ill client who may have a clouded sensorium or the presence of nasogastric tubes or artificial airways may require the nurse to ask specific directive questions that the client can answer with a nod of the head or by writing out a response. If the client speaks a different language, pain assessment will be difficult. A family member or interpreter may be necessary to describe the client's feelings and sensations. Assessment tools such as the visual analog scale (VAS) has been translated into several languages to aid the nurse

when an interpreter or family is not present (McCaffery and Pasero, 1999).

Characteristics of Pain.
A client's self-report of pain is the single most reliable indicator of the existence and intensity of pain and any related discomfort (NIH, 1986). Pain is individualistic. Assessment of common characteristics of pain helps the nurse form an understanding of the pattern of pain and the type of interventions that may bring relief. Use of instruments to quantify the extent and degree of pain depends on a client's being cognitively alert and able to understand a nurse's instructions.

Onset and Duration.
The nurse asks questions to determine the onset, duration, and sequence of pain. When did the pain begin? How long has it lasted? Does it occur at the same time each day? How often does it recur?

Certain types of headaches can be characterized by the time of day when they occur. The onset of sudden and severe pain is easier to assess than is gradual, mild discomfort. An understanding of the time cycle of pain helps the nurse to know when to intervene before the pain occurs or worsens (Table 42-6).

Location.
To assess pain location, the nurse asks the client to tell or to point to all areas of discomfort. The site or multiple sites can be documented on a body diagram (Figure 42-6). This can be useful as a baseline if the pain should change.

When describing pain location, the nurse uses anatomical landmarks and descriptive terminology. The state-

---

Possible Sources for Error in Pain Assessment   Box 42-6

- Bias, which causes nurses to consistently overestimate or underestimate the pain that clients experience
- Vague or unclear assessment questions, which lead to unreliable assessment data
- Use of pain assessment tools that have not been proved reliable and valid with identical clients (a reliable assessment tool focuses only on pain cues that provide a reliable measure of relevant clinical changes)
- Clients who do not always provide complete, pertinent, and accurate pain information
- Cognitively impaired older clients who are unable to use pain scales

---

Table 42-6	Implications of Pain Assessment for Nursing Interventions
Assessment Criteria	Nursing Interventions
Onset and duration	Administer analgesics so that peak action occurs when pain is most acute (e.g., during dressing change or exercise therapy).
Location	Position client off of affected area. Apply local treatments (e.g., elastic bandage and splinting) directly over painful site.
Intensity	Change or revise interventions, depending on success of one intervention.
Precipitating or aggravating factors	Avoid activities that cause or aggravate pain. Teach client or family to avoid same activities.
Relief measures	Use measures that client uses to relieve pain, as long as they are safe and appropriate, including nonpharmacological interventions.

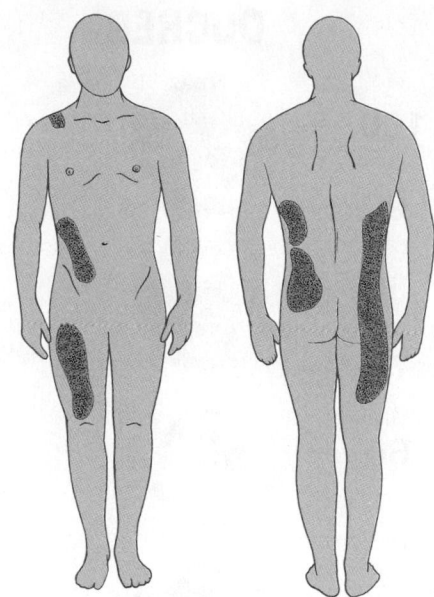

Figure 42-6   Body diagrams to locate a client's pain

ment, "The pain is localized in the upper right abdominal quadrant, is more specific than "The client states the pain is in the abdomen." Pain, classified by location, may be superficial or cutaneous, deep or visceral, or referred or radiating (Table 42-7).

Intensity.   One of the most subjective, and therefore most useful, characteristics for the reporting of pain may be its severity, or intensity. Clients are often asked to describe pain as mild, moderate, or severe. However, the meaning of these terms differs for the nurse and client. This type of information is also difficult to verify over time.

Descriptive scales are a more objective means of measuring pain intensity (Figure 42-7). A verbal descriptor scale (VDS) consists of a line with three- to five-word descriptors equally spaced along the line. The descriptors are ranked from "no pain" to "unbearable pain." The nurse shows the client the scale and asks the client to choose the current intensity of pain. The nurse also asks how much the pain hurts at its worst and how much it hurts at its best. The VDS enables a client to choose a category for describing pain. A numerical rating scale (NRS) may be used instead of word descriptors. In this case clients rate pain on a scale of 0 to 10. The scales work best when assessing pain intensity before and after therapeutic interventions.

Table 42-7   Classification of Pain by Location

Location	Characteristics	Examples of Causes
Superficial or Cutaneous Pain resulting from stimulation of skin	Pain is of short duration and is localized. It usually is a sharp sensation.	Needlestick; small cut or laceration
Deep Visceral Pain resulting from stimulation of internal organs	Pain is diffuse and may radiate in several directions. Duration varies but it usually lasts longer than superficial pain. Pain may be sharp, dull, or unique to organ involved.	Crushing sensation (e.g., angina pectoris); burning sensation (e.g., gastric ulcer)
Referred Common phenomenon in visceral pain because many organs themselves have no pain receptors; entrance of sensory neurons from affected organ into same spinal cord segment as neurons from areas where pain is felt; perception of pain in unaffected areas	Pain is felt in part of body separate from source of pain and may assume any characteristic.	Myocardial infarction, which may cause referred pain to jaw, left arm, and left shoulder; kidney stones, which may refer pain to groin
Radiating Sensation of pain extending from initial site of injury to another body part	Pain feels as though it travels down or along body part. It may be intermittent or constant.	Low back pain from ruptured intravertebral disk accompanied by pain radiating down leg from sciatic nerve irritation

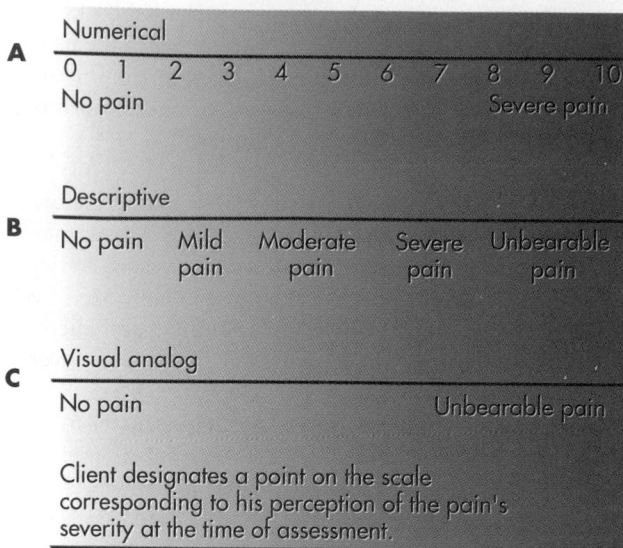

Figure 42-7   Sample pain scales. **A,** Numerical. **B,** Verbal descriptive. **C,** Visual analog.

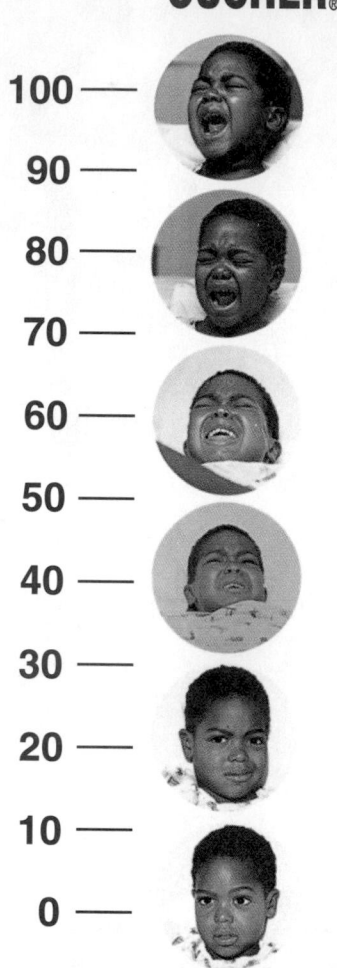

Figure 42-8   African-American version of the Oucher Pain Scale.

Copyright Denyes Villarruel, 1990.

When scales are used to rate pain, a 10-cm (4-inch) baseline is recommended (AHCPR, 1992; Willens, 1996).

The VAS does not have labeled subdivisions. It consists of a straight line, representing a continuum of intensity, and has verbal descriptors at each end. This scale gives the client total freedom in identifying the severity of pain. The VAS may not be as practical for daily use as an NMS (McCaffery and Pasero, 1999). However, Mottola (1993) argues that the VAS is a more sensitive measure of pain severity, because clients mark at any point on the continuum rather than choosing one word or number.

There are some unique tools available to measure pain intensity in children. Beyer and others (1992) have developed the "Oucher," which consists of two separate scales: a 0 to 100 scale on the left for older children and a six-picture photographic scale on the right for younger children. Photographs of the face of a child (in increasing levels of discomfort) are designed to cue children into understanding what pain is and its severity. A child merely points to the selection, thus simplifying the task of describing the pain. New ethnic versions of the tool have also been developed (Figure 42-8). Wong and Baker (1988) developed the FACES scale to assess pain in children (Figure 42-9). The scale consists of six cartoon faces ranging from a smiling face ("no pain") to increasingly less happy faces, to a final sad, tearful face ("worst pain"). Children as young as 3 years of age can use the scale.

A pain scale should be designed so that it is easy to use and is not time consuming for the client to complete. If the client can read and understand the scale, the description of pain should be more accurate. Descriptive scales are useful not only in assessing the severity of pain, but also in evaluating changes in a client's condition. The nurse can use the scales after an intervention or when

symptoms become aggravated to evaluate whether the pain has decreased or increased. It is important for every nurse to select and consistently use one scale when assessing a client. A pain scale cannot be used to compare the pain of one client to that of another client.

Quality.   Another subjective characteristic of pain is its quality. Because there is no common or specific pain vocabulary in general use, the words a client may choose to describe pain can apply to any number of things. Often, a client describes pain as crushing, throbbing, sharp, or dull. For example, the nurse might say, "Tell me what your pain feels like." The nurse offers to list descriptive terms when the client cannot describe the pain. The terms *pricking*, *burning*, and *aching* are useful to describe pain initially. Later the client may choose more descriptive terms.

There is some consistency in the way people describe

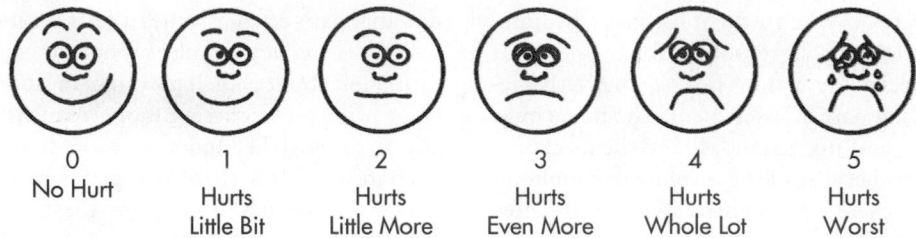

Figure 42-9   Wong-Baker FACES Pain Rating Scale.
From Wong DL and others: *Whaley and Wong's nursing care of infants and children,* ed 6, St. Louis, 1999, Mosby.

certain types of pain. The pain associated with a myocardial infarction is often described as crushing or viselike, whereas the pain of a surgical incision is often described as sharp and stabbing. Neuropathic pain is described as burning. When the client's descriptions fit the pattern forming in the nurse's assessment, a clearer analysis can be made of the nature and type of pain.

Pain Pattern.   Various factors affect the character of pain. It helps to assess specific events or conditions that precipitate or aggravate pain. The nurse asks the client to describe activities that cause pain, such as physical movement, coffee ingestion, or urination. The nurse may also ask the client to demonstrate actions that cause a painful response, such as coughing or turning a certain way. In the example of a ruptured intravertebral disk, the low back pain and radiation down the leg is usually aggravated by bending over or lifting objects. Swallowing and talking typically aggravate the pain of pharyngitis. After the nurse identifies precipitating or aggravating factors, it is easier to plan interventions to prevent pain from occurring or worsening.

Relief Measures.   It is useful to know whether a client has an effective way of relieving pain, such as changing position, using ritualistic behavior (pacing, rocking, rubbing), eating, meditation, or applying heat or cold to the painful site. The client's methods often work best for the nurse, too. Clients gain comfort from knowing that the nurse is willing to try their relief measures. Copp (1990) discovered that clients develop methods to reduce the intensity of oncoming pain. They used a range of muscular activities, verbal methods (prayer and cursing), and concentration exercises. In the home, the nurse must be sure that relief measures (such as a heating pad) are used safely. Assessment of relieving factors should also include identification of practitioners (e.g., internist, orthopedist, acupuncturist, chiropractor, dentist) whose services the client has used.

Concomitant Symptoms.   Concomitant symptoms are those that often occur with pain (e.g., nausea,

headache, dizziness, urge to urinate, constipation, and restlessness). Certain types of pain have predictable accompanying symptoms. For example, severe rectal pain often results in constipation. The pain of an inflamed gallbladder or a kidney stone frequently causes nausea and vomiting. Concomitant symptoms may be as much a treatment priority as the pain itself.

Effects of Pain on the Client.   Pain is a stressful event that can alter a person's lifestyle and affect psychological well-being. In the case of cancer and chronic nonmalignant pain, it can cause suffering, loss of control, and impaired quality of life throughout the client's course of care. By recognizing the effects pain has on clients, the nurse can better identify the nature and existence of pain.

When a client has acute pain, the nurse should assess vital signs, conduct a focused physical examination, and observe for autonomic nervous system involvement. Physiological signs can reveal pain in a client who tries not to complain or admit discomfort. There is no predictable level or extent of change in a client's condition that indicates pain.

At the onset of acute pain, the heart and respiratory rates and blood pressure increase. The nurse compares vital signs with baseline measurements recorded before onset. Any change in vital signs is significant, so the nurse should take into account all signs and symptoms before determining that pain is the cause. The nurse should not confuse signs and symptoms of pain with other pathological changes. For example, a client who is highly anxious also has elevated heart and respiratory rates. The nurse performs a physical and neurological assessment based on the client's pain history. The painful area should be examined to see if palpation or manipulation of the site increases pain (Jacox and others, 1994). During a general overview, the nurse looks for cues indicating pain (e.g., posturing or guarding a painful area). If pain is unrelieved, the nurse looks for signs of physical exhaustion. Decreasing vital sign values indicate parasympathetic nerve response. The client becomes less responsive to stimuli within the environment. The nurse should measure vital signs more often if the client's condition deteriorates.

Behavioral Effects. When a client has pain, the nurse assesses verbalization, vocal response, facial and body movements, and social interaction (Box 42-7). A verbal report of pain is a vital part of assessment. The nurse must be willing to listen and understand. Many clients cannot verbalize discomfort because of the inability to communicate. An infant or a client who is unconscious, disoriented or confused, or aphasic, or who speaks a foreign language is unable to explain the pain experience. In these cases it is especially important for the nurse to be alert for behaviors that indicate pain (Box 42-8).

Groaning, grunting, and crying are examples of vocalizations used to express pain. Certain vocalizations may be involuntary and may occur without warning when acute pain occurs. For some clients, vocalizations are culturally acceptable ways to communicate and do not necessarily indicate a higher severity of pain or reduced tolerance.

Subtle facial expressions or body movements often reveal more about the character of pain than does precise questioning. For example, the client may grimace or begin to toss and turn at regular intervals. The amount of restlessness or protective movement may increase as the assessment progresses. Some nonverbal expressions characterize sources of pain. The client with chest pain often grabs or holds the chest. A child or adult with severe abdominal pain often assumes a fetal position. The nonverbal expression of pain may support or contradict other information about pain. If a woman in labor reports that her labor pains are occurring more frequently, and if she begins to massage her abdomen more frequently, her report is confirmed. If a client complains of severe abdominal pain but continues to grasp the chest, a more detailed assessment may be necessary.

The nature of a person's pain causes the person to attend to the discomfort and fight it or give in to the discomfort and withdraw socially. The extent to which a client interacts with the environment can provide a clue for the nurse about the intensity or nature of the pain. Severe pain can seriously hamper a person's lifestyle.

Influence on Activities of Daily Living. Clients who live with daily pain are less able to participate in routine activities. Assessment of these changes reveals the extent of the client's disability and adjustments necessary to help clients participate in self-care.

The nurse asks whether pain interferes with sleep. There may be initial difficulty falling asleep. Sleeping pills or other medications may be needed to induce sleep. The

---

Behavioral Indicators of Effects of Pain   Box 42-7

VOCALIZATIONS
Moaning
Crying
Gasping
Grunting

FACIAL EXPRESSIONS
Grimace
Clenched teeth
Wrinkled forehead
Tightly closed or widely opened eyes or mouth
Lip biting

BODY MOVEMENT
Restlessness
Immobilization
Muscle tension
Increased hand and finger movements
Pacing activities
Rhythmic or rubbing motions
Protective movement of body parts

SOCIAL INTERACTION
Avoidance of conversation
Focus only on activities for pain relief
Avoidance of social contacts
Reduced attention span

Research HIGHLIGHT   Box 42-8

RESEARCH ABSTRACT
Confused, disoriented, or nonverbal older clients frequently suffer from painful conditions. A sample of 26 clients from the Alzheimer's unit of a large Midwestern nursing home was studied for behaviors that indicated pain. Each client's medical record confirmed the presence of a painful disorder such as cancer or degenerative joint disease. A pain assessment was performed on each client by a certified nurse practitioner. Most clients had no pain behaviors despite their diagnosis. Only three clients showed typical pain behaviors. Staff were surveyed and found to be surprised that the identified clients were in pain. Further review resulted in staff being able to describe client's pain behaviors. Clients who normally moaned and rocked became quiet and withdrawn when in pain. Clients who were friendly and outgoing became agitated and combative. Clients who were outgoing and easily involved in activities began to cry easily and withdraw when pain developed. Some clients refrained from eating when in pain.

IMPLICATIONS FOR PRACTICE
- There is lack of objective assessment tools and criteria for assessing pain in nonverbal older clients.
- Nurses must become very familiar with the "normal behavior" of this population to detect pain.
- Family can be a source to help identify behavioral changes.

REFERENCE
Marzinski LR: The tragedy of dementia: clinically assessing pain in the confused, nonverbal elderly, *J Gerontol Nurs* 17(6):25, 1991.

pain may awaken the client during the night and create difficulty in falling back to sleep (see Chapter 41).

Depending on the location of the pain, the client may have difficulty performing normal hygiene measures. The nurse determines whether the client can perform hygiene and dressing/grooming activities independently. The pain may restrict mobility to the point that the client is no longer able to bathe in a bathtub. The client may have problems performing other activities of daily living. For example, a client with severe arthritis may find it painful to grasp eating utensils. The nurse assesses the client's need for assistance with self-care activities and collaborates with members of the health care team (e.g., physical therapy and occupational therapy). The nurse also considers the need for family members or friends to assist the client with basic hygiene.

Pain can impair the ability to maintain normal sexual relations. Conditions such as arthritis, degenerative diseases of the hip, and chronic back pain make it difficult for a person to assume usual positions during intercourse. Prolonged use of opioids for cancer pain is known to affect sexual function and libido in men and women (Jacox and others, 1994). The nurse should assess the extent to which pain has affected sexual activity. It also helps to learn whether a client is physically unable to participate or if the desire for sexual intercourse has been reduced by the pain.

The ability of people to work can be seriously threatened by pain. The more physical activity required in a job, the greater the risk of discomfort when the pain is associated with musculoskeletal and certain visceral alterations. Pain related to emotional stress is probably increased in individuals whose jobs involve tension-laden decision making. The nurse assesses the work that clients do and their abilities to function in regular jobs. The daily chores of homemakers are assessed in the same manner as the duties involved in jobs outside the home. The nurse assesses whether it is necessary for clients to stop activity occasionally because of pain. Often the nurse can help clients select ways of minimizing or controlling the pain so that they can remain productive.

It is also important to include an assessment of the effect of pain on social activities. The pain may be so debilitating that the client becomes too exhausted to socialize. The nurse identifies the client's normal social activities, the extent to which they have been disrupted, and the client's wish to participate.

A client's neurological function can easily influence the pain experience. Any factor that interrupts or influences normal pain reception or perception affects the client's awareness and response to pain. For example, a client who has a spinal cord injury; peripheral neuropathy, as in the case of diabetes mellitus; or a neurological disease, such as multiple sclerosis, has an altered sensation of pain. Certain pharmacologic agents influence pain perception and response. Analgesics, sedatives, and anesthetics depress

functions of the central nervous system. It is important for the nurse to conduct a neurological assessment (see Chapter 32) of a client at risk for being insensitive to pain. This client could suffer injury easily and thus requires preventive nursing care.

Client Expectations.   A recent national survey states that the public views pain as a "part of life" and would rather bear it than take action to relieve it (Bostrom, 1997). Clients who seek treatment with pain as a major symptom may have experienced this pain for many hours or days before seeking health care assistance. They may expect and even accept a certain amount of pain while hospitalized. Asking the client the comfort level that is acceptable to him or her is an initial step in encouraging the client to regain control. Assessing previous pain experiences and what interventions were effective at home provides a foundation on which the nurse can build. Clients expect that nurses will be prompt in meeting their pain needs.

NURSING DIAGNOSIS

The development of an accurate nursing diagnosis for a client in pain results from thorough data collection and analysis (Box 42-9). A nurse must not diagnose pain simply because it is presumed that a client will be uncomfortable. Too often a nurse may choose the diagnosis of pain because a client is about to have surgery or a specific disease condition implies pain.

An accurate diagnosis is made only after a complete assessment has been performed. In the example of the diagnosis of pain, the nurse may assess the client's withdrawal from communication, grimacing, and moaning, as well as the client's verbalization of discomfort. In contrast, the diagnosis of anxiety may be made by observing a client's facial tension and appearance, poor eye contact, restlessness, and verbalizations of feeling scared. The two diagnoses have similar defining characteristics. The nurse sorts out patterns of data to identify pain as the correct diagnosis.

The nursing diagnosis should focus on the specific nature of the pain to help the nurse identify the most useful types of interventions for alleviating pain and minimizing its effect on the client's lifestyle and function. Pain related to physical trauma versus pain related to natural childbirth processes require very different nursing interventions. Accurate identification of related factors ensures that appropriate nursing interventions will be chosen.

The nurse may make diagnoses other than that of *pain* (Box 42-10). The extent to which pain affects a client's lifestyle and general state of health determines whether other nursing diagnoses are relevant. For example, the nurse's assessment may reveal that a client suffers from pain of the hands and shoulders as a result of crippling arthritis that the client has had for over 3 years. As a result, the client is unable to remove or fasten necessary items of

SAMPLE NURSING DIAGNOSTIC PROCESS   Box 42-9
CHRONIC PAIN

Assessment Activities	Defining Characteristics	Nursing Diagnosis
Have client describe pain intensity.	Pain is constant; rated as 5 on a scale of 0 to 10.	Chronic pain related to chronic physical disability
Assess onset and location of pain.	Pain has been present for 7 months; localized in lower lumbar area, radiates down to right.	
Observe client behaviors.	Client moves slowly, stays in bed during much of day, has a blank facial expression.	
Assess influence pain has had on daily activities.	Client's appetite is reduced; unable to complete dressing without pain increasing. Spouse reports client awakens frequently during night, gets little sleep.	
Review medical history.	Client is diagnosed with previous traumatic injury to lumbar area.	

NURSING DIAGNOSES Box 42-10
CLIENTS IN PAIN

Anxiety
Hopelessness
Mobility, impaired physical
Pain
Pain, chronic
Self-care deficit
Sexual dysfunction
Sleep pattern disturbance

clothing. The nursing diagnoses for this client would be that of *self-care deficit: dressing/grooming* and *chronic pain.* The diagnosis of *self-care deficit* would lead the nurse to involve members of the health care team to provide the client with assistive devices for performing self-care.

PLANNING

During planning the nurse again synthesizes information from multiple resources. Critical thinking ensures that the client's plan of care integrates all that the nurse knows about the individual client, as well as key critical thinking elements (Figure 42-10). Professional standards are especially important to consider when the nurse develops a plan of care. These standards often establish scientifically proven guidelines for selecting effective nursing interventions.

Together the nurse and client discuss realistic expectations for an individualized plan of care. This consists of a comprehensive assessment, identification of appropriate nursing diagnoses, outcomes and interventions (see care plan). Planned interventions must be appropriate for the nature and type of pain. For example, pain related to acute incisional pain usually responds to analgesics, whereas pain related to early labor contractions can often be reduced with relaxation exercises.

An intervention that works for one client will not work for all. In the home, the nurse uses some of the remedies that the client has adopted. However, the nurse cannot use interventions that are unsafe. When developing a plan of care, the nurse selects priorities based on the client's level of pain and its effect on the client's condition. For acute, severe pain it is important to provide relief as soon as possible. Analgesics can provide relatively rapid relief and lessen the chance of pain worsening. After a client gains some relief from the pain, the nurse plans other interventions such as relaxation or the application of heat to enhance the effect of analgesics.

A comprehensive plan includes a variety of resources for pain control. Resources available include nurse specialists, physical therapists, and occupational therapists. An oncology nurse specialist is very familiar with the pharmacological and nonpharmacological interventions that are most effective for chronic and cancer pain. Physical therapists can plan exercises that strengthen muscle groups and lessen pain in affected areas. Occupational therapists may devise splints to support painful body parts. It is also important to involve the family in the plan of care because

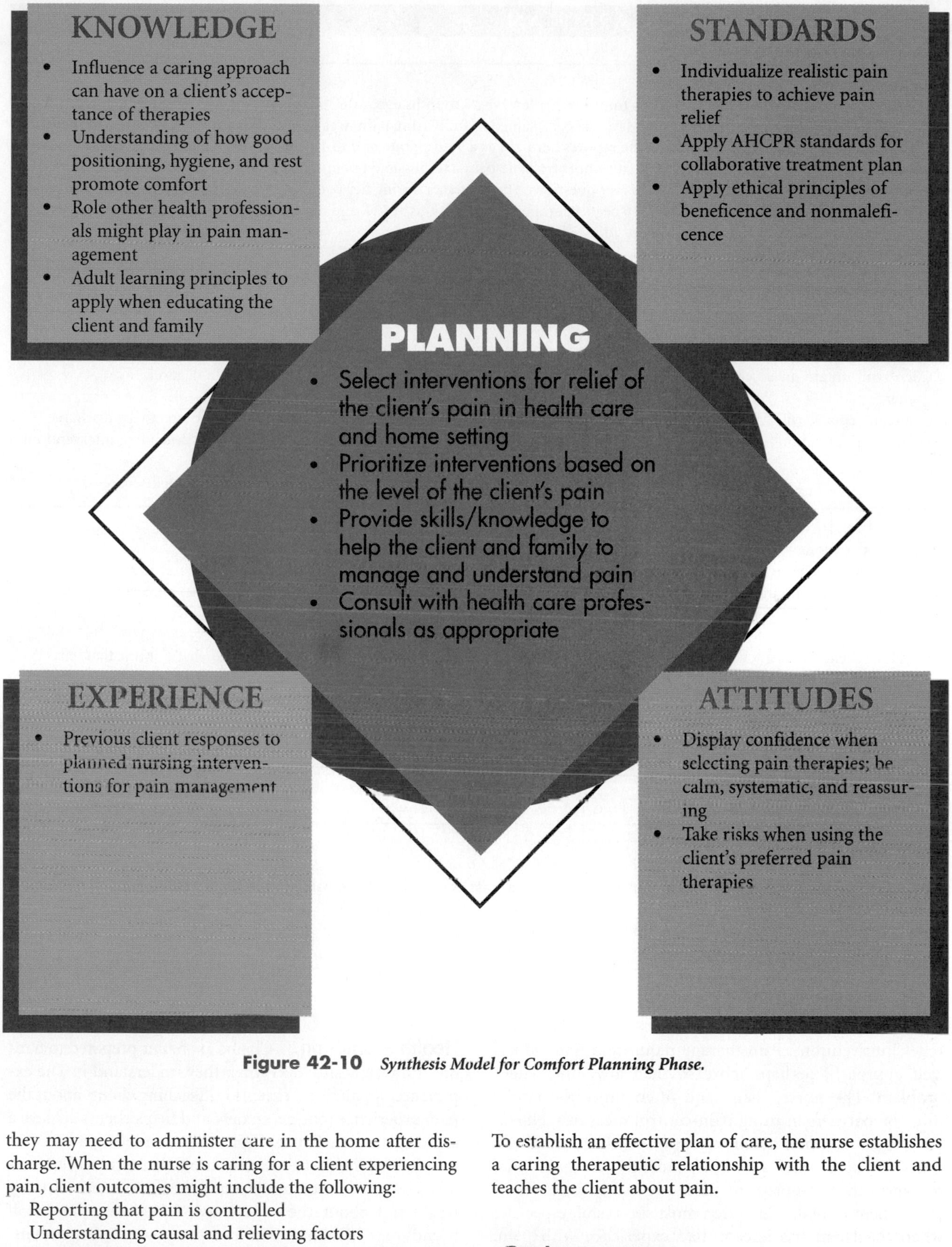

KNOWLEDGE

- Influence a caring approach can have on a client's acceptance of therapies
- Understanding of how good positioning, hygiene, and rest promote comfort
- Role other health professionals might play in pain management
- Adult learning principles to apply when educating the client and family

STANDARDS

- Individualize realistic pain therapies to achieve pain relief
- Apply AHCPR standards for collaborative treatment plan
- Apply ethical principles of beneficence and nonmaleficence

PLANNING

- Select interventions for relief of the client's pain in health care and home setting
- Prioritize interventions based on the level of the client's pain
- Provide skills/knowledge to help the client and family to manage and understand pain
- Consult with health care professionals as appropriate

EXPERIENCE

- Previous client responses to planned nursing interventions for pain management

ATTITUDES

- Display confidence when selecting pain therapies; be calm, systematic, and reassuring
- Take risks when using the client's preferred pain therapies

Figure 42-10 *Synthesis Model for Comfort Planning Phase.*

they may need to administer care in the home after discharge. When the nurse is caring for a client experiencing pain, client outcomes might include the following:

Reporting that pain is controlled

Understanding causal and relieving factors

Maintaining existing physical and psychosocial function

Maintaining the ability to perform self-care

Using pain relief measures safely

To establish an effective plan of care, the nurse establishes a caring therapeutic relationship with the client and teaches the client about pain.

IMPLEMENTATION

The nature of the pain and the extent to which it affects a person's well-being determine the choice of pain-

SAMPLE NURSING CARE PLAN

ALTERATION IN COMFORT

ASSESSMENT*

Mrs. Mays was diagnosed with a cancerous tumor in her left lung 8 months ago. After treatment, she was taking oral analgesics on a prn basis. During the past 2 weeks Mrs. Mays has complained of **increasing pain, weakness,** uncontrollable cough, and **inability to complete her own hygiene activities. She reports her pain as a 9 on a scale of 0 to 10** and, **crying,** states, "The pain pills aren't working." She is admitted to the hospital with uncontrollable pain and possible pneumonia. She is **restless** during the admission interview and **unable to stay focused** to answer questions. She **grimaces** during her coughing episodes. **Blood pressure and pulse rate are elevated** at 190/100, and pulse is 110 beats per minute. Respirations are 24, and temperature is 37.2° C (99° F). She is started on slow-release morphine bid with the dose adjusted according to her prn use.

*Defining characteristics are shown in bold type.

NURSING DIAGNOSIS: Acute pain related to a biological injuring agent (tumor).

PLANNING

GOALS

Client will obtain an acceptable level of comfort before discharge.

Client and spouse will actively participate in pain management plan in preparation for discharge.

EXPECTED OUTCOMES

Client will report pain at an acceptable level.

Spouse will use slow-stroke massage correctly by discharge.

Client will maintain a daily log of pain-control interventions and responses obtained.

Client is able to complete own hygiene by discharge.

INTERVENTIONS†

Pain Management

- Administer slow-release morphine as ordered. Explain to client and spouse the use of the medication; potential side effects, including constipation; and the method to treat breakthrough pain.
- Have client select interventions that have relieved pain in the past (e.g. distraction, music, simple relaxation therapy)
- Have client complete a pain diary of the type of pain, measures used to control pain, and responses obtained.

- Teach spouse how to perform slow-stroke back massage.

RATIONALE

Client is experiencing an acute episode of her chronic cancer pain. This route continuously releases analgesia so as to control pain around the clock (ATC) with decreased side effects (Jacox and others, 1994).

Personal control allows a client to shape immediate circumstances through own actions (Salerno and Willens, 1996).

Recording pain experiences and relief measures allows for systematic evaluation of pain management interventions (McCaffery and Pasero, 1999).

Slow-stroke back massage is easy to do, takes a brief time, and has been shown to induce relaxation (Meek, 1993)

†Intervention Classification labels from McCloskey JC, Bulechek GM: *Nursing interventions classification (NIC),* ed 3, St. Louis, 2000, Mosby.

EVALUATION

Ask client to identify an acceptable level of comfort on a scale of 0 to 10.

Following analgesia and massage, ask client to rate pain on a scale of 0 to 10 and compare with her acceptable level.

Observe client performing hygiene.

Observe spouse performing slow-stroke massage for the client.

Discuss with the client if nonpharmacological interventions are effective.

---

relief interventions. Pain therapy requires an individualized approach, perhaps more so than any other client problem. The nurse, client, and often times the family must be partners in using pain-control measures. Nurses administer and monitor interventions ordered by physicians for pain relief and independently use pain-relief measures that complement those prescribed by a physician. Client remedies are often most successful, especially when the client has already had experience with pain. Generally, the least invasive or safest therapy should be tried first. If there is doubt about a nursing therapy, the nurse should consult with a physician.

Health Promotion.   Clients are better prepared to handle almost any situation when they understand it. The experience of pain is no exception. Teaching clients about the pain experience reduces anxiety and helps clients achieve a sense of control. For example, clients entering a clinic or hospital for the first time may know that tests will be performed but do not understand them. As a result, they might fret about the experience. Fears are enhanced if friends have had unpleasant experiences in similar circumstances. Fear increases the perception of painful stimuli.

During the anticipatory phase of the pain experience, the nurse needs to teach clients about the procedures and associated discomfort. Explaining the procedure in a confident tone conveys a sense that the nurse will care for the client correctly. When clients receive instruction about an upcoming painful experience, they often perceive the actual experience as less unpleasant.

Relevant play is a type of teaching that works well with children. Play reduces anxiety that might otherwise be created if the nurse tried to explain complicated procedures. For example, if a child is to have a laceration of the arm sutured, it helps to let the child put sutures into a doll's arm. Almost any procedure or situation can be acted out with dolls or other appropriate toys.

Because comfort affects a person's physical and mental functioning, holistic health approaches are becoming important interventions for maintaining a person's wellness. Holistic health is an ongoing state of wellness that involves taking care of the physical self, expressing emotions appropriately and effectively, using the mind constructively, being creatively involved with others, and becoming aware of higher levels of consciousness (Association for Holistic Health, 1981). The use of holistic health approaches assumes a person's own capacity for healing and returns responsibility for health back to the individual (Edelman and Mandle, 1998). The concept of holistic health parallels the values nursing has always had in maintaining the integrity of the whole person.

Holistic health is more than just self-care. It also is a process of personal inquiry. Individuals learn to look at the emotional meaning of any health problems they might have and the significance of the problem in light of their purpose in life (Edelman and Mandle, 1998). A person becomes consciously aware of the relationship between emotional health and physical health. The role of clients is to participate actively in their own well-being. Common holistic health approaches include wellness education, regular exercise, rest, attention to good hygiene practices and nutrition, and management of interpersonal relationships. When a person develops pain or other symptoms of discomfort, there are tools the nurse can offer.

Failure of clinicians to assess a client's pain, accept the findings, and treat the report of pain is a common cause of unrelieved pain and suffering (McCaffery and Pasero, 1999). Thorough assessments and use of nonpharmacological and/or pharmacological interventions leads to improved client outcomes.

Nonpharmacological Pain-Relief Interventions.
There are a number of nonpharmacological interventions that might lessen pain and that can be used in acute and tertiary care, as well as in the home and restorative care settings. These interventions can also be used in combination with pharmacological measures. Nonpharmacological interventions include cognitive-behavioral and physical approaches. The goals of cognitive-behavioral interventions are to change clients' perceptions of pain, to alter pain behavior, and to provide clients with a greater sense of con-

trol. Relaxation and guided imagery are examples. Physical agents have the goal of providing comfort, correcting physical dysfunction, altering physiological responses, and reducing fears associated with pain-related immobility. The AHCPR guidelines for acute pain management (1992) cite nonpharmacological interventions to be appropriate for clients who meet the following criteria:

Find such interventions appealing

Express anxiety or fear

May benefit from avoiding or reducing drug therapy

Are likely to experience and need to cope with a prolonged interval of postoperative pain

Have incomplete pain relief after use of pharmacological interventions.

Acupressure.   Based on the theory of Asian medicine that a life force, in the form of energy, circulates throughout the body in well-defined cycles, **acupressure** opens congested energy pathways to promote a healthier state. Nurse therapists learn the energy pathways or body meridians and apply pressure over particular points along the pathways. For example, if a client has a headache, pressure over the Hoku point (Figure 42-11) will relieve the discomfort. As the pressure points are touched, the nurse begins to feel a subtle sensation or pulse under the fingers. At first, the pulses at various points will feel different, but as they continue to be held, they come into balance. Once the points are balanced, the nurse gently removes the fingers. Many simple acupressure techniques can be taught to clients for primary pain prevention. A complete acupressure session takes about 1 hour.

Relaxation and Guided Imagery.   Clients can alter affective-motivational and cognitive pain perception through relaxation and guided imagery. **Relaxation** is mental and physical freedom from tension or stress. Relaxation techniques provide individuals with self-control when discomfort or pain occurs, reversing the physical and emotional stress of pain. Relaxation techniques can be used at any phase of health or illness.

Clients who use relaxation techniques successfully experience several physiological and behavioral changes (Box 42-11). Relaxation techniques include meditation, yoga, Zen, guided imagery, and progressive relaxation exercises.

For effective relaxation, the individual's participation and cooperation are needed. Relaxation techniques are taught only when the client is not in acute discomfort because the inability to concentrate makes the exercise ineffective. The nurse explains the technique in detail and describes common sensations the client may experience (e.g., a decrease in temperature or numbness of a body part). The client should use these sensations as feedback.

The nurse is a coach, guiding the client slowly through steps of the exercise. The environment should be free of noises or other irritating stimuli. The client may sit in a

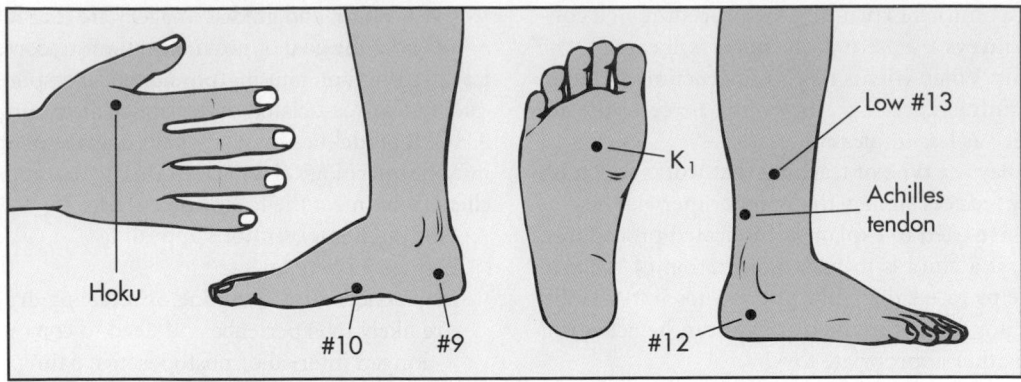

Figure 42-11 Examples of pressure points used in acupressure.
From Edelman CL, Mandle CL: *Health promotion throughout the lifespan,* ed 4, St. Louis, 1998, Mosby.

Effects of Relaxation	Box 42-11

Decreased pulse, blood pressure, and respirations
Decreased oxygen consumption
Decreased muscle tension
Decreased metabolic rate
Heightened global awareness
Lack of attention to environmental stimuli
No voluntary change of position
Sense of peace and well-being
Deep, wakeful, restful period of alertness

Body Positions for Relaxation	Box 42-12

SITTING
Sit with entire back resting against back of chair.
Place feet flat on floor.
Keep legs separated.
Hang arms at the side or rest on chair arms.
Keep head aligned with spine.

LYING
Keep legs separated with toes pointed slightly outward.
Rest arms at sides without touching sides of body.
Keep head aligned with spine.
Use thin, small pillow under head.

comfortable chair or lie in bed (Box 42-12). A light sheet or blanket for warmth often helps the client feel more comfortable. The client may use guided imagery and relaxation exercises together or separately.

In **guided imagery** the client creates an image in the mind, concentrates on that image, and gradually becomes less aware of pain. The nurse coaches the client in forming the image and concentrating on the sensory experience. Initially the nurse asks the client to think of a pleasant scene or experience that promotes the use of all the senses. The client describes the image and the nurse records it so that it can be used during later exercises. The nurse uses specific information given by the client and does not make changes in the client's image. The following is an example of a portion of a guided imagery exercise:

> Imagine yourself lying on a cool bed of grass with the sounds of rushing water from a nearby stream. It's a balmy day. You turn to see a patch of blue wildflowers in bloom and can smell their fragrance.

The nurse sits closely enough to the client to be heard but is not intrusive. The nurse's calm, soft voice helps the client focus more completely on the suggested image. While relaxing, the client focuses on the image, and it becomes unnecessary for the nurse to speak continuously. If the client shows signs of agitation, restlessness, or discomfort, the nurse should stop the exercise and begin later when the client is more at ease.

Progressive relaxation of the entire body takes about 15 minutes. The client pays attention to the body, noting areas of tension. Tense areas are replaced with warmth and relaxation. Some clients relax better with their eyes closed. Soft background music can help.

Progressive relaxation exercise involves a combination of controlled breathing exercises and a series of contractions and relaxation of muscle groups. The client begins by breathing slowly and diaphragmatically, allowing the abdomen to rise slowly and the chest to expand fully. When the client establishes a regular breathing pattern, the nurse coaches the client to locate any area of muscular tension, to think about how it feels, to tense muscles fully, and then completely to relax them. This creates the sensation of removing all discomfort and stress. Gradually the client can relax the muscles without first tensing them. When full relaxation is achieved, pain perception is lowered and anxiety toward the pain experience becomes minimal. The following is an example of how a nurse coaches a client:

> Let's begin by finding as comfortable a position as possible. Arms at your side . . . legs uncrossed. . . . Move until you feel at ease. . . . Take a deep breath. Feel your stomach and chest slowly rise. . . . Relax. . . . Now breathe out slowly . . . slowly . . . and relax.
>
> Count to 4, inhaling on 1 and 2, exhaling on 3 and 4. . . . Continue to breathe slowly. . . . Your body is beginning to relax. . . . Think "relax." . . . Feel the parts of your body. . . . Notice any tension in your muscles. . . . Continue to breathe slowly . . . and relax.
>
> Concentrate on your face . . . your jaws . . . your neck. . . . Notice any tightness. . . . Breathe in warmth and relaxation. . . . Concentrate on any tension in your hands. . . . Notice how it feels. . . . Now make a fist, a tight fist! As you begin to exhale, relax your fist. . . . Good! Notice how your hand feels. . . . Think "relax." . . . Your hand feels warm . . . heavy or light. . . . Just relax more . . . and more. Now focus on your forearms. . . . Notice any tension. . . . Relax your arms. . . . Feel your body relaxing. . . . Let the feelings of relaxation spread from your fingers and hands through the muscles of your arms.

If the client becomes agitated or uncomfortable, the nurse stops the exercise. If the client seems to have difficulty relaxing any part of the body, the nurse slows the progression of the exercise and concentrates on the tensed body part. The client must also know from the beginning that the exercise can be stopped at any time. With practice the client can soon perform relaxation exercises independently.

Distraction. The reticular activating system inhibits painful stimuli if a person receives sufficient or excessive sensory input. With meaningful sensory stimuli, a person can ignore or become unaware of pain. Pleasurable stimuli cause the release of endorphins. Persons who are bored or in isolation have only their pain to think about and thus perceive it more acutely. Distraction directs a client's attention to something else and thus can reduce the awareness of pain and even increase tolerance. There is one disadvantage. If it works, health care personnel or family may question the existence or severity of the pain. Distraction may work best for short, intense pain lasting a few minutes, such as during an invasive procedure or while waiting for an analgesic to work.

The nurse assesses activities enjoyed by the client that may act as distractions. These might include singing, praying, describing photos or pictures aloud, listening to music, and playing games. Most distractions can be used in a hospital, home, or long-term care facility.

Music. One effective distraction is music, which decreases physiological pain, stress, and anxiety by diverting the person's attention away from the pain and creating a relaxation response. The nurse can use music creatively in many clinical situations. Clients generally prefer to perform (play an instrument or sing a song) or listen to mu-

sic. Music that initially matches a person's mood is usually best. Classical, popular, and nontraditional music (music with no vocals, periods of silence) is used in music therapy. Popular music does not usually produce a deep level of relaxation because it is short with a steady beat and words. Music produces an altered state of consciousness through sound, silence, space, and time. It must be listened to for at least 15 minutes to be therapeutic. In an acute care setting, listening to music can be highly effective in reducing a client's postoperative pain (Box 42-13).

Biofeedback. **Biofeedback** is a behavioral therapy that involves giving individuals information about physiological responses (e.g., blood pressure or tension) and ways to exercise voluntary control over those responses (NIH, 1986). The therapy is used to produce deep relaxation and is especially effective for muscle tension and migraine headaches. When headaches are treated, electrodes are attached externally over each temple. The electrodes measure skin tension in microvolts. A polygraph machine visibly records the tension level for the client to see. The client learns to achieve optimal relaxation using feedback from the polygraph while lowering the actual level of tension experienced. The therapy takes several weeks to learn. Biofeedback can stop headaches and lessen the risk of development of future headaches.

Self-Hypnosis. Hypnosis can help alter pain perception through the influence of positive suggestion. A holistic health approach, self-hypnosis uses self-suggestion and images of relaxation and peace. The person enters the relaxation state using a variety of seed thoughts and then conditions a certain response to them (Edelman and Mandle, 1998). Self-hypnosis is like daydreaming. The intense concentration reduces apprehension and stress as a person concentrates on only one thought.

Using Music to Control Pain   Box 42-13

Match musical selections to the client's taste. Consider age and background.

Use earphones to avoid annoying other clients or staff and help client to concentrate on music.

Be sure controls on the radio, CD, or tape player are easy to press, manipulate, and distinguish.

Have family members bring tapes or CDs from home.

If pain is acute, increase the volume of the music. As pain decreases, reduce the volume.

If background music is provided, select general types suited to the client's preferences.

Have the client concentrate on the music and emphasize rhythm by tapping fingers or patting the thigh.

Avoid interruptions by dimming lights and closing the drapes or door.

Leave clients alone as they listen to the music.

Reducing Pain Perception. One simple way to promote comfort is by removing or preventing painful stimuli (Box 42-14). This is especially important for clients who are immobilized or unable to sense discomfort. Pain can also be prevented by anticipating painful events. For example, a client who is allowed to become constipated may suffer from distention and abdominal cramping. The nurse actively intervenes to ensure that the normal elimination process continues. Before performing procedures, the nurse considers the client's condition, aspects of the procedure that may be uncomfortable, and techniques to avoid causing pain. For example, in a client with severe arthritic knee pain, the nurse knows that any extreme flexion of the knee causes much pain. Before walking the client to the bathroom, the nurse makes sure that an elevated toilet seat is available. The client can then be seated and can rise with minimal discomfort. It takes only simple consideration of the client's comfort and a little extra time to avoid pain-producing situations.

Cutaneous Stimulation. **Cutaneous stimulation** is the stimulation of the skin to relieve pain. A massage, warm bath, ice bag, and transcutaneous electrical nerve stimulation (TENS) are simple ways to reduce pain perception. The specific way in which cutaneous stimulation works is unclear. One suggestion is that it causes release of endorphins, thus blocking the transmission of painful stimuli. The gate-control theory suggests that cutaneous stimulation activates larger, faster-transmitting A-beta sensory nerve fibers. This decreases pain transmission through small-diameter A-delta and C fibers. Synaptic gates close to the transmission of pain impulses. Meek (1993) suggests that touch and massage are sensory integration techniques that influence autonomic nervous system activity. When a person perceives touch to be relaxing, the relaxation response is elicited.

Controlling Painful Stimuli in the Client's Environment   Box 42-14

Tighten and smooth wrinkled bed linen.

Position tubing on which client is lying.

Loosen constricting bandages (unless specifically applied as a pressure dressing).

Change wet dressings and linens.

Position client in anatomical alignment.

Check temperature of hot or cold applications, including bathwater.

Lift client in bed—do not pull.

Position client correctly on bed pan.

Avoid exposing skin or mucous membranes to irritants (e.g., urine, stool, wound drainage).

Prevent urinary retention by keeping Foley catheters patent and free flowing.

Prevent constipation with fluids, diet, and exercise.

An advantage to cutaneous stimulation is that the measures can be used in the home, giving clients and families some control over pain symptoms and treatment. The proper use of cutaneous stimulation can reduce pain perception and help to reduce muscle tension that might otherwise increase pain.

When using cutaneous stimulation methods, the nurse eliminates sources of environmental noise, helps the client to assume a comfortable position, and explains the purpose of the therapy. Cutaneous stimulation should not be used directly on sensitive skin areas (e.g., burns, bruises, skin rashes, inflammation, and underlying bone fractures).

Cold and heat applications (see Chapter 47) relieve pain and promote healing. The selection of heat versus cold interventions varies with clients' conditions. For example, moist heat can help relieve the pain from a tension headache, and cold applications can reduce the acute pain from inflamed joints. When using any form of heat or cold application, the nurse instructs the client to avoid injury to the skin by checking the temperature and avoiding direct application of the cold or hot surface to the skin. Especially at risk are clients with spinal cord or other neurological injury, older adults, and confused clients.

Ice massage and application of cold packs are two types of cold therapy that are particularly effective for pain relief. Ice massage involves the use of a large ice cube or a small paper cup filled with water and frozen (water rises out of the cup as it freezes to create a smooth surface of ice for massage). The massage is simple. A nurse or the client can apply the ice with firm pressure to the skin, followed by a slow, steady, circular massage over the area. Cold may be applied near the pain site, on the opposite side of the body corresponding to the pain site, or on a site located between the brain and the pain site. It takes 5 to 10 minutes to apply cold. Each client responds differently to the site of application that is most effective. Application near the actual site of pain tends to work best. A client feels cold, burning, and aching sensations and numbness. When numbness occurs, the ice should be removed. Cold is particularly effective for tooth or mouth pain when ice is placed on the web of the hand between the thumb and index finger. This point on the hand is an acupuncture point that apparently influences nerve pathways to the face and head. Cold applications are also effective before invasive needle punctures.

Another form of cutaneous stimulation, sometimes called counterstimulation, is **transcutaneous electrical nerve stimulation (TENS),** involving stimulation of the skin with a mild electrical current passed through external electrodes. The therapy requires a physician's order. The TENS unit consists of a battery-powered transmitter, lead wires, and electrodes. The electrodes are placed directly over or near the site of pain. Hair or skin preparations should be removed before attaching the electrodes. When a client feels pain, the transmitter is turned on and a buzzing or tingling sensation is created. The client may adjust the intensity and quality of skin stimulation. The tingling sensation can be applied until pain relief occurs. TENS is effective for postsurgical pain control and reduction of pain caused by postoperative procedures.

Acute Care

Pharmacological Pain-Relief Interventions.   There are several pharmacological agents that provide pain management, and all require a physician's order to administer.

The nurse's judgment in the use and management of these medications helps ensure the best pain relief possible.

Acute Pain Management.   Nurses care for clients who have acute pain due to invasive procedures (e.g., surgery, endoscopy) or trauma. The AHCPR (1992) has established a pain treatment flow chart (Figure 42-12) for the aggressive treatment of postoperative pain and pain from medical procedures and trauma. The systematic approach

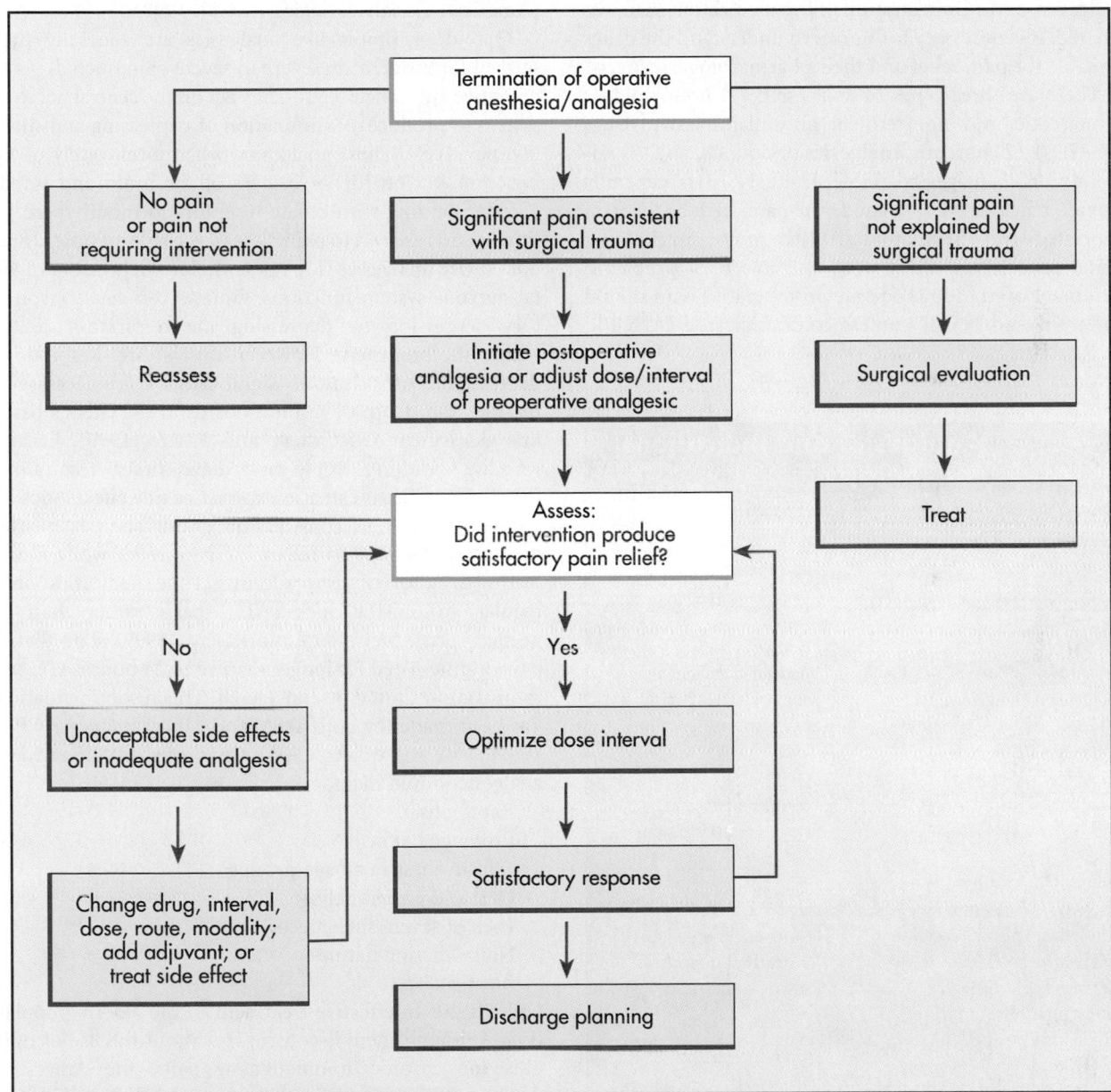

Figure 42-12   Pain treatment flow chart: postoperative phase.
From Agency for Health Care Policy and Research, Acute Pain Management Guideline Panel: *Acute pain management: operative or medical procedures and trauma*, Clinical Practice Guideline, AHCPR Pub No. 92-0032, Rockville, Md, 1992, Agency for Health Care Policy and Research, Public Health Service, U.S. Department of Health and Human Services.

ensures quick response on the part of caregivers to client discomfort. The key to success is ongoing evaluation of interventions: Is relief obtained? Are there any unacceptable side effects from the medications? It is the responsibility of the health care team to collaborate to find the combination of therapy that works best for a client.

Analgesics. **Analgesics** are the most common method of pain relief. Although analgesics can effectively relieve pain, nurses and physicians still tend to undertreat clients because of incorrect drug information, concerns about addiction, anxiety over errors in using narcotic analgesics, and administration of less medication than was ordered. It is necessary for nurses to understand the drugs available for pain relief and their pharmacological effects.

There are three types of analgesics: (1) nonopioid or nonnarcotic and nonsteroidal antiinflammatory drugs (NSAIDs), (2) **narcotic analgesics** or **opioids,** and (3) adjuvants or coanalgesics (Table 42-8). NSAIDs generally provide relief for mild to moderate pain, such as the pain associated with rheumatoid arthritis, minor surgical and dental procedures, episiotomy, and low back problems. Treatment of mild to moderate postoperative pain should begin with an NSAID unless contraindicated (AHCPR,

1992). Although the exact mechanism of action is unknown, NSAIDs are believed to act by inhibiting the synthesis of prostaglandins (Paice, 1994) and by inhibiting the cellular responses during inflammation. Most NSAIDs act on peripheral nerve receptors to reduce transmission and reception of pain stimuli. Unlike opioids, NSAIDs do not cause sedation or respiratory depression, nor do they interfere with bowel or bladder function (AHCPR, 1992). Chronic NSAID use in the older client, though, is associated with more frequent adverse effects and should be avoided. Mild to moderate musculoskeletal pain in older adults is effectively managed with acetaminophen (American Geriatrics Society [AGS], 1998).

Opioid or opioid-like analgesics are generally prescribed for moderately severe to severe pain, such as postoperative and cancer pain. They act on the central nervous system to produce a combination of depressing and stimulating effects. These analgesics, when given orally or by injection, act on higher centers of the brain and spinal cord by binding with opiate receptors to modify perception of and reaction to pain. One of the risks of opioid and opioid-like analgesics is the potential for depression of vital nervous system functions. Opiates can cause respiratory depression by depressing the respiratory center within the brainstem. However, this is rare. Respiratory depression is only clinically significant if it is a decrease in the rate and depth of respirations from the client's baseline assessment (McCaffery and Pasero, 1999). Clients who are breathing deeply rarely have clinical respiratory depression. Clients can also experience side effects such as nausea, vomiting, constipation, and altered mental processes. One way to maximize pain relief while minimizing drug toxicity is to administer the medication on a regular around-the-clock (ATC) basis rather than as needed (prn). McCaffery and Pasero (1999) state that if pain is anticipated for longer than 12 to 24 hours, ATC administration should be considered. This recommendation has been made for both acute and cancer pain (AHCPR, 1992; Jacox and others, 1994). Characteristics of an ideal analgesic should include:

Rapid onset
Prolonged effectiveness
Effectiveness in all age-groups
Oral and parenteral use
Lack of severe side effects
Nonaddicting nature
Inexpensive

Opioids are an effective treatment in the elderly population. Although there is controversy about the use of opioids for chronic nonmalignant pain, the American Geriatrics Society (AGS, 1998) does feel that opioids are probably not used enough with older persons. The AGS suggests a "start low" and "go slow" philosophy.

The proper use of analgesics requires careful assessment, application of pharmacological principles, and common sense (Box 42-15). A person's response to an

Table 42-8	**Analgesics and Indications for Therapy**
Drug Category	**Indications**
Nonnarcotic Analgesics	
Acetaminophen (Tylenol)	Mild postoperative pain
Acetylsalicylic acid (aspirin)	Fever
NSAIDs	Dysmenorrhea
Ibuprofen (Motrin, Nuprin)	Vascular headaches
Naproxen (Naprosyn)	Rheumatoid arthritis
Indomethacin (Indocin)	Soft tissue athletic injury
Tolmetin (Tolectin)	Gout
Piroxicam (Feldene)	
Ketorolac (Toradol)	Postoperative pain
	Severe traumatic pain
Narcotic Analgesics	
Meperidine (Demerol)	Cancer pain (except
Methylmorphine (codeine)	meperidine)
Morphine sulfate	Myocardial infarction
Fentanyl (Sublimaze)	Postoperative pain
Butorphanol (Stadol)	
Hydromorphone HCL (Dilaudid)	
Adjuvants	
Amitriptyline (Elavil)	Anxiety
Hydroxyzine (Vistaril)	Depression
Chlorpromazine (Thorazine)	Nausea
Diazepam (Valium)	Vomiting

| Nursing Principles for Administering Analgesics | Box 42-15 |

KNOW THE CLIENT'S PREVIOUS RESPONSE TO ANALGESICS

Determine whether relief was obtained.

Ask whether a nonnarcotic was as effective as a narcotic.

Identify previous doses and routes of administration to avoid undertreatment.

Determine whether the client has allergies.

SELECT PROPER MEDICATIONS WHEN MORE THAN ONE IS ORDERED

Use nonnarcotic analgesics or milder narcotics for mild to moderate pain.

Know that nonnarcotics can be alternated with narcotics.

In older adults, avoid combinations of narcotics.

Remember that morphine and hydromorphone are the narcotics of choice for long-term management of severe pain.

Know that injectable medications act quicker and can relieve severe, acute pain within 1 hour and that oral medication may take as long as 2 hours to relieve pain.

Use a narcotic with a nonnarcotic analgesic for severe pain because such combinations treat pain peripherally and centrally.

For chronic pain, give an oral drug for sustained relief.

KNOW THE ACCURATE DOSAGE

Remember that doses at the upper end of normal are generally needed for severe pain.

Adjust doses, as appropriate, for children and older clients.

ASSESS THE RIGHT TIME AND INTERVAL FOR ADMINISTRATION

Administer analgesics as soon as pain occurs and before it increases in severity.

Do not give analgesics only by ordered schedules. Remember that an around-the-clock (ATC) administration schedule is usually best.

Give analgesics before pain-producing procedures or activities.

Know the average duration of action for a drug and the time of administration so that the peak effect occurs when the pain is most intense.

---

analgesic is highly individualized. An NSAID may be as effective as a potent opioid for some clients, or an orally administered analgesic may bring the same relief as an injectable form. Nurses must stay familiar with comparative doses of different analgesics. In addition, nurses must know the route of administration most effective for a client so that controlled, sustained pain relief is achieved.

The nurse should always know the comparative potencies of analgesics in oral and injectable form. If nurses on succeeding shifts choose different routes for the same doses, the client will not receive the same level of analgesia, and pain control will be poor. Nurses must provide controlled, sustained pain relief. Equianalgesic charts that convert recommended adult doses to children's doses are available. These charts consider age and body size. Older adults also require special considerations

Adjuvants such as sedatives, antianxiety agents, and muscle relaxants enhance pain control or relieve other symptoms associated with pain, such as depression and nausea. They may be given alone or with analgesics. Sedatives are often prescribed to chronic pain sufferers. These drugs can cause drowsiness and impairment of coordination, judgment, and mental alertness. Misuse of sedatives and antianxiety agents is a serious health problem that can cause disabling illness behaviors.

Patient-Controlled Analgesia.   Clients benefit from having control over pain therapy. When clients depend on nurses for **analgesia,** an erratic cycle of alternating pain and analgesia often occurs. The client feels pain and asks for medication, but the nurse must first assess the client and then prepare the medication. Within an hour, analgesia finally occurs, but pain relief may last only 30 minutes, and the client may be sedated as long as an hour. Then, gradually, the client again feels discomfort, and the cycle begins again.

A drug delivery system called **patient-controlled analgesia (PCA)** is a safe method for postoperative, traumatic, and cancer pain management that most clients prefer to intermittent injections. It is a drug delivery system that allows clients to self-administer pain medications without risk of overdose. The goal is to maintain a constant plasma level of analgesic so that the problems of as-needed (prn) dosing are avoided. Systemic PCA usually involves IV drug administration, but it can also be given subcutaneously. PCAs are portable infusion pumps (usually computerized), containing a chamber for a syringe (Figure 42-13) or bag that delivers a small, preset dose of medication. To receive a dose, the client pushes a button attached to the PCA device. The system is designed to deliver no more than a specified number of doses either every hour or every 4 hours (depending on the pump) to avoid overdoses. A typical PCA prescription relies on a series of "loading" doses (e.g., 3 to 5 mg of morphine) repeated every 5 minutes until initial postoperative pain diminishes. A low-dose infusion (basal rate) of 0.5 to 1 mg/hr may be programmed to deliver a steady dose of continuous medication. On-demand doses typically add 1 mg morphine every 6 minutes, with a total hourly limit of 10 mg (AHCPR, 1992). Most pumps have locked safety sys-

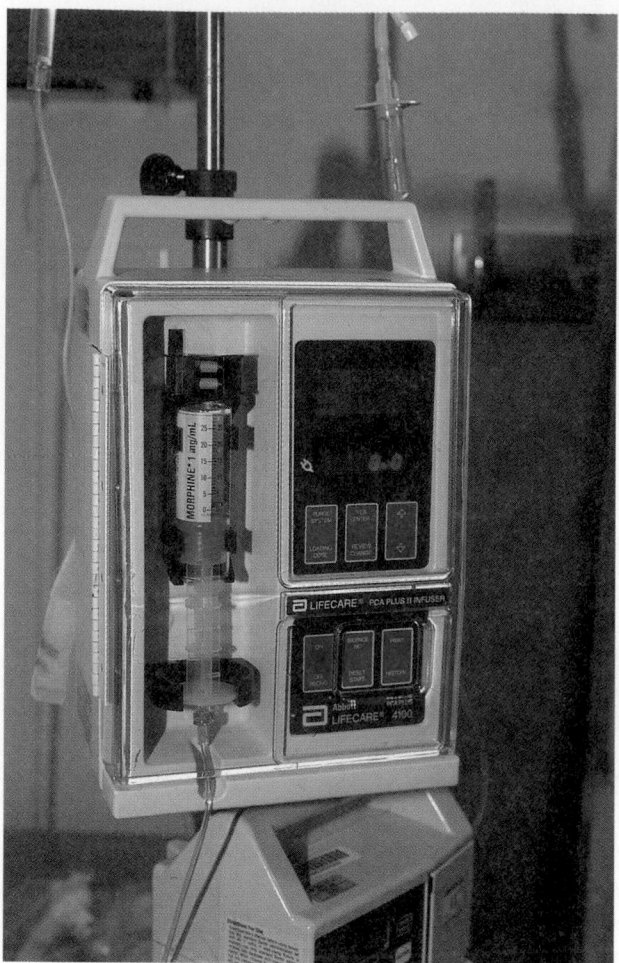

Figure 42-13 PCA infusion pump.

tems that prevent tampering by clients or their family members and are generally safe to be managed in the home.

There are many benefits to PCA use. The client gains control over pain, and pain relief does not depend on nurse availability. Clients can also access medication when they need it. This can decrease anxiety and lead to decreased medication use. Small doses of medications are delivered at short intervals, stabilizing serum drug concentrations for sustained pain relief. Client preparation and teaching is critical to the safe and effective use of PCA devices (Box 42-16). Clients must be able to understand the use of the equipment and be physically able to locate and press the button to deliver the dose. Clients who are confused and unresponsive, those with neurological disease, and those with impaired renal or pulmonary function are not candidates for PCA.

Nurses must check the IV line and PCA device regularly to ensure proper functioning. Even though clients control administration of analgesics, the nurse must routinely check that the PCA device operates correctly. The

nurse also documents drug dosages and tracks any waste of medications.

Local and Regional Anesthetics.   **Local anesthesia** is the loss of sensation to a localized body part. Physicians use local anesthesia while suturing a wound, delivering an infant, and performing simple surgery. Local anesthetics can be applied topically on skin and mucous membranes or injected to anesthetize a body part. The drugs produce temporary loss of sensation by inhibiting nerve conduction; they also block motor and autonomic functions when administered as nerve blocks. Local anesthetics block the function of sensory, motor, and autonomic neurons supplying the affected area. Thus when the client temporarily loses sensation in a body part, motor and autonomic function is also lost. Smaller sensory nerve fibers are more sensitive to local anesthetics than are large motor fibers. As a result, the client loses sensation before losing motor function, and conversely, motor activity returns before sensation.

Local anesthetics can cause side effects, depending on their absorption into the circulation. Itching or burning of the skin or a localized rash is common after topical applications. Application to vascular mucous membranes increases the chance of systemic effects, such as a change in heart rate. Injection of anesthetics increases the risk of systemic side effects, depending on the amount of drug used and the area injected.

Table 42-9 summarizes the types of local anesthesia by injection. Each produces a different level of anesthesia as a result of the amount of anesthetic used and location of the spinal nerve affected.

The nurse provides emotional support to clients receiving local anesthesia by explaining insertion sites and warning clients that they will temporarily lose sensory function. It is common for clients to fear paralysis because epidural and spinal injections come close to the spinal cord. Autonomic function (bowel and bladder control) may also be temporarily lost. To reassure the client, the nurse explains application of the anesthetic and the sensations experienced. Injection can be painful unless the physician numbs the injection site. The nurse prepares clients for such discomfort. Before a client receives an anesthetic, the nurse checks for allergies. To monitor systemic effects, the nurse assesses blood pressure and pulse. Spinal anesthesia may also cause respiratory changes.

After administration of a local anesthetic, the nurse protects the client from injury until full sensory and motor function return. Pain is a protective mechanism. Until a local anesthetic is absorbed and metabolized, the client must be careful in using an anesthetized body part. Clients can easily injure themselves without knowing it. For example, after an injection into a joint, the nurse warns the client to avoid using the joint until function returns. For clients with topical anesthesia, the nurse avoids applying heat or cold to numb areas. After spinal anesthesia the

OBJECTIVES
- Client will be able to explain purpose of PCA in managing pain.
- Client will use the PCA device correctly.
- Client achieves pain control.

TEACHING STRATEGIES
- Teach the use of PCA before any procedure so that clients can understand how to use it after awakening from anesthesia or sedation. Reinforce as needed.
- Instruct client on the purpose of PCA, emphasizing that the client controls medication delivery.

- Explain that the pump prevents the risk of overdose.
- Tell family members or friends that they should not operate the PCA device for the client.
- Have the client demonstrate use of the PCA delivery button.

EVALUATION
- Ask client to tell you the purpose of the PCA device.
- Observe the client administering a dose.
- Evaluate the severity of the client's pain 15 to 20 minutes after use of the PCA device.

Table 42-9   Local Anesthesia Techniques

Type	Area of Injection	Area Anesthetized	Indications for Use
Infiltration	In superficial area under skin or mucous membranes	Small peripheral nerves to area infiltrated	Small incisions of skin, insertion of sutures to close cuts or wounds, minor dental repairs
Peripheral nerve block	In area surrounding large peripheral nerve at point above bifurcation of nerve	Wider area than with infiltration, numbing entire body part (e.g., hand, upper gums, foot)	Major dental repairs, manipulation or reduction of extremity fractures, minor hand and foot surgery
Epidural or peridural nerve block	In lumbosacral region of spinal cord, around major nerve roots exiting base of spinal cord at site outside dura mater	Lower trunk and extremities	Delivery of newborn, major surgery to lower trunk and extremities (e.g., hemorrhoidectomy, appendectomy, vascular repair)
Spinal nerve block	Around major nerve root within subarachnoid space of spinal cord	Lower trunk and extremities	Major surgery to lower trunk and extremities, clients at risk with general anesthesia

client stays in bed until sensory and motor function return. The nurse assists the client during the first attempt at getting out of bed.

Epidural Analgesia.   Epidural analgesia is a form of local anesthesia and an effective therapy for the treatment of acute postoperative pain, labor and delivery pain, and chronic pain, especially that associated with cancer (McNair, 1990). It permits control or reduction of severe pain without the more serious sedative effects of parenteral or oral narcotics. (However, intraspinal morphine can produce the same side effects of nausea, mental clouding, and sedation, since it is absorbed into the circulation of the epidural vascular plexus.) Epidural analgesia can be short or long term, depending on the client's condition and life expectancy. Short-term therapy is used for pain after intrathoracic, abdominal, and orthopedic surgery. Long-term therapy is used for intractable pain in the

lower part of the body, particularly when it is bilateral (DuPen and Williams, 1992). McNair (1990) lists several advantages of epidural analgesia, including the following:

Production of excellent analgesia

Occurrence of minimal sedation

Action of long duration

Facilitation of early ambulation

Avoidance of repeated injections

No significant effect on sensation

Little effect on blood pressure or heart rate

Epidural analgesia is administered into the spinal **epidural space.** The physician inserts a blunt-tip needle into the level of the vertebral interspace nearest to the area requiring analgesia. When the needle reaches the space, solutions may be freely injected and small catheters may be passed into it. Once a catheter is advanced into the epidural space (Figure 42-14) and the needle is removed, the remainder of the catheter is secured with a dressing and taped up the back of

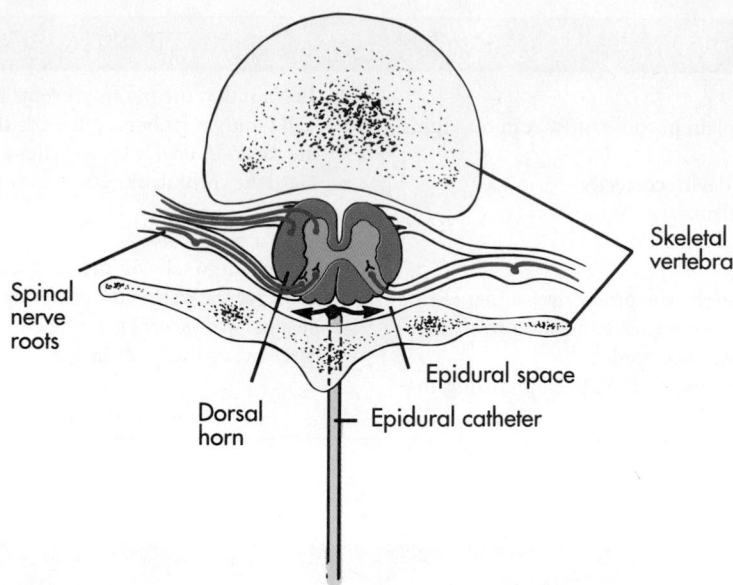

Figure 42-14   Anatomical drawing of epidural space.

the client (Figure 42-15). If the catheter is only temporary, it is connected to tubing positioned along the spine and over the client's shoulder. The end of the catheter can then be placed on the client's chest for the nurse's access.

The catheter is connected to a continuous epidural infusion pump, a port, or reservoir or is capped off for bolus injections. To reduce the risk of accidental epidural injection of drugs intended for IV use, the catheter should be clearly labeled "epidural catheter." Continuous infusions must be administered through electronic infusion devices for proper control. Because of the catheter location, strict surgical asepsis is needed to prevent a serious and potentially fatal infection. Physicians are notified immediately of any signs or symptoms of infection or pain at the insertion site. Thorough nursing care is needed during hygiene procedures to keep the catheter system clean and dry.

Nurses receive special training for the administration of epidural analgesia. Opioids used commonly for epidural analgesia include preservative-free morphine sulfate, fentanyl, sufentanil, and hydromorphone. The medications act like the neurotransmitter enkephalin, an endorphin, blocking transmission of pain stimuli in the spinal cord (McNair, 1990).

Frequently a local anesthetic such as bupivacaine is also administered. The anesthetic blocks pain conduction through local peripheral nerve fibers around the site of insertion. Bupivacaine also blocks the sympathetic nervous system, causing side effects such as hypotension, reduced intestinal peristalsis, and bladder dysfunction.

The nursing implications for managing epidural analgesia are numerous (Table 42-10). Monitoring of medications' effects differs, depending on whether infusions are intermittent or continuous. Complications of epidural

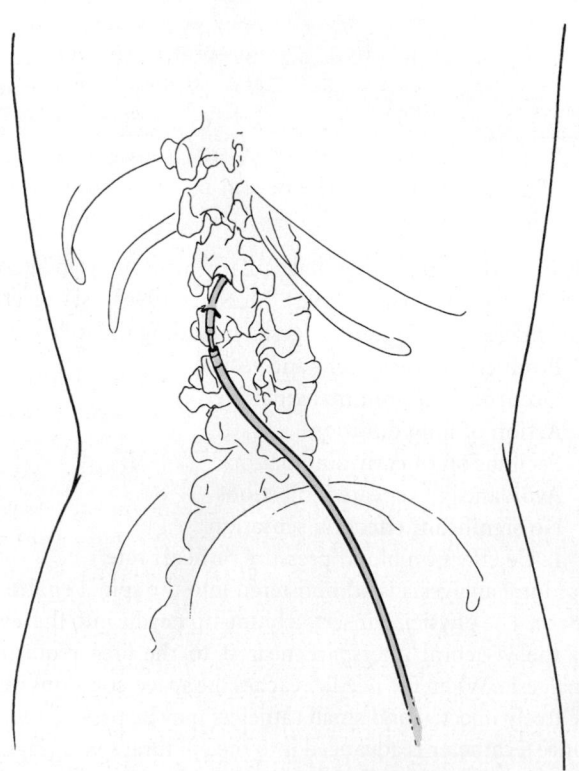

Figure 42-15   Epidural catheter.

Table 42-10 Nursing Care for Clients With Epidural Infusions

Goal	Actions
Prevent catheter displacement.	Secure catheter (if not connected to implanted reservoir) carefully to outside skin.
Maintain catheter function.	Check external dressing around catheter site for dampness or discharge. (Leak of cerebrospinal fluid may develop.)
	Use transparent, adhesive dressing to aid inspection.
	Inspect catheter for breaks.
Prevent infection.	Use strict aseptic technique when caring for catheter (see Chapter 33).
	Do not routinely change dressing over site.
	Change tubing every 24 hours.
Monitor for respiratory depression.	Monitor vital signs, especially respirations, per policy.
	Pulse oximetry and apnea monitoring may be used.
Prevent undesirable complications.	Assess for pruritis (itching) and nausea and vomiting.
	Administer antiemetics as ordered.
Maintain urinary and bowel function.	Monitor intake and output.
	Assess for bladder and bowel distention.
	Assess for discomfort, frequency, and urgency.

opioid use include nausea and vomiting, urinary retention, constipation, respiratory depression, and **pruritus.** When clients are receiving epidural analgesia, monitoring occurs as often as every 15 minutes, including assessment of respiratory rate, respiratory effort, and skin color. Once stabilized, monitoring can move to every hour (refer to agency policy). The client must receive thorough education about epidural analgesia in terms of the action of the medication and its advantages and disadvantages. Clients should know about the potential for side effects and should be instructed to notify a health care provider if they develop. If the client requires long-term epidural use, a permanent catheter may be tunneled through the skin and exit at the client's side. A client on long-term therapy can be taught to safely administer infusions in the home with minimal ongoing intervention by the nurse.

Surgical Interventions for Pain Relief.   When a client's pain persists despite medical treatment, surgical interventions may give relief. Neurosurgical treatment is appropriate for clients in whom more conservative treatment is neither tolerated nor effective (Jacox and others, 1994). The risks include new pain symptoms from nerve damage or nerve division, recurrence of pain, and postoperative neurological impairment. Surgery involves resection of either peripheral nerve roots or pain pathways in the spinothalamic tract. For example, a **dorsal rhizotomy** involves surgically cutting the dorsal (posterior) nerve roots as they enter the spinal cord. It is effective for relieving localized acute pain in the area supplied by the nerve root and deep visceral pain. The client loses sensation of pain but retains full motor function. A **chordotomy** is more extensive and involves resection of the spinothalamic tract. The procedure is used to treat unrelieved pain. The risks of the procedure are great because permanent paralysis may result from edema of the spinal cord or ac-

cidental resection of motor nerves. After the procedure, the client has a permanent loss of pain and temperature sensation in the affected areas.

When nurses care for these clients, they need to be aware of the area of resection to assess for paresthesia, change in temperature sensation, and loss of motor function. When performed correctly, these procedures can relieve persistent pain without causing serious neurological deficits.

Cancer Pain Management.   Cancer pain can be chronic or acute. The AHCPR released clinical practice guidelines for the management of cancer pain (Jacox and others, 1994). The guidelines are designed to treat cancer pain in a more comprehensive and aggressive manner. Similarly, they provide clients and families more options for pain relief. Figure 42-16 is a flow chart depicting cancer pain management from assessment to various treatment options. The best choice of treatment often changes as the client's condition and the characteristics of pain change. Nonpharmacological interventions, as well as pharmacological interventions, can be used together.

Various medications and routes of administration can provide some relief for clients with cancer pain. There are relatively new oral analgesics with fewer side effects. Long-acting or controlled-release medications have been very successful in managing cancer pain. These controlled-released medications (MS Contin, Roxanol SR, and Oxycontin) can provide pain relief for 6 to 12 hours.

Although most cancer pain can be managed by using oral medications, there are times when other routes are needed. Epidural analgesia and intrathecal infusions (administration of opioids via catheters placed within the brain's ventricles) have been highly effective with select clients.

Studies show that drug dependence is low among

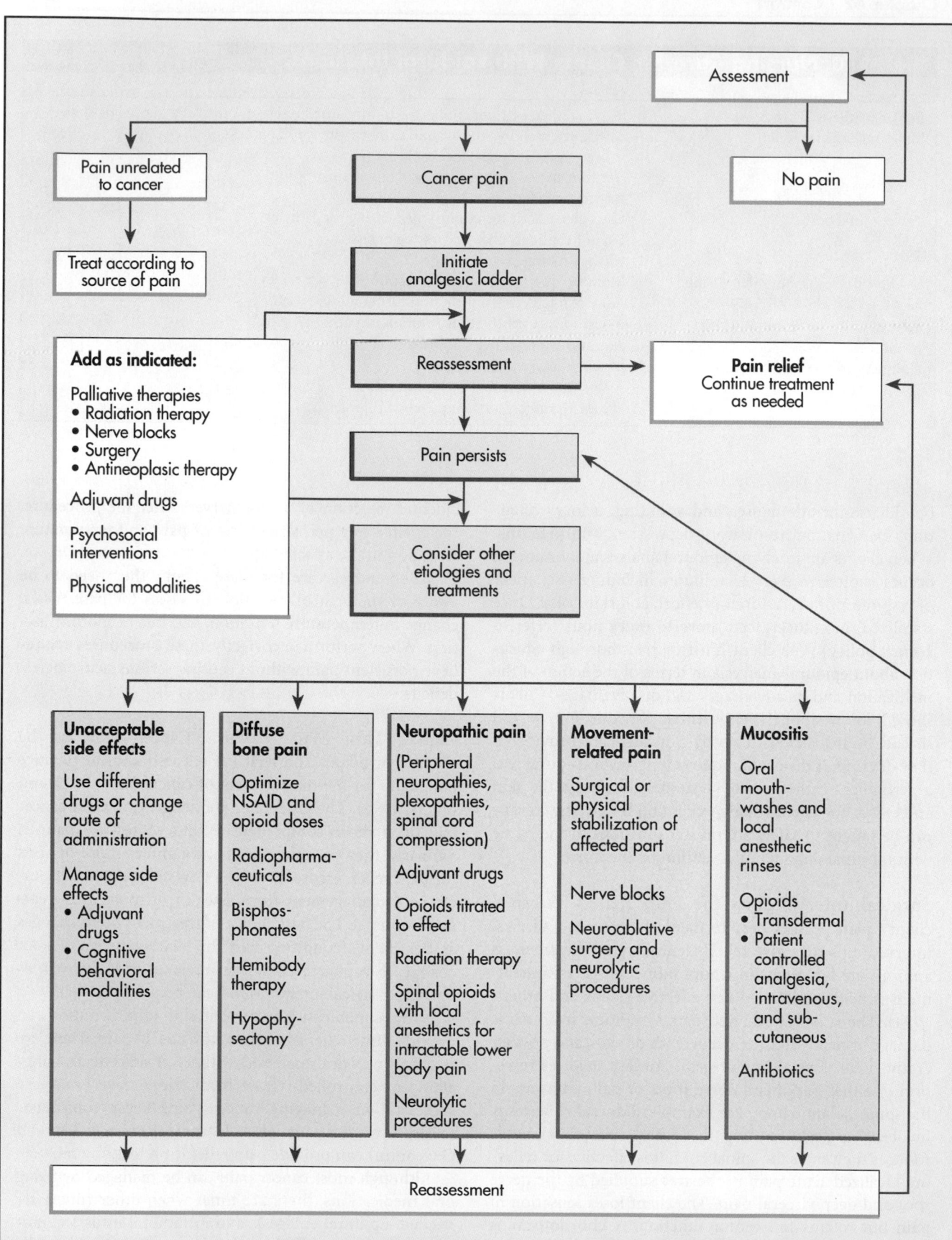

Figure 42-16 Flow chart: continuing pain management in patients with cancer.
From Jacox A and others: *Management of cancer pain*, Clinical Practice Guideline No. 9, AHCPR Pub
No. 94-0592, Rockville, Md, 1994, Agency for Health Care Policy and Research, Public Health
Service, U.S. Department of Health and Human Services.

clients with cancer-related pain. It has also been shown that terminally ill clients with prolonged pain can develop a tolerance to analgesics. As a result, clients require higher doses of analgesics to attain pain relief. Higher analgesic doses in clients who have become tolerant to narcotics are not lethal because these clients also develop a tolerance to life-threatening side effects.

For clients with cancer, the aim of drug therapy may be to anticipate and minimize pain rather than cure it. It is therefore necessary to give required doses on a regular basis. Prescribing analgesics on a prn basis for cancer clients is ineffective and causes more suffering. The cancer client must take an analgesic regularly, even when the pain, nausea, and other symptoms subside. Regular administration maintains blood levels for ongoing pain control.

Administering analgesics to treat cancer-related pain requires applying principles different from those used to treat acute pain. The World Health Organization (WHO, 1990) recommends a three-step approach to managing cancer pain (Figure 42-17). Basically, therapy begins with using NSAIDs and/or adjuvants and progresses to strong opioids if pain persists. When a client with cancer first experiences pain, it is best to begin with a higher dosage than will be needed for relief. The physician can slowly decrease the dosage to the amount needed, thus providing the client with immediate pain relief. In addition, there is aggressive treatment of the side effects of analgesia, such as nausea and constipation, so that analgesia can be continued. Clients can become tolerant to the side effects of nausea but not to the constipating effects of analgesics. Therefore clients should have prescribed medication routinely administered both to prevent and to treat constipation.

Transdermal drug systems administer drugs such as fentanyl at predetermined rates for up to 48 to 72 hours.

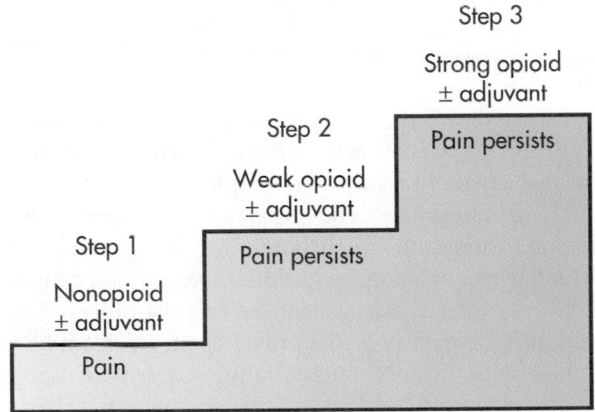

Figure 42-17 WHO analgesic ladder is a three-step approach to using drugs in cancer pain management. ± *adjuvant*, With or without adjuvant medications.
From World Health Organization: *Cancer pain relief and palliative care: report of a WHO expert committee*, WHO Tech Rep Series No. 804, Geneva, 1990, The Organization.

This route is useful when clients are unable to take drugs orally. Clients find these systems easy to use, and they allow for continuous opioid administration without needles or pumps. Self-adhesive patches release the medication slowly over time, achieving effective analgesia. Caution is needed in administering transdermal patches to clients who are hyperthermic. Hyperthermia causes more rapid drug absorption. A transmucosal fentanyl has been developed that is placed in the client's mouth between the cheek and lower gum. Medication is absorbed over a 15-minute period and needs to be left intact and not chewed.

Analgesics may be given rectally when clients have nausea and vomiting or are fasting before or after surgery (Jacox and others, 1994). The route is contraindicated if clients have diarrhea or if cancerous lesions involve the anus or rectum. Morphine, hydromorphone, and oxymorphone are available in suppositories. Pharmacies may be able to put other medication in a gel capsule for rectal use.

Another way to treat severe cancer pain is morphine sulfate administered by continuous IV drip or intermittently by a PCA pump. Continuous infusions or a basal rate on a PCA device provide improved, uniform pain control with fewer peaks and valleys in plasma concentration, more effective drug action, and lower drug dosages overall. The intramuscular route should be rarely used for controlling cancer pain. Candidates for continuous infusions include clients with severe pain, for whom oral and injectable medications provide minimal relief; clients with severe nausea and vomiting; and clients unable to swallow oral medications.

Continuous-drip morphine sulfate is given in acute care settings and in the home. The morphine sulfate is delivered by an infusion-control pump to ensure a safe, accurate, and steady rate of infusion. Each agency has guidelines for morphine dose and infusion rates. The drug can cause numerous side effects that initially require the nurse's ongoing assessment. Clients receiving the drug at home are taught how to monitor the drug's effects.

Adjuvant drugs, such as antiemetics, corticosteroids, anticonvulsants, neuroleptics, biphosphonates, calcitonin (given for bone pain), or antidepressants may be needed to enhance pain control and prevent side effects (Paice, 1991; Jacox and others, 1994).

When a client is first given continuous-drip morphine sulfate, it is essential that the IV access be patent and that the IV site be without complications (see Chapter 40). A central line catheter such as a Groshong or Hickman catheter, an implanted venous access port, or a peripherally inserted central catheter is usually best suited for long-term IV infusion. When IV access is poor, the subcutaneous route with a concentrated dose is possible. When infusions begin, the client continues to be monitored. Clients who are placed on continuous analgesic infusions are not usually opioid naive, and thus respiratory depression is rare.

In the home, clients may use ambulatory infusion

pumps. State-of-the-art ambulatory pumps are small devices, often no larger than a deck of cards, that contain a 1- to 30-day supply of medication. The pumps are lightweight and allow free movement. The pump is battery powered and worn in a pouch attached to a belt or harness. The bag of medication and IV fluid fits inside the pump.

Although the pumps are programmed by physicians, pharmacists, or nurses, clients or families must be highly motivated to care for the pump properly. The client must show the capacity to learn the procedures and to assume responsibility for proper pump operation (Bernstein and others, 1993). In addition, it is important that the client have the physical capabilities to make adjustments to the pump (e.g., change batteries). The client and family learn to manage the pump, to observe for side effects, and to maintain function of the central venous catheter. Because the client is initially managed with opioids in the hospital before going home, the risk of side effects is not as great unless the client or family member increases the dosage. A home health care nurse makes routine visits to ensure that the client manages the pump correctly. The IV fluid bag and tubing are changed routinely by the nurse. This maintains the sterility of the system.

The nurse uses all available pain-relief measures for the client with cancer. The nurse-client relationship can help the client adapt to chronic pain. The client must feel that those responsible for managing the pain are competent and dependable.

The barriers to effective pain management can be complex, as in the case of a lack of organizational commitment to pain work. Similarly pain management can be as simple as providing health care workers with formal education about pain. One of the deep-seeded and often inappropriate fears shared by health care providers and clients is the fear of addiction when long-term opioid use is prescribed to manage pain. There is a difference between dependence, tolerance, and addiction. There needs to be continued clarification of the differences. Experiencing a physical dependency does not necessarily imply addiction, and tolerance in and of itself does not constitute addiction (Box 42-17) (McCaffery and Pasero, 1999).

Restorative Care
Pain Clinics and Hospices.
During the last decade, health professionals from the United States and Canada have recognized pain as a significant health problem. With an increased awareness of the multiple problems that pain can cause for clients, programs have been designed for pain management. Pain clinics may offer several options. A comprehensive pain center can treat persons on an inpatient or outpatient basis. Staff members representing all health care disciplines, such as nursing, medicine, physical therapy, pastoral care, and dietetics, work with clients to find the most effective pain-relief measures. A comprehensive clinic can provide not only diverse therapy but also research into new treatments and training for professionals.

Definitions Related to the Use of Opioids in Pain Treatment   Box 42-17

The Committee on Pain of the American Society of Addiction Medicine recognizes the following definitions as appropriate and clinically useful definitions and recommends their use when assessing the use of opioids in the context of pain treatment.

PHYSICAL DEPENDENCE

Physical dependence on an opioid is a physiological state in which abrupt cessation of the opioid, or administration of an opioid antagonist, results in a withdrawal syndrome. Physical dependency on opioids is an expected occurrence in all individuals in the presence of continuous use of opioids for therapeutic or for nontherapeutic purposes. It does not, in and of itself, imply addiction.

TOLERANCE

Tolerance is a form of neuroadaptation to the effects of chronically administered opioids (or other medications), which is indicated by the need for increasing or more frequent doses of the medication to achieve the initial effects of the drug. Tolerance may occur both to the analgesic effects of opioids and to the unwanted side effects such as respiratory depression, sedation or nausea. The occurrence of tolerance is variable, but it does not, in and of itself, imply addiction.

ADDICTION

Addiction in the context of pain treatment with opioids is characterized by a persistent pattern of dysfunctional opioid use that may involve any or all of the following:
Adverse consequences associated with the use of opioids
Loss of control over the use of opioids
Preoccupation with obtaining opioids despite the presence of adequate analgesia

From McCaffery M, Pasero C: *Pain: clinical manual, ed 2*, St. Louis, 1999, Mosby; modified from Hoffman NG, Halikas J, Mee-Lee Y: *Patient placement criteria for the treatment of psychoactive substance use disorders*, Chevy Chase, Md, 1991, American Society of Addiction Medicine.

Hospices are programs for care of the terminally ill. The term *hospice* comes from the Latin word *hospes,* which means "a place to rest." Often, hospice programs are affiliated with hospitals. The programs help terminally ill clients continue to live at home in comfort and privacy with the help of a hospice health care team. Pain control is a priority for hospices. Clients receive the proper dosage and form of analgesics that provide pain relief. Under the guidance of hospice nurses, families learn to monitor clients' symptoms and become the primary caregivers. A hospice client may become hospitalized in the event of a brief, acute care crisis or family problem.

EVALUATION
Client Care.   The evaluation of pain is one of many nursing responsibilities that requires effective criti-

cal thinking (Figure 42-18). The client's behavioral responses to pain-relief interventions are not always obvious. The nurse must be an intent observer and know what responses to anticipate on the basis of the type of pain, the intervention, the timing of the interventions, the physiological nature of the injury or disease, and the client's previous responses.

If the nurse assesses that a client continues to have discomfort after an intervention, it may be necessary to try a different approach. For example, if an analgesic provides only partial relief, the nurse may add relaxation exercises or guided-imagery exercises. The nurse may also consult with the physician about increasing the dosage, decreasing the interval between doses, or trying different analgesics.

The nurse also evaluates the client's perceptions of the effectiveness of interventions. The client may help decide the best times to attempt a treatment. In essence, the client is the best judge of whether an intervention works.

The nurse also assesses tolerance to therapy and the overall relief obtained. For example, if a nurse administers an analgesic, side effects from the medication and the client's reported pain relief must be assessed. Similarly, after turning a client, the nurse should return to determine whether the client is tolerating the new position and whether pain has subsided. If an intervention aggravates discomfort, the nurse stops it immediately and seeks an alternative. Time and patience are necessary to maximize the effectiveness of pain management. The nurse evaluates the entire pain experience to determine interventions that are most effective and times that they should be administered.

Client Expectations. The client, if able, is the best resource for evaluating the effectiveness of pain-relief measures. The nurse must continually assess whether the char-

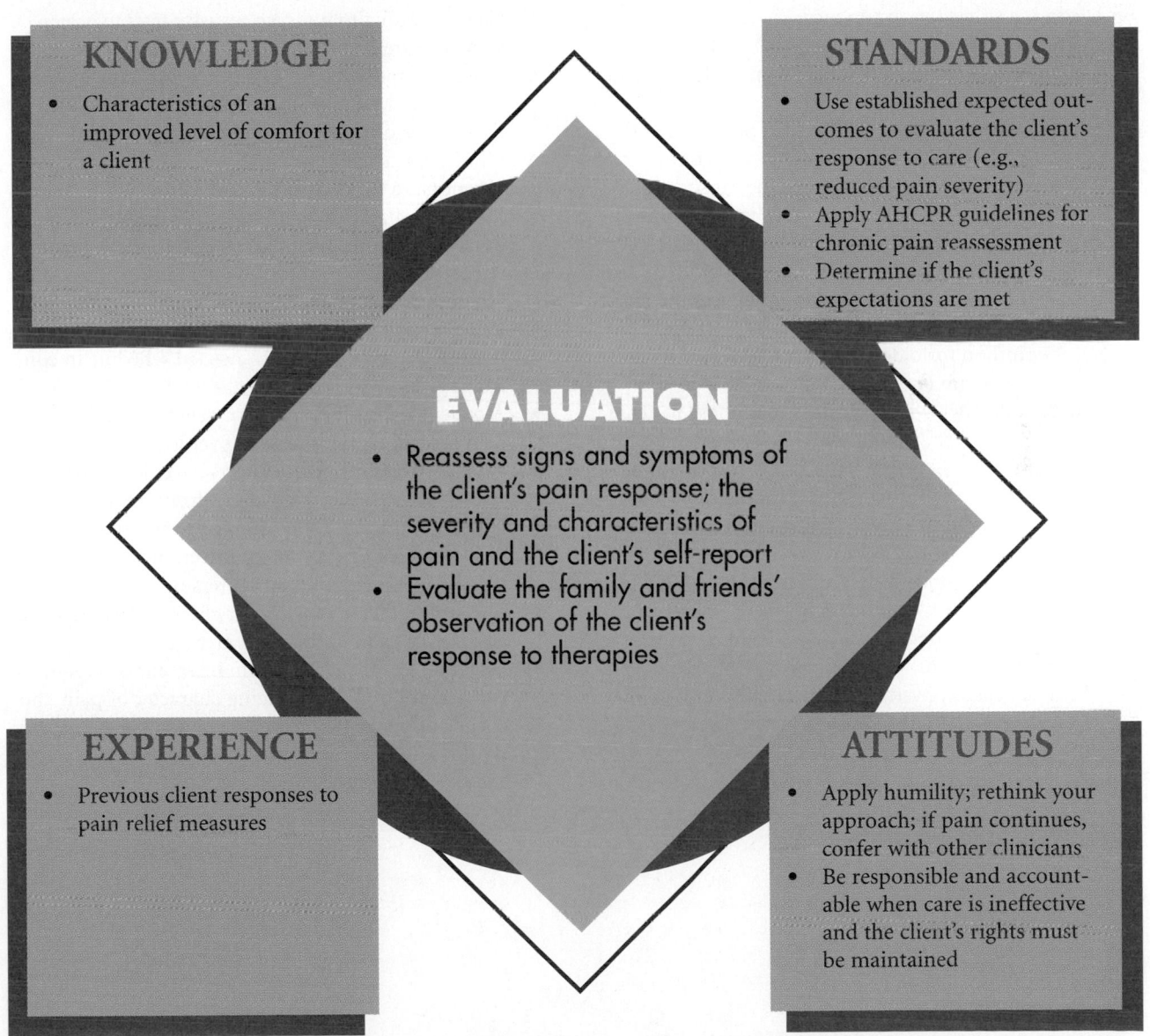

KNOWLEDGE

- Characteristics of an improved level of comfort for a client

STANDARDS

- Use established expected outcomes to evaluate the client's response to care (e.g., reduced pain severity)
- Apply AHCPR guidelines for chronic pain reassessment
- Determine if the client's expectations are met

EVALUATION

- Reassess signs and symptoms of the client's pain response; the severity and characteristics of pain and the client's self-report
- Evaluate the family and friends' observation of the client's response to therapies

EXPERIENCE

- Previous client responses to pain relief measures

ATTITUDES

- Apply humility; rethink your approach; if pain continues, confer with other clinicians
- Be responsible and accountable when care is ineffective and the client's rights must be maintained

Figure 42-18 *Synthesis Model for Comfort Evaluation Phase.*

acter of the client's pain changes and whether individual interventions are effective. The family often is another valuable resource, particularly in the case of the client with cancer who may not be able to express discomfort during the latter stages of terminal illness. The nurse is successful in treating pain when the client's expectations of pain relief are met. The nurse uses evaluative criteria in determining the outcome of pain-relief interventions.

Effective communication of a client's assessment of pain and his or her response to intervention is facilitated by accurate and thorough documentation. This communication needs to transpire from nurse to nurse, shift to shift, and nurse to other health care providers. It is the professional responsibility of the nurse caring for the client to report what has been effective for managing the client's pain. The client is not responsible for ensuring that this information is accurately transmitted. A variety of tools such as a pain flow sheet or diary will help centralize information about pain management. The client expects the nurse to be sensitive to his or her pain and to be diligent in attempts to manage that pain.

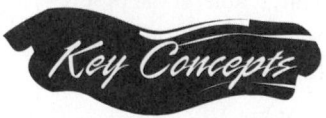

Key Concepts

- Pain is a subjective experience.
- A nurse's misconceptions about pain often result in doubt about the degree of the client's suffering and unwillingness to provide relief.
- Knowledge of the nociceptive pain processes of the pain experience—transmission, transduction, perception, and modulation—provides the nurse with guidelines for determining pain-relief measures.
- An interaction of psychological and cognitive factors affects pain perception.
- A person's cultural background influences the meaning of pain and how it is expressed.
- It is common for older clients not to report pain.
- Clients who are in chronic pain are likely to show more subtle behavioral changes than those in acute pain.
- The difference between acute and chronic pain involves duration of discomfort, physical signs and symptoms, and the client's perceptions regarding pain relief.
- The nurse does not collect an in-depth pain history when the client is experiencing severe discomfort.
- Pain scales are used to evaluate the effectiveness of pain interventions.
- Pain can cause physical signs and symptoms similar to the signs and symptoms of certain disease processes.

- Clients waiting to undergo invasive tests may gain some pain relief by anticipatory guidance.
- The nurse individualizes pain interventions by collaborating closely with the client, using assessment findings, and trying a variety of interventions.
- Eliminating sources of painful stimuli is a basic nursing measure for promoting comfort.
- Proper administration of analgesics requires the nurse to know the client's response to the drugs, to select the proper medication, and to administer an accurate dose in a timely manner.
- Using a regular schedule for analgesic administration is more effective than an as-needed schedule in controlling pain.
- A patient-controlled analgesic device gives clients pain control with low risk of overdose.
- While caring for a client who receives local anesthesia, the nurse protects the client from injury.
- Nursing implications for administering epidural analgesia include preventing infection and monitoring closely for respiratory depression.
- The aim of therapy for cancer clients is to anticipate and prevent pain rather than treat it.
- Evaluation of the client's pain interventions requires consideration of the changing character of pain, the client's response to interventions, and the client's perceptions of a therapy's effectiveness.

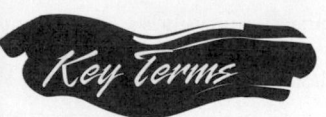

Key Terms

Critical Thinking Exercises

1. John is a 32-year-old construction worker who sustained an injury to the lumbar region of his back during a fall approximately 8 months ago. John is 6 feet tall and weighs 280 pounds. He continues to report pain intensity as a 5 (on a scale of 0 to 10), increasing with activity; he has limited flexibility and is unable to return to work. He has recently been admitted for treatment at a comprehensive pain clinic. What interventions might the health care team employ?

2. Alexis is a 3-year-old admitted to the pediatric unit for a third-degree burn to her right lower extremity. What tools might be useful when assessing this child's pain?

3. You are caring for an unconscious client who was involved in an automobile accident and sustained multiple injuries. The client has several lacerations, wounds, and surgical incisions, as well as multiple lines and tubes. What measures might you take to promote the client's comfort?

4. Mary Beth Jones, a 55-year-old woman with metastatic breast cancer to the bone, has been receiving IV morphine sulfate (MSO_4) for a week for severe back and leg pain. Her frequently increased infusion of MSO_4 is not reducing her pain to an acceptable level, and she is becoming increasingly sedated. What other pharmacological interventions might be considered?

References

Agency for Health Care Policy and Research, Acute Pain Management Guideline Panel: *Acute pain management: operative or medical procedures and trauma,* Clinical Practice Guideline, AHCPR Pub No. 92-0032, Rockville, Md, 1992, Agency for Health Care Policy and Research, Public Health Service, U.S. Department of Health and Human Services.

American Geriatrics Society Panel on Chronic Pain in Older Persons: Clinical practice guidelines, *J Am Geriatr Soc* 46(5):636, 1998.

Anand KJS: The applied physiology of pain. In Anand KJS, McGrath PJ, editors: *Pain in neonates,* Amsterdam, 1993, Elsevier.

Anand KJS: Analgesia and sedation in ventilated neonates, *Neonatal Respir Dis* 5:1, 1995.

Anand KJS, Craig KD: New perspectives on the definition of pain, *Pain* 67:3, 1996.

Association for Holistic Health: *Statement on holistic health practitioners,* San Diego, Calif, 1981, The Association.

Bernstein LH and others: Portable medicine pumps in primary care, *Patient Care* 27:91, 1993.

Beyer JE and others: The creation, validation, and continuing development of the Oucher: a measure of pain intensity in children, *J Pediatr Nurs* 7(5):335, 1992.

Bostrom M: Summary of the Mayday fund survey: public attitudes about pain and analgesics, *J Pain Symptom Manage* 13(3):166, 1997.

Butler RN, Gastel B: Care of the aged: perspectives on pain and discomfort. In Ng LK, Bonica J, editors: *Pain, discomfort and humanitarian care,* New York, 1980, Elsevier.

Calvillo ER, Flaskerud JH: Review of literature on culture and pain of adults with focus on Mexican-Americans, *J Transcult Nurs* 2(2):16, 1991.

Clarke EB and others: Pain management knowledge, attitudes, and clinical practice: the impact of nurses' characteristics and education, *J Pain Symptom Manage* 11(1):18, 1996.

Copp LA: The spectrum of suffering, *Am J Nurs* 90:35, 1990.

Craig KD: The facial display of pain in infants and children. In Finley GA, McGrath PJ, editors: Measurement of pain in infants and children, *Prog Pain Res Manage* 10:103, 1998.

Donahue P: *Nursing: the finest art,* St. Louis, 1989, Mosby.

DuPen SL, Williams AR: Management of patients receiving combined epidural morphine and bupivacaine for the treatment of cancer pain, *J Pain Symptom Manage* 7(2):125, 1992.

Edelman CL, Mandle CL: *Health promotion throughout the lifespan,* ed 4, St. Louis, 1998, Mosby.

Foley KM: Pain syndromes in patients with cancer. In Bonica JJ, Ventafriddaz V, editors: *International symposium on pain of advanced cancer, Venice, 1978: advances in pain research and therapy,* New York, 1979, Raven Press.

Gil K: Psychologic aspects of acute pain, *Anesthesiol Rep* 2(2):246, 1990.

Grunau RVE, Whitfield M, Petrie J: Pain sensitivity and temperament in extremely low-birth-weight premature toddlers and preterm and full-term controls, *Pain* 58:341, 1994.

Grunau RVE and others: Early pain experience, child and family factors, as precursors of somatization: a prospective study of extremely premature and full-term children, *Pain* 56:353, 1994.

Harkins SW, Price DD: Assessment of pain in the elderly. In Turk DC, Malzack R, editors: *The handbook of pain assessment,* New York, 1992, Guilford Press.

Harkins SW, Price DD: Are there special needs for pain assessment in the elderly? *APS Bull* 3:1, January/February 1993.

Harkins SW and others: Geriatric pain. In Wall PD, Melzack R, editors: *Textbook of pain,* London, 1994, Churchill Livingstone.

Hoffman NG, Halikas J, Mee-Lee Y: *Patient placement criteria for the treatment of psychoactive substance use disorders,* Chevy Chase, Md, 1991, American Society of Addiction Medicine.

Horgas AL, Tpai PF: Analgesic prescription and use in cognitively impaired nursing home residents, *Nurs Res* 47(4):235, 1998.

International Association for the Study of Pain, Subcommittee on Taxonomy: Pain terms: a list with definitions and notes on usage, *Pain* 6:249, 1979.

Jacox A and others: *Management of cancer pain,* Clinical Practice Guideline No. 9, AHCPR Pub No. 94-0592, Rockville, Md, 1994, Agency for Health Care Policy and Research, Public Health Service, U.S. Department of Health and Human Services.

Kolcaba KY: Holistic comfort: operationalizing the construct as a nurse-sensitive outcome, *Adv Nurs Sci* 15(1):1, 1992.

Mahon SM: Concept analysis of pain: implications related to nursing diagnoses, *Nurs Diag* 5(1):14, 1994.

Marzinski LR: The tragedy of dementia: clinically assessing pain in the confused, nonverbal elderly, *J Gerontol Nurs* 17(6):25, 1991.

Max MB, Portenoy RK: Methodological challenges for clinical trials of cancer pain treatments. In Chapman CR, Foley KM editors: *Current and emerging issues in cancer pain: research and practice,* New York, 1993, Raven Press.

McCaffery M: *Nursing management of the patient with pain,* ed 2, Philadelphia, 1979, JB Lippincott.

McCaffery M, Pasero C: *Pain: clinical manual,* ed 2, St. Louis, 1999, Mosby.

McCance KL, Huether SE: *Pathophysiology: the biologic basis for disease in adults and children,* ed 3, St. Louis, 1998 Mosby.

McCloskey JC, Bulechek GM: *Nursing interventions classification (NIC),* ed 3, St. Louis, 2000, Mosby.

McGuire DB: Comprehensive and multidimensional assessment and measurement of pain, *J Pain Symptom Manage* 7(5):312, 1992.

McMillian SC: Pain and pain relief experienced by hospice patients with cancer, *Cancer Nurs,* 19:298, 1996.

McNair ND: Epidural narcotics for postoperative pain: nursing implications, *J Neurosci Nurs* 22(5):275, 1990.

Meek SS: Effects of slow-stroke back massage on relaxation in hospice clients, *Image J Nurs Sch* 25(1):17, 1993.

Melzack R, Wall PD: Pain mechanisms: a new theory, *Science* 150:971, 1965.

Mottola C: Measurement strategies: the visual analog scale, *Decubitus* 6(5):56, 1993.

National Institutes of Health Consensus Development Panel: New gains against pain, *Emerg Med,* p 143, November 1986.

Paice JA: Unraveling the mystery of pain, *Oncol Nurs Forum* 18(5):843, 1991.

Paice JA: *The physiology and pharmacologic management of pain: physiology of pain: unraveling the mystery,* Baltimore, 1994, Williams & Wilkins.

Portenoy RK: Neuropathic pain. In Portenoy RK, Kanner RM, editors: *Pain management: theory and practice,* Philadelphia, 1996, FA Davis.

Ryan P, Vortherms R, Ward S: Cancer pain: knowledge, attitudes of pharmacologic management, *J Gerontol Nurs* 20(1):7, 1994.

Salerno E, Willens JS: *Pain management handbook: an interdisciplinary approach,* St. Louis, 1996, Mosby.

Stevens B: Pain assessment in children: birth through adolescence. In Weisman S, editor: Pain management in children, *Child Adolesc Psychiatr Clin North Am,* p 725, 1997.

Stevens B: Composite measures of pain. In Finley GA, McGrath PJ editors: Measurement of pain in infants and children, *Prog Pain Res Manage* 10:161, 1998.

Taddio A and others: Effect of circumcision on pain responses during vaccination in male infants, *Lancet* 345:291, 1995.

Taddio A and others: Neonatal circumcision and pain response during routine vaccination 4 to 6 months later, *Lancet* 349:599, 1997.

Vallerand AH: Gender differences in pain, *Image J Nurs Sch* 27(3), 235, 1995.

Villarruel AM: Mexican-American cultural meanings, expressions, self-care and dependent-care actions associated with experiences of pain, *Res Nurs Health* 18:427, 1995.

Walker AC and others: Impact of culture on pain management: an Australian nursing perspective, *Holistic Nurs Pract* 9(2):48, 1995.

Willens J: Introduction to pain management. In Salerno E, Willens J, editors: *Pain management handbook: an interdisciplinary approach.* St. Louis, 1996, Mosby.

Wong DL and others: *Whaley and Wong's nursing care of infants and children,* ed 6, St. Louis, 1999, Mosby.

Wong DL, Baker CM: Pain in children: comparison of assessment scales, *Okla Nurse* 33(1):8, 1988.

World Health Organization: *Cancer pain relief and palliative care, report of a WHO expert committee,* WHO Tech Rep Series No. 804, Geneva, 1990, The Organization

Yaster M and others: *Pediatric pain management and sedation handbook,* St. Louis, 1997, Mosby.

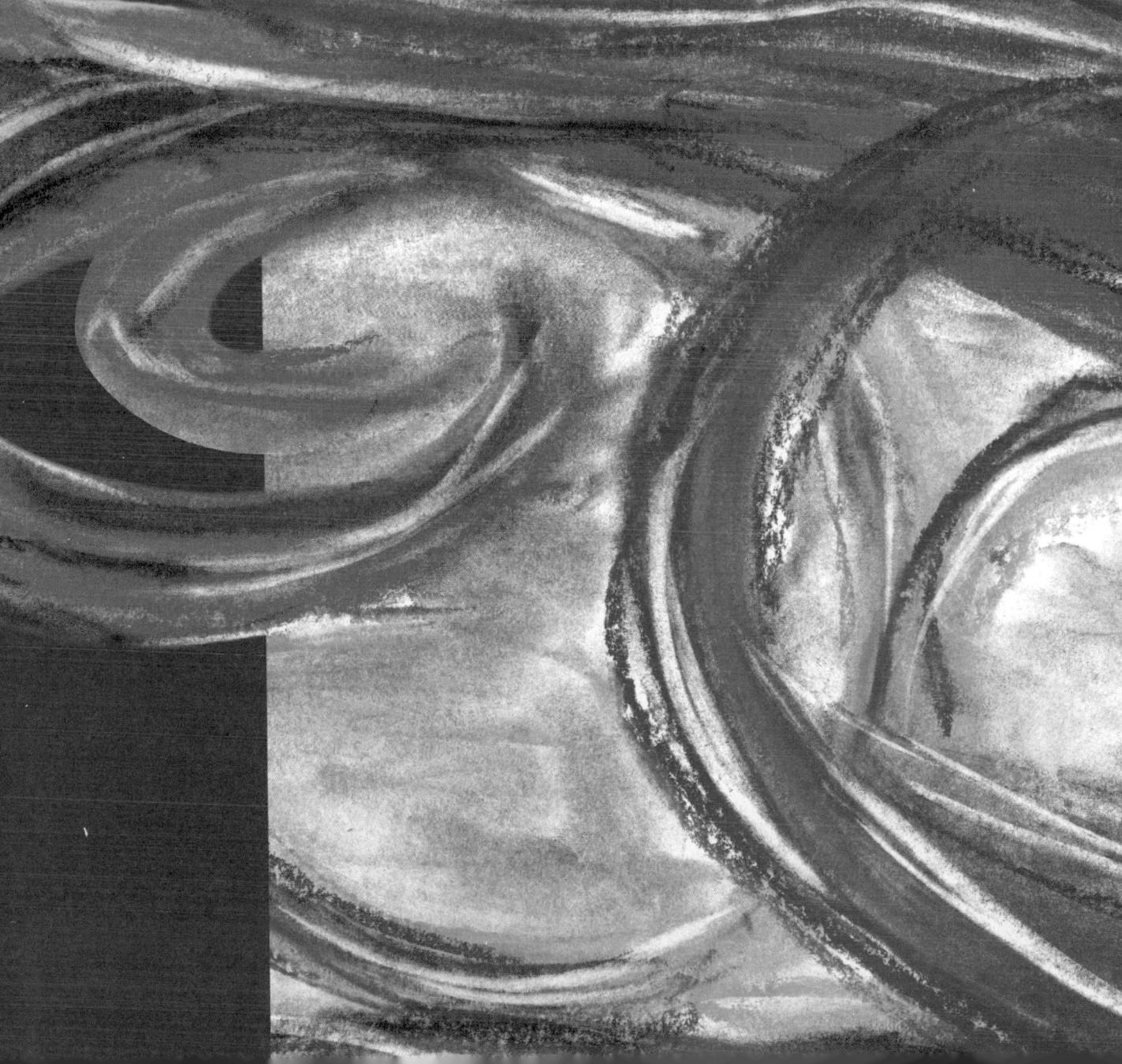

43

Nutrition

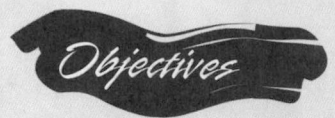

Objectives

Mastery of content in this chapter will enable the student to:

- Define the key terms listed.
- Explain why each major nutrient is necessary for nutrition.
- Explain the importance of a balance between energy intake and energy requirements.
- List the end products of carbohydrate, protein, and fat metabolism.
- Explain the significance of saturated, unsaturated, and polyunsaturated fats.
- Describe the food guide pyramid and the healthy eating index and discuss their value in planning meals for good nutrition.
- Explain dietary reference intakes.
- List seven dietary guidelines for health promotion.
- Explain the variance in nutritional requirements throughout growth and development.
- Discuss the major methods of nutritional assessment.
- Identify three major nutritional problems and describe clients at risk.
- State the goals of enteral and parenteral nutrition.
- Describe the procedure for initiating and maintaining tube feedings.
- Describe the methods to avoid complications of tube feedings.
- Describe the methods to avoid complications of parenteral nutrition.
- Discuss medical nutrition therapy in relation to three medical conditions.
- Discuss diet counseling and client teaching in relation to client expectations.

Food provides sustenance and also holds symbolic meaning. The giving or taking of food is part of ceremonies, social gatherings, holiday traditions, religious events, the celebration of birth, and the mourning of death. The difficulty of the decision to withdraw food in a terminal illness, even in the form of intravenous (IV) nutrients, is a testament to the symbolic power of food and feeding.

Florence Nightingale understood the importance of nutrition, stressing the nurse's role in the science and art of feeding during the mid-1800s (Dossey, 1999). Since then, the nurse's role in nutrition and diet therapy has changed. In the early nineteenth century, the description of a calorie as a unit of energy obtained from food moved nutrition into the realm of science (Stacey, 1994). Medical nutrition therapy (MNT) is now recognized as a disease-specific treatment modality when clients are at risk for malnutrition (American Academy of Family Physicians, 1997; Inman-Felton and Smith, 1997). In some illnesses, such as Type 1 diabetes mellitus or mild hypertension, diet therapy may be the major treatment for disease control. Other conditions, such as inflammatory bowel disease, may require specialized nutrition support such as enteral nutrition (EN) or parenteral nutrition (PN). Standards now exist that clearly designate the standard of care for promotion of optimal nutrition in all health care clients.

The authors acknowledge the contribution of Marsha Evans Orr to this chapter in the previous edition of this text.

Scientific Knowledge Base

NUTRIENTS: THE BIOCHEMICAL UNITS OF NUTRITION

The body requires fuel to provide energy for cellular metabolism and repair, organ function, growth, and body movement. An individual's energy requirements are influenced by several factors. The energy requirement of a person at rest is called the **basal metabolic rate (BMR)**. This is the energy needed to maintain life-sustaining activities (breathing, circulation, heart rate, and temperature) for a specific period of time. Factors such as age, body mass, gender, fever, starvation, menstruation, illness, injury, infection, activity level, or thyroid function affect energy requirements. The **resting energy expenditure (REE)** is a measurement that accounts for BMR plus energy to digest meals and perform mild activity. Resting energy expenditure (Table 43-1) is a baseline of energy requirement that accounts for approximately 60% to 75% of our daily needs. Factors that affect metabolism include illness, pregnancy, lactation, and activity level. In hospitals, energy requirements may be estimated by measuring oxygen consumption, carbon dioxide production, and nitrogen excretion by means of a metabolic chart.

In general, when energy requirements are completely met by kilocalorie (kcal) intake in food, weight does not change. When the kilocalories ingested exceed energy demands, a person gains weight. If the kilocalories ingested fail to meet energy requirements, a person loses weight.

Nutrients are the elements necessary for body processes and function. Energy needs are met from six cat-

Table 43-1	Resting Energy Expenditure (REE*), Median Heights/Weights, and Recommended Energy Intake						
Category	Age (years) Condition	Weight (kg)	Weight (lb)	Height (cm)	Height (in)	REE (kcal/day)	Multiples of REE†	Average Daily Allowance (kcal‡/day§)
Infants	0.0-0.5	6	13	60	24	320		650
	0.5-1.0	9	20	71	28	500		850
Children	1-3	13	29	90	35	740		1300
	4-6	20	44	112	44	950		1800
	7-10	28	62	132	52	1130		2000
Males	11-14	45	99	157	62	1440	1.70	2500
	15-18	66	145	176	69	1760	1.67	3000
	19-24	72	160	177	70	1780	1.67	2900
	25-50	79	174	176	70	1800	1.60	2900
	51+	77	170	173	68	1530	1.50	2300
Females	11-14	46	101	157	62	1310	1.67	2200
	15-18	55	120	163	64	1370	1.60	2200
	19-24	58	128	164	65	1350	1.60	2200
	25-50	63	138	163	64	1380	1.55	2200
	51+	65	143	160	63	1280	1.50	1900
Pregnant	First trimester							+0
	Second and third trimester							+300
Lactating								+500
Severe injury/illness								
	Burns ≥40% total body surface area							+750
	Sepsis, trauma, or head injury							

Modified from Grodner M, Anderson S, DeYoung S: *Foundations and clinical applications of nutrition: a nursing approach*, ed 2, St. Louis, 2000, Mosby.

*Resting energy expenditure is calculated based on United Nations Food and Agriculture Organization (FAO) equations, then rounded.

†Multiples of REE are factors of exercise, health status, or illness to multiply REE by to determine daily kilocalorie requirements.

‡Range of moderate activity, the coefficient of variation is ± 20%.

§Figure is rounded.

egories of nutrients: carbohydrates, proteins, fats, water, vitamins, and minerals. Water is a vital body component that acts as a solvent for metabolic processes. Vitamins and minerals do not provide energy but are essential to metabolic processes, including acid-base balance.

Foods are sometimes described according to their **nutrient density,** the proportion of essential nutrients to the number of kilocalories. High-nutrient-density foods, such as fruits and vegetables, provide a large number of nutrients in relationship to kilocalories. Low-nutrient-density foods, such as alcohol or sugar, are high in kilocalories but are nutrient poor.

Carbohydrates.
Carbohydrates are the main source of energy in the diet. Each gram of carbohydrate produces 4 kcals and serve as the main source of fuel (glucose) for the brain, skeletal muscles during exercise, erythrocyte and leukocyte production, and cell function of the renal medulla. Carbohydrates are obtained primarily from plant foods, except for lactose (milk sugar). Carbohydrates are classified according to their carbohydrate units, or **saccharides.** Monosaccharides such as glucose (dextrose) or

fructose cannot be broken down into a more basic carbohydrate unit. Disaccharides such as sucrose, lactose, and maltose are composed of two monosaccharides and water. Both monosaccharides and disaccharides are classified as **simple carbohydrates** and are found primarily in sugars. Polysaccharides such as glycogen are composed of many carbohydrate units and are classified as **complex carbohydrates.** They are insoluble in water and are digested to varying degrees. Starches are polysaccharides. Starch digestion consists of several steps (Table 43-2).

Some polysaccharides cannot be digested because humans do not have enzymes capable of breaking them down. **Fiber** has received attention as a dietary factor in disease prevention and treatment and prevention of diarrhea in tube-fed clients. Insoluble fibers are not digestible and include cellulose, hemicellulose, and lignin. Soluble fibers include pectin, guar gum, and mucilage.

Proteins.
Although proteins may provide a source of energy (4 kcal/g), they are essential for synthesis (building) of body tissue in growth, maintenance, and repair. Collagen, hormones, enzymes, immune cells, DNA, and

Table 43-2 **Summary of Carbohydrate Digestion**		
	Enzyme	Action
Mouth	Salivary:	
	1. Amylase	Starch........Dextrins.......Maltose
	2. Ptyalin	Starch........Dextrins.......Maltose
Stomach	None	Starch hydrolysis continues briefly.
Small intestine	Pancreatic:	
	1. Amylase	Starch........Dextrins......Maltose
	2. Amylopsin	Starch........Dextrins......Maltose
	Disaccharides:	
	1. Sucrase	Sucrose......Glucose + Fructose
	2. Lactase	Lactose......Glucose + Galactose
	3. Maltase	Maltose......Glucose + Glucose

From Williams SR: *Nutrition and diet therapy*, ed 8, St. Louis, 1997, Mosby.

RNA are all composed of protein. In addition, blood clotting, fluid regulation, and acid-base balance require proteins. Nutrients and many pharmacological substances are transported in the blood by proteins.

The simplest form of protein is the amino acid. **Essential amino acids** are those that the body cannot synthesize but must have provided in the diet. Others can be synthesized and are classified as **nonessential amino acids** (Table 43-3). **Amino acids** can be linked together to form dipeptides, tripeptides and oligopeptides. Albumin and insulin are simple proteins because they contain only amino acids or their derivatives. The combination of a simple protein with a nonprotein substance produces a complex protein, such as lipoprotein, formed by a combination of a lipid and a simple protein.

A complete protein contains all essential amino acids in sufficient quantity to support growth and maintain nitrogen balance. Ingestion of proteins is not primary for meeting energy needs but is most important for continued positive nitrogen balance. Complete proteins are also referred to as high-quality proteins. Incomplete proteins lack one or more of the nine essential amino acids and include cereals, legumes (beans, peas), and vegetables. **Complementary proteins** are pairs of incomplete proteins that when combined supply the total amount of protein provided by complete protein sources. Protein is 16% nitrogen and serves as the only source of nitrogen for the body. **Nitrogen balance** is achieved when the intake and output of nitrogen are equal. When the intake of nitrogen exceeds the output, the body is in positive nitrogen balance, which is required for growth, normal pregnancy, maintenance of lean muscle mass and vital organs, and wound healing. The nitrogen retained by the body is used for building, repair, and replacement of body tissues. Negative nitrogen balance occurs when the body loses more nitrogen than the body gains, for example, with infection, sepsis, burns, fever, starvation, head injury, and trauma. The increased nitrogen loss is the result of body-tissue destruction or loss of nitrogen-containing body flu-

Table 43-3 **Amino Acids Required in Nutrition**	
Essential Amino Acids	Nonessential Amino Acids
Arginine	Alanine
Histidine	Asparagine
Isoleucine	Aspartic acid
Leucine	Cystine (cysteine)
Lysine	Glutamic acid
Methionine	Glutamine
Phenylalanine	Glycine
Threonine	Hydroxylysine
Tryptophan	Proline
	Serine
	Tyrosine

From Williams SR: *Nutrition and diet therapy*, ed 8, St. Louis, 1997, Mosby.

ids. Nutrition during this period must provide nutrients to put patients into positive balance for healing.

Protein can be used to provide energy, but because of protein's essential role in growth, maintenance, and repair, adequate kilocalories should be provided in the diet from nonprotein sources. Protein is spared as an energy source when there is sufficient carbohydrate in the diet to meet the energy needs of the body. The required dietary intake of protein for adults is shown in Table 43-4. Additional protein is required during pregnancy and lactation (Food and Nutrition Board, 1992a).

Fats.   Fats (**lipids**) are the most calorically dense nutrient since they provide 9 kcal/g. Fats are composed of triglycerides and fatty acids. **Triglycerides** circulate in the blood and are made up of three fatty acids attached to a glycerol. **Fatty acids** are composed of chains of carbon and hydrogen atoms with an acid group on one end of the chain and a methyl group at the other. Synthesis of fatty acids is called **lipogenesis.** Fatty acids can be **saturated,** in

	Recommended Dietary Allowances and Adequate Intakes: Protein and Fat Soluble Vitamins									

Table 43-4

Age/Group	Weight (kg)	Weight (lb)	Height (cm)	Height (in)	Kcal per day	Protein (g)	Vitamin A RE	Vitamin D μg	Vitamin E mgαTE	Vitamin K μg
Infants										
0-6 mo	7	16	64	25	650	13	375	5	3	5
7-12 mo	9	20	72	28	850	14	375	5	4	10
Children										
1-3 yr	13	29	91	36	1300	16	400	5	6	15
4-8 yr	22	48	118	46	1800	24	500	5	7	20
Males										
9-13 yr	40	88	147	58	2500	45	1000	5	10	45
14-18 yr	64	142	174	68	3000	59	1000	5	10	65
19-30 yr	76	166	176	69	2900	58	1000	5	10	70
31-50 yr	79	174	176	69	2900	63	1000	5	10	80
Over 50 yr	77	170	173	68	2300	63	1000	10	10	80
Females										
9-13 yr	40	88	148	58	2200	46	800	5	8	45
14-18 yr	57	125	163	64	2200	44	800	5	8	55
19-30 yr	61	133	163	64	2200	46	800	5	8	60
31-50 yr	63	138	163	64	2200	50	800	5	8	65
Over 50 yr	65	143	160	63	1900	50	800	10	8	65
Pregnant					2200	60	800	5	10	65
Lactating					2700	65	1300	5	12	65

Data from Food and Nutrition Board: *Recommended dietary allowances*, ed 10, Washington, DC, 1989, National Academy Press; Food and Nutrition Board: *Dietary reference intakes for calcium, phosphorus, magnesium, vitamin D, and fluoride*, Washington, DC, 1997, National Academy Press; and Food and Nutrition Board: *Dietary reference intakes: thiamin, riboflavin, niacin, vitamin B6, folate, vitamin B12, pantothenic acid, biotin, and choline*, Washington, DC, 1998, National Academy Press.

which each carbon in the chain has two attached hydrogen atoms, or **unsaturated,** in which an unequal number of hydrogen atoms are attached and the carbon atoms attach to each other with a double bond. **Monounsaturated** fatty acids have one double bond, whereas **polyunsaturated** fatty acids have two or more double carbon bonds. The various types of fatty acids have significance for health and the incidence of disease and are referred to in dietary guidelines.

Fatty acids are also classified as essential or nonessential. Linoleic acid, an unsaturated fatty acid, is the only essential fatty acid in humans. Linolenic acid and arachidonic acid (also unsaturated fatty acids) are important for metabolic processes but can be manufactured by the body when linoleic acid is available. Deficiency occurs when fat intake falls below 10% of daily nutrition. Most animal fats have high proportions of saturated fatty acids, whereas vegetable fats have higher amounts of unsaturated and polyunsaturated fatty acids. See Figure 43-1 for a summary.

Olestra is a fat replacer approved by the Food and Drug Administration (FDA) for public consumption. Olestra (brand name Olean) is created from sucrose and fatty acids and shares many properties of regular fat sources in regard to taste and texture. Because of the body's inability to digest olestra, the intestines cannot absorb it, hence it is calorie free. The fact that human intestines cannot absorb olestra causes some persons to experience cramping, nausea, or diarrhea after ingestion of this product.

Benecol is a product now available in foods such as margarine, and salad dressing. It is claimed to have cholesterol-lowering properties when taken consistently in three servings per day for 1 year (Raloff, 1998). First developed in the early 1990s, Benecol is composed of stanol esters derived from plant relatives of cholesterol that are not absorbed in the gut due to structural differences from actual cholesterol.

Water. Water is a critical component of the body because cell function depends on a fluid environment. Water

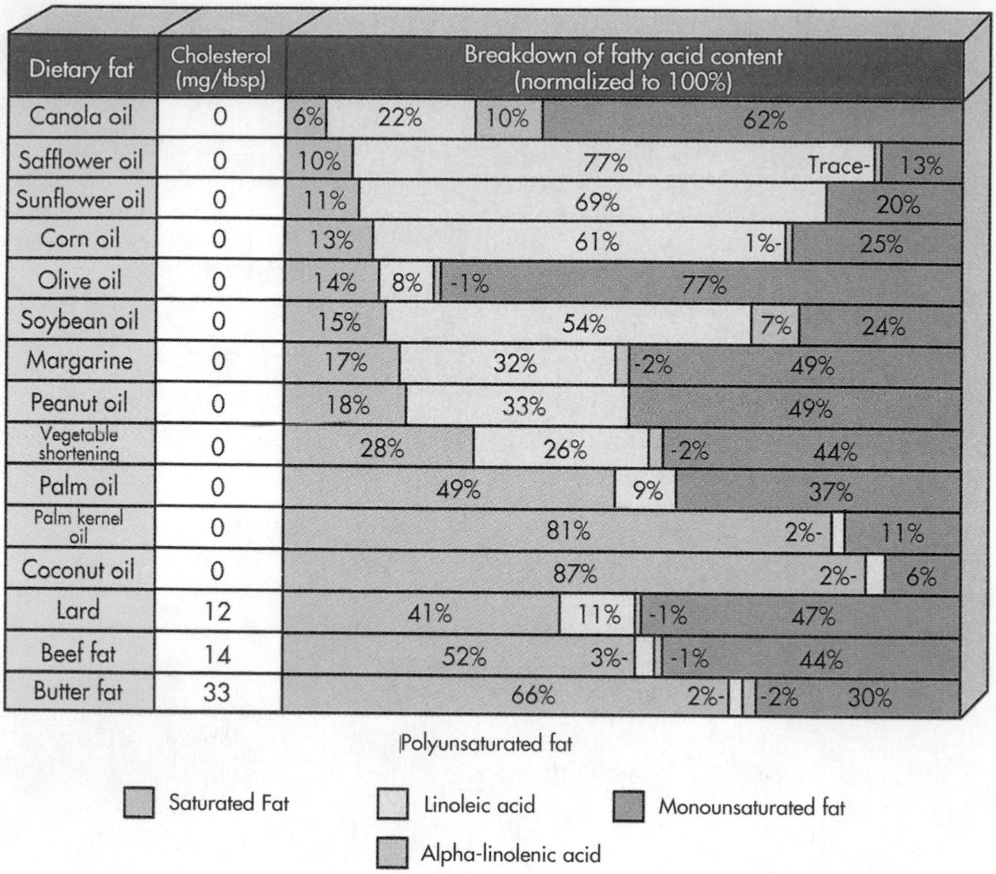

Dietary fat	Cholesterol (mg/tbsp)	Breakdown of fatty acid content (normalized to 100%)			
Canola oil	0	6%	22%	10%	62%
Safflower oil	0	10%	77%	Trace-	13%
Sunflower oil	0	11%	69%		20%
Corn oil	0	13%	61%	1%-	25%
Olive oil	0	14%	8%	-1%	77%
Soybean oil	0	15%	54%	7%	24%
Margarine	0	17%	32%	-2%	49%
Peanut oil	0	18%	33%		49%
Vegetable shortening	0	28%	26%	-2%	44%
Palm oil	0	49%	9%		37%
Palm kernel oil	0	81%	2%-		11%
Coconut oil	0	87%	2%-		6%
Lard	12	41%	11%	-1%	47%
Beef fat	14	52%	3%-	-1%	44%
Butter fat	33	66%	2%-	-2%	30%

Polyunsaturated fat

☐ Saturated Fat   ☐ Linoleic acid   ☐ Monounsaturated fat

☐ Alpha-linolenic acid

Figure 43-1   Comparison of fats in terms of cholesterol, saturated, and unsaturated dietary intake.
From Wardlaw GM, Insell PM: *Perspectives in nutrition,* ed 2, New York, 1993, McGraw-Hill.

composes 60% to 70% of total body weight. The percent of total body water is greater for lean people than obese people because muscle contains more water than any other tissue except blood. Infants have the greatest percentage of total body water, and older people have the least. When deprived of water, a person cannot survive for more than a few days.

Fluid needs are met by ingesting liquids and solid foods high in water content, such as fresh fruits and vegetables. Water is also produced during digestion when food is oxidized. In a healthy individual, fluid intake from all sources equals fluid output through elimination, respiration, and sweating (see Chapters 40 and 44). An ill person can have an increased need for fluid (e.g., with fever or gastrointestinal losses). By contrast, an ill person can also have a decreased ability to excrete fluid (e.g., with cardiopulmonary or renal disease), which may lead to the need to restrict fluid intake.

Vitamins.   **Vitamins** are organic substances present in small amounts in foods that are essential to normal metabolism. The body is unable to synthesize vitamins in the required amounts and depends on dietary intake. Vitamins are affected by processing, storage, and preparation. Vitamin content is usually highest in fresh foods that are used quickly after minimal exposure to heat, air, or water. Vitamins are classified as fat soluble and water soluble.

Fat-Soluble Vitamins.   The **fat-soluble vitamins** (A, D, E, and K) can be stored in the body. With the exception of vitamin D, these vitamins are provided through dietary intake. Olestra may decrease absorption of vitamins A, D, E, K when these vitamins are eaten at the same time as foods containing olestra. Olestra does not affect fat-soluble vitamins previously eaten. To offset these losses, companies producing snacks with olestra supplement foods with specific amounts of these essential vitamins (American Dietetic Association, 1998). **Hypervitaminosis** of fat-soluble vitamins can result from megadoses (intentional or unintentional) of supplemental vitamins, excessive amounts in fortified food, and large intake of fish oils. Table 43-4 summarizes the fat-soluble vitamins.

Certain vitamins are currently of considerable interest in their role as antioxidants that neutralize substances called free radicals, which are thought to produce oxidative damage to body cells and tissues. These vitamins include beta-carotene and vitamins A, C, and E (Williams, 1997).

Water-Soluble Vitamins.   The **water-soluble vitamins** are vitamin C and B complex (which consists of eight vitamins). Water-soluble vitamins cannot be stored in the body and must be provided in the daily food intake. Although water-soluble vitamins are not stored, toxicity may still occur. Vitamins are chemicals used as catalysts in biochemical reactions. When there is enough of any specific vitamin to meet the catalytic demands, the rest of the vitamin supply acts as a free chemical and may be toxic to the body. Table

43-5 summarizes the recommended dietary allowances and adequate intakes of water-soluble vitamins.

Minerals.   **Minerals** are inorganic elements essential to the body as catalysts in biochemical reactions. Minerals are classified as **macrominerals** when the daily requirement is 100 mg or more and microminerals or **trace elements** when less than 100 mg is needed daily. Both macrominerals and trace element requirements are summarized in Table 43-6. Selenium is a trace mineral that also has antioxidant properties. Silicon, vanadium, nickel, tin, cadmium, arsenic, aluminum, and boron may play an unidentified role in nutrition. Toxic effects of arsenic, aluminum, and cadmium are documented.

Table 43-5   Recommended Dietary Allowances and Adequate Intakes: Water Soluble Vitamins

Age/Group	Vitamin C (mg)	Thiamin (mg)	Riboflavin (mg)	Vitamin B_6 $(mg)^d$	Niacin (mg)	Folate μg^e	Vitamin B_{12} μg^f	Pantothenic acid (mg)	Choline (mg)	Biotin μg
Infants										
0.6 mo	30	0.2	0.3	2	0.1	65*	0.4	1.7	125	5
7-12 mo	35	0.3	0.4	4	0.3	80*	0.5	1.8	150	6
Children										
1-3 yr	40	0.5	0.5	6	0.5	150	0.9	2.0	200	8
4-8 yr	45	0.6	0.6	8	0.6	200	1.2	3.0	250	12
Males										
9-13 yr	50	0.9	0.9	12	1.0	300	1.8	4.0	375	20
14-18 yr	60	1.2	1.3	16	1.3	400	2.4	5.0	550	25
19-30 yr	60	1.2	1.3	16	1.3	400	2.4	5.0	550	30
31-50 yr	60	1.2	1.3	16	1.3	400	2.4	5.0	550	30
Over 50 yr	60	1.2	1.3	16	1.7	400	2.4	5.0	550	30
Females										
9-13 yr	50	0.9	0.9	12	1.0	300	1.8	4.0	375	20
14-18 yr	60	1.0	1.0	14	1.2	400^h	2.4	5.0	400	25
19-30 yr	60	1.1	1.1	14	1.3	400^h	2.4	5.0	425	30
31-50 yr	60	1.1	1.1	14	1.3	400^h	2.4	5.0	425	30
Over 50 yr	60	1.1	1.1	14	1.5	400	2.4	5.0	425	30
Pregnant	70	1.4	1.4	18	1.9	600	2.6	6.0	450	30
Lactating	95	1.5	1.6	17	2.0	500	2.8	7.0	550	35

Data from Food and Nutrition Board: *Recommended dietary allowances,* ed 10, Washington, DC, 1989, National Academy Press; Food and Nutrition Board: *Dietary reference intakes for calcium, phosphorus, magnesium, vitamin D, and fluoride,* Washington, DC, 1997, National Academy Press; and Food and Nutrition Board: *Dietary reference intakes: thiamin, riboflavin, niacin, vitamin B₆, folate, vitamin B₁₂, pantothenic acid, biotin, and choline,* Washington, DC, 1998, National Academy Press.

Table 43-6	Recommended Dietary Allowances and Adequate Intakes: Minerals							
Age/Group	Calcium (mg)	Phosphorus (mg)	Magnesium (mg)	Fluoride (mg)	Iron (mg)	Iodine (μg)	Selenium (μg)	Zinc (mg)
Infants								
0-6 mo	210	100*	30*	0.01	6	40	10	5
7-12 mo	270	275*	75*	0.5	10	50	15	5
Children								
1-3 yr	500	460	80	0.7	10	70	20	10
4-8 yr	800	500	130	1.0	10	90	25	10
Males								
9-13 yr	1300	1250	240	2.0	12	150	40	15
14-18 yr	1300	1250	410	3.0	12	150	50	15
19-30 yr	1000	700	400	4.0	10	150	70	15
31-50 yr	1000	700	420	4.0	10	150	70	15
Over 50 yr	1200	700	420	4.0	10	150	70	15
Females								
9-13 yr	1300	1250	240	2.0	15	150	45	12
14-18 yr	1300	1250	360	3.0	15	150	50	12
19-30 yr	1000	700	310	3.0	15	150	55	12
31-50 yr	1000	700	320	3.0	15	150	55	12
Over 50 yr	1200	700	320	3.0	10	150	55	12
Pregnant								
Under 19 yr	1300	1250	400	3.0	30	175	65	15
19-50 yr	1000	700	350	3.0	30	175	65	15
Lactating[d]								
Under 19 yr	1300	1250	360	3.0	15	200	75	19
19-50 yr	1000	700	310	3.0	15	200	75	19

Data from Food and Nutrition Board: *Recommended dietary allowances,* ed 10, Washington, DC, 1989, National Academy Press; Food and Nutrition Board: *Dietary reference intakes for calcium, phosphorus, magnesium, vitamin D, and fluoride,* Washington, DC, 1997, National Academy Press; and Food and Nutrition Board: *Dietary reference intakes: thiamin, riboflavin, niacin, vitamin B₆, folate, vitamin B₁₂, pantothenic acid, biotin, and choline,* Washington, DC, 1998, National Academy Press.

ANATOMY AND PHYSIOLOGY OF DIGESTIVE SYSTEM

Digestion. Digestion of food consists of mechanical breakdown that results from chewing, churning, and mixing with fluid, as well as chemical reactions by which food is reduced to its simplest form. Each part of the gastrointestinal (GI) system has an important digestive or absorptive function. Enzymes are an essential component of the chemistry of digestion. **Enzymes** are the proteinlike substances that act as catalysts to speed up chemical reactions.

Most enzymes have one specific function. Each enzyme functions best at a specific pH. The secretions of the GI tract have vastly different pH levels. For example, saliva is relatively neutral, gastric juice is highly acidic, and the secretions of the small intestine are alkaline. For anatomical reference of the digestive system see Figure 43-2.

The mechanical, chemical, and hormonal activities of digestion are interdependent. Enzyme activity depends on the mechanical breakdown of food to increase its surface area for chemical action. Hormones regulate the flow of digestive secretions needed for enzyme supply, and digestion may also be decreased or increased by strong emotional states. The secretion of digestive juices and the motility of the GI tract are also regulated by physical, chemical, and hormonal factors, as they are bound to psychological, emotional, and nervous system alterations. Gastrointestinal tract action is increased by nerve stimulation from the parasympathetic nervous system (e.g., the vagus nerve).

Digestion begins in the mouth, where food is mechanically broken down by chewing. The food is mixed with saliva, which contains ptyalin (salivary amylase), an en-

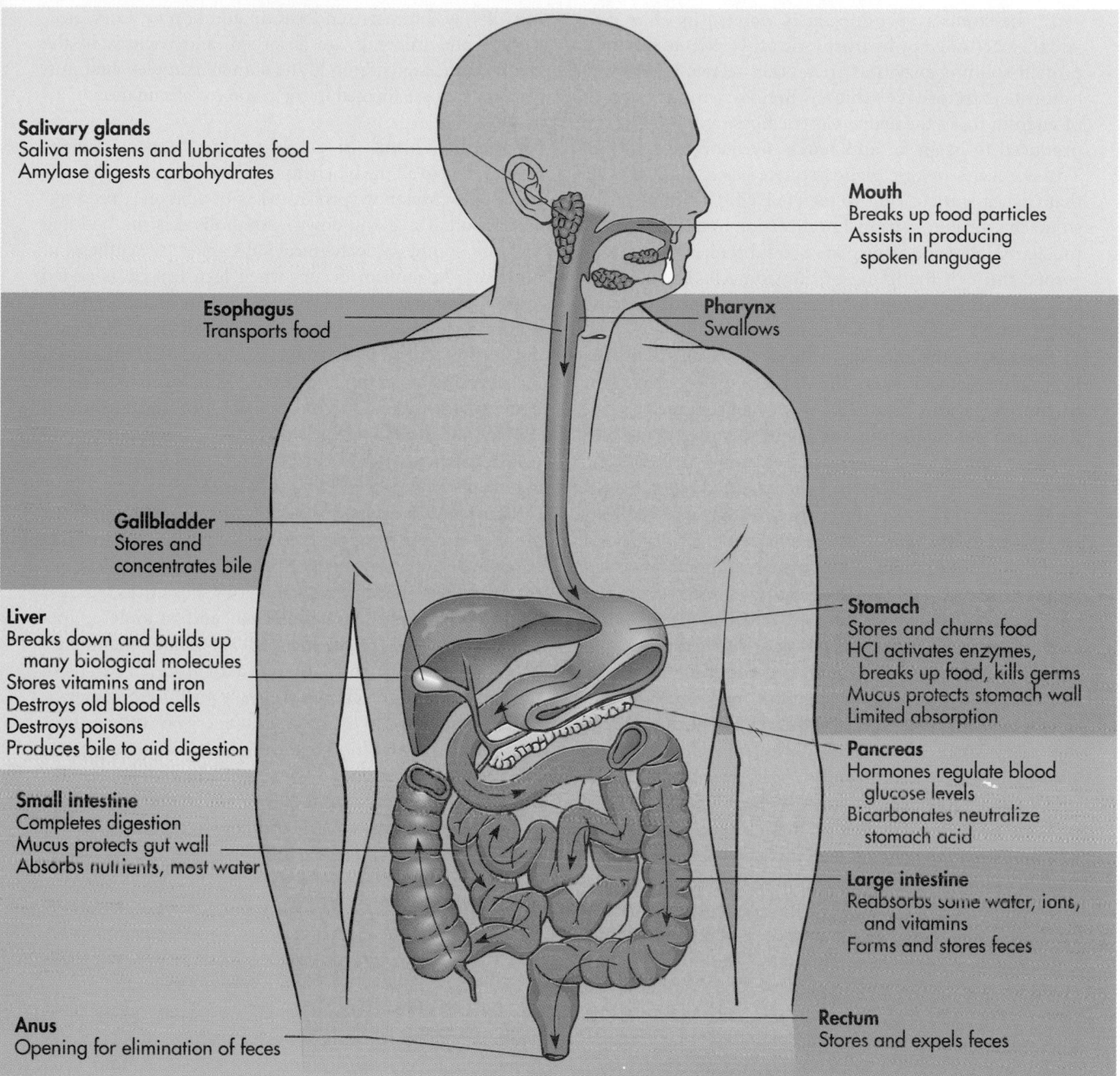

Salivary glands
Saliva moistens and lubricates food
Amylase digests carbohydrates

Mouth
Breaks up food particles
Assists in producing
    spoken language

Esophagus
Transports food

Pharynx
Swallows

Gallbladder
Stores and
concentrates bile

Stomach
Stores and churns food
HCl activates enzymes,
    breaks up food, kills germs
Mucus protects stomach wall
Limited absorption

Liver
Breaks down and builds up
    many biological molecules
Stores vitamins and iron
Destroys old blood cells
Destroys poisons
Produces bile to aid digestion

Pancreas
Hormones regulate blood
    glucose levels
Bicarbonates neutralize
    stomach acid

Small intestine
Completes digestion
Mucus protects gut wall
Absorbs nutrients, most water

Large intestine
Reabsorbs some water, ions,
    and vitamins
Forms and stores feces

Anus
Opening for elimination of feces

Rectum
Stores and expels feces

Figure 43-2   Summary of digestive system anatomy/organ function.
From Rolin Graphics.

zyme that acts on cooked starch to begin its conversion to maltose. The longer food is chewed, the more starch digestion occurs in the mouth. Proteins and fats are broken down physically but remain unchanged chemically because enzymes in the mouth do not react with these nutrients. Chewing reduces food particles to a size suitable for swallowing, and saliva provides lubrication to further ease swallowing of the food. The epiglottis is a flap of skin that closes over the trachea as we swallow to prevent aspiration. Swallowed food enters the esophagus and is moved along by wavelike muscular contractions (**peristalsis**) to the base of the esophagus, above the cardiac sphincter. Pressure from a bolus of food at the cardiac sphincter causes it to relax, allowing the food to enter the fundus, or uppermost portion, of the stomach. Difficulty swallowing is referred to as **dysphagia.**

In the stomach, pepsinogen is secreted by chief cells and then activated by hydrochloric acid (HCl) to pepsin, a protein-splitting enzyme. Parietal cells secrete HCl as well as intrinsic factor (IF), which is necessary for absorption of vitamin B_{12} in the ileum. Gastric lipase and amylase are produced to begin fat and starch digestion, respectively. The stomach's pyloric glands secrete gastrin, a hormone that triggers parietal cells to secrete HCl. The lining of the stomach is protected from autodigestion by a thick layer of mucus. Alcohol and aspirin are two substances directly absorbed through the lining of the stomach. The stomach acts as a reservoir where food remains for approximately 3 hours, with a range of 1 to 7 hours.

Food leaves the antrum, or distal stomach, via the pyloric sphincter and enters the duodenum. Food has now become an acidic, liquified mass called **chyme.** Chyme flows into the duodenum and is quickly mixed with bile, intestinal juices, and pancreatic secretions. Secretin and cholecystokinin (CCK) are hormones secreted by the small intestine mucosa. Secretin activates release of bicarbonate from the pancreas, raising the pH of chyme. Cholecystokinin inhibits further gastrin secretion and initiates release of additional digestive enzymes from the pancreas and gallbladder.

Bile is manufactured in the liver and stored in the gallbladder. Bile acts as a detergent, as it emulsifies fat to permit enzyme action while suspending fatty acids in solution. Pancreatic secretions contain six enzymes: amylase to digest starch; lipase to break down emulsified fats; and trypsin, elastase, chymotrypsin, and carboxypeptidase to break down proteins.

Peristalsis continues in the small intestine, mixing the secretions with the chyme. The mixture becomes increasingly alkaline, inhibiting the action of the gastric enzymes and promoting the action of the duodenal secretions. The epithelial cells of the small intestinal brush border microvilli secrete enzymes to facilitate digestion. These include sucrase, lactase, maltase, lipase, and peptidase. The major portion of digestion occurs in the small intestine, producing glucose, fructose, and galactose from carbohydrates (see Table 43-2); amino acids and dipeptides from proteins; and fatty acids, glycerides, and glycerol from lipids. Approximately 5 hours are required to pass food through the small intestine via peristalsis.

Absorption.   The small intestine is the primary absorption site for nutrients. It is lined with fingerlike projections called villi, which increase the surface area available for absorption. Nutrients are absorbed by means of passive diffusion, osmosis, active transport, and pinocytosis. Table 43-7 describes the means and route of absorption of major nutrients.

The main source of water absorption is via the intestine. Approximately 8.5 L of GI secretions and 1.5 L of oral intake, totaling 10 L of fluid, must be managed daily within the GI tract. The small intestine reabsorbs 9.5 L, and approximately 0.4 L is reabsorbed in the colon. The remaining 0.1 L is eliminated in feces. In addition to water, electrolytes and minerals are absorbed, and bacteria in the colon synthesize vitamin K and some B complex vitamins. Finally, feces are formed in the colon for elimination.

Metabolism and Storage of Nutrients.   **Metabolism** refers to all the biochemical reactions within the cells of the body. Metabolic processes can be anabolic (building) or catabolic (breaking down). **Anabolism** is the building of more complex biochemical substances by synthesis of nutrients. Anabolism occurs when lean muscle is added through diet and exercise. Amino acids are anabolized into tissues, hormones, and enzymes. **Catabolism** is the breakdown of biochemical substances into simpler substances. Starvation is an example of catabolism, when wasting of body tissues occurs. Normal metabolism and anabolism are physiologically possible when the body is in positive nitrogen balance, whereas catabolism occurs during physiologic states of negative nitrogen balance.

Nutrients absorbed in the intestines, including water, are transported through the circulatory system to body tissues. Through the chemical changes of metabolism nutrients are converted into a number of substances required by the body. Carbohydrates, protein, and fat undergo metabolism to produce chemical energy and to maintain a balance between anabolism and catabolism. To carry out the body's work, the chemical energy produced by metabolism is converted to other types of energy by different tissues. Muscle contraction involves mechanical energy, nervous system function involves electrical energy, and the mechanisms of heat production involve thermal energy. All of these forms of energy originate in metabolism. The interrelationships of protein, carbohydrate, and fat metabolism are depicted in Figure 43-3.

Some of the nutrients required by the body are stored in tissues. The body's major form of reserve energy is fat, stored as adipose tissue. Protein is stored in muscle mass. When the body's energy requirements exceed the energy supplied by ingested nutrients, stored energy is used. Monoglycerides from the digested portion of fats can be converted to glucose by gluconeogenesis. Amino acids can also be converted to fat and stored or catabolized into energy via gluconeogenesis. All body cells except red blood cells and neurons can oxidize fatty acids into **ketones** for energy in the absence of dietary carbohydrates (glucose). Glycogen, synthesized from glucose, provides energy during brief periods of fasting. Glycogen is stored in small reserves in liver and muscle tissue. For example, blood glucose levels are maintained by this mechanism as we sleep. Nutrient metabolism consists of three main processes:

1. Catabolism of glycogen into glucose, carbon dioxide, and water (**glycogenolysis**)
2. Anabolism of glucose into glycogen for storage (**glycogenesis**)
3. Catabolism of amino acids and glycerol into glucose for energy (**gluconeogenesis**)

Table 43-7   Intestinal Absorption of Major Nutrients

Nutrient	From	Absorption Method	Control Agent/ Cofactor	Route
Carbohydrate†	Monosaccharides (glucose and galactose)	Competitive	—	Blood
		Selective	—	Blood
		Active transport (via sodium pump)	Sodium	Blood
Fat‡	Fatty acids	Fatty acid-bile complex (micelles)	Bile	Lymph
	Glycerides (mono, di)		—	Lymph
	Triglycerides (few) (neutral fat)	Pinocytosis	—	Lymph
Protein	Amino acids	Selective	—	Blood
	Dipeptides (some)	Carrier transport systems	Pyridoxine (pyridoxal phosphate)	Blood
	Whole protein (rare)	Pinocytosis	—	Blood
Minerals	Sodium	Active transport via sodium pump	—	Blood
	Calcium	Active transport	Vitamin D	Blood
	Iron	Active transport	Ferritin mechanism (as transferritin)	Blood
Vitamins§	B$_{12}$	Carrier transport	IF	Blood
	A	Bile complex	Bile	Blood
	K	Bile complex	Bile	From large intestine to blood
Water[11]	H$_2$O	Osmosis		Blood, lymph, interstitual fluid

Modified from Williams SR: *Nutrition and diet therapy*, ed 8, St. Louis, 1997, Mosby.

†Carbohydrates, protein, minerals, and water-soluble vitamins are absorbed by villus capillaries within the small intestine, processed within the liver, and released via the portal vein circulatory means.

‡Fatty acids are absorbed into the lymphatic circulatory system via lacteal ducts at the center of each microvilli found within the small intestine.

§Exceptions to vitamin absorption are listed (i.e., B$_{12}$, A, and K). Vitamins A and K are fat soluble and are transported via bile to the blood. Vitamin B$_{12}$ is water soluble, but requires specialized transport factor for absorption.

[11]Water is reabsorbed in the large intestine through capillaries to the blood, also flows to the lymphatic system by absorption via large intestinal lymphatic ducts, and serves as a source of interstitial fluid per osmosis.

Elimination.   Chyme is moved by peristaltic action through the ileocecal valve into the large intestine, where it becomes feces. As feces move toward the rectum, water is absorbed in the mucosa. The longer the material stays in the large intestine, the more water is absorbed, causing the feces to become firmer. Exercise and fiber stimulate peristalsis, and water maintains consistency. Feces contain cellulose and similar indigestible substances, sloughed epithelial cells from the GI tract, digestive secretions, water, and microbes.

DIETARY GUIDELINES

Dietary Reference Intakes.   In 1997 the Food and Nutrition Board of the National Institute of Medicine/ National Academy of Sciences, in partnership with Health Canada, initiated **Dietary reference intakes (DRIs).** This new format presents a range of acceptable intake in place of absolute values. Dietary reference intakes will serve as a generic term referring to four different values that include the estimated average requirement, recommended dietary allowance, adequate intake, and tolerable upper intake level. The **estimated average requirement (EAR)** serves as a minimum indicator, meeting the nutrient needs of only 50% of any gender- or age-specific group. The **recommended dietary allowance (RDA)** continues to be a sufficient average indicator, necessary for all healthy people. When the RDA is not known, **adequate intake (AI)** is presented. Average intake values are derived from expert judgment, are less evidence based, but are deemed to meet nutrient needs of all individuals in a group. Finally, the **tolerable upper intake level (UL)** is the maximum level of daily nutrient intake that is evidenced to be unlikely to induce toxicity (Food and Nutrition Board, 1997, 1998). Figure 43-4 depicts the meaning of these four different reference values.

As research has expanded the scientific body of nutrition knowledge, absolute values are no longer sufficient. Studies addressing the reduction of risk of chronic diseases such as cardiovascular disease, cancer, and osteoporosis have launched a need for expanded nutrient infor-

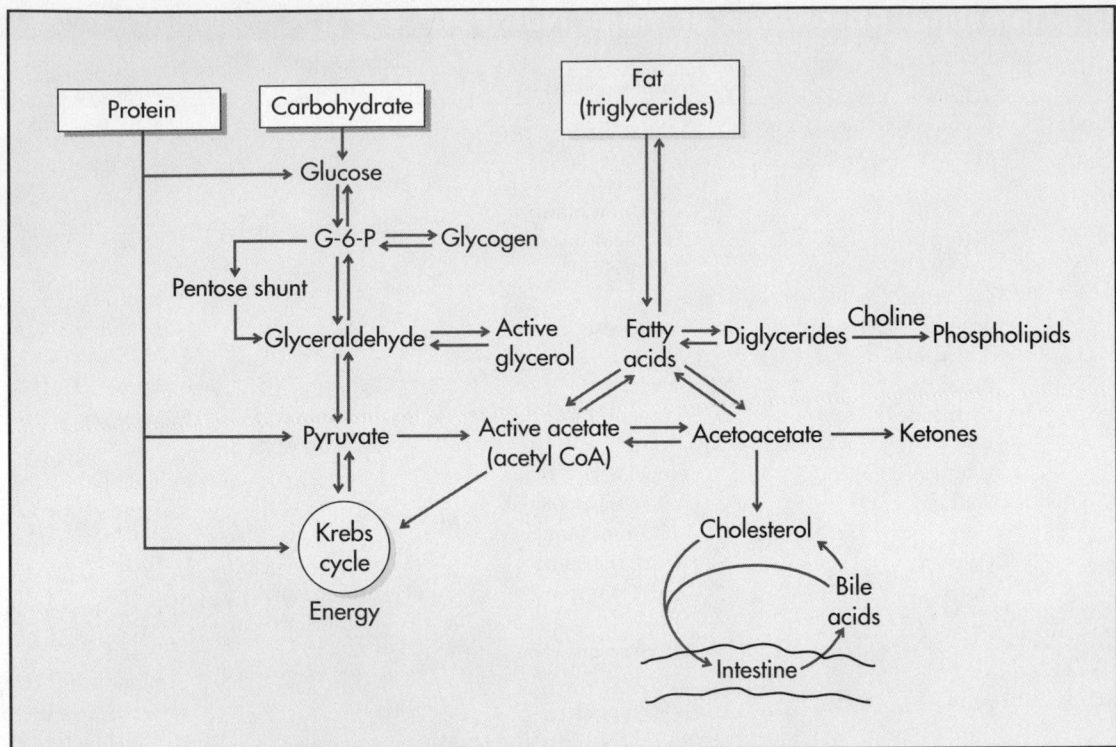

Figure 43-3   Interrelationship of macronutrient metabolism.
From Williams SR: *Nutrition and diet therapy,* ed 8, St. Louis, 1997, Mosby.

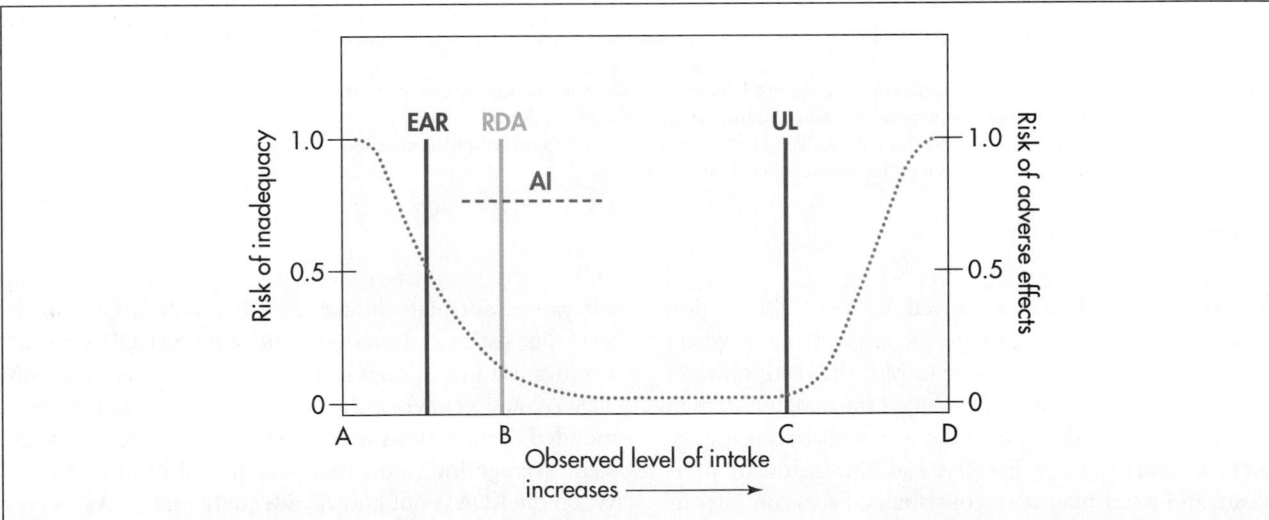

Dietary Reference Intakes. This figure shows that the Estimated Average Requirement (EAR) is the intake at which the risk of inadequacy is 0.5 (50%). The Recommended Dietary Allowance (RDA) is the intake at which the risk of inadequacy is very small—only 0.02 to 0.03 (2% to 3%). The Adequate Intake (AI) does not bear a consistent relationship to the EAR or the RDA because it is set without being able to estimate the requirement. At intakes between the RDA and the Tolerable Upper Intake Level (UL), the risks of inadequacy and of adverse effects are both close to 0. The UL is the highest level of daily nutrient intake that is likely to pose no risks of adverse health effects to almost all individuals in the general population. At intakes above the UL, the risk of adverse effects increases. A dashed line is used for the AI because the actual shape of the curve has not been determined experimentally. The distances between points A and B, B and C, and C and D may differ much more than is depicted in this figure. Thus, the AI may be greater or less than the RDA, if it were known.

Figure 43-4   Summary of dietary reference intakes.
Source: Food and Nutrition Board: *Dietary reference intakes: thiamin, riboflavin, niacin, vitamin B_6, folate, vitamin B_{12}, pantothenic acid, biotin, and choline,* Washington, DC, 1998, National Academy Press.

mation. Specifically, seven nutrient groups are being reevaluated: calcium, vitamin D, phosphorus, magnesium, and fluoride; folate and other B complex vitamins; antioxidants (vitamins C and E, selenium); macronutrients (protein, fat, carbohydrates); trace elements (iron, zinc); electrolytes and water; and other food components (fiber, phytoestrogens). Updated recommendations are currently available for thiamin, riboflavin, niacin, folate, vitamin B_6, vitamin B_{12}, pantothenic acid, choline, biotin, calcium, phosphorus, vitamin D, magnesium, and fluoride as depicted in Tables 43-4, 43-5, and 43-6.

Food Guidelines.   The United States and Canadian health organizations have developed food guide models designed to represent a daily diet (Figure 43-5). The United States developed *USDA's Food Guide Pyramid,*

(USDA, 1996) whereas the Canadian model is *Food Guide to Healthy Eating* (Health & Welfare Canada, 1992). These basic plans provide for diets ranging from 1600 to 1800 kcal/day. Additional foods to round out meals and meet energy requirements can be selected from enriched cereals, complex carbohydrates, and additional grains. To further augment the food pyramid, the U.S. Department of Agriculture (USDA) and the U.S. Department of Health and Human Services (USDHHS) have published *Nutrition and Your Health: Dietary Guidelines for Americans* (1995) and *Healthy Eating Index* (1995), which gives recommended servings per day for age- and gender-specific groups. Table 43-8 shows the dietary guidelines, and Table 43-9 summarizes the healthy eating index.

Daily Values.   **Daily values** for food labels were created by the FDA in response to the 1990 Nutrition Labeling and Education Act (NLEA). The FDA first established two sets of reference values. The reference daily intakes (RDI) are the first set, comprising protein, vitamins, and minerals based upon the RDA. The daily reference values (DRV) make up the second set and consist of nutrients such as total fat, saturated fat, cholesterol, carbohydrates, fiber, sodium, and potassium. Combined, both sets make up the daily values used on food labels (FDA, 1995). Daily values did not replace RDAs but provided a separate, more understandable format for the public. Daily values are based on percentages of 2000 kcal/day (Figure 43-6). Serving sizes were set by the FDA, and terms to describe food products, such as low calorie, diet, and lite, were changed to universal terms with legal definitions. Nurses should be familiar with the changes in food labeling and their meanings.

Table 43-8	1995 Dietary Guidelines

Eat a variety of foods.

Maintain a healthy weight; balance your food with physical activity.

Choose a diet low in fat, saturated fat, and cholesterol.

Choose a diet with plenty of vegetables, fruits, and grain products.

Use sugar in moderation.

Use salt and sodium in moderation.

Drink alcoholic beverages in moderation, if at all.

Data from U.S. Department of Agriculture and U.S. Department of Health and Human Services: *Nutrition and your health: dietary guidelines for Americans,* ed 4, USDA/DHHS Home and Garden Bulletin No. 232, Washington, DC, 1995, U.S. Government Printing Office.

Table 43-9	Healthy Eating Index Summary: Recommended Number of Servings per Day for Age/Gender Groups						
Age/Gender Group	Total Kilocalories	Grains	Vegetables	Fruits	Milk	Meat	Unsaturated Fats
Children 1-2	1300	6.0*	3.0*	2.0*	2.0*	2.0*	1
Children 2-3	1600	6.0	3.0	2.0	2.0	2.0	1
Children 4-6	1800	7.0	3.3	2.3	2.0	2.1	1
Children 7-10	2000	7.8	3.7	2.7	2.0	2.3	1
Females 11-24	2200	9.0	4.0	3.0	3.0	2.4	1-2
Males 11-14	2500	9.9	4.5	3.5	3.0	2.6	1-2
Males 15-18	3000	11.0	5.0	4.0	2.0	2.8	1-2
Males 19-24	2900	11.0	5.0	4.0	3.0	2.8	1-2
Females 25-50	2200	9.0	4.0	3.0	2.0	2.4	1-2
Males 25-50	2900	11.0	5.0	4.0	2.0	2.8	1-2
Females Over 50	1900	7.4	3.5	2.5	2.0	2.2	1-2
Males Over 50	2300	9.1	4.2	3.2	2.0	2.5	1-2
Pregnant or Lactating	2700	11.0	9.0	4.0	4.0	3.0	1-2

*Refers to smaller than regular serving sizes.

Modified from U.S. Department of Agriculture: *Healthy eating index,* Washington, DC, October 1995, USDA; and Williams SR: *Nutrition and diet therapy,* ed 8, St. Louis, 1997, Mosby.

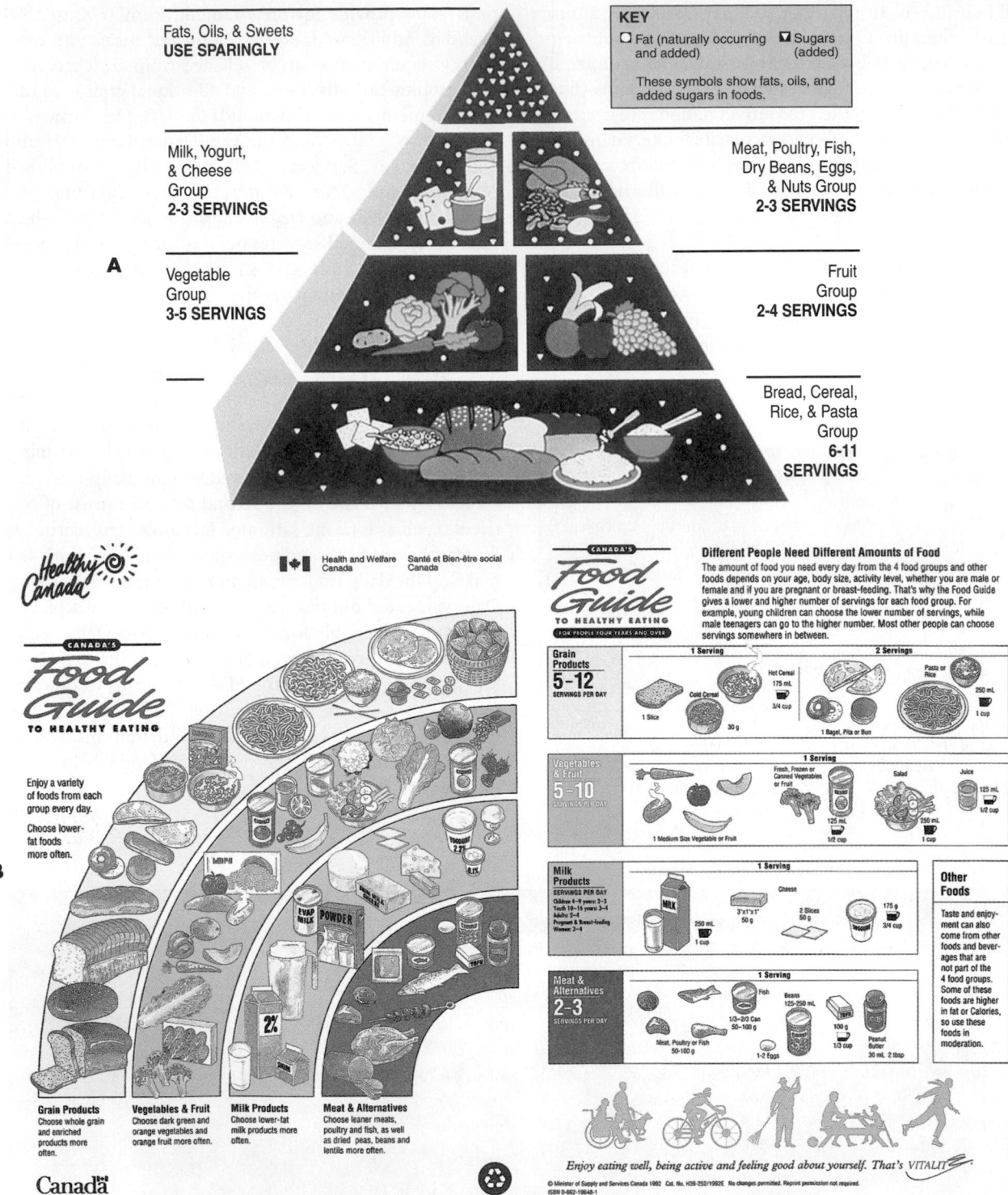

Figure 43-5 A, U.S. food guide pyramid. **B,** Canada's food guide to healthy eating.
From U.S. Department of Agriculture: *USDA's food guide pyramid,* USDA Human Nutrition
Information Service Pub No. 249, Washington, DC, 1996, U.S. Government Printing Office; and
Health and Welfare Canada, Minister of Supply and Services Canada: Catalogue H39-252/1992,
Ottawa, 1992.

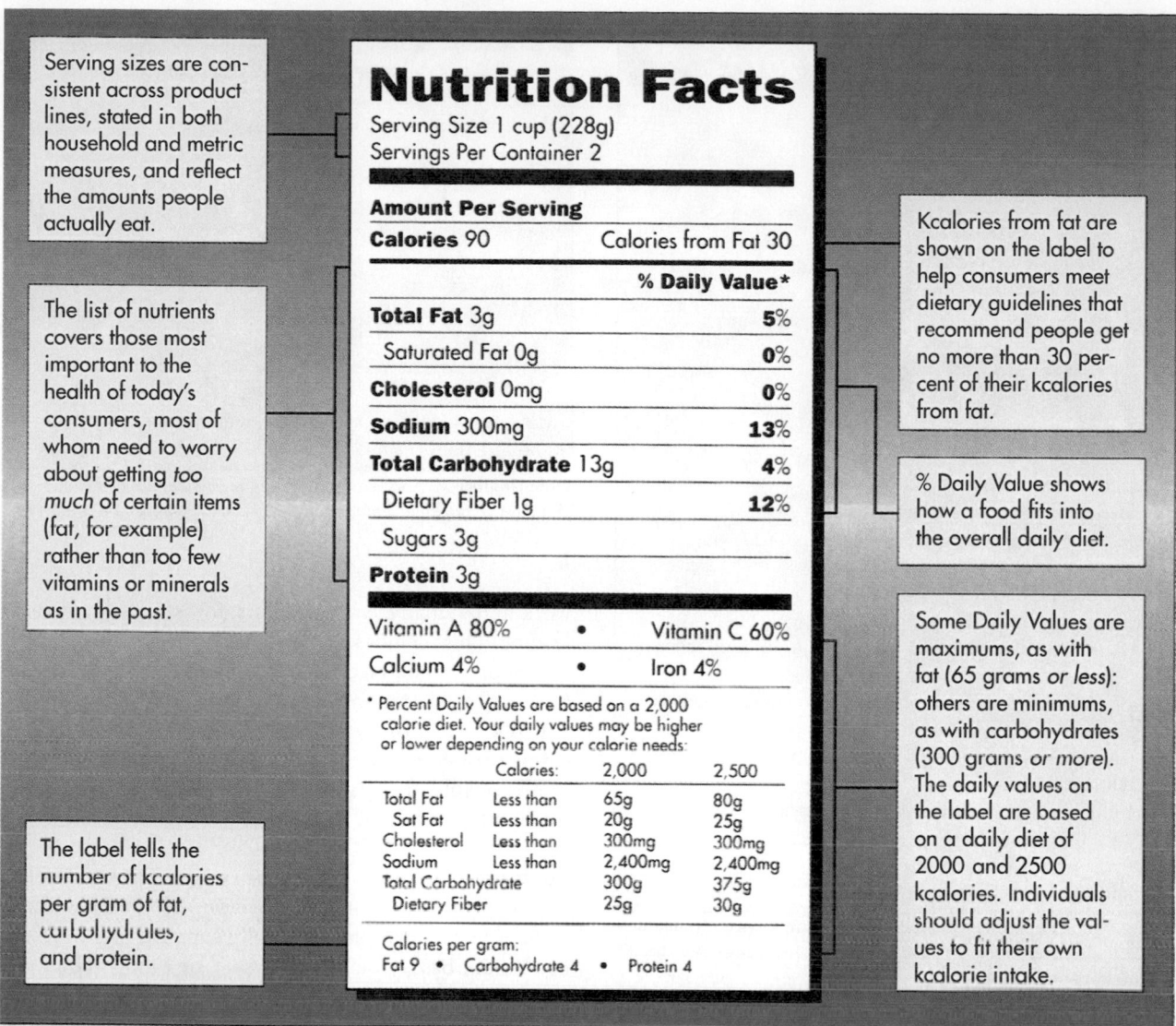

Serving sizes are consistent across product lines, stated in both household and metric measures, and reflect the amounts people actually eat.

The list of nutrients covers those most important to the health of today's consumers, most of whom need to worry about getting *too much* of certain items (fat, for example) rather than too few vitamins or minerals as in the past.

The label tells the number of kcalories per gram of fat, carbohydrates, and protein.

Kcalories from fat are shown on the label to help consumers meet dietary guidelines that recommend people get no more than 30 percent of their kcalories from fat.

% Daily Value shows how a food fits into the overall daily diet.

Some Daily Values are maximums, as with fat (65 grams *or less*): others are minimums, as with carbohydrates (300 grams *or more*). The daily values on the label are based on a daily diet of 2000 and 2500 kcalories. Individuals should adjust the values to fit their own kcalorie intake.

Nutrition Facts

Serving Size 1 cup (228g)
Servings Per Container 2

Amount Per Serving

Calories 90   Calories from Fat 30

                                    % Daily Value*

Total Fat 3g   5%

  Saturated Fat 0g   0%

Cholesterol 0mg   0%

Sodium 300mg   13%

Total Carbohydrate 13g   4%

  Dietary Fiber 1g   12%

  Sugars 3g

Protein 3g

Vitamin A 80%   •   Vitamin C 60%

Calcium 4%   •   Iron 4%

* Percent Daily Values are based on a 2,000 calorie diet. Your daily values may be higher or lower depending on your calorie needs:

		Calories:	2,000	2,500
Total Fat	Less than		65g	80g
Sat Fat	Less than		20g	25g
Cholesterol	Less than		300mg	300mg
Sodium	Less than		2,400mg	2,400mg
Total Carbohydrate			300g	375g
Dietary Fiber			25g	30g

Calories per gram:
Fat 9 • Carbohydrate 4 • Protein 4

Figure 43-6 FDA daily values for food labels.
From Food and Drug Administration: *Daily values for food labels*, Washington, DC, 1995, U.S. Government Printing Office.

Healthy People 2010.   In 1997 the USDHHS and the Public Health Service (PHS) began a consensus process, establishing nutritional goals and objectives for *Healthy People 2010: National Health Promotion and Disease Prevention Objectives. Healthy People 2010* is the United States' contribution to the World Health Organization's (WHO's) "Health for All" strategy. The report defines national goals to be met to increase the proportion of Americans who live long, healthy lives (Table 43-10). *Healthy People 2010* continues goals initiated previously in *Healthy People 2000.* All nutrition-related goals include baseline data, from which progress is measured. The challenge remains to motivate consumers to put these dietary recommendations into practice. Many target goals of *Healthy People 2000* show positive indicators, including

decreasing fat consumption and death rates from coronary heart disease. An increase in overall life expectancy has also occurred; however, obesity remains problematic. Health professionals can play a key role in promoting healthy dietary practices.

Nursing Knowledge Base

NUTRITION DURING HUMAN GROWTH AND DEVELOPMENT

Infants.   Infancy is marked by rapid growth and high protein, vitamin, mineral, and energy requirements. The average birth weight of an American baby is 3.2 to 3.4 kg (7 to 7½ pounds). The infant usually doubles birth weight at 4 to 5 months and triples it at 1 year. An energy intake

Table 43-10	**Nutrition Objectives for Healthy People 2010**

Healthy weight

Reduction of obesity in adults

Reduction of obesity in children (6 to 11) and adolescents (12 to 19)

Decrease in growth retardation to <10% in low-income children <5 years

Decrease in fat intake to <30% daily intake

Decrease in saturated fat intake to <10% daily intake

Vegetable and fruit intake of five daily servings in 75% of people

Grain products intake of six daily servings in 80% of people

Calcium RDA met in 90% of people

Sodium daily intake no more than 2400 mg in 65% of people

Reduction of prevalence of iron deficiency in children and childbearing women

Reduction of prevalence of anemia in pregnant women to <23%

Nutrient-dense meals and snacks at school for children and adolescents

Nutrition education required in elementary schools

Nutrition education required in middle/junior high schools

Nutrition education required in senior high schools

Work-site nutrition education and weight management programs

Nutrition assessment and individualized planning at primary care sites

Nutritional education and counseling services for diabetics at primary care sites

Increase in prevalence of food security to 94% of households

Data from U.S. Department of Health and Human Services: *Healthy people 2010 objectives: draft for public comment,* 1998, http://web.health.gov./healthypeople.

Table 43-11	**Benefits of Breast-Feeding**

Immunologic protection conferred (especially GI tract and respiratory)

Nutrient composition is of ideal composition with high bioavailability

Food allergy risk reduction

Oral motor development promoted

Convenience, always correct temperature, available, and fresh

Economical, as is less expensive than formula

Bonding between mother and infant promoted

Chronic disease protection, may guard against development of IDDM and childhood leukemia

Uterine contractions facilitated, helps control postpartum bleeding

Maternal weight loss promoted, to prepregnant weight due to increased kcal utilization

From Grodner M, Anderson S, DeYoung S: *Foundations and clinical applications of nutrition: a nursing approach,* ed 2, St. Louis, 2000, Mosby.

of approximately 108 kcal/kg of body weight is need in the first half of infancy and 98 kcal/kg in the second half (Food and Nutrition Board, 1992b).

Commercial formulas and human breast milk both provide approximately 20 kcal/oz. A full-term newborn is able to digest and absorb simple carbohydrates, proteins, and a moderate amount of emulsified fat. Amylase, the starch-splitting enzyme, is not present until approximately $2\frac{1}{2}$ to $3\frac{1}{2}$ months. Infants need about 100 to 150 ml/kg/day of fluid because a large portion of total body weight is water.

Breast-Feeding. The American Academy of Pediatrics (1997a) strongly recommends breast-feeding. Table 43-11 summarizes the benefits of breast-feeding. Breast-fed infants need supplemental vitamin D. Other possible supplements include vitamin K, iron, and fluoride, although their use remains controversial.

Multidisciplinary promotion of breast-feeding has resulted in 50% to 60% of mothers electing to breast-feed. Many hospitals now have nurse lactation consultants who work individually with mothers for successful breast-feeding. This includes home visitation as well. The recent advent of portable electric breast pumps has made breast-feeding feasible for working mothers. Infection with hepatitis C, HIV, or cytomegalovirus (CMV) contraindicates breast-feeding, since these viruses have been isolated in breast milk, increasing the chance of infectious transmission to the infant.

Formula. Infant formulas are designed to contain the approximate nutrient composition of human milk. Protein in the formula is typically supplied as whey, soy, cow's milk base, casein hydrolysate, or elemental amino acids. The American Academy of Pediatrics (1997b) has set standards for the level of nutrients in infant formulas. The addition of nucleotides to infant formula is a new area of research, intending to more closely parallel human milk and boost immune function (Pickering and others, 1998).

Regular cow's milk should not be used for infant formula during the first year of life. It may cause gastrointestinal bleeding and is too concentrated for the infant's kidneys to manage. The American Academy of Pediatrics (1994) issued a policy statement citing research supporting a possible relationship between cow's milk given in the first year of life and later development of Type 1 diabetes mellitus. Honey and corn syrup are potential sources of botulism toxin and should not be used in the infant's diet. The toxin can be fatal in children under 1 year of age (Williams, 1997).

Introduction to Solid Food. Breast milk or formula provides sufficient nutrition for the first 4 to 6 months of life. The development of fine motor skills of the hand and fingers parallels the infant's interest in food and self-feeding. Iron-fortified cereals are typically the first semisolid food to be introduced.

Table 43-12 presents a suggested sequence for introducing new foods. The addition of foods to an infant's diet should be governed by the infant's nutrient needs, physical readiness to handle different forms of foods, and the need to detect and control allergic reactions. New foods should be introduced one at a time, approximately 4 to 7 days apart to identify allergies. It is best to introduce new foods before milk or other foods to avoid satiety (Wong, 1997).

Toddlers and Preschoolers.   The growth rate slows during toddler years (1 to 3). The toddler needs fewer kilocalories but an increased amount of protein in relation to body weight; consequently appetite may decrease at 18 months of age. Toddlers exhibit strong food preferences and become picky eaters. Small frequent meals consisting of breakfast, lunch, and dinner with three interspersed high-nutrient-density snacks may improve nutritional intake (Wong, 1997). Calcium and phosphorus are impor-

Table 43-12   Introduction of Solid Foods to Infants

Age/Food Group	Foods	Daily Servings	Suggested Serving Size	Feeding Tips
0 to 4 mo				Nurse baby 5 to 10 min on each breast.
Milk	Breast milk or	8-12 or on demand		Six wet diapers per day is good.
	Formula* 0-1 mo	6-8	2-5 oz	There is no need to force baby to finish bottles.
	1-2 mo	5-7	3-6 oz	Putting baby to bed with bottle could cause choking.
	2-3 mo	4-7	4-7 oz	
	3-4 mo	4-6	6-8 oz	Microwave heating of formula is not recommended.
4 to 6 mo				
Milk	Breast milk or	4-6		Offer baby extra water.
	Formula*	4-6	6-8 oz	May start baby cereal* (iron fortified).
Grain	Baby cereal (iron fortified)	2	1-2 T	Feed one new cereal a week.†
				No need to add salt/sugar to cereal.
6 to 8 mo				
Milk	Breast milk or	3-5		Add strained fruits/vegetables first.
	Formula*	3-5	6-8 oz	Progress to finely chopped fruits and cooked vegetables.
Grain	Baby cereal (iron fortified)	2	2-4 T	Introduce one new food a week.†
	Bread, bagel, bun	Offer	½	Remove from jar needed food serving
	Crackers		2	and refrigerate remainder.
Fruit/Vegetable	Fruit or vegetables	3-4	2-3 T	Try using cup for fruit juice.
	Baby fruit juice	1	3 oz	Only when baby has teeth, offer foods that require chewing.
				Always monitor child for choking (grapes, popcorn, hot dogs).
8 to 12 mo				
Milk	Breast milk or	3-4		Ask your doctor before giving whole milk to baby.
	Formula*	3-4	6-8 oz	
	Cheese	Offer	½ oz	Add strained and finely chopped meats.
	Plain yogurt		½ cup	Feed only one new food a week.†
	Cottage cheese		¼ cup	No egg whites until 12 months; however, egg yolks are okay.
Grain	Baby cereal	2	2-4 T	
	Bread, bagel, bun	2	½	Messes are normal, so be patient.
	Crackers		2	Temperature of food should be checked carefully.
Fruit/Vegetable	Fruit or vegetables	4-5	3-4 T	
	Baby fruit juice	1	3 oz	Give beverages in cup.
Meat	Chicken, beef, pork	2	3-4 T	
	Cooked dried beans or egg yolks			

Modified from National Dairy Council: *Feeding guide for first two years*, Rosemont, Ill, 1990, The Council.
*Based on infant's physical readiness; consult physician.
†Assists in identification or control of food allergies.

tant for healthy bone growth. See Table 43-6 for a summary of recommended dietary intake.

Toddlers who consume more than 24 ounces of milk daily in lieu of other foods may develop milk anemia, since milk is a poor source of iron. Whole milk should be used until the toddler reaches 2 years of age to help ensure adequate intake of fatty acids necessary for brain and neurological development. Fat replacers, such as olestra, should not be given to children under 2 years of age for this reason. Certain foods such as hot dogs, candy, nuts, grapes, raw vegetables, and popcorn have been implicated in choking deaths and should be avoided.

Preschoolers' (3 to 5 years) dietary requirements are similar to toddlers. They consume slightly more than toddlers, and nutrient density is more important than quantity.

School-Age Children. School-age children, 6 to 12 years old, grow at a slower and steadier rate, with a gradual decline in energy requirements per unit of body weight. The school-age child gains 3 to 5 kg (6½ to 11 pounds) in weight and 6 cm (2½ inches) in height per year until puberty.

Despite better appetites and more varied food intake, school-age children's diets should be carefully assessed for adequate protein and vitamins A and C (see Tables 43-4, 43-5, and 43-9). School-age children frequently fail to eat a proper breakfast and have unsupervised intake at school. High fat, sugar, and salt can result from too-liberal intake of snack foods. Kennedy-Caldwell (1998) notes that children are spending more time away from home, as do parents, further compounding this modern-day problem. There is a consistent increase in childhood obesity statistics from three consecutive National Health and Nutrition Examination Surveys (NHANES, 1990). Greater prevalence of cardiovascular risk for school-age children calls for more nursing input (Kennedy and Caldwell, 1998).

Adolescents. During adolescence, physiological age is a better guide to nutritional needs than chronological age. Energy needs increase to meet greater metabolic demands of growth. Daily requirement of protein also increases. Calcium is essential for the rapid bone growth of adolescence, and girls need a continuous source of iron to replace menstrual losses. Boys also need adequate iron for muscle development. Iodine supports increased thyroid activity, and use of iodized table salt assures availability. B complex vitamins are needed to support heightened metabolic activity (see Tables 43-4 and 43-5).

The adolescent's diet is influenced by many factors other than nutritional needs, including concern about body image and appearance, desire for independence, and fad diets. Nutritional deficiencies may occur in adolescent girls as a result of dieting and use of oral contraceptives (Table 43-13). The adolescent boy's diet may be inadequate in total kilocalories, protein, iron, folic acid, B vitamins, and iodine. Snacks provide approximately 25% of the teenager's total dietary intake. Fast food is common and adds extra salt, fat, and kilocalories. Skipping meals or eating meals with wrong choices of snacks contributes to nutrient deficiency and obesity (Wong, 1997).

Fortified foods (nutrients added) are important sources of vitamins and minerals. Snack food from the dairy and fruit and vegetable groups are good choices. To counter obesity, increasing physical activity is often more important than curbing intake. The onset of eating disorders such as **anorexia nervosa** or **bulimia nervosa** is often during adolescence. Recognition of eating disorders (Table 43-14) is essential for early intervention.

Sports and regular moderate-to-intense exercise necessitate dietary modification to meet increased energy needs for adolescents. Carbohydrates, both simple and complex, should be the main source of energy, providing 55% to 60% of total daily kilocalories. Protein needs are increased to 1.0 to 1.5 g/kg/day. Fat needs are not increased. Adequate hydration is very important for all athletes. Water should be ingested before and after exercise to prevent dehydration, especially in hot humid environments. Vitamin and mineral supplements are not required, but intake of iron-rich foods is required to prevent anemia.

Parents often have more influence on the adolescent diet than they believe. Effective strategies include limiting the amount of unhealthy food choices kept at home and enhancing the appearance and taste of healthy foods. Making healthy food choices more convenient and available and working to change social norms of what foods are "cool" are also ways to promote optimal nutritional health in adolescents (Neumark-Sztainer and others, 1999)

Pregnancy occurring within 4 years of menarche may place mother and fetus at risk because of anatomical and physiological immaturity. Malnutrition at the time of conception increases risk to the adolescent and her fetus. Most teenage girls do not want to gain weight. Counseling related to nutritional needs of pregnancy may be difficult, and suggestions are better tolerated than rigid directions. The diet of pregnant adolescents is often deficient in calcium, iron, and vitamins A and C. Prenatal vitamin and mineral supplements are recommended.

Young and Middle Adults. The demands for most nutrients are reduced as the growth period ends. Mature adults need nutrients for energy, maintenance, and repair. Energy needs usually decline over the years. Obesity may become a problem due to decreased physical exercise, dining out more often, and increased ability to afford more luxury foods. Adult women who use oral contraceptives may need extra vitamins (Table 43-13). Iron and calcium intake continues to be important. Table 43-9 addresses required servings of each food group per day.

Maintaining good oral health is significant throughout adulthood. A position paper of the American Academy of Periodontology identified periodontal disease as a potential risk factor for systemic diseases such as bacteremia, en-

Table 43-13 Sample of Drug-Nutrient Interactions[*]

Drug	Effect
Analgesic/Narcotic	
Acetaminophen	Decreased drug absorption with food; overdose associated with liver failure
Aspirin	Absorbed directly through stomach; decreased drug absorption with food; decreased folic acid, vitamins C and K, and iron absorption
Opiates	Decreased peristalsis; constipation
Antacid	
Aluminum hydroxide	Decreased phosphate absorption
Sodium bicarbonate	Decreased folic acid absorption
Antiarrhythmic	
Amiodarone	Taste alteration
Digitalis	Anorexia, decreased renal clearance in older persons
Propranolol	Increased drug absorption with food
Antiarthritic	
Methotrexate	Decreased drug absorption with food, decreased folic acid
Penicillamine	Taste alteration
Antibiotic	
Amoxicillin	Decreased drug absorption with food
Ampicillin	Taste alteration, decreased drug absorption with food
Cephalosporin	Decreased vitamin K
Clarithromycin	Taste alteration
Doxycycline	Decreased drug absorption with food
Gentamicin	Anorexia, decreased renal excretion in older persons
Metronidazole	Anorexia
Neomycin	Decreased fat, nitrogen, vitamin B_{12}, lactose, sucrose, sodium, potassium, iron, calcium
Nitrofurantoin	Increased drug absorption with food
Penicillin	Decreased drug absorption with food
Rifampin	Decreased vitamin B_6, niacin, vitamin D
Tetracycline	Decreased drug absorption with milk and antacids, decreased nutrient absorption of calcium, riboflavin, vitamin C due to binding
Trimethoprim/sulfamethoxazole	Decreased folic acid
Anticoagulant	
Coumarin	Acts as antagonist to vitamin K
Anticonvulsant	
Carbamazepine	Increased drug absorption with food
Phenobarbital	Decreased drug absorption with food, decreased vitamin D
Phenytoin	Decreased calcium absorption; decreased vitamins D and K and folic acid; taste alteration; decreased drug absorption with food
Primidone	Decreased calcium absorption, increased metabolism of vitamins D and K
Antidepressant	
Amitriptyline	Appetite stimulant
Clomipramine	Taste alteration, appetite stimulant
Fluoxetine (selective serotonin reuptake inhibitors [SSRIs])	Taste alteration, anorexia
Antifungal	
Amphotericin B	Anorexia
Griseofulvin	Taste alteration, enhanced absorption with food

[*]Not intended to be an exhaustive or all-inclusive list. Always check pharmacology references before administering medications.

Continued

Table 43-13   **Sample of Drug-Nutrient Interactions**—cont'd

Drug	Effect
Antigout	
Allopurinol	Taste alteration
Colchicine	Decreased vitamin B_{12}, vitamin A (carotene), lactose, sodium, potassium
Antihistamine	
Astemizole	Increased appetite, decreased drug absorption with food
Cyproheptadine	Increased appetite
Antihypertensive	
Captopril	Taste alteration, anorexia
Hydralazine	Enhanced drug absorption with food, decreased vitamin B_6
Labetalol	Taste alteration (weight gain for all beta-blockers)
Methyldopa	Decreased vitamin B_{12}, folic acid, iron
Antiinflammatory	
All steroids	Increased appetite and weight, increased folic acid, decreased calcium (osteoporosis with long-term use), promotes gluconeogenesis of protein
Indomethacin	Decreased iron absorption
Salicylazosulfapyridine (Azulfidine)	Decreased folic acid
Antimanic	
Lithium carbonate	Anorexia, nausea, vomiting, diarrhea, mucositis, decreased folic acid
Antiparkinson	
Levodopa	Taste alteration, decreased vitamin B_6 and drug absorption with food
Antipsychotic	
Chlorpromazine	Increased appetite
Thiothixene	Decreased riboflavin, increased need
Antituberculosis	
Isoniazid	Decreased calcium, niacin, vitamins B_6 and D
Para-aminosalicylic acid	Decreased fat, folic acid, vitamin B_{12}
Bronchodilator	
Albuterol sulfate	Appetite stimulant
Theophylline	Anorexia
Cholesterol Lowering	
Cholestyramine	Decreased fat-soluble vitamins (A, D, E, K); vitamin B_{12}; iron
Diuretic	
Furosemide	Decreased drug absorption with food
Spironolactone	Increased drug absorption with food
Thiazides	Decreased magnesium, zinc, and potassium
Triamterene	Decreased folic acid
Estrogen/Progestin	
Oral contraceptive Hormone replacement therapy (HRT)	Decreased vitamin B_6, B_{12}, folic acid, zinc; increased transferrin as above

Table 43-13 **Sample of Drug-Nutrient Interactions**—cont'd

Drug	Effect
Laxative	
Mineral oil	Decreased absorption of fat-soluble vitamins (A, D, E, K), carotene
Phenolphthalein	Decreased calcium, potassium, vitamin D
Muscle Relaxant	
Baclofen	Taste alteration
Dantrolene	Taste alteration, anorexia
Platelet Aggregate Inhibitor	
Dipyridamole	Decreased drug absorption with food
Potassium Replacement	
Potassium chloride	Decreased vitamin B_{12}
Stimulant	
Dextroamphetamine	Taste alteration, anorexia
Methylphenidate	Anorexia, decreased weight, decreased growth
Tranquilizer	
Benzodiazepines	Increased appetite

Table 43-14 **Diagnostic Criteria for Eating Disorders**

Anorexia Nervosa

A. Refusal to maintain body weight over a minimal normal weight for age and height, e.g., weight loss leading to maintenance of body weight less than 85% of IBW; or failure to make expected weight gain during period of growth, leading to body weight less than 85% of that expected.

B. Intense fear of gaining weight or becoming fat, although underweight.

C. Disturbance in the way in which one's body weight, size, or shape is experienced, e.g., the person claims to "feel fat" even when emaciated, believes that one area of the body is "too fat" even when obviously underweight.

D. In females, absence of at least 3 consecutive menstrual cycles when otherwise expected to occur (primary or secondary amenorrhea). (A woman is considered to have amenorrhea if her periods occur only following hormone, e.g., estrogen, administration.)

Bulimia Nervosa

A. Recurrent episodes of binge eating (rapid-consumption of a large amount of food in a discrete period of time).

B. A feeling of lack of control over eating behavior during the eating binges.

C. The person regularly engages in either self-induced vomiting, use of laxatives or diuretics, strict dieting or fasting, or vigorous exercise in order to prevent weight gain.

D. A minimum average of 2 binge eating episodes a week for at least 3 months.

From American Psychiatric Association: *Diagnostic and statistical manual of mental disorders*, ed 4-revised, Washington, DC, 1994, The Association.

docarditis, cardiopulmonary disease, diabetes mellitus, and adverse outcomes in pregnancy (Scannapieco, 1998).

Pregnancy. Poor nutrition during pregnancy can cause low birth weight in infants and decreased chances of survival. Generally the fetus's needs are met at the expense of the mother. However, if nutrient sources are not available, both suffer. The nutritional status of the mother at the time of conception is important. Significant aspects of fetal growth and development often occur before pregnancy is even suspected.

The energy requirements of pregnancy are related to the mother's body weight and activity. An average weight gain of 11 to 14 kg (25 to 30 pounds) occurs during pregnancy. Rigid recommendations about weight gain should be avoided. Pregnant women should be cautioned against fasting as a method of weight control, because fasting may lead to **ketoacidosis** (metabolic acidosis caused by excess buildup of ketone bodies), which can be dangerous to the fetus as well as the mother. The quality of nutrition during pregnancy is more important than weight gain per se or kilocalories consumed per day. Food intake in the first trimester should include balanced portions of essential nutrients with emphasis on quality (see Table 42-9). Protein intake throughout pregnancy is increased to 60 g (Table 43-4).

Calcium intake is especially critical in the third trimester, when fetal bones are mineralized. Iron may be supplemented to provide for increased maternal blood volume, for fetal blood storage, and for blood loss during delivery. Iodine needs increase 15% to 17% because of increased activity of the thyroid gland. Folic acid intake is particularly important for DNA synthesis and the growth of red blood cells. Inadequate intake may lead to fetal neural tube defects, anencephaly, or maternal megaloblastic anemia (Daly and others, 1997; Food and Nutrition Board, 1992a). In 1998 the FDA began requiring that grain products be fortified with folic acid. Prenatal care usually includes vitamin and mineral supplementation to ensure daily intakes; however, pregnant women should not take additional supplements beyond prescribed amounts. For example, vitamin A is essential to maternal and fetal health but is teratogenic when consumed in excess (Kessler, 1995).

Pregnant women should drink at least eight glasses of water daily. They should avoid artificial sweeteners, alcohol, excessive caffeine, and all drugs not specifically ordered. Adequate fluid and fiber intake, in addition to moderate exercise, helps prevent constipation commonly associated with pregnancy.

Lactation. The lactating woman needs 500 kcal/day above the usual allowance. The production of milk increases energy requirements. Protein requirements increase to 65 g/day. The need for calcium remains the same as during pregnancy. There is an increased need for vitamins A and C. Daily intake of water-soluble vitamins (B and C) is needed to ensure adequate levels in breast milk (Tables 43-5 and 43-9). Fluid intake should be adequate but need not be excessive. Caffeine, alcohol, and drugs are excreted in breast milk and should be avoided. Tobacco use can decrease milk production (Food and Nutrition Board, 1992a).

Older Adults. Adults 65 years and older have a decreased need for energy as metabolic rate slows with age. However, vitamin and mineral requirements remain unchanged from middle adulthood. Numerous factors influence the nutritional status of the older adult. Income is significant because living on a fixed income may reduce the amount of money available to buy food. Health is another important influence. The older adult may be on a therapeutic diet or have difficulty eating because of physical symptoms, lack of teeth, or dentures or be at risk for

drug-nutrient interactions (Table 43-13). A review of these factors is given in Box 43-1. Thirst sensation may diminish, leading to inadequate fluid intake or dehydration (see Chapter 40). Some symptoms of dehydration in older adults may include confusion, weakness, hot dry skin, furrowed tongue, rapid pulse, and high urinary sodium. Meats may be avoided because of cost or because they are difficult to chew. Cream soups and meat-based vegetable soups are nutrient-dense sources of protein. Cheese, eggs, and peanut butter are also useful high-protein alternatives. Milk continues to be an important food for older women (and men) who need adequate calcium to protect against osteoporosis (a decrease of bone mass density). Research has shown that older men lag behind women in developing osteoporosis by approximately a decade. Therefore screening and treatment are also necessary for older men as well as older women (Ybarra, Ade, and Romeo, 1996). The diet of older adults should contain choices from all food groups and may require a vitamin and mineral supplement.

The USDHHS's Administration on Aging (AOA) now requires states to provide nutritional screening services to elderly clients who benefit from home-delivered or congregate meal services. Reports of findings are sent to AOA. An estimated 2.5 million community-dwelling older adults suffer from food inadequacies within any 6-month period, and 40% to 50% of this group have a moderate-to-high risk of malnutrition. A public-private partnership with the USDHHS and General Mills was recently formed to provide breakfast as a second meal to older homebound adults in a Morning Meals on Wheels program (USDHHS, 1997).

The Nutrition Screening Initiative is a multidisciplinary effort begun in 1991 to identify warning signs of malnutrition in older adults. A three-tiered approach was designed for the nutritional assessment of older adults. Ten key risk factors are shown in the checklist to determine nutritional health (Fig. 43-7), which serves as the first tier. Second-tier screening aims at prevention, and the third tier involves diagnosis and intervention (Nutrition Screening Initiative, 1992; Grindel and Costello, 1996).

ALTERNATIVE FOOD PATTERNS

Long before recommended allowances and guidelines were issued, many people followed special patterns of food intake based on religion (Table 43-15), cultural background (Box 43-2), ethics, health beliefs, personal preference, or concern for the efficient use of land to produce food. Such special diets are not necessarily more or less nutritious than diets based on the food pyramid or other nutritional guidelines, because good nutrition depends on a balanced intake of all required nutrients. A common alternative dietary pattern is the vegetarian diet.

Vegetarianism is the consumption of a diet consisting predominantly of plant foods. Vegetarians may be ovolactovegetarian (avoid meat, fish, and poultry but eat eggs

The Warning Signs of poor nutritional health are often overlooked. Use this checklist to find out if you or someone you know is at nutritional risk.

Read the statements below. Circle the number in the yes column for those that apply. For each yes answer, score the number in the box. Total the nutritional score.

DETERMINE YOUR NUTRITIONAL HEALTH

	YES
I have an illness or condition that made me change the kind and/or amount of food I eat.	2
I eat fewer than 2 meals per day.	3
I eat few fruits or vegetables, or milk products.	2
I have 3 or more drinks of beer, liquor or wine almost every day.	2
I have tooth or mouth problems that make it hard for me to eat.	2
I don't always have enough money to buy the food I need.	4
I eat alone most of the time.	1
I take 3 or more different prescribed or over-the-counter drugs a day.	1
Without wanting to, I have lost or gained 10 pounds in the last 6 months.	2
I am not always physically able to shop, cook and/or feed myself.	2
TOTAL	

Total Your Nutritional Score. If it's –

0–2   **Good!** Recheck your nutritional score in 6 months.

3–5   **You are at moderate nutritional risk.** See what can be done to improve your eating habits and lifestyle. Your office on aging, senior nutrition program, senior citizens center or health department can help. Recheck your nutritional score in 3 months.

6 or more   **You are at high nutritional risk.** Bring this checklist the next time you see your doctor, dietitian or other qualified health or social service professional. Talk with them about any problems you may have. Ask for help to improve your nutritional health.

These materials developed and distributed by the Nutritional Screening Initiative, a project of:

AMERICAN ACADEMY
OF FAMILY PHYSICIANS

THE AMERICAN
DIETETIC ASSOCIATION

NATIONAL COUNCIL
ON THE AGING

Remember that warning signs suggest risk, but do not represent diagnosis of any condition.

Figure 43-7   Nutrition screening tool for older adults.
From the Nutrition Screening Initiative (1998), a project of the American Academy of Family Physicians, the American Dietetic Association, and the National Council of the Aging, Inc. and funded in part by a grant from Ross Products Division, Abbott Laboratories.

and milk), lactovegetarians (drink milk but avoid eggs), or vegans (consume only plant foods). Vegan, zen macrobiotic (eat primarily brown rice, other grains, and herb teas), and fruitarian (eat only fruit, nuts, honey, and olive oil) diets are nutrient poor and can result in malnutrition. Knowledge related to complementary use of complete and incomplete proteins is necessary (Table 43-16). Children who follow a vegetarian diet are especially at risk for protein and vitamin deficiencies, such as vitamin B_{12}.

Alternative therapies are now becoming more accepted (see Chapter 35). Many involve nutrition. Increased attention to alternative therapies is evidenced by the recent formation by the National Institutes of Health of the National Center for Complementary and Alternative Medicine.

KNOWLEDGE

- Normal nutrition parameters
- Anatomy and physiology of gastrointestinal system
- Cultural influences on nutrition
- Developmental factors affecting nutrition
- Effects of medications on nutrition

STANDARDS

- Apply intellectual standards of accuracy, completeness, and significance when obtaining a health history for clients with altered nutrition
- Compare gathered data with established nutritional standards, (e.g., dietary reference intake, food pyramid, food guidelines, and healthy eating index)

ASSESSMENT

- Identify the signs and symptoms associated with altered nutrition
- Gather data from clients regarding nutritional practices
- Determine clients' nutritional energy needs (REE $\times$ activity or illness factor)
- Obtain clients' dietary history

EXPERIENCE

- Caring for clients with altered nutrition
- Observation of nutritional practices of friends and family
- Personal assessment of nutritional practices

ATTITUDES

- Be open minded about the client's nutritional practices when obtaining nutritional assessment
- Display confidence when collecting data related to culture, socioeconomic status, physical functioning, dietary restrictions, and personal preferences as necessary to a complete nutritional assessment

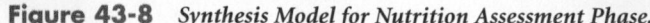

Figure 43-8 *Synthesis Model for Nutrition Assessment Phase.*

Critical Thinking Synthesis

Successful critical thinking requires a synthesis of knowledge, experience, information collected from clients, critical thinking attitudes, and intellectual and professional standards. Clinical judgments require the nurse to anticipate the required information, analyze the data, and make decisions regarding client care. Critical thinking is a dynamic process. During assessment (Figure 43-8) the nurse must consider all elements that build toward making appropriate nursing diagnoses.

In the case of nutrition, the nurse must integrate knowledge from nursing and other disciplines, previous experiences, and information gathered from clients and families regarding customary food preferences, as well as recent dietary history. The use of professional standards, such as the DRIs developed by the Food and Nutrition Board (see Tables 43-4, 43-5, and 43-6), the USDA's food

---

Gerontological NURSING PRACTICE | Box 43-1

FACTORS AFFECTING FOOD CHOICE
Income
Educational level
Nutrition knowledge
  Reading food labels
  Nutrient value of foods
  Number of required servings per day
Physical functional level to meet activities of daily living (ADLs)
Dentition
Socialization versus isolation
Loss of spouse
Depression
Disease or pathological process
Transportation

FACTORS AFFECTING NUTRIENT ABSORPTION
Alcohol consumption oz/day
Decreased liver mass
Decreased renal function
Decreased gastrointestinal peristalsis
Decreased HCl and digestive enzymes
Gastrointestinal disorder/malabsorption
Polypharmacy/chronic medications
Disease/pathological process

FACTORS AFFECTING NUTRIENT NEEDS
Calcium, vitamin D, or phosphorus for basic metabolic demand (BMD)
B_{12} may not be synthesized because of lack of intrinsic factor in terminal ileum
Decreased lean muscle mass, lower basic energy expenditure (BEE)

Modified from Lueckenotte AG: *Gerontologic nursing*, ed 2, St. Louis, 2000, Mosby.

Table 43-15 Religious Dietary Restrictions

Islam	Christianity	Hinduism	Judaism	Church of Jesus Christ of Latter-Day Saints (Mormons)	Seventh-Day Adventists Church
Pork	Minimal or no alcohol	All meats	Pork	Alcohol	Pork
Alcohol	Holy day observances may restrict meat		Predatory fowl	Tobacco	Shellfish
Caffeine			Shellfish (eat only fish with scales)	Caffeine	Alcohol
Ramadan fasting sunrise to sunset for month			Rare meats		Vegetarian diet encouraged
Ritualized methods of animal slaughter required for meat ingestion			Blood (blood sausage, etc.)		
			Mixing of milk or dairy products with meat dishes		
			Must adhere to kosher food preparation methods		
			24 hr of fasting on Yom Kippur, a day of atonement		
			No leavened bread eaten during Passover (8 days)		
			No cooking on the Sabbath (Saturday)		

Nutrition

The incidence of lactose intolerance around the world occurs from high to low in the following ethnic or racial groups: Asian-Pacific, African and African-American, Native American, Mexican-American, Middle Eastern, followed by white Caucasian. This condition affects nutrient absorption, and calcium deficiency results. Calcium is necessary for maintaining bone mass density. Alternative sources of calcium with low lactose are aged cheddar or Swiss cheese, green leafy vegetables, legumes, tofu, sardines, nuts, and low-lactose milk products.

The theory of hot and cold foods predominates in many cultures. The origin appears to be from Hippocratic beliefs concerning health and the four humors. Arabs were keepers of this knowledge during the Dark Ages and later influenced the Spanish to adopt this belief system in the later Middle Ages. The foundation is keeping harmony with nature by balancing "cold," "hot," "wet," and "dry." Filipinos, Caribbean Islanders, Mexicans, and Latinos may plan their meals based upon these beliefs. Immigrants to the United States and Canada have assimilated to varying degrees. Food classification as hot or cold varies slightly from one culture to another.

Mexicans believe hot is warmth, strength, and reassurance, whereas cold is menacing and weak. Classification has nothing to do with spiciness but is a symbolic representation of temperature. Hot foods include rice, grain cereals, alcohol, beef, lamb, chili peppers, chocolate, cheese, Temperate Zone fruits, eggs, peas, goat's milk, cornhusks, oils, onions, pork, radishes, and tamales. By contrast, cold foods encompass beans, citrus fruits, tropical fruits, dairy products, most vegetables, honey, raisins, chicken, fish, and goat. Foods can be made hot or cold through methods of preparation. A blending of hot and cold balances food. Menstruation, cancer, pneumonia, earache, colds, paralysis, headache, and rheumatism are cold illnesses requiring hot foods. Pregnancy, fever, infections, diarrhea, rashes, ulcers, liver problems, constipation, kidney problems, and sore throats are believed to be hot conditions; thus cold foods may be eaten during these times.

guide pyramid (see Figure 43-5), dietary guidelines (see Table 43-8), and healthy eating index (see Table 43-9) provide assistance in maintaining clients' positive nutritional status. The World Health Organization (WHO/Food and Agriculture Organization of the United Nation (FAO), 1994, 1996, 1998a, 1998b) also offers nutrition guidelines. Other professional standards by the American Heart Association (1996), the American Diabetic Association, and the American Society for Parenteral and Enteral Nutrition (ASPEN) (1993, 1996) are available. These standards are research based and are regularly updated for optimal client care.

Nursing Process and Nutrition

Nurses are in an excellent position to recognize signs of poor nutrition and to take steps to initiate change. Close contact with clients and their families enables nurses to make observations about physical status, food intake, weight changes, and response to therapy.

ASSESSMENT

Early recognition of malnourished or at-risk clients has a strong positive influence on both short- and long-term health outcomes (Evans-Stoner, 1997). Studies have identified 40% to 55% of adult hospitalized clients as being either malnourished or at risk for malnutrition and have also found a relationship between malnutrition and adverse outcomes, including mortality (Gallagher-Allred and others, 1996). Nutrition assessment forms used to identify clients in need or at risk are useful. Hennessy and Orr (1996), Kovacevich and others (1997), and Costello and Todd-Magel, (1997) are sources of useable forms. Assessment of nutritional status is essential due to the common need of all human beings for nutrients, energy, and fluids. Nutrition assessment centers on five major areas: anthropometry, laboratory tests, dietary and health history, clinical observation, and client expectations.

Anthropometry. **Anthropometry** is a measurement system of the size and makeup of the body. Height and weight should be obtained for each client on hospital admission or entry into any health care setting. If possible, the client should be weighed at the same time each day, on the same scale, and with the same clothing or linen. Rapid weight gain usually reflects fluid shifts. One pint of fluid equals one pound. Height and weight can be compared to standards for height-weight relationships. Recent weight changes should be documented.

Body mass index (BMI) measures weight corrected for height and serves as an alternative to traditional height-weight relationships. Calculation of BMI is achieved by dividing the client's weight in kilograms by his or her height in meters squared $\frac{\text{Weight (Kg)}}{\text{Height}^2 \text{ (M}^2)}$. A BMI of less than 20 places a client at higher medical risk of respiratory disease, tuberculosis, digestive disease, and some cancers. By contrast, a BMI of greater than 35 places a client at higher medical risk of coronary heart disease, some cancers, diabetes mellitus, and hypertension (Grodner, Anderson, and DeYoung, 2000).

An **ideal body weight (IBW)** provides an estimate of what a person should weigh. This can be calculated by use of the rule of "5s and 6s." For women IBW equals 100 pounds plus 5 additional pounds for each inch of height over 60 inches (5 feet). Males' IBW can be estimated by a baseline of 106 pounds plus 6 additional pounds for each

Table 43-16 Complete Versus Incomplete Protein Sources

Foods Containing Complete Proteins	Foods Containing Incomplete Proteins
Meat	**Cereals**
Fish, shellfish	Ready to eat
Chicken	Oatmeal
Turkey	
Duck	**Grains**
Beef	Wheat
Lamb	Rice
Pork	Corn
	Oats/oatmeal
Eggs	Barley
	Pasta
Soybeans (tofu)	Bagels
	Bread
Cheese	
Hard Cheeses	**Legumes**
Muenster	Black-eyed peas
Swiss cheese	Lentils
Soft Cheeses	Beans
Cottage cheese	Peanuts/peanut butter
Ricotta	Chick peas
	Split peas
Milk	
Ice cream	**Vegetables**
Yogurt	Potatoes
Frozen yogurt	Green peas
	Leafy green vegetables
	Broccoli

Food Combinations That Provide Complete Protein

A. GRAINS + LEGUMES = COMPLETE PROTEIN	B. GRAINS OR LEGUMES + SMALL AMOUNT ANIMAL PROTEIN = COMPLETE PROTEIN
Peanut butter sandwich	Chili with beans and cornbread
Tacos with refried beans	Ready to eat cereal with skim milk
Rice and beans	Cheese sandwich
Split pea soup with croutons	Pasta with cheese
Falafel (chick-pea balls) on pita bread	Rice pudding
Lentil soup with rye bread	French toast
Baked beans with bread	Pancakes (made with milk and/or eggs)
	Tuna casserole

From Grodner M, Anderson S, DeYoung S: *Foundations and clinical applications of nutrition: a nursing approach*, ed 2, St. Louis, 2000, Mosby.

inch of height over 60 inches. Addition of 10% for large-boned frame or subtraction of 10% for small-boned frame is also applied. Other useful measures include current body weight (CBW) and usual body weight (UBW). Percentage of weight loss is calculated by subtracting the CBW from the UBW, dividing the difference by the UBW, and multiplying that quotient by 100.

If height cannot be measured with the client standing, position the client lying flat in bed as straight as possible,

arms folded on the client's chest, and measure the client lengthwise.

Anthropometric measurements that aid in identifying nutritional problems include the ratio of height to wrist circumference, mid-upper arm circumference (MAC), triceps skinfold (TSF), and mid-upper arm muscle circumference (MAMC). Significant variation may result unless the examiner is skilled and has proper equipment. Values for MAC, TSF, and MAMC are compared to standards and calculated as a percentage of the standard. Changes in values for an individual over time are of greater significance than isolated measurements. For more information see Williams (1997).

Bioelectrical impedance analysis (BIA) is noninvasive and increasingly replacing traditional anthropometric methods, but it is not available in all health care settings. Assessment is derived from measurement of an innocuous electrical current that travels from one (of four) externally attached poles to another (one on each distal arm and leg). The speed of current is different for lean versus fat tissue. BIA is considered to be a more direct and immediate measure of lean body mass (Bioelectrical Impedance Analysis, 1996).

Laboratory and Biochemical Tests.

No single laboratory or biochemical test is diagnostic for malnutrition. Factors that may alter test results include fluid balance, liver function, kidney function, and the presence of disease. Common laboratory tests used to study nutritional status include measures of plasma proteins such as albumin, transferrin, prealbumin, retinol binding protein, total iron-binding capacity, and hemoglobin. After feeding, the response time for changes in these proteins ranges from hours to weeks. The metabolic half-life of albumin is 21 days, transferrin is 8 days, prealbumin is 2 days, and retinol binding protein is 12 hours. This range demonstrates why albumin level, for example, is not an accurate short-term indicator of serum protein status (Pagana and Pagana, 1999). Furthermore, serum albumin levels are affected by the following factors: hydration; hemorrhage; renal or hepatic disease; high-output drainage of wounds, drains, burns, or the gut; steroid administration; exogenous albumin infusions; age; and trauma, burns, stress, or surgery. In summary, albumin level is a better indicator for chronic illnesses, whereas prealbumin level is preferred for acute conditions.

Nitrogen balance is important to establish serum protein status (see the discussion of protein in this chapter). Nitrogen intake is calculated by dividing 6.25 into the total grams of protein ingested in a day (24 hours). The output of nitrogen is established through laboratory analysis of a 24-hour urinary urea nitrogen (UUN). For clients with diarrhea or fistula drainage, a further addition of 2 to 4 g of nitrogen output is estimated. Nitrogen balance is found by subtracting the nitrogen output from the nitrogen intake. A positive (more nitrogen is taken in than is put out) 2- to 3-g nitrogen balance is ideal for anabolism. By contrast, negative (more nitrogen is put out than is taken in) nitrogen balance is present when catabolic states exist, seen in either starvation or physiologic stress.

Dietary History and Health History.

In addition to the general nursing history, the nurse obtains a more specific diet history to assess the client's actual or potential needs. The diet history focuses on the client's habitual intake of foods and liquids, as well as information about preferences, allergies, and other relevant areas, such as the client's ability to obtain food. The nurse gathers information about the client's illness/activity level to determine energy needs (see Table 43-1) and compares food intake. Nursing assessment of nutrition includes health status; age; cultural background (see Box 43-2); religion (see Table 43-15); socioeconomic status; personal preference; psychological factors; use of alcohol or illegal drugs; vitamin, mineral, or herbal supplements; prescription or over-the-counter (OTC) drugs (see Table 43-13); and nutrition knowledge (Evans-Stoner, 1997).

In outpatient settings, a 3- to 7-day food diary may be kept by the client. This allows the nurse to calculate nutritional intake and to compare it with DRIs to see if dietary habits are adequate. Food-frequency questionnaires may be used to establish patterns over time.

Clinical Observation.

Clinical observations can be among the most important aspects of a nutritional assessment. As in other kinds of nursing assessment, the nurse observes the client for signs of nutritional alterations. Because improper nutrition affects all body systems, clues to malnutrition may be observed during physical assessment (see Chapter 32). When the general physical assessment of body systems is complete, the nurse can recheck pertinent areas to evaluate the client's nutritional status. The clinical signs of nutritional status (Table 43-17) provide guidelines for observation during physical assessment.

Client Expectations.

Clients rely on health care professionals to identify problems of which they may not be aware. Most nutritional problems tend to develop insidiously over weeks and months, not overnight. Lindseth (1997) studied graduate nurses and found scores of 50% to 60% on nutrition knowledge. The poorest scores were for topics related to nutrient requirements for specific populations, body weight versus energy intake, and food sources of specific nutrients. In a similar study Weigley (1995) found several specific nutrition tasks that were performed least by nurses. These tasks included development of nutrition plans, reference to diet manuals and research literature, use of nutritional materials in teaching, and use of resources to learn about clients' cultural food habits. A firm knowledge base is important to meet client expectations.

NURSING DIAGNOSIS

Assessment enables the nurse to determine existence of actual or potential nutrition problems (Box 43-3). Knowledge of normal nutrition parameters, anatomy and physiology of the GI system, and cultural, developmental, pharmacological, and dietary guidelines is necessary for complete assessment. A problem may occur when overall intake is significantly decreased or increased

Table 43-17   Clinical Signs of Nutritional Status

Body Area	Signs of Good Nutrition	Signs of Poor Nutrition
General appearance	Alert: responsive	Listless, apathetic, cachexia, cachectic appearance
Weight	Weight normal for height, age, body build	Obesity or underweight appearance (special concern for underweight)
Posture	Erect posture; straight arms and legs	Sagging shoulders; sunken chest; humped back
Muscles	Well-developed, firm muscles; good tone; some fat under skin	Flaccid appearance, poor tone, underdeveloped tone; tenderness; edema; wasted appearance; inability to walk properly
Nervous system control	Good attention span; lack of irritability or restlessness; normal reflexes; psychological stability	Inattention; irritability; confusion; burning and tingling of hands and feet (paresthesia); loss of position and vibratory sense; weakness and tenderness of muscles (may result in inability to walk); decrease or loss of ankle and knee reflexes; absent vibratory sense
Gastrointestinal function	Good appetite and digestion; normal regular elimination; no palpable organs or masses	Anorexia; indigestion; constipation or diarrhea; liver or spleen enlargement
Cardiovascular function	Normal heart rate and rhythm; lack of murmurs; normal blood pressure for age	Rapid heart rate (above 100 beats/min), enlarged heart; abnormal rhythm; elevated blood pressure
General vitality	Endurance; energy, good sleep habits; vigorous appearance	Easily fatigued; lack of energy; falling asleep easily, tired and apathetic appearance
Hair	Shiny, lustrous appearance; firmness; strands not easily plucked, healthy scalp	Stringy, dull, brittle, dry, thin, and sparse, depigmented appearance; strands that can be easily plucked
Skin (general)	Smooth and slightly moist skin with good color	Rough, dry, scaly, pale, pigmented, irritated appearance; bruises; petechiae; subcutaneous fat loss
Face and neck	Uniform color; smooth, pink, healthy appearance; lack of swelling	Greasy, discolored, scaly, swollen appearance; dark skin over cheeks and under eyes; lumpiness or flakiness of skin around nose and mouth
Lips	Smoothness; good color; moist (not chapped or swollen) appearance	Dry, scaly, swollen appearance; redness and swelling (cheilosis); angular lesions at corners of mouth; fissures or scars (stomatitis)
Mouth, oral membranes	Reddish pink mucous membranes in oral cavity	Swollen, boggy oral mucous membranes
Gums	Good pink color; healthy and red appearance; lack of swelling or bleeding	Spongy gums that bleed easily; marginal redness, inflammation; receding gums
Tongue	Good pink or deep reddish color; lack of swelling; smoothness, presence of surface papillae; lack of lesions	Swelling, scarlet and raw appearance; magenta color, beefiness (glossitis); hyperemic and hypertrophic papillae; atrophic papillae
Teeth	Lack of cavities and pain; bright, straight appearance; lack of crowding; well-shaped jaw; clean appearance with no discoloration	Unfilled caries; absent teeth; worn surfaces; mottled (fluorosis), malpositioned appearance
Eyes	Bright, clear, shiny appearance; lack of sores at corner of membranes; eyelids; moist and healthy pink color; prominent blood vessels or lack of mound of tissue or sclera; lack of fatigue circles beneath eyes	Pale eye membranes (pale conjunctivas); redness of membrane (conjunctival injection); dryness; signs of infection; Bitot's spots, redness and fissuring of eyelid corners (angular palpebritis); dryness of eye membrane (conjunctival xerosis); dull appearance of cornea (corneal xerosis); soft cornea (keratomalacia)
Neck (glands)	Lack of enlargement	Thyroid enlargement
Nails	Firm, pink appearance	Spoon shape (koilonychia); brittleness; ridges
Legs, feet	Lack of tenderness, weakness, or swelling; good color	Edema; tender calf; tingling; weakness
Skeleton	Lack of malformations	Bowlegs; knock-knees; chest deformity at diaphragm; prominent scapulae and ribs

From Williams SR: *Nutrition and diet therapy,* ed 8, St. Louis, 1997, Mosby.

or when one or more nutrients are not ingested, completely digested, or completely absorbed. Specific diagnoses are related to the actual nutrition problem (e.g., inadequate intake) but may also involve problems that place the client at risk for nutritional deficiencies, such as oral trauma, severe burns, or infections.

NURSING DIAGNOSES   Box 43-3
NUTRITION RELATED

Aspiration, risk for in enteral nutrition (EN) therapy
Breastfeeding, effective
Breastfeeding, ineffective
Breastfeeding, interrupted
Constipation
Diarrhea
Fluid volume deficit
Fluid volume excess
Health maintenance, altered
Health-seeking behaviors (nutrition)
Infant feeding pattern, ineffective
Infection, risk for
Knowledge deficit (nutrition)
Management of therapeutic regimen, individuals: ineffective
Nutrition, altered: less than body requirements
Nutrition, altered: more than body requirements
Self-care deficit, feeding
Skin integrity, impaired
Skin integrity, impaired, risk for
Ventilatory weaning response, dysfunctional

The nursing diagnostic statement is based on defining characteristics present in the assessment database (Box 43-4). In addition, the suspected health problem related to the nursing diagnosis is stated.

PLANNING

Planning to maintain optimal nutritional status requires a higher level of care than simply correction of problems. Synthesis of client information from multiple sources is necessary (Figure 43-9). Critical thinking application is the best way to ensure that all data sources are considered in developing a client's plan of care. Referring to professional standards for nutrition is especially important during this step, since published standards are based on scientific findings. The identification of clients at risk for nutritional problems should result in a care plan that will prevent or minimize nutritional problems (see care plan, pp. 1354-1355).

The intake of food is often altered in the perioperative period. Preoperative nutrition support should be administered to clients with malnutrition. The resumption of food intake postoperatively depends upon the return of bowel function, the extent of the surgical procedure, and the presence of any complications (see Chapter 49).

Clients who have had oral and throat surgery must chew and swallow food in the presence of excision sites, sutures, or otherwise manipulated tissue. The ingestion of food causes discomfort, so clients are usually reluctant to eat or drink. Fluids are usually offered first. The use of a

SAMPLE NURSING DIAGNOSTIC PROCESS   Box 43-4
NUTRITION

Assessment Activities	Defining Characteristics	Nursing Diagnosis
BMI	BMI = 17	Altered nutrition: less than body requirements
Body weight within gender/age/height range	72-year-old female Ht = 5'6" (167.6 cm), Wt = 106 lb (48.08 kg) 20% below IBW (130 lb)	

24-hr food history	Inadequate intake reported
	    Early satiety
	    Lack of interest in food	

Fluid intake	Low fluid intake, mostly coffee Low evening intake due to nocturia	
Physical assessment	Pale conjunctivae and mucous membranes, dry scaly skin, dull thinning hair, and taste change 2 + pitting ankle edema bilaterally	
Laboratory values	Serum albumin, 2.6 g/dl; total lymphocyte count, 750	
Knowledge of nutrition	Unfamiliar with food pyramid or dietary guidelines	

Review medical history
    Medication
    Diagnoses
	
	Sertraline, captopril
	Depression	

Review social history	Death of spouse 6 mo ago	

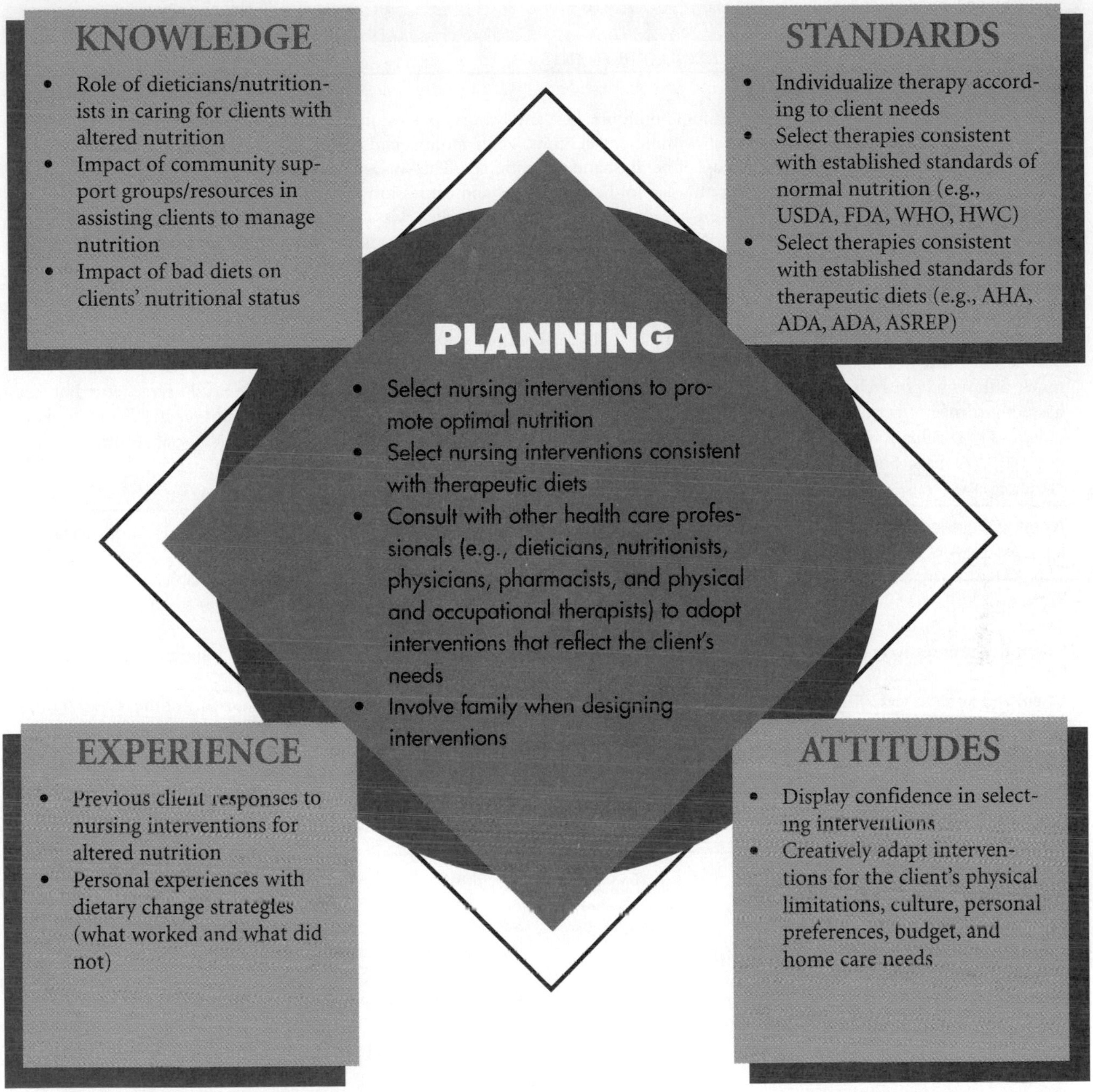

KNOWLEDGE

- Role of dieticians/nutritionists in caring for clients with altered nutrition
- Impact of community support groups/resources in assisting clients to manage nutrition
- Impact of bad diets on clients' nutritional status

STANDARDS

- Individualize therapy according to client needs
- Select therapies consistent with established standards of normal nutrition (e.g., USDA, FDA, WHO, HWC)
- Select therapies consistent with established standards for therapeutic diets (e.g., AHA, ADA, ADA, ASREP)

PLANNING

- Select nursing interventions to promote optimal nutrition
- Select nursing interventions consistent with therapeutic diets
- Consult with other health care professionals (e.g., dieticians, nutritionists, physicians, pharmacists, and physical and occupational therapists) to adopt interventions that reflect the client's needs
- Involve family when designing interventions

EXPERIENCE

- Previous client responses to nursing interventions for altered nutrition
- Personal experiences with dietary change strategies (what worked and what did not)

ATTITUDES

- Display confidence in selecting interventions
- Creatively adapt interventions for the client's physical limitations, culture, personal preferences, budget, and home care needs

Figure 43-9 *Synthesis Model for Nutrition Planning Phase.*

straw may help in some cases, but it is specifically contraindicated in others such as dental extractions, dental surgeries, and cleft palate repairs. Soft foods are sometimes easier to swallow than liquids. Hot fluids, tart juices, and coarse food that is difficult to chew should be avoided after throat or mouth surgery. Parenteral or enteral nutrition may be required.

Nasogastric suction is often used following GI surgery to prevent distention and pressure on resected areas (see Chapter 45). When oral intake is restricted, fluids are usually given intravenously, but these fluids are characteristically nutrient poor. Standard 5% dextrose solutions contain only 170 kcal/L. Gastric resections may limit the amount of food that can be ingested per meal if the remaining gastric pouch is small. Frequent small meals may be advised. Other surgeries on the stomach and intestines may require an alternative method of feeding. Intestinal surgery may interfere with absorption of nutrients (**malabsorption**) or the amount of stool losses if large portions of the intestine are resected or bypassed or if an ileostomy or mucous fistula is created (see Chapter 45). Clients with ileostomies may lose ability to absorb vitamin B_{12} since the ileum is the site of absorption for this vitamin.

Extended immobilization can result in deossification

SAMPLE NURSING CARE PLAN

ALTERED NUTRITION: LESS THAN BODY REQUIREMENTS

ASSESSMENT*

Marie walked with Mrs. Cooper into an examination room. As a family nurse practitioner, Marie worked with Dr. Harris to deliver client care. Mrs. Cooper's vital signs were all within normal limits. Three months had passed since Mrs. Cooper had been started on sertraline for depression related to the loss of her husband 6 months ago. This was an initial episode of depression. Mrs. Cooper had also been referred for counseling 3 months ago for help with grief and depression through a local senior service agency. After checking Mrs. Cooper's weight and reviewing her chart, Marie realized her client was **20% below her IBW** and had a **low BMI of 17.** This weight loss had occurred in **6 months' time, down 24 pounds.** Mrs. Cooper said "I'm just **not interested in food.** It has **no taste."** Mrs. Cooper also said she **gets full quickly.** Marie observed **dull, thinning hair, dry scaling skin, pale conjunctivae and mucous membranes** in addition to **⁺2 pitting edema bilaterally in the ankles.** Mrs. Cooper complained of chronic constipation and said she, **tires easily.** Marie noted generalized poor muscle tone and a stooped posture. Laboratory data revealed a **low serum albumin level** of 2.6 g/dl and a **TLC** of 750 (see Table 43-19). Laboratory values also suggested dehydration. Mrs. Cooper said she drinks some juice in the morning and 2 or 3 cups of coffee. Mrs. Cooper complained of loneliness, and said she does not get out much, although her psychologist recommended more socializing. She said she likes her counselor and that she feels better but just has not returned to her old self. Her friends at church call her to come back to meetings, but she is just not ready. When Marie inquired as to her financial situation, Mrs. Cooper responded that it was tight living on a small pension and Social Security, but she was able to manage. She thanked Marie for finding a psychologist that she could afford.

*Defining characteristics are shown in bold type.

NURSING DIAGNOSIS:

Altered nutrition: less than body requirements related to an inability to ingest food as a result of psychological depression

PLANNING

GOALS	EXPECTED OUTCOMES
Client will progressively gain weight.	Client will gain 1 to 2 pounds per month until goal of 130 pounds is reached.
Client will learn to verbalize key nutritional concepts.	Client will demonstrate an understanding of the food pyramid and dietary guidelines.
Client will consume adequate nourishment each day.	Client will ingest 1900 kcal/day, including 50 g of protein per day.
Client will exhibit no signs of malnutrition.	Physical assessment and laboratory values will be within normal limits.

INTERVENTIONS†

Nutritional Counseling
- Coordinate plan of care with physician, psychologist, client, and dietitian.
- Individualize menu plans.
- Frequent small meals.
- Review food pyramid.
- Review dietary guidelines.

Nutritional Monitoring
- Monitor client monthly for weight gain, anemia, serum albumin level, and TLC.

- Perform physical assessment of hair, eyes, mouth, skin, and muscle tone.

Nutritional Management
- Promote optimal oral hygiene before and after meals.

- Alternate rest with activity, resting before meals and after for 30 min.
- Consider medication (sertraline)-induced anorexia and diminished taste.
- Encourage fluid intake.

RATIONALE

Successful nutrition care planning is a multidisciplinary approach throughout the continuum of care.
Individualized meal planning is more useful to the client.
Frequent small meals offset early satiety.
USDA (1998) and USDA and USDHHS (1997) recommendations for optimal nutrition.

Weight gain should be slow and progressive. Serum albumin of >4.0 g/dl and TLC >1500/mm³ are within normal limits (Grodner, Anderson, and DeYoung, 2000).

Consistent oral hygiene promotes taste sensation (Chernoff, 1991).
This allow for necessary energy for eating and digestion (Williams, 1997).
SSRIs diminish taste and appetite.

Older adults need eight 8-ounce glasses per day of fluid from beverage and food sources. Concentrating intake in morning and early afternoon is acceptable to prevent nocturia.

†Intervention Classification labels from McCloskey JC, Bulechek GM: *Nursing interventions classification (NIC),* ed 3, St. Louis, 2000, Mosby.

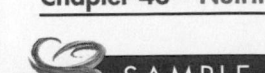

SAMPLE NURSING CARE PLAN — cont'd

ALTERED NUTRITION: LESS THAN BODY REQUIREMENTS

INTERVENTIONS†	RATIONALE
Nutritional Management	
• Encourage fiber intake.	Adequate fluid, fiber, and exercise deter constipation.
• Consult with client about referral for congregate meals (lunch at senior center) 5 times per week.	Congregate meal participation would encourage good nutrition and promote socialization with peers.

†Intervention Classification labels from McCloskey JC, Bulechek GM: *Nursing interventions classification (NIC)*, ed 3, St. Louis, 2000, Mosby.

EVALUATION

Ask client to identify groups depicted in the food pyramid and representative food choices.

Ask client to restate number of servings from each group necessary for her optimal nutrition.

Ask client to verbalize amount of kilocalories and protein she needs each day.

Observe and monitor physical nutrition status (weight, biochemical indicators).

Ask client about appetite and taste status.

---

and osteoporosis of bones, in addition to hypercalcemia (see Chapter 46), since without weight-bearing activity calcium leaves the bones. Hypercalcemia predisposes clients to kidney and bladder stones. It is a particular problem in children and adolescents because of their rapid bone growth. Ambulation is the best way to prevent demineralization of bone from immobility. When ambulation is not possible, adequate quantities of high-biological-value proteins help prevent skin breakdown and infections, and high phosphorus intake in the early weeks of immobilization reduces serum calcium levels. Generous fluid intake also safeguards against kidney stones. Range-of-motion exercises for uninvolved joints provides some protection.

Nutritional education and counseling are important for clients on regular diets to prevent disease and promote health. Clients on therapeutic diets who understand the rationale for the diet are more likely to be compliant. For this group of clients the care plan is based on one or more of the following goals:

Client will return to appropriate BMI height-weight range or within 10% of IBW.

Client will maintain fluid and electrolyte balance within normal limits.

Client will ingest or have administered a nutrition that, at a minimum, meets the DRIs.

No complications will result from nutritional therapies.

Individualized client planning cannot be overemphasized. Mutually planned goals negotiated between the client, dietitian, and nurse will ensure success. For example, obese clients will usually respond better to smaller obtainable goals of weight loss accomplished in a series over time than to one large overwhelming goal (Foster and others, 1997).

Health care personnel supervised by the nurse are of invaluable assistance in planning and delivering nutritional care. Meal trays should be delivered while hot, and ill clients may need assistance with tray setup or feeding.

Oral care before meals and after enhances appetite. Clients may need help getting up to a chair, where they may feel more like eating. Collaboration with a registered dietitian ensures appropriate nutrition treatment plans. Calorie counts are frequently ordered, and assistance is necessary in obtaining accurate data. Laboratory tests such as UUNs require urine to be consistently saved for 24 hours. Weights and heights should consistently be on each chart. Assistive health care personnel are also important sources of information regarding client observation and assessment. Two-way communication is essential between the registered nurse and assistive personnel, in addition to communication with personnel in other disciplines.

Meeting nutritional goals requires multidisciplinary input. Knowledge of each discipline's role in provision of nutrition support is necessary to maximize nutritional outcomes. As with any health care team, the physician directs the overall plan of care: ordering diets, laboratory tests, diagnosing, monitoring, and prescribing. A good plan of care requires accurate exchange of information between disciplines.

The nurse is responsible for coordinating and administering that plan of care. The nurse's role in physical assessment of nutritional status is vital. Documentation of client response to therapy is also essential.

The dietitian monitors the client's nutritional status and intake and makes recommendations for changes, based primarily upon data documented in the client's chart. Dietitians are expert in choice of enteral formulas and dietary modifications required for specific disease states.

The pharmacist is expert in drug-nutrient interactions and mixture of total parenteral nutrition (TPN). In addition, occupational therapists work with clients and families to identify assistive devices that aid clients in eating or in rearranging food preparation areas in an effort to maximize the client's functional capacity.

〜 IMPLEMENTATION

Ill or debilitated clients often have poor appetites **(anorexia).** The ketosis that accompanies starvation is an appetite suppressant, and surgical procedures and trauma cause pain. Deficiencies in certain vitamins and minerals can cause anorexia. Nurses can help clients to understand the factors that cause anorexia and use creative approaches to stimulate appetite. During hospitalizations diagnostic testing disrupts many mealtimes or requires nothing by mouth (NPO) status before tests. Clients worried about families, finances, employment, or illnesses are often not able to eat an adequate diet. Both physiological stress due to illness and emotional stress influence dietary need and intake (Table 43-18). Medications may interfere with taste, cause nausea, interfere with absorption, or affect metabolism (see Table 43-13).

A nurse can help stimulate the client's appetite. The environment may be adapted by minimizing odors, attending to oral hygiene, removing reminders of treatment, and positioning the client before meals. Consultation with a dietitian is necessary. Interviewing the client for a dietary history helps in provision of special diets with food preferences the client is more likely to eat. Assessing clients for the need for pharmacological agents to stimulate appetite such as Cyproheptadine (Periactin), Megestrol (Megace), or Dronabinol (Marinol) or to manage symptoms that interfere with nutrition may require physician consultation (see Box 43-4).

Health Promotion.   Nurses are in a key position to educate clients about good nutrition habits. Incorporating knowledge of nutrition into lifestyle serves as prevention against the development of many diseases. Outpatient and community-based settings may be optimal locations for nursing assessment of nutritional practices and status. Early identification of potential or actual problems is the best way to avoid more serious problems. Similarly, in other health care settings, clients with nutritional problems such as obesity may require assistance in menu planning and compliance strategies. The nurse's role as educator often includes educating families and providing information about community resources. A means, such as telephone numbers, of contacting a dietitian or nurse for follow-up questions should always be part of counseling.

Meal planning must take into account the family's budget and different preferences of family members. Specific foods are chosen on the basis of the dietary prescription and food groups. For families on limited budgets, substitutes can be used. For example, bean or cheese dishes can often replace meat in a meal, and evaporated milk or dry skim milk can be used for cooking. The method of preparation may also be modified when it is necessary to minimize certain substances. Baking rather than frying reduces fat intake, and lemon juice or spices can be used to add flavor to low-sodium diets.

Planning menus a week in advance has several benefits. It helps ensure good nutrition or compliance with a specific diet and helps the family stay within the allotted budget. Menus may in turn be checked by a nurse or dietitian for content. Often a simple tip can be of value in meal planning, such as advice to avoid grocery shopping when hungry, which can lead to spontaneous purchases of more expensive or less nutritional foods that are not included in meal plans. The USDA (1998) provides sample weekly meal planning services for a range of sample budgets accessible on the USDA Web site. Food safety is also an important public health issue. Nurses should be aware of the factors related to food safety (Boxes 43-5 and 43-6).

Table 43-18 **Metabolic Responses to Severe Stress**	
Ebb Phase (onset)	Flow Phase (36-48 hours post injury)
Decreased oxygen consumption	Increased oxygen consumption
Cardiac output	Cardiac output
Plasma volume	Plasma volume
Hypothermia	Hyperthermia
Decreased insulin levels	Increased nitrogen excretion
Hyperglycemia	Elevated insulin levels
Hypovolemia	Hyperglycemia
Hypotension	Increased gluconeogenesis
Increased lactate	Normal lactate
Free fatty acids	Increased free fatty acids
Catecholamines	Catecholamines
Glucagon	Glucagon
Cortisol	Cortisol
Insulin resistance	Increased insulin resistance

From Grodner M, Anderson S, DeYoung S: *Foundations and clinical applications of nutrition: a nursing approach,* ed 2, St. Louis, 2000, Mosby.

Food Safety — Box 43-5

Food-Borne Disease	Organism	Food Source	Symptoms*
Botulism	C. botulinum	Improperly home-canned foods, smoked and salted fish, ham, sausage, shellfish	Symptoms are varied from mild discomfort to death in 24 hours, initially nausea, dizziness, progressing to motor (respiratory) paralysis
Escherichia coli	Escherichia coli 0157:H7	Undercooked meat (ground beef)	Severe cramps, nausea, vomiting, diarrhea (may be bloody), renal failure. Appears 1-8 days after eating, lasts 1-7 days
Listeriosis	Listeria L. monocytogenes	Soft cheese, meat (hot dogs, pate, lunch meats), unpasteurized milk, poultry, seafood	Severe diarrhea, fever, headache, pneumonia, meningitis, endocarditis, appears 3-21 days after infection
Perfringens enteritis	Clostridium C. perfringens	Cooked meats, meat dishes held at room or warm temperature	Mild diarrhea, vomiting. Appears 8-24 hours after eating, lasts 1-2 days
Salmonellosis	Salmonella S. typhi S. paratyphi	Milk, custards, egg dishes, salad dressings, sandwich fillings, polluted shellfish	Mild to severe diarrhea, cramps, vomiting. Appears 12 to 24 hours after ingestion, lasts 1-7 days
Shigellosis	Shigella S. dysenteriae	Milk, milk products, seafood, salads	Mild diarrhea to fatal dysentery. Appears 7-36 hours after ingestion. Lasts 3-14 days.
Staphylococcus	Staphylococcus S. aureus	Custards, cream fillings, processed meats, ham, cheese, ice cream, potato salad, sauces, casseroles	Severe abdominal cramps, pain, vomiting, diarrhea, perspiration, headache, fever, prostration. Appears 1-6 hrs after ingestion, lasts 1-2 days

From Williams SR: *Nutrition and diet therapy,* ed 8, St. Louis, 1997, Mosby.
*Symptoms are generally most severe for youngest and oldest age groups.

Client Teaching FOR FOOD SAFETY — Box 43-6

OBJECTIVES
- Client will be able to verbalize measures to protect from food-borne illness.
- Client will understand the primary types of illness and how they are transmitted.
- Client will not experience food-borne illness.

TEACHING STRATEGIES
- Food safety has become an important public health issue in recent years. Populations particularly at risk are older and younger persons, as well as immunosuppressed individuals. See Box 43-5 for specific information on food-borne illnesses.
- Precautionary Measures
  - Wash hands with hot, soapy water before touching or eating food.
  - Cook meat, poultry, fish, and eggs until they are well done.
  - Wash fresh fruits and vegetables thoroughly.
  - Do not eat raw meats or unpasteurized milk.
  - Do not buy or consume food that has passed the expiration date.
  - Keep foods properly refrigerated at 40° F and frozen at 0° F.
  - Wash dishes and cutting boards with hot soapy water.
  - Do not save leftovers for more than 2 days in refrigerator
  - Wash dishrags, towels, and sponges regularly, or use paper towels.
  - Clean the inside of refrigerator and microwave regularly to prevent microbial growth.

EVALUATION
- Ask client to verbalize measures to prevent food-borne illnesses.
- Observe the client at home for safe practices, if making home visit.

Modified from Keithley JK, Swanson B: Minimizing HIV/AIDS malnutrition, *MedSurg Nurs* 7(5):256, 1998.

Acute Care.   Clients who are NPO and receive only standard IV fluids for more than 7 days are at nutritional risk. In addition, nutritional problems commonly occur in conditions such as HIV infection, cancer, eating disorders, gastrointestinal disease, critical illness, malabsorption problems, metabolic diseases, obesity, renal disease, and diseases of the liver, pancreas, and gallbladder.

Table 43-19 gives an overview of the immune system and how it relates to nutrient intake. The normal course of dietary advancement and a basic description of each type of therapeutic diet for hospitalized patients are summarized in Table 43-20.

Enteral Tube Feeding.   **Enteral nutrition (EN)** refers to nutrients given via the GI tract. Enteral nutrition is the preferred method of meeting nutritional needs if the client's GI tract is functioning by providing physiological, safe, and economical nutrition support. Enterally fed clients receive formula via nasogastric, jejunal, or gastric tubes. Gastric feedings may be given to clients with a low risk of aspiration; however, if there is a risk of aspiration, jejunal feeding is preferred. Table 43-21 lists indications for tube feeding. Enteral tube feedings are easily given in the home setting by either the nurse or the family. Regardless of the setting, the principles in Skill 43-1 for gastrostomy and jejunostomy enteral feedings must be maintained.

Tube feedings are typically started at full strength at slow rates of 20 to 50 ml/hr. The hourly rate is increased by 25-ml increments every 12 to 24 hours if no signs of intolerance appear (nausea, cramping, vomiting, diarrhea).

Studies have demonstrated a beneficial effect of enteral feedings compared with parenteral nutrition. Feeding by the enteral route may reduce sepsis, blunt the hypermetabolic response to trauma, and maintain intestinal structure and function (Guenter, Ericson, and Jones, 1997). Enteral nutrition has been used successfully within 24 to 48 hours after surgery or trauma to provide fluids, electrolytes, and nutritional support. Gastric ileus may prevent nasogastric feedings, whereas nasointestinal or jejunal tubes allow successful postpyloric feeding, where formula is placed directly into the small intestine or jejunum or beyond the pyloric sphincter of the stomach (Kudsk, 1994).

Aspiration of enteral formula into the lungs irritates the bronchial mucosa, resulting in decreased blood supply to affected pulmonary tissue. This then leads to necrotizing infection, pneumonia, and potential abscess formation. The high glucose content serves as a bacterial medium for growth, promoting infection. Adult respiratory distress syndrome (ARDS) is also an outcome frequently associated with pulmonary aspiration (Goodwin, 1996).

Enteral nutrition formulas vary in composition and nutrient density. General categories of EN formulas include standard whole protein formulas, hydrolized protein (elemental or peptide), and disease-specific formulas or crystalline amino acids (see Box 43-7, p. 1364).

Table 43-19 Nutrition and the Immune System

Immune/Physiological Component	Malnutrition Effect	Vital Nutrient
Antibodies	Decreased amount	Protein, vitamins A, C, B_{12}, B_6, folic acid, thiamin, biotin, riboflavin, niacin
GI tract	Translocation of bacteria to systemic bodily areas	Arginine, glutamine, omega-3 fatty acids
Granulocytes and macrocytes	Longer time for phagocytosis kill time and lymphocyte activation	Protein, vitamins A, C, B_{12}, B_6, folic acid, thiamin, riboflavin, niacin, zinc, iron
Mucus	Flat microvilli in GI tract, decreased antibody secretion	Vitamins B_{12}, B_6, C, biotin
Skin	Integrity compromised, density reduced, wound healing slowed	Protein, vitamins A, B_{12}, C, niacin, copper, zinc
T-lymphocytes	Depressed T-cell distribution	Protein, arginine, iron, zinc, omega-3 fatty acids, vitamins A, B_{12}, B_6, folic acid, thiamin, riboflavin, niacin, pantothenic acid

Total Lymphocyte Count (TLC)
TLC = % lymphocytes $\times$ WBC count $\div$ 100*

Modified from Grodner M, Anderson S, DeYoung S: *Foundations and clinical applications of nutrition: a nursing approach,* ed 2, St. Louis, 2000, Mosby.

*Results <2000 cells/mm³ suggest impaired immunocompetence; results <1500 cells/mm³ are associated with greater morbidity and mortality.

Table 43-20 Diet Progression of Hospitalized Clients

Clear Liquid
Broth, bouillon, coffee, tea, carbonated beverages, clear fruit juices, gelatin, popsicles

Full Liquid
As above with addition of smooth textured dairy products, custards, refined cooked cereals, vegetable juice, pureed vegetables, all fruit juices

Pureed
All of above with addition of scrambled eggs, pureed meats, vegetables, fruits, mashed potatoes and gravy

Mechanical Soft
All of above with addition of ground or finely diced meats, flaked fish, cottage cheese, cheese, rice, potatoes, pancakes, light breads, cooked vegetables, cooked or canned fruits, bananas, soups, peanut butter

Soft
All of above with addition of moist tender meat, poultry, fish, soft casseroles, lettuce, tomatoes, soft fresh fruit, cake, cookies without nuts or coconut

Regular
No restrictions, unless specified

From Grodner M, Anderson S, DeYoung S: *Foundations and clinical applications of nutrition: a nursing approach*, ed 2, St. Louis, 2000, Mosby.

Table 43-21 Indications for Enteral and Parenteral Nutrition

Enteral Nutrition	Parenteral Nutrition
CANCER	NONFUNCTIONAL GI TRACT
Head and neck	Massive small bowel resection/GI surgery
Upper GI	Paralytic ileus
Critical illness/trauma	Intestinal obstruction
	Trauma to abdomen, head, or neck
	Severe malabsorption
NEUROLOGICAL AND MUSCULAR DISORDERS	Intolerance to enteral feeding (established by trial)
Brain neoplasm	Chemotherapy, radiation therapy, bone marrow
Cerebrovascular accident	transplantation
Dementia	
Myopathy	EXTENDED BOWEL REST
Parkinson's disease	Enterocutaneous fistula
	Inflammatory bowel disease exacerbation
GASTROINTESTINAL DISORDER	Severe diarrhea
Enterocutaneous fistula	Moderate to severe pancreatitis
Inflammatory bowel disease	
Mild pancreatitis	PREOPERATIVE TPN
	Preoperative bowel rest
RESPIRATORY FAILURE WITH PROLONGED INTUBATION	Treatment for comorbid severe malnutrition in patients with nonfunctional GI tracts
	Severely catabolic clients when GI tract nonusable for >4
INADEQUATE ORAL INTAKE	to 5 days
Continuous feedings	
Supine positioning	
Cerebral vascular accident	
Local trauma	
Anorexia nervosa	
Difficulty chewing, swallowing	
Severe depression	

Skill 43-1   Inserting a Small-Bore Nasoenteric Tube for Enteral Feedings

Delegation Considerations

This skill requires problem solving and knowledge application unique to a professional nurse. For this reason, delegation of this skill to assistive personnel is inappropriate.

Equipment

- Nasogastric or nasointestinal tube (8 to 12 Fr) with guide wire or stylet
- 60-ml or larger Luer-Lok or catheter-tip syringe
- Hypoallergenic tape and tincture of benzoin
- pH indicator strip
- Glass of water and straw
- Emesis basin
- Safety pin

- Rubber band
- Towel
- Facial tissues
- Clean gloves
- Suction equipment in case of aspiration
- Penlight to check placement in nasopharynx
- Tongue blade

STEPS	RATIONALE
1. Assess client for the need for enteral tube feeding: NPO or insufficient intake for more than 5 days, functional GI tract, unable to ingest sufficient nutrients.	Identifying clients who need tube feedings before they become nutritionally depleted may help to prevent complications related to malnutrition.
2. Assess client for appropriate route of administration:	Evaluates nares for patency.
a. Close each nostril alternately, and ask client to breathe	Nares may be obstructed. Assessment determines which naris to use.
b. Assess for gag reflex.	Identifies ability to swallow and risk of aspiration.
c. Inspect nares for any irritation or obstruction.	
d. Review client's medical history for nasal problems and risk of aspiration.	Nurse may seek physician's order to change route of nutritional support or to place tube past the stomach into the intestine with increased risk of aspiration.
3. Review physician's order for type of tube and enteral feeding schedule.	Procedure and tube feedings require a physician's order.
4. Wash hands.	Reduces transfer of microorganisms.
5. Explain procedure to client.	Reduces anxiety and helps client to assist in insertion.
6. Stand on same side of bed as naris for insertion, and assist client to high-Fowler's position unless contraindicated. Place pillow behind head and shoulders.	Allows easier manipulation of tube. Fowler's position reduces risk of aspiration and promotes effective swallowing.
7. Place bath towel over chest. Keep facial tissues within reach.	Prevents soiling of gown. Insertion of tube may produce tearing.
8. Determine length of tube to be inserted and mark with tape:	Length approximates distance from nose to stomach in 98% of clients. For duodenal or jejunal placement, an additional 20 to 30 cm is required.
a. Traditional method: measure distance from tip of nose to earlobe to xiphoid process of sternum (see illustration).	
9. Prepare nasogastric or nasointestinal tube for intubation:	
a. Plastic tubes should not be iced.	Tubes will become stiff and inflexible, causing trauma to mucous membranes.
b. Inject 10 ml of water from 30-ml or larger Luer-Lok or catheter-tip syringe into the tube.	Aids in guide wire or stylet insertion.
c. Make certain that guide wire is securely positioned against weighted tip and that both Luer-Lok connections are snugly fitted together.	Promotes smooth passage of tube into GI tract. Improperly positioned stylet can induce serious trauma.
10. Cut tape 10 cm (4 in) long.	
11. Put on clean gloves.	Reduces transmission of microorganisms.
12. Dip tube with surface lubricant into glass of water.	Activates lubricant to facilitate passage of tube into naris to GI tract.
13. Insert tube through nostril to back of throat (posterior nasopharynx). Aim back and down toward ear.	Natural contours facilitate passage of tube into GI tract and reduces gagging by client.

STEPS	RATIONALE
14. Flex client's head toward chest after tube has passed through nasopharynx.	Closes off glottis and reduces risk of tube entering trachea.

Critical Decision Point: Encourage client to swallow by giving small sips of water or ice chips when possible. Advance tube as client swallows. Rotate tube 180 degrees while inserting.

15. Emphasize need to mouth breathe and swallow during the procedure.	Helps facilitate passage of tube and alleviates client's fears during the procedure.
16. Advance tube each time client swallows until desired length has been passed. Do not force tube. If resistance is met or client starts to cough, choke, or become cyanotic, stop advancing the tube and pull tube back.	Reduces discomfort and trauma to client.
17. Check for position of tube in back of throat with penlight and tongue blade.	Tube may be coiled, kinked, or entering trachea.

18. Perform measures to verify placement of tube:
  a. Inject 30 ml of air into the tube, and aspirate GI contents with a syringe.
  b. Measure pH of aspirated GI contents (see illustration).
	Gastric contents are usually cloudy and grassy green or tan to off-white; in contrast, intestinal fluid is usually deep golden yellow and is more clear than gastric fluid (See Figure 43-10). Fasting gastric pH is usually in a range of 1 to 4; only infrequently is it greater than 6. In contrast, intestinal sites usually have a pH of 7 or greater (Metheny and others, 1998).

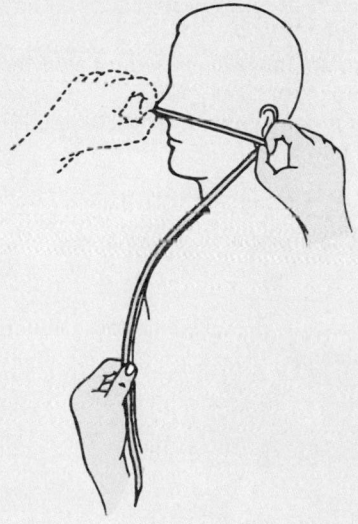

Step 8a

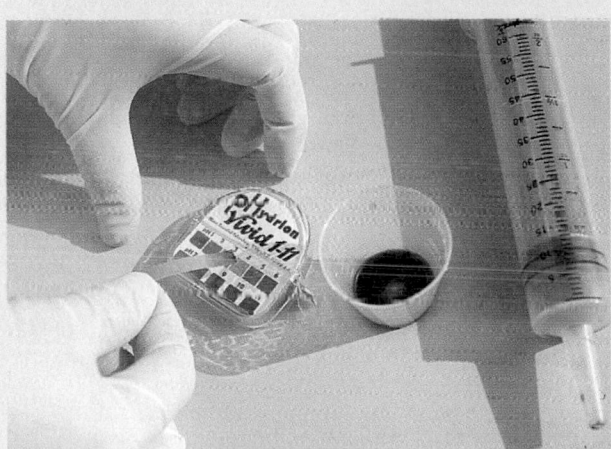

Step 18b

Figure 43-10   Gastrointestinal contents: **A,** Stomach.
B, Stomach. **C,** Intestinal.
Courtesy Dr. Norma Metheny, Professor, St. Louis University
School of Nursing.

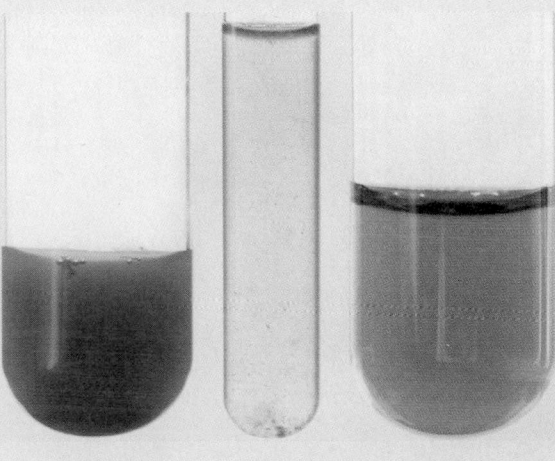

A   B   C

Obtaining GI Fluid for pH Measurement, Large- and Small-Bore Feeding Tubes: Bolus and Continuous Feeding
Timing of pH testing:
- Wait at least 1 hr after oral or tube-administered medications.
- Wait as long as possible after last feeding; this is important because formula elevates the pH of gastric contents.
- For intermittent feedings, test pH immediately prior to administration of new feeding (usually at least 3 hr after previous feeding).
- For continuous feedings, plan pH testing at times when feedings may be withheld, such as for chest physical therapy, transport off the division for tests, or avoidance of medication interaction.

Flush tube with 30 ml of air.
Aspirate GI contents.
- If unable to aspirate GI contents during the first attempt, reposition client to allow tip of tube to rest in a pool of GI fluid. Flush tube with an additional 30 ml of air, and attempt to aspirate.

Modified from Metheny N and others: Effectiveness of pH measurements in predicting feeding tube placement: an update, *Nurs Res* 42(6):324, 1993.

Critical Decision Point: Auscultation is no longer considered a reliable method for verification of tube placement because a tube inadvertently placed in the lungs, pharynx, or esophagus can transmit a sound similar to that of air entering the stomach (Metheny and others, 1990b; Chang and others, 1982).

---

19. Apply tincture of benzoin or other skin adhesive on tip of client's nose and tube. Allow to dry.	Helps tape adhere better. Protects skin.
20. Remove gloves, and secure tube with tape, avoiding pressure on naris.	A properly secured tube allows the client more mobility and prevents trauma to nasal mucosa.
a. Split one end of tape lengthwise 5 cm (2 inches). Place the intact end of tape over bridge of client's nose. Wrap each of the 5-cm strips around tube as it exits nose (see illustrations).	Securing tape to nares prevents tissue necrosis.
b. Fasten end of nasogastric tube to client's gown by looping rubber band around tube in slip knot. Pin rubber band to gown.	Reduces traction on the naris if tube moves.
21. For intestinal placement, position client on right side when possible until radiological confirmation of correct placement has been verified. Otherwise, assist client to a comfortable position.	Promotes passage of the tube into the small intestine (duodenum or jejunum).

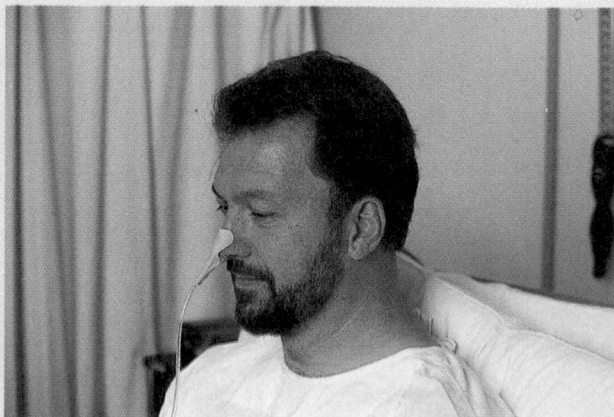
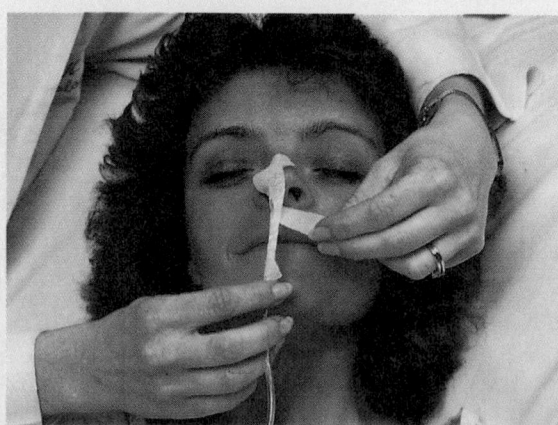

Step 20a

STEPS	RATIONALE

Critical Decision Point: Leave guide wire or stylet in place until correct position is ensured by x-ray film. Never attempt to reinsert partially or fully removed guide wire or stylet while feeding tube is in place.

STEPS	RATIONALE
22. Obtain x-ray film of abdomen.	Placement of tube is verified by x-ray examination (Metheny, 1988).
23. Apply gloves, and administer oral hygiene (see Chapter 38). Cleanse tubing at nostril.	Promotes client comfort and integrity of oral mucous membranes.
24. Remove gloves, dispose of equipment, and wash hands.	Reduces transmission of microorganisms.
25. Inspect naris and oropharynx for any irritation after insertion.	If insertion was difficult, irritation of naris or oropharynx may have occurred.
26. Ask if client feels comfortable.	Evaluates client's level of comfort.
27. Observe client for any difficulty breathing or gagging.	Malposition of the tube may cause these symptoms.

Recording and Reporting

- Record and report type and size of tube placed, location of distal tip of tube, client's tolerance of procedure, pH value, and confirmation of tube position by x-ray.

Home Care Considerations

- Placement may be verified on the basis of pH recordings. A small amount of water may be instilled via the feeding tube while the client is carefully observed for coughing or gagging.
- The client and care provider should be instructed to report pH values that fall outside of an established range and to report any difficulties that occur during the feeding.

Standard formulas are suitable for clients who do not have altered digestion or absorption; elemental and peptide formulas are used for clients who have impaired digestion or absorption; and disease-specific formulas have modifications in the content of specific nutrients or in caloric density. Nearly all tube-feeding formulas are lactose free. Specialty enteral products tend to be very costly, and their use is generally reserved for specific indications (Matarese, 1994). Research is examining nutrients such as glutamine, arginine, nucleotides, and omega-3 fatty acids for enteral formulas.

Enteral Access Tubes. When the client is unable to ingest food but is still able to digest and absorb nutrients, enteral tube feeding is indicated. Feeding tubes can be inserted through the nose (nasogastric or nasointestinal), surgically (gastrostomy or jejunostomy), or endoscopically (percutaneous endoscopic gastrostomy or jejunostomy [PEG or PEJ]). If EN therapy is for less than 4 weeks total, nasogastric or nasojejunal feeding tubes may be used. Surgical or endoscopically placed tubes are preferred for long-term feeding (more than 4 weeks) to reduce the discomfort of a nasal tube and to provide a more secure, reliable access (Bowers, 1996). Clients with gastroparesis (decreased or absent innervation to the stomach that results in delayed gastric emptying) or esophageal reflux, at risk for aspiration, or with a history of aspiration pneumonia require placement of tubes beyond the stomach into the intestine (Sweed, Guenter, and Jones, 1995).

Nursing research has investigated the problems associated with nasoenteric tube placement, type of feeding instilled, rate of feeding, and complications associated with tube feeding. Small-bore feeding tubes create less discomfort for the client and are currently most often used (Figure 43-11). For the adult, most of these tubes are 8 to 12 Fr and 36 to 43 inches long. A stylet is often used during insertion of a small-bore tube to stiffen it. The stylet is removed when the correct position of the feeding tube is confirmed. Skills 43-2 and 43-3 describe the procedure for inserting a small-bore nasoenteric tube and initiating enteral feedings.

Text continued on p. 1367.

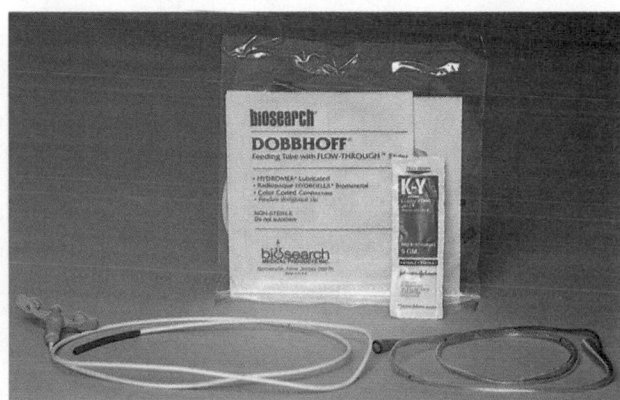

Figure 43-11 Enteral tubes, small bore.

Classification of Enternal Nutrition Products   Box 43-7

Classification	Formula Characteristics	Sample Products
Intact protein		
Blenderized	Isotonic; nutritionally complete; contain fiber; lactose containing and lactose free	Compleat Regular, Vitaneed, Compleat Modified
Low-residue	Isotonic; nutritionally complete; lactose free	Entrition 1.0, Isocal, Isosource, Isolan, Osmolite, Resource
Standard protein		
Intermediate-high protein	Isotonic; nutritionally complete; lactose free	Entrition HN, Isocal HN, Osmolite HN, Isosource HN
Concentrated	Calorically dense (1.5-2.0 cal/ml); lactose free; nutritionally complete; hyperosmolar	Isocal HCN, Magnacal, TwoCal HN, Nutren 2.0
Fiber-supplemented	Isotonic; nutritionally complete; lactose free; fiber ranges from 5-14.4 g/L; standard to intermediate protein	Fibersource, Jevity, Ultracal, Fiberian
Disease specific		
Renal	Low and standard protein; low mineral, vitamin A, and vitamin D content; lactose free; calorically dense; hyperosmolar	Nepro, Suplena
Glucose intolerant	Low CHO, high fat; lactose free; isotonic; contain fiber; nutritionally complete	Glucema
Pulmonary	Low CHO, high fat; lactose free; nutritionally complete; hyperosmolar; calorically dense	Nutrivent, Pulmocare, Respalor
Trauma/stress	High protein; isotonic to hyperosmolar; lactose free; nutritionally complete; some contain fiber, hydrolyzed protein, supplemental amino acids (BCAA, arginine, glutamine), and β-carotene; low to high fat	AlitraQ, Impact, Impact with Fiber, Immun-Aid, Isotein HN, Replete, Replete with Fiber, Traumacal, Promote
Hydrolized protein		
Very low fat	Nutritionally complete, lactose free, fewer than 10% of the calories from fat, hyperosmolar, vary in peptide length, contain amino acids	Accupep HPF, Criticare HN, Vital HN
Low fat	Nutritionally complete, lactose free, 11%-30% of the calories from fat, hyperosmolar, vary in peptide length, contain amino acids	Travasorb HN, Travasorb STD
Moderate fat	Nutritionally complete, lactose free, 30%-35% of the calories from fat (high MCT); hyperosmolar, vary in peptide length, contain amino acids	Peptamen, Reabilan
Disease specific:	Nutritionally complete, lactose free, intermediate to high protein content, 25%-35% of the calories from fat (high MCT), vary in peptide length, contain amino acids, may contain supplemental arginine and β-carotene	Perative, Reabilan HN
Trauma		
Crystalline amino acids	Nutritionally complete, lactose free, low fat (1%-3% of the total calories), low to standard protein content, hyperosmolar	Tolerex, Vivonex TEN
Disease specific	High BCAA, nutritionally incomplete, lactose free, low to moderate fat	Hepatic Aid II, Travasorb Hepatic
Hepatic failure	Essential amino acids plus histidine, nutritionally incomplete, lactose free, hyperosmolar, low fat	Amin-Aid
Renal failure	Essential and nonessential amino acids, nutritionally incomplete but contain water-soluble vitamins, hyperosmolar, lactose free, low fat	Travasorb Renal

From Hopkins B: Enteral formulas. In Zaloga G, editor: *Nutrition in critical care*, St. Louis, 1994, Mosby.
MCT = medium-chain triglyceride; BCAA = branched-chain amino acid; LCT = long-chain triglyceride.

Administering Enteral Feedings via Nasoenteric Tubes | Skill 43-2

Delegation Considerations

Administration of enteral tube feeding via nasogastric tube is a procedure that can be delegated to assistive personnel.

- The professional nurse should verify tube placement before the feeding and establish patency of the tube by flushing it with water.

- The nurse should also ensure that the client is sitting upright in a chair or in bed and instruct assistive personnel to infuse the feeding slowly.
- Assistive personnel should be instructed to report any difficulty infusing the feeding or any discomfort voiced by the client.

EQUIPMENT

- Disposable feeding bag and tubing or ready-to-hang system
- 30-ml or larger Luer-lok or catheter-tip syringe
- Stethoscope
- pH indicator strip
- Infusion pump (required for intestinal feedings): use pump designed for tube feedings

- Prescribed enteral feedings
- Gloves
- Equipment to obtain blood glucose by finger stick

STEPS	RATIONALE
1. Assess client's need for enteral tube feedings: impaired swallowing, decreased level of consciousness, head or neck surgery, facial trauma, surgeries of upper alimentary canal.	Identify clients who need tube feedings before they become nutritionally depleted.
2. Auscultate for bowel sounds before feeding.	Absent bowel sounds may indicate decreased ability of GI tract to digest or absorb nutrients.
3. Obtain baseline weight and laboratory values. Assess client for fluid volume excess or deficit, electrolyte abnormalities, and metabolic abnormalities such as hyperglycemia.	Enteral feedings are to restore or maintain a client's nutritional status. Provides objective data to measure effectiveness of feedings.
4. Verify physician's order for formula, rate, route, and frequency. Laboratory data and bedside assessments, such as finger-stick blood glucose measurement, are also ordered by the physician.	Tube feedings, laboratory tests, and bedside tests must be ordered by physician.
5. Explain procedure to client.	Well-informed client is more cooperative and at ease.
6. Wash hands.	Reduces transmission of microorganisms.
7. Prepare feeding container to administer formula:	
a. Have tube feeding at room temperature.	Cold formula may cause gastric cramping and discomfort because the liquid is not warmed by mouth and esophagus.
b. Connect tubing to container as needed or prepare ready-to-hang container.	Tubing must be free of contamination to prevent bacterial growth.
c. Shake formula container well, and fill container and tubing with formula (see illustration, p. 1366).	Filling the tubing with formula prevents excess air from entering GI tract.
8. Place client in high-Fowler's position, or elevate head of bed 30 degrees.	Elevated head helps prevent aspiration.
9. Determine tube placement:	
a. Aspirate gastric contents to check for gastric residual (see illustration, p. 1366). Return aspirated contents to stomach unless the volume exceeds 150 ml.	Presence of gastric secretions indicates that the distal end of the tube is in the stomach. Residual volume indicates if gastric emptying is delayed. Delayed gastric emptying may be reflected by 150 ml or more remaining in the client's stomach.
b. Measure pH of aspirated GI contents.	Fasting gastric pH is usually equal to or less than 4; it is only infrequently greater than 6; in contrast, intestinal aspirates usually have a pH equal to or greater than 7 (Metheny and others, 1998).
c. Observe the aspirate's appearance.	Gastric fluid is usually cloudy and grassy green or tan to off-white in color; in contrast, intestinal fluid is usually deep golden yellow and is more clear than gastric contents.
d. Consider the results from pH testing and the aspirate's appearance together.	An aspirate with a low pH and a typical gastric fluid color indicates a high probability of gastric placement; in contrast, a golden-colored aspirate with a high pH indicates a high probability of intestinal placement.

STEPS	RATIONALE

Critical Decision Point: Auscultation is no longer considered a reliable method for verification of placement of tube because air in tube inadvertently placed in lungs, pharynx, or esophagus can transmit sound similar to that of air entering stomach (Metheny and others, 1990a, 1990b; Chang and others, 1982).

10.   Initiate feeding:

A.   **Bolus or intermittent feeding**

(1)   Pinch proximal end of the feeding tube.

Prevents air from entering client's stomach.

(2)   Remove plunger from syringe and attach barrel of syringe to end of tube.

(3)   Fill syringe with measured amount of formula. Release tube and hold syringe high enough to allow it to empty gradually by gravity, refill; repeat until prescribed amount has been delivered to the client.

(4)   If feeding bag is used, hang feeding bag on an IV pole. Fill bag with prescribed amount of formula, and allow bag to empty gradually over at least 30 min.

Gradual emptying of tube feeding by gravity from syringe or feeding bag reduces risk of abdominal discomfort, vomiting, or diarrhea induced by bolus or too-rapid infusion of tube feedings.

B.   **Continuous-drip method** (see illustration)

(1)   Hang feeding bag and tubing on IV pole.

Continuous feeding method is designed to deliver prescribed hourly rate of feeding. This method reduces risk of abdominal discomfort. Clients who receive continuous drip feedings should have residuals checked every 4 hr and tube placement verified.

(2)   Connect distal end of tubing to the proximal end of the feeding tube.

(3)   Connect tubing through infusion pump and set rate.

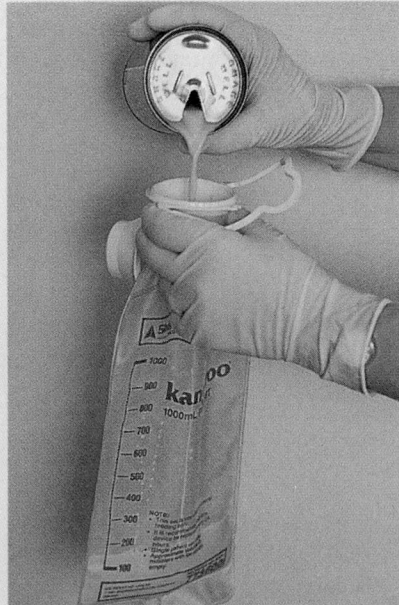

Step 7c

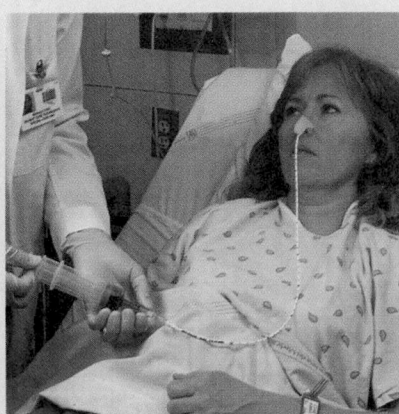

Step 9a

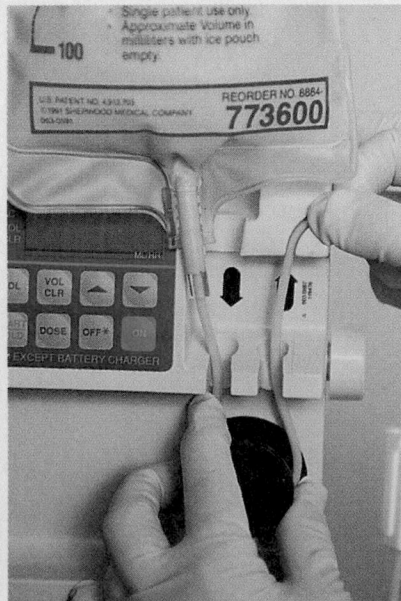

Step 10B

STEPS	RATIONALE
11. Advance tube feeding gradually (see box).	Tube feedings should be advanced gradually to prevent diarrhea and gastric intolerance to formula.

Advancing the Rate of Tube Feeding

Intermittent

1. Start formula at full strength for isotonic formulas (300 to 400 mOsm) or diluted to isotonicity.
2. Infuse formula over at least 20 to 30 min via syringe or feeding container.
3. Begin feedings with no more than 150 to 250 ml at one time. Increase by 50 ml per feeding per day to achieve needed volume and calories in six to eight feedings.

Continuous

1. Start formula at full strength for isotonic formulas (300 to 400 mOsm) or diluted to isotonicity.
2. Begin infusion rate at 30 to 50 ml/hr.
3. Advance rate by 10 to 20 ml/hr per day to target rate if tolerated.

STEPS	RATIONALE
12. When tube feedings are not being administered, cap or clamp the proximal end of the feeding tube.	Prevents air from entering stomach between feedings.
13. Administer water via feeding tube as ordered with diluted formula.	Provides client with source of water to help maintain fluid and electrolyte balance.
14. Rinse bag and tubing with warm water whenever feedings are interrupted.	Rinsing bag and tubing with warm water clears old tube feedings and reduces bacterial growth.
15. Measure amount of aspirate (residual) every 4 hr.	Evaluates tolerance of tube feeding.
16. Monitor finger-stick blood glucose every 6 hr until maximum administration rate is reached and maintained for 24 hr.	Alerts nurse to client's tolerance of glucose.
17. Monitor intake and output every 24 hr.	Intake and output are indications of fluid balance or fluid volume excess or deficit.
18. Weigh client daily until maximum administration rate is reached and maintained for 24 hr; then weigh client 3 times per week.	Weight gain is indicator of improved nutritional status; however, sudden gain of more than 2 lb in 24 hr usually indicates fluid retention.
19. Observe return of normal laboratory values.	Improving laboratory values (e.g., albumin, transferrin, and pre-albumin) indicate an improved nutritional status.

Recording and Reporting

- Record amount and type of feeding, client's response to tube feeding, patency of tube, and any side effects. Report client's tolerance and adverse effects.

Home Care Considerations

- Ask client or care provider about any symptoms or discomfort during enteral feedings. Reinforce instruction to contact nurse if symptoms or discomfort occurs.

Upon insertion, the placement of small-bore feeding tubes is verified by x-ray examination. The tube should then be marked where it exits the nose and taped securely. Historically, feeding tube placement was checked by injecting air through the tube while auscultating the stomach for a gurgling or bubbling sound, or asking the client to speak (Metheny and others, 1998). These methods have a high degree of inaccuracy. Rombeau and Rolandelli (1997) report that clients have been able to speak despite placement of feeding tubes in the lung. Auscultation has repeatedly been shown to be ineffective in detecting tubes accidentally placed in the lung; further, it is not effective in distinguishing between gastric and intestinal placement for stationary feeding tubes (Metheny and others, 1997, 1998). Thus the nurse must suspect tube displacement in clients at risk and use meticulous assessment skills. Metheny, Aud, and Ignatavicius (1998) reported several cases in which nasoenteral feeding tube displacement in the lung went undetected by auscultation.

At present, the most reliable method is radiographic verification, which is cost prohibitive for ongoing placement verification. The measurement of pH of secretions withdrawn from the feeding tube may help to differentiate the location of the tube (see Box 43-8). For accurate pH measurements, 30 ml of air is injected into the tube before measurement to flush out formula, medications, flush so-

Skill 43-3

Administering Enteral Feedings via Gastrostomy or Jejunostomy Tube

Delegation Considerations

Administration of enteral tube feeding via a gastrostomy or jejunostomy tube or a jejunal tube is a procedure that can be delegated to assistive personnel.

- The professional nurse should verify tube placement before the feeding and establish patency of the tube by flushing it with water.

- The nurse should also ensure that the client is sitting upright in a chair or in bed and instruct the assistive personnel to infuse the feeding slowly.
- Assistive personnel should be instructed to report any difficulty infusing the feeding or any discomfort voiced by the client.

EQUIPMENT

- Disposable feeding container or ready-to-hang bag
- 30-ml or larger Luer-Lok or catheter-tip syringe
- Formula
- Infusion pump: use pump designed for tube feedings

- pH indicator strips
- Stethoscope
- Gloves
- Equipment to obtain blood glucose by finger stick

STEPS	RATIONALE
1. Assess client's need for enteral tube feedings (see Skill 43-2): impaired swallowing, decreased level of consciousness, surgeries of upper alimentary tract, need for long-term enteral nutrition.	Identifies clients who need tube feedings before they become nutritionally depleted. Enteral feeding preserves the function and mass of the gut, promotes wound healing, diminishes hypermetabolism in burn injuries, and may decrease infection in critically ill clients (Zaloga, 1994).
2. Auscultate for bowel sounds before feeding. Consult physician if bowel sounds are absent.	Absence of bowel sounds may indicate decreased or absent peristalsis and increased risk of aspiration or abdominal distention.
3. Obtain baseline weight and laboratory values.	Enteral feedings are to restore or maintain nutritional status. Provides objective data to measure effectiveness of feedings.
4. Verify physician's order for formula, rate, route, and frequency.	Tube feedings must be ordered by physician.
5. Explain procedure to client.	Well-informed client is more cooperative and feels more at ease.
6. Prepare feeding container to administer formula:	
a. Have tube feeding at room temperature.	Cold formula may cause gastric cramping and discomfort because the liquid is not warmed by mouth and esophagus.
b. Connect tubing to container as needed, or prepare ready-to-hang bag.	Tubing must be free of contamination to prevent bacterial growth.
c. Fill container and tubing with formula.	Placement of formula through tubing prevents excess air from entering gastrointestinal tract.
7. Elevate head of bed 30 to 45 degrees.	Elevating client's head helps prevent chance of aspiration.
8. Verify tube placement:	
A. **Gastrostomy tube:** Aspirate gastric secretions; observe their appearance and check pH; return aspirated contents to stomach unless the volume exceeds 150 ml.	Gastric fluid is usually cloudy and grassy green or tan to off-white in color; in contrast, intestinal fluid is usually deep golden yellow and more clear than gastric fluid.
B. **Jejunostomy tube:** Aspirate intestinal secretions, observe their appearance and check pH.	Presence of intestinal fluid indicates that the end of the tube is in the small intestine (i.e., duodenum or jejunum). Generally the intestinal residual is very small (10 ml or less). If fluid tests acidic on pH test, looks like gastric fluid, or the residual volume is large (more than 10 ml), displacement of the tube into the stomach may have occurred.
9. Flush with 30 ml of water.	
10. Initiate feedings:	Usually gastrostomy and jejunostomy feedings are given continuously to ensure proper absorption. However, initial feedings may be given by bolus to assess client's tolerance to formula. See Skill 43-2 for guidelines to advance enteral feedings.
A. **Syringe feedings**	
(1) Pinch proximal end of gastrostomy tube.	
(2) Remove plunger and attach barrel of syringe to end of tube, then fill syringe with formula.	
(3) Allow syringe to empty gradually. Refill until prescribed amount has been delivered to client.	

STEPS	RATIONALE

B. **Continuous drip method**
   (1) Fill feeding container with enough formula for 4 hr of feeding.
   (2) Hang container on IV pole, and clear tubing of air.
   (3) Thread tubing on pump according to manufacturer's directions.
   (4) Connect tubing to end of feeding tube.
   (5) Begin infusion at prescribed rate.

STEPS	RATIONALE
11. Assess skin around tube exit site. The skin around the tube should be cleansed daily with warm water and mild soap. Dressings around the exit site are not recommended.	Report any drainage, redness, swelling, or displacement of the tube to the physician.
12. Dispose of supplies, and wash hands.	Prevents transmission of microorganisms.
13. Measure the amount of aspirate (residual) every 4 hr.	Evaluates tolerance of tube feeding.
14. Monitor finger-stick blood glucose every 6 hr until maximum administration rate is reached and maintained for 24 hr.	Alerts nurse to client's tolerance of glucose.
15. Monitor intake and output every 24 hr.	Intake and output are indications of fluid balance or fluid volume excess.
16. Weigh client daily until maximum administration rate is reached and maintained for 24 hr; then weigh client 3 times per week.	Weight gain is indicator of improved nutritional status; however, a sudden gain of more than 2 lb in 24 hr usually indicates fluid retention.
17. Observe return of normal laboratory values.	Improving laboratory values (albumin, transferrin, prealbumin) indicate an improved nutritional status.
18. Inspect site for signs of pressure.	Enteral tubes can cause uncomfortable pressure areas on client's nares.

Recording and Reporting
- Record amount and type of feeding and client's response to tube feeding, patency of tube, and any side effects.
- Report to oncoming nursing staff: type of feeding, status of feeding tube, client's tolerance, adverse effects.

Home Care Considerations
- Ask client or care provider about any symptoms or discomfort during enteral feeding. Reinforce instruction to contact nurse if symptoms or discomfort occur.
- Instruct client or care provider in how to care for gastrostomy or jejunostomy tube site and symptoms to report.

lutions, or other substances (Metheny and others, 1994). Addition of blue food coloring to enteral formula (0.2/250 ml) assists with the detection of formula aspirated into the lung, presumably by staining the tracheobronchial secretions. However, the absence of blue-stained tracheobronchial secretions does not rule out pulmonary aspiration (Davis, 1995; Metheny, Aud, and Wuderlich, 1999). Another method sometimes advocated for detecting pulmonary aspiration of enteral formula is testing the tracheobronchial secretions for the presence of glucose (using glucose reagent strips) (Davis, 1995).

Checking samples of fluid withdrawn from newly inserted feeding tubes for acidic (gastric) or alkaline (intestinal) values prior to use and before intermittent feedings is perhaps the most sensitive bedside indicator of tube placement at this time (Metheny and others, 1998). X-ray verification remains the "gold standard." Concurrent use of acid-inhibitor medications alters gastric pH; however, in clients who have fasted for at least 4 hours, gastric pH continues to be 4 or less in slightly over

half the cases. When acid inhibitors are used, fasting gastric pH is equal to or less that 6 in about three fourths of the cases (Metheny and others, 1998). Acid inhibitors have no effect on intestinal pH, which is usually 7 or greater. For a continuously tube-fed client, gastric pH is expected to be higher because most enteral formulas have pH values close to 6. Thus, although pH is a helpful indicator of tube location, additional markers are needed to help differentiate between gastric and intestinal fluids. Metheny and others have investigated the feasibility of developing indicator strips for pepsin and trypsin (1997) and bilirubin (1999) to measure these substances in fluid aspirated from feeding tubes as a means to detect tube placement (Box 43-8).

Major complications of enteral nutrition are outlined in Table 43-22. Of special note, severely malnourished clients are at risk for electrolyte disturbances from refeeding syndrome as cations such as potassium, magnesium, and phosphate move intracellularly during EN or PN therapy.

Research HIGHLIGHT   Box 43-8

RESEARCH ABSTRACT

Background. Two possible adverse outcomes of enteral nutrition are accidental placement of a nasoenteric feeding tube into the lung and pulmonary aspiration of gastric contents. No one knows the precise incidence of accidental tube misplacements into the lung, but estimates of close to 5% have been cited; clients at highest risk are those with a decreased level of consciousness (LOC), confusion, uncooperativeness, agitation, presence of an endotracheal tube, recent extubation, and poor gag reflex. A feeding tube accidentally inserted into the lung may end in the tracheobronchial tree or perforate into the pleural space. In either event, efforts are made to detect the misplacement prior to the introduction of tube feedings; inadvertent infusion of formula into the lung promotes tissue consolidation, pneumonia, and respiratory failure. The most accurate method for checking feeding tube placement is x-ray examination; the most effective nonradiological methods include aspirating fluid from the feeding tube and measuring its pH and describing its appearance. Far less reliable methods include auscultating for air that is insufflated through the feeding tube and checking for bubbles when the end of the tube is held under water. Although observing for respiratory distress is helpful in alert clients (especially when firm large-diameter tubes are used), it is of little benefit in those who have a decreased LOC and when small-bore tubes are used. Risk factors for pulmonary aspiration in tube-fed clients include feeding into the stomach when gastric atony is present (resulting in high gastric residual volumes), poor gag reflexes, mechanical ventilation, and flat positioning in bed. Bedside methods used to detect pulmonary aspiration are not well defined.

Study One. A survey of 281 intensive care units (ICUs) throughout the United States was conducted by telephone. One ICU nurse per facility was interviewed as to the method used for assessing for pulmonary aspiration in intubated tube-fed clients. Although many authors indicate that using glucose strips to test for glucose in fluid suctioned from the tracheobronchial tree of intubated tube-fed clients is superior to adding blue food dye to the formula and observing for dye-stained secretions, it was found that 73% of the respondents preferred the dye method. Presumably this was because it is easier to perform. Although the dye method is most frequently used, there is little consensus as to the amount of dye needed. Only 1% of the respondents reported using only the glucose method; 13% did not use either method. Further research is required to identify the most effective bedside protocols for identifying pulmonary aspiration of enteral feedings (Metheny and others, 1999).

Study Two. The aim of this study was to examine bilirubin concentrations in pulmonary, gastric, and intestinal regions and to determine the degree to which these findings could add to the ability of the pH method to verify the position of newly inserted nasoenteric tubes. Fluid was withdrawn from 587 feeding tubes at the time of x-ray verification. The average pH in the lung (7.73) and intestine (7.35) was much higher than gastric pH (3.90). As expected, bilirubin was essentially absent from the lung. Also as expected, bilirubin was far more plentiful in intestinal fluid than in gastric fluid (12.73 mg/dl versus 1.28 mg/dl, respectively, $p < .001$). The results strongly support the potential use of bilirubin levels for tube verification (Metheny and others, 1999).

IMPLICATIONS FOR PRACTICE

- X-ray verification of feeding tube placement is the most reliable method available to confirm correct feeding tube location and is required in most acute care facilities when small-bore tubes are initially inserted.

- When the x-ray method is not feasible, the next best method involves testing the feeding tube aspirate's pH and observing its appearance. A properly obtained pH of 0 to 4, is a good indication of gastric placement; a pH of 6 or higher could indicate placement in the lung, intestine, or even the stomach when gastric pH is unusually high. Intestinal fluid is usually bile-stained (dark golden yellow); in contrast, gastric fluid is usually grassy green, off-white to tan, or clear and colorless.

- The auscultatory method should not be the sole or primary method used to determine tube location.

- If the dye method is used to detect aspiratory of enteral feedings, the dye should be sterile to reduce the risk of pulmonary infection in the event of aspiration.

REFERENCES

Metheny N, Aud M, Ignatavicius D: Detection of improperly placed feeding tubes, *J Healthcare Risk Manage* p 37, summer, 1998.

Metheny NA, Aud MA, Wunderlich RJ: A survey of bedside methods used to detect pulmonary aspiration of enteral formula in intubated tube-fed patients, *Am J Crit Care* 8(3): 160, 1999. Metheny NA and others: pH and concentrations of bilirubin in feeding tube aspirates as predictors of tube placement, *Nurs Res* 48(4):189, 1999.

Table 43-22 Enteral Tube Feeding Complications

Problem	Possible Cause	Intervention*
Pulmonary aspiration	Regurgitation of formula Feeding tube displaced Client in supine position Deficient gag reflex Gastroesophageal reflux disease (GERD) Delayed gastric emptying	Check tube placement before feeding (q4-8h during continuous). Elevate head of bed 30 to 45 degrees during feedings and for 2 hours afterwards. Add sterile (blue) food coloring to formula for easier formula detection. (See delayed gastric emptying below.)
Diarrhea	Hyperosmolar formula or medications Allergy to elixir ingredients (sorbitol) Malnutrition/hypoalbuminemia Antibiotic therapy Bacterial contamination Malabsorption	Deliver formula continuously, lower rate, dilute, or change to isotonic EN. Liquid medications are often sweetened with sorbitol, consider as possible cause. Albumin, 2.5 g/dl lessens oncotic pressure equilibrium. Antibiotics may destroy normal intestinal flora; physician may change medication; treat symptoms with Lomotil, Kaopectate. Do not hang formula longer than 4-8 hours in bag, wash bag out well when refilling, change tube feeding bags q24h, and use aseptic practices. Check expiration dates. Check for pancreatic insufficiency, use low-fat, lactose-free formula, and continuous feedings.
Constipation	Lack of fiber Lack of free water Medications Inactivity	Select a formula containing fiber. Add water as needed as flushes.* Evaluate side effects; suggest stool softener or bulk-forming laxative. Monitor client's ability to ambulate; collaborate with physician for activity order or physical therapy.
Tube occlusion	Pulverized medications given per tube Insufficient tube irrigation Sedimentation of formula Reaction of incompatible medications or formula	Irrigate with 20 ml water before and after each medication per tube.* Dilute crushed medications if not liquid. Avoid crushed medications, if liquid available. Shake cans well before administering (read label). Read pharmacological information on compatibility of drugs and formula.
Tube displacement	Coughing, vomiting Not taped securely	Replace tube and confirm placement before restarting tube feeding. With placement verification, check that tape is secure (nasoenteric).
Abdominal cramping, nausea/vomiting	High osmolality of formula Rapid increase in rate/volume Delayed gastric emptying Lactose intolerance Intestinal obstruction High-fat formula used Cold formula used	Suggest an isotonic formula, or dilute current formula. Lower rate of delivery to increase tolerance. Suggest use of lactose-free formula. Stop feeding with GI obstruction. Use greater proportion of carbohydrate. Warm formula to room temperature.
Delayed gastric emptying	Diabetic gastroparesis Prematurity Serious illnesses Inactivity	Consult with physician regarding medication for increasing gastric motility (e.g., metoclopramide or cisapride). Check for residual (see agency policy). Consult physician regarding advancing tube to intestinal placement (if gastric). Monitor medications and pathologic conditions that may affect GI motility. Monitor for increase of client activity.

*Check first for fluid-restricted conditions that would affect volume of water given.

Table 43-22 **Enteral Tube Feeding Complications**—cont'd		
Problem	Possible Cause	Intervention*
Serum electrolyte imbalance	Excess GI losses Dehydration Cirrhosis Renal insufficiency Congestive heart failure, edema Diabetes mellitus	Monitor serum electrolyte levels daily. Know of links with specific pathologic condition. Monitor blood glucose level in diabetics or clients receiving insulin.
Increased respiratory quotient	Overfeeding of carbohydrates	Balance kilocalorie needs provided from fat, protein, and carbohydrate with greater proportion of fat in formula (to decrease CO_2 production).
Fluid overload	Refeeding syndrome in malnutrition Excess free water or diluted (hypotonic) formula	Restrict fluids if necessary and used either a specialized formula or a diluted enteral formula at first. Monitor levels of serum proteins and electrolytes. Use a more concentrated formula with fluid volume excess without risk of refeeding syndrome.
Hyperosmolar dehydration	Hypertonic formula with insufficient free water	Slow rate of delivery, dilute, or change to isotonic formula.

Parenteral Nutrition.   **Parenteral nutrition (PN)** is a form of specialized nutrition support in which nutrients are provided intravenously. Safe administration of this form of nutrition depends on appropriate assessment of nutrition needs, meticulous management of the central venous catheter (CVC), and careful monitoring to prevent or treat metabolic complications. Parenteral nutrition is administered in a variety of settings, including the client's home. Regardless of the setting, the nurse adheres to the same principles of asepsis and infusion management to ensure safe nutrition support.

Clients who are unable to digest or absorb enteral nutrition benefit from PN. Clients in highly stressed physiological states such as sepsis, head injury, or burns are candidates for PN therapy (see Table 43-18). Table 43-21 outlines indications for PN.

Clinical and laboratory monitoring by a multidisciplinary team is required throughout PN therapy (Table 43-23). The need for continued PN is consistently reevaluated. The goal to move toward use of the GI tract is constant (ASPEN, 1993, 1996). Disuse of the GI tract has been associated with villus atrophy and generalized cell shrinkage. Translocation of bacteria from the local gut to systemic regions has been noted in relation to GI cell shrinkage, resulting in gram-negative septicemia (Panigrahi and others, 1997).

Lipid emulsions provide supplemental kilocalories and prevent essential fatty acid deficiencies. These emulsions can be administered through a separate peripheral line, through the central line by Y-connector tubing (see Chapter 40), or as an admixture to the PN solution. The addition of lipid emulsion to the PN solution is called a 3-in-1 admixture and is given over a 24-hour period. The admixture should not be used if oil droplets are observed or if an oil or creamy layer is observed on the surface of the admixture. This observation indicates that the emulsion has broken into large lipid droplets that can cause fat emboli if administered. Lipid emulsions are white and opaque; thus care should be taken to avoid confusing enteral formula with parenteral lipids.

Initiating PN.   Solutions of less than 10% dextrose may be given in a peripheral vein in combination with amino acids and lipids. Peripheral solutions are not as calorically dense and therefore are usually temporary. Parenteral nutrition with greater than 10% dextrose requires a CVC that is placed into a high-flow central vein such as the superior vena cava by a physician under sterile conditions (Figure 43-12). Nurses who have special training insert peripherally inserted central catheters (PICCs) that are started in a vein of the forearm and threaded into the subclavian or superior vena cava vein.

After CVC placement, the catheter is flushed with saline or heparin until the position is radiographically confirmed. The physician sutures the catheter in place and covers the site with a sterile dressing. A chest x-ray examination identifies any complications.

Beginning an Infusion.   Before beginning an infusion, the nurse compares the physician's order with the solution prepared by the pharmacy and checks the solution for particulate matter or a break in the lipid emulsion. An infusion pump is always used.

Infusion Flow Rate.   Clients initially receive PN solutions at a moderate rate such as 40 to 60 ml/hr. The rate is gradually increased until the target energy needs are being supplied. Too-rapid administration of hypertonic dex-

Table 43-23 **Monitoring Parenteral Nutrition (PN)**

Parameter	Baseline	Routine
Weight	Daily	Daily
Glucose (bedside)	Every 6 hours	Every 6 hours
Vital signs/temperature	Once a shift when necessary (prn)	Once a shift/prn
Intake/output	Daily	Daily
Electrolytes	Daily first 3 days	Biweekly
Creatinine blood urea nitrogen (BUN)	Baseline	Biweekly
Albumin, prealbumin, transferrin	Baseline	Weekly
Cholesterol	Baseline	As ordered
Triglycerides	Baseline	As ordered
Liver enzymes (LFTs)	Baseline	Weekly
Complete blood count (CBC)	Baseline	Weekly
Prothrombin time (PT)/partial thromboplastin time (PTT)†	Baseline Baseline	Weekly As ordered
Platelets	1-2 days after PN started	Weekly
Nitrogen balance (24-hour UUN)	Baseline	As ordered
Serum trace minerals and vitamins	Baseline	As needed
Estimate energy requirements		

Modified from Grodner M, Anderson S, DeYoung S: *Foundations and clinical applications of nutrition: a nursing approach,* ed 2, St. Louis, 2000, Mosby.
*Clients at home often adapt to less frequent monitoring.
†Give intramuscular vitamin K once weekly while on TPN and NPO.

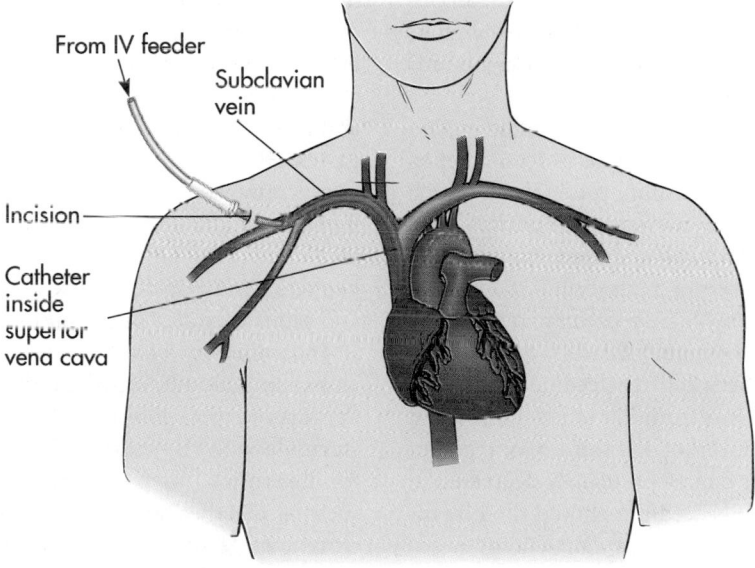

Figure 43-12   Central venous catheter placement.
From Rolin Graphics.

trose can result in an osmotic diuresis and dehydration (see Chapter 40). If an infusion falls behind schedule, the nurse should not increase the rate in an attempt to catch up. Sudden discontinuation of the solution can cause hypoglycemia. Usually, 5% to 10% dextrose is infused when PN solution is suddenly discontinued. Diabetic clients are more at risk.

Clients who receive PN at home on a long-term basis are frequently acclimated to a system of delivering 1 to 3 L of PN over 12 hours at night. The CVC is flushed each morning for independent mobility during daytime hours. Nocturnal administration of PN is accomplished by tapering the flow rate up at the beginning and down when ending. This individualized routine is tested during hospital stays for success.

Preventing Complications.   Complications of PN include mechanical complications from insertion of the CVC, infection, and metabolic aberrations (Table 43-24). Pneumothorax results from a puncture insult to the pulmonary system and results in accumulation of air in the pleural cavity with subsequent impaired breath. Pneumothorax is usually accompanied by symptoms of sudden sharp chest pain, dyspnea, and coughing. In relation to PN, pneumothorax most often occurs during CVC placement.

Air embolus can occur during insertion of the catheter or when changing the tubing or cap. Having the client perform a Valsalva maneuver (hold his or her breath and "bear down") while assuming a left lateral decubitus position can prevent air embolus.

To avoid infection, the infusion tubing should be changed every 24 hours with lipids and every 48 hours when lipids are not infused. During CVC dressing changes sterile mask and gloves are always used and insertion sites should be assessed for signs and symptoms of infection (see Chapter 40).

The PN solution contains most of the major electrolytes, vitamins, and minerals. Supplemental vitamin K must be given as ordered throughout therapy. Vitamin K can be synthesized by microflora found in the jejunum and ileum with normal use of the GI tract; however, since PN circumvents GI use, exogenous vitamin K must be administered.

Electrolyte and mineral imbalances may occur. Administration of concentrated glucose is accompanied by increases in endogenous insulin production, which causes cations (potassium, magnesium, and phosphorus) to move intracellularly. In malnourished or cachectic clients the resulting low serum (extracellular) levels of electrolytes and edema may cause cardiac arrythmias, congestive heart failure, respiratory distress, convulsions, coma, or death. This has been called refeeding syndrome.

The goal is to move clients from PN to EN and/or oral feeding. Once clients are meeting one third to one half of their kilocalorie needs per day, PN is usually decreased to half the original volume. EN feedings should then be increased to meet needs. When 75% of daily energy needs are consistently met with tube feeding, PN may be discontinued. Clients who make the transition from PN to oral feedings typically have early satiety and decreased appetite. Parenteral nutrition should be gradually decreased in response to increased oral intake. If oral intake is inadequate, small frequent meals may prove helpful. Calorie/protein counts are recommended when clients begin taking soft foods. When 75% of needs are being met by reliable dietary intake, PN therapy may be discontinued.

Medical Nutrition Therapy.   Optimal nutrition is important in health and illness, but the specific dietary intake pattern that results in optimal nutrition must be modified for clients with particular diseases. **Medical nutrition therapy (MNT)** is the use of specific nutritional therapies to treat an illness, injury, or condition. Medical nutrition therapy may be necessary to assist the body's ability to metabolize certain nutrients, correct nutritional deficiencies related to the disease, and eliminate foods that may exacerbate disease symptoms. Sheils, Rubin, and Stapleton (1999) examined the cost savings generated by MNT and found specific savings associated with diabetes and cardiovascular disease and an overall decrease in physician office visits of 23.5%. This section provides a summary of MNT for a variety of diseases.

Restorative and Continuing Care.   Clients discharged from a hospital with diet prescriptions often need dietary education to plan meals that meet specific therapeutic requirements. Restorative care includes both immediate postsurgical care and routine medical care and therefore includes hospitalized and home care clients. The following sections address nutritional interventions for some common disease states.

Gastrointestinal Diseases.   Peptic ulcers are controlled with regular meals and medications such as cimetidine. Cimetidine is one of a class of drugs that are histamine receptor antagonists that block secretion of hydrochloric acid. *Helicobacter pylori* was first identified by Marshall and Warren in 1984 and is a bacteria that causes peptic ulcers. This is confirmed by laboratory tests and treated with antibiotics. Stress and overproduction of gastric HCl also contribute to peptic ulcer disease. Clients are encouraged to avoid foods that increase stomach acidity, such as caffeine, decaffeinated coffee, frequent milk intake, citric acid juices, and certain seasonings (hot chili peppers, chili powder, black pepper). Smoking, alcohol, and aspirin are also discouraged.

Inflammatory bowel disease includes Crohn's disease and idiopathic ulcerative colitis. Treatment of acute inflammatory bowel disease may include elemental diets (formula with the nutrients in their simplest form ready for absorption) or parenteral nutrition when symptoms such as diarrhea and weight loss are prevalent. In the chronic stage of the disease a regular highly nourishing diet is appropriate. Vitamins and iron supplements may be required to correct or prevent anemia. Irritable bowel syndrome is managed by increasing fiber, reducing fat, avoiding large meals, and avoiding lactose or sorbitol-containing foods for susceptible individuals.

The treatment of malabsorption syndromes, such as celiac disease, includes a gluten-free diet. Gluten is present in wheat, rye, barley, and oats. Short-bowel syndrome results from extensive resection of bowel after which clients suffer from malabsorption due to lack of intestinal surface area. These clients may require lifetime feeding with either elemental enteral formulas or parenteral nutrition.

Diverticulitis is nutritionally treated with a moderate-

Table 43-24 Complications of Parenteral Nutrition (PN)

Problem	Signs/Symptoms	Intervention
Air embolism	Tachypnea, apnea, wheezing, hypotension, cyanosis	Turn client to left lateral decubitus position, instruct client to perform Valsalva maneuver, and lower head of bed. Cap open end of catheter or tape perforation in catheter wall. Administer oxygen; notify physician. Maintain integrity of closed system to prevent, and have client perform Valsalva maneuver when changing cap.
Catheter occlusion	No flow or sluggish flow through the catheter	Temporarily stop infusion and flush with heparin, if effort to flush is unsuccessful, attempt to aspirate a clot; if still unsuccessful, follow protocol for use of thrombolytic agent (e.g., urokinase).
Catheter sepsis	Fever, chills, glucose intolerance, positive blood culture	To prevent, change catheter site dressing if it becomes wet or contaminated, use aseptic technique when changing dressing or handling IV tubing, catheter caps, or PN containers. Do not hang a single container of PN for more than 24 hours, or lipids more than 12 hours; use an in-line .22-micron filter to remove bacteria.*
Electrolyte imbalance	Monitor Na, Ca, K, Cl, PO$_4$, Mg, and CO$_2$ levels	See Chapter 40 signs of deficiency/toxicity. Check TPN for supplemental electrolyte levels. Notify physician of imbalances.
Fatty liver	LFT and bilirubin elevation, jaundice, upper abdominal pain	To prevent, do not overfeed carbohydrates, check history of hepatic dysfunction, chronic alcoholism, biliary disease. A maximum 200:1 kilocalorie to protein ratio and cycling TPN 12 hours on/off may help reduce elevated liver enzymes.
Hypercapnia	Increased oxygen consumption, increased CO$_2$, respiratory quotient >1.0, minute ventilation	To prevent, ventilator-dependent clients are at risk; monitor parameters; provide 30% to 60% of energy requirements as fat.
Hypoglycemia	Diaphoresis, shakiness, confusion, loss of consciousness	To prevent, do not abruptly discontinue TPN but taper rate down to within 10% of infusion rate 1 to 2 hours before stopping. If hyperglycemia is suggested, test blood glucose, administer IV bolus of dextrose per physician order if necessary.
Hyperglycemia	Thirst, headache, lethargy, increased urination	Monitor blood glucose level daily until stable, then as ordered or prn. TPN is initiated slowly and tapered up to maximal infusion rate. Additional insulin may be required during therapy if problem persists (or if client has diabetes mellitus).
Hyperglycemic hyperosmolar nonketotic dehydration/coma (HHNC)	Hyperglycemia (>500 mg%/dl), glycosuria, serum osmolarity >350 mOsm/L, confusion, azotemia, headache, severe signs of dehydration (see Chapter 40) hypernatremia, metabolic acidosis, convulsions, coma	To prevent, monitor blood glucose, BUN, serum osmolarity, glucose in urine, and fluid losses; administer insulin as ordered; replace fluids as needed; maintain consistent infusion rate; and provide 30% of daily energy needs as fat. Clients at risk are hypermetabolic, receiving steroids, elderly, diabetic, have impaired renal or pancreatic function, or are septic.
Pneumothorax	Severe dyspnea, cyanosis, x-ray confirmation	Complication that occurs upon catheter insertion, may evolve slowly afterwards. Monitor for first 24 hours for pulmonary distress.
Thrombosis of central vein	Unilateral edema of neck, shoulder, and arm, pain	Repeated or traumatic catheter insertions place clients at risk; notify physician.

*With 3-in-1-admixture TPN, filtration is not possible due to large lipid molecules.

or low-residue diet until the infection subsides. Afterward, a high-fiber diet is generally prescribed for chronic diverticulosis.

Diabetes Mellitus. Type 1 diabetes mellitus (DM) requires both insulin and dietary restrictions for optimal control, beginning with diagnosis. By contrast, type 2 diabetes mellitus may initially be controlled solely by exercise and diet therapy. If these measures prove ineffective, it is common to add oral medications. Insulin injections may follow if type 2 diabetes worsens or fails to respond to these initial interventions. In both cases the diet is individualized according to the client's age, build, weight, and activity level. Fats are moderately controlled (30% or less), and complex carbohydrates make up the majority (50% to 60%) of the diet, rather than simple carbohydrates. Protein comprises 10% to 20% of daily intake. Foods that contain soluble fiber are recommended, with a daily intake of 40 g of fiber. Foods for dietary planning are classified into two exchange groups: the carbohydrate group and the meat and meat substitute group. Foods from within the same group can be exchanged, but it is not recommended to exchange a carbohydrate food for a meat item. Each item has about the same nutrient value as other foods in the group (for more information, see Williams, 1997). The strategies used for Type 1 versus Type 2 diabetes are summarized in Table 43-25. The goal of treatment is normal glycemic levels, and hemoglobin A_{Ic} level of less than 7%, with resultant minimization of complications of ophthalmic, vascular, renal, and neuropathic damage (Lipkin, 1999). Nurses also need to be aware of signs and symptoms of hypoglycemia and hyperglycemia.

Cardiovascular Diseases. The American Heart Association's (AHA's) dietary guidelines are given in Table 43-26 and are intended to reduce risk factors for the development of coronary artery disease. Dietary therapy following an acute myocardial infarction includes initial reduction in kilocalories, soft-textured foods, and amounts of fat, sodium, and cholesterol that conform to AHA recommendations. Magnesium, folic acid, and vitamin B_6 appear to be important for primary prevention of coronary heart disease. Increases in folic acid are associated with a decrease in homocysteine, which is associated with greater risk of coronary artery disease (Rimm and others, 1998).

Nutritional therapy for hypertension includes kilocalorie reduction to promote weight loss as appropriate, decreased sodium intake, and potassium-rich foods if potassium-wasting diuretics are part of the treatment.

Pulmonary Disease. Macronutrients are digested and metabolized to form CO_2 and water. The ratio of CO_2 produced to O_2 consumed is the respiratory quotient (RQ). The RQ of carbohydrate digestion is 1.0, whereas for fat the RQ is 0.7. Clients with pulmonary disease generally maintain healthier RQs with higher dietary intake fat and less carbohydrate source. This is relevant when weaning clients from ventilators in acute care settings or counseling chronic obstructive pulmonary disease (COPD) clients for self-care.

Renal Disease. The dietary treatment of acute glomerulonephritis depends on the client's symptoms and is designed to maximize nutritional intake. Fluid, salt, and protein are not restricted unless indicated by symptoms such as edema, uremia, or oliguria.

Acute renal failure (ARF) is related to low blood pressure or cellular damage within the nephron. Low blood pressure results from trauma, hemorrhage, or shock and indirectly damages the nephrons. Other causes of ARF are nephrotoxic drugs, septicemia, or streptococcal infection that directly damage the nephrons. Acute renal failure usually consists of three stages: oliguric, diuretic, and recovery. Treatment of ARF changes according to these stages. The oliguric stage (from 7 to 21 days) requires that fluids be restricted to the client's output (typically 400 to 500 ml per day) plus an additional 400 ml to 500 ml per day. By contrast, diuresis (which ranges in duration from 7 to 14 days) requires large amounts of fluid replacement to make up for high urinary output. Protein is restricted to 0.6 to 0.8 g/kg/day, and parenteral amino acids may be required. A balanced mixture of essential and nonessential

Table 43-25 Dietary Strategies for Type 1 Versus Type 2 Diabetes Mellitus

Dietary Strategy	Type 1 DM (Nonobese)	Type 2 DM (Usually Obese)
Decrease energy intake (kilocalories)	No	Yes
Increase frequency and number meals	Yes	Usually no
Regular daily intake of kilocalories, carbohydrates, protein, and fat	Very important	Not as important as low average kcals intake
Consistent daily ratio of protein, carbohydrates, and fat per meal	Desirable	Not necessary
Plan ahead for food to treat or prevent hypoglycemia	Very important	Not necessary
Use extra food for exercise	Yes	Not usually necessary
Illnesses require small, frequent feeding of carbohydrates to prevent starvation ketosis	Important	Not usually necessary due to resistance to ketosis

From Williams SR: *Nutrition and diet therapy*, ed 8, St. Louis, 1997, Mosby.

American Heart Association
Table 43-26 Dietary Guidelines
Reduce dietary fat to 30% daily energy intake.
10% to 15% of total daily fat intake should be unsaturated fatty acids.
Carbohydrates should comprise 55% to 60% of total daily intake.
Use protein in moderation, with less emphasis on animal sources.
Limit cholesterol to 300 mg or less per day.
Sodium should not exceed 2400 mg per day.

From American Heart Association: AHA scientific position: "dietary guidelines for healthy American adults," *Circulation,* 94(7): 1795, 1996.

amino acids is provided along with concentrated dextrose and lipids. If the GI tract is functional, special enteral products are also available (Box 43-7). Finally, the recovery stage occurs over 3 to 12 months and is highly individual. Some residual kidney damage is common (Grodner, Anderson, and DeYoung, 2000).

Chronic renal failure treatment typically consists of a diet that restricts protein, potassium, phosphate, sodium, and fluid. Adequate carbohydrates spare the use of protein for energy. As dialysis is begun, protein ingestion may increase. Calcium intake varies according to serum levels. Leung and Dwyer (1998) have developed a method for detection of malnutrition in renal clients using the Renal DETERMINE screening tool, which is also useful for client teaching in renal disease. In 1993 the American Dietetic Association (ADA) published the National Renal Diet, developed by the Renal Dietitians Practice Group and the National Kidney Foundation Council on Renal Nutrition. The renal diet also works with exchange groups to develop diet guidelines and meal plans.

Dietary treatment for renal calculi depends on the stone composition. For calcium phosphate stones the diet is low in calcium and high in acid ash. For uric acid stones the diet is low in purines. For calcium oxalate stones the diet avoids all foods high in calcium and oxalates (Grodner, Anderson, and DeYoung, 2000).

Cancer and Cancer Treatment.   Malignant cells compete with normal cells for nutrients, increasing the metabolic needs of the client. Most cancer treatments cause nutritional problems. Clients with cancer typically complain of anorexia and taste distortions. Malnutrition in cancer is associated with increased morbidity and mortality. Enhanced nutritional status may improve the client's quality of life.

Radiation therapy is intended to destroy rapidly dividing malignant cells; however, other normal rapidly dividing cells, such as the epithelial lining of the GI tract, are often affected. Radiation therapy can cause anorexia, stomatitis, severe diarrhea, strictures of the intestine, and

pain. Radiation treatment of the head and neck region can cause taste and smell disturbances, decreased salivation, and dysphagia.

Nutrition management of the client with cancer focuses on maximizing intake of nutrients and fluids. The nurse should use creative approaches to manage alterations in taste and smell.

Human Immunodeficiency Virus (HIV).   Human immunodeficiency virus (HIV)-infected clients typically experience body wasting and severe weight loss. The wasting can be related to anorexia, stomatitis, oral thrush infection, nausea, or recurrent vomiting, all resulting in inadequate intake. Factors associated with weight loss and malnutrition are severe diarrhea, GI malabsorption, and altered metabolism of nutrients. Systemic infection results in hypermetabolism from cytokine elevation. Often the medications taken to treat HIV infection cause side effects that alter nutritional status.

Restorative care of acquired immunodeficiency syndrome (AIDS) malnutrition focuses upon maximizing kilocalories and nutrients. Each cause of nutritional depletion should be diagnosed and addressed in the care plan. Individually tailored nutrition support should progress in stages from oral, to enteral, and lastly to parenteral. Good hand washing and food safety (see Boxes 43-5 and 43-6) are essential, including minimization of exposure to *Cryptosporidium* in drinking water, lakes, or swimming pools. Low-fat diets and small frequent nutrient-dense meals may be better tolerated (Keithley and Swanson, 1998).

EVALUATION

Care plans should reflect achievable goals. Nurses need to evaluate outcomes of nursing actions and be alert for signs that goals are being met. Adequate time should be allowed to test each nursing approach to a problem. Multidisciplinary collaboration remains essential in provision of nutrition support.

Client Care.   Effectiveness of nutritional interventions is best measured by meeting the client's expected outcomes and goals of care (Figure 43-13). Nutrition therapy does not always produce rapid results. Ongoing comparisons may be made with baseline measures of weight, serum albumin or prealbumin, and protein and kilocalorie intake. Enteral nutrition therapy is frequently interrupted. Medications may produce unwanted side effects. If gradual weight gain is not observed, or if weight loss continues, the prescription may need to be increased. Changes in condition may also indicate a need to change the nutritional plan of care. Multidisciplinary members of the health care team should be consulted in an effort to better individualize the client's plan of care. The client should be an active participant whenever possible. In the end, the

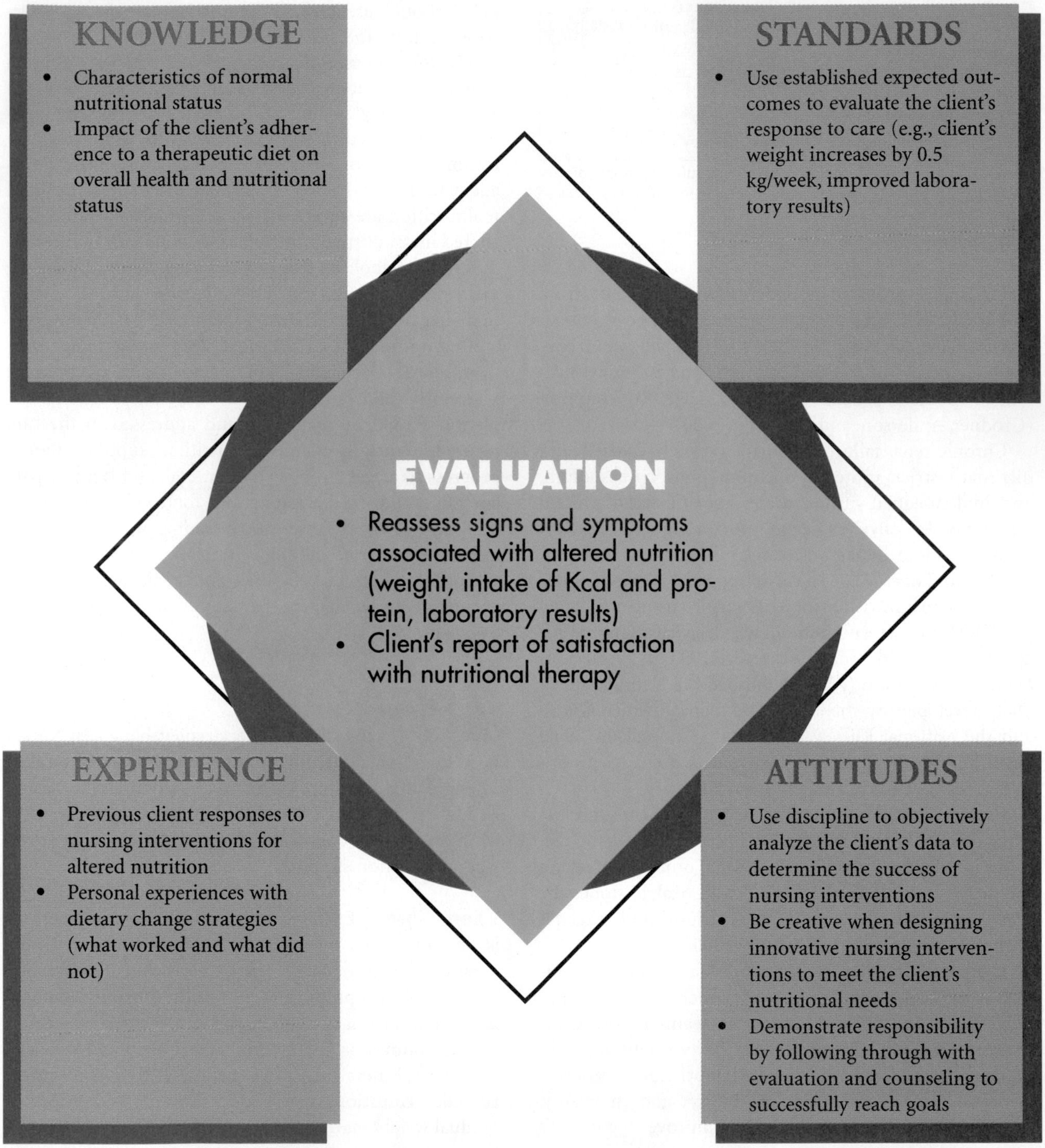

KNOWLEDGE

- Characteristics of normal nutritional status
- Impact of the client's adherence to a therapeutic diet on overall health and nutritional status

STANDARDS

- Use established expected outcomes to evaluate the client's response to care (e.g., client's weight increases by 0.5 kg/week, improved laboratory results)

EVALUATION

- Reassess signs and symptoms associated with altered nutrition (weight, intake of Kcal and protein, laboratory results)
- Client's report of satisfaction with nutritional therapy

EXPERIENCE

- Previous client responses to nursing interventions for altered nutrition
- Personal experiences with dietary change strategies (what worked and what did not)

ATTITUDES

- Use discipline to objectively analyze the client's data to determine the success of nursing interventions
- Be creative when designing innovative nursing interventions to meet the client's nutritional needs
- Demonstrate responsibility by following through with evaluation and counseling to successfully reach goals

Figure 43-13   *Synthesis Model for Nutrition Evaluation Phase.*

client's ability to incorporate dietary changes into his or her lifestyle with the least amount of stress or disruption will ensure that outcome measures are successfully met.

Client Expectations.

Clients expect competent and accurate care. If ongoing nutritional therapies are not resulting in successful outcomes, clients expect nurses to recognize this fact and alter the plan of care accordingly. Expectations held by nurses may differ from those held by clients. For example, Young, Minnick, and Marcantonio (1996) found discrepancies between nursing staff, nursing managers, and clients regarding health care values. Oscar (1996) writes that "an expectation is an anticipation of something that may occur" and stresses the importance of beginning all client teaching with a clear understanding of the client's present knowledge and expectations. Successful interventions and outcomes depend on recognition of this concept in addition to nursing knowledge and skill. Working closely with the client will enable the nurse to redefine those expectations that can be realistically met within the limits of the client's conditions and treatment.

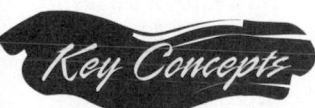

- Essential amino acids and essential fatty acids must be supplied by dietary intake since the body is unable to synthesize them from other ingested substances.
- Through digestion, food is broken down into its simplest form for absorption. Digestion and absorption occur mainly in the small intestine.
- Dietary reference intakes provide a range of values that address the needs of both groups (estimated average requirement) and individuals (adequate intakes, recommended dietary allowances, and tolerable upper intake level).
- Guidelines for dietary change advocate reduced fat, saturated fat, sodium, refined sugar, and cholesterol and increased intake of complex carbohydrates and fiber.
- Age affects the requirements for essential nutrients. Periods of rapid growth increase the need for protein, vitamins, and minerals.
- Because improper nutrition can affect all body systems, nutritional assessment includes a review of total physical assessment.
- Multidisciplinary collaboration is essential to optimal nutrition.

- Nurses can improve food intake of clients by thoughtful attention to the preparation of the client and environment before meals are served.
- Tube feedings can be used for clients who are unable to ingest food but are able to digest and absorb food.
- Enteral nutrition may protect intestinal structure and function and enhance immunity.
- Total parenteral nutrition supplies essential nutrients in appropriate amounts to support life through the introduction of a concentrated nutrient solution into the superior vena cava near the right atrium of the heart.
- Medical nutrition therapy is a recognized treatment modality for both acute and chronic disease states.
- Special diets alter the composition, texture, digestibility, and residue of foods to suit the client's particular needs.
- Evaluation of the outcomes of nursing intervention in the area of nutrition support is essential to revise, update, or continue nursing activities.
- Nutritional research is a dynamic process. Results of studies and new recommendations by expert sources need to be followed for future changes in practice standards.

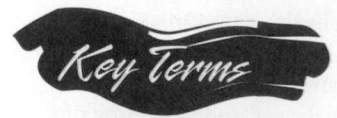

Key Terms

Adequate intake (AI), *p. 1333*

Amino acids, *p. 1326*

Anabolism, *p. 1332*

Anorexia, *p. 1356*

Anorexia nervosa, *p. 1340*

Anthropometry, *p. 1348*

Basal metabolic rate (BMR), *p. 1324*

Bioelectrical impedance analysis (BIA), *p. 1350*

Body mass index (BMI), *p. 1348*

Bulimia nervosa, *p. 1340*

Carbohydrates, *p. 1325*

Catabolism, *p. 1332*

Chyme, *p. 1332*

Complex carbohydrates, *p. 1325*

Complementary proteins, *p. 1326*

Daily values, *p. 1335*

Dietary reference intakes (DRIs), *p. 1333*

Dysphagia, *p. 1331*

Enteral nutrition (EN), *p. 1358*

Enzymes, *p. 1330*

Essential amino acids, *p. 1326*

Estimated average requirement (EAR), *p. 1333*

Fat-soluble vitamins, *p. 1328*

Fatty acids, *p. 1326*

Fiber, *p. 1325*

Gluconeogenesis, *p. 1332*

Glycogenesis, *p. 1332*

Glycogenolysis, *p. 1332*

Hypervitaminosis, *p. 1328*

Ideal body weight (IBW), *p. 1348*

Ketoacidosis, *p. 1343*

Ketones, *p. 1332*

Lipids, *p. 1326*

Lipid emulsions, *p. 1372*

Lipogenesis, *p. 1326*

Macrominerals, *p. 1329*

Malabsorption, *p. 1353*

Medical nutrition therapy (MNT), *p. 1374*

Metabolism, *p. 1332*

Minerals, *p. 1329*

Monounsaturated (fatty acids), *p. 1327*

Nitrogen balance, *p. 1326*

Nonessential amino acids, *p. 1326*

Nutrient density, *p. 1325*

Nutrients, *p. 1324*

Parenteral nutrition (PN), *p. 1372*

Peristalsis, *p. 1331*

Polyunsaturated (fatty acids), *p. 1327*

Recommended dietary allowance (RDAs), *p. 1333*

Resting energy expenditure (REE), *p. 1324*

Saccharides, *p. 1325*

Saturated (fatty acids), *p. 1326*

Simple carbohydrates, *p. 1325*

Tolerable upper intake level (UL), *p. 1333*

Trace elements, *p. 1329*

Triglycerides, *p. 1326*

Unsaturated (fatty acids), *p. 1327*

Vegetarianism, *p. 1344*

Vitamins, *p. 1328*

Water-soluble vitamins, *p. 1329*

Critical Thinking Exercises

1. Jean, age 35, has just had surgery for a bowel obstruction. Her medical history includes Crohn's disease. Before this exacerbation, 3 months ago, Jean's weight was 123 pounds (55.8 kg). Admission weight was 115 pounds (52.2 kg), 3 days after surgery she now weighs 108 pounds (49.0 kg). Her height is 5'5" (165 cm). Reported laboratory values are white blood cell count, 8.3; % lymphocytes 13; albumin, 2.3 g/dl. What is Jean's BMI? What is her percent weight loss? What is her total lymphocyte count? Jean remains NPO with nasogastric suction; what intervention(s) would you discuss with her physician?

2. During a well-child check-up, Mrs. Grosboll asks if she should be concerned about John, her 20-month-old son. She complains that his appetite was good until a few months ago, when he became a picky eater. She worries that he is not getting adequate nutrition. What is your response?

3. Roberta is being treated for breast cancer with chemotherapy as adjunct to a lumpectomy. She has maintained a positive attitude as well as possible but is concerned about the side effects of the medication. Roberta has bleeding gums, stomatitis, nausea, and diarrhea. As a result she has no desire to eat. She is 85% of her UBW at present. How could you assist Roberta to improve her nutritional status?

4. Mrs. Caine is 85 years old. She has been hospitalized for a fractured left hip and is now ready for discharge. She has always been active, living alone. She has no family nearby, but a few close friends. What arrangements would you make to continue her nutritional intake at home while she recovers?

References

American Academy of Family Physicians: *A position paper on disease state management,* http://www.aafp.org/family/managed/disease, (November 7, 1997).

American Academy of Pediatrics: Infant feeding practices and their possible relationship to the etiology of diabetes mellitus (RE9430), *Pediatrics* 94(5):752, 1994.

American Academy of Pediatrics: Breastfeeding recommendations, *Pediatrics* 100(6):1035, 1997a.

American Academy of Pediatrics: Pediatrician's responsibility for infant nutrition, *Pediatrics* 99(5):749, 1997b.

American Dietetic Association: *Facts about Olestra,* http://www.eatright.org, (December 22, 1998).

American Heart Association: AHA scientific position: "dietary guidelines for healthy American adults," *Circulation* 94(7):1795, 1996.

American Psychiatric Association: *Diagnostic and statistical manual of mental disorders,* ed 4-revised, Washington, DC, 1994, The Association.

American Society of Parenteral and Enteral Nutrition: Guidelines for the use of parenteral and enteral nutrition in adult and pediatric patients, *J Parenter Enteral Nutr* 17(suppl 4), 1SA, 1993.

American Society of Parenteral and Enteral Nutrition: Standards of practice, nutrition support nurse, *Nutr Clin Prac,* 11(3), 127, 1996.

Bioelectrical impedance analysis in body composition measurement: National Institutes of Health Technology Assessment Conference statement, *Am J Clin Nutr* 64 (suppl 3):524S, 1996.

Bowers S: Tubes: a nurse's guide to enteral feeding devices, *MedSurg Nurs* 5(5):313, 1996.

Chang J and others: Inadvertent endobrachial intubation with nasogastric tube, *Arch Otolaryngol* 108:528, 1982.

Chernoff R: *Geriatric nutrition: the health professional's handbook,* Gaithersburg, Md, 1991, Aspen.

Costello MC, Todd-Magel C: Bridging the gap: hospital to home nutrition support, *MedSurg Nurs* 6(6):328, 1997.

Daly S and others: Minimum effective dose of folic acid for food fortification to prevent neural tube defects, *Lancet* 347, 657, 1997.

Davis AE and others: Preventing feeding-associated aspiration, *MedSurg Nurs* 4(2):111, 1995.

Dossey B: *Florence Nightingale: mystic, visionary, and healer,* Philadelphia, 1999, Springhouse.

Evans-Stoner N: Nutritional assessment: a practical approach, *Nurs Clin North Am* 32(4):637, 1997.

Food and Drug Administration: *Daily values for food labels,* Washington, DC, 1995, US Government Printing Office.

Food and Nutrition Board: *Recommended dietary allowances,* ed 10, Washington DC, 1989, National Academy Press.

Food and Nutrition Board: *Nutrition during pregnancy and lactation: an implementation guide,* Washington, DC, 1992a, National Academy Press.

Food and Nutrition Board: *Nutrition services in perinatal care,* ed 2, 1992b, National Academy Press.

Food and Nutrition Board: *Dietary reference intakes for calcium, phosphorus, magnesium, vitamin D, and fluoride,* Washington, DC, 1997, National Academy Press.

Food and Nutrition Board: *Dietary reference intakes: thiamin, riboflavin, niacin, vitamin B_6, folate, vitamin B_{12}, pantothenic acid, biotin, and choline,* Washington, DC, 1998, National Academy Press.

Foster GD and others: What is a reasonable weight loss? Patient expectations of obesity treatment, *J Consult Clin Psychol,* 65(1):79, 1997.

Gallagher-Allred CR and others: Malnutrition and clinical outcomes: the case for medical nutrition therapy, *J Am Diet Assoc* 96(4):361, 1996.

Giger JN, Davidhizar RE: *Transcultural nursing: assessment and intervention,* ed 2, St. Louis, 1995, Mosby.

Goodwin RS: Prevention of aspiration pneumonia: a research based protocol, *Dimens Crit Care Nurs* 15(4):58, 1996.

Grindel CG, Costello MC: Nutrition screening: an essential assessment parameter, *MedSurg Nurs* 5(3):145, 1996.

Grodner M, Anderson S, DeYoung S: *Foundations and clinical applications of nutrition: a nursing approach,* ed 2, St. Louis, 2000, Mosby.

Guenter P, Ericson M, Jones S: Enteral nutrition therapy, *Nurs Clin North Am,* 32(4):651, 1997.

Health and Welfare Canada, Minister of Supply and Services Canada: Catalogue H39-252/1992, Ottawa, 1992.

Hennessy KA, Orr ME: *Nutrition support core curriculum,* ed 3, Silver Spring, Md. 1996, American Society of Parenteral and Enteral Nutrition.

Hopkins B: Enteral formulas. In Zaloga G, editor: *Nutrition in critical care,* St. Louis, 1994, Mosby.

Inman-Felton A, Smith K: *Medical nutrition therapy across the continuum of care: Supplement 1,* Chicago, 1997, American Dietetic Association and Morrison Health Care, Inc.

Keithley K, Swanson B: Minimizing HIV/AIDS malnutrition, *MedSurg Nurs* 7(5):256, 1998.

Kennedy-Caldwell CM: Childhood nutrition, *Annu Rev Nurs Res* 16:3, 1998.

Kessler DA: The evolution of national nutrition policy, *Annu Rev Nutr* 15:xiii, 1995.

Kovacevich DS and others: Nutrition risk classification: a reproducible and valid tool for nurses, *Nutr Clin Pract,* 12(1):20, 1997.

Kudsk K: Clinical applications of enteral nutrition, *Nutr Clin Pract* 9(5):165, 1994.

Leung J, Dwyer J: Renal DETERMINE nutrition screening tools for the identification and treatment of malnutrition, *J Ren Nutr* 8(2):95, 1998.

Lindseth F: Factors affecting graduating nurses' nutritional knowledge: implications for continuing education, *J Contin Educ Nurs* 28:245, 1997.

Lipkin E: New strategies for the treatment of type 2 diabetes, *J Am Diet Assoc* 99(3):329, 1999.

Lueckenotte AG: *Gerontologic nursing,* ed 2, St. Louis, 2000, Mosby.

Marshall BJ, Warren JR: Unidentified curved bacilli in the stomach of patients with gastritis and peptic ulcerations, *Lancet* 2(8397):281, 1984.

Matarese LE: Rationale and efficiency of specialized enteral nutrition, *Nutr Clin Pract* 9(2):58, 1994.

McCloskey JC, Bulechek GM: Nursing interventions classification (NIC), ed 3, St. Louis, 2000, Mosby.

Metheny N, Aud M, Ignatavicius D: Detection of improperly placed feeding tubes, *J Healthcare Risk Manage* 18(3):37, 1998.

Metheny N, Aud MA, Wunderlich RJ: A survey of bedside methods used to detect pulmonary aspiration of enteral formula in intubated tube-fed patients, *Am J Crit Care* 8(3):160, 1999.

Metheny N and others: Measures to test placement of nasogastric and nasointestinal feeding tubes: a review, *Nurse Res* 37:324, 1988.

Metheny N and others: Detection of inadvertent respiratory placement of small-bore feeding tubes: a report of 10 cases, *Heart Lung* 19(6):631, 1990a.

Metheny N and others: Effectiveness of the auscultatory method in predicting feeding tube location, *Nurse Res* 39(5):262, 1990b.

Metheny N and others: Effectiveness of pH measurements in predicting feeding tube placement: an update, *Nurs Res* 42(6):324, 1993.

Metheny N and others: Visual characteristics of aspirates from feeding tubes as a method for predicting tube location, *Nurs Res* 43:282, 1994.

Metheny N and others: pH and concentrations of pepsin and trypsin in feeding tube aspirates as predictors of tube placement, *J Parenter Enteral Nutr* 21(5):279, 1997.

Metheny N and others: pH, color, and feeding tubes, *RN* 61(1):277, 1998.

Metheny N and others: Testing feeding tube placement: auscultation vs. pH method, *Am J Nurs* 98:37, 1998.

Metheny N and others: pH and concentrations of bilirubin in feeding tube aspirates as predictors of tube placement, *Nurs Res* 48(4):189, 1999.

National Center for Health Statistics: *National Health and Nutrition Examination Survey (NHANES) III,* Hyattsville, Md, 1990, Centers for Disease Control and Prevention.

National Dairy Council: *Feeding guide for the first two years,* Rosemont, Ill, 1990, The Council.

Neumark-Sztainer D and others: Factors influencing food choices of adolescents: findings from focus-group discussions with adolescents, *J Am Diet Assoc* 99(8):929, 1999.

Nutrition Labeling and Education Act, PL 100-535, 104 Stat 2353, 21 USC §301 (1990).

Nutrition Screening Initiative: *Nutrition interventions manual for professionals caring for older Americans,* Washington, DC, 1992, Greer, Margolis, Mitchell, Grunwald & Associates.

Nutrition Screening Initiative: A project of the American Academy of Family Physicians, the American Dietetic Association, and the National Council of the Aging, Inc. and funded in part by a grant from Ross Products Division, Abbott Laboratories, 1998.

Oscar G: The influence of patient expectations on learning experience, *J CANNT* 6(2):23, 1996.

Pagana KD, Pagana TJ: *Mosby's diagnostic and laboratory test reference,* ed 4, St. Louis, 1999, Mosby.

Panigrahi P and others: Role of glutamine in bacterial transcytosis and epithelial cell injury, *J Parenter Enteral Nutr* 21:75, March-April 1997.

Pickering LK and others: Modulation of the immune system by human milk and infant formula containing nucleotides, *Pediatrics* 101:242, 1998.

Raloff J: Cholesterol-busting products provoke FDA, *Science News* 154(20):311, 1998.

Rimm EB and others: Folate and vitamin B$_6$ from diet and supplements in relation to risk of coronary heart disease among women, *JAMA* 279(5):359, 1998.

Rombeau JL, Rolandelli RH, editors: *Enteral feeding and tube feeding,* Philadelphia, 1997, WB Saunders.

Scannapieco FA: Position paper of the American Academy of Periodontology: periodontal disease as a potential risk factor for systemic diseases, *J Periodontol* 69(7):841, 1998.

Sheils JF, Rubin R, Stapleton DC: The estimated costs and savings of medical nutrition therapy: the medicare population, *J Am Diet Assoc* 99(4):428, 1999.

Stacey M: *Consumed: why Americans love, hate, and fear food,* New York, 1994, Simon & Schuster.

Sweed MR, Guenter P, Jones S: Nursing implications for the adult receiving nutritional support, *MedSurg Nurs* 4(2):1995.

U.S. Department of Agriculture: *USDA's food guide pyramid,* USDA Human Nutrition Information Service Pub No. 249, Washington, DC, 1996, U.S. Government Printing Office.

U.S. Department of Agriculture and U.S. Department of Health and Human Services: *Nutrition and your health: dietary guidelines for Americans,* ed 4, USDA/DHHS Home and Garden Bulletin No. 232, Washington, DC, 1995, U.S. Government Printing Office.

U.S. Department of Agriculture: *Healthy eating index,* Washington, DC, October 1995, U.S. Department of Agriculture.

U.S. Department of Agriculture: *Official USDA food plans: cost of food at home at four levels, U.S. average,* October 1998, http://www.usda.gov/cnpp.

U.S. Department of Health and Human Services: *Healthy people 2010 objectives: draft for public comment,* 1998, http://web.health.gov./healthypeople.

U.S. Department of Health and Human Services: *Morning Meals on Wheels program initiative announced,* March 19, 1997, http://www.hhs.gov.

Wardlaw GM, Insell PM: *Perspectives in nutrition,* ed 2, New York, 1993, McGraw-Hill.

Weigley ES: Nutrition-related activities of entry level nurses, *Nurse Educ* 20:3, 1995.

World Health Organization/Food and Agriculture Organization of the United Nations: *Fats and oils in human nutrition,* Rome, 1994, Food and Agriculture Organization of the United Nations.

World Health Organization/Food and Agriculture Organization of the United Nations/IAEA: *Trace elements in human nutrition and health,* Geneva, 1996, World Health Organization.

World Health Organization/Food and Agriculture Organization of the United Nations: *Carbohydrates in human nutrition,* Rome, 1998a, Food and Agriculture Organization of the United Nations, World Health Organization.

World Health Organization/Food and Agriculture Organization of the United Nations: *Preparation and use of food-based dietary guidelines,* Technical report series, No. 880, #1100880, Geneva, 1998b, World Health Organization.

Williams SR: *Nutrition and diet therapy,* ed 8, St. Louis, 1997, Mosby.

Wong DL: *Whaley & Wong's essentials of pediatric nursing,* ed 5, St. Louis, 1997, Mosby.

Ybarra J, Ade R, Romeo JH: Osteoporosis in men: a review, *Nurs Clin North Am* 31(4):805, 1996.

Young WB, Minnick AF, Marcantonio R: How wide is the gap in defining quality care? Comparison of patient and nurse perceptions of important aspects of patient care, *J Nurs Adm* 26(2):15, 1996.

Zaloga G: Frontiers in critical care nutrition, *New Horizons* 2(2):121, 1994.

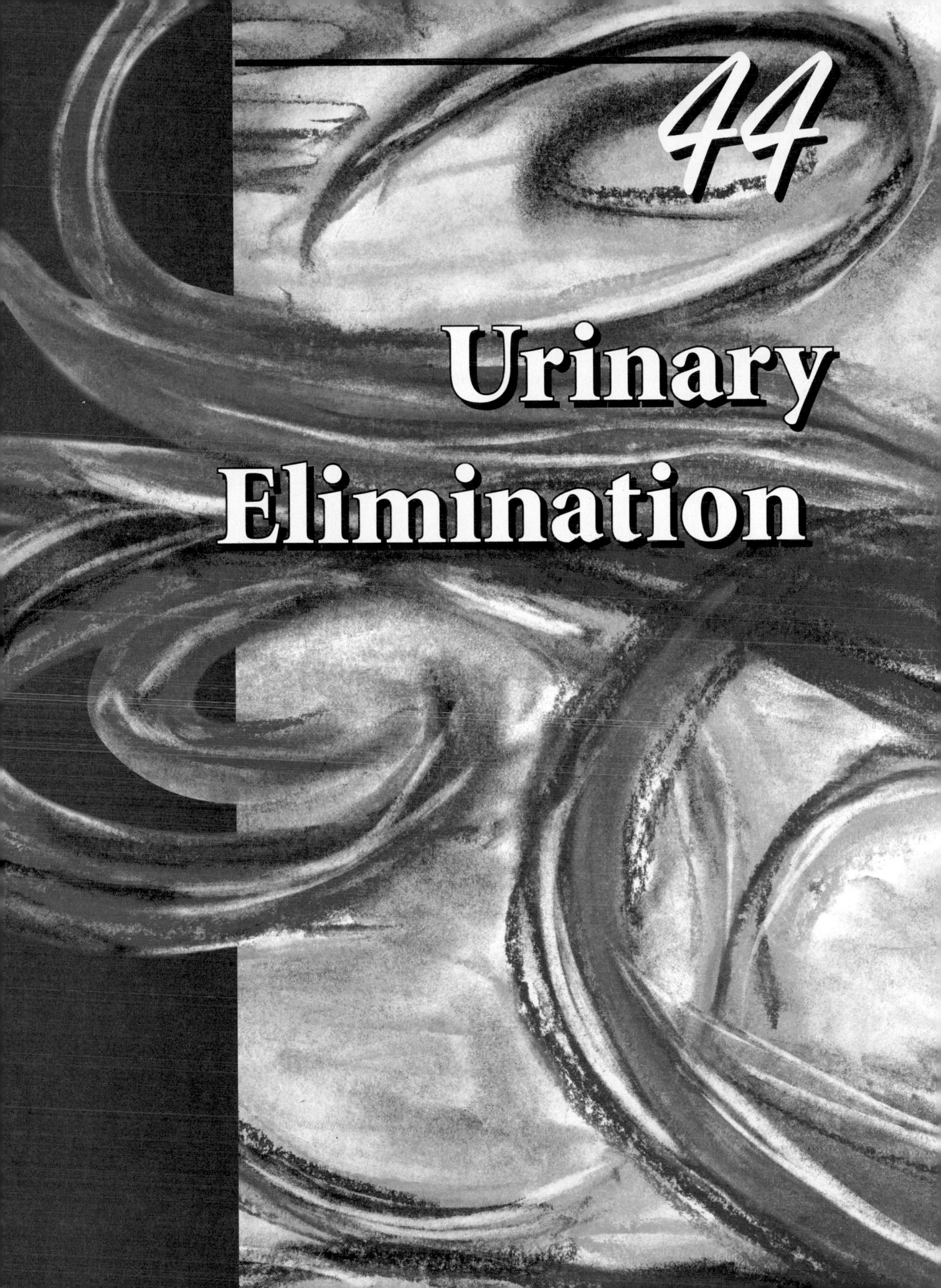

44

Urinary Elimination

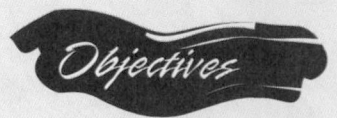
Objectives

Mastery of content in this chapter will enable the student to:

- Define the key terms listed.
- Describe the process of urination.
- Identify factors that commonly influence urinary elimination.
- Compare and contrast common alterations in urinary elimination.
- Obtain a nursing history for a client with urinary elimination problems.
- Identify nursing diagnoses appropriate for clients with alterations in urinary elimination.
- Obtain urine specimens.
- Describe characteristics of normal and abnormal urine.
- Describe the nursing implications of common diagnostic tests of the urinary system.
- Discuss nursing measures to promote normal micturition and reduce episodes of incontinence.
- Insert a urinary catheter.
- Discuss nursing measures to reduce urinary tract infection.
- Irrigate a urinary catheter.
- Identify two modalities of renal replacement therapy.

Normal elimination of urinary wastes is a basic function most people take for granted. When the urinary system fails to function properly, virtually all organ systems will be eventually affected. Clients with alterations in urinary elimination may also suffer emotionally from body image changes. The nurse provides understanding and a sensitivity to all clients' needs. The nurse must understand the reasons for problems and find acceptable solutions.

Scientific Knowledge Base

Urinary elimination depends on the function of the kidneys, ureters, bladder, and urethra. Kidneys remove wastes from the blood to form urine. Ureters transport urine from the kidneys to the bladder. The bladder holds urine until the urge to urinate develops. Urine leaves the body through the urethra. All organs of the urinary system must be intact and functional for successful removal of urinary wastes (Figure 44-1).

KIDNEYS

Kidneys are paired, reddish brown, bean-shaped organs that lie on either side of the vertebral column posterior to the peritoneum and against deep muscles of the back. The kidneys extend to the twelfth thoracic and third lumbar vertebrae. Normally the left kidney is 1.5 to 2 cm ($^6/_{10}$ to $^8/_{10}$ inch) higher than the right because of the anatomical position of the liver. Each kidney typically measures approximately 12 by 7 cm (5 by 3 inches) and weighs 120 to 150 g. Each kidney is covered by a tough capsule and surrounded by a cushion of fat.

Waste products of metabolism that collect in the blood are filtered in the kidneys. Blood reaches each kidney by a renal (kidney) artery that branches from the abdominal aorta. The renal artery enters the kidney at the hilum. Approximately 20% to 25% of the cardiac output circulates each minute through the kidneys. The **nephron,** the functional unit of the kidney, forms the urine. The nephron is composed of the glomerulus, Bowman's capsule, proximal convoluted tubule, loop of Henle, distal tubule, and collecting duct (Figure 44-2).

Blood reaches nephrons through the afferent arterioles. A cluster of these blood vessels forms the capillary network of the glomerulus, which is the initial site of filtration of the blood and the beginning of urine formation. The glomerular capillaries are porous and permit filtration of water and substances such as glucose, amino acids, urea, creatinine, and major electrolytes into Bowman's capsule. Large proteins and blood cells do not normally filter through the glomerulus. The presence of large proteins in the urine (**proteinuria**) is a sign of glomerular injury. The glomerulus filters approximately 125 ml of filtrate per minute. Initially the filtrate closely approximates blood plasma minus the large proteins.

Not all of the glomerular filtrate is excreted as urine. About 99% of the filtrate is reabsorbed into the plasma, with the remaining 1% excreted as urine. Thus the kidneys play a key role in fluid and electrolyte balance (see Chapter 40). Although output does depend on intake, the normal adult 24-hour output of urine is about 1500 to 1600 ml. An output of less than 30 ml per hour may indicate renal alterations. The kidneys also produce several hormones

The authors acknowledge the contribution of Dr. Elizabeth A. Ayello to this chapter in the previous edition of this text.

vital to production of red blood cells (RBCs), blood pressure regulation, and bone mineralization.

The kidneys are responsible for maintaining a normal RBC volume by producing **erythropoietin.** As a hormone erythropoietin functions within the bone marrow to stimulate red blood cell production and maturation (McCance and Huether, 1998). Erythropoietin also prolongs the life of mature RBCs. Clients with chronic alterations in kidney function cannot produce sufficient quantities of this hormone; therefore they are prone to anemia.

Renin is another hormone produced by the kidneys. Its major role is the regulation of blood flow in times of renal ischemia (decreased blood supply). Renin is released from juxtaglomerular cells (Figure 44-3).

Renin functions as an enzyme to convert angiotensinogen (a substance synthesized by the liver) into angiotensin I. As angiotensin I circulates through the lungs, it is converted to angiotensin II and angiotensin III. Angiotensin II exerts its effect on vascular smooth muscle to cause vasoconstriction and stimulates aldosterone release from the adrenal cortex. Aldosterone causes retention of water, which increases blood volume. Angiotensin III exerts similar effects but to a lesser degree. The net effect of both of these mechanisms is an increase in arterial blood pressure and renal blood flow (McCance and Huether, 1998).

The kidneys also play a role in calcium and phosphate regulation. They are responsible for producing a substance that converts vitamin D into its active form. Clients with chronic alterations in kidney function do not make suffi-

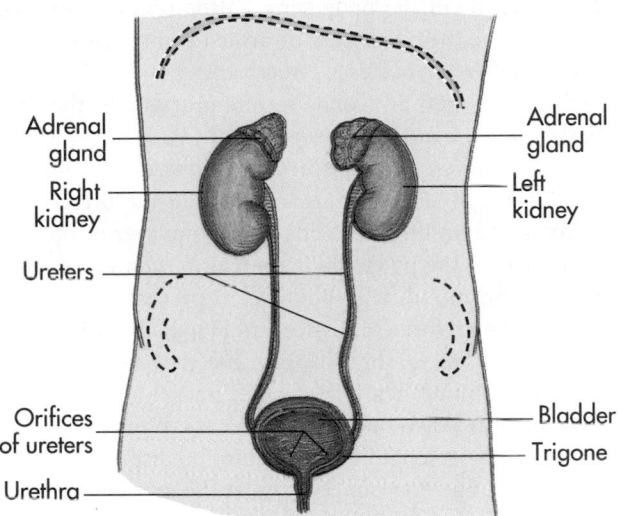

Figure 44-1   Organs of the urinary system.

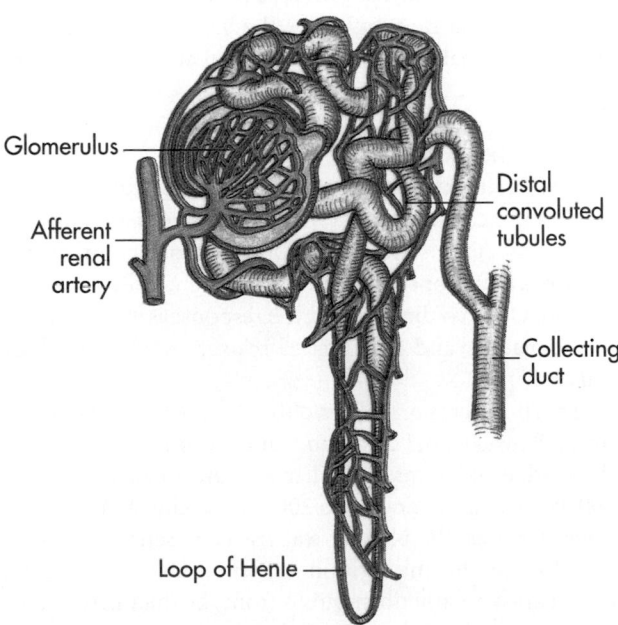

Figure 44-2   Renal nephron.

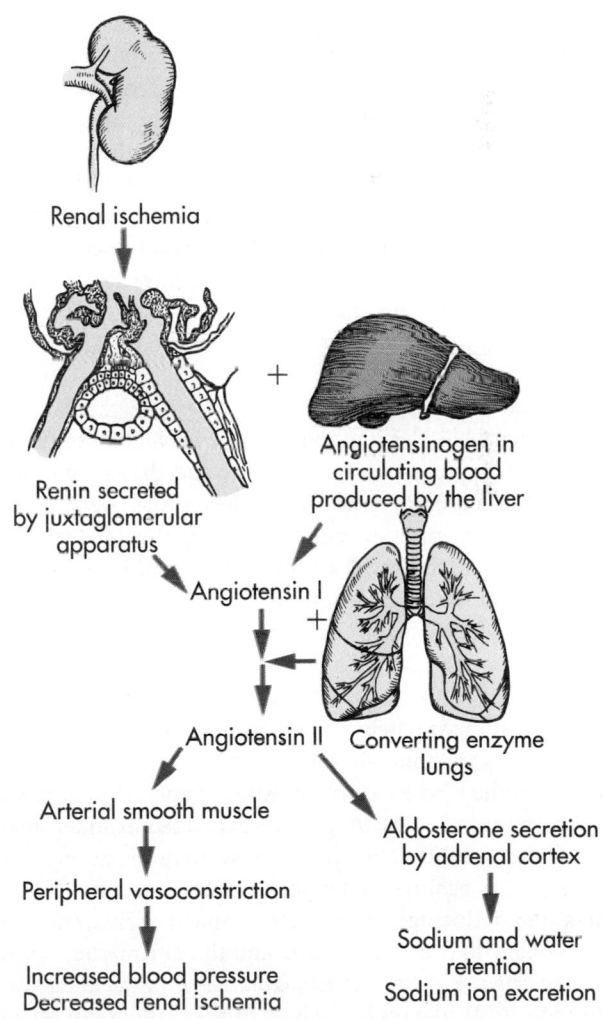

Figure 44-3   Physiological effects of renin-angiotensin mechanism.

cient amounts of the active vitamin D metabolite. Therefore they are prone to develop renal bone disease resulting from the demineralization of bone secondary to impaired intestinal calcium absorption unless the active form of vitamin D is supplied.

URETERS

Urine enters the renal pelvis from the collecting ducts. A ureter joins each renal pelvis to the urinary bladder. Ureters are tubular structures measuring 25 to 30 cm (10 to 12 inches) in length and 1.25 cm (½ inch) in diameter in the adult. They extend retroperitoneally to enter the urinary bladder in the pelvic cavity at the ureterovesical junction. Urine draining from the ureters to the bladder is usually sterile.

Three layers of tissue form the wall of the ureter. The inner layer is a mucous membrane continuous with the lining of the renal pelvis and urinary bladder. The middle layer consists of smooth muscle fibers that transport urine through the ureters by peristaltic waves stimulated by distention with urine. An outer layer of fibrous connective tissue supports the ureters.

Peristaltic waves cause the urine to enter the bladder in spurts rather than steadily. The ureters enter obliquely through the posterior bladder wall. This arrangement normally prevents the reflux of urine from the bladder into the ureters during the act of **micturition** by the compression of the ureter at the ureterovesical junction (the juncture of the ureters with the bladder). An obstruction within a ureter, such as a kidney stone (**renal calculus**), results in strong peristaltic waves that attempt to move the obstruction into the bladder. These strong peristaltic waves result in pain often referred to as renal colic.

BLADDER

The urinary bladder is a hollow, distensible, muscular organ that is both a reservoir for urine and the organ of excretion. When empty, the bladder lies in the pelvic cavity behind the symphysis pubis. In men the bladder lies against the anterior wall of the rectum and in women it rests against the anterior wall of the uterus and vagina.

The bladder expands as it becomes filled with urine. Pressure within the bladder is usually low, even when partly full, a factor that protects against infection. The capacity is approximately 600 ml of urine, although a normal voiding is about 300 ml.

When the bladder is full, it expands and extends above the symphysis pubis. A greatly distended bladder may reach the umbilicus. In a pregnant woman the developing fetus pushes against the bladder, causing a feeling of fullness and reducing the bladder's capacity. This effect is more likely to occur in the first and third trimester.

The trigone (a smooth triangular area on the inner surface of the bladder) is at the base of the bladder. An opening exists at each of the trigone's three angles. Two are for the ureters, and one is for the urethra.

The wall of the bladder has four layers: the inner mucous coat, a submucous coat of connective tissue, a muscular coat, and an outer serous coat. The muscular layer has bundles of muscle fibers that form the detrusor muscle. Parasympathetic nerve fibers stimulate the detrusor muscle during urination. The internal urethral sphincter, made of a ringlike band of muscle, is at the base of the bladder where it joins the urethra. The sphincter prevents escape of urine from the bladder and is under voluntary control.

URETHRA

Urine travels from the bladder through the urethra and passes outside of the body through the urethral meatus. Normally the turbulent flow of urine through the urethra washes it free of bacteria. Mucous membrane lines the urethra, and urethral glands secrete mucus into the urethral canal. The mucus is believed to be bacteriostatic and forms a mucous plug to prevent entrance of bacteria. Thick layers of smooth muscle surround the urethra. In addition, the urethra descends through a layer of skeletal muscle called the pelvic floor muscles. When these muscles are contracted, it is possible to prevent urine flow through the urethra (McCance and Huether, 1998).

In women the urethra is approximately 4 to 6.5 cm (1½ to 2½ inches) long. The external urethral sphincter, located about halfway down the urethra, permits voluntary flow of urine. The short length of the urethra predisposes women to infection. Bacteria can easily enter the urethra from the perineal area. In men the urethra, which is both a urinary canal and a passageway for cells and secretions from reproductive organs, is 20 cm (8 inches) long. The male urethra has three sections: the prostatic urethra, the membranous urethra, and the cavernous or penile urethra.

In a female the urinary **meatus** (opening) is located between the labia minora, above the vagina and below the clitoris. In a male the meatus is located at the distal end of the penis.

ACT OF URINATION

Several brain structures influence bladder function, including the cerebral cortex, thalamus, hypothalamus, and brain stem. Together they suppress contraction of the bladder's detrusor muscle until a person wishes to urinate or void. Once voiding occurs, the response is a contraction of the bladder and coordinated relaxation of pelvic floor muscles.

The bladder normally holds as much as 600 ml of urine. However, the desire to urinate can be sensed when the bladder contains a smaller amount of urine (150 to 200 ml in an adult and 50 to 200 ml in a child). As the volume increases, the bladder walls stretch, sending sensory impulses to the micturition center in the sacral spinal cord. Parasympathetic impulses from the micturition center stimulate the detrusor muscle to contract rhythmically. The internal urethral sphincter also relaxes so that urine may enter the urethra, although voiding does not yet occur. As the bladder contracts, nerve impulses travel up the spinal cord to the pons and cerebral cortex. A person is thus conscious of the need to urinate. Older children and adults can respond to or ignore this urge, thus making urination under voluntary control. If the person chooses not to void, the external urinary sphincter remains contracted, and the micturition reflex is inhibited. However, when a person is ready to void, the external sphincter relaxes, the micturition reflex stimulates the detrusor muscle to contract, and efficient emptying of the bladder occurs.

If the urge to void has been ignored repeatedly, the bladder capacity may be reached and the resulting pressure on the sphincter may make continued voluntary control impossible.

Damage to the spinal cord above the sacral region causes loss of voluntary control of urination, but the micturition reflex pathway may remain intact, allowing urination to occur reflexively. This condition is called a **reflex bladder.** If bladder emptying is hindered by chronic obstruction such as prostate enlargement, over time the micturition reflex becomes nonfunctional and severe urinary retention occurs.

Factors Influencing Urination.

Many factors influence the volume and quality of urine and the client's ability to urinate. Some pathophysiological conditions may be acute and reversible (urinary tract infection) whereas others may be chronic and irreversible (slow, progressive development of renal dysfunction). Sociocultural factors and psychological factors may influence the client's expectation of the degree of privacy and location for attending to urinary needs. Growth and development factors determine the client's ability to control the act of urination during the lifespan. Problems related to the act of urination may be the result of cognitive, functional, or physical means resulting in incontinence, retention, or infection.

Disease Conditions.

Disease processes that primarily affect renal function (changes in urine volume or quality) are generally categorized as prerenal, renal, or postrenal in origin (Box 44-1).

Prerenal alterations in urinary elimination decrease circulating blood flow to and through the kidneys with subsequent decreased perfusion to renal tissue. In other words, the alterations are outside of the urinary system. The decrease in renal perfusion leads to **oliguria** (diminished capacity to form urine) or, less commonly, **anuria** (inability to produce urine). Renal alterations result from factors that cause injury directly to the glomeruli or renal tubule, interfering with their normal filtering, reabsorptive, and secretory functions. Postrenal alterations result from obstruction to the urinary collecting system anywhere from the calyces (drainage structures within the kidney) to the urethral meatus (that is, outside of the kidney but within the urinary system). Urine is formed by the

---

Conditions Causing Alterations in Renal Function Box 44-1

PRERENAL CONDITIONS
Decreased intravascular volume: dehydration, hemorrhage, burns, shock
Altered peripheral vascular resistance: sepsis, anaphylactic (allergic) reactions
Cardiac pump failure: congestive heart failure, myocardial infarction, hypertensive heart disease, valvular disease, pericardial tamponade

RENAL CONDITIONS
Nephrotoxic agents (e.g., gentamycin)
Transfusion reactions
Diseases of the glomeruli (e.g., glomerulonephritis)
Renal neoplasms
Systemic diseases (e.g., diabetes mellitus)
Hereditary diseases (e.g., polycystic kidney disease)
Infections

POSTRENAL CONDITIONS
Ureteral, bladder, or urethral obstruction: calculi, blood clots, tumors, stricture
Prostatic hypertrophy or tumor
Neurogenic bladder
Pelvic tumors

---

urinary system but cannot be eliminated by normal means.

Several diseases can affect the ability to micturate. Any lesion of peripheral nerves leading to the bladder causes loss of bladder tone, reduced sensation of bladder fullness, and difficulty in controlling urination. For example, diabetes mellitus and multiple sclerosis cause neuropathic conditions that alter bladder function.

Diseases that slow or hinder physical activity interfere with the ability to void. Rheumatoid arthritis, degenerative joint disease, and parkinsonism are examples of conditions that make it difficult to reach and use toilet facilities. A client with rheumatoid arthritis often cannot sit on or rise from a toilet without an elevated seat.

Diseases that cause irreversible damage to the glomerulus or tubules result in permanent alterations in renal function. Chronic or end-stage renal disease (ESRD) are the terms used to describe the resulting decline in kidney function from these processes. The client with ESRD manifests numerous metabolic disturbances that require treatment for survival. The associated symptoms experienced by the client occur as a result of the **uremic syndrome.** This syndrome is characterized by an increase in nitrogenous wastes in the blood, altered regulatory functions (causing marked fluid and electrolyte abnormalities), nausea, vomiting, headache, coma, and convulsions. Treatment options include methods to correct these biochemical derangements. The problem may be managed conservatively with medications and a regimen of dietary and fluid restrictions. However, as worsening of the uremic symptoms becomes evident, more aggressive treatment is indicated. These treatments are known as **renal replacement therapies.** Dialysis and organ transplantation are the two methods of renal replacement. The two methods of dialysis are peritoneal and hemodialysis (Box 44-2).

Peritoneal dialysis is an indirect method of cleansing the blood of waste products using the processes of osmosis and diffusion. The peritoneum is the serous membrane in the peritoneal cavity that functions as a semipermeable membrane. Excess fluid and waste products are readily removed from the bloodstream when a sterile electrolyte solution (dialysate) is instilled into the peritoneal cavity by gravity via a surgically placed catheter. The dialysate is left in the cavity for a prescribed time interval and then is drained out by gravity, taking accumulated wastes and excess fluid and electrolytes with it.

Hemodialysis involves using a machine equipped with a semipermeable filtering membrane (artificial kidney) that removes accumulated waste products from the blood. In the dialysis machine, dialysate fluid is pumped through one side of the filter membrane (artificial kidney) while the client's blood passes through the other side. The processes of diffusion, osmosis, and ultrafiltration cleanse the client's blood, and it is returned through a specially placed vascular access device (Gore-Tex graft). Both dialysis modalities can be applied for a short or long time, and they require specialized equipment and trained nurses.

Organ transplantation is the replacement of the client's diseased kidneys with a healthy one from a living or cadaveric donor of compatible blood and tissue type. After the client (recipient) is deemed medically and psychosocially suitable, the organ is surgically implanted. Special medications (immunosuppressives) are administered for life to prevent the body from rejecting the transplanted organ. Unlike the other treatments, successful organ transplantation offers the client the potential for restoration of normal kidney function.

Growth and Development.   Infants and young children cannot effectively concentrate urine. Their urine thus appears light yellow or clear. In relation to their small

body size, infants and children excrete large volumes of urine. For example, a 6-month-old infant who weighs 6 to 8 kg (13 to 18 pounds) excretes 400 to 500 ml of urine daily.

A child cannot control micturition voluntarily until age 18 to 24 months. A child must be able to recognize the feeling of bladder fullness, to hold urine for 1 to 2 hours, and to communicate the sense of urgency to an adult. The young child needs parents' understanding, patience, and consistency. A child may not gain full control of micturition until age 4 or 5. Daytime control of micturition is easier to accomplish than nighttime control and occurs earlier in the child's development, usually by 2 years of age.

The adult normally voids 1500 to 1600 ml of urine daily. The kidney concentrates urine, producing a normal, amber-colored urine. A person does not normally wake to void during sleep because of reduction of renal blood flow during rest and the kidney's ability to concentrate urine.

Aging impairs micturition. Problems of mobility sometimes make it difficult for the older adult to reach a toilet in time. An older person may be too weak to rise from a toilet seat without assistance. Chronic neurological disease such as parkinsonism or cerebrovascular accident (stroke) impairs the sense of balance and makes it difficult for a man to stand while voiding or a woman to walk to the toilet. If an older person loses control of thought processes such as with Alzheimer's disease, the ability to control micturition is unpredictable. The person may lose the ability to sense a full bladder or be unable to recall the procedure for voiding.

Changes in kidney and bladder function also occur with aging. The glomerular filtration rate declines, but the kidney's ability to concentrate urine also declines. Thus the older adult often experiences **nocturia** (excessive urination at night). The bladder loses its muscle tone and capacity to hold urine, resulting in increased **urinary frequency.** Because the bladder cannot contract as effectively, an older person often retains urine in the bladder after voiding (**residual urine**). Older men may also suffer from benign prostatic hypertrophy, which makes them prone to urinary retention and incontinence. These changes increase the risk for bacterial growth and development of urinary tract infections (UTIs). Another factor related to urine elimination difficulties is constipation. Constipation and resulting bowel fullness may put external pressure on the bladder, reducing the effective capacity, causing frequency or even incontinence.

Sociocultural Factors.   Cultural norms vary on the privacy of urination. North Americans expect toilet facilities to be private, whereas some European cultures accept communal toilet facilities. Social expectations (e.g., school recesses) influence the time of urination. Indoor plumbing for toilet facilities may be rare in many poor rural areas such as Appalachia and other remote mountain communities.

Indications for Dialysis   Box 44-2

Renal failure that can no longer be controlled by conservative management (i.e., dietary modifications and administration of medications to correct electrolyte abnormalities)

Worsening of uremic syndrome associated with ESRD (i.e., nausea, vomiting, neurological changes, pericarditis)

Severe electrolyte and/or fluid abnormalities that cannot be controlled by simpler measures (e.g., hyperkalemia, pulmonary edema)

The nurse's approach to a client's elimination needs must consider cultural, social, and gender habits. If a client prefers privacy, the nurse tries to prevent interruptions as the client voids. A client with less need for privacy should be treated with understanding and acceptance. Place clients in the position that is best for them. Men generally urinate best in a standing position whereas women generally sit on a toilet. In some cultures the client would squat over a receptacle rather than on one.

Psychological Factors.   Anxiety and emotional stress may cause a sense of urgency and increased frequency of urination. An anxious person may have the urge to void even after voiding only a few minutes earlier. Anxiety may also prevent a person from being able to urinate completely. Emotional tension makes it difficult to relax abdominal and perineal muscles. If the external urethral sphincter is not completely relaxed, voiding may be incomplete, and urine is retained in the bladder. Attempting to void in a public restroom may result in a temporary inability to void. Privacy and adequate time to urinate are usually important to most people. Some people need distractions (e.g., reading) to relax.

Muscle Tone.   Weak abdominal and pelvic floor muscles impair bladder contraction and control of the external urethral sphincter. Poor control of micturition can result from muscle wasting caused by prolonged immobility, stretching of muscles during childbirth, menopausal muscle atrophy, and damage to muscles from trauma. Continuous drainage of urine through an indwelling catheter causes loss of bladder tone and/or damage to urethral sphincters. When a catheter is removed, the client may have difficulty regaining urinary control.

Fluid Balance.   The kidneys maintain a sensitive balance between retention and excretion of fluids (see Chapter 40). If fluids and the concentration of electrolytes and solutes are in equilibrium, an increase in fluid intake causes an increase in urine production. Ingested fluids increase the body's circulating plasma and thus increase the volume of glomerular filtrate and urine excreted.

This amount varies with food and fluid intake. The volume of urine formed at night is about half that formed during the day because both intake and metabolism decline. This results in a decline in renal blood flow. Nocturia can be a sign of renal alteration. In a healthy person, the intake of water in food and fluids balances the output of water in urine, feces, and insensible losses in perspiration and respiration. An excessive output of urine is known as **polyuria.**

Ingestion of certain fluids directly affects urine production and excretion. Coffee, tea, cocoa, and cola drinks that contain caffeine promote increased urine formation (**diuresis**). Alcohol inhibits the release of antidiuretic hormone (ADH), resulting in increased water loss in urine.

Foods that contain a high fluid content, such as fruits and vegetables, may also increase urine production.

Febrile conditions affect urine production. The client who becomes diaphoretic loses a large amount of fluids through insensible water loss, which decreases urine production. However, the increased body metabolism associated with fever increases accumulation of body wastes. Although urine volume may be reduced, it is highly concentrated.

Surgical Procedures.   The stress of surgery initially triggers the general adaptation syndrome (see Chapter 30). The posterior pituitary gland releases an increased amount of ADH, which increases water reabsorption and reduces urine output. The surgical client is often in an altered state of fluid balance before surgery due to the disease process or preoperative fasting, which aggravates the reduction in urine output. The stress response also elevates the level of aldosterone, resulting in reduction of urine output in an effort to maintain circulatory fluid volume.

Anesthetic and narcotic analgesics may slow the glomerular filtration rate, reducing urine output. These pharmacological agents also impair sensory and motor impulses traveling between the bladder, spinal cord, and brain. Clients recovering from anesthesia and deep analgesia are often unable to sense bladder fullness and are unable to initiate or inhibit micturition. Spinal anesthetics, in particular, create the risk of urinary retention because of an inability to sense the need to void and a possible inability of the bladder muscles and sphincters to respond (Beare and Myers, 1998).

Surgery of lower abdominal and pelvic structures can impair urination because of local trauma to surrounding tissues. The edema and inflammation associated with healing may obstruct the flow of urine from the kidneys to the bladder or from the bladder or urethra, interfere with relaxation of pelvic and sphincter muscles, or cause discomfort during voiding. After returning from surgery involving the ureters, bladder, and urethra, clients routinely have urinary catheters.

The surgical formation of a **urinary diversion** temporarily or permanently bypasses the bladder and urethra as the exit routes for urine. Permanent urinary diversions may be needed in the client with cancer of the bladder. The client with a urinary diversion has a **stoma** (artificial opening) on the abdomen to drain urine.

Medications.   Diuretics prevent reabsorption of water and certain electrolytes to increase urine output. Urinary retention may be caused by use of anticholinergics (e.g., atropine), antihistamines (e.g., Sudafed), antihypertensives (e.g., Aldomet), or beta-adrenergic blockers (e.g., Inderal). Some medications change the color of urine. Pyridium colors the urine a bright orange to rust, amitriptyline causes a green or blue discoloration, while levodopa may discolor the urine to brown or black.

Cancer chemotherapy drugs may also color the urine and be toxic to the kidneys or the bladder. Clients with alterations in kidney function require dosage adjustments in medications excreted by the kidneys.

Diagnostic Examination.   Examination of the urinary system can influence micturition. Procedures such as an intravenous pyelogram or urogram may require that the client omit fluids or greatly limit fluids before the test. A restriction in fluid intake commonly lowers urine output. Diagnostic examinations (e.g., cystoscopy) that involve direct visualization of urinary structures may cause localized edema of the urethral passageway and spasm of the bladder sphincter. The client often has urinary retention after such a procedure and may pass red or pink urine because of bleeding resulting from trauma to the urethral or bladder mucosa.

Alterations in Urinary Elimination.   Clients with
urinary problems most commonly have disturbances in the act of micturition that involve a failure to store urine or a failure to empty urine. These disturbances result from impaired bladder function, obstruction to urine outflow, or inability to voluntarily control micturition. Some clients may have permanent or temporary changes in the normal pathway of urinary excretion. The client with a urinary diversion has special problems because urine drains to the outside through a stoma.

Urinary Retention.   **Urinary retention** is the marked accumulation of urine in the bladder as a result of the inability of the bladder to empty. Urine continues to collect in the bladder, stretching its walls and causing feelings of pressure, discomfort, tenderness over the symphysis pubis, restlessness, and diaphoresis (sweating).

Normally urine production slowly fills the bladder and prevents activation of stretch receptors until it distends to a certain level of stretch. The micturition reflex occurs, and the bladder empties. In urinary retention the bladder becomes unable to respond to the micturition reflex and thus unable to empty.

As retention progresses, retention with overflow may develop. Pressure in the bladder builds to a point where the external urethral sphincter is unable to hold back urine. The sphincter temporarily opens to allow a small volume of urine (25 to 60 ml) to escape. As urine exits, the bladder pressure falls enough to allow the sphincter to regain control and close. With retention overflow the client voids small amounts of urine 2 or 3 times an hour with no real relief of discomfort. The nurse should be aware of the volume and frequency of voiding to assess this condition in the client. The nurse should assess the abdomen for evidence of bladder distention. Bladder spasms may occur with voiding.

In acute retention key signs are bladder distention and absence of urine output over several hours. The client un-

der the influence of anesthetics or analgesics may feel only pressure, but the alert client has severe pain as the bladder distends beyond its normal capacity. In severe urinary retention the bladder may hold as much as 2000 to 3000 ml of urine. Retention occurs as a result of urethral obstruction, surgical trauma, alterations in motor and sensory innervation of the bladder, medication side effects, or anxiety.

Lower Urinary Tract Infections.   Urinary tract infections are responsible for more than 7 million physician visits a year and are the most common hospital-acquired (nosocomial) infections in the United States (Buscheller and Bernstein, 1997). Many cases result from catheterization or surgical manipulation. Bacteria in the urine (**bacteriuria**) may lead to the spread of organisms into the bloodstream and kidneys, leading to **urosepsis** (Travis and Lampley-Dallas, 1997). Microorganisms most commonly enter the urinary tract through the ascending urethral route. Bacteria inhabit the distal urethra, external genitalia, and vagina in women. Organisms enter the urethral meatus easily and travel up the inner mucosal lining to the bladder. Women are more susceptible to infection because of the proximity of the anus to the urethral meatus and because of the short urethra. Older adults and clients with progressive underlying disease or decreased immunity are also at increased risk. In men, prostatic secretions that contain an antibacterial substance and the length of the urethra reduce the susceptibility to UTIs. It is estimated that 40% to 50% of hospitalized older adults have significant bacteriuria (Travis and Lampley-Dallas, 1997).

In a healthy person with good bladder function, organisms are flushed out during voiding. However, bladder distention reduces blood flow to the mucosal and submucosal layers, and tissues become more susceptible to bacteria. Residual urine in the bladder becomes more alkaline and is an ideal site for microorganism growth.

The most common cause of infection is the introduction of instruments into the urinary tract. For example, the introduction of a catheter through the urethra provides a direct route for microorganisms. With an indwelling bladder catheter, bacteria ascend along the outside of the catheter on the urethral wall or travel up the catheter's lumen. The catheter interferes with the normal voiding mechanism that acts as a defense against organisms entering the urethra. Local irritation to the urethra or bladder further predisposes tissues to bacterial invasion.

Poor perineal hygiene is a common cause of UTIs in women. Inadequate hand washing, failure to wipe from front to back after voiding or defecating, and frequent sexual intercourse predispose women to infection. Any interference with the free flow of urine can cause infection. A kinked, obstructed, or clamped catheter and any condition resulting in urinary retention increase the risk of a bladder infection.

Clients with lower UTIs have pain or burning during

urination (**dysuria**) as urine flows past inflamed tissues. Fever, chills, nausea and vomiting, and malaise develop as the infection worsens. An irritated bladder causes a frequent and urgent sensation of the need to void. Irritation to bladder and urethral mucosa results in blood-tinged urine (**hematuria**). The urine appears concentrated and cloudy because of the presence of white blood cells (WBCs) or bacteria. If infection spreads to the upper urinary tract (kidneys—**pyelonephritis**), flank pain, tenderness, fever, and chills are common.

Urinary Incontinence.   Urinary incontinence is the involuntary loss of urine that is sufficient to be a problem (Urinary Incontinence Guideline Panel [UGIP], 1996). It may be temporary or permanent. The client can no longer control the act of micturition. Leakage of urine may be continuous or intermittent. Urinary incontinence can be identified as functional, overflow, reflex, stress, or urge (Table 44-1).

Incontinence should not be associated only with older adults. It may develop in people of every age, although it is more common in older adults. It is estimated that 12% of community-dwelling older adults and as many as 50% of institutionalized older adults have some degree of incontinence (Hutchinson, Leger-Krall, and Wilson, 1996). Incontinence can impair body image. Clothing may become wet with urine, and the accompanying odor adds to embarrassment. As a result clients with this problem often avoid social activities.

Older adults may have special problems with incontinence because of physical limitations and the environments in which they live. Older persons with restricted mobility have greater chances of being incontinent because of their inability to reach toilet facilities in time. Low-set chairs and beds raised well above the floor may be obstacles for older adults who must get up to reach a toilet. Older clients who have difficulty undoing buttons or manipulating zippers face another obstacle. Older clients often lack the energy to walk very far at one time. The toilet may be too far away for clients with urge incontinence.

Continued episodes of incontinence create the potential for skin breakdown. The acidic character of urine is ir-

Table 44-1 **Types of Urinary Incontinence**		
Description	Causes	Symptoms
Functional Involuntary, unpredictable passage of urine in a client with intact urinary and nervous system	Change in environment: sensory, cognitive, or mobility deficits	Urge to void that causes loss of urine before reaching appropriate receptacle. The client with cognitive changes may have forgotten what to do.
Overflow Voluntary or involuntary loss of a small amount of urine (20-30 ml) from an overdistended bladder	Hypotonic or underactive detrussor secondary to drugs, fecal impaction, diabetes, spinal cord injury; men—prostate enlargement, women—severe uterine prolapse	Symptoms may vary from dribbling of a few drops of urine to larger amounts with urgency and frequency.
Reflex Involuntary loss of urine occurring at somewhat predictable intervals; large or small volume	Spinal cord dysfunction (either inhibition of cerebral awareness or impairment of the reflex arc)	Unawareness of bladder filling, lack of urge to void, uninhibited bladder spasm contraction.
Stress Leakage of small volumes of urine caused by sudden increase in intraabdominal pressure	Coughing, laughing, sneezing, or lifting with a full bladder; obesity; full uterus in third trimester; incompetent bladder outlet; weak pelvic musculature	Loss of urine with increased intraabdominal pressure, urinary urgency and frequency.
Urge Involuntary passage of urine after a strong sense of urgency to void	Decreased bladder capacity; irritation of bladder stretch receptors; alcohol or caffeine ingestion; increased fluid intake; infection	Urinary urgency, often with frequency (more often than every 2 hours); bladder spasm or contraction; voiding in either small amounts (<100 ml) or large amounts (>500 ml).

Modified from Kim MJ, McFarland GK, McLane AM: *Pocket guide to nursing diagnoses*, ed 7, St. Louis, 1997, Mosby.

ritating to skin. The immobilized client who has frequent incontinence is especially at risk for pressure ulcers (see Chapter 46).

Urinary Diversions.　A urinary stoma to divert the flow of urine from the kidneys directly to the abdominal surface is created for several reasons (Box 44-3). Such a urinary diversion may be temporary or permanent. Figure 44-4 illustrates several approaches to urinary diversion.

The ileal loop or conduit involves separating a loop of intestinal ileum with its blood supply intact. The surgeon implants the ureters into the isolated segment of ileum, which is then an outlet for urine drainage. The remaining ileum is reconnected to the rest of the digestive tract. The ileal segment can then be used as a conduit for continuous urine drainage or fashioned into a continent reservoir (McCance and Huether, 1998). The continent pouch is constructed to provide urinary flow in a nonrefluxing manner. The portion of the ileum connected to the abdominal wall acts as a continent nipple, requiring intermittent catheterization for emptying. The disadvantage of either an ileal conduit or reservoir is that if urine outflow becomes obstructed, irreversible damage to the kidneys can occur secondary to chronic infections or hydronephrosis.

A **ureterostomy** involves bringing the end of one or both ureters to the abdominal surface. To avoid the need for two collecting devices, a transureteroureterostomy connects the ureters and brings one out through the abdominal wall. In some cases a tube may need to be placed directly into the renal pelvis to provide urinary drainage. This procedure is called a **nephrostomy.**

The client with an incontinent urinary diversion must wear a stomal pouch continuously because there is no sphincter control for regulation of urine flow. Local irritation and skin breakdown occur when urine comes in contact with the skin for long periods.

A urinary diversion poses threats to a client's body image. The client must wear an artificial device to collect urine and must learn to manage it. However, the client can wear normal clothing, engage in physical activity, travel, and have sexual relations.

A client with a urinary diversion should be referred to the enterostomal therapist (a nurse with specialized training in this area). The therapist can be an invaluable resource to assist the client with matters pertaining to all aspects of care. The enterostomal therapist will often meet with the client before surgery. The client should also be referred to the United Ostomy Association. This organization may help in providing information regarding support groups to enhance coping and adaptation to lifestyle and body-image changes.

Nursing Knowledge Base

Urinary elimination is a basic function of humans that is usually a private process. Many clients may need physiological and psychological assistance from the nurse. Whether the client has an actual or potential urinary problem, the nurse must be sensitive to the client's urinary function needs. The nurse will need knowledge of concepts beyond the anatomy and physiology of the urinary system to give appropriate care. Other concepts that must be understood are infection control, hygiene measures, growth and development, and psychosocial influences.

INFECTION CONTROL AND HYGIENE

The urinary tract is usually considered sterile but is a common site for infections. The nurse must use infection-control principles to help prevent the development and spread of urinary tract infections, as well as to treat existing infections (see Chapter 33). Many UTIs are caused by *Escherichia coli,* a common bacteria found in feces. Infection can occur in any location of the urinary tract

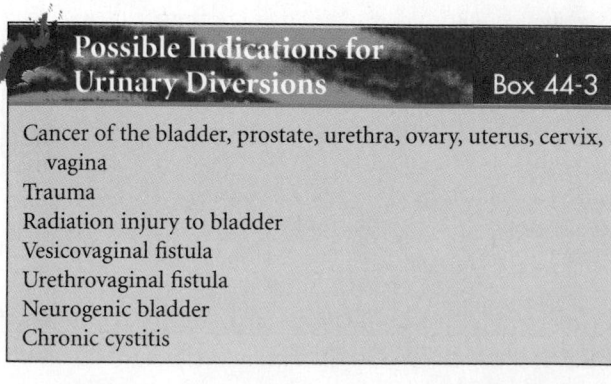

Possible Indications for Urinary Diversions　　　　　Box 44-3

Cancer of the bladder, prostate, urethra, ovary, uterus, cervix, vagina
Trauma
Radiation injury to bladder
Vesicovaginal fistula
Urethrovaginal fistula
Neurogenic bladder
Chronic cystitis

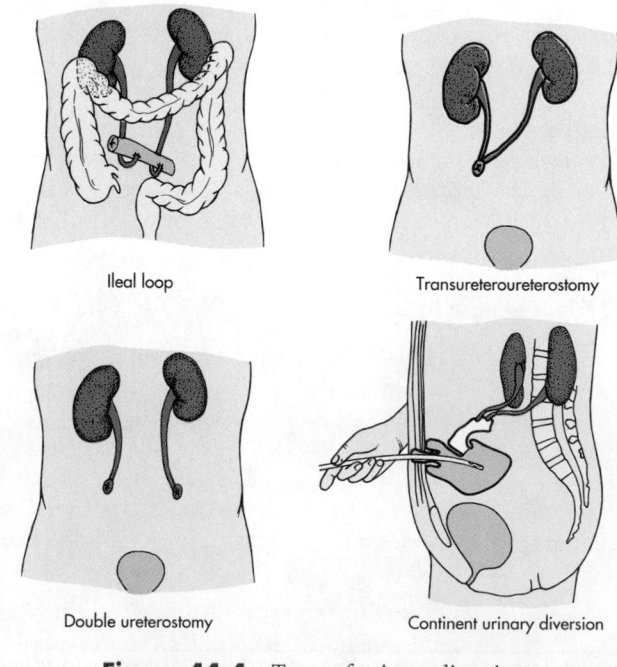

Ileal loop

Transureteroureterostomy

Double ureterostomy

Continent urinary diversion

Figure 44-4　Types of urinary diversions.

from the urethra to the kidneys. Hospital-acquired UTIs are often related to poor hand washing, improper catheter care, or faulty catheterization technique (Buscheller and Bernstein, 1997).

Knowledge of both medical and surgical asepsis must be applied meticulously when providing care involving the urinary tract or external genitalia (see Chapter 33). Any invasive procedure of the urinary tract such as catheterization requires sterile technique. Procedures such as perineal care or examination of the genitalia require medical asepsis.

DEVELOPMENTAL CONSIDERATIONS

In the infant, urination (voiding) is a reflex response that occurs as a result of filling and stretch. As the neurological system matures, a toddler of 2 or 3 years is able to associate the sensations of bladder filling and urination. Many toddlers may then be able to control the external sphincter, and toilet training will begin. Bladder control is often accomplished by age 3, but occasional daytime accidents or nocturnal enuresis may continue until age 5 (see Chapter 10).

Advancing age also causes changes that may result in voiding problems. In the male, prostate enlargement may begin during the 40s and continue throughout life, resulting in urinary frequency and possible urinary retention. In the female, childbearing and/or hormonal changes of menopause may cause changes that lead to urinary difficulties. During a pregnancy urinary frequency is common, and susceptibility to urinary tract infection is increased. Temporary or permanent changes that result from repeated deliveries or hormonal changes may result in decreased perineal muscle tone, leading to urgency and stress incontinence (see Chapter 12). The changes in the urethral mucosa associated with loss of estrogen during and after menopause also contribute to increased susceptibility to infection (McCance and Huether, 1998).

PSYCHOSOCIAL CONSIDERATIONS

The nurse must consider that urinary elimination problems may result in alterations of self-concept and sexuality, and culture may influence the choice of appropriate nursing interventions. Self-concept, which includes body image, self-esteem, roles, and identity, develops over a lifespan. Children may not want to urinate to avoid losing part of themselves (see Chapter 10). Gender influences positioning for urination: males stand, whereas females sit. Culture dictates when and where it is appropriate to urinate. Culture determines whether it is proper for a male to care for the urinary needs of a female (see Chapter 7).

Critical Thinking Synthesis

Successful critical thinking requires a synthesis of knowledge, experience, information gathered from clients, critical thinking attitudes, and intellectual and professional standards. Clinical judgments require the nurse to anticipate the information necessary, analyze the data, and make decisions regarding client care. Critical thinking is always changing. During assessment the nurse must consider all elements that build toward making appropriate nursing diagnoses.

In the case of urinary elimination, the nurse must integrate knowledge from nursing and other disciplines, previous experiences, and information gathered from clients to understand the process of urinary elimination and the impact on the client and family. In addition, the use of critical thinking attitudes such as perseverence is needed to find a plan of care to provide successful management of urinary elimination problems. Professional standards, such as those developed by the Agency for Health Care Policy and Research (AHCPR), (UIGP, 1996), provide valuable guidelines for management.

Nursing Process and Alterations in Urinary Function

ASSESSMENT

To identify a urinary elimination problem and gather data for a care plan, the nurse uses scientific and nursing knowledge, obtains information by a nursing history, performs a physical assessment, assesses the client's urine, and reviews information from diagnostic tests and examinations. The nurse uses critical thinking to synthesize this information as assessment proceeds (Figure 44-5). Adequate assessment should result in the formulation of nursing diagnoses appropriate for alterations in urinary elimination. Box 44-4 illustrates the factor of culture and language in the assessment process.

Nursing History.   The nursing history includes a review of the client's elimination patterns and symptoms of urinary alterations and an assessment of other factors that may be affecting the ability to urinate normally.

Pattern of Urination.   The nurse asks the client about daily voiding patterns, including frequency and times of day, normal volume at each voiding, and any recent changes. Frequency varies among individuals and varies with intake and other types of fluid losses. The common times for urination are on awakening, after meals, and before bedtime. Most people void an average of 5 or more times a day. The client who voids frequently during the night may have renal disease or prostate enlargement. Information about the pattern of urination establishes a baseline for comparison.

Symptoms of Urinary Alterations.   Certain symptoms specific to urinary alterations may occur in more

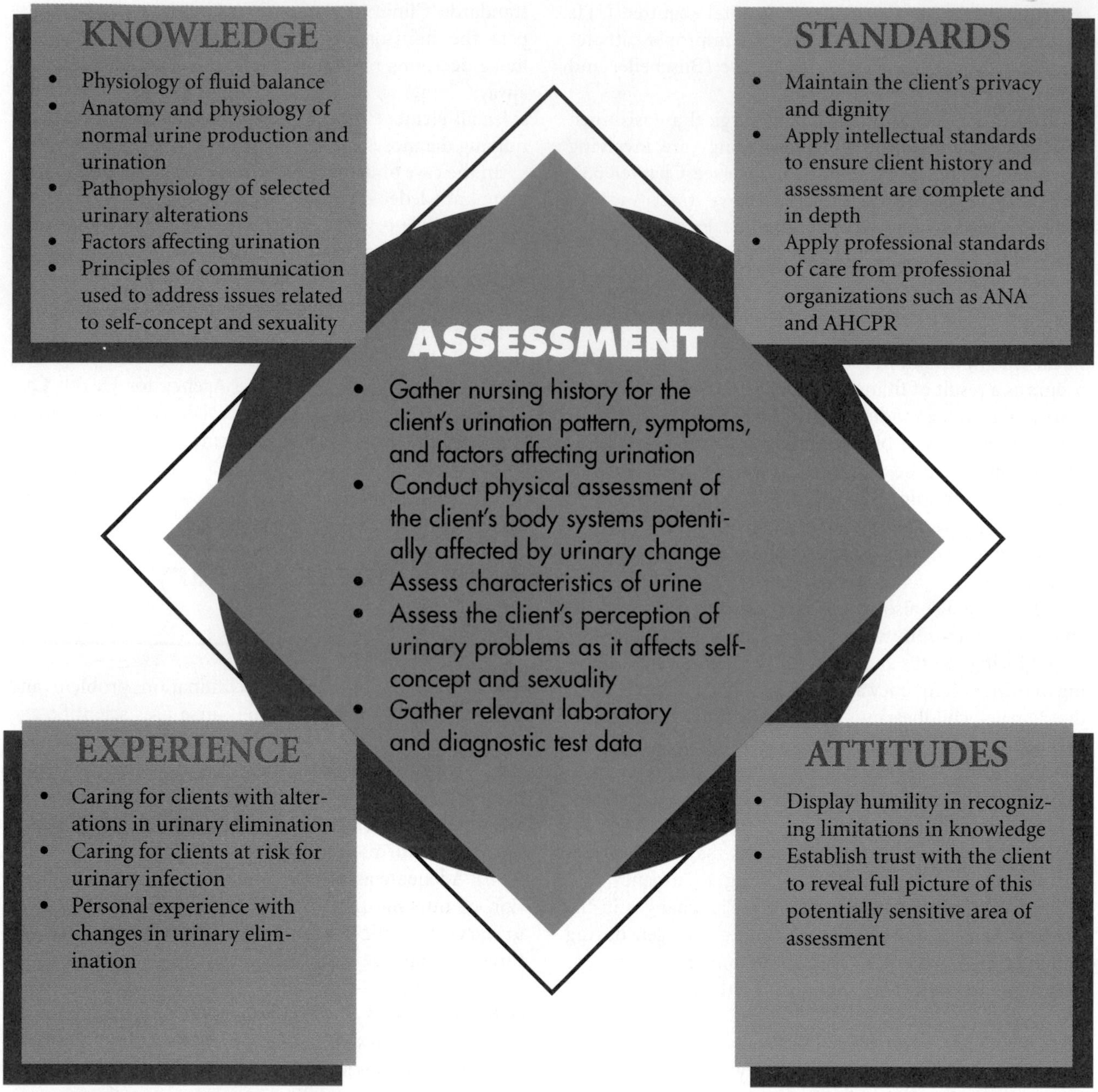

KNOWLEDGE

- Physiology of fluid balance
- Anatomy and physiology of normal urine production and urination
- Pathophysiology of selected urinary alterations
- Factors affecting urination
- Principles of communication used to address issues related to self-concept and sexuality

STANDARDS

- Maintain the client's privacy and dignity
- Apply intellectual standards to ensure client history and assessment are complete and in depth
- Apply professional standards of care from professional organizations such as ANA and AHCPR

ASSESSMENT

- Gather nursing history for the client's urination pattern, symptoms, and factors affecting urination
- Conduct physical assessment of the client's body systems potentially affected by urinary change
- Assess characteristics of urine
- Assess the client's perception of urinary problems as it affects self-concept and sexuality
- Gather relevant laboratory and diagnostic test data

EXPERIENCE

- Caring for clients with alterations in urinary elimination
- Caring for clients at risk for urinary infection
- Personal experience with changes in urinary elimination

ATTITUDES

- Display humility in recognizing limitations in knowledge
- Establish trust with the client to reveal full picture of this potentially sensitive area of assessment

Figure 44-5   *Synthesis Model for Urinary Elimination Assessment Phase.*

than one type of disorder. During assessment the nurse asks the client about the symptoms listed in Table 44-2, p. 1396. The nurse also assesses whether the client is aware of conditions or factors that precipitate or aggravate symptoms.

Factors Affecting Urination.   The nurse summarizes factors in the client's history that normally affect urination such as age, environmental factors, and medication history. Knowledge of the influence of growth and development on urination is important. Older adults require care-

ful assessment. Normal changes of aging predispose older adults to certain elimination problems (Box 44-5). Another factor to consider is the bowel elimination pattern. Constipation often may interfere with normal urine elimination. The name, amount, and frequency of prescription drugs should be noted. Over-the-counter drugs and exposure to cleaning solvents, pesticides, or other nephrotoxic agents are also important aspects of the history. Environmental barriers at home or in a health care setting are also evaluated. The client may need an elevated toilet seat, grab bars, or a portable commode. The nurse

Nguyen thi Hung, an elderly Vietnamese woman, has been admitted with a diagnosis of urosepsis. Her daughter, who speaks some English, is with her. In completing the nursing history the nurse attempts to find out about the client's urinary elimination habits. The daughter appears uncomfortable and does not translate but rather just smiles and nods her head.

NURSING IMPLICATIONS

- In an attempt to gather assessment data it may be necessary to use a bicultural medical translator. With a female client a female translator is to be preferred when a physical examination is to be done or questions are of an intimate nature.

The client's granddaughter arrives and is able to translate effectively that her grandmother and mother did not want to tell the nurse their beliefs about what caused the disease. The daughter was hesitant to explain about the "wind" that is believed to have caused the problem.

Vietnamese do not wish to disappoint, upset, or embarrass others and so may choose to not answer questions from the nurse at all. The mention of a Vietnamese health belief may have been seen as unacceptable, and therefore no answer was preferred. The Vietnamese client will often not express anger or discomfort.

NURSING IMPLICATIONS

- It is important for the nurse to anticipate the likelihood of need and acknowledge it through action. For example, rather than asking "Do you need to go to the bathroom?" state "I'll take you to the bathroom now."

The nurse was able to successfully assess the client. After establishing rapport with the client and her family, the nurse was able to plan appropriate interventions that conveyed acceptance of the client's culture and beliefs.

NURSING IMPLICATIONS

- Family continues to be the cohesive unit of Vietnamese society even in the United States. This source of strength is important to the health of the client, and family must be included in the plan of care.

Modified from Giger JN, Davidhizer RE: *Transcultural nursing: assessment and intervention*, ed 3, St. Louis, 1999, Mosby.

- High-quality nursing care is essential in care of the older adult. When older adults become dependent on others for personal care, maintenance of their urinary health falls into the domain of nursing practice (Travis and Lampley-Dallas, 1997).
- Dilute urine discourages bacterial growth, so older adults should be encouraged to drink at least six to eight glasses of fluids a day, unless medically contraindicated.
- Fluids such as cranberry juice that promote an acidic urine should be made available as part of the client's fluid intake, as an acidic urine also inhibits bacterial growth (Jackson and Hicks, 1997).
- Indwelling catheters should not be used routinely in older adults or if used, for no longer than 3 days. The risk of infection increases dramatically for catheterized clients (Buscheller and Bernstein, 1997).
- The nurse should note that incontinence is not a normal part of aging, and efforts should be made to assess incontinence and provide interventions to promote return to continence.

client has a urinary diversion, the nurse determines the rationale for its creation, the type of diversion, and usual methods for management (type of appliance or pouch, type of skin barriers or applications, methods used to reduce skin irritation, frequency of appliance changes, and the type of nighttime drainage system). Personal habits also affect urination. If a client is hospitalized, the nurse assesses the extent to which personal habits are altered. Privacy is often difficult to accomplish in a health care setting, particularly if a client must use a bedpan, but it is necessary to ensure maintenance of dignity.

The nurse assesses for the presence of an indwelling catheter. A client recovering from major surgery or suffering critical illness or disability often has an indwelling catheter to aid urinary drainage and provide a measurement of urine output. The presence of a catheter places a client at risk for infection. A client's physical condition affects the frequency with which the nurse monitors fluid intake (see Chapter 40). Regular intake and output (I&O) measurements help assess a client's overall fluid balance.

Physical Assessment.   A physical examination (see Chapter 32) provides the nurse with data to determine the presence and severity of urinary elimination problems. The primary structures reviewed include the skin and mucosal membranes, kidneys, bladder, and urethral meatus.

Skin and Mucosal Membranes.   The nurse assesses the condition of the skin and mucosal membranes. Problems with urinary elimination are often associated with fluid and electrolyte disturbances. By assessing skin turgor and the oral mucosa the nurse assesses the client's

observes for sensory restrictions, such as clients with visual problems who may have trouble reaching toilet facilities. If the client has difficulty with hand coordination, the nurse assesses the type of clothing and ease in using clothing fasteners.

Knowledge of past illness such as UTI or urinary tract surgery that increases the risk for recurrent problems is important also. Chronic diseases (e.g., multiple sclerosis) that impair bladder function require the nurse to consider preventive care measures such as frequent toileting to keep a client's skin dry and free from irritation. The nurse asks the client about the presence of urinary diversion. If the

Table 44-2   Common Types of Urinary Alterations

Symptoms	Description	Causes or Associated Factors
Urgency	Feeling of need to void immediately	Full bladder, bladder irritation or inflammation from infection, incompetent urethral sphincter, psychological stress
Dysuria	Painful or difficult urination	Bladder inflammation, trauma or inflammation of urethral sphincter
Frequency	Voiding at frequent intervals (<2 hr)	Increased fluid intake, bladder inflammation, increased pressure on bladder (pregnancy, psychological stress)
Hesitancy	Difficulty initiating urination	Prostate enlargement, anxiety, urethral edema
Polyuria	Voiding large amounts of urine	Excess fluid intake, diabetes mellitus or insipidus, use of diuretics, postobstructive diuresis
Oliguria	Diminished urinary output relative to intake (usually <400 ml/24 hr)	Dehydration, renal failure, UTI, increased ADH secretion, congestive heart failure
Nocturia	Urination, particularly excessive or frequent, at night	Excessive fluid intake before bed (especially coffee or alcohol), renal disease, aging process, prostate enlargement
Dribbling	Leakage of urine despite voluntary control of urination	Stress incontinence, overflow from urinary retention
Incontinence	Involuntary loss of urine	Multiple factors: unstable urethra, loss of pelvic muscle tone, estrogen depletion, fecal impaction, neurological impairment
Hematuria	Blood in the urine	Neoplasms of the kidney or bladder, glomerular disease, infection of kidney or bladder, trauma to urinary structures, calculi, bleeding disorders
Retention	Accumulation of urine in the bladder, with inability of bladder to empty fully	Urethral obstruction, bladder inflammation, decreased sensory activity, neurogenic bladder, prostate enlargement, postanesthesia effects, side effects of medications (e.g., anticholinergics, antidepressants)
Residual urine	Volume of urine remaining after voiding (>100 ml)	Inflammation or irritation of bladder mucosa from infection, neurogenic bladder, prostate enlargement, trauma, or inflammation of urethra

hydration status. Urinary incontinence increases the risk of skin breakdown.

Kidneys.   If the kidneys become infected or inflamed, flank pain typically develops. The nurse can assess for flank tenderness early in the disease by percussing the costovertebral angle (the angle formed by the spine and the twelfth rib). Inflammation of the kidney results in pain during percussion. Auscultation is also performed to detect the presence of a renal artery bruit (sound resulting from turbulent blood flow through a narrowed artery).

Nurses with advanced examination skills learn to palpate the kidneys during abdominal examination. Their position, shape, and size can reveal problems such as tumors.

Bladder.   In adults the bladder rests below the symphysis pubis and cannot be examined by the nurse. When distended, the bladder rises above the symphysis pubis at the midline of the abdomen and may extend to just below the umbilicus. On inspection the nurse may note a swelling or convex curvature of the lower abdomen. The nurse lightly palpates the lower abdomen. The partially filled bladder normally feels smooth and rounded. As the nurse applies light pressure to the bladder, the client may feel tenderness or even pain. Even when the bladder is not visible palpation may cause the urge to urinate. Percussion of a full bladder yields a dull percussion note.

Urethral Meatus.   The nurse assesses the urinary meatus to note the presence of discharge, inflammation, and lesions. This assessment screens for infections and other abnormalities. To examine the female, a dorsal recumbent position provides full exposure of the genitalia. While wearing gloves, the nurse retracts the labial folds to see the urethral meatus. Normally the meatus is pink and appears as a small slitlike opening below the clitoris and above the vaginal orifice. There is normally no discharge from the meatus. If present, specimens of urethral discharge should be obtained before the client voids.

Women with vaginal infections are susceptible to UTIs because the vaginal discharge may travel easily to the urethral meatus. Older women commonly have vaginitis as a result of hormonal deficiencies. The nurse inspects the vaginal orifice carefully and describes any drainage. Infection may also be indicated by reddened, inflamed vaginal mucosa.

A man's urethral meatus is normally a small opening at the tip of the penis. The nurse inspects the meatus for discharge, inflammation, and lesions. It may be necessary to retract the foreskin in uncircumcised men to see the meatus.

Assessment of Urine.   Assessment of urine involves measuring the client's fluid intake and urine output and observing characteristics of the client's urine.

Intake and Output.   The nurse assesses the client's average daily fluid intake. If an accurate measurement of fluid intake is needed from the client who is at home, the nurse may ask the client to show a commonly used glass or cup on which the intake estimate is based.

In a health care setting the nurse measures a client's fluid intake either when the physician orders I&O measurements (see Chapter 40) or when nursing judgment warrants a more precise measurement. The nurse includes all sources, including oral intake, intravenous fluid infusions, tube feedings, and fluid instilled into nasogastric or gastric tubes.

Because it is often difficult for the client to estimate volumes of urine voided, the nurse must obtain measurements. A change in urine volume is a significant indicator of fluid alterations or kidney disease. While caring for the client, the nurse assesses volume by measuring (with plastic receptacles, bedpans, or urinals) urinary output with each voiding. Special receptacles (urimeters) attach between indwelling catheters and drainage bags and are a convenient means of accurately measuring urine volume. A urimeter holds 100 to 200 ml of urine. After measuring urine from a urimeter, the nurse can drain the cylinder into the urinary drainage bag or into a receptacle for disposal. Urimeters are indicated when precise hourly measurements of urine are needed.

When urine from a drainage bag is measured, it is best to use a separate plastic graduated measuring receptacle (Figure 44-6). Scales on the bags offer only an approximate volume. Each client should have a graduated receptacle for his or her exclusive use to prevent potential cross contamination.

The nurse reports any extreme increase or decrease in volume. An hourly output of less than 30 ml for more than 2 hours is cause for concern. Similarly, consistently high volumes of urine (polyuria), over 2000 to 2500 ml daily, should be reported to a physician.

Characteristics of Urine.   The nurse inspects the client's urine for color, clarity, and odor.

Color.   Normal urine ranges from a pale, straw color to amber, depending on its concentration. Urine is usually more concentrated in the morning or with fluid volume deficits. As the person drinks more fluids, urine becomes less concentrated.

Bleeding from the kidneys or ureters causes urine to become dark red; bleeding from the bladder or urethra causes a bright red urine. Various medications also change urine color. Eating beets, rhubarb, or blackberries may cause red urine. Special dyes used in intravenous diagnostic studies eventually discolor urine. Dark amber urine may be the result of high concentrations of bilirubin caused by liver dysfunction. The nurse documents and reports any abnormal color or sediment, especially if the cause is unknown.

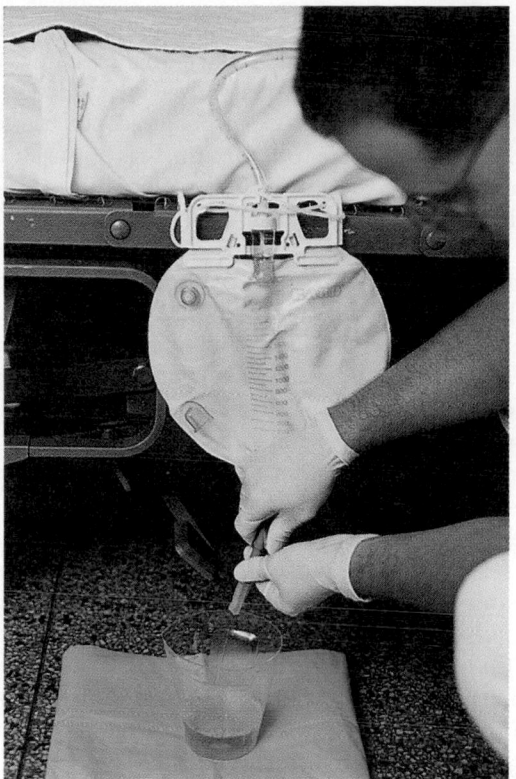

Figure 44-6   Urine drainage bag.

Clarity.   Normal urine appears transparent at voiding. Urine that stands several minutes in a container becomes cloudy. Freshly voided urine in clients with renal disease may appear cloudy or foamy because of high protein concentrations. Urine also appears thick and cloudy as a result of bacteria.

Odor.   Urine has a characteristic odor. The more concentrated the urine, the stronger the odor. Stagnant urine has an ammonia odor, which is common in clients who are repeatedly incontinent. A sweet or fruity odor occurs from acetone or acetoacetic acid (by-products of incomplete fat metabolism) seen with diabetes mellitus or starvation.

Urine Testing.   The nurse often collects urine specimens for laboratory testing. The type of test determines the method of collection. All specimens are labeled with the client's name, date, and time of collection. Specimens should be transported to the laboratory in a timely fashion to ensure accuracy of test results. Agency infection-control policies require the adherence to standard precautions by all personnel during specimen handling (see Chapter 33).

Specimen Collection.   The nurse collects random, clean-voided or midstream, sterile, and timed specimens.

Random Specimen.   A random routine urine specimen can be collected with a client voiding naturally or from a Foley catheter or urinary diversion collection bag. The specimen should be clean but need not be sterile. Random specimens are used for urinalysis testing or measurements of specific gravity, pH, or glucose levels.

The client voids into a clean urine cup, urinal, or bedpan. Many clients are able to do this independently. However, mobility restrictions or poor vision may require the nurse to assist. It is easier to collect a specimen if the client drinks a glass of fluid 30 minutes before the procedure. A client should void before defecating so that feces do not contaminate the specimen. Female clients are also instructed not to place toilet tissue in the bedpan. Only 120 ml (4 ounces) of urine is needed for accurate testing. After the specimen is collected the nurse places the lid tightly on the specimen container, washes off any urine that splashed on the outside of the container, places the container in a plastic bag, and sends the labeled specimen promptly to the laboratory.

Clean-Voided or Midstream Specimen.   To obtain a specimen relatively free of the microorganisms growing in the lower urethra, the nurse instructs the client on the method for obtaining a clean-voided specimen (Skill 44-1). This type of specimen is needed to test urine for culture and sensitivity. After appropriate cleansing of the external genitalia, a client begins the urinary stream, allowing the initial portion to escape; then during the middle portion of voiding, the client collects the specimen. The initial stream of urine cleans or flushes the urethral orifice and meatus of resident bacteria. It is easiest for a client to obtain clean-voided specimens while using toilet facilities.

Sterile Specimen.   Another method for collecting a urine specimen for culture is to obtain it from an indwelling catheter. It is no longer recommended to catheterize a client just to obtain a specimen because of the high risk of causing an infection. A urine specimen is also not collected for culture from a urine drainage bag unless it is the first urine drained into a new sterile bag. Bacteria grow rapidly in the drainage bags and could cause a false measurement.

For an indwelling retention catheter, the nurse uses a sterile syringe to withdraw urine. The nurse washes hands and applies nonsterile gloves to prevent transmission of microorganisms. A 3-ml syringe with a small-gauge needle (23- or 25-gauge) is best to prevent creation of a permanent hole in the catheter port. However, if blood is suspected in the urine, a large-bore needle prevents breakdown of RBCs during withdrawal of the specimen. Most urinary catheters have special ports to withdraw specimens (Figure 44-7). First, the nurse clamps the tubing just below the site chosen for withdrawal, allowing fresh, uncontaminated urine to collect in the tube. The nurse then wipes the catheter or port with an antimicrobial swab. Inserting the needle at a 30-degree angle ensures entrance into the catheter lumen.

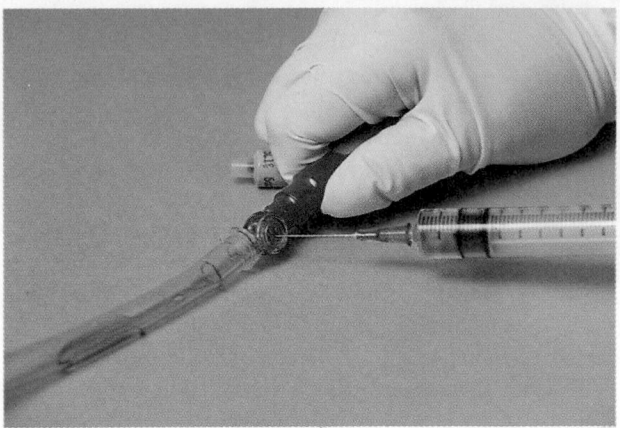

Figure 44-7   Urine specimen collection: aspiration from a collection port in drainage tubing of an indwelling catheter.

While aspirating 3 to 5 ml of urine the nurse must be careful not to raise the tubing, which would cause urine to flow back into the bladder.

After obtaining the specimen the nurse transfers the urine into a sterile container using sterile aseptic technique (see Chapter 33). The nurse removes the gloves, properly disposes of equipment, and washes hands to reduce the transfer of microorganisms to other clients and health care workers. The laboratory requisition should indicate the method of collection.

Timed Urine Specimens.   Some tests of renal function and urine composition, such as measuring levels of adrenocortical steroids or hormones, creatinine clearance, or protein quantitation tests, require collection of urine over 2-, 12-, or 24-hour intervals.

The timed collection period begins after the client urinates. The nurse discards the sample and indicates the starting time on the collection container and on the laboratory requisition (check agency policy). The client then collects all urine voided in the timed period.

Each voiding is collected in a clean container and immediately emptied into the larger container. Some tests require the client to void at specific times. Each specimen must be free of feces or toilet tissue.

Any missed specimens will make test results inaccurate. The nurse should remind the client to void before defecating so that urine is not contaminated by feces. The collection container may contain a preservative or require refrigeration. The laboratory should be consulted for instructions. The client should void the last specimen at the end of the timed period.

Urine Collection in Children.   Specimen collection from infants and children is often difficult. Adolescents and school-age children are usually able to cooperate, although they may be embarrassed. Preschool children and toddlers have difficulty voiding on request. Offering a young child fluids 30 minutes before requesting a specimen may help.

Collecting Midstream (Clean-Voided) Urine Specimen | Skill 44-1

Delegation Considerations

Selected specimen collections may be delegated to assistive personnel. If appropriate, an alert client who is physically able may be instructed to collect the specimen. Be aware of agency policy regarding specimen collection.

EQUIPMENT

- Soap or cleansing solution, washcloth, and towel
- Commercial kit for clean-voided specimen or individual supplies as listed
  - Sterile cotton balls or sterile 2 × 2 or 4 × 4 gauze pads
  - Antiseptic solution (e.g., providone-iodine); check for client allergy, if allergic provide an alternative
  - Sterile water
- Sterile specimen collection cup or jar
- Sterile and nonsterile gloves
- Bedpan, bedside commode, or specimen hat
- Completed specimen label

STEPS	RATIONALE
1. Assess status of client.	
a. When client last voided	May indicate bladder fullness.
b. Level of awareness or developmental stage	Reveals client's ability to cooperate during procedure.
c. Mobility, balance, and physical limitations	Determines level of assistance.
2. Assess client's understanding of purpose of test and method of collection.	Information allows you to clarify misunderstandings and promotes client cooperation.
3. Explain procedure to client:	
a. Reason midstream specimen is needed	Helps client understand the procedure.
b. Ways client and family can assist	
c. Ways to obtain specimen free of feces	Feces change characteristics of urine and may cause abnormal values.
4. Provide fluids to drink 1/2 hour before collection unless contraindicated (i.e., fluid restriction) if client does not feel urge to void.	Improves likelihood of client being able to void.
5. Provide privacy for client by closing door or bed curtain.	Privacy allows client to relax and produce specimen more quickly.
6. Give client or family members soap, washcloth, and towel to cleanse perineal area.	Client may prefer to wash own perineal area.
7. Apply nonsterile gloves and assist nonambulatory clients with perineal care. Assist female client onto bedpan.	Prevents transmission of microorganisms to nurse, provides easy access to perineal area to collect specimen.
8. Change gloves if necessary.	Reduces transfer of infection.

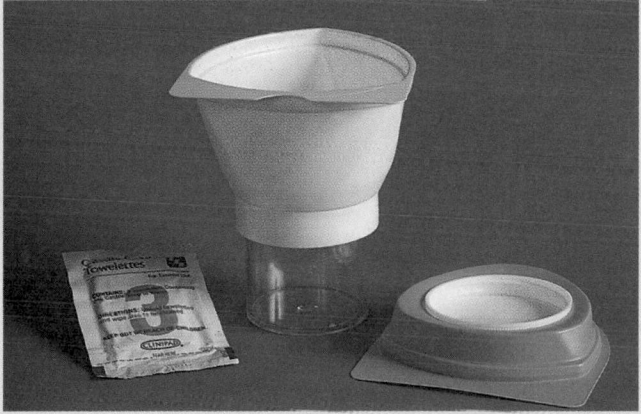

Step 9

STEPS	RATIONALE
9. Using surgical asepsis, open sterile kit (see illustration) or prepare sterile supplies. Apply sterile gloves after opening sterile specimen cup, placing cap with sterile inside surface up, and do not touch inside of container or cap (see Chapter 33).	Sterile technique is essential to maintain sterility of equipment and specimen. Sterile gloves prevent the transmission of microorganisms to the specimen from the nurse or from the client to the nurse. Contaminated specimen is most frequent reason for inaccurate reporting of urine cultures and sensitivities.
10. Pour antiseptic solution over cotton balls or gauze pads unless kit contains prepared gauze pads in antiseptic solution.	Cotton balls or gauze pads will be used to further cleanse the perineum.
11. Assist or allow client to independently cleanse perineum and collect specimen:	
A. **Female**	
(1) Spread labia with thumb and forefinger of non-dominant hand.	Provides access to urethral meatus.
(2) Cleanse area with cotton ball or gauze, moving from front (above urethral orifice) to back (towards anus) (see illustration).	Cleanse from area of least contamination to area of greatest contamination to decrease bacterial levels.
(3) If agency policy indicates, rinse area with sterile water, and dry with dry cotton ball or gauze.	Prevents contamination of specimen with antiseptic solution.
(4) While continuing to hold labia apart, client should initiate stream and after stream is achieved, pass container into stream and collect 30 to 60 ml (see illustration).	Initial stream flushes out microorganisms that accumulate at urethral meatus and prevents transfer into specimen.
B. **Male**	
(1) Hold penis with one hand and using circular motion and antiseptic swab, cleanse end of penis, moving from center to outside (see illustration). In uncircumscribed men, the foreskin should be retracted prior to cleansing.	Cleanse from area of least contamination to area of greatest contamination to decrease bacterial levels.

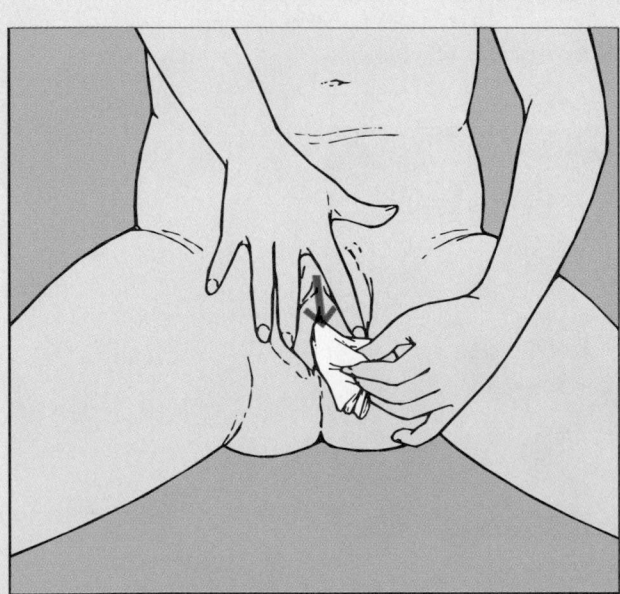

Step 11A(2)

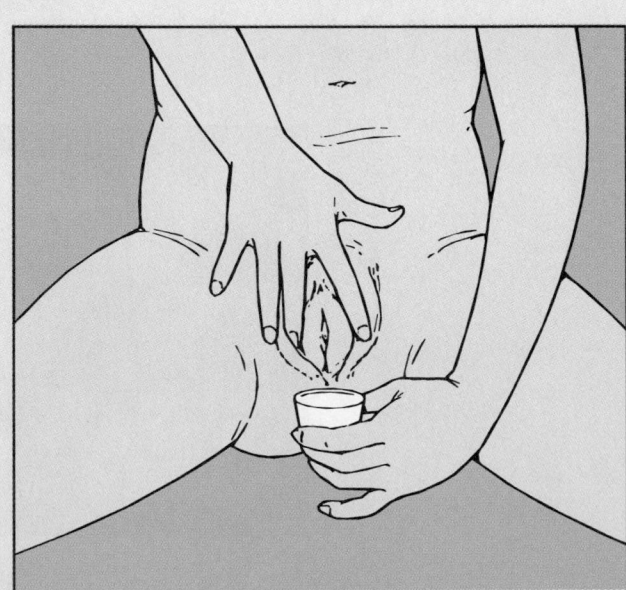

Step 11A(4)

STEPS	RATIONALE
(2) If agency procedure indicates, rinse area with sterile water, and dry with cotton or gauze.	Prevents contamination of specimen with antiseptic solution.
(3) After client has initiated urine stream, pass specimen collection container into stream, and collect 30 to 60 ml (see illustration).	Initial stream flushes out microorganisms that accumulate at urethral meatus and prevents transfer into specimen.
12. Remove specimen container before flow of urine stops and before releasing labia or penis. Client finishes voiding in bedpan or toilet. If foreskin was retracted for specimen collection, it must be replaced over the glans.	Prevents contamination of specimen with skin flora. If foreskin not replaced, swelling and constriction may occur, causing pain and possible obstruction to urine flow.
13. Replace cap securely on specimen container (touch outside only).	Retains sterility of inside of container and prevents spillage of urine.
14. Cleanse any urine from exterior surface of container, and place in a plastic specimen bag.	Prevents transfer of microorganisms to others.
15. Remove bedpan (if applicable), and assist client to comfortable position.	Promotes relaxing environment.
16. Label specimen, and attach laboratory requisition.	Prevents inaccurate identification that could lead to errors in diagnosis or treatment.

Critical Decision Point: If client is menstruating, indicate information on laboratory requisition.

---

17. Remove gloves, dispose in proper receptacle, and wash hands.	Reduces transmission of infection.
18. Transport specimen to laboratory within 15 minutes or refrigerate immediately.	Bacteria grow quickly in urine, and specimen should be analyzed immediately to obtain correct results.

Recording and Reporting

- Record date and time urine specimen was obtained, and place information in nurses' notes.

Home Care Considerations

- If client is to collect specimen as outpatient, proper instruction for collection needs to be given.
- Appropriate equipment will need to be given to client and family.
- Information on storing specimen until time for delivery to doctor's office or hospital laboratory needs to be given.

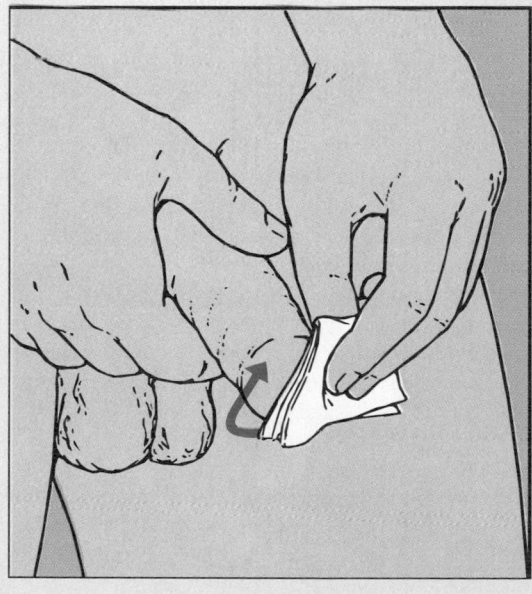

Step 11B(1)

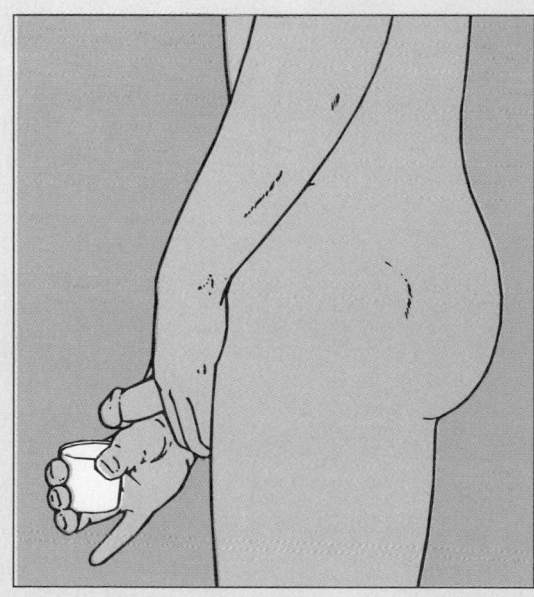

Step 11B(3)

The nurse must use terms for urination that the child can understand. A young child may be reluctant to void in unfamiliar receptacles. A potty chair or specimen hat placed under the toilet seat is usually effective. The nurse must use special collection devices for infants or toddlers who are not toilet trained. Clear plastic, single-use bags with self-adhering material can be attached over the child's urethral meatus. Specimens should not be obtained by squeezing urine from the diaper material.

Common Urine Tests.   Urine tests include **urinalysis,** specific gravity, and urine culture.

Urinalysis.   The laboratory performs a urinalysis on a specimen obtained by any of the previously described methods. Table 44-3 lists normal values for a urinalysis. The specimen should be examined as soon as possible, preferably within 2 hours. It should be the first voided specimen in the morning to ensure a uniform concentration of constituents. For a quick screening the nurse can perform certain portions of the urinalysis with special reagent strips. The nurse dips the strips into the urine and then observes for a color change in the time interval designated on the package (Figure 44-8).

Specific Gravity.   The **specific gravity** is the weight or degree of concentration of a substance compared with an equal volume of water. To measure specific gravity a urinometer and cylinder are used. The urinometer has a specific gravity scale at the top and a weighted mercury bulb at the bottom. A urine specimen is poured into a special clean, dry cylinder. The weighted urinometer is suspended in the cylinder of urine. The concentration of dissolved substances in the urine aids in determination of a client's fluid balance. This measurement is always done as part of a complete urinalysis. The nurse in a critical care unit may be responsible for doing periodic measurement of specific gravity of urine as part of complete client assessment.

The specific gravity of a morning urine specimen voided by a fasting client reflects the kidney's maximum concentrating ability. A specific gravity below 1.010 reflects an inability of the kidneys to concentrate urine or an insufficient secretion of ADH. An elevated specific gravity can indicate dehydration. Radiopaque substances or high molecular weight substances in the urine (e.g., protein or glucose) may cause a falsely high specific gravity.

If questions regarding the accuracy of specific gravity measurements arise, a urine osmolality test should be obtained. Although both tests measure urine concentration, the osmolality test is more accurate because it measures the total number of particles in a solution (see Chapter 40).

Urine Culture.   A urine culture requires a sterile or clean-voided sample of urine. It takes approximately 48 hours before the laboratory can report findings of bacterial growth. While awaiting results, a broad spectrum antibiotic may be ordered as soon as a culture has been ob-

Table 44-3 **Routine Urinalysis**	
Measurement and Normal Value	Interpretation
pH (4.6-8.0) average 6.0	pH helps indicate acid-base balance. Urine that stands for several hours becomes alkaline. An acid pH helps protect against bacterial growth.
Protein (none or up to 8 mg/100 ml)	Normally protein is not present in urine. It is seen in renal disease because damage to glomeruli or tubules allow protein to enter urine.
Glucose (none)	Diabetic clients have glucose in urine as a result of inability of tubules to reabsorb high glucose concentrations (>180 mg/100 ml). Ingestion of high concentrations of glucose may cause some glucose to appear in urine of healthy persons.
Ketones (none)	Clients whose diabetes mellitus is poorly controlled experience breakdown of fatty acids. End products of fat metabolism are ketones. Clients with dehydration, starvation, or excessive aspirin usage also may have **ketonuria.**
Blood (up to 2 RBCs)	Damage to glomeruli or tubules may allow RBCs to enter the urine. Trauma, disease, or surgery of the lower urinary tract also may cause blood to be present. In women, blood in a routine urine specimen may be contaminated with menstrual fluid.
Specific gravity (1.010-1.025)	Specific gravity measures concentration of particles in urine. High specific gravity reflects concentrated urine, and low specific gravity reflects diluted urine. Dehydration, reduced renal blood flow, and increased ADH secretion elevate specific gravity. Overhydration, early renal disease, and inadequate ADH secretion reduce specific gravity.
Microscopic Examination	
WBCs (0 to 4 per low-power field)	Greater numbers may indicate urinary tract infection.
Bacteria (none)	Bacteria indicate urinary tract infection. (Client may or may not have symptoms.)
Casts (none)	Casts are cylindrical bodies whose shapes take on likeness of objects within the renal tubule. Types include hyaline, WBCs, RBCs, granular cells, and epithelial cells. Their presence is always an abnormal finding and indicates renal alterations.

Modified from Pagana KD, Pagana TJ: *Mosby's diagnostic and laboratory test reference,* ed 4, St. Louis, 1999, Mosby.

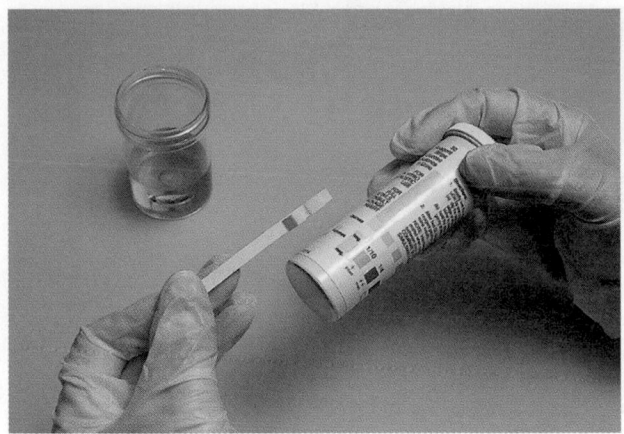

Figure 44-8   Checking results of a chemical reagent strip dipped in urine.

tained. The test for sensitivity determines which specific antibiotics are effective. The results (sensitivities) of a urine culture may indicate a change in choice of medication.

Diagnostic Examinations.   The urinary system is one of the few organ systems amenable to accurate diagnostic study by several radiographic techniques. The two approaches for visualization of urinary structures, direct and indirect techniques, can be quite simple or very complex, requiring extensive nursing intervention. These procedures are further subdivided into invasive or noninvasive categories.

Noninvasive Procedures

Abdominal Roentgenogram.   Abdominal roentgenogram, also referred to as plain film, KUB, or flat plate, of the abdomen is commonly used to assess the gross structures of the urinary tract for abnormalities. It can determine size, symmetry, shape, and location of the kidneys, ureters, and bladder structures. It is also useful in visualizing calculi (if calcified) or tumors in these organs. In addition, the ribs or other surrounding support structures can be assessed for fractures or abnormalities. Lack of positive findings on the roentgenogram does not rule out the possibility of abnormalities in the urinary tract. Additional diagnostic studies may be needed.

The nursing implications for clients undergoing this procedure include explanation of the procedure and alleviation of client anxiety. No special bowel preparation is needed unless the physician chooses otherwise.

Intravenous Pyelogram.   To view the entire urinary system, the physician orders the excretory urogram or intravenous pyelogram (IVP). This procedure visualizes the collecting ducts and renal pelvis and outlines the ureters, bladder, and urethra. Although this procedure is noninvasive, it requires the client to receive an intravenous injec-

tion of a radiopaque dye. Because the kidneys and ureters lie behind the intestines, it is necessary that the client receive a bowel preparation to empty the intestines before the procedure.

During the IVP, x-ray studies are taken at specific intervals over 30 to 60 minutes as the dye concentrates. The client may also be asked to void during the procedure to measure bladder emptying. Diseases or disorders of the urinary tract that should be investigated by this means include renal artery occlusion, tumors, cysts or calculi, vesicoureteral reflux, and traumatic injuries.

Nursing implications before the test include recognizing clients at risk for alterations in renal function as a result of the intravenous injection of the contrast dye. Any client with renal insufficiency is at risk. Older clients are prone to the nephrotoxic effects of contrast dye because of the fluid loss during bowel preparation. Nursing assessment of volume status and its maintenance before this procedure is of utmost importance (see Chapter 40). Additional nursing implications follow:

Obtain signed informed consent (if agency policy).

Assess client for history of shellfish (iodine) allergy, which predicts allergies to the IVP dye.

Administer cathartic on evening before test.

Ensure that client follows the appropriate intake restriction prior to the test. (May be nothing by mouth [NPO] after midnight or clear liquids only after a clear liquid supper.)

Explain that facial flushing is normal during dye injection and that client may feel dizzy or warm.

Explain that an intravenous infusion for dye injection is started before the test.

Explain that the test involves x-ray studies taken at several intervals and that client will void near the end of the test.

Not all agencies employ nurses in the radiology department. If a nurse is not present, the physician or radiology technician assumes these responsibilities. Implications during the test include the following:

Assess intravenous site for signs of infiltration of dye into tissues (e.g., swelling, redness, and pain).

Observe for signs of allergic reaction to dye (e.g., respiratory distress, fall in blood pressure, and hives).

Remind client of normal sensations caused by dye injection.

Nursing implications after the test include the following:

Ensure that client receives usual diet afterward.

Encourage fluid intake to minimize dehydration caused by bowel prep and to avoid the potential nephrotoxic effects of the contrast material.

Monitor I&O and promptly report alterations to physician.

Observe for possible delayed allergic reactions.

Renal Scan.   Radionuclide tests such as renal scans allow indirect visualization of urinary tract structures after an intravenous injection of radioactive isotopes. The emissions from the radionuclides can be photographed by special cameras. The isotope can be detected without the need of bowel preparation. A very low dose of radioisotope is used. No precautions against radioactive exposure are needed except for the use of disposable gloves if the client uses a bedpan or urinal to void. Rinse bedpan or urinal and double flush urine down the toilet to dilute any possible remaining radiation hazard.

After a radionuclide is injected, it circulates through the kidneys and is excreted. The renal scan measures radioactive concentrations. Except for the venipuncture, it is painless. The scanning procedure is completed in about 1 hour. Information pertaining to renal blood flow, anatomical structures, and their excretory function can be obtained from this procedure. The physician can diagnose abnormalities such as renal artery occlusion, urinary obstruction, and many other diseases of the kidney. This procedure is indicated for clients unable to receive IVP dyes. The nurse does not routinely give a sedative before the test unless the physician views the client as highly anxious. Nursing implications before the test include the following:

    Obtain signed informed consent (if agency policy).

    Explain that radioisotope is injected intravenously through an existing IV line or needle.

    Explain that the machine measuring the isotope uptake is similar to a Geiger counter.

    Explain that client will feel no discomfort but must lie still.

    Explain that there is no risk of radioactive exposure.

Nursing implications during the test include the following:

    Assist the client in changing positions during the test. (Technician may do this.)

No specific nursing implications after the test.

Computerized Axial Tomography.   Computerized tomography (CT) is a computerized x-ray procedure used to obtain detailed images of structures within a selected plane of the body. The tomographic scanner is a large machine that contains specialized computers and x-ray detector systems that function simultaneously to photograph internal structures in thin, transverse cross sections (Figure 44-9). The computer, through a series of complex manipulations, is able to "reconstruct" the cross-sectional image as a recognizable photograph on the television monitor. With this procedure it is possible to visualize abnormal pathological conditions such as tumors, obstructions, retroperitoneal masses, and lymph node enlargement. Although this procedure is noninvasive, in some examinations oral or intravenous contrast material is used to enhance the areas under study. If intravenous contrast is used, it may be necessary to administer a bowel cleansing solution orally (such as GoLYTELY) or an enema, especially if additional organs in the abdominal cavity will be examined. The nursing implications before, during, and after this test are the same as those listed under the

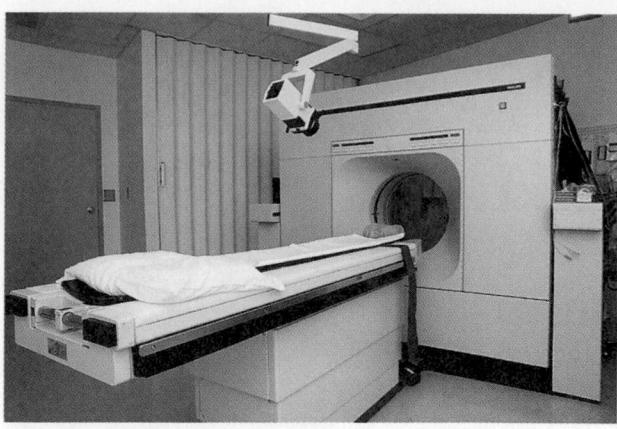

Figure 44-9   CT equipment.
From Brundage DJ: *Renal disorders,* St. Louis, 1992, Mosby.

IVP examination. However, the nurse explains that the client will be placed in a large machine, which may cause feelings of claustrophobia in susceptible individuals.

Renal Ultrasound.   Ultrasonography is a valuable noninvasive diagnostic tool in the assessment of urinary disorders. It makes use of high-frequency, inaudible sound waves that reflect off tissue structures. Some of the sound waves are reflected back to the transducer as echoes. The velocity of the sound waves varies with tissue density. The client is usually prone during the procedure but can be positioned in a sitting position. Ultrasound is frequently used to identify gross renal structures and structural abnormalities of the kidneys or lower urinary tract and to assist with percutaneous biopsy. Abnormalities such as tumors or cysts in the kidney are easily identified. If a Doppler is used with the transducer, examination of blood flow through the kidney can also be performed. This procedure is painless.

Nursing implications before the procedure involve explanation of the test and possibly encouraging the client to ingest oral fluids to cause bladder distention. No specific client care is indicated after the test.

Invasive Procedures

Endoscopy.   Endoscopy is the visualization of a hollow body organ with the aid of a fiber-optic instrument. A cystoscopy allows the physician to view the interior of the bladder and urethra. The cystoscope looks much like a urinary catheter, although it is not as flexible and is generally larger. It is inserted through the client's urethra. The instrument has an outer plastic or rubber sheath, an obturator that keeps the scope rigid during insertion, a telescope for viewing the bladder and urethra, and a channel for inserting catheters or special surgical instruments.

The procedure is painful during instrument insertion. There is risk of bladder perforation if the client is not relaxed and cooperative. Local, spinal, or general anesthesia may be given. Because the test requires insertion of a foreign object into a sterile cavity, the client receives large amounts of fluids (intravenously or orally) before and during the procedure to maintain a continuous urine flow and to flush out any bacteria. Antibiotics may also be administered intravenously. During the test, urine and tissue specimens may be collected.

Special cystoscopy tables minimize the stress and fatigue that clients may experience from maintaining one position for a prolonged time. Nursing implications before the test include the following:

Obtain signed informed consent.

Perform a bowel preparation or enema or administer a cathartic on the evening before the test if ordered.

If local anesthetic will be used, encourage intake of oral fluids.

If general anesthetic is to be used, instruct client to take nothing by mouth after midnight.

Explain that insertion of the cystoscope is similar to insertion of urethral catheter.

Explain the importance of lying still during the test.

Explain that an intravenous line will be started to give fluids during the test.

Administer a sedative and analgesic per the physician's orders.

Nursing implications during the test include the following:

Assist client to assume a lithotomy position.

Prepare perineal area with antiseptic solution.

Explain (if client is awake) that insertion of cystoscope causes an urge to void.

Remind client to lie still if awake.

Nursing implications after the test include the following:

Instruct the client to remain in bed as ordered.

Assess for signs of possible urinary retention and time of first voiding.

Observe volume and characteristics of urine, including bloody or cloudy urine for each voiding.

Encourage increased fluid intake and monitor I&O.

Observe for fever, dysuria, or change in blood pressure.

Administer medications to alleviate bladder spasms and/or low back pain.

Angiography (Arteriogram).

A renal angiogram is an invasive radiographical procedure that evaluates the renal arterial system. The arteriogram is most often used to examine the main renal artery or its branches to detect any narrowing or occlusion. In addition, this procedure evaluates masses (e.g., neoplasms or cysts) to determine changes in blood flow. The arteriogram is performed by placing a catheter into one of the femoral arteries and advancing it to the level of the renal arteries. Radiopaque contrast material is injected through the catheter while x-ray images are taken in rapid succession.

Nursing implications before the test include the following:

Obtain signed informed consent.

Assess for iodine allergy, which predicts allergy to the dye used in angiograms.

Ensure client takes nothing by mouth after midnight.

Explain that facial flushing is normal during dye injection and that client may feel dizzy or warm.

Explain that the test involves x-ray studies to be taken at several intervals after the dye is injected.

Nursing implications after an arteriogram include the following:

Monitor vital signs hourly until client is stable, and then advance intervals to every 2 hours and 4 hours, respectively.

Ensure that the client maintains bed rest for 8 to 12 hours.

Check pulse, assess the circulation in the cannulated extremity, and ensure that the extremity is kept in straight alignment.

Observe for bleeding, increased tenderness, and hematoma formation at the catheter insertion site for 24 hours.

Maintain a pressure dressing over the site for 24 hours (check agency policy).

Observe client for possible delayed reactions to the contrast material.

Monitor the client's I&O and report abnormalities in urine volume to the physician. Fluids are usually increased either intravenously or by mouth after the test to help flush the dye and minimize the nephrotoxic effects of the dye.

Urodynamic Testing.

A variety of studies may be done to measure the transport, storage, and elimination of urine in the lower urinary tract. Cystometrogram (CMG) is one such test that determines the level of function of the detrusor muscle. This test is used to rule out causes of incontinence. A catheter is inserted, residual volume is measured and discarded, and the bladder is filled with either sterile saline or carbon dioxide gas in predetermined increments. Pressure readings are taken at those increments. During the filling time the client's perceptions related to bladder fullness, urge to void, and the ability to inhibit voiding are documented.

Nursing implications before the test involve explanation of the procedure and the need to report sensations as they occur. After the test is completed the client should be instructed to report the following sensations: sweating, pain, nausea, bladder fullness, or a strong urge to void.

Client Expectations.

Clients are dependent on their caregivers to recognize and meet their needs. Nurses need to use a skilled and caring approach, to be creative in using a variety of assessment techniques, and to serve as a client advocate. A caring nurse will be creative in meeting the client's needs in a way that is acceptable and individualized for the client and family situation. The client having needs related to urinary function expects that the nurse will be respectful of privacy needs and sensitive to the impact of urinary impairments on sexuality and self-concept. The nurse should always include the client in the plan of care and develop goals that are mutually acceptable. Cultural practices and personal preferences should also be considered. Clients expect that assistance from the nurse will be prompt. Once children and adults have achieved continence, urinary incontinence is often a source of embarrassment and shame.

NURSING DIAGNOSIS

A thorough assessment of the client's urinary elimination function reveals patterns of data that allow the nurse to make relevant and accurate nursing diagnoses. The nurse thinks critically by reflecting on knowledge of previous clients, the influence of urinary elimination alterations on such areas as self-concept and sexuality, reviewing defining characteristics identified, applying knowledge of urinary function, and then making a specific diagnosis. The diagnosis may be an actual problem or a problem that the client is at risk of developing (Box 44-6).

The diagnosis may focus on a specific urinary elimination alteration or associated problems such as *impaired*

skin integrity related to urinary incontinence. Identification of defining characteristics leads the nurse to select an appropriate diagnosis (Box 44-7). Specifying related factors for each diagnosis allows selection of individualized nursing interventions (Ackley, 1997). For the nursing diagnosis of *stress incontinence* the nursing interventions are primarily long term as time will be needed to strengthen the pelvic floor muscles. In contrast, a nursing diagnosis of *urinary retention* will need different interventions. For the client with permanent neurological impairment such as multiple sclerosis the nurse needs to plan for alternative methods of bladder emptying such as long-term catheter placement. The client with urinary retention with overflow related to anesthesia probably has no need of any intervention after a single catheter insertion empties the bladder. Full recovery from the anesthesia eliminates the problem.

PLANNING

During planning the nurse again synthesizes information from multiple resources (Figure 44-10). Critical thinking ensures that the client's plan of care integrates all that the nurse knows about the individual as well as key critical thinking elements. Professional standards are especially important to consider when the nurse develops a plan of care. These standards often establish scientifically proven guidelines for selecting effective nursing interventions.

The nurse develops an individualized plan of care for each nursing diagnosis (see care plan). The nurse and the client set realistic expectations for care. Goals are to be individualized and realistic with measurable outcomes.

The plan incorporates health promotion activities and therapeutic interventions for clients with urinary elimination problems. Preventive interventions may be required for clients at risk for urinary problems. The nurse also plans therapies according to the severity of risks to the client. It is important in the nursing process to consider the client's home environment and normal elimination

---

NURSING DIAGNOSES   Box 44-6

URINARY ELIMINATION

Body image disturbance
Incontinence, stress
Incontinence, urge
Incontinence, urinary, functional
Pain
Self-care deficit, toileting
Skin integrity, impaired
Urinary elimination, altered
Urinary retention

SAMPLE NURSING DIAGNOSTIC PROCESS   Box 44-7

STRESS INCONTINENCE

Assessment Activities	Defining Characteristics	Nursing Diagnosis
Have client describe situations that accompany urine leakage (Skoner, Thompson, and Caron, 1994).	Client states that she "loses a little urine" whenever she sneezes, coughs, or laughs. Client states she has been having problems for the past year.	Stress incontinence related to decreased pelvic muscle tone and urethral sphincter trauma
Observe client behavior.	Client is wearing a menstrual minipad continuously. Client is reluctant to interact with others and tries not to cough or laugh.	
Review medical history.	Client is postmenopausal after three vaginal births.	

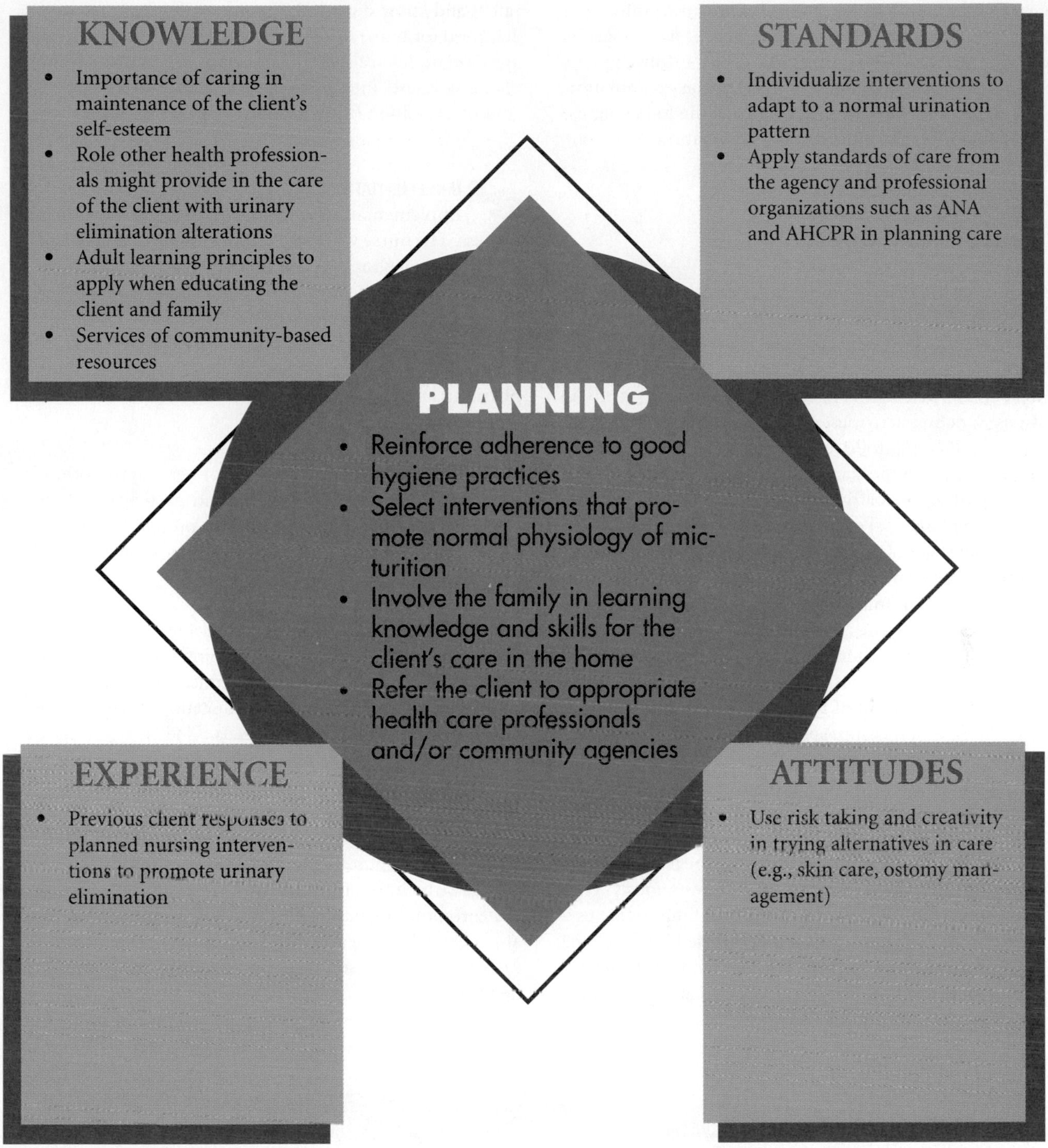

KNOWLEDGE

- Importance of caring in maintenance of the client's self-esteem
- Role other health professionals might provide in the care of the client with urinary elimination alterations
- Adult learning principles to apply when educating the client and family
- Services of community-based resources

STANDARDS

- Individualize interventions to adapt to a normal urination pattern
- Apply standards of care from the agency and professional organizations such as ANA and AHCPR in planning care

PLANNING

- Reinforce adherence to good hygiene practices
- Select interventions that promote normal physiology of micturition
- Involve the family in learning knowledge and skills for the client's care in the home
- Refer the client to appropriate health care professionals and/or community agencies

EXPERIENCE

- Previous client responses to planned nursing interventions to promote urinary elimination

ATTITUDES

- Use risk taking and creativity in trying alternatives in care (e.g., skin care, ostomy management)

Figure 44-10   *Synthesis Model for Urinary Elimination Planning Phase.*

routines when planning therapies. In planning the care for some clients, consultation with other health care professionals may be needed. For example, the physical therapist can design an exercise plan to increase strength and endurance so the client will be able to ambulate to the bathroom. Reinforcement of good health habits that are already followed improves compliance with the care plan.

The alert client with actual or risks for alterations in urinary elimination learns to recognize signs of change and may be able to prevent serious problems. Alterations in urinary elimination pose a high risk to a client's overall state of health.

Planning care also involves an understanding of the client's need to control body function. Alterations in urinary elimination can be embarrassing, uncomfortable, and often frustrating. The nurse and client work together to establish ways of maintaining client involvement in nursing care and to maintain normal urinary elimination. General goals for the client may include the following:

Understanding normal urinary elimination
Promoting normal micturition
Achieving complete bladder emptying
Preventing infection
Maintaining skin integrity
Gaining a sense of comfort

When delegating care to nurse aides or other patient care personnel it is important for the nurse to assure that the client's needs for safety, privacy, and dignity are met. Assistive caregivers need to be aware of medical asepsis when giving personal care and when assisting clients in urinary function activities. Attention to appropriate communication during toileting of the client may need to be stressed to protect the client's dignity, and simple measures such as closing the bathroom door or pulling the curtain during use of a urinal or bedpan will protect privacy.

Associated problems such as anxiety may require interventions that often have no direct effect on urinary elimination. Unless the nurse intervenes, however, associated problems are likely to continue. Problems involved with urinary elimination alterations are often interrelated and complex. The nurse must also anticipate problems that may develop as a result of therapy. For example, diagnosis of *risk for infection* is appropriate when a client has an indwelling catheter.

For hospitalized clients, planning should include preparations for discharge (Figure 44-11). The nurse determines any assistive devices that will be required and the client's educational needs. Teaching throughout the hospital stay is important. Teaching for self-care is continuously reinforced, and return demonstrations of important psychomotor and self-care skills are performed by the client. For example, a client being discharged with an indwelling catheter will need to perform catheter care, understand ways to empty the drainage bag safely, measure urine accu-

rately, and know signs and symptoms of urinary infection. The need for home health services should be explored, and appropriate referrals should be made. The nurse's role in planning these interventions will result in the client's smooth transition from health care agency to home.

IMPLEMENTATION

Implementation is the action phase of the nursing process. The nurse will carry out the independent and collaborative behaviors needed to assist the client in achieving the desired outcomes and goals. The independent activities are those in which nurses use their own judgment. An example of this is teaching self-care activities to the client. Collaborative activities are those prescribed by the physician and carried out by the nurse, such as medication administration.

Health Promotion. The focus of health promotion is to assist the client to understand and participate in self-care practices that will preserve and protect healthy urinary system function. This focus can be achieved using several means.

Client Education. Success of therapies aimed at eliminating or minimizing urinary elimination problems depends in part on successful client education. Box 44-8 describes an example of nursing education related to one area of urinary elimination needs. The nurse instructs clients on their specific elimination problems. For example, clients who practice poor hygiene benefit from learning about normal sterility of the urinary tract and ways to prevent infection. It may also be useful to discuss the basic mechanism for urine production and voiding for clients with elimination alterations. Knowledge of factors that promote normal urine production and voiding can also help. Clients learn the significance of symptoms of urinary alterations so that early preventive health care can be initiated.

The nurse can easily incorporate teaching when giving

Client Teaching FOR URINARY ELIMINATION PROBLEMS RELATED TO SPHINCTER DYSFUNCTION   Box 44-8

OBJECTIVES
• Client will achieve continence through increased sphincter control.

TEACHING STRATEGIES (UIGP, 1996)
• Have client attempt to tighten urinary sphincter during urination to feel the sensations associated with urinary sphincter contraction.
• Teach client progressive use of pelvic floor exercises (PFEs).
  • Provide written instructions.
  • Have client sit or stand without tensing muscles of legs, buttocks, or abdomen.

• Have client contract and relax circumvaginal muscles and urinary and anal sphincters for 3 to 4 seconds and repeat in quick succession.
• Have client repeat these cycles for 25 to 30 times 3 times a day for 6 months.
• Teach and monitor use of a voiding record.

EVALUATION
• Monitor voiding record to identify changes in patterns of urinary elimination.
• Ask client to tell you of the degree of satisfaction related to control achieved in urinary elimination.

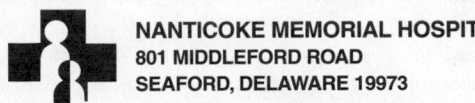

This product has been developed and licensed in association with The Center for Case Management, Inc. and is considered a CareMap® tool. For more information re: licensure, contact The Center at (508) 651-2600. CareMap® tools and systems provide guidance in case management and coordinated care for a specified patient population. Using CareMap® tools and systems in actual practice demands consideration of the individual patient care needs and discretionary clinical judgment.

NANTICOKE MEMORIAL HOSPITAL
801 MIDDLEFORD ROAD
SEAFORD, DELAWARE 19973

adapted from CareMap with permission
of The Center for Case Management,
South Natick, MA

UTI WITH SYSTEMIC INVOLVEMENT (PYELONEPHRITIS)

DRG 320   LOS 5 DAYS

Admit Date: _____

Discharge Date: _____

Pathway	Day 1		Day 2	Day 3-4	Day 5
Critical Path Implemented (initial):					
Diagnostic Studies	•CBC •UA, Urine C&S •Chem 7 •CXR •Blood Culture x____	•Consider: KUB/ABD Xray if flank pain present	•Consider: •CBC •Lytes	Consider: •CBC •Lytes •Repeat Blood Culture If pain and fever persist past 72 Hrs of therapy Consider: Ultrasound or CT to R/O urological pathology, otherwise D/C	•Repeat urine culture 2 weeks p therapy as O.P.
Treatments	•Strain all urine if flank pain present				
IV/Meds	•IV____@____cc/hr •Antibiotics •Analgesic/Antipyretic •Antiemetic			•Transition to p.o. meds if afebrile X48H•Heplock IV	
Consults	•Social Services if ind				
Nursing	•Physical assessment Q Shift/PRN, esp fluid volume parameters (turgor, lytes, I&O, mucous membranes) •VS Q2HX6H, then Q4HX24H, then Q8H, monitor temp & notify physician of spike >____° •I&O Q4H X 24H, then Q shift, notify MD of UO <600cc/24H, adm weight •Skin care, assist with ADL's, daily re-evaluation of skin risk assessment with appropriate interventions, obtain skin care evaluation if indicated •Collaborate with pt on pain management, use 1-5 pain scale •Provide emotional support to pt/family to help reduce anxiety				
Diet	•Clear liquids, advance as tolerated				
Activity & Safety	•OOB as tolerated •Routine safety measures		•OOB as tolerated	•Consider discharge if stable	•Discharge
Teaching Patient & Family	•Teach 1-5 pain scale •Orient to environment •Explain tests/procedures to pt/family •Explain diet, meds, activity		•Explain relationship between disease process, resulting symptoms & therapy prescribed •Implement UTI teaching plan •Implement related procedural teaching plans		
Discharge Planning	•Initial assessment •Advance Directives reviewed •Assess educational needs		•Facilitate phys/RN/family conference for discharge planning & medical follow up		

new 11/94

Figure 44-11 CareMap® for urinary tract infections.
Courtesy Nanticoke Memorial Hospital, Seaford, Del, and the Center for Case Management, South Natick, Mass.

SAMPLE NURSING CARE PLAN
FUNCTIONAL INCONTINENCE

ASSESSMENT*

When Judi was home from college on break she went to visit her grandmother. After entering the living room she noted that her grandmother's favorite chair was covered with plastic. The three-room apartment was neat and clean, but the distinct odor of ammonia was present. She asked about the plastic, and her grandmother became embarrassed and started to cry. "I'm so ashamed, Judi, **I wet myself. I** just **can't get to the bathroom in time.**" Judi remembered that lately her grandmother had not been attending some family functions, saying that she was **too tired** or that **she walked too slowly** to keep up. After the grandmother regained her composure she explained to Judi that she had her neighbor get her those "adult diapers" at the store. "I really need them at night so I don't wet the bed. **I lose urine** just trying to get up to the bathroom, and I don't want a wet bed. Sometimes I get to the bathroom, but when I'm trying to lift my nightgown the urine starts and I can't stop it." Judi does notice that her grandmother's arthritis must be worse as she is **moving very slowly.**

*Defining characteristics are shown in bold type.

NURSING DIAGNOSIS: Functional incontinence related to impaired mobility

PLANNING

GOALS

Client will have reduced episodes of incontinence within 1 week.

Client will ambulate with less discomfort within 2 weeks.

EXPECTED OUTCOMES

Client will report less frequent episodes of incontinence following initiation of a pattern of timed voiding.

Client will demonstrate ability to walk with a steady gait to bathroom within 2 weeks.

INTERVENTIONS†

Urinary Incontinence Care

- Have client complete a 24-hr bladder log of urination.

- Begin prompted voiding program to anticipate need for voiding toileting based on bladder log data.

- Assess the client for mobility, including the ability to rise from a chair and a bed, ability to ambulate, ability to transfer to toilet.
- Use aggressive continence management for clients living in the community by working with the client and the family.

RATIONALE

The bladder log provides objective verification of urine elimination pattern and patterns of urine leakage and provides a baseline for evaluation of effectiveness of management plans.

Timed voiding (habit training) will empty the bladder prior to the usual stimuli (bladder stretch) and avoid association with inability to get to bathroom facilities in time (UIGP, 1996).

Functional continence requires the ability to gain access to a toilet facility either independently or with assistive devices (UIGP, 1996).

Uncontrolled incontinence can lead to institutionalization of older adults who prefer to remain in their own homes and contributes to increased illness (urinary tract infections, skin breakdown).

†Intervention Classification labels from McCloskey JC, Bulechek GM: *Nursing interventions classification (NIC)*, ed 3, St. Louis, 2000, Mosby.

EVALUATION

Evaluate the change in frequency of incontinence episodes after using timed voiding (habit training).

Ask the client about satisfaction with bladder control.

Observe the client's ability to ambulate, rise from chair and bed, and transfer to toilet.

---

nursing care. For example, if the nurse is attempting to increase the client's fluid intake, a good time to discuss the benefits is while giving fluids with medications or meals. The nurse may be more successful in teaching about perineal hygiene while giving a bath or performing catheter care.

Promoting Normal Micturition.   Maintaining normal urinary elimination will help to prevent many urination problems. Many nursing measures have been designed to promote normal voiding in clients at risk for

urination difficulties and in clients with established urination problems. The nurse can initiate many of these measures independently.

Stimulating Micturition Reflex.   The client's ability to void depends on feeling the urge to urinate, being able to control the urethral sphincter, and being able to relax during voiding. The nurse can help a client learn to relax and stimulate the reflex to void by assuming the normal position for voiding. A woman is better able to void in a squatting or sitting position. This position promotes contraction of the pelvic and intraabdominal muscles that assist in sphincter control and bladder contraction. If the client is unable to use toilet facilities, the nurse positions the client in a squatting position on a bedpan (see Chapter 45) or bedside commode. A man voids more easily in the standing position. If the man cannot reach toilet facilities, he may stand at the bedside and void into a urinal (a metal or plastic receptacle for urine) (Figure 44-12). At times it may be necessary for one or more nurses to assist a man to stand.

Other measures that promote relaxation and the ability to void include sensory stimuli. The sound of running water helps many clients void through the power of suggestion. Stroking the inner aspect of the thigh may stimulate sensory nerves and promote the micturition reflex. Placing the client's hand in a pan of warm water often promotes voiding. It is easier for a person to relax and void when sitting on a bedpan that has been warmed. The nurse can also pour warm water over the client's perineum and create the sensation to urinate. If urine output is to be measured, the nurse must first measure the volume of water to be poured over the perineal area. Offering fluids the client will drink may also promote voiding.

Maintaining Elimination Habits. Many clients follow routines to promote normal voiding. In a hospital or long-term care facility the nurse's routines may conflict with those of clients. Integrating clients' habits into the care plan fosters normal voiding and will assist in preventing problems related to urination.

Maintaining Adequate Fluid Intake. A simple method of promoting normal micturition is maintaining good fluid intake. A client with normal renal function who does not have heart disease or alterations requiring fluid restriction should drink 2000 to 2500 ml of fluid daily. However, an average daily intake of 1200 to 1500 ml of fluids is usually adequate.

When fluid intake is increased, the excreted urine

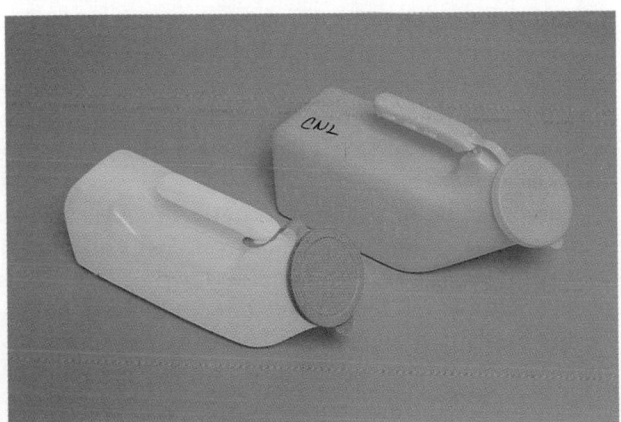

Figure 44-12 Types of male urinals.

flushes out solutes or particles that may collect in the urinary system. Because a client may be unwilling to drink 2500 ml of water daily, the nurse should encourage fluids that the client prefers. Many vegetables and fruits also have a high fluid content. At home it may help to set a schedule for drinking fluids (e.g., with meals or medications). To minimize nocturia, fluids should be avoided 2 hours before bedtime.

Promoting Complete Bladder Emptying. Under normal conditions, a small amount of the client's urine remains in the bladder after voiding because urinary sphincters close (residual urine). The sphincters provide more pressure than the pressure of urine remaining in the bladder. Thus persons normally remain continent and dry. Urinary incontinence may occur because pressure in the bladder is too great or because the sphincters are too weak. Urinary retention occurs from a strong or contracted sphincter or a weak detrusor muscle that prevents normal bladder emptying.

Measures that promote micturition may help clients with incontinence or retention. Additional measures are used to promote and control bladder emptying so that clients gain a sense of elimination control (Table 44-4).

Preventing Infection. One of the most important considerations for a client with urinary alterations is the need to prevent infection of the urinary system. Good perineal hygiene that includes cleansing the urethral meatus after each voiding or bowel movement is essential. A daily fluid intake of 2000 to 2500 ml dilutes urine and promotes regular micturition, which flushes the urethra of microorganisms.

Acidifying Urine. Urine is normally acidic and tends to inhibit growth of microorganisms. Meats, eggs, whole-grain breads, cranberries, prunes, and plums increase urine acidity. These foods metabolize into acid end products that eventually enter the urine. Cranberry juice has been shown to lower urine pH (Box 44-9) High doses of ascorbic acid may also lower urine pH.

Acute Care
Maintaining Elimination Habits. Clients usually require time to void. Asking clients to void quickly so that they can be transported to x-ray testing or requesting a urine specimen as soon as possible does not contribute to relaxation and normal voiding habits. Clients should be given at least 30 minutes to provide a specimen. The nurse learns the times when clients normally void, such as on awakening or before meals, and offers the opportunity to use toilet facilities then. Also important is the need to respond to clients' urges to urinate. Delay in assisting clients to the bathroom may interfere with normal micturition and contribute to incontinence.

Privacy is essential for normal voiding. If the client

Table 44-4 Treatment Options for Urinary Incontinence

Primary Treatment	Other Treatments/Interventions
Functional Incontinence	
Habit training	Environmental alterations
	Scheduled toileting
	Skin care
	Protective undergarments
	Condom catheters (men)
Overflow Incontinence	
Intermittent catheterization	Credé's method
Surgery	Indwelling or condom catheter
Reflex Incontinence	
Anticholinergic medications	Credé's method
Surgery	Indwelling or condom catheter
Intermittent catheterization	Estrogen replacement
Stress Incontinence	
Pelvic floor exercises (Kegel)	Artificial sphincter
Surgery	Biofeedback
Urge Incontinence	
Anticholinergic drug therapy	Biofeedback
Bladder retraining	
Treatment of associated UTI or vaginitis	

Modified from Urinary Incontinence Guideline Panel (UIGP): *Urinary incontinence in adults: clinical practice guideline,* ed 2, Rockville, Md, 1996, Agency for Health Care Policy and Research.

cannot reach the bathroom, the nurse makes sure that the bedside area is enclosed by a curtain. In the home the debilitated client may prefer using a bedside commode enclosed behind a partition or room divider. Some clients are embarrassed by the sound of voiding. Running water or flushing the toilet masks the sound. Young children are often unable to void in the presence of persons other than their parents.

If the client typically uses special measures to void, the nurse should encourage their continued use at home and, when possible, in the institution. The client may be able to relax and void more easily while reading or listening to music. Having a cup or glass of fluids may also promote urination.

Medications. Drug therapy given alone or with other therapies can help problems of incontinence and retention. There are three types of medications. One relaxes a spastic bladder, thereby increasing bladder capacity; one stimulates the bladder to contract, thus improving emptying; and one causes relaxation of the prostatic smooth muscle, reducing obstruction to urethral flow.

The bladder is innervated by the parasympathetic nervous system. Uncontrolled bladder contractions may be caused by local bladder irritants such as calculi or infection. Drugs that depress the neurotransmitter acetylcholine, which stimulates the bladder, reduce inconti-

nence caused by bladder irritation. Examples of these anticholinergic drugs include propantheline (Pro-Banthine) and oxybutynin chloride (Ditropan). The anticholinergics can cause cardiac dysrhythmias and should be used with caution in clients with heart disease. Anticholinergics may also cause constipation and a dry mouth (McKenry and Salerno, 1998).

When the bladder empties, the detrusor muscle contracts in response to parasympathetic stimulation. Incomplete bladder emptying results from impaired innervation or weakness of the detrusor muscle. The client experiences retention and possible overflow incontinence. Cholinergic drugs increase contraction of the bladder and improve emptying. Bethanechol (Urecholine) stimulates parasympathetic nerves to increase bladder wall contraction and relax the sphincter. Bethanechol can be given by subcutaneous or oral routes. Cholinergic drugs may cause diarrhea as a side effect.

The dribbling or overflow incontinence seen in men with prostatic enlargement can be treated with an alpha-1 adrenergic blocker, such as terazosin (Hytrin). Terazosin is given orally and relaxes prostatic smooth muscle, thus relieving obstructive symptoms. This drug may cause hypotension as it is also used in treatment of hypertension.

Catheterization. **Catheterization** of the bladder involves introducing a rubber or plastic tube through the

Research HIGHLIGHT   Box 44-9

RESEARCH ABSTRACT

Cranberry juice has long been claimed to reduce urinary pH. The importance of this claim is that most bacterial growth is inhibited in an acidic urine. The ingestion of cranberry juice has also been noted to decrease urine odor and to promote bladder emptying. A study using cranberry juice was conducted in a veterans' home with 21 men. All the men were 65 years or older either with a previous history of UTI or at risk for UTI (stroke, decreased mobility, or indwelling catheter). The men remained on their usual diets; the only change was the replacement of other fluids with cranberry juice during the middle part of the study. The men served as their own controls. During the first 4 weeks the first urine of the day was tested for pH to serve as the baseline measurements for each man. The second 4 weeks saw the replacement of other fluids with two individual juice boxes of cranberry juice drink (25% juice) consumed at each of three meals. The pH of the first morning urine was measured. The study was completed by a second 4-week period of no cranberry juice use and continued measurement of first morning urine specimens for pH. Although the difference in urine pH when drinking cranberry juice and not drinking it was not statistically significant, the urine pH was markedly lower when drinking the juice.

IMPLICATIONS FOR NURSING

- Since urosepsis is a leading cause of death in persons over 70, the use of cranberry juice may be an easy way to decrease bacterial growth in the urine.
- Nurses can support the use of cranberry juice in client teaching for promoting urinary health for community-based and institutionalized older adults.
- Cranberry juice ingestion will help to decrease urine odor if leakage does occur. For clients with concern about odor this strategy may increase their ability to socialize with increased confidence.

REFERENCE

Jackson B, Hicks LE: Effect of cranberry juice on urinary pH in older adults, *Home Health Nurse* 15(3):198, 1997.

urethra and into the bladder. The catheter provides a continuous flow of urine in clients unable to control micturition or those with obstructions. It also provides a means of assessing hourly urine outputs in hemodynamically unstable clients. Because bladder catheterization carries the risk of UTI and trauma to the urethra, it is preferable to rely on other measures for either specimen collection or management of incontinence.

Types of Catheterization. Intermittent and indwelling retention catheterization are the two forms of catheter insertion. With the intermittent technique a straight single-use catheter (Figure 44-13, *A*) is introduced long enough to drain the bladder (5 to 10 minutes). When the bladder is empty, the nurse immediately withdraws the catheter. Intermittent catheterization can be repeated as necessary, but repeated use increases the risks of trauma and infection. An indwelling or Foley catheter remains in place for a longer period until a client is able to void completely and voluntarily or as long as accurate hourly measurements are needed. It may be necessary to change indwelling catheters periodically.

The straight single-use catheter has a single lumen with a small opening about 1.3 cm (½ inch) from the tip. Urine drains from the tip, through the lumen, and to a receptacle. An indwelling Foley catheter has a small inflatable balloon that encircles the catheter just below the tip. When inflated, the balloon rests against the bladder outlet to anchor the catheter in place. The indwelling retention catheter also has two or three lumens within the body of the catheter (Figure 44-13, *B*). One lumen drains urine through the catheter to a collecting tube. A second lumen carries sterile water to and from the balloon when it is inflated or deflated. A third (optional) lumen may be used to instill fluids or medications into the bladder. It is easy to determine the number of lumens by the number of drainage and injection ports at the catheter's end.

A third type of catheter has a curved tip. A Coudé catheter is used on male clients who may have enlarged prostates that partly obstruct the urethra. The Coudé catheter is less traumatic during insertion because it is stiffer and easier to control than the straight-tip catheter.

Catheters come in many diameters to fit the size of a client's urethral canal. Suggestions on how to make appropriate decisions regarding catheter selection are provided in Box 44-10.

Indications for Catheterization. Catheterization may be indicated for many reasons. When catheterization time will be short and minimizing infection is a priority, the intermittent method is best. Intermittent catheterization is also preferred for persons with spinal cord injuries who have no bladder control. By intermittently draining the bladder on a routine basis, these clients have fewer infections. Indwelling catheterization is used when long-term bladder emptying is necessary. Box 44-11 outlines specific indications for catheterization.

Catheter Insertion. Urethral catheterization requires a physician's order. The nurse must use strict aseptic technique (see Chapter 33). Organizing equipment before the procedure prevents interruptions. The steps for inserting indwelling and single-use straight catheters are basically the same. The difference lies in the procedure taken to inflate the indwelling catheter balloon and secure the catheter. Skill 44-2 lists steps for performing female and male urethral catheterization.

Closed Drainage Systems. After inserting an indwelling catheter, the nurse maintains a closed urinary

Text continued on p. 1422.

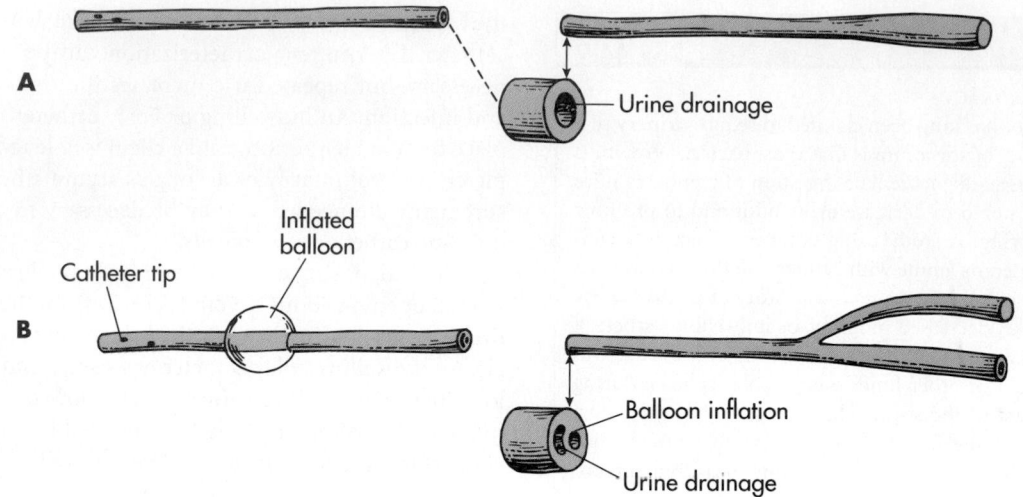

Figure 44-13   Types of urinary catheters. **A,** Straight catheter. **B,** Indwelling (Foley).

Guidelines for Appropriate Catheter Selection   Box 44-10

- The catheter size should be determined by the size of the client's urethral canal. When the French system is used, the larger the gauge number, the larger the catheter size. Generally, children require an 8 to 10 Fr, women require a 14 to 16 Fr, whereas men require a 16 to 18 Fr (Lewis, Collier, and Heitkemper, 1996). To prevent trauma, the smallest effective catheter size is preferred.
- The expected time required for the catheterization will determine the catheter material selection.
- Plastic catheters are suitable only for intermittent use due to their inflexibility.
- Latex and rubber catheters are recommended for use up to 3 weeks. Be aware of allergies to either of these materials.
- Pure silicon or teflon catheters are best suited for long-term use (2 to 3 months) as they cause less encrustation at the urethral meatus.
- Balloon size is also important in selecting an indwelling catheter. Balloon sizes range from 3 ml (pediatric) to large postoperative volumes (75 ml). In adults, the 5-ml and 30-ml sizes are the most common: The 5-ml size allows for optimal drainage, whereas the 30-ml size is used after prostatectomies to provide hemostasis of the prostatic bed (Beare and Myers, 1998).
- Only sterile water should be used to inflate the balloon as saline may crystallize, resulting in incomplete deflation of the balloon at the time of removal.
- If leakage should occur around the catheter, a change in lumen size or use of antispasmodic medication may be warranted.

Indications for Catheterization   Box 44-11

INTERMITTENT CATHETERIZATION
Relief of discomfort of bladder distention, provision of decompression
Obtaining sterile urine specimen
Assessment of residual urine after urination
Long-term management of clients with spinal cord injuries, neuromuscular degeneration, or incompetent bladders

SHORT-TERM INDWELLING CATHETERIZATION
Obstruction to urine outflow (e.g., prostate enlargement)
Surgical repair of bladder, urethra, and surrounding structures
Prevention of urethral obstruction from blood clots
Measurement of urinary output in critically ill clients
Continuous or intermittent bladder irrigations

LONG-TERM INDWELLING CATHETERIZATION
Severe urinary retention with recurrent episodes of UTI
Skin rashes, ulcers, or wounds irritated by contact with urine
Terminal illness when bed linen changes are painful for client

Inserting a Straight or Indwelling Catheter | Skill 44-2

Delegation Considerations

Catheterization is not usually delegated to assistive personnel; however, agency policy is to be followed. This procedure may be delegated to personnel who have been properly instructed.

Catheterization requires problem solving and knowledge ap-

plication unique to a professional nurse. Assistive personnel routinely may empty urine from the collection bag, provide perineal care, and report specific abnormal findings to the nurse.

EQUIPMENT

- Catheterization kit containing the following sterile items:
  - Gloves (extra pair optional)
  - Drapes, one fenestrated
  - Lubricant
  - Antiseptic cleansing solution
  - Cotton balls
  - Forceps
  - Prefilled syringe with sterile water to inflate the balloon of indwelling catheter

- Catheter of correct size and type for procedure (i.e., intermittent or indwelling)
- Sterile drainage tubing with collection bag and multipurpose tube holder or tape, safety pin, and elastic band for securing tubing to bed if client is bed bound (for indwelling catheter)
- Receptacle or basin (usually bottom of catheterization tray)
- Specimen container
- Blanket

STEPS	RATIONALE
1. Assess status of client:	
a. Time of last urination by asking client, checking I&O flow sheet, or by palpating bladder	Bladder fullness may be detected with deep palpation above the symphysis pubis.
b. Level of awareness or developmental stage	Reveals the client's ability to cooperate and level of explanation needed.
c. Mobility and physical limitations of client	Affect way the nurse positions client.
d. Client's gender and age	Determines catheter size: 8 to 10 Fr is generally used for children, 14 to 16 Fr is indicated for women, 12 Fr may be considered for young girls, and 16 to 18 Fr is used for male clients unless larger size is ordered by physician.
e. Distended bladder	Causes pain. Can indicate need to insert catheter if client is unable to void independently.
f. Perineum erythema, drainage, and odor	Determines condition of the perineum.
g. Any pathological condition that may impair passage of catheter (i.e., enlarged prostate in men)	Obstruction prevents passage of catheter through urethra into the bladder.
h. Allergies	Determines allergy to antiseptic, tape, latex, and lubricant. Betadine allergies are common; if the client is unaware of allergy, ask if allergic to shellfish.
2. Review client's medical record, including physician's order and nurses' notes.	Determines purpose of inserting catheter: preparation for surgery, urinary irrigations, collection of sterile specimens, or measurement of residual urine. Assess for previous catheterization, including catheter size, response of client, and time of last catheterization.
3. Assess client's knowledge of the purpose for catheterization.	Reveals need for client instruction.
4. Explain procedure to client.	Promotes cooperation.
5. Arrange for extra nursing personnel to assist as necessary.	Client may be unable to assume positioning for procedure.
6. Begin monitoring I&O.	Catheterized clients are at risk for urinary complications.
7. Wash hands.	Reduces transmission of microorganisms.
8. Close curtain or door.	Offers privacy, reduce embarrassment, and aids in relaxation during procedure.
9. Raise bed to appropriate working height.	Promotes use of proper body mechanics.
10. Facing client, stand on left side of bed if right-handed (on right side of bed if left-handed). Clear the bedside table and arrange equipment.	Successful catheter insertion requires nurse to assume comfortable position with all equipment easily accessible.
11. Raise side rail on opposite side of bed, and put side rail down on working side.	Promotes client safety.
12. Place waterproof pad under client.	Prevents soiling of bed linen.

STEPS	RATIONALE

13. Position client.

    A. **Female client**

      (1) Assist to dorsal recumbent position (supine with knees flexed). Ask client to relax thighs so the hips can be externally rotated.

      (2) Position female client in side-lying (Sims') position with upper leg flexed at hip if unable to be supine. If this position is used, nurse must take extra precautions to cover rectal area with drape to reduce chance of cross contamination.

    B. **Male client**

      (1) Assist to supine position with thighs slightly abducted.

14. Drape client.

    A. **Female client** (see illustration)

      (1) Drape with bath blanket. Place blanket diamond fashion over client, with one corner at client's neck, side corners over each arm and side, and last corner over perineum.

    B. **Male client** (see illustration)

      (1) Drape upper trunk with bath blanket, and cover lower extremities with bedsheets, exposing only genitalia.

RATIONALE column:

Provides good visualization of perineal structures.

Legs may be supported with pillows to reduce muscle tension and promote comfort.

This alternate position is used if client cannot abduct leg at hip joint (e.g., if client has arthritic joints). Also, this position may be more comfortable for client. Support client with pillows if necessary to maintain position.

Comfortable position for client that aids in visualization.

Avoids unnecessary exposure of body parts and maintains client's comfort.

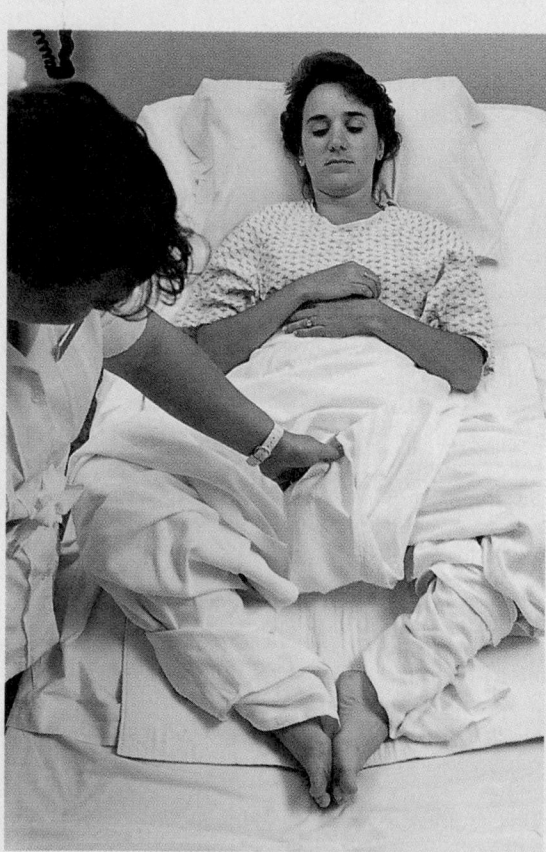

Step 14A

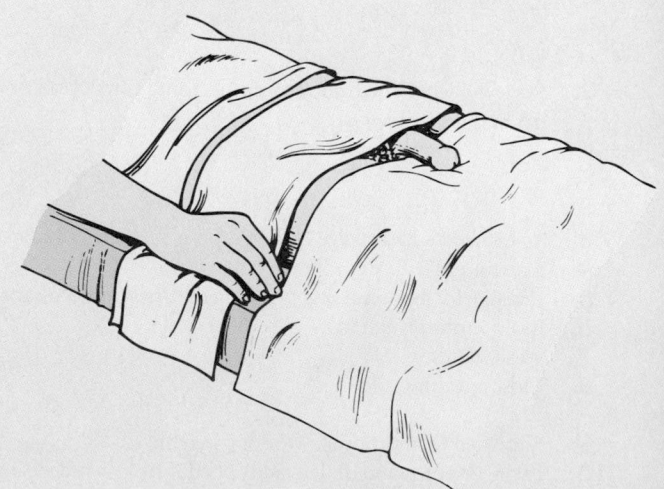

Step 14B

STEPS	RATIONALE
15. Wearing disposable gloves, wash perineal area with soap and water as needed; dry.	Reduces microorganisms near urethral meatus and allows further opportunity to visualize perineum and landmarks.
16. Remove and discard gloves; wash hands.	
17. Position lamp to illuminate perineal area. (When using flashlight have an assistant hold it.)	Permits accurate identification and good visualization of urethral meatus.
18. Open package containing drainage system; place drainage bag over edge of bottom bed frame, and bring drainage tube up between side rails and mattress (indwelling catheter only).	
19. Open catheterization kit according to directions, keeping bottom of container sterile.	Prevents transmission of microorganisms from table or work area to sterile supplies. The materials in the kit are arranged in sequence of use.
20. Apply sterile gloves (see Chapter 33).	Allows nurse to handle sterile supplies without contamination.
21. Organize supplies on sterile field. Open inner sterile package containing catheter. Pour sterile antiseptic solution into correct compartment containing sterile cotton balls. Open packet containing lubricant. Remove specimen container (lid should be placed loosely on top) and prefilled syringe from collection compartment of tray, and set them aside on sterile field.	Maintains principles of surgical asepsis and organizes work area.
22. Before inserting indwelling catheter, test balloon by injecting fluid from prefilled syringe into balloon port (see illustration).	Checks integrity of balloon. Do not use the catheter if the balloon does not inflate or leaks.
23. Lubricate 2.5 to 5 cm (1 to 2 in) of catheter for women and 12.5 to 17.7 cm (5 to 7 in) for men.	
24. Apply sterile drape:	
A. Female client	
(1) Allow top edge of drape to form a cuff over both hands. Place drape down on bed between client's thighs. Slip cuffed edge just under buttocks, taking care not to touch contaminated surface with gloves.	Outer surface of drape covering hands remains sterile. Sterile drape against sterile gloves is sterile.
(2) Pick up fenestrated sterile, and allow it to unfold without touching an unsterile object. Apply drape over perineum, exposing labia, and being sure not to touch contaminated surface.	Maintains sterility of work surface.

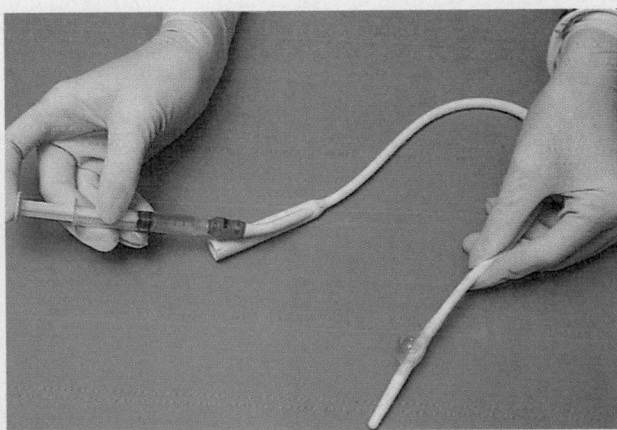

Step 22

STEPS	RATIONALE

B. **Male client**

(1) Two methods are used for draping depending on preference. *First method:* Apply drape over thighs and under penis without completely opening fenestrated drape. *Second method:* Apply drape over thighs just below penis. Pick up fenestrated sterile drape, allow it to unfold, and drape it over penis with fenestrated slit resting over penis.

Maintains sterility of work surface.

25. Place sterile tray and contents on sterile drape. Open specimen container.

Provides easy access to supplies during catheter insertion. Maintains aseptic technique during procedure.

26. Cleanse urethral meatus:

A. **Female client**

(1) With nondominant hand, carefully retract labia to fully expose urethral meatus. Maintain position of nondominant hand throughout procedure.

Full visualization of urethral meatus is provided. Full retraction prevents contamination of urethral meatus during cleansing.

(2) Using forceps in sterile dominant hand, pick up cotton ball saturated with antiseptic solution and clean perineal area, wiping from front to back from clitoris toward anus. Using a new cotton ball for each area, wipe along the far labial fold, near labial fold, and directly over center of urethral meatus (see illustration)

Cleansing reduces number of microorganism at urethral meatus. Use of a single cotton ball for each wipe prevents transfer of microorganisms. Cleansing proceeds from area of least contamination to that of most contamination. Dominant hand remains sterile.

B. **Male client**

(1) If client is not circumcised, retract foreskin with nondominant hand. Grasp penis at shaft just below glans. Retract urethral meatus between thumb and forefinger. Maintain nondominant hand in this position throughout procedure.

Accidental release of foreskin or dropping of penis during cleansing requires process to be repeated because area has become contaminated.

(2) With dominant hand, pick up cotton ball with forceps and clean penis. Move in a circular motion from urethral meatus down to base of glans. Repeat cleansing three more times, using a clean cotton ball each time (see illustration).

Reduces number of microorganisms at urethral meatus and moves from area of least to most contamination. Dominant hand remains sterile.

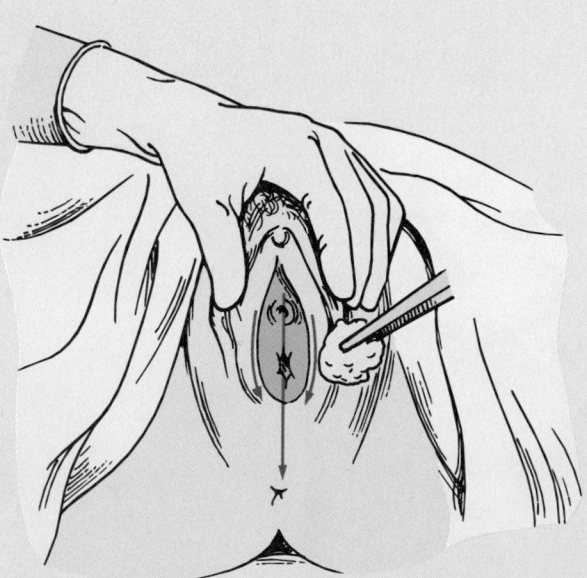

Step 26A(2)

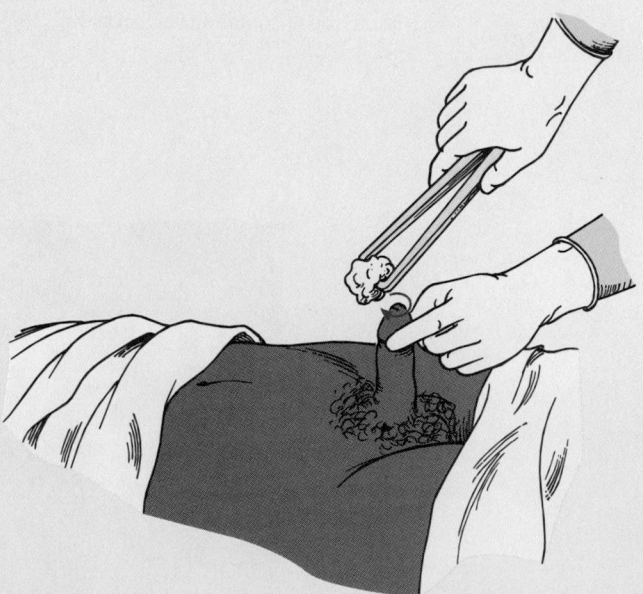

Step 26B(2)

STEPS	RATIONALE

Critical Decision Point: Closure of labia during cleansing requires that the cleansing procedure be repeated because the area has become contaminated.

---

27. Pick up catheter with gloved dominant hand 7.5 to 10 cm (3 to 4 in) from catheter tip. Hold end of catheter loosely coiled in palm of dominant hand (optional: may grasp catheter with forceps).

28. Insert catheter:

A. **Female client**

    (1) Ask client to bear down gently as if to void, and slowly insert catheter through urethral meatus (see illustration).

                      Relaxation of external sphincter aids in insertion of catheter.

    (2) Advance catheter a total of 5 to 7.5 cm (2 to 3 in) in adult or until urine flows out of catheter's end. When urine appears, advance catheter another 2.5 to 5 cm (1 to 2 in). Do not force against resistance.

                      Female urethra is short. Appearance of urine indicates that catheter tip is in bladder or lower urethra. Advancement of catheter ensures bladder placement.

Critical Decision Point: If no urine appears, check if catheter is in vagina. If misplaced, leave catheter in vagina as landmark indicating where not to insert, and insert another.

---

    (3) Release labia, and hold catheter securely with nondominant hand. Inflate balloon if retention catheter is used (see illustrations).

                      Bladder or sphincter contraction may cause accidental expulsion of catheter.

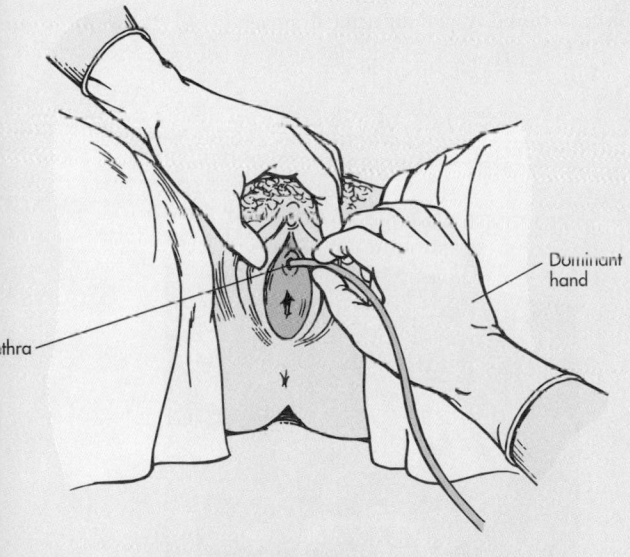

Step 28A(1)

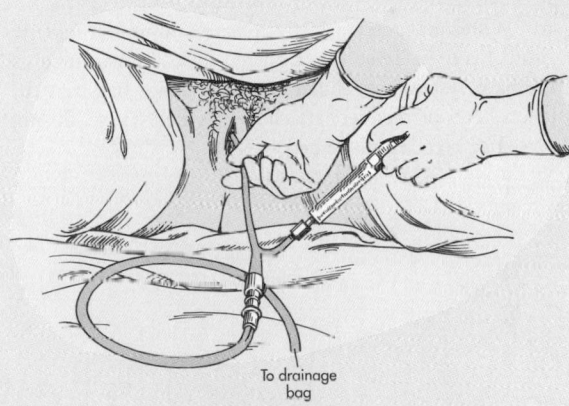

Step 28A(3)

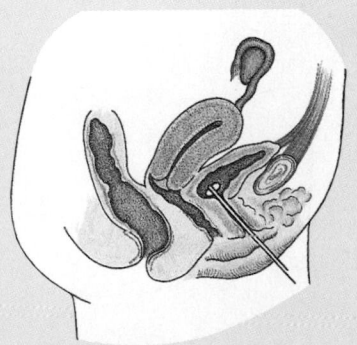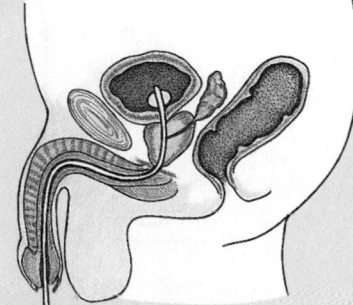

Step 28A(3)

STEPS	RATIONALE

B. **Male Client**

(1) Lift penis to position perpendicular to client's body and apply light traction (see illustration).

Straightens urethral canal to ease catheter insertion.

(2) Ask client to bear down as if to void, and slowly insert catheter through urethral meatus.

Relaxation of external sphincter aids in insertion of catheter.

(3) Advance catheter 17 to 22.5 cm (7 to 9 in) in adult or until urine flows out catheter's end. If resistance is felt, withdraw catheter; do not force it through urethra. When urine appears, advance catheter another 2.5 to 5 cm (1 to 2 in).

The adult male urethra is long. It is normal to meet resistance at the prostatic sphincter. When resistance is met, nurse should hold catheter firmly against sphincter without forcing catheter. After a few seconds, the sphincter relaxes, and the catheter is advanced. Appearance of urine indicates catheter tip is in bladder or urethra. Further advancement of catheter ensures proper placement.

(4) Lower penis and hold catheter securely in non-dominant hand. Place end of catheter in urine tray. Inflate balloon if retention catheter is used.

Catheter may be accidentally expelled by bladder or urethral contraction. Collection of urine prevents soiling and provides output measurement.

(5) Reduce (or reposition) the foreskin.

Paraphimosis (retraction and constriction of the foreskin behind the glans penis) secondary to catheterization may occur if foreskin is not reduced.

29. Collect urine specimen as needed. Fill specimen cup or jar to desired level (20 to 30 ml) by holding end of catheter in dominant hand over cup.

Allows sterile specimen to be obtained for culture analysis.

30. Allow bladder to empty fully (about 800 to 1000 ml) unless institution policy restricts maximal volume of urine to drain with each catheterization. Check institution policy before beginning catheterization. If a restriction is in place, the range is often 800 to 1000 ml.

There is no limit to the amount of urine that can be drained (Sueppel, 1995; Williams and others, 1993). As always the nurse should monitor the client's condition, and if the vital signs change or bleeding occurs, temporarily stop the flow of urine and continue when the client's condition warrants. Retained urine may serve as a reservoir for growth of microorganisms.

31. Remove straight, single-use catheters:

a. Withdraw catheter slowly but smoothly until removed.

Minimizes discomfort to client.

32. Attach end of retention catheter to collecting tube of drainage system (see illustration). Drainage bag must be below level of bladder; attach bag to bed frame, do not place bag on side rails of bed.

Establishes a closed system for urine drainage.

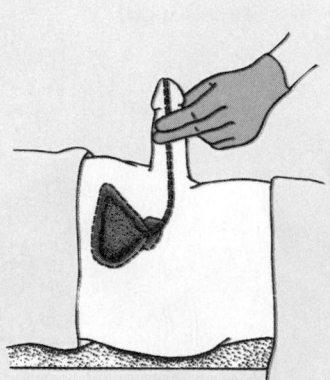

Step 28B(1)

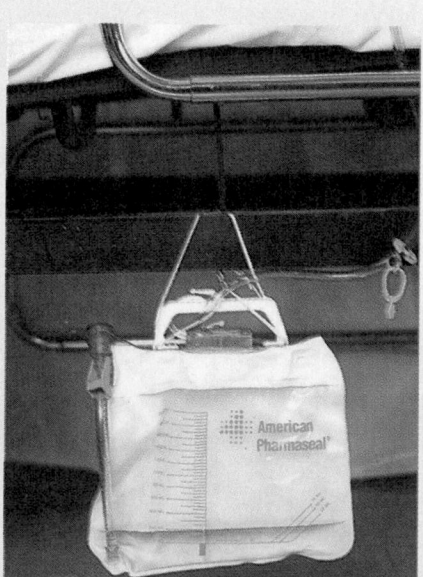

Step 32

STEPS	RATIONALE

33. Anchor catheter:

  A. **Female client**

    (1) Secure catheter tubing to inner thigh with strip of nonallergenic tape (or multipurpose tube holders with a Velcro strap). Allow for slack so movement of thigh does not create tension on catheter (see illustration).

Anchoring catheter to inner thigh reduces pressure on urethra, thus reducing possibility of tissue injury.

  B. **Male client**

    (1) Secure catheter tubing to top of thigh or lower abdomen (with penis directed toward chest). Allow slack in catheter so movement does not create tension on catheter (see illustration).

Anchoring catheter to lower abdomen reduces pressure on urethra at junction of penis and scrotum, thus reducing possibility of tissue injury.

34. Assist client to comfortable position. Wash and dry perineal area as needed.

Maintains comfort and security.

35. Remove gloves, and dispose of equipment, drapes, and urine in proper receptacles.

Reduces transmission of microorganisms.

36. Wash hands.

Reduces transmission of microorganisms.

37. Palpate bladder.

Determines if distention is relieved.

38. Ask about client's comfort.

Determines if client's sensation of discomfort or fullness has been relieved.

39. Observe character and amount of urine in drainage system.

Determines if urine is flowing adequately.

40. Determine that there is no urine leaking from catheter or tubing connections.

Prevents injury to client's skin.

Recording and Reporting

- Report and record type and size of catheter inserted, amount of fluid used to inflate the balloon, characteristics of urine, amount of urine, reasons for catheterization, specimen collection if appropriate, and client's response to procedure and teaching concepts.
- Initiate I&O record.
- If catheter is definitely in bladder and no urine is produced within an hour, absence of urine should be immediately reported to physician.

Home Care Considerations

- Clients who are at home may use a leg bag during the day and switch to a large-volume bag at night so sleep can be uninterrupted.
- Clients may catheterize themselves at home using a clean technique.

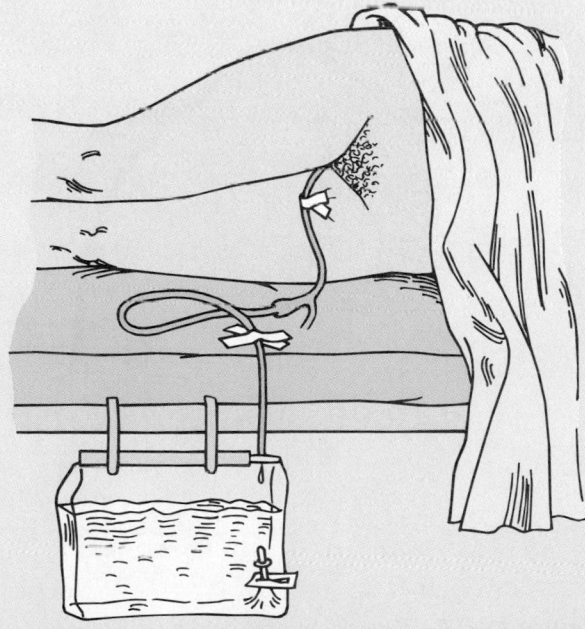

Step 33A(1)

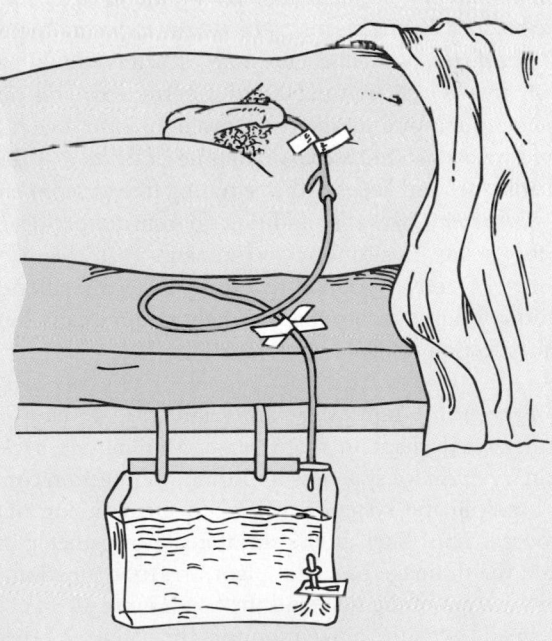

Step 33B(1)

drainage system to minimize the risk of infection. Urinary drainage bags are plastic and can hold about 1000 to 1500 ml of urine. The bag should hang on the bed frame or wheelchair without touching the floor. Never hang the bag on the bed rail as it can be accidentally raised above the level of the bladder.

When the client ambulates, the nurse or client carries the bag below the client's waist. The drainage bag should never be raised above the level of the client's bladder. Urine in the bag and tubing can become a medium for bacteria, and infection is likely to develop if urine flows back into the bladder.

Most drainage bags contain an antireflux valve to prevent urine in the bag from reentering the drainage tubing and contaminating the client's bladder. A spigot at the base of the bag provides a means for emptying the bag. The spigot should always be clamped, except during emptying, and tucked into the protective pouch on the side of the bag. To keep the drainage system patent the nurse checks for kinks or bends in the tubing, avoids positioning the client on the drainage tubing, and observes for clots or sediment that may occlude the collecting tubing.

Routine Catheter Care. Clients with indwelling catheters have a number of special care needs. Nursing measures are directed at preventing infection and maintaining unobstructed flow of urine through the catheter drainage system.

Perineal Hygiene. Buildup of secretions or encrustation at the catheter insertion site is a source of irritation and potential infection. Nurses provide perineal hygiene (see Chapter 38) at least twice daily or as needed for a client with a retention catheter. Soap and water are effective in reducing the number of organisms around the urethra. The nurse must not accidentally advance the catheter up into the bladder during cleansing or risk introducing bacteria.

Fluid Intake. All clients with catheters should have a daily intake of 2000 to 2500 ml if permitted. This can be met through oral intake or intravenous infusion. A high fluid intake produces a large volume of urine that flushes the bladder and keeps catheter tubing free of sediment.

Catheter Care. In addition to routine perineal hygiene, many institutions recommend that clients with catheters receive special care 3 times a day and after defecation or bowel incontinence to help minimize discomfort and infection (Skill 44-3).

Preventing Infection. Infection can develop in a catheterized client in many ways. Maintaining a closed urinary drainage system is important in infection control. A break in the system can lead to introduction of microorganisms. Sites at risk are the site of catheter insertion, the drainage bag, the spigot, the tube junction, and the junction of the tube and the bag (Figure 44-14).

In addition, the nurse monitors the patency of the system to prevent pooling of urine within the tubing. Urine

in the drainage bag is an excellent medium for microorganism growth. Bacteria can travel up drainage tubing to grow in pools of urine. If this urine flows back into the client's bladder, an infection will likely develop (Buscheller and Bernstein, 1997). Suggestions for ways to prevent infections in catheterized clients are provided in Box 44-12.

Catheter Irrigations and Instillations. To maintain the patency of indwelling urinary catheters, it sometimes becomes necessary to irrigate or flush a catheter. Blood, pus, or sediment can collect within tubing and result in bladder distention and the buildup of stagnant urine. Instillation of a sterile solution ordered by the physician clears the tubing of accumulated material. For clients with bladder infections, a physician may order bladder irrigations to include instillation of antiseptic or antibiotic solutions to wash out the bladder or treat local infection. In both irrigations, sterile aseptic technique is followed.

Before performing an irrigation, the nurse assesses the catheter for blockage. If the amount of urine in the drainage bag is less than the client's intake or less than the output during the previous shift, blockage can be expected. If urine does not drain freely, the nurse milks the tubing. Milking is done by gently squeezing then releasing the drainage tube in an alternating fashion. The nurse should always milk from the client to the drainage bag so a clot or sediment will not be forced back into the catheter.

Maintenance of a closed system is recommended during intermittent irrigations or instillations. This technique is effective for irrigating a partially blocked catheter or for bladder instillations. Steps for using this closed system are in Skill 44-4.

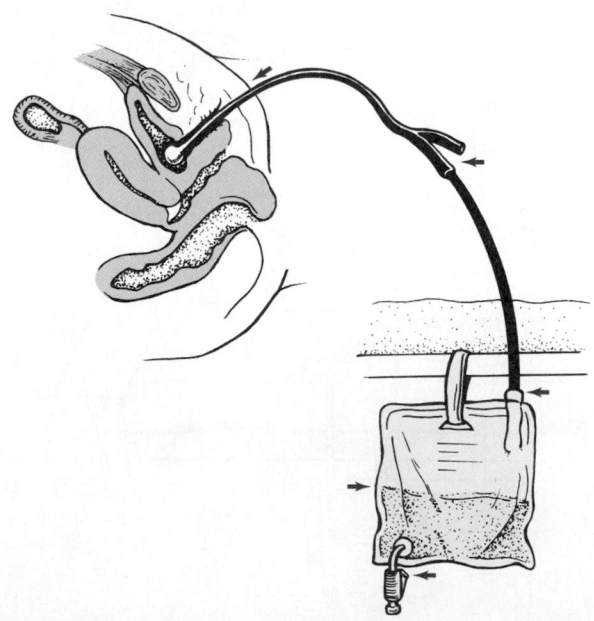

Figure 44-14 Potential sites for introduction of infectious organisms into a urinary drainage system.

Indwelling Catheter Care Skill 44-3

Delegation Considerations

Perineal care is often part of routine hygiene care that is delegated to assistive personnel. With instruction, indwelling catheter care can be incorporated with perineal care by assistive personnel. If client has had trauma or surgical procedures that involve the perineal area, this care should not be delegated. Proper assessment and care of the perineal area will need professional clinical judgment.

EQUIPMENT
- Catheter care kit or individual supplies
  - Nonsterile gloves
  - Cotton balls or large swabs
  - Clean washcloth and towel
  - Warm water and soap
  - Antibiotic ointment (if agency policy)
- Bath blanket
- Waterproof absorbant pad

STEPS	RATIONALE
1. Assess for episode of bowel incontinence or client discomfort or provide care as per agency routine as part of hygiene measures.	Accumulation of secretions or feces causes irritation to perineal tissues and acts as a source of bacterial growth.
2. Explain procedure to client. Offer opportunity to perform self-care to able client.	Reduces anxiety and promotes cooperation. Embarrassment may motivate client to perform own hygiene.
3. Close door or bedside curtain.	Maintains client privacy.
4. Wash hands.	Reduces transmission of infection.

5. Position client:
  A. **Female**
    (1) Dorsal recumbent position
  B. **Male**
    (1) Supine or Fowler's position
	Ensures easy access to perineal tissues.

6. Place waterproof pad under client.	Protects bed linens from soiling.
7. Drape bath blanket on client so that only perineal area is exposed.	Prevents unnecessary exposure of body parts.
8. Apply gloves.	
9. Remove anchor device to free catheter tubing.	

10. With nondominant hand:
  A. **Female**
    (1) Gently retract labia to fully expose urethral meatus and catheter insertion site, maintaining position of hand throughout procedure.
	Provides full visualization of urethral meatus. Full retraction prevents contamination of meatus during cleansing.

B. **Male** (1) Retract foreskin if not circumscribed, and hold penis at shaft just below glans, maintaining position throughout procedure.	Accidental closure of labia or dropping of penis during cleansing requires procedure to be repeated.
11. Assess urethral meatus and surrounding tissue for inflammation, swelling, and discharge. Note amount, color, odor, and consistancy of discharge. Ask client if any burning or discomfort is felt.	Determines presence of local infection and status of hygiene.

12. Cleanse perineal tissue:
  A. **Female**
    (1) Use clean cloth, soap, and water. Cleanse around urethral meatus and catheter. Cleaning from pubis toward anus, clean labia minora. Use a clean side of cloth for each wipe. Finally clean around anus. Dry each area well.
	Reduces the number of microorganisms at urethral meatus. Use of clean cloth prevents transfer of microorganisms.

B. **Male** (1) While spreading urethral meatus, cleanse around catheter first, and then wipe in circular motion around meatus and glans.	Cleansing moves from area of least to most contamination.

STEPS	RATIONALE
13. Reassess urethral meatus for discharge.	Determines if cleansing is complete.
14. With towel, soap, and water, wipe in a circular motion along length of catheter for 10 cm (4 in).	Reduces presence of secretions or drainage on exterior of catheter surface.
15. Apply an antibiotic ointment at urethral meatus and along 2.5 cm (1 in) of catheter if ordered by physician or part of agency policy.	Further reduces growth of microorganisms at insertion site.
16. In male client reduce (or reposition) the foreskin.	
17. Place client in a safe, comfortable position.	Promotes comfort.
18. Dispose of contaminated supplies, remove gloves, and wash hands.	Prevents spread of infection.

Recording and Reporting

- Report and record presence and characteristics of drainage, condition of perineal tissue, and any discomfort reported by client.
- If infection is suspected, report findings to physician.

Home Care Considerations

- If client is discharged with indwelling catheter, the client and family should be taught catheter care and signs and symptoms to report to nurse or physician.

Tips for Preventing Infection in Catheterized Clients   Box 44-12

Follow good hand-washing techniques (see Chapter 33).

Do not allow the spigot on the drainage system to touch a contaminated surface.

Do not open the drainage system at connecting points to collect specimens.

If the drainage tube becomes disconnected, do not touch the ends of the catheter or tubing. Wipe the end of the tubing and catheter with an antimicrobial solution before reconnecting.

Ensure that each client has a separate receptacle for measuring urine to prevent cross contamination.

Prevent pooling of urine in the tubing and reflux of urine into the bladder.

   Avoid raising the drainage bag above the level of the bladder.

   If it becomes necessary to raise the bag during transfer of the client to a bed or stretcher, clamp the tubing or empty the tubing contents to the drainage bag first.

   Avoid allowing large loops of tubing to lie on the bed.

   Provide for drainage of urine from the tubing to the bag by positioning the tubing.

   Before exercise or ambulation drain all urine from the tubing into the drainage bag.

Avoid prolonged kinking or clamping of the tubing.

Empty the drainage bag at least every 8 hours. If large outputs are noted, empty more frequently.

Remove the catheter as soon as clinically warranted.

Tape or secure the catheter appropriately for the client (see Skill 44-2).

Perform routine perineal hygiene per agency policy and after defecation or bowel incontinence (see Skill 44-3).

A single intermittent irrigation is safer and less likely to introduce infections into the urinary tract than repeated irrigations. There are two additional methods for catheter irrigation. One is a closed bladder irrigation system (Skill 44-4). This system provides for frequent intermittent irrigations or continuous irrigation without disruption of the sterile catheter system through use of a three-way catheter. This method is used most often in clients who have had genitourinary surgery and are at risk for blood clots and mucus fragments occluding the catheter. The other system involves opening the closed drainage system to instill bladder irrigations (Skill 44-4). This technique poses greater risk for causing infection. However, it may be needed when catheters become blocked and it is undesirable to change the catheter (e.g., after recent prostate surgery).

Removal of Indwelling Catheter.   When removing an indwelling catheter, the nurse promotes normal bladder function and prevents trauma to the urethra.

To remove a catheter the nurse requires a clean, disposable towel; a trash receptacle; and a sterile syringe the same size as the volume of solution within the catheter's inflated balloon. Disposable gloves are also recommended. The end of each catheter contains a label that denotes the volume of solution (5 to 30 ml) within the balloon.

The nurse positions the client in the same position as during catheterization. Some institutions recommend collecting a sterile urine specimen at this time or sending the catheter tip for culture and sensitivity tests. After removing the tape, the nurse places the towel between a female

Closed and Open Catheter Irrigation   Skill 44-4

Delegation Considerations

Although closed catheter irrigation carries less risk of infection, neither closed nor open catheter irrigation is usually delegated to assistive personnel. Catheter irrigation is usually done in clients with complications such as urinary tract infections or postsurgically after prostatectomy. Professional nursing judgment is indicated for safe client care.

EQUIPMENT

- **Closed intermittent method**
  - Sterile irrigation solution at room temperature
  - Sterile graduated container
  - Sterile 30-50 ml syringe
  - Sterile 19-22-gauge 1-in needle
  - Antiseptic swab
  - Clamp for catheter or tubing
  - Bath blanket
- **Closed continuous method**
  - Sterile irrigation solution at room temperature
  - Irrigation tubing and clamp (with or without Y connector)
  - IV pole
  - Antiseptic swab

- Y connector (optional)
- Bath blanket
- **Open method**
  - Sterile irrigation set with tray
  - Bulb syringe or 60-ml piston-type syringe
  - Sterile collection basin
  - Waterproof drape
  - Sterile solution container
  - Antiseptic swabs
  - Sterile gloves
  - Sterile correct irrigation solution at room temperature
  - Tape or elastic band to resecure catheter
  - Bath blanket

STEPS	RATIONALE
1. Assess physician's order for type of irrigation and irrigation solution to use.	Ensures proper selection of equipment.
2. Assess color of urine and presence of mucus or sediment.	Determines if client is bleeding, has infection, or is sloughing tissue.
3. Determine type of catheter in place: a. Triple lumen (one lumen to inflate balloon, one to instill irrigation solution, one to allow outflow of urine). b. Double lumen (one lumen to inflate balloon, one to allow outflow of urine).	Indicates method for irrigation.
4. Determine patency of drainage tubing.	Ensures that drainage tubing is not kinked, clamped incorrectly, or looped.
5. Assess amount of urine in drainage bag (may want to empty drainage bag prior to irrigation).	If not empty, will need to subtract urine volume from amount drained to determine if all irrigant returned.
6. Explain procedure and purpose to client.	Helps client relax and cooperate during procedure.
7. Wash hands and apply clean gloves for closed methods.	Prevents transmission of microorganisms.
8. Provide privacy by pulling bed curtains closed. Fold back covers so that catheter is exposed. Cover client's upper torso with bath blanket.	Promotes client comfort.
9. Assess lower abdomen for bladder distention.	Detects whether catheter is malfunctioning or blocking urinary drainage.
10. Position client in dorsal recumbent or supine position.	Promotes client comfort and provides easy access to catheter. Promotes flow of irrigating solution into bladder.
11. Closed intermittent irrigation: a. Prepare prescribed sterile solution in sterile graduated cup. b. Draw sterile solution into syringe using aseptic technique. c. Clamp indwelling retention catheter just below soft injection port. d. Cleanse injection port with antiseptic swab (same port used for specimen collection). e. Insert needle of syringe through port at 30-degree angle towards bladder.	Ensures that irrigating fluid remains sterile. Occlusion of catheter provides resistance against which irrigant can be forcefully instilled into catheter. Reduces transmission of infection. Ensures that needle tip enters lumen of catheter and flow is directed into bladder.

STEPS	RATIONALE
f. Slowly inject fluid into catheter and bladder.	Slow, continuous pressure dislodges clots and sediment without traumatizing bladder wall.
g. Withdraw syringe, remove clamp, and allow solution to drain into drainage bag. If ordered by physician, keep clamped to allow solution to remain in bladder for short time (20-30 min).	Allows drainage by gravity.

Critical Decision Point: If solution is to remain in bladder, do not forget to unclamp tubing at specified time!

---

12. Closed continuous irrigation (see illustration):

a. Using aseptic technique, insert tip of sterile irrigation tubing into bag of sterile irrigating solution.

Prevents entrance of microorganisms.

b. Close clamp on tubing and hang bag of solution on IV pole.

c. Open clamp and allow solution to flow through tubing, keeping end of tubing sterile. Close clamp.

Removes air from tubing.

d. Wipe off irrigation port of triple lumen catheter, or attach sterile Y connector to double lumen catheter and then attach to irrigation tubing.

Third lumen or Y connector provides means for irrigation solution to enter bladder. System must remain sterile.

e. Be sure that drainage bag and tubing are securely connected to drainage port of triple lumen catheter or other arm of Y connector.

Ensures that urine and irrigation solution will drain from bladder.

f. For intermittent flow, clamp tubing on drainage system, open clamp on irrigation tubing, and allow prescribed amount of fluid to enter bladder (100 ml is normal for adults).

Fluid instills through catheter into bladder, flushing system. Fluid drains out after irrigation is completed.

Close irrigation clamp, and then open drainage tubing clamp. (Optional: Leave clamp closed for 20-30 min if ordered. See previous Critical Decision Point.)

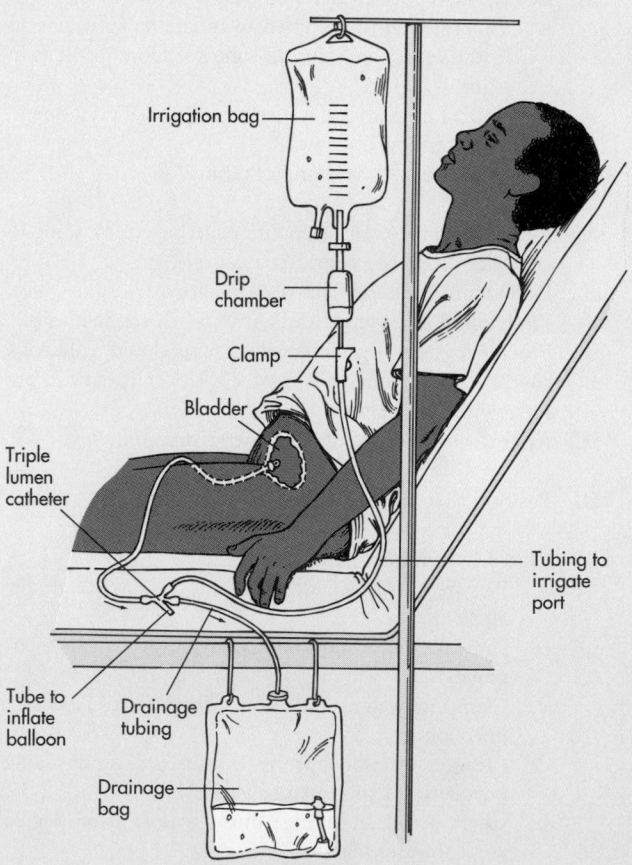

Irrigation bag

Drip chamber

Clamp

Bladder

Triple lumen catheter

Tube to inflate balloon

Drainage tubing

Drainage bag

Tubing to irrigate port

Step 12

STEPS	RATIONALE
g. For continuous drainage, calculate drip rate and adjust clamp on irrigation tubing accordingly. Be sure that clamp on drainage tubing is open, and check volume of drainage in drainage bag. Make sure drainage tubing is patent, and avoid kinks.	Ensures continuous, even irrigation of catheter system. Prevents accumulation of solution in bladder, which may cause bladder distention and possible injury.
13. Open irrigation (when double lumen catheter is in place):	
a. Open sterile irrigation tray, establish sterile field, pour required volume of sterile solution into sterile container, and replace cap on large container of solution.	Adheres to principles of surgical asepsis (see Chapter 33).
b. Apply sterile gloves.	Reduces transmission of infection.
c. Position sterile waterproof drape under catheter.	Prevents soiling of bed linens.
d. Aspirate 30 ml of solution into sterile irrigating syringe.	Prepares irrigant for instillation into catheter.
e. Move sterile collection close to client's thighs.	Prevents soiling of bed linen and prohibits reaching over sterile field.
f. Disconnect catheter from drainage tubing, allowing urine from catheter to flow into collection basin. Allow urine in tubing to flow into drainage bag. Cover end of tubing with sterile protective cap. Position tubing in a safe place.	Maintains sterility of inner aspect of catheter and drainage tubing and reduces potential of introducing pathogens into bladder.
g. Insert tip of syringe into catheter lumen, and gently instill solution.	Gentle instillation reduces incidence of bladder spasm but clears catheter of obstruction.

Critical Decision Point: If resistance is noted, do not force the irrigation.

---

h. Withdraw syringe, lower catheter, and allow solution to drain into basin. Repeat instillation until prescribed solution has been used or until drainage is clear (will depend on purpose of irrigation).	Allows drainage to flow by gravity. Provides for adequate flushing of catheter.
i. If solution does not return, have client turn onto side facing you. If changing position does not help, reinsert syringe and gently aspirate solution.	Change of position may move catheter tip in bladder, increasing likelihood that fluid instilled will flow out.
j. After irrigation is complete, remove protector cap from tubing, cleanse end with alcohol swab (or recommended agency solution), and reestablish drainage system.	Reduces entrance of microorganisms into system.
14. Reanchor catheter to client with tape or elastic tube holder.	Prevents trauma to urethral tissue
15. Assist client to comfortable position.	Promotes relaxation and rest.
16. Lower bed to lowest position. Put side rails up if appropriate.	Promotes client safety.
17. Dispose of contaminated supplies, remove gloves, and wash hands.	Prevents spread of infection.
18. Calculate fluid used to irrigate bladder and catheter and subtract from total output.	Determines accurate urinary output.
19. Assess characteristics of output: viscosity, color, and presence of matter (e.g., sediment, clots, blood).	Evaluates results of irrigation.

Recording and Reporting

- Record type and amount of irrigation solution used, amount returned as drainage, and the character of drainage.
- Record and report any findings such as complaints of bladder spasms, inability to instill fluid into bladder, and/or presence of blood clots.

Home Care Considerations

- If client is discharged with indwelling catheter and requires bladder irrigations, either the client and or the family must be properly instructed.
- In the home it is most likely that open irrigation will be required. As this method carries the highest risk of contamination, the nurse must assess the level of understanding of surgical asepsis by the client and family.

client's thighs or over a male client's thighs. The nurse inserts the syringe into the injection port. Most ports are self-sealing and require that only the tip of the syringe be inserted. The nurse slowly withdraws all of the solution to deflate the balloon totally. If a portion of the solution remains, the partially inflated balloon will traumatize the urethral canal as the catheter is removed. After deflation the nurse explains that the client may feel a burning sensation as the catheter is withdrawn. The nurse then pulls the catheter out smoothly and slowly.

It is normal for the client to experience some dysuria, especially if the catheter has been in place several days or weeks. The catheter causes inflammation of the urethral canal. Until the bladder regains full tone, the client may also experience frequency of urination or urinary retention.

The nurse assesses the client's urinary function by noting the first voiding after catheter removal and documents the time and amount of voiding for the next 24 hours. If amounts are small, frequent assessment of bladder distention is necessary. If over 8 hours elapse without voiding, it may become necessary to reinsert the catheter.

Alternatives to Urethral Catheterization.   To avoid the risks associated with catheters inserted through the urethra, there are two alternatives for urinary drainage.

Suprapubic Catheterization.   Suprapubic catheterization involves surgical placement of a catheter through the abdominal wall above the symphysis pubis and into the urinary bladder. The physician performs the procedure under local or general anesthesia. The catheter is anchored in place with sutures, a commercially prepared body seal, or both. Urine drains into a urinary drainage bag. The suprapubic catheter is relatively painless and reduces the incidence of infection commonly seen with retention catheters. Women who have undergone a vaginal hysterectomy may also benefit temporarily from the insertion of a suprapubic catheter after surgery.

The suprapubic catheter can become blocked by sediment, clots, or the abdominal wall itself. Nurses must monitor the client's I&O carefully, observe for signs of kidney infection (e.g., flank tenderness, chills, and fever), and monitor the appearance of urine. Spread of infection to the kidneys may indicate removal of the catheter. Adequate fluid intake will help to minimize risk of blockage by sediment or infection due to stagnation. The suprapubic catheter must remain patent at all times. The nurse also administers skin care around the insertion site.

Condom Catheter.   The second alternative to catheterization is the condom catheter (Skill 44-5). It is suitable for incontinent or comatose men who still have complete and spontaneous bladder emptying. The condom is a soft, pliable, rubber sheath that slips over the penis. It may be worn at night only or continuously, depending on the client's needs. There are three general methods of securing the condom catheter. One method uses a strip of elastic tape or rubber that encircles the top of the condom to secure it in place. Another condom uses a self-adhesive inside the sheath. The third method uses an inflatable ring within the condom to secure placement. Care must be taken to ensure that whatever type or size is used, blood supply to the penis is not impaired. Standard adhesive tape should never be used to secure a condom catheter because it does not expand with change in penis size and is painful to remove.

The end of the condom fits into a plastic drainage tubing. A drainage bag can be attached to the side of the bed or strapped to the client's leg. The condom catheter itself poses little risk of infection. Infections with condom catheters usually result from buildup of secretions around the urethra, trauma to the urethral meatus, or buildup of pressure in the outflow tubing.

If the condom catheter is made of opaque material, the nurse should remove the condom catheter daily to check for skin irritation. Some new condom catheters are more transparent, and the skin may be observed through them more easily. With each catheter change the nurse cleans the urethral meatus and penis thoroughly. Twisting of the condom at the drainage tube attachment irritates the skin and obstructs urine outflow. The drainage tubing must be checked often for patency.

For a man with a retracted penis, maintaining a conventional condom catheter may prove difficult. Special devices are available to help alleviate this problem (Figure 44-15). Manufacturers' guidelines for product application should be consulted.

There are no collection devices for women as effective as the condom catheter, so frequently the only incontinent devices used are pads and protective clothing. To maintain dignity, pads and protective clothing should not be referred to as adult diapers and should be changed frequently to control odor. These devices should be only used temporarily while treatment methods are being used to minimize or prevent episodes of incontinence. Clients should be monitored frequently and good skin care given to prevent irritation caused by urine.

Restorative Care.   The client may regain normal urinary voiding function through special activities such as bladder retraining or habit training. If either of those activities is not possible, then self-catheterization may restore a measure of control to the client.

Strengthening Pelvic Floor Muscles.   Clients who have difficulty starting or stopping the urine stream may benefit from **pelvic floor exercises** (PFEs). Pelvic floor exercises, also known as Kegel exercises, improve the strength of pelvic floor muscles and consist of repetitive contractions of muscle groups (UIGP, 1996). A client begins these exercises during voiding to learn the technique. They are then practiced at nonvoiding times. Improvement is usu-

Applying a Condom Catheter | Skill 44-5

Delegation Considerations

The skill of applying a condom catheter can be delegated to assistive personnel.

- Ensure that caregiver knows standard precautions guidelines relating to body fluids.
- Caution caregiver to be sensitive to the privacy needs of clients.

- Clarify that skin of penile shaft is intact and free from swelling, redness, or open lesions before condom catheter is applied.
- Clarify the caregiver's understanding of how to apply the adhesive strip that secures the condom catheter.

EQUIPMENT

- Condom catheter kit
  - Rubber/latex condom sheath (proper size) (Check for possible rubber or latex allergy)
  - Strip of elastic tape (if needed)
  - Skin preparation solution or swab
- Urinary collection bag with tubing or leg bag with straps

- Basin with warm water and soap
- Towels and washcloths
- Nonsterile disposable gloves
- Bath blanket
- Scissors and/or safety razor

STEPS	RATIONALE
1. Assess urinary elimination patterns, client's ability to voluntarily urinate, and continence.	Clients who are incontinent are at high risk of skin breakdown.
2. Assess mental status of client so appropriate teaching related to condom catheter can be implemented.	Some male clients may be incontinent only at night. Teaching can be implemented to instruct client on self-application.
3. Assess condition of penis.	Provides a baseline to compare changes in condition of skin after condom application.
4. Assess client's knowledge of the purpose of a condom catheter.	Reveals need for client instruction.
5. Explain procedure to client.	Reduces anxiety and promotes cooperation.
6. Arrange for extra nursing personnel to assist with moving dependent client.	Promotes client safety and proper use of body mechanics by nurse.
7. Wash hands.	Reduces transmission of microorganisms.
8. Provide privacy by closing door or bed curtains.	Maintains client's self-esteem.
9. Raise bed to appropriate working height. Raise side rail on opposite side of bed, and lower side on working side.	Promotes use of good body mechanics and client safety.
10. Assist client into supine position. Place bath blanket over upper torso. Fold bedsheets so that lower extremities are covered; only genitalia should be exposed.	Promotes client comfort and prevents unnecessary exposure of body parts.
11. Prepare urinary drainage collection or leg bag for connection to condom catheter. Clamp off all drainage exit ports. Secure collection bag to bed frame; bring drainage tubing up through side rails onto bed. Prepare leg bag for connection to condom if necessary.	Provides easy access to drainage equipment after condom is applied.
12. Apply disposable gloves. Provide perineal care (see Skill 44-3), and dry thoroughly.	Removes irritating secretions. Rubber/latex sheath rolls onto dry skin more easily. Be aware of possible latex allergy!

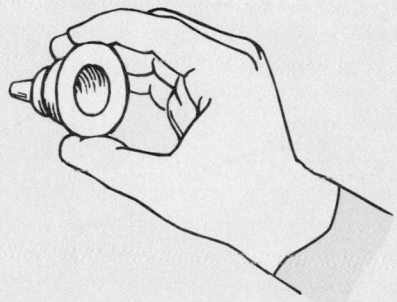 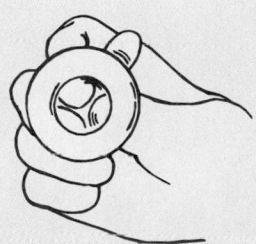 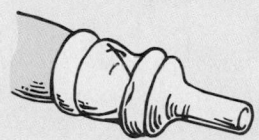

Step 15

STEPS	RATIONALE
13. Clip hair at base of penis. In some cases shaving the hair at the base of the penis may be necessary.	Hair adheres to condom and is pulled during condom removal or may get caught as condom catheter is applied.
14. Apply skin preparation to shaft of penis, and allow to dry. If client is uncircumscised, return foreskin to normal position.	Prepares penis for easy condom placement.
15. With nondominant hand, grasp penis along shaft. With dominant hand hold condom sheath at tip of penis, and smoothly roll sheath onto penis (see illustrations).	Prepares penis for easy condom placement.

Critical Decision Point: Allow 2.5 to 5 cm (1 to 2 in) of space between tip of glans penis and end of condom catheter (see illustration).

STEPS	RATIONALE
16. Spiral wrap penile shaft with strip of elastic adhesive. With some brands of catheters the adhesive is applied before the condom is applied. Do not use any tape because it may impede circulation.	Condom must be secured so that it is snug and will stay on but not so tight as to cause constriction of blood flow. Strip should be spiral wrapped and not overlap itself. Tapes other than those provided by manufacturer will not provide the flexibility needed for the spiral wrap and may impair circulation to the penis.
17. Connect drainage tubing to end of condom catheter. Be sure condom is not twisted. Catheter can be attached to large-volume bag or leg bag (see illustrations).	Allows urine to be collected and measured. Keeps client dry. Twisted condom obstructs urine flow.
18. Place excess coiling of tubing on bed, and secure to bottom sheet.	Promotes free drainage of urine.
19. Place client in a safe, comfortable position. Lower bed, and place side rails accordingly.	Promotes safety and comfort.
20. Dispose of contaminated supplies. Remove gloves, and wash hands.	Reduces spread of microorganisms.
21. Observe urinary drainage.	Determines if normal voiding is occurring.
22. Inspect penis with condom catheter in place within 30 min after application. Look for swelling and discoloration, and ask client if there is any discomfort.	Determines if catheter has been applied incorrectly.
23. Remove and change condom and inspect skin on penile shaft for signs of breakdown or irritation at least daily when hygiene is performed and when condom is reapplied.	Indicates if condom or urine is causing irritation or if adhesive is too restrictive. Frequent assessment of circulation of glans penis is important to determine if condom has been applied too tightly.

Recording and Reporting
- Record and report pertinent information: condom application, condition of skin, voiding pattern.
- Monitor I&O as indicated.

Home Care Considerations
- If leg bag is used, assess leg for circulatory impairment. Switch to a large-volume drainage bag at night.
- Teach client that a collection bag that fills completely may put unnecessary tension on the catheter and contribute to problems keeping the catheter intact.

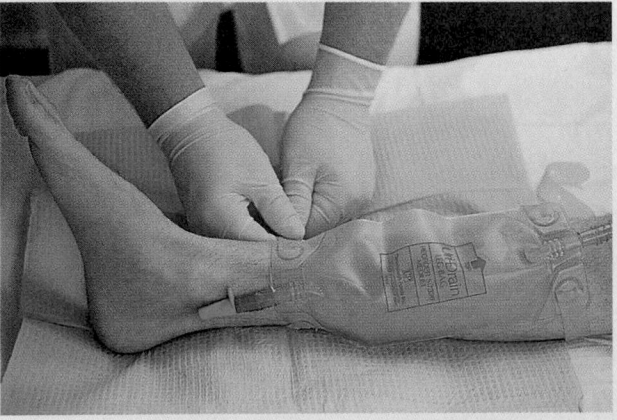

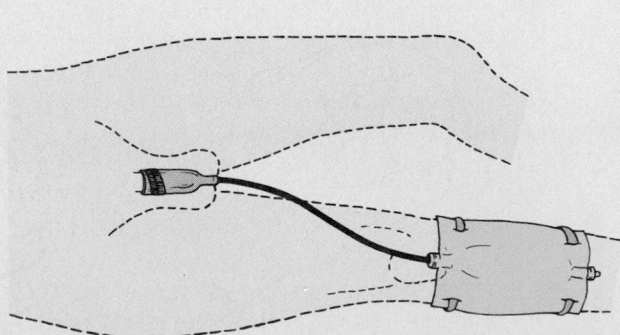

Step 17

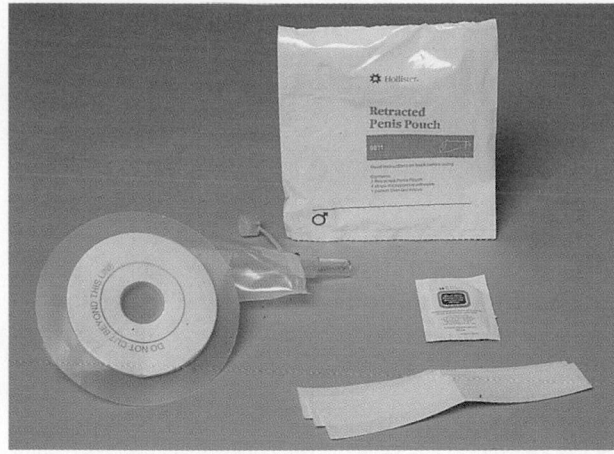

Figure 44-15 Retracted penis pouch external urinary device.

ally gradual. Clients should be alert and motivated to perform the exercises. The client must continue to use these exercises to maintain effectiveness (see Box 44-8).

Bladder Retraining. The goal of bladder retraining is to restore a normal pattern of voiding by inhibiting or stimulating voiding (UIGP, 1996). For bladder retraining to be successful, clients must be alert and physically able to follow a training program. The program includes education, scheduled voiding, and positive reinforcement. Bladder function may be temporarily disrupted after a period of catheterization.

The nurse first assesses the client's current pattern of urination. This information allows the nurse to plan a program that often takes 2 weeks or more to learn. Although the program may be started in the hospital or rehabilitation unit it may need to be continued in an extended care facility or at home. If the client has an underlying UTI, this should be treated at the same time. The following measures may help the incontinent client gain control over urination and are part of restorative and rehabilitative care:

Learning exercises to strengthen the pelvic floor

Initiating a toileting schedule on awakening, at least every 2 hours during the day and evening, before getting into bed, and every 4 hours at night (individualizing time frame as needed)

Using methods to initiate voiding (e.g., running water and stroking the inner thigh)

Using methods to relax to aid complete bladder emptying (e.g., reading and deep breathing)

Never ignoring the urge to void (only if problem involves infrequent voidings that result in retention)

Minimizing tea, coffee, alcohol, and other caffeine drinks

Taking prescribed diuretic medication or fluids that increase diuresis (such as tea or coffee) early in the morning

Progressively lengthening or shortening periods between voiding as appropriate for control of specific cause of incontinence

Offering protective undergarments to contain urine and reduce the client's embarrassment (not diapers)

Following a weight-control program if obesity is a problem

Providing positive reinforcement when continence is maintained

These guidelines help the client to establish a routine for voiding and control factors that might increase the number of incontinent episodes.

Habit Training. A client with functional incontinence may benefit from habit training, which helps clients improve voluntary control over urination. A flexible toileting schedule based on the client's pattern is established.

The nurse helps the client to the bathroom before incontinent episodes occur. Fluids and medications are timed to prevent interference with the toileting schedule. Clients with moderate or severe mental or physical dysfunction can benefit. When combined with positive reinforcement to reward successful voiding, this approach is also called prompted voiding.

Self-Catheterization. Some clients with chronic disorders such as spinal cord injury learn to perform self-catheterization. The client must be able to physically manipulate equipment and assume a position for successful catheterization. The nurse teaches the client the structures of the urinary tract, clean versus sterile technique, the importance of adequate fluid intake, and the frequency of self-catheterization. Generally, the goal is to have clients perform self-catheterizations every 6 to 8 hours, but the schedule should be individualized.

Maintenance of Skin Integrity. The normal acidity of urine is irritating to skin. Urine allowed to be in contact with the skin becomes alkaline, causing encrustations or precipitates to collect on the skin, fostering breakdown. Continuous exposure of the perineal area or skin around an ostomy leads to gradual maceration and excoriation (see Chapter 47). Washing with mild soap and warm water is the best way to remove urine from skin. Body lotion keeps skin moisturized and petroleum-based ointments provide a barrier to the urine. Clients who wet their clothing should receive partial baths and dry clothing after voiding.

When the skin becomes irritated or inflamed, the physician may prescribe a cream or spray containing steroids (e.g., Kenalog) to reduce inflammation. If fungal growth develops, the antifungal drug nystatin (Mycostatin), available in cream or powder, is effective.

For clients with urinary diversion special nursing care is required to prevent complications related to the collection devices. It is important that the device fit snugly against the skin surface to prevent constant exposure to urine. Urine that remains in contact with the skin causes breakdown and denuding of the skin surface. When this happens, the device will not adhere and leakage becomes a major problem. Urine is constantly produced so the pouch may need frequent emptying throughout the day and may need to be hooked to a larger drainage bag for nighttime use.

The client with an ostomy has a special hygiene problem because urine drains continuously from the ostomy site. Skin barriers provide a layer of protection between the client's skin and ostomy pouch. It is important that the appliance fit snugly against the skin's surface around the stoma to prevent constant exposure to urine. Abdominal skin that remains in contact with urine for extended periods of time will break down. If breakdown occurs, the pouch system will not adhere to the denuded tissue, and leakage becomes a major problem, causing additional skin breakdown. Urine is constantly produced, so the pouch may need frequent emptying throughout the day and may need to be connected to a larger drainage bag for nighttime use.

Promotion of Comfort.   Clients with urinary alterations become uncomfortable as a result of the symptoms of urinary problems. Frequent or unpredictable voiding, dysuria, and painful distention are sources of discomfort.

The incontinent client gains comfort from having clean, dry clothing. When stress incontinence is the problem, a protective pad offers protection against soiling. Wet clothing adheres to the skin and can cause rubbing and irritation.

Dysuria may be relieved by giving urinary analgesics that act on the urethral and bladder mucosa. Phenazopyridine (Pyridium) helps relieve dysuria, burning, and itching. This medication may also be found with sulfonamide antibiotics in preparations such as Azo-Gantanol and Azo-Gantrisin. The sulfonamide provides additional antibacterial action. Clients taking drugs with phenazopyridine should be aware that their urine may appear orange. They must drink large amounts of fluids to prevent toxicity from the sulfonamides and to maintain optimal flow through the urinary system.

If the client has local discomfort from an inflamed urethra, a warm sitz bath may provide pain relief. The warm water soothes inflamed tissues near the urethral meatus by improving blood supply. The client is often relaxed after a sitz bath, so voiding occurs easily. Pain of distention cannot be relieved unless the client is able to empty the bladder. Interventions that stimulate micturition or intermittant catheterization may be the only sources of pain relief.

EVALUATION

Client Care.   The client is the best source of evaluation of outcomes and responses to nursing care (see Figure 44-16). Although most clients will be able to assess for themselves whether their goals have been met, the nurse will also evaluate the effectiveness of nursing interventions through comparisons with baseline data. The nurse evaluates for change in the client's voiding pattern, presence of urinary tract alteration, and physical condition. Outcomes are compared with expected outcomes to determine the client's health status. Continuous evaluation allows the nurse to determine whether new or revised therapies are required or if any new nursing diagnoses have developed.

Client Expectations.   If the nurse has developed a trust relationship with a client, indications of the client's degree of satisfaction with his or her care is evident. The client may smile or nod in appreciation. However, the nurse needs to confirm whether the client's expectations have been met to full satisfaction. The nurse may need to ask specifically about the client's degree of urinary control and comfort. If just asked "How are you feeling today?" the client may reply with a noncommittal "OK." The nurse needs specific information about how well an intervention has met the need in order to continue or revise the plan of care. The nurse can also assist the client in redefining unrealistic client goals when an impairment in function is not likely to be altered as completely as the client might like.

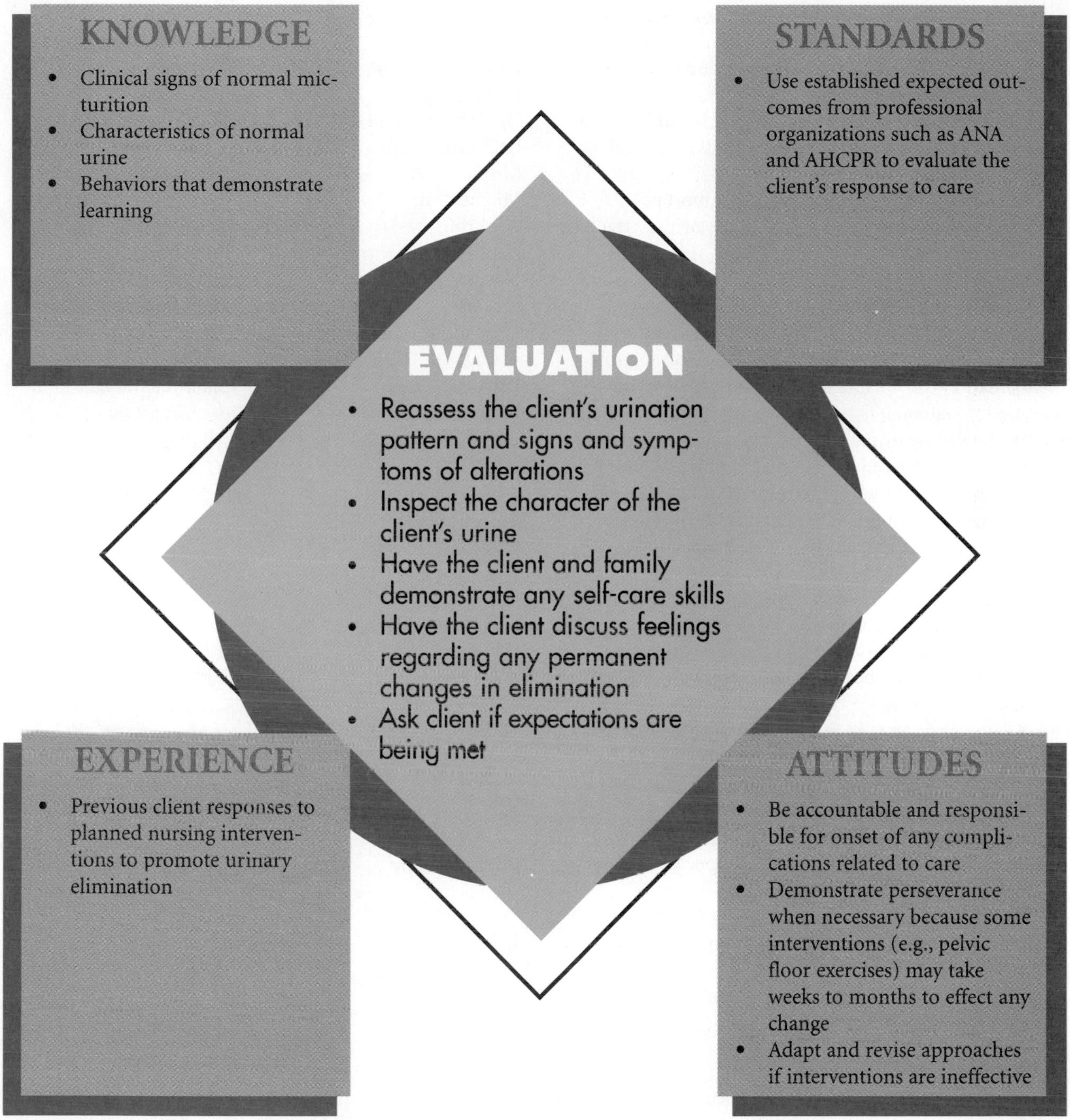

KNOWLEDGE

- Clinical signs of normal micturition
- Characteristics of normal urine
- Behaviors that demonstrate learning

STANDARDS

- Use established expected outcomes from professional organizations such as ANA and AHCPR to evaluate the client's response to care

EVALUATION

- Reassess the client's urination pattern and signs and symptoms of alterations
- Inspect the character of the client's urine
- Have the client and family demonstrate any self-care skills
- Have the client discuss feelings regarding any permanent changes in elimination
- Ask client if expectations are being met

EXPERIENCE

- Previous client responses to planned nursing interventions to promote urinary elimination

ATTITUDES

- Be accountable and responsible for onset of any complications related to care
- Demonstrate perseverance when necessary because some interventions (e.g., pelvic floor exercises) may take weeks to months to effect any change
- Adapt and revise approaches if interventions are ineffective

Figure 44-16 *Synthesis Model for Urinary Elimination Evaluation Phase.*

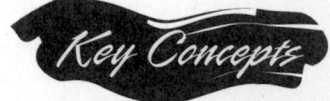

Key Concepts

- The act of micturition or voiding is influenced by voluntary control from higher brain centers and involuntary control from the spinal cord.
- Symptoms common to urinary disturbances include urgency, dysuria, polyuria, oliguria, and difficulty in starting the urinary stream.
- When collected properly, a clean-voided urine specimen does not contain bacteria from the urethral meatus.
- A client can better understand the importance of perineal hygiene by knowing that the urinary tract is normally sterile.
- Methods of promoting the micturition reflex assist clients in sensing the urge to urinate and controlling urethral sphincter relaxation.
- An increased fluid intake results in increased urine formation that flushes particles and solutes from the urinary system.
- An indwelling urinary catheter remains in the bladder for an extended period, making the risk of infection greater than with intermittent catheterization.
- Because urine drains almost continuously from a ureterostomy, there is a risk of skin breakdown around a stoma site.
- A primary function of the elimination process is fluid and electrolyte balance.
- Catheter irrigation becomes necessary when the catheter becomes occluded with sediment or blood clots.
- A catheter drainage system should be positioned to allow free drainage of urine by gravity.
- Condom catheters are applied snugly but not so tightly as to constrict blood flow.
- Incontinence is classified as functional, overflow, stress, urge, or total. Each type has specific nursing interventions.
- Specific guidelines for catheter selection should be followed so that the catheter does not cause harm during insertion.
- Alterations in the urinary system can cause alterations in other organ systems.

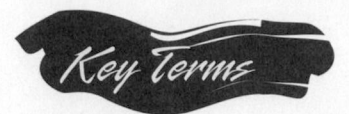

Key Terms

Anuria, *p. 1387*
Bacteriuria, *p. 1390*
Catheterization, *p. 1412*
Diuresis, *p. 1389*
Dysuria, *p. 1391*
Erythropoietin, *p. 1385*
Hematuria, *p. 1391*
Ketonuria, *p. 1402*
Meatus, *p. 1386*
Micturition, *p. 1386*
Nephron, *p. 1384*
Nephrostomy, *p. 1392*
Nocturia, *p. 1388*
Oliguria, *p. 1387*
Pelvic floor exercises, *p. 1428*
Polyuria, *p. 1389*
Proteinuria, *p. 1384*

Pyelonephritis, *p. 1391*
Reflex bladder, *p. 1387*
Renal calculus, *p. 1386*
Renal replacement therapies, *p. 1388*
Renin, *p. 1385*
Residual urine, *p. 1388*
Specific gravity, *p. 1402*
Stoma, *p. 1389*
Uremic syndrome, *p. 1387*
Ureterostomy, *p. 1392*
Urinalysis, *p. 1402*
Urinary diversion, *p. 1389*
Urinary frequency, *p. 1388*
Urinary incontinence, *p. 1391*
Urinary retention, *p. 1390*
Urosepsis, *p. 1390*

Critical Thinking Exercises

1. Mr. Miller is a 75-year-old widower who has had prostate surgery for benign prostatic hypertrophy. He thought his problems would be over, but now he is experiencing continual dribbling of urine. He has been attempting to deal with the problem by using an absorbant pad in his underwear but he feels as though everyone knows his problem. The embarrassment of having an odor often keeps him at home. He has given up attending his senior citizen center.
   a. How can the nurse help him regain control of his urinary elimination?
   b. What are the actual nursing diagnoses that apply to Mr. Miller?
   c. For one diagnosis give one goal/outcome and two nursing interventions.
2. Mrs. Luis is a 37-year-old woman who has been admitted with hematuria. She has noticed blood in her urine for a week, but she was hoping it would go away. She is to undergo a cystoscopy in 4 hours.
   a. What is the purpose of the cystoscopy?
   b. What nursing care is needed before she goes to the operating room?
   c. Give at least two nursing responsibilities for care of the client after undergoing a cystectomy.
3. Mrs. Joseph is a 70-year-old woman with cognitive changes associated with Alzheimer's disease. Her daughter, with whom she lives, has brought her to her family practitioner's office. You are the family nurse practitioner in the practice. As you assess Mrs. Joseph, you ask her daughter how she is coping with her mother. The daughter replies that her mother does not seem to remember how to go to the bathroom. Mrs. Joseph will go into the bathroom but forget to pull down her underwear before going to the bathroom. After the incident her mother becomes upset and blames the daughter for her wetness. She asks you for suggestions on how to manage, as she noticed that her mother's perineal skin is reddened and sore. What assessments does the nurse need to complete before planning interventions for Mrs. Joseph's care?

References

Ackley BJ, Ludwig GB: *Nursing diagnosis handbook: a guide to planning care,* St. Louis, 1997, Mosby.

Beare PG, Myers JL: *Adult health nursing,* ed 3, St. Louis, 1998, Mosby.

Brundage DJ: *Renal disorders,* St. Louis, 1992, Mosby.

Buscheller CD, Bernstein J: Urinary tract infection, *Med Clin North Am* 81(3):1997.

Giger JN, Davidhizer RE: *Transcultural nursing: assessment and intervention,* ed 3, St. Louis, 1999, Mosby.

Hutchinson S, Leger-Krall S, Wilson HS: Toileting: a biobehavioral challenge in Alzheimer's dementia care, *J Gerontol Nurs* 22(10):18, 1996.

Jackson, B, Hicks, LE: Effect of cranberry juice on urinary pH in older adults, *Home Health Nurse* 15(3):198, 1997.

Kim MJ, McFarland GK, McLane AM: *Pocket guide to nursing diagnoses,* ed 7, St. Louis, 1997, Mosby.

Lewis S, Collier IC, Heitkemper MM: *Medical-surgical nursing,* ed 4, St. Louis, 1996.

McCance KL, Huether SE: *Pathophysiology: the biological basis for disease in adults and children,* St. Louis, 1998, Mosby.

McCloskey JC, Bulechek GM: *Nursing interventions classification (NIC),* ed 3, St. Louis, 2000, Mosby.

McKenry LM, Salerno E: *Mosby's pharmacology in nursing,* ed 20, St. Louis, 1998, Mosby.

Pagana KD, Pagana TJ: *Mosby's diagnostic and laboratory test reference,* ed 4, St. Louis, 1999, Mosby.

Skoner MM, Thompson WD, Caron VA: Factors associated with risk of stress urinary incontinence in women, *Nurs Res* 43(5):301, 1994.

Sueppel C: Rapid or slow decompression, *Urol Nurs* 15(2):64, 1995.

Travis SS, Lampley-Dallas V: Nursing management of elderly patients with asymptomatic bacteriuria, *Geriatr Nurs* 18(3):103, 1997.

Urinary Incontinence Guideline Panel (UIGP): *Urinary incontinence in adults: clinical practice guideline,* ed 2, Rockville, Md, 1996, Agency for Health Care Policy and Research.

Williams M and others: Urinary retention in hospitalized women, *J Gerontol Nurs* 19(2):7, 1993.

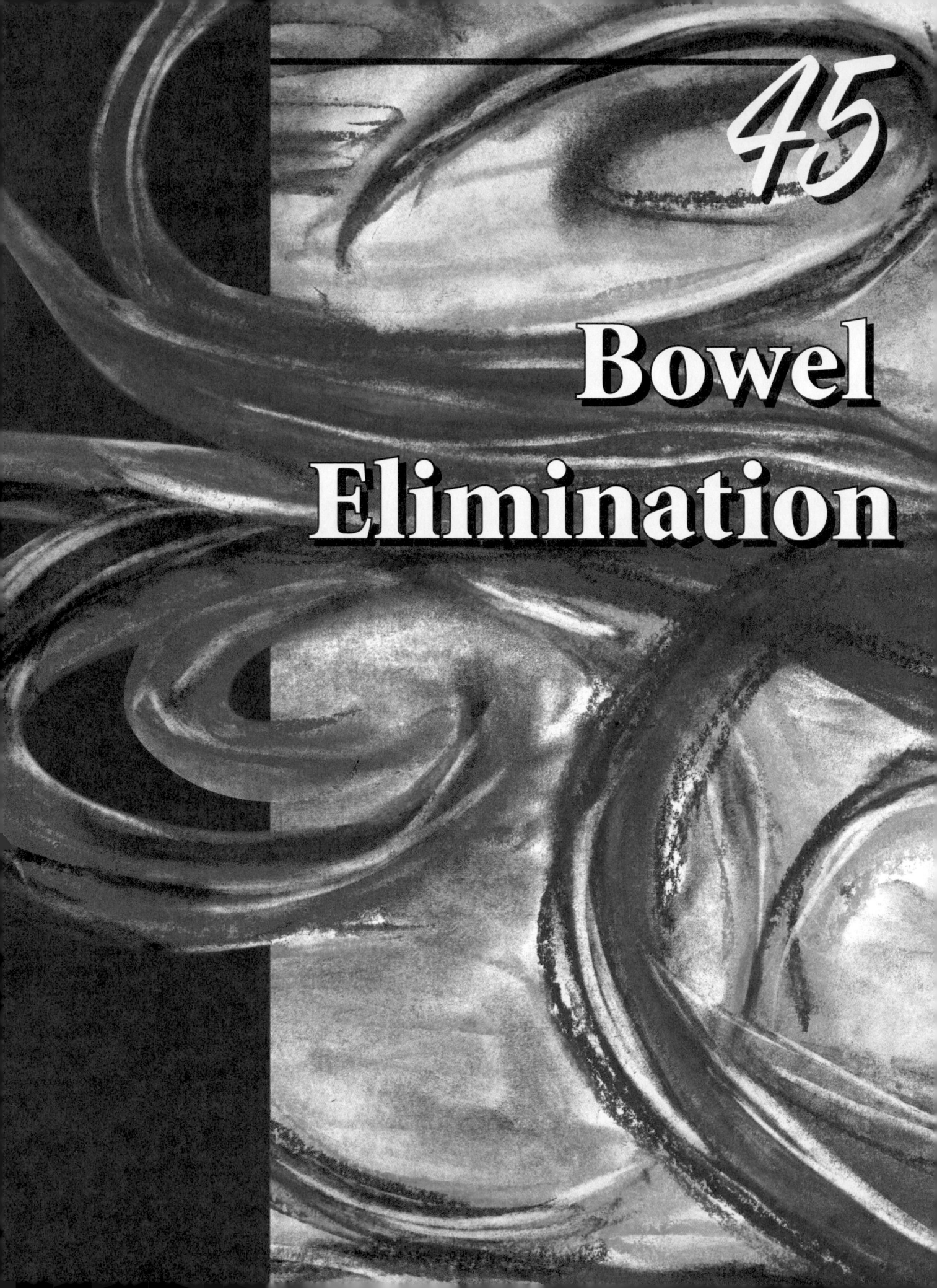

45

Bowel Elimination

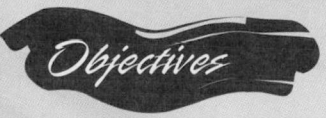

Mastery of content in this chapter will enable the student to:

- Define the key terms listed.
- Discuss the role of gastrointestinal organs in digestion and elimination.
- Describe four functions of the large intestine.
- Explain the physiological aspects of normal defecation.
- Discuss psychological and physiological factors that influence the elimination process.
- Describe common physiological alterations in elimination.
- Assess a client's elimination pattern.
- List nursing diagnoses related to alterations in elimination.
- Describe nursing implications for common diagnostic examinations of the gastrointestinal tract.
- Administer an enema.
- List nursing measures that promote normal elimination.
- List nursing measures included in bowel training.
- Discuss the relationship between the structure and function of bowel diversions and nursing care required.
- Utilize critical thinking in the provision of care to clients with alterations in bowel elimination.

Regular elimination of bowel waste products is essential for normal body functioning. Alterations in elimination are often early signs or symptoms of problems within the gastrointestinal or other body systems. Because bowel function depends on the balance of several factors, elimination patterns and habits vary among individuals.

To manage clients' elimination problems, the nurse must understand normal elimination and factors that promote, impede, or cause alterations in elimination. Supportive nursing care respects the client's privacy and emotional needs. Measures designed to promote normal elimination should also minimize discomfort.

Scientific Knowledge Base

The gastrointestinal (GI) tract is a series of hollow mucous membrane-lined muscular organs. The purposes of these organs are to absorb fluid and nutrients, prepare food for absorption and use by the body's cells, and provide for temporary storage of feces (Figure 45-1). The volume of fluids absorbed by the GI tract is high, making fluid balance a key function of the GI system. In addition to ingested fluids and foods, the GI tract also receives many secretions from organs such as the gallbladder and the pancreas. Any condition that seriously impairs normal absorption or secretion of GI fluids could cause fluid imbalance.

The authors acknowledge the contribution of Dr. Elizabeth A. Ayello to this chapter in the previous edition of this text.

MOUTH

Digestion begins in the mouth, where mechanical and chemical breakdown of nutrients occurs. The teeth **masticate** (chew) food, breaking it down to a suitable size for swallowing. Salivary secretions contain enzymes, such as ptyalin, that initiate digestion of certain food elements. Saliva dilutes and softens the **bolus** of food in the mouth for easier swallowing.

ESOPHAGUS

As food enters the upper esophagus, it passes through the upper esophageal sphincter, which is a circular muscle that prevents air from entering the esophagus and food from **refluxing** (moving backward) into the throat. The bolus of food travels approximately 25 cm (10 inches) down the esophagus. Food is pushed along by slow **peristalsis** produced by alternating involuntary contractions and relaxations of smooth muscle. As a portion of the esophagus contracts above the food bolus, the circular muscle below (or in front) of the bolus relaxes. This alternate contraction-relaxation of smooth muscle propels food toward the next wave (Figure 45-2).

In 15 seconds the bolus of food moves down the esophagus and reaches the lower esophageal sphincter. The lower esophageal sphincter, or cardiac sphincter, lies between the esophagus and stomach and prevents backward movement of fluids from the stomach to the esophagus. Factors influencing cardiac sphincter pressure include antacids, which minimize reflux, and fatty foods and nicotine, which increase reflux.

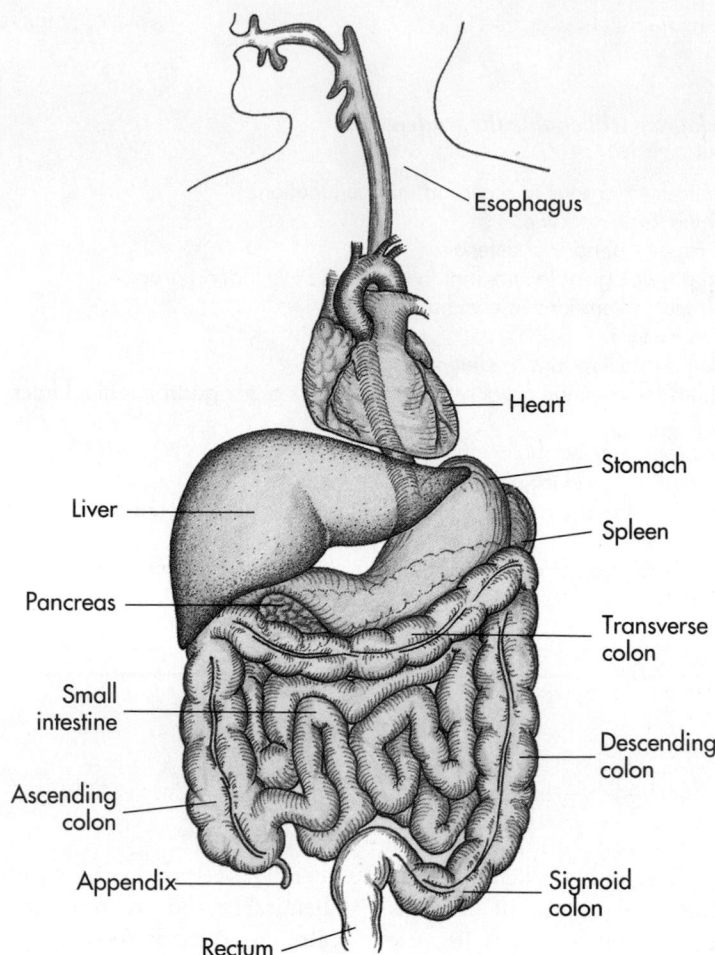

Figure 45-1   Organs of the gastrointestinal tract (with the heart as a reference point).

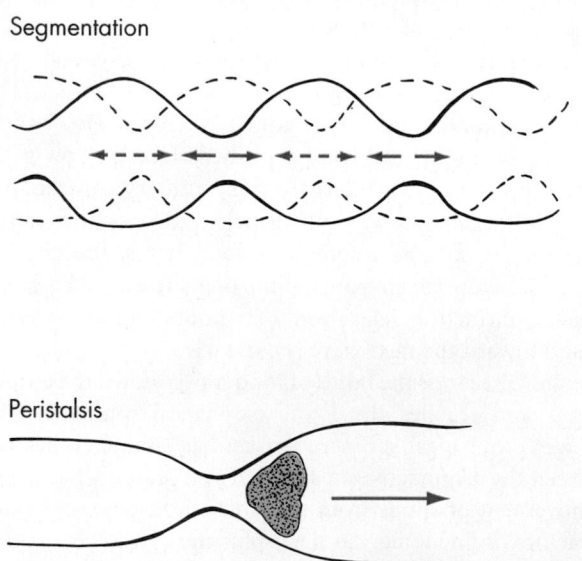

Figure 45-2   Segmented and peristaltic waves.

STOMACH

In the stomach, food is temporarily stored and mechanically and chemically broken down for digestion and absorption (see Chapter 43). The stomach secretes hydrochloric acid (HCl), mucus, the enzyme pepsin, and intrinsic factor. The concentration of HCl influences stomach acidity and the body's acid-base balance (see Chapter 40) and helps mix and break down food. Prostaglandins assist in the formation of mucus, which protects the stomach mucosa from acidity and enzyme activity. Pepsin digests proteins, although not much digestion occurs in the stomach. Intrinsic factor is the essential component needed for vitamin B_{12} absorption in the intestine and subsequent normal red blood cell formation. Lack of this intrinsic factor results in pernicious anemia.

Before food leaves the stomach, it is changed into a semifluid material called **chyme.** Chyme is more easily digested and absorbed than solid food. Clients who have portions of their stomachs removed, have had a gastroplasty, or have rapid stomach emptying (as with gastritis) may have serious digestive problems because food is not broken down into chyme.

SMALL INTESTINE

During normal digestion, chyme leaves the stomach and enters the small intestine. The small intestine is a tube about 2.5 cm (1 inch) in diameter and 6 m (20 feet) long. It contains three divisions: duodenum, jejunum, and ileum. Chyme mixes with digestive enzymes (e.g., bile and amylase) while traveling through the small intestine. Segmentation (alternating contraction and relaxation of smooth muscle) churns the chyme, further breaking down food for digestion (see Figure 45-2). These alternating contractions occur about a dozen times a minute. As chyme mixes, forward peristaltic movement temporarily ceases, permitting absorption. Chyme travels slowly through the small intestine to allow absorption of nutrients and electrolytes.

Enzymes from the pancreas (e.g., amylase) and bile from the gallbladder are released into the duodenum. The enzymes in the small intestine break down fats, proteins, and carbohydrates into basic elements (see Chapter 43). Nutrients are almost entirely absorbed by the duodenum and jejunum. The ileum absorbs certain vitamins, iron, and bile salts. If its function is impaired, the digestive process is greatly altered. For example, inflammation, surgical resection, or obstruction can disrupt peristalsis, reduce the area of absorption, or block passage of chyme.

LARGE INTESTINE

The lower GI tract is called the large intestine (**colon**) because it is larger in diameter than the small intestine. However, its length of 1.5 to 1.8 m (5 to 6 feet) is much shorter. The large intestine is divided into the cecum, colon, and rectum (Figure 45-3). It is responsible for the absorption of water and is the primary organ of bowel elimination.

Cecum.
Unabsorbed chyme enters the large intestine at the cecum through the ileocecal valve. This valve is a circular muscle layer that prevents colon contents from **regurgitating** and returning to the small intestine. Located at the end of the cecum is the appendix. Inflammation of this area can result in blockage of the appendix, leading to appendicitis.

Colon.
Although watery chyme enters the colon, the volume of water lessens as chyme moves along it. The colon is divided into the ascending, transverse, descending, and sigmoid colon. The colon is made of muscular tissue, which allows it to accommodate and thus eliminate large quantities of waste.

The colon has four interrelated functions: absorption, protection, secretion, and elimination. A large volume of water and significant amounts of sodium and chloride are absorbed by the colon daily. As food passes through the

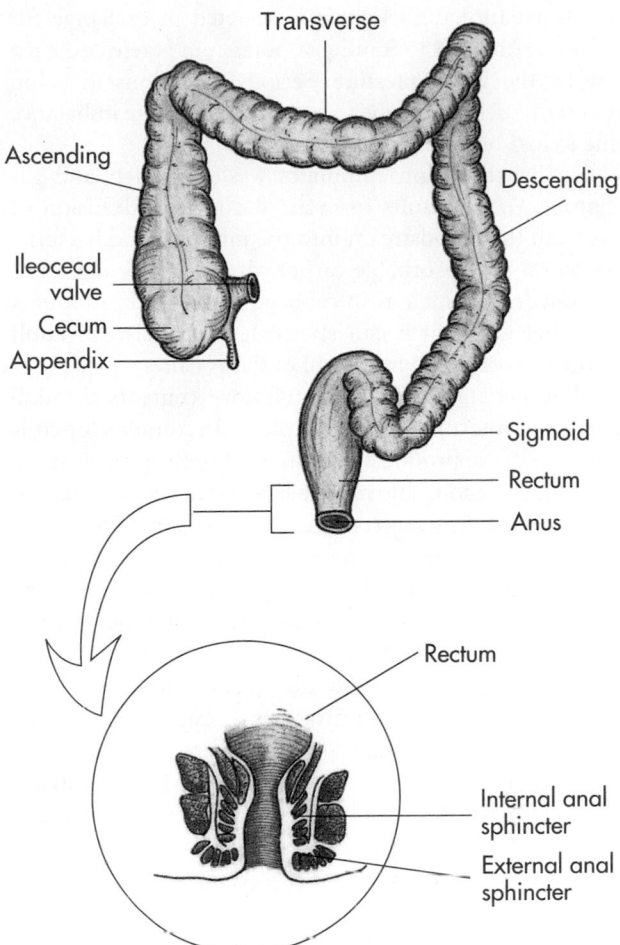

Figure 45-3   Divisions of the large intestine.

colon, **haustral contractions** occur. These are similar to segmental contractions of the small intestine but last longer, up to 5 minutes. The contractions produce large sacs in the colon's wall, providing a large surface area for absorption.

As much as 2.5 L of water can be absorbed by the colon in 24 hours. On the average, 55 mEq of sodium and 23 mEq of chloride are absorbed daily. The amount of water absorbed from chyme depends on the speed at which colonic contents move. Chyme is normally a soft, formed mass. If the speed of peristaltic contractions is abnormally fast, there is less time for water to be absorbed and the stool will be watery. If peristaltic contractions slow down, water continues to be absorbed and a hard mass of stool forms, resulting in constipation.

The colon protects itself by releasing a supply of mucus. Mucus is normally clear to opaque with a stringy consistency. Mucus lubricates the colon, preventing trauma to its inner walls. Lubrication is especially important near the distal end of the colon, where contents become more dry and hard. The secretory function of the colon aids in electrolyte balance. Bicarbonate is secreted in exchange for chloride. About 4 to 9 mEq of potassium is released each day by the large intestine. Serious alterations in colon function, such as diarrhea, can cause electrolyte imbalance due to loss of potassium and chloride.

Finally, the colon eliminates waste products and gas (**flatus**). Flatus results from air swallowing, diffusion of gas from the bloodstream into the intestine, and bacterial action on nonabsorbable carbohydrates. Fermentation of carbohydrates (such as in cabbage and onions) produces intestinal gas, which can stimulate peristalsis. An adult normally forms 400 to 700 ml of flatus daily.

Slow peristaltic contractions move contents through the colon. Intestinal content is the main stimulus for contraction. Waste products and gas exert pressure against the walls of the colon. The muscle layer stretches, stimulating the reflex that initiates contraction. Mass peristaltic movements push undigested food toward the rectum. These movements occur only three or four times daily, unlike the frequent peristaltic waves in the small intestine (usually heard during auscultation).

When these mass peristaltic movements occur, large segments of the colon contract as a result of gastrocolic and duodenocolic reflex responses. These occur when the stomach or duodenum is filled with food. Filling initiates nerve impulses that stimulate the colon's muscular walls. Mass peristalsis is strongest during the hour after mealtime.

Rectum.   Waste products that reach the sigmoid portion of the colon are called **feces.** The sigmoid stores feces until just before defecation. The rectum is the final division of the GI tract. Its length varies according to age:

Infant	2.5 to 3.8 cm (1 to 1.5 inches)
Toddler	5 cm (2 inches)
Preschooler	7.5 cm (3 inches)
School-ager	10 cm (4 inches)
Adult	15 to 20 cm (6 to 8 inches)

Normally the rectum is empty of feces until defecation. It contains vertical and transverse folds of tissue. Each vertical fold contains an artery and veins. If the veins become distended from pressure during the straining, hemorrhoids form. Hemorrhoids can make defecation painful.

When the fecal mass or gas moves into the rectum to distend its walls, **defecation** begins. The process involves involuntary and voluntary control. The internal sphincter is a smooth muscle innervated by the autonomic nervous system.

As the rectum distends, sensory nerves are stimulated and carry impulses that cause the internal sphincter to relax, allowing more feces to enter the rectum. At the same time, impulses travel to the brain to create awareness of the need to defecate.

As the internal sphincter relaxes, so does the external sphincter. Adults and toilet-trained children can voluntarily control the external sphincter. If the time for defecation is not right, constriction of the levator ani muscles closes the anus and defecation is delayed. At the time of defecation, the external sphincter relaxes. Pressure can be exerted to expel feces through an increase in intraabdominal pressure, or a Valsalva maneuver. A **Valsalva maneuver** is voluntary contraction of abdominal muscles during forced expiration with a closed glottis (holding one's breath while straining). Because the Valsalva maneuver can cause changes in heart rate and rhythm, it is contraindicated in some clients, such as those experiencing heart problems.

Nursing Knowledge Base

FACTORS AFFECTING BOWEL ELIMINATION

Many factors influence the process of bowel elimination. Knowledge of these factors enables the nurse to anticipate measures required to maintain a normal elimination pattern.

Age.   Developmental changes that affect elimination occur throughout life. An infant has a small stomach capacity and less secretion of digestive enzymes. Some foods such as complex starches are tolerated poorly. Food passes quickly through an infant's intestinal tract because of rapid peristalsis. The infant is unable to control defecation because of a lack of neuromuscular development. This development usually does not take place until 2 to 3 years of age. During adolescence, there is rapid growth of the large intestine. The secretion of HCl increases, particularly in boys. Adolescents typically eat more. Older adults often experience changes in the GI system that impair digestion and elimination (Ebersole and Hess, 1998). These changes in the GI tract that occur with aging are listed in Table 45-1.

In addition, peristaltic action declines with age, and esophageal emptying slows. Sluggish emptying of the esophagus can cause discomfort in the epigastric section of the abdomen. Absorptive properties of the intestinal mucosa change, causing protein, vitamin, and mineral deficiencies. Older adults also lose muscle tone in the perineal floor and anal sphincter. Although the integrity of the external sphincter may remain intact, older adults may have difficulty controlling bowel evacuation. Because of slowing of nerve impulses, some are less aware of the need to defecate and are likely to become constipated.

Infection.   Some studies estimate that the etiology of 95% of duodenal ulcers may be related to infection with the bacteria *Helicobacter pylori* (Ciociola and others, 1999). These ulcers are treated with antibiotic therapy with successful results.

Diet.   The food that a person eats influences elimination. Regular daily food intake helps maintain a regular pattern of peristalsis in the colon. **Fiber,** the undigestible residue in the diet, provides the bulk in fecal material.

Table 45-1   Normal Changes in the Gastrointestinal Tract From Aging

Portion of GI Tract	Changes	Causes
Mouth	Decreased chewing and decreased salivation, including oral dryness	Degeneration of cells, medications.
Esophagus	Reduced motility, especially in lower third	Degeneration of neural cells.
Stomach	Decrease in:	Degeneration of gastric mucosa.
	Acid secretions	Alkaline gastric medium contributes to malabsorption of iron. Although digestive enzymes are decreased, enough remain available for digestion.
	Motor activity	Delayed gastric emptying and fewer hunger contractions.
	Mucosal thickness	Loss of parietal cells also leads to loss of intrinsic factor, which is needed for vitamin B_{12} absorption.
Small intestine	Fewer absorbing cells	Absorption not significantly affected.
Large intestine	Weakened musculature	Increase in pouches on the weakened intestinal wall called diverticulosis.
	Decreased peristalsis	Constipation.
	Duller nerve sensations	Missed defecation signal.
Liver	Size decreased	Reduced storage capacity and ability to synthesize protein.

Data from Lueckenotte AG: *Pocket guide to gerontologic assessment,* ed 3, St. Louis, 1998, Mosby.

Bulk-forming foods absorb fluids, thereby increasing stool mass. The bowel walls are stretched, creating peristalsis and initiating the defecation reflex. An infant's immature bowel cannot usually tolerate fiber-containing foods until several months of age. By stimulating peristalsis, bulk foods pass quickly through the intestines, keeping the stool soft (Ouellet, 1996). The following foods contain a high amount of fiber, more commonly called bulk (Clark, 1998):

Raw fruits (apples, bananas, oranges)
Cooked fruits (prunes, apricots)
Greens (spinach, kale, cabbage)
Raw vegetables (celery, green beans, zucchini)
Whole grains (cereal, bran flakes, breads)

Ingestion of a high-fiber diet improves the likelihood of a normal elimination pattern if other factors are normal. Gas-producing foods such as onions, cauliflower, and beans also stimulate peristalsis. The gas formed distends intestinal walls, increasing colon motility. Some spicy foods can increase peristalsis but can also cause indigestion and watery stools.

Some foods, such as milk and milk products, are difficult or impossible for some people to digest. This is caused by a **lactose intolerance,** which bears a genetic link. Lactose, a simple form of sugar found in milk, is normally broken down by the enzyme lactase. Intolerance to lactose-containing foods may result in diarrhea, gaseous distention, and cramping (Mishkin, 1997).

Fluid Intake.   An inadequate intake of fluids or disturbances resulting in loss of fluid (such as vomiting) affect the character of feces. Fluid liquefies intestinal contents, easing its passage through the colon. Reduced fluid intake slows passage of food through the intestine and can result in hardening of stool contents. An adult should drink 6 to 8 glasses (1400 to 2000 ml) of fluid daily. An increase in fluid intake with the use of fruit juices softens stool and increases peristalsis. A large ingestion of milk or milk products may slow peristalsis in some persons and cause constipation (Anti and others, 1998).

Physical Activity.   Physical activity promotes peristalsis, whereas immobilization depresses peristalsis. Early ambulation as illness begins to resolve or as soon as possible after surgery is encouraged to promote maintenance of peristalsis and normal elimination. Maintaining tone of skeletal muscles used during defecation is important. Weakened abdominal and pelvic floor muscles impair the ability to increase intraabdominal pressure and to control the external sphincter. Muscle tone may be weakened or lost as a result of long-term illness or neurological disease that impairs nerve transmission.

Psychological Factors.   The function of almost all body systems can be impaired by prolonged emotional stress (see Chapter 30). If an individual becomes anxious, afraid, or angry, the stress response is initiated, which allows the body to restore defenses. The digestive process is accelerated, and peristalsis is increased to provide nutrients needed for defense. Side effects of increased peristalsis are diarrhea and gaseous distention. If a person becomes depressed, the autonomic nervous system slows impulses and peristalsis can decrease. A number of diseases of the GI tract may be associated with stress. These include ulcerative **colitis,** gastric and duodenal ulcers, and **Crohn's disease.** Repeated research endeavors have failed to prove the myth that clients with such diseases have underlying psychopathological conditions.

Personal Habits.

Personal elimination habits influence bowel function. Most people benefit from being able to use their own toilet facilities at a time that is most effective and convenient for them. A busy work schedule may prevent the individual from responding appropriately to the urge to defecate, disrupting regular habits and causing possible alterations such as constipation. A person should learn the best time for elimination. The **gastrocolic reflex** is most easily stimulated to cause defecation after meals.

Hospitalized clients can rarely maintain privacy during defecation. Bathroom facilities are often shared with a roommate whose hygienic habits might be quite different. The client's illness often limits physical activity and requires the use of a bedpan or bedside commode. The sights, sounds, and odors associated with sharing toilet facilities or using bedpans are often embarrassing. Embarrassment prompts clients to ignore the urge to defecate, which can begin a vicious cycle of constipation and discomfort.

Position During Defecation.

Squatting is the normal position during defecation. Modern toilets are designed to facilitate this posture, allowing the person to lean forward, exert intraabdominal pressure, and contract the thigh muscles. For the client immobilized in bed, defecation is often difficult. In a supine position it is impossible to contract the muscles used during defecation. If allowable within the client's condition, raise the head of the bed, this assists the client to a more normal sitting position on a bedpan, enhancing the ability to defecate.

Pain.

Normally the act of defecation is painless. However, a number of conditions, including hemorrhoids, rectal surgery, rectal fistulas, and abdominal surgery, can result in discomfort. In these instances the client often suppresses the urge to defecate to avoid pain. Constipation is a common problem for clients with pain during defecation.

Pregnancy.

As pregnancy advances and the size of the fetus increases, pressure is exerted on the rectum. A temporary obstruction created by the fetus impairs passage of feces. Slowing of peristalsis during the third trimester often leads to constipation. A pregnant woman's frequent straining during defecation or delivery can result in formation of permanent hemorrhoids.

Surgery and Anesthesia.

General anesthetic agents used during surgery cause temporary cessation of peristalsis (see Chapter 49). Inhaled anesthetic agents block parasympathetic impulses to the intestinal musculature. The anesthetic's action slows or stops peristaltic waves. The client who receives local or regional anesthesia is less at risk for elimination alterations because bowel activity is affected minimally or not at all.

Surgery that involves direct manipulation of the bowel temporarily stops peristalsis. This condition, called **paralytic ileus,** usually lasts about 24 to 48 hours. If the client remains inactive or is unable to eat after surgery, return of normal bowel function may be further delayed.

Medications.

Medications are available for promoting defecation (Table 45-2). **Laxatives** and **cathartics** soften the stool and promote peristalsis. Although similar, laxatives are milder in action than cathartics. When used correctly, laxatives and cathartics safely maintain normal elimination patterns. However, chronic use of cathartics causes the large intestine to lose muscle tone and become less responsive to stimulation by laxatives. Laxative overuse can also cause serious diarrhea that can lead to dehydration and electrolyte depletion. Mineral oil, a common laxative, decreases fat-soluble vitamin absorption. Laxatives can influence the efficacy of other medications by altering the **transit time** (i.e., the time the medication remains in the GI tract).

Several medications have side effects that can impair elimination. Medications such as dicyclomine HCl (Bentyl) suppress peristalsis and can decrease gastric emptying. Narcotic analgesics slow peristalsis and segmental contractions, often resulting in constipation. Anticholinergic drugs, such as atropine or glycopyrrolate (Robinul) inhibit gastric acid secretion and depress GI motility (McKenry and Salerno, 1998). Although useful in treating hyperactive bowel disorders, anticholinergics can cause constipation. Antibiotics may produce diarrhea by disrupting the normal bacterial flora in the GI tract, especially if administered orally. If the diarrhea and associated abdominal cramping become severe, the client might need to change medications. Nonsteroidal antiinflammatory drugs promote gastrointestinal irritation that can range from dyspepsia to life-threatening hemorrhage (Cooke, 1996). Aspirin, a prostaglandin inhibitor, can interfere with the formation and production of protective mucus and can predispose clients to gastritis.

Diagnostic Tests.

Diagnostic examinations involving visualization of GI structures often require that portions of the bowel be empty of contents. A client is not allowed to eat or drink after midnight of the day preceding examinations such as a meglumine diatrizoate (Gastrografin) enema, endoscopy of the lower GI tract, or an upper GI (UGI) series. In the case of evaluation through the use of an enema or endoscopy, the client usually receives cathartics and an enema until the bowel contents that are expelled are clear. Such emptying of the bowel can interfere with elimination until normal eating is resumed.

Table 45-2 Medications and the Gastrointestinal System

Medications	Action
Dicyclomine HCl (Bentyl)	Suppresses peristalsis and can decrease gastric emptying.
Narcotic analgesics	Slow peristalsis and segmental contractions, often resulting in constipation.
Anticholinergic drugs, such as atropine or glycopyrrolate (Robinul)	Inhibit gastric acid secretion and depress GI motility (McKenry and Salerno, 1998). Although useful in treating hyperactive bowel disorders, anticholinergics can cause constipation.
Antibiotics	May produce diarrhea by disrupting the normal bacterial flora in the GI tract, especially if administered orally. If the diarrhea and associated abdominal cramping become severe, the client might need to change medications.
Nonsteroidal antiinflammatory drugs	Promote gastrointestinal irritation that can range from dyspepsia to life-threatening hemorrhage (Cooke, 1996).
Aspirin	A prostaglandin inhibitor, it can interfere with the formation and production of protective mucus and can predispose clients to gastritis.
Histamine$_2$ (H$_2$) antagonists	Suppress the secretion of hydrochloric acid and may interfere with the digestion of some foods.
Iron	Can cause discoloration of the stool (black) and lead to constipation.

COMMON BOWEL ELIMINATION PROBLEMS

The nurse might care for clients who have or are at risk for elimination problems because of emotional stress (anxiety or depression), physiological changes in the GI tract, surgical alteration of intestinal structures, other prescribed therapy, or disorders impairing defecation.

Constipation. **Constipation** is a symptom, not a disease. It is a decrease in frequency of bowel movements, accompanied by prolonged or difficult passage of hard, dry stools (Clark, 1998). Straining during defecation is an associated sign. When intestinal motility slows, the fecal mass becomes exposed over time to the intestinal walls and most of the fecal water content is absorbed. Little water is left to soften and lubricate stool. Passage of a dry, hard stool may cause rectal pain.

Each person has an individual defecation pattern that the nurse must assess (Box 45-1). It is important to remember that not every adult has a daily bowel movement (Ebersole and Hess, 1998). A bowel movement only every 4 or more days may be considered normal, if it is not associated with pain or bloating (Abyad and Mourad, 1996). A usual bowel movement pattern of every 2 to 3 days without any difficulty, pain, or bleeding may be normal for an older adult (Ebersole and Hess, 1998). If daily records start to suggest an altered frequency of defecation, there is cause for concern.

Constipation is a significant hazard to health. Straining during defecation may cause problems to the client with recent abdominal, gynecological, or rectal surgery. The effort to pass a stool can cause sutures to separate, reopening the wound. In addition, clients with histories of cardiovascular disease, diseases causing elevated intraocular pressure (glaucoma), and increased intracranial pressure should prevent constipation and avoid using the Valsalva maneuver (see Chapter 31). Exhaling through the mouth

Common Causes of Constipation   Box 45-1

- Irregular bowel habits and ignoring the urge to defecate can cause constipation.
- Clients who have a low-fiber diet high in animal fats (e.g., meats, dairy products, eggs) and refined sugars (rich desserts) often have constipation problems. Also, low fluid intake slows peristalsis.
- Lengthy bed rest or lack of regular exercise causes constipation.
- Heavy laxative use causes loss of normal defecation reflex. In addition, the lower colon is completely emptied, requiring time to refill with bulk.
- Tranquilizers, opiates, anticholinergics, iron, diuretics, antacids with calcium or aluminum, and antiparkinsonism drugs can cause constipation.
- Older adults experience slowed peristalsis, loss of abdominal muscle elasticity, and reduced intestinal mucus secretion. Older adults often eat low-fiber foods.
- Constipation is also caused by GI abnormalities such as bowel obstruction, paralytic ileus, and diverticulitis.
- Neurological conditions that block nerve impulses to the colon (e.g., spinal cord injury, tumor) can cause constipation.
- Organic illnesses such as hypothyroidism, hypocalcemia, or hypokalemia can cause constipation.

during straining avoids a Valsalva maneuver (Stewart, 1998). Older adults may have constipation from certain medications that they are taking. Some of these medications are aspirin, antihistamines, diuretics, tranquilizers, hypnotics, antacids with aluminum or calcium, and drugs used to control Parkinson's disease.

Impaction. Fecal **impaction** results from unrelieved constipation. It is a collection of hardened feces, wedged in the rectum, which cannot be expelled. In cases of severe impaction, the mass can extend up into the sigmoid colon. Clients who are debilitated, confused, or unconscious are most at risk for impaction. They are too weak or unaware of the need to defecate, or they may be dehydrated so that the stool becomes too hard and dry to pass.

An obvious sign of impaction is the inability to pass a stool for several days, despite a repeated urge to defecate. When a continuous oozing of diarrheal stool develops, impaction should be suspected. The liquid portion of feces located higher in the colon seeps around the impacted mass. Loss of appetite (anorexia), abdominal distention and cramping, and rectal pain may accompany the condition. The nurse who suspects an impaction can gently perform a digital examination of the rectum and palpate the impacted mass.

Diarrhea. **Diarrhea** is an increase in the number of stools and the passage of liquid, unformed feces. It is a symptom of disorders affecting digestion, absorption, and secretion in the GI tract. Intestinal contents pass through the small and large intestine too quickly to allow the usual absorption of fluid and nutrients. Irritation within the colon can result in an increased mucus secretion. As a result, feces become watery and the client may be unable to control the urge to defecate.

It is often difficult to assess diarrhea in infants. An infant who is bottle-fed may have one firm stool every second day, whereas a breast-fed baby may pass five to eight small, soft stools daily. The mother or nurse should note any sudden increase in the number of stools, any reduction in fecal consistency with an increase in fluid content, and a tendency for feces to be greenish.

Excess loss of colonic fluid can result in serious fluid and electrolyte or acid-base imbalances. Infants and older adults are particularly susceptible to associated complications (see Chapter 40). Because repeated passage of diarrheal stools also exposes the skin of the perineum and buttocks to irritating intestinal contents, meticulous skin care is needed to prevent skin breakdown (see Chapter 38), and containment of fecal drainage is needed.

Many conditions cause diarrhea (Table 45-3). The aims of treatment are to remove precipitating conditions and to slow peristalsis. Box 45-2 lists nursing responsibilities for managing the client with diarrhea.

Incontinence. Fecal **incontinence** is the inability to control passage of feces and gas from the anus. Physical conditions that impair anal sphincter function or control can cause incontinence. Conditions that create frequent, loose, large-volume, watery stools also predispose to incontinence.

Incontinence can harm a client's body image (see Chapter 26). In many situations the client is mentally alert

---

> ### Summary of Nursing Responsibilities in the Management of Diarrhea   Box 45-2
>
> Provide general supportive measures to maintain fluid status and electrolyte balance.
> Observe systemic manifestations such as fever, leukocytosis, fluid volume deficits, hypokalemia, and metabolic acidosis.
> Identify relationship between onset of diarrhea and initiation of enteral feeding.
> Report symptoms promptly and look for association of occurrence of diarrhea with either initiation or continuous consumption of hyperosmolar medications.
> Consult dietitians and pharmacists regarding drug-nutrient interactions and alternative regimens.
> Maintain perianal skin integrity.

From Fruto LV: Current concepts: management of diarrhea in acute care, *J Wound Ostomy Continence Nurs* 21(5):199, 1994.

---

but physically unable to avoid defecation. The embarrassment of soiling clothes can lead to social isolation. The client must depend on the nurse for a basic need.

Flatulence. As gas accumulates in the lumen of the intestines, the bowel wall stretches and distends (**flatulence**). It is a common cause of abdominal fullness, pain, and cramping. Normally, intestinal gas escapes through the mouth (belching) or the anus (passing of flatus). However, if there is a reduction in intestinal motility resulting from opiates, general anesthetics, abdominal surgery, or immobilization, flatulence can become severe enough to cause abdominal distention and severe sharp pain.

Hemorrhoids. **Hemorrhoids** are dilated, engorged veins in the lining of the rectum. They are either external or internal. External hemorrhoids are clearly visible as protrusions of skin. If the underlying vein is hardened, there can be a purplish discoloration (thrombosis). This causes increased pain and may need to be excised. Internal hemorrhoids have an outer mucous membrane. Increased venous pressure from straining at defecation, pregnancy, congestive heart failure, and chronic liver disease can cause hemorrhoids.

BOWEL DIVERSIONS

Certain diseases cause conditions that prevent normal passage of feces through the rectum. This creates the need for a temporary or permanent artificial opening (**stoma**) in the abdominal wall. Surgical openings (ostomies) are most commonly formed in the ileum (**ileostomy**) or colon (**colostomy**) (Figure 45-4). Ends of the intestines are brought through a surgical opening in the abdominal wall to create the stoma (Thompson, 1998). Depending on the type of surgical procedure done, the client will either

Table 45-3   Conditions That Cause Diarrhea

Condition	Physiological Effects
Emotional stress (anxiety)	Increased intestinal motility
Intestinal infection (streptococcal or staphylococcal enteritis)	Inflammation of intestinal mucosa, increased mucus secretion in colon
Food allergies	Reduced digestion of food elements
Food intolerance (greasy foods, coffee, alcohol, spicy foods)	Increased intestinal motility, increased mucus secretion in colon
Tube feedings	Hyperosmolarity of some enteral solutions results in diarrhea, because hyperosmolar fluids draw fluids into the gastrointestinal tract
Medications	
Iron	Irritation of intestinal mucosa
Antibiotics	Superinfection allowing overgrowth of normal flora, inflammation and irritation of mucosa
Laxatives (short term)	Increased intestinal motility
Colon disease (colitis, Crohn's disease)	Inflammation and ulceration of intestinal walls, reduced absorption of fluids, increased intestinal motility
Surgical alterations	
Gastrectomy	Loss of reservoir function of stomach, improper absorption because food is moved into duodenum too quickly
Colon resection	Reduced size of colon, reduced amount of absorptive surface

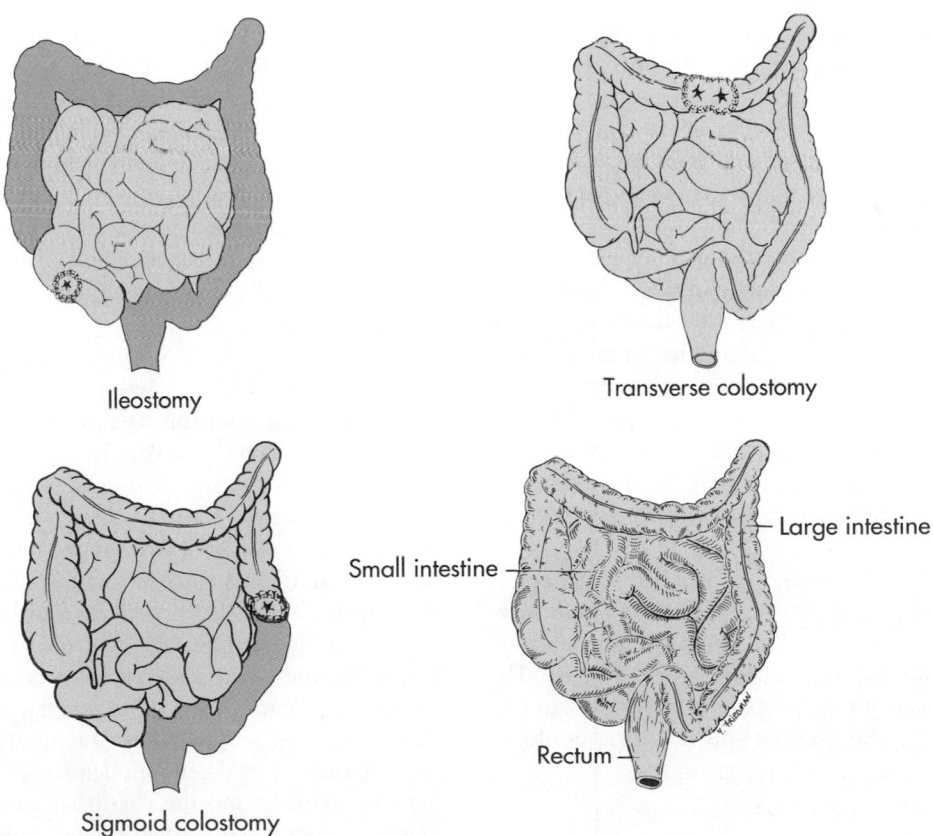

Figure 45-4   Normal intestines (bottom right) and three types of ostomies. Shaded areas indicate excised tissue.

have no control over when the fecal material exits the stoma (incontinent ostomy) or will have control (continent ostomy). For incontinent ostomies, the stoma is covered with a pouch (appliance) or what clients refer to as "a bag" to collect fecal material.

Incontinent Ostomies.   The location of the ostomy determines the consistency of stool. An ileostomy bypasses the entire large intestine. As a result, stools are frequent and liquid. The same is true for a colostomy of the ascending colon. A colostomy of the transverse colon generally results in a more solid, formed stool. The sigmoid colostomy emits near-normal stool. The location of a colostomy is determined by the client's medical problem and general condition. There are three types of colostomy construction: loop colostomy, end colostomy, and double-barrel colostomy.

Loop Colostomy.   A loop colostomy is usually performed in a medical emergency when closure of the colostomy is anticipated. These are usually temporary large stomas constructed in the transverse colon (Figure 45-5, *A-D*). The surgeon pulls a loop of bowel onto the abdomen (Figure 45-5, *E*). An external supporting device such as a plastic rod, bridge (Figure 45-5, *C* and *D*), or rubber catheter (Figure 45-5, *A*) is temporarily placed under the bowel loop to keep it from slipping back (Figure 45-5, *A*). The surgeon then opens the bowel and sutures it to the skin of the abdomen (Figure 45-5, *F*). A communicating wall remains between the proximal and distal bowel. The loop ostomy has two openings through the stoma (Figure 45-5, *D* and *G*). The proximal end drains stool, whereas the distal portion drains mucus. Within 7 to 10 days the external supporting device is removed.

End Colostomy.   The end colostomy consists of one stoma formed from the proximal end of the bowel with the distal portion of the GI tract either removed or sewn closed (called Hartmann's pouch) and left in the abdominal cavity. For many clients, end colostomies are a result of surgical treatment of colorectal cancer. In such cases the rectum might also be removed. Clients with diverticulitis who are treated surgically often have a temporary end colostomy with a Hartmann's pouch (Figure 45-6).

Double-Barrel Colostomy.   Unlike the loop colostomy, the bowel is surgically severed in a double-barrel colostomy (Figure 45-7, *A*), and the two ends are brought out onto the abdomen (Figure 45-7, *B*). The double-barrel colostomy consists of two distinct stomas: the proximal functioning stoma and the distal nonfunctioning stoma.

. . .

Ostomies that emit frequent liquid stools (e.g., ileostomy) create a management challenge. A pouch must

always be worn. Control of defecation cannot be achieved because of a continuous oozing of liquid stool. The pouch must be emptied, washed, and if a two-piece ostomy system is being used, even replaced throughout the day. Skin care is vital to prevent exposure to fecal irritants.

A colostomy in the transverse or sigmoid colon needs less frequent emptying of the pouch. Although some clients might choose to not wear a pouch at all times, most clients with sigmoid colostomies wear a pouch at all times even though bowel movements may occur only once or twice daily. Selected foods can be eaten at prescribed intervals so that bowel movements occur at a convenient time.

A physician might order ostomy irrigations similar to an enema for clients with a transverse, descending, or sigmoid colostomy. This allows the person to empty the bowel regularly and regain control as to the time of elimination of feces from the stoma.

Since the late 1980s, some progress has been made toward the development and successful use of a colostomy plug, which can provide continence for up to 28 hours. This two-piece system consists of an adhesive base plate that is put around the stoma and a soft, pliable, carbon-filtered plug that is inserted into the stoma. Usually the client does an irrigation before inserting the plug. This increases the length of time that the client has fecal continence. The plug is not usually used by clients who have frequent, liquid ostomy stools, excessive gas, or abdominal cramping.

Continent Ostomies.   Certain types of surgery may provide continence for select colectomy clients. These continent ostomies are also called continent diversions or continent reservoirs. In a procedure called an ileoanal pull-through, the colon is removed and the ileum is anastomosed or connected to an intact anal sphincter. Not every colectomy client is a candidate for this procedure. Selection criteria require close coordination between the client and surgeon.

Ileoanal Reservoir.   A newer surgical procedure based on the ileoanal pull-through is the ileoanal reservoir (IAR). The ileoanal reservoir is also called a restorative proctocolectomy, ileal pouch-anal anastomosis, or pelvic pouch. In this procedure, the client has no permanent external stoma and therefore does not need to wear an ostomy pouch. Clients have an internal pouch created from their ileum. These ileum pouches can be constructed in various configurations such as in a lateral, S, J, or W shape. The end of the pouch is then sewn or anastomosed to the anus (Figure 45-8). The surgery is done in several stages, and the client may have a temporary ostomy until the surgically created ileum pouch has healed. When healing has occurred and the client has successfully learned Kegel exercises to strengthen the pelvic floor, the temporary ostomy is removed. The client then has bowel movements from only the anal area. Nursing care for clients

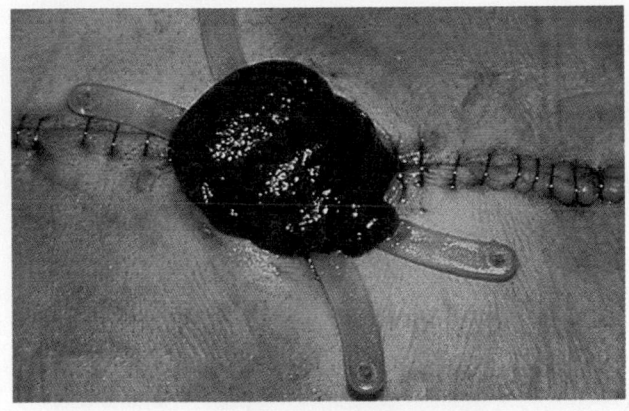

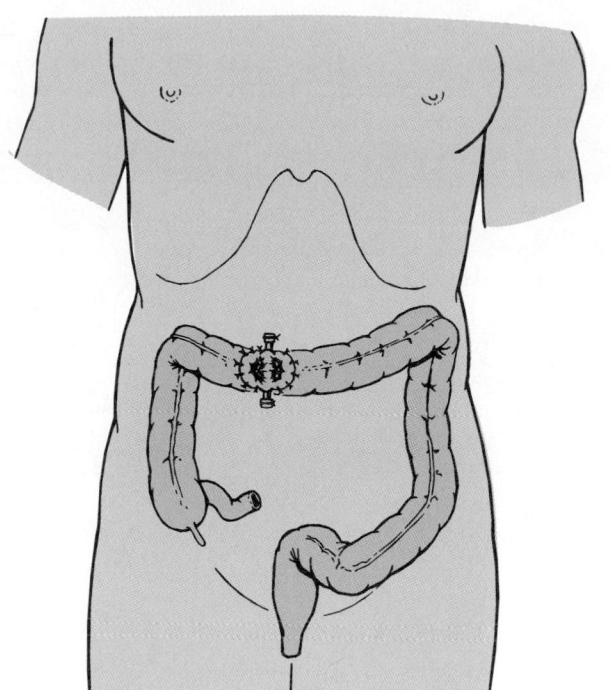

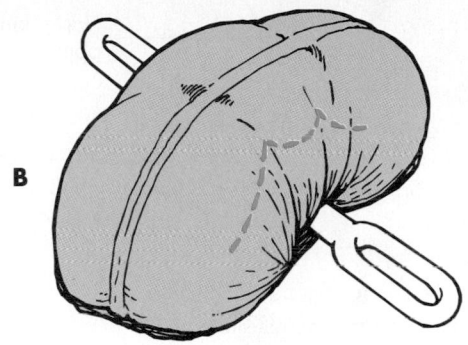

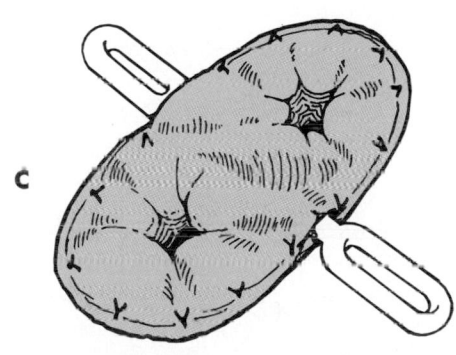

Figure 45-5   **A,** Transverse loop colostomy supported with a flexible red rubber catheter. **A, B,** Abdominal view of loop colostomy in transverse colon. **C,** Loop colostomy construction is much the same as construction of loop ileostomy. Stoma is created with longitudinal incision through sacculations in colon. **D,** Loop colostomy matured. **E,** Loop ostomy construction, loop of bowel exteriorized. **F,** Support device placed to maintain position of bowel on abdominal surface. Distal bowel of ileum is incised, mesentery. Stitch placed to designate proximal bowel. **G,** Loop ileostomy matured with protruding functional limb.
Courtesy Hollister, Inc., Libertyville, Ill; **B** to **G** From Hampton BG, Bryant RA: *Ostomies and continent diversions: nursing management,* St. Louis, 1992, Mosby.

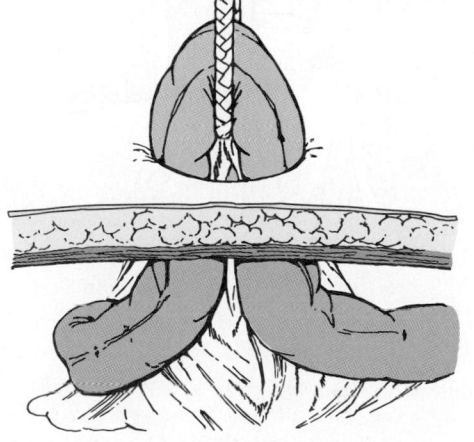

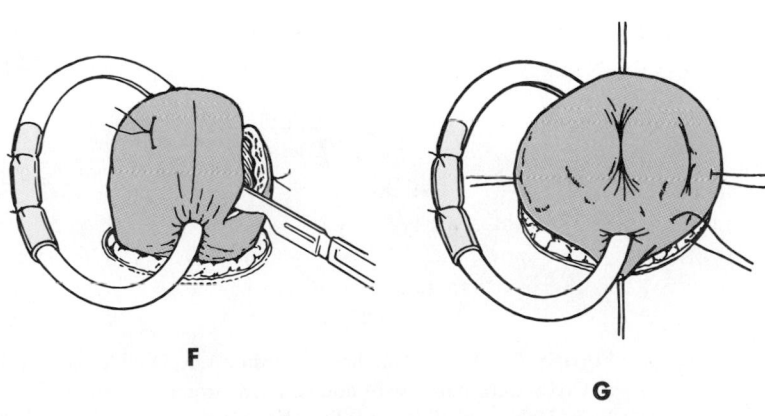

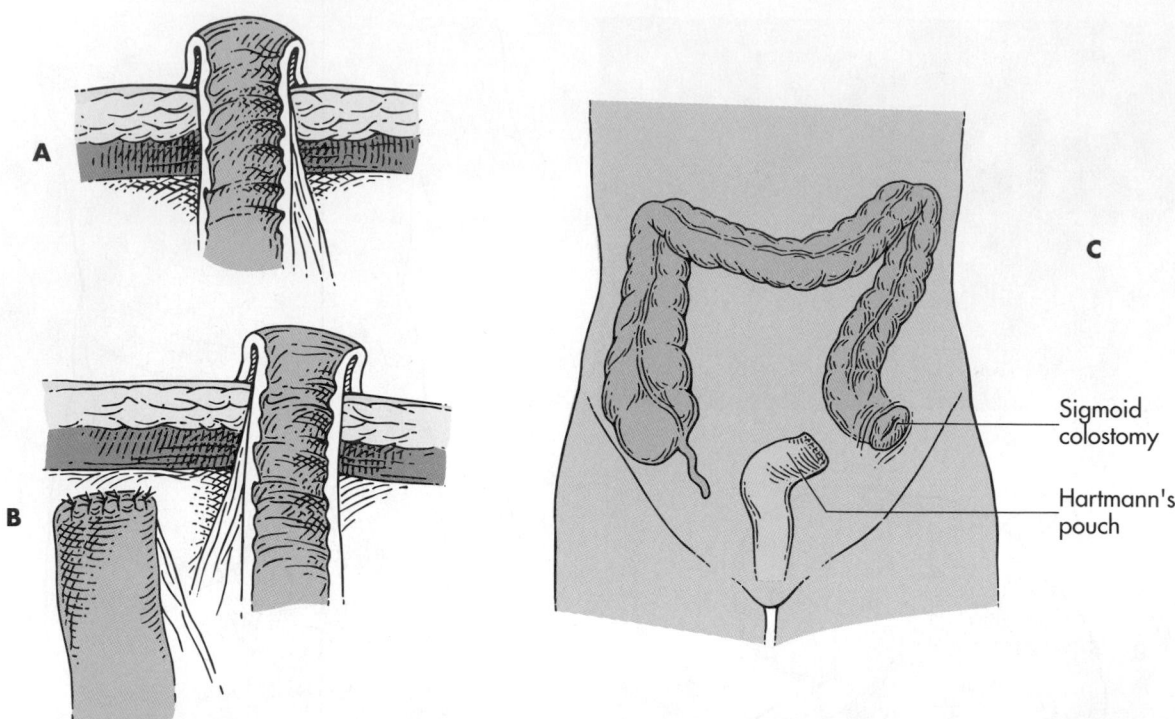

Figure 45-6   End colostomy. **A,** Cross-sectional view of end stoma. **B,** Cross-sectional view of end stoma with distal bowel oversewn and secured to anterior peritoneum at stoma site. **C,** Sigmoid colostomy. Distal bowel is oversewn and left in place to create Hartmann's pouch. From Hampton BG, Bryant RA: *Ostomies and continent diversions: nursing management,* St. Louis, 1992, Mosby.

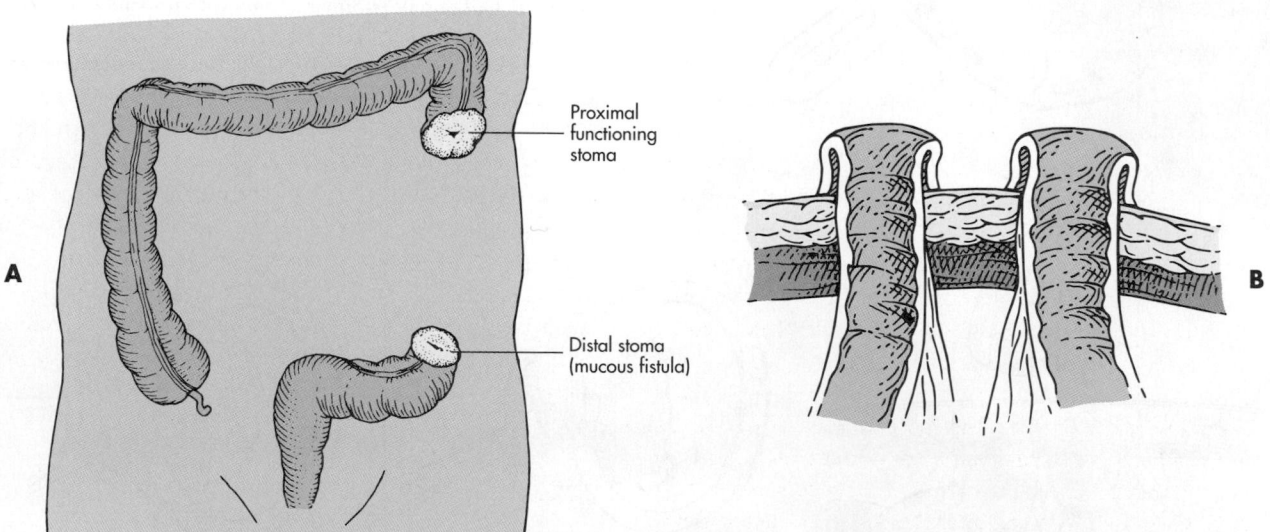

Figure 45-7   Double-barrel colostomy. **A,** Double-barrel colostomy in the descending colon. **B,** Cross-sectional view of double-barrel stoma. From Hampton BG, Bryant RA: *Ostomies and continent diversions: nursing management,* St. Louis, 1992, Mosby.

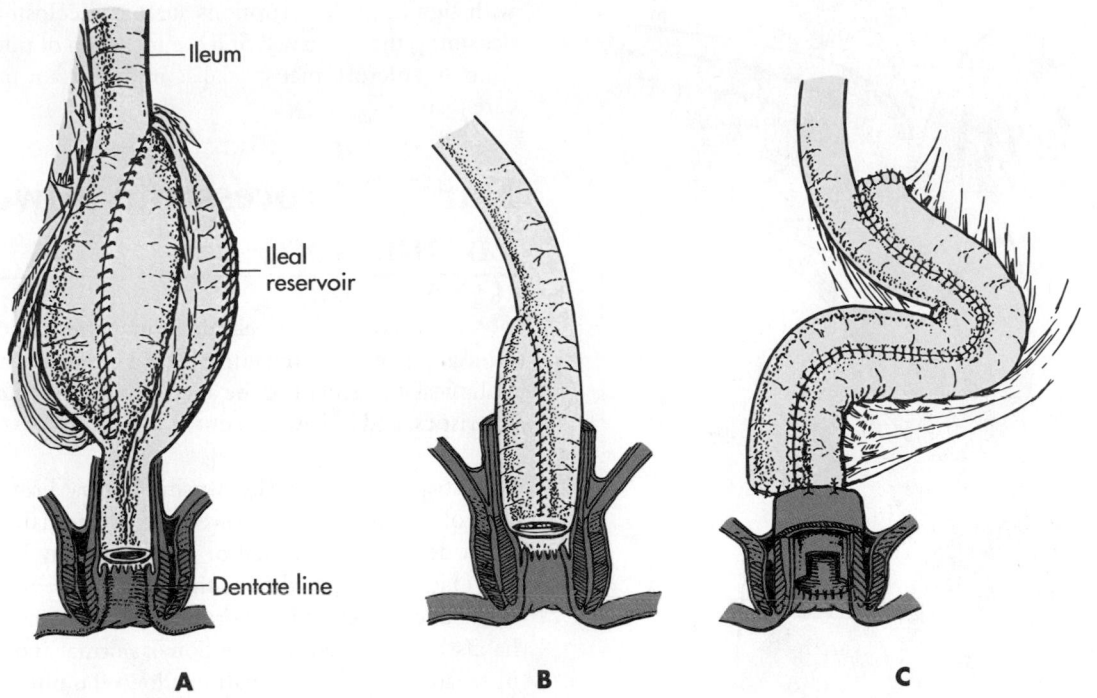

Figure 45-8   Ileoanal reservoirs (IARs). **A,** S-shaped configuration for IAR. Three 10-cm limbs of ileum are used, antimesenteric surface of each limb opened, and adjacent bowel walls anastomosed. **B,** J-shaped configuration for IAR. Distal ileum is aligned in J shape; antimesenteric surface of J shape is opened, and adjacent bowel walls anastomosed. Side-to-end anastomosis of bowel to dentate line is evident. **C,** Lateral or side-by-side ileoanal pouch configuration. From Hampton BG, Bryant RA: *Ostomies and continent diversions: nursing management,* St. Louis, 1992, Mosby.

with an ileoanal reservoir should focus on emotional support, perianal skin care, use of medications, sphincter reeducation, and prompt recognition of complications (Beitz, 1994).

Kock Continent Ileostomy.   The Kock continent ileostomy is yet another new type of continent ostomy. In this procedure an internal reservoir or pouch is created from a piece of the client's small intestine (Figure 45-9, *A*). Part of the pouch is brought out onto the client's abdomen as an enteral stoma (Figure 45-9, *B*). Unlike other ostomy stomas, the external stoma from a Kock continent ileostomy is usually very low on the client's abdomen; usually below the line of the client's underpants. At the end of the internal part of the pouch is a one-way nipple valve, which is how continence is accomplished (see Fig 45-9, *B*). This valve only allows fecal contents to drain from the pouch when an external catheter is intermittently placed into the stoma. As fecal contents are only eliminated from the Kock pouch when intubated with the catheter, unlike other people with an ostomy, the client does not have to wear an ostomy pouch. Nursing care of clients with a Kock reservoir focuses on emotional support, teaching self-intubation technique, determining an intubation schedule, diet teaching, and recognizing complications.

Psychological Considerations.   A stoma can cause serious body image changes, particularly if it is permanent. A study reported by Walsh and others (1995) measured the perception of body image in clients who had a stoma. Clients who had a long-standing history of chronic bowel disease such as Crohn's disease or ulcerative colitis had improved quality of life, but a lower body image. Conversely, clients who needed an ostomy because of cancer had a higher body image but a reduced quality of life. Clients often perceive a stoma as a form of mutilation. Even though clothing conceals the ostomy, the client feels different. Many clients have difficulty maintaining or initiating normal sexual relations (see Chapter 27). An important factor in the client's reactions is the character of fecal secretions and the ability to control them. Foul odors, spillage, or leakage of liquid stools and inability to regulate bowel movements give the client a loss of self-esteem.

Critical Thinking Synthesis

Successful critical thinking requires a synthesis of knowledge, experience, information gathered from clients, critical thinking attitudes, and intellectual and professional standards. Clinical judgments require the nurse to anticipate the information necessary, analyze the data, and

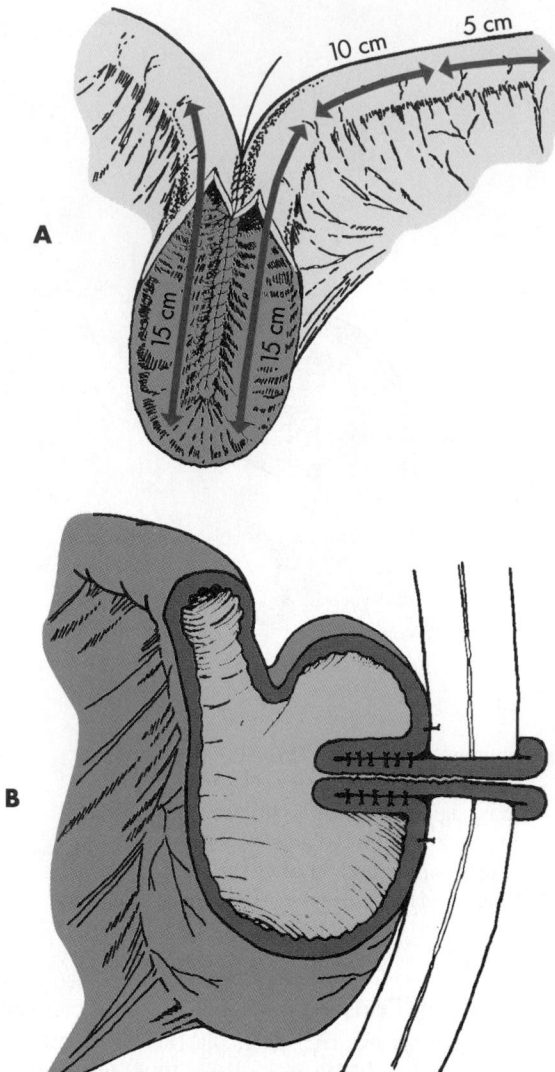

Figure 45-9 Construction of Kock continent ileostomy—Kock pouch. **A,** Two 15-cm limbs are used to create pouch, and one 15-cm limb is used to fashion a nipple valve and stoma. **B,** Distal limb is intussuscepted into reservoir to create one-way valve and accomplish continence. Sutures or staples, or both, are placed to stabilize and maintain intussuscepted nipple. Anterior surface of reservoir is anchored to anterior peritoneal wall. From Hampton BG, Bryant RA: *Ostomies and continent diversions: nursing management,* St. Louis, 1992, Mosby.

make decisions regarding client care. Critical thinking is always changing. During assessment (Figure 45-10) the nurse must consider all elements that build toward making appropriate diagnoses.

In the case of bowel elimination, the nurse must integrate the knowledge from nursing and other disciplines to better understand the client's response to bowel elimination interruptions. Often clients respond to disruptions in bowel elimination with fright and embarrassment. Sensitivity on the part of the nurse is essential. For clients

with significant interruptions such as a colostomy or an ileostomy, the nurse will find the inclusion of information from an enterostomal specialist an important part of the care plan.

Nursing Process and Bowel Elimination

ASSESSMENT

To assess bowel elimination patterns and determine abnormalities, the nurse takes a nursing history, does a physical assessment of the abdomen, inspects fecal characteristics, and reviews pertinent test results.

Nursing History.   The nursing history provides a review of the client's usual bowel pattern and habits. What a client describes as normal or abnormal may be different from factors and conditions that tend to promote normal elimination. Identifying normal and abnormal patterns, habits, and the client's perception of normal and abnormal in regard to bowel elimination allows the nurse to determine the client's problems. Much of the nursing history can be organized around the factors that affect elimination:

- *Determination of the usual elimination pattern:* Frequency and time of day are included. Accurate assessment of a client's current bowel elimination pattern can be enhanced by having the client or caregiver complete a bowel elimination or defecation diary. As with any client teaching, the nurse must make sure that the person completing the diary understands what information must be recorded.
- *Identification of routines followed to promote normal elimination:* Examples are drinking hot liquids, using laxatives, eating specific foods, or taking time to defecate during a certain part of the day.
- *Description of any recent change in elimination pattern:* This information is perhaps the most significant because elimination patterns are variable and the client can best detect change.
- *Client's description of usual characteristics of stool:* The nurse determines whether the stool is usually watery or formed or soft or hard, as well as the typical color.
- *Diet history:* The nurse determines the client's dietary preferences for a day. The nurse measures servings of fruits, vegetables, cereals, and breads.
- *Description of daily fluid intake:* This includes the type and amount of fluid. The client might have to estimate the amount using common household measurements.
- *History of exercise:* The nurse asks the client to specifically describe the type and amount of daily exercise.
- *Assessment of the use of artificial aids at home:* The nurse assesses whether the client uses enemas, laxatives, or special foods before having a bowel movement.
- *History of surgery or illnesses affecting the GI tract:* This information can often help explain symptoms.

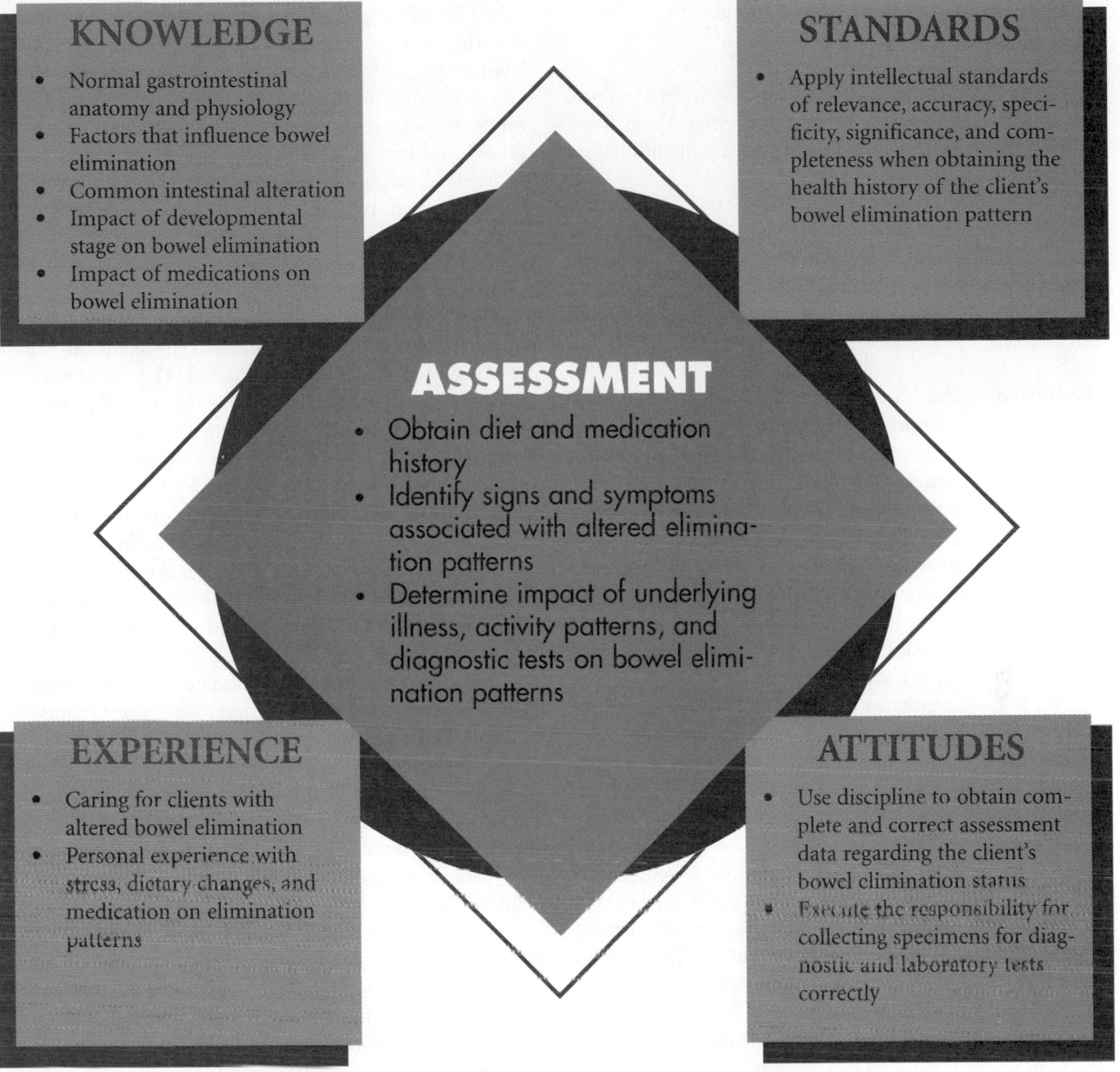

Figure 45-10 *Synthesis Model for Bowel Elimination Assessment Phase.*

- *Presence and status of bowel diversions:* If the client has an ostomy, the nurse assesses frequency of fecal drainage, character of feces, appearance and condition of the stoma (color, swelling, and irritation), type of appliance used, and methods used to maintain the ostomy's function.
- *Medication history:* The nurse asks whether the client takes medications (such as laxatives, antacids, iron supplements, and analgesics) that might alter defecation or fecal characteristics.
- *Emotional state:* The client's emotions can significantly alter frequency of defecation. During assessment, observation of the client's emotions, tone of

voice, and mannerisms can reveal significant behaviors that indicate stress.
- *Social history:* Clients have many different living arrangements. Where clients live may affect their toileting habits. If the client is sharing living quarters, how many bathrooms are there? Do clients have their own bathroom, or do they need to share and thus adjust the time they use the bathroom to accommodate others? If clients live alone, are they capable of ambulating to the toilet safely? If the client is not independent in bowel management, the nurse determines who assists the client and how.
- *Mobility and dexterity:* The client's mobility and dex-

terity need to be evaluated to determine if the client needs assistive devices or personnel.

Physical Assessment.
The nurse conducts a physical assessment (see Chapter 32) of body systems and functions likely to be influenced by the presence of elimination problems.

Mouth.
An assessment includes inspection of the client's teeth, tongue, and gums. Poor dentition or poorly fitting dentures influence the ability to chew (see Chapter 43). Sores in the mouth can make eating not only difficult, but painful.

Abdomen.
The nurse inspects all four abdominal quadrants for contour, shape, symmetry, and skin color. Inspection also includes noting masses, peristaltic waves, scars, venous patterns, stomas, and lesions. Normally, peristaltic waves are not visible. However, observable peristalsis can be a sign of intestinal obstruction.

Abdominal distention appears as an overall outward protuberance of the abdomen. Intestinal gas, large tumors, or fluid in the peritoneal cavity may cause distention. A distended abdomen feels tight, like a drum, and the skin appears taut, as if stretched.

The nurse auscultates the abdomen with the stethoscope to assess bowel sounds in each quadrant (see Chapter 32). Normal bowel sounds occur every 5 to 15 seconds and last a second to several seconds. While auscultating, the nurse notes the character and frequency of bowel sounds. An increase in pitch or a tinkling sound may be heard with abdominal distention. Absent or hypoactive sounds (less than five sounds per minute) occur with paralytic ileus, such as after abdominal surgery. High-pitched and hyperactive bowel sounds (35 or more sounds per minute) occur with small intestine obstruction and inflammatory disorders.

The nurse palpates the abdomen for masses or areas of tenderness (see Chapter 32). It is important for the client to relax. Tensing abdominal muscles interferes with palpating underlying organs or masses.

Percussion detects lesions, fluid, or gas within the abdomen. Familiarity with the five percussion notes (see Chapter 32) also permits identification of underlying abdominal structures. Gas or flatulence creates a tympanic note. Masses, tumors, and fluid are dull to percussion.

Rectum.
The nurse inspects the area around the anus for lesions, discolorations, inflammation, and hemorrhoids. Abnormalities should be carefully recorded (see Chapter 32).

Laboratory Tests.
Laboratory and diagnostic examinations yield useful information concerning elimination problems. Laboratory analysis of fecal contents can detect pathological conditions such as tumors, hemorrhage, and infection.

Fecal Specimens.
The nurse is directly responsible for ensuring that specimens are accurately obtained, properly labeled in appropriate containers, and transported to the laboratory on time. Institutions provide special containers for fecal specimens. Some tests require specimens to be placed in chemical preservatives.

Medical aseptic technique should be used during collection of stool specimens (see Chapter 33). Because about 25% of the solid portion of a stool is bacteria from the colon, the nurse should wear disposable gloves when handling specimens.

Hand washing is necessary for anyone who might come in contact with the specimen. Often the client can obtain the specimen if properly instructed. The nurse explains that feces cannot be mixed with urine or water. For this reason the client must defecate into a clean, dry bedpan or special container placed under the toilet seat.

Tests performed by the laboratory for occult (microscopic) blood in the stool and stool cultures require only a small sample. The nurse collects about an inch of formed stool or 15 to 30 ml of liquid diarrheal stool. Tests for measuring the output of fecal fat require a 3- to 5-day collection of stool. All fecal material must be saved throughout the test period.

After obtaining a specimen, the nurse labels and tightly seals the container and completes laboratory requisition forms. The nurse then records specimen collections in the client's medical record. It is important to avoid delays in sending specimens to the laboratory. Some tests such as measurement for ova and parasites require the stool to be warm. When stool specimens are allowed to stand at room temperature, bacteriological changes that alter test results can occur.

Guaiac Test.
A common laboratory test that can be done at home or at the client's bedside is the **guaiac test,** or fecal occult blood testing (FOBT), which measures microscopic amounts of blood in feces. Guaiac tests help reveal visually undetectable blood. It is useful as a diagnostic screening test for colon cancer (Box 45-3). There are client characteristics, especially cultural, that must be considered when nurses plan colon cancer screening programs (Box 45-4).

Clients who are receiving anticoagulants or who have a bleeding disorder or a GI disorder known to cause bleeding (e.g., intestinal tumors, bowel inflammation, or ulcerations) should be guaiac tested. The most common guaiac test is the Hemoccult slide test. This test is typically performed in the laboratory; the nurse will assist in collection of specimens.

Fecal Characteristics.
Inspection of fecal characteristics (Table 45-4) reveals information about the nature of elimination alterations. Several factors can influence each characteristic. A key to assessment is knowing whether there have been any recent changes. The client can best provide this information.

<table>
<tr><td colspan="2">

Screening for Colon Cancer   Box 45-3

RISK FACTORS
Age: over 50
Family history: colon polyps or colorectal cancer
History of inflammatory bowel disease (colitis, Crohn's
 disease)
Living in urban area
Diet: high intake of fats, low fiber intake

WARNING SIGNS
Change in bowel habits
Rectal bleeding

SCREENING TESTS
Digital rectal examination every year after age 40
Guaiac test for occult blood every year after 50
Proctoscopy every 3-5 years after age 50, after two annual
 negative examinations

</td><td>

Cultural ASPECTS OF CARE   Box 45-4

Colorectal cancer is one of the most frequently occurring cancers among older adult African-Americans. Although the use of fecal occult blood testing (FOBT) to detect colorectal cancer early has decreased mortality rates in the general population, the mortality rate in African-Americans has increased. This may be because older adult African-Americans are least likely to participate in early detection and therefore when they are diagnosed their cancers are at an advanced stage. Increasing the participation in FOBT by older adult African-Americans is a national nursing priority and must be part of African-American clients' primary prevention screening activities.

</td></tr>
</table>

Modified from Powe BD: Fatalism among elderly African Americans: effects on colorectal cancer screening, *Cancer Nurs* 18(5):385, 1995.

Table 45-4 Fecal Characteristics

Characteristic	Normal	Abnormal	Abnormal Cause
Color	Infant: yellow; adult: brown	White or clay	Absence of bile
		Black or tarry (melena)	Iron ingestion or upper GI bleeding
		Red	Lower GI bleeding, hemorrhoids
		Pale with fat	Malabsorption of fat
Odor	Pungent; affected by food type	Noxious change	Blood in feces or infection
Consistency	Soft, formed	Liquid	Diarrhea, reduced absorption
		Hard	Constipation
Frequency	Varies: Infant 4 to 6 times daily (breast-fed) or 1 to 3 times daily (bottle-fed); adult daily or 2 to 3 times a week	Infant more than 6 times daily or less than once every 1-2 days; adult more than 3 times a day or less than once a week	Hypomotility or hypermotility
Amount	150 g per day (adult)		
Shape	Resembles diameter of rectum	Narrow, pencil shaped	Obstruction, rapid peristalsis
Constituents	Undigested food, dead bacteria, fat, bile pigment, cells lining intestinal mucosa, water	Blood, pus, foreign bodies, mucus, worms	Internal bleeding, infection, swallowed objects, irritation, inflammation

Diagnostic Examinations.   A client may have a diagnostic test as an outpatient or inpatient. Visualization of GI structures may be by direct or indirect approach. Many facilities employ the use of conscious sedation during these procedures. Midazolam (Versed) is often the sedative drug of choice with possible augmentation with merperidine (Demerol) or morphine. It is essential for the nurse to understand the safety precautions involved concerning the use of this form of anesthesia. In many institutions special training will be required (Clark, 1998). A crash cart must be present at the bedside, and the patient be must monitored continuously with pulse oximetry.

Direct Visualization.   Instruments introduced through the mouth (upper GI viewing, or UGI) or the rectum (lower GI viewing) allow the physician to inspect the integrity of mucosa, blood vessels, and organ parts. A colonoscopy is the usually the test of choice and employs the use of a **fiber optic endoscope** with a lens viewer, a long flexible tube, and a light source at the end. It allows viewing of structures at the tip of the tube and insertion of special instruments for biopsy. Proctoscopes and sigmoidoscopes are rigid, tube-shaped instruments with attached light sources. The proctoscope looks like a speculum with a light. These instruments are less flexible than fiber optic scopes and more capable of causing discomfort. Many times procedures involving these instruments are performed in the health care provider's office.

UGI **endoscopy** or **gastroscopy** allows visualization of the esophagus, stomach, and duodenum. The physician inspects for tumors, vascular changes, mucosal inflammation, ulcers, hernias, and obstructions. A gastroscope enables the physician to remove tissue specimens (or **biopsy**), remove abnormal tissue growth (**polyps**), and coagulate sources of bleeding. Nursing implications before diagnostic procedures concerning the gastrointestinal system include the following:

1. Client signs informed consent.
2. Client performs any necessary bowel preparations.
3. For procedures involving the upper GI tract, client takes nothing by mouth after midnight.
4. If conscious sedation is not utilized, the nurse explains that the client may feel fullness in the throat and a sense of gagging during the test.
5. Nurse explains that the client will be unable to speak as the endoscope enters the esophagus.
6. Nurse positions the client in the left Sims' or left lateral position.

For procedures involving the lower GI tract:

7. For procedures involving the lower bowel, the client may eat a light breakfast.
8. Nurse explains that the client will feel discomfort and the urge to defecate as the instruments are inserted.
9. During the test the physician uses air to distend the bowel for better visualization; the nurse explains that the client will feel "gas pains."
10. Nurse positions the client in a knee-chest position face down; Sims' position on the left side is acceptable. If a proctoscope table is being used, the nurse has the client kneel and lean over the table.
11. Nurse drapes the client to avoid unnecessary exposure and minimize embarrassment.

Nursing implications during the test include the following:

12. Nurse describes steps of the test to the client.
13. Nurse places tissue specimens in a properly labeled container that is sealed tightly.
14. Nurse has emergency equipment available in case of respiratory complications.

Following the test:

15. The nurse instructs the client to avoid eating or drinking until the gag reflex returns (2 to 4 hours). To check for the gag reflex the nurse places a tongue blade at the back of the client's tongue.
16. Nurse explains that hoarseness and a sore throat are normal for several days; cool fluids and normal saline gargling relieve soreness.
17. Nurse observes for bleeding, fever, abdominal pain, blood in the stool, difficulty with swallowing, and difficulty breathing.

Indirect Visualization.   When direct visualization is impossible (as with deeper GI structures), the physician relies on indirect x-ray examination. The client ingests a **contrast medium** or has the medium given as an enema. One of the most common media is barium, a white,

chalky, radiopaque substance that the client drinks like a milkshake. It is used in UGI studies and barium enemas. Contrast media usually contain a flavoring agent for better taste.

The upper GI study is an x-ray study of an ingested contrast medium that allows the physician to visualize the lower esophagus, stomach, and duodenum. The physician notes ulcerations, inflammation, tumors, and anatomical malposition of organs. The patency of organs and the pyloric valve are also observed. Nursing implications before the test include the following:

1. Client signs an informed consent.
2. Client takes nothing by mouth after midnight.
3. Nurse explains that the test might take several hours and requires frequent position changes; nurse explains that discomfort is minimal except for lying on a hard examination table.
4. Nurse explains that meglumine diatrizoate (Gastrografin) may have a chalky taste and that the client can resume eating after the test.

Small bowel follow-through (continuation of UGI) allows the physician to examine the small intestine. The flow of meglumine through the intestine may suggest motility problems. A barium enema allows indirect visualization of the lower colon to reveal location of tumors, polyps, and **diverticula.** The physician can also detect positional abnormalities.

Client Expectations.

Clients expect the nurse to be able to answer all of their questions regarding diagnostic tests and the preparation for those tests. Clients will be concerned about discomfort and exposure of their more personal areas. Fear of loss of control over bowel elimination is especially worrisome. Clients will need reassurance that their needs will be met and that the nurse will be supportive. Constipation is more of a problem as people age (Abyad and Mourad, 1996). Some older clients who may fail to recognize their elimination needs will need the nurse to monitor elimination patterns so that negative consequences will not occur. It is important for the nurse to remember that the client brings to any situation an individual perception of what is "right" for them. In the area of bowel elimination the client will expect a knowledgeable nurse who can teach them methods of promoting and maintaining a normal bowel elimination pattern.

NURSING DIAGNOSIS

The nurse's assessment of the client's bowel function reveals data that may indicate an actual or potential elimination problem or a problem resulting from elimination alterations (Box 45-5). Associated problems, such as body-image changes or skin breakdown, require interventions unrelated to bowel function impairment. However, in some instances the nurse must direct as much attention to the elimination problem as to the associated problem.

The nurse's ability to identify the correct diagnosis depends not only on the thoroughness of assessment but also on recognition of defining characteristics and factors that can impair elimination (Box 45-6). The nurse determines the client's risk and institutes measures to ensure maintenance of normal bowel function.

PLANNING

During the planning of care the nurse synthesizes information from multiple resources (Figure 45-11). Critical thinking ensures that the plan of care integrates all the nurse knows about the client and the clinical problem. The nurse relies on professional standards. The guidelines on incontinence (see Chapter 44) can assist the nurse in protecting the client's skin, promoting continence, and reducing the embarrassment associated with incontinence. In addition, the Agency for Health Care Policy and Research (AHCPR) guidelines on reduction of pressure ulcers also assist in developing care for clients with bowel incontinence (see Chapter 47).

The care plan establishes goals and outcomes by incorporating the client's elimination habits or routines as much as possible. If the habits caused the elimination problem, the nurse helps the client learn new ones. Defecation patterns vary among individuals. For this reason, the nurse and client must work together closely to plan effective interventions (see care plan).

When clients are disabled or debilitated by illness, it is necessary to include the family in the plan of care. Often family members have the same ineffective elimination habits as the client. Thus client and family teaching is an important part of the care plan. Other health team members such as dietitians and enterostomal therapists (ET nurses) can be valuable resources. When clients require surgical intervention, a critical pathway may be used to coordinate the activities of the multidisciplinary health care team (Figure 45-12).

The goals of care for clients with elimination problems include the following:
Understanding normal elimination
Attaining regular defecation habits
Understanding and maintaining proper fluid and food intake
Achieving a regular exercise program
Achieving comfort
Maintaining skin integrity
Maintaining self-concept

The client with alterations in bowel elimination will require intervention from many members of the health care team. Certain tasks, such as assisting clients onto the bedpan or bedside commode, are appropriate to delegate to assistive personnel. It will be important for the nurse to remind the assistant to report any abnormal findings or difficulties encountered during the elimination process. Many of the diagnostic tests for evaluation of the gas-

NURSING DIAGNOSES Box 45-5
CLIENTS WITH ALTERATION IN BOWEL ELIMINATION

Bowel incontinence
Constipation
Constipation, colonic
Constipation, perceived
Diarrhea
Skin integrity, impaired

SAMPLE NURSING DIAGNOSTIC PROCESS Box 45-6
DIARRHEA

Assessment Activities	Defining Characteristics	Nursing Diagnosis
Auscultate bowel sounds.	Bowel sounds will be hyperactive and may be audible without a stethescope.	Diarrhea related to infection, changes in diet, or alteration in gastrointestinal functioning
Assess frequency of stools.	Frequency is an early indication of increased risk for fluid and electrolyte imbalance, which is further indicated by muscle cramps.	
Assess hydration status.	Loss of skin turgor and dry mucous membranes indicate fluid deficit.	
Have clients describe pain, cramping, or any associated factors.	Pain is colicky in nature and spasmodic.	
Evaluate perianal area for redness and irritation.	Frequent stools lead to breakdown of perianal tissues.	

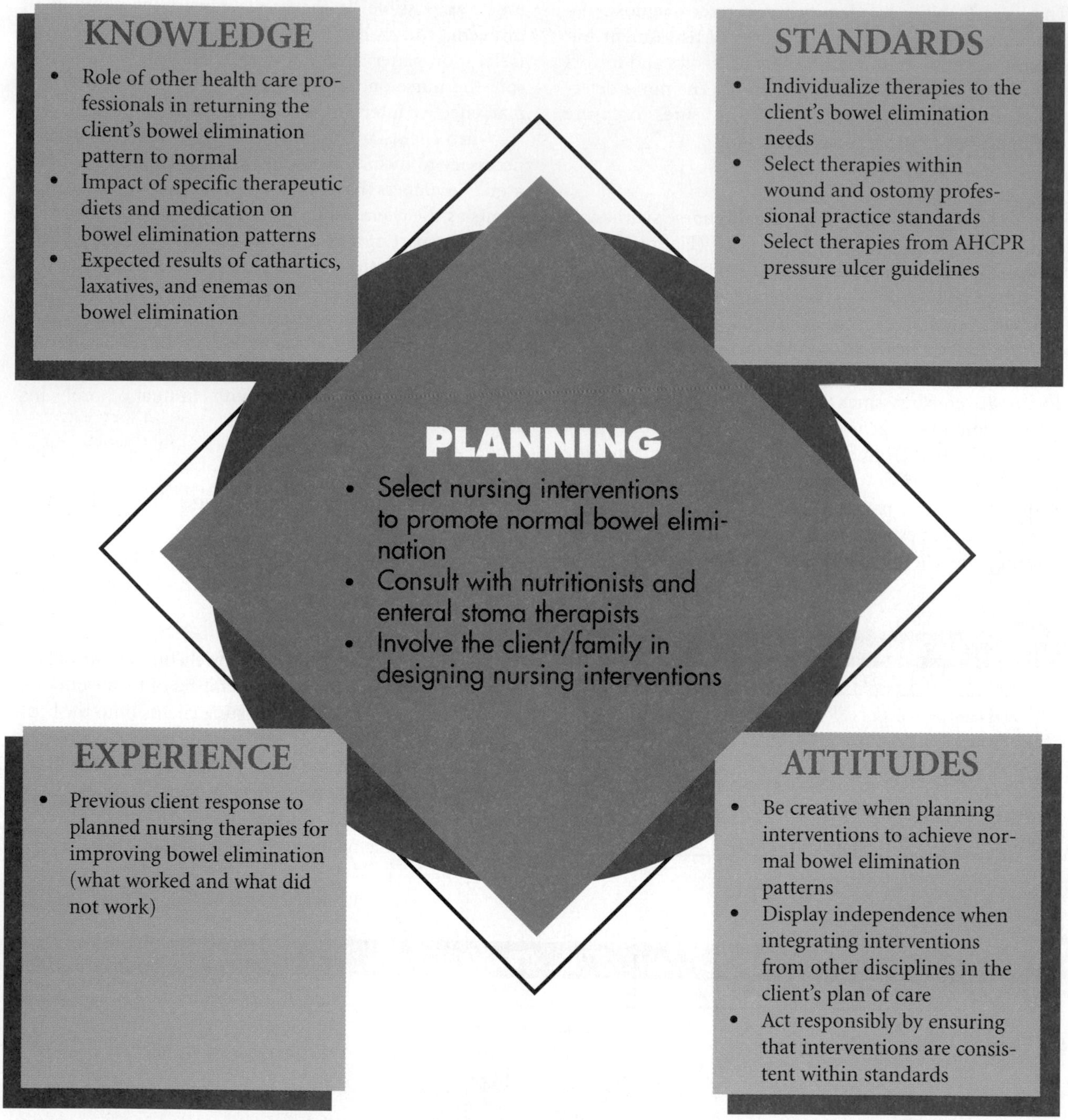

KNOWLEDGE

- Role of other health care professionals in returning the client's bowel elimination pattern to normal
- Impact of specific therapeutic diets and medication on bowel elimination patterns
- Expected results of cathartics, laxatives, and enemas on bowel elimination

STANDARDS

- Individualize therapies to the client's bowel elimination needs
- Select therapies within wound and ostomy professional practice standards
- Select therapies from AHCPR pressure ulcer guidelines

PLANNING

- Select nursing interventions to promote normal bowel elimination
- Consult with nutritionists and enteral stoma therapists
- Involve the client/family in designing nursing interventions

EXPERIENCE

- Previous client response to planned nursing therapies for improving bowel elimination (what worked and what did not work)

ATTITUDES

- Be creative when planning interventions to achieve normal bowel elimination patterns
- Display independence when integrating interventions from other disciplines in the client's plan of care
- Act responsibly by ensuring that interventions are consistent within standards

Figure 45-11   *Synthesis Model for Bowel Elimination Planning Phase.*

trointestinal system will be performed by nonnursing personnel. The nurse must maintain ongoing communication with these caregivers to ensure that the client's needs, wants, and concerns are addressed.

IMPLEMENTATION

Success of the nurse's interventions depends on improving the clients and family members' understanding of bowel elimination. In the home, hospital, or long-term care facility, clients capable of learning can be taught effective bowel habits.

The nurse should teach the client and family about proper diet, adequate fluid intake, and factors that stimulate or slow peristalsis, such as emotional stress. This often can best be done during the client's mealtime. The client should also learn the importance of establishing regular bowel routines and regular exercise and taking appropriate measures when elimination problems develop.

SAMPLE NURSING CARE PLAN

BOWEL ELIMINATION ALTERATIONS

ASSESSMENT*

Javier is visiting Larry at his home on one of the local cattle ranches. Larry lives 20 miles from town. He is 22 years old and **had surgery 6 days ago for repair of a badly broken right leg.** Larry tells Javier that **he has not had a bowel movement since he left the hospital** 4 days ago and that he **feels like his abdomen is tight and sore.** While auscultating for bowel sounds, Javier hears **decreased bowel sounds throughout.** While Javier is palpating Larry's abdomen, Larry tells Javier, **"It really hurts."** While reviewing the care plan, Javier also notices that Larry has been prescribed **Loritabs for pain.** Larry says he is taking one tablet every 6 hours, up to 3 a day. Larry also tells Javier that he **"Just doesn't feel good."** Javier asks Larry to do a 24-hour diet recall. Larry has eaten eggs, bacon, and toast and had soup for lunch. For supper Larry had chicken, rice and corn.

*****Defining characteristics** are shown in bold type.

NURSING DIAGNOSIS: Constipation related to opiate-containing pain medication

PLANNING

GOALS

Client will pass a soft, formed stool within the next 24 hours.
Client will voice relief from constipation.
Client will identify measures that will prevent constipation.

EXPECTED OUTCOMES

Client will drink at least 1500 ml of fluid over the next 8 hours.
Client will report passage of soft stool without straining.
Client will increase the fiber content of his diet.
Client discusses effect of exercise on elimination.

INTERVENTIONS†

Constipation/Impaction Management
- Encourage fluid intake of appropriate fluids, fruit juice, water.
- Encourage activity within the limits of client's mobility regimen.
- Add bran flakes or bran to the diet.
- Provide laxative or stool softeners as ordered

- Provide privacy.

RATIONALE

Adequate fluid intake is necessary to prevent hard, dry stool.

Even minimal activity (such as leg lifts) increases peristalsis.

The number of bowel movements are increased with bran.
Medications can soften the stool and prevent straining (Thompson, 1997).
Clients should feel relaxed when moving bowels (Stewart, 1998).

†Intervention Classification labels from McCloskey JC, Bulechek GM: *Nursing interventions classification (NIC),* ed 3, St. Louis, 2000, Mosby.

EVALUATION

Ask client to identify foods high in fiber.
Observe client's activity.
Ask client to plan menus to increase fiber.
Observe client's subsequent stool for characteristics such as consistency and color.

Health Promotion.   One of the most important habits a nurse can teach regarding bowel habits is to take time for defecation. To establish regular bowel habits, a client must know when the urge to defecate normally occurs. The nurse advises the client to begin establishing a routine during a time when defecation is most likely to occur, usually an hour after a meal. If a client is restricted to bed or requires assistance in ambulating, the nurse should offer a bedpan or help the client reach the bathroom.

Many clients have established rituals for defecation. In a hospital or long-term care facility, the nurse should make certain that treatment routines do not interfere with these schedules. It is also important to provide privacy. When clients forced to use a bedpan share rooms with other persons, the nurse should pull the curtain around the area so

that clients can relax, knowing that interruptions will not occur. The call light should always be placed within clients' reach. Bathroom doors should be closed, although the nurse may stand close in case clients need assistance.

Promotion of Normal Defecation.   To help clients evacuate bowel contents normally and without discomfort, a number of interventions can stimulate the defecation reflex, affect the character of feces, or increase peristalsis.

Squatting Position.   The nurse might need to assist clients who have difficulty squatting because of muscular weakness and mobility problems. Regular toilets are too low for clients unable to lower themselves to a squatting position because of joint- or muscle-wasting diseases.

BARNES

CARE PATH® 550
MAJOR SMALL & LARGE
BOWEL PROCEDURE

SERVICE		PHYSICIAN		1
PRIMARY NURSE		PRIMARY NURSE		
DC DATE	ADM DATE	DATE OF SURGERY	A-8	

Problem Number	PATIENT PROBLEMS / NURSING DIAGNOSES
#1	ALTERATION IN COMFORT RELATED TO ABDOMINAL SURGERY
#2	ALTERATION IN BOWEL ELIMINATION RELATED TO ABDOMINAL SURGERY
#3	ALTERATION IN SKIN INTEGRITY RELATED TO ABDOMINAL INCISION AND RECOVERY FROM SURGERY
#4	LACK OF KNOWLEDGE RELATED TO HOSPITALIZATION AND SURGICAL PROCEDURE
#5	ALTERATION IN BODY IMAGE RELATED TO ABDOMINAL SURGERY AND OSTOMY

* IF APPROPRIATE

#	1, 2, 3	3, 4, 5	4	4	1, 4
	ASSESSMENT / MONITORING	CONSULTS	PROCEDURES / TEST	TREATMENT	ACTIVITY
DAY 1 PRE OP	Assessment: Nursing Admission lab results Monitoring: VS routine O₂ saturation x1 I & O	Nurse specialist (if ostomy is a consideration).	CBC, 6, 12, PT, PTT T & C x2 units (admission labs) EKG ≥ 40 years old CXR ≥ 50 years old UA with micro *Mark ostomy site	Antithrombolytic stockings Mechanical bowel preparation	UAL
DAY 2 DOS	Assessment: Wound/dressing q 4 hrs. Bowel function q 4 hrs. Stoma appearance q 4 hrs. Pulmonary status q 2 hrs. Comfort level q 2 hrs. Braden score x1 Patency of tubes and characteristics of drainage q 8 hrs. IV patency & site appearance q 8 hrs. Fall risk factors Monitoring: VS q 1 hr. x 2 q 2 hrs. x2 then q 4 hrs. I & O q 4 hrs. O₂ saturation x1 x2	Respiratory Therapy for O₂		Antithrombolytic stockings O₂ to maintain O₂ saturation ≥ 92% Oral care q 4 hrs. Assist with Incentive Spirometer and TCDB q 2 hrs. Gastric decompression and tube irrigation	Bedrest
DAY 3 POD 1	Assessment: Wound/dressing q 4 hrs. Bowel function q 4 hrs. Stoma appearance q 4 hrs. Pulmonary status q 2 hrs. Comfort level q 2 hrs. Braden score x1 Patency of tubes and characteristics of drainage q 8 hrs. IV patency & site appearance q 8 hrs. Fall risk factors Lab results **O₂ saturation ≥ 92%** Monitoring: VS q 4 hrs. I & O q 8 hrs. Room air O₂ saturation x1 x2	Social Work Respiratory (if O₂ or tx needed) Nurse specialist (if ostomy placed).	CBC, 6	Antithrombolytic stockings Oral care q 4 hrs. Assist with Incentive Spirometer q 2 hrs. Gastric decompression and tube irrigation d/c foley d/c O₂	Up in chair with assist x1 x2 x3 Ambulate in room with assist x1 x2 Bed bath
DAY 4 POD 2	Assessment: Wound/dressing q 4 hrs. Bowel function q 4 hrs. Stoma appearance q 4 hrs. Pulmonary status q 2 hrs. Comfort level q 2 hrs. Braden score x1 Patency of tubes and characteristics of drainage q 8 hrs. IV patency & site appearance q 8 hrs. Fall risk factors Lab results **Voiding without difficulty (UO ≥ 240 cc q 8 hrs.)** Monitoring: VS q 4 hrs. I & O q 8 hrs.	Dietary screening		Antithrombolytic stockings Oral care q 4 hrs. Assist with Incentive Spirometer q 2 hrs. Gastric decompression and tube irrigation *Abdominal wound wet to dry dressing Change TID	Up in chair with assist x1 x2 x3 Ambulate in room with assist x1 x2 Bed bath

SIGNATURE	INIT.	SIGNATURE	INIT.	SIGNATURE	INIT.

Figure 45-12   Example of a portion of a care path for major small and large bowel procedure. Courtesy Barnes-Jewish Hospital, St. Louis, Mo.

Clients can purchase elevated toilet seats for the home. With such a seat, less effort is needed to sit or stand.

Positioning on Bedpan. Clients restricted to bed must use bedpans for defecation. Women use bedpans to pass both urine and feces, whereas men use bedpans only for defecation. Sitting on a bedpan can be extremely uncomfortable. The nurse should help position clients comfortably. Two types of bedpans are available (Figure 45-13). The regular bedpan, made of metal or hard plastic, has a curved smooth upper end and a sharp-edged lower end and is about 5 cm (2 inches) deep. A fracture pan, designed for clients with body or leg casts, has a shallow upper end about 1.3 cm (½ inch) deep. The upper end of the pan fits under the buttocks toward the sacrum, with the lower end just under the upper thighs. The pan should be high enough so that feces enter the pan. A metal bedpan should be warmed with water first, then dried.

When positioning a client, it is important to prevent muscle strain and discomfort. A client should never be placed on a bedpan and then left with the bed flat unless activity restrictions demand it. If the bed is flat, the hips remain hyperextended. It may be necessary to have the bed flat when placing the client on the bedpan. After the client is on it, the nurse raises the head of the bed 30 degrees. Raising the client to a 90-degree angle makes positioning difficult. In a sitting position, the client must rise straight up while using the strength of the arms as the nurse positions the pan. Most clients are too weak to accomplish this. Clients who have had abdominal surgery are hesitant to exert strain on suture lines. Furthermore, the nurse risks injury in trying to lift the client onto the bedpan.

Figure 45-14 shows proper and improper positions on bedpans. The best method is to be sure the client is positioned high in bed. The nurse raises the client's head about 30 degrees, to prevent hyperextension of the back and to provide support to the upper torso, as the client raises the hips by bending the knees and lifting the hips upward. The nurse places a hand palm up under the client's sacrum, resting the elbow on the mattress and using it as a lever to help in lifting, while slipping the pan under the client. Gloves should always be worn by the nurse when handling a bedpan.

If the client is immobile or it is unsafe to allow the client to exert such effort, the client can roll onto the bedpan by using the following steps:

1. Lower the head of the bed flat and assist the client to roll onto one side, backside toward you.
2. Apply powder lightly to back and buttocks to prevent skin from sticking to the pan
3. Place the bedpan firmly against the buttocks, down into the mattress with the open rim toward the client's feet (Figure 45-15).
4. Keeping one hand against the bedpan, place the other around the client's far hip. Ask the client to roll back onto the pan, flat in bed. Do not shove the pan under the client.
5. With the client positioned comfortably, raise the head of the bed 30 degrees.
6. Place a rolled towel or small pillow under the lumbar curve of the client's back for added comfort.
7. Raise the knee gatch or ask the client to bend the knees to assume a squatting position. Do not raise the knee gatch if contraindicated.

The nurse should maintain the privacy of a client using a bedpan. The call light and a supply of toilet paper should be within easy reach. When the client finishes, the nurse responds to the call signal immediately and removes the pan. The client might require assistance with wiping. To remove the pan the nurse asks the client to roll off to the side or raise the hips. The nurse holds the pan steady to avoid spilling. The nurse should avoid pulling or shoving

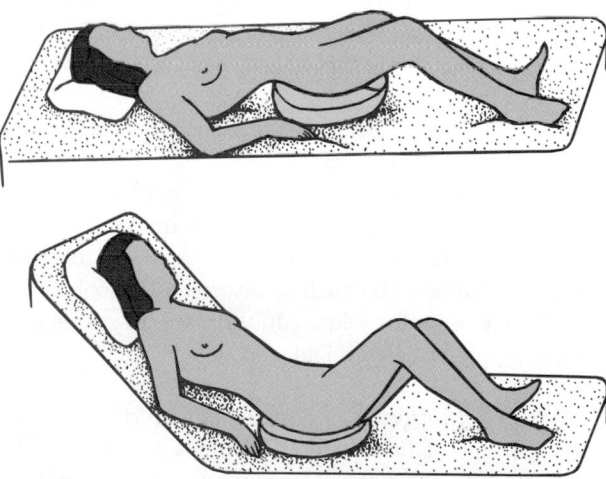

Figure 45-14 Positions on a bedpan. Top, Improper positioning of client. Bottom, Proper position reduces client's back strain.

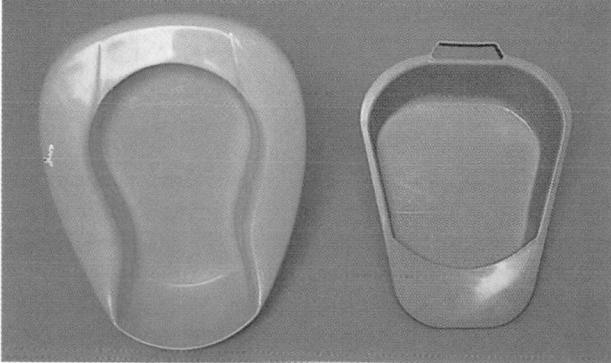

Figure 45-13 Types of bedpans. From left, regular bedpan and fracture bedpan.

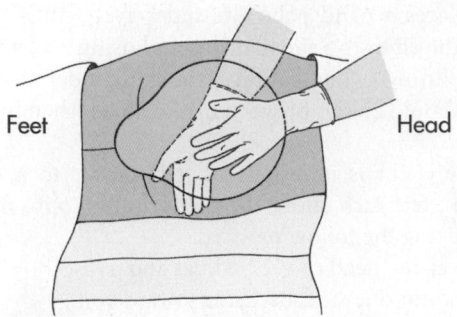

Figure 45-15   Positioning an immobilized client on a bed-pan.

the pan from under the client's hips because this can pull the client's skin and cause tissue injury such as a pressure ulcer (see Chapter 47). After the pan is removed, the nurse, while wearing gloves, cleans the anal and perineal areas.

After assessing the stool, the nurse should immediately empty the bedpan's contents into the toilet or in a special receptacle in the utility room. A spray faucet attached to most toilets allows the nurse to rinse the bedpan thoroughly. The client uses the same bedpan each time. The nurse should chart the characteristics of the feces.

The nurse should offer the bedpan often. Clients may accidentally soil bedclothes if forced to wait. Many clients try to avoid using a bedpan because it is embarrassing and uncomfortable. They may try to get to the bathroom even though their conditions prohibit ambulation. The nurse must warn clients about the risk of falls or accidents.

Cathartics and Laxatives.

Often a client is unable to defecate normally because of pain, constipation, or impaction. Cathartics and laxatives have the short-term action of emptying the bowel. They are also used in bowel evacuation for clients undergoing GI tests and abdominal surgery. Although the terms cathartic and laxative are often used interchangeably, cathartics have a stronger effect on the intestines. Five types of laxatives and cathartics are available (Table 45-5).

Cathartics and laxatives are available in oral, tablet, and powder suppository dosage forms (see Chapter 34). Although the oral route is most commonly used, cathartics that come prepared as suppositories are more effective because of their stimulant effect on the rectal mucosa. Cathartic suppositories such as bisacodyl (Dulcolax) can act within 30 minutes. Older adults often get a strong sudden urge to defecate with Dulcolax.

Antidiarrheal Agents.

For clients with diarrhea, frequent passage of liquid stools becomes a problem. The most effective antidiarrheal agents are opiates such as codeine phosphate, opium tincture (paregoric), and diphenoxylate (Lomotil). Antidiarrheal opiate agents decrease intestinal muscle tone to slow passage of feces.

Opiates inhibit peristaltic waves that move feces forward, but they also increase segmental contractions that mix intestinal contents. As a result, more water is absorbed by the intestinal walls. Antidiarrheal agents should be used with caution because opiates are habit forming.

Acute Care

Enemas.   An **enema** is the instillation of a solution into the rectum and sigmoid colon. The primary reason for an enema is to promote defecation by stimulating peristalsis. The volume of fluid instilled breaks up the fecal mass, stretches the rectal wall, and initiates the defecation reflex. Enemas are also given as a vehicle for drugs that exert a local effect on rectal mucosa.

The most common use for an enema is temporary relief of constipation. Other indications include removing impacted feces; emptying the bowel before diagnostic tests, surgery, or childbirth; and beginning a program of bowel training.

Cleansing Enemas.   Cleansing enemas promote the complete evacuation of feces from the colon. They act by stimulating peristalsis through the infusion of a large volume of solution or through local irritation of the colon's mucosa. Suggested maximum volumes follow:

Infant	150 to 250 ml
Toddler	250 to 350 ml
School-ager	300 to 500 ml
Adolescent	500 to 750 ml
Adult	750 to 1000 ml

Cleansing enemas include tap water, normal saline, soapsuds solution, and low-volume hypertonic saline. Each solution exerts a different osmotic effect (see Chapter 40), influencing the movement of fluids between the colon and interstitial spaces beyond the intestinal wall. Infants and children should receive only normal saline because they are at risk for fluid imbalance.

Tap Water.   Tap water is hypotonic and exerts a lower osmotic pressure than fluid in interstitial spaces. After infusion into the colon, tap water escapes from the bowel lumen into interstitial spaces. The net movement of water is low. The infused volume stimulates defecation before large amounts of water leave the bowel. Tap water enemas should not be repeated because water toxicity or circulatory overload can develop if large amounts of water are absorbed.

Normal Saline.   Physiologically normal saline is the safest solution to use because it exerts the same osmotic pressure as fluids in interstitial spaces surrounding the bowel. The volume of infused saline stimulates peristalsis. Giving saline enemas does not create the danger of excess fluid absorption. If prepared saline is not available at home, the client may be instructed by the physician or nurse to mix 500 ml (1 pint) of tap water with 1 teaspoon of table salt.

Table 45-5   Common Types of Laxatives and Cathartics

Agent/Brand Name	Action	Indications	Risks
Bulk Forming Methylcellulose (Cologel, Hydrolose) Psyllium (Metamucil, Naturacil)	High-fiber content absorbs water and increases solid intestinal bulk. Agents stretch intestinal wall to stimulate peristalsis.	Agents are least irritating, most natural, and safest cathartics. Agents are drugs of choice for chronic constipation (e.g., pregnancy, low-residue diet). Agents may also be used to relieve mild, watery diarrhea.	Agents can cause obstruction if not mixed with at least 240 ml of water or juice and swallowed quickly. Caution is used with bulk-forming laxatives that also contain stimulants. Agents are not used in clients for whom large fluid intake is contraindicated.
Emollient or Wetting Docusate sodium (Colace, Disonate) Docusate calcium (Surfak) Docusate potassium (Dialose)	Stool softeners are detergents that lower surface tension of feces, allowing water and fat to penetrate. They may increase secretion of water by intestine.	Agents are used for short-term therapy to relieve straining on defecation (e.g., hemorrhoids, perianal surgery, pregnancy, recovery from myocardial infarction).	Agents are of little value for treatment of chronic constipation.
Saline Magnesium citrate or citrate of magnesia (Citroma) Magnesium hydroxide (Milk of Magnesia) Sodium phosphate (Fleet Phospho-Soda, Fleet Enema)	Agents contain salt preparation not absorbed by intestines. Osmotic effect increases pressure in bowel to act as stimulant for peristalsis. Agents may also lubricate feces.	Agents are used only for acute emptying of bowel (e.g., endoscopic examination, suspected poisoning, acute constipation).	Agents are not used in long-term management of constipation. Agents are not used in clients with kidney dysfunction (toxic buildup of magnesium). Phosphate salts are not used for clients on fluid restriction.
Stimulant Cathartics Bisacodyl (Dulcolax) Castor oil (Neoloid, Purge) Casanthranol (Dialose Plus, Peri-Colace) Danthron (Modane Bulk) Phenolphthalein (Doxidan, Correctol, Ex-Lax)	Agents irritate intestinal mucosa to increase motility. Agents decrease absorption in small bowel and colon. Phenolphthalein and danthron may cause pink or red urine.	Agents may be used to prepare bowel for diagnostic procedures.	Agents may cause severe cramping. Agents are not for long-term use. Chronic use may cause fluid and electrolyte imbalances. Agents are avoided during pregnancy and lactation.
Lubricants Mineral oil (Haley's M-O, Petrogalar Plain)	Agents coat fecal contents, allowing easier passage of stool. Agents reduce water absorption in colon.	Agents are used to prevent straining on defecation (e.g., hemorrhoids, perianal surgery).	Agents decrease absorption of fat-soluble vitamins (A, D, E, and K). Agents can cause dangerous form of pneumonia if aspirated into lungs. Mineral oil when taken with emollients can increase risk for fat emboli.

Hypertonic solutions infused into the bowel exert osmotic pressure that pulls fluids out of interstitial spaces. The colon fills with fluid, and the resultant distention promotes defecation. Clients unable to tolerate large volumes of fluid benefit most from this type of enema, which is, by design, low volume. Contraindications for this type of enema are clients who are dehydrated and young infants. A hypertonic solution of 120 to 180 ml (4 to 6 oz) is usually effective. The commercially prepared Fleets Enema is the most commonly used.

Soapsuds.   Soapsuds may be added to tap water or saline to create the effect of intestinal irritation to stimulate peristalsis. This soap is called castile and comes in a liquid form included in most soapsuds enema kits. Harsh soaps or detergents can cause serious bowel inflammation. The recommended ratio of soap to solution is 5 ml (1 teaspoon) of castile soap to 1000 ml of warm water or saline.

A physician may order a high or low cleansing enema. The terms *high* and *low* refer to the height from which and hence the pressure with which the fluid is delivered. High enemas are given to cleanse the entire colon. Fluid is delivered at a high pressure by raising the enema container to a high level. During administration of a regular enema, the enema can or bag is held 30 cm (12 inches) above the client's hips. With a high enema the bag or can is raised to 30 to 45 cm (12 to 18 inches) or slightly higher above the hips. The client is asked to turn from the left lateral to the dorsal recumbent, over to the right lateral position. The position change ensures that fluid reaches the large intestine. With a low enema the nurse holds the bag 7.5 cm (3 inches) or less above the client's hips. A low enema cleans only the rectum and sigmoid colon.

Oil Retention.   Oil-retention enemas lubricate the rectum and colon. The feces absorb the oil and become softer and easier to pass. To enhance action of the oil, the client retains the enema for several hours if possible.

Other Types of Enemas.   Carminative enemas provide relief from gaseous distention. They improve the ability to pass flatus. An example of a carminative enema is MGW solution, which contains 30 ml of magnesium, 60 ml of glycerin, and 90 ml of water.

A return-flow enema, or Harris flush, is a mild colonic irrigation that helps expel flatus. The nurse first administers a small amount (100 to 200 ml) of mild enema solution into the client's rectum and colon. Then the nurse lowers the enema container to allow the solution to flow back through the rectal tube and into the container. Repeating this process several times aids in reducing flatus and promoting peristalsis.

Medicated enemas contain drugs. An example is sodium polystyrene sulfonate (Kayexalate), used to treat clients with dangerously high serum potassium levels. This drug contains a resin that exchanges sodium ions for potassium ions in the large intestine. Another medicated enema is neomycin solution, an antibiotic used to reduce bacteria in the colon before bowel surgery.

Enema Administration.   The nurse administers enemas in commercially packaged, disposable units or with reusable equipment prepared before use. Sterile technique is unnecessary because the colon normally contains bacteria. However, the nurse wears gloves to prevent the transmission of fecal microorganisms.

The nurse should explain the procedure, including the position to assume, precautions to take to avoid discomfort, and the length of time necessary to retain the solution before defecation. If the client is to receive the enema at home, the nurse explains the procedure to a family member.

Often the physician orders "enemas till clear." This means that the enema is repeated until the client passes fluid that is clear and contains no fecal material. It may be necessary to give as many as three enemas, but the nurse should caution the client against using more than three. Excess enema use seriously depletes fluids and electrolytes. If the enema fails to return a clear solution after three times (check agency policy) or if the client seems to not be tolerating the rigors of repeated enemas, the physician should be notified.

Giving an enema to a client who is unable to contract the external sphincter can pose difficulties. The nurse gives the enema with the client positioned on the bedpan. Giving the enema with the client sitting on the toilet is unsafe because the curved rectal tubing can abrade the rectal wall. Skill 45-1 outlines the steps for an enema administration.

Digital Removal of Stool.   For clients with an impaction, the fecal mass may be too large to be passed voluntarily. If enemas fail, the nurse must break up the fecal mass with the fingers and remove it in sections. The procedure can be very uncomfortable for the client. Excess rectal manipulation may cause irritation to the mucosa, bleeding, and stimulation of the vagus nerve, which results in a reflex slowing of the heart rate. Because of the procedure's potential complications, a physician's order is necessary for the nurse to remove a fecal impaction.

The steps for removing stool digitally follow:

1. Explain the procedure. Take baseline vital signs prior to the procedure. Help the client lie on the side with knees flexed and back toward you.
2. Drape the trunk and lower extremities with a bath blanket and place a waterproof pad under the buttocks. Keep a bedpan next to the client.
3. Apply disposable gloves and lubricate the index finger of your dominant hand with lubricating jelly.
4. Gently insert the gloved index finger into the rectum and advance the finger slowly along the rectal wall toward the umbilicus.
5. Gently loosen the fecal mass by massaging around it. Work the finger into the hardened mass.
6. Work the feces downward toward the end of the rectum. Remove small pieces at a time and discard into bedpan.
7. Reassess the client's heart rate and look for signs of

Text continued on p. 1466.

Administering a Cleansing Enema   Skill 45-1

Delegation Considerations

The skill of administering an enema can be delegated to assistive personnel.

- Inform and assist caregiver in proper way to position clients who have mobility restrictions.
- Caution caregiver about transmission of pathogens.
- Inform caregiver about how to position clients who also have therapeutic equipment present, such as drains, intravenous catheters, or traction.
- Inform caregiver regarding signs and symptoms of client not tolerating the procedure, and when it must be stopped.

EQUIPMENT

- Disposable gloves
- Water-soluble lubricant
- Waterproof, absorbent pads
- Bath blanket
- Toilet tissue
- Bedpan, bedside commode, or access to toilet
- Washbasin, washcloths, towel, and soap
- Intravenous pole
- Enema bag administration
    - Enema container
    - Tubing and clamp (if not already attached to container)
    - Appropriate size rectal tube:
        Adult: 22 to 30 Fr
        Child: 12 to 18 Fr
- Correct volume of warmed solution:
    Adult: 750 to 1000 ml
    Child:
        150 to 250 ml, infant
        250 to 350 ml, toddler
        300 to 500 ml, school-age child
        500 to 750 ml, adolescent
- Prepackaged enema
    - Prepackaged enema container with rectal tip

STEPS	RATIONALE
1. Assess status of client: last bowel movement, normal bowel patterns, hemorrhoids, mobility, external sphincter control, abdominal pain.	Determines factors indicating need for enema and influencing the type of enema used.
2. Assess for presence of increased intracranial pressure, glaucoma, or recent rectal or prostate surgery.	Conditions contraindicate use of enemas.
3. Determine client's level of understanding of purpose of enema.	Allows nurse to plan for appropriate teaching measures.
4. Check client's medical record to clarify the rationale for the enema.	Determines purpose of enema administration: preparation for special procedure or relief of constipation.
5. Review physician's order for enema.	Order by physician is required. Determines number and type of enema to be given.
6. Collect appropriate equipment.	
7. Correctly identify client and explain procedure.	Information promotes client cooperation and reduces anxiety.
8. Assemble enema bag with appropriate solution and rectal tube.	
9. Wash hands and apply gloves.	Reduces transmission of microorganisms.
10. Provide privacy by closing curtains around bed or closing door.	Reduces embarrassment for client.
11. Raise bed to appropriate working height for nurse: raise side rail on opposite side.	Promotes good body mechanics and client safety.
12. Assist client into left side-lying (Sims') position with right knee flexed. Children may also be placed in dorsal recumbent position.	Allows enema solution to flow downward by gravity along natural curve of sigmoid colon and rectum, thus improving retention of solution.

Critical Decision Point: If client is suspected of having poor sphincter control, position on bedpan. Client will have difficulty retaining enema solution.

13. Place waterproof pad under hips and buttocks.	Prevents soiling of linen.
14. Cover client with bath blanket, exposing only rectal area, clearly visualizing anus.	Provides warmth, reduces exposure of body parts, and allows client to feel more relaxed and comfortable.

STEPS	RATIONALE
15. Place bedpan or commode in easily accessible position. If client will be expelling contents in toilet, ensure that toilet is free. (If client will be getting up to bathroom to expel enema, place client's slippers and bathrobe in easily accessible position.)	Used in case client is unable to retain enema solution.
16. Administer enema:	
A. **Prepackaged disposable container**	
(1) Remove plastic cap from rectal tip. Tip is already lubricated, but more jelly can be applied as needed.	Lubrication provides for smooth insertion of rectal tube without causing rectal irritation or trauma.
(2) Gently separate buttocks and locate rectum. Instruct client to relax by breathing out slowly through mouth.	Breathing out promotes relaxation of external rectal sphincter.
(3) Insert tip of bottle gently into rectum. 　　Adult: 7.5 to 10 cm (3 to 4 in) 　　Child: 5 to 7.5 cm (2 to 3 in) 　　Infant: 2.5 to 3.75 cm (1 to 1 ½ in)	Gentle insertion prevents trauma to rectal mucosa.
(4) Squeeze bottle until all of solution has entered rectum and colon. Instruct client to retain solution until the urge to defecate occurs, usually 2 to 5 minutes.	Hypertonic solutions require only small volumes to stimulate defecation.
B. **Enema bag**	
(1) Add warmed solution to enema bag: warm tap water as it flows from faucet, place saline container in basin of hot water before adding saline to enema bag, check temperature of solution with bath thermometer or by pouring small amount of solution over inner wrist.	Hot water can burn intestinal mucosa. Cold water can cause abdominal cramping and is difficult to retain.
(2) Raise container, release clamp, and allow solution to flow long enough to fill tubing.	Removes air from tubing.
(3) Reclamp tubing.	Prevents further loss of solution.
(4) Lubricate 6 to 8 cm (2½ to 4 in) of tip of rectal tube with lubricating jelly.	Allows smooth insertion of rectal tube without risk of irritation or trauma to mucosa.
(5) Gently separate buttocks and locate anus. Instruct client to relax by breathing out slowly through mouth.	Breathing out promotes relaxation of external anal sphincter.
(6) Insert tip of rectal tube slowly by pointing tip in direction of client's umbilicus (see illustration). Length of insertion varies: 　　Adult: 7.5 to 10 cm (3 to 4 in) 　　Child: 5 to 7.5 cm (2 to 3 in) 　　Infant: 2.5 to 3.75 cm (1 to 1 ½ in)	Careful insertion prevents trauma to rectal mucosa from accidental lodging of tube against rectal wall. Insertion beyond proper limit can cause bowel perforation.
(7) Hold tubing in rectum constantly until end of fluid instillation.	Bowel contraction can cause expulsion of rectal tube.
(8) Open regulating clamp and allow solution to enter slowly with container at client's hip level.	Rapid instillation can stimulate evacuation of rectal tube.
(9) Raise height of enema container slowly to appropriate level above anus: 30 to 45 cm (12 to 18 in) for high enema, 30 cm (12 in) for regular enema, 7.5 cm (3 in) for low enema.	Allows for continuous, slow instillation of solution. Raising container too high causes rapid instillation and possible painful distention of colon. High pressure can cause rupture of bowel in infant.
(10) Lower container or clamp tubing if client complains of cramping or if fluid escapes around rectal tube.	Temporary cessation of instillation prevents cramping, which may prevent client from retaining all fluid, altering effectiveness of enema.
(11) Clamp tubing after all solution is instilled.	Prevents entrance of air into rectum.

STEPS	RATIONALE
17. Place layers of toilet tissue around tube at anus and gently withdraw rectal tube.	Provides client's comfort and cleanliness.
18. Explain to client that feeling of distention is normal. Ask client to retain solution as long as possible while lying quietly in bed. (For infant or young child, gently hold buttocks together for a few minutes.)	Solution distends bowel. Length of retention varies with type of enema and client's ability to contract rectal sphincter. Longer retention promotes more effective stimulation of peristalsis and defecation.
19. Discard enema container and tubing in proper receptacle or rinse out thoroughly with warm soap and water if container is to be reused.	Reduces transmission and growth of microorganisms.
20. Assist client to bathroom or help to position client on bedpan.	Normal squatting position promotes defecation.
21. Observe character of feces and solution (caution client against flushing toilet before inspection).	

Critical Decision Point: When enemas are ordered "until clear," observe contents of solution passed. Return is "clear" when no solid fecal material exists, but solution may be colored.

---

22. Assist client as needed to wash anal area with warm soap and water (if nurse administers perineal care, use gloves).	Fecal contents can irritate skin. Hygiene promotes client's comfort.
23. Remove and discard gloves and wash hands.	Reduces transmission of microorganisms.
24. Inspect color, consistency, amount of stool, and fluid passed.	Determines if stool is evacuated or fluid is retained. Note abnormalities such as presence of blood or mucus.
25. Assess condition of abdomen; cramping, rigidity, or distention can indicate a serious problem.	Determines if distention is relieved. Excess volume can distend or perforate the bowel.

Recording and Reporting
- Record type and volume of enema given and characteristics of results.
- Report failure of client to defecate to physician.

Home Care Considerations
- For clients who require enemas for bowel preparation at home, instruct family not to exceed recommended fluid volume levels or number of enemas. Encourage family about the need for slow administration of warmed fluid.
- Instruct family about the negative side effects of tap water enemas.

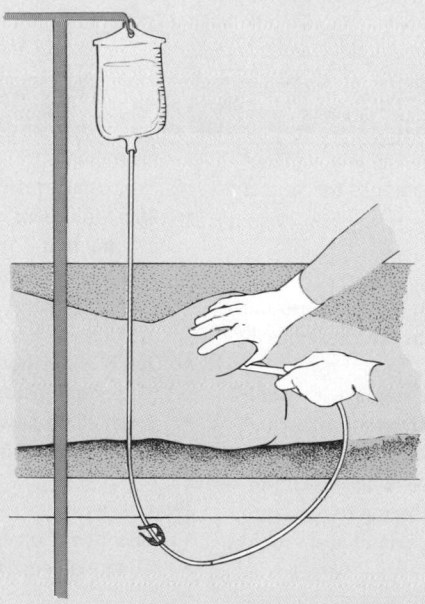

Step 16B(6)

fatigue. Stop the procedure if the heart rate drops significantly or the rhythm changes.

8. Continue to clean feces and allow the client to rest at intervals.

9. Once completed, offer a washcloth and towel to wash and dry the buttocks and anal area. Assist as needed.

10. Remove bedpan and dispose of feces. Remove gloves by turning them inside out, then discard.

11. Assist client to toilet or clean bedpan if urge to defecate develops.

12. Wash hands. Record results of disimpaction by describing fecal characteristics.

13. The procedure may be followed by enemas or cathartics.

14. Reassess client's vital signs.

Care of Ostomies. Clients who have temporary or permanent bowel diversions face unique health care problems. Their patterns of bowel elimination differ from those of clients with intact colons. Persons with incontinent ostomies must wear pouches or appliances to collect stool emitted from the stomas. Some clients learn to irrigate their ostomies to establish regular bowel elimination routines. Clients with ostomies must also follow good health practices such as maintaining proper dietary habits and exercising regularly to maintain normal elimination patterns. Clients with an ostomy have many education needs (Box 45-7).

Pouching Ostomies. An incontinent ostomy requires a pouch to collect fecal material. An effective pouching system protects the skin, contains fecal material, remains odor free, and is comfortable and inconspicuous. A person wearing a pouch should feel secure in participating in any activity.

Many pouching systems are available. To ensure that a pouch fits well and meets the client's needs, the nurse considers the location of the ostomy, type and size of the stoma, type and amount of ostomy drainage, size and contour of the abdomen, condition of the skin around the stoma, physical activities of the client, client's personal preference, age, and dexterity, and cost of equipment. An **enterostomal therapist (ET)** is a nurse trained to care for ostomy clients. The staff nurse collaborates with the ET to be sure the correct pouching system is used. For example, referral to an ET nurse would be appropriate to plan the care of a client who has a high-output ostomy that requires a pouch modification.

A pouching system consists of a pouch and skin barrier. Some pouching systems, such as Squibb-Convatec, Hollister, Coloplast, and Smith & Nephew, are attached to the client's skin from the product's adhesive surface, whereas other pouching systems, such as VIP, are nonadhesive systems. Pouches come in one- and two-piece systems that are disposable or reusable. Some pouches have the opening precut by the manufacturer; others require the stoma opening to be custom cut by someone to the client's specific stoma size.

Skin barriers include wafers, pastes, powders, and liquid film that are applied to the skin around the stoma. Some wafer skin barriers are permanently attached to the ostomy pouch. These are called one-piece pouch systems. In a two-piece system, the pouch can be detached from the skin barrier for emptying or changing. This allows the skin barrier to remain around the client's stoma for several days, thus minimizing the chance of skin damage from too-frequent removal of the skin barrier from the peris-

---

Client Teaching FOR STOMAL CARE (INCONTINENT OSTOMY)   Box 45-7

OBJECTIVE
• Client will demonstrate the correct procedure for stomal care.

TEACHING STRATEGIES
• Instruct client to avoid using alcohol in cleansing around the stoma. Alcohol dilates capillaries and can cause bleeding of the stomal margin.
• Demonstrate how to wash around the stoma with water and a mild soap or with a commercial preparation, such as Peri-Wash. Pat the skin dry, but do not rub.
• Instruct client not to use cold cream on skin because it prevents the pouch or skin barrier from adhering to the skin.
• Explain to the client that peroxide is an irritant and should not be used.
• Instruct the client that if a yeast infection occurs, thorough cleansing, followed by patting the area dry and applying

triamcinolone acetonide (Kenalog) spray or nystatin (Mycostatin) usually resolves the infection.
• Show the client how to inspect the stoma daily and observe a stoma that is moist, shiny, and dark pink to red.
• Teach client to observe for and report excessive bleeding, edema, or abnormal discharge or color to the nurse or physician.
• Teach client how to select and apply correctly sized skin barrier and ostomy pouch.
• Teach client how to empty pouch.
• Teach client techniques to reduce odor.

EVALUATION
• Client will correctly state skin care procedures.
• Client will correctly perform stoma skin care procedure.

tomal skin. When using a two-piece pouching system, it is important to remember that the skin barrier and pouch must be the same corresponding size and from the same manufacturer. The pouch from one manufacturer will not fit correctly on the skin barrier from another manufacturer. The nurse must be sure to use an ostomy pouch made for collecting fecal matter (colostomy or ileostomy) and not one for collecting urine.

It is important to measure the stoma size carefully when selecting and cutting out the opening on the wafer skin barrier. A good skin barrier protects the skin, prevents irritation from repeated removal of the pouch, and is comfortable for the client to wear. Skill 45-2 describes steps for applying one type of pouch system.

Irrigating a Colostomy. To establish a pattern of regular defecation, clients with descending and sigmoid colostomies often irrigate their ostomy. The muscular quality of the colon allows it to be safely irrigated with a relatively large volume of water or saline. The irrigation acts like an enema, distending the bowel and stimulating peristalsis. Fluid is instilled into the colon via the stoma. Elimination thus occurs at a time chosen by the client. The irrigation also cleans the colon of gas and odor. Only specific equipment for irrigating an ostomy should be used. NEVER use an enema set to irrigate an ostomy. Gentle irrigation using the correct equipment is performed to reduce the risk of bowel perforation.

Surgical creation of a colostomy can seriously change a person's body image. Regaining control of fecal elimination through irrigation helps emotional adjustment. The client can also gain freedom without the need to wear a stomal pouch continuously, although most clients prefer to wear a smaller pouch over the stoma between irrigations in case of any fecal spillage.

The physician recommends when to begin irrigations and their frequency. Eventually clients develop their own schedules. However, it is usually necessary to perform the procedure the same way, at the same time of day, and with the same frequency (e.g., every day or every other day, 3 times a week). Some clients have physical or mental limitations that make colostomy irrigations unwise; these include ascending colostomies, recent colostomy formation,

presence of disease in the remainder of the colon, and a prolapsed stoma. Young children and infants should not receive colostomy irrigations. Infants are at risk for bowel perforation. Young children often cannot sit still for the procedure.

Clients may find irrigation a problem. The procedure is time consuming (45 to 60 minutes), and clients may be unwilling to interrupt their lifestyles. For many, irrigation is unpleasant. The nurse's emotional support can help clients make a choice. Alternate methods of ostomy management are available such as dietary control or laxative use. If a client initially decides against irrigations, the decision can be changed later. Skill 45-3 outlines the steps for an ostomy irrigation.

Inserting and Maintaining a Nasogastric Tube. A client's condition or situation may warrant special interventions to decompress the GI tract. Such conditions include surgery (see Chapter 49), infections of the GI tract, trauma to the GI tract, and conditions in which peristalsis is absent.

A nasogastric (NG) tube is a pliable tube that is inserted through the client's nasopharynx into the stomach. The tube has a hollow lumen that allows removal of gastric secretions and introduction of solutions into the stomach. Nasogastric intubation has several purposes (Table 45-6).

The Levin and Salem sump tubes are the most common for stomach decompression. The Levin tube is a single-lumen tube with holes near the tip. It may be connected to a drainage bag or to an intermittent suction device to drain stomach secretions.

The Salem sump tube is preferable for stomach decompression. The tube has two lumina: one for removal of gastric contents and one to provide an air vent. A blue "pigtail" is the air vent that connects with the second lumen. When the sump tube's main lumen is connected to suction, the air vent permits free, continuous drainage of secretions. The air vent should never be clamped off, connected to suction, or used for irrigation.

Nasogastric tube insertion (Skill 45-4) does not require sterile technique. The nurse simply uses clean technique. The procedure is uncomfortable. The client experiences a

Text continued on p. 1480.

Table 45-6	**Purposes of Nasogastric Intubation**	
Purpose	Description	Type of Tube
Decompression	Removal of secretions and gaseous substances from gastrointestinal tract; prevention or relief of abdominal distention	Salem sump, Levin, Miller-Abbott
Feeding (gavage) (see Chapter 43)	Instillation of liquid nutritional supplements or feedings into stomach for clients unable to swallow fluid	Duo, Dobhoff, Levin
Compression	Internal application of pressure by means of inflated balloon to prevent internal esophageal or gastrointestinal hemorrhage	Sengstaken-Blakemore
Lavage	Irrigation of stomach in cases of active bleeding, poisoning, or gastric dilation	Levin, Ewald, Salem sump

Skill 45-2   Pouching an Ostomy

Delegation Considerations

The skill of pouching an ostomy, especially a newly established ostomy, requires problem solving and knowledge application unique to a professional nurse. Delegation is inappropriate. Pouching of an established ostomy can be delegated to assistive personnel.

- Assist caregiver in selecting appropriate pouch and skin barrier.
- Inform caregiver of the signs of stomal and peristomal skin changes that should be reported to a registered professional

nurse (RN).

- Have caregiver monitor and report characteristics and volume of ostomy output.

EQUIPMENT (SEE ILLUSTRATION)

- Pouch, clear drainable colostomy/ileostomy in correct size for two-piece system or custom cut-to-fit one-piece type with attached skin barrier
- Pouch closure device, such as clamp
- Adhesive remover (optional)
- Clean disposable gloves
- Deodorant

- Gauze pads or washcloth
- Towel or disposable waterproof barrier
- Basin with warm tap water
- Scissors
- Skin barrier such as sealant wipes or wafer
- Tape or ostomy belt

STEPS	RATIONALE
1. Auscultate for bowel sounds.	Documents presence of peristalsis.
2. Observe skin barrier and pouch for leakage and length of time in place. Depending on type of pouching system used (such as with an opaque pouch), the nurse may have to remove the pouch to fully observe the stoma. Clear pouches permit the viewing of the stoma without their removal.	May indicate need for different type of pouch or sealant.
3. Observe stoma for color, swelling, trauma, and healing, stoma should be moist and reddish-pink. Assess type of stoma. Stomas can be flush with the skin or be a budlike protrusion on the abdomen (see illustration for a normal bud stoma).	Stoma characteristics should be one of the factors to consider when selecting an appropriate pouching system.

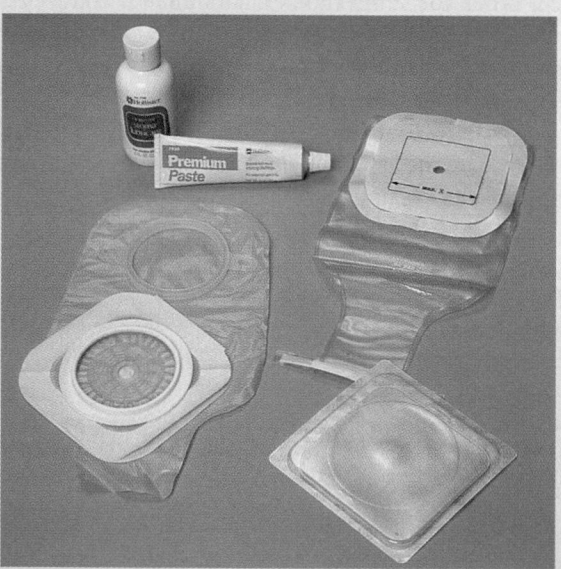

Equipment

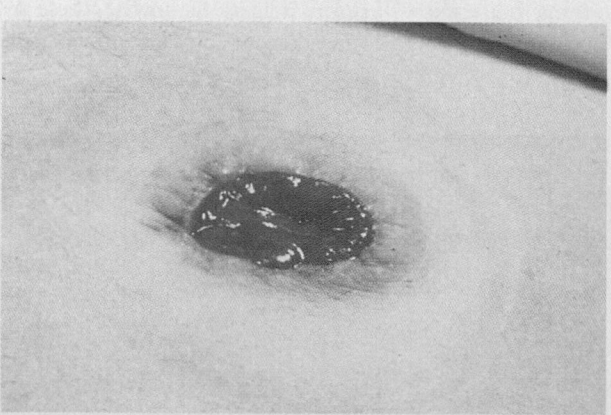

Step 3

Courtesy Hollister, Inc., Libertyville, Ill.

STEPS	RATIONALE
4. Measure the stoma with each pouching change. Follow pouch manufacturer's directions and measuring guide as to which pouch to use based on client's stoma size.	Determines correct size equipment, preventing trauma to stoma.
5. Observe abdominal incision (if present).	Relationship to stoma determines proper placement of pouch.
6. Observe effluent from stoma and keep a record of intake and output. Ask client about skin tenderness.	
7. Avoid unnecessary changing of the entire pouching system. A one-piece pouch with attached skin barriers or the skin barrier of a two-piece pouching system should be changed every 3 to 7 days, *not* daily.	Pouches should be emptied when one-third to one-half full, because the weight of contents may dislodge the skin seal, and ostomy drainage is irritating to the skin. Also, pouches collect flatus (gas), which needs to be expelled because it can disrupt the skin seal.

Critical Decision Point: Do not put holes in ostomy pouch for flatus to escape.

STEPS	RATIONALE

8. Assess abdomen for best type of pouching system to use. Consider:
  a. Contour and peristomal plane
  b. Presence of scars, incisions
  c. Location and type of stoma
	Determines pouching system selection and need for other equipment.

9. Assess the client's self-care ability to determine the best type of pouching system to use.	Clients who have difficulty using their hands or who have limited vision may find a one-piece system or a precut pouch and skin barrier more desirable to use; others prefer being able to keep the skin barrier in place for several days, changing just the pouch, and therefore prefer the two-piece system.
10. After skin barrier and pouch removal, assess skin around stoma, noting scars, folds, skin breakdown, and peristomal suture line, if present.	Determines need for barrier paste to increase adherence of pouch to skin or to fill in irregularities.
11. Determine client's emotional response and knowledge and understanding of an ostomy and its care.	Assists in determining extent to which client is able to participate in care and need for teaching and information clarification.
12. Explain procedure to client; encourage client's interaction and questions.	Lessens anxiety and promotes client's participation.
13. Assemble equipment and close room curtains or door.	Optimizes use of time; conserves client's and nurse's energy. Provides privacy.
14. Position client either standing or supine and drape. If seated, position either on or in front of the toilet.	When client is supine, fewer wrinkles allow for ease of application of pouching system; maintains client's dignity.
15. Wash hands and put on disposable gloves.	Reduces transmission of microorganisms.
16. Place towel or disposable waterproof barrier under the client.	Protects bed linen.
17. Remove used pouch and skin barrier gently by pushing the skin away from the barrier. An adhesive remover may be used to facilitate removal of the skin barrier.	Reduces trauma; jerking irritates the skin and can cause tears.
18. Cleanse peristomal skin gently with warm tap water using gauze pads or clean washcloth; do not scrub the skin; dry completely by patting the skin with gauze or towel.	Avoid use of soap because it leaves a residue on the skin that interferes with pouch adhesion to the skin. Skin must be as dry as skin barrier; pouch does not adhere to wet skin. If blood appears on the gauze pad, do not be alarmed; the stoma, if rubbed, may ooze some blood from the cleaning process. Bleeding into the pouch is abnormal. The stoma's surface is a highly vascular mucous membrane.
19. Measure the stoma for correct size of pouching system needed, using the manufacturer's measuring guide (see illustration).	Ensures accuracy in determining correct pouch size needed. Stoma shrinks and does not reach usual size for 6 to 8 wk.

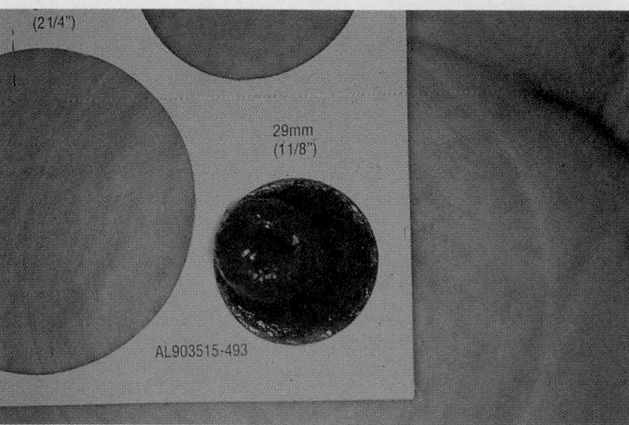

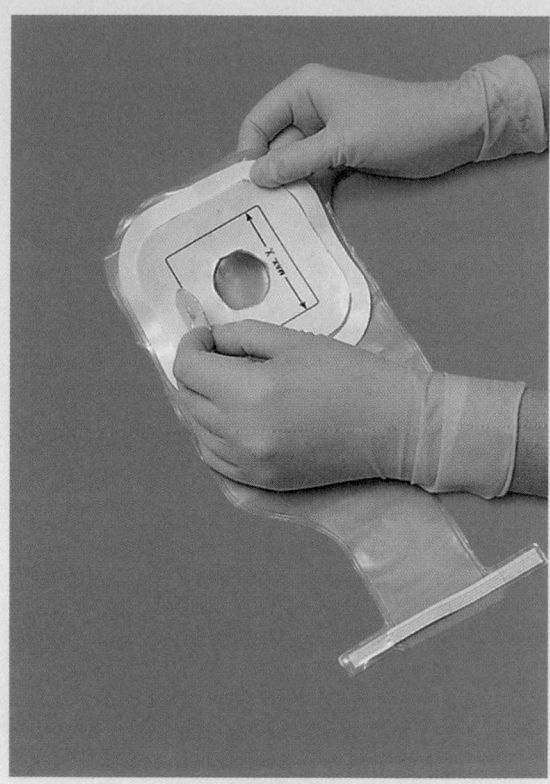

Step 19   **Step 20**

20. Select appropriate pouch for client based on client assessment. With a custom cut-to-fit pouch, use an ostomy guide to cut opening on the pouch $\frac{1}{16}$ to $\frac{1}{8}$ inch larger than stoma before removing backing. Prepare pouch by removing backing from barrier and adhesive (see illustration). With ileostomy, apply thin circle of barrier paste around opening in pouch; allow to dry.

The paste facilitates seal and protects skin. Size of pouch opening keeps drainage off skin and lessens risk of damage to stoma during peristalsis or activity. Pouch and skin barrier are changed whenever leaking. Can also be changed before or after tub bath or shower. Stool is alkaline and this irritates the skin; fecal bacteria can colonize on the skin and increase risk of infection. Change when client is comfortable; before a meal is better, because this avoids increased peristalsis and chance of evacuation during the pouch change.

21. Apply the skin barrier and pouch. If creases next to stoma occur, use barrier paste to fill in; let dry 1 to 2 min.

Critical Decision Point: If client has surgical incision near stoma, the skin barrier may have to be trimmed for fit.

A. **For one-piece pouching system**
   (1) Use skin sealant wipes on skin directly under adhesive skin barrier or pouch; allow to dry. Press the adhesive backing of the pouch and/or skin barrier smoothly against the skin, starting from the bottom and working up and around the sides.
   (2) Hold pouch by barrier, center over stoma, and press down gently on barrier, bottom of pouch should point toward client's knees.

STEPS	RATIONALE
(3) Maintain gentle finger pressure around the barrier for 1 to 2 min.	
B. **For two-piece pouching system**	
(1) Apply flange (barrier with adhesive) as in steps above for one-piece system. Then snap on pouch and maintain finger pressure.	Creates wrinkle-free, secure seal; decreases irritation from the adhesive on skin.
22. Apply nonallergic paper tape around the pectin skin barrier in a "picture frame" method. Half of the tape should be on the skin barrier and half on the client's skin. Some clients may prefer a belt attached to the pouch for extra security rather than tape.	"Picture framing" the pectin skin barrier adds to the security of keeping the pouch system attached securely.

Critical Decision Point: Be sure belt is not too tight by placing two fingers between belt and skin.

STEPS	RATIONALE
23. Although many ostomy pouches are odorproof, some nurses and clients like to put a small amount of ostomy deodorant into the pouch. Do not use "home remedies," such as aspirin, to control ostomy odor.	Aspirin or other substances can harm the stoma.
24. Fold bottom of drainable open-ended pouches up once and close using a closure device such as a clamp (or follow manufacturer's instructions for closure).	Maintains secure seal to prevent leaking.
25. Properly dispose of old pouch and soiled equipment. Consider spraying deodorant in room if needed.	Lessens odors in room.
26. Remove gloves and wash hands.	Reduces transmission of microorganisms.
27. Change pouch every 3 to 7 days unless leaking; pouch can remain in place for tub bath or shower; after bath, pat adhesive dry.	Avoids unnecessary trauma to skin from too frequent changes. Drying ensures adhesion of pouch.
28. Ask if client feels discomfort around stoma.	Determines presence of skin irritation.
29. Note appearance of stoma around skin and existing incision (if present) while pouch is removed and skin is cleansed. Reinspect condition of skin barrier and adhesive.	Determines condition of tissues and progress of healing. Determines presence of leaks.
30. Auscultate bowel sounds and observe characteristics of stool.	Determines return of peristalsis and bowel elimination.
31. Observe client's nonverbal behaviors as pouch is applied. Ask if client has any questions about pouching.	May indicate emotional response to stoma and readiness for teaching. Determines level of understanding of procedure.

Recording and Reporting

- Chart type of pouch and skin barrier applied.
- Record amount and appearance of stool, texture, condition of peristomal skin, and sutures.
- Report any of the following to the charge nurse and/or physician.
  - Abnormal appearance of stoma, suture line, peristomal skin, character of output, absence of bowel sounds.
  - No flatus in 24 to 36 hours and no stool by third day.
- Document abdominal distention and excessive tenderness, nature of bowel sounds.
- Record client's level of participation and need for teaching.

Home Care Considerations

- Evaluate the client's home toileting facilities. This includes presence of adequate toileting facilities, flushable toilet, and number and location of toilets.
- Caution the client that most ostomy pouches and barriers cannot be flushed down the toilet; they clog the system. Dispose of used ostomy pouch according to local sanitation regulations.
- Instruct client to use a washcloth or any soft material to cleanse around stoma.

Skill 45-3   Irrigating a Colostomy

Delegation Considerations
The skill of irrigating a colostomy requires problem solving and knowledge application unique to the professional nurse. Delegation is inappropriate.

EQUIPMENT
- Graduated container
- Tubing with regulatory clamp
- Cone
- Irrigation sleeve, with or without belt
- Water-soluble lubricant
- Clamps or closure device
- New appliance with skin barrier
- Disposable gloves
- Bedpan, commode, or toilet
- Washcloth, towel, washbasin
- Intravenous pole
- Liquid cleaner

STEPS	RATIONALE
1. Assess frequency of defecation and character of stool.	Unrelieved constipation characterized by hardened feces can indicate need to irrigate colon.
2. Assess time when client normally irrigates ostomy or obtain physician's order.	Maintains established routine for bowel emptying.
3. Assess client's understanding of procedure and ability to perform techniques.	Determines level of client participation.
4. Prepare client by explaining procedure.	Allays client fears by explaining stoma is not painful. Ensures cooperation.
5. Choose proper time for irrigation, about 1 hr after meal.	Coordinates irrigation during normal time of duodenocolic reflex.
6. Assist client with positioning. If ambulatory, have client sit on chair in front of toilet; if confined to bed, have client lie on side.	Allows for directing sleeve into toilet for drainage of fecal contents and irrigant.
7. Wash hands and apply gloves.	Reduces transmission of infection.
8. Close bathroom door or room curtains.	Provides privacy.
9. Remove appliance and cleanse skin as normally done in changing enterostomy pouch.	Allows access to stoma.
10. Apply irrigation sleeve. Roll up so that bottom just touches water in toilet. (For client confined to bed, clip bottom of drain sleeve.)	Directs flow of stool into toilet. Rolling up sleeve prevents it from stopping up plumbing when commode is flushed. Also keeps end of sleeve clean.
11. Fill graduated container with required solution (usually 500-1000 ml tepid water or saline). Hang on intravenous pole so that bottom of container is level with client's shoulder.	Volume of 500-1000 ml is sufficient to distend colon and trigger effective emptying. Cold water results in syncope, and hot water could damage stoma or intestine. Height of bag creates pressure gradient for fluid to enter colon.
12. Attach cone to irrigating tube. Allow enough fluid to run through entire length of tube.	Flushes air out of tube. Air is expelled from tubing because it causes air lock and will not let solution flow.
13. Apply lubricant to cone.	Prevents trauma to stoma.
14. Insert cone through top of irrigation sleeve.	Ensures containment of stool within sleeve.
15. Insert cone gently but firmly into stoma (see illustration). Stoma should be dilated before first irrigation with gloved, lubricated finger to determine direction of bowel lumen.	Stoma is easily injured. Inserting tube toward direction of bowel facilitates introduction of solution.
16. Begin flow of solution and readjust position of cone as necessary (see illustration).	To get sufficient distention, solution must not leak around cone. Client or you may need to redirect cone and slowly increase firmness against stoma until solution flows in easily and leakage around cone ceases.
17. Adjust flow of solution by raising or lowering irrigating container. To aid in this, bottom of irrigator bag should be hung 18 in above stoma.	Too-rapid administration results in cramping and inability to hold sufficient volume for adequate results.
18. Administer 500-1000 ml of solution slowly over 15 min, pausing when client cramps but not removing cone until above amount is given.	Usually 500-1000 ml is required to empty colon. Pauses prevent premature leakage of solution because cone replaces sphincter.

STEPS	RATIONALE

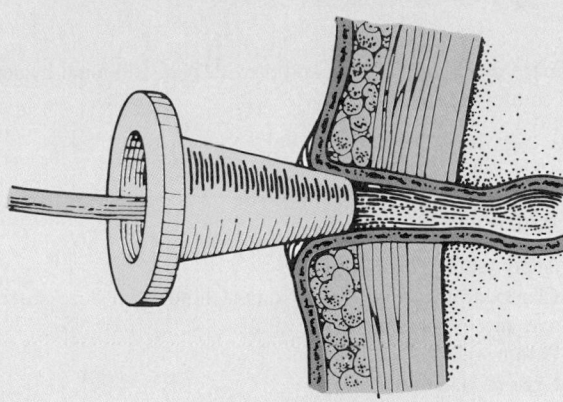

Step 15

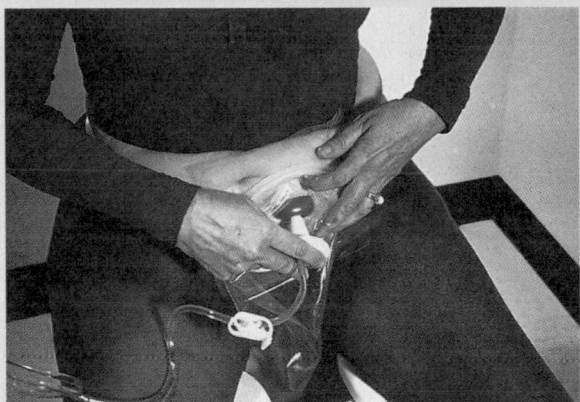

Step 16

STEPS	RATIONALE
19. When solution runs in, clamp tubing and remove cone, making sure sleeve fits around stoma, close top of irrigation sleeve. Should obtain small gush of fluid, then returns in spurts.	Clamping tubing prevents return of results into irrigator. Sleeve should be placed properly to avoid gush of solution over top of sleeve. If colon was distended sufficiently, contracting of bowel musculature results in return of solution in intermittent spurts.
20. Clamp top of sleeve.	Prevents leakage at top.
21. When most of solution has returned (15-20 min), rinse sleeve with water, fold end up, fasten it to top, and have client ambulate (unless restricted to bed).	Allows ambulation. Prevents leakage. Entire procedure takes about 1 hr, and client may become tired of sitting.
22. When all of feces have returned, rinse sleeve out with water and special liquid cleanser and remove. Then wash sleeve out with soap and water, rinse, and air dry. Do not throw irrigation sleeve away—it is reusable.	Prevents sleeve from deteriorating, permitting reuse. Controls odor.
23. Apply new pouch according to procedure (see Skill 45-2).	Avoids leakage and skin problems.
24. Dispose of equipment no longer needed. Remove gloves by turning them inside out and dispose in receptacle.	Reduces transmission of microorganisms.
25. Wash hands.	Prevents cross contamination.
26. Inspect volume and character of fecal material and fluid that returns after irrigation.	Determines whether irrigant is retained (serious fluid imbalances can occur if retained). Character and amount of stool reveal success of cleaning bowel.
27. Note client's response during irrigant infusion. Ask if client feels cramping or abdominal pain.	Reveals client's tolerance of irrigation.
28. Palpate and auscultate abdomen after return of irrigant.	Evaluates for potential complication of bowel perforation.
29. Assist client to comfortable position.	Ensures client comfort.
30. If regular evaluation of client irrigations are being done, assess whether there is any fecal drainage or distention between irrigation procedures.	With time, feces will be eliminated only at time of irrigations and not in between irrigations.

Recording and Reporting

- Chart type of pouch and skin barrier applied.
- Record amount and appearance of stool or drainage in pouch, size of stoma, color of stool, texture, condition of peristomal skin, and sutures, and abdominal tenderness.
- Record client's level of participation and need for teaching.
- Report any of the following to the charge nurse and/or physician:
  a. Abnormal appearance of stoma, suture line, peristomal skin, character of output, absence of bowel sounds.
  b. No flatus in 24 to 36 hours and no stool by third day.

Home Care Considerations

- Evaluate the client's home toileting facilities.
- Evaluate the client's ostomy routine in relationship to usual lifestyle after discharge.
- Caution the client that most ostomy pouches and barriers cannot be flushed down the toilet; they clog the system. Dispose of used ostomy pouch according to local sanitation regulations.
- Client should understand that while the nurse may have used sterile gauze to clean the stoma, it is *not* necessary to use sterile gauze. In fact, gauze is not needed at all; a washcloth or any soft material can be used.

Skill 45-4 Inserting and Maintaining a Nasogastric Tube

Delegation Considerations

The skill of inserting and maintaining the NG tube requires problem solving and knowledge application unique to a professional nurse. Assistive personnel may measure and record the drainage from the NG tube and provide oral and nasal hygiene and comfort measures.

EQUIPMENT

- No. 14 or no. 16 Fr NG tube (smaller-lumen catheters are not used for decompression in adults because they must be able to remove thick secretions)
- Water-soluble lubricating jelly
- pH test strips (measure gastric aspirate acidity)
- Tongue blade
- Flashlight
- Asepto bulb or catheter-tipped syringe
- 1-in (2.5-cm) wide hypoallergenic tape

- Safety pin and rubber band
- Clamp, drainage bag, or suction machine or pressure gauge if wall suction is to be used
- Bath towel
- Glass of water with straw
- Facial tissues
- Normal saline
- Tincture of benzoin (optional)
- Disposable gloves

STEPS	RATIONALE
1. Inspect condition of client's nasal and oral cavity.	Baseline condition of nasal and oral cavity determines need for special nursing measures for oral hygiene after tube placement.
2. Ask if client has had history of nasal surgery and note if deviated nasal septum is present.	Nurse should insert tube into uninvolved nasal passage. Procedure may be contraindicated if surgery is recent.
3. Palpate client's abdomen for distention, pain, and rigidity. Auscultate for bowel sounds.	Baseline determination of level of abdominal distention later serves as comparison once tube is inserted.
4. Assess client's level of consciousness and ability to follow instructions.	Determines client's ability to assist in procedure.

Critical Decision Point: If client is confused, disoriented, or unable to follow commands, obtain assistance from another staff member to insert the tube.

STEPS	RATIONALE
5. Check medical record for surgeon's order, type of NG tube to be placed, and whether tube is to be attached to suction or drainage bag.	Procedure requires physician's order. Adequate decompression depends on NG suction.
6. Prepare equipment at the bedside. Have a 2- to 3-in piece of tape ready with one end split in half.	
7. Identify client and explain procedure.	Identification prevents error of placing tube in wrong client. Explanation gains client's cooperation and lessens possibility that client will remove tube.
8. Wash hands and apply disposable gloves.	Reduces transmission of microorganisms.
9. Position client in high Fowler's position with pillows behind head and shoulders. Raise bed to a horizontal level comfortable for the nurse.	Promotes client's ability to swallow during procedure. Good body mechanics prevent injury to nurse or client.
10. Pull curtain around the bed or close room door.	Provides privacy.
11. Stand on client's right side if right-handed, left side if left-handed.	Allows easiest manipulation of tubing.
12. Place bath towel over client's chest; give facial tissues to client.	Prevents soiling of client's gown. Tube insertion through nasal passages may cause tearing and coughing with increased salivation.
13. Instruct client to relax and breathe normally while occluding one naris. Then repeat this action for other naris. Select nostril with greater air flow.	Tube passes more easily through naris that is more patent.

STEPS	RATIONALE

14. Measure distance to insert tube:

   A. **Traditional method:** Measure distance from tip of nose to earlobe to xiphoid process (see illustration).

              Tube should extend from nares to stomach; distance varies with each client.

   B. **Hanson method:** First mark 50-cm point on tube, then do traditional measurement. Tube insertion should be to midway point between 50 cm (20 in) and traditional mark.

15. Mark length of tube to be inserted with small piece of tape placed so it can easily be removed.

              Marks amount of tube to be inserted from nares to stomach.

16. Cut a 10-cm (4-in) piece of tape. Split one end down the middle lengthwise 5 cm (2 in). Place on bed rail or bedside table.

              Tape will be used after tube insertion to anchor the tube securely.

17. Curve 10 to 15 cm (4 to 6 in) of end of tube tightly around index finger, then release.

              Curving tube tip aids insertion and decreases stiffness of tube.

18. Lubricate 7.5 to 10 cm (3 to 4 in) of end of tube with water-soluble lubricating jelly.

              Minimizes friction against nasal mucosa and aids insertion of tube.

19. Alert client that procedure is to begin.

              Decreases client anxiety and increases client cooperation.

20. Initially instruct client to extend neck back against pillow; insert tube slowly through naris with curved end pointing downward (see illustration).

              Facilitates initial passage of tube through naris and maintains clear airway for open naris.

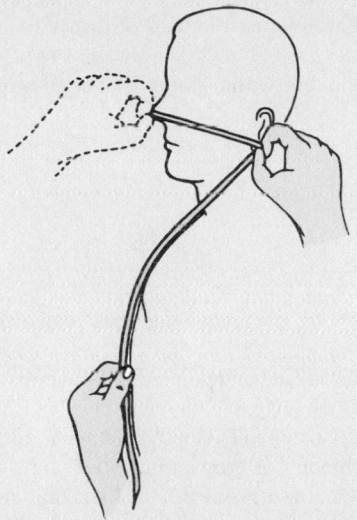

Step 14A

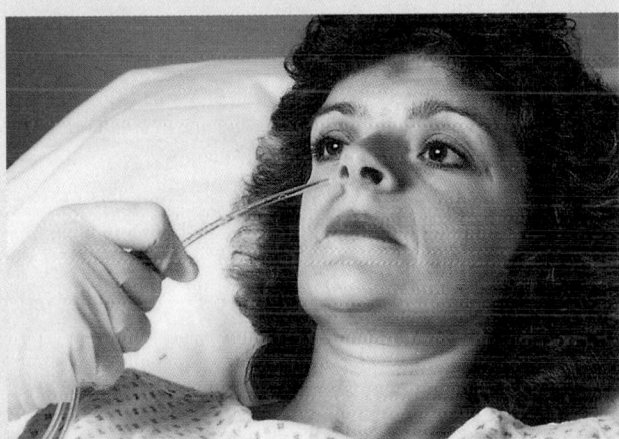

Step 20

21. Continue to pass tube along floor of nasal passage, aiming down toward ear. When resistance is felt, apply gentle downward pressure to advance tube (do not force past resistance).

              Minimizes discomfort of tube rubbing against upper nasal turbinates. Resistance is caused by posterior nasopharynx. Downward pressure helps tube curl around corner of nasopharynx

22. If resistance is met, try to rotate the tube and see if it advances. If still resistant, withdraw tube, allow client to rest, relubricate tube, and insert into other naris.

              Forcing against resistance can cause trauma to mucosa. Helps relieve client's anxiety.

Critical Decision Point: If unable to insert tube in either naris, stop procedure and notify physician.

STEPS	RATIONALE
23. Continue insertion of tube until just past nasopharynx by gently rotating tube toward opposite naris.	
a. Stop tube advancement, allow client to relax, and provide tissues.	Relieves client's anxiety; tearing is natural response to mucosal irritation, and excessive salivation may occur because of oral stimulation.
b. Explain to client that next step requires that client swallow. Give client glass of water unless contraindicated.	Slipping of water aids passage of NG tube into esophagus.
24. With tube just above oropharynx, instruct client to flex head forward, take a small sip of water, and swallow. Advance tube 2.5 to 5 cm (1 to 2 in) with each swallow of water. If client is not allowed fluids, instruct to dry swallow or suck air through straw. Advance tube with each swallow.	Flexed position closes off upper airway to trachea and opens esophagus. Swallowing closes epiglottis over trachea and helps move the tube into the esophagus. Swallowing water reduces gagging or choking. Water can be removed later from stomach by suction.
25. If client begins to cough, gag, or choke, withdraw slightly and stop tube advancement. Instruct client to breathe easily and take sips of water.	Tubing may accidentally enter larynx and initiate cough reflex. Gaging is eased by swallowing water. Risk for aspiration increases if vomiting occurs.

Critical Decision Point: If vomiting occurs, assist client in clearing airway; oral suctioning may be needed. Do not proceed until airway is cleared.

STEPS	RATIONALE
26. If client continues to cough during insertion, pull tube back slightly.	Tube may enter larynx and obstruct airway.
27. If client continues to gag, check back of pharynx using flashlight and tongue blade.	Tube may coil around itself in back of throat and stimulate gag reflex.
28. After client relaxes, continue to advance tube desired distance.	Tip of tube should be within stomach to decompress properly.
29. Once tube is correctly advanced, remove tape used to mark length of tube and place the prepared split tape with nonsplit side on nose. Anchor with one of split ends while checking tube placement.	Tube should be partially anchored before placement is checked.
30. Checking tube placement: check institutional policy for preferred methods for checking tube placement.	
a. Ask client to talk.	Client is unable to talk if NG tube has passed through vocal cords.
b. Inspect posterior pharynx for presence of coiled tube.	Tube is pliable and can coil up in back of pharynx instead of advancing into esophagus.
c. Aspirate gently back on syringe to obtain gastric contents, observing color (see illustration).	Gastric contents are usually cloudy and green, but may be off-white, tan, bloody, or brown in color. Aspiration of contents provides means to measure fluid pH and thus determine tube tip placement in gastrointestinal tract. Other common aspirate colors include the following: Duodenal placement (yellow or bile stained), esophagus (may or may not have saliva-appearing aspirate).
d. Measure pH of aspirate with color-coded pH paper with range of whole numbers 1 to 11 (see illustration).	Gastric aspirates have decidedly acidic pH values, preferably 4 or less, compared with intestinal aspirates, which are usually greater than 4, or respiratory secretions, which are usually greater than 5.5 (Metheny and others, 1993, 1994, 1998).

Critical Decision Point: Be sure to use gastric (Gastrocult) pH test and not Hemoccult test.

STEPS	RATIONALE
e. If tube is not in stomach, advance another 2.5 to 5 cm (1 to 2 in) and repeat steps, 30C, D, and E to check tube position.	Tube must be in stomach to provide decompression.

31. Anchoring tube:

    a. After tube is properly inserted and positioned, either clamp end or connect it to drainage bag or suction machine.

Drainage bag is used for gravity drainage. Intermittent suction is most effective for decompression. Client going to the operating room often has tube clamped.

    b. Tape tube to nose; avoid putting pressure on nares.

Prevents tissue necrosis. Tape anchors tube securely.

       (1) Before taping tube to nose, apply small amount of tincture of benzoin to lower end of nose and allow to dry (optional). Be sure top end of tape over nose is secure.

Benzoin prevents loosening of tape if client perspires.

       (2) Carefully wrap two split ends of tape around tube (see illustration).

       (3) Alternative: Apply tube fixation device using shaped adhesive patch (see illustration).

    c. Fasten end of NG tube to client's gown by looping rubber band around tube in slip knot. Pin rubber band to gown (provides slack for movement).

Reduces pressure on the nares if tube moves.

    d. Unless physician orders otherwise, head of bed should be elevated 30 degrees.

Helps prevent esophageal reflux and minimizes irritation of tube against posterior pharynx.

    e. Explain to client that sensation of tube should decrease somewhat with time.

Adaptation to continued sensory stimulus.

    f. Remove gloves and wash hands.

Reduces transmission of microorganisms.

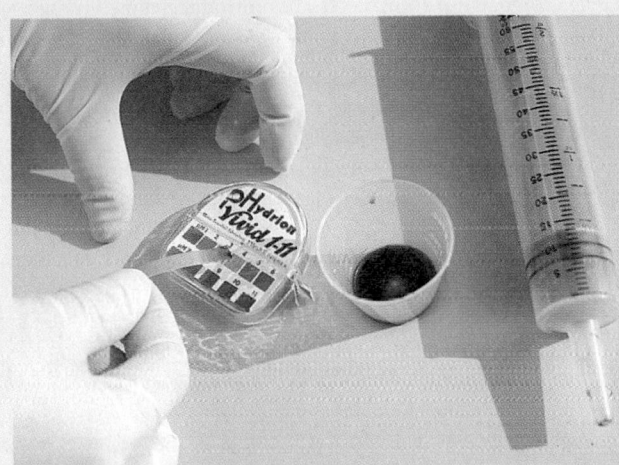

Step 30e

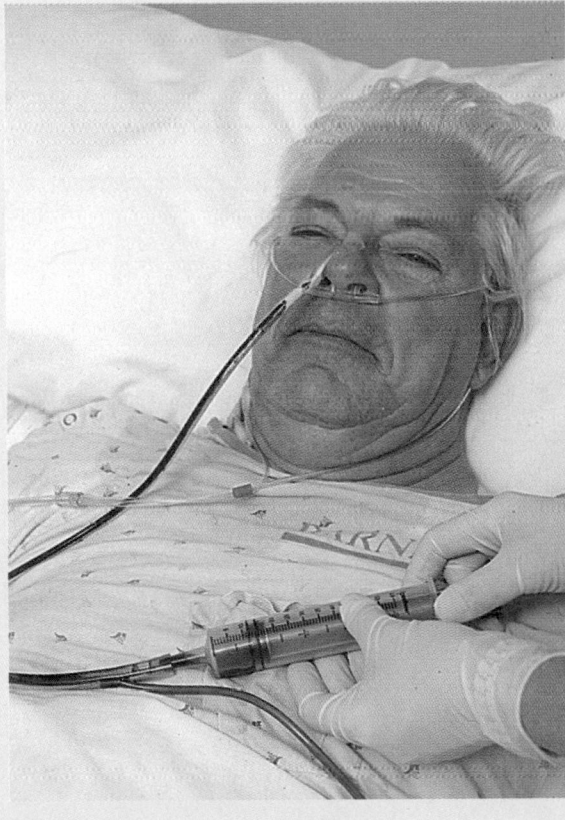

Step 30c

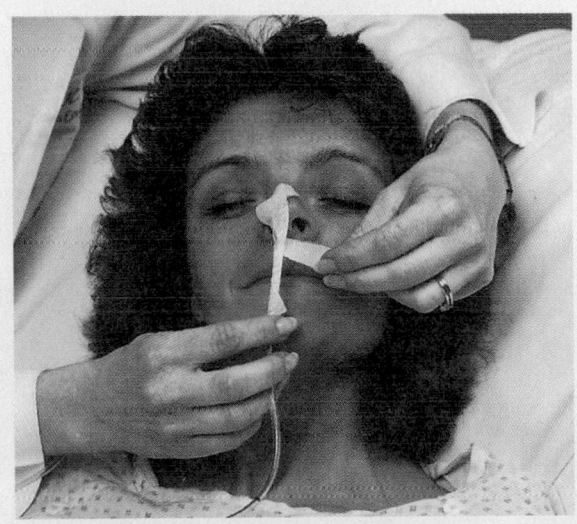

Step 31b(2)

STEPS	RATIONALE

32. Safety:

   a. Once placement is confirmed, place a mark, either a red mark or tape, on the tube to indicate where the tube exists in the nose.

                The mark or tube length is to be used as a guide to indicate whether displacement may have occurred.

   b. Measurement of the tube length from nares to connector is an alternate method.

   c. If tube length is the method used, document the tube length in the client record.

33. Tube irrigation:

   a. Wash hands and apply gloves.   Reduces transmission of microorganisms.

   b. Check for tube placement in stomach (see Step 30). Reconnect NG tube to connecting tube.   Prevents accidental entrance of irrigating solution into lungs.

   c. Draw up 30 ml of normal saline into Asepto or catheter-tipped syringe.   Use of saline minimizes loss of electrolytes from stomach fluids.

   d. Clamp NG tube. Disconnect from connection tubing and lay end of connection tubing on towel.   Reduces soiling of client's gown and bed linen.

   e. Insert tip of irrigating syringe into end of NG tube. Remove clamp. Hold syringe with tip pointed at floor and inject saline slowly and evenly. Do not force solution.   Position of syringe prevents introduction of air into vent tubing, which could cause gastric distention. Solution introduced under pressure can cause gastric trauma.

Critical Decision Point: Do not introduce saline through blue colored "pigtail" air vent of Salem sump tube.

---

   f. If resistance occurs, check for kinks in tubing. Turn client onto left side. Repeated resistance should be reported to surgeon.   Tip of tube may lie against stomach lining. Repositioning on left side may dislodge tube away from the stomach lining. Buildup of secretions will cause distention.

   g. After instilling saline, immediately aspirate or pull back slowly on syringe to withdraw fluid. If amount aspirated is greater than amount instilled, record the difference as output. If amount aspirated is less than amount instilled, record the difference as intake.   Irrigation clears tubing, so stomach should remain empty. Fluid remaining in stomach is measured as intake.

   h. Reconnect NG tube to drainage or suction. (If solution does not return, repeat irrigation.)   Reestablishes drainage collection; may repeat irrigation or repositioning of tube until NG tube drains properly.

   i. Remove gloves and wash hands.   Reduces transmission of microorganisms.

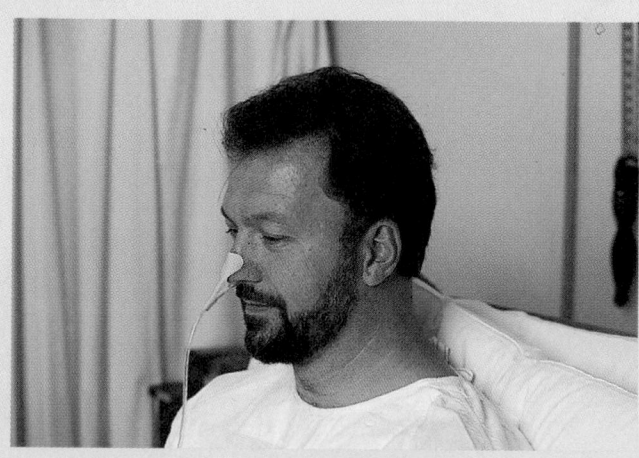

Step 31b(3)

STEPS	RATIONALE
34. Discontinuation of NG tube:	
a. Verify order to discontinue NG tube.	Physician's order required for procedure.
b. Explain procedure to client and reassure that removal is less distressing than insertion.	Minimizes anxiety and increases cooperation. Tube passes out smoothly.
c. Wash hands and apply disposable gloves.	Reduces transmission of microorganisms.
d. Turn off suction and disconnect NG tube from drainage bag or suction. Remove tape from bridge of nose and unpin tube from gown.	Have tube free of connections before removal.
e. Stand on client's right side if right-handed, left side if left-handed.	Allows easiest manipulation of tube.
f. Hand the client facial tissue; place clean towel across chest. Instruct client to take and hold a deep breath.	Client may wish to blow nose after tube is removed. Towel may keep gown from getting soiled. Airway will be temporarily obstructed during tube removal.
g. Clamp or kink tubing securely and then pull tube out steadily and smoothly into towel held in other hand while client holds breath.	Clamping prevents tube contents from draining into oropharynx. Reduces trauma to mucosa and minimizes client's discomfort. Towel covers tube, which can be an unpleasant sight. Holding breath helps to prevent aspiration.
h. Measure amount of drainage and note character of content. Dispose of tube and drainage equipment.	Provides accurate measure of fluid output. Reduces transfer of microorganisms.
i. Clean nares and provide mouth care.	Promotes comfort.
j. Position client comfortably and explain procedure for drinking fluids, if not contraindicated.	Depends on physician's order. Sometimes clients are allowed nothing by mouth (NPO) for up to 24 hours. When fluids are allowed, the order usually begins with a small amount of ice chips each hour and increases as client is able to tolerate more.
35. Clean equipment and return to proper place. Place soiled linen in utility room or proper receptacle.	Proper disposal of equipment prevents spread of microorganisms and ensures proper exchange procedures.
36. Remove gloves and wash hands.	Reduces transmission of microorganisms.
37. Observe amount and character of contents draining from NG tube. Ask if client feels nauseated.	Determines if tube is decompressing stomach of contents.
38. Palpate client's abdomen periodically, noting any distention, pain, and rigidity and auscultate for the presence of bowel sounds. Turn off suction while auscultating.	Determines success of abdominal decompression and the return of peristalsis. The sound of the suction apparatus may be transmitted to abdomen and be misinterpreted as bowel sounds.
39. Inspect condition of nares and nose.	Evaluates onset of skin and tissue irritation.
40. Observe position of tubing.	Determines if tension is being applied to nasal structures.
41. Ask if client feels sore throat or irritation in pharynx.	Evaluates level of client's discomfort.

Recording and Reporting

- Record in nurses' notes time and type of NG tube inserted, client's tolerance of procedure, confirmation of placement, character of gastric contents, pH value, and whether tube is clamped or connected to drainage device.
- Record in nurses' notes and/or flow sheet amount and character of contents draining from NG tube every shift, unless ordered more frequently by physician.

burning sensation as the tube passes through the sensitive nasal mucosa. When the tube reaches the back of the pharynx, the client may begin to gag. The nurse must help the client relax to make tube insertion easier. Some institutions allow xylocaine jelly to be used when inserting the tube as it increases client comfort during the procedure.

One of the greatest problems in caring for a client with an NG tube is maintaining comfort. The tube is a constant irritation to nasal mucosa. The nurse must assess the condition of the nares and mucosa for inflammation and excoriation. The tape used to anchor the tube often becomes soiled. The nurse changes it every day to lessen irritation. Frequent lubrication of the nares also minimizes excoriation. With one naris occluded, the client may breathe through the mouth. Frequent mouth care (at least every 2 hours) helps minimize dehydration. A glass of cool water for rinsing is useful, but the client who is allowed nothing by mouth (NPO) should not swallow the water. The client will frequently complain of a sore throat. An ice bag applied externally to the throat sometimes helps. Gargling with topical xylocaine jelly and/or lozenges may be used if ordered by the physician.

After the tube is inserted, the nurse must maintain its patency. If the tip of the tubing rests against the stomach wall or if the tube becomes blocked with thick secretions, regular irrigation is necessary. Flushing the tube with normal saline by way of a cone-tipped syringe clears blockage within the tube (see Skill 45-4). If an NG tube continues to drain improperly after irrigation, the nurse must reposition it by advancing or withdrawing it slightly. Any change in tube position requires the nurse to reassess the placement of the tube in the client's GI tract.

The NG tube can cause distention. The presence of the tube causes many clients to swallow large volumes of air. Channels of gastric secretions also form along the walls of the stomach and bypass the suction holes. Turning the client regularly helps to collapse the channels and promote emptying of stomach contents.

Restorative and Continuing Care
Bowel Training. The client with incontinence is unable to maintain bowel control. A **bowel training** program can help some clients achieve normal defecation, especially those who still have some neuromuscular control.

The training program involves setting up a daily routine. By attempting to defecate at the same time each day and using measures that promote defecation, the client gains control of bowel reflexes. The program requires time, patience, and consistency. The physician determines the client's physical readiness and ability to benefit from bowel training. A successful program includes the following:
- Assessing the normal elimination pattern and recording times when the client is incontinent
- Incorporating principles of gerontologic nursing when providing bowel retraining programs for the older adult client (Box 45-8)

- Choosing a time in the client's pattern to initiate defecation-control measures
- Giving stool softeners orally every day or a cathartic suppository at least half an hour before the selected defecation time (lower colon must be free of stool so that suppository contacts intestinal mucosa)
- Offering a hot drink (hot tea) or fruit juice (prune juice) (or whatever fluids normally stimulate peristalsis for the client) before the defecation time
- Assisting the client to the toilet at the designated time
- Avoiding medications, such as analgesics, that may increase constipation
- Providing privacy and setting a time limit for defecation (15 to 20 minutes)
- Instructing the client to lean forward at the hips while sitting on the toilet, to apply manual pressure with the hands over the abdomen, and to bear down but not strain to stimulate colon emptying
- Not criticizing or conveying frustration if the client is unable to defecate
- Providing regular meals with adequate fluids and fiber
- Maintaining normal exercise within the client's physical ability

Maintenance of Proper Fluid and Food Intake. In choosing a diet for promoting normal elimination, the nurse should consider the frequency of defecation, characteristics of feces, and types of foods that impair or promote defecation. The client with frequent constipation or impaction requires an increased intake of high-fiber foods and more fluids. However, the client should realize that diet therapy provides only long-term relief of elimination problems and may not give immediate relief from problems such as constipation (Box 45-9).

Research HIGHLIGHT   **Box 45-9**

RESEARCH ABSTRACT

Orthopedic clients are at greater risk for becoming constipated because of limitations of their mobility. Narcotic analgesics also contribute to this risk. A quasi-experimental design, a study and a control group, was designed to test the
effectiveness of wheat bran as a measure to prevent constipation in postoperative orthopedic clients who had undergone
elective joint replacement. The addition of wheat bran to the
diet of the orthopedic surgical clients promoted spontaneous
bowel movements. This reduced the incidence of constipation. In fact the bowel output of clients who had received
wheat bran added to their diet was 5 times better than that of
the control group. Water intake and activity were the same in
both groups.

IMPLICATIONS FOR PRACTICE
- The effectiveness of bran is well documented.
- A combination of natural bran and All Bran worked
  more effectively.
- The incidence of constipation decreased.

REFERENCE
Ouellet LL: Dietary fiber and laxation in postop orthopedic
patients, *Clin Nurs Res* 5(4):428, 1996.

When diarrhea is a problem, the nurse can recommend
foods with a low fiber content and discourage foods that
typically cause gastric upset or abdominal cramping.
Diarrhea caused by illness can be debilitating. If the client
cannot tolerate foods or liquids orally, intravenous therapy (with potassium supplements) is necessary. The client
returns to a normal diet slowly, often beginning with fluids. Excessively hot or cold fluids stimulate peristalsis,
causing abdominal cramps and further diarrhea. As the
tolerance to liquids improves, solid foods are ordered.

Diet therapy is important for clients with ostomies.
During the first weeks after surgery, many physicians recommend low-fiber diets, particularly for ileostomy clients
because the small bowel requires time to adapt to the diversion. Low-fiber foods include bread, noodles, rice,
cream cheese, eggs (not fried), strained fruit juices, lean
meats, fish, and poultry. As ostomies heal, clients can eat
almost any food. High-fiber foods such as fresh fruits and
vegetables help ensure a more solid stool needed to
achieve success at irrigation. Blockage must be avoided.
The stoma's surgical construction can affect the likelihood
of blockage. Ileostomy clients should eat slowly and chew
food completely. Drinking 10 to 12 glasses of water daily
also prevents blockage. High-fiber foods that may cause
problems include stringy meats, mushrooms, popcorn,
fruits such as cherries, and some seafood such as shrimp
and crab. Ostomy clients may benefit from avoiding foods
that cause gas and odor, including broccoli, cauliflower,
dried beans, and brussels sprouts.

Promotion of Regular Exercise.   A daily exercise
program helps prevent elimination problems. Walking,
riding a stationary bicycle, or swimming stimulates peristalsis. Clients who are sedentary at work are most in need
of regular exercise.

For a client temporarily immobilized, the nurse should
attempt ambulation as soon as possible. If the condition
permits, the nurse assists a postoperative client in walking
to a chair on the evening of the day of surgery. The client
should walk farther each day.

Some clients have difficulty passing stool because of
weak abdominal and pelvic floor muscles. Exercises help
bedridden clients using a bedpan. The client can practice
the exercises as follows:

Lie supine; tighten the abdominal muscles as though
pushing them to the floor. Hold them tight to the count of
three; relax. Repeat 5 to 10 times as tolerated.

Flex and contract the thigh muscles by raising one knee
slowly toward the chest. Repeat for each leg at least 5 times
and increase frequency as tolerated.

Promotion of Comfort.   Many clients have discomfort from alterations in elimination. Pain results when he-
morrhoidal tissues are directly irritated. Flatulence can
also create discomfort, particularly if distention develops.

The primary goal for the client with hemorrhoids is to
have soft-formed, painless stools. Proper diet, fluids, and
regular exercise improve the likelihood of stools being
soft. If the client becomes constipated, passage of hard
stools may cause bleeding and irritation. Local heat provides temporary relief to swollen hemorrhoids. A sitz bath
is the most effective means of heat application (see
Chapter 47).

To relieve the discomfort of flatulence, the nurse should
use measures that reduce flatus or promote its escape. Air
swallowing increase flatus. The client can reduce the
amount of air swallowed by not drinking carbonated beverages, not using straws for drinking, and not chewing gum
or hard candies. When flatulence becomes severe as a result
of reduced peristalsis, a nasogastric tube is often used.

When flatulence results in abdominal cramping, ambulation promotes passage of flatus. Having the client
walk down the hall may be enough to stimulate peristalsis
and relieve gas. When conservative measures fail, flatulence can be relieved by insertion of a rectal tube. The
client assumes a side-lying position while the nurse inserts
the tube in the same manner as for an enema (see Skill
45-1). Because fluid is not instilled into the bowel, the
nurse can advance the tube deeper to reach areas where
flatus has accumulated (15 cm or 6 inches in an adult, 5 to
10 cm or 2 to 4 inches in a child).

After inserting the tube the nurse instructs the client to
lie quietly in bed. To prevent the tube from being dislodged, the nurse may tape it to one of the buttocks. A
gauze dressing or waterproof pad placed around the open
end of the rectal tube will catch liquid fecal material.

Continual use of rectal tubes can cause irritation and eventual **excoriation** of the anus and rectal mucosa. A rectal tube should not remain in place longer than 30 minutes. The physician determines the frequency with which the tube can be inserted. If flatulence persists, the nurse should notify the physician.

Maintenance of Skin Integrity. The client with diarrhea or fecal incontinence is at risk for skin breakdown when fecal contents remain on the skin. The same problem exists for the client with an ostomy that drains liquid stool. Liquid stool is usually acidic and contains digestive enzymes. Irritation from repeated wiping with toilet tissue

aggravates skin breakdown. Bathing the skin after soiling helps but may result in more breakdown unless the skin is thoroughly dried.

When caring for a debilitated, incontinent client who is unable to ask for assistance, the nurse should check often for defecation. The anal areas can be protected with petrolatum, zinc oxide, or another ointment that holds moisture in the skin, preventing drying and cracking. Yeast infections of the skin can develop easily. Several powdered antifungal agents are effective against yeast. Baby powder or cornstarch should not be used because they have no medical properties and they frequently cake on the skin and become difficult to remove.

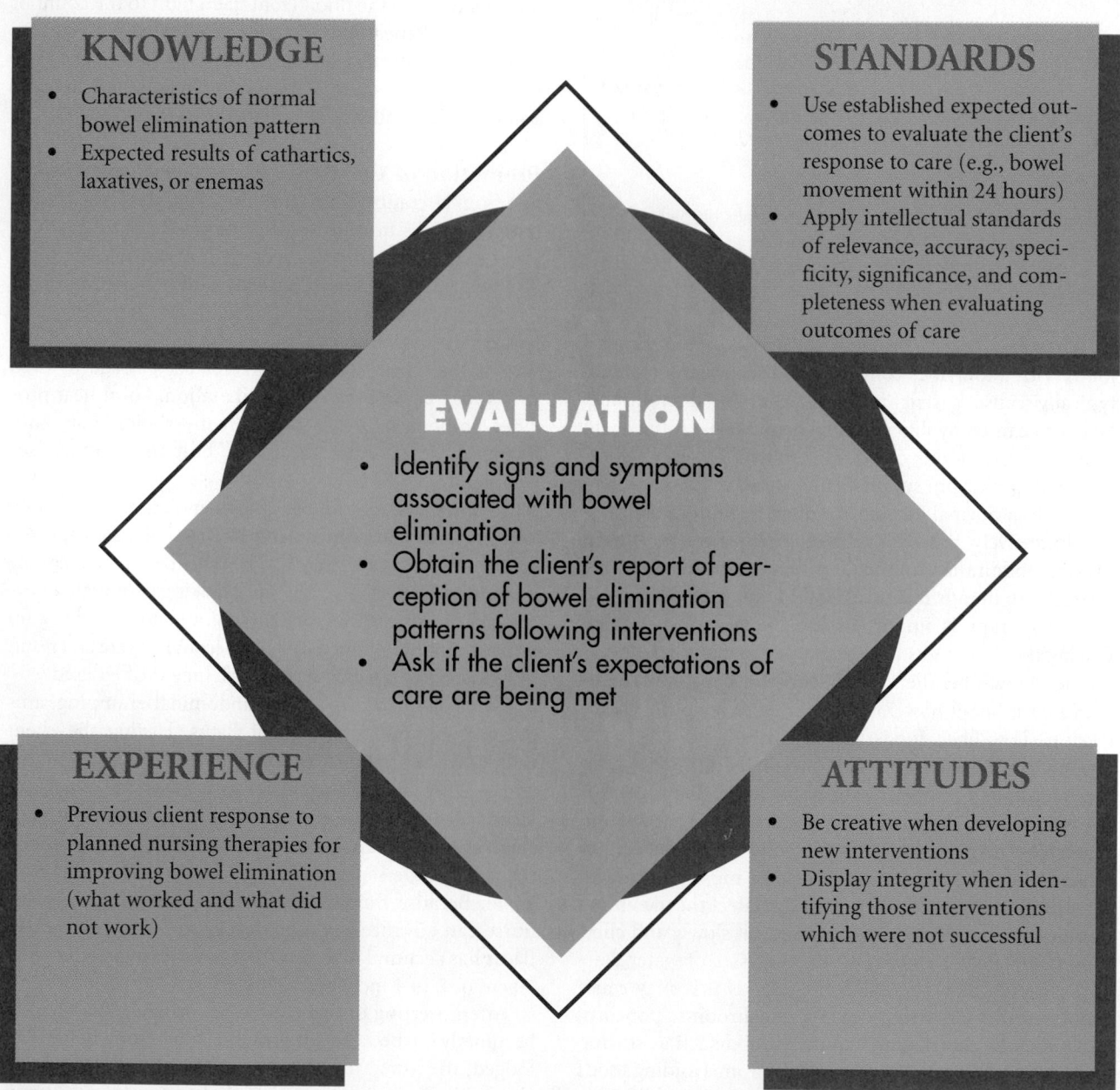

Figure 45-16 *Synthesis Model for Bowel Elimination Evaluation Phase.*

Promotion of Self-Concept. When a client has a bowel elimination problem, a threat to self-concept may be experienced. Frequent incontinence, foul odorous stools, and an ostomy appliance are just a few factors that may cause a client to perceive a change in body image. The result could be a client who avoids socializing with others or who is unwilling to assume responsibility for self-care. The nurse can play an important role in restoring a client's self-concept through the following interventions:

- Give the client an opportunity to discuss concerns or fears about elimination problems.
- Provide the client and family with information to understand and manage the elimination problem.
- Give positive feedback when the client attempts self-care measures.
- Help the client manage the condition but do not expect the client to like it.
- Provide privacy during care.
- Show acceptance and understanding. Remember that the client will be watching the nurse during ostomy care and pouch changes for facial expressions and other nonverbal clues that demonstrate acceptance of the ostomy.

EVALUATION

Client Care. The effectiveness of care depends on success in meeting the goals and expected outcomes of care. Optimally the client will be able to regularly defecate soft-formed, painless stools. The client is the only one who is able to determine if the bowel elimination problems have been relieved and which therapies were the most effective (Figure 45-16). The client will also be able to demonstrate information gained regarding establishment of a normal elimination pattern. The client will be able to demonstrate any skills learned such as ostomy protocols and skin protection. The client will be able to accomplish normal defecation by manipulating natural components of daily living such as diet, fluid intake, and exercise. The client will have minimal reliance on artificial means of defecation such as enemas and laxative use.

Client Expectations. If the nurse has been successful in establishing a therapeutic relationship with the client, the client will feel comfortable in discussing the intimate details often associated with bowel elimination. The client will not be fearful of embarrassment as the nurse assists the client with elimination needs. The client will relate a feeling of comfort and freedom from pain as elimination needs are met within the limits of the client's condition and treatment.

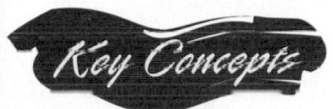

Key Concepts

- A primary function of the elimination process is fluid balance.
- Mechanical breakdown of food elements, gastrointestinal motility, and selective absorption and secretion of substances by the large intestine influence the character of feces.
- Food high in fiber content and an increased fluid intake keep feces soft.
- Ongoing use of laxatives to promote elimination can lead to constipation.
- Vagal stimulation, which slows the heart rate, may occur during straining while defecating, taking rectal temperatures, and enemas.
- The greatest danger from diarrhea is development of fluid and electrolyte imbalance.
- The location of an ostomy influences consistency of the stool.
- Assessment of elimination patterns should focus on bowel habits, factors that normally influence defecation, recent changes in elimination, and a physical examination.

- Indirect and direct visualization of the lower gastrointestinal tract requires cleansing of the bowel before the procedure.
- The nurse should consider frequency of defecation, fecal characteristics, and effect of foods on gastrointestinal function when selecting a diet promoting normal elimination.
- Proper positioning on a bedpan allows the client to assume a position similar to squatting without experiencing muscle strain.
- Proper selection and use of an ostomy pouching system is necessary to prevent damage to the skin around the stoma. Irrigation of an ostomy follows the same principles as an enema administration except a special irrigating tube is needed and the client cannot control passage of feces.
- Dangers during digital removal of stool include traumatizing the rectal mucosa and promoting vagal stimulation.
- Skin breakdown can occur after repeated exposure to liquid stool.

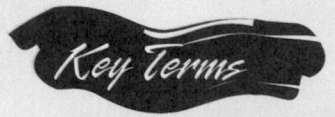

Key Terms

Biopsy, *p. 1454*
Bolus, *p. 1437*
Bowel training, *p. 1480*
Cathartics, *p. 1442*
Chyme, *p. 1438*
Colitis, *p. 1442*
Colon, *p. 1439*
Colostomy, *p. 1444*
Constipation, *p. 1443*
Contrast medium, *p. 1454*
Crohn's disease, *p. 1442*
Defecation, *p. 1440*
Diarrhea, *p. 1444*
Diverticula, *p. 1454*
Endoscopy, *p. 1453*
Enema, *p. 1460*
Enterostomal therapist (ET), *p. 1466*
Excoriation, *p. 1482*
Feces, *p. 1440*
Fiber, *p. 1440*
Fiber optic endoscope, *p. 1453*

Flatulence, *p. 1444*
Flatus, *p. 1440*
Gastrocolic reflex, *p. 1442*
Gastroscopy, *p. 1453*
Guaiac test, *p. 1452*
Haustral contractions, *p. 1439*
Hemorrhoids, *p. 1444*
Ileostomy, *p. 1444*
Impaction, *p. 1444*
Incontinence, *p. 1444*
Lactose intolerance, *p. 1441*
Laxatives, *p. 1442*
Masticate, *p. 1437*
Paralytic ileus, *p. 1442*
Peristalsis, *p. 1437*
Polyps, *p. 1454*
Refluxing, *p. 1437*
Regurgitating, *p. 1439*
Stoma, *p. 1444*
Transit time, *p. 1442*
Valsalva maneuver, *p. 1440*

Critical Thinking Exercises

1. A 17-year-old man with a history of good health and regular exercise is seen by the school nurse. He complains of increasing diarrhea and abdominal cramping. He states that on rare occasions he had noticed blood on the toilet paper he has used. What additional pieces of assessment data do you need?
2. The nursing long-term care center has invited you to come and do a presentation concerning prevention of constipation in their residents. What points of information would you want to include in your presentation?
3. A 22-year-old man is to undergo surgery for Crohn's disease. He will have a new, pouching ileostomy. He and his mother need teaching about what this means for his future elimination needs. What would you tell them?

References

Abyad A, Mourad F: Constipation: common-sense care of the older patient, *Geriatrics* 51(12):28, 1996.

Anti M and others: Water supplementation enhances the effect of high-fiber diet on stool frequency and laxative consumption in adult patients with functional constipation, *Hepatogastroenterology* 45(21):727, 1998.

Beitz JM: The ileoanal reservoir: an alternative to ileostomy, *J Wound Ostomy Continence Nurs* 21(3):120, 1994.

Ciociola AA and others: Helicobacter pylori infection rates in duodenal ulcer patients in the United States may be lower than previously estimated, *Am J Gastroenterol* 94(7):1834, 1999.

Clark BA: A new approach to assessment and documentation of conscious sedation during endoscopic examination, *Gastroenterol Nurs,* 21(2):59, 1998.

Cooke CE: Disease management: prevention of NSAID induced gastropathy, *Drug Benefit Trends* 8(3):14, 1996.

Ebersole P, Hess P: *Toward healthy aging: human needs and nursing response,* St. Louis, 1998, Mosby.

Fruto LV: Current concepts: management of diarrhea in acute care, *J Wound Ostomy Continence Nurs* 21(5):199, 1994.

Hampton BG, Bryant RA: *Ostomies and continent diversions: nursing management,* St. Louis, 1992, Mosby.

Lueckenotte AG: *Pocket guide to gerontologic assessment,* ed 3, St. Louis, 1998, Mosby.

McCloskey JC, Bulechek GM: *Nursing interventions classification (NIC),* ed 3, St. Louis, 2000, Mosby.

McKenry LM, Salerno E: *Pharmacology in nursing,* ed 20, St. Louis, 1998, Mosby.

Metheny N and others: Effectiveness of pH measurements in predicting feeding tube placement: an update, *Nurs Res* 42(6):324, 1993.

Metheny N and others: Visual characteristics of aspirates from feeding tubes as a method for predicting tube location, *Nurs Res* 43:282, 1994.

Metheny N and others: pH, color, and feeding tubes, *RN* 61(1):277, 1998.

Mishkin S: Dairy sensitivity, lactose malabsorption, and elimination diets in inflammatory bowel disease, *Am J Clin Nutr* 65(2):564, 1997.

Morrisson SG: Feeding the elderly population, *Nurs Clin North Am* 32(4):791, 1997.

Ouellet LL: Dietary fiber and laxation in postop orthopedic patients, *Clin Nurs Res* 5(4):428, 1996.

Powe BD: Fatalism among elderly African Americans: effects on colorectal cancer screening, *Cancer Nurs* 18(5):385, 1995.

Stewart KB: Helping your patient contend with constipation, *Nursing* 28(9 Hosp Nurs):32hn 22-3, September, 1998.

Thompson I: Teaching the skills to cope with a stoma, *Nurs Times* 94(4):62, 1998.

Thompson JM and others: *Clinical nursing,* ed 4, St. Louis, 1997, Mosby.

Walsh BA and others: Psychometric evaluation of body image and quality of life following ostomy surgery, oral abstract presented at the Wound, Ostomy, Continence Nurses (WOCN) Society 27th Annual Conference, Denver, May 1995.

Mobility and Immobility

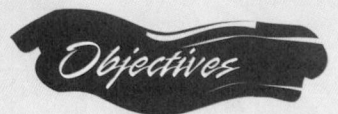

Mastery of content in this chapter will enable the student to:

- Define the key terms listed.
- Describe the functions of the musculoskeletal (skeleton, skeletal muscles) and nervous systems in the regulation of movement.
- Discuss physiological and pathological influences on body alignment and joint mobility.
- Identify changes in physiological and psychosocial function associated with mobility and immobility.
- Assess for correct and impaired body alignment and mobility.
- State correct nursing diagnoses for impaired body alignment and mobility.
- Develop nursing care plans for clients with impaired body alignment and mobility.
- Describe essential techniques when helping a client to move up in bed, repositioning a client, assisting a client to a sitting position, and transferring a client from a bed to a chair or from a bed to a stretcher.
- Describe active/passive range-of-motion exercises.
- Describe essential techniques when helping a client to safely use crutches.
- Evaluate the nursing plan for maintaining body alignment and mobility.

Mobility serves many purposes, such as expression of an emotion with a nonverbal gesture, self-defense, satisfaction of basic needs, and performance of activities of daily living (ADLs) and recreational activities. Many functions of the body need mobility to function optimally. To maintain optimal physical mobility, the musculoskeletal and nervous systems of the body must be intact and functioning.

Clinical nursing practice related to mobility requires incorporating knowledge and skills related to body mechanics to provide competent care. *Body mechanics* is a term used to describe coordinated efforts of the musculoskeletal and nervous systems in moving and lifting the body. Knowing the movements and functions of muscles in maintaining posture and movement is vital to safe production and maintenance of motion for nurses, as well as for clients.

Scientific Knowledge Base

PHYSIOLOGY AND PRINCIPLES OF BODY MECHANICS

Body mechanics are the coordinated efforts of the musculoskeletal and nervous systems to maintain balance, posture, and body alignment during lifting, bending, moving, and performing ADLs. Use of proper body mechanics reduces risk of injury to the musculoskeletal system, facilitates ease of body movement, and allows for more efficient use of energy.

Use of proper body mechanics is important to the safety and well-being of the nurse and of clients. The nurse uses a variety of muscle groups for each nursing activity, such as walking during nursing rounds, administering medications, lifting and transferring clients, and moving objects. The physical forces of weight and friction can influence body movement. Correctly used, these forces increase the nurse's efficiency. Incorrect use can impair the nurse's ability to lift, transfer, and position clients and cause serious injury. Knowledge of the basic structures and functions of the neuromuscular system and knowledge of physiological and pathological influences on mobility and body alignment are important to a full understanding of body mechanics (see Table 36-1 in Chapter 36).

Alignment. The terms *body alignment* and *posture* are analogous and refer to the positioning of the joints, tendons, ligaments, and muscles while standing, sitting, and lying. Correct body alignment reduces strain on musculoskeletal structures and risk for injury, aids in maintaining adequate muscle tone, and contributes to balance and conservation of energy.

Balance. **Body alignment** contributes to body balance, "whereby the body's state of equilibrium is controlled for a given purpose" (Kreighbaum and Barthels, 1996). Without balance control, the center of gravity is displaced, thus creating a risk for falls and subsequent injuries. Balance is enhanced with a wide base of support and correct body posture, and when the body's center of gravity is kept low and within the base of support.

Balance is required for maintaining a static position such as sitting, for performing ADLs, and for moving freely in the community. The ability to balance can be compromised by disease, injury, pain, physical development (e.g., age), life changes (e.g., pregnancy), medications (e.g., in which dizziness is a side effect), and prolonged immobility, which may cause deconditioning. Nurses must be alert to impaired balance, since it is a ma-

---

The authors acknowledge the contribution of Jana L. Weindel Dees to this chapter in the previous edition of this text.

jor threat to physical safety. Impaired balance can also lead to a client's fear of falls and self-imposed restrictions on activity.

Gravity and Friction.

Weight is the force exerted on a body by gravity. To lift safely, the lifter must overcome the weight of the object to be lifted and know its center of gravity. In symmetrical objects the center of gravity is located at the exact center of the object. Nurses do not just lift symmetrical objects, they often lift people. People are not geometrically perfect; their centers of gravity are usually at 55% to 57% of standing height and are located in the midline. The force of weight is always directed downward, which is why an unbalanced object falls. Clients or nurses who are unsteady can fall as their centers of gravity become unbalanced because of the gravitational pull of their weight. Therefore nurses are responsible for protecting clients from falling and ensuring the safety of clients and themselves (see Chapter 36).

Friction is a force that occurs in a direction to oppose movement. As the nurse turns, transfers, or moves a client up in bed, friction must be overcome. A nurse can reduce friction by following some basic principles. The greater the surface area of the object to be moved, the greater the friction. A larger object produces greater resistance to movement. To decrease surface area and reduce friction when a client is unable to assist in moving up in bed, the client's arms should be placed across the chest. This decreases surface area and reduces friction.

Whenever possible, the nurse should use some of the client's strength when lifting, transferring, or moving clients. This can be done by explaining the procedure and telling the client when and what body parts to move. The result should be a synchronized movement in which the client can participate and friction is decreased. Involving the client may have the added bonus of increasing participation in self-care, thus promoting a sense of accomplishment.

Friction can also be reduced by lifting rather than pushing a client. Lifting has an upward component and decreases the pressure between the client and the bed or chair. Placing the client on a sheet or blanket (pull sheet, or lift sheet) and then pulling this sheet to move the client reduces friction because the client is more easily moved along the bed's surface.

REGULATION OF MOVEMENT

Coordinated body movement involves integrated functioning of the skeletal system, skeletal muscle, and nervous system. Because these three systems cooperate so closely in mechanical support of the body, they are discussed as a single functional unit.

Skeletal System.

The skeleton is the body's supporting framework and comprises four types of bones: long, short, flat, and irregular. **Long bones** contribute to height (e.g., the femur, fibula, and tibia in the leg) and length (e.g., the phalanges of the fingers and toes). **Short bones** occur in clusters and, when combined with ligaments and cartilage, permit movement of the extremities. Two examples of short bones are the carpal bones in the foot and the patella in the knee. **Flat bones** provide structural contour, such as bones in the skull and the ribs in the thorax. **Irregular bones** make up the vertebral column and some bones of the skull, such as the mandible.

The skeleton provides attachments for muscles and ligaments and provides the leverage necessary for movement. **Leverage** is an inducing or compelling force. Leverage occurs when specific bones, such as the humerus, ulna, and radius, and the associated joint, such as the elbow, act together as a lever. Thus force is applied to one end of the bone to lift a weight as another point tends to rotate the bone in the direction opposite that of the applied force.

The skeletal system has several functions. It protects vital organs (e.g., the skull around the brain; the ribs around the heart and lungs), and bones aid in calcium regulation. Bones store calcium and release it into the circulation as needed. Clients with decreased calcium regulation and metabolism are at risk for developing osteoporosis and **pathological fractures** (fractures caused by weakened bone tissue). In addition, the internal structure of bones contains bone marrow, participates in red blood cell (RBC) production, and acts as a reservoir for blood. Clients with altered bone marrow function or diminished RBC production are usually weakened and fatigue easily, which decreases their mobility and places them at risk of falling.

Characteristics of Bone.

The characteristics of bone include firmness, rigidity, and elasticity. Firmness results from inorganic salts, such as calcium and phosphate, that are laid down in the bone matrix. Firmness is related to the bone's rigidity, which is necessary to keep long bones straight, and enables bones to withstand weight bearing. In addition, bones have a degree of elasticity and skeletal flexibility that changes with age. For example, the newborn has a large amount of cartilage and is highly flexible but is unable to support weight. The toddler's bones are more pliable than those of an older person and are better able to withstand falls. Older adults, especially women, are more susceptible to bone loss (resorption) and osteoporosis (see Skeletal Effects, p. 1495).

Joints.

Joints are the connections between bones. Each joint is classified according to its structure and degree of mobility. There are four classifications of joints: synostotic, cartilaginous, fibrous, and synovial.

The **synostotic joint** refers to bones jointed by bones. No movement is associated with this type of joint, and the bony tissue that forms between the bones provides strength and stability. The classic example of this type of joint is the sacrum, in which vertebrae are joined (Figure 46-1, *A*).

The **cartilaginous joint,** or synchondrodial joint, has little movement but is elastic and uses cartilage to unite body surfaces. Cartilaginous joints are found when bones are exposed to constant pressure, such as the costosternal joints between the sternum and ribs (Figure 46-1, *B*).

The **fibrous joint,** or syndesmodial joint, is a joint in which two bony surfaces are united by a ligament or membrane. The fibers of ligaments are flexible and stretch, permitting a limited amount of movement. For example, the paired bones of the lower leg (tibia and fibula) are syndesmotic joints (McCance and Huether, 1998) (Figure 46-1, *C*).

The **synovial joint,** or true joint, is a freely movable joint in which contiguous bony surfaces are covered by articular cartilage and connected by ligaments lined with a synovial membrane. Joining of the humeral radius and ulna by cartilage and ligaments forms a pivotal joint (Figure 46-1, *D*). Other types of synovial joints are the ball-and-socket joints, such as the hip joint, and the hinge joints, such as the interphalangeal joints of the fingers.

Ligaments.   **Ligaments** are white, shiny, flexible bands of fibrous tissue binding joints together and connecting bones and cartilages. Ligaments are elastic and aid joint flexibility and support (Figure 46-2). In addition, some ligaments have a protective function. For example, ligaments between the vertebral bodies and the ligamentum flavum prevent damage to the spinal cord during movement of the back.

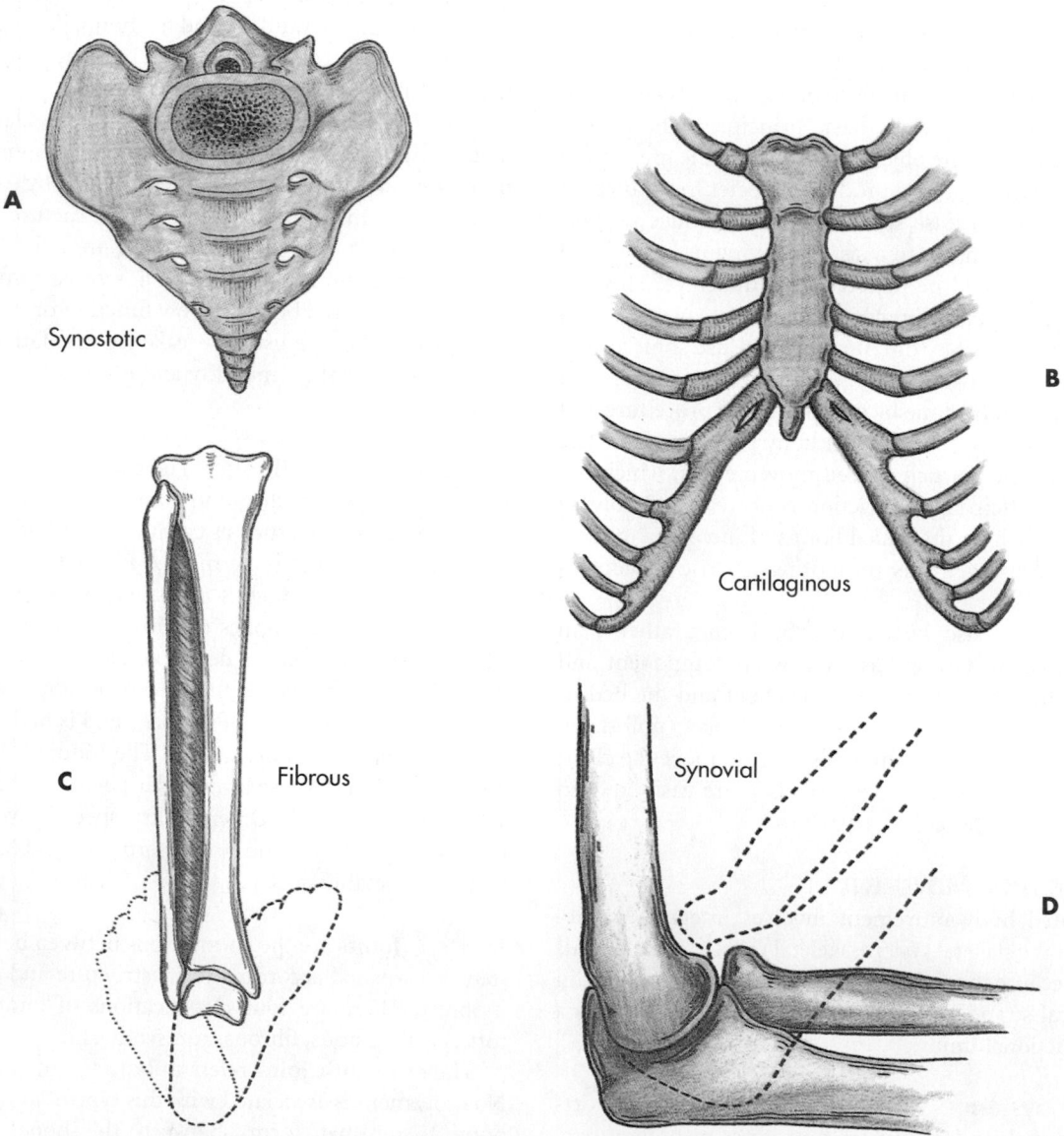

A Synostotic

B Cartilaginous

C Fibrous

D Synovial

Figure 46-1   Joint types.

Tendons.   **Tendons** are white, glistening, fibrous bands of tissue that connect muscle to bone. Tendons are strong, flexible, and inelastic, and they occur in various lengths and thicknesses. The Achilles tendon (tendo calcaneus) is the thickest and strongest tendon in the body. It begins near the middle of the posterior of the leg and attaches the gastrocnemius and soleus muscles in the calf to the calcaneal bone in the back of the foot (Figure 46-3).

Cartilage.   **Cartilage** is nonvascular, supporting connective tissue located chiefly in the joints and thorax, trachea, larynx, nose, and ear. The fetus has a large amount of temporary cartilage, which is replaced by bone developed during infancy. Permanent cartilage is unossified except in advanced age and diseases such as osteoarthritis.

Joints, ligaments, tendons, and cartilage permit strength and flexibility of the skeleton. Strength enables the skeletal system to support the body. A person's flexibility is demonstrated through range of motion (ROM). However, strength and flexibility do not result entirely from these four structures. Adequate skeletal muscle is also necessary.

Skeletal Muscle.   Movement of bones and joints involves active processes that must be carefully integrated to achieve coordination. Skeletal muscles, because of their ability to contract and relax, are the working elements of movement. Contractile elements of the skeletal muscle are enhanced by anatomical structure and attachment to the skeleton.

Muscles are made of fibers that contract when stimulated by an electrochemical impulse that travels from the nerve to the muscle across the neuromuscular junction. The electrochemical impulse causes the filaments (pre-

dominantly protein molecules of myosin and actin) within the fiber to slide past each other, with the filaments changing length. This theory of muscle shortening and lengthening is called the sliding filament theory (Latash, 1998).

Muscle contractions can be categorized by functional purpose: moving, resisting, or stabilizing body parts. In **concentric tension,** increased muscle contraction results in muscle shortening with movement resulting, such as when a client uses an overhead trapeze to pull up in bed. **Eccentric tension** helps control the speed and direction of movement. In the example of the overhead trapeze, the client should slowly lower to the bed. The lowering is controlled when the antagonistic muscles lengthen. Concentric and eccentric muscle actions are necessary for active movement and are therefore referred to as dynamic or **isotonic contraction. Isometric contraction** (static contraction) causes an increase in muscle tension or muscle work but no shortening or active movement of the muscle (e.g., instructing the client in tightening and relaxing a muscle group, as in quadriceps set exercises or pelvic floor exercises). Voluntary movement is a combination of isotonic

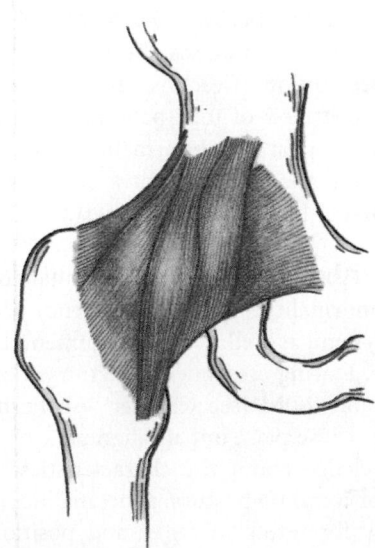

Figure 46-2   Ligaments of the hip joint.

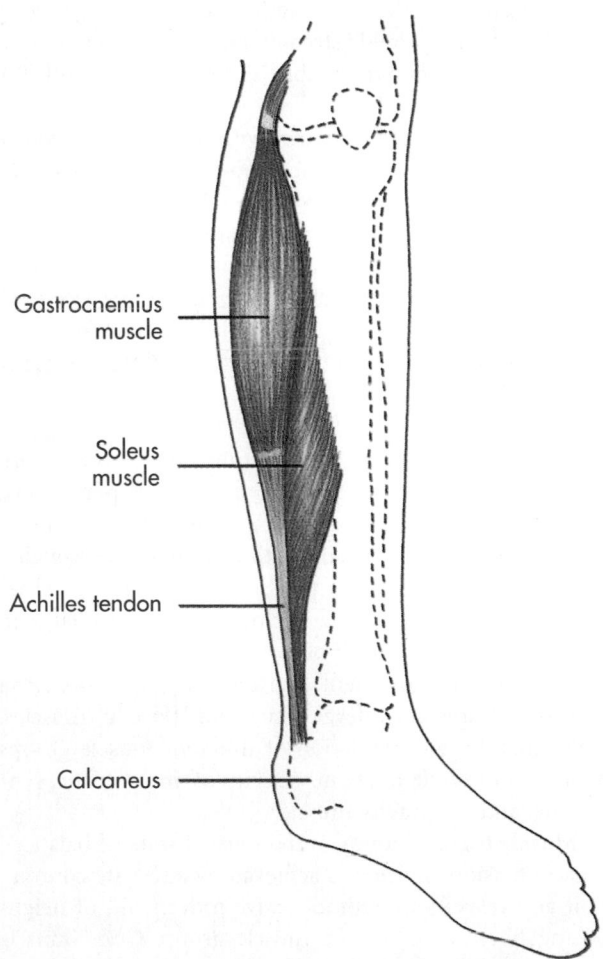

Figure 46-3   Tendons and muscles of the lower leg.

Gastrocnemius muscle

Soleus muscle

Achilles tendon

Calcaneus

and isometric contractions. For example, when the nurse lifts a client up in bed, the client's weight causes increased tension in the muscles of the nurse's arms until the tension (isometric) is equal to the weight to be lifted and the weight of the lower arm. When this equilibrium is reached, continued stimulation to the muscles results in muscle shortening (isotonic) and bending of the elbow (active movement), and the client is lifted off the bed.

Although isometric contractions do not result in muscle shortening, energy expenditure is increased. This type of muscle work is comparable to having a car in neutral with the driver continually depressing the accelerator and racing the engine. The driver is not going anywhere but expends a large amount of energy. The nurse must recognize the energy expenditure (increased respiratory rate and increased work on the heart) associated with isometric exercises because they may be contraindicated in certain clients' illnesses (e.g., myocardial infarction or chronic obstructive pulmonary disease).

Muscle Movement and Posture.

Muscles that attach to bones of leverage provide necessary strength to move an object. Leverage is characteristic of movements of the upper extremities. Arm muscles are parallel to one another and extend the full length of the bones. The long parallel muscles provide strength and work together with the bones and joints to enable lifting an object with the arms.

Muscles associated primarily with maintaining posture are short and featherlike in appearance because they converge obliquely at a common tendon. Muscles of the lower extremities, trunk, neck, and back are concerned primarily with **posture** (the position of the body in relation to the surrounding space). These muscle groups work together to stabilize and support body weight standing or sitting, and they allow an individual to maintain a sitting or standing posture.

Muscle Regulation of Posture and Movement.

Posture and movement can be reflections of personality, discomfort, and mood, as well as musculoskeletal function. For example, a person with a dramatic personality gestures with the hands, a person who is fatigued or depressed may slouch, and a person with abdominal pain may curl into a fetal-like position.

Posture and movement also depend on the skeleton and the shape and development of skeletal muscles. Coordination and regulation of different muscle groups depend on muscle tone and activity of antagonistic, synergistic, and antigravity muscles.

Muscle tone, or tonus, is the normal state of balanced muscle tension. Tension is achieved by alternate contraction and relaxation, without active movement, of neighboring fibers of a specific muscle group. Good muscle tone helps maintain functional positions such as sitting or standing without excess muscle fatigue. Muscle tone is maintained through continual use of muscles. ADLs require muscle action and help maintain muscle tone. As a result of immobility or prolonged bed rest, activity level, activity tolerance, and muscle tone decrease.

The antagonistic, synergistic, and antigravity muscle groups are coordinated by the nervous system and work together to maintain posture and initiate movement (see Chapter 36).

Nervous System.

Movement and posture are regulated by the nervous system. The major voluntary motor area, located in the cerebral cortex, is the precentral gyrus, or motor strip. A majority of motor fibers descend from the motor strip and cross at the level of the medulla. Thus the motor fibers from the right motor strip initiate voluntary movement for the left side of the body, and motor fibers from the left motor strip initiate voluntary movement for the right side of the body.

During voluntary movement, impulses descend from the motor strip to the spinal cord. An impulse exits the spinal cord through efferent motor nerves and travels through the nerves to the muscles, where movement occurs. This impulse is controlled by synapses, which keep the impulse traveling in one direction.

Transmission of the impulse from the nervous system to the musculoskeletal system is an electrochemical event and requires a neurotransmitter. Through a complex process, **neurotransmitters,** or chemicals such as acetylcholine, transfer electric impulses from the nerve across the neuromuscular junction to the muscle. The neurotransmitter reaches a muscle and stimulates it, causing movement. Movement can be impaired by disorders that alter neurotransmitter production, transfer from the nerve to the muscle, or activation of muscle activity. Parkinsonism is an example of such a disorder (see Chapter 36).

PATHOLOGICAL INFLUENCES ON MOBILITY

Many pathological conditions affect mobility. Although a complete description of each is beyond the scope of this chapter, an overview of four pathological influences are presented here: postural abnormalities, impaired muscle development, damage to the central nervous system, and direct trauma to the musculoskeletal system.

Postural Abnormalities.

Congenital or acquired postural abnormalities affect the efficiency of the musculoskeletal system, as well as body alignment, balance, and appearance. During assessment, the nurse observes body alignment and ROM (see Chapter 36). Postural abnormalities can cause pain, impair alignment or mobility, or both. Knowledge about the characteristics, causes, and treatment of common postural abnormalities (Table 46-1) is necessary for lifting, transfer, and positioning. Some postural abnormalities may limit ROM. Nurses intervene to maintain maximum ROM in unaffected joints and then

Table 46-1   Postural Abnormalities

Abnormality	Description	Cause	Possible Treatments*
Torticollis	Inclining of head to affected side, in which sternocleidomastoid muscle is contracted	Congenital or acquired condition	Surgery, heat, support, or immobilization, depending on cause and severity, gentle ROM
Lordosis	Exaggeration of anterior convex curve of lumbar spine	Congenital condition Temporary condition (e.g., pregnancy)	Spine-stretching exercises (based on cause)
Kyphosis	Increased convexity in curvature of thoracic spine	Congenital condition Rickets, osteoporosis Tuberculosis of spine	Spine-stretching exercises, sleeping without pillows, using bed board, bracing, spinal fusion (based on cause and severity)
Kypholordosis	Combination of kyphosis and lordosis	Congenital condition	Similar to methods used in kyphosis or lordosis (based on cause)
Scoliosis	Lateral curvature of spine, unequal heights of hips and shoulders	Congenital condition Poliomyelitis Spastic paralysis Unequal leg length	Immobilization and surgery (based on cause and severity)
Kyphoscoliosis	Abnormal anteroposterior and lateral curvature of spine	Congenital condition Poliomyelitis Cor pulmonale	Immobilization and surgery (based on cause and severity)
Congenital hip dysplasia	Hip instability with limited abduction of hips and, occasionally, adduction contractures (head of femur does not articulate with acetabulum because of abnormal shallowness of acetabulum)	Congenital condition (more common with breech deliveries)	Maintenance of continuous abduction of thigh so that head of femur presses into center of acetabulum Abduction splints, casting, surgery
Knock-knee (genu valgum)	Legs curved inward so that knees knock together as person walks	Congenital condition Rickets	Knee braces, surgery if not corrected by growth
Bowlegs (genu varum)	One or both legs bent outward at knee, which is normal until 2 to 3 years of age	Congenital condition Rickets	Slowing rate of curving if not corrected by growth With rickets, increase of vitamin D, calcium, and phosphorus intake to normal ranges
Clubfoot	95%: medial deviation and plantar flexion of foot (equinovarus) 5%: lateral deviation and dorsiflexion (calcaneovalgus)	Congenital condition	Casts, splints such as Denis-Browne splint, and surgery (based on degree and rigidity of deformity)
Footdrop	Inability to dorsiflex and invert foot because of peroneal nerve damage	Congenital condition Trauma Improper position of immobilized client	None (cannot be corrected) Prevention through physical therapy Bracing with ankle-foot orthotic (AFO)
Pigeon-toes	Internal rotation of forefoot or entire foot, common in infants	Congenital condition Habit	Growth, wearing reversed shoes

Data from McCance KL, Huether SE: *Pathophysiology: the biologic basis for disease in adults and children,* ed 3, St. Louis, 1998, Mosby.
*Severity of condition and cause will dictate treatment, which must be individualized.

may design interventions to strengthen affected muscles and joints, improve the client's posture, and adequately use affected and unaffected muscle groups. Referral to and/or collaboration with a physical therapist may enhance the nurse's interventions for a client with a postural abnormality.

Impaired Muscle Development.

Injury and disease can lead to numerous alterations in musculoskeletal function. The muscular dystrophies are a group of familial disorders that cause degeneration of skeletal muscle fibers. The most prevalent of the muscle diseases in childhood, the muscular dystrophies are characterized by progressive, symmetrical weakness and wasting of skeletal muscle groups, with increasing disability and deformity (McCance and Huether, 1998).

Damage to the Central Nervous System.

Damage to any component of the central nervous system that regulates voluntary movement results in impaired body alignment and mobility. The motor strip in the cerebrum can be damaged by trauma from a head injury, ischemia from a cerebrovascular accident (stroke), or bacterial infection from meningitis. Motor impairment is directly related to the amount of destruction of the motor strip. For example, a person with a right-sided cerebral hemorrhage with complete necrosis will likely have destruction of the right motor strip and left-sided hemiplegia.

Because voluntary motor fibers descend from the motor strip in the cerebrum down the spinal cord, trauma to the spinal cord also impairs mobility. The most common trauma is transection of the spinal cord in which motor fibers are cut. If the injury is complete, it will likely cause a complete bilateral loss of voluntary motor control below the level of the trauma. Spinal cord trauma frequently results from diving or automobile accidents or gunshot or knife wounds to the neck and back.

Direct Trauma to the Musculoskeletal System.

Direct trauma to the musculoskeletal system can result in bruises, contusions, sprains, and fractures. A **fracture** is a disruption of bone tissue continuity. Fractures most commonly result from direct external trauma, but they can also occur as a consequence of some deformity of the bone (e.g., pathological fractures of osteoporosis, Paget's disease, or osteogenesis imperfecta). As the fracture heals, bone begins to repair. The fractured bone initiates a cellular process that results in bone formation. Young children are able to form new bone more easily than adults and, as a result, have few complications after a bone fracture. Treatment includes positioning the fractured bone in proper alignment and immobilizing it to promote healing and restore function. Immobilization results in some muscle atrophy, loss of tone, and joint stiffness.

Acquired or congenital conditions that affect the structure of the musculoskeletal or nervous system impair body alignment or joint mobility. Impairment can be temporary or permanent. Regardless of the duration of the impairment, the nursing care plan includes interventions that maintain the present level of alignment and joint mobility and/or increase the client's level of motor function.

Nursing Knowledge Base

MOBILITY-IMMOBILITY

Fully understanding mobility requires more than an overview of body mechanics and the regulation of movement by the musculoskeletal and nervous systems. The nurse must be knowledgeable about how mobility and immobility affect the systems of the body and the psychosocial and developmental aspects of clients.

Mobility refers to a person's ability to move about freely, and **immobility** refers to the inability to move about freely. Mobility and immobility are best understood as the end points of a continuum, with many degrees of partial immobility between. Some clients move back and forth on this continuum, but for other clients, immobility is absolute and continues indefinitely. The terms *bed rest* and *impaired physical mobility* are frequently used when discussing clients on the mobility-immobility continuum.

Bed rest is an intervention that restricts clients to bed for therapeutic reasons. This intervention is most often prescribed by nurses and physicians. Bed rest has many different interpretations among health care professionals. Clients with a wide variety of conditions are placed on bed rest. The duration of bed rest depends on the illness or injury and the client's prior state of health (Box 46-1).

Impaired physical mobility is defined by the North American Nursing Diagnosis Association (NANDA) as a state in which the individual experiences or is at risk of experiencing limitation of physical movement (Kim, McFarland, and McLane, 1997). Alterations in the level of physical mobility can result from prescribed restriction of movement in the form of bed rest, physical restriction of movement because of external devices (e.g., a cast or skeletal traction), voluntary restriction of movement, or impairment of motor or skeletal function.

The effects of muscular deconditioning associated with lack of physical activity may be apparent in a matter of days. The normal individual on bed rest loses muscle

---

General Objectives of Bed Rest   Box 46-1

Reducing physical activity and the oxygen needs of the body
Reducing pain, including postoperative pain, and the need for large doses of analgesics
Allowing ill or debilitated clients to rest
Allowing exhausted clients the opportunity for uninterrupted rest

strength from baseline levels at a rate of 3% a day. Bed rest also is associated with cardiovascular, skeletal, and other organ changes. The term *disuse atrophy* has been used to describe the pathological reduction in normal size of muscle fibers after prolonged inactivity from bed rest, trauma, casting, or local nerve damage (McCance and Huether, 1998).

In a classic study, Deitrick and others (1948) found that even young healthy men put on bed rest had physiological problems. Periods of immobility or prolonged bed rest can cause major physiological and psychological effects. These effects can be gradual or immediate and vary from client to client. The greater the extent and the longer the duration of immobility, the more pronounced the consequences. The client with complete mobility restrictions is continually at risk for hazardous system-wide effects.

Systemic Effects.
All body systems work more efficiently with some form of movement. Exercise has been shown to have positive outcomes for all major systems of the body. Therefore when there is an alteration in mobility, each body system is at risk for impairment. The severity of the impairment depends on the client's overall health, degree and length of immobility, and age. For example, older adults with chronic illnesses develop pronounced effects of immobility more quickly than do younger clients with the same immobility problem.

Metabolic Changes.
Endocrine metabolism, calcium resorption, and functioning of the gastrointestinal system are altered by changes in mobility.

The endocrine system, made up of hormone-secreting glands, helps to maintain and regulate vital functions such as (1) response to stress and injury, (2) growth and development, (3) reproduction, (4) ionic homeostasis, and (5) energy metabolism. When injury or stress occurs, the endocrine system triggers a series of responses aimed at maintaining blood pressure and preserving life. The endocrine system is important in maintenance of ionic homeostasis. Humans live in an external environment that changes constantly, but tissues and cells live in an internal environment that must remain constant. The endocrine system participates in the regulation of this internal environment through maintenance of sodium, potassium, water, and acid-base balance. Finally, the endocrine system acts as a regulator of energy metabolism. The basal metabolic rate (BMR) is increased by thyroid hormone, and energy is made available to cells through the integrated action of gastrointestinal and pancreatic hormones (Price and Wilson, 1997).

Immobility disrupts normal metabolic functioning, including decreasing the metabolic rate; altering the metabolism of carbohydrates, fats, and proteins; causing fluid, electrolyte, and calcium imbalances; and causing gastrointestinal disturbances such as decreased appetite and slowing of peristalsis. However, in the presence of an infectious process, immobilized clients may have an increased BMR as a result of fever or wound healing. Fever and repair of wounds increase cellular oxygen requirements (McCance and Huether, 1998).

A deficiency in calories and protein is characteristic of clients with a decreased appetite secondary to immobility. Proteins are constantly being synthesized and broken down into amino acids in the body to be reformed into other proteins. Amino acids that are not used are excreted. The body can synthesize certain amino nonessential acids but depends on ingested proteins to supply the eight essential amino acids. When more nitrogen (the end product of amino acid breakdown) is excreted than is ingested in proteins, the body is said to have a **negative nitrogen balance** (Figure 46-4), and weight loss, decreased muscle mass, and weakness result from tissue catabolism (tissue breakdown). Protein loss leads to muscle loss.

Another metabolic change is calcium resorption (loss) from bones. As a result, urinary excretion of calcium increases because immobility causes the release of calcium into the circulation. Normally the kidneys can excrete the excess calcium. However, if the kidneys are unable to respond appropriately, hypercalcemia results (Beare and Myers, 1998). (See also Skeletal Effects, p. 1495, and Urinary Elimination Changes, p. 1496.)

Impairments of gastrointestinal functioning, resulting from decreased gastrointestinal motility that develops subsequent to decreased mobility, vary. Difficulty in passing stools (constipation) is a common symptom, although diarrhea may result from a fecal impaction (accumulation of hardened feces). The nurse must be aware that this finding is not normal diarrhea, but rather liquid stool passing around the area of impaction (see Chapter 45).

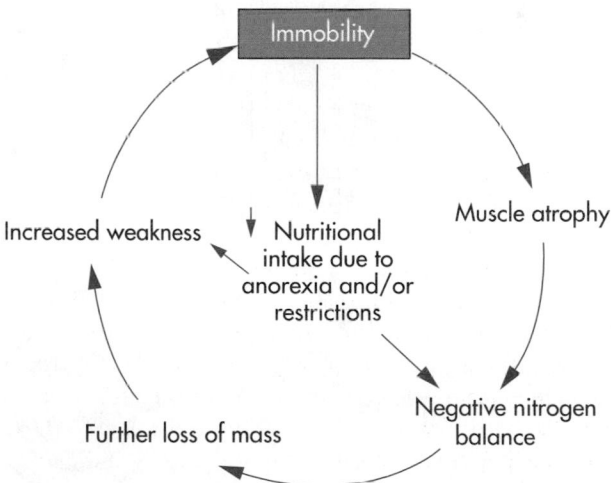

Figure 46-4 Factors contributing to negative nitrogen balance associated with immobility.
From Gröer MW, Shekleton ME: *Basic pathophysiology: a holistic approach*, ed 3, St. Louis, 1989, Mosby.

Left untreated, fecal impaction can result in a mechanical bowel obstruction that may partially or completely occlude the intestinal lumen, blocking normal propulsion of liquid and gas. The resulting fluid in the intestine produces distention and increases intraluminal pressure. Over time, intestinal function becomes depressed, dehydration occurs, absorption ceases, and fluid and electrolyte disturbances worsen.

Respiratory Changes. Regular aerobic exercise is known to enhance respiratory functioning. Lack of movement and exercise places clients at higher risk for respiratory complications. Postoperative and immobile clients are at high risk for developing pulmonary complications. The most common respiratory complications are **atelectasis** (collapse of alveoli) and **hypostatic pneumonia** (inflammation of the lung from stasis or pooling of secretions). Both decrease oxygenation, prolong recovery, and add to the client's discomfort (Long, Phipps, and Cassmeyer, 1993). In atelectasis a bronchiole or a bronchus becomes blocked by secretions and the distal lung tissue (alveoli) collapses as the existing air is absorbed, producing hypoventilation. The extent of atelectasis is determined by the site of the blockage. A lung lobe or a whole lung may even be collapsed. At some point in the development of these complications, there is a proportional decline in the client's ability to cough productively. Ultimately the distribution of mucus in the bronchi increases, particularly when the client is in the supine, prone, or lateral position (Figure 46-5). Mucus accumulates in the dependent regions of the airways (Figure

46-6). Because mucus is an excellent medium for bacterial growth, hypostatic pneumonia may result.

Cardiovascular Changes. The cardiovascular system is also affected by immobilization. The three major changes are orthostatic hypotension, increased cardiac workload, and thrombus formation.

Orthostatic hypotension is a drop of 25 mm Hg in systolic blood pressure and of 10 mm Hg in diastolic blood pressure when the client rises from a lying or sitting position to a standing position. In the immobilized client, decreased circulating fluid volume, pooling of blood in the lower extremities, and decreased autonomic response occur. These factors result in decreased venous return, followed by a decrease in cardiac output, which is reflected by a decline in blood pressure (McCance and Huether, 1998).

As the workload of the heart increases, its oxygen consumption does, too. The heart therefore works harder and less efficiently during periods of prolonged rest. As immobilization increases, cardiac output falls, further decreasing cardiac efficiency and increasing workload.

Clients are also at risk for thrombus formation. A **thrombus** is an accumulation of platelets, fibrin, clotting factors, and the cellular elements of the blood attached to the interior wall of a vein or artery, sometimes occluding the lumen of the vessel (Figure 46-7).

There are three factors that contribute to venous thrombus formation: (1) loss of integrity of the vessel wall (e.g., injury), (2) abnormalities of blood flow (e.g., slow blood flow in calf veins associated with bed rest), and (3) alterations in blood constituents (e.g., a change in clot-

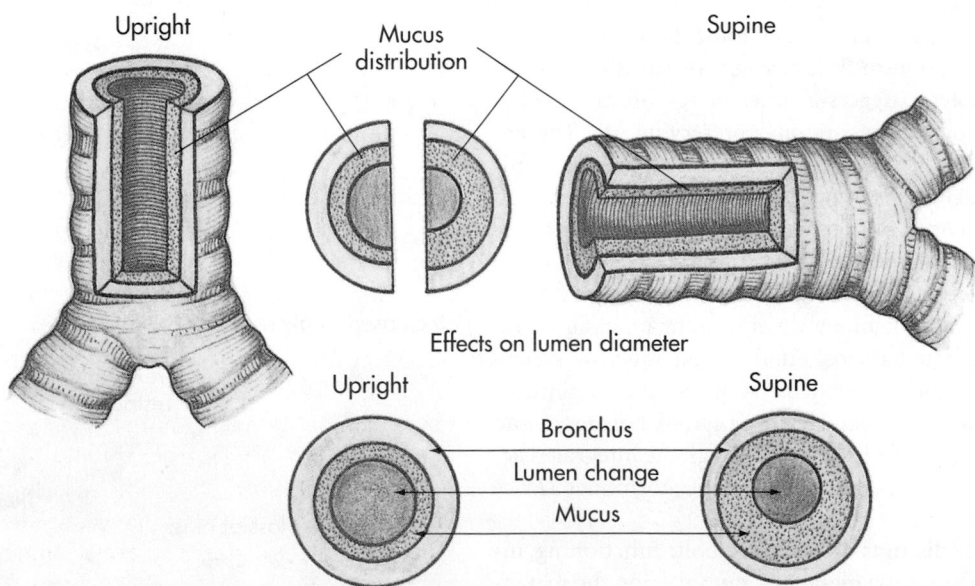

Figure 46-5 Effect of recumbency and gravity on distribution of respiratory tract and diameter of bronchiolar lumen.
From Gröer MW, Shekleton ME: *Basic pathophysiology: a holistic approach,* ed 3, St. Louis, 1989, Mosby.

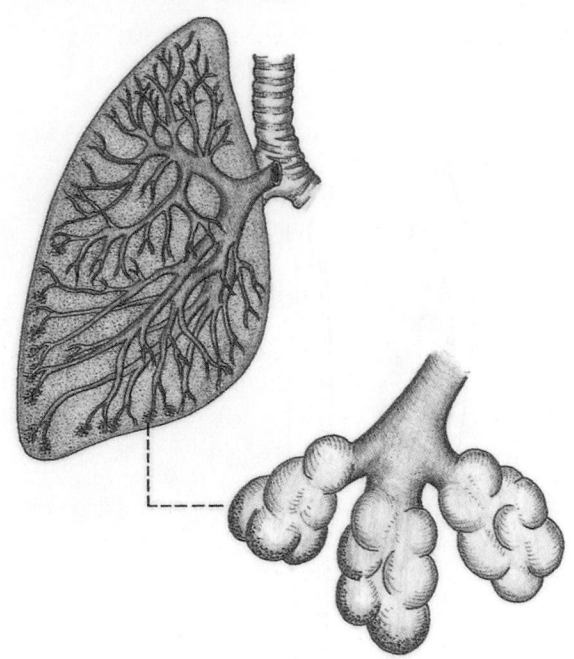

Figure 46-6 Pooling of secretions in dependent regions of the lungs in the supine position.

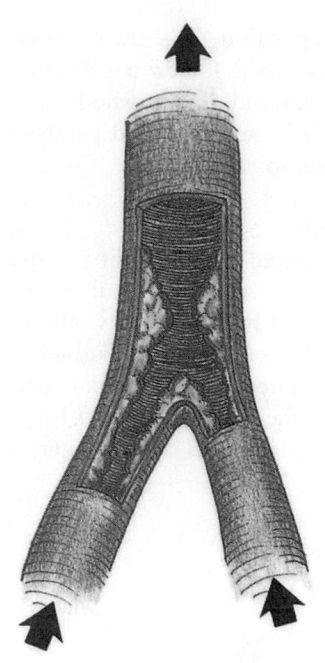

Figure 46-7 Thrombus formation in a vessel.

ting factors or increased platelet activity) (McCance and Huether, 1998).

Musculoskeletal Changes. The effects of immobility on the musculoskeletal system can include permanent impairment of mobility. Restricted mobility may result in loss of endurance, strength, and muscle mass. Other effects of restricted mobility affecting the skeletal system are impaired calcium metabolism and impaired joint mobility.

Muscle Effects. Because of protein breakdown, the client loses lean body mass, which is composed partially of muscle. Therefore the reduced muscle mass is unable to sustain activity without increased fatigue. The muscle mass is decreased from metabolic causes and disuse. As immobility continues and the muscles are not exercised, there is continued decrease in mass.

Decreased mobility and **muscle atrophy,** or loss of muscle tissue, may occur with immobility. Atrophy is a phenomenon widely observed in response to illness, decreased ADLs, and immobilization (Kasper, Maxwell, and White, 1996). Loss of endurance, decreased muscle mass and strength, and joint instability subsequent to immobility put clients at risk for falls (see Chapter 37).

Skeletal Effects. Immobilization causes two skeletal changes: impaired calcium metabolism (see also Metabolic Changes, p. 1493) and joint abnormalities. Because immobilization results in bone resorption, the bone tissue is less dense, or is atrophied, and **osteoporosis**

results. When osteoporosis occurs, the client is at risk for pathological fractures. Immobilization and non-weight-bearing activities increase the rate of bone resorption. Bone resorption also causes calcium to be released in the blood, and hypercalcemia results.

Osteoporosis is a major health concern in this country. Most affected are women; 20% are men. Galsworthy and Wilson (1996) report that predictions are that one out of two women will suffer the severe consequence of a pathological fracture as a result of primary osteoporosis. Although primary osteoporosis is different in origin from the osteoporosis that results from immobility, it is imperative for nurses to recognize that immobilized clients may be at high risk for accelerated bone loss if they have primary osteoporosis. Early client evaluation and consultation and referral with physicians, dietitians, and physical therapists are important interventions for preventing disability in clients with primary osteoporosis who become immobilized.

Immobility can lead to joint contractures. A **joint contracture** is an abnormal and possibly permanent condition characterized by fixation of the joint (Figure 46-8). It is caused by disuse, atrophy, and shortening of the muscle fibers. When a contracture occurs, the joint cannot obtain full ROM. Contractures may leave a joint(s) in a nonfunctional position, as seen in some clients who are permanently curled in a fetal position.

One common and debilitating contracture is footdrop (Figure 46-9). When **footdrop** occurs, the foot is permanently fixed in plantar flexion. Ambulation is difficult with the foot in this position, since the client cannot dorsiflex the foot. The client with footdrop is therefore unable to lift the toes off the ground. Clients who have suffered strokes with resulting left- or right-sided paralysis (hemiplegia) are susceptible to footdrop.

Urinary Elimination Changes.   The client's urinary elimination is altered by immobility. In the upright position, urine flows out of the renal pelvis and into the ureters and bladder because of gravitational forces. When the client is recumbent or flat, the kidneys and the ureters move toward a more level plane. Urine formed by the kidney must enter the bladder unaided by gravity. Because the peristaltic contractions of the ureters are insufficient

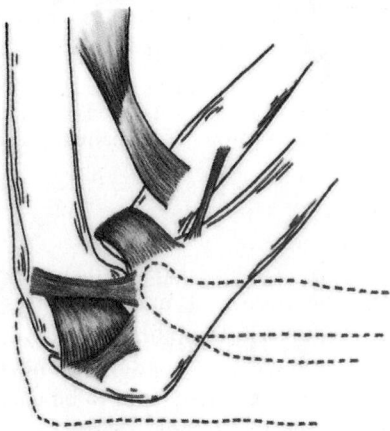

Figure 46-8   Contracture of the elbow is able to extend to a 90-degree angle (*dotted line*) and to a 180-degree angle (not illustrated).

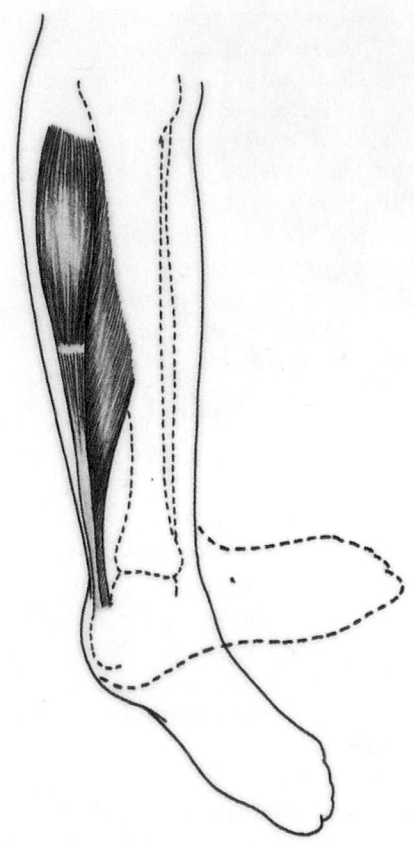

Figure 46-9   Footdrop. Ankle is fixed in a plantar flexion. Normally the ankle is able to flex (*dotted line*), which eases walking.

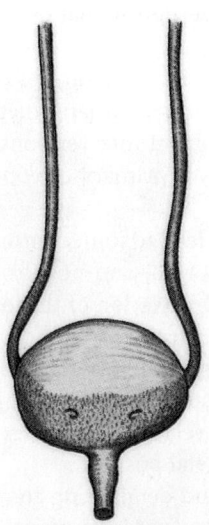

Figure 46-10   Stasis of urine with reflux to ureters.

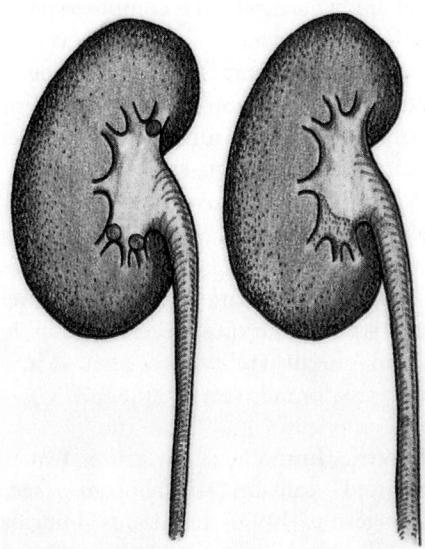

Figure 46-11   Types of renal calculi in the renal pelvis.

to overcome gravity, the renal pelvis may fill before urine enters the ureters (Figure 46-10). This condition is called **urinary stasis** and increases the risk of urinary tract infection and renal calculi (see Chapter 44).

Renal calculi are calcium stones that lodge in the renal pelvis and pass through the ureters (Figure 46-11). Immobilized clients are at risk for calculi because of altered calcium metabolism and the resulting hypercalcemia.

As the period of immobility continues, fluid intake can diminish, and other causes, such as fever, increase the risk for dehydration. As a result, urinary output declines on or about the fifth or sixth day. The urine that is produced is usually highly concentrated.

This concentrated urine increases the risk for calculi formation and infection. Poor perineal care after bowel movements, particularly in women, increases the risk of urinary tract contamination by *Escherichia coli* bacteria. Another cause of urinary tract infections in immobilized clients is the use of an indwelling urinary catheter.

Integumentary Changes.

The direct effect of pressure on the skin by immobility is compounded by the changes in metabolism that accompany immobility. Older adult clients and clients with paralysis have a greater risk for developing pressure ulcers. Any break in the skin's integrity is difficult to heal in the immobilized client. Preventing a pressure ulcer is much less expensive than treating one (Helme, 1994).

A **pressure ulcer** is an impairment of the skin as a result of prolonged ischemia (decreased blood supply to an area) in tissues (see Chapter 47). The ulcer is characterized initially by inflammation and usually forms over a bony prominence. Ischemia develops when the pressure on the skin is greater than the pressure inside the small peripheral blood vessels supplying blood to the skin.

Tissue metabolism depends on the body's receipt of oxygen and nutrients from the blood supply and the elimination of metabolic wastes. Any factor that interferes with this process affects cellular metabolism and, as a result, the function or life of the cell. Pressure affects cellular metabolism by decreasing or obliterating tissue circulation. When a client lies in bed or sits in a chair, the weight of the body is on bony prominences. The longer the pressure is applied, the longer the period of ischemia and therefore the greater the risk of skin breakdown.

Psychosocial Effects.

Immobilization may lead to emotional and behavioral responses, sensory alterations, and changes in coping. These changes are individualized to each client. In addition, immobilized clients may also have social and family difficulties.

The most common emotional changes are depression, behavioral changes, sleep-wake disturbances, and impaired coping. The immobilized client can become depressed because of changes in role, self-concept, and other factors. Depression is an affective disorder characterized by exaggerated feelings of sadness, melancholy, dejection, worthlessness, emptiness, and hopelessness out of proportion to reality. Depression can result from worrying about present and future levels of health, finances, and family needs. Because immobilization removes the client from a daily routine, he or she has more time to worry about disability. Worrying can quickly increase the client's depression, causing withdrawal. Assessing behavioral changes throughout restricted mobility helps the nurse to identify changes in self-concept, recognize early signs of depression, and develop nursing interventions.

Behavioral changes resulting from immobilization vary widely, depending on the client. Common behavioral changes include hostility, belligerence, giddiness, fear, and anxiety. Early in the nursing process the nurse should interview the client's family and friends about normal behavioral patterns to gain baseline data. If unexpected behaviors are observed later, the nurse can intervene to reduce the effects of immobilization on the client's behavioral patterns.

The immobilized client requires constant nursing care. Because of physiological hazards, the client cannot be allowed to sleep for 8 hours without a change of position or other nursing care. Disruption of normal sleeping patterns can further cause behavioral changes. Nursing interventions should be used to ensure that the client receives sufficient sleep (see Chapter 41). The client who is on bed rest and is able to change position during sleep does not require continuous physical nursing care directed at reducing the hazards of immobility. Unless other treatment activities are required during the night, the care plan for the physiologically stable client on bed rest should provide for uninterrupted sleep.

Long-term immobility or bed rest can affect usual coping patterns. Such a client may withdraw and become passive. The passive client allows nurses to provide care but is not interested in increasing independence or involvement in care. Early in the care of an immobilized client, the nurse should assess the client's normal coping mechanisms. The nurse then designs a nursing care plan that will allow the client to continue to use these coping abilities or will help him or her develop new ones.

Developmental Changes.

More developmental changes tend to be associated with immobility in the very young and in older adults. The immobilized young or middle-age adult who has been healthy may experience few, if any, developmental changes. However, there are exceptions, and clients must be fully assessed for developmental implications. One exception might be a mother who has complications at childbirth and as a result cannot interact with the newborn as expected.

Infants, Toddlers, and Preschoolers.

The newborn infant's spine is flexed and lacks the anteroposterior curves of the adult (see Chapter 10). As the baby grows, musculoskeletal development permits support of weight for standing and walking. Posture is awkward because the head and upper trunk are carried forward. Because body weight is not evenly distributed along a line of gravity, posture is off balance, and falls occur often. When the infant, toddler, or preschooler is immobilized, it is usually because of trauma or the need to correct a congenital skeletal abnormality. Prolonged immobilization can delay the child's gross motor skills and intellectual development. Nurses caring for immobilized children should plan activities that provide physical and psychosocial stimuli.

Adolescents.   The adolescence stage is usually initiated by a tremendous growth spurt (see Chapter 10). Growth is frequently uneven. Prolonged immobilization may alter adolescent growth patterns. In addition, the adolescent may lag behind peers in gaining independence. When immobilization occurs, social isolation must be a concern for this age-group.

Adults.   An adult who has correct posture and body alignment feels good, looks good, and generally appears self-confident. The healthy adult also has the necessary musculoskeletal development and coordination to carry out ADLs (see Chapter 11). When periods of prolonged immobility occur, all physiological systems are at risk. In addition, the role of the adult may change with regard to the family or social structure. The adult may lose identity associated with a job.

Older Adults.   A progressive loss of total bone mass occurs with the older adult. Some of the possible causes of this loss include decreased physical activity, hormonal changes, and actual bone resorption. The effect of bone loss is weaker bones. Older adults may walk more slowly and flexed, take smaller steps, and appear less coordinated. Thus balance is impaired, and they are at greater risk for falls and injuries (see Chapter 12). The outcomes of a fall include not only possible injury, but also hospitalization, loss of independence, and psychological effects (Rawsky, 1998)

Older adults may experience functional status changes secondary to hospitalization and altered mobility status (Box 46-2). Immobilization of older adults may increase their physical dependence on others and accelerate functional losses. Immobilization of some older adults results from a degenerative disease, neurological trauma, or chronic illness. For some older adults, immobilization occurs gradually and progressively, whereas for others—especially those who have had a stroke—immobilization is sudden. When providing nursing care for an older adult, the nurse should develop a care plan that encourages the client to perform as many self-care activities as possible, thereby maintaining the highest level of mobility. Blair (1995) points out that nurses may inadvertently contribute to a client's immobility by providing unnecessary help with activities such as bathing and transferring.

Hazards of Hospitalization of the Older Adult   Box 46-2

For many older persons, hospitalization results in functional decline, despite cure or repair of the condition for which they were admitted. Hospitalization can result in complications unrelated to the problem that caused admission or to its specific treatment and for reasons that are explainable and avoidable.

Usual aging is often associated with functional change, such as a decline in muscle strength and aerobic capacity; vasomotor instability; reduced bone density; diminished pulmonary ventilation; altered sensory continence, appetite, and thirst; and a tendency toward urinary incontinence. Hospitalization and bed rest superimpose factors such as enforced immobilization, reduction of plasma volume, accelerated bone loss, increased closing volume, and sensory deprivation. Any of these factors may thrust vulnerable older persons into a state of irreversible functional decline.

The relationships among physicians, nurses, and other health care professionals must reflect the importance of interdisciplinary care and the implementation of shared objectives.

Modified from Creditor MC: Hazards of hospitalization of the elderly, *Ann Intern Med* 118(3):219, 1993.

Critical Thinking Synthesis

Critical thinking requires the nurse to combine information from new knowledge, experiences, client data, critical thinking attitudes, and intellectual and professional standards. Each of these sources must be weighed for its validity and applicability to the client who is facing impaired mobility. The immobile client's needs are multiple, and by integrating these sources the nurse can best judge appropriate nursing diagnoses and subsequent care.

To understand the impact of immobility on the client and family, the nurse must integrate knowledge from nursing and other disciplines, previous experiences, and information gathered from clients. In addition, the use of critical thinking attitudes such as creativity is needed to devise a plan to provide successful interventions for immobility. Professional standards such as those developed by the Agency for Health Care Policy and Research (AHCPR) and intellectual standards such as accuracy provide valuable guides for mobility management (Figure 46-12).

Nursing Process for Impaired Body Alignment and Mobility

The use of the nursing process, critical application of anatomy and physiology, and experience with clients enables the nurse to develop individualized care plans for clients with preexisting mobility impairments and for those who are at risk. A care plan is designed to improve the client's functional status, promote self-care, maintain

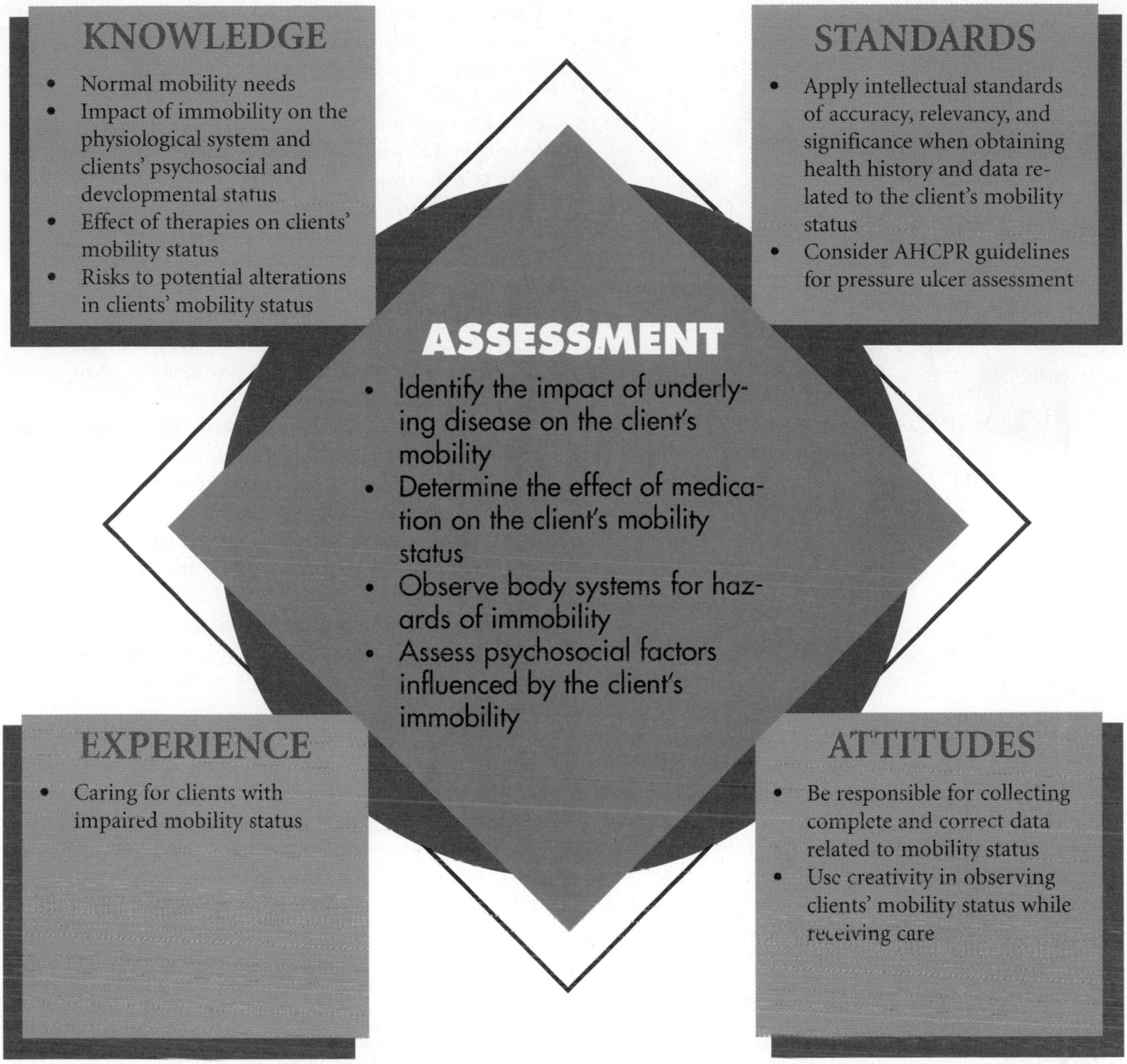

KNOWLEDGE

- Normal mobility needs
- Impact of immobility on the physiological system and clients' psychosocial and developmental status
- Effect of therapies on clients' mobility status
- Risks to potential alterations in clients' mobility status

STANDARDS

- Apply intellectual standards of accuracy, relevancy, and significance when obtaining health history and data related to the client's mobility status
- Consider AHCPR guidelines for pressure ulcer assessment

ASSESSMENT

- Identify the impact of underlying disease on the client's mobility
- Determine the effect of medication on the client's mobility status
- Observe body systems for hazards of immobility
- Assess psychosocial factors influenced by the client's immobility

EXPERIENCE

- Caring for clients with impaired mobility status

ATTITUDES

- Be responsible for collecting complete and correct data related to mobility status
- Use creativity in observing clients' mobility status while receiving care

Figure 46-12   *Synthesis Model for Immobility Assessment Phase.*

psychological well-being, and reduce the hazards of immobility.

ASSESSMENT

Nursing assessment is presented in two sections: mobility and immobility. Both areas are usually assessed during the complete physical examination.

Mobility.   Assessment of client mobility focuses on ROM, gait, exercise and activity tolerance, and body alignment. When unsure of the client's abilities, the nurse should begin assessment of mobility with the client in the most supportive position and move to higher levels of mobility according to the client's tolerance. Generally, the nurse starts assessing movement while the client is lying, then proceeds to assessing sitting positions in bed, transfers to chair, and finally gait. This helps to protect the client's safety.

Range of Motion.   **Range of motion (ROM)** is the maximum amount of movement available at a joint in one of the three planes of the body: sagittal, frontal, or transverse (Figure 46-13). The sagittal plane is a line that passes through the body from front to back, dividing the body into a left and a right side. The frontal plane passes through the body from side to side and divides the body into front and back. The transverse plane is a horizontal

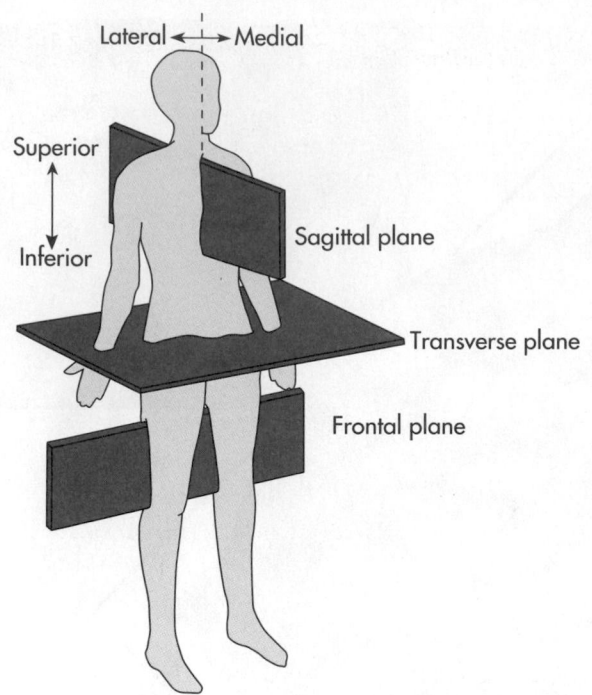

Figure 46-13 Planes of the body.

line that divides the body into upper and lower portions.

Joint mobility in each of the planes is limited by ligaments, muscles, and the nature of the joint. However, some joint movements are specific to each plane. In the sagittal plane, movements are flexion and extension (fingers and elbows), dorsiflexion and plantar flexion (feet), and extension (hip). In the frontal plane, movements are abduction and adduction (arms and legs), and eversion and inversion (feet). In the transverse plane, movements are pronation and supination (hands), and internal and external rotation (hips).

When assessing ROM, the nurse asks questions about and physically examines the client for stiffness, swelling, pain, limited movement, and unequal movement. Clients whose mobility is restricted because of illness, disability, or trauma require ROM to reduce the hazards of immobility. ROM exercises may be active (the client is able to move all joints through their ROM unassisted), passive (the client is unable to move independently, and the nurse moves each joint through its ROM), or somewhere in between (Table 46-2). With a weak client, for example, the nurse may merely provide support while the client performs most of the movement, or the client may be able to move some joints actively while the nurse passively moves others. The nurse first assesses the client's ability to engage in active ROM exercises and the need for assistance, teaching, or reinforcement. In general, exercises should be as active as health and mobility allow. Contractures may develop in joints not moved periodically through their full ROM.

Gait. The term **gait** is used to describe a particular manner or style of walking. The gait cycle begins with the heel strike of one leg and continues to the heel strike of the same leg. Assessing a client's gait allows the nurse to draw conclusions about balance, posture, safety, and ability to walk without assistance. The mechanics of human gait involve coordination of the skeletal, neurological, and muscular systems of the human body.

Exercise and Activity Tolerance. **Exercise** is physical activity for conditioning the body, improving health, and maintaining fitness. It can be used as therapy to correct a deformity or restore the overall body to a maximal state of health. When a person exercises, physiological changes occur in body systems (see Chapter 36).

Assessment of the client's energy level includes the physiological effects of exercise and activity tolerance. **Activity tolerance** is the kind and amount of exercise or work that a person is able to perform. Assessment of activity tolerance is necessary when planning activity such as walking, ROM exercises, or ADLs such as bathing for clients with acute or chronic illness. Activity tolerance assessment includes data from physiological, emotional, and developmental domains (see Chapter 36). This assessment is applicable in all clinical settings and is quickly completed by the nurse.

As activity is begun, clients should be monitored for symptoms such as dyspnea, fatigue, or chest pain, and/or for a change in vital signs from baseline. The weak or debilitated client is unable to sustain activity because the greater energy needed to complete the activity creates fatigue and generalized weakness. Even seemingly simple tasks such as eating and moving in bed may need to be monitored. When decreased activity tolerance is noted, the nurse should assess the time needed by the client to recover. Decreasing recovery time may indicate improving activity tolerance.

People who are depressed, worried, or anxious are frequently unable to tolerate exercise. Depressed clients are usually not motivated to participate. Clients who are worried or anxious fatigue easily because they expend a great deal of energy in worry and anxiety. Thus they may experience physical and emotional exhaustion.

Developmental changes also affect activity tolerance. As the infant enters the toddler stage, the activity level increases and the need for sleep declines. The child entering nursery school, preschool, or primary grades expends mental energy in learning and may require more rest after school or before strenuous play. The adolescent going through puberty may require more rest because much of the body's energy is expended for growth and hormone changes.

Changes may still occur through the adult years, but many of these changes are related to work and lifestyle choices. Pregnancy may cause fluctuations in a woman's energy tolerance; especially during the first and third

Text continued on p. 1505.

Table 46-2   Range-of-Motion Exercises

Body Part	Type of Joint	Type of Movement	Range (Degrees)	Primary Muscles
Neck, cervical spine	Pivotal	*Flexion:* Bring chin to rest on chest	45	Sternocleidomastoid
		Extension: Bend head back as far as possible	10	Trapezius
		Lateral flexion: Tilt head as far as possible toward each shoulder	40-45	Sternocleidomastoid
		Rotation: Turn head as far as possible in circular movement	180	Sternocleidomastoid, trapezius
Shoulder	Ball and socket	*Flexion:* Raise arm from side position forward to position above head	170-180	Coracobrachialis, deltoid,
		Extension: Move arm behind body, keeping elbow straight	45-60	Latissimus dorsi, teres major, deltoid
		Abduction: Raise arm to side to position above head with palm away from head	170-180	Deltoid, supraspinatus
		Adduction: Lower arm sideways and across body as far as possible		Pectoralis major

Continued

Body Part	Type of Joint	Type of Movement	Range (Degrees)	Primary Muscles
Shoulder, cont'd		*Internal rotation:* With elbow flexed, rotate shoulder by moving arm until thumb is turned inward and toward back.	70-80	Pectoralis major, latissimus dorsi, teres major, subscapularis
		External rotation: With elbow in full circle, move arm until thumb is upward and lateral to head	81-90	Infraspinatus, teres major
		Circumduction: Move arm in full circle (Circumduction is combination of all movements of ball-and-socket joint.)	360	Deltoid, coracobrachialis, latissimus dorsi, teres major
Elbow	Hinge	*Flexion:* Bend elbow so that lower arm moves toward its shoulder joint and hand is level with shoulder	150	Biceps brachii, brachialis, brachioradialis
		Extension: Straighten elbow by lowering hand	150	Triceps brachii
Forearm	Pivotal	*Supination:* Turn lower arm and hand so that palm is up	70-90	Supinator, biceps brachii
		Pronation: Turn lower arm so that palm is down	70-90	Pronator teres, pronator quadratus
Wrist	Condyloid	*Flexion:* Move palm toward inner aspect of forearm	80-90	Flexor carpi ulnaris, flexor carpi radialis

Table 46-2   Range-of-Motion Exercises—cont'd

Table 46-2   Range-of-Motion Exercises—cont'd

Body Part	Type of Joint	Type of Movement	Range (Degrees)	Primary Muscles
		Extension: Bring dorsal surface of hand back as far as possible	89-90	Extensor carpi radialis brevis, extensor carpi radialis longus, extensor carpi ulnaris
		Abduction (radial deviation): Bend wrist medially toward thumb	Up to 30	Flexor carpi radialis, extensor carpi radialis brevis, extensor carpi radialis longus
		Adduction (ulnar deviation): Bend wrist laterally toward fifth finger	30-50	Flexor carpi ulnaris, extensor carpi ulnaris
Fingers	Condyloid hinge	*Flexion:* Make fist	90	Lumbricales, interosseus volaris, interosseus dorsalis
		Extension: Bend fingers back as far as possible	30-60	Extensor digiti quinti proprius, extensor digitorum communis, extensor indicis proprius
		Abduction: Spread fingers apart	30	Interosseus dorsalis
		Adduction: Bring fingers together	30	Interosseus volaris
Thumb	Saddle	*Flexion:* Move thumb across palmar surface of hand		Flexor pollicis brevis
		Extension: Move thumb straight away from hand		Extensor pollicis longus, extensor pollicis brevis
		Abduction: Extend thumb laterally (usually done when placing fingers in abduction and adduction)	70-80	Abductor pollicis brevis and longus
		Adduction: Move thumb back toward hand	70-80	Adductor pollicis obliquus, adductor pollicis transversus
		Opposition: Touch thumb to each finger of same hand		Opponeus pollicis, opponeus digiti minimi
Hip	Ball and socket	*Flexion:* Move leg forward and up	120-130	Psoas major, iliacus, sartorius
		Extension: Move back beside other leg	120-130	Gluteus maximus, semitendinodud, semimembranosus

Continued

Table 46-2   Range-of-Motion Exercises—cont'd

Body Part	Type of Joint	Type of Movement	Range (Degrees)	Primary Muscles
Hip, cont'd		*Hyperextension:* Move leg behind body	10-20	Gluteus maximus, semitendinosus, semimembranosus
		Abduction: Move leg laterally away from body	30-50	Gluteus medius, gluteus minimus
		Adduction: Move leg back toward medial position and beyond if possible	20-30	Adductor longus, adductor brevis, adductor magnus
		Internal rotation: Turn foot and leg toward other leg	35-40	Gluteus medius, gluteus minimus, tensor fasciae latae
		External rotation: Turn foot and leg away from other leg	40-50	Obturatorius internus, oburatorius externus, quadratus femoris, piriformis, gemellus superior and inferior, gluteus maximus
		Circumduction: Move leg in circle		Psoas major, gluteus maximus, gluteus medius, adductor magnus
Knee	Hinge	*Flexion:* Bring heel back toward back of thigh	135-145	Biceps femoris, semitendinosus, semimembranosus, sartorius
		Extension: Return leg to floor	0	Rectus femoris, vastus lateralis, vastus medialis, vastus intermedius

Table 46-2   **Range-of-Motion Exercises**—cont'd

Body Part	Type of Joint	Type of Movement	Range (Degrees)	Primary Muscles
Ankle	Hinge	*Dorsal flexion:* Move foot so that toes are pointed upward	20-30	Tibialis anterior
		Plantar flexion: Move foot so that toes are pointed downward	45-50	Gastrocnemius, soleus
Foot	Gliding	*Inversion:* Turn sole of foot medially	30-40	Tibialis anterior, tibialis posterior
		Eversion: Turn sole of foot laterally	15-25	Peroneus longus, peroneus brevis
Toes	Condyloid	*Flexion:* Curl toes downward	30-60	Flexor digitorum, lumbricalis pedis, flexor hallucis brevis
		Extension: Straighten toes	30-60	Extensor digitorum longus, extensor digitorum brevis, extensor hallucis longus
		Abduction: Spread toes apart	15 or less	Abductor hallucis, interosseus dorsalis
		Adduction: Bring toes together	15 or less	Adductor hallucis, interosseus plantaris

trimesters, she may have increased fatigue. Hormonal changes and fetal development use body energy, and the woman may be unable or unmotivated to carry out physical activities. During the last trimester, fetal development consumes a great deal of the mother's energy, and the size and location of the fetus may limit the ability to take a deep breath, resulting in less oxygen being available for physical activities.

As the person grows older, activity tolerance changes. Muscle mass is reduced, posture changes, and the composition of bones is altered. There are often changes in the cardiorespiratory system, such as decreased maximum heart rate and decreased lung compliance, that affect the intensity of exercise. As age progresses, the older individual may still exercise but will do so at a reduced intensity.

There is an overall improvement of physiological functioning as a result of exercise. All systems become stronger and function more efficiently. Therefore nurses may plan interventions directed at increasing exercise. However, nurses in rehabilitation and acute care hospitals often care for clients whose mobility is restricted and, as a result, must develop nursing therapies designed to minimize the hazards of immobility.

Body Alignment.   Assessment of body alignment can be carried out with the client standing, sitting, or lying down. This assessment has the following objectives:

Determining normal physiological changes in body alignment resulting from growth and development for each individual client

Identifying deviations in body alignment caused by poor posture

Providing opportunities for clients to observe their posture

Identifying learning needs of clients for maintaining correct body alignment

Identifying trauma, muscle damage, or nerve dysfunction

Obtaining information concerning other factors that contribute to poor alignment, such as fatigue, malnutrition, and psychological problems

The first step in assessing body alignment is to put clients at ease so that unnatural or rigid positions are not assumed. When the body alignment of an immobilized or unconscious client is assessed, pillows and positioning supports should be removed from the bed and the client placed in the supine position.

Standing.   The nurse should focus assessment of body alignment for the standing client on the following points:

1.   The head is erect and midline.
2.   When observed posteriorly, the shoulders and hips are straight and parallel.
3.   When observed posteriorly, the vertebral column is straight.
4.   When the client is observed laterally, the head is erect and the spinal curves are aligned in a reversed S pattern. The cervical vertebrae are anteriorly convex, the thoracic vertebrae are posteriorly convex, and the lumbar vertebrae are anteriorly convex.
5.   When observed laterally, the abdomen is comfortably tucked in and the knees and ankles are slightly flexed. The person appears comfortable and does not seem conscious of the flexion of knees or ankles.
6.   The arms hang comfortably at the sides.
7.   The feet are placed slightly apart to achieve a base of support, and the toes are pointed forward.
8.   When the client is viewed anteriorly, the center of gravity is in the midline, and the line of gravity is from the middle of the forehead to a midpoint between the feet. Laterally the line of gravity runs vertically from the middle of the skull to the posterior third of the foot (Figure 46-14).

Sitting.   The nurse assesses alignment of the sitting client by the following observations:

1.   The head is erect, and the neck and vertebral column are in straight alignment.
2.   The body weight is evenly distributed on the buttocks and thighs.
3.   The thighs are parallel and in a horizontal plane.
4.   Both feet are supported on the floor (Figure 46-15). With clients of short stature, a footstool is used and the ankles are comfortably flexed.
5.   A 2- to 4-cm (1- to 2-inch) space is maintained between the edge of the seat and the popliteal space on the posterior surface of the knee. This space ensures that there is no pressure on the popliteal artery or nerve to decrease circulation or impair nerve function.
6.   The client's forearms are supported on the armrest, in the lap, or on a table in front of the chair.

It is particularly important to assess alignment when sitting if the client has muscle weakness, muscle paralysis, or nerve damage. Because of these alterations, the client has diminished sensation in the affected area and is unable to perceive pressure or decreased circulation. Proper alignment while sitting reduces the risk of musculoskeletal system damage in such a client. The client with severe respiratory disease may assume a posture of leaning on the table in front of the chair in an attempt to breathe more easily.

Lying.   People who are conscious have voluntary muscle control and normal perception of pressure. As a result, they usually assume a position of comfort when lying down. Because their ROM, sensation, and circulation are within normal limits, they change positions when they perceive muscle strain and decreased circulation.

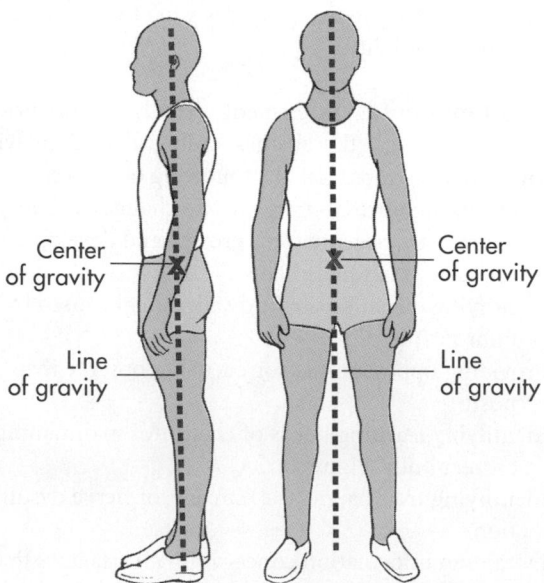

Figure 46-14   Correct body alignment when standing.

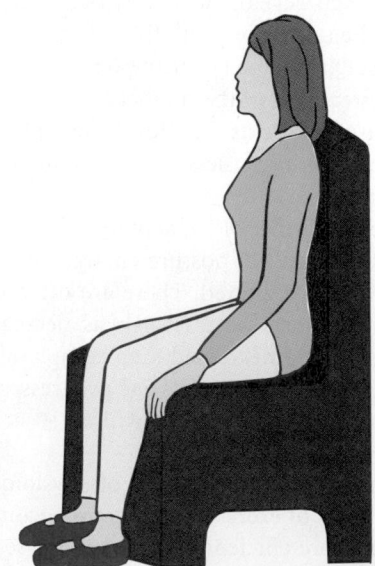

Figure 46-15   Correct body alignment when sitting.

Assessment of body alignment is best done with the client in the lateral position when the client is restricted to bed and not able to move well. All positioning supports should be removed from the bed except for the pillow under the head, and the body should be supported by an adequate mattress (Figure 46-16). This position allows for full view of the spine and back and will help provide other baseline body alignment data, such as whether the client can remain positioned without aid. The vertebrae should be in straight alignment without observable curves. The position should not cause discomfort. Conditions that create a risk of damage to the musculoskeletal system when lying down include clients with impaired mobility, such as those in traction or with arthritis; clients with decreased sensation, such as those with hemiparesis (one-sided weakness) following stroke; clients with impaired circulation, such as those with diabetes; and clients with lack of voluntary muscle control, such as those with spinal cord injuries.

Immobility.   The nurse assesses the immobilized client for hazards of immobility by performing a head-to-toe physical assessment (see Chapter 32). In addition, the nursing assessment should focus on certain physiological areas, as well as the client's psychosocial and developmental dimensions.

Physiological Factors.   The physiological hazards of immobility that may be identified during a nursing assessment are summarized in Table 46-3.

Metabolic System.   When assessing metabolic functioning, the nurse uses **anthropometric measurements** (measures of height, weight, and skinfold thickness) to evaluate muscle atrophy (see Chapter 32). In addition, the nurse may analyze intake and output records for balance. Does intake equal output? Intake and output measurements assist the nurse in determining whether a fluid imbalance exists (see Chapter 40). Dehydration and edema can increase the rate of skin breakdown in an immobilized client. Monitoring laboratory data such as electrolytes, serum protein (albumin and total protein) levels, and blood urea nitrogen (BUN) aid the nurse in determining metabolic functioning.

Assessing wound healing to evaluate alterations in the exchange of nutrients and monitoring food intake and elimination patterns will help to determine altered gastrointestinal functioning and potential metabolic problems. If an immobilized client has a wound, the rate of healing indicates how well nutrients are being delivered to tissues. Normal progression of healing indicates that metabolic needs of injured tissues are being met. Anorexia occurs commonly in immobilized clients. The client's food intake should be assessed before the tray is removed to determine the amount eaten. Nutritional imbalances

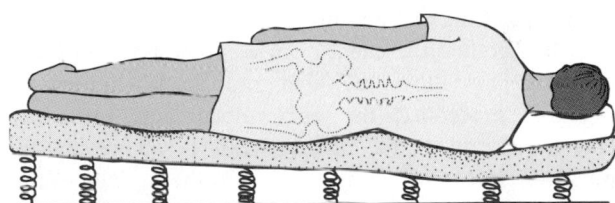

Figure 46-16   Correct body alignment when lying down.

Table 46-3	**Physiological Hazards of Immobility**	
System	Assessment Techniques	Abnormal Findings
Metabolic	Inspection	Slowed wound healing, abnormal laboratory data
	Inspection	Muscle atrophy
	Anthropometric measurements (mid-upper arm circumference, triceps skinfold measurement)	Decreased amount of subcutaneous fat
	Palpation	Generalized edema
Respiratory	Inspection	Asymmetrical chest wall movement, dyspnea, increased respiratory rate
	Auscultation	Crackles, wheezes
Cardiovascular	Auscultation	Orthostatic hypotension
	Auscultation, palpation	Increased heart rate, third heart sound, weak peripheral pulses, peripheral edema
Musculoskeletal	Inspection, palpation	Decreased ROM, erythema, increased diameter in calf or thigh
	Palpation	Joint contracture
	Inspection	Activity intolerance, muscle atrophy, joint contracture
Skin	Inspection, palpation	Break in skin integrity
Elimination	Inspection	Decreased urine output, cloudy or concentrated urine, decreased frequency of bowel movements
	Palpation	Distended bladder and abdomen
	Auscultation	Decreased bowel sounds

can be avoided if the nurse assesses the client's dietary patterns and food preferences early in immobilization (see Chapter 43).

Respiratory System. A respiratory assessment should be performed at least every 2 hours for clients with restricted activity. The nurse inspects chest wall movements during the full inspiratory-expiratory cycle. If a client has an atelectatic area, chest movement may be asymmetrical. In addition, the nurse auscultates the entire lung region to identify diminished breath sounds, crackles, or wheezes. Auscultation should focus on the dependent lung fields because pulmonary secretions tend to collect in these lower regions. A complete respiratory assessment identifies the presence of secretions and can be used to determine nursing interventions necessary for optimal respiratory function.

Cardiovascular System. Cardiovascular nursing assessment of the immobilized client includes blood pressure monitoring, evaluation of apical and peripheral pulses, and observation for signs of venous stasis (e.g., edema and poor wound healing). Although not all clients will experience orthostatic hypotension, clients should have their vital signs monitored during the first few attempts at sitting or standing.

When getting the client from a supine position into a chair, the nurse moves the client gradually. When performing this procedure, the nurse documents orthostatic changes. The nurse first obtains baseline blood pressure and pulse measurements with the client in the supine position (Roper, 1996). The nurse then raises the client to a high-Fowler's position and measures blood pressure and pulse again to detect decreases in blood pressure or elevations in pulse. The nurse remains with the client in the high-Fowler's position for a few moments to allow the body to adapt. The nurse continually monitors the client for dizziness or light-headedness. Then the nurse has the client sit at the side of the bed with the feet on the floor. If there is no dizziness or drop in blood pressure (greater than 10 mm/Hg), the nurse assists the client to a chair and retakes the blood pressure for comparison with the baseline.

The nurse also assesses the apical and peripheral pulses. Recumbency increases cardiac workload and results in an increased pulse rate. In some clients, particularly older adults, the heart may not tolerate the increased workload, and a form of cardiac failure may develop. A third heart sound, heard at the apex, can be an early indication of congestive heart failure. Monitoring peripheral pulses allows the nurse to evaluate the heart's ability to pump blood. The absence of a peripheral pulse in the lower extremities, particularly one that was previously present, should be documented and reported to the client's physician.

Edema may indicate the heart's inability to handle the increased workload. Because edema moves to dependent body regions, assessment of the immobilized client should include the sacrum, legs, and feet. If the heart is unable to tolerate the increased workload, peripheral body regions, such as the hands, feet, nose, and earlobes, will be colder than central body regions.

Finally, the nurse assesses the venous system, because deep vein thrombosis is a hazard of restricted mobility. A dislodged thrombus, called an **embolus,** may travel through the circulatory system to the lungs or brain and impair circulation. Venous emboli may travel to the lungs, where they are life threatening. Better than 90% of all pulmonary emboli begin in the legs or pelvis (Christie, 1998).

To assess for a deep vein thrombosis, the nurse removes the client's elastic stockings and/or sequential compression devices (SCDs) every 8 hours and observes the calves for redness, warmth, and tenderness. Homans' sign, or calf pain on dorsiflexion of the foot, indicates a probable thrombus, but this sign is not always present (Nunnelee, 1995). In addition, calf circumference should be measured daily. To do this, the nurse marks a point on each calf 10 cm from the midpatella. The circumference is measured each day using the mark for placement of the tape measure. One-sided increases in calf diameter can be an early indication of thrombosis. Because deep vein thrombosis can also occur in the thigh, thigh measurements should be taken daily if the client is prone to thrombosis. In many clients, deep vein thrombosis can be prevented by active exercise and compression devices in conjunction with prescribed anticoagulant treatment.

Musculoskeletal System. Major musculoskeletal abnormalities that may be identified during nursing assessment include decreased muscle tone and strength, loss of muscle mass, and contractures. The anthropometric measurements described previously may indicate losses in muscle tone and muscle mass. Muscle atrophy is a common complication that arises from the lack of weight bearing found with bed rest (St. Pierre and Flaskerud, 1995).

Assessment of ROM is important as a baseline against which later measurements can be compared to evaluate whether a loss in joint mobility has occurred. ROM can be measured with a goniometer (see Figure 36-10).

Disuse osteoporosis cannot be identified by physical assessment. However, postmenopausal women, clients taking steroids, and persons with increased serum and urine calcium levels probably have a greater risk for bone demineralization. The risk of disuse osteoporosis should be considered when planning nursing interventions. Not only may falls result in injury, but falls may occur because of pathological fractures secondary to osteoporosis. Clients who are at risk for osteoporosis should have their diet assessed for calcium intake. Some clients have a lactose intolerance and need dietary teaching about alternative sources of calcium (Box 46-3).

Lactose intolerance, the deficiency in digestion and absorption of the disaccharide in milk, is thought to be related to ethnic background. This problem is more frequent in Native Americans, and descendants from Africa, Asia, India, and Mexico. It is less common in ethnic groups from Northern Europe. Although lactose intolerance can occur at any age, it is common for symptoms of the intolerance to develop in adulthood (Beare and Myers, 1998).

Lactose is a simple sugar found in milk and milk-based food products. Lactose is normally broken down by lactase, an enzyme found in the intestines. Lactose intolerance may cause diarrhea, gaseous distention, and cramping.

It is important to identify foods rich in calcium for clients who are at risk for not getting enough calcium. Foods high in calcium include some vegetables, particularly leafy green vegetables; fish like sardines and canned salmon; oysters; tofu; and yogurt (Tresolini and others, 1996). In suggesting calcium-rich foods, the nurse must consider culture. Clients of Asian descent may find dark green leafy vegetables and fish acceptable.

Integumentary System. The nurse must continually assess the client's skin for breakdown and color changes such as pallor or redness. The skin should be observed when the client is turned, hygiene measures are performed, or elimination needs are provided for. At a minimum, assessment should occur every 2 hours (see Chapter 47).

Elimination System. The client's elimination status should be evaluated on each shift, and total intake and output should be evaluated every 24 hours. The nurse should determine that the client is receiving the correct amount and type of fluids orally or parenterally (see Chapter 44). Inadequate intake and output or fluid and electrolyte imbalances can increase the risk for renal system impairment, ranging from recurrent infections to kidney failure. Dehydration can also increase the risk for skin breakdown, thrombus formation, respiratory infections, and constipation.

Assessment of elimination status should also include the adequacy of dietary choices and the frequency and consistency of bowel movements (see Chapter 45). Accurate assessment enables the nurse to intervene before constipation and fecal impaction occur.

Psychosocial Assessment. Many alterations in physiological, sociocultural, and developmental functioning are related to immobility. Often, these problems are interrelated, and it is imperative that nursing care focus on all dimensions. Often the focus of immobility is on the easily visible physical problems, such as skin impairment, but the psychosocial and developmental aspects of immobility should not be overlooked.

Changes in a client's psychosocial status often occur slowly and may be overlooked by health care personnel. Abrupt changes in personality may have a physiological cause, such as a medication reaction, a pulmonary embolus, or an acute infection. For example, compromised older clients have confusion as their main symptom when experiencing a pulmonary emboli or an acute urinary tract infection. Confusion in older adults is not normal and should be thoroughly examined (Miller and others, 1997).

Common reactions to immobilization include boredom, feelings of isolation, depression, and anger. The nurse should observe for changes in emotional status. Examples of change that may indicate psychosocial concerns are a cooperative client who becomes less cooperative or an independent client who asks for more help than is necessary. The nurse should try to determine the reasons for such alterations. Identifying how the client usually copes with loss is vital (see Chapters 29 and 30). A change in mobility status, whether permanent or not, may cause a grief reaction. Families are a key resource for information about behavior changes.

Unexplained changes in the sleep-wake cycle must be identified and corrected. Most can be prevented or minimized, such as those occurring because of nursing activities, a noisy environment, or discomfort. They may also occur because of medications such as analgesics, sleeping pills, or cardiovascular drugs (see Chapter 41).

Because psychosocial changes usually occur gradually, the nurse should observe the client's behavior on a daily basis. If behavioral changes occur, the nurse should determine the causes and evaluate the changes as short or long term. Identifying the cause helps the nurse design appropriate nursing interventions.

Developmental Assessment. Assessment of the immobilized client should include developmental considerations to ensure that the client's needs are identified. The nurse determines whether the young child can meet developmental tasks and is progressing normally. The child's development may regress or be slowed because of immobilization. By identifying a child's overall developmental needs, the nurse can design nursing therapies to maintain normal development. The nurse may also need to assure the parents that developmental delays are usually temporary.

Immobilization of a family member changes the family's functioning. The family's response to this change may lead to problems, stress, and anxieties. Children seeing parents who are immobile may have difficulty understanding what is happening.

Immobility can have a significant effect on the older adult's levels of health, independence, and functional status. Nursing assessment enables the nurse to determine the older client's ability to meet needs independently and to adapt to developmental changes such as declining physical functioning and altered family and peer relationships. A decline in developmental functioning needs prompt investigation to determine why the change occurred and what can be done to return the client to an optimal level of functioning as soon as possible. Assessment also includes the client's home and community to identify factors that are risks to the client's mobility and safety (see Chapter 37).

Client Expectations. Clients may have unrealistic expectations of themselves or their caregivers. They may agree with the staff and understand their limitations, or they may set their expectations of themselves too high or too low. Since clients may rely on caregivers to provide personal care that they have not received from another since early childhood, it is vital that the caregivers take the time to assess the client's expectations.

Some clients may expect to be waited on, and other clients may want to do as much for themselves as possible. Key to understanding these expectations is the client's psychosocial reaction, knowledge about his or her condition, and developmental level. Asking clients to explain what they know about their mobility status, what questions they and their families have, and how the immobility is affecting their goals will help the nurse and other caregivers more fully appreciate and incorporate clients' expectations into care planning.

NURSING DIAGNOSIS

An immobilized or partially immobilized client may have one or more nursing diagnoses. The two diagnoses most directly related to mobility problems are *impaired physical mobility* and *risk for disuse syndrome*. The diagnosis of *impaired physical mobility* is used for the client who has some limitation but is not completely immobile. The diagnosis of *risk for disuse syndrome* should be considered for the client who is immobile and at risk for multisystem pathophysiology because of inactivity. Beyond these diagnoses, the list of potential diagnoses is extensive, since immobility affects multiple body systems (Box 46-4).

Assessment reveals clusters of data that indicate whether a client is at risk or if a problem exists. Assessment also identifies pertinent defining characteristics that support the diagnostic label and probable cause of the diagnosis. Locating the probable cause of the diagnosis (based on assessment data) is important to planning client-centered goals and subsequent nursing interventions that will best help the client.

Impaired physical mobility related to bed rest would require slightly different interventions than *impaired physical mobility related to pain in the left shoulder*. Thus it is critical that nursing assessment activities identify and cluster defining characteristics that ultimately support the nursing diagnosis selected (Box 46-5). The diagnosis re-

---

NURSING DIAGNOSES Box 46-4

IMMOBILITY

Activity intolerance
Airway clearance, ineffective
Breathing pattern, ineffective
Coping, ineffective individual
Disuse syndrome, risk for
Fluid volume deficit, risk for
Gas exchange, impaired
Infection, risk for
Injury, risk for
Mobility, impaired physical
Skin integrity, impaired
Skin integrity, impaired, risk for
Sleep pattern disturbance
Social isolation
Tissue perfusion, altered (peripheral)
Urinary elimination, altered

---

lated to bed rest would require interventions aimed at keeping the client as mobile as possible and encouraging the client to do self-care and ROM in bed. The diagnosis related to pain would require the nurse to assist the client with comfort measures so that the client would then be willing and more able to move. In both situations the nurse would explain the importance of activity to healthy body functioning.

Often the physiological dimension is the major focus of nursing care for clients with impaired mobility. Thus the psychosocial and developmental dimensions are neglected. Yet they are important to health. For example, during immobilization, social interaction and stimuli are decreased. Ultimately the client may become isolated, withdrawn, and bored. Such clients may frequently use the nurse's call bell to request minor physical attention when their real need is greater socialization. Nursing diagnoses for health needs in developmental areas reflect changes from the client's normal activities. Immobility can lead to a developmental crisis if the client is unable to resolve problems and continue to mature.

Immobility may also lead to complications such as pulmonary emboli or pneumonia. If these conditions develop, the nurse will collaborate with the physician or nurse practitioner for prescribed therapy to intervene. The nurse is alert for these potential complications and works to prevent them.

PLANNING

During planning the nurse synthesizes information from resources such as knowledge of the role of respiratory and physical therapy, standards such as skin care guidelines from the AHCPR, protocols for clients at risk for falls, attitudes such as creativity and perseverance, and past experiences with immobilized clients (Figure 46-17). Critical

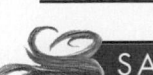

SAMPLE NURSING DIAGNOSTIC PROCESS   Box 46-5

IMPAIRED PHYSICAL MOBILITY

Assessment Activities	Defining Characteristics	Nursing Diagnosis
Measure ROM during exercises of extremities.	Limited ROM with left shoulder Reluctance to attempt movement with left shoulder Impaired coordination while attempting to perform ROM with left shoulder	Impaired physical mobility related to left shoulder pain
Ask client about perception of pain.	Client complains of sharp pain in shoulder	
Ask client about endurance and activity tolerance.	Client reports decreased muscle strength in left shoulder	

KNOWLEDGE

- Benefit of mobility on body system functioning
- Role of physical, occupational, or respiratory therapists or dieticians in reducing hazards of immobility
- Effect of new medications on the client's mobility status

STANDARDS

- Individualize therapies for the client's mobility needs
- Apply skin care therapies consistent with AHCPR standards
- Apply cardiopulmonary reconditioning therapies consistent with AHCPR standards
- Protocols for fall prevention

PLANNING

- Consult with member of the health care team for resources to improve the client's mobility status
- Identify nursing interventions designed to reduce hazards of immobility to increase mobility status
- Involve the client and family in care activities
- Determine the client's ability to increase activity level

EXPERIENCE

- Previous client responses to planned nursing therapies for improving mobility (what worked and what did not work)

ATTITUDES

- Use creativity to design interventions that improve mobility
- Display perseverance to adapt interventions to multiple health care settings

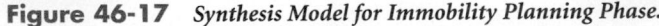

Figure 46-17 *Synthesis Model for Immobility Planning Phase.*

 SAMPLE NURSING CARE PLAN

IMMOBILITY

ASSESSMENT*

Miss Barbara Adams, an 84-year-old client, has been admitted for rehabilitation after a **total hip replacement (THR) for osteoarthritis.** The wound is clean, dry, and intact. Staples will be removed in 2 days. She is **not able to transfer with help from chair to bed.** She states that she is **"afraid of falling"** and **frequently refuses to get out of bed.** She rates her pain as a 2 on a scale of 1 to 10. She has a **history of smoking.** She states that she needs pain medication to help her sleep during the night but does not need any during the day. She is to start physical therapy tomorrow.

*Defining characteristics are shown in bold type.

NURSING DIAGNOSIS: Impaired mobility related to musculoskeletal impairment secondary to THR and fear of falling.

PLANNING

GOALS
Client will remain free of complications of immobility.

EXPECTED OUTCOMES
Client's skin will remain intact.

Client's calf diameters will remain within 1 cm of baseline through discharge.

Client will transfer to chair with assistance 3 times per day within 2 days.

Client will state fear of falling is less within 2 days.

INTERVENTIONS†

Circulatory Care
- Administer low-dose heparin as ordered.

- Apply intermittent compression stockings as ordered and remove each shift for hygiene.
- Reinforce antiembolic exercises while awake.
- Assist client out of bed slowly.

Skin Surveillance
- Instruct client to shift position every 1 to 1½ hours while awake.
- When recumbent, place client in 30-degree lateral position.

- Keep client's heels off of the bed by placing a pad under the lower legs.

Positioning
- Explain positioning procedure to client.
- Refer to physical therapy for transfer training.
- Encourage client to assist in transfer and positioning.

RATIONALE

Administration of low-dose heparin has shown reduction in risk for vein thrombosis (Proctor, Greenfield, and Marsh, 1997)

Application increases venous tone, improving venous return and reducing venous stasis (Proctor, Greenfield, and Marsh, 1997).

Moving slowly will decrease the likelihood of orthostatic hypotension. Moving the client slowly will also avoid the perception by the client of being rushed, which may cause the client to become more fearful.

The 30-degree lateral position reduces pressure from the sacral area and reduces the risk of skin breakdown (AHCPR, 1994).

Using a thin pad under the lower legs raises the heel just enough so that a paper can slide between the heels and the bed, thereby reducing the pressure on the heels so that tissue blood flow is maintained (AHCPR, 1994).

Reduces anxiety.

Helps to strengthen muscles used in transfer.

†Intervention Classification labels from McCloskey JC, Bulechek GM: *Nursing interventions classification (NIC)*, ed 3, St. Louis, 2000, Mosby.

EVALUATION
Measure calves daily.

Perform circulatory assessment of extremities every shift.

Observe skin integrity each shift.

Observe client transfer from bed to chair.

Ask client to rate her fear of falling on a scale of 1 to 10.

thinking ensures that the client's plan of care integrates all that the nurse knows about the individual, as well as key critical thinking elements. Professional standards are especially important to consider when the nurse develops a plan of care. These standards often establish scientifically proven guidelines for selecting effective nursing interventions.

The nurse develops an individualized plan of care for each nursing diagnosis (see care plan). The nurse and client set realistic expectations for care. Goals are set that are individualized, realistic, and measurable.

The nurse plans therapeutic interventions for clients with actual problems or risks to body alignment and mobility. The nurse plans therapies according to severity of risks to the client, and the plan is individualized according to the client's developmental stage, level of health, and lifestyle. Care planning must take into consideration priority setting, so that immediate needs are attended to first. The immediacy of any problem is determined by the effect the problem has on the client's mental and physical health.

The interventions planned for the client may be done directly by the nurse or delegated to assistive personnel (AP). AP can reinforce leg exercises, use of the incentive spirometer, and coughing and deep breathing (see Chapter 39). They may turn and position clients, apply elastic stockings, and assess leg circumferences and height and weight.

Because many of the skills associated with care of the immobile can be delegated, it may be easy for the nurse to overlook the potential complications of immobility until they occur. Therefore the nurse must be vigilant in monitoring the client, reinforcing prevention techniques, and supervising AP in carrying out activities aimed at preventing immobility complications. Maintaining body alignment is especially important for clients with actual or potential limitations in mobility. Although turning and positioning of a comatose client may be delegated, the nurse must ensure that it is done correctly and that the position is changed frequently to reduce the risk of poor alignment and future injury to the skin and musculoskeletal system. The frequency of turning is based on client assessment for risk of pressure ulcer development (see Chapter 47).

The nurse may need the help of another health team member such as a physical or occupational therapist when considering mobility needs. For example, physical therapists are a resource for planning ROM or strengthening exercises, and occupational therapists are a resource for planning ADLs that clients need to modify or relearn. Discharge planning is begun when a client enters the health care system. In anticipation of the client's discharge from an institution, a referral may be made to help the client remain mobile or regain mobility at home. Therefore, consideration must be given to the client's home environment when planning therapies to maintain or improve body alignment and mobility.

IMPLEMENTATION

Nursing interventions related to immobility are classified into health promotion activities, acute care–based implementations, and restorative and continuing care services.

Health Promotion.   Health promotion activities include a variety of interventions that can be divided into education, prevention, and early detection. Respectively, some examples of these health promotion activities are how to lift correctly, preventing falls (see Chapter 37), and early detection of scoliosis (see Chapter 32). Most health promotion interventions related to mobility will be educative and preventive. In this section lifting correctly and exercise are emphasized.

Lifting.   The rate of injuries in occupational settings has increased in recent years. Back pain is the costliest job-related injury (Neal, 1997). Back injuries are often the direct result of improper lifting and bending. The most common back injury is strain on the lumbar muscle group, which includes the muscles around the lumbar vertebrae. Injury to these areas affects the ability to bend forward, backward, and from side to side and limits the ability to rotate the hips and lower back.

Nurses and AP are especially at risk for injury to lumbar muscles when lifting, transferring, or positioning immobilized clients. Therefore nurses need to be cognizant of good lifting techniques to protect themselves, those they supervise, and the clients being cared for. Therefore when lifting, the nurse should assess the weight to be lifted and what assistance, if any, is needed. If help is needed, the nurse should determine if a second person or mechanical assistance is needed.

The nurse should know the maximum weight that is safe to carry. The nurse should not lift an object if its weight is 35% or more of his or her body weight. Therefore a nurse who weighs 130 pounds (59.1 kg) should not try to lift an immobilized 100-pound (45.5-kg) person. Although the nurse may be able to do it, there is a risk of dropping the client or causing injury to the nurse's back. Another consideration is the condition of the client and whether he or she can provide help while being moved. Once the amount of assistance is determined, these steps are followed:

1.   Keep the weight to be lifted as close to the body as possible; this action places the object in the same plane as the lifter and close to the center of gravity for balance.
2.   Bend at the knees; this helps to maintain the center of gravity and uses the stronger leg muscles to do the lifting (Figure 46-18).
3.   Avoid twisting. Twisting can overload the spine and lead to serious injury.
4.   Tighten abdominal muscles and tuck the pelvis; this provides balance and helps protect the back.

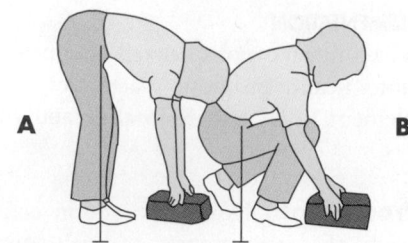

Figure 46-18 Incorrect (**A**) and correct (**B**) body position for lifting.

Research HIGHLIGHT   **Box 46-6**

RESEARCH ABSTRACT

Often exercise programs offered to older adults focus on traditional Western exercises such as walking, stretching, or swimming. This study examined the outcomes of tai chi chuan in a group of 24 community-based older adults who were 55 years of age or older. A volunteer group of 22 older adults served as the control group. The control group maintained their usual routines. A pretest-posttest design was used, and the following measures were evaluated: balance, flexibility, mood, health status, and blood pressure. The subjects exercised for 60 minutes once a week and also practiced their exercises at home. A significant difference was found in the balance of those who used tai chi chuan.

IMPLICATIONS FOR PRACTICE
- The authors assert that tai chi chuan is safe and enjoyable.
- Tai chi chuan might help balance, which may help older adults maintain their mobility.
- Nurses can use a variety of means to introduce exercise into the lives of clients.

REFERENCE
Schaller KJ: Tai Chi Chih: an exercise option for older adults, *J Gerontol Nurs* 22(10):12, 1996.

5. Maintain the trunk erect and knees bent so that multiple groups work together in a coordinated manner (Gassett and others, 1996).

Exercise. Although many diseases and physical problems can cause or contribute to immobility, it is important to remember that exercise programs can enhance feelings of well-being, as well as improve endurance, strength, and health. Exercise is known to reduce the risk of many health problems such as cardiovascular disease, diabetes, and osteoporosis.

Exercise should be a key prescription given by nurses who work with health promotion of clients. Functional decline from disuse is a major concern as aging occurs. Nurses can contribute to promoting health for many types of clients by encouraging or starting managed exercise programs. Research has shown that older adults can enjoy and benefit from exercises other than traditional Western exercises such as walking or swimming (Box 46-6). Even hospitalized clients can be encouraged to do stretching, ROM, and light walking within the limits of their condition (see Chapter 36).

Acute Care. In the acute care setting, specific interventions are designed to reduce the impact of immobility on the client by reducing the hazards of immobility and by positioning and transferring clients correctly.

Immobility Hazards. Clients in acute care settings may demonstrate some problems associated with prolonged immobility, such as impaired respiratory status, orthostatic hypotension, and impaired skin integrity. For these clients, nursing interventions are designed to reduce the impact of immobility on body systems and prepare the client for the restorative phase of care.

Metabolic System. The immobilized client requires a high-protein, high-calorie diet with vitamin B and C supplements. Protein is needed to repair injured tissue and rebuild depleted protein stores. A high-calorie intake provides sufficient fuel to meet metabolic needs and to replace subcutaneous tissue. Supplementation with vita-

min C is necessary to replace protein stores. Vitamin B complex is needed for skin integrity and wound healing.

If the client is unable to eat, nutrition must be provided parenterally or enterally. Enteral feedings include delivery through a nasogastric, gastrostomy, or jejunostomy tube of high-protein, high-calorie solutions with complete requirements of vitamins, minerals, and electrolytes (see Chapter 43). Total parenteral nutrition refers to delivery of nutritional supplements through a central or peripheral intravenous catheter.

Respiratory System. Nursing interventions for the respiratory system are aimed at promoting expansion of the chest and lungs, preventing stasis of pulmonary secretions, maintaining a patent airway, and promoting adequate exchange of respiratory gases.

Promoting Expansion of the Chest and Lungs. The nurse promotes chest expansion with several interventions. Changing the position of the client at least every 2 hours allows the dependent lung regions to reexpand. Reexpansion maintains the elastic recoil property of the lungs and clears the dependent lung regions of pulmonary secretions.

The nurse should encourage the client to deep breathe and cough every 1 to 2 hours. Alert clients can be taught to deep breathe or yawn every hour or to use an incentive spirometer (see Chapter 39). The nurse instructs the client to take in three deep breaths and cough with the third exhalation. This technique produces a more forceful, productive cough without excessive fatigue. These respiratory interventions will aid alveolar expansion and prevent atelectasis. Coughing reduces the stasis of pulmonary secretions. For unconscious clients with an artificial airway, the nurse can expand the chest and lungs by using an Ambubag (see Chapter 39).

If abdominal binders or rib supports are required, they should be removed every 2 hours to allow the client to breathe deeply. Binders must be assessed for correct positioning and adjusted as necessary to prevent interference with respirations. Often clients will wear the binder only when ambulating. Specific physician instructions for the use of binders will vary.

Preventing Stasis of Pulmonary Secretions.

Stagnant secretions accumulating in the bronchi and lungs may lead to growth of bacteria and subsequent development of pneumonia. Stagnation of secretions can be reduced by changing the client's position every 2 hours. This change rotates the dependent lung, mobilizing secretions.

The immobile client should take in a minimum of 2000 ml of fluid a day, if not contraindicated, to help keep mucociliary clearance normal. In clients free from infection and with adequate hydration, pulmonary secretions will appear thin, watery, and clear. The client can easily remove the secretions with coughing. Without adequate hydration the secretions are thick and tenacious and difficult to remove. Encouraging fluids also benefits in helping with bowel and urine elimination and aids in maintaining circulation and skin integrity.

Chest physiotherapy (CPT) (percussion and positioning) is an effective method for preventing pulmonary secretion stasis. CPT techniques help the client to drain secretions from specific segments of the bronchi and lungs into the trachea so that the client can cough and expel the secretions. Respiratory assessment findings identify areas of the lungs requiring CPT (see Chapter 39).

Maintaining a Patent Airway.

Immobilized clients and those on bed rest are generally weakened. If weakness progresses, the cough reflex gradually becomes inefficient. The stasis of secretions in the lungs may be life threatening for an immobilized client because hypostatic pneumonia can easily develop. Dislodging and mobilizing the stagnant secretions reduce the risk of pneumonia. Assessment findings that indicate this condition include productive cough with greenish yellow sputum; fever; pain on breathing; and crackles, wheezes, and dyspnea. The nurse should actively work with the client to deep breathe and cough every 1 to 2 hours as described in promoting chest expansion.

In the immobilized client an obstructed airway is usually a result of a mucous plug. The nurse can implement several therapies, such as CPT, to reduce the risk of mucous plugs and to maintain a patent airway. Nasotracheal or orotracheal suction techniques may be used to remove secretions in the upper airways of a client who is unable to cough productively. This procedure must be performed aseptically.

The nurse places a suction catheter in the client's nose or through the mouth and applies suction. The nurse can also suction secretions from an artificial airway such as an endotracheal or tracheal tube. The nurse inserts a catheter into the artificial airway in a sterile procedure. This removes pulmonary secretions from the upper and lower airways (see Chapter 39 for suctioning techniques).

Cardiovascular System.

The effects of bed rest or immobilization on the cardiovascular system include orthostatic hypotension, increased cardiac workload, and thrombus formation. Nursing therapies are designed to minimize or prevent these alterations.

Reducing Orthostatic Hypotension.

After bed rest, clients usually have an increased pulse rate, a decrease in pulse pressure, and an increase in fainting in response to a tilting or an erect posture (Roper, 1996). Interventions should be directed toward reducing or eliminating the effects of orthostatic hypotension. The nurse attempts to get the client moving as soon as the physical condition allows, even if this only involves dangling at the bedside or moving to a chair. This activity maintains muscle tone and increases venous return. Isometric exercises, those activities that involve muscle tension without muscle shortening, do not have any beneficial effect on preventing orthostatic hypotension but may improve activity tolerance. When getting an immobile client up for the first time, the nurse should usually be assisted by at least one other person. This is a precautionary step. The client will still be expected to do as much of the transfer as the condition allows.

Reducing Cardiac Workload.

The nurse designs interventions to reduce cardiac workload, which is increased by immobility. A primary intervention is to discourage the client from using the Valsalva maneuver. When using this maneuver, the client holds his or her breath, which increases intrathoracic pressure. This decreases venous return and cardiac output. When the strain is released, venous return and cardiac output immediately increase and systolic blood pressure and pulse pressure rise. These pressure changes produce a reflex bradycardia and a possible decrease in blood pressure that may cause sudden cardiac death in clients with heart disease. The nurse teaches the client to breathe out while moving or being lifted up in bed.

Preventing Thrombus Formation.

The most cost-effective way to address the deep vein thrombosis (DVT) problem is through an aggressive program of prophylaxis. It begins with identification of clients at risk and continues throughout the time clients are immobile or otherwise at risk. This is clearly a collaborative role between nurses and physicians. Risk factors can be easily identified by the nurse during an admission nursing assessment. Many interventions reduce the risk of thrombus formation in the immobilized client. Leg exercises, encouraging fluids, position changes, and teaching should begin when the client becomes immobile. Preoperative clients should be given this information before surgery (see Chapter 49). Other interventions such as medications and intermittent pneumatic compression (IPC) devices require a physician's order. Maintenance and administration of prophylaxis is a nursing role, and nurses can determine when the client is fully mobile postoperatively, decreasing the continued risk for DVT.

Heparin is the most widely used drug in the prophylaxis of DVT and is the gold standard for treatment because it has been well studied and validated (Nunnelee, 1995). Common dosage for low-dose heparin (LDH) therapy is 5000 units given subcutaneously 2 hours before surgery and repeated every 8 to 12 hours until the client is fully mobile or discharged. Heparin is an anticoagulant, and it suppresses clot formation. Because of the action of this medication, the nurse must continually assess the client for signs of bleeding, such as increased bruising, guaiac-positive stools, and bleeding gums. Although the majority of clients receiving LDH do not experience side effects, the risk remains present.

IPC devices (also referred to as sequential compression devices (SCDs) consist of sleeves or stockings, made of fabric or plastic that are wrapped around the leg and secured with Velcro (Box 46-7). The sleeves are then connected to a pump that alternately inflates and deflates the stocking around the leg. A typical cycle is inflation for 10 to 15 seconds and deflation for 45 to 60 seconds. Inflation pressures average 40 mm Hg. Use of IPC/SCDs on the legs decreases venous stasis by increasing venous return through the deep veins of the legs. For optimal results, use of IPC/SCDs is begun as soon as possible and maintained until the client becomes fully ambulatory. Graded compression stockings can help prevent DVT, but clients must receive the right size, and the IPC/SCDs must be used correctly.

Elastic stockings (sometimes called TED hose) also aid in maintaining external pressure on the muscles of the lower extremities and thus may promote venous return (Skill 46-1). When considering applying graded compression stockings, the nurse first needs to assess the client's suitability for wearing them. The stockings should not be applied if there is any local condition affecting the leg (e.g., any skin lesion, gangrenous condition, or recent vein ligation), as application may compromise circulation. The stockings must be applied properly, and they must be removed and reapplied (see Skill 46-1) at least twice a day. In addition, the stockings should always be clean and dry, and it may be useful for the client to have two pairs.

Positioning techniques aid in reducing compression of the leg veins. Proper positioning used with other therapies (e.g., heparin or elastic stockings) aid in reducing the client's risk of thrombus formation. When positioning clients, the nurse uses caution to prevent pressure on the posterior knee and deep veins in the lower extremities. Client teaching should include avoiding crossing the legs, not sitting for prolonged periods of time, not wearing clothing that constricts the legs or waist, not putting pillows under the knees, and avoiding massaging the legs.

ROM exercises are designed to reduce the risk of contractures but may also aid in preventing thrombi. Activity causes contraction of the skeletal muscles, which in turn exerts pressure on the veins to promote venous return, thereby reducing venous stasis. Specific exercises that help prevent thrombophlebitis are ankle pumps, foot circles, and knee flexion. Ankle pumps, sometimes called calf pumps, include alternating plantar flexion and dorsiflexion. Foot circles require the client to rotate the ankle. This can be done by instructing the client to make the letters of the alphabet with the feet. Knee flexion involves alternately extending and flexing the knee. These exercises are sometimes referred to as antiembolic exercises and should be done hourly while awake.

When DVT is suspected, the nurse should report it immediately. The leg should be elevated with no pressure on the thrombus. The family, client, and all health care personnel should be instructed not to massage the area because of the danger of dislodging the thrombus.

Musculoskeletal System. The immobilized client must receive some exercise to prevent excessive muscle atrophy and joint contractures. If the client is unable to move part or all of the body, the nurse must perform passive ROM exercises for all immobilized joints while bathing the client and at least 2 or 3 more times a day. If

---

Box 46-7	**Procedural Guidelines**

For Application of Sequential Compression Stockings

1. Measure client for proper-size stocking by measuring around the largest part of the client's thigh.
2. Place a protective stockinette over the client's leg.
3. Wrap the stocking around the leg, starting at the ankle, with the opening over the patella (see illustration).
4. Attach the stockings to the insufflator and verify that the intermittent pressure is between 35 and 45 mm Hg.

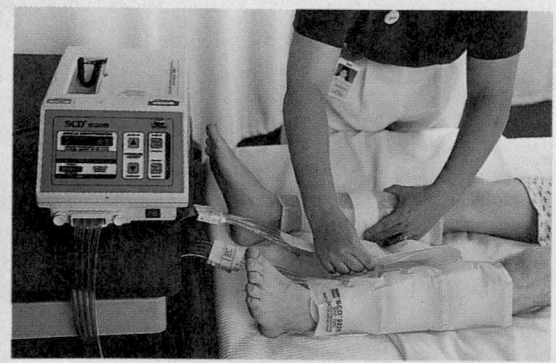

Application of sequential compression stockings.

Applying Elastic Stockings | Skill 46-1

Delegation Considerations

The skill of applying elastic stockings can be delegated to assistive personnel. The following information is needed when delegating this skill:

- Avoid activities that promote venous stasis (e.g., crossing legs, wearing garters, or elevating legs on pillows).
- When possible, elevate legs to improve venous return.

- Do not massage legs.
- Elevate legs before applying stockings.
- Avoid wrinkles in the stockings.
- Observe for allergic reactions, skin irritation, and thrombophlebitis.

EQUIPMENT

- Tape measure
- Talcum powder
- Elastic support stockings (proper size)

STEPS	RATIONALE
1. Assess client for risk factors in Virchow's triad to determine need for elastic stockings:	Potential candidates for elastic stockings are clients who have an alteration in one of the elements of Virchow's triad (Bright and Georgi, 1992; Von Rueden and Harris, 1995).
a. *Hypercoagulability:* all clients with clotting disorders, fever, or dehydration; during pregnancy and first 6 weeks postpartum if the woman was confined to bed; and with oral contraceptive use (especially if client smokes)	
b. *Venous wall abnormalities:* local trauma, orthopedic surgeries, major abdominal surgery, varicose veins, atherosclerosis	
c. *Blood stasis:* immobility, obesity, pregnancy	
2. Observe for signs, symptoms, and conditions that might contraindicate use of elastic stockings:	
a. Dermatitis or open skin lesion	Elastic stockings may aggravate skin condition or cause it to spread. Also, physician may want medication and dressing applied to lesion.
b. Recent skin graft	Continuous pressure is necessary to keep graft adherent to recipient bed, but pressure should not be so firm as to cause death of graft.
c. Disproportionately large thighs	Elastic stockings may not fit correctly, causing excessive pressure and constriction around thighs, thereby reducing venous return (Phipps, 1995).
d. Decreased circulation in lower extremities as evidenced by cyanotic, cool extremities	Elastic stockings may further impede circulation.
3. Obtain physician's order.	May be needed for legal or reimbursement reasons.
4. Assess client's or caregiver's understanding of application of elastic stockings.	Identifies potential educational needs of client or caregiver.
5. Assess and document condition of client's skin and circulation to legs (i.e., presence of pedal pulses, edema, discoloration of skin, temperature, lesions, or cuts).	Identifies a baseline for skin integrity and quality of peripheral pulses in lower extremities.
6. Explain procedure and reasons for applying stockings.	Reduces anxiety and encourages client cooperation.
7. Use tape measure to measure client's legs to determine proper stocking size.	Stockings must be measured according to manufacturer's directions. Elastic stockings come in two lengths: knee length and thigh length. The choice of length depends on physician's order.

Critical Decision Point: Compare client's measurements with the manufacturer's sizing chart. If too large, stockings will not adequately support extremities. If too small, stockings may impede circulation. The optimum stocking pressure is 20 to 30 mm Hg at the ankle, decreasing to 8 mm Hg at the middle to upper thigh. This change in pressure produces the greatest increase in venous flow velocity that is both safe and practical (Bright and Georgi, 1992).

STEPS	RATIONALE
8. Wash hands.	Reduces transmission of microorganisms.
9. Position client in supine position. Elevate head of bed to comfortable level.	Promotes good body mechanics for nurse. Client position eases application. Also, the stockings should be applied before standing to prevent stagnation of blood in lower extremities. If client has been standing, client should sit in chair or lie in bed for 15 minutes with legs elevated before applying elastic stockings (Bright and Georgi, 1992).
10. After legs are cleansed, apply small amount of talcum powder to legs and feet, provided that client does not have sensitivity to talcum powder.	Talcum powder reduces friction and allows for easier application of stockings.
11. Apply stockings.	
a. Turn elastic stocking inside out by placing one hand into sock, holding toe of sock with other hand, and pulling (see illustration).	Allows easier application of stocking.
b. Place client's toes into foot of elastic stocking, making sure that sock is smooth (see illustration).	Wrinkles in sock can impede circulation to lower region of extremity (Bright and Georgi, 1992).
c. Slide remaining portion of sock over client's foot, being sure that the toes are covered. Make sure the foot fits into the toe and heel position of the sock. Sock will now be right side out (see illustration).	If toes remain uncovered, they will become constricted by elastic and their circulation can be reduced.
d. Slide sock up over client's calf until sock is completely extended. Be sure sock is smooth and no ridges are present (see illustration).	Ridges impede venous return and can counteract overall purpose of elastic stocking (Bright and Georgi, 1992).
e. Instruct client not to roll socks partially down.	Rolling sock partially down has a constricting effect and can impede venous return.

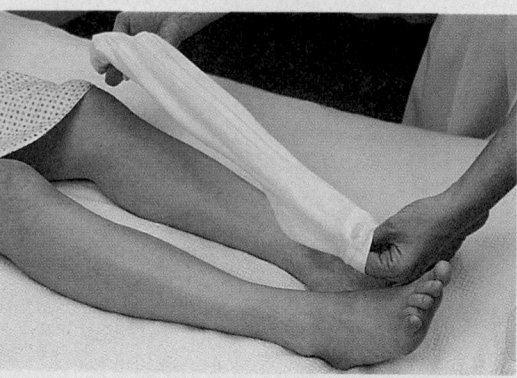

Step 11a

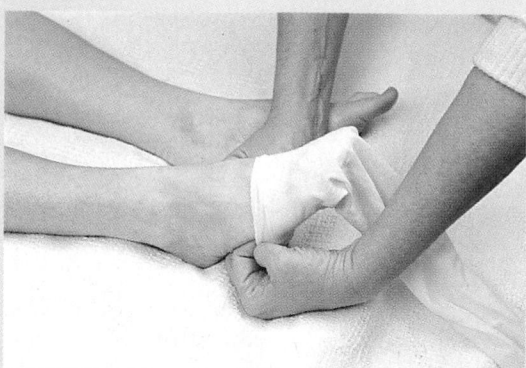

Step 11b

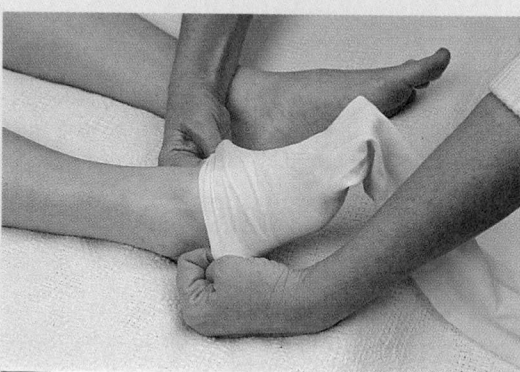

Step 11c

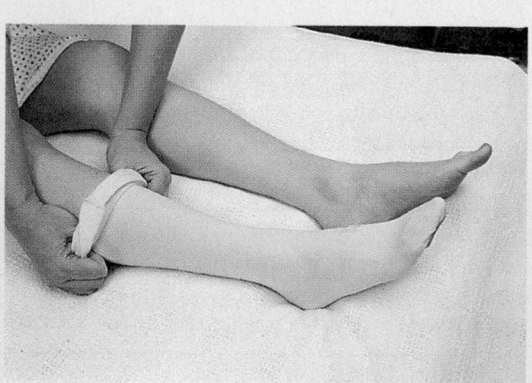

Step 11d

STEPS	RATIONALE
12. Reposition client to position of comfort, and wash hands.	Maintains proper body alignment and promotes comfort. Reduces transmission of microorganisms.
13. Inspect stocking to make sure there are no wrinkles or binding at top of stocking.	Wrinkles lead to increased pressure and alter circulation.
14. Observe client's reaction to stockings.	Ensures client is adapting to stockings and is not experiencing any discomfort from stockings.
15. Observe client or caregiver apply stockings.	Determines ability to perform skill accurately.
16. Remove stockings at least once a shift, and assess skin and circulatory status.	Stockings may shift or be too tight, and this step ensures skin and circulation are intact.

Recording and Reporting

- Record date and time of stocking application and stocking length and size in nurses' notes (flow sheet may be used).
- Record condition of skin and circulatory assessment, including pulses, temperature, sensation, movement, capillary refill, and calf circumference at application and each shift.
- Report changes indicating a decline in circulation.

Home Care Considerations

- Instruct clients to have two pairs of stockings—one pair to wear, the other to wash.
- Instruct clients that if there are weight changes greater than 10 lb, stockings should be remeasured.
- Remind clients to put on stockings before getting up for the morning or sitting for prolonged periods. As the day progresses, leg swelling may increase and may make stocking application difficult. (It may be helpful to remind clients that they may have noticed this swelling when wearing shoes.)

---

one extremity is paralyzed, the client can be taught to put each joint independently through its ROM. Clients on bed rest should have active ROM exercises incorporated into their daily schedules. Nurses can teach clients to integrate exercises during ADLs (see Box 36-11).

Some orthopedic conditions require more frequent passive ROM exercises to restore the injured joint's function after surgery. Clients with such conditions may use automatic equipment for passive ROM exercises (Figure 46-19). The equipment moves an extremity to a prescribed angle for a prescribed period. This is beneficial when the client must gradually increase the degree and duration of flexion and extension.

Active ROM exercises maintain function of the musculoskeletal system. The nurse should also plan interventions for the gradual return of mobility for clients who will be able to resume normal activity. The best nursing intervention is establishing an individualized progressive exercise program. A progressive exercise program gradually increases the client's physical activity to reverse the deconditioning associated with immobility. Progressive exercise programs are used for clients with musculoskeletal, neurological, cardiopulmonary, renal, and other chronic diseases.

When working with older adults, the nurse must keep in mind gerontological principles that enhance the effectiveness of exercise programs and limit injuries (Box 46-8).

Teaching, referral, and interdisciplinary collaboration are important for clients with limited mobility. Depending on the setting and resources available, the nurse may want

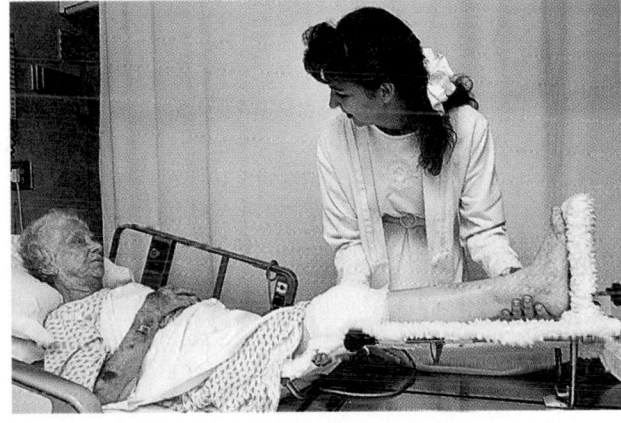

Figure 46-19 Continuous passive range-of-motion machine.

to refer the client for physical therapy. The therapist would set up the specific exercise program, and the nurse would reinforce it.

Integumentary System. The major risk to the skin from restricted mobility is the formation of pressure ulcers. Nursing interventions therefore focus on preventing or treating these ulcers (see Chapter 47). Early identification of high-risk clients and their risk factors aids the nurse in preventing pressure ulcers. Interventions aimed at prevention are positioning, skin care, and the use of therapeutic devices to relieve pressure. The immobilized

Gerontological NURSING PRACTICE   Box 46-8

- Ensure low exercise intensity of 40% to 70% maximum predicted heart rate and very gentle exercise progression.
- Use perceived exertion versus exercise heart rate to monitor exercise intensity.
- Perform a gradual, extended exercise warm-up and cooldown to decrease risk of postural hypotension and cardiac dysrhythmias.
- Use correct body mechanics, appropriate clothing, exercise-specific shoes, and sufficient hydration.
- Avoid sudden twisting movements, rapid movements, and rapid transitions from one movement to the next.
- Avoid exercises that tax vision and balance.
- Avoid sustained isometric contractions of greater than 10 seconds.
- Avoid exercise during acute viral infections.
- Stop exercising if angina, premature ventricular contractions, or excessive breathlessness occurs.
- Obtain physician approval and written orders for specific exercise restrictions before onset of an exercise program.
- Engage in brisk walking for 10 to 15 minutes to tone the extremities and provide aerobic activity for older adults (Ebersole and Hess, 1998).
- Older adults may perform both strenuous and less strenuous activities. Activities may range from gardening, to chair-based exercises and tai chi chih (Ebersole and Hess, 1998; Schaller, 1996).

client's position should be changed according to the client's activity level, perceptual ability, treatment protocols, and daily routines. Although turning every 1 to 2 hours is recommended for preventing ulcers, it may also be necessary to use devices for relieving pressure. The time that a client sits uninterrupted in a chair should be limited to 1 hour or less, but this time interval is individualized. The client should be repositioned frequently because uninterrupted pressure will cause skin breakdown. The nurse should teach clients who are able to do so, to shift their weight every 15 minutes. Chair-bound clients should have a device for the chair that reduces pressure (AHCPR, 1994).

Elimination System. The nursing interventions for maintaining optimal urinary functioning are directed at keeping the client well hydrated and preventing urinary stasis, calculi, and infections without causing bladder distention.

Adequate hydration (e.g., 2000 to 3000 ml of fluids per day) helps prevent renal calculi and urinary tract infections. The well-hydrated client should void large amounts of dilute urine that is approximately equal to fluid intake. If the client is incontinent, the nurse should modify the care plan to include toileting aids and a hygiene schedule so that the increased urinary output does not cause skin breakdown.

To prevent bladder distention, the nurse assesses the frequency and amount of urinary output. A client who continually dribbles urine and whose bladder is distended may have reflex incontinence. If the immobilized client does not have voluntary control of bladder elimination, bladder retraining may be necessary. If the client experiences bladder distention, the nurse may be required to insert a straight catheter or an indwelling Foley catheter (see Chapter 44).

The nurse must also record the frequency and consistency of bowel movements. A diet rich in fluids, fruits, vegetables, and fiber can facilitate normal peristalsis. If a client is unable to maintain regular bowel patterns, the physician may order stool softeners, cathartics, or enemas (see Chapter 45).

Psychosocial Changes. Assessment can identify effects of prolonged immobilization on the client's psychosocial dimension. People who have a tendency toward depression or mood swings are at greater risk for developing psychosocial effects during bed rest or immobilization. There are many nursing interventions to meet the client's psychosocial needs.

The nurse should anticipate changes in the client's psychosocial status. The nurse can provide routine and informal socialization. Nursing activities can be planned so that the client can talk and interact with staff. If possible, the client should be placed in a room with others who are mobile and interactive. If a private room is required, staff members should be asked to visit throughout the shift to provide meaningful interaction.

The nurse also provides stimuli to maintain orientation. A daily newspaper helps the client keep track of events and time. Bedside chats at appropriate moments orient the client to nursing activities, meals, and visiting hours. Books help occupy the client when he or she is alone. The client can participate in craft activities. Radio, television, and videotapes provide stimulation and help pass the time.

Clients should also be involved in their care whenever possible. For example, the nurse should encourage the client to determine when the bed should be made. Some clients rest better during the night when fresh sheets are put on in the evening rather than in the morning. The client should provide as much self-care as possible. Hygiene and grooming articles should be kept within easy reach. Clients should be encouraged to wear their glasses or artificial teeth and to shave or apply makeup. These are activities through which people maintain their body images. Maintenance of body image can help improve the client's outlook.

In institutional health care settings, nursing care given between 10:00 PM and 7:00 AM should be scheduled to minimize interruptions of sleep. For example, the nurse may administer medications and assess vital signs at the time when the client is turned or receives special skin care.

The nurse should also observe the client's failure to cope with restricted mobility. If the nursing care plan is not improving coping patterns, a clinical nurse specialist, counselor, social worker, spiritual adviser, or other consultant may be needed. Their recommendations should be incorporated into the care plan.

Developmental Changes.   Ideally, immobilized clients continue normal development. Nursing interventions can help. Nursing care should provide mental and physical stimulation, particularly for a young child. Play activities can be incorporated into the care plan. Completing puzzles, for example, helps a child to develop fine motor skills, and reading helps the child to develop cognitively. An immobilized child should be placed with children of the same age who are not immobilized, unless a contagious disease is present. Nursing activities, such as dressing changes, cast care, and care of traction, can be designed to require the child's participation. The nurse must recognize significant changes from normal behavioral patterns. If these continue, the nurse should consult with a clinical nurse, counselor, or other health care professional whose specialty is children.

Restricted mobility of older clients presents unique nursing problems. Older clients who are frail or have chronic illnesses may be at increased risk for the psychosocial hazards of immobility. Maintaining a calendar and clock with a large dial, conversing about current events and family members, and encouraging visits from significant others may reduce the risk of social isolation.

Nursing care should encourage older immobilized clients to perform as many ADLs as independently as possible. Clients should continue to perform personal grooming if they did so before their mobility was restricted.

Positioning Techniques.

Clients with impaired nervous, skeletal, or muscular system functioning and increased weakness and fatigability often require help from the nurse to attain proper body alignment while in bed or sitting. Several positioning devices are available for maintaining good body alignment for clients (Table 46-4).

Pillows are a positioning aid that may or may not be readily available. Before using a pillow, the nurse should determine whether it is the proper size. A thick pillow under the client's head increases cervical flexion. A thin pillow under body prominences may be inadequate to protect skin and tissue from damage caused by pressure. When additional pillows are unavailable, or if they are an improper size, the nurse can use folded sheets, blankets, or towels as positioning aids. The 30-degree lateral position is strongly recommended in clients at risk for pressure ulcer development (see Chapter 47).

A footboard is placed perpendicular to the mattress, parallel to and touching the plantar surfaces of the client's feet. The footboard prevents footdrop by maintaining the feet in dorsiflexion. After placing it on the bed, the nurse needs to determine that it is correctly placed, with the client's feet placed firmly against the board. Another common technique is the use of high-top tennis shoes or an ankle-foot orthotic (AFO) to help maintain dorsiflexion.

A **trochanter roll** prevents external rotation of the hips when the client is in a supine position. To form a trochanter roll, a cotton bath blanket is folded lengthwise to a width that will extend from the greater trochanter of the femur to the lower border of the popliteal space (see Figure 46-20). The blanket is placed under the buttocks and then rolled counterclockwise until the thigh is in neutral position or in inward rotation. When correct alignment of the hip is achieved, the patella faces directly upward. Sandbags are sand-filled plastic tubes or bags that can be shaped to body contours. Sandbags can be used in place of or in addition to trochanter rolls. They immobilize an extremity or maintain body alignment.

Hand rolls maintain the thumb in slight adduction and in opposition to the fingers. A hand roll maintains the hand, thumb, and fingers in a functional position. The nurse evaluates the hand roll to make sure that the hand is indeed in a functional position. Hand rolls are most often used for clients whose arms are paralyzed or who are unconscious. Rolled washcloths should not be used as hand rolls, since they do not keep the thumb well abducted, especially in clients who have a spastic paralysis.

Hand-wrist splints are individually molded for the client to maintain proper alignment of the thumb (slight adduction) and the wrist (slight dorsiflexion). These splints should be used only by the client for whom the splint was made.

The **trapeze bar** is a triangular device that descends from a securely fastened overhead bar that is attached to the bed frame. It allows the client to pull with the upper

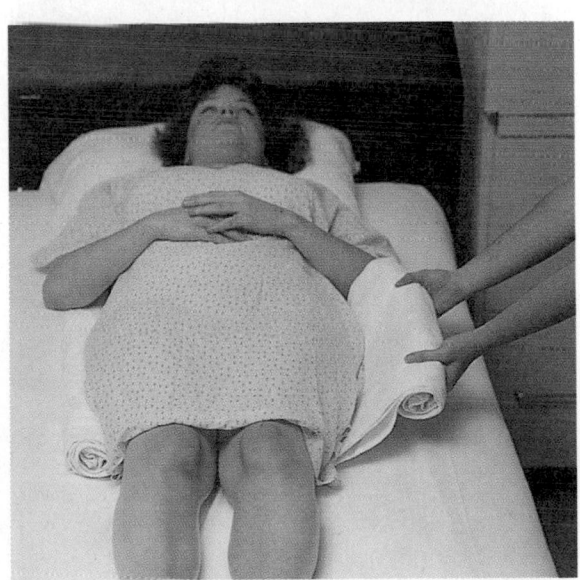

Figure 46-20   Trochanter roll.

Table 46-4   Devices Used for Proper Positioning

Devices	Uses and Descriptions
Pillows	Pillows are readily available in most health care facilities, including the home. They should be of appropriate size for the body part to be positioned. Pillows provide support, elevate body parts, and can splint incisional areas, reducing postoperative pain during activity or coughing and deep breathing.
Foot boots	Foot boots maintain feet in dorsiflexion. Boots are made of rigid plastic or heavy foam and keep the foot flexed at the proper angle. The nurse should remove the foot boots 2 or 3 times a day to assess skin integrity and joint mobility.
Trochanter rolls	Trochanter rolls prevent external rotation of legs when clients are in the supine position. To form a trochanter roll, a cotton bath blanket or a sheet is folded lengthwise to a width extending from the greater trochanter of the femur to the lower border of the popliteal space (Figure 46-20). The blanket is placed under the buttocks and then rolled away from the client until the thigh is in the neutral position or an inward position with the patella facing upward.
Sandbags	Sandbags provide support and shape to body contours; they immobilize extremities and maintain specific body alignment. Sandbags are filled plastic tubes that can be shaped to body contours. They can be used in place of, or in addition to, trochanter rolls.
Hand rolls	Hand rolls maintain the thumb slightly adducted and in opposition to the fingers; they maintain fingers in a slightly flexed position. The nurse evaluates the position of the hand roll to make certain the hand is indeed in a functional position.
Hand-wrist splints	Hand-wrist splints are individually molded for the client to maintain proper alignment of the thumb in slight adduction and the wrist in slight dorsiflexion. These splints should be used only for the client for whom the splint was made.
Trapeze bar	The trapeze bar descends from a securely fastened overhead bar attached to the bed frame (Figure 46-21). The trapeze allows the client to use upper extremities to raise the trunk off the bed, to assist in transfer from bed to wheelchair, or to perform upper arm strengthening exercises.
Side rails	Side rails are bars positioned along the sides of the length of the bed. They ensure client safety and are useful for increasing mobility. In addition, they provide assistance in rolling from side to side or sitting up in bed.
Bed boards	Bed boards are plywood boards placed under the entire surface area of the mattress. They are useful for increasing back support and alignment, especially with a soft mattress.
Wedge pillow	A wedge or abductor pillow is a triangular-shaped pillow made of heavy foam. It is used to maintain the legs in abduction following total hip replacement surgery (Figure 46-22).

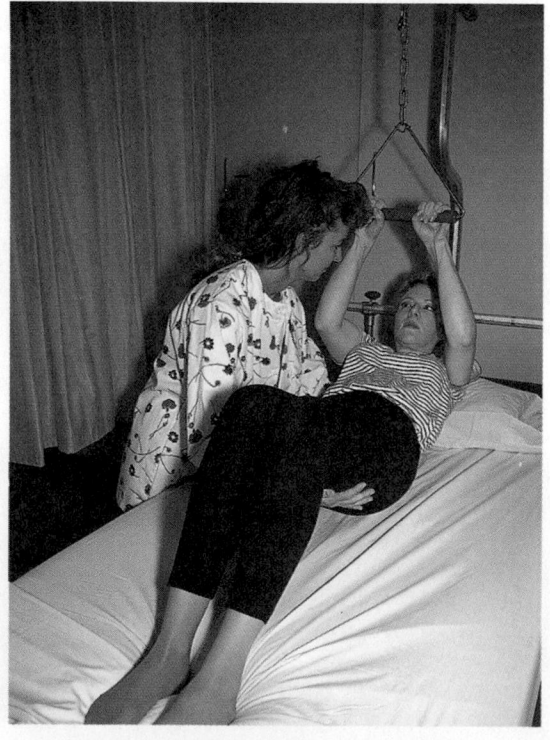

Figure 46-21   Client using a trapeze bar.

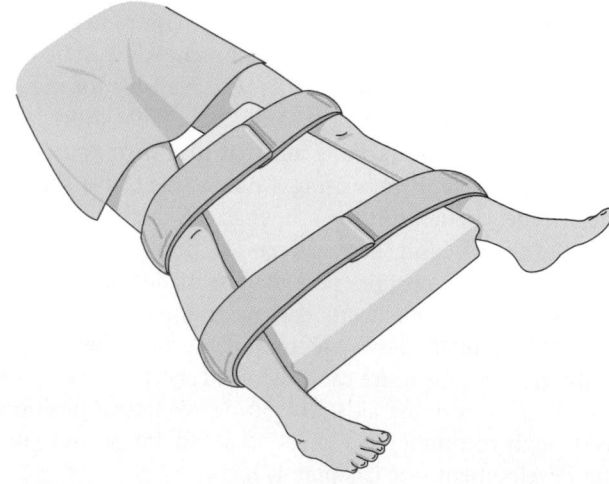

Figure 46-22   Abduction pillow used after total hip replacement.
From Beare PG, Myers JL: *Adult health nursing,* ed 3, St. Louis, 1998, Mosby.

extremities to raise the trunk off the bed, to assist in transfer from bed to wheelchair, or to perform upper arm exercises (see Figure 46-21). It is a useful device for helping to increase independence, maintain upper body strength, and decrease the shearing action from sliding across or up and down in bed.

Although each procedure for positioning has specific guidelines, there are some universal steps the nurse should follow for clients who require positioning assistance (Skill 46-2). Following the guidelines reduces the risk of injury to the musculoskeletal system when the client is sitting or lying. When joints are unsupported, their alignment is impaired. Likewise, if joints are not positioned in a slightly flexed position, their mobility is decreased. During positioning, the nurse also assesses for pressure points (see Figure 47-13). When actual or potential pressure areas exist, nursing interventions involve removal of the pressure, thus decreasing the risk for development of pressure ulcers and further trauma to the musculoskeletal system. In these clients the 30-degree lateral position should be used.

Supported Fowler's Position. In the supported Fowler's position, the head of the bed is elevated 45 to 60 degrees and the client's knees are slightly elevated without pressure to restrict circulation in the lower legs. The angle of head and knee elevation and the length of time that the client should remain in the supported Fowler's position are influenced by the client's illness and overall condition. Supports must permit flexion of the hips and knees and proper alignment of the normal curves in the cervical, thoracic, and lumbar vertebrae. The following are common trouble areas for the client in the supported Fowler's position:

Increased cervical flexion because the pillow at the head is too thick and the head thrusts forward

Extension of the knees, allowing the client to slide to the foot of the bed

Pressure on the posterior aspect of the knees, decreasing circulation to the feet

External rotation of the hips

Arms hanging unsupported at the client's sides

Unsupported feet or pressure on the heels

Unprotected pressure points at the sacrum and heels

Increased shearing force on the back and heels when the head of the bed is raised greater than 60 degrees

Supine Position. The supine position, in which the client rests on the back, is also called the dorsal recumbent position. In the supine position the relationship of body parts is essentially the same as in good standing alignment except that the body is in the horizontal plane. Pillows, trochanter rolls, and hand rolls or arm splints are used to increase comfort and reduce injury to the skin or musculoskeletal system. The mattress should be firm enough to support the cervical, thoracic, and lumbar vertebrae. Shoulders are supported, and the elbows are slightly flexed

to control shoulder rotation. A foot support is used to prevent footdrop and maintain proper alignment. The following are some common trouble areas for clients in the supine position:

Pillow at the head that is too thick, increasing cervical flexion

Head flat on the mattress

Shoulders unsupported and internally rotated

Elbows extended

Thumb not in opposition to the fingers

Hips externally rotated

Unsupported feet

Unprotected pressure points at the occiput region of the head, vertebrae, coccyx, elbows, and heels

Prone Position. The client in the prone position is lying face or chest down. Often the client's head is turned to the side, but if a pillow is under the head, it should be thin enough to prevent cervical flexion or extension and maintain alignment of the lumbar spine. Placing a pillow under the lower leg permits dorsiflexion of the ankles and some knee flexion, which promotes relaxation. If a pillow is unavailable, the ankles should be in dorsiflexion over the end of the mattress. The nurse should assess for and correct any of the following potential trouble points:

Neck hyperextension

Hyperextension of the lumbar spine

Plantar flexion of the ankles

Unprotected pressure points at the chin, elbows, hips, knees, and toes

Side-Lying Position. In the side-lying (or lateral) position the client is resting on the side with the major portion of body weight on the dependent hip and shoulder. Therefore in clients at risk for pressure ulcers, a 30-degree lateral position may be used (see Chapter 47). Trunk alignment should be the same as in standing. For example, the structural curves of the spine should be maintained, the head should be supported in line with the midline of the trunk, and rotation of the spine should be avoided. The following trouble points are common in the side-lying position:

Lateral flexion of the neck

Spinal curves out of normal alignment

Shoulder and hip joints internally rotated, adducted, or unsupported

Lack of support for the feet

Lack of protection for pressure points at the ear, shoulder, anterior iliac spine, trochanter, and ankles

Excessive lateral flexion of the spine if the client has large hips and a pillow is not placed superior to the hips at the waist

Sims' Position. Sims' position differs from the side-lying position in the distribution of the client's weight. In Sims' position the weight is placed on the anterior ilium,

Text continued on p. 1530.

Skill 46-2   Positioning Clients in Bed

Delegation Considerations

The skills of moving and positioning clients in bed can be delegated to assistive personnel. Clients who have spinal cord trauma usually require transfer and moving by professional nurses.

- Caution caregiver about level of the bed for selected skills.
- Caution caregiver to maintain proper body mechanics.
- Instruct caregiver on moving and positioning in bed.

EQUIPMENT

- Pillows
- Footboard (optional)
- High-top sneakers
- Trochanter roll

- Sandbag
- Hand rolls
- Side rails
- Drawsheet

STEPS	RATIONALE
1. Assess client's body alignment and comfort level while client is lying down.	Provides baseline data for later comparisons. Determines ways to improve position and alignment.
2. Assess for risk factors that may contribute to complications of immobility:	Increased risk factors require client to be repositioned more frequently.
a. Paralysis: hemiparesis resulting from cerebrovascular accident (CVA); decreased sensation	Paralysis impairs movement; muscle tone changes; sensation is affected. Because of difficulty in moving and poor awareness of involved body part, client is unable to protect and position body part for self.
b. Impaired mobility: traction or arthritis or other contributing disease processes	Traction or arthritic changes of affected extremity result in decreased range of joint motion (ROJM).
c. Impaired circulation	Decreased circulation predisposes client to pressure sores.
d. Age: very young, older adults	Premature and young infants require frequent turning because their skin is fragile. Normal physiological changes associated with aging predispose older adults to greater risks for developing complications of immobility.
e. Client's level of consciousness	Determines need for special aids or devices. Clients with altered levels of consciousness may not understand instructions and may be unable to help.
3. Assess client's physical ability to help with moving and positioning.	Enables nurse to use client's mobility and strength. Determines need for additional help. Ensures client and nurse safety.
4. Raise level of bed to comfortable working height.	Raises level of work toward nurse's center of gravity.
5. Remove all pillows and devices used in previous position.	Reduces interferences from bedding during positioning procedure.
6. Get extra help as needed.	Provides for client and nurse safety.
7. Explain procedure to client.	Helps to decrease anxiety and increase cooperation.
8. Position client in bed.	
A. Move immobile client up in bed (one nurse):	
(1) Place client on back with head of bed flat. Stand on one side of bed.	Enables nurse to assess body alignment. Reduces gravity's pull on client's upper body.
(2) Remove pillow from under head and shoulders and place pillow at head of bed.	Prevents striking client's head against head of bed.
(3) Begin at client's feet. Face foot of bed at 45-degree angle. Place feet apart with foot nearest head of bed behind other foot (forward-backward stance) (see illustration). Flex knees and hips as needed to bring arms level with client's legs. Shift weight from front to back leg, and slide client's legs diagonally toward head of bed.	Positioning is begun at client's legs because they are lighter and easier to move. Facing direction of movement ensures proper balance. Shifting nurse's weight reduces force needed to move load. Diagonal motion permits pull in direction of force. Flexing knees lowers nurse's center of gravity and uses thigh muscles rather than back muscles.
(4) Move parallel to client's hips. Flex knees and hips as needed to bring arms level with client's hips.	Maintains nurse's correct body alignment. Brings nurse closer to object to be moved and lowers center of gravity. Uses thigh muscles rather than back muscles.
(5) Slide client's hips diagonally toward head of bed.	Aligns client's hips and feet.
(6) Move parallel to client's head and shoulders. Flex knees and hips as needed to bring arms level with client's body.	Maintains nurse's proper body alignment. Brings nurse closer to object to be moved. Lowers nurse's center of gravity. Uses thigh muscles rather than back muscles.

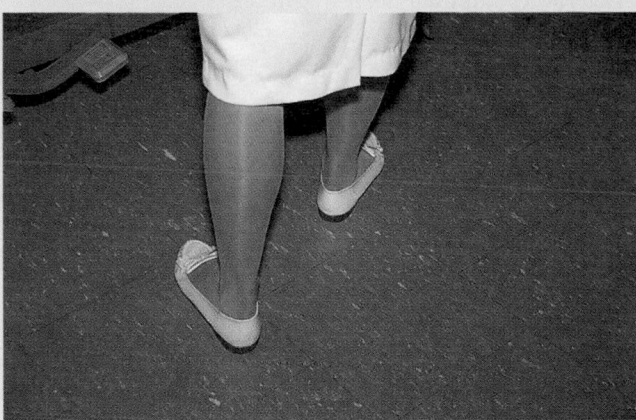

Step 8A(3)

STEPS	RATIONALE
(7) Slide arm closest to head of bed under client's neck, with hand reaching under and supporting client's shoulder.	Supports client's head and neck, maintaining alignment and preventing injury during movement.
(8) Place other arm under client's upper back.	Supports client's body weight and reduces friction during movement.
(9) Slide client's trunk, shoulders, head, and neck diagonally toward head of bed.	Realigns client's body on one side of bed.
(10) Elevate side rail. Move to other side of bed and lower side rail.	Protects client from falling out of bed.
(11) Repeat procedure, switching sides until client reaches desired position in bed.	
(12) Center client in middle of bed, moving body in same three sections.	Maintains proper body alignment. Provides ample room for turning, positioning, and other nursing activities.
B. **Assist client to move up in bed (one or two nurses):**	
(1) Place client on back with head of bed flat.	Enables nurse to assess body alignment. Reduces gravity's pull on client's upper body.
(2) Remove pillow from under head and shoulders and place pillow at head of bed.	Prevents striking client's head against head of bed.
(3) Face head of bed.	Facing direction of movement prevents twisting of nurse's body while moving client.
(a) Each nurse should have one arm under client's shoulders and one arm under client's thighs.	
(b) *Alternative position:* Position one nurse at client's upper body. Nurse's arm nearest head of bed should be under client's head and opposite shoulder; other arm should be under client's closest arm and shoulder. Position other nurse at client's lower torso. Second nurse's arms should be under client's lower back and torso.	Prevents trauma to client's musculoskeletal system by supporting shoulder and hip joints and evenly distributing weight.
(4) Place feet apart, with foot nearest head of bed behind other foot (forward-backward stance).	Wide base of support increases nurse's balance. Stance enables nurse to shift body weight as client is moved up in bed, thereby reducing force needed to move load.
(5) Flex knees and hips. Shift weight from front to back leg, and move client and drawsheet or pull sheet to desired position in bed.	Facing direction of movement ensures proper balance. Shifting weight reduces force needed to move load. Flexing knees lowers nurses' center of gravity and uses thighs instead of back muscles.

STEPS	RATIONALE
C. **Position client in supported Fowler's position (see illustration):**	Increases comfort, improves ventilation, and increases client's opportunity to socialize or relax.
(1) Elevate head of bed 45 to 60 degrees.	Prevents flexion contractures of cervical vertebrae.
(2) Rest head against mattress or on small pillow.	Prevents shoulder dislocation from effect of downward pull of unsupported arms, promotes circulation by preventing venous pooling, and prevents flexion contractures of arms and wrists.
(3) Use pillows to support arms and hand if client does not have voluntary control or use of hands and arms.	Supports lumbar vertebrae and decreases flexion of vertebrae.
(4) Position pillow at lower back.	Prevents hyperextension of knee and occlusion of popliteal artery from pressure from body weight.
(5) Place small pillow or roll under thigh.	Prevents prolonged pressure of mattress on heels.
(6) Place small pillow or roll under ankles.	

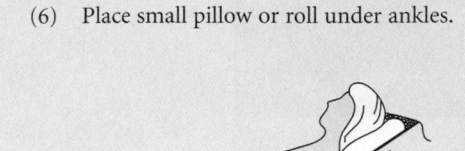

45°

Step 8C

Critical Decision Point: To keep feet in proper alignment, place footboard at bottom of client's feet or apply high-top sneakers on client's feet.

STEPS	RATIONALE
D. **Position hemiplegic client in supported Fowler's position:**	
(1) Elevate head of bed 45 to 60 degrees.	Increases comfort, improves ventilation, and increases client's opportunity to relax.
(2) Position client in sitting position as straight as possible. With support for affected shoulder (see Table 46-5).	Counteracts tendency to slump toward affected side. Improves ventilation and cardiac output; decreases intracranial pressure. Improves client's ability to swallow and helps to prevent aspiration of food, liquids, and gastric secretions.
(3) Position head on small pillow with chin slightly forward. If client is totally unable to control head movement, hyperextension of the neck must be avoided.	Prevents hyperextension of neck. Too many pillows under head may cause or worsen neck flexion contracture.
(4) Provide support for involved arm and hand on overbed table in front of client. If transfer is to wheelchair, arms of chair can provide support. Place arm away from client's side and support elbow with pillow.	Paralyzed muscles do not automatically resist pull of gravity as they do normally. As a result, shoulder subluxation, pain, and edema may occur.
(a) Position *flaccid* hand in normal resting position with wrist slightly extended, arches of hand maintained, and fingers partially flexed; may use section of rubber ball cut in half; clasp client's hands together.	Maintains hand in functional position. Prevents contractures.
(b) Position *spastic* hand with wrist in neutral position or slightly extended; fingers should be extended with palm down or may be left in relaxed position with palm up.	Maintains hand in functional position. Inhibits flexor spasticity.
(5) Flex knees and hips by using pillow or folded blanket under knees.	Ensures proper alignment. Flexion prevents prolonged hyperextension, which could impair joint mobility.
(6) Support feet in dorsiflexion with firm pillow, footboard, or high-top sneakers.	Prevents footdrop. Stimulation of ball of foot by hard surface has tendency to increase muscle tone in client with extensor spasticity of lower extremity.

STEPS	RATIONALE

E. **Position client in supine position:**

(1) Place client on back with head of bed flat. — Necessary for placing client in supine position.

(2) Place small rolled towel under lumbar area of back. — Provides support for lumbar spine.

(3) Place pillow under upper shoulders, neck, or head. — Maintains correct alignment and prevents flexion contractures of cervical lumbar spine.

(4) Place trochanter rolls or sandbags parallel to lateral surface of client's thighs. — Reduces external rotation of hip.

(5) Place small pillow or roll under ankle to elevate heels. — Reduces pressure on heels, helping to prevent pressure sores.

(6) Support feet in dorsiflexion with firm pillow, footboard, or high-top sneakers. — Prevents footdrop.

(7) Place pillows under pronated forearms, keeping upper arms parallel to client's body (see illustrations). — Reduces internal rotation of shoulder and prevents extension of elbows. Maintains correct body alignment.

(8) Place hand rolls in client's hands. Consider physical therapy referral for use of hand splints. — Reduces extension of fingers and abduction of thumb. Maintains thumb slightly adducted and in opposition to fingers.

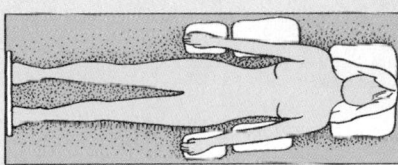
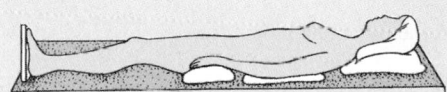
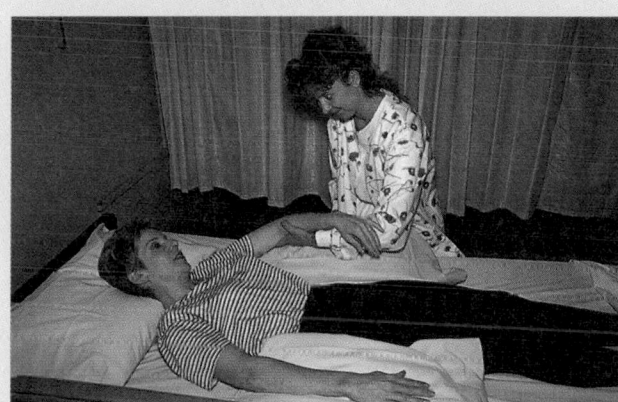

Step 8E(7)

F. **Position hemiplegic client in supine position:**

(1) Place head of bed flat. — Necessary for positioning in supine position.

(2) Place folded towel or small pillow under shoulder or affected side. — Decreases possibility of pain, joint contracture, and subluxation. Maintains mobility in muscles around shoulder to permit normal movement patterns.

(3) Keep affected arm away from body with elbow extended and palm up. (Alternative is to place arm out to side, with elbow bent and hand toward head of bed.) — Maintains mobility in arm, joints, and shoulder to permit normal movement patterns. (Alternative position counteracts limitation of ability of arm to rotate outward at shoulder [external rotation]. External rotation must be present to raise arm overhead without pain.)

(4) Place folded towel under hip of involved side. — Diminishes effect of spasticity in entire leg by controlling hip position. Slight flexion breaks up abnormal extension pattern of leg. Extensor spasticity is most severe when client is supine.

(5) Support feet with soft pillows at right angle to leg, and keep heels off bed or use heel protectors (see Chapter 47). — Maintains foot in dorsiflexion and prevents footdrop. Pillows prevent stimulation to ball of foot by hard surface, which has tendency to increase muscle tone in client with extensor spasticity extremity.

G. **Position client in prone position:**

(1) Roll client over arm positioned close to body, with elbow straight and hand under hip. Position on abdomen in center of bed. — Positions client correctly so alignment can be maintained.

|

(2) Turn client's head to one side and support head with small pillow (see illustration).

Reduces flexion or hyperextension of cervical vertebrae.

(3) Place small pillow under client's abdomen below level of diaphragm (see illustration).

Reduces pressure on breasts of some female clients and decreases hyperextension of lumbar vertebrae and strain on lower back. Improves breathing by reducing mattress pressure on diaphragm.

(4) Support arms in flexed position level at shoulders.

Maintains proper body alignment. Support reduces risk of joint dislocation.

(5) Support lower legs with pillow to elevate toes (see illustration).

Reduces external rotation of legs and mattress pressure on toes.

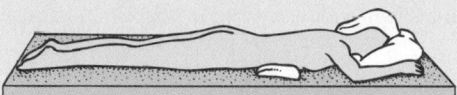

Step 8G(2)

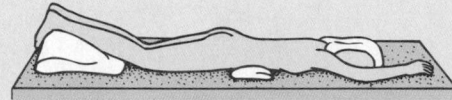

Step 8G(3)

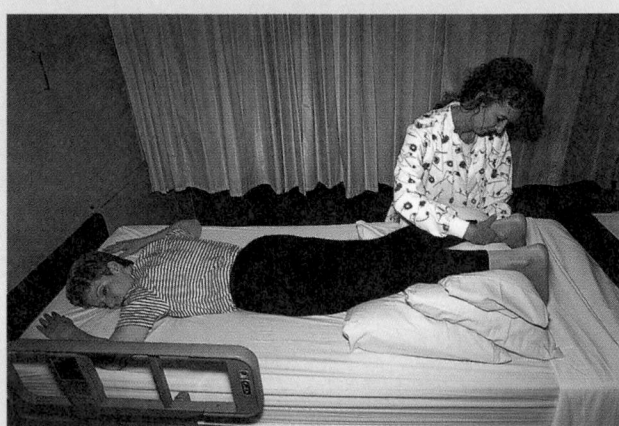

Step 8G(5)

H. **Position hemiplegic client in prone position:**

(1) Move client toward unaffected side.

Ensures proper client alignment in center of bed when client is rolled onto abdomen.

(2) Roll client onto side.

(3) Place pillow on client's abdomen.

Prevents sagging of abdomen when client is rolled over; decreases hyperextension of lumbar vertebrae and strain on lower back.

(4) Roll client onto abdomen by positioning involved arm close to client's body, with elbow straight and hand under hip. Roll client carefully over arm.

Prevents injury to affected side.

(5) Turn head toward involved side.

Promotes development of neck and trunk extension, which is necessary for standing and walking.

(6) Position involved arm out to side, with elbow bent, hand toward head of bed, and fingers extended (if possible).

Counteracts limitation of arm's ability to rotate outward at shoulder (external rotation). External rotation must be present to raise arm over head without pain.

(7) Flex knees slightly by placing pillow under legs from knees to ankles.

Flexion prevents prolonged hyperextension, which could impair joint mobility.

(8) Keep feet at right angle to legs by using pillow high enough to keep toes off mattress and use high-top sneakers.

Maintains feet in dorsiflexion.

I. **Position client in lateral (side-lying) position:**

(1) Lower head of bed completely or as low as client can tolerate.

Provides position of comfort for client and removes pressure from bony prominence on back.

(2) Position client supine toward side of bed.

Provides room for client to turn to side.

Critical Decision Point: Clients at risk for pressure ulcer development require the 30-degree lateral position (see Chapter 47).

STEPS	RATIONALE
(3) Roll client onto side toward nurse by flexing client's knees and placing one hand on client's hip and one hand on client's shoulder.	Client is positioned so leverage on hip makes turning easy. Rolling client toward nurse lessens trauma to tissues.
(4) Place pillow under client's head and neck.	Maintains alignment. Reduces lateral neck flexion. Decreases strain on sternocleidomastoid muscle.
(5) Bring shoulder blade forward.	Prevents client's weight from resting directly on shoulder joint.
(6) Position both arms in slightly flexed position. Upper arm is supported by, pillow level with shoulder; other arm, by mattress.	Decreases internal rotation and adduction of shoulder. Supporting both arms in slightly flexed position protects joint. Ventilation is improved because chest is able to expand more easily.
(7) Place tuck-back pillow behind client's back. (Make by folding pillow lengthwise. Smooth area is slightly tucked under client's back.).	Provides support to maintain client on side.
(8) Place pillow under semiflexed upper leg level at hip from groin to foot (see illustrations).	Flexion prevents hyperextension of leg. Maintains leg in correct alignment. Prevents pressure on bony prominence.
(9) Place sandbag parallel to plantar surface of dependent foot. Place high-top sneakers on client's feet.	Maintains dorsiflexion of foot. Prevents footdrop.

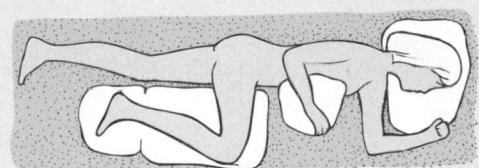

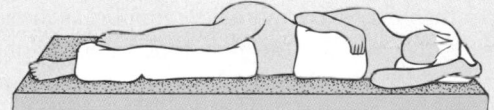

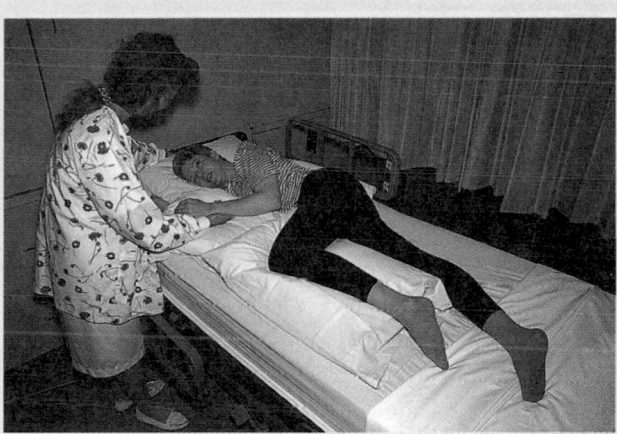

Step 8I(8)

J. **Position client in Sims' (semiprone) position:**	
(1) Lower head of bed completely.	Provides for proper body alignment while client is lying down.
(2) Place client in supine position.	Prepares client for position.
(3) Position client in lateral position, lying partially on abdomen.	Client is rolled only partially on abdomen.
(4) Place small pillow under client's head.	Maintains proper alignment and prevents lateral neck flexion.
(5) Place pillow under flexed upper arm, supporting arm level with shoulder.	Prevents internal rotation of shoulder. Maintains alignment.
(6) Place pillow under flexed upper legs, supporting leg level with hip.	Prevents internal rotation of hip and adduction of leg. Flexion prevents hyperextension of leg. Reduces mattress pressure on knees and ankles.
(7) Place sandbags parallel to plantar surface of foot (see illustration).	

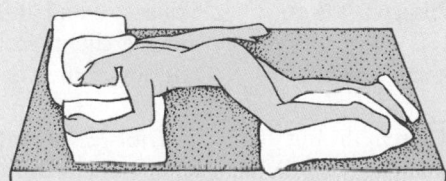

Step 8J(7)

STEPS	RATIONALE
(8) Place high-top sneakers on client's feet.	Maintains foot in dorsiflexion. Prevents footdrop.
(9) Wash hands.	Reduces transmission of infection.
(10) Lower bed and raise side rails.	Provides for client safety.
(11) Observe client's body alignment, position, and level of comfort.	Determines effectiveness of positioning. Additional supports (e.g., pillows, bath blankets), may be added or removed to promote comfort and correct body alignment.
(12) Assess for areas of erythema or breakdown involving skin.	Provides ongoing observation regarding client's skin and musculoskeletal systems. Indicates complications of immobility or improper positioning of body part.

Recording and Reporting

- Record each position change, including amount of assistance needed and client's response and tolerance.
- Record and report any signs of redness in areas such as over bony prominences.

Home Care Considerations

- For clients who need positioning at home, teach family the importance of body mechanics for themselves and the client.
- Teach family about the signs of skin breakdown and the importance of safety during positioning for clients with decreased sensation.

humerus, and clavicle. Trouble points common in Sims' position include the following:

Lateral flexion of the neck

Internal rotation, adduction, or lack of support to the shoulders and hips

Lack of support for the feet

Lack of protection for pressure points at the ilium, humerus, clavicle, knees, and ankles

Transfer Techniques.   Nurses often provide care for immobilized clients whose position must be changed, who must be moved up in bed, or who must be transferred from a bed to a chair or from a bed to a stretcher. Use of proper body mechanics enables the nurse to move, lift, or transfer clients safely and also protects the nurse from injury to the musculoskeletal system. Although nurses use many transfer techniques, the following general guidelines should be followed in any transfer procedure:

Raising the side rail on the side of the bed opposite the nurse to prevent the client from falling out of bed

Elevating the level of the bed to a comfortable height

Assessing the client's mobility and strength to determine what assistance the client can offer during transfer

Determining the need for assistance

Explaining the procedure and describing what is expected of the client

Assessing for correct body alignment and pressure areas after each transfer

The nurse should recognize personal strength and its limits. Moving a completely immobilized client alone is difficult and dangerous. The nurse who is attempting transfer or moving techniques for the first time should request help to reduce the risk of injury to client and nurse.

Moving Clients.   Clients require various levels of assistance to move up in bed, move to the side-lying position, or sit up at the side of the bed. For example, a young, healthy woman may need only a little support as she sits at the side of the bed for the first time after childbirth, whereas an older man may need help from one or more nurses to do the same task 1 day after abdominal surgery.

The nurse should always enlist the client's help to the fullest extent possible. To determine what the client is able to do alone and how many people are needed to help move the client in bed, the nurse assesses the client to determine whether the illness contradicts exertion (e.g., cardiovascular disease). Next, the nurse determines whether the client comprehends what is expected. For example, a client recently medicated for postoperative pain may be too lethargic to understand instruction; thus to ensure safety, two nurses are needed to move the client in bed. The nurse then determines the comfort level of the client. The nurse also evaluates personal strength and knowledge of the procedure. Finally, the nurse determines whether the client is too heavy or immobile for the nurse to complete the procedure alone. In doubtful cases the nurse should always request assistance from another person. Skills 46-2 and 46-3 describe the steps commonly used in moving clients in bed and transferring them to a sitting position at the side of the bed.

Transferring a Client From a Bed to a Chair.   Transfer of a client from a bed to a chair by one nurse requires assistance from the client and should not be attempted with a client who cannot help (see Skill 46-3). The nurse

Transfer Techniques | Skill 46-3

Delegation Considerations

The skills of safe and effective transfer techniques can be delegated to assistive personnel. Clients who have spinal cord trauma usually require transfer and moving by professional nurses.

- Caution caregiver about level of the bed for selected skills.
- Caution caregiver to maintain proper body mechanics.
- Instruct caregiver on safe transfer techniques.

EQUIPMENT

- Transfer belt (if needed), sling or lap board (as needed), nonskid shoes, bath blankets, pillows.
- Wheelchair: position chair at 45-degree angle to bed, lock brakes, remove footrests, lock bed brakes.

- Stretcher: position at right angle (90 degrees) to bed, lock brakes on stretcher, lock brakes on bed.
- Mechanical/hydraulic lift: use frame, canvas strips or chains, and hammock or canvas strips.

STEPS	RATIONALE

1. Assess the client for the following:
  a. Muscle strength
  b. Joint mobility
  c. Presence of paralysis or paresis
  d. Orthostatic hypotension
  e. Activity tolerance
  f. Level of consciousness
  g. Level of comfort
  h. Ability to follow instructions
	Provides information relative to client's abilities, physical status, ability to comprehend, and the number of individuals needed to provide safe transferring.

2. Identify clients at greatest risk for problems with transferring.	Provides information relative to clients who may require intervention beyond the assistive care provider (e.g., physical therapy department).
3. Explain procedure to client.	Promotes cooperation, encourages assistance, and enhances understanding of procedure.
4. Close door or curtain.	Maintains privacy.
5. Wash hands.	Reduces transfer of microorganisms.
6. Transfer client. A. **Assist client to sitting position (bed at waist level):**	
(1) Place client in supine position.	Enables nurse to assess client's body alignment continually and to administer additional care, such as suctioning or hygiene needs.
(2) Face head of bed and remove pillows.	Proper positioning reduces twisting of nurse's body when moving client. Pillows may cause interference when client is sitting up in bed.
(3) Place feet apart with foot nearer bed behind other foot.	Improves nurse's balance and allows transfer of body weight as client is moved to sitting position.
(4) Place hand farther from client under shoulders, supporting client's head and cervical vertebrae.	Maintains alignment of head and cervical vertebrae and allows for even lifting of client's upper trunk.
(5) Place other hand on bed surface.	Provides support and balance.
(6) Raise client to sitting position by shifting weight from front to back leg.	Improves nurse's balance, overcomes inertia, and transfers weight in direction in which client is moved.
(7) Push against bed using arm that is placed on bed surface.	Divides activity between nurse's arms and legs and protects back from strain. By bracing one hand against mattress and pushing against it as client is lifted, part of weight that would be lifted by nurse's back muscles is transferred through nurse's arms onto mattress.
B. **Assist client to sitting position on side of bed with bed in low position:**	
(1) With client in supine position, raise head of bed 30 degrees.	Decreases amount of work needed by client and nurse to raise client to sitting position.
(2) Turn client to side, facing nurse on side of bed on which client will be sitting (see illustration, p. 1532).	Prepares client to move to side of bed and protects client from falling.
(3) Stand opposite client's hips. Turn diagonally so that nurse faces client and far corner of foot of bed.	Places nurse's center of gravity nearer client. Reduces twisting of nurse's body because nurse is facing direction of movement.

STEPS	RATIONALE
(4) Place feet apart with foot closer to head of bed in front of other foot.	Increases balance and allows nurse to transfer weight as client is brought to sitting position on side of bed.
(5) Place arm nearer head of bed under client's shoulder, supporting head and neck.	Maintains alignment of head and neck as nurse brings client to sitting position.
(6) Place other arm nearer head and neck (see illustration).	Supports hip and prevents client from falling backward during procedure.
(7) Move client's lower legs and feet over side of bed. Pivot toward rear leg, allowing client's upper legs to swing downward.	Decreases friction and resistance. Weight of client's legs when off of bed provides gravity to lower legs, and weight of legs assists in pulling upper body into sitting position.
(8) At same time, shift weight to rear leg and elevate client (see illustration).	Allows nurse to transfer weight in direction of motion.
(9) Remain in front of client until client regains balance.	Reduces risk of falling.
C. **Transfer client from bed to chair with bed in low position:**	
(1) Assist client to sitting position on side of bed. Have chair in position at 45-degree angle to bed.	Positions chair within easy access for transfer.
(2) Apply transfer belt or other transfer aids, if needed.	Transfer belt allows nurse to maintain stability of client during transfer and reduces risk of falling. Client's arm should be in sling if flaccid paralysis is present.

Critical Decision Point: If client has immobile lower leg (i.e., cast, paralysis) transfer toward the stronger leg.

---

(3) Ensure that client has stable, nonskid shoes. Weight-bearing, or stronger, leg is placed forward, with weaker foot back.	Nonskid soles decrease risk of slipping during transfer. Always have clients wear shoes during transfer; bare feet increase risk of falls. Client will stand on weight-bearing, or stronger, leg.
(4) Spread feet apart.	Ensure balance with wide base of support.
(5) Flex hips and knees, aligning knees with client's knees (see illustration).	Flexion of knees and hips lowers nurse's center of gravity to object to be raised; aligning knees with client's allows for stabilization of knees when client stands.
(6) Grasp transfer belt from underneath, if used, or reach through client's axillae and place hands on client's scapulae.	Lifting client with hands on scapulae reduces pressure on axillae and maintains client stability. Clients with upper extremity paralysis or paresis should never be lifted by or under arms. Transfer belt is grasped at each side to provide movement of client at center of gravity.
(7) Rock client up to standing position on count of three while straightening hips and legs and keeping knees slightly flexed (see illustration). Client may be instructed to use hands to push up if applicable.	Rocking motion gives client's body momentum and requires less muscular effort to lift client.

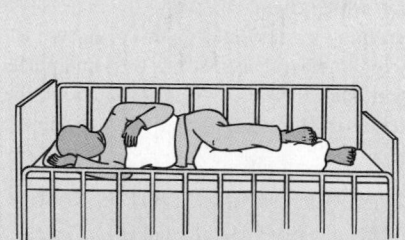

Step 6B(2)

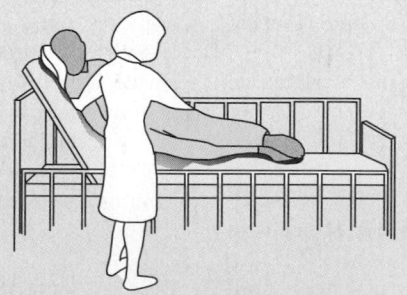

Step 6B(6)

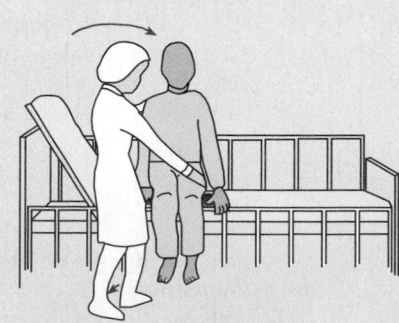

Step 6B(8)

STEPS	RATIONALE
(8) Maintain stability of client's weak or paralyzed leg with knee.	Ability to stand can often be maintained in paralyzed or weak limb with support of knee to stabilize.
(9) Pivot on foot farther from chair.	Maintains support of client while allowing adequate space for client to move.
(10) Instruct client to use armrests on chair for support and ease into chair (see illustration).	Increases client stability.
(11) Flex hips and knees while lowering client into chair (see illustration).	Prevents injury to nurse from poor body mechanics.
(12) Assess client for proper alignment for sitting position. Provide support for paralyzed extremities. Lap board or sling will support flaccid arm. Stabilize leg with bath blanket or pillow.	Prevents injury to client from poor body alignment.
(13) Praise client's progress, effort, performance.	Continued support and encouragement provide incentive for client perseverance.
D. Perform three-person carry from bed to stretcher (bed at stretcher level):	
(1) Three nurses stand side by side facing side of client's bed. Individuals performing the procedure should be of equal height.	Prevents twisting of nurses' bodies. Client's alignment is maintained.
(2) Each person assumes responsibility for one of three areas: head and shoulders, hips, and thighs and ankles.	Distributes client's body weight evenly.
(3) Each person assumes wide base of support with foot closer to stretcher in front and knees slightly flexed.	Increases balance and lowers center of gravity of person lifting.
(4) Arms of lifters are placed under client's head and shoulders, hips, and thighs and ankles, with fingers securely around other side of client's body (see illustration, p. 1534).	Distributes client's weight over forearms of lifters.

Critical Decision Point: Spinal cord injuries must be stabilized before transfer.

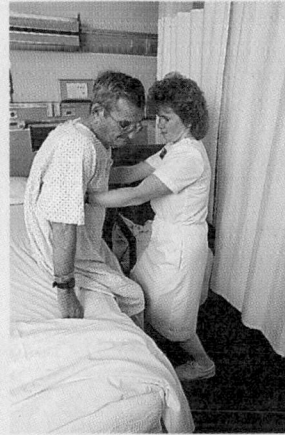
Step 6C(5)

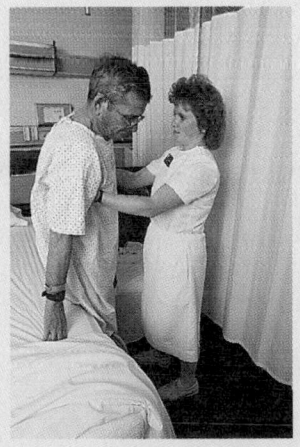
Step 6C(7)

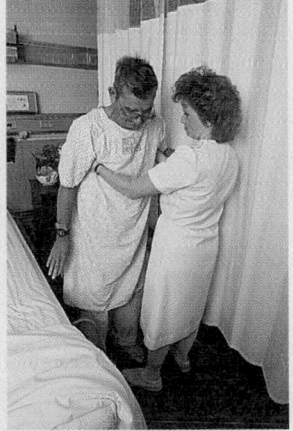
Step 6C(10)

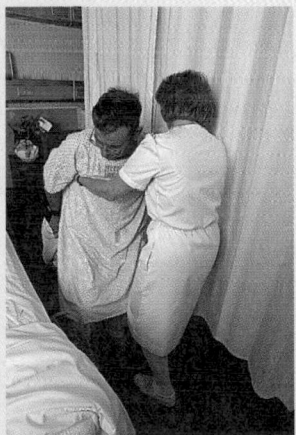
Step 6C(11)

STEPS	RATIONALE

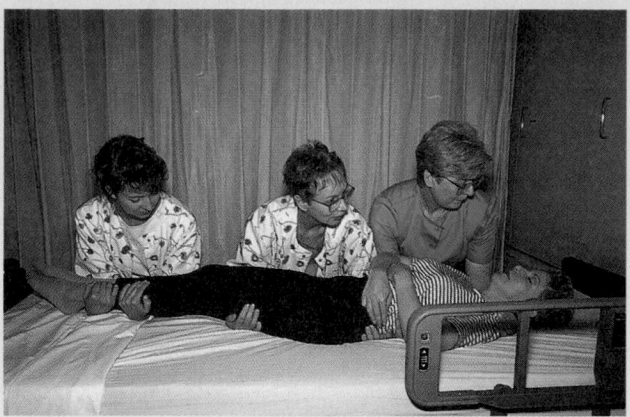

Step 6D(4)

STEPS	RATIONALE
(5) Lifters roll client toward their chests. On count of three, client is lifted and held against nurses chests.	Moves workload over lifters' base of support. Enables lifters to work together and safely lift client.
(6) On second count of three, nurses step back and pivot toward stretcher, moving forward if needed.	Transfers weight toward stretcher.
(7) Nurses gently lower client onto center of stretcher by flexing knees and hips until elbows are level with edge of stretcher.	Maintains nurses' alignment during transfer.
(8) Nurses assess client's body alignment, place safety straps across body, and raise side rails.	Reduces risk of injury from poor alignment or falling.

E. **Use mechanical/hydraulic lift to transfer client from bed to chair:**

STEPS	RATIONALE
(1) Bring lift to bedside.	Ensures safe elevation of client off bed. (Before using lift, be thoroughly familiar with its operation.)
(2) Position chair near bed and allow adequate space to maneuver lift.	Prepares environment for safe use of lift and subsequent transfer.
(3) Raise bed to high position with mattress flat. Lower side rail.	Allows nurse to use proper body mechanics.
(4) Keep bed side rail up on side opposite nurse.	Maintains client safety.

Critical Decision Point: Assess all tubes, making sure that they are not inadvertently pulled, tangled, or strained during transfer.

STEPS	RATIONALE
(5) Roll client away from nurse.	Positions client for use of lift sling.
(6) Place hammock or canvas strips under client to form sling (see illustration, p. 1535). With two canvas pieces, lower edge fits under client's knees (wide piece), and upper edge fits under client's shoulders (narrow piece).	Two types of seats are supplied with mechanical/hydraulic lift: hammock style is better for clients who are flaccid, weak, and need support; canvas strips can be used for clients with normal muscle tone. Hooks should face away from client's skin. Place sling under client's center of gravity and greatest portion of body weight.
(7) Raise bed rail.	Maintains client safety.
(8) Go to opposite side of bed and lower side rail.	
(9) Roll client to opposite side and pull hammock (strips) through.	Completes positioning of client on mechanical/hydraulic sling.
(10) Roll client supine onto canvas seat.	Sling should extend from shoulders to knees (hammock) to support client's body weight equally.

STEPS	RATIONALE
(11) Remove client's glasses, if appropriate.	Swivel bar is close to client's head and could break eyeglasses.
(12) Place lift's horseshoe bar under side of bed (on side with chair).	Positions lift efficiently and promotes smooth transfer.
(13) Lower horizontal bar to sling level by releasing hydraulic valve. Lock valve.	Positions hydraulic lift close to client. Locking valve prevents injury to client.
(14) Attach hooks on strap (chain) to holes in sling. Short chains or straps hook to top holes of sling; longer chains hook to bottom of sling.	Secures hydraulic lift to sling.
(15) Elevate head of bed.	Positions client in sitting position.
(16) Fold client's arms over chest.	Prevents injury to paralyzed arms.
(17) Pump hydraulic handle using long, slow, even strokes until client is raised off bed.	Ensures safe support of client during elevation.
(18) Use steering handle to pull lift from bed and maneuver to chair.	Moves client from bed to chair.
(19) Roll base around chair.	Positions lift in front of the chair in which client is to be transferred.
(20) Release check valve slowly (turn to left) and lower client into chair (see illustration).	Safely guides client into back of chair as seat descends.
(21) Close check valve as soon as client is down and straps can be released.	If valve is left open, boom may continue to lower and injure client.
(22) Remove straps and mechanical/hydraulic lift.	Prevents damage to skin and underlying tissues from canvas or hooks.
(23) Check client's sitting alignment.	Prevents injury from poor posture.
7. Wash hands.	Reduces transmission of microorganisms.
8. With each transfer, assess client's tolerance and level of tiredness.	Increased activity may elevate heart rate and blood pressure.
9. With each transfer, evaluate client's alignment.	

Recording and Reporting

- Record each transfer and position change, including amount of assistance needed and client's response.
- Record and report any signs of redness over areas such as bony prominences.

Home Care Considerations

- For clients who need head of bed elevated at home, teach family about use of pillows or bed blocks.
- Teach family the importance of body mechanics for themselves and the client.

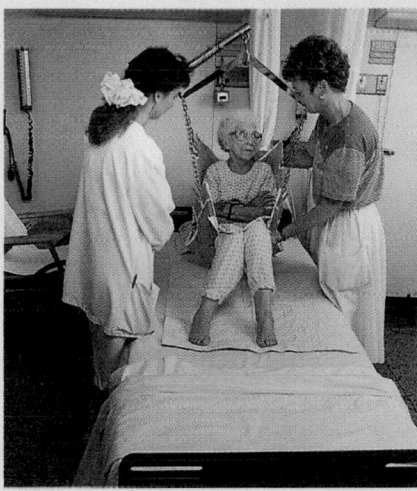

Step 6E(6)

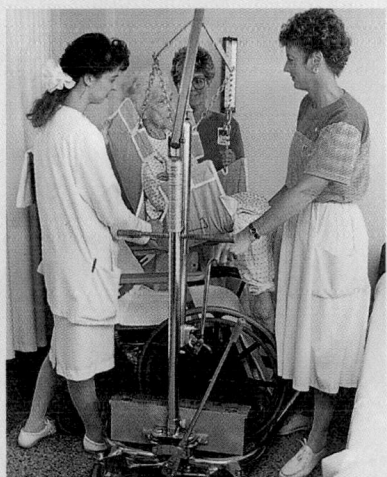

Step 6E(20)

explains the procedure to the client before the transfer. The environment is also prepared by moving obstacles out of the way. The chair is placed next to the bed with the chair back in the same plane as the head of the bed. Placement of the chair allows the nurse to pivot with the client and to transfer the client's weight quickly.

A safe transfer is the first priority. The nurse who is doubtful about personal strength or the client's ability to help should request assistance. Often a hydraulic lift can be used to transfer clients (see Skill 46-3). The client should sit and dangle the feet at the side of the bed for a minute before standing. The client should then stand at the side of the bed for another minute so that the client can quickly be lowered back into it in case of dizziness or fainting. When moving an immobilized client from a bed to a wheelchair, both nurses must use proper body mechanics (Figure 46-23). If a client has an immobile lower extremity from a cast or paralysis, the transfer should be toward the unaffected leg.

Transferring a Client From a Bed to a Stretcher.   An immobilized client who must be transferred from a bed to a stretcher or from a bed to another bed often requires a three-person carry (see Skill 46-3). This technique is best implemented when personnel who are doing the lifting are similar in height. If their centers of gravity are within the same plane, they can lift as a team. Another way to transfer a client is by using a lift sheet or a quilted transfer pad placed under the client (Figure 46-24). The lift sheet serves as a "cradle" while the client is being transferred to the stretcher. In this technique, nurses need to be on opposite sides of the bed and holding onto the lift sheet when transferring the client to the stretcher. The stretcher and the bed are placed side by side so that the client can be transferred quickly and easily using the lift sheet. As with all procedures, safety is the priority. Safety is increased in the three-person team if the lifters work together. Therefore one person should assume the leadership role.

Caution is used when the client has or is suspected of having spinal cord trauma. If the client must be moved, a transfer board should be placed under the client to maintain spinal alignment before transferring the client to a stretcher. The client should be prepared for the transfer and asked to help when possible (e.g., by folding the arms over the chest). The environment should be free from obstacles, and unnecessary equipment should be removed from the bed.

Restorative Care.   The goal of restorative care for the client who is immobile is to maximize functional mobility and independence and reduce residual functional deficits such as impaired gait and decreased endurance. The focus in restorative care is not only on ADLs that relate to physical self-care, but also on **instrumental activities of daily living (IADLs).** IADLs are activities that are necessary to be independent in society beyond eating, grooming, transferring, and toileting and include such skills as shopping, preparing meals, banking, and taking medications.

The nurse uses many of the same interventions as described in the health promotion and acute care sections, but the emphasis is on working collaboratively with clients and their significant others and with other health care professionals. The emphasis is on facilitating the client's return to maximal functional ability in both ADLs and IADLs so that quality of life is enhanced.

Intensive specialized therapy such as occupational or physical therapy is common. The client, if in an institution, will likely go to the therapy department 2 to 3 times a day. The nurse's role is to work collaboratively with these professionals and reinforce exercises and teaching done. For example, after a complete stroke, a client will likely receive gait training from a physical therapist, speech reha-

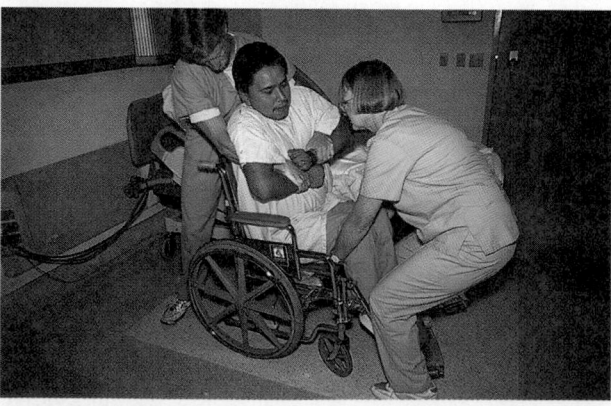

Figure 46-23   Transferring an immobile client from bed to wheelchair.

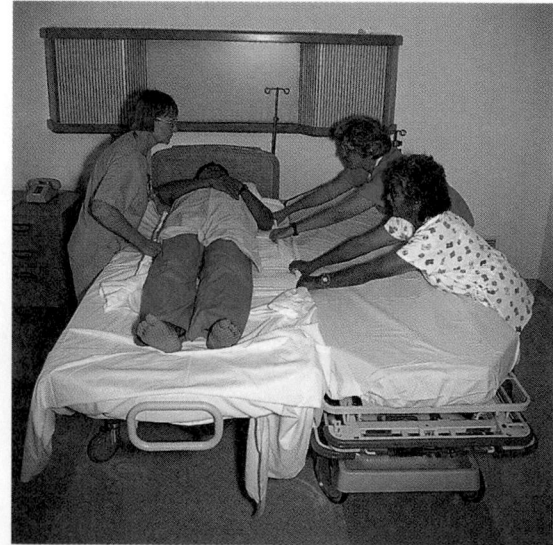

Figure 46-24   Use of a draw or pull sheet to transfer a client from bed to stretcher.

bilitation from a speech therapist, and training from an occupational therapist on food preparation or other household chores. The therapy may not be able to restore total functional health but may help the client adapt to the mobility limitations or complications.

Restorative care is carried out in a variety of settings for the client who has mobility limitations. The site of the care depends on the level of care needed, the amount and frequency of care required, and the types of care that are available in a geographical area. Long-term care refers to a variety of supportive care services that are provided to clients who have lost the ability for some aspect of self-care. The term *long-term care* is somewhat misnamed, however, since the time frame for restorative care services that a client requires may range from several weeks to years. After a total knee replacement it is not unusual for a client to move from the acute care setting to a restorative care setting such as a nursing home or a rehabilitation hospital or to a rehabilitative unit at the same hospital where acute care was provided. Restorative care may also take place at home. The client may go from hospital to nursing home to home or go directly home from a hospital. The client may receive care in the home by professionals or make outpatient visits to therapists' offices.

Common restorative interventions are focused on regaining mobility. Performing exercises to maintain or regain joint mobility and teaching the use of assistive devices for walking are common restorative nursing interventions. Items frequently used to help adapt to mobility limitations include walkers, canes, wheelchairs, and assistive devices such as toilet seat extenders, reaching sticks, special silverware, and clothing with Velcro closures.

Joint Mobility. To ensure adequate joint mobility, the nurse can teach the client about ROM exercises. When the client does not have voluntary motor control, the nurse institutes passive ROM exercises. Joint mobility is also increased by walking. Occasionally clients need to use assistive devices such as crutches or walkers to help them walk.

Range-of-Motion Exercises. Clients with restricted mobility are unable to perform some or all ROM exercises independently. This limitation can be identified in clients in whom one extremity has limited movement or in completely immobilized clients. When caring for clients with actual or potential impaired mobility, the nurse designs interventions directed at maintaining maximum joint mobility. One such nursing intervention is ROM exercises.

To ensure that clients routinely receive these exercises, the nurse should schedule them at specific times, perhaps with another nursing activity, such as during the client's bath. This enables the nurse to systematically assess and improve the client's ROM. In addition, bathing usually requires that extremities and joints are put through complete ROM.

ROM exercises may be active (the client is able to move all joints through their ROM unassisted), passive (the client is unable to move independently and the nurse moves each joint through its ROM), or somewhere in between. With a weak client, for example, the nurse may provide support while the client performs the movement, or the client may be able to move some joints actively while the nurse passively moves others. The nurse first assesses the client's ability to engage in active ROM exercises and the need for assistance from the nurse. In general, exercises should be as active as health and mobility allow. Contractures may develop in joints not moved periodically through their full ROM.

Unless contraindicated, the care plan should include moving the client's extremities through the fullest ROM possible. Passive ROM exercises should begin as soon as the client's ability to move the extremity or joint is lost. Movements are carried out slowly and smoothly, just to the point of resistance, and should not cause pain. The nurse should never force a joint beyond its capacity. Each movement should be repeated 5 times during the session.

When performing passive ROM exercises, the nurse stands at the side of the bed closest to the joint being exercised. If an extremity is to be moved or lifted, the nurse places a cupped hand under the joint to support it (Figure 46-25), supports the joint by holding the adjacent distal and proximal areas (Figure 46-26), or supports the joint with one hand and cradles the distal portion of the extremity with the remaining arm (Figure 46-27).

The following sections describe movements for major joints in the body. See Table 46-3 for detailed ROM and illustrated motion for each joint.

Neck. ROM for the neck is permitted by the flexibility of the cervical vertebrae and the pivotal connection between the head and neck. Unless contraindicated because of spinal surgery, spinal cord trauma, or other central nervous system trauma, ROM exercises should be performed by clients with limited neck mobility. When flexion contracture of the neck occurs, the client's neck is perma-

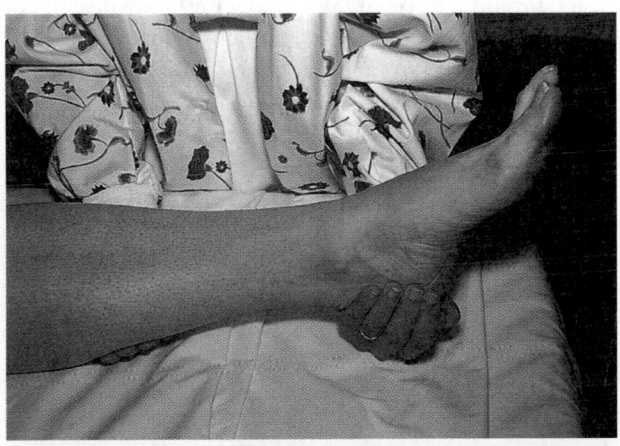

Figure 46-25 Using a cupped hand to support a joint.

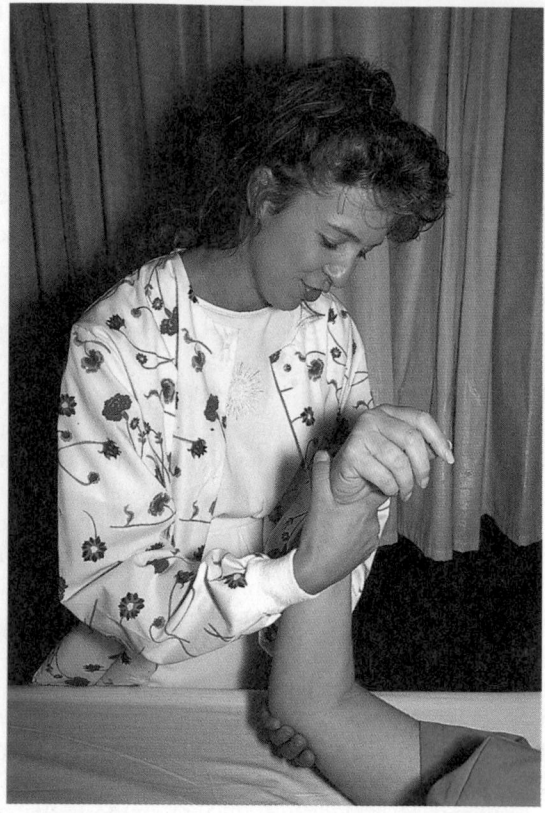

Figure 46-26   Supporting the joint by holding the distal and proximal areas adjacent to the joint.

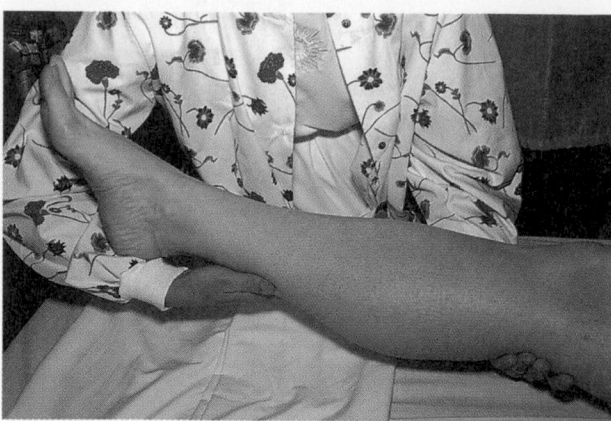

Figure 46-27   Cradling the distal portion of an extremity.

nently flexed with the chin close to or actually touching the chest. Ultimately, the client's body alignment is altered, the visual field is changed, and the level of independent functioning is decreased.

Shoulder.   One feature of the shoulder that sets it apart from other joints in the body is that the strongest muscle controlling it, the deltoid, is in complete elongation in the normal position. No other muscle exerts its full strength when in complete elongation. The goal of action in the shoulder is full ROM. Shoulder movements include flexion, extension, abduction, adduction, internal and external rotation, and circumduction. The full ROM must be maintained or regained to avoid pain.

When caring for a client with limited shoulder mobility, the nurse may need to design support devices for the shoulder, such as slings when the client is standing or sitting or pillows when the client is in bed. Correctly positioning the shoulder prevents pain, joint dislocation, and further changes in body alignment.

Elbow.   The elbow functions optimally at an angle of about 90 degrees. An elbow fixed in full extension is disabling and limits the client's independence.

Forearm.   Most functions of the hand are best carried out with the forearm in moderate pronation. When the forearm is fixed in a position of full supination, the client's use

of the hand is limited. For optimal functioning, the forearm must be able to rotate from supination to pronation.

Wrist.   The primary function of the wrist is to place the hand in slight dorsiflexion, the position of functioning. Therefore full ROM is not as great a priority as maintaining the wrist in a functional position. When the wrist is fixed in even a slightly flexed position, the grasp is weakened. In the immobilized client the functional position of the wrist can be achieved by using splints.

Fingers and Thumb.   The ROM in the fingers and thumb enables the client to perform ADLs and activities requiring fine motor skills, such as carpentry, needlework, drawing, and painting. The functional position of the fingers and thumb is slight flexion of the thumb in opposition to the fingers. In clients with restricted mobility, hand rolls help maintain this position.

Hip.   Because the lower extremities are concerned chiefly with locomotion and weight bearing, stability of the hip joint may be more important than its mobility. For example, if one hip has no mobility but is fixed in a neutral position and fully extended, it is possible to walk without a significant limp.

However, contractures often fix the hip in positions of deformity. Excessive abduction makes the affected leg appear too short, whereas excessive adduction makes the affected leg appear too long. In either case the client has limited locomotion and walks with an obvious limp. Internal and external rotation contractures cause an abnormal and unbalanced gait.

Knee.   A primary function of the knee is stability, which is achieved by ROM, ligaments, and muscles. However, the knees cannot remain stable under weight-bearing conditions unless there is adequate quadriceps power to maintain the knee in full extension. ROM exercises should include pulling the knee into full extension.

An immobile knee joint can result in serious disability. The degree of disability depends on the position in which the knee is stiffened. If the knee is fixed in full extension, the person must sit with the leg thrust out in front. When the knee is flexed, the person limps while walking. The greater the flexion, the greater the limp. Complete flexion contractures prevent the person from walking without a walker or crutches.

Ankle and Foot. Ankle ROM is important; without full ROM there will be gait deviations. The joint must be stabile and able to bear weight, or the person will fall. If joint mobility is diminished, the nurse should maintain the joint in a position in which walking can be carried out with a forward rolling motion from the heel onto the forefoot.

When the person relaxes as in sleep or coma, the foot relaxes and assumes a position of plantar flexion. This results from relaxation of the gastrocnemius and soleus muscles, which maintain dorsiflexion. If the foot remains in plantar flexion without support, these two muscles shorten and the dorsiflexion muscles try to compensate by overstretching. As a result, the foot becomes fixed in plantar flexion (footdrop), which impairs the ability to walk. Inversion and eversion must also be avoided to allow the foot to rest flat on the floor. The foot must be flat to allow weight bearing and proper walking.

Toes. Excessive flexion of the toes results in clawing. When this is a permanent deformity, the foot is unable to rest flat on the floor and the client is unable to walk properly. Flexion contractures are the most common foot deformity associated with reduced joint mobility.

• • •

Adequate ROM gives the necessary mobility to carry out ADLs and exercise and to engage in relaxing activities. In addition, adequate ROM in the lower extremities allows walking.

Walking. In the normal walking posture the head is erect; the cervical, thoracic, and lumbar vertebrae are aligned; the hips and knees have appropriate flexion; and the arms swing freely with the legs. Illness or trauma can reduce activity tolerance, so assistance in walking is required. In addition, temporary or permanent damage to the musculoskeletal and nervous systems may necessitate use of a assistive device for walking.

Helping a Client to Walk. Like other procedures, helping a client to walk requires preparation. When a client's mobility has been restricted, the nurse must assess the client's activity tolerance, tolerance to the upright position (orthostatic hypotension), strength, presence of pain, coordination, and balance to determine the amount of assistance needed.

The nurse explains how far the client should try to walk, who is going to help, when the walk will take place, and why walking is important. In addition, the nurse and client determine how much independence the client can assume.

The nurse also checks the environment to be sure that there are no obstacles in the client's path. Chairs, over-the-bed tables, and wheelchairs are cleared out of the way so that the client has ample room to walk safely. Before starting, rest points should be established in case activity tolerance is less than estimated or the client becomes dizzy. For example, a chair might be placed in the hall for the client to rest if needed.

To prevent orthostatic hypotension, the client should be assisted to a position of sitting at the side of the bed and should rest for 1 to 2 minutes before standing. Likewise, after standing, the client should remain stationary for 1 to 2 minutes before moving. The client's balance must stabilize before walking. Thus the nurse can quickly ease a dizzy client back to bed. The longer the period of immobility, the greater the risk of hypotension when the client stands.

The nurse should provide support at the waist so that the client's center of gravity remains midline. This can be achieved when the nurse places both hands at the client's waist or uses a gait belt. A **gait belt** is a leather belt that encircles the waist and has handles attached for the nurse to hold. While walking, the client should not lean to one side because this alters the center of gravity, distorts balance, and increases the risk of falling.

A client who at any point appears unsteady or complains of dizziness should be returned to a nearby bed or chair. If the client faints or begins to fall, the nurse should assume a wide base of support with one foot in front of the other, thus supporting the body weight. Then the nurse should gently lower the client to the floor, protecting the head. Although lowering a client to the floor is not difficult, the student should practice this technique with a friend or classmate before attempting it in a clinical setting.

Clients with **hemiplegia** (one-sided paralysis) or **hemiparesis** (one-sided weakness) often need assistance to walk. The nurse always stands on the client's affected side and supports the client by holding one arm around the client's waist (or uses a gait belt once the client's stability is ensured) and the other arm around the inferior aspect of the client's upper arm so that the nurse's hand is under the client's axilla. Providing support by holding the client's arm is incorrect because the nurse cannot easily support the weight to lower the client to the floor if the client faints or falls. In addition, if the client falls with the nurse holding an arm, a shoulder joint may be dislocated.

A nurse who does not have a lot of strength and who is unable to ambulate a client alone should request help. The two-nurse method helps distribute the client's weight evenly. The two nurses stand on either side of the client. Each nurse's near arm is around the client's waist, and the other arm is around the inferior aspect of the client's arm so that both nurses' hands are supporting the client's axillae.

Using Assistive Devices for Walking. Clients who are recovering from a lengthy illness that required bed rest and whose mobility is impaired frequently require assistive devices to assist in ambulation. These devices include canes, walkers, crutches, and assistive personnel to teach and assist the client and family in the use of these devices. Chapter 36 provides descriptions and detailed use of each of these devices.

EVALUATION

Client Care.   To evaluate outcomes and response to nursing care, the nurse measures the effectiveness of all interventions. The outcomes are compared with the selected outcomes, such as the client's ability to maintain or improve body alignment, joint mobility, walking, moving, or transferring, or to prevent the hazards of immobility. The nurse evaluates specific interventions designed to promote body alignment, improve mobility, and protect the client from the hazards of immobility. Client

and family teaching to prevent future risks to body alignment and hazards of immobility is also evaluated (Figure 46-28). Evaluation is summative and continuous. The continuous or formative nature of evaluation allows the nurse to determine whether new or revised therapies are required and if new nursing diagnoses have developed.

Client Expectations.   Movement is often taken for granted until it is lost. Lack of movement is often associated with punishment in Western society. Children are given "time-outs," teens are "grounded," and criminals are jailed. It is therefore important to recognize that immobility may lead to fear, anger, grief, withdrawal, or hostility. Whether the nurse is sensitive to these reactions and helps the client work through them or responds negatively will greatly influence clients' expectations.

Clients who are immobile and dependent on others for

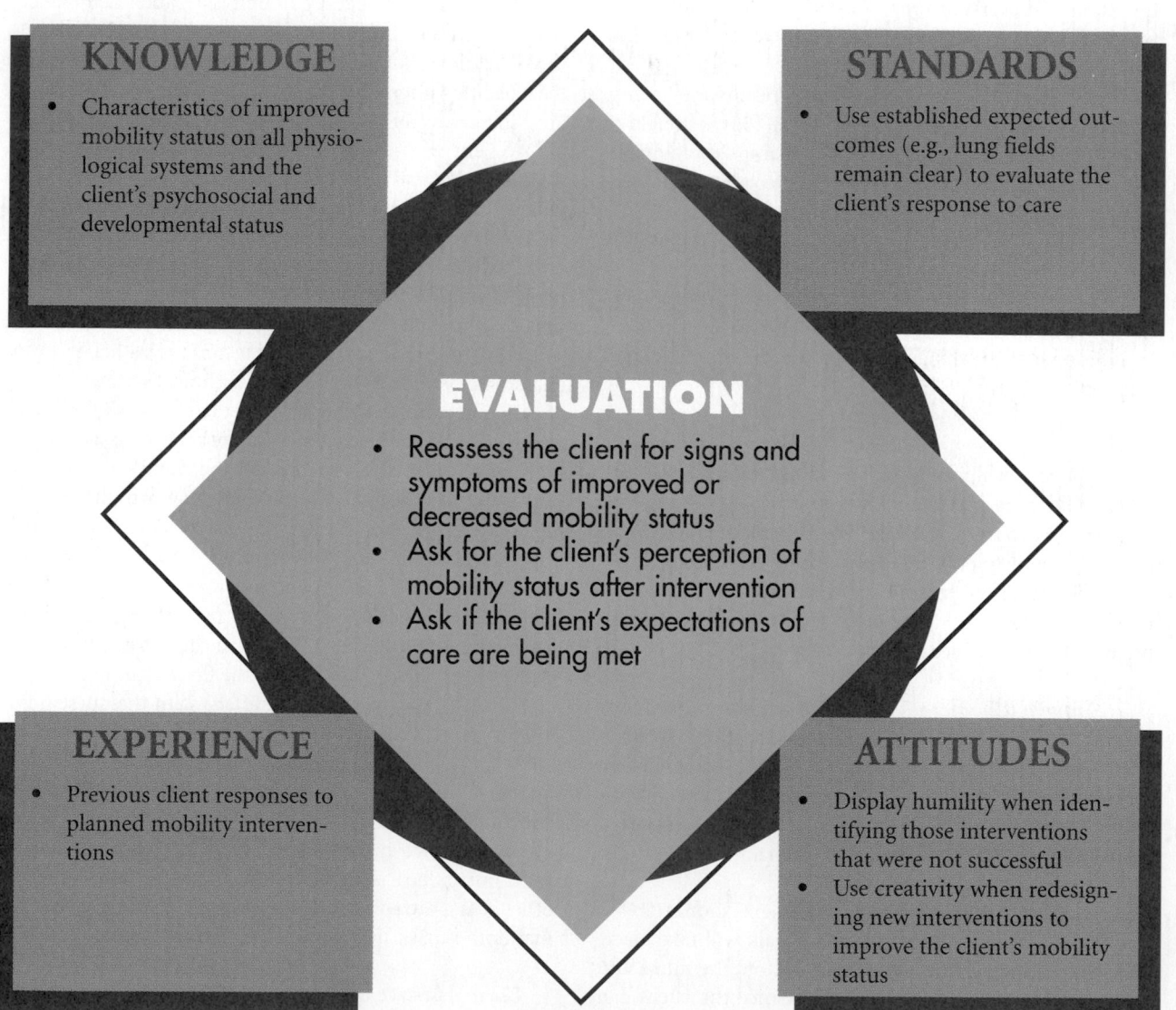

Figure 46-28   *Synthesis Model for Immobility Evaluation Phase.*

some or all of their needs can become overly dependent or try to do too much themselves too early. Finding the interdependent balance between independence and dependence is a difficult task. Clients will want control over their mobility that is personally satisfactory. In the client who is completely dependent on others for care, control over how and when things are done may be very important. Do clients feel they are treated with dignity? Do caregivers treat them as adults? Are they given opportunities to make meaningful choices? Clients who are dependent on others for care may see their demands as the only control they have over their life. Humility is an important attitude in critical thinking when assessing clients' expectations. Humility helps the nurse to identify modifications that may be needed in care planning.

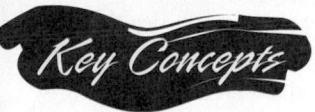

Key Concepts

- Body mechanics are the coordinated efforts of the musculoskeletal and nervous systems as the person moves, lifts, bends, stands, sits, lies down, and completes daily activities.
- Coordinated body movement requires integrated functioning of the skeletal system, skeletal muscles, and nervous system.
- The skeletal system provides bony support structure for movement, attachment of ligaments and muscles, protection of vital organs, some of the regulation of calcium, and production of red blood cells.
- The nervous system provides initiation and voluntary control of movement.
- Coordination and regulation of muscle groups depend on muscle tone; activity of antagonistic, synergistic, and antigravity muscles; and neural input to muscles.
- Balance is assisted through nervous system control by the cerebellum and inner ear.
- Body alignment is the condition of joints, tendons, ligaments, and muscles in various body positions.
- Balance is achieved when there is a wide base of support, the center of gravity falls within the base of support, and a vertical line falls from the center of gravity through the base of support.
- Developmental stages influence body alignment and mobility; the greatest impact of physiological changes on the musculoskeletal system is observed in children and older adults.

- Normal physical mobility depends on intact and functioning nervous and musculoskeletal systems.
- The risk of disabilities related to immobilization depends on the extent and duration of immobilization and the client's premorbid condition.
- Immobility may result from illness or trauma or may be prescribed for therapeutic reasons.
- Immobility presents hazards in the physiological, psychological, and developmental dimensions.
- The nurse uses the nursing process and critical thinking synthesis to provide care for clients who are experiencing or are at risk for the adverse effects of impaired body alignment and immobility.
- After identifying nursing diagnoses, the nurse plans and implements interventions to prevent or minimize the hazards and complications of impaired body alignment and immobilization.
- Clients with impaired body alignment require nursing interventions to maintain them in the supported Fowler's, supine, prone, side-lying, and Sims' positions.
- Range-of-motion exercises include one or all of the body joints.
- Assistive devices to promote walking include canes, walkers, and crutches.

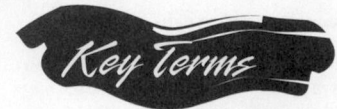
Key Terms

Atelectasis, *p. 1494*

Activity tolerance, *p. 1500*

Anthropometric measurements, *p. 1507*

Bed rest, *p. 1492*

Body alignment, *p. 1486*

Body mechanics, *p. 1486*

Cartilage, *p. 1489*

Cartilaginous joint, *p. 1488*

Chest physiotherapy (CPT), *p. 1515*

Concentric tension, *p. 1489*

Eccentric tension, *p. 1489*

Embolus, *p. 1508*

Exercise, *p. 1500*

Fibrous joint, *p. 1488*

Flat bones, *p. 1487*

Footdrop, *p. 1495*

Fracture, *p. 1492*

Friction, *p. 1487*

Gait, *p. 1500*

Gait belt, *p. 1539*

Hemiparesis, *p. 1539*

Hemiplegia, *p. 1496*

Hypostatic pneumonia, *p. 1494*

Immobility, *p. 1492*

Impaired physical mobility, *p. 1492*

Instrumental activities of daily living (IADLs), *p. 1536*

Irregular bones, *p. 1487*

Isometric contraction, *p. 1489*

Isotonic contraction, *p. 1489*

Joint contracture, *p. 1495*

Joints, *p. 1487*

Leverage, *p. 1487*

Ligaments, *p. 1488*

Long bones, *p. 1487*

Mobility, *p. 1486*

Muscle atrophy, *p. 1495*

Muscle tone, *p. 1490*

Negative nitrogen balance, *p. 1493*

Neurotransmitters, *p. 1490*

Orthostatic hypotension, *p. 1494*

Osteoporosis, *p. 1495*

Pathological fractures, *p. 1487*

Posture, *p. 1490*

Pressure ulcer, *p. 1497*

Range of motion (ROM), *p. 1499*

Renal calculi, *p. 1497*

Short bones, *p. 1487*

Synostotic joint, *p. 1487*

Synovial joint, *p. 1488*

Tendons, *p. 1489*

Thrombus, *p. 1494*

Trapeze bar, *p. 1521*

Trochanter roll, *p. 1521*

Urinary stasis, *p. 1497*

Critical Thinking Exercises

1. You are caring for a 57-year-old male client who has just had a bilateral total knee replacement for osteoarthritis. He is 2 days postoperative and beginning to transfer to a chair with help. He is 100 pounds overweight and has a history of deep vein thrombosis. He has compression stockings, continuous passive range of motion, and a heparin lock. Make a list of potential nursing diagnoses.

2. When doing a home visit for a 75-year-old female client, the client's granddaughter runs in and says, "Did you show the nurse the sore on your leg that you got from falling yesterday?" What questions about mobility are important to ask the client? How do you begin your assessment?

3. Your clinical experience is in long-term care. You are working in assisted living. The nurse in charge of the assisted living wing asks you to help her with a program titled, "Lifestyle Choices: Living Life to Its Fullest." She asks you to participate and discuss how regular exercise can improve overall health and to show how exercise can be incorporated into activities of daily living. Develop a content outline and a time frame for your presentation.

4. You are caring for a 20-year-old female college student who is immobilized after spinal cord trauma. You note that she is becoming increasingly depressed and withdrawn. What skill is important at this point in the client's care?

References

Agency for Health Care Policy and Research: *Treating pressure sores: consumer guide,* Clinical Practice Guideline, No. 15, Rockville, Md, 1994, U.S. Department of Health and Human Services.

Beare PG, Myers JL: *Adult health nursing,* ed 3, St. Louis, 1998, Mosby.

Blair C: Combining behavior management and mutual goal setting to reduce physical dependency in nursing home residents, *Nurs Res* 44(3):160, 1995.

Bright LD, Georgi S: How to protect your patient from DVT . . . deep vein thrombosis, *Am J Nurs* 94(12):28, 1992.

Christie F: Clinical snapshot: pulmonary embolism, *Am J Nurs* 98(11):36, 1998.

Creditor MC: Hazards of hospitalization of the elderly, *Am Coll Physicians* 118(3):219, 1993.

Deitrick JE and others: Effects of immobilization upon various metabolic and physiological functions of normal men, *Am J Med* 4:3, 1948.

Ebersole P, Hess P: *Toward healthy aging: human needs and nursing response,* ed 5, St. Louis, Mosby, 1998.

Galsworthy T, Wilson P: Osteoporosis: it steals more than bones, *Am J Nurs* 96(6):27, 1996.

Gassett RS and others: Ergonomics and body mechanics in the work place, *Orthop Clin North Am* 27(4):861, 1996.

Gröer MW, Shekleton ME: *Basic pathophysiology: a holistic approach,* ed 3, St. Louis, 1989, Mosby.

Helme T: Position changes for residents in long-term care, *Adv Wound Care* 7(5):57, 1994.

Kasper C, Maxwell L, White T: Alterations in skeletal muscle related to short-term impaired physical mobility: an empirical model, *Res Nurs Health* 19:133, 1996.

Kim MJ, McFarland GK, McLane AM: *Pocket guide to nursing diagnoses,* ed 7, St. Louis, 1997, Mosby.

Kreighbaum E, Barthels KM: *Biomechanics: a qualitative approach for studying human movement,* Boston, 1996, Allyn & Bacon.

Latash ML: *Neurophysiological basis of movement,* Champaign, Ill, 1998, Human Kinetics.

Long BC, Phipps WJ, Cassmeyer VL: *Medical-surgical nursing: a nursing process approach,* ed 3, St. Louis, 1993, Mosby.

McCance KL, Huether SE: *Pathophysiology: the biologic basis for disease in adults and children,* ed 3, St. Louis, 1998, Mosby.

McCloskey JC, Bulechek GM: *Nursing interventions classification (NIC),* ed 3, St. Louis, 2000, Mosby.

Miller J and others: The assessment of acute confusion as part of nursing care, *Appl Nurs Res* 10(3):143, 1997.

Neal C: The assessment of knowledge and application of proper body mechanics in the workplace, *Orthop Nurs* 16(1):66, 1997.

Nunnelee J: Minimize the risk of DVT, *RN* 58(12):28, 1995.

Phipps WI and others: *Medical-surgical nursing,* ed 5, St. Louis, 1995, Mosby.

Price SA, Wilson LM: *Pathophysiology: clinical concepts of disease processes,* ed 5, St. Louis, 1997, Mosby.

Proctor M, Greenfield L, Marsh E: Prophylaxis for thromboembolism in elective orthopaedic surgery, *Orthop Nurs* 16(5):51, 1997.

Rawsky E: Review of the literature on falls among the elderly, *Image J Nurs Sch* 30(1):47, 1998.

Roper M: Back to basics: assessing orthostatic vital signs, *Am J Nurs* 96(8):43, 1996.

St. Pierre B, Flaskerud J: Clinical nursing implications for recovery of atrophied skeletal muscle following bed rest, *Rehabil Nurs* (20)6:314, 1995.

Schaller KJ: Tai Chi Chih: an exercise option for older adults, *J Gerontol Nurs* 22(10):12, 1996.

Tresolini C and others, editors: *Working with patients to prevent, treat, and manage osteoporosis: a curriculum guide for health professions,* San Francisco; 1996, National Fund for Medical Education.

Von Rueden KT, Harris JR: Pulmonary dysfunction related to immobility in the trauma patient, *AACN Clin Issues* 6(2):212, 1995.

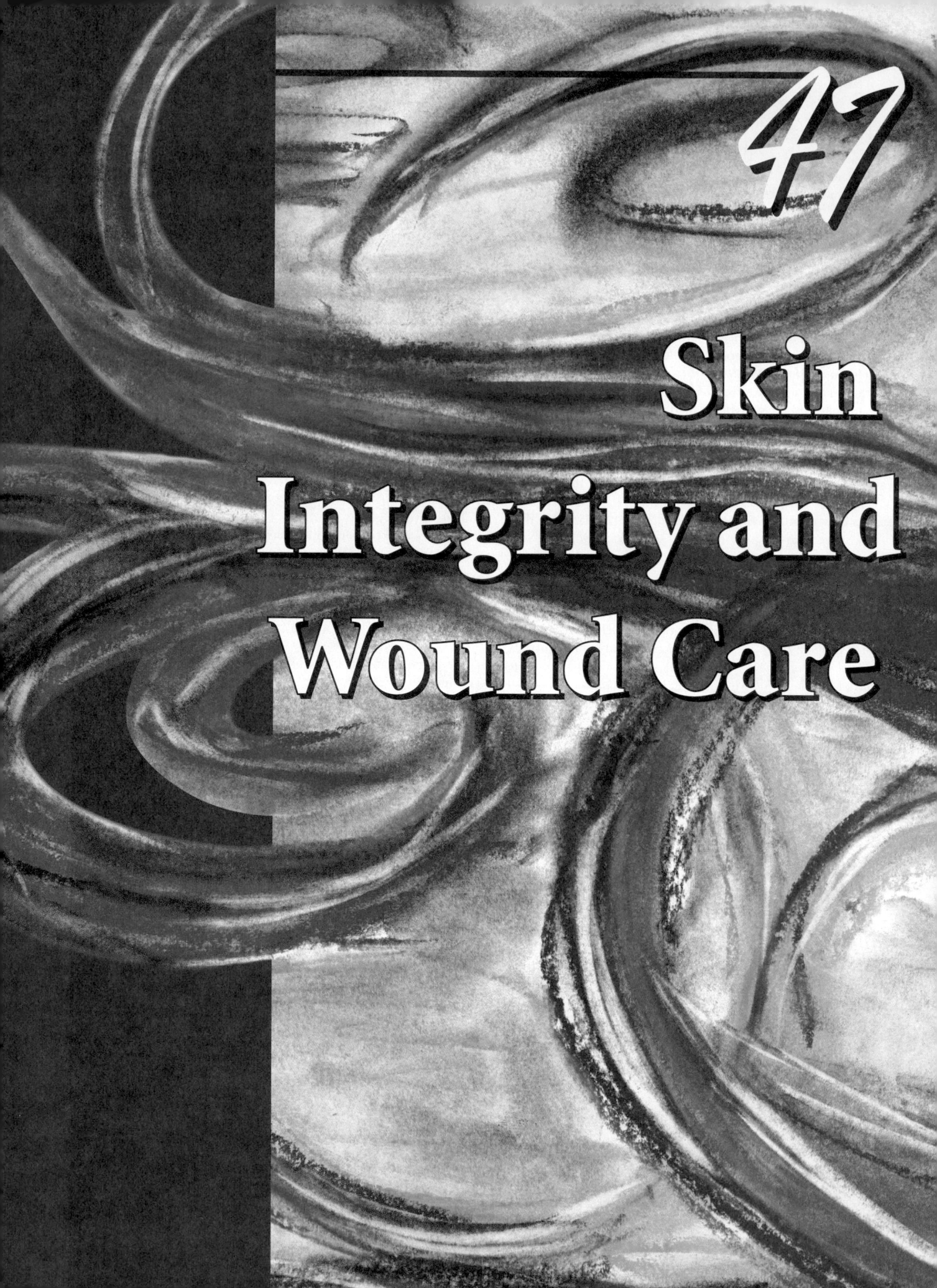

47

Skin Integrity and Wound Care

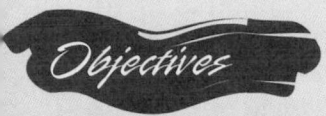
Mastery of content in this chapter will enable the student to:

- Define the key terms listed.
- Discuss the risks and contributing factors to pressure ulcer formation.
- List the four stages of pressure ulcers.
- Define the four stages for classification of pressure ulcers.
- Discuss normal processes of wound healing.
- Describe the differences among wounds healing by primary or secondary intention.
- Describe complications of wound healing and their usual time of occurrence.
- Explain the factors that impair or promote wound healing.
- Describe the differences between nursing care of acute and chronic wounds.
- Complete an assessment for a client with impaired skin integrity.
- List nursing diagnoses associated with impaired skin integrity.
- Develop a nursing care plan for a client with impaired skin integrity.
- List appropriate nursing interventions for a client with impaired skin integrity.
- State evaluation criteria for a client with impaired skin integrity.

The skin, or the integumentary system, is the body's largest organ. It composes one sixth of the total body weight (Wysocki, 1995). The integument is a protective barrier against disease-causing organisms; is a sensory organ for pain, temperature, and touch; and can synthesize vitamin D. Injury to the integument poses risks to safety and triggers a complex healing response. Knowing the normal healing pattern helps the nurse to recognize alterations that require intervention.

Scientific Knowledge Base

NORMAL INTEGUMENT
In relation to wound healing, the integument has two principal layers: the epidermis and the dermis (Figure 47-1). These two layers are separated by a basement membrane, which is often referred to as the dermal-epidermal junction. The **epidermis,** or outer layer, has several layers. The stratum corneum is the thin, outermost layer of the epidermis. It consists of flattened, dead, keratinized cells. The cells originate from the epidermal layer, the stratum basale. Cells in the stratum basale divide, proliferate, and migrate toward the epidermal surface. After cells reach the stratum corneum, they flatten and die. This constant movement ensures replacement of surface cells sloughed off during normal **desquamation.** The thin stratum corneum protects underlying cells and tissues from dehydration and prevents entrance of certain chemical agents. However, the stratum corneum does allow evaporation of water from the skin and permits absorption of certain topically applied medications.

The **dermis** is the inner layer of the skin, which provides the tensile strength, mechanical support, and protection to the underlying muscles, bones, and organs. It differs from the epidermis in that it contains mostly connective tissue and few skin cells. **Collagen** (a tough, fibrous protein), blood vessels, and nerves compose it. Fibroblasts, which are responsible for collagen formation, are the only distinctive cell type within the dermis.

Understanding the integument's layers helps the nurse promote wound healing. The epidermis functions to resurface wounds and restore the barrier against invading organisms. The dermis responds to restore the structural integrity (collagen) and the physical properties of the skin. Even though a wound may close in the upper epidermal layer, the client is at risk for infection, circulatory impairment, and tissue breakdown if the underlying dermis fails to heal. A summary of the normal changes in aging skin can be found in Box 47-1.

PRESSURE ULCERS
Pressure ulcer, pressure sore, decubitus ulcer, and *bedsore* are terms used to describe impaired skin integrity. The most current terminology is **pressure ulcer** (Figure 47-2), which is consistent with the recommendations of the National Pressure Ulcer Advisory Panel (NPUAP) and the pressure ulcer guidelines panel of the Agency for Health Care Policy and Research (AHCPR) (AHCPR, 1992a; Maklebust and Margolis, 1995; Margolis, 1995). Any client experiencing decreased mobility, impaired neurological functioning, decreased sensory perception, or decreased circulation is at risk for pressure ulcer development.

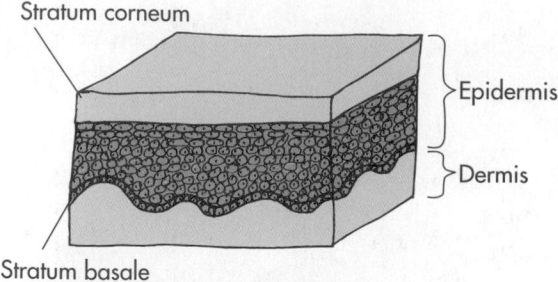

Figure 47-1   Layers of the integument.

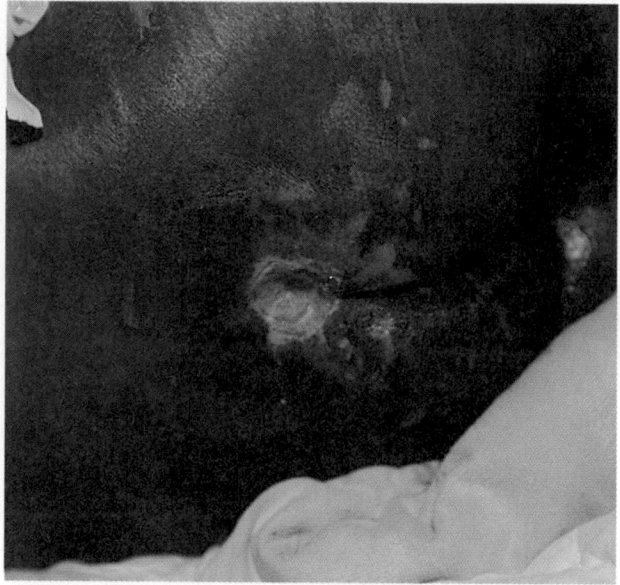

Figure 47-2   Pressure ulcer with tissue necrosis.

Gerontological NURSING PRACTICE   **Box 47-1**

- Diminished epidermal cell activity in older adult skin increases the epidermal cell renewal time by one third. For example, in a young adult, the epithelium renews itself in about 20 days; after the age of 50, epithelium renewal takes 30 or more days. Slow replacement of epithelial cells means that older adults have slower wound healing.
- Aging causes atrophy and thinning of both layers of the skin. The nurse should monitor the older client's skin in the buttock area. The sacrum is the most common site of pressure ulcers. With the thinning of the epidermis the skin's barrier function is diminished, so chemicals can easily get into the body. Because the dermis is thinner and flatter, the skin wrinkles.
- There is less surface area in the skin of older people as compared with younger skin; there is also a weakening in the epidermis and dermis attachment. Because in older adults the attachment between these two layers of the skin (dermal-epidermal junction) is weakened, the epidermis can "slide"; therefore the skin can tear more easily.
- Aging causes impaired immune function of cells located in the skin. Altered immune function of older adult skin means the ability to fight infection is decreased in older adults.
- The hypodermis ("the insulator of the skin") is decreased in size with age. Older clients have little subcutaneous padding over bony prominences, so they are more at risk for skin breakdown and heat stroke.
- Structural changes in collagen occur in older adult skin. Collagen fibers come together as bundles. Also, there is a loss in the amount of collagen. Older clients have decreased skin turgor, so they are at greater risk for shearing and tearing injuries.

Tissues receive oxygen and nutrients and eliminate metabolic wastes via the blood. Any factor that interferes with this affects cellular metabolism and the function or life of the cell. Pressure affects cellular metabolism by decreasing or obliterating tissue circulation, resulting in tissue ischemia.

Tissue ischemia is the localized absence of blood or a major reduction of blood flow resulting from mechanical obstruction (Pires and Muller, 1991). The reduction in blood flow causes blanching. **Blanching** is seen when the normal red tones of the light-skinned client are absent. Blanching does not occur in clients with darkly pigmented skin. The Task Force on the Implications for Darkly Pigmented Intact Skin in the Prediction and Prevention of Pressure Ulcers (Bennett, 1995) defined **darkly pigmented skin** as skin that "remains unchanged (does not blanch) when pressure is applied over a bony prominence, irrespective of the client's race or ethnicity." Characteristics of intact dark skin that might alert nurses to the potential for pressure ulcers have been identified (Box 47-2).

Characteristics of Intact Dark Skin   Box 47-2

COLOR
Appears darker than surrounding skin
May be purplish/bluish hue
Natural or halogen light source best for assessing skin
Fluorescent light source, to be avoided, since it casts a bluish hue, making accurate assessment difficult

TEMPERATURE
Initial warmth when compared with surrounding skin
Later coolness as tissue is devitalized

TOUCH	APPEARANCE
Indurated	Taut
Edema	Shiny
Soft, boggy	Itchy

Tissue damage occurs when the pressure exerted on the capillaries is high enough to close the capillaries (capillary closing pressure). **Capillary closing pressure** is the pressure needed to close the capillaries (e.g., when the pressure exceeds the normal capillary pressure range of 16 to 32 mm Hg).

After a period of ischemia, light-toned skin can undergo one of two hyperemic changes. **Normal reactive hyperemia** (redness) is the visible effect of localized vasodilation, the body's normal response to lack of blood flow to the underlying tissue (Figure 47-3, *A*). The area blanches with fingertip pressure (Figure 47-3, *B*), and reactive hyperemia lasts less than 1 hour. **Abnormal reactive hyperemia** is an excessive vasodilation and induration in response to pressure. The skin appears bright pink to red. The **induration** is an area of localized edema under the skin. Abnormal reactive hyperemia (Figure 47-4) can last more than 1 hour up to 2 weeks after the removal of pressure (Pires and Muller, 1991).

When a client is lying or sitting, the body weight is placed on bony prominences. The longer unrelieved pressure is applied, the greater the risk of skin breakdown. Pressure causes a decrease in blood supply to the tissues, and ischemia occurs. When the pressure is removed, there is a period of reactive hyperemia, or a sudden increase in blood flow to the region. Reactive hyperemia is a compensatory response and is effective only if the pressure on the skin is removed before necrosis or damage occurs.

Risk Factors for Pressure Ulcer Development.

A variety of factors can predispose a client to pressure ulcer formation. These factors can be directly related to disease, such as decreased level of consciousness; related to the aftereffects of trauma, such as the presence of a cast; or secondary to an illness, such as decreased sensory input following a cerebrovascular accident.

Impaired Sensory Input.

Clients with altered sensory perception for pain and pressure are at greater risk for impaired skin integrity than are clients with normal sensation. Clients whose sensory perception of pain and pressure is intact can feel when a portion of their body senses too much pressure or pain. In turn, when clients are

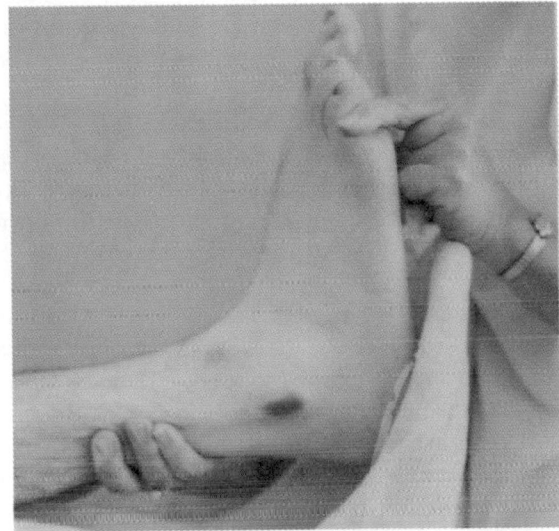
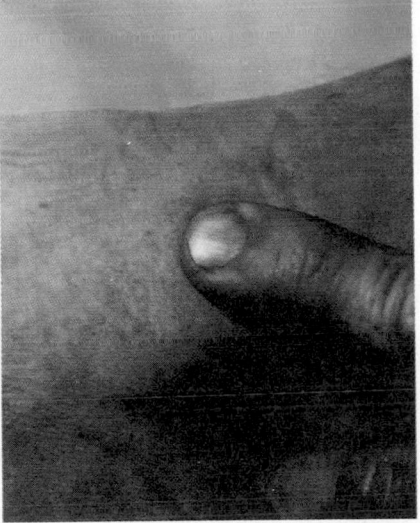
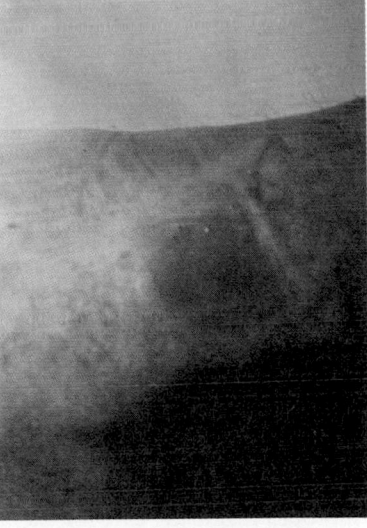

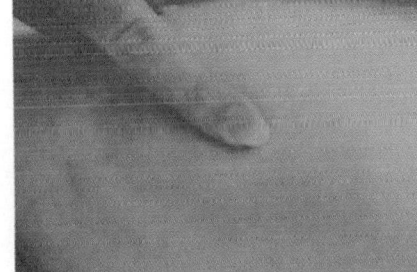
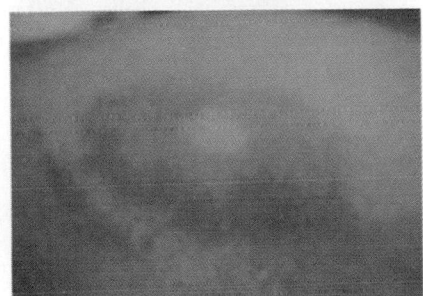

Figure 47-3   **A**, Reactive hyperemia. **B**, Blanches with fingertip pressure. From Pires M, Muller A: Detection and management of early tissue pressure indicators: pictorial essay, *Progressions* 3(3):3, 1991.

Figure 47-4   **A**, Abnormal reactive hyperemia. **B** and **C**, In abnormal reactive hyperemia the area is much darker than the surrounding skin and does not blanch with fingertip pressure. From Pires M, Muller A: Detection and management of early tissue pressure indicators: pictorial essay, *Progressions* 3(3):3, 1991.

alert and oriented, they can change positions or request assistance in changing positions.

Impaired Motor Function.

Clients unable to independently change positions are at greater risk for pressure ulcers. These clients can perceive the pressure but are unable to independently change positions to relieve it. Thus the chance of pressure ulcer development increases. In clients with spinal cord injuries there is motor and sensory impairment. A recent survey found that 62.4% of respondents had at least one pressure ulcer since their paralysis (Salzberg and others, 1998).

Alterations in Level of Consciousness.

Clients who are confused or disoriented, or who have changing levels of consciousness are unable to protect themselves from pressure ulcers. Clients who are confused or disoriented may be able to feel the pressure, but they may not be able to understand how to relieve it. Clients who are in a coma may not perceive pressure and are unable to move voluntarily into a more protective position. In addition, clients whose levels of consciousness change may easily become confused. Some examples are clients in the operating room and intensive care units who are sedated.

Orthopedic Devices.

Casts and traction reduce mobility of the client or of an extremity. A client with a cast has an increased risk of pressure ulcer development because of the mechanical external force of friction from the surface of the cast rubbing against the skin. A second mechanical force is the pressure exerted by the cast on the skin if the cast dries too tightly or if the extremity swells.

Orthotic devices such as cervical collars are used in the treatment of clients with fractures of the upper cervical spine. Pressure ulcers are a potential complication of these cervical collars. A study by Plaisier and others (1994) examined the amount of pressure exerted on the scalp and face by four different cervical collars with the subjects in both the supine and upright positions. Results showed that for some of the cervical collars, the capillary closing pressure was exceeded. Nurses need to be aware of the risk of skin breakdown in clients wearing these cervical collars. Nurses must assess skin beneath cervical collars, braces, or other orthotic devices to observe for signs of skin breakdown.

Any equipment that exerts pressure on a client's skin can lead to the development of a pressure ulcer. Oxygen tubing and nasogastric tubes are just two common examples of equipment that may cause pressure ulcers. Appropriate nursing care for clients with such equipment includes frequent assessment of the client's skin beneath the tube to identify any signs of skin breakdown.

Pathogenesis of Pressure Ulcers.

Three elements are the cornerstone of pressure ulcer development: (1) intensity of pressure and capillary closing pressure (Landis, 1930), (2) duration and sustenance of pressure (Koziak, 1959), and (3) tissue tolerance (Trumble, 1930; Husain, 1953). Some of the most common sites where pressure ulcers develop are the sacrum, heels, elbows, lateral malleoli, greater trochanter, and ischial tuberosities (Barczak and others, 1997).

A pressure ulcer occurs as a result of a time-pressure relationship. The greater the pressure and the duration of the pressure, the greater the incidence of ulcer formation. The skin and subcutaneous tissue can tolerate some pressure. However, externally applied pressure greater than the pressure in the capillary bed decreases or obliterates blood flow to adjacent tissues. These tissues become hypoxic, and ischemic injury results. If this pressure is greater than 32 mm Hg and remains unrelieved to the point of hypoxia, the vessels collapse and thrombose (develop a clot) (Maklebust and Sieggreen, 1996). If the pressure is relieved before the critical point, circulation to the affected tissues is restored through the physiological mechanism of reactive hyperemia. Because the skin has greater ability to tolerate ischemia than does muscle, true pressure ulcers begin at the bone, with pressure-related muscle ischemia eventually declaring itself at the epidermis (Maklebust, 1995).

Pressure ulcers also form as a result of shearing force that occurs when moving the client up in bed. The sacral areas and heels are the most susceptible. The effect of pressure can also be increased by unequal distribution of body weight. Because of gravity, a person is subjected to constant pressures of the body against any surface on which it rests. If the pressure is unevenly distributed on the body, a pressure gradient is increased on tissues receiving the pressure. The cellular metabolism of the skin is altered at the point of pressure.

The compensatory response of the tissues to ischemia—reactive hyperemia—permits ischemic tissue to be flooded with blood when pressure is removed. Increased blood flow increases delivery of oxygen and nutrients to tissue. The metabolic debt resulting from pressure can then be met. Healthy equilibrium is restored, and necrosis of the compressed tissue is avoided (Pires and Muller, 1991). Reactive hyperemia is effective only if pressure is removed before damage occurs. Some researchers feel that the interval before damage occurs can be between 1 and 2 hours. However, this is a subjective time interval and it is not based on client assessment data.

CLASSIFICATION OF PRESSURE ULCER STAGING OR COLOR

One of the earliest ways to classify pressure ulcers was by using a grading or staging system. Staging systems for pressure ulcers are based on describing the depth of tissue destroyed (Maklebust, 1995). An ulcer that is covered with necrotic tissue such as eschar cannot be staged until it is debrided and the depth of the tissue destroyed in the pressure ulcer can be observed (AHCPR, 1992a, 1994).

Orthopedic devices and braces can make assessment difficult (AHCPR, 1992a, 1994).

There are several different staging systems that are used clinically (AHCPR, 1994). It is important to note that the definitions are different for each of these staging systems. Therefore the same pressure ulcer could have a different stage number, depending on the staging system used. The stages below are from the NPUAP system (Cuddigan and Frantz, 1998), and some of them are also used in the AHCPR guidelines (1994). In 1998 the NPUAP stage I definition was changed to reflect assessment characteristics of clients with dark skin tones (Box 47-3). Indicators other than skin color, such as temperature, "orange peel" pore appearance, firmness or tightness, hardness, and laboratory data, may be helpful when assessing clients with dark skin (Henderson and others, 1997).

Bennett (1995) suggests that when assessing clients with darkly pigmented skin, proper lighting is important to accurately assess the skin. Either natural or a halogen light is recommended. This prevents the blue tones that are produced by fluorescent light sources on darkly pigmented skin, which can interfere with accurate assessment. A comparison of stage I pressure ulcers in lightly and darkly pigmented skin can be seen in Figure 47-5.

I   A stage I pressure ulcer is an observable pressure-related alteration of intact skin whose indicators, as compared

with an adjacent or opposite area on the body, may include changes in one or more of the following: skin temperature (warmth or coolness), tissue consistency (firm or beefy feel), and/or sensation (pain, itching). The ulcer appears as a defined area of persistent redness in lightly pigmented skin, whereas in darker skin tones the ulcer may appear with persistent red, blue, or purple hues (Figure 47-6, *A*).

II   Partial-thickness skin loss involving epidermis and/or dermis. The ulcer is superficial and presents clinically as an abrasion, blister, or shallow crater (Figure 47-6, *B*).

III   Full-thickness skin loss involving damage or necrosis of subcutaneous tissue that may extend down to, but not through, underlying fascia. The ulcer presents clinically as a deep crater with or without undermining of adjacent tissue (Figure 47-6, *C*).

IV   Full-thickness skin loss with extensive destruction; tissue necrosis; or damage to muscle, bone, or supporting structures (e.g., tendon, joint capsules) (Figure 47-6, *D*).

Some problems with the use of sequential numbers in staging systems were raised again at the 1995 NPUAP Fourth National Conference. Pressure ulcers do not progress from a stage I to a stage IV (NPUAP, 1995b). Maklebust (1995) cautions clinicians to remember that although staging systems use sequential numbers to describe pressure ulcers, this does not mean that there is a progression in pressure ulcer severity. It is important to remember that the staging systems are a method of classification of pressure ulcers that signify "wounding" or tissue destruction; they are not designed to describe healing of a pressure ulcer. Some clinicians have used the staging numbers in reverse order to measure improvement in a pressure ulcer. It is incorrect to do this, since staging is a method of "wounding," and a healing pressure ulcer is "filled in" with granulation tissue rather than the original tissue that was destroyed (NPUAP, 1995 a,b). There are several tools available to measure pressure ulcer healing, such as the Pressure Sore Status Tool (PSST) (Bates-Jensen, 1990) and the Pressure Ulcer Scale for Healing (PUSH) (Thomas and others, 1997).

Another method of wound classification is by the color of the wound, which identifies its healing phase. Wounds

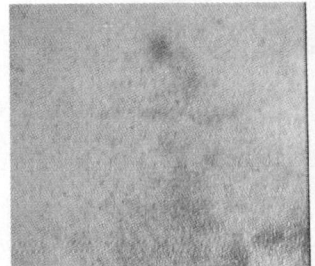

Figure 47-5 Comparison of stage I pressure ulcers in clients with lightly and darkly pigmented skin. Courtesy Convatec.

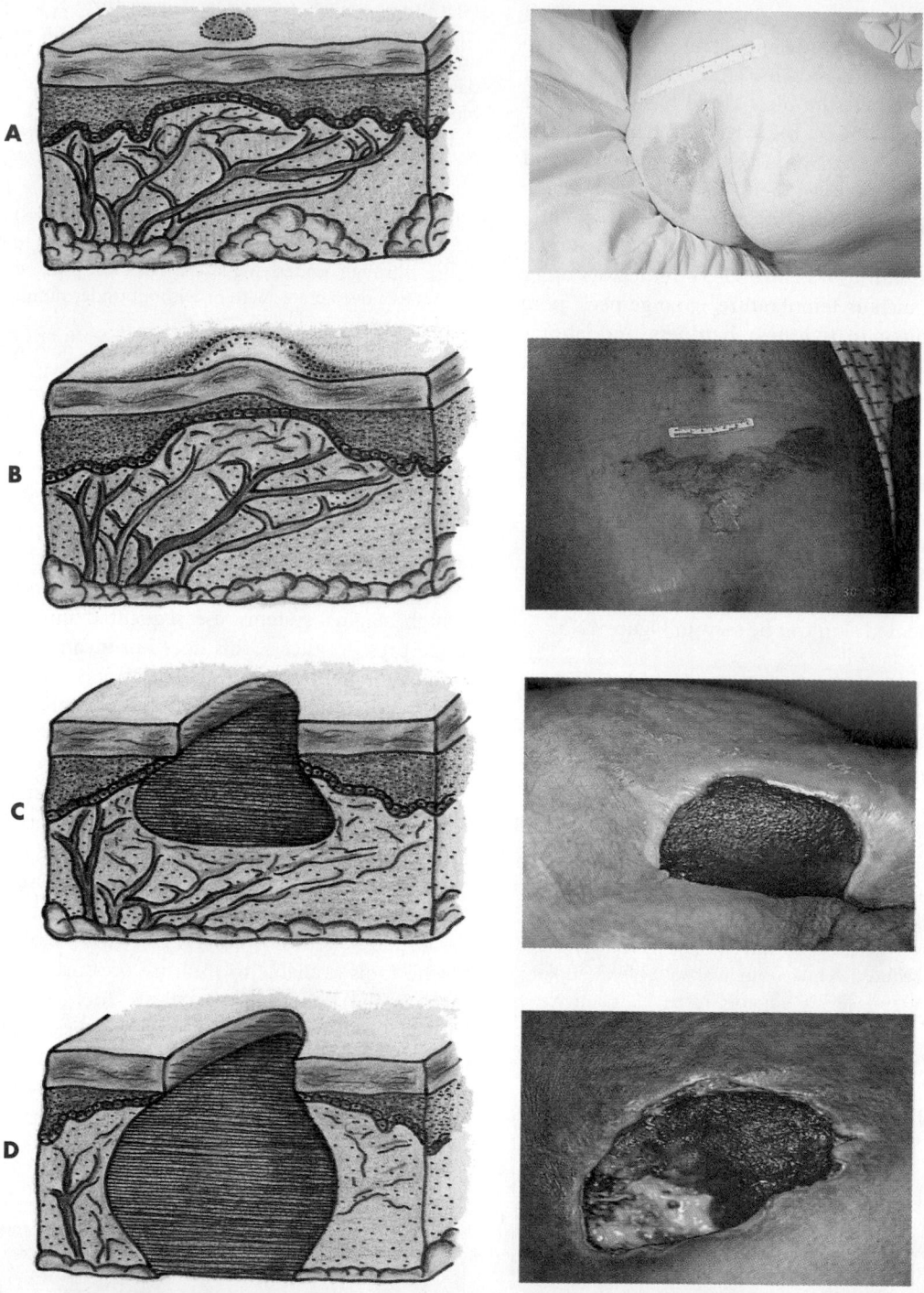

Figure 47-6   Diagram of stages. **A,** Stage I pressure ulcer. **B,** Stage II pressure ulcer. **C,** Stage III pressure ulcer. **D,** Stage IV pressure ulcer.
Courtesy Laurel Wiersma, RN, MSN, Clinical Nurse Specialist, Barnes-Jewish Hospital, St. Louis, Mo.

that are necrotic are classified as black wounds (Figure 47-7, *A*); wounds with exudate and yellow fibrous debris are classified as yellow wounds (Figure 47-7, *B*); and wounds that are in the active healing phase and are clean with pink to red granulation and epithelial tissue are classified as red wounds (Figure 47-7, *C*). Wounds may be a mixture of colors (e.g., 25% yellow and 75% red) (Figure 47-7, *D*). Clinicians may find this color method of classifying wounds to be quick and easy (Krasner, 1995b).

There is no consensus about the best way to classify pressure ulcers (NPUAP, 1995b). However, it is generally agreed that more than staging or color classification should be used to fully describe the pressure ulcer and to give it a comprehensive description (Rodeheaver and Stotts, 1995) and that staging systems should not be used to measure healing.

WOUND CLASSIFICATIONS

A **wound** is a disruption of normal anatomical structure and function that results from pathological processes beginning internally or externally to the involved organ(s) (Lazarus and others, 1994). Although at first assessment a wound may look like any other wound, it is imperative for the nurse to know that *all wounds are not created equal.* Understanding the etiology of a wound is important, since the treatment for the wound varies depending on the underlying disease process. Some treatments may even be harmful to certain wounds, so the nurse should always know the complete history, including the etiology of the wound. Stotts and Cavanaugh (1999) suggest that five questions (regarding wound etiology, occurrence, chronology, aggravating and alleviating factors, and associated symptoms) be included in the nursing assessment of a wound's history (Box 47-4, p. 1554).

There are many ways to classify wounds. Wound classification systems describe the status of skin integrity, cause of the wound, severity or extent of tissue injury or damage, cleanliness of the wound, or descriptive qualities of the wound such as color (Table 47-1; see also Figure 47-7). These classifications overlap. For example, a penetrating knife wound is also an open wound, and a contused wound is a closed wound.

Wound classifications enable the nurse to understand the risks associated with a wound and implications for its

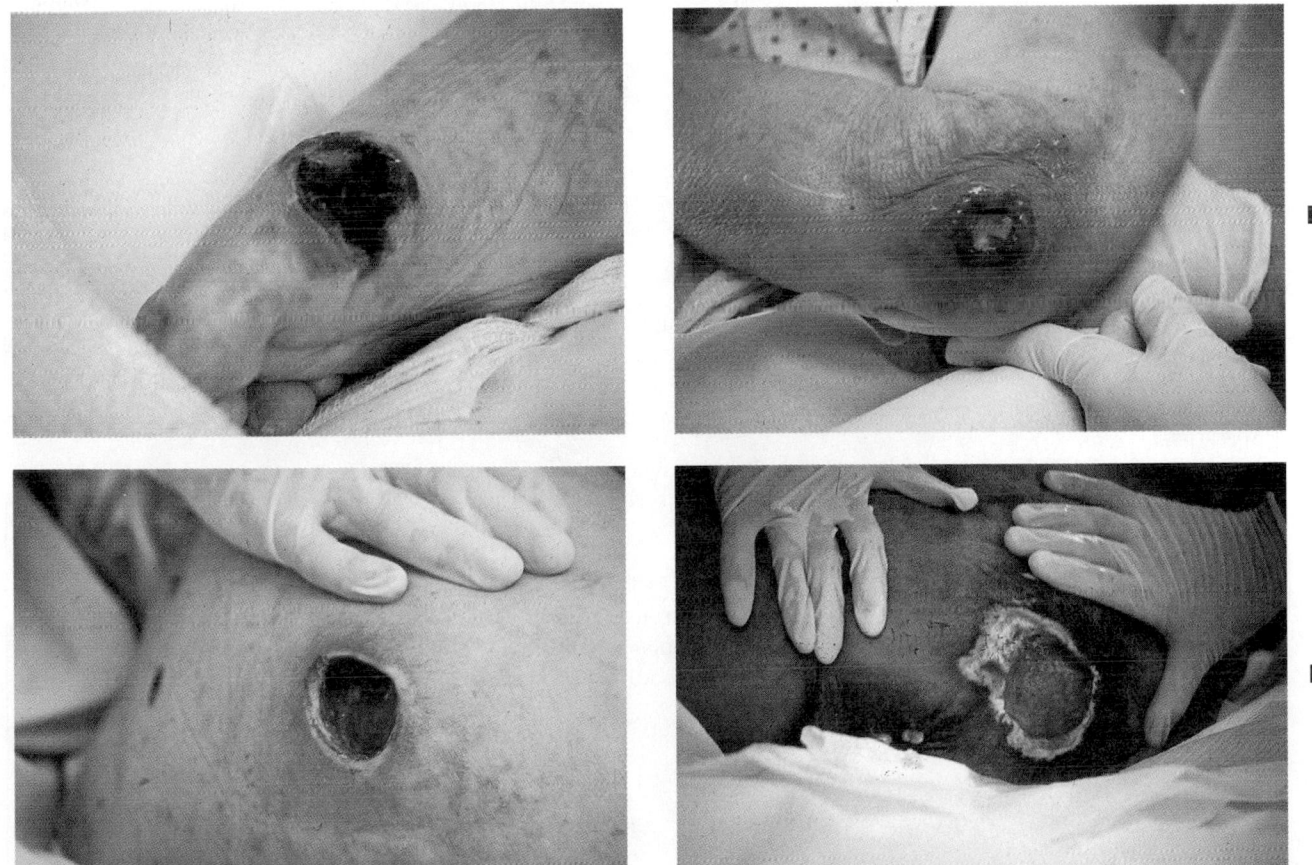

Figure 47-7 Wounds classified by color assessment. **A,** A "black" wound. **B,** A "yellow" wound. **C,** A "red" wound. **D,** A mixed-color wound. Courtesy Scott Health Care—A Molnlyche Company, Philadelphia.

Table 47-1   Wound Classification

Description	Causes	Implications for Healing
Status of Skin Integrity		
OPEN		
Wound involving a break in skin or mucous membranes	Trauma by sharp object or blow (surgical incision, venipuncture, gunshot wound)	Break in skin exposes body to invasion by microorganisms. Loss of blood and body fluids through wound occurs. Function of body part is reduced.
CLOSED		
Wound involving no break in skin	Part of body being struck by blunt object; twisting, straining, or deceleration force against body (bone fracture, tear of visceral organ)	Wound may predispose person to internal hemorrhage. Function of affected body part is reduced.
ACUTE		
Wound that proceeds through an orderly and timely reparative process that results in sustained restoration of anatomical and functional integrity	Trauma from a sharp object	Wounds are usually easily cleaned and repaired. Wound edges are clean and intact.
CHRONIC		
Wound that fails to proceed through an orderly and timely process to produce anatomical and functional integrity	Ulcers, sores exposed to friction, secretions, pressure	Continued exposure to pressure, friction, and secretions impedes wound healing. Wound edges may be necrotic, and drainage may be present.
Cause		
INTENTIONAL		
Wound resulting from therapy	Surgical incision; introduction of needle into body part	Incision is usually performed under aseptic technique to minimize chance of infection. Wound edges are usually smooth and clean.
UNINTENTIONAL		
Wound that occurs unexpectedly	Traumatic injury (knife wound, burn)	Wound occurs under unsterile conditions. Wound edges are often jagged.
Severity of Injury		
SUPERFICIAL		
Wound that involves only epidermal layer of skin	Result of friction applied to skin surface (abrasion, first-degree burn, shearing)	Break creates risk of infection. Wound does not involve underlying injury to tissues or organs. Blood supply to area is intact.
PENETRATING		
Wound involving break in epidermal skin layer, as well as dermis and deeper tissues or organs	Foreign object or instrument entering deep into body tissues; usually unintentional (gunshot wound, stab wound)	There is high risk of infection because foreign object is contaminated. Wound may cause internal and external hemorrhage; damage to organs causes temporary or permanent loss of function.
PERFORATING		
Penetrating wound in which foreign object enters and exits an internal organ	(See above entry.)	There is high risk of infection. Nature of injury depends on organ perforated (lung, compromised oxygenation; major vessel, hemorrhage; intestine, contamination of abdominal cavity by feces).

Table 47-1 **Wound Classification**—cont'd

Description	Causes	Implications for Healing
Cleanliness		
CLEAN		
Wound containing no pathogenic organisms	Closed surgical wound not entering gastrointestinal, respiratory, genital, or uninfected urinary tract or oropharyngeal cavity	There is low risk of infection.
CLEAN-CONTAMINATED		
Wound made under aseptic conditions but involving body cavity that normally harbors microorganisms	Surgical wound entering gastrointestinal, respiratory, genital, or urinary tract or oropharyngeal cavity under controlled conditions	There is greater risk of infection than with clean wound.
CONTAMINATED		
Wound existing under conditions in which presence of microorganisms is likely	Open, traumatic, accidental wounds; surgical wound in which break in asepsis occurred	Tissues are often not healthy and show inflammation. There is high risk of infection.
INFECTED		
Bacterial organisms present in wound site, usually above 10^5 organisms per gram of tissue	Any wound that does not properly heal and grows organisms, old traumatic wound, surgical incision into area infected (e.g., ruptured bowel)	Wound presents signs of infection (inflammation, purulent drainage, skin separation).
COLONIZED		
Wound containing microorganisms (usually multiple)	Chronic wound (vascular stasis ulcer, pressure ulcer)	Wound healing is slow, and high risk of infection exists.
Descriptive Qualities		
LACERATION		
Tearing of tissues with irregular wound edges	Severe traumatic injury (knife wound, industrial accident involving machinery, tissues cut by broken glass)	Wound is usually created by contaminated object. Depth of wound determines other complications.
ABRASION		
Superficial wound involving scraping or rubbing of skin's surface	Wound often resulting from fall (skinned knee or elbow); wound also resulting from dermatological procedure for removing scar tissue	Wound is painful from exposure of superficial nerves; deeper tissues are not involved. There is risk of infection from exposure to contaminated surface.
CONTUSION		
Closed wound caused by a blow to body by blunt object; contusion or bruise characterized by swelling, discoloration, and pain	Bleeding in underlying tissues caused by blunt force against body part	Wound is more severe if internal organ is contused. Wound may cause temporary loss of function of body part. Localized bleeding into tissues may form hematoma (collection of blood).

Modified from Stotts NA, Cavanaugh CE: Assessing the patient with a wound, *Home Healthcare Nurse* 17(1):27, 1999.

care. An open wound, for example, presents a greater risk of infection than a closed wound, whereas an abrasion requires less extensive dressings than a deeply penetrating wound. It is important for the nurse to understand the difference between acute and chronic wounds. Acute wounds follow the normal healing process in an orderly and timely way (Krasner, 1999). Examples of some acute wounds are those caused by trauma or surgery. In chronic wounds the healing trajectory is delayed, repair fails to occur, and return to normal function is slowed (Krasner, 1999). Chronic wounds such as peripheral vascular venous ulcers, peripheral vascular arterial ulcers, neuropathic ulcers, and pressure ulcers take much longer to heal and can be a nursing challenge.

Process of Wound Healing.

Wound healing involves integrated physiological processes. The nature of healing is the same for all wounds, with variations depending on the location, severity, and extent of injury. The ability of cells and tissues to regenerate or return to normal structure by cell growth also affects healing. Cells of the liver, renal tubules, and neurons of the central nervous system typically regenerate slowly or not at all.

There are two types of wounds: those with loss of tissue and those without. A clean surgical incision is an example of a wound with little tissue loss. The surgical wound heals by **primary intention.** The skin edges **approximate,** or close together, and the risk of infection is low. Healing occurs quickly; drainage stops by day 3 of closure (unless a drain is present), the wound is epithelialized by day 4, inflammation is present up to day 5, and the healing ridge is present by day 9 (Stotts and Cavanaugh, 1999). In contrast, a wound involving loss of tissue, such as a burn, pressure ulcer, or severe laceration, heals by **secondary intention.** The wound edges do not approximate. The wound is left open until it becomes filled by scar tissue. It takes longer for a wound to heal by secondary intention, and thus the chance of infection is greater. If scar-

ring from secondary intention is severe, there may be permanent loss of tissue function.

Healing by Primary Intention.

An example of the normal healing process is repair of a clean surgical wound. Healing occurs in several stages, described as inflammatory, proliferative, and maturation, or as the three *R*s: reaction, regeneration, and remodeling (Krasner, 1995a).

Inflammatory Phase (Reaction). The inflammation stage is the body's reaction to wounding and begins within minutes of injury and lasts about 3 days. Reparative processes control bleeding (hemostasis), deliver blood and cells to the injured area (inflammation), and form epithelial cells at the injury site, or **epithelialization.** During **hemostasis,** injured blood vessels constrict, and platelets gather to stop bleeding. Clots form a **fibrin** matrix that later provides a framework for cellular repair. Damaged tissue and mast cells secrete histamine, resulting in vasodilation of surrounding capillaries and exudation of serum and white blood cells into damaged tissues. This results in localized redness, edema, warmth, and throbbing. The inflammatory response is beneficial, and there is no value in attempting to cool the area or reduce the swelling unless the swelling occurs within a closed compartment (e.g., ankle or neck).

Leukocytes (white blood cells) reach the wound within a few hours. The primary acting white blood cell is the neutrophil, which begins to ingest bacteria and small debris. The neutrophils die in a few days and leave behind an enzyme **exudate** that attacks bacteria or interferes with tissue repair. In chronic inflammation the dying neutrophils create pus. The second important leukocyte is the monocyte, which transforms into macrophages. The macrophages are the "garbage cells" that clean a wound of bacteria, dead cells, and debris by phagocytosis. The macrophages also digest and recycle substances, such as amino acids and sugars, that aid in wound repair. Macrophages continue the process of clearing the wound of debris, attracting further macrophages, and stimulating the formation of **fibroblasts,** the cells that synthesize collagen. Collagen can be found as early as the second day and is the main component of scar tissue.

After the macrophages clean the wound and make it ready for tissue repair, epithelial cells move from the wound margins under the base of the clot or scab. Epithelial cells continue to gather under the wound space for about 48 hours. Eventually a thin layer of epithelial tissue forms over the wound as a barrier against infectious organisms and toxic materials. Growth hormones are released by platelets and macrophages. There is increasing evidence that these factors promote wound healing.

The inflammatory phase is prolonged and repair processes are slowed if too little inflammation occurs, as in debilitating disease or after administration of steroids. Too much inflammation also prolongs healing because arriving cells compete for available nutrients.

Proliferative Phase (Regeneration). With the appearance of new blood vessels as reconstruction progresses, the proliferative phase begins and lasts from 3 to 24 days. The main activities during this regeneration phase are the filling in of the wound with new connective or granulation tissue and the closing of the top of the wound by epithelization. Fibroblasts are the cells that synthesize collagen, which will close the wound. Fibroblasts require vitamins B and C, oxygen, and amino acids to function properly. Collagen provides strength and structural integrity to a wound. During this period the wound begins to close with new tissue. As reconstruction progresses, the tensile strength of the wound increases and the risk of wound separation or rupture is less likely. The degree of stress on a wound influences the amount of scar tissue formed. For example, more scar tissue forms in an extremity wound than in a less mobile area such as the scalp or chest. Impairment of healing during this stage usually results from systemic factors such as age, anemia, hypoproteinemia, and zinc deficiency.

Maturation (Remodeling). Maturation, the final stage of healing, may take more than a year, depending on the depth and extent of the wound. The collagen scar continues to reorganize and gain strength for several months. However, a healed wound usually does not have the strength of the tissue it replaces (tensile strength). Collagen fibers undergo remodeling or reorganization before assuming their normal appearance. Usually scar tissue contains fewer pigmented cells (melanocytes) and has a lighter color than normal skin.

Healing by Secondary Intention.

When tissue loss in a wound is extensive, wound healing takes longer. A large open wound typically drains more fluid than a closed wound. Inflammation is often chronic, and tissue defects become filled with fragile granulation tissue rather than collagen. **Granulation tissue** is a form of connective tissue that has a more abundant blood supply than collagen. Because the wound is larger, the amount of connective tissue scarring is larger.

When epithelial and connective tissue cells are unable to close a wound defect, contraction may occur. **Wound contraction** involves movement of the dermis and epidermis on each side of the wound. The mechanism of contracture is not completely understood. It is known, however, that collagen is not essential and that any event that interferes with cell viability at the wound margin inhibits contraction. Wound contraction begins on about the fourth day and occurs simultaneously with epithelization. The cell that provides the motive force is the myofibroblast. Wound contraction results in thinning of surround-ing tissues, and the size and shape of the final scar correspond to tension lines in the damaged area. For example, a square wound in the abdomen assumes the shape of two Ys, end to end. There are areas of the body where contraction gives poor results, such as wounds on the face, sternum, and anterior lower leg. Wound contraction is not the same as a contracture or deformity resulting from muscle shortening and joint fixation.

Complications of Wound Healing

Hemorrhage. **Hemorrhage,** or bleeding from a wound site, is normal during and immediately after the initial trauma. Hemostasis occurs within several minutes unless large blood vessels are involved or the client has poor clotting function. Hemorrhage occurring after hemostasis indicates a slipped surgical suture, a dislodged clot, infection, or erosion of a blood vessel by a foreign object (e.g., a drain). Hemorrhage may occur externally or internally. For example, if a surgical suture slips off a blood vessel, bleeding occurs internally within the tissues, and there are no visible signs of blood unless a surgical drain is present, which is inserted into tissues beneath a wound to remove fluid that collects in underlying tissues. The nurse can detect internal bleeding by looking for distention or swelling of the affected body part, a change in the type and amount of drainage from a surgical drain, or signs of **hypovolemic shock.** A **hematoma** is a localized collection of blood underneath the tissues. It appears as a swelling or mass that often takes on a bluish discoloration. A hematoma near a major artery or vein is dangerous because pressure from the expanding hematoma may obstruct blood flow.

External hemorrhaging is more obvious. The nurse observes dressings covering the wound for bloody drainage. If bleeding is extensive, the dressing soon becomes saturated, and frequently blood escapes along the sides of the dressing and pools beneath the client. The nurse observes all wounds closely, particularly surgical wounds, in which the risk of hemorrhage is great during the first 24 to 48 hours after surgery.

Infection. Wound infection is the second most common **nosocomial** (hospital-related) **infection** (see Chapter 33). According to the Centers for Disease Control and Prevention (CDC) (Garner, 1985), a wound is infected if purulent material drains from it, even if a culture is not taken or has negative results. A sample of drainage from an infected wound may not reveal bacteria due to poor culture technique or administration of antibiotics. Positive culture findings do not always indicate an infection because many wounds contain colonies of noninfective resident bacteria. In fact, all chronic dermal wounds are considered contaminated with bacteria. What differentiates contaminated wounds from infected wounds is the amount of bacteria present. It is generally agreed that wounds with more than 100,000 (10^5) organisms per milliliter are infected. The only exception is when the organism is beta-hemolytic streptococcus; the presence of this organism in colony counts of less than 100,000 (10^5) organisms per milliliter is considered an infection (Doughty, 1992). The chances of wound infection are greater when the wound contains dead or necrotic tissue, there are foreign bodies in or near the wound, and the blood supply and local tissue defenses are reduced. Bacterial wound infection inhibits wound healing.

A contaminated or traumatic wound may show signs of infection early, within 2 to 3 days. A surgical wound infection usually does not develop until the fourth or fifth postoperative day. The client has a fever, tenderness and pain at the wound site, and an elevated white blood cell count. The edges of the wound may appear inflamed. If drainage is present, it is odorous and **purulent,** which causes a yellow, green, or brown color, depending on the causative organism (Table 47-2).

Dehiscence.   When a wound fails to heal properly, the layers of skin and tissue may separate. This most commonly occurs before collagen formation (3 to 11 days after injury). **Dehiscence** is the partial or total separation of wound layers. A client who is a risk for poor wound healing (e.g., poor nutritional status, infection, obesity) is at risk for dehiscence. However, obese clients have a higher risk because of the constant strain placed on their wounds and the poor healing qualities of fatty tissue. Dehiscence often involves abdominal surgical wounds and occurs after a sudden strain, such as coughing, vomiting, or sitting up in bed. Clients often report feeling as though something has given way. When there is an increase in serosanguineous drainage from a wound, the nurse should be alert for the potential for dehiscence.

Evisceration.   With total separation of wound layers, **evisceration** (protrusion of visceral organs through a wound opening) may occur. The condition is a medical emergency that requires surgical repair. When evisceration occurs, the nurse places sterile towels soaked in sterile saline over the extruding tissues to reduce chances of bacterial invasion and drying. If the organs protrude through the wound, blood supply to the tissues is compromised. The client should be kept NPO, observed for signs and symptoms of shock, and prepared for emergency surgery.

Fistulas.   A **fistula** is an abnormal passage between two organs or between an organ and the outside of the body. A surgeon may create a fistula for therapeutic purposes (e.g., making an opening between the stomach and the outer abdominal wall to insert a gastrostomy tube for feeding). Most fistulas, however, form as a result of poor wound healing or as a complication of disease, such as Crohn's disease or regional enteritis. Trauma, infection, radiation exposure, and diseases such as cancer prevent tissue layers

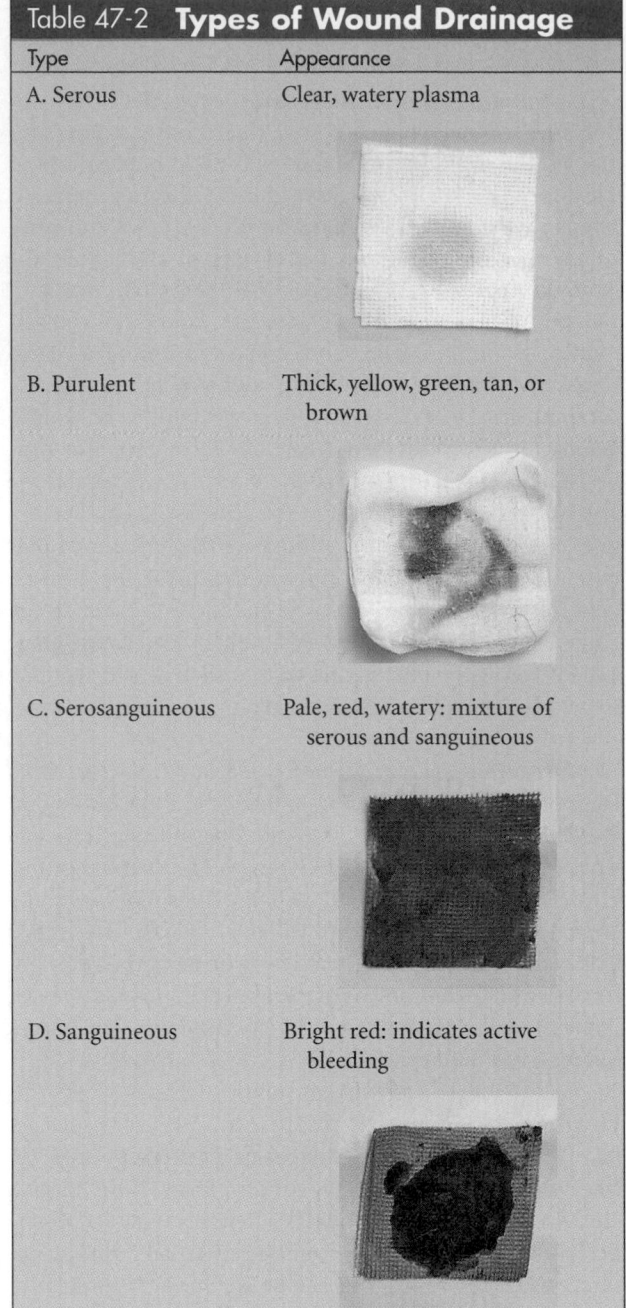

Table 47-2	**Types of Wound Drainage**
Type	Appearance
A. Serous	Clear, watery plasma
B. Purulent	Thick, yellow, green, tan, or brown
C. Serosanguineous	Pale, red, watery: mixture of serous and sanguineous
D. Sanguineous	Bright red: indicates active bleeding

from closing properly and allow the fistula tract to form. Fistulas increase the risk of infection and fluid and electrolyte imbalances from fluid loss. Chronic drainage of fluids through a fistula can also predispose a person to skin breakdown (Box 47-5).

Delayed Wound Closure.   Sometimes referred to as third-intention wound healing, delayed wound closure is a deliberate attempt by the surgeon to allow effective drainage and cleansing of a clean-contaminated or contaminated wound. The wound is not closed until all evidence of edema and wound debris has been removed. A

NPO do not take by mouth

Risks for Skin Breakdown From Body Fluids	Box 47-5
LOW RISK Saliva Serosanguineous drainage **HIGH RISK** Gastric drainage Pancreatic drainage	**MODERATE RISK** Bile Stool Urine Ascitic fluid Purulent exudate

dressing is used to prevent bacterial contamination of the wound. Then the wound is closed as in primary closure, or first intention. Experimentally, it has been demonstrated that scarring or delayed healing does not significantly increase when this technique is used (Cooper, 1992a, b).

Nursing Knowledge Base

PREDICTION AND PREVENTION OF PRESSURE ULCERS

A major aspect of nursing care is the maintenance of skin integrity. Consistent, planned skin care interventions are critical to ensuring high quality in care (Hoff, 1989). Nurses constantly observe their clients' skin for breaks or impairment in skin integrity. Impaired skin integrity occurs from prolonged pressure, irritation of the skin, or immobility, leading to the development of pressure ulcers.

A pressure ulcer is a localized area of tissue necrosis (death) that tends to develop when soft tissue is compressed between a bony prominence and an external surface for a prolonged period (NPUAP, 1989a). Nursing care interventions aimed at the prevention, assessment, and treatment of pressure ulcers should be based on research (AHCPR, 1992a, 1994).

Risk Assessment.   There are several instruments for assessing clients who are at high risk for developing a pressure ulcer. Clients with little risk for pressure ulcer development are spared the unnecessary and sometimes costly preventive treatments and the related risk of complications (Stotts, 1988). Prevention and treatment of pressure

ulcers are major nursing priorities. The ability to identify clients at risk helps contain health care costs (Norton, McLaren, and Exon-Smith, 1962; Gosnell, 1973). Several risk assessment scales (Norton, McLaren, and Exon-Smith, 1962; Gosnell, 1973; Bergstrom and others, 1987) developed by nurses enable them to systematically assess their clients. Both the Norton Scale and the Braden Scale are mentioned in the AHCPR guidelines (1992a) as being valid tools to use for pressure ulcer risk assessment. Each tool has a different number of risk factors (5 to 8 items) that are ranked by number. The client's risk assessment score is obtained by adding the individual number given for each risk factor. Interpretation of the meaning of the numerical score differs with each scale.

Norton Scale.   The first scale reported in the literature is the Norton Scale (Norton, McLaren, and Exon-Smith, 1962) (Table 47-3). It scores five risk factors: physical condition, mental condition, activity, mobility, and incontinence. The total score ranges from 5 to 20; a lower score indicates a higher risk for pressure ulcer development.

Gosnell Scale.   Based on the Norton Scale, the original Gosnell Scale (Gosnell, 1973) was developed from research on 30 clients in a nursing home. *Nutrition* replaced Norton's category of *physical condition*, and *incontinence* was renamed *continence*. Demographic data, clinical items, and narrative criteria guidelines were also added. The scale scores five factors: mental status, continence, mobility, activity, and nutrition (Table 47-4). The total score ranges from 5 to 20; a higher total score indicates risk for pressure ulcer development (Gosnell, 1987, 1989a, 1989b).

Braden Scale.   The last instrument is the Braden Scale (Table 47-5), which was developed based on risk factors in a nursing home population (Bergstrom and others, 1987). The Braden Scale is composed of six subscales: sensory perception, moisture, activity, mobility, nutrition, friction and shear. The total score ranges from 6 to 23; a lower total score indicates a higher risk for pressure ulcer development (Braden and Bergstrom, 1989). The cutoff score for

Table 47-3 **Norton Scale**											
		Physical Condition		Mental Condition		Activity		Mobility		Incontinent	
		Good	4	Alert	4	Ambulant	4	Full	4	Not	4	
		Fair	3	Apathetic	3	Walk/help	3	Slightly limited	3	Occasional	3	
		Poor	2	Confused	2	Chair bound	2	Very limited	2	Usually/urine	2	TOTAL
Name	Date	Very bad	1	Stupor	1	Bed	1	Immobile	1	Doubly	1	SCORE

Modified from Centre for Policy on Ageing: London, England, 1962.

Table 47-4   Gosnell Score: Pressure Sore Risk Assessment (Part1)

I.D. _____   Medical Diagnosis: _____

Age _____ Sex _____   Primary _____

Height _____ Weight _____   Secondary _____

Date of Admission _____   Nursing Diagnosis: _____

Date of Discharge _____   _____

Instructions: Complete all categories within 24 hours of admission and every other day thereafter. Refer to the accompanying guidelines for specific rating details.

Date	Mental Status*	Continence*	Mobility*	Activity*	Nutrition*	TOTAL SCORE
	1. Alert 2. Apathetic 3. Confused 4. Stuporous 5. Unconscious	1. Fully controlled 2. Usually controlled 3. Minimally controlled 4. Absence of control	1. Full 2. Slightly limited 3. Very limited 4. Immobile	1. Ambulatory 2. Walks with assistance 3. Chairfast 4. Bedfast	1. Good 2. Fair 3. Poor	

Pressure Sore Risk Assessment Medication Profile

Medication	Dosage	Frequency†	Route	Date Begun	Date Discontinued

Courtesy Davina Gosnell, RN, PhD.

*See Part 3, p. 1560, for guidelines for rating.

†If prn, record pattern for past 48 hours.

onset of risk with the Braden Scale varies depending on the population. Hospitalized adults with a score of 16 or below and older clients with a score of 17 or 18 are considered at risk (Bryant, 1992; Braden and Bergstrom, 1994). For black and Latino clients with darkly pigmented skin, a score of 17 or 18 has been suggested (Lyder and others, 1998). The Braden Scale is highly reliable when used to identify clients at greatest risk for pressure ulcers (Bergstrom and others, 1987; Braden and Bergstrom, 1994). The Braden Scale is the most widely used scale for pressure ulcer risk.

Prevention.   The prevention of pressure ulcers is a priority in caring for clients and is not limited to clients with restrictions in mobility. Impaired skin integrity may not be a problem in healthy, immobilized individuals but is a serious and potentially devastating problem in ill or debilitated clients (AHCPR, 1992a).

Economic Consequences of Pressure Ulcers. Pressure ulcers are a continual problem in acute and restorative care settings. Prevalence refers to the "number of cases present in a population at one point in time" (AHCPR, 1994). The prevalence rates vary among different client settings. Reported prevalence rates in the acute hospital setting range between 3% and 11% (Allman, 1989), 14% (Langemo and others, 1989), and 20% (Leshem and Skelskey, 1994). Prevalence rates in the restorative and long-term care settings have ranged from 3.5% (Leshem and Skelskey, 1994), to 23% (Langemo and others, 1989; Young, 1989). There is a lack of clarity about the prevalence of pressure ulcers among persons being cared for in the home without supervision or assistance of professionals (AHCPR, 1994). In the home care setting, prevalence rates have been reported to be 12.9% (Hentzen, Bergstrom, and Pozehl, 1993) and 19% (Hanson and others, 1993).

Table 47-4   Gosnell Scale: Pressure Sore Risk Assessment—cont'd (Part 2)

	Vital Signs				Diet	24-Hour Fluid Balance		Color 1. Pallor 2. Mottled 3. Pink 4. Ashen 5. Ruddy 6. Cyanotic 7. Jaundice 8. Other	General Skin Appearance				Interventions		
									Moisture 1. Dry 2. Damp 3. Oily 4. Other	Temperature 1. Cold 2. Cool 3. Warm 4. Hot	Texture 1. Smooth 2. Rough 3. Thin/transparent 4. Scaly 5. Crusty 6. Other				
Date	T	P	R	BP	Diet	Intake	Output						No	Yes	Describe

Vital signs: The temperature, pulse, respiration, and blood pressure to be taken and recorded at the time of every assessment rating.

Skin appearance: A description of observed skin characteristics: color, moisture, temperature, and texture.

Diet: Record the specific diet order.

24-hour fluid balance: The amount of fluid intake and output during the previous 24-hour period should be recorded.

Interventions: List all devices, measures, and/or nursing care activity being used for the purpose of pressure sore prevention.

Medications: List name, dosage, frequency, and route for all prescribed medications. If a prn order, list the pattern for the period since last assessment.

Comments: Use this space to add explanation or further detail regarding any of the previously recorded data, patient condition, etc.
                       or
                       Describe anything that you believe to be of importance but not accounted for previously.

NOTE: For any item marked "other," please describe.

If any signs of pressure, etc., on bony prominences or other body parts are observed, please describe in detail the location, color, temperature, moisture, texture, and size and any other pertinent items.

Continued

Table 47-4 **Gosnell Scale: Pressure Sore Risk Assessment**—cont'd (Part 3)

Guidelines for Numerical Rating of the Defined Categories

Rating	1	2	3	4	5
Mental Status An assessment of one's level of response to the environment.	**Alert** Oriented to time, place, and person. Responsive to all stimuli and understands explanations.	**Apathetic** Lethargic, forgetful, drowsy, passive, and dull. Sluggish, depressed. Able to obey simple commands. Possibly disoriented to time.	**Confused** Partial and/or intermittent disorientation to time, place and person. Purposeless response to stimuli. Restless, aggressive, irritable, anxious, and may require tranquilizers or sedatives.	**Stuporous** Total disorientation. Does not respond to name, simple commands, or verbal stimuli.	**Unconscious** Nonresponsive to painful stimuli.
Continence The amount of bodily control or urination and defecation.	**Fully Controlled** Total control of urine and feces.	**Usually Controlled** Incontinent of urine and/or of feces not more often than once every 48 hours or has Foley catheter and is incontinent of feces.	**Minimally Controlled** Incontinent of urine or feces at least once every 24 hours.	**Absence of Control** Consistently incontinent of both urine and feces.	
Mobility The amount and control of movement of one's body.	**Full** Able to control and move all extremities at will. May require the use of a device but turns, lifts, pulls, balances, and attains sitting position at will.	**Slightly Limited** Able to control and move all extremities but a degree of limitation is present. Requires assistance of another person to turn, pull, balance, and/or attain a sitting position at will but self-initiates movement or requests for help to move.	**Very Limited** Can assist another person, who must initiate movement via turning, lifting, pulling, balancing, and/or attaining a sitting position (contractures, paralysis may be present).	**Immobile** Does not assist self in any way to change position. Is unable to change position without assistance. Is completely dependent on others for movement.	
Activity The ability of an individual to ambulate.	**Ambulatory** Is able to walk unassisted. Rises from bed unassisted. With the use of a device such as cane or walker is able to ambulate without the assistance of another person.	**Walks With Help** Able to ambulate with assistance of another person, braces, or crutches. May have limitation of stairs.	**Chairfast** Ambulates only to a chair, requires assistance to do so or is confined to a wheelchair.	**Bedfast** Is confined to bed during entire 24 hours of the day.	
Nutrition The process of food intake.	Eats some food from each basic food category every day and the majority of each meal served or is on tube feeding.	Occasionally refuses a meal or frequently leaves at least half of a meal.	Seldom eats a complete meal and only a few bites of food at a meal.		

Table 47-5 Braden Scale for Predicting Pressure Sore Risk

Patient's Name _____ Evaluator's Name _____ Date of Assessment

Sensory Perception Ability to respond meaningfully to pressure-related discomfort	1. **Completely limited** Unresponsive (does not moan, flinch, or grasp) to painful stimuli due to diminished level of consciousness or sedation. OR Limited ability to feel pain over most of body surface.	2. **Very limited** Responds only to painful stimuli. Cannot communicate discomfort except by moaning or restlessness. OR Has a sensory impairment which limits the ability to feel pain or discomfort over ½ of body.	3. **Slightly limited** Responds to verbal commands, but cannot always communicate discomfort or need to be turned. OR Has some sensory impairment that limits ability to feel pain or discomfort in 1 or 2 extremities.	4. **No impairment** Responds to verbal commands. Has no sensory deficit that would limit ability to feel or voice pain or discomfort.
Moisture Degree to which skin is exposed to moisture	1. **Constantly moist** Skin is kept moist almost constantly by perspiration, urine, etc. Dampness is detected every time patient is moved or turned.	2. **Very moist** Skin is often, but not always, moist. Linen must be changed at least once a shift.	3. **Occasionally moist** Skin is occasionally moist, requiring an extra linen change approximately once a day.	4. **Rarely moist** Skin is usually dry, linen only requires changing at routine intervals.
Activity Degree of physical activity	1. **Bedfast** Confined to bed.	2. **Chairfast** Ability to walk severely limited or nonexistent. Cannot bear own weight and/or must be assisted into chair or wheelchair.	3. **Walks occasionally** Walks occasionally during day, but for very short distances, with or without assistance. Spends majority of each shift in bed or chair.	4. **Walks frequently** Walks outside the room at least twice a day and inside room at least once every 2 hours during waking hours.
Mobility Ability to change and control body position	1. **Completely immobile** Does not make even slight changes in body or extremity position without assistance.	2. **Very limited** Makes occasional slight changes in body or extremity position but unable to make frequent or significant changes independently.	3. **Slightly limited** Makes frequent though slight changes in body or extremity position independently.	4. **No limitations** Makes major and frequent changes in position without assistance.

Courtesy Barbara Braden and Nancy Bergstrom.

Continued

Table 47-5   Braden Scale for Predicting Pressure Sore Risk—cont'd

Nutrition *Usual* food intake pattern	1. Very poor Never eats a complete meal. Rarely eats more than ⅓ of any food offered. Eats 2 servings or less of protein (meat or dairy products) per day. Takes fluids poorly. Does not take a liquid dietary supplement. OR Is NPO and/or maintained on clear liquids or IVs for more than 5 days.	2. Probably inadequate Rarely eats a complete meal and generally eats only about ½ of any food offered. Protein intake includes only 3 servings of meat or dairy products per day. Occasionally will take a dietary supplement. OR Receives less than optimum amount of liquid diet or tube feeding.	3. Adequate Eats over half of most meals. Eats a total of 4 servings of protein (meat, dairy products) each day. Occasionally will refuse a meal, but will usually take a supplement if offered. OR Is on a tube feeding or total parenteral nutrition regimen that probably meets most of nutritional needs.	4. Excellent Eats most of every meal. Never refuses a meal. Usually eats a total of 4 or more servings of meat and dairy products. Occasionally eats between meals. Does not require supplementation.	
Friction and Shear	1. Problem Requires moderate to maximum assistance in moving. Complete lifting without sliding against sheets is impossible. Frequently slides down in bed or chair, requiring frequent repositioning with maximum assistance. Spasticity, contractures, or agitation leads to almost constant friction.	2. Potential problem Moves feebly or requires minimum assistance. During a move skin probably slides to some extent against sheets, chair, restraints, or other devices. Maintains relatively good position in chair or bed most of the time but occasionally slides down.	3. No apparent problem Moves in bed and in chair independently and has sufficient muscle strength to lift up completely during move. Maintains good position in bed or chair at all times.		
				TOTAL SCORE	

When a pressure ulcer occurs, the length of stay in a hospital and the overall cost of health care increase (AHCPR, 1994). The actual cost of treatment is difficult to approximate. Ranges are between $5000 and $27,000, depending on the number and severity of ulcers (Stotts, 1988; Hoff, 1989; Bryant, 1992). Although treatment of pressure ulcers is more costly than prevention (Oot-Giromini and others, 1989), the preventive measures themselves are expensive. Extra equipment, such as special beds and mattresses, and increased nursing time are needed to administer these measures. When an ulcer develops, mean hospital costs ($37,288 versus $13,924) and length of stay (30.4 versus 12.8 days) are increased (Allman and others, 1999).

The AHCPR Clinical Practice Guideline No. 3 (1992a) recommends strategies for identifying at-risk individuals, implementing preventive measures, and treating early (stage I) pressure ulcers. The AHCPR Clinical Practice Guideline No. 15 (1994) provides a comprehensive plan for treating stage II, III, and IV pressure ulcers in adults by clinicians who examine and treat individuals in all health care settings. The recommendations in both guidelines are supported by research, literature, and expert opinion.

FACTORS INFLUENCING PRESSURE ULCER FORMATION AND WOUND HEALING

Impaired skin integrity resulting in pressure ulcers is primarily the result of pressure. However, additional factors can further increase the client's risk for pressure ulcer development. These include shearing and friction forces, moisture, poor nutrition, anemia, infection, fever, impaired peripheral circulation, obesity, cachexia, and age.

In addition, once a pressure ulcer is present, there are a number of factors that can influence the rate of wound healing. A client with any factors listed in Table 47-6 is at risk for wound complications. The nurse's knowledge of factors influencing healing helps in providing preventive care and selecting appropriate wound care therapies.

Shearing Force.
Shearing force is the pressure exerted against the skin in a direction parallel to the body's surface (AHCPR, 1994). It can occur when a client is moved or repositioned in bed by being pulled or being allowed to slide down in bed while in a high-Fowler's position (Figure 47-8). When a shearing force is present, the skin and subcutaneous layers adhere to the surface of the bed, and the layers of muscle and even the bones slide in the direction of body movement. The client's bone slides down into the skin and exerts a force onto the skin (Maklebust and Sieggreen, 1996). The underlying tissue capillaries are compressed and severed by the pressure. As a result, minute layers of bleeding and necrosis occur deep within the tissue layers. In addition, there is a decrease in capillary blood flow from the external pressure against the skin. Subcutaneous fat is more vulnerable to the effects of shearing and the resultant pressure from the underlying bony structure. Eventually a tract can open to the skin to allow drainage from the necrotic area. It is important to remember that shearing force injuries usually occur over bony prominences such as the sacral and coccygeal areas. These injuries involve deep tissue layers and are most often initially the size of the outline of the bone located beneath the destroyed tissue. Keeping the head of the bed be-

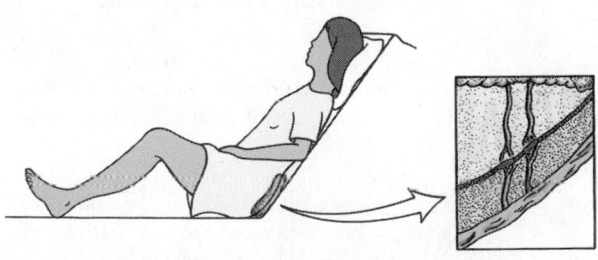

Figure 47-8 Diagrammatic sketch of shearing force exerted against sacral area.

low 30 degrees can avoid injuries from shearing forces (AHCPR, 1992a, 1994).

Friction.
Friction is the mechanical force exerted when skin is dragged across a coarse surface such as bed linens (AHCPR, 1994). Unlike shearing injuries, friction injuries affect the epidermis or top layer of the skin, which is rubbed away as the client is repositioned. They are frequently shallow abrasion injuries seen on the elbows or heels. Because of the way these wounds occur, nurses often refer to them as sheet burns (Bryant and others, 1992). They can occur in clients who are restless; in those who have uncontrollable movements, such as spastic conditions; and in those whose skin is dragged rather than lifted from the bed surface during position changes (Maklebust and Sieggreen, 1996). Nursing measures to prevent friction injuries include the following: proper transfer of clients using correct lifting techniques; using products on the elbows and heels such as sheepskin protectors, skin sealants, and transparent membrane or hydrocolloid dressings to protect the skin; and applying moisturizers to maintain the hydration of the epidermis.

Moisture.
The presence and duration of moisture on the skin increases the risk of ulcer formation. Moisture reduces the skin's resistance to other physical factors such as pressure or shearing force. Immobilized clients, who are unable to perform their own hygiene needs, depend on the nurse to keep the skin dry and intact. The nurse must therefore incorporate hygiene into the care plan. Moisture on the skin can originate from wound drainage, perspiration, condensation from humidified oxygen-delivery systems, vomitus, and incontinence. Certain body fluids (e.g., urine, stool, and wound drainage) cause skin erosion, and in the presence of pressure, the client's risk increases.

Nutrition.
For clients weakened or debilitated by illness, nutritional therapy is especially important. A client who has undergone surgery (see Chapter 49) and is well nourished still requires at least 1500 kcal/day for nutritional maintenance. Alternatives such as enteral feedings (see Chapter 43) and parenteral nutrition (see Chapter 40) are made available for clients unable to maintain normal food intake.

Normal wound healing requires proper nutrition (Table 47-7). Physiological processes of wound healing depend on the ready availability of protein, vitamins (especially A and C), and the trace minerals zinc and copper. Collagen is a protein formed from amino acids acquired by fibroblasts from protein ingested in food. Vitamin C is needed for synthesis of collagen. Vitamin A reduces the negative effects of steroids on wound healing. Trace elements are also needed, zinc is needed for epithelization and collagen synthesis, and copper is necessary for collagen fiber linking. Supplementation of vitamins and minerals to accelerate wound healing without a deficiency

Table 47-6   Factors That Impair Wound Healing

Physiological Effects	Nursing Implications
Age Aging alters all phases of wound healing. Vascular changes impair circulation to wound site. Reduced liver function alters synthesis of clotting factors. Inflammatory response is slowed. Formation of antibodies and lymphocytes is reduced. Collagen tissue is less pliable. Scar tissue is less elastic.	Instruct client on safety precautions to avoid injuries. Be prepared to provide wound care for longer period. Teach support persons in home wound care techniques.
Malnutrition All phases of wound healing are impaired. Stress from burns or severe trauma increases nutritional requirements.	Provide balanced diet rich in protein, carbohydrates, lipids, vitamins A and C, and minerals (e.g., zinc, copper). Provide adequate amounts of calories and fluid.
Obesity Fatty tissue lacks adequate blood supply to resist bacterial infection and deliver nutrients and cellular elements for healing.	Observe obese client for signs of wound infection and evisceration.
Impaired Oxygenation Low arterial oxygen tension alters synthesis of collagen and formation of epithelial cells. If local circulating blood flow is poor, tissues fail to receive needed oxygen. Decreased hemoglobin in blood (anemia) reduces arterial oxygen levels in capillaries and interferes with tissue repair.	Provide diet adequate in iron, Vitamin B_{12}, and folic acid. Monitor hematocrit and hemoglobin levels of clients with wounds.
Smoking Smoking reduces amount of functional hemoglobin in blood, thus decreasing tissue oxygenation. Smoking may increase platelet aggregation and cause hypercoagulability. Smoking interferes with normal cellular mechanisms that promote release of oxygen to tissues.	Discourage client from smoking by explaining its effects on wound healing.
Drugs Steroids reduce inflammatory response and slow collagen synthesis. Antiinflammatory drugs suppress protein synthesis, wound contraction, epithelization, and inflammation. Prolonged antibiotic use may increase risk of superinfection. Chemotherapeutic drugs can depress bone marrow function, lower number of leukocytes, and impair inflammatory response.	Carefully observe clients receiving these drugs because signs of inflammation may not be obvious. Vitamin A can counteract effects of steroids.
Diabetes Chronic disease causes small blood vessel disease that impairs tissue perfusion. Diabetes causes hemoglobin to have greater affinity for oxygen, so it fails to release oxygen to tissues. Hyperglycemia alters ability of leukocytes to perform phagocytosis and also supports overgrowth of fungal and yeast infection.	Instruct diabetic clients to take preventive measures to avoid cuts or breaks in skin. Provide preventive foot care. Control blood sugar to reduce the physiological changes associated with diabetes.
Radiation Fibrosis and vascular scarring eventually develop in irradiated skin layers. Tissues become fragile and poorly oxygenated.	Closely observe clients who have surgery after radiation for wound complications.
Wound Stress Vomiting, abdominal distention, and respiratory effort may stress suture line and disrupt wound layer. Sudden, unexpected tension on incision inhibits formation of endothelial cell and collagen networks.	Control nausea with ordered antiemetics. Keep nasogastric tubes patent and draining to avoid accumulation of secretions. Instruct and help client to splint abdominal wound during coughing.

Table 47-7	**Role of Selected Nutrients in Wound Healing**		
Nutrient	Role	Recommendations	Sources
Calories	Fuel for cell energy "Protein protection"	30-35 kcal/kg/day, or enough to maintain positive nitrogen balance	
Protein	Building block for cells and tissues	1.25-1.50 g/kg/day, or enough to maintain positive nitrogen balance	
Vitamin C (ascorbic acid)	Hydroxylation of proline and lysine in collagen synthesis	RDA = 60 mg Supplement if deficient 500 mg bid Need long time to develop clinical scurvy from vitamin C deficiency Low toxicity	Citrus fruits, tomatoes, potatoes, fortified fruit juices
Vitamin A	Enhances epithelialization, collagen synthesis, and cross-linking Can reverse steroid effects on skin and delayed healing	RDA = 4000 IU Supplement if deficient 20,000U × 10 days	Green leafy vegetables (spinach), broccoli, carrots, sweet potatoes, liver
Vitamin E	No known role in wound healing	None	
Zinc	Cell mitosis and cell proliferation	RDA = 12-15 mg Correct deficiencies No improvement in wound healing with supplementation unless zinc deficient Use with caution—large doses can be toxic May inhibit copper metabolism and impair immune function	Fish, oysters, liver, dark meat, eggs, legumes
Fluid	Essential fluid environment for all cell function	30-35 ml/kg/day Increase by another 10-15 ml/kg if patient is on an air-fluidized bed Use noncaffeine, nonalcoholic fluids without sugar Water is best—6-8 glasses/day	

Modified from Ayello EA, Thomas DR, Litchford MA: Nutritional aspects of wound healing, *Home Healthcare Nurse*, (in press).

state is controversial (Ayello, Thomas, and Litchford, in press).

Clients with poor nutrition often experience serious muscle atrophy and decreases in subcutaneous tissue (see Chapter 43). Because of these changes, less tissue is present to serve as padding between the skin and underlying bone. Therefore the effects of pressure are increased on remaining tissue. Malnutrition is second only to excessive pressure in the etiology, pathogenesis, and nonhealing of pressure ulcers (NPUAP, 1989a, 1989b; Hanan and Scheele, 1991). The malnourished client can also have protein deficiency and negative nitrogen balance and have an inadequate intake of vitamin C (Shekleton and Litwack, 1991). Poor nutritional status may be overlooked if the client has a weight equal to or above the ideal body weight (IBW). The client with poor nutritional status frequently has hypoalbuminemia (serum albumin levels below 3 g/100 ml) and anemia (Steinberg, 1990).

Albumin is a frequently measured variable used to evaluate the client's protein status. A client with a serum albumin level below 3 g/100 ml is at greater risk for pressure ulcers than a client with a higher albumin level. In addition, low albumin levels are associated with poor wound healing (Pinchcofsky-Devin and Kaminski, 1989; Hanan and Scheele, 1991). Although serum albumin levels are slow to reflect changes in visceral proteins, they are good predictors of malnutrition in all age groups (Hanan and Scheele, 1991). Because of its shorter half life and less sensitivity to hydration status, prealbumin is used in some settings to monitor a client's nutritional status (Ayello, Thomas, and Litchford, in press).

Total protein levels are also correlated with pressure ulcer development. Total protein levels below 5.4 g/100 ml decrease colloid osmotic pressure, which leads to interstitial edema and decreased oxygen to the tissues (Hanan and Scheele, 1991). Edema decreases the skin and underlying tissue's tolerance to pressure, friction, and shearing force. In addition, the decreased oxygen levels increase the speed of ischemic injury to the tissue.

Poor nutrition also alters fluid and electrolyte balance. In clients with severe protein loss, hypoalbuminemia leads to a shift of fluid from the extracellular fluid volume to the tissues, resulting in edema. **Edema** increases the affected tissue's risk for pressure ulcers. The blood supply to the edematous tissue is decreased, and waste products remain because of the changing pressures in the capillary circulation and capillary bed (Shekleton and Litwack, 1991).

Clients with **anemia** are at risk for pressure ulcer formation. Decreased levels of hemoglobin reduce the oxygen-carrying capacity of the blood and the amount of oxygen available to tissues. Anemia also alters cellular metabolism and impairs wound healing.

Cachexia is generalized ill health and malnutrition, marked by weakness and emaciation. It is usually associated with severe diseases such as cancer and end-stage cardiopulmonary diseases. This condition increases the client's risk for pressure ulcers. Basically the cachexic client has lost the adipose tissue necessary to protect bony prominences from pressure.

Obesity can accelerate pressure ulcer development. Adipose tissue in small quantities protects the skin by cushioning bony prominences against pressure. However, in moderate to severe obesity, adipose tissue is poorly vascularized, and the adipose and underlying tissues are more susceptible to ischemic damage.

Infection. Infection results from the presence of pathogens in the body. A client with an infection usually has a fever. Infection and fever increase the metabolic needs of the body, making already-hypoxic (decreased oxygen) tissue more susceptible to ischemic injury (Shekleton and Litwack, 1991). In addition, fever results in diaphoresis (sweating) and increased skin moisture, which further predispose the client to skin breakdown.

Impaired Peripheral Circulation. Impaired peripheral circulation is also related to pressure ulcer development. With decreased circulation the tissue becomes hypoxic and more susceptible to ischemic damage. Impaired circulation occurs in clients who have peripheral vascular diseases, who are in shock, or who are receiving vasopressor-type medications.

Age. Older adults have a more frequent occurrence of pressure ulcers. There is a greater incidence of ulcer development in people over 75 years of age (Stotts, 1995). Some of the normal changes in aging skin account for the increased risk of pressure ulcers in older adults (see Chapter 12).

Although the rates for the stages of wound healing among older clients may be slowed, the physiological aspects of healing are unchanged from those in the younger adult. Problems that arise during healing may be difficult to assign to the aging process or to other possible causes, such as poor nutrition, environment, or individual response to stress. Before surgery, the nurse assesses any factors that may influence or alter wound healing in older clients (see Tables 47-1 and 47-2).

PSYCHOSOCIAL IMPACT OF WOUNDS

The psychosocial impact of wounds on the physiological process of healing is unknown. The client's psychological response to any wound is part of the nurse's assessment. Body image changes may impose a great stress on the client's adaptive mechanisms. In addition, body image changes influence self-concept (see Chapter 26) and sexuality (see Chapter 27). The client's personal and social resources for adaptation should also be a part of the assessment. Factors that may affect the client's perception of the wound include the presence of scars, drains (drains may be necessary for weeks or even months after certain procedures), odor from drainage, and temporary or permanent prosthetic devices.

Critical Thinking Synthesis

Successful critical thinking requires a synthesis of knowledge, experience, information gathered from clients, critical thinking attitudes, and intellectual and professional standards. Clinical judgments require the nurse to anticipate the information necessary, analyze the data, and make decisions regarding client care. Critical thinking is always changing. During assessment (Figure 47-9) the nurse must consider all elements that build toward making appropriate nursing diagnoses.

When caring for clients who have impaired skin integrity and chronic wounds, the nurse must integrate knowledge from nursing and other disciplines, previous experiences, and information gathered from clients to understand the risk to skin integrity and wound healing. Knowledge of normal musculoskeletal physiology, the pathogenesis of pressure ulcers, normal wound healing, and the pathophysiology of underlying diseases enables the nurse to have a scientific basis for care. The AHCPR guidelines for assessment of risk for impaired skin integrity, prevention measures, and interventions to promote wound healing (AHCPR, 1992a, 1994), as well as other standards of practice, should be applied. Past experience with clients at risk for impaired skin integrity or with clients with wounds increases the experiential knowledge base from which the nurse can identify interventions. Finally, the nurse must be disciplined during assessment to obtain comprehensive and correct assessment data. Another attitude that the nurse must demonstrate is one of creativity. Since chronic wounds are difficult to heal, the nurse must be diligent in evaluating nursing interventions and determining which interventions are effective and which need to be modified.

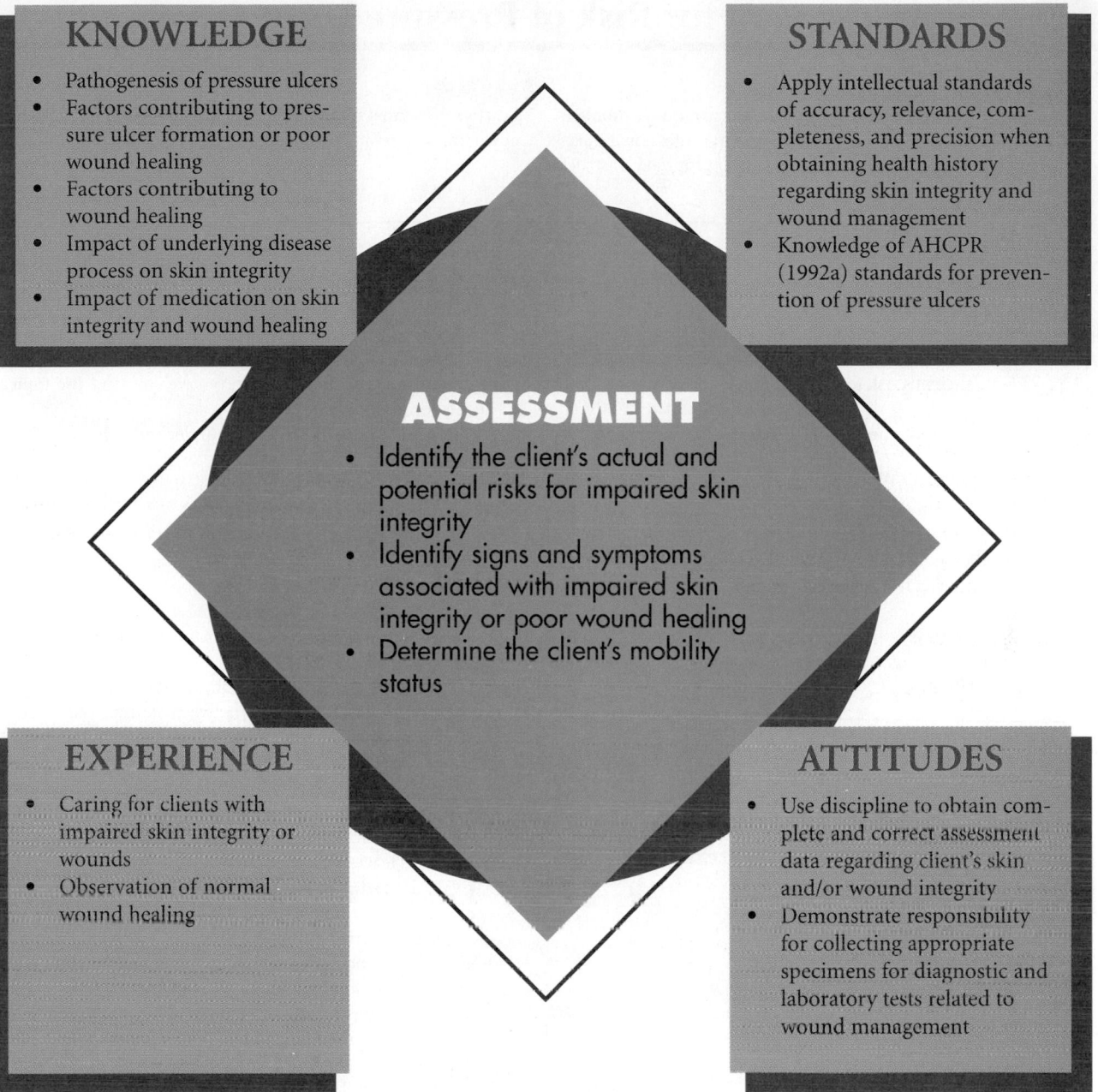

Figure 47-9 *Synthesis Model for Skin Integrity and Wound Care Assessment Phase.*

Nursing Process

ASSESSMENT

Baseline and continual assessment data provide critical information about the client's skin integrity and the increased risk for pressure ulcer development.

Pressure Ulcers.   Because pressure ulcers have multiple etiological factors, assessment for pressure ulcers (Skill 47-1) is not limited to the skin. Therefore, the initial assessment of clients with pressure ulcers has several dimensions (AHCPR, 1994).

Predictive Measures.   On admission to acute care and rehabilitation hospitals, nursing homes, home care programs, and other health care facilities, individuals should be assessed for risk of pressure ulcer development (AHCPR, 1992a). Pressure ulcer risk assessment should be done systematically (NPUAP, 1989; AHCPR, 1992a). An assessment tool that is validated for a specific type of client population is recommended (see Tables 47-3 to 47-5). Interpretation of the meaning of the total numerical scores differs with each risk assessment scale. A low numerical score on the Braden Scale or the Norton Scale in-

Skill 47-1   Assessment for Risk of Pressure Ulcer Development

Delegation Considerations

Assessment of adults for risk of pressure ulcers requires problem solving and knowledge application unique to professional nursing. For this procedure delegation is not appropriate. Instruct assistive personnel to report any changes in skin integrity to the nurse immediately.

EQUIPMENT
- Risk assessment tool
- Documentation record
- Body chart or tracing film and/or camera

STEPS	RATIONALE
1. Identify client's risk for pressure ulcer formation:	Determines need to administer preventive care and use topical agents for existing ulcers.
a. Paralysis or immobilization caused by restrictive devices	Client is unable to turn or reposition independently.
b. Sensory loss	Client feels no discomfort from pressure.
c. Circulatory disorders	Reduce perfusion of skin's tissue layers.
d. Decreased level of consciousness, sedation, or anesthesia	Client is unable to perceive pressure to turn or reposition independently.
e. Shearing force, friction	Causes skin and underlying subcutaneous layers to adhere to surface of bed. Trauma occurs to underlying tissues.
f. Moisture: incontinence, perspiration, wound drainage, or vomitus	Reduces skin's resistance to pressure from shearing force.
g. Malnutrition	Can lead to weight loss, muscle atrophy, and reduced tissue mass. Less tissue is available to pad between skin and underlying bone. Poor protein, vitamin, and caloric intake limit wound-healing capabilities.
h. Anemia	Decreased hemoglobin level reduces oxygen-carrying capacity of blood and amount of oxygen available to tissues.
i. Infection	Causes increase in metabolic demands of tissues. Accompanying diaphoresis leaves skin moist.
j. Obesity	Poorly vascularized excess adipose tissue is more susceptible to pressure. Body weight against bony prominences places underlying skin at risk for breakdown.
k. Cachexia	Causes loss of adipose tissue that protects bony prominences from pressure.
l. Hydration: edema or dehydration	Edematous tissue has decreased blood supply and thereby is less tolerant of pressure, friction, and shearing force. Dehydrated skin is less elastic, and skin turgor is poor.
m. Older adulthood	Skin is less elastic and drier; tissue mass is reduced.
n. Existing pressure ulcers	Limits surfaces available for position changes, placing available tissues at increased risk.
2. Assess condition of skin over regions of pressure. Look for the following characteristics:	
a. Normal or abnormal reactive hyperemia lasting less than 1 hour	May indicate that tissue was under pressure. Normal reactive hyperemia is normal physiological response to hypoxemia. In dark-skinned persons, skin that was under pressure will appear darker than surrounding skin and may even take on purplish hue (Pires and Muller, 1991; Bennett, 1995).
	In light-skinned client, affected area blanches at fingertip pressure (Pires and Muller, 1991).
	Abnormal reactive hyperemia lasts longer than 1 hour. Surrounding tissue does not blanch (Pires and Muller, 1991).
b. Blanching	Blanching is a normal, expected response in light-skinned clients.
c. Induration	Localized edema beneath the skin surface; induration commonly occurs with abnormal reactive hyperemia (Pires and Muller, 1991).

STEPS	RATIONALE
d. Pallor and mottling	Persistent hypoxia in tissues that were under pressure is an abnormal physiological response.
e. Absence of superficial skin layers	Represents early pressure ulcer formation.
f. Scabs, blisters, or pimples	Early signs of skin damage, but damage to underlying tissue may be more progressive (Pires and Muller, 1991).
3. Assess client for areas of potential pressure:	Clients at high risk have multiple sites of pressure necrosis.
a. Nares	Pressure can occur from nasogastric tube or nasal O_2 cannula.
b. Tongue, lips	Oral airway and endotracheal tube are high-risk locations.
c. Intravenous sites (especially long-term access sites)	Stress occurs at catheter exit sites.
d. Drainage tubes	There is stress against tissue at exit site.
e. Foley catheter	There is pressure against labia, especially with edema.
4. Observe client for preferred positions when in bed or chair	Weight of body will be placed on bony prominences. Contractures (flexion and fixation of joint) may result in pressure exerted in unexpected places. Phenomenon is best assessed through observation.
5. Observe client's mobility and ability to initiate and assist with position changes.	Potential for friction and shear increases when client is completely dependent for position changes.

6. Obtain risk score and compare with established scores.
a. Braden Scale (see Table 47-5)
     ≤ 16 = high risk
     ≤ 18 = high risk in older black and Latino adults
b. Norton Scale
     ≤ 16 = risk
	Risk score depends on instrument used and predicts client's need for preventive care (AHCPR, 1992a).

7. Help client to change position. Use the following positions: a. Supine b. Prone c. 30-degree lateral (see Figure 47-18)	Avoid positions that place client directly on an area of existing ulceration. It may be helpful to use a schedule for position changes. Achieved with one pillow under shoulder and one pillow under leg on same side. Protects sacrum and trochanters.
8. Palpate any area of discoloration or mottling. Skin temperature changes may be an important early indicator of a stage I (see Figure 47-5) pressure ulcer in clients with darkly pigmented skin (Bennett, 1995).	Early detection of pressure indicates need for more frequent position changes.
9. Monitor length of time any area of discoloration persists:	In clients with lightly pigmented skin, redness usually persists for half of time hypoxia occurred. For example, redness lasts 15 minutes, so hypoxia lasted approximately 30 minutes.
a. Determine appropriate turning interval, which should be (turning interval − hypoxia time = suggested interval).	For example, turning interval is 2 hours, and hypoxia time is 30 minutes (2 hours − 30 minutes = $1\frac{1}{2}$ hours suggested turning interval).
b. Use pressure-relief device, if indicated.	Short turning intervals (e.g., 1 to 2 hours) may not be realistic. Therefore use of device is recommended.
10. Obtain nutritional assessment data, including serum albumin level, total protein level, hemoglobin level, and IBW percentage.	Poor nutritional status decreases skin's and underlying tissue's tolerance to pressure, friction, and shearing force (AHCPR, 1994).
11. Assess client's and family's understanding of risks for pressure ulcers.	Provides opportunity to begin prevention education (Ayello, 1993, 1995).
12. Observe client's skin for areas at risk for change in color or texture.	Enables the nurse to evaluate success of prevention techniques.
13. Observe tolerance of client for position change.	Position changes may interfere with client's sleep and rest pattern.
14. Compare subsequent risk assessment scores.	Provides ongoing comparison of client's risk level to facilitate appropriateness of care plan.

Recording and Reporting
- Record client's risk score.
- Record appearance of skin under pressure.
- Describe positions, turning intervals, pressure-relieving support devices, and other prevention measures.
- Report any need for additional consultations for the high-risk client.

Home Care Considerations
- The 30-degree lateral and prone positions may be useful at night to prolong the time between position changes, resulting in less sleep disruption for the client and caregiver.
- Pressure-relief maneuvers must be customized for the independent client. The individual may find a watch with a timer, even or odd hours, and television commercials helpful in remembering to complete pressure-relief techniques.

dicates that a client is at high risk for skin breakdown. A high numerical score on the Gosnell Scale indicates high risk for skin breakdown.

A benefit of the predictive instruments is to increase the nurse's early detection of clients at greatest risk for ulcer development. Once these clients are identified, appropriate interventions are instituted to maintain skin integrity. Reassessment for pressure ulcer risk should be done periodically. Once a client is identified to be at risk for developing pressure ulcers, prevention strategies should be implemented (AHCPR, 1992a; NPUAP, 1992).

Skin. The nurse must continually assess the skin for signs of ulcer development. The neurologically impaired client; the chronically ill client in long-term care; the client with diminished mental status; and the intensive care unit (ICU), oncology, hospice, or orthopedic client have increased potential for developing pressure ulcers.

Assessment for tissue pressure indicators includes visual and tactile inspection of the skin. Baseline assessment is performed to determine the client's normal skin characteristics and any actual or potential areas of breakdown. Assessment characteristics of a client's skin should be individualized, depending on the client's skin tone (Bennett, 1995; Henderson and others, 1997). Assessment characteristics of darkly pigmented skin are described earlier (see Boxes 47-2 and 47-3). The nurse pays particular attention to areas under casts, traction, splints, braces, collars, or other orthopedic devices. The frequency of pressure checks depends on the schedule of appliance application and the skin's response to the external pressure (Figures 47-10 and 47-11).

When hyperemia is noted, the nurse documents the location, size, and color and reassesses the area after 1 hour (Figure 47-12, *A*). When abnormal reactive hyperemia is suspected, the nurse can outline the affected area with a marker to make reassessment easier. Another early warning sign of pressure damage is a blister or pimple over the weight-bearing area with possible hyperemia. Pires and Muller (1991) report that a frequently overlooked sign of early pressure is scabbing over of the weight-bearing areas in the absence of trauma (Figure 47-12, *B*). All of these signs are very early indicators of impaired skin integrity, but damage to the underlying tissue may be more progressive (Figure 47-12, *C*). Tactile assessment enables the nurse to use palpation to acquire further data about induration and the damage to the skin and underlying tissues.

The nurse palpates the tissue adjacent to the observed area of hyperemia, assessing for blanching with return to normal skin tones in clients with light-toned skin. In addition, the nurse palpates for induration, noting the size in millimeters or centimeters of the induration around the injured area. The nurse also notes changes in temperature of the surrounding skin and tissues.

The nurse includes visual and tactile inspection over the body areas most frequently at risk for pressure ulcer development (Figure 47-13). When a client lies in bed or sits in a chair, body weight is heavily placed on certain bony prominences. Body surfaces subjected to the greatest weight or

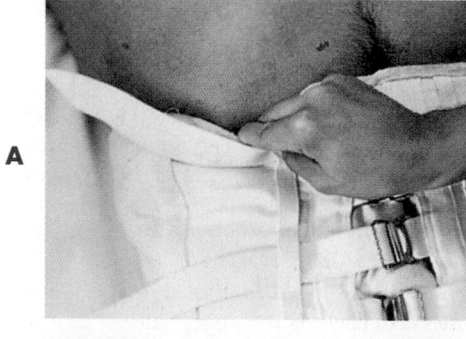

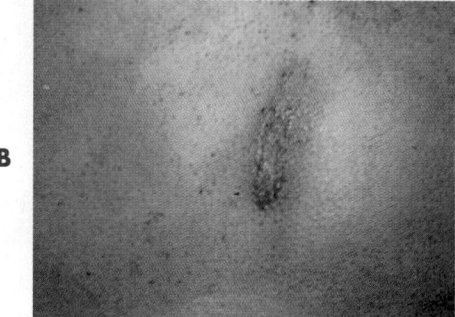

Figure 47-10   Benign devices such as this corset, **A,** may result in scabbing or blistering, **B,** resulting from external pressure.
From Pires M, Muller A: Detection and management of early tissue pressure indicators: a pictorial essay, *Progressions* 3(3):3, 1991.

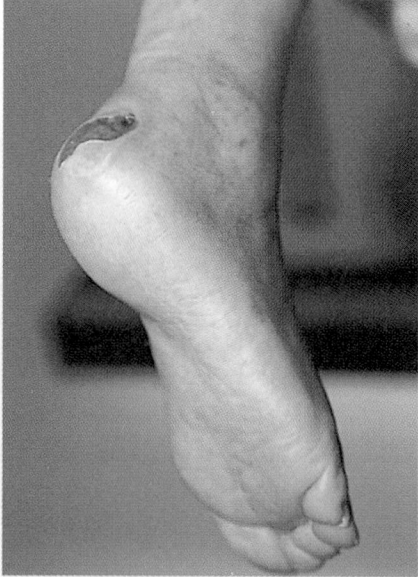

Figure 47-11   Formation of pressure ulcer on heel resulting from external pressure from mattress of bed.

pressure are at greatest risk for pressure ulcer formation. Remember that "time wounds all heels" (Helt, 1991).

Mobility.   Assessment includes documenting the level of mobility and the potential effects of impaired mobility on skin integrity. Assessment of mobility should also in-

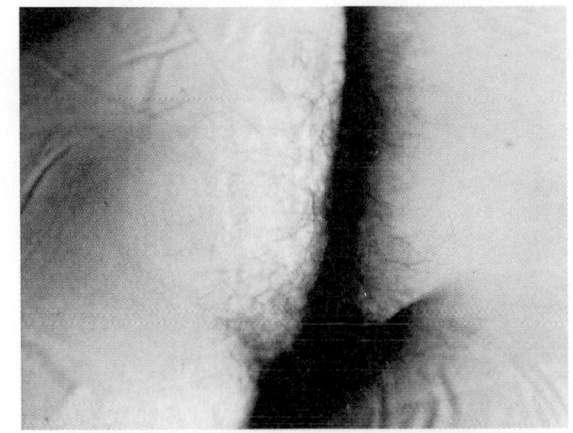

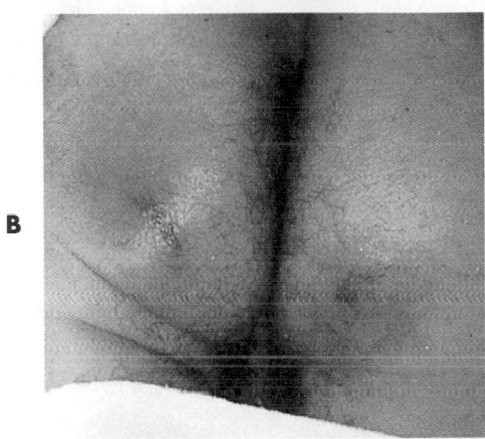

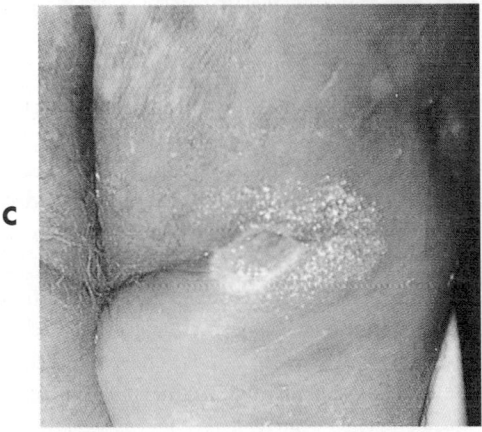

Figure 47-12   **A,** Hyperemia on ischial tuberosities. **B,** Scabbing over bony prominence is a sign of excessive pressure. **C,** Deeper stages of ulceration.
From Pires M, Muller A: Detection and management of early tissue pressure indicators: a pictorial essay, *Progressions* 3(3):3, 1991.

clude obtaining data regarding the quality of muscle tone and strength. For example, the nurse determines whether the client can lift the weight off of the ischial tuberosities and roll the body to a side-lying position. The client may have adequate range of motion (ROM) to move independently into a more protective position. Finally, the nurse notes the client's activity tolerance (see Chapter 36).

Mobility must be assessed as part of baseline data. If the client has some degree of independence in mobility, the nurse reinforces the frequency of position changes and measures to relieve pressure. The frequency of position changes is based on ongoing skin assessment and is revised as data change. The nurse must be meticulous when assessing pressure sites. Normal reactive hyperemia must be present, because once abnormal reactive hyperemia occurs, it may take as long as 2 weeks of non-weight bearing or total pressure relief to heal completely (Pires and Muller, 1991). As a result, if attention is not paid to skin integrity, the lost work time for the client can increase by an additional 2 weeks beyond the normal postoperative course of treatment.

Nutritional Status.   An assessment of the client's nutritional status should be an integral part of the initial assessment data for clients at risk for impaired skin integrity and wounds (Breslow and Bergstrom, 1994; Finucane, 1995; Thomas, 1997a,b; Ayello, Thomas, and Litchford, in press). A client who is malnourished or cachexic and whose body weight is less than 90% of IBW, or a client whose body weight is greater than 110% of IBW has an increased risk for the development of pressure ulcers (Hanan and Scheele 1991). The percentage of IBW alone is not a good predictor; however, when used with a low serum albumin or total protein level, the client's percentage of IBW can have an impact on the occurrence of pressure ulcers.

Pain.   Until recently, little has been written or researched about pain and pressure ulcers. The AHCPR (1994) has recommended that the assessment and management of pain be included in the care of clients with pressure ulcers (Dallam and others, 1995).

Wounds.   The nurse often assesses wounds under two conditions: at the time of injury before treatment and after therapy when the wound is relatively stable. Each condition requires the nurse to make different observations and to take different actions.

Emergency Setting.   The nurse may see wounds in any setting, including a clinic, emergency department, rural youth camp, or the nurse's own backyard. The type of wound determines the criteria for inspection. For example, the nurse need not inspect for signs of internal bleeding after an abrasion but should do so in the event of a puncture wound.

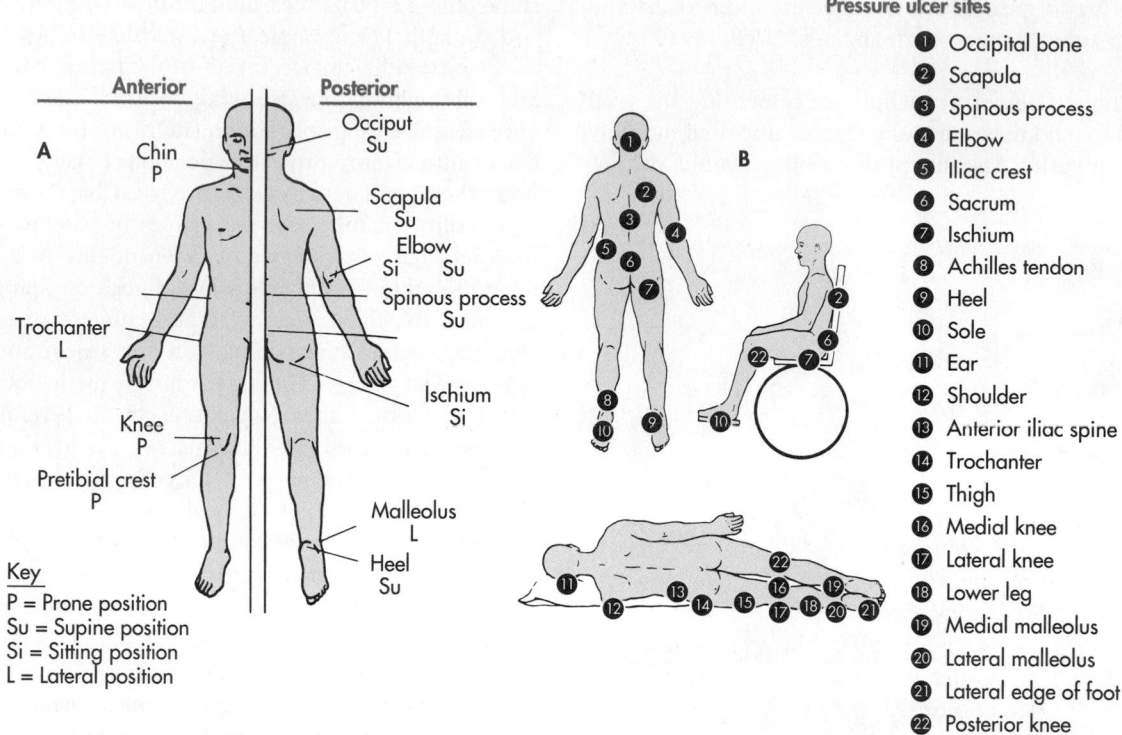

Figure 47-13 **A,** Bony prominence most frequently underlying pressure ulcer. **B,** Pressure ulcer sites.
From Trelease CC: *Ostomy/Wound Manage* 20:46, 1988.

When a client's condition is judged to be stable because of the presence of spontaneous breathing, a clear airway, and a strong carotid pulse (see Chapter 39), the nurse inspects the wound for bleeding. An **abrasion** is usually superficial with little bleeding. The wound may appear "weepy" because of plasma leakage from damaged capillaries. A **laceration** may bleed more profusely, depending on the wound's depth and location. For example, minor scalp lacerations tend to bleed profusely because of the rich blood supply to the scalp. Lacerations greater than 5 cm (2 inches) long or 2.5 cm (1 inch) deep can cause serious bleeding. **Puncture** wounds bleed in relation to the depth and size of the wound; for example, a nail puncture does not cause as much bleeding as a knife wound. The primary dangers of puncture wounds are internal bleeding and infection.

The nurse next inspects the wound for foreign bodies or contaminant material. Most traumatic wounds are dirty. Soil, broken glass, shreds of cloth, and foreign substances clinging to penetrating objects can become embedded in the wound.

The size of the wound is the next criterion for inspection. A deep laceration requires suturing by a physician. A large, open wound may expose bone or tissue that should be protected.

When the injury is a result of trauma from a dirty pen-

etrating object, the nurse determines when the client last received a tetanus toxoid injection. Tetanus bacteria reside in soil and in the gut of humans and animals. A tetanus antitoxin injection is necessary if the client has not had one within 5 years.

Stable Setting. When the client's condition is stabilized (e.g., after surgery or treatment) the nurse assesses the wound to determine its progress toward healing. If the wound is covered by a dressing and the physician has not ordered it changed, the nurse should not directly inspect the wound unless serious complications are suspected. In such a situation the nurse should inspect only the dressing and any external drains. If the physician prefers to change the dressing, the physician will assess the wound at least daily. When the nurse removes dressings, care is taken to avoid accidental removal or displacement of underlying drains. Because removal of dressings can be painful, it may help to give an analgesic at least 30 minutes before exposing a wound.

Wound Appearance. The nurse notes whether wound edges are closed. A surgical incision healing by primary intention should have clean, well-approximated edges. Crusts often form along the wound edges from exudate. A puncture wound is usually a small, circular

Table 47-8	Assessment of Abnormal Healing in Primary and Secondary Intention Wounds	
Primary Wounds	Secondary Wounds
Incision line poorly approximated	Pale or fragile granulation tissue, granulation tissue bed may be excessively dry or moist
Drainage present more than 3 days after closure	Exudate present
Inflammation decreased in first 3-5 days after injury	Necrotic or slough tissue present
No epithelialization of wound edges by day 4	Epithelialization not continuous
No healing ridge by day 9	Fruity, earthy, or putrid odor present
	Presence of fistula(s), tunneling, undermining

Modified from Stotts NA, Cavanaugh CE: Assessing the patient with a wound, *Home Healthcare Nurse* 17(1):27, 1999.

wound with the edges coming together toward the center. If a wound is open, the wound edges are separated, and the nurse inspects the condition of underlying tissue such as adipose and connective tissue. The nurse also looks for complications such as dehiscence and evisceration. The outer edges of a wound normally appear inflamed for the first 2 to 3 days, but this slowly disappears. Within 7 to 10 days a normally healing wound fills with epithelial cells, and edges close. Table 47-8 lists assessment characteristics for abnormal wound healing in primary and secondary wounds. If infection develops, the wound edges become brightly inflamed and swollen.

Skin discoloration usually results from bruising of interstitial tissues or hematoma formation. Blood collecting beneath the skin first takes on a bluish or purplish appearance. Gradually, as the clotted blood is broken down, shades of brown and yellow appear.

Character of Wound Drainage. The nurse notes the amount, color, odor, and consistency of drainage. The amount of drainage depends on the location and extent of the wound. For example, drainage is minimal after a simple appendectomy. In contrast, wound drainage is moderate for 1 to 2 days after resection of a portion of the small bowel. If the nurse needs an accurate measurement of the amount of drainage within a dressing, the dressing can be weighed and compared with the weight of the same dressing when clean and dry. A rule of thumb is that 1 g by weight of drainage equals 1 ml of volume of drainage. The color and consistency of drainage vary depending on the components. Types of drainage include the following: **serous, sanguineous, serosanguineous,** and purulent (see Table 47-3).

If the drainage has a pungent or strong odor, an infection should be suspected. The nurse should describe the wound's appearance according to characteristics observed. An example of accurate recording follows:

abdominal incision is 5 cm long across RLQ (right lower quadrant); edges well approximated without inflamma-

tion or exudate. 1.2-cm diameter circle of serous drainage present on one 4 × 4 gauze.

Drains. The physician inserts a drain into or close to a surgical wound if a large amount of drainage is expected and if keeping wound layers closed is especially important. Some drains are sutured in place. Caution should be exercised when changing the dressing over drains that are not sutured in place to prevent their being accidentally removed. A drain such as a Penrose may lie under a dressing, extend through a dressing, or be connected to a drainage bag or a suction apparatus. The physician often places a pin or clip through the drain to prevent it from slipping farther into a wound (Figure 47-14). It is usually the physician's responsibility to pull or advance the drain as drainage decreases to permit healing deep within the drain site.

The nurse assesses the number of drains, drain placement, character of drainage, and condition of collecting apparatus. First the nurse observes the security of the drain and its location with respect to the wound. Next the nurse notes the character of drainage. If there is a collecting device, the nurse measures the drainage volume. Because a drainage system must be patent, the nurse looks for drainage flow through the tubing, as well as around the tubing. A sudden decrease in drainage through the tubing may indicate a blocked drain, and the physician should be notified. When a drain is connected to suction, the nurse

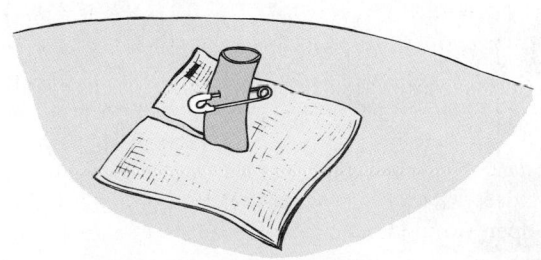

Figure 47-14   Penrose drain.

assesses the system to be sure that the pressure ordered is being exerted. Evacuator units such as a Hemovac or Jackson-Pratt (Figure 47-15) exert a constant low pressure as long as the suction device (bladder or bag) is fully compressed. These types of drainage devices are often referred to as self-suction. When the evacuator device is unable to maintain a vacuum on its own, the nurse notifies the surgeon, who can then order a secondary vacuum system (such as wall suction). If fluid is allowed to accumulate within the tissues, wound healing will not progress at an optimal rate, and the risk of infection is increased.

Wound Closures.   Surgical wounds are closed with staples, sutures, or wound closures. A popular skin closure is the stainless-steel staple. The staple provides more strength than nylon or silk sutures and tends to cause less irritation to the skin. The nurse looks for irritation around staple or suture sites and notes whether closures are intact. The nurse may choose to count sutures when the physician has removed a portion of them. Normally for the first 2 to 3 days after surgery the skin around sutures or staples is swollen. Continued swelling may indicate that the closures are too tight. The skin can be cut by overly tight suture material, leading to wound separation. Sutures that are too tight are a common cause of wound dehiscence. Early suture removal reduces formation of defects along the suture line and minimizes chances of unattractive scar formation.

Palpation of Wound.   When inspecting a wound, the nurse may observe swelling or separation of wound edges. While wearing gloves, the nurse lightly palpates wound edges, detecting localized areas of tenderness or drainage collection. The nurse gently applies the fingertips along the wound edges. If pressure causes fluid to be expressed, the nurse notes the character of the drainage. It may be necessary to collect the drainage for culture. The client is normally sensitive to palpation of wound edges. Extreme tenderness may indicate infection.

Wound Cultures.   If the nurse detects purulent or suspicious-looking drainage, collecting a specimen for culture may be necessary (see Chapter 33). The nurse never collects a wound culture sample from old drainage. Resident colonies of bacteria from the skin grow within exudate and may not be the true causative organisms of a wound infection. The nurse cleans a wound first with normal saline to remove skin flora. Aerobic organisms grow in superficial wounds exposed to the air, and anaerobic organisms tend to grow within body cavities. The nurse uses a different method of specimen collection for each type of organism.

To collect an aerobic specimen, the nurse uses a sterile swab from a culturette tube (Figure 47-16). If wound edges are separated, the nurse slowly and gently inserts the tip of the swab into the wound to collect deeper secretions. The nurse needs to apply sufficient pressure with the swab to cause some tissue fluid to be expressed in an area the size of 1 cm^2 and collected onto the tip of the swab (Stotts, 1995). After collecting the specimen, the nurse returns the swab to the culturette tube, caps the tube, and crushes the inner ampule containing the medium for organism growth. The medium must moisten and coat the swab tip. The nurse immediately sends the labeled specimen to the laboratory for quantitative bacterial cultures rather than swab cultures (AHCPR, 1994).

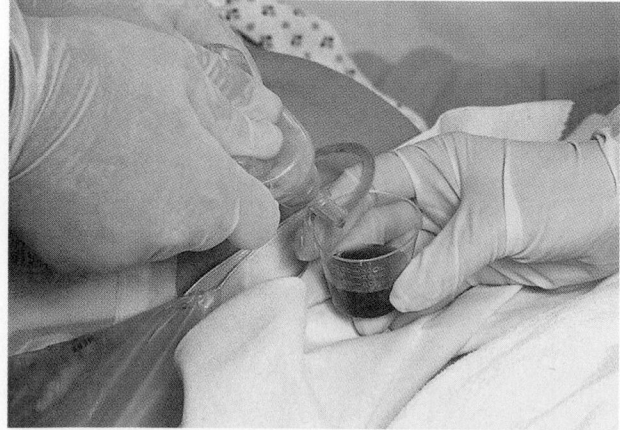

Figure 47-15   Jackson-Pratt drainage device. **A,** Drainage tubes and reservoir. **B,** Emptying drainage reservoir.

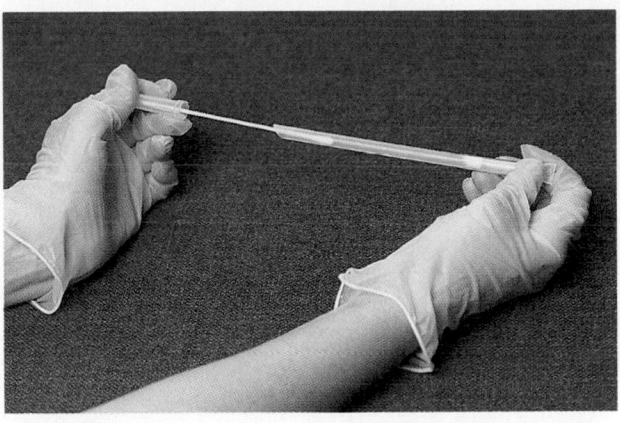

Figure 47-16 Wound culturette tube.

If drainage from a deep body cavity has a foul odor, there is a chance of anaerobic organism growth. The nurse uses a sterile syringe tip to aspirate drainage from the inner wound. Afterward the nurse applies a sterile needle to the syringe, expels air from the syringe and needle, and places a cork over the needle to prevent entrance of air. In some institutions the nurse may inject the specimen into a special vacuum container with a culture medium.

Gram stains are often performed as well. This test often allows the physician to order appropriate treatment earlier than when only cultures are done. No additional specimens are usually required. The microbiology laboratory needs only to be notified to perform the additional test.

Client Expectations. When clients have pressure ulcers or chronic wounds, their course of treatment is lengthy and costly. Because the client and family must be involved with wound care management, it is important to know the client's expectations. A client who has realistic goals and is informed about the length of time for wound healing is more likely to adhere to the specific therapies designed to promote wound healing and prevent further skin breakdown.

NURSING DIAGNOSIS

Assessment reveals clusters of data that indicate whether an actual or high risk for *impaired skin integrity* exists. After gathering appropriate assessment data, the nurse clusters defining characteristics to establish nursing diagnoses (Box 47-6). In addition, the data may support more than one diagnostic label. For example, a postoperative client has purulent drainage from a surgical wound and reports tenderness around the area of the wound. These data would support a nursing diagnoses of *infection*. After completing an assessment of the client's wound, the nurse identifies nursing diagnoses that will direct supportive and preventive care.

The client may be at risk for poor wound healing because of previously defined factors that impair healing. Thus even though the client's wound may appear normal, the nurse identifies nursing diagnoses, such as *altered nutrition* or *altered tissue perfusion,* that direct nursing care toward support of wound repair.

The nature of a wound can cause problems unrelated to wound healing. Alteration in comfort and impaired mobility are problems that have implications for the client's eventual recovery. For example, a large abdominal incision can cause enough pain to interfere with the client's ability to turn in bed effectively. Box 47-7 lists nursing diagnoses related to problems of wound healing.

PLANNING

After identifying nursing diagnoses, the nurse develops a care plan for the client who has actual or is at high risk for impaired skin integrity. During planning the nurse again synthesizes information from multiple resources (Figure 47-17). Critical thinking ensures that the client's plan of care integrates all that the nurse knows about the individual, as well as key critical thinking elements. Professional standards are especially important to consider when the nurse develops a plan of care. The plan is based on the client's identified needs and priorities. Goals and expected outcomes are established, and from the goals the nurse plans therapies ac-

cording to the severity and type of wound and the presence of any complicating conditions (e.g., infection, poor nutrition, immunosuppression, and diabetes) that may affect wound healing.

With early acute care discharges, it is important to consider the client's home when planning therapies to promote skin integrity and wound healing. Clients and their families may need to continue the objectives of wound management after discharge. The ability of the caregiver and the amount of time needed to change a particular dressing need to be considered when selecting a dressing that will be used by the client after discharge. For example, in the home setting, caregivers may choose more expen-

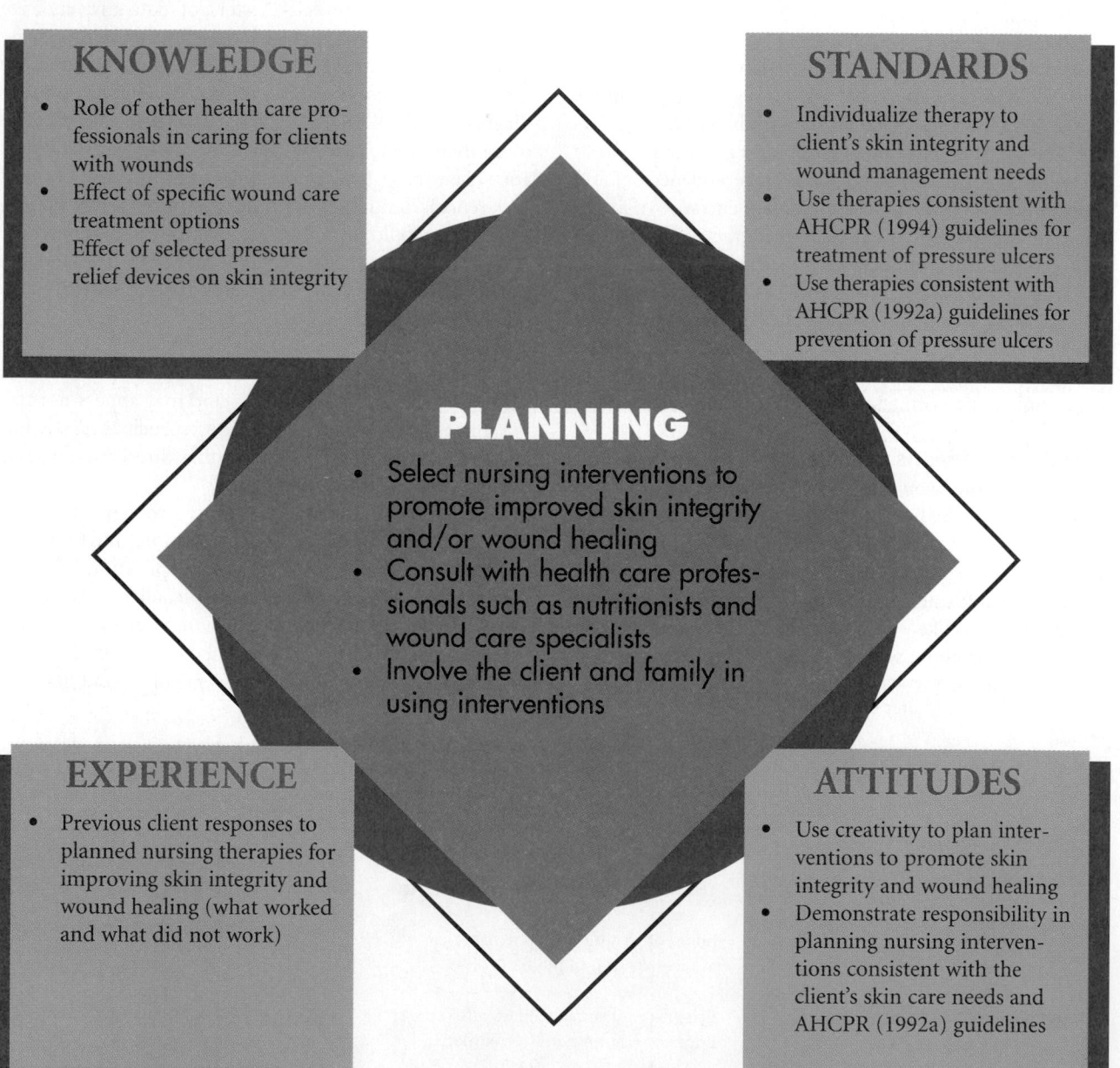

KNOWLEDGE

- Role of other health care professionals in caring for clients with wounds
- Effect of specific wound care treatment options
- Effect of selected pressure relief devices on skin integrity

STANDARDS

- Individualize therapy to client's skin integrity and wound management needs
- Use therapies consistent with AHCPR (1994) guidelines for treatment of pressure ulcers
- Use therapies consistent with AHCPR (1992a) guidelines for prevention of pressure ulcers

PLANNING

- Select nursing interventions to promote improved skin integrity and/or wound healing
- Consult with health care professionals such as nutritionists and wound care specialists
- Involve the client and family in using interventions

EXPERIENCE

- Previous client responses to planned nursing therapies for improving skin integrity and wound healing (what worked and what did not work)

ATTITUDES

- Use creativity to plan interventions to promote skin integrity and wound healing
- Demonstrate responsibility in planning nursing interventions consistent with the client's skin care needs and AHCPR (1992a) guidelines

Figure 47-17 *Synthesis Model for Skin Integrity and Wound Care Planning Phase.*

sive dressing materials to reduce the frequency of dressing changes (AHCPR, 1994). The nurse and client work together to establish ways of maintaining client involvement in nursing care and to promote wound healing whether the client is in the hospital or home.

The nurse's priorities in wound care depend on whether the client's condition is stable or emergent. The type of wound care administered depends on the type of wound, its size and location, and complications. Nursing interventions will be both dependent and independent (see care plan). Goals of care for clients with wounds include the following:

Promoting wound hemostasis
Preventing infection
Promoting wound healing
Maintaining skin integrity
Gaining comfort

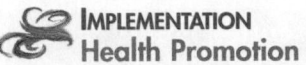 **IMPLEMENTATION**
Health Promotion

Prevention of Pressure Ulcers. When the client is immobile, the major risk to the skin is the formation of pressure ulcers. Nursing interventions focus on prevention or wound management. The first step in prevention is to assess the client's risk factors. The nurse then reduces environmental factors that accelerate pressure ulcer formation, such as high room temperature, which causes diaphoresis.

Early identification of clients at risk and their risk factors aids the nurse in preventing pressure ulcers. Skill 47-1 identifies frequent pressure ulcer sites. Prevention minimizes the impact that risk factors or contributing factors may have on pressure ulcer development. Box 47-8 and Table 47-9 provide some universal preventive measures. Three major areas of nursing interventions for prevention

 ## SAMPLE NURSING CARE PLAN

Skin Integrity and Wound Care

ASSESSMENT*
Mrs. Stein is 3 weeks postoperative for a total hip replacement. She has developed a severe postoperative wound infection. She is **febrile and has limited activity tolerance. She does not tolerate position changes or sitting out of bed; she wants to stay in a semi-Fowler's position at all times.** She does not complain of discomfort in the operative site; however, she complains of **a painful, burning sensation in the sacral region.** On inspection, **reactive hyperemia remains for a period of greater than 2 hours. A 1 × 2 inch open area is present, and serous drainage is noted.** On palpation, **underlying skin is soft and indurated.**
*Defining characteristics are shown in bold type.

NURSING DIAGNOSIS: Impaired skin integrity related to pressure on the bony prominence in the sacral region.

PLANNING

GOALS
Injury to skin and underlying tissue resulting from pressure on the bony prominence will be reduced within 2 to 4 weeks.

EXPECTED OUTCOMES
Wound will decrease in size by 12/01.
Wound drainage will be reduced by 11/27.
Reactive hyperemia to surrounding tissue will remain within normal limits.

INTERVENTIONS†
Pressure Management
- Reposition client every 90 minutes. Turning interval: 120 minutes − 30 minutes hypoxia time = 90 minutes.

- Place client on an egg crate-style mattress.

RATIONALE

Repositioning removes pressure and allows normal hyperemic response. Frequency of turning is based on initial assessment (Maklebust, 1991; AHCPR, 1994).
Clients with pressure ulcer development are at greater risk for new ulcers and need preventive measures to prevent ulcer progression (AHCPR, 1994; NPUAP, 1995a, 1995b).

Wound Care
- Apply dressing to wound.

- Maintain sterile technique when doing wound care.

Dressings protect underlying skin and remove drainage from surface of wound (Makelebust, 1991; NPUAP, 1995a).
Reduces the risk of nosocomial wound infections.

†Intervention Classification labels from McCloskey JC, Bulechek GM: *Nursing interventions classification (NIC)*, ed 3, St. Louis, 2000, Mosby.

EVALUATION
Measure wound size daily.
Observe color and amount of drainage with each dressing change.
Observe and time the duration of reactive hyperemia after each position change.
Palpate underlying and adjacent tissues after each position change.

Pressure Ulcer Prevention Points

Box 47-8

A. Risk assessment

1. Consider all bed-bound or chair-bound persons, or those whose ability to reposition is impaired, to be at risk for pressure ulcers.

2. Select and use a method of risk assessment, such as the Norton Scale or the Braden Scale, that ensures systematic evaluation of individual risk factors.

3. Assess all at-risk clients at the time of admission to health care facilities and at regular intervals thereafter.

4. Identify all individual risk factors (decreased mental status, moisture, incontinence, nutritional deficits) to direct specific preventive treatments. Modify care according to the individual factors.

B. Skin care and early treatment

1. Inspect the skin at least daily, and document assessment results.

2. Individualize bathing frequency. Use a mild cleansing agent. Avoid hot water and excessive friction.

3. Assess and treat incontinence. When incontinence cannot be controlled, cleanse skin at time of soiling, use a topical moisture barrier, and select underpads or briefs that are absorbent and provide a quick drying surface to the skin.

4. Use moisturizers for dry skin. Minimize environmental factors leading to dry skin such as low humidity and cold air.

5. Do not massage over bony prominences.

6. Use proper positioning, transferring, and turning techniques to minimize skin injury caused by friction and shear forces.

7. Use dry lubricants (cornstarch) or protective coverings to reduce friction injury.

8. Identify and correct factors compromising protein/caloric intake, and consider nutritional supplementation/support for nutritionally compromised persons.

9. Institute a rehabilitation program to maintain or improve mobility/activity status.

10. Monitor and document interventions and outcomes.

C. Mechanical loading and support surfaces

1. Reposition bed-bound persons at least every 2 hours, chair-bound persons every hour.

2. Use a written repositioning schedule.

3. Place at-risk persons on a pressure-reducing mattress/chair cushion. Do not use donut-type devices.

4. Consider postural alignment, distribution of weight, balance and stability, and pressure relief when positioning persons in chairs or wheelchairs.

5. Teach chair-bound persons, who are able, to shift weight every 15 minutes.

6. Use lifting device (e.g., trapeze or bed linen) to move rather than drag persons during transfer and position changes.

7. Use pillows or foam wedges to keep bony prominences such as knees and ankles from direct contact with each other.

8. Use devices that totally relieve pressure on the heels (e.g., place pillows under the calf to raise the heels off the bed).

9. Avoid positioning directly on the trochanter when using the side-lying position (use the 30-degree lateral inclined position).

10. Elevate the head of the bed as little (maximum 30-degree angle) and for as short a time as possible.

D. Education

1. Implement educational programs for the prevention of pressure ulcers that are structured, organized, comprehensive, and directed at all levels of health care providers, clients, family, and caregivers.

2. Include information on:

    a. Etiology of and risk factors for pressure ulcers

    b. Risk assessment tools and their application

    c. Skin assessment

    d. Selection/use of support surfaces

    e. Development/implementation of individualized programs of skin care

    f. Demonstration of positioning to decrease risk of tissue breakdown

    g. Accurate documentation of pertinent data

3. Include built-in mechanisms to evaluate program effectiveness in preventing pressure ulcers.

Modified from National Pressure Ulcer Advisory Panel, 1989.

of pressure ulcers are (1) skin care, which includes hygiene and skin care; (2) mechanical loading and support devices, which include proper positioning and the use of therapeutic beds and mattresses; and (3) education (AHCPR, 1992a).

Hygiene and Skin Care. The nurse must keep the client's skin clean and dry. In this initial line of defense for preventing skin breakdown, the client's skin is continually assessed by nurses, rather than being delegated to other personnel. In addition, the types of products available for

skin care are numerous, and their uses need to be matched to the specific needs of the client (Hess, 1995).

When the skin is cleansed, soaps and hot water are avoided. Soaps and alcohol-based lotions cause drying and leave an alkaline residue. The alkaline residue discourages the growth of normal skin bacteria, thus promoting an overgrowth of opportunistic bacteria, which can then enter an open wound (AHCPR, 1992a).

After the skin is cleaned and completely dried, protective moisturizer should be applied to keep the epidermis well lubricated but not oversaturated. Cornstarch is a dry

Table 47-9	A Quick Guide to Pressure Ulcer Prevention
Risk Factor	**Nursing Interventions**
Immobility	Establish individualized turning schedule.
	Reduce shear and friction.
Inactivity	Provide pressure-relief surface.
	Provide assistive devices to increase activity.
Incontinence	Assess need for incontinence management.
	Clean and dry skin after soiling.
Malnutrition	Provide adequate nutritional and fluid intake.
	Consult dietitian for nutritional evaluation.
Diminished sensation, decreased mental status	Assess client's and family's ability to provide care.
	Educate caregiver regarding pressure ulcer prevention.
Impaired skin integrity	Avoid pressure.
	Do not use donut-shaped cushions.
	Lubricate skin.
	Do not massage red areas.
	Do not use heat lamps.

Modified from Maklebust J, Sieggreen M: *Pressure ulcers: guidelines for prevention and nursing management*, West Dundee, Ill, 1996, S-N Publications.

lubricant and helps to reduce friction. A & D, Unicare, and Pericare are some examples of bland, water-repellent ointments that protect the skin from moisture (AHCPR, 1992a). In addition, these ointments are easily cleansed from the skin. When using any water-repellent ointment, the nurse must completely clean the area on a routine basis. Ointment, when left in place too long, can be a medium for bacteria and can cause further skin problems, such as maceration, yeast, and other infections.

Efforts should be made to control, contain, or correct incontinence, perspiration, or wound drainage. Clinicians may find the AHCPR guidelines on urinary incontinence (1992b) helpful (see Chapter 44). Clients who are incontinent of bowel and who are also receiving enteral tube feeding provide another challenge to the nurse. When clients are incontinent, the area should be cleansed and a skin barrier applied. These barriers protect the skin from excessive moisture and toxin from urine or stool.

The expertise of an advanced practice nurse with a focus on enterostomal therapy, wound care, or management of incontinence should be used in caring for at-risk clients. Methods for controlling or containing incontinence vary. Urinary incontinence may be treated with behavioral techniques, medication, and surgery. Behavioral techniques are used to help clients learn ways to control their bladder and sphincter muscles. Two examples are bladder training and habit training, which is also called time voiding.

Use of absorbent pads and garments should be considered only after the above incontinent measures have been tried. Although controversial, absorbent products, such as absorptive underpads and garments, may be part of the treatment plan for an incontinent client. The nurse should use only products that drain moisture away from the client's skin (AHCPR, 1992b). Absorptive garments have a quilted lining and contain a polymer filling. Disposable, plastic-lined underpads should not be placed directly under the client, because they do not drain moisture away from the client's skin. These products protect the bed, not the client. The plastic lining also increases diaphoresis. Moist, macerated skin is more at risk for pressure ulcer development. If it is necessary to use a plastic-lined product, it should be placed in a pillow case or under a drawsheet.

Positioning.   Positioning interventions are designed to reduce pressure and shearing force to the skin. Keeping the head of the bed to 30 degrees or less will decrease the chance of pressure ulcer development from shearing forces (AHCPR, 1992a). The immobilized client's position should be changed according to activity level, perceptual ability, and daily routines (Pajk and others, 1986; Bergstrom and others, 1987). Therefore a standard turning interval of 1½ to 2 hours may not prevent pressure ulcer development in some clients. The AHCPR guidelines (1992a) recommend that a written turning and positioning schedule be used. Clients should be repositioned at least every 2 hours. When doing full position changes, positioning devices should be used to protect bony prominences (AHCPR, 1992a, 1994; Jacobs, 1994). A 30-degree lateral position is recommended in the AHCPR guidelines (1992a) (Figure 47-18). To prevent friction injuries, lift rather than drag the client when changing positions.

Clients able to sit in a chair should be limited to sitting for 2 hours or less. Again, the exact time is individualized, but the nurse should not allow the client to sit for a period longer than the recommended time that was calculated during assessment (see Skill 47-1). Thus if the interval is every 1½ hours, the client should remain in a sitting position for less than 1½ hours. In the sitting position, the pressure on the ischial tuberosities is greater than when in the supine position (Pajk and others, 1986). In addition, for a client at risk such as an individual with a spinal cord injury, sitting in a chair should be taught or the client should be helped to shift weight every 15 minutes (AHCPR, 1992a). Shifting weight provides short-term relief on the ischial tuberosities. A client should also sit on foam, gel, or an air cushion to redistribute weight so that it is not all on the ischium. Rigid and donut-shaped cushions are contraindicated because they reduce blood supply to the area, resulting in wider areas of ischemia (AHCPR, 1992a, 1994).

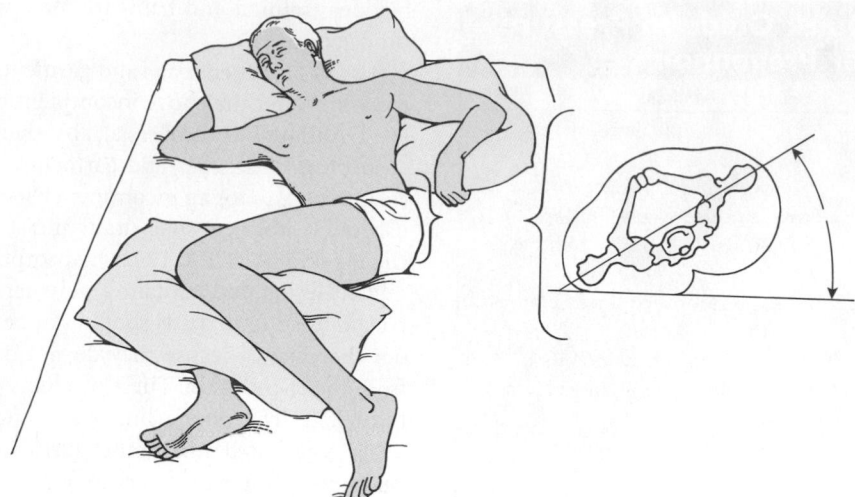

Figure 47-18   Thirty-degree lateral position to avoid pressure points.
From Bryant RA and others: Pressure ulcers. In Bryant RA, editor: *Acute and chronic wounds: nursing management,* St. Louis, 1992, Mosby.

After the client is repositioned, the nurse reassesses the skin. Identifying characteristics that might indicate early signs of tissue ischemia in darkly pigmented skin can be found in Boxes 47-2 and 47-3. For clients with light-toned skin, the nurse observes for normal reactive hyperemia and blanching. The reddened areas should never be massaged. This change in practice is a result of nursing research (AHCPR, 1992a). Massaging the reddened areas increases breaks in the capillaries in the underlying tissues and increases the risk of pressure ulcer formation.

Support Surfaces (Therapeutic Beds and Mattresses).
A variety of support surfaces, including specialty beds and mattresses, have been designed to reduce the hazards of immobility to the skin and musculoskeletal system. However, none eliminates the need for meticulous nursing care. No single device eliminates the effects of pressure on the skin.

It is important to understand the difference between a pressure-reducing and a pressure-relieving support surface or device. A device that is **pressure relieving** reduces the interface pressure (the pressure between the body and the support surface) below 32 mm Hg (capillary closing pressure). Devices that are **pressure reducing** also reduce the interface pressure, but not necessarily below the capillary closing pressure (AHCPR, 1994).

When selecting specialty beds, the nurse must thoroughly assess the client's needs. A flow diagram (Figure 47-19) and table of support surface characteristics (Table 47-10) assists the nurse in clinical decision making. In selecting a support surface, the nurse should know its purpose. The Support Surface Consensus Panel identified three purposes of support surfaces: comfort, postural control, and pressure management (Krouskop and van Rijswijk, 1995). Furthermore, they identified nine para-

> ### AHCPR Support Surface Recommendations   Box 47-9
>
> Assess all clients with existing pressure ulcers to determine their risk for developing additional pressure ulcers. If the client remains at risk, use a pressure-reducing surface.
>
> Use a static support surface if a client can assume a variety of positions without bearing weight on a pressure ulcer and without "bottoming out."
>
> Use a dynamic support surface if the client cannot assume a variety of positions without bearing weight on a pressure ulcer, if the client fully compresses the static support surface, or if the pressure ulcer does not show evidence of healing.
>
> If a client has large stage III or stage IV pressure ulcers on multiple turning surfaces, a low-air-loss bed or an air-fluidized bed may be indicated.
>
> When excess moisture on intact skin is a potential source of maceration and skin breakdown, a support surface that provides air flow can be important in drying the skin and preventing additional pressure ulcers.

Modified from Agency for Health Care Policy and Research, Panel for Treatment of Pressure Ulcers in Adults: *Treatment of pressure ulcers,* Clinical Practice Guideline No. 15, AHCPR Pub No. 95-0653, Rockville, Md, 1994, Agency for Health Care Policy and Research, Public Health Service, U.S. Department of Health and Human Services.

meters to use when evaluating support surfaces and their relationship to each of the three purposes: life expectancy, skin moisture control, skin temperature control, redistribution of pressure, product service requirements, fall safety, infection control, flammability, and client-product friction (Krouskop and van Rijswijk, 1995). A summary of AHCPR recommendations (1994) regarding the use of support surfaces is found in Box 47-9. In addition, Table

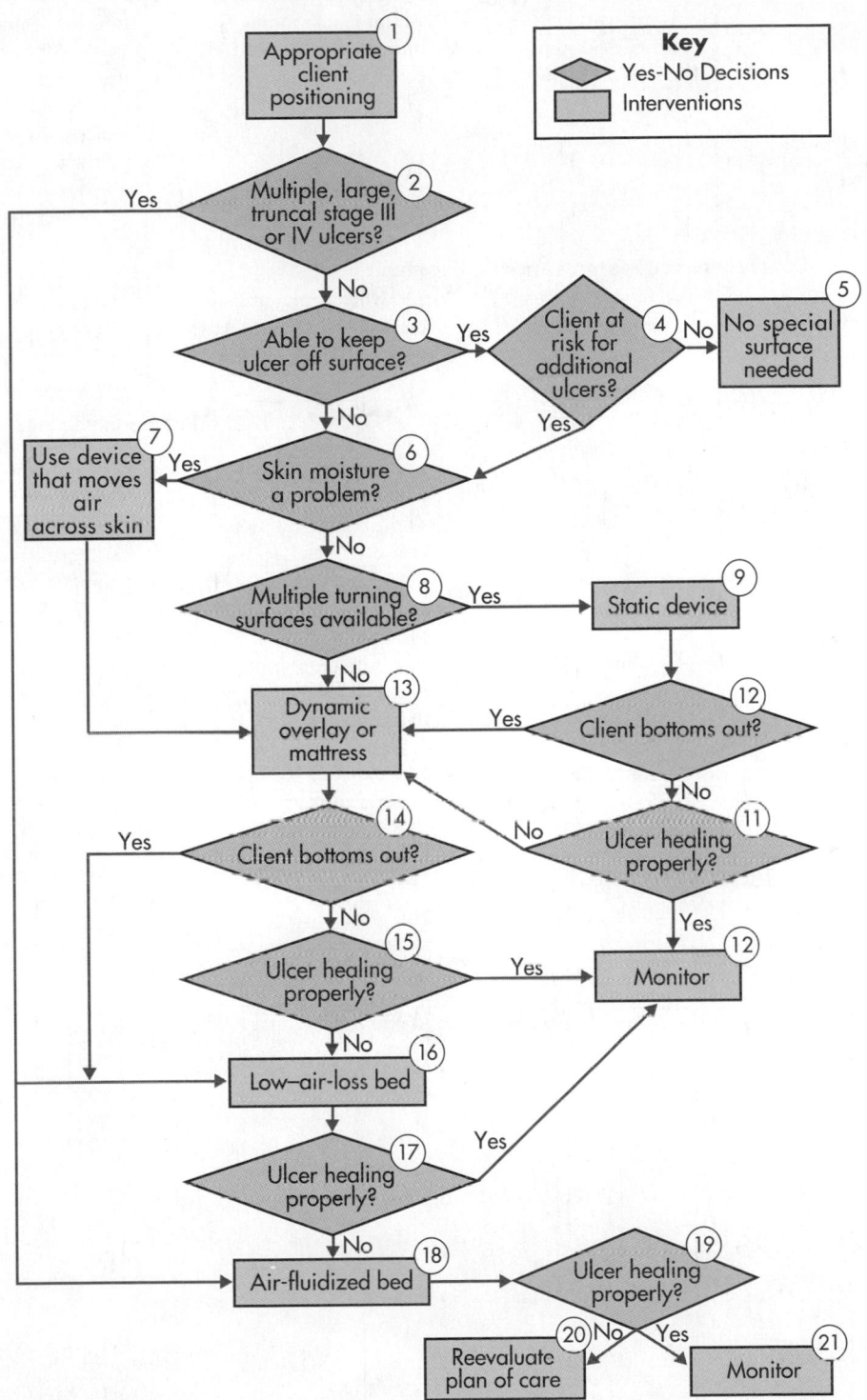

Figure 47-19 Support surfaces diagram.
From Agency for Health Care Policy and Research, Panel for Treatment of Pressure Ulcers in
Adults: *Treatment of pressure ulcers*, Clinical Practice Guideline No. 15, AHCPR Pub No.
95-0653, Rockville, Md, 1994, Agency for Health Care Policy and Research, Public Health Service,
U.S. Department of Health and Human Services.

Table 47-10 Support Beds and Mattresses

Brand Names (Examples)	Manufacturer	Indications	Comments
Low-Air-Loss System			
Flexicair KinAir Mediscus	Hill-Rom Gaymar Industries Kinetic Concepts Mediscus Group	Pressure relief in clients in whom repositioning is difficult or contraindicated	Nurse must consider need for built-in or underbed scales (may cost extra and be optional feature). Nurse should use only incontinence pads recommended by manufacturer. Nurse cannot adjust temperature to cool feverish client.
Oscillating Low-Air-Loss Frame and Maintenance Replacement			
BioDyne Pulmonair-40	Kinetic Concepts Mediscus Group	Hemodynamically unstable clients who cannot tolerate sudden changes in position Clients with documented pneumonia and unmanageable secretions requiring frequent position changes to mobilize secretions	If client has small frame, it is difficult to prevent sliding, and there is higher risk of falls. Movement of bed may contribute to agitation or cause motion sickness in some clients. Nurse cannot adjust temperature to cool feverish client. Nurse should use only incontinence pads recommended by manufacturer.
Oscillating Support Surface			
Keane Mobility System RotoRest Pressure Guard Turn Select Tilt and Turn Paragon 9000	Hill-Rom Kinetic Concepts Span-America Egerton Hospital Equipment, UK	Clients who require frequent turning but have unstable spines	Movement of bed raises risk of skin shearing on support surface. Movement of bed may contribute to agitation or cause motion sickness in some clients. Bed does not have built-in scales.
Air-Fluidized System			
Air Plus Therapy System Clinitron II (ELEXIS, Rite-hite) FluidAir Elite Skytron	Air Plus Hill-Rom Kinetic Concepts Skytron	Clients who require minimal movement to prevent skin damage by shearing forces (e.g., posterior grafts, flaps)	Several people or lifts are required to transfer client to and from bed. Airflow increases evaporative water loss and can contribute to dehydration. Foam wedge is needed for head elevation. Bed requires routine cleaning of beads (check with manufacturer for frequency). Nurse should use only incontinence pads recommended by manufacturer.
Obese Clients			
Burke Bariatric Treatment System Pressure Guard CFT	Kinetic Concepts Span-America	Clients over 300 pounds	Pressure-relief capabilities may vary from client to client.

Modified from Willey T: High tech beds and mattress overlays: a decision guide, *Am J Nurs* 89:1142, 1989.

Table 47-10   Support Beds and Mattresses—cont'd

Brand Names	Manufacturer	Indications	Comments
Special Function			
TheraPulse II	Support Systems	Same as low-air-loss beds,	No evidence yet exists to support
Rescue	International	plus pulsation	therapeutic effect of pulsation.
		Clients needing low-air-loss therapy, oscillating therapy, or pulsation therapy	
Foam Product			
Bio Gard	Bio Clinic	Reduction of pressure in	Nurse should check with manu-
Geo Mattress (Plus, Pro, Wings)	Span-America	clients at risk	facturer regarding flammabil-
High Float	Pre-Foam	Adjunct to care of clients	ity of product and to deter-
Comfortline (Basic ultimate)	Hill-Rom	with established ulcer if client can be turned frequently and positioned off ulcer	mine whether flame retardation is removed with washing or sterilization.
Static Air Mattress			
Sof-Care	Gaymar Industries		Nurse should avoid puncturing it
Roho (see illustration)	Roho		(requires mattress replacement
First Step Plus	Kinetic Concepts		with some models).
KoalaKair	Pharmaseal		Nurse follows manufacturer's instructions for checking inflation level (every 8 hours and as needed).
Mattress Replacement			
Flexicair Eclipse	Hill-Rom		Nurse checks for increased perspiration because of plastic surface.

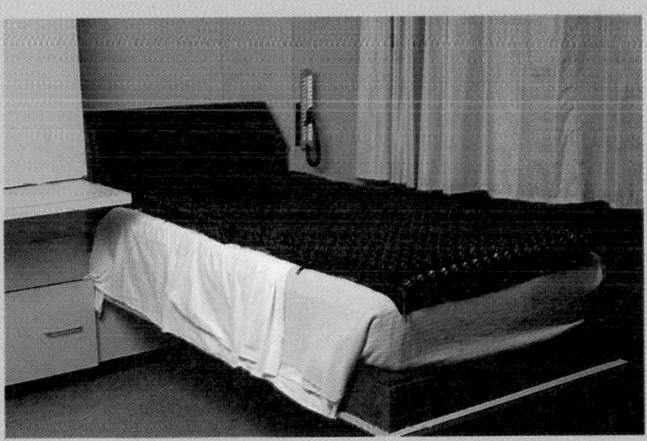

Brand Names	Manufacturer	Indications	Comments
Alternating Air Mattress			
Bio Flote	Bio Clinic		Nurse should follow manufac-
Grant PCA Systems	Grant		turer's instructions for proper
Pressure Guard (APM, Site Select)	Span-America		functioning of equipment; it may require some assembly.
Water Mattress			
Lotus Water Flotation Mattress	Lotus		Nurse should avoid puncturing it (check every shift and as needed for water leakage).

47-10 lists the specific device, client assessment, and pertinent nurse alerts for using the equipment safely. Clients and families need to be taught the reason for and proper use of the beds or mattresses (Box 47-10). Some common errors with support surfaces are placing the wrong side of the support surface toward the client, not plugging support surfaces into the electrical source, not turning on the power source for some support surfaces, failing to do "hand checks" for some support surfaces, and improperly inflating some support surfaces. When used correctly, these mattresses and specialty beds assist in reducing pressure ulcers in clients at risk.

Research suggests that clients on air-fluidized beds may have increased fluid losses and decreased urinary nitrogen losses (Breslow, 1994; Breslow and others, 1993). Clients on air-fluidized beds should have increased amounts of fluid to prevent dehydration and may need increased protein intake (Breslow, 1994; Breslow and others, 1993).

Acute Care

Management of Pressure Ulcers. Treatment of clients with pressure ulcers requires a holistic approach that uses the expertise of several multidisciplinary health care professionals (AHCPR, 1994). In addition to the nurse, this can include the physician, physical therapist, occupational therapist, nutritionist, and pharmacist. Aspects of pressure ulcer treatment include local care of the wound and supportive measures such as adequate nutrients and relief of pressure.

When treating a pressure ulcer, the wound should be reassessed for location, stage, size, sinus tracts, undermining, tunneling, exudate, necrotic tissue, and the presence or absence of granulation tissue and epithelialization (AHCPR, 1994). Pressure ulcers should be reassessed at least daily (AHCPR, 1994). This may be modified in the home care setting (Box 47-11), since weekly assessment by health care providers may not always be feasible (AHCPR, 1994). A clean pressure ulcer should show evidence of some healing within 2 to 4 weeks (AHCPR, 1994).

A thorough reassessment in the management of a pressure ulcer provides the basis for clinical decision making for the treatment plan (AHCPR, 1994; Maklebust and Sieggreen, 1996). In the literature there are two tools that may provide a useful means for consistent assessment and reassessment of pressure ulcers. Exploration of the Bates-Jensen (1990) (Figure 47-20) and Ayello (1992, 1996) (Box 47-12) tools may prove helpful. This would enhance communication and collaboration among team members for more focused treatment of these ulcers.

Skin. In addition to removing all pressure from the affected area and keeping pressure from the area, cleanliness of the ulcer area and all skin surfaces is essential (Skill 47-2). Maintaining cleanliness may be extremely difficult with incontinent, feverish, or confused clients.

Moisture in and around an area of skin breakdown can cause further ulceration and infection. Many products are available for the care of pressure ulcers (Table 47-11). Before instituting treatment measures, the nurse must thoroughly assess the client's pressure ulcer and determine the correct dressing based on the stage of ulcer development.

Principles of local wound care include debridement, cleansing, and dressing application (Figure 47-21). An ulcer that has necrotic tissue or eschar or shows signs of sloughing must be debrided. **Eschar** is the scab or dry crust that results from death of the skin. **Sloughing** is the shedding of dead tissue as a result of skin ulceration.

Debridement is the removal of necrotic tissue so that healthy tissue can regenerate. Removal of necrotic tissue is necessary to rid the ulcer of a source of infection, to enable visualization of the wound bed to accurately stage the ulcer, and to provide a clean base necessary for healing (Rodeheaver and others, 1994). An exception to the rule that all eschar be debrided is a dry necrotic heel pressure ulcer. According to the AHCPR guidelines (1994), "heel ulcers with dry eschar need not be debrided if they do not have edema, erythema, fluctuance, or drainage."

The method of debridement used should depend on which is most appropriate to the client's condition and care goals (AHCPR, 1994). It is important to remember that during the debridement process some normal wound observations that may occur are an increase in wound ex-

Text continued on p. 1593.

Client Teaching FOR THERAPEUTIC BEDS AND MATTRESSES | Box 47-10

OBJECTIVE
- Client will demonstrate understanding of the purposes and basic operations of the therapeutic bed.

TEACHING STRATEGIES
- Explain to client the reasons for the therapeutic bed.
- Explain proper body mechanics while using the therapeutic bed.
- Educate family about the use and care of the therapeutic bed.

- Explain to client and family about additional pressure-relief measures.
- Give client and family a copy of each of the AHCPR booklets for clients on prevention and treatment of pressure ulcers.

EVALUATION
- Client and family will state basic purposes for the therapeutic mattresses.
- Client and family will be able to describe the function of the therapeutic bed.

Home Care Recommendations   Box 47-11

ASSESSMENT

"Assessment and documentation [of the pressure ulcer] should be carried out at least weekly, unless there is evidence of deterioration, in which case both the pressure ulcer and the client's overall management must be reassessed immediately. In the home setting, this may require the assistance of the client and family because weekly assessment by health care providers is not always feasible."

PSYCHOSOCIAL ASSESSMENT AND MANAGEMENT

Assess resources (e.g., availability and skill of caregivers, finances, equipment) of individuals being treated for pressure ulcers in the home.

A successful treatment program requires adequate caregiver and equipment resources. Caregivers need to be evaluated for their ability to comprehend and implement the treatment requirements. Caregivers should also be evaluated for their level of strength and endurance. Economic factors should be considered, because they may limit the supply and availability of equipment, as well as opportunities to relieve caregivers.

ULCER CARE DRESSINGS

Consider caregiver time when selecting a dressing.

In the home setting, caregivers may choose more expensive dressing materials to reduce the frequency of dressing changes.

INFECTION CONTROL

Clean dressing may also be used in the home setting. Disposal of contaminated dressings in the home should be done in a manner consistent with local regulations.

Clean dressings, as opposed to sterile ones, are recommended for home use until research demonstrates otherwise. This recommendation is in keeping with principles regarding nosocomial infections and with past success of clean urinary catheterization in the home setting, and it takes into account the expense of sterile dressings and the dexterity required to apply them. The "no-touch" technique can be used for dressing changes. This technique is a method of changing surface dressings without touching the wound or the surface of any dressing that might be in contact with the wound. Adherent dressings should be grasped by the corner and removed slowly, whereas gauze dressings can be pinched in the center and lifted off.

The Environmental Protection Agency recommends that soiled dressings be placed in securely fastened plastic bags before being added to other household trash. Local regulations vary, however, and home care agencies and clients are advised to follow procedures that are consistent with local laws.

Modified from Agency for Health Care Policy and Research, Panel for the Treatment of Pressure Ulcers in Adults: *Treatment of pressure ulcers*, Clinical Practice Guideline No. 15, AHCPR Pub No. 95-0653, Rockville, Md, 1994, Agency for Health Care Policy and Research, Public Health Service, U.S. Department of Health and Human Services.

Ayello's Assessment   Box 47-12

A	natomical location, age of wound	A	Chronic wounds heal slower. Wounds near the anus need more frequent observation of dressings.
S	ize, shape, stage	S	taging of the wound will help in selecting the appropriate healing treatments and dressing. Measuring guides can assist in determining the length and width of the ulcer. A sterile cotton-tipped applicator can be used to measure the depth of the ulcer.
S	inus tract	S	Gently use a sterile cotton-tipped applicator to locate any sinus tracts. Use a clock as a reference to describe location.
E	xudate	E	Wound drainage must be contained to protect the surrounding skin. Note amount, color, and characteristic of the drainage.
S	epsis	S	All pressure ulcers are considered colonized. Wounds with bacterial counts $>10^5$ are infected. Observe for signs and symptoms of local infection: purulent exudate, odor, erythema, warmth, tenderness, edema, pain, fever, and elevated white count. Systemic infection such as osteomyelitis must be treated. Routine swab culturing of all pressure ulcers is not recommended.
S	urrounding skin	S	Protect the surrounding skin from breakdown from moisture.
M	argins, maceration	M	Identify condition of wound margins and if they are contracting. Evaluate for maceration if present. Institute measures to protect skin.
E	rythema, epithelialization, eschar	E	valuate for wound healing as evidenced by these changes in the ulcer, skin tone. Changes in dark-skinned clients are best assessed with good lighting.
N	ecrotic, nose, neovascularization	N	ecrotic tissue must be removed to stage and heal the ulcer. If an odor is present, more frequent cleansing and maybe debridement are needed.
T	issue bed, tenderness to touch, tension	T	Identify tissue bed and medicate for pain.

From Ayello EA, 1992 (revised 1995).

PRESSURE SORE STATUS TOOL   NAME_____

Complete the rating sheet to assess pressure sore status. Evaluate each item by picking the response that best describes the wound and entering the score in the item score column for the appropriate date.

Location: Anatomic site. Circle, identify right (**R**) or left (**L**) and use "**X**" to mark site on body diagrams:

_____ Sacrum & coccyx	_____ Lateral ankle
_____ Trochanter	_____ Medial ankle
_____ Ischial tuberosity	_____ Heel Other Site _____

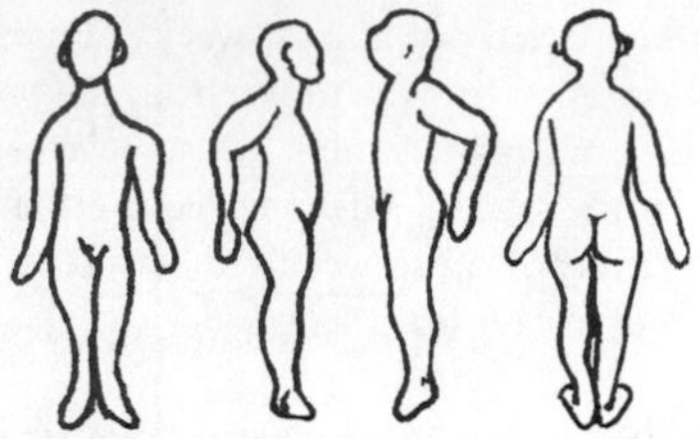

Shape: Overall wound pattern; assess by observing perimeter and depth.
Circle and <u>date</u> appropriate description:

_____ Irregular	_____ Linear or elongated
_____ Round/oval	_____ Bowl/boat
_____ Square/rectangle _____	_____ Butterfly Other Shape _____

Item	Assessment	Date	Date	Date
		Score	**Score**	**Score**
1. Size	1 = Length x width < 4 sq cm 2 = Length x width 4 -16 sq cm 3 = Length x width 16.1 - 36 sq cm 4 = Length x width 36.1 - 80 sq cm 5 = Length x width > 80 sq cm			
2. Depth	1 = Non-blanchable erythema on intact skin 2 = Partial thickness skin loss involving epidermis &/or dermis 3 = Full thickness skin loss involving damage or necrosis of subcutaneous tissue; may extend down to but not through underlying fascia; &/or mixed partial & full thickness &/or tissue layers obscured by granulation tissue 4 = Obscured by necrosis 5 = Full thickness skin loss with extensive destruction, tissue necrosis or damage to muscle, bone or supporting structures			
3. Edges	1 = Indistinct, diffuse, none clearly visible 2 = Distinct, outline clearly visible, attached, even with wound base 3 = Well-defined, not attached to wound base 4 = Well-defined, not attached to base, rolled under, thickened 5 = Well-defined, fibrotic, scarred or hyperkeratotic			
4. Under-mining	1 = Undermining < 2 cm in any area 2 = Undermining 2-4 cm involving < 50% wound margins 3 = Undermining 2-4 cm involving > 50% wound margins 4 = Undermining > 4 cm in any area 5 = Tunneling &/or sinus tract formation			
5. Necrotic Tissue Type	1 = None visible 2 = White/grey non-viable tissue &/or non-adherent yellow slough 3 = Loosely adherent yellow slough 4 = Adherent, soft, black eschar 5 = Firmly adherent, hard, black eschar			
6. Necrotic Tissue Amount	1 = None visible 2 = < 25% of wound bed covered 3 = 25% to 50% of wound covered 4 = > 50% and < 75% of wound covered 5 = 75% to 100% of wound covered			

c 1990 Barbara Bates-Jensen

Figure 47-20 Pressure Sore Status Tool (PSST).
Courtesy Barbara Bates-Jensen.

Item	Assessment	Date	Date	Date
		Score	Score	Score
7. Exudate Type	1 = None or bloody 2 = Serosanguineous: thin, watery, pale red/pink 3 = Serous: thin, watery, clear 4 = Purulent: thin or thick, opaque, tan/yellow 5 = Foul purulent: thick, opaque, yellow/green with odor			
8. Exudate Amount	1 = None 2 = Scant 3 = Small 4 = Moderate 5 = Large			
9. Skin color Surrounding Wound	1 = Pink or normal for ethnic group 2 = Bright red &/or blanches to touch 3 = White or grey pallor or hypopigmented 4 = Dark red or purple &/or non-blanchable 5 = Black or hyperpigmented			
10. Peripheral Tissue Edema	1 = Minimal swelling around wound 2 = Non-pitting edema extends < 4 cm around wound 3 = Non-pitting edema extends $\geq$ 4 cm around wound 4 = Pitting edema extends < 4 cm around wound 5 = Crepitus &/or pitting edema extends $\geq$ 4 cm			
11. Peripheral Tissue Induration	1 = Minimal firmness around wound 2 = Induration < 2 cm around wound 3 = Induration 2-4 cm extending < 50% around wound 4 = Induration 2-4 cm extending $\geq$ 50% around wound 5 = Induration > 4 cm in any area			
12. Granulation Tissue	1 = Skin intact or partial thickness wound 2 = Bright, beefy red; 75% to 100% of wound filled &/or tissue overgrowth 3 = Bright, beefy red; < 75% & > 25% of wound filled 4 = Pink, &/or dull, dusky red &/or fills $\leq$ 25% of wound 5 = No granulation tissue present			
13. Epithelialization	1 = 100% wound covered, surface intact 2 = 75% to <100% wound covered &/or epithelial tissue extends >0.5cm into wound bed 3 = 50% to <75% wound covered &/or epithelial tissue extends to <0.5cm into wound bed 4 = 25% to < 50% wound covered 5 = < 25% wound covered			
TOTAL SCORE				
SIGNATURE				

PRESSURE SORE STATUS CONTINUUM

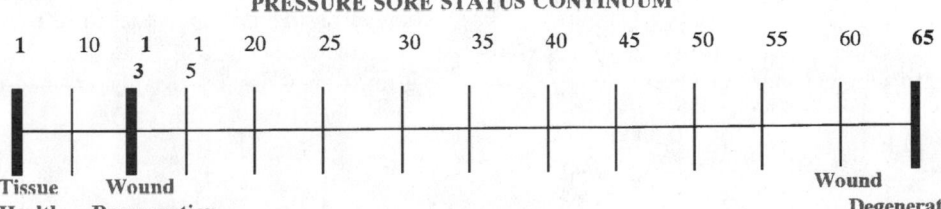

Plot the total score on the Pressure Sore Status Continuum by putting an "X" on the line and the date beneath the line. Plot multiple scores with their dates to see-at-a-glance regeneration or degeneration of the wound.

c 1990 Barbara Bates-Jensen

Figure 47-20, cont'd   Pressure Sore Status Tool (PSST).

PRESSURE SORE STATUS TOOL

Instructions for use

<u>General Guidelines:</u>

Fill out the attached rating sheet to assess a pressure sore's status after reading the definitions and methods of assessment described below. Evaluate once a week and whenever a change occurs in the wound. Rate according to each item by picking the response that best describes the wound and entering that score in the item score column for the appropriate date. When you have rated the pressure sore on all items, determine the total score by adding together the 13-item scores. The HIGHER the total score, the more severe the pressure sore status. Plot total score on the Pressure Sore Status Continuum to determine progress.

<u>Specific Instructions:</u>

1.   Size: Use ruler to measure the longest and widest aspect of the wound surface in centimeters; multiply length x width.

2.   Depth: Pick the depth, thickness, most appropriate to the wound using these additional descriptions:
    1 =   tissues damaged but no break in skin surface.
    2 =   superficial, abrasion, blister or shallow crater. Even with, &/or elevated above skin surface (e.g., hyperplasia).
    3 =   deep crater with or without undermining of adjacent tissue.
    4 =   visualization of tissue layers not possible due to necrosis.
    5 =   supporting structures include tendon, joint capsule.

3.   Edges: Use this guide:

Indistinct, diffuse	=	unable to clearly distinguish wound outline.
Attached	=	even or flush with wound base, <u>no</u> sides or walls present; flat.
Not attached	=	sides or walls <u>are</u> present; floor or base of wound is deeper than edge.
Rolled under, thickened	=	soft to firm and flexible to touch.
Hyperkeratosis	=	callous-like tissue formation around wound & at edges.
Fibrotic, scarred	=	hard, rigid to touch.

4.   Undermining: Assess by inserting a cotton tipped applicator under the wound edge; advance it as far as it will go without using undue force; raise the tip of the applicator so it may be seen or felt on the surface of the skin; mark the surface with a pen; measure the distance from the mark on the skin to the edge of the wound. Continue process around the wound. Then use a transparent metric measuring guide with concentric circles divided into 4 (25%) pie-shaped quadrants to help determine percent of wound involved.

5.   Necrotic Tissue Type: Pick the type of necrotic tissue that is <u>predominant</u> in the wound according to color, consistency and adherence using this guide:

White/gray non-viable tissue	=	may appear prior to wound opening; skin surface is white or gray.
Non-adherent, yellow slough	=	thin, mucinous substance; scattered throughout wound bed; easily separated from wound tissue.
Loosely adherent, yellow slough	=	thick, stringy, clumps of debris; attached to wound tissue.
Adherent, soft, black eschar	=	soggy tissue; strongly attached to tissue in center or base of wound.
Firmly adherent, hard/black eschar	=	firm, crusty tissue; strongly attached to wound base <u>and</u> edges (like a hard scab).

c 1990 Barbara Bates-Jensen

Figure 47-20, cont'd   Pressure Sore Status Tool (PSST).

6. **Necrotic Tissue Amount**: Use a transparent metric measuring guide with concentric circles divided into 4 (25%) pie-shaped quadrants to help determine percent of wound involved.

7. **Exudate Type**: Some dressings interact with wound drainage to produce a gel or trap liquid. Before assessing exudate type, gently cleanse wound with normal saline or water. Pick the exudate type that is <u>predominant</u> in the wound according to color and consistency, using this guide:

Bloody	=	thin, bright red
Serosanguineous	=	thin, watery pale red to pink
Serous	=	thin, watery, clear
Purulent	=	thin or thick, opaque tan to yellow
Foul purulent	=	thick, opaque yellow to green with offensive odor

8. **Exudate Amount**: Use a transparent metric measuring guide with concentric circles divided into 4 (25%) pie-shaped quadrants to determine percent of dressing involved with exudate. Use this guide:

None	=	wound tissues dry.
Scant	=	wound tissues moist; no measurable exudate.
Small	=	wound tissues wet; moisture evenly distributed in wound; drainage involves $\leq$ 25% dressing.
Moderate	=	wound tissues saturated; drainage may or may not be evenly distributed in wound; drainage involves > 25% to $\leq$ 75% dressing.
Large	=	wound tissues bathed in fluid; drainage freely expressed; may or may not be evenly distributed in wound; drainage involves > 75% of dressing.

9. **Skin Color Surrounding Wound**: Assess tissues within 4cm of wound edge. Dark-skinned persons show the colors "bright red" and "dark red" as a deepening of normal ethnic skin color or a purple hue. As healing occurs in dark-skinned persons, the new skin is pink and may never darken.

10. **Peripheral Tissue Edema**: Assess tissues within 4cm of wound edge. Non-pitting edema appears as skin that is shiny and taut. Identify pitting edema by firmly pressing a finger down into the tissues and waiting for 5 seconds, on release of pressure, tissues fail to resume previous position and an indentation appears. Crepitus is accumulation of air or gas in tissues. Use a transparent metric measuring guide to determine how far edema extends beyond wound.

11. **Peripheral Tissue Induration**: Assess tissues within 4cm of wound edge. Induration is abnormal firmness of tissues with margins. Assess by gently pinching the tissues. Induration results in an inability to pinch the tissues. Use a transparent metric measuring guide with concentric circles divided into 4 (25%) pie-shaped quadrants to determine percent of wound and area involved.

12. **Granulation Tissue**: Granulation tissue is the growth of small blood vessels and connective tissue to fill in full thickness wounds. Tissue is healthy when bright, beefy red, shiny and granular with a velvety appearance. Poor vascular supply appears as pale pink or blanched to dull, dusky red color.

13. **Epithelialization**: Epithelialization is the process of epidermal resurfacing and appears as pink or red skin. In partial thickness wounds it can occur throughout the wound bed as well as from the wound edges. In full thickness wounds it occurs from the edges only. Use a transparent metric measuring guide with concentric circles divided into 4 (25%) pie-shaped quadrants to help determine percent of wound involved and to measure the distance the epithelial tissue extends into the wound.

Table 47-11 **Dressing by Ulcer Stage**

Dressing	Comments*
Stage I	
Film dressing (Tegadern, Bioclusive, Op-site, Uniflex)	Protects from shearing force
	May be left in place up to 7 days if occlusive seal remains
	Will facilitate softening of eschar on deeper-ulcers
	Traps serous exudate and provides moist wound environment
Hydrocolloid dressing (such as DuoDERM, Comfeel, IntraSite)	Is absorbent
	May be left in place up to 7 days, if occlusive seal remains (Nurse is unable to assess wound with dressing in place.)
	Reacts with wound fluid to create a soft gel that promotes granulation and epithelialization
Stage II	
Hydrocolloid dressing	See stage I
Composite dressing (such as Viasorb, film dressing over Telfa)	Provides absorbent, nonadherent layer over wound with occlusive cover
Hydrogel dressing (such as Vigilon, Geliperm, J&J Gel)	Is absorbent for draining ulcers
	Usually requires gauze dressing cover
Absorptive dressing (such as Exu-dry, Bard absorption dressing)	Is absorbent and nonadherent
	Protects from shearing force
	May be used with topical agents
	Is not occlusive dressing
	Absorbs exudate and debris while maintaining moist environment*
Stage III	
Polyurethane foam (Lyofoam, Allevyn)	Absorbs exudate
	Maintains moist wound environment*
Hydrocolloid dressing (see stage I)	Increases absorbency and wear time when hydrocolloid granules or paste is used
	Can cause damage because of frequent removal (every day or more often) (Recommend other dressing.)
Hydrogel dressing (see stage II)	May be used as carrier for topical agents, including topically applied growth factors
Absorptive dressing	See stage II
Stage IV	
Hydrocolloid dressing (see stages I to III)	May be contraindicated because of location of ulcer, exposed bone, and amount of drainage
Hydrogel dressing	See stages II to III
Gauze dressing	*Kerlix type:*
	Is absorbent but not occlusive
	Generally requires dressing changes every 8 to 12 hr
	Dry gauze:
	Removes drainage away from wound surface†
	Moist gauze:
	Maintains moist wound environment while removing drainage away from surface†
	Moist-to-dry:
	Debrides necrotic and healthy tissue nonselectively

*As with *all* occlusive dressing, wounds should *not* be clinically infected.

†Data from Maklebust J: Pressure ulcer update, *RN* 41(12):56, 1991.

Treating Pressure Ulcers Skill 47-2

Delegation Considerations

Treatment of pressure ulcers requires problem solving and knowledge application unique to professional nursing. For this procedure delegation is not appropriate. Instruct assistive personnel to report changes in skin integrity to the nurse immediately. In some states and practice settings, *nonsterile* dressing application may be delegated to others for chronic, established wounds where the protocol has been evaluated and designated by a professional nurse.

EQUIPMENT

- Disposable gloves (clean)
- Goggles and cover gown
- Plastic bag for dressing disposal
- Measuring device (tape measure)
- Cotton-tipped applicators
- Camera and tracing film (optional)
- Topical cleansing agent
- Sterile solution container
- Washbasin, washcloths, towels
- Dressing of choice (see Table 47-11)
- Skin protectant
- Hypoallergenic tape (if needed)
- 35-ml syringe with 19-gauge needle
- Documentation records (e.g., graph paper)
- Scale for assessing wound healing

STEPS	RATIONALE
1. Assess client's level of comfort and need for pain medication.	Dressing change procedure is better tolerated if pain is controlled.
2. Determine if client has allergies to topical agents.	Topical agents may cause localized skin reactions.
3. Review physician's order for topical agent or dressing (in many cases physician follows nurse's recommendation for pressure ulcer care).	Ensures that proper medication and treatment are administered.
4. Wash hands and apply clean gloves. Close room door or bedside curtains.	Reduces transmission of microorganisms and prevents accidental exposure to body fluids.
5. Position client to allow dressing removal.	Area should be accessible for dressing change.
6. Assess pressure ulcer and surrounding skin to determine ulcer stage (see Figure 47-5).	Assessment of a pressure ulcer should be comprehensive (Ayello, 1996).
a. Note color, moisture, and appearance of skin around ulcer and of ulcer itself.	
b. Measure two maximum perpendicular diameters.	Skin condition may indicate progressive tissue damage. Provides an objective measure of wound size. May influence size and type of dressing selected.
	Surface area = length $\times$ width

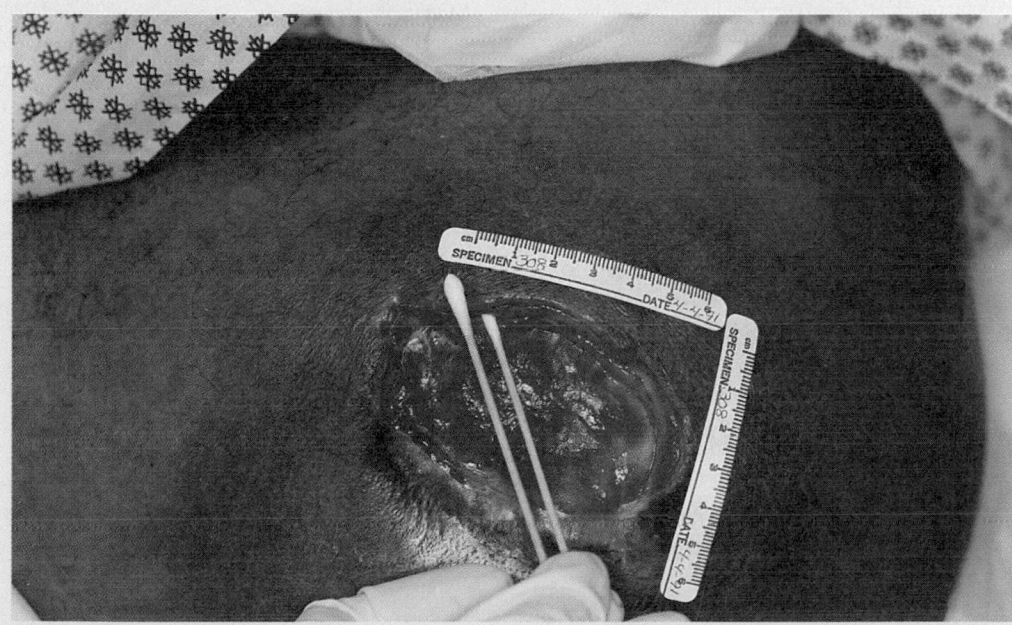

Step 6c

STEPS	RATIONALE
c. Measure depth of pressure ulcer using sterile cotton-tipped applicator or other device that will allow measurement of wound depth (see illustration).	Depth measure is important for determining wound volume. While surface area adequately represents tissue loss in stage I and II ulcers, volume more adequately represents tissue loss in deeper stage III and IV wounds. $$\text{Volume} = 2(L \times D) + 2(W \times D) + (L + D)$$
d. Measure depth (D) of undermining skin by lateral tissue necrosis. Use a cotton-tipped applicator and gently probe under skin edges.	Undermining represents the loss of the underlying tissue (subcutaneous and muscle) to a greater extent than the skin (see illustration). Undermining may indicate progressive tissue necrosis.
7. Wash skin around ulcer gently with warm water and rinse area thoroughly with water.	Reduces number of resident bacteria. Soap can be irritating to skin.
8. Gently dry skin thoroughly by patting lightly with towel.	Retained moisture causes maceration of skin layers.
9. Change to sterile gloves (check agency policy).	Aseptic technique must be maintained during cleansing, measuring, and application of dressings. Refer to institutional policy regarding use of clean or sterile gloves.
10. Cleanse ulcer thoroughly with normal saline or cleansing agent: a. Use irrigating syringe for deep ulcers. b. Cleansing in the shower may be done with a hand-held shower head.	Removes wound debris. Previously applied enzymes may require soaking for removal.
11. Apply topical agents, as prescribed:	Topical agents should be changed as wound heals or worsens.
A. **Enzymes**	
(1) Apply thin, even layer of ointment over necrotic areas of ulcer only. Do not apply enzyme to surrounding skin.	Thick layer of ointment is not necessary. Thin layer absorbs and acts more effectively. Excess medication can irritate surrounding skin. Some enzymes can cause burning, paresthesia, and dermatitis to surrounding skin. Check manufacturer's direction for frequency of application.
(2) Apply gauze dressing directly over ulcer. (3) Tape securely in place.	Protects wound. Prevents bacteria from entering wound.
B. **Hydrogel agents**	
(1) Cover surface of ulcer with Hydrogel using applicator or gloved hand.	Provides maintenance of wound humidity while absorbing excess drainage. May be used as carrier for topical agents.
(2) Apply dry fluffy gauze or hydrocolloid or transparent dressing over gel to completely cover ulcer.	Holds Hydrogel against wound surface; is absorbent.
C. **Calcium alginates**	
(1) Pack wound with alginate using applicator or gloved hand.	Provides maintenance of wound humidity while absorbing excess drainage.
(2) Apply dry gauze, foam, or hydrocolloid over alginate.	Holds alginate against wound surface.
12. Reposition client comfortably off of pressure ulcer.	Avoids accidental removal of dressings.
13. Remove gloves and dispose of soiled supplies. Wash hands.	Reduces transmission of microorganisms.

Critical Decision Point: A clean pressure ulcer should show evidence of some healing within 2 to 4 weeks.

14. Observe skin surrounding ulcer for inflammation, edema, and tenderness.	Contact dermatitis may result from exposure to certain topical agents. Without proper preventive care, ulcer can spread to involve neighboring tissue.
15. Inspect dressings and exposed ulcer, observing for drainage, foul odor, and tissue necrosis. Monitor client for signs and symptoms of infection, including fever and elevated white blood cell count.	Ulcers can become infected. Dressings and wound care products should be changed as the wound characteristics change (e.g., necrotic ulcer requires certain products; ulcers with large amounts of drainage require others).
16. Complete ulcer information required for one of wound-healing scales.	Allows comparison of serial measurements to assess wound healing. It is helpful to plot surface area and volume measurements on graph paper.

STEPS	RATIONALE
17. Compare subsequent ulcer measurements.	Wound-healing scales such as the PUSH or the PSST (see Figure 47-20) can be used to quantify and measure pressure ulcer healing.
18. Do *not* use the pressure ulcer staging system to measure pressure ulcer healing (NPUAP, 1995a,b).	System measures "wounding," not healing.

Recording and Reporting
- Record appearance of ulcer in client's record.
- Describe type of topical agent used, dressing applied, and client's response.
- Report any deterioration in ulcer appearance to nurse in charge or physician.

Home Care Considerations
- Cost can be a factor. Some clients have more time than financial resources. They may choose a less expensive treatment option such as dressing material, especially if there is no third-party reimbursement.
- "Disposal of contaminated dressings in the home should be done in a manner consistent with local regulations" (AHCPR, 1994).
- Discuss need for home pressure-relief surface or bed.

udate, odor, and size. Pain that occurs with debridement needs to be assessed and prevented or effectively managed (AHCPR, 1994).

Methods of debridement include mechanical, autolytic, chemical/enzymatic, and sharp/surgical. Mechanical debridement may use wet-to-dry saline gauze dressings. The dressing must be allowed to dry thoroughly before the nurse "pulls" the gauze that has adhered to the tissue out of the pressure ulcer. This is a nonselective method of debridement, since devitalized and viable tissue are both removed. It should never be used in a clean, granulating wound. Other methods of mechanical debridement are wound irrigation and whirlpool treatments (AHCPR, 1994). Whirlpool treatments are performed by physical therapists.

Autolytic debridement uses synthetic dressings over a wound to allow the eschar to be self-digested by the action of enzymes that are present in wound fluids (AHCPR, 1994). It can be accomplished by using some of the newer dressing materials over the pressure ulcer. Some examples of dressings used are transparent synthetic membrane dressings and hydrocolloid dressings. The dressing will interact with the pressure ulcer tissue surface. Eschar is softened because the devitalized tissue is self-digested from the enzymes that are normally found in wound fluid. Autolytic debridement is contraindicated for infected wounds (AHCPR, 1994).

Enzymatic debridement is the application of topical debriding enzymes to the devitalized tissue on the wound surface. These drugs require a physician's order. It is important to remember that the techniques for use and the properties of each of the enzymatic debriding agents are different. Clinicians should follow the manufacturer's specific directions. Of all the enzymatic debriding agents, only collagenase (Santyl) is mentioned in the AHCPR

guidelines (1994) as promoting debridement and growth of granulation tissue.

Surgical debridement is the removal of devitalized tissue by using a scalpel, scissors, or other sharp instrument. Physicians and, in some states, specially educated nurses can perform surgical debridement of a pressure ulcer. Nurses should check the Nurse Practice Act for their state to see if surgical debridement is covered as a nursing function. It is the quickest method of debridement. It is usually indicated when the client has signs of cellulitis or sepsis. Clean, dry dressings should be used for 8 to 24 hours after sharp debridement associated with bleeding. Afterward, moist dressings can be reinstituted to promote wound healing (AHCPR, 1994).

Moist Wound Healing. In the past, choices for wound care management have been based on superstition and magic (Levine, 1992) and clinician preference (Doughty, 1992). Clinicians previously believed that a dry environment was necessary to heal a wound. Studies of the wound-healing process have shown that a moist rather than a dry wound environment (e.g., when a heat lamp is used) is necessary for wound healing. A **moist wound-healing environment** is of prime importance for wound healing because it affects both the rate of epithelialization and the amount of scar formation. A moist wound-healing environment provides the optimum condition for rapid healing. When a barrier, such as a dressing, is placed over the wound (either semioccluded or occluded), the surface of the wound remains moist with wound fluid. This allows epidermal cells to migrate more readily and rapidly. A moist wound environment can be promoted with the use of appropriate dressings.

Once a pressure ulcer has been successfully debrided and has a clean granulating base, the goal of local care is to

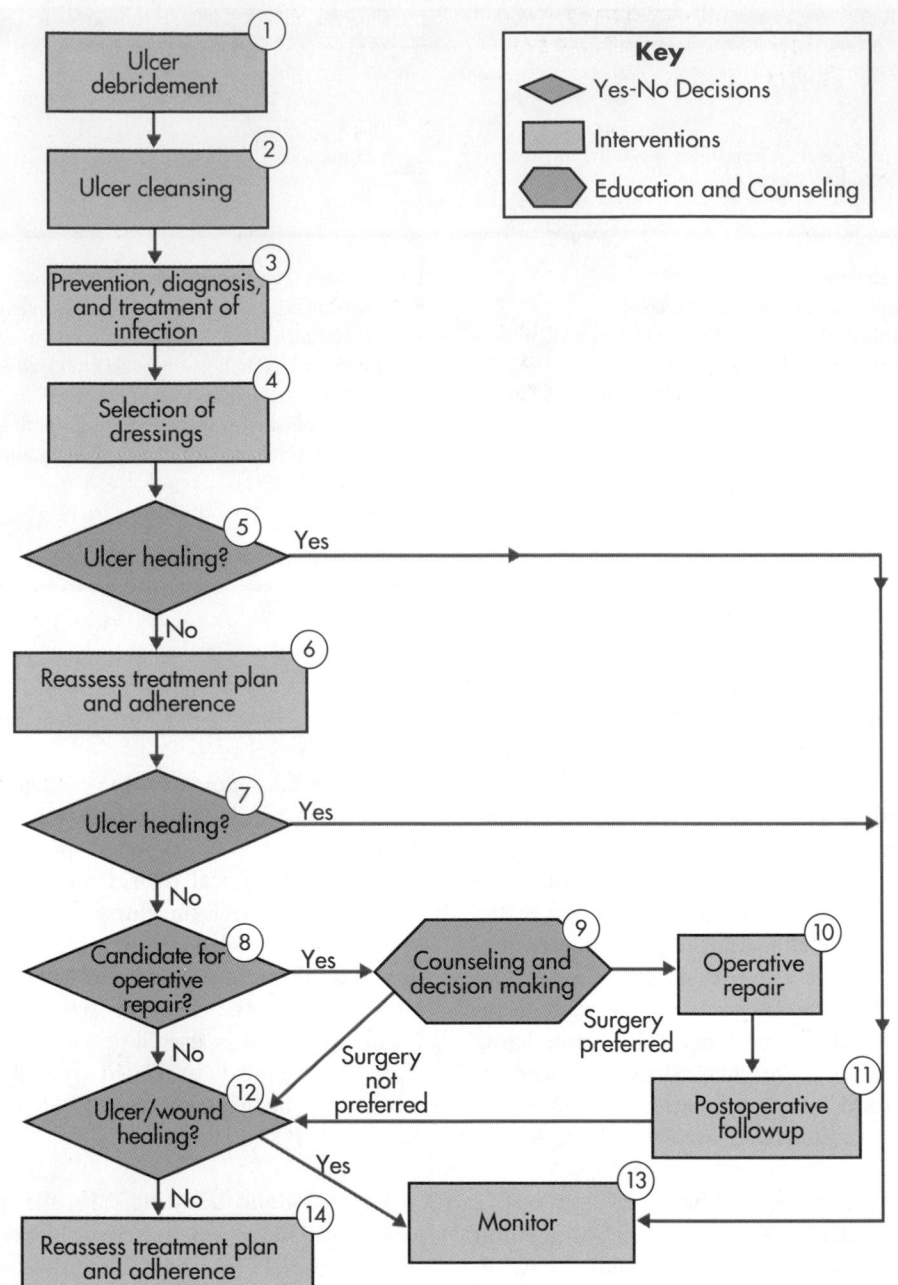

Figure 47-21   Ulcer care.
From Agency for Health Care Policy and Research, Panel for Treatment of Pressure Ulcers in
Adults: *Treatment of pressure ulcers,* Clinical Practice Guideline No. 15, AHCPR Pub No.
95-0653, Rockville, Md, 1994, Agency for Health Care Policy and Research, Public Health Service,
U.S. Department of Health and Human Services.

provide an appropriate environment for moist wound
healing and to support the newly formed granulation tissue. Wounds should be cleansed initially and at each
dressing change (AHCPR, 1994). Pressure ulcers should
be cleansed only with wound cleansers such as normal
saline or some commercial wound cleansers that are not
cytotoxic (will not damage or kill cells, such as fibroblasts
and healing tissue) (AHCPR, 1994). Research has reported

that some commercial wound cleansers are cytotoxic
(Foresman and others, 1993; Wright and Orr, 1993). Skin
cleaners are not the same as wound cleansers. *Do not clean
uninfected or necrotic ulcer wounds with skin cleaners or antiseptic agents* (AHCPR, 1994). Some commonly used solutions that are cytotoxic and therefore should not be used
to clean granulating wounds are Dakin's solution (sodium
hypochlorite solution), acetic acid, povidone iodine, hy-

drogen peroxide, and some commercial wound cleansers.

Besides using the correct type of solution, it is important to use enough irrigation pressure to clean the pressure ulcer without causing trauma to the wound bed (Barr, 1995; Rodeheaver, 1999). The AHCPR guidelines (1994) state that 4 to 15 psi is a safe and effective pressure for cleaning a granulating pressure ulcer. A 19-gauge needle or an angiocatheter and a 35-cc syringe delivers saline to a pressure ulcer at 8 psi (Figure 47-22). A bulb syringe has an irrigation pressure below 4 psi and therefore will not adequately clean the pressure ulcer (AHCPR, 1994). A list of different types of systems used to clean pressure ulcers and a list of their pressures can be found in Table 47-12.

The cleansed pressure ulcer needs a dressing. The goal of dressings is to protect the pressure ulcer, to maintain a moist healing environment, and to prevent maceration of the surrounding wound skin. There are many dressings available today from which the clinician can choose to use on pressure ulcers (Baranoski, 1999; Krasner, 1992). Some factors to consider when selecting a dressing are maintenance of a moist environment, prevention of wound desiccation (drying out), ability to absorb the wound drainage, location of the wound, elimination of dead space, amount of caregiver time, cost, and clean versus sterile dressings. Studies of different types of moist wound dressings showed no differences in pressure ulcer healing outcomes (AHCPR, 1994).

The treatment plan will change as the ulcer heals. For example, for a necrotic wound, a membrane dressing may be used initially to debride the wound by autolysis. Afterward, pressure ulcers that have large amounts of exudate (stage III or IV) require a dressing with absorptive ability. For reddened areas or areas of broken skin integrity, skin care products that lubricate and protect and promote wound healing are recommended. When the ulcer is pink with granulation tissue throughout, a dressing is indicated to promote healing. A clean, moist environment promotes migration of epithelial cells across the ulcer surface (Kloth, McCulloch, and Feedar, 1990).

There have been many practice changes as a result of the AHCPR guidelines (1994). Clean dressings, especially in the home setting, can be used on pressure ulcers. Clean gloves can be used for pressure ulcer care. If a client has more than one pressure ulcer, one pair of clean gloves can be used to do all of the dressing changes. The nurse must clean the least contaminated pressure ulcer first. For example, if a client has a pressure ulcer near the anus, it should be cleaned last. After the nurse completes all of the dressing changes for a particular client, the nurse can remove the gloves, wash hands, and put on clean gloves to care for the next clients wounds. All pressure ulcers are considered contaminated or colonized with bacteria; therefore routine swab cultures are not recommended. According to the AHCPR guidelines (1994), quantitative swab cultures may be indicated in a clean pressure ulcer that is not healing. Stotts (1995) believes that quantitative bacterial cultures can be performed by either needle biopsy or quantitative swab culture. Furthermore, a standardized technique for performing these two types of cul-

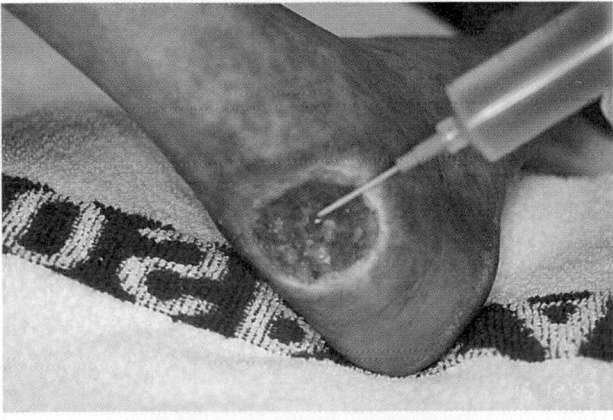

Figure 47-22 Wound irrigation.

Table 47-12	Irrigation Pressures Delivered by Various Devices	
Device		Irrigation Impact Pressure (PSI)
Spray Bottle—Ultra Klenz* (Carrington Laboratories, Inc., Dallas, Tex.)		1.2
Bulb Syringe* (Davol Inc., Cranston, R.I.)		2.0
Piston Irrigation Syringe (60-ml) with catheter tip (Premium Plastics, Inc., Chicago, Ill.)		4.2
Saline Squeeze Bottle (250-ml) with irrigation cap (Baxter Healthcare Corp., Deerfield, Ill.)		4.5
Water Pik at lowest setting (No. 1) (Teledyne Water Pik, Fort Collins, Col.)		6.0
Irrijet DS Syringe with tip (Ackrad Laboratories, Inc., Cranford, N.J.)		7.6
35-ml syringe with 19-gauge needle or angiocatheter		8.0
Water Pik at middle setting (No. 3)† (Teledyne Water Pik, Fort Collins, Col.)		42
Water Pik at highest setting (No. 5)† (Teledyne Water Pik, Fort Collins, Col.)		>50
Pressurized Cannister-Dey-Wash† (Dey Laboratories, Inc., Napa, Calif.)		>50

From Agency for Health Care Policy and Research, Panel for Treatment of Pressure Ulcers in Adults: *Treatment of pressure ulcers*, Clinical Practice Guideline No. 15, AHCPR Pub No. 95-0653, Rockville, Md, 1994, Agency for Health Care Policy and Research, Public Health Service, U.S. Department of Health and Human Services.

*These devices may not deliver enough pressure to adequately cleanse wounds.

†These devices may cause trauma and drive bacteria into wounds. They are not recommended for cleansing of soft tissue wounds.

tures is recommended (Box 47-13). Some authors have suggested some changes in practice from the AHCPR guidelines regarding infection-control management of pressure ulcers (Brown and Smith, 1999; Krasner, 1999).

In addition to local wound treatment, other methods, including electromagnetic energy, have been used to foster ulcer healing (Itoh and others, 1991). The AHCPR guidelines (1994) recommend considering a course of treatment with electrotherapy for stage III and IV pressure ulcers that are unresponsive to conventional therapies. The guidelines state that other adjunctive therapies (e.g., hyperbaric oxygen; infrared, ultraviolet, and low-energy laser irradiation; ultrasound; platelet-derived growth factors; miscellaneous topical agents; and systemic drugs other than antibiotics) require more research before a recommendation can be made regarding their use in the treatment of pressure ulcers. Some other new modalities for healing wounds are living skin equivalents, vacuum-assisted healing, and warming up the wound environment.

Education. Education of the client and caregivers/family is an important nursing function (Ayello, 1993, 1995; Ayello, Mezey, and Amella, 1997). There are a variety of educational tools, including videotapes and written materials, that can be used by the nurse when teaching clients and caregivers/family to prevent and treat pressure ulcers. Written materials are available on a variety of topics, including dressing changes; there are also guides for measuring wounds and charts for positioning clients. A step-by-step outline of practical pointers for nurses who will be developing their own client teaching materials has been written by Doak, Doak, and Root (1996). AHCPR (1992a, 1994) has booklets for clients on pressure ulcer prevention and treatment that can be helpful when teaching clients and their caregivers/family. These booklets are available in English and in Spanish. Teaching should be individualized for each client, especially with older clients (Box 47-14). A review of these booklets with suggestions on how to use them in the teaching plan of clients can be found in the literature (Ayello, 1993, 1995).

Understanding and assessment of the experience of the client and support person are also important dimensions in the treatment of people with pressure ulcers (AHCPR, 1994). Clinicians are only just now exploring through research the caregiver's perspective of the concerns and issues faced by frail older spouses caring for their loved ones with pressure ulcers (Baharestani, 1994). Interventions should be planned to meet the identified psychosocial needs of clients and their support persons (AHCPR, 1994).

Nutritional Status. Maintaining adequate protein intake and hemoglobin levels is important in the treatment of pressure ulcers (Kaminski, Pinchocofsky-Devin, and Williams, 1989). An algorithm provided by AHCPR (1994) can be used to help clinicians meet the goals of nutritional assessment and management for clients with pressure ulcers. The AHCPR guidelines (1994) recommend that an abbreviated nutritional assessment be done every 3 months for individuals at risk for malnutrition

---

Recommedations for Standardized Techniques for Wound Cultures   Box 47-13

NEEDLE ASPIRATION PROCEDURE

Clean intact skin with an antimicrobial solution. Allow it to dry.

Insert the needle through the client's skin while maintaining adequate *negative* pressure in the syringe and while pulling back on the syringe.

When performing the aspiration culture technique, it is essential to probe two to four areas when obtaining the culture.

QUANTITATIVE SWAB PROCEDURE

Clean the wound surface with a nonantimicrobial solution. Allow it to dry.

Swabbing of the wound should encompass a 1- to 2-cm area. Enough pressure needs to be used so that fluid is expressed from the wound tissue.

The culture can be processed during either a quantitative or semiquantitative method, depending on the microbiological expertise of the laboratory.

Modified from Stotts NA: Determination of bacterial burden in wounds. NPUAP Proceedings 1995, *Adv Wound Care* 7(4):28, 1995.

Client Teaching FOR IMPAIRED SKIN INTEGRITY   Box 47-14

OBJECTIVE
- Risks for impaired skin integrity will be reduced.

TEACHING STRATEGIES
- Demonstrate measures to reduce pressure, moisture, and friction on the skin.
- Explain how to evaluate and select proper incontinence control devices.
- Provide written materials that explain skin care procedures in clear, easy-to-understand, nontechnical language.

- Explain to client whom to contact and what to do if a break in skin integrity occurs.

EVALUATION
- Observe client perform proper positioning and skin care measures.
- Assess skin for breaks in integrity.
- Ask client how an incontinence control device was selected.
- Ask client what to do if a break in skin integrity occurs.

(Box 47-15). This includes individuals who are unable to take food by mouth or who have experienced an involuntary change in weight. Parameters for clinically significant malnutrition have been defined (AHCPR, 1994) (Box 47-16). The client's mouth and skin should be assessed for signs of nutritional deficiencies (see Chapter 43). Vitamin and mineral supplements should be given if deficiencies are confirmed or suspected. The client's hydration status, especially the amount of fluids and the weight pattern, should also be assessed (Ayello, Thomas, and Litchford, in press).

Protein Status. Clients with a potential for or actual decreased serum albumin levels or poor protein intake need a nutritional evaluation to ensure proper caloric intake (AHCPR, 1994). A client can lose as much as 50 g of protein per day from an open, weeping pressure ulcer. While the RDA of protein for adults is 0.8 g/kg, a higher intake of protein up to 1.8 g/kg/day may be needed for healing (Ayello, Thomas, and Litchford, in press). Increased protein intake helps rebuild epidermal tissue. Increased caloric intake helps replace subcutaneous tissue. Vitamin C promotes protein synthesis and tissue repair.

Hemoglobin. A low hemoglobin level decreases delivery of oxygen to the tissues and leads to further ischemia. When possible, hemoglobin should be maintained at 12 g/100 ml.

First Aid for Wounds. In an emergency setting the nurse uses first aid measures for wound care. Under more stable conditions the nurse uses a variety of interventions to ensure wound healing. When a client suffers a traumatic wound, first aid interventions include stabilizing cardiopulmonary function (see Chapter 39), promoting hemostasis, cleansing the wound, and protecting the wound from further injury.

Hemostasis. After assessing the type and extent of the wound, the nurse controls bleeding of a laceration by applying direct pressure on the wound with a sterile or clean dressing, such as a washcloth. After bleeding subsides, an adhesive bandage strip or gauze dressing taped over the laceration allows skin edges to close and a blood clot to form. If a dressing becomes saturated with blood, the nurse adds another layer of dressing, continues to apply pressure, and elevates the affected part. Further disruption of skin layers should be avoided. More serious lacerations should be sutured by a physician. Pressure dressings used during the first 24 to 48 hours after trauma help maintain hemostasis.

A puncture wound is allowed to bleed to remove dirt and other contaminants, such as saliva from a dog bite. When a penetrating object, such as a knife blade, is present, it is not removed. Removal could cause massive, uncontrolled bleeding. Except for skull injuries, the nurse may apply pressure around the penetrating object, but not on it, and the client should be transported to an emergency facility.

Cleansing. The process of cleansing a wound involves selecting both an appropriate cleansing solution and using a mechanical means of delivering that solution without causing injury to the healing wound tissue (AHCPR, 1994). Gentle cleansing of a wound removes contaminants that might serve as sources of infection. However, vigorous cleaning using a method with too much mechanical force can cause bleeding or further injury. For abrasions, minor lacerations, and small puncture wounds, the nurse first rinses the wound in running water, cleans it with mild soap and water, and may apply an over-the-counter antiseptic. Topical antibiotics applied to wound edges may slow microorganism growth. However, prolonged application of topical antibiotics can foster growth of nonsusceptible organisms. When a laceration is

---

Clinically Significant Malnutrition Box 47-15

Serum albumin is less than 3.5 mg/100 ml.
Total lymphocyte count is less than 1800/mm³.
Body weight has decreased more than 15%.

Modified from Agency for Health Care Policy and Research, Panel for Treatment of Pressure Ulcers in Adults: *Treatment of pressure ulcers,* Clinical Practice Guideline No. 15, AHCPR Pub No. 95-0653, Rockville, Md, 1994, Agency for Health Care Policy and Research, Public Health Service, U.S. Department of Health and Human Services.

AHCPR Recommendations for Nutritional Assessment and Management of Pressure Ulcers Box 47-16

Ensure adequate dietary intake to prevent malnutrition to the extent that this is compatible with the individual's wishes.
Perform an abbreviated nutritional assessment, as defined by the Nutritional Screening Initiative, at least every 3 months for individuals who are unable to take food by mouth or who experience an involuntary change in weight.
Encourage dietary intake or supplementation if an individual with a pressure ulcer is malnourished. If dietary intake continues to be inadequate, impractical, or impossible, nutritional support (usually tube feeding) should be used to place the client into positive nitrogen balance (approximately 30 to 35 calories/kg/day and 1.25 to 1.50 g of protein/kg/day) according to the goals of care.
Give vitamin and mineral supplements if deficiencies are confirmed or suspected.

Modified from Agency for Health Care Policy and Research, Panel for Treatment of Pressure Ulcers in Adults: *Treatment of pressure ulcers,* Clinical Practice Guideline No. 15, AHCPR Pub No. 95-0653, Rockville, Md, 1994, Agency for Health Care Policy and Research, Public Health Service, U.S. Department of Health and Human Services.

bleeding profusely, the nurse should only brush away surface contaminants and concentrate on hemostasis until the client can be cared for in a clinic or hospital.

Topical Agents for Cleansing Wounds.   According to the AHCPR guidelines (1994), normal saline is the preferred cleansing agent. It is physiological and will not harm tissue. Many topical agents that in the past were used to clean wounds, including povidone-iodine solutions, Dakin's solution (sodium hypochlorite solution), acetic acid solution, and hydrogen peroxide, are toxic to fibroblasts and therefore should not be used to clean wounds. The type of cleansing solution selected is based on such factors as the wound type, drainage, and presence or absence of infection.

Gentle cleansing with normal saline and the application of saline dressings (wet-to-wet, wet-to-damp) are often used in healing wounds and to debride wounds (wet-to-dry). The nurse uses saline to maintain the moist surface needed to promote the development and migration of epithelial tissue. Damp (wet-to-dry) saline dressings should be used only to debride wounds. They should never be used in a clean granulating wound.

Growth Factors.   Topical and parenteral growth factors have been used to treat nonhealing wounds and fistula formation. The growth hormone preparation Regranex is approved by the Food and Drug Administration only for use in diabetic foot ulcers. The nurse may be responsible for the use of this treatment modality after the physician determines that it may provide a benefit for the client's wound care. Teaching the client or significant other about the use of growth factors is also the nurse's responsibility. The nurse teaches the use of the medication, wound care, and the prevention of wound breakdown and recurrence.

Protection.   Regardless of whether bleeding has stopped, the nurse protects the wound from further injury by applying sterile or clean dressings and immobilizing the body part. A light dressing applied over minor wounds prevents entrance of microorganisms. In the case of small abrasions, it is acceptable to leave the wound open to air so that a scab can form.

Dressings.   The more extensive the wound, the larger the dressing required. In the home a clean towel or diaper may be the best dressing. A bulky dressing applied with pressure minimizes movement of underlying tissues and helps immobilize the entire body part. A bandage or cloth wrapped around a penetrating object should immobilize it adequately.

There are alternative dressings that can be used to cover and protect certain types of wounds. Examples are large wounds, wounds with drainage tubes or suction catheters in the wound, wounds that need frequent changing, and fistulas. In these wounds, pouches or special wound collection systems are now used to cover the wound. Some of these newer devices even have a plastic door on the front of the wound pouch so that the nurse can change the wound packing without removing the wound pouch from the skin.

The use of dressings requires an understanding of wound healing. A variety of dressing material is commercially available. Unless a dressing is suited to the characteristics of a wound, the dressing can hinder wound repair (Erwin-Toth and Hocevar, 1995; Krasner, 1995a; Motta, 1995; Baranoski, 1999).

The choice of dressings and the method of dressing a wound influence the progress of wound healing. The proper dressing should not allow a draining wound to become overly dry (desiccated) with extensive scab formation. When this occurs, the dermis dehydrates and crusts. As a result, a barrier forms against normal epidermal cell growth, leaving a depression or defect in the new epidermal surface. Furthermore, dryness of the wound may increase the client's discomfort. Ideally, a dressing leaves a wound slightly moist to promote epithelial cell migration. The dressing should also absorb drainage to prevent pooling of exudate that may promote bacterial growth, as well as maceration of surrounding skin from wound exudate (Erwin-Toth and Hocevar, 1995; Krasner, 1995a; Motta, 1995; Baranoski, 1999).

For surgical wounds that heal by primary intention, it is common to remove dressings as soon as drainage stops. In contrast, when the nurse dresses an open wound healing by secondary intention, the dressing material becomes a means for mechanically removing exudate and necrotic tissue.

Purposes of Dressings.   A dressing may serve several purposes:

Protecting a wound from microorganism contamination

Aiding hemostasis

Promoting healing by absorbing drainage and debriding a wound

Supporting or splinting the wound site

Protecting the client from seeing the wound (if perceived as unpleasant)

Promoting thermal insulation of the wound surface

Providing maintenance of high humidity between the wound and dressing

When the skin becomes broken, a dressing helps reduce exposure to microorganisms. However, when wound drainage is minimal, the healing process forms a natural fibrin seal that can eliminate the need for a dressing. A dressing is always needed for extensive wounds.

Pressure dressings promote hemostasis. Applied with elastic bandages, a pressure dressing exerts localized downward pressure over an actual or potential bleeding site. A pressure dressing eliminates dead space in underlying tissues so that wound healing progresses normally. The nurse checks pressure dressings to be sure that they do not interfere with circulation to a body part. The nurse assesses skin color, pulses in distal extremities, the client's comfort, and changes in sensation. Pressure dressings are not routinely removed.

A primary function of a dressing on a healing wound is to absorb drainage. Most traditional surgical dressings have three layers: a contact or primary layer, an absorbent layer, and an outer protective layer. The contact dressing covers the incision and part of the adjacent skin. Fibrin, blood products, and debris adhere to the contact dressing's surface. A problem occurs if the wound drainage dries, causing the dressing to stick to the suture line. Improper removal of the dressing can cause tearing of the healing epidermal surface. The nurse must either remove the dressing gently and moisten the attached area with sterile normal saline before removal or leave the dressing unchanged for several days.

The dressing technique will vary depending on the goal of the treatment plan for the wound. For example, if the goal is to maintain a moist environment for a clean granulating wound, it is important for the nurse to prevent the saline-moistened gauze dressing from drying and sticking to the healing wound. This is in direct contrast to the dressing technique that should be used if the goal of care is to mechanically debride the wound using a saline wet-to-dry dressing. When wounds require **debriding,** such as infected or necrotic wounds, the contact dressing debrides necrotic tissue and debris. In this case the contact dressing must be allowed to dry so that it sticks to underlying tissue, and debridement occurs during removal.

Dressings applied to a draining wound require frequent changing to prevent microorganism growth and skin breakdown. Bacteria grow readily in the dark, warm, moist environment under a dressing. Skin surfaces become macerated and irritated. Skin breakdown can be minimized by keeping the skin clean and dry and reducing the use of tape.

The absorbent dressing layer serves as a reservoir for additional secretions. The wicking action of woven gauze dressings pulls excess drainage into the dressing and away from the wound.

The final outer layer of a dressing helps prevent bacteria and other external contaminants from reaching the wound surface. Usually the outer dressing is made of a thicker dressing material.

A firmly taped or wrapped dressing supports or immobilizes a body part, minimizing movement of the underlying incision and injured tissues. Finally, a dressing insulates and keeps a wound's surface well hydrated. The humidity between a dressing and the client's skin surface promotes normal epithelial cell growth.

Types of Dressings.   Dressings vary by type of material and mode of application (wet or dry) (Skill 47-3). They should be easy to apply, comfortable, and made of materi-als that promote wound healing. The AHCPR guidelines (1994) are helpful when selecting dressings based on the goal of wound treatment (Box 47-17).

Woven gauze sponges are the oldest and most common dressing. They are absorbent and are especially useful in wounds to wick away the wound exudate (Aronovitch, 1995). They do not interact with wound tissues and thus cause little wound irritation. Gauze is available in different textures and in squares of 10 × 10 cm (4 × 4 inches) or 5 × 5 cm (2 × 2 inches), rectangles of 10 × 20 cm (4 × 8 inches), and rolls of various lengths. These dressings should not be confused with nonwoven sponges. Nonwoven dressings are a blend of synthetic fibers such as rayon and polyester. Because they do not adhere to the skin, they are used to wipe and clean wounds. They are not as useful as woven sponges for packing wounds and wicking away wound exudate (Aronovitch, 1995).

Wet-to-dry dressings are used in treating wounds that require debridement. The nurse moistens the contact dressing layer, increasing the gauze's ability to collect exudate and wound debris, and then applies a dry second layer of absorbent dressing. This wet-to-dry dressing effectively debrides infected and necrotic wounds.

Nonadherent gauze dressings such as Telfa are used over clean wounds. Telfa gauze has a shiny, nonadherent surface that does not stick to incisions or wound openings but allows drainage to pass through to the softened gauze above.

AHCPR Dressing Recommendations   Box 47-17

Use a dressing that will keep the ulcer bed continuously moist. Wet-to-dry dressings should be used only for debridement and are not considered continuously moist saline dressings.

Use clinical judgment to select a type of moist wound dressing suitable for the ulcer. Studies of different types of moist wound dressings showed no differences in pressure ulcer healing outcomes.

Choose a dressing that keeps the surrounding intact (periulcer) skin dry while keeping the ulcer bed moist.

Choose a dressing that controls exudate but does not desiccate the ulcer bed.

Consider caregiver time when selecting a dressing.

Eliminate wound dead space by loosely filling all cavities with dressing material. Avoid overpacking the wound.

Monitor dressings applied near the anus, since they are difficult to keep intact.

Modified from Agency for Health Care Policy and Research, Panel for Treatment of Pressure Ulcers in Adults: *Treatment of pressure ulcers,* Clinical Practice Guideline No. 15, AHCPR Pub No. 95-0653, Rockville, Md, 1994, Agency for Health Care Policy and Research, Public Health Service, U.S. Department of Health and Human Services.

Skill 47-3 Applying Dry and Wet-to-Dry Moist Dressings

Delegation Considerations

Controversy about delegating wound care to other personnel exists. All nurses should check their specific State Practice Act as to what interventions are considered within the scope of nursing practice and which can be delegated to others, including assistive personnel. In some states, aspects of wound care such as dressing change can be delegated. This may include the changing of dressings using *clean* technique for chronic wounds. The care of acute new wounds and those that require sterile technique for dressing change generally remain within the domain of professional nursing practice. The *assessment* of the wound remains within the scope of the professional nurse even if the dressing change is delegated to others.

EQUIPMENT

- Sterile gloves
- Dressing set (sterile), scissors, forceps
- Sterile drape (optional)
- Variety of gauze dressings and pads
- Fine mesh gauze (wet-to-dry only)
- Sterile basin
- Antiseptic ointment (optional)
- Cleansing solution
- Sterile solution (wet-to-dry only)

- Clean, disposable gloves
- Tape, ties, or bandage as needed
- Waterproof bag
- Extra gauze dressings, Surgipads, or ABD pads
- Bath blanket
- Adhesive remover (optional)
- Disposable mask (optional)
- Moisture-proof gown (optional)
- Goggles (optional)

STEPS	RATIONALE
1. Assess size and location of wound to be dressed.	Helps nurse to plan for proper type and amount of supplies needed. Alerts nurse when assistance is needed to hold dressings in place.
2. Assess client's level of comfort.	Removal of dry dressing can be painful; client may require pain medication.
3. Review medical orders for dressing change procedure.	Indicates type of dressing or applications to use.
4. Explain procedure to client and instruct client not to touch wound area or sterile supplies.	Decreases anxiety. Sudden, unexpected movement on client's part could result in contamination of wound and supplies.
5. Close room or cubicle curtains and windows.	Provides privacy and reduces airborne microorganisms.
6. Position client comfortably and drape with bath blanket to expose only wound site.	Provides access to wound, yet minimizes unnecessary exposure.
7. Place disposable bag within reach of work area. Fold top of bag to make cuff.	Ensures easy disposal of soiled dressings. Prevents soiling of bag's outer surface.
8. Apply face mask and protective eyewear, if required, and wash hands thoroughly.	Reduces transmission of pathogens to exposed tissues. Protects nurse from splashes.
9. Put on clean, disposable gloves and remove tape, bandage, or ties.	Prevents transmission of infectious organisms from soiled dressings to nurse's hands.
10. Remove tape: pull parallel to skin; pull toward dressing; remove remaining adhesive from skin.	Pulling tape toward dressing reduces stress on suture line or wound edges.
11. With gloved hand carefully remove gauze dressings one layer at a time, taking care not to dislodge drains or tubes. Keep soiled undersurface away from client's sight.	Appearance of drainage may be upsetting to client. Removal of one layer at a time reduces the chance of accidental removal of underlying drains.
a. If dressing sticks on a wet-to-dry dressing, do not moisten it; instead gently free dressing and alert client of potential discomfort.	Wet-to-dry dressing should debride wound. Do not wet the dressing to remove it. It is supposed to be dry so that as it is removed from the wound, it also removes necrotic tissue from the wound. *Never use a wet-to-dry dressing in a clean granulating wound. Use only for debridement.*
12. Observe character and amount of drainage on dressing and appearance of wound.	Provides estimate of drainage amount and assessment of wound's condition.
13. Dispose of soiled dressings in disposable bag.	Reduces transmission of microorganisms.
14. Remove gloves by pulling them inside out. Dispose of in bag.	Prevents contact of nurse's hands with material on gloves.

STEPS	**RATIONALE**
15. Open sterile dressing tray or individually wrapped sterile supplies. Place on bedside table (see illustration).	Sterile dressings remain sterile while on or within sterile surface. Preparation of supplies prevents break in technique during dressing change.
16. Apply dressing:	
A. **Dry dressing**	
(1) Open bottle of solution (if ordered) and pour into sterile basin.	Keeps supplies sterile.
(2) Apply sterile gloves.	Allows handling of sterile supplies without contamination.
(3) Inspect wound for appearance, drains, drainage, and integrity. Avoid contact with contaminated material.	Indicates status of wound healing.
(4) Cleanse wound with solution:	Prevents contamination of previously cleaned area.
(a) Use separate swab for each cleansing stroke.	
(b) Clean from least-contaminated area to most-contaminated area.	Prevents introduction of organisms into wound.
(5) Use dry gauze to swab in same manner as in Step 16A(4) to dry wound.	Reduces excess moisture, which could eventually harbor microorganisms.
(6) Apply antiseptic ointment if ordered, using same technique as for cleansing.	Helps to reduce growth of microorganisms. Ointment may be applied to dressing if direct application causes discomfort.
(7) Apply dry sterile dressings to incision or wound:	
(a) Apply loose, woven gauze as contact layer.	Promotes proper absorption of drainage.
(b) Cut 4 × 4 gauze flat to fit around drain, if present. Precut gauze is also available.	Secures drain and promotes drainage absorption at site.
(c) Apply second layer of gauze.	Protects wound from microorganisms.
(d) Apply thicker woven pad.	Protects wound from external environment.
B. **Wet-to-dry dressing**	
(1) Pour prescribed solution into sterile basin and add fine-mesh gauze.	Contact layer must be totally moistened to increase dressing's absorptive abilities.
(2) Apply sterile gloves.	Allows handling of sterile supplies without contamination.
(3) Inspect wound for color, character of drainage, type of sutures, and drains (see illustration).	Provides assessment of wound healing.
(4) Cleanse wound with prescribed antiseptic solution or normal saline. Clean from least to most contaminated area.	Assists in debridement and cleanses wound of debris.

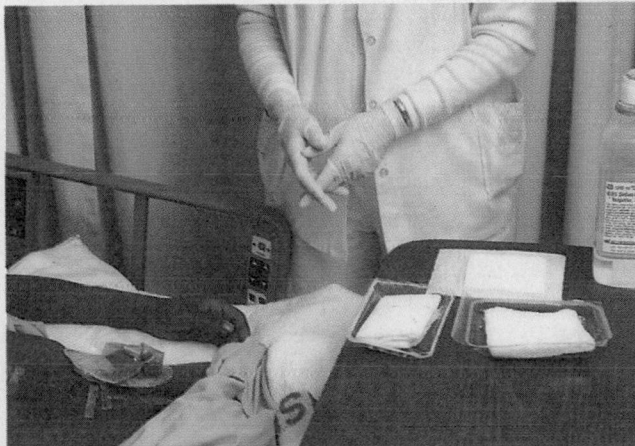

Step 15

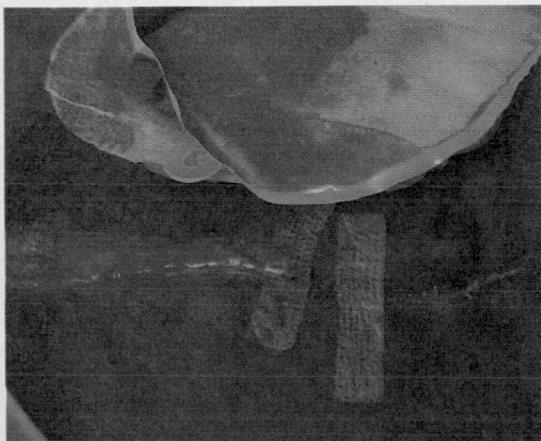

Step 16B(3)

STEPS	RATIONALE
(5) Apply moist fine-mesh gauze as a single layer directly onto wound surface. If wound is deep, gently pack gauze into wound with forceps until all wound surfaces are in contact with moist gauze (see illustrations).	Absorbs drainage and adheres to debris. Wound should be loosely packed to facilitate wicking of drainage into absorbent outer layer of dressing.
(6) Apply dry, sterile 4 × 4 gauze over wet gauze.	Pulls moisture from wound.
(7) Cover with ABD pad, Surgipad, or gauze.	Protects wound from entrance of microorganisms.

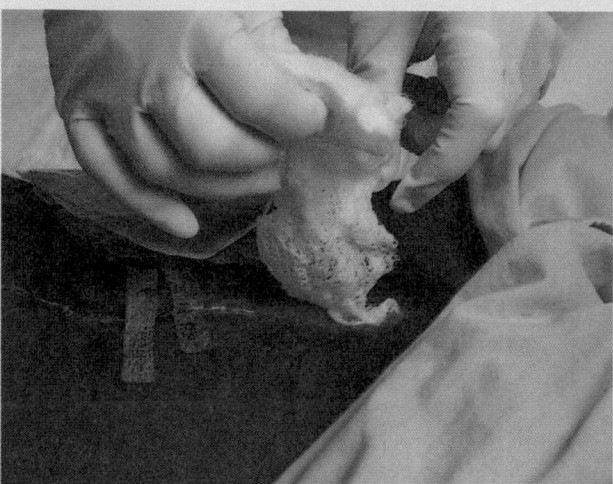
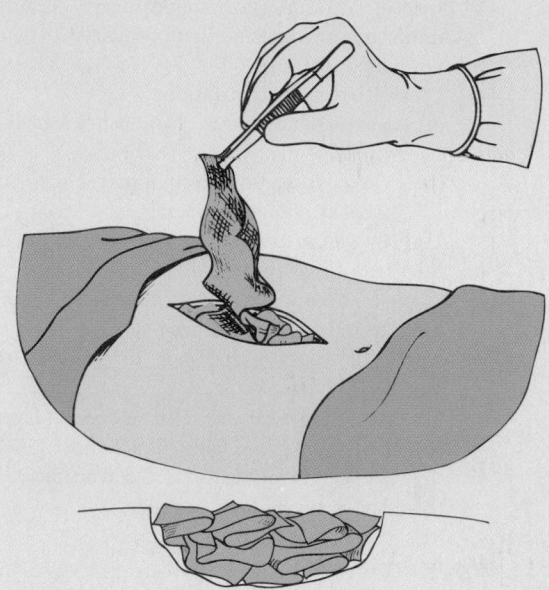

Step 16B(5)

17. Apply tape over dressing, Kling roll (for circumferential dressings), or Montgomery ties. For application of Montgomery ties (see Figure 47-24):	Secures dressing in place.
a. Expose adhesive surface of tape on end of each tie.	Montgomery tie allows for frequent dressing changes without removal of adhesive tape.
b. Place ties on opposite sides of dressing.	
c. Place adhesive directly on skin or use skin barrier.	
d. Secure dressing by lacing ties across it.	Ensures that dressing remains intact and covers wound.
18. Remove gloves and dispose of in bag. Remove mask and eyewear.	Reduces transmission of infection.
19. Assist client to comfortable position.	Promotes client's sense of well-being. Enhances comfort.
20. Dispose of supplies and wash hands.	Reduces transmission of infection.

Recording and Reporting

- Report brisk, bright red bleeding or evidence of wound dehiscence or evisceration to physician immediately.
- Report wound appearance and characteristics of drainage at shift change.
- Record wound appearance, color, presence and characteristics of exudate, type and amount of dressings used, and tolerance of client to procedure.

- Write date and time dressing applied on tape in ink (not marker).

Home Care Considerations

- More expensive specialty dressings may be used, because they decrease the frequency of dressing changes.
- Clean dressings may also be used in the home setting.
- Disposal of contaminated dressings in the home should be done in a manner consistent with local regulations.

Another type of dressing is a self-adhesive, transparent film that acts as a temporary second skin (Figure 47-23). Some examples of these film dressings are Bioclusive, Blisterfilm, Mefilm, Op-Site, Polyskin, Tegaderm, and Uniflex. The transparent dressing is ideal for small, superficial wounds such as partial-thickness wounds, donor sites, stage I and II pressure ulcers, and superficial burns. Film dressings can also be used as a secondary dressing, as well as for autolytic debridement of small wounds. It has the following advantages:

It adheres to undamaged skin.

It serves as a barrier to external fluids and bacteria but still allows the wound surface to "breathe," since oxygen can pass through the film dressing.

It promotes a moist environment that speeds epithelial cell growth.

It can be removed without damaging underlying tissues.

It permits viewing the wound.

It does not require a secondary dressing.

Hydrocolloid dressings are dressings with complex formulations of colloids, elastomeric, and adhesive components. Some examples are Comfeel, DuoDERM, Intrasite, Restore, Tegasorb, and Ultec. These dressings are occlusive. The wound contact layer of this dressing swells in the presence of exudate and maintains a moist healing environment. Hydrocolloids can be used to heal clean granulating wounds as well as to autolytically debride necrotic wounds. These dressings come in a variety of sizes and shapes. This type of dressing has the following functions:

It absorbs drainage through the use of exudate absorbers beneath the dressing.

It maintains wound humidity.

It slowly liquefies necrotic debris.

It provides protective cushioning.

It is impermeable to bacteria and other contaminants.

It is self-adhesive and molds well.

It can be used as a preventive dressing for high-risk friction areas.

It may be left in place for 3 to 5 days, minimizing skin trauma and disruption of healing.

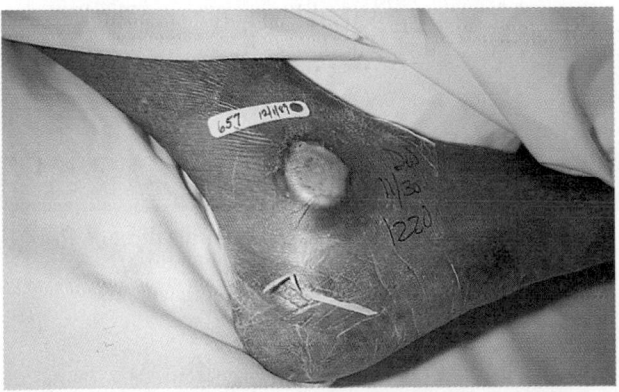

Figure 47-23   Transparent film dressing.

This type of dressing is most useful on shallow to moderately deep dermal ulcers. A disadvantage of hydrocolloid dressings is that most are opaque, most cannot absorb the amount of drainage from heavily draining wounds, and some are contraindicated for use in full-thickness and infected wounds. Some hydrocolloids may leave a residue in the wound bed that can be confused with pus.

Hydrogel dressings are water or glycerin-based amorphous gel-impregnated gauze or sheet dressings. They have a high water content and can absorb some but not large amounts of exudate. Hydrogel dressings are used on partial thickness and full-thickness wounds, deep wounds with some exudate, necrotic wounds, burns, and radiation-damaged skin. They are very useful in painful wounds, since they are very soothing to the client and do not adhere to the wound bed and thus cause little trauma during dressing removal. A disadvantage is that some hydrogels require a secondary dressing and that care must be taken so that periwound skin is not macerated. Some examples of these dressings are Aquasorb, Carrasyn Hydrogel wound dressing, ClearSite, Curasol, Elaso-Gel, HyperGel, IntraSite Gel, Nu-Gel, Restore, SoloSite, Tegagel, Transorb, and Vigilon.

Hydrogel has the following advantages:

It is very soothing and reduces pain in the wound.

It provides a moist environment.

It can debride the wound.

It does not stick to the wound and can be removed easily.

There are many other types of dressings available. Foam dressings, alginate dressings, and exudate absorbers are used in wounds with large amounts of exudate and in wounds that need packing. Calcium alginate dressings are manufactured from seaweed and come in sheet and rope form. The alginate forms a soft gel when it comes in contact with wound fluid. These highly absorbent dressings can be used on infected wounds and do not cause trauma when removed from the wound. They should not be used in dry wounds and require a secondary dressing. Nurses need to know that the dressing may smell like "low tide" when it is changed as the seaweed component of the dressing forms a gel with the wound fluid; this is a normal occurrence and should not be confused with the foul odor of a wound infection. Some examples of alginates are Algiderm, Curasorb, Dermacea, Kaltostat, Melgisorb, and Sorbsan. Foam dressings are also used around drainage tubes to absorb drainage. Several manufacturers produce composite dressings. These dressings combine two different dressing types into one dressing. Much research is being done on what type of dressing is best for what type of wound at what point in the healing process.

Changing Dressings.   To prepare for changing a dressing, the nurse must know the type of dressing, the presence of underlying drains or tubing, and the type of supplies needed for wound care. Poor preparation may cause a break in aseptic technique (see Chapter 33) or accidental dislodging of a drain. The nurse's judgment in modifying a dressing change procedure is important during wound care, particularly if the character of a wound changes. Notifying the physician of any change is essential.

The physician's order for changing a dressing should indicate the dressing type, the frequency of changing, and any solutions or ointments to be applied to the wound. An order to "reinforce dressing prn" (add dressings without removing the original one) is common right after surgery, when the physician does not want accidental disruption of the suture line or bleeding. The medical or operating room record usually tells whether drains are present and from what body cavity they drain. After the first dressing change, the nurse describes the location of drains and the type of dressing materials and solutions to use in the client's care plan. The CDC (Garner, 1985) recommends the following during the dressing change procedure:

> The nurse should perform thorough hand washing before and after wound care.
>
> Personnel should not touch an open or fresh wound directly without wearing sterile gloves (see Chapter 33).
>
> If a wound is sealed, dressings may be changed without gloves.
>
> Dressings over closed wounds should be removed or changed when they become wet or if the client has signs or symptoms of infection.

There is a growing body of literature about sterile versus clean dressings (Faller, 1999). The AHCPR guidelines (1994) recommend that clean dressings and gloves be used on pressure ulcers. For surgical wounds, preliminary research indicates no difference in the healing rate of wounds when clean rather than sterile dressing change technique is used (Box 47-18).

To prepare a client for a dressing change, the nurse does the following:

> Administers required analgesics so that peak effects occur during the dressing change
>
> Describes steps of the procedure to lessen client anxiety
>
> Recognizes normal signs of healing
>
> Answers questions about the procedure or the wound

Often the physician orders clients to learn how to change dressings so that they will be prepared for home care. In this situation the nurse must demonstrate dressing changes to the client and family and then provide an opportunity for the client or family member to practice (Box 47-19). Usually in this situation wound healing has progressed to the point that risks of complications such as dehiscence or evisceration are minimal. The client should be able to change a dressing independently or with assistance from a family member before discharge. The AHCPR guidelines (1994) state that "clean dressing may also be used in the home setting for pressure ulcers. Disposal of contaminated dressings in the home should be done in a manner consistent with local regulations". Skill 47-1 outlines the steps for changing dry and wet-to-dry dressings.

Research HIGHLIGHT   **Box 47-18**

RESEARCH ABSTRACT

The purpose of this research was to determine if there was a difference in the rate of wound healing and cost of supplies when clean or sterile dressing change techniques were used in open surgical wounds in postoperative clients. In this pilot study, the subjects were 15 men and 15 women who had gastrointestinal surgery. The mean age of subjects was 40.6 years (SD 13). The wounds were healing by secondary intention. Subjects were randomized as to either clean or sterile techniques. Dressing changes were begun on the first day postoperative. They were repeated three times a day until discharge from the hospital. Subjects were studied for 3 to 9 days. Results showed that there was no difference between the groups in the rate of wound healing. However, the mean cost for the clean dressing technique group was significantly less than for the sterile dressing technique group. The authors caution that the findings of this pilot study need to be confirmed using a large sample size.

IMPLICATIONS FOR PRACTICE

- Evaluate which wounds can be managed with a *clean* dressing technique.
- Determine which clients must *always* have sterile dressing changes (e.g., clients who are immunosuppressed, and clients receiving radiation).

REFERENCE

Stotts NA and others: Sterile vs clean technique in wound care of patients with open surgical wounds in the post-op period: a pilot study, *Adv Wound Care* 8(2):13, 1995.

Client Teaching FOR DRESSING APPLICATION   Box 47-19

OBJECTIVE

- Client (or family member) will demonstrate the correct technique for the application of dressing.

TEACHING STRATEGIES

- Discuss with client and significant other the importance of infection control.

- Demonstrate the correct technique for the dressing change for the client and the family member.
- Discuss signs and symptoms of wound infection.

EVALUATION

- Observe family member performing the dressing change.
- Client and family state symptoms of wound infection.

Packing a Wound.   The first step in packing a wound is to assess the size, depth, and shape of the wound. These wound characteristics are important in determining the size and type of dressing used to pack a wound. The dressing should be flexible and must be able to be in contact with all of the wound's surface. The nurse must make sure that the type of material being used to pack the wound is appropriate. Nonwoven sponges are usually not used to pack wounds. There are many new dressing materials such as alginates that are also used to pack wounds. Because of their ability to absorb wound exudate and conform to the shape of the wound, woven gauze sponges are commonly used to pack wounds that need mechanical debridement (Aronovitch, 1995). After removing the woven gauze from the package, it is essential to fluff the gauze before putting it into the wound (see Skill 47-3). Fluffing (opening up the gauze) increases the amount of surface area of the sponge that can be in contact with the wound surface. The woven gauze sponges should be moistened with normal saline only, since cytotoxic solutions cannot be used in wounds.

Using sterile technique, the wound should gently be filled with the saline-moistened woven gauze. As the wound is being filled, the packing material is held above the wound so that it does not touch the surrounding wound tissue before being packed into the wound. The sterile packing material must not drag across the surrounding wound tissue. The AHCPR guidelines (1994) recommend that wound dead space be eliminated by loosely filling all of the wound cavity with the dressing material. Dead space is "a cavity remaining in a wound" (AHCPR, 1994). It is important to remember that the wound cavity needs to be filled so that areas are not "walled off," to prevent abscesses (AHCPR, 1994).

It is important to remember that the wound should not be packed too tightly. Overpacking the wound may cause pressure on the tissue in the wound bed. The wound should be packed only until the packing material reaches the surface of the wound; there should never be so much packing material in the wound that it extends higher than the wound surface. Wound packing that overlaps onto the wound edges can cause maceration of the tissue surrounding the wound (Hess and Miller, 1990). It can also impede the proper healing and closing of the wound.

Securing Dressings.   The nurse may use tape, ties, or bandages, or a secondary dressing and cloth binders to secure a dressing over a wound site. The choice of anchoring depends on the wound size and location, the presence of drainage, the frequency of dressing changes, and the client's level of activity.

The nurse most often uses strips of tape to secure dressings if the client is not allergic to tape. Nonallergenic paper and plastic tapes minimize skin reactions. Common adhesive tape adheres well to the skin's surface, whereas elastic adhesive tape compresses closely around pressure bandages and permits more movement of a body part.

Skin sensitive to adhesive tape can become severely inflamed and excoriated and may even slough when the tape is removed.

Tape is available in various widths such as 1.2, 2.5, 5, and 7.5 cm, ½, 1, 2, and 3 inches). The nurse chooses the size that sufficiently secures the dressing. For example, a large abdominal wound dressing must remain secure over a large area despite frequent stress from movement, respiratory effort, and possibly abdominal distention. Strips of 7.5-cm (3-inch) adhesive better stabilize such a large dressing so that it does not continually slip off. When applying tape, the nurse ensures that it adheres to several inches of skin on both sides of the dressing and that it is placed across the middle of the dressing. When securing the dressing, the nurse presses the tape gently, exerting pressure away from the wound. This way, tension occurs in both directions away from the wound, minimizing skin distortion and irritation. Tape is never applied over irritated or broken skin. Some nurses protect the skin beneath the tape with a skin sealant product.

To remove tape safely, the nurse loosens the tape ends and gently pulls the outer end parallel with the skin surface toward the wound. The nurse applies light traction to the skin away from the wound as the tape is loosened and removed. Adhesive remover can also be used to loosen the tape from the skin. The traction minimizes pulling of the skin. If tape covers an area of hair growth, the client experiences less discomfort if the nurse pulls the tape in the direction of hair growth.

To avoid repeated removal of tape from sensitive skin, the nurse can secure dressings with pairs of reusable Montgomery ties (Figure 47-24). Each tie consists of a long strip; half contains an adhesive backing to apply to the skin, and the other half folds back and contains a cloth tie or a safety pin and rubber band combination to be fastened across a dressing and untied at dressing changes. A large, bulky dressing may require two or more sets of Montgomery ties. Another method to protect the surrounding skin on wounds that need frequent dressing changes is to place strips of hydrocolloid dressings on either side of the wound edges, cover the wound with a dressing, and then apply the tape to the hydrocolloid dressing. To provide even support to a wound and immobilize a body part, the nurse may apply elastic gauze or cloth bandages and binders over a dressing.

Comfort Measures.   A wound can be painful, depending on the extent of tissue injury. The nurse uses several techniques to minimize discomfort during wound care. Careful removal of tape, gentle cleansing of wound edges, and careful manipulation of dressings and drains minimize stress on sensitive tissues. Careful turning and positioning also reduce strain on a wound. Administration of analgesic medications 30 to 60 minutes before dressing changes (depending on a drug's time of peak action) also reduces discomfort.

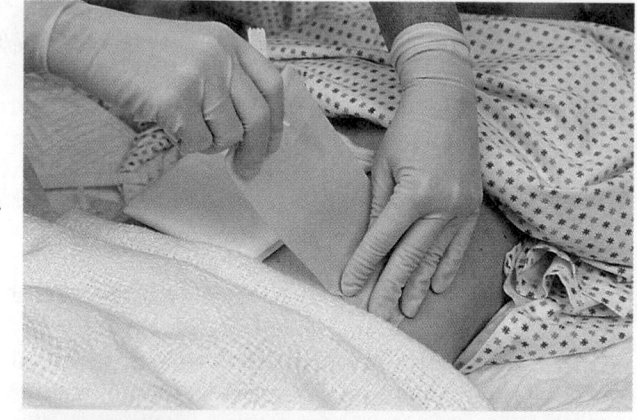

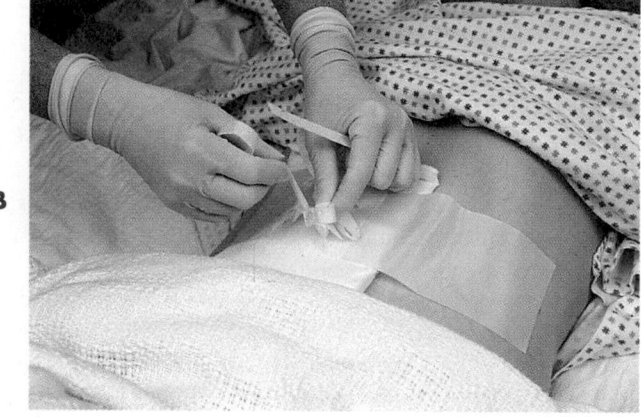

Figure 47-24   Montgomery ties. **A,** Each tie is placed at side of dressing. **B,** Securing ties encloses dressing.

Cleansing Skin and Drain Sites.   Although a moderate amount of wound exudate promotes epithelial cell growth, the physician may order cleansing of a wound or drain site if a dressing does not properly absorb drainage or if an open drain deposits drainage onto the skin. Wound cleansing requires good hand-washing and aseptic techniques (see Chapter 33). The nurse may use irrigation to remove debris.

Basic Skin Cleansing.   The nurse cleanses surgical or traumatic wounds by applying noncytotoxic solutions with sterile gauze or by irrigation. The following three principles are important when cleansing an incision or the area surrounding a drain:

1. Cleanse in a direction from the least contaminated area, such as from the wound or incision to the surrounding skin (Figure 47-25) or from an isolated drain site to the surrounding skin (Figure 47-26).
2. Use gentle friction when applying solutions locally to the skin.
3. When irrigating, allow the solution to flow from the least to most contaminated area.

A wound is thought to be less contaminated than the surrounding skin. After applying a solution to sterile gauze, the nurse cleanses away from the wound. The nurse never uses the same piece of gauze to cleanse across an incision or wound twice.

A drain site is highly contaminated because the moist drainage harbors microorganisms. If a wound has a dry incisional area and a moist drain site, cleansing moves from the incisional area toward the drain. The nurse uses two separate swabs, one to cleanse from the top of the incision toward the drain and one to cleanse from the bot-

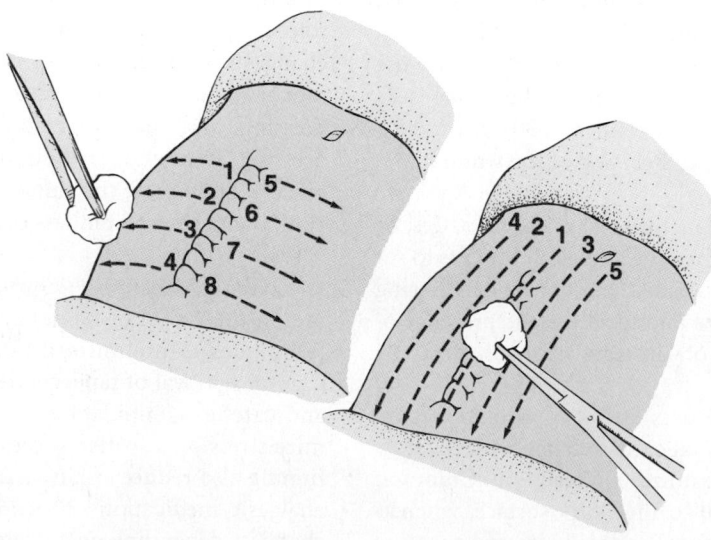

Figure 47-25   Methods for cleansing a wound site.

tom of the incision toward the drain. To cleanse the area of an isolated drain site, the nurse swabs around the drain, moving in circular rotations outward from a point closest to the drain. In this situation the skin near the site is more contaminated than the site itself. To cleanse circular wounds, the nurse uses the same technique as in cleansing around a drain.

Irrigations.   Irrigations are a special way of cleansing wounds. The nurse uses an irrigating syringe to flush the area with a constant low-pressure flow of solution. The gentle washing action of the irrigation cleanses a wound of exudate and debris. Irrigations are particularly useful for open, deep wounds involving an inaccessible body part, such as the ear canal, or when cleansing sensitive body parts, such as the conjunctival lining of the eye.

In addition to wound cleansing, irrigations serve to apply heat to an affected area and apply locally acting medications in the form of sterile solutions. The prescribed solution is usually sterile water or saline. Administration of irrigating solutions at body temperature enhances comfort and provides the added benefit of local heat application.

Wound Irrigations.   Irrigation of an open wound requires sterile technique. The nurse uses a 35-cc syringe with a 19-gauge needle (AHCPR, 1994) to deliver the solution, using an irrigation system that has a safe pressure and will not damage healing wound tissue. It is important to never occlude a wound opening with a syringe, because this results in the introduction of irrigating fluid into a closed space. The pressure of the fluid could cause tissue damage and discomfort. A wound should always be irrigated with the syringe tip over but not in the drainage site. Fluid should flow directly into the wound and not over a contaminated area before entering the wound. Skill 47-4 lists steps for wound irrigation.

Suture Care.   A surgeon closes a wound by bringing the wound edges as close together as possible to reduce scar formation. Proper wound closure involves minimal trauma and tension to tissues with control of bleeding.

Sutures are threads or wire used to sew body tissues together (Figure 47-27). The client's history of wound healing, the site of surgery, the tissues involved, and the purpose of the sutures determine the suture material to be used. For example, if the client has had repeated surgery for an abdominal hernia, the physician might choose wire sutures to provide greater strength for wound closure. In contrast, a small laceration of the face calls for the use of very fine Dacron (polyester) sutures to minimize scar formation.

Sutures are available in a variety of materials, including silk, steel, cotton, linen, wire, nylon, and Dacron. Sutures come with or without sharp surgical needles attached. Commonly seen are steel staples, a type of outer skin closure that causes less trauma to tissues than sutures, yet provides extra strength. It is also common to see wounds closed with Steri-Strips. A **Steri-Strip** is a sterile butterfly tape applied along both sides of a wound to keep the edges closed.

Sutures are placed within tissue layers in deep wounds and superficially as the final means for wound closure. The deeper sutures are usually an absorbable material that disappears in several days. Sutures are foreign bodies and thus are capable of causing local inflammation. The surgeon can minimize tissue injury by using the finest suture possible and the smallest number necessary.

Policies vary within institutions as to who may remove sutures. If the nurse is allowed to remove them, a physician's order is required. An order for suture removal is not written until the physician believes that the wound has closed (usually in 7 to 10 days). Special scissors with

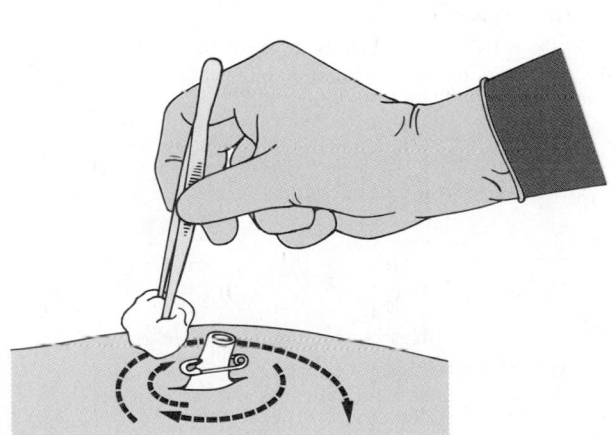

Figure 47-26   Cleansing a drain site.

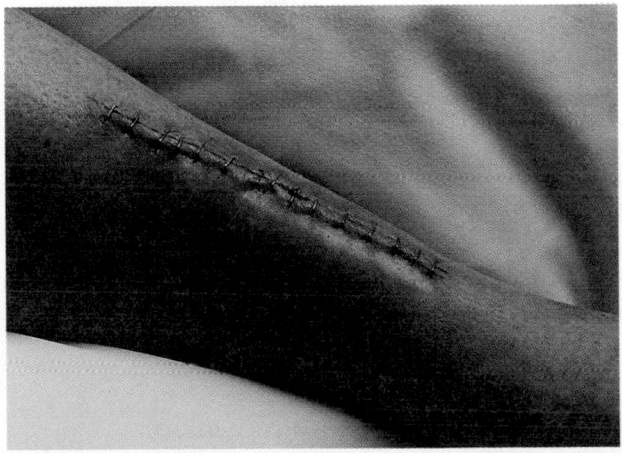

Figure 47-27   Incision closed with wire staples.

| Skill 47-4 | **Performing Wound Irrigations** |

Delegation Considerations

Check institutional policy and the state's Nurse Practice Act regarding which wound care interventions can be delegated to assistive personnel. The skill of wound irrigation requires problem solving and knowledge application unique to a professional nurse, particularly regarding the assessment of any wounds and care of acute new wounds. However, cleansing of chronic wounds using *clean* technique can be delegated to assistive personnel. In this situation, instruct staff on what to report when a wound is cleansed. Assistive personnel must also know how to use clean technique to avoid cross contamination from irrigation syringes and equipment.

EQUIPMENT

- Irrigant/cleansing solution (volume 1.2 to 2 times the estimated wound volume)
- Irrigation delivery system depending on amount of pressure desired:
    Sterile irrigation 35-ml syringe with sterile soft angiocatheter or 19-gauge needle (AHCPR, 1994) *or*
    Handheld shower or whirlpool

- Clean gloves
- Sterile gloves
- Waterproof underpad, if needed
- Dressing supplies
- Disposable waterproof bag
- Gown, if risk of spray
- Goggles, if risk of spray

STEPS	RATIONALE
1. Assess client's level of pain. Administer prescribed analgesic 30 to 45 minutes before starting wound irrigation procedure.	Discomfort may be related directly to wound or indirectly to muscle tension or immobility. Increased comfort level permits client to move more easily and be positioned to facilitate wound irrigation.
2. Review medical record for physician's prescription for irrigation of open wound and type of solution to be used.	Open wound irrigation requires medical order, including type of solutions to use.
3. Assess recent recording of signs and symptoms related to client's open wound:	Data are used as baseline to indicate change in condition of wound.
a. Condition of skin and wound	
b. Elevation of body temperature	May indicate response to infection.
c. Drainage from wound (amount, color)	Amount will decrease as healing takes place.
d. Odor	Strong odor indicates infectious process.
e. Consistency of drainage	Leukocytes produce thick drainage.
f. Size of wounds, including depth, length, and width	Determines stage of healing.
4. Explain procedure of wound irrigation and cleansing.	Information will reduce client's anxiety.
5. Position client comfortably to permit gravitational flow of irrigating solution through wound and into collection receptacle. Position client so that wound is vertical to collection basin.	Directing solution from top to bottom of wound and from clean to contaminated area prevents further infection. Positioning client during planning stage provides bed surfaces for later preparation of equipment.
6. Warm irrigation solution to approximate body temperature.	Warmed solution increases comfort and reduces vascular constriction response in tissues.
7. Wash hands.	Reduces transmission of microorganisms.
8. Form cuff on waterproof bag and place it near bed.	Cuffing helps to maintain large opening, thereby permitting placement of contaminated dressing without touching refuse bag itself.
9. Close room door or bed curtains.	Maintains privacy.
10. Apply gown and goggles if needed.	Protects nurse from splashes or sprays of blood and body fluids.
11. Put on clean gloves and remove soiled dressing and discard in waterproof bag. Discard gloves.	Reduces transmission of microorganisms.
12. Prepare equipment; open sterile supplies.	
13. Put on sterile gloves.	
14. To irrigate wound with wide opening:	
a. Fill 35-ml syringe with irrigation solution.	Flushing wound helps remove debris and facilitates healing by secondary intention.
b. Attach 19-gauge needle or angiocatheter (see Figure 47-22, p. 1595).	Provides ideal pressure for cleansing and removal of debris.

STEPS	RATIONALE
c. Hold syringe tip 2.5 cm (1 inch) above upper end of wound and over area being cleansed.	Prevents syringe contamination. Careful placement of the syringe prevents unsafe pressure of the flowing solution.
d. Using continuous pressure, flush wound; repeat Steps 15a, b, and c until solution draining into basin is clear.	Clear solution indicates that all debris has been removed.
15. To irrigate deep wound with very small opening:	
a. Attach soft angiocatheter to filled irrigating syringe.	Catheter permits direct flow of irrigant into wound. Expect wound to take longer to empty when opening is small.
b. Lubricate tip of catheter with irrigating solution; then gently insert tip of catheter and pull out about 1 cm ($^1/_2$ inch).	Removes tip from fragile inner wall of wound.
c. Using slow, continuous pressure, flush wound.	

Critical Decision Point: CAUTION: Splashing may occur during this step.

---

d. Pinch off catheter just below syringe while keeping catheter in place.	Avoids contamination of sterile solution.
e. Remove and refill syringe. Reconnect to catheter and repeat until solution draining into basin is clear.	
16. To cleanse wound with handheld shower:	Useful for clients able to shower with assistance or independently. May be accomplished at home. A shower table is helpful for bed-bound or acutely ill clients.
a. With client seated comfortably in shower chair, adjust spray to gentle flow; water temperature should be warm.	
b. Cover showerhead with clean washcloth if needed.	
c. Shower for 5 to 10 minutes with showerhead 12 inches (30 cm) from wound.	

Critical Decision Point: Consider culturing a wound if it has a foul, purulent odor; inflammation surrounds the wound; a nondraining wound begins to drain; or client is febrile.

---

17. Obtain cultures, if needed, after cleansing with nonbacteriostatic saline.	Routine culturing of open wounds is not recommended in the AHCPR guidelines (1994). They recommend using quantitative bacterial cultures (tissue biopsy or wound fluid by needle aspiration) rather than swab cultures, which often detect only surface bacterial contaminants.
18. Dry wound edges with gauze; dry client if shower or whirlpool is used.	Prevents maceration of surrounding tissue from excess moisture.
19. Apply appropriate dressing (see Skill 47-2).	Maintains protective barrier and healing environment for wound.
20. Remove gloves and, if worn, mask, goggles, and gown.	Prevents transfer of microorganisms.
21. Assist client to comfortable position.	
22. Dispose of equipment and soiled supplies. Wash hands.	Reduces transmission of microorganisms.
23. Assess type of tissue in the wound bed.	Identifies wound-healing progress and determines type of wound cleansing needed.
24. Inspect dressing periodically.	Determines client's response to wound irrigation and need to modify plan of care.
25. Evaluate skin integrity.	Determines if extension of wound has occurred.
26. Observe client for signs of discomfort.	Client's pain should not increase as a result of wound irrigation.
27. Observe for presence of retained irrigant.	Retained irrigant is a medium for bacterial growth and subsequent infection.

Recording and Reporting

- Record wound irrigation and client response on progress notes.
- Immediately report any evidence of fresh bleeding, sharp increase in pain, retention of irrigant, or signs of shock to attending physician.
- At change of shift, report expected and unexpected outcomes that have actually occurred.

Home Care Considerations

- Teach client and caregiver how to make normal saline, especially if cost is an issue. Normal saline can be made by using 2 teaspoons of salt in 1 liter (1 quart) of boiling water (Barr, 1995).
- Tell client and caregiver that because normal saline has no preservatives, it should be thrown out 24 to 48 hours after it is first opened or made (Barr, 1995).

curved cutting tips or special staple removers slide under the skin closures for suture removal (Figure 47-28). The physician usually signifies the number of sutures or staples to remove. If the suture line appears to be healing in certain locations better than in others, the physician may choose to have only some sutures removed (e.g., every other one).

To remove staples, the nurse simply inserts the tips of the staple remover under each wire staple. While slowly closing the ends of the staple remover together, the nurse squeezes the center of the staple with the tips, freeing the staple from the skin.

To remove sutures, the nurse first checks the type of suturing used (Figure 47-29). With intermittent suturing, the surgeon ties each individual suture made in the skin. Continuous suturing, as the name implies, is a series of sutures with only two knots, one at the beginning and one at the end of the suture line. Retention sutures are placed more deeply than skin sutures and may or may not be removed by the nurse, depending on agency policy. The

manner in which the suture crosses and penetrates the skin determines the method for removal. The most important principle in suture removal is to never pull the visible portion of a suture through underlying tissue. Sutures on the skin's surface harbor microorganisms and debris. The portion of the suture beneath the skin is sterile. Pulling the contaminated portion of the suture through tissues may lead to infection. The nurse clips suture materials as close to the skin edge on one side as possible and then pulls the suture through from the other side (Figure 47-30).

Drainage Evacuation.   When drainage interferes with healing, drainage evacuation can be achieved by using either a drain alone or a drainage tube with continuous suction. The nurse may apply special skin barriers, including

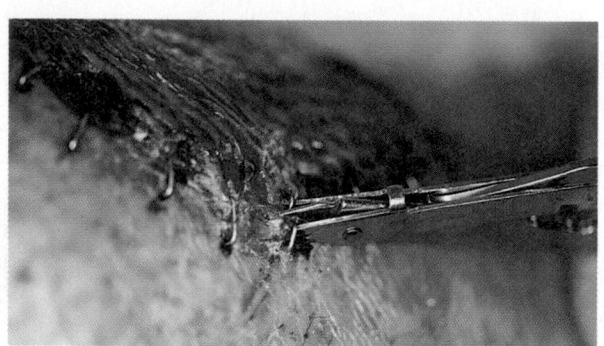

Figure 47-28   Staple remover.

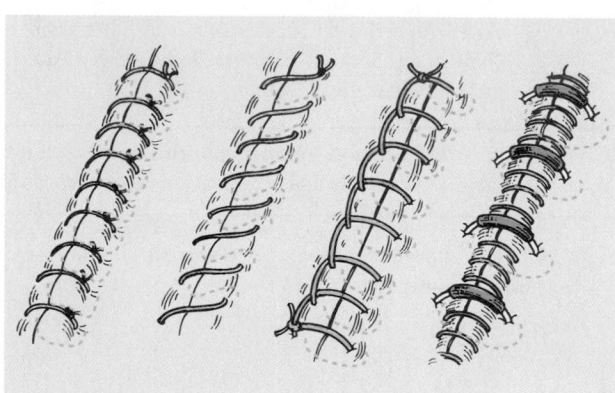

Figure 47-29   Examples of suturing methods. **A,** Intermittent. **B,** Continuous. **C,** Blanket continuous. **D,** Retention.

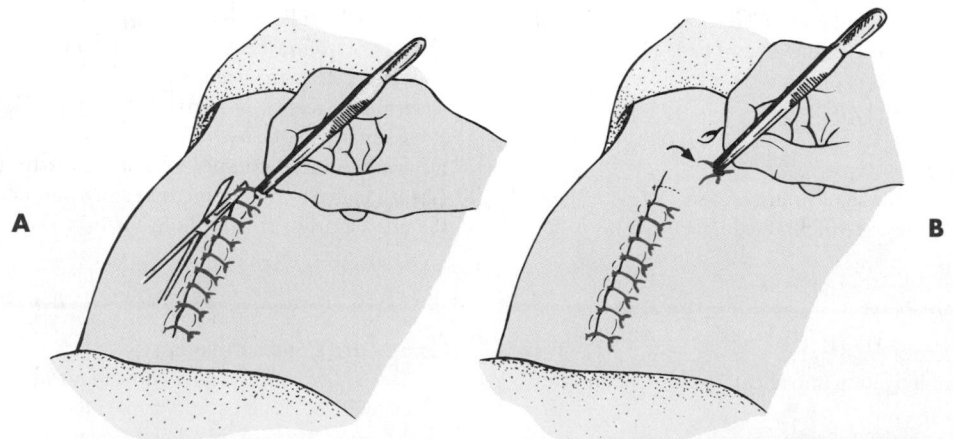

Figure 47-30   Removal of intermittent suture. **A,** The nurse cuts the suture as close to the skin as possible, away from the knot. **B,** The nurse removes the suture and never pulls the contaminated stitch through tissues.

hydrocolloid dressings, similar to those used with ostomies (see Chapter 45), around drain sites. The **skin barriers** are soft, waferlike, plastic materials that are applied to the skin with adhesive. Drainage flows on the barrier but not directly on the skin. **Drainage evacuators** (Figure 47-31) are convenient, portable units that connect to tubular drains lying within a wound bed and exert a safe, constant, low-pressure vacuum to remove and collect drainage. The nurse ensures that suction is exerted and that connection points between the evacuator and tubing are intact. The evacuator collects drainage that the nurse assesses for volume and character every shift and as needed. When the evacuator fills, the nurse measures output by emptying the contents into a graduated cylinder and immediately resets the evacuator to apply suction.

Bandages and Binders.

A simple gauze dressing is often not enough to immobilize or provide support to a wound. **Binders** and bandages applied over or around dressings can provide extra protection and therapeutic benefits by:

1. Creating pressure over a body part (e.g., an elastic pressure bandage applied over an arterial puncture site)
2. Immobilizing a body part (e.g., an elastic bandage applied around a sprained ankle)
3. Supporting a wound (e.g., an abdominal binder applied over a large abdominal incision and dressing)
4. Reducing or preventing edema (e.g., a well-supporting bra to minimize breast discomfort after delivery of a baby)
5. Securing a splint (e.g., a bandage applied around hand splints for correction of deformities)

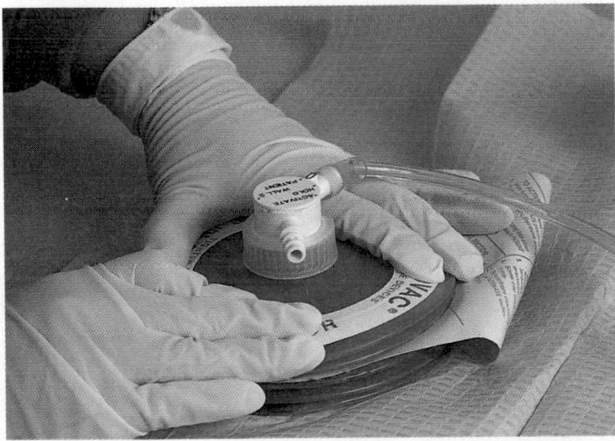

Figure 47-31 Setting the suction on a drainage evacuator. 1. With the drainage port open, the level on the diaphragm is raised. 2. The nurse pushes straight down on the lever to lower the diaphragm. 3. Closure of the port prevents escape of air and creates vacuum pressure.

6. Securing dressings (e.g., elastic webbing applied around leg dressings after a vein stripping)

Bandages are available in rolls of various widths and materials, including gauze, elasticized knit, elastic webbing, flannel, and muslin. Gauze bandages are lightweight and inexpensive, mold easily around contours of the body, and permit air circulation to prevent skin maceration. Elastic bandages conform well to body parts but can also be used to exert pressure over a body part. Flannel and muslin bandages are thicker than gauze and thus stronger for supporting or applying pressure. A flannel bandage also insulates to provide warmth.

Binders are bandages that are made of large pieces of material to fit a specific body part. Most binders are made of elastic, cotton, muslin, or flannel. An abdominal binder and a breast binder are examples.

Principles for Applying Bandages and Binders.

Correctly applied bandages and binders do not cause injury to underlying and nearby body parts or create discomfort for the client. For example, a chest binder must not be so tight as to restrict chest wall expansion. Before a bandage or binder is applied, the nurse's responsibilities include the following:

Inspecting the skin for abrasions, edema, discoloration, or exposed wound edges

Covering exposed wounds or open abrasions with a sterile dressing

Assessing the condition of underlying dressings and changing them if soiled

Assessing the skin of underlying body parts and parts that will be distal to the bandage for signs of circulatory impairment (coolness, pallor or cyanosis, diminished or absent pulses, swelling, numbness, and tingling) to provide a means for comparing changes in circulation after bandage application

Table 47-13 outlines the principles of bandage and binder application. After a bandage is applied, the nurse assesses, documents, and immediately reports changes in circulation, skin integrity, comfort level, and body function (e.g., ventilation or movement). The nurse who applies a bandage can loosen or readjust it as necessary. The nurse should have a physician's order before loosening or removing a bandage applied by a physician. The nurse explains to the client that any bandage or binder feels relatively firm or tight. A bandage should be carefully assessed to be sure that it is properly applied and is providing therapeutic benefit, and soiled bandages should be replaced. Like a damp dressing, a bandage or binder can harbor microorganisms.

Binder Application.

Binders are especially designed for the body part to be supported. The most common types of binders are the abdominal binder, and T binder (Skill 47-5). Breast binders, used to provide support after breast surgery or to exert pressure to reduce lactation in a

Table 47-13 **Types of Bandage Turns**

Type	Description	Purpose or Use
Circular	Bandage turn overlapping previous turn completely	Anchors bandage at the first and final turn; covers small part (finger, toe)
Spiral	Bandage ascending body part, with each turn overlapping previous one by one-half or two-thirds width of bandage	Covers cylindrical body parts such as wrist or upper arm
Spiral-reverse	Turn requiring twist (reversal) of bandage halfway through each turn	Covers cone-shaped body parts such as forearm, thigh, or calf; useful with nonstretching bandages such as gauze or flannel
Figure eight	Oblique overlapping turns alternately ascending and descending over bandaged part; each turn crossing previous one to form figure eight	Covers joints; snug fit provides excellent immobilization
Recurrent	Bandage first secured with two circular turns around proximal end of body part; half turn made perpendicular up from bandage edge; body of bandage brought over distal end of body-part to be covered with each turn folded back over on itself	Covers uneven body parts such as head or stump

Applying an Abdominal, T, or Breast Binder   Skill 47-5

Delegation Considerations

The skills of applying a binder (abdominal, T, or breast) can be delegated to assistive personnel.

- Be sure personnel are competent to perform procedures.
- The nurse should complete an assessment of the client's ability to breathe deeply, cough effectively, and move independently; of skin for irritation/abrasion; of incision/wound and dressing; and of comfort level before a binder or sling is applied for the first time.
- The nurse should evaluate the client's response to binder application.

EQUIPMENT

- Gloves, if wound drainage is present.
- Abdominal binder:
    Correct size cloth/elastic straight binder
    Safety pins (unless Velcro closure or metal fasteners are attached): six to eight safety pins are usually adequate for abdominal binders
- T and double-T binders:
    Correct size binder
    Safety pins: two pins for T binder; three pins for double-T binder
- Breast binder:
    Correct size binder
    Safety pins (approximately 12) unless Velcro closure is attached

STEPS	RATIONALE
1. Observe client with need for support of thorax or abdomen. Observe ability to breathe deeply and cough effectively.	Baseline assessment determines client's ability to breathe and cough. Impaired ventilation of lung can lead to alveolar atelectasis and inadequate arterial oxygenation.
2. Review medical record if medical prescription for particular binder is required and reasons for application.	Application of supportive binders may be used on nursing judgment. In some situations, physician input is required.
3. Inspect skin for actual or potential alterations in integrity. Observe for irritation, abrasion, skin surfaces that rub against each other, or allergic response to adhesive tape used to secure dressing.	Actual impairments in skin integrity can be worsened with application of a binder. Binder can cause pressure and excoriation.
4. Inspect any surgical dressing.	Dressing replacement or reinforcement precedes application of any binder.

Critical Decision Point: Dressing should be clean and dry, and incision/wound should be entirely covered by dressing.

5. Assess client's comfort level, using analog scale of 0 to 10 (see Chapter 42) and noting any objective signs and symptoms.	Data will determine effectiveness of binder placement.

Critical Decision Point: Expect client in moderate-to-severe pain to have diaphoresis, tachycardia, and elevated blood pressure.

6. Gather necessary data regarding size of client and appropriate binder.	Ensures proper fit of binder.
7. Explain procedure to client.	Promotes client's understanding and cooperation.
8. Teach skill to client or significant other.	Reduces anxiety and ensures continuity of care after discharge.
9. Wash hands and apply gloves (if likely to contact wound drainage).	Reduces transmission of microorganisms.
10. Close curtains or room door.	Maintains client's comfort and dignity.
11. Apply binder.	
A. **Abdominal binder**	
(1) Position client in supine position with head slightly elevated and knees slightly flexed.	Minimizes muscular tension on abdominal organs.
(2) Fanfold far side of binder toward midline of binder.	Reduces time client remains in uncomfortable position.
(3) Instruct and help client to roll away from nurse toward raised side rail while firmly supporting abdominal incision and dressing with hands.	Reduces pain and discomfort.

STEPS	RATIONALE
(4) Place fanfolded ends of binder under client.	Permits placement and centering of binder with minimal discomfort.
(5) Instruct or assist client to roll over folded ends.	
(6) Unfold and stretch ends out smoothly on far side of bed.	Maintains skin integrity and comfort.
(7) Instruct client to roll back into supine position.	Facilitates chest expansion and adequate wound support when binder is closed.
(8) Adjust binder so that supine client is centered over binder using symphysis pubis and costal margins as lower and upper landmarks.	Centers support from binder over abdominal structures, which reduces incidence of decreased lung expansion.

Critical Decision Point: Cover any exposed areas of an incision or wound with sterile dressing.

---

(9) Close binder. Pull one end of binder over center of client's abdomen. While maintaining tension on that end of binder, pull opposite end of binder over center and secure with Velcro closure tabs, metal fasteners, or horizontally placed safety pins (see Figure 47-32).	Provides continuous wound support and comfort.
(10) Assess client's comfort level.	Helps determine effectiveness of binder placement.
(11) Adjust binder as necessary.	Promotes comfort and chest expansion.

B. Single-T and double-T binders (Figure 47-33)

(1) Assist client to dorsal recumbent position, with lower extremities slightly flexed and hips rotated slightly outward.	Minimizes muscular tension on perineal organs.
(2) Have client raise hips and place horizontal band around client's waist (or above iliac crests) with vertical tails extending past buttocks. Overlap waistband in front and secure with safety pins.	Permits placement of binder. Secures binder around client.
(3) Complete binder application:	
(a) T binder: Bring remaining vertical strip over perineal dressing and continue up and under center front of horizontal band. Bring ends over waistband and secure all thicknesses with safety pin.	Single-T and double-T binders provide support to perineal muscles and organs and help maintain placement of perineal or suprapubic dressing.
(b) Double-T binder: Bring remaining vertical strips over perineal or suprapubic dressing with each tail supporting one side of scrotum and proceeding upward on either side of penis. Continue drawing ends behind and then downward in front of horizontal band. Secure all thicknesses with one horizontally placed safety pin.	
(4) Assess client's comfort level with client in lying, sitting, and standing positions. Readjust front pins and tails as necessary, ensuring that tails are not too tight. Increase padding if any area rubs against surrounding tissues.	Determines efficacy of binder to maintain dressings and support perineal structures.

Critical Decision Point: Binder should hold perineal or suprapubic dressing in place as client ambulates without applying pressure to urethra or scrotum.

---

(5) Instruct client regarding removal of binder before defecating or urinating and need to replace binder after performing these bodily functions.	Cleanliness of binder reduces infection risk.

STEPS	RATIONALE
C. **Breast binder**	
(1) Assist client in placing arms through binder's armholes.	Eases binder placement process.
(2) Assist client to supine position in bed.	Supine positioning facilitates normal anatomical position of breasts; facilitates healing and comfort.
(3) Pad area under breasts if necessary.	Prevents skin contact with undersurface.
(4) Using Velcro closure tabs or horizontally placed safety pins, secure binder at nipple level first. Continue closure process above and then below nipple line until entire binder is closed.	Horizontal placement of pins may reduce risk of uneven pressure or localized irritation.
(5) Make appropriate adjustments, including individualizing fit of shoulder straps and pinning waistline darts to reduce binder size.	Maintains support to client's breasts.
(6) Instruct and observe skill development in self-care related to reapplying breast binder.	Self-care is integral aspect of discharge planning. Skin integrity and comfort level goals are ensured.
12. Remove gloves and wash hands.	Prevents cross infections.
13. Observe site for skin integrity, circulation, and characteristics of the wound. (Periodically remove binder and surgical dressing to assess wound characteristics.)	Determines that binder has not resulted in complication to skin, wound, or underlying organs.
14. Assess comfort level of client, using analog scale of 0 to 10 and noting any objective signs and symptoms.	Binders should not increase discomfort.
15. Assess client's ability to ventilate properly, including deep breathing and coughing.	Identifies any impaired ventilation and potential pulmonary complications.
16. Identify client's need for assistance with activities such as hair combing, dressing, and ambulating.	Mobility of upper extremities may be limited, depending on severity and location of incision.

Recording and Reporting

- Report any skin irritation to nurse at between-shift report.
- Record application of binder, condition of skin, circulation, integrity of dressing, and client's comfort level.
- Report ineffective lung expansion to physician immediately.

Home Care Considerations

- Abdominal, T, and breast binders are washable and are placed over a line to dry.
- Instruct caregiver to avoid excessive pressure with binder application.

woman after childbirth, are now being replaced with well-fitting bras.

Abdominal Binders.   An abdominal binder supports large abdominal incisions that are vulnerable to tension or stress as the client moves or coughs (Figure 47-32). The nurse secures an abdominal binder with safety pins, Velcro strips, or metal stays.

T Binders.   As the name implies, the T binder looks like the letter T (Figure 47-33) and is used to secure rectal or perineal dressings. The single T is for female clients, and the double T fits male clients.

The belt of the binder fits securely around the client's waist with the tail passing between the client's legs from back to front and attaching to the belt's front. The nurse must be sure that the tail fits smoothly and against the dressing. T binders become soiled easily and require frequent changing. Irritation to the urethra or scrotum must be avoided.

Slings.   Slings support arms with muscular sprains or fractures. A commercially made sling consists of a long sleeve that extends above the elbow, with a strap that fits around the neck. In the home a large triangular piece of cloth can be used. The client may sit or lie supine during sling application (Figure 47-34). The nurse instructs the client to bend the affected arm, bringing the forearm straight across the chest. The open sling fits under the client's arm and over the chest, with the base of the triangle under the wrist and the triangle's point at the client's elbow. One end of the sling fits around the back of the client's neck. The nurse brings the other end up and over the affected arm while supporting the extremity. The

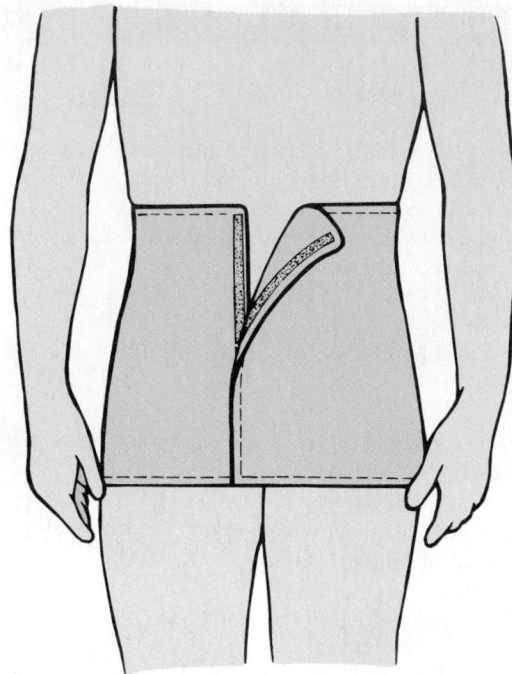

Figure 47-32   Securing an abdominal binder with Velcro.

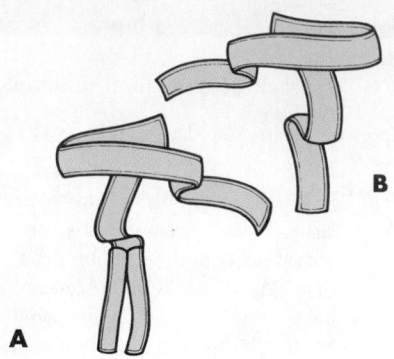

Figure 47-33   T binders. **A,** Male. **B,** Female.

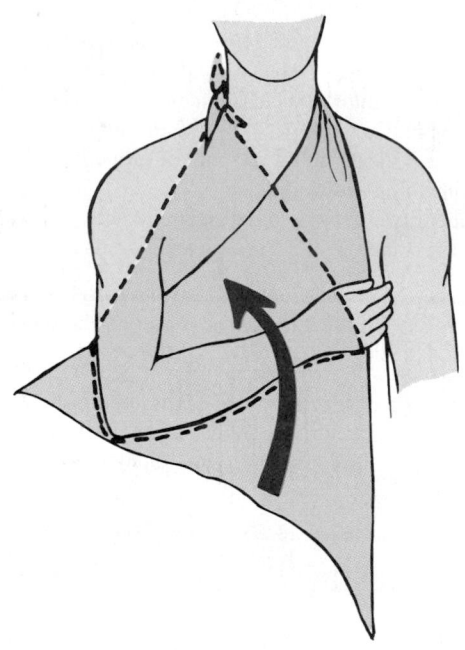

Figure 47-34   Application of a sling.

nurse ties the two ends at the side of the neck so that the knot does not press against the cervical spine. The loose material at the elbow can be folded evenly around the elbow and pinned. The lower arm and hand should always be supported at a level above the elbow to prevent the formation of dependent edema.

Bandage Application.   Rolls of bandage can secure or support dressings over irregularly shaped body parts. Each roll has a free outer end and a terminal end at the center of the roll. The rolled portion of the bandage is its body, and its outer surface is placed against the client's skin or dressing. Skill 47-6 describes the steps for applying an elastic bandage. The nurse may use a variety of bandage turns, depending on the body part to be bandaged (Table 47-13).

Heat and Cold Therapy.   Local application of heat and cold to an injured body part can be therapeutic. Before using these therapies, however, the nurse must understand normal body responses to local temperature variations, assess the integrity of the body part, determine the client's ability to sense temperature variations, and ensure proper operation of equipment. The nurse is legally responsible for safe administration of heat and cold applications.

Bodily Responses to Heat and Cold.   Exposure to heat and cold can cause systemic and local responses. Systemic responses occur through heat-loss mechanisms (sweating and vasodilation) or mechanisms promoting heat conser-

vation (vasoconstriction and piloerection) and heat production (shivering) (see Chapter 32). Local responses to heat and cold occur through stimulation of temperature-sensitive nerve endings within the skin. This stimulation sends impulses from the periphery to the hypothalamus, which becomes aware of local temperature sensations and triggers adaptive responses for maintenance of normal body temperature. If alterations occur along temperature sensation pathways, the reception and eventual perception of stimuli will be altered.

The body can tolerate wide variations in temperature. The normal temperature of the skin's surface is 34° C (93.2° F), but temperature receptors usually adapt quickly to local temperatures between 45° and 15° C (113° and 59° F). Pain develops when local temperatures exceed this

Applying an Elastic Bandage   Skill 47-6

Delegation Considerations

The application of an elastic bandage can be delegated to assistive personnel.

- Be sure personnel are trained in application of elastic bandages.

- The nurse should completely assess the client's wound and distal extremity circulation before and after bandage application.

EQUIPMENT

- Correct width and number of bandages
- Safety pins, clips, or adhesive tape

- Disposable gloves, if wound drainage is present

STEPS	RATIONALE
1. Inspect skin for alterations in integrity as indicated by abrasions, discoloration, chafing, or edema. (Look carefully at bony prominences.)	Altered skin integrity contraindicates the use of elastic bandages.
2. Inspect surgical dressing.	Surgical dressing replacement or reinforcement precedes application of any bandage.
3. Observe adequacy of circulation (distal to bandage) by noting surface temperature, skin color, and sensation of body parts to be wrapped.	Comparison of area before and after application of bandage is necessary to ensure continued adequate circulation. Impairment of circulation may result in coolness to touch when compared with opposite side of body, cyanosis or pallor of skin, diminished or absent pulses, edema or localized pooling, and numbness or tingling of part.
4. Review medical record for specific orders related to application of elastic bandage. Note area to be covered, type of bandage required, frequency of change, and previous response to treatment.	Specific prescription may direct procedure, including factors such as extent of application (e.g., toe to knee, toe to groin) and duration of treatment.
5. Identify client's and primary caregiver's present knowledge level of skill if bandaging will be continued at home.	Ensures that planning and teaching are individualized.
6. Explain procedure to client.	Increased knowledge promotes cooperation and reduces anxiety.
7. Teach skill to client or significant other.	Reduces anxiety and ensures continuity of care after discharge.
8. Wash hands and apply gloves if drainage is present.	Reduces transmission of microorganisms.
9. Close room door or curtains.	Maintains client's comfort and dignity.
10. Help client to assume comfortable, anatomically correct position.	Maintains alignment. Prevents musculoskeletal deformity.

Critical Decision Point: Bandages applied to lower extremities are applied before client sits or stands. Elevation of dependent extremities for 20 minutes before bandage application will enhance venous return.

11. Hold roll of elastic bandage in dominant hand and use other hand to lightly hold beginning of bandage at distal body part. Continue transferring roll to dominant hand as bandage is wrapped.	Maintains appropriate and consistent bandage tension.

Critical Decision Point: Toes or fingertips should be visible for follow-up circulatory assessment.

12. Apply bandage from distal point toward proximal boundary using variety of turns to cover various shapes of body parts (see Table 47-13).	Bandage is applied in manner that conforms evenly to body part and promotes venous return.
13. Unroll and very slightly stretch bandage.	Maintains uniform bandage tension.
14. Overlap turns by one-half to two-thirds width of bandage roll.	Prevents uneven bandage tension and circulatory impairment.

STEPS	RATIONALE
15. Secure first bandage with clip or tape before applying additional rolls.	
a. Apply additional rolls without leaving any uncovered skin surface. Secure last bandage applied.	Prevents wrinkling or loose ends.
16. Remove gloves if worn and wash hands.	Reduces transmission of microorganisms.
17. Assess distal circulation when bandage application is complete and at least twice during 8-hour period.	Early detection and management of circulatory impairment ensures healthy neurovascular status.
a. Observe skin color for pallor or cyanosis.	
b. Palpate skin for warmth.	
c. Palpate pulses and compare bilaterally.	
d. Ask if client is aware of pain, numbness, tingling, or other discomfort.	Neurovascular changes indicate impaired venous return.
e. Observe mobility of extremity.	Determines if bandage is too tight, which restricts movement, or determines if joint immobility is attained.
18. Have client demonstrate bandage application.	Return demonstration documents learning.

Recording and Reporting

- Document condition of wound, integrity of dressing, application of bandage, circulation, and client's comfort level.
- Report any changes in neurological or circulatory status to nurse in charge or physician.

Home Care Considerations

- Instruct client or caregiver not to make bandages too tight, which interferes with circulation.
- Elastic bandages that are used to reduce swelling are best applied to the feet in the morning, before getting out of bed.
- Always remove an elastic bandage daily and inspect skin beneath it.

range. Excessive heat causes a burning sensation. Cold produces a numbing sensation before pain.

The body's adaptive ability creates the major problem in protecting clients from injury resulting from temperature extremes. A person initially feels an extreme change in temperature but within a short time hardly notices it. This can be dangerous because a person insensitive to heat and cold extremes can suffer serious tissue injury. The nurse must recognize clients most at risk for injuries from heat and cold applications (Table 47-14).

Local Effects of Heat and Cold. Heat and cold stimuli create different physiological responses. The choice of heat or cold therapy depends on local responses desired for wound healing.

Effects of Heat Application. Table 47-15 summarizes the benefits of heat application. Heat generally is quite therapeutic, improving blood flow to an injured part. If heat is applied for 1 hour or more, however, blood flow is reduced by a reflex vasoconstriction as the body attempts to control heat loss from the area. Periodic removal and reapplication of local heat restores vasodilation. Continuous exposure to heat damages epithelial cells, causing redness, localized tenderness, and even blistering.

Effects of Cold Application. Table 47-16 also summarizes the benefits of cold application. Prolonged exposure

of the skin to cold results in a reflex vasodilation. The cell's inability to receive adequate blood flow and nutrients results in tissue ischemia. The skin initially takes on a reddened appearance, followed by a bluish purple mottling with numbness and a burning type of pain. The skin's tissues can freeze from exposure to extreme cold.

Factors Influencing Heat and Cold Tolerance. The body's response to heat and cold therapies depends on the following factors:

Duration of application. A person is better able to tolerate short exposure to temperature extremes.

Body part. Certain areas of the skin are more sensitive to temperature variations. These include the neck, inner aspect of the wrist and forearm, and perineal region. The foot and palm of the hand are less sensitive.

Damage to body surface. Exposed skin layers are more sensitive to temperature variations.

Prior skin temperature. The body responds best to minor temperature adjustments. If a body part is cool and a hot stimulus touches the skin, the response is greater than if the skin were already warm.

Body surface area. A person has less tolerance to temperature changes to which a large area of the body is exposed.

Age and physical condition. Tolerance to temperature

Table 47-14 Conditions That Increase Risk of Injury from Heat and Cold Application

Condition	Risk Factors
Very young clients or older clients	Thinner skin layers in children increase risk of burns. Older clients have reduced sensitivity to pain.
Open wounds, broken skin, stomas	Subcutaneous and visceral tissues are more sensitive to temperature variations. They also contain no temperature and fewer pain receptors.
Areas of edema or scar formation	Reduced sensation to temperature stimuli occurs because of thickening of skin layers from fluid buildup or scar formation.
Peripheral vascular disease (e.g., diabetes, arteriosclerosis)	Body's extremities are less sensitive to temperature and pain stimuli because of circulatory impairment and local tissue injury. Cold application further compromises blood flow.
Confusion or unconsciousness	Perception of sensory or painful stimuli is reduced.
Spinal cord injury	Alterations in nerve pathways prevent reception of sensory or painful stimuli.
Abscessed tooth or appendix	Infection is highly localized. Application of heat may cause rupture with spread of microorganisms systemically.

Table 47-15 Therapeutic Effects of Heat and Cold Applications

Physiological Response	Therapeutic Benefit	Examples of Conditions Treated
Heat		
Vasodilation	Improves blood flow to injured body part; promotes delivery of nutrients and removal of wastes; lessens venous congestion in injured tissues	Inflamed or edematous body part; new surgical wound; infected wound; arthritis, degenerative joint disease; localized joint pain, muscle strains; low back pain; menstrual cramping, hemorrhoidal, perianal, and vaginal inflammation; local abscesses
Reduced blood viscosity	Improves delivery of leukocytes and antibiotics to wound site	
Reduced muscle tension	Promotes muscle relaxation and reduces pain from spasm or stiffness	
Increased tissue metabolism	Increases blood flow; provides local warmth	
Increased capillary permeability	Promotes movement of waste products and nutrients	
Cold		
Vasoconstriction	Reduces blood flow to injured body part, preventing edema formation; reduces inflammation	Direct trauma (sprains, strains, fractures, muscle spasms); superficial laceration or puncture wound; minor burn; suspected malignancy in area of injury or pain; injections; arthritis and joint trauma
Local anesthesia	Reduces localized pain	
Reduced cell metabolism	Reduces oxygen needs of tissues	
Increased blood viscosity	Promotes blood coagulation at injury site	
Decreased muscle tension	Relieves pain	

Table 47-16 Choice of Dry or Moist Applications

Advantages	Disadvantages
Moist Applications	
Moist application reduces drying of skin and softens wound exudate.	Prolonged exposure can cause maceration of skin.
Moist compresses conform well to body area being treated.	Moist heat will cool rapidly because of moisture evaporation.
Moist heat penetrates deeply into tissue layers.	Moist heat creates greater risk for burns to skin because moisture conducts heat.
Warm moist heat does not promote sweating and insensible fluid loss.	
Dry Applications	
Dry heat has less risk of burns to skin than moist applications.	Dry heat increases body fluid loss through sweating.
Dry application does not cause skin maceration.	Dry applications do not penetrate deep into tissues.
Dry heat retains temperature longer because it is not influenced by evaporation.	Dry heat causes increased drying of skin.

variations changes with age. Clients who are very young and old are most sensitive to heat and cold. If a client's physical condition reduces the reception or perception of sensory stimuli, tolerance to temperature extremes is high, but the risk of injury is also high.

Assessment for Temperature Tolerance.   Before applying heat or cold therapies, the nurse assesses the client's physical condition for signs of potential intolerance to heat and cold. The nurse first observes the area to be treated. Alterations in skin integrity, such as abrasions, open wounds, edema, bruising, bleeding, or localized areas of inflammation, increase the client's risk of injury. Because the physician commonly orders heat and cold applications to be placed on traumatized areas, the baseline assessment provides a guide for evaluating skin changes that might occur during therapy.

Assessment includes identification of conditions that contraindicate heat or cold therapy. An active area of bleeding should not be covered by a warm application because bleeding will continue. Warm applications are contraindicated when the client has an acute, localized inflammation such as appendicitis because the heat could cause the appendix to rupture. If a client has cardiovascular problems, it is unwise to apply heat to large portions of the body because the resulting massive vasodilation may disrupt blood supply to vital organs.

Cold is contraindicated if the site of injury is already edematous. Cold further retards circulation to the area and prevents absorption of the interstitial fluid. If the client has impairment in circulation (e.g., arteriosclerosis), cold further reduces blood supply to the affected area. Cold therapy is also contraindicated in the presence of neuropathy, since the client is unable to perceive temperature change and damage resulting from temperature extremes. One other contraindication for cold therapy is shivering. Cold applications may intensify shivering and dangerously increase body temperature. The nurse also assesses the client's response to stimuli. Sensation to light touch, pinprick, and mild temperature variations (see Chapter 32) reveals the ability of the client to recognize when heat or cold becomes excessive. If a client has peripheral vascular disease, the nurse pays particular attention to the integrity of extremities. For example, if the physician's order is to apply a cold compress to a lower extremity, the nurse should assess circulation to the leg by observing skin color and palpating skin temperatures, distal pulses, and edematous areas. If signs of circulatory inadequacy are present, the nurse should question the order.

Level of consciousness influences the ability to perceive heat, cold, and pain. If a client is confused or unresponsive, the nurse must make frequent observations of skin integrity after therapy begins.

The nurse must also assess the condition of equipment being used. Electrical equipment should be checked for cracked cords, frayed wires, damaged insulation, and exposed heating components. Equipment containing circulating fluids should not have leaks. The nurse also checks equipment for evenness of temperature distribution. Uneven temperature distribution suggests that the equipment is functioning improperly.

Client Education and Safety.   Before application of heat or cold therapy the client should understand its purpose, the symptoms of temperature exposure, and precautions taken to prevent injury. Box 47-20 provides hints for safely applying heat and cold therapy.

Application of Heat and Cold Therapies.   A prerequisite to using any heat or cold application is a physician's order, which should include the body site to be treated and the type, frequency, and duration of application. The nurse should consult the agency's procedure manual for correct temperatures to use.

Choice of Moist or Dry.   Heat and cold applications can be administered in dry or moist forms. The type of wound or injury, the location of the body part, and the presence of drainage or inflammation are factors considered in selecting dry or moist applications. Table 47-16 summarizes advantages and disadvantages of both.

Hot, Moist Compresses.   For open wounds, sterile, hot, moist compresses improve circulation, relieve edema, and promote consolidation of pus and drainage. A **compress** is a piece of gauze dressing moistened in a prescribed warmed solution. A **pack** is a larger cloth or dressing applied to a larger body area.

Heat from hot compresses dissipates quickly. To maintain a constant temperature, the nurse must change the compress often or apply a warm aquathermic pad or wa-

---

Safety Suggestions for Applying Heat or Cold Therapy   Box 47-20

Do explain to the client sensations to be felt during the procedure.

Do instruct the client to report changes in sensation or discomfort immediately.

Do provide a timer, clock, or watch so that the client can help the nurse time the application.

Do keep the call light within the client's reach.

Do refer to the institution's policy and procedure manual for safe temperatures.

Do not allow the client to adjust temperature settings.

Do not allow the client to move an application or place hands on the wound site.

Do not place the client in a position that prevents movement away from the temperature source.

Do not leave unattended a client who is unable to sense temperature changes or move from the temperature source.

Applying a Hot, Moist Compress to an Open Wound   Skill 47-7

Delegation Considerations

This skill can be delegated to assistive personnel.

- Ensure that caregiver can perform skill competently.
- Caution caregiver to maintain proper temperature of application during duration of treatment.

- Caution caregiver to keep application in place for only the length of time specified in physician's orders.
- Have caregiver notify the nurse when treatment is complete so that an evaluation of client's response can be made.

EQUIPMENT

- Prescribed solution warmed to appropriate temperature
- Sterile gauze dressings or commercially prepared compresses
- Sterile container for solution
- Dry bath towel
- Disposable gloves

- Sterile gloves
- Waterproof pad
- Ties or tape
- Aquathermia or heating pad (optional)
- Bath blanket

STEPS	RATIONALE
1. Refer to physician's order for type of compress, location and duration of application, desired temperature, and institutional policies regarding temperature of compress.	Ensures safe and correct application.
2. Inspect condition of exposed skin and wound on which compress is to be applied.	Provides baseline to determine changes in skin during heat application.

Critical Decision Point: Very thin or damaged skin is more susceptible to injury from heat. Nonintact skin and drainage from wounds are indications to wear gloves.

3. Assess client's extremities for sensitivity to temperature and pain by measuring light touch, pin-prick, and temperature sensation.	Clients insensitive to heat or cold sensations must be monitored closely during treatment.

Critical Decision Point: Diabetic clients, victims of stroke, and clients with peripheral neuropathy are particularly at risk for thermal injury.

4. Refer to medical record to identify any systemic contraindications to heat application.	Heat causes vasodilation, which aggravates active bleeding. Heat applied to localized area of acute inflammation or tumor may cause rupture or activate cell growth.
5. Assemble equipment and supplies.	Organization of supplies prevents unnecessary delays in the procedure.
6. Explain steps of procedure and purpose to client. Describe sensations to be felt, such as decreasing warmth and wetness. Explain precautions to prevent burning.	Minimizes client's anxiety and promotes cooperation during the procedure.
7. Close door and bedside curtains.	Decreases drafts, thus decreasing the transmission of microorganisms. Provides for client privacy.
8. Assist client in assuming comfortable position in proper body alignment and place waterproof pad under area to be treated.	Compress remains in place for several minutes. Limited mobility in uncomfortable position causes muscular stress. Pad prevents soiling of bed linen.
9. Expose body part to be covered with compress and drape client with bath blanket.	Prevents unnecessary cooling and exposure of body part.
10. Wash hands.	Reduces transmission of microorganisms.
11. Prepare compress:	Ensures orderly procedure.
a. Pour solution into sterile container.	
b. If using portable heating source, warm solution. Commercially prepared compresses may remain under infrared lamp until just before use. Open sterile packages and drop gauze into container to become immersed in solution.	Compresses must retain warmth for therapeutic benefit.

STEPS	RATIONALE

Critical Decision Point: Temperature must be tested by applying sterile solution to nurse's forearm (without contaminating solution).

c. Adjust temperature of aquathermia pad (if needed).	
12. Apply disposable gloves. Remove any existing dressing covering wound. Dispose of gloves and dressings in proper receptacle.	Reduces transmission of microorganisms.
13. Assess condition of wound and surrounding skin. Inflamed wound appears reddened, but surrounding skin is less red in color.	Provides baseline to determine skin changes following compress application.

Critical Decision Point: If skin surrounding wound is reddened, application may be contraindicated.

14. Apply sterile gloves.	Allows nurse to manipulate sterile dressing and touch open wound.
15. Pick up one layer of immersed gauze, wring out any excess solution, and apply it lightly to open wound.	Excess moisture macerates skin and increases risks of burns and infection. Skin is sensitive to sudden change in temperature.
16. In a few seconds, lift edge of gauze to assess for redness.	Increased redness indicates burn.
17. If client tolerates compress, pack gauze snugly against the wound. Be sure all wound surfaces are covered by hot compress.	Packing of compress prevents rapid cooling from underlying air currents.
18. Cover moist compress with dry sterile dressing and bath towel. If necessary, pin or tie in place. Remove sterile gloves.	Dry sterile dressing will prevent transfer of microorganisms to wound via capillary action caused by moist compress. Towel insulates compress to prevent heat loss.
19. Apply aquathermic or waterproof heating pad over towel (optional). Keep it in place for desired duration of application.	Provides constant temperature to compress.
20. If an aquathermia pad is *not* used to maintain temperature of application, change hot compress using sterile technique every 5 minutes or as ordered during duration of therapy.	Prevents cooling and maintains therapeutic benefit of compress.
21. After prescribed time, apply disposable gloves and remove pad, towel, and compress. Reassess wound and condition of skin, and replace dry sterile dressing as ordered.	Continued exposure to moisture will macerate skin. Prevents entrance of microorganisms into wound site.
22. Assist client to preferred comfortable position.	Maintains client's comfort.
23. Dispose of equipment and soiled compress. Wash hands.	Reduces transmission of microorganisms.
24. Inspect affected area covered by compress and heating pad every 5 to 10 minutes.	Assists in determining effects of application.
25. Ask every 5 to 10 minutes if client notices any unusual burning sensation not felt before application.	It may be difficult to assess burn merely by color changes if wound is inflamed or drainage is present.
26. Have client explain and demonstrate application.	Evaluates client's understanding of and ability to perform procedure.

Recording and Reporting

- Record type, location, and duration of application. Note solution and temperature.
- Describe condition of wound and skin before and after treatment, as well as client's response to therapy.
- Describe any instructions given and client's ability to explain and perform procedure.
- Report unusual findings to nurse in charge or physician.

Home Care Considerations

- When necessary, assess availability of primary caregivers to assist clients in application of compress, their understanding of purpose of procedure, and their willingness to comply with procedure and not leave client with compress in place beyond prescribed time limit.
- Assess physical environment to determine existence of adequate facilities to prepare hot compress and provide for sterile technique.

terproof heating pad over the compress. Because moisture conducts heat, any device's temperature setting should be lower for a moist compress than for a dry application. A layer of plastic wrap or a dry towel can also be used to insulate the compress and retain heat. Moist heat promotes vasodilation and evaporation of heat from the skin's surface. For this reason, a client may feel chilly. The nurse controls drafts within the room and keeps the client covered with a blanket or robe. Skill 47-7 describes the steps for applying a hot, moist compress.

Warm Soaks.   Immersion of a body part in a warmed solution promotes circulation, lessens edema, increases muscle relaxation, and can provide a means to debride wounds and apply medicated solution. A soak can also be accompanied by wrapping the body part in dressings and saturating them with the warmed solution.

The nurse positions the client comfortably, places waterproof pads under the area to be treated, and heats the solution to about 40.5° to 43° C (105° to 110° F). After immersing the body part, the nurse covers the container and extremity with a towel to reduce heat loss. It is usually necessary to remove the cooled solution and add heated solution after about 10 minutes. The problem is to keep the solution at a constant temperature. The nurse never adds a hotter solution while the body part remains immersed. After any soak, the nurse dries the body part thoroughly to prevent maceration.

Sitz Baths.   The client who has had rectal surgery, an episiotomy during childbirth, painful hemorrhoids, or vaginal inflammation may benefit from a **sitz bath,** a bath in which only the pelvic area is immersed in warm fluid. The client sits in a special tub or chair or in a basin that fits on the toilet seat so that the legs and feet remain out of the water. Immersing the entire body causes widespread vasodilation and nullifies the effect of local heat application to the pelvic area.

The desired temperature for a sitz bath depends on whether the purpose is to promote relaxation or to clean a wound. It may be necessary to add warm water during the procedure, which normally lasts 20 minutes, to maintain a constant temperature. Agency procedure manuals recommend safe water temperatures. A disposable sitz basin contains an attachment resembling an enema bag that allows gradual introduction of warmer water (Figure 47-35).

The nurse prevents overexposure of the client by draping bath blankets around the client's shoulders and thighs and controlling drafts. The client should be able to sit in the basin or tub with feet flat on the floor and without pressure on the sacrum or thighs. Because exposure of a large portion of the body to heat can cause extensive vasodilation, the nurse should assess the pulse and facial color and ask whether the client feels light-headed or nauseated.

Aquathermia (Water-Flow) Pads.   A popular device in health care institutions is the **aquathermia pad,** or water-flow pad (Figure 47-36), used for treating muscle sprains and areas of mild inflammation or edema. The aquathermia unit consists of a waterproof plastic or rubber pad connected by two hoses to an electrical control unit that has a heating element and motor.

Distilled water circulates through hollowed channels within the pad to the control unit where water is heated or cooled (depending on temperature setting). Some pads have an absorbent surface to apply moist heat. The units are safer than conventional heating pads. However, the nurse should still check for equipment malfunctions. The temperature setting is fixed by inserting a plastic key into

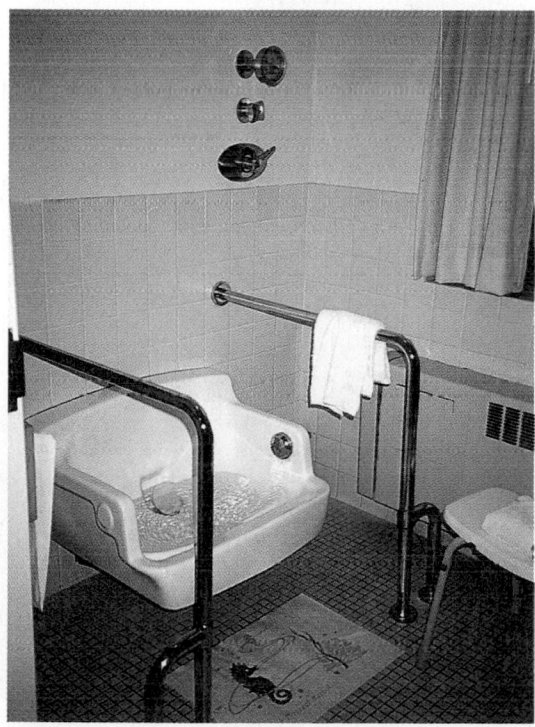

Figure 47-35 Sitz bath.

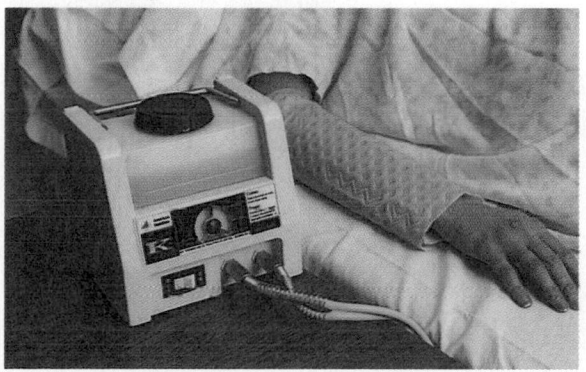

Figure 47-36 Aquathermia pad.

the temperature regulator. In many institutions the central supply room sets the regulators to the recommended temperature (40.5° to 43° C [105° to 110° F]). If the distilled water in the unit runs low, the nurse simply fills the reservoir two-thirds full. Plain tap water is never added, because it might leave mineral deposits in the unit.

To avoid burning the client's skin, the nurse does not place the pad directly on it. A thin towel or pillow case fits easily over the heating pad. Tape, ties, or a gauze roll holds the pad in place. Pins are never used, because they might cause a leak. The nurse checks the client's skin often for signs of burning. An application should last only 20 to 30 minutes. The nurse does not allow a client to lie on a pad. Pressure against a mattress prevents normal heat dissipation. If the pad is to be applied to a region of the back, the client should lie prone or on one side.

Warm Air Blower. When wounds require drying (such as the donor site in split-thickness skin grafting), the nurse may use a hair dryer. The hair dryer is set on medium warm setting and held about 8 to 10 inches from the wound. The nurse then gently waves the device over the site for about 5 minutes or the time prescribed by the surgeon. This procedure is repeated 3 or 4 times a day until the wound is completely dry.

Commercial Hot Packs. Commercially prepared, disposable hot packs apply warm, dry heat to an injured area. By striking, kneading, or squeezing the pack, chemicals are mixed and release heat. Package directions recommend the time for heat application.

Electric Heating Pads. Another conventional form of heat therapy is the heating pad, an electric coil enclosed within a waterproof pad covered with cotton or flannel cloth. The pad is connected to an electric cord that has a temperature-regulating unit for a high, medium, or low setting. Nurses should advise clients to avoid using the high setting and to never lie on the pad. Another precau-

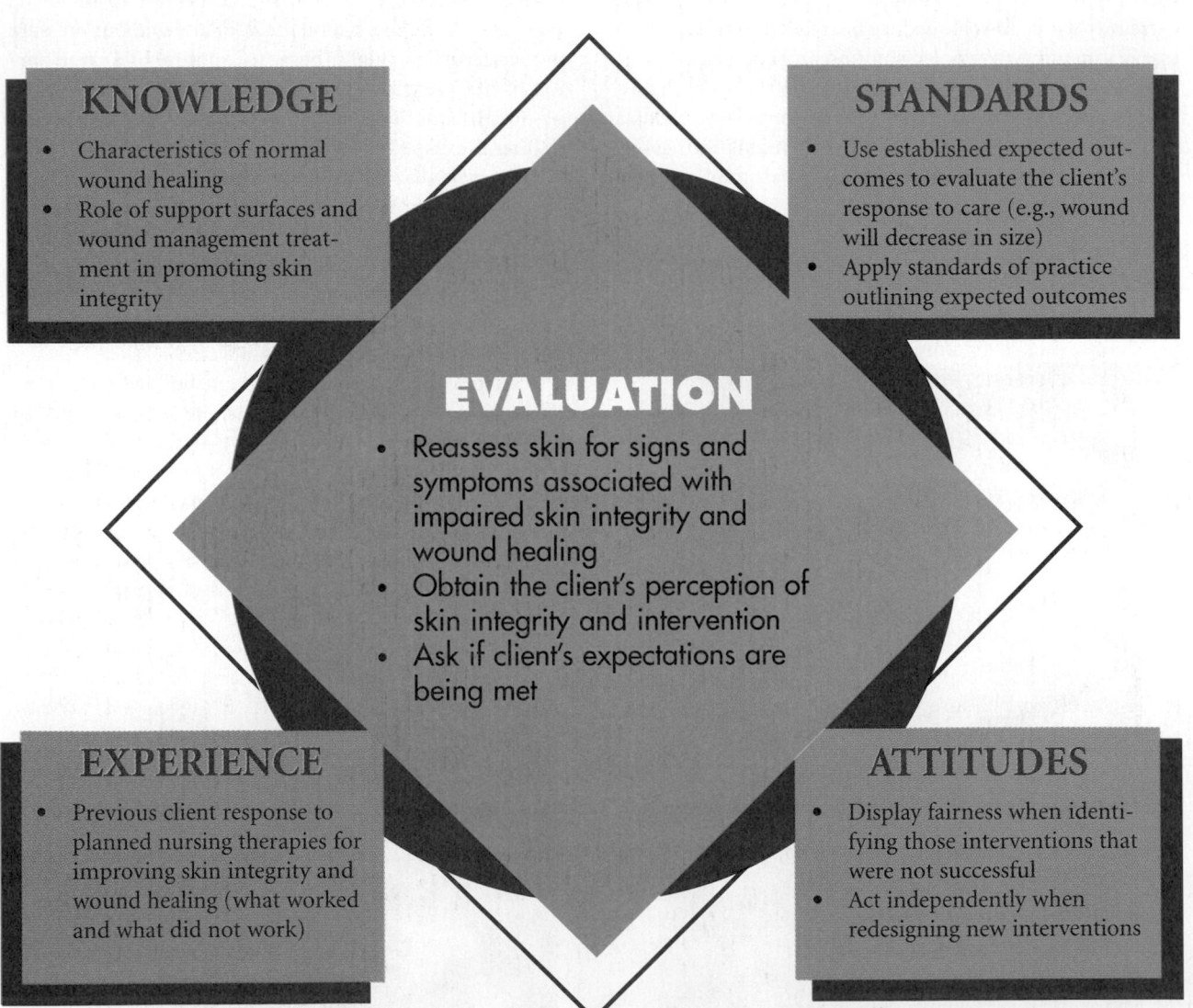

KNOWLEDGE

- Characteristics of normal wound healing
- Role of support surfaces and wound management treatment in promoting skin integrity

STANDARDS

- Use established expected outcomes to evaluate the client's response to care (e.g., wound will decrease in size)
- Apply standards of practice outlining expected outcomes

EVALUATION

- Reassess skin for signs and symptoms associated with impaired skin integrity and wound healing
- Obtain the client's perception of skin integrity and intervention
- Ask if client's expectations are being met

EXPERIENCE

- Previous client response to planned nursing therapies for improving skin integrity and wound healing (what worked and what did not work)

ATTITUDES

- Display fairness when identifying those interventions that were not successful
- Act independently when redesigning new interventions

Figure 47-37 *Synthesis Model for Skin Integrity and Wound Care Evaluation Phase.*

tion to note is that a safety pin inserted through a pad can result in an electrical shock.

Cold, Moist, and Dry Compresses. The procedure for applying cold, moist compresses is the same as that for warm compresses. Cold compresses should be applied for 20 minutes at a temperature of 15° C (59° F) to relieve inflammation and swelling. They may be clean or sterile.

There are commercially prepared cold packs that are similar to the disposable hot packs for dry applications. They come in various shapes and sizes to fit different body parts. When using cold compresses, the nurse observes for adverse reactions such as burning or numbness, mottling of the skin, redness, extreme paleness, and a bluish skin discoloration.

Cold Soaks. The procedure for preparing cold soaks and immersing a body part is the same as for warm soaks. The desired temperature for a 20-minute cold soak is 15° C (59° F). The nurse controls drafts and uses outer coverings to protect the client from chilling. It may be necessary to add cold water during the procedure to maintain a constant temperature.

Ice Bags or Collars. For a client who has a muscle sprain, localized hemorrhage, or hematoma or who has undergone dental surgery, an ice bag is ideal to prevent edema formation, control bleeding, and anesthetize the body part. Proper use of the bag requires the following steps:

1. Fill the bag with water, secure the cap, invert to check for leaks, and pour out the water.
2. Fill the bag two-thirds full with crushed ice so that the bag can mold easily over a body part.
3. Release any air from the bag by squeezing its sides before securing the cap, because excess air interferes with conduction of cold.
4. Wipe off excess moisture.
5. Cover the bag with a flannel cover, towel, or pillow case.
6. Apply the bag to the injury site for 30 minutes; the bag can be reapplied in an hour.

✎ EVALUATION

Client Care. Nursing interventions for reducing and treating pressure ulcers are evaluated by determining the client's response to nursing therapies and by determining whether each goal was achieved. To evaluate outcomes and responses to care, the nurse measures the effectiveness of interventions. The optimal outcomes are to prevent injury to the skin and tissues, reduce injury to the skin and underlying tissues, and restore skin integrity.

Because each client has different risk factors for impaired skin integrity, nursing interventions must be individualized. Clients with minimal mobility impairments or relatively stable health status may need only a few measures. Nursing interventions for reducing and treating pressure ulcers are evaluated by determining the client's response to nursing therapies and by determining whether each goal was achieved (see Figure 47-37).

To evaluate outcomes and responses to care, the nurse measures the effectiveness of interventions. This often occurs over an extended period of time, requiring the nurse to make careful ongoing measurements of an ulcer's condition. The nurse also evaluates specific interventions designed to promote skin integrity and to teach the client and family to reduce future threats to skin integrity.

The nurse also evaluates specific interventions designed to promote skin integrity and to teach the client and family to reduce future threats to skin integrity. The AHCPR panel (1992a) produced a client's guide for pressure ulcers that is short with clear illustrations (Ayello, 1993). The nurse also evaluates the client's and family's need for additional support services (e.g., home health care, physical therapy, and counseling) and initiates the referral process.

Finally, the nurse evaluates the need for additional referrals to other experts in pressure ulcers, such as enterostomal and wound care nurses and physical therapists (PTs) when indicated. Care of the client with a pressure ulcer requires a multidisciplinary team approach.

Client Expectations. The client and caregiver need to understand how to prevent or treat pressure ulcers. Helping them understand the content in the AHCPR consumer version of the prevention and treatment guidelines is helpful. Clients may enter into the wound-healing phase with unrealistic expectations with regard to the duration of care. The nurse needs to collect evaluation data about the client's perception of wound care management. Clients with chronic wounds are often cared for in their home settings and have certain expectations about their level of comfort, lifestyle, independence, and privacy. Therefore, the nurse must determine from the client whether his or her expectations were respected and met.

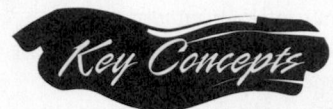

- Pressure ulcers increase the length of stay in hospitals and extended care settings, as well as the overall cost of nursing care needed to manage the wound.
- The Agency for Health Care Policy and Research developed guidelines for future research directions and for the prevention and treatment of pressure ulcers.
- Improvement of a healing pressure ulcer can be measured by several of the newly developed healing scales (PUSH, PSST); the staging systems for wounding should not be used for this purpose.
- Prediction for development of pressure ulcers must focus on clients having the greatest risk for developing impaired skin integrity.
- Alterations in mobility, sensory perception, level of consciousness, and nutrition; the use of orthopedic devices such as casts; and the presence of severe infection or other debilitating diseases increase the risk for pressure ulcer development.
- The risk of impaired skin integrity related to immobilization depends on the extent and duration of immobilization.
- External pressure, shearing force, moisture, impaired peripheral circulation, edema, and obesity are also contributing factors to the development of pressure ulcers.
- When the external pressure against the skin is greater than the pressure in the capillary bed, blood flow decreases to the adjacent tissues.
- Meticulous assessment of the skin and underlying tissue, and identification of risk factors are important in decreasing the opportunity for pressure ulcer development.
- Preventive skin care is aimed at controlling external pressure on bony prominences and keeping the skin clean, well lubricated and hydrated, and free of excess moisture.
- Proper positioning should reduce the effects of pressure and guard against the shearing force.
- Therapeutic beds and mattresses reduce the effects of pressure; however, selection is based on assessment data to identify the best bed for individual needs.

- Cleansing and topical agents used to treat pressure ulcers vary according to the stage of the pressure ulcer and condition of the wound bed. Assessment of the ulcer enables the nurse to select proper skin care agents.
- Nutritional interventions are directed at improving wound healing through increasing protein, calorie, and hemoglobin levels.
- Wound assessment requires a description of the appearance of the wound; palpation of the area; and information regarding the character of drainage, drains and wound closures, and pain.
- Healing by primary intention proceeds through three stages: inflammation, proliferation, and maturation.
- When there is extensive tissue loss, a wound heals by secondary intention.
- In normal wound healing, the epidermal skin layer resurfaces wounds and the dermis restores the structural integrity and physical properties of the skin.
- The chances of wound infection are greater when the wound contains dead or necrotic tissue, when foreign bodies lie on or near the wound, and when the blood supply and tissue defenses are reduced.
- Principles of wound first aid include control of bleeding, cleansing, and protection.
- The layers of a dry dressing protect the wound edges, absorb drainage, and prevent entrance of bacteria.
- The wet-to-dry dressing mechanically removes dead tissue and wound exudate to debride the wound.
- When cleansing wounds or drain sites, the nurse cleans from the least to most contaminated area, away from wound edges.
- A bandage or binder should be applied in a manner that does not impair circulation or irritate the skin.
- An acute sprain, fracture, or bruise responds best to cold applications.
- The choice of moist or dry applications depends on the type of wound, location of the body part, and presence of drainage or inflammation.
- Warm applications are effective for improving circulation to wound sites and promoting muscle relaxation.

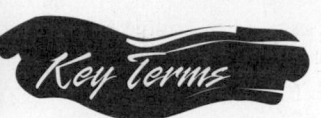

Key Terms

Abnormal reactive hyperemia, *p. 1547*
Abrasion, *p. 1572*
Anemia, *p. 1566*
Approximate, *p. 1554*
Aquathermia pad, *p. 1623*
Binders, *p. 1611*
Blanching, *p. 1546*
Cachexia, *p. 1566*
Capillary closing pressure, *p. 1547*
Collagen, *p. 1545*
Compress, *p. 1620*
Darkly pigmented skin, *p. 1546*
Debridement, *p. 1584*
Debriding, *p. 1599*
Dehiscence, *p. 1556*
Dermis, *p. 1545*
Desquamation, *p. 1545*
Drainage evacuators, *p. 1611*
Edema, *p. 1566*
Epidermis, *p. 1545*
Epithelialization, *p. 1554*
Eschar, *p. 1584*
Evisceration, *p. 1556*
Exudate, *p. 1554*
Fibrin, *p. 1554*
Fibroblasts, *p. 1554*
Fistula, *p. 1556*
Friction, *p. 1563*
Granulation tissue, *p. 1554*

Hematoma, *p. 1555*
Hemorrhage, *p. 1555*
Hemostasis, *p. 1554*
Hypovolemic shock, *p. 1555*
Induration, *p. 1547*
Laceration, *p. 1572*
Moist wound-healing environment, *p. 1593*
Normal reactive hyperemia, *p. 1547*
Nosocomial infection, *p. 1555*
Pack, *p. 1620*
Pressure reducing, *p. 1580*
Pressure relieving, *p. 1580*
Pressure ulcer, *p. 1545*
Primary intention, *p. 1554*
Puncture, *p. 1572*
Purulent, *p. 1556*
Sanguineous, *p. 1573*
Secondary intention, *p. 1554*
Serosanguineous, *p. 1573*
Serous, *p. 1573*
Shearing force, *p. 1563*
Sitz bath, *p. 1623*
Skin barriers, *p. 1611*
Sloughing, *p. 1584*
Steri-Strip, *p. 1607*
Sutures, *p. 1607*
Tissue ischemia, *p. 1546*
Wound, *p. 1551*
Wound contraction, *p. 1555*

Critical Thinking Exercises

1. When removing a wet-to-dry dressing, you note that the underlying gauze is wet with saline. The skin surrounding the wound is macerated. What conclusions can you make about the previous dressing? What would you do to avoid recurrence of this type of wet-to-dry application?

2. After changing a client's position, you observe redness over the bony prominences. What type of assessment must you perform to obtain correct information regarding pressure ulcer risk?

3. You have just admitted a client from a nursing home to your division. On initial assessment, you assess a stage III pressure ulcer. How do you determine the type of care and dressing to use with this particular pressure ulcer?

4. You are providing care to an elderly incontinent Hispanic man who is bed-bound. How will you assess for pressure ulcers in this client? What measures can you take to prevent his skin from breaking down?

References

Agency for Health Care Policy and Research, Panel for the Prediction and Prevention of Pressure Ulcers in Adults: *Pressure ulcers in adults: prediction and prevention,* Clinical Practice Guideline No. 3, AHCPR Pub No. 92-0047, Rockville, Md, 1992a, Agency for Health Care Policy and Research, Public Health Service, U.S. Department of Health and Human Services.

Agency for Health Care Policy and Research, Panel for Treatment of Pressure Ulcers in Adults: *Treatment of pressure ulcers,* Clinical Practice Guideline No. 15, AHCPR Pub No. 95-0653, Rockville, Md, 1994, Agency for Health Care Policy and Research, Public Health Service, U.S. Department of Health and Human Services.

Agency for Health Care Policy and Research, Panel for Urinary Incontinence Guideline: *Urinary incontinence in adults,* Clinical Practice Guideline, AHCPR Pub No. 92-0038, Rockville, Md, 1992b, Agency for Health Care Policy and Research, Public Health Service, U.S. Department of Health and Human Services.

Allman RM: Epidemiology of pressure sores in different populations, *Decubitus* 2(20):30, 1989.

Allman RM and others: Pressure ulcers, hospital complications, and disease severity: impact on hospital costs and length of stay, *Adv Wound Care* 12:22, 1999.

Aronovitch S: Selecting the best dressing sponge, *Nurs 95* 25(7):52, 1995.

Ayello EA: Teaching the assessment of patients with pressure ulcers, *Decubitus* 5(4):53, 1992.

Ayello EA: A critique of the AHCPR's "Preventing pressure ulcers patient's guide" as a written instructional tool, *Decubitus* 6(3):44, 1993.

Ayello EA: Critique of AHCPR's consumer guide "Treating pressure sores," *Adv Wound Care* 7(5):18, 1995.

Ayello EA: Keeping pressure ulcers in check, *Nursing* 26(10):62, 1996.

Ayello EA, Mezey M, Amella EA: Educational assessment and teaching of older clients with pressure ulcers, *Clin Geriatr Med* 13(3):483, 1997.

Ayello EA, Thomas DR, Litchford MA: Nutritional aspects of wound healing, *Home Healthcare Nurse* (in press).

Baharestani MM: The lived experience of wives caring for their frail, homebound, elderly husbands with pressure ulcers, *Adv Wound Care* 7(3):40, 1994.

Baranoski S: Wound assessment and dressing selection, *Ostomy/Wound Manage* 41(7A):7S, 1995.

Baranoski S: Wound dressings: Challenging decisions, *Home Healthcare Nurse,* 17(1):18, 1999.

Barczak CA and others: Fourth National Pressure Ulcer Prevalence Survey, *Adv Wound Care* 10(4):18, 1997.

Barr JE: Principles of wound cleansing, *Ostomy/Wound Manage* 41(7A):15S, 1995.

Bates-Jensen B: New pressure ulcer status tool, *Decubitus* 3(3):14, 1990.

Bennett MA: Report of the Task Force on the Implications for Darkly Pigmented Intact Skin in the Prediction and Prevention of Pressure Ulcers, *Adv Wound Care* 8(6):34, 1995.

Bergstrom N, Demuth PJ, Branden B: A clinical trial of the Braden scale for predicting pressure sore risk, *Nurs Clin North Am* 22(2):417, 1987.

Bergstrom N and others: The Braden Scale for predicting pressure sore risk, *Nurs Res* 36:205, 1987.

Braden BJ, Bergstrom N: Clinical utility of the Braden Scale for predicting pressure sore risk, *Decubitus* 2:3, 1989.

Braden BJ, Bergstrom N: Predictive validity of the Braden Scale for pressure sore risk in a nursing home population, *Res Nurs Health* 17(6):459, 1994.

Breslow RA: Nutrition and air-fluidized beds: a literature review, *Adv Wound Care* 7(3):57, 1994.

Breslow RA, Bergstrom N: Nutritional prediction of pressure ulcers, *J Am Diet Assoc* 94(11):1301, 1994.

Breslow RA and others: The importance of dietary protein in healing pressure ulcers, *J Am Geriatr Soc* 41(4):357, 1993.

Brown DL, Smith, DJ: Bacterial colonization/infection and the surgical management of pressure ulcers, *Ostomy/Wound Manage* 45(suppl 1A):109S, 1999.

Bryant RA: *Acute and chronic wounds: nursing management*, St. Louis, 1992, Mosby.

Bryant RA and others: Pressure ulcers. In Bryant RA, editor: *Acute and chronic wounds: nursing management*, St. Louis, 1992, Mosby.

Centre for Policy on Ageing: London, England, 1962.

Cooper DM: Acute surgical wounds. In Bryant RA, editor: *Acute and chronic wounds: nursing management*, St. Louis, 1992a, Mosby.

Cooper DM: Wound assessment and evaluation of healing. In Bryant RA, editor: *Acute and chronic wounds: nursing management*, St. Louis, 1992b, Mosby.

Cuddigan J, Frantz RA: Pressure ulcer research: pressure ulcer treatment, National Pressure Ulcer Advisory Panel Monograph, *Adv Wound Care* 11(6):294, 1998.

Dallam L and others: *Pressure ulcer pain: assessment and quantification*. Poster session presented at the National Pressure Ulcer Advisory Panel Fourth National Conference, Washington, DC, February 24-25, 1995.

Doak CC, Doak LG, Root JH: *Teaching patients with low literacy skills*, ed 2, Philadelphia, 1996, JB Lippincott.

Doughty DB: Principles of wound healing and wound management. In Bryant RA, editor: *Acute and chronic wounds: nursing management*, St. Louis, 1992, Mosby.

Erwin-Toth P, Hocevar BJ: Wound care: selecting the right dressing, *Am J Nurs* 95(2):46, 1995.

Faller NA: Clean versus sterile: a review of the literature, *Ostomy/Wound Manage* 45(5):56, 1999.

Finucane TE: Malnutrition, tube feeding and pressure sores: data are incomplete, *Am Geriatr Soc* 43(4):447, 1995.

Foresman PA and others: A relative toxicity index for wound cleansers, *Wounds* 5(5):226, 1993.

Garner JS: *Guidelines for prevention of surgical wound infections*, Atlanta, 1985, Centers for Disease Control.

Gaskin FC: Detection of cyanosis in the person with dark skin, *J Natl Black Nurses Assoc* 1:52, 1986.

Gosnell DJ: An assessment tool to identify pressure sores, *Nurs Res* 22(1):55, 1973.

Gosnell, DJ: Pressure sore risk assessment: a critique. I. The Gosnell Scale, *Decubitus* 2:3, 1989a.

Gosnell DJ: Pressure sore risk assessment. IIa. Analysis of risk factors, *Decubitus* 2:3, 1989b.

Gosnell DJ: Assessment and evaluation of pressure sores, *Nurs Clin North Am* 22(2):399, 1987.

Hanan K, Scheele L: Albumin vs. weight as a predictor of nutritional status and pressure ulcer development, *Ostomy/Wound Manage* 33:22, 1991.

Hanson D and others: The prevalence and incidence of pressure ulcers in home care: are patients at risk? *J Home Health Care* 5(3):25, 1993.

Helt J: Foot care and footwear to prevent amputation, *J Vasc Nurs* 9(4):2, 1991.

Henderson CT and others: Draft definition of stage I pressure ulcers: inclusion of persons with darkly pigmented skin, *Adv Wound Care* 10(5):16, 1997.

Hentzen B, Bergstrom N, Pozehl B: *Prevalence and incidence of pressure ulcers and associated risk factors in rural-based home health population*. Poster presentation at the 17th Annual Meeting of the Midwest Nursing Research Society, Cleveland, Ohio, March 28-30, 1993.

Hess CT: *Nurse's clinical guide: wound care*, Philadelphia, 1995, Springhouse.

Hess CT, Miller P: The management of open wounds: acute and chronic, *Ostomy/Wound Manage* 31:58, 1990.

Hoff J: Effecting a change in nursing practice: pressure ulcer prevention, *J Nurs Qual Assur* 3(4):56, 1989.

Husain T: An experimental study of some pressure effects on tissues, with reference to the bedsore problem, *J Pathol Bacteriol* 66:347, 1953.

Itoh M and others: Accelerated wound healing of pressure ulcers by pulsed high peak power electromagnetic energy (Diapulse), *Decubitus* 4(1):24, 1991.

Jacobs BW: Working on the right moves, *Nurs 94* 24:58, 1994.

Kaminski MV, Pinchocofsky-Devin G, Williams SD: Nutritional management of decubitus ulcers in the elderly, *Decubitus* 2(4):20, 1989.

Kloth LC, McCulloch JM, Feedar JA: *Wound healing: alternatives in management*, Philadelphia, 1990, FA Davis.

Koziak M: Etiology and pathology of ischemic ulcers, *Arch Phys Med Rehabil* 40:62, 1959.

Krasner D: The twelve commandments of wound care, *Nurs 92* 22(12):34, 1992.

Krasner D: The chronic wound pain experience: a conceptual model, *Ostomy/Wound Manage* 42:20, 1995a.

Krasner D: Wound care: how to use the red-yellow-black system, *Am J Nurs* 5:44, 1995b.

Krasner D: The AHCPR pressure ulcer infection control recommendations revisited, *Ostomy/Wound Manage* 45(suppl 1A):88S, 1999.

Krouskop T, van Rijswijk L: Standardizing performance-based criteria for support surfaces, *Ostomy/Wound Manage* 41(1):34, 1995.

Landis EM: Micro-injection studies of capillary blood pressure in human skin, *Heart* 15:209, 1930.

Langemo DK and others: Incidences of pressure sores in acute care, rehabilitation, extended care, home health, and hospice in one locale, *Decubitus* 2(2):42, 1989.

Lazarus GS and others: Definitions and guidelines for assessment of wounds and evaluation of healing, *Wound Repair Regen* 2:165, 1994.

Leshem OA, Skelskey C: Pressure ulcers: quality management, prevalence, and severity in a long-term care setting, *Adv Wound Care* 7(2):50, 1994.

Levine JM: Historical notes on pressure ulcers: the cure of Ambrose Pare, Decubitus 5(2):23, 1992.

Lyder, CH and others: Validating the Braden Scale for the prediction of pressure ulcer risk in blacks and Latino/Hispanic elders: a pilot study, *Ostomy/Wound Manage* 44(3A suppl):42S, 1998.

Maklebust J: Pressure ulcer update, *RN* 41(12):56, 1991.

Maklebust J: Pressure ulcer staging systems. NPUAP Proceedings 1995, *Adv Wound Care* 7(4):28, 1995.

Maklebust J, Sieggreen M: *Pressure ulcers: guidelines for prevention and nursing management,* West Dundee, Ill, 1996, S-N Publications.

Maklebust J, Margolis D: Pressure ulcers: definition and assessment parameters. NPUAP Proceedings 1995, *Adv Wound Care* 7(4):28, 1995.

Margolis DJ: Definition of a pressure ulcer. NPUAP Proceedings 1995, *Adv Wound Care* 7(4):28, 1995.

McCloskey JC, Bulechek GM: *Nursing interventions classification (NIC),* ed 3, St. Louis, 2000, Mosby.

Motta GJ: Moistening up for good healing, *Nurs 95* 25:32H, 1995.

National Pressure Ulcer Advisory Panel: Pressure ulcer prevalence, cost and risk assessment: consensus development conference statement, *Decubitus* 2(2):24, 1989a.

National Pressure Ulcer Advisory Panel: *Pressure ulcer research: etiology, assessment, and early intervention,* Buffalo, New York, 1995a, The Panel.

National Pressure Ulcer Advisory Panel: *NPUAP proceedings of the Fourth National NPUAP Conference,* Washington, DC, February 24-25, 1995b.

Norton D: Calculating the risk: reflections on the Norton Scale, *Decubitus* 2:3, 1989.

Norton D, McLaren R, Exon-Smith AN: *An investigation of geriatric nursing problems in hospital,* 1962, Edinburgh, Churchill Livingstone.

Oot-Giromini BA and others: Pressure ulcer prevention versus treatment: comparative product cost study, *Decubitus* 2(3):52, 1989.

Pajk M and others: Investigating the problem of pressure sores, *J Gerontol Nurs* 12(7):11, 1986.

Pinchcofsky-Devin GD, Kaminski MV: Correlation of pressure sores and nutritional status, *J Am Geriatr Soc* 34:435, 1989.

Pires M, Muller A: Detection and management of early tissue pressure indicators: a pictorial essay, *Progressions* 3(3):3, 1991

Plaisier B and others: Prospective evaluation of craniofacial pressure in four different cervical orthoses, *J Trauma* 37(5):714, 1994.

Rodeheaver GT: Pressure ulcer debridement and cleaning: a review of current literature, *Ostomy/Wound Manage* 45(suppl 1A):80S, 1999.

Rodeheaver GT, Stotts NA: Methods for assessing change in pressure ulcer status. NPUAP Proceedings 1995, *Adv Wound Care* 7(4):28, 1995.

Rodeheaver G and others: Wound healing and wound management: focus on debridement, *Adv Wound Care* 7(1):22, 1994.

Salzberg CA and others: Predicting and preventing pressure ulcers in adults with paralysis, *Adv Wound Care* 11(5):237, 1998.

Shekleton ME, Litwack K: *Critical care nursing of the surgical patient,* Philadelphia, 1991, WB Saunders.

Steinberg J: Prevalence of decubitus ulcers: issues of concern, *Decubitus* 2(2):50, 1990.

Stotts NA: Predicting pressure ulcer development in surgical patients, *Heart Lung* 17(6):641, 1988.

Stotts NA: Determination of bacterial burden in wounds. NPUAP Proceedings 1995, *Adv Wound Care* 7(4):28, 1995.

Stotts NA, Cavanaugh CE: Assessing the patient with a wound, *Home Healthcare Nurse* 17(1):27, 1999.

Stotts NA and others: Sterile vs clean technique in wound care of patients with open surgical wounds in the post-op period: a pilot study, *Adv Wound Care* 8(2):13, 1995.

Thomas DR: The role of nutrition in prevention and healing of pressure ulcers, *Clin Geriatr Med* 13(3):497, 1997a.

Thomas DR: Specific nutritional factors in wound healing, *Adv Wound Care* 10(4):40-43, 1997b.

Thomas DR and others: Pressure Ulcer Scale for Healing: derivation and validation of the PUSH tool, *Adv Wound Care* 10(5):96, 1997.

Trelease CC: Developing standards for wound care, *Ostomy Wound Manage* 20:46, 1988.

Trumble HC: The skin tolerance for pressure and pressure sores, *Med J Aust* 2.724, 1930.

Willey T: High tech beds and mattress overlays: a decision guide, *Am J Nurs* 89:1142, 1989.

Wright RW, Orr R: Fibroblast cytotoxicity and blood cell integrity following exposure to dermal wound cleaners, *Ostomy/Wound Manage* 39(7):33, 1993.

Wysocki AB: A review of the skin and its appendages, *Adv Wound Care* 8:53, 1995.

Young L: Pressure ulcer prevalence and associated patient characteristics in one long-term care facility, *Decubitus* 2(2):52, 1989.

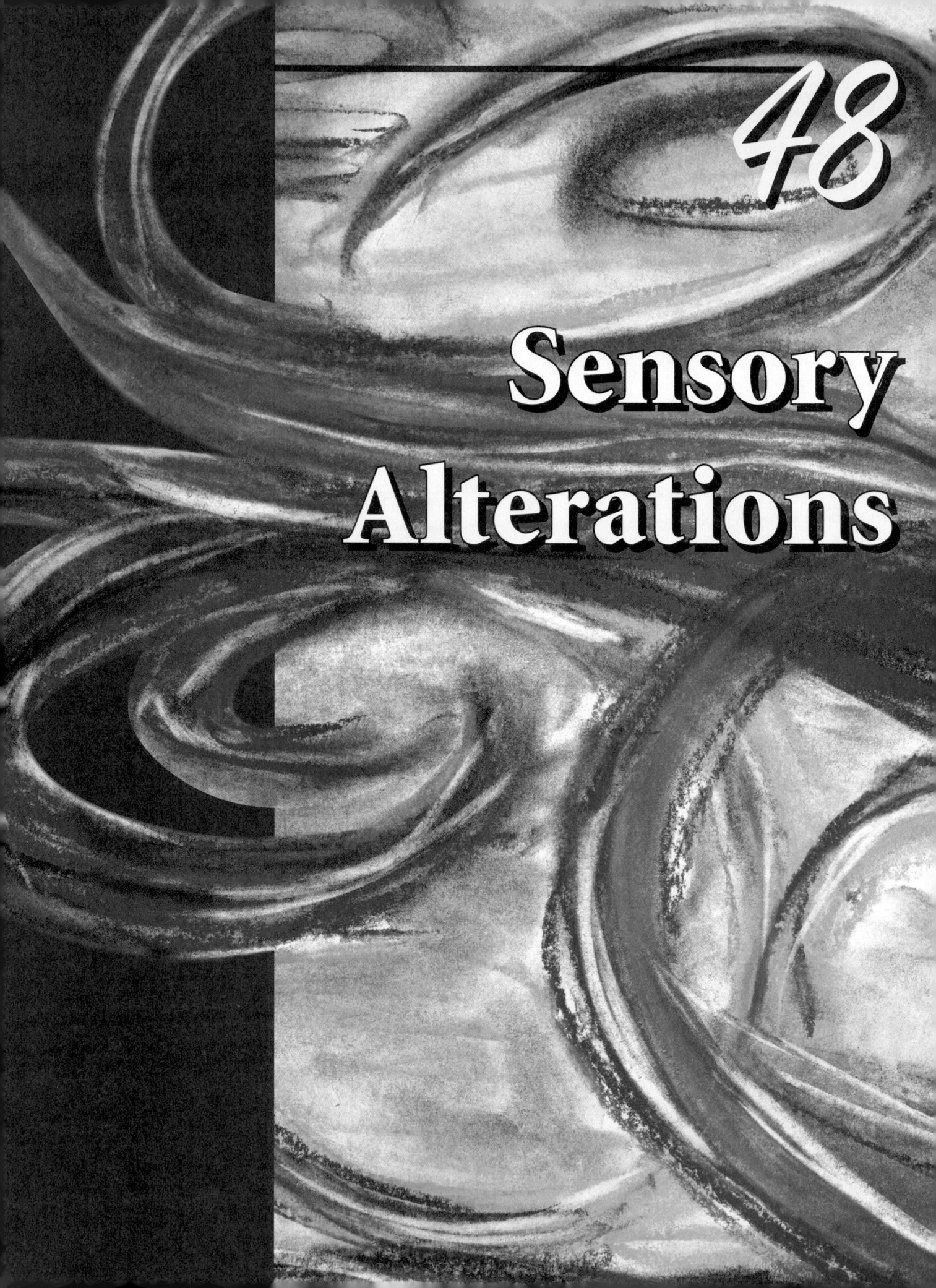

48

Sensory Alterations

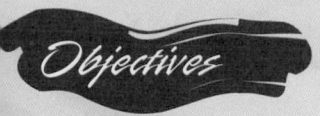

Mastery of content in this chapter will enable the student to:

- Define the key terms listed.
- Differentiate among the processes of reception, perception, and reaction to sensory stimuli.
- Discuss the relationship of sensory function to an individual's level of wellness.
- Discuss common causes and effects of sensory alterations.
- Discuss common sensory changes that normally occur with aging.
- Identify factors to assess in determining a client's sensory status.
- Identify nursing diagnoses relevant to clients with sensory alterations.
- Develop a plan of care for clients with visual, auditory, tactile, speech, and olfactory deficits.
- List interventions for preventing sensory deprivation and controlling sensory overload.
- Describe conditions in the health care agency or client's home that can be adjusted to promote meaningful sensory stimulation.
- Discuss ways to maintain a safe environment for clients with sensory deficits.

Imagine the world without sight, hearing, or the ability to feel objects or sense aromas around you. Human beings rely on a variety of sensory stimuli to give meaning and order to events occurring in their environment. The senses are tightly interwoven in forming the perceptual base of our world (Ebersole and Hess, 1998). Stimulation comes from many sources in and outside the body, particularly through the senses of sight (visual), hearing (**auditory**), touch (**tactile**), smell (**olfactory**), and taste (**gustatory**). The body also has a **kinesthetic** sense that enables a person to be aware of the position and movement of body parts without seeing them. **Stereognosis** is a sense that allows a person to recognize an object's size, shape, and texture. The ability to speak is not considered a sense but it is similar in that the client may lose the ability to interact meaningfully with other human beings. Meaningful stimuli allow a person to learn about the environment and are necessary for healthy functioning and normal development. When sensory function is altered, the person's ability to relate to and function within the environment changes drastically.

Many clients seeking health care have preexisting sensory alterations. Others may develop sensory alterations as a result of medical treatment (e.g., hearing loss from antibiotic use). The environment of a health care setting (e.g., a noisy intensive care unit) can cause sensory alterations. Clients who have partial or complete loss of a major sense may have developed or may need to find alternative ways to function safely within the environment. If sensory alterations occur early in life, clients often have developmental and socialization problems because of difficulty in responding to people and the environment. A health care setting is often a place of unfamiliar sights, sounds, and smells, as well as minimal contact with family and friends. If clients feel depersonalized and are unable to receive meaningful stimuli, serious sensory alterations can develop.

The nurse must understand and help meet the needs of clients with sensory alterations, as well as recognize clients most at risk for developing sensory problems. The nurse helps clients learn to interact and react safely and effectively in their environment.

Scientific Knowledge Base

NORMAL SENSATION

Normally the nervous system continually receives thousands of bits of information from sensory nerve organs, relays the information through appropriate channels, and integrates the information into a meaningful response. Sensory stimuli reach the sensory organs and can elicit an immediate reaction or present information to the brain to be stored for future use. The nervous system must be intact for sensory stimuli to reach appropriate brain centers and for the individual to perceive the sensation. After interpreting the significance of a sensation, the person can then react to the stimulus. Table 48-1 summarizes normal hearing and vision.

Reception, perception, and reaction are the three components of any sensory experience (see Chapter 42). Reception begins with stimulation of a nerve cell called a receptor, which is usually designed for only one type of stimulus, such as light or sound. In the case of special senses, the receptors are grouped close together or located in specialized organs (Thibodeau and Patton, 1999) such as the taste buds of the tongue or the retina of the eye.

Table 48-1 **Normal Hearing and Vision**	
Function	Anatomy and Physiology
The Ear	
Transmits to the brain an accurate pattern of all sounds received from the environment, the relative intensity of these sounds, and the direction from which they originate	Two ears provide stereophonic hearing to judge sound direction.
	The external ear canal shelters the eardrum and maintains relatively constant temperature and humidity to maintain elasticity.
	The middle ear is an air-containing space between the eardrum and oval window. It contains three small bones (ossicles).
	The eardrum and ossicles transfer sound to the fluid-filled inner ear.
	Movement of the stapes in the oval window creates vibrations in the fluid that bathes the membranous labyrinth, which contains the end organs of hearing and balance.
	The union of the vestibular (balance) and cochlear (hearing) portions of the labyrinth explains the combination of hearing and balance symptoms of inner ear disorders.
	Vibration of the eardrum is transmitted through the bony ossicles. Vibrations at the oval window are transmitted in perilymph within the inner ear to stimulate hair cells that send impulses along the eighth cranial nerve to the brain.
	Light rays enter the convex cornea and begin to converge.
The Eye	
Transmits to the brain an accurate pattern of light reflected from solid objects in the environment and transformed into color and hue	Fine adjustment of light rays occurs as they pass through the pupil and through the lens.
	Change in the shape of the lens focuses light on the retina.
	The retina has a pigmented layer of cells to enhance visual acuity.
	The sensory retina contains the rods and cones—photoreceptor cells sensitive to stimulation from light.
	Photoreceptor cells send electrical potentials by way of the optic nerve to the brain.

When a nerve impulse is created, it travels along pathways to the spinal cord or directly to the brain. For example, sound waves stimulate hair cell receptors within the organ of Corti, which causes impulses to travel along the eighth cranial nerve to the acoustic area of the temporal lobe. Sensory nerve pathways usually cross over to send stimuli to opposite sides of the brain. The actual perception or awareness of unique sensations depends on the receiving region of the cerebral cortex, where specialized brain cells interpret the quality and nature of sensory stimuli. When the person becomes conscious of the stimuli and receives the information, perception takes place. Perception includes integration and interpretation of the stimuli based on the person's experiences. A person's level of consciousness influences how well stimuli are perceived and interpreted. Any factors lowering consciousness impair sensory perception. If sensation is incomplete, such as blurred vision, or if past experience is inadequate for understanding stimuli such as pain, the person may react inappropriately to the sensory stimulus.

It is impossible to react to all of the multiple stimuli entering the nervous system. The brain prevents sensory bombardment by discarding or storing sensory information. A person will usually react to stimuli that are most meaningful or significant at the time. After continued reception of the same stimulus, however, a person stops responding and the sensory experience goes unnoticed. For example, a person concentrating on reading a good book may not be aware of music in the background. This adapt-

ability phenomenon occurs with most sensory stimuli except for those of pain.

The balance between sensory stimuli entering the brain and those actually reaching a person's conscious awareness maintains a person's well-being. If an individual attempts to react to every stimulus within the environment or if there is insufficient variety and quality of stimuli, sensory alterations will occur.

SENSORY ALTERATIONS

Many factors change the capacity to receive or perceive sensations (Box 48-1), thus causing sensory alterations. The types of sensory alterations commonly seen by the nurse are sensory deficits, sensory deprivation, and sensory overload. When a client suffers from more than one sensory alteration, the ability to function and relate effectively within the environment is seriously impaired.

Sensory Deficits.   A deficit in the normal function of sensory reception and perception is a **sensory deficit.** A client may not be able to receive certain stimuli (e.g., a client who is blind or deaf), or stimuli may become distorted (e.g., a client with blurred vision from cataracts). A sudden loss can cause fear, anger, or feelings of helplessness. When senses are impaired, the sense of self is impaired. Initially a person may withdraw by avoiding communication or socialization with others in an attempt to cope with the sensory loss. It becomes difficult for the person to interact safely with the environment until new skills

Factors That Influence Sensory Function   Box 48-1

AGE

Infants are unable to discriminate sensory stimuli. Nerve pathways are immature.

Visual changes during adulthood include presbyopia (inability to focus on near objects) and the need for glasses for reading (usually occurring from ages 40 to 50).

Hearing changes, which begin at age 30, include decreased hearing acuity, speech intelligibility, pitch discrimination, and hearing threshold. Tinnitus often accompanies a hearing loss as a side effect of drugs. Older adults hear low-pitched sounds the best but have difficulty hearing conversation over background noise.

Older adults have reduced visual fields, increased glare sensitivity, impaired night vision, reduced accommodation and depth perception, and reduced color discrimination.

Older adults have difficulty discriminating the consonants (*f, s, th, ch*). Speech sounds are garbled, and there is a delayed reception and reaction to speech.

Gustatory and olfactory changes include a decrease in the number of taste buds in later years and reduction of olfactory nerve fibers by age 50. Reduced taste discrimination and reduced sensitivity to odors are common.

Proprioceptive changes after age 60 include increased difficulty with balance, spatial orientation, and coordination.

Older adults experience tactile changes, including declining sensitivity to pain, pressure, and temperature.

MEDICATIONS

Some antibiotics (e.g., streptomycin, gentamicin) are **ototoxic** and can permanently damage the auditory nerve; chloramphenicol can irritate the optic nerve. Narcotic analgesics, sedatives, and antidepressant medications can alter the perception of stimuli.

ENVIRONMENT

Excessive environmental stimuli (e.g., equipment noise and staff conversation in an intensive care unit [ICU]) can result in sensory overload, marked by confusion, disorientation, and the inability to make decisions. Restricted environmental stimulation (e.g., with protective isolation) can lead to sensory deprivation. Poor-quality environmental stimuli (e.g., reduced lighting, narrow walkways, background noise) can worsen sensory impairment.

COMFORT LEVEL

Pain and fatigue alter the way a person perceives and reacts to stimuli.

PREEXISTING ILLNESS

Peripheral vascular disease can cause reduced sensation in the extremities and impaired cognition. Chronic diabetes mellitus can lead to reduced vision, blindness, or peripheral neuropathy. Strokes often produce loss of speech. Some neurological disorders impair motor function and sensory reception.

SMOKING

Chronic tobacco use can cause the taste buds to atrophy, lessening the perception of flavors.

NOISE LEVELS

Constant exposure to high noise levels (e.g., on a construction job site) can cause hearing loss.

ENDOTRACHEAL INTUBATION

Temporary loss of speech results from insertion of an endotracheal tube through the mouth or nose into the trachea.

---

relying on existing functions are learned. When a deficit develops gradually or when considerable time has passed since the onset of an acute sensory loss, the person learns to rely on unaffected senses. Some senses may even become more acute to compensate for an alteration. For example, a blind client often develops an acute sense of hearing.

Clients with sensory deficits may change behavior in adaptive or maladaptive ways. For example, one client with a hearing impairment may turn the unaffected ear toward the speaker to hear better, whereas another client may shun other people to avoid the embarrassment of not being able to understand their speech. Box 48-2 summarizes common sensory deficits and their influence on those affected.

Sensory Deprivation. The reticular activating system in the brain stem mediates all sensory stimuli to the cerebral cortex, so even in deep sleep, clients are able to receive stimuli. Sensory stimulation must be of sufficient quality and quantity to maintain a person's awareness. The sensory deprivation that clients experience relate to the need for a comforting touch. Clients in intensive care units (ICUs) are often exposed to physical touch, but it is usually associated with technical intervention rather than personal, comforting touch (Thelan and others; 1998). When a person experiences an inadequate quality or quantity of stimulation, such as monotonous or meaningless stimuli, **sensory deprivation** occurs. Three types of sensory deprivation are reduced sensory input (sensory deficit from visual or hearing loss), elimination of order or meaning from input (e.g., exposure to strange environments), and restriction of the environment (e.g., bed rest or reduced environmental variation) that produces monotony and boredom (Ebersole and Hess, 1998).

Individuals at risk for sensory deprivation are commonly those living in a confined environment such as a nursing home. Although most quality nursing homes offer meaningful stimulation through group activities, environmental design, and mealtime gatherings, there are exceptions. The older adult who is confined to a wheelchair,

Common Sensory Deficits

Box 48-2

VISUAL DEFICITS

Presbyopia: A gradual decline in the ability of the lens to accommodate or to focus on close objects. Individual is unable to see near objects clearly.

Cataract: Cloudy or opaque areas in part or all of the lens that interfere with passage of light through the lens. Cataracts usually develop gradually, without pain, redness, or tearing in the eye.

Dry eyes: Result when tear glands produce too few tears. Common in older adults and resulting in itching, burning, or even reduced vision.

Open-angle glaucoma: An increase in intraocular pressure caused by an obstruction to the normal flow of aqueous humor through Schlemm's canal. Causes progressive pressure against the optic nerve, resulting in visual field loss, decreased visual acuity, and a halo effect around the eyes if untreated.

Diabetic retinopathy: Pathological changes occur in the blood vessels of the retina, resulting in decreased vision or vision loss.

Senile macular degeneration: Condition in which the macula (specialized portion of the retina responsible for central vision) loses its ability to function efficiently. First signs may include blurring of reading matter, distortion or loss of central vision, and distortion of vertical lines.

HEARING DEFICITS

Presbycusis: A common progressive hearing disorder in older adults.

Cerumen accumulation: Buildup of ear wax in the external auditory canal. Cerumen, which is normally absorbed in a younger person's ear, becomes hard and collects in the canal and causes a conduction deafness.

BALANCE DEFICIT

Dizziness and disequilibrium: Common condition in older adulthood, usually resulting from vestibular dysfunction. Frequently an episode of vertigo or disequilibrium is precipitated by a change in position of the head.

TASTE DEFICIT

Xerostomia: Decrease in salivary production that leads to thicker mucus and a dry mouth. Can interfere with the ability to eat and leads to appetite and nutritional problems.

NEUROLOGICAL DEFICITS

Peripheral neuropathy: Disorder of the peripheral nervous system. Commonly caused in older adults by diabetes, Guillain-Barré syndrome, and neoplasms (Ebersole and Hess, 1998). Symptoms include numbness and tingling of the affected area and stumbling gait.

Stroke: Cerebrovascular accident caused by clot, hemorrhage, or emboli affecting a blood vessel leading to or within the brain. Creates altered proprioception with marked incoordination and imbalance. Loss of sensation and motor function in extremities controlled by the affected area of the brain also occurs.

---

suffers from poor hearing and/or vision, has decreased energy, and avoids contact with others is at significant risk for sensory deprivation (Figure 48-1). If the environment creates monotony, the nursing home resident has a reduced capacity to learn and to think.

There are many effects of sensory deprivation (Box 48-3). The symptoms can easily cause nurses and physicians to believe that a client is psychologically ill and confused, is suffering from severe electrolyte imbalance, or is under the influence of psychotropic drugs. Therefore the nurse must always be aware of the client's existing sensory function and the quality of stimuli within the environment.

Sensory Overload. When a person receives multiple sensory stimuli and cannot perceptually disregard or selectively ignore some stimuli, **sensory overload** occurs. Excessive sensory stimulation prevents the brain from appropriately responding to or ignoring certain stimuli. Because of the multitude of stimuli leading to overload, the person no longer perceives the environment in a way that makes sense. Overload prevents meaningful response by the brain; the person's thoughts race, attention moves in many directions, and anxiety and restlessness occur. As a result, overload causes a state similar to that produced by sensory deprivation. However, in contrast to deprivation,

overload is individualized. The amount of stimuli needed for healthy function varies with each individual. Persons may be subject to environmental overload more at one time than at another. A person's tolerance to sensory overload may vary by level of fatigue, attitude, and emotional and physical well-being.

The acutely ill client may fall victim to sensory overload. The constant pain from the disease process, the nurse's frequent monitoring of vital signs, and the irritation from drainage tubes protruding from the body combine to cause overload. Even if the nurse offers a comforting word or provides a gentle back rub, clients may not benefit because their attention and energy are focused on more stressful stimuli. Another example is the client who is hospitalized in an ICU. There the activity is constant. Lights are always on. Sounds can be heard from monitoring equipment, staff conversations, equipment alarms, and the activities of people entering the unit. Even at night, an ICU can be very noisy.

The behavioral changes associated with sensory overload can easily be confused with mood swings or simple disorientation. The nurse must look for symptoms such as racing thoughts, scattered attention, restlessness, and anxiety. Clients in ICUs sometimes resort to constantly fingering tubes and dressings. Constant reorientation and

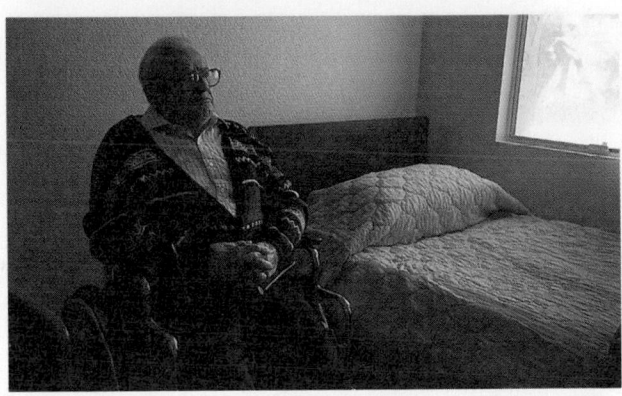

Figure 48-1   Isolation contributes to sensory deprivation.

Effects of Sensory Deprivation	Box 48-3

COGNITIVE
Reduced capacity to learn
Inability to think or problem solve
Poor task performance
Disorientation
Bizarre thinking
Regression
Increased need for socialization, altered mechanisms of attention

AFFECTIVE
Boredom
Restlessness
Increased anxiety
Emotional lability
Panic
Increased need for physical stimulation

PERCEPTUAL
Visual/motor coordination
Color perception
Apparent movement
Tactile accuracy
Ability to perceive size and shape
Spatial and time judgment

Modified from Ebersole P, Hess P: *Toward healthy aging: human needs and nursing response*, ed 5, St. Louis, 1998, Mosby.

control of excessive stimuli become an important part of the client's care.

Nursing Knowledge Base

FACTORS AFFECTING SENSORY FUNCTION

There are multiple factors that may affect an individual's sensory functioning. These factors relate to the quality and quantity of sensory stimuli. Other influences are family, environmental, and cultural factors that affect the client.

Persons at Risk.   A nurse assesses sensory function for clients most at risk. Older adults are a high-risk group because of normal physiological changes involving sensory organs. The nurse must be careful to not automatically assume that an older adult's hearing problem is related to advancing age. Adult sensorineural hearing loss can be due to metabolic, vascular, and other systemic lesions. A problem with age-related hearing loss is that some individuals who are affected may not even be aware of their deficit (Tolson, 1997). A client may benefit from a referral to an audiologist or otolaryngologist if the assessment reveals serious problems.

Meaningful Stimuli.   Meaningful stimuli reduce the incidence of sensory deprivation. In the home, meaningful stimuli include pets, a record player or television, pictures of family members, and a calendar and clock. The same types of items should be present in a nursing home. In a health care setting the nurse notes whether clients have roommates or visitors. The presence of others can offer positive stimulation. However, a roommate who constantly watches television, persistently tries to talk, or continuously keeps lights on can contribute to sensory overload. A client can become disoriented in a barren environment that gives few signals for normal sensory perception. The presence or absence of meaningful stimuli influences alertness and the ability to participate in care. In the home or health care setting the environment should

be decorated with bright colors and have comfortable furnishings, adequate lighting, good ventilation, and clean surroundings.

Amount of Stimuli.   Excessive stimuli in an environment can cause sensory overload. The frequency of observations and procedures performed in an acute care setting may be stressful. If the client is in pain, has many tubes and dressings, or is restricted by casts or traction, overstimulation can be a problem. A client's room may be near repetitive or loud noises (e.g., an elevator, stairwell, or nurses' station), which may contribute to sensory overload.

Family Factors.   The amount and quality of contact with supportive family members and significant others can influence the degree of isolation the client feels. Whether a client lives alone or whether family and friends frequently visit influences client reactions. The absence of visitors during hospitalization or residency in a nursing home or extended care facility can also affect sensory status. This is a common problem in hospital intensive care settings, where visitation is often restricted. A pattern of social isolation can contribute to sensory changes. The ability to discuss fears or concerns with loved ones is an important coping mechanism for most people. Therefore the absence of meaningful conversation can cause a person to become sensorially deprived, and the nurse may not be alerted until behavioral changes occur.

Clients with hearing loss tend to decrease time spent with social activities and with verbal communication (Resnick, Fries, and Verbrugge, 1997). Children with hearing deficits will be inattentive, uncooperative, or easily bored (Wong and others, 1999). Often a client becomes embarrassed by needing to continually ask another person to repeat what he or she has said. So instead, they initiate little communication. Clients who find their lifestyles influenced by a hearing loss experience loneliness and lowered self-esteem. Social difficulties caused by hearing loss further contribute to the feeling of loneliness.

It is important for the nurse to know the client's social skills and level of satisfaction with the support given by family and friends. Is the client satisfied with the support made available from friends? Is the client able to solve problems with family members? Does the family offer the support needed when the client requires assistance as a result of a sensory loss? The long-term effects of sensory alterations can influence family dynamics and a client's willingness to remain active in society.

Environmental Factors.

A person's occupation can place him or her at risk for visual, hearing, and peripheral nerve alterations (Box 48-4). Individuals who are exposed to loud noises at work or who have occupations involving risk of exposure to chemicals or flying objects should be screened for hearing and visual problems. Clients who use their hands in a repetitive fashion, causing trauma to the median nerve, can develop carpal tunnel syndrome. Carpal tunnel syndrome is one of the most common industrial or work-related injuries. Occupations that involve continuous wrist movement may cause the client to develop swelling or inflammation, which creates pressure on the nerve as it passes through the narrow area in the wrist. The client experiences numbness, tingling, pain, and weakness in the hand while performing fine hand movements (Ruda, 1999).

A hospitalized client can be at risk for sensory alterations due to exposure to environmental stimuli or a change in sensory input. Clients who are immobilized because of bed rest or physical encumbrances (e.g., casts or traction) are at risk, since they are unable to experience all of the normal sensations of free movement. Another group at risk includes clients isolated in a health care setting or at home. For example, the client placed in isolation because of tuberculosis (see Chapter 33) is often restricted to a hospital room and is unable to enjoy normal interactions with visitors. A hospital environment is full of sensory stimuli. Therapeutic isolation, the sounds of electrical monitors and equipment, bright lighting, and the odors of body fluids are just some examples. A healthy person can change an environment or seek a different one.

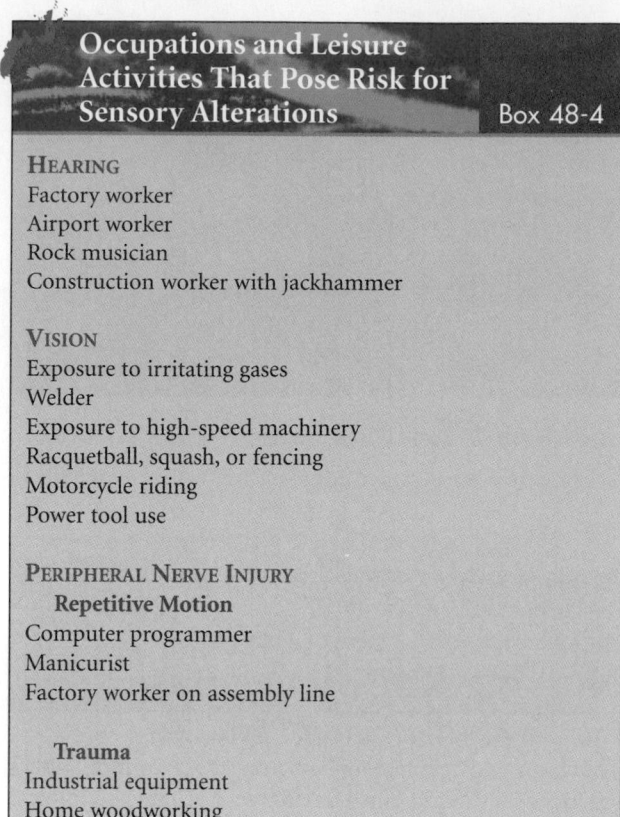

Occupations and Leisure Activities That Pose Risk for Sensory Alterations   Box 48-4

HEARING
Factory worker
Airport worker
Rock musician
Construction worker with jackhammer

VISION
Exposure to irritating gases
Welder
Exposure to high-speed machinery
Racquetball, squash, or fencing
Motorcycle riding
Power tool use

PERIPHERAL NERVE INJURY
  Repetitive Motion
Computer programmer
Manicurist
Factory worker on assembly line

  Trauma
Industrial equipment
Home woodworking

As a result of illness or hospitalization, a client is often confined to an unfamiliar and unresponsive environment. This does not mean that all hospitalized clients have sensory alterations. However, the nurse must assess more carefully those clients subjected to continued sensory stimulation (e.g., ICU settings, long-term hospitalization, multiple therapies). The environment can either minimize or heighten sensory alterations. In some cases the environment (e.g., ICU setting) is the cause of the problem. The nurse assesses the client's environment, both within the health care setting and the home, looking for factors that pose risks or that need adjustment to provide safety and more stimulation.

Hazards.

A client with sensory alterations is at risk for injury if the living environment is unsafe. For example, a client with visual impairment cannot see potential hazards clearly. A client with proprioceptive problems may lose balance easily. The condition of the home, the rooms, and the front and back entrances can be problematic to the client with sensory alterations. Some of the more common hazards include the following:

Uneven, cracked walkways leading to front/back door
Doormats with slippery backing
Extension and phone cords in the main route of walking traffic
Loose area rugs and runners placed over carpeting
Bathrooms without shower or tub grab bars

Water faucets unmarked to designate hot and cold

Bathroom floor with slippery surface

Absence of smoke detectors in rooms

Unlit stairways

Cluttered furniture, including footstools

Kitchen equipment (e.g., ovens, irons, toasters) with control knobs with hard-to-read settings

In the hospital environment, caregivers often forget to rearrange furniture and equipment to keep paths from the bed and chair to the bathroom and entrance clear. Walking into a client's room and looking for safety hazards can be a useful exercise:

Are intravenous (IV) poles on wheels and easy to move?

Are footstools in the middle of the room?

Are suction machines, IV pumps, or drainage bags positioned so that a client can rise from a bed or chair easily?

An additional problem faced by the visually impaired is the inability to read medication labels and syringe gauges. The nurse asks the client to read a label to determine if the client can read the dosage and frequency. If a client has a hearing impairment, the nurse checks to see whether the sounds of a doorbell, telephone, smoke alarm, and alarm clock are easy to discriminate.

Cultural Factors. The nurse needs to be aware of cultural and ethnic considerations that may contribute to hearing and visual problems. For example, the frequency and severity of glaucoma is higher in African-Americans as compared with Caucasians. Other statistics have shown that the incidence of hearing impairment is greater in Caucasians than in either African-Americans or Asian-Americans (Smith and Wilbur, 1999).

The client with sensory alterations expects that the nurse will assess for family, environmental, cultural, and other risk factors that might affect sensory functioning so as to plan for early intervention.

Critical Thinking Synthesis

Successful critical thinking requires a synthesis of knowledge, experience, information gathered from clients, critical thinking attitudes, and intellectual and professional standards. Clinical judgments require the nurse to anticipate the information necessary, analyze the data, and make decisions regarding client care. Critical thinking is always changing. During assessment (Figure 48-2) the nurse must consider all critical thinking elements that build toward making appropriate nursing diagnoses.

In the case of sensory alterations the nurse must integrate knowledge of the pathophysiology of sensory deficits, factors that affect sensory function, and therapeutic communication principles. This positions the nurse to be able to anticipate what to recognize when a client describes a sensory problem and to be able to then make a clinical judgment of any abnormalities. For example, knowing the normal symptoms of a cataract helps the nurse recognize the pattern of visual changes a client with a cataract will report.

The use of communication knowledge improves the nurse's ability to acquire a thorough nursing assessment. Previous experiences in caring for clients with sensory deficits enables the nurse to recognize limitations in function in each new client and how limitations might affect the client's ability to carry out daily activities. For example, after caring for a client with a hearing impairment, the nurse will be able to conduct a more effective assessment of the next client by using approaches that promote the client's ability to hear the nurse's questions.

Critical thinking attitudes and standards, when applied during assessment, ensure a thorough and accurate database from which to make decisions. For example, perseverance is needed to learn details as to how visual changes influence a client's ability to socialize. Standards of care and practice, such as those from the American Academy of Ophthalmology, provide criteria for screening sensory problems and for establishing standards for competent practice. Using critical thinking, the nurse can conduct a thorough assessment and then plan and implement care that will enable the client to function safely and effectively.

Nursing Process

ASSESSMENT

When assessing clients with or at risk for sensory alterations, it is important to consider any pathophysiology of existing deficits, as well as all of the factors influencing sensory function (see Box 48-1), to anticipate how to approach a given client's assessment. For example, if the client has a hearing disorder, the nurse will adjust his or her communication style and then focus the assessment on relevant criteria related to hearing deficits. The nurse collects a history that also assesses the client's current sensory status and the degree to which a sensory deficit affects the client's lifestyle, psychosocial adjustment, developmental status, self-care ability, and safety. The assessment must also focus on the quality and quantity of environmental stimuli.

Mental Status. Mental status assessment is an important component of any evaluation of sensory function (Box 48-5). Observation of the client during history taking, during the physical examination, and during care provides valuable data that can serve as the basis for evaluation of mental status. An assessment of mental status is valuable particularly if the nurse suspects sensory deprivation or overload. Observation of the client can provide data that reveal key client behaviors. The nurse will observe the client's physical appearance and behavior, measure cognitive ability, and assess the client's emotional status. The Mini-Mental Status Examination (MMSE) is an

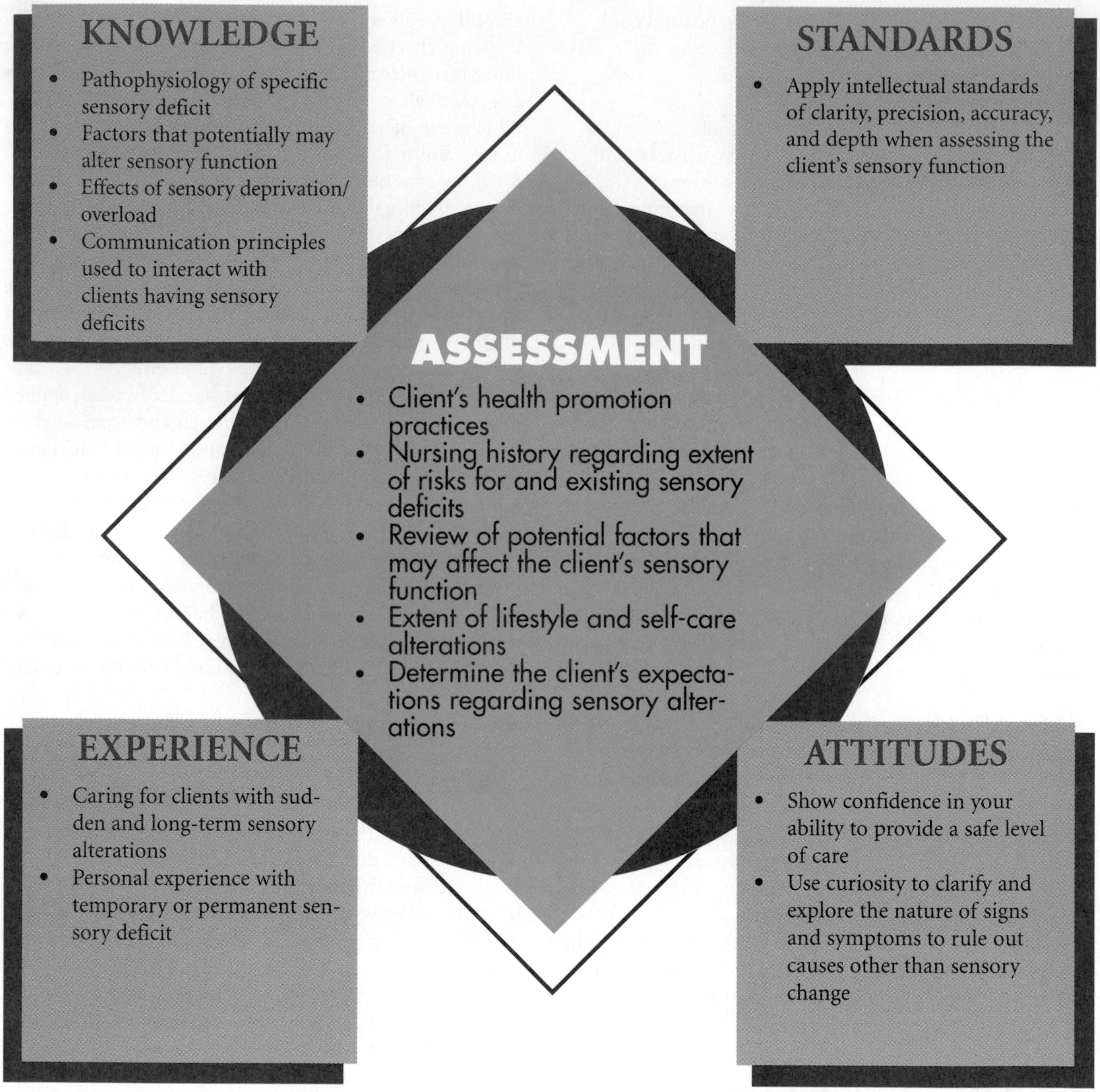

KNOWLEDGE

- Pathophysiology of specific sensory deficit
- Factors that potentially may alter sensory function
- Effects of sensory deprivation/ overload
- Communication principles used to interact with clients having sensory deficits

STANDARDS

- Apply intellectual standards of clarity, precision, accuracy, and depth when assessing the client's sensory function

ASSESSMENT

- Client's health promotion practices
- Nursing history regarding extent of risks for and existing sensory deficits
- Review of potential factors that may affect the client's sensory function
- Extent of lifestyle and self-care alterations
- Determine the client's expectations regarding sensory alterations

EXPERIENCE

- Caring for clients with sudden and long-term sensory alterations
- Personal experience with temporary or permanent sensory deficit

ATTITUDES

- Show confidence in your ability to provide a safe level of care
- Use curiosity to clarify and explore the nature of signs and symptoms to rule out causes other than sensory change

Figure 48-2   *Synthesis Model for Sensory Alterations Assessment Phase.*

example of a tool that can *formally* be used to measure disorientation, altered conceptualization and abstract thinking, and change in problem-solving abilities (see Chapter 32). For example, a client with severe sensory deprivation may not be able to carry on a conversation, remain attentive, or display recent or past memory.

Physical Assessment.   To identify sensory deficits and their severity, the nurse assesses vision, hearing, olfaction, taste, and the ability to discriminate light touch, temperature, pain, and position (see Chapter 32). Table 48-2

summarizes assessment techniques for identifying sensory deficits. In all examples the nurse will gather more accurate data if the examination room is private, quiet, and comfortable for the client.

The typical physical tests used to screen for hearing impairment rely on an examiner's whispered voice or a tuning fork. The Welch-Allyn audioscope is very effective for measuring hearing acuity. The handheld instrument includes an ear speculum that is placed within the external ear canal. The examiner can view the tympanic membrane to ensure that cerumen is not blocking the canal. A tonal

Assessment of Mental Status   Box 48-5

PHYSICAL APPEARANCE AND BEHAVIOR
Motor activity
Posture
Facial expression
Hygiene

COGNITIVE ABILITY
Level of consciousness
Abstract reasoning
Calculation
Attention
Judgment
Ability to carry on conversation
Ability to read, write, and copy figure
Recent and remote memory

EMOTIONAL STABILITY
Agitation, euphoria, irritability, hopelessness, or wide mood
    swings
Auditory, visual, or tactile hallucinations
Illusions
Delusions

Cultural ASPECTS OF CARE   Box 48-6

Caucasians have more hearing impairment problems than African-Americans and Asian-Americans.

Eskimos are more vulnerable to developing primary narrow-angle glaucoma, and it is more often seen in older adults and in women (Giger and Davidhizar, 1999).

The percentage and acuity of glaucoma is higher in African-Americans as compared with Caucasians.

The incidence of astigmatism is higher for both African-Americans and Native Americans than for Caucasians.

Otitis media is more prevalent among Native Americans than among Caucasians (Smith and Wilbur, 1999).

Jewish Americans have a greater incidence of myopia, and it is more prevalent in boys than in girls (Lewis, Collier, and Heitkemper, 1999).

sequence is initiated by pressing a button on the audioscope. The instrument is highly sensitive to detecting hearing loss.

Ability to Perform Self-Care. The nurse assesses clients' functional abilities in their home environment or health care setting, including feeding, dressing, grooming, and toileting activities. For example, the nurse assesses whether a client with altered vision can find items on a meal tray and can read directions on a prescription. The nurse also determines a visually impaired client's ability to perform daily routines such as reading bills and writing checks, differentiating money denominations, and driving a vehicle at night. If a client seems sensorially deprived, is concern shown for grooming? Does a client's loss of balance prevent rising from a toilet seat safely? Can the client with a stroke manipulate buttons or zippers for dressing? Any impairment in the ability to perform self-care has implications for planning discharge from a health care setting and in providing resources within the home.

Sensory Alterations History. The nursing history allows assessment of the nature and characteristics of sensory alterations or any problem related to an alteration. It is important to remember that many older adults are sensitive about admitting losses and may hesitate to share information (Ebersole and Hess, 1998). When taking the sensory alterations history, the nurse should consider the ethnic or cultural background of the client, since certain alterations are higher in some cultural groups (Box 48-6).

The nurse begins by asking the client to describe the sensory deficit. For example:
Describe your hearing loss for me.
Describe how your vision is affected.
Explain how use of your hands has changed.
Knowledge about the onset and duration of the sensory alteration can be helpful. The nurse begins to learn how long the client has taken measures to adjust to the alteration:
How long have you had a visual problem?
When did you begin to feel numbness in your legs?
How long have you noticed being unable to hear conversations clearly?
It is also useful to assess the client's self-rating for a sensory deficit. Lewis-Cullinan and Janken (1990) found that a client's self-rating for hearing was one of the most important defining characteristics for the nursing diagnosis of *sensory/perceptual alterations (auditory)*. The nurse can simply say, "Rate your hearing as either excellent, good, fair, poor, or bad." Then, based on the client's self-rating, the nurse may explore more fully the client's perception of a sensory loss. This provides a more in-depth look at how the client's quality of life has been influenced. In the specific case of hearing problems, a screening tool developed by Ventry and Weinstein (1986) has been found to be effective in identifying clients needing audiological intervention. The screening version of the Hearing Handicap Inventory for the Elderly (HHIE-S) is a 5-minute, 10-item questionnaire (Figure 48-3) designed to assess how a client perceives the emotional and social effects of hearing loss (Weinstein, 1994).

A nursing history can also reveal any recent changes in a client's behavior. Frequently friends or family are the best resources for this information, since the client may be unaware of any change:
Has the client shown any recent mood swings (e.g., outbursts of anger, nervousness, fear, or irritability)?
Have you noticed the client avoiding social activities?

Table 48-2   Assessment of Sensory Function

Assessment	Behavior Indicating Deficit (Children)	Behavior Indicating Deficit (Adults)
Vision Ask client to read newspaper, magazine, or lettering on menu. Measure visual acuity with Snellen chart (see Chapter 32). Assess visual fields and depth perception. Assess pupil size and accommodation to light. Ask client to identify colors on color chart or crayons.	Self-stimulation, including eye rubbing, body rocking, sniffing or smelling, arm twirling; hitching (using legs to propel while in sitting position) instead of crawling	Poor coordination, squinting, underreaching or overreaching for objects, persistent repositioning of objects, impaired night vision, accidental falls
Hearing Perform conventional assessment, including ticking watch, whisper, and tuning fork (see Chapter 32). Perform audiometry. Observe client conversing with others. Compare client's ability to recognize consonants with ability to distinguish vowels. Assess client's perception of hearing ability and history of tinnitus. Inspect ear canal for hardened cerumen.	Frightened when unfamiliar people approach, no reflex or purposeful response to sounds, failure to be awakened by loud noise, slow or absent development of speech, greater response to movement than to sound, avoidance of social interaction with other children	Blank looks, decreased attention span, lack of reaction to loud noises, increased volume of speech, positioning of head toward sound, smiling and nodding of head in approval when someone speaks, use of other means of communication such as lipreading or writing, complaints of ringing in ears
Touch Assess client for sensitivity to light touch and temperature (see Chapter 32). Check client's ability to discriminate between sharp and full stimuli. Assess whether client can distinguish objects (coin or safety pin) in the hand with eyes closed. Ask whether client feels unusual sensations.	Inability to perform developmental tasks related to grasping objects or drawing, repeated injury from handling of harmful objects (e.g., hot stove, sharp knife)	Clumsiness, overreaction or underreaction to painful stimulus, failure to respond when touched, avoidance of touch, sensation of pins and needles, numbness
Smell Have client close eyes and identify several nonirritating odors (e.g., coffee, vanilla).	Difficult to assess until child is 6 or 7 years old, difficulty discriminating noxious odors	Failure to react to noxious or strong odor, increased body odor, increased sensitivity to odors
Taste Ask client to sample and distinguish different tastes (e.g., lemon, sugar, salt). (Have client drink or sip water and wait 1 minute between each taste.) Ask client if recent weight change has occurred.	Inability to tell whether food is salty or sweet, possible ingestion of strange-tasting things	Change in appetite, excessive use of seasoning and sugar, complaints about taste of food, weight change
Position Sense Perform conventional tests for balance and position sense (see Chapter 32).	Clumsiness, extraneous movement, excessive arm swinging in those with hyperactivity or learning difficulty	Poor balance and spatial orientation, shuffling gait, reduced response to brace self when falling, more precise and deliberate movements

---

Screening version of the Hearing Handicap Inventory for the Elderly (HHIE-S)

ITEM		YES (4 pts)	NO (0 pts)	SOMETIMES (2 pts)
E-1	Does a hearing problem cause you to feel embarrassed when you meet new people?	_____	_____	_____
E-2	Does a hearing problem cause you to feel frustrated when talking to members of your family?	_____	_____	_____
S-3	Do you have difficulting hearing when someone speaks in a whisper?	_____	_____	_____
E-4	Do you feel handicapped by a hearing problem?	_____	_____	_____
S-5	Does a hearing problem cause you difficulty when visiting friends, relatives, or neighbors?	_____	_____	_____
S-6	Does a hearing problem cause you to attend religious services less often than you would like?	_____	_____	_____
E-7	Does a hearing problem cause you to have arguments with family members?	_____	_____	_____
S-8	Does a hearing problem cause you difficulty when listening to TV or radio?	_____	_____	_____
E-9	Do you feel that any difficulty with your hearing limits or hampers your personal or social life?	_____	_____	_____
S-10	Does a hearing problem cause you difficulty when in a restaurant with relatives or friends?	_____	_____	_____

RAW SCORE _____ (sum of the points assigned each of the Items)

INTERPRETING THE RAW SCORE
0 to 8 = 13% probability of hearing impairment (no handicap/no referral)
10 to 24 = 50% probability of hearing impairment (mild moderate handicap)
26 to 40 = 84% probability of hearing impairment (severe handicap)

E = Emotional items
S = Social/situational items

Figure 48-3   Screening version of the Hearing Handicap Inventory for the Elderly (HHIE-S). Redrawn from Ventry I, Weinstein B: The hearing handicap inventory for the elderly: a new tool, *Ear Hearing* 3:133, 1986.

Health Promotion Habits. It is important for the nurse to assess the daily routines clients follow to maintain sensory function. What type of eye and ear care is incorporated into daily hygiene? For those individuals who participate in sports (e.g., racquetball) or recreational activities (e.g., motorcycle riding), or who work in a setting where ear or eye injury is a possibility (e.g., chemical exposure, welding, glass or stone polishing, or constant exposure to loud noise), the nurse determines if safety glasses or hearing protective devices (HPDs) are worn. Do clients who use assistive devices such as eyeglasses, contact lenses, or hearing aids know how to provide daily care (see Chapter 38)? Are the devices in proper working order?

The nurse also assesses the client's compliance with routine health screening. When was the last time the client had an eye examination or hearing evaluation? Recommended screening guidelines are usually structured on the basis of age. When a client begins to show a hearing

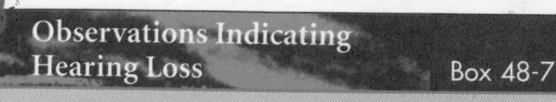

Observations Indicating Hearing Loss   Box 48-7

Client seems inattentive to others.
Client responds with inappropriate anger when spoken to.
Client believes people are talking about him or her.
Client has trouble following clear directions.
Client asks to have something repeated.
Client has monotonous or unusual voice quality and speaks unusually loud or soft.
Client has TV unusually loud.

Modified from Ebersole P, Hess P: *Toward healthy aging: human needs and nursing response,* ed 5, St. Louis, 1998, Mosby.

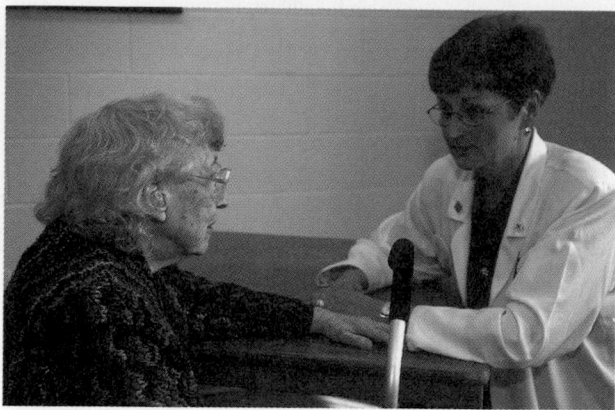

Figure 48-4   Nurse sits at eye level so that client with hearing impairment can communicate.

deficit, routine screening should be incorporated in regular examinations.

• • •

Finally, the nurse must often rely on personal observation of the client to detect sensory alterations. Ebersole and Hess (1998) have identified some typical observations indicating hearing loss (Box 48-7).

Communication Methods.   Clients with existing sensory deficits often develop alternative ways of communicating. To interact with the client and to promote interaction with others (Figure 48-4), the nurse must understand the client's method of communication. A deaf or hearing-impaired client may read lips, use sign language, listen with the help of a hearing aid, or read and write notes. Vision becomes almost a primary sense for the hearing impaired.

Visually impaired clients are unable to observe facial expressions and other nonverbal behaviors that clarify the content of spoken communication. Instead, they rely on voice tones and inflections to detect the emotional tone of communication. Clients with visual deficits often learn to read Braille.

Clients with **aphasia** may be unable to produce or understand language. **Expressive aphasia,** a motor type of aphasia, is the inability to name common objects or to express simple ideas in words or writing. For example, a client may understand a question but be unable to express an answer. Sensory or **receptive aphasia** is the inability to understand written or spoken language. The client may be able to express words but is unable to understand questions or comments of others. Global aphasia is the inability to understand language or communicate orally.

The temporary or permanent loss of the ability to speak is extremely traumatic to an individual. The nurse assesses a client's alternative communication method and whether it causes anxiety in the client. Clients who have undergone laryngectomies often write notes, use communication boards, speak with mechanical vibrators, or use esophageal speech. Clients with endotracheal or tra-

cheostomy tubes have a temporary loss of speech. Most use a notepad to write their questions and requests. However, the client may become incapacitated and unable to write messages. The nurse needs to determine whether the client has developed a sign language or system of symbols to communicate needs.

To understand the nature of a communication problem, the nurse must know whether a client has trouble speaking, understanding, naming, reading, or writing. Depending on the nature of the problem, the nurse selects the best way to interact with the client.

Other Factors Affecting Perception.   The nurse should remember that factors other than sensory deprivation or overload may cause impaired perception (e.g., medications, pain, and reduced oxygenation). The nurse assesses the client's medication history, which includes prescribed and over-the-counter medications. This history includes gaining information regarding the frequency, dose, method of administration, and last time these medications were taken. The nurse should also assess the use of caffeine and other remedies or assistive devices (e.g., use of a hearing aid) and the sensory effects for the client. When the nurse identifies that the client has a hearing aid, it is also important to remember that just because the individual has the assistive device, it does not mean that it works or that the client uses it or benefits from it (Tolson, 1997).

Client Expectations.   Clients depend on their senses to provide them with information so as to respond or react to a specific situation or problem. Therefore clients expect caregivers to recognize and appropriately manage and adjust the client's environment to meet their sensory needs. This would include assisting the individual client in learning and adapting to a changed lifestyle based on the specific sensory impairment. The nurse should determine from the client exactly what the client expects to achieve

SAMPLE NURSING DIAGNOSTIC PROCESS

Box 48-8

SENSORY ALTERATIONS

Assessment Activities	Defining Characteristics	Nursing Diagnosis
Assess client's visual acuity.	Has reduced ability to see objects clearly. Needs brighter light to read. Has trouble distinguishing edges of stairs.	Risk for injury related to visual impairment from cataract formation
Visit home setting and inspect for any hazards that may pose risks to client.	Lighting in rooms, hallways, and stairwells is very dim. Carpet in living room is old, and edges are curled up. Steps lead up to front entrance of home.	
Review medical record from clinic visit.	Client has been diagnosed as having senile cataracts in both eyes.	

NURSING DIAGNOSES   Box 48-9

SENSORY ALTERATIONS

Adjustment, impaired
Communication, impaired verbal
Injury, risk for
Mobility, impaired physical
Self-care deficit, bathing/hygiene
Self-care deficit, dressing/grooming
Self-care deficit, toileting
Self-esteem disturbance
Sensory/perceptual alterations (visual, auditory, kinesthetic, gustatory)
Social isolation
Thought processes, altered

and what interventions have been helpful in the past in the management of the client's limitation. The nurse should remember that clients with sensory alterations have strengthened their other senses and expect the caregivers to anticipate their needs (e.g., for safety and security).

NURSING DIAGNOSIS

After assessment, the nurse reviews all available data and critically looks for patterns and trends suggestive of a health problem relating to sensory alterations (Box 48-8). For example, a client's advanced age, apathy, inattentiveness during conversations, and self-rating of hearing as "poor" are all defining characteristics for the nursing diagnosis of *sensory/perceptual alterations (auditory)* (Lewis-Cullinan and Janken, 1990). The nurse validates findings to ensure accuracy of the diagnosis. For example, the diagnosis of *altered thought processes* could mistakenly be made if the nurse does not confirm the client's hearing deficit and perception of poor hearing.

The nurse determines the factor that likely causes the client's health problem. In the previous example impacted cerumen is the etiology for the client's hearing alteration. The etiology, or related factor, of a nursing diagnosis is a condition that can be affected by nursing interventions. The etiology must be accurate; otherwise, nursing therapies will be ineffective. For a client with impacted cerumen, regular irrigations of the ear canal have the potential for improving auditory perception (Wong and others, 1999). In contrast, if the client's auditory alteration was related to hearing loss from nerve deafness, nursing interventions for alternative communication methods would be necessary.

The client may also have health care problems for which sensory alteration is the etiology, such as with the diagnosis of *risk for injury*. The nurse may also select nursing diagnoses by recognizing the way that sensory alterations will affect a client's ability to function (e.g., self-care deficit). The nurse must recognize patterns of data that reveal health problems created by the client's sensory alteration (Box 48-9).

PLANNING

During planning the nurse again synthesizes information from multiple resources (Figure 48-5). The nurse reflects on knowledge gained from the assessment and knowledge of how sensory deficits affect normal functioning. In this way the nurse can recognize the extent of the client's deficit and know the type of interventions most likely to be helpful. The nurse also considers the role that health professionals can play in planning care and the available community resources that may be useful. The nurse's previous experience in caring for clients with sensory alterations can be invaluable. Caring for a client, for example, with a visual loss should assist the nurse in knowing how to plan nursing approaches that ensure the client's safety while maximizing the client's independence.

Critical thinking ensures that the client's plan of care

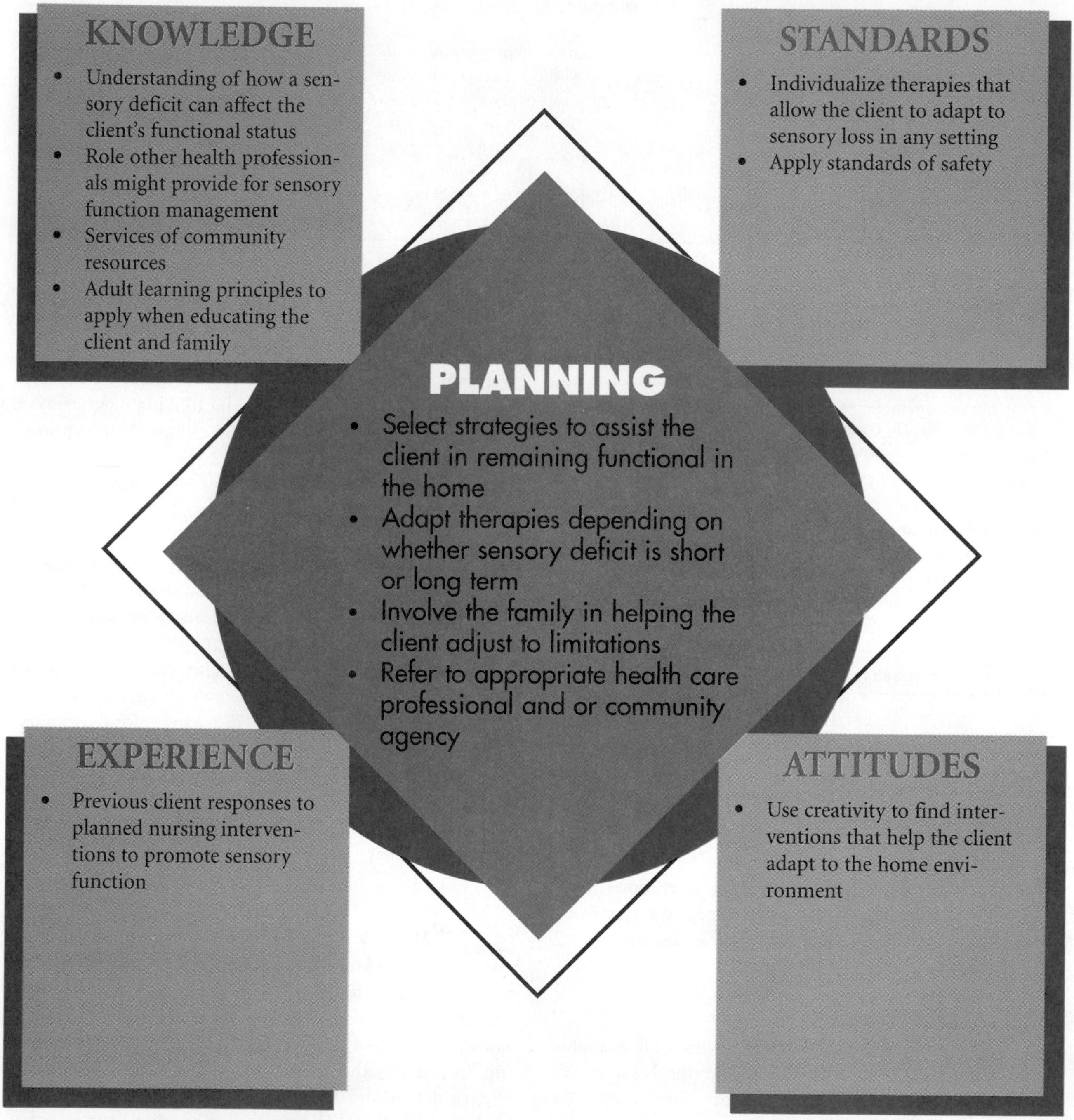

KNOWLEDGE

- Understanding of how a sensory deficit can affect the client's functional status
- Role other health professionals might provide for sensory function management
- Services of community resources
- Adult learning principles to apply when educating the client and family

STANDARDS

- Individualize therapies that allow the client to adapt to sensory loss in any setting
- Apply standards of safety

PLANNING

- Select strategies to assist the client in remaining functional in the home
- Adapt therapies depending on whether sensory deficit is short or long term
- Involve the family in helping the client adjust to limitations
- Refer to appropriate health care professional and or community agency

EXPERIENCE

- Previous client responses to planned nursing interventions to promote sensory function

ATTITUDES

- Use creativity to find interventions that help the client adapt to the home environment

Figure 48-5   *Synthesis Model for Sensory Alterations Planning Phase.*

integrates all that the nurse knows about the individual, as well as information applied through the critical thinking elements. Professional standards are especially important to apply when the nurse develops the plan of care. These standards, in the form of clinical pathways (see Chapter 2) or evidenced-based treatment protocols, often recommend scientifically proven interventions for the client's condition. For example, clients who have visual deficits

and are hospitalized may be placed on a fall prevention protocol that will incorporate research-based precautions to ensure client safety.

The nurse develops an individualized plan of care for each nursing diagnosis (see care plan). The nurse and client partner in setting realistic expectations for care. Goals are to be individualized and realistic with measurable outcomes.

SAMPLE NURSING CARE PLAN

SENSORY/PERCEPTUAL ALTERATIONS

ASSESSMENT*
Judy Long, a 70-year-old receptionist for a college dormitory, complains to the community health nurse that lately it seems that a **film** has formed over her **left eye, making her vision blurred.** She notices that in some lighting there is a **glare.** She comments that she is having **increasing difficulty seeing to drive.** Specifically, she **cannot tolerate driving at night**—the oncoming **headlights are blurred.** Judy has had her neighbor drive her places, but this makes her feel as though **she is losing her independence. She reports that she has always worked and managed her home, and has volunteered at a local library.** She indicates that since this problem with her vision, she has been **reluctant to use the stairs in her home.** Judy visited an opthamologist, who told her **she has a cataract,** and she is scheduled for **surgery in 3 weeks.**
*Defining characteristics are shown in bold type.

NURSING DIAGNOSIS: Sensory/perceptual alterations (visual) related to altered sensory reception of senile cataract.

PLANNING
GOALS
Client will maintain independence in a safe home environment.

Client will continue to seek alternate transportation until eye condition has been corrected.

EXPECTED OUTCOMES
Client will verbalize changes made to protect and maintain visual acuity for indoor and outdoor activities in 1 week. A safety check of the client's home will show up safety hazards in 1 week.
Client will explain plans for alternate transportation to work and social activities.

INTERVENTIONS†
Environmental Management
- Instruct client to keep walking area in home and work area free of clutter, footstools, and electric cords, and to avoid rearranging furniture.
- Instruct client to reduce glare by wearing dark-colored sunglasses for outside and light-colored glasses for inside.
- Teach client to use a light over the shoulder for reading and writing.

Emotional Support
- Encourage client to express feelings regarding loss of vision and lifestyle changes.

Family Involvement
- Confer with client on selecting a family member, friend, or community resource who can provide them with transportation until after the eye condition has been corrected.

RATIONALE

Keeping the area clutter free reduces the risk of injury, and these measures help promote a safe environment (Beaver and Mann, 1995).
Clients have better visual acuity when they protect their eyes from bright light (Cleary, 1995).
People with cataracts see better with wider illumination (Cleary, 1995).

People who experience visual loss grieve over loss of independence (Vader, 1992).

An alternate means of transportation will foster safety (Beaver and Mann, 1995).

†Intervention Classification labels from McCloskey JC, Bulechek GM: *Nursing interventions classification (NIC),* ed 3, St. Louis, 2000, Mosby.

EVALUATION
Ask client to describe the changes that have made the home environment safer. During a home visit, observe the home environment for safety hazards.
Observe client's verbal and nonverbal responses to the lifestyle adaptations.
Ask if client is able to maintain a degree of independence with the environmental and lifestyle modifications.
Ask client to identify source of transportation.

Priorities of care must be set with regard to the extent that a sensory alteration affects a client. Safety is a top priority. The client can also help prioritize aspects of care. For example, the client may wish to learn ways to communicate more effectively or to participate in favorite hobbies given his or her limitation.

Some sensory alterations are short term (e.g., a client suffering sensory/perceptual alterations as a result of sensory overload in an ICU). Appropriate interventions are thus likely to be temporary (e.g., frequent reorientation or introduction of intimate and pleasant stimuli such as a back rub). Sensory alterations such as permanent visual loss require long-term goals of care for clients to adapt. However, clients who have sensory alterations at the time of entering a health care setting are usually most informed about how to adapt interventions to their lifestyles. The blind in particular need to control whatever part of their care they can. Sometimes it becomes necessary for the client to make major changes in self-care activities, communication, and socialization.

When developing a plan of care, the nurse considers all resources available to clients. The family can play a key role in providing meaningful stimulation and learning ways to help the client adjust to any limitations. The nurse may also refer the client to other health care professionals. Early referrals to occupational or speech therapists, for example, can speed a client's recovery. There are also numerous community-based resources (e.g., local chapter of the Society for the Blind and Visually Impaired, Area on Aging, and the National Council on Independent Living Programs). The nurse may be able to arrange a volunteer to visit a client or have printed materials made available that describe ways to cope with sensory problems.

The goals of care for a client with actual or potential sensory alterations may include the following:

The client maintains current functioning of existing senses.

The client's environment contains meaningful sensory stimuli.

The client interacts in a safe environment.

The client experiences no additional sensory loss.

The client communicates effectively with existing sensory alterations.

The client is able to perform self-care.

The client engages in regular social activities.

The client understands the nature and implications of sensory loss.

IMPLEMENTATION

Nursing interventions involve the client and family so that a safe, pleasant, and stimulating sensory environment can be maintained. The most effective interventions enable the client with sensory alterations to function safely with existing deficits. The client generally is able to continue a normal lifestyle. Learning to adjust to sensory

impairments can occur at an early age. However, every person begins to develop sensory changes as he or she ages. Nursing interventions are chosen depending on the nursing diagnosis identified and the related factors contributing to the client's problem. There are measures to take to maintain sensory function at the highest level possible. This ensures a stimulating environment for the client and an improved level of health.

Health Promotion.   Good sensory function begins with prevention. Almost everyone becomes exposed to risks in the environment that may cause sensory alterations. When clients enter primary care settings, the nurse can take the opportunity to review commonsense approaches for reducing risk of sensory loss.

Screening.   The prevention of visual impairment in children requires appropriate screening (Wong and others, 1999). There are three recommended interventions: (1) screening for rubella or syphilis in women who are considering pregnancy; (2) adequate prenatal care to prevent premature birth (with the danger of exposure of the infant to excessive oxygen); and (3) periodic screening of all children, especially newborns through preschoolers, for congenital blindness and visual impairment caused by refractive errors and **strabismus.**

Visual impairments are common during childhood. The most common visual problem is a **refractive error** such as nearsightedness. The nurse's role is one of detection and referral. Parents must know signs suggesting visual impairment (e.g., failure to react to light and reduced eye contact from the infant). These signs should be reported to a physician immediately. Vision screening of school-age children and adolescents can detect problems early. The school nurse is usually responsible for vision testing.

Hearing impairment is one of the most common disabilities in the United States. It is estimated that over 28 million Americans have a hearing, speech, or language impairment (Smith and Wilbur, 1999). Children at risk include those with a family history of childhood hearing impairment, perinatal infection (rubella, herpes, cytomegalovirus), low birth weight, chronic ear infection, and Down syndrome. Nurses should advise pregnant women of the importance of early prenatal care, avoidance of ototoxic drugs, and testing for syphilis or rubella.

Children with chronic middle ear infections, a common cause of impaired hearing, should receive periodic auditory testing. Parents must be warned of the risks and should seek medical care when the child has symptoms of earache or respiratory infection.

Hearing loss from noise-induced environments was once thought to affect primarily older individuals, however, this is now being observed in 20- to 30-year-olds. This loss is attributed to exposure to noise at constantly high levels, such as from portable music devices, automobile music systems, concerts, and aerobic classes. School nurses should participate in providing hearing conservation classes for teachers and students alike (Lukes and Johnson, 1998).

For adults, routine screening of visual and hearing function is imperative to detect problems early. This is especially true in the case of glaucoma, which if undetected can lead to permanent visual loss. In the United States, glaucoma is the second leading cause of blindness in the general population and the primary cause of blindness in African-Americans. It is important to recommend that clients between the ages of 40 and 64 have an eye examination every 2 to 4 years. Examinations should occur every 1 to 2 years if there is a family history of glaucoma or if the client is of African ancestry, has had a serious eye injury in the past, is taking steroid medications, or is over 65 years of age (Smith and Wilbur, 1999).

The guidelines for hearing screening for adults are less prescriptive. Generally, if a client works or lives in an environment where there is a high noise level, routine screening is highly recommended. Nurses in occupational settings can assess for symptoms of tinnitus and make prompt referrals. Early detection may prevent hearing disabilities in millions of individuals (Griest and Bishop, 1998). The most important thing for adults to understand is to not accept hearing loss as a natural part of aging. Once hearing loss becomes acknowledged by a client, it is important to have regular hearing testing. Nurses should encourage older adults to follow through with recommendations for hearing aids.

Preventive Safety.   Trauma is a common cause of blindness in children. Penetrating injury from propulsive objects such as firecrackers, slingshots, or rocks, or from penetrating wounds from sticks, scissors, or toy weapons are just a few examples. Parents and children require counseling on ways to avoid eye trauma (Box 48-10). Safety equipment can easily be found in most sports shops and large department stores.

Adults are at risk for eye injury while playing sports and working in jobs involving exposure to chemicals or flying objects. The Occupational Safety and Health Administration has guidelines for safety in the workplace. Employers are required to have employees wear eye goggles and/or use equipment such as HPDs to reduce the risk of injury. Nurses in occupational health settings can reinforce use of protective devices (Box 48-11).

Tips for Preventing Eye Injury in Children   Box 48-10

INFANTS AND TODDLERS
Avoid toys with long, pointed handles or projections.
Do not allow child to walk or run with pointed object in hand.
Keep pointed instruments and tools out of reach.

PRESCHOOLERS
Supervise use of sharp or pointed objects such as scissors.
Teach child to walk carefully when carrying pointed objects.
Keep child away from projectile activities.
Begin to teach respect for firearms and fireworks.

SCHOOL-AGE CHILDREN AND ADOLESCENTS
Teach proper use of potentially dangerous equipment such as power tools, fireworks, and sports equipment (hockey sticks).
Stress use of eye protection when playing ball and racquet sports, shooting, using power tools, or riding motorcycles.
Warn children not to look directly at the sun even when wearing sunglasses.
Be sure corrective lenses are made of safety glass, which is shatterproof.

Research HIGHLIGHT   Box 48-11

RESEARCH ABSTRACT

Noise-induced hearing loss (NIHL) is a consequence of exposure to constant high noise levels. Approximately 30 million workers are in occupational environments with noise levels that are potentially harmful to hearing. Two hundred fifty-five noise-exposed and 195 non-noise-exposed male subjects working at a large metropolitan airport were studied. The subjects responded to an occupational hearing questionnaire and participated in a hearing evaluation. The researchers recorded the noise levels of the work areas. The subjects in the noise group experienced tinnitus as the main symptom, as well as headache and fullness in the ears. The individuals who also experienced low-frequency hearing loss reported having difficulty understanding speech. The results showed that those who consistently wore hearing protective devices (HPDs) had significantly lower occurrences of hearing loss than those who used them infrequently or not at all.

IMPLICATIONS FOR PRACTICE
- Assess clients who work in environments with high noise levels for symptoms of tinnitus and encourage audiometric testing.
- Control background noise when interacting with the hearing impaired.
- Teach varied age-groups (especially school-age children) the danger of permanent ear damage from high noise levels.
- Teach clients the value of HPDs to prevent hearing loss.
- Teach at schools, at outreach programs, and at work settings with high noise levels the impact of high noise levels on hearing.
- Refer clients with suspected hearing impairment to a hearing clinic or to an audiologist for testing.

REFERENCE
Hong OS, Chen SC, Conrad KM: Noise induced hearing loss among male airport workers in Korea, *Am Assoc Occup Health Nurs J* 46(2):67, 1998.

Preventing hearing loss requires individuals to avoid exposure to continuous high noise levels and brief loud impulse noise. HPDs should be worn by clients who must work around noise. Earplugs and earphones are useful in blocking high-decibel sounds.

Another means of prevention involves regular immunization of children against diseases capable of causing hearing loss (e.g., rubella, mumps, and measles). Nurses who work in physicians' offices, schools, and community clinics should reinforce the importance of early and timely immunization. When a child or an adult develops any type of health problem, caution should be used in prescribing drugs that are ototoxic.

Use of Assistive Devices.   Health promotion requires appropriate use of assistive aids and good, routine hygiene measures. A client who wears corrective contact lenses, eyeglasses, or hearing aids should make sure they are kept clean, accessible, and functional (see Chapter 38). It is helpful to have a family member or friend also know how to clean an assistive aid (Box 48-12).

It is critical for contact lens wearers to frequently clean lenses (see Chapter 38) and to use the appropriate solutions for cleaning and disinfection. With the rise in use of soft contact lenses, particularly extended-wear lenses, some clients have become casual with regard to both the care and wearing time of the contacts; as a result, there has been an increase in serious corneal infections. Infrequent lens disinfection, contamination of lens storage cases and contact lens solutions, and use of homemade saline adds to a client's risk. Swimming while wearing lenses also creates a serious risk of infection.

Wearing a hearing aid no longer has to be a social stigma. There are a wide variety of aids that not only successfully enhance a person's hearing, but can also be cosmetically acceptable. Chapter 38 summarizes the types of hearing aids available and tips for proper care and use.

Smith and Wilbur (1999) identify factors that determine a person's likelihood for wearing a hearing aid: perceived need for improved hearing, attitude toward the hearing problem, and motivation to seek solutions. Acknowledging a need to improve hearing is a person's first step. The nurse can give clients useful information on the benefits of wearing a hearing aid. It is also important to have a significant other available to assist with hearing aid adjustment. Federal regulations require medical clearance from a physician before a person can be fitted with a hearing aid (Ebersole and Hess, 1998). If a client has any of the following ear conditions, a hearing aid cannot be used: visible congenital or traumatic deformity of the ear, active drainage in the last 90 days, sudden or progressive hearing loss within the last 90 days, acute or chronic dizziness, unilateral sudden hearing loss within the last 90 days, visible cerumen accumulation or a foreign body in the ear canal, pain or discomfort in the ear, or an audiometric air-bone gap of 15 decibels or greater. The nurse can detect the first seven conditions on physical examination and should refer the client to an **otolaryngologist** for further counseling (Ebersole and Hess, 1998).

Promoting Meaningful Stimulation.   Life becomes much more enriching and satisfying when meaningful and pleasant stimuli exist within the environment. There are many ways that the nurse can help clients make adjustments to their environment so that it becomes more stimulating. This is best done when the nurse considers the normal physiological changes that accompany sensory deficits.

Vision.   As a result of the normal changes of aging, the pupil's ability to adjust to light is diminished. As a result, older adults can be very sensitive to glare. The nurse can suggest ways for the client to minimize glare by selecting satin and nongloss finishes for walls and countertops in the home and choosing sheer curtains, tinted windows, or adjustable shades to reduce outdoor light. Wearing sunglasses outside obviously can reduce the glare of direct sunlight.

The ability to read is important to everyone. Therefore clients should be allowed to use their glasses whenever

---

Client Teaching FOR TROUBLESHOOTING HEARING AID MALFUNCTION   Box 48-12

OBJECTIVES
- Family member will identify source of malfunction in hearing aid.
- Family member will demonstrate hearing aid care.

TEACHING STRATEGIES
- Show family member locations on hearing aid device where damage (e.g., cracks, fraying) is likely to occur: ear mold or case, earphone, dials, cord, and connection plugs.
- Demonstrate battery replacement: match + on battery to + on compartment. Have extra set of unused batteries available.

- Review method to check volume: turn dial to maximum gain to check. Is voice clear?
- Consult manufacturer's directions for specific care measures for cleaning battery case and ear mold.
- Review factors to report to hearing aid laboratory: static, distortion of sound, poor volume quality.

EVALUATION
- Have family member describe types of common malfunctions with hearing aid.
- Have family demonstrate battery removal and cleaning.

possible (e.g., during procedures and client instruction); it helps clients to remain oriented, maintain some control, and retain their dignity (Larsen, Hazen, and Hootmartin, 1997). Clients with reduced visual acuity may need more than corrective lenses. A pocket magnifier can help a client read most printed material. Telescopic lens eyeglasses are smaller, easier to focus, and have a greater range. Learning to adjust to sensory impairments can occur at an early age. However, every person begins to develop sensory changes as he or she ages. There are measures to take to maintain sensory function at the highest level possible. This ensures a stimulating environment for the client and an improved level of health. (Figure 48-6). There are also books and other publications available in larger print. If a client has a legal or other important document he or she wishes to read, standard copying machines have enlarging capabilities. There are now closed-circuit television magnifying units that enlarge written characters up to 45 times (Ebersole and Hess, 1998).

With aging, a person experiences a change in color perception. Perception of the colors blue, violet, and green usually declines. Brighter colors such as red, orange, and yellow are easier to see. The nurse can offer suggestions of ways the client may decorate a room and paint hallways or stairwells so that differentiations can be made in surfaces and objects in a room.

Hearing. One way to help an older adult with a hearing loss is to ensure that the problem is not impacted cerumen. With aging, cerumen thickens and builds up in the ear canal. Excessive cerumen occluding the ear canal can cause a **conductive hearing loss.** Irrigation of the canal with tepid water in a 60-ml syringe (see Chapter 38) will remove cerumen. Removal of cerumen can significantly improve the client's hearing ability. Lewis-Cullinan and Janken (1990) conducted a study involving 226 older adults. They found improvement in the hearing test scores in 75% of the subjects after cerumen removal.

To maximize residual hearing function, the nurse suggests ways to modify the environment. Telephones and televisions can be amplified. Alarm clocks that shake the bed or activate a flashing light are useful adaptive devices. An innovative way to enrich the lives of the hearing impaired is recorded music. Music recorded in the low-frequency sound cycles can be heard by clients with severe hearing loss.

Taste and Smell. The nurse can easily promote the sense of taste by using measures to enhance remaining taste perception. Good oral hygiene keeps the taste buds well hydrated. Taste perception is heightened if foods are well seasoned, differently textured, and eaten separately. Vinegar or lemon juice can add tartness to food. The nurse should always ask the client what foods are the most taste appealing. If taste perception is improved, food intake and appetite will also improve.

Stimulation of the sense of smell with aromas such as brewing coffee and baking bread can heighten taste sensation. The client should avoid blending or mixing foods, because these actions make it difficult to identify tastes. Older persons should chew food thoroughly to allow more food to contact remaining taste buds.

Smell can be improved by strengthening pleasant olfactory stimulation. A client's environment can be made more pleasant with smells such as cologne, mild room deodorizers, fragrant flowers, and sachets. The nurse also encourages clients to sniff food before eating. When the nurse assists clients with eating or sets up a meal tray in a health care setting, naming the foods may help clients imagine the aromas. The client is again an important resource. Certain aromas may actually cause clients to lose their appetites.

Removal of unpleasant odors improves the quality of a person's environment. The nurse should keep a client's room clean, empty bedpans or urinals, remove and dispose of soiled dressings, and keep bathroom doors closed.

Touch. Clients with reduced tactile sensation usually have the impairment over a limited portion of their bodies. The nurse can stimulate existing function by providing touch therapy. If the client is willing to be touched, hair brushing and combing, a back rub, and touching of the arms or shoulders are ways of increasing tactile contact. When sensation is reduced, a firm pressure may be necessary for the client to feel the nurse's hand. Turning and repositioning can also improve the quality of tactile sensation. When invasive procedures are being performed, it is important to use touch, hold clients hands, and keep them warm and dry.

If a client is overly sensitive to tactile stimuli (**hyperesthesia**), the nurse must minimize irritating stimuli. Keeping bed linens loose to minimize direct contact with the client and protecting the skin from exposure to irritants are helpful measures. If the client has numbness and

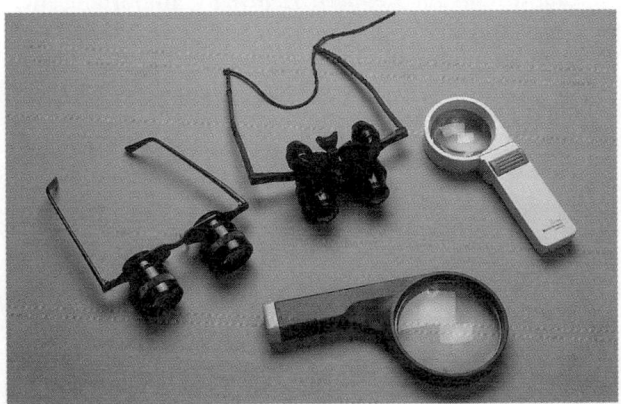

Figure 48-6 A variety of telescopic lenses aid the visually impaired.

tingling or pain in the hands, as with carpal tunnel syndrome, special wrist splints may be worn to dorsiflex the wrist to relieve the nerve pressure. For those clients who use computers, there are special keyboards available to decrease the pressure on the median nerve and aid in relief of pain and promote healing.

Establishing Safe Environments. When sensory function becomes impaired, individuals become less secure, and the world around them becomes smaller. Older adults in particular find it important to feel secure about their immediate environment. This is necessary for the person to have a sense of independence. Feeling safe allows a person to function within the home. The nurse can make recommendations to assist clients in making their living environment safer without restricting their independence. During a home visit or while completing an examination in the clinic, the nurse can offer several useful suggestions for home safety. The nature of the actual or potential sensory loss determines the safety precautions taken.

Adaptations for Visual Loss.   Whether a visual alteration is a result of injury, eye disease, or the changes of aging, safety becomes a factor if visual acuity, peripheral vision, adaptation to the dark, and depth perception are permanently reduced. With reduced peripheral vision a client cannot see panoramically, since the outer visual field is less discrete. This creates a special hazard for driving. Older adults with reduced adaptation to the dark require three times as much light to see objects as they did as young adults. With reduced depth perception a person cannot see how far away objects are located. This is a special danger as an older adult attempts to walk down stairs.

To create a safe environment, the nurse begins by looking at the results of the home environment assessment (see Chapter 37). What hazards exist in the client's living areas? Clutter such as footstools, children's toys, and electrical cords in walking paths should be removed. Electrical cords should be placed under furniture, rugs, or carpeting. Furniture should be arranged so that a client can move about easily without fear of tripping or running into objects.

Because of reduced depth perception, an older adult can trip on throw rugs, runners, or the edge of stairs. All flooring or carpeting should be kept in good repair. The nurse can advise the client to use low-pile rather than shag carpeting. Thresholds between rooms should be level with the floor. Any stairwell should have a securely fastened banister or handrail extending the full length of the stairs.

Front and back entrances to the home, work areas, and stairwells can be dangerous if improperly lighted. The nurse encourages the client to have a repairman install lights with higher wattage and wider illumination. Fluorescent lighting should be avoided. A light switch should be located at the top and bottom of stairwells. It is also important to be sure lighting on the stairs does not cast shadows. Be sure the client can clearly see the edge of each step, especially the first and last. When possible, steps inside and outside the home should be replaced with ramps.

Driving can be a particular safety hazard for older adults. The changes in the lens cause the older adult to be highly sensitive to glare during night driving. Reduced peripheral vision may prevent a driver from seeing a car in an adjacent lane. Vision is a primary consideration for safety, but there are other factors as well. Older clients may have decreased reaction time, reduced hearing, and decreased strength in the legs and arms. All of these factors can affect an older adult's driving skills. Box 48-13 summarizes tips for older adults who continue to drive.

The inability to see visual contrast can be a problem for an older adult. Sometimes settings on electrical appliances and equipment are only highlighted in black and white or shades of gray. Color contrasts help to distinguish settings. Colored tape, paint, or nail enamel can be used to color code appliance dials. Color can also be useful to highlight the edge of stairs. Painting the edge of stairs with bright orange paint or applying a broad strip of colored tape at the stair edge can help a person see the edges of stairs more clearly. The nurse can help the client tour the home to find opportunities for color coding.

If a client is partially or totally blind, fire hazards should be removed from the home. Flammable items, such as paper and cloth, should be kept away from the stove. A client who smokes must learn to discard ashes frequently into an ashtray. Water in the bottom of an ashtray helps ensure that cigarette butts are extinguished.

An added consideration for the visually impaired is the assurance that eye medications are administered safely. For conditions such as glaucoma, clients must closely adhere to regular medication schedules. Older adults may have some difficulty manipulating eye droppers. A friend or spouse should always be familiar with dosage schedules in case a client is unable to self-administer a medication.

Adaptations for Reduced Hearing.   Important environmental sounds (e.g., doorbells and alarm clocks) may best be heard if amplified or changed to a lower-pitched, buzzerlike sound. There are also sound lamps that re-

---

Gerontological NURSING PRACTICE   **Box 48-13**

- Drive in familiar areas.
- Do not drive during rush hour.
- Drive defensively—use rear-view and side-view mirrors when changing lanes.
- Avoid driving at dusk or night.
- Go slow, but not too slow.
- Keep the car in good working condition.

spond with light to sounds such as doorbells, burglar alarms, smoke detectors, and babies crying. These can be purchased from hearing aid dealers, telephone companies, and appliance stores (Ebersole and Hess, 1998). Signaling devices allow the deaf person greater independence. Family members or anyone who calls the client regularly should learn to let the phone ring for a longer period. There are amplified receivers for telephones and telephone communications devices (TTDs) that use a computer and printer to transfer words over the telephone for the hearing impaired. Both sender and receiver must have the special device to complete a call.

Adaptations for Reduced Olfaction. A reduced sensitivity to odors means that the client may be unable to smell leaking gas, a smoldering cigarette or fire, or tainted food. The client should use smoke detectors and other alternative precautions such as checking ashtrays or placing cigarette butts in water. A client can learn to check dates on food packages and the color and texture of food. Pilot gas flames should be checked visually.

Adaptations for Reduced Tactile Sensation. When clients have reduced sensation in their extremities, they are at risk for injury from exposure to temperature extremes. The nurse should caution them on the use of wa-

ter bottles or heating pads (see Chapter 47). The temperature setting on the home water heater should be no higher than 48.8° C (120° F). If a client also has a visual impairment, it is important to be sure that water faucets are clearly marked "hot" and "cold," or color codes (i.e., red for hot and blue for cold) can be used.

Promoting Communication. A sensory deficit can cause a person to feel isolated because of an inability to communicate with others. It is important for individuals to be able to interact with people whom they encounter. This problem can complicate a nurse's effectiveness in teaching clients information and skills. The nature of the sensory loss influences the methods and styles of communication that nurses can use (Box 48-14). Communication methods can also be taught to family members and significant others.

When beginning a conversation with a client who has a hearing deficit, it helps to reduce any background noise by turning off or lowering the volume of any TV, appliance, or radio. It is also helpful to have conversations in settings where there are better acoustics, which aid in controlling and muffling extraneous background noises. In a group setting it is better to form a semicircle in front of the client so that the client can see who is speaking next; this helps foster group involvement. The client with a hearing im-

---

Communication Methods   Box 48-14

CLIENTS WITH APHASIA
Listen to the client and wait for the client to communicate.
Do not shout or speak loudly (hearing loss is not the problem).
If the client has problems with comprehension, use simple, short questions and facial gestures to give additional clues.
Speak of things familiar and of interest to the client.
If the client has problems speaking, ask questions that require simple yes or no answers or blinking of the eyes. Offer pictures or a communication board so that the client can point.
Give the client time to understand; be calm and patient.
Do not pressure or tire the client.
Avoid patronizing and childish phrases.

CLIENTS WITH AN ARTIFICIAL AIRWAY
Use pictures, objects, or word cards so that the client can point.
Offer a pad and pencil or Magic Slate for the client to write messages.
Do not shout or speak loudly.
Give the client time to write messages, since these clients become easily fatigued.
Provide an artificial voice box (vibrator) for the client with a laryngectomy to use to speak words or phrases.

CLIENTS WITH HEARING IMPAIRMENT
Get the client's attention. Do not startle the client when entering the room. Do not approach a client from behind. Be sure the client knows you wish to speak.

Face the client and stand or sit on the same level. Be sure your face and lips are illuminated to promote lipreading. Keep hands away from mouth.
If the client wears glasses, be sure they are clean so that your gestures and face can be seen.
If the client wears a hearing aid, make sure it is in place and working.
Speak slowly and articulate clearly. Older adults may take longer to process verbal messages.
Use a normal tone of voice and inflections of speech. Refrain from speaking with something in your mouth.
When you are not understood, rephrase rather than repeat the conversation.
Use visible expressions. Speak with your hands, your face, and your eyes.
Do not shout. Loud sounds are usually higher pitched and may impede hearing by accentuating vowel sounds and concealing consonants. If it is necessary to raise your voice, speak in lower tones.
Talk toward the client's best or normal ear.
Use written information to enhance the spoken word.
Do not restrict a deaf client's hands. Never have IV lines in both of the client's hands if the preferred method of communication is sign language.
Avoid eating, chewing, or smoking while speaking.
Avoid speaking from another room or while walking away.

pairment may be able to speak normally. However, the deaf client's inability to hear self-spoken words may cause serious speech alterations. Clients may use sign language or lipreading, write with a pad and pencil, or learn to use a computer for communication. Special communication boards contain common terms used in nursing care and help clients express their needs.

Client instruction is one aspect of communication. There are teaching booklets available in large print for clients with visual loss. The client who is blind may require more frequent and detailed verbal descriptions of information. This is particularly true if there are no instructional booklets written in Braille. The visually impaired can learn by listening to audiotapes or the sound portion of a televised teaching session. Clients with hearing impairment may benefit from written instructional materials and visual teaching aids (e.g., posters and graphs). Demonstrations by the nurse are very useful. Hospitals are required to make interpreters available to read sign language of deaf clients.

Acute Care. When clients enter acute care settings for therapeutic management of sensory deficits or as a result of traumatic injury, the nurse uses approaches to maximize sensory function existing at the time. Safety again is an obvious priority until the client's sensory status is either stabilized or improved. For example, clients with sensory deficits have a high risk for falls in the acute care environment. It also becomes very important to know the extent of any existing sensory impairment before the acute episode of illness so that the nurse can reinforce what the client already knows about self-care or plan for more instruction before and following discharge.

Another group of clients who are at risk for developing sensory alterations while hospitalized are those in ICUs and the acutely ill. The constant activity within an ICU and the frequent monitoring of the acutely ill can easily cause clients to experience sensory overload. The nurse's main challenge becomes introducing regular, meaningful stimulation so that clients maintain a clearer perception of their immediate environment.

Orientation to the Environment. The client with recent sensory impairment requires a complete orientation to the immediate environment. Reorientation to the institutional environment may be provided by ensuring that name tags on uniforms are visible, addressing the client by name, explaining where the client is (especially if clients are transported to different areas for treatment), and using conversational cues to time or location. The tendency for clients to become confused can be reduced by offering short and simple, repeated explanations and reassurance. Family members and visitors can also help orient clients to the hospital surroundings.

A client with serious visual impairment must feel comfortable in knowing the boundaries of the immediate environment. Normally we see physical boundaries within a room. The blind or severely visually impaired must touch the boundaries or objects to gain a sense of their surroundings. The client needs to walk through a room and feel the walls to establish a sense of direction. The nurse can help by explaining objects within the room, such as furniture or equipment. It takes time for the client to absorb a room's arrangement. The client may need to reorient again, with the nurse explaining the location of key items (e.g., call light, telephone, chair). It also helps to always approach a blind client from the front to avoid startling him or her.

It is important to keep all objects in the same position and place. After an object is moved even a short distance, it no longer exists for a blind person. Simply moving a chair aside may create a dangerous safety hazard. The nurse should ask the client if any item should be arranged to make ambulation easier. Traffic patterns should be kept clear, and use of furniture with sharp edges avoided. The client who is blind always needs extra time to perform any task. The client needs a detailed description of how to perform an activity and will move slowly to remain safe.

Bedridden clients are at risk for sensory deprivation. Normally movement gives an integrated awareness of the self through vestibular and tactile stimulation. A person's sensory perception is influenced by movement patterns. The limited movement of bed rest changes how a person interprets the environment; surroundings seem different, and objects seem to assume shapes different from normal. A person who is on bed rest requires routine stimulation through range-of-motion exercises, positioning, and participation in self-care activities (as appropriate). Comfort measures such as washing the face and hands and providing back rubs can help to improve the quality of stimulation and lessen the chance of sensory deprivation. Planning time to talk with clients is also essential. The nurse should explain unfamiliar environmental noises and sensations. A calm, unhurried approach during contact with a client gives the nurse quality time to help reorient and familiarize the client with care activities. The client who is well enough to read will benefit from a variety of reading material.

Communication. The most common language disorder following a stroke is aphasia. As a result of a disruption in blood flow to the brain, the speech center becomes damaged, altering a person's ability to either use or understand spoken words. Depending on the type of aphasia, the inability to communicate can be frustrating and frightening (see Box 48-14). The nurse should initially establish very basic communication and recognize that aphasia does not indicate intellectual impairment or degeneration of personality. The nurse explains situations and treatments that are pertinent to the client, since he or she may understand (Ebersole and Hess, 1998). Because a stroke often causes partial or complete paralysis of one side of the client's body, an aphasic client may need special assistive devices. There are communication boards that have been developed for several levels of disability. Sensitive pressure switches, activated by the touch of an ear, nose, or chin, can control electronic communication boards (Ebersole and Hess, 1998). Clients who have had a stroke usually acquire referrals to speech therapists to develop appropriate rehabilitation plans.

In acute care hospitals or long-term care facilities, nurses often care for clients with artificial airways (see Chapter 39). For example, an endotracheal tube is inserted into the oropharynx and down through the vocal cords of the larynx into the upper bronchus. The placement of the tube prevents a client from speaking. In this case the nurse must use special communication methods to facilitate the client's ability to express needs (see Box 48-14). The client may be completely alert and able to hear and see the nurse normally. Giving the client time to convey any needs or requests is very important. Creative communication techniques (e.g., a board or a laptop computer) can be used to foster and strengthen the client's interactions with health care personnel, family, and friends.

Controlling Sensory Stimuli.

The nurse controls excessive stimuli for clients at risk for sensory overload. Clients need time for rest and freedom from stress caused by frequent monitoring and repeated tests. The nurse can reduce sensory overload by organizing the care plan. Combining activities such as dressing changes, bathing, and vital sign measurement in one visit prevents the client from becoming overly fatigued. The client also needs scheduled time for rest and quiet. Planning for rest periods often requires cooperation from family and visitors. Coordination with laboratory and radiology departments may help minimize the number of procedures the client must undergo. The nurse may encourage a family member to sit quietly with a client or involve the client in an undemanding repetitive activity such as combing hair or brushing teeth. Helping clients to become as mobile and independent as possible within prescribed limits provides meaningful stimulation.

When clients experience sensory overload or deprivation, the resultant behavior can be difficult for family or friends to accept. The nurse encourages the family not to argue with or contradict the confused client, but to calmly explain location, identity, and time of day. Engaging the client in a normal discussion about familiar topics may assist in reorientation. Prearranging tests and procedures with departments reduces the amount of time needed for tests and examinations. Anticipating client needs such as voiding helps reduce uncomfortable stimuli.

The nurse can also try to control extraneous noise in and around the client's room. It may be necessary to ask a roommate to lower the volume on a television or to move the client to a quieter room. Equipment noise should be kept to a minimum. Bedside equipment not in use, such as suction and oxygen equipment, should be turned off. The nurse also avoids abrupt loud noises, such as dropping objects or causing the overbed table to adjust to the lowest level suddenly. Nursing staff should also try to control laughter or conversation at the nurses' station. Nurses should allow clients to close room doors.

When the client leaves an acute care setting for the home environment, nurses should communicate with colleagues in the home care setting about the interventions that helped the client adapt to sensory problems. Similarly, information describing the client's existing sensory deficits should be reported. Continuity of care is achieved when the client is required to make only minimal changes in the home setting.

Safety Measures.

The client with recent visual impairment often requires help with walking. The presence of an eye patch, frequently instilled eye drops, or the swelling of eyelid structures following surgery are just a few factors that cause a client to need more assistance than usual. A sighted guide can give confidence to the visually impaired and ensure safe mobility. Ebersole and Hess (1998) list four suggestions for a sighted guide:

1. Ask the blind client if he or she wants a "sighted guide."
2. If assistance is accepted, offer an elbow or arm. Instruct the client to grasp your arm just above the elbow. If necessary, physically assist the person by guiding his or her hand to your arm or elbow (Figure 48-7).
3. Go one half step ahead and slightly to the side of the blind person. The shoulder of the person should be directly behind your shoulder. If the person is frail, place the hand on your forearm.
4. Relax and walk at a comfortable pace. Warn the client when you approach doorways or narrow spaces.

While walking the client, describe the course of movement and ensure that obstacles have been removed. A client with visual impairment should never be left standing alone in an unfamiliar area. For clients who undergo eye surgery, it is important to teach family members techniques for assisting with ambulation.

A visually impaired client who spends considerable time in bed should have a call light nearby. Necessary objects should be placed in front of the client to prevent falls caused by reaching over the bedside. Side rails are also important in this regard. At night a night-light with a red bulb can help reduce falls. The red light reduces the time required for the eyes to adapt to the dark and allows the client to see well enough to function without keeping the regular light on (Matteson and McConnell, 1988).

Nurses may rely on clients in health care settings to report unusual sounds, such as a suction apparatus running improperly or an IV pump alarm. However, the client with a hearing loss may not hear such sounds and thus requires

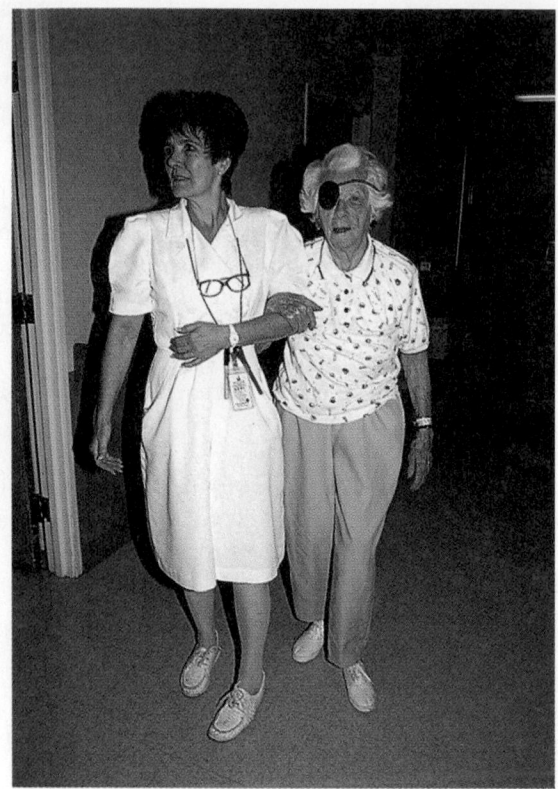

Figure 48-7   Nurse assists in the ambulation of a client wearing an eye patch.

more frequent visits by the nurse. The client can also benefit from learning to use vision to discover sources of danger. The nurse should never restrict both arms of deaf or hearing-impaired clients (e.g., with restraints or IV lines), since they need their hands to communicate. It is wise to note on the intercom button and a client's chart if the client is deaf and/or blind.

A client lacking the ability to speak cannot call out for assistance. Clients with aphasia, a laryngectomy, or an artificial airway must have alternative means of communication, such as message boards, close at hand. In the hospital a call light should always be near the client.

Clients with reduced tactile sensation risk injury when their conditions confine them to bed, because they are unable to sense pressure on bony prominences or the need to change position. These clients rely on nurses for timely repositioning, moving tubes or devices the client may lie on, and turning to avoid skin breakdown. When the ability to sense temperature variations is reduced, the nurse should use extra caution in applying heat and cold therapies (see Chapter 47) and preparing bathwater. The nurse must frequently check the condition of the client's skin.

Restorative and Continuing Care
Maintaining Healthy Lifestyles.   After a client has experienced a sensory loss, it becomes important to un-

derstand the implications of the loss and to make the adjustments needed to continue a normal lifestyle. Sensory impairments need not prevent a person from leading an active, rewarding life. Many of the interventions applicable to health promotion, such as adapting the home environment, can be used after a client leaves an acute care setting.

Understanding Sensory Loss.   Clients who have experienced a recent loss must understand how to adapt so that living environments can be safe and appropriately stimulating. All family members should understand the way that a client's sensory impairment affects normal daily activities. Family and friends can be more supportive when they understand sensory deficits and the types of elements that worsen or lessen sensory problems. For example, family and friends need to learn how to communicate with someone who has a hearing loss. There are resources within a community that provide information that assists clients with personal management needs. The American Foundation for the Blind, American National Red Cross, and National Association for Speech and Hearing offer resource materials and product information.

Socialization.   The ability to communicate is gratifying. It tests our intellect, opens opportunities, and allows us to exchange the feelings we have about others (Figure 48-8). When interactions are hindered by sensory alterations, a person can feel ineffective and lose self-esteem. If clients feel socially unaccepted, they will perceive sensory losses as seriously impairing the quality of life.

Interacting with others can become a burden for many clients with sensory alterations. Asking people to continuously repeat what they say is both embarrassing and exhausting for a client with hearing loss. Many clients lose the motivation to engage in social situations. As a person withdraws from interaction, a deep sense of loneliness can develop. The nurse can introduce therapies to reduce loneliness, particularly for older clients (Box 48-15). In addition, family members must learn to focus on a person's ability to interact rather than on the person's disability. It should not be assumed, for example, that a person who is hard of hearing does not wish to speak. A blind person can still enjoy a walk through a park with a companion describing the sights around them.

Promoting Self-Care.   The ability to perform self-care is essential for self-esteem. Frequently, family members and nurses believe that sensorially impaired persons require assistance, when in fact they can help themselves. Useful guidelines assist clients with visual or tactile impairment when help is required with activities of daily living.

A meal tray can be set up as though food on the tray and condiments and drinks around the tray are numbers on the face of a clock. The visually impaired client can easily become oriented to the items after the nurse or family member explains each item's location.

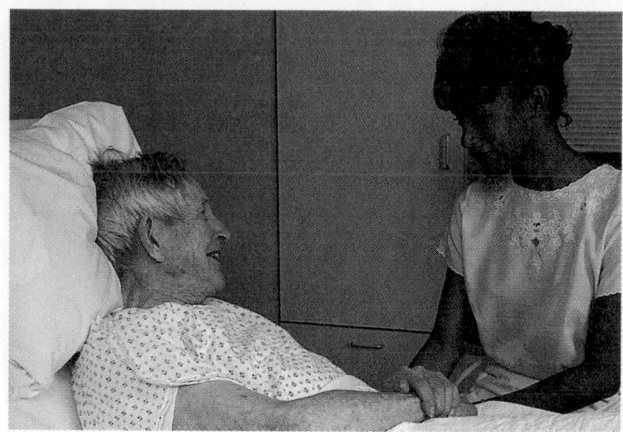

Figure 48-8   Conversation with nurse can reduce loneliness and sense of isolation.

- Spend time with a person in silence or conversation.
- Use physical contact—holding a hand, embracing a shoulder—to convey caring.
- Help recommend alterations in living arrangements if physical isolation is a factor.
- Assist older adults in keeping contact with people important to them.
- Help obtain information about mutual help groups.
- Arrange for security escort services as needed.
- Bring a pet that is easy to care for into the home.
- Link a person with religious organizations attuned to the social needs of older adults.

If tactile sense is diminished, the client can dress more easily with zippers or Velcro strips, pullover sweaters or blouses, and elasticized waists. If a client has partial paralysis and reduced sensation, the affected side should be dressed first. Family members responsible for selecting clothing for visually impaired clients should be encouraged to follow the client's preferences. Any sensory impairment has a significant influence on body image, and it is important for the client to feel well groomed and attractive. A client may need assistance with basic grooming such as brushing, combing, and shampooing hair. The client also may need assistance with medication selection, clothing identification, and learning to manage routine procedures such as blood pressure and glucose monitoring (Cleary, 1995). It is important to assist clients in maintaining a degree of independence and in having as much control over the management of their care and lifestyle as possible.

The client with visual problems needs assistance in reaching toilet facilities safely. Safety bars should be installed near the toilet. It may be helpful to have the bar a different color than the wall for easier visibility. Towels should never be placed on safety bars, since they may interfere with a person's grasp. Toilet paper should be within easy reach.

Clients with proprioceptive problems may lose their balance easily. Bathrooms should have nonskid surfaces in the tub and shower. Grab bars should be installed either vertically or horizontally in tubs and showers, depending on how the client is able to grasp or hold onto the bar. The nurse can instruct family members to supervise ambulation and sitting, make frequent checks to prevent falls, and caution the client against leaning forward.

EVALUATION
Client Care.   With regard to problems with sensory alterations, the client is the source for evaluating outcomes. The client is the only one who will know if his or her sensory abilities are improved and which specific interventions or therapies are most successful in facilitating a change in the client's performance (Figure 48-9). To evaluate the effectiveness of nursing interventions, the nurse uses critical thinking and makes comparisons with the baseline sensory assessment data to evaluate if sensory alterations have changed.

The nurse determines if the expected outcomes have been met. For example, the nurse uses evaluative data to determine whether care measures improve or at least maintain a client's ability to interact and function within the environment. The nature of a client's sensory alterations influences the way a nurse evaluates the outcome of care. For example, the nurse uses proper communication techniques with a client with a hearing deficit and then evaluates whether the client has gained the ability to hear or interact more effectively. When expected outcomes have not been achieved, there may be a need to change interventions or alter the client's environment. Family members may need to become more involved in support of the client.

If nursing care has been directed at improving sensory acuity, the nurse evaluates the integrity of the sensory organs and the client's ability to perceive stimuli. Any interventions designed to relieve problems associated with sensory alterations are evaluated on the basis of the client's ability to function normally without injury. When the nurse attempts to directly or indirectly (through education) alter the client's environment, evaluation is directed at observing whether the client makes environmental changes. When client teaching is designed to improve a client's sensory function, it is important to determine whether the client is following recommended therapies. Asking the client to explain or demonstrate self-care skills evaluates the level of learning that has occurred. It may be necessary to reinforce previous instruction if learning has not taken place.

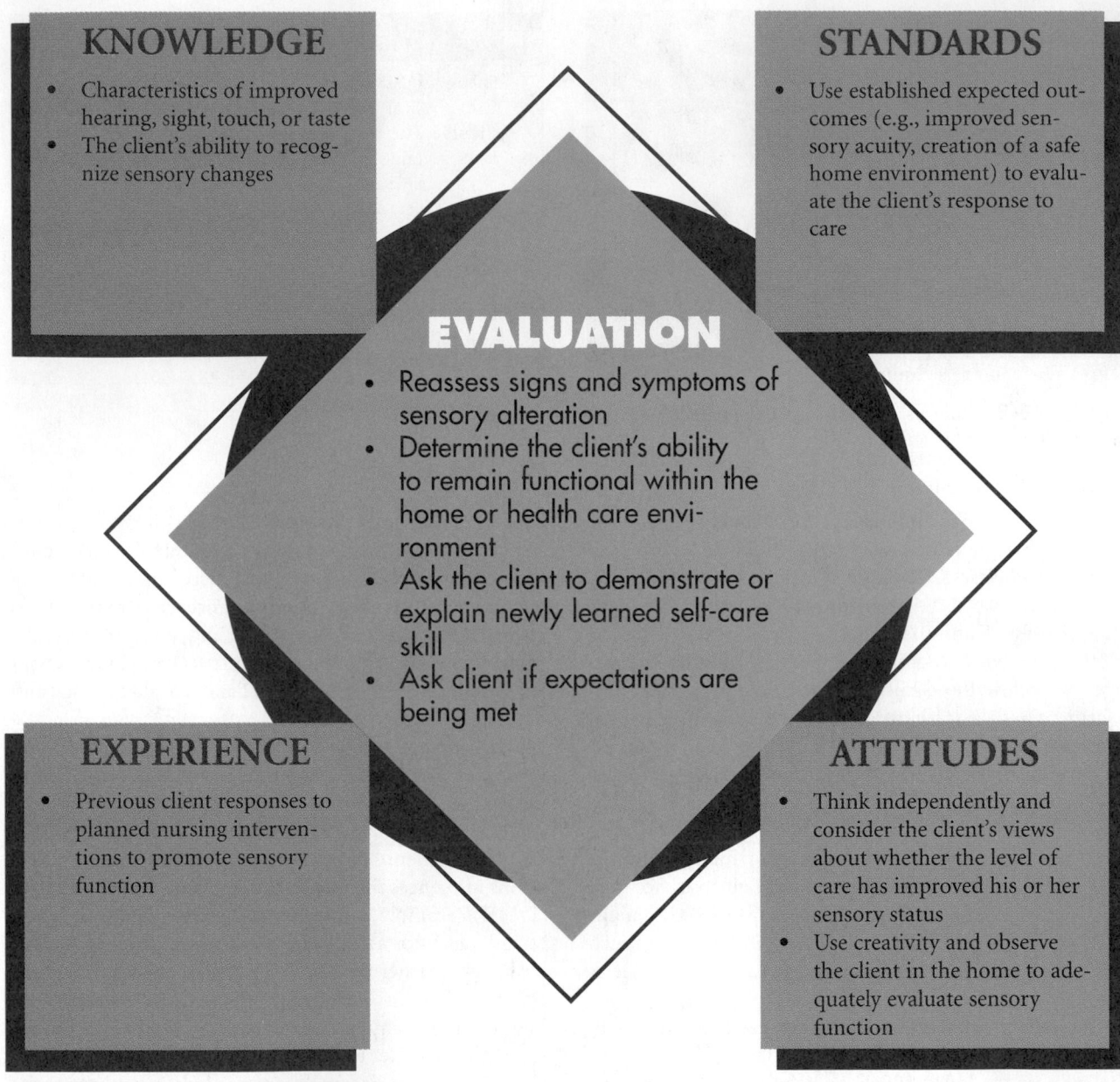

KNOWLEDGE

- Characteristics of improved hearing, sight, touch, or taste
- The client's ability to recognize sensory changes

STANDARDS

- Use established expected outcomes (e.g., improved sensory acuity, creation of a safe home environment) to evaluate the client's response to care

EVALUATION

- Reassess signs and symptoms of sensory alteration
- Determine the client's ability to remain functional within the home or health care environment
- Ask the client to demonstrate or explain newly learned self-care skill
- Ask client if expectations are being met

EXPERIENCE

- Previous client responses to planned nursing interventions to promote sensory function

ATTITUDES

- Think independently and consider the client's views about whether the level of care has improved his or her sensory status
- Use creativity and observe the client in the home to adequately evaluate sensory function

Figure 48-9   *Synthesis Model for Sensory Alterations Evaluation Phase.*

Client Expectations.   If the nurse has successfully developed a good relationship with a client and has a therapeutic plan of care, subtle behaviors often indicate the level of the client's satisfaction. The nurse may note that the client responds appropriately, such as by smiling. The nurse may observe that the client interacts more with family or with the nurse and is not asking to have information repeated. However, it is important for the nurse to ask the client if his or her sensory needs have been met. For example, the nurse may ask the client, "Can you tell me if you feel we have done all we can do to help improve your ability to hear?" If the client's expectations have not been met, then the nurse needs to spend more time understanding the client's needs and specific preferences. Working closely with the client and family will enable the nurse to redefine those expectations that can be realistically met within the limits of the client's condition and therapies. The nurse is effective when the client's goals and expectations have been met.

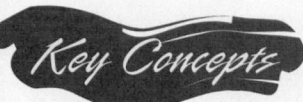

Key Concepts

- Sensory reception involves the stimulation of sensory nerve fibers and the transmission of impulses to higher centers within the brain.
- When sensory function is impaired, the sense of self is impaired.
- Sensory deprivation results from an inadequate quality or quantity of sensory stimuli.
- Aging results in a gradual decline of acuity in all senses.
- Clients in intensive care units are at risk for sensory deprivation as a result of the lack of personal, comforting touch.
- Clients who are older, immobilized, or confined in isolated environments are at risk for sensory alterations.
- The extent of support from family members and significant others can influence the quality of sensory experiences.
- Assessment of a client's health promotion habits helps to reveal risks for sensory impairment.
- An older adult often will not admit to a sensory loss.
- An assessment of hazards in the environment requires the nurse to tour living areas in the home and to look for conditions that increase the chances of injury such as falls.
- The plan of care for clients with sensory alterations should include participation by family members.
- Hearing loss should not be accepted as a natural part of aging.
- Clients with sensory deficits develop alternative ways of communicating that rely on other senses.
- Eye injuries can occur while participating in contact sports.
- Care of clients at risk for sensory deprivation includes introducing meaningful and pleasant stimuli for all senses.
- Sensory losses can impair a person's ability to socialize.
- To prevent sensory overload, the nurse controls stimuli and orients the client to the environment.
- To improve communication with the hearing impaired, the nurse speaks clearly, stands in front of the client, and makes sure that lip and facial movements are visible.
- Clients with artificial airways can communicate effectively with communication boards and written messages.

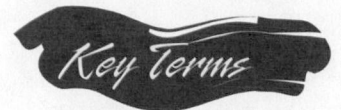

Key Terms

Aphasia, *p. 1642*
Auditory, *p. 1631*
Conductive hearing loss, *p. 1649*
Expressive aphasia, *p. 1642*
Gustatory, *p. 1631*
Hyperesthesia, *p. 1649*
Kinesthetic, *p. 1631*
Olfactory, *p. 1631*
Otolaryngologist, *p. 1648*

Ototoxic, *p. 1633*
Proprioceptive, *p. 1633*
Receptive aphasia, *p. 1642*
Refractive error, *p. 1642*
Sensory deficit, *p. 1632*
Sensory deprivation, *p. 1633*
Sensory overload, *p. 1634*
Stereognosis, *p. 1631*
Strabismus, *p. 1646*
Tactile, *p. 1631*

Critical Thinking Exercises

1. Mr. Michaels is 84 years old and is the primary caregiver for his 83-year-old wife. During an initial home visit to the wife, the nurse observed that Mr. Michaels would only respond when he was looking directly at the nurse or was standing close. Otherwise, he would not respond to questions or would seem to ignore what was happening or what was being said. What follow-up assessments should be gathered? What interventions would be helpful?

2. The school nurse learns from the fifth-grade teacher that 10-year-old Sue Pieper has been having difficulty with following simple written directions and homework assignments. She seems disinterested when they are assigned to use the computer. The teacher also reports that Sue is showing difficulty with sports such as baseball and soccer—her timing is off—and previously that was not the case. The nurse identifies that Sue has decreased visual acuity. What nursing actions are important to ensure her safety?

3. Mrs. Jones is admitted to the emergency department after being involved in a motor vehicle accident. Assessment reveals severe visual impairment due to bilateral cataracts. Currently she is in stable condition but requires admission. To promote optimal sensory function, what nursing measures should be considered?

References

Beaver K, Mann W: Overview of technology for low vision, *Am J Occup Ther* 49:913, 1995.

Cleary ME: Helping the person who is visually impaired: concerns, questions, remedies, and resources, *J Ophthalmic Nurs Technol* 14(5):205, 1995.

Ebersole P, Hess P: *Toward healthy aging: human needs and nursing response,* ed 5, St. Louis, 1998, Mosby.

Giger JN, Davidhizar RE: *Transcultural nursing: assessment and intervention,* ed 3, St. Louis, 1999, Mosby.

Griest SE, Bishop PM: Tinnitus as an early indicator of permanent hearing loss, *Am Assoc Occup Health Nurs J* 46(7):325, 1998.

Hong OS, Chen SC, Conrad KM: Noise induced hearing loss among male airport workers in Korea, *Am Assoc Occup Health Nurs J* 46(2):67, 1998.

Larsen PD, Hazen SE, Hootmartin JL: Assessment and management of sensory loss in elderly patients, *AORN J* 65(2):432 1997.

Lewis SM, Collier IC, Heitkemper MM, editors: *Medical-surgical nursing: assessment and management of clinical problems,* ed 5, St. Louis, 1999, Mosby.

Lewis-Cullinan C, Janken JK: Effect of cerumen removal on the hearing ability of geriatric patients, *J Adv Nurs* 15:594, 1990.

Lukes E, Johnson M: Hearing conservation, *Am Assoc Occup Health Nurs J* 46(7):340, 1998.

Matteson MA, McConnell ES: *Gerontological nursing: concepts and practice,* Philadelphia, 1988, WB Saunders.

McCloskey JC, Bulechek GM: Nursing interventions classification (NIC), ed 3, St. Louis, 2000, Mosby.

Resnick HE, Fries BE, Verbrugge LM: Windows to their world: the effects of sensory impairments on social engagement and activity time in nursing home residents, *J Gerontol Soc Sci* 52(3):S135, 1997.

Ruda SC: Nursing assessment: musculoskeletal system. In Lewis SM, Collier IC, Heitkemper MM, editors: *Medical-surgical nursing: assessment and management of clinical problems,* ed 5, St. Louis, 1999, Mosby.

Smith SC, Wilbur ME: Vision and hearing problems. In Lewis SM, Collier IC, Heitkemper MM, editors: *Medical-surgical nursing: assessment and management of clinical problems,* ed 5, St. Louis, 1999, Mosby.

Thelan, LA and others: *Critical care nursing: diagnosis and management,* ed 3, St. Louis, 1998, Mosby.

Thibodeau GA, Patton KT: *Anatomy and physiology,* ed 3, St. Louis, 1999, Mosby.

Tolson D: Age-related hearing loss: a case for nursing intervention, *J Adv Nurs* 26(6):1150, 1997.

Vader L: Vision and vision loss, *Nurs Clin North Am* 27:705, 1992.

Ventry I, Weinstein B: The hearing handicap inventory for the elderly: a new tool, *Ear Hearing* 3:133, 1986.

Weinstein BE: Age-related hearing loss: how to screen for it, and when to intervene, *Geriatrics* 49(8):40, 1994.

Wong DL and others: *Whaley and Wong's nursing care of infants and children,* ed 6, St. Louis, 1999, Mosby.

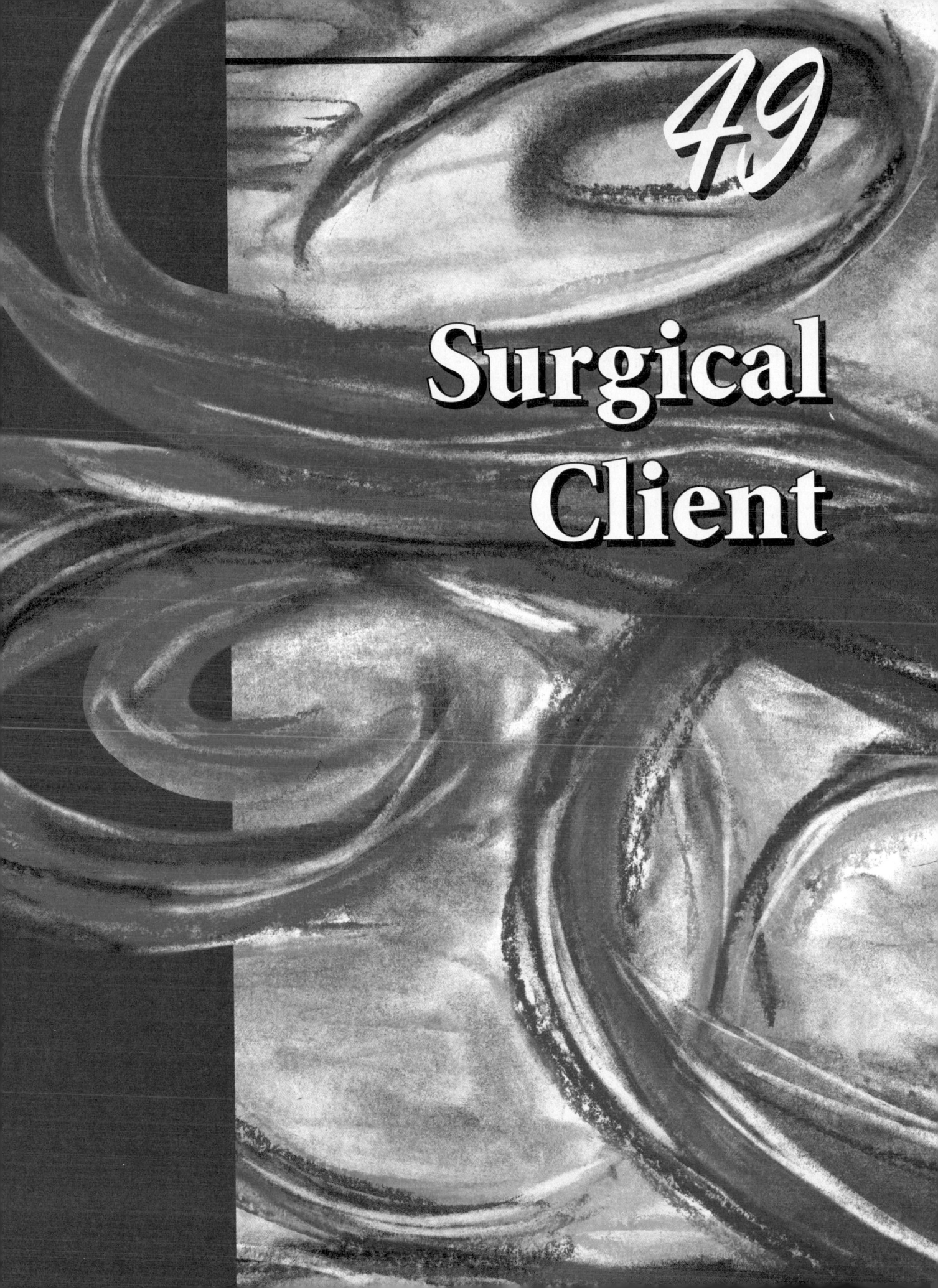

49

Surgical Client

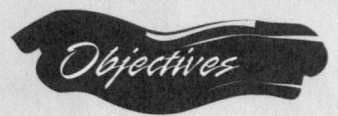

Objectives

Mastery of content in this chapter will enable the student to:

- Define the key terms listed.
- Explain the concept of perioperative nursing care.
- Differentiate between classifications of surgery.
- List factors to include in the preoperative assessment of a surgical client.
- Describe how to correctly witness a client's informed consent for surgery.
- Demonstrate postoperative exercises: diaphragmatic breathing, coughing, turning, and leg exercises.
- Provide a client with preoperative instruction.
- Prepare a client for surgery.
- Compare and contrast the actions and side effects of general, regional, and local anesthesia.
- Explain the nurse's role in the operating room.
- Describe the nurse's role in phase I and phase II recovery.
- Identify factors to include in the postoperative assessment of a client in recovery.
- Describe the rationale for nursing interventions designed to prevent postoperative complications.
- Explain the difference and similarities in caring for outpatient versus inpatient surgical clients.

Perioperative nursing care includes nursing care given before (preoperative), during (intraoperative), and after surgery (postoperative). It may take place in the hospital, in a surgical center attached to a hospital, in a free-standing surgical center, or in a physician's office. Perioperative nursing is a fast-paced, changing, and challenging field in which to work. It is based on the nurse's understanding of several important characteristics, including high-quality, multidisciplinary teamwork; effective and therapeutic communication and collaboration with the client, the client's family, and the surgical team; effective and efficient client assessment and intervention in all phases; advocacy for the client and the client's family; and understanding of cost containment. The nurse must practice good surgical asepsis, thoroughly document care, and emphasize client safety in all phases. Effective teaching and discharge planning are needed to prevent or minimize complications and ensure quality outcomes. The nursing process provides a basis for **perioperative nursing,** with the nurse individualizing strategies throughout the perioperative period so that the client has a smooth course from admission into the health care system through convalescence. The continuity of care is stressed in the perioperative model.

A client experiences a variety of stressors when facing surgery. Anticipating surgery leads to fear and anxiety for clients who associate surgery with pain, possible disfigurement, dependence, and perhaps even death. As a result of hospitalization, the client may be concerned about loss of income or insurance coverage. Family members often fear a disruption in lifestyle and may experience a sense of powerlessness as the surgery date approaches. The ability to quickly establish rapport with clients and actively listen to them so that their concerns are addressed is important to the outcome of surgery. The continuing care of the surgical client has shifted from hospital-based convalescence to home-based convalescence, with the majority of responsibility shifting to the client and/or family. As the length of hospital stay decreases, the educational needs of the client undergoing a surgical procedure increases. Clients are sent home with complex medical/surgical conditions that require both education and follow-up. Proper client education is essential to ensure positive surgical outcomes (Gershenson, and others, 1999).

In today's health care environment, surgery is not confined to the hospital setting. By 1998 over 60% of surgical procedures were completed in ambulatory care centers, and this number continues to rise (Federated Ambulatory Surgery Association, 1998). Clients who are admitted for surgical inpatient hospital stays experience much shorter lengths of stay as well. This presents a challenge to nurses working in the perioperative setting to adjust preoperative and postoperative care to afford clients the best possible surgical experience and outcome.

History of Surgical Nursing

It was not until the twentieth century that the discipline of surgery truly progressed as a science. Surgery gave physicians the means to treat conditions that were difficult or impossible to manage only by pure medicine. Early sur-

The authors acknowledge the contribution of Lynne Dearing to this chapter in the previous edition of this text.

geons had little knowledge of the principles of asepsis, and anesthesia techniques were primitive and unsafe. Indeed, a surgeon's success was based on speed. The discovery of anesthesia in the 1840s revolutionized the surgical process. Anesthesia provided for the combination of analgesia, muscle relaxation, and amnesia, which allowed the surgical procedure time to be extended (Greenfield and others, 1997). The value of hand washing in the 1800s, along with the development of the germ theory (Pasteur), triggered the study of aseptic technique, which reduced postoperative infections and mortality. Nursing played a major role in disease prevention, beginning with Florence Nightingale's belief that the environment was a key factor in disease prevention (Atkinson and Fortunato, 1996). Nurses working in the first operating rooms cleaned the rooms and equipment, performed technical tasks such as obtaining supplies, and occasionally accompanied the client to the surgical ward to deliver nursing care. Massachusetts General Hospital provided the first operating room education for nurses in 1876. This trend continued into the 1900s as nursing schools included operating room experience in each nurse's clinical instruction.

During the 1970s a change occurred in nursing education. A focus on the importance of nurses acquiring a broad knowledge base resulted in less emphasis on operating room techniques. Many schools eliminated operating room experience from the curriculum. However, today many nursing schools have reinstituted clinical operating room experience.

In 1956 the **Association of Operating Room Nurses (AORN)** was formed to gain knowledge of surgical principles and explore methods to improve nursing care of surgical clients. The organization developed standards of nursing practice that outline the scope of responsibility of the perioperative nurse. AORN was the first nursing organization to develop structure, process, and outcome standards as defined by the American Nurses Association (ANA). The standards of perioperative nursing include (1) administrative practice, (2) clinical practice, (3) professional performance, (4) quality improvement, and (5) client outcomes (AORN, 1999). AORN continues to be a driving force for the practice of perioperative nursing.

AMBULATORY SURGERY

A recent change in the surgery setting is the advent of **ambulatory surgery,** also referred to as outpatient surgery, short-stay surgery, or same-day surgery. Centers providing these services may be hospital based or freestanding centers (surgicenters). The first surgicenters opened in the 1970s. By 1982, surgicenters became Medicare approved, and expansion throughout the United States occurred. At least half of all surgical procedures are conducted on an outpatient basis (around 5 million procedures). These procedures include ophthalmic (27%), gynecological (16%), eye-ear-nose-throat (7%), orthopedic (9%), cosmetic/restorative (8%), and general procedures (7%)

(Atkinson and Fortunato, 1996; Federated Ambulatory Surgery Association, 1998). One-day surgery in which the client is admitted the day of surgery and observed overnight (23-hour admission) has also increased in popularity.

There are distinct benefits for the client who has ambulatory surgery. Anesthetic drugs that metabolize rapidly with few aftereffects allow shorter operative times. Nurses recognize the benefit of early postoperative ambulation and encourage clients to assume an active role in recovery. Ambulatory surgery also offers cost savings by eliminating the need for hospital stays. It also reduces the possibility of acquiring nosocomial infections, since once clients are hospitalized, their normal skin flora changes and they soon become colonized with bacteria found in the hospital setting (Morales and Andrews, 1993).

Procedures such as tumor biopsies and gallbladder removal (**cholecystectomy**) can now be done using laser procedures. For example, a laser or laparoscopic cholecystectomy involves only a few hours to a 24-hour hospital stay and a recovery period of a week. By contrast, a traditional cholecystectomy usually involves a 3- to 5-day hospitalization and at least a 4-week recovery period. Thus many surgeons use laser procedures instead of traditional surgical procedures, thereby decreasing the length of surgery, hospitalization, and associated costs.

Scientific Knowledge Base

CLASSIFICATION OF SURGERY

The types of surgical procedures are classified according to seriousness, urgency, and purpose (Table 49-1). A procedure may fall into more than one classification. For example, surgical removal of a disfiguring scar is minor in seriousness, elective in urgency, and reconstructive in purpose. Frequently the classes overlap. An urgent procedure is also considered major in seriousness. The same operation may be performed for different reasons on different clients. For example, a gastrectomy may be performed as an emergency procedure to resect a bleeding ulcer or as an urgent procedure to remove a cancerous growth. The classification indicates to the nurse the level of care a client might require.

RISK FACTORS

Various conditions and factors increase a person's risk in surgery. Knowledge of risk factors enables the nurse to take necessary precautions in planning care.

The American Society of Anesthesiologists (ASA) assigns classification based on a client's physiological condition independent of the proposed surgical procedure (Table 49-2). Intraoperative difficulties occur more frequently with clients who have a poor physical status classification (Meeker and Rothrock, 1999). ASA physical status class I and class II and also stable class III are now acceptable for ambulatory surgery. Class IV and class V are

Table 49-1 Classification for Surgical Procedures

Type	Description	Example
Seriousness		
Major	Involves extensive reconstruction or alteration in body parts; poses great risks to well-being	Coronary artery bypass, colon resection, removal of larynx, resection of lung lobe
Minor	Involves minimal alteration in body parts; often designed to correct deformities; involves minimal risks compared with major procedures	Cataract extraction, facial plastic surgery, skin graft, tooth extraction
Urgency		
Elective	Is performed on basis of client's choice; is not essential and may not be necessary for health	Bunionectomy, facial plastic surgery, hernia repair, breast reconstruction
Urgent	Is necessary for client's health, may prevent additional problems from developing (e.g., tissue destruction or impaired organ function); not necessarily emergency	Excision of cancerous tumor, removal of gallbladder for stones, vascular repair for obstructed artery (e.g., coronary artery bypass)
Emergency	Must be done immediately to save life or preserve function of body part	Repair of perforated appendix, repair of traumatic amputation, control of internal hemorrhaging
Purpose		
Diagnostic	Is surgical exploration that allows physician to confirm diagnosis; may involve removal of tissue for further diagnostic testing	Exploratory laparotomy (incision into peritoneal cavity to inspect abdominal organs), breast mass biopsy
Ablative	Is excision or removal of diseased body part	Amputation, removal of appendix, cholecystectomy
Palliative	Relieves or reduces intensity of disease symptoms; will not produce cure	Colostomy, debridement of necrotic tissue, resection of nerve roots
Reconstructive/ Restorative	Restores function or appearance to traumatized or malfunctioning tissues	Internal fixation of fractures, scar revision
Procurement for transplant	Removal of organs and/or tissues from a person pronounced brain dead for transplantation into another person	Kidney, cornea, or liver transplant
Constructive	Restores function lost or reduced as result of congenital anomalies	Repair of cleft palate, closure of atrial septal defect in heart
Cosmetic	Performed to improve personal appearance	Blepharoplasty to correct eyelid deformities; rhinoplasty to reshape nose

Table 49-2 Physical Status Classification of the American Society of Anesthesiologists

Class	Description	Characteristics
PS-1	A normal healthy client	No physiological, biological, organic disturbance
PS-2	A client with a mild systemic disease	Cardiovascular (CV) disease with minimal restriction on activity
PS-3	A client with a severe systemic disease that limits activity but is not incapacitating	Hypertension (HTN), obesity, diabetes mellitus (DM)
PS-4	A client with a severe systemic disease that is a constant threat to life	CV or pulmonary disease that limits activity; severe diabetes with systemic complications; history of myocardial infarction (MI), angina pectoris, or poorly controlled HTN
PS-5	A **moribund** client who is not expected to survive 24 hours with/without the operation	Severe cardiac, pulmonary, renal, hepatic, or endocrine dysfunction
PS-6	A client declared brain dead whose organs are being removed for donor purpose	Surgery is done as a last recourse of resuscitative effort; major multisystem or cerebral trauma, ruptured aneurysm, or large pulmonary embolus
E	Emergency operation	

Data from Meeker MH, Rothrock JC: *Alexander's care of the patient in surgery,* ed 11, St. Louis, 1999, Mosby; and Greenfield L and others: *Surgery: scientific principles and practice,* ed 2, Philadelphia, 1997, Lippincott-Raven.

completed on an inpatient basis (Atkinson and Fortunato, 1996).

Age.

Very young and old clients are at risk during surgery because of immature or declining physiological status. Mortality rates are higher in the very young and very old client. During surgery, nurses and physicians are especially concerned with maintaining an infant's normal body temperature. The infant's shivering reflex is underdeveloped, and often wide temperature variations occur. Anesthesia adds to the risk because anesthetics can cause vasodilation and heat loss.

During surgery an infant has difficulty maintaining a normal circulatory blood volume. The total blood volume of an infant is considerably less than that of an older child or an adult. Even a small amount of blood loss can be serious. A reduced circulatory volume makes it difficult for the infant to respond to the need for increased oxygen during surgery. Thus the infant is highly susceptible to dehydration. However, if blood or fluids are replaced too quickly, overhydration may occur. Other important aspects of a child's surgical care include airway management, fluid maintenance, treatment of seizures, treatment of temperature alterations, identification and treatment of emergence delirium and delayed emergence from anesthesia, treatment of pain and agitation, and availability of appropriate emergency equipment and medication (Sabiston and Lyerly, 1997).

With advancing age, a client's physical capacity to adapt to the stress of surgery is hampered because of deterioration in certain body functions. Despite the risk, the majority of clients undergoing surgery are older adults. Table 49-3 summarizes physiological factors that place older clients at risk during surgery

Nutrition.

Normal tissue repair and resistance to infection depend on adequate nutrients. Surgery intensifies this need. After surgery a client requires at least 1500 kcal/day to maintain energy reserves. Increased protein, vitamins A and C, and zinc facilitate wound healing (see Chapters 43 and 47). A malnourished client is prone to poor tolerance to anesthesia, negative nitrogen balance, delayed blood clotting mechanisms, infection, poor wound healing, and the potential for multiple organ failure. It is estimated that half of hospitalized clients display some degree of malnourishment (Atkinson and Fortunato, 1996). If a client has elective surgery, attempts to correct nutritional imbalances before surgery should be made. However, if a malnourished client must undergo an emergency procedure, efforts to restore nutrients occur after surgery.

Obesity.

Obesity increases surgical risk by reducing ventilatory and cardiac function. Hypertension, coronary artery disease, diabetes mellitus, and congestive heart failure are common in the **bariatric** population. Embolus, atelectasis, and pneumonia are also more frequent postoperative complications in the obese client. The client has difficulty resuming normal physical activity after surgery. The obese client is susceptible to poor wound healing and wound infection because of the structure of fatty tissue, which contains a poor blood supply. This slows delivery of essential nutrients, antibodies, and enzymes needed for wound healing (see Chapter 47). It is often difficult to close the surgical wound of an obese client because of the thick adipose layer. An obese client is also at risk for **dehiscence** (opening of the suture line).

Radiotherapy.

For the client with cancer, radiotherapy is often given to reduce the size of the cancerous tumor so that it can be removed surgically. Radiation has some unavoidable effects on normal tissue, such as excess thinning of skin layers, destruction of collagen, and impaired vascularization of tissue. Ideally, the surgeon waits to perform surgery 4 to 6 weeks after completion of radiation treatments. Otherwise, the client may face serious wound-healing problems.

Fluid and Electrolyte Balance.

The body responds to surgery as a form of trauma. As a result of the adrenocortical stress response, hormonal reactions cause sodium and water retention and potassium loss within the first 2 to 5 days after surgery. Severe protein breakdown causes a negative nitrogen balance. The severity of the stress response influences the degree of fluid and electrolyte imbalance. The more extensive the surgery, the more severe the stress. A client who is hypovolemic or who has serious preoperative electrolyte alterations is at significant risk during and after surgery. For example, an excess or depletion of potassium increases the chance of dysrhythmia during or after surgery. If the client has preexisting renal, gastrointestinal, or cardiovascular abnormalities, the risk of fluid and electrolyte alterations is even greater.

Pregnancy.

The perioperative plan of care must address not one, but two clients: the mother and the developing fetus. Surgery is performed on the pregnant client on an emergent or urgent basis. All major systems of the mother are affected during pregnancy. Cardiac output significantly increases as does respiratory tidal volume to accommodate the increase in metabolic rate. Gastrointestinal motility decreases, hormone levels increase, and energy levels decrease with advancing pregnancy. Laboratory and hemodynamic values change. Fibrinogen levels increase, so pregnant clients are more susceptible to the development of deep vein thrombosis due to increased coagulability. Hemoglobin and hematocrit levels decrease, mostly as a result of the effects of hemodilution (increased circulating volume). Blood urea nitrogen (BUN) and albumin levels decrease as well. The white blood cell (WBC) count is elevated when the woman is near term and postpartum without the presence of infection. General anesthesia is administered with caution because

Table 49-3   Physiological Factors That Place the Older Adult at Risk During Surgery

Alterations	Risks	Nursing Implications
Cardiovascular System		
Degenerative change in myocardium and valves	Change reduces cardiac reserve.	Assess baseline vital signs.
Rigidity of arterial walls and reduction in sympathetic and parasympathetic innervation to heart	Alterations predispose client to post-operative hemorrhage and rise in systolic and diastolic blood pressure.	
Increase in calcium and cholesterol deposits within small arteries; thickened arterial walls	Problems predispose client to clot formation in lower extremities.	Instruct client on techniques for performing leg exercises and proper turning.
		Apply elastic stockings; sequential compression devices (SCDs).
Integumentary System		
Decreased subcutaneous tissue and increased fragility of skin	Client is prone to pressure ulcers and tears.	Assess skin every 4 hours; pad all bony prominences during surgery. Turn or reposition.
Pulmonary System		
Rib cage stiffened and reduced in size	Complication reduces vital capacity.	Instruct client on proper technique for coughing, deep breathing, and use of spirometers.
Reduced range of movement in diaphragm	Greater residual capacity of volume of air is left in lung after normal breath increases, reducing amount of new air brought into lungs with each inspiration.	When possible, have client ambulate and sit in chair frequently.
Stiffened lung tissue and enlarged air spaces	Alteration reduces blood oxygenation.	
Renal System		
Reduced blood flow to kidneys	Reduced flow increases danger of shock when blood loss occurs.	For clients hospitalized before surgery, determine baseline urinary output for 24 hours.
Reduced glomerular filtration rate and excretory times	Problem limits ability to eliminate drugs or toxic substances.	
Reduced bladder capacity	Voiding frequency increases, and larger amount of urine stays in bladder after voiding.	Instruct client to notify nurse immediately when sensation of bladder fullness develops.
	Sensation of need to void may not occur until bladder is filled.	Keep call light and bedpan within easy reach.
Neurological System		
Sensory losses, including reduced tactile sense and increased pain tolerance	Client is less able to respond to early warning signs of surgical complications.	Orient client to surrounding environment. Observe for nonverbal signs of pain.
Decreased reaction time	Client becomes easily confused after anesthesia.	
Metabolic System		
Lower basal metabolic rate	Lower rate reduces total oxygen consumption.	
Reduced number of red blood cells and hemoglobin levels	Ability to carry adequate oxygen to tissues is reduced.	Administer necessary blood products. Monitor blood test results.
Change in total amounts of body potassium and water volume	Greater risk for fluid or electrolyte imbalance occurs.	Monitor electrolyte levels.

of the increased risk of fetal death and preterm labor. Psychological considerations for mother and family are essential (Atkinson and Fortunato, 1996).

Nursing Knowledge Base

To meet the holistic needs of the client, nurses base their knowledge on multiple factors. The nursing plan of care is not based entirely on the client's disease process and surgical procedure but on multiple factors that concern the client's health. The formation of nursing knowledge is multifaceted, taking into consideration such things as client's developmental factors, cultural influences, family factors, lifestyle issues, and emotional issues.

Perioperative nursing involves the nursing process of assessment, diagnosis, planning, treatment, and evaluation of problems resulting from the administration of anesthesia and medical interventions. In the preoperative or preanesthetic phase the nurse's role centers on (1) identifying actual or potential problems through assessment and interview techniques, (2) validating existing information, and (3) preparing the client both emotionally and physically for the surgical event (American Society of PeriAnesthesia Nurses [ASPAN] 1998). In the postoperative or postanesthesia phase the nurse's responsibilities include the transition of the client from total anesthesia to a state in which less nursing and medical intervention is required (phase I), preparation of the family and client to assume self-care or for transfer into another care environment (phase II), and the provision of ongoing care for clients requiring extended observation and interventions, as well as preparation to assume self-care (phase III) (ASPAN, 1998).

Critical Thinking Synthesis

Successful critical thinking requires a synthesis of knowledge, experience, information gathered from clients, critical thinking attitudes, and intellectual and professional standards. Clinical judgments require the nurse to anticipate the information necessary, analyze the data, and make decisions regarding client care. Critical thinking is always changing. During assessment (Figure 49-1) the nurse must consider all of the elements that build toward making appropriate nursing diagnoses.

In the case of caring for the perioperative client, the nurse integrates knowledge from anatomy and physiology, pathophysiology, and the surgical stress response, along with previous experiences in caring for surgical clients and information gathered from the specific client, to make clinical decisions for the client's care. The use of critical thinking attitudes such as perseverance is needed to find a plan of care that provides successful perioperative care (e.g., airway management, infection control, pain management, and discharge planning). The use of professional standards as developed by the Agency for Health Care Policy and Research (AHCPR, AORN, and the **American Society of PeriAnesthesia Nurses (ASPAN)** provide valuable guidelines for perioperative management and evaluation of process and outcomes.

The Nursing Process in the Preoperative Surgical Phase

Surgical clients enter the health care setting in different stages of health. A client may enter the hospital or ambulatory satellite unit on a predetermined day feeling relatively healthy and prepared to face elective surgery. In contrast, a victim of a motor vehicle accident may face emergency surgery with no time to prepare. The ability to establish rapport and maintain a professional relationship is an essential component of the preoperative phase. Nurses must do this quickly, but compassionately and effectively.

The surgical client may undergo tests and procedures to confirm or rule out alterations requiring surgery. Most testing is performed before the day of surgery. Usually clients scheduled for ambulatory surgery have tests done several days before surgery. Testing done the day of surgery is usually limited to such things as glucose monitoring for the diabetic client. Nurses must be familiar with the tests, their purpose, and how to monitor results.

The client meets many health care personnel, including surgeons, nurse anesthetists or anesthesiologists, therapists, and nurses. All play a role in the client's care and recovery. Family members attempt to provide support through their presence but face many of the same stressors as the client. The nurse must effectively communicate with the client and family because the nurse-client relationship is the foundation of care (see Chapter 22). The nurse assesses the client's physical, emotional, and spiritual well-being; recognizes the degree of surgical risk; coordinates diagnostic tests; identifies nursing diagnoses and nursing interventions; and establishes outcomes in collaboration with the client and the client's family. Pertinent data and the plan of care are communicated to the surgical team.

ASSESSMENT

Assessment of the surgical client can be extensive. Ambulatory and same-day surgical programs provide challenges in gathering a complete assessment in a limited time. A multidisciplinary team approach is essential. Clients are admitted only hours before the surgical event, so nurses must organize and verify data obtained preoperatively to implement a perioperative plan of care. This occurs not only with the ambulatory care client, but also with the client who will require a more prolonged hospital stay. It has become common practice for clients to be admitted the day of surgery, even for such major procedures as open heart surgery or craniotomy.

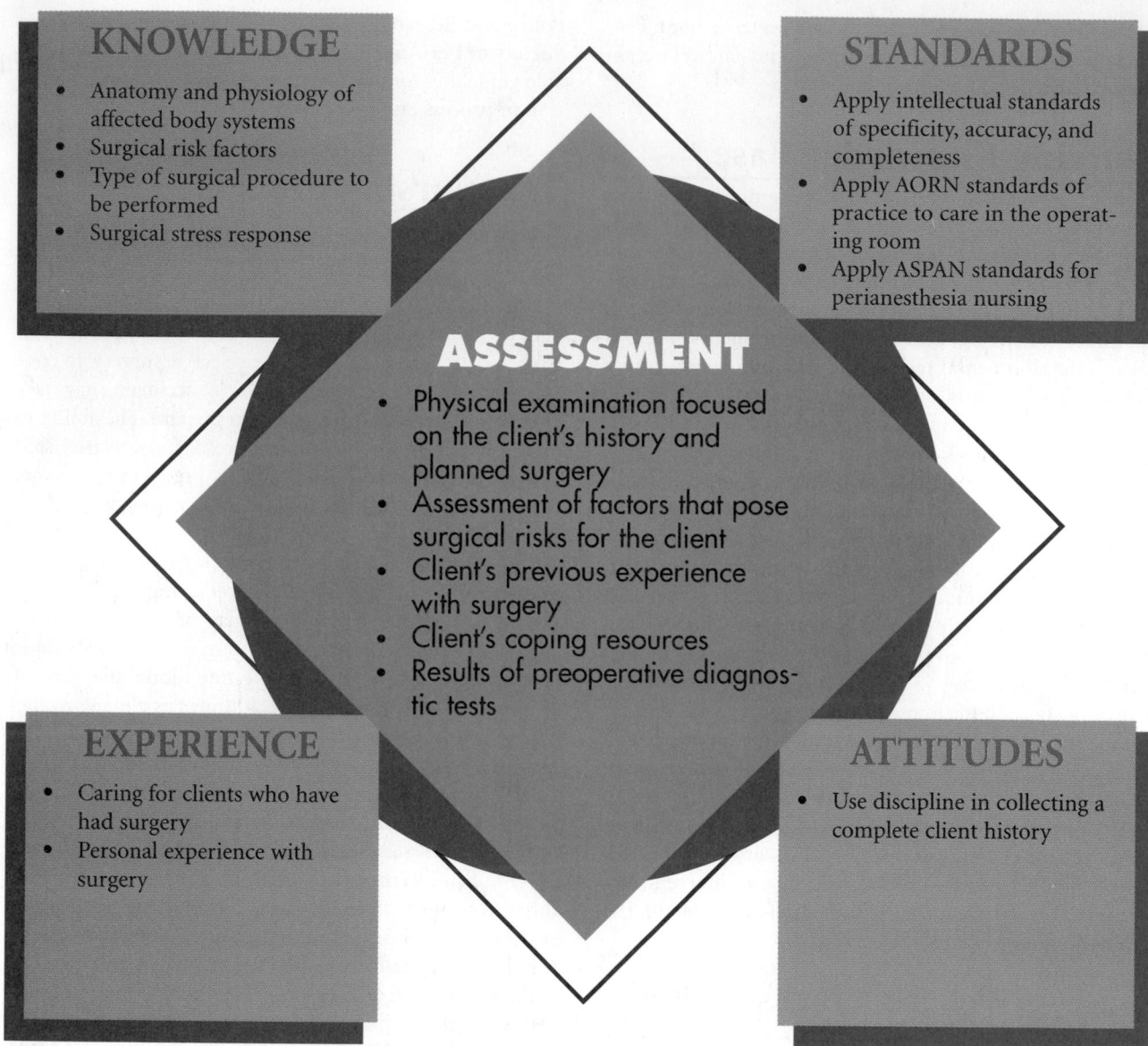

KNOWLEDGE

- Anatomy and physiology of affected body systems
- Surgical risk factors
- Type of surgical procedure to be performed
- Surgical stress response

STANDARDS

- Apply intellectual standards of specificity, accuracy, and completeness
- Apply AORN standards of practice to care in the operating room
- Apply ASPAN standards for perianesthesia nursing

ASSESSMENT

- Physical examination focused on the client's history and planned surgery
- Assessment of factors that pose surgical risks for the client
- Client's previous experience with surgery
- Client's coping resources
- Results of preoperative diagnostic tests

EXPERIENCE

- Caring for clients who have had surgery
- Personal experience with surgery

ATTITUDES

- Use discipline in collecting a complete client history

Figure 49-1   *Synthesis Model for Surgical Client Assessment Phase.*

The majority of assessments begin before admission for surgery—in the physician's office, preadmission clinic, anesthesia clinic, or by telephone. Clients may answer a self-report inventory, a rudimentary physical examination may be completed by a surgical nurse, laboratory tests may be drawn or completed, teaching is begun, questions are answered, and paperwork is initiated. This streamlines the care required by the client on the day of surgery. Nurses in the immediate preoperative period must assess the client's understanding of previous teaching and individualize client and family care.

A comprehensive history and physical examination is performed by the physician with follow-up by the preadmission testing nurse. In this case the nurse needs to review assessments and testing already completed so as not

to waste time duplicating information. The nurse focuses on key measurements for all body systems to ensure that no obvious problems are overlooked and that the client has understood education previously provided. Even though the surgeon will screen the client before scheduling surgery, preoperative assessment occasionally reveals an abnormality that delays or cancels surgery. For example, the client may have a cough and low-grade temperature on admission. This may indicate the onset of infection, and the surgeon will need to be notified immediately. Further education regarding the procedure may also be required.

The intention of the assessment of the surgical client is the same no matter what the setting is. The intent is to establish the client's normal preoperative function to assist the nurse in preventing and recognizing possible postoperative complications.

Nursing History.
The nurse conducts an initial interview to collect a client history similar to that described in Chapter 32. If a client is unable to relate all of the necessary information, the nurse relies on family members as resources.

Medical History.
A review of the client's medical history should include past illnesses and the primary reason for seeking medical care. The client's medical record is an excellent source. Another valuable source of data is medical records from past hospitalizations.

Preexisting illnesses can influence the choice of anesthetic agents used, as well as the client's ability to tolerate surgery and reach full recovery (Table 49-4). Candidates for ambulatory surgery must be carefully screened for medical conditions that may increase the risk for complications during or after surgery. For example, a client who has a history of congestive heart failure (CHF) may experience a further decline in cardiac function both intraoperatively and postoperatively. IV fluids may need to be administered at a slower rate, or a diuretic may need to be given after blood transfusions.

Previous Surgeries.
A client's past experience with surgery can influence physical and psychological responses to a procedure. The previous type of surgery, level of discomfort, extent of disability, and overall level of care provided are factors the nurse asks the client to recall. The nurse assesses any complications that the client experienced. Prior anesthesia records may be useful if any previous problems occurred. This information helps the nurse anticipate the client's preoperative and postoperative needs.

Previous surgery may also influence the level of physical care required after a surgical procedure. For example, a client who has had a previous thoracotomy for resection of a lung lobe has a greater risk for postoperative pulmonary complications than a client with intact normal lungs.

Perceptions and Understanding of Surgery.
The surgical experience affects not only the client, but the family unit as a whole. What affects the client will affect the family and vice versa. The nurse, therefore, must prepare both the client and the family for the surgical experience. Identification of client's and family's knowledge, expectations, and perceptions allows the nurse to plan teaching and emotional preparation measures.

Each client brings fears to the surgical setting. Some are due to past hospital experiences, warnings from friends

Table 49-4 Medical Conditions That Increase the Risks of Surgery

Type of Condition	Reason for Risk
Bleeding disorders (thrombocytopenia, hemophilia)	Disorders increase risk of hemorrhaging during and after surgery.
Diabetes mellitus	Diabetes increases susceptibility to infection and may impair wound healing from altered glucose metabolism and associated circulatory impairment. Fluctuating blood levels may cause central nervous system (CNS) malfunction during anesthesia. Stress of surgery may cause increases in blood glucose levels.
Heart disease (recent myocardial infarction, dysrhythmias, congestive heart failure) and peripheral vascular disease	Stress of surgery causes increased demands on myocardium to maintain cardiac output. General anesthetic agents depress cardiac function.
Upper respiratory infection	Infection increases risk of respiratory complications during anesthesia (e.g., pneumonia and spasm of laryngeal muscles).
Liver disease	Liver disease alters metabolism and elimination of drugs administered during surgery and impairs wound healing and clotting time because of alterations in protein metabolism.
Fever	Fever predisposes client to fluid and electrolyte imbalances and may indicate underlying infection.
Chronic respiratory disease (emphysema, bronchitis, asthma)	Respiratory disease reduces client's means to compensate for acid-base alterations (see Chapter 40). Anesthetic agents reduce respiratory function, increasing risk for severe hypoventilation.
Immunological disorders (leukemia, acquired immunodeficiency syndrome [AIDS], bone marrow depression, and use of chemotherapeutic drugs)	Immunological disorders increase risk of infection and delay wound healing after surgery.
Abuse of street drugs	Persons abusing drugs may have underlying disease (HIV/hepatitis) and altered wellness, which affect healing.
Chronic pain	Regular use of pain medications may result in higher tolerance. Increased doses of narcotics/analgesics may be required to achieve postoperative pain control.

and family, or lack of knowledge. The nurse faces an ethical dilemma when a client is misinformed or unaware of the reason for surgery. The nurse asks for a description of the client's understanding of the planned surgery and its implications. The nurse might ask questions such as "Tell me what you think will happen before and after surgery" or "Explain what you know about surgery." The nurse should confer with the physician if the client has an inaccurate perception or knowledge of the surgical procedure before the client is sent to the surgical suite. The nurse also determines whether the physician explained routine preoperative and postoperative procedures. When a client is well prepared and knows what to expect, the nurse reinforces the client's knowledge and maintains accuracy and consistency.

Medication History.   If a client regularly uses prescription or over-the-counter drugs, the surgeon or anesthesiologist/anesthetist may temporarily discontinue the drugs before surgery or adjust the dosages (Table 49-5). Certain drugs have special implications for the surgical client, creating greater risks for complications. Clients should also be asked if any herbal preparations are used, since many clients do not view herbs as medications and may omit them from their medication history. There are herbs that may interfere with the action of other medications (consult the pharmacist). For hospitalized clients, prescription drugs taken preoperatively are automatically discontinued postoperatively unless the physician reorders them.

Allergies.   The nurse is alert for allergies to drugs that may be given during a phase of the surgical experience. In addition, it is also critical to assess for latex, food, and contact allergies (e.g., to tape, ointments, or solutions). A client may be too young or have too few exposures to drugs to know if he or she has allergies. However, a client who has other allergies is at risk for drug allergies. The type of allergic response is also important. Allergies need to be delineated from unpleasant side effects. For example, the client may state that codeine causes nausea (a side effect), or it may cause hypotension and confusion (an allergy). It is critical that the client specifically be asked about latex allergies (see p. 1692), since a latex-free environment must be provided for clients with latex allergies. Once these clients come in contact with latex gloves used by the surgical team, serious reactions can develop. The nurse makes sure that a list of the client's allergies is noted appropriately in the client's chart and/or the hospital computer system, as well as any other places designated by institutional policy.

Smoking Habits.   The client who smokes is at greater risk for postoperative pulmonary complications than a client who does not. The chronic smoker already has an increased amount and thickness of mucous secretions in the lungs. General anesthetics increase airway irritation and stimulate pulmonary secretions, which are retained as a result of reduction in ciliary activity during anesthesia. After surgery the client who smokes has greater difficulty

Table 49-5 Drugs With Special Implications for the Surgical Client	
Drug Class	**Effects During Surgery**
Antibiotics	Antibiotics potentiate action of anesthetic agents. If taken within 2 weeks before surgery, aminoglycosides (gentamicin, tobramycin, neomycin) may cause mild respiratory depression from depressed neuromuscular transmission.
Antidysrhythmics	Antidysrhythmics can reduce cardiac contractility and impair cardiac conduction during anesthesia.
Anticoagulants	Anticoagulants alter normal clotting factors and thus increase risk of hemorrhaging. They should be discontinued at least 48 hours before surgery. Aspirin is a commonly used medication that can alter clotting mechanisms.
Anticonvulsants	Long-term use of certain anticonvulsants (e.g., phenytoin [Dilantin] and phenobarbital) can alter metabolism of anesthetic agents.
Antihypertensives	Antihypertensives interact with anesthetic agents to cause bradycardia, hypotension, and impaired circulation. They inhibit synthesis and storage of norepinephrine in sympathetic nerve endings.
Corticosteroids	With prolonged use, corticosteroids cause adrenal atrophy, which reduces body's ability to withstand stress. Before and during surgery, dosages may be temporarily increased.
Insulin	Diabetic client's need for insulin after surgery is reduced because client's nutritional intake is decreased. Stress response and intravenous (IV) administration of glucose solutions can increase dosage requirements after surgery.
Diuretics	Diuretics potentiate electrolyte imbalances (particularly potassium) after surgery.
Nonsteroidal antiinflammatory drugs (NSAIDs)	NSAIDs inhibit platelet aggregation and may prolong bleeding time, increasing susceptibility to postoperative bleeding.

clearing the airways of mucous secretions and needs emphasis on the importance of postoperative deep breathing and coughing (see Chapter 39).

Alcohol Ingestion and Substance Use and Abuse.

Habitual use of alcohol predisposes the client to adverse reactions to anesthetic drugs. The client also experiences a cross-tolerance to anesthetic drugs, necessitating higher-than-normal doses. In addition, the physician may need to increase postoperative dosages of analgesics. Excessive alcohol ingestion can also lead to malnutrition, which may contribute to delayed wound healing, as well as liver disease, portal hypertension, and esophageal varices (predisposing the client to bleeding disorders). The client who will remain in the hospital longer than 24 hours is also at risk for acute alcohol withdrawal and its more severe form, delirium tremens (DTs). The surgeon and anesthesiologist should be made aware of the client's history of alcohol use so that measures to prevent or treat withdrawal can be taken (Phipps, Sands, and Marek, 1999). Use of prescription narcotics or barbiturates, and abuse of street drugs may impair the ability of the client to manage pain following surgery, as well as affect the level and amount of anesthesia required during surgery. Intravenous (IV) drug use may impair the vascular system and may make venous access difficult. The client is more likely to be exposed to diseases such as human immunodeficiency virus (HIV) infection and hepatitis.

Family Support.

It is important for the nurse to determine the extent of the client's support from family members or friends. Because family not be defined by blood relations, it is best to have the client identify his or her support (or "family"). Surgery often results in temporary or permanent disability that requires added assistance during recovery. The client usually cannot immediately assume the same level of physical activity enjoyed before an illness. Often a client returns home with dressings to change or exercises to perform. With ambulatory surgery, clients and families assume responsibility for postoperative care. The family is an important resource for the client with physical limitations and provides the emotional support needed to motivate the client to return to a previous state of health. The family may better remember preoperative and postoperative teaching as well.

Occupation.

Surgery may result in physical alterations that hinder or prevent a person from returning to work. Ideally, the nurse assesses the client's occupational history to anticipate the possible effects of surgery on recovery and eventual work performance. This prepares the nurse to explain any restrictions before a client returns to work. When a client is unable to return to a job, the nurse confers with a social worker and/or occupational therapist to refer the client to job-training programs or to help the client seek economic assistance.

Preoperative Pain Assessment.

Surgical manipulation of tissues, treatments, and positioning on the operating room table may result in postoperative pain for the client. Pain is a very personal experience and requires an individualized plan of care. Preoperatively the nurse should conduct a comprehensive pain assessment (see Chapter 42), including the client's and family's expectations for pain management following surgery (Miaskowski, 1993). Clients may believe mistakenly that the nurse will detect their pain and treat it or that pain medication, if ordered, will be given on a schedule. Box 49-1 explores the issue of postoperative pain control and the perspective of the client as well as the nurse and physician. The client needs to be told that he or she must ask for pain medication. Preoperative education should include the use of a pain scale to rate the presence and severity of pain (see Chapter 42). Frequent pain assessments are necessary to alert the nurse to treat the pain and assess the adequacy (outcome) of pain interventions.

Review of Emotional Health.

Surgery is psychologically stressful. The client may be anxious about the

---

Research HIGHLIGHT   **Box 49-1**

RESEARCH ABSTRACT

The purpose of this study was to identify pain experience in the postsurgical client; identify discrepancies in reports of pain intensity between client, nurse, and physician; and describe the documentation of the client's pain. This was a descriptive study of 100 clients over a 3-month period. A two-part questionnaire was used for data collection. The first part of the questionnaire collected information regarding demographics, analgesics ordered and given at 24 and 72 hours, and effectiveness of postanalgesic administration. A structured client interview was conducted (part 2 of the questionnaire). Results of the study included the following: (1) 74% of clients reported experiencing pain during the interview, (2) 87% reported pain in the previous 24 hours, and (3) 90% reported pain in the past 72 hours. On average, only 17% of the total analgesic amounts ordered were given. Documentation of pain in the nursing progress note took place 94% of the time, and documentation of the effect of administered analgesics took place 70% of the time. Documentation of the intensity, quality, and pattern of pain ranged from 7% to 14%.

IMPLICATIONS FOR PRACTICE
- Despite new technology (new medications, patient-controlled analgesia [PCA], epidural analgesia), clients continue to experience pain following surgery.
- Nurses are administering insufficient amounts of medications to treat pain.
- Pain assessment and documentation by both nurses and physicians is not done frequently enough to determine a client's clinical status.

REFERENCE
Price J, Mahon, S, Faut-Callahan M: Pain control in hospitalized postsurgical patients, *MedSurg Nurs* 4(5):367, 1995.

surgery and its implications. Clients often feel that they are powerless over their situation. Family members may perceive the client's surgery as a disruption of their lifestyle. Hospitalization and the recovery period at home may be lengthy. The family is usually concerned about the client returning to a normal, productive life. When the client has chronic illness, the family may be fearful that surgery may result in further disability or hopeful that it may improve their lifestyle. To understand the impact of surgery on a client's and family's emotional health, the nurse assesses the client's feelings about surgery, self-concept, body image, and coping resources.

Feelings. The nurse may observe the client's feelings about surgery as expressed through mannerisms or behavior. A fearful client often asks many questions, seems uneasy when strangers enter the room, or actively seeks the company of friends and relatives. The nurse, however, must not assume to know the client's feelings. Questions such as "Can you tell me what you are thinking about regarding your surgery?" or "Are there any concerns about surgery we can talk about?" will help clients share their views.

It is often difficult to assess feelings thoroughly when ambulatory surgery is scheduled. The nurse usually has less time to establish a relationship with the client. In some outpatient surgical programs the nurse may visit with a client in the home or on the telephone before surgery. In a hospital room the nurse should choose a time for discussion after admitting procedures or diagnostic tests are completed. The nurse should explain that it is normal to have fears and concerns. The client's ability to share feelings depends on the nurse's willingness to listen, be supportive, and clarify misconceptions.

If the client feels powerless, the nurse determines the reason. The medical diagnosis may generate apprehension of increased dependence and loss of physical or mental function. The thought of being "put to sleep" under anesthesia may create concern about loss of control. Many clients feel the need to retain the power to make decisions about treatment. The nurse must assure clients of their right to ask questions and seek information.

A client may be angry about the need for surgery. For example, a young person may feel that it is unfair to have a disorder that typically affects older people. Surgery may occur at a time when it is inconvenient or potentially disruptive. The client may occasionally express anger by verbally attacking the nurse or physician. Being argumentative or overly demanding, refusing to cooperate, and criticizing the nurse's efforts to provide care are manifestations of anger and anxiety.

Self-Concept. Clients with a positive self-concept are more likely to approach surgical experiences appropriately. The nurse assesses self-concept by asking clients to identify personal strengths and weaknesses (see Chapter 26). Clients who are quick to criticize or scorn personal characteristics may have little self-regard or may be testing the nurse's opinion of their characters. Poor self-concept hinders the ability to adapt to the stress of surgery and aggravates feelings of guilt or inadequacy.

Body Image. Surgical removal of any diseased body part often leaves permanent disfigurement, alteration in body function, or concern over mutilation. Loss of certain body functions (e.g., with a colostomy or urostomy) compounds a client's fears. The nurse assesses for the body image alterations that clients perceive will result from surgery. Individuals will react differently depending on their self-concept and degree of self-esteem (see Chapter 26).

Often surgery changes the physical or psychological aspects of client's sexuality. Excision of breast tissue, colostomies, ureterostomies, hysterectomy, or removal of prostate glands may affect client's perceptions of their sexuality. Surgery such as hernia repair or cataract extraction forces clients to temporarily refrain from sexual intercourse until they return to normal physical activity.

The nurse should encourage clients to express concerns about sexuality. The client facing even temporary sexual dysfunction requires understanding and support. Discussions about the client's sexuality should be held with the client's sexual partner so that they can gain a shared understanding of how to cope with limitations in sexual function.

Coping Resources. Assessment of feelings and self-concept helps reveal whether the client can cope with the stress of surgery. The physiological effects of stress are well documented. Activation of the endocrine system results in the release of hormones and catecholamines (epinephrine, norepinephrine), which result in increases in blood pressure, heart rate, and respiration. Platelet aggregation also occurs, along with a myriad of other physiological responses. The nurse must be aware of these responses and assist with stress management. The nurse also asks the client about past stress management. If the client has had previous surgery, the nurse determines behaviors that helped resolve any tension or nervousness. The nurse may instruct the client on relaxation exercises that can help control anxiety (see Chapter 30).

The nurse should ask if family members or friends can provide support. The client may want someone else present when the nurse provides instructions or explanations. Family presence should be encouraged when feasible, especially for clients in the ambulatory setting. Often a family member can become the client's coach, offering valuable support during the postoperative period, when the client's participation in care is vital.

Culture. Culture is a system of beliefs that have developed over time and subsequently been passed on through many generations (Lipson, Dibble, and Minarik, 1996).

Americans come from diverse cultural and religious backgrounds. These backgrounds affect the way each client perceives and reacts to the surgical experience. If cultural, ethnic, and religious differences are not acknowledged and planned for in the perioperative plan of care, desired surgical outcomes may not be achieved. Therefore the acquisition of knowledge regarding cultural and ethnic groups assists the nurse in caring for the perioperative client. Examples of cultural differences (Lipson, Dibble, and Minarik, 1996) that may influence perioperative care are summarized in Table 49-6. The boxed information provides only a few examples of cultural care in perioperative nursing. Although it is important to recognize and plan for differences based on culture, it is also necessary to recognize that members of the same culture are individuals and may not hold these shared beliefs.

Physical Examination. The nurse conducts a partial or complete physical examination, depending on the amount of time available and the client's preoperative condition. Chapter 32 describes techniques used in physical assessment. Assessment focuses on findings related to the client's medical history and on body systems that will likely be affected by the surgery.

General Survey. The nurse observes the client's general appearance. Gestures and body movements may reflect weakness caused by illness. The client may appear malnourished to the nurse. Height and body weight are important indicators of nutritional status.

Preoperative assessment of vital signs, including blood pressure while sitting and standing, provides important baseline data with which to compare alterations that occur during and after surgery. Some institutions request that blood pressure be obtained in both arms for comparison. Anxiety and fear commonly cause elevations in heart rate and blood pressure. Anesthetic agents typically depress all vital functions. However, adverse drug reactions may include elevations in heart rate and blood pressure. As the effects of the anesthesia diminish after surgery, the nurse closely monitors vital signs and compares findings with the preoperative baseline.

Preoperative assessment of vital signs is also important to rule out fluid and electrolyte abnormalities (see Chapter 40). An elevated heart rate may result from a plasma-fluid volume deficit, potassium deficit, or sodium excess. If the pulse is full and bounding, a fluid volume excess may be the cause. Cardiac dysrhythmias are commonly caused by electrolyte imbalances, especially potassium, magnesium, and calcium.

An elevated temperature before surgery is a cause for concern. If the client has an underlying infection, the surgeon may choose to postpone surgery until the infection has been treated. An elevated body temperature increases the risk of fluid and electrolyte imbalance after surgery.

Head and Neck. The condition of oral mucous membranes reveals the level of hydration. A dehydrated client is at risk for developing serious fluid and electrolyte imbalances during surgery. Inspection of the soft palate and nasal sinuses can reveal sinus drainage indicative of respiratory or sinus infection. To rule out the possibility of local or systemic infection, the nurse palpates for cervical lymph node enlargement.

The nurse inspects the jugular veins for distention. Excess fluid within the circulatory system or failure of the heart to contract efficiently may lead to jugular vein distention and reveal a risk for cardiovascular complications during surgery.

Integument. The nurse carefully inspects the skin overlying all body parts. Particular attention is paid to bony prominences, such as the heels, elbows, sacrum, and scapula. During surgery, a client must lie in a fixed position, often for several hours. Thus a client is susceptible to pressure ulcers (see Chapter 47) if the skin is thin and dry and has poor turgor. Chronic use of steroids also increases the client's susceptibility to skin tears. The overall condition of the skin also reveals the client's level of hydration. An older adult is at high risk for alteration in skin integrity

Table 49-6 **Cultural Differences That May Influence the Surgical Experience**	
Ethnicity	General Considerations
Native Americans	Generally stoic when ill. Complaints of pain to nurse may be in general terms such as "I am uncomfortable." Under-treatment of pain is common. May have a basic lack of trust.
Arab-Americans	Verbal consent has more meaning than written consent because it is based on trust. Must explain fully the need for written consent. Very expressive regarding pain; pain may cause intense fear. Prepare client for painful procedures and develop a plan of care to prevent pain from occurring.
African-Americans	Generally are open to expression of pain but may avoid medication because of fear of addiction. If terminal diagnosis, news is best expressed through a family care conference or speaking with client's minister.
Vietnamese-Americans	Having an interpreter is very important. May need to be a hired interpreter, depending on sensitivity of subject being discussed (because of modesty). A female family member is expected to be at bedside for care and comfort. Men are the decision makers and support for the family.

from positioning and sliding on the operating room table, causing shear and pressure.

Thorax and Lungs.   Assessment of the client's breathing pattern and chest excursion aids in assessing ventilatory capacity. Clients are encouraged to deep breathe and cough postoperatively. A decline in ventilatory function may place the client at risk for respiratory complications. For example, a client who has high abdominal surgery will have difficulty breathing deeply because of a painful abdominal incision. Auscultation of breath sounds will indicate whether the client has pulmonary congestion or narrowing of airways. Assessment of the client's color for pallor or cyanosis will also point to possible respiratory problems. As a general rule, central cyanosis may indicate a respiratory problem, whereas peripheral cyanosis may indicate a cardiovascular problem (Price and Wilson, 1997).

Existing atelectasis or moisture in the airways will be aggravated during surgery. Serious pulmonary congestion may cause postponement of the surgery. Certain anesthetics can cause laryngeal muscle spasm; thus if the nurse auscultates wheezing in the airways preoperatively, the client is at risk for further airway narrowing during surgery and after extubation (removal of the endotracheal tube). The nurse should assess for clubbing of the fingers, which may indicate lung disease and possible postanesthetic difficulty (Price and Wilson, 1997).

Heart and Vascular System.   If the client has cardiac disease, the nurse assesses the character of the apical pulse. After surgery the nurse compares the rate and rhythm of the pulse with preoperative baselines. Anesthetic agents, alterations in fluid and electrolyte balance, and stimulation from the surgical stress response can cause cardiac dysrhythmias.

The nurse assesses peripheral pulses, capillary refill time, and the color and temperature of extremities to determine a client's circulatory status. If peripheral pulses are not palpable, a Doppler instrument should be used for assessment of their presence. Acceptable capillary refill occurs in less than 3 seconds. Sluggish capillary refill is refill time greater than 3 seconds.

Measurement of capillary refill and assessment of peripheral pulses are particularly important for the client having vascular surgery or for a client who may have casts or constricting bandages applied to the extremities after surgery. Postoperative development of a weak or absent pulse in a client who had adequate circulation before surgery indicates impaired circulation.

Abdomen.   The nurse assesses the abdomen for size, shape, symmetry, and distention. If the client has abdominal surgery, the nurse makes frequent postoperative assessments of the abdominal incision and compares findings with preoperative data. Distention may indicate postoperative alterations in gastrointestinal function. The

nurse should know whether the client has a protuberant abdomen or whether the abdomen has become distended after surgery.

Assessment of preoperative bowel sounds is useful as a baseline. The nurse also determines whether the client has regular bowel movements and the color and consistency of stools. If the surgery requires manipulation of the gastrointestinal tract or if a general anesthetic is used, normal peristalsis will not return and bowel sounds will be absent or diminished for several days after surgery.

Neurological Status.   Preoperative assessment of neurological status is imperative for all clients receiving general anesthesia. The baseline neurological status assists with the assessment of ascent from anesthesia. During the health history and physical assessment, the nurse observes the client's level of orientation, alertness, and mood, noting whether the client answers questions appropriately and can recall recent and past events. A client who will have surgery for neurological disease (e.g., brain tumor or aneurysm) is likely to demonstrate an impaired level of consciousness or altered behavior. Level of consciousness changes as a result of general anesthesia. However, after the effects of anesthesia disappear, the client should return to the preoperative level of responsiveness.

If the client will have spinal anesthesia, preoperative assessment of gross motor function and strength is important. Spinal anesthesia causes temporary paralysis of the lower extremities (see Chapter 42). The nurse should be aware of a client entering surgery with weakness or impaired mobility of the lower extremities to avoid becoming alarmed when full motor function does not return as the spinal anesthetic wears off.

Risk Factors.   It is necessary for the nurse to assess the client for the presence of risk factors. Risk factors are obtained by client or family interview, as well as present and past medical records. Risk factors help the nurse to establish a perioperative plan of care that addresses immediate and potential problems.

Diagnostic Screening.   Before a client has surgery, the surgeon may order diagnostic tests to screen for preexisting abnormalities. Historically, it was routine to do standard baseline diagnostic studies no matter what the surgical procedure or health of the client was. A CBC, electrolytes, urinalysis, BUN, creatinine level, chest x-ray study, and electrocardiogram (ECG) were commonly done on many surgical clients, even those categorized as PS-1 (the normal healthy client). Tests now are determined by the client's history and physical assessment (Greenfield and others, 1997). Table 49-7 contains common diagnostic tests drawn preoperatively based on the client's medical history. For example, the client with a history of renal insufficiency may require a recent BUN and creatinine level to determine preoperative renal function.

Also, a hemoglobin (Hgb) and hematocrit (Hct) may be necessary, since clients with renal disease are frequently anemic from decreased levels of erythropoietin. Tests are also determined by the procedure itself. Since blood loss frequently occurs with hip and knee replacements, a type and crossmatch would be indicated preoperatively. Table 49-8 gives the purpose and normal values for the more common blood tests. If diagnostic tests reveal severe problems, the surgeon may cancel surgery until the condition stabilizes.

The nurse is responsible for the preparation of clients for diagnostic studies and for coordinating completion of

Table 49-7   Common Diagnostic Tests Performed Preoperatively Based on Client History

History	Tests
Hepatic disease	Prothrombin time/partial thromboplastin time (PT/PTT); liver enzymes, such as serum glutamic-oxaloacetic transaminase (SGOT); alkaline phosphatase
Medications:	
Diuretics	Blood urea nitrogen (BUN), creatinine, electrolytes
Steroids	Electrolytes, glucose
Cardiovascular disease	BUN, creatinine, CBC, chest x-ray study, electrocardiogram (ECG)
Pulmonary disease	Complete blood count (CBC), chest x-ray study, ECG
Central nervous system disease	White blood cell (WBC) count, electrolytes, BUN, creatinine, glucose, and ECG

Table 49-8   Diagnostic Screening for Surgical Clients

Type of Test	Purpose/Significance	Common Values

Complete blood count (CBC)	Peripheral venous sample of blood measures red blood cells (RBCs), white blood cells (WBCs), hemoglobin (Hgb), and hematocrit (Hct). May reveal infection, low blood volume, and potential for oxygenation problems. Surgeon may order blood replacement.	RBC:
		  Men: 4.7-6.1 million/mm³
		  Women: 4.2-5.4 million/mm³
		Hgb:
		  Men: 14.7-16.1 g/100 ml
		  Women: 12-16 g/100 ml
		Hct:
		  Men: 42%-52%
		  Women: 37%-47%
		WBC: Adults and children >2 yrs:
		  5000-10,000/mm³

Serum electrolytes	Peripheral venous sample of blood reveals significant fluid and electrolyte imbalances preoperatively. Attention is given to Na, K, and Cl levels. IV fluid replacement may be indicated preoperatively.	Sodium (Na⁺): 135-145 mEq/L Potassium (K⁺): 3.5-5.0 mEq/L Chloride (Cl⁻): 100-106 mEq/L Bicarb (HCO₃⁻): 24-32 mEq/L
Coagulation studies	Prothrombin time (PT), partial thromboplastin time (PTT), and platelet counts reveal clotting ability of blood. Reveals clients at risk for bleeding tendencies and thrombus formation.	PT: Less than 2-second deviation from control PTT: 25-27 seconds Platelets: 150,000-350,000/mm³
Serum creatinine	Ability of kidneys to excrete creatinine, by-product of muscle metabolism, assesses renal function. Elevated level can indicate renal failure.	Creatinine: 0.5-1.5 mg/100 ml
Blood urea nitrogen (BUN)	Ability of kidneys to excrete urea and nitrogen indicates renal function. BUN becomes elevated if client is dehydrated. Preoperative IV fluid replacement may be needed.	BUN: 7-22 mg/100 ml
Glucose	Finger stick or peripheral blood sample. Clients may require treatment of low or high levels preoperatively and postoperatively.	Fasting: 70-105 Random: 70-140

the tests. The nurse also reviews diagnostic results as they become available to alert physicians to findings and to assist with planning appropriate therapy.

Additional Screening Tests.

If a client is over the age of 40 or has heart disease, the physician may order a chest x-ray study or an ECG. The chest x-ray study is an examination of the condition of the heart and lungs. If the physician detects lung abnormalities, a different type and dosage of sedatives or anesthetic agents may be used. The female client requiring radiographic studies needs to be asked if there is a possibility that she is pregnant, since exposure to radiation may cause injury to a fetus. If the client is unsure, serum or urine B-Hcg levels will need to be ordered. Some institutions routinely use lead aprons placed over the client's abdomen in this population. An ECG measures the heart's electrical activity to determine whether the heart rate, rhythm, and other factors are normal. The procedure takes less than 5 minutes and requires the client simply to lie flat and relax.

Depending on the type of surgery the client will undergo, there are several diagnostic tests for specific anatomical structures and physiological functions. Pulmonary function testing and occasionally arterial blood gas analysis may be performed on clients with preexisting lung disease. Blood glucose levels are measured preoperatively on diabetic clients. If the client is likely to lose a large amount of blood during surgery, the physician orders a blood specimen for type and crossmatching to determine the proper blood type and Rh factor. The surgeon usually designates the number of blood units to have available during surgery.

Autogolous infusions are an option for some clients who choose to donate their own blood before surgery to reduce the risk of transfusion-related infections. The donation usually must be made several weeks before the scheduled surgery. Autotransfusion via the use of a cell-saver device in surgery may be possible if physicians are anticipating large blood loss (e.g., open heart surgery). The cell saver, although expensive, returns washed red blood cells to the client and decreases the risk of HIV infection and hepatitis B by using the client's own blood and has created positive outcomes in terms of length of client stay (Meeker and Rothrock, 1999).

Client Expectations.

Clients rely on their caregivers for information, comfort, pain control, adequate monitoring, and performance of interventions that ensure their safety throughout the surgical experience. This involves having a caring attitude, serving as an advocate for the client, being skilled in surgical assessment and interventions, and anticipating the client's needs throughout the perioperative period. Each plan of care must be individualized to the client, which makes it essential to understand the client's expectations. Do they expect full pain relief or simply to have their pain reduced? Do they expect to be independent immediately after surgery, or do they expect to be fully dependent on the nurse or family? These are only a few of the questions that need to be asked of the surgical client to establish a plan of care congruent with the client's needs and expectations.

❧ NURSING DIAGNOSIS

The nurse clusters patterns of defining characteristics gathered during assessment to identify nursing diagnoses for the surgical client (Box 49-2). The client with preexisting health problems is likely to have a variety of risk diagnoses (Box 49-3). For example, a client with preexisting bronchitis who has abnormal breath sounds and a productive cough will be at risk for *ineffective airway clearance*. The nature of the surgery and the client's health status provide defining characteristics for a number of nursing diagnoses. For example, a client who undergoes a surgical procedure is at risk for developing infection at either the surgical site, the IV site, or the bloodstream (sepsis). A diagnosis of *risk for infection* will require the nurse's attention from admission through convalescence.

The related factors for each diagnosis establish directions for nursing care that will be provided during one or all surgical phases. For example, the diagnosis of *risk for infection related to an invasive procedure* will require different interventions than if the related factors were inadequate immune response. Preoperative nursing diagnoses allow the nurse to take precautions and actions so that care provided during the intraoperative and postoperative phases is consistent with the client's needs.

Nursing diagnoses made preoperatively may also focus on the potential risks a client may face after surgery.

❧ SAMPLE NURSING DIAGNOSTIC PROCESS   Box 49-2
CLIENTS FACING SURGERY

Assessment Activities	Defining Characteristics	Nursing Diagnosis
Ask client to describe previous surgical experiences.	Apprehension	Fear related to knowledge deficit and previous surgical experience
Ask client about preoperative education/preparation before admission.	Frightened	
Observe client's nonverbal behavior.	Identifies fear of surgery	
Assess vital signs.	Unaware of preoperative testing	
	Increased tension	
	Increased heart rate	

NURSING DIAGNOSES   Box 49-3
SURGICAL CLIENTS

Airway clearance, ineffective
Breathing pattern, ineffective
Constipation, risk for
Coping, family: potential for growth
Fear
Fluid volume deficit, risk for
Infection, risk for
Knowledge deficit (specify)
Latex allergy response, risk for
Management of therapeutic regimen, individual: effective
Mobility, impaired physical
Pain
Powerlessness
Skin integrity, impaired, risk for
Surgical recovery, delayed

Preventive care is essential so that the surgical client can be managed effectively.

PLANNING

During planning the nurse again synthesizes information from multiple resources (Figure 49-2). For example, knowledge pertaining to adult learning principles, coupled with the client's unique needs, will ensure a well-designed **preoperative teaching** plan. Critical thinking ensures that the client's plan of care integrates all that the nurse knows about the individual, as well as key critical thinking elements. Previous experience in caring for surgical clients helps the nurse anticipate how to approach client care (e.g., complications to look for and methods to reduce anxiety). Professional standards are especially important to consider when the nurse develops a plan of care. These standards often establish scientifically proven guidelines for selecting effective nursing interventions. For example, ANA and AORN (1972) have established criteria to demonstrate client understanding of the surgical procedure following preoperative education.

The nurse develops an individualized plan of care for each nursing diagnosis (see care plan). The nurse and client set realistic expectations for care. Goals are to be individualized and realistic with measurable outcomes.

Successful critical thinking requires the involvement of the surgical client and family in establishing the plan of care. The nurse must provide the client and family with necessary information to assist in decision making regarding care. Involving the client early when developing the surgical care plan minimizes surgical risks and postoperative complications. For example, nursing research has shown that structured preoperative teaching can reduce the length of the client's hospital stay (Dalayon, 1994). A client informed about the surgical experience is less likely to be fearful and can prepare to participate in the postop-

erative recovery phase so that outcomes can be met. It is important to include the client and family in developing the plan of care and establishing outcomes. Diagnosis, interventions, and outcomes are established to ensure recovery or maintenance of the preoperative state.

For ambulatory surgery clients and clients admitted the day of their scheduled surgery, preoperative planning occurs (ideally) days before admission to the hospital or surgical center. Frequently, preoperative education begins in the physician's office, continues during the scheduled preadmission testing visit, and is reinforced by the nurse the day of admission. Preoperative information and instructions may include follow-up telephone calls, mailings from the physician's office or hospital, or the use of videotapes or client pathways (Figure 49-3). Preoperative instruction gives the client time to think about the surgical experience, make necessary physical preparations (e.g., altering diet or discontinuing medication use), and ask questions about postoperative procedures. The ambulatory surgical client usually returns home on the day of surgery. Thus well-planned preoperative care ensures that the client is well informed and able to be an active participant during recovery. The family or spouse can also play an active supportive role for the client.

The preoperative care plan is based on individualized nursing diagnoses. However, each client must undergo basic preparations. Goals of care for the surgical client include the following:

Understanding physiological and psychological responses to surgery
Understanding intraoperative and postoperative events
Achieving emotional comfort and relaxation
Achieving a return of normal physiological function after surgery (e.g., return of normal vital signs, temperature, and muscle function)
Maintaining a normal fluid and electrolyte balance
Achieving comfort and rest
Remaining free of surgical wound infection
Remaining safe from harm during the perioperative period

IMPLEMENTATION

Preoperative nursing interventions provide the client with a complete understanding of the surgery and prepare the client physically and psychologically for surgical intervention.

Informed Consent.   Surgery cannot be legally or ethically performed until a client understands the need for a procedure, the steps involved, risks, expected results, and alternative treatments. To operate without **informed consent** is battery (see Chapter 21). The primary responsibility for informing the client rests with the physician. Consent is not informed if the client is confused, uncon-

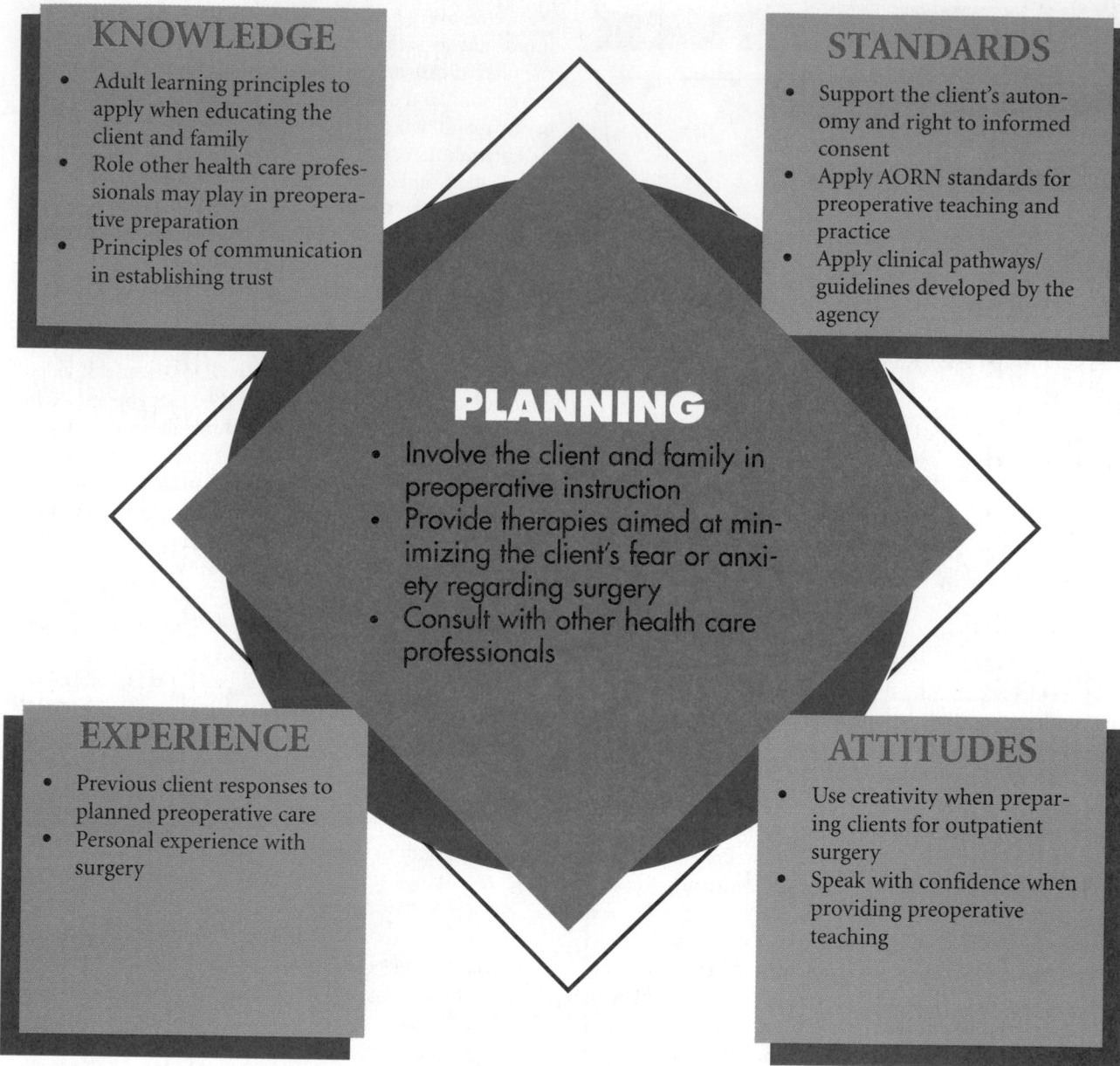

KNOWLEDGE

- Adult learning principles to apply when educating the client and family
- Role other health care professionals may play in preoperative preparation
- Principles of communication in establishing trust

STANDARDS

- Support the client's autonomy and right to informed consent
- Apply AORN standards for preoperative teaching and practice
- Apply clinical pathways/guidelines developed by the agency

PLANNING

- Involve the client and family in preoperative instruction
- Provide therapies aimed at minimizing the client's fear or anxiety regarding surgery
- Consult with other health care professionals

EXPERIENCE

- Previous client responses to planned preoperative care
- Personal experience with surgery

ATTITUDES

- Use creativity when preparing clients for outpatient surgery
- Speak with confidence when providing preoperative teaching

Figure 49-2   *Synthesis Model for Surgical Client Planning Phase.*

scious, mentally incompetent, or under the influence of sedatives or narcotics. All consent forms must be signed by the client *before* the nurse administers preoperative medications that will sedate the client. Ideally, a physician obtains consent before the client is admitted to the hospital or satellite ambulatory surgical setting. Each organization has a surgical consent form that includes a description of the procedure to be performed, risks, and a statement that the procedure has been explained by the physician.

The surgeon's explanation should be witnessed by a qualified member of the health care team. The form's structure allows the physician to write information related to the surgery. A client's signature on a consent form implies that the client has been thoroughly informed about

the procedure. The nurse frequently witnesses signing of the form and examines the document for the correct date, time, and signature, which must be in ink. A client who is illiterate can sign by making a mark, as long as it is properly witnessed. As a witness the nurse is able to attest that the client's signature is on the form but not that the client was properly informed. In many institutions a time limit is placed on consent forms (e.g., 30 days).

In emergencies the client may be unable to sign and family members or a legal guardian may be unavailable. The physician is legally permitted to perform surgery without consent in such a case. However, every effort must be made to obtain permission from a responsible family member by telephone, by telegram, or in some states by court order. A

SAMPLE NURSING CARE PLAN

PERIOPERATIVE CLIENT

ASSESSMENT*

Mrs. Campana is an 80-year-old client scheduled to be admitted in 5 days for elective bowel resection. Joe Marrero is the nurse in the clinic surgery service assigned to prepare Mrs. Campana for surgery. During Joe's initial discussion with Mrs. Campana, he observes her to be alert and oriented. Mrs. Campana has severely reduced visual acuity but is able to hear Joe's questions clearly. Mrs. Campana last **had surgery over 20 years ago.** She says to Joe, **"It is my understanding that I will probably be in the hospital for quite a while."** Joe clarifies that hospitalization for surgery is shorter than what was expected 20 years ago. After further questioning, Joe learns that **Mrs. Campana has not received instruction on the surgical procedure and the routines for postoperative recovery.** Mrs. Campana shows **interest in Joe's questions** and **asks what to expect following surgery.**

*Defining characteristics are shown in bold type.

NURSING DIAGNOSIS: Knowledge deficit regarding preoperative and postoperative care requirements related to lack of exposure to information.

PLANNING

GOALS

Client will participate actively in postoperative recovery activities by day 1 following surgery.

Client will understand the postoperative routines of surgical care by day before surgery

EXPECTED OUTCOMES

Client will successfully perform postoperative exercises by morning of surgery.

Client will discuss monitoring routines following surgery by morning of surgery.

Client will be able to describe importance of postoperative exercises by morning of surgery.

Client will be able to describe schedule for activity and nutritional management following surgery by day 1 postoperatively.

INTERVENTIONS†

Teaching: Preoperative

- Provide client with audiotape program that explains preoperative and postoperative routines. Supply instruction booklet designed for visually impaired. Make a follow-up call to give client opportunity to ask questions and voice concerns.

- On admission to hospital, demonstrate to client performance of postoperative exercises and how to get out of bed.
- Explain sensations to be expected postoperatively (e.g., incisional pain, IV, nasogastric tube, wound care solutions).
- Give client opportunity to return demonstrate postoperative exercises before surgery.
- Correct any unrealistic expectations client may have of surgery.

RATIONALE

Greater effects are gained when preoperative education involves individual rather than group teaching (Hathaway, 1986). Preadmission education can require less teaching time and better performance of exercises on admission (Rice and others, 1992). Education has a beneficial effect in reducing postoperative anxiety (Shuldham, 1999).

Demonstration is an effective method to reinforce didactic instruction.

Teaching about sensory aspects (what the client sees, feels, smells) should be structured (Shuldham, 1999).

Return demonstration measures client learning and provides opportunity to reinforce instruction.

Unrealistic expectations, when unmet, can contribute to client's anxiety. Psychologic preparation for surgery reduces anxiety (Devine and Cook, 1992).

†Intervention Classification labels from McCloskey JC, Bulechek GM: *Nursing interventions classification (NIC),* ed 3, St. Louis, 2000, Mosby.

EVALUATION

Ask client to describe typical monitoring and care activities following surgery.

Observe client's demonstration of postoperative exercises.

Plan a discussion asking client to express any remaining fears or concerns.

---

telephone consent must be witnessed by two persons who hear the family member's verbal consent. The two witnesses sign the consent with the name of the family member, noting that a verbal consent was obtained. Informed consent is critical to protect the client's legal rights.

After the consent form has been completed, the nurse makes sure that the form is placed in the client's medical record. The record goes to the operating room with the client. Chapter 21 discusses in detail the nurse's responsibilities for informed consent.

Preoperative Teaching.   Client education is an important aspect of the client's surgical experience (Fortner, 1998). Preoperative teaching concerning a client's expected postoperative behavior, provided in a systematic and structured format with teaching and learning princi-

	DAY OF SURGERY—BEFORE GOING TO SURGERY	SURGICAL INTENSIVE CARE UNIT (SICU)	DAY 1 - ON PROGRESSIVE CARDIOVASCULAR UNIT (PCVU)
OBSERVATIONS & TREATMENTS	You will take your second shower with special soap before leaving home or with the nurse's help if you are in the hospital. Do not use lotions, powders, or deodorants. Put on your blood bracelet, if not already done. In the hospital, your height, weight, blood pressure, pulse, breathing rate, and temperature will be measured. Give your glasses and jewelry to your family. You will wear a hospital gown. An IV may be started in a vein in your arm.	You will come straight to the SICU after surgery. You will have several different IVs, tubes, and wires connected to various pieces of equipment. Each has a specific purpose that allows us to watch your progress closely. We will monitor your temperature, blood pressure, pulse, heart rhythm, heart function, breathing, and oxygen level. Your breathing will be controlled by a machine through a tube in your mouth until it is safe for you to breathe on your own. Tubes will drain excess fluid and blood from your chest and urine from your bladder. You may have a tube in your nose that goes into your stomach to keep it empty. You will have bandages over your incisions. Chest x-rays and blood tests will be taken as needed. Once the breathing tube is removed, you will begin your breathing exercises. We will encourage you to do a lot of deep breathing. The morning after surgery, most of the IVs, tubes, and wires will be removed and you will transfer to the PCCU.	Your blood pressure, pulse, temperature, breathing rate, and oxygen level will be checked at least every 4 hours. Your heart rhythm is constantly watched on a monitor. If you are diabetic, your blood sugar will be checked before meals and at bedtime until you go home. You will continue the breathing exercises that you started in the SICU—20 times every 2 hours. Deep breathing is very important! Some patients need other breathing treatments, which will be given by the pulmonary staff. You will be weighed every day before breakfast. Your bandages will be changed and might come off entirely today. Some drainage is normal. You will wear white elastic stockings to increase circulation and decrease swelling. They may be taken off at night while you sleep. It is important to keep your legs up on a stool (even with your hips) or up on the recliner footrest whenever you sit for more than 30 minutes.
ACTIVITY	You may be up walking until the preoperative medication is given.	After the breathing tube has been removed for a few hours, we will help you to sit on the edge of the bed. Starting the day after surgery, you will sit in the chair for meals.	You will sit in the chair for 1 hour at mealtimes. You may walk to the bathroom with help. The cardiac rehab staff will walk with you today (Step 1). The first 2 days after surgery are very busy, and your rest is very important.
DIET	You should have nothing to eat or drink.	After the breathing tube has been removed, and if you don't have any nausea, your nurse will give you clear liquids or ice chips in small amounts.	Today you will get a soft diet with small servings. It is important to eat, even if your appetite is poor. We will limit the amount of fluids that you drink to 2 quarts each day.
MEDICATIONS	One of your doctors will order a pill or shot to make you sleepy before surgery. Oxygen will be started after the medication is given.	Medications will be given to you as ordered by your doctor. Intravenous fluids and medications will be infusing as needed. You will take pain pills and other medications by mouth after the breathing tube is out.	You will be taking several different medications. Good pain control is important so you feel like doing the activity needed for recovery. Your nurse will ask you to describe your pain level on a 0-10 scale with 0 = no pain, and 10 = worst pain. It is important to take your pain medication every 3-4 hours. If you are nauseated, let your nurse know so medication can be given to help. You will have an IV in your neck or arm for medications, if needed.
EDUCATION	Preadmission patients should follow their preadmission instructions sheet. The nurses will be explaining and reinforcing information you have already heard. Please ask questions. Your family will be given directions to the waiting room. They will be notified when you have gone to the SICU.	The SICU is a busy place, and your nurse will explain noises, IVs, tubes, and equipment to you and your family. The nurses will discuss and answer any questions you or your family may have regarding your progress and plan of care. Visiting time will be discussed with you and your family. Please read the ICU visitor's brochure.	We will teach you and reinforce the following: • Proper ways to move in and out of bed • Pain control • Breathing exercises • Supporting your chest incision • 5-pound weight limit • Importance of eating • Fluid restriction You and/or your family members or visitors may attend class at 1:30 PM, Monday, Tuesday, or Wednesday each week.
GOING HOME			

Figure 49-3　Client pathway for coronary artery bypass graft (CABG). The first day of a 6-day pathway highlights what the client can expect the day of surgery. Courtesy Genesis Medical Center, Davenport, Iowa.

ples, has a positive influence on the client's recovery. Structured preoperative teaching can influence postoperative factors such as the following:

Ventilatory function. Demonstrating the technique of deep breathing and coughing will assist the client in performing these exercises postoperatively.

Physical functional capacity. Teaching the client leg exercises and turning will improve the client's ability to ambulate and resume activities of daily living early.

Sense of well-being. Clients who are prepared for surgery experience less anxiety and report a greater sense of psychological well-being (Shuldham, 1999).

Length of hospital stay. Structured preoperative teaching has reduced the length of stay. However, it becomes increasingly difficult to effect a reduction, since the length of stay shortens because of financial pressures (Shuldham, 1999).

Pain control. Anxiety about pain and amount of pain medication needed for comfort. Clients who undergo teaching about pain and ways to relieve it are less anxious about pain, ask for what they need, and actually need lesser amounts of pain medication.

The most effective teaching program for surgical clients is planned so that all clients receive the same information. Detailed discussion and demonstration of postoperative exercises is vital. If the client understands why these exercises are important to postoperative recovery and knows how to perform them correctly, the recovery period will be less complicated.

Preadmission nurses may call clients up to 1 week before surgery to clarify questions and reinforce explanations. Educational strategies that meet the needs of clients in today's surgical settings of ambulatory surgery, same-day admission, and shortened lengths of stay need to be devised. Lookinland and Pool (1998) found that clients who received structured education before admission had better clinical outcomes and were more satisfied. However, despite the education being provided to clients, client retention following discharge is poor, especially in the elderly population (Bean and Waldron, 1995). Lee and others (1998) conducted postdischarge surveys of 206 clients hospitalized over a 6-week period. Results from this study indicated that continuity of care was enhanced if education was provided before, during, and after discharge. They found that half of the clients who were contacted requested additional education. Therefore it seems ideal to attempt perioperative education before admission, during the hospital stay, and after discharge. Most ambulatory care centers conduct follow-up surveys on clients through telephone interview at 24 hours following discharge.

Including family members in perioperative preparation is advised. Often a family member is the coach for postoperative exercises when the client returns from surgery. If anxious relatives do not understand routine postoperative events, it is likely that their anxiety will heighten the client's fears and concerns. Perioperative preparation of family members before surgery minimizes anxiety and misunderstanding.

The nurse should provide clients with information about sensations typically experienced after surgery. Preparatory information helps clients anticipate the steps of a procedure and thus helps them form realistic images of the surgical experience. When events occur as predicted, clients are better able to cope and attend to the experiences. For example, in the operating room the anesthesiologist may apply ointment to clients' eyes to prevent corneal damage. Warning clients about sensations of blurred vision will reduce their anxiety on awakening from surgery. Sensations that the nurse may describe include the expected pain at the surgical site, the tightness of dressings, dryness of the mouth, or the sensation of a sore throat resulting from an endotracheal tube.

Anxiety and fear are barriers to learning, and both emotions are heightened as surgery approaches. The nurse assesses the surgical client's readiness and ability to learn. If the client is capable of and receptive to learning, the nurse presents information in a logical sequence, beginning with preoperative events and advancing to intraoperative and postoperative routines. If possible, the family or significant others should be present during teaching. Preoperative teaching guidelines and checklists give nurses useful practice standards for presenting comprehensive instructions.

The following standards have been established by ANA and AORN (1972) to demonstrate client understanding of the surgical experience.

Client Cites Reasons for Preoperative Instructions and Exercises.   Given a rationale for preoperative and postoperative procedures, the client is better prepared to participate in care. Every preoperative teaching program includes explanation and demonstration of the five postoperative exercises: diaphragmatic breathing, incentive spirometry, positive expiratory pressure (PEP) therapy, coughing, turning, and leg exercises. These exercises are designed to prevent postoperative complications (Skill 49-1).

When a client is under general anesthesia, the lungs do not ventilate fully. After surgery the client has a reduced lung volume and needs greater effort to breathe. Diaphragmatic breathing improves lung expansion and oxygen delivery without using excess energy. The client learns to use the diaphragm during deep breathing to take slow, deep, and relaxed breaths. Eventually the client's lung volume improves. Deep breathing also helps clear out anesthetic gases remaining in the airways. To facilitate deep breathing, the physician may order an *incentive spirometer* for the client, which encourages effective deep breathing through sustained maximal inspiration (see Chapter 39). During surgery, venous blood flow to the legs

Skill 49-1 Demonstrating Postoperative Exercises

Delegation Considerations

This skill requires problem solving and knowledge application unique to a professional nurse. For this reason, delegation of this skill to assistive personnel is inappropriate. The registered nurse can educate assistive personnel to encourage clients to practice exercises regularly following instruction.

EQUIPMENT
- Pillow or wrapped towel (optional)
- Incentive spirometer
- Positive expiratory pressure (PEP) device and nose clip

STEPS	RATIONALE
1. Assess client's risk for postoperative respiratory complications. Review medical history to identify presence of chronic pulmonary conditions (e.g., emphysema, asthma), any condition that affects chest wall movement, history of smoking, and presence of reduced hemoglobin.	General anesthesia predisposes client to respiratory problems because lungs are not fully inflated during surgery; cough reflex is suppressed, so mucus collects within airway passages. After surgery, client may have reduced lung volume and require greater efforts to cough and deep breathe; inadequate lung expansion can lead to atelectasis and pneumonia. Client is at greater risk to develop respiratory complications if other chronic lung conditions are present. Smoking damages ciliary clearance and increases mucus secretion. Reduced hemoglobin level can lead to inadequate oxygenation.
2. Assess ability to cough and deep breathe by having client take deep breath and observing movement of shoulders and chest wall. Measure chest excursion during deep breath. Ask client to cough after taking deep breath.	Reveals maximum potential for chest expansion and ability to cough forcefully; serves as baseline to measure ability to perform exercises after surgery.
3. Assess risk for postoperative thrombus formation. (Older and immobilized clients are most at risk.) Observe for positive Homans' sign by monitoring calf pain when dorsiflexing client's foot with knee flexed. Observe for calf pain, redness, warmth, swelling, or vein distention.	After general anesthesia, circulation is slowed, and when rate of blood flow is slowed, there is greater tendency for clot formation. Immobilization results in decreased muscular contraction in lower extremities, which promotes venous stasis.
4. Explain postoperative exercises to client, including importance to recovery and physiological benefits.	Information allows client to attend and can motivate learning. Persons tend to learn new skills when benefits can be gained.
5. Demonstrate exercises.	
A. **Diaphragmatic breathing**	
(1) Assist client to comfortable sitting or standing position. If client chooses to sit, assist to side of bed or to upright position in chair.	Upright position facilitates diaphragmatic excursion.
(2) Stand or sit facing client.	Allows client to observe breathing exercise.

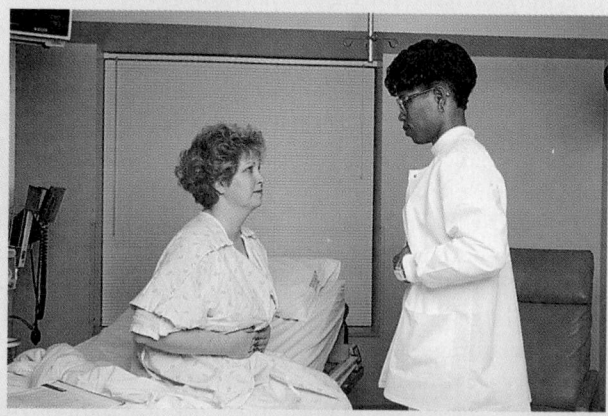

Step 5A(3)

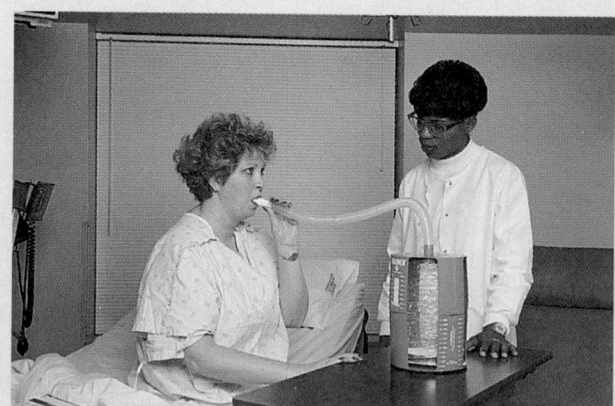

Step 5B(3)

STEPS	RATIONALE

(3) Instruct client to place palms of hands across from each other, down and along lower borders of anterior rib cage. Place tips of third fingers lightly together (see illustration). Demonstrate for client.

Position of hands allows client to feel movement of chest and abdomen as diaphragm descends and lungs expand.

(4) Have client take slow, deep breaths, inhaling through nose. Tell client to feel middle fingers separate during inhalation. Demonstrate.

Taking slow, deep breaths prevents panting or hyperventilation. Inhaling through nose warms, humidifies, and filters air.

(5) Explain that client will feel normal downward movement of diaphragm during inspiration. Explain that abdominal organs descend and chest wall expands.

Explanation and demonstration focus on normal ventilatory movement of chest wall. Client develops understanding of how diaphragmatic breathing feels.

(6) Avoid using chest and shoulders while inhaling and instruct client in same manner.

Using auxiliary chest and shoulder muscles increases useless energy expenditure.

(7) Have client hold slow, deep breath for count of three and then slowly exhale through mouth. Tell client middle fingertips will touch as chest wall contracts.

Allows for gradual expulsion of all air.

(8) Repeat breathing exercise 3 to 5 times.

Allows client to observe slow, rhythmic breathing pattern.

(9) Have client practice exercise. Instruct client to take 10 slow, deep breaths every 2 hours while awake during postoperative period until mobile.

Repetition of exercise reinforces learning. Regular deep breathing prevents postoperative complications.

B. **Incentive spirometry**

(1) Wash hands.

Reduces transmission of microorganisms.

(2) Instruct client to assume semi-Fowler's or high-Fowler's position.

Promotes optimal lung expansion during respiratory maneuver.

(3) Either set or indicate to client on the device scale, the volume level to be attained with each breath (see illustration).

Establishes goal to volume level necessary for lung expansion.

(4) Demonstrate to client how to place mouthpiece of spirometer so that lips completely cover mouthpiece (see illustration for Step 5B[3]).

Demonstration is reliable technique for teaching psychomotor skill and enables client to ask questions.

(5) Instruct client to inhale slowly and maintain constant flow through unit. When maximal inspiration is reached, client should hold breath for 2 to 3 seconds (see illustration) and then exhale slowly. Number of breaths should not exceed 10 to 12/min (Dettenmeier, 1992).

Maintains maximal inspiration and reduces risk of progressive collapse of individual alveoli. Slow breath prevents or minimizes pain from sudden pressure changes in chest (Dettenmeier, 1992).

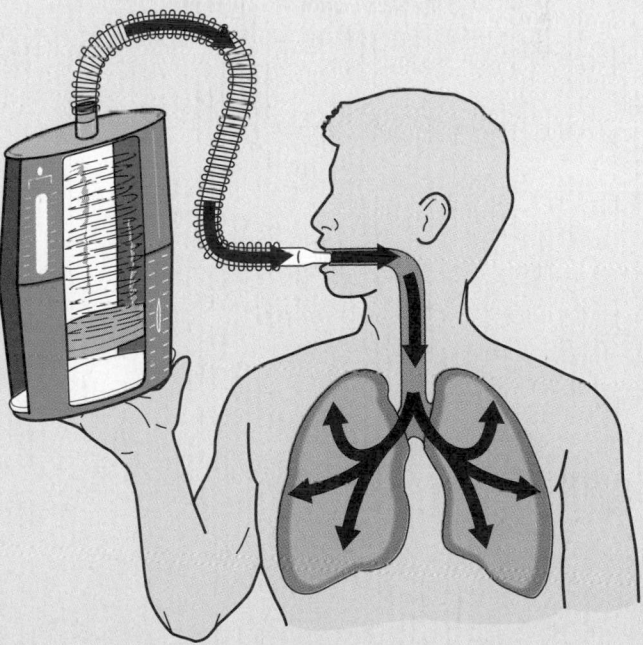

Step 5B(5)

Steps	**Rationale**
(6) Instruct client to breathe normally for short period.	Prevents hyperventilation and fatigue.
(7) Have client repeat maneuver until volume goals are achieved.	Ensures correct use of spirometer.
(8) Wash hands.	Reduces transmission of microorganisms.

C. **Positive expiratory pressure therapy and "huff" coughing**

(1) Wash hands.	Reduces transmission of microorganisms.
(2) Set PEP device for the setting ordered.	The higher the setting, the more effort will be required by the client.
(3) Instruct client to assume semi-Fowler's or high-Fowler's position and place nose clip on client's nose (illustration).	Promotes optimal lung expansion and expectoration of mucus.
(4) Have client place lips around mouthpiece. Client should take a full breath and then exhale 2 to 3 times longer than inhalation. Pattern should be repeated for 10 to 20 breaths.	Ensures that all breathing is done through the mouth and that the device is used properly.
(5) Remove device from mouth and have client take a slow, deep breath and hold for 3 seconds.	Promotes lung expansion before coughing.
(6) Instruct client to exhale in quick, short, forced exhalations.	"Huff" coughing, or forced expiratory technique, promotes bronchial hygiene by increased expectoration of secretions.

D. **Controlled coughing**

(1) Explain importance of maintaining upright position.	Position facilitates diaphragm excursion and enhances thorax expansion.
(2) Demonstrate coughing. Take two slow, deep breaths, inhaling through nose and exhaling through mouth.	Deep breaths expand lungs fully so that air moves behind mucus and facilitates effects of coughing.
(3) Inhale deeply third time and hold breath to count of three. Cough fully for two or three consecutive coughs without inhaling between coughs. (Tell client to push all air out of lungs.)	Consecutive coughs help remove mucus more effectively and completely than one forceful cough.
(4) Caution client against just clearing throat instead of coughing.	Clearing throat does not remove mucus from deep in airways.
(5) If surgical incision will be abdominal or thoracic, teach client to place one hand over incisional area and other hand on top of first. During breathing and coughing exercises, client presses gently against incisional area to splint or support it. Pillow over incision is optional (see illustration).	Surgical incision cuts through muscles, tissues, and nerve endings. Deep breathing and coughing exercises place additional stress on suture line and cause discomfort. Splinting incision with hands provides firm support and reduces incisional pulling. (Some clients prefer to have pillow to place over incision.)

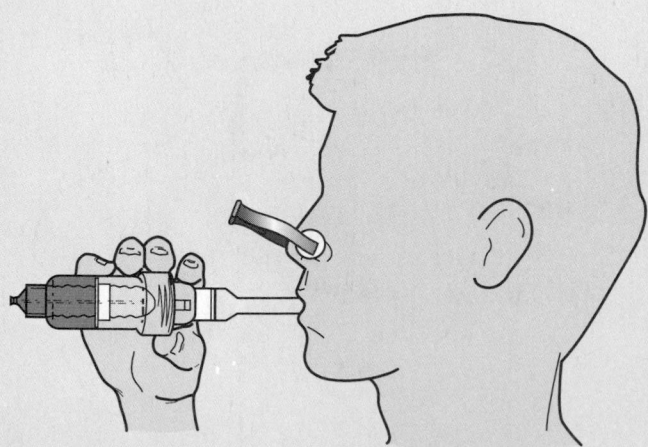

Step 5C(3)

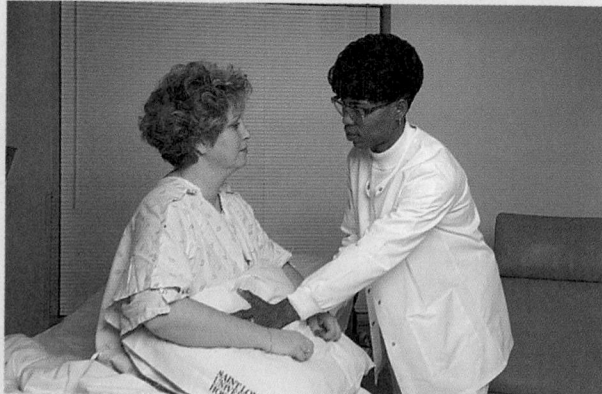

Step 5D(5)

STEPS	RATIONALE
(6) Client continues to practice coughing exercises, splinting imaginary incision. Instruct client to cough 2 to 3 times every 2 hours while awake.	Value of deep coughing with splinting is stressed to effectively expectorate mucus with minimal discomfort.
(7) Instruct client to examine sputum for consistency, amount, and color changes.	Sputum consistency, amount, and color changes may indicate presence of pulmonary complication, such as pneumonia.
E. Turning	
(1) Instruct client to assume supine position to right side of bed if permitted by surgery. Side rails on both sides of bed should be in up position.	Positioning begins on right side of bed so that turning to left side will not cause client to roll toward bed's edge.
(2) Instruct client to place left hand over incisional area to splint it.	Supports and minimizes pulling on suture line during turning.
(3) Instruct client to keep left leg straight and flex right knee up and over left leg (If back surgery was performed, client will need to logroll).	Straight leg stabilizes client's position. Flexed right leg shifts weight for easier turning.
(4) Have client grab left side rail with right hand, pull toward left, and roll onto left side.	Pulling toward side rail reduces effort needed for turning.
(5) Instruct client to turn every 2 hours while awake.	Reduces risk of vascular and pulmonary complications.
F. Leg exercises	
(1) Have client assume supine position in bed. Demonstrate leg exercises by performing passive range-of-motion exercises and simultaneously explaining exercise.	Provides normal anatomical position of lower extremities.
(2) Rotate each ankle in complete circle. Instruct client to draw imaginary circles with big toe. Repeat 5 times.	Leg exercises maintain joint mobility and promote venous return to prevent thrombi.
(3) Alternate dorsiflexion and plantar flexion of both feet. Direct client to feel calf muscles contract and relax alternately (see illustration). Repeat 5 times.	Stretches and contracts gastrocnemius muscles.
(4) Have client continue leg exercises by alternately flexing and extending knees. Repeat 5 times (see illustration).	Contracts muscles of upper legs and maintains knee mobility.
(5) Have client alternately raise each leg straight up from bed surface, keeping legs straight. Repeat 5 times.	Promotes contraction and relaxation of quadricep muscles.

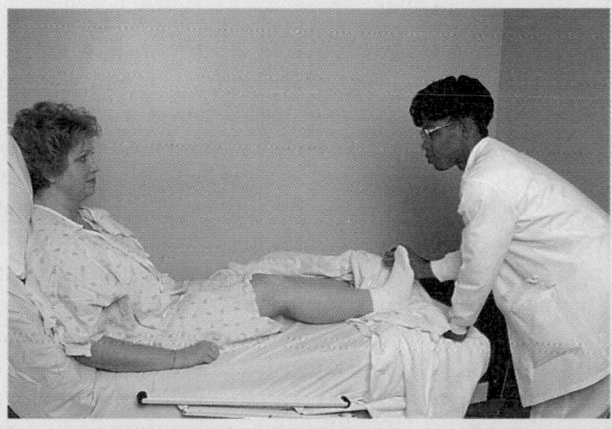

Step 5F(3)

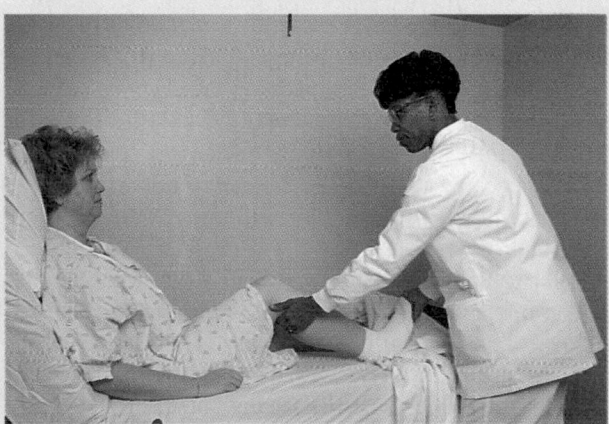

Step 5F(4)

STEPS	RATIONALE
6. Have client practice exercises at least every 2 hours while awake. Instruct client to coordinate turning and leg exercises with diaphragmatic breathing, incentive spirometry, and coughing exercises.	Repetition of sequence reinforces learning. Establishes routine for exercises that develops habit for performance. Sequence of exercises should be leg exercises, turning, breathing, incentive spirometry, and coughing.
7. Observe client's ability to perform all five exercises independently.	Ensures that client has learned correct technique.
8. Record exercises demonstrated and client's ability to perform them independently.	Documents client's education and provides data for instructional follow-up.

slows. Stasis of circulation may lead to thrombi or clots. A clot that breaks off is referred to as an embolus. An embolus from the leg usually lodges in the lungs but may also lodge in the heart or brain. Emboli are potentially fatal complications.

Clients undergoing cardiothoracic procedures or who may have preexisting lung disease may use *PEP therapy* postoperatively. PEP therapy assists with bronchial hygiene and may be used as a substitute for chest physiotherapy. After use of the device, the client inhales deeply; holds for 3 seconds; and exhales in short, rapid, forced exhalations ("huff" coughing) (AARC Clinical Practice Guideline, 1993). Coughing assists in removing retained mucus in the airways. A deep, productive cough is more beneficial than merely clearing the throat. Aerosol treatments with bronchodilating medications (such as albuterol [Proventil]), ipratropium [Atrovent] may also be ordered to assist with mucous expectoration. Postoperative incisional pain makes coughing difficult. The client must anticipate the pain and understand the importance of coughing. The nurse demonstrates methods for splinting the incision to minimize pain during coughing. Nurses direct clients to cough and deep breathe at least every 2 hours while awake.

Leg exercises and turning improve blood flow to the extremities and thus reduce stasis. Contraction of lower leg muscles promotes venous return, making it difficult for clots to form. The nurse encourages the client to perform exercises at least every 2 hours while awake. If the client is measured for elastic stockings or pneumatic compression devices, teaching about the purposes and nursing care that will be required following application is necessary (see Chapter 46).

After explaining each exercise, the nurse demonstrates it. The nurse acts as a coach, guiding the client through each exercise. For example, the nurse assesses whether the client is sitting properly and helps the client place the hands in the proper position during breathing. The nurse then allows the client time for independent practice and returns to evaluate effectiveness before surgery.

Client States the Time of Surgery.   The client and family should be told the approximate time that surgery will begin. If the hospital has a busy operating room schedule, it is best to let them know how many procedures are scheduled before the client's. The surgeon usually informs the client and family of the anticipated length of surgery. Unanticipated delays may occur for many reasons. The family needs to be aware that delays occur for various reasons and does not necessarily indicate a problem. Family members wait in the surgical waiting area during the operative procedure.

Client States the Postoperative Unit and Location of the Family During Surgery and Recovery.   The unit to which the client is admitted before surgery may be different from the postoperative unit. The family needs to know where the client will be taken after surgery. The nurse also explains where the family can wait and where the surgeon will attempt to find family members after surgery. Many institutions have implemented programs in which the circulating nurse gives periodic reports to the family in the waiting room for surgeries that are expected to be prolonged. If the client will be taken to a special unit, it helps to orient the client and family members to the unit's environment before surgery.

Client Discusses Anticipated Postoperative Monitoring and Therapies.   The client and family want to know about postoperative events. If they understand the frequency of postoperative vital sign monitoring before surgery occurs, they will be less apprehensive when nurses assess vital signs. The nurse can also explain whether the client is likely to have IV lines, monitoring lines, dressings, or drainage tubes or will require ventilator support. The nurse should neither overprepare nor underprepare the client and family. The nurse cannot predict all of the client's postoperative therapies because each surgeon follows different practices for each type of surgery. Although the nurse becomes familiar with each surgeon's preferences, a client could be misinformed about a therapy that may not be initiated. Contradictions between the nurse's explanations and postoperative reality can cause confusion and anxiety.

Client Describes Surgical Procedures and Postoperative Treatment.   After the surgeon has explained the basic purpose of a surgical procedure, the client may ask the nurse additional questions to clarify misunderstandings. Preestablished teaching standards, such as those integrated in **clinical pathways** for preoperative and postoperative care (Figure 49-4), give the nurse an excellent guide for instruction. One way to avoid problems is to first ask what the client has been told. When the client has little or no understanding about the surgery, the physician will need to be notified to reinform the client. The nurse can augment the physician's explanations. Before surgery certain predictable aspects of the client's treatment plan (e.g., dressing changes and respiratory therapy) and level of supportive nursing care are explained.

Client Describes Postoperative Activity Resumption.   The type of surgery a client undergoes affects the speed with which normal physical activity and regular eating habits can be resumed. The nurse explains that it is normal to progress gradually in activity and eating. If the client tolerates activity and diet well, activity levels will progress more quickly.

Client Verbalizes Pain-Relief Measures.   One of the surgical client's greatest fears is pain. The family is also concerned for the client's comfort. Pain after surgery is expected. The nurse informs the client and family of interventions available for pain relief (e.g., analgesics, positioning, splinting, and relaxation exercises) (see Chapter 42). The client needs to know the schedule for analgesic drugs, the route of administration, and their effects.

Many surgical clients often avoid taking pain-relief drugs for fear of becoming dependent. The nurse should encourage the client to use analgesics as needed. Unless the pain is controlled, it will be difficult for the client to participate in postoperative therapy. Hospitalized clients may initially receive IV medication depending on the nature of the surgery. As they become able to tolerate food, the physician replaces IV analgesics with oral forms.

The client should be encouraged to inform nurses before the pain becomes a constant discomfort. If a client waits until pain becomes excruciating, an analgesic may not provide relief at the dose ordered. Clients who will have patient-controlled analgesia (PCA) after surgery should know how to push the button, know to push the button when beginning to feel discomfort, and understand that use of PCA will not cause overmedication. The client should also know the length of time that it takes for the drug to begin working. Epidural analgesia is also a measure used for pain control in the surgical client. Epidural analgesia is discussed in Chapter 42. The use of a pain scale can be a helpful tool for the client to express the intensity and presence of pain, as well as evaluating effectiveness of pain-control interventions. Information from preoperative pain assessment will be helpful to the nurse when teaching about pain-relief measures.

Client Expresses Feelings Regarding Surgery.   The client may feel like part of an assembly line during the preoperative surgical phase. Frequent visits by staff, diagnostic testing, and physical preparation for surgery consume a lot of time, and the client has few opportunities to reflect on the surgical experience. The nurse makes sure that the client feels like an individual. The client and family need time to express feelings about surgery. The client's level of anxiety influences the frequency of discussions. While delivering routine care, the nurse can encourage expression of concerns. The family may wish to discuss concerns without the client so that their fears will not frighten the client and vice versa. The establishment of a trusting and therapeutic relationship with the client and family allows this to happen.

Physical Preparation.   The degree of preoperative physical preparation depends on the client's health status, the surgery to be performed, and the surgeon's preferences. A seriously ill client receives more supportive care in the form of medications, IV fluid therapy, and monitoring than the client facing a minor elective procedure. The nurse explains the purpose of all procedures.

Maintenance of Normal Fluid and Electrolyte Balance.   The surgical client is vulnerable to fluid and electrolyte imbalances as a result of inadequate preoperative intake or excessive fluid losses during surgery (see Chapter 40). A client traditionally takes nothing by mouth (NPO) after midnight on the morning of surgery, although this concept has been steadily changing over the past 10 years (Box 49-4). The nurse removes fluids and solid foods from the client's bedside and posts a sign over the bed to alert hospital personnel and family members about fasting restrictions. After 6 to 8 hours of fasting, the client's stomach will be relatively empty, so the risks of vomiting or aspirating emesis during surgery are reduced. The client may be allowed clear liquids up to 3 hours before the scheduled surgery. The nurse reviews the physician's orders carefully. General anesthetics typically cause slowing of gastrointestinal peristalsis. The client may be instructed to take specific medications (e.g., anticoagulants, cardiovascular medications, and anticonvulsants) with a sip of water as ordered by the physician.

A client who is at home the evening before surgery must understand the importance of not taking food for at least 8 hours before surgery and be willing to follow restrictions on fluids as ordered. The nurse can allow the client to rinse the mouth with water or mouthwash and brush the teeth immediately before surgery as long as the

OPEN HEART CLINICAL PATHWAY   PROCEDURE _____
GENESIS MEDICAL CENTER, Davenport, Iowa

	PAS / Day prior to OR Date/Time	ADMISSION / Day of OR Date/Time	SICU Date	Date
ASSESSMENT/ REASSESSMENT	N _____ WNL D_____ E _____ Pulm screen / protocol parameters Send old charts including cath report to PCCU Send all x-rays to OR	N _____ WNL D_____ E _____ Braden _____ Weight_____Height_____	2400 _____ 0400 _____ 0800 _____ 1200 _____ 1600 _____ 2000 _____ Weight _____ Notify surgeon per parameters	2400 _____ 0400 _____ 0800 _____ 1200 _____ 1600 _____ 2000 _____
ACTIVITY	As Tolerated	As Tolerated	Bedrest reposition every 2 hours Dangle 5 minutes within 2 hours post extubation Up in chair post extubation, CXR / meals <u>FAST TRACK</u>: <u>Nsg</u>: Walk in place 1 minute before breakfast. Page Cardiac Rehab 15 minutes before PCCU transfer	
DIET	NAS, low cholesterol then NPO midnight before surgery	NPO	NPO while intubated Open Heart Progressive Diet-ADA if diabetic	
MEDICATIONS	Hold medications per physician orders	Preoperative medications per anesthesia PRN	No Atropine Central/peripheral IV (lock at transfer) Antibiotic ASA (hold if valve) Analgesic IV PRN. Add analgesic po when extubated Nitroglycerin IV, begin weaning at 0500 POD 1 Renew/start beta blockers	
TESTS	PA/Lateral CXR, EKG, Comprehensive Metabolic Panel, CBC, INR, PTT, U/A, Type & Cross , 4 units RBCs PFT per protocol	Review test results and ensure availability on chart	Admission stat ABG, K+, CBC, PT/PTT, CA++, Mg, CXR 4 hour ABG, K+, CBC, CA++ \12 hour CPK 0500 ABG, CMP, CBC, & EKG 0500 daily CXR while in SICU 0500 daily INR if valve K+, ABG PRN. CBC every 4 hours PRN	
TREATMENTS	DVT screen Chlorhexidine shower night before surgery	Chlorhexidine shower morning before surgery	Extubation Protocol at_____O2 Protocol PEP Therapy Protocol TEDs (Remove at hs)	

INTERVENTIONS	• Discharge Planning
	• Nutritional Management
	• Preop Coordination
	• Risk Identification
	• Teaching: Preoperative
	• Teaching: Individual
	• Teaching: Procedure/ Treatment
		• Admission Care
		Discharge Planning
		• Fall Prevention
		• Infection Control
		• Nutritional Monitoring
		• Surgical Preparation
		Teaching: Individual
			• Analgesic Administration: Infection Control
			  Intraspinal • Invasive Hemodynamic
			• Autotransfusion Monitoring
			• Bleeding Precautions • Mech. Ventilation
			• Cardiac Care Weaning
			Discharge Planning • Nutritional Monitoring
			• ET Extubation • Pain Management
			Fall Prevention • Physical Restraints
			• Fl/Electrolyte Teaching :Individual
			  Management • Tube Care	

TEACHING	Able to read and write ☐Y ☐N Readiness to learn barriers☐Y ☐N Other☐vision ☐hearing☐language Learns best ☐see ☐hear ☐do Initiate clinical pathway Initial Learner = Pt Method = 1:1, H/O, PAS class	Review clinical pathway Learner = Pt Method = 1:1	Review clinical pathway D____ E____ N____ D____ E____ N____ Learner = Pt. Method = 1:1	
DISCHARGE PLANNING	Screen/ Notify MSS	Date_____Time_____ Transferred to OR per cart in stable condition with staff	Date_____Time_____ Transferred to PCCU per wheelchair/ambulate/bed in stable condition with staff. Day of OR 24hour I/O:_____ Transfer I/O information: Night I/O_____ Day I/O_____ Evening I/O_____	
CONSULT/ OTHER	Cardiac Rehab Dietitian OR RN RT	Notify of admission Cardiologist _____ Surgeon _____ Family physician _____	Pulmonary artery line removed_____ Arterial line removed_____ Foley removed_____ MCTs removed_____ Other removed_____	

Learner:		**Method:**	
Pt = Patient	A/V	= Audio/Visual	
Par = Parent	1:1	= One to One	
Sp = Spouse	Demo	= Demonstrates	
S.O. = Significant other	H/O	= Handouts	
	P/I	= Phone Interview	
	G	= Group	

2

Figure 49-4   Open heart clinical pathway.
Courtesy Genesis Medical Center, Davenport, Iowa.

OPEN HEART CLINICAL PATHWAY
GENESIS MEDICAL CENTER, Davenport, Iowa

	PCCU/Day 1 Date/Time	PCCU/Day 2 Date/Time	PCCU/Day 3 Date/Time	PCCU/Day 4 Date/Time	PCCU/Day 5-Discharge Date/Time
ASSESSMENT/ REASSESSMENT	N_____ WNL D_____ E_____ Weight _____	N_____ WNL D_____ E_____ Weight _____	N_____ WNL D_____ E_____ Braden _____ Weight_____	N_____ WNL D_____ E_____ Weight _____	N_____ WNL D_____ E_____ Weight _____
ACTIVITY	Nsg: Up in chair for meals, BRP with assist Cardiac Rehab: Step 1 Step 1 FAST TRACK Nsg: walk in place 1 minute before meals(1 2 3) Cardiac Rehab: walk 4-8 minutes BID (1 2)	Nsg: Up in chair for meals, Up ad lib in room, Shower Cardiac Rehab: Step 2 Step 2 FAST TRACK Nsg: walk in hall BID(1 2) Cardiac Rehab: walk 8-10 minutes BID(1 2)	Nsg: Up in chair for meals, Up ad lib in room, Walk in hall BID, Shower Cardiac Rehab: Step 3 Step 3 FAST TRACK Nsg: walk TID 2-4-minutes (1 2 3) Cardiac Rehab: walk 10-12 minutes BID with stairs PRN (1 2)	Nsg: Up in chair for meals, Up ad lib in room, Walk in hall independently, Shower Cardiac Rehab: Step 4 Step 4 FAST TRACK Nsg: walk TID 4-5 minutes (1 2 3) Cardiac Rehab: walk 12-15 minutes BID with stairs PRN (1 2)	Nsg:Up ad lib in room, Walk in hall independently, Shower Cardiac Rehab: Step 5 Step 5
DIET	open heart progressive (ADA if diabetic)	open heart progressive (ADA if diabetic)	open heart progressive (ADA if diabetic)	open heart progressive (ADA if diabetic)	open heart progressive (NAS, low cholesterol, 2000 cc fluid restriction) 1800 ADA if diabetic)
MEDICATIONS	Central/periph IV lock Analgesic IV/po ASA (hold if valve)	Central / periph IV lock Analgesic IV/po PRN ASA (hold if valve)	Central / periph IV lock Analgesic po PRN ASA (hold if valve)	Central / periph IV lock Analgesic po PRN ASA (hold if valve)	D/C central/periph IV lock Analgesic po PRN ASA (hold if valve)
TESTS	INR if valve K+ PRN	INR if valve CXR if on O2 K+ PRN	INR if valve K+ PRN	INR if valve K+ PRN	INR if valve K+ PRN
TREATMENTS	O2 Protocol PEP Therapy Protocol TEDs, remove at hs	O2 Protocol PEP Therapy Protocol TEDs, remove at hs	O2 Protocol PEP Therapy Protocol TEDs, remove at hs	O2 Protocol PEP Therapy Protocol TEDs, remove at hs	O2 Protocol PEP Therapy Protocol TEDs, remove at hs
INTERVENTIONS	Cardiac Care • Card Care: Rehab Discharge Planning Fall Prevention Fluid/Electrolyte Management Infection Control Nutritional Monitoring Pain Management Teaching: Individual Tube Care	Cardiac Care Card Care: Rehab Discharge Planning Fall Prevention Fluid/Electrolyte Management Infection Control Nutritional Monitoring Pain Management Teaching: Individual Tube Care	Cardiac Care Card Care: Rehab Discharge Planning Fall Prevention Fluid/Electrolyte Management Infection Control Nutritional Monitoring Pain Management Teaching: Individual	Cardiac Care Card Care: Rehab Discharge Planning Fall Prevention Fluid/Electrolyte Management Infection Control Nutritional Monitoring Pain Management Teaching: Individual	Cardiac Care Card Care: Rehab Discharge Planning Fall Prevention Fluid/Electrolyte Management Infection Control Nutritional Monitoring Pain Management Teaching: Individual
TEACHING	review patient pathway Learner = Pt Method = 1:1	review patient pathway Learner = Pt Method = 1:1	review patient pathway Learner = Pt Method = 1:1	review patient pathway Discharge Class Learner = Pt Method = 1:1 Food/drug interaction H/O	review patient pathway Learner = Pt Method = 1:1
DISCHARGE PLANNING				FAST TRACK may discharge	Discharge
CONSULT/ OTHER	1st void _____ Straight cath if no void 12 hrs post foley d/c		Pull pacer wires (MD) consider TSU if <100 feet	Phase II Referral	

Learner:		**Method:**	
Pt = Patient		A/V	= Audio/Visual
Par = Parent		1:1	= One to One
Sp = Spouse		Demo	= Demonstrates
S.O. = Significant other		H/O	= Handouts
		P/I	= Phone Interview
		G	= Group

Figure 49-4, cont'd   Open heart clinical pathway.

472-001   6/98 mw bn

Research HIGHLIGHT   **Box 49-4**

RESEARCH ABSTRACT

This study provided an extensive review of current literature regarding NPO guidelines. Most studies support the liberalization of policies for preoperative fluids. Although a 2-hour fast is safe, a 3-hour fast is recommended to accommodate last-minute operating room changes. Solid food should not be consumed at least 8 hours before surgery. The most common clear fluids allowed are water, apple juice, carbonated beverages, broth, black tea, and coffee. In addition, a national survey conducted by Green, Pandit, and Schork (1996) found that 57% of the responding institutions had liberalized NPO guidelines. Anesthesiologists were more likely to liberalize fluids for children than for adults.

IMPLICATIONS FOR PRACTICE

- Conduct discussions with surgeons to explore the feasibility of changing NPO guidelines.
- Conduct a quality improvement or research study that examines whether a change in the time frame for allowing fluids results in adverse client outcomes.

REFERENCE

Pandit VA, Pandit SK: Fasting before and after ambulatory surgery, *J PeriAnesth Nurs* 12(3):181, 1997.

---

client does not swallow water. The nurse notifies the surgeon if the client eats or drinks during the fasting period.

During surgery, normal mechanisms for controlling fluid and electrolyte balance, including respiration, digestion, circulation, and elimination, are disturbed. The surgical procedure may cause extensive losses of blood and other body fluids. The surgical stress response aggravates any fluid and electrolyte imbalance. The client's preoperative diet should include foods high in protein, with sufficient carbohydrates, fat, and vitamins. If a client cannot eat because of gastrointestinal alterations or impairments in consciousness, an IV route for fluid replacement is started. The physician relies on serum electrolyte levels to determine the type of IV fluids and electrolyte additives to administer. Clients with severe nutritional imbalances may require supplements with concentrated protein and glucose (see Chapter 43).

Reduction of Risk of Surgical Wound Infection.
The risk of developing a surgical wound infection is determined by the amount and type of microorganisms contaminating a wound, susceptibility of the host, and condition of the wound at the end of the operation (largely determined by the surgeon's operative technique). All three factors may interact to cause infection.

The skin is a favorite site for microorganisms to grow and multiply. Without proper skin preparation, the risk of postoperative wound infection is high. Many surgeons

have clients bathe or shower the evening before surgery. Some physicians may request clients to bathe or shower more than once, whereas others may have clients give special attention to cleansing the proposed operative site. This attention could include use of an antibacterial soap. Depending on the surgical procedure, a client may also shower the morning of surgery.

If the surgical procedure involves the head, neck, or upper chest area, the client may also be required to shampoo the hair. Cleansing and trimming of fingernails and toenails may also be necessary.

Hair removal is ordered only if the hair has the potential to interfere with exposure, closure, or dressing of the surgical site (AORN, 1996). Hair removal can damage and cause breaks in the client's skin, which may allow for the entry of microorganisms. A nick in the skin made up to 30 minutes before a surgical procedure is considered a clean wound. If the skin near the surgical site has been disrupted for longer than this, the client is at higher risk for developing a wound infection. Electric clippers are usually used, since they cut close to the skin without nicks. **Depilatories** remove hair chemically and can cause skin irritation. They should be used before arrival in the OR area. Some hospitals and surgical clinics still require shaving. Frequently this job is performed by a member of the surgical team. If the nurse is to perform this job, he or she should consult the institution's policy and procedure manual regarding the use of razors.

Short hospital stays are known to reduce the chance of a **nosocomial** infection (hospital acquired). Respiratory, urinary tract, and wound infections can all be acquired during hospitalization. This is one advantage to having ambulatory surgical procedures, since the client usually returns home when the surgery has been completed.

Prevention of Bowel and Bladder Incontinence.
The client may not receive a bowel preparation (e.g., a cathartic or enema) unless surgery involves the gastrointestinal system. Manipulation of portions of the gastrointestinal tract during surgery results in absence of peristalsis for 24 hours and sometimes longer. Enemas and cathartics such as Golytely cleanse the gastrointestinal tract to prevent intraoperative incontinence and postoperative constipation. An empty bowel reduces risk of injury to the intestines and prevents contamination of the operative wound in case a portion of the bowel is incised or opened accidentally, or if colon surgery is planned. The surgeon's order may read "give enemas until clear." This means that the nurse is to administer enemas until the enema return contains no solid fecal material (see Chapter 45). Too many enemas given over a short time, however, can cause serious fluid and electrolyte imbalances. Most agencies recommend a limit to the number of enemas (usually three) a nurse may administer successively and/or a recheck of potassium levels after bowel preparation has been completed.

The bladder is not prepared until the morning of surgery. The nurse instructs the client to void just before leaving for the operating room and before giving preoperative medications. An empty bladder prevents a client from being incontinent during surgery. This is important during abdominal surgery, when it may become necessary for the surgeon to manipulate the bladder. An empty bladder also makes abdominal organs more accessible during surgery. The nurse in the operating room often inserts a Foley catheter to maintain an empty bladder.

Promotion of Rest and Comfort. Rest is essential for normal healing. Anxiety about surgery can easily interfere with the ability to relax or sleep. The underlying condition requiring surgery may be painful, further impairing rest.

The nurse should attempt to make the client's environment quiet and comfortable. Frequently the physician orders a sedative-hypnotic or antianxiety agent for the night before surgery. Sedative-hypnotics (e.g., temazepam [Restoril]) affect and promote sleep. Antianxiety agents (e.g., alprazolam [Xanax], midazolam [Versed], diazepam [Valium], lorazepam [Ativan]) act on the cerebral cortex and limbic system to relieve anxiety.

An advantage to ambulatory surgery or same-day surgical admissions is that the client is able to sleep at home the night before surgery. The client is likely to get more rest in a familiar environment. The nonhospitalized client may also have medication ordered by the physician if apprehension about surgery interferes with a good night's rest.

Preparation on the Day of Surgery.
On the morning before surgery the nurse completes a number of routine procedures before releasing the client for surgery.

Checking Medical Record Contents and Completing Recording. Before the client goes to the operating room, the nurse checks the contents of the medical record to be sure that pertinent laboratory results are present. The nurse checks consent forms for accuracy of information. A preoperative checklist (Figure 49-5) provides the nurse with guidelines for ensuring completion of nursing interventions. The nurse also checks the nurse's notes to be sure that documentation of care is current. This is especially important if the hospitalized client experienced unpredicted problems the night before surgery.

Checking Vital Signs. The nurse makes a final preoperative assessment of vital signs. The anesthesiologist uses these values as a baseline for intraoperative vital signs. If preoperative vital signs are abnormal, surgery may need to be postponed. For example, an elevated temperature may indicate an infection, which may increase the client's surgical risk. The nurse notifies the physician of abnormalities before sending the client to surgery.

Providing Hygiene. Basic hygiene measures provide additional comfort before surgery. If the hospitalized client is unwilling to take a complete bath, a partial bath is refreshing and removes irritating secretions or drainage from the skin. Because the client cannot wear personal nightwear to the operating room, the nurse provides a clean hospital gown. If the client has been NPO throughout the night, the client's mouth may be very dry. The nurse may offer the client mouthwash and toothpaste, again cautioning the client not to swallow water.

Checking Hair and Cosmetics. During surgery with the client under general anesthesia, the anesthesiologist positions the client's head to introduce an endotracheal tube into the airway (see Chapter 39). This procedure may involve manipulation of the client's hair and scalp. To avoid injury, the nurse asks the client to remove hairpins or clips before leaving for surgery. Hairpieces or wigs should also be removed. Long hair can be braided to keep it in place. The client will wear a paper hair cover before entering the operating room.

During and after surgery the anesthesiologist and nurses assess skin and mucous membranes to determine the client's level of oxygenation and circulation. Therefore all makeup (lipstick, powder, blush, nail polish) should be removed to expose normal skin and nail coloring. Pulse oximetry is capable of recording accurate measurements through nail polish colors, but removal is still considered good practice.

Checking for Removal of Prostheses. It is easy for any type of prosthetic device to become lost or damaged during surgery. The client must remove all prostheses, including partial or complete dentures, artificial limbs, artificial eyes, and contact lenses. Hearing aids, false eyelashes, and eyeglasses must also be removed. If a client has a brace or splint, the nurse checks with the physician to determine whether it should remain with the client.

For many clients it is embarrassing to remove dentures, wigs, or other devices that enhance personal appearance. Privacy should be offered as the personal items are removed. Clients may be allowed to keep personal items until they reach the preoperative area. Dentures must be placed in special containers for safekeeping to prevent loss or breakage, then the client is assessed for any loose teeth. A broken tooth can become dislodged during insertion of an endotracheal tube and obstruct the airway.

In many agencies nurses must document an inventory of all prosthetic devices or personal items and have them locked away for safekeeping according to agency policy. It is also common practice for nurses to give prostheses to family members or to keep the devices at the client's bedside. Documentation in the nursing notes or the surgical checklist should reflect these actions.

A-1c PREOPERATIVE/PREPROCEDURAL CHECKLIST

• File with other A-1c's of same date. •

PROCEDURE: _____

DATE OF PROCEDURE: _____

1. Place initials in appropriate box: YES, NO, N/A (not applicable, or was not ordered). Each item must have an entry.
2. Explain any "No." This can be done in the space after the item or in the "Comments" section. Use back of form, if needed.
3. To give more information on any item, use the space after the item. If more space is needed, use the "Comments" section or back of form.

DATE

HOSP. NO.

NAME

BIRTHDATE

ADDRESS

IF NOT IMPRINTED, PLEASE PRINT DATE, HOSP. NO., NAME AND LOCATION.

YES	NO	N/A	
			Special information (e.g., blind, O$_2$, combative)
			Preoperative orders written.
			(If "NO", Dr. _____ notified at _____ date/time.)
			Consent complete and in medical record.
			Allergies (or NKA) labelled on cover of medical record.
			Specify Allergies:
			Isolation label on cover of medical record. Specify type.
			Ordered lab results in medical record.
			Urinalysis results in medical record.
			Chest x-ray completed. (Report in medical record: Yes____ No____)
			EKG in medical record.
			Type and cross/screen (circle) done. Date drawn:
			History and physical in medical record.
			Forms complete and in medical record:
			1. Nursing documentation with assessment, VS, and wt./ht.
			2. IV Solution Administration Cardex.
			3. Medication Administration Cardex.
			Addressograph plate on cover of medical record. All volumes to procedure, if required.

COMMENTS:

YES	NO	N/A	
			Blood band on patient and legible. Specify location _____ and blood band #_____
			Identification band on patient and legible. Specify location:
			Bathed and in proper attire.
			Nail polish, makeup, and hairpins removed.
			Jewelry removed. Specify item(s) removed and disposition:
			Prosthesis removed: hearing aid, dentures, eye glasses, contact lenses (circle).
			Other: Disposition:
			Anti-embolism stockings on.
			Sequential compression device sleeves on and controller to OR.
			NPO since:
			Teaching completed and documented.
			Preps/tests completed as ordered. Specify:
			Voided/catheterized (circle). Time:
			Medication(s) given.
			Medication(s)/article(s) sent with patient. Specify:

COMMENTS:

Date	Initials	Signature and Title of Individuals Filling Out Form
Date	Initials	Signature of RN Sending Patient to Procedure

41006/4-93/H7528   **THE UNIVERSITY OF IOWA HOSPITALS AND CLINICS**

Figure 49-5   Preoperative/procedural checklist.
Courtesy University of Iowa Hospitals and Clinics.

Safeguarding Valuables. If a client has any valuables, the nurse should give them to family members or secure them for safekeeping. Many hospitals require clients to sign a release to free the institution of responsibility for lost valuables. Valuables can usually be stored and locked in a designated location. Often clients are reluctant to remove wedding rings or religious medals. A wedding band can be taped in place. However, if there is a risk that the client will experience swelling of the hand or fingers (mastectomy, hand surgery, fluid shifts), the band should be removed. Many hospitals allow clients to pin religious medals to their gowns, although the risk of loss increases. For safety, other metal items, such as for pierced areas, should also be removed. The location of valuables is documented per hospital policy.

Preparing the Bowel and Bladder. The client may require an enema or cathartic the morning of surgery to ensure that the colon is empty. If so, it should be given at least an hour before the client is scheduled to leave, allowing time for the client to defecate without rushing. The client should void before surgery. If the client is unable to void, it should be noted on the preoperative checklist.

Applying Antiembolism Stockings or Pneumatic Compression Devices. Many physicians prefer clients to wear **antiembolism stockings** during surgery. These are designed to support the lower extremities and maintain compression of small veins and capillaries. The constant compression forces blood into larger vessels, thus promoting venous return and preventing circulatory stasis. When correctly sized and properly applied, antiem bolism stockings can reduce the risk of thrombi. Chapter 46 reviews the procedure for sizing and application. **Pneumatic compression devices** may be applied to the lower extremities for the same purpose (see Skill 46-1 in Chapter 46). These stockings promote circulation by sequentially compressing the legs from the ankle upward, promoting venous return. Stockings may be applied intraoperatively (especially for long cases) or postoperatively according to agency policy and the procedure manual. Documentation of application, capillary refill, and client tolerance should be in the nursing notes.

Performing Special Procedures. A client's condition may warrant special interventions before surgery. The surgeon's orders inform nurses of the need to start IV infusions, insert Foley catheters, or administer medications. Occasionally, a nasogastric tube may be inserted before leaving for surgery or in the preoperative area, but this is usually done in the operating room if needed (see Chapter 45).

Administering Preoperative Medications. The advent of ambulatory surgery has reduced the use of preoperative medications. However, the anesthesiologist or surgeon may order preanesthetic drugs ("on-call medications," "preops") to reduce the client's anxiety, the amount of general anesthesia required, the risk of nausea and vomiting (aspiration), and respiratory tract secretions (Litwack, 1995) (Table 49-9).

Typically the physician orders preoperative medications to be administered when the client leaves for the operating room or at an earlier prescribed time. The nurse provides all nursing care measures before giving the client

Table 49-9 **Preoperative Medications and Their Purpose**	
Medication	Purpose
Benzodiazepine	Reduce anxiety and/or provide sedation.
Midazolam (Versed)	
Diazepam (Valium)	
Lorazepam (Ativan)	
Barbiturates	Provide sedation with minimal cardiopulmonary depressant effects.
Secobarbital	
Pentobarbital	
H_2 receptor blocking agents	Increase gastric pH and/or promote gastric emptying (decreasing risk of aspiration).
Ranitidine (Zantac)	
Cimetidine (Tagamet)	
Famotidine (Pepcid)	
Metoclopramide (Reglan)	
Antacids	Decrease gastric acidity.
Anticholinergics	Dry secretions and decrease risk of aspiration and airway irritability.
Atropine	
Scopolamine	
Glycopyrrolate	
Opioids	Decrease intraoperative anesthesia requirements and facilitate induction.
Antibiotics	Minimize risk of wound infection.

From Litwack K: *Post anesthesia care nursing,* ed 2, St. Louis, 1995, Mosby.

preoperative medications. The consent form needs to be signed before the administration of these medications. In addition, the client should be helped to void. Because the drugs cause sedation, the client should not be allowed to leave the bed or stretcher until surgical personnel arrive to transport the client to the operating room. The client should be warned to expect drowsiness and a dry mouth. The side rails should be raised and the bed or stretcher kept in the low position for client safety.

Latex Sensitivity/Allergy.

Latex sensitivity or allergy has become a hot topic in the past several years. As the incidence and prevalence of latex allergy increases, the need for recognition of potential sources of latex is extremely critical. Federal regulations enacted in September 1998 mandate that all medical supplies contain a label notifying the consumer of the latex content (Doepke, 1998).

The operating room and postanesthesia care unit (PACU) contain innumerable products that contain latex. Some common sources include gloves, IV tubing, syringes, and rubber stoppers on bottles and vials. Latex is also present in objects that may be overlooked, including adhesive tape, disposable electrodes, endotracheal tube cuffs, protection sheets, and ventilator equipment. Those most at risk include persons with genetic predisposition to latex allergy, children with spina bifida, clients with urogenital abnormalities or spinal cord injury (because of a long history of catheter use), clients with a history of multiple surgeries, health care professionals, and workers who manufacture rubber products (Paquet, 1998)

Signs and symptoms of a latex reaction can include local effects ranging from urticaria and flat or raised red patches to vesicular, scaling, or bleeding eruptions. Acute dermatitis may also be present. Rhinitis and/or rhinorrhea are other common reactions in both mild and severe latex reactions. Immediate hypersensitivity reactions can be life threatening, leading to focal or generalized urticaria, edema, bronchospasm, and mucous hypersecretion, which can compromise respiratory status. Vasodilation compounded by vascular leakiness can lead to circulatory collapse and eventual death. Since the client may be draped during surgery, any unexplained acute deterioration in a previously healthy client should be investigated for possible latex allergy (Shoup, 1998).

The American Association of Nurse Anesthetists (AANA), as well as many other nursing organizations, has developed a protocol to provide safe, competent care to the client identified as being at risk for latex allergy (AANA, 1995). A latex allergy cart should be available when needed. All of the contents must be latex free. A reference binder is kept with the cart that indicates supplies, medications, and appropriate care options for latex-sensitive clients. It is recommended that the client with a latex allergy be scheduled as the first case of the day in the operating room. The room should be thoroughly cleaned, including all equipment, and all unnecessary items removed (Doepke, 1998). The client can then be safely accommodated by using appropriate latex-free items during the perioperative period and recovery.

EVALUATION

Client Care.   The admitting nurse and the nurse in the preoperative area will be the source for evaluating outcomes (Figure 49-6). With regard to the preoperative client's plan of care, there is usually limited time to evaluate the outcomes. To determine the effectiveness of the preoperative interventions, the nurse may have the client review an understanding of the surgical procedure to determine the client's knowledge level. Careful observation and dialogue with the client may identify the presence of fear or anxiety, which can then be treated with reassurance, compassion, information, and possibly medication. The nurse can also evaluate the client's knowledge of postoperative care, which can include such things as use of PCA, exercises, and a pain scale. The client's current status is compared with expected outcomes to determine whether new or revised interventions and/or nursing diagnoses need to be implemented.

The nurse's interventions may continue during and after surgery, so that evaluation does not occur until after surgery. For example, the nurse will not be able to evaluate the success of reducing postoperative wound infection or promoting return of normal physiological function until a few days after surgery. If the client is having ambulatory surgery, the client will return home, and nursing may not be able to assess the effectiveness of certain interventions.

Client Expectations.   It may be difficult to determine whether the client's expectations have been met regarding preoperative teaching. The nurse is evaluating the client in a "hurried" atmosphere, since there are many things that need to be accomplished in a short amount of time. The client's surgery may be an emergency, or performance of various procedures may make it difficult for the nurse to find time for evaluation. The client may feel somewhat depersonalized by the need to complete tasks. It is important that the nurse remember to attend to the personal needs of the client, as well as the tasks at hand (privacy, fear, anxiety). The client should be given an opportunity to state whether expectations have been met. If expectations are unmet, the nurse will need to work closely with the client to redefine expectations that can be realistically met within the time limits imposed by this particular setting.

Transport to the Operating Room

Personnel in the operating room notify the nursing division or ambulatory surgical waiting area when it is time for surgery. In many hospitals a nursing orderly or trans-

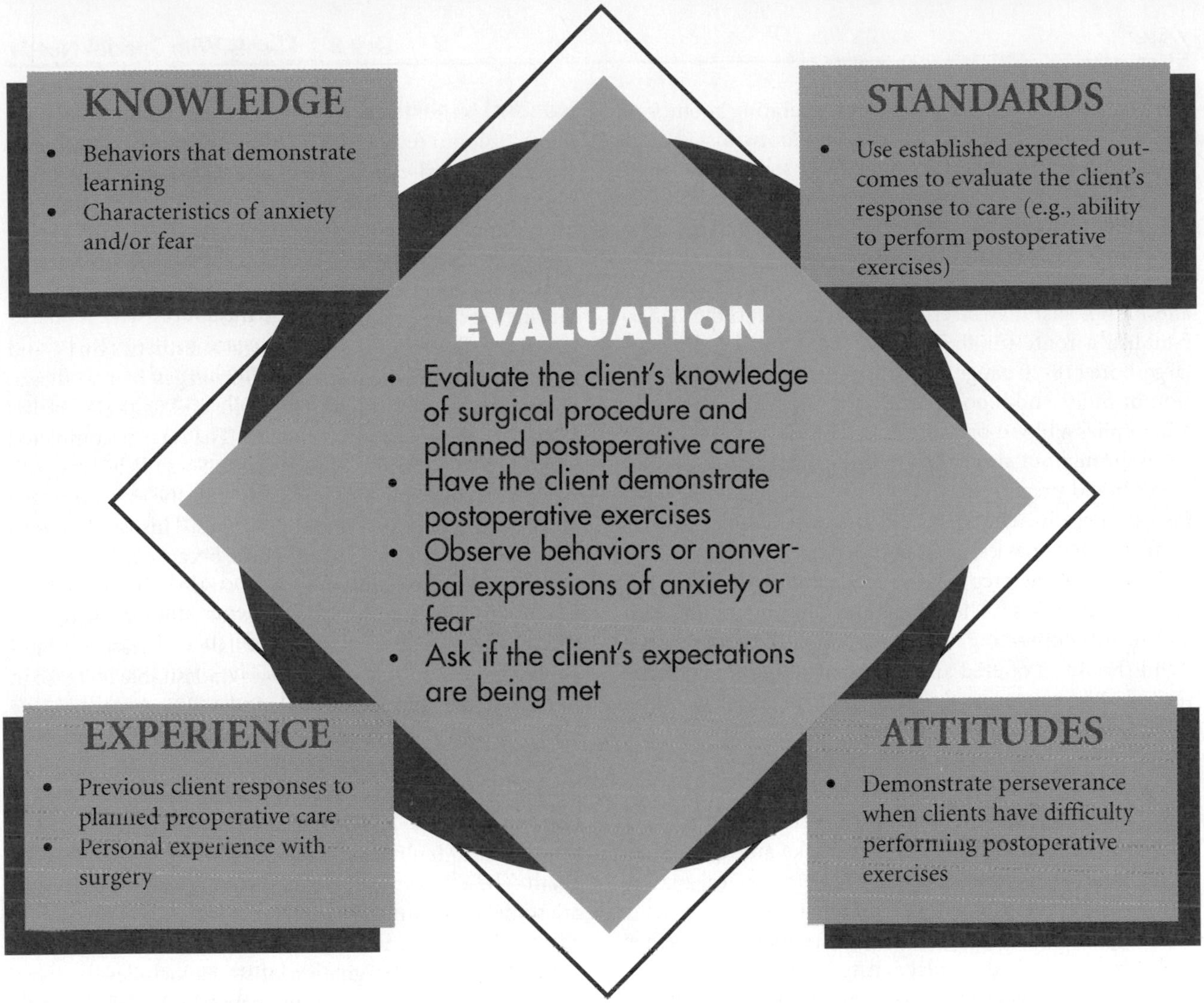

KNOWLEDGE
- Behaviors that demonstrate learning
- Characteristics of anxiety and/or fear

STANDARDS
- Use established expected outcomes to evaluate the client's response to care (e.g., ability to perform postoperative exercises)

EVALUATION
- Evaluate the client's knowledge of surgical procedure and planned postoperative care
- Have the client demonstrate postoperative exercises
- Observe behaviors or nonverbal expressions of anxiety or fear
- Ask if the client's expectations are being met

EXPERIENCE
- Previous client responses to planned preoperative care
- Personal experience with surgery

ATTITUDES
- Demonstrate perseverance when clients have difficulty performing postoperative exercises

Figure 49-6 *Synthesis Model for Surgical Client Evaluation phase.*

porter brings a stretcher for transporting the client. The transporter checks the client's identification bracelet against the client's chart to be sure that the right person is going to surgery. Because the client has already received preoperative drugs, the nurses and transporter assist the client in transferring from bed to stretcher to prevent falls. The family gets one last opportunity to visit before the client is transported to the operating room. Nurses then direct the family to a waiting area. In some hospitals the family may be allowed to wait with the client in the operating room holding area until they are transported into the operating room.

After the client leaves the nursing division, the nurse prepares the bed and room for the client's return if the client is returning to the same nursing division. A postoperative bedside unit should include the following:

1. Sphygmomanometer, stethoscope, and thermometer
2. Emesis basin
3. Clean gown
4. Washcloth, towel, and facial tissues
5. IV pole
6. Suction equipment (if needed)
7. Oxygen equipment (if needed)
8. Extra pillows for positioning the client comfortably
9. Bed pads to protect bed linen from drainage
10. Bed raised to stretcher height with bed linens pulled back and furniture moved to accommodate the gurney and equipment (such as IV lines)

The nurse will be better prepared to care for the client after surgery if the room is readied before the client's return.

Intraoperative Surgical Phase

Care of the client during surgery requires careful preparation and knowledge of the events that occur during the surgical procedure.

PREOPERATIVE (HOLDING) AREA

In most hospitals the client enters a holding area outside the operating room. There the nurse explains the steps to be taken in preparing the client for surgery. Nurses in the holding area are usually part of the operating room staff and wear surgical scrub suits, hats, and footwear in accordance with infection-control policies. In some ambulatory surgical settings a perioperative primary nurse admits the client, circulates for the operative procedure, and manages the client's recovery and discharge.

In the preoperative area the nurse, nurse anesthetist, or anesthesiologist may insert an IV catheter into the arm to establish a route for fluid replacement and IV drugs. A large-bore (18-20 gauge) IV catheter is used for easy infusion of fluids and blood products if necessary. The nurse also applies a blood pressure cuff. The cuff will remain in place throughout surgery so that the anesthesiologist can assess blood pressure readings. The nurse usually reviews the preoperative checklist, and the anesthesiologist may perform a client assessment at this time.

Because of the preoperative medications, the client begins to feel drowsy. The temperature in the holding area and adjacent operating room suites is usually cool, and the client should be offered an extra blanket. Conscious sedation may be started at this time. The client's stay in the holding area is usually brief.

ADMISSION TO THE OPERATING ROOM

Nurses transfer the client to the operating room via a stretcher. The client is usually still awake and will notice nurses and physicians wearing complete surgical masks, gowns, and eyewear. The staff carefully transfers the client to the operating room table, being sure that the stretcher and table are locked in place. After the client is on the table, the nurse fastens a safety strap around the client.

The operating room nurse checks the client's identification and chart; reviews consent forms, medical history, physical assessment findings, and test results; makes sure that prosthetic devices and valuables have been removed; and reviews the preoperative care plan to establish an intraoperative care plan.

The nurse may apply monitoring devices to the client before surgery. Clients receiving general and regional anesthesia undergo continuous ECG monitoring during surgery. Small plastic electrodes are placed on the chest and extremities to record electrical activity of the heart. A monitor in the operating room displays the heart's electrical activity. Pulse oximetry will be used to monitor oxygen saturation as an index of ventilation quality.

Many ambulatory surgical clients remain awake during the procedure because only local anesthesia is used. Conscious sedation may also be used with local or regional anesthesia. The nurse supports the client by explaining procedures and encouraging the client to ask questions. Sights and sounds in the surgical suite can frighten clients.

INTRODUCTION OF ANESTHESIA

Clients undergoing surgical procedures receive one of four types of anesthesia: general, regional, local, or conscious sedation.

General Anesthesia.   Modern anesthetic agents are much easier to reverse and allow the client to recover with fewer untoward effects. **General anesthesia** results in an immobile, quiet client who does not recall the surgical procedure. The client's amnesia acts as a protective measure from the unpleasant events of the procedure. Surgery using general anesthesia involves major procedures requiring extensive tissue manipulation.

An anesthesiologist gives general anesthetics by IV and inhalation routes through the four stages of anesthesia. Stage I begins with the client awake and as the administration of anesthetic agents begins. The stage is completed when the client loses consciousness. Stage II begins with the loss of consciousness and ends with the onset of regular breathing and loss of eyelid reflexes. This is referred to as the excitement or delirium phase because it is often accompanied by involuntary motor activity. The client must not receive any auditory or physical stimulation during this period, because it can stimulate a release of catecholamines, which can result in an undesirable increase in heart rate and blood pressure. Stage III begins with the onset of regular breathing and ends with the cessation of respirations. This stage is known as the operative or surgical phase. Stage IV begins with the cessation of respirations and must be avoided, or it will necessitate the initiation of cardiopulmonary resuscitation and may lead to death. These stages were defined with the use of ether and are sometimes difficult to ascertain with newer anesthetic agents (Atkinson and Fortunato, 1996).

A more useful designation of stages includes the three phases of induction, maintenance, and emergence. Induction includes the administration of agents and endotracheal intubation. The maintenance phase includes positioning the client, preparation of the skin for incision, and the surgical procedure itself. Appropriate levels of anesthesia are maintained during this phase. During emergence, anesthetics are decreased and the client begins to awaken. Because of the short half-life of today's medications, emergence is often in the operating room.

To induce anesthesia, an IV agent is often given, although an inhalation agent may be used (Table 49-10). Unconsciousness is achieved in 10 to 20 seconds after the dose. Barbiturates provide sedation, amnesia, and hypnosis but must be used in combination with other agents to achieve pain relief and muscle relaxation (Atkinson and Fortunato, 1996). To prevent possible aspiration and other respiratory complications, the anesthesiologist puts an endotracheal tube into the client's airway. Endotracheal intubation is usually performed following administration of short-acting or, occasionally, long-acting muscle relaxants.

An anesthesia provider or operating room nurse may assist with cricoid pressure and endotracheal cuff inflation during intubation. In clients at risk for aspiration, cricoid pressure can prevent silent regurgitation and aspiration of gastric contents during induction and intubation. The maneuver is begun while the client is awake. Client reassurance is important, to provide support during this period of mild

Table 49-10 Commonly Used Anesthetic Gases and Drugs

	Common Usage	Advantages	Disadvantages	Comments
Inhalation Gases				
Air	Maintenance with O$_2$; laser surgery near airway	Less support of combustion than N$_2$O	No anesthetic qualities	Possibly less nausea than N$_2$O
Oxygen (O$_2$)	Essential for life	Can slightly ↑ O$_2$ available to tissues in low-cardiac-output states	Can cause retinopathy in premature infants	High concentrations hazardous with lasers in surgery of head, neck, and pulmonary areas
Nitrous oxide (N$_2$O)	Maintenance; frequently for induction	Rapid induction and recovery; additive effects to other anesthetics	No relaxation; can depress myocardium	Hypoxia if overdose given; ↑ uptake of other volatile agents
Enflurane (Ethrane)	Maintenance; occasionally for induction	Good relaxation; allows more epinephrine to be used than with halothane; 2.4% metabolized	Can cause ↑ heart rate (HR) and ↓ blood pressure (BP); lowers seizure threshold; slightly irritating odor	Abnormal electroencephalogram (EEG) at high concentrations; used less often today
Desflurane (Suprane)	Maintenance in shorter cases	Very rapid emergence; good relaxation: 0.02% metabolized	May cause transient ↑ HR and ↓ BP; airway irritation; requires heated vaporizer	Rapid recovery phase; can use for emergence after maintenance with another volatile agent; expensive
Halothane (Fluothane)	Maintenance; frequently for induction in pediatrics	Rapid induction and recovery; pleasant, nonirritating odor; fair relaxation	Narrow margin of safety; sensitizes myocardium to epinephrine; rare cause of liver damage; 15% to 20% metabolized	May cause ↓ HR and ↓ BP; premature ventricular contractions (PVCs) and ventricular fibrillation may occur with epinephrine
Isoflurane (Forane)	Maintenance; occasionally for induction	Good relaxation; allows more epinephrine to be used than with halothane; maintains cardiac output; 0.2% metabolized	↑ HR; slightly irritating odor	Isomer of enflurane; probably most common agent used today
Sevoflurane (Ultane)	Induction and maintenance	Very rapid induction and emergence; good relaxation; ~5% metabolized	A metabolite (compound A) is nephrotoxic in rats; effect in humans unknown	Very rapid and smooth mask induction in children or adults; expensive
Opioid Analgesics				
Morphine sulfate (MS)	Perioperative pain; premedication	Inexpensive; duration of action 4 to 5 hours; euphoria; good cardiovascular stability	Nausea and vomiting; histamine release; postural hypotension (↓ BP) [decreased systemic vascular resistance (↓ SVR)]	Used intrathecally and epidurally for postoperative pain; elimination half-life 3 hours
Alfentanil (Alfenta)	Surgical analgesia in ambulatory patients	Duration of action 0.5 hour; used as bolus or infusion		Potency: 750 μg = 10 mg morphine sulfate; elimination half-life 1.6 hours

Data from Meeker MH, Rothrock JC: Alexander's care of the patient in surgery, ed 11, St. Louis, 1999, Mosby.

Continued

Table 49-10 Commonly Used Anesthetic Gases and Drugs—cont'd

	Common Usage	Advantages	Disadvantages	Comments
Opioid Analgesics—cont'd				
Fentanyl (Sublimaze)	Surgical analgesia: epidural infusion for postoperative analgesia	Good cardiovascular stability; duration of action 0.5 hour		Most commonly used opioid; potency: 100 μg = 10 mg morphine sulfate; elimination half-life 3.6 hours
Remifentanil (Ultiva)	0.25 to 1.0 μg/kg/min infusion for surgical analgesia; small boluses for brief, intense pain	Easily titratable; metabolized by blood and tissue esterases; very short duration; good cardiovascular stability	New; expensive; requires mixing	Potency: 25μg = 10 mg morphine sulfate; 20 to 30 times potency of alfentanil; elimination half-life 3 to 10 minutes
Sufentanil (Sufenta)	Surgical analgesia	Good cardiovascular stability; duration of action 0.5 hour; prolonged analgesia	Prolonged respiratory depression	Potency: 15 μg = 10 mg morphine sulfate; elimination half-life 2.7 hours
Depolarizing Muscle Relaxants				
Succinylcholine (Anectine, Quelicin)	Intubation; short cases	Rapid onset; short duration	Requires refrigeration; may cause fasciculations, postoperative myalgias, and arrhythmias; ↑ serum K$^+$ with burns, tissue trauma, paralysis, and muscle diseases; slight histamine release	Prolonged muscle relaxation with serum cholinesterase deficiency and certain antibiotics; trigger agent for malignant hyperthermia
Nondepolarizing Muscle Relaxants—Intermediate Onset and Duration				
Atracurium (Tracrium)	Intubation; maintenance of relaxation	No significant cardiovascular or cumulative effects; good with renal failure	Requires refrigeration; slight histamine release	Breakdown by Hofmann elimination and ester hydrolysis
Cisatracurium (Nimbex)	Intubation; maintenance of relaxation	Similar to atracurium	No histamine release	Similar to atracurium
Mivacurium (Mivacron)	Intubation; maintenance of relaxation	Short acting; rapid metabolism by plasma cholinesterase; used as bolus or infusion	Expensive in longer cases	New; rarely need to reverse; prolonged effect with plasma cholinesterase deficiency
Rocuronium (Zemuron)	Intubation; maintenance of relaxation	Rapid onset; elimination via kidney and liver	Vagolytic; may ↑ HR	Duration similar to atracurium and vecuronium
Vecuronium (Norcuron)	Intubation; maintenance of relaxation	No significant cardiovascular or cumulative effects; no histamine release	Requires mixing	Mostly eliminated in bile, some in urine
Nondepolarizing Muscle Relaxants—Longer Onset and Duration				
d-Tubocurarine	Maintenance of relaxation		May cause histamine release and transient ganglionic blockade	Mostly used for pretreatment with succinylcholine
Metocurine (Metubine)	Maintenance of relaxation	Good cardiovascular stability	Slight histamine release	Large bolus may cause ↓ BP
Pancuronium (Pavulon)	Maintenance of relaxation		May cause ↑ HR and ↑ BP	Mostly renal elimination

	Use			
Intravenous Anesthetics				
Etomidate (Amidate)	Induction	Good cardiovascular stability; fast, smooth induction and recovery	May cause pain with injection and myotonic movements	Residual effects for 20 to 90 hours; ↑ effect with alcohol
Diazepam (Valium, Dizac)	Amnesia; hypnotic; preoperative medication	Good sedation	Prolonged duration	
Ketamine (Ketalar)	Induction, occasional maintenance (IV or IM)	Short acting; patient maintains airway; good in small children and burn patients	Large doses may cause hallucinations and respiratory depression	Need darkened, quiet room for recovery; often used in trauma cases
Midazolam (Versed)	Hypnotic; anxiolytic; sedation; often used as adjunct to induction	Excellent amnesia; water soluble (no pain with IV injection); short acting	Slower induction than thiopental	Often used for amnesia with insertion of invasive monitors or regional anesthesia
Propofol (Diprivan)	Induction and maintenance; sedation with regional anesthesia or MAC	Rapid onset; awakening in 4 to 8 minutes	May cause pain when injected into small veins	Short elimination half-life (34 to 64 minutes)
Sodium methohexital (Brevital)	Induction	Ultrashort-acting barbiturate	May cause hiccups	Can be given rectally
Thiopental sodium (Pentothal)	Induction	Smooth induction and recovery	Large doses may cause apnea and cardiovascular depression	May cause laryngospasm; can be given rectally
Local Anesthetics				
Bupivacaine (Marcaine, Sensorcaine)	Epidural, spinal, or local infiltration	Good relaxation; long acting	Overdose can cause cardiac collapse	Max. dose: 200 and 150 mg/70 kg with and without epinephrine respectively
Chloroprocaine (Nesacaine)	Epidural anesthesia	Ultrashort acting; good relaxation	May cause neurotoxicity if injected into cerebrospinal fluid (CSF)	Max. dose: 1000 and 800 mg/70 kg with and without epinephrine respectively
Lidocaine (Xylocaine)	Epidural, spinal, peripheral, IV anesthesia, and local infiltration	Short acting; good relaxation; low toxicity	Overdose can cause convulsions; possible transient neurologic changes with spinal anesthesia	Also used for ventricular arrhythmias Max. dose: 7 and 5 mg/kg with and without epinephrine respectively
Tetracaine (Pontocaine)	Spinal anesthesia	Long acting; good relaxation		Max. dose: 1 to 1.5 mg/kg (epinephrine rarely used)
Anticholinergics				
Atropine	Block effects of acetylcholine; ↓ vagal tone; reverse muscle relaxants; treat sinus bradycardia	↑ HR; suppresses salivation, bronchial and gastric secretions	Depresses sweating; may cause dry mouth, flushing, dizziness, CNS symptoms	Quite selective at muscarinic receptor in smooth and cardiac muscle and exocrine glands
Glycopyrrolate (Robinul)	Similar to atropine	Small ↑ HR; does not cross blood-brain barrier; can ↑ gastric pH > atropine	Prolonged duration of effects	Lower incidence of arrhythmias than atropine

discomfort. Once initiated, pressure must be held constant until the cuff has been inflated or aspiration can happen rapidly (Gruendemann and Fernsebner, 1995).

When induction is completed, anesthesia may be maintained through a combination of inhalation and IV medications. The client also receives a continuous supply of oxygen and adjunct medications such as opioid analgesics (analgesia) and muscle relaxants. A combination of smaller amounts of several medications allows a significant reduction in the dose that would be required to produce anesthesia with a single medication (Gruendemann and Fernsebner, 1995).

The duration of anesthesia depends on the length of surgery. Surgical risks influence the duration of surgery. The greatest risks from general anesthesia are the side effects of anesthetic agents, including cardiovascular depression or irritability, respiratory depression, and liver and kidney damage.

The emergence from anesthesia occurs when the procedure is completed and reversal agents are given. The oropharynx is suctioned to decrease the risk of aspiration and laryngeal spasm following extubation. Extubation is often accomplished before transfer to the PACU.

Regional Anesthesia.
Induction of **regional anesthesia** results in loss of sensation in an area of the body. The method of induction influences the portion of sensory pathways that is anesthetized. There is no loss of consciousness with regional anesthesia, but the client is usually sedated. The anesthesiologist gives regional anesthetics by infiltration and local application. Figure 49-7 demonstrates common locations for the introduction of medication to achieve the regional block. Infiltration of anesthetic agents may involve one of the following induction methods:

- *Nerve block:* Local anesthetic is injected into a nerve (e.g., brachial plexus in the arm), blocking the nerve supply to the operative site.
- *Spinal anesthesia:* The anesthesiologist performs a lumbar puncture and introduces local anesthetic into the cerebrospinal fluid in the spinal subarachnoid space. Anesthesia can extend from the tip of the xiphoid process down to the feet. Positioning of the client influences movement of the anesthetic agent up or down the spinal cord. This is often used for lower abdominal, pelvic, and lower extremity procedures; urologic procedures; or surgical obstetrics.
- *Epidural anesthesia:* This is a safer procedure than spinal anesthesia because the anesthetic agent is injected into the epidural space outside the dura mater and the depth of anesthesia is not as great as that with spinal anesthesia. Because epidural anesthesia provides an effective loss of sensation in the vaginal and perineal areas, it is often used for obstetrical procedures. The epidural catheter may be left in so that the client may receive medication via continuous epidural infusion following surgery (see Chapter 42).

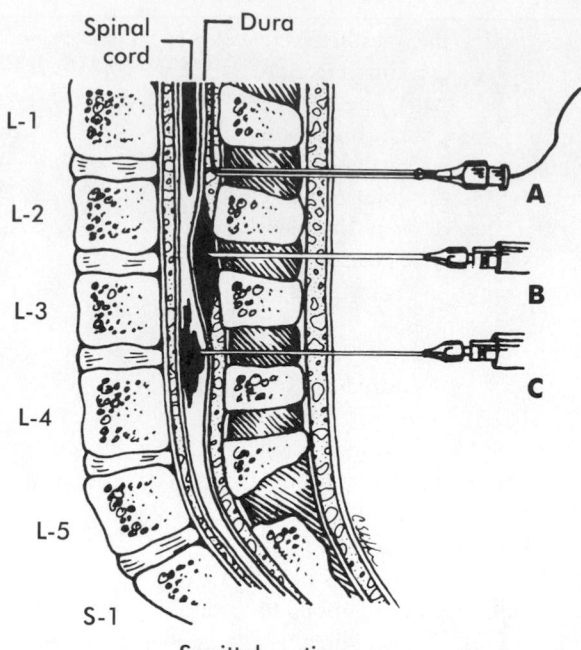

Figure 49-7 Spinal column—side view with spinal and epidural anesthesia needle placement. **A,** Epidural catheter. **B,** Single injection epidural. **C,** Spinal anesthesia. (Interspaces most commonly used are L4-5, L3-4, and L2-3.) From Meeker MH, Rothrock JC: *Alexander's care of the patient in surgery,* ed 11, St. Louis, 1999, Mosby.

- *Intravenous regional anesthesia (Bier Block):* Local anesthetic is injected via an IV line into an extremity below the level of a tourniquet after blood has been withdrawn. The drug is allowed to infiltrate only tissues in the intended surgical area. The extremity is pain free while the tourniquet is in place. Advantages include a short onset and short recovery time. However, the tourniquet may only be inflated for 2 hours or tissue damage will occur.

There are risks involved with infiltrative anesthetics, particularly in the case of spinal anesthesia, because the level of anesthesia may rise, which means that the anesthetic agent moves upward in the spinal cord and breathing may be affected. This migration of anesthetic depends on the drug type, amount, and client position. The client may have a sudden fall in blood pressure, which results from extensive vasodilation caused by the anesthetic block to sympathetic vasomotor nerves and pain and motor nerve fibers. If the level of anesthesia rises, respiratory paralysis may develop, requiring resuscitation by the anesthesiologist. Elevation of the upper body prevents respiratory paralysis. The client requires careful monitoring during and immediately after surgery.

The client under regional anesthesia is awake throughout the surgery unless the physician orders a tranquilizer that promotes sleep and/or amnesia. Because the client is responsive and capable of breathing voluntarily, it is unnecessary for the anesthesiologist to use an endotracheal tube. Operating room personnel often gain a false sense of security because of the client's relative alertness. Nurses must remember that burns and other trauma can occur on the anesthetized part of the body without the client being aware of the injury. It is therefore necessary to frequently observe the position of extremities and the condition of the skin. It is also important that operating room staff use caution regarding topics discussed in surgery.

Local Anesthesia.

Local anesthesia involves loss of sensation at the desired site (e.g., a growth on the skin or the cornea of the eye). The anesthetic agent (e.g., lidocaine) inhibits nerve conduction until the drug diffuses into the circulation. It may be injected or applied topically. The client experiences a loss in pain sensation and touch, and in motor and autonomic activities (e.g., bladder emptying). Local anesthesia is commonly used for minor procedures performed in ambulatory surgery. Physicians may infiltrate the operative area with local anesthetics to promote postoperative pain relief.

Conscious Sedation.

Conscious sedation is routinely used for procedures that do not require complete anesthesia but rather a depressed level of consciousness. A client under conscious sedation must independently retain a patent airway and airway reflexes and be able to respond appropriately to physical and verbal stimuli (Litwack, 1999).

Advantages of conscious sedation include adequate sedation and reduction of fear and anxiety with minimal risk, amnesia, relief of pain and noxious stimuli, mood alteration, elevation of pain threshold, enhanced client cooperation, stable vital signs, and rapid recovery. A variety of diagnostic and therapeutic procedures are appropriate for conscious sedation (burn dressing changes, cosmetic surgery, pulmonary biopsy and bronchoscopy, and many others) (Litwack, 1999).

Nurses assisting with the administration of conscious sedation must demonstrate competency in the care of these clients. Knowledge of anatomy, physiology, cardiac dysrhythmias, procedural complications, and pharmacological principles related to the administration of individual conscious agents is essential. Nurses must also be able to assess, diagnose, and intervene in the event of untoward reactions and demonstrate skill in airway management and oxygen delivery. Resuscitation equipment must be readily available if conscious sedation is being used (Litwack, 1999).

POSITIONING THE CLIENT FOR SURGERY

During general anesthesia the nursing personnel and surgeon often do not position the client until the stage of complete relaxation is achieved. The choice of position is usually determined by the surgical approach. Ideally the client's position provides good access to the operative site and sustains adequate circulatory and respiratory function. It should not impair neuromuscular structures. The client's comfort and safety must be considered. The team must take into account age, weight, height, nutritional status, physical limitations, and preexisting conditions and document them for staff who care for the client postoperatively (Atkinson and Fortunato, 1996).

It is sometimes difficult for nurses in postoperative divisions to appreciate the discomfort a client may feel after surgery (e.g., discomfort of the left arm or side of a client whose right kidney was removed). Normal range of joint motion is maintained in an alert person by pain and pressure receptors. If a joint is extended too far, pain stimuli provide a warning that muscle and joint strain is too great. In a client who is anesthetized, normal defense mechanisms cannot guard against joint damage, muscle stretch, and strain. The muscles are so relaxed that it is relatively easy to place the client in a position the individual normally could not assume while awake. The client often remains in a given position for several hours. Although it may be necessary to place a client in an unusual position, the nurse should attempt to maintain correct alignment and protect the client from pressure, abrasion, and other injuries (corneal abrasion). Attachments to the operating room table allow protection and padding of extremities and bony prominences. Positioning should not impede normal movement of the diaphragm or interfere with circulation to body parts. If restraints are necessary, the nurse pads the area to be restrained to prevent skin trauma.

NURSE'S ROLE DURING SURGERY

The nurse assumes one of two roles during the surgical procedure: scrub nurse or circulating nurse. The **scrub nurse** wears surgical attire and provides the surgeon with instruments and supplies, which requires strict surgical asepsis (see Chapter 33) and familiarity with surgical instruments. Each instrument is designed for a specific purpose during a phase or step in surgery. It takes knowledge and skill to anticipate which instrument the surgeon requires and to pass it quickly and smoothly. The scrub nurse also disposes of soiled gauze sponges and accounts for sponges, needles, and instruments on the surgical field and in body cavities. This role may be assumed by a scrub technician who is not a nurse.

The **circulating nurse** is an assistant to the scrub nurse and surgeon and is not required to wear sterile attire. A circulating nurse is a registered nurse. When the client first enters the operating room the circulator helps position the client and applies necessary equipment and surgical drapes. During surgery the circulator provides the scrub nurse with supplies, disposes of soiled equipment and sponges, and keeps a count of instruments, needles, and sponges used. If there is a need to help reposition the client or move the operating room lights, the circulating nurse is available to assist. Like all members of the surgical team, the circulator follows surgical aseptic technique.

If a break in asepsis occurs, the circulator assists team members with regowning and regloving.

At the end of each surgical procedure the scrub and circulating nurses count the number of used instruments, needles, and gauze sponges. This procedure prevents the accidental loss of such items within the client's surgical wound. It is not difficult for a sponge saturated with blood to be overlooked within a wound. Careful monitoring of items is essential for the client's safety. The nurse who fails to make accurate counts can be held legally accountable. If a client is injured by a misplaced needle or instrument, the nurse may be judged negligent.

Documentation of Intraoperative Care. During the intraoperative phase the nursing staff continues the preoperative care plan. For example, strict asepsis must be followed to minimize the risk of surgical wound infection. IV fluid infusion and monitoring of urinary and nasogastric output are actions the nurse takes to maintain fluid balance. Throughout the surgical procedure the nurse keeps an accurate record of client care activities and procedures performed by operating room personnel. Documentation of intraoperative care provides useful data for the nurse who cares for the client postoperatively.

Postoperative Surgical Phase

After surgery a client's care can become complex as a result of physiological changes that may occur. Clients who have undergone general anesthesia are more likely to face complications than those who have had only local anesthesia. The client who requires general anesthesia usually has undergone extensive surgery as well. In contrast, an ambulatory surgical client who has had local anesthesia with no sedation and has stable vital signs may be immediately discharged. A client who has undergone regional or general anesthesia usually is transferred to the PACU to be stabilized before discharge, whereas a client who has had local anesthesia may go directly to the nursing unit or back to the ambulatory surgery center.

To assess a client's postoperative condition, the nurse applies critical thinking while relying on information from the preoperative nursing assessment, knowledge regarding the surgical procedure performed, and events occurring during surgery. This information helps the nurse to detect change and make decisions about the client's care. A variation from the client's norm may indicate the onset of surgically related complications. Along with the anesthetist or anesthesiologist, the circulating nurse may accompany the client to the PACU and report to the nurse to provide continuity of care.

A client's postoperative course involves two phases: the immediate recovery period and postoperative convalescence. For an ambulatory surgical client, **recovery** normally lasts only 1 to 2 hours, and **convalescence** takes place at home. For a hospitalized client, recovery may last a few hours, and convalescence takes 1 or more days depending on the extent of surgery and the client's response.

IMMEDIATE POSTOPERATIVE RECOVERY

Before the arrival of the client in the PACU, the PACU nurse obtains data from the surgical team in the operating room regarding the client's general status and need for special equipment and nursing care. Careful planning allows the nursing staff to consider placement of clients in the PACU. For example, clients who undergo spinal anesthesia are aware of their surroundings and may benefit from being in a quieter part of the PACU, away from clients needing frequent monitoring. The client with a serious infection such as tuberculosis should be isolated from other clients. Standard precautions (see Chapter 33) are used for all clients.

When the client is admitted to the PACU, the personnel notify the client care area of the client's arrival. This allows the nursing staff to inform family members of the client's operative course and possible reasons for any delays that may have occurred. The nurse usually advises family members to remain in the designated waiting area so that they can be found when the surgeon arrives to explain the client's condition. *It is the surgeon's responsibility to describe the client's status, the results of surgery, and any complications that may have been encountered.* The nurse can be a valuable resource to the family if complications have arisen in the operative phase.

When the client enters the PACU (Figure 49-8), the nurse and members of the surgical team confer about the client's status. The surgical team's report includes a review of anesthetic agents administered so that the PACU nurse can anticipate how quickly a client should regain consciousness or anticipate analgesic needs. A report on IV fluids or blood products administered during surgery alerts the nurse to the fluid and electrolyte balance. The surgeon often reports special concerns (e.g., whether the client is at risk for hemorrhaging or infection). The oper-

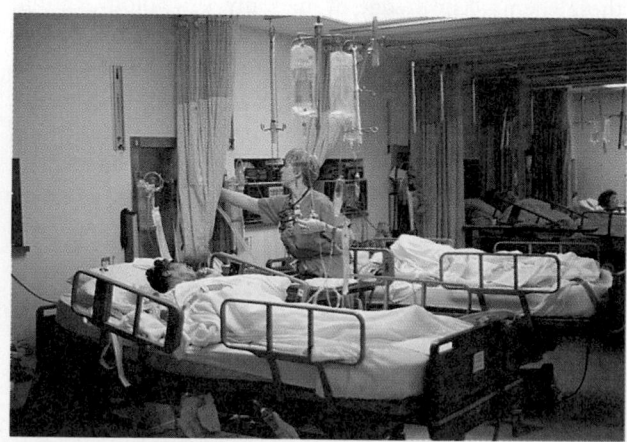

Figure 49-8   Postanesthesia care unit.

ating room nurse or anesthesia provider discusses whether there were complications during surgery, such as excessive blood loss or cardiac irregularities. Frequently this report takes place while PACU staff are admitting the client. The nurse will attach the client to monitoring equipment such as the noninvasive blood pressure monitor, ECG monitor, and pulse oximeter. Clients often receive some form of oxygen in this immediate recovery period.

After reviewing events in the operating room, the PACU nurse makes a complete assessment of the client's status. The assessment should be performed rapidly and thoroughly and be targeted to the needs of the postsurgical client (Litwack, 1995). The standards of care of the American Society of PeriAnesthesia Nurses (ASPAN, 1998) outlines the urgent nature and components of the admission assessment. A systems approach to assessment is discussed in a later section outlining the nursing process in postoperative care.

DISCHARGE FROM THE PACU

The nurse evaluates readiness for discharge from the PACU on the basis of vital sign stability in comparison with the preoperative data. Other outcomes for discharge include body temperature control, good ventilatory function, orientation to surroundings, absence of complications, minimal pain and nausea, controlled wound drainage, adequate urine output, and fluid and electrolyte balance. Clients with more extensive surgery requiring

anesthesia of longer duration usually recover more slowly. Many PACU staffs use an objective scoring system that helps delineate when clients may be discharged. The Aldrete score or the **Postanesthesia Recovery Score (PARS)** is the most widely used scoring tool (Table 49-11). It measures various criteria, including oxygen saturation, level of consciousness, circulation, activity, and respiration. The client must receive a composite score of 8 to 10 before discharge from the PACU (Aldrete, 1998). If the client's condition is still poor after 2 to 3 hours, the stay lengthens or the surgeon may transfer the client to an intensive care unit (ICU).

When the client is ready to be discharged from the PACU, the nurse calls the nursing unit to report vital signs, the type of surgery and anesthesia performed, blood loss, level of consciousness, general physical condition, and presence of IV lines or drainage tubes. The PACU nurse's report helps the nurse on the acute patient care area to anticipate special client needs and obtain necessary equipment.

Personnel, which may include nurses, return the client on a stretcher. Staff members assist in safely transferring the client to a bed (see Chapter 36). The PACU nurse, if helping to transport the client, shows the acute care area nurse the recovery room record and reviews the client's condition and course of care. The PACU nurse also points out physician orders that require attention. *Before the PACU nurse leaves the acute care area, the staff nurse assuming care for the client takes a complete set of vital signs*

Table 49-11 Modified Aldrete Score

		Admission	5 Min	15 Min	30 Min	45 Min	60 Min	Discharge
Able to move four extremities voluntarily or on command 2 Able to move two extremities voluntarily or on command 1 Unable to move extremities voluntarily or on command 0	Activity							
Able to breathe deeply and cough freely 2 Dyspnea or limited breathing 1 Apneic 0	Respiratory							
BP + 20% of preanesthetic level 2 BP + 20%-49% of preanesthetic level 1 BP + 50% of preanesthetic level 0	Circulation							
Fully awake 2 Arousable on calling 1 Not responding 0	Consciousness							
Able to maintain O_2 saturation >92% on room air 2 Needs O_2 inhalation to maintain O_2 saturation >90% 1 O_2 saturation <90% even with O_2 supplement 0	O_2 saturation							
	TOTALS							

Modified from Aldrete JA, Kroulik D: A post-anesthetic recovery score, *Anesth Analg* 49:924, 1970; and Aldrete JA: Modifications to the post anesthesia score for use in ambulatory surgery, *J PeriAnesth Nurs* 13(3): 148, 1998.
BP, Blood pressure.

to compare with PACU findings. Minor vital sign variations normally occur after transporting the client.

RECOVERY IN AMBULATORY SURGERY

The thoroughness and extent of postoperative assessment depends on the ambulatory client's condition, type of surgery, and anesthesia. In many cases the assessment is identical to that conducted for hospitalized clients. However, if the client has undergone minor surgery (e.g., cosmetic removal of a mole), the postoperative recovery phase requires minimal assessment.

If an ambulatory client has received general or regional anesthesia or intensive IV sedation, the client will be transferred to the recovery room. In phase I recovery, clients in need of close monitoring are frequently assessed for vital sign changes, respiratory and circulatory status, level of consciousness, condition of the surgical wound, and pain level. The PARS may be used, with a score of 8 to 10 determining discharge from the PACU.

The time that a client spends in phase I recovery depends on several factors. Outpatient anesthesia is gauged to provide a quick recovery time, few aftereffects, and a speedy return to daily routines. The average time spent in phase I (without complications) is 1 hour. Clients are encouraged to gradually sit up on the stretcher or bed and begin to take ice chips or sips of water while regaining full alertness. After clients become stable and no longer require close monitoring, the nurse transfers them to phase II recovery. Clients who have undergone minor surgery may be transferred directly to phase II recovery.

Phase II recovery may consist of a room equipped with medical recliner chairs, side tables, and foot rests. Kitchen facilities for preparing light snacks and beverages are usually located in the area, along with bathrooms. Aldrete (1998) has added five more areas of functional assessment for the ambulatory surgery client, which makeup the **Postanesthesia Recovery Score for Ambulatory Patients (PARSAP).** The five additional areas of assessment include the condition of the dressing, intensity and location of pain, ability to stand and ambulate, tolerance of oral fluids and/or food, and ability to urinate spontaneously (Table 49-12). The phase II environment is designed to promote the client's and family's comfort and well-being until discharge. The nurse monitors clients but not at the same intensity as during phase I. In phase II recovery, nurses initiate postoperative teaching with clients and family members (Box 49-5).

POSTOPERATIVE CONVALESCENCE

Ambulatory surgical clients are discharged to home when they meet certain criteria; for example, they are able to void (if applicable) and ambulate, they are alert and oriented, they have minimal nausea/vomiting, they have received no pain medication for 1 hour, they have minimal postoperative pain and no excess bleeding or drainage, they have received written postoperative instructions and

prescriptions, they verbalize understanding of these instructions, and they are being discharged to a responsible adult (Litwack, 1999). A client being monitored by the PARSAP must achieve a score of 18 or higher before he or she can be discharged. An exception may be allowed if the client was unable to walk or use extremities before surgery (Aldrete, 1998). Good judgment should be used in determining the appropriate discharge status. In contrast, inpatient clients are kept in the PACU until their condition stabilizes; they are then returned to the postoperative nursing division.

Nursing care focuses on returning the client to a relatively functional level of wellness as soon as possible. The speed of convalescence depends on the type or extent of surgery, risk factors, postoperative complications, and the client's plan of care. Nursing care in the PACU focuses on monitoring and maintaining respiratory, circulatory, and neurological status and on managing pain.

The Nursing Process in Postoperative Care

Nursing care in the PACU focuses on monitoring and maintaining respiratory, circulatory, fluid and electrolyte, and neurological status, as well as the management of pain. Other important factors to assess include temperature control, skin and incision/wound status, and genitourinary and gastrointestinal function. These factors are not, however unique to the PACU setting. The nurse on the acute care division continues assessment of these critical factors on a less intensive basis until the client's discharge from the acute care facility.

ASSESSMENT

After the initial assessment on the client's arrival to recovery, the nurse repeats evaluation of vital signs and other key observations at least every 15 minutes or more frequently, depending on the client's condition and unit policy. This assessment usually continues until discharge from the PACU. Vital sign monitoring should initially be hourly for 4 hours and then every 4 hours. As the client's condition stabilizes, frequency of assessment will usually decrease to once a shift until discharge. Frequency of assessment should always be based on the client's current condition. *A nurse should not assume that further monitoring is unnecessary if the client appears normal during the initial assessment.* A client's condition can change rapidly, especially during the postoperative period.

The nurse thoroughly documents the initial assessment, including vital signs, level of consciousness, condition of dressings and drains, comfort level, IV fluid status, and urinary output measurements. Client data can be entered on flowsheets, a computerized client record, or

Table 49-12 Expanded Postanesthetic Recovery Score for Ambulatory Patients

Indices	Task	Score	Time in Minutes						
			0	5	10	15	30	45	60
Activity	Able to move four extremities voluntarily or on command	2							
	Able to move two extremities voluntarily or on command	1							
	Unable to move extremities voluntarily or on command	0							
Respiration	Able to breathe deeply and cough freely	2							
	Dyspnea, limited breathing, or tachypnea	1							
	Apneic or on mechanical ventilator	0							
Circulation	BP ± 20% of preanesthetic level	2							
	BP ± 20-49% of preanesthetic level	1							
	BP ± 50% of preanesthetic level	0							
Consciousness	Fully awake	2							
	Arousable on calling	1							
	Not responding	0							
O_2 saturation	Able to maintain O_2 saturation >92% on room air	2							
	Needs O_2 inhalation to maintain O_2 saturation >90%	1							
	O_2 saturation <90% even with O_2 supplement	0							
Dressing	Dry and clean	2							
	Wet but marked and not increasing	1							
	Growing area of wetness	0							
Pain	Pain free	2							
	Mild pain handled by oral medication	1							
	Severe pain requiring parenteral medication	0							
Ambulation	Able to stand up and walk straight*	2							
	Vertigo when erect	1							
	Dizziness when supine	0							
Fasting-feeding	Able to drink fluids	2							
	Nauseated	1							
	Nausea and vomiting	0							
Urine output	Has voided	2							
	Unable to void but comfortable	1							
	Unable to void and uncomfortable	0							
TOTALS									

Modified from Aldrete JA, Kroulik D: A post-anesthetic recovery score, *Anesth Analg* 49:924, 1970; and Aldrete JA: Modifications to the post anesthesia score for use in ambulatory surgery, *J PeriAnesth Nurs* 13(3): 148, 1998.

NOTE: Total score must be at least 18 for client to be discharged to home.

BP, Blood pressure.

*May be substituted by Romberg's test, or picking up 12 clips in one hand.

Client Teaching of Postoperative Instructions for Ambulatory Surgical Client   Box 49-5

OBJECTIVE
- Client will verbalize resources to contact for assistance.
- Client will describe signs and symptoms of postoperative problems.
- Client will list the name and dose of medications.
- Client will describe guidelines related to specific surgery.

TEACHING STRATEGIES
- Give instruction sheet with physician's telephone number, surgery center's number, and follow-up appointment date and time. Allow client and family to ask questions.
- Explain to family member the signs and symptoms of infection for which to observe.
- Explain name, dose, schedule, and purpose of medications. Provide drug information leaflets.
- Explain activity restrictions, diet progression, and any special wound care related to specific surgery. Provide instruction sheet with clear, focused explanations.

EVALUATION
- Client is able to explain when to call physician with problems.
- Client is able to recite date for follow-up appointment.
- Client and family member describe signs and symptoms of infection.
- Client recites name of drug, dose, and when to take.
- Client demonstrates proper activity/movement and wound care.

progress notes. The initial findings are a baseline for comparing postoperative changes.

After the first assessment is completed on the acute care area and immediate needs are attended to, the family is allowed to visit. The nurse can explain the purpose of postoperative procedures or equipment and how the client is doing. The family should know that the client will fall in and out of sleep for most of the rest of the day from the effects of general anesthesia and pain medication. The family should also be reminded that frequent assessments are to be expected and that loss of sensation and movement in the extremities remains for several hours if the client had spinal or epidural anesthesia.

Respiration.   Certain anesthetic agents may cause respiratory depression. Thus the nurse is especially alert for shallow, slow breathing and a weak cough. The nurse assesses respiratory rate, rhythm, depth of ventilation, symmetry of chest wall movement, breath sounds, and color of mucous membranes. If breathing is unusually shallow, placement of the hand over the client's face or mouth allows the nurse to feel exhaled air. Pulse oximetry should reflect 92% to 100% saturation.

The client often has an oral or nasal airway (see Chapter 39) inserted in the operating room after extubation to maintain a patent airway until comfortable breathing at a normal rate resumes. As respiratory function returns, the nurse asks the client to spit out the airway. The ability to do so signifies the return of a normal gag reflex.

One of the nurse's greatest concerns is airway obstruction. A number of factors can contribute to obstruction, including weak pharyngeal/laryngeal muscle tone from anesthetics; secretions in the pharynx, bronchial tree, or trachea; and laryngeal or subglottic edema (Litwack, 1999). In the postanesthetic client the tongue causes the majority of airway obstructions. The following measures maintain airway patency:

- The client may be turned on one side to facilitate a forward movement of the tongue and the flow of mucous secretions out of the mouth. However, in most cases, the head of the bed is slightly elevated and the client's neck slightly extended, with the head turned to the side. The client should never be positioned with the arms over or across the chest, because this position reduces maximal chest expansion. The nurse may perform a jaw thrust maneuver and/or chin lift continuously to maintain the airway in some clients.
- The nurse suctions artificial airways and the oral cavity for mucous secretions (see Chapter 39). Care must be taken to avoid continually eliciting the gag reflex, which might cause vomiting. Before the nurse or client removes an airway, the back of the airway should be suctioned so that mucous plugs and secretions are not retained.

- The nurse begins coughing and deep breathing exercises as soon as the client is responsive and the endotracheal tube has been removed. This decreases the risk of atelectasis, a collapsed or airless portion of the lung, developing as a result of a mucous plug or fluid.
- The nurse administers oxygen as ordered and monitors oxygen saturation with a pulse oximeter.

The nurse providing acute care continues respiratory assessment by auscultating for effective lung sounds. Older clients, smokers, and clients with a history of respiratory disease are prone to developing complications such as atelectasis or pneumonia. The client is also assessed for any signs of shortness of breath or difficulty with endurance. A pulmonary infection caused by aspiration in the operating room or PACU setting may not be evident until several days later. Clients should also be instructed to report any of these symptoms to the physician after discharge, since the length of stay in acute care may be quite short.

Circulation.   The client is at risk for cardiovascular complications resulting from actual or potential blood loss from the surgical site, side effects of anesthesia, electrolyte imbalances, and depression of normal circulatory regulating mechanisms. Careful assessment of heart rate and rhythm, along with blood pressure, reveals the client's cardiovascular status. A rhythm strip is usually obtained, compared with preoperative ECG tracings, and mounted on the PACU record. The values are monitored at least every 15 minutes throughout the recovery phase. The nurse compares preoperative vital signs with postoperative values. The surgeon's postoperative orders may specify when vital sign changes should be reported. For example, a heart rate above 140 beats per minute or below 60 beats per minute should be reported immediately. However, the nurse must use judgment in reporting vital sign changes. If the client's blood pressure drops progressively after each check or if the heart rate becomes more irregular, the physician should be notified.

The nurse assesses circulatory perfusion by noting capillary refill, pulses, and the color of the nail beds and skin. If the client has had vascular surgery or has casts or constricting devices that may impair circulation, the nurse assesses peripheral pulses distal to the site of surgery. For example, after surgery to the femoral artery, the nurse assesses posterior tibial and dorsalis pedis pulses. The nurse also compares pulses in the affected extremity with those in the nonaffected extremity. A complaint of pain or swelling, especially in a lower extremity, could be an indication of deep vein thrombosis (DVT).

A common early circulatory problem is hemorrhage. Blood loss may occur externally through a drain or incision or internally within the surgical wound. Either type of hemorrhage may result in a fall in blood pressure; elevated heart and respiratory rate; thready pulse; cool, clammy, pale skin; and restlessness. If hemorrhage is external, the nurse observes increased bloody drainage on dressings or through drains. If a dressing becomes saturated, the blood oozes down the client's sides and collects in a pool under bedclothes. *An alert nurse always checks under the client for drainage even if the dressing is not saturated.* When hemorrhage is internal, the operative site becomes swollen and tight. For example, if a client bleeds within the abdomen, the abdomen becomes tight and distended. The first signs of suspected hemorrhaging should be reported to the physician immediately. The nurse maintains IV fluid infusion and monitors the client's vital signs every 15 minutes or more frequently until the client's condition stabilizes. Oxygen may be continued and the client's legs and head elevated to promote venous return and increase the volume of blood available for supplying oxygen and nutrients to vital organ systems. Medications and volume replacement may be considered.

The potential for cardiovascular complications remains when the client is transferred to the acute care area. The nurse continues to assess the same factors that were identified in the PACU. If the client is on prolonged bed rest, low-dose heparin may be given, in addition to the use of pneumatic compression stockings, for the prevention of DVT. The risk for DVT decreases when the client begins to mobilize.

Temperature Control.

The operating room and recovery room environments are extremely cool. The client's anesthetically depressed level of body function results in a lowering of metabolism and fall in body temperature. When clients begin to awaken, they complain of feeling cold and uncomfortable. The length of time spent in the operating room and laminar flow rooms contributes to heat loss (Litwack, 1995). Surgeries that require an open body cavity also contribute to heat loss. Older adults and pediatric clients are at higher risk for developing problems associated with hypothermia.

The nurse measures the client's body temperature and provides warmed blankets. If the temperature is 35.6° C (96° F) or below, a warming mattress or convective warming device may be used. Increasing body warmth causes the client's metabolism to rise and circulatory and respiratory functions to improve.

Shivering may not be a sign of hypothermia but rather a side effect of certain anesthetic agents. Meperidine (Demerol) may be given in small increments to decrease shivering. Deep breathing and coughing help expel retained anesthetic gases.

In rare instances **malignant hyperthermia,** a life-threatening complication of anesthesia, develops. Malignant hyperthermia causes tachypnea, tachycardia, premature ventricular contractions (PVCs), unstable blood pressure, cyanosis, skin mottling, and muscular rigidity. Despite the name, an elevated temperature is a late sign

(Atkinson and Fortunato, 1996). Although it is often seen during the induction phase of anesthesia, symptoms may recur 24 to 72 hours postoperatively (Karlet, 1998). Without proper treatment, it can be fatal. Immediate administration of dantrolene sodium is the most critical treatment.

Temperature is monitored closely in the acute care area. Since an elevated temperature may be the first indication of an infection, if the temperature is elevated, the nurse evaluates the client for a potential source of infection, including the IV site (if present), the surgical incision/wound, and the respiratory and urinary tracts. The physician must be notified, since a further evaluation, including blood, sputum and urinary specimens, will likely be needed.

Fluid and Electrolyte Balance.

Because of the surgical client's risk for fluid and electrolyte abnormalities, the nurse assesses the hydration status and monitors cardiac and neurological function for signs of electrolyte alterations (see Chapter 40). Fluids are especially important as the client recovers from regional anesthesia. Laboratory values will be monitored and compared with the client's baseline values. If a nasogastric tube is in place, any irrigation should be with normal saline to preserve electrolyte balance.

An important responsibility is maintaining patency of IV infusions. The client's only source of fluid intake immediately after surgery is through IV catheters. The nurse inspects the catheter insertion site to be sure that the catheter is properly positioned within a vein so that fluid flows freely. The physician orders a prescribed rate for each infusion. To ensure adequate fluid intake, the nurse should not allow infusion of fluids to fall behind. As the client begins to take oral fluids, the IV rate will be decreased. When the client no longer needs a continuous IV infusion, the IV line may be saline locked to preserve the site for antibiotics or other use (see Chapter 40). This usually takes place on the acute care floor the day after surgery. The client may also receive blood products after surgery, depending on blood loss during surgery.

Accurate recording of intake and output helps assess renal and circulatory function. The nurse measures all sources of output, including urine, surgically placed drains, gastric drainage, and drainage from wounds, and notes any insensible loss from diaphoresis. Mucus suctioned from airways is not included in output measurements.

Although the measurement of intake and output is important and should continue in the acute care area, the most accurate measurement of a client's fluid status is weight (Welsh, Arzoukman, and Holm, 1996). The nurse should assess daily weight for the first several days after surgery and compare it with the preoperative weight. If the client has a known cardiac history such as congestive heart failure, daily weights may be continued. It is important to use a consistent scale, amount of clothing, and time of day to obtain accurate weight measurement.

Neurological Functions.

A client should at least be oriented to self and the hospital before discharge from the PACU. As the effects of anesthesia wear off, the client's reflexes return, muscle strength is regained, and a normal level of orientation returns. The nurse can easily check for pupillary and gag reflexes (see Chapter 32) and assess hand grips and movement of extremities. If a client has had surgery involving a portion of the neurological system, the nurse conducts a more thorough neurological assessment. For example, if the client has had low back surgery, the nurse assesses leg movement, sensation, and strength. Clients with regional anesthesia begin to experience a return in motor function before tactile sensation returns. **Dermatome** (a segmental skin area innervated by segments of spinal cord) assessment of the spinal nerves is completed (Figure 49-9). Typically the nurse assesses the dermatome level by touching the client bilaterally and documenting where the client feels touch. The touch can be with hand pressure or a gentle pinch of the skin.

Orientation to the environment is important in main-

taining the client's alertness. The nurse reorients the client, explains that surgery is completed, and describes procedures and nursing measures. The client who was properly prepared before surgery is less likely to be anxious when nurses begin their care.

Unless the client has undergone neurological surgery, the focus of the nursing assessment will be on a basic neurological examination. Of primary importance is the client's level of consciousness. An altered level of alertness may be one of the first indications that there may be something untoward happening to the client. Although the client may still be drowsy from anesthesia, the nurse should be able to assess the client's ability to follow commands and answer orientation questions. Extremity strength assessment continues to be important if spinal or epidural anesthesia has been given, although the client should remain in the PACU until sensation and voluntary movement of the lower extremities have been reestablished.

Skin Integrity and Condition of the Wound.

In the PACU the nurse assess the condition of the client's skin, noting rashes, petechiae, abrasions, or burns. A rash may indicate a drug sensitivity or allergy. Abrasions or pe-

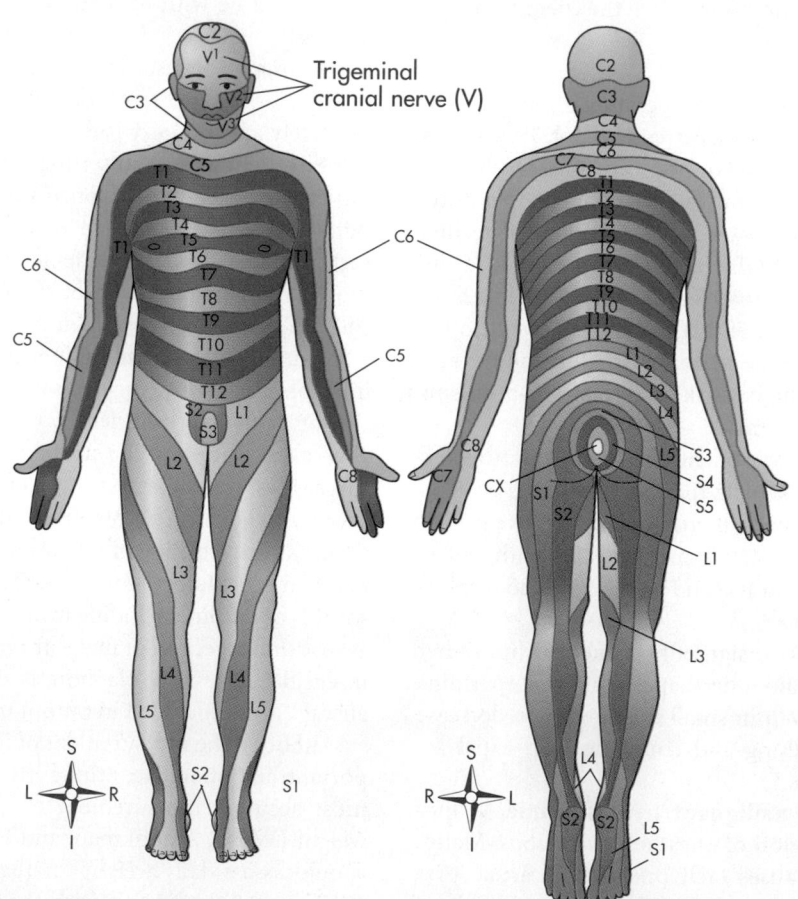

Figure 49-9 Segmental dermatome distribution of spinal nerves. *C,* Cervical segments; *T,* thoracic segments; *L,* lumbar segments; *S* sacral segments.
From Thibodeau G, Patton K: *Anthony's textbook of anatomy and physiology,* ed 15, St. Louis, 1996, Mosby.

techiae may result from inappropriate positioning or restraining that injures skin layers, or from a clotting disorder. The nurse should also note if the client is complaining of any burning or pain in the eye that could indicate a corneal abrasion. Burns may indicate that an electrical cautery grounding pad was incorrectly placed on the client's skin. Burns or serious injury to the skin should be documented by an incident report (see Chapter 24).

After surgery most surgical wounds are covered with a dressing that protects the wound site and collects drainage. The nurse observes the amount, color, odor, and consistency of drainage on dressings. The nurse estimates the amount of drainage by noting the number of saturated gauze sponges. If drainage appears on the outer surface of a dressing, another way of assessing drainage is by drawing a circle around the outer perimeter of the drainage and dating it with the time noted. This way the nurse can easily note if drainage is increasing (see Chapter 47). However, this is not the most accurate measure of volume of fluid lost.

Many physicians prefer to change surgical dressings the first time so that they can inspect the incisional area. The nurse on the acute care area will usually have the first opportunity to view and thoroughly assess and document the status of the incision/wound. This assessment is especially important, since it forms the baseline for continued monitoring during the client's hospital stay.

It is important to assess the client's mobility level at this time. If the client is unable or unwilling to turn, pressure ulcer development is a concern. The nurse should institute the use of the Braden Scale or some other means to determine the risk of developing pressure ulcers. Preventive measures such as a turning schedule and pressure reduction devices can then be instituted (see Chapter 47).

Genitourinary Function.

Depending on the surgery, a client may not regain voluntary control over urinary function for 6 to 8 hours after anesthesia. An epidural or spinal anesthetic may prevent the client from feeling bladder fullness or distention. The nurse palpates the lower abdomen just above the symphysis pubis for bladder distention. Clients need to be helped to void if they are unable to void in 8 hours or if the bladder becomes distended. Because a full bladder can be painful and often causes restlessness in recovery, it may become necessary to insert a catheter. If the client has a Foley catheter, there should be a continuous flow of urine of at least 1 ml/kg/hr in adults. The nurse observes the color and odor of urine. Surgery involving portions of the urinary tract normally causes bloody urine for at least 12 to 24 hours, depending on the type of surgery. The acute care nurse will provide ongoing assessment of genitourinary function. If the client has a Foley catheter, the goal should be to have it removed as soon as possible. Clients with a Foley catheter are at high risk to develop a nosocomial bladder or urinary tract infection. This will contribute to increased client cost and an increase in the length of hospitalization.

Gastrointestinal Function.

Anesthetics slow gastrointestinal motility and cause nausea. Normally during the immediate recovery phase, faint or absent bowel sounds are auscultated in all four quadrants. Inspection of the abdomen rules out distention that may be caused by accumulation of gas. In a client who has had abdominal surgery, distention will develop if internal bleeding occurs. Distention may also occur in the client who develops a **paralytic ileus** from handling of the bowel in surgery. This paralysis of intestines with distention and symptoms of acute obstruction may also be related to the administration of anticholinergic drugs. This usually does not occur for 24 hours. The acute care nurse must be aware of its potential development and include observation for distention and auscultation for bowel sounds during routine assessment.

To minimize nausea, sudden movement of the client should be avoided. If the client has a nasogastric tube, the nurse keeps it patent by regular normal saline irrigations as ordered. Occlusion of nasogastric tubes results in accumulation of gastric contents within the stomach. Because stomach emptying slows with the client under anesthesia, the accumulated contents cannot escape and nausea and vomiting develop. Normally a client does not receive fluids to drink in the PACU because of bowel sluggishness, with the risk of nausea and vomiting, and because of grogginess from general anesthesia.

The client will likely begin taking ice chips or sips of fluids when arriving on the acute care unit. If these are tolerated, a clear liquid meal will usually be ordered. The acute care nurse closely monitors the client's initial oral intake for potential aspiration or the presence of nausea and vomiting. The client's diet will be liberalized as tolerated beginning the day after surgery for many operative procedures. In cases of abdominal surgery, the bowel may need to rest and oral intake will not be started for several days.

Comfort.

As clients awaken from general anesthesia, the sensation of pain becomes prominent. Pain can be perceived before full consciousness is regained. Acute incisional pain causes clients to become restless and may be responsible for changes in vital signs. It is difficult for clients to begin coughing and deep breathing exercises when they experience pain. The client who had regional or local anesthesia usually does not experience pain initially, because the incisional area is still anesthetized.

Assessment of the client's discomfort and evaluation of pain-relief therapies are essential nursing functions. Pain scales are an effective method for nurses to assess postoperative pain, evaluate response to analgesics, and objectively document pain severity (see Chapter 42). Using preoperative pain assessments as a baseline, the nurse is able to evaluate the effectiveness of interventions throughout the client's recovery.

It is common to administer narcotic analgesics immediately after surgery for pain relief and to maximize the client's ability to perform respiratory exercises such as coughing and deep breathing. Initial analgesic doses are usually given by IV infusion in the PACU and titrated to client comfort. After an anesthetized client is awake and aware, PCA may be used. This is given by IV infusion or via an epidural, as with fentanyl or morphine. Many clients receive epidural analgesia that may be continued throughout the recovery period (see Chapter 42).

The acute care nurse continues pain assessment and assessment of the effectiveness of interventions. If the client has a PCA and is using it much more frequently than what it is programmed, for the nurse should contact the physician to increase the amount of medication the client can receive. The PCA gives the nurse a useful monitor of the effectiveness of pain medication. As oral intake is tolerated, the nurse facilitates changing the client's pain medication from IV to oral administration. The importance of nonpharmacological interventions should not be overlooked. The nurse should assess what care routines contribute to pain and use nonpharmacological measures to treat them. An example would be to lower the head of the bed and use a pillow for incisional splinting while turning a client with recent abdominal surgery.

NURSING DIAGNOSIS

The nurse determines the status of problems identified from preoperative nursing diagnoses and clusters new relevant data to identify new diagnoses. Previously defined diagnoses, such as *impaired skin integrity,* may continue as a postoperative problem. The nurse may also identify new risk factors leading to identification of nursing diagnoses (Box 49-6). For example, an older client who has undergone major abdominal surgery and who has a preexisting problem of reduced hip mobility resulting from arthritis will likely have the diagnosis of *impaired physical mobility.* The surgery itself may add risk factors for the client. The nurse also considers needs of a client's family when making diagnoses. For example, the inability of the family to cope with the client's condition requires the nurse's intervention.

PLANNING

During the convalescent phase the nurse has much information for planning the client's care. Current physical assessment data and analysis of the preoperative nursing history allow the nurse to plan specific nursing interventions. The surgeon's postoperative orders also offer guidelines. Typical postoperative orders include the following:

Frequency of vital sign monitoring and special assessments

Types of IV fluids and rates of infusion

Postoperative medications (especially those for pain and nausea)

Fluids and food allowed by mouth

Level of activity that the client is allowed to resume

Position that the client is to maintain while in bed

Intake and output

Laboratory tests and x-ray studies

Special directions

The nurse considers the effects of the stress of surgery and limitations it produces when establishing expected outcomes and interventions for the individual client. Measurable outcomes help to ensure aggressive but appropriate recovery from surgery. For example, the client at risk for impaired mobility should have specific outcomes selected that may include ambulation and range of joint movement. After each outcome is met, the client will ultimately achieve the goal of independent mobility at a preoperative level or better. The nurse carefully considers all goals of care established during the preoperative surgical phase. Typical broad goals of postoperative care include the following:

Demonstrating return or maintenance of normal physiological function, including respiratory, circulatory, elimination, and nutritional status

Demonstrating absence of postoperative surgical wound infection

Achieving rest and comfort

Maintaining or enhancing self-concept

IMPLEMENTATION

Regaining Normal Physiological Function. A surgical wound, the effects of prolonged immobilization during surgery and convalescence, and the influence of anesthesia and analgesics are the principal causes for postoperative complications. Nursing interventions are directed at preventing complications so that the client returns to the highest level of functioning possible. Failure of the client to become actively involved in recovery adds to the risk of complications (Table 49-13). Virtually any body system can be affected. The nurse must consider the interrelationship of all systems and therapies provided.

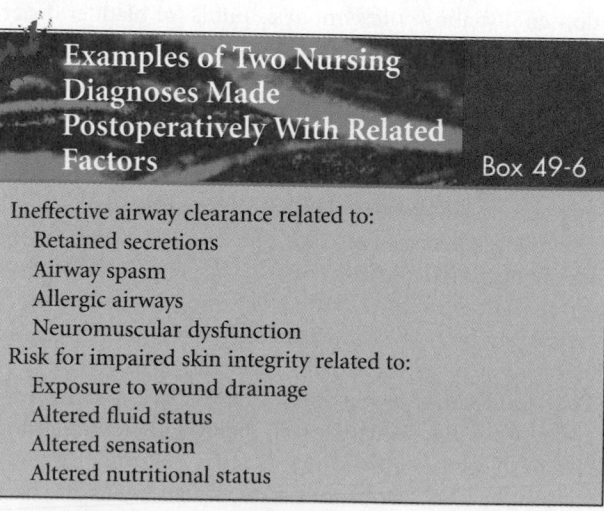

Examples of Two Nursing Diagnoses Made Postoperatively With Related Factors   Box 49-6

Ineffective airway clearance related to:
  Retained secretions
  Airway spasm
  Allergic airways
  Neuromuscular dysfunction
Risk for impaired skin integrity related to:
  Exposure to wound drainage
  Altered fluid status
  Altered sensation
  Altered nutritional status

Table 49-13 Postoperative Complications

Complication	Cause
Respiratory System **Atelectasis** is collapse of alveoli with retained mucous secretions. Signs and symptoms include elevated respiratory rate, dyspnea, fever, crackles auscultated over involved lobes of lungs, and productive cough.	Atelectasis is caused by inadequate lung expansion. Anesthesia, analgesia, and immobilized position prevent full lung expansion. There is greater risk in clients with upper abdominal surgery who have pain during inspiration and repress deep breathing.
Pneumonia is inflammation of alveoli caused by infectious process. It may involve one or several lobes of lung. Development of pneumonia in lower dependent lobes of lung is common in immobilized surgical client. Signs and symptoms include fever, chills, productive cough, chest pain, purulent mucus, and dyspnea.	Pneumonia is caused by poor lung expansion with retained secretions. Common resident bacterium in respiratory tract is *Diplococcus pneumoniae*, which causes most cases of pneumonia.
Hypoxia is inadequate concentration of oxygen in arterial blood. Signs and symptoms include restlessness, dyspnea, high blood pressure, tachycardia, diaphoresis, and cyanosis.	Respirations are depressed by anesthetics or analgesics. Increased retention of mucus with impaired ventilation occurs because of pain or poor positioning.
Pulmonary embolism is embolus blocking pulmonary artery and disrupting blood flow to one or more lobes of lung. Signs and symptoms include dyspnea, sudden chest pain, cyanosis, tachycardia, and drop in blood pressure.	Same factors lead to formation of thrombus or embolus. Immobilized surgical client with preexisting circulatory or coagulation disorders is at risk.
Circulatory System *Hemorrhage* is loss of large amount of blood externally or internally in short period of time. Signs and symptoms are same as for hypovolemic shock.	Hemorrhage is caused by slipping of suture or dislodged clot at incisional site. Clients with coagulation disorders are at greater risk.
Hypovolemic shock is perfusion of tissues and cells from loss of circulatory fluid volume. Signs and symptoms include hypotension, weak and rapid pulse, cool and clammy skin, rapid breathing, restlessness, and reduced urine output.	In surgical client, hypovolemic shock is usually caused by hemorrhage.
Thrombophlebitis is inflammation of vein often accompanied by clot formation. Veins in legs are most commonly affected. Signs and symptoms include swelling and inflammation of involved site and aching or cramping pain. Vein feels hard, cordlike, and sensitive to touch. Pain in calf occurs when client walks or dorsiflexes foot (Homans' sign).	Venous stasis is aggravated by prolonged sitting or immobilization. Trauma to vessel wall and hypercoagulability of blood increase risk of vessel inflammation.
Thrombus is formation of clot attached to interior wall of a vein or artery, which can occlude the vessel lumen.	Thrombus is caused by venous stasis (see thrombophlebitis) and vessel trauma. Venous injury is common after surgery of legs, abdomen, pelvis, and major vessels.
Embolus is piece of thrombus that has dislodged and circulates in bloodstream until it lodges in another vessel, commonly lungs, heart, or brain.	Thrombi also form from increased coagulability of blood (e.g., polycythemia and use of birth control pills containing estrogen).
Gastrointestinal System *Abdominal distention* is retention of air within intestines. Signs and symptoms include increased abdominal girth and tympanic percussion over abdominal quadrants. Client complains of fullness and "gas pains."	Distention is caused by slowed peristalsis from anesthesia, bowel manipulation, or immobilization.
Constipation is infrequent passage of stools. It should not be immediate concern after surgery, especially if client has preoperative bowel preparation. After client resumes solid diet, failure to pass stool within 48 hours is cause for concern.	Slowed peristalsis (see causes of distention) and delay in resuming normal diet cause constipation.
Nausea and vomiting are symptoms of improper gastric emptying or chemical stimulation of vomiting center. Client complains of gagging or feeling full or sick to stomach.	Nausea and vomiting are caused by severe pain, abdominal distention, fear, medications, eating or drinking before peristalsis returns, and initiation of gag reflex.

Continued

Table 49-13 **Postoperative Complications**—cont'd

Complication	Cause
Genitourinary System	
Urinary retention is involuntary accumulation of urine in bladder as result of loss of muscle tone. Signs and symptoms include inability to void, restlessness, and bladder distention. It appears 6-8 hours after surgery.	Retention is caused by effects of anesthesia and narcotic analgesics. Local manipulation of tissues surrounding bladder and edema interfere with bladder tone. Poor positioning of client impairs voiding reflexes.
Integumentary System	
Wound infection is an invasion of deep or superficial wound tissues by pathogenic microorganisms; signs and symptoms include warm, red, and tender skin around incision. Client may have fever and chills. Purulent material may exit from drains or from separated wound edges. It appears 3-6 days after surgery.	Infection is caused by poor aseptic technique and contaminated wound before surgical exploration.
Wound dehiscence is separation of wound edges at suture line. Signs and symptoms include increased drainage and appearance of underlying tissues. It usually occurs 6-8 days after surgery.	Malnutrition, obesity, preoperative radiation to surgical site, old age, poor circulation to tissues, and unusual strain on suture line from coughing cause dehiscence.
Wound evisceration is protrusion of internal organs and tissues through incision. It usually occurs 6-8 days after surgery.	See Wound Dehiscence. Client with dehiscence is at risk for developing evisceration.
Surgical mumps (parotitis) is swelling of parotid glands due to poor mouth care	Surgical mumps is caused by obstruction of the parotid gland.
Nervous System	
Pain that is intractable	Intractable pain may be related to the wound or dressing; anxiety, or positioning.

Maintaining Respiratory Function. To prevent respiratory complications, the nurse begins aggressive pulmonary hygiene measures early. The benefits of thorough preoperative teaching are realized when clients are able to participate actively. The following measures promote expansion of the lungs:

- Encourage diaphragmatic breathing exercises at least every 2 hours while clients are awake. Maximal inspirations lasting 3 to 5 seconds open up alveoli.
- Instruct clients to use an incentive spirometer for maximum inspiration.
- Encourage early ambulation. Walking causes clients to assume a position that does not restrict chest wall expansion and stimulates an increased respiratory rate.
- Help clients who are restricted to bed to turn on their sides every 1 to 2 hours while awake and to sit when possible. Turning permits expansion of the lungs. Sitting causes lowering of abdominal organs, thus facilitating diaphragmatic movement and lung expansion.
- Keep the client comfortable. A client who is comfortable will be able to participate in the postoperative regimen. Assess, document, treat, and evaluate the client's pain.

The following measures promote removal of pulmonary secretions if they are present:

- Encourage coughing exercises every 2 hours while clients are awake and maintain pain control to promote a deep, productive cough. For clients who have had eye, intracranial, or spinal surgery, coughing may be contraindicated because of the potential increase in intraocular or intracranial pressure.
- Provide oral hygiene to expectorate mucus. Oral mucosa become dry when clients are NPO or are placed on limited fluid intake.
- Initiate orotracheal or nasotracheal suction for clients who are too weak or are unable to cough (see Chapter 39).

Preventing Circulatory Stasis. Early measures directed at preventing circulatory complications prevent circulatory stasis. Some clients are at greater risk of venous stasis because of the nature of their surgery. The following measures promote normal venous return and circulatory blood flow:

- Encourage clients to perform leg exercises at least every hour while awake. Exercise may be contraindicated in an affected extremity involving vascular repair or realignment of fractured bones and torn cartilage.
- Apply elastic antiembolism stockings as ordered by the physician. The stockings should be removed every 8 hours and left off for 1 hour (see Chapter 46).
- Apply pneumatic compression stockings as ordered. Each stocking wraps around a client's leg and is kept in place with a Velcro attachment. Compressed air in-

flates the padded plastic stocking systematically from ankle to calf to thigh and then deflates. The alternating inflation and deflation of the stocking reduces venous stasis.

- Encourage early ambulation. Most clients are expected to ambulate the evening of surgery, depending on the severity of the surgery and their condition. Even if a client has an epidural catheter or PCA device, ambulation should be encouraged. The degree of activity allowed progresses as the condition improves. Before ambulation, assess vital signs. Abnormalities may contraindicate ambulation. If vital signs are normal, first help the client to sit on the side of the bed. Client complaints of dizziness are a sign of postural hypotension. A recheck of blood pressure determines whether ambulation is safe. Assist with ambulation by standing at the client's side and making sure that the client can walk steadily. The first few times out of bed, clients may be able to walk only a few feet. This improves each time. Evaluate tolerance to activity by periodically assessing the pulse rate.
- Avoid positioning clients in a manner that interrupts blood flow to extremities. While in bed, clients should not have pillows or rolled blankets placed under the knees. Compression of the popliteal vessels can cause thrombi. When clients sit in chairs, their legs should be elevated on footstools. A client should never be allowed to sit with one leg crossed over the other.
- Administer anticoagulant drugs as ordered. Physicians often order small doses of anticoagulants, such as heparin, for clients at greatest risk for thrombus formation. Orthopedic clients often receive aspirin, warfarin (Coumadin), or enoxaparin (Lovenox) for anticoagulation.
- Promote adequate fluid intake orally or intravenously. Adequate hydration prevents concentrated buildup of formed blood elements, such as platelets and red blood cells. When the plasma volume is low, these elements may gather and form small clots within blood vessels.

Promoting Normal Elimination and Adequate Nutrition. Interventions for preventing gastrointestinal complications promote return of normal elimination and faster return of normal nutritional intake. It takes several days for a client who has had surgery on gastrointestinal structures (e.g., a colon resection) to resume a normal diet. Normal peristalsis may not return for 2 to 3 days. In contrast, the client whose gastrointestinal tract is unaffected directly by surgery can resume dietary intake after recovering from the effects of anesthesia. The following measures promote return of normal elimination:

- Assess for return of peristalsis every 4 to 8 hours. Routinely auscultate the abdomen to detect return of

normal bowel sounds; 5 to 30 loud gurgles per minute over each quadrant indicates that peristalsis has returned. High-pitched tinkling sounds accompanied by abdominal distention suggest that the bowel is not functioning properly. Ask if the client is passing gas (flatus). This is an important sign indicating normal bowel function.

- Maintain a gradual progression in dietary intake. For the first few hours after surgery a client receives only IV fluids. If bowel sounds are active and the physician orders a normal diet the first evening after surgery, first provide clear liquids, such as water, apple juice, broth, or tea, after nausea subsides. Overloading with large amounts of fluids may lead to distention and vomiting. If the client tolerates liquids without nausea, advance the diet as ordered. Clients who have had abdominal surgery are usually NPO the first 24 to 48 hours. As peristalsis returns, provide clear liquids, followed by full liquids, a light diet of solid foods, and finally a regular diet.
- Promote ambulation and exercise. Physical activity stimulates a return of peristalsis. The client who suffers abdominal distention and "gas pain" will obtain relief while walking.
- Maintain an adequate fluid intake. Fluids keep fecal material soft for easy passage. Fruit juices and warm liquids are especially effective.
- Administer enemas, rectal suppositories, and rectal tubes as ordered. If constipation or distention develops, the physician attempts to stimulate peristalsis with cathartics or enemas. A rectal tube or return-flow enema promotes passage of flatus (see Chapter 45).

The following measures maintain an adequate dietary intake:

- Remove sources of noxious odors.
- Assist the client to a comfortable position during mealtime. The client should sit if possible to minimize pressure on the abdomen.
- Provide desired servings of food. For example, a client may be more willing to face the first meal when servings are not large.
- Provide frequent oral hygiene. Adequate hydration and cleansing of the oral cavity eliminate dryness and bad tastes.
- Provide meals when the client is rested and free from pain. Often a client loses interest in eating if mealtime has been preceded by exhausting activities, such as ambulation, coughing and deep breathing exercises, or extensive dressing changes. When a client has pain, the associated nausea often causes a loss of appetite.

Promoting Urinary Elimination. The depressant effects of anesthetics and analgesics impair the sensation of bladder fullness. If bladder tone is reduced, the client has difficulty starting urination. However, clients should void within 8 to 12 hours after surgery. Clients who undergo surgery of the urinary system frequently have Foley catheters inserted to maintain free urinary flow until voluntary control of urination returns. The following measures promote normal urinary elimination (see Chapter 44):

- Help the client to assume normal positions during voiding. The male client may need assistance to stand to void. Bedpans make voiding difficult. A female client will have better results if she is able to use a toilet or bedside commode.
- Check the client frequently for the need to void. A surgical client restricted to bed needs assistance in handling and using bedpans or urinals. Often the client acquires a sudden feeling of bladder fullness and urgency to void and will need help quickly.
- Assess for bladder distention. If a client does not void within 8 hours of surgery or bladder distention is present, it may be necessary to insert a urinary catheter. A physician's order is needed.
- Monitor intake and output. An accepted level of urinary output is at least 1 ml/kg/hr for adults. If the urine is dark, concentrated, and low in volume, the physician should be notified. A client can easily become dehydrated as a result of fluid loss from the surgical wound. Measure intake and output for several days after surgery until normal fluid intake and urinary output are achieved.

Promoting Wound Healing.

A surgical wound undergoes considerable stress during convalescence. The stress of inadequate nutrition, impaired circulation, and metabolic alterations increase the risk for delayed healing (see Chapter 47). A wound may also undergo considerable physical stress. Strain on sutures from coughing, vomiting, distention, and movement of body parts can disrupt the wound layers. The nurse protects the wound and promotes healing. A critical time for wound healing is 24 to 72 hours after surgery, after which a seal is established. If a wound becomes infected, it usually occurs 3 to 6 days after surgery. A clean surgical wound usually does not regain strength against normal stress for 15 to 20 days after surgery. The nurse uses aseptic technique during dressing changes and wound care (see Chapters 33 and 47). Surgical drains must remain patent so that accumulated secretions can escape from the wound bed. Ongoing observation of the wound identifies early signs and symptoms of infection.

Achieving Rest and Comfort.

A surgical client's pain increases as anesthesia wears off. The client becomes more aware of the surroundings and more perceptive of discomfort. The incisional area may be only one source of pain. Irritation from drainage tubes, tight dressings or casts, and the muscular strains caused from positioning on the operating room table can make the client feel miserable.

Pain can significantly slow recovery. The client becomes reluctant to cough, breathe deeply, turn, ambulate, or perform necessary exercises. The nurse assesses the client's pain thoroughly (see Chapter 42). *It should not be assumed that the pain is incisional.* When the client asks for pain medication, the nurse determines the location, intensity, and character of the pain. The nurse should provide analgesics as often as allowed, around the clock, the first 24 to 48 hours after surgery to improve pain control (AHCPR, 1992). The PCA system allows clients to administer their own IV analgesics from a specially prepared IV pump (see Chapter 42). If clients gain a sense of control over their pain, they usually have fewer postoperative problems. If pain medications are not relieving discomfort, the nurse should notify the physician for additional orders after completing a thorough assessment. The nurse can also use other methods of promoting pain relief, such as positioning, back rubs, distraction, or imagery.

Epidural infusion of narcotics, such as morphine or fentanyl, via PCA is also a popular method of postoperative analgesia for many surgical clients (see Chapter 42). These medications may be delivered at a basal rate, preprogrammed bolus dose or interval, or both. Epidural narcotics relieve severe pain, often without the central nervous system depression that can occur with systemic narcotics. Recognizing potential complications and what to do if they occur is an important role for the postoperative nurse (see Chapter 42).

Maintaining/Enhancing Self-Concept.

The appearance of wounds, bulky dressings, and extruding drains and tubes threatens a client's self-concept. The effects of surgery, such as disfiguring scars, may create permanent changes in the client's body image. If surgery leads to impairment in body function, the client's role within the family can change significantly.

The nurse observes clients for alterations in self-concept. Clients may show a revulsion toward their appearance by refusing to look at incisions, carefully covering dressings with bedclothes, or refusing to get out of bed because of tubes and devices. The fear of not being able to return to a functional role in their families may even cause clients to avoid participating in the care plan.

The family becomes an important part of the efforts to improve the client's self-concept. The nurse explains the client's appearance to the family and ways to avoid nonverbal expressions of revulsion or surprise. The family needs to be accepting of the client's needs and still encourage the client's independence. If the condition is permanent, the family learns to assist the client through the grieving process so that the client can reach a stage of acceptance. The following measures maintain the client's self-concept:

- Provide privacy during dressing changes or inspection of the wound. Keep room curtains closed around the bed, and drape the client so that only the dressing or incisional area is exposed.
- Maintain the client's hygiene. Wound drainage and

antiseptic solutions from the surgical skin preparation dry on the skin's surface and cause irritation. A complete bath the first day after surgery can make the client feel renewed. When the gown becomes soiled by wound drainage, offer a clean gown and washcloth. Keep the client's hair neatly combed and offer frequent oral hygiene, especially for the client who is NPO. Room deodorizers may be useful if the odor from drainage seems particularly troublesome to the client and family.

- Prevent drainage sets from overflowing. Typically the physician orders contents of drainage sets to be measured every 8 hours for output recording. The client sometimes becomes preoccupied with observing the gradual collection of drainage, and some drainage sets can leak contents if they become too full. Empty the sets periodically to prevent accidental spills and hampering of the client's movement.

- Maintain a pleasant environment. Self-concept is heightened by being in pleasant, comfortable surroundings. Frequently the room of a surgical client becomes cluttered with extra dressings, rolls of tape, and bottles of antiseptic solution. If the client requires frequent dressing changes, the room may take on the appearance of a supply room. Store or remove unused supplies and keep the client's bedside orderly and clean.

- Offer opportunities for the client to discuss feelings about appearance. A client who avoids looking at an incision may need to discuss fears or concerns. A client having surgery for the first time is often more anxious than one who has had multiple surgeries. Both male and female clients may worry about permanent scarring. A client is more apt to look at an incision several days after surgery, when healing is occurring and energy and well-being are increased. When the client chooses to look at an incision for the first time, the area should be clean. Eventually the client should be able to care for the incision site by applying simple dressings or bathing the affected area.

- Provide the family with opportunities to discuss ways to promote the client's self-concept. Encouraging independence can be difficult for a family member who has a strong desire to assist the client in any way. By knowing about the appearance of a wound or incision, family members can be supportive during dressing changes. The topic or tone of a conversation can also help family members distract a client from dwelling on fears and concerns. Family members should not avoid discussing the future. However, they need help to know when it is appropriate to discuss future plans.

Then the client and family can work together to discuss realistic plans for the client's return home.

EVALUATION

Client Care. The nurse evaluates the effectiveness of care provided to the surgical client on the basis of expected outcomes following nursing interventions. In all surgical settings the nurse consults with the client and family to gather evaluation data. The nurse can evaluate the ambulatory surgical client's outcomes by making a telephone call to the client's home, asking if complications have developed and if the client understands restrictions or medications. The call is usually placed 24 hours after surgery, which allows the nurse to evaluate the progress of recovery.

In an acute care setting the evaluation of a surgical client is ongoing. If a client fails to progress as expected, the nurse revises the client's plan of care based on the priorities of the client's needs. Every effort is made to assist the client in returning to as healthy and functional a state as possible.

Part of the nurse's evaluation is determining the extent to which the client and family have learned self-care measures. A client often has to continue dressing care, follow activity restrictions, continue medication therapy, and observe for signs and symptoms of complications on returning home. A referral to home health care assists clients unable to perform self-care activities. It is useful to have a home health nurse in attendance at discharge to know what a client can effectively perform.

Client Expectations. With short hospital stays and ambulatory surgery, it is especially important to evaluate client expectations early in the postoperative process. Pain relief is usually a priority in the surgical population. Asking the client if everything possible has been done to alleviate pain, including nonpharmacological measures, can determine if the client's needs have been met. Timeliness of response to the client's needs, such as scheduled times for pain medication and prompt answering of a call light, may increase satisfaction. The client usually wants to be discharged from acute care as soon as possible and when indicated by the physician. Ensuring that discharge plans are in place facilitates that process and enhances the client's satisfaction with care. A phone call to the client 24 hours after ambulatory surgery or after discharge from acute care provides reassurance that the nurse has been sincere and is truly concerned with progress toward a return to the presurgical state of wellness.

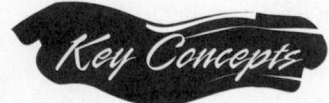

- Perioperative nursing is professional nursing care afforded the surgical client before, during, and after surgery.
- Surgery is classified by level of severity, urgency, and purpose.
- Previous illnesses, past surgeries, and the nature of nursing care provided influence the client's ability to tolerate surgery.
- The preoperative period may be several days or only a few hours long.
- All medications taken before surgery are automatically discontinued after surgery unless a physician reorders the drugs.
- Family members are important in assisting clients with any physical limitations and in providing emotional support during postoperative recovery.
- Preoperative assessment of vital signs and physical findings provides an important baseline with which to compare postoperative assessment data.
- A client's feelings about surgery can have a significant impact on relationships with the nursing staff and the client's ability to participate in care.
- Surgical removal of a body part may permanently alter a person's body image and sexuality.
- Nursing diagnoses of the surgical client may pose implications for nursing care during one or all phases of surgery.
- Primary responsibility for informed consent rests with the client's surgeon.
- Informed consent cannot be obtained if a client is confused, unconscious, mentally incompetent, or under the influence of sedatives.
- Structured preoperative teaching has a positive influence on postoperative recovery.
- Basic to preoperative teaching is explanation of all preoperative and postoperative routines and demonstration of postoperative exercises.
- Clipping hair on a surgical site should be done as close as possible to the time of surgery to minimize infection.
- In ambulatory surgery, nurses must use the limited time available to educate clients, assess their health status, and prepare them for surgery.
- A routine preoperative checklist is a guide for final preparation of the client before surgery.
- Many responsibilities of nurses within the operating room focus on protecting the client from potential harm.
- Assessment of the postoperative client centers on the body systems most likely to be affected by anesthesia, immobilization, and surgical trauma.

- The PACU nurse reports to the nurse on the postoperative division information pertaining to the client's current physical status and risk for postoperative complications.
- Accurate pain assessment and intervention are necessary for healing.

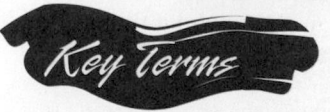

Ambulatory surgery, *p. 1661*

American Society of PeriAnesthesia Nurses (ASPAN), *p. 1665*

Antiembolism stockings, *p. 1691*

Association of Operating Room Nurses (AORN), *p. 1661*

Atelectasis, *p. 1709*

Bariatric, *p. 1663*

Cholecystectomy, *p. 1661*

Circulating nurse, *p. 1699*

Clinical pathways, *p. 1685*

Conscious sedation, *p. 1699*

Convalescence, *p. 1700*

Dehiscence, *p. 1663*

Depilatories, *p. 1688*

Dermatome, *p. 1706*

General anesthesia, *p. 1694*

Informed consent, *p. 1675*

Latex sensitivity, *p. 1692*

Local anesthesia, *p. 1699*

Malignant hyperthermia, *p. 1705*

Moribund, *p. 1662*

Nosocomial, *p. 1688*

Paralytic ileus, *p. 1707*

Perioperative nursing, *p. 1660*

Pneumatic compression device, *p. 1691*

Postanesthesia Recovery Score (PARS), *p. 1701*

Postanesthesia Recovery Score for Ambulatory Patients (PARSAP), *p. 1702*

Preoperative teaching, *p. 1675*

Recovery, *p. 1700*

Regional anesthesia, *p. 1698*

Scrub nurse, *p. 1699*

Critical Thinking Exercises

1. Your 82-year-old client is admitted after a fall for repair of a fractured hip. What postoperative complications are seen in the older client undergoing this type of surgery?

2. Mr. B. is a 52-year-old client who will have thoracic surgery. He has a 30-year history of smoking one pack of cigarettes per day. What type of pulmonary preventive measures would you expect Mr. B to need postoperatively?

3. Your client is of Native American descent. He will be having a cholecystectomy. Describe a potential problem related to pain control and how the problem can be avoided through preoperative teaching.

4. Mrs. C. was admitted for ambulatory surgery for an inguinal hernia repair. What discharge criteria would be used for Mrs. C. and what discharge instructions would she require?

References

AARC Clinical Practice Guideline: Use of positive airway pressure adjuncts to bronchial hygiene therapy, *Respir Care* 38(5):515, 1993.

Agency for Health Care Policy and Research: *Acute pain management: operative or medical procedures and trauma,* Clinical Practice Guideline, AHCPR Pub No. 92-0032, Rockville, Md, 1992, Public Health Service, U.S. Department of Health and Human Services.

Aldrete JA: Modifications to the post anesthesia score for use in ambulatory surgery, *J PeriAnesth Nurs* 13(3):148, 1998.

Aldrete JA, Kroulik D: A post-anesthetic recovery score, *Anesth Analg* 49:924, 1970.

American Association of Nurse Anesthetists, Infection/Environmental Control Task Force: *Latex allergy protocol,* Park Ridge, Ill, 1995, The Association.

American Nurses Association, Association of Operating Room Nurses: Standards of perioperative nursing care, Kansas City, Mo, 1972, The Associations.

American Society of PeriAnesthesia Nurses: *Standards of periAnesthesia nursing practice,* Thorofare, NJ, 1998, The Society.

Association of Operating Room Nurses: Recommended practices for skin preparation of patients, *AORN J* 64(5):813, 1996.

Association of Operating Room Nurses: *Standards, recommended practices, and guidelines,* Denver, 1999, The Association.

Atkinson LJ, Fortunato N: *Berry and Kohn's operating room technique,* ed 8, St. Louis, 1996, Mosby.

Bean P, Waldron K: Readmission study leads to continuum of care, *Nurs Manage* 26:65, 1995.

Dalayon A: Components of preoperative patient teaching in Kuwait, *J Adv Nurs* 19:537, 1994.

Dettenmeier P: *Pulmonary nursing care,* St. Louis, 1992, Mosby.

Devine EC, Cook TD: Clinical and cost saving effects of psychoeducational interventions with surgical patients: a meta-analysis, *Res Nurs Health* 9:89, 1992.

Doepke S: Identifying the risk, *Semin Periop Nurs* 7(4):226, 1998.

Federated Ambulatory Surgery Association: *Most common outpatient procedures* (on line), 1998, http://fasa.org/procedures.html.

Fortner P: Preoperative patient preparation: psychological and educational aspects, *Semin Periop Nurs* 7(1):3, 1998.

Gershenson A and others: Tilling the soil: nurturing the seeds of patient and family education, *J Nurs Care Qual* 13(6):83, 1999.

Green C, Pandit S, Schork M: Preoperative fasting time: is traditional policy changing? Results of a national survey, *Anesth Analg* 83:123, 1996.

Greenfield L and others: *Surgery: scientific principles and practice,* ed 2, Philadelphia, 1997, Lippincott-Raven.

Gruendemann B, Fernsebner B: *Comprehensive perioperative nursing,* Boston, 1995, Jones & Bartlett.

Hathaway D: Effect of pre-operative instruction on post-operative outcomes: a meta-analysis, *Nurs Res* 35(5):269, 1986.

Karlet MC: Malignant hyperthermia consideration for ambulatory surgery, *J Perianesthesia Nurs* 13(5):304, 1998.

Lee N and others: A survey of patient education postdischarge, *J Nurs Care Qual* 13(1):63, 1998.

Lipson J, Dibble S, Minarik P: *Culture and nursing care: a pocket guide,* San Francisco, 1996, UCSF Nursing Press.

Litwack K: *Post anesthesia care nursing,* ed 2, St. Louis, 1995, Mosby.

Litwack K: *Core curriculum for perianesthesia nursing practice,* ed 4, Philadelphia, 1999, WB Saunders.

Lookinland S, Pool M: Study on effect of methods of preoperative education in women, *AORN J* 67(1):203, 1998.

McCloskey JC, Bulechek GM: *Nursing interventions classification (NIC),* ed 3, St. Louis, 2000, Mosby.

Meeker MH, Rothrock JC: *Alexander's care of the patient in surgery,* ed 11, St. Louis, 1999, Mosby.

Miaskowski C: Current concepts in the assessment and management of acute pain, *MedSurg Nursing* 2(1):28, 1993.

Morales C, Andrews J: Postoperative wound care: nursing assessment and management, *Semin Perioperative Nurs* 2(4):231, 1993.

Pandit VA, Pandit SK: Fasting before and after ambulatory surgery, *J PeriAnesth Nurs* 12(3):181, 1997.

Paquet J: Latex hypersensitivity: the IgE response, *Semin Periop Nurs* 7(4):203, 1998.

Phipps WJ, Sands JK, and Marek JF: *Medical-surgical nursing: concepts and clinical practice,* ed 6, St. Louis, 1999, Mosby.

Price J, Mahon S, Faut-Callahan M: Pain control in hospitalized postsurgical patients, *MedSurg Nurs* 4(5):367, 1995.

Price SA, Wilson LM: *Pathophysiology: clinical concepts of disease processes,* ed 5, St. Louis, 1997, Mosby.

Rice VH and others: Pre-admission self-instruction effect on post-admission and post-operative indicators in CABG patients: partial replication and extension, *Res Nurs Health* 15:253, 1992.

Sabiston D, Lyerly H: *Textbook of surgery: the biological basis of modern surgical practice,* ed 5, Philadelphia, 1997, WB Saunders.

Shoup A: Why latex allergy now? *Semin Periop Nurs* 7(4):222, 1998.

Shuldham C: A review of the impact of pre-operative education on recovery from surgery, *Int J Nurs Stud* 36:171, 1999.

Thibodeau G, Patton K: *Anthony's textbook of anatomy and physiology,* ed 15, St. Louis, 1996, Mosby.

Welsh JR, Arzoukman JMR, Holm K: Nurse's assessment and documentation of peripheral edema, *Clin Nurse Spec* 10(1):7, 1996.

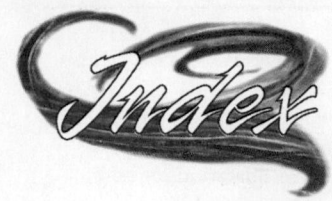

A

A-beta fiber, 1286
A-delta fiber, 1284-1286
Abbreviations, dosage, 893
Abdellah's theory of nursing, 94, 95
Abdomen
  assessment of bowel function and, 1452
  isometric exercises for, 1005
  of middle adult, 236
  of older adult, 253
  physical examination of, 800-805
  preoperative assessment of, 1672
  ventilatory rhythm and, 702
Abdominal binder, 1613-1615, 1616
Abdominal cramping, enteral nutrition-
      related, 1371
Abdominal distention, 1452
  nasogastric tube-related, 1480
  postoperative, 1707, 1709
  before surgery, 1672
Abdominal pain, 800
Abdominal reflex, 830
Abdominal respiratory muscles, 1131
Abdominal x-ray, 1403
Abducens nerve, 826
Abduction, 818
  of finger, 1503
  of hip, 1504
  of shoulder, 1501
  of thumb, 1503
  of toe, 1505
  of wrist, 1503
Abduction pillow, 1522
Ability to learn, 480-482
Ablative surgery, 1662
Abnormal reactive hyperemia, 1547
ABO system, 1242
Abortion, 571
  decisional issues in, 573
  legal implications in, 435
Abrasion, 1062, 1553, 1572
  child abuse and, 190
Absorption
  of medication, 889-890, 910
  of nutrients, 1332, 1333
Absorptive dressing, 1590
Abstinence from sexual intercourse, 570
Abstract, 534
Abstract thinking, 825
Abuse
  clinical indicators of, 738
  community-based nursing and, 55
  sexual, 573-574, 579
Acceptance
  death and dying and, 633
  life satisfaction and, 599-600
  psychosocial adaptation to illness and, 480
Access to health care, 36
Accessory muscles of respiration, 1130, 1131
Accident
  adolescent and, 217
  fire, 1044-1045
  in health care agency, 1025-1026
  infant, toddler, and preschooler and, 1023
  older adult and, 261, 1024

Accident—cont'd
  poisoning, 1046, 1047
  school-age child and, 207
Accommodation, 618, 633, 757
Accountability, 73, 381
  critical thinking and, 283-284
  ethics and, 404-405
  medication administration and, 902-903
Accreditation
  documentation and, 501
  of nursing program, 382
Accuracy of documentation, 504-505
Acetaminophen, 1310, 1341
Acetylsalicylic acid, 1310
Achilles reflex, 830
Achilles tendon, 1489
Acid-base balance, 1202-1203
  hyperventilation and, 1139
  interventions for imbalances, 1243-1245
  regulation of, 1199-1200
  risk factors for imbalances, 1205
  types of imbalances, 1203-1205
Acidifying of urine, 1411
Acidosis, 1203, 1204, 1205, 1214
Acne, 1062, 1066
Acquired immunodeficiency syndrome,
      571-572
  adolescent and, 219
  African-Americans and, 125
  concerns facing family, 142
  Hispanics and, 129
  legal implications in, 436
  Native Americans and, 134
  nutritional interventions in, 1377
  pathologic responses of, 842
  respiratory tract infections and, 1146
  transmission of, 1022
Acromegaly, 752
Active immunity, 1022
Active listening, 459
Active participation in learning, 479-480
Active strategies of health promotion, 11,
      1029
Active transport, 1196
Activities of daily living
  assisting with, 355-356
  body mechanics and, 990
  continuing care and, 1007
  incorporation of active exercise into, 1004
  pain and, 1300-1301
  restorative care and, 269-270
Activity, 989-1017
  acute care and, 1004-1007
  assessment of, 998-1000
  assistive devices for walking and,
      1007-1013
  behavioral aspects of, 995
  body mechanics and, 990-992
    lifting techniques, 1004, 1005
    pathologic influences on, 993-994
  bowel elimination and, 1441
  chronic obstructive pulmonary disease
      and, 1013-1014
  coronary heart disease and, 1013
  critical thinking and, 997-998

Activity—cont'd
  cultural and ethnic influences on, 996
  developmental changes and, 994-995
  diabetes mellitus and, 1014
  environmental issues in, 995-996
  evaluation of, 1014-1015
  family and social support for, 996
  health promotion and, 1001-1004
  hypertension and, 1013
  metabolic rate and, 672
  nursing diagnosis in, 1000
  older adult and, 264
  planning and, 1000-1001, 1002-1003
  Postanesthetic Recovery Score for
      Ambulatory Patients, 1703
  pressure sore risk and, 1560, 1561
  regulation of movement and, 992-993
  temperament and, 165
Activity reinforcer, 490-491
Activity theory of aging, 248
Activity tolerance, 991, 999-1000, 1500-1505
Actual health problem, 317
Actual loss, 615
Actual nursing diagnosis, 317
Acuity recording, 513
Acupoints, 981
Acupressure, 971, 1305, 1306
Acupuncture, 970, 981-982
Acute care
  activity and exercise and, 1004-1007
  bowel elimination and, 1460-1480
    enemas in, 1460-1466
    inserting and maintaining nasogastric
        tube, 1467, 1474-1479, 1480
    ostomy care and, 1466-1467
  in cardiopulmonary disease, 1161-1181
    airway maintenance, 1162-1164, 1165
    artificial airways, 1166, 1171-1172
    cardiopulmonary resuscitation, 1181,
        1184-1188
    dyspnea management, 1161
    maintenance of lung expansion,
        1172-1176
    oxygen therapy, 1176-1181
    suctioning techniques, 1164-1166,
        1167-1171
  family and, 150-151
  in fluid, electrolyte, and acid-base imbal-
      ances, 1206-1247
    daily weights and intake and output
        measurement, 1218
    enteral replacement and, 1218
    intravenous therapy and, 1218-1243; see
        also Intravenous administration
    restriction of fluids and, 1218
  hygiene and, 1074-1110
    artificial eye and, 1104
    back rub and, 1086, 1087-1088
    bag baths and, 1082
    bathing and skin care, 1074-1082
    bathing infant and, 1086-1089
    contact lenses and, 1103-1104,
        1105-1109
    ear care, 1104
    eye care, 1102-1103